MW00846725

Harper's
Textbook of Pediatric Dermatology

Harper's Textbook of Pediatric Dermatology

IN TWO VOLUMES

VOLUME 2

FOURTH EDITION

EDITED BY

Peter Hoeger
Veronica Kinsler
Albert Yan

EDITORIAL ADVISORS

John Harper
Arnold Oranje

ASSOCIATE EDITORS

Christine Bodemer
Margarita Larralde
David Luk
Vibhu Mendiratta
Diana Purvis

WILEY Blackwell

Edition History
Blackwell Publishing Ltd (1e, 2000 2e, 2006; 3e, 2011)

Registered Offices
John Wiley & Sons, Inc., 111 River Street, Hoboken, NJ 07030, USA
John Wiley & Sons Ltd, The Atrium, Southern Gate, Chichester, West Sussex, PO19 8SQ, UK

Editorial Office
9600 Garsington Road, Oxford, OX4 2DQ, UK

For details of our global editorial offices, customer services, and more information about Wiley products visit us at www.wiley.com.

Wiley also publishes its books in a variety of electronic formats and by print-on-demand. Some content that appears in standard print versions of this book may not be available in other formats.

Library of Congress Cataloging-in-Publication Data
Names: Hoeger, Peter H., editor. | Kinsler, Veronica, editor. | Yan, Albert C., editor.
Title: Harper's textbook of pediatric dermatology / edited by Peter Hoeger, Veronica Kinsler, Albert Yan ; editorial advisors, John Harper, Arnold Oranje ; associate editors, Christine Bodemer, Margarita Larralde, David Luk, Vibhu Mendiratta, Diana Purvis.
Other titles: Textbook of pediatric dermatology
Description: Fourth edition. | Hoboken, NJ : Wiley-Blackwell, 2020. | Includes bibliographical references and index.
Identifiers: LCCN 2019031032 (print) | ISBN 9781119142195 (hardback) | ISBN 9781119142805 (adobe pdf) | ISBN 9781119142737 (epub)
Subjects: MESH: Skin Diseases | Child | Infant
Classification: LCC RJ511 (print) | LCC RJ511 (ebook) | NLM WS 265 | DDC 618.92/5–dc23
LC record available at https://lccn.loc.gov/2019031032
LC ebook record available at https://lccn.loc.gov/2019031033

Cover image: CP Photo Art/Getty Images
Cover design by Wiley

Set in 9.5/11.5pt Palatino by SPi Global, Pondicherry, India
Printed and bound in Singapore by Markono Print Media Pte Ltd

10 9 8 7 6 5 4 3 2 1

Contents

List of Contributors, xi

Preface to the Fourth Edition, xxiv

Dedication to Arnold P. Oranje, xxv

Acknowledgements, xxvi

List of Abbreviations, xxvii

VOLUME 1

Section 1 Development, Structure and Physiology of the Skin

1 Embryogenesis of the Skin, 1
Lara Wine Lee & Karen A. Holbrook

2 Molecular Genetics in Paediatric Dermatology, 36
Anna C. Thomas & Veronica A. Kinsler

3 Cutaneous Microbiome, 46
Carrie C. Coughlin & William H. McCoy IV

4 Physiology of Neonatal Skin, 56
Peter H. Hoeger

Section 2 Skin Disorders of the Neonate and Young Infant

5 Neonatal Skin Care, 63
Peter H. Hoeger

6 Transient Skin Disorders in the Neonate and Young Infant, 72
Margarita Larralde & Maria Eugenia Abad

7 Congenital and Acquired Infections in the Neonate, 84
Scott H. James, Nico G. Hartwig, David W. Kimberlin & Peter H. Hoeger

8 Transplacentally Acquired Dermatoses, 93
Paula Carolina Luna

9 Developmental Anomalies, 101
Marion Wobser & Henning Hamm

10 Differential Diagnosis of Neonatal Erythroderma, 121
Hagen Ott & Peter H. Hoeger

11 Vesiculopustular, Bullous and Erosive Diseases of the Neonate, 134
Caroline Mahon & Anna E. Martinez

12 Iatrogenic Disorders of the Newborn, 154
Elia F. Maalouf & Wilson Lopez

Section 3 Atopic Dermatitis and Related Disorders

13 Epidemiology of Atopic Dermatitis, 167
Carsten Flohr, Jonathan I. Silverberg, Joy Wan & Sinéad M. Langan

14 Genetics and Aetiology of Atopic Dermatitis, 184
Elke Rodriguez & Stephan Weidinger

15 Clinical Features and Diagnostic Criteria of Atopic Dermatitis, 193
Sinéad M. Langan & Hywel C. Williams

16 Severity Scoring and Quality of Life Assessment in Atopic Dermatitis, 212
Christian Apfelbacher, Cecilia A.C. (Sanna) Prinsen, Daniel Heinl & Hywel C. Williams

17 Atopic Dermatitis and Related Disorders: Special Types of Presentation, 228
Nawaf Almutairi

18 Atopic Dermatitis: Complications, 245
Kevin B. Yarbrough & Eric L. Simpson

19 Management of Atopic Dermatitis, 253
Lea Solman & Mary Glover

Section 4 Other Types of Dermatitis

20 Napkin Dermatitis, 265
Arnold P. Oranje, Ernesto Bonifazi, Paul J. Honig & Albert C. Yan

21 Adolescent Seborrhoeic Dermatitis, 279
Roselyn Kellen & Nanette Silverberg

22 Irritant Contact Dermatitis, 287
David Luk

23 Allergic Contact Dermatitis, 300
Sharon E. Jacob, Hannah Hill & Alina Goldenberg

24 Hypereosinophilic Disorders, 316
Eirini E. Merika & Nerys Roberts

25 Juvenile Plantar Dermatosis, 335
John C. Browning & Margaret Brown

26 Perioral Dermatitis, 338
Marius Rademaker

Section 5 Psoriasis

27 Psoriasis: Epidemiology, 343
Matthias Augustin & Marc Alexander Radtke

28 Psoriasis: Aetiology and Pathogenesis, 350
Jonathan Barker

29 Psoriasis: Clinical Features and Comorbidities, 354
Derek H. Chu & Kelly M. Cordoro

30 Psoriasis: Classification, Scores and Diagnosis, 362
Nirav Patel & Megha Tollefson

31 Psoriasis: Management, 368
Marieke M.B. Seyger

Section 6 Other Papulosquamous Disorders

32 Pityriasis Rubra Pilaris, 377
Liat Samuelov & Eli Sprecher

33 Lichen Planus, 390
Vibhu Mendiratta & Sarita Sanke

34 Lichen Nitidus, 403
Jasem M. Alshaiji

35 Lichen Striatus, 408
Franck Boralevi & Alain Taïeb

36 Pityriasis Rosea, 416
Antonio A.T. Chuh & Vijay Zawar

Section 7 Bacterial Skin Infections

37 Pyodermas and Bacterial Toxin-mediated Syndromes, 423
James R. Treat, Christian R. Millett, Warren R. Heymann & Steven M. Manders

38 Cutaneous Manifestations of Gram-negative Infections, 434
Saul N. Faust, Diane Gbesemete & Robert S. Heyderman

39 Pitted Keratolysis, Erythrasma and Erysipeloid, 456
Zhe Xu, Yuanyuan Xiao, Ying Xiu & Lin Ma

40 Lyme Borreliosis, 463
Susan O'Connell

41 *Bartonella* Infections, 475
Sonia Kamath & Minnelly Luu

42 Mycobacterial Skin Infections, 485
G. Sethuraman, Tanvi Dev & V. Ramesh

43 Rickettsial Disease, 503
Arun C. Inamadar & Aparna Palit

44 Endemic Treponematoses: Yaws, Pinta and Endemic Syphilis, 515
Herman Jan H. Engelkens

45 Tropical Ulcer, 523
Vibhu Mendiratta & Soumya Agarwal

Section 8 Fungal Skin Infections

46 Superficial Fungal Infections, 527
Peter Mayser & Yvonne Gräser

47 Deep Fungal Infections, 560
María Teresa García-Romero

Section 9 Viral Skin Infections and Opportunistic Infections

48 Molluscum Contagiosum, 579
Joachim J. Bugert, Ali Alikhan & Tor Shwayder

49 Human Papillomavirus Infection, 588
Yun Tong, Stephen K. Tyring & Zsuzsanna Z. Szalai

50 Herpes Simplex Virus Infections, 598
Manuraj Singh, Helen M. Goodyear & Judith Breuer

51 Varicella Zoster Virus Infections, 612
Manuraj Singh & Judith Breuer

52 Poxvirus Infections, 624
Susan Lewis-Jones & Jane C. Sterling

53 HIV and HTLV-1 Infection, 649
Neil S. Prose, Ncoza C. Dlova, Rosalia A. Ballona & Coleen K. Cunningham

54 Viral Exanthems, 660
Jusleen Ahluwalia, Pamela Gangar & Sheila Fallon Friedlander

55 Eruptive Hypomelanosis, 681
Vijay Zawar & Antonio A.T. Chuh

56 Cutaneous Infections in Immunocompromised Children, 684
Miriam Weinstein, Hagen Ott & Peter H. Hoeger

Section 10 Parasitic Skin Infestations and Sting Reactions

57 Leishmaniasis, 693
Bernardo Gontijo & Carolina Talhari

58 Helminthic Infections, 702
Héctor Cáceres-Ríos & Felipe Velasquez

59 Scabies and Pseudoscabies, 711
Wingfield E. Rehmus & Julie S. Prendiville

60 Pediculosis and Cimicosis, 723
Sandipan Dhar & Sahana M. Srinivas

61 Noxious and Venomous Creatures, 733
Kam Lun Ellis Hon, Theresa Ngan Ho Leung & Ting Fan Leung

62 Aquatic Dermatoses, 746
Sarah Hill

Section 11 Urticaria, Erythemas and Drug Reactions

63 Urticaria, 751
Bettina Wedi

64 Annular Erythemas, 764
Kimberly A. Horii

65 Gianotti–Crosti Syndrome, 771
Carlo M. Gelmetti

66 Erythema Multiforme, Stevens–Johnson Syndrome and Toxic Epidermal Necrolysis, 777
Benjamin S. Daniel, Lizbeth Ruth Wheeler & Dédée F. Murrell

67 Hypersensitivity Reactions to Drugs, 785
Mohannad Abu-Hilal & Neil Shear

Section 12 Acne and Acneiform Disorders

68 Acne, 803
Marissa J. Perman, Bodo C. Melnik & Anne W. Lucky

69 Childhood Rosacea, 821
Clio Dessinioti & Andreas Katsambas

70 Hidradenitis Suppurativa, 825
Peter Theut Riis & Gregor B.E. Jemec

Section 13 Nutritional Disorders

71 Skin Manifestations of Nutritional Disorders, 831
Carola Durán McKinster & Luz Orozco-Covarrubias

72 Skin Manifestations of Paediatric Metabolic Syndrome, 841
Gregor Holzer & Beatrix Volc-Platzer

Section 14 Blistering Disorders

73 Differential Diagnosis of Vesiculobullous Lesions, 859
Sharleen F. Hill & Dédée F. Murrell

74 Autoimmune Bullous Diseases, 868
Nina van Beek & Enno Schmidt

75 Childhood Dermatitis Herpetiformis, 898
Carmen Liy Wong & Irene Lara-Corrales

76 Epidermolysis Bullosa and Kindler Syndrome, 907
Jemima E. Mellerio, Anna E. Martinez & Christina Has

Section 15 Photodermatoses, Photoprotection and Environmental Skin Disorders

77 The Idiopathic Photodermatoses and Skin Testing, 943
Erhard Hölzle & Robert Dawe

78 The Porphyrias, 957
Jorge Frank

79 Photoprotection, 969
Lachlan Warren & Genevieve Casey

80 Skin Reactions to Plants, Cold, Heat and Chemicals, 983
Tuyet A. Nguyen, Christopher Lovell & Andrew C. Krakowski

Section 16 Granulomatous Diseases

81 Sarcoidosis, 995
Lisa M. Arkin, Julie L. Cantatore-Francis & Julie V. Schaffer

82 Granuloma Annulare, 1006
Annalisa Patrizi & Iria Neri

83 Orofacial Granulomatosis, 1017
Lisa Weibel & Martin Theiler

Section 17 Neutrophilic Dermatoses

84 Sweet Syndrome, 1023
Peter von den Driesch

85 Pyoderma Gangrenosum, 1027
Karolina Gholam

Section 18 Lymphocytic Disorders

86 Pityriasis Lichenoides, 1035
Christine T. Lauren & Maria C. Garzon

87 Jessner Lymphocytic Infiltrate of the Skin, 1040
R.M. Ross Hearn

88 Primary Cutaneous Lymphoma, 1044
Rebecca Levy & Elena Pope

89 Childhood Leukaemias and Lymphomas, 1063
Keith Morley & Jennifer Huang

Section 19 Histiocytic Disorders

90 Langerhans Cell Histiocytosis, 1071
Sylvie Fraitag & Jean Donadieu

91 Juvenile Xanthogranuloma and Other Non-Langerhans Cell Histiocytoses, 1078
Gudrun Ratzinger & Bernhard W.H. Zelger

Section 20 Mastocytosis

92 Paediatric Mastocytosis, 1097
Laura Polivka & Christine Bodemer

Section 21 Disorders of Connective Tissue

93 Ehlers–Danlos Syndromes, 1111
Nigel P. Burrows

94 Pseudoxanthoma Elasticum and Cutis Laxa, 1125
Sean D. Reynolds & Lionel Bercovitch

95 Buschke–Ollendorff Syndrome, Marfan Syndrome and Osteogenesis Imperfecta, 1139
Marc Lacour

96 Anetodermas and Atrophodermas, 1151
Marc Lacour

97 Hyalinoses, Stiff Skin Syndrome and Restrictive Dermopathy, 1164
David G. Paige

98 Striae in Children and Adolescents, 1172
Marcelo Ruvertoni

99 Morphoea (Localized Scleroderma), 1175
Despina Eleftheriou & Lindsay Shaw

100 Systemic Sclerosis in Childhood, 1183
Christopher P. Denton & Carol M. Black

Index, i1

VOLUME 2

Section 22 Disorders of Fat Tissue

101 Lipoma and Lipomatosis, 1195
Siriwan Wananukul & Susheera Chatproedprai

102 Panniculitis in Children, 1207
Christine Bodemer

103 Lipodystrophies, 1221
Robert K. Semple

Section 23 Mosaic Disorders, Naevi and Hamartomas

104 An Introduction to Mosaicism, 1229
Veronica A. Kinsler

105 Melanocytic Naevi, 1237
Veronica A. Kinsler

106 Epidermal Naevi, 1260
Leopold M. Groesser & Christian Hafner

107 Other Naevi and Hamartomas, 1276
Jonathan A. Dyer

108 Proteus Syndrome and Other Localized Overgrowth Disorders, 1283
Veronica A. Kinsler

109 Mosaic Disorders of Pigmentation, 1296
Veronica A. Kinsler

Section 24 Nonvascular Skin Tumours

110 Differential Diagnosis of Skin Nodules and Cysts, 1313
Susanne Abraham & Peter H. Hoeger

111 Adnexal Disorders, 1325
Andrew Wang & Robert Sidbury

112 Calcification and Ossification in the Skin, 1338
Amanda T. Moon, Albert C. Yan & Eulalia T. Baselga

113 Angiolymphoid Hyperplasia with Eosinophilia, 1350
Jasem M. Alshaiji

114 Fibromatoses, 1356
Jenna L. Streicher, Moise L. Levy & Albert C. Yan

115 Carcinomas of the Skin, 1370
Karen Agnew

116 Childhood Melanoma, 1377
Birgitta Schmidt & Elena B. Hawryluk

117 Other Malignant Skin Tumours, 1382
Andrea Bettina Cervini, Marcela Bocian, María Marta Bujan & Paola Stefano

Section 25 Vascular Tumours and Malformations

118 Vascular Malformations, 1399
Laurence M. Boon & Miikka Vikkula

119 Infantile Haemangiomas, 1425
Anna L. Bruckner, Ilona J. Frieden & Julie Powell

120 Other Vascular Tumours, 1440
Ann M. Kulungowski, Taizo A. Nakano & Anna L. Bruckner

121 Disorders of Lymphatics, 1452
Arin K. Greene & Jeremy A. Goss

Section 26 Disorders of Pigmentation

122 Inherited and Acquired Hyperpigmentation, 1463
Leslie Castelo-Soccio & Alexis Weymann Perlmutter

123 Vitiligo, 1476
Julien Seneschal, Juliette Mazereeuw-Hautier & Alain Taïeb

124 Albinism, 1486
Fanny Morice-Picard & Alain Taïeb

125 Disorders of Hypopigmentation, 1492
M.W. Bekkenk & A. Wolkerstorfer

126 Dyschromatosis, 1499
Liat Samuelov & Eli Sprecher

Section 27 Disorders of Keratin and Keratinization

127 Review of Keratin Disorders, 1515
Maurice A.M. van Steensel & Peter M. Steijlen

128 Mendelian Disorders of Cornification (MEDOC): The Keratodermas, 1524
Edel A. O'Toole

129 Mendelian Disorders of Cornification (MEDOC): The Ichthyoses, 1549
Angela Hernández, Robert Gruber & Vinzenz Oji

130 Keratosis Pilaris and Darier Disease, 1599
Flora B. de Waard-van der Spek & Arnold P. Oranje

131 The Erythrokeratodermas, 1608
Juliette Mazereeuw-Hautier, S. Leclerc-Mercier & E. Bourrat

132 Netherton Syndrome, 1613
Wei-Li Di & John Harper

133 Porokeratosis, 1623
Leslie Castelo-Soccio

Section 28 Focal or Generalized Hypoplasia and Premature Ageing

134 Ectodermal Dysplasias, 1629
Cathal O'Connor, Yuka Asai & Alan D. Irvine

135 Focal Dermal Hypoplasia, 1706
Bret L. Bostwick, Ignatia B. Van den Veyver & V. Reid Sutton

136 Incontinentia Pigmenti, 1718
Elizabeth A. Jones & Dian Donnai

137 Premature Ageing Syndromes, 1725
Helga V. Toriello & Caleb P. Bupp

Section 29 Genetic Diseases Predisposing to Malignancy

138 Xeroderma Pigmentosum and Related Diseases, 1743
Steffen Schubert & Steffen Emmert

139 Gorlin (Naevoid Basal Cell Carcinoma) Syndrome, 1769
Kai Ren Ong & Peter A. Farndon

140 Rothmund–Thomson Syndrome, Bloom Syndrome, Dyskeratosis Congenita, Fanconi Anaemia and Poikiloderma with Neutropenia, 1786
Lisa L. Wang & Moise L. Levy

141 Other Genetic Disorders Predisposing to Malignancy, 1802
Julie V. Schaffer

Section 30 Neurofibromatosis, RASopathies and Hamartoma-Overgrowth Syndromes

142 The Neurofibromatoses, 1823
Amy Theos, Kevin P. Boyd & Bruce R. Korf

143 Tuberous Sclerosis Complex, 1837
Francis J. DiMario Jr

144 Other RASopathies, 1857
Fanny Morice-Picard

Section 31 Vasculitic and Rheumatic Syndromes

145 Cutaneous Vasculitis, 1865
Joyce C. Chang & Pamela F. Weiss

146 Purpura Fulminans, 1891
Michael Levin, Brian Eley & Saul N. Faust

147 Kawasaki Disease, 1906
Wynnis L. Tom & Jane C. Burns

148 Polyarteritis Nodosa, Granulomatosis with Polyangiitis and Microscopic Polyangiitis, 1918
Paul A. Brogan

149 Juvenile Idiopathic Arthritis, Systemic Lupus Erythematosus and Juvenile Dermatomyositis, 1933
Elena Moraitis & Despina Eleftheriou

150 Behçet Disease and Relapsing Polychondritis, 1952
Sibel Ersoy-Evans, Ayşen Karaduman & Seza Özen

151 Erythromelalgia, 1961
Nedaa Skeik

Section 32 Cutaneous Manifestations of Systemic Disease

152 Metabolic Disorders and the Skin, 1965
Fatma Al Jasmi, Hassan Galadari, Peter T. Clayton & Emma J. Footitt

153 Cystic Fibrosis, 1988
Roderic J. Phillips

154 Cutaneous Manifestations of Endocrine Disease, 1993
Devika Icecreamwala & Tor A. Shwayder

155 Autoinflammatory Diseases and Amyloidosis, 2010
Antonio Torrelo, Sergio Hernández-Ostiz & Teri A. Kahn

156 Immunodeficiency Syndromes, 2028
Julie V. Schaffer, Melanie Makhija & Amy S. Paller

157 Graft-Versus-Host Disease, 2067
John Harper & Paul Veys

Section 33 The Oral Cavity

158 The Oral Mucosa and Tongue, 2079
Jane Luker & Crispian Scully

Section 34 Hair, Scalp and Nail Disorders

159 Hair Disorders, 2103
Elise A. Olsen & Matilde Iorizzo

160 Alopecia Areata, 2139
Kerstin Foitzik-Lau

161 Nail Disorders, 2147
Antonella Tosti & Bianca Maria Piraccini

Section 35 Anogenital Disease in Children

162 Genital Disease in Children, 2159
Gayle O. Fischer

163 Sexually Transmitted Diseases in Children and Adolescents, 2195
Arnold P. Oranje, Robert A.C. Bilo & Nico G. Hartwig

Section 36 Cutaneous Signs of Child Maltreatment and Sexual Abuse

164 Maltreatment, Physical and Sexual Abuse, 2219
Bernhard Herrmann

Section 37 Psychological Aspects of Skin Disease in Children

165 Assessing and Scoring Life Quality, 2241
Andrew Y. Finlay

166 Coping with the Burden of Disease, 2255
Sarah L. Chamlin

167 Physiological Habits, Self-Mutilation and Factitious Disorders, 2262
Arnold P. Oranje, Jeroen Novak & Robert A.C. Bilo

Section 38 Principles of Treatment in Children

168 Topical Therapy, 2275
Johannes Wohlrab

169 Systemic Therapy in Paediatric Dermatology, 2282
Blanca Rosa Del Pozzo-Magana & Irene Lara-Corrales

170 New Genetic Approaches to Treating Diseases of the Skin, 2301
Stephen Hart & Amy Walker

171 Surgical Therapy, 2310
Julianne A. Mann & Jane S. Bellet

172 Laser Therapy, 2319
Samira Batul Syed, Maria Gnarra & Sean Lanigan

173 Sedation and Anaesthesia, 2330
Brenda M. Simpson, Yuin-Chew Chan & Lawrence F. Eichenfield

Section 39 Diagnostic Procedures in Dermatology

174 Approach to the Paediatric Patient, 2341
Diana Purvis

175 Dermoscopy of Melanocytic Lesions in the Paediatric Population, 2357
Maria L. Marino, Jennifer L. DeFazio, Ralph P. Braun & Ashfaq A. Marghoob

176 The Role of Histopathology and Molecular Techniques in Paediatric Dermatology, 2378
Lori Prok & Adnan Mir

Section 40 Nursing Care of Cutaneous Disorders in Children

177 Nursing Care of the Skin in Children, 2393
Bisola Laguda, Hilary Kennedy, Jackie Denyer, Heulwen Wyatt, Jean Robinson & Karen Pett

Index, i1

List of Contributors

Maria Eugenia Abad, MD
Dermatology Department
Hospital Alemán
Pediatric Dermatology Department
Hospital Ramos Mejía
Buenos Aires, Argentina

Susanne Abraham, MD
Department of Dermatology
Medical Faculty Carl-Gustav-Carus
Technical University of Dresden
Dresden, Germany

Mohannad Abu-Hilal, MD
Assistant Professor
Division of Dermatology
Department of Medicine
McMaster University
Hamilton, ON, Canada

Soumya Agarwal, MD
Senior Resident
Department of Dermatology
Lady Hardinge Medical College and Associated Hospitals
New Delhi, India

Karen Agnew, MBChB, FRACP, FNZDS
Consultant Dermatologist
Starship Children's and Auckland City Hospitals
Auckland, New Zealand

Jusleen Ahluwalia, MD
Resident Physician
Department of Pediatric and Adolescent Dermatology
Rady Children's Hospital
San Diego, CA, USA

Fatma Al Jasmi, MBBS, FRCPC, FCCMG
Associate Professor
College of Medicine and Health Science
United Arab Emirates University
Al Ain, United Arab Emirates

Ali Alikhan
University of Cincinnati
Department of Dermatology
Cincinnati, OH, USA

Nawaf Almutairi, MD
Professor
Department of Medicine
Faculty of Medicine
Kuwait University
Kuwait

Jasem M. Alshaiji, MD
Head of Dermatology Department
Head of Pediatric Dermatology Unit
Amiri Hospital
Kuwait

Christian Apfelbacher, PhD
Medical Sociology
Institute of Epidemiology and Preventive Medicine
University of Regensburg
Regensburg, Germany

Lisa M. Arkin, MD
Department of Dermatology
University of Wisconsin School of Medicine and Public Health
Madison, WI, USA

Yuka Asai, MSc, PhD, MD
Assistant Professor
Division of Dermatology
Queen's University
Kingston, ON, Canada

Matthias Augustin, MD
Professor
Institute for Health Services Research in Dermatology and Nursing (IVDP)
University Medical Center Hamburg-Eppendorf (UKE)
Hamburg, Germany

Rosalia A. Ballona
Division of Dermatology
Instituto del Salud del Niño
Lima, Peru

Jonathan Barker, MD, FRCP, FRCPath
Professor of Dermatology
St John's Institute of Dermatology (King's College)
Guy's Hospital
London, UK

Eulalia T. Baselga, MD
Pediatric Dermatology Unit
Hospital de la Santa Creu I Sant Pau
Universitat Autònoma de Barcelona
Spain

M.W. Bekkenk, MD, PhD
Dermatologist
Netherlands Institute for Pigment Disorders
Amsterdam University Medical Centers
Amsterdam, The Netherlands

Jane S. Bellet, MD
Associate Professor of Dermatology and Pediatrics
Duke University Medical Center
Durham, NC, USA

Lionel Bercovitch, MD
Professor of Dermatology
Warren Alpert Medical School of Brown University
Director of Pediatric Dermatology
Hasbro Children's Hospital
Providence, RI, USA
Medical Director
PXE International, Inc.
Washington, DC, USA

Robert A.C. Bilo
Department of Forensic Medicine
Section on Forensic Pediatrics
Netherlands Forensic Institute
The Hague, The Netherlands

Carol M. Black, DBE, MD, FRCP, MACP, FMedSci
Principal of Newnham College Cambridge, Expert Adviser on Health and Work to NHS England and Public Health England, Chair of Think Ahead, Chair of the British Library
Centre for Rheumatology
Royal Free Hospital and UCL Division of Medicine
London, UK

Christine Bodemer, MD, PhD
Professor of Dermatology
Department of Dermatology
Imagine Institute
Necker-Enfants Malades Hospital
Paris, France

Marcela Bocian, MD
Assistant Physician
Dermatology Department
Hospital de Pediatría 'Prof. Dr. Juan P. Garrahan'
Buenos Aires, Argentina

Ernesto Bonifazi, MD
Professor of Dermatology
Dermatologia Pediatrica Association
Bari, Italy

Laurence M. Boon, MD, PhD
Coordinator of the Center for Vascular Anomalies
Division of Plastic Surgery
Cliniques Universitaires Saint Luc and Human Molecular Genetics
de Duve Institute
University of Louvain
Brussels, Belgium

Franck Boralevi, MD, PhD
Pediatric Dermatology Unit
Hôpital Pellegrin-Enfants
Bordeaux, France

Bret L. Bostwick, MD
Assistant Professor
Department of Molecular and Human Genetics
Baylor College of Medicine and Texas Children's Hospital
Houston, TX, USA

E. Bourrat, MD
Reference Center for Inherited Skin Disease
Dermatology Department
CHU Saint Louis
Paris, France

Kevin P. Boyd, MD
Clinical Assistant Professor
University of Alabama at Birmingham
Birmingham, AL, USA

Ralph P. Braun, MD
Dermatology Clinic
University Hospital Zürich
Zürich, Switzerland

Judith Breuer, MBBS, MD, FRCPath
Professor of Virology
UCL
Honorary Consultant Virologist
Great Ormond Street Hospital
UCL Division of Infection and Immunity
London, UK

Paul A. Brogan, MBChB, FRCPCH, PhD
Professor of Vasculitis and Honorary Consultant Paediatric Rheumatologist
Section Head: Infection and Inflammation and Rheumatology
Co-Director of Education (Clinical Academics)
UCL Institute of Child Health
Great Ormond Street Hospital NHS Foundation Trust
London, UK

Margaret Brown, MD
Division of Dermatology
The University of Texas Health Science Center at San Antonio
San Antonio, TX, USA

John C. Browning, MD, FAAD, FAAP
Assistant Professor
Baylor College of Medicine
Chief of Dermatology
Children's Hospital of San Antonio
San Antonio, TX, USA

Anna L. Bruckner, MD, MSCS
Associate Professor of Dermatology and Pediatrics
University of Colorado School of Medicine
Section Head
Division of Dermatology
Children's Hospital Colorado
Aurora, CO, USA

Joachim J. Bugert, MD, PhD
Lab Group Leader
Institut für Mikrobiologie der Bundeswehr
München, Germany

María Marta Bujan, MD
Assistant Physician
Dermatology Department
Hospital de Pediatría 'Prof. Dr. Juan P. Garrahan'
Buenos Aires, Argentina

Caleb P. Bupp, MD
Medical Geneticist
Spectrum Health Medical Group
Grand Rapids, MI, USA

Jane C. Burns, MD
Professor of Pediatrics
Director, Kawasaki Disease Research Center
University of California, San Diego
Rady Children's Hospital
La Jolla, CA, USA

Nigel P. Burrows, MBBS, MD, FRCP
Consultant Dermatologist and Associated Lecturer
Department of Dermatology
Addenbrooke's Hospital
Cambridge University Hospitals NHS Foundation Trust
Cambridge, UK

Héctor Cáceres-Ríos, MD
Consultant in Pediatric Dermatology
Department of Pediatric Dermatology
Instituto de Salud del Niño
Lima, Peru

Julie L. Cantatore-Francis, MD
Dermatology Physicians of Connecticut
Shelton, CT, USA

Genevieve Casey
Specialist Registrar
Department of Dermatology
Women's & Children's Hospital
Adelaide, SA, Australia

Leslie Castelo-Soccio, MD, PhD
Professor of Pediatrics and Dermatology
Department of Pediatrics
Section of Pediatric Dermatology
University of Pennsylvania Perelman School of Medicine and Children's Hospital of Philadelphia
Philadelphia, PA, USA

Andrea Bettina Cervini, MD
Dermatologist, Pediatric Dermatologist
Head of Dermatology Department
Hospital de Pediatría 'Prof. Dr. Juan P. Garrahan'
Buenos Aires, Argentina

Sarah L. Chamlin, MD
Professor of Pediatrics and Dermatology
The Ann and Robert H. Lurie Children's Hospital of Chicago and Northwestern University
Feinberg School of Medicine
Chicago, IL, USA

Yuin-Chew Chan
Dermatologist
Dermatology Associates
Gleneagles Medical Centre
Singapore

Joyce C. Chang, MD
Instructor
Division of Rheumatology
The Children's Hospital of Philadelphia
Philadelphia, PA, USA

Susheera Chatproedprai, MD
Associate Professor of Paediatrics
Head of Division of Paediatric Dermatology
Department of Paediatrics
Faculty of Medicine
Chulalongkorn University,
Bangkok, Thailand

Derek H. Chu, MD
Clinical Assistant Professor of Dermatology and Pediatrics
Stanford University School of Medicine
Palo Alto, CA, USA

Antonio A.T. Chuh, MD
Department of Family Medicine and Primary Care
The University of Hong Kong and Queen Mary Hospital
Pokfulam, Hong Kong
JC School of Public Health and Primary Care
The Chinese University of Hong Kong and the Prince of Wales Hospital
Shatin, Hong Kong

Peter T. Clayton, BA, MBBS, MSc, MRCP
Professor
Institute of Child Health
University College London with Great Ormond Street Hospital for Children NHS Trust
London, UK

Kelly M. Cordoro, MD
Associate Professor of Dermatology and Pediatrics
University of California San Francisco
San Francisco, CA, USA

Carrie C. Coughlin, MD
Assistant Professor
Division of Dermatology
Department of Medicine and Department of Pediatrics
Washington University School of Medicine
St Louis, MO, USA

Coleen K. Cunningham
Department of Pediatrics and Dermatology
Duke University Medical Center
Durham, NC, USA

Benjamin S. Daniel
Department of Dermatology
St George Hospital and University of New South Wales
Sydney, NSW, Australia

Robert Dawe, MBCh, MD, FRCPE
Photodermatology Unit
Department of Dermatology
Ninewells Hospital and Medical School
Dundee, UK

Jennifer L. DeFazio, MD
Department of Dermatology
Memorial Sloan-Kettering Cancer Center
New York, NY, USA

Blanca Rosa Del Pozzo-Magana
London Health Sciences Center and Western University
London, ON, Canada

Christopher P. Denton, PhD, FRCP
Professor of Experimental Rheumatology
Centre for Rheumatology
Royal Free Hospital and UCL Division of Medicine
London, UK

Jackie Denyer
Clinical Nurse Specialist in Paediatric Dermatology
Great Ormond Street Hospital
London, UK

Clio Dessinioti
Department of Dermatology
Andreas Syggros Hospital
University of Athens
Greece

Tanvi Dev, MD
Senior Resident (Fellow)
Department of Dermatology
All India Institute of Medical Sciences
New Delhi, India

Flora B. de Waard-van der Spek, MD, PhD
Paediatric Dermatologist
Department of Dermatology
Franciscus Gasthuis and Vlietland
Rotterdam/Schiedam, The Netherlands

Sandipan Dhar, MBBS, MD, DNB, FRCP(Edin)
Professor and Head
Department of Pediatric Dermatology
Institute of Child Health
Kolkata, West Bengal, India

Wei-Li Di, MBBS, PhD
Associate Professor in Skin Biology
Infection, Immunity and Inflammation Programme
Immunobiology Section
Institute of Child Health
University College London
London, UK

Francis J. DiMario Jr, MD
Professor of Pediatrics and Neurology
University of Connecticut School of Medicine
Farmington, CT, USA
Associate Chair for Academic Affairs,
Department of Pediatrics,
Director, Neurogenetic-Tuberous Sclerosis Clinic
Division of Pediatric Neurology
Connecticut Children's Medical Center
Hartford, CT, USA

Ncoza C. Dlova
Department of Dermatology
University of Kwazulu-Natal
Durban, South Africa

Jean Donadieu, MD, PhD
Service d'Hémato-Oncologie Pédiatrique
Registre des Histiocytoses
Centre de Référence des Histiocytoses
Hopital Trousseau
Paris, France

Dian Donnai, CBE, FMedSci, FRCP, FRCOG
Professor of Medical Genetics
Manchester Centre for Genomic Medicine
St Mary's Hospital
Manchester University NHS Foundation Trust
Manchester, UK
Division of Evolution and Genomic Sciences
Faculty of Biology Medicine and Health
University of Manchester
Manchester, UK

Carola Durán McKinster, MD
Paediatric Dermatologist and Professor of Pediatric Dermatology
Universidad Nacional Autonoma de México
Head of the Department of Pediatric Dermatology
National Institute of Paediatrics of Mexico
Mexico City, Mexico

Jonathan A. Dyer, MD
Associate Professor of Dermatology and Child Health
Departments of Dermatology and Child Health
University of Missouri
Columbia, MO, USA

Lawrence F. Eichenfield, MD
Professor of Clinical Dermatology
Pediatric and Adolescent Dermatology
Rady Children's Hospital
San Diego University of California
San Diego School of Medicine
San Diego, CA, USA

Despina Eleftheriou, MBBS, PhD, MRCPCH
Associate Professor in Paediatric Rheumatology
Infection, Inflammation and Rheumatology Section
UCL Institute of Child Health
Paediatric Rheumatology Department, Great Ormond Street Hospital for Children NHS Foundation Trust
Arthritis Research UK Centre for Adolescent Rheumatology
London, UK

Brian Eley, BSc (Hons) (Med Biochem), MBChB (Cape Town), FCP (SA)
Professor of Paediatric Infectious Diseases
University of Cape Town
South Africa

Steffen Emmert, MD
Professor of Dermatology
Director
Clinic for Dermatology and Venereology
University Medical Center Rostock
Rostock, Germany

Herman Jan H. Engelkens, MD, PhD
Department of Dermatology and Venereology
Ikazia Hospital
Rotterdam, The Netherlands

Sibel Ersoy-Evans, MD
Professor of Dermatology
Hacettepe University School of Medicine
Department of Dermatology
Ankara, Turkey

Peter A. Farndon, MSc, MD, FRCP
Professor of Clinical Genetics (Retired)
University of Birmingham
Birmingham, UK

Saul N. Faust, FRCPCH, PhD
Professor of Paediatric Immunology and Infectious Diseases and Director of the NIHR Southampton Clinical Research Facility
University of Southampton and University Hospital Southampton NHS Foundation Trust
Southampton, UK

Andrew Y. Finlay, CBE, FRCP (Lond. and Glasg.)
Professor of Dermatology
Division of Infection and Immunity
Cardiff University School of Medicine
Cardiff, UK

Gayle O. Fischer, MBBS, FACD, MD
Associate Professor in Dermatology
The Northern Clinical School
The University of Sydney
Sydney, NSW, Australia

Carsten Flohr, MD, PhD
Professor of Dermatology
Unit for Population-Based Dermatology Research
St John's Institute of Dermatology
Guy's and St Thomas' NHS Foundation Trust and King's College
London, UK

Kerstin Foitzik-Lau, MD
Physician
Skin and Vein Clinic Winterhude
Hamburg, Germany

Emma J. Footitt, MB, BS, BSc, PhD
Institute of Child Health
University College London with Great Ormond Street Hospital for Children NHS Trust
London, UK

Sylvie Fraitag, MD
Dermatopathologie Pédiatrique
Service d'Anatomo-Pathologie
Hôpital Necker-Enfants Malades
Paris, France

Jorge Frank, MD
Professor of Dermatology
Department of Dermatology, Venereology and Allergology
University Medical Center Göttingen
Göttingen, Germany

Ilona J. Frieden, MD
Professor of Dermatology and Pediatrics
Division of Pediatric Dermatology
San Francisco School of Medicine
University of California
San Francisco, CA, USA

Sheila Fallon Friedlander, MD
Professor of Dermatology and Pediatrics
Department of Pediatric and Adolescent Dermatology
Rady Children's Hospital
San Diego, CA, USA

Hassan Galadari, MD
Associate Professor
College of Medicine and Health Science
United Arab Emirates University
Al Ain, United Arab Emirates

Pamela Gangar, MD
Resident Physician
University of Arizona Department of Pediatrics
Tucson, AZ, USA

María Teresa García-Romero, MD, MPH
Attending Physician
Department of Dermatology
National Institute for Pediatrics
Member of the National System of Researchers
Mexico City, Mexico

Maria C. Garzon, MD
Columbia University Medical Center
New York, NY, USA

Diane Gbesemete, BM, MRCPCH, PGDipID
Clinical Research Fellow
NIHR Southampton Clinical Research Facility
University of Southampton and University Hospital Southampton NHS Foundation Trust
Southampton, UK

Carlo M. Gelmetti
Professor of Dermatology and Venereology
Department of Pathophysiology and Transplantation
Università degli Studi di Milano
Head
Unit of Pediatric Dermatology
Fondazione IRCCS Ca' Granda 'Ospedale Maggiore Policlinico'
Milan, Italy

Karolina Gholam, MBSS, MSc, FRCPCH, SCEderm
Consultant Paediatric Dermatologist
Great Ormond Street Hospital
London, UK

Mary Glover, MA, FRCP, FRCPCH
Consultant Paediatric Dermatologist
Great Ormond Street Hospital for Children NHS Foundation Trust
London, UK

Maria Gnarra, MD, PhD
Research Fellow
Paediatric Dermatology
Great Ormond Street Hospital for Children NHS Trust
London, UK

Alina Goldenberg, MD
Resident in-training
Department of Dermatology
University of California
San Diego, CA, USA

Bernardo Gontijo, MD, PhD
Professor of Dermatology
Federal University of Minas Gerais
Medical School
Belo Horizonte, MG, Brazil

Helen M. Goodyear, MB, ChB, FRCP, FRCPCH, MD, MMEd, MA
Health Education England (West Midlands)
Associate Postgraduate Dean
Heart of England NHS Foundation Trust
Birmingham, UK

Jeremy A. Goss, MD
Research Fellow
Department of Plastic and Oral Surgery
Vascular Anomalies Center
Boston Children's Hospital
Harvard Medical School
Boston, MA, USA

Yvonne Gräser, PhD
Professor of Molecular Mycology
The National Reference Laboratory for Dermatophytes
Universitätsmedizin – Charité
Institute of Microbiology and Hygiene
Berlin, Germany

Arin K. Greene, MD, MMSc
Professor of Surgery
Department of Plastic and Oral Surgery
Vascular Anomalies Center
Boston Children's Hospital
Harvard Medical School
Boston, MA, USA

Leopold M. Groesser, Dr med.
Department of Dermatology
University of Regensburg
Regensburg, Germany

Robert Gruber, MD
Department of Dermatology and Division of Human Genetics
Medical University of Innsbruck
Innsbruck, Austria

Christian Hafner, Dr med.
Professor of Dermatology
Department of Dermatology
University of Regensburg
Regensburg, Germany

Henning Hamm, MD
Professor of Dermatology
Department of Dermatology, Venereology and Allergology
University Hospital Würzburg
Würzburg, Germany

John Harper, MBBS, MD, FRCP, FRCPCH
Honorary Professor of Paediatric Dermatology
Great Ormond Street Hospital for Children NHS Trust
London, UK

Stephen Hart, PhD
Professor in Molecular Genetics
Experimental and Personalised Medicine
UCL Great Ormond Street Institute of Child Health
London, UK

Nico G. Hartwig, MD, PhD
Department of Paediatrics
Franciscus Gasthuis & Vlietland
Rotterdam, The Netherlands

Christina Has, MD
Consultant Dermatologist and Professor
Molecular Dermatology
Medical Center
University of Freiburg
Freiburg, Germany

Elena B. Hawryluk, MD, PhD
Department of Dermatology
Massachusetts General Hospital
Harvard Medical School;
Dermatology Program
Division of Allergy and Immunology
Department of Medicine
Boston Children's Hospital
Harvard Medical School
Boston, MA, USA

R.M. Ross Hearn
Department of Dermatology and Photobiology
Ninewells Hospital and Medical School
Dundee, UK

Daniel Heinl, MD
Medical Sociology
Institute of Epidemiology and Preventive Medicine
University of Regensburg
Regensburg, Germany

Angela Hernández, MD
Department of Dermatology
Hospital Infantil del Niño Jesús
Madrid, Spain

Sergio Hernández-Ostiz, MD
Department of Dermatology
Hospital Infantil del Niño Jesús
Madrid, Spain

Bernhard Herrmann, MD
Consultant
Child Protection Center
Pediatric and Adolescent Gynecology
Department of Pediatrics
Klinikum Kassel
Kassel, Germany

Robert S. Heyderman, PhD, FRCP, DTM & H
Professor of Infectious Diseases
University College London
London, UK

Warren R. Heymann, MD
Head, Division of Dermatology,
Clinical Professor of Dermatology
University of Pennsylvania School of Medicine
Professor of Medicine and Paediatrics
University of Medicine and Dentistry of New Jersey
Robert Wood Johnson Medical School
Camden, NJ, USA

Hannah Hill, MD
Resident in-training
Department of Dermatology
Mayo Clinic
Scottsdale, AZ, USA

Sarah Hill, MBChB, FRACP
Paediatric and General Dermatologist
Department of Dermatology
Waikato Hospital
Hamilton, New Zealand

Sharleen F. Hill, BM BSc MRCP
Dermatology Clinical Research Fellow
St George Hospital
Conjoint Associate Lecturer
University of New South Wales
Sydney, NSW, Australia

Peter H. Hoeger, MD
Professor of Paediatrics and Dermatology (University of Hamburg)
Head, Departments of Paediatrics and Dermatology
Catholic Children's Hospital, Wilhelmstift
Hamburg, Germany

Karen A. Holbrook, MD
(Retired)
Department of Physiology and Cell Biology
Ohio State University
Columbus, OH, USA

Gregor Holzer, MD
Department of Dermatology
Donauspital SMZ Ost
Vienna, Austria

Erhard Hölzle, MD
Professor of Dermatology
Director
Department of Dermatology and Allergology
University Hospital
Oldenburg, Germany

Kam Lun Ellis Hon, MBBS, MD, FAAP, FCCM, FHKCPaed, FHKAM(Paed)
Honorary Professor
Department of Paediatrics, The Chinese University of Hong Kong
Consultant
The Hong Kong Children's Hospital
Hong Kong

Paul J. Honig, MD
Division of Dermatology
Denver Children's Hospital
Denver, CO, USA
Department of Pediatrics
Perelman School of Medicine at the University of Pennsylvania
Philadelphia, PA, USA

Kimberly A. Horii, MD
Associate Professor of Pediatrics
Division of Dermatology
University of Missouri-Kansas City School of Medicine
Children's Mercy-Kansas City
Kansas City, MO, USA

Jennifer Huang, MD
Assistant Professor of Dermatology
Dermatology Program
Boston Children's Hospital
Boston, MA, USA

Devika Icecreamwala, MD
Pediatric Dermatology Fellow
Department of Dermatology
Henry Ford Health System
Detroit, MI, USA

Ying Liu, MD, PhD
Associate Chief Physician
Department of Dermatology
Beijing Children's Hospital
Capital Medical University
National Center for Children's Health
Beijing, China

Arun C. Inamadar, MD, FRCP
Professor and Head
Department of Dermatology, Venereology & Leprosy
Sri B.M.Patil Medical College
Hospital & Research Centre
BLDE University
Vijayapur, Karnataka, India

Matilde Iorizzo, MD
Private Dermatology Practice
Bellinzona and Lugano
Switzerland

Alan D. Irvine, MD, FRCPI, FRCP
Professor
Paediatric Dermatology
Trinity College Dublin and Our Lady's Children's Hospital
Dublin, Ireland

Sharon E. Jacob, MD
Professor
Department of Dermatology
Loma Linda University
Loma Linda, CA, USA

Scott H. James, MD
Department of Paediatrics
Division of Infectious Diseases
University of Alabama
Birmingham, AL, USA

Gregor B.E. Jemec, MD, DMSc
Department of Dermatology
Roskilde Hospital
Roskilde, Denmark

Elizabeth A. Jones, MA MB, BChir, FRCP, PhD
Consultant Clinical Geneticist
Manchester Centre for Genomic Medicine
St Mary's Hospital
Manchester University NHS Foundation Trust
Manchester, UK
Division of Evolution and Genomic Sciences
Faculty of Biology Medicine and Health
University of Manchester
Manchester, UK

Teri A. Kahn, MD, MPH
Associate Professor
Department of Dermatology
University of Maryland
Baltimore, MD, USA

Sonia Kamath, MD
Resident Physician
Department of Dermatology
Keck School of Medicine of University of Southern California
Los Angeles, CA, USA

Ayşen Karaduman, MD
Professor of Dermatology
Hacettepe University School of Medicine
Department of Dermatology
Ankara, Turkey

Andreas Katsambas
Professor of Dermatology
Department of Dermatology
Andreas Syggros Hospital
University of Athens
Greece

Roselyn Kellen, MD
Resident Physician
Icahn School of Medicine at Mount Sinai
New York, NY, USA

Hilary Kennedy
Clinical Nurse Specialist in Paediatric Dermatology
Great Ormond Street Hospital
London, UK

David W. Kimberlin, MD
Department of Pediatrics
Division of Infectious Diseases
University of Alabama
Birmingham, AL, USA

Veronica A. Kinsler, MA, MB, BChir, FRCPCH, PhD
Professor of Paediatric Dermatology and Dermatogenetics
Paediatric Dermatology Department
Great Ormond Street Hospital for Children NHS Foundation Trust
Genetics and Genomic Medicine
UCL Great Ormond Street Institute of Child Health
London, UK

Bruce R. Korf, MD, PhD
Professor and Chairman of Department of Genetics
University of Alabama at Birmingham
Birmingham, AL, USA

Andrew C. Krakowski, MD
Chief
Department of Dermatology
St Luke's University Health Network
Easton, PA, USA

Ann M. Kulungowski, MD
Assistant Professor of Surgery and Pediatrics
University of Colorado School of Medicine
Surgical Director
Vascular Anomalies Center
Children's Hospital Colorado
Aurora, CO, USA

Marc Lacour, MD
Paediatrician
Pediatric Dermatology Clinic
Carouge, Switzerland

Bisola Laguda
Consultant
Paediatric Dermatology
Chelsea and Westminster Hospital
London, UK

Sinéad M. Langan, MD, PhD
Associate Professor of Epidemiology
Faculty of Epidemiology and Population Health
London School of Hygiene and Tropical Medicine
London, UK

Sean Lanigan, MD, FRCP, DCH
Regional Medical Director
sk:n Limited
Birmingham, UK

Irene Lara-Corrales, MD
Associate Professor of Pediatrics
Pediatric Dermatology Fellow
Section of Dermatology
Division of Paediatric Medicine
Hospital for Sick Children
University of Toronto
Toronto, ON, Canada

Margarita Larralde, PhD, MD
Head
Dermatology Department
Hospital Alemán
Head
Pediatric Dermatology Department
Hospital Ramos Mejía
Buenos Aires, Argentina

Christine T. Lauren, MD
Assistant Professor of Dermatology and Pediatrics
Columbia University Medical Center
New York, NY, USA

S. Leclerc-Mercier, MD
Reference Center for Rare and Inherited Skin Diseases (MAGEC)
Departments of Dermatology and Pathology
CHU Necker-Enfants Malades
Paris, France

Theresa Ngan Ho Leung, MBBS, FRCPCH, FHKCPaed, FHKAM(Paed)
Clinical Associate Professor
Department of Paediatrics and Adolescent Medicine
The University of Hong Kong
Hong Kong

Ting Fan Leung, MBChB(CUHK), MD(CUHK), MRCP(UK), FRCPCH, FAAAAI, FHKCPaed, FHKAM(Paediatrics)
Chairman and Professor
Department of Paediatrics
The Chinese University of Hong Kong
Hong Kong

Michael Levin, FRCPCH, PhD
Professor of Paediatrics and International Child Health
Imperial College London
London, UK

Moise L. Levy, MD
Professor
Department of Pediatrics
Texas Children's Hospital
Baylor College of Medicine
Houston, TX, USA
Department of Pediatrics
Dell Medical School/University of Texas and Dell Children's Medical Center
Austin, TX, USA

Rebecca Levy, MD, FRCPC
Clinical Fellow
Pediatric Dermatology
University of Toronto
The Hospital for Sick Children
Toronto, ON, Canada

Susan Lewis-Jones, FRCP, FRCPCH
Honorary Consultant Dermatologist
Ninewells Hospital & Medical School
Dundee, UK

Carmen Liy Wong
Pediatric Dermatology Fellow
Section of Dermatology
Division of Paediatric Medicine
Hospital for Sick Children
Toronto, ON, Canada

Wilson Lopez, MBBS, MD, MRCP, FRCPCH, DCH, MSc
Consultant Neonatologist
Neonatal Unit
Barking, Havering and Redbridge University Hospitals NHS Trust
UK

Christopher Lovell
Consultant Dermatologist
Kinghorn Dermatology Unit
Royal United Hospital
Bath, UK

Anne W. Lucky, MD
Adjunct Professor of Pediatrics and Dermatology
Divisions of General and Community Pediatrics and Pediatric Dermatology
Cincinnati Children's Hospital
Cincinnati, OH, USA

David Luk, FHKAM(Paed), FHKCPaed, FRCPCH
Consultant Paediatrician
United Christian Hospital, Hong Kong
Hong Kong Children's Hospital
Honorary Clinical Assistant Professor
The Chinese University of Hong Kong
The University of Hong Kong
President
Hong Kong Paediatric and Adolescent Dermatology Society

Jane Luker, BDS, PhD, FDSRCS Eng @ Edin DDR, RCR
Consultant Dental Surgeon
Bristol Dental Hospital
University Hospitals Bristol NHS Foundation Trust
Bristol, UK

Paula Carolina Luna, MD
Dermatology Department
Hospital Alemán
Buenos Aires, Argentina

Minnelly Luu, MD
Assistant Professor of Clinical Dermatology
Department of Dermatology
Keck School of Medicine of University of Southern California
Los Angeles, CA, USA
Division of Pediatric Dermatology
Children's Hospital Los Angeles
Los Angeles, CA, USA

Lin Ma, MD, PhD
Professor, Director
Department of Dermatology
Beijing Children's Hospital
Capital Medical University
National Center for Children's Health
Beijing, China

Elia F. Maalouf, MBChB, MRCP, FRCPCH, MD
Consultant in General Paediatrics and Neonatal Medicine
Neonatal Unit
Homerton University Hospital NHS Foundation Trust
London, UK

Caroline Mahon, MD
Consultant Paediatric Dermatologist
Department of Dermatology
Bristol Royal Infirmary
University Hospitals Bristol NHS Foundation Trust
Bristol, UK

Melanie Makhija, MD, MSc
Assistant Professor of Pediatrics
Department of Pediatrics
Northwestern University
Feinberg School of Medicine,
Chicago, IL, USA

Steven M. Manders, MD
Professor of Medicine and Paediatrics
Division of Dermatology
University of Medicine and Dentistry of New Jersey
Robert Wood Johnson Medical School
Camden, NJ, USA

Julianne A. Mann, MD
Assistant Professor of Dermatology
Dartmouth-Hitchcock Medical Center
Lebanon, NH, USA

Ashfaq A. Marghoob, MD
Department of Dermatology
Memorial Sloan-Kettering Cancer Center
New York, NY, USA

Maria L. Marino, MD
Department of Dermatology
Memorial Sloan-Kettering Cancer Center
New York, NY, USA

Anna E. Martinez, FRCPCH
Consultant Paediatric Dermatologist
Paediatric Dermatology Department
Great Ormond Street Hospital for Children
NHS Trust
London, UK

Peter Mayser, MD
Professor of Dermatology
Clinic of Dermatology, Allergology and Venereology
Justus Liebig University (UKGM)
Giessen, Germany

Juliette Mazereeuw-Hautier, MD, PhD
Professor of Dermatology
Reference Center for Rare Skin Diseases
Department of Dermatology
CHU Larrey
Toulouse, France

William H. McCoy IV, MD, PhD
Resident Physician
Division of Dermatology
Department of Medicine
Washington University School of Medicine
St Louis, MO, USA

Jemima E. Mellerio, MD, FRDP
Consultant Dermatologist and Honorary Professor
Paediatric Dermatology Department
Great Ormond Street Hospital for Children
NHS Trust
and St John's Institute of Dermatology
Guy's and St Thomas' NHS Foundation Trust
London, UK

Bodo C. Melnik, MD
Adjunct Professor of Dermatology
Department of Dermatology, Environmental Medicine and Health Theory
University of Osnabrück
Osnabrück, Germany

Vibhu Mendiratta, MD
Director and Professor
Department of Dermatology
Lady Hardinge Medical College and associated hospitals
New Delhi, India

Eirini E. Merika, MBBS, iBSc, MRCP Derm
Consultant Paediatric Dermatologist
Chelsea and Westminster Hospital
London, UK

Christian R. Millett, MD
Forefront Dermatology
Vienna, VA, USA

Adnan Mir, MD, PhD
Assistant Professor of Dermatology
University of Texas Southwestern Medical Center and Children's Medical Center Dallas
Dallas, TX, USA

Amanda T. Moon, MD
Departments of Pediatrics and Dermatology
Perelman School of Medicine at the University of Pennsylvania
Philadelphia, PA, USA
Section of Dermatology
Children's Hospital of Philadelphia
Philadelphia, PA, USA

Elena Moraitis, MBBS, PhD
Consultant in Paediatric Rheumatology
Infection, Inflammation and Rheumatology Section
UCL Institute of Child Health
London, UK
Paediatric Rheumatology Department
Great Ormond Street Hospital for Children
NHS Foundation Trust
London, UK

Fanny Morice-Picard, MD, PhD
Department of Dermatology and Paediatric Dermatology
Reference Center for Rare Skin Diseases
Hôpital Saint André
Bordeaux, France

Keith Morley, MD
Paediatric Dermatology Fellow
Dermatology Program
Boston Children's Hospital
Boston, MA, USA

Dédée F. Murrell, MA(Cambridge), BMBCh (Oxford), FAAD(USA), MD (UNSW), FACD, FRCP(Edin)
Head
Department of Dermatology
St George Hospital
Professor of Dermatology
University of New South Wales
Sydney, NSW, Australia

Taizo A. Nakano, MD
Assistant Professor of Pediatrics
University of Colorado School of Medicine
Medical Director
Vascular Anomalies Center
Children's Hospital Colorado
Aurora, CO, USA

Iria Neri
Professor of Dermatology
Department of Specialized, Diagnostic and Experimental Medicine
Division of Dermatology
University of Bologna
Bologna, Italy

Tuyet A. Nguyen, MD
Kaiser Permanente Dermatology
Los Angeles, CA, USA

Jeroen Novak
GGZ Momentum
Breda, The Netherlands

Susan O'Connell, MD
Formerly Lyme Borreliosis Unit
Health Protection Agency Microbiology Laboratory
Southampton University Hospitals NHS Trust
Southampton, UK

Cathal O'Connor, MD
Paediatric Dermatology
Trinity College Dublin and Our Lady's Children's Hospital
Dublin, Ireland

Vinzenz Oji, MD
Department of Dermatology
University Hospital Münster
Münster, Germany

Elise A. Olsen, MD
Professor of Dermatology and Medicine
Director, Cutaneous Lymphoma Research and Treatment Center
Director, Hair Disorders Research and Treatment Center
Director, Dermatopharmacology Study Center
Departments of Dermatology and Medicine
Duke University Medical Center
Durham, NC, USA

Kai Ren Ong, MD, MRCP
Consultant Clinical Geneticist
West Midlands Regional Clinical Genetics Service
Birmingham Women's Hospital
Birmingham, UK

Arnold P. Oranje, MD, PhD
(Deceased)
Professor of Pediatric Dermatology
Kinderhuid.nl, Rotterdam, The Netherlands
Hair Clinic, Breda, The Netherlands
Dermicis Skin Clinic, Alkmaar, The Netherlands

Luz Orozco-Covarrubias, MD
Paediatric Dermatologist and Associated Professor of Pediatric Dermatology
Universidad Nacional Autonoma de México
Attending Physician
Department of Pediatric Dermatology
National Institute of Paediatrics of Mexico
Mexico City, Mexico

Edel A. O'Toole, MB, PhD, FRCP, FRCPI
Professor of Molecular Dermatology and Honorary Consultant Dermatologist
Department of Dermatology
Royal London Hospital
Barts Health NHS Trust and Centre for Cell Biology and Cutaneous Research
Barts and the London School of Medicine and Dentistry
London, UK

Hagen Ott, MD
Head of the Division of Pediatric Dermatology and Allergology
Epidermolysis Bullosa Centre Hannover
Children's Hospital AUF DER BULT
Hannover, Germany

Seza Özen, MD
Professor of Pediatrics
Hacettepe University School of Medicine
Department of Pediatric Rheumatology
Ankara, Turkey

David G. Paige, MBBS, MA, FRCP
Consultant Dermatologist
Department of Dermatology,
Bart's and The London NHS Trust
London, UK

Aparna Palit, MD
Professor
Department of Dermatology
Venereology and Leprosy
Sri B.M.Patil Medical College
Hospital & Research Centre
BLDE University
Vijayapur, Karnataka, India

Amy S. Paller, MD, MSc
Walter J. Hamlin Professor and Chair of Dermatology, Professor of Pediatrics
Departments of Pediatrics and Dermatology
Northwestern University
Feinberg School of Medicine
Chicago, IL, USA

Nirav Patel, MD
Departments of Dermatology and Pediatrics
Mayo Clinic
Rochester, MN, USA

Annalisa Patrizi, MD
Professor
Head of Dermatology
Department of Specialized, Diagnostic and Experimental Medicine,
Division of Dermatology
University of Bologna
Bologna, Italy

Marissa J. Perman, MD
Assistant Professor of Pediatrics and Dermatology
Children's Hospital of Philadelphia and The University of Pennsylvania
Philadelphia, PA, USA

Karen Pett
Clinical Nurse Specialist in Paediatric Dermatology
West Hertfordshire Hospitals NHS Trust
St Albans, UK

Roderic J. Phillips, BSc(Hons), MBBS, PhD, FRACP, AMAM, CIRF
Associate Professor
Paediatric Dermatologist
Royal Children's Hospital
Honorary Research Fellow
Murdoch Children's Research Institute
Adjunct Professor
Paediatrics
Monash University
Melbourne, VIC, Australia

Bianca Maria Piraccini, MD, PhD
Dermatology
Department of Experimental, Diagnostic and Specialty Medicine
University of Bologna
Bologna, Italy

Laura Polivka, MD, PhD
Department of Dermatology
Imagine Institute
Necker-Enfants Malades Hospital
Paris, France

Elena Pope, MSc, FRCPC
Professor of Paediatrics
University of Toronto
Fellowship Director and Section Head
Paediatric Dermatology
The Hospital for Sick Children
Toronto, ON, Canada

Julie Powell, MD, FRCPC
Director
Pediatric Dermatology
Professor of Dermatology (Pediatrics)
Division of Dermatology
Department of Pediatrics
CHU Sainte-Justine
University of Montreal
Montreal, QC, Canada

Julie S. Prendiville, MBBCH, DCH, BAO, FRCPC
Chief
Pediatric Dermatology
Sidra Medicine
Doha, Qatar

Cecilia A.C. (Sanna) Prinsen, PhD
VU University Medical Center
Department of Epidemiology and Biostatistics
Amsterdam Public Health Research Institute
Amsterdam, The Netherlands

Lori Prok, MD
Associate Professor of Dermatology and Pathology
University of Colorado Denver and Children's Hospital Colorado
Denver, CO, USA

Neil S. Prose, MD
Professor
Department of Pediatrics and Dermatology
Duke University Medical Center
Research Professor of Global Health, Duke Global Health Institute
Co-Director, Duke Health Humanities Lab
Durham, NC, USA

Diana Purvis, MB ChB, MRCPCH, FRACP
Paediatric Dermatologist
Starship Children's Hospital
Honorary Senior Lecturer
Department of Paediatrics
University of Auckland
Auckland, New Zealand

Marius Rademaker, BM, FRCP(Edin), FRACP, DM
Clinical Director
Dermatology Department
Waikato District Health Board
Hon Associate Professor
Waikato Clinical Campus
Faculty of Medical and Health Sciences
The University of Auckland
Hamilton, New Zealand

Marc Alexander Radtke, MD
Professor
Institute for Health Services Research in Dermatology and Nursing (IVDP)
University Medical Center Hamburg-Eppendorf (UKE)
Hamburg, Germany

V. Ramesh, MD
Professor of Dermatology
Department of Dermatology
Vardhman Mahavir Medical College & Safdarjung Hospital
New Delhi, India

Gudrun Ratzinger, MD
Professor of Dermatology
Department of Dermatology, Venereology and Allergology
Medical University Innsbruck
Austria

Wingfield E. Rehmus, MD
Clinical Assistant Professor
Department of Pediatrics
University of British Columbia and British Columbia's Children's Hospital
Vancouver, BC, Canada

Sean D. Reynolds, MB BCh, BAO
Department of Dermatology
Warren Alpert Medical School of Brown University
Providence, RI, USA

Nerys Roberts, MD, FRCP, MRCPCH, BSc
Consultant Paediatric Dermatologist
Chelsea & Westminster Hospital
London, UK

Jean Robinson
Clinical Nurse Specialist in Paediatric Dermatology
Royal London Hospital
London, UK

Elke Rodriguez, PhD
Senior Researcher
Department of Dermatology, Allergology and Venereology
University Hospital Schleswig-Holstein
Campus Kiel
Kiel, Germany

Marcelo Ruvertoni, MD
Paediatric Dermatologist and Paediatrician
British Hospital
Montevideo, Uruguay

Liat Samuelov, MD
Vice Chair
Department of Dermatology
Tel Aviv Sourasky Medical Center
Tel Aviv, Israel

Sarita Sanke, MD Dermatology and STD
Lady Hardinge Medical College and associated hospitals
New Delhi, India

Julie V. Schaffer, MD
Associate Professor of Pediatrics
Division of Pediatric and Adolescent Dermatology
Hackensack University Medical Center
Hackensack, NJ, USA

Birgitta Schmidt, MD
Department of Pathology
Boston Children's Hospital
Harvard Medical School
Boston, MA, USA

Enno Schmidt, MD, PhD
Professor of Dermatology
Lübeck Institute of Experimental Dermatology (LIED)
Lübeck, Germany

Steffen Schubert
Department of Dermatology, Venereology and Allergology
University Medical Center Göttingen
Göttingen, Germany

Crispian Scully, CBE, DSc, DChD, DMed (HC), Dhc (multi), MD, PhD, PhD (HC), FMedSci, MDS, MRCS, BSc, FDSRCS, FDSRCPS, FFDRCSI, FDSRCSEd, FRCPath, FHEA
(Deceased)
Emeritus Professor of Oral Medicine at UCL
Bristol Dental Hospital
University Hospitals Bristol NHS Foundation Trust
Bristol, UK
University College London
London, UK

Robert K. Semple, PhD, FRCP
Professor of Translational Molecular Medicine
Centre for Cardiovascular Sciences, Queens Medical Research Institute
University of Edinburgh
Edinburgh, UK

Julien Seneschal, MD, PhD
Professor
Department of Dermatology and Paediatric Dermatology
Reference Center for Rare Skin Diseases
Hôpital Saint André
Bordeaux, France

G. Sethuraman, MD
Professor of Dermatology
Department of Dermatology
All India Institute of Medical Sciences
New Delhi, India

Marieke M.B. Seyger, MD, PhD
Associate Professor of Dermatology
Department of Dermatology
Radboud University Medical Center
Nijmegen, The Netherlands

Lindsay Shaw, MBBS, MRCPCH
Consultant in Paediatric Rheumatology
Paediatric Dermatology
Great Ormond Street Hospital for Children NHS Foundation Trust
London and Bristol Children's Hospital
Bristol UK

Neil Shear, MD, FRCPC, FACP
Professor of Medicine and Pharmacology
Division of Dermatology
Sunnybrook Health Sciences Center and University of Toronto
Toronto, ON, Canada

Tor A. Shwayder, MD
Director
Pediatric Dermatology
Department of Dermatology
Henry Ford Hospital
Detroit, MI, USA

Brenda M. Simpson
Dermatologist
El Paso Dermatology Center
El Paso, TX, USA

Robert Sidbury, MD, MPH
Professor
Department of Pediatrics
Chief
Division of Dermatology
Seattle Children's Hospital
University of Washington School of Medicine
Seattle, WA, USA

Jonathan I. Silverberg, MD, PhD
Associate Professor of Dermatology
Northwestern University Feinberg School of Medicine
Chicago, IL, USA

Nanette Silverberg, MD
Clinical Professor of Dermatology
Icahn School of Medicine at Mount Sinai
Chief
Pediatric Dermatology
Mount Sinai Health System
Director
Pediatric and Adolescent Dermatology
Department of Dermatology
New York, NY, USA

Eric L. Simpson, MD
Professor of Dermatology
School of Medicine
Department of Dermatology
Oregon Health and Science University
Portland, OR, USA

Manuraj Singh, MBBS, MRCP, PhD, DipRCPath (Dermpath)
Consultant Dermatologist and Dermatopathologist
St George's University Hospitals
London, UK

Nedaa Skeik, MD, FACP, FSVM, RPVI
Associate Professor of Medicine
Section Head, Vascular Medicine Department
Medical Director, Thrombophilia & Anticoagulation Clinic
Medical Director, Hyperbaric Medicine
Medical Director, Vascular Laboratories
Minneapolis Heart Institute at Abbott Northwestern Hospital – part of Allina Health
Minneapolis, MN, USA

Lea Solman, MD, FRCPCH
Consultant Paediatric Dermatologist
Department of Paediatric Dermatology
Great Ormond Street Hospital for Children NHS Trust
London, UK

Eli Sprecher, MD, PhD
Professor and Chair
Department of Dermatology and Deputy Director General for Patient Safety
Tel Aviv Sourasky Medical Center
Frederick Reiss Chair of Dermatology
Sackler Faculty of Medicine
Tel Aviv University
Tel Aviv, Israel

Sahana M. Srinivas, DNB, DVD, FRGUHS (Paediatric Dermatology)
Consultant Paediatric Dermatologist
Department of Pediatric Dermatology
Indira Gandhi Institute of Child Health
Bangalore, Karnataka, India

Paola Stefano, MD
Assistant Physician
Dermatology Department
Hospital de Pediatría 'Prof. Dr. Juan P. Garrahan'
Buenos Aires, Argentina

Peter M. Steijlen, MD, PhD
Professor of Dermatology and Chair
Department of Dermatology
Maastricht University Medical Center
Maastricht, The Netherlands

Jane C. Sterling, MB, BChir, MA, FRCP, PhD
Consultant Dermatologist
Department of Dermatology
Cambridge University Hospitals NHS Foundation Trust
Addenbrooke's Hospital
Cambridge, UK

Jenna L. Streicher, MD
Clinical Assistant Professor
Department of Pediatrics, Dermatology Section
Children's Hospital of Philadelphia
Departments of Pediatrics and Dermatology
Perelman School of Medicine at the University of Pennsylvania
Philadelphia, PA, USA

V. Reid Sutton, MD
Professor
Department of Molecular and Human Genetics
Baylor College of Medicine and Texas Children's Hospital
Houston, TX, USA

Samira Batul Syed, MBBS, DCH, DCCH, RCPEd, RCGP, FCM, BTEC Adv LASER, DPD
Associate Specialist in Paediatrics Dermatology
Great Ormond Street Hospital for Children NHS Trust
London, UK

Zsuzsanna Z. Szalai, MD
Professor and Head
Department of Pediatric Dermatology
Heim Pál Children's Hospital
Budapest, Hungary

Alain Taïeb, MD, PhD
Professor of Dermatology
Department of Dermatology and Paediatric Dermatology, Reference Center for Rare Skin Diseases
Hôpital Saint André
Bordeaux, France

Carolina Talhari, MD, PhD
Adjunct Professor of Dermatology
Amazon State University
Manaus, AM, Brazil

Martin Theiler, MD
Paediatric Dermatology Department
University Children's Hospital Zurich
Switzerland

Amy Theos, MD
Associate Professor of Department of Dermatology
University of Alabama at Birmingham
Birmingham, AL, USA

Peter Theut Riis, MD
Department of Dermatology
Roskilde Hospital
Roskilde, Denmark

Anna C. Thomas, BSc, PhD
Post-doctoral Research Associate
Genetics and Genomic Medicine
UCL Great Ormond Street Institute of Child Health
London, UK

Megha Tollefson, MD
Departments of Dermatology and Pediatrics
Mayo Clinic
Rochester, MN, USA

Wynnis L. Tom, MD
Associate Clinical Professor of Dermatology and Pediatrics
University of California, San Diego
Rady Children's Hospital
San Diego, CA, USA

Yun Tong, MD
Clinical Research Fellow
Department of Dermatology, University of California San Diego
San Diego, CA, USA

Helga V. Toriello, PhD
Professor
Department of Pediatrics/Human Development
Michigan State University College of Human Medicine
Grand Rapids, MI, USA

Antonio Torrelo, MD
Head
Department of Dermatology
Hospital Infantil del Niño Jesús
Madrid, Spain

Antonella Tosti, MD
Department of Dermatology and Cutaneous Surgery
Miller Medical School University of Miami
Miami, FL, USA

James R. Treat, MD
Associate Professor of Clinical Pediatrics and Dermatology
Fellowship Director, Pediatric Dermatology
Education Director, Pediatric Dermatology
Children's Hospital of Philadelphia
Dermatology Section
Perelman School of Medicine at the University of Pennsylvania
Philadelphia, PA, USA

Stephen K. Tyring, MD, PhD
Clinical Professor
Department of Dermatology
University of Texas Health Science Center at Houston
Houston, TX, USA

Nina van Beek, MD
Department of Dermatology
University of Lübeck
Lübeck, Germany

Ignatia B. Van den Veyver, MD
Professor
Departments of Obstetrics and Gynecology and Molecular and Human Genetics
Director of Clinical Prenatal Genetics
BCM and Texas Children's Hospital Pavilion for Women
Investigator
Jan and Dan Duncan Neurological Research Institute at Texas Children's Hospital
Baylor College of Medicine
Houston, TX, USA

Maurice A.M. van Steensel, MD, PhD
Professor of Dermatology and Skin Biology
Lee Kong Chian School of Medicine
Singapore
Research Director
Skin Research Institute of Singapore
Singapore

Felipe Velasquez, MD
Consultant in Pediatric Dermatology
Department of Pediatric Dermatology
Instituto de Salud del Niño
Lima, Peru

Paul Veys
Director
Bone Marrow Transplantation Unit
Great Ormond Street Hospital for Children NHS Trust
London, UK

Miikka Vikkula, MD, PhD
Head of Laboratory of Human Molecular Genetics
de Duve Institute
University of Louvain
Brussels, Belgium

Beatrix Volc-Platzer, MD
Professor of Dermatology
Department of Dermatology
Donauspital SMZ Ost
Vienna, Austria

Peter von den Driesch, MD
Professor of Dermatology
Head
Center for Dermatology
Klinikum Stuttgart
Stuttgart, Germany

Amy Walker, MRes, BSc
Experimental and Personalised Medicine
UCL Great Ormond Street Institute of Child Health
London, UK

Lachlan Warren
Consultant Dermatologist
Department of Dermatology
Women's & Children's Hospital
Adelaide, SA, Australia

Joy Wan, MD, MSCE
Postdoctoral Fellow of Dermatology
Department of Biostatistics and Epidemiology
University of Pennsylvania Perelman School of Medicine
Philadelphia, PA, USA

Siriwan Wananukul, MD
Professor of Paediatrics
Head of Department of Paediatrics
Faculty of Medicine
Chulalongkorn University
Bangkok, Thailand

Andrew Wang, MD
Brookline Dermatology Associates
West Roxbury
MA, USA

Lisa L. Wang, MD
Associate Professor
Department of Pediatrics
Texas Children's Hospital
Baylor College of Medicine
Houston, TX, USA

Bettina Wedi, MD, PhD
Professor of Dermatology
Department of Dermatology and Allergology
Hannover Medical School
Hannover, Germany

Lisa Weibel, MD
Paediatric Dermatology Department
University Children's Hospital Zurich
Switzerland

Stephan Weidinger, MD
Professor of Dermatology
Deputy Head
Department of Dermatology, Allergology and Venereology
University Hospital Schleswig-Holstein
Campus Kiel
Kiel, Germany

Miriam Weinstein, BSc, BScN, MD, FRCPC (Paediatrics) FRCPC (Dermatology)
Department of Paediatrics
Hospital for Sick Children
Toronto, ON, Canada

Pamela F. Weiss, MD, MSCE
Associate Professor of Pediatrics and Epidemiology
Divison of Rheumatology
Children's Hospital of Philadelphia
Center for Clinical Epidemiology and Biostatistics
University of Pennsylvania
Philadelphia, PA, USA

Alexis Weymann Perlmutter, MD
Resident
Department of Dermatology
Geisinger Medical Center
PA, USA

Lizbeth Ruth Wheeler
Department of Dermatology
St George Hospital and University of New South Wales
Sydney, NSW, Australia

Hywel C. Williams, MD, PhD
Director of the NIHR Health Technology Assessment Programme
Co-Director of the Centre of Evidence Based Dermatology
University of Nottingham
Nottingham, UK

Lara Wine Lee, MD, PhD
Departments of Dermatology and Pediatrics
Medical University of South Carolina
Charleston, SC, USA

Marion Wobser, MD
Department of Dermatology, Venereology and Allergology
University Hospital Würzburg
Würzburg, Germany

Johannes Wohlrab, MD
Professor of Dermatology
Department of Dermatology and Venereology and Institute of Applied Dermatopharmacy
Martin-Luther-University Halle-Wittenberg
Halle (Saale), Germany

A. Wolkerstorfer, MD, PhD
Netherlands Institute for Pigment Disorders
Amsterdam University Medical Centers
Amsterdam, The Netherlands

Heulwen Wyatt
Clinical Nurse Specialist in Paediatric Dermatology
Dermatology Unit
St Woolos Hospital,
Newport, UK

Yuanyuan Xiao, MD
Associate Chief Physician
Department of Dermatology
Beijing Children's Hospital
Capital Medical University
National Center for Children's Health
Beijing, China

Zhe Xu, MD, PhD
Chief Physician
Department of Dermatology
Beijing Children's Hospital
Capital Medical University
National Center for Children's Health
Beijing, China

Albert C. Yan, MD, FAAP, FAAD
Section of Dermatology
Children's Hospital of Philadelphia
Philadelphia, PA, USA
Departments of Pediatrics and Dermatology
Perelman School of Medicine at the University of Pennsylvania
Philadelphia, PA, USA

Kevin B. Yarbrough, MD
Staff Physician
Department of Pediatric Dermatology
Phoenix Children's Hospital
Phoenix, AZ, USA

Vijay Zawar, MD
Skin Diseases Centre
Nashik, India
Professor
Department of Dermatology
MVP's Dr Vasantrao Pawar Medical College and Research Centre
Nashik, Maharashtra, India

Bernhard W.H. Zelger, MD, MSc
Professor of Dermatology
Department of Dermatology, Venereology and Allergology
Medical University Innsbruck
Austria

Preface to the Fourth Edition

It is with much delight and pride that we present the fourth edition of this textbook. The new edition continues to provide state-of-the-art information on all aspects of skin disease in children. Existing content has been refreshed and fully updated to reflect emerging thinking and to incorporate the latest in research and clinical data – especially at the genetic level. The three Editors, two Editorial Advisors and five Associate Editors from across the world bring a truly global perspective to the work. Some 31 countries are represented by 313 contributors, of whom 192 are new contributors, who have extensively updated or completely rewritten the 177 chapters. The book represents a definitive reference text for dermatologists, paediatricians, clinician scientists, research workers and all other individuals involved in the care of children with skin disease.

The fourth edition appears at a time when digital instant access to information, retrievable anywhere and at anytime, is the norm. Nevertheless, the value of having a physical textbook to read and study remains an integral part of clinical practice and academia; but, in order to keep up to date, the book will also be accessible online on an interactive platform via laptops and smartphones. The book's virtue is, in our opinion, its comprehensiveness and in-depth information written by international experts on each subject.

We hope that this fourth edition will be as warmly received as its three predecessors and will contribute to the improved care of children with skin diseases.

PH
VK
AY
JIH

Dedication

In memory of Arnold P. Oranje, 1948–2016

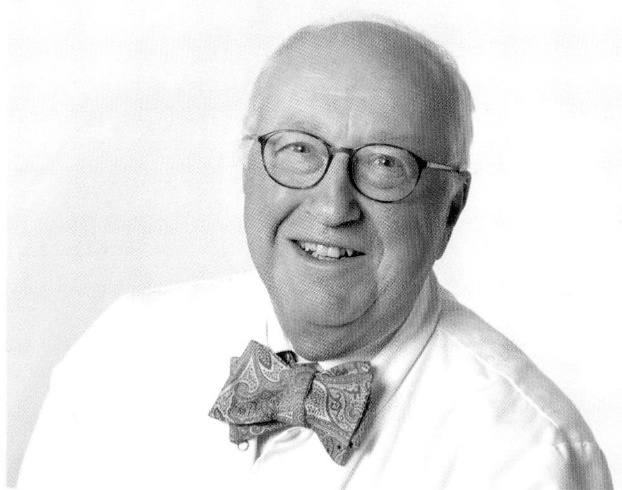

This 4th edition of the textbook is dedicated to my dear friend and colleague Arnold Oranje. Arnold's untimely death shocked us all and is a great loss to the world of paediatric dermatology. He was one of the three original editors of this book, with Neil Prose and myself, and was working on this edition at the time of his death.

On a personal note, my collaboration with Arnold was unique: his enthusiasm, passion for the subject, expertise and exuberant laughter made him a joy to work with. I hope that Arnold would be immensely proud of this new edition.

John Harper

Taïeb A, Stalder J-F, de Waard-van der Spek F, Harper J. In Memoriam: Arnold P. Oranje. Pediatr Dermatol 2017; 34: 231–4.

Acknowledgements

We wish to thank the following people: the Associate Editors and chapter authors for their invaluable contribution to the book; the editorial staff and production staff at Wiley-Blackwell, freelance project editor, Alison Nick, project manager, Nik Prowse, and the copy-editors for their tireless efforts; the families who gave permission for the photographs of their children to be used in this book and our own families for their understanding and support.

However, the biggest thank you has to be to our patients who provide the inspiration and motivation for our work on a daily basis.

PH
VK
AY
JIH

List of Abbreviations

AA alopecia areata
AA amyloid A
AAD American Academy of Dermatology
AAV adeno-associated virus
AAV antineutrophil cytoplasmic antibody (ANCA)-associated vasculitides
ABC ATP-binding cassette
ACA acrodermatitis chronica atrophicans
ACA anticentromere antibodies
ACC aplasia cutis congenita
ACD allergic contact dermatitis
ACD amyloidosis cutis dyschromica
ACE angiotensin-converting enzyme
aCGH array-comparative genomic hybridization
ACR American College of Rheumatology
ACS Aicardi–Goutiéres syndrome
ACTH adrenocorticotropic hormone
AD atopic dermatitis
AD autosomal dominant
ADA adenosine deaminase
ADCL autosomal dominant cutis laxa
ADCL anergic diffuse cutaneous leishmaniasis
ADHD attention deficit hyperactivity disorder
ADR adverse drug reaction
ADM atypical dermal melanocytosis
ADULT acro-dermato-ungual-lacrimal-tooth
ADWH autosomal-dominant woolly hair
AEC ankyloblepharon, ectodermal defects and cleft lip/palate
AEDS atopic eczema/dermatitis syndrome
AEI annular epidermolytic ichthyosis
AFB acid-fast bacilli
AGA androgenetic alopecia
AGEP acute generalized exanthematous pustulosis
aGVHD acute GVHD
AGL acquired generalized lipoatrophy
AGM acrylate gelling material
AHA American Heart Association
AHA antihistone antibody
AHEI acute haemorrhagic oedema of infancy
AHO Albright hereditary osteodystrophy
AHT abusive head trauma
AID autoinflammatory disease
AIDS acquired immune deficiency syndrome
AIP acute intermittent porphyria
ALHE angiolymphoid hyperplasia with eosinophilia
ALL acute lymphoblastic leukaemia
ALN actinic lichen nitidus
ALP actinic lichen planus
ALT alanine transaminase
ALU aphthous-like ulceration
AML acute myeloid leukaemia
AMMoL acute myelomonocytic leukaemia
AMN acquired melanocytic naevi
AMoL acute monocytic leukaemia
AMP antimicrobial peptide
AMPK adenosine monophosphate-activated protein kinase
AN acanthosis nigricans
ANA antinuclear antibody
ANCA antineutrophilic cytoplasmic antibody
AP actinic prurigo
AP adaptor protein complex
AP anteroposterior
APC antigen-presenting cell
APECED autoimmune polyendocrinopathy–candidiasis–ectodermal dystrophy (syndrome)
APL acquired partial lipoatrophy
APL atrichia with papular lesions
APP atrophoderma of Pasini and Pierini
APS antiphospholipid antibody syndrome
APSS acral peeling skin syndrome
AR androgen receptor
AR autosomal recessive
ARC arthrogryposis–renal dysfunction–cholestasis (syndrome)
ARCI autosomal recessive congenital ichthyosis
ARCL autosomal recessive cutis laxa
ARD adult Refsum disease
AR-HIES autosomal recessive hyperimmunoglobulin E syndrome
ARKID autosomal recessive keratoderma ichthyosis and deafness (syndrome)
ARMS amplification-refractory mutation system
ASD autism spectrum disorders
ASM aggressive systemic mastocytosis
ASO antistreptolysin O
ASPS alveolar soft part sarcoma
ASST autologous serum skin test
AST aspartate transaminase
AST aspartate aminotransferase
AT ataxia telangiectasia
ATG anti-thymocyte globulin
ATGL adipose triglyceride lipase
ATP adenosine triphosphate
ATPase adenosine triphosphatase
ATS arterial tortuosity syndrome
ATT antitubercular therapy
AUC area under the concentration-time curve
AUG acute ulcerative gingivitis
AV arteriovenous
AVF arteriovenous fistula
AVM arteriovenous malformations
AV atrophoderma vermiculata
AZA azathioprine

BAL bronchoalveolar lavage
BB β-blockers
BCC basal cell carcinoma
BCG bacillus Calmette–Guérin
BCIE bullous congenital ichthyosiform erythroderma
BD Behçet disease
BDCS Bazex–Dupré–Christol syndrome
BDD blistering distal dactylitis
BDNG British Dermatological Nursing Group
BER base excision repair
BGS Baller–Gerold syndrome
BHDS Birt–Hogg–Dubé syndrome
BHPR British Health Professionals in Rheumatology
BMD bone mineral density
BMI body mass index
BMP bone morphogenetic protein
BMT bone marrow transplantation
BO branchio-otic
BOR branchio-oto-renal
BOS Buschke–Ollendorff syndrome
BP blood pressure
BP bullous pemphigoid
BRBN blue rubber bleb naevus
BRRS Bannayan–Riley–Ruvalcaba syndrome
BS Bloom syndrome
BSA body surface area
BSCL Berardinelli–Seip congenital lipodystrophy
BSI bathing suit ichthyosis
BSLE benign summer light eruption
BSR British Society for Rheumatology
BSS Brooke–Spiegler syndrome
BTK Bruton tyrosine kinase
BV bacterial vaginitis
BWS Beckwith–Wiedemann syndrome
CA condyloma acuminata
CAD chronic actinic dermatitis
CADIS Childhood Atopic Dermatitis Impact Scale
C-ALCL cutaneous anaplastic large cell lymphoma
CALM café-au-lait macules
CAM cell adhesion molecule
CA-MRSA community-associated meticillin-resistant *Streptococcus aureus*
CAN child abuse and neglect
c-ANCA cytoplasmic antineutrophil cytoplasmic antibody
CANDLE chronic atypical neutrophilic dermatosis with lipodystrophy and elevated temperature
CAPS cryopyrin-associated autoinflammatory syndromes
CAT cutaneovisceral angiomatosis with thrombocyopenia
CAVB complete atrioventricular block
CAVM capillary–arteriolovenular malformations
CBCL cutaneous B-cell lymphoma
CBS cystathionine β-synthase
CCA congenital contractural arachnodactyly
CCC congenital cutaneous candidiasis
CCTN cerebriform connective tissue naevi
CD coeliac disease
CDLQI Children's Dermatology Life Quality Index
CDP chondrodysplasia punctata
CDPX2 X-linked dominant chondrodysplasia punctata
CDS Chanarin–Dorfman syndrome
CE cell envelope
CEA carcinoembryonic antigen
CEDNIK cerebral dysgenesis, neuropathy, ichthyosis, keratoderma (syndrome)
CEP congenital erythropoietic porphyria
CEVD congenital erosive and vesicular dermatosis (with reticulated supple scarring)
CFCS cardiofaciocutaneous syndrome
CFTR cystic fibrosis transmembrane conductance regulator
CFU colony-forming unit
CGD chronic granulomatous disease
CGH comparative genomic hybridization
CGL congenital generalized lipodystrophy
CGRP calcitonin gene-related product
CGS contiguous gene syndrome
cGVHD chronic graft versus host disease
CH congenital haemangiomas
CHAND curly hair, ankyloblepheron, nail dysplasia (syndrome)
CHCC Chapel Hill Consensus Conference
CHH Conradi–Hünermann–Happle syndrome
CHH cartilage hair hypoplasia
CHIKV Chikungunya virus
CHILD congenital hemidysplasia with ichthyosiform erythroderma and limb defect (syndrome)
CHIME colobomas, congenital heart disease, early-onset ichthyosiform dermatosis, mental retardation and ear abnormalities
CHP cytophagic histiocytic panniculitis
CHRPE congenital hypertrophy of the retinal pigment epithelium
CHS Chédiak–Higashi syndrome
CI congenital ichthyoses
CIAD Childhood Impact of Atopic Dermatitis
CID combined immunodeficiency
CIE congenital ichthyosiform erythroderma
CIL-F congenital infiltrating lipomatosis of the face
CL cutaneous leishmaniasis
CLM cutaneous larva migrans
CLOVE congenital lipomatous overgrowth, vascular malformations and epidermal naevi (syndrome)
CLQI Children's Life Quality Index
CLSM confocal laser scanning microscopy
CM capillary malformation
CM cutaneous mastocytosis
CM-AVM capillary malformation-arteriovenous malformation
CMC chronic mucocutaneous candidiasis
CML chronic myeloid leukaemia
CMN congenital melanocytic naevi
CMN congenital mesoblastic nephroma
CMO carotenoid 15,15′-mono-oxygenase
CMRDS constitutional mismatch repair deficiency syndrome
CMTC cutis marmorata telangiectatica congenita
CMV cytomegalovirus
CNS central nervous system
CNTP connective tissue naevus of the proteoglycan type
CNV copy number variations
CoA co-enzyme A
C1-INH C1-esterase inhibitor
CoNS coagulase-negative *Staphylococcus*
COFS cerebro-oculo-facio-skeletal
CPAP continuous positive airway pressure
CRP C-reactive protein
CRIE congenital reticular ichthyosiform erythroderma
CRISPR clustered regularly interspaced palindromic repeats
CPD cyclobutanepyrimidine dimers
CS Cockayne syndrome
CS Costello syndrome
CSA child sexual abuse
CSD cat scratch disease
CSF cerebrospinal fluid
CSMH congenital smooth muscle hamartoma
CST Christ–Siemens–Touraine
CT *Chlamydia trachomatis*
CT computed tomography
CTCL cutaneous T-cell lymphoma
CTGF connective tissue growth factor
CTN connective tissue naevi

CTL cytotoxic T-lymphocyte
CTLA-4 cytotoxic T-lymphocyte antigen-4
CVG cutis verticis gyrata
CVID common variable immunodeficiency
CVS chorionic villus sampling
CVS congenital varicella syndrome
CVST cerebral venous sinus thrombosis
Cx connexin
DADA2 deficiency of adenosine deaminase type 2
DASI Dyshidrotic Eczema Area and Severity Index
DBPCDC double-blind placebo-controlled drug challenge
DBS DeBarsy syndrome
DC dyskeratosis congenita
DCM diffuse cutaneous mastocytosis
dcSSc diffuse cutaneous systemic sclerosis
DD Darier disease
DDD Dowling–Degos disease
DDEB dominant dystrophic epidermolysis bullosa
DE dermoepidermal
DEB dystrophic epidermolysis bullosa
DEJ dermoepidermal junction
DEPPK diffuse epidermolytic palmoplantar keratoderma
DFA direct fluorescent antibody
DFI Dermatitis Family Impact
DFSP dermatofibrosarcoma protuberans
DG1 DGI disseminated gonoccocal infection
DGS DiGeorge syndrome
DH dermatitis herpetiformis
DHEA dihydroepiandrosterone
DHEAS dihydroepiandrosterone sulphate
DI dentinogenensis imperfecta
DIF direct immunofluorescence
DIHS/AHS drug-induced or anticonvulsant hypersensitivity syndrome
DIRA deficiency of the IL-1 receptor antagonist
DKS dyskeratosis congenita
DLE discoid lupus erythematosus
DMARD disease modifying antirheumatic drugs
DMEG dysplastic megalencephaly
DMSA dimercaptosuccinic acid
DMSO dimethyl sulphoxide
DNEPPK diffuse nonepidermolytic palmoplantar keratoderma
DOC disorders of cornification
DOPA dihydroxyphenylalanine
DP dyschromatosis ptychotropica
DPR dermatopathia pigmentosa reticularis
DRESS drug rash with eosinophilia and systemic symptoms
DSAP disseminated superficial actinic porokeratosis
DSH dyschromatosis symmetrica hereditaria
DSP disseminated superficial porokeratosis
DTE desmoplastic trichoepithelioma
DUH dyschromatosis universalis hereditaria
DVA developmental venous anomaly
DVT deep vein thrombosis
EAACI European Academy of Allergy and Clinical Immunology
EASI Eczema Area and Severity Index
EB epidermolysis bullosa
EBA epidermolysis bullosa acquisita
EBP emopamil binding protein
EBV Epstein–Barr virus
EBS epidermolysis bullosa simplex
EBS-DM epidermolysis bullosa simplex Dowling–Meara
EBS-MP epidermolysis bullosa simplex with mottled pigmentation
ECCL encephalocraniocutaneous lipomatosis
ECF eosinophil chemotactic factor
ECG electrocardiogram
ECHO enteric cytopathic human orphan
ECM1 extracellular matrix protein 1
ECP eosinophil cationic protein
ECP extracorporeal photopheresis
ED ectodermal dysplasia
EDA ectodysplasin-A
EDP erythema dyschromicum perstans
EDS Ehlers–Danlos syndrome
EDTA ethylenediaminetetraacetic acid
EDV epidermodysplasia verruciformis
EEC ectrodactyly, ectodermal dysplasia and cleft lip/palate
EED erythema elevatum diutinum
EEG electroencephalogram
EF eosinophilic fasciitis
EGA estimated gestational age
EGF epidermal growth factor
EGFR epidermal growth factor receptor
EGPA eosinophilic granulomatosis with polyangiitis
EGW external genital wart
EH eczema herpeticum
EH epithelioid haemangioma
EHK epidermolytic hyperkeratosis
EI epidermolytic ichthyosis
EIA enzyme immunoassay
EIB erythema induratum of Bazin
EKA erythrokeratoderma with ataxia
EKC erythrokeratoderma en cocardes
EKV erythrokeratoderma variabilis
EKVP erythrokeratoderma variabilis progressiva
ELISA enzyme-linked immunosorbent assay
EM erythema migrans
EM erythema multiforme
EMG electromyogram
EMLA eutectic mixture of local anaesthetics
EMS electromagnetic spectrum
EN epidermal naevus
EN erythema nodosum
EN-D epidermal naevus – Darier type
ENDA European Network for Drug Allergy
ENS epidermal naevus syndrome
ENT ear, nose and throat
EORTC European Research and Treatment of Cancer
EOS early-onset sarcoidosis
EP eccrine poroma
EPDS erosive pustular dermatosis of the scalp
EPI eosinophilic pustulosis of infancy
EPF eosinophilic pustular folliculitis
EPP erythropoietic protoporphyria
ER endoplasmic reticulum
ERA enthesitis-related arthritis
ES epithelioid sarcoma
ESPD European Society of Pediatric Dermatology
ESR erythrocyte sedimentation rate
ESRD end-stage renal disease
ET exfoliative toxin
ETN erythema toxicum neonatorum
EULAR European League Against Rheumatism
EV eczema vaccinatum
EV enteroviruses
EV epidermodysplasia verruciformis
EV-HPV epidermodysplasia verruciformis-associated human papillomavirus
FADH fatty alcohol dehydrogenase
FAE fumaric acid ester
FALDH fatty aldehyde dehydrogenase
FAP familial adenomatous polyposis
FAO fibroadipose hyperplasia or overgrowth
FATP fatty acid transport protein
FC familial cylindromatosis

FDA US Food and Drug Administration
FDE fixed drug eruptions
FDEIA food-dependent exercise-induced urticaria/anaphylaxis
FDH focal dermal hypoplasia
FFD Fox–Fordyce disease
FFDD focal facial dermal dysplasias
FFM focus-floating microscopy
FFP fresh frozen plasma
FFPE formalin-fixed paraffin-embedded
FGFR fibroblast growth factor receptor
FH familial hypercholesterolaemia
FHL familial haemophagocytic lymphohistiocytosis
FII fabricated or induced illness
FISH fluorescence *in situ* hybridization
FITC fluorescein isothiocyanate
5-FU 5-fluorouracil
FMF familial Mediterranean fever
FML familial multiple lipomatosis
FNAC fine needle aspiration cytology
FOP fibrodysplasia ossificans progressiva
FPHH familial progressive hyperpigmentation and hypopigmentation
FPLD familial partial lipodystrophies
FSH follicle-stimulating hormone
FTC familial tumoural calcinosis
FTG full-thickness skin graft
FTI farnesyltransferase inhibitors
FVC forced vital capacity
GA granuloma annulare
GABA γ-aminobutyric acid
GACI generalized arterial calcification of infancy
GAS Group A *Streptococcus*
GBFDE generalized bullous fixed drug eruption
GCDFP gross cystic disease fluid protein
GCS Giannott—Crosti syndrome
GD Gaucher disease
GFR glomerular filtration rate
GGR global genome repair
GGT gamma-glutamyl transpeptidase
GH growth hormone
GI gastrointestinal
GLA generalized lymphatic anomaly
GM-CSF granulocyte macrophage colony-stimulating factor
GMS Gomori's methenamine silver
GNCST granular nerve cell sheath tumour
GO geroderma osteodysplastica
GOSH Great Ormond Street Hospital for Children
GPA granulomatosis with polyangiitis
GPP generalized pustular psoriasis
GPS Griscelli–Prunieras syndrome
GS Griscelli syndrome
GSD Gorham–Stout disease
GSE gluten-sensitive enteropathy
G6PD glucose-6-phosphate dehydrogenase
GSS granulomatous slack skin
GVHD graft-versus-host disease
GVHR graft-versus-host reaction
GVL graft-versus-leukaemia
GVM glomuvenous malformation
GWAS genome-wide association study
HAART highly active antiretroviral therapy
HAE hereditary angioedema
HA-MRSA hospital-associated meticillin-resistant *Streptococcus aureus*
H&E haematoxylin and eosin
HBD human β-defensin
HBT hereditary benign telangiectasia
HBV hepatitis B virus
HCC harlequin colour change
HCG human chorionic gonadotropin
HCP hereditary coproporphyria
HCT haemopoietic cell transplantation
HDL high-density lipoprotein
HDN haematodermic neoplasm
HE hypereosinophilia
HED hypohidrotic ectodermal dysplasia
HEP hepatoerythropoietic porphyria
HES hypereosinophilic syndrome
HFMD hand, foot and mouth disease
HFS hyaline fibromatosis syndrome
HGA homogentisic acid
HGPS Hutchinson–Gilford progeria syndrome
HHD Hailey–Hailey disease
HHML hemihyperplasia–multiple lipomatosis syndrome
HHT hereditary haemorrhagic telangiectasia
HHV human herpesvirus
HI haemangioma of infancy
HI harlequin ichthyosis
HI hypomelanosis of Ito
HID hystrix-like ichthyosis with deafness (syndrome)
HIES hyperimmunoglobulin E syndrome
HIF hypoxia inducible factor
HIMS hyperimmunoglobulin M syndrome
HIP helix initiation peptide
HIV human immunodeficiency virus
HJMD hypotrichosis with juvenile macular dystrophy
HLA human leucocyte antigen
HLH haemophagocytic lymphohistiocytosis
HLRCC hereditary leiomyomatosis and renal cell cancer
HMG high mobility group
HMS Haim–Munk syndrome
HOME Harmonising Outcome Measures for Eczema
HOPP hypotrichosis–osteolysis–periodontitis–palmoplantar keratoderma
HP hydroxylysylpyridinoline
HPC haemangiopericytoma
HPS Hermansky–Pudlak syndrome
HPETE hydroperoxyeicosatetraenoic acid
HPV human papillomavirus
HR H_1-receptor
HRCT high resolution computed tomography
HRM high-resolution melt PCR
HS hidradenitis suppurativa
HSCT haematopoietic stem cell transplantation
HSD holocarboxylase synthetase deficiency
HSP heat shock proteins
HSP Henoch–Schönlein purpura
HSV herpes simplex virus
HTLV human T-lymphotropic virus
HTP helix termination peptide
HUV hypocomplementemic urticarial vasculitis
HUVS hypocomplementemic urticarial vasculitis syndrome
HV hydroa vacciniforme
IA infantile acropustulosis
IBD inflammatory bowel disease
IBIDS ichthyosis, brittle hair, intellectual impairment, decreased fertility and short stature
IBS ichthyosis bullosa of Siemens
ICAM intracellular adhesion molecule
ICD irritant contact dermatitis
IC1/IC2 imprinting centre 1/2
ID infective dermatitis
IDQoL Infants' Dermatitis Quality of Life Index
IEM inborn errors of metabolism
IF immunofluorescence
IF infantile fibrosarcoma
IF intermediate filament

IFA	indirect fluorescence assay
IFAP	ichthyosis follicularis, alopecia and photophobia
IFM	immunofluorescence mapping
IFN	interferon
Ig	immunoglobulin
IgA_1	IgA subtype 1
Ig ε RI	high-affinity IgE receptor
IGF	insulin-like growth factor
IGFBP	insulin-like growth factor binding protein
IgM	immunoglobulin M
IGRA	interferon-γ release assay
IH	infantile haemangiomas
IHCM	ichthyosis hystrix of Curth–Macklin
IHS	ichthyosis hypotrichosis syndrome
IHSC	ichthyosis–hypotrichosis–sclerosing cholangitis (syndrome)
IIF	indirect immunofluorescence
IL	interleukin
ILAR	International League of Associations for Rheumatology
ILC	ichthyosis linearis circumflexia
ILVEN	inflammatory linear verrucous epidermal naevus
IMF	immunofluorescence
IM	infectious mononucleosis
IM	intramuscular
IP	incontinentia pigmenti
iPCS	inducible pluripotential stem cells
IPEX	immune dysregulation, polyendocrinopathy, enteropathy, X-linked
IPP	infantile perineal protrusion
IPS	ichthyosis prematurity syndrome
IR	insulin resistance
IRAK-4	IL-1 receptor associated kinase-4
IRIS	immune reconstitution inflammatory syndrome
IS	infantile spasms
ISAAC	International Study of Asthma and Allergies in Childhood
ISD	infantile seborrhoeic dermatitis
ISH	infantile systemic hyalinosis
ISM	indolent systemic mastocytosis
ISSVA	International Society for the Study of Vascular Anomalies
ISU	idiopathic solar urticaria
IV	ichthyosis vulgaris
IVF	*in vitro* fertilization
IVIG	intravenous immunoglobulin
JAK	janus kinase
JDM	juvenile dermatomyositis
JEB	junctional epidermolysis bullosa
JHF	juvenile hyaline fibromatosis
JIA	juvenile idiopathic arthritis
JLI	Jessner lymphocytic infiltrate
JPD	juvenile plantar dermatosis
JSPD	Japanese Society for Pediatric Dermatology
JSLE	juvenile systemic lupus erythematosus
JSSc	juvenile-onset systemic sclerosis
JXG	juvenile xanthogranuloma
KD	Kawasaki disease
KEN	keratinocytic epidermal naevus
KFSD	keratosis follicularis spinulosa decalvans
KHE	kaposiform haemangioendothelioma
KID	keratitis, ichthyosis and deafness (syndrome)
KIF	keratin intermediate filaments
KLA	Kaposiform lymphangiomatosis
KLICK	keratosis linearis-ichthyosis congenita-keratoderma
KLK	kallikrein
KMP	Kasabach–Merritt phenomenon
KPI	keratinopathic ichthyoses
KS	Kaposi sarcoma
KS	Kindler syndrome
KTS	Klippel–Trenaunay syndrome
KWE	keratolytic winter erythema
LABD	linear immunoglobulin IgA bullous dermatosis
LAD	leucocyte adhesion deficiency
LAD	linear IgA dermatosis
LAH	localized autosomal recessive hypotrichosis
LAM	linear atrophoderma of Moulin
LAM	lymphangiomyomatosis
LAS	loose anagen syndrome
LB	Lyme borreliosis
LCD	liquor carbonis detergens
LCH	Langerhans cell histiocytosis
LCR	locus control region
lcSSC	limited cutaneous systemic sclerosis
LED	light-emitting diode
LIC	localized intravascular coagulopathy
LD	linkage disequilibrium
LD	lymphoedema-distichiasis
LDF	laser Doppler flowmetry
LDH	lactate dehydrogenase
LDL	low-density lipoprotein
LDS	Loeys–Dietz syndrome
LE	lupus erythematosus
LEC	lymphatic endothelial cells
LEKTI	lymphoepithelial Kazal-type inhibitor
LET	lidocaine/epinephrine/tetracaine
LFA-3	lymphocyte function-associated antigen-3
LH	luteinizing hormone
LI	lamellar ichthyosis
LJ	Lowenstein–Jensen (medium)
LM	lymphatic malformation
LMP	last menstrual period
LMP1	latent membrane protein 1
LMS	Lenz–Majewski syndrome
LMS	limb–mammary syndrome
LMX	liposomal lidocaine
LN	lichen nitidus
LOH	loss of heterozygosity
LOSSI	localized scleroderma severity index
LOX	lipoxygenase
LP	lichen planus
LP	lupus panniculitis
LP	lysylpyridinoline
LPL	lipoprotein lipase deficiency
LPP	lichen planopilaris
LPS	lipopolysaccharide
LS	lichen sclerosus
LS	lichen scrofulosorum
LS	lichen striatus
LSC	lichen simplex chronicus
LSc	localized scleroderma
LT-β	lymphotoxin-β
LTT	lymphocyte transformation test
LV	lentiviral vector
LV	livedoid vasculopathy
LV	lupus vulgaris
LyP	lymphomatoid papulosis
MAC	membrane attack complex
MACS	macrocephaly-alopecia-cutis laxa-scoliosis
MACS	magnetic-activated cell sorting
MAD	mandibuloacral dysplasia
MAIC	*M. avium-intracellulare* complex
MALDI-TOF	matrix-assisted laser desorption/ionization time-of-flight
MALT	mucosa-associated lymphoid tissue
MAPK	mitogen-activated protein kinase
MAS	macrophage activation syndrome
MAS	McCune–Albright syndrome

MBL mannose-binding lectin
MBP major basic protein
MBTPS2 membrane-bound transcription factor protease, site 2
MC mast cells
MC molluscum contagiosum
MCAS mast cell activation symptoms
MC&S microscopy, culture and (antibiotic) sensitivity
MCL mast cell leukaemia
MCL mucocutaneous leishmaniasis
M-CM megalencephaly-capillary malformation
MCS mast cell lymphoma
MCV molluscum contagiosum virus
MDM minor determinant mixture
MDP mandibular hypoplasia, deafness and progeria (syndrome)
MDR multidrug-resistant
MED minimal erythema dose
MEDNIK mental retardation, enteropathy, deafness, peripheral neuropathy, ichthyosis, keratoderma
MeDOC mendelian disorders of cornification
MEN-1 multiple endocrine neoplasia type-1
MetS metabolic syndrome
MF mycosis fungoides
MFS Marfan syndrome
MFT multiple familial trichoepitheliomas
mHA minor histocompatibility antigen
MHC major histocompatibility complex
MIDAS microphthalmia, dermal aplasia and sclerocornea (syndrome)
MKD mevalonate kinase deficiency
MLPA multiplex ligation-dependent probe amplification
MLT multifocal lymphangioendotheliomatosis with thrombocyopenia
MMA methylmalonic acidaemia
MMF mycophenolate mofetil
MMP matrix metalloproteinases
MMP mucous membrane pemphigoid
MMPH multifocal micronodular pneumocyte hyperplasia
MMR mismatch repair
MODY maturity-onset diabetes of the young
MPA microscopic polyangiitis
MPCM maculopapular cutaneous mastocytosis
MPDE maculopapular drug eruptions or exanthems
MPE maculopapular exanthems
MPNST malignant peripheral nerve sheath tumour
MPO myeloperoxidase
MPS mucopolysaccharidoses
MRA magnetic resonance angiography
MRI magnetic resonance imaging
MRSA meticillin-resistant *Staphylococcus aureus*
MRSS modified Rodnan skin score
MSD multiple sulphatase deficiency
MSF Milton sterilizing fluid
MSH melanocyte-stimulating hormone
MSL multiple symmetric lipomatosis
MSS Mulvihill–Smith syndrome
MSUD maple syrup urine disease
MTC *Mycobacterium tuberculosis* complex
mtDNA mitochondrial DNA
mTOR mammalian target of rapamycin
MTS Muir–Torre syndrome
MTX methotrexate
MUGA multiple uptake gated acquisition angiography
MUHH Marie–Unna hereditary hypotrichosis
MVP mitral valve prolapse
MWS Muckle–Wells syndrome
NA naevus anaemicus
NAC N-acetylcysteine
NADPH nicotinamide adenine dinucleotide phosphate
NBCC naevoid basal cell carcinoma
NBD nucleotide-binding domain
NBS Nijmegen breakage syndrome
NBT nitroblue tetrazolium
NB-UVB narrow-band UVB
NC naevus comedonicus
NCAM neural cell adhesion molecule
NCIE nonbullous congenital ichthyosiform erythroderma
NCP neonatal cephalic pustulosis
NCV nerve conduction velocity
ND naevus depigmentosus
Nd:YAG neodymium:yttrium aluminium garnet
NEP neonatal eosinophilic pustulosis
NEPPK nonepidermolytic palmoplantar keratoderma
NER nucleotide excision repair
NET neutrophil extracellular trap
NF necrotizing fasciitis
NFJ Naegeli-Franceschetti-Jadassohn (syndrome)
NF-κB nuclear factor κB
NF1 neurofibromatosis type 1
NGCO non-gestational ovarian choriocarcinoma
NGF nerve growth factor
NGFR nerve growth factor receptor
NGS next-generation sequencing
NHL non-Hodgkin lymphoma
NICE National Institute for Health and Care Excellence (UK)
NICH noninvoluting congenital haemangioma
NICU neonatal intensive care unit
NIH National Institutes of Health (USA)
NISCH neonatal ichthyosis-sclerosing cholangitis (syndrome)
NK natural killer (cell)
NL necrobiosis lipoidica
NL neonatal lupus
NLCH non-Langerhans cell histiocytosis
NLCS naevus lipomatosus cutaneous superficialis
NLD necrobiosis lipoidica
NLP nail lichen planus
NLS naevus lipomatosus superficialis
NLS Neu-Laxova syndrome
NLSD neutral lipid storage disease
NLSDI neutral lipid storage disease with ichthyosis
NMF natural moisturizing factor
NOMID neonatal onset multisystemic inflammatory disorder
N_2O nitrous oxide
NPSA National Patient Safety Agency (UK)
NP-SLE neuropsychiatric systemic lupus erythematosus
NPY neuropeptide Y
NS naevus sebaceus
NS Netherton syndrome
NS Noonan syndrome
NSML Noonan syndrome with multiple lentigines
NSAIDs nonsteroidal anti-inflammatory drugs
NSIP nonspecific interstitial pneumonia
NSV nonsegmental vitiligo
NTM nontuberculous mycobacteria
NUV normocomplementemic urticarial vasculitis
OA ocular albinism
OC osteoma cutis
OCA oculocutaneous albinism
OCCS oculocerebrocutaneous syndrome
OES oculoectodermal syndrome
OFC oral food challenge
OFG orofacial granulomatosis
OI osteogenesis imperfecta
OL-EDA-ID osteopetrosis, lymphoedema, anhidrotic ectodermal dysplasia and immune deficiency
OMIM Online Mendelian Inheritance in Man
OODD odonto-onycho-dermal dysplasia

OPG optic pathway glioma
OPK osteopoikilosis
ORF open reading frame
OS Omenn syndrome
OSD occult spinal dysraphism
OTU operational taxonomic unit
O/W oil in water
PA pityriasis alba
PA phytanic acid
PABA *para*-aminobenzoic acid
PAF platelet-activating factor
PAH phenylalanine hydroxylase
PAHX phytanoyl CoA hydroxylase
PAI-1 plasminogen activator inhibitor 1
PAN polyarteritis nodosa
p-ANCA perinuclear antineutrophilic cytoplasmic antibody
PAP peak arterial pressure
PAPA pyogenic arthritis, pyoderma gangrenosum and acne
PAR2 protease-activated receptor 2
PAS periodic acid–Schiff
PASI Psoriasis Area and Severity Index
PC pachyonychia congenita
PCFCL primary cutaneous follicle-centre lymphoma
PCFH precalcaneal congenital fibrolipomatous hamartoma
PCL primary cutaneous lymphoma
PCLBCL primary cutaneous diffuse large B-cell lymphoma
PCMZL primary cutaneous marginal zone B-cell lymphoma
PCNA proliferating cell nuclear antigen
PCOS polycystic ovarian syndrome
PCR polymerase chain reaction
PCT porphyria cutanea tarda
PCT primary care trust
PDGF platelet-derived growth factor
PDL pulsed-dye laser
PDT photodynamic therapy
PE pulmonary embolism
PEG polyethylene glycol
PEH palmoplantar eccrine hidradenitis
PELVIS perianal haemangioma, external genitalia malformations, lipomyelomeningocoele, vesicorenal abnormalities, imperforate anus and skin tags
PEP postexposure prophylaxis
PEPD paroxysmal extreme pain disorder
PEN porokeratotic eccrine naevus
PENS papular epidermal naevus with skyline basal cell layer
PEODDN porokeratotic eccrine ostial and dermal duct naevus
PET positron emission tomography
PF pemphigus foliaceus
PFT pulmonary function tests
PG pyoderma gangrenosum
PG pyogenic granuloma
PGA Physician Global Assessment
PGD preimplantation genetic diagnosis
PGP 9.5 protein gene product 9.5
PGRP peptidoglycan recognition protein
PH palmoplantar hidradenitis
PH pulmonary hypertension
PHA phytohaemagglutinin
PHACES posterior fossa brain malformations, large or complex haemangiomas of the face, arterial anomalies, cardiac anomalies and eye abnormalities
PHP pseudo-hypoparathyroidism
PHTS PTEN hamartoma tumour syndrome
PhyH phytanoyl-CoA2-hydroxylase
PICH partially involuting congenital haemangioma
PID pelvic inflammatory disease
PID primary immunodeficiency
PILA papillary intralymphatic angioendothelioma
PJS Peutz–Jeghers syndrome
PKDL post-kala-azar dermal leishmaniasis
PKS Pallister–Killian syndrome
PKU phenylketonuria
pI isoelectric point
PI3 proteinase inhibitor 3
PIP proximal interphalangeal
PL pityriasis lichenoides
PLC pityriasis lichenoides chronica
PLCA primary localized cutaneous amyloidosis
PLE polymorphous light eruption
PLEVA pityriasis lichenoides et varioliformis acuta
PLS Papillon–Lefèvre syndrome
PM porokeratosis of Mibelli
PML progressive multifocal leucoencephalopathy
PMLE polymorphous light eruption
PMN polymorphonuclear cell
PN poikiloderma with neutropenia
PN prurigo nodularis
PNET peripheral neuroectodermal tumour
PNF plexiform neurofibroma
POC point of care
P1cp procollagen type 1 carboxy-terminal peptide
PNT papulonecrotic tuberculid
POEM Patient-Oriented Eczema Measure
POEMS polyneuropathy, organomegaly, endocrinopathy, M protein, skin changes (syndrome)
POH progressive osseous heteroplasia
PP prurigo pigmentosa
PPAR peroxisome proliferator-activated receptor
PPGSS papular-purpuric gloves-and-socks syndrome
PPi inorganic pyrophosphate
PPK palmoplantar keratoderma
PPK phacomatosis pigmentokeratotica
PPKN palmoplantar keratoderma Nagashima
PPL penicilloyl-polylysine
PPP palmoplantar pustulosis
PPV phakomatosis pigmentovascularis
PPPD porokeratosis palmaris et plantaris disseminata
PPT positive patch test
PPTR positive patch test reaction
PR pagetoid reticulosis
PRES Paediatric Rheumatology European Society
PRINTO Paediatric Rheumatology International Trials Organization
PRIS propofol-related infusion syndrome
PRNT plaque-reduction neutralization test
PRO patient-reported outcome
PROM patient-reported outcome measure
PROS PIK3CA-related overgrowth spectrum disorders
PRP pityriasis rubra pilaris
PRR pathogen recognition receptors
PR3 proteinase 3
PS Proteus syndrome
PSEK progressive symmetric erythrokeratoderma
PSH premature sebaceous hyperplasia
PSS peeling skin syndromes
PT prothrombin time
PTC premature termination codon
PTEN phosphatase and TENsin homologue
PTH parathyroid hormone
PTHrP parathyroid-hormone-related peptide
PTT partial thromboplastin time
PUVA psoralens plus UVA
PV pemphigus vulgaris
PV psoriasis vulgaris
PVL Panton–Valentine leukocidin
PWS port wine stain
PXE pseudoxanthoma elasticum
QoL quality of life

qPCR	quantitative polymerase chain reaction
qRT-PCR	quantitative real-time PCR
QUADAS	Quality Assessment of Diagnostic Accuracy tool
RAK	reticulate acropigmentation of Kitamura
RAMBA	retinoic acid metabolism blocking agent
RAS	recurrent aphthous stomatitis
RAST	radio-allergosorbent test
RBP	retinol-binding protein
RCC	renal cell carcinoma
RCDP	rhizomelic chondrodysplasia punctata
RCT	randomized controlled trial
RD	restrictive dermopathy
RDD	Rosai–Dorfman disease
RDEB	recessive dystrophic epidermolysis bullosa
RICH	rapidly involuting congenital haemangioma
RF	rheumatoid factor
RF	rib fracture
RFC	replication factor C
RFLP	restriction fragment length polymorphism
RH	retinal haemorrhage
RMH	rhabdomyomatous mesenchymal hamartoma
RMS	rhabdomyosarcoma
RNP	ribonucleoprotein
ROAT	repeated open application test
ROS	reactive oxygen species
RP	relapsing polychondritis
RPA	replication protein A
RPE	recurrent toxin-mediated perineal erythema
RRP	recurrent respiratory papillomatosis
RSC	respiratory syncytial virus
RT-PCR	reverse transcription polymerase chain reaction
RTS	Rothmund–Thomson syndrome
RTX	rituximab
RV	retroviral vector
RXLI	recessive X-linked ichthyosis
SA	*Streptococcus aureus*
SAA	serum amyloid A
SAM	severe dermatitis, multiple allergies and metabolic wasting
SAPHO	synovitis, acne, pustulosis, hyperostosis and osteitis
SASSAD	six-area, six-sign atopic dermatitis (score)
SC	stratum corneum
SC	subcutaneous
SCALP	sebaceous naevus, central nervous system abnormalities, aplasia cutis, limbal dermoid and pigmented naevus (syndrome)
SCAP	syringocystadenoma papillifera
SCC	squamous cell carcinoma
SCCE	stratum corneum chymotryptic enzyme
SCE	sister chromatid exchange
SCF	stem cell factor
SCFN	subcutaneous fat necrosis
SCH	spindle cell haemangioma
SCID	severe combined immunodeficiency
SCLE	subacute cutaneous lupus erythematosus
SCORAD	SCORing Atopic Dermatitis
SCT	stem cell transplantation
SCTE	stratum corneum tryptic enzyme
SD	seborrhoeic dermatitis
SDA	Sabouraud dextrose agar
SDH	subdural haematoma
SEGA	subependymal giant cell astrocytoma
SegPD	segmental pigmentary disorder
SEI	superficial epidermolytic ichthyosis
SEN	scalp–ear–nipple (syndrome)
SEN	subependymal nodules
SERCA2	sarco/endoplasmic reticulum ATPase type 2
SFD	scrofuloderma
SFT	solitary fibrous tumour
SGC	Shprintzen–Goldberg craniosynostosis
SHBG	sex hormone-binding globulin
SHCB	self-healing collodion baby
SHH	Sonic Hedgehog
SHFM	split hand–split foot syndrome
SHP	Schönlein–Henoch purpura
SIB	self-injurious behaviour
SICI	self-improving congenital ichthyosis
SID	sudden infant death (syndrome)
sIgE	drug-specific IgE antibodies
siRNA	small interfering RNA
SIRS	systemic inflammatory response syndrome
6-4PP	pyrimidine-6,4-pyrimidone photoproducts
SJIA	systemic juvenile idiopathic arthritis
SJS	Stevens–Johnson syndrome
SLADP	Latin American Society for Pediatric Dermatology
S-LAM	spontaneous lymphangiomyomatosis
SLC27	solute carrier family 27
SLE	systemic lupus erythematosus
SLICC	Systemic Lupus International Collaborating Clinics
SLN	speckled lentiginous naevus
SLOS	Smith–Lemli–Opitz syndrome
SLPI	secretory leucocyte protease inhibitor
SLS	Sjögren–Larsson syndrome
SLS	sodium lauryl sulphate
SM	systemic mastocytosis
SM-AHN	systemic mastocytosis with an associated haematological neoplasm
SMO	smoothened
SNA	spherical nucleic acid
SNP	single nucleotide polymorphism
SNV	single nucleotide variant
SP	syringocystadenoma papilliferum
SPD	Society for Pediatric Dermatology
SPECT	single-photon emission computed tomography
SPF	sun protection factor
SPINK	serine protease inhibitor Kazal type
SPRR	small proline-rich proteins
SPTCL	subcutaneous panniculitis-like T-cell lymphoma
SR	systemic retinoids
SS	Sézary syndrome
SS	Sjögren syndrome
SS	Sweet syndrome
SSc	systemic sclerosis
SSG	split-thickness skin graft
SSKI	saturated solution of potassium iodide
SSLR	serum sickness-like reaction
SSM	smouldering systemic mastocytosis
SSP	Schöpf–Schulz–Passarge
SSPE	subacute sclerosing panencephalitis
SSRI	selective serotonin reuptake inhibitors
SSS	stiff skin syndrome
SSSS	staphylococcal scalded skin syndrome
SSTI	skin and soft tissue infection
STD	sexually transmitted disease
STI	sexually transmitted infection
STS	sodium thiosulfate
STS	steroid sulphatase
STS	soft tissue sarcoma
STSS	streptococcal toxic shock syndrome
SWS	Sturge–Weber syndrome
TA	tufted angioma
TA	teichoic acid
TAC	tetracaine/adrenaline/cocaine
TBE	tickborne encephalitis
TBSA	total body surface area
TCC	triple-combination cream

TCI	topical calcineurin inhibitors
TCR	T-cell receptor
TCS	topical corticosteroids
TDO	trichodento-osseous
TEN	toxic epidermal necrolysis
TEWL	transepidermal water loss
TFIIH	transcription factor IIH
TG	transglutaminase
TG	triacylglycerol
TGF	transforming growth factor
TG1	transglutaminase-1
TIMP	tissue inhibitor of metalloproteinase
TJ	tight junction
TLR	toll-like receptor
TMD	transmembrane domains
TMEP	telangiectasia macularis eruptiva perstans
TMP-SMX	trimethoprim-sulfamethoxazole
TND	twenty-nail dystrophy
TNF	tumour necrosis factor
TNFR	tumour necrosis factor receptor
TNPM	transient neonatal pustular melanosis
tPA	tissue plasminogen activator
TPM	transient pustular melanosis
TPMT	thiopurine methyltransferase
TPN	total parenteral nutrition
TRAPS	TNF receptor superfamily 1A-associated periodic fever syndrome
TREC	T-cell receptor excision circle
TRPS	trichorhinophalangeal syndrome
TRT	thermal relaxation time
TS	tuberous sclerosis
TSC	tuberous sclerosis complex
TSC-IS	TSC-associated infantile spasms
TSH	thyroid-stimulating hormone
TSS	toxic shock syndrome
TST	tuberculosis skin test
TTD	trichothiodystrophy
TU	tropical ulcer
TV	*Trichomonas vaginalis*
UD	unrelated donor
uE3	unconjugated oestriol
UNT	unilateral naevoid telangiectasia
UP	urticaria pigmentosa
UPD	uniparental disomy
URDS	Urban–Rifkin–Davis syndrome
US	ultrasound
US/LS	upper to lower segment
UTR	untranslated region
UV	ultraviolet
UVA	ultraviolet A
UVB	ultraviolet B
UV-DDB	UV-damaged DNA-binding
UVSS	UV-sensitive syndrome
UVR	ultraviolet radiation
VACTERL	vertebral anomalies, anal atresia, congenital cardiac anomalies, tracheo-oesophageal fistula and/or oesophageal atresia, renal anomalies, radial dysplasia and other limb defects
VDLR	Venereal Disease Research Laboratory
VEGF	vascular endothelial growth factor
VEGFR3	vascular endothelial growth factor receptor 3
VIG	vaccinia immune globulin
VIT	venom immunotherapy
VL	visceral leishmaniasis
VL	visible light
VLBW	very low birthweight
VLCFA	very-long-chain fatty acid
VLDL	very low-density lipoproteins
VM	venous malformation
VMCM	cutaneomucosal venous malformation
VS	Vohwinkel syndrome
VZIG	varicella zoster immunoglobulin
VZV	varicella zoster virus
WAO	World Allergy Organization
WAS	Wiskott–Aldrich syndrome
WGS	whole-genome shotgun
WHO	World Health Organization
W/O	water in oil
WPWS	Wolff–Parkinson–White syndrome
WRS	Wiedemann–Rautenstrauch syndrome
WS	Werner syndrome
XD	X-linked dominant
XLA	X-linked agammaglobulinaemia
XLI	X-linked ichthyosis
XLMR	X-linked mental retardation
XP	xeroderma pigmentosum
XPV	xeroderma pigmentosum variant
XR	X-linked recessive
YNS	yellow nail syndrome
ZIKV	Zika virus
ZNS	Zunich neuroectodermal syndrome

CHAPTER 101
Lipoma and Lipomatosis

Siriwan Wananukul & Susheera Chatproedprai
Department of Paediatrics, Faculty of Medicine, Chulalongkorn University, Pathumwan, Bangkok, Thailand

Lipoma, 1195
Lipoblastoma, 1196
Hibernoma, 1197
Liposarcoma, 1197
Other variants of neoplasms of subcutaneous fat, 1198
Lipomatosis, 1198
Congenital infiltrating lipomatosis of the face, 1198
Encephalocraniocutaneous lipomatosis, 1200
***PTEN* hamartoma tumour syndrome, 1201**
Cowden syndrome, 1201
Bannayan–Riley–Ruvalcaba syndrome, 1201
Proteus syndrome, 1202
Hemihyperplasia–multiple lipomatosis syndrome, 1202
Multiple symmetric lipomatosis, 1203
Familial multiple lipomatosis, 1204

Abstract

Benign soft tissue tumours are relatively uncommon in children. They present as painless, slow-growing, movable subcutaneous masses with a soft or rubbery consistency. The most common in this group are lipomas, which are composed of mature fat cells. Lipoblastomas are rare benign tumours composed of a mixture of mature and immature fat cells that occur mostly in young children. In lipoblastomatosis, the tumours are more diffuse and infiltrate deeper into adjacent structures, becoming symptomatic because of compression on adjacent structures. Liposarcomas are rare malignant soft tissue tumours in children, the severity depending on the cell type and extent of the lesion. Lipomatosis consists of multiple masses or diffuse lesions infiltrating existing structures. It is regarded as a developmental abnormality or a mesenchymal malformation that presents with other, associated findings. Syndromes that present with lipomatosis are very rare and may present at birth or later in adulthood. Histopathology is very important in distinguishing these soft tissue tumours.

Lipoma

Key points

- **Lipomas are benign soft tissue tumours of mature fat cells.**
- **These lesions are less common in children than in adults.**
- **Lipomas present as subcutaneous painless soft tissue nodules.**
- **Typical histology reveals a circumscribed mass composed of lobules of mature adipocytes.**

Introduction. Lipomas are benign soft tissue tumours composed of mature fat cells. They are more common in adults and usually present as a soft, subcutaneous movable painless mass. Subcutaneous lipomas on the lumbosacral area should be investigated for spina bifida and spinal lipoma [1].

Epidemiology and pathogenesis. Lipomas are the most common benign soft tissue tumours in adults. They can occur at any age but are most commonly encountered between the ages of 40 and 60 years [1]. Lipoma in childhood is relatively uncommon [2]. According to Coffin and colleagues [1], 15% of adipose tumours in children are ordinary lipomas. Little is known about the pathogenesis of lipoma. The cytogenetic hallmarks are structural rearrangements of chromosomes 12q13-15 and 6p21, involving the high mobility group subfamily A1 (*HMGA*1) gene and the *HMGA*2 gene [3–7].

Clinical features. Lipoma usually presents as a painless, slow-growing, movable, soft or rubbery subcutaneous mass. Although the size is variable, most lesions are smaller than 5 cm. Lesions can be either single or multiple lesions. The trunk is the most common site, and lesions can occur at the neck, shoulder, back or abdomen [1,2]. Children presenting with subcutaneous lipomas in the midline lumbosacral area should be investigated for occult spina bifida and spinal cord (lumbosacral) lipoma. Reports indicate that 47% of spinal cord (lumbosacral) lipomas in children are subcutaneous [8]. Other cutaneous abnormalities associated with spinal cord lipoma include skin tags, dimples, dermal sinus tracts, haemangiomas, and hairy patches [8,9]. Spinal cord lipoma is a common cause of spinal cord tethering, even in apparently asymptomatic patients [9]. There are reports of lipomas arising in children in deeper structures, including intramuscular [5,10,11] and intraoral lipomas [12,13]. The differential diagnosis of a subcutaneous lipoma includes other subcutaneous soft tissue masses and tumours of fat cells (Table 101.1), as well as other subcutaneous tumours

Harper's Textbook of Pediatric Dermatology, Fourth Edition. Edited by Peter Hoeger, Veronica Kinsler and Albert Yan.

Table 101.1 Characteristics and histological features of adipocyte tumours in children

	Onset	Genetic abnormality	Common presentation	Key histological features
Lipoma	All ages	Chromosome 12q13-15, (*HMGA1* and *HMGA2*)	Painless, soft to rubbery consistency subcutaneous slow-growing mass	Circumscribed mass composed of lobules of mature adipocytes
Lipoblastoma	Infants up to 5 years	Chromosome 8q11-13 (*PLAG1*), polysomy of chromosome 8	Painless, solitary subcutaneous rapidly enlarging mass	Well-circumscribed lobulated tumour with fibrous septa, composed of mature and immature adipocytes
Hibernoma	All ages, rare in children	Chromosome 11q13 (*MEN1* and *AIP*)	Slowly growing tumour	Multivacuolated adipocyte with centrally placed nuclei and eosinophilic granular cytoplasm
Angiolipoma	Young adult	Small number of familial cases has been reported	Painful subcutaneous nodules with a predilection for the forearm	Well-circumscribed tumour composed of mature adipocytes and small venules
Spindle cell lipoma	Middle-age	Chromosome 13q	Asymptomatic subcutaneous nodule at the posterior neck, upper back and shoulder	Well-circumscribed tumour composed of mature adipocytes, spindle cells and strands of dense collagen
Liposarcoma Myxoid (OMIM #613488)	Mostly adult	Chromosome 12q13.3 (*CHOP/DDIT3*) with translocation partners 16p11 (*FUS-TLS*) or 22p11 (*EWS*)	Large deep subcutaneous mass of the extremities, especially the thigh and retroperitoneum that can extend to skin and muscles	Incomplete lobulation of highly variable lipoblast cells with hyperchromatic and mitotic figures
Lipomatosis	All ages	See Table 101.2	Multiple or diffuse lipomas	Multiple masses or diffuse, infiltrating pre-existing structures such as skeletal muscle and bone

AIP, aryl hydrocarbon receptor interaction protein; *CHOP*, CCAAT/enhancer-binding protein-homologous protein; *DDIT3*, DNA damage-inducible transcript 3; *FUS-TLS*, fused in sarcoma-translocated in liposarcoma; *EWS*, Ewing's sarcoma gene; *HMGA1*, high mobility group subfamily A1; *HMGA2*, high mobility group subfamily A2; *MEN1*, multiple endocrine neoplasia gene 1; OMIM, Online Mendelian Inheritance in Man; *PLAG1*, pleomorphic adenoma gene 1.

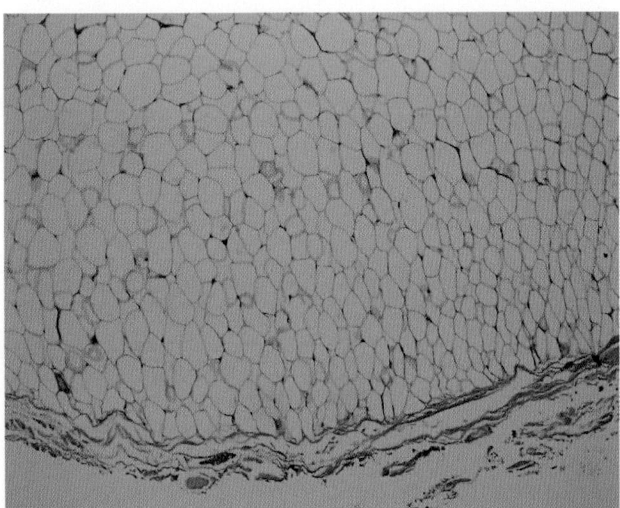

Fig. 101.1 Lipoma: the tumour shows thin fibrous encapsulation with diffuse mature adipocyte proliferation. Cells have eccentric nuclei and vacuolated cytoplasm. Source: Courtesy of Assoc. Prof. Dr. Voranuch Thanakit.

including deep or subcutaneous granuloma annulare, deep infantile haemangiomas, neurofibromas and leiomyomas.

Laboratory and histological findings. The histopathology of lipoma is an encapsulated nodule composed of lobules of mature adipocytes, a fibrous septum and thin-walled capillary-sized vessels (Fig. 101.1).

In those where the diagnosis is uncertain, such as multiple or large lesions, magnetic resonance imaging (MRI) shows a discrete encapsulated homogeneous fatty mass. MRI is reliable in distinguishing both simple lipomas and well-differentiated liposarcomas in order to plan management [14].

Treatment and prevention. Lipomas are benign and slow-growing. Treatment can include observation or, in cases where there is doubt regarding the diagnosis or a desire for cosmetic improvement, excision can be performed. Generally, the prognosis is excellent.

Lipoblastoma

Key points

- **Lipoblastoma is a rare, benign tumour composed of mature and immature fat cells.**
- **Most lipoblastomas occur in young children.**
- **Lipoblastomatosis is more diffuse and infiltrates tissues.**

Introduction. Lipoblastomas are rare benign tumours of infants and children, composed of mature and immature fat cells. Lipoblastomatosis is more diffuse and infiltrates deeper into adjacent muscles. Most lipoblastomas present in young children.

Epidemiology and pathogenesis. Lipoblastoma occurs predominantly in children under 5 years of age [1,15–18], but has been found in 30% of adipose tumours in children and adolescents [1].

The pathogenesis of lipoblastoma is unclear. Molecular cytogenetic studies reveal predominantly chromosomal alterations at the 8q11-13 region, leading to rearrangements of the transcription factor of pleomorphic adenoma gene 1 (*PLAG1*) [7,19]. Some have reported that the tumour possesses polysomy of chromosome 8 with or without *PLAG1* rearrangements [20,21]. A small number of patients (13%) lack a chromosome 8 abnormality [21].

Clinical features. Lipoblastoma presents as a painless, well-circumscribed rapidly enlarging soft tissue mass, frequently located on the extremities [22]. The clinical features of lipoblastoma are no different from those of lipoma, but lipoblastomas present at a younger age. Cervical lipoblastomas typically present as a rapid enlarging painless mass, which can cause respiratory problems in children [23–25]. There are also reports of lipoblastoma involving the thorax, mediastinum and mesentery [18,26,27]. In lipoblastomatosis the tumours are more diffuse and infiltrate deeper into adjacent structures, becoming symptomatic as a result of compression.

The differential diagnosis of lipoblastoma includes lipoma, liposarcoma and hibernoma. The differential diagnosis of cervical lipoblastoma includes cystic hygroma, vascular malformation, deep infantile haemangioma and thyroglossal duct cyst.

Laboratory and histological findings. The histopathology of lipoblastoma is one of lobules of mature and immature fat cells separated by a fibrous septum, and numerous capillaries and venules, and no abnormal mitoses [1] (Fig. 101.2). MRI is extremely useful for delineating the extent of the mass so as to allow planning surgical removal.

Treatment. For lipoblastoma complete resection is curative and the prognosis is excellent. Malignant transformation has not been reported [7]. In lipoblastomatosis, recurrences are common owing to incomplete resection. Long-term follow up is recommended.

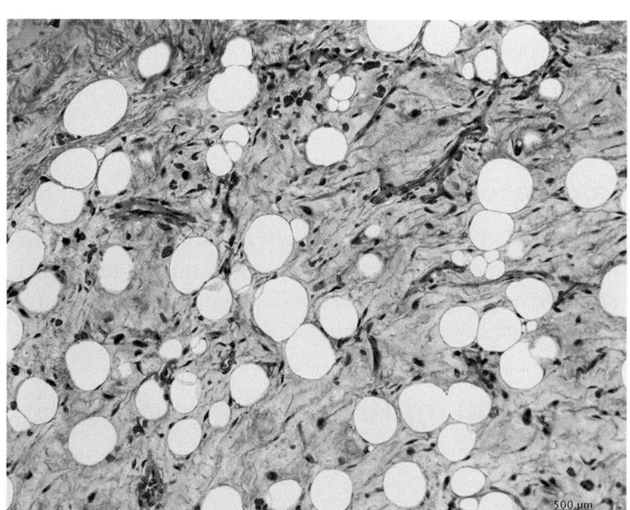

Fig. 101.2 Lipoblastoma: the tumour shows irregular lobular arrangement, composed of immature adipocytes separated by connective tissue septae and loose myxoid material. These lipoblasts are in different stages of development. In this image the cells are composed of stellate- and spindle-shaped cells, so called preadipocytes, together with uni- and multivacuolated adipocytes. Source: Courtesy of Assoc. Prof. Dr. Voranuch Thanakit.

Hibernoma

Key points

- Hibernoma is a very rare, benign soft tissue tumour of brown fat tissue in children.
- Presents as an asymptomatic slow-growing progressively enlarging soft subcutaneous tumour.

Introduction. Hibernoma is a rare, benign soft tissue tumour of brown fat which usually presents in young adults.

Epidemiology and pathogenesis. Hibernoma is very rare in children, presenting mostly in young adults [1]. According to Furlong and colleagues [28], only 5% of hibernomas present in children. The pathogenesis is still unclear. The cytogenetic alteration involves the region of chromosome 11q13, leading to the rearrangement of tumour suppressor gene multiple endocrine neoplasia (*MEN*) 1 and aryl hydrocarbon receptor interaction protein (*AIP*) [7,29].

Clinical features. Hibernoma presents as an asymptomatic, slow-growing, progressively enlarging soft subcutaneous tumour. The clinical features are indistinguishable from those of lipoma [26,30]. The thigh is the most common location, followed by the shoulder, scapular area, neck, chest, arm and abdomen [28,30]. There are also reports of intramuscular hibernomas [31].

The differential diagnosis includes subcutaneous soft tissue masses such as lipoma, lipoblastoma and neurofibroma.

Laboratory and histological findings. The histopathology of hibernoma is one of a well-circumscribed multilobulated mass consisting of multivacuolated adipocytes with small, centrally located nuclei having an eosinophilic granular cytoplasm of brown fat admixed with mature adipose tissue (Fig. 101.3). MRI reveals a well-circumscribed heterogeneous mass with diffusely hypointense surrounding subcutaneous fat which may mimic liposarcoma [14,32].

Treatment. Complete surgical excision is curative and recurrences are rare [33]. The prognosis is excellent.

Liposarcoma

Key points

- Liposarcoma is a rare, malignant soft tissue tumour in children.
- Severity depends on cell type and the extent of the lesion.

Introduction. Liposarcoma is a rare, malignant soft tissue tumour in children. It has many variants and may be locally invasive to metastatic, depending on cell type. The most common type encountered in children and adolescents is the myxoid liposarcoma [1].

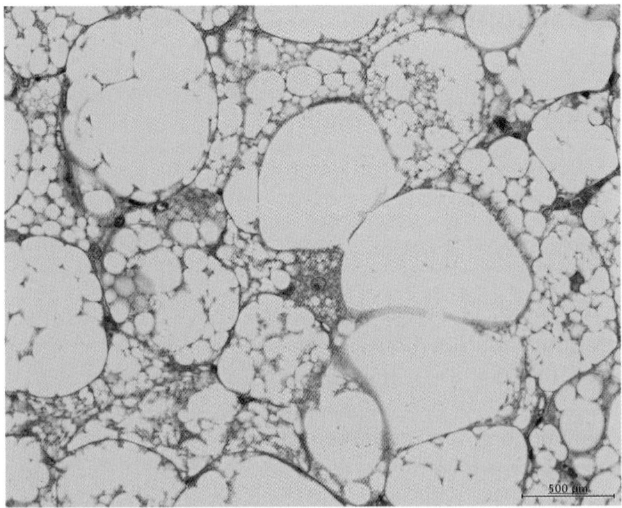

Fig. 101.3 Hibernoma: the tumour shows a lobular arrangement, composed of cells with a varying degree of differentiations. This image demonstrates cells with granular eosinophilic cytoplasm in the middle whereas the surrounding cells are large cells with centrally located nuclei and multiple small lipid droplets in the cytoplasm. Frequently, blood vessels are seen in association. Source: Courtesy of Assoc. Prof. Dr. Voranuch Thanakit.

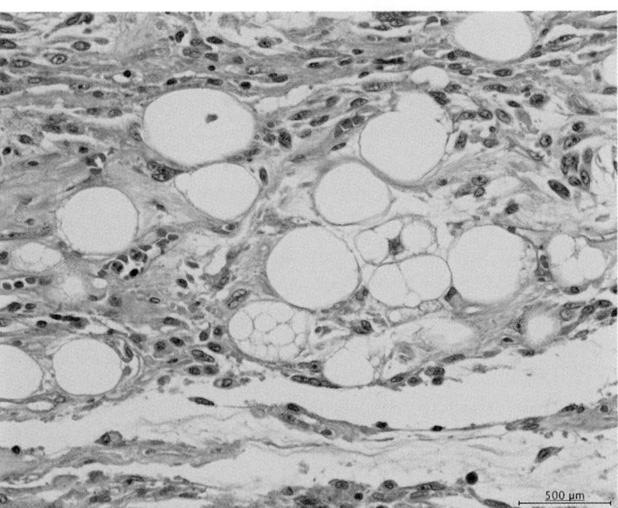

Fig. 101.4 Liposarcoma: the tumour shows adipocyte proliferation scatter lipoblasts. The stromal cells demonstrate moderately pleomorphic and hyperchromatic nuclei with visible nucleoli. The lipoblasts, which are immature fat cells, have multivacuolated cytoplasm and indented nuclei. Source: Courtesy of Assoc. Prof. Dr. Voranuch Thanakit.

Epidemiology and pathogenesis. Liposarcoma is very rare in children, occurring in only 5% of adipose tumours in children; most patients range from 10 to 22 years of age [1,28,34–36]. Myxoid liposarcoma is the most common liposarcoma in children, followed by pleomorphic–myxoid and spindle–myxoid [36]. The cytogenetic alteration involves chromosome 12q13 (*CHOP/DDIT3*) with translocation partners 16p11 (*FUS-TLS*) or 22p11 (*EWS*) [7,37–41].

Clinical features. The most common presentation of liposarcoma in children and adolescents is a deep soft tissue mass of the extremities, especially the thigh. Other sites of involvement include the retroperitoneum, pelvic and inguinal areas. According to Alaggio and colleagues [36], myxoid liposarcoma is locally invasive and distant metastases have not been reported. The spindle–myxoid variant is a low-grade malignancy, local invasiveness being common. Pleomorphic–myxoid liposarcoma is a high-grade variant with local invasion and metastases, and has a marked predilection for the mediastinum [36]. Other subtypes reported in children and adolescents include atypical lipomatous tumour (well-differentiated liposarcoma), dedifferentiated liposarcoma and myxoid–round cell liposarcoma [1,36,38].

The differential diagnosis of liposarcoma includes lipoma and lipoblastoma.

Laboratory and histological findings. The histopathology of myxoid liposarcoma is one of partially encapsulated mature adipocytes at the periphery and nuclear atypia and mitoses in the middle of lobules dispersed in a myxoid matrix (Fig. 101.4). Spindle–myxoid liposarcoma has significant numbers of spindle cells within a myxoid liposarcoma. Pleomorphic–myxoid liposarcoma has hyperchromatic tumour cells intermingled with large pleomorphic lipoblasts, and cells with atypical mitosis.

MRI is very useful in identifying and defining the extent of liposarcoma [14].

Treatment. Complete surgical excision is curative. The prognosis depends on cell type and the extent of the lesion. Myxoid liposarcoma has good prognosis, although local recurrence is common. The prognosis for pleomorphic liposarcoma with distant metastasis is guarded.

Other variants of neoplasms of subcutaneous fat

There are many subcutaneous masses that contain adipocytes, including angiolipoma, chondroid lipoma, lipofibroma, fibrolipoma, and spindle cell lipoma [1,28]. Most of these tumours arise in adults and the clinical manifestations are generally indistinguishable from each other. However, pain within a clinically recognized lipoma would indicate an angiolipoma which are characteristically painful. Imaging studies are not reliable and a definitive diagnosis depends on the histopathology.

Lipomatosis

Lipomatosis is a condition in which adipocytes form an infiltrative mass or multifocal masses on the body. It is regarded as a developmental abnormality or a mesenchymal malformation [1] (Table 101.2).

Congenital infiltrating lipomatosis of the face

Key points

- **Presents with hemifacial soft tissue and skeletal overgrowth, precocious dental development, macrodontia, hemimacroglossia and mucosal neuroma.**
- **Histological findings show nonencapsulated tumours.**

Table 101.2 Characteristics and clinical features of lipomatosis

Lipomatosis	Age at presentation	Inheritance pattern	Presentation	Additional findings
Congenital infiltrating lipomatosis of the face	Birth	AD	Facial asymmetry at birth; hemifacial soft tissue and skeletal overgrowth	Early eruption of deciduous, permanent teeth; macrodontia; ipsilateral hemimacroglossia, eyelid ptosis; mucosal neuroma
Encephalocraniocutaneous lipomatosis (OMIM #613001)	Birth	Sporadic	Cutaneous findings: unilateral lipomatous hamartoma of the scalp (naevus psiloliparus) Ophthalmological findings: ipsilateral epibulbar choristoma; small skin nodules around eyelids. Neurological findings: cerebral/intraspinal lipoma	Possible psychomotor and mental retardation; seizures; congenital heart abnormalities; lytic bone lesions; hypospadias; cryptorchidism
PTEN hamartoma tumour syndrome (OMIM #601728)	Birth/childhood	Chromosome 10q23.31	Phenotypically diverse disorders	
Cowden syndrome (OMIM #158350)		AD; chromosome 10q23.31	Facial trichilemmomas; acral keratosis; mucosal papillomas	Macrocephaly; dermal fibromas; scrotal tongue; mental retardation; malignancies; GI polyps
Bannayan–Riley–Ruvulcaba syndrome (OMIM #158350)		AD; chromosome 10q23.31	Pigmented macules of the penile shaft; cutaneous lipomas; vascular and lymphatic anomalies	Macrocephaly; GI polyps; Hashimoto thyroiditis
Proteus syndrome (OMIM #176920)		Sporadic chromosome 14q32.33	Lipomas; asymmetric, distorting overgrowth; cerebriform CNT naevi	Epidermal naevi; vascular malformation; skeletal deformities
Hemihyperplasia multiple lipomatosis syndrome		Sporadic	Asymmetric, nonprogressive, nondistorting overgrowth; lipomas	Occasional superficial vascular malformation; mild macrodactyly; thickened plantar skin; prominent creases
Nasopalpebral lipoma coloboma syndrome (OMIM #167730)	Childhood	AD, sporadic (some cases)	Nasopalpebral lipomatous growth; eyelid colobomas; telecanthus; maxillary hypoplasia	Broad forehead; widow's peak; outflaring of medial eyebrow; malpositioning of the lacrimal punctae
Gardner syndrome (OMIM #175100)		AD (chromosome 5q22.2)	Congenital hypertrophy of the retinal pigment epithelium; lipomas; fibromas; epidermoid cysts	Osteomas; dental abnormalities (odontomas); desmoid tumours; leiomyomas
Multiple symmetric lipomatosis; benign symmetric lipomatosis; Madelung's disease; Launois–Bensaude syndrome (OMIM #151800)	Adulthood (age 30–50 years)	Sporadic (predominantly)	Two variants: Localized form: diffuse, symmetrical nonencapsulated fat deposition at cervical area Diffuse form: obesity-like	Polyneuropathy; macrocytic anaemia; dysphonia; dysphagia; obstructive sleep apnoea; gustatory sweating; hyperhidrosis
Familial multiple lipomatosis, hereditary multiple lipomas (OMIM #151900)	Adulthood (age 30–50 years)	AD (chromosome 12q14; 3)	Solitary numerous discrete encapsulated lipomas	May have associated family history

AD, autosomal dominant; CNT, connective tissue naevi; GI, gastrointestinal tract; PTEN, Phosphatase and TENsin homologue.

Introduction. Congenital infiltrating lipomatosis of the face (CIL-F), also known as facial infiltrating lipomatosis, is a rare autosomal-dominant genetic disorder [42] characterized by a diffuse fatty infiltration of the facial soft tissue, generally noted at birth or shortly after [43].

Epidemiology and pathogenesis. The pathogenesis of CIL-F remains uncertain. Possible hypotheses include a somatic mutation in the phosphatidylinositide-3 kinase (*PIK3CA*) gene [44,45], alterations in chromosome 12 [44,46] and somatic mosaicism [47]. Deletion of chromosome 1q24.3q31.1 was reported in a 6-year-old girl with this syndrome and pituitary deficiency [48]. There is no gender predilection [43].

Clinical features. CIL-F presents with hemifacial soft tissue and skeletal overgrowth, precocious dental development, macrodontia, hemimacroglossia and mucosal neuroma [45]. It can present as either a rapidly progressive form (arising rapidly within a year), especially in the first year of life, or a more indolent form (evolving over decades). Facial asymmetry at birth is a common clinical manifestation [44]. Lipomatous masses are always unilateral and accompanied by enlargement of the ipsilateral side of the face [49]. Other associated findings include an increasing density of facial hair on the affected side, eyelid ptosis and ipsilateral faint cutaneous capillary staining [44,46].

Differential diagnosis. Lipoma is often well defined and encapsulated, whereas CIL-F is often nonencapsulated and infiltrative [43].

Laboratory and histological findings. Histological findings show a nonencapsulated tumour containing mature adipocytes, the presence of fibrous elements, and hypertrophy of subjacent bone [50].

Treatment and prevention. Surgery and palliative treatments such as antiangiogenic agents or anti-inflammatory therapy are the mainstay of treatment. However, recurrence is likely, probably because of diffuse infiltration [42].

Encephalocraniocutaneous lipomatosis

Key points

- **Characterized by unilateral naevus psiloliparus, ipsilateral ophthalmic (choristoma, skin tags) and cerebral malformation.**
- **Histological findings reveal well-circumscribed mature adipocytes.**
- **In some patients, mutations in KRAS have been associated.**

Introduction. Encephalocraniocutaneous lipomatosis (ECCL), also known as Haberland syndrome or Fishman syndrome [51], is a rare congenital hamartomatous and neurocutaneous disorder characterized by unilateral lipomatous hamartomas of the scalp, ipsilateral ophthalmia (eyelid, and outer globe of the eye) and cerebral malformation [52]. It was first described in 1970 by Haberland and Perou [53].

Epidemiology and pathogenesis. The incidence is rare and sporadic. No geographical, gender or racial predilection has been reported [52]. The syndrome is caused by somatic mosaic activating mutations in genes within the RAS-MAPK signalling pathway. Mutations in both *FGFR1* and *KRAS* have been identified as aetiological in several reported patients [54,55]. In one patient, mutations in the neurofibromatosis-1 (*NF1*) gene were speculated to be the cause in one patient [56]. However, it is unclear whether mutations in *NF1* were causative because no other patients with ECCL have been reported with such mutations since, and this patient was not screened for mutations in *FGFR1* or *KRAS* at the time.

Clinical features. The clinical features are typically present at birth. Cutaneous manifestations vary from significant skin lesions to less prominent skin involvement [57]. Nonscarring alopecia, with or without underlying fatty tissue, accompanied by subcutaneous fatty masses, is the most important skin anomaly [58]. The characteristic skin lesion is naevus psiloliparus [51,59], a fatty tissue naevus localized on the scalp with an irregular border, a flat smooth surface, absence of hair follicles [58,59], and often covered by telangiectasia [60]. However, this naevus has also been reported in nonsyndromic patients [58,61].

Choristoma is a benign ocular tumour including epibulbar or limbal dermoids (dermolipomas) or lipodermoids. Small nodular skin tags representing fibromas, lipomas, fibrolipomas or choristomas on the eyelids or following a line from the outer canthus to the tragus are common ophthalmological findings [58].

The spectrum of central nervous system anomalies is very broad and may be variably associated with psychomotor and mental retardation, and seizures [52,58]. The intracranial malformations include cerebral lipoma, porencephalic cysts, cortical atrophy and cranial asymmetry [62–65]. Compressive cervical myeloradiculopathy caused by intraspinal lipoma and low-grade astrocytomas has been documented [51,66].

Other reported abnormalities are congenital heart malformations, especially coarctation of the aorta [58], lytic bone lesions, hypospadias and cryptorchidism [58,62–64].

The diagnosis is based on the involvement of different systems, including the skin, eyes, central nervous system and others, and in 2009 the diagnostic criteria were revised by Moog [58].

Differential diagnosis. Sebaceous naevus syndrome [64] is a group of congenital neurocutaneous disorders characterized by sebaceous naevi in association with cerebral, ocular, skeletal, and sometimes cardiac and renal abnormalities. A feature that is shared between naevus sebaceus and naevus psiloliparus is the lack of hair, but naevus psiloliparus presents with a smooth surface, unlike the peau d'orange or cobblestoned surface of naevus sebaceus.

Oculocerebrocutaneous syndrome (OCCS) [58] is characterized by the triad of congenital brain, eye and skin anomalies, as in ECCL. Both syndromes can have focal aplastic or hypoplastic skin lesions and microphthalmia. However, the most typical cutaneous sign in ECCL is naevus psiloliparus, as opposed to a postauricular almond-shaped hypoplastic skin defect in OCCS. In addition, the ocular hallmark in ECCL is the epibulbar choristoma, whereas in OCCS it is cystic microphthalmia. The brain anomalies in ECCL, which primarily affect the tissue surrounding the brain and the vessels, are very different from the characteristic pattern of primary brain malformations seen in OCCS, including frontal-predominant polymicrogyria, agenesis of the corpus callosum, asymmetrically enlarged lateral ventricles or hydrocephalus, and a unique malformation of the mid-hindbrain.

Laboratory and histological findings. Both subcutaneous fat tumours and intracranial tumours are typical lipomas.

Treatment and prevention. Treatment focuses on the associated symptoms and abnormalities. ECCL is at risk of the development of certain neoplasms, such as gingival angiofibroma, papillary glioneuronal tumour and low-grade glioma/astrocytoma. Screening for these conditions is recommended during the follow-up period [52].

The prognosis seems to correlate with intracerebral malformations or with drug and surgical therapies for neurological symptoms [52].

PTEN hamartoma tumour syndrome

Key point

- **Phenotypically diverse disorders caused by mutations of the germline *PTEN* gene on chromosome 10q23.31.**

Introduction. *PTEN* (Phosphatase and TENsin homologue) hamartoma tumour syndrome is a collection of phenotypically diverse disorders that share overlapping clinical features, including Cowden syndrome and Bannayan–Riley–Ruvalcaba syndrome. Proteus syndrome was traditionally classified as a *PTEN*-associated disorder, but subsequent studies have identified mutations in *AKT1* as being aetiological for Proteus syndrome.

Epidemiology and pathogenesis. These disorders are caused by mutations in the germline *PTEN* gene on chromosome 10q23.31. *PTEN* acts as a tumour suppressor gene through the action of its phosphatase protein product. This phosphatase is involved in the regulation of the cell cycle, preventing cells from growing and dividing too rapidly [67]. Mutations responsible for these syndromes cause the resulting protein to be nonfunctional or absent. The defective protein allows the cell to divide uncontrollably and prevents damaged cells from dying, thereby leading to the growth of tumours [68]. For further details on PTEN-hamartoma, Cowden syndrome and Bannayan–Ruvalcalba syndrome see Chapter 141.

Cowden syndrome

Key points

- **Characterized by lipomas, facial trichilemmomas, acral keratoses and mucosal papillomas.**
- **Increased risk of both malignant and benign tumours.**

Clinical features. Cowden syndrome is a rare multisystem disorder with autosomal dominant inheritance. It carries an increased risk of tumours, both malignant (thyroid, breast, gastrointestinal tract, female reproductive system) and benign hamartomatous overgrowths of tissues (including but not limited to skin, colon, thyroid) [69]. The mucocutaneous findings include multiple facial trichilemmomas (at least three), especially on the central portions [69], acral keratoses either on the palmoplantar surfaces or the dorsal sides, oral papillomas, and mucocutaneous neuromas. Lipomas affect approximately 30–40% of cases [70,71]. Other important signs are macrocephaly (40–80%), dermal fibromas (24%), scrotal tongue (20%) and multiple skin tags (16%) [72].

Differential diagnosis. Trichilemmomas are clinically indistinguishable from trichoepitheliomas, fibrofolliculomas, trichodiscomas, or other benign lesions involving the pilosebaceous unit [69].

Bannayan–Riley–Ruvalcaba syndrome

Key point

- **Characterized by pigmented macules on the penis or vulva, macrocephaly, lipomas, vascular and lymphatic anomalies.**

Clinical features. Bannayan–Riley–Ruvalcaba syndrome is an allelic genetic disorder to Cowden syndrome with an autosomal dominant pattern. It is characterized by macrocephaly, multiple cutaneous lipomas, vascular and lymphatic anomalies such as haemangiomas, lymphangiomas, multiple intestinal hamartomatous polyps limited to the distal ileum and colon, and pigmented macules on the genital area [69].

Differential diagnosis. Peutz–Jeghers syndrome presents with benign hamartomatous polyps in the gastrointestinal tract, usually the jejunum and ileum, and hyperpigmented macules on the lips and oral mucosa. However, it is rarely associated with macrocephaly and lipoma.

Proteus syndrome

Key points

- Characterized by progressive, distorting, segmental overgrowth of multiple tissues and multiple hamartomas, and vascular malformations.
- Associated with activating mutations in *AKT1*.

Clinical features. Proteus syndrome occurs sporadically with a highly variable phenotype [73]. It is characterized by progressive, distorting segmental overgrowth of multiple tissues, and multiple hamartomatous and vascular malformations [73,74]. Cerebriform connective tissue naevi are highly specific and common in patients with Proteus syndrome [75,76]. Patients occasionally have epidermal naevi, partial lipohypoplasia and patchy dermal hypoplasia [75] (Fig. 101.5). The aetiology is a mosaic-activating mutation in *AKT1* [73,77].

Differential diagnosis. The progressive and distorting overgrowth in Proteus syndrome differs from that in hemihyperplasia–multiple lipomatosis syndrome [78].

Treatment and prevention. Treatment focuses on the associated symptoms and abnormalities. For further details see Chapter 108.

Hemihyperplasia–multiple lipomatosis syndrome

Key points

- Characterized by multiple lipomas and an asymmetric, nonprogressive and nondistorting overgrowth.
- Higher risk for intraabdominal embryonal malignancies.

Introduction. Hemihyperplasia–multiple lipomatosis syndrome (HHML) was first documented by Biesecker in 1998 [79]. It is characterized by subcutaneous lipomatosis and an asymmetric, nonprogressive overgrowth [78].

Epidemiology and pathogenesis. HHML is a sporadic disorder which is differentiated from Proteus syndrome by Biesecker [79]. The aetiology of this syndrome is associated with mutations in *PIK3CA* [74].

Clinical features. HHML presents as moderately asymmetric, nonprogressive nondistorting overgrowth accompanied by multiple subcutaneous lipomas and occasional superficial vascular malformations [74]. In addition, in some cases mild macrodactyly, thickened plantar skin and prominent creases have also been noted. HHML has a higher risk for intra-abdominal embryonal malignancies, including Wilms tumour,

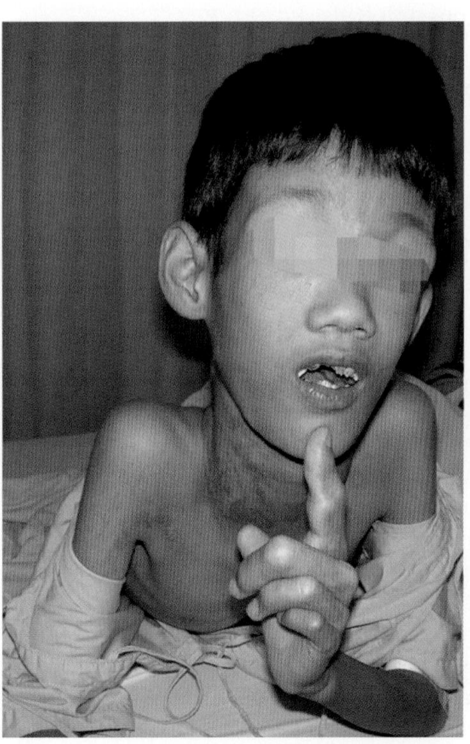
(a)

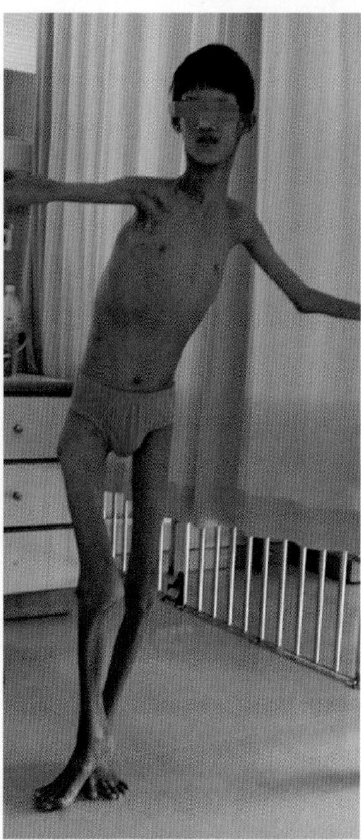
(b)

Fig. 101.5 (a) Lipomas at left upper eyelid, left index finger and linear epidermal naevi at right side of neck and right shoulder in Proteus syndrome. (b) Hemihypertrophy of right side of body in Proteus syndrome.

adrenal cell carcinoma and hepatoblastoma. The incidence of these tumours begins before puberty, so that routine surveillance via abdominal ultrasonography has been recommended [80].

Differential diagnosis. Clinically, HHML shares similar features to a number of PIK3CA-related overgrowth syndromes such as CLOVES syndrome (congenital lipomatous overgrowth, vascular malformations and epidermal naevi), and must be differentiated from other overgrowth syndromes such as Proteus syndrome and SOLAMEN syndrome (segmental overgrowth, lipomatosis, arteriovenous malformation and epidermal naevi).

Treatment and prevention. Except for screening with serial abdominal ultrasonography, treatment of the associated lipomas is controversial because of a high risk of recurrence and a significant incidence of postoperative scarring.

Multiple symmetric lipomatosis

Key points

- **Characterized by multiple diffuse symmetrical fat deposition on the cervical area, polyneuropathy and related metabolic diseases.**
- **Histological findings are nonencapsulated and infiltrative.**

Introduction. Multiple symmetric lipomatosis (MSL), also termed Madelung's disease, benign symmetric lipomatosis or Launois–Bensaude syndrome, is characterized by multiple diffuse symmetrical fat deposition on the cervical area. MSL was first documented by Brodie in 1846 [81], and in 1888 Madelung described a series of 35 patients with cervical lipomatosis and gave his name to the disease [82].

Epidemiology and pathogenesis. MSL begins after the age of 20 and is commonest at around 30–60 years of age [81]. Nevertheless, MSL was reported in a 9-year-old girl in association with severe obesity, developmental delay, mild mental retardation, peripheral neuropathy and latent hypothyroidism, and a 13-year-old boy with severe obesity, mild mental retardation and insulin-dependent diabetes mellitus [83]. It presents predominantly in males, with a ratio of 15 : 1–30 : 1 [84]. MSL is markedly associated with a history of increased alcohol intake, with a reported incidence of 88% [42].

The aetiology of most cases of MSL remains unclear. Some believe it is caused by mutations in the mitochondrial DNA gene or a signalling dysfunction in brown adipocytes, but others think it is caused by a local defect in catecholamine-induced lipolysis [42,81]. Some patients with MSL have also been documented with partial lipodystrophy and myopathy, cases of which have been linked to chromosome 19 that correspond to mutations in the hormone sensitive lipase (*LIPE*) gene [85].

Clinical features. There have been two reported variants: a 'localized form' described by symmetrical distributed fat deposits on the upper part of the body with sparing of the distal aspects of the extremities (Fig. 101.6); and a more 'diffuse form', presenting as generalized simple obesity [81]. The cutaneous features are multiple extensive symmetrical nonencapsulated fat deposits that are infiltrative, plus irreversible tumour growth [82]. The predilection sites for adipocyte accumulation in subcutaneous and skeletal muscles are the face, neck, shoulders and proximal upper limbs.

The common associated finding is polyneuropathy, including sensory, motor and autonomic function. Sensory dysfunction ranges from disturbances in vibratory sensory loss to severe trophic ulcers. In cases of autonomic dysfunction, gustatory sweating, hyperhidrosis and tachycardia at rest may be present [81]. In addition, mediastinal involvement with tracheal and vena cava compression is possible [81], so that the patient might encounter dysphagia, dysphonia and obstructive sleep apnoea caused by endopharyngeal growth [81,82]. Other related diseases are diabetes, hyperlipidaemia (types I, IV), hyperthyroidism, hyperuricaemia [81] and macrocytic anaemia [81]. Malignant transformation is extremely rare [42].

The diagnosis of MSL is made by a combination of physical examination, location, distribution of the adipose tissue, age, gender and history of alcohol abuse [42].

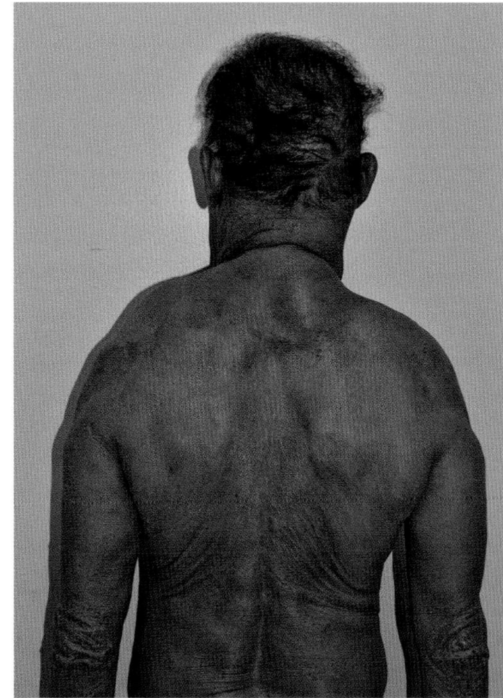

Fig. 101.6 Symmetrical distributed fat deposits on the neck and shoulders in Madelung's disease. Source: Courtesy of Dr. Panlop Chakkavittumrong.

The course of the disease is variable. Palmar and Blackburn [81] have reported that the typical course is fast growing during the initial years, followed by slow growth over a long period.

Differential diagnosis. Both MSL and familial multiple lipomas present during adulthood, but the location of lipomas in familial multiple lipomatosis is usually on the forearms and thighs, sparing the neck and shoulders, the common sites found in MSL [42,81,86]. In cases of more diffuse patterns, simple obesity, Cushing syndrome should be differentiated.

Laboratory and histological findings. Histologically the tumours of MSL are nonencapsulated and infiltrative.

Treatment and prevention. Treatment is difficult because of the pattern of infiltration to deep-seated structures, including major nerves and vessels. Preoperative computed tomography (CT) is crucial to assess the extent of the lesions and their proximity to vital structures [87]. Treatment options include medication (oral $ß_2$-agonists, fibrate drugs [87]) and surgical intervention (liposuction [87], lipectomy [87], mesotherapy [88] and debulking surgery [42]). However, complications such as haematoma and seroma are commonly described after surgery [42]. Also, lipoma has a tendency to recur after surgical treatment [82].

Familial multiple lipomatosis

Key points

- **Characterized by numerous discrete painless lipomas with a possible associated family history.**
- **Histological findings show a well circumscribed and encapsulated tumour.**

Introduction. Familial multiple lipomatosis (FML), also termed multiple familial lipomatosis, hereditary multiple lipomas or multiple circumscribed lipomas, is characterized by numerous discrete encapsulated painless lipomas with a possible associated family history.

Epidemiology and pathogenesis. FML is a predominantly inherited autosomal-dominant syndrome with a reported incidence of 2:100000 [42]. No geographic predilection has been noted, but there is an increased prevalence in males of 76% [42]. The aetiology is still unclear. Reports suggest that translocation of 12q14 and its partner gene on chromosome 3 could be responsible for this condition [89] and one case report described familial multiple subcutaneous lipomatosis with a predilection to malignancy (breast, uterine, pancreatic, ovarian) in association with a mutation in the *PALB2* gene [90].

Clinical features. FML develops as an asymptomatic clinical manifestation during adulthood, usually between the third and fifth decades. Lipomas can present as solitary lesions or in clusters of over 100 [91], with sizes varying from a few millimetres in diameter to 25 cm [89]. Tumours are benign [42] and found predominantly at the mid-level of the body (the lower arms, forearms, lower chest, abdomen and lumbar region, with sparing of the neck and shoulders) (Fig. 101.7). A family history is not always present [42].

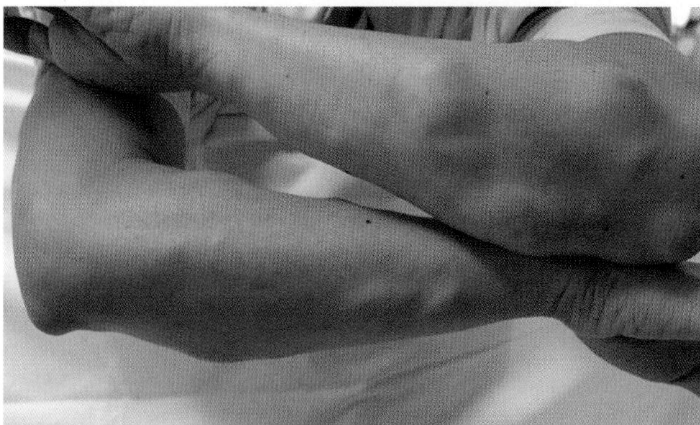

Fig. 101.7 Multiple lipomas on both forearms in familial multiple lipomatosis.

Differential diagnosis. FML is both clinically and histologically different from Madelung's disease [86].

Laboratory and histological findings. Pathological biopsy is the most definitive test, demonstrating in the benign condition well-circumscribed and encapsulated spindle cell lipomas [91], pleomorphism or angiolipomas [42]. Diagnostic imaging may help evaluate the borders and dimensions of the tumour, and CT is the most used modality [42].

Treatment and prevention. The standard treatment is surgical excision. Total excision may be difficult and recurrence is frequent because of late clinical presentation [42]. Malignant transformation has not been reported in FML. However, one report documented an association of this condition with certain malignancies, including breast, uterine, pancreatic and ovarian cancer.

References

1 **Coffin CM, Alaggio R. Adipose and myxoid tumors of childhood and adolescence. Pediatr Dev Pathol 2012;15:239–54.**

2 Rydholm A, Berg NO. Size, site and clinical incidence of lipoma. Factors in the differential diagnosis of lipoma and sarcoma. Acta Orthop Scand 1983;54:929–34.

3 Sandberg AA. Updates on the cytogenetics and molecular genetics of bone and soft tissue tumors: lipoma. Cancer Genet Cytogenet 2004;150:93–115.

4 Ligon AH, Moore SD, Parisi MA et al. Constitutional rearrangement of the architectural factor HMGA2: a novel human phenotype including overgrowth and lipomas. Am J Hum Genet 2005;76:340–8.

5 Pierron A, Fernandez C, Saada E et al. HMGA2-NFIB fusion in a pediatric intramuscular lipoma: a novel case of NFIB alteration in a large deep-seated adipocytic tumor. Cancer Genet Cytogenet 2009; 195:66–70.

6 Bartuma H, Hallor KH, Panagopoulos I et al. Assessment of the clinical and molecular impact of different cytogenetic subgroups in a series of 272 lipomas with abnormal karyotype. Genes Chromosomes Cancer 2007;46:594–606.

7 **Dadone B, Refae S, Lemarie-Delaunay C et al. Molecular cytogenetics of pediatric adipocytic tumors. Cancer Genet 2015;208:469–81.**
8 Xenos C, Sgouros S, Walsh R, Hockley A. Spinal lipomas in children. Pediatr Neurosurg 2000;32:295–307.
9 Wykes V, Desai D, Thompson DN. Asymptomatic lumbosacral lipomas--a natural history study. Childs Nerv Syst 2012;28:1731–9.
10 Shiraki K, Kamo M, Sai T, Kamo R. Rare site for an intramuscular lipoma. Lancet 2002;359:2077.
11 Lee YH, Jung JM, Baek GH, Chung MS. Intramuscular lipoma in thenar or hypothenar muscles. Hand Surg 2004;9:49–54.
12 Venkateswarlu M, Geetha P, Srikanth M. A rare case of intraoral lipoma in a six year-old child: a case report. Int J Oral Sci 2011;3:43–6.
13 Manor E, Sion-Vardy N, Joshua BZ, Bodner L. Oral lipoma: analysis of 58 new cases and review of the literature. Ann Diagn Pathol 2011; 15:257–61.
14 Gaskin CM, Helms CA. Lipomas, lipoma variants, and well-differentiated liposarcomas (atypical lipomas): results of MRI evaluations of 126 consecutive fatty masses. Am J Roentgenol 2004;182:733–9.
15 Chung EB, Enzinger FM. Benign lipoblastomatosis. An analysis of 35 cases. Cancer 1973;32:482–92.
16 Mentzel T, Calonje E, Fletcher CD. Lipoblastoma and lipoblastomatosis: a clinicopathological study of 14 cases. Histopathology 1993; 23:527–33.
17 Hicks J, Dilley A, Patel D et al. Lipoblastoma and lipoblastomatosis in infancy and childhood: histopathologic, ultrastructural, and cytogenetic features. Ultrastruct Pathol 2001;25:321–33.
18 Jung SM, Chang PY, Luo CC et al. Lipoblastoma/lipoblastomatosis: a clinicopathologic study of 16 cases in Taiwan. Pediatr Surg Int 2005;21:809–12.
19 Brandal P, Bjerkehagen B, Heim S. Rearrangement of chromosomal region 8q11-13 in lipomatous tumours: correlation with lipoblastoma morphology. J Pathol 2006;208:388–94.
20 **Coffin CM, Lowichik A, Putnam A. Lipoblastoma (LPB): a clinicopathologic and immunohistochemical analysis of 59 cases. Am J Surg Pathol 2009;33:1705–12.**
21 Gisselsson D, Hibbard MK, Dal Cin P et al. PLAG1 alterations in lipoblastoma: involvement in varied mesenchymal cell types and evidence for alternative oncogenic mechanisms. Am J Pathol 2001; 159:955–62.
22 Chien AL, Song DH, Stein SL. Two young girls with lipoblastoma and a review of the literature. Pediatr Dermatol 2006;23:152–6.
23 Brodsky JR, Kim DY, Jiang Z. Cervical lipoblastoma: case report, review of literature, and genetic analysis. Head Neck 2007;29: 1055–60.
24 Lorenzen JC, Godballe C, Kerndrup GB. Lipoblastoma of the neck: a rare cause of respiratory problems in children. Auris Nasus Larynx 2005;32:169–73.
25 Choi HJ, Lee YM, Lee JH et al. Pediatric lipoblastoma of the neck. J Craniofac Surg 2013;24:e507–10.
26 Whyte AM, Powell N. Mediastinal lipoblastoma of infancy. Clin Radiol 1990;42:205–6.
27 Kerkeni Y, Sahnoun L, Ksia A et al. Lipoblastoma in childhood: about 10 cases. Afr J Paediatr Surg 2014;11:32–4.
28 Furlong MA, Fanburg-Smith JC, Miettinen M. The morphologic spectrum of hibernoma: a clinicopathologic study of 170 cases. Am J Surg Pathol 2001;25:809–14.
29 Nord KH, Magnusson L, Isaksson M et al. Concomitant deletions of tumor suppressor genes MEN1 and AIP are essential for the pathogenesis of the brown fat tumor hibernoma. Proc Natl Acad Sci U S A 2010;107:21122–7.
30 Beals C, Rogers A, Wakely P et al. Hibernomas: a single-institution experience and review of literature. Med Oncol 2014;31:769.
31 Naik R, Panda KM, Kushwaha AK, Agrawal PC. Intramuscular hibernoma: a rare tumour in buttock. J Clin Diagn Res 2015;9:ED01–02.
32 Lee JC, Gupta A, Saifuddin A et al. Hibernoma: MRI features in eight consecutive cases. Clin Radiol 2006;61:1029–34.
33 Ahmed SA, Schuller I. Pediatric hibernoma: a case review. J Pediatr Hematol Oncol 2008;30:900–1.
34 La Quaglia MP, Spiro SA, Ghavimi F et al. Liposarcoma in patients younger than or equal to 22 years of age. Cancer 1993;72:3114–19.
35 Ferrari A, Casanova M, Spreafico F et al. Childhood liposarcoma: a single-institutional twenty-year experience. Pediatr Hematol Oncol 1999;16:415–21.
36 **Alaggio R, Coffin CM, Weiss SW et al. Liposarcomas in young patients: a study of 82 cases occurring in patients younger than 22 years of age. Am J Surg Pathol 2009;33:645–58.**
37 Turc-Carel C, Limon J, Dal Cin P et al. Cytogenetic studies of adipose tissue tumors. II. Recurrent reciprocal translocation t(12;16)(q13;p11) in myxoid liposarcomas. Cancer Genet Cytogenet 1986;23:291–9.
38 Willmore-Payne C, Holden J, Turner KC et al. Translocations and amplifications of chromosome 12 in liposarcoma demonstrated by the LSI CHOP breakapart rearrangement probe. Arch Pathol Lab Med 2008;132:952–7.
39 Sreekantaiah C, Karakousis CP, Leong SP, Sandberg AA. Cytogenetic findings in liposarcoma correlate with histopathologic subtypes. Cancer 1992;69:2484–95.
40 Gibas Z, Miettinen M, Limon J et al. Cytogenetic and immunohistochemical profile of myxoid liposarcoma. Am J Clin Pathol 1995;103:20–6.
41 Tallini G, Akerman M, Dal Cin P et al. Combined morphologic and karyotypic study of 28 myxoid liposarcomas. Implications for a revised morphologic typing, (a report from the CHAMP Group). Am J Surg Pathol 1996;20:1047–55.
42 **Tadisina KK, Mlynek KS, Hwang LK et al. Syndromic lipomatosis of the head and neck: a review of the literature. Aesthetic Plast Surg 2015;39:440–8.**
43 **Langhans L, Frevert SC, Andersen M. Lipomatous tumours of the face in infants: diagnosis and treatment. J Plast Surg Hand Surg 2015:1–5.**
44 Mahadevappa A, Raghavan VH, Ravishankar S, Manjunath GV. Congenital infiltrating lipomatosis of the face: a case report. Case Rep Pediatr 2012;2012:134646.
45 Maclellan RA, Luks VL, Vivero MP et al. PIK3CA activating mutations in facial infiltrating lipomatosis. Plast Reconstr Surg 2014; 133:12e–19e.
46 Sahai S, Rajan S, Singh N, Arora H. Congenital infiltrating lipomatosis of the face with exophytic temporomandibular joint ankylosis: a case report and review of the literature. Dentomaxillofac Radiol 2013;42:16128745.
47 Padwa BL, Mulliken JB. Facial infiltrating lipomatosis. Plast Reconstr Surg 2001;108:1544–54.
48 Capra V, Severino M, Rossi A et al. Pituitary deficiency and congenital infiltrating lipomatosis of the face in a girl with deletion of chromosome 1q24.3q31.1. Am J Med Genet A 2014;164A:495–9.
49 Singh K, Sen P, Musgrove BT, Thakker N. Facial infiltrating lipomatosis: a case report and review of literature. Int J Surg Case Rep 2011; 2:201–5.
50 Slavin SA, Baker DC, McCarthy JG, Mufarrij A. Congenital infiltrating lipomatosis of the face: clinicopathologic evaluation and treatment. Plast Reconstr Surg 1983;72:158–64.
51 Chiang CC, Lin SC, Wu HM et al. Clinical manifestation and neurosurgical intervention of encephalocraniocutaneous lipomatosis – a case report and review of the literature. Childs Nerv Syst 2014; 30:13–17.
52 Borgognoni L, Brandani P, Reali F et al. Encephalocraniocutaneous lipomatosis: congenital alopecia treatment in a rare neurocutaneous syndrome. J Plast Surg Hand Surg 2014;48:449–51.
53 Haberland C, Perou M. Encephalocraniocutaneous lipomatosis. A new example of ectomesodermal dysgenesis. Arch Neurol 1970; 22:144–55.
54 Bennett JT, Tan TY, Alcantara D et al. Mosaic activating mutations in FGFR1 cause encephalocraniocutaneous lipomatosis. Am J Hum Genet 2016;98:579–87.
55 Boppudi S, Bogershausen N, Hove HB et al. Specific mosaic KRAS mutations affecting codon 146 cause oculoectodermal syndrome and encephalocraniocutaneous lipomatosis. Clin Genet 2016;90:334–42.
56 Legius E, Wu R, Eyssen M et al. Encephalocraniocutaneous lipomatosis with a mutation in the NF1 gene. J Med Genet 1995;32:316–19.
57 Barbagallo JS, Kolodzieh MS, Silverberg NB, Weinberg JM. Neurocutaneous disorders. Dermatol Clin 2002;20:547–60.
58 Moog U. Encephalocraniocutaneous lipomatosis. J Med Genet 2009;46:721–9.
59 Happle R, Kuster W. Nevus psiloliparus: a distinct fatty tissue nevus. Dermatology 1998;197:6–10.
60 Sofiatti A, Cirto AG, Arnone M et al. Encephalocraniocutaneous lipomatosis: clinical spectrum of systemic involvement. Pediatr Dermatol 2006;23:27–30.
61 Happle R, Horster S. Nevus psiloliparus: report of two nonsyndromic cases. Eur J Dermatol 2004;14:314–16.
62 Dhouib A, Hanquinet S, La Scala GC. Encephalocraniocutaneous lipomatosis: magnetic resonance imaging findings in a child. J Pediatr 2013;163:297.
63 Kim DH, Park SB, Lee Y et al. Encephalocraniocutaneous lipomatosis without neurologic anomalies. Ann Dermatol 2012;24:476–8.

64 Rubegni P, Risulo M, Sbano P et al. Encephalocraniocutaneous lipomatosis (Haberland syndrome) with bilateral cutaneous and visceral involvement. Clin Exp Dermatol 2003;28:387–90.

65 Moog U, Jones MC, Viskochil DH et al. Brain anomalies in encephalocraniocutaneous lipomatosis. Am J Med Genet A 2007;143A:2963–72.

66 Brassesco MS, Valera ET, Becker AP et al. Low-grade astrocytoma in a child with encephalocraniocutaneous lipomatosis. J Neurooncol 2010;96:437–41.

67 Chu EC, Tarnawski AS. PTEN regulatory functions in tumor suppression and cell biology. Med Sci Monit 2004;10:RA235–41.

68 Pilarski R, Eng C. Will the real Cowden syndrome please stand up (again)? Expanding mutational and clinical spectra of the PTEN hamartoma tumour syndrome. J Med Genet 2004;41:323–6.

69 Pilarski R, Burt R, Kohlman W et al. Cowden syndrome and the PTEN hamartoma tumor syndrome: systematic review and revised diagnostic criteria. J Natl Cancer Inst 2013;105:1607–16.

70 Starink TM, van der Veen JP, Arwert F et al. The Cowden syndrome: a clinical and genetic study in 21 patients. Clin Genet 1986;29:222–33.

71 Salem OS, Steck WD. Cowden's disease (multiple hamartoma and neoplasia syndrome). A case report and review of the English literature. J Am Acad Dermatol 1983;8:686–96.

72 Pilarski R. Cowden syndrome: a critical review of the clinical literature. J Genet Couns 2009;18:13–27.

73 Lindhurst MJ, Wang JA, Bloomhardt HM et al. AKT1 gene mutation levels are correlated with the type of dermatologic lesions in patients with Proteus syndrome. J Invest Dermatol 2014;134:543–6.

74 Keppler-Noreuil KM, Sapp JC, Lindhurst MJ, et al. Clinical delineation and natural history of the PIK3CA-related overgrowth spectrum. Am J Med Genet A. 2014;164(7):1713–33.

75 Nguyen D, Turner JT, Olsen C et al. Cutaneous manifestations of proteus syndrome: correlations with general clinical severity. Arch Dermatol 2004;140:947–53.

76 Biesecker LG. The multifaceted challenges of Proteus syndrome. JAMA 2001;285:2240–3.

77 Lindhurst MJ, Sapp JC, Teer JK et al. A mosaic activating mutation in AKT1 associated with the Proteus syndrome. N Engl J Med 2011; 365:611–19.

78 Schulte TL, Liljenqvist U, Gorgens H et al. Hemihyperplasia-multiple lipomatosis syndrome (HHML): a challenge in spinal care. Acta Orthop Belg 2008;74:714–19.

79 Biesecker LG, Peters KF, Darling TN et al. Clinical differentiation between Proteus syndrome and hemihyperplasia: description of a distinct form of hemihyperplasia. Am J Med Genet 1998;79:311–18.

80 Hoyme HE, Seaver LH, Jones KL et al. Isolated hemihyperplasia (hemihypertrophy): report of a prospective multicenter study of the incidence of neoplasia and review. Am J Med Genet 1998;79:274–8.

81 Parmar C, Blackburn C. Madelung's disease: an uncommon disorder of unknown aetiology? Br J Oral Maxillofac Surg 1996;34:467–70.

82 Guilemany JM, Romero E, Blanch JL. An aesthetic deformity: Madelung's disease. Acta Otolaryngol 2005;125:328–30.

83 Kratz C, Lenard HG, Ruzicka T, Gartner J. Multiple symmetric lipomatosis: an unusual cause of childhood obesity and mental retardation. Eur J Paediatr Neurol 2000;4:63–7.

84 Gonzalez-Garcia R, Rodriguez-Campo FJ, Sastre-Perez J, Munoz-Guerra MF. Benign symmetric lipomatosis (Madelung's disease): case reports and current management. Aesthetic Plast Surg 2004; 28:108–12.

85 Zolotov S, Xing C, Mahamid R et al. Homozygous LIPE mutation in siblings with multiple symmetric lipomatosis, partial lipodystrophy, and myopathy. Am J Med Genet A 2017;173:190–4.

86 Abbasi NR, Brownell I, Fangman W. Familial multiple angiolipomatosis. Dermatol Online J 2007;13:3.

87 Sia KJ, Tang IP, Tan TY. Multiple symmetrical lipomatosis: case report and literature review. J Laryngol Otol 2012;126:756–8.

88 Hasegawa T, Matsukura T, Ikeda S. Mesotherapy for benign symmetric lipomatosis. Aesthetic Plast Surg 2010;34:153–6.

89 Toy BR. Familial multiple lipomatosis. Dermatol Online J 2003;9:9.

90 Reddy N, Malipatil B, Kumar S. A rare case of familial multiple subcutaneous lipomatosis with novel PALB2 mutation and increased predilection to cancers. Hematol/Oncol Stem Cell Ther 2016; 9:154–6.

91 Fanburg-Smith JC, Devaney KO, Miettinen M, Weiss SW. Multiple spindle cell lipomas: a report of 7 familial and 11 nonfamilial cases. Am J Surg Pathol 1998;22:40–8.

CHAPTER 102
Panniculitis in Children

Christine Bodemer

Department of Dermatology, Imagine Institute, Necker-Enfants Malades Hospital, Paris, France

Subcutaneous fat necrosis of the newborn, 1209
Sclerema neonatorum, 1210
Poststeroid panniculitis, 1210
Cold panniculitis, 1211
Panniculitis and monogenic autoinflammatory diseases and primary immune deficiency, 1211
Pannicultis and monogenic autoinflammatory diseases, 1212
Erythema nodosum, 1213
Panniculitis associated with connective tissue diseases and vasculitis, 1215
Cytophagic histiocytic panniculitis, 1216
Subcutaneous panniculitis-like T-cell lymphoma, 1217
α_1-Antitrypsin deficiency, 1218
Pancreatic panniculitis, 1219
Calciphylaxis, 1219
Infective panniculitis, 1220
Factitial, iatrogenic or traumatic panniculitis, 1220

Abstract

Pediatric panniculitis is a group of rare disorders characterized by inflammation of the subcutaneous fat, characterized clinically by nodules and indurated plaques with a frequent discolouration of the overlying skin. Panniculitides are often classified as septal versus lobular, with or without vasculitis and with an infiltrate comprising of a wide variety of inflammatory cells. This classification guides the aetiological investigation. However, the same specimen may show a mixed lobular and septal infiltrate, and variable histological features. Panniculitis can be a primary disease but is most often a secondary process related to different underlying disorders. Some types are more specific to the paediatric population, such as subcutaneous fat necrosis of the newborn, or occur in a specific context, such as poststeroid panniculitis and cold panniculitis. Other recognized associations in adults are infections, connective tissue diseases, subcutaneous lymphoma-like panniculitis, metabolic conditions and trauma. However, in many paediatric patients no specific aetiology can be identified.

Key points

- Panniculitis, characterized by inflammation of the subcutaneous fat, can be a primary disease, but is most often a secondary process.
- A histological classification, distinguishing predominant lobular or septal panniculitis, with or without vasculitis, guides the aetiological investigations. However, the same specimen may show a mixed aspect with lobular and septal infiltrate, and variable histological features.
- Under the age of 2 years specific aetiologies have to be considered, such as: subcutaneous fat necrosis of the newborn, sclerema neonatorum, cold panniculitis, poststeroid panniculitis, monogenic autoinflammatory diseases and primary immune deficiencies.
- All the aetiologies described in adults can be observed in children but remain rare in this population.

Introduction and history. Panniculitis in children is a group of rare disorders characterized by inflammation of the subcutaneous fat. Histopathology is required to confirm the diagnosis because lesions can have different presentations as either erythematous nodules or large infiltrated plaques. A histological classification has been proposed distinguishing mostly lobular, mostly septal or mixed panniculitis, depending on the distribution of the dominant subcutaneous inflammatory infiltrate, with or without vasculitis [1–3]. This classification guides the aetiological investigations (Table 102.1). However, the same specimen may show a mixed aspect with lobular and septal infiltrate, and variable histological features.

Epidemiology and pathogenesis. Panniculitis can be a primary disease but is most often a secondary process related to different underlying disorders. Some types of panniculitis are specific to children, including those only seen in neonates, such as subcutaneous fat necrosis (SCFN) of the newborn (Figs 102.1 and 102.2), or occur in a particular context such as poststeroid panniculitis and cold panniculitis. All the other recognized aetiologies described in adults may be observed in children but are less frequent or rare in the paediatric population, such as infections, connective tissue disease, subcutaneous lymphoma-like, metabolic and drug- and trauma-induced panniculitis [4]. In many paediatric patients no classical specific aetiology can be identified and the interim term of 'idiopathic panniculitis' has been used. However, currently there is improved characterization of the large group of autoinflammatory diseases and primary immune deficiencies, and paediatric panniculitis has been reported as one of the first presenting symptoms in some of these

Harper's Textbook of Pediatric Dermatology, Fourth Edition. Edited by Peter Hoeger, Veronica Kinsler and Albert Yan.

Table 102.1 Classification of panniculitis

Predominantly septal panniculitis without vasculitis[a]
Erythema nodosum
Predominantly septal panniculitis with vasculitis
Cutaneous polyarteritis nodosa
Superficial thrombophlebitis
Predominantly lobular panniculitis without vasculitis
Cold panniculitis
Post-steroid panniculitis
Subcutaneous fat necrosis of the newborn
Sclerema neonatorum
Panniculitis associated with connective tissue diseases
Lupus panniculitis (lupus erythematosus profundus)
Panniculitis in dermatomyositis
Lipodystrophy and lipoatrophy[a]
Pancreatic panniculitis
α_1-Antitrypsin deficiency panniculitis
Calciphylaxis
Infective panniculitis
Factitial, iatrogenic or traumatic panniculitis
Sclerosing panniculitis (lipodermatosclerosis)[b]
Cytophagic histiocytic panniculitis
Subcutaneous panniculitis-like T-cell lymphoma
Predominantly lobular panniculitis with vasculitis
Erythema induratum of Bazin (nodular vasculitis)
Erythema nodosum leprosum[c]

[a] Lipodystrophy and lipoatrophy are discussed in Chapter 103.
[b] Sclerosing panniculitis occurs primarily in middle-aged or elderly patients with chronic venous insufficiency of the lower extremities [3].
[c] Erythema nodosum leprosum is immune complex-mediated cutaneous small vessel vasculitis that is a type II reaction seen in leprosy patients usually undergoing treatment. Although exceedingly rare, erythema nodosum leprosum does occur in children and may precede the diagnosis of leprosy [8].
Source: Modified from Requena and Yus (2001) [1].

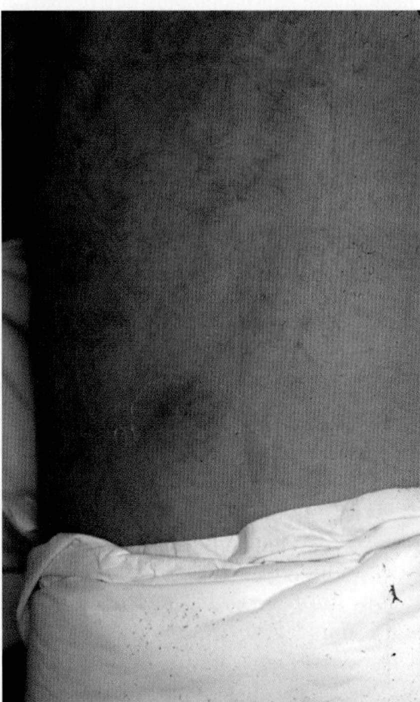

Fig. 102.1 An Inflammatory nodule on the back of a neonate, related to a subcutaneous fat necrosis of the newborn (SCFN). Source: Photo courtesy of Dermatology Department, Hôpital Necker – Enfants Malades, Paris, France.

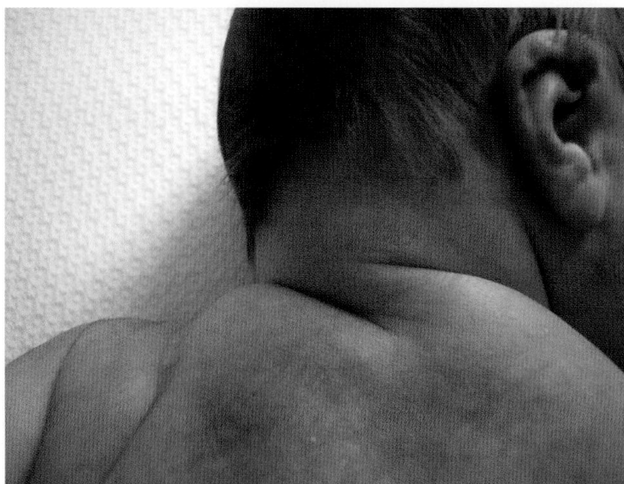

Fig. 102.2 Large inflammatory, infiltrated back in a newborn on the neck and the back related to SCFN. Source: Photo courtesy of Dermatology Department, Hôpital Necker – Enfants Malades, Paris, France.

Table 102.2 Main aetiologies of paediatric panniculitis according to the age of onset

Neonates
Subcutaneous fat necrosis of newborns
Sclerema neonatorum
Infants
Cold panniculitis
Post-steroid panniculitis
Autoinflammatory diseases
Primary immune deficiencies
Children and adolescents
Erythema nodosum
Panniculitis with connective disease
Lupus panniculitis, dermatomyositis
Cytophagic histiocytic panniculitis
Subcutaneous panniculitis-like T-cell lymphoma
Lipodystrophy and lipoatrophy[a]
Pancreatic panniculitis
α_1-Antitrypsin deficiency panniculitis
Calciphylaxis
Infective panniculitis
Factitial, iatrogenic or traumatic
Sclerosing panniculitis

[a] Lipodystrophy and lipoatrophy are discussed in Chapter 103.

diseases. These clinical cases remain exceptional. However, because the clinical manifestations of such monogenic disorders usually occur early in life it is necessary to consider the possibility of such aetiologies when we are confronted by unexplained panniculitis in young children.

The main aetiologies of paediatric panniculitis, according to the age of onset of the cutaneous lesions, are summarized in Table 102.2.

Clinical features and differential diagnosis. The clinical diagnosis of paediatric panniculitis can be a challenge because of the spectrum of presenting signs. Nodules are the most frequent, classical clinical manifestation. Plaques of thickened skin can also be seen, usually but not always with discolouration of the overlying skin. The lesions can be painful, and occur mostly on the legs, thighs, buttocks and cheeks where fat tissue is more prominent. Their size is variable from 1 to 5 cm. The lesions can resolve spontaneously but they can relapse. Necrosis is possible during evolution and lipoatrophy is frequent after healing. A skin biopsy of adequate depth is required for accurate diagnosis and can be helpful for the aetiological diagnosis (Table 102.1). Although most forms of panniculitis have the same clinical and histological appearance, in some cases the clinical characteristics, the evolution and the accompanying signs depend on the aetiology. For example, panniculitis without systemic manifestations can be the result of trauma or cold, whereas panniculitis with systemic manifestations is usually associated with an underlying systemic disease, mostly autoinflammatory diseases in infants and children and connectivitis or lymphoproliferation in children and adolescents.

In this chapter, we will detail only the more specific or unusual aetiologies observed in the paediatric population, excluding some, such as lipodystrophy and lipoatrophy, that are covered in other chapters. When panniculitis appears as the secondary process the characteristics of the underlying pathologies are also discussed in other corresponding chapters (e.g. dermatomyositis and systemic lupus erythematosus).

References

1 **Requena L, Yus ES. Panniculitis. Part I. Mostly septal panniculitis. J Am Acad Dermatol 2001;45:163–83.**
2 Diaz Cascajo C, Borghi S, Weyers W. Panniculitis: definition of terms and diagnostic strategy. Am J Dermatopathol 2000;22:530–49.
3 **Requena L, Sanchez Yus E. Panniculitis. Part II. Mostly lobular panniculitis. J Am Acad Dermatol 2001;45:325–61.**
4 Torrelo A, Hernandez A. Panniculitis in children. Dermatol Clin 2008; 26:491.

Subcutaneous fat necrosis of the newborn

Epidemiology and pathogenesis. SCFN is a rare condition, characterized by erythematous or skin-coloured nodules (Fig. 102.1) or plaques occurring in the neonatal period on the back, buttocks and limbs, or as large hardened areas (Fig. 102.2) [1–3]. It occurs usually in full-term or post-term infants, often associated with perinatal risk factors including hypoxaemia, gestational diabetes, maternal toxaemia and drug exposure (such as calcium channel-blockers or cocaine) [2–4]. The pathogenesis is not completely understood. One hypothesis is that it may be related to a deficiency of brown fat or to an underlying defect in fat composition coupled with a stressful event. With hypothermia this neonatal subcutaneous fat may undergo crystallization, with adipocyte damage leading to a granulomatous reaction.

Clinical features and differential diagnosis. Multiple indurated, nonpitting, painful, subcutaneous plaques or nodules are observed with a predilection for areas of the body with the most fat tissue. The overlying skin may be normal, or erythematous to hyperpigmented (Fig. 102.3). Associated signs depend on the circumstances surrounding the onset [5]. Usually the cutaneous lesions resolve spontaneously in several weeks but can persist for up to 6 months. Residual subcutaneous atrophy is frequent [2]. The lesions may become calcified or fluctuant with liquefied fat in their evolution, and in the case of large plaques or diffuse skin involvement moderate fever can be observed. Metabolic complications can occur and should be looked for. Hypercalcaemia is the most frequent metabolic complication and can be observed even after the resolution of the skin lesions [6,7]. This can lead to dystrophic calcification, and rarely to seizures, renal failure or cardiac arrest. It may be also asymptomatic, highlighting the importance of screening all infants with SCFN for hypercalcaemia. Severe hypercalcaemia is usually observed during the first six weeks of life.

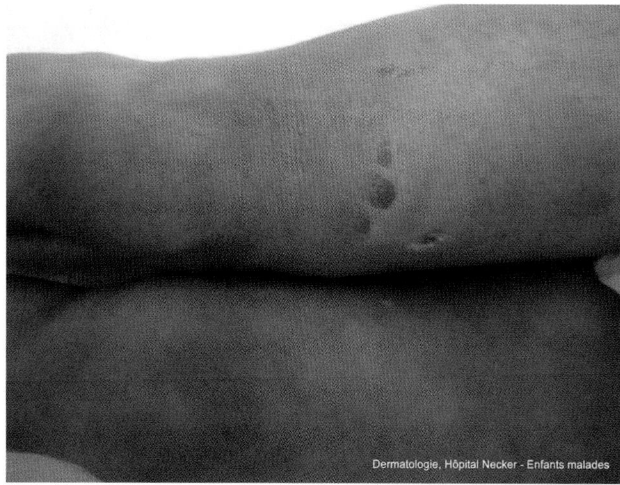

Fig. 102.3 Plaques of thickened skin, on the legs with skin discoloration, superficial necrosis and some areas of lipoatrophy. Source: Photo courtesy of Dermatology Department, Hôpital Necker – Enfants Malades, Paris, France.

It is suggested that hypercalcaemia is caused by increased renal production of 1,25-dihydroxyvitamin D_3 by macrophages, calcium release from resolving subcutaneous lesions, or bone resorption stimulated by elevated parathyroid hormone and prostaglandin E_2 [7,8]. Other rare but described metabolic associations are hypoglycaemia and thrombocytopenia, which precede the onset of skin lesions and may be related to underlying factors. Hypertriglyceridaemia is very unusual and could be related to the release of fatty acids from necrotic adipocytes [8]. The diagnosis is based on the clinical history, and if in doubt a skin biopsy is required.

Histology. Biopsy of an early lesion is characteristic, showing a dense inflammatory lobular infiltrate composed of lymphocytes, histiocytes and possible eosinophils, and multinucleated giant cells with necrosis of the fat. Radially arranged needle-shaped clefts, representing crystallized fatty acids dissolved during processing, are found within adipocytes and giant cells [9]. Fine-needle aspiration can also be useful, showing typical cells [10].

Treatment and prevention. The subcutaneous lesions resolve spontaneously. The most important part of management is to monitor and treat potential metabolic complications. Because hypercalcaemia can be a late complication, parents should be instructed to look for clinical signs of hypercalcaemia, and serum calcium levels should be checked at regular intervals. Prevention of hypercalcaemia includes adequate hydration and restriction of calcium and vitamin D_3 intake. Loop diuretics such as frusemide may be used with caution so as not to cause dehydration, which will exacerbate hypercalcaemia. Glucocorticoids, bisphosphonates, calcitonin or citrate may be required to treat resistant cases of hypercalcaemia associated with SCFN [11].

References

1 Burden AD, Krafchik BR. Subcutaneous fat necrosis of the newborn: a review of 11 cases. Pediatr Dermatol 1999;16:384–7.
2 Mahe E, Girszyn N, Hadj-Rabia S et al. Subcutaneous fat necrosis of the newborn: a systematic evaluation of risk factors, clinical manifestations, complications and outcome of 16 children. Br J Dermatol 2007;156:709–15.
3 Torrelo A, Hernandez A. Panniculitis in children. Dermatol Clin 2008;26:491–500, vii.
4 Del Pozzo-Magaña BR, Ho N. Subcutaneous fat necrosis of the newborn: a 20-year retrospective study. Pediatr Dermatol 2016;33:e353–e355.
5 Oza V, Treat J, Cook N et al. Subcutaneous fat necrosis as a complication of whole-body cooling for birth asphyxia. Arch Dermatol 2010;146:882–5.
6 Borgia F, De Pasquale L, Cacace C et al. Subcutaneous fat necrosis of the newborn: be aware of hypercalcaemia. J Paediatr Child Health 2006;42:316–18.
7 Shumer DE, Thaker V, Taylor GA, Wassner AJ. Severe hypercalcaemia due to subcutaneous fat necrosis: presentation, management and complications. Arch Dis Child Fetal Neonatal Ed 2014;99:F419–21.
8 Tran JT, Sheth AP. Complications of subcutaneous fat necrosis of the newborn: a case report and review of the literature. Pediatr Dermatol 2003;20:257–61.
9 Friedman SJ, Winkelmann RK. Subcutaneous fat necrosis of the newborn: light, ultrastructural and histochemical microscopic studies. J Cutan Pathol 1989;16:99–105.
10 Gupta RK, Naran S, Selby RE. Fine needle aspiration cytodiagnosis of subcutaneous fat necrosis of newborn. A case report. Acta Cytol 1995;39:759–61.
11 Rice AM, Rivkees SA. Etidronate therapy for hypercalcemia in subcutaneous fat necrosis of the newborn. J Pediatr 1999;134:349–51.

Sclerema neonatorum

Sclerema neonatorum is a very rare and life-threatening condition, with diffuse hardening of the skin, that generally affects ill, preterm neonates in the first few days of life.

Epidemiology and aetiology. It is observed in low-weight premature newborns with a wide variety of severe illnesses [1–3]. Pathogenesis remains unclear. The higher concentration of saturated fatty acids in neonatal fat is, once more, believed to play a key role. Alternative hypotheses of decreased ability to mobilize fatty acids from adipose tissue, or of thickening resulting from oedema affecting the connective tissue septa, have also been proposed.

Clinical features. The cutaneous involvement occurs during the first week of life in premature and small-for-dates babies with severe underlying illness, particularly severe infections, congenital heart disease and other major developmental defects. It presents clinically with woody induration of the skin of the buttocks, thighs or calves, and extends rapidly and symmetrically to involve almost the whole surface except palms, soles and genitalia [1,2,4]. Prognosis is poor with up to 75% mortality. Respiratory function becomes severely restricted caused by the skin hardening, with fatal consequences. Because of the clinical and histopathological overlap with SCFN of the newborn, some authors consider that they represent the same disease but with a spectrum of severity, sclerema neonatorum being the most severe [5]. Others consider that they are distinct entities with specific clinical features and prognosis. There have been reports of sclerema neonatorum and SCFN of the newborn occurring in the same patient [5].

Histology. The histopathology of sclerema neonatorum shows a sparse (if any) inflammatory infiltrate without fat necrosis. The characteristic feature is needle-shaped clefts radially arranged within adipocytes. Identical needle-shaped clefts have been found in visceral fat in autopsy studies [4].

Treatment. Treatment of any underlying or associated illness is critical for neonates with sclerema neonatorum, although the diagnosis carries a poor prognosis [6]. Exchange transfusion may reduce mortality [7,8]. In a few cases, treatment with IVIG led to marked but short-term clinical improvement [9].

References

1 Zeb A, Darmstadt GL. Sclerema neonatorum: a review of nomenclature, clinical presentation, histological features, differential diagnoses and management. J Perinatol 2008;28:453–60.
2 Torrelo A, Hernandez A. Panniculitis in children. Dermatol Clin 2008; 26:491–500, vii.
3 Battin M, Harding J, Gunn A. Sclerema neonatorum following hypothermia. J Paediatr Child Health 2002;38:533–4.
4 Requena L, Sanchez Yus E. Panniculitis. Part II. Mostly lobular panniculitis. J Am Acad Dermatol 2001;45:325–61.
5 Jardine D, Atherton DJ, Trompeter RS. Sclerema neonatorum and subcutaneous fat necrosis of the newborn in the same infant. Eur J Pediatr 1990;150:125–6.
6 Kwon EJ, Emanuel PO, Gribetz CH et al. Poststeroid panniculitis. J Cutan Pathol 2007;34(Suppl. 1):64–7.
7 Sadana S, Mathur NB, Thakur A. Exchange transfusion in septic neonates with sclerema: effect on immunoglobulin and complement levels. Indian Pediatr 1997;34:20–5.
8 Vain NE, Mazlumian JR, Swarner OW, Cha CC. Role of exchange transfusion in the treatment of severe septicemia. Pediatrics 1980;66:693–7.
9 Buster KJ, Burford HN, Stewart FA et al. Sclerema neonatorum treated with intravenous immunoglobulin: a case report and review of treatments. Cutis 2013;92:83–7.

Poststeroid panniculitis

Poststeroid panniculitis is a complication of systemic corticosteroid therapy, which develops within days or weeks following rapid tapering or cessation of the drug. Only a few cases have been reported in the literature, the majority in children.

Epidemiology and pathogenesis. Poststeroid panniculitis is a rare condition, observed mostly in children. One hypothesis is that the withdrawal of systemic corticosteroids leads to abnormal lipid metabolism, resulting in the elevation of the saturated to unsaturated fatty acid ratio, resulting in crystal formation.

Clinical features. The lesions consist of erythematous subcutaneous nodules and plaques that appear 1–10 days after stopping high doses of systemic corticosteroids [1–3]. The lesions develop mostly in those areas in which steroids induce the greatest accumulation of fat: mostly on the cheeks, posterior neck and upper trunk. However, nodules can also occur on arms, forearms, thighs and leg [2–4]. The lesions are usually painless with sometimes moderate pruritus. They resolve slowly over weeks to months without residual scarring unless, rarely, ulceration occurs. The diagnosis is based on the clinical history but a skin biopsy may be necessary to eliminate other causes of subcutaneous nodules, particularly in the context of an underlying systemic disease treated by steroids.

Histology findings. Poststeroid panniculitis presents as lobular panniculitis with a mixed inflammatory infiltrate without vasculitis. Needle-shaped crystals within adipocytes are present and foreign body giant cells may surround the clefts [4,5]. This aspect is similar to that observed in the skin biopsy of SCFN in neonates and sclerema neonatorum.

Treatment. Whereas some authors have suggested reinstitution of systemic corticosteroids with a more gradual taper, others have suggested that no treatment is necessary.

References

1 Torrelo A, Hernandez A. Panniculitis in children. Dermatol Clin 2008;26:491–500, vii.
2 Reichel M, Diaz Cascajo C. Bilateral jawline nodules in a child with a brain-stem glioma. Poststeroid panniculitis. Arch Dermatol 1995;131:1448–9, 1451–2.
3 Silverman RA, Newman AJ, LeVine MJ, Kaplan B. Poststeroid panniculitis: a case report. Pediatr Dermatol 1988;5:92–3.
4 Kwon EJ, Emanuel PO, Gribetz CH et al. Poststeroid panniculitis. J Cutan Pathol 2007;34(Suppl. 1):64–7.
5 Requena L, Sanchez Yus E. Panniculitis. Part II. Mostly lobular panniculitis. J Am Acad Dermatol 2001;45:325–61.

Cold panniculitis

Epidemiology and pathogenesis. Cold panniculitis is an acute, nodular, erythematous eruption usually limited to areas exposed to the cold [1,2]. It is more frequent in infants and children than in adults. It is related to the crystallization of subcutaneous fat with subsequent inflammation in response to cold injury. It is thought to be caused by the higher concentration of saturated fat in an infant than in adults.

Clinical features and differential diagnosis. Inflammatory nodules or plaques occur in an infant or young child around 48 hours after a prolonged cold injury to cheeks, limbs and chest. The classical circumstances are prolonged environmental cold, therapeutic application of cold (e.g. during cardiac surgery), or other cold exposure (e.g. from an ice lolly) [1,3–5]. Similar lesions have been described in prepubertal boys after swimming in cold water (scrotal cold panniculitis) [6], or on the upper-lateral thighs of women who ride horses ('equestrian panniculitis') [7]. The clinical history in an otherwise well child is the best argument for the aetiological history.

Histology findings. A skin biopsy is usually not necessary for the diagnosis. It reveals a predominantly lobular infiltrate of lymphocytes and histiocytes [8]. There may be overlying dermal oedema, with a superficial and deep perivascular lymphocytic infiltrate resembling perniosis.

Treatment and prevention. The lesions resolve spontaneously in a few days to weeks, without scarring, and may leave postinflammatory hyperpigmentation. The best treatment is preventive against further episodes.

References

1 Baruchin AM, Scharf S. Cold panniculitis in children (Haxthausen's disease). Burns Incl Therm Inj 1988;14:51–2.
2 Epstein EH Jr, Oren ME. Popsicle panniculitis. N Engl J Med 1970; 282:966–7.
3 Craig JE, Scholz TA, Vanderhooft SL, Etheridge SP. Fat necrosis after ice application for supraventricular tachycardia termination. J Pediatr 1998;133:727.
4 Ter Poorten JC, Hebert AA, Ilkiw R. Cold panniculitis in a neonate. J Am Acad Dermatol 1995;33:383–5.
5 Quesada-Cortes A, Campos-Munoz L, Diaz-Diaz RM, Casado-Jimenez M. Cold panniculitis. Dermatol Clin 2008;26:485–9, vii.
6 Versini P, Varlet F, Blanc P et al. [Scrotal panniculitis due to cold: a pseudo-tumoral lesion in the prepubertal child. Report of a case]. Ann Pathol 1996;16:282–4.
7 Beacham BE, Cooper PH, Buchanan CS, Weary PE. Equestrian cold panniculitis in women. Arch Dermatol 1980;116:1025–7.
8 Requena L, Sanchez Yus E. Panniculitis. Part II. Mostly lobular panniculitis. J Am Acad Dermatol 2001;45:325–61.

Panniculits and monogenic autoinflammatory diseases and primary immune deficiency

Adipose tissue appears to be an active participant in the immunity and inflammation process, and macrophages and adipocytes are known to be two essential cells of adipose tissue. Until now, panniculitis has been described as an expression of a spectrum of monogenic autoinflammatory diseases in five diseases [1–5]. Aseptic panniculitis was also recently reported in association with primary inherited immunodeficiency [6,7]. Currently, the clinical spectrum of a new group of diseases overlapping between autoinflammation and immunodeficiency is under consideration and is expanding. The first clinical manifestations of these monogenic disorders occur usually early in life, before the age of 2–3 years. Therefore, it is important to consider systematically the possibility of such a group of aetiologies, with underlying autoinflammatory disorders, underlying primary immune deficiency or underlying intricate autoinflammatory and primary immune deficiency disorders, in infants with unexplained, usually recurrent, aseptic panniculitis (Table 102.3).

Table 102.3 Potential work-up for infants (under 2 years) with unexplained panniculitis

Clinical evaluation	Familial history History (age of onset, accompanying signs, infectious episodes, fever and its characteristics) Vaccination (family tree) Physical examination (with curves of growth)
Laboratory investigation (at least)	Blood cell counts Inflammatory markers (C-reactive protein concentrations, erythrocyte sedimentation rate), Autoantibodies (ANA) Serum immunoglobulin (Ig) levels Phenotype of B and T lymphocytes
Other more specific tests/ investigations according to presentation	
Highly specialized multidisciplinary approach	

Panniculitis and monogenic autoinflammatory diseases

Epidemiology and pathogenesis. Autoinflammatory diseases are rare. In the last 15 years the focus has been on the central role of interleukin (IL)-1 in driving autoinflammatory phenotypes. Recent discoveries highlighted other key inflammatory mediators and pathways, with notably the discovery of interferon (IFN) deregulation causing the autoinflammatory phenotype. Many of these discoveries highlight the intricate interconnections between autoinflammation, autoimmunity, immunodeficiency and lymphoproliferation. Panniculitis has been described as an expression of a spectrum of monogenic autoinflammatory diseases in five diseases: (i) tumour necrosis factor receptor associated periodic syndrome (TRAPS) [1], (ii) chronic atypical neutrophilic dermatosis with lipodystrophy and elevated temperature (CANDLE) [2], (iii) familial Mediterranean fever (FMF) [3] (neutrophilic panniculitis), (iv) otupulinemia (neutrophilic panniculitis or predominantly septal panniculitis with vasculitis of small and medium-sized blood vessels) [4], and (v) infantile-onset granulomatous panniculitis (with an underlying molecular defect not yet defined) [5].

Clinical features. In these diseases the whole clinical picture needs to be taken into consideration, because signs other than panniculitis are variable between diseases. The diagnosis of an autoinflammatory disease may be suspected when cutaneous lesions are associated with either: periodic or chronic systemic inflammation, or a frequent unexplained fever, without evidence of high-titer autoantibodies or autoantigen-specific T cells. Cutaneous lesions can be present at the onset of the disease with relapsing nodules coinciding with febrile attacks (Fig. 102.4). The semiology of panniculitis lesions is not specific. The aetiological diagnosis is based on the global clinical context and molecular investigations. The characteristics of autoinflammatory diseases are covered in another chapter (Chapter 155). The possibility of an underlying primary immune deficiency also has to be considered according to the clinical history of the infant with investigations in a specialized laboratory for paediatric immune deficiencies.

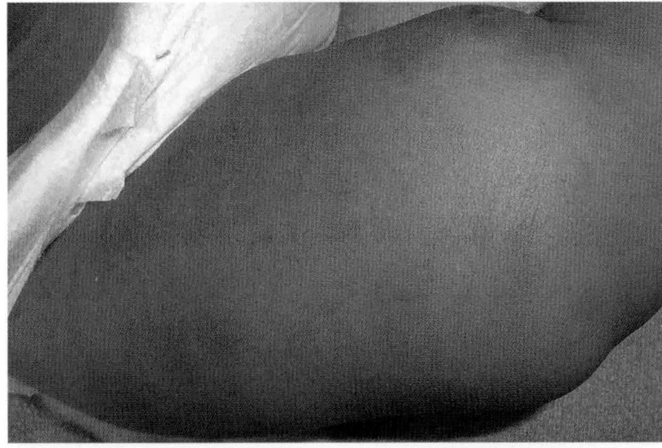

(a)

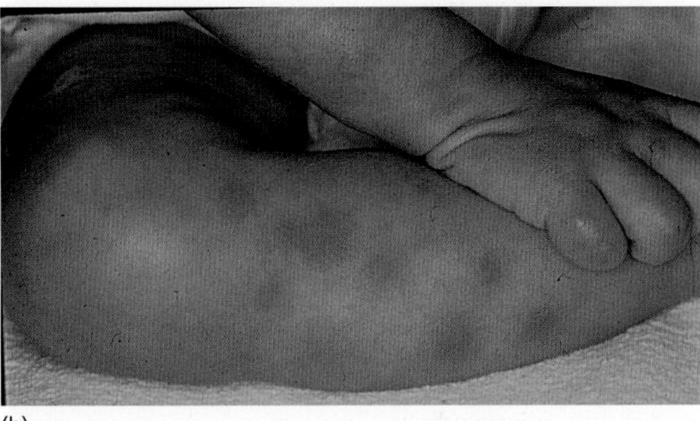

(b)

Fig. 102.4 Several inflammatory (a) subtle or (b) marked nodules on the legs in children with autoinflammatory disorders. Source: Photo courtesy of Dermatology Department, Hôpital Necker – Enfants Malades, Paris, France.

Histology. The histological findings are not specific to the aetiology. Panniculitis is mostly lobular, but not always and the predominant infiltrate is mostly composed of neutrophils (FMF, CANDLE syndrome), lymphocytes (TRAPS), or histiocytes (infantile-onset granulomatous panniculitis). The histological findings have to be interpreted in the light of the clinical characteristics of each patient.

Treatment. Treatment depend on the underlying aetiology. Anti-IL-1 and anti-tumour necrosis factor (TNF) medications should be considered in each situation.

Panniculitis and primary immune deficiency

Aseptic panniculitis was reported in association with inherited immunodeficiency related to mutations in haematopoietic transcription factor GATA2 and in *CECR1* (recently renamed *ADA2*). GATA2 underlies monocytopaenia, mycobacterial infections and a broad spectrum of other manifestations [6]. Mutations in *CECR1* result in adenosine deaminase-2 deficiency (DADA2) and are associated with a spectrum of vascular and inflammatory phenotypes, ranging from early onset recurrent stroke to systemic vasculopathy or vasculitis, associated with hypogammaglobulinaemia in some patients [7].

References

1 Lamprecht P, Moosig F, Adam-Klages S et al. Small vessel vasculitis and relapsing panniculitis in tumour necrosis factor receptor associated periodic syndrome (TRAPS). Ann Rheum Dis 2004;63:1518–20.
2 Liu Y, Ramot Y, Torrelo A et al. Mutations in proteasome subunit β type 8 cause chronic atypical neutrophilic dermatosis with lipodystrophy and elevated temperature with evidence of genetic and phenotypic heterogeneity. Arthritis Rheum 2012;64:895–907.
3 Leiva-Salinas M, Betlloch I, Arribas MP, Francés L, Pascual JC. Neutrophilic lobular panniculitis as an expression of a widened spectrum of familial mediterranean fever. JAMA Dermatol 2014;150:213–4.
4 Zhou Q, Yu X, Demirkaya E, Deuitch N et al. Biallelic hypomorphic mutations in a linear deubiquitinase define otulipenia, an early-onset autoinflammatory disease. Proc Natl Acad Sci U S A 2016;113;10127–32.
5 Wouters CH, Martin TM, Stichweh D et al.Infantile onset panniculitis with uveitis and systemic granulomatosis: a new clinicopathologic entity. J Pediatr 2007;151:707–9.
6 Spinner MA, Sanchez LA, Hsu AP et al. GATA2 deficiency: a protean disorder of hematopoiesis, lymphatics, and immunity. Blood 2014;123:809–21.
7 Zhou Q, Yang D, Ombrello AK et al. Early-onset stroke and vasculopathy associated with mutations in ADA2. N Engl J Med 2014;370:911–20.

Erythema nodosum

Erythema nodosum (EN) is the most common type of panniculitis, observed usually during the third decade of life although it can occur at any age. Histopathologically, EN is the prototypical septal panniculitis without true vasculitis.

Epidemiology and pathogenesis. Overall, EN occurs in approximately one to five per 100 000 persons. In adults, it is more common among women, with a male-to-female ratio of 1:6. In children, the sex ratio is 1:1 [1–9]. EN appears as a nonspecific cutaneous reaction pattern to a variety of antigens. Most direct and indirect evidence supports the involvement of a type IV delayed hypersensitivity response to numerous antigens. There have been many reported causes of EN (Table 102.4) but no specific cause can be identified in up to one-third of cases of childhood EN [4–23], Streptococcal infections are the most common identifiable aetiology, especially in children [4–8]. Noninfectious aetiologies including sarcoidosis, inflammatory bowel disease and drugs are rare in children, but should still be considered. Malignancy has been rarely associated with EN, both in children and adults.

Table 102.4 Potential causes of erythema nodosum in childhood [4–23]

Idiopathic	
Infectious	β-Haemolytic streptococcus, usually pharyngitis
	Nonstreptococcal respiratory infections
	Yersinia, *Salmonella* or *Campylobacter* gastroenteritis
	Pneumonia (*Mycoplasma* or *Chlamydia*)
	Cat-scratch disease
	Tuberculosis or other mycobacterium[a]
	Tularemia
	Leptospirosis
	Epstein–Barr virus
	Parvovirus
	Dermatophytosis (e.g. kerion)
	Histoplasmosis, coccidiomycosis or blastomycosis
Inflammatory diseases	Crohn disease
	Ulcerative colitis
	Sarcoidosis
	Behçet disease[b]
	Ankylosing spondylitis
	Acne fulminans
Drugs/immunizations	Oral contraceptive pills[c]
	Antibiotics (e.g. penicillins, sulphonamides)[c]
	Amfepramone (anorexigenic)
	BCG vaccination
Malignancy	Leukaemia
	Hodgkin lymphoma
	Langerhans cell histiocytosis

[a] Erythema nodosum leprosum is a different disease that is a form of cutaneous small vessel vasculitis and is a type II reaction seen in leprosy patients undergoing treatment.
[b] The histopathology of erythema nodosum-like lesions associated with Behçet disease may be distinct from the findings in classic erythema nodosum [25].
[c] Reported primarily in adults [2,11,21,22].

Clinical features and differential diagnosis. The main clinical features of EN are the sudden onset of painful, erythematous nodules, from 1 to 10 cm in diameter, with a symmetric location. Pretibial involvement is most common, although the extensor surfaces of the forearm, the thighs and the trunk also may be affected. The nodules are initially firm, and usually become more fluctuant during evolution, without leading to ulceration. Individual nodules resolve spontaneously within two to six weeks with a bruise-like appearance. New lesions may continue to arise for up to six weeks, and complete healing is usually observed within two months without atrophy or scarring. Recurrences are possible but they are usually observed in patients with an underlying chronic condition such as sarcoidosis or Crohn disease, and so they are less frequent in children. Associated symptoms such as fever, malaise, arthralgia, headache, upper respiratory symptoms, abdominal pain, vomiting or diarrhoea are possible, sometimes preceding the subcutaneous nodules. They are variable, rare in children and depend on the underlying pathology. A skin biopsy is usually not necessary, but it should be undertaken in patients with an atypical presentation or an abnormal disease course (Table 102.5).

Behçet disease can present with EN-like lesions, but the diagnosis should be made based on associated symptoms that meet the criteria for diagnosis of Behçet disease. Erysipelas-like lesions on the lower legs may be mistaken for EN, but the episodic nature, associated symptoms that characterize familial Mediterranean fever, family history and histopathology are distinctive.

Laboratory and histological findings. Laboratory findings depend on the aetiology. The hallmark histopathological feature of EN is a septal panniculitis without vasculitis. There is inflammation and thickening of the

SECTION 22: DISORDERS OF FAT TISSUE

Table 102.5 Potential work-up for children with erythema nodosum of unknown aetiology

Initial evaluation	History and physical examination Skin biopsy if needed to confirm diagnosis Complete blood count with differential Erythrocyte sedimentation rate C-reactive protein Liver function tests Throat culture +/– rapid streptococcal antigen test Antistreptolysin O titer Tuberculin skin test[a] Chest X-ray
Additional studies to consider as indicated	Serologies for prevalent or endemic bacterial, viral, fungal or protozoal infections Stool culture for *Yersinia*, *Salmonella* or *Campylobacter* Inflammatory bowel disease panel (ASCA IgA, ASCA IgG, anti-OmpC, anti-CBlr1, IBD-specific pANCA) Serum immunoglobulins

[a] Patients with erythema nodosum and a positive tuberculin skin test do not always have evidence of active underlying tuberculosis [23].

fibrous septa of the subcutaneous fat. The inflammatory infiltrate varies with the stage of the lesion, ranging from neutrophils in early lesions to lymphoctyes, giant cells and granulation tissue in late-stage lesions. Miescher radial granulomas are composed of histiocytes distributed in a rosette-like fashion around a central cleft and are considered a classic feature in EN, but can be seen in other conditions such as erythema induratum or necrobiosis lipoidica. Late-stage lesions may have fibrotic septa [24].

Children with Behçet disease can present with EN-like lesions, usually showing lobular or mixed panniculitis with leukocytoclastic or lymphocytic vasculitis, distinct from the findings in classical EN [25,26].

A differential diagnosis of palmoplantar EN in children is palmoplantar eccrine hidradenitis (PEH) mostly observed in the paediatric population. In this condition, painful erythematous plaques or nodules occur suddenly, unilaterally or bilaterally on the palms and/or soles, in an otherwise healthy child [27–29]. The nodules are occasionally accompanied by low-grade fever, and the condition is transient and often recurrent. The histological hallmark of this disease is a deep dermal mixed infiltrate with abundant neutrophils surrounding eccrine sweat glands. Biopsy is rarely necessary because in a child in good general health, PEH is the main clinical diagnosis.

Treatment. When an associated or underlying condition is identified, treatment should be directed at that condition. In mild cases, bed rest may be sufficient to result in spontaneous resolution of the lesions. Nonsteroidal anti-inflammatory drugs are often used to decrease inflammation and pain. Systemic steroids should only be used once an underlying infection has been ruled out. Potassium iodide is used to treat adults with EN and other inflammatory dermatoses, but its use in children is limited by its potential side-effects [30].

References

1 Diaz Cascajo C, Borghi S, Weyers W. Panniculitis: definition of terms and diagnostic strategy. Am J Dermatopathol 2000;22:530–49.

2 **Cribier B, Caille A, Heid E, Grosshans E. Erythema nodosum and associated diseases. A study of 129 cases. Int J Dermatol 1998;37: 667–72.**

3 Tay YK. Erythema nodosum in Singapore. Clin Exp Dermatol 2000;25:377–80.

4 Garty BZ, Poznanski O. Erythema nodosum in Israeli children. Isr Med Assoc J 2000;2:145–6.

5 Hassink RI, Pasquinelli-Egli CE, Jacomella V et al. Conditions currently associated with erythema nodosum in Swiss children. Eur J Pediatr 1997;156:851–3.

6 Kakourou T, Drosatou P, Psychou F et al. Erythema nodosum in children: a prospective study. J Am Acad Dermatol 2001;44;17–21.

7 Labbe L, Perel Y, Maleville J, Taieb A. Erythema nodosum in children: a study of 27 patients. Pediatr Dermatol 1996;13:447–50.

8 Picco P, Gattorno M, Vignola S et al. Clinical and biological characteristics of immunopathological disease-related erythema nodosum in children. Scand J Rheumatol 1999;28:27–32.

9 Doxiadis SA. Aetiology of erythema nodosum in children. Br Med J 1949;2:844.

10 Laurance B, Stone DGH, Philpott MG et al. Aetiology of erythema nodosum in children. A study by a group of paediatricians. Lancet 1961;ii:14–16.

11 Bonci A, Di Lernia V, Merli F, Lo Scocco G. Erythema nodosum and Hodgkin's disease. Clin Exp Dermatol 2001;26:408–11.

12 Kone-Paut I, Yurdakul S, Bahabri SA et al. Clinical features of Behcet's disease in children: an international collaborative study of 86 cases. J Pediatr 1998;132:721–5.

13 Erntell M, Ljunggren K, Gadd T, Persson K. Erythema nodosum – a manifestation of Chlamydia pneumoniae (strain TWAR) infection. Scand J Infect Dis 1989;21:693–6.

14 Ozols, II, Wheat LJ. Erythema nodosum in an epidemic of histoplasmosis in Indianapolis. Arch Dermatol 1981;117:709–12.

15 Martinez-Roig A, Llorens-Terol J, Torres JM. Erythema nodosum and kerion of the scalp. Am J Dis Child 1982;136:440–2.

16 Kellett JK, Beck MH, Chalmers RJ. Erythema nodosum and circulating immune complexes in acne fulminans after treatment with isotretinoin. Br Med J (Clin Res Ed) 1985;290:820.

17 Reizis Z, Trattner A, Hodak E et al. Acne fulminans with hepatosplenomegaly and erythema nodosum migrans. J Am Acad Dermatol 1991;24:886–8.

18 Modgil G, Bridges S. Erythema nodosum associated with Shigella colitis in a 7-year-old boy. Int J Infect Dis 2007;11:556–7.

19 La Spina M, Russo G. Presentation of childhood acute myeloid leukemia with erythema nodosum. J Clin Oncol 2007;25:4011–12.

20 Akdis AC, Kilicturgay K, Helvaci S et al. Immunological evaluation of erythema nodosum in tularaemia. Br J Dermatol 1993;129:275–9.

21 Psychos DN, Voulgari PV, Skopouli FN et al. Erythema nodosum: the underlying conditions. Clin Rheumatol 2000;19:212–16.

22 Salvatore MA, Lynch PJ. Erythema nodosum, estrogens, and pregnancy. Arch Dermatol 1980;116:557–8.

23 Nicol MP, Kampmann B, Lawrence P et al. Enhanced anti-mycobacterial immunity in children with erythema nodosum and a positive tuberculin skin test. J Invest Dermatol 2007;127:2152–7.

24 Requena L, Yus ES. Panniculitis. Part I. Mostly septal panniculitis. J Am Acad Dermatol 2001;45:163–83.

25 Kim B, LeBoit PE. Histopathologic features of erythema nodosum-like lesions in Behcet disease: a comparison with erythema nodosum focusing on the role of vasculitis. Am J Dermatopathol 2000;22: 379–90.

26 Chun SI, Su WP, Lee S, Rogers RS 3rd. Erythema nodosum-like lesions in Behcet's syndrome: a histopathologic study of 30 cases. J Cutan Pathol 1989;16:259–65.

27 Suarez SM, Paller AS. Plantar erythema nodosum: cases in two children. Arch Dermatol 1993;129:1064–5.

28 Hern AE, Shwayder TA. Unilateral plantar erythema nodosum. J Am Acad Dermatol 1992;26:259–60.

29 Ohtake N, Kawamura T, Akiyama C et al. Unilateral plantar erythema nodosum. J Am Acad Dermatol 1994;30:654–5.

30 Sterling JB, Heymann WR. Potassium iodide in dermatology: a 19th century drug for the 21st century – uses, pharmacology, adverse effects, and contraindications. J Am Acad Dermatol 2000; 43:691–7.

Panniculitis associated with connective tissue diseases and vasculitis

Panniculitis has been described in association with various connective tissue diseases [1]. It can be the sole manifestation or occur along with the underlying disease process of connective tissue diseases. The best described forms are lupus panniculitis and lupus erythematosus profundus, panniculitis associated with dermatomyositis, and involvement of the fat tissue during a sclerodermiform process (such as morphoea and systemic scleroderma). Although rare, it can occur in children, mostly (and not exclusively) reported in cases of paediatric lupus panniculitis and juvenile dermatomyositis [2].

Lupus panniculitis (lupus erythematosus profundus)

Lupus panniculitis (LP), also called lupus erythematosus profundus, is an uncommon clinical variant of cutaneous lupus erythematosus. The prevalence of LP associated with systemic lupus erythematosus ranges from 2% to 5%, and this presentation may occur before or after the disease onset, and more frequently in females [3–5]. LP has been reported only rarely in children [6,7] and occurs more frequently in females.

Clinical features. LP usually presents clinically as tender subcutaneous nodules or plaques, which may develop on the shoulders, upper arms, hips and trunk with a lack of involvement of the distal extremities. A predilection for facial involvement has been underlined in paediatric cases [3,7]. A case report has been reported in an infant with neonatal lupus erythematosus [6]. The subcutaneous nodules or plaques resolve with characteristic lipoatrophy. The overlying epidermis may be normal or have features of discoid lupus erythematosus including erythema, poikiloderma, atrophy, scale, follicular plugging or even ulceration. Linear lesions following Blaschko's lines have been described in children [8–10]. Other clinical manifestations have been described associated with LP, such as pericarditis and fever [7].

Laboratory and histology findings. Histopathology shows a predominantly lobular lymphocytic infiltrate in the subcutaneous fat, sometimes with lymphoid follicles, and with or without overlying changes of discoid lupus erythematosus in the dermis and epidermis [4,5]. Direct immunofluorescence will often show a linear deposition of IgM and C3 along the dermoepidermal junction. The laboratory findings are variable with no specific serological findings. It is unclear what proportion of children with LP has abnormal laboratory findings or other features of systemic lupus erythematosus. Although there are no specific serological findings in LP, some studies suggest a high probability of systemic involvement in patients with LP and a positive antinuclear antibody titre [11]. A generalized lupus panniculitis and antiphospholipid syndrome has been described in a child without complement deficiency [12]. Because systemic involvement is possible, careful follow-up is advised.

Treatment. Treatment for LP includes antimalarials, corticosteroids (topical, intralesional or systemic), dapsone, or other immunosuppressants, as well as sun protection. Topical corticosteroids are generally ineffective. Attempted treatments for refractory cases have included thalidomide, and immunosuppressive drugs such as methotrexate, mycophenolate mofetil, cyclosporin and intravenous cyclophosphamide [7,13]. Rituximab was the only therapy to induce skin improvement in a patient, after thalidomide and immunosuppressive drugs, including mycophenolate mofetil, cyclosporin and intravenous cyclophosphamide, in a few patients [7].

Panniculitis in dermatomyositis

Frank panniculitis is rare in both adult and juvenile dermatomyositis, but may be a more common subclinical or incidental histopathological finding.

Clinical features. The onset of panniculitis has been described concurrently or subsequent to the diagnosis of dermatomyositis, ranging from 14 months before to 5 years after the diagnosis of dermatomyositis. Panniculitis in dermatomyositis may be the only cutaneous manifestation [13–16]. The majority of reported cases occur in females. In this condition, panniculitis is often associated with calcification of muscle or subcutaneous tissue. The painful erythematous lesions typically occur on the buttocks, thighs, arms and abdomen, and are usually attributed to a flare of the underlying disease and treated with increased immunosuppression. Interestingly, multiple reports of generalized, partial or focal acquired lipodystrophy have been described in patients with juvenile dermatomyositis [17]. Like other connective tissue panniculitides, the cause is unknown. However, descriptions of a parallel flare and remission of panniculitis and myositis point to a single underlying process [18]. A paediatric case has been reported with the development of panniculitis secondary to *Staphylococcus aureus*. Patients with juvenile dermatomyositis and panniculitis should have extensive testing for infectious aetiologies before increasing their immunosuppressive regimens [19]. Thus far there are no reports of panniculitis in patients with amyopathic dermatomyositis.

Laboratory and histological findings. Histopathology shows a mostly lobular panniculitis with an infiltrate of lymphocytes and plasma cells, often with endothelial swelling of subcutaneous vessels, vasculitis and calcification. Overlying characteristic findings of dermatomyositis, such as vacuolar change at the dermoepidermal junction, are sometimes seen. Some reported cases describe positive antinuclear antibodies, cytopenia, increased mucin deposition and positive direct immunofluorescence in vessels pointing towards overlap with LP [5,15].

Treatment. The panniculitis of dermatomyositis does not appear to resolve spontaneously, and the primary treatments are those for the underlying disease such as systemic corticosteroids and immunosuppressives, after extensive testing to exclude infectious aetiologies.

Other autoimmune disorders

Panniculitis has also been described in association with other autoimmune disorders, such as morphoea (deep morphea) and vasculitis (polyarteritis nodosa). The so-called 'connective tissue panniculitis' are discussed in Chapter 149. Panniculitis associated with juvenile idiopathic arthritis and autoimmune thyroiditis has also been reported in children [20,21].

References

1 Winkelmann RK. Panniculitis in connective tissue disease. Arch Dermatol 1983;119:336–44.
2 Torrelo A, Hernandez A. Panniculitis in children. Dermatol Clin 2008;26:491–500
3 Fraga J, García-Díez A. Lupus erythematosus panniculitis. Dermatol Clin 2008;26:453–63.
4 Massone C, Kodama K, Salmhofer W et al. Lupus erythematosus panniculitis (lupus profundus): clinical, histopathological, and molecular analysis of nine cases. J Cutan Pathol 2005;32:396–404.
5 Requena L, Sánchez Yus E. Panniculitis. Part II. Mostly lobular panniculitis. J Am Acad Dermatol 2001;45:325–61.
6 Nitta Y. Lupus erythematosus profundus associated with neonatal lupus erythematosus. Br J Dermatol 1997;136:112–14.
7 Guissa VR, Trudes G, Jesus AA et al. Lupus erythematosus panniculitis in children and adolescents. Acta Reumatol Port 2012;37:82–5.
8 Heid E. A 17-year old Italian boy with a linear lupus erythematosus profundus. Eur J Dermatol 1998;8:69.
9 Nagai Y, Ishikawa O, Hattori T, Ogawa T. Linear lupus erythematosus profundus on the scalp following the lines of Blaschko. Eur J Dermatol 2003;13:294–6.
10 Tada J, Arata J, Katayama H. Linear lupus erythematosus profundus in a child. J Am Acad Dermatol 1991;24:871–4.
11 Ng PP, Tan SH, Tan T. Lupus erythematosus panniculitis: a clinicopathologic study. Int J Dermatol 2002;41:488–90.
12 Nousari HC, Kimyai-Asadi A, Santana HM et al. Generalized lupus panniculitis and antiphospholipid syndrome in a patient without complement deficiency. Pediatr Dermatol 1999;16:273–6.
13 Hansen CB, Callen JP. Connective tissue panniculitis: lupus panniculitis, dermatomyositis, morphea/scleroderma. Dermatol Ther 2010;23:341–9.
14 Ghali FE, Reed AM, Groben PA, McCauliffe DP. Panniculitis in juvenile dermatomyositis. Pediatr Dermatol 1999;16:270–2.
15 Chao YY, Yang LJ. Dermatomyositis presenting as panniculitis. Int J Dermatol 2000;39:141–4.
16 Neidenbach PJ, Sahn EE, Helton J. Panniculitis in juvenile dermatomyositis. J Am Acad Dermatol 1995;33:305–7.
17 Bingham A, Mamyrova G, Rother KI et al. Predictors of acquired lipodystrophy in juvenile-onset dermatomyositis and a gradient of severity. Medicine (Baltimore) 2008;87:70–86.
18 Solans R, Cortes J, Selva A, et al. Panniculitis: a cutaneous manifestation of dermatomyositis. J Am Acad Dermatol 2002;46:S148–50.
19 Spalding SJ, Meza MP, Ranganathan S, Hirsch R. Staphylococcus aureus panniculitis complicating juvenile dermatomyositis. Pediatrics 2007;119:e528–30.
20 Dyer JA, Guitart J, Klein-Gitelman M, Mancini AJ. Neutrophilic panniculitis in infancy: a cutaneous manifestation of juvenile rheumatoid arthritis. J Am Acad Dermatol 2007;57:S65–8.
21 Mirza B, Muir J, Peake J, Whitehead K. Connective tissue panniculitis in a child with vitiligo and Hashimoto's thyroiditis. Australas J Dermatol 2006;47:49–52.

Cytophagic histiocytic panniculitis

Cytophagic histiocytic panniculitis (CHP) is a rare disease, first described in 1980 by Winkelmann and Bowie, characterized by infiltration of subcutaneous adipose tissue by benign-appearing T lymphocytes and phagocytic histiocytes [1]. CHP may be an isolated skin disease or associated with nonmalignant conditions such as infections, as well as with malignancies, including subcutaneous panniculitis-like T-cell lymphoma, a rare form of lymphoma infiltrating into subcutaneous adipose tissue (Fig. 102.5) [2]. Subcutaneous panniculitis has also been reported in a small number of patients with haemophagocytic lymphohistiocytosis (HLH), a life-threatening condition characterized by uncontrolled activation and proliferation of T cells resulting in proliferation of histiocytes and hemophagocytosis [3,4]. The familial form of HLH (FHL) is a genetically heterogeneous disorder caused by mutations in genes involved in the granule-dependent exocytosis pathway. The spectrum of mutations involved in FHL has expanded since the original report of perforin defect in 1999, with mutations identified in the *UNC13D* (FHL3), *STX11* (FHL4) and *STXBP2* (FHL5) genes [5]. Patients with FHL are unable to cope with common pathogens.

Epidemiology and pathogenesis. CHP is a very rare form of panniculitis. In more than 50% of cases, the disease occurs in immunocompromised patients (those with immunodeficiency, autoimmune disease or haematological disease) and is triggered by an infection (mainly with a virus from the herpes virus family). The release of cytokines by T lymphocytes is thought to play a role in pathogenesis. In HLH, the ever expanding population of cytotoxic lymphocytes produces large quantities of cytokines, such as IFN-γ, which sustain macrophage activation. In addition, TNF-α- and IL-6 are inflammatory cytokines, which induce changes akin to the clinical and laboratory findings that characterize HLH. A study of liver biopsies from patients with

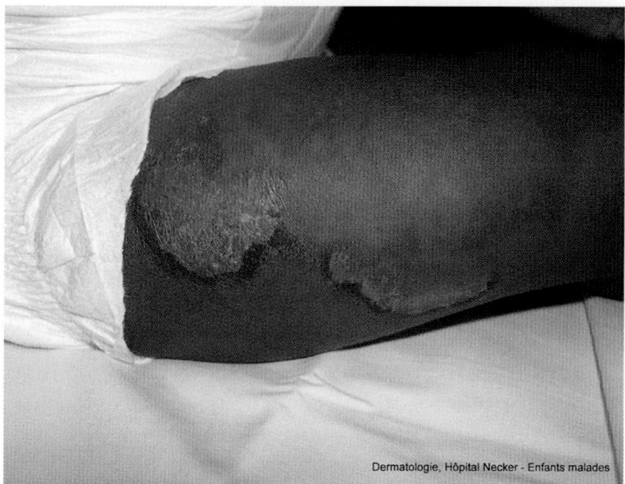

Fig. 102.5 Infiltrated and ulcerative plaques in a child with an exceptional subcutaneous panniculitis-like T-cell lymphoma. Source: Photo courtesy of Dermatology Department, Hôpital Necker – Enfants Malades, Paris, France.

different types of haemophagocytic syndromes has documented the *in situ* involvement of activated, IFN-γ-producing cytotoxic T lymphocytes and of TNF-α- and IL-6 producing macrophages whatever the cause of macrophagic activating syndromes [6].

Clinical features. Subcutaneous erythematous nodules are located predominantly on the trunk and extremities, usually associated with fever. The course of the disease is chronic and recurrent over years. Patients with CHP may follow one of three clinical courses, mainly depending on whether the presentation is isolated or in association with HLH. In the first reviews of paediatric CHP, most cases demonstrated fever, generalized lymphadenopathy, hepatosplenomegaly, pancytopenia, liver enzyme elevation and subcutaneous cytophagic panniculitis. HLH syndrome can be seen in various different disorders including infections, especially Epstein–Barr virus (EBV), connective tissue diseases and lymphomas (notably subcutaneous panniculitis-like T-cell lymphoma) [7–15]. The diseases usually follow a long, chronic, fatal course with terminal hemophagocytic syndrome. In the third group, recurrent episodes of CHP occur, but the patient may survive for years. Other patients respond well to treatment and may have a normal life expectancy.

Histopathology. Histopathology is characterized by an infiltrate of cytologically benign histiocytes and mature T lymphocytes in the lobules of the subcutaneous fat. Cytophagic histiocytes that engulf erythrocytes, lymphocytes, platelets or nuclear debris, giving them a characteristic 'beanbag cell' appearance, are a consistent feature. CHP is usually polyclonal, even when fatal [15–18].

Treatment. Treatment includes systemic corticosteroids, ciclosporin and/or other immunosuppressive agents. The choice depends on the clinical context and has to be discussed carefully for each patient. Chemotherapy and peripheral stem cell transplantation have been used for more aggressive cases [19,20].

References

1 Winkelmann RK, Bowie EJ. Hemorrhagic diathesis associated with benign histiocytic, cytophagic panniculitis and systemic histiocytosis. Arch Intern Med 1980;140:1460–3.

2 Aronson IK, Worobec SM. Cytophagic histiocytic panniculitis and hemophagocytic lymphohistiocytosis: an overview. Dermatol Ther 2010;23:389–402.

3 Gupta S, Weitzman S. Primary and secondary hemophagocytic lymphohistiocytosis: clinical features, pathogenesis and therapy. Expert Rev Clin Immunol 2010;6:137–54.

4 Aricò M, Janka G, Fischer A et al. Hemophagocytic lymphohistiocytosis. Report of 122 children from the International Registry. FHL Study Group of the Histiocyte Society. Leukemia 1996;10:197–203.

5 Cetica V, Pende D, Griffiths GM, Aricò M. Molecular basis of familial hemophagocytic lymphohistiocytosis. Haematologica 2010;95:538–41.

6 Billiau AD, Roskams T, Van Damme-Lombaerts R et al. Macrophage activation syndrome: characteristic findings on liver biopsy illustrating the key role of activated, IFN-gamma-producing lymphocytes and IL- and TNF-alpha-producing macrophages. Blood 2005;105:1648.

7 Garcia-Consuegra J, Barrio MI, Fonseca E et al. Histiocytic cytophagic panniculitis: report of a case in a 12-year-old girl. Eur J Pediatr 1991;150:468–9

8 Schuval SJ, Frances A, Valderrama E et al. Panniculitis and fever in children. J Pediatr 1993;122:372–8.

9 Secmeer G, Sakalli H, Gok F et al. Fatal cytophagic histiocytic panniculitis. Pediatr Dermatol 2004;21:246–9.

10 Pettersson T, Kariniemi AL, Tervonen S, Franssila K. Cytophagic histiocytic panniculitis: a report of four cases. Br J Dermatol 1992; 127:635–40.

11 Pasqualini C, Jorini M, Carloni I et al. Cytophagic histiocytic panniculitis, hemophagocytic lymphohistiocytosis and undetermined autoimmune disorder: reconciling the puzzle. Ital J Pediatr 2014;40:17.

12 Bader-Meunier B, Fraitag S, Janssen C et al. Clonal cytophagic histiocytic panniculitis in children may be cured by cyclosporine A. Pediatrics 2013;132:e545–9.

13 Gallardo F, Pujol RM. Subcutaneous panniculitic-like T-cell lymphoma and other primary cutaneous lymphomas with prominent subcutaneous tissue involvement. Dermatol Clin 2008;26:529–40, viii.

14 Marzano AV, Berti E, Paulli M, Caputo R. Cytophagic histiocytic panniculitis and subcutaneous panniculitis-like T-cell lymphoma: report of 7 cases. Arch Dermatol 2000;136:889–96.

15 Willemze R, Jansen PM, Cerroni L et al. Subcutaneous panniculitis-like T-cell lymphoma: definition, classification, and prognostic factors: an EORTC Cutaneous Lymphoma Group Study of 83 cases. Blood 2008;111:838–45.

16 Yung A, Snow J, Jarrett P. Subcutaneous panniculitic T-cell lymphoma and cytophagic histiocytic panniculitis. Australas J Dermatol 2001;42: 183–7.

17 Gallardo F, Pujol RM. Subcutaneous panniculitic-like T-cell lymphoma and other primary cutaneous lymphomas with prominent subcutaneous tissue involvement. Dermatol Clin 2008;26:529–40, viii.

18 Requena L, Sanchez Yus E. Panniculitis. Part II. Mostly lobular panniculitis. J Am Acad Dermatol 2001;45:325–61

19 Craig AJ, Cualing H, Thomas G et al. Cytophagic histiocytic panniculitis – a syndrome associated with benign and malignant panniculitis: case comparison and review of the literature. J Am Acad Dermatol 1998;39:721–36.

20 Yung A, Snow J, Jarrett P. Subcutaneous panniculitic T-cell lymphoma and cytophagic histiocytic panniculitis. Australas J Dermatol 2001;42:183–7.

Subcutaneous panniculitis-like T-cell lymphoma

Subcutaneous panniculitis-like T-cell lymphoma (SPTCL) was described in 1992 as a new type of cutaneous T-cell lymphoma mimicking panniculitis. In the classification of primary cutaneous lymphomas by WHO/European Research and Treatment of Cancer (EORTC), only SPTCLs expressing an α/β phenotype were referred to as SPTCL [1,2]. The cases with a γ/δ phenotype were included in the group of peripheral T-cell lymphomas, unspecified, referred to as cutaneous γ/δ T-cell lymphomas [3]. SPTCLs differ from other cutaneous lymphoma by the incidence of autoimmune manifestations. The presence of autoantibodies should ask the question of autoimmune disease with T-cell lymphoproliferation rather than the diagnosis of SPTCL.

Epidemiology and pathogenesis. SPTCL mostly affects adults, with 70% of patients presenting between 18 and 60 years of age, and is extremely rare in children [4]. The aetiology and pathogenesis of SPTCL are unknown. In children, three cases were diagnosed after an infectious process [5]. One suggested hypothesis is that SPTCL could be the consequence of a deregulation of T-cell response after auto- or infectious antigen recognition. SPTCL can be associated with CHP. The distinction between these two conditions is a therapeutic challenge because benign CHP often improves with cyclosporine A and prednisone without chemotherapy. Some authors have postulated that EBV may play a role

SECTION 22: DISORDERS OF FAT TISSUE

in the pathogenesis of haemophagocytic syndrome associated with SPTCL.

Clinical features. Few cases have been reported in children [5–9]. Patients present with multiple erythematous subcutaneous nodules or plaques ranging from less than 1 cm to greater than 10 cm in diameter which may ulcerate. Facial lesions and systemic symptoms such as fever and malaise appear to be more common in children. Systemic signs of macrophagic activating syndromes can be observed: fever, hepatosplenomegaly, lymphadenopathy, pancytopaenia, liver dysfunction, disseminated intravascular coagulation, hypofibrinogenaemia, hyperferritinaemia, and hypertriglyceridaemia.

Histopathology. Biopsy reveals a lobular or diffuse infiltrate of pleomorphic, atypical T cells in the subcutaneous fat. Rimming of individual adipocytes with neoplastic lymphocytes with a ring-like appearance is considered a characteristic histopathological feature but may be seen in other lymphomas. Reactive histiocytes with engulfment of nuclear debris or blood cells (cytophagocytosis) may be seen.

Numerous infiltrating small lymphocytes with macrophages are observed. Immunohistochemical staining shows mostly cytotoxic T lymphocytes (T CD8+ cells) with an activated phenotype (human leukocyte antigen-DR+), and expressed IFN-γ and the cytotoxic proteins granzyme B and TIA-1, but are negative for CD56, a marker of natural killer (NK) T cells. Reactive histiocytes with engulfment of nuclear debris or blood cells (cytophagocytosis) may be seen. Clonal rearrangement of T-cell receptor genes in biopsy specimens is often detected by polymerase chain reaction, although this finding should be interpreted with caution because benign conditions can demonstrate clonality, and in addition clonality is not required for a diagnosis of lymphoma. Extensive necrosis may also lead to negative results. Some cases originally diagnosed as LP may indeed have consisted of cases of SPTCL (α/β). Absence of epidermal and dermal involvement, of lymphoid follicles, of B or plasma cells, presence of cellular atypia or monoclonal rearrangement of the T-cell receptor are generally used to distinguished lupus panniculitis and SPTCL. But none of these criteria is specific to one disease and overlapping diseases have already been described.

Treatment. In a recent study reporting the analysis of 27 SPTCL patients (24 adults and three children) it was concluded that immunosuppressive drugs should be considered as first-line therapy for patients with SPTCL, even if some could still benefit from conventional chemotherapy in case of treatment failure [5]. The efficiency of immunosuppressive drugs in this pathology and the frequency of autoimmune biological abnormalities or the occurrence of infections before their onset in children, suggest that SPTCL may be considered rather as a reactive T-cell lymphoproliferation syndrome than as a true T-cell lymphoma, even in adults.

References

1 Gonzalez CL, Medeiros LJ, Braziel RM, Jaffe ES. T-cell lymphoma involving subcutaneous tissue. A clinicopathologic entity commonly associated with hemophagocytic syndrome. Am J Surg Pathol 1991; 15:17–27.
2 Willemze R, Jaffe ES, Burg G et al. WHO-EORTC classification for cutaneous lymphomas. Blood 2005;105:3768–85.
3 Jaffe ES, Ralfkiaer E. Subcutaneous panniculitis-like T-Cell lymphoma. In: Jaffe ES, Harris N, Stein H, Vardiman JW (eds) World Health Organization Classification of Tumours: Pathology and Genetics of Tumours of Haematopoietic and Lymphoid Tissues. Lyon, France: IARC, 2001: 212–13.
4 **Michonneau D, Petrella T, Ortonne N et al. Subcutaneous panniculitis-like T cell lymphoma: immunosuppressive drugs induce better response than polychemotherapy. Acta Derm Venereol 2016:97;358–64.**
5 Bader-Meunier B, Fraitag S, Janssen C et al. Clonal cytophagic histiocytic panniculitis in children may be cured by cyclosporine A. Pediatrics 2013;132:e545–9.
6 Chan YF, Lee KC, Llewellyn H. Subcutaneous T-cell lymphoma presenting as panniculitis in children: report of two cases. Pediatr Pathol 1994;14:595–608.
7 Shani-Adir A, Lucky AW, Prendiville J et al. Subcutaneous panniculitic T-cell lymphoma in children: response to combination therapy with cyclosporine and chemotherapy. J Am Acad Dermatol 2004;50:S18–22.
8 Thomson AB, McKenzie KJ, Jackson R, Wallace WH. Subcutaneous panniculitic T-cell lymphoma in childhood: successful response to chemotherapy. Med Pediatr Oncol 2001;37:549–52.
9 Yim JH, Kim MY, Kim HO et al. Subcutaneous panniculitis-like T-cell lymphoma in a 26-month-old child with a review of the literature. Pediatr Dermatol 2006;23:537–40.

α_1-Antitrypsin deficiency

This is a very rare cause of panniculitis, and extremely rare in children.

Epidemiology and pathogenesis. α_1-Antitrypsin deficiency is classically a disease of adulthood (third decade) and remains very unusual in children [1–3]. α_1-Antitrypsin is the primary serine protease inhibitor that inactivates trypsin, chymotrypsin, neutrophilic elastase, pancreatic elastase, collagenase, factor VII, plasmin, thrombin, kallikrein, urokinase and cathepsin C [4]. The association of panniculitis and α_1-antitrypsin deficiency occurs most commonly in those homozygous for the Z allele of the α_1-antitrypsin gene *SERPINA1*. The pathogenesis of panniculitis is unclear because it is an uncommon and sometimes isolated manifestation of enzyme deficiency [1]. Triggering factors such as trauma may be essential.

Clinical features. Manifestations include emphysema, hepatitis, cirrhosis, vasculitis, urticaria, angioedema and in some cases panniculitis. The age of onset of the skin lesions in children, ranges from 7 to 16 years [4]. A history of a trauma is common and the lesions of panniculitis develop on the traumatized areas. Lesions have a predilection for the lower extremities and buttocks, but may be widespread on the arms, trunk or face. The initial appearance is of an erythematous plaque, often mimicking cellulitis. The lesions evolve into painful ulcerated subcutaneous nodules, with the exudation of an oily substance resulting from necrosis of adipocytes. The lesions usually heal with atrophic scarring. The condition is usually chronic and relapsing.

Histopathology. Early lesions may show neutrophils splaying through collagen of the reticular dermis. The neutrophilic infiltrate is thought to progress to the fibrous septa of the subcutaneous fat and then to the fat lobules [5]. The resulting severe necrosis of adipocytes may be focal with interspersed large areas of adjacent normal fat. Vasculitis is usually only seen in areas of dense neutrophilic inflammation or necrosis.

Treatment. Avoiding trauma is potentially helpful to prevent the onset of new lesions but this remains difficult in children. Dapsone (1–2 mg/kg/day) is often considered first-line treatment. Tetracyclines (doxycycline and minocycline), colchicine, corticosteroids and cyclophosphamide have been reported to be effective in some but not all patients [6,7]. Severe α_1-antitrypsin deficiency can be treated with intravenous infusions of α_1-antitrypsin, plasma exchange or liver transplantation. The role of gene therapy is being studied.

References

1 Loche F, Tremeau-Martinage C, Laplanche G et al. Panniculitis revealing qualitative alpha 1 antitrypsine deficiency (MS variant). Eur J Dermatol 1999;9:565–7.
2 Edmonds BK, Hodge JA, Rietschel RL. Alpha 1-antitrypsin deficiency-associated panniculitis: case report and review of the literature. Pediatr Dermatol 1991;8:296–9.
3 Hendrick SJ, Silverman AK, Solomon AR, Headington JT. Alpha 1-antitrypsin deficiency associated with panniculitis. J Am Acad Dermatol 1988;18:684–92.
4 Valverde R, Rosales B, Ortiz-de Frutos FJ et al. Alpha-1-antitrypsin deficiency panniculitis. Dermatol Clin 2008;26:447–51
5 Requena L, Sanchez Yus E. Panniculitis. Part II. Mostly lobular panniculitis. J Am Acad Dermatol 2001;45:325–61.
6 Smith KC, Pittelkow MR, Su WP. Panniculitis associated with severe alpha 1-antitrypsin deficiency. Treatment and review of the literature. Arch Dermatol 1987;123:1655–61.
7 Ortiz PG, Skov BG, Benfeldt E. Alpha1-antitrypsin deficiency-associated panniculitis: case report and review of treatment options. J Eur Acad Dermatol Venereol 2005;19:487–90.

Pancreatic panniculitis

Pancreatic panniculitis is an uncommon form of panniculitis, rarely reported in children [1,2].

Epidemiology and pathogenesis. This form is associated with acute or chronic pancreatic disease. The development of the skin lesions may be related to an alteration of the permeability of the tissue blood vessels by trypsin, allowing lipase to hydrolyse lipids in the adipocyte, with lipocyte degeneration of the tissue.

Clinical features. Purple–red tender nodules or plaques occur on the extremities, trunk and buttocks and may later become fluctuant and spontaneously ulcerate and drain an oily substance from liquefactive necrosis of adipocytes. Panniculitis may be associated with arthritis, pleural effusion, pericardial effusion, gastrointestinal bleeding, ascites and mesenteric thrombosis [3,4].

Histopathology. Histopathology is distinctive, showing a predominantly lobular panniculitis with coagulative necrosis of adipocytes leading to 'ghost cells' with thick shadowy walls and no nucleus [4,5]. Dystrophic calcification results from saponification of fat by pancreatic enzymes.

Treatment. Treatment of pancreatic panniculitis usually requires diagnosis and treatment of the underlying pancreatic pathology. Supportive measures include rest, elevation of the legs and compression stockings. Nonsteroidal anti-inflammatory drugs may be helpful. One child with panniculitis, pancreatitis and aplastic anaemia responded to treatment with cyclosporine [2].

References

1 Suwattee P, Cham PM, Pope E, Ho N. Pancreatic panniculitis in a 4-year-old child with nephrotic syndrome. Pediatr Dermatol 2007;24: 659–60.
2 Holstein T, Horneff G, Wawer A et al. Panniculitis, pancreatitis and very severe aplastic anemia in childhood: a challenge to treat. Ann Hematol 2000;79:631–4.
3 Dahl PR, Su WP, Cullimore KC, Dicken CH. Pancreatic panniculitis. J Am Acad Dermatol 1995;33:413–17.
4 Garcia-Romero D, Vanaclocha F. Pancreatic panniculitis. Dermatol Clin 2008;26:465–70, vi.
5 Requena L, Sanchez Yus E. Panniculitis. Part II. Mostly lobular panniculitis. J Am Acad Dermatol 2001;45:325–61.

Calciphylaxis

Calciphylaxis is a poorly understood and highly morbid syndrome of vascular calcification and skin necrosis. It is observed in end-stage renal disease. The pathogenesis of calciphylaxis remains obscure and is likely the result of a multiplicity of comorbid factors or events. Disorders that are most often implicated in the pathogenesis of calciphylaxis include chronic renal failure, obesity, diabetes mellitus, hypercalcaemia, hyperphosphatemia, an elevated calcium–phosphate product, secondary hyperparathyroidism, and perhaps a variety of hypercoagulable states. The distal limbs are the most common areas involved, with legs being the most common site. Lesions start with tender red areas developing into a livedoid pattern. Solitary or multiple indurated plaques and/or nodules are then seen. Patients may subsequently develop an eschar followed by frank ulceration, gangrene or sepsis. When calcium deposition is limited to the subcutaneous tissue, the term 'calcifying panniculitis' has been used [1]. The process is associated with an elevated calcium–phosphate product and hyperparathyroidism. 'Calcifying panniculitis' has only rarely been reported in children [2], but it should be considered in the differential diagnosis in patients with chronic renal failure who develop subcutaneous nodules.

Systemic corticosteroids are of no benefit and may exacerbate arteriolar calcification. Furthermore, corticosteroids may cause calcium and phosphorous abnormalities from a dynamic bone disease [3]. Bisphosphonate therapy with etidronate disodium has been shown to be effective in treating patients with calciphylaxis. A possible mechanism may involve removing arterial calcification. A dose of 200 mg/day for 14 days has been used with success, effectively lowering the calcium–phosphorus levels [4].

Sodium thiosulfate (STS) has been used for many years for the treatment of cyanide and cisplatin intoxication [5]. The half-life of STS in patients with normal renal function is 15 minutes. The exact mechanism of STS in calciphylaxis is unknown; however, it may play a role in chelating calcium from tissue deposits. A successful use of STS has been reported in three patients between 12 and 21 years of age [6].

References

1 Koch Nogueira PC, Giuliani C, Rey N et al. Calcifying panniculitis in a child after renal transplantation. Nephrol Dial Transplant 1997;12:216–18.
2 Feng J, Gohara M, Lazova R, Antaya RJ. Fatal childhood calciphylaxis in a 10-year-old and literature review. Pediatr Dermatol 2006;23:266–72.
3 Weenig RH, Sewell LD, Davis MD et al. Calciphylaxis: natural history, risk factor analysis, and outcome. J Am Acad Dermatol 2007;56: 569–79.
4 Hanafusa T, Yamaguchi Y, Tani M et al. Intractable wounds caused by calcific uremic arteriolopathy treated with bisphosphonates. J Am Acad Dermatol 2007;57:1021–5
5 Meissner M, Kaufmann R, Gille J. Sodium thiosulphate: a new way of treatment for calciphylaxis? Dermatology 2007;214:278–82.
6 Araya CE, Fennell RS, Neiberger RE et al. Sodium thiosulfate treatment for calcific uremic arteriolopathy in children and young adults. Clin J Am Soc Nephrol 2006;1:1161–6.

Infective panniculitis

Infection-induced panniculitis may result from a number of microbes including bacteria, fungi and parasites, and even viruses. This type of panniculitis can occur as a primary infection by direct inoculation of infectious microorganisms into the subcutaneous tissue, or secondarily via microbial haematogenous dissemination with subsequent infection of the subcutaneous tissue [1]. Infective panniculitis is mostly a lobular panniculitis. However, a mixed lobular and septal inflammation has also been observed, and occasionally a septal process may predominate [2]. The infiltrate is predominantly neutrophilic, with frequent findings of suppurative granulomas, necrosis and haemorrhage, and rarely vasculitis may be seen. Microorganisms are sometimes identified on histopathology, particularly in immunosuppressed patients, or grown in tissue culture from biopsy specimens. Infection should be considered in any case of panniculitis, particularly in immunocompromised patients, but also in immunocompetent children [3,4]

References

1 Delgado-Jimenez Y, Fraga J, Garcia-Diez A. Infective panniculitis. Dermatol Clin 2008;26:471–80, vi.
2 Requena L, Sanchez Yus E. Panniculitis. Part II. Mostly lobular panniculitis. J Am Acad Dermatol 2001;45:325–61.
3 Patterson JW, Brown PC, Broecker AH. Infection-induced panniculitis. J Cutan Pathol 1989;16:183–93.
4 Pao W, Duncan KO, Bolognia JL et al. Numerous eruptive lesions of panniculitis associated with group A streptococcus bacteremia in an immunocompetent child. Clin Infect Dis 1998;27:430–3.

Factitial, iatrogenic or traumatic panniculitis

Factitial panniculitides are subcutaneous tissue injuries produced by external agents or actions, including injection, blunt trauma, and temperature change [1–3]. In most cases, factitial panniculitis is caused by self-injection of different substances. The clinical features of factitial panniculitis are variable, depending on the inciting agent. The histopathology of factitial panniculitis usually shows a pattern of an acute lobular panniculitis associated with fat necrosis and an abundant inflammatory infiltrate predominantly composed of neutrophils [4]. Membranous fat necrosis and haemorrhage typical of traumatic panniculitis may be found. A search for foreign materials under regular and polarized light is recommended for cases showing neutrophilic panniculitis, and is absolutely essential when foreign body giant cells or granulomas are present. Treatment ranges from supportive care to surgical debridement, requires avoidance of the responsible agent if known, and should include social and psychological care when intentional factitial panniculitis is suspected [5,6].

Acknowledgement

The author acknowledges the work of the previous authors, Heather A. Brandling-Bennett and Maria C. Garzon, and for the reuse of some text and for the reuse or adaptation of Tables 1, 2 and 3 from their chapter in the 3rd edition.

References

1 Oh C, Ginsberg-Fellner F, Dolger H. Factitial panniculitis and necrotizing fasciitis in juvenile diabetes. Diabetes 1975;24:856–8.
2 Prendiville J, Thiessen P, Mallory SB. Neutrophilic dermatoses in two children with idiopathic neutropenia: association with granulocyte colony-stimulating factor (G-CSF) therapy. Pediatr Dermatol 2001;18: 417–21.
3 Buswell WA. Traumatic fat necrosis of the face in children. Br J Plast Surg 1979;32:127–8.
4 Requena L, Sanchez Yus E. Panniculitis. Part II. Mostly lobular panniculitis. J Am Acad Dermatol 2001;45:325–61.
5 Sanmartin O, Requena C, Requena L. Factitial panniculitis. Dermatol Clin 2008;26:519–27, viii.
6 Moreno A, Marcoval J, Peyri J. Traumatic panniculitis. Dermatol Clin 2008;26:481–3, vii.

CHAPTER 103
Lipodystrophies

Robert K. Semple

Centre for Cardiovascular Sciences, Queens Medical Research Institute, University of Edinburgh, Edinburgh, UK

Abstract

Lipodystrophy refers to a heterogeneous group of genetic and acquired conditions defined by regional or global lack of adipose tissue. Generalized lipodystrophy and limb lipodystrophy are usually associated with severe insulin resistance, diabetes, fatty liver and dyslipidaemia, and clinical and biochemical detection of these, and their early treatment, are essential to prevent major premature morbidity and mortality. Many autosomal recessive and autosomal dominant molecular subtypes of lipodystrophy are now known, some of which may be recognized by associated clinical features. In some genetic disorders lipodystrophy is only one component of a pleiotropic syndrome. Acquired lipodystrophies are commonly immunologically mediated, with detectable derangement of immunoglobulin levels or complement, and often are associated with other autoimmune diseases. Many localized forms of lipodystrophy also exist. Knowledge of such complex syndromes, and understanding of the metabolic implications of lipodystrophy, is important in offering early diagnosis and optimal management.

Key points

- Adipose tissue is critical for metabolic health and for establishment of normal body contours.
- Lipodystrophy refers to localized, regional or global anatomical deficits in adipose tissue.
- It is often cosmetic distress which leads to clinical presentation of lipodystrophy, but it is commonly complicated by serious metabolic sequelae including severe insulin resistance, diabetes, fatty liver and extreme hypertriglyceridaemia with risk of acute pancreatitis.
- Lipodystrophy may be congenital or acquired.
- Congenital generalized lipodystrophy is rare, shows autosomal recessive inheritance, and in most cases is attributable to biallelic mutations in the *BSCL2* or *AGPAT2* genes.
- Familial partial lipodystrophy is commonly autosomal dominant, and the commonest known causative genetic defects lie in the *LMNA* and *PPARG* genes.
- Lipodystrophy is also a component of many more complex Mendelian syndromes including several featuring defects in DNA replication and repair.
- Acquired lipodystrophy presents in many forms, some relating to local tissue damage, and some relating to systemic insults such as irradiation, human immunodeficiency virus infection and highly active antiretroviral therapy.
- Acquired lipodystrophy may also be autoimmune, presenting as progressive multifocal panniculitis, or as generalized loss of adipose tissue with hypergammaglobulinaemia, complement activation, and often co-occurring autoantibody-mediated disease.
- Management of lipodystrophy centres on accurate diagnosis and screening for known associated systemic conditions and complications. In patients with associated severe metabolic disease, offloading adipose tissue with behavioural and pharmacological treatments focusing on reducing positive energy balance are critical.

Introduction. Fat, or adipose tissue, is critical for health. It shapes body contours, cushions body prominences, and protects vital organs mechanically and thermally. Both subcutaneous and visceral adipose tissue are also richly invested with primary immunological cell types, and express genes encoding complement components that are involved in innate immunity [1]. This reflects the anatomical location of much adipose tissue, which means that it plays a role in the early response to external trauma or perforating gastrointestinal pathologies. Adipose tissue is above all, however, critical for metabolic health, buffering fluctuating nutritional intake by storing excess ingested energy in times of plenty, only to release it later at times of privation.

Adipose tissue is heterogenous in terms of development, anatomy, gene expression and function across different anatomical sites, and engages in complex metabolic dialogue with viscera involved in metabolic regulation such as muscle, liver and heart. Lipodystrophy may generally be defined as a visible, pathological deficit of adipose tissue in all or part of the body. In keeping with the complexity of adipose tissue itself, lipodystrophies, too, are highly variable, and many genetic and acquired forms are known (Table 103.1). Some acquired forms are localized and asymmetrical, and relate to insults such as radiotherapy, subcutaneous drug administration or trauma, or to circumscribed inflammatory processes, often autoimmune. Other acquired forms are symmetrical, and are caused by systemic insults, including human immunodeficiency virus (HIV) infection and antiretroviral therapies, whole body irradiation or systemic autoimmunity, usually with evidence of deranged humoral immunity and complement activation. Inflammatory forms of localized

Harper's Textbook of Pediatric Dermatology, Fourth Edition. Edited by Peter Hoeger, Veronica Kinsler and Albert Yan.

Table 103.1 Classification of lipodystrophies

	Inherited	Acquired
Localized		Secondary lipoatrophies Centrifugal lipoatrophy Atrophy of the ankles Semicircular lipoatrophy Annular lipoatrophy Naevoid disorders
Partial	Familial partial lipodystrophies Complex syndromes, e.g. mandibuloacral dysplasia, MDP syndrome, Werner syndrome	Acquired partial lipoatrophy HIV/HAART-related
Generalized	Congenital generalized lipodystrophy	Acquired generalized lipoatrophy

lipodystrophy are discussed in other chapters, so in this chapter the focus is predominantly on noninflammatory, primary lipodystrophies.

Lipodystrophies are important to diagnose not only because precise diagnosis offers an explanation to patients and families worried by a change in appearance, but also because they may be associated with systemic disease. The manifest harm caused by excess adiposity, or obesity, should not be taken to imply that constrained ability to make adipose tissue is a healthy state. Indeed, individuals with many forms of lipodystrophy, far from being protected from the adverse consequences of obesity, exhibit the full spectrum of metabolic complications of obesity, often to an extremely severe degree and at young ages [2]. Thus presentation to a dermatologist with altered appearance may be a sentinel event that prompts more detailed systemic investigation.

Clinical features and differential diagnosis. Lipodystrophy is a diagnosis made by observation of anatomical deficiency of adipose tissue from all or part of the body. The major challenge in clinical diagnosis lies in the normal variability of whole body adipose stores. Adipose tissue is highly dynamic, fluctuating across the lifespan according to energy balance, which in turn is determined by environmental conditions, psychological factors, systemic illness, and hormonal milieu. In general, pathological deficiency of adipose tissue is easiest to identify where there is a clear difference between an affected body site or region and unaffected sites with replete adipose tissue. It is difficult to identify when normal adipose tissue is delipidated by negative energy balance, minimizing the visible difference between affected and unaffected adipose tissue. Even generalized lipodystrophy may be very difficult to discriminate from global leanness, especially in prepubertal children with low body fat mass.

In cases where discriminating lipodystrophy and leanness for other reasons is difficult, important clues may be clinical and biochemical features of complications of lipodystrophy. In generalized lipodystrophy, and partial lipodystrophies affecting femorogluteal adipose tissue in particular, loss of adipose energy buffering capacity leads to 'spillover' of lipid to liver, muscle, pancreatic beta cells and elsewhere. As a consequence, insulin resistance, dyslipidaemia and diabetes develop. General clinical features of severe insulin resistance include ovulatory dysfunction, and ovarian hyperandrogenism, often leading to pronounced hirsutism in postpubertal girls, as well as acanthosis nigricans and sometimes pseudoacromegaloid soft tissue overgrowth [3]. Insulin-resistant diabetes appears when pancreatic beta cell insulin production begins to fail. Other complications seen particularly in lipodystrophy include severe hypertriglyceridaemia that is exquisitely sensitive to dietary fat intake and that commonly causes recurrent attacks of acute pancreatitis and/or eruptive xanthomata if not controlled. Fatty liver disease is also a major component of lipodystrophic syndromes, and is often severe even in childhood, with advanced liver disease a major cause of later mortality (Box 103.1). However, such collateral evidence of 'adipose failure' may be absent in patients with lipodystrophy who are in negative energy balance, because this offloads adipose tissue and may mask lipodystrophy.

It follows from the above that the main differential diagnosis of lipodystrophy is any disorder that leads to negative energy balance, including anorexia nervosa, systemic illnesses, malabsorption, or neglect and malnourishment. Specific, very rare disorders that should be considered in children with absent or globally poorly developed adipose tissue, but which are not considered to be primary lipodystrophies, are Donohue Syndrome, an infantile extreme form of insulin resistance caused by biallelic mutations in the insulin receptor gene, and diencephalic syndrome. The near total absence of adipose tissue from limbs, trunk and

Box 103.1 Clinical findings in genetic lipodystrophy syndromes

- Lipoatrophy (*sine qua non*)
- Acanthosis nigricans (common)
- Hirsutism/hyperandrogenism (common)
- Fatty liver (common)
- Eruptive xanthomata (usually only if diet poorly controlled)
- Muscular hypertrophy (common)
- Pseudoacromegaly or soft tissue overgrowth (common)
- Syndrome-specific features (e.g. myopathy, premature ageing)

face in congenital generalized lipodystrophy (CGL) coupled to abdominal protruberance can be mistaken for the wrinkled appearance and distended abdomen seen in Donohue syndrome. However, reduced muscle bulk, absence of fatty liver or dyslipidaemia, and other dysmorphic features of Donohue syndrome permit its clinical discrimination [4]. Diencephalic syndrome, caused by tumours in the region of the hypothalamus, may also produce generalized loss of adipose tissue, but without features of insulin resistance, fatty liver and muscular hypertrophy, and the global loss of adipose tissue may be the presenting symptom of the underlying tumour, and may precede neurological symptoms by several years [5].

Epidemiology and pathogenesis. Congenital and acquired lipodystrophies will be considered in turn.

Autosomal recessive lipodystrophies

The most severe form of lipodystrophy is CGL, sometimes called Berardinelli–Seip congenital lipodystrophy (BSCL) in recognition of 1950s descriptions of the syndrome in Brazil and Norway [6,7]. CGL is invariably autosomal recessive, is extremely rare and is usually easily recognized in infancy because of failure of infants to develop a normal 'plump' appearance. Affected infants are often described as 'wrinkled', or 'aged' (Fig. 103.1).

In most cases a genetic aetiology can be established. The first gene implicated, *BSCL2*, was identified in 2001 [8]. *BSCL2* encodes an endoplasmic reticulum protein named seipin, which is implicated in triglyceride metabolism, lipid droplet function and adipocyte differentiation, although many questions remain [9]. Biallelic mutations in a second gene, *AGPAT2,* were reported in CGL soon afterwards [10]. *AGPAT2* encodes the enzyme 1-acylglycerol-3-phosphate O-acyltransferase 2 (AGPAT2), which catalyses a key step in the biosynthesis of triglycerides.

It is clinically difficult to distinguish CGL caused by mutations in *AGPAT2* and *BSCL2*, but differences have been described, including preserved 'mechanical' adipose depots (e.g. in periarticular regions, palms and soles) and increased prevalence of lytic bone lesions in patients with *AGPAT2* mutations. *BSCL2*-related CGL has been suggested to feature more mental retardation and cardiomyopathy. However, in practice genetic screening for both *AGPAT2* and *BSCL2* simultaneously is often appropriate in CGL.

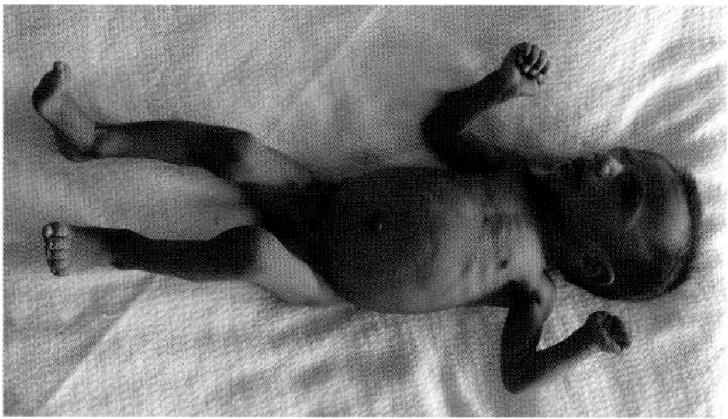

Fig. 103.1 Characteristic appearance of congenital generalized lipoatrophy in an infant. There is lack of subcutaneous fat, producing a somewhat 'wrinkly' appearance, with a distended abdomen caused by engorgement of the liver with triglyceride, and some soft tissue overgrowth including acanthosis nigricans. Muscularity is prominent.

Mutations in *BSCL2* and *AGPAT2* account for around 95% of CGL. However, very rare mutations in a handful of other genes has also been described. Two of these genes, *CAV1* [11] and *PTRF* [12], are required for the formation of caveolae, specialized plasma membrane invaginations involved in key signalling pathways, and that are abundant in adipocytes. Patients with *PTRF* mutations may be discriminated clinically because of co-occurrence of myopathy with CGL.

Partial lipodystrophies are generally transmitted as autosomal dominant traits. However, rare examples of recessive partial lipodystrophies have been described. A single case of lipodystrophy caused by a homozygous early truncation mutation in the lipid droplet protein *CIDEC* has been reported [13], whereas partial lipodystrophy has also recently been attributed in rare cases to biallelic mutations in *PCYT1A*, which encodes phosphate cytidyl transferase 1 alpha, which plays a critical role in the synthesis of the essential phospholipid phosphatidylcholine [14].

Autosomal dominant lipodystrophies

Partial lipodystrophies are defined by sparing of some regions or depots of adipose tissue, particularly visceral and head and neck adipose tissue. Such remaining depots may show compensatory excess fat deposition. Familial partial lipodystrophies (FPLD) are far more common than CGL, and usually show autosomal dominant inheritance, although around 40% of patients remain without a genetic diagnosis. Involvement of femorogluteal subcutaneous adipose tissue is the norm, with different subtypes showing variable extents of fat loss elsewhere. Clinical presentation is usually peripubertal, because pathological deficits in adipose tissue are difficult to discriminate in lean prepubertal children. Failure of normal adipose accretion in girls is frequently noticed, often with features of severe insulin resistance including oligomenorrhoea and hirsutism. Lean boys are commonly undiagnosed, and often are identified only later in mid life when diabetes has developed. Several genes have been shown to harbour mutations causing autosomal dominant FPLD.

LMNA

Heterozygous mutations in *LMNA,* encoding lamins A and C (structural components of the lamina that runs under the nuclear membrane of cells), are the most common cause of FPLD, referred to as FPLD2 or Dunnigan-type familial partial lipodystrophy [15]. Patients with lamin A/C-associated lipodystrophy have preservation of fat in the neck, chin, face, viscera and labia majora. Residual fat depots in the head and neck and intra-abdominally commonly increase in size leading to a 'Cushingoid' adipose topography, and give the erroneous impression of normal or increased adipose tissue in clothed patients.

LMNA mutations are associated with other clinical syndromes including Emery–Dreyfuss myopathy, Charcot–Marie–Tooth neuropathy, various progeroid syndromes,

SECTION 22: DISORDERS OF FAT TISSUE

and cardiomyopathy and cardiac conduction disorders [16]. Ninety percent of 'isolated' Dunnigan-type lipodystrophy is caused by a mutation at arginine 482. However, some overlap among syndromes is well recognized, especially for minor FPLD mutations, and so cardiomyopathy or skeletal myopathy should be sought in FPLD2.

PPARG

Heterozygous mutations in *PPARG*, which encodes the receptor for the thiazolidinedione class of insulin-sensitizing drugs, were identified to cause severe insulin resistance in 1999 [17], and it later became clear that this was associated with FPLD [18,19]. This subgroup is sometimes labelled FPLD3. Patients with *PPARG* mutations show preserved visceral fat and usually also some subcutaneous abdominal adipose tissue. Indeed, it is not uncommon for patients with FPLD3 to have some degree of centripetal obesity, although relative limb lipodystrophy is invariable. Like other types of FPLD, FPLD3 is often discerned at the onset of puberty. The presentation is more subtle anatomically than in FPLD2. However, unusually severe dyslipidaemia, fatty liver, insulin resistance or early onset hypertension should prompt *PPARG* testing.

LMNA or *PPARG* mutations account for most FPLD where a pathogenic mutation is identified. However, mutations in the lipid droplet protein Perilipin 1 (encoded by *PLIN1*), were recently identified in a small group of patients [20]. Subcutaneous fat loss has been more uniform than in FPLD2 in patients described to date, and have been accompanied by early adult onset diabetes mellitus, acanthosis nigricans, and hyperandrogenism. PLIN1 has a crucial role on the outer membrane of the lipid droplet, inhibiting lipolysis of triacylglycerol [21].

'Insulin signalling' genes

Mutations in proximal components of the insulin signalling pathway have also been shown to cause lipodystrophy. One of these is *PIK3R1*, encoding catalytic subunits of phosphatidylinositol-3-kinase. Mutations in *PIK3R1* produce SHORT syndrome (Short stature, Ocular depression, Rieger anomaly, delayed Tooth loss) [22–24] which also frequently features femorogluteal lipodystrophy, but not not fatty liver or dyslipidaemia [25]. In a single four generation family described to date, a mutation in the downstream signalling gene *AKT2* also caused lipodystrophic insulin resistance. However, this resembled other types of FPLD metabolically with severe dyslipidaemia and fatty liver [26].

Lipodystrophy in complex syndromes

Lipodystrophy and severe insulin resistance are also encountered in several, rare complex syndromes. The first group are caused by perturbation of *LMNA* function or processing. Mandibuloacral dysplasia (MAD) describes small mandibles and clavicles, acro-osteolysis, delayed closure of cranial sutures, joint contractures, early ageing, and a mottled pigmentation [27]. This may be caused by biallelic mutations in *LMNA* that are distinct from those causing FPLD2. Another rare laminopathy is Hutchinson–Gilford syndrome, in which a particular *de novo* point mutation in *LMNA* produces lipodystrophy with MAD, as well as premature ageing and early death [28]. The lipodystrophy involves global childhood loss of fat with no face and neck sparing. Another form of MAD is caused by mutations in *ZMPSTE24*, encoding a zinc metalloproteinase that cleaves prelamin A during maturation. Fat loss in these patients includes the face, leading to a progeroid appearance [29].

Other syndromes that feature dyslipidaemic severe insulin resistance with lipodystrophy are caused by defects in DNA replication or damage repair. The lipodystrophy is most clearly described for Werner's syndrome, a premature ageing syndrome caused by biallelic mutation of a DNA helicase involved in many pathways of DNA repair [30,31], and in the MDP (Mandibular hypoplasia, Deafness and Progeria) syndrome [32]. Patients with MDP syndrome have normal birth weight and appearance, but progressive fat loss starts in early childhood and is accompanied by increased visceral adipose tissue and marked insulin resistance. Other common features include atrophy of limb muscles, sensorineural deafness, mandibular hypoplasia, hypogonadism, scleroderma and joint contractures. MDP syndrome is caused by heterozygous mutation of the polymerase active site of DNA polymerase delta [33]. How such fundamental defects in DNA replication and repair produce tissue-selective dysfunction is currently being studied. Biallelic mutations in several other genes have been shown to cause rare syndromic forms of lipodystrophy, including *PSMB8*, associated with a progressive and striking autoinflammatory form of lipodystrophy, and *FBN1*, associated with neonatal progeroid lipodystrophy. However, these are beyond the scope of this chapter.

Acquired lipodystrophies

Many forms of lipodystrophy are acquired, and may present at any age. Most localized lipodystrophy is attributable to a local insult, which is often inflammatory. Such inflammatory disorders are considered elsewhere.

Autoimmune lipodystrophies

Acquired generalized lipoatrophy (AGL) is the most severe form of acquired lipodystrophy, characterized by global loss of adipose tissue after normal early development [34]. This often begins in adolescence or early adulthood. In 25% of cases multifocal panniculitis heralds onset of lipoatrophy, whereas in another subgroup patients show autoimmune diseases such as hepatitis or haemolytic anaemia [34], and polyclonal hypergammaglobulinaemia with suppression of complement factor C4, consistent with the presence of circulating immune complexes, is common [1]. Juvenile dermatomyositis has a particularly strong association with acquired subcutaneous lipodystrophy [35]. AGL may lead to all the metabolic complications of CGL. However, associated autoimmune diseases may dominate the clinical picture.

Acquired partial lipoatrophy (APL) usually presents in the second decade of life although earlier onset is well described. APL shows female predominance and has a fairly sudden onset, with symmetrical disappearance of facial fat the first sign, giving a gaunt facial appearance.

A preceding febrile illness is commonly reported [36]. Adipose loss progresses caudally, but does not usually extend below the umbilicus. Compensatory increase in femorogluteal adipose tissue may be seen. Ninety percent of cases have low C3 levels caused by the presence of C3 nephritic factor, an antibody which stabilizes C3 convertase, and about 50% of patients develop membranoproliferative glomerulonephritis. Screening for this is an important facet of clinical management. The prevalence of metabolic complications and diabetes is much lower than seen in partial lipodystrophies affecting femorogluteal adipose tissue.

Lipodystrophy in HIV-infected patients

Lipodystrophy is well recognized as a complication in HIV patients, with highly active antiretroviral therapy (HAART) including protease inhibitors being most strongly implicated as the cause. Prevalence is variable but may reach 50% in patients treated for more than 1 year with protease inhibitors, and children can be affected. HIV-related lipodystrophy usually presents with selective loss of fat from the face and extremities, but may also feature adipose remodeling with increased adiposity in the dorsocervical region, abdomen and trunk. Like many other forms of lipodystrophy it is associated with dyslipidaemic insulin resistance [37].

Whole body irradiation

Lipodystrophy is also sometimes seen in patients who underwent whole body irradiation during cancer treatment in early childhood, most likely because irradiation damages the proliferative potential of adipose precursor cells [38]. This is not a limiting factor in the prepubertal state. However, when adipose tissue is called upon to increase in mass around the time of puberty under the influence of sex hormones, the prior damage may be unmasked, and a highly dyslipidaemic form of insulin resistance may ensue, sometimes accompanied by absolute lipodystrophy, and sometimes accompanied by a relatively reduced ability to lay down adipose tissue in femorogluteal depots, leading to centripetal adipose remodeling. Awareness of this phenomenon is important in assessing patients who received childhood cancer treatment.

Localized lipodystrophies

Localized lipodystrophies are a heterogenous group of disorders generally not associated with systemic metabolic derangement. They often resolve spontaneously. In childhood they may roughly be divided into those which feature involutional lipoatrophy, for example linked to repeated trauma, pressure or drug injection, those which follow panniculitides, primarily associated with connective tissue disease, and centrifugal lipodystrophy or lipodystrophia centrifugalis abdominalis infantilis (Box 103.2). Panniculitides are discussed in Chapter 102, so consideration here will be limited to one form of drug-induced lipoatrophy, namely that caused by local insulin injection, and centrifugal lipodystrophy.

Lipoatrophy following subcutaneous insulin injections was a common cause of localized fat atrophy when bovine–porcine insulin preparations were widely used, and its prevalence greatly decreased with the availability first of highly purified porcine insulins [39], and later human insulins. It was considered to be an immunological reaction to impurities in the insulin preparations and/or to the nonhuman insulin [40]. It is still seen in the modern era of human and analogue insulins, however, and is a cosmetically distressing complication, presenting as a painless dimple at insulin injection sites (Fig. 103.2). Most cases are associated with higher levels of insulin requirements, because insulin absorption can be variable caused by the formation of avascular, fibrous scar tissue. Lipoatrophic lesions distant from the sites of injection may occur, as well as the coexistence of both fat atrophy and hypertrophy. Skin biopsies show a loss of fat tissue and sometimes an increase is found in insulin-binding capacity on the edge of the lesions. Although histological studies are relatively rare, insulin-induced lipoatrophy may sometimes be seen in association with high circulating titres of anti-insulin antibodies.

Box 103.2 Causes of localized lipoatrophy

- Injections (e.g. insulin, corticosteroids, vaccinations)
- Neonatal subcutaneous necrosis
- Subcutaneous calcification/ossification
- Lipoatrophic panniculitis
- Trauma
- Radiation
- Infections (bacterial, fungal or parasitic)
- Connective tissue diseases (lupus erythematosus, dermatomyositis, scleroderma)
- Lipodermatosclerosis
- Granuloma annulare, necrobiosis lipoidica, rheumatic nodules
- Lymphoma, leukaemia, neoplasia

Centrifugal lipoatrophy features localized loss of abdominal subcutaneous fat, usually before 8 years of age, with centrifugal enlargement of the affected area to leave a central part of lipoatrophy, where subcutaneous veins become easily visible [41]. Most cases have been in Japanese patients, with a female preponderance. Erythematous, bluish macules or ecchymoses with lymph node enlargement are seen at presentation in about half of cases. Histology shows inflammatory cells in the surrounding area, sometimes involving the dermis as well as the subcutaneous tissue, but no vasculitis is seen. Enlargement arrests within 3 years in 50% of patients and within 8 years in 90%, followed by spontaneous resolution in most cases [41]. Systemic signs of inflammation are usually absent, corticosteroids do not stop the progressive enlargement of centrifugal lipoatrophy, and the aetiopathogenesis remains largely a subject of speculation.

Laboratory and imaging findings.

Endocrine and metabolic

Lipodystrophy is a clinical diagnosis, and no reliable laboratory surrogates exist. However, biochemical evidence may support a clinical diagnosis. Plasma leptin is severely reduced or absent in CGL, but is more variable in FPLD,

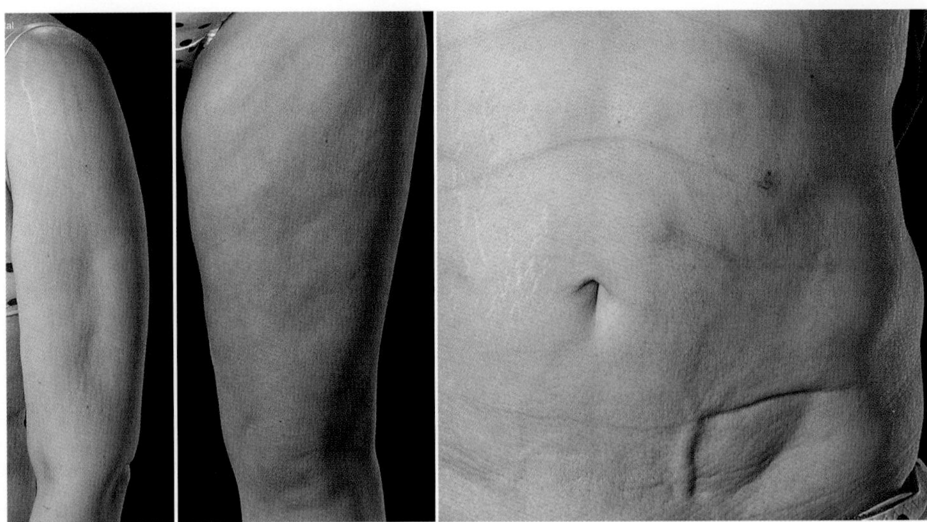

Fig. 103.2 Typical appearance of insulin-induced lipoatrophy. Patchy lipoatrophy with some lipohypertrophy and localized inflammation at recent injection sites can be seen on the upper arm, abdomen and thigh of a patient with high levels of anti-insulin autoantibodies.

depending on the overall size of whole body adipose depots. It is also very low in thin healthy people, especially in prepubertal boys, and thus does not serve as a reliable marker of lipodystrophy. Biochemical evidence of insulin resistance and dyslipidaemia is common in CGL and often FPLD, and so fasting glucose, insulin and triglyceride determinations are an important part of evaluation. Collateral markers of insulin resistance include low serum sex hormone-binding globulin (SHBG) and insulin-like growth factor binding protein 1 (IGFBP1), and adiponectin concentrations [42].

Haematological and autoimmune markers

A blood count, immunoglobulin profile, complement components C3 and C4 (and C3 nephritic factor if C3 is low), and sometimes specific testing for autoantibodies guided by the presenting clinical problems are of value in the diagnostic work-up of suspected autoimmune lipodystrophy, given the high prevalence of associated organ-specific autoimmune disorders.

Imaging

Various methods have been applied to standardized imaging or quantifying of adiposity in the context of lipodystrophy including magnetic resonance imaging or computed tomography, dual energy X-ray absorptiometry, or standardized assessment of skinfold thickness. However, these remain predominantly research tools. Imaging may be indicated, however, to investigate organs affected by associated autoimmune disease, or to assess for the presence of steatohepatitis and/or liver fibrosis in those with longstanding dyslipidaemic insulin resistance related to lipodystrophy.

Treatment and prevention.

Endocrine and metabolic

The major morbidity and early mortality associated with lipodystrophies arise from poorly controlled diabetes mellitus and dyslipidaemia as well as to acute pancreatitis and advanced liver disease related to non-alcoholic steatohepatitis. These metabolic derangements are thought to be caused by a lack of buffering capacity for dietary caloric excess, compounded in some patients with lipodystrophy by deficiency of leptin, which erroneously indicates to the brain that energy stores are critically low and thus drives hyperphagia. A low fat, hypocaloric diet and promotion of exercise is critical, and in patients with leptin deficiency subcutaneous leptin therapy may be a valuable adjunct in reducing appetite and facilitating achievement of neutral energy balance [43]. Where these measures are ineffective, use of treatments commonly regarded as 'obesity therapies' is rational, though guided only by clinical experience and case reports at present.

Metabolic control is frequently not achieved with these measures alone, in which case an insulin sensitizer such as metformin is of value. Severe hypertriglyceridaemia may be treated with conventional therapies if needed, including fibrates and dietary supplementation with n–3 polyunsaturated fatty acids. Glycaemic control can be difficult to achieve in some patients with very high requirements for exogenous insulin. The use of high concentration (U500) insulin can be beneficial both to prevent injection-site reactions and to increase glycaemic control [43].

Acknowledgements

RKS is supported by a Senior Research Fellowship from the Wellcome Trust (Grant WT 210752/Z/18/Z). Professor Semple has received speaker fees from Novo Nordisk and Sandoz.

References

1 Savage DB, Semple RK, Clatworthy MR et al. Complement abnormalities in acquired lipodystrophy revisited. J Clin Endocrinol Metab 2009;94:10–6.

2 **Patni N, Garg A. Congenital generalized lipodystrophies – new insights into metabolic dysfunction. Nat Rev Endocrinol 2015;11: 522–34.**

3 **Semple RK, Savage DB, Cochran EK et al. Genetic syndromes of severe insulin resistance. Endocr Rev 2011;32:498–514.**

4 de Bock M, Hayes I, Semple R. 'Donohue syndrome'. J Clin Endocrinol Metab 2012;97:1416–7.

5 Patni N, Alves C, von Schnurbein J et al. A novel syndrome of generalized lipodystrophy associated with pilocytic astrocytoma. J Clin Endocrinol Metab 2015;100:3603–6.

6 Berardinelli W. An undiagnosed endocrinometabolic syndrome: report of 2 cases. J Clin Endocrinol Metab 1954;14:193–204.

7 Seip M, Trygstad O. Generalized lipodystrophy. Arch Dis Child 1963;38:447–53.

8 Magre J, Delepine M, Khallouf E et al. Identification of the gene altered in Berardinelli-Seip congenital lipodystrophy on chromosome 11q13. Nat Genet 2001;28:365–70.

9 Wee K, Yang W, Sugii S, Han W. Towards a mechanistic understanding of lipodystrophy and seipin functions. Biosci Rep 2014;34:e000141.

10 Agarwal AK, Arioglu E, De Almeida S et al. AGPAT2 is mutated in congenital generalized lipodystrophy linked to chromosome 9q34. Nat Genet 2002;31:21–3.

11 Kim CA, Delepine M, Boutet E et al. Association of a homozygous nonsense caveolin-1 mutation with Berardinelli-Seip congenital lipodystrophy. J Clin Endocrinol Metab 2008;93:1129–34.

12 Hayashi YK, Matsuda C, Ogawa M et al. Human PTRF mutations cause secondary deficiency of caveolins resulting in muscular dystrophy with generalized lipodystrophy. J Clin Invest 2009;119:2623–33.

13 Rubio-Cabezas O, Puri V, Murano I et al. Partial lipodystrophy and insulin resistant diabetes in a patient with a homozygous nonsense mutation in CIDEC. EMBO Mol Med 2009;1:280–7.

14 Payne F, Lim K, Girousse A et al. Mutations disrupting the Kennedy phosphatidylcholine pathway in humans with congenital lipodystrophy and fatty liver disease. Proc Natl Acad Sci U S A 2014;111:8901–6.

15 Shackleton S, Lloyd DJ, Jackson SN et al. LMNA, encoding lamin A/C, is mutated in partial lipodystrophy. Nat Genet 2000;24:153–6.

16 Worman HJ, Bonne G. 'Laminopathies': a wide spectrum of human diseases. Exp Cell Res 2007;313:2121–33.

17 Barroso I, Gurnell M, Crowley VE et al. Dominant negative mutations in human PPARgamma associated with severe insulin resistance, diabetes mellitus and hypertension. Nature 1999;402(6764):880–3.

18 Semple RK, Chatterjee VK, O'Rahilly S. PPAR gamma and human metabolic disease. J Clin Invest 2006;116:581–9.

19 Agarwal AK, Garg A. A novel heterozygous mutation in peroxisome proliferator-activated receptor-gamma gene in a patient with familial partial lipodystrophy. J Clin Endocrinol Metab 2002;87:408–11.

20 Gandotra S, Le Dour C, Bottomley W et al. Perilipin deficiency and autosomal dominant partial lipodystrophy. N Engl J Med 2011;364:740–8.

21 Kozusko K, Patel S, Savage DB. Human congenital perilipin deficiency and insulin resistance. Endocr Dev 2013;24:150–5.

22 Chudasama KK, Winnay J, Johansson S et al. SHORT syndrome with partial lipodystrophy due to impaired phosphatidylinositol 3 kinase signaling. Am J Hum Genet 2013;93:150–7.

23 Dyment DA, Smith AC, Alcantara D et al. Mutations in PIK3R1 cause SHORT syndrome. Am J Hum Genet 2013;93:158–66.

24 Thauvin-Robinet C, Auclair M, Duplomb L et al. PIK3R1 mutations cause syndromic insulin resistance with lipoatrophy. Am J Hum Genet 2013;93:141–9.

25 Huang-Doran I, Tomlinson P, Payne F et al. Insulin resistance uncoupled from dyslipidemia due to C-terminal PIK3R1 mutations. JCI Insight 2016;1:e88766.

26 George S, Rochford JJ, Wolfrum C et al. A family with severe insulin resistance and diabetes due to a mutation in AKT2. Science 2004; 304(5675):1325–8.

27 Young LW, Radebaugh JF, Rubin P et al. New syndrome manifested by mandibular hypoplasia, acroosteolysis, stiff joints and cutaneous atrophy (mandibuloacral dysplasia) in two unrelated boys. Birth Defects Orig Artic Ser 1971;7:291–7.

28 Prokocimer M, Barkan R, Gruenbaum Y. Hutchinson-Gilford progeria syndrome through the lens of transcription. Aging Cell 2013;12: 533–43.

29 Simha V, Agarwal AK, Oral EA et al. Genetic and phenotypic heterogeneity in patients with mandibuloacral dysplasia-associated lipodystrophy. J Clin Endocrinol Metab 2003;88:2821–4.

30 Oshima J, Sidorova JM, Monnat RJ, Jr. Werner syndrome: clinical features, pathogenesis and potential therapeutic interventions. Ageing Res Rev 2017;33:105–14.

31 Imura H, Nakao Y, Kuzuya H et al. Clinical, endocrine and metabolic aspects of the Werner syndrome compared with those of normal aging. Adv Exp Med Biol 1985;190:171–85.

32 Shastry S, Simha V, Godbole K et al. A novel syndrome of mandibular hypoplasia, deafness, and progeroid features associated with lipodystrophy, undescended testes, and male hypogonadism. J Clin Endocrinol Metab 2010;95(10):E192–7.

33 Weedon MN, Ellard S, Prindle MJ et al. An in-frame deletion at the polymerase active site of POLD1 causes a multisystem disorder with lipodystrophy. Nat Genet 2013;45:947–50.

34 Misra A, Garg A. Clinical features and metabolic derangements in acquired generalized lipodystrophy: case reports and review of the literature. Medicine 2003;82:129–46.

35 Bingham A, Mamyrova G, Rother KI et al. Predictors of acquired lipodystrophy in juvenile-onset dermatomyositis and a gradient of severity. Medicine 2008;87:70–86.

36 Misra A, Peethambaram A, Garg A. Clinical features and metabolic and autoimmune derangements in acquired partial lipodystrophy: report of 35 cases and review of the literature. Medicine 2004;83: 18–34.

37 Galescu O, Bhangoo A, Ten S. Insulin resistance, lipodystrophy and cardiometabolic syndrome in HIV/AIDS. Rev Endocr Metab Disord 2013;14:133–40.

38 Mayson SE, Parker VE, Schutta MH et al. Severe insulin resistance and hypertriglyceridemia after childhood total body irradiation. Endocr Pract 2013;19:51–8.

39 Young RJ, Steel JM, Frier BM, Duncan LJ. Insulin injection sites in diabetes--a neglected area? Br Med J (Clin Res Ed) 1981;283(6287):349.

40 Reeves WG, Allen BR, Tattersall RB. Insulin-induced lipoatrophy: evidence for an immune pathogenesis. Br Med J 1980;280(6230):1500–3.

41 Imamura S, Yamada M, Yamamoto K. Lipodystrophia centrifugalis abdominalis infantilis. A follow-up study. J Am Acad Dermatol 1984;11:203–9.

42 Semple RK, Cochran EK, Soos MA et al. Plasma adiponectin as a marker of insulin receptor dysfunction: clinical utility in severe insulin resistance. Diabetes Care 2008;31(5):977–9.

43 Brown RJ, Araujo-Vilar D, Cheung PT et al. The Diagnosis and Management of Lipodystrophy Syndromes: A Multi-Society Practice Guideline. J Clin Endocrinol Metab 2016;101:4500–11.

CHAPTER 104
An Introduction to Mosaicism

Veronica A. Kinsler

Paediatric Dermatology Department, Great Ormond Street Hospital for Children NHS Foundation Trust, London, UK and Genetics and Genomic Medicine, UCL Great Ormond Street Institute of Child Health, London, UK

Definition of mosaic abnormalities of the skin, 1229
Classification of mosaic abnormalities by inheritance potential, 1229
Genetic mechanisms underlying cutaneous mosaicism, 1231
Conditions mimicking mosaicism, 1231
Principles governing the phenotype of mosaic disorders, 1232
Patterns of mosaic disorders, 1233
Genetic investigation of mosaic disorders, 1234

Abstract

Cutaneous mosaicism has become an increasingly important field in paediatric dermatology. This has been triggered by the advent of next generation sequencing, a new technique in molecular genetics which has been able to detect mutations present at low levels in the skin, and which were previously undetectable or unsuspected. A fascinating sequela of these findings is the confirmation of what we recognize as a cutaneous mosaic phenotype, surpassing the initial descriptions of Blaschko lines to include many other phenotypic patterns. This chapter explains the concept of cutaneous mosaicism in understandable terms, and addresses the clinically important concepts of inheritance of these genetic defects in a manner practically relevant to the paediatric dermatologist. The genetic mechanisms leading to mosaicism are explored using clear diagrams, and examples of the different mechanisms from paediatric skin disease are given throughout the text.

Definition of mosaic abnormalities of the skin

The common definition of mosaicism is 'the presence in an individual of two or more cell lines that are karyotypically or genotypically distinct and are derived from a single zygote' [1]. Mosaicism in paediatric dermatology has until now been a term used synonymously with a disease state caused by this genetic phenomenon, or for the spontaneous genetic rescue of a disease state (revertant mosaicism). However, it has become clear that the frequency of mutations during pre- and postnatal life is very high, and all individuals are by this traditional definition mosaic [2–7]. Therefore, whilst the traditional definition stands as an accurate description of a genetic state, it is no longer adequate as a definition of a mosaic abnormality of the skin.

A mosaic abnormality of the skin can be better defined as the coexistence of cells with at least two genotypes, at least one of which is pathological, by the time of birth, in an individual derived from a single zygote, and which leads to a disease phenotype. Importantly, this includes conditions where the phenotype does not develop fully until the first few years of life, but is clearly embryonic in pattern or size, such as inflammatory linear verrucous epidermal nevus, or tardive congenital melanocytic naevi. Also importantly, very common occurrences such as a single small congenital melanocytic naevus, or a single nonlinear sebaceous naevus would be generally considered to be in the normal range for the normal population, rather than a disease phenotype. These would therefore not be considered to be mosaic abnormalities.

Revertant mosaicism is the phenomenon of self-correction of part of a pre-existing disease phenotype. This can be pre- or postnatal, and theoretically can occur in the context of either a germline or mosaic genetic disorder, although thus far has only been published in germline conditions. Although the unifying principle of revertance thus far is of a new genetic event correcting or compensating for the mutant genotype, the exact mechanisms depend upon the condition, they are often complex, and they can be variable even within an individual.

Classification of mosaic abnormalities by inheritance potential

Mosaicism has traditionally been classified by the tissue type affected by the mutation, divided into somatic (nongamete tissues only), gonadal (gametes only) or somatic and gonadal (affecting both). This is an important concept, because it alerts the physician to the possibility that a mosaic disorder in a parent can be passed on to subsequent offspring in the germline (Fig. 104.1a). In practice, however, it is often not possible to be certain whether a proband with a mosaic disorder affecting the skin also has gamete involvement and is therefore at risk of passing on the mutation. Genetic counselling is therefore usually undertaken on the basis of what is known in the literature and in clinical practice about

Harper's Textbook of Pediatric Dermatology, Fourth Edition. Edited by Peter Hoeger, Veronica Kinsler and Albert Yan.

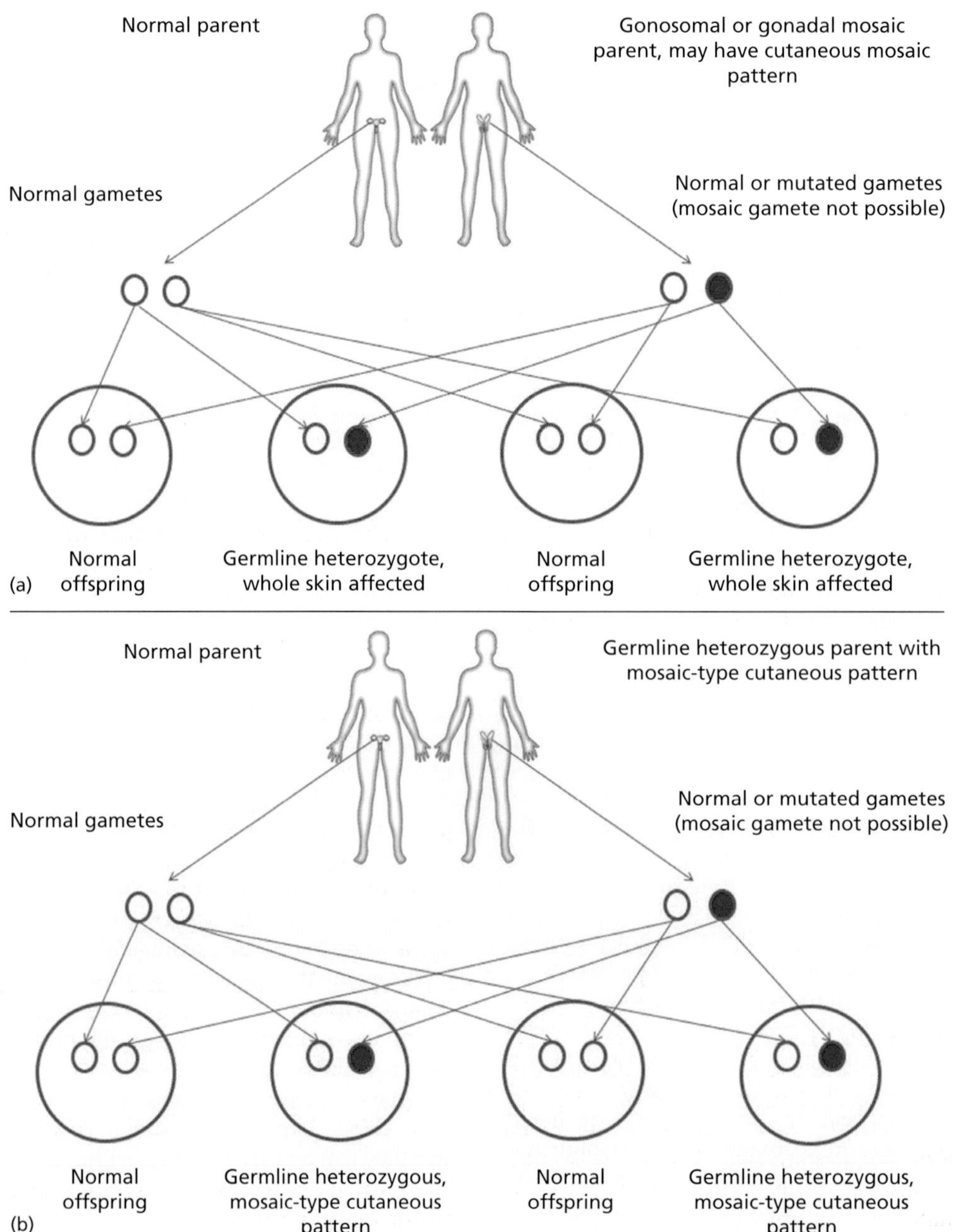

Fig. 104.1 The principles of inheritance of disorders with a mosaic cutaneous pattern. (a) A parent who has gonadal or gonosomal mosaicism can pass on the disorder if it is not lethal to the embryo, but it will then be passed on in a germline heterozygote form. The proportion of germline heterozygote offspring will depend on the proportion of mutated gametes. However, this proportion is not known to be predictable from the extent of the cutaneous mosaicism. Examples of this type of inheritance are mosaic neurofibromatosis type 1 (NF1) leading to germline NF1 in the offspring, or epidermolytic epidermal naevus in a parent leading to germline epidermolytic ichthyosis in the offspring. (b) The inheritance of a cutaneous mosaic pattern means that the disorder must in fact be a germline disorder, but with a mosaic pattern of expression, thus far only known in X-linked dominant disorders such as CHILD (congenital hemidyslasia with ichthhyosiform erythroderma and limb defects) syndrome, or Goltz syndrome.

possible inheritance of individual disorders, and increasingly of individual mutations.

A much more practical classification based on inheritance is therefore between sporadic mosaic disorders, which have not been described as being passed on in a germline state, and mosaic forms of Mendelian disorders which can be. The list of mosaic forms of Mendelian disorders which can be passed on in this way in paediatric dermatology is growing. Classically, it includes mosaic neurofibromatosis type 1 (NF1), which can be passed on as germline NF1 [8–10], or epidermolytic epidermal naevi caused by *KRT1* or *KRT10* mutations which can be passed on in the germline as epidermolytic ichthyosis [11,12]. Recent additions are mosaic dominant dystrophic epidermolysis bullosa [13], and porokeratotic eccrine and ostial dermal duct naevus with the potential to be passed on as keratitis-ichthyosis-deafness (KID) syndrome [14], adding to the list of diagnoses in which it is important to consider screening parents of apparently *de novo* cases [15]. This list will certainly increase over time with better mutation detection methods.

Sporadic mosaic disorders currently make up the majority of known cutaneous mosaic disorders and are, or at least behave as though they are, somatic only. This could be because the mutations truly do not appear in the gametes. However, it could be that mutated gametes do not survive or do not compete well when carrying the mutation, or because the mutation is embryonic lethal when passed on in the germline. The concept of mosaic mutations 'surviving' by mosaicism was proposed by Happle in 1987 [16]; and is strongly supported by the absence of a germline heterozygote state for many of the cutaneous mosaic mutations which have been solved at molecular level [17–22].

It is worth iterating that mosaic abnormalities cannot be passed on in a mosaic form (Fig. 104.1). Where a mosaic-type cutaneous pattern appears in a parent and a child, or in two siblings, this is likely to be a germline condition which has a mosaic pattern (Fig. 104.1b, and see Conditions mimicking mosaicism), or could be a chance occurrence, or theoretically there could be an unknown inherited germline predisposition to somatic mutation in that family.

Genetic mechanisms underlying cutaneous mosaicism

To complement the classification by inheritance potential, a mechanistic classification is useful for understanding the genetic mechanisms of cutaneous mosaicism [15]. This mechanistic classification was begun by Rudolf Happle with type 1 and type 2 (segmental) mosaic disorders [23], where it forms part of a larger classification by cutaneous pattern.

Sporadic mosaic disorders

During embryogenesis a single dominant mutation occurs in a single cell, on the background of an apparently healthy inherited genome, and leads to a cutaneous phenotype in a mosaic pattern (Fig. 104.2a). This is the mechanism responsible for many mosaic disorders in paediatric dermatology. Examples are congenital melanocytic naevus syndrome, Schimmelpenning syndrome, Proteus syndrome, phakomatosis pigmentovascularis and Sturge–Weber syndrome.

Mosaicism in the context of Mendelian disorders

Mosaicism in the context of Mendelian disorders is expressed in two ways. Firstly, a single dominant mutation occurring in a single cell, on the background of a healthy inherited genome, leads to a mosaic manifestation of Mendelian disease. This subset of mosaic disease has been termed type 1 mosaicism by Happle [24]. Secondly, in the context of an inherited heterozygous mutation it is possible for there to be a postzygotic mutation affecting the other (normal) allele (Fig. 104.2b). Usually this relates to inherited/germline autosomal dominant mutations and postzygotic mutations leading to loss of function or actual loss of the normal allele. This presents clinically as a mosaic pattern area of skin with the autosomal dominant phenotype, apparent either congenitally or earlier in life than expected, and/or more severe. This has been termed type 2 segmental mosaicism by Happle [24]. Proof of this mechanism has been demonstrated in various cutaneous conditions including Hailey–Hailey disease [25], Darier disease [26], Cowden syndrome [27], and Gorlin syndrome [28].

It is also possible to have a postzygotic mutation in the normal allele where the individual has a germline heterozygous pathogenic mutation in a gene with an autosomal recessive pattern of expression, leading to a mosaic autosomal recessive phenotype, and this has recently been described in the context of ectodermal dysplasia skin fragility syndrome [29].

Revertant mosaicism

Revertant mosaicism was originally described in autosomal recessive forms of epidermolysis bullosa where both alleles are mutated in the germline, and are loss-of-function. There is then a postzygotic or somatic corrective DNA mutation to one allele [30–33] (Fig. 104.2c). The restoration of function to one allele is enough to rescue the phenotype. Revertant mosaic skin has been hypothesized to be, and being trialled as, a source of cells for culture and grafting back to the patient, in an autonomous cell therapy [34–36].

Revertant mosaicism can also occur with a postzygotic or somatic single allele mutation where there is one autosomal dominant allele mutated in the germline (Fig. 104.2c). This mechanism is responsible for the phenotype of ichthyosis with confetti, an autosomal dominant condition characterized by the progressive appearance of scattered small islands of normal skin. Here somatic mutation (in this case recombination events) leading to loss of the mutant allele leads to phenotypic rescue [37,38].

Conditions mimicking mosaicism

Germline conditions with a mosaic-type cutaneous pattern

Currently all known germline conditions which have a mosaic-type cutaneous pattern are X-linked dominant, are lethal in XY males, and the pattern is caused in females by the normal process of X-inactivation. Where the mutated X chromosome is inactivated the skin is phenotypically normal, and where the normal X is inactivated the skin is affected. The only patterns described so far which can be included in this group are Blaschko-linear, but this is likely only because other patterns are not so easily recognizable as mosaic. Classic examples are incontinentia pigmenti, Goltz syndrome, CHILD (congenital hemidyslasia with ichthhyosiform erythroderma and limb defects) syndrome and Conradi–Hünermann–Happle syndrome.

Chimaerism

Chimaerism is the coexistence of cells with at least two genotypes in one individual who has derived from more than one zygote. Chimaeric individuals can present with

SECTION 23: MOSAIC DISORDERS

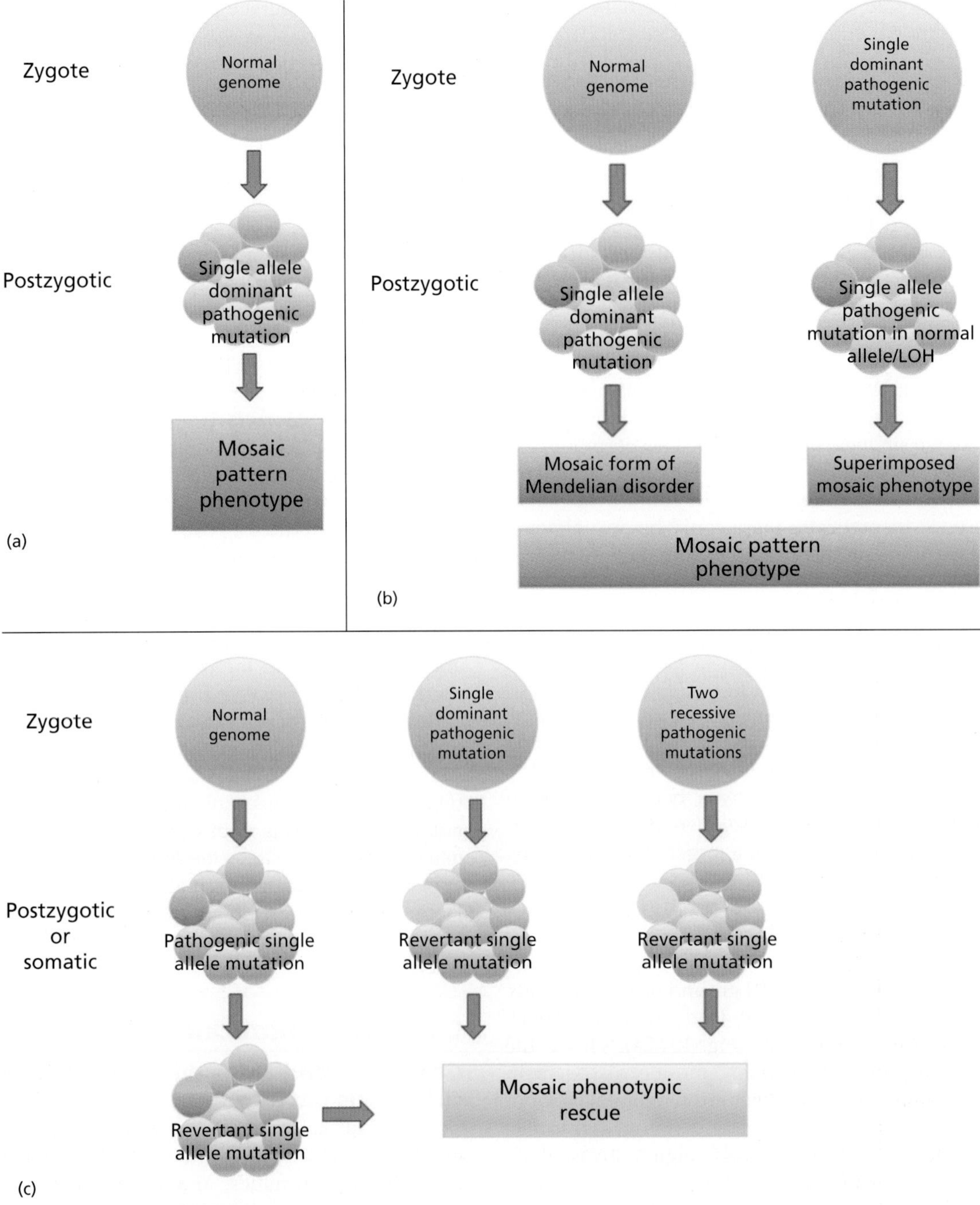

Fig. 104.2 Genetic mechanisms underlying different forms of cutaneous mosaicism. (a) Sporadic mosaic disorders. (b) Mosaicism in the context of Mendelian disorders. (c) Revertant mosaicism.

the same cutaneous appearances as mosaicism [39,40] and as the genetics of individual rare mosaic disorders are not routinely investigated in normal clinical services, it is likely that it is underdiagnosed. Even when investigated, a diagnosis of chimaerism in paediatric dermatology is most likely to be made in the case of fusion of a female and male zygote, with other fusions much less likely to be recognized as chimaeras. In cases of female/male chimaerism it is important to refer the child to clinical genetics and to relevant paediatric services such as endocrinology to assess for other sequelae.

Principles governing the phenotype of mosaic disorders

For a diagrammatic representation see Fig. 104.3.

Timing of the mutation

The timing of a postzygotic mutation is critical to the resultant phenotype. On the simplest level we would expect an identical mutation earlier in embryogenesis to result in a more severe phenotype than the same mutation occurring later in pregnancy. This has been demonstrated

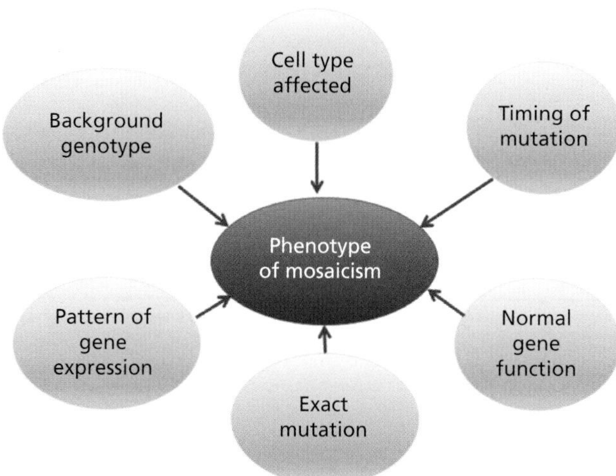

Fig. 104.3 Key factors governing the phenotype of mosaic disorders. These factors are likely to have varying importance in different disorders, and in different individuals, resulting in the wide spectrum of phenotypes in mosaic disorders.

to be correct in conditions such as sebaceous naevi, where the commonest mutation found is responsible for both the common round single sebaceous naevus, and for full-blown Schimmelpenning syndrome where Blaschko-linear sebaceous naevi are associated with neurological, ophthalmological and bony abnormalities [18]. In some conditions the number of skin lesions is related to the chances of extracutaneous complications, almost certainly because of the same reason. For example, single congenital melanocytic naevi are not usually associated with neurological abnormalities whereas two or more can be [41], suggesting that a mutation that can produce two skin lesions is in a precursor cell that could differentiate into or migrate to other organ types.

Cell type affected by the mutation

The cell type affected by the mutation is also crucial in development of the phenotype. This has been proven by the finding of the same mutation in different mosaic disorders, for example one of the mutations leading to Schimmelpenning syndrome – *KRAS* p.G12D – can also cause vascular malformations [42]. The mutations presumably occurred in two different cell types in these cases, although potentially at similar stages of development.

Germline genotype of the affected individual

Germline mutations or variants are known to affect the clinical phenotype of genetically separate germline disorders, for example *MC1R* variants in the germline affect the phenotype of oculocutaneous albinism [43]. This type of phenomenon is thought to be caused by an interaction between *in utero* effects of both changes. Such an interaction has also been shown between germline genotype and a mosaic genotype in the context of congenital melanocytic naevi, where certain *MC1R* variants modify the phenotype resultant from the postzygotic mutation [44]. Furthermore, there is evidence that ethnicity modifies the phenotype of *GNA11/GNAQ* mosaicism [45]. This type of interaction is likely to be extremely common in mosaic disease, and to be responsible for some of the phenotypic variability seen between patients.

Spatial and temporal patterns of gene expression

The normal pattern of expression of the gene involved is important in the phenotypic characteristics of a condition. For example, if a mosaic mutation is present within an organ where a gene is not expressed at all there will be no phenotype in that organ. Similarly, if the mutation occurs during embryogenesis but the gene is not expressed antenatally there will be no congenital phenotype, but there could be a postnatal phenotype if the gene expression is important in that tissue after birth. This phenomenon can be recognized in overgrowth conditions, where for example *PIK3CA*-related overgrowth syndromes present with overgrowth at birth, whereas *AKT1*-related overgrowth as in the Proteus syndrome generally does not develop until after birth [46,47]. This suggests that *PIK3CA* is expressed in tissues involved in growth antenatally more than *AKT1*, or has a more important role at that time.

Specificity of the mutated genotype

In some mosaic disorders there are highly specific genotype–phenotype interactions. For example, the naevus spilus subtype of multiple congenital melanocytic naevi is caused by different missense mutations in the same codon of the gene *NRAS*, when compared with the non-naevus spilus phenotype [48]. In other conditions such as Schimmelpenning syndrome, however, currently indistinguishable phenotypes can be caused by mutations in different genes [18].

Patterns of mosaic disorders

For a diagrammatic representation see Fig. 104.4.

The best-known cutaneous mosaic pattern is Blaschko's lines, first described by Blaschko in 1901 [49], and suggested to be a sign of mosaicism by Jackson in 1976 [50]. The pattern of the lines were detailed on the scalp by Happle in 1984 [51], and suggested to be a visible representation of normal embryological development [52]. Blaschko's original treatise in fact also described some segmental mosaic patterns, not just the famous fine lines. Happle delineated between five and seven patterns he considered to be caused by mosaicism, fine Blaschko-linear, broad Blaschko-linear, chequerboard, phylloid, patchy pattern without midline separation [52], lateralization [53] and sash-like [54,55], six of which have so far been shown to be caused by genetic mosaicism (sash-like being the outstanding seventh). Typical patterns are shown in Fig. 104.4. Other patterns exist, such as multiple small round lesions, as in some cases of congenital melanocytic naevi.

SECTION 23: MOSAIC DISORDERS

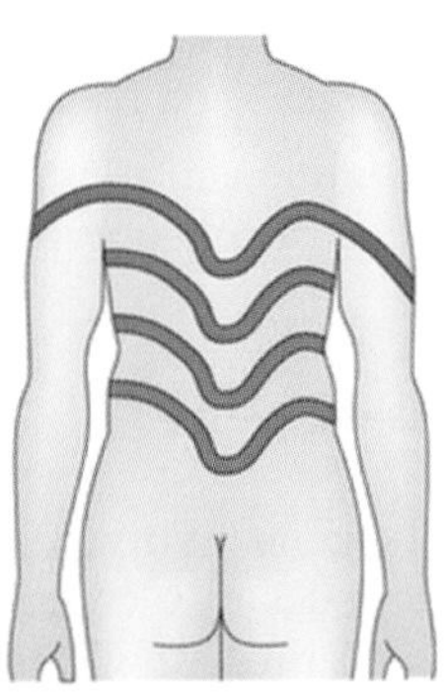
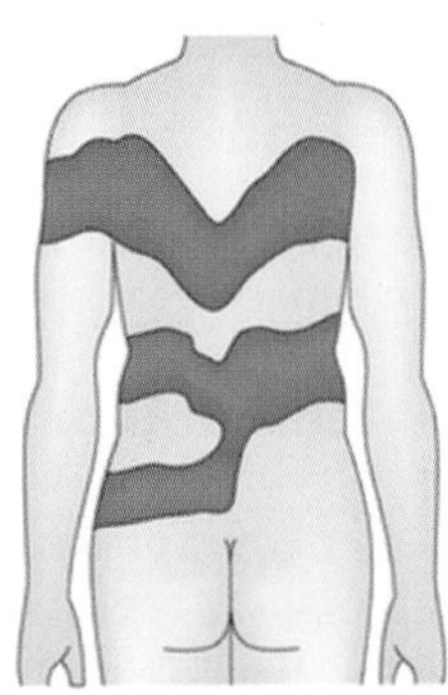
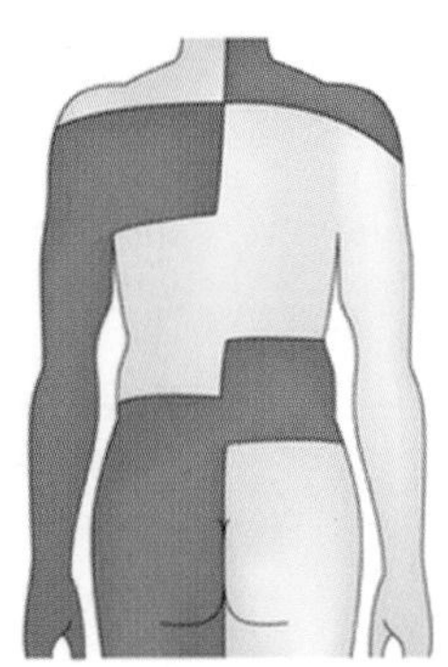
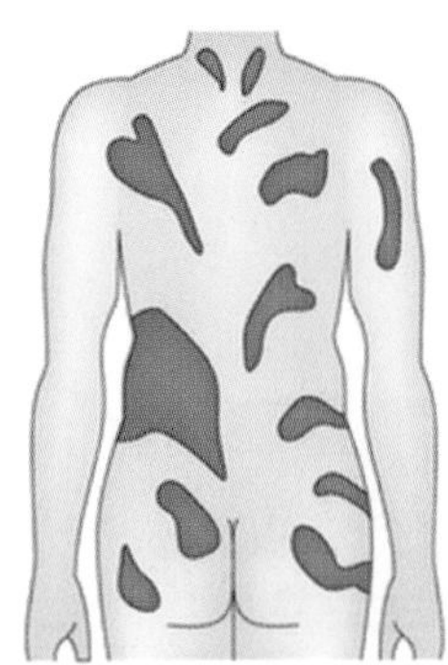
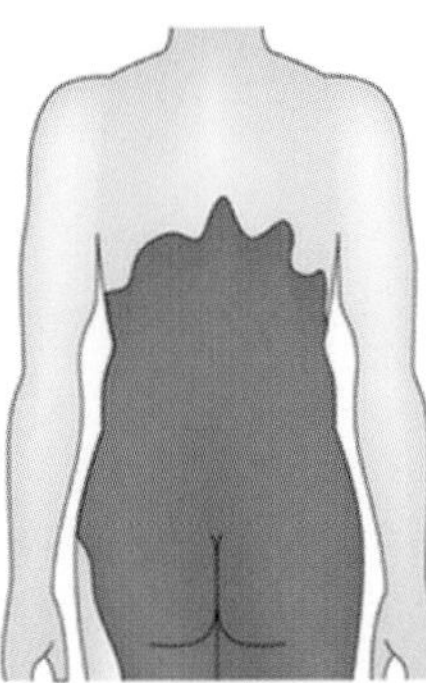

Fig. 104.4 Known patterns of cutaneous mosaic disorders. The original five described patterns of cutaneous mosaicism, from left to right, fine or narrow band lines of Blaschko, broad lines of Blaschko, chequerboard, phylloid, and patchy pattern without midline separation. Source: Adapted from Biesecker and Spinner [57]. Reprinted by permission from Macmillan Publishers Ltd.

Genetic investigation of mosaic disorders

The investigation of mosaic disorders has been revolutionized in recent years with the advent of next generation sequencing and whole genome techniques for detection of copy number changes below the resolution of the traditional karyotype. Key to investigation of mosaic disorders is the sampling and testing of affected cells, and the use of sufficiently sensitive techniques to detect low mutant allele frequencies.

Sampling and testing the right tissue

For germline-inherited disorders that have a mosaic pattern or component only a blood sample is required for testing. For all other mosaic abnormalities, a skin biopsy will be required, and it is worth taking blood for DNA extraction at the same time, because some mosaic mutations will also be present in the blood. If the patient's presentation does not fit with a known diagnosis it is always worth sampling both blood and affected skin, and if possible also taking parental blood, because these can be used as control negatives when trying to identify a new gene in a child.

Blood samples

Blood samples for extraction of DNA from lymphocytes should generally be taken into a vial containing ethylenediaminetetraacetic acid (EDTA), but it is worth checking with the local laboratory on their protocol. For children 5mL of blood is adequate for sufficient DNA to be extracted for all standard tests, but again this may depend on the laboratory's methods. In practice, many laboratories need substantially less than this and if a smaller sample is all that is obtained it is always worth checking whether it is still usable. A blood sample taken in this way is stable at room temperature while it is transferred to the relevant laboratory.

Skin biopsy

If a skin biopsy is to be taken for DNA extraction a 4mm punch is adequate, and it can be sent fresh to the laboratory on a saline-soaked gauze. If DNA cannot be extracted straightaway or is not needed immediately, then the skin biopsy sample can be snap-frozen, or put into a medium which preserves nucleic acids. The sample can then be stored in the freezer until DNA extraction is required.

If requesting either DNA sequencing or copy number analysis then as standard practice DNA should be extracted directly from the biopsy rather than first culturing cells from the sample, and the laboratory needs to be informed of this requirement. The reason for this is that when skin samples are cultured the default cell grown will be fibroblasts, which may or may not carry the mutation. Furthermore, the process of culture can alter genotype. There are conditions, however, where the affected cell type is known, and where culture of that cell type (rather than default fibroblast culture) may assist mutation detection, for example melanocyte culture of the café-au lait macules in McCune–Albright syndrome or mosaic NF1 is performed in some diagnostic laboratories. This requires expertise in the local laboratory.

If requesting tests which require cells to be in a particular stage of the cell cycle, such as for chromosomal mosaicism detection by karyotype, then culture of the biopsy with preservation of whole cells is needed rather than direct DNA extraction.

Formalin-fixed paraffin-embedded tissue

DNA can be extracted from formalin-fixed paraffin-embedded tissue (FFPE) tissue. However, the quantities and quality are generally very low, the DNA is highly fragmented, and the fixation process is known to cause DNA sequencing artefacts [56]. In many cases it is possible to use FFPE extracted DNA to identify specific genotypes, for example for short-read polymerase chain reactions (PCRs) for single hotspots, and it can also be used for some types of next generation sequencing if the samples pass quality control stages, with the caveat that there is a reduction in sensitivity compared with fresh tissue samples, particularly for mosaic disorders.

Choosing the right test

This depends largely on what is available in the local laboratory, but it is good to have an understanding of which test might be most suitable for a particular condition so that a negative result can be viewed within the limitations of the test. For germline disorders which present with a mosaic type pattern then standard Sanger sequencing of lymphocyte DNA is still the test of choice in many laboratories, particularly where there are mutation 'hotspots' associated with that disease (i.e. the whole gene does not need to be sequenced). For mosaic disorders Sanger sequencing is often not sensitive enough and next generation sequencing is the test of choice. With adequate depth a sensitivity down to 1% mutant allele frequency can be provided. Where this is not available, or again where there are well-known mutation 'hotspots', individual laboratories may have worked up other techniques such as touchdown PCR, high-resolution-melt (HRM) PCR, amplification-refractory mutation system (ARMS), restriction-fragment-length polymorphism (RFLP) detection or Cold PCR. These will generally have a detection limit of 1–10% allele frequency, which should be stated on the test report.

References

1 Dorland's Medical Dictionary for Health Consumers. Elsevier, 2007.
2 Laurie CC, Laurie CA, Rice K et al. Detectable clonal mosaicism from birth to old age and its relationship to cancer. Nat Genet 2012;44:642–50.
3 Vattathil S, Scheet P. Extensive hidden genomic mosaicism revealed in normal tissue. Am J Hum Genet 2016;98:571–8.
4 Tomasetti C, Vogelstein B, Parmigiani G. Half or more of the somatic mutations in cancers of self-renewing tissues originate prior to tumor initiation. Proc Natl Acad Sci U S A 2013;110:1999–2004.
5 Forsberg LA, Rasi C, Razzaghian HR et al. Age-related somatic structural changes in the nuclear genome of human blood cells. Am J Hum Genet 2012;90:217–28.
6 Bruder CE, Piotrowski A, Gijsbers AA et al. Phenotypically concordant and discordant monozygotic twins display different DNA copy-number-variation profiles. Am J Hum Genet 2008;82:763–71.
7 Ju YS, Martincorena I, Gerstung M et al. Somatic mutations reveal asymmetric cellular dynamics in the early human embryo. Nature 2017;543:714–18.
8 Tinschert S, Naumann I, Stegmann E et al. Segmental neurofibromatosis is caused by somatic mutation of the neurofibromatosis type 1 (NF1) gene. Eur J Hum Genet 2000;8:455–9.
9 Zlotogora J. Mutations in von Recklinghausen neurofibromatosis: an hypothesis. Am J Med Genet 1993;46:182–4.
10 Rasmussen SA, Colman SD, Ho VT et al. Constitutional and mosaic large NF1 gene deletions in neurofibromatosis type 1. J Med Genet 1998;35:468–71.
11 Paller AS, Syder AJ, Chan YM et al. Genetic and clinical mosaicism in a type of epidermal nevus. N Engl J Med 1994;331:1408–15.
12 Nomura K, Umeki K, Hatayama I, Kuronuma T. Phenotypic heterogeneity in bullous congenital ichthyosiform erythroderma: possible somatic mosaicism for keratin gene mutation in the mildly affected mother of the proband. Arch Dermatol 2001;137:1192–5.
13 van den Akker PC, Pasmooij AM, Meijer R et al. Somatic mosaicism for the COL7A1 mutation p.Gly2034Arg in the unaffected mother of a patient with dystrophic epidermolysis bullosa pruriginosa. Br J Dermatol 2015;172:778–81.
14 Levinsohn JL, McNiff JM, Antaya RJ, Choate KA. A somatic p.G45E GJB2 mutation causing porokeratotic eccrine ostial and dermal duct nevus. JAMA Dermatol 2015;151:638–41.
15 Kinsler VA, Boccara O, Fraitag S et al. Mosaic abnormalities of the skin - review and guidelines from the European Reference Network for rare skin diseases (ERN-Skin). Br J Dermatol 2019;doi: 10.1111/bjd.17924 [epub ahead of print].
16 Happle R. Lethal genes surviving by mosaicism: a possible explanation for sporadic birth defects involving the skin. J Am Acad Dermatol 1987;16:899–906.
17 Kinsler VA, Thomas AC, Ishida M et al. Multiple congenital melanocytic nevi and neurocutaneous melanosis are caused by postzygotic mutations in codon 61 of NRAS. J Invest Dermatol 2013;133:2229–36.
18 Groesser L, Herschberger E, Ruetten A et al. Postzygotic HRAS and KRAS mutations cause nevus sebaceous and Schimmelpenning syndrome. Nat Genet 2012;44:783–7.
19 Groesser L, Herschberger E, Sagrera A et al. Phacomatosis pigmentokeratotica is caused by a postzygotic HRAS mutation in a multipotent progenitor cell. J Invest Dermatol 2013;133:1998–2003;.
20 Lindhurst MJ, Sapp JC, Teer JK et al. A mosaic activating mutation in AKT1 associated with the Proteus syndrome. N Engl J Med 2011;365: 611–19.
21 Thomas AC, Zeng Z, Riviere JB et al. Mosaic activating mutations in GNA11 and GNAQ are associated with phakomatosis pigmentovascularis and extensive dermal melanocytosis. J Invest Dermatol 2016;136:770–8.
22 Shirley MD, Tang H, Gallione CJ et al. Sturge–Weber syndrome and port-wine stains caused by somatic mutation in GNAQ. N Engl J Med 2013;368:1971–9.
23 Happle R. The categories of cutaneous mosaicism: a proposed classification. Am J Med Genet Part A 2016;170:452–9.
24 Happle R. The categories of cutaneous mosaicism: a proposed classification. Am J Med Genet Part A 2016;170A;452–9.
25 Poblete-Gutierrez P, Wiederholt T, Konig A et al. Allelic loss underlies type 2 segmental Hailey–Hailey disease, providing molecular confirmation of a novel genetic concept. J Clin Invest 2004;114:1467–74.
26 Folster-Holst R, Nellen RG, Jensen JM et al. Molecular genetic support for the rule of dichotomy in type 2 segmental Darier disease. Br J Dermatol 2012;166:464–6.
27 Loffeld A, McLellan NJ, Cole T et al. Epidermal naevus in Proteus syndrome showing loss of heterozygosity for an inherited PTEN mutation. Br J Dermatol 2006;154:1194–8.
28 Torrelo A, Hernandez-Martin A, Bueno E et al. Molecular evidence of type 2 mosaicism in Gorlin syndrome. Br J Dermatol 2013;169: 1342–5.
29 Vazquez-Osorio I, Chmel N, Rodriguez-Diaz E et al. (2017). A case of mosaicism in ectodermal dysplasia-skin fragility syndrome. Br J Dermatol 2017;177:e101–2.
30 Schuilenga-Hut PH, Scheffer H, Pas HH et al. Partial revertant mosaicism of keratin 14 in a patient with recessive epidermolysis bullosa simplex. J Invest Dermatol 2002;118:626–30.
31 Jonkman MF, Castellanos Nuijts M, van Essen AJ. Natural repair mechanisms in correcting pathogenic mutations in inherited skin disorders. Clin Exp Dermatol 2003;28: 625–31.
32 Pasmooij AM, Pas HH, Bolling MC, Jonkman MF. Revertant mosaicism in junctional epidermolysis bullosa due to multiple correcting second-site mutations in LAMB3. J Clin Invest 2007;117:1240–8.
33 Kiritsi D, He Y, Pasmooij AM et al. Revertant mosaicism in a human skin fragility disorder results from slipped mispairing and mitotic recombination. J Clin Invest 2012;122:1742–6.
34 Umegaki-Arao N, Pasmooij AM, Itoh M et al. Induced pluripotent stem cells from human revertant keratinocytes for the treatment of epidermolysis bullosa. Sci Transl Med 2014;6:264ra164.
35 Gostynski A, Pasmooij AM, Jonkman MF. Successful therapeutic transplantation of revertant skin in epidermolysis bullosa. J Am Acad Dermatol 2014;70:98–101.
36 Tolar J, McGrath JA, Xia L et al. Patient-specific naturally gene-reverted induced pluripotent stem cells in recessive dystrophic epidermolysis bullosa. J Invest Dermatol 2014;134:1246–54.
37 Choate KA, Lu Y, Zhou J et al. Mitotic recombination in patients with ichthyosis causes reversion of dominant mutations in KRT10. Science 2010;330:94–7.
38 Choate KA, Lu Y, Zhou J et al. Frequent somatic reversion of KRT1 mutations in ichthyosis with confetti. J Clin Invest 2015;125:1703–7.
39 Thomas IT, Frias JL, Cantu ES et al. Association of pigmentary anomalies with chromosomal and genetic mosaicism and chimerism. Am J Hum Genet 1989;45:193–205.
40 Taibjee SM, Bennett DC, Moss C. Abnormal pigmentation in hypomelanosis of Ito and pigmentary mosaicism: the role of pigmentary genes. Br J Dermatol 2004;151:269–82.
41 Kinsler VA, Chong WK, Aylett SE, Atherton DJ. Complications of congenital melanocytic naevi in children: analysis of 16 years' experience and clinical practice. Br J Dermatol 2008;159:907–14.
42 Al-Olabi L, Polubothu S, Dowsett K et al. Mosaic RAS/MAPK variants cause sporadic vascular malformations which respond to targeted therapy. J Clin Invest 2018;128:5185.
43 King RA, Willaert RK, Schmidt RM et al. MC1R mutations modify the classic phenotype of oculocutaneous albinism type 2 (OCA2). Am J Hum Genet 2003;73:638–45.
44 Kinsler VA, Abu-Amero S, Budd P et al. Germline melanocortin-1-receptor genotype is associated with severity of cutaneous phenotype in congenital melanocytic nevi: a role for MC1R in human fetal development. J Invest Dermatol 2012;132:2026–32.
45 Polubothu S, Kinsler VA. The ethnic profile of patients with birthmarks reveals interaction of germline and postzygotic genetics. Br J Dermatol 2017;176:1385–7.
46 Biesecker LG, Happle R, Mulliken JB et al. Proteus syndrome: diagnostic criteria, differential diagnosis, and patient evaluation. Am J Med Genet 1999;84:389–95.

47 Keppler-Noreuil, KM, Sapp JC, Lindhurst MJ et al. Clinical delineation and natural history of the PIK3CA-related overgrowth spectrum. Am J Med Genet Part A 2014;164A: 1713–33.

48 Kinsler VA, Krengel S, Riviere JB et al. Next-generation sequencing of nevus spilus-type congenital melanocytic nevus: exquisite genotype-phenotype correlation in mosaic RASopathies. J Invest Dermatol 2014;134:2658–60.

49 Blaschko A. Die Nervenverteilung in der Haut in ihrer Beziehung zu den Erkrankungen der Haut. In Bericht erstattet dem VII Congress der Deutschen Dermatologischen Gesellschaft. Breslau, 1901

50 Jackson R. The lines of Blaschko: a review and reconsideration: observations of the cause of certain unusual linear conditions of the skin. Br J Dermatol 1976;95:349–60.

51 Happle R, Fuhrmann-Rieger A, Fuhrmann W. [How are the Blaschko lines arranged on the scalp?]. Der Hautarzt; Zeitschrift fur Dermatologie, Venerologie, und verwandte Gebiete 1984;35:366–9.

52 Happle R. Mosaicism in human skin. Understanding the patterns and mechanisms. Arch Dermatol 1993;129:1460–70.

53 Happle R. [Patterns on the skin. New aspects of their embryologic and genetic causes]. Der Hautarzt; Zeitschrift fur Dermatologie, Venerologie, und verwandte Gebiete 2004;55:960–1, 964–8.

54 Ruggieri M, Roggini M, Kennerknecht I et al. Spectrum of skeletal abnormalities in a complex malformation syndrome with "cutis tricolor" (Ruggieri–Happle syndrome). Acta Paediatr 2011;100:121–7.

55 Happle R. Mosaicism in Human Skin. Berlin: Springer-Verlag, 2013.

56 Do H, Dobrovic A. Sequence artifacts in DNA from formalin-fixed tissues: causes and strategies for minimization. Clin Chem 2015;61: 64–71.

57 Biesecker LG, Spinner NB. A genomic view of mosaicism and human disease. Nat Rev Genet 2013;14:307–20.

CHAPTER 105
Melanocytic Naevi

Veronica A. Kinsler

Paediatric Dermatology Department, Great Ormond Street Hospital for Children NHS Foundation Trust, London, UK and Genetics and Genomic Medicine, UCL Great Ormond Street Institute of Child Health, London, UK

Congenital melanocytic naevi, 1237

Acquired melanocytic naevi in childhood, 1252

Abstract

The topic of melanocytic naevi in children incorporates both congenital and acquired melanocytic naevi, as well as other distinct pigment cell naevi such as Spitz, blue, naevus spilus and halo naevi. The presentation and behaviour of such naevi is often very different from that of adult melanocytic naevi, and a good knowledge of paediatric dermatology is required to avoid anxiety over intrinsic differences. In addition, the awareness of the association of some types of melanocytic naevi with extracutaneous abnormalities, and of 'who, how and when' to investigate further, is a key role of the paediatric dermatologist. Major advances in the understanding of the pathogenesis of naevi in the past decade are contributing to management, particularly in those instances where progression to malignancy is suspected.

Key points

- **Small single congenital melanocytic naevi (CMN) are common birthmarks which are not associated with extracutaneous complications and have an extremely low risk of melanoma in childhood.**
- **Multiple CMN is defined as two or more at birth, and these are rare birthmarks which can be associated with extracutaneous complications, and an increased risk of melanoma in certain phenotypic groups.**
- **Risk of all adverse outcomes in multiple CMN is currently most strongly predicted by the outcome of a single screening magnetic resonance image of the central nervous system in the first year of life, rather than by examination of the skin only.**
- **Multiple CMN and CMN syndrome (CMN with extracutaneous complications) is caused by a postzygotic mutation in the gene *NRAS* in 70% of cases.**
- **Acquired melanocytic naevi in childhood do not necessarily conform to the same rules of ABCDE as adult melanocytic naevi, and a 'watch and wait' approach is often appropriate when a naevus has changed, particularly around puberty.**
- **Atypical naevus syndrome can present in childhood or teenage years and should be managed in the same way as for adults.**

Congenital melanocytic naevi

Introduction. A congenital melanocytic naevus (CMN) is a congenital, abnormal but benign collection of naevus cells [1] within the skin, for which the clinical diagnosis is usually straightforward. The term, however, covers a broad spectrum of clinical presentations, ranging from the frequent occurrence of small isolated CMN, to the rare occurrence of extensive or numerous CMN, which can be accompanied by extracutaneous abnormalities. The study of this disease contributes to the understanding of naevogenesis and progression to melanoma, and in particular allows insights into the genetics of this process because of the lack of involvement of ultraviolet radiation in the formation of CMN. There have been substantial advances in the understanding of the pathogenesis and natural behavior of CMN in recent years, and this has begun to contribute to the management of affected children.

Clinical features. Examples of the clinical spectrum of CMN are shown in Fig. 105.1.

Colour and lightening

CMN are usually brown or black in colour, and are usually darkest at birth. In some cases, however, they may appear pink, purple or red in the neonatal period, leading to diagnostic confusion with vascular malformations or other tumours. Large or extensive CMN are often highly heterogeneous in colour. CMN often lighten after birth, occasionally dramatically [2,3], and their final colour is related to the underlying pigmentary phenotype of the patient [4]. In other words, children with fairer skin, experience more lightening of the CMN than those who are more darkly pigmented [4]. This lightening process occurs over a period of years in childhood and then stabilizes.

CMN surface characteristics and benign proliferations

CMN are usually palpable. A useful diagnostic feature for very small lesions which are not palpable is that they will usually have increased skin surface markings. For large or extensive CMN the surface is often heterogeneous [5],

Harper's Textbook of Pediatric Dermatology, Fourth Edition. Edited by Peter Hoeger, Veronica Kinsler and Albert Yan.

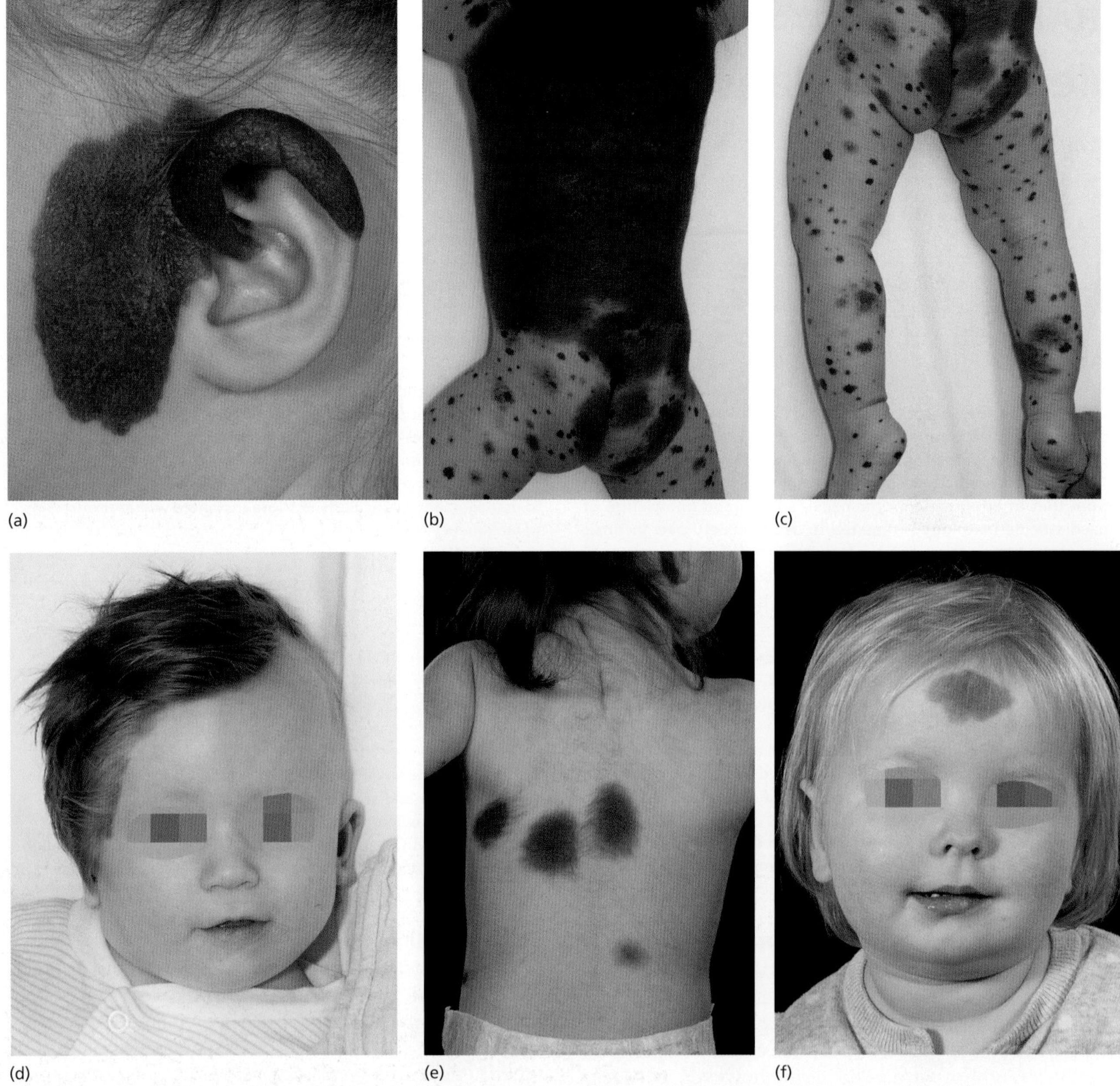

Fig. 105.1 Clinical photographs demonstrating the range of severity of cutaneous phenotype seen in patients with congenital melanocytic naevus (CMN). (a) Single CMN of the ear helix. (b), (c) Multiple CMN in a single patient, with the largest overlying the back. (d) Multiple CMN, with the largest (shown) overlying the scalp and forehead. (e) Multiple medium-sized CMN with no one larger naevus. (f) Single CMN of the forehead.

and nodules or other types of benign proliferation are not an unusual finding. In addition, although localized hypertrichosis is a very common finding in CMN and can occur in all sizes, it is also commoner in larger naevi [5]. For CMN not on the scalp the overlying hair is often not present at birth and can develop later. For CMN on the scalp there is usually thicker, more luxuriant, and more deeply pigmented hair in the affected region at birth. This can persist throughout childhood. However, sometimes the colour of the hair reverts to the surrounding hair tone, and occasionally the hair colour is lighter than on the surrounding scalp. Depigmented hairs within a scalp CMN can start to appear in childhood and can become increasingly common with age. If these are a cosmetic issue they can be dyed individually. Patchy alopecia within scalp CMN can sometimes be evident at birth or can develop later in life.

Benign proliferations arising within a CMN can be present at birth, or can develop thereafter [6,7]. Their appearance can cause anxiety and can cause clinical and histological difficulties in differentiation from melanoma [8]. Many clinical variants of proliferation exist, but two are recurrent and to some extent definable. These can be termed 'classical' proliferative nodules and diffuse neuroid proliferations (Fig. 105.2).

Classic proliferative nodules are well circumscribed, easily visible nodules, which are symmetrical, round or oval, soft to firm, and usually of uniform colour. They are

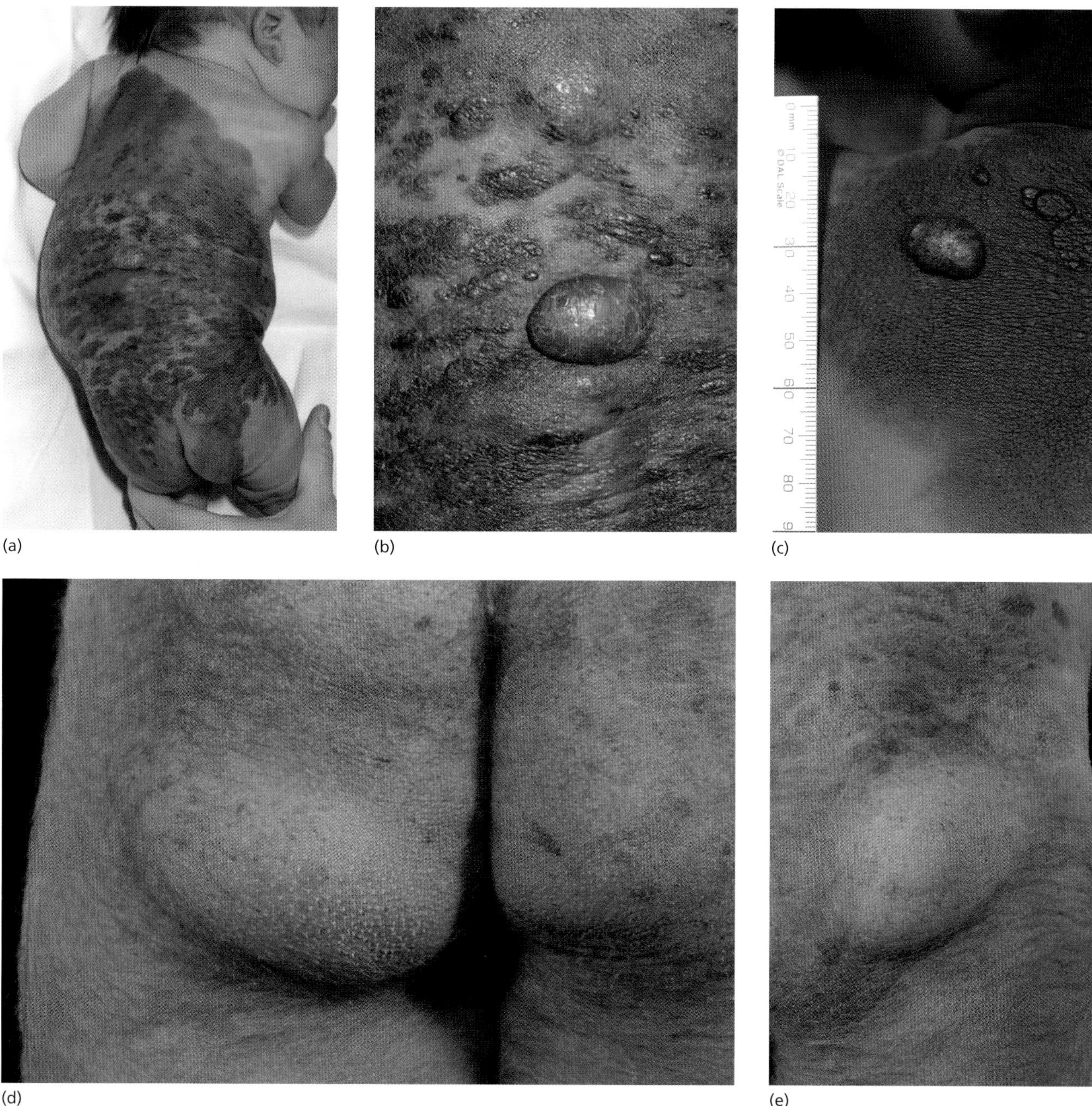

Fig. 105.2 Examples of benign proliferations arising in congenital melanocytic naevus (CMN). (a), (b) Classical proliferative nodule arising in a limb CMN in a single patient. (c) Classical proliferative nodule arising in a CMN on the back. (d), (e) Diffuse neuroid proliferations arising on the buttocks within bathing trunk CMN in two different patients.

usually present at birth. The colour is most often less pigmented than the surrounding CMN, appearing pink or red, but can be the same as the background CMN. They are approximately 0.5 cm to several centimetres in diameter, and if not present at birth are seen to grow over a period of weeks before stabilizing. They commonly catch and bleed, increasing anxiety, but are not usually ulcerated unless traumatized at birth. If polypoid or very prominent they often need to be resected for practical reasons, and are usually easy to remove. They do not usually regrow, and indeed regrowth would be a worrying clinical sign. Management and histology of lumps in a CMN are detailed below.

Diffuse neuroid proliferations are entirely different in clinical appearance. They are not usually present at birth and can develop at any point during childhood. They are slow-growing but may increase in size around puberty. They are characteristically found in the loin areas on the back within bathing trunk CMN, or on the buttocks or genitalia. They are round or more commonly fusiform in gross outline, have poorly defined edges, are soft or firm to touch, never hard, and are the same colour as the surrounding CMN. They are between a few centimetres to up to 20 cm in diameter, and when large they become pendulous. They can be difficult to resect as the margins are indistinct, and frequently regrow after resection, but this is not intrinsically a worrying clinical sign. Histology usually shows neuroid differentiation.

Rarely CMN can be associated with collocated vascular malformations, which from the recent descriptions thus far have been low flow [9,10].

CMN number and satellites

CMN can be single, or multiple, defined as two or more at birth. When multiple they can number hundreds in one individual. Smaller CMN in association with a larger CMN are often termed satellite lesions. This term was probably borrowed from use in melanoma, where a malignant lesion seeds new colonies at its peripheries. In patients with multiple CMN, however, these smaller lesions are usually not geographically connected with the larger naevus, and therefore this term is not ideal [11]. However, developmentally they would have originated from the same parent cell. In children with multiple CMN apparently new naevi can continue to appear after birth, and this process is largely unpredictable. In some individuals it can continue throughout childhood [5]. Families of new babies with multiple CMN should therefore be warned that they may develop new (small) naevi, and that this is not a concerning feature *per se*. In a small number of cases patients have multiple CMN without a main naevus. This can be multiple medium or multiple small CMN, or a mixture.

Phenotypic subtypes

Tardive CMN

A small percentage of CMN are invisible or barely visible at the time of birth. These then appear after birth, developing over a period of a year to approximately 5 years, and eventually appear indistinguishable from a typical CMN. This delayed appearance has led to the name 'tardive' CMN. A tardive component can sometimes be seen in typical CMN present at birth, where a paler area often at the periphery gradually appears as CMN tissue over the first year or so (Fig. 105.3). This has led to the idea that CMN can sometimes 'grow' out of proportion to the child after birth. However, retrospective review of clinical photography from the time of birth usually reveals the pale outline of the tardive component.

Naevus spilus-type CMN

Another subtype which is not fully developed phenotypically at birth is the naevus spilus-type CMN. This subtype has a macular café-au-lait background, with superimposed areas of more typical CMN on top, with or without other melanocytic lesions (Fig. 105.3). The background area is often entirely invisible at birth and can only be inferred by the agmination of the superimposed naevi. It should, however, be anticipated and usually appears over a period of years. Importantly, if the CMN is a naevus spilus-type it is not possible to enumerate the total number of CMN at birth. This is because the associated smaller ('satellite') naevi will also be fundamentally café-au-lait macular in nature, and often do not have superimposed naevi on their surface, at least not initially. They are therefore entirely invisible at birth and will appear only over the first few years. It is safer to assume that there are associated invisible smaller naevus spilus lesions, and manage the patient as multiple CMN, rather than confidently assuming only a single naevus is present, unless this is small.

The superimposed naevi on medium or large CMN are probably subject to the same phenotypic intralesional variability as normal CMN. However, this is more striking in the context of naevus spilus-type because it is easier to see. Often, but not always, there is an extraordinary range of sizes, type and colour of the superimposed lesions, which led to the term 'melanocytic garden' to describe this appearance [12]. They are most commonly a mixture of different sizes and colours, ranging from a millimeter to up to 10 cm. However, in some cases they are much more uniform and in these cases are generally a few millimetres across (very similar to or even the same as the description of naevus spilus papulosus). The causal genotype of these different phenotypes of naevus spilus can be identical [15], and other patient-specific factors must be governing these phenotypic variations.

Neurological abnormalities have not thus far been described with naevus spilus CMN. However, because this is a relatively rare subtype this may just be because of small numbers of published cases. Melanoma arising in naevus spilus-type CMN has been described and has been fatal [17], and management of this subtype should therefore be the same as for more typical CMN. Naevus spilus-type CMN has a subtly different causal genotype from more typical CMN (see Pathogenesis).

Classification. The classification of CMN is performed for two reasons. Firstly, classification for the purposes of research is important to standardize phenotype data collection, because this allows comparison of publications and improves communication between groups of clinicians and researchers. Secondly, classification is performed for the purposes of practical clinical management and the production of management guidelines. In most cases, therefore, only the second classification will be necessary on a day-to-day basis, whilst realizing it is based on the distillation of knowledge from the research classification.

Classification for research, publication and accurate sharing of data

In line with the classification of all types of congenital naevi [19], classification is based on cutaneous features, extracutaneous features and genotype.

Cutaneous features

There have been various suggested classifications of cutaneous phenotype over the last decades, mainly based around the size of the largest naevus and the total number of naevi [13,14]. The most recent published version which builds on these previous systems [16] is shown in outline in Table 105.1 (full details in the reference) and is based on size, site, number and surface characteristics. Of note, the term 'giant' naevus in this type of classification is not

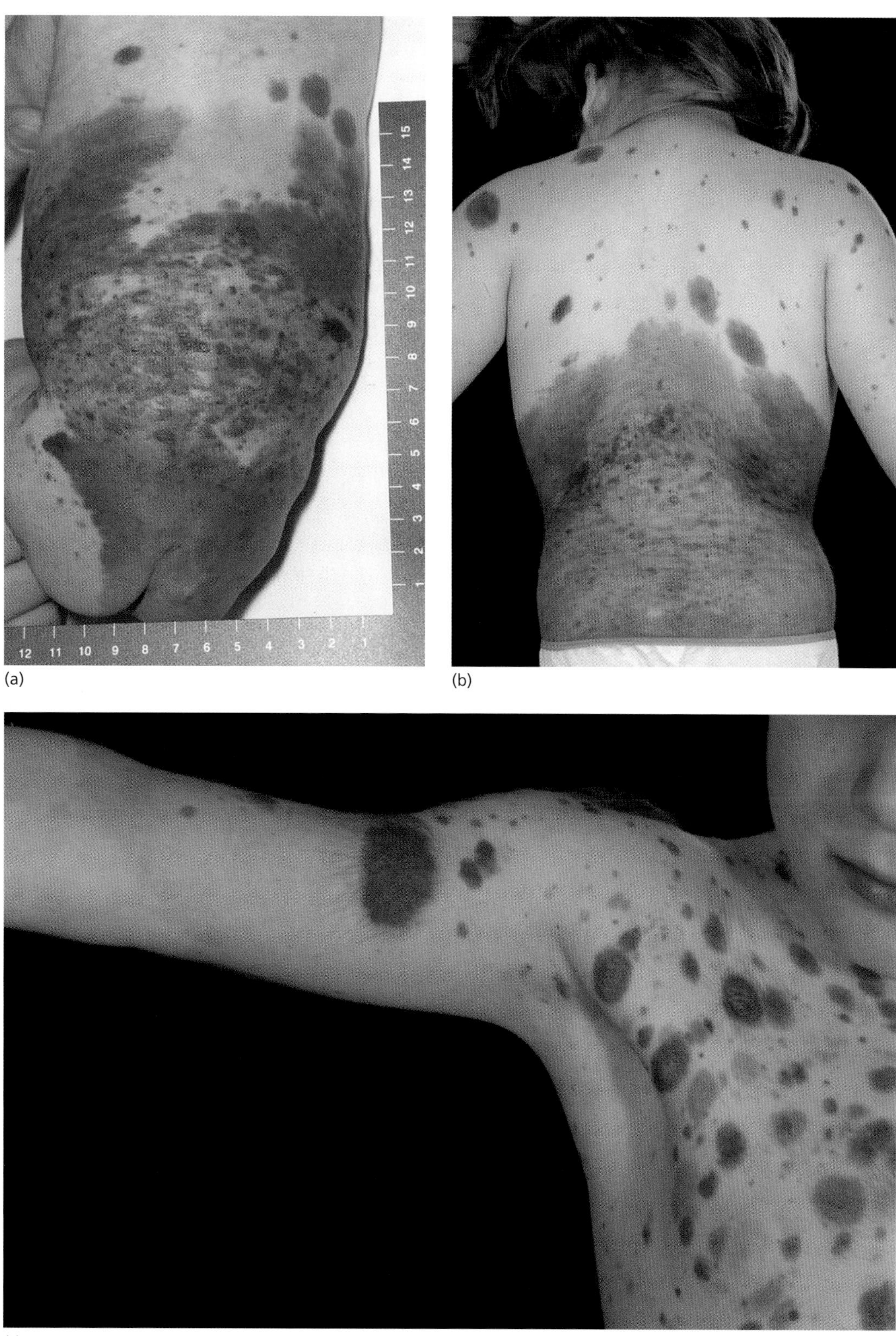

Fig. 105.3 Clinical photographs demonstrating the same child (a) after birth and (b) 5 years later, showing at the upper border of the largest congenital melanocytic naevus (CMN) a tardive area which later becomes pigmented. (c) A naevus spilus type CMN demonstrating the café-au-lait macular background border on the upper arm.

always appreciated by patients and families, particularly when coupled with other older terms such as 'giant hairy naevus', and it is more sensitive to use the terms 'extensive' or 'large' during patient interaction.

One concept which needs some explanation is that of projected adult size. This is an inaccurate and frequently subjective estimate of the size that the largest CMN will be when the individual affected is fully grown. The

Table 105.1 The most recently published cutaneous classification of congenital melanocytic naevus (CMN) for research and publication purposes. Each row is scored using the letter/number codes shown, producing for example, G1/Head/S1/C0/R1/N0/H2. Source: Adapted from Krengel et al. [16]. Reproduced with permission of Elsevier.

Projected adult size of largest CMN	Small (<1.5 cm) Medium (M1) (1.5–10 cm) Medium M2) (>10–20 cm) Large (L1) (>20–30 cm) Large (L2) (>30–40 cm) Giant (G1) (>40–60 cm) Giant (G2) (>60 cm) Multiple medium CMN (three or more medium CMN without an obvious predominant-sized CMN)
Number of 'satellites' (CMN other than the largest)	0 (S0) 1–20 (S1) >20–50 (S2) >50 (S3)
Location of largest CMN	Head Trunk Extremities
Colour heterogeneity of largest CMN	None (C0) Moderate (C1) Marked (C2)
Rugosity of largest CMN	None (R0) Moderate (R1) Marked (R2)
Nodules within largest CMN	None (N0) Moderate (N1) Marked (N2)
Hypertrichosis of largest CMN	None (H0) Moderate (H1) Marked (H2)

limitations of this measurement cannot be overstated. However, it has been demonstrated to be associated with adverse outcome measures in many studies (see later), and even to have a reasonable degree of concordance between observers [18]. It can be measured in two main ways. The first is by multiplying the longest diameter of a CMN by a growth factor for the body part affected, which has most recently been produced in graphical form [16]. The main limitation of this method is that, very frequently, extensive CMN affect more than one body part, which grow at different rates. The second is by drawing the largest CMN on a standard adult body map, and estimating the maximum longitudinal diameter based on average adult height. The main limitation of both these methods is inaccuracy.

Extracutaneous features – CMN syndrome

Other than for small single CMN the classification of the extracutaneous associations is an important part of the full description of phenotype. Where extracutaneous features are present the term CMN syndrome is appropriate [20], in line with the classification of other congenital naevi [19,21]. Known features of CMN syndrome, which will be detailed later, are characteristic facial features, clinical and radiological neurological abnormalities, endocrinological and metabolic abnormalities (including measurement of growth parameters in children), skeletal abnormalities, and the occurrence of malignancy (cutaneous and noncutaneous melanoma, and very occasionally other types).

Genotype

If available, include the mutational status of the *NRAS* gene, and if negative for the *BRAF* gene, for a full classification of CMN (see later for genotyping details).

Classification for practical clinical management

This classification is much more streamlined and is based on published knowledge of which of the previously described phenotypic factors have been demonstrated to be associated with clinical outcome. In other words, this is a classification which allows prognosis and management to be determined. The adverse medical outcomes for patients born with CMN are: (i) clinical abnormalities of neurology or neurodevelopment; (ii) development of melanoma; and (iii) death.

Early studies which associated cutaneous classification variables to abnormalities of neurology or neurodevelopment were retrospective and statistical analysis was often not performed to look for confounding interactions between the clinical variables. One of the early suggestions therefore was that the site of the largest CMN over the head or spine (posterior axial location) was an important factor in determining risk of neurological abnormalities [22]. In more recent analyses, however, site was unconnected to any outcome measure. It is known, however, that the largest naevi are often found over the back, and larger naevi are usually associated with a higher number of total naevi. In statistical modelling where all these variables were included it transpired that projected adult size [17] or total number [23] of naevi were a better indicator of neurological risk than site, and that the largest naevi located in sites such as a limb can just as likely be associated with neurological problems if the size or number was high [24]. When both size and number of naevi were combined, projected adult size was the more significant variable [7,25]. In essence, however, increasing size is correlated to increasing number, so the two variables confound each other. Other cutaneous phenotypic variables (e.g. rugosity, hairiness, nodularity) have not yet been shown to be associated with any outcome measures.

Thereafter, neuroradiological phenotyping was added as a variable when modelling adverse outcome measures. Seminal work in the 1990s demonstrated a characteristic signal for melanin on magnetic resonance imaging (MRI) [26], and studies of children with CMN delineated the characteristic features of congenital melanocytic disease [27]. A large prospective study which combined the neuroradiological results of a single screening MRI of the central nervous system (CNS) in the first year of life with the clinical phenotyping variables listed previously, showed that an abnormal MRI is more strongly associated with clinical abnormalities in neurology (seizures) and neurodevelopment, and with the development of any-site melanoma [28]. The MRI result was also correlated with risk of death, as might be expected [25]. However, the

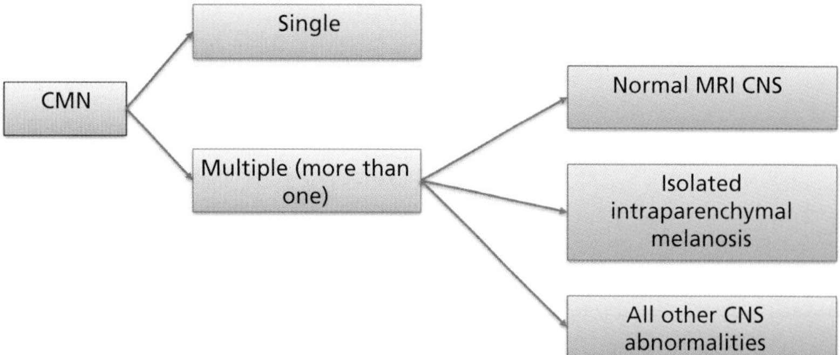

Fig. 105.4 Practical classification of patients with congenital melanocytic naevus for use in clinic. This classification alters the resultant clinical management.

number of patients who died in this cohort was too small to be adequately powered.

Amalgamating this knowledge we can say that for the purposes of determining clinical outcome for new babies with CMN, the key decision in clinic is whether or not to perform an MRI. Critically, individuals with a single CMN at birth (independent of size or site) who do not have another concurrent diagnosis have not so far been described as having radiological neurological abnormalities, or serious neurodevelopmental abnormalities, whereas children with two CMN at birth have rarely been described with neurological abnormalities after a MRI scan [17]. Although two CMN at birth can therefore be seen as an arbitrary cut-off for performing a scan, it is at the moment the only cut-off with any evidence base, and serves therefore as a guideline for management. In addition, there are theoretical reasons for a clinical difference between a single CMN at birth and two CMN, in that two distinct CMN generated from a single cell mutation (as is known to be the case) may imply that the cell still had embryonic migratory potential and could therefore also be a neural precursor. As with all guidelines, however, this can be interpreted by clinicians as they see fit on an individual basis.

For practical classification in clinic, individuals with CMN can be divided into two groups: (i) single CMN (of any size or site) who do not routinely need an MRI of the CNS; and (ii) multiple CMN (two or more at birth of any size or site) who do, and thereafter they are classified on the basis of their neuroradiological phenotype. This practical classification is shown in Fig. 105.4.

Epidemiology. The incidence of CMN varies with the severity of the cutaneous phenotype. The incidence of single small CMN has been found consistently to be 1–2% [29–31]. The incidence of CMN of greater than 20 cm projected adult size in one study was one in 20 000 births (0.005%) [32]. However, there was only one positive case in this cohort. The incidences of multiple CMN and CMN syndrome have not been studied; for multiple CMN the incidence is likely to lie somewhere between these figures.

Most epidemiological data on CMN show a slightly increased number of affected females to males, with a ratio of 1.2 : 1 [4,33,34]. However, no difference was found in one large prospective study [32]. The incidence of small CMN in all ethnic groups studied so far appears to be similar, and CMN can be seen in all ethnic groups. A small increase in incidence in infants of Black African descent was suggested on analysis in the large prospective study [32].

Associations. The cutaneous findings of CMN can be associated with a variety of extracutaneous features and malignancy.

Neurological

Neurological abnormalities in the context of CMN were first described by Rokitansky in 1861 at postmortem [35]. This led to the term 'neurocutaneous melanosis' to describe the coexistence of cutaneous and CNS melanocytic disease, which was later defined by Kadonaga and Frieden [36]. However, with the advent of MRI screening of neurologically asymptomatic children it became apparent that CNS disease in CMN patients could take a wide variety of forms both radiologically and clinically [22,26,27,37,38], and it has taken large prospective cohorts and new genetic techniques to dissect the situation fully.

What is now understood is that CNS disease in this condition is highly analogous to the cutaneous disease – in the skin there are benign congenital naevi at birth, and it is possible to develop cutaneous melanoma; in the CNS there can be benign congenital CNS lesions, and it is possible to develop CNS melanoma. It is crucial to differentiate between the benign congenital and the acquired malignant CNS disease, rather than placing both of these under the same heading of 'neurocutaneous melanosis'. A previous attempt to differentiate was by using the terms 'asymptomatic' and 'symptomatic' neurocutaneous melanosis [36], with multiple papers recycling the message that symptomatic neurocutaneous melanosis was associated with death. However, this is not sufficiently accurate because many patients are symptomatic from their benign congenital CNS disease (with seizures or neurodevelopmental delay) but do not have a reduced life expectancy. A further reason for limiting the use of the term neurocutaneous melanosis is that a substantial number of the congenital CNS abnormalities are not melanotic. For these reasons, and because of the other more recently described associations of CMN described later, the term 'CMN syndrome' is preferable to neurocutaneous melanosis when describing the association of CMN and any congenital benign neurological disease, with primary CNS melanoma being used for malignant CNS disease.

Congenital disease of the CNS in individuals with CMN is caused by the same mutation which leads to the CMN itself [39]. This type of disease has not thus far been described in individuals with a single CMN, and therefore all types of congenital CNS disease described here are seen only in the context of multiple CMN. A recent long-term prospective cohort study was able to classify the findings on MRI and relate these to clinical outcome measures [25]. This has resulted in differential management strategies depending on the MRI findings. It has also reinforced the previously published guidelines that all children with multiple CMN at birth (two or more, independent of size or site), should have a single screening MRI of the whole CNS with gadolinium contrast, under the age of 6 months if possible [17,25]. Children with a single CMN (independent of size or site) are not recommended to have a routine scan assuming they are well neurologically.

Intraparenchymal melanosis

Isolated intraparenchymal melanosis is the commonest type of congenital CNS disease in CMN syndrome [26,27], occurring in approximately 20% of cases in one large prospectively collected cohort of patients with multiple CMN [22]. Intraparenchymal melanosis is the presence of collections of melanin-containing cells within the parenchyma of the brain, and is identifiable on MRI by characteristic hyperintensity on T1 weighting [26]. These cell collections are by far most commonly seen in the temporal lobes, particularly in the amygdala [17,26,27]. However, they can also be seen in the brainstem, the cerebellum and the cerebral cortex. Histology of these lesions reveal that there is not only melanin but melanosomes within these cells, and that the cells are neurons and astrocytes, not naevus cells. There can also be subtle associated cortical dysplasia [40,41]. Interestingly, histological evidence has revealed that foci are not necessarily visible on MRI [42], presumably because small collections are below current levels of imaging resolution. Importantly, however, intraparenchymal melanosis is diagnosed on the basis of the MRI findings, and does not need a biopsy to confirm it. Children with this finding on MRI do have an increased risk of neurodevelopmental abnormalities and seizures. However, importantly, they do not have an increased risk of melanoma in childhood (cutaneous or CNS primary) compared with children with a normal MRI [25]. As a result, this finding in a newborn should trigger a referral for paediatric neurodevelopmental assessment, to pick up on and address any neurodevelopmental issues that arise. The MRI does not need to be repeated routinely, because these lesions are usually clinically stable, and a recent small study of repeated scans demonstrated a diminution of intraparenchymal melanosis over time in most cases [43]. However, it is known that the signal for melanin can be obscured by increasing CNS myelination in early childhood.

Other abnormalities of the CNS

Many of the individuals described in the literature who fall under this heading have unique presentations and so it is important to treat each case individually. In general, however, although these 'other' abnormalities of the CNS are much less common than isolated intraparenchymal melanosis, as a group they have a much higher incidence of serious adverse outcomes [25,28,44] and are therefore important to identify. This group often have intraparenchymal melanosis as part of their MRI findings, but it is associated with other features such as leptomeningeal disease (diffuse or focal), hydrocephalus, benign tumours, Dandy–Walker malformation, Arnold–Chiari malformation, or spinal syrinx [17,44–46]. Repeat MRI is often required to assess the stability or behaviour of these cases, and all children in this group should be looked after in a multidisciplinary team setting, with input as required from paediatric neurology and neurosurgery specialists. In particular diffuse leptomeningeal melanocytosis is always a concerning finding [25,36,44], because the vast majority of these cases are, or become, leptomeningeal melanoma [47]. Diffuse leptomeningeal melanocytosis manifests radiologically as thickening/enhancement of the leptomeninges surrounding the brain, spine and ventricles, and manifests clinically as hydrocephalus in a baby, or raised intracranial pressure in an older child. Of note, a clinical presentation of hydrocephalus in a child with multiple CMN should be assumed to be caused by diffuse leptomeningeal melanocytosis or melanoma even if the initial MRI is normal. Gadolinium enhancement increases the pick-up rate of leptomeningeal disease, but if negative the scan should be repeated within a few weeks.

Unfortunately, there are as yet no clear cutaneous phenotyping features at birth which discriminate these children with complex congenital neurological disease from those with normal MRI or isolated intraparenchymal melanosis, hence the current recommendation to screen all children with multiple CMN (two or more) in the first year of life and preferably within the first 6 months. During childhood as a group they have a high requirement for neurosurgery, more serious neurodevelopmental abnormalities and seizures, and a higher risk of melanoma. Primary CNS melanoma appears to be the most common type in children generally, and is much more common in this group than in any other MRI result group [25,28].

Facial

Children with CMN often have characteristic facial features [20]. This has so far only been studied in a White Caucasian population because of the difficulties in standardization of morphological facial characteristics across different ethnic groups. The characteristic features were ascertained in comparison with a large control cohort using standardized definitions of facial morphological terms; three or more features were found in 70% of the cohort studied. The commonest facial features are wide or prominent forehead, hypertelorism, eyebrow variants, periorbital fullness, small/short nose, narrow nasal ridge, broad nasal tip, broad or round face, full cheeks, prominent premaxilla, prominent/long philtrum and everted lower lip [20]. There was no relationship found between facial features and cutaneous or neurological phenotype.

Characteristic facial features are likely to result from the influence of the *NRAS* mutation on the embryonic development of the bones and cartilage of the face. Inherited mutations in *NRAS* and other RAS-pathway genes are known to affect facial development [48]. In addition, there are increasing numbers of mosaic syndromes known to have characteristic facial features, including Cornelia de Lange syndrome [49] and Pallister–Killian syndrome [50].

Endocrinological and metabolic

Disorders of these systems are quite common in the germline RASopathies, implying that the RAS signalling pathway is involved in postnatal endocrinological and metabolic pathways. These features are newly described associations of CMN in one large childhood cohort [51]. Unsurprisingly for a mosaic disorder the presentation of endocrinological and metabolic abnormalities can vary substantially between individuals. However, when the cohort was examined as a whole it was clear that prenatal growth was normal, but there was a tendency to gain weight in childhood, which was a gain of adiposity rather than lean or bone mass. The tendency to weight gain was significantly more than contemporary statistics for the general childhood population, and was associated with indicators of insulin resistance [51]. The cause of weight gain or the relationship with insulin resistance are not yet known and could be connected to environmental as well as genetic factors. It is, however, clinically relevant to monitor growth parameters in children with CMN, and to start appropriate dietary and exercise interventions as for all overweight individuals. These interventions appear to be generally effective.

Other clinical abnormalities which can present in these systems are premature thelarche variant in girls, undescended testes in boys and localized underdevelopment of fat and/or muscle underneath large or extensive CMN. Measurement of anterior pituitary hormones often demonstrate subtle abnormalities of G-protein coupled receptor hormones, most typically marked suppression of luteinizing hormone (LH) [51]. These findings may be related to the clinical features seen, but do not seem to have a long-term effect on progression to puberty, or anecdotally to fertility.

Metabolic bone disease caused by a FGF23-associated phosphaturic state is a complication much more commonly seen with epidermal naevus syndromes [52,53], and has recently been termed cutaneous skeletal hypophosphataemia syndrome [54,55]. It has been only described in two cases of CMN syndrome thus far, and in both there was a co-occurring epidermal naevus [56,57]. *NRAS* mutations have not yet been tested for in the bone itself of the two affected patients. Because it is exceptionally rare in CMN, a suggested guideline would be that if an epidermal naevus is also present in patients with CMN, or if there is a clinical presentation of bone disease, a metabolic bone profile should be performed on blood and urine. Subsequent management guidelines have been proposed [54].

Melanoma in CMN

Primary melanoma of the CNS

The study of melanoma in CMN is hampered by the rarity of the occurrence, because the overall incidence in the skin or CNS is around 1–2% in childhood across all cutaneous phenotypes. Cutaneous melanoma has historically been considered to be more common than primary CNS melanoma, but this is likely to have been confounded by the use of the term neurocutaneous melanosis for both benign and malignant CNS disease. CNS melanoma is, in fact, overrepresented in children with complex congenital neurological disease on MRI, and very rare in those without [25]. Primary melanoma can arise either within the brain parenchyma, or more commonly within the leptomeninges in individuals with multiple CMN. An abnormal MRI has been shown to be the most significant predictor of all-site melanoma [28]. However, the numbers are still small and more data will be analysed over time. It is not clear why this association exists, but it is likely either to be caused by the number or presence of melanocytic cells in the CNS leading to increased risk of malignant transformation, or more likely because the congenital neurological abnormalities are reflective of a more aggressive phenotype in general.

Importantly, independent of what the screening MRI shows, any child with CMN who presents with new neurological signs or symptoms at any age should have a full history and examination. Clinicians should have a low threshold for repeating an MRI of the whole CNS with gadolinium contrast. Symptoms of primary CNS melanoma at presentation are typically raised intracranial pressure and/or a focal space-occupying lesion (e.g. seizures). Neuroradiologists should be alerted to look for: (i) communicating hydrocephalus without an apparent tumour – this is typically diffuse leptomeningeal disease which may not be visible initially; (ii) leptomeningeal enhancement or thickening; (iii) a new space-occupying lesion compared with the early screening scan, or if no screening scan is available intraparenchymal melanoma can be distinguished from intraparenchymal melanosis by typical radiological features [58,59]. Sometimes a parenchymal space-occupying lesion can also be accompanied by leptomeningeal disease, and the two may be in communication or may be separate [25,44,60]. In suspected CNS melanoma, a CNS biopsy should be performed for both histopathology and genetic studies. Copy number measurement by whole genome array comparative genetic hybridization (CGH), SNP array, exome sequencing, or fluorescent *in-situ* hybridization (FISH), is very useful in distinguishing benign from malignant CNS disease in addition to histology [28,61,62]. Karyotyping or RNAseq would be required to look for translocations if so wished.

Other tumours in CMN

Rhabdomyosarcoma (RMS) is the most commonly described non-melanoma tumour to arise within a CMN [63–66]. Genetic studies on these tumours in CMN patients have so far not been published. It is likely that *NRAS* hotspot mutations could be a driver mutation for

SECTION 23: MOSAIC DISORDERS

RMS in this context, because RAS mutations (and including in *NRAS)* have been found in RMS when not in the context of CMN [67]. Very rarely non-melanoma primary CNS tumours arise in children with CMN, for example astrocytoma, meningioma and ependymoma [17,25].

Histopathology. In general terms it is important to involve a specialist dermatopathologist in the interpretation of biopsies from CMN, particularly where there is a query of malignancy, because histology of these lesions can be very difficult. The pathology of CMN varies with the size of the lesion and can vary also with age. Smaller naevi are more commonly junctional, whereas larger or extensive CMN are often dermal with a Grenz zone of separation in the papillary dermis or compound. CMN typically show nesting of bland melanocytes. However, in undifferentiated areas of large or extensive naevi, nesting is not seen. Naevus cells typically extend around and into the adnexae and blood vessels and can also be seen in underlying muscle and fat. There is generally no cytological atypia, and the mitotic index is low (<1%). Melanocyte morphology classically varies with depth, sometimes termed 'maturation with depth'. However, the more superficial cells are in fact more differentiated towards the melanocyte lineage, being more spindle-shaped or ovoid in the deep dermis, and non-pigmented (Fig. 105.5), and this concept has therefore been challenged.

Histology of benign proliferative nodules can be difficult to differentiate from melanoma, because very occasionally these proliferations have a high mitotic index. They are, however, generally very well circumscribed, with no signs of infiltration, and little or no cellular atypia. Melanoma on the other hand is identified by poorly circumscribed, infiltrating proliferations sometimes with focal necrosis, and cells demonstrate marked atypia with a high mitotic index (Fig. 105.6).

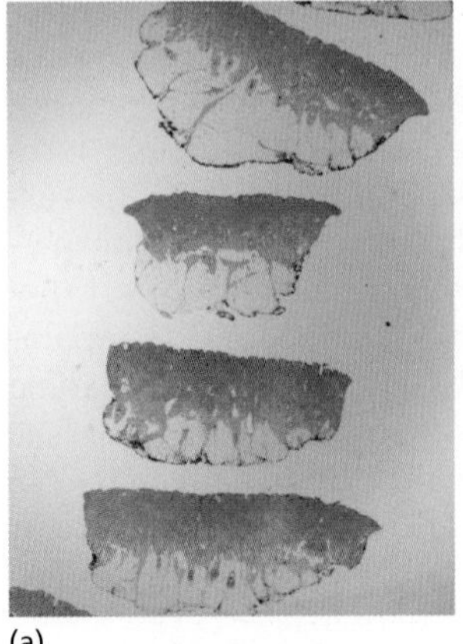

(a)

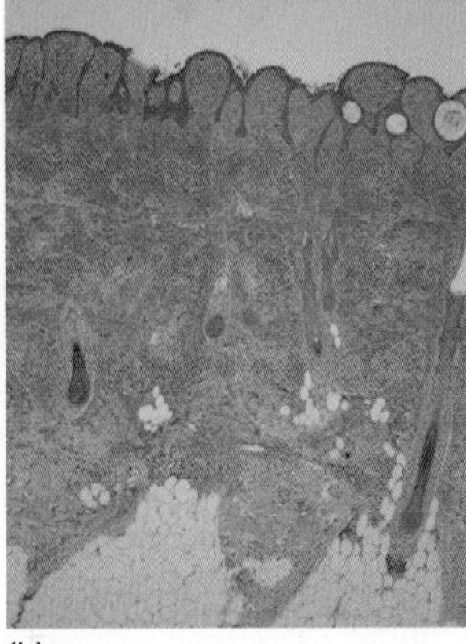

(b)

Fig. 105.5 Photomicrographs of a typical congenital melanocytic naevus demonstrating a predominantly dermal lesion composed of bland naevus cells that extend around adnexal structures with no cytological atypia. Original magnifications (a) ×20 and (b) ×40 (H&E).Source: Kinsler and Sebire 2016 [19]. Reproduced with permission of John Wiley & Sons and courtesy of Professor N. J. Sebire.

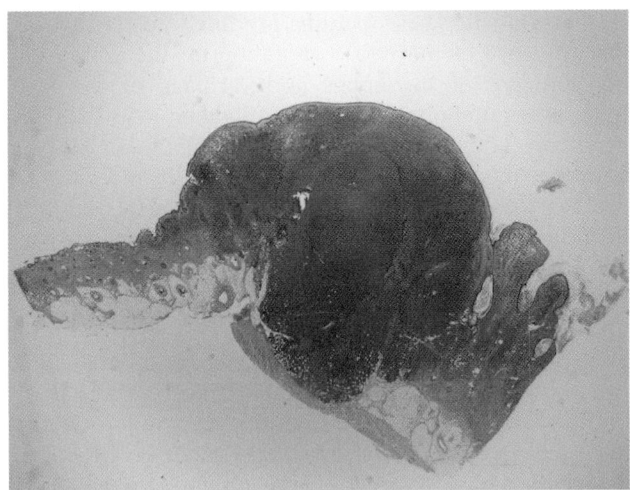

Fig. 105.6 Photomicrograph of a melanoma developing within a congenital melanocytic naevus demonstrating a proliferative subpopulation, which infiltrates widely and distorts the surrounding architecture, associated with cytological atypia. Original magnification ×20 (H&E). Source: Kinsler and Sebire 2016 [19]. Reproduced with permission of John Wiley & Sons and courtesy of Professor N. J. Sebire.

It is not yet clear which cell type naevus cells derive from embryologically, or what they were destined to be before they were mutated [1,68–72]. Many dermal CMN have a normal overlying population of dermal–epidermal junctional melanocytes [73], suggesting perhaps that they were not destined for that fate. Proposed candidate cell types include mature melanocytes, immature melanocytes, neural crest stem cells and dermal or melanocyte stem cells [73–78].

Pathogenesis. Environmental factors have not been shown to be important in the development of CMN. A large retrospective questionnaire study looked at potential environmental factors during pregnancy of mothers who had children with CMN, as compared with a control cohort [5]. Smoking during pregnancy appeared to be associated with a small excess risk. However, medications, radiography, alcohol, sunbed use, maternal infections and anaesthetics were not found to be different. Significantly more common in the CMN mothers were threatened miscarriage, severe nausea or vomiting and raised blood pressure [5]. Whether these factors are the cause or effect of the mutation, or due to a common independent factor is not known.

CMN are caused by a postzygotic mutation leading to mosaicism. In line with the principles outlined in Chapter 104, a likely explanation for a single rather than multiple CMN phenotype is that the mutation probably occurs later in development, at a time when the cells are already fate-determined and destined for one area of skin. A mutation is assumed to be the cause of the phenotype if it is found in more than one physically distinct lesion (cutaneous or extracutaneous). Multiple CMN and CMN syndrome was found to be caused in approximately 70–80% of cases because of postzygotic mutations in the gene *NRAS* [39]. Mutations in *NRAS* had been previously described in individual samples of CMN [80–85], along with mutations in *BRAF* [80,81,86–90], *MC1R* [80,91], *TP53* [80] and *GNAQ* [84]. However, there were no data as to causality at this stage, and the disease was considered to be of unknown cause. In the delineation of postzygotic mosaicism two different missense mutations were found to lead to an amino acid change at codon 61 (p.Q61K is the commonest and p.Q61R less frequent). Within any one patient the same mutation was found in different affected tissues, both in naevi or CNS abnormalities, and was not detectable in blood or unaffected skin or CNS tissue [39]. *NRAS* mutations were absent from a proportion of cases in two studies [39,90], indicating that there were other genes as yet unidentified which lead to a very similar phenotype. In another study, however, *NRAS* mutations were found in all samples analysed [92]. Naevus spilus-type CMN has a subtly different genotype, being caused by different *NRAS* missense mutations. The commonest of these [15] causes a p.Q61H amino acid change, with p.G13R and p.Q61L [15,93] also described in single patients. The codon 61 hotspot is also the driver mutation responsible in 15–20% of nonsyndromic melanoma [94], and is known to lead to constitutive activation of the *NRAS* GTPase and downstream signalling pathways.

Subsequently, *BRAF* mutations have been described as a second and rare cause of multiple CMN/CMN syndrome, leading to the classic melanoma amino acid change p.V600E [10]. In this case, a nodular phenotype within the largest CMN were described [10]. *BRAF* mutations had also previously been described in single samples of CMN [80,81,86–90], including from patients with multiple CMN, but causality had not been proven. In a large genotype-phenotype cohort study, *BRAF* was found in 7% of cases, implying that it is a rare but important cause, and a distinct multinodular phenotype was again described clinically and histologically in the majority of these [79]. Importantly, the same study did not highlight any differences in clinical outcome measures between *NRAS*, *BRAF*, and double wild-type patients, and routine genotyping is not therefore required for standard day to day management. Genotyping for *NRAS* and *BRAF* should, however, be undertaken in cases of suspected malignancy because it directs therapy [95,96].

Single patients have been described with potentially causative gene fusions in multiple CMN, one *ZEB2-ALK* and one *SOX5-RAF1* [97]. Whether these are recurrent causes of CMN is not yet known. The patterns of CMN have recently been evaluated with an embryological perspective, which may lead to insights into pathogenesis [72].

Potential germline predisposition

Despite the fact that the ultimate cause of CMN is a postzygotic mutation, a family history of CMN (of any size) in a first or second degree relative has been found in 25–30% of cases in one UK cohort [98,99]. This is more than expected statistically, because the incidence of small single CMN is approximately 1%. One germline genetic factor has been identified in this cohort as being associated with CMN and linked to the positive family history. This is an enrichment of familial variants in the gene responsible for red hair, *MC1R*, with an increase in compound heterozygosity and homozygosity in children with CMN compared with controls [91]. This again mirrors the genetics of nonsyndromic melanoma, and suggests that CMN may be a good genetic model for some types of melanoma. There are very likely to be other predisposing genetic influences, which may be different in different ethnic groups.

Genetic testing.

In the absence of malignancy

Currently genetic testing in CMN in the absence of suspected malignancy does not alter management, and there is no current clinical need for it [4]. Patients and families are, however, increasingly interested to know the genotype of their naevi, and subtyping of the phenotype in this way is likely to prove useful from a clinical research perspective. In particular, there appears to be an increase in nodularity in non-*NRAS* mutant CMN, including a specific phenotypic and histological type in *BRAF*-mutant CMN [10,79,100]. A punch biopsy can be taken from a single representative naevus, or from a naevus removed for cosmetic reasons. DNA should be extracted directly from the skin rather than from fibroblast culture, because the mutation may not be present outside naevus cells. *NRAS* mutations should be looked for using sensitive laboratory techniques appropriate for mosaic disorders (see Chapter 109). If wildtype at *NRAS*, *BRAF* p.V600E mutations can also be screened for [10].

In suspected malignancy

Genetic testing in suspected cutaneous or neurological malignancy should be performed where at all possible. This is because management in melanoma is now framed in the context of which driver mutations are present, and because copy number analysis is highly correlated with lesion behaviour in the skin and in the CNS. Clinically relevant tests divide into driver mutation genotyping and copy number measurement.

Driver mutation genotyping is currently for *NRAS* and *BRAF* hotspots. This is widely available in diagnostic laboratories for other cancers, and the required techniques are the same. Fresh tissue is always preferred. However, hotspot genotyping can be performed on formalin-fixed paraffin-embedded tissue.

If heterozygosity for *NRAS* codon 61 mutations is found in the suspected melanoma, this does not assign the lesion as benign or malignant (because these mutations are found in most CMN). However, it does inform medical management. In particular, *BRAF* inhibitors are contraindicated in *NRAS*-mutated melanoma caused by the paradoxical activation effects of these drugs in that context [101,102], and MEK inhibition is a possible therapy [28,103–106]. Homozygosity for *NRAS* codon 61 mutations has been described in one case of melanoma arising in a CMN, and in the context of a heterozygous CMN this may be suggestive of malignant progression [39]. Although no cases of melanoma arising in *BRAF*-mutant multiple CMN have yet been described, a recent cohort study suggests that this is not a significant finding, and likely due to the rarity of the *BRAF* causative genotype and the number of published cases of melanoma [79].

Whole genome copy number analysis was the first genetic test to differentiate between benign CMN and melanoma arising within it [107]. This can be done by array CGH, or single nucleotide polymorphism (SNP) arrays, or if whole genome analysis is not available, by melanoma-specific FISH. In general terms, benign CMN have no or few copy number changes, as would a normal tissue, classic proliferative nodules can demonstrate single abnormalities, usually of whole chromosomes, and melanoma demonstrates multiple gains and/or losses of whole or parts of chromosomes [107]. In some cases, amplification of mutant *NRAS* can occur, which can be detected by these methods or by specific quantitative real time polymerase chain reaction (PCR) [108]. The pattern of copy number alteration in malignancy in the context of CMN has been demonstrated to hold true also for CNS melanoma, including progressive leptomeningeal disease where the histology is not necessarily malignant [61,62]. This test therefore seems to be helpful clinically in distinguishing the rare cases of diffuse leptomeningeal melanocytosis which are not malignant [61].

Management.

Skin care of CMN

For reasons which are not yet clear the skin of a CMN is somewhat fragile, and susceptible to splitting or tearing with relatively minor trauma. As a result, at birth erosions are not uncommon in large CMN, particularly over the spine or sacrum where the skin is stretched thinly over bone, or over proliferative nodules. These neonatal erosions should be allowed to heal over for the first month or so, treated conservatively with cleaning and nonadherent dressings, and not considered to be indicators of malignancy. During early childhood, skin fragility can be a problem if the CMN covers areas prone to injury, such as the knees, elbows, or sometimes forehead. Simple protective measures with clothing during the period of learning to walk or when playing particular sports is usually all that is required. Skin fragility does not limit normal choice of activities. CMN do not appear to bleed more than would be expected from other areas of skin, and tears or cuts can be dealt with by pressure in the usual way. If a superficial area of CMN has been lost it usually heals by secondary intention and with loss of pigment in that area which gradually repigments over a period of years. If an injury heals by primary closure the scar is usually barely visible.

CMN are prone to xerosis, again for reasons which are not yet clear. From birth it is useful to avoid soaps and shampoos, and if necessary to use moisturizers. A minority of children with CMN have substantial problems with pruritus, which may or may not be associated with active eczema in the CMN, or exacerbated in the areas of CMN. These usually improve to some degree with the addition of topical steroids, even if eczema is not in evidence. However, in a very small number of cases the pruritus is resistant to all topical therapies. There is evidence of increased mast cells in the skin of CMN, which could potentially contribute to this clinical symptom [109]. Pruritus usually improves with age during the first decade. Very rarely severe and intractable pruritus is seen with indurated and inflamed (desmoplastic) CMN [110], and sometimes with a multinodular phenotype [4]. In these cases, extending medical management to oral medication for pruritus control is worth trying, and surgical excision if technically feasible is an option.

In very rare cases CMN are or can become cerebriform in superficial appearance, a cause of cutis verticis gyrata. This is usually but not always in scalp CMN. Resultant problems are difficulty in cleaning the naevus, and hair loss on the tops of the gyrate areas. Shampoos which contain an antifungal can be helpful, as can antibacterial moisturizing washes although neither should be overused because they can irritate the CMN. Sometimes these naevi are also multinodular. Where surgical excision or partial excision is possible currently this would be the management of choice.

Single CMN and natural lightening

Management of a patient with a single CMN involves a full history and examination, particularly to check there are no pale multiple CMN or café-au-lait macules which have not been detected, and to examine neurology and neurodevelopment. If the examination is normal no routine investigations need to be undertaken. Baseline photography is useful for future reference if needed. Single CMN do not need to be removed for medical reasons. Once the family have understood this point, if surgical excision is possible and desired for cosmetic reasons the patient can be referred to the plastic surgery department from the age of 3 years old, in line with the current recommendations for avoidance of general anaesthesia for nonurgent procedures [111,112]. Another increasingly popular option, however, is to wait until the child is old enough to participate in the decision. Possible methods of excision dependent on size and site are serial excision, tissue expansion or grafting, all of which have advantages and disadvantages and can be discussed with the surgical team. Superficial removal techniques such as curettage, dermabrasion and laser are not recommended from either a medical or cosmetic perspective, despite prevalent beliefs that such techniques can lighten the CMN. Recent data has explained the basis of this impression, by systematic measurement of CMN colour over time in untreated naevi, and by the comparison of the final colour of adjacent treated and untreated areas in the same patient [4]. This cohort study was able to unravel the interacting effects of two key concepts – firstly that the natural history of CMN in many patients is to lighten over time, and secondly that repigmentation follows superficial removal. It transpires that the final colour of a CMN is related to the baseline skin colour of the patient, to the genetically determined normal pigmentary phenotype, and not to that of the CMN colour at birth. In other words, the final colour of the CMN will be lighter in those with lighter skin (and blonde or red hair), than in those with darker skin. In addition, the final colour of the CMN is not at all related to the colour at birth (which is often very dark), likely in the same way that all pigmentation at birth seems to be affected by maternal and other factors. These facts were strikingly demonstrated in patients where partial superficial removal has been performed (for example sparing the genital or buttocks areas), and the final colour of the treated CMN after repigmentation was exactly the same as the untreated area after natural lightening. The ultimate colour of the CMN is therefore not affected by superficial removal, but is related instead to the genetic pigmentary phenotype of the individual [4].

Multiple CMN

Management of a patient with multiple CMN (two or more at birth) should also start with a full history and examination. Because an MRI of the CNS is currently a better predictor of all adverse outcomes than clinical phenotyping, it is recommended that all children with multiple CMN have a scan within the first 6 months. This scan should be of the brain and whole spine with gadolinium contrast injection, rather than either brain or spine alone, because it is not possible to predict from the cutaneous phenotype which part of the CNS will be affected. Contrast is required because it improves the visualization of particularly leptomeningeal lesions. Up to the end of the first year it is usually possible to perform the MRI without a general anaesthetic, using either the 'feed-and-wrap' technique for very young infants, or using sedation. This has been demonstrated in a cohort study of MRI scans in infants with CMN, and sedation protocols for the appropriate ages have been published recently [113].

The single screening MRI scan of the CNS allows for practical management stratification, and rather than leading to anxiety, is in fact vastly reassuring to both families and clinicians in approximately 90% of cases, as well as identifying the 10% who should have close monitoring. On the basis of the scan results patients are divided into three groups [25] – those with a normal scan (approximately 80%), those with isolated intraparenchymal melanosis (approximately 10%), and those with all other CNS abnormalities (approximately 10%). Those with a normal MRI are at low risk of any neurological or developmental problems (around 10% at most) and these issues where they arise are usually mild. In addition, they are at very low risk of all-type melanoma in childhood. Arguably, therefore, these children do not need medical follow up, but they do need access to a paediatric dermatologist for skin care advice, help with pruritus if it arises and access to psychological support services for parents or children where required. Figure 105.7 recommends initial management but discretion must be used depending on individual circumstances. Those children with isolated intraparenchymal melanosis are at higher risk of neurological or neurodevelopmental abnormalities and require yearly follow up with a developmental paediatrician to detect and manage any issues which arise. However, they are still at very low risk of all-site melanoma in childhood and dermatological follow up can be the same as for those with a normal scan. For those children with any other CNS abnormality, management needs to be individually tailored to their needs, and should be in a multidisciplinary team setting at least until it is clear how their disease is behaving.

The current published recommendation for what to do in the case of an older child presenting for the first time with multiple CMN, is that if they are 2 years old or more and neurologically well they do not need to go through a screening MRI of the CNS [17,25]. Despite the fact that the all-site melanoma risk has now been linked to the outcome of this MRI, this still seems a reasonable practical recommendation, given that these older children would be required to have a general anaesthetic for the MRI, and complex CNS abnormalities should have presented symptomatically by 2 years old. However, because there is no clear data on this it would be at the clinician's discretion to decide on individual cases.

A new lump or cutaneous change within a CMN

New lumps arising in large or extensive CMN are common, particularly in some individuals. It is therefore neither practical nor necessarily good for the patient to remove every lump, particularly if they are stable. The following suggestions are a guideline (Fig. 105.8); individual cases have to be managed at the clinician's discretion.

When taking the history it is important to establish if the lump was congenital, whether it has changed, whether it has now stabilized, and how long it is since it was growing actively. Melanoma is rare at birth, whereas proliferative nodules are quite common. In addition, melanoma at any stage will not stabilize in its growth whereas classical proliferative nodules do. As a basis of assessment, a good quality photograph of all new lumps or changes should be taken, with colour and size references, and thorough examination of the patient's neurology, abdominal system and lymph nodes should be undertaken. Dermoscopy can be performed for small lesions. If the change is thought to be malignant it should be excised if feasible as soon as possible, rather than biopsied. If it is thought to be benign, the patient can be seen again within 4 weeks and appearances compared with previous photographs. It is reassuring if there has been no change in this time frame, but the patient should be seen again within another month or two. However, if there has been a clear change at this first check within 4 weeks from presentation then excision should be performed. If a suspected malignant lesion is being excised, it is very important that the sample is not only sent for

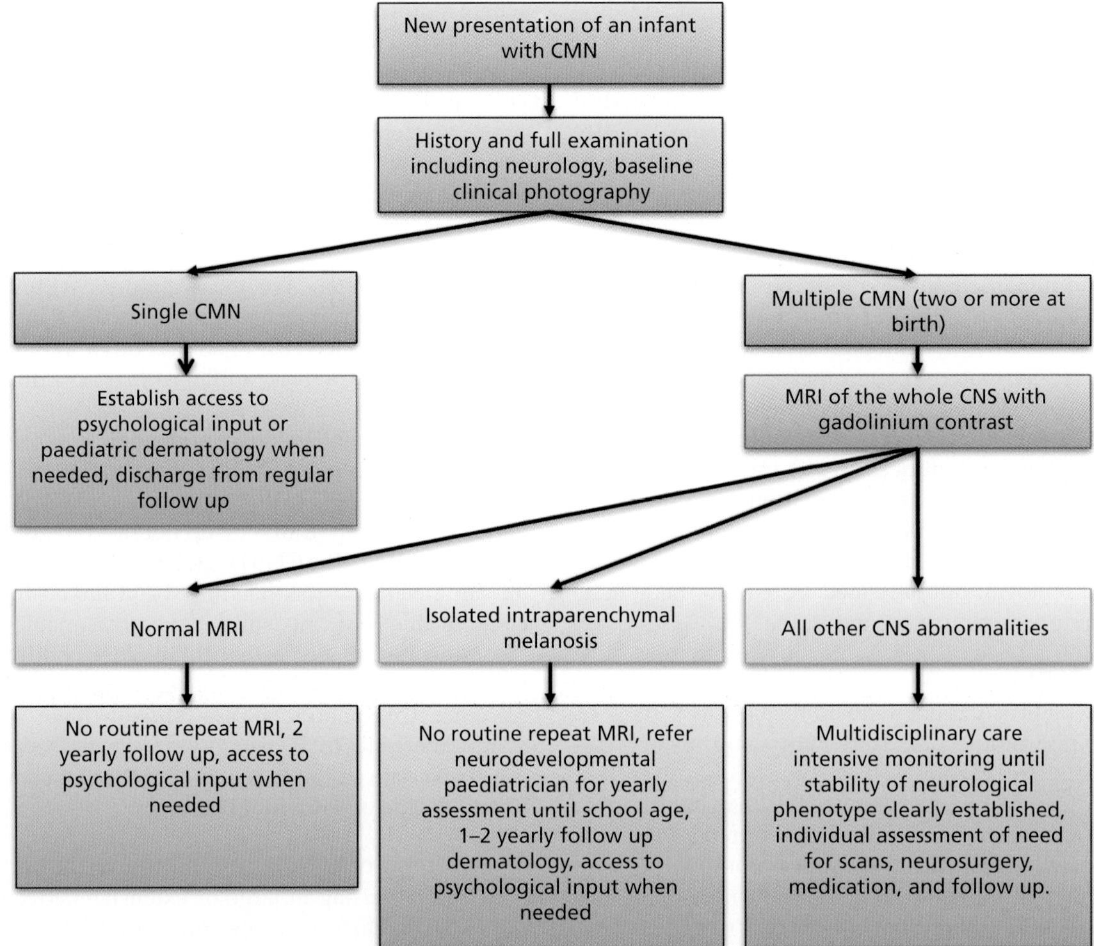

Fig. 105.7 Clinical management of a new infant with congenital melanocytic naevus (CMN). CNS, central nervous system; MRI, magnetic resonance imaging.

histology, but some tissue also sent fresh or snap frozen for genetic analysis, as the last is at least as important as the first.

A new neurological presentation in a patient with CMN

New neurological symptoms or signs in a child with CMN which have been persistent over a period of weeks should prompt a full history and examination by a paediatrician or neurologist, and there should be a low threshold for performing an MRI of the whole CNS with contrast enhancement (Fig. 105.9). This is independent of the results of the initial screening MRI, and is to look for a primary CNS melanoma or other tumour.

Melanoma arising in the skin

Very little hard data exist on management of melanoma in CMN. What follows is the distillation of the author's experience of this disease, and a recent review of the existing literature [28]. Currently, melanoma in the context of CMN is almost universally fatal: this is not caused by publishing bias because it is seen even in prospective cohorts [28]. However, striving for accurate diagnosis and targeted therapy where possible, may in the longer term help to improve the outcome of this disease.

If a diagnosis of cutaneous melanoma is established from the clinical findings, histology and/or genetic testing, multidisciplinary management should be instituted. Suggested baseline investigations are listed in Table 105.2. In particular positron emission tomography (PET-CT) scanning is recommended, because benign CMN do not appear on PET-CT, allowing discrimination of malignant deposits. This is also important for assessment of lymphatic involvement, because histology of lymph nodes can reveal naevus cells in benign congenital disease. Very early malignancies in theory can be completely excised, and in small CMN in adulthood this may be a practical option. In children, however, cutaneous melanoma usually arises in those with multiple CMN and usually in large lesions, and complete excision leading to recovery has not been clearly described. It should, however, be attempted, and local lymph node clearance performed if there is clinical or imaging evidence of lymph node involvement. There is no evidence for sentinel node biopsy in this disease and it is generally not undertaken in paediatric melanoma.

Melanoma arising in the CNS

If a diagnosis of primary CNS melanoma is established multidisciplinary management should be initiated and it

New change/lump in CMN
Full clinical examination of patient, high quality photography with colour and size scale, review within 4 weeks
Resolved, or unchanged compared with photographs, and normal full examination
Clinical progression or abnormal examination (e.g. new localized lymphadenopathy)
Regular review until certain of stability
Histopathology, driver mutation genotyping, copy number measurement
Nonmalignant
Malignant

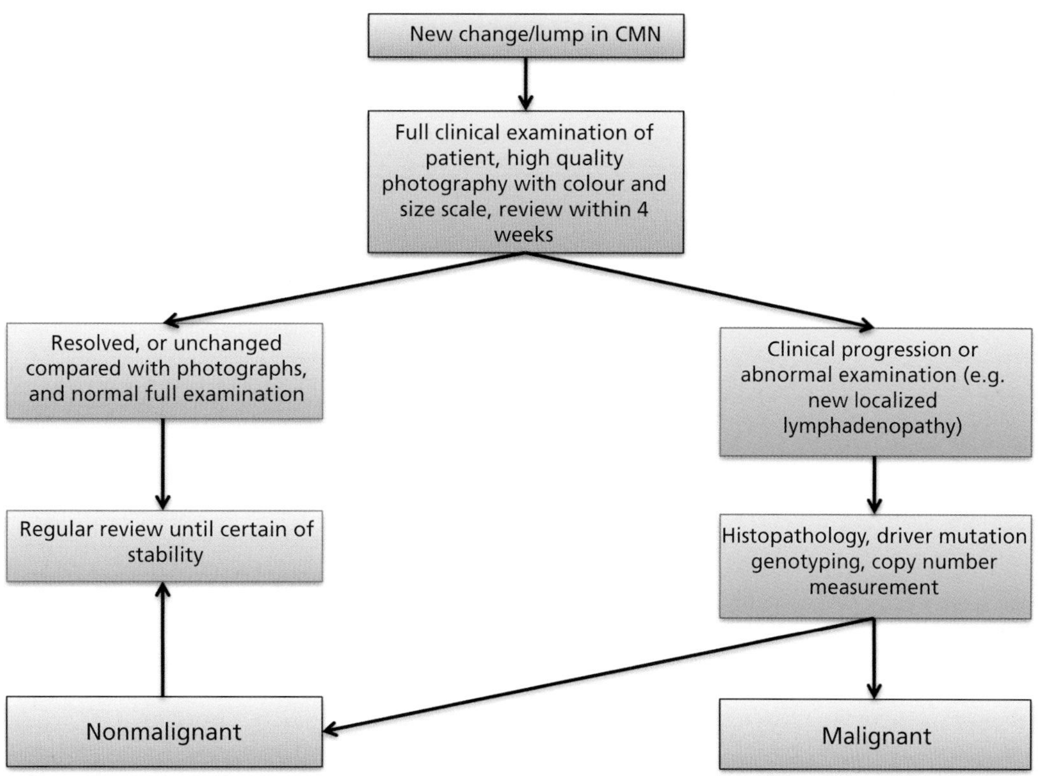

Fig. 105.8 Management of a new lump in a patient with congenital melanocytic naevus (CMN). Source: Adapted from Kinsler et al. 2017 [28]. Reproduced with permission of John Wiley & Sons.

New neurological symptoms or signs
MRI of brain and spine with contrast
Normal, or unchanged from screening MRI after birth
Abnormal, new leptomeningeal enhancement, or hydrocephalus with no visible cause
Abnormal, intraparenchymal solid tumour
Regular neurological review, low threshold for repeating scan if clinical progression
Repeat MRI within 1 month to look for progression
No clinical or radiological progression
Progression
Biopsy of CNS lesion
Histopathology, driver mutation genotyping, copy number measurement
Nonmalignant
Malignant

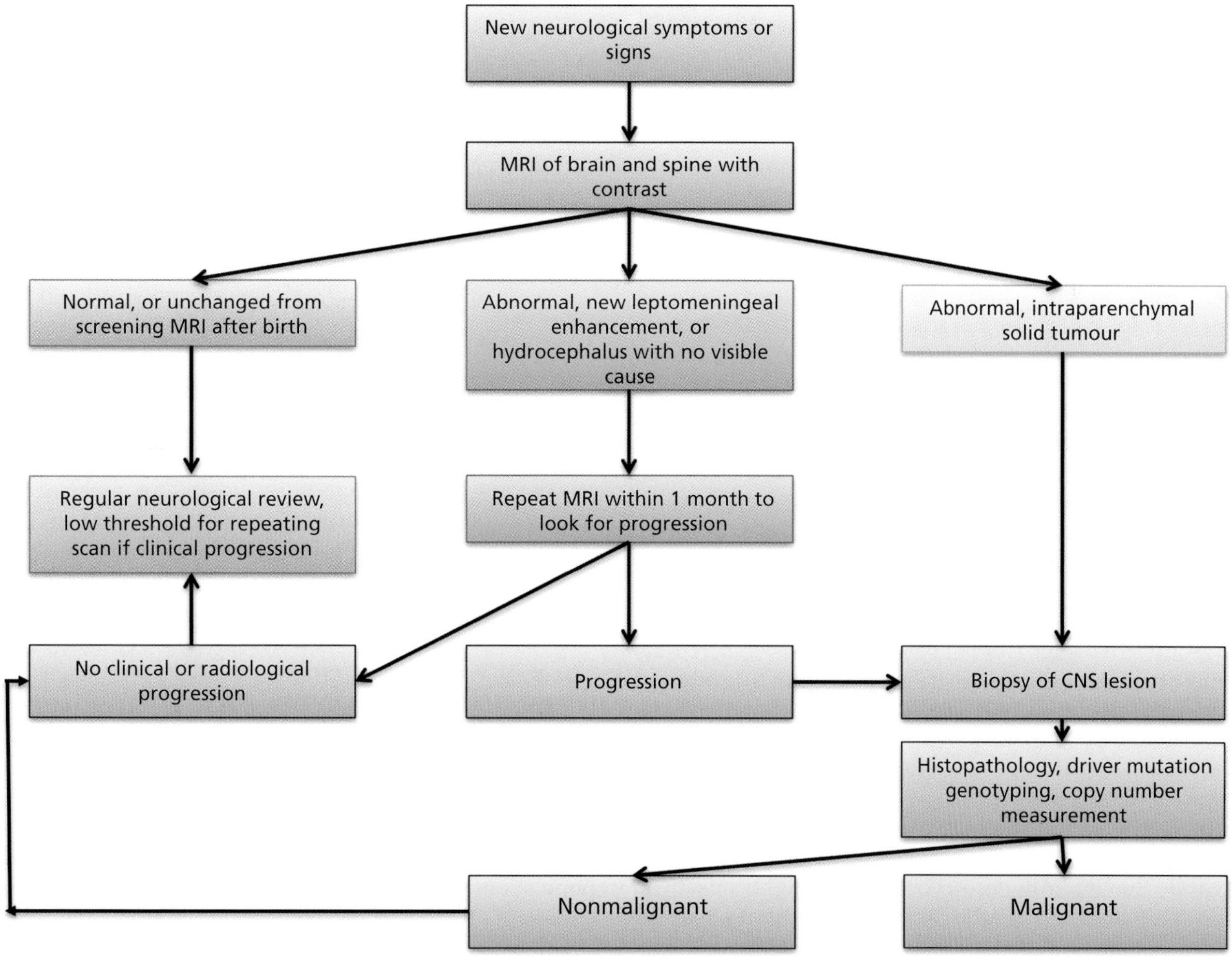

Fig. 105.9 Management of a new neurological presentation in a patient with congenital melanocytic naevus. CNS, central nervous system; MRI, magnetic resonance imaging. Source: Adapted from Kinsler et al. 2017 [28]. Reproduced with permission of John Wiley & Sons.

Table 105.2 Suggested investigations once diagnosis of melanoma is confirmed. Specific pretreatment investigations may be required for particular therapies

Bloods	Imaging	Tissue	Other
Full blood count Urea and electrolytes Liver function tests Lactate dehydrogenase Lipid profile Vitamin D level and bone profile Thyroid function Creatine kinase HbA1c Total protein and glucose	CNS MRI with gadolinium contrast Whole body PET-CT scan Echocardiogram Plain radiograph of wrist and tibial growth plate	Biopsy of suspected primary Histopathology, preferably with at least two expert opinions *NRAS/BRAF* hotspot genotyping Copy number measurement	Urinalysis Ophthalmology assessment

CNS, central nervous system; MRI, magnetic resonance imaging; PET-CT, positron emission computed tomography.

should involve neurosurgery and neuro-oncology teams. A central venous catheter is usually needed to minimize repeated phlebotomy and for intravenous drug administration. If leptomeningeal disease is present then a ventriculoperitoneal shunt is always required to manage symptoms of raised intracranial pressure. Oral corticosteroids can be helpful symptomatically as can local radiotherapy as a palliative measure. Recent data on oral MEK inhibition in *NRAS*-mutant melanoma has been provisionally encouraging, giving symptomatic relief and no significant side-effects in a small cohort [106]. Ipilimumab has been tried in two cases with no beneficial effect [28,114].

Cosmetic aspects of CMN

The aesthetic aspects of CMN should not be underestimated, both for the patient and at least initially for their parents; every family deals with this aspect in a different way. This problem should be addressed early on and continue to be discussed at all appointments. It is known that children with facial differences (at least) are subject to stigmatization [115,116], and that good support of a stigmatized child can help improve psychological outcomes [117]. Patient support groups are a key factor in helping with this aspect of CMN, because practical advice from people who are also affected and have lived through the same issues can be more useful than from clinicians. Excellent support groups exist in many countries (a full list of known worldwide support groups is accessible via www.naevusinternational.com) and often give advice to international patients. However, access to clinical psychologists is a vital part of caring for children and families with CMN, and should be offered where available early in life to parents, and from the age of 7 to 16 years for children. Access to these measures at the time of changing schools or moving home can be particularly useful.

Simple measures to improve cosmetic appearance include shaving of hypertrichosis. This is highly effective, and often does not need to be done more than weekly. A beard-trimmer is suggested to avoid pruritus on regrowth; hair removal creams are not recommended because they can induce irritation in the CMN.

Genetic counselling

Genetic counselling of families with CMN is similar to that for other sporadic disorders. This would be that the recurrence rate is expected to be extremely low, and should be of the same order of magnitude as the risk in the first pregnancy. For individuals severely affected by CMN themselves the advice would be the same. As stated above, however, some families have a loose family history of CMN of some size in first or second degree relatives, but even in these cases recurrence should be extremely low. Very rarely there are families with an apparently Mendelian inheritance pattern, who are presumably either carrying a strong predisposing mutation to somatic mutation in the skin [118] or have an entirely different origin for their CMN. In these very rare cases, referral to a clinical geneticist would be advisable.

Acquired melanocytic naevi in childhood

Introduction. Acquired melanocytic naevi (AMN) in childhood, and particularly those in the first decade of life and during puberty, frequently do not follow the rules of appearance and behaviour we expect of melanocytic naevi in adults. A knowledge of these differences in this age group is very helpful in avoiding anxiety in most cases, whilst allowing a sensible approach to monitoring or biopsy where it is required. Entities such as Spitz naevi and blue naevi also have specific features in childhood, and again a knowledge of these can allow safe conservative management in many cases [119].

Epidemiology and pathogenesis. New AMN can develop from birth and continue throughout childhood and adolescence [120]. Mean numbers of AMN in children vary between ethnic groups, being commonest in white-skinned populations and particularly in fair-haired and freckled children [121]. For White European origin children ages 6–10 a mean number of 20 has been recorded [120,132].

The pathogenesis of AMN is in part caused by genetic factors, and in part environmental [121], the latter somehow related to ultraviolet radiation (UVR) exposure from the sun [123]. Genetics, however, play a larger role in determination of naevus count than sun exposure, as determined by twin studies [124–127]. In recent years identification of many genetic loci for AMN susceptibility has contributed greatly to the understanding of this genetic trait [128–134], and has helped to explain the association between naevus count and lifetime susceptibility to melanoma.

The somatic mutations in AMN may also support a genetic susceptibility rather than a UVR -triggered mechanism of naevogenesis. The commonest mutations in AMN are *BRAF* p.V600E mutations, and these do not bear a typical UVR-damage signature. In further support of this, the mutation signature of naevi and melanoma in xeroderma pigmentosum is not the same as in the normal population [135].

Clinical features and natural history. AMN are brown to black, typically uniformly pigmented naevi, and display increased surface markings. Junctional naevi are usually impalpable. However, dermal and compound naevi are usually palpable, with a smooth surface. Generally, AMN will be symmetrical and round or ovoid in outline, but those acquired early in life do not always follow these rules, and stability of phenotype is very important in assessing naevi in children. In addition, individual children often have a 'signature' type of naevus which predominates [136,137], and thorough examination of the whole child rather than just a single naevus can therefore be reassuring (Fig. 105.10).

AMN are typically 1–5 mm in diameter in childhood, with only 5% of naevi being bigger than 5 mm in early adolescence in one study [138] (Fig. 105.10). At the time of puberty, however, not only do they increase in number [138,139], but individual naevi grow with the child, or even more than in proportion with the child [140]. This type of change is a common trigger for referral to dermatology services, but is not a reliable sign of malignant change in children of this age [141]; a change in a naevus is not sufficient to lead to excision in children, particularly those in the first decade of life [140]. Not uncommonly naevi in children can disappear [139]. Rarely AMN occur on the mucosal and acral surfaces, and in the latter locations can be more difficult to assess because of the distortion of the outline by the thicker palmo-plantar skin (Fig. 105.10).

Associations. Atypical naevus syndrome (or familial atypical multiple mole melanoma syndrome, FAMMM) can present in the first or more usually second decade of life and can therefore present to the paediatric dermatologist. This syndrome is characterized by a large number and/or atypia of AMN, a family history of multiple atypical naevi, and an associated increased risk of melanoma and pancreatic cancer [142]. Approximately 40% of these families will carry germline mutations in the gene *CDKN2A* [143–145], the commonest known highly penetrant gene for familial melanoma. Mutations in *CDK4* are far rarer [146]. Affected children should be monitored regularly and should be aware of the need to present to a paediatric dermatologist if changes are noticed.

A specific variant of an atypical naevus syndrome is that associated with germline mutations in the gene *BAP1*. This leads to a phenotype of multiple atypical melanocytic naevi and a predisposition to cutaneous and uveal melanoma [147,148]. In addition, somatic loss of

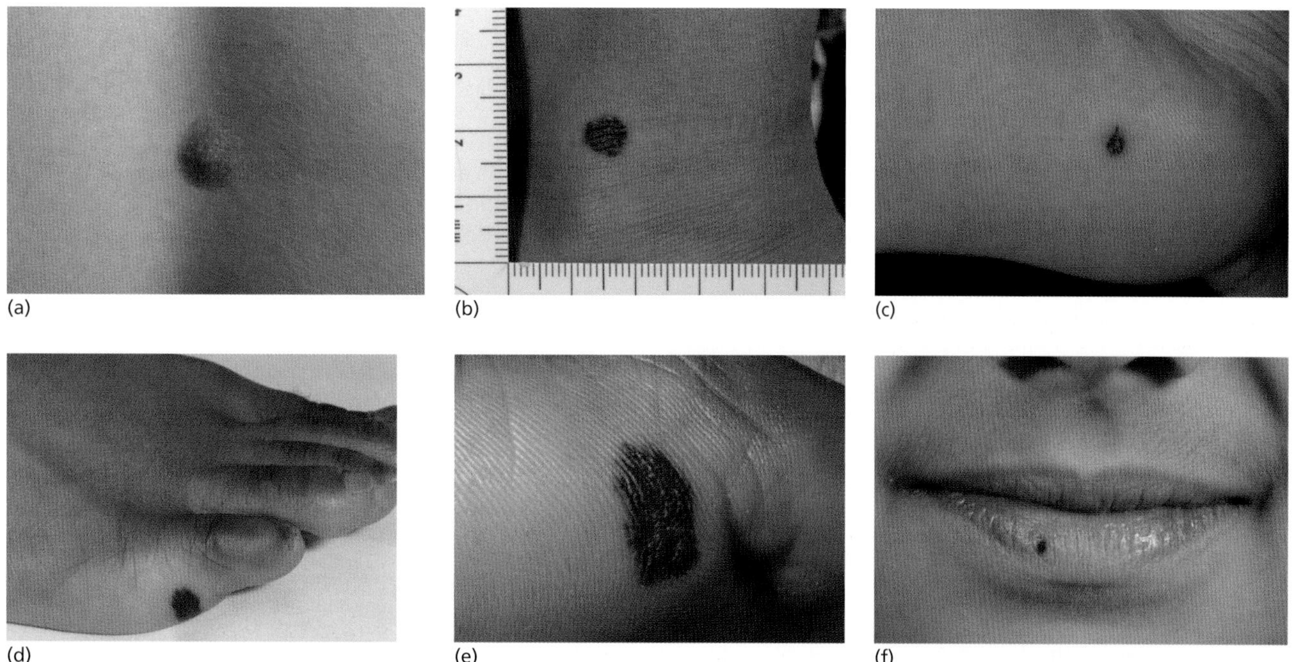

Fig. 105.10 Clinical photographs of acquired melanocytic naevi (AMN) in children. (a) Typical benign AMN in the mid back. (b) Benign AMN demonstrating irregular outline. (c) Benign AMN on the sole of the foot, with distortion of the outline by the thickened epidermis. (d), (e) AMN of the sole of the foot demonstrating hyperlinearity of the surface because of the location. (f) Benign AMN of the lower lip.

BAP1 can lead to an atypical naevus without the inherited disorder component [147]. Clinically these naevi appear skin-coloured and raised above the skin, and their clinical appearance may not be particularly concerning. Histologically, however, they show a spectrum of changes from epithelioid change to atypia overlapping with melanoma, similar to atypical Spitz naevi [147,149]. If these histological changes are seen in one naevus it is worth considering whether the patient may have a germline mutation, because pathogenic loss-of-function mutations, although rare, are associated with a high penetrance of a melanoma phenotype [150].

Multiple AMN can be a sign of a RASopathy, a germline disorder of the RAS pathway (see Chapter 144), particularly Noonan syndrome, or of Turner syndrome (monosomy X). In general, the naevi in this condition are not frankly atypical, but they can be higher in number than might be expected for the age of the child, and would be associated with other clinical features of Noonan syndrome.

Children who have been given immunosuppressive treatment, particularly those after chemotherapy or bone marrow transplant, can present with either a high number of AMN or a rapid increase in number. Again, generally these naevi are not frankly atypical, and there is no evidence that these eruptive naevi confer any additional risks.

Histopathology. AMN are divided into junctional, dermal and compound naevi. Junctional naevi occupy the epidermo–dermal junction, dermal naevi the dermis, and compound naevi have both components. Nests of naevus cells are present in the upper dermis, and show the same 'maturation' with increasing depth as is seen in CMN [6]. Histopathological features of dysplastic AMN have been delineated [151].

Management. AMN which appear to grow or change at puberty, or AMN at unusual sites such as the palms and soles, should be monitored using baseline photographs and dermoscopy until it is clear they are stable.

AMN in childhood in otherwise normal children have an extremely low risk of malignant transformation, and prophylactic excision is generally not required. In general, excision of AMN should only be undertaken if melanoma is suspected. In this case it is advisable to excise the whole lesion rather than to biopsy part of it, and to have the whole lesion examined by histology. Driver mutations in *BRAF* can be tested for if melanoma is suspected, as detailed previously under CMN, because if mutated this permits targeted BRAF therapy to be employed in treatment if appropriate. *NRAS* can also be mutated in AMN but less commonly.

Multiple AMN can be a sign of excessive sun exposure or sunbed use in teenagers and should be addressed with education on sun protection measures.

Other subtypes of pigmented naevi seen in children.

Blue naevi

Blue naevi in children are rare, and can be congenital or acquired. Acquired blue naevi are generally indistinguishable from those in later life. Congenital blue naevi are divided into common, cellular and epithelioid blue naevus types. All types have the characteristic dark blue or slate grey appearance of a deep dermal pigmented lesion. Congenital common blue naevi are usually less than 0.5 cm in diameter, round and symmetrical in outline, and palpable with a smooth dome-shaped surface (Fig. 105.11). These are very similar to the acquired common blue naevus which have been associated with somatic mutations in the genes *GNAQ* [152] and *GNA11*. Where typical these do not need to be resected for medical reasons. Congenital cellular blue naevi, however, can be larger, and are most frequently seen on the scalp. This type has been associated with underlying scalp and neurological defects [153,154], and with transformation to malignancy [155]. Multiple congenital blue naevi have been described very rarely [156,157], and can be familial [158].

Spitz naevi

Spitz naevi were first described by Sophie Spitz in the 1940s [159] and were thought to be juvenile melanoma. As the natural history became recognized they were reclassified as a type of benign melanocytic naevus.

Acquired Spitz naevi are known as difficult lesions in clinical practice, because they are relatively uncommon

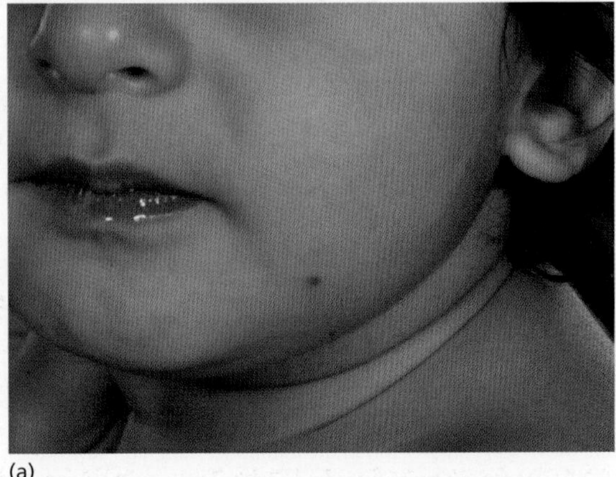

(a)

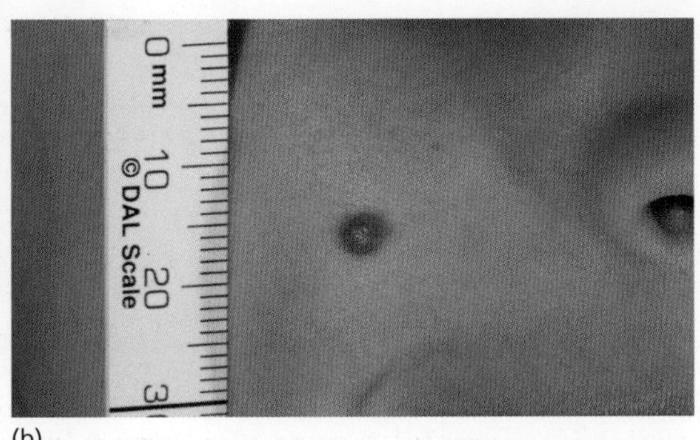

(b)

Fig. 105.11 Clinical photographs of other types of pigment cell naevus. (a) Congenital common blue naevus on the cheek. (b) Spitz naevus on the cheek.

compared with AMN, and cause anxiety both clinically and histologically about the possibility of melanoma. The vast majority of paediatric dermatologists, however, recognize and believe that these naevi are benign [160], and nonsurgical management of the common Spitz naevus is recommended [161]. The natural history of Spitz naevi is to grow rapidly for around 6 months, to be stable over a period of years, and then to resolve spontaneously. They have a typical clinical appearance of a pink, red or brown coloured dome, up to 1 cm across, and most commonly seen on the head, neck or limbs (Fig. 105.11). Dermoscopy can be particularly useful in the diagnosis of Spitz naevi [162–164], and recent evidence suggests that confocal microscopy may add additional diagnostic power for some subsets [165]. In the phase of rapid growth, however, it can be very difficult to be completely confident of a clinical and dermoscopic diagnosis, particularly given that paediatric melanoma is often amelanotic and usually raised [166,167]. Each patient should therefore be treated on their individual presentation at the clinician's discretion.

The classical histological features are of large epithelioid and/or spindle cells [8,159]. Where the histology is of a classical Spitz naevus, patients and clinicians can be reassured as to the benign nature of the lesion. Where the histological diagnosis is of an atypical Spitz naevus, or Spitzoid tumour of unknown malignant potential, the prognosis should be much more guarded, and management recommendations (including those on controversy of sentinel lymph node biopsy) in children have been produced based on reviews of the latest literature [119,161,168].

Congenital Spitz naevi are very rare, but can also mimic melanoma [169,170]. The diagnosis is often made after excisional biopsy, because histopathological features are typical of Spitz [171]. However, congenital melanocytic naevi can also exhibit Spitzoid changes [171]. The chance of malignant transformation in congenital Spitz naevi is not known. Agminated or eruptive Spitz naevi can rarely be seen at birth [172], or as an acquired feature in childhood on the background of a café-au-lait macule or naevus spilus [173–175].

The genetics of Spitz naevi are complex, with interactions between copy number changes, fusion proteins and point mutations. Copy number changes are primarily seen in *HRAS*, which also frequently carries missense mutations [176]. Fusions involving *ALK, MET, ROS1, NTRK1, BRAF, RET* and *NTRK3* have all been described [177–180]. There is some correlation between the genetics and histopathological findings [145,176,181], and an increased understanding of the variation in clinical behaviour of these lesions is likely to result from stratification of patients by the molecular characteristics of their naevi, for example no *HRAS*-mutated Spitz have yet been described as behaving in a malignant fashion [182].

Naevus spilus

Naevus spilus (or speckled lentiginous naevi) are pigmented lesions with a café-au-lait macular background with small more deeply pigmented speckles within it (see Chapter 109). These can be congenital or acquired, and it has been suggested that they can be divided into two phenotypes: naevus spilus maculosus and papulosus [181]. The clinical difference is said to be that in the former the speckles are macular and relatively regular in spacing and size, whereas in the latter they are papular and more irregularly spaced and sized. However, this clinical distinction is not always clear cut, and in particular the suggestion that the two types segregate with clinical diagnosis has not been confirmed. Naevus spilus usually vary from 1 cm in diameter to covering a whole limb in a segmental or zosteriform distribution for single lesions. Large naevus spilus can be a part of the syndrome phakomatosis pigmentovascularis spilorosea, or speckled lentiginous naevus syndrome. The latter includes hyperhidrosis, dysaesthesia, neurological abnormalities and underlying muscular defects [184,185]. Large naevus spilus are also seen in phakomatosis pigmentokeratotica [183,186]. HRAS mutations have been found in this context and in smaller naevus spilus [187,188]. This may partly explain the predilection for these lesions to develop agminated Spitz naevi [189,190], also known to harbour *HRAS* mutations [191] (Fig. 105.11).

This type of naevus spilus can usually be differentiated from naevus spilus type CMN by the much more varied size, colour, and texture of the superimposed pigmented naevi in the latter [15]. However, occasionally the phenotype of the very large naevus spilus type CMN caused by *NRAS* mutation is indistinguishable from a very large naevus spilus [15]. There is therefore heterogeneity of genotype–phenotype association in this group.

Halo naevi

Halo naevus is the term given to a melanocytic naevus surrounded by an area of hypo- or depigmentation. This is generally assumed to be a local immunological reaction to the naevus, and in adults this often heralds the regression of the central naevus. In children regression does not necessarily follow the appearance of the halo, for example in the context of congenital melanocytic naevi. Halo naevi may be more commen in Turner syndrome [192,193], although this could be a function of the fact that AMN are more common in Turner syndrome.

References

1 Cramer SF. What are nevus cells? Am J Dermatopathol 1990;12:629–30.
2 Strauss RM, Newton Bishop JA. Spontaneous involution of congenital melanocytic nevi of the scalp. J Am Acad Dermatol 2008;58:508–11.
3 Kinsler V, Bulstrode N. The role of surgery in the management of congenital melanocytic naevi in children: a perspective from Great Ormond Street Hospital. J Plast Reconstr Aesthet Surg 2009;62:595–601.
4 Polubothu S, Kinsler VA. Longitudinal study of congenital melanocytic naevi reveals that final colour is determined by normal skin colour, and is unaltered by superficial removal techniques. Br J Dermatol 2019; doi:10.1111/bjd.18149.
5 Kinsler VA, Birley J, Atherton DJ. Great Ormond Street Hospital for Children Registry for congenital melanocytic naevi: prospective study 1988–2007. Part 1 – epidemiology, phenotype and outcomes. Br J Dermatol 2009;160:143–50.
6 Herron MD, Vanderhooft SL, Smock K et al. Proliferative nodules in congenital melanocytic nevi: a clinicopathologic and immunohistochemical analysis. Am J Surg Pathol 2004;28:1017–25.

7 Phadke PA, Rakheja D, Le LP et al. Proliferative nodules arising within congenital melanocytic nevi: a histologic, immunohistochemical, and molecular analyses of 43 cases. Am J Surg Pathol 2011;35:656–69.
8 Barnhill RL, Piepkorn MW, Busam KJ. Pathology of Melanocytic Nevi and Malignant Melanoma. Berlin: Springer, 2004.
9 Al-Olabi L, Polubothu S, Dowsett K et al. Mosaic RAS/MAPK variants cause sporadic vascular malformations which respond to targeted therapy. J Clin Invest 2018;128:5185.
10 Etchevers HC, Rose C, Kahle B et al. Giant congenital melanocytic nevus with vascular malformation and epidermal cysts associated with a somatic activating mutation in BRAF. Pigment Cell Melanoma Res 2018;31:437–41.
11 Kinsler, V. Satellite lesions in congenital melanocytic nevi–time for a change of name. Pediatr Dermatol 2011;28(2):212–13.
12 Schaffer JV, Orlow SJ, Lazova R, Bolognia, JL. Speckled lentiginous nevus: within the spectrum of congenital melanocytic nevi. Arch Dermatol 2001;137(2):172–8.
13 Kinsler VA, Krengel S, Riviere JB et al. Next-generation sequencing of nevus spilus-type congenital melanocytic nevus: exquisite genotype-phenotype correlation in mosaic RASopathies. J Invest Dermatol 2014;134:2658–60.
14 Kinsler VA, Chong WK, Aylett SE, Atherton DJ. Complications of congenital melanocytic naevi in children: analysis of 16 years' experience and clinical practice. Br J Dermatol 2008;159:907–14.
15 Kinsler VA, Sebire NJ. congenital naevi and other developmental abnormalities affecting the skin. In: Griffiths C, Barker J, Bleiker T, Chalmers R, Creamer D (eds) Rook's Textbook of Dermatology. Oxford: John Wiley & Sons, 2016.
16 Ruiz-Maldonado, R. Measuring congenital melanocytic nevi. Pediatr Dermatol 2004;21: 178–9.
17 Kopf AW, Bart RS, Hennessey P. Congenital nevocytic nevi and malignant melanomas. J Am Acad Dermatol 1979;1:123–30.
18 Krengel S, Scope A, Dusza SW et al. New recommendations for the categorization of cutaneous features of congenital melanocytic nevi. J Am Acad Dermatol 2013;68: 441–51.
19 Price HN, O'Haver J, Marghoob A et al. Practical application of the new classification scheme for congenital melanocytic nevi. Pediatr Dermatol 2015;32:23–7.
20 Kinsler V, Shaw AC, Merks JH, Hennekam RC. The face in congenital melanocytic nevus syndrome. Am J Med Genet A 2012;158A:1014–19.
21 Happle R. How many epidermal nevus syndromes exist? A clinicogenetic classification. J Am Acad Dermatol 1991;25:550–6.
22 DeDavid M, Orlow SJ, Provost N et al. Neurocutaneous melanosis: clinical features of large congenital melanocytic nevi in patients with manifest central nervous system melanosis. J Am Acad Dermatol 1996;35:529–38.
23 Marghoob AA, Dusza S, Oliveria S, Halpern AC. Number of satellite nevi as a correlate for neurocutaneous melanocytosis in patients with large congenital melanocytic nevi. Arch Dermatol 2004;140:171–5.
24 Becher OJ, Souweidane M, Lavi E et al. Large congenital melanotic nevi in an extremity with neurocutaneous melanocytosis. Pediatr Dermatol 2009;26:79–82.
25 Waelchli R, Aylett SE, Atherton D et al. Classification of neurological abnormalities in children with congenital melanocytic naevus syndrome identifies MRI as the best predictor of clinical outcome. Br J Dermatol 2015;173:739–50.
26 Barkovich AJ, Frieden IJ, Williams ML. MR of neurocutaneous melanosis. Am J Neuroradiol 1994;15:859–67.
27 Frieden IJ, Williams ML, Barkovich AJ. Giant congenital melanocytic nevi: brain magnetic resonance findings in neurologically asymptomatic children. J Am Acad Dermatol 1994;31:423–9.
28 Kinsler VA, O'Hare P, Bulstrode N et al. Melanoma in congenital melanocytic naevi. Bri J Dermatol 2017;176:1131–43.
29 Alper JC, Holmes LB. The incidence and significance of birthmarks in a cohort of 4,641 newborns. Pediatr Dermatol 1983;1:58–68.
30 Chaithirayanon S, Chunharas A. A survey of birthmarks and cutaneous skin lesions in newborns. J Med Assoc Thai 2013; 96(Suppl 1):S49–53.
31 Jacobs AH, Walton RG. The incidence of birthmarks in the neonate. Pediatrics 1976;58: 218–22.
32 Castilla EE, da Graca DM, Orioli-Parreiras IM. Epidemiology of congenital pigmented naevi: I. Incidence rates and relative frequencies. Br J Dermatol 1981;104:307–15.
33 Ruiz-Maldonado R, Tamayo L, Laterz AM, Duran C. Giant pigmented nevi: clinical, histopathologic, and therapeutic considerations. J Pediatr 1992;120:906–11.
34 Bittencourt FV, Marghoob AA, Kopf AW et al. Large congenital melanocytic nevi and the risk for development of malignant melanoma and neurocutaneous melanocytosis. Pediatrics 2000;106: 736–41.
35 Rokitansky J. Ein ausgezeichneter Fall von Pigment-mal mit ausgebreiteter Pigmentierung der inneren Hirn- und Ruchenmarkshaute. Allg Wien Med 1861;Z6:113–16.
36 Kadonaga JN, Frieden IJ. Neurocutaneous melanosis: definition and review of the literature. J Am Acad Dermatol 1991;24:747–55.
37 Kadonaga JN, Barkovich AJ, Edwards MS, Frieden IJ. Neurocutaneous melanosis in association with the Dandy-Walker complex. Pediatr Dermatol 1992;9:37–43.
38 Kinsler VA, Aylett SE, Coley SC et al. Central nervous system imaging and congenital melanocytic naevi. Arch Dis Child 2001;84:152–5.
39 Kinsler VA, Thomas AC, Ishida M et al. Multiple congenital melanocytic nevi and neurocutaneous melanosis are caused by postzygotic mutations in codon 61 of NRAS. J Invest Dermatol 2013;133:2229–36.
40 Kinsler VA, Paine SM, Anderson GW et al. Neuropathology of neurocutaneous melanosis: histological foci of melanotic neurones and glia may be undetectable on MRI. Acta Neuropathol 2012; 123:453–6.
41 Fu YJ, Morota N, Nakagawa A et al. Neurocutaneous melanosis: surgical pathological features of an apparently hamartomatous lesion in the amygdala. J Neurosurg Pediatr 2010;6:82–6.
42 Kinsler V. Letters to the editor: Neurocutaneous melanosis. J Neurosurg Pediatr 2013;12:307–8.
43 Bekiesinska-Figatowska M, Sawicka E, Zak K, Szczygielski O. Age related changes in brain MR appearance in the course of neurocutaneous melanosis. Eur J Radiol 2016;85:1427–31.
44 Ramaswamy V, Delaney H, Haque S et al. Spectrum of central nervous system abnormalities in neurocutaneous melanocytosis. Dev Med Child Neurol 2012;54: 563–8.
45 Arai M, Nosaka, K, Kashihara K, Kaizaki Y. Neurocutaneous melanosis associated with Dandy-Walker malformation and a meningohydroencephalocele. Case report. J Neurosurg 2004; 100:501–5.
46 Kadonaga JN, Barkovich AJ, Edwards MS, Frieden IJ. Neurocutaneous melanosis in association with the Dandy-Walker complex. Pediatr Dermatol 1992;9:37–43.
47 Kinsler VA, Polubothu S, Calonje JE et al. Copy number abnormalities in new or progressive 'neurocutaneous melanosis' confirm it to be primary CNS melanoma. Acta Neuropathol 2017;133:329–31.
48 Tidyman WE, Rauen KA. Expansion of the RASopathies. Curr Genet Med Rep 2016;4: 57–64.
49 Huisman SA, Redeker EJ, Maas SM et al. High rate of mosaicism in individuals with Cornelia de Lange syndrome. J Med Genet 2013; 50:339–44.
50 Hunter AG, Clifford B, Cox DM. The characteristic physiognomy and tissue specific karyotype distribution in the Pallister-Killian syndrome. Clin Genet 1985;28:47–53.
51 Waelchli R, Williams J, Cole T et al. Growth and hormone profiling in children with congenital melanocytic naevi. Br J Dermatol 2015;173: 1471–8.
52 Ivker R, Resnick SD, Skidmore RA. Hypophosphatemic vitamin D-resistant rickets, precocious puberty, and the epidermal nevus syndrome. Arch Dermatol 1997;133: 1557–61.
53 Heike CL, Cunningham ML, Steiner RD et al. Skeletal changes in epidermal nevus syndrome: does focal bone disease harbor clues concerning pathogenesis? Am J Med Genet A 2005;139A:67–77.
54 Ovejero D, Lim YH, Boyce AM et al. Cutaneous skeletal hypophosphatemia syndrome: clinical spectrum, natural history, and treatment. Osteoporos Int 2016;27:3615–26.
55 Lim YH, Ovejero D, Derrick KM et al. Cutaneous skeletal hypophosphatemia syndrome (CSHS) is a multilineage somatic mosaic RASopathy. J Am Acad Dermatol 2016;75: 420–7.
56 Ramesh R, Shaw N, Miles EK et al. Mosaic NRAS Q61R mutation in a child with giant congenital melanocytic naevus, epidermal naevus syndrome and hypophosphataemic rickets. Clin Exp Dermatol 2017;42:75–9.
57 Lim YH, Ovejero D, Sugarman JS et al. Multilineage somatic activating mutations in HRAS and NRAS cause mosaic cutaneous and skeletal lesions, elevated FGF23 and hypophosphatemia. Hum Mol Genet 2014;23:397–407.
58 Waelchli R, Aylett SE, Atherton D et al. Classification of neurological abnormalities in children with congenital melanocytic naevus

syndrome identifies MRI as the best predictor of clinical outcome. Br J Dermatology 2015;173:739–50.
59 Barkovich AJ, Frieden IJ, Williams ML. MR of neurocutaneous melanosis. Am J Neuroradiol 1994;15:859–67.
60 Reyes-Mugica M, Chou P, Byrd S et al. Nevomelanocytic proliferations in the central nervous system of children. Cancer 1993;72:2277–85.
61 Kinsler VA, Polubothu S, Calonje JE et al. Copy number abnormalities in new or progressive 'neurocutaneous melanosis' confirm it as primary CNS melanoma. Acta Neuropathol 2017;133:329–31.
62 van Engen-van Grunsven AC, Rabold K, Kusters-Vandevelde HV et al. Copy number variations as potential diagnostic and prognostic markers for CNS melanocytic neoplasms in neurocutaneous melanosis. Acta Neuropathol 2017;133:333–5.
63 Cohen MC, Kaschula RO, Sinclair-Smith C et al. Pluripotential melanoblastoma, a unifying concept on malignancies arising in congenital melanocytic nevi: report of two cases. Pediatr Pathol Lab Med 1996;16:801–12.
64 Hendrickson MR, Ross JC. Neoplasms arising in congenital giant nevi: morphologic study of seven cases and a review of the literature. Am J Surg Pathol 1981;5:109–35.
65 Hoang MP, Sinkre P, Albores-Saavedra J. Rhabdomyosarcoma arising in a congenital melanocytic nevus. Am J Dermatopathol 2002; 24:26–9.
66 Ilyas EN, Goldsmith K, Lintner R, Manders SM. Rhabdomyosarcoma arising in a giant congenital melanocytic nevus. Cutis 2004;73:39–43.
67 Stratton MR, Fisher C, Gusterson BA, Cooper CS. Detection of point mutations in N-ras and K-ras genes of human embryonal rhabdomyosarcomas using oligonucleotide probes and the polymerase chain reaction. Cancer Res 1989;49:6324–7.
68 Cramer SF. The origin of epidermal melanocytes. Implications for the histogenesis of nevi and melanomas. Arch Pathol Lab Med 1991;115:115–19.
69 Cramer SF. Dermal melanocytes in nevi. Am J Dermatopathol 1994; 16:350–1.
70 Cramer SF. Possible neural basis for the field effect in local recurrence of melanoma in situ. Arch Dermatol 1996;132:971–2.
71 Cramer SF, Fesyuk A. On the development of neurocutaneous units – implications for the histogenesis of congenital, acquired, and dysplastic nevi. Am J Dermatopathol 2012;34:60–81.
72 Kinsler VA, Larue L. The patterns of birthmarks suggest a novel population of melanocyte precursors arising around the time of gastrulation. Pigment Cell Melanoma Res 2018; 31:95–109.
73 Kinsler VA, Anderson G, Latimer B et al. Immunohistochemical and ultrastructural features of congenital melanocytic naevus cells support a stem-cell phenotype. Br J Dermatol 2013;169:374–83.
74 Cramer SF. The histogenesis of acquired melanocytic nevi. Based on a new concept of melanocytic differentiation. Am J Dermatopathol 1984;6(Suppl):289–98.
75 Cramer SF. The melanocytic differentiation pathway in congenital melanocytic nevi: theoretical considerations. Pediatr Pathol 1988;8: 253–65.
76 Adameyko I, Lallemend F, Aquino JB et al. Schwann cell precursors from nerve innervation are a cellular origin of melanocytes in skin. Cell 2009;139:366–79.
77 Barnhill RL, Chastain MA, Jerdan MS et al. Angiotropic neonatal congenital melanocytic nevus: how extravascular migration of melanocytes may explain the development of congenital nevi. Am J Dermatopathol 2010;32:495–9.
78 Dupin E, Calloni G, Real C et al. Neural crest progenitors and stem cells. C R Biol 2007;330:521–9.
79 Polubothu S, McGuire N, Al-Olabi L et al. Does the gene matter? Genotype-phenotype and genotype-outcome associations in congenital melanocytic naevi. Br J Dermatol 2019;doi:10.1111/bjd. 18106 [epub ahead of print].
80 Papp T, Pemsel H, Zimmermann R et al. Mutational analysis of the N-ras, p53, p16INK4a, CDK4, and MC1R genes in human congenital melanocytic naevi. J Med Genet 1999;36:610–14.
81 Papp T, Schipper H, Kumar K et al. Mutational analysis of the BRAF gene in human congenital and dysplastic melanocytic naevi. Melan Res 2005;15:401–7.
82 Bauer J, Curtin JA, Pinkel D, Bastian BC. Congenital melanocytic nevi frequently harbor NRAS mutations but no BRAF mutations. J Invest Dermatol 2007;127:179–82.
83 Dessars B, De Raeve LE, Morandini R et al. Genotypic and gene expression studies in congenital melanocytic nevi: insight into initial steps of melanotumorigenesis. J Invest Dermatol 2009;129:139–47.
84 Phadke PA, Rakheja D, Le LP et al. Proliferative nodules arising within congenital melanocytic nevi: a histologic, immunohistochemical, and molecular analyses of 43 cases. Am J Surg Pathol 2011;35:656–69.
85 Wu D, Wang M, Wang X et al. Lack of BRAF(V600E) mutations in giant congenital melanocytic nevi in a Chinese population. Am J Dermatopathol 2011;33:341–4.
86 Pollock PM, Harper UL, Hansen KS et al. High frequency of BRAF mutations in nevi. Nature Genet 2003;33:19–20.
87 Kumar R, Angelini S, Snellman E, Hemminki K. BRAF mutations are common somatic events in melanocytic nevi. J Invest Dermatol 2004;122:342–8.
88 Ichii-Nakato N, Takata M, Takayanagi S et al. High frequency of BRAFV600E mutation in acquired nevi and small congenital nevi, but low frequency of mutation in medium-sized congenital nevi. J Invest Dermatol 2006;126:2111–18.
89 Dessars B, De Raeve LE, El Housni H et al. Chromosomal translocations as a mechanism of BRAF activation in two cases of large congenital melanocytic nevi. J Invest Dermatol 2007;127: 1468–70.
90 Salgado CM, Basu D, Nikiforova M et al. BRAF mutations are also associated with neurocutaneous melanocytosis and large/giant congenital melanocytic nevi. Pediatr Dev Pathol 2015;18:1–9.
91 Kinsler VA, Abu-Amero S, Budd P et al. Germline melanocortin-1-receptor genotype is associated with severity of cutaneous phenotype in congenital melanocytic nevi: a role for MC1R in human fetal development. J Invest Dermatol 2012;132:2026–32.
92 Charbel C, Fontaine RH, Malouf GG et al. NRAS mutation is the sole recurrent somatic mutation in large congenital melanocytic nevi. J Invest Dermatol 2014;134:1067–74.
93 Krengel S, Widmer DS, Kerl K et al. Naevus spilus-type congenital melanocytic naevus associated with a novel NRAS codon 61 mutation. Br J Dermatol 2016;174:642–4.
94 Forbes SA, Beare D, Gunasekaran P et al. COSMIC: exploring the world's knowledge of somatic mutations in human cancer. Nucleic Acids Res 2015;43:D805–11.
95 Kinsler VA, O'Hare P, Bulstrode N et al. Melanoma in congenital melanocytic naevi. Br J Dermatol 2017;176:1131–43.
96 Kinsler VA. O'Hare P, Jacques T et al. MEK inhibition appears to improve symptom control in primary NRAS-driven CNS melanoma in children. Br J Cancer 2017;116:990–3.
97 Martins da Silva V, Martinez-Barrios E, Tell-Marti G et al. Genetic abnormalities in large to giant congenital nevi: beyond NRAS mutations. J Invest Dermatol 2018; doi: 10.1016/j.jid.2018.07.045.
98 Kinsler VA, Birley J, Atherton DJ. Great Ormond Street Hospital for Children Registry for congenital melanocytic naevi: prospective study 1988–2007. Part 1 – epidemiology, phenotype and outcomes. Br J Dermatol 2009;160:143–50.
99 Kinsler VA, Abu-Amero S, Budd P et al. Germline melanocortin-1-receptor genotype is associated with severity of cutaneous phenotype in congenital melanocytic nevi: a role for MC1R in human fetal development. J Invest Dermat 2012;132:2026–32.
100 Salgado CM, Basu D, Nikiforova M et al. BRAF mutations are also associated with neurocutaneous melanocytosis and large/giant congenital melanocytic nevi. Pediatr Dev Pathol 2015;18:1–9.
101 Weeraratna AT. RAF around the edges – the paradox of BRAF inhibitors. N Engl J Med 2012;366:271–3.
102 Long GV, Fung C, Menzies AM et al. Increased MAPK reactivation in early resistance to dabrafenib/trametinib combination therapy of BRAF-mutant metastatic melanoma. Nature Comm 2014;5:5694.
103 Johnson DB, Puzanov I. Treatment of NRAS-mutant melanoma. Curr Treatment Options Oncol 2015;16;330.
104 Pawlikowski JS, Brock C, Chen SC et al. Acute inhibition of MEK suppresses congenital melanocytic nevus syndrome in a murine model driven by activated NRAS and Wnt signaling. J Invest Dermatol 2015;135:2902.
105 Kusters-Vandevelde HV, Willemsen AE, Groenen PJ et al. Experimental treatment of NRAS-mutated neurocutaneous melanocytosis with MEK162, a MEK-inhibitor. Acta Neuropathol Comm 2014;2:41.
106 Kinsler VA, O'Hare P, Jacques T et al. MEK inhibition appears to improve symptom control in primary NRAS-driven CNS melanoma in children. Br J Cancer 2017;116:990–3.
107 Bastian BC, Xiong J, Frieden IJ et al. Genetic changes in neoplasms arising in congenital melanocytic nevi: differences between nodular proliferations and melanomas. Am J Pathol 2002;161:1163–9.

108 Salgado CM, Basu D, Nikiforova M et al. Amplification of mutated NRAS leading to congenital melanoma in neurocutaneous melanocytosis. Melanoma Res 2015;25:453–60.

109 Salgado CM, Silver RB, Bauer BS et al. Skin of patients with large/giant congenital melanocytic nevi shows increased mast cells. Pediatr Dev Pathol 2014;17:198–203.

110 Feng J, Sethi A, Reyes-Mugica M, Antaya R. Life-threatening blood loss from scratching provoked by pruritus in the bulky perineal nevocytoma variant of giant congenital melanocytic nevus in a child. J Am Acad Dermatol 2005;53S:139–42.

111 Rappaport B, Mellon RD, Simone A, Woodcock J. Defining safe use of anesthesia in children. N Engl J Med 2011;364:1387–90.

112 Rappaport BA, Suresh S, Hertz S et al. Anesthetic neurotoxicity – clinical implications of animal models. N Engl J Med 2015;372:796–7.

113 Plumptre I, Stuart G, Cerullo A, Kinsler VA. Sedation for screening MRI in patients with congenital melanocytic naevi under the age of one is a successful, safe and economical first-line approach. Br J Dermatol 2019;180:668–9.

114 Volejnikova J, Bajciova V, Sulovska L et al. Bone marrow metastasis of malignant melanoma in childhood arising within a congenital melanocytic nevus. Biomed Pap Med Fac Univ Palacky Olomouc Czech Repub 2016;160:456–60.

115 Masnari O, Landolt MA, Roessler J et al. Self- and parent-perceived stigmatisation in children and adolescents with congenital or acquired facial differences. J Plast Reconstr Aesthet Surg 2012;65: 1664–70.

116 Masnari O, Schiestl C, Weibel L et al. How children with facial differences are perceived by non-affected children and adolescents: perceiver effects on stereotypical attitudes. Body Image 2013;10: 515–23.

117 Masnari O, Schiestl C, Rossler J et al. Stigmatization predicts psychological adjustment and quality of life in children and adolescents with a facial difference. J Pediatr Psychol 2013;38: 162–72.

118 de Wijn RS, Zaal LH, Hennekam RC, van der Horst CM. Familial clustering of giant congenital melanocytic nevi. J Plast Reconstr Aesthet Surg 2010;63:906–13.

119 Schaffer JV. Update on melanocytic nevi in children. Clin Dermatol 2015;33:368–86.

120 Crane LA, Mokrohisky ST, Dellavalle RP et al. Melanocytic nevus development in Colorado children born in 1998: a longitudinal study. Arch Dermatol 2009;145:148–56.

121 Baron AE, Asdigian NL, Gonzalez V et al. Interactions between ultraviolet light and MC1R and OCA2 variants are determinants of childhood nevus and freckle phenotypes. Cancer Epidemiol Biomarkers Prev 2014;23:2829–39.

122 Buendia-Eisman A, Palau-Lazaro MC, Arias-Santiago S et al. Prevalence of melanocytic nevi in 8- to 10-year-old children in Southern Spain and analysis of associated factors. J Eur Acad Dermatol Venereol 2012;26:1558–64.

123 Dulon M, Weichenthal M, Blettner M et al. Sun exposure and number of nevi in 5- to 6-year-old European children. J Clin Epidemiol 2002;55:1075–81.

124 Easton DF, Cox GM, Macdonald AM, Ponder BA. Genetic susceptibility to naevi – a twin study. Br J Cancer 1991;64:1164–7.

125 Duffy DL, Macdonald AM, Easton DF et al. Is the genetics of moliness simply the genetics of sun exposure? A path analysis of nevus counts and risk factors in British twins. Cytogenet Cell Genet 1992;59:194–6.

126 Zhu G, Duffy DL, Eldridge A et al. A major quantitative-trait locus for mole density is linked to the familial melanoma gene CDKN2A: a maximum-likelihood combined linkage and association analysis in twins and their sibs. Am J Hum Genet 1999;65:483–92.

127 McGregor B, Pfitzner J, Zhu G et al. Genetic and environmental contributions to size, color, shape, and other characteristics of melanocytic naevi in a sample of adolescent twins. Genet Epidemiol 1999;16:40–53.

128 Falchi M, Bataille V, Hayward NK et al. Genome-wide association study identifies variants at 9p21 and 22q13 associated with development of cutaneous nevi. Nature Genet 2009;41:915–19.

129 Duffy DL, Iles MM, Glass D et al. IRF4 variants have age-specific effects on nevus count and predispose to melanoma. Am J Hum Genet 2010;87:6–16.

130 Newton-Bishop JA. Chang YM, Iles MM et al. Melanocytic nevi, nevus genes, and melanoma risk in a large case-control study in the United Kingdom. Cancer Epidemiol Biomarkers Prev 2010;19:2043–54.

131 Zhu G, Duffy DL, Turner DR et al. Linkage and association analysis of radiation damage repair genes XRCC3 and XRCC5 with nevus density in adolescent twins. Twin Res 2003;6:315–21.

132 Zhu G, Montgomery GW, James MR et al. A genome-wide scan for naevus count: linkage to CDKN2A and to other chromosome regions. Eur J Hum Genet 2007;15: 94–102.

133 Yang XR, Liang X, Pfeiffer RM et al. Associations of 9p21 variants with cutaneous malignant melanoma, nevi, and pigmentation phenotypes in melanoma-prone families with and without CDKN2A mutations. Famil Cancer 2010;9:625–33.

134 Nan H, Xu M., Zhang J et al. Genome-wide association study identifies nidogen 1 (NID1) as a susceptibility locus to cutaneous nevi and melanoma risk. Hum Mol Genet 2011;20:2673–9.

135 Masaki T, Wang Y, DiGiovanna JJ et al. High frequency of PTEN mutations in nevi and melanomas from xeroderma pigmentosum patients. Pigment Cell Melanoma Res 2014;27:454–64.

136 Suh KY, Bolognia JL. Signature nevi. J Am Acad Dermatol 2009; 60:508–14.

137 Hurwitz RM, Buckel LJ. Signature nevi: individuals with multiple melanocytic nevi commonly have similar clinical and histologic patterns. Dermatol Pract Concept 2011;1:13–17.

138 Siskind V, Darlington S, Green L, Green A. Evolution of melanocytic nevi on the faces and necks of adolescents: a 4 y longitudinal study. J Invest Dermatol 2002;118:500–4.

139 Scope A. Dusza SW, Marghoob AA et al. Clinical and dermoscopic stability and volatility of melanocytic nevi in a population-based cohort of children in Framingham school system. J Invest Dermatol 2011;131:1615–21.

140 Kittler H, Seltenheim M, Dawid M et al. Frequency and characteristics of enlarging common melanocytic nevi. Arch Dermatol 2000;136: 316–20.

141 Cheng H, Oakley A, Rademaker M. Change in a child's naevus prompts referral to a dermatology service. J Prim Health Care 2014; 6:123–8.

142 Chamlin SL, Williams ML. Pigmented lesions in adolescents. Adolesc Med 2001;12: 195–212.

143 Goldstein AM, Chan M, Harland M et al. Features associated with germline CDKN2A mutations: a GenoMEL study of melanoma-prone families from three continents. J Med Genet 2007;44:99–106.

144 Kamb A, Shattuck-Eidens D, Eeles R et al. Analysis of the p16 gene (CDKN2) as a candidate for the chromosome 9p melanoma susceptibility locus. Nature Genet 1994;8:23–6.

145 Hussussian CJ, Struewing JP, Goldstein AM et al. Germline p16 mutations in familial melanoma. Nature Genet 1994;8:15–21.

146 Ward KA, Lazovich D, Hordinsky MK. Germline melanoma susceptibility and prognostic genes: a review of the literature. J Am Acad Dermatol 2012;67:1055–67.

147 Wiesner T, Obenauf AC, Murali R et al. Germline mutations in BAP1 predispose to melanocytic tumors. Nature Genet 2011;43:1018–21.

148 Harbour JW, Onken MD, Roberson ED et al. Frequent mutation of BAP1 in metastasizing uveal melanomas. Science 2010;330:1410–13.

149 Wiesner T, Murali R, Fried I et al. A distinct subset of atypical Spitz tumors is characterized by BRAF mutation and loss of BAP1 expression. Am J Surg Pathol 2012;36:818–30.

150 O'Shea SJ, Robles-Espinoza CD, McLellan L et al. A population-based analysis of germline BAP1 mutations in melanoma. Hum Mol Genet 2017;26:717–28.

151 Duncan LM, Berwick M, Bruijn JA et al. Histopathologic recognition and grading of dysplastic melanocytic nevi: an interobserver agreement study. J Invest Dermatol 1993;100:318S–321S.

152 Van Raamsdonk CD, Bezrookove V, Green G et al. Frequent somatic mutations of GNAQ in uveal melanoma and blue naevi. Nature 2009;457:599–602.

153 Marano SR, Brooks RA, Spetzler RF, Rekate HL. Giant congenital cellular blue nevus of the scalp of a newborn with an underlying skull defect and invasion of the dura mater. Neurosurgery 1986; 18:85–9.

154 Micali G, Innocenzi D, Nasca MR. Cellular blue nevus of the scalp infiltrating the underlying bone: case report and review. Pediatr Dermatol 1997;14:199–203.

155 Nakamura Y, Shibata-Ito M, Nakamura Y et al. Malignant blue nevus arising in a giant congenital cellular blue nevus in an infant. Pediatr Dermatol 2012;29:651–5.

156 Serarslan G, Yaldiz M, Verdi M. Giant congenital cellular blue naevus of the scalp with disseminated common blue naevi of the body. J Eur Acad Dermatol Venereol 2009;23:190–1.

157 Shi G, Zhou Y, Li SJ, Fan YM. Clinicopathologic features of an infant with generalized congenital epithelioid blue nevi. Pediatr Dev Pathol 2013;16:442–6.
158 Hawkes JE, Campbell J, Garvin D et al. Lack of GNAQ and GNA11 germ-line mutations in familial melanoma pedigrees with uveal melanoma or blue nevi. Frontiers Oncol 2013;3:160.
159 Spitz S. Melanomas of childhood. Am J Pathol 1948;24:591–609.
160 Tlougan BE, Orlow SJ, Schaffer JV. Spitz nevi: beliefs, behaviors, and experiences of pediatric dermatologists. JAMA Dermatol 2013; 149:283–91.
161 Luo S, Sepehr A, Tsao H. Spitz nevi and other Spitzoid lesions part II. Natural history and management. J Am Acad Dermatol 2011;65: 1087–92.
162 Brunetti B, Nino M, Sammarco E, Scalvenzi M. Spitz naevus: a proposal for management. J Eur Acad Dermatol Venereol 2005;19: 391–3.
163 Haliasos EC, Kerner M, Jaimes N et al. Dermoscopy for the pediatric dermatologist part III: dermoscopy of melanocytic lesions. Pediatr Dermatol 2013;30:281–93.
164 Marghoob AA. Practice gaps. Underuse of dermoscopy in assessing Spitz nevi in children: comment on 'Spitz nevi: beliefs, behaviors, and experiences of pediatric dermatologists'. JAMA Dermatol 2013;149:291–2.
165 Guida S, Pellacani G, Cesinaro AM et al. Spitz naevi and melanomas with similar dermoscopic patterns: can confocal microscopy differentiate? Br J Dermatol 2016;174:610–16.
166 Ferrari A, Bono A, Baldi M et al. Does melanoma behave differently in younger children than in adults? A retrospective study of 33 cases of childhood melanoma from a single institution. Pediatrics 2005;115:649–54.
167 Ferrari A, Bisogno G, Cecchetto G et al. Cutaneous melanoma in children and adolescents: the Italian rare tumors in pediatric age project experience. J Pediatr 2014;164:376–382.
168 166Tom WL, Hsu JW, Eichenfield LF, Friedlander SF. Pediatric 'STUMP' lesions: evaluation and management of difficult atypical Spitzoid lesions in children. J Am Acad Dermatol 2011;64:559–72.
169 Zaenglein AL, Heintz P, Kamino H et al. Congenital Spitz nevus clinically mimicking melanoma. J Am Acad Dermatol 2002;47:441–4.
170 Palazzo JP, Duray PH. Congenital agminated Spitz nevi: immunoreactivity with a melanoma-associated monoclonal antibody. J Cutan Pathol 1988;15:166–70.
171 Harris MN, Hurwitz RM, Buckel LJ, Gray HR. Congenital spitz nevus. Dermatol Surg 2000;26:931–5.
172 Feito-Rodriguez M, de Lucas-Laguna R, Bastian BC et al. Nodular lesions arising in a large congenital melanocytic nevus in a newborn with eruptive disseminated spitz nevi (nodular lesions arising in a congenital melanocytic nevus and eruptive spitz nevi). Br J Dermatol 2011;165:1138–42.
173 Bullen R, Snow SN, Larson PO et al. Multiple agminated Spitz nevi: report of two cases and review of the literature. Pediatr Dermatol 1995;12:156–8.
174 Glasgow MA, Lain EL, Kincannon JM. Agminated Spitz nevi: report of a child with a unique dermatomal distribution. Pediatr Dermatol 2005;22:546–9.
175 Aida K, Monia K, Ahlem S et al. Agminated Spitz nevi arising on a nevus spilus after chemotherapy. Pediatr Dermatol 2010;27: 411–13.
176 Bastian BC, LeBoit PE, Pinkel D. Mutations and copy number increase of HRAS in Spitz nevi with distinctive histopathological features. Am J Pathol 2000;157:967–72.
177 Wiesner T, He J, Yelensky R et al. Kinase fusions are frequent in Spitz tumours and spitzoid melanomas. Nature Comm 2014;5:3116.
178 Yeh I, Botton T, Talevich E et al. Activating MET kinase rearrangements in melanoma and Spitz tumours. Nature Comm 2015;6:7174.
179 Yeh I, Tee MK, Botton T et al. NTRK3 kinase fusions in Spitz tumours. J Pathol 2016;240:282–90.
180 Wu G, Barnhill RL, Lee S et al. The landscape of fusion transcripts in spitzoid melanoma and biologically indeterminate spitzoid tumors by RNA sequencing. Modern Pathol 2016;29:359–69.
181 Kiuru M, Jungbluth A, Kutzner H et al. Spitz tumors: comparison of histological features in relationship to immunohistochemical staining for ALK and NTRK1. Int J Surg Pathol 2016;24:200–6.
182 van Engen-van Grunsven AC, van Dijk MC, Ruiter DJ et al. HRAS-mutated Spitz tumors: A subtype of Spitz tumors with distinct features. Am J Surg Pathol 2010;34: 1436–41.
183 Happle R. Speckled lentiginous naevus: which of the two disorders do you mean? Clin Exp Dermatol 2009;34:133–5.
184 Happle R. Speckled lentiginous nevus syndrome: delineation of a new distinct neurocutaneous phenotype. Eur J Dermatol 2002;12: 133–5.
185 Torchia D, Schachner LA. Speckled lentiginous nevus syndrome: central nervous system abnormalities as a critical diagnostic feature. Pediatr Dermatol 2011;28:749.
186 Happle R, Hoffmann R, Restano L et al. Phacomatosis pigmentokeratotica: a melanocytic-epidermal twin nevus syndrome. Am J Med Genet 1996;65:363–5.
187 Groesser L, Herschberger E, Sagrera A et al. Phacomatosis pigmentokeratotica is caused by a postzygotic HRAS mutation in a multipotent progenitor cell. J Invest Dermatol 2013;133: 1998–2003.
188 Sarin KY, McNiff JM, Kwok S et al. Activating HRAS mutation in nevus spilus. J Invest Dermatol 2014;134:1766–8.
189 Betti R, Inselvini E, Palvarini M, Crosti C. Agminated intradermal Spitz nevi arising on an unusual speckled lentiginous nevus with localized lentiginosis: a continuum? Am J Dermatopathol 1997:19: 524–7.
190 Aloi F, Tomasini C, Pippione M. Agminated Spitz nevi occurring within a congenital speckled lentiginous nevus. Am J Dermatopathol 1995;17:594–8.
191 Bastian BC, LeBoit PE, Pinkel D. Mutations and copy number increase of HRAS in Spitz nevi with distinctive histopathological features. Am J Pathol 2000;157:967–72.
192 Brazzelli V, Larizza D, Martinetti M et al. Halo nevus, rather than vitiligo, is a typical dermatologic finding of turner's syndrome: clinical, genetic, and immunogenetic study in 72 patients. J Am Acad Dermatol 2004;51:354–8.
193 Bello-Quintero CE, Gonzalez ME, Alvarez-Connelly E. Halo nevi in Turner syndrome. Pediatr Dermatol 2010;27:368–9.

CHAPTER 106
Epidermal Naevi

Leopold M. Groesser & Christian Hafner
Department of Dermatology, University of Regensburg, Regensburg, Germany

Introduction, 1260 | Organoid epidermal naevi, 1261 | Nonorganoid epidermal naevi, 1267

Abstract

'Epidermal naevus' is a general term for various clinically different circumscribed ectodermal lesions reflecting genetic mosaicism. The term epidermal naevus syndrome (ENS) indicates the association of an epidermal naevus with extracutaneous abnormalities. Depending on the skin compartment affected, nonorganoid epidermal naevi (EN), displaying epidermal changes only, is differentiated from organoid EN, which show (additional) abnormal adnexal structures. Advances in molecular biology have rapidly expanded the knowledge of the genetic basis of various epidermal naevi and their respective syndromes in recent years. This chapter elaborates on the pathogenesis, the clinical and histopathological hallmarks as well as the treatment options of all previously described nonorganoid and organoid epidermal naevi.

Introduction

In recent years advances in molecular biology have rapidly expanded the knowledge of the genetic basis of various epidermal naevi (EN), which altogether have an incidence estimated at one to three per 1000 live births. 'Epidermal naevus' is a general term for various clinically different circumscribed ectodermal lesions which reflect genetic mosaicism. Some EN are visible at birth, others manifest in the first years of life. Depending on the skin compartment affected nonorganoid EN, displaying epidermal changes only, is differentiated from organoid EN, which show (additional) abnormal adnexal structures.

Cutaneous mosaicism

In 1987 Happle hypothesized that the phenotypic consequences of some activating mutations in the germline may be so fundamental that they are not compatible with development and life. Because of this, these mutations may only survive in a mosaic state with a limited number of affected tissues and cells [1]. Indeed, some of the mutations identified in EN, have not been described in the germline yet, whereas others have been described in the germline as well as in a mosaic state [2]. The fact that the occurrence of the respective mutations in a mosaic state often leads to a phenotype that is not merely an incomplete manifestation of the corresponding germline mutation is not fully understood. However, the cell types affected by the mutation, as well as timing of the mutational event and subsequent cross talk with the tissue microenvironment, is likely to be what crucially determines the respective phenotype.

Genetic mosaicism is defined as the presence of genetically distinct populations of cells in a given organism. It may be caused by DNA mutations, chromosomal abnormalities, epigenetic alterations of DNA and the spontaneous reversion of inherited mutations [3]. Single small- or medium-sized naevi may produce different shapes in the form of 'round or oval', 'patchy indented' and 'teardrop/triangular' configurations. Extensive naevi, however, demonstrate a Blaschko-linear, block/flag-like, phylloid (leaf-like), garment-like, agminated, diffuse patchy or lateralization pattern [4]. A review of 1188 cases found that epidermal naevi show a tendency to be round/oval or triangular and to follow the lines of Blaschko [4].

Epidermal naevus syndromes

The term epidermal naevus syndrome (ENS) indicates the association of an epidermal naevus with extracutaneous abnormalities and was coined in 1968 by Solomon et al. [5]. Whereas the first comprehensive review on epidermal naevi and epidermal naevus syndromes emphasized that EN are mere variants of each other [6], molecular investigations of recent years have often confirmed the validity of the clinical differentiation of various EN and ENS subtypes. The extent and clinical phenotype of the respective epidermal naevus as well as the degree of extracutaneous involvement seems to be determined by the timing of the specific mutation during embryogenesis, the level of pathway activation, as well as the affected postzygotic (pluripotent) cell.

Despite new insights and the falsification of established unitizing EN classification systems, a new comprehensive

Harper's Textbook of Pediatric Dermatology, Fourth Edition. Edited by Peter Hoeger, Veronica Kinsler and Albert Yan.

EN classification system based on clinical and molecular data does not yet exist.

Organoid epidermal naevi

Key points

- **Naevus sebaceous, Schimmelpenning syndrome and phacomatosis pigmentokeratotica are variants of a continuous clinical spectrum caused by activating mosaic mutations affecting the RAS–MAPK pathway (mosaic RASopathies).**
- **Naevus comedonicus and 'acne naevus/Munro naevus' are clinically and genetically two different entities, the former caused by somatic mutations in *NEK9*, the latter by somatic mutations in *FGFR2*.**
- **Porokeratotic eccrine ostial and dermal duct naevus presents as linear, spiky, hyperkeratotic papules and plaques and is caused by somatic mutations in *GJB2*.**
- **Becker naevus is characterized by a well-demarcated irregularly bordered, tan-coloured patch covered with coarse dark hairs.**
- **Woolly hair naevus presents as an area of tightly curled scalp hair and is caused by activating mosaic mutations affecting the RAS–MAPK pathway (mosaic RASopathies).**

Organoid epidermal naevi are naevus sebaceous, naevus comedonicus, porokeratotic eccrine and ostial dermal duct naevus, Becker naevus, woolly hair naevus, eccrine naevus, angora hair naevus, naevus trichilemmocysticus, and segmentally arranged basaloid follicular hamartomas.

Naevus sebaceous

Introduction and history. Naevus sebaceous is an organoid EN consisting of epidermal, sebaceous and apocrine elements with the predominant component being the sebaceous glands. This naevus was first described by the dermatologist Josef Jadassohn in 1895 [7].

Epidemiology and pathogenesis. Naevus sebaceous has an incidence of 1 in 1000 live births and thus represents approximately one half of all EN [8]. In 2012 it was elucidated that sebaceous naevi are caused by activating postzygotic hotspot mutations in the *HRAS* and *KRAS* genes. About 90% of sebaceous naevi habour mutations in *HRAS*, whereas *KRAS* mutations are found in approximately 5% of the lesions. Interestingly, some naevi showed double mutations of *RAS* genes [9]. Several papers have confirmed the *HRAS* c.37G>C (p.Gly13Arg) mutation as the predominant mutation, present in about 90% of the sebaceous naevi [10,11]. Recently a rare distinct subtype of sebaceous naevi, the papillomatous pedunculated sebaceous naevus, has been shown to be caused by a postzygotic *FGFR2* mutation [12].

A meta-analysis of 4900 sebaceous naevi ascertained the secondary development of mostly benign tumours (syringocystadenoma papilliferum, trichoblastoma and trichilemmoma) in about 25% of lesions during life. Molecular analyses suggest that secondary tumours arising within sebaceous naevi derive directly from the sebaceous naevus cells, because tumour cells were demonstrated to carry the same oncogenic *HRAS* mutation as the respective naevus [9]. Interestingly, somatic activating *HRAS/KRAS* mutations could be detected in two of 18 sporadic trichoblastoma and seven of 23 sporadic syringocystadenoma papillifera (SCAP). Furthermore, the *BRAF* p.V600E mutation in SCAP could be validated in 12 of 23 lesions, with *BRAF* and *RAS* mutations being mutually exclusive. Of note, *BRAF* mutations were not found in SCAP arising within naevus sebaceous [13]. The finding of a single somatic mutation without loss of heterozygosity causing SCAP could later be confirmed using whole exome sequencing [14] and may point to auxiliary stimuli required for secondary tumour formation in naevus sebaceous [15].

Clinical features and differential diagnosis. Single sebaceous naevi are preferentially localized in the head and neck region and present as a yellowish, greasy, hairless plaque of varying size and shape seen at birth or shortly thereafter [8] (Fig. 106.1). Intraoral lesions may be seen, presenting as papillomatous plaques, which may be linear [16].

Mehregan and Pinkus have defined three overlapping stages in the natural development of sebaceous naevi. Whereas lesions in infancy and childhood are flat because of an underdevelopment of hairs and sebaceous glands, they typically thicken during adolescence secondary to hormonal stimulation. The third stage is characterized by the complicating development of neoplasms in the original naevus [17]. These neoplasms include benign lesions such as syringocystadenoma papilliferum, trichoblastoma (Fig. 106.2) and trichilemmoma as well as far less

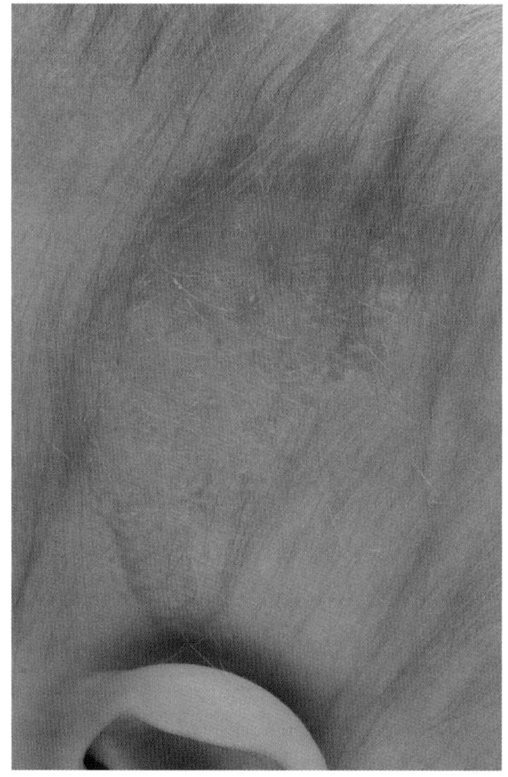

Fig. 106.1 Sebaceous naevus appearing as a hairless yellowish plaque.

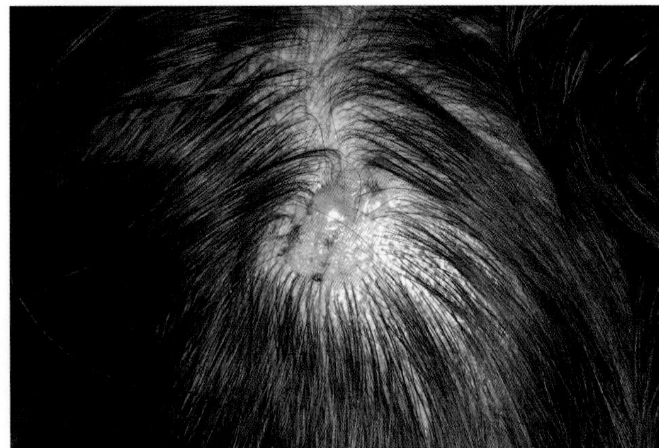

Fig. 106.2 Sebaceous naevus with associated trichoblastoma.

likely malignant lesions such as basal cell carcinoma, squamous cell carcinoma and sebaceous carcinoma [18].

A rare distinct subtype of sebaceous naevus is characterized by large, pink papillomatous and pedunculated nodules in neonates and fetuses [12,19]. For differential diagnosis keratinocytic epidermal naevus, naevus comedonicus and naevus psiloliparus should be considered [20].

Histopathology. The histopathology of sebaceous naevi varies with the patient's age. Although the sebaceous component may be prominent in the neonatal period as a result of androgenic stimulation, they often regress and appear relatively undeveloped in childhood, when they may exhibit cords of undifferentiated cells similar to embryonic hair follicles. With the onset of puberty, glandular enlargement and epidermal proliferation often occur in addition to proliferation and hyperkeratosis of the epidermis as well as papillomatosis. In histological sections, large mature sebaceous glands abnormally high in the dermis, effectively replacing hair follicles, are noted, some of which empty directly to the skin surface. Ectopic apocrine glands may be present as well as persistence of the primordial follicular structures.

Treatment. The only definitive treatment for naevus sebaceous is full thickness excision. Superficial ablative treatments like cryotherapy, electrodessication, CO_2-laser and photodynamic therapy carry a very high risk of recurrence of the naevus with its associated risk of secondary malignancy and thus cannot be recommended. There is a difference of opinion in the literature regarding the surgical management of naevus sebaceous. It is the opinion of the author that the decision to excise should be on a case by case basis. Prophylactic excision may be justified for cosmetic reasons or to avoid the formation of tumours [21]. If the decision is made to excise the naevus sebaceous prophylactically, excision should be performed before puberty, because this removes the naevus sebaceous before possible lesion enlargement and development of secondary tumours [17].

The recent identification of the genetic basis of naevus sebaceous may lead to the development of new medical treatments that target the aberrant signalling pathway.

Associated syndromes: Schimmelpenning syndrome, phacomatosis pigmentokeratotica and cutaneous skeletal hypophosphatemia syndrome

The *Schimmelpenning syndrome* was first described in 1957 by Gustav Schimmelpenning [22] and is defined as the association of a Blaschko-linear sebaceous naevus with extracutaneous abnormalities in the neurological, ocular and/or skeletal systems (Fig. 106.3). CNS abnormalities may manifest as seizures, mental deficiency, hemimegalencephaly, agyria, microgyria, pachygyria, dysplasia of brain vessels, Dandy–Walker malformation or cerebral heterotopia [20]. In a series of 196 patients with sebaceous naevus, 7% revealed neurological defects, particularly those with extensive naevi and naevi located on the central face [23]. Ocular abnormalities include colobomas, epibulbar lipodermoids, corneal opacities as well as optic nerve defects. Skeletal impairments comprise craniofacial defects, frontal bossing, kyphoskoliosis, deformities of limbs as well as hypophosphataemic rickets [20]. Importantly, however, although there are many reports on the association of neurological, ocular and skeletal anomalies in ENS, these reports do not distinguish between the EN subtypes, and do not necessarily distinguish between small single lesions and Blaschko-linear lesions which are likely to have arisen earlier in development. Given that that sebaceous naevi represent approximately one half of all EN, ocular and skeletal anomalies may have an incidence of 20–50% in patients with Schimmelpenning syndrome [24]. In 2012, somatic activating *HRAS* and *KRAS* mutations have been reported in two patients with Schimmelpenning syndrome [9], a finding that has been confirmed in further patients since then.

Phacomatosis pigmentokeratotica (PPK) was defined in 1996 as a distinct type of epidermal naevus syndrome by Rudolf Happle and is characterized by the coexistence of a sebaceous or verrucous (keratinocytic) epidermal naevus and a speckled lentiginous naevus (Fig. 106.4) [25]. With more than 30 cases of PPK reported in the literature, PPK has been described in association with skeletal (vitamin D-resistant hypophosphataemic rickets, scoliosis), ocular (coloboma, strabism), vascular (aortic stenosis)

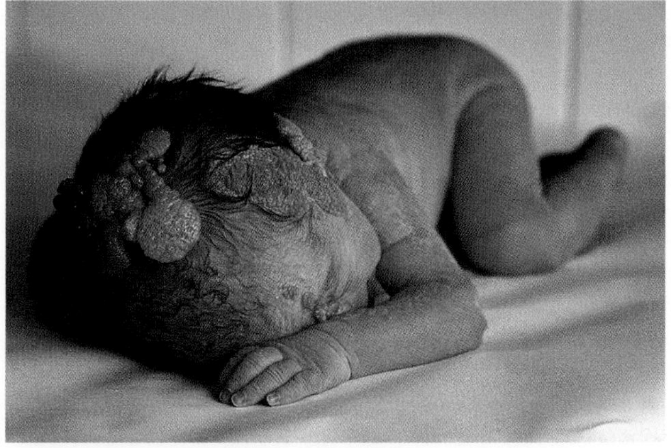

Fig. 106.3 Extensive sebaceous naevus, elevated from birth.

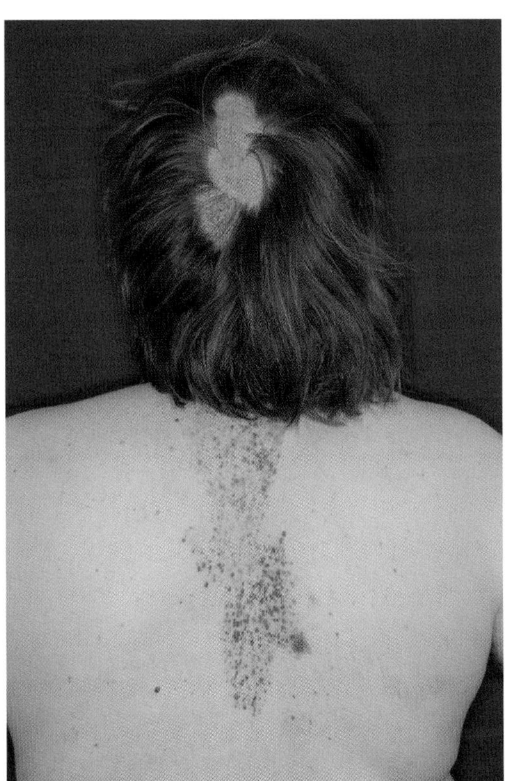

Fig. 106.4 Phacomatosis pigmentokeratotica.

and particularly neurological abnormalities (seizures, mental deficiency, sensory/motor neuropathy) [26].

Historically, PPK was thought to be a 'didymosis' (or twin-spotting phenomenon) with early postzygotic recombination as the cause of two different birthmarks in one individual. However, recently this concept was refuted at molecular level, and a new explanation provided. In 2013, heterozygous postzygotic activating mutations in exon 1 and 2 of the *HRAS* gene were reported in both the sebaceous naevus and naevus spilus cells in PPK, suggesting an early mutational event in a common progenitor cell [27]. Beside *HRAS* alterations, somatic activating *BRAF* mutations affecting exon 15 have also been reported as causative in a few PPK cases [28], and a single case of *NRAS* p.Q61R mutation [29].

With respect to the extracutaneous associations mentioned above, patients with Schimmelpenning syndrome and PPK should undergo complete physical examination and clinical evaluation. Specifically, they should be evaluated for neurological, ophthalmological, skeletal, endocrinological and vascular abnormalities. Intervention in the case of developmental delay should start as early as possible. Because the naevi themselves may develop secondary neoplasms, close clinical monitoring with biopsy of suspicious or changing lesions is advised.

From a genetic point of view Schimmelpenning syndrome and PPK may be viewed as variants of a continuous clinical spectrum caused by activating mosaic mutations affecting the RAS–MAPK pathway (mosaic RASopathies). Within this spectrum lies the only recently described disorder *cutaneous skeletal hypophosphatemia syndrome*, which is caused by somatic *RAS* mutations and is defined by the association of epidermal and/or very rarely melanocytic naevi in association with epidermal naevi, mosaic skeletal dysplasia and FGF23-mediated hypophosphatemia [30–32]. The different phenotypes of these syndromes may best be explained by a mutated progenitor cell, which results in mutated cell populations with variable developmental potential and subsequently different clinical phenotypes [27].

Naevus comedonicus

Introduction and history. Naevus comedonicus (NC) was first described in 1895 by Kofmann [33]. It is a rare organoid epidermal naevus, occurring before the age of 10 in the great majority of cases. The estimated prevalence is one in 45 000 to one in 100 000 [34]. Historically, there has been some debate over whether NC consisting of comedo-like dilated follicular orifices and 'acne naevus' are two different entities [20,35]. Recent molecular data have proven the concept of two different entities.

Pathogenesis. Recently whole exome sequencing helped identify postzygotic *NEK9* mutations as the cause of NC [36]. The *NEK9* mutations detected in a small series of three NC are gain-of-function mutations, resulting in an increased NEK9 kinase activity. Interestingly the respective *NEK9* mutations could be found in DNA isolated from the follicle tissue as well as from the interfollicular epidermis. This finding argues for a follicle-specific effect of *NEK9* mutations, because no clinical or histological phenotype is found in the interfollicular epidermis [36].

By way of contrast, 'acne naevus' is caused by postzygotic *FGFR2* mutations [37]. In an elegant approach revealing the precise topography of *FGFR2* mosaicism in this particular form of acne, keratinocytes around the dilated infundibulum were identified as carriers of the *FGFR2* mutation. Perilesional epidermal keratinocytes, the keratin plug, the sebaceous gland or the surrounding dermis were found to carry a *FGFR2* wildtype status [38].

Clinical features. NC is characterized by grouped dilated infundibula, which have dark, hyperkeratotic plugs in their centre (Fig. 106.5). NC may present at different extents unilaterally, bilaterally and in a linear, interrupted, segmental or blaschkoid fashion [34]. Generally, NC is an asymptomatic lesion. However, it may be complicated by the development of deeper nodulocystic lesions resolving with scarring. Segmentally arranged basaloid follicular hamartomas, may clinically resemble NC [39] and must be separated. Tumours described in association with NC are mostly benign and include trichoepithelioma, pilar sheath tumour, keratoacanthoma, syringocystadenoma papilliferum and hidradenoma papilliferum. Only very rarely basal cell carcinoma and squamous cell carcinoma have been reported [34].

Histopathology. NC exhibits deep wide epidermal invaginations derived from follicular structures, which contain keratin. Small sebaceous glands may be seen opening into the lower portion of the structure. Hair is rarely formed.

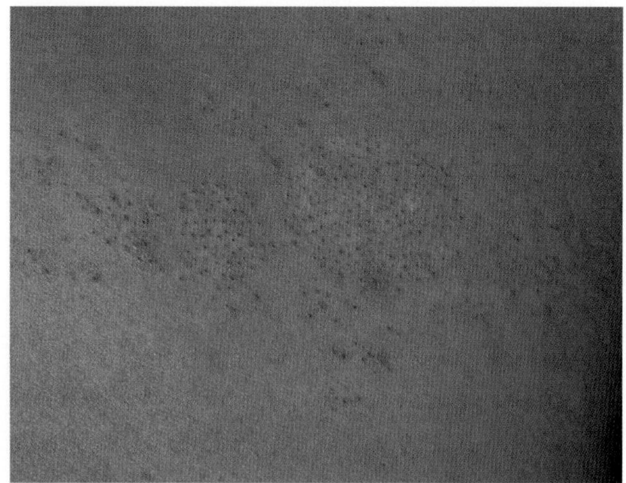

Fig. 106.5 Naevus comedonicus demonstrating multiple horny plugs.

The epidermis between comedones may exhibit hyperkeratosis, papillomatosis and acanthosis typical of nonorganoid EN. Some lesions resemble a collection of dilated pores of Winer [40].

Treatment. Except for aesthetic reasons, NC does not require aggressive treatment. Keratolytics such as salicylic acid or 12% ammonium lactate may be beneficial in some patients. Topical and oral retinoids are mostly found to be ineffective and may only show some benefit in the treatment of the 'acne naevus' [34]. Ablative lasers like erbium YAG or CO_2 lasers have shown improvements in single patients [41]. However, surgical full-thickness excision is the only definite treatment option. Previous to excision, implantation of a tissue expander may be needed for defect closure [42]. Alternatively, skin transplantation may be an option.

Associated syndrome

The NC syndrome was delineated in 1978 by Engber [43]. The most characteristic extracutaneous abnormality associated with NC is ipsilateral cataract. Other extracutaneous manifestations associated with NC include neurological defects such as electroencephalographic (EEG) abnormalities and seizures, microcephaly, dysgenesis of corpus callosum and cognitive defects. Skeletal anomalies comprise scoliosis, polysyndactyly or clinodactyly, vertebral defects and absence of a ray of hand bones [20,34].

Porokeratotic eccrine and ostial dermal duct naevus

Introduction and history. Porokeratotic eccrine ostial and dermal duct naevus (PEODDN) is also known as porokeratotic eccrine naevus (PEN). The term was coined in 1980 by Abell and Read to describe a hard verrucous epidermal naevus.

Pathogenesis. In 2012 somatic mutations in *GJB2*, which codes for the gap junction protein connexin 26 which permits intercellular ion and macromolecule flux, were identified as the cause of PEODDN [44]. By using whole-exome sequencing, another group later confirmed that somatic GJB2 mutations alone are sufficient to cause PEODDN [45]. Interestingly, dominantly inherited (germline) *GJB2* mutations are known to cause the severe multisystem disorder keratitis–ichthyosis–deafness (KID) syndrome.

Clinical features. PEODDN present as linear, spiky, hyperkeratotic papules and plaques, which may resemble verrucous epidermal naevi (Figs 106.6 and 106.7). In the palmoplantar region a comedo-like appearance (keratotic

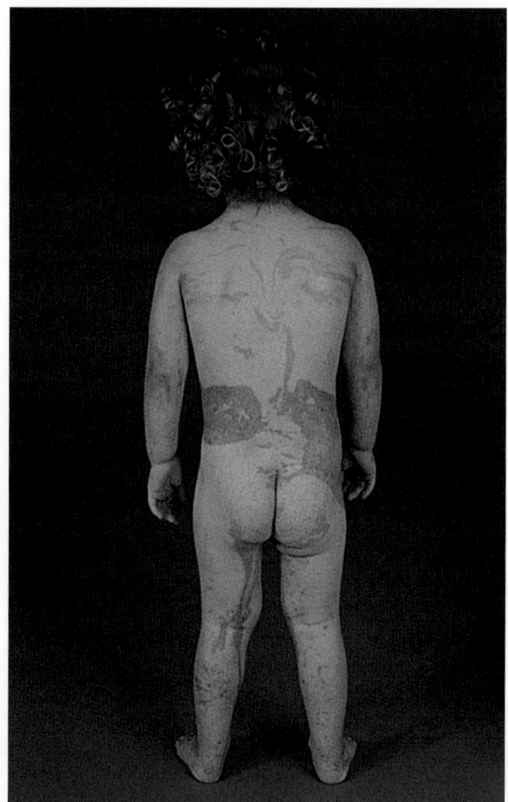

Fig. 106.6 Extensive porokeratotic eccrine naevus.

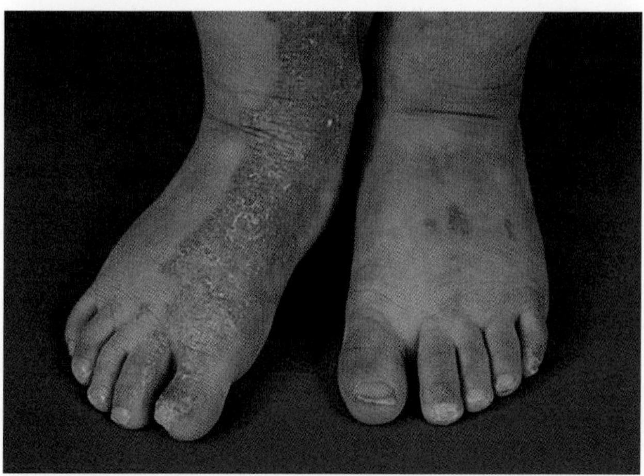

Fig. 106.7 Detail of porokeratotic eccrine naevus in the patient depicted in Fig. 106.6.

plugs within central pits) can be found [44]. The keratinous plug cannot be extracted with manual pressure. The lesions are usually asymptomatic, although mild pruritus is rarely noted [46]. Although PEODDN may be considered as a congenital hamartoma of eccrine origin, late-onset variants have been described [47]. The differential diagnosis of PEODDN comprises naevus comedonicus, (linear verrucous) keratinocytic epidermal naevus, inflammatory linear verrucous epidermal naevus and congenital unilateral punctate porokeratosis.

Histopathology. The histopathological hallmark of PEODDN is the finding of multiple ortho-/parakeratotic plugs resembling cornoid lamellae protruding from dilated and hyperplastic eccrine acrosyringia. In addition, hyper(para)keratosis and wavy psoriasiform epidermal acanthosis can also be present [44].

Treatment. PEODDN may respond to topical treatment with tazarotene gel, dithranol and topical photodynamic therapy. However, CO_2 laser or CO_2/erbium laser treatments seem to be the more promising therapeutic modality in most but not all patients. Topical steroids and topical tretinoin are ineffective [48]. Becasue *GJB2* mutations cause PEODDN when postzygotic, and KID syndrome when germline, all individuals with PEODDN lesions should be counselled regarding the potential risk of having a child with KID syndrome.

Associated syndrome

Extracutaneous findings reported in association with widespread PEN include seizures, polyneuropathy, hemiparesis, deafness and scoliosis, unilateral breast hypoplasia and developmental delay [48].

Becker naevus

Introduction and history. Becker naevus (BN) was first described in 1949 by S.W. Becker as 'concurrent melanosis and hypertrichosis in the distribution of naevus unius lateris' [49].

Pathogenesis. In 2017 whole exome sequencing helped identify postzygotic *ACTB* mutations as the cause of BN and BN syndrome. The *ACTB* p.R147C and p.R147S hotspot mutations were detected in 61% of BN and found to potentiate Hedgehog pathway signalling, thereby probably disrupting hair follicle and pilar muscle development. Laser capture microdissection identified pilar muscle as cell linage containing the *ACTB* mutation [50].

Clinical features. BN is observed in both sexes and is characterized by a well-demarcated irregularly bordered, tan-coloured patch covered with coarse dark hairs (Fig. 106.8). Three varieties of BN have been suggested: melanotic, hypertrichotic and mixed types [51]. Of note, BN in children are often hairless with the characteristic hypertrichosis particularly developing in postpubertal men. When rubbed, BN become more elevated/infiltrated (pseudo-Darier's sign). In contrast to other epidermal naevi, BN is characteristically arranged in a segmental, flag or chequerboard pattern with midline cut-off [20]. BN may rarely be present at birth but may also have its onset later in childhood or in adolescence [52]. The lesion is typically observed on the trunk, especially on the scapular and chest region. In a series of 118 cases a conspicuous association with other pigmentary anomalies such as congenital melanocytic naevi and café-au-lait spots was noted [52].

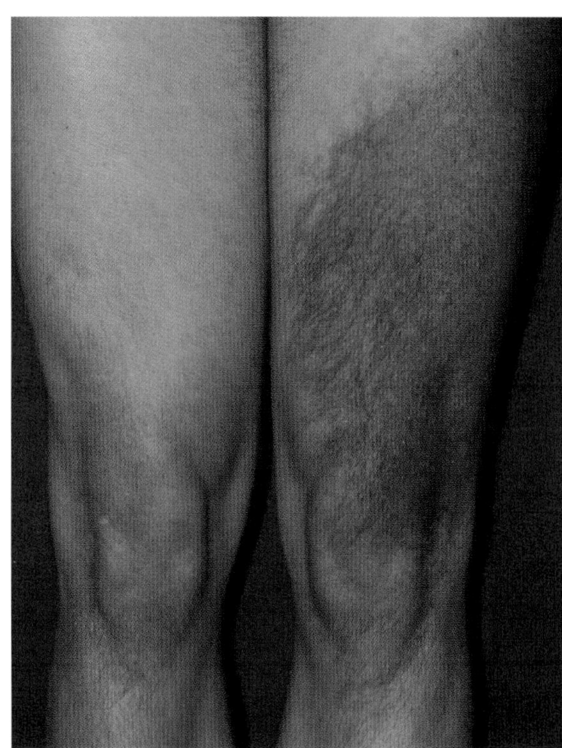

Fig. 106.8 Becker naevus presenting as an irregularly bordered tan-coloured patch, covered with coarse dark hairs.

Differential diagnoses, especially in children, are congenital smooth muscle hamartomas, congenital melanocytic naevi and large solitary café-au lait-spots. Congenital smooth muscle hamartomas appear as a skin-coloured or mildly hyperpigmented and irregularly shaped patch or plaque with prominent vellus hairs [53].

Histopathology. The general histopathological features of BN skin are acanthosis, papillomatosis, keratotic plugging and irregular elongated rete ridges, which show a characteristic fusion of two or more adjacent rete ridges. In the dermis, mild superficial perivascular lymphohistiocytic infiltration and an increase of smooth muscle bundles, which are not associated with hair follicles, may be observed [54].

Treatment. BN are generally asymptomatic, but they may represent a distressing cosmetic handicap. In a prospective comparative study of 11 patients with 2 years follow up and histological evaluation, one pass of Er:YAG laser treatment resulted in a complete clearance (100%) in six patients, whereas clearance of more that 50% was obtained in all subjects. Repigmentation was mild because of total ablation of the epidermis and partial ablation of the papillary dermis. In the same study 11 patients were treated with a Q-switched Nd:YAG system. However, in terms of pigment removal after 2 years, one pass with Er:YAG proved to be superior to three treatment sessions with the Nd:YAG system [55]. Fractional CO_2-laser treatment of 11 patients showed only moderate effectiveness in a prospective randomized controlled, observer-blinded split-lesion trial [56]. Hair removal may be achieved using long-pulsed ruby, Nd:YAG and alexandrite lasers, or intense pulsed light technology but requires 10–15 treatment sessions [57].

Associated syndrome

BN have been associated with ipsilateral hypoplasia of the breast, supernumerary nipples, hypoplasia of underlying musculature, scoliosis, vertebral defects, fused or accessory cervical ribs, pectus excavatum or carinatum, short limb and segmental odontomaxillary hypoplasia or dysplasia [20].

Woolly hair naevus

This naevus entity is characterized by distinct areas of tightly curled scalp hair and may present as an isolated lesion or in association with keratinocytic EN at other sites (Fig. 106.9). Recently, mosaic *HRAS* c.34G>A and mosaic *BRAF* c.1803A>T mutations were identified as genetic causes of woolly hair naevi [28,58]. In both publications the same mutation could be detected in the woolly hair naevus as well as in the associated keratinocytic epidermal naevi. Woolly hair is also frequently found in Costello syndrome, which results from germline heterozygous *HRAS* mutations. These data exemplify the above-mentioned concept that the extent and clinical phenotype of the respective naevus is determined by the timing of the specific mutation during embryogenesis, the level of pathway activation as well as the affected postzygotic (pluripotent) cell.

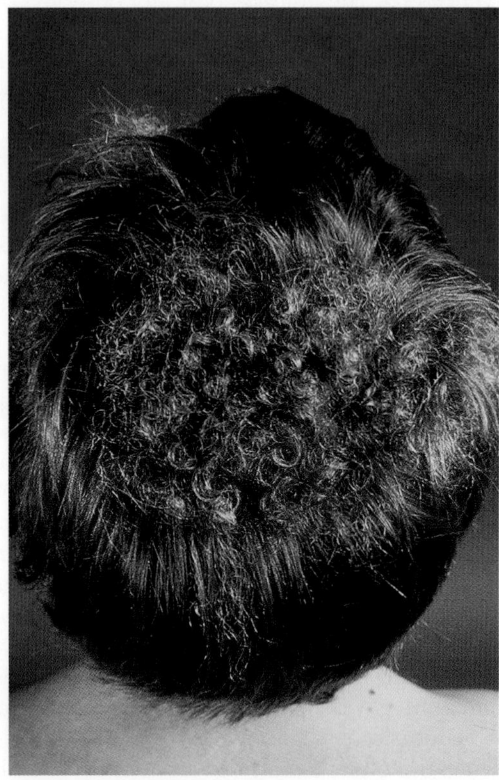

Fig. 106.9 Woolly hair naevus.

Important differential diagnoses are the Naxos syndrome caused by alterations in the *JUP* gene encoding placoglobin, as well as the Caravajal syndrome, which is associated with mutations in desmoplakin. Clinically, both syndromes are characterized by woolly hair, palmoplantar keratoderma and cardiomyopathy [59].

Although there are no definitive treatments for woolly hair naevus, treatment with nonablative fractional lasers may help promote normal hair growth [60].

Eccrine naevus/mucinous eccrine naevus

The pathogenesis of eccrine naevus is not yet known. Eccrine naevi are very rare congenital lesions most commonly presenting on the forearms as a hyperhidrotic area without any epidermal changes. However, solitary or multiple brown patches or plaques may also be a part of the clinical presentation [61]. Of note, eccrine naevi without associated hyperhidrosis as well as naevi appearing at an advanced age have been reported. Histology shows an increased number of normal-appearing eccrine coils or an increase in the size of coils within the superficial dermis. Surgical excision is the usual treatment of eccrine naevus. Intralesional botulinum toxin has been described as an alternative therapy [62].

Mucinous eccrine naevus is an extremely rare variant of eccrine naevi. The most common clinical presentation is a unilateral, solitary, brownish nodule on the legs with facultative localized hyperhidrosis.

The histopathological features comprise both eccrine proliferation and abundant mucin deposition surrounding the eccrine glands and ducts. The main treatment options are no intervention or surgical excision [63].

Angora hair naevus

The angora hair naevus was first described in 2000 by Schauder and colleagues and may be deemed to be exceedingly rare. Its genetic basis is still unknown. Clinically this organoid epidermal naevus is characterized by rather broad linear areas of lanugo-like depigmented hypertrichosis along Blaschko lines. Histological evaluation reveals dilated follicular pores and dermal acanthosis [64]. Associated extracutaneous features may include ocular defects (e.g. iris coloboma, iridocorneal adhesions) and craniocerebral anomalies (e.g. dilated ventricles, porencephaly, seizures) [20].

Naevus trichilemnocysticus

This rare organoid epidermal naevus entity was delineated in 2007. Its hallmark is the linear arrangement of trichilemnal cysts which are accompanied by hyperkeratotic plaques covered with multiple filiform hyperkeratoses [65]. Histopathology of the nodules is typical of trichilemmal cysts, which are characterized by a flat stratified epithelium with abrupt keratinization without the presence of a granular layer. The filiform hyperkeratoses show follicular dilation with parakeratotic plugging. Skeletal abnormalities like frontal bossing and juvenile idiopathic arthritis have been described in association with this naevus entity. However, in the majority of reported cases no extracutaneous anomalies are described [65–67].

Segmentally arranged basaloid follicular hamartomas

Segmentally arranged basaloid follicular hamartomas associated with osseous, dental and cerebral anomalies were described as a distinct entity in 2008 by Happle and Tinschert [39]. This syndrome is clinically characterized by segmentally and rather densely arranged skin-coloured papules and nodules, dark comedones and pits. Furthermore, the affected segments may show hypo- or hyperpigmentation, hypo- or hypertrichosis and atrophodermia. Histopathology reveals squamoid or basaloid cells emanating from the follicular infundibulum and forming horn cysts and anastomoses. An activating mutation in *smoothened (SMO)* encoding a receptor for sonic hedgehog has only recently been reported in a patient with segmentally arranged basaloid follicular hamartomas, basal cell carcinomas, pits and comedones, thus conforming with the entity delineated by Happle and Tinschert [68,69]. The coincidental finding of basaloid follicular hamartomas and basal cell carcinomas in this patient, which has previously led to some debate, may best be explained by various degrees of pathway activation.

Nonorganoid epidermal naevi

Key points

- **Keratinocytic epidermal naevi manifest as linear or whorled skin-coloured or brownish papules or plaques. Somatic *HRAS*, *KRAS*, *NRAS*, *FGFR3*, *FGFR2*, *PIK3CA* and rarely *AKT1* mutations have been described as aetiological in this naevus entity.**
- **Congenital lipomatous overgrowth, vascular malformations and epidermal naevi (CLOVE) and Proteus syndrome are associated with keratinocytic epidermal naevi and are caused by somatic heterocygous *PIK3CA* and *AKT1* mutations respectively.**
- **The epidermolytic hyperkeratotic epidermal naevus is only histologically distinguishable from other keratinocytic epidermal naevi (KEN) and is caused by somatic heterocygous *KRT1* and *KRT10* mutations.**
- **Dyskeratotic and acantholytic epidermal naevi present as pruritic warty follicular and nonfollicular brown papules and plaques arranged in a linear fashion. Somatic mosaic mutations in *ATP2A2* have been identified as the genetic basis of these naevi.**
- **Inflammatory linear verrucous epidermal naevi manifest as unilateral, Blaschko-linear, intensely pruritic flesh-coloured papules and may be caused by somatic heterocygous mutations in *GJA1*.**
- **The CHILD (congenital hemidysplasia with ichthyosiform erythroderma and limb defects) naevus consists of circumscribed inflammatory plaques surmounted by prominent wax-like scales. CHILD naevus and the associated syndrome is caused by missense or nonsense mutations in the *NSDHL* gene.**
- **Naevus marginatus combines elements of both: an organoid naevus sebaceous and a nonorganoid keratinocytic epidermal naevus and is caused by *HRAS* mutations.**

Nonorganoid epidermal naevi comprise the common keratinocytic epidermal naevus, the keratinocytic epidermal naevus in Proteus and Cowden syndrome, the papular epidermal naevus with skyline basal cell layer (PENS), the epidermolytic hyperkeratotic epidermal naevus, the inflammatory linear verrucous epidermal naevus (ILVEN) as well as the congenital hemidysplasia with ichthyosiform erythroderma and limb defects (CHILD) naevus.

Keratinocytic epidermal naevus

Introduction and history. The common keratinocytic epidermal naevus (KEN), which shows differentiation exclusively to keratinocytes, is the most frequent nonorganoid epidermal naevus and has an incidence of about 1 in 1000 live births [70].

Pathogenesis. Approximately 40% of KEN have been shown to harbour postzygotic activating mutations in *FGFR3* and *PIK3CA* [71,72]. Another 40% result from mosaic activating *HRAS*, *KRAS* and very rarely *NRAS* mutations. Of note, *AKT1* mutations were absent in a series of 47 randomly assembled KEN [73], but have been described in individual cases [74]. Only recently the mutational spectrum has been expanded by somatic embryonic *FGFR2* mutations, which cause 5–10% of KEN [75]. Interestingly, *HRAS* or *FGFR3* mutations may co-occur with *PIK3CA* mutations; however, *HRAS* and *FGFR3* mutations are mutually exclusive. Within this mutational spectrum, there is a predominance of the *FGFR3* p.R248C and the *HRAS* p.G13R mutation, which together account for 30–40% of KEN [73]. Despite these hotspots, the mutational spectrum in KEN is much more diverse than in organoid epidermal naevi, e.g. in sebaceous naevi.

Clinical features and differential diagnosis. KEN are usually present at birth or manifest in early infancy as linear or whorled skin-coloured or brownish papules or plaques, following the lines of Blaschko (Figs 106.10 and 106.11). Lesions in infancy and childhood are commonly flat but can thicken and darken over time [6]. Some lesions can exhibit striking hyperkeratosis leading to a verrucous appearance. KEN primarily present on the trunk or the extremities, with the extent and distribution varying greatly from small to large, and unilateral to bilateral, with strict midline demarcation. Acral lesions tend to have a warty appearance with ensuing nail dystrophy if the nail matrix is involved. Body fold lesions are apt to be softer.

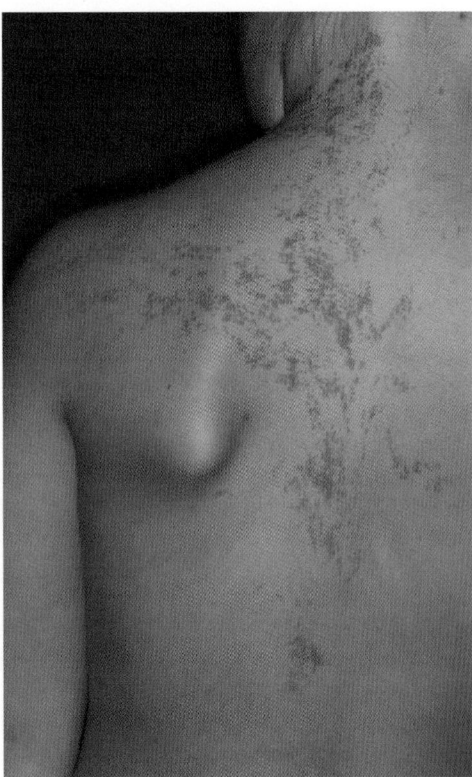

Fig. 106.10 Keratinocytic naevus on the trunk with multiple curved lines and midline demarcation.

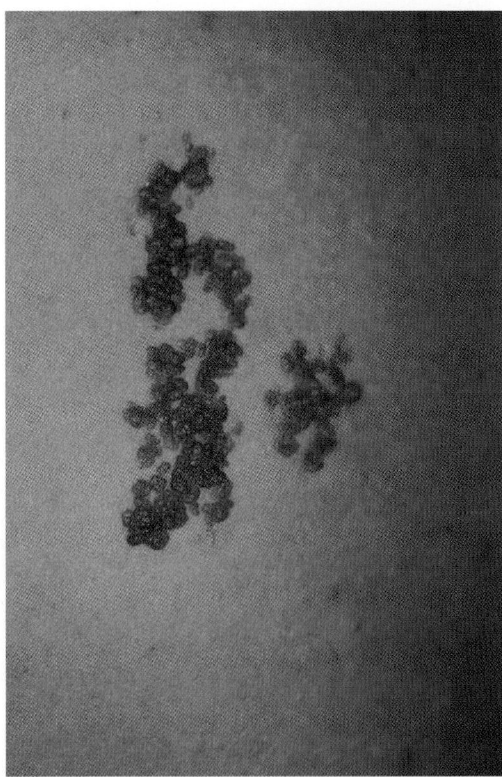

Fig. 106.11 Keratinocytic naevus, comprising an array of small papillomas.

Histopathology. The keratinocytic epidermal naevus is histologically characterized by acanthosis with elongation of rete ridges, papillomatosis, orthohyperkeratosis and possibly basal hyperpigmentation. These epidermal changes are sharply demarcated from the surrounding unaffected skin [76].

Treatment. Surgical excision where possible is a straightforward definite treatment. Superficial destructive treatment modalities with a reasonable chance of success are ablative laser treatments, shave excisions, electroplaning and cryotherapy. In a series of 71 verrucous (keratinocytic) epidermal naevi, cryotherapy resulted in 75–100% clearance rates in approximately 90% of patients with small localized naevi. All the lesions were treated by two freeze–thaw cycles using spray cryosurgery until clinical frosting was sustained for 5–10 seconds depending on body area and thickness of the lesion. After defrosting, a second cycle was performed. Small lesions required three to four, larger lesions seven to eight treatments in 6–8-week intervals. Of the six patients with extensive naevi included in the study, all responded poorly to cryotherapy. The major adverse event after cryotherapy was hypopigmentation in about 40% of cases. CO_2 laser treatment was performed in nine patients with insufficient response to cryotherapy leading to 75–100% clearance rates in four patients [77]. In a series of 15 patients with KEN, CO_2 laser therapy resulted in 50–75% clearance in 50% of cases and more than 75% clearance in 30% of cases. Recurrence was primarily observed in patients with epidermal naevi exceeding 100 cm^2. The side effects were hypopigmentation in 25% and scarring in 20% of patients [78].

Associated syndromes

The keratinocytic epidermal naevus syndrome is characterized by a keratinocytic epidermal naevus, whose underlying mosaic mutation has spread to other organs. The extracutaneous abnormalities in KEN syndrome may comprise neuronal (e.g. seizures, mental retardation, hemimegalencephaly, ventricular abnormalities, cortical atrophy and hemiparesis), skeletal (e.g. incomplete bone formation, hypertrophy or hypoplasia of bones, bone cysts, kyphoscoliosis and vitamin D-resistant rickets) and ocular defects (e.g. colobomas, corneal opacities, macrophthalmia and microphthalmia) [2,79]. Particular attention has to be paid to the occurrence of urothelial carcinomas in patients with KEN syndrome, whose correlation with KEN is nonstochastic [80].

A general problem in the delineation of 'the KEN syndrome' is the fact that extracutaneous abnormalities associated with KEN have been grouped with extracutaneous defects associated with other EN in the past. From a genetic point of view, the genetic heterogeneity of KEN makes the delineation of one all-encompassing 'KEN syndrome' seem unreasonable, even though the clinical appearance of KEN with varying genetic background is the same. Therefore, 'the KEN syndrome' will probably be subdivided in the future, with the correlation of genetic defect and extracutaneous features worked out. An example of this reasonable subdivision is the congenital lipomatous overgrowth, vascular malformations and epidermal naevi (CLOVE) syndrome.

CLOVE syndrome

CLOVE is an acronym for congenital lipomatous overgrowth, vascular malformations and epidermal naevus. Another acronym used is CLOVES syndrome (congenital lipomatous overgrowth with vascular, epidermal and skeletal anomalies). This disorder shares some features with the Proteus syndrome, but was separated from it by Sapp in 2007 by the criterion of nonprogressive proportionate overgrowth, which is not distorting, in contrast to the Proteus syndrome [81]. In 2012 this syndrome could also genetically be separated from Proteus syndrome as somatic *PIK3CA* mutations could be identified as the underlying genetic cause of CLOVES syndrome [82]. CLOVES thus adds to a growing list of overgrowth syndromes that result from somatic activation of the PI3K-AKT pathway, and as such comes under the term PIK3CA-related overgrowth spectrum disorders (PROS) [83].

As the name CLOVES encompasses, this syndrome clinically comprises beside a keratinocytic epidermal naevus, progressive, complex and mixed truncal vascular and lymphatic malformations, dysregulated adipose tissue, varying degrees of scoliosis and enlarged bony structures without progressive bony overgrowth [82]. Patients with CLOVES syndrome have a low but important susceptibility to various adult onset cancers, including gastrointestinal tract, brain, breast, bladder, kidney, lung and thyroid [35].

Therapeutically, patients with CLOVES syndrome require ongoing surgical care for the progressive overgrowth of truncal lipomas as well as for the complex vascular malformations. Close interdisciplinary monitoring with respect to the increased cancer risk is warranted.

Proteus syndrome

The Proteus syndrome (PS) has an incidence of less than one case per 1 million and was described in 1979 by Cohen and Hayden [84], and clearly delineated in 1999 by Biesecker and colleagues [85]. In 2011 the somatic activating mutation p.E17K in the oncogene *AKT1*, encoding the AKT1 kinase, was identified as the genetic cause in at least 90% of PS patients [86]. The cutaneous PS phenotype is characterized by a flat, soft and velvety epidermal naevus, vascular malformations (especially capillary malformations) and cerebriform hyperplasia of palmar or plantar connective tissue [20]. *AKT1* mutations in keratinocytes were identified as the key determinant of KEN formation. Moreover, *AKT1* mutations could be identified in fibroblasts isolated from cerebriform connective tissue naevi (CCTN), whereas the mutant allele was not detected in the keratinocytes of CCTN. Because mutant cells were found in dermal fibroblasts of both CCTN and normal appearing skin, the presence of mutant cells in the dermis appears necessary but not sufficient to drive the formation of CCTN [87]. As mentioned above, *AKT1* mutations are a rare cause of KEN [73]. The overgrowth of skin is most commonly associated with patchy or segmental disproportionate and progressive overgrowth of bones, connective tissue and fat. However, the manifestations of Proteus syndrome may include any tissue of the body. Most patients with PS are born without significant asymmetry and the rapid asymmetric overgrowth starts at the age of 6–18 months. Patients with PS appear to have an increased susceptibility to the development of tumours, with the two types of tumours most specifically associated with PS being monomorphic adenomas of the parotid glands and bilateral ovarian cystadenomas [88]. The management of PS patients is challenging and requires early and aggressive treatment of overgrowth with multiple orthopaedic procedures over years. Because one of the most common causes of death for patients with PS is deep venous thrombosis and pulmonary embolism, perioperative anticoagulant prophylaxis is strongly recommended. In contrast to this, chronic anticoagulation is not recommended [88].

Linear Cowden naevus

Linear Cowden naevus is associated with type 2 segmental Cowden disease, a term coined in 2007 by Happle to denote a multisystem birth defect, for which the acronym SOLAMEN syndrome (segmental overgrowth, lipomatosis, arteriovenous malformation and epidermal naevus) has also been proposed [89,90]. Linear Cowden naevus is a keratinocytic epidermal naevus caused by loss of heterozygosity in the context of a heterozygous *PTEN* germline mutation [89] and is clinically characterized with a rather thick and papillomatous surface, reminiscent of the structure of a common wart. Type 2 segmental Cowden disease clinically comprises cutaneous and extracutaneous vascular anomalies, cutaneous and extracutaneous lipomas, polyps of the jejunum or colon, skeletal (e.g. asymmetric growth of limbs) and neurological anomalies (seizures, macrocephaly) [20]. As for patients with CLOVES and Proteus syndrome, patients with type 2 segmental Cowden disease require ongoing surgical care and close interdisciplinary monitoring with respect to the polyps of the jejunum and colon.

Note: Clinical similarity of CLOVES, Proteus and type 2 segmental Cowden disease are reflected genetically, because *PIK3CA*, *AKT* and *PTEN* mutations all affect the same growth regulatory pathway (IP3/AKT/MTOR).

Papular epidermal naevus with skyline basal cell layer (PENS)

Pathogenesis. In the first report delineating the papular epidermal naevus with skyline basal cell layer (PENS) as a variant of epidermal naevus, genetic testing for *PIK3CA* and *FGFR3* mutations has been performed on two naevus samples, revealing a wildtype sequence [91]. Since this initial report the pathogenesis of PENS remains to be elucidated.

Clinical features and differential diagnosis. PENS is visible at birth or develops shortly thereafter. The lesions are asymptomatic and of variable shapes. They appear as small hyperkeratotic papules and plaques with a rough, flat surface and a randomized asymmetric distribution [91]. However, PENS following a Blaschko-linear pattern have also been described [92].

SECTION 23: MOSAIC DISORDERS

Histopathology. PENS characteristically shows a compact orthokeratotic hyperkeratosis, acanthosis and a perfectly delineated basal cell layer with palisaded arrangement ('skyline') of basal cell nuclei. No dermal or appendiceal changes can be observed [91].

Treatment. To date there are no specific reports on how to treat PENS. Principally all methods used in the treatment of common KEN may be applied.

Associated syndromes

Rarely PENS may be associated with neurological anomalies like mild developmental delay, epilepsy or autism. Peculiar facies, bilateral Achilles tendon shortening, hypospadias and curved penis have been observed in single reports [93].

Epidermolytic hyperkeratotic epidermal naevus

The epidermolytic hyperkeratotic epidermal naevus represents approximately 5–10% of KEN.

Pathogenesis. In 1994 somatic *KRT10* gene mutations were identified as the genetic basis of this naevus in four patients [94]. In 2007 a somatic mutation in the *KRT1* gene was reported to result in an epidermolytic hyperkeratotic epidermal naevus in one patient [95].

Clinical features and differential diagnosis. Clinically, the epidermolytic hyperkeratotic epidermal naevus is only barely distinguishable from other KEN and appears as a yellowish-greyish-brown, thin, soft and scaly plaque, which may follow the lines of Blaschko. Because keratin 1 and 10 are only expressed in the epidermis, no extracutaneous manifestations are expected with this epidermal naevus type. However, in the case of gonosomal mosaicism, the offspring of patients with epidermolytic hyperkeratotic epidermal naevus may have generalized epidermolytic hyperkeratosis.

Histopathology. As the name encompasses, the histopathological hallmark of this keratinocytic EN is epidermolytic hyperkeratosis, which is accompanied by irregularly shaped keratohyaline granules and perinuclear vacuolization [76].

Treatment. There are reports on the improvement of epidermolytic hyperkeratotic epidermal naevi when treated with topical calcipotriol/betametasone dipropionate combination ointment or topical application of the topical vitamin D3 analogue maxacalcitol [96,97]. In this respect the recent incidental observation of an excellent clinical response with regard to skin scaling and stiffness in children with congenital ichthyosis after short-term high-dose vitamin D supplementation is highly interesting. Patients were given 60 000 IU of oral cholecalciferol daily for 10 days with subsequent daily doses of 400– 600 IU of cholecalciferol [98]. From a series of 16 patients from 12 families with generalized or naevoid epidermolytic hyperkeratosis nine patients had been treated with systemic retinoids (etretinate, acitretin, isotretinoin or alitretinoin), but only three patients had acceptable treatment responses. Two patients worsened during treatment [99].

Dyskeratotic and acantholytic epidermal naevus

Introduction and history. Reviewing 32 cases of linear or zosteriform epidermal lesions with the clinical and histological characteristics of Darier's disease, Starink and Woerdeman proposed the term 'acantholytic dyskeratotic epidermal naevi' for these kinds of lesions [100].

Pathogenesis. Dyskeratotic and acantholytic epidermal naevi represent about 1% of EN [76]. In 2000 Sakuntabhai *et al.* identified somatic mosaic mutations in *ATP2A2* as the genetic basis of acantholytic dyskeratotic naevi in two patients. *ATP2A2* encodes the sarco/endoplasmic reticulum calcium ATPase isoform 2 (SERCA2), a calcium pump, which plays an important part in Ca^{2+} signal transduction. Because acantholytic dyskeratotic naevi can thus arise from a somatic mutation in the same gene that is causative in Darier's disease; the term segmental Darier's disease has been proposed for this EN. In some patients with EN showing acantholysis and dyskeratosis, no *ATP2A2* mutations or mutations in similar genes such as *ATP2C1* could be detected [101].

Clinical features and differential diagnosis, Dyskeratotic and acantholytic epidermal naevi may present as pruritic confluent warty follicular as well as nonfollicular, pink or brown papules and plaques arranged in a linear fashion. As a peculiarity of this naevus and consistent with (systemic) Darier´s disease, delayed onset at an age of 20 years or later is commonly observed. Lesions may be aggravated by sunlight, heat, sweating and friction [100].

Histopathology. The histological hallmark of this form of epidermal naevus is acantholytic dyskeratosis, i.e. loss of adhesion between keratinocytes (acantholysis) with dyskeratotic cells (corps ronds and grains) in the upper epidermis [102].

Treatment. Mild cases require emollients and sun protection. In severer cases oral (acictretin and isotretinoin) and topical retinoids (tretinoin and adapalene) have proved to be quite useful in the treatment of (localized) Darier´s disease and may thus be applied. Ablative lasers (CO_2 and Erbium:YAG lasers) have also proved to be effective [103].

ILVEN

Introduction and history. Unlike the noninflammatory keratinocytic epidermal naevus, the ILVEN is far less common and was first described in 1971 by Altman and Mehregan.

Pathogenesis. In a single case of ILVEN, whole exome sequencing helped identify a somatic heterocygous mutation in *GJA1*, a gene encoding a gap junction protein and causatively involved in erythrokeratodermia variabilis et progressiva [104]. Mutation screening of epidermal connexins could be promising for identifying other causative mutations of ILVEN in future studies.

Clinical features and differential diagnosis. ILVEN show a predilection for the buttock and legs and initially present as unilateral, Blaschko-linear, intensely pruritic cutaneous lesions consisting of dense flesh-coloured papules which later form dark red to brown plaques with verrucous surface (Fig. 106.12). About half of the lesions are congenital with the remainder occurring early in life. However, onset during adulthood has also been reported [105]. No associated syndromes have been reported for ILVEN.

Differential diagnoses include keratinocytic epidermal naevi, linear psoriasis, CHILD naevus and lichen striatus. Lichen striatus is less pruritic than ILVEN and transient, typically lasting for 2–4 years and then resolving. CHILD naevus histologically shows verruciform xanthomatous changes and may safely be differentiated. Linear psoriasis (Fig. 106.13) typically occurs in patients with existing psoriasis elsewhere [106].

Histopathology. ILVEN demonstrates a characteristic alternating pattern of hypogranulosis with parakeratosis and hypergranulosis with orthohyperkeratosis. Frequently the epidermis is acanthotic with psoriasiform changes and shows exaggerated rete ridges. The dermis contains a perivascular and interface T cell predominate lymphocytic inflammatory infiltrate. In attempts to differentiate histologically ILVEN from psoriasis, immunohistochemical analyses have demonstrated increased numbers of keratin-10 positive cells and greater HLA-DR expression in ILVEN compared with psoriatic lesions [107]. However, to date no immunohistochemical marker may conclusively differentiate ILVEN from psoriasis.

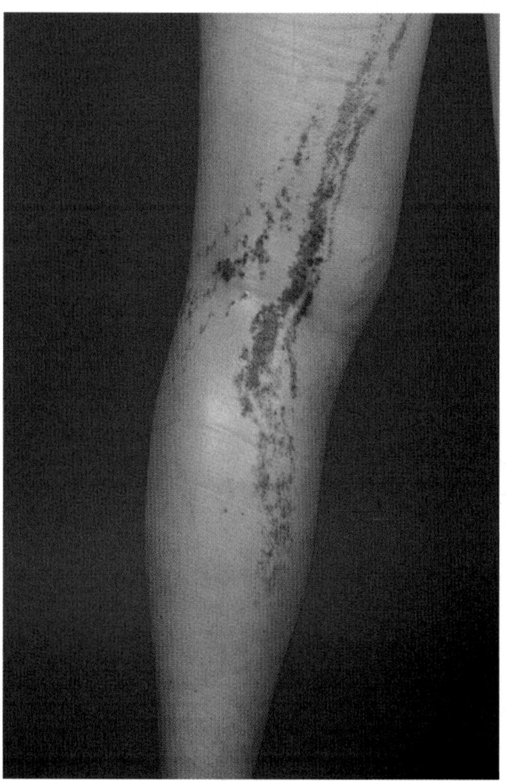

Fig. 106.12 Inflammatory linear verrucous naevus on the lower limb.

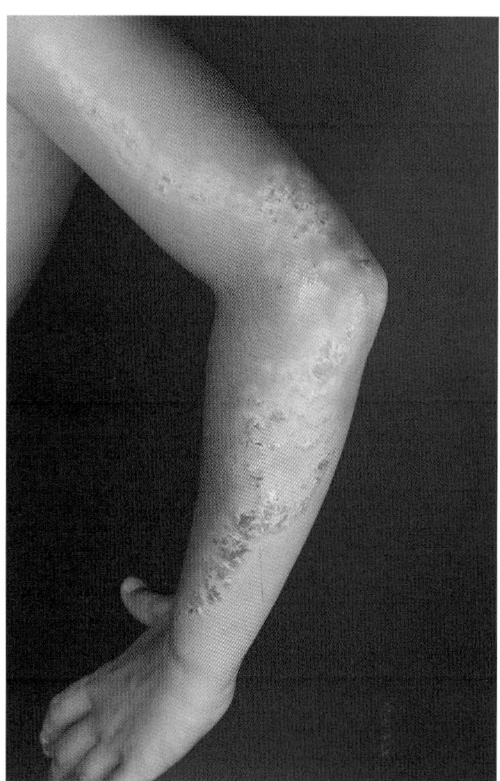

Fig. 106.13 Segmental psoriasis.

Treatment. Although ILVEN has been reported to be resistant to various topical therapies including corticosteroids, tazaroten, dithranol and fluorouracil, medical management is still considered first-line therapy. In some patients topical application of 0.005% calcipotriol ointment twice daily or corticosteroids plus tacrolimus 0.1% has been reported to be effective [108,109]. In ILVEN recalcitrant to medical management, photodynamic therapy or CO_2 laser may be tried, because these modalities have shown promising results in several cases [78,110].

The only definitive treatment is full-thickness surgical excision. To achieve primary closure, tissue expansion as an adjunct or serial excision may be required. Alternatively, split-thickness skin grafts are an option [111]. Another effective therapeutic modality with good cosmetic outcome is liquid nitrogen. Deep dermabrasion is effective, but produces substantial hypertrophic scarring [112].

CHILD syndrome

Introduction and history. CHILD is an acronym for congenital hemidysplasia with ichthyosiform naevus and limb defects. It was coined in 1980 by Happle [113].

Pathogenesis. CHILD syndrome is inherited as an X-linked dominant condition caused by missense or nonsense mutations in the *NSDHL* gene (NADH steroid dehydrogenase-like), which encodes an enzyme in the distal cholesterol biosynthesis pathway [114]. In rare cases, deletions of exons 6,7 and 8 of the *NSDHL* gene have been identified, confirming that loss of function of the NAD(P)H steroid dehydrogenase-like protein causes CHILD syndrome [115]. Mechanisms proven to be responsible for the cutaneous manifestations are the cholesterol deficiency itself, which impairs the proper formation of the corneocyte membrane, and the toxic accumulation of steroid precursors.

Clinical features and differential diagnosis. The CHILD naevus consists of circumscribed inflammatory plaques surmounted by prominent wax-like scales and may either follow Blaschko lines or in more severe cases diffusely affect one side of the body with strict midline demarcation. Bilateral cutaneous lesions have rarely been described [116].

Peculiarly, the inflammatory plaques may wax and wane and show a marked affinity to the body folds (which has been termed ptychotropism), where the lesions represent a therapeutic challenge [117]. In the majority of cases reported, the right half of the body is affected. Extracutaneous features in CHILD syndrome may involve ipsilateral hypoplasia of the brain, of all skeletal structures with shortness or absence of limbs, as well as of lungs, heart or kidneys.

Differential diagnoses include ILVEN, ichthyosis and psoriasis. Histologically, verruciform xanthoma and CHILD naevus are indistinguishable. However, as verruciform xanthoma present as solitary, raised or polypoid lesions, CHILD naevus and verruciform xanthoma may be confidently separated clinically.

Histopathology. The CHILD naevus is characterized by verrucous acanthosis of the epidermis, hyperkeratosis with focal parakeratosis and an infiltrate of foamy xanthoma cells expressing CD68 and adipophilin in the dermal papillae [118]. In some cases xanthoma cells may be absent.

Treatment. Topical treatment with lovastatin and cholesterol has been shown to clear skin lesions within 3 months [119]. This pathogenesis-based approach was published in 2011 by Paller and colleagues [11] and has been reproduced by other groups. Because simvastatin has a higher absorption capacity as lovastatin, 2% simvastatin and 2% cholesterol in Unguentum Cordes® may be viewed as improved formulation compared with the original [120]. Because lesions in the body folds continue to represent a therapeutic challenge even under targeted medical therapy, excision or dermabrasion followed by skin grafts obtained from a contralateral unaffected donor region poses a promising treatment option for these areas [121]. With respect to the extracutaneous associations mentioned previously, patients with CHILD syndrome should undergo complete physical examination and clinical evaluation by appropriate specialists.

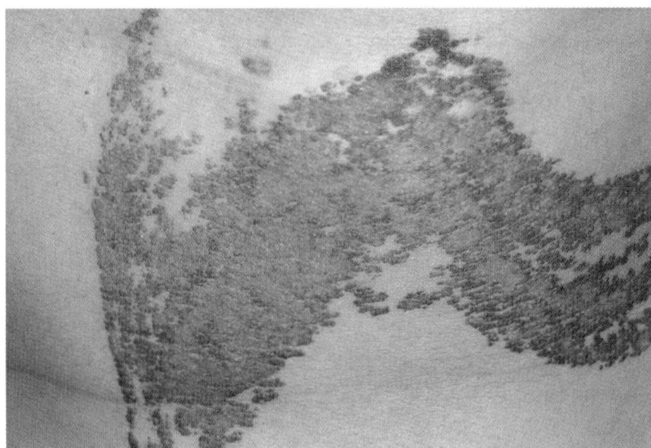

Fig. 106.14 Naevus marginatus.

Naevus marginatus

Naevus marginatus is a peculiar type of naevus, combining elements of both an organoid naevus sebaceous and a nonorganoid keratinocytic epidermal naevus (Fig. 106.14). It was delineated in 2008 by Hafner and Happle. Although there are only two reports published on this peculiar type of naevus, lots of published photographs show epidermal naevi which have to be classified as naevus marginatus [122]. Genetic analysis revealed the postzygotic *HRAS* p.G13R mosaic mutation both in the organoid and nonorganoid portion of one naevus marginatus [123]. Similarly to phakomatosis pigmentokeratotica, naevus marginatus thus highlights the meaning of a mutated multipotent progenitor cell, which results in mutated cell populations with variable developmental potential and subsequently different clinical phenotypes. Clinically and histologically, naevus marginatus presents with an elevated brown margin reflecting acanthopapillomatosis of the epidermis in the absence of abundant sebaceous glands and an erythematous central area caused by abundant sebaceous glands. Therapeutic options are as for naevus sebaceous.

References

1 **Happle R. Lethal genes surviving by mosaicism: a possible explanation for sporadic birth defects involving the skin. J Am Acad Dermatol 1987;16:899–906.**

2 **Hafner C, Groesser L. Mosaic RASopathies. Cell Cycle 2013;12:43–50.**

3 Youssoufian H, Pyeritz RE. Mechanisms and consequences of somatic mosaicism in humans. Nat Rev Genet 2002;3:748–58.

4 Torrelo A, Baselga E, Nagore E et al. Delineation of the various shapes and patterns of nevi. Eur J Dermatol 2005;15:439–50.

5 Solomon LM, Fretzin DF, Dewald RL. The epidermal naevus syndrome. Arch Dermatol 1968;97:273–85.

6 Solomon LM, Esterly NB. Epidermal and other congenital organoid nevi. Curr Probl Pediatr 1975;6:1–56.

7 Weyers W. Josef Jadassohn – an appreciation on the occasion of his 150th birthday. Am J Dermatopathol 2013;35:742–51.

8 Rogers M. Epidermal nevi and the epidermal naevus syndromes: a review of 233 cases. Pediatr Dermatol 1992;9:342–4.

9 **Groesser L, Herschberger E, Ruetten A et al. Postzygotic HRAS and KRAS mutations cause naevus sebaceous and Schimmelpenning syndrome. Nat Genet 2012;44:783–7.**

10 Levinsohn JL, Tian LC, Boyden LM et al. Whole-exome sequencing reveals somatic mutations in HRAS and KRAS, which cause naevus sebaceus. J Invest Dermatol 2013;133:827–30.

11 Sun BK, Saggini A, Sarin KY et al. Mosaic activating RAS mutations in naevus sebaceus and naevus sebaceus syndrome. J Invest Dermatol 2013;133:824–7.

12 Kuentz P, Fraitag S, Gonzales M et al. Mosaic activating FGFR2 mutation in two foetuses with papillomatous pedunculated sebaceous naevus. Br J Dermatol 2017;176:204–8.

13 Shen AS, Peterhof E, Kind P et al. Activating mutations in the RAS/mitogen-activated protein kinase signaling pathway in sporadic trichoblastoma and syringocystadenoma papilliferum. Hum Pathol 2015; 46:272–6.

14 Levinsohn JL, Sugarman JL, Bilguvar K et al. Somatic V600E BRAF mutation in linear and sporadic syringocystadenoma papilliferum. J Invest Dermatol 2015;135:2536–8.

15 Page ME, Lombard P, Ng F et al. The epidermis comprises autonomous compartments maintained by distinct stem cell populations. Cell Stem Cell 2013;13:471–82.

16 Warnke PH, Russo PA, Schimmelpenning GW et al. Linear intraoral lesions in the sebaceous naevus syndrome. J Am Acad Dermatol 2005;52:62–4.

17 Mehregan AH, Pinkus H. Life History of organoid nevi. special reference to naevus sebaceus of jadassohn. Arch Dermatol 1965;91:574–88.

18 Moody MN, Landau JM, Goldberg LH. Naevus sebaceous revisited. Pediatr Dermatol 2012;29:15–23.

19 Correale D, Ringpfeil F, Rogers M. Large, papillomatous, pedunculated naevus sebaceus: a new phenotype. Pediatr Dermatol 2008;25: 355–8.

20 **Happle R. The group of epidermal naevus syndromes Part I. Well defined phenotypes. J Am Acad Dermatol 2010;63:1–22;quiz 23–24.**

21 Barkham MC, White N, Brundler MA et al. Should naevus sebaceus be excised prophylactically? A clinical audit. J Plast Reconstr Aesthet Surg 2007;60:1269–70.

22 Schimmelpenning GW. [Clinical contribution to symptomatology of phacomatosis]. Fortschr Geb Rontgenstr Nuklearmed 1957; 87:716–20.

23 Davies D, Rogers M. Review of neurological manifestations in 196 patients with sebaceous naevi. Australas J Dermatol 2002;43:20–3.

24 Grebe TA, Rimsza ME, Richter SF et al. Further delineation of the epidermal naevus syndrome: two cases with new findings and literature review. Am J Med Genet 1993;47:24–30.

25 Happle R, Hoffmann R, Restano L et al. Phacomatosis pigmentokeratotica: a melanocytic-epidermal twin naevus syndrome. Am J Med Genet 1996;65:363–5.

26 Chantorn R, Shwayder T. Phacomatosis pigmentokeratotica: a further case without extracutaneous anomalies and review of the condition. Pediatr Dermatol 2011;28:715–19.

27 **Groesser L, Herschberger E, Sagrera A et al. Phacomatosis pigmentokeratotica is caused by a postzygotic HRAS mutation in a multipotent progenitor cell. J Invest Dermatol 2013;133:1998–2003.**

28 Kuentz P, Mignot C, St-Onge J et al. Postzygotic BRAF p.Lys601Asn mutation in phacomatosis pigmentokeratotica with woolly hair naevus and focal cortical dysplasia. J Invest Dermatol 2016;136:1060–2.

29 Kuroda Y, Ohashi I, Enomoto Y et al. A postzygotic NRAS mutation in a patient with Schimmelpenning syndrome. Am J Med Genet A 2015;167A:2223–5.

30 Ovejero D, Lim YH, Boyce AM et al. Cutaneous skeletal hypophosphatemia syndrome: clinical spectrum, natural history, and treatment. Osteoporos Int 2016;27:3615–26.

31 **Lim YH, Ovejero D, Derrick KM et al. Cutaneous skeletal hypophosphatemia syndrome (CSHS) is a multilineage somatic mosaic RASopathy. J Am Acad Dermatol 2016;75:420–7.**

32 Lim YH, Ovejero D, Sugarman JS et al. Multilineage somatic activating mutations in HRAS and NRAS cause mosaic cutaneous and skeletal lesions, elevated FGF23 and hypophosphatemia. Hum Mol Genet 2014;23:397–407.

33 Kofmann S. [A case of rare localization and spreading of comedones.] Arch Dermatol Syphilol (Berlin) 1895;32:177–8.

34 **Tchernev G, Ananiev J, Semkova K et al. Naevus comedonicus: an updated review. Dermatol Ther (Heidelb) 2013;3:33–40.**

35 **Asch S, Sugarman JL. Epidermal naevus syndromes. Handb Clin Neurol 2015;132:291–316.**

36 **Levinsohn JL, Sugarman JL, Yale Center for Mendelian Genomics et al. Somatic mutations in NEK9 cause naevus comedonicus. Am J Hum Genet 2016;98:1030–7.**

37 Munro CS, Wilkie AO. Epidermal mosaicism producing localised acne: somatic mutation in FGFR2. Lancet 1998;352:704–5.

38 **Kiritsi D, Lorente AI, Happle R et al. Blaschko line acne on preexistent hypomelanosis reflecting a mosaic FGFR2 mutation. Br J Dermatol 2015;172:1125–7.**

39 **Happle R, Tinschert S. Segmentally arranged basaloid follicular hamartomas with osseous, dental and cerebral anomalies: a distinct syndrome. Acta Derm Venereol 2008;88:382–7.**

40 Nabai H, Mehregan AH. Naevus comedonicus. A review of the literature and report of twelve cases. Acta Derm Venereol 1973;53:71–4.

41 Sardana K, Garg VK. Successful treatment of naevus comedonicus with ultrapulse CO2 laser. Indian J Dermatol Venereol Leprol 2009;75:534–5.

42 Marcus J, Esterly NB, Bauer BS. Tissue expansion in a patient with extensive naevus comedonicus. Ann Plast Surg 1992;29:362–6.

43 Engber PB. The naevus comedonicus syndrome: a case report with emphasis on associated internal manifestations. Int J Dermatol 1978;17:745–9.

44 **Easton JA, Donnelly S, Kamps MA et al. Porokeratotic eccrine naevus may be caused by somatic connexin26 mutations. J Invest Dermatol 2012;132:2184–91.**

45 Levinsohn JL, McNiff JM, Antaya RJ, Choate KA. A somatic p.G45E GJB2 mutation causing porokeratotic eccrine ostial and dermal duct naevus. JAMA Dermatol 2015;151:638–41.

46 Masferrer E, Vicente MA, Bassas-Vila J et al. Porokeratotic eccrine ostial and dermal duct naevus: report of 10 cases. J Eur Acad Dermatol Venereol 2010;24:847–51.

47 Valks R, Abajo P, Fraga J et al. Porokeratotic eccrine ostial and dermal duct naevus of late onset: more frequent than previously suggested? Dermatology 1996;193:138–40.

48 Llamas-Velasco M, Hilty N, Kempf W. Porokeratotic adnexal ostial naevus: review on the entity and therapeutic approach. J Eur Acad Dermatol Venereol 2015;29:2032–7.

49 Becker SW. Concurrent melanosis and hypertrichosis in distribution of naevus unius lateris. Arch Derm Syphilol 1949;60:155–60.

50 Cai ED, Sun BK, Chiang A et al. Postzygotic mutations in beta-actin are associated with Becker's nevus and Becker's nevus syndrome. J Invest Dermatol 2017;137:1795–8.

51 Panizzon R, Brungger H, Vogel A. [Becker naevus. A clinicohistologic-electron microscopy study of 39 patients]. Hautarzt 1984; 35:578–84.

52 Patrizi A, Medri M, Raone B et al. Clinical characteristics of Becker's naevus in children: report of 118 cases from Italy. Pediatr Dermatol 2012;29:571–4.

53 Schmidt CS, Bentz ML. Congenital smooth muscle hamartoma: the importance of differentiation from melanocytic nevi. J Craniofac Surg 2005;16:926–9.

54 Kim YJ, Han JH, Kang HY et al. Androgen receptor overexpression in Becker naevus: histopathologic and immunohistochemical analysis. J Cutan Pathol 2008;35:1121–6.

55 Trelles MA, Allones I, Moreno-Arias GA, Velez M. Becker's naevus: a comparative study between erbium: YAG and Q-switched neodymium:YAG; clinical and histopathological findings. Br J Dermatol 2005;152:308–13.

56 Meesters AA, Wind BS, Kroon MW et al. Ablative fractional laser therapy as treatment for Becker naevus: a randomized controlled pilot study. J Am Acad Dermatol 2011;65:1173–9.

57 Greve B, Raulin C. [Medical dermatologic laser therapy. A review]. Hautarzt 2003;54:594–602.

58 **Levinsohn JL, Teng J, Craiglow BG et al. Somatic HRAS p.G12S mutation causes woolly hair and epidermal nevi. J Invest Dermatol 2014;134:1149–52.**

59 Bolling MC, Jonkman MF. Skin and heart: une liaison dangereuse. Exp Dermatol 2009;18:658–68.

60 Singh G, Miteva M. Prognosis and management of congenital hair shaft disorders without fragility-part II. Pediatr Dermatol 2016; 33:481–7.

61 Vazquez MR, Gomez de la Fuente E, Fernandez JG et al. Eccrine naevus: case report and literature review. Acta Derm Venereol 2002; 82:154–6.

62 Lera M, Espana A, Idoate MA. Focal hyperhidrosis secondary to eccrine naevus successfully treated with botulinum toxin type A. Clin Exp Dermatol 2015;40:640–3.

63 Tempark T, Shwayder T. Mucinous eccrine naevus: case report and review of the literature. Clin Exp Dermatol 2013;38:1–4;quiz 5–6.

64 Schauder S, Hanefeld F, Noske UM, Zoll B. Depigmented hypertrichosis following Blaschko's lines associated with cerebral and ocular malformations: a new neurocutaneous, autosomal lethal gene syndrome from the group of epidermal naevus syndromes? Br J Dermatol 2000;142:1204–7.

65 Tantcheva-Poor I, Reinhold K, Krieg T, Happle R. Trichilemmal cyst naevus: a new complex organoid epidermal naevus. J Am Acad Dermatol 2007;57:S72–7.

66 Ferreira PS, Valente NY, Nico MM. Multiple filiform keratoses and nodules in a 10-year-old girl. Naevus trichilemmocysticus. Pediatr Dermatol 2013;30:261–2.

67 Larralde M, Boggio P, Abad ME et al. Naevus trichilemmocysticus: report of a new case of a recently recognized entity. Pediatr Dermatol 2011;28:286–9.

68 Khamaysi Z, Bochner R, Indelman M et al. Segmental basal cell naevus syndrome caused by an activating mutation in smoothened. Br J Dermatol 2016;175:178–81.

69 Happle R, Tinschert S. Happle-Tinschert syndrome can be caused by a mosaic SMO mutation and is suggested to be a variant of Curry-Jones syndrome. Br J Dermatol 2016;175:1108.

70 Alper JC, Holmes LB. The incidence and significance of birthmarks in a cohort of 4,641 newborns. Pediatr Dermatol 1983;1:58–68.

71 Hafner C, van Oers JM, Vogt T et al. Mosaicism of activating FGFR3 mutations in human skin causes epidermal nevi. J Clin Invest 2006;116:2201–7.

72 Hafner C, Lopez-Knowles E, Luis NM et al. Oncogenic PIK3CA mutations occur in epidermal nevi and seborrheic keratoses with a characteristic mutation pattern. Proc Natl Acad Sci U S A 2007;104: 13450–4.

73 Hafner C, Toll A, Gantner S et al. Keratinocytic epidermal nevi are associated with mosaic RAS mutations. J Med Genet 2012;49:249–53.

74 Polubothu S, Al-Olabi L, Wilson L et al. Extending the spectrum of AKT1 mosaicism: not just the Proteus syndrome. Br J Dermatol 2016; 175:612–14.

75 Toll A, Fernandez LC, Pons T et al. Somatic embryonic FGFR2 mutations in keratinocytic epidermal nevi. J Invest Dermatol 2016; 136:1718–21.

76 Su WP. Histopathologic varieties of epidermal naevus. A study of 160 cases. Am J Dermatopathol 1982;4:161–70.

77 Lapidoth M, Israeli H, Ben Amitai D, Halachmi S. Treatment of verrucous epidermal naevus: experience with 71 cases. Dermatology 2013;226:342–6.

78 Alonso-Castro L, Boixeda P, Reig I et al. Carbon dioxide laser treatment of epidermal nevi: response and long-term follow-up. Actas Dermosifiliogr 2012;103:910–18.

79 Vujevich JJ, Mancini AJ. The epidermal naevus syndromes: multisystem disorders. J Am Acad Dermatol 2004;50:957–61.

80 Hafner C, Toll A, Real FX. HRAS mutation mosaicism causing urothelial cancer and epidermal naevus. N Engl J Med 2011;365:1940–2.

81 Sapp JC, Turner JT, van de Kamp JM et al. Newly delineated syndrome of congenital lipomatous overgrowth, vascular malformations, and epidermal nevi (CLOVE syndrome) in seven patients. Am J Med Genet A 2007;143A:2944–58.

82 Kurek KC, Luks VL, Ayturk UM et al. Somatic mosaic activating mutations in PIK3CA cause CLOVES syndrome. Am J Hum Genet 2012;90:1108–15.

83 Keppler-Noreuil KM, Sapp JC, Lindhurst MJ et al. Clinical delineation and natural history of the PIK3CA-related overgrowth spectrum. Am J Med Genet A 2014;164A:1713–33.

84 Cohen MM, Jr, Hayden PW. A newly recognized hamartomatous syndrome. Birth Defects Orig Artic Ser 1979;15:291–6.

85 Biesecker LG, Happle R, Mulliken JB et al. Proteus syndrome: diagnostic criteria, differential diagnosis, and patient evaluation. Am J Med Genet 1999;84:389–95.

86 Lindhurst MJ, Sapp JC, Teer JK et al. A mosaic activating mutation in AKT1 associated with the Proteus syndrome. N Engl J Med 2011; 365:611–19.

87 Lindhurst MJ, Wang JA, Bloomhardt HM et al. AKT1 gene mutation levels are correlated with the type of dermatologic lesions in patients with Proteus syndrome. J Invest Dermatol 2014;134:543–6.

88 Biesecker L. The challenges of Proteus syndrome: diagnosis and management. Eur J Hum Genet 2006;14:1151–7.

89 Caux F, Plauchu H, Chibon F et al. Segmental overgrowth, lipomatosis, arteriovenous malformation and epidermal naevus (SOLAMEN) syndrome is related to mosaic PTEN nullizygosity. Eur J Hum Genet 2007;15:767–73.

90 Happle R. Type 2 segmental Cowden disease vs Proteus syndrome. Br J Dermatol 2007;156:1089–90.

91 Torrelo A, Colmenero I, Kristal L et al. Papular epidermal naevus with 'skyline' basal cell layer (PENS). J Am Acad Dermatol 2011; 64:888–92.

92 Faure E, Tadini G, Brena M, Cassulini LR. Papular epidermal naevus with 'skyline' basal cell layer (PENS) following a Blaschko linear pattern. Pediatr Dermatol 2013;30:e270–1.

93 Luna PC, Pannizardi AA, Martin CI et al. Papular epidermal naevus with skyline basal cell layer (PENS): three new cases and review of the literature. Pediatr Dermatol 2016;33:296–300.

94 Paller AS, Syder AJ, Chan YM et al. Genetic and clinical mosaicism in a type of epidermal naevus. N Engl J Med 1994;331:1408–15.

95 Tsubota A, Akiyama M, Sakai K et al. Keratin 1 gene mutation detected in epidermal naevus with epidermolytic hyperkeratosis. J Invest Dermatol 2007;127:1371–4.

96 Koh MJ, Lee JS, Chong WS. Systematized epidermal naevus with epidermolytic hyperkeratosis improving with topical calcipotriol/ betametasone dipropionate combination ointment. Pediatr Dermatol 2013;30:370–3.

97 Umekoji A, Fukai K, Ishii M. A case of mosaic-type bullous congenital ichthyosiform erythroderma successfully treated with topical maxacalcitol, a vitamin D3 analogue. Clin Exp Dermatol 2008; 33:501–2.

98 Sethuraman G, Marwaha RK, Challa A et al. Vitamin D: A New promising therapy for congenital ichthyosis. Pediatrics 2016;137:.

99 Bygum A, Virtanen M, Brandrup F et al. Generalized and naevoid epidermolytic ichthyosis in Denmark: clinical and mutational findings. Acta Derm Venereol 2013;93:309–13.

100 Starink TM, Woerdeman MJ. Unilateral systematized keratosis follicularis. A variant of Darier's disease or an epidermal naevus (acantholytic dyskeratotic epidermal naevus)? Br J Dermatol 1981; 105:207–14.

101 Huh WK, Fujiwara K, Takahashi H, Kanitakis J. Congenital acantholytic dyskeratotic epidermal naevus following Blaschko's lines versus segmental Darier's disease. Eur J Dermatol 2007;17:130–2.

102 Mazereeuw-Hautier J, Thibaut I, Bonafe JL. Acantholytic dyskeratotic epidermal naevus: a rare histopathologic feature. J Cutan Pathol 2002;29:52–4.

103 Sehgal VN, Srivastava G. Darier's (Darier-White) disease/keratosis follicularis. Int J Dermatol 2005;44:184–92.

104 Umegaki-Arao N, Sasaki T, Fujita H et al. Inflammatory linear verrucous epidermal naevus with a postzygotic GJA1 mutation is a mosaic erythrokeratodermia variabilis et progressiva. J Invest Dermatol 2017;137:967–70.

105 Lee SH, Rogers M. Inflammatory linear verrucous epidermal naevi: a review of 23 cases. Australas J Dermatol 2001;42:252–6.

106 Lenormand C, Cribier B, Lipsker D. Blaschko-linear manifestations of polygenic inflammatory diseases: analysis of 17 cases. Eur J Dermatol 2013;23:671–6.

107 Vissers WH, Muys L, Erp PE et al. Immunohistochemical differentiation between inflammatory linear verrucous epidermal naevus (ILVEN) and psoriasis. Eur J Dermatol 2004;14:216–20.

108 Zvulunov A, Grunwald MH, Halvy S. Topical calcipotriol for treatment of inflammatory linear verrucous epidermal naevus. Arch Dermatol 1997;133:567–8.

109 Mutasim DF. Successful treatment of inflammatory linear verrucous epidermal naevus with tacrolimus and fluocinonide. J Cutan Med Surg 2006;10:45–7.

110 Parera E, Gallardo F, Toll A et al. Inflammatory linear verrucous epidermal naevus successfully treated with methyl-aminolevulinate photodynamic therapy. Dermatol Surg 2010;36:253–6.

111 Lee BJ, Mancini AJ, Renucci J et al. Full-thickness surgical excision for the treatment of inflammatory linear verrucous epidermal naevus. Ann Plast Surg 2001;47:285–92.

112 Fox BJ, Lapins NA. Comparison of treatment modalities for epidermal naevus: a case report and review. J Dermatol Surg Oncol 1983;9:879–85.

113 Happle R, Koch H, Lenz W. The CHILD syndrome. Congenital hemidysplasia with ichthyosiform erythroderma and limb defects. Eur J Pediatr 1980;134:27–33.

114 Konig A, Happle R, Bornholdt D et al. Mutations in the NSDHL gene, encoding a 3beta-hydroxysteroid dehydrogenase, cause CHILD syndrome. Am J Med Genet 2000;90:339–46.

115 Kim CA, Konig A, Bertola DR et al. CHILD syndrome caused by a deletion of exons 6–8 of the NSDHL gene. Dermatology 2005;211: 155–8.
116 Estape A, Josifova D, Rampling D et al. Congenital hemidysplasia with ichthyosiform naevus and limb defects (CHILD) syndrome without hemidysplasia. Br J Dermatol 2015;173:304–7.
117 Happle R. Ptychotropism as a cutaneous feature of the CHILD syndrome. J Am Acad Dermatol 1990;23:763–6.
118 Gantner S, Rutten A, Requena L et al. CHILD syndrome with mild skin lesions: histopathologic clues for the diagnosis. J Cutan Pathol 2014;41:787–90.
119 Paller AS, van Steensel MA, Rodriguez-Martin M et al. Pathogenesis-based therapy reverses cutaneous abnormalities in an inherited disorder of distal cholesterol metabolism. J Invest Dermatol 2011;131:2242–8.
120 Kiritsi D, Schauer F, Wolfle U et al. Targeting epidermal lipids for treatment of Mendelian disorders of cornification. Orphanet J Rare Dis 2014;9:33.
121 Konig A, Skrzypek J, Loffler H et al. Donor dominance cures CHILD naevus. Dermatology 2010;220:340–5.
122 Hafner C, Landthaler M, Happle R, Vogt T. Naevus marginatus: a distinct type of epidermal naevus or merely a variant of naevus sebaceus? Dermatology 2008;216:236–8.
123 Groesser L, Vogt T, Happle R et al. Naevus marginatus revisited: a combined organoid and nonorganoid epidermal naevus caused by HRAS mutation. Br J Dermatol 2013;168:892–4.

CHAPTER 107
Other Naevi and Hamartomas

Jonathan A. Dyer
Departments of Dermatology and Child Health, University of Missouri, Columbia, MO, USA

Connective tissue naevi, 1276
Buschke–Ollendorf syndrome, 1278
Smooth muscle hamartoma, 1279
Other hamartomas, 1280

Abstract

A variety of naevoid lesions of dermal tissues are recognized. Benign and typically congenital, they are traditionally characterized by the cell type or material of which they are composed. Typically isolated, some are related to underlying genetic disorders. This chapter will review those naevi most commonly recognized in the paediatric population.

Key points

- **Naevoid lesions composed of a variety of different cell types or tissue components have been described and are named accordingly.**
- **Although many naevoid lesions are isolated, some are associated with underlying disorders.**
- **Dermatofibrosis lenticularis disseminata may be composed of focal excess elastin or collagen and is classically associated with the autosomal dominant Buschke–Ollendorf syndrome. Osteopoikilosis is often noted in these patients.**
- **Cutaneous collagenomas, although often isolated, may be a prominent feature of tuberous sclerosis. They have also been noted in multiple endocrine neoplasia type 1 and Proteus syndrome.**
- **Fibroblastic connective tissue naevi may mimic dermatofibrosarcoma protuberans.**
- **Mutations in beta-actin are associated with Becker naevi**

Connective tissue naevi

Brief introduction and history. A variety of naevoid lesions of dermal tissues are recognized. Connective tissue naevi (CTN) are among the most common. These naevi are benign, and most often congenital. They are typically characterized by the cell type or material of which they are composed. Some are clinically similar, presenting as variably firm, slow-growing, skin or pink coloured painless papules or plaques.

Epidemiology and pathogenesis. CTN are typically sporadic and solitary; however, multiple, segmental and symmetric lesions may occur. In a recent review of over 100 cases, 85% of lesions were solitary and 15% were multiple [1]. CTN may be noted at birth though many subtle lesions are only first noted during childhood.

Collagenomas, composed of excess dermal collagen, and elastomas, similarly composed of excess elastin, are the most common forms of CTN. Collagenomas may be sporadic or multiple collagenomas may be inherited in an autosomal dominant (AD) pattern (OMIM #115250). Although the aetiology of most CTN is unknown, causal mutations have been identified in familial and syndromic cases.

Collagenomas can also occur as part of an underlying genetic syndrome. The classic shagreen patch and fibrous forehead plaque of tuberous sclerosis (OMIM #191100; see Chapter 143) are collagenomas. Additionally, collagenomas are noted as one of the skin findings in multiple endocrine neoplasia type I (MEN1; OMIM #131100). Large progressive cerebriform collagenomas of the extremities are a key feature of Proteus syndrome (OMIM #176920; see Chapter 108). A familial form of collagenoma associated with cardiac disease (cardiomyopathy) and testicular failure has been reported [2]. Patients with Cowden disease exhibit 'storiform' collagenomas (sclerotic fibroma) [3].

Elastomas may also occur as part of a syndrome, most classically Buschke–Ollendorf syndrome (OMIM #166700; see later) an AD genodermatosis characterized by multiple cutaneous elastomas (dermatofibrosis lenticularis disseminata) along with radiographic findings of opacities, especially at the end of long bones (termed osteopoikilosis) (see Chapter 95).

Mucinous naevi are very rare, with approximately 25 cases reported in the literature. The literature regarding these lesions is quite variable and there is debate regarding whether they are a variant of cutaneous mucinosis or CTN. However, they are included here based on recent classification criteria and their frequent clinical resemblance to other forms of CTN [4]. Familial and acquired forms are described.

Harper's Textbook of Pediatric Dermatology, Fourth Edition. Edited by Peter Hoeger, Veronica Kinsler and Albert Yan.

Clinical features and differential diagnosis. The various subtypes of CTN often exhibit similar clinical features. CTN typically present as variably firm, slow-growing, skin or pink coloured painless papules or plaques. CTN are most commonly located on the trunk or extremities. Collagenomas are often skin coloured (Fig. 107.1). Elastomas can exhibit a yellowish appearance (Fig. 107.2). The overlying surface is smooth to lobulated. Solitary lesions are typically static. Patients with multiple lesions may note the development of new lesions over time.

The shagreen patch of tuberous sclerosis (Fig. 107.3) is typically located on the lower back and derives its name from the resemblance of the lesional skin surface to the coarse granular appearance of shagreen leather. Both shagreen patches and the fibrous forehead plaque of tuberous sclerosis are cutaneous collagenomas.

A recent report proposes a subtype of CTN which is rare, progressive and typically involves the lower extremity. This aggressive subtype often initially clinically resembles segmental morphoea. Lesions typically began as papules on the buttock and lumbar areas that rapidly merge, progressing to become segmental lesions with deep infiltration. Histological findings are typical of mixed CTN. Unlike typical, relatively static CTN, these lesions progress rapidly to involve the entire lower limb leading to significant functional impairment. The relationship of these lesions to more typical CTN remains unclear [5].

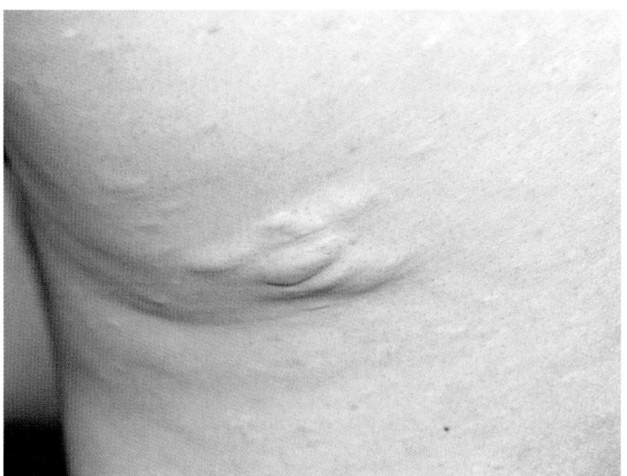

Fig. 107.1 Cutaneous collagenoma.

Fig. 107.2 Cutaneous elastoma: collection of yellowish papules.

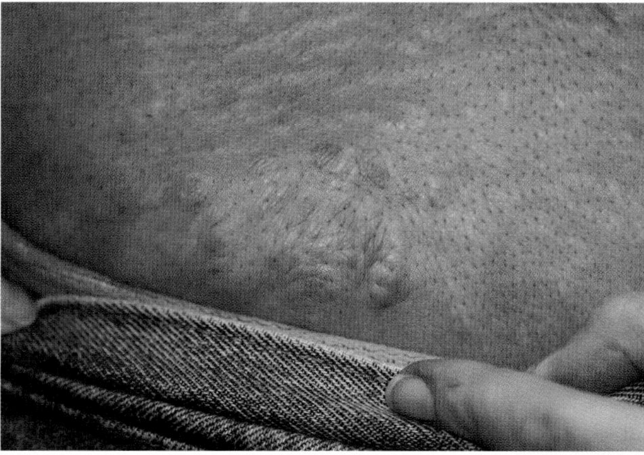

Fig. 107.3 Typical shagreen patch of tuberous sclerosis.

Fibroblastic connective tissue nevi (FCTN) are a rare, newly appreciated subtype of CTN. They may present in childhood, although adult cases are reported. One report suggests a female predominance. They most commonly present on the trunk and the head/neck of children. FCTN typically present as solitary, slow growing papules, nodules or plaques. They are painless, smooth, firm and vary from slightly tan–brown to tan–white in colour [6].

Mucinous naevi often resemble other forms of CTN. They can present as skin to slightly tan–brown coloured individual or grouped papules and plaques. A recent review of the literature suggests a male predominance. The back (most often lower back) was the typical location and the majority of lesions were linear and unilateral in distribution. They are often separated into two main clinical forms – CTN of the proteoglycan type (CTNP), which exhibit normal epidermis and excess proteoglycan in the dermis and CTN of the combined epidermal–CTNP type, in which the typical dermal changes are associated with overlying epidermal hyperkeratosis and acanthosis typical for epidermal naevi. Reports exist describing clinical resemblance to naevus lipomatosis superficialis [4,7].

Histology is typically used to differentiate between these clinically similar lesions.

Laboratory and histological findings. CTN are typically separated by their histological appearance, namely, which type of connective tissue is present in excess. Biopsy is necessary only to define progressive lesions more accurately or if a specific diagnosis is required. Histological diagnosis can be difficult, because CTN often exhibit subtle excesses of normal appearing connective tissue. It is often helpful to compare histological features of CTN lesional skin with an accompanying biopsy taken from clinically normal skin from the same patient which allows appreciation of subtle increases in connective tissue. Alternatively, a larger 5–6 mm biopsy taken from the edge of a lesion including clinically normal skin may be performed.

In typical collagenoma the epidermis is normal. Dermal thickening may be noted, with thickened collagen bundles haphazardly arranged. Elastic fibres may be decreased in density although this may be a dilution artefact as a result of the increased collagen. Although some lesions exhibit clear excess of collagen or elastin, mixed lesions exhibiting roughly equal increases in both also occur.

Special stains are often used to highlight and differentiate specific types of excess connective tissue. Haematoxylin phloxine saffron stains collagen bundles yellow and elastic fibres red [1]. Masson's trichrome stain differentiates smooth muscle from collagen. The abnormal collagen in collagenomas is reported to exhibit different polarization characteristics under polarization microscopy when stained with picosirius red when compared with normal dermal collagen [8].

Cutaneous elastomas often exhibit a relatively normal histological appearance with standard tissue stains such as haematoxylin and eosin. Specific elastic tissue stains, such as Verhoeff–Van Gieson or Orcein and Weigert, highlight elastic fibres and demonstrate broadened, branched interwoven elastic fibres predominantly in the mid and lower dermis [9].

Fibroblastic CTN exhibit a disorderly CD34-positive spindle cell proliferation within the deeper dermis and superficial subcutaneous tissues. The fibroblastic/myofibroblastic cells exhibit no atypia and the lesions are typically poorly circumscribed and are not encapsulated. Unlike other CTN, overlying epidermal papillomatous hyperplasia as well as adipose tissue in the reticular dermis is frequently present. FCTN can resemble dermatofibrosarcoma protuberans (DFSP) clinically and histologically and differentiation between these two entities is important given their differing clinical behaviour. DFSP typically exhibit uniform, only slightly atypical fibroblasts arrayed in a storiform pattern, compared with a more disordered fascicular pattern of growth typical of FCTN. In cases where differentiation is difficult, findings which favour DFSP include: lack of epidermal papillomatous hyperplasia; a hypocellular zone just below the epidermis; uniform but slightly atypical nuclei; and diffuse, strong positivity of CD34 staining of lesional cells.

Mucinous naevi exhibit diffuse mucin deposition in the upper dermis associated with sparse spindle cells [4]. These cells were noted to be CD34 positive in one study [10]. Acanthosis and variable hyperkeratosis are reported in approximately 50%. A recent case was noted to have superficially placed adipose tissue.

Treatment and intervention. Most isolated CTN require no intervention. For patients with larger lesions or those that cause local impairment, treatment is on a case by case basis.

Appropriate work-up and evaluation in patients with CTN involves a thorough personal and family history, including screening for skin lesions or bone issues. Historical questions should include screening for any history of epilepsy, mental retardation or deafness in the patient or their family, as well as for any history of endocrinopathies or hypogonadism. A thorough physical examination should screen for subtle clinical lesions, as well as additional cutaneous stigmata or findings suggestive of underlying syndromic disorders. When necessary, skin biopsy (see previously) and radiography (see section on Buschke–Ollendorf syndrome) are obtained. The physical examination in appropriate cases should include a black light examination for ash leaf spots to detect subtle cases of tuberous sclerosis, as well as other cutaneous findings of MEN1 or Proteus syndrome.

FCTN are thought to be localized nevoid anomalies. They tend not to recur after resection and metastatic lesions are not reported. Although there can be clinical and histological similarity to DFSP, DFSP are locally aggressive and have a tendency to recur if not completely excised, thus differentiating FCTN from DFSP has clinical relevance [6]. Treatment is unnecessary unless there are cosmetic implications of individual lesions [11]. For patients with progressive CTN involving a lower extremity, lesions persist over time. The only beneficial intervention noted was physiotherapy [5].

Mucinous naevi typically require no intervention. Larger lesions with similarity to naevus lipomatosus could be treated surgically on a case by case basis.

Buschke–Ollendorf syndrome

Brief introduction and history. The autosomal dominant association of cutaneous elastomas (dermatofibrosis lenticularis disseminata) with multiple round to oval or linear osteosclerotic bony lesions (osteopoikilosis; 'spotted bone') was first described in 1928 by Buschke and Ollendorf [12].

Epidemiology and pathogenesis. The estimated incidence is 1 : 20 000 live births [1]. Familial studies have clarified the wide phenotypic variability in affected individuals with some patients exhibiting minimal cutaneous lesions. Loss of function mutations in the *LEMD3* (MAN1; OMIM # 607844) gene have been identified, both in families with Buschke–Ollendorf syndrome (BOS) as well as individual sporadic lesions of osteopoikilosis as well as melorheostosis (OMIM #155950). *LEMD3* participates in controlling signalling both in the bone morphogenetic protein (BMP) and transforming growth factor-beta (TGFβ) pathways. Decreased levels of *LEMD3* leads to increased signalling through both BMP and TGFβ pathways which increases formation of bone tissue. The pathomechanism for the development of CTN in BOS is not clear.

Clinical features. Skin lesions typical of BOS are often first noted during childhood, before puberty, and increase in number over time. They appear as subtle skin-coloured to yellowish papules or plaques on otherwise normal skin (Fig. 107.4). They can appear anywhere although truncal lesions are common. Importantly, osteopoikilosis develops

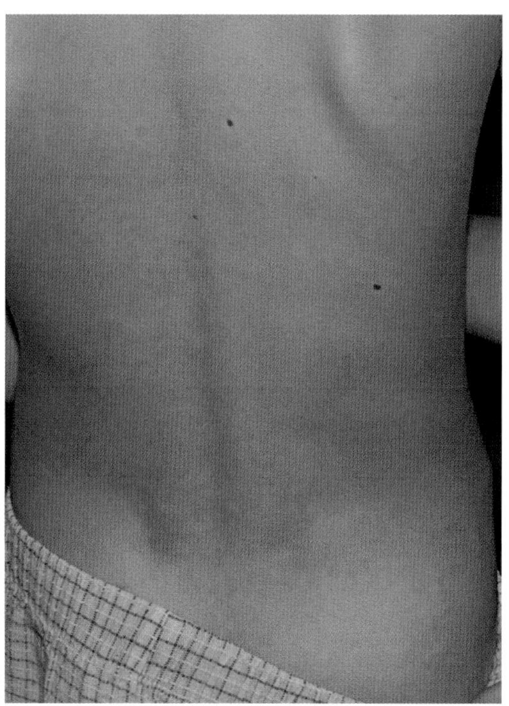

Fig. 107.4 Dermatofibrosis lenticularis disseminata. Multiple cutaneous elastomas in a patient with Buschke–Ollendorf syndrome. LEMD3 mutation positive.

over time and may not be detected initially during childhood when the skin lesions are first noted. It is often noted in carpal and tarsal bones, the phalanges, epiphyses and metaphyses of long bones and the pelvis.

Differential diagnosis. The cutaneous lesions resemble isolated elastomas or collagenomas of the skin. However, when larger numbers of lesions are present it suggests BOS. Because lesions of osteopoikilosis may resemble bony metastasis, recognition of their benign nature can prevent costly and elaborate work-ups in BOS patients [1].

Importantly, close study of BOS patients and families has revealed that in some cases osteopoikilosis is associated with cutaneous collagenoma or mixed CTN rather than exclusively elastoma. This has led to the resurrection of the term dermatofibrosis lenticularis disseminata for describing the cutaneous lesions of BOS, to incorporate both collagenous and elastic tissue lesions.

Treatment. No intervention is necessary in BOS.

Smooth muscle hamartoma

Smooth muscle hamartoma was first described in 1923.

Epidemiology and pathogenesis. Smooth muscle hamartoma are rare and are typically congenital lesions, although they may be first noted during infancy. They are local areas of hyperplastic dermal smooth muscle [13].

Clinical features and differential diagnosis. Smooth muscle hamartoma may be skin coloured or exhibit a faint overlying hyperpigmentation along with increased hairs, which may be terminal or vellus (Fig. 107.5). Localized lesions are most common. Rarely, however, individuals exhibit diffuse follicular papules or circumscribed patches of follicular papules. Diffuse cutaneous infiltration leading to a circumferential ring (Michelin tyre baby) phenotype in infancy has also been rarely described [13]. These patients also exhibited diffuse hypertrichosis and occasionally slight hyperpigmentation. The skin folds often improve over time [14].

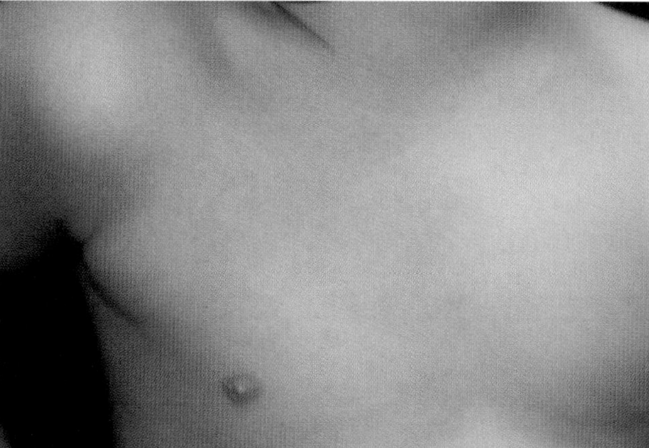

Fig. 107.5 Smooth muscle hamartoma: slightly hyperpigmented patch with positive pseudo-Darier's sign and follicular prominence.

Composed of excess arrector pili muscles, changes in temperature or rubbing the smooth muscle hamartoma often triggers contractions of the muscles leading to increased firmness or a 'goose-flesh' appearance of the lesion, termed a 'pseudo-Darier sign'. Spontaneous movement (myokymia) has been described [15] and may aid diagnosis.

Becker naevi exhibit many clinical and histological similarities with smooth muscle hamartoma. Becker naevi typically exhibit adolescent onset with hyperpigmentation and hypertrichosis. They are most common in males, on the upper chest or back. However, they may be located on other body sites. Recently, lethal mutations in *ACTB*, which encodes beta-actin, were detected in Becker naevi. The causative mutations appear to occur only in pilar musculature from lesional areas [16]. How these mutations lead to the other clinical findings of Becker naevi is unknown at present [17]. They are more extensively described Chapter 106.

Laboratory and histology findings. Histology of smooth muscle hamartomas is typically consistent. Well-defined smooth muscle bundles exhibiting variable orientation are present in the dermis. Often some, but not all, of these bundles attach to hair follicles. The overlying epidermis often exhibits slight rete ridge elongation with mild basal layer hypermelanosis. Becker naevi exhibit essentially identical hypertrophic smooth muscle fibres. The smooth muscle fibres stain clearly with Masson trichrome [18–21].

Treatment and prevention. No treatment is necessary.

Other hamartomas

Naevus lipomatosus superficialis/naevus lipomatosus cutaneous superficialis

First described in 1921, naevus lipomatosus superficialis (NLS) are rare cutaneous lesions that are typically congenital, although acquired lesions are described. Typically they manifest as flesh-coloured to yellow papules, which may coalesce into plaques (often linear or segmental). Some larger lesions exhibit a cerebriform appearance. Two main forms are described: multiple (classic; Hoffman–Zurhelle type) and solitary [22]. The classic form occurs in the first decades of life and the NLS are commonly located in the pelvic region. The solitary form is often pedunculated, may present at any age and appear anywhere on the body.

Histological examination of NLS typically reveals mature adipose tissue between dermal collagen bundles in the reticular dermis. Increased vascularity and increased numbers of spindle and/or mononuclear cells have also been described. Thickening of the epidermis overlying NLS has been described [23]. Widespread naevus lipomatosus has also been noted to lead to a circumferential ring (Michelin tyre) phenotype in infancy [13].

NLS with associated folliculosebaceous cystic hamartomas have been reported as well as lesions exhibiting hyperplastic hair follicles and sebaceous glands [24–26]. Additional neoplasms associated with NLS include cylindromas and fibrofolliculomas [27]. Patients with the X-linked dominant genodermatoses focal dermal hypoplasia (FDH; Goltz syndrome; OMIM #305600) exhibit areas of dermally located adipose tissue which clinically resemble NLS [28].

Although typically isolated, cases with associated pigmentary abnormalities (café-au-lait macules; focal leukoderma) are reported [22]. The underlying cause of NLS is unclear. A 2p24 chromosomal deletion has been reported in one case of NLS and 2p deletions have been reported in sporadic lipomas [29].

Although no treatment is necessary for naevus lipomatosus cutaneous superficialis (NLCS), problematic pedunculated or cerebriform lesions can be excised [30]. Carbon dioxide laser has also been used with variable results [31,32]. Intralesional injection with phosphatidylcholine and sodium deoxycholate has also been reported with some success at flattening the NLS. However, the visible skin lesions remain [33,34].

Basaloid follicular hamartoma

Basaloid follicular hamartomas present clinically as skin-coloured or brownish papules, often with a central os or plug. Histologically they resemble basal cell carcinoma, with basaloid/squamous cells forming a network arising from the follicle infundibulum. Horn cysts may be seen surrounded by slight stroma. Staining with bcl-2 (strongly positive in basal cell carcinoma) is minimal in basaloid follicular hamartoma and may aid in differentiating the lesions. The involved skin areas may exhibit hypo- or hyperpigmentation. Atrophoderma as well as other associated skin abnormalities have been reported. Lesions are typically congenital. A variety of different clinical forms of basaloid follicular hamartoma have been described: solitary or multiple papules with no apparent associated distribution; unilateral Blaschkolinear lesions (see later); plaque-like lesions with associated alopecia (typical for scalp involvement); generalized lesions (typically autosomal dominant); and generalized lesions with associated alopecia. Associated myasthenia gravis (acquired) or cystic fibrosis (congenital) have also been reported in some cases [35,36].

Happle–Tinschert syndrome is characterized by segmentally distributed basaloid follicular hamartomas, with associated linear atrophoderma, hypo- and hyperpigmentation, dental enamel defects (hypoplastic teeth), ipsilateral hypertrichosis, and bony and cerebral abnormalities. The skin lesions, characterized by linear hypopigmentation, are typically noted in early infancy. Patients with this constellation of phenotypic findings had traditionally been included under the designation of basal cell naevus syndrome. However, *PTCH* gene testing is negative and the cutaneous lesions are basaloid follicular hamartomas rather than true basal cell carcinomas [37,38]. The underlying causative genetic defect remains unclear.

Mixed hamartomas

The literature describes occasional cases of mixed hamartomas composed of a variety of different cell types. In some cases the hamartomatous tissue is distributed similarly to better recognized developmental anomalies, such as accessory digits, accessory tragi or lumbosacral spinal dysraphism. The relationship of these mixed hamartomas to such developmental anomalies is unclear [39].

Encephalocraniocutaneous lipomatosis

Encephalocraniocutaneous lipomatosis (ECCL; Haberland syndrome; OMIM #613001) is a rare sporadic disorder exhibiting unilateral lipomatous hamartomas of the scalp, eyelid and outer globe of the eye [40] with associated ipsilateral hairlessness and neurological malformations including hemiatrophy, enlarged ventricles, lipomas, calcifications, porencephalic cysts, dysplastic cortex, arachnoid cysts and leptomeningeal angiomatosis [41]. There is significant clinical overlap between ECCL and oculoectodermal syndrome (OES, OMIM #600268). A skin lesion considered specific for ECCL, naevus psiloliparus, presents as unilateral, alopecic, often slightly raised plaques, with relatively well-defined borders and colouring ranging from yellowish to skin coloured. These lesions are typically located in the frontal or frontoparietal region of the scalp. Histology of naevus psiloliparus exhibits abundant mature nonencapsulated adipose tissue, few to absent hair follicles and arrector pili muscle bundles that are normal in quantity but unassociated with hair follicles [42]. Despite frequent widespread neurological abnormalities, symptomatology is often mild, characterized by seizures and mild intellectual disability. A variety of other abnormalities are reported including angiolipomas, fibrolipomas, connective tissue naevi, poorly defined protuberances of the skull, as well as cartilage, fat and connective tissue hamartomas [43]. Recently mosaic activating mutations in *FGFR1* were identified as a cause of encephalocraniocutaneous lipomatosis [44]. Specific mosaic KRAS mutations have recently been identified in patients apparently meeting criteria for both ECCL and OES [45].

Apocrine naevi

Apocrine naevi have also been termed apocrine gland hamartoma. Isolated apocrine naevi are very rare. They may be congenital and some occur in association with naevus sebaceous. They are composed of a proliferation of mature apocrine glands that are thicker and more numerous than normal axillary skin. Often skin coloured, they are commonly located in the axilla and may be pedunculated. Others have occurred on the face, scalp, chest and inguinal region. They are typically asymptomatic though tenderness can occur. There appears to be a male predominance. Apocrine naevi are benign. There are a few reports, however, of progression to apocrine carcinoma within these lesions [46].

Eccrine naevi

Eccrine naevi are very rare skin hamartomas characterized by an excess of normal eccrine sweat glands within the dermis. Fewer than 30 cases are described in the literature and there is significant clinical variability. Eccrine naevi may present as red or brownish patches, brown variable nodules and patches of hypopigmentation. Although the forearms are a common location for eccrine naevi, they have also been described on the hands and feet as well as the extremities, trunk, neck and forehead. Patients may note hyperhidrosis [47].

Although typically isolated, syndromic forms may exist. A recently described patient exhibited broad Blaschkolinear indurated, depressed, slightly hyperpigmented skin lesions on the extremities in addition to a constellation of other defects. These skin lesions were composed of a proliferation of both immature and well-formed eccrine duct-like structures in the deep dermis embedded within an abundant fibrous stroma which was composed of thickened collagen oriented relatively parallel to the skin surface. The hyperpigmentation was within basal layer keratinocytes. This patient also exhibited facial and intraoral depressed pox-like scarring, gingival synechiae, asymmetry of the body, blepharophimosis and mental retardation. A causative genetic defect was not reported [48].

Mucinous eccrine naevi are very rare variants of eccrine naevi. They most commonly present before puberty as solitary brownish lesions (papule, nodule, plaque) typically on the legs. Blaschkolinear lesions are reported [49]. They may exhibit hyperhidrosis. Histology reveals lobulated eccrine glands increased in both number and diameter as well as positive Alcian blue staining of mucin deposited around the glands [49–51]. Blood vessels in the areas adjacent to the glands are typically thicker than in uninvolved areas, in contrast to standard eccrine naevi which do not exhibit changes in vascular structures and are negative for Alcian blue staining.

Eccrine angiomatous hamartomas exhibit proliferation of capillary-like vascular elements as well as eccrine glands within the dermis. The aetiology is unknown. Clinically they often resemble nodular or plaque-like vascular proliferations, typically on the distal extremities. Some resemble capillary malformations and they may be linear, following a broad Blaschkolinear pattern. They are often noted in childhood and may be congenital. Some have exhibited focal hyperhidrosis and even pain. Cases occurring in adulthood or developing after injury or surgery are also described. Histology reveals the association of eccrine glands and thin walled vascular elements within the dermis. Some cases have grown or expanded rapidly with hormonal stimulation [52].

Isolated eccrine naevi are benign and are typically observed. Symptomatic lesions may be treated with topical aluminium chloride, topical glycopyrrolate [53], systemic anticholinergics or intralesional botulinum toxin [54,55].

References

1 **McCuaig CC, Vera C, Kokta V et al. Connective tissue nevi in children: institutional experience and review. J Am Acad Dermatol 2012:67:890–7.**

2 Sacks HN, Crawley IS, Ward JA, Fine RM. Familial cardiomyopathy, hypogonadism, and collagenoma. Ann Intern Med 1980;93:813–7.

3 Al-Daraji WI, Ramsay HM, Ali RB. Storiform collagenoma as a clue for Cowden disease or PTEN hamartoma tumour syndrome. J Clin Pathol 2007;60:840–2.

4 Cobos G, Braunstein I, Abuabara K et al. Mucinous nevus: report of a case and review of the literature. JAMA Dermatol 2014;150:1018–9.

5 **Saussine A, Marrou K, Delanoé P et al. Connective tissue nevi: an entity revisited. J Am Acad Dermatol 2012;67:233–9.**

6 **de Feraudy S, Fletcher CD. Fibroblastic connective tissue nevus: a rare cutaneous lesion analyzed in a series of 25 cases. Am J Surg Pathol 2012;36:1509–15.**

7 Kim EJ, Jo SJ, Cho KH. A case of mucinous nevus clinically mimicking nevus lipomatosus superficialis. Ann Dermatol 2014;26:549–50.

8 Trau H, Dayan D, Hirschberg A et al. Connective tissue nevi collagens. Study with picrosirius red and polarizing microscopy. Am J Dermatopathol 1991:13:374–7.

9 Patterson JW.Weedon's Skin Pathology, 4th edn. Philadelphia: Elsevier, 2016.

10 Tardio JC, Granados R. The cellular component of the mucinous nevus consists of CD34-positive fibroblasts. J Cutan Pathol 2010;37:1019–20.

11 Velez MJ, Billings SD, Weaver JA. Fibroblastic connective tissue nevus. J Cutan Pathol 2016;43:75–9.

12 Buschke A, Ollendorff H. Ein Fall von Dermatofibrosis lenticularis disseminata. Derm Wochenschr 1928;86:257–62.

13 Rothman IL. Michelin tire baby syndrome: a review of the literature and a proposal for diagnostic criteria with adoption of the name circumferential skin folds syndrome. Pediatr Dermatol 2014;31:659–63.

14 Holland KE, Galbraith SS. Generalized congenital smooth muscle hamartoma presenting with hypertrichosis, excess skin folds, and follicular dimpling. Pediatr Dermatol 2008 25:236–9.

15 Kienast A, Maerker J, Hoeger PH. Myokymia as a presenting sign of congenital smooth muscle hamartoma. Pediatr Dermatol 2007; 24:628–31.

16 **Cai ED, Sun BK, Chiang A, et al. Postzygotic mutations in beta-actin are associated with Becker's nevus and Becker's nevus syndrome. J Invest Dermatol 2017;137:1795–8.**

17 Happle R. Becker's nevus and lethal beta-actin mutations. J Invest Dermatol 2017;137:1619–21.

18 Berger TG, Levin MW. Congenital smooth muscle hamartoma. J Am Acad Dermatol 1984;11:709–12.

19 Huffman DW, Mallory SB. Congenital smooth muscle hamartoma. Am Fam Physician 1989;39:117–20.

20 Metzker A, Merlob P. Congenital smooth muscle hamartoma. J Am Acad Dermatol 1986;14:691.

21 Prendiville J, Esterly NB. Congenital smooth muscle hamartoma. J Pediatr 1987;110:742–4.

22 Jones EW, Marks R, Pongsehirun D. Naevus superficialis lipomatosus. A clinicopathological report of twenty cases. Br J Dermatol 1975;93:121–33.

23 Kim RH, Stevenson ML, Hale CS et al. Nevus lipomatosus superficialis. Dermatol Online J 2015;20(12). https://escholarship.org/uc/item/2cb3c5t3.
24 Bancalari E, Martinez-Sanchez D, Tardio JC. Nevus lipomatosus superficialis with a folliculosebaceous component: report of 2 cases. Patholog Res Int 2011:105973.
25 Inoue M, Ueda K, Hashimoto T. Nevus lipomatosus cutaneus superficialis with follicular papules and hypertrophic pilo-sebaceous units. Int J Dermatol 2002;41:241–3.
26 Kang H Kim SE, Park K et al. Nevus lipomatosus cutaneous superficialis with folliculosebaceous cystic hamartoma. J Am Acad Dermatol 2007;56(2 Suppl):S55–7.
27 Anzai A, Halpern I, Rivitti-Machado MC. Nevus lipomatosus cutaneous superficialis with perifollicular fibromas. Am J Dermatopathol 2015;37:704–6.
28 Ishii N, Baba N, Kanaizuka I et al. Histopathological study of focal dermal hypoplasia (Goltz syndrome). Clin Exp Dermatol 1992; 17:24–6.
29 Cardot-Leccia N, Italiano A, Monteil MC et al. Naevus lipomatosus superficialis: a case report with a 2p24 deletion. Br J Dermatol 2007;156:380–1.
30 Akoglu G, Dincer N, Metin A. Giant polypoid mass on thigh: a child with nevus lipomatosus cutaneous superficialis. An Bras Dermatol 2016;91:554–5.
31 Fatah S, Ellis R, Seukeran DC, Carmichael AJ. Successful CO_2 laser treatment of naevus lipomatosus cutaneous superficialis. Clin Exp Dermatol 2010;35:559–60.
32 Kim YJ, Choi JH, Kim H et al. Recurrence of nevus lipomatosus cutaneous superficialis after CO_2 laser treatment. Arch Plast Surg 2012; 39:671–3.
33 de Paula Mesquita T, de Almeida HL, Jr, de Paula Mesquita MC. Histologic resolution of naevus lipomatosus superficialis with intralesional phosphatidylcholine. J Eur Acad Dermatol Venereol 2009; 23:714–5.
34 Kim HS, Park YM, Kim HO, Lee JY. Intralesional phosphatidylcholine and sodium deoxycholate: a possible treatment option for nevus lipomatosus superficialis. Pediatr Dermatol 2012;29:119–21.
35 Gumaste P, Ortiz AE, Patel A et al. Generalized basaloid follicular hamartoma syndrome: a case report and review of the literature. Am J Dermatopathol 2015;37:e37–40.
36 Saxena A, Shapiro M, Kasper DA et al. Basaloid follicular hamartoma: a cautionary tale and review of the literature. Dermatol Surg 2007;33:1130–5.
37 Happle R, Tinschert S. Segmentally arranged basaloid follicular hamartomas with osseous, dental and cerebral anomalies: a distinct syndrome. Acta Derm Venereol 2008; 88:382–7.
38 Itin PH. Happle-Tinschert syndrome. Segmentally arranged basaloid follicular hamartomas, linear atrophoderma with hypo- and hyperpigmentation, enamel defects, ipsilateral hypertrichosis, and skeletal and cerebral anomalies. Dermatology 2009; 218:221–5.
39 Choo JY, Lee JH, Lee JY, Park YM. Congenital cutaneous solitary mixed hamartoma: an unusual case containing eccrine, neural, and lipomatous components. JAAD Case Rep 2015;1:88–90.
40 Happle R, Kuster W. Nevus psiloliparus: a distinct fatty tissue nevus. Dermatology 1998;197:6–10.
41 Levy ML, Massey C. Encephalocraniocutaneous lipomatosis. Handb Clin Neurol 2015; 132:265–9.
42 Llamas-Velasco M, Hernández A, Colmenero I, Torrelo A. [Nevus psiloliparus in a child with encephalocraniocutaneous lipomatosis]. Actas Dermosifiliogr 2011;102:303–5.
43 Ruggieri M, Pratico AD. Mosaic neurocutaneous disorders and their causes. Semin Pediatr Neurol 2015;22:207–33.
44 Bennett JT, Tan TY, Alcantara D et al. Mosaic activating mutations in FGFR1 cause encephalocraniocutaneous lipomatosis. Am J Hum Genet 2016;98:579–87.
45 Boppudi S, Bögershausen N, Hove HB et al. Specific mosaic KRAS mutations affecting codon 146 cause oculoectodermal syndrome and encephalocraniocutaneous lipomatosis. Clin Genet 2016;90:334–42.
46 Cordero SC, Royer MC, Rush WL et al. Pure apocrine nevus: a report of 4 cases. Am J Dermatopathol 2012; 34:305–9.
47 Kawaoka JC, Gray J, Schappell D, Robinson-Bostom L. Eccrine nevus. J Am Acad Dermatol 2004;51:301–4.
48 Castori M, Annessi G, Castiglia D et al. Systematized organoid epidermal nevus with eccrine differentiation, multiple facial and oral congenital scars, gingival synechiae, and blepharophimosis: a novel epidermal nevus syndrome. Am J Med Genet A 2010;152a:25–31.
49 Espana A, Marquina M, Idoate MA. Extensive mucinous eccrine naevus following the lines of Blaschko: a new type of eccrine naevus. Br J Dermatol 2006;154:1004–6.
50 Chen J, Sun JF, Zeng XS et al. Mucinous eccrine nevus: a case report and literature review. Am J Dermatopathol 2009;31:387–90.
51 Man XY, Cai SQ, Zhang AH, Zheng M. Mucinous eccrine naevus presenting with hyperhidrosis: a case report. Acta Derm Venereol 2006; 86:554–5.
52 Patterson AT, Kumar MG, Bayliss SJ et al. Eccrine angiomatous hamartoma: a clinicopathologic review of 18 cases. Am J Dermatopathol 2016;38:413–7.
53 Dua J, Grabczynska S. Eccrine nevus affecting the forearm of an 11-year-old girl successfully controlled with topical glycopyrrolate. Pediatr Dermatol 2014;31:611–2.
54 Lera M, Espana A, Idoate MA. Focal hyperhidrosis secondary to eccrine naevus successfully treated with botulinum toxin type A. Clin Exp Dermatol 2015;40:640–3.
55 Honeyman JF, Valdés R, Rojas H, Gaete M. Efficacy of botulinum toxin for a congenital eccrine naevus. J Eur Acad Dermatol Venereol 2008;22:1275–6.

CHAPTER 108

Proteus Syndrome and Other Localized Overgrowth Disorders

Veronica A. Kinsler

Paediatric Dermatology Department, Great Ormond Street Hospital for Children NHS Foundation Trust, London, UK, and Genetics and Genomic Medicine, UCL Great Ormond Street Institute of Child Health, London, UK

Introduction, 1283
Proteus syndrome and the spectrum of *AKT1* mosaicism, 1284
PIK3CA-related overgrowth spectrum, 1289
Other causes of localized overgrowth with cutaneous features, 1293

Abstract

Our understanding of localized or segmental overgrowth disorders has been revolutionized in recent years. This is as a result of both accurate in-depth clinical phenotyping separating out distinct phenotypes, and the availability of high sensitivity DNA sequencing techniques revealing the genetic basis of many of these disorders. The resultant understanding has led to a new appreciation of this spectrum of mosaic disorders, and to a regrouping of disorders within classifications. In addition, it has allowed the first steps into targeted therapies for localized overgrowth, with clinical trials beginning to report results. This chapter reviews the latest knowledge of the clinical and genetic aspects of the mosaic causes of localized overgrowth which have a cutaneous phenotype, including Proteus syndrome and the *PIK3CA*-related overgrowth syndromes.

Key points

- Localized overgrowth syndromes with cutaneous features present with overgrowth of one or more body parts, either at birth or in childhood.
- Cutaneous features are connective tissue naevi, epidermal naevi, vascular malformations and dysregulated adipose tissue.
- These rare disorders are caused by different mosaic mutations, which occur at any time during *in utero* development, affecting any cell type or body part. As a result, a whole spectrum of phenotypes can be seen, from very localized to extensive, and from mild to severe.
- The clinical distinction between a largely noncongenital presentation with disproportionate postnatal overgrowth, and a congenital presentation with proportionate overgrowth, is generally useful in distinguishing between the extremely rare *AKT1*-related Proteus syndrome, and the commoner *PIK3CA*-related overgrowth spectrum respectively.
- There is a substantial risk of deep vein thrombosis and pulmonary embolism in Proteus syndrome which leads to a high mortality in the first two decades.
- The risk of associated cancers in localized overgrowth syndromes is real but appears to be low.
- Mutations are detectable in affected tissues but usually not in blood.
- Targeted medical therapies are being trialled in these conditions instead of, or as an adjunct to, surgical management.

Introduction

Localized or segmental overgrowth disorders can be defined as the disproportionate growth of one or more body parts either pre- or postnatally. From the perspective of the paediatric dermatologist, overgrowth presents in the context of associated skin findings, most commonly vascular malformations, epidermal naevi, lipomatous overgrowth and/or connective tissue naevi. Due to the mosaic nature of the segmental overgrowth disorders the definition and classification has been difficult over the years, but accurate clinical phenotyping and genetic advances have now helped to distinguish major diagnoses from each other in recent times. As a result of this history, however, a literature search will not only identify references for what is now known to be, for example, Proteus syndrome, but will also contain reports of many other now distinct conditions previously published as Proteus. It is important therefore to rely on recent or recently updated texts for knowledge and management of this group of conditions.

This chapter will describe the key clinical and genetic features of the segmental overgrowth disorders as they relate to paediatric dermatology. However, from the patients' perspective, the importance is in the enormous impact these clinical features have on their lives and the lives of their families. The extent of this has not been

Harper's Textbook of Pediatric Dermatology, Fourth Edition. Edited by Peter Hoeger, Veronica Kinsler and Albert Yan.

studied systematically, although it is clear to clinicians working in the field that it is substantial. Recent data on the impact of vascular malformations on quality of life have identified a very substantial negative impact via pain and psychosocial mental health [1].

A major shift in the approach to these patients has occurred in the last few years, with the introduction of medical therapies as an alternative or an adjunct to surgery. Publications from clinical trial cohorts and case reports are increasing in number, and results in many instances have been promising. As matters currently stand, in order to prognosticate about and treat such patients most effectively, both clinical and genetic information about the individual patient is likely to be required. With the advent of new treatments, it is likely that our role as paediatric dermatologists will be to diagnose as accurately as possible, and direct to appropriate treatment as early as possible. This is, however, an ideal which can be difficult to achieve in practice in many healthcare systems, and ongoing trials may be helpful in designing clinically based management guidelines.

The diagnosis and management of epidermal naevi and vascular malformations are covered in detail in Chapters 106 and 118 respectively.

Proteus syndrome and the spectrum of *AKT1* mosaicism

Introduction. Proteus syndrome (PS) was first described as a distinct clinical entity in 1979 by Cohen [2], and the name Proteus syndrome was coined by Wiedemann in 1993 [3], after the prophetic god of Greek mythology Proteus who was able to assume different shapes at will. Subsequently it was concluded that this was the correct diagnosis for the famous case of Joseph Merrick, sometimes known as the 'Elephant Man', who had previously been thought to have neurofibromatosis [4]. Segmental or localized overgrowth is the cardinal feature of PS. It is characteristically either absent or of limited presentation at birth, but disproportionate and unrelenting in postnatal life, and most commonly affects the bones, skin, adipose tissue and the central nervous system (CNS) [5]. Cutaneous features are cerebriform connective tissue naevi, epidermal naevi, vascular malformations and dysregulation of adipose tissue.

Epidemiology. PS is a very rare disease, with an incidence estimated to be approximately 1 in 1 000 000–1 in 10 000 000 new births [6]. The sex ratio is not completely clear, with a review of published cases diagnosed under the clinical criteria suggesting there was a male preponderance [7]. However, a published cohort study reports an equal sex ratio and this is more likely to be accurate [8]. PS has been described in all races.

Pathogenesis. Postzygotic activating mutations in *AKT1* were identified in 2011 as causing PS, using next generation sequencing. The variant identified was the same missense change *AKT1* c.49G>A, p.(Glu17Lys) in the affected tissues of 26 of 29 patients who met the clinical diagnostic criteria for PS [9]. The amino acid change leads to abnormal localization of the AKT protein to the plasma membrane, which leads to autonomous activation [10], with downstream effects via the mTOR complex, a pathway known to be important in the regulation of cellular proliferation and apoptosis. No other mutations have thus far been implicated in this phenotype.

The tight phenotype–genotype correlation validated the clinical delineation of PS as a separate entity in the localized overgrowth syndromes, and confirmed that full-blown PS is usually (possibly always) caused by this specific *AKT1* mutation. However, the reverse is not necessarily true. As with all mosaic syndromes, there is a spectrum of phenotypes associated with the genotype, and more limited cases of *AKT1* mosaicism caused by the same mutation do not necessarily fulfil the criteria for PS [11]. Importantly though, the characteristics of the overgrowth in the milder cases are the same as for Proteus, with postnatal, progressive, disproportionate growth being the hallmark. This suggests that the role of *AKT1* in bony and soft tissue overgrowth is primarily postnatal (as opposed to prenatal for *PIK3CA*). This is echoed by the natural history of the connective tissue naevi, which grow through adolescence and then appear to halt [12]. In contrast, epidermal naevi and cutaneous vascular malformations can be present at birth and remain largely stable throughout childhood [12,13], suggesting that *AKT1* in keratinocytes and cutaneous vasculature is involved in the pre- and postnatal periods.

An in-depth study of phenotype, histology and genotype in different affected and unaffected tissues in one patient at postmortem, revealed that tissues which appear clinically and histopathologically unaffected may still harbour high mosaic levels of the *AKT1* mutation [14]. This study also revealed that the overgrowth in PS can be caused by either cellular proliferation or overgrowth of extracellular matrix [14].

Clinical features.

Diagnostic criteria

Diagnostic criteria for PS are well defined and are based on detailed clinical phenotyping. First published in 1999 [5], these are regularly curated and full details are freely available online [6].

A summary of these criteria is listed in Box 108.1.

Cutaneous features

The characteristic connective tissue naevus of PS is a skin-coloured or pinkish, firm, pronounced exophytic overgrowth of dermal connective tissue, which leads to a marked cerebriform appearance with deep 'sulci' over the surface, and a smooth appearance of the intervening 'gyri'. They typically affect the palms or soles, but can also be seen on the alae nasi, the ear helix and the lacrimal puncta [6] and can occur anywhere, for example rarely covering the whole anterior chest wall [15]. These lesions are not present at birth, appearing in childhood and progressing in adolescence, but thereafter appearing to

Box 108.1 A summary of diagnostic criteria for Proteus syndrome

- *General* characteristics of the disease which must all be fulfilled
  (A) Sporadic (nonfamilial) occurrence
  (B) A mosaic distribution
  (C) A progressive course

Plus

- *Specific* clinical characteristics which are divided into three groups
  (A) One from group A
  (B) Or two from group B
  (C) Or three from group C

Group A

- This group only contains the classical cerebriform connective tissue naevus

Group B

- Blaschkolinear epidermal naevus (keratinocytic)
- Asymmetric disproportionate growth of one or more defined body parts (limbs, hyperostosis of skull, hyperostosis of external auditory canal, vertebrae or either spleen or thymus)
- Specific tumours with onset before the second decade (bilateral ovarian cystadenoma or parotid monomorphic adenoma)

Group C

- Dysregulated growth of adipose tissue, increased or decreased
- Vascular malformation
- Typical facial features (all of: dolichocephaly, long face, downslanting palpebral fissures and/or minor ptosis, depressed nasal bridge, wide or anteverted nares, open mouth at rest)

stabilize [12]. These are almost pathognomonic of PS. They can usually be distinguished from the deep palmar or plantar creases seen with *PIK3CA* mutation mosaicism, as the latter are softer and not clearly cerebriform [16]. This distinction, however, may not be absolute. Connective tissue naevi are frequently symptomatic, leading to pain, bleeding, pruritus and infection, and this can lead to functional impairment particularly when on the sole [13].

Epidermal naevi in PS are common, found in 72% of cases fulfilling clinical criteria in a literature review [7] and 26% of a cohort study of 31 patients [13]. These demonstrate fine Blaschkolinear patterning (Fig. 108.1d,e), and in all descriptions thus far are keratinocytic in origin. They present therefore with a palpable hyperkeratosis which varies from mild to verrucous, and from skin-coloured to darkly pigmented (Figure 108.1d,e). Unlike many of the other features they are usually present at birth or soon after, and do not progress postnatally [12,17]. Unlike some types of epidermal naevi they are primarily a mild cosmetic rather than a symptomatic problem [13].

Cutaneous vascular malformations are common in PS, and present with capillary malformations, visible venous vessels and/or lymphatic malformation. Typically, capillary and venous malformations present at birth or in the first few months of life and behave in a relatively stable manner thereafter [13]. Lymphatic malformations can affect any body part and can be progressive [6]. Arteriovenous malformations have not so far been described in genetically confirmed cases of PS. Importantly, a recent study demonstrated that hepatosplenic involvement by vascular malformations was not seen in PS patients where there were no cutaneous vascular malformations [18].

Dysregulated adipose tissue is a hallmark of PS. This encompasses lipomas and lipohypoplasia. Lipomas in PS can be subcutaneous, but can also occur internally, and are in fact overgrowth of fat tissue rather than a well-encapsulated localized tumour of fat [19]. Subcutaneous lipomas are usually not present at birth, appearing in the first year of life, and although most common on the trunk, can arise on the head or limbs [13]. This fatty overgrowth can be severe. Lipohypoplasia includes decreased or absent fat and tends to occur on the trunk or limbs [15]. Dysregulation of adipose tissue, however, can occur anywhere that tissue is found, including myocardial fat overgrowth [20]. The latter is a common finding on an echocardiogram, but does not seem to have functional implications for the heart [20].

Skeletal overgrowth

Skeletal overgrowth is not present at birth, other than congenital megalencephaly, and typically presents between 6 and 18 months of life, although occasionally it can present later in childhood [6,21]. It typically progresses rapidly and relentlessly thereafter (Fig. 108.1d,e). Bony overgrowth in the limbs can be bilateral but is usually asymmetrical, and is a severe feature [6], with leg length discrepancy of more than 10 cm not unusual by the age of 10 years [21]. Scoliosis is a very common feature due to megaspondylodysplasia (overgrowth of individual vertebrae) and the resultant distortion of vertebral column growth [19,21]. Involvement of the skull often affects the frontal bone asymmetrically, leading to characteristic facial distortion, with frontal prominence, and often trigonocephaly (Fig. 108.1a,b). In this situation there can be accompanying hyperostosis affecting the external auditory canal [7,21,22], and/or intracranial mengiomas [23].

Radiological appearances of skeletal overgrowth are very unusual and are characteristic of PS. These include hyperostosis, which eventually destroys the basic architecture of the bone, and striking connective tissue calcification around the epiphyses, which can lead to joint immobility [19,21].

Pulmonary disease

Pulmonary disease is a common problem in PS [19], mainly due to extrinsic factors such as compression of the thorax due to skeletal deformity and problems of immobility, and more rarely due to intrapulmonary disease. Intrapulmonary disease includes vascular malformations involving the lungs, or bullous pulmonary degeneration [7,19,24]. Pulmonary embolism (PE) should also always be considered in the differential diagnosis of pulmonary symptoms in PS.

Neurological disease

CNS abnormalities are a common feature of PS [6], seen in approximately 40% of cases in a literature review [7]. Hemimegalencephaly is a common abnormality within

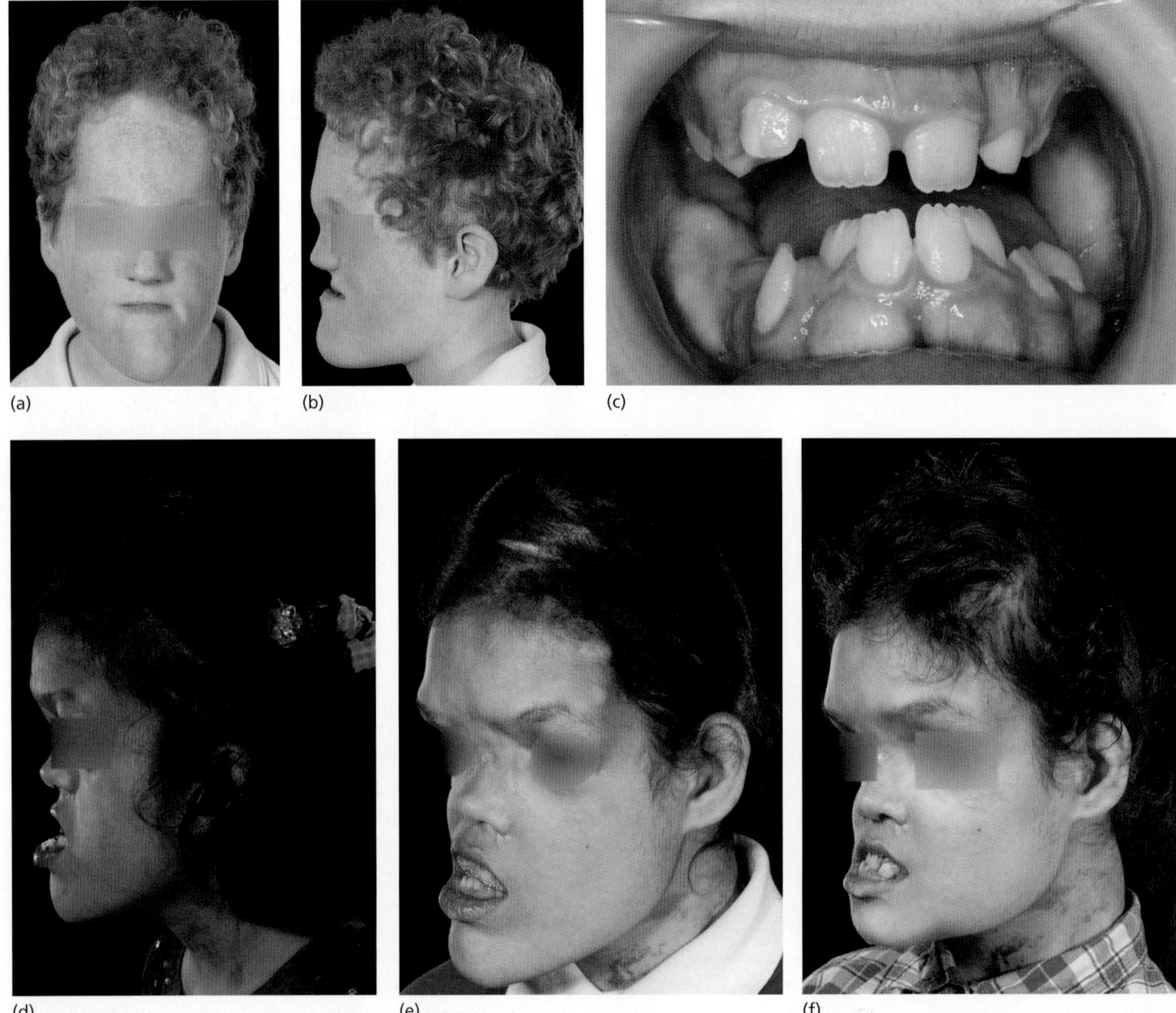

Fig. 108.1 Clinical images of *AKT1*-mosaic patients. Bony overgrowth of skull bones in a characteristic pattern leading to trigonocephaly and prominence of the mandible (a,b), with resultant dental crowding (c). Progressive bony overgrowth is demonstrated over time in the same patient over a decade (d,e,f), and a pigmented Blaschkolinear keratinocytic epidermal naevus is visible on the left neck (e,f)

this group and unlike many of the features of PS can be present at birth [7]. Hemimegalencephaly can be associated with neuronal migration defects and with developmental delay and/or seizures [6].

Dental abnormalities

Dental abnormalities are relatively common, seen in 18% in a literature review [7]. The main issues arise from hyperostosis and asymmetric overgrowth of the jaws (Fig. 108.1a,b,d,e), with resultant malocclusion and overcrowding (Fig. 108.1c). In addition, there can be enamel or dental hypoplasia or dental dysplasia with overgrowth of individual teeth [7].

Other abnormalities

The eye, ENT (ear, nose and throat), renal, reproductive tract and indeed any other system can be affected in PS, but are beyond the scope of this chapter. Appropriate referrals should be made on a case by case basis.

The spectrum of AKT1-mosaicism

Descriptions of limited *AKT1*-mosaicism which does not fulfil the diagnostic criteria for PS include a case of bilateral cerebriform collagenomas with varicose veins without evidence of overgrowth [11]. In contrast, very mild clinical cases of *AKT1*-mosaicism can nonetheless fulfil the diagnostic criteria for PS [17], and these are perhaps more likely to present to the paediatric dermatologist than any other specialty.

Complications.

Thromboembolic disease

Deep vein thrombosis (DVT) and PE can occur in PS [25,26]. The risk is now known to be high, and it is the leading cause of death in this condition [8,27]. The basis for the prothrombotic state appears to be multifaceted. A recent review of the NIH cohort confirmed that surgical procedures were a significant risk factor and that prothrombotic genetic abnormalities such as Factor V

Leiden and protein C and S deficiencies were occasionally seen but were not likely to be a major cause [27]. The authors further concluded that the risk appeared to be out of proportion to what might be expected simply from the vascular malformations, and that therefore there may be a prothrombotic effect of AKT/PI3K pathway activation [27]. Although overall patient numbers were small there was a trend between the occurrence of a DVT and the absolute level of D-dimers, which is a measurement of fibrinolysis and a known association with DVT in the general population. The clinically relevant level of D-dimers, however, may not be the same as in the general population, where 0.5 μg/dL (for the STA-Liatest D-dimer assay) is taken as the threshold for further investigation for a DVT, as in PS this level appeared possibly to be more correctly set at 1.0 μg/dL [27].

Overall from the literature it is possible to conclude the following about PS and thromboembolic disease:

1 That the risk is high, and the outcome can be fatal;
2 That the risk may not be related only to vascular malformations;
3 That surgery increases the risk and anticoagulation prophylaxis should be given to cover surgical procedures;
4 That patients with PS should be referred to a paediatric haematologist for consideration of their thromboembolic risk due to immobility (if relevant) and personal coagulation profile; and
5 That D-dimers should be measured regularly to have a baseline, and acutely if DVT or PE is suspected, and that a level of more than 0.5 μg/dL (for the STA-Liatest D-dimer assay) should trigger further investigation for DVT or PE.

Tumour risk

As with many of the cutaneous mosaic syndromes, the mutation in *AKT1* has been described as a somatic mutation in the context of cancers [10,28]. Although there is an excess risk of benign and malignant tumour formation in *AKT1* mosaicism, again as is seen with other mosaic syndromes, this is not a high absolute risk. The commonest cancer described with PS is meningioma, which is particularly prevalent (approximately 13%) in patients with a characteristic pattern of cranial hyperostosis [23], and *AKT1* mutations are known to be present in a proportion of nonsyndromic meningiomas [28]. Meningiomas can also be present in the spinal cord [29]. Other described cancers in PS include ovarian cystadenomas and parotid monomorphic adenoma (included in the clinical criteria), breast cancer and male reproductive tumours [7]. At present, given the high degree of variability of clinical presentation between patients there are currently no standard recommendations for monitoring for tumours, and patients are recommended to be monitored clinically, by history and examination, rather than by routine imaging [6].

Life expectancy

A confirmed diagnosis of PS is associated with a reduced life expectancy. In a recent study of survival in the largest cohort of 64 patients in the literature, 11 had died; 10 of the 11 had died by the age of 22 years, equating to a 25% mortality in this age range, and with a mean and median age at death of 14–15 years [8]. However, 68% of the cohort still alive were under the age of 22 years, and the early mortality might therefore be expected to increase further in the future. The authors suggested that the statistics imply peak disease severity in adolescence with a stabilization or lessening thereafter. Importantly, the cause of death in seven of the 11 cases was a PE, or likely PE. There were no deaths from cancer [8]. However, this has previously been described.

Laboratory findings.

Genetics

Biopsy of affected tissue is key to the genetic diagnosis, as the mutation will not be detectable in blood. Skin biopsy from an epidermal naevus or vascular malformation is the easiest method, unless the child is having surgery to remove or debulk an overgrowth body part or a mass of tissue. Primary culture of individual cell types from skin biopsies has demonstrated that in epidermal naevi the mutation is usually present in the keratinocytes as opposed to dermal fibroblasts [30]. DNA should therefore be extracted directly from the tissue without initial tissue culture and sequenced for the hotspot mutation in *AKT1*. It is important that the diagnostic laboratory is aware that they are looking for a mosaic mutation with a low allele load, to allow correct interpretation of results. Sanger sequencing is adequate in many instances to detect the mutation, but if this is negative and the clinical suspicion of *AKT1* mosaicism is strong, next generation sequencing is far superior and the sample should be retested.

Histopathology

The epidermal naevi are keratinocytic or nonorganoid, demonstrating hyperkeratosis and acanthosis. The connective tissue naevi consist of highly collagenized fibrous connective tissue [15,31]. Subcutaneous lipomas are not atypical on histology, but are generally nonencapsulated [15].

General management. Management of PS is extremely challenging, owing to the combination of the individuality of each case, the severity of the disease, and the risks of complications from procedures. Consultation with international experts in the field is strongly recommended to obtain the best possible management plans for individual patients.

- Advice on the signs and symptoms of DVT and PE should be given as soon as the diagnosis is established. Doppler ultrasound and clotting parameters including D-dimers are suggested as important measurements. However, there are no clear guidelines on how to interpret the results of these, and individuals with vascular malformations can have complex clotting profiles with a difficult balance between coagulation and bleeding. Anticoagulation is however recommended under expert guidance from a haematologist for any surgical procedures carried out [19,21].
- Early referral to a paediatric orthopaedic surgeon is important in the setting of PS where limbs, extremities and/or spine are involved, as it is predictable that the bony overgrowth will continue relentlessly throughout

childhood and adolescence, and that deformity will worsen [19,21,32]. A baseline skeletal survey is recommended for all patients with a diagnosis of PS [6]. Monitoring of disease progression has been debated by an expert workshop panel who recommend a combination of annual clinical assessment and plain radiography, with bone scanning and magnetic resonance imaging (MRI) or computed tomography (CT) as needed on an individual basis [21]. The degree of disability due to bony deformity ultimately can be very severe and therefore orthopaedic intervention is often essential to maintain quality of life or functionality. However, the risks of intervention are substantial, particularly from the thromboembolic complications. Careful assessment of the timing of surgery should be undertaken on a case-by-case basis in consultation with international experts in the field [21]. Surgical intervention to reduce leg length discrepancy, however, has been demonstrated to be effective [32]. Referrals to orthotics are important.

- Early referral to a craniofacial surgeon is advisable where there is craniofacial involvement, as well as to ophthalmology, dental and ENT departments. An MRI of the CNS is indicated at diagnosis where there is clear craniofacial involvement.
- Pulmonary function tests and referral to a respiratory paediatrician is important at baseline, and for anyone thereafter with skeletal involvement of the truncal area. High resolution CT of the chest is recommended for those where bullous pulmonary disease is suspected [6].
- Consultation with a clinical genetics team and genetic counsellor is recommended once the diagnosis is established. Transmission of PS from a patient to the next generation has not been described and would not be expected. Re-occurrence in a sibling of an affected proband has also not been described and would not be expected other than by chance.
- Neurological assessment and neurodevelopmental follow-up are recommended for those with hemimegalencephaly at birth, or any evidence of neurodevelopmental issues at any stage [19].
- Epidermal naevi can be managed symptomatically if this issue arises, with general skin care advice and moisturisers.
- Connective tissue naevi are frequently symptomatic. Surgical debulking, however, has not been found to be useful, leading to complications, and current recommendations are to manage these nonsurgically, with skin care measures and as careful cleaning as possible [13].
- Referral to psychosocial support teams and patient support groups with specialist knowledge, are important for both patients and families.

Targeted medical therapy. The discovery of the causative mutation in PS [9] led to the idea that AKT inhibitors, designed to combat cancers with an AKT gene driver mutation, could be repurposed for use in PS [33] (Fig. 108.2). *In vitro* studies demonstrated that patient cells treated with the pan-AKT inhibitor ARQ092 had reduced activation of the AKT-PI3K-mTOR pathway [33]. Clinical trials of this drug in PS are in progress.

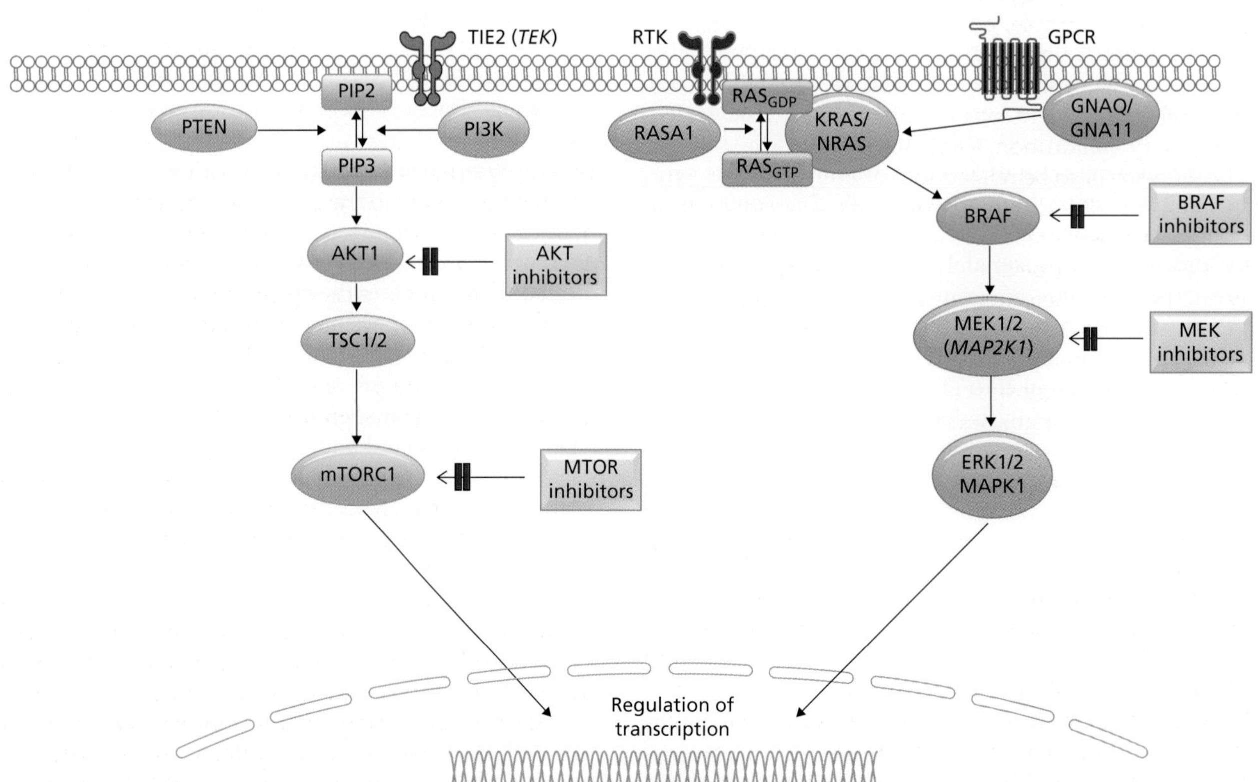

Fig. 108.2 Schematic of the cell signalling pathways involved in overgrowth and potential positions for medical therapeutic targets.

PIK3CA-related overgrowth spectrum

Introduction. *PIK3CA* mutations were first described in the skin in keratinocytic epidermal naevi and seborrhoeic keratoses [34], without an overgrowth phenotype. This study revealed mutations in *PIK3CA* in 27% of EN tested, which resulted in the p.(E545G) amino acid change, rarely found in cancers. On the other hand, seborrhoeic keratoses harboured classical oncogenic hotspot mutations [28,35] p.(E542K), p.(E545K), and p.(H1047R). *PIK3CA* mutations have also recently been described in isolated venous and lymphatic malformations without overgrowth [36–38]. Although with single lesions it is very difficult to demonstrate causality of a mutant genotype, particularly as they often carry multiple somatic mutations, the causative role of *PIK3CA* in epidermal naevi and vascular malformations has since been confirmed by the multifocal mosaic phenotypes described later. Epidermal naevi and vascular malformations are covered in detail in Chapters 106 and 118.

The term *PIK3CA*-related overgrowth spectrum (PROS) was coined in 2014 in an attempt to unify multiple clinical diagnoses which had been found to have the same genetic basis [39]. These previously distinct diagnoses were fibroadipose hyperplasia or overgrowth (FAO), hemihyperplasia multiple lipomatosis (HHML), fibroadipose infiltrating lipomatosis, CLOVE(S) syndrome (Congenital Lipomatous Overgrowth, Vascular malformations, Epidermal nevi, Scoliosis/skeletal and spinal), isolated macrodactyly, megalencephaly-capillary malformation (MCAP or M-CM) and dysplastic megalencephaly (DMEG) [39]. These different clinical presentations are a result of the timing, cell type and body part affected by the mutation. For example, patients with MCAP have likely had a mutation involving the head at an embryonic stage where this was compatible with life, whereas those with CLOVES have had a mutation more focused on the trunk/body. In addition, there is some evidence that the diagnosis may also be related to the activating strength of the mutation [39–41]. While groups of patients with these clinical diagnoses are discernible within the spectrum of *PIK3CA*-related mosaicism, and it is clear that these groupings can be helpful in directing genetic diagnosis to *PIK3CA* mutation testing, in many instances patients do not fit into any one clinical diagnosis, and it is not yet clear that the clinical diagnosis is able to direct management. In general, therefore, management has still to be considered on a case-by-case basis and should be based where possible on both clinical assessment and genotype.

Epidemiology and pathogenesis. PROS is a spectrum of clinical presentations unified by a common genetic cause – namely a postzygotic *in utero* mutation in the gene *PIK3CA*. This gene encodes a protein p110α, a catalytic subunit of one of the phosphatidylinositol 3-kinases (PI3Ks), key enzymes involved in intracellular signalling pathways which control growth, differentiation and apoptosis of tissues [42]. A role for *PIK3CA* in overgrowth was first described in 2012 and 2013, with a series of papers from different groups working on the different clinical presentations uncovering the same molecular pathogenesis [43–48].

Although certain mutational hotspots are more common in PROS, pathogenic mutations in *PIK3CA* can occur anywhere in the gene, and novel mutations continue to be described [40,41]. This underlines the need to sequence the whole of the coding sequence of the gene in these conditions. Importantly also, germline mutations in *PIK3CA* are seen in a small proportion of patients with segmental overgrowth [40,41,44], and rarely as a cause of megalencephaly and macrosomia without the classic segmental phenotype [49]. This clearly has implications for genetic counselling surrounding the rare possibility of passing on *PIK3CA*-related disease to future generations.

Recent cohort studies have attempted to tackle the difficult area of genotype–phenotype interactions [39–41]. This is fraught with difficulty, as classification of the clinical phenotype is not straightforward, with many patients not conforming to a clear disease category and many competing classifications already in the literature. In addition, the wide range of mutations makes genotypic classification difficult. Some recent data on this, however, has given an indication of the activating strength of a proportion of the genetic changes [50], and some assumptions can be made from the somatic cancer profile [28]. Overall, there is definitely some evidence that less activating mutations are more commonly seen in disease involving the brain, and in patients with germline mutations, with more strongly activating mutations more commonly seen in truncal or limb phenotypes [39–41,45].

The prevalence at birth of PROS taken as a whole is not known, partly because of the recent delineation of the spectrum. What can be said is that it is far commoner than PS, perhaps in the region of 50 times as common, which would put the figure at approximately 1 in 20000 at lowest estimate, but the true figure remains to be established. Presentation with segmental overgrowth of this type appears to be roughly equal between the sexes in both primarily non-neurological and neurological cohorts [40,51]. However, details on sex balance in those with a *PIK3CA* mutant genotype have not always been published. Where the data are published there was a 4:3 female:male ratio in one study [39]. PROS has been described in all ethnic groups.

Clinical features. The clinical features of this spectrum of diseases vary enormously, as can be seen from the range of clinical diagnoses included under this umbrella [52]. Cutaneous features include epidermal naevi, vascular malformations and dysregulation of adipose tissue (Fig. 108.3a,b). There is a large degree of overlap with PS in that the essential criteria of sporadic nature, mosaic distribution and progressive overgrowth are frequently fulfilled. However, some key differences were discerned in a review of a PROS cohort, most notably the congenital nature of overgrowth in the vast majority of cases, the

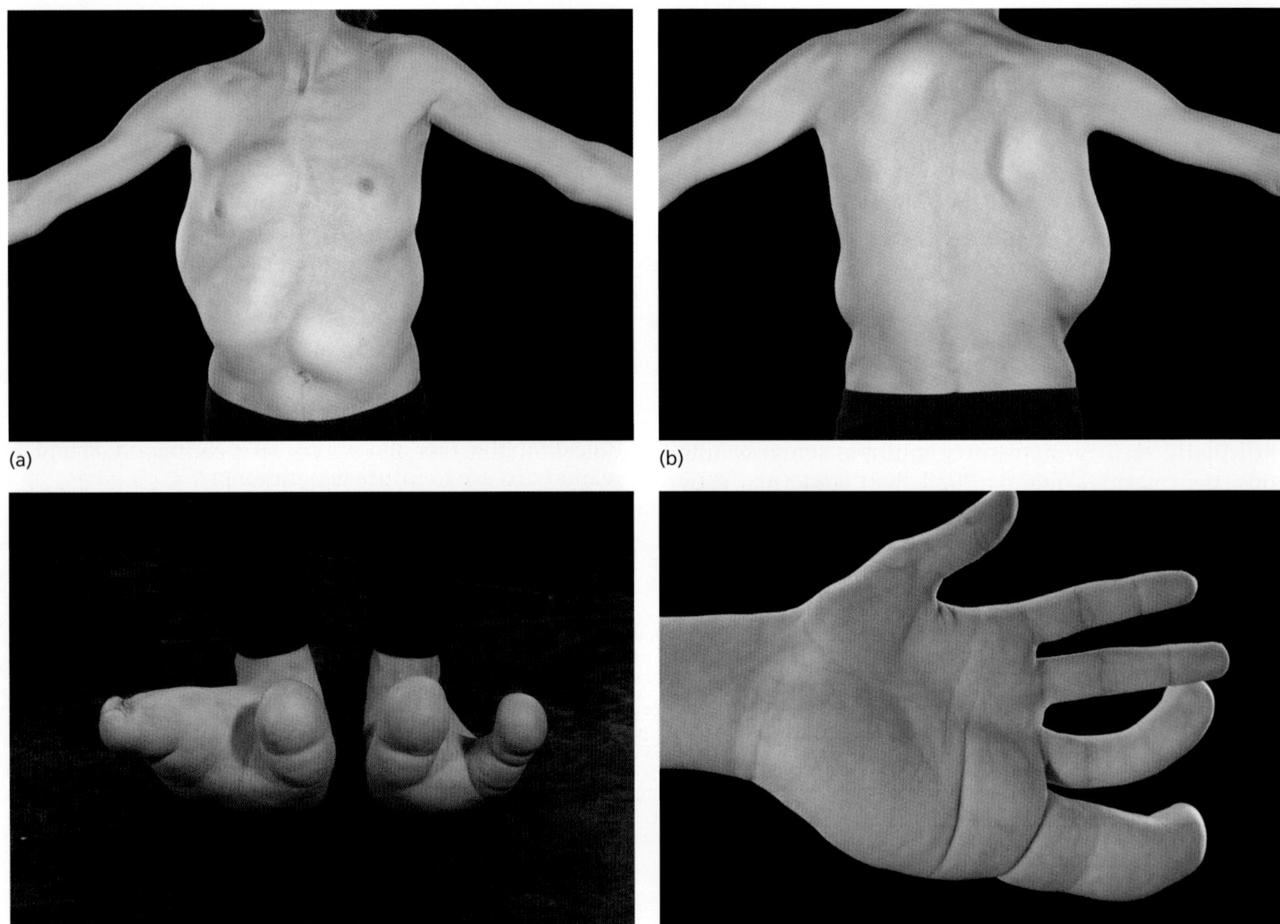

Fig. 108.3 Clinical images of a *PIK3CA*-mosaic patient. Widespread lipomatous overgrowth on the trunk is visible on anterior and posterior surfaces (a,b). Macrodactyly and splaying of hands and feet (c,d) has resulted in amputation of some toes to allow functionality.

overgrowth of lower limbs more than upper and left side more than right, and the prominence of adipose dysregulation, which included both adipose hyperplasia in affected areas and a decrease in adiposity in unaffected areas [39]. A workshop of experts later led to the formulation of proposed diagnostic criteria for PROS, which are currently as shown in Box 108.2 [52].

Since this publication [52] other isolated features which could be added are small venous or lymphatic malformations [36–38].

Box 108.2 Proposed diagnostic criteria for PROS [52]

Required features:
- The detection of a somatic *PIK3CA* mutation
- Congenital or early childhood onset
- Sporadic or mosaic pattern of overgrowth

Plus

Clinical features for diagnosis of PROS – two or more of:
- Overgrowth of adipose (Fig. 108.3a,b), muscle, nerve, or skeletal tissue
- Vascular malformations (capillary, venous, arteriovenous, lymphatic)
- Epidermal naevus

Or

Clinical features for diagnosis of isolated abnormality due to *PIK3CA* mutation:
- Large isolated lymphatic malformation
- Isolated macrodactyly, splayed feet/hands (Fig. 108.3c,d), overgrown limbs
- Truncal adipose overgrowth (Fig. 108.3a,b)
- Hemimegalencephaly, dysplastic megalencephaly, focal cortical dysplasia
- Epidermal naevus
- Seborrhoiec keratosis (not applicable in children)
- Benign lichenoid keratosis (not applicable in children)

Specific syndromic clinical diagnoses within PROS.

CLOVES syndrome

Congenital Lipomatous Overgrowth, Vascular malformations and Epidermal naevus (CLOVE) syndrome was first delineated in 2007 [16], as a distinct entity from PS. The acronym has since been expanded to include Scoliosis/Skeletal and spinal anomalies, hence CLOVES. This entity is an overgrowth disorder centred on truncal involvement by vascular malformations and lipomatous overgrowth (Fig. 108.1a,b). Subsequently, hemimegalencephaly, neuronal migration defects, and agenesis of the corpus callosum, with ensuing neurodevelopmental problems and seizures, have been described in association with CLOVES [53].

MCAP syndrome
Megalencephaly CAPillary malformation syndrome (MCAP, previously known as Macrocephaly-Capillary Malformation M-CM), is the association of megalencephaly (brain overgrowth), with vascular anomalies and/or digital anomalies (polydactyly/syndactyly), in addition to connective tissue laxity and variable body overgrowth [41,51]. Importantly, megalencephaly is almost always congenital, and is progressive, with the head circumference increasing more than expected with normal growth [51]. Radiological imaging frequently demonstrates cortical brain malformations, most commonly polymicrogyria [51]. Neurological features include seizures in approximately one-third of cases and some degree of neurodevelopmental delay in the majority [51]. Vascular anomalies are usually capillary malformations affecting any body part, but frequently involving the midline of the face, and are often telengiectatic in nature [41,51]. Larger vessel abnormalities have occasionally been described [51]. In a study of 131 patients with the MCAP phenotype, 38% were *PIK3CA*-mutation positive [41]. Importantly, in this cohort other described features were complex congenital heart defects, arrythmias, hypoglycaemia, endocrine disorders and rhizomelic limb shortening [41].

Klippel–Trenaunay syndrome
Klippel–Trenaunay syndrome (KTS) is classically defined as the association of a capillary malformation of a limb, in association with deep venous anomaly, and overgrowth of the same limb. However, the term has frequently been used to describe either overgrowth of a limb, or a vascular anomaly on a limb without overgrowth, causing some degree of confusion in the literature. KTS is probably no longer a useful clinical subdivision in the context of PROS, although this could change with refinement of outcome measures and genotypic characterization. Several studies have demonstrated *PIK3CA* mutations in the context of what could be defined as KTS [43,54,55].

CLAPO syndrome
This acronym represents the constellation of features described originally as a Capillary malformation of the lower lip, a Lymphatic malformation of the face and/or neck, and Partial or generalized Overgrowth [56]. It has very recently been described as being caused by mutations in *PIK3CA* in six of nine patients genotyped [57]. As expected not all the features are always present, with a recent description in the absence of overgrowth [58] reinforcing the message that *PIK3CA* mosaicism does not always lead to overgrowth.

Complications. The complication profile may vary with specific genotype, or with the tissue type affected, but this level of detail is not yet available in this new field. An outline of what is currently known of complications in general in PROS is delineated here.

Thromboembolic disease
There is a risk of thromboembolic disease in PROS. However, the level of risk is not known [39]. A risk of pulmonary embolism was described in a study of 12 CLOVES patients, where two patients developed severe postoperative PE, fatal in one [59]. In this study 11 of 12 patients had central and thoracic phlebectasia. Other sites of thrombosis have also been described in PROS, including the jugular vein [41], neonatal cerebral infarcts [39] and spinal thrombosis, the latter in the absence of vascular anomalies [39]. It has been suggested that due to this and the parallels with PS, it is advisable to consider anticoagulation for surgical and other high risk procedures [39,59].

Tumour risk
As with many genes involved in cutaneous mosaic disorders, *PIK3CA* was first discovered in the context of cancer, and was found to be very commonly mutated across a range of malignant tumours [35]. Despite this, the risk of tumour development in *PIK3CA* mosaicism as is seen in paediatric dermatology practice is low. The first description of malignancy in association with PROS was of Wilm's tumour [43], and including this case there are now a total of four cases in the literature with Wilm's tumour or nephroblastomatosis (premalignant). Genotypically, three of these patients had mutations affecting codon 1047 (however, this is the commonest mutation site), and phenotypically two had CLOVES, one had fibroadipose hyperplasia, and one had hemihyperplasia [60]. The same mutation was present in the tumour as in other affected tissues of one patient tested, demonstrating a direct link between the *PIK3CA* mosaicism and the oncogenic process [61]. Two further cases of Wilm's tumour in cases with a clinical diagnosis of CLOVES, but no genotypic diagnosis, were reported recently [62]. One case of nonmalignant ovarian cystadenoma has also been described [52]. It has been suggested that this may be sufficient evidence on which to undertake surveillance screening by abdominal ultrasound imaging every 3–4 months until the age of 8 years [52,60], as is recommended for hyperplasia in Beckwith–Wiedemann syndrome. However, there is clear evidence that *PIK3CA* mutations *per se* are not oncogenic, from their high prevalence in keratinocytic epidermal naevi and seborrhoeic keratoses [34], and in animal models with physiological levels of expression of mutant *PIK3CA* affecting codon 1047 there was no ovarian tumour formation after 1 year [63]. Furthermore, the incidence of Wilm's/nephroblastomatosis in PROS is fewer than 1% in one literature review [60], with 3.3% in a cohort study determined on a clinical diagnosis of CLOVES without genotypic characterization relating these patients to *PIK3CA* [62]. This is in contrast to the incidence in Beckwith–Wiedemann syndrome of embryonic tumours of 7.5% [64]. Therefore, more data are really required before such high-intensity screening recommendations can be implemented in routine clinical practice. Recent data have demonstrated detection of *PIK3CA* mutation in the urine of a patient with CLOVES and a Wilm's tumour [61], and a significant association between detection of cell-free DNA in the urine of patients with PROS and nephroblastomatosis [65]. Such tests may therefore be useful biomarkers for screening for renal tumours in the future.

Other complications

It has been suggested that patients with PROS may be more likely to develop hypertrophic scarring after surgical intervention in affected tissues, which was described in four of six patients with *PIK3CA* mutations who had undergone a surgical procedure [66]. However, it remains to be clarified in larger studies whether this observation is related to genotype more than to the procedure or clinical problems.

Hypoinsulinaemic, hypoketotic hypoglycaemia presents with neonatal hypoglycaemia, and has rarely been described in *PIK3CA* mosaicism, in association with hemimegalencephaly and asymmetric overgrowth. This manifestation is thought to be related to a high allele load of mutation within the liver [67].

Life expectancy in PROS

The life expectancy in PROS is not known. The phenotypic spectrum is so broad that it is likely to be more appropriate to study complications and life expectancy in the context of the outline clinical diagnoses, rather than in PROS taken as a whole. There have, however, been deaths due to both thromboembolic disease [59] and tumours [60], and therefore life expectancy is not normal. It does not appear anecdotally, however, to be as severely reduced as in PS.

Laboratory findings.

Genetics

Biopsy of affected tissue is key to the genetic diagnosis, as the mutation will usually not be detectable in blood, and tissue should be obtained in the same manner as for PS (see previously). In cases of MCAP, however, it is possible in some cases to detect the mutation in the buccal mucosa, using a DNA cheek swab kit. Therefore, if tissue is difficult to obtain in patients with MCAP it is worth doing a cheek swab initially. In addition, recent data demonstrate that mutation detection is possible from the urine of a proportion of patients with CLOVES [61]. In all instances, DNA should be extracted directly from the tissue or sample without initial tissue culture, and the whole coding sequence of the gene *PIK3CA* sequenced. In some laboratories, a couple of hotspots will be sequenced first. However, it is possible in this disease spectrum to have mutations at any position in this gene, and if the hotspots are negative, the rest of the gene should be sequenced. Again, it is important that the diagnostic laboratory is aware that they are looking for a mosaic mutation with a low allele load, to allow correct interpretation of results. Sanger sequencing in this condition is not adequate, because of the relative frequency of non-hotspot mutations, and high-depth next generation sequencing or another high sensitivity method should be used [52].

Histopathology

Epidermal naevi carrying *PIK3CA* mutations demonstrate acanthosis, papillomatosis and hyperkeratosis. However, these are typical findings in keratinocytic epidermal naevi and are not specific to this genotype [34].

General management.

- Suggested imaging guidelines [52]:
  - Truncal overgrowth or involvement (including scoliosis) merits whole body MRI scan, plus spinal radiographs if scoliosis is present, and a baseline spinal canal ultrasound scan in neonates with truncal involvement for cord tethering or lipomeningomyelocoele;
  - Facial or neurological involvement merits a cranial MRI scan;
  - Plain radiography of any affected area;
- Referral to a paediatric orthopaedic surgeon is important where limbs, extremities and/or spine are involved. Surgical intervention to reduce leg length discrepancy may be required. Referrals to orthotics and to occupational therapy are important, particularly where there is digital involvement;
- Neurological assessment and neurodevelopmental follow-up are recommended for those with megalencephaly or any symptoms of neurological disease;
- Advice on the signs and symptoms of DVT and PE should be given. Doppler ultrasound and clotting parameters including D-dimers are often used for patients with extensive vascular malformations (see Chapter 118). However, there are no clear guidelines on how to interpret the results of these. Consideration should be given to anticoagulant prophylaxis to cover procedures such as surgery which increase the risk of thromboembolism, with consultation with a paediatric haematologist to assess the balance of pro- and anticoagulation in such patients;
- Referral to psychosocial support teams and patient support groups are important for both probands and families, particularly where there are substantial issues surrounding disfigurement;
- Epidermal naevi can be managed symptomatically with general skin care advice and moisturisers;
- Consideration should be given to screening for Wilm's tumour/nephroblastomatosis with 3–4 monthly abdominal ultrasound scans until the age of 8 years (for a discussion see previously);
- Consultation with a clinical genetics team and genetic counsellor is recommended once the diagnosis is established. Transmission of PROS from a patient to the next generation has not been described, and in general would not be expected. Very rare cases of germline *PIK3CA* mutations, however, have been described, and theoretically in these cases, or in mosaic cases of these specific mutations, the mutation could be passed on to future generations in the germline. Reoccurrence in a sibling of an affected proband has not been described and would not be expected other than by chance.

Targeted medical therapy. As *PIK3CA* mutations are known to activate the PI3K-AKT-mTOR pathway, drug therapy targeted at inhibition of this pathway could theoretically be used for some or all of the features of PROS. This is supported by evidence from patient cell [67,68] and animal models of PROS [37,38,69]. There is ongoing debate about whether the congenital features in patients are malformations and therefore irreversible, and the answer to this question is not yet known. However, there is evidence that progressive overgrowth can be slowed or reversed at least in some cases [67].

Evidence of successful treatment of clinical presentations which might be expected to be due to *PIK3CA* mutations is helpful to some degree, but in the absence of genotype it is difficult to draw conclusions about the treatment of PROS *per se*. Such reports include the treatment of various types of vascular anomaly with high dose over the period of a year (mean trough levels 10–15 ng/mL), which had high levels of effectiveness, with 47 of 57 patients demonstrating partial response or stabilization after 6 months [70]. The safety profile in the same study demonstrated a relatively high level of abnormalities in blood indices (27%), but only two patients had to be removed from treatment due to adverse effects, and there were no drug-related deaths [70]. Another approach has also demonstrated good effect and safety, with a clinically relevant response in a case of generalized lymphatic malformation with low dose sirolimus over a longer period of 5 years (mean trough level approximately 5 ng/mL) [71]. A recent prospective open label phase II trial of low dose rapamycin in *PIK3CA*-mosaic patients with overgrowth, demonstrated a slight decrease in affected tissue volume after 6 months. However, a substantial proportion of patients experienced side effects which may have been attributable to the drug [72]. A compassionate use study with an inhibitor aimed directly at p110α activity (the protein encoded by *PIK3CA*), demonstrated promising results [73].

Other causes of localized overgrowth with cutaneous features

Vascular malformations of many types can be associated with overgrowth, but in general are considered to be related directly to the presence of the vascular malformation. This may or not may be correct and remains to be determined. However, in some cutaneous mosaic syndromes, overgrowth is definitely a feature which appears to be over and above what would be expected from the extent of the vascular malformation. In these conditions, it is generally not the presenting feature, and not the most pressing clinical problem, but may require intervention and may help diagnostically.

Sturge–Weber syndrome and phakomatosis pigmentovascularis

Patients with Sturge–Weber syndrome (SWS) (Chapter 118) or phakomatosis pigmentovascularis (PPV) (Chapter 109) often get a degree of overgrowth of soft tissues and or bone [74]. This is usually not evident or not particularly prominent at birth, but does progress slowly over time. It can lead to noticeable facial asymmetry, or functionally significant limb asymmetry, and associated functional scoliosis if the lower limb is involved. In one series of SWS, 23% of cases had surgical intervention related to the effects of tissue overgrowth [74]. SWS and some types of PPV are usually caused by mosaic mutations in one of the homologous genes *GNAQ* [75,76] or *GNA11* [76]. This type of overgrowth has been described with both PPV cesioflammea type, and with spilorosea type.

RAS gene associated mosaicism

A recently described rare cause of vascular malformations with overgrowth are those due to core *RAS* family gene mutations [77]. These patients present with capillary or deep venous malformations, with mild and apparently nonprogressive overgrowth in the affected limb. Possible distinguishing diagnostic features of the capillary malformations were a brown-red discolouration, very subtle outline and superimposed telangiectasia. In addition, pain in the affected area appeared to be a more prominent feature than would have been expected. However, the numbers of these patients published are currently very low. Mutations described were in known oncogenic hotspots of *KRAS* and *NRAS*, detectable only in affected tissue [77].

SECTION 23: MOSAIC DISORDERS

References

1 Nguyen HL, Bonadurer GF, 3rd, Tollefson MM Vascular malformations and health-related quality of life: a systematic review and meta-analysis. JAMA Dermatol 2018;154:661–9.

2 Cohen MM, Jr, Hayden PW. A newly recognized hamartomatous syndrome. Birth Defects Orig Artic Ser 1979;15:291–6.

3 Wiedemann HR Burgio GR, Aldenhoff P et al. The proteus syndrome. Partial gigantism of the hands and/or feet, nevi, hemihypertrophy, subcutaneous tumors, macrocephaly or other skull anomalies and possible accelerated growth and visceral affections. Eur J Pediatr 1983;140:5–12.

4 Tibbles JA, Cohen MM, Jr. The Proteus syndrome: the Elephant Man diagnosed. Br Med J (Clin Res Ed) 1986;293:683–5.

5 Biesecker LG, Happle R, Mulliken JB et al. Proteus syndrome: diagnostic criteria, differential diagnosis, and patient evaluation. Am J Med Genet 1999;84:389–95.

6 Biesecker LG, Sapp JC. Proteus syndrome. In: Pagon RA et al. (eds) GeneReviews(R). Seattle, 1993–2018.

7 Turner JT, Cohen MM, Jr, Biesecker LG. Reassessment of the Proteus syndrome literature: application of diagnostic criteria to published cases. Am J Med Genet A 2004;130A:111–22.

8 Sapp JC, Hu L, Zhao J et al. Quantifying survival in patients with Proteus syndrome. Genet Med 2017;19:1376–9.

9 Lindhurst MJ, Sapp JC, Teer JK et al. A mosaic activating mutation in AKT1 associated with the Proteus syndrome. N Engl J Med 2011;365:611–9.

10 Carpten JD, Faber AL, Horn C et al. A transforming mutation in the pleckstrin homology domain of AKT1 in cancer. Nature 2007; 448:439–44.

11 Wee JS, Mortimer PS, Lindhurst MJ et al. A limited form of proteus syndrome with bilateral plantar cerebriform collagenomas and varicose veins secondary to a mosaic AKT1 mutation. JAMA Dermatol 2014;150:990–3.

12 Beachkofsky TM, Sapp JC, Biesecker LG, Darling TN. Progressive overgrowth of the cerebriform connective tissue nevus in patients with Proteus syndrome. J Am Acad Dermatol 2010;63:799–804.

13 Twede JV, Turner JT, Biesecker LG, Darling TN. Evolution of skin lesions in Proteus syndrome. J Am Acad Dermatol 2005;52:834–8.

14 Doucet ME, Bloomhardt HM, Moroz K et al. Lack of mutation-histopathology correlation in a patient with Proteus syndrome. Am J Med Genet A 2016;170:1422–32.

15 Cohen MM, Jr. Proteus syndrome review: molecular, clinical, and pathologic features. Clin Genet 2014;85:111–9.

16 Sapp JC, Turner JT, van de Kamp JM et al. Newly delineated syndrome of congenital lipomatous overgrowth, vascular malformations, and epidermal nevi (CLOVE syndrome) in seven patients. Am J Med Genet A 2007;143A:2944–58.

17 Polubothu S, Al-Olabi L, Wilson L et al. Extending the spectrum of AKT1 mosaicism – not just the Proteus syndrome. Br J Dermatol 2016;176:612–4.

18 Takyar V, Khattar T, Ling A *et al*. Characterization of the hepatosplenic and portal venous findings in patients with Proteus syndrome. Am J Med Genet A 2018;176:2677–84.
19 Biesecker L. The challenges of Proteus syndrome: diagnosis and management. Eur J Hum Genet 2006;14:1151–7.
20 Hannoush H, Sachdev V, Brofferio A et al. Myocardial fat overgrowth in Proteus syndrome. Am J Med Genet A 2015;167A:103–10.
21 Tosi LL, Sapp JC, Allen ES et al. Assessment and management of the orthopedic and other complications of Proteus syndrome. J Child Orthop 2011;5:319–27.
22 Jamis-Dow CA, Turner J, Biesecker LG, Choyke PL. Radiologic manifestations of Proteus syndrome. Radiographics 2004;24:1051–68.
23 Keppler-Noreuil KM, Baker EH, Sapp JC et al. Somatic AKT1 mutations cause meningiomas colocalizing with a characteristic pattern of cranial hyperostosis. Am J Med Genet A 2016;170:2605–10.
24 Lim GY, Kim OH, Kim HW et al. Pulmonary manifestations in Proteus syndrome: pulmonary varicosities and bullous lung disease. Am J Med Genet A 2011;155A:865–9.
25 Slavotinek AM, Vacha SJ, Peters KF, Biesecker LG. Sudden death caused by pulmonary thromboembolism in Proteus syndrome. Clin Genet 2000;58:386–9.
26 Eberhard DA. Two-year-old boy with Proteus syndrome and fatal pulmonary thromboembolism. Pediatr Pathol 1994;14:771–9.
27 Keppler-Noreuil KM, Lozier JN, Sapp JC, Biesecker LG. Characterization of thrombosis in patients with Proteus syndrome. Am J Med Genet A 2017;173: 2359–65.
28 Forbes SA, Beare D, Gunasekaran P et al. COSMIC: exploring the world's knowledge of somatic mutations in human cancer. Nucleic Acids Res 2015;43:D805–11.
29 Asahina A, Fujita H, Omori T et al. Proteus syndrome complicated by multiple spinal meningiomas. Clin Exp Dermatol 2008;33:729–32.
30 Lindhurst MJ, Wang JA, Bloomhardt HM et al. AKT1 gene mutation levels are correlated with the type of dermatologic lesions in patients with Proteus syndrome. J Invest Dermatol 2014;134:543–6.
31 Cohen MM, Jr. Overgrowth syndromes: an update. Adv Pediatr 1999;46:441–91.
32 Crenshaw MM, Goerlich CG, Ivey LE et al. Orthopaedic management of leg-length discrepancy in proteus syndrome: a case series. J Pediatr Orthop 2018;38:e138–e144.
33 Lindhurst MJ, Yourick MR, Yu Y et al. Repression of AKT signaling by ARQ 092 in cells and tissues from patients with Proteus syndrome. Sci Rep 2015;5:17162.
34 Hafner C, López-Knowles E, Luis NM et al. Oncogenic PIK3CA mutations occur in epidermal nevi and seborrheic keratoses with a characteristic mutation pattern. Proc Natl Acad Sci U S A 2007;104:13450–4.
35 Samuels Y, Wang Z, Bardelli A et al. High frequency of mutations of the PIK3CA gene in human cancers. Science 2004;304:554.
36 Limaye N, Kangas J, Mendola A et al. Somatic activating PIK3CA mutations cause venous malformation. Am J Hum Genet 2015; 97:914–21.
37 Castillo SD, Tzouanacou E, Zaw-Thin M et al. Somatic activating mutations in Pik3ca cause sporadic venous malformations in mice and humans. Sci Transl Med 2016;8:332ra43.
38 Castel P, Carmona FJ, Grego-Bessa J et al. Somatic PIK3CA mutations as a driver of sporadic venous malformations. Sci Transl Med 2016;8:332ra42.
39 Keppler-Noreuil KM, Sapp JC, Lindhurst MJ et al. Clinical delineation and natural history of the PIK3CA-related overgrowth spectrum. Am J Med Genet A 2014;164A:1713–33.
40 Kuentz P, St-Onge J, Duffourd Y et al. Molecular diagnosis of PIK3CA-related overgrowth spectrum (PROS) in 162 patients and recommendations for genetic testing. Genet Med 2017;19:989–97.
41 Mirzaa G, Timms AE, Conti V et al. PIK3CA-associated developmental disorders exhibit distinct classes of mutations with variable expression and tissue distribution. JCI Insight 1 2016;1: pii: e87623.
42 Vivanco I, Sawyers CL. The phosphatidylinositol 3-Kinase AKT pathway in human cancer. Nat Rev Cancer 2002;2:489–501.
43 Kurek KC, Luks VL, Ayturk UM et al. Somatic mosaic activating mutations in PIK3CA cause CLOVES syndrome. Am J Hum Genet 2012;90:1108–15.
44 Riviere JB, Mirzaa GM, O'Roak BJ et al. De novo germline and postzygotic mutations in AKT3, PIK3R2 and PIK3CA cause a spectrum of related megalencephaly syndromes. Nat Genet 2012;44: 934–40.
45 Lindhurst MJ, Parker VE, Payne F et al. Mosaic overgrowth with fibroadipose hyperplasia is caused by somatic activating mutations in PIK3CA. Nat Genet 2012;44:928–33.
46 Lee JH, Huynh M, Silhavy JL et al. De novo somatic mutations in components of the PI3K-AKT3-mTOR pathway cause hemimegalencephaly. Nat Genet 2012;44:941–5.
47 Mirzaa GM, Riviere JB, Dobyns WB. Megalencephaly syndromes and activating mutations in the PI3K-AKT pathway: MPPH and MCAP. Am J Med Genet C Semin Med Genet 2013;163C:122–30.
48 Rios JJ, Paria N, Burns DK et al. Somatic gain-of-function mutations in PIK3CA in patients with macrodactyly. Hum Mol Genet 2013; 22:444–51.
49 Di Donato N, Rump A, Mirzaa GM et al. Identification and characterization of a novel constitutional PIK3CA mutation in a child lacking the typical segmental overgrowth of 'PIK3CA-related overgrowth spectrum'. Hum Mutat 2016;37:242–5.
50 Dogruluk T, Tsang YH, Espitia M et al. Identification of variant-specific functions of PIK3CA by rapid phenotyping of rare mutations. Cancer Res 2015;75:5341–54.
51 Mirzaa GM, Conway RL, Gripp KW et al. Megalencephaly-capillary malformation (MCAP) and megalencephaly-polydactyly-polymicrogyria-hydrocephalus (MPPH) syndromes: two closely related disorders of brain overgrowth and abnormal brain and body morphogenesis. Am J Med Genet A 2012;158A:269–91.
52 Keppler-Noreuil KM, Rios JJ, Parker VE et al. PIK3CA-related overgrowth spectrum (PROS): diagnostic and testing eligibility criteria, differential diagnosis, and evaluation. Am J Med Genet A 2015; 167A:287–95.
53 Gucev ZS, Tasic V, Jancevska A et al. Congenital lipomatous overgrowth, vascular malformations, and epidermal nevi (CLOVE) syndrome: CNS malformations and seizures may be a component of this disorder. Am J Med Genet A 2008;146A:2688–90.
54 Luks VL, Kamitaki N, Vivero MP et al. Lymphatic and other vascular malformative/overgrowth disorders are caused by somatic mutations in PIK3CA. J Pediatr 2015;166:1048–54, e1–5.
55 Vahidnezhad H, Youssefian L, Uitto J. Klippel-Trenaunay syndrome belongs to the PIK3CA-related overgrowth spectrum (PROS). Exp Dermatol 2016;25:17–9.
56 Lopez-Gutierrez JC, Lapunzina P. Capillary malformation of the lower lip, lymphatic malformation of the face and neck, asymmetry and partial/generalized overgrowth (CLAPO): report of six cases of a new syndrome/association. Am J Med Genet A 2008;146A:2583–8.
57 Rodriguez-Laguna L, Ibañez K, Gordo G et al. CLAPO syndrome: identification of somatic activating PIK3CA mutations and delineation of the natural history and phenotype. Genet Med 2018;20:882–9.
58 Downey C, Lopez-Gutierrez JC, Roe-Crespo E et al. Lower lip capillary malformation associated with lymphatic malformation without overgrowth: part of the spectrum of CLAPO syndrome. Pediatr Dermatol 2018;35:e243–4.
59 Alomari AI, Burrows PE, Lee EY et al. CLOVES syndrome with thoracic and central phlebectasia: increased risk of pulmonary embolism. J Thorac Cardiovasc Surg 2010;140:459–63.
60 Gripp KW, Baker L, Kandula V et al. Nephroblastomatosis or Wilms tumor in a fourth patient with a somatic PIK3CA mutation. Am J Med Genet A 2016;170:2559–69.
61 Michel ME, Konczyk DJ, Yeung KS et al. Causal somatic mutations in urine DNA from persons with the CLOVES subgroup of the PIK3CA-related overgrowth spectrum. Clin Genet 2018;93:1075–80.
62 Peterman CM, Fevurly RD, Alomari AI et al. Sonographic screening for Wilms tumor in children with CLOVES syndrome. Pediatr Blood Cancer 2017;64.
63 Kinross KM, Montgomery KG, Kleinschmidt M et al. An activating Pik3ca mutation coupled with Pten loss is sufficient to initiate ovarian tumorigenesis in mice. J Clin Invest 2012;122:553–7.
64 Weksberg R, Shuman C, Beckwith JB. Beckwith-Wiedemann syndrome. Eur J Hum Genet 2010;18:8–14.
65 Biderman Waberski M, Lindhurst M, Keppler-Noreuil KM et al. Urine cell-free DNA is a biomarker for nephroblastomatosis or Wilms tumor in PIK3CA-related overgrowth spectrum (PROS). Genet Med 2018;20:1077–81.
66 Steiner JE, Cottrell CE, Streicher JL et al. Scarring in patients with PIK3CA-related overgrowth syndromes. JAMA Dermatol 2018;154:452–5.
67 Leiter SM, Parker VER, Welters A et al. Hypoinsulinaemic, hypoketotic hypoglycaemia due to mosaic genetic activation of PI3-kinase. Eur J Endocrinol 2017;177:175–86.
68 Ranieri C, Di Tommaso S, Loconte DC et al. In vitro efficacy of ARQ 092, an allosteric AKT inhibitor, on primary fibroblast cells derived from patients with PIK3CA-related overgrowth spectrum (PROS). Neurogenetics 2018;19:77–91.

69 Roy A, Skibo J, Kalume F et al. Mouse models of human PIK3CA-related brain overgrowth have acutely treatable epilepsy. Elife 2015;4:p.ii:e12703.
70 Adams DM, Trenor CC 3rd, Hammill AM et al. Efficacy and safety of sirolimus in the treatment of complicated vascular anomalies. Pediatrics 2016;137:e20153257.
71 Dvorakova V, Rea D, O'Regan GM, Irvine AD. Generalized lymphatic anomaly successfully treated with long-term, low-dose sirolimus. Pediatr Dermatol 2018;25:533–4.
72 Parker VER, Keppler-Noreuil KM, Faivre L et al. Safety and efficacy of low-dose sirolimus in the PIK3CA-related overgrowth spectrum. Genet Med 2018: doi: 10.1038/s41436-018-0297-9.
73 Venot Q, Blanc T, Rabia SH *et al*. Targeted therapy in patients with PIK3CA-related overgrowth syndrome. Nature 2018;558:540–6.
74 Greene AK, Taber SF, Ball KL et al. Sturge-Weber syndrome: soft-tissue and skeletal overgrowth. J Craniofac Surg 2009;20(Suppl 1): 617–21.
75 Shirley MD, Tang H, Gallione CJ et al. Sturge-Weber syndrome and port-wine stains caused by somatic mutation in GNAQ. N Engl J Med 2013;368:1971–9.
76 Thomas AC, Zeng Z, Rivière JB et al. Mosaic activating mutations in GNA11 and GNAQ are associated with phakomatosis pigmentovascularis and extensive dermal melanocytosis. J Invest Dermatol 2016;136:770–8.
77 Al-Olabi L, Polubothu S, Dowsett K et al. Mosaic RAS/MAPK variants cause sporadic vascular malformations which respond to targeted therapy. J Clin Invest 2018;128:1496–508.

CHAPTER 109
Mosaic Disorders of Pigmentation

Veronica A. Kinsler

Paediatric Dermatology Department, Great Ormond Street Hospital for Children NHS Foundation Trust, London, UK and Genetics and Genomic Medicine, UCL Great Ormond Street Institute of Child Health, London, UK

Introduction, 1296
Fine and whorled Blaschkolinear hypo- and hyperpigmentation (incorporating hypomelanosis of Ito, and linear and whorled naevoid hypermelanosis), 1297
Phylloid hypo- and hypermelanosis, 1300
McCune–Albright syndrome, 1300
Phakomatosis pigmentovascularis, 1301
Extensive or atypical dermal melanocytosis, including naevus of Ota and naevus of Ito, 1303
Phakomatosis pigmentokeratotica, 1304
Congenital melanocytic naevi (CMN) and CMN syndrome, 1304
Becker naevi and Becker naevus syndrome, 1304
Speckled lentiginous naevi, 1304
Naevus depigmentosus, 1306
Mosaic neurofibromatosis type 1, 1306

Abstract

Mosaic disorders of pigmentation has traditionally been a complex field from the clinical perspective. This is partly because of the intrinsic variability in phenotype seen in mosaic disorders, and, as is becoming more apparent, partly because of the wide array of genetic defects which can influence skin pigmentation, whether directly or indirectly. Although certain phenotypes are well defined, some like hypomelanosis of Ito are descriptive umbrella terms rather than diagnoses, which has led to conflicting literature on the incidences of extracutaneous manifestations with such phenotypes. Furthermore, many clinical presentations remain unclassifiable. With the advent of next generation sequencing techniques the genetic basis of increasing numbers of these disorders is being defined. Fascinatingly, this is improving the phenotypic recognition of distinct disorders which were previously unrecognizable, demonstrating that both clinical and molecular examination can be beneficial to patients. In this chapter we will delineate current knowledge of phenotypic and genetic classification of known diseases, and review management in the light of evolution of this field.

Key points

- **Mosaic disorders affecting pigmentation are not restricted to genes which govern melanin production or melanocyte biology, but can be thought of simply as a sign of mosaicism.**
- **Clinical diagnostic terms continue to be useful, but these can encompass a large number of genetic causes, with highly variable associated features and prognosis.**
- **Full history and systems examination are vital in assessing the patient's individual phenotype, and for framing individual management.**
- **Genetic investigation where indicated usually involves a blood sample and fresh skin biopsy from an affected area, and both chromosomal and single gene abnormalities can be looked for.**

Introduction

Arguably, any mosaic cutaneous condition can affect skin pigmentation to some degree. This is witnessed by such diverse examples as the decrease in skin pigmentation in epidermolysis bullosa compared with revertant mosaic patches, by the increased background skin colour of mosaic neurofibromatosis type 1, or by the entire spectrum of light to dark brought about by innumerable chromosomal changes in Blaschkolinear pigmentary mosaicism. As increasing numbers of genes are discovered to alter pigment levels in the skin, the concept of a 'pigmentary gene' has become obsolete to a large degree, with the possible exception of the core genes of the melanin synthesis pathway. This phenomenon can be explained by the complexity of the processes which either directly or indirectly affect pigmentation, and supports what we already know of the high degree of variability in the normal pigmentary phenotype between siblings. In addition, it helps to understand why this field has been a complex area from a clinical view point. For the purposes of this chapter we will be focusing on disorders where a necessary feature for clinical diagnosis is the abnormal pigmentation, and where DNA level genetic mosaicism has either been demonstrated in the literature, or is highly likely based on sporadic occurrence and clinical pattern of the condition.

Harper's Textbook of Pediatric Dermatology, Fourth Edition. Edited by Peter Hoeger, Veronica Kinsler and Albert Yan.

Fine and whorled Blaschkolinear hypo- and hyperpigmentation (incorporating hypomelanosis of Ito, and linear and whorled naevoid hypermelanosis)

Fine and whorled Blaschkolinear hypo- and hyperpigmentation are grouped together here, because the clinical approach to children with alterations in pigmentation in this pattern, with no preceding history suggestive of incontinentia pigmenti (see Chapter 136), is currently the same. In addition, it can occasionally be difficult to tell whether the abnormal skin colour is the increased or decreased pigmentation, and in other cases there can be a mixture of both increased and decreased pigmentation in this pattern.

A note on terminology

The original description of Blaschko's lines in 1901 [1] did not include cases of hypopigmentation in that pattern, and it is not clear if it included cases of hyperpigmentation where this was macular (unassociated with epidermal naevi). The first clearly identifiable description of fine and whorled Blaschkolinear hypopigmentation was of a single case in 1951 by Ito [2], and the term hypomelanosis of Ito was proposed thereafter [3] (NB, the old term incontinentia pigmenti achromians should not now be used, because this disease is not connected to the X-linked condition incontinentia pigmenti). Linear and whorled naevoid hyperpigmentation was first described as two case reports [4], with further cases under the same diagnostic label reported thereafter [5].

The term hypomelanosis of Ito was later understood to be a description, rather than a unique diagnosis, and in fact one that encompasses a very broad range of genetic diagnoses [6]. Much of the older literature on either hypomelanosis of Ito and linear and whorled naevoid hypermelanosis understandably combines all different genetic causes into single clinical study groups. In addition, there is evidence that patients with patchy abnormalities of pigmentation rather than fine and whorled Blaschkolinear abnormalities of pigmentation were included in some of these publications [7,8]. Furthermore, studies from neurology centres [9,10] often report higher incidences of neurological complications than those from dermatology centres [5], although with more mixed clinical phenotypes this is not always the case [8]. As a result, the literature is relatively unhelpful in managing individual patients in a clinical setting, and in particular, giving confident or accurate advice on the risk of neurological and other extracutaneous associations is extremely difficult. Prognostication will only be improved once better genetic dissection of the causes is achieved, and the individual diagnoses separated into cohorts with good phenotypic characterization and follow up.

Epidemiology. Fine and whorled Blaschkolinear hypo- or hyperpigmentation is rare, but no systematic evaluation of incidence in the general population has been performed. It is likely that mild phenotypic cases go unrecognized or at least unreported. An estimate from the author's clinical experience in a paediatric pigmentary service would be approximately 1 in 20 000 new births, and all ethnicities appear to be affected. Estimates from hospital attendance were that it was the third most common neurocutaneous condition, after neurofibromatosis type 1 and tuberous sclerosis, diagnosed in approximately 1 in 8000–10 000 general paediatric outpatient visits [8,9]. The quoted male to female ratio is highly variable, with both male preponderance [9] and female preponderance [8] reported. Again, this is likely to be caused by the amalgamation of different genetic diagnoses and even different clinical phenotypes into single clinical cohorts.

Clinical features. The cardinal skin finding is fine and whorled Blaschkolinear hypo- or hyperpigmentation (Fig. 109.1), which is present at birth or develops in the early years [8]. This rather wordy description is to distinguish this pattern from other linear patterns with are sometimes given the epithets 'Blaschkoid', or 'broad Blaschkolinear'. It is clear that many skin diseases can produce a linear pattern, particularly on the limbs, but this does not mean they are Blaschkolinear. In the pattern discussed here there should be fine (generally less than a centimetre in diameter on an infant) lines on limbs, and/or fine and whorled patterns on the trunk, which show a midline dip both anteriorly and posteriorly, and a wavy, whorled or serpiginous pattern around the trunk (Fig. 109.1).

For specific associations as part of known genotypic diagnoses see later. Noncutaneous associated features which have been described in association with fine and whorled Blaschkolinear hypo- or hyperpigmentation are highly variable, affecting many different body systems, and likely caused by a differing genetic basis in different conditions. Further clearly delineated syndromes are likely to become apparent over the next few years.

Management. The recognized genotypic diagnoses listed later should be looked for on clinical examination, and if suspected can be tested for specifically using sensitive methods (see Chapter 104 Introduction to Mosaicism, and under individual conditions). Where no known diagnosis is clinically apparent on thorough history and examination, then investigation can proceed in collaboration with the clinical genetics team. In general, in the absence of a diagnosis it is appropriate to investigate only where there are clinical symptoms or signs, rather than to do screening investigations. For example, a magnetic resonance image (MRI) of the brain would be clinically indicated in the presence of neurodevelopmental problems, but not if the child is developing normally. If, however, a genetic diagnosis is made, and particularly if this is chromosomal or chimaeric, there may be screening tests which are appropriate depending upon the particular abnormality.

It is important to consider not only the child's own state of health, but also potential implications for the child's offspring. In this regard, it is worth excluding chromosomal mosaicism and chimaerism on a blood

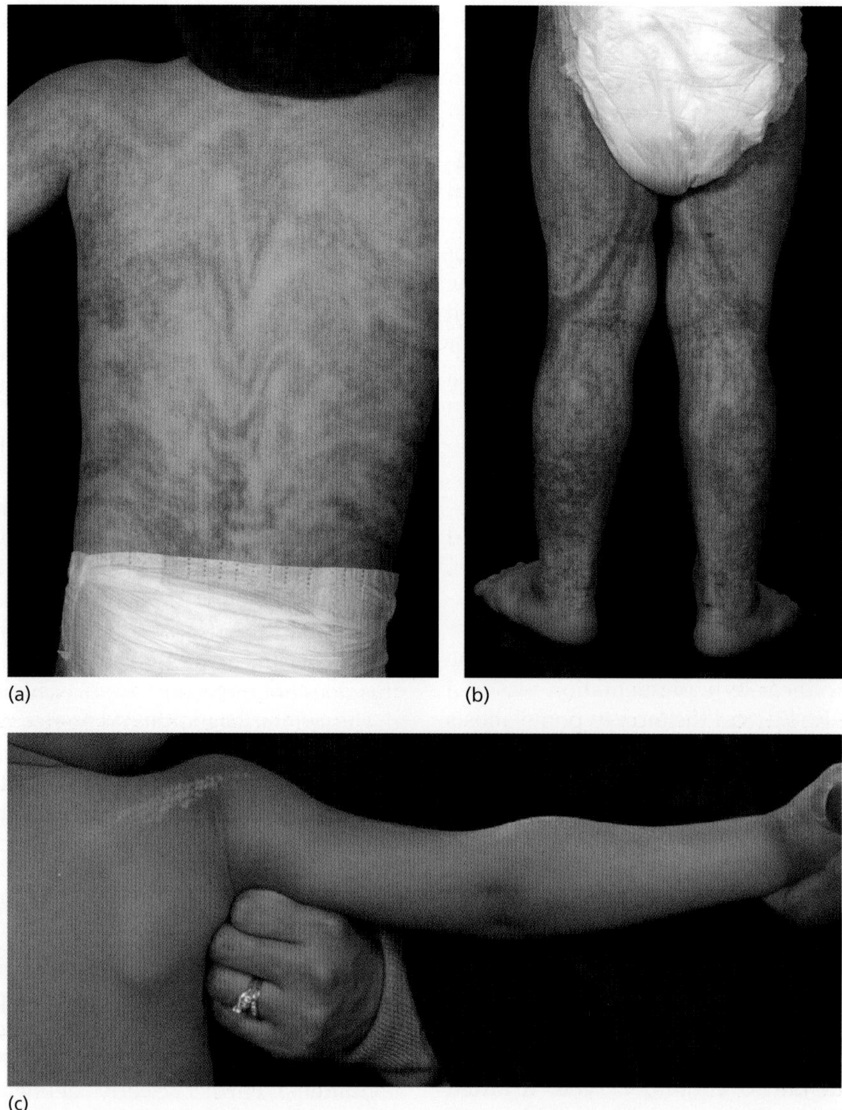

Fig. 109.1 Clinical appearences of (a,b) extensive fine and whorled Blaschkolinear hyperpigmentation and (c) lichen striatus on the arm, part of the differential diagnosis for fine and whorled Blaschkolinear hypopigmentation.

sample (a combined cytogenetics and molecular genetics approach is usually best), and if normal also on DNA from a skin biopsy. The cytogenetic parts of the tests can only be performed on cultured cells, and currently most laboratories will only be able to culture fibroblasts from skin, which may not carry the mutation [11]. However, chromosomal mosaicism can be detected in fibroblasts when it is not detectable in blood, and until keratinocyte culture becomes routinely available this is a reasonable first step. If chromosomal mosaicism and chimaerism have been excluded to the best of the local services' ability in these ways, then further management can be dictated by the child's clinical presentation. In particular, if there are any neurological or neurodevelopmental concerns an MRI of the brain is advisable. Follow up of children with this clinical presentation where there is no known genetic diagnosis is advised at least until school age, with thorough examinations of full systems undertaken. This could be undertaken by a paediatrician if the dermatological picture is stable.

Histology. Currently, the histological and ultrastructural features of fine and whorled Blaschkolinear changes in pigmentation is not diagnostic of any particular condition. Changes described in a large series but with highly variable phenotypes were a decrease in epidermal melanocytes and of their melanin content, with an increase in numbers of large epidermal clear cells and Langerhans cells, and a decrease in melanosomes [8]. Histopathological evidence from two cases of hypomelanosis of Ito was interpreted also as a primary abnormality of the epidermis [11]. However, the illustrations of the abnormal pigmentation in that study are not clearly of fine and whorled Blaschkolinear hypopigmentation.

Pathogenesis. As mentioned previously, this pattern can be caused by a wide variety of mosaic causes, from chimaerism through to single gene mutations. The unifying cause of fine and whorled Blaschkolinear changes in pigmentation, however, has been proposed to be a melanocyte non-cell-autonomous effect, or in other words a change in pigmentation not caused by a primary abnormality affecting melanocytes [12]. This was based on a systematic examination of mosaic conditions known to affect melanocytes directly, not revealing this pattern in any case [12]. This pattern is therefore most likely to represent the pattern of development of epidermal structures, not including melanocytes. This proposal is supported by single gene mutations leading to linear and whorled naevoid hypermelanosis, namely *TP63* mosaicism [13] and *KITLG* mosaicism [14], because both p63 and KITLG are known to be predominantly expressed in ectodermal/keratinocytic cells rather than in melanocytes.

Differential diagnosis. Lichen striatus in the hypopigmented phase may be considered as a differential diagnosis for Blaschkolinear hypopigmentation (see Chapter 35) (Fig. 109.1). Similarly, incontinentia pigmenti in either the hypopigmented or the hyperpigmented phase could present as a differential (see Chapter 136).

Specific genotypic diagnoses within or overlapping with this group

Chromsomal mosaicism and chimaerism

Fine and whorled Blaschkolinear pigmentary changes have been described in association with a very wide variety of chromosomal mosaicism [6,8,15–18], with these responsible for approximately 50% of cases of this skin phenotype in the literature in two large reviews [6,17]. The commonest changes were aneuploidy and unbalanced translocations [6]. Mosaic trisomy 18 [6,15,19–24] and mosaic trisomy 20 [25–29] have been described repeatedly as a cause of fine and whorled Blaschkolinear pigmentary changes, in some clearly as both hyper- and hypopigmentation. Chimaerism appears to be a much rarer cause of this phenotype, present in approximately 6–7% of cases [6,17]. In all cases where chromosomal mosaicism and chimaerism is detected, and particularly where chimaerism involves sex chromosomes, it is very important that the child has a thorough paediatric review and clinical genetics counselling.

Pallister–Killian syndrome

Pallister–Killian syndrome (PKS) is dealt with separately because the pigmentary findings are an important part of both the clinical phenotype and the diagnosis. PKS is a rare sporadic mosaic disorder first described in 1977 [30], and described separately in 1981. It is a well-defined clinical entity usually caused by mosaic tetrasomy 12p (four copies of the short arm of chromosome 12), which in turn is usually caused by the mosaic presence of an isochromosome 12p (i12p, an extra chromosome made from two identical copies of 12p, with no long arm) [31]. This is often caused by gonadal mosaicism in a parent. Less commonly the syndrome is not caused by tetrasomy 12p but other genetic mechanisms involving chromosome 12 [32,33]. The incidence is approximately 1 in 200 000 live births [34], and it affects both sexes equally [35].

The skin findings in PKS can be fine and whorled Blaschkolinear hypopigmentation. However, very often they are more disordered than this, and in particular with disrespect of the midline [36,37]. Some papers cite hyperpigmentation as a feature but in the largest review of cases only hypopigmentation has been found [35]. Hair is often sparse, particularly bitemporally [38,39], but can improve with age. Anyhydrosis or hypohydrosis can be a feature [34].

The clinical diagnosis in a paediatric dermatology clinic would usually be made because of the facial dysmorphism, and the presence of extracutaneous abnormalities. These are variable because of the mosaic nature of the condition. Facial features include a high forehead, hypertelorism, broad nasal bridge, short nose, wide mouth with a thin upper lip, large tongue and abnormal ears, with 'coarsening' of features with age. Children have neurological abnormalities including mild to severe intellectual disability, infantile hypotonia and seizures, and may have high birth weight, congenital diaphragmatic hernia, cleft or high-arched palate, seizures, hearing and/or visual impairment or abnormalities, cardiac anomalies, renal abnormalities, gastrointestinal abnormalities, extra digits and/or broad toes, other skeletal abnormalities, extra nipples, and genitourinary abnormalities [35].

The genetic diagnosis was classically made from affected skin fibroblast culture and cytogenetic chromosomal analysis. However, nowadays with more sensitive detection methods for mosaic copy number changes this can often be made on either lymphocyte or buccal swab DNA [40]. If strongly suspected and not apparent by these latter methods, biopsy of the affected skin can still be used.

Single gene mosaicism

Mosaic TP63 mutations

Two cases of *TP63* mutations have been described in association with fine and whorled Blaschkolinear hyperpigmentation. In the first, mosaicism was shown at cellular level from blood DNA, suggesting relatively high levels of mosaicism and an early mutation. In the second mosaicism was not demonstrated, but seems highly likely from the clinical phenotype, the de novo presentation, and the parallels with the first case.

Mosaic MTOR mutations

A recurrent mosaic mutation in the gene *MTOR* (c.5930C>T (p.Thr1977Ile)) has recently been described as a cause of fine and whorled Blaschkolinear hypopigmentation, with asymmetric megalencephaly and polymicrogyria [41]. In these three patients with very similar phenotypic presentation the skin findings were described as being Blaschkolinear cutis tricolor. However, the predominant feature in the images demonstrated seems to be hypopigmentation. The mutation was detectable in high levels in the affected skin, and also detectable at lower levels in blood or saliva [41]. Recently a similar fourth case has been described where the mutation was only detectable in cultured fibroblasts [42].

Mosaic KITLG mutations

This has been described in a single case only so far, presenting as fine and whorled Blaschkolinear hyperpigmentation (linear and whorled naevoid hypermelanosis) on the skin, with no associated abnormalities [14]. The mutation (*KITLG* c.329A>G (p.(Asp110Gly)) was detectable in blood and skin in the patient reported. *KITLG* mutations in the germline are known to be associated with familial progressive hyper- and hypopigmentation [43]. Although this particular mutation has not previously been described in a heterozygous state, given the levels it is likely that it could be transmitted to offspring, with the theoretical potential for familial progressive hyper- and hypopigmentation in the next generation.

Phylloid hypo- and hypermelanosis

Macular phylloid patterning was first described by Happle as distinct from Blaschko's lines, defined as leaf-like or floral patterns on the skin [44], which can take either hypo- or hyperpigmented forms. Hypopigmented phylloid patterns have been most frequently found to be associated with mosaic abnormalities of chromosome 13 [45–52], most commonly mosaic trisomy 13. Associated clinical features are variable, but include neurodevelopmental delay, conductive hearing loss, short stature, skeletal abnormalities and asymmetric growth, craniofacial abnormalities, and choroidal and retinal coloboma [45,53]. Hyperpigmented phylloid patterns have also been described with mosaicism involving chromosome 13 [54] but also with 5p mosaicism (although this pattern did not clearly respect the midline) [55] or no diagnosed chromosomal mosaicism [56]. Associated features described include craniofacial dysmorphism, neurological abnormalities, both structural and developmental, skeletal abnormalities, eye anomalies, sensorineural hearing loss, cicatricial alopecia and tooth abnormalities.

Children diagnosed with these patterns should have blood and skin biopsies taken for karyotype and chromosomal mosaicism analysis. Further investigation of systems should be dictated by the clinical presentation and examination, given the relatively small number of cases so far described.

McCune–Albright syndrome

Epidemiology. McCune–Albright syndrome (MAS) is estimated to have a prevalence of between 1 in 100 000 and 1 in 1 million [57]. It is commoner in females than males but there is no evidence of differences in incidence between ethnic groups [58].

Clinical features. MAS was originally described as a sporadic disease characterized by the triad of café-au-lait macular hyperpigmentation, polyostotic fibrous dysplasia and autonomous endocrine over-function [59]. The diagnosis can be made by the finding of two of the three clinical features, or one feature with a confirmed genetic diagnosis [58]. It has been suggested that fibrous dysplasia is the commonest manifestation and should be considered the primary diagnostic criterion [57]. However, there is good evidence that the syndrome can exist with any single feature and a genetic diagnosis [58,60]. In addition, no systematic genetic studies of cohorts of patients with isolated typical café-au-lait macules and no other clinical features have been published in the dermatology literature, and therefore it is not clear what the prevalence of MAS is in this group. Clinically, the cafe-au lait macular pigmentation is usually present at birth and occurs in a distribution which respects the midline anteriorly and posteriorly, with either segmental patterns or in broad Blaschkolinear bands [57–61]. The edges of the pigmentation are said to resemble the coast of Maine, in other words irregular rather than smooth, in contrast to the typical outline of the café-au-lait macules in neurofibromatosis. Pigmentation can be found on the oral mucosae later in childhood or adulthood [62]. Where fibrous dysplasia exists, the teeth can be affected, with an increase in caries and malocclusion as frequent dental complications [63]. Interestingly, an exaggerated wheal-and-flare response has been documented in the skin of MAS patients [64].

Where bony involvement is symptomatic it presents with deformity, bone or joint pain, or pathological fracture [65]. Endocrinological disease is caused by autonomous hyperfunctioning of endocrine glands, and therefore a wide range of endocrinopathies can occur. The commonest is gonadotrophin-independent precocious puberty, which tends to have an earlier onset in girls than in boys where it occurs [66], but hyperthyroidism, growth hormone excess, Cushing syndrome, hyperprolactinism [67], and hyperparathyroidism have all been described [68].

Management. If there is typical café-au-lait pigmentation only, with no symptoms or signs of other disease, there is little evidence base for management. Alerting parents to the possibility of endocrinological and bony associations is a sensible precaution. It is arguable that screening should be considered for polyostotic fibrous dysplasia using plain radiographs of the skull, mandible, pelvis and long bones, and baseline endocrinological blood tests. If there is no bony involvement and no signs of endocrine dysfunction the patient can be discharged. If bony involvement is suspected from radiographs referral to a paediatric endocrinologist is recommended as per published guidelines for monitoring for osteosarcoma [69]. Similarly, if endocrinological disease is suspected, or if the diagnosis of MAS has been established by other criteria, referral to a paediatric endocrinologist is appropriate. Some degree of renal involvement is present in approximately 50% of patients with MAS [70], and manifests as FGF23-induced renal phosphate wasting [70–72]. Urinary and blood indices relating to renal function and bone metabolism are therefore key investigations where the diagnosis is suspected. Arguably, mutation hotspot screening of a typical birthmark is less invasive than X-rays and bloods.

It is worth remembering that there is a long-term risk of benign and malignant tumours in MAS [57,58,73], and diagnosis should therefore be considered seriously by the paediatric dermatologist, even if the child is well at presentation.

Histology. The histology of café-au lait macules in MAS has not been well characterized, and has not thus far been documented to demonstrate macromelanosomes which are seen in a large proportion of café-au lait macules in neurofibromatosis.

Pathogenesis. MAS was the first pigmentary mosaic disorder characterized at molecular level, and is caused by mosaicism for activating mutations in the *GNAS* gene [74]. This finding was because of insightful clinical extrapolation from the phenotypic overlap with Albright's hereditary osteodystrophy, which had been found to be caused by mutations in the same gene [75]. *GNAS* encodes one of the G-alpha subunits of the heterotrimeric G-proteins, and the activating mutation in MAS leads to autonomous activation of G-protein coupled receptor signalling pathways. Genetic diagnosis is subject to the same requirement for high sensitivity detection techniques as for other mosaic disorders (see Chapter 104), but in MAS the mutation can fairly frequently be detected in leukocyte DNA [58], with the chance increasing with the number of clinical features present [58]. It is therefore worth testing blood and skin to maximize detection. Although mutation detection is traditionally thought to have had a low pick up in skin particularly, with next generation sequencing the sensitivity detection limit is now below 1% allele load [76].

Phakomatosis pigmentovascularis

Clinical features and epidemiology. Phakomatosis pigmentovascularis (PPV) is the phenotypic diagnosis given to the co-occurrence of different pigmentary and vascular birthmarks of particular types. The original phenotypic subclassification of this group delineated five types, reclassified as three types subsequently. However, new phenotypic subtypes are still being described. The two original classifications are shown in Table 109.1 [77–79]. Another addition to the Happle (second) classification is PPV melanorosea [80], the combination of a capillary malformation and café-au-lait macular pigmentation without the naevus spilus type component. All types have been described in association with naevus anaemicus, and indeed this led to the subclassification of each of types I–V into a and b, with or without naevus anaemicus respectively. Rarely, some cases have been associated with hypopigmentation of skin or hair [80–82].

Originally the term PPV referred to one particular phenotype, that of type 2 or cesioflammea [83], which is the co-occurrence of dermal melanocytosis (mongolian blue spots) and a port-wine stain/naevus flammeus type capillary malformation (Fig. 109.2). Because this phenotype appears to be substantially more common than all others under this diagnostic umbrella it has been argued that it alone should be called PPV [84]. The prevalence of this type has been estimated in a large Mexican hospital population at approximately 6 per 100 000 patients [85], with no other types documented in a 5-year period. However, although it is possible that this is the commonest phenotype in Mexico, other phenotypic subsets are well described and recurrent, and there is recent evidence that some at least may be genotypically separate [85]. There may also be differences in incidence between different racial groups, because most cases of PPV have so far been described in those of Afro-Caribbean, Hispanic or Asian ancestry [77,85–88]. A recent analysis of self-designated ethnicity in patients with different types of birthmarks in a tertiary centre supported this observation [89]. This pattern, however, may not apply to all phenotypic subtypes of PPV and more numbers are needed for further study in this area.

Associated abnormalities and management. There are many described associations and complications of PPV other than naevus anaemicus, but because the numbers of patients are small there are no clear evidence-based guidelines for investigation and management. Previously the diagnosis has been said to be 'co-occurring' with Sturge–Weber (SWS) and Klippel–Trenaunay syndromes [84,90–93], but with genetic resolution this is now recognized to be phenotypic overlap rather than a dual diagnosis. However, it does allow lessons from these other syndromes to be used to some degree as evidence for clinical management in PPV.

Principal amongst the associated abnormalities are ocular and neurological abnormalities. In the eye, the problems can be vascular, pigmentary or malignant. Abnormalities described are congenital or acquired glaucoma, choroidal angioma, congenital or acquired

Table 109.1 Phenotypic subclassifications of phakomatosis pigmentovascularis

Pigmentary birthmark	Vascular birthmark	Classification 1 Ota [77]	Classification 2 Happle [78]
Linear epidermal naevus	Capillary malformation (port-wine stain/ naevus flammeus type)	Type I	Deemed not to exist in this classification but cases have been described [77,84]
Dermal melanocytosis	Capillary malformation (port-wine stain/ naevus flammeus type)	Type II	Cesioflammea type
Naevus spilus	Capillary malformation (port-wine stain/ naevus flammeus in classification 1, pale pink telengiectatic naevus in classification 2)	Type III	Spilorosea type
Dermal melanocytosis and naevus spilus	Capillary malformation (port-wine stain/ naevus flammeus type)	Type IV	Extremely rare, unclassifiable in this classification
Dermal melanocytosis	Capillary malformation (cutis marmorata telengiectatica congenital type)	Type V	Cesiomarmorata type

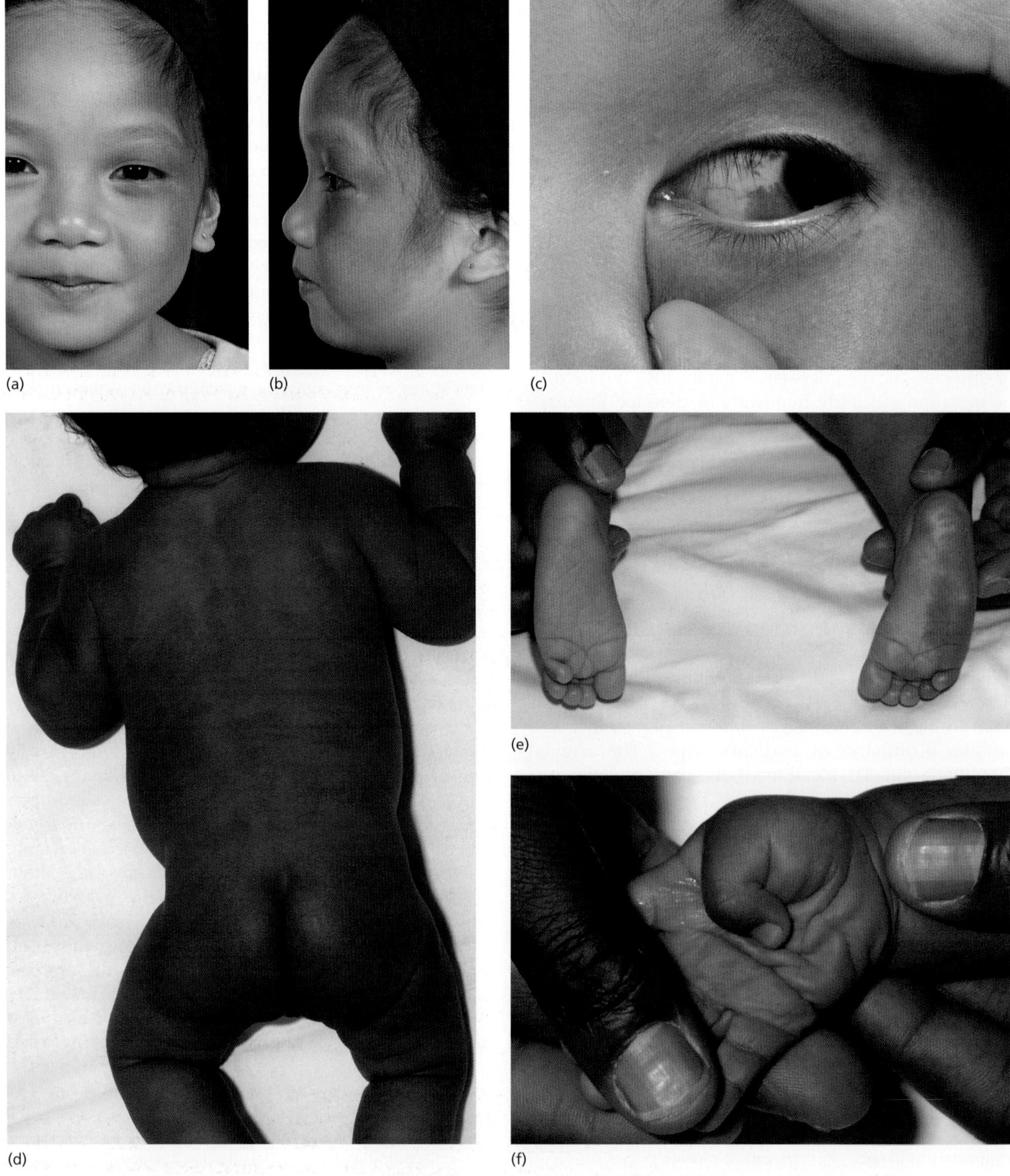

Fig. 109.2 Clinical appearances of different types of dermal melanocytosis: (a,b,c) naevus of Ota with scleral melanocytosis; (d,e,f) in the context of phakomatosis pigmentovascularis type II or cesioflammea, where there are associated areas of capillary malformation on the hand and foot. Were these vascular lesions not present on careful examination this child would otherwise have a diagnosis of extensive or atypical dermal melanocytosis.

scleral or ocular melanosis, iris mammillations or pigmentation, and tumours including choroidal melanoma, optic disc melanocytoma and conjunctival melanoma [84,90,94]. Importantly, eye involvement may not be evident without a slit-lamp examination and therefore referral to ophthalmology is always advised [94]. Central nervous system (CNS) abnormalities include those of SWS, such as leptomeningeal angioma, cortical atrophy, cognitive deficit and seizures, in addition to hydrocephalus, Arnold–Chiari malformation and polymicrogryria [85,86,92,95]. A paediatric neurology examination is therefore advised along with an electroencephalogram, and an MRI of the brain following guidelines as for those with SWS [96,97]. Other described associations include lipohypoplasia [98], hypospadias [99], hemihypertophy with interdigital gaps and scoliosis [100], hemifacial, hemicorporal, or limb hypertrophy without venous insufficiency [84], thumb hypoplasia, hydronephrosis, coronal synostosis, three to four finger syndactyly [86], and triangular alopecia [101].

Pathogenesis. The genetic cause of PPV has recently been established in the majority of cases studied thus far. In subtypes where there is dermal melanocytosis the majority of patients tested have mosaic mutations in the genes *GNA11* or *GNAQ* [85]. Only one patient with cesiomarmorata has so far been tested, and was positive. In all cases where biopsies from the vascular and pigmentary birthmarks were available the same mutation was present in both, suggesting that the mutation occurs in a single common precursor cell [85]. Twin spotting is therefore not the mechanism which underlies the co-occurrence of two birthmarks in this condition. The mutation has not been reported in blood so far.

GNA11 is highly homologous to *GNAQ*, and mosaic mutations in the latter are the commonest cause of SWS [102]. Furthermore, both genes are known to be somatically mutated in ocular melanoma. In general (although not always) the cancer-associated mutations affect codons 209, and those in PPV and in SWS (*GNAQ*) affect codon 183.

Extensive or atypical dermal melanocytosis, including naevus of Ota and naevus of Ito

Clinical features, differential diagnosis and epidemiology. Mongolian blue spots, or dermal melanocytosis, are very common birthmarks seen in infants of all ethnic backgrounds, but with a much higher incidence in Afro-Caribbean, Hispanic and Asian populations than in White Caucasians [103–108], and a higher incidence in brown-haired rather than blonde-haired children within the same population [109]. Thus, it seems that the clinical phenotype is altered by ethnic background, and that this may be related to pigmentary phenotype rather than another aspect of genetic ethnic differences. Typical Mongolian blue spots are macular, with no increase in skin markings, blue-grey-black in colour, and homogeneous. They are typically seen over the lumbosacral region, are from 1 to 20 cm roughly in diameter, have ill-defined edges, and resolve spontaneously over a period of a few years [103–106,110–112]. One study clearly demonstrated disappearance by the age of six [105]. Because Mongolian blue spots are so common, dermal melanocytosis is often not noted in hospital records [103], which has led to difficulties in establishing the difference between these transient birthmarks and extensive dermal melanocytosis as a mosaic pigmentary disorder.

Congenital extensive or atypical dermal melanocytosis (EDM) can be defined as involving areas of the skin other than just the lumbosacral region, and/or more strongly pigmented with well-defined edges, and/or persistent past the age of 6 years [85,112] (Fig. 109.2). Although EDM frequently persists longer than common Mongolian blue spots, in the author's experience it can also gradually lighten over time. The clinical pattern of melanocytosis can be either segmental or nonsegmental [12], and there can be single or multiple lesions. Historically, some anatomically defined areas of EDM have been given a separate label, namely congenital naevus of Ota and naevus of Ito. Naevus of Ota is dermal melanocytosis in the forehead/temporal/periocular regions of the face [113] (Fig. 109.2), whereas naevus of Ito affects the neck/shoulder/upper trunk [114]. In practice, these conditions are often seen together, and in association with EDM at other sites on the body [85,115–117]. EDM at different sites probably does have different implications for involvement of other organs (see later), however such variation within a cutaneous diagnostic grouping is very much in line with other pigmentary mosaic disorders, and not a reason *per se* to continue to separate these two anatomical areas from the rest of the condition. There is also histopathological and early genetic evidence to support a common origin, as will be reviewed later.

There is evidence for a difference in incidence in EDM in different ethnic groups, to some extent mirroring that seen with Mongolian blue spots and isolated scleral melanocytosis (see later). Naevus of Ota is documented to be commoner in Asian populations [110], whereas EDM in other areas seems also be more common in Afro-Caribbean and Asian ethnic groups compared with White Caucasian populations [89,108].

Histology. Histologically, EDM is characterized by dermal melanocytes, which can be dendritic and/or spindle-shaped, with or without dermal melanophages [113,114,118–120]. Histological subclassification of naevus of Ota suggested that deeper melanocytosis was commoner on the forehead, temple and upper eyelid, whereas more superficial ones were seen on the cheeks [121].

Associated abnormalities and management. EDM can be associated with capillary malformations in the context of PPV (see earlier). EDM can be associated with pigmentary abnormalities in other organs, most commonly ocular melanocytosis, which can affect the conjunctiva, sclera, cornea, iris, fundus, optic disc, and even the extraocular muscles and optic nerve [122–125]. Of note, isolated scleral melanocytosis is very common in at least some populations, for example in a Chinese study of more than 2000 children of all ages, almost 50% had acquired evidence of scleral melanocytosis by the age of six, with the prevalence diminishing thereafter [126]. This may be the ocular correlate of simple Mongolian blue spots, or at least classifiable as a physiological phenomenon. In the same cohort only one case of oculodermal melanocytosis was seen, and other dermal melanocytosis not looked for. Melanocytosis can also be found on the oral, palatal, nasopharyngeal and auricular mucosae and the tympanic membrane [124,127–130].

As in PPV and SWS an important association in the eye is congenital or acquired glaucoma [123,131], and early referral to ophthalmology should be undertaken in the same way. Whether this is only seen with periorbital dermal melanocytosis is not yet clear. Malignancies, unlike in SWS, are described in EDM and in PPV. Tumours described include melanoma arising in naevus of Ota [132,133], naevus of Ito [134,135], in the dura and CNS [125,136,137], and in the orbit [124,125,138–140].

A progressively worsening phenotype of EDM which is often more patchy or spotty is seen with metabolic storage disorders, particularly GM1-gangliosidosis and Hurler syndrome [141–146], and this possibility should be considered even in the absence of other suggestive features in a very young child. A metabolic screen of urinary glycosaminoglycans or referral to paediatrics can be performed if suspected. Other rarely described associations of EDM are cleft lip underlying the cutaneous abnormality [147] and aplasia cutis congenita [148].

Pathogenesis. In some cases, the proportion as yet to be established by larger studies, EDM can be caused by mosaic mutations in *GNAQ* [85]. Mutations in both codons 183 and 209 have been described. These mutations are again detectable in affected skin by next generation sequencing and other high sensitivity techniques, but not thus far in blood [85]. A single case of naevus of Ota (whether associated with other EDM was not clear) has also been described as carrying a *GNAQ* mutation [149], which is supportive evidence that these phenotypes are part of the same clinical spectrum. Although it has not yet been demonstrated at molecular level, patients with these mutations are likely to be those or amongst those at risk of ocular melanoma. Whether the chance of ocular involvement is related to the pattern of the cutaneous lesions is not yet clear.

Phakomatosis pigmentokeratotica

Phakomatosis pigmentokeratotica (PPK) is covered in detail in Chapter 106. Briefly, PPK is the association of congenital linear sebaceous naevi and naevus spilus (Fig. 109.3), and can be accompanied by a variety of extracutaneous manifestations. This condition is caused by mosaicism for mutations in the gene *HRAS* [150], or more rarely *BRAF* [151], which can be detected in the skin.

Congenital melanocytic naevi (CMN) and CMN syndrome

Congenital melanocytic naevi (CMN) are covered in detail in Chapter 105. Briefly, CMN can be single or multiple, and if associated with extracutaneous features are then termed CMN syndrome [152]. The commonest associated features are neurological abnormalities of various types. There is an increased risk of melanoma which varies with the cutaneous and neuroradiological phenotype [153–156]. The diagnosis can usually be made clinically on the basis of well-defined areas of increased pigmentation and increased skin markings, often with a palpable component and/or hypertrichosis, and with the most typical pattern in multiple CMN being one larger naevus and multiple other smaller naevi. The genetic basis of multiple CMN and CMN syndrome is mosaicism for mutations in the gene *NRAS* in 80% of cases [157].

Becker naevi and Becker naevus syndrome

Becker naevi are covered in detail in Chapter 106. These are slightly pigmented and often hypertrichotic naevi which develop in the first two decades, classically around puberty but frequently also in early childhood. Rarely there are signs at birth. The most typical site is a unilateral segmental distribution involving the upper chest or upper back/shoulder, with indistinct edges. It can be associated with various extracutaneous abnormalities, then termed Becker naevus syndrome, and these are most typically ipsilateral underdevelopment of the pectoral muscles and/or breast tissue. Becker naevi can usually be diagnosed clinically by a variable combination of the noncongenital history, increased pigmentation, overlying hypertrichosis and the characteristic upper truncal/upper limb site. The genetic basis of this naevus and the associated syndrome has recently been described in 60% of cases tested as somatic mutations in *ACTB*, the gene encoding the cytoskeletal protein beta-actin or actin, cytoplasmic 1 [158]. Mutations were found in the myocyte lineage, including in the pilar muscles, but not in the epidermis or stromal tissue [158]. Because of the sporadic occurrence and large segmental distribution of Becker naevi these must represent a mosaic mutation occurring *in utero*, but which does not become expressed phenotypically until the first or, more commonly, the second decade of life.

Speckled lentiginous naevi

Speckled lentiginous naevus (SLN), or naevus spilus, is an entity in which multiple small areas of hyperpigmentation (of the order of millimetres) appear progressively on the background of a café-au-lait macule (Fig. 109.3). This general description, however, includes various distinguishable phenotypes, which both look and probably behave in different manners, and which are beginning to be distinguished genetically. The café-au lait macular background in congenital lesions may not be visible at birth, developing only slowly over the first few years of life.

Small isolated SLN are covered in Chapter 105 and have been found to carry mutations in the gene *HRAS* (c.37G>C, p.Gly13Arg) [159]. Large or multiple SLN are a feature of PPK (see Chapter 106 and later), and in that context has been shown to carry *HRAS* mutations in codons 13 and 61 [150]. They can also be a feature of phakomatosis pigmentovascularis spilorosea type (see later) [77,78] and speckled lentiginous naevus syndrome. The latter is extremely rare and constitutes the association of extensive and/or multiple naevus spilus maculosus with extracutaneous manifestations, including scoliosis and skeletal muscular weakness. The genetic basis of these conditions has not yet been pinpointed. What has been

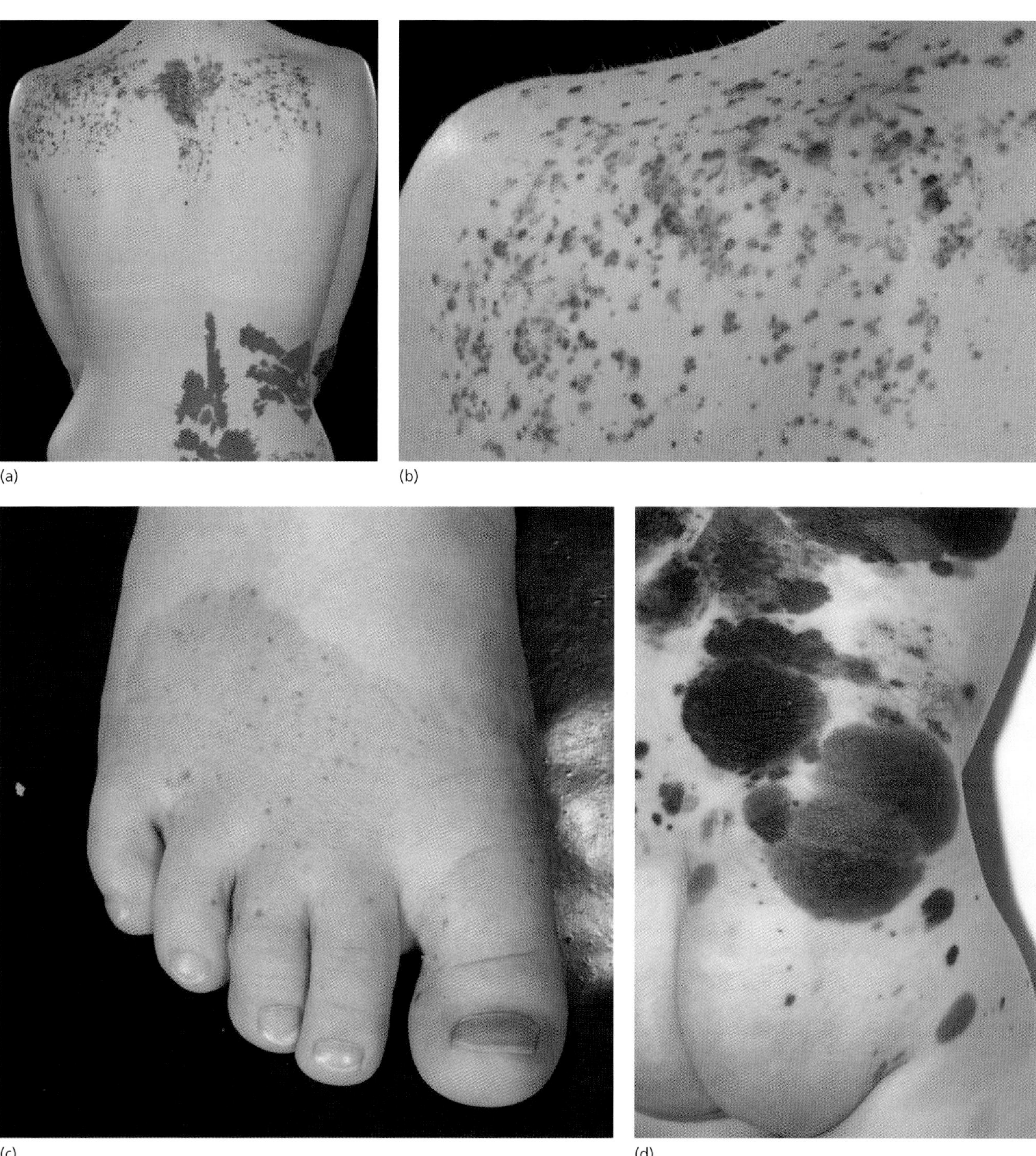

(a) (b) (c) (d)

Fig. 109.3 Clinical appearances of different types of naevus spilus: (a,b) naevus spilus papulosus on the upper back in the context of phakomatosis pigmentokeratotica (the pigmented Blaschkolinear sebaceous naevus is seen on the lower back), (c) naevus spilus maculosus on the foot in the context of speckled lentiginous naevus syndrome, and (d) naevus spilus type of congenital melanocytic naevus.

proposed but is not yet clear is if there is an association with the clinically recognizable subtypes and syndromes. Instead, interpersonal variation may be responsible for the differences in the clinical subtype of large SLN.

A further naevus spilus phenotype is naevus spilus-type congenital melanocytic naevus (Fig. 109.3). Although it can be difficult to distinguish these in every case, generally this phenotype can be distinguished from the large SLN described here by the nonsegmental pattern, and usually by the much larger size (of the order of centimetres) and clear CMN phenotype of the superimposed hyperpigmented areas [161]. Because these lesions are CMN they are often hairy, which is not a typical feature of the other types of large SLN described here. Genetically they are also different, being caused by specific *NRAS* mutations [162]. These are covered in Chapter 105.

Secondary melanocytic proliferations can arise within SLN. However, exactly which SLN types give rise to which proliferations is somewhat unclear because of the difficulties with terminology in this area. It may well become clearer once the causative mutation is published consistently. Spitz naevi are a relatively common finding within large SLN [160,163,164], producing an agminated Spitz naevus phenotype; however, the subtype is not always clear from the literature. It has been suggested that these tend to arise in naevus spilus maculosus rather than papulosus [161], and in the author's experience they do not commonly arise in CMN-type naevus spilus. Sometimes the café-au-lait macular background is not in evidence early in life but the agmination of Spitz naevi should alert the clinician to an underlying lentiginous naevus. The Spitz naevi have been shown in one study to carry the same *HRAS* mutation in codon 13, although the underlying SLN was not tested [164]. Melanoma arising in SLN is described [165–174], including in all phenotypes described here, and further work will need to be done to ascertain whether some types of lesion are at higher risk.

Naevus depigmentosus

Naevus depigmentosus (ND) is a descriptive term which correlates with a distinct clinical phenotype, which has also been termed achromic naevus. The cause is currently unknown, and the condition is not yet known on a molecular level to be mosaic. It is included in this chapter, however, because the phenotype and sporadic nature suggest that it will be found to be so. There are discrepancies in the literature about what constitutes a ND, with some studies including Blaschkolinear hypopigmentation as a form of ND. Currently, however, it is more generally accepted to be defined as a single area of congenital (or early onset) hypopigmentation, with more than 90% of cases in one study appearing by the age of 3 years [175]. The naevus can be round/ovoid or frequently in a segmental pattern with midline cutoff either anteriorly or posteriorly, has relatively well-defined edges, and once developed does not progress over life. Within the hypopigmented area there are frequently islands of normal-coloured skin. Overlying hair may show hypopigmentation [176]. Other cutaneous associations described with naevus depigmentosus are vitiligo [177,178], naevus spilus [179,180], naevus of Ito [181], segmental lentiginosis [182–184], naevus flammeus [185], Becker naevus [179,186], generalized milia [187] and inflammatory linear epidermal naevus [188]. Extracutaneous abnormalities are extremely rare. However, descriptions include ipsilateral breast hypoplasia [183], CNS abnormalities [189] and hemihypertrophy [190,191]. Management therefore does not involve routine investigations, unless there are clinical concerns about an individual patient. Photography, reassurance, referral for camouflage make up if this is wished for, and psychological and/or patient group support for both parents and child are the mainstay of care. Advice can be given on additional sun protection in that area if it is felt to be sufficiently hypopigmented to be at risk. Long-term follow up is not generally required.

Histology and electron microscopy of ND show a normal population density of melanocytes, and a normal size of melanosomes, suggesting that the defect in pigmentation is caused by abnormal melanin synthesis or transfer of melanosomes [175,192,193]. Expression of cKIT was found to be strong in one study [194].

Mosaic neurofibromatosis type 1

Classification and epidemiology. Mosaic neurofibromatosis type 1 (NF1) has been divided into two categories: mosaic generalized and mosaic localized [195]. The skin signs in mosaic generalized NF1 are not restricted to one body part, whereas mosaic localized NF1 is equivalent to what used to be termed 'segmental'. The incidence of mosaic NF1 is not known, and was estimated in 2001 as 1 in 36–40 000 live births [196]. Given the high *de novo* mutation rate and the much higher incidence of germline NF1, it is, however, very likely to be underdiagnosed.

Pathogenesis. The genetic basis of mosaic generalized NF1 was first demonstrated in 1996 as a loss of function mutation in the gene *NF1* in the blood [197], and in mosaic localized NF1 in 2000, when a mutation was detected in affected skin fibroblasts, but absent from unaffected skin and leukocytes [198]. The difference between the two categories is the timing of the mutation in embryogenesis, with the generalized mosaic mutation preceding the localized. It is important to be aware of these categories, however, because publications may or may not include both in their definition.

Cutaneous features. The classical presentation of localized mosaic NF1 is of a restricted part of the body exhibiting one or more signs of NF1, with no other evidence of disease. Skin signs may be café-au-lait macules only, cutaneous neurofibromas only, or both combined. Elegant dissection of these on a molecular level demonstrated that these different clinical presentations were dependent on which embryonic cell type had been hit by the mutation, either melanocyte, Schwann cell or a common precursor. In the same study the mechanism behind the appearance of the skin signs was shown to be a second hit in those same cells [199]. Where café-au-lait macules are present there is a background macular hyperpigmentation in the affected area and this, however, must be attributable to the first hit.

Associated features and management. Two large cohort studies have recently been published. In the first a cohort of 40 patients from a paediatric dermatology service with mosaic localized NF1 multiple café-au-lait macules and freckling were confirmed as the recurrent skin signs, with a single case of associated cutaneous neurofibromas and no juvenile xanthogranuloma or naevus anaemicus reported [200]. Extracutaneous likely associations, however, were seen in four patients (10%), with two having epilepsy and two developing a malignancy. In the second large cohort study of 60 patients with mosaic localized NF1, associated neurofibromas and isolated neurofibromas featured in 16% and 15% of the cohort respectively, although pigmentary changes remained the primary presenting feature [201]. In this cohort there were no reported malignancies; however, neurodevelopmental delay and bony abnormalities were seen in 12% and 10% respectively [201]. Both studies conclude that regular follow up of patients with mosaic localized NF1 is advisable. A recent review of the literature identified 320 cases of mosaic NF1, where 76% of cases were localized, and where the extracutaneous complications rate was 29% [202]. Cohorts presenting to nondermatological services unsurprisingly have a lower rate of cutaneous features and a higher rate of plexiform neurofibroma and bony abnormalities [203].

Differential diagnosis. Differential diagnosis for mosaic localized NF1 can be a large naevus spilus, or isolated large segmental café-au-lait macule. The former will generally contain either freckling only (no substantial separate café-au-lait macules) or melanocytic naevi, whereas the latter will not contain any other melanocytic lesions.

Genetic investigation and risk to offspring

Mosaic NF1 is an important diagnosis to make because it has implications not only for the health of the affected individual, but also for their offspring, because the mosaic mutation can be passed on in germline form. In a study of 23 half-siblings fathered by a single unsuspected case of mosaic NF1 who was a sperm donor, 9 of 23 (39%) were found to have germline NF1, with varying severity of clinical phenotypes [204]. The clinical examination of this donor was only described in the literature, with no photos. The description is of four 'naevi' between 1.5 and 6 cm in diameter, all on the back, but the largest was described as grey-brown. It is not clear if any of these are café-au-lait macules. However, importantly no other clinical features were found, and in particular nothing outside of the skin. The level of gonosomal mosaicism from sperm was found to be 20% and was not measured in blood. The paper concludes that the transmission rate of 39% is not significantly different from transmission of a heterozygous autosomal dominant trait and provides other references to support this discrepancy between relatively low measured mosaicism and high rate of transmission in NF1.

Genetic diagnosis of mosaic localized disease is best done on skin biopsy from an affected area, and melanocyte or Schwann cell culture before DNA sequencing. Melanocyte culture and occasionally Schwann cell culture is offered in specialist NF1 centres, and if the diagnosis is strongly suspected and has been excluded on lymphocyte DNA sequencing, it is worth contacting a specialist centre for this. If genetic diagnosis of this type is not available then management of the patient as for germline NF1 is most appropriate, with genetic counselling from clinical geneticists.

The rate of transmission is in accordance with two previous reports where three of six and two of three siblings had NF1 in spite of a germline mosaicisms of 10% and 10–17%, respectively [22,23].

Mosaic Legius syndrome

Because Legius syndrome is much rarer than NF1, and particularly because mosaic NF1 can present with only skin features, it is always worth testing for mosaic NF1 if considering mosaic Legius syndrome. Diagnosis would be as for mosaic NF1, by skin biopsy, culture of melanocytes if possible and sequencing of the *SPRED1* gene. Management of the patient should involve reassurance that the phenotype is highly likely only to affect the skin and, on current knowledge, should not confer an excess cancer risk. If a genetic diagnosis is established, no further routine investigations should be required.

References

1 Blaschko A. Die Nervenverteilung in der Haut in ihrer Beziehung zu den Erkrankungen der Haut. In: Bericht erstattet dem VII. Congress der Deutschen Dermatologischen Gesellschaft. Breslau, 1901.

2 Ito M. Incontinentia pigmenti achromians: a singular case of nevus depigmentosus systematicus bilateralis. Japan J Dermatol 1951; 61:31–2.

3 Jelinek JE, Bart RS, Schiff SM. Hypomelanosis of Ito ('incontinentia pigmenti achromians'). Report of three cases and review of the literature. Arch Dermatol 1973;107:596–601.

4 Kalter DC, Griffiths WA, Atherton DJ. Linear and whorled nevoid hypermelanosis. J Am Acad Dermatol 1988;19:1037–44.

5 Nehal KS, PeBenito R, Orlow SJ. Analysis of 54 cases of hypopigmentation and hyperpigmentation along the lines of Blaschko. Arch Dermatol 1996;132:1167–70.

6 Sybert VP. Hypomelanosis of Ito: a description, not a diagnosis. J Invest Dermatol 1994;103:141S–3S.

7 Ruggieri M, Pavone L. Hypomelanosis of Ito: clinical syndrome or just phenotype? J Child Neurol 2000;15:635–44.

8 Ruiz-Maldonado R, Toussaint S, Tamayo L et al. Hypomelanosis of Ito: diagnostic criteria and report of 41 cases. Pediatr Dermatol 1992;9:1–10.

9 Pascual-Castroviejo I, Lopez-Rodriguez L, de la Cruz Medina M et al. Hypomelanosis of Ito. Neurological complications in 34 cases. Can J Neurol Sci 1988;15:124–9.

10 Pascual-Castroviejo I, Roche C, Martinez-Bermejo A et al. Hypomelanosis of ITO. A study of 76 infantile cases. Brain Dev 1998;20:36–43.

11 Moss C, Larkins S, Stacey M et al. Epidermal mosaicism and Blaschko's lines. J Med Genet 1993;30:752–5.

12 Kinsler VA, Larue L. The patterns of birthmarks suggest a novel population of melanocyte precursors arising around the time of gastrulation. Pigment Cell Melanoma Res 2018;31:95–109.

13 Kosaki R, Naito Y, Torii C et al. Split hand foot malformation with whorl-like pigmentary pattern: phenotypic expression of somatic mosaicism for the p63 mutation. Am J Med Genet Part A 2008; 146A:2574–7.

14 Sorlin A, Maruani A, Aubriot-Lorton MH et al. Mosaicism for a KITLG mutation in linear and whorled nevoid hypermelanosis. J Invest Dermatol 2017;137:1575–8.

15 Sybert VP, Pagon RA, Donlan M et al. Pigmentary abnormalities and mosaicism for chromosomal aberration: association with clinical features similar to hypomelanosis of Ito. J Pediatr 1990;116:581–6.

16 Lombillo VA, Sybert VP. Mosaicism in cutaneous pigmentation. Curr Opin Pediatr 2005;17:494–500.

17 Taibjee SM, Bennett DC, Moss C. Abnormal pigmentation in hypomelanosis of Ito and pigmentary mosaicism: the role of pigmentary genes. Br J Dermatol 2004;151:269–82.

18 Thomas IT, Frias JL, Cantu ES et al. Association of pigmentary anomalies with chromosomal and genetic mosaicism and chimerism. Am J Hum Genet 1989;45:193–205.

19 Chemke J, Rappaport S, Etrog R. Aberrant melanoblast migration associated with trisomy 18 mosaicism. J Med Genet 1983;20:135–7.

20 Chitayat D, Friedman JM, Johnston MM. Hypomelanosis of Ito – a nonspecific marker of somatic mosaicism: report of case with trisomy 18 mosaicism. Am J Med Genet 1990;35:422–4.

21 Murano I, Ohashi H, Tsukahara M et al. Pigmentary dysplasias in long survivors with mosaic trisomy 18: report of two cases. Clin Genet 1991;39:68–74.

22 Grazia R, Tullini A, Rossi PG et al. Hypomelanosis of Ito with trisomy 18 mosaicism. Am J Med Genet 1993;45:120–1.

23 Ukita M, Hasegawa M, Nakahori T. Trisomy 18 mosaicism in a woman with normal intelligence, pigmentary dysplasia, and an 18 trisomic daughter. Am J Med Genet 1997;68:240–1.

24 Komine M, Hino M, Shiina M et al. Linear and whorled naevoid hypermelanosis: a case with systemic involvement and trisomy 18 mosaicism. Br J Dermatol 2002;146:500–2.

25 Girard C, Guillot B, Rivier F et al. [Trisomy 20 mosaicism revealed by pigmentary mosaicism of the Ito-type]. Ann Dermatol Venereol 2005;132:151–3.

26 Taibjee SM, Hall D, Balderson D et al. Keratinocyte cytogenetics in 10 patients with pigmentary mosaicism: identification of one case of trisomy 20 mosaicism confined to keratinocytes. Clin Exp Dermatol 2009;34:823–9.

27 Hartmann A, Hofmann UB, Hoehn H et al. Postnatal confirmation of prenatally diagnosed trisomy 20 mosaicism in a patient with linear and whorled nevoid hypermelanosis. Pediatr Dermatol 2004; 21:636–41.

28 Ensenauer RE, Shaughnessy WJ, Jalal SM et al. Trisomy 20 mosaicism caused by a maternal meiosis II error is associated with normal intellect but multiple congenital anomalies. Am J Med Genet Part A 2005;134A:202–6.

29 Menke J, Pauli S, Sigler M et al. Uniparental trisomy of a mutated HRAS proto-oncogene in embryonal rhabdomyosarcoma of a patient with Costello syndrome. J Clin Oncol 2015;33:e62–5.

30 Pallister PD, Meisner LF, Elejalde BR et al. The pallister mosaic syndrome. Birth Defects Orig Artic Ser 1977;13:103–10.

31 Warburton D, Anyane-Yeboa K, Francke U. Mosaic tetrasomy 12p: four new cases, and confirmation of the chromosomal origin of the supernumerary chromosome in one of the original Pallister-Mosaic syndrome cases. Am J Med Genet 1987;27:275–83.

32 Vogel I, Lyngbye T, Nielsen A et al. Pallister-Killian syndrome in a girl with mild developmental delay and mosaicism for hexasomy 12p. Am J Med Genet Part A 2009;149A:510–4.

33 Yeung A, Francis D, Giouzeppos O et al. Pallister-Killian syndrome caused by mosaicism for a supernumerary ring chromosome 12p. Am J Med Genet Part A 2009;149A:505–9.

34 Blyth M, Maloney V, Beal S et al. Pallister-Killian syndrome: a study of 22 British patients. J Med Genet 2015;52:454–64.

35 Wilkens A, Liu H, Park K et al. Novel clinical manifestations in Pallister-Killian syndrome: comprehensive evaluation of 59 affected individuals and review of previously reported cases. Am J Med Genet Part A 2012;158A:3002–17.

36 Alesi V, Dentici ML, Restaldi F et al. Unclassifiable pattern of hypopigmentation in a patient with mosaic partial 12p tetrasomy without Pallister-Killian syndrome. Am J Med Genet Part A 2017.

37 Happle R. Mosaicism in Human Skin. Berlin: Springer-Verlag, 2014.

38 Reynolds JF, Daniel A, Kelly TE et al. Isochromosome 12p mosaicism (Pallister mosaic aneuploidy or Pallister-Killian syndrome): report of 11 cases. Am J Med Genet 1987;27:257–74.

39 Schinzel A. Tetrasomy 12p (Pallister-Killian syndrome). J Med Genet 1991;28:122–5.

40 Theisen A, Rosenfeld JA, Farrell SA et al. aCGH detects partial tetrasomy of 12p in blood from Pallister–Killian syndrome cases without invasive skin biopsy. Am J Med Genet Part A 2009;149A:914–8.

41 Mirzaa GM, Campbell CD, Solovieff N et al. Association of MTOR mutations with developmental brain disorders, including megalencephaly, focal cortical dysplasia, and pigmentary mosaicism. JAMA Neurol 2016;73:836–45.

42 Handoko M, Emrick LT, Rosenfeld JA et al. Recurrent mosaic MTOR c.5930C > T (p.Thr1977Ile) variant causing megalencephaly, asymmetric polymicrogyria, and cutaneous pigmentary mosaicism: case report and review of the literature. Am J Med Genet A 2019;179:475–9.

43 Amyere M, Vogt T, Hoo J et al. KITLG mutations cause familial progressive hyper- and hypopigmentation. J Invest Dermatol 2011; 131:1234–9.

44 Happle R. Mosaicism in human skin. Understanding the patterns and mechanisms. Arch Dermatol 1993;129:1460–70.

45 Horn D, Rommeck M, Sommer D et al. Phylloid pigmentary pattern with mosaic trisomy 13. Pediatr Dermatol 1997;14:278–80.

46 Pillay T, Winship WS, Ramdial PK. Pigmentary abnormalities in trisomy of chromosome 13. Clin Dysmorphol 1998;7:191–4.

47 Happle R. Phylloid hypomelanosis is closely related to mosaic trisomy 13. Eur J Dermatol 2000;10:511–12.

48 Schepis C, Failla P, Siragusa M et al. An additional case of macular phylloid mosaicism. Dermatology 2001;202:73.

49 Ribeiro Noce T, de Pina-Neto JM, Happle R. Phylloid pattern of pigmentary disturbance in a case of complex mosaicism. Am J Med Genet 2001;98:145–7.

50 Yakinci C, Kutlu NO, Alp MN et al. Hypomelanosis of ito with trisomy 13 mosaicism [46, XY, der (13;13) (q10;q10), +13/46,xy]. Turk J Pediatr 2002;44:152–5.

51 Gonzalez-Ensenat MA, Vicente A, Poo P et al. Phylloid hypomelanosis and mosaic partial trisomy 13: two cases that provide further evidence of a distinct clinicogenetic entity. Arch Dermatol 2009;145: 576–8.

52 Dhar SU, Robbins-Furman P, Levy ML et al. Tetrasomy 13q mosaicism associated with phylloid hypomelanosis and precocious puberty. Am J Med Genet Part A 2009;149A:993–6.

53 Happle R. [Phylloid hypomelanosis and mosaic trisomy 13: a new etiologically defined neurocutaneous syndrome]. Der Hautarzt; Zeitschrift fur Dermatologie, Venerologie, und verwandte Gebiete 2001;52:3–5.

54 Oiso N, Tsuruta D, Imanishi H et al. Phylloid hypermelanosis and melanocytic nevi with aggregated and disfigured melanosomes: causal relationship between phylloid pigment distribution and chromosome 13 abnormalities. Dermatology 2010;220:169–72.

55 Hansen LK, Brandrup F, Rasmussen K. Pigmentary mosaicism with mosaic chromosome 5p tetrasomy. Br J Dermatol 2003;149:414–6.

56 Happle R, Franco-Guio MF, Santacoloma-Osorio G. Phylloid hypermelanosis: a cutaneous marker of several different disorders? Pediatr Dermatol 2014;31:504–6.

57 Dumitrescu CE, Collins MT. McCune-Albright syndrome. Orphanet J Rare Dis 2008;3:12.

58 Lumbroso S, Paris F, Sultan C. Activating Gsalpha mutations: analysis of 113 patients with signs of McCune–Albright syndrome–a European Collaborative Study. J.Clin.Endocrinol.Metab 2004; 89:2107–13.

59 Albright F, Butler, A. M., Hampton, A. O., Smith, P. Syndrome characterized by osteitis fibrosa disseminata, areas of pigmentation and endocrine dysfunction, with precocious puberty in females: report of five cases. New England Journal of Medicine 1937;216:727–46.

60 Jung AJ, Soskin S, Paris F et al. [McCune–Albright syndrome revealed by Blaschko–linear cafe-au-lait spots on the back]. Ann Dermatol Venereol 2016;143:21–6.

61 Rieger E, Kofler R, Borkenstein M et al. Melanotic macules following Blaschko's lines in McCune–Albright syndrome. Br J Dermatol 1994;130:215–20.

62 Pichard DC, Boyce AM, Collins MT et al. Oral pigmentation in McCune–Albright syndrome. JAMA Dermatol 2014;150:760–3.

63 Akintoye SO, Lee JS, Feimster T et al. Dental characteristics of fibrous dysplasia and McCune–Albright syndrome. Oral Surg Oral Med Oral Pathol Oral Radiol Endod 2003;96:275–82.

64 Jacobson JD, Turpin AL, Sands SA. Allergic manifestations and cutaneous histamine responses in patients with McCune Albright syndrome. World Allergy Organ J 2013;6:9.

65 Leet AI, Chebli C, Kushner H et al. Fracture incidence in polyostotic fibrous dysplasia and the McCune–Albright syndrome. J Bone Miner Res 2004;19:571–7.

66 Wasniewska M, Matarazzo P, Weber G et al. Clinical presentation of McCune–Albright syndrome in males. Journal of pediatric endocrinology & metabolism: JPEM 2006;19 Suppl 2:619–22.

67 Volkl TM, Dorr HG. McCune–Albright syndrome: clinical picture and natural history in children and adolescents. Journal of pediatric endocrinology & metabolism: JPEM 2006;19 Suppl 2:551–9.

68 Diaz A, Danon M, Crawford J. McCune–Albright syndrome and disorders due to activating mutations of GNAS1. J Pediatr Endocrinol. Metab 2007;20:853–80.

69 Bousson V, Rey-Jouvin C, Laredo JD et al. Fibrous dysplasia and McCune–Albright syndrome: Imaging for positive and differential diagnoses, prognosis, and follow-up guidelines. European journal of radiology 2014;83:1828–42.

70 Collins MT, Chebli C, Jones J et al. Renal phosphate wasting in fibrous dysplasia of bone is part of a generalized renal tubular dysfunction similar to that seen in tumor-induced osteomalacia. J Bone Miner Res 2001;16:806–13.

71 Riminucci M, Collins MT, Fedarko NS et al. FGF-23 in fibrous dysplasia of bone and its relationship to renal phosphate wasting. J Clin Invest 2003;112:683–92.

72 Kobayashi K, Imanishi Y, Koshiyama H et al. Expression of FGF23 is correlated with serum phosphate level in isolated fibrous dysplasia. Life Sci 2006;78:2295–301.

73 Collins MT, Sarlis NJ, Merino MJ et al. Thyroid carcinoma in the McCune–Albright syndrome: contributory role of activating Gs alpha mutations. The Journal of clinical endocrinology and metabolism 2003;88:4413–7.

74 Weinstein LS, Shenker A, Gejman PV et al. Activating mutations of the stimulatory G protein in the McCune–Albright syndrome. N Engl J Med 1991;325:1688–95.

75 Patten JL, Johns DR, Valle D et al. Mutation in the gene encoding the stimulatory G protein of adenylate cyclase in Albright's hereditary osteodystrophy. N Engl J Med 1990;322:1412–9.

76 Narumi S, Matsuo K, Ishii T et al. Quantitative and sensitive detection of GNAS mutations causing mccune–albright syndrome with next generation sequencing. PloS one 2013;8:e60525.

77 Ota M, Kawamura T, Ito N. Phakomatosis pigmentovascularis. Japan J Dermatol 1947;52:1–31.

78 Happle R. Phacomatosis pigmentovascularis revisited and reclassified. Arch Dermatol 2005;141:385–8.

79 Hasegawa Y, Yasuhara, M. A variant of phakomatosis pigmentovascularis. Skin Research 1979;21:178–86.

80 Almeida H, Jr., Happle R, Jr., Reginatto F, Jr. et al. Phacomatosis melanorosea with heterochromia of scalp hair. Eur J Dermatol 2011; 21:598–9.

81 Torchia D, Happle R. Segmental hypomelanosis and hypermelanosis arranged in a checkerboard pattern are distinct naevi: flag-like hypomelanotic naevus and flag-like hypermelanotic naevus. Journal of the European Academy of Dermatology and Venereology: JEADV 2015.

82 Boente Mdel C, Obeid R, Asial RA et al. Cutis tricolor coexistent with cutis marmorata telangiectatica congenita: 'phacomatosis achromico-melano-marmorata'. Eur J Dermatol 2008;18:394–6.

83 Ota M, Kawamura T, Ito N. Phakomatosis pigmentovascularis. Japan J Dermatol 1947;52:1–31.

84 Vidaurri-de la CH, Tamayo-Sanchez L, Duran-Mckinster C et al. Phakomatosis pigmentovascularis II A and II B: clinical findings in 24 patients. J.Dermatol. 2003;30:381–8.

85 Thomas AC, Zeng Z, Riviere JB et al. Mosaic Activating Mutations in GNA11 and GNAQ Are Associated with Phakomatosis Pigmentovascularis and Extensive Dermal Melanocytosis. J Invest Dermatol 2016;136(4):770–8.

86 Hall BD, Cadle RG, Morrill-Cornelius SM et al. Phakomatosis pigmentovascularis: Implications for severity with special reference to Mongolian spots associated with Sturge–Weber and Klippel–Trenaunay syndromes. Am J Med Genet Part A 2007;143A:3047–53.

87 Hasegawa Y, Yasuhara M. Phakomatosis pigmentovascularis type IVa. Arch Dermatol 1985;121:651–5.

88 Tsuruta D, Fukai K, Seto M et al. Phakomatosis pigmentovascularis type IIIb associated with moyamoya disease. Pediatr Dermatol 1999;16:35–8.

89 Polubothu S, Kinsler VA. The ethnic profile of patients with birthmarks reveals interaction of germline and postzygotic genetics. Br J Dermatol 2017;176:1385–7.

90 Teekhasaenee C, Ritch R. Glaucoma in phakomatosis pigmentovascularis. Ophthalmology 1997;104:150–7.

91 Saricaoglu MS, Guven D, Karakurt A et al. An unusual case of Sturge–Weber syndrome in association with phakomatosis pigmentovascularis and Klippel–Trenaunay–Weber syndrome. Retina 2002;22:368–71.

92 Lee CW, Choi DY, Oh YG et al. An infantile case of Sturge–Weber syndrome in association with Klippel–Trenaunay–Weber syndrome and phakomatosis pigmentovascularis. J Korean Med Sci 2005;20: 1082–4.

93 Diociaiuti A, Guidi B, Aguilar Sanchez JA et al. Phakomatosis pigmentovascularis type IIIb: a case associated with Sturge–Weber and Klippel–Trenaunay syndromes. J Am Acad Dermatol 2005;53: 536–9.

94 Shields CL, Kligman BE, Suriano M et al. Phacomatosis pigmentovascularis of cesioflammea type in 7 patients: combination of ocular pigmentation (melanocytosis or melanosis) and nevus flammeus with risk for melanoma. Arch Ophthalmol 2011;129:746–50.

95 Chen LW, Tsai YS, Lee JS et al. Extensive subarachnoid venous angiomatosis with hydrocephalus in phacomatosis pigmentovascularis. Neurology 2013;81:1020–1.

96 Bachur CD, Comi AM. Sturge–Weber syndrome. Curr Treat Options Neurol 2013;15:607–17.

97 Waelchli R, Aylett SE, Robinson K et al. New vascular classification of port-wine stains: improving prediction of Sturge–Weber risk. Br J Dermatol 2014;171:861–7.

98 Castori M, Rinaldi R, Angelo C et al. Phacomatosis cesioflammea with unilateral lipohypoplasia. Am J Med Genet Part A 2008;146A:492–5.

99 Kaur T, Sharma N, Sethi A et al. Phacomatosis cesiomarmorata with hypospadias and phacomatosis cesioflammea with Sturge–Weber syndrome, Klippel–Trenaunay syndrome and aplasia of veins – case reports with rare associations. Dermatol Online J 2015;21.

100 Jeon SY, Ha SM, Ko DY et al. Phakomatosis pigmentovascularis Ib with left-sided hemihypertrophy, interdigital gaps and scoliosis: a unique case of phakomatosis pigmentovascularis. J Dermatol 2013;40:78–9.

101 Kim HJ, Park KB, Yang JM et al. Congenital triangular alopecia in phakomatosis pigmentovascularis: report of 3 cases. Acta Dermato-Venereol 2000;80:215–6.

102 Shirley MD, Tang H, Gallione CJ et al. Sturge–Weber syndrome and port-wine stains caused by somatic mutation in GNAQ. N Engl J Med 2013;368:1971–9.

103 Cordova A. The Mongolian spot: a study of ethnic differences and a literature review. Clin Pediatr 1981;20:714–9.

104 Leung AK. Mongolian spots in Chinese children. Int J Dermatol 1988;27:106–8.

105 Onayemi O, Adejuyigbe EA, Torimiro SE et al. Prevalence of Mongolian spots in Nigerian children in Ile-Ife, Nigeria. Niger J Med 2001;10:121–3.

106 Reza AM, Farahnaz GZ, Hamideh S et al. Incidence of Mongolian spots and its common sites at two university hospitals in Tehran, Iran. Pediatr Dermatol 2010;27:397–8.

107 Goss BD, Forman D, Ansell PE et al. The prevalence and characteristics of congenital pigmented lesions in newborn babies in Oxford. Paediatr Perinat Epidemiol 1990;4:448–57.

108 Kanada KN, Merin MR, Munden A et al. A prospective study of cutaneous findings in newborns in the United States: correlation with race, ethnicity, and gestational status using updated classification and nomenclature. J Pediatr 2012;161:240–5.

109 Egemen A, Ikizoglu T, Ergor S et al. Frequency and characteristics of mongolian spots among Turkish children in Aegean region. Turkish J Pediatr 2006;48:232–6.

110 Kikuchi I, Inoue S. Natural history of the Mongolian spot. J Dermatol 1980;7:449–50.

111 Jimbow M, Jimbow K. Pigmentary disorders in oriental skin. Clin Dermatol 1989;7:11–27.

112 Gupta D, Thappa DM. Mongolian spots – a prospective study. Pediatr Dermatol 2013;30:683–8.

113 Ota M, Tanino H. Japan J Dermatol and Urology 1939;45:119.

114 Ito M. Studies on melanin XXII. Nevus fuscocaeruleus acromiodeltoideus. Tohoku J Exp Med 1954;60:10.

115 Tanyasiri K, Kono T, Groff WF et al. Mongolian spots with involvement of mandibular area. J Dermatol 2007;34:381–4.

116 Mukhopadhyay AK. Unilateral nevus of Ota with bilateral nevus of Ito and palatal lesion: a case report with a proposed clinical modification of Tanino's classification. Indian J Dermatol 2013;58:286–9.

117 Namiki T, Takahashi M, Nojima K et al. Phakomatosis pigmentovascularis type IIb: a case with Klippel–Trenaunay syndrome and extensive dermal melanocytosis as nevus of Ota, nevus of Ito and ectopic Mongolian spots. J Dermatol 2017;44:e32–e33.

118 Bashiti HM, Blair JD, Triska RA et al. Generalized dermal melanocytosis. Arch Dermatol 1981;117:791–3.

119 Velez A, Fuente C, Belinchon I et al. Congenital segmental dermal melanocytosis in an adult. Arch Dermatol 1992;128:521–5.

120 Goncharuk V, Mulvaney M, Carlson JA. Bednar tumor associated with dermal melanocytosis: melanocytic colonization or neuroectodermal multidirectional differentiation? J Cutan Pathol 2003; 30:147–51.

121 Hirayama T, Suzuki T. A new classification of Ota's nevus based on histopathological features. Dermatologica 1991;183:169–72.

122 Gupta GP, Gangwa DN. Naevus of Ota. Br J Ophthalmol 1965; 49:364–8.

123 Teekhasaenee C, Ritch R, Rutnin U et al. Ocular findings in oculodermal melanocytosis. Arch Ophthalmol 1990;108:1114–20.

124 Shields CL, Qureshi A, Mashayekhi A et al. Sector (partial) oculo(dermal) melanocytosis in 89 eyes. Ophthalmology 2011;118: 2474–9.

125 Koca MR, Rummelt V, Fahlbusch R et al. [Orbital, osseous, meningeal and cerebral findings in oculodermal melanocytosis (nevus of Ota). Clinico-histopathologic correlation in 2 patients]. Klinische Monatsblatter fur Augenheilkunde 1992;200:665–70.

126 Leung AK, Kao CP, Cho HY et al. Scleral melanocytosis and oculodermal melanocytosis (nevus of Ota) in Chinese children. J Pediatr 2000;137:581–4.

127 Kannan SK. Oculodermal melanocytosis – nevus of Ota (with palatal pigmentation). Indian J Dental Res 2003;14:230–3.

128 Guledgud MV, Patil K, Srivathsa SH et al. Report of rare palatal expression of nevus of Ota with amendment of Tanino's classification. Indian J Dental Res 2011;22:850–2.

129 Shetty SR, Subhas BG, Rao KA et al. Nevus of ota with buccal mucosal pigmentation: a rare case. Dent Res J (Isfahan) 2011;8:52–5.

130 Rathi SK. Bilateral nevus of ota with oral mucosal involvement. Indian J Dermatol Venereol Leprol 2002;68:104.

131 Sinha S, Cohen PJ, Schwartz RA. Nevus of Ota in children. Cutis 2008;82:25–9.

132 Dompmartin A, Leroy D, Labbe D et al. Dermal malignant melanoma developing from a nevus of Ota. Int J Dermatol 1989;28:535–6.

133 Shaffer D, Walker K, Weiss GR. Malignant melanoma in a Hispanic male with nevus of Ota. Dermatology 1992;185:146–50.

134 Martinez-Penuela A, Iglesias ME, Mercado MR et al. [Malignant transformation of a nevus of Ito: description of a rare case]. Actas Dermo-Sifiliograficas 2011;102:817–20.

135 Tse JY, Walls BE, Pomerantz H et al. Melanoma arising in a nevus of Ito: novel genetic mutations and a review of the literature on cutaneous malignant transformation of dermal melanocytosis. J Cutan Pathol 2016;43:57–63.

136 Hartmann LC, Oliver GF, Winkelmann RK et al. Blue nevus and nevus of Ota associated with dural melanoma. Cancer 1989;64:182–6.

137 Balmaceda CM, Fetell MR, O'Brien JL et al. Nevus of Ota and leptomeningeal melanocytic lesions. Neurology 1993;43:381–6.

138 Shields CL, Kaliki S, Livesey M et al. Association of ocular and oculodermal melanocytosis with the rate of uveal melanoma metastasis: analysis of 7872 consecutive eyes. JAMA Ophthalmol 2013;131: 993–1003.

139 Bordon AF, Wray ML, Belfort R et al. Choroidal malignant melanoma in association with oculodermal melanocytosis in a black patient. Br J Ophthalmol 1995;79:191–2.

140 Infante de German-Ribon R, Singh AD, Arevalo JF et al. Choroidal melanoma with oculodermal melanocytosis in Hispanic patients. Am J Ophthalmol 1999;128:251–3.

141 Hanson M, Lupski JR, Hicks J et al. Association of dermal melanocytosis with lysosomal storage disease: clinical features and hypotheses regarding pathogenesis. Arch Dermatol 2003;139:916–20.

142 Weissbluth M, Esterly NB, Caro WA. Report of an infant with GM1 gangliosidosis type I and extensive and unusual mongolian spots. Br J Dermatol 1981;104:195–200.

143 Rybojad M, Moraillon I, Ogier de Baulny H et al. [Extensive Mongolian spot related to Hurler disease]. Ann Dermatol Venereol 1999;126:35–7.

144 Bloch LD, Matsumoto FY, Belda W, Jr et al. Dermal melanocytosis associated with GM1-gangliosidosis type 1. Acta Dermato-Venereol 2006;86:156–8.

145 Armstrong-Javors A, Chu CJ. Child neurology: exaggerated dermal melanocytosis in a hypotonic infant: a harbinger of GM1 gangliosidosis. Neurology 2014;83:e166–8.

146 Vedak P, Sells R, De Souza A et al. Extensive and progressing congenital dermal melanocytosis leading to diagnosis of GM1 gangliosidosis. Pediatr Dermatol 2015;32:e294–5.

147 Igawa HH, Ohura T, Sugihara T et al. Cleft lip mongolian spot: mongolian spot associated with cleft lip. J Am Acad Dermatol 1994; 30:566–9.

148 Fujita Y, Yokota K, Akiyama M et al. Two cases of atypical membranous aplasia cutis with hair collar sign: one with dermal melanocytosis, and the other with naevus flammeus. Clin Exp Dermatol 2005;30:497–9.

149 Van Raamsdonk CD, Bezrookove V, Green G et al. Frequent somatic mutations of GNAQ in uveal melanoma and blue naevi. Nature 2009;457:599–602.

150 Groesser L, Herschberger E, Sagrera A et al. Phacomatosis pigmentokeratotica is caused by a postzygotic HRAS mutation in a multipotent progenitor cell. J Invest Dermatol 2013;133:1998–2003.

151 Kuentz P, Mignot C, St-Onge J et al. Postzygotic BRAF p.Lys601Asn mutation in phacomatosis pigmentokeratotica with woolly hair nevus and focal cortical dysplasia. J Invest Dermatol 2016; 136:1060–2.

152 Kinsler V, Shaw AC, Merks JH et al. The face in congenital melanocytic nevus syndrome. Am J Med Genet Part A 2012;158A: 1014–9.

153 DeDavid M, Orlow SJ, Provost N et al. A study of large congenital melanocytic nevi and associated malignant melanomas: review of cases in the New York University Registry and the world literature. J Am Acad Dermatol 1997;36:409–16.

154 Ka VS, Dusza SW, Halpern AC et al. The association between large congenital melanocytic naevi and cutaneous melanoma: preliminary findings from an Internet-based registry of 379 patients. Melanoma Res 2005;15:61–7.

155 Kinsler VA, Birley J, Atherton DJ. Great Ormond Street Hospital for Children Registry for congenital melanocytic naevi: prospective study 1988–2007. Part 1 –epidemiology, phenotype and outcomes. Br J Dermatol 2009;160:143–50.

156 Waelchli R, Aylett SE, Atherton D et al. Classification of neurological abnormalities in children with congenital melanocytic naevus syndrome identifies MRI as the best predictor of clinical outcome. Br J Dermatol 2015;173739–50.

157 Kinsler VA, Thomas AC, Ishida M et al. Multiple congenital melanocytic nevi and neurocutaneous melanosis are caused by postzygotic mutations in codon 61 of NRAS. J Invest Dermatol 2013; 133:2229–36.

158 Cai ED, Sun BK, Chiang A et al. Postzygotic mutations in beta-actin are associated with Becker's nevus and Becker's nevus syndrome. J Invest Dermatol 2017;137:1795–8.

159 Sarin KY, McNiff JM, Kwok S et al. Activating HRAS mutation in nevus spilus. J Invest Dermatol 2014;134:1766–8.

160 Happle R. Speckled lentiginous naevus: which of the two disorders do you mean? Clin Exp Dermatol 2009;34:133–5.

161 Schaffer JV, Orlow SJ, Lazova R et al. Speckled lentiginous nevus – classic congenital melanocytic nevus hybrid not the result of 'collision'. Arch Dermatol 2001;137:1655.

162 Kinsler VA, Krengel S, Riviere JB et al. Next-generation sequencing of nevus spilus-type congenital melanocytic nevus: exquisite genotype-phenotype correlation in mosaic RASopathies. J Invest Dermatol 2014;134:2658–60.

163 Zayour M, Bolognia JL, Lazova R. Multiple Spitz nevi: a clinicopathologic study of 9 patients. J Am Acad Dermatol 2012;67:451–8, 8 e1–2.

164 Sarin KY, Sun BK, Bangs CD et al. Activating HRAS mutation in agminated Spitz nevi arising in a nevus spilus. JAMA Dermatol 2013;149:1077–81.

165 Haenssle HA, Kaune KM, Buhl T et al. Melanoma arising in segmental nevus spilus: detection by sequential digital dermatoscopy. J Am Acad Dermatol 2009;61:337–41.

166 Piana S, Gelli MC, Grenzi L et al. Multifocal melanoma arising on nevus spilus. Int J Dermatol 2006;45:1380–1.

167 Zeren-Bilgin I, Gur S, Aydin O et al. Melanoma arising in a hairy nevus spilus. Int J Dermatol 2006;45:1362–4.

168 Abecassis S, Spatz A, Cazeneuve C et al. [Melanoma within naevus spilus: 5 cases]. Ann Dermatol Venereol 2006;133:323–8.

169 Livory M, Descamps V, Pelletier F et al. [Melanoma in invisible naevus spilus]. Ann Dermatol Venereol 2008;135:48–52.

170 Meguerditchian AN, Cheney RT, Kane JM, 3rd. Nevus spilus with synchronous melanomas: case report and literature review. J Cutan Med Surg 2009;13:96–101.

171 Corradin MT, Zattra E, Fiorentino R et al. Nevus spilus and melanoma: case report and review of the literature. J Cutan Med Surg 2010;14:85–9.

172 Angit C, Khirwadkar N, Azurdia RM. Malignant melanoma arising in a nevus spilus. Dermatol Online J 2011;17:10.

173 Karam SL, Jackson SM. Malignant melanoma arising within nevus spilus. Skinmed 2012;10:100–2.

174 Corradin MT, Giulioni E, Fiorentino R et al. In situ malignant melanoma on nevus spilus in an elderly patient. Acta Dermatovenerol Alp Pannonica Adriat 2014;23:17–9.

175 Lee HS, Chun YS, Hann SK. Nevus depigmentosus: clinical features and histopathologic characteristics in 67 patients. J Am Acad Dermatol 1999;40:21–6.

176 Dhar S, Kanwar AJ, Ghosh S. Leucotrichia in nevus depigmentosus. Pediatr Dermatol 1993;10:198–9.

177 Gupta N, Shenoi SD. Nevus depigmentosus with segmental vitiligo. Indian J Dermatol Venereol Leprol 1999;65:152–3.

178 Hwang SW, Kang JH, Jung SY et al. Vitiligo coexistent with nevus depigmentosus: this was treated with narrow-band UVB and these lesions were followed using the Mexameter(R), a pigment-measuring device. Ann Dermatol 2010;22:482–5.
179 Chokoeva A, Wollina U, Lotti T et al. Nevus depigmentosus associated with nevus spilus: first report in the world literature. Georgian Med News 2015:73–6.
180 Yamamoto T, Hirano M, Ueda K. Eccrine angiomatous hamartoma in a patient with nevus depigmentosus and nevus spilus. Indian J Dermatol 2017;62:99–100.
181 Singh N, Chandrashekar L, Thappa DM et al. Nevus depigmentosus and nevus of Ito: pigmentary twin spotting. Int J Dermatol 2014; 53:1005–7.
182 Baba M, Akcali C, Seckin D et al. Segmental lentiginosis with ipsilateral nevus depigmentosus: another example of twin spotting? Eur J Dermatol 2002;12:319–21.
183 Jagia R, Mendiratt V, Koranne RV et al. Colocalized nevus depigmentosus and lentigines with underlying breast hypoplasia: a case of reverse mutation? Dermatol Online J 2004;10:12.
184 In SI, Kang HY. Partial unilateral lentiginosis colocalized with naevus depigmentosus. Clin Exp Dermatol 2008;33:337–9.
185 Dippel E, Utikal J, Feller G et al. Nevi flammei affecting two contralateral quadrants and nevus depigmentosus: a new type of phacomatosis pigmentovascularis? Am J Med Genet Part A 2003;119A:228–30.
186 Afsar FS, Aktas S, Ortac R. Becker's naevus and segmental naevus depigmentosus: an example of twin spotting? Australas J Dermatol 2007;48:224–6.
187 Taniguchi S, Tsuruta D, Higashi J et al. Coexistence of generalized milia and naevus depigmentosus. Br J Dermatol 1995;132:317–8.
188 Ogunbiyi AO, Ogunbiyi JO. Nevus depigmentosus and inflammatory linear epidermal nevus – an unusual combination with a note on histology. Int J Dermatol 1998;37:600–2.
189 Paul M, Shenoi SD. CNS abnormality in nevus depigmentosus. Indian J Dermatol Venereol Leprol 1999;65:40–1.
190 Di Lernia V. Segmental nevus depigmentosus: analysis of 20 patients. Pediatr Dermatol 1999;16:349–53.
191 Dawn G, Dhar S, Handa S et al. Nevus depigmentosus associated with hemihypertrophy of the limbs. Pediatr Dermatol 1995;12:286–7.
192 Jimbow K, Fitzpatrick TB, Szabo G et al. Congenital circumscribed hypomelanosis: a characterization based on electron microscopic study of tuberous sclerosis, nevus depigmentosus, and piebaldism. J Invest Dermatol 1975;64:50–62.
193 Xu AE, Huang B, Li YW et al. Clinical, histopathological and ultrastructural characteristics of naevus depigmentosus. Clin Exp Dermatol 2008;33:400–5.
194 Dippel E, Haas N, Grabbe J et al. Expression of the c-kit receptor in hypomelanosis: a comparative study between piebaldism, naevus depigmentosus and vitiligo. Br J Dermatol 1995;132:182–9.
195 Hardin J, Behm A, Haber RM. Mosaic generalized neurofibromatosis 1: report of two cases. J Cutan Med Surg 2014;18:271–4.
196 Ruggieri M, Huson SM. The clinical and diagnostic implications of mosaicism in the neurofibromatoses. Neurology 2001;56: 1433–43.
197 Colman SD, Rasmussen SA, Ho VT et al. Somatic mosaicism in a patient with neurofibromatosis type 1. Am J Hum Genet 1996; 58:484–90.
198 Tinschert S, Naumann I, Stegmann E et al. Segmental neurofibromatosis is caused by somatic mutation of the neurofibromatosis type 1 (NF1) gene. Eur J Hum Genet 2000;8:455–9.
199 Maertens O, De Schepper S, Vandesompele J et al. Molecular dissection of isolated disease features in mosaic neurofibromatosis type 1. Am J Hum Genet 2007;81:243–51.
200 Vazquez-Osorio I, Duat-Rodriguez A, Garcia-Martinez FJ et al. Cutaneous and systemic findings in mosaic neurofibromatosis type 1. Pediatr Dermatol 2017;34:271–6.
201 Lara-Corrales I, Moazzami M, Garcia-Romero MT et al. Mosaic neurofibromatosis type 1 in children: a single-institution experience. J Cutan Med Surg 2017;21:379–82.
202 Garcia-Romero MT, Parkin P, Lara-Corrales I. Mosaic neurofibromatosis type 1: a systematic review. Pediatr Dermatol 2016;33:9–17.
203 Pascual-Castroviejo I, Pascual-Pascual SI, Velazquez-Fragua R et al. [Segmental neurofibromatosis in children. Presentation of 43 patients]. Rev Neurol 2008;47:399–403.
204 Ejerskov C, Farholt S, Skovby F et al. Clinical presentations of 23 half-siblings from a mosaic neurofibromatosis type 1 sperm donor. Clin Genet 2016;89:346–50.

CHAPTER 110
Differential Diagnosis of Skin Nodules and Cysts

Susanne Abraham[1] *& Peter H. Hoeger*[2]

[1] Department of Dermatology, Medical Faculty Carl-Gustav-Carus, Technical University of Dresden, Dresden, Germany
[2] Department of Paediatric Dermatology, Catholic Children's Hospital Wilhelmstift, Hamburg, Germany

Differential diagnosis, 1313
Individual skin tumours, 1316
Nonvascular nodules and cysts, 1316
Vascular neoplasms, 1322

Abstract

The occurrence of nodules and cysts in a child is often a matter of great concern to the parents because of the threat of malignancy. Fortunately, malignancy is very rare in childhood. Although it is often difficult to make a diagnosis based on clinical grounds alone, and most if not all lumps that do not resolve spontaneously over time will eventually be excised, it is helpful to limit the wide range of possible diagnoses using clinical criteria. In this chapter the differential diagnosis of nonvascular nodules such as pilomatricoma, dermatofibroma and granular cell tumour is discussed. Skin cysts are very common; epidermal and trichilemmal cysts, dermoid cysts and eruptive vellus hair cysts are also elucidated. Finally, the clinical features and the recommended treatment of vascular neoplasms such as pyogenic granuloma and glomus tumour are discussed.

Key points

- The occurrence of nodules and cysts in a child is often a matter of great concern to the parents because of the threat of malignancy. Fortunately, malignancy is very rare in childhood.
- Pilomatricoma is a benign tumour of hair matrix cells that does not regress spontaneously.
- Following trauma (insect bites, excoriations), dermatofibroma, also known as histiocytoma, represents a benign proliferation of oval cells resembling histiocytes, and of spindle-shaped cells resembling fibroblasts in the dermis. Usually no treatment is necessary.
- Epidermal cysts are common intradermal or subcutaneous tumours that grow slowly and occur on the face, neck, back and scrotum. Trichilemmal cysts are clinically indistinguishable from epidermal cysts but are less common in children. They are mainly located on the scalp.
- Dermoid cysts are present at birth, mainly on the head, and arise from entrapment of skin along the lines of embryonic fusion. In the case of dermoid cysts located on the anterior or posterior midline, magnetic resonance imaging should be performed before surgical therapy.
- Eruptive vellus hair cysts are characterized by the occlusion and cystic dilation of vellus hair follicles. Eruptive vellus hair cysts are a benign condition. Some may resolve spontaneously, but most tend to persist for many years.
- The term 'granular cell tumour', also known as Abricosoff tumour, comprises a variety of rare dermal tumours with nerve sheath-like features: granular nerve cell sheath tumour (GNCST), malignant granular cell tumour and granular cell epulis of infancy. Granular nerve cell sheath tumours are locally invasive; malignant granular cell tumours very seldom are.
- Pyogenic granuloma is a common benign proliferative vascular tumour of the skin and mucous membranes that often follows a minor injury or infection. Pyogenic granulomas persist without treatment and tend to bleed.
- Glomus tumours are rare benign vascular neoplasms usually found on hands, forearm or feet. They are tender and persist without treatment.

Differential diagnosis

A nodule is a solid circumscribed mass with a diameter of more than 5 mm in infants and more than 10 mm in older children. A cyst is a hollow mass that is surrounded by an epithelium-lined wall and is well demarcated from the adjacent tissue. It may or may not contain serous liquid. Vesicles, pustules and bullae, by contrast, do not have a complete epithelial lining and are therefore less well demarcated.

The occurrence of nodules and cysts in a child is often a matter of great concern to the parents because of the threat of malignancy. Fortunately, malignancy is very rare in childhood. The histological diagnoses of a series of 775 superficial lumps excised in children are listed in Table 110.1 [1].

Although it is often difficult to make a diagnosis based on clinical grounds alone, and most if not all lumps that do not resolve spontaneously over time will eventually be excised, it is helpful to limit the wide range of possible

Harper's Textbook of Pediatric Dermatology, Fourth Edition. Edited by Peter Hoeger, Veronica Kinsler and Albert Yan.

Table 110.1 Histological diagnoses of 775 superficial lumps excised in children

Histological diagnosis	Number per diagnosis	Total number per group	Percent of all lesions
Squamous epithelial cysts		459	59
Presumed post-traumatic epithelial implantation	38		
Uncertain aetiology, most probably congenital	421		
Congenital malformations		117	15
Pilomatricoma	79		
Lymphangioma/haemolymphangioma	22		
Branchial cleft/cyst without sinus	10		
Juvenile haemangioendothelioma	5		
Other hamartoma	1		
Benign neoplasms		56	7
Neurofibroma, neurolemmoma	27		
Lipoma, angiolipoma	25		
Sweat gland tumour	2		
Other benign tumours	2		
Lesions of ill-defined aetiology		50	6
Xanthoma, xanthogranuloma	18		
Aggressive fibromatosis; recurrent digital fibromas	15		
Fibroma	12		
Histiocytoma	5		
Probably self-limited processes		47	6
Pseudo-rheumatoid nodules and granuloma annulare	22		
Urticaria pigmentosa	17		
Persistent insect bite reaction	8		
Malignant tumours		11	1.4
Rhabdomyosarcoma	5		
Neurofibrosarcoma	1		
Fibrosarcoma	2		
Malignant fibrous histiocytoma	1		
Malignant pleomorphic adenoma	1		
Basal cell carcinoma	1		
Miscellaneous lesions		35	4
Pseudo-sarcomatous lesions (myositis ossificans, degenerating schwannoma)	3		
Granular cell myoblastoma	8		
Traumatic neuroma	1		
Miscellaneous cysts without epithelial lining			
Sterile abscess, organizing haematoma, etc.	23		

Source: Adapted from Knight and Reiner (1983) [1].

diagnoses using clinical criteria. Criteria that may serve this purpose are:

1 Age of onset;
2 Location and distribution of the lesion;
3 Colour of the lesion (Table 110.2);
4 Surface appearance of the lesion (Table 110.3); and
5 Texture of the lesion (Table 110.4) [2].

In addition to these criteria, tenderness (Box 110.1) and itchiness (Box 110.2) are important features that are associated with certain lesions.

Sometimes imaging modalities are necessary as further diagnostic methods [3]. Ultrasound is widely available, noninvasive and performed without radiation and without the need for sedation. However, ultrasound is highly user dependent. Further imaging modalities such as plain radiography, computed tomography and magnetic resonance imaging are essential only in a few cases.

See also Table 110.5 for the differential diagnosis of most common skin papules and cysts in childhood.

References

1 Knight PJ, Reiner CB. Superficial lumps in children: what, when, and why? Pediatrics 1983;72:147–53.
2 Price HN, Zaenglein AL. Diagnosis and management of benign lumps and bumps in childhood. Curr Opin Pediatr 2007;19:420–4.
3 Morrow MS, Oliveira AM. Imaging of lumps and bumps in pediatric patients: an algorithm for appropriate imaging and pictorial review. Semin Ultrasound CT MR 2014;35:415–29.

Table 110.2 Differential diagnosis of cutaneous lumps by colour

Colour	Lesion
Blue	Cavernous haemangioma Pigmented histiocytoma/dermatofibroma Angiokeratoma Blue rubber bleb naevus Glomus tumour Pilomatricoma Eccrine/apocrine hidrocystoma
Red	Folliculitis/furunculosis/carbunculosis, abscess Pyogenic granuloma Haemangioma Spitz naevus Erythema nodosum Keloid Acne conglobata Langerhans cell histiocytosis Leukaemia cutis Leishmaniasis Merkel cell tumour Atypical mycobacteriosis
Yellowish	Xanthelasma Xanthoma Juvenile xanthogranuloma Xanthomatized histiocytoma Langerhans cell histiocytosis Naevus lipomatosus Epidermal, follicular cysts Scrotal cyst/calcinosis Disseminated lipogranulomatosis (Farber) Nodular amyloidosis
Brown	Melanocytic naevus Epidermal naevus Malignant melanoma Mastocytoma Dermatofibrosarcoma protuberans Deep mycoses
Black	Melanocytic naevus Pigmented dermatofibroma Thrombosed haemangioma Malignant melanoma
Skin-coloured	Dermoid Granuloma annulare Dermal melanocytic naevus Neurofibroma Fibroma Lipoma Epidermal follicular cyst Steatocystoma
Translucent nodules	Giant molluscum contagiosum Syringoma Apocrine/eccrine hidrocystoma Trichoepithelioma

Table 110.3 Differential diagnosis of cutaneous lumps by surface appearance

Surface	Lesion
Indented	Large molluscum contagiosum Giant comedo Keratoacanthoma
Exophytic	(Filiform) verruca vulgaris Fibroma Pyogenic granuloma
Erosive/ulcerated	Leishmaniasis Pyogenic granuloma Ecthyma contagiosum (milker's nodule) Atypical mycobacteriosis Malignant melanoma Furunculosis/carbunculosis Cutaneous tuberculosis Mycetoma Chromomycosis Cryptococcosis Blastomycosis Sporotrichosis Necrobiotic xanthogranuloma

Table 110.4 Differential diagnosis of cutaneous lumps by texture

Texture	Lesion
Hard	Exostosis Osteoma cutis Calcinosis cutis Chondroma Pilomatricoma
Firm	Dermatofibroma Keloid Prurigo nodularis Fibroma Dermoid Fibrosarcoma Trichoepithelioma Rheumatoid nodule Syringoma Angiofibroma Lymphangioma Juvenile xanthogranuloma Histiocytosis Leukaemia cutis Neuroblastoma Lymphoma
Soft	Lipoma Neurofibroma Angiolipoma Connective tissue naevus
Keratotic	Verruca vulgaris Condyloma acuminatum Angiokeratoma
Cystic	Follicular cyst Epidermoid Dermoid Steatocystoma multiplex Milia

Box 110.1 Skin lumps that may be tender/painful

Glomus tumour
Granular cell tumour
Blue rubber bleb naevus
Eccrine spiradenoma
Neurofibroma
Angiolipoma, leiomyoma
Foreign body granuloma
Clavus (corn)
Erythema nodosum
Superficial thrombophlebitis
Thrombosis within a haemangioma

Box 110.2 Skin lumps that are itchy

Prurigo
Insect bites
Scabetic nodule
Mastocytoma

Individual skin tumours

The many different individual skin nodules and cysts are described in the relevant chapters. The following are covered in detail in this chapter.

Nonvascular nodules and cysts

Pilomatricoma (also pilomatrixoma)

Definition. Pilomatricoma, also known as trichomatricoma and previously referred to as calcifying epithelioma of Malherbe, is a benign tumour of hair matrix cells. Pilomatricomas are thought to be the second most common superficial tumour to be removed in children [1]. Although they show typical features, such as the rock-hard appearance, the clinical accuracy of primary care physicians in diagnosing a pilomatricoma is low [1].

Pathogenesis. The tumour is derived from immature hair matrix cells. It shows evidence of keratinization and frequently (75%) undergoes calcification. Histopathology reveals a sharply demarcated, frequently encapsulated tumour in the lower dermis, embedded in islands of epithelial cells. Among these, basophilic and shadow cells can be recognized [2]. Chan et al. [3] identified activating mutations of β-catenin in a high percentage of pilomatricomas. The cytological features of pilomatricomas seem to be characteristic and allow a conclusive diagnosis bearing in mind the diagnostic traps that can mislead a cytopathologist [4].

Clinical features. Pilomatricomas are firm, solitary, asymptomatic papules or nodules in the dermis or subcutaneous tissue covered by normal skin (Fig. 110.1). If more superficially located, they can appear with a blue–red discolouration. A rare variant with a bullous appearance was reported [5]; pigmented pilomatricoma can also occur [6]. The nodules typically measure 0.2–5.2 cm in diameter with an average diameter of 1.4 cm [7]. Pilomatricomas are mainly located on the head and neck (50–55%), on the upper extremities (25–30%) and, rarely (15–25%), on the trunk and legs. Most cases (60%) occur in childhood and adolescence, and two thirds of these occur before the age of 10 years. There is a 2 : 1 female preponderance [1,8]. Multiple and familial cases are rare [9,10]. The presence of multiple pilomatricomas has been reported in association with Gardner syndrome [10], myotonic dystrophy [10,11], Turner syndrome [12], Rubinstein–Taybi syndrome [13], familial Sotos syndrome [14] and *MYH*-positive familial adenomatous polyposis [15]. Possible associations also have been reported in sarcoidosis, HIV and trisomy 9 [16,17].

Course and prognosis. Most pilomatricomas increase slowly in size; some cease to grow at a small size, whereas others can occasionally grow up to a size of 15 cm [8]. They can rupture spontaneously and discharge a chalky material. Haemorrhage within a pilomatricoma can lead to rapid enlargement of a blue–red tumour. Pilomatrix carcinoma, a malignant variant of pilomatricoma, is extremely rare; it occurs at an average age of 45 years and more commonly in men, but has also been reported in children [18,19]. Pilomatrix carcinoma was mainly reported to develop in large pilomatricomas that had been present for years. It shows locally aggressive (invasive) growth and tends to recur if excised incompletely. Pulmonary metastasis can occur [18,19].

Treatment. Since pilomatricomas do not spontaneously regress, surgical excision is the treatment of choice. Incomplete excision may lead to local recurrence [1,20].

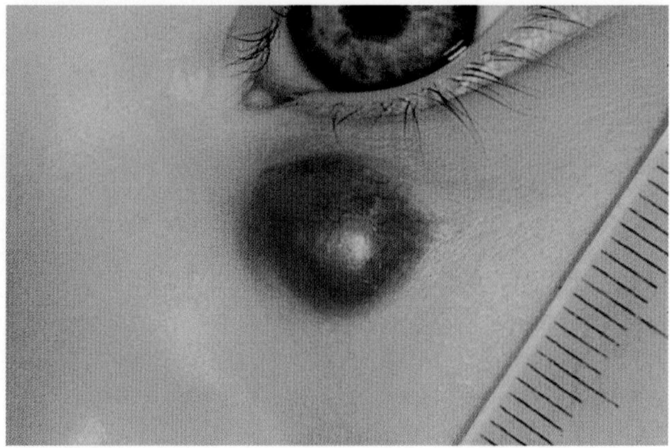

Fig. 110.1 Pilomatricoma.

Table 110.5 Differential diagnosis of most common skin papules and cysts in childhood

	Mastocytoma (see Chapter 92)	Pilomatricoma	Juvenile xanthogranuloma (see Chapter 91)	Dermatofibroma	Epidermal cyst	Pyogenic granuloma	Spitz naevus (see Chapter 105)
Synonym	Mast cell tumour	Former name: epithelioma calcificans Malherbe	Naevo-xanthoendothelioma, xanthoma multiplex, juvenile xanthoma	Histiocytoma, benign fibrous histiocytoma, sclerosing haemangioma	Epithelial or infundibular cysts	Lobular capillary haemangioma	Pigmented variant: Reed naevus
Clinical findings	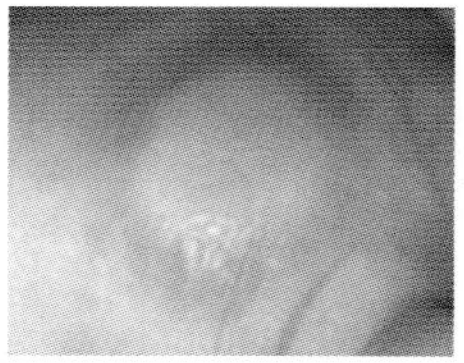	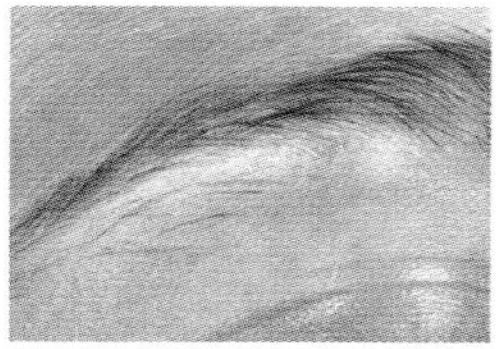	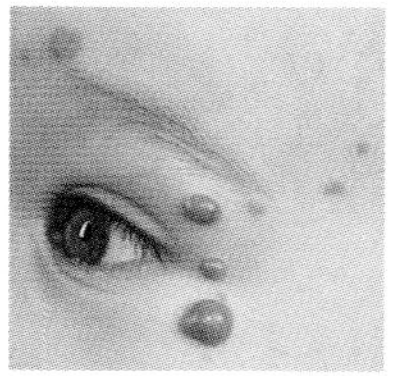	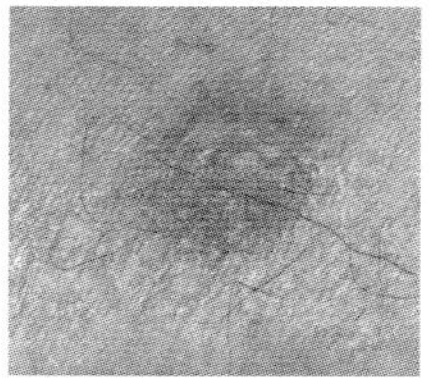	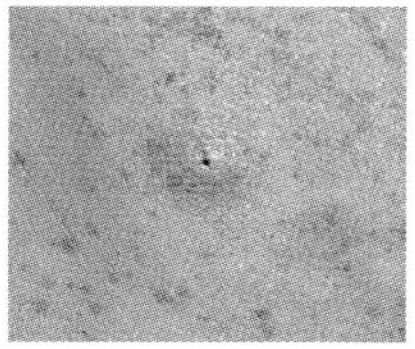	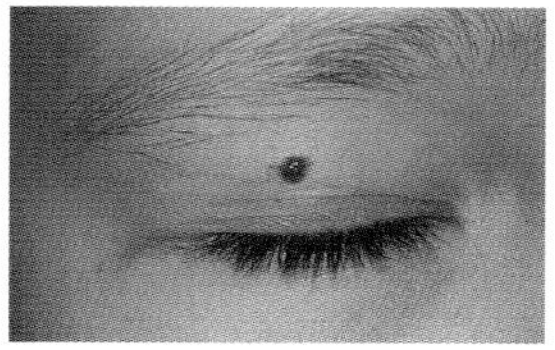	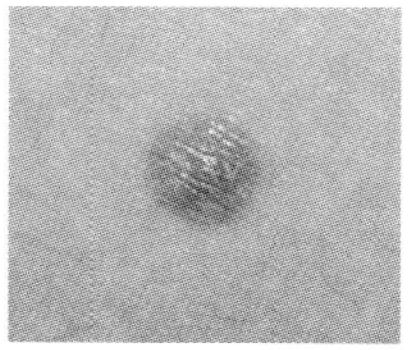
Localization	Whole integument	Head, neck, upper extremities	Face, chest	Limbs	Face, neck, back and scrotum	Skin and mucous membranes; most often on the head and upper limbs	Face
Age	Infancy	Childhood/adolescence	Infancy	Young adults, possible at any age	Around puberty, possible at any age	Often in childhood <5 years, in all ages	Childhood
Occurrence	Common	Multiple appearance: association with syndrome possible	Multiple appearance: ophthalmological control recommended	Very common	Sometimes autosomal dominant trait	Common	Sudden appearance
Course	Spontaneous regression	No spontaneous regression	Spontaneous regression	Remain unchanged for years	Rupture of cysts possible	No regression; frequently recurs after treatment	Grows rapidly for a few months
Treatment	No treatment	Excision	No treatment	Excision if unclear	Complete extirpation of proliferationg cysts and if the cysts are cosmetically impairing	Shave excision or coagulation	Complete excision if diagnosis is clinically unclear

References

1 Price HN, Zaenglein AL. Diagnosis and management of benign lumps and bumps in childhood. Curr Opin Pediatr 2007;19:420–4.

2 Klein W, Chan E, Seykora JT. Tumors of the epidermal appendages. In: Elder D, Elenitsas R, Johnson BL et al. (eds) Lever's Histopathology of the Skin, 9th edn. Philadelphia: Lippincott-Raven, 2005:867–926.

3 Chan EF, Gat U, McNiff JM et al. A common human skin tumour is caused by activating mutations in beta-catenin. Nat Genet 1999;21:410–13.

4 Bansal C, Handa U, Mohan H. Fine needle aspiration cytology of pilomatrixoma. J Cytol 2011;28:1–6.

5 DiGiorgio CM, Kaskas NM, Matherne RJ et al. Bullous pilomatricoma: a rarely reported variant of pilomatricoma. Dermatol Online J 2015;21.

6 Ishida M, Okabe H. Pigmented pilomatricoma: an underrecognized variant. Int J Clin Exp Pathol 2013;6:1890–3.

7 Kwon D, Grekov K, Krishnan M, Dyleski R. Characteristics of pilomatrixoma in children: a review of 137 patients. Int J Pediatr Otorhinolaryngol 2014;78:1337–41.

8 Agarwal RP, Handler SD, Matthews MR et al. Pilomatrixoma of the head and neck in children. Otolaryngol Head Neck Surg 2001;125:510–15.

9 Pujol RM, Casanova JM, Egido R et al. Multiple familial pilomatricomas: a cutaneous marker for Gardner syndrome? Pediatr Dermatol 1995;12:331–5.

10 Chan JJ, Tey HL. Multiple pilomatricomas: case presentation and review of the literature. Dermatol Online J 2010;16:4.

11 Schwartz BK, Peraza JE. Pilomatricoma associated with muscular dystrophy. J Am Acad Dermatol 1987;16:887–9.

12 Noguchi H, Kayashima K, Nishiyama S et al. Two cases of pilomatricoma in Turner's syndrome. Dermatology 1999;199:338–40.

13 Cambiaghi S, Ermacora E, Brusasco A et al. Multiple pilomatricomas in Rubinstein–Taybi syndrome: a case report. Pediatr Dermatol 1994;11:21–5.

14 Gilaberte Y, Ferrer-Lozano M, Oliván MJ et al. Multiple giant pilomatricoma in familial Sotos syndrome. Pediatr Dermatol 2008;25:122–5.

15 Baglioni S, Melean G, Gensini F et al. A kindred with MYH-associated polyposis and pilomatricomas. Am J Medical Genet A 2005;134:212–14.

16 Matsuura H, Hatamochi A, Nakamura Y et al. Multiple pilomatricomas in trisomy 9. Dermatology 2002;204:82–3.

17 Blaya B, Gonzalez-Hermosa, Hardeazabal J et al. Multiple pilomatricomas in association with trisomy 9. Pediatr Dermatol 2009;26:482–4.

18 Sau P, Lupton GP, Graham JH. Pilomatrix carcinoma. Cancer 1993;71:2491–8.

19 Herrmann JL, Allan A, Trapp KM, Morgan MB. Pilomatrix carcinoma: 13 new cases and review of the literature with emphasis on predictors of metastasis. J Am Acad Dermatol 2014;71:38–43.

20 Yencha MW. Head and neck pilomatricoma in the pediatric age group: a retrospective study and literature review. Int J Pediatr Otorhinolaryngol 2001;57:123–8.

Dermatofibroma

Definition. Dermatofibroma, also known as histiocytoma, benign fibrous histiocytoma or sclerosing haemangioma, represents a benign proliferation of oval cells resembling histiocytes, and of spindle-shaped cells resembling fibroblasts in the dermis. It occurs at any age and is the most common cutaneous neoplasm in adults [1,2]. There is an ongoing debate whether dermatofibromas represent clonal proliferation or are brought about by a reactive inflammatory process [3].

Pathogenesis. Following trauma (insect bites, excoriations), a proliferation of fibroblastic spindle cells and histiocytic cells is observed in the dermis, and this is accompanied by excessive deposition of collagen and pronounced hyperplasia of the overlying epidermis [1].

Clinical features. Dermatofibromas are firm, indolent, single or multiple dermal nodules (Fig. 110.2). They are most frequently located on the limbs, shoulder and pelvic girdles, although they can occur anywhere; 0.5% of dermatofibromas are found on a digit [4]. The size usually does not exceed 5 mm, but they can occasionally measure up to 2–3 cm in diameter (Fig. 110.3) and rarely 'giant' lesions (>5 cm in diameter) can be observed. Dermatofibromas are mostly red or red–brown but can also be blue–black when haemosiderin is deposited within the tumour. The characteristic 'dimple sign' can be induced by squeezing the overlying epidermis; it is attributable to tethering of the epidermis to the underlying lesion. Dermatofibromas are most common in young adults and are only occasionally seen in children. Multiple dermatofibromas are not uncommon [5]. Eruptive variants have been described in familial cases [6] and in immunocompromised patients (human

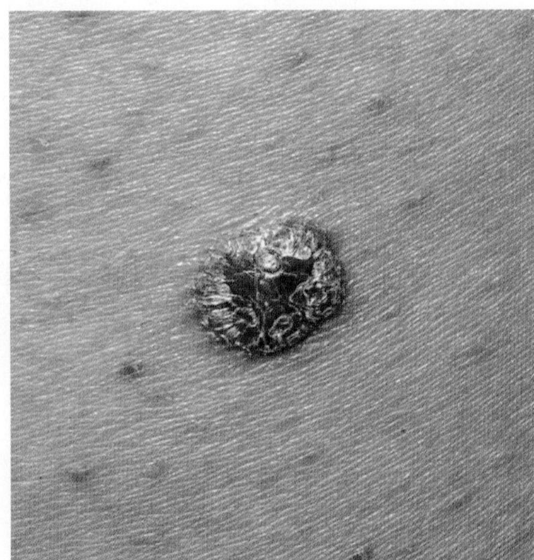

Fig. 110.2 Dermatofibroma.

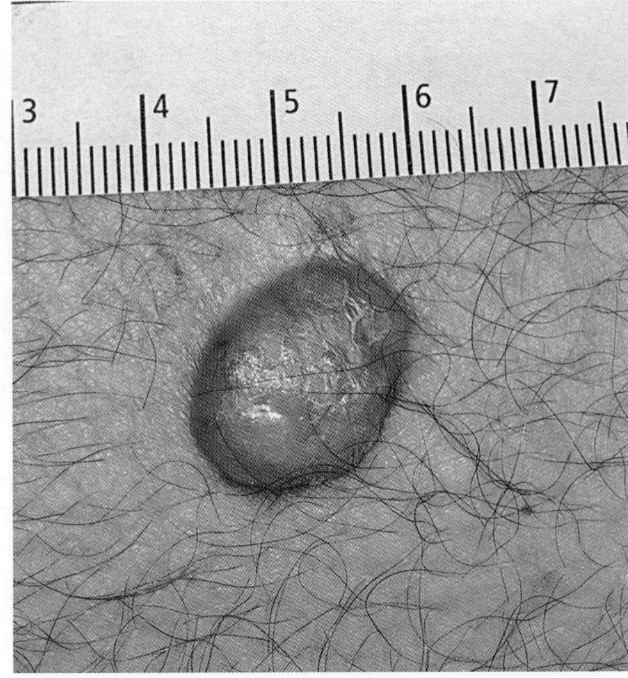

Fig. 110.3 Dermatofibroma.

immunodeficiency virus [HIV], systemic lupus erythematosus, malignancy) [7]. Multiple clustered dermatofibroma is a distinct entity and occurs in healthy individuals of both sexes in the first to third decades on the lower half of the body [8].

Course and prognosis. After an initial period of enlargement the lesions tend to remain unchanged for years.

Treatment. Usually no treatment is required, but excision may be indicated for cosmetic or diagnostic reasons as in some cases the differential diagnosis from other papular lesions can be difficult.

References

1 **Li D-F, Iwasaki H, Kikuchi M et al. Dermatofibroma: superficial fibrous proliferation with reactive histiocytes – a multiple immunostaining analysis. Cancer 1994;74:66–73.**
2 Tardío JC, Azorín D, Hernández-Núñez A et al. Dermatomyofibromas presenting in pediatric patients: clinicopathologic characteristics and differential diagnosis. J Cutan Pathol 2011;38:967–72.
3 Calonje E. Dermatofibroma (fibrous histiocytoma): an inflammatory or neoplastic disease? Histopathology 2001;39:213.
4 Lehmer LM, Ragsdale BD. Digital dermatofibromas – common lesion, uncommon location: A series of 26 cases and review of the literature. Dermatol Online J 2011;17.
5 **Gonzáles S, Duarte I. Benign fibrous histiocytoma of the skin: a morphologic study of 290 cases. Pathol Res 1982;174:379–91.**
6 Yazici AC, Baz K, Ikizoglu G et al. Familial eruptive dermatofibromas in atopic dermatitis. J Eur Acad Dermatol Venereol 2006;20:90–2.
7 **Niiyama S, Katsuoka K, Happle R et al. Multiple eruptive dermatofibromas: a review of the literature. Acta Derm Venereol 2002;82:241–4.**
8 Gershtenson PC, Krunic AL, Chen HM. Multiple clustered dermatofibroma: case report and review of the literature. J Cutan Pathol 2010;37:e42–5.

Epidermal and trichilemmal cysts

Definition. Epidermal cysts, also known as epithelial or infundibular cysts, are common intradermal or subcutaneous tumours that grow slowly and occur on the face, neck, back and scrotum (Fig. 110.4). Trichilemmal cysts, also referred to as pilar cysts, are clinically indistinguishable from epidermal cysts but less common in children. They can occur as sporadic lesions or in hereditary-familial settings with autosomal dominant transmission [1]. Trichilemmal cysts are mainly (>90%) located on the scalp

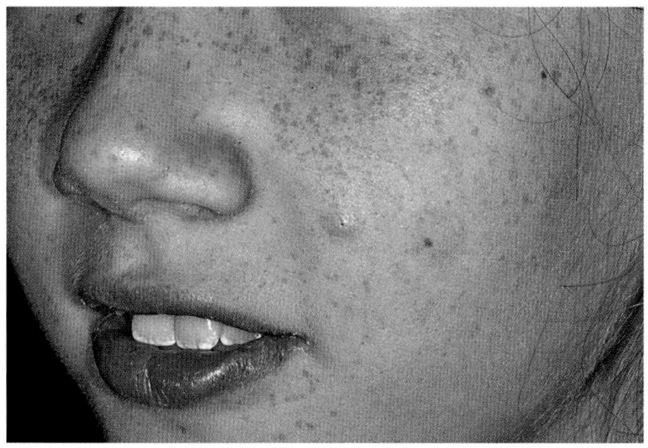

Fig. 110.4 Epidermal cyst.

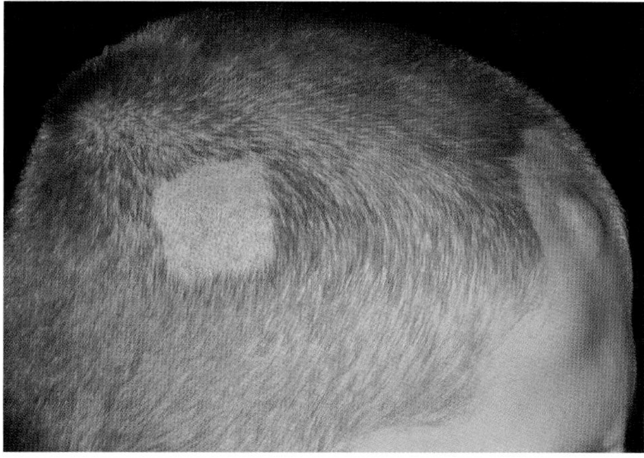

Fig. 110.5 Trichilemmal cysts.

(Fig. 110.5); they were formerly called sebaceous cysts but contain keratinous rather than sebaceous material.

Pathogenesis. Epidermal cysts result from the proliferation of epidermal cells within the dermis. These are derived from either the skin surface or the infundibular section of the hair follicle. Epidermal cysts arise from occluded pilosebaceous ducts or, in nonfollicular regions such as the palms and soles, from traumatic engulfment of epidermal cells. Whereas the wall of the epidermal cyst conserves the epidermal layers, the wall of the trichilemmal cysts, which arise from the external root sheath, shows palisading of unlayered epithelial cells. Homogeneous horny material that is further degraded to fat and cholesterol forms within both types of cysts.

Clinical features. The cysts are nontender, round and firm, but slightly compressible, intradermal or subcutaneous nodules measuring 0.5–5 cm in diameter. They usually appear at or around puberty. Epidermal cysts are solitary (or few); sometimes a central pore can be seen [2]. The presence of a pore in a subcutaneous nodule allows the diagnosis of epidermal cyst to be made [3]. In the autosomal dominant Gardner syndrome with almost complete penetrance, numerous large epidermal cysts of the skin and adenomatous polyposis of the gastrointestinal tract are observed [4]. Trichilemmal cysts are usually multiple and are often inherited as an autosomal dominant trait [5]. A case of multiple blaschkolinear trichilemmal cysts associated with filiform hyperkeratosis and termed trichilemmal cyst naevus has been described [6].

Course and prognosis. Rupture of the cyst and release of its contents into the epidermis leads to an inflammatory foreign body reaction (keratin granuloma). Focal calcification is seen in 25% of trichilemmal cysts. Malignant transformation (basal cell epithelioma, squamous cell carcinoma, Bowen disease) has rarely been observed [7].

Treatment. In proliferating cysts and if the cysts cause cosmetic impairment, complete extirpation is necessary.

References

1 **Seidenari S, Pellacani G, Nasti S et al. Hereditary trichilemmal cysts: a proposal for the assessment of diagnostic clinical criteria. Clin Genet 2013;84:65–9.**
2 **Solanki A, Narang S, Kathpalia R, Goel A. Scrotal calcinosis: pathogenetic link with epidermal cyst. BMJ Case Rep 2015;23.**
3 Ghigliotti G, Cinotti E, Parodi A. Usefulness of dermoscopy for the diagnosis of epidermal cyst: the 'pore' sign. Clin Exp Dermatol 2014;39:649–50.
4 Cristofaro MG, Giudice A, Amantea M et al. Gardner's syndrome: a clinical and genetic study of a family. Oral Surg Oral Med Oral Pathol Oral Radiol 2013;115:e1–6.
5 **Kirkham N. Tumours and cysts of the epidermis. In: Elder D, Elenitsas R, Johnson BL et al. (eds) Lever's Histopathology of the Skin, 9th edn. Philadelphia: Lippincott-Raven, 2005:805–66.**
6 Tantcheva-Poor I, Reinhold K, Krieg T et al. Trichilemmal cyst nevus: a new complex organoid epidermal nevus. J Am Acad Dermatol 2007;57:572–5.
7 Haas N, Audring H, Sterry W. Carcinoma arising in a proliferating trichilemmal cyst expresses fetal and trichilemmal hair phenotype. Am J Dermatopathol 2002;24:340–4.

Dermoid cysts

Definition. Dermoid cysts are congenital subcutaneous cysts.

Pathogenesis. Dermoid cysts arise from entrapment of skin along the lines of embryonic fusion. Unlike epidermal cysts, dermoid cysts are therefore hamartomas and often contain various adnexal structures (hair, sebaceous, eccrine or apocrine glands) and, rarely, other tissues such as bone, teeth and nerves.

Clinical features. At birth, indolent, firm, deep, subcutaneous nodules are observed mainly on the head, especially periorbitally (Fig. 110.6), most commonly in the area of the anterolateral frontozygomatic suture [1] as well as the parieto-occipital scalp, and neck, and rarely in the anogenital area. The incidence of midline frontonasal dermoid cysts is one in 20 000 to one in 40 000 [2]. Dermoid cysts are slowly progressive and can grow to a size of 1–4 cm. Dermoid cysts on the scalp are often adherent to the periosteum, or form a bulging mass over the anterior fontanelle [3].

Course and prognosis. Dermoid cysts remain stable for years, but they can become symptomatic as a result of enlargement and rupture or, more rarely, as a result of extension into surrounding tissues [4]. Untreated dermoid cysts persist and can later grow. Malignant transformation is extremely rare [5,6]. Midline frontonasal dermoid cysts can be connected to underlying structures, communicate with the ventricular system or represent brain tissue (encephalocoele) [7]. This is explained by the anatomy and embryology of nasofrontal development [2]. On the back, dermoid tumours can be associated with a dermal sinus communicating with the spinal canal, giving rise to recurrent meningitis [8–11].

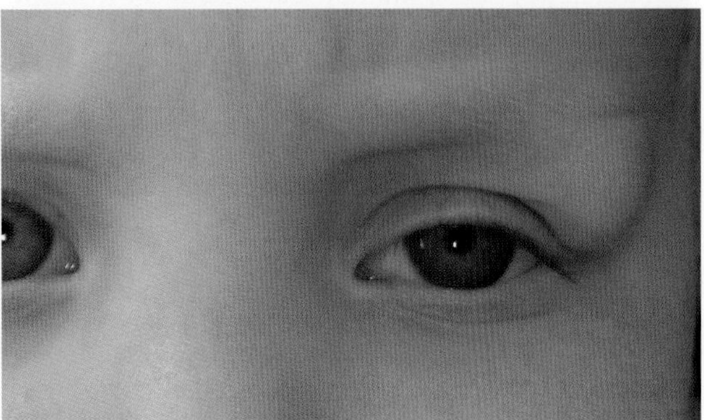

Fig. 110.6 Dermoid cyst.

Treatment. Complete excision without rupture of the cyst is required. In the case of dermoid cysts located on the anterior or posterior midline, magnetic resonance imaging studies should be performed preoperatively to rule out the possibility of intracranial or intraspinal connections of the tumour [1,4,12].

References

1 **Ahuja R, Azar NF. Orbital dermoids in children. Semin Ophthalmol 2006;21:207–11.**
2 **Moses MA, Green BC, Cugno S et al. The management of midline frontonasal dermoids: a review of 55 cases at a tertiary referral center and a protocol for treatment. Plast Reconstr Surg 2015;135:187–96.**
3 Tan E-C, Takagi T. Congenital inclusion cysts over the anterior fontanel in Japanese children: a study of five cases. Childs Nerv Syst 1993;9:81–3.
4 **Orozco-Covarrubias L, Lara-Carpio R, Saez-De-Ocariz M et al. Dermoid cysts: a report of 75 pediatric patients. Pediatr Dermatol 2013;30:706–11.**
5 Adouani A, Chennoufi M, Hammoud M et al. [Malignant transformation of a dermoïd cyst of the scalp. A case report]. Tunis Med 2004;82:972
6 Göl IH, Kiyici H, Yildirim E et al. Congenital sublingual teratoid cyst: a case report and literature review. J Pediatr Surg 2005;40:e9–12.
7 **Paller AS, Pensler JM, Tomita T. Nasal midline masses in infants and children. Arch Dermatol 1991;127:362–6.**
8 Raqbi F, Zerah M, Bodemer C et al. Dermoid cysts revealed by meningitis with medullary compression. Arch Pediatr 2001;8:499–503.
9 Kriss TC, Kriss VM, Warf BC. Recurrent meningitis: the search for the dermoid or epidermoid tumor. Pediatr Infect Dis J 1995;14:697–700.
10 Drolet BA. Cutaneous signs of neural tube dysraphism. Pediatr Clin North Am 2000;47:813–23.
11 Maaloul I, Hsairi M, Fourati H et al. Occipital dermoid cyst associated with dermal sinus complicated with meningitis: A case report. Arch Pediatr 2016;23:197–200.
12 **Sorenson EP, Powel JE, Rozzelle CJ et al. Scalp dermoids: a review of their anatomy, diagnosis, and treatment. Childs Nerv Syst 2013;29:375–80.**

Eruptive vellus hair cysts

Definition. Eruptive vellus hair cysts are characterized by the occlusion and cystic dilation of vellus hair follicles.

Pathogenesis. They are seen as a developmental abnormality of the vellus hair follicle resulting in occlusion and subsequent retention of hairs [1]. Histology reveals a mid-dermal cyst containing keratinous material and vellus hair; the cyst is lined by squamous epithelium. Eruptive vellus hair cysts, steatocystoma multiplex and persistent milia are considered subtypes of multiple pilosebaceous cysts distinguished mainly, if not exclusively, by the different level at which the pilosebaceous duct is affected [2–5].

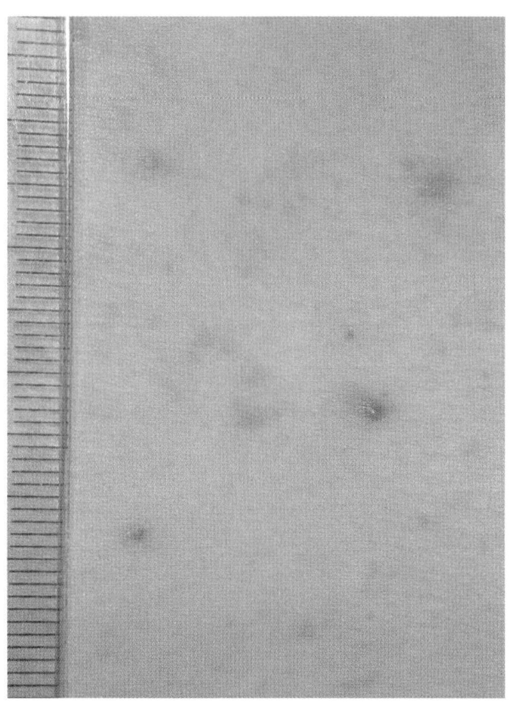

Fig. 110.7 Eruptive vellus hair cysts. Source: Courtesy of Professor John Harper.

Clinical features. Eruptive vellus hair cysts generally present in a monomorphous fashion with small (1–2 mm in diameter), asymptomatic follicular papules that are usually skin coloured but may have a reddish or brownish tinge (Fig. 110.7) [5,6]. They appear suddenly and are most commonly located on the chest, but can also be found on the extremities. Eruptive vellus hair cysts can occur at any age, but are seen predominantly in children and adolescents between the ages of 4 and 18 years. The average age of diagnosis is 24 years, with 90% being under the age of 35 [7]. Familial occurrence [5,8–10] and autosomal dominant cases with manifestation at birth [11] have been described. Vellus hair cysts seem to be more common in patients with pachyonychia congenita [12].

Pathology. Vellus hair cysts contain vellus hair and keratin; they are located in mid-dermis and lined by squamous epithelium. Based on keratin expression, it is likely that eruptive vellus hair cysts are derived from the infrainfundibulum and sebaceous duct [13].

Course and prognosis. Eruptive vellus hair cysts are a benign condition. Some may resolve spontaneously, but most tend to persist for many years.

Treatment. Treatment, if desired for cosmetic reasons, may include topical retinoic or lactic acid, incision and gentle curettage of the cyst content, cauterization, Erbium:YAG laser or CO_2 laser treatment [6,7]; these procedures should be chosen and performed with great caution in order to avoid scarring.

References

1 **Esterly NB, Fretzin DF, Pinkus H. Eruptive vellus hair cysts. Arch Dermatol 1977;113:500–3.**
2 **Ohtake N, Kubota Y, Takayama O et al. Relationship between steatocystoma multiplex and eruptive vellus hair cysts. J Am Acad Dermatol 1992;26:876–8.**
3 Patrizi A, Neri I, Guerrini V et al. Persistent milia, steatocystoma multiplex and eruptive vellus hair cysts: variable expression of multiple pilosebaceous cysts within an affected family. Dermatology 1998;196:392–6.
4 Cho S, Chang SE, Choi JH et al. Clinical and histologic features of 64 cases of steatocystoma multiplex. J Dermatol 2002;29:152–6.
5 **Torchia D, Vega J, Schachner LA. Eruptive vellus hair cysts: a systematic review. Am J Clin Dermatol 2012;13:19–28.**
6 Grimalt R, Gelmetti C. Eruptive vellus hair cysts: case report and review of the literature. Pediatr Dermatol 1992;9:98–102.
7 **Patel U, Terushkin V, Fischer M et al. Eruptive vellus hair cysts. Dermatol Online J 2012;18:7.**
8 Mayron R, Grimwood RE. Familial occurrence of eruptive vellus hair cysts. Pediatr Dermatol 1988;5:94–6.
9 Pauline G, Alain H, Jean-Jaques R et al. Eruptive vellus hair cysts: an original case occurring in twins. Int J Dermatol 2015;54:e209–12.
10 Rodgers SA, Kitagawa K, Selim MA, Bellet JS. Familial eruptive vellus hair cysts. Pediatr Dermatol 2012;29:367–9.
11 Piepkorn MW, Clark L, Lombardi DL. A kindred with congenital vellus hair cysts. J Am Acad Dermatol 1981;5:661–5.
12 Lee HT, Chang SH, Yoon TY. Eruptive vellus hair cysts in a patient with pachyonychia congenita. J Dermatol 1999;26:402–4.
13 Shi G, Zhou Y, Cai YX et al. Clinicopathological features and expression of four keratins (K10, K14, K17 and K19) in six cases of eruptive vellus hair cysts. Clin Exp Dermatol 2014;39:496–9.

Granular cell tumour

Definition. The term 'granular cell tumour', also known as Abricosoff tumour or granular cell myoblastoma, comprises a variety of rare dermal tumours with nerve sheath-like features: granular nerve cell sheath tumour (GNCST), malignant granular cell tumour and granular cell epulis of infancy.

Pathogenesis. Granular cell tumours have been previously classified as granular cell myoblastomas and granular cell schwannomas [1]. The tumours are mostly extraneural. Tumour cells appear large and polygonal with cytoplasmic granules and spread neurotrophically along peripheral nerves. Like nerve sheath tumours such as schwannomas and neurofibromas, granular cell tumours are positive for S100 protein; a Schwann cell origin for nongingival GNCST has been suggested [2].

Clinical features. GNCSTs of the skin are firm circumscribed nodules with a raised and sometimes verrucous surface. Their diameter ranges from 0.5 to 3.0 cm. GNCSTs can be either congenital [3,4] or acquired [5,6]. They are usually solitary [3], but in 10% of cases may be multiple or multifocal [4–7]. The tumours are mostly located in the oral cavity (gingiva and tongue, 40%), skin and subcutaneous tissue, but can also involve many internal organs [1,8,9]. Dermoscopy shows a yellowish centre surrounded by a light-brown subtle pigment network and tiny circles [10]. Patients sometimes complain of tenderness or pruritus. Multiple subcutaneous nodules can mimic neurofibromatosis type I. In fact, as a result of their common neuroectodermal origin, an association between the two entities has been suggested [7]. Malignant granular cell tumour is very rare. It affects skin and subcutaneous tissue but can also, like GNCST, affect visceral organs. It is characterized clinically as a rapidly growing, nodular mass that may undergo ulceration [11].

Course and prognosis. GNCSTs are locally invasive. They can infiltrate the skeletal muscle. Recurrences are common after incomplete excision. Malignant granular cell tumours are very rare (less than 2% of granular cell tumours); they metastasize to the skin, lymph nodes, muscles and visceral organs [11,12].

Treatment. Complete excision is recommended.

References

1 **Reed RJ, Argenyi Z. Tumor of neural tissue. In: Elder D, Elenitsas R, Johnson BL et al. (eds) Lever's Histopathology of the Skin, 9th edn. Philadelphia: Lippincott-Raven, 2005:1109–48.**

2 **Mazur MT, Shultz JJ, Myers JL. Granular cell tumor. Immunohistochemical analysis of 21 benign tumors and one malignant tumor. Arch Pathol Lab Med 1990;114:692–6.**

3 **Belal MS, Ibricevic H, Madda JP et al. Granular congenital cell tumor in the newborn: a case report. J Clin Pediatr Dent 2002;26:315–17.**

4 Zaenglein AL, Meehan SA, Orlow SJ. Congenital granular cell tumors localized to the arm. Pediatr Dermatol 2001;18:234–7.

5 De Raeve L, Rosseuw D, Otten J. Multiple cutaneous granular cell tumours in a child in remission for Hodgkin's disease. J Am Acad Dermatol 2002;47:S180–2.

6 Dorta S, Sanchez R, Garcia-Bustinduy M et al. Multiple granular cell tumours in a teenager. Br J Dermatol 2000;143:892–3.

7 Sahn EE, Dunlavey ES, Parsons JL. Multiple cutaneous granular cell tumors in a child with possible neurofibromatosis. J Am Acad Dermatol 1997;36:327–30.

8 López V, Santonja N, Jordá E. Granular cell tumor on the sole of a child: a case report. Pediatr Dermatol 2011;28;473–4.

9 Barbieri M, Musizzano Y, Boggio M, Carcuscia C. Granular cell tumour of the tongue in a 14-year-old boy: case report. Acta Otorhinolaryngol Ital 2011;31:186–9.

10 **Popadić M, Dermoscopy of cutaneous Abrikossoff tumor (granular cell tumor) in a pediatric patient. J Am Acad Dermatol 2015;73:137–8.**

11 Pérez-González YC, Pagura L, Llamas-Velasco M et al. Primary cutaneous malignant granular cell tumor: an immunohistochemical study and review of the literature. Am J Dermatopathol 2015;37:334–40.

12 Price MA, Horwitz P, Tschen JA et al. Malignant granular cell tumor. Dermatol Surg 1995;21:820–1.

Vascular neoplasms

Pyogenic granuloma (Lobular capillary haemangioma)

Definition. Pyogenic granuloma, also known as lobular capillary haemangioma, is a common benign proliferative vascular tumour of the skin and mucous membranes that often follows a minor injury or infection [1,2].

Pathogenesis. Although it was previously thought that pyogenic granuloma was caused by pyogenic infections, the histopathological findings of early lesions are characterized by angiomatous tissue resembling capillary haemangioma without evidence of inflammation [2]. Therefore the term 'lobular capillary haemangioma' has been suggested [2]. Recently, *BRAF* mutations were identified in 8 of 10 secondary pyogenic granulomas arising on port-wine stains [3].

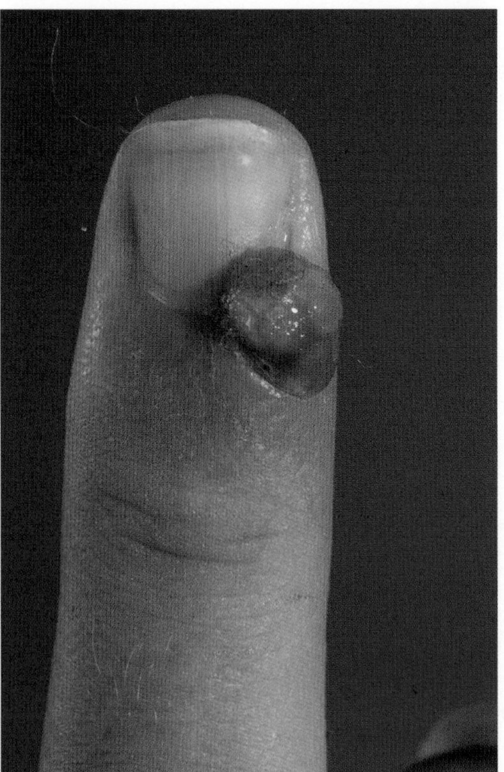

Fig. 110.8 Pyogenic granuloma.

Clinical features. In about 28% a preceding lesion is evident prior to the occurrence of pyogenic granuloma [4]. A bright-red indolent nodule grows rapidly within 1–3 weeks up to a final size of 0.5–2.0 cm in diameter (Fig. 110.8). It often becomes pedunculated. Older lesions are frequently eroded or crusted and bleed easily. Pyogenic granulomas are usually solitary and preferentially located on the head and especially the gingiva, followed by the upper limbs, trunk and lower limbs [2,4–6]. They are most common in children under 5 years of age but can also occur in older children and young adults [1,2,7,8]. The male to female ratio is 1.5 : 1.0 [4].

Pyogenic granulomas are sometimes observed within port-wine stains [9]. Certain drugs, particularly retinoids, favour their formation [10].

Course and prognosis. Pyogenic granulomas persist without treatment; spontaneous regression is quite rare. They bleed easily on minor trauma. Recurrence after treatment is not uncommon [1–3]. A histological examination is reasonable to distinguish pyogenic granuloma from a malignant tumour that may mimic it [11].

Treatment. Treatment consists of curettage with cauterization or thermal coagulation of the tumour base [2,7]. Pedunculated granulomas can be ligated at the base. However, pyogenic granulomas frequently recur unless they are excised, and sometimes multiple satellites (satellitosis) can be seen [4,12]. Other alternatives are cryosurgery or laser therapy (Nd:YAG, pulsed-dye laser, CO_2 laser) [4,7].

References
1 **Mooney MA, Janniger CK. Pyogenic granuloma. Cutis 1995;55:133–6.**
2 **Patrice SJ, Wiss K, Mulliken JB. Pyogenic granuloma (lobular capillary hemangioma): a clinicopathologic study of 178 cases. Pediatr Dermatol 1994;8:267–76.**
3 **Groesser L, Peterhof E, Evert M et al. BRAF and RAS mutations in sporadic and secondary pyogenic granuloma. J Invest Dermatol 2016;136:481–6.**
4 **Akamatsu T, Hanai U, Kobayashi M, Miyasaka M. Pyogenic granuloma: a retrospective 10-year analysis of 82 cases. Tokai J Exp Clin Med 2015;40:110–14.**
5 Al-Khateeb T, Ababneh K. Oral pyogenic granuloma in Jordanians: a retrospective analysis of 108 cases. J Oral Maxillofac Surg 2003;61:1285–8.
6 Gordón-Núñez MA, de Vasconcelos Carvalho M, Benevenuto TG et al. Oral pyogenic granuloma: a retrospective analysis of 293 cases in a Brazilian population. J Oral Maxillofac Surg 2010;68:2185–8.
7 Tay YK, Weston WL, Morelli JG. Treatment of pyogenic granuloma in children with the flashlamp-pumped pulsed dye laser. Pediatrics 1997;99:368–70.
8 **Pagliai KA, Cohen BA. Pyogenic granuloma in children. Pediatr Dermatol 2004;2:10–13.**
9 Sheehan DJ, Lesher JL. Pyogenic granuloma arising within a portwine stain. Cutis 2004;73:175–80.
10 Exner JH, Dahod S, Pochi PE. Pyogenic granuloma-like acne lesions during isotretinoin therapy. Arch Dermatol 1983;119:808–11.
11 Tashiro J, Perlyn CA, Melnick SJ et al. Non-pigmented melanoma with nodal metastases masquerading as pyogenic granuloma in a 1-year old. J Pediatr Surg 2014;49:653–5.
12 **Hoeger PH, Colmenero I. Vascular tumours in infants. Part I: benign vascular tumours other than infantile haemangioma. Br J Dermatol 2014;171:466–73.**

Glomus tumour (glomuvenous malformation)

Definition. Glomus tumours, also known as glomangioma or glomangiomyoma, are rare benign vascular neoplasms derived from the myoarterial glomus. They can occur either as a solitary nodule or as inherited glomangiomatosis.

Pathogenesis. Glomus tumours are derived from the glomus body, a temperature-sensitive corpuscle of modified perivascular smooth muscle cells involved in the vascular regulation of acral skin temperature. They are composed of glomus cells, blood vessels and smooth muscle cells, and are classified according to the prevailing cell type into solid glomus tumours (25%), glomangioma (60%) (Fig. 110.9) and glomangiomyoma (15%) [1]. Recent evidence suggests that these different forms might represent transitional variants of the same tumour [2], which is attributable to a mutation in the glomulin gene located on chromosome 1p22–p21 [3,4].

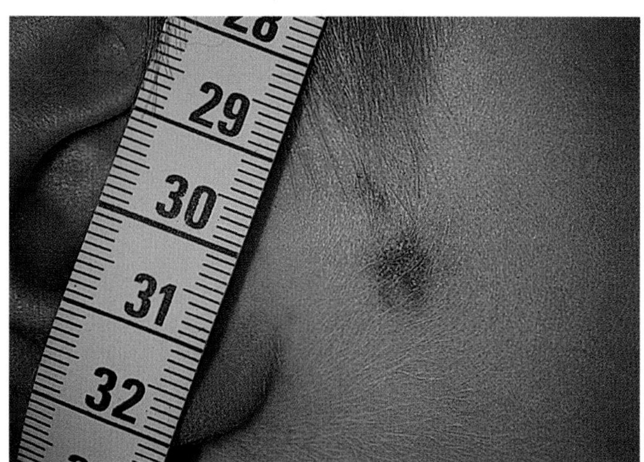

Fig. 110.9 Glomangioma.

Clinical features. Glomus tumours are quite uncommon. They usually present as solitary bluish-red cutaneous patches, papules and nodules. Solitary glomus tumours are typically located on the hands (subungual and palmar), forearm or feet; other locations, including mucous membranes, are less common [5,6]. Their size varies between one and several centimetres. They are extremely tender; cold temperature can often elicit pain attacks. The cause of pain is disproportionate to their mostly tiny size [7]. Multiple glomus tumours are less common. Their number varies from a few to several hundred lesions; they are larger, not painful and less restricted to the extremities. Although solitary glomus tumours are most prevalent in adolescents and young adults, multiple glomus tumours often manifest in younger children [8,9]. Multiple glomus tumours are mostly glomangiomas; they can be disseminated, regional (e.g. affecting only one extremity) or present as a congenital plaque-like lesion [8–10]. Unlike the solitary glomus tumour in adults, glomangiomas are not painful on palpitation [11]. Autosomal dominant inheritance and a newly recognized association with neurofibromatosis have been described [2,12,13]. Multiple glomus tumours can be confused with the blue rubber bleb naevus syndrome.

Course and prognosis. The lesions persist without treatment. Rare cases of glomangiosarcoma evolving from solitary glomus tumours have been described [8].

Treatment. Surgical excision is the treatment of choice and allows complete regression of pain with significant patient satisfaction. Local recurrence is possible, but less common than with electrocoagulation. Argon and CO_2 and Nd:YAG laser therapy can improve pain and superficial appearance [8,14].

References
1 **Calonje E, Wison-Jones E. Vascular tumours and tumour-like conditions of blood vessels and lymphatics. In: Elder D, Elenitsas R, Johnson BL et al. (eds) Lever's Histopathology of the Skin, 9th edn. Philadelphia: Lippincott-Raven, 2005:1015–60.**
2 **Calduch L, Monteagudo C, Martine-Ruiz E et al. Familial generalized multiple glomangiomyoma: report of a new family, with immunohistochemical and ultrastructural studies and review of the literature. Pediatr Dermatol 2002;19:402–8.**
3 Brouillard P, Boon LM, Mulliken JB et al. Mutations in a novel factor, glomulin, are responsible for glomuvenous malformations ('glomangiomas'). Am J Hum Genet 2002;70:866–74.
4 Mounayer C, Wassef M, Enjolras O et al. Facial 'glomangiomas': large facial venous malformations with glomus cells. J Am Acad Dermatol 2001;45:239–45.
5 **Sandoval M, Carrasco-Zuber J, Gonzalez S. Extradigital symplastic glomus tumor of the hand: report of 2 cases and literature review. Am J Dermatopathol 2015;37:560–2.**
6 Chirila M, Rogojan L Glomangioma of the nasal septum: a case report and review. Ear Nose Throat J 2013;92:E7–9.
7 Lauretti L, Coli A, Signorelli F et al. Skin glomic tumors referred for local pain and cured by surgical removal. Acta Neurochir 2016;158:761–6.

8 **Glick SA, Markstein EA, Herreid P. Congenital glomangioma: case report and review of the world literature. Pediatr Dermatol 1995;12:242–4.**

9 **Cavalli R, Milani GP, Chelleri C et al. Plaque-type glomuvenous malformations in a child. Lancet 2015;386:e61.**

10 Landthaler M, Braun-Falco E, Eckert F et al. Congenital multiple plaque-like glomus tumors. Arch Dermatol 1990;126:1203–7.

11 **Hoeger PH, Colmenero I. Vascular tumours in infants. Part I: benign vascular tumours other than infantile haemangioma. Br J Dermatol 2014;171:466–73.**

12 Tran LP, Velanovich V, Kaufmann CR. Familial multiple glomus tumors: report of a pedigree and literature review. Ann Plast Surg 1994;32:89–91.

13 Kumar MG, Emnett RJ, Bayliss SJ, Gutmann DH. Glomus tumors in individuals with neurofibromatosis type 1. J Am Acad Dermatol 2014;71:44–8.

14 Rivers JK, Rivers CA, Li MK, Martinka M. Laser therapy for an acquired glomuvenous malformation (glomus tumour): a nonsurgical approach. J Cutan Med Surg 2016;20:80–3.

CHAPTER 111
Adnexal Disorders

Andrew Wang[1] *& Robert Sidbury*[2]
[1] Brookline Dermatology Associates, West Roxbury, MA, USA
[2] Department of Pediatrics, Division of Dermatology, Seattle Children's Hospital, University of Washington School of Medicine, Seattle, WA, USA

Introduction, 1325
Inflammatory diseases, 1325
Tumours, 1329

Abstract

Skin appendages, or adnexae, are structures associated with thermoregulation, cutaneous homeostasis and sensation. A wide array of disorders develop from adnexal tissues ranging from inflammatory dermatoses such as hidradenitis suppurativa to neoplastic conditions such as trichoepitheliomas. This chapter describes both common and uncommon paediatric presentations of adnexal disorders with emphasis on clinical and histological presentation, differential diagnosis, aetiology and management.

Key points

- Palmoplantar hidradenitis should be in the differential diagnosis for new-onset painful palm and sole lesions. Perniosis can be a clinical mimic and both may be triggered by cold exposure.
- Hidradenitis suppurativa can have a tremendous impact on quality of life. A careful history with attention to psychosocial factors should be a part of the complete assessment. Clinicians must be mindful of associated comorbidities such as metabolic syndrome.
- Syringocystadenoma papilliferum (SP) is the most common benign neoplasm in naevus sebaceus. Mutations in *HRAS*, *KRAS*, *BRAF* and *PTCH* genes have been found in SP.

Introduction

Adnexal disorders relate to abnormalities of cutaneous appendages such as hair follicles, sebaceous, eccrine and apocrine glands. These structures serve critical roles in thermoregulation, homeostasis and sensation. Most adnexal disorders are very uncommon in general, and particularly rare in the paediatric population. They run the gamut from benign self-limiting conditions such as sebaceous hyperplasia that afflicts most healthy newborns, to potentially devastating inflammatory conditions such as hidradenitis suppurativa. This chapter reviews both common and uncommon presentations with emphasis on clinical and histological presentation, differential diagnosis, aetiology and management.

Inflammatory diseases

Palmoplantar hidradenitis

First described in 1988 by Metzker and Brodsky under the name 'traumatic plantar urticaria' [1], palmoplantar hidradenitis (PH) is a benign and self-limiting inflammatory disease of the eccrine sweat gland. Primarily a disease of children, PH presents as distinct tender erythematous papules and nodules involving the soles of the feet or the palms of the hands. Palmoplantar hidradenitis has also been called idiopathic recurrent palmoplantar hidradenitis [2], palmoplantar eccrine hidradenitis, idiopathic palmoplantar hidradenitis, idiopathic plantar hidradenitis, recurrent palmoplantar hidradenitis [3] and plantar erythema nodosum [4].

Epidemiology. Palmoplantar hidradenitis primarily affects healthy children of the younger paediatric age group. A mean age of 6 years with an age range of 1.5–15 years was published in a report of 22 cases [5]. Seasonal peaks in the autumn and spring have also been reported [2].

Aetiology. The precise aetiology of PH is unknown. Histological findings of a perieccrine neutrophilic infiltrate imply a reaction pattern similar to the direct toxic effect seen in cases of malignancy-associated neutrophilic eccrine hidradenitis [4]. Proposed mechanisms include local mechanical or thermal trauma through strenuous activity [5], wet footwear [4], hyperhidrosis [6] or recent infection. Implicated infectious agents include group A β-haemolytic streptococci, *Mycoplasma pneumoniae*, *Yersinia enterocolitica* and pseudomonal infections [2]. In cases involving the palmar surface, a history of hand trauma (baseball camp, hockey practice and ice skating [7]) or thermal trauma (hot tub use) have been reported [8].

Harper's Textbook of Pediatric Dermatology, Fourth Edition. Edited by Peter Hoeger, Veronica Kinsler and Albert Yan.

Clinical and histological observations support the belief that mechanical or thermal trauma can lead to rupture of the palmoplantar eccrine glands. The release of glandular secretion into the surrounding tissue subsequently promotes an inflammatory response that manifests as palmoplantar papules and nodules.

Clinical presentation. Palmoplantar hidradenitis typically presents with rapid onset of tender erythematous papules and nodules on the palms of the hands and, more commonly, on the plantar and lateral aspects of the feet, usually bilaterally, with resultant significant difficulty walking [3]. Pustules were reported in one patient, with the proposed aetiology of massive invasion of the acrosyringium by the neutrophils [2]. Patients may also present with a low-grade fever [4], but constitutional symptoms are typically absent [2]. The clinical features and course are usually sufficient to establish a diagnosis of PH. White blood cell count, erythrocyte sedimentation rate, serum C-reactive protein level and blood chemistry tests have been reported as within normal limits in patients with PH [9].

Differential diagnosis. The differential diagnosis of acral, tender, erythematous lesions includes insect bites, chilblains, atypical panniculitis or plantar erythema nodosum, thrombophlebitis, vasculitis, embolic phenomenon, cellulitis, migratory angioedema [4], traumatic plantar urticaria, Sweet syndrome, Behçet disease, sarcoidosis, periarteritis nodosa, pool palms [5] and neutrophilic eccrine hidradenitis [2].

Histology. Palmoplantar hidradenitis presents with a distinctly focal and nodular perieccrine inflammatory infiltrate composed primarily of neutrophils [5]. The infiltrate is most dense around the ductal component of the coil, sparing the secretory segment. Neutrophilic abscesses next to the eccrine coils are also common [2]. A superficial and deep perivascular infiltrate of neutrophils, lymphocytes and histiocytes is also observed. Septal panniculitis has been reported [3]. Despite these characteristic histological findings, skin biopsy is generally not necessary to establish the diagnosis in a patient with typical skin lesions.

Management. Palmoplantar hidradenitis is a benign self-limiting condition with most patients responding to bedrest, with the intention of decreasing both trauma and sweat secretion. Other therapies include systemic antibiotics, topical and systemic steroids, nonsteroidal anti-inflammatory drugs and potassium iodide solution, drips and soaks, although they offer no clear or consistent benefit. Gradual resumption of normal activity after resolution of symptoms is recommended. Despite rapid resolution, with most reporting clearance within 1 month, relapse has been reported in 50% of patients [5].

References

1 Metzker A, Brodsky F. Traumatic plantar urticaria: an unrecognized entity? J Am Acad Dermatol 1988;18:144–6.

2 Hernandez-Martin A, Pinedo F, Perez-Lescure J. Pustular idiopathic recurrent palmoplantar hidradenitis: an unusual clinical feature. J Am Acad Dermatol 2002;47(5 suppl):S263–5.

3 Esler-Brauer L, Rothman I. Tender nodules on the palms and soles: palmoplantar eccrine hidradenitis. Arch Dermatol 2007;143:1201–6.

4 Naimer SA, Zvulunov A, Ben-Amitai D, Landau M. Plantar hidradenitis in children induced by exposure to wet footwear. Pediatr Emerg Care 2000;16:182–3.

5 Simon M Jr, Cremer H, von den Driesch P. Idiopathic recurrent palmoplantar hidradenitis in children: report of 22 cases. Arch Dermatol 1998;134:76–9.

6 Landau M, Metzker A, Gat A et al. Palmoplantar eccrine hidradenitis: three new cases and review. Pediatr Dermatol 1998;15:97–102.

7 Tlougan BE, Mancini AJ, Mandell JA et al. Skin conditions in figure skaters, ice-hockey players and speed skaters: part II - cold-induced, infectious and inflammatory dermatoses. Sports Med 2011;41:967–84.

8 Shehan JM, Clowers-Webb HE, Kalaaji AN. Recurrent palmoplantar hidradenitis with exclusive palmar involvement and an association with trauma and exposure to aluminum dust. Pediatr Dermatol 2004;21:30–2.

9 Rubinson R, Larralde M, Santos-Muñoz A et al. Palmoplantar eccrine hidradenitis: seven new cases. Pediatr Dermatol 2004;21:466–8.

Hidradenitis suppurativa (acne inversa)

Hidradenitis suppurativa (HS) is a chronic inflammatory disease of the hair follicle, most commonly affecting the intertriginous areas. Initially thought to be a primary disorder of the apocrine gland, HS is most likely caused by inflammation of the apocrine glands secondary to follicular plugging, placing the disease in the follicular occlusion tetrad along with acne conglobata, dissecting cellulitis and pilonidal sinuses [1]. The term 'acne inversa' is sometimes used to reflect this mechanism. A burgeoning literature has demonstrated the tremendous impact HS has on quality of life [2]

Epidemiology. HS has long been perceived as a rare disease. Prevalence estimates ranging from 0.33 to 4 patients per 1000 inhabitants suggest HS is more common than originally thought [3]. HS is more common in women of reproductive age, implicating hormonal factors in the pathogenesis. HS is rare before puberty and decreases in incidence after the fifth decade of life [4].

The median age has been reported as 42 years for men and 39 years for women. Hidradenitis suppurativa has been observed in association with metabolic syndrome [5], arthritis, Crohn disease, Down syndrome, Graves disease, Hashimoto thyroiditis, herpes simplex virus, irritable bowel syndrome and Sjögren syndrome [6]. While rare, prepubertal HS has been reported [7,8].

Aetiology. As evidenced by the varied terminology used to identify this disorder, the aetiology of HS/acne inversa is unclear. While affected areas reflect the anatomical distribution of apocrine sweat glands, histology suggests that apocrine glands are not the primary source of pathology. HS has rather been identified as a follicular hyperkeratosis with plugging and dilation of the hair follicle, precipitating inflammation, abscess and sinus tract formation. Involvement of the apocrine glands is secondary, resulting in deeper granulomatous inflammation.

The aetiology of follicular plugging is unclear. Proposed mechanisms such as hypersecretion of sebum, proliferation of *Propionibacterium acnes* in the setting of an alteration of innate immunity, and inflammatory reactions mirror those implicated in the pathogenesis of acne vulgaris [9].

HS has a clear genetic component with multiple familial cases being reported, implying an autosomal dominant inheritance pattern [10]. A recent genome-wide association study has identified mutations in γ-secretase linked to HS in some kindreds [11]. A report from two case-control studies in France also identified two risk factors significantly associated with HS: current smoking and obesity [3]. An active area of investigation relates to similarities between the inflammation seen in HS and that in inflammatory bowel disease and psoriasis. Accordingly there is some early evidence that HS patients, like those with psoriasis, may have increased risk of cardiovascular events and all-cause mortality [12]. A recent report suggested a possible paradoxical induction of HS by biologic agents in some patients. As in psoriasis, where biologics can both treat and cause inflammation, providers should remain mindful of similar effects in HS [13].

Clinical presentation. Hidradenitis suppurativa presents as tender cutaneous and subcutaneous nodular inflammation, fistula formation and discharge of foul-smelling secretions in apocrine-bearing regions, most commonly the intertriginous areas including the axillae, inguinal, anogenital and mammary areas (Fig. 111.1). Relapses and chronicity cause significant impact on quality of life [3].

Differential diagnosis. At the initial stages, the differential diagnosis should include infectious lesions such as furuncles and carbuncles, deep fungal infections, actinomycosis and sporotrichosis. Lesions in the anogenital region are reminiscent of lymphogranuloma venereum and granuloma inguinale. Sweat gland abscesses, vegetating pyoderma, cutaneous tuberculosis, irritated sebaceous gland retention cysts and cutaneous fistulas in Crohn disease should also be ruled out [4,10].

Histology. Early histopathological changes in HS are follicular hyperkeratosis of a dilated infundibulum with plugging. Subsequent bacterial superinfection and rupture of the follicle is then seen, resulting in inflammation of the connective tissue. A mixed perifollicular lymphohistiocytic infiltrate with plasma cells, mononuclear cells and neutrophilic granulocytes is seen, with an acanthotic and anastomosing interfollicular epithelium [4,11].

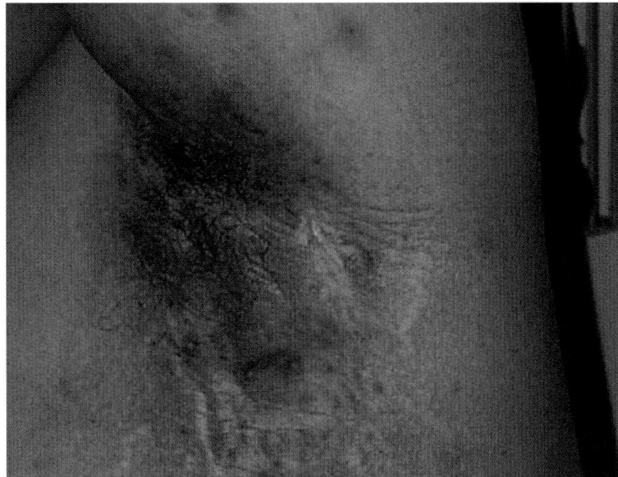

Fig. 111.1 Hidradenitis suppurativa. Axillary draining nodules with scarring in an obese adolescent female with associated acanthosis nigricans.

Management. More than 50 interventions have been described in HS, leading to therapeutic uncertainty in some settings. A recent Cochrane review helpfully grades the available evidence but acknowledges a dearth of high-quality studies [14]. First-line treatment consists of lifestyle modification including appropriate hygiene, loose-fitting clothing, smoking cessation and weight loss when relevant [15]. Drainage incisions parallel to skinfolds will aid in the resolution of the acute inflammation secondary to infection. Short-course antibiotics should be used for cases complicated by cellulitis. Topical clindamycin and systemic tetracycline-class antibiotics have been used with success. Adjunctive therapies include the use of retinoids, intralesional injection of triamcinolone acetonide suspension, antiandrogens, anakinra [16] and infliximab [17]. Excision to fascia can be effective in chronic or refractory disease [6].

Prognosis. Healing of areas affected by HS with scarring can lead to contractures and significant limitation in mobility. There is a recurrence rate of 2.5% after wide surgical excision. Ninety percent of patients with HS will continue to have symptomatic disease years after initial presentation. There is a 3% prevalence of squamous cell carcinoma in patients with longstanding perianal HS [6].

References

1 Ingram JR. Hidradenitis suppurativa: an update. Clin Med (London) 2016;16:70–3.
2 Deckers IE, Kimball AB. The handicap of hidradenitis suppurativa. Dermatol Clin 2016;34:17–22.
3 Revuz JE, Canoui-Poitrine F, Wolkenstein P et al. Prevalence and factors associated with hidradenitis suppurativa: results from two case–control studies. J Am Acad Dermatol 2008;59:596–601.
4 Meixner D, Schneider S, Krause M, Sterry W. Acne inversa. J Dtsch Dermatol Ges 2008;6:189–96.
5 **Miller IM, Ellervik C, Vinding GR et al. Association of metabolic syndrome and hidradenitis suppurativa. JAMA Dermatol 2014; 150:1273–80.**
6 Golladay ES. Outpatient adolescent surgical problems. Adolesc Med Clin 2004;15:503–20.
7 Mengesha YM, Holcombe TC, Hansen RC. Prepubertal hidradenitis suppurativa: two case reports and review of the literature. Pediatr Dermatol 1999;16:292–6.
8 Palmer RA, Keefe M. Early-onset hidradenitis suppurativa. Clin Exp Dermatol 2001;26:501–3.
9 Kurzen H, Kurokawa I, Jemec GB et al. What causes hidradenitis suppurativa? Exp Dermatol 2008;17:455–6; discussion 457–72.
10 Prasad PV, Kaviarasan PK, Joseph JM et al. Familial acne inversa with acne conglobata in three generations. Indian J Dermatol Venereol Leprol 2008;74:283–5.
11 Liu M, Davis JW, Idler KB et al. Genetic analysis of the NCSTN gene for potential association to hidradenitis suppurativa in familial and non-familial subjects. Br J Dermatol 2016;175:414–16.
12 Egeberg A, Gislason GH, Hansen PR. Risk of major adverse cardiovascular events and all-cause mortality in patients with hidradenitis suppurativa. JAMA Dermatol 2016;152:429–34.
13 Faivre C, Villani AP, Aubin F et al; French Society of Dermatology and Club Rheumatisms and Inflammation. Hidradenitis suppurativa (HS): An unrecognized paradoxical effect of biologic agents (BA) used in chronic inflammatory diseases. J Am Acad Dermatol 2016;74:1153–9.

14 **Ingram JR, Woo PN, Chua SL et al. Interventions for hidradenitis suppurativa. Cochrane Database Syst Rev 2015;10:CD010081.**
15 Slade DE, Powell BW, Mortimer PS. Hidradenitis suppurativa: pathogenesis and management. Br J Plast Surg 2003;56:451–61.
16 Tzanetakou V, Kanni T, Giakatrou S et al. Safety and efficacy of anakinra in severe hidradenitis suppurativa: a randomized clinical trial. JAMA Dermatol 2016;152:52–9.
17 Antonucci A, Negosanti M, Negosanti L et al. Acne inversa treated with infliximab: different outcomes in 2 patients. Acta Derm Venereol 2008;88:274–5.

Fox–Fordyce disease

Fox–Fordyce disease (FFD) or apocrine miliaria is a rare and chronic disorder characterized by inflammation of the apocrine sweat glands causing pruritic follicular papules confined to apocrine gland-bearing areas.

Epidemiology. FFD is an extremely rare disease, most common in women between 13 and 35 years of age [1]. Cases in prepubescent girls have been reported [1,2], highlighting the fact that hormonal factors may not be operative in all cases. Pregnancy has been found to be protective.

Aetiology. FFD is caused by obstruction of the apocrine duct at the entrance into the follicular wall [3]. Subsequent apocrine sweat retention leads to rupture of the duct causing a secondary inflammatory reaction within the dermis. Alternative theories hypothesize an inflammatory process inducing a reactive hyperkeratosis. Proposed influences include emotional factors, hormonal influences and chemical changes in sweat composition. The role of regional trauma and follicular disruption has been considered and FFD has been reported after laser destruction of axillary hair [4]. Although no genetic basis has been identified, FFD has been reported in monozygotic twins [5].

Presentation. FFD is characterized by pruritic small 1–3 mm conical skin-coloured to slightly yellow follicular papules on a slightly erythematous base in the apocrine gland-bearing region (axillae, groins, pubic region, perineum, labia majora, areolae mammae and umbilicus) (Fig. 111.2). The regions most commonly affected are the axillae and areolae [6]. Hairs are usually sparse in affected areas, probably because of rubbing and scratching. Lesions are often refractory to treatment and spontaneous resolution is not expected.

Diagnosis. FFD is diagnosed based on its characteristic clinical features. Histopathological features of FFD, while well described, are less consistently observed.

Differential diagnosis. While the clinical features of FFD are characteristic and unique, folliculitis, lichen nitidus, miliaria rubra, lichen simplex, lichen planus and syringoma should be considered [3,7].

Pathology. The histopathological findings of FFD have been traditionally described as infundibular plugging, acanthosis, parakeratosis and spongiosis, with a nonspecific inflammatory infiltrate [6]. The 'sweat retention vesicle' described by Shelley and Levy has been proposed as a singular diagnostic feature [8]. Additional findings of scattered infundibular dyskeratotic cells, vacuolar alteration at the junction between the infundibular epithelium and its adventitia, and cornoid lamella-like parakeratosis within the infundibular plug have been reported by Boer [9]. Recently, perifollicular xanthomatosis has been proposed as a representative hallmark of FFD. Perifollicular mucin, adventitial fibrosis and increased mast cell density may also be used as clues to aid in diagnosis [6].

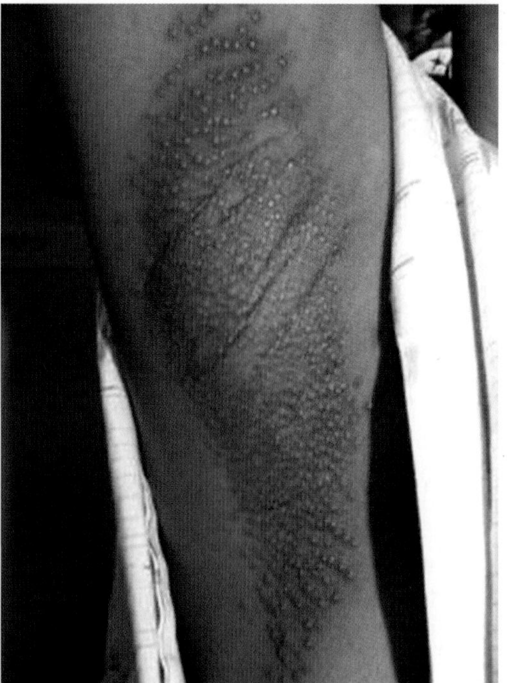

Fig. 111.2 Fox–Fordyce disease.

Treatment. Treatment of FFD has been uniformly unsatisfactory. Goals are to improve pruritus and decrease the size and number of the lesions. Reported treatments include oral antihistamines, topical steroids, propylene glycol, ultraviolet light treatment, oral contraceptives, topical clindamycin [10], topical tretinoin, isotretinoin and topical 5% benzoyl peroxide in combination with loratadine [3]. Pimecrolimus has also been reported to have benefit [11]. Surgical treatment, electrocoagulation, laser therapy, dermabrasion and liposuction-assisted curettage [12] have all been tried with variable results.

References

1 Ranalletta M, Rositto A, Drut R. Fox–Fordyce disease in two prepubertal girls: histopathologic demonstration of eccrine sweat gland involvement. Pediatr Dermatol 1996;13:294–7.
2 Sandhu K, Gupta S, Kanwar AJ. Fox–Fordyce disease in a prepubertal girl. Pediatr Dermatol 2005;22:89–90.
3 **Yost J, Robinson SM, Meehan M. Fox Fordyce disease. Dermatol Online J 2012;18:28.**
4 **Tetzlaff MT, Evans K, DeHoratius DM et al. FFD following axillary laser hair removal. Arch Dermatol 2011;147:573–6.**
5 Guiotoku MM, Lopes PT, Marques ME et al. FFD in monozygotic female twins. J Am Acad Dermatol 2011;65:229–30.
6 Bormate AB Jr, Leboit PE, McCalmont TH. Perifollicular xanthomatosis as the hallmark of axillary Fox–Fordyce disease: an evaluation of histopathologic features of 7 cases. Arch Dermatol 2008;144:1020–4.

7 Kineston DP, Martin KO. Pruritic axillary papules: Fox–Fordyce disease. Am Fam Physician 2008;77:1735–6.
8 Shelley WB, Levy EJ. Apocrine sweat retention in man. II. Fox–Fordyce disease (apocrine miliaria). AMA Arch Derm 1956;73:38–49.
9 Boer A. Patterns histopathologic of Fox Fordyce disease. Am J Dermatopathol 2004;26:482–92.
10 Miller ML, Harford RR, Yeager JK. Fox–Fordyce disease treated with topical clindamycin solution. Arch Dermatol 1995;131:1112–3.
11 Pock L, Svrcková M, Machácková R, Hercogová J. Pimecrolimus is effective in Fox–Fordyce disease. Int J Dermatol 2006;45:1134–5.
12 Chae KM, Marschall MA, Marschall SF. Axillary Fox–Fordyce disease treated with liposuction-assisted curettage. Arch Dermatol 2002; 138:452–4.

Tumours

Follicular differentiation

Trichofolliculoma

Trichofolliculoma is a rare benign adnexal hamartoma of hair follicle origin with differentiation towards hair production [1,2].

Epidemiology. While trichofolliculoma is generally perceived as a disorder of the adult population, a single case of congenital trichofolliculoma has been reported in the literature [3]. A review of 29 cases reported a mean age at time of removal of 44 years [2].

Aetiology. Trichofolliculoma is considered an intermediate differentiation between a hair follicle naevus, simple hyperplasia of the hair follicle and trichoepithelioma, which usually lacks mature hair follicles [4]. Studies examining cytokeratin expression in trichofolliculoma reveal differentiation towards the hair bulge and the outer root sheath in the isthmus [5]. After examining multiple lesions, Hartschuh and Schulz [2] developed the concept of trichofolliculoma as a lesion that undergoes great morphological changes that correspond to the normal hair follicle.

Presentation. Trichofolliculoma typically presents as a single 2–5 mm skin-coloured nodule on the head or neck, especially in the area of the nose, cheek, scalp and eyeline [1]. Occasionally, wool-like wisps of immature hairs emerge from a central orifice [1].

Diagnosis. Diagnosis is based upon histopathology.

Differential diagnosis. Differential diagnosis of this disorder includes hair follicle naevus, trichoepithelioma, fibrous papule and fibrofolliculomas.

Pathology. Histology reveals one or several keratin-filled cysts or sinuses in the dermis (primary follicle) that are lined by squamous epithelium. Many small, well-differentiated hair follicles (secondary follicles) radiate from the wall of these sinuses. Trichofolliculoma generally differentiates in the direction of the outer root sheath [5]. Merkel cell hyperplasia can be a diagnostic aid, helping to differentiate later-stage trichofolliculomas from fibrofolliculomas and fibrous papules.

Treatment. Surgical excision is standard of care.

Prognosis. Trichofolliculoma has a generally benign course [4]. Extraction of associated hairs may promote inflammatory reactions [1].

References

1 Thompson CB, Hossler EW. Trichofolliculoma. Cutis 2012;90:284, 289–90.
2 Hartschuh W, Schulz T. Immunohistochemical investigation of the different developmental stages of trichofolliculoma with special reference to the Merkel cell. Am J Dermatopathol 1999;21:8–15.
3 Ishii N, Kawaguchi H, Takahashi K, Nakajima H. A case of congenital trichofolliculoma. J Dermatol 1992;19:195–6.
4 Mizutani H, Senga K, Ueda M. Trichofolliculoma of the upper lip: report of a case. Int J Oral Maxillofac Surg 1999;28:135–6.
5 Misago N, Kimura T, Toda S et al. A revaluation of trichofolliculoma: the histopathological and immunohistochemical features. Am J Dermatopathol 2010;32:35–43.

Desmoplastic trichoepithelioma

Trichoepitheliomas are rare benign adnexal tumours of follicular differentiation. Three distinct subtypes of trichoepitheliomas have been described: solitary, multiple and desmoplastic [1]. The solitary variant, usually seen only in the adult population, has been described as a skin-coloured 5–8 mm diameter perinasal papule. Multiple trichoepitheliomas, morphologically identical to the solitary variants, are seen in various genetic disorders including cylindromatosis and Rombo syndrome, and usually appear during adolescence. The third variant, desmoplastic trichoepithelioma (DTE), first described by Brownstein and Shapiro in 1977 [2], presents as firm annular asymptomatic 3–8 mm diameter plaques. This section will address solitary DTE.

Epidemiology. DTE has an incidence of 1 in 5000 skin biopsies in adults. DTE most commonly occurs in middle-aged women [3]; patients range in age at diagnosis from 8 to 70 years with a median age of 46, and 85% of cases are seen in females. Familial DTE is extremely rare [4]. Cases of DTE have been reported in infants with improvement of the physical appearance of the lesions with the ageing of the child [5,6].

Aetiology. Histological examination of DTE has provided clues as to the aetiology of this disorder. The presence of Merkel cells indicates a bulge of isthmus-derived origin. The cells in DTE are suggested to be in close association with the basal cells in the outer root sheath which can subsequently differentiate into parts of the folliculosebaceous unit [4]. Reports of familial DTE imply an unknown genetic influence.

Presentation. Desmoplastic trichoepitheliomas are firm, symmetrical, oval, asymptomatic white to yellow papules or plaques. Lesions are indurated with depressed nonulcerated centres and raised or rolled borders. They are predominantly found on the face (cheeks, chin and forehead) but have also been seen on the scalp, neck and upper trunk areas [3]. Lesions enlarge slowly over many years and rarely are observed larger than 2 cm. DTE is associated with intradermal

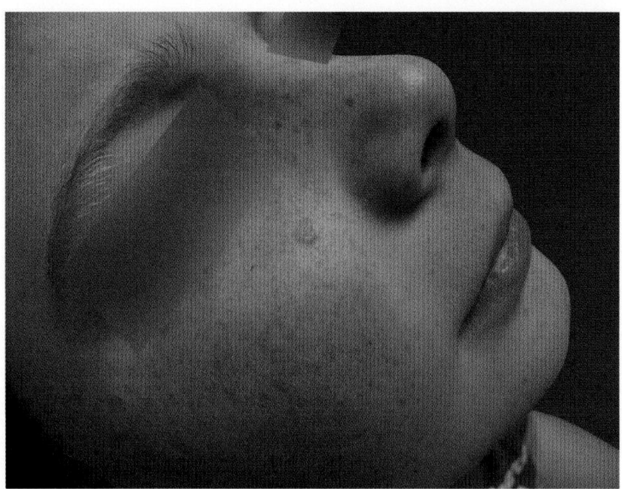

Fig. 111.3 Desmoplastic trichoepithelioma.

naevus at a frequency of 10% [4]. Milia-like components may also surround the lesions [5] (Fig. 111.3).

Diagnosis. Diagnosis is based on clinical and histological features. Dermoscopy may aid in the diagnosis, revealing lesions with a distinctive pearl-white to ivory white colour and prominent, large, arborizing vessels but no ovoid nests or leaf-life structures, distinct from basal cell carcinoma (BCC) [1].

Differential diagnosis. The clinical and histological features of DTE are most similar to those of morpheaform BCC. One must also consider sebaceous hyperplasia, conventional trichoepithelioma, granuloma annulare, scar tissue, scleroderma and cutaneous sarcoidosis [3,4].

Pathology. Histologically, DTE shares some features with BCC. The following triad describes DTE: narrow strands of trichoblast tumour cells, keratinaceous cysts and desmoplastic stroma [2]. Other characteristics include horn cysts, epidermal hyperplasia, foreign body keratin granulomas and calcification. In some cases epidermal change may lead to confusion with squamous cell carcinoma [7]. Sebaceous and apocrine differentiation is occasionally seen along with the usual follicular differentiation. Aggregations are rimmed by thin bundles of collagen that are separated from the surrounding dermis by a cleft [8]. Absence of androgen receptor expression in DTE helps to differentiate this lesion from BCC [9].

Treatment. DTEs do not require treatment. However, many patients undergo treatment for cosmetic reasons. Standard treatment is surgical excision [4]. DTEs are benign lesions but their tendency towards growth and facial predilection can make watchful waiting challenging. Curettage and electrodessication have also been used with no recurrence reported [5]. Dermabrasion with laser surgery has been reported to have success [3].

References

1 **Khelifa E, Masouyé I, Kaya G et al. Dermoscopy of desmoplastic trichoepithelioma reveals other criteria to distinguish it from basal cell carcinoma. Dermatology 2013;226:101–4.**
2 Brownstein MH, Shapiro L. Desmoplastic trichoepithelioma. Cancer 1977;40:2979–86.
3 Koay JL, Ledbetter LS, Page RN, Hsu S. Asymptomatic annular plaque of the chin: desmoplastic trichoepithelioma. Arch Dermatol 2002; 138:1091–6.
4 Mamelak AJ, Goldberg LH, Katz TM et al. Desmoplastic trichoepithelioma. J Am Acad Dermatol 2010;62:102–6.
5 Nuno-Gonzalez A. Desmoplastic trichoepithelioma: An infrequent entity not to be missed. A report of 2 cases. Pediatr Dermatol 2015; 32:e208–9.
6 Chuo CB, Slator R, Brown RM, Anderson KD. Management of desmoplastic trichoepithelioma in an infant. J Plast Reconstr Aesthet Surg 2008;61:1241–4.
7 Rossi AM, Busam KJ, Mehrara B, Nehal KS. Desmoplastic trichoepithelioma with overlying pseudoepitheliomatous hyperplasia mimicking squamous cell carcinoma in a pediatric patient. Dermatol Surg 2014; 40:477–9.
8 Costache M, Bresch M, Boer A. Desmoplastic trichoepithelioma versus morphoeic basal cell carcinoma: a critical reappraisal of histomorphological and immunohistochemical criteria for differentiation. Histopathology 2008;52:865–76.
9 Arits AH, Van Marion AM, Lohman BG et al. Differentiation between basal cell carcinoma and trichoepithelioma by immunohistochemical staining of the androgen receptor: an overview. Eur J Dermatol 2011; 21:870–3.

Hair follicle naevus

Hair follicle naevi are rare, benign, often congenital hamartomas of follicular differentiation composed of multiple vellus hairs.

Epidemiology. Hair follicle naevi are often congenital, presenting most commonly in infancy as a single nondescript 3–7 mm skin-coloured papule [1]. Although it is generally considered a congenital lesion, cases of acquired lesions have been reported [2,3].

Aetiology. The aetiology of hair follicle naevi is unknown. Reports of multiple lesions following the lines of Blaschko suggest that this hamartoma might have resulted from a somatic mutation that occurred early in gestation [4]. The presence of hair follicle naevi with leptomeningeal angiomatosis raises the possibility of a neurocutaneous disorder [5].

Presentation. Hair follicle naevus most commonly presents as a nodule on the face within the distribution of the first branchial arch [2]. Although it is usually a solitary lesion, reports of multiple lesions have been described [6], including those that follow the lines of Blaschko [4]. Association with leptomeningeal angiomatosis [6] and other epidermal lesions [4–6] has also been reported.

Diagnosis. Diagnosis is made clinically and pathologically. Dermoscopic evaluation may also aid in diagnosis. Dermoscopic findings include many uniform hair follicles and an interfollicular pseudo-pigment network within the nodules [7].

Differential diagnosis. Hair follicle naevus should be distinguished from dilated pore of Winer, accessory tragus, pilar sheath acanthoma, naevus sebaceus, woolly hair naevus, fibroma and trichofolliculoma. In contrast to these other hair follicle hamartomas, pathological differentiating characteristics of hair follicle naevi include lack of a central keratin-filled pore and the presence of well-developed hair follicles.

Pathology. Histologically, hair follicle naevus is composed of an excessive concentration of normal vellus or small telogen hairs haphazardly arranged at different stages of maturation with thickened perifollicular sheaths. Lesions are occasionally accompanied by a few small sebaceous glands, eccrine glands and pilar muscles [2,3].

Treatment. Treatment of choice is simple excision [2].

Prognosis. Hair follicle naevus has a benign course.

References

1 **Larson KN, O'Shea P, Zedek DC, Morrell D. Hair follicle nevus located on the chin of an infant: case report and review of literature. Pediatr Dermatol 2016;33:e106–8.**
2 Davis DA, Cohen PR. Hair follicle nevus: case report and review of the literature. Pediatr Dermatol 1996;13:135–8.
3 Motegi S, Amano H, Tamura A, Ishikawa O. Hair follicle nevus in a 2-year old. Pediatr Dermatol 2008;25:60–2.
4 Germain M, Smith KJ. Hair follicle nevus in a distribution following Blaskho's lines. J Am Acad Dermatol 2002;46(suppl):125–7.
5 Okada Y, Hamano K, Iwasaki N et al. Leptomeningeal angiomatosis accompanied by hair follicle nevus. Childs Nerv Syst 1998;14:218–21.
6 Ikeda S, Kawada J, Yaguchi H, Ogawa H. A case of unilateral, systematized linear hair follicle nevi associated with epidermal nevus-like lesions. Dermatology 2003;206:172–4.
7 Okada J, Moroi Y, Tsujita J et al. Hair follicle nevus: a dermoscopic approach. Eur J Dermatol 2008;18:185–7.

Apocrine differentiation

Apocrine hidrocystoma

Apocrine hidrocystoma is a rare, benign, adenomatous, cystic proliferation of the apocrine gland.

Epidemiology. An analysis of 167 cases revealed no predilection towards a specific sex or any age group, with cases occurring from <10 years of age to >80 years of age. In contrast with eccrine hidrocystomas, there is no relationship between the size or presentation of apocrine hidrocystomas with climate [1].

Aetiology. Apocrine hidrocystomas are benign skin neoplasms derived from the secretory portion of the apocrine gland [2]. Accordingly, most lesions are limited to the head, chest, axilla, groin and periareolar areas. In contrast to simple retention cysts, apocrine hidrocystomas are considered to be cystic proliferations of apocrine gland tufts.

Presentation. Apocrine hidrocystomas are slow-growing tumours generally found on the head and neck, especially in the periorbital region (61% of lesions [3]). Despite a predominance of periorbital lesions, appearance in other locations, including the penis [4,5] and finger [6], has also been reported [3]. Apocrine hidrocystomas are typically 1–2 mm in diameter, but have been reported up to 30–40 mm [1,3]. Lesions may be painful to touch [6]. While apocrine hidrocystoma most commonly presents as a single lesion, cases of multiple lesions have been observed [1,7]. The colour varies from skin-coloured to light-red, brown, blue or purple. Puncture of larger lesions may result in extravasation of a straw-coloured fluid [3,8].

Diagnosis. Diagnosis of apocrine hidrocystoma is based on pathological examination with special stains.

Differential diagnosis. This lesion must be distinguished from apocrine cystadenoma [2], eccrine hidrocystoma, cystic basal cell epithelioma, milium and epidermoid or pilar cysts [3].

Pathology. Histological examination reveals cystic spaces in the mid-dermis with some papillary projections. The epithelial lining of the cysts is composed of columnar cells showing a 'decapitation' secretion that is indicative of apocrine secretion [3] and underlying myoepithelial cells. Periodic acid–Schiff (PAS) stain demonstrates PAS-positive granules within the cells. Lesions stain negatively for S100, and positively for gross cystic disease fluid protein 15 (GCDFP-15), a marker of apocrine epithelium [5]. Adenomatous cysts with florid Ki-67-positive papillary projections into the cystic cavity, however, should be labelled apocrine cystadenomas and deserve more aggressive management [2].

Treatment. Simple excision is the treatment of choice for solitary lesions [6]. For lesions less than 1 cm in size, electrodessication has been reported to be effective, and may be more practical in individuals with multiple lesions [1]. The periorbital location of the majority of these lesions brings additional concern for complications of compromising lid function and causing ectropion through surgical excision. *En bloc* lower eyelid blepharoplasty has been reported as an effective means of excising apocrine hidrocystomas in close proximity to the eye [8].

Prognosis. In contrast to apocrine cystadenomas, apocrine hidrocystomas are benign lesions with no potential for malignant transformation [2].

References

1 Gupta S, Handa U, Handa S, Mohan H. The efficacy of electrosurgery and excision in treating patients with multiple apocrine hidrocystomas. Dermatol Surg 2001;27:382–4.
2 **Sugiyama A, Sugiura M, Piris A et al. Apocrine cystadenoma and apocrine hidrocystoma: examination of 21 cases with emphasis on nomenclature according to proliferative features. J Cutan Pathol 2007;34:912–17.**
3 Anzai S, Goto M, Fujiwara S, Da T. Apocrine hidrocystoma: a case report and analysis of 167 Japanese cases. Int J Dermatol 2005;44:702–3.
4 Mataix J, Bañuls J, Blanes M et al. Translucent nodular lesion of the penis: apocrine hidrocystoma of the penis. Arch Dermatol 2006;142:1221–6.
5 Samplaski MK, Somani N, Palmer JS. Apocrine hidrocystoma on the glans penis of a child. Urology 2009;73:800–1.

6 Santos-Juanes J, Galache Osuna C, Sánchez Del Río J et al. Apocrine hidrocystoma on the tip of a finger. Br J Dermatol 2005;152:379–80.
7 Vignes JR, Franco-Vidal V, Eimer S, Liguoro D. Intraorbital apocrine hidrocystoma. Clin Neurol Neurosurg 2007;109:631–3.
8 Henderer JD, Tanenbaum M. Excision of multiple eyelid apocrine hidrocystomas via an en bloc lower eyelid blepharoplasty incision. Ophthalmic Surg Lasers 2000;31:157–61.

Syringocystadenoma papilliferum

Syringocystadenoma papilliferum (SP) is a rare adnexal neoplasm of apocrine or apo-eccrine differentiation with characteristic histopathological findings despite a varied clinical appearance.

Epidemiology. SP is generally considered a congenital lesion. Between 45% and 51% of SP lesions are noted at birth, with another 13–15% appearing during infancy and childhood [1]. Linear plaque variants present at birth or during infancy, with the less common solitary nodular form appearing during puberty [2].

Aetiology. SP is derived from apocrine glands, although eccrine glands are also occasionally seen. Current consensus posits that SP derives from pluripotential appendageal cells or primitive apocrine glands [3,4]. SP arising with naevus sebaceus has been linked to somatic mutations in *HRAS* and *KRAS* [5]; however, mutations have also been identified in *PTCH* and v600E *BRAF* in certain contexts [6].

Presentation. SP typically appears as one of two different well-established primary lesions: a solitary skin-coloured to dark brown less than 4 cm in diameter hairless plaque, or one to several skin-coloured to pink papules less than 1 cm in diameter (Fig. 111.4). Lesions are most commonly found on the head or neck region (75%) and less commonly on the trunk (20%) or extremities (5%), along with other unusual locations including the breast, buttock, inguinal and perianal regions, and the scrotum [1,7]. Surface appearances range from flat and smooth to raised and exophytic. The smaller papular primary lesions are less common and are typically arranged in a linear pattern [8]. Solitary forms are seen predominantly as 1 cm domed or umbilicated nodules with a friable or crusted surface on the shoulders [2]. SP is the most common benign neoplasm found in naevus sebaceus. A recent retrospective analysis of 450 patients with naevus sebaceus found SP in 2.7% [9]. Between 30% and 40% of SP lesions occur within a naevus sebaceus. In this setting, multiple other benign adnexal neoplasms may be associated [1]. Associations with apocrine naevus [10], BCC, giant comedo and condyloma acuminatum have also been reported [2]. Larger ulcerated lesions may produce serous drainage or keratinous debris.

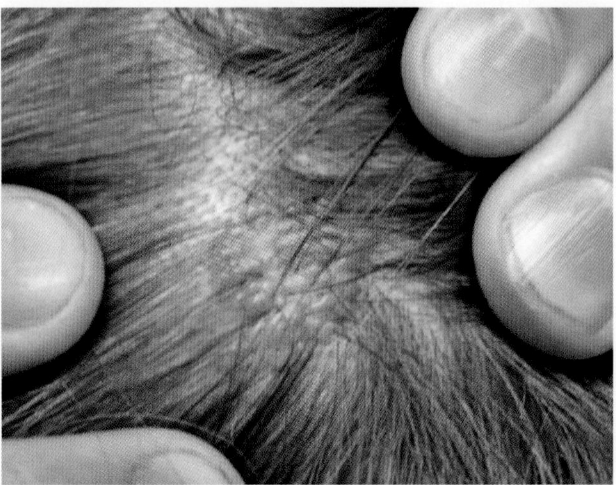

Fig. 111.4 Syringocystadenoma papilliferum. A flesh-coloured to pink alopecic plaque on the scalp.

Diagnosis. Because of the wide variety of morphological presentations, SP is generally a histological diagnosis.

Differential diagnosis. The differential diagnosis for the papular form includes molluscum contagiosum and BCC. The plaque type may suggest naevus sebaceus, verrucae vulgaris, seborrhoeic keratosis, extramammary Paget disease and hidradenoma papilliferum.

Pathology. Despite the morphological heterogeneity, SP has the distinctive histopathological characteristic of the presence of duct-like invaginations and cyst-like cavities extending from the epidermal surface into the body of the lesion. The papillary invaginations are lined by a two-layered epithelium: the luminal layer composed of columnar cells with oval nuclei and abundant eosinophilic cytoplasm, and the outer layer composed of small cuboidal cells with oval nuclei and scanty cytoplasm with 'capitation' secretion [1]. The stroma of the tumour often contains a dense infiltration of numerous plasma cells and lymphoid cells consistent with chronic inflammation. Histopathological differentiation from its malignant counterpart, syringocystadenocarcinoma papilliferum, is based on lack of cellular atypia, mitotic figures or invasive growth patterns.

Treatment. Standard treatment of SP is surgical excision into the subcutaneous layer with primary closure. CO_2 laser resurfacing has been proposed with some efficacy [11]. Prophylactic excision for diagnosis confirmation in the paediatric patient is of uncertain benefit because of the low risk of malignancy. Indications for surgical excision would include cosmesis as well as indications of malignant transformation: a rapid increase in size or number, ulceration with drainage, pruritus or pain [1,8].

Prognosis. While most lesions are benign, cases of syringocystadenocarcinoma papilliferum have been reported in the adult patient population [7]. Such malignant transformation is more common in cases of SP arising from naevus sebaceus. Ten per cent of SP lesions arising from naevus sebaceus also develop secondary BCC [2]. The time of malignant transformation from onset of syringocystadenoma papilliferum ranges from 20 to 50 years [8].

References

1 Townsend TC, Bowen AR, Nobuhara KK. Syringocystadenoma papilliferum: an unusual cutaneous lesion in a pediatric patient. J Pediatr 2004;145:131–3.
2 Saricaoglu H, Baskan EB, Ozuysal S, Tunali S. A case of syringocystadenoma papilliferum: an unusual localization on postoperative scar. J Eur Acad Dermatol Venereol 2002;16:534–6.
3 Dawn G, Gupta G. Linear warty papules on the neck of a young woman: syringocystadenoma papilliferum (SP) in a sebaceous nevus (SN). Arch Dermatol 2002;138:1091–6.
4 Chi CC, Tsai RY, Wang SH. Syringocystadenocarcinoma papilliferum: successfully treated with Mohs micrographic surgery. Dermatol Surg 2004;30:468–71.
5 Groesser L, Herschberger E, Ruetten A et al. Postzygotic HRAS and KRAS mutations cause nevus sebaceous and Schimmelpenning syndrome. Nat Genet 2012;44:783–7.
6 Levinsohn JL, Sugarman JL, Bilguvar K. Somatic V600E BRAF mutation in linear and sporadic syringocystadenoma papilliferum. J Invest Dermatol 2015;135:2536–8.
7 Gonul M, Soylu S, Gül U et al. Linear syringocystadenoma papilliferum of the arm: a rare localization of an uncommon tumor. Acta Derm Venereol 2008;88:528–9.
8 Narang T, De D, Dogra S et al. Linear papules and nodules on the neck: syringocystadenoma papilliferum (SP). Arch Dermatol 2008;144:1509–14.
9 Hsu MC, Liau JY, Hong JL. Secondary neoplasms arising from nevus sebaceous: a retrospective study of 450 cases in Taiwan. J Dermatol 2016;43:175–80.
10 Misago N, Narisawa Y. Syringocystadenoma papilliferum with extensive apocrine nevus. J Dermatol 2006;33:303–5.
11 Jordan JA, Brown OE, Biavati MJ, Manning SC. Congenital syringocystadenoma papilliferum of the ear and neck treated with the CO2 laser. Int J Pediatr Otorhinolaryngol 1996;38:81–7.

Apocrine naevus

The apocrine naevus is an extremely rare benign congenital tumour of the apocrine gland.

Epidemiology. While the presenting age of patients reporting lesions ranges from 19 to 68 years [1,2], the apocrine naevus is presumed to be congenital.

Aetiology. Immunohistochemical staining patterns of apocrine naevus lesions indicate an aetiology of these lesions as pure proliferations of mature well-differentiated apocrine glands [1].

Presentation. Very few cases of apocrine naevi have been reported in the literature. Clinical presentations have included alopecia, large fleshy nontender masses, infiltrated plaques, small solitary papules, multiple papules or nodules. While lesions are generally found in apocrine gland-rich areas, including the axillae and scalp [1,3,4], cases on non-apocrine gland-rich areas including the chest, cheek and abdominal skin have also been reported [2]. More commonly, this lesion is an associated finding of either naevus sebaceus or syringocystadenoma papilliferum [5].

Diagnosis. Despite a varied clinical appearance, the histological findings in apocrine naevi are distinct and diagnostic.

Differential diagnosis. Differential diagnosis includes hidradenitis suppurativa for lesions presenting in the axilla.

Pathology. Histological evaluation of the lesions reveals characteristic multiple mature apocrine glands with apical snouts arranged in lobules divided by thin fibrous septa. Luminal layers are composed of cuboidal or columnar secretory cells with cytoplasm and apical caps projecting into the lumen and the outer cell layer consisting of myoepithelial cells [1]. No cell atypia or mitotic figures are observed. There is no connection of the tumour to the normal overlying epidermis, fibrous capsules, cystic spaces or papillary projections, differentiating the tumour from other apocrine growths. Immunohistochemical studies of the glandular epithelium stain positively for low-molecular-weight cytokeratin, epithelial membrane antigen and GCDFP-15, and negatively for high-molecular-weight cytokeratin and S100 protein reactivity.

Carcinoembryonic antigen reactivity is found in the duct epithelium [4]. Cytokeratin 19 is positive in luminal cells but not in basal cells, consistent with maturated apocrine glands [2].

Treatment. Surgical excision is an effective treatment for these lesions [5].

References

1 Ando K, Hashikawa Y, Nakashima M et al. Pure apocrine nevus: a study of light-microscopic and immunohistochemical features of a rare tumor. Am J Dermatopathol 1991;13:71–6.
2 Numata Y, Okuyama R, Terui T et al. Apocrine nevus in abdominal skin. Dermatology 2006;213:46–7.
3 Kim JH, Hur H, Lee CW, Kim YT. Apocrine nevus. J Am Acad Dermatol 1988;18:579–81.
4 Neill JS, Park HK. Apocrine nevus: light microscopic, immunohistochemical and ultrastructural studies of a case. J Cutan Pathol 1993; 20:79–83.
5 Misago N, Narisawa Y. Syringocystadenoma papilliferum with extensive apocrine nevus. J Dermatol 2006;33:303–5.

Eccrine differentiation

Syringoma

Syringoma is a relatively common benign adnexal tumour derived from the eccrine duct. Although it is most often seen on the periorbital skin of middle-aged women, syringoma may manifest in many other clinical variants differing in age of onset, location and clinical appearance. Four principal clinical variants have been proposed in the medical literature: localized including the clear cell variant; familial; a form associated with Down syndrome; and a generalized form that encompasses multiple and eruptive syringomas. Despite the wide variety in clinical presentation, the underlying histological findings are identical [1].

Epidemiology. Syringomas affect 0.6% of the population with a female : male ratio of 6.6: 1 [2], and are equally common before and after puberty [3]. The eruptive form is more commonly seen in adolescent patients [4,5]. Familial syringoma is thought to be inherited in an autosomal dominant pattern [3,6]. Syringomas are seen in higher frequency in those with Down syndrome [1]. The clear cell variant of syringoma is associated with diabetes mellitus [7].

Aetiology. Immunohistochemical expression patterns suggest syringomas are derived from the eccrine duct [1,8]. The histogenesis is most related to pluripotent stem

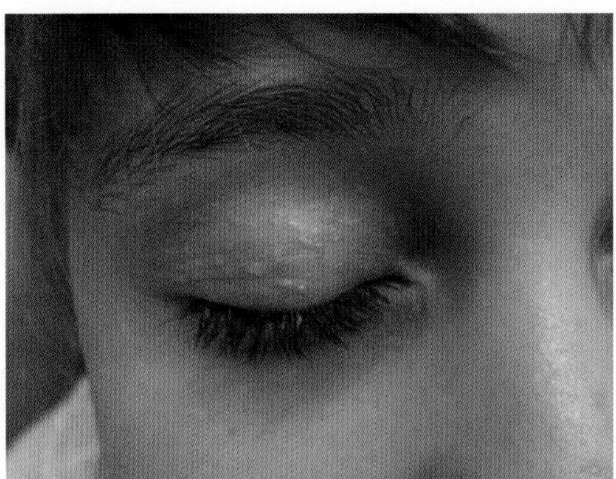

Fig. 111.5 Syringoma.

cells. Clear cell syringoma is considered a metabolic variant of ordinary syringoma [7].

Presentation. Syringomas present as single or multiple, small, soft, flesh-coloured to yellow-brown papules (Fig. 111.5). Lesions are firm, smooth and approximately 1–3 mm in diameter. They are most commonly found on the eyelids and upper aspects of the cheeks. Other sites include the face, neck, axillae, abdomen, vulva and penis [9]. Lesions on the scalp may present as a nonscarring alopecia [3]. Eruptive syringomas present as successive crops of small skin-coloured papules on the anterior of body surfaces [5].

Diagnosis. Because of the wide variety in clinical presentations of syringomas, diagnosis is based on histological examination.

Differential diagnosis. The differential diagnosis for syringoma should include multiple BCC, pigmented naevi, trichoepithelioma, angiofibroma, cylindroma, lichen planus-like lesions, keratosis pilaris, cutaneous sarcoidosis and sebaceous hyperplasia [1,10]. Penile lesions may be clinically similar to condyloma, lichen nitidus, lichen planus and bowenoid papulosis [9]. Lesions around the eyelid should be differentiated from xanthelasma and tuberous xanthomas. The differential diagnosis for axillary, vulvar or inguinal lesions would include Fox–Fordyce disease, epidermal inclusion cysts, lichen simplex chronicus and steatocystoma multiplex. Eruptive syringoma may be clinically mistaken for acne vulgaris, sebaceous hyperplasia, milia, lichen planus, eruptive xanthoma, urticaria pigmentosa or hidrocystoma [5].

Pathology. The histological findings of syringomas are characteristic and diagnostic. Examination of pathology reveals a proliferation of small cysts, lined by a double layer of epithelium, set in a fibrous stroma. Cysts are often described as comma-like or tadpole-like in shape, with this finding being reported in 56% of lesions [2]. Immunohistochemical staining patterns show expression of CK6 on inner ductal cells and CK10 on intermediate or middle ductal cells. These lesions also stain positively for CD34 but negatively for smooth muscle actin and CD10 [8].

Treatment. Treatment of syringomas is generally considered cosmetic. Effective methods include surgical excision, cryotherapy with liquid nitrogen, CO_2 laser [11], dermabrasion, chemical peeling with tattoo and laser, electrocoagulation at low voltage [12] and chemical therapy with agents such as topical or systemic retinoids [12]. Topical atropine has been reported to alleviate the pruritus in symptomatic eruptive syringoma [2].

Prognosis. Syringomas are benign lesions with no malignant potential and limited proliferative capacity [8]. Recurrence frequently occurs following treatment. Rarely, tumours may regress spontaneously in adulthood [5].

References

1 Friedman SJ, Butler DF. Syringoma presenting as milia. J Am Acad Dermatol 1987;16:310–14.
2 Lee JH, Chang JY, Lee KH. Syringoma: a clinicopathologic and immunohistologic study and results of treatment. Yonsei Med J 2007;48:35–40.
3 Draznin M. Hereditary syringomas: a case report. Dermatol Online J 2004;10:19.
4 Patrizi A, Neri I, Marzaduri S et al. Syringoma: a review of twenty-nine cases. Acta Derm Venereol 1998;78:460–2.
5 Teixeira M, Ferreira M, Machado S et al. Eruptive syringomas. Dermatol Online J 2005;11:34.
6 Ribera M, Servitje O, Peyri J, Ferrándiz C. Familial syringoma clinically suggesting milia. J Am Acad Dermatol 1989;20:702–3.
7 Shimizu A, Nagai Y, Ishikawa O. Guess what! Clear cell syringoma. Eur J Dermatol 2000;10:633–4.
8 Missall TA, Burkemper NM, Jensen SL, Hurley MY. Immunohistochemical differentiation of four benign eccrine tumors. J Cutan Pathol 2009; 36:190–6.
9 Olson JM, Robles DT, Argenyi ZB et al. Multiple penile syringomas. J Am Acad Dermatol 2008;59(suppl 1):46–7.
10 Gordon D, Barankin B. Question: can you identify this condition? Can Fam Physician 2008;54:1114, 1122.
11 Park HJ, Lee DY, Lee JH et al. The treatment of syringomas by CO(2) laser using a multiple-drilling method. Dermatol Surg 2007;33:310–3.
12 Al Aradi IK. Periorbital syringoma: a pilot study of the efficacy of low-voltage electrocoagulation. Dermatol Surg 2006;32:1244–50.

Eccrine poroma

Eccrine poroma (EP) is a benign tumour of the eccrine sweat duct. Eccrine sweat gland tumours represent about 1% of all primary skin lesions, of which only 10% are EP [1].

Epidemiology. While EP generally occurs in patients over the age of 40 years, with a peak incidence in the seventh decade of life, a few cases have also been reported in children [1–3] with a single congenital case currently in the literature [4]. There does not seem to be any sexual, racial or familial predisposition for these lesions [5,6].

Aetiology. Comparative observations of immunohistochemical staining between EP and normal eccrine glands revealed a staining pattern of poroma cells similar to that of basal cells of the eccrine gland dermal duct [7]. Additionally, the lack of expression of the secretory coil marker CK7 suggests derivation from the outer portion of the eccrine duct [8]. Recent reports of histological findings of elongated 'clefts', hair follicles and other appendageal structures in poromas, however, suggest a mixed eccrine and apocrine origin [2]. Radiation, trauma and hormonal influence during pregnancy have all been suggested as

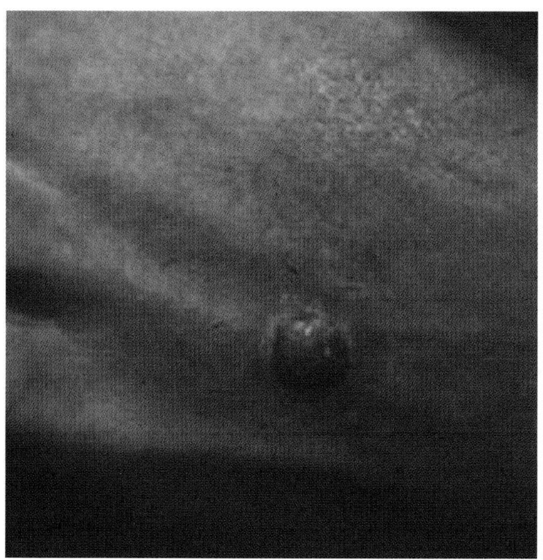

Fig. 111.6 Eccrine poroma. Solitary circumscribed red papule on foot. Source: Courtesy of Dr Marilyn Liang.

potential pathogenic triggers for EP [9]. Intrauterine trauma has been proposed as a possible mechanism for the single case of congenital EP [4].

Presentation. Morphologically, EP exhibit a polymorphic gross appearance, presenting most commonly as solitary, sharply demarcated, nontender (though sometimes painful), skin-coloured papules or nodules less than 3 cm in diameter. Eccrine poroma may also be protuberant, sessile or pedunculated, and is often verrucous or lobulated [10]. Lesions may also be pigmented or erythematous (Fig. 111.6). Reported surface changes include bleeding, erosion and ulceration, probably secondary to trauma. While historically perceived as acral lesions restricted to hairless eccrine (plantar or palmar) surfaces, EP can also present on the fingers, trunk, head and neck [1,2]. Eccrine poroma can rarely present as clusters, referred to as poromatosis [5].

Diagnosis. Because of the wide variety in clinical presentations of EP, diagnosis is based on histological examination.

Differential diagnosis. Because of the clinical heterogeneity exhibited by EP, a wide differential is often considered. Verruca vulgaris, pyogenic granuloma, fibroma, intradermal naevus, papillomatous naevus, benign haemangioma, Kaposi sarcoma, molluscum contagiosum, seborrhoeic keratosis, squamous cell carcinoma and BCC have been described as potential differential diagnoses [1,3,6,10,11].

Pathology. The histological features of EP are distinctive and diagnostic. EP are located superficially in the dermis. They are composed of solid bands of monomorphic basaloid cells with varying numbers of cystic or ductal structures, in a richly vascularized stroma. The nuclei of these cells are small, dark and centrally located. Surface tumour cells undergoing keratinization form keratohyalin granules. Cells are connected by intercellular bridges and glycogen is unevenly distributed among the cells, causing some cells to appear paler than others [6,10,11].

Treatment. Malignant transformation of pre-existing EP is rare. Indications for treatment would include cosmesis and signs of malignant transformation: ulceration, bleeding, pain or itching. While malignant transformation is generally restricted to longstanding EP, a single case of malignant transformation in a child illustrates the potential for an aggressive course in these lesions [3]. Definitive treatment for EP is complete local surgical excision.

Prognosis. EP has the potential for malignant transformation. Local recurrence is common after incomplete resection.

References

1 Orlandi C, Arcangeli F, Patrizi A, Neri I. Eccrine poroma in a child. Pediatr Dermatol 2005;22:279–80.
2 Betti R, Bombinates C, Cerri A et al. Unusual sites for poromas are not very unusual: a survey of 101 cases. Clin Exp Dermatol 2014;39:119–22.
3 Valverde K, Senger C, Ngan BY, Chan HS. Eccrine porocarcinoma in a child that evolved rapidly from an eccrine poroma. Med Pediatr Oncol 2001;37:412–14.
4 Wang SH, Tsai TF. Congenital polypoid pigmented eccrine poroma of a young woman. J Eur Acad Dermatol Venereol 2008;22:366–8.
5 Navi D, Fung M, Lynch PJ. Poromatosis: the occurrence of multiple eccrine poromas. Dermatol Online J 2008;14:3.
6 Hyman AB, Brownstein MH. Eccrine poroma. An analysis of forty-five new cases. Dermatologica 1969;138:29–38.
7 Watanabe S, Mogi S, Ichikawa E et al. Immunohistochemical analysis of keratin distribution in eccrine poroma. Am J Pathol 1993;142:231–9.
8 Missall TA, Burkemper NM, Jensen SL, Hurley MY. Immunohistochemical differentiation of four benign eccrine tumors. J Cutan Pathol 2009;36:190–6.
9 Nemoto I, Akiyama N, Aoyagi S et al. Eccrine porocarcinoma and eccrine poroma arising in a scar. Br J Dermatol 2004;150:1232–3.
10 Moeller CA, Welch RH, Kaplan DL. An enlarging tumor of the foot. Eccrine poroma. Arch Dermatol 1987;123:653–4, 656.
11 Johnson RC, Rosenmeier GJ, Keeling JH 3rd. A painful step: eccrine poroma. Arch Dermatol 1992;128:1530, 1533.

Eccrine naevus

Eccrine naevi are extremely rare hamartomas characterized histologically by an increase in the number and/or size of structurally normal eccrine sweat glands without vascular proliferation [1]. A subtype of eccrine naevus, mucinous eccrine naevus, contains both eccrine and mucinous elements.

Epidemiology. Eccrine naevus most commonly presents at birth or at an early age with no gender predilection [1]. While there have reports of symptoms occurring at an advanced age, most cases present at birth or in childhood [2]. Cases of congenital mucinous eccrine naevi have been reported [3]. The age range of mucinous eccrine naevi in the medical literature is between 2 and 47 years [4–6].

Aetiology. The pathogenesis of eccrine naevi is unknown. Trauma and a potential defect in embryogenesis have both been proposed as potential aetiologies for this disorder [4]. Its predominant appearance on the forearm has been hypothesized to be phylogenetically related to the *Lemur catta* antebrachial organ formed by the sudoriparous glands to delimit its territory [7].

Presentation. Clinical manifestations of eccrine naevi include localized hyperhidrosis, nonspecific skin surface changes, or both. Most patients present with localized hyperhidrosis with no overlying skin abnormality. Occasionally, skin changes accompanying the hyperhidrosis can occur, most commonly as a hyperpigmented patch overlying a hyperhidrotic area, but also as a single sweat-discharging pore [3]. Additionally, a variant of eccrine naevi without hyperhidrosis has been reported with the presenting lesions described as skin-coloured papules [2], slightly brown papules, depressed brown macules [8], coccygeal polypoid mass or perianal skin tag [9,10]. Fifty per cent of eccrine naevi present on the forearm [1]. Other locations include the back or the trunk. It has been observed that eccrine naevi follow the lines of Blaschko [5]. Clinical manifestations of mucinous eccrine naevi have been described as brown nodules or patches. Involved sites include the lower extremities, buttock and toes. As with eccrine naevi, hyperhidrosis is not always seen with the clinical lesions [4–6].

Diagnosis. Diagnosis of eccrine naevus is based on histological examination.

Differential diagnosis. Differential diagnosis should include other aetiologies of localized hyperhidrosis including eccrine angiomatous hamartoma, sudoriparous angioma or idiopathic hyperhidrosis (in which no changes are identified upon histological examination) [1].

Pathology. Eccrine naevus is defined by the histological findings of an increase in size and/or number of normally structured mature eccrine secretory coils without vascular proliferation. The mucinous variant is characterized by a proliferation of normally structured eccrine sweat glands surrounded by abundant mucinous material [4].

Prognosis. Eccrine naevi follow a benign course.

Treatment. First-line treatment for localized hyperhidrosis consists of topical aluminium chloride and anticholinergic medications. Other treatments include botulinum toxin [7] and iontophoresis. Systemic anticholinergics and antidepressants with anticholinergic properties have also been reported as potential treatments. Surgical excision of the affected skin or sympathectomy are other treatment modalities. Intralesional steroids have been reported as effective in cases of mucinous eccrine naevi [6].

References

1 Kawaoka JC, Gray J, Schappell D, Robinson-Bostom L. Eccrine nevus. J Am Acad Dermatol 2004;51:301–4.

2 Morris ES, Scheel MM, Lundquist KF, Raimer SS. Grouped papules on the arm of an infant: eccrine nevus. Arch Dermatol 2000;136:549, 552.

3 Tempark T, Schwayder T. Mucinous eccrine naevus: case report and review of the literature. Clin Exp Dermatol 2013;38:1–4.

4 Chen CW, Tsai TF, Chen YF, Hung CM. Congenital mucinous eccrine nevus in a 5-month-old girl with frequent intertriginous dermatitis. Pediatr Dermatol 2008;25:573–4.

5 Espana A, Marquina M, Idoate MA. Extensive mucinous eccrine naevus following the lines of Blaschko: a new type of eccrine naevus. Br J Dermatol 2006;154:1004–6.

6 Lee WJ, Chang SE, Lee MW et al. Bilateral mucinous eccrine nevus in an adult. J Dermatol 2008;35:552–4.

7 Honeyman JF, Valdés R, Rojas H, Gaete M. Efficacy of botulinum toxin for a congenital eccrine naevus. J Eur Acad Dermatol Venereol 2008;22:1275–6.

8 Hong CE, Lee SH. Multiple eccrine nevus with depressed patches. Yonsei Med J 1997;38:60–2.

9 Mahdavy M, Smoller BR. Eccrine nevus presenting as a perianal skin tag: a case report and review of the literature. Am J Dermatopathol 2002;24:361–3.

10 Oh SW, Kang TW, Kim YC, Lew W. Coccygeal polypoid eccrine naevus. Br J Dermatol 2007;157:614–15.

Porokeratotic eccrine ostial and dermal duct naevus (PEODDN)

A porokeratotic eccrine ostial and dermal duct naevus (PEODDN) is a rare hamartoma of eccrine origin typically present at birth but occasionally presenting later on the palms or soles [1].

Epidemiology. PEODDN typically presents at birth but may appear later in life. There is no gender predilection and PEODDN has been described occasionally in association with deafness, seizure disorder, developmental delay, breast hypoplasia and squamous cell carcinoma [2].

Aetiology. Cases of PEODDN in patients with keratitis, ichthyosis and deafness (KID) syndrome [3] suggested the possibility of connexin mutations being related to causation, and recent work has confirmed the role of p.G45E *GJB2* mutations in both sporadic and KID-related cases of PEODDN [4].

Presentation. PEODDN presents with a linear array of keratotic pits on the palms or soles. Lesions can occur later in life and are variably itchy.

Diagnosis. Diagnosis of PEODDN is typically clinical with consistent supportive histology.

Differential diagnosis. Clinically, PEODDN looks like a naevus comedonicus but it occurs on the palms and soles. Other considerations could include linear porokeratosis, linear lichen planus and linear Darier disease.

Pathology. Histopathology shows hyperkeratosis and acanthosis with a cornoid lamella overlying a dilated hyperkeratinized acrosyringium [1].

Prognosis. PEODDN follow a benign course.

Treatment. Treatment can be challenging but good results have been achieved with CO_2 laser. Topical modalities including keratolytics, retinoids and steroids as well as locally destructive techniques such as cryotherapy or electrocautery have generally been unsatisfactory [5].

References

1 Masferrer E, Vicente MA, Bassas-Vila J et al. PEODDN: a report of 10 cases. J Eur Acad Dermatol Venereol 2010;24:847–51.

2 Goddard DS, Rogers M, Frieden IJ et al. Widespread PEODDN: Clinical features and a proposal for a new name unifying PEODDN and porokeratotic eccrine and hair follicle nevus. JAAD 2009;61:1060.

3 Criscione V, Lachiewicz A, Robinson-Bostom L et al. Porokeratotic eccrine duct and hair follicle nevus (PEHFN) associated with keratitis-ichthyosis-deafness (KID) syndrome. Pediatr Dermatol 2010;27:514–17.
4 Levinsohn JL, McNiff JM, Antaya RJ, Choate KA. A somatic p.G45E GJB2 mutation causing porokeratotic eccrine ostial and dermal duct nevus. JAMA Dermatol 2015;151:638–41.
5 Jain S, Sardana K, Garg VK. Ultrapulse carbon dioxide laser treatment of porokeratotic eccrine ostial and dermal duct nevus. Pediatr Dermatol 2013;30:264–6.

Sebaceous differentiation

Sebaceous hyperplasia

Sebaceous hyperplasia describes benign skin lesions that are most commonly seen in middle-aged men. Sebaceous glands are aggregates of acini that empty into networks of ducts around hair follicles to produce sebum on the skin surface. Activity and size of the glands varies with age: they are large at birth, smaller in childhood and increase in activity during puberty along with increased androgen production. Gland size and activity peak at 20–30 years [1]. A normal variant of transient sebaceous hyperplasia occurs in most neonates, prominently around the nose, in response to maternal androgens. The present focus will be on a subset of patients who present with persistent skin lesions called premature sebaceous hyperplasia (PSH) [2].

Epidemiology. PSH presents from birth through puberty and up to 26 years of age. There is no gender predominance [2,3].

Aetiology. Case reports of familial PSH, including one where a five-consecutive-generation pedigree was described, suggest autosomal dominant inheritance with incomplete penetrance. A lesser degree of involvement in one female family member in the setting of normal serum testosterone levels suggests that the disease is not caused by an overproduction of testosterone, but rather a presumed hyper-responsiveness of the sebaceous gland to testosterone [4].

Presentation. The clinical appearance of PSH consists of scattered or sometimes confluent soft umbilicated papules or plaques. There is selective localization on the face, neck and upper thorax, mirroring the anatomical locations where sebaceous glands are most abundant. Cases have also been described on genital skin [5]. Lesions worsen with age [2,3]. The eruption is chronic and has no seasonal variations [3].

Traditional sebaceous hyperplasia, which is seen most commonly in middle-aged men, in contrast, is suspected to be caused by a reduced cellular turnover secondary to decreased androgen levels with age and the subsequent crowding of undifferentiated sebaceous cells in sebaceous gland lobules [6]. Systemic corticosteroids and haemodialysis have been implicated among the various causes of sebaceous hyperplasia.

Other than the familial form, sebaceous hyperplasia has been reported at earlier ages in the immunosuppressed, as part of Muir–Torre syndrome, pachydermoperiostosis, and in association with X-linked hypohidrotic ectodermal dysplasia [6].

Diagnosis. The distinct visual characteristics of this disease make the diagnosis a clinical one. Because of distinguishing changes seen in pathology, biopsy can be performed to confirm a diagnosis.

Differential diagnosis. Differential diagnosis of this condition includes rosacea, multiple sebaceous adenomas, trichoepitheliomas, angiofibromas of tuberous sclerosis [3], sebaceous epithelioma and BCC [6].

Histologically, these lesions should be differentiated from naevus sebaceus, sebaceous adenoma, basal cell epithelioma with sebaceous differentiation and sebaceous carcinoma [3].

Pathology. Histological findings of PSH are the same as those of senile sebaceous hyperplasia. Pathological examination reveals normal epidermis overlying sebaceous gland hypertrophy with normal cellular and glandular maturation [3]. Some sebaceous lobules may contain a central large dilated follicular channel [2].

Treatment. Successful response to oral isotretinoin has been reported [3]. Surgical excision, topical chemicals, cryotherapy and bichloroacetic acid, electrodessication and curettage, intralesional desiccation and lasers have all been described as potential treatments for sebaceous hyperplasia. Photodynamic therapy with 5-aminolaevulinic acid has also been described as a safe and effective treatment [6].

Prognosis. Sebaceous hyperplasia is considered a benign lesion and treatment is most commonly pursued for cosmetic reasons.

References

1 Zouboulis CC, Boschnakow A. Chronological ageing and photoageing of the human sebaceous gland. Clin Exp Dermatol 2001;26:600–7.
2 Oh ST, Kwon HJ. Premature sebaceous hyperplasia in a neonate. Pediatr Dermatol 2007;24:443–5.
3 Grimalt R, Ferrando J, Mascaro JM. Premature familial sebaceous hyperplasia: successful response to oral isotretinoin in three patients. J Am Acad Dermatol 1997;37:996– 8.
4 Boonchai W, Leenutaphong V. Familial presenile sebaceous gland hyperplasia. J Am Acad Dermatol 1997;36:120–2.
5 Al-Daraji WI, Wagner B, Ali RB, McDonagh AJ. Sebaceous hyperplasia of the vulva: a clinicopathological case report with a review of the literature. J Clin Pathol 2007;60:835–7.
6 Richey DF. Aminolevulinic acid photodynamic therapy for sebaceous gland hyperplasia. Dermatol Clin 2007;25:59–65.

CHAPTER 112
Calcification and Ossification in the Skin

Amanda T. Moon[1,2], *Albert C. Yan*[1,2] *& Eulalia T. Baselga*[3]

[1] Departments of Pediatrics and Dermatology, Perelman School of Medicine at the University of Pennsylvania, Philadelphia, PA, USA
[2] Section of Dermatology, Children's Hospital of Philadelphia, Philadelphia, PA, USA
[3] Pediatric Dermatology Unit, Hospital de la Santa Creu I Sant Pau, Universitat Autònoma de Barcelona, Spain

Introduction, 1338
Calcium regulation and phosphate regulation, 1338
Aberrant calcification and ossification of the skin, 1339
Idiopathic calcification, 1340
Dystrophic calcification, 1343
Metastatic calcification, 1345
Iatrogenic calcinosis cutis, 1346
Cutaneous ossification, 1346

Abstract

Disorders of calcium regulation can result in aberrant deposition of calcium in the skin, resulting in cutaneous forms of calcification or ossification. This chapter focuses on explaining the regulation of calcium by regulatory hormones, and the disorders that can arise from mutations affecting enzymes involved in this regulation. We focus specifically on classifying cutaneous calcification into the traditional categories of idiopathic, dystrophic, metastatic and iatrogenic forms, and then discuss specific entities associated with cutaneous ossification. The principal forms of cutaneous ossification – progressive osseous heteroplasia, Albright hereditary osteodystrophy and plate-like osteoma cutis – are all derived from inactivating mutations in *GNAS*, with the specific phenotype manifesting attributed to genomic imprinting.

Key points

- Calcium levels in the serum and body fluids are tightly regulated by the action of a series of regulatory hormones. Disorders of calcium regulation by these hormones can result in aberrant deposition of calcium in the skin and lead to calcification or ossification.
- Calcification is the deposition of insoluble calcium salts; when it occurs in the skin it is termed calcinosis cutis.
- Ossification is the formation of true bony tissue by deposition of a proteinaceous matrix by osteoblasts; calcium salts are then deposited within this proteinaceous matrix as in normal bone formation.
- Cutaneous calcification can be divided into four main groups: dystrophic, metastatic, idiopathic and iatrogenic.
- The principal forms of cutaneous ossification – progressive osseous heteroplasia, Albright hereditary osteodystrophy and plate-like osteoma cutis – result from inactivating mutations in *GNAS*, with the specific phenotype manifesting attributed to genomic imprinting.

Introduction

Calcium is an essential divalent cation involved in diverse cellular functions, including keratinocyte proliferation and differentiation, and cell–cell adhesion. Because of its central role in physiology, calcium levels in the serum and body fluids are tightly regulated by the action of a series of regulatory hormones. The balance of serum and extracellular calcium with respect to phosphates is close to their saturation points, so deviations in concentrations of either can cause precipitation. Despite this tight regulation, various disorders can result in aberrant deposition of calcium in the skin as either crystalline deposits of calcium or bone.

Calcium regulation and phosphate regulation

The three major regulators of calcium are parathyroid hormone (PTH), vitamin D and calcitonin. Both PTH and the active metabolite of vitamin D ($1,25[OH]_2D_3$) act to increase serum calcium, whereas calcitonin acts to decrease serum calcium. There is growing evidence that other factors, such as phosphatonins, play a role in regulating phosphate and calcium homeostasis as well.

Parathyroid hormone

PTH is an 84-amino-acid polypeptide that is synthesized in the parathyroid gland. A decrease in serum calcium

Harper's Textbook of Pediatric Dermatology, Fourth Edition. Edited by Peter Hoeger, Veronica Kinsler and Albert Yan.

or 1,25(OH)$_2$D$_3$ stimulates PTH synthesis and secretion. PTH acts directly to increase renal tubular resorption of calcium and to enhance bone reabsorption. PTH also stimulates 1α-hydroxylase activity in the kidney, causing an increase in the plasma concentration of 1,25(OH)$_2$D$_3$, which, in turn, increases intestinal absorption of calcium. A protein related to PTH, PTH-related peptide (PTHrP), has been isolated from malignant cells, particularly of epithelial origin, as well as normal keratinocytes. It acts through the same receptor as PTH, although its role in normal physiology is not well understood. It is believed to be responsible for hypercalcaemia of malignancy. Elevated levels of PTH have been found in various keratinization disorders including ichthyosis vulgaris, Darier disease, epidermolytic hyperkeratosis, autosomal recessive congenital ichthyoses, pityriasis rubra pilaris and ichthyosis linearis circumflexa [1]. The significance of this finding is unclear; however, PTH/PTHrP type I receptors have been identified in skin fibroblasts [2], and a novel receptor has been identified in keratinocytes [3], suggesting that PTH may have hormonal effects on these cells in addition to its classic targets.

Vitamin D

Vitamin D, or cholecalciferol, is a secosteroid formed by the opening of the β-ring of 7-dehydrocholesterol in the skin after exposure to ultraviolet B light. Chemical photolysis produces a thermally labile provitamin D$_3$ that undergoes thermal isomerization to form vitamin D$_3$. Vitamin D$_3$ is hydroxylated at C-25 in the liver and C-1 in the kidney to become the biologically active 1,25(OH)$_2$D$_3$. The C-1 hydroxylation is inhibited by calcium, phosphate and 1,25(OH)$_2$D$_3$, whereas PTH and calcitonin stimulate it. The main action of 1,25(OH)$_2$D$_3$ is to increase intestinal absorption of calcium and phosphate. 1,25(OH)$_2$D$_3$ is also necessary for PTH-induced bone resorption. In addition to these actions, 1,25(OH)$_2$D$_3$ has a major role in the growth and differentiation of tissues, including the skin. 1,25(OH)$_2$D$_3$ receptors have been found in keratinocytes, pilosebaceous structures and dermal fibroblasts. 1,25(OH)$_2$D$_3$ causes a dose-dependent decrease in proliferation and an increase in differentiation in human keratinocytes. Whether the effect of 1,25(OH)$_2$D$_3$ on keratinocytes is mediated via its effects on calcium and calcium-binding proteins or whether it is a hormonal effect through interaction with the vitamin D receptor remains unknown.

Calcitonin

Calcitonin is a 32-amino-acid polypeptide synthesized by parafollicular cells of the thyroid gland. Calcitonin in pharmacological doses acts to decrease serum calcium by decreasing bone resorption and tubular calcium reabsorption. Calcitonin levels are much higher in children than adults; however, the role of this hormone in normal physiology is speculative because thyroidectomized patients maintain normal serum calcium levels.

Phosphatonins

A growing body of evidence now suggests that in addition to PTH and vitamin D there are other factors that have a role in phosphate homeostasis. The term phosphatonins has been introduced to describe these endocrine factors that induce renal phosphate wasting and a phosphaturic response [4], independent of PTH. Phosphatonins include fibroblast growth factor (FGF-23), secreted frizzled related protein (sFRP-4) and matrix extracellular phosphoglycoprotein (MEPE).

References

1 Milstone LM, Ellison AF, Insogna KL. Serum parathyroid hormone level is elevated in some patients with disorders of keratinization. Arch Dermatol 1992;128:926–30.
2 Hanafin NM, Chen TC, Heinrich G et al. Cultured human fibroblasts and not cultured human keratinocytes express a PTH/PTHrP receptor mRNA. J Invest Dermatol 1995;105:133–7.
3 Orloff JJ, Kats Y, Urena P et al. Further evidence for a novel receptor for amino-terminal parathyroid hormone-related protein on keratinocytes and squamous carcinoma cell lines. Endocrinology 1995;136:3016–23.
4 Berndt T, Kumar R. Novel mechanisms in the regulation of phosphorus homeostasis. Physiology (Bethesda) 2009;24:17–25.

Aberrant calcification and ossification of the skin

Calcification is the deposition of insoluble calcium salts; when it occurs in the skin it is termed calcinosis cutis. Ossification is the formation of true bony tissue by deposition of a collagen I proteinaceous matrix by osteoblasts; calcium salts are then deposited within this proteinaceous matrix as in normal bone formation [1–3].

Cutaneous calcification can be divided into four main groups: dystrophic, metastatic, idiopathic and iatrogenic (Box 112.1). Dystrophic calcification refers to calcium deposition secondary to trauma or local tissue inflammation

Box 112.1 Causes (or classification) of cutaneous calcification

Idiopathic calcification

Subepidermal calcified nodule
Idiopathic calcinosis of the scrotum
Milia-like idiopathic calcinosis cutis
Tumoral calcinosis

Dystrophic

Connective tissue diseases
Panniculitis
Pseudoxanthoma elasticum
Ehlers–Danlos syndrome
Werner syndrome
Rothmund–Thomson syndrome
Cutaneous neoplasms
Infections
Trauma

Metastatic

Chronic renal insufficiency
Primary hyperparathyroidism
Hypervitaminosis D

(Continued)

Box 112.1 *Continued*

Milk–alkali syndrome
Sarcoidosis
Neoplasms
Osteomyelitis

Iatrogenic

Intravenous calcium solution/infusions
Subcutaneous heparin
Electroencephalography/electromyography/evoked potential
Liver transplantation
Intramuscular injection of vitamin E

in patients with normal calcium and phosphate metabolism. Dystrophic calcification is the most common cause of calcinosis cutis. Metastatic calcification is the result of an underlying derangement in calcium or phosphorus metabolism. It can affect any organ, including the skin. In idiopathic calcification, there is neither local tissue injury nor abnormal calcium and/or phosphate metabolism. Finally, cutaneous calcinosis may be iatrogenic.

Histologically, calcium deposits stain deep blue with haematoxylin and eosin, and black with von Kossa stain. In the dermis, calcium deposits are small and finely granular, whereas they are often much larger in the subcutaneous tissue. Cutaneous ossification usually occurs in a previously calcified focus or after local tissue injury. Any calcifying disorder of the skin may secondarily ossify. Primary ossification with spontaneous new bone formation occurs in a few instances and has been referred to as osteoma cutis (OC).

References

1 Orlow SJ, Watsky KL, Bolognia JL. Skin and bones. II. J Am Acad Dermatol 1991;25:447–62.

2 **Walsh JS, Fairley JA. Calcifying disorders of the skin. J Am Acad Dermatol 1995;33:693–706.**

3 **Mehregan AH. Calcinosis cutis: a review of the clinical forms and report of 75 cases. Semin Dermatol 1984;3:53–61.**

Idiopathic calcification

Subepidermal calcified nodule

Subepidermal calcified nodule [1], also known as solitary congenital nodular calcification or Winer's nodular calcinosis, is a form of localized calcinosis cutis that occurs in infancy or early childhood. The lesions may be present at birth.

Epidemiology and pathogenesis. The male to female ratio is 2:1. The pathogenesis remains unknown. Calcification of a pre-existing milium, eccrine duct, sweat duct hamartoma or naevus cells has been proposed. Degranulation of mast cells with secondary calcification has also been suggested. Since they are frequently located on the ears, trauma may play a role.

Clinical features. Solitary, firm, white, verrucous 3–10 mm papules are found most commonly on the head and neck

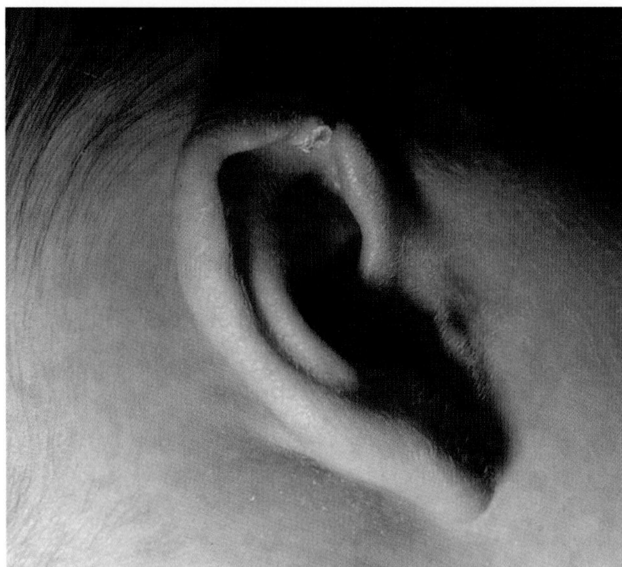

Fig. 112.1 Subepidermal calcified nodule on the ear of a child. Source: Courtesy of Dr Nancy Esterly.

area, especially on the ears (Fig. 112.1) and eyelids. They may also occur on limbs and the sides of the fingers and soles. Lesions have also been reported in the oral mucosa [2]. The lesions may ulcerate and extrude chalky material, but are typically asymptomatic.

Differential diagnosis. Subepidermal calcified nodules may be confused with verruca vulgaris and pilomatricomas. On the eyelids in an elderly patient they may occasionally be confused with xanthelasma.

Histopathology. Focal globular or large amorphous collections of calcium are found in the dermis with a variable degree of histiocytic infiltration and foreign body granuloma formation [1]. Epidermal ulceration with transepidermal elimination of calcium can be seen.

Treatment. Surgical excision is the treatment of choice.

Idiopathic calcinosis of the scrotum/vulva

Calcinosis of the scrotum is a rare disease characterized by calcified nodules of the scrotal wall. Most patients present between 20 and 40 years of age, but patients as young as 5 years old have been reported [3].

Epidemiology and pathogenesis. The pathogenesis remains controversial. Many believe that the condition is truly idiopathic. Others maintain that it represents dystrophic calcification of pre-existing epidermal cysts [4], foreign bodies, dartoic muscle or eccrine ducts or is secondary to trauma [5]. Idiopathic calcinosis of the vulva may be the female counterpart [6].

Clinical features. Firm, painless, yellow-to-white papules or nodules on the scrotal wall range from pinhead to walnut size, and can number between 1 and over 100. Associated symptoms include pruritus and a sensation of scrotal heaviness. The nodules may ulcerate and discharge a cheese-like material.

Differential diagnosis. Idiopathic calcinosis of the scrotum is usually misdiagnosed clinically as epidermal cysts.

Histopathology. Deposits of calcium are seen either as solitary large nodules or multiple small deposits scattered throughout the dermis. There is often a band of compressed collagen and fibrous tissue surrounding the deposits. A true epithelial cyst wall is extremely unusual. There is a variable degree of inflammatory infiltration and foreign body reaction.

Treatment. Full excision or 'pinch–punch' excision, mainly for cosmetic reasons, is the treatment of choice [7]. Recurrences are rare.

Milia-like idiopathic calcinosis cutis

In milia-like idiopathic calcinosis cutis, multiple 1–2 mm white papules develop during childhood.

Epidemiology and pathogenesis. The male to female ratio is approximately equal. Reported cases range in age from 6 months to adolescence, and most resolve by adulthood [8]. An association with Down syndrome has been reported in two thirds of patients [9,10].

Clinical features. Multiple 1–2 mm white papules develop during early childhood. Classically, they occur on the dorsum of the hands, although they may be seen on face, knees, elbows, and soles of the feet. In a few cases they may represent calcification of pre-existing syringomas. A perforating variety has been described occurring on the pubic and groin area of healthy children [11]. In rare instances, patients with pilomatricomas present with a clinical picture of milia-like calcinosis cutis. Pilomatricomas may heal spontaneously before adulthood, with or without scarring.

Tumoral calcinosis

Tumoral calcinosis is a rare disease characterized by the development of multiple large calcified periarticular nodules [12,13]. Tumoral calcinosis can be either primary (Fig. 112.2) or secondary in association with an underlying condition such as chronic renal failure, hyperparathyroidism, hypervitaminosis D, sarcoidosis and milk–alkali syndrome. Secondary tumoral calcinosis is thus a form of metastatic calcification. Primary tumoral calcinosis can be sporadic or familial with an autosomal recessive inheritance. Familial tumoral calcinosis (FTC) is further subdivided into normophosphataemic (OMIM610456) and hyperphosphataemic (OMIM211900) types [14]. Although these two disorders were initially considered part of a clinical continuum, they represent distinct entities. Hyperphosphataemic FTC has been shown to result from

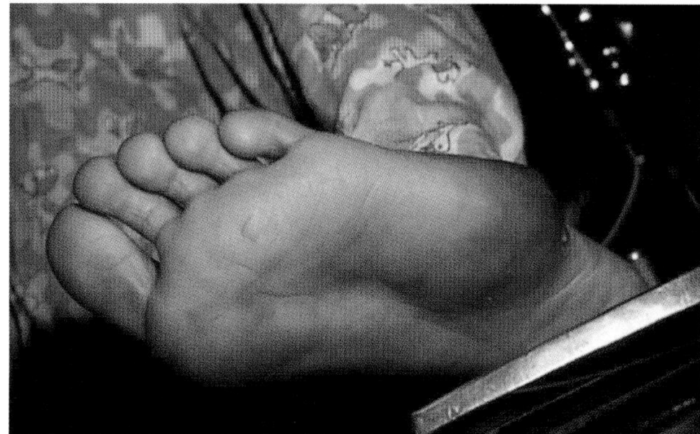

Fig. 112.2 Primary tumoral calcinosis without an identifiable defect in calcium or phosphorus metabolism.

a mutation in one of three genes: fibroblast growth factor-23 (*FGF23*), coding for a potent phosphaturic protein; KL encoding Klotho, which serves as a co-receptor for *FGF23*; and *GALNT3*, which encodes a glycosyltransferase responsible for *FGF23 O*-glycosylation [12,13,15–20]. Defective function of any one of these three proteins results in hyperphosphataemia and ectopic calcification. Normophosphataemic FTC has been linked to mutations in the *SAMD9* gene which encodes a putative tumour suppressor and anti-inflammatory protein, and is upregulated by tumour necrosis factor α (TNF-α) [21].

Epidemiology and pathogenesis. In tumoral calcinosis, the calcium is deposited as calcium pyrophosphate crystals. In the hyperphosphataemic variant, increased renal reabsorption of phosphate independent of PTH leads to hyperphosphataemia and therefore tumoral calcinosis may represent a form of metastatic calcification with trauma as a precipitating factor. However, unlike other disorders of metastatic calcification, no other organs are involved. The pathogenesis of the normophosphataemic variant is more obscure.

Clinical features. Hyperphosphataemic FTC has been mainly reported in Africa and the Middle East [13,22]. Calcified nodules usually develop during the first or second decade of life [23] although they may develop in infancy [24]. Slowly growing calcified masses develop mainly at periarticular locations, with a predilection for skin areas overlying large joints. The hips are most often involved. The lesions may be solitary but are usually multiple. These calcified masses are initially asymptomatic and are often incidentally diagnosed in patients undergoing radiographic investigation for unrelated reasons. The nodules progressively increase in size to reach several centimetres and interfere with movements or cause compression neuropathy. The overlying skin is usually normal, but ulceration, draining sinuses and dermal calcinosis cutis may occur. In some affected individuals, extracutaneous signs may predominate. Dental abnormalities, including hypoplasia and pulp calcifications, may be a prominent feature in some families [20,25]. Angioid streaks and corneal calcifications, as well as testicular microlithiasis, have been described [24,26]. Hyperphosphataemic FTC has been reported in association with pseudoxanthoma elasticum (PXE) [27]. The prognosis of the disease is good although patients often undergo many surgical procedures to remove the calcified tumours [22].

Normophosphataemic FTC is less prevalent than the hyperphosphataemic variant [21,28]. Calcified tumour formation is generally preceded by a vasculitis-like rash during the first year of life and is associated with inflammatory manifestations, mostly evident in mucosal tissues [23]. This eruption heralds the progressive, and rapid, development of small, acrally located calcified nodules, which very often ulcerate.

Tumoral calcinosis appears radiologically as dense multilocular calcific masses without bony or joint abnormalities.

Histopathology and laboratory studies. Histopathologically, there is a multilocular structure containing solid calcified material and chalky pasty fluid surrounded by a fibrous wall and a foreign body granuloma reaction. The calcified masses are mainly composed of calcium hydroxyapatite with amorphous calcium carbonate and calcium phosphate.

In the normophosphataemic type serum concentrations of calcium and phosphate are normal, whereas in the hyperphosphataemic type the serum calcium concentration is normal but the phosphate concentration is slightly high. Serum 1,25-dihydroxyvitamin D may be elevated or inappropriately normal, PTH levels are low to low-normal and the circulating *FGF23* level is increased. Subtle biochemical abnormalities may be seen in heterozygous carriers of hyperphosphataemic FTC [29].

Treatment. Surgical excision is the primary form of treatment although recurrences are frequent. Phosphate deprivation and oral aluminium hydroxide administration have been met with some success. Acetazolamide and sevelamer hydrochloride, a non-calcium phosphate binder, have been used in a few patients [19].

References

1 Evans MJ, Blessing K, Gray ES. Subepidermal calcified nodule in children: a clinicopathologic study of 21 cases. Pediatr Dermatol 1995;12:307–10.
2 Afzal MN, Dancea S, de Nanassy J. Mucosal calcified nodule of the hard palate in an infant: case report and review of the literature. Pediatr Pathol Lab Med 1997;17:611–15.
3 Shapiro L, Platt N, Torres-Rodriguez VM. Idiopathic calcinosis of the scrotum. Arch Dermatol 1970;102:199–204.
4 Yuyucu Karabulut Y, Kankaya D, Şenel E et al. Idiopathic scrotal calcinosis: the incorrect terminology of scrotal calcinosis. G Ital Dermatol Venereol 2015;150:495–9.
5 Shah V, Shet T. Scrotal calcinosis results from calcification of cysts derived from hair follicles: a series of 20 cases evaluating the spectrum of changes resulting in scrotal calcinosis. Am J Dermatopathol 2007;29:172–5.
6 Bernardo BD, Huettner PC, Merritt DF, Ratts VS. Idiopathic calcinosis cutis presenting as labial lesions in children: report of two cases with literature review. J Pediatr Adolesc Gynecol 1999;12:157–60.
7 Chang CH, Yang CH, Hong HS. Surgical pearl: pinch–punch excisions for scrotal calcinosis. J Am Acad Dermatol 2004;50:780–1.
8 Menni S, Gualandri L, Boccardi D. Youngest case of idiopathic calcinosis cutis not associated with Down syndrome. Int J Dermatol 2008;47:870–1.
9 Becuwe C, Roth B, Villedieu MH et al. Milia-like idiopathic calcinosis cutis. Pediatr Dermatol 2004;21:483–5.
10 Schepis C, Siragusa M, Palazzo R et al. Perforating milia-like idiopathic calcinosis cutis and periorbital syringomas in a girl with Down syndrome. Pediatr Dermatol 1994;11:258–60.
11 Eng AM, Mandrea E. Perforating calcinosis cutis presenting as milia. J Cutan Pathol 1981;8:247–50.
12 Joseph L, Hing SN, Presneau N et al. Familial tumoral calcinosis and hyperostosis-hyperphosphataemia syndrome are different manifestations of the same disease: novel missense mutations in GALNT3. Skeletal Radiol 2010;39:63–8.
13 Sprecher E. Familial tumoral calcinosis: from characterization of a rare phenotype to the pathogenesis of ectopic calcification. J Invest Dermatol 2010;130:652–60.
14 Smack D, Norton SA, Fitzpatrick JE. Proposal for a pathogenesis based classification of tumoral calcinosis. Int J Dermatol 1996;35: 265–71.
15 Araya K, Fukumoto S, Backenroth R et al. A novel mutation in fibroblast growth factor 23 gene as a cause of tumoral calcinosis. J Clin Endocrinol Metab 2005;90:5523–7.
16 Barbieri AM, Filopanti M, Bua G, Beck-Peccoz P. Two novel nonsense mutations in GALNT3 gene are responsible for familial tumoral calcinosis. J Hum Genet 2007;52:464–8.
17 Chefetz I, Heller R, Galli-Tsinopoulou A et al. A novel homozygous missense mutation in FGF23 causes familial tumoral calcinosis associated with disseminated visceral calcification. Hum Genet 2005;118: 261–6.
18 Garringer HJ, Mortazavi SM, Esteghamat F et al. Two novel GALNT3 mutations in familial tumoral calcinosis. Am J Med Genet A 2007;143A:2390–6.
19 Lammoglia JJ, Mericq V. Familial tumoral calcinosis caused by a novel FGF23 mutation: response to induction of tubular renal acidosis with acetazolamide and the non-calcium phosphate binder sevelamer. Horm Res 2009;71:178–84.
20 Specktor P, Cooper JG, Indelman M, Sprecher E. Hyperphosphatemic familial tumoral calcinosis caused by a mutation in GALNT3 in a European kindred. J Hum Genet 2006;51:487–90.
21 Chefetz I, Ben AD, Browning S et al. Normophosphatemic familial tumoral calcinosis is caused by deleterious mutations in SAMD9, encoding a TNF-alpha responsive protein. J Invest Dermatol 2008;128:1423–9.
22 Carmichael KD, Bynum JA, Evans EB. Familial tumoral calcinosis: a forty-year follow-up on one family. J Bone Joint Surg Am 2009;91:664–71.
23 Metzker A, Eisenstein B, Oren J, Samuel R. Tumoral calcinosis revisited: common and uncommon features – report of ten cases and review. Eur J Pediatr 1988;147:128–32.
24 Polykandriotis EP, Beutel FK, Horch RE, Grünert J. A case of familial tumoral calcinosis in a neonate and review of the literature. Arch Orthop Trauma Surg 2004;124:563–7.
25 Frishberg Y, Topaz O, Bergman R et al. Identification of a recurrent mutation in GALNT3 demonstrates that hyperostosishyperphosphatemia syndrome and familial tumoral calcinosis are allelic disorders. J Mol Med 2005;83:33–8.
26 Campagnoli MF, Pucci A, Garelli E et al. Familial tumoral calcinosis and testicular microlithiasis associated with a new mutation of GALNT3 in a white family. J Clin Pathol 2006;59:440–2.
27 Mallette LE, Mechanick JI. Heritable syndrome of pseudoxanthoma elasticum with abnormal phosphorus and vitamin D metabolism. Am J Med 1987;83:1157–62.
28 Topaz O, Indelman M, Chefetz I et al. A deleterious mutation in SAMD9 causes normophosphatemic familial tumoral calcinosis. Am J Hum Genet 2006;79:759–64.
29 Ichikawa S, Lyles KW, Econs MJ. A novel GALNT3 mutation in a pseudoautosomal dominant form of tumoral calcinosis: evidence that the disorder is autosomal recessive. J Clin Endocrinol Metab 2005;90:2420–3.

Dystrophic calcification

Dystrophic calcification has been reported in a variety of disorders (Box 112.1).

Connective tissue diseases

Cutaneous calcification can occur in all connective tissue diseases. The mechanism for dystrophic calcification in connective tissue diseases is unknown [1].

Dermatomyositis is the disorder most frequently associated with calcification in children (Fig. 112.3). Between 50% and 70% of children with dermatomyositis will develop calcinosis compared to only 20% of adults [2]. A high incidence of staphylococcal infection in children with dermatomyositis who subsequently develop calcinosis has been noted [3]. Calcinosis cutis tends to develop 2–3 years after the onset of dermatomyositis, and rarely is the presenting sign. Calcifications may range from small asymptomatic skin nodules which rarely interfere with function (calcinosis circumscripta) to large tumoral masses in the muscles or sheet-like deposits in the intermuscular fascial planes (calcinosis universalis). In a few children, often those with early onset erythroderma and diffuse cutaneous vasculitis, the calcification may be severe resembling an 'exoskeleton'. Nodular calcium deposits are seen primarily in the most severely involved muscular groups (i.e. the shoulder and pelvic girdles, followed by the elbows and knees). Episodes of ulceration, calcium extrusion and cellulitis accompanied by severe systemic symptoms are common. After expulsion of calcium, the ulcerations usually heal promptly. Calcium deposits typically increase over a period of several months and then stabilize for a few months before slowly resolving. The degree of calcinosis seems to correlate with the degree of muscle involvement and a longer time to diagnosis and treatment (and longer disease duration) [2,4]. Generally, calcinosis develops in those patients who are most seriously ill but who will ultimately survive. For this reason, although it can be severely incapacitating, it is viewed as a good prognostic sign for survival. Children with autoantibodies to anti-NXP2 and to anti-MDA5 have been shown to have a higher incidence of calcinosis, as well as more severe disease [5,6]. B-cell lymphoma arising from foci of calcinosis has been described in a girl with dermatomyositis [7].

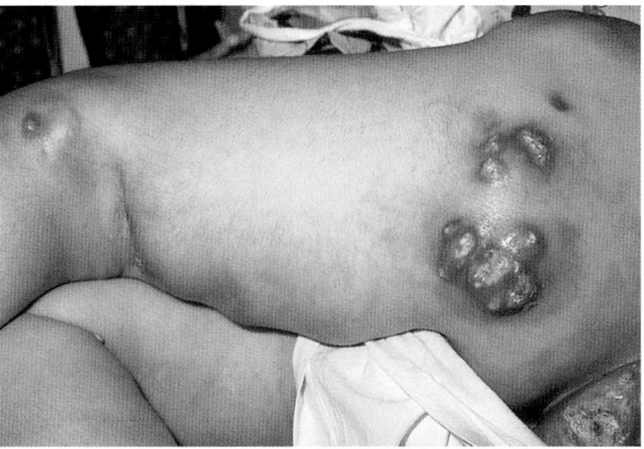

Fig. 112.3 Localized calcinosis cutis in a child with dermatomyositis.

Calcinosis is also frequent in scleroderma and CREST syndrome (calcinosis, Raynaud phenomenon, oesophageal involvement, sclerodactyly and telangiectasia), an association that has been recognized as the Thibierge–Weissenbach syndrome. Calcification occurs in 27% of patients with acrosclerosis, developing an average of 10 years after disease onset. It is not commonly seen during childhood. Calcium deposits are usually more limited than in dermatomyositis, and calcinosis universalis is rare. The sites of predilection are the hands (finger fat pads) and upper extremities, pre-existing areas of sclerosis, and periarticular areas [8]. Paraspinal and intraspinal calcifications may be seen [9]. Cutaneous calcification, although rare, may occur in morphoea and linear scleroderma [10].

Calcinosis is less common in systemic subacute cutaneous and chronic cutaneous lupus and is extremely rare in children [11]. The lesions may be located underneath the cutaneous lesions of lupus or elsewhere. Calcification usually develops an average of 8 years after the disease onset, although it can precede other symptoms.

Dystrophic calcinosis in connective tissue disease runs an independent course from that of the underlying disease. However, there is some evidence that aggressive management of dermatomyositis results in decreased incidence of calcinosis [4]. Several forms of treatment have been attempted, including diets high in phosphate and low in calcium, calcium-chelating agents, such as disodium ethylenediamine tetra-acetic acid (EDTA) and diphosphonates and oral aluminium hydroxide, which is a phosphate chelator [1]. These treatments are associated with significant side-effects and in general have yielded unimpressive results. In a few patients, probenecid and colchicine have appeared to be beneficial. Warfarin has been shown to decrease the tissue levels of the calcium-binding amino acid, γ-carboxyglutamic acid, by inhibition of the vitamin K-dependent γ-carboxylase [12]. Low-dose warfarin only improves the findings on bone scans without any clinically significant effect. Diltiazem has been effective in a few patients [13]. The presumed mechanism of action is its inhibitory effect on calcium transport into the cells. Treatment of the underlying disease with intravenous immunoglobulin has had variable results [14,15]. Intralesional administration of steroids may be beneficial for localized deposits. Surgical removal of the calcium deposits is indicated when deposits are large, painful or recurrently ulcerated. Postoperative recurrences are possible. Spontaneous regression of calcinosis has been described.

Panniculitis

Lobular panniculitis may lead to significant fat necrosis and dystrophic calcification. Subcutaneous fat necrosis of the newborn is one example. Calcifications are usually discrete and detected as an incidental finding on radiographs. In rare instances extensive widespread gritty plaques occur. Spontaneous resolution over a period of months is the rule. As the lesions resolve, symptomatic hypercalcaemia may ensue and routine serum calcium determination has been recommended.

Pancreatic enzyme panniculitis and panniculitis associated with systemic lupus erythematosus (lupus profundus), which are rare in children, are other panniculitides that occasionally calcify.

Inherited disorders

Dystrophic calcification is also observed in pseudoxanthoma elasticum (PXE) [16]. The skin changes usually begin in the second decade. Yellow-orange discrete or confluent papules and linear plaques occur in the skin creases and flexural folds. Calcification is invariably present at a microscopic level although it may not be clinically evident. Calcium deposits are seen in association with dystrophic and frayed elastic fibres in the mid and lower dermis. PXE is caused by mutations in the ABCC6 membrane transporter, but the mechanism of elastic fibre calcification is not clear. Some patients with PXE develop tumoral calcinosis in association with hyperphosphataemia with or without hypercalcaemia and elevated 1,25-dihydroxyvitamin D levels, suggesting an additional inborn error in calcium, phosphate and vitamin D metabolism [17]. In addition, one report highlights the association of *ABCC6* mutations normally associated with PXE as also being associated with manifestations consistent with generalized arterial calcification of infancy. These patients may have clinical features of PXE but characteristically have more severe vascular phenotypes predisposing to arterial stenoses and myocardial ischaemia caused by vascular calcifications in early infancy [18].

In Ehlers–Danlos syndrome, subcutaneous nodules, so-called spherules or spheroids, may calcify. They are pea-sized, freely movable subcutaneous nodules, thought to represent fat herniations. They are barely visible but, when calcified, are demonstrable radiologically. Calcified haematomas are another basis for calcinosis cutis in Ehlers–Danlos syndrome.

In Werner premature ageing syndrome, the skin is scleroderma-like in appearance and subcutaneous calcification has been reported [19]. Calcinosis cutis presenting as numerous small yellow papules on the extremities has also been reported to occur in association with Rothmund–Thomson syndrome [20]. A case of calcinosis cutis with secondary ossification, poikiloderma and metaphyseal changes in the bones has been reported under the acronym COPS syndrome [21].

Tumours

Many benign and malignant neoplasms may calcify. The classic example is a pilomatricoma (calcifying epithelioma of Malherbe). Calcification occurs in approximately 81% of these tumours and ossification in 15–25%. Some pilomatricomas will perforate and extrude calcified material. Histologically, calcium is seen either as granules within the cytoplasm of shadow cells or as large amorphous deposits replacing the shadow cells. Calcification usually occurs in the connective tissue surrounding the tumour. The mechanism of calcification in pilomatricomas is not known but it may involve osteopontin, a bone matrix protein with high affinity for hydroxyapatite. Epidermal cysts in Gardner syndrome may show pilomatricoma-like changes with calcification and ossification. Pilar cysts and, less often, epidermal cysts may show calcification. Basal cell carcinoma, especially in the setting of the naevoid basal cell carcinoma syndrome, is another neoplasm that may calcify and ossify. Psammoma bodies and foci of calcification and/or ossification have been noted in melanocytic naevi. Psammoma bodies are laminated hyaline bodies with varying degrees of calcification that may be seen in the skin in cutaneous meningioma, intradermal naevi and juvenile xanthogranuloma. Chondroid syringomas may show calcification and ossification. However, unlike other neoplasms, the ossification occurs within the tumour via ossification of the chondroid cells (endochondral ossification) [22]. Other neoplasms rarely associated with calcification and/or ossification include pyogenic granuloma, haemangioma, neurilemmomas, trichoepitheliomas, ossifying plexiform tumour and seborrhoeic keratoses.

Infections

Parasitic infections are another cause of dystrophic calcification. In cysticercosis (*Taenia solium*) and hydatid disease (*Echinococcus* spp.), calcified cysts may be found in the subcutaneous tissue. In onchocerciasis, the larvae of *Onchocerca volvulus* remain in the subcutaneous tissue and skin, producing nodules that may calcify. Congenital annular plaques of calcinosis cutis have been observed in a newborn infant with intrauterine herpes simplex infection.

Trauma

Dystrophic calcifications have been described in a variety of situations in which local tissue injury occurs. Infantile calcinosis cutis of the heel, otherwise known as heelstick calcification, is a classic example in which calcified nodules and plaques develop in infants requiring multiple heelsticks. Calcinosis cutis has also been reported in burns, toxic epidermal necrolysis, surgical scars, keloids and areas of repetitive trauma.

References

1 Boulman N, Slobodin G, Rozenbaum M, Rosner I. Calcinosis in rheumatic diseases. Semin Arthritis Rheum 2005;34:805–12.

2 Bowyer SL, Blane CE, Sullivan DB, Cassidy JT. Childhood dermatomyositis: factors predicting functional outcome and development of dystrophic calcification. J Pediatr 1983;103:882–8.

3 Moore EC, Cohen F, Douglas SD, Gutta V. Staphylococcal infections in childhood dermatomyositis: association with the development of calcinosis, raised IgE concentrations and granulocyte chemotactic defect. Ann Rheum Dis 1992;51:378–83.

4 Fisler RE, Liang MG, Fuhlbrigge RC et al. Aggressive management of juvenile dermatomyositis results in improved outcome and decreased incidence of calcinosis. J Am Acad Dermatol 2002;47:505–11.

5 Gunawardena H, Wedderburn LR, Chinoy H et al. Autoantibodies to a 140-kd protein in juvenile dermatomyositis are associated with calcinosis. Arthritis Rheum 2009;60:1807–14.

6 Groh M, Rogowska K, Monsarrat O et al. Interleukin-1 receptor antagonist for refractory anti-MDA5 clinically amyopathic dermatomyostitis. Clin Exp Rheumatol 2015;33:904–5.

7 Morris P, Herrera-Guerra A, Parham D. Lymphoma arising from a calcinotic lesion in a patient with juvenile dermatomyositis. Pediatr Dermatol 2009;26:159–61.

SECTION 24: NONVASCULAR SKIN TUMOURS

8 Nielsen AO, Brun B, Secher L. Calcosis in generalized scleroderma. Acta Derm Venereol 1980;60:301–7.
9 Nagai Y, Sogabe Y, Ishikawa O. Tumoral calcinosis of the ribs and lumbar spine in systemic sclerosis. Eur J Dermatol 2008;18:473–4.
10 Yamamoto A, Morita A, Shintani Y et al. Localized linear scleroderma with cutaneous calcinosis. J Dermatol 2002;29:112–14.
11 Tristano AG, Villarroel JL, Rodriguez MA, Millan A. Calcinosis cutis universalis in a patient with systemic lupus erythematosus. Clin Rheumatol 2006;25:70–4.
12 Berger RG, Featherstone GL, Raasch RH et al. Treatment of calcinosis universalis with low-dose warfarin. Am J Med 1987;83:72–6.
13 Palmieri GM, Sebes JI, Aelion JA et al. Treatment of calcinosis with diltiazem. Arthritis Rheum 1995;38:1646–54.
14 Kalajian AH, Perryman JH, Callen JP. Intravenous immunoglobulin therapy for dystrophic calcinosis cutis: unreliable in our hands. Arch Dermatol 2009;145:334.
15 Schanz S, Ulmer A, Fierlbeck G. Response of dystrophic calcification to intravenous immunoglobulin. Arch Dermatol 2008;144:585–7.
16 Reeve EB, Neldner KH, Subryan V, Gordon SG. Development and calcification of skin lesions in thirty-nine patients with pseudoxanthoma elasticum. Clin Exp Dermatol 1979;4:291–301.
17 Mallette LE, Mechanick JI. Heritable syndrome of pseudoxanthoma elasticum with abnormal phosphorus and vitamin D metabolism. Am J Med 1987;83:1157–62.
18 LeBoulanger G, Labreze C, Schurgers LJ et al. An unusual severe vascular case of pseudoxanthoma elasticum presenting as generalized arterial calcification of infancy. Am J Med Genet 2010;152A: 118–23.
19 Honjo S, Yokote K, Fujimoto M et al. Clinical outcome and mechanism of soft tissue calcification in Werner syndrome. Rejuvenation Res 2008;11:809–19.
20 Aydemir EH, Onsun N, Ozan S, Hatemi HH. Rothmund–Thomson syndrome with calcinosis universalis. Int J Dermatol 1988;27:591–2.
21 Oranje AP, de Muinck Keizer-Schrama SM, Vuzevski VD, Meradji M. Calcinosis cutis, osteoma cutis, poikiloderma and skeletal abnormalities (COPS syndrome): a new entity? Eur J Pediatr 1991;150:343–6.
22 Roth SI, Stowell RE, Helwig EB. Cutaneous ossification: report of 120 cases and review of the literature. Arch Pathol 1963;76:44–54.

Metastatic calcification

Metastatic calcification is a less common cause of calcinosis cutis [1]. It occurs in a variety of systemic disorders with abnormal calcium and/or phosphate metabolism (Box 112.1). The calcification is widespread and affects predominantly blood vessels, kidneys, lungs and gastric mucosa. In the skin, metastatic calcification takes the form of either benign nodular calcification or calciphylaxis. In benign nodular calcification (also termed secondary or uraemic tumoral calcinosis), there are large calcific masses in the skin and subcutaneous tissue, usually in periarticular sites similar to those seen in tumoral calcinosis. The lesions are usually asymptomatic unless they impair mobility of the joint. Calciphylaxis is characterized by vascular calcification of small and medium-sized arteries with thrombosis, and ischaemic necrosis of the skin and subcutaneous tissue [2,3]. Clinically, it manifests as firm, extremely painful, well-demarcated, violaceous plaques with ulceration. The lesions may initially have a livedo reticularis-like pattern.

Chronic renal insufficiency is the most common cause of metastatic calcification. Decreased phosphate excretion and impaired synthesis of 1,25-dihydroxyvitamin D are the two main factors of abnormal calcification. Impaired production of 1,25-dihydroxyvitamin D leads to decreased intestinal calcium absorption. The resultant hypocalcaemia leads to secondary hyperparathyroidism. Elevated PTH levels normalize serum calcium by bone resorption but at the expense of higher phosphate levels and a higher calcium/phosphate solubility product. Soft-tissue calcifications occur in 60% of children with uraemia, but calciphylaxis is extremely rare in children [4]. Calciphylaxis has been increasingly recognized in patients with normal renal function and normal calcium/phosphate product [5]. Therefore the pathogenesis of calciphylaxis remains unclear and factors independent of calcium/phosphate levels may contribute to thrombosis and calcium deposits [3].

Primary hyperparathyroidism is rare in children. Tumoral calcinosis, calciphylaxis and benign nodular calcification may all occur in this setting.

Chronic ingestion of excessive amounts of vitamin D (50 000–100 000 U/day) results in hypervitaminosis D, with hypercalcaemia and hypercalciuria which leads to chronic renal insufficiency and metastatic calcification. Oral alendronate sodium has been used with success in an infant with vitamin D intoxication [6].

Milk–alkali syndrome results from excessive ingestion of calcium-containing antacids or calcium supplements (calcium carbonate). It is extremely rare in children, especially with the advent of nonabsorbable antacids. Acute manifestations of hypercalcaemia are most common, but metastatic calcifications may occur. Cutaneous calcification is exceptional [7].

Hypercalcaemia occurs in 30–50% of children with sarcoidosis, but cutaneous calcification is extremely rare. Hypercalcaemia in sarcoidosis is secondary to ectopic production of 1,25-dihydroxyvitamin D by activated macrophages. Bone destruction by haematological or metastatic malignancies and osteomyelitis is another infrequent cause. Metastatic calcification has been reported in association with cytomegalovirus infection.

Treatment of metastatic calcification should be directed to correcting the calcium/phosphate product. Benign nodular calcification may resorb after normalization of calcium and phosphate, but surgical removal may be necessary for lesions that interfere with function. Treatment of calciphylaxis includes surgical debridement of skin ulcers and adequate wound care to prevent infection and sepsis. Parathyroidectomy is recommended if possible in patients with secondary hyperthyroidism [8]. Sodium thiosulfate, a calcium-chelating agent, as well as bisphosphonates, and cinacalcet, a calcimimetic shown to lower PTH, have been used with some success [9]. Despite treatment, calciphylaxis has a poor prognosis with a high rate of death from gangrene and sepsis.

References

1 Khafif RA, DeLima C, Silverberg A, Frankel R. Calciphylaxis and systemic calcinosis: collective review. Arch Intern Med 1990;150:956–9.
2 Dauden E, Onate MJ. Calciphylaxis. Dermatol Clin 2008;26:557–68, ix.
3 Weenig RH. Pathogenesis of calciphylaxis: Hans Selye to nuclear factor kappa-B. J Am Acad Dermatol 2008;58:458–71.
4 Feng J, Gohara M, Lazova R, Antaya RJ. Fatal childhood calciphylaxis in a 10-year-old and literature review. Pediatr Dermatol 2006;23: 266–72.
5 Kalajian AH, Malhotra PS, Callen JP, Parker LP. Calciphylaxis with normal renal and parathyroid function: not as rare as previously believed. Arch Dermatol 2009;145:451–8.

6 Bereket A, Erdogan T. Oral bisphosphonate therapy for vitamin D intoxication of the infant. Pediatrics 2003;111:899–901.
7 Duthie JS, Solanki HP, Krishnamurthy M, Chertow BS. Milk–alkali syndrome with metastatic calcification. Am J Med 1995;99:102–3.
8 Low TH, Clark J, Gao K et al. Outcome of parathyroidectomy for patients with renal disease and hyperparathyroidism: predictors for recurrent hyperparathyroidism. ANZ J Surg 2009;79:378–82.
9 Araya CE, Fennell RS, Neiberger RE, Dharnidharka VR. Sodium thiosulfate treatment for calcific uremic arteriolopathy in children and young adults. Clin J Am Soc Nephrol 2006;1:1161–6.

Iatrogenic calcinosis cutis

Calcinosis cutis may occur after parenteral administration of calcium- or phosphate-containing solutions with or without extravasation (Fig. 112.4) [1]. The mechanism of calcification is multifactorial. Calcium solutions are strong irritants and, when extravasated, can cause extensive local tissue necrosis, which may calcify secondarily. The elevated local concentration of calcium must have a contributing role because calcification may also occur after minor extravasation. The development of skin lesions may be rapid, occurring within a few hours. Most often, however, the appearance is delayed for 1–2 weeks. Initial lesions resemble abscesses or cellulitis. The calcium deposits may be papular, plaque-like, nodular, annular or linear, following the blood vessels. Radiography can demonstrate the calcification along the muscular fascial planes or blood vessels. However, it is not useful in diagnosing extravasation because the calcium solutions used in clinical practice are radiolucent. Gradual resolution, with or without extrusion of calcium, follows. Sodium thiosulfate has been successfully used to treat iatrogenic calcinosis resulting from extravasation of calcium gluconate [2].

Calcinosis cutis can also occur at the site of electrode placement in patients who have undergone electroencephalography, electromyography or brainstem auditory-evoked potentials with calcium chloride-containing electrode-conducting paste [3]. The lesions occur at the sites of prolonged electrode placement as skin trauma or abrasion seems to be necessary for calcium deposition.

Transient calcification of the skin has been reported following liver transplantation [4]. The onset is usually within a week or two following transplantation and resolution occurs spontaneously over several months. Various causes have been hypothesized, including intraoperative use of calcium-containing fluid and metabolic abnormalities in the perioperative period.

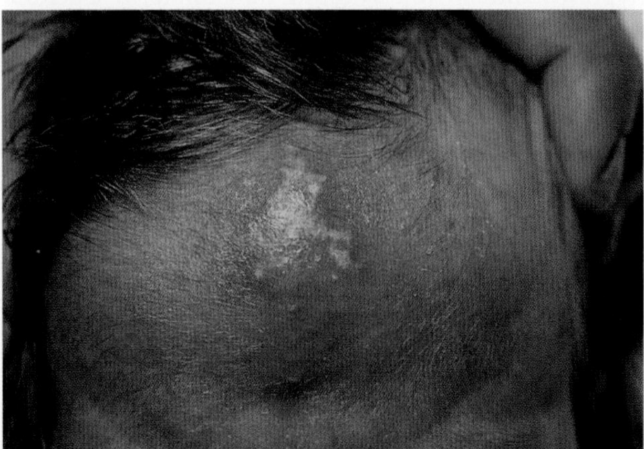

Fig. 112.4 Iatrogenic calcinosis cutis in a child resulting from extravasation of a calcium-containing intravenous solution.

Massive subcutaneous calcification and ossification have been described after intramuscular injection of vitamin E in premature newborns [5]. Subcutaneous administration of calcium heparin or low-molecular-weight heparins, usually in the setting of chronic renal failure, can also lead to iatrogenic calcification [6].

References
1 Goldminz D, Barnhill R, McGuire J, Stenn KS. Calcinosis cutis following extravasation of calcium chloride. Arch Dermatol 1988;124:922–5.
2 Raffaella C, Annapaola C, Tullio I et al. Successful treatment of severe iatrogenic calcinosis cutis with intravenous sodium thiosulfate in a child affected by T-acute lymphoblastic leukemia. Pediatr Dermatol 2009;26:311–15.
3 Puig L, Rocamora V, Romani J et al. Calcinosis cutis following calcium chloride electrode paste application for auditory-brainstem evoked potentials recording. Pediatr Dermatol 1998;15:27–30.
4 Larralde M, Giachetti A, Kowalczuk A et al. Calcinosis cutis following liver transplantation in a pediatric patient. Pediatr Dermatol 2003;20:225–8.
5 Barak M, Herschkowitz S, Montag J. Soft tissue calcification: a complication of vitamin E injection. Pediatrics 1986;77:382–5.
6 Giorgini S, Martinelli C, Massi D et al. Iatrogenic calcinosis cutis following nadroparin injection. Int J Dermatol 2005;44:855–7.

Cutaneous ossification

Cutaneous ossification is most often a secondary phenomenon to local tissue alteration or pre-existing calcification. Any calcifying disorder may thus ossify secondarily. Primary ossification of the skin and subcutaneous tissue is exceedingly rare [1]. There are four main genetic disorders of primary cutaneous or subcutaneous ossification: progressive osseous heteroplasia (POH); Albright hereditary osteodystrophy (AHO); fibrodysplasia ossificans progressiva (FOP); and plate-like osteoma cutis (OC). In addition, there is an acquired form of primary ossification of the skin without known genetic background: miliary osteoma of the face.

FOP rarely presents to dermatologists as ossification affects deeper tissues and only affects the skin as an extension.

POH, AHO and OC probably represent a spectrum of diseases caused by heterozygous inactivating mutations of *GNAS*, the gene encoding the α-subunit of the G-stimulatory protein of adenylyl cyclase [2]. In fact, some patients may present overlapping clinical features between these entities. There is no known genotype–phenotype correlation although it has been shown that genomic imprinting may determine the clinical phenotype. POH is due to mutations in the paternal allele of *GNAS*, while AHO is due to mutations in the maternal allele.

Two mechanisms have been proposed for heterotopic bone formation:

1 Persistence of primitive mesenchymal cells differentiating into osteoblasts (hamartomas); or
2 Transformation of extraskeletal mesenchymal cells into bone-forming cells (metaplasia).

Ossification in the skin manifests clinically as hard, red to bluish papules, nodules and plaques with a gritty consistency that range in size from a few millimetres to several centimetres. Ulceration with extrusion of ossified material is possible. Histologically, there are spicules or sheets of bone in the dermis and sometimes subcutaneous tissues with osteocytes, and a peripheral layer of osteoblasts. Osteoclasts, which resemble multinucleated foreign body cells, are only rarely seen. Mature fat cells and occasionally haematopoietic cells may be seen between the spicules. The ossification in POH and AHO primary ossifying disorders is intramembranous, without identifiable cartilage, and in FOP it is endochondral [3].

Progressive osseous heteroplasia

This genetic condition is characterized by progressive heterotopic ossification that progresses from skin and subcutaneous tissues into deep skeletal muscle [4,5]. POH is most often sporadic, but familial occurrence has been reported. It affects predominantly females.

Epidemiology and pathogenesis. Most cases of POH are caused by heterozygous inactivating mutations of the paternal allele of *GNAS*, the gene encoding the α-subunit of the G-stimulatory protein of adenylyl cyclase [2]. POH is one of several disorders associated with *GNAS* mutation, including AHO, pseudo-hypoparathyroidism (PHP) and OC. These disorders may represent a clinical spectrum because there are a few case reports of patients with POH with additional features of AHO or with plate-like OC [4,6]. There are no genotype–phenotype correlations in *GNAS* mutation disorders and therefore POH, AHO, PHP and OC can be distinguished solely by clinical criteria. It has been demonstrated that the phenotypic expression of *GNAS* mutations is regulated by genomic imprinting. Paternally inherited mutations are associated with POH, whereas maternally inherited mutations lead to PHP and most cases of AHO [2,4].

Clinical features. Skin lesions are characterized by plaques with small papules resembling rice grains and small hard papules (Fig. 112.5) [4]. The plaques have a gritty consistency. The lesions are usually present at birth or develop shortly thereafter, although later age of onset has also been described [4]. In infancy, the ossification is limited to the superficial dermis but it characteristically progresses during childhood to involve deep connective tissue and skeletal muscle. The osteomas are asymmetrically distributed although patients with unilateral involvement have been reported [7–10]. Extensive ossification of the deep connective tissues results in ankylosis of affected joints and focal growth retardation of involved limbs. The lesions progress to extensive coalescing ossified plaques. The major complication is joint ankylosis, which may cause severe growth retardation, limb length discrepancies and limitation of motion. A small subset of patients with POH share some features of AHO or PHP.

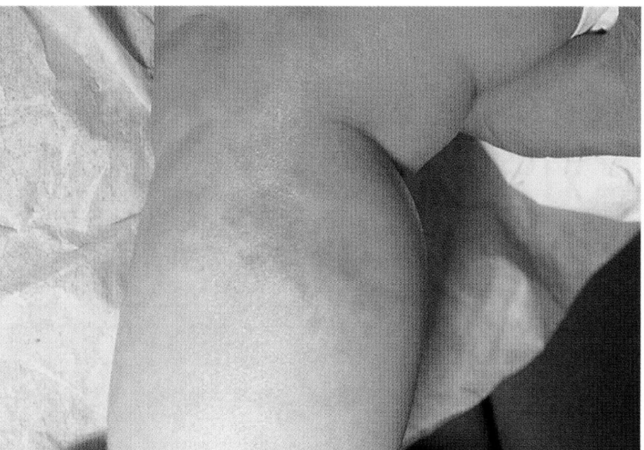

Fig. 112.5 Cutaneous lesions in progressive osseous heteroplasia (POH). Clinically, the lesions are subtle but may have what has been described as a 'rice grain' feel on palpation. Source: Courtesy of Dr Nancy Esterly.

Differential diagnosis. POH has to be differentiated from AHO, PHP, OC and FOP. In AHO, PHP and OC, the ossification is superficial, limited to the skin and does not progress to deeper tissues. In addition, patients with POH do not have the dysmorphic features (short stature, round face, brachydactyly, mental retardation) seen in AHO and the endocrine abnormalities seen in PHP, except for the small subset of patients with overlapping clinical features (Table 112.1). FOP is an ossifying disorder characterized also by progressive heterotopic ossification in the deep connective tissue and muscle but it spares the skin. Moreover, the type of ossification in FOP is endochondrial. Malformed toes are another feature of FOP not seen in POH.

Histopathology and laboratory studies. The ossification is initially located in the dermis and with time extends to affect the subcutaneous tissue, tendons and muscle. Superficial biopsy specimens may only show calcification. In half of patients the ossification is intramembranous, in 20% endochondral and in 30% of both types [4].

There may be elevated serum levels of alkaline phosphatase, reflecting active ossification, and elevated muscle enzymes secondary to muscle involvement [10]. In a small subset of patient there may be endocrine abnormalities with PTH resistance or thyroid-stimulating hormone (TSH) resistance (POH/PHP overlap). Therefore, endocrine evaluation including calcium, phosphorus, TSH and PTH blood levels is recommended (Table 112.1).

Treatment. Attempts to remove the osteomas surgically have been followed by recurrences.

Albright hereditary osteodystrophy

AHO is a congenital genetic syndrome characterized by short stature, obesity, round face, neurobehavioural problems, brachydactyly and cutaneous ossification. AHO is usually associated with end-organ resistance to PTH (pseudo-hypoparathyroidism type 1a) or other hormones. Patients who exhibit AHO features without

Table 112.1 Disorders of heterotopic ossification

Disease	Depth of ossification	AHO dysmorphic features[a]	Endocrine abnormalities[b]
POH	Superficial (only dermis) and deep	No	No
POH–AHO overlap	Superficial (only dermis) and deep	Yes	No
POH–PHP overlap	Superficial (only dermis) and deep	Yes	Yes
Osteoma cutis	Superficial (only dermis)	No	No
AHO	Superficial (only dermis)	Yes	No
PHP	Superficial (only dermis)	Yes	Yes

AHO, Albright hereditary osteodystrophy; PHP, pseudo-hypoparathyroidism; POH, progressive osseous heteroplasia.
[a]AHO features include short stature, obesity, round face, brachydactyly and neurobehavioural abnormalities.
[b]Endocrine evaluation should include calcium, phosphorus, thyroid-stimulating hormone (TSH) and parathyroid hormone (PTH) blood levels.

evidence for hormone resistance are said to have pseudo-pseudo-hypoparathyroidism. PHP is subclassified into types 1a, 1b and 1c [11]. Clinically, PHP 1a and 1c are identical and can present with AHO features. PHP 1a is distinguished from PHP 1c by the presence of inactivating *GNAS* mutation or reduced activity of the α-subunit of the stimulatory G protein (Gsα). In PHP 1b there is end-organ resistance to PTH but without AHO features or reduced activity of Gsα-subunit.

Epidemiology and pathogenesis. AHO is known to be caused by an inactivating mutation in the gene for the α-subunit of the stimulatory G protein of the adenylate cyclase on chromosome 20 termed *GNAS*. The decreased activity of the stimulatory G protein leads to resistance to PTH and other hormones whose action is mediated by activation of adenylate cyclase. AHO is only one of the disorders associated with *GNAS* mutation which include POH (AHO), PHP and OC [4]. AHO is more frequently associated with maternally inherited mutations, whereas paternally inherited mutation is more commonly associated with pseudo-pseudo-hypoparathyroidism (AHO with normal target-organ response to PTH). The osteomas are apparently a phenotypic feature of the syndrome unrelated to the calcium and phosphorus levels.

Clinical features. The phenotypic features of AHO include obesity, short stature, round face, short neck, short fingers (especially the fourth and fifth fingers), dimpling over the metacarpophalangeal joints (Albright's sign) and abnormal dentition [12]. Ossification is limited to the skin and subcutaneous tissue, is a frequent early clinical manifestation and may be the presenting sign of AHO. It does not progress to involve fascia or muscle. The osteomas are usually multiple and asymmetrical. They may occur in any part of the body as blue-tinged stony-hard papules, plaques or nodules. Apart from the dysmorphic features, there may be signs and symptoms of hypocalcaemia or other endocrine abnormalities.

Laboratory studies. Hypocalcaemia, hyperphosphataemia with increased phosphate tubular reabsorption and normal to elevated PTH levels may be seen. Serum calcium may be normal at birth and other signs of PHP may precede the development of hypocalcaemia. There is a blunted rise in urinary cyclic adenosine monophosphate and phosphate excretion in response to exogenous PTH administration. In AHO with PHP (PHP 1a) there may be end-organ resistance to TSH, and gonadotropins and growth hormone-releasing hormone [13]. Genetic analysis of α-subunit of stimulatory G protein is useful.

Differential diagnosis. The associated dysmorphic characteristics differentiate AHO from other ossifying disorders (Table 112.1).

Treatment. The treatment is directed to obtain adequate calcium–phosphate control and to correct the multiple hormonal resistance, when present. Treatment includes the use of vitamin D active metabolites (alfacalcidol and calcitriol, 20–50 mg/kg per day given in two doses) and calcium supplementation. The goal is to maintain blood calcium at 2.2–2.7 mmol/L (8.8–10.8 mg/dL), urinary calcium excretion <4 mg/kg per day and the urinary calcium : urinary creatinine ratio <0.2. Surgical excision is the only form of treatment for the osteomas.

Plate-like osteoma cutis and other primary osteomas

The term plate-like osteoma cutis was coined by Worret and Burgdorf [14] in 1978 to describe cutaneous osteomas that satisfied the following criteria:
1 Present at birth or within the first year of life;
2 No evidence of abnormal calcium/phosphate metabolism;
3 Absence of trauma or any predisposing event; and
Presence of at least one bony plate with or without other cutaneous osteomas [15].

Most of the cases of limited or isolated primary OC reported in the literature previous to that description meet these diagnostic criteria. Conversely, although widespread plate-like OC may occur, in many instances this probably represents a more limited form of POH [16]. In fact, inactivating mutations of the *GNAS1* gene, as in POH, have been detected in some cases of plate-like OC [4] and there is at least one reported family in which two members had plate-like OC and one had POH [17].

Plate-like OC clinically manifests as hard plaques with a gritty consistency, varying in size from one to several centimetres. The lesions may be multiple or solitary and are more common on the scalp, face and limbs. The ossified plaques slowly increase in size and a few new lesions may develop with time. Familial occurrence has been reported. Transepidermal elimination of bony spicules has been described [18]. The ossification is superficial and does not progress to affect deeper connective tissue, muscle or fascia. The superficial nature is the main distinction from POH. There are no associated dysmorphic features of AHO or PHP. Surgical excision is the only form of treatment.

There is still a subset of patients with single or multiple primary OC in which the lesions are not congenital or plate-like and do not conform to the diagnosis of any ossifying syndrome [19]. Primary OC has been seen in association with multiple exostosis and unilateral linear basal cell naevus with unilateral anodontia [20].

Miliary osteoma cutis of the face

Miliary OC of the face most commonly occurs as multiple small firm blue-red nodules on the faces of young women with a history of acne vulgaris [21]. In a minority of patients there is no history of preceding acne [22]. Pigmentation of miliary OC of the face after long-term use of tetracyclines for acne has been described [23]. Treatment of miliary OC includes surgical excision, curettage and laser (CO_2 continuous-wave laser, erbium or Nd:YAG laser) [24,25]. For small and superficial lesions, topical application of tretinoin cream may be beneficial [26].

Acknowledgement

We thank Janet A. Fairley for her contribution to the previous edition.

References

1 Roth SI, Stowell RE, Helwig EB. Cutaneous ossification: report of 120 cases and review of the literature. Arch Pathol 1963;76:44–54.

2 Shore EM, Ahn J, Jan de BS et al. Paternally inherited inactivating mutations of the GNAS1 gene in progressive osseous heteroplasia. N Engl J Med 2002;346:99–106.

3 Kaplan FS, Tabas JA, Gannon FH et al. The histopathology of fibrodysplasia ossificans progressiva: an endochondral process. J Bone Joint Surg Am 1993;75:220–30.

4 Adegbite NS, Xu M, Kaplan FS et al. Diagnostic and mutational spectrum of progressive osseous heteroplasia (POH) and other forms of GNAS-based heterotopic ossification. Am J Med Genet A 2008; 146A:1788–96.

5 Kaplan FS, Shore EM. Progressive osseous heteroplasia. J Bone Miner Res 2000;15:2084–94.

6 Eddy MC, Jan De Beur SM, Yandow SM et al. Deficiency of the alpha subunit of the stimulatory G protein and severe extraskeletal ossification. J Bone Miner Res 2000;15:2074–83.

7 Milstone LM, Ellison AF, Insogna KL. Serum parathyroid hormone level is elevated in some patients with disorders of keratinization. Arch Dermatol 1992;128:926–30.

8 Evans MJ, Blessing K, Gray ES. Subepidermal calcified nodule in children: a clinicopathologic study of 21 cases. Pediatr Dermatol 1995;12:307–10.

9 Afzal MN, Dancea S, de Nanassy J. Mucosal calcified nodule of the hard palate in an infant: case report and review of the literature. Pediatr Pathol Lab Med 1997;17:611–15.

10 Shapiro L, Platt N, Torres-Rodriguez VM. Idiopathic calcinosis of the scrotum. Arch Dermatol 1970;102:199–204.

11 Bastepe M. The GNAS locus and pseudohypoparathyroidism. Adv Exp Med Biol 2008;626:27–40.

12 Kacerovska D, Nemcova J, Pomahacova R et al. Cutaneous and superficial soft tissue lesions associated with Albright hereditary osteodystrophy: clinicopathological and molecular genetic study of 4 cases, including a novel mutation of the GNAS gene. Am J Dermatopathol 2008;30:417–24.

13 Mantovani G, Spada A. Resistance to growth hormone releasing hormone and gonadotropins in Albright's hereditary osteodystrophy. J Pediatr Endocrinol Metab 2006;19(suppl 2):663–70.

14 Worret WI, Burgdorf W. Angeborenes plattenartiges Osteoma cutis bei einem Saugling. Hautarzt 1978;29:590–6.

15 Sanmartin O, Alegre V, Martinez-Aparicio A et al. Congenital plate-like osteoma cutis: case report and review of the literature. Pediatr Dermatol 1993;10:182–6.

16 Lim MO, Mukherjee AB, Hansen JW. Dysplastic cutaneous osteomatosis: a unique case of true osteoma. Arch Dermatol 1981;117:797–9.

17 Urtizberea JA, Testart H, Cartault F et al. Progressive osseous heteroplasia: report of a family. J Bone Joint Surg Br 1998;80:768–71.

18 Haro R, Revelles JM, Angulo J et al. Plaque-like osteoma cutis with transepidermal elimination. J Cutan Pathol 2009;36:591–3.

19 Cottoni F, Dell'Orbo C, Quacci D, Tedde G. Primary osteoma cutis: clinical, morphological, and ultrastructural study. Am J Dermatopathol 1993;15:77–81.

20 Aloi FG, Tomasini CF, Isaia G, Grazia BM. Unilateral linear basal cell nevus associated with diffuse osteoma cutis, unilateral anodontia, and abnormal bone mineralization. J Am Acad Dermatol 1989;20: 973–8.

21 Thielen AM, Stucki L, Braun RP et al. Multiple cutaneous osteomas of the face associated with chronic inflammatory acne. J Eur Acad Dermatol Venereol 2006;20:321–6.

22 Bowman PH, Lesher JL Jr. Primary multiple miliary osteoma cutis and exogenous ochronosis. Cutis 2001;68:103–6.

23 Burford C. Pigmented osteoma cutis secondary to long-term tetracyclines. Australas J Dermatol 2007;48:134–6.

24 Ochsendorf FR, Kaufmann R. Erbium:YAG laser ablation of osteoma cutis: modifications of the approach. Arch Dermatol 1999;135:1416.

25 Altman JF, Nehal KS, Busam KJ, Halpern AC. Treatment of primary miliary osteoma cutis with incision, curettage, and primary closure. J Am Acad Dermatol 2001;44:96–9.

26 Cohen AD, Chetov T, Cagnano E et al. Treatment of multiple miliary osteoma cutis of the face with local application of tretinoin (all-trans-retinoic acid): a case report and review of the literature. J Dermatolog Treat 2001;12:171–3.

CHAPTER 113
Angiolymphoid Hyperplasia with Eosinophilia

Jasem M. Alshaiji
Dermatology Department and Pediatric Dermatology Unit, Amiri Hospital, Kuwait

Abstract

Angiolymphoid hyperplasia with eosinophilia (ALHE) or epithelioid haemangioma (EH) is a rare benign vascular proliferative disorder of unknown aetiology. It affects mostly Asian and Caucasian men and women between 20 and 50 years old. It presents with persistent and recurrent reddish-brown dome-shaped dermal papules or subcutaneous nodules, which can be pruritic or painful, affecting mostly the periauricular area, forehead and scalp. Histologically, it is characterized by the prominent proliferation of plump histiocytoid endothelial cells and the accompanying eosinophilic and lymphocytic inflammation with the occasional formation of lymphoid follicles. Although the pathogenesis is still unclear, there have been many hypotheses, which include reactive, neoplastic and infectious mechanisms. No definitive treatment is reported, but surgical excision, intralesional corticosteroid injection and pulsed-dye laser are the mainstays of treatment.

Key points

- Angiolymphoid hyperplasia with eosinophilia (ALHE) is a rare chronic benign disorder of vascular origin.
- It is more commonly seen in Asians and Caucasians.
- Young and middle-aged men and women are mostly affected.
- The pathogenesis is still unclear and controversial.
- The periauricular area, forehead and scalp are the predominant sites.
- Lesions are usually pruritic, but may be painful, haemorrhagic, pulsatile or even asymptomatic.
- Mostly solitary, red to brown dome-shaped firm mobile smooth-surfaced intradermal papules or subcutaneous nodules range in size from 0.2 cm up to 10 cm.
- Regional lymphadenopathy is noted in 5–10% of cases.
- Kimura disease is the main differential diagnosis.
- Peripheral eosinophilia is present in only 20% of cases.
- The histopathological findings are characteristic.
- Treatment remains challenging with a high rate of recurrence (30–50%).
- Surgical excision, intralesional corticosteroid and pulsed-dye laser therapy are the mainstays of treatment.

Definition. Angiolymphoid hyperplasia with eosinophilia (ALHE) is defined as a rare chronic benign skin disorder of vascular origin with characteristic histopathological findings.

History. ALHE was first described by Wells and Whimster in 1969 [1] who presented nine cases in asymptomatic young adults, seven of whom had peripheral eosinophilia. The lesions were solitary or multiple and were located in the subcutaneous tissue of the head and neck region. Although recurrence after excision was observed in some, all cases followed a benign course. Weiss and Enzinger introduced the term epithelioid haemangioma in 1982, as they believed the lesion was neoplastic in nature and wanted to delineate it clearly from the malignant vascular tumour, epithelioid haemangioendothelioma [2,3].

The other names given to ALHE are pseudo- or atypical pyogenic granuloma, subcutaneous angioblastic lymphoid hyperplasia with eosinophilia, inflammatory angiomatous nodules, lymphofolliculosis, intravenous atypical vascular proliferation, histiocytoid haemangioma, inflammatory arteriovenous haemangioma and papular angioplasia [4–6].

Kimura disease was originally described by Kim and Szeto in 1937 in the Chinese literature and later by Kimura et al. in 1948 [7,8].

Epidemiology. ALHE is a rare benign chronic acquired vascular skin disease affecting more commonly young and middle-aged (20–50 years old) men and women. It occurs more frequently in Asians, followed by Caucasians, but can occur in any race [9,10]. On the other hand, Kimura disease affects mainly young boys and men of Asian origin and it is uncommon in western countries [10].

Children and the elderly are rarely affected, with only a few cases of ALHE in these age groups reported in the literature [11–21].

Pathogenesis. The exact aetiology of ALHE is still unknown. There has been a debate on whether ALHE is a reactive disorder or a true vascular neoplasm, with the former receiving more support [22].

Many reports also indicate the possibility that ALHE might be secondary to infections/infestations such as human immunodeficiency virus (HIV), hepatitis B virus (HBV), hepatitis C virus (HCV), human herpesvirus 8 (HHV8),

Harper's Textbook of Pediatric Dermatology, Fourth Edition. Edited by Peter Hoeger, Veronica Kinsler and Albert Yan.

human T-cell lymphotropic virus (HTLV), and scabies [3,18,22–24]. Human polyomavirus-6 infecting lymph nodes of a patient with ALHE or Kimura disease has been recently reported [25].

The response of the endothelial cells and eosinophils to proliferative stimuli such as vascular endothelial growth factor (VEGF) and interleukin-5 (IL-5) generated by the accompanying inflammatory cells (such as mast cells) and immunological allergic reactions (such as after immunization or insect bites) may contribute to the vascular proliferation and disease formation [4,16].

Arteriovenous shunting/malformation, local trauma (surgery, friction, injection, penetrating injury and venipuncture), autoimmune disorders and elevated serum oestrogen levels (due to pregnancy or long-term use of oral contraceptive pills) are possible contributory factors [26–29].

There are anecdotal case reports of ALHE development following a welding burn, blunt trauma to the scalp, scabietic infestation and otitis externa [18,27].

A mutation in the *TEK* gene, which encodes the endothelial cell tyrosine kinase receptor Tie-2, is found and might be another contributory factor [3]. Although ALHE is a benign condition, various lymphoproliferative disorders (e.g. peripheral T-cell lymphoma) have been reported in association with ALHE, reflecting that in some cases ALHE may represent a monoclonal T-cell process [3,30]. There are also cases of ALHE in which T-cell receptor gene (TCR) rearrangement and monoclonality have been detected [3].

The expression of angiotensin-converting enzyme and angiotensin II receptors 1 and 2 by the endothelial cells of an ALHE lesion that developed within a port-wine stain has recently been reported and thus there might be a possible role of the renin–angiotensin system in the pathogenesis of ALHE [31].

Clinical features. ALHE manifests clinically as solitary or multiple red to brown dome-shaped firm mobile intradermal papules or subcutaneous nodules with a smooth surface, ranging in size from 0.2 up to 10 cm in diameter with average of 0.5–3 cm [11] (Fig. 113.1). The lesions are usually pruritic, but can be painful, haemorrhagic (either spontaneously or after minor trauma), pulsatile or even asymptomatic. They occur predominantly on the head and neck region, especially on auricular and periauricular areas.

On the face, ALHE tends to occur on the forehead and nose, while on the scalp it tends to occur on the temporoparietal, occipital, frontal and posterior cervical region [32–34].

Cases of ALHE in the submental region and the angle region of the mandible have been reported [35,36].

ALHE developing within a port-wine stain on the base of the neck in a 19-year-old male has been reported [31].

The extremities are the next most common site and very rarely the trunk (including pubic and infra-axillary regions), back and genitalia (penis/scrotum) [15,17,30,37–41]. Kurihara et al. reported a rare manifestation of ALHE on the lower back in a zosteriform distribution consistent

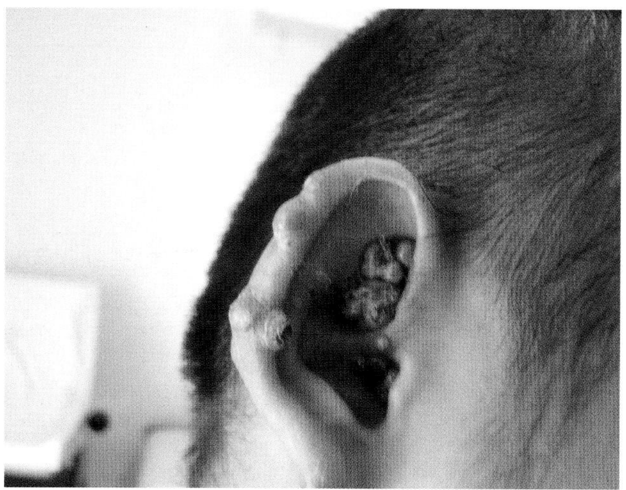

Fig. 113.1 Multiple vascular papules of AHLE on a young boy's ear. Source: Courtesy of Dr Bernice Krafchik.

with the area served by histologically aberrant vessels (AV shunt) [42]. Recently, a case of congenital ALHE in a 2-year-old girl presenting with unilateral lesions in a blaschkoid segmental distribution in the anogenital region has been reported [12].

Skin lesions of ALHE tend to present as solitary papules with very clearly defined margins and with a superficial crust or ulcer. However, in the temporoparietal region, it tends to present in groups and to coalesce into large plaques with an irregular smooth surface [22].

Extracutaneous sites with various signs and symptoms including oral (lips, tongue, buccal mucosa, palate), genital or colonic mucosae, parotid glands, lacrimal glands, bone, breast, liver, spleen, heart, conjunctiva, orbits, ocular adnexa and many muscular arteries have been reported. Regional lymphadenopathy is noted in 5–10% of the cases [4,5,11,19,21,27,39,43–49].

Tokoro et al. reported a rare case of ALHE on the head that arose within the aponeurosis of the trapezius muscle [50].

If ALHE affects the orbit and ocular adnexa, patients usually present with a variety of nonspecific symptoms, such as blurred vision, proptosis, ptosis (most common), diplopia and lid swelling [19,45].

The reported muscular arteries involved include the temporal artery, radial artery, facial artery, postauricular artery, popliteal artery, brachial artery, occipital artery, ulnar artery and axillary artery [4,5].

Differential diagnosis. Kimura disease is the main disease to be differentiated from ALHE. In the past, ALHE and Kimura disease were believed to be subsets of one disease process [51]. Currently, ALHE is considered a separate disease entity from Kimura disease with its distinct clinical and histological features (Table 113.1). Both disorders belong to the group of eosinophilic dermatoses [11].

Kimura disease manifests with a painless large subcutaneous nodule, usually unilateral, in the head and neck region. Salivary gland (parotid or submandibular) enlargement may also occur [10].

Table 113.1 Comparison between angiolymphoid hyperplasia with eosinophilia (ALHE) and Kimura disease

	ALHE	Kimura disease
Age	20–50 years old	8–64 years old
Sex	Men = women	Men > women
Ethnicity	Asians and Caucasians mostly	Asians
Location	Head and neck	Head and neck
Appearance	Superficial papules and nodules	Tumour-like mass with deep soft tissues involved
Size	0.2–10 cm	3–10 cm
Lymphadenopathy	Cervical (5–10% of cases)	Posterior auricular, cervical, inguinal and epitrochlear (frequently noted)
Blood findings	Peripheral eosinophilia present in 20% of cases Serum IgE normal, but can be raised	Peripheral eosinophilia present in ≥75% of cases Serum IgE usually elevated
Histopathological findings	Proliferating vessels with florid intimal proliferation with plump epithelioid endothelial cells, eosinophils, lymphocytes and plasma cells with occasional lymphoid follicles Fibrosis absent or minimal Mast cells commonly increased	Vessels not prominent Fibrosis prominent surrounding lymphoid follicles with reactive germinal centres, lymphocytes, plasma cells, mast cells with IgE, eosinophils and eosinophilic microabscesses Mast cells rarely increased
Immunohistochemistry	CD34, CD31, factor VIII	IgE reticular staining
Associated disorders	Rare	Nephrotic syndrome, Raynaud phenomenon, asthma, ulcerative colitis, temporal arteritis, coronary spasm/aneurysm, atopic dermatitis, lichen amyloidosis
Treatment	Surgical excision, intralesional corticosteroid, pulsed-dye laser	Surgical excision

Regional lymph node enlargement is frequently noted. Nephrotic syndrome has been reported more often in association with Kimura disease than ALHE [51]. Raynaud phenomenon, asthma, ulcerative colitis, coronary spasm/aneurysms and temporal arteritis, atopic dermatitis and lichen amyloidosis are other possible associated features of Kimura disease [35,52–55]. A few case reports of ALHE and Kimura disease coexisting in the same patient have been published [51,56–58].

Other differential diagnoses include angiosarcoma (epithelioid variant), epithelioid haemangioendothelioma, nodular Kaposi sarcoma, cutaneous epithelioid angiomatous nodule, skin metastases, accessory tragus, lymphoma cutis, extranodal lymphoma, sarcoidosis, insect bite reaction, Mikulicz disease (IgG4-related disease), bacillary angiomatosis, organized thrombosis, granuloma faciale, cylindromas, epidermoid cyst, pilar cyst, cavernous haemangioma, eosinophilic granulomatosis with polyangiitis (Churg–Strauss syndrome) and pyogenic granuloma [4,6,11,22,27–29,42,59,60].

Dermoscopic features

Dermoscopic examination of the lesion shows a lacunar pattern similar to the characteristic pattern seen in haemangiomas [37] or a polymorphous vascular pattern composed of dotted, corkscrew and irregular linear vessels arranged radially with a regular distribution over a diffuse pale-reddish to light-pink background [61].

Laboratory tests

Peripheral eosinophilia of 6–34% is present in only 20% of cases and this is not required to make the diagnosis of ALHE. Elevated serum IgE levels are not commonly found. On the other hand, there is marked peripheral eosinophilia and a significant increase in serum immunoglobulin E levels in Kimura disease.

Radiological examination

The ultrasonographic findings of ALHE are also characteristic. It consists of a dermal or subcutaneous mass with poorly defined borders composed of intertwined hyperechoic and hypoechoic bundles, forming an image of a 'ball of wool' surrounded by a hyperechoic halo along with increased vascularization in Doppler studies [62].

Radiological examinations such as Doppler ultrasonography, magnetic resonance imaging (MRI) or angiography may be required to determine the extent and margins of the lesions and to evaluate for arteriovenous shunt and intravascular proliferation as both seem to be correlated with a high rate of local recurrences after treatment [11].

Histology

The histopathological findings of ALHE are quite characteristic: vascular proliferation of varying sizes and types (capillaries, arterioles, venules as well as lymphatic vessels) is present, and the vessels are lined by plump histiocytoid or epithelioid endothelial cells. There are perivascular and interstitial inflammatory infiltrates with numerous eosinophils (5–15% of the infiltrate), lymphocytes with occasional lymphoid follicle formation, as well as plasma cells, mast cells and histiocytes.

The endothelial cells frequently demonstrate atypia, enlarged cuboidal cells with abundant eosinophilic or clear cytoplasm containing vacuoles, occasionally causing cytoplasmic protrusion into lumina (i.e. hobnail or cobblestone appearance) and large vesicular nuclei [3,19].

The vascular proliferations accumulate in loosely lobular patterns with a surrounding fibromyxoid stroma [63]. Early lesions show more vascular proliferation than older lesions, which demonstrate more prominent lymphoid tissue with a flatter vascular endothelium. The concurrent occurrence of ALHE and follicular mucinosis in the same biopsy specimen has been rarely reported [64].

Immunohistochemical studies show positive staining for CD31, CD34 and von Willebrand factor (VWF)/factor VIII of endothelial cells, and the main lymphocytes are T-helper (Th) cells expressing CD3, CD4, CD43 and CD45RO [11], with a few B cells expressing CD20, BCL-2 and MT2 [6,63]. Direct immunofluorescence testing reveals granular deposits of IgA, IgM and C3 around small blood vessels in the centre of the lesion [65].

The histopathology for Kimura disease differs from ALHE: there are florid lymphoid follicles with germinal centre formation, the vascular proliferations are mostly capillaries and their endothelial cells are flat and do not demonstrate atypia, there is massive infiltration of eosinophils, which may extend to the muscular fascia, and eosinophilic microabscesses, eosinophilic folliculosis, fibrosis and IgE deposits may be present [3,10,11,19].

Treatment. The treatment of ALHE remains challenging given the high rate of recurrence (30–50%) due to incomplete resection of the lesion (identifying the margins is difficult), and due to unexcised arteriovenous shunt [26,42].

In general, smaller lesions usually require no treatment because they can undergo spontaneous regression, but larger lesions tend to persist and require therapy.

Surgical excision, intralesional corticosteroid and pulsed-dye laser (PDL) therapy are the mainstays of treatment [66]. Surgical excision is the most effective and commonly used treatment modality for small, few and persistent lesions, and laser therapies are promising and more appropriate for elderly or debilitated patients [33].

There are many other therapeutic modalities that have been anecdotally tried with variable levels of success [6,11,26,33,37,49,51,56,67–83] (Table 113.2).

Table 113.2 Other therapeutic modalities that have been anecdotally tried with variable levels of success

Other surgical procedures	Electrosurgery (electrodessication or electrocoagulation), cryotherapy, curettage, Mohs micrographic surgery, intra-arterial embolization, radiofrequency ablation and sclerotherapy
Other intralesional therapies	Alpha-2a/2b interferon, chemotherapeutic agents (bleomycin, vinblastine, fluorouracil), radiofrequency
Other laser therapies	Carbon dioxide, copper vapour, argon, Nd:YAG
Topical therapies	Corticosteroid, tacrolimus, timolol, antibiotics, imiquimod
Systemic therapies	Corticosteroid, NSAIDs (indometacin farnesil), antibiotics, dapsone, pentoxifylline, oral retinoids (isotretinoin, acitretin), methotrexate, levamisole, propranolol, thalidomide, suplatast tosilate
Biologic therapies	Bevacizumab, mepolizumab
Phototherapy	
Photodynamic therapy	
Radiotherapy	

Adapted from [6,11,26,33,37,49,51,56,67–83].

Singh et al. reported a case of nodular ALHE on the forehead successfully treated with intralesional radiofrequency ablation with cosmetically acceptable results, no recurrence and minimal side-effects [80].

IL-5-based treatments, such as imiquimod and mepolizumab, represent an interesting approach and were reported to be effective because they inhibit either the production or interaction of IL-5 with its receptor respectively, thus inhibiting the production or activation of eosinophils. Imiquimod also decreases tumour cell proliferation, increases tumour apoptosis and increases expression of tissue inhibitor of matrix metalloproteinase-I, which is an inhibitor of angiogenesis and cell motility [11,81].

Propranolol appears to be another interesting and novel therapeutic option that has been reported to be effective, probably due to its anti-angiogenic properties [82]. Rongioletti et al. reported a case of refractory ALHE on the occipital region in a 58-year-old Caucasian woman successfully treated with thalidomide, without recurrence after 3 months of follow-up. Thalidomide has anti-angiogenic, anti-inflammatory and antitumour effects [69].

Bito et al. reported a case of ALHE on the leg of a 63-year-old man successfully treated with the oral Th2 cytokine inhibitor, suplatast tosilate. It exerts an inhibitory effect on IL-4 and IL-5 production by Th2 cells and reduces IgE production by B cells [83].

Although many treatment options are available, as listed in Table 113.2, there is no consensus on the treatment of choice due to a lack of studies [37]. The majority of the previously mentioned treatment options for ALHE are not suitable for use in children due to safety issues, with the exception of a few: surgical modalities (e.g. excision, curettage, cryotherapy), laser therapy (e.g. PDL), topical therapy (e.g. corticosteroids, tacrolimus, timolol, antibiotics) and some systemic therapies (e.g. corticosteroids, NSAIDs, systemic antibiotics, propranolol).

Given that ALHE is a benign condition and follows a chronic, recurrent course with possible spontaneous resolution, the best approach in the majority of cases, especially in areas where extensive resection may be disfiguring, is a simple follow-up 'watch and wait' for 3–6 months before surgical excision or other treatment options are attempted [11,15,19,20,37].

Treatment failure (defined as incomplete resolution of disease or recurrence after treatment) is high among all modalities, but is lowest for surgical excision and laser therapy (PDL and CO_2 laser) and highest for systemic and topical corticosteroids [33].

Prognosis. ALHE is a rare benign chronic disorder with no evidence of malignant transformation and no tendency to metastasize. The general health of the patient is unaffected. Although the lesions generally tend to persist and recur, they can undergo spontaneous remission without any intervention within 1–4 years compared to Kimura disease, which can last up to 25 years [9,19]. Higher rates of recurrence post excision have been associated with earlier age of onset, longer duration of disease, multiple lesions, bilateral lesions, associated pruritus, pain and bleeding [33].

References

1 **Wells GC, Whimster IW. Subcutaneous angiolymphoid hyperplasia with eosinophilia. Br J Dermatol 1969;81:1–15.**

2 **Weiss SW, Enzinger FM. Epithelioid hemangioendothelioma: a vascular tumor often mistaken for a carcinoma. Cancer 1982;50:970–81.**

3 Guo R, Gavino AC. Angiolymphoid hyperplasia with eosinophilia. Arch Pathol Lab Med 2015;139:683–6.

4 Amin A, Umashankar T, Dsouza CO. Intra-arterial angiolymphoid hyperplasia with eosinophilia: A rare case report of peripheral medium sized muscular artery involvement. J Clin Diagn Res 2015;9:16–17.

5 Kukreja N, Koslowski M, Insall R. Angiolymphoid hyperplasia with eosinophilia presenting as an axillary artery aneurysm. BMJ Case Rep 2011:1–4.

6 Kamath MP, Bhojwani KM, Bhandarkar AM et al. Angiolymphoid hyperplasia with eosinophilia of root of nose: A rare phenomenon. J Clin Diagn Res 2014;8:144–5.

7 **Kimm HT, Szeto C. Eosinophilic hyperplastic lymphogranuloma, comparison with Mikulicz's disease. Proc Chin Med Soc 1937;23:699–700.**

8 **Kimura T, Yoshimura S, Ishikawa E. On the unusual granulation combined with hyperplastic changes of lymphatic tissues. Trans Soc Pathol Jpn 1948;37:179–80.**

9 **Chitrapu P, Patel M, Readinger A, Menter A. Angiolymphoid hyperplasia with eosinophilia. Proc (Bayl Univ Med Cent) 2014;27:336–7.**

10 Esteves P, Barbalho M, Lima T et al. Angiolymphoid hyperplasia with eosinophilia: A case report. Case Rep Dermatol 2015;7:113–16.

11 **Zaraa I, Mlika M, Chouk S et al. Angiolymphoid hyperplasia with eosinophilia: A study of 7 cases. Dermatol Online J 2011;17:1.**

12 Su HH, Shan SJ, Elston DM et al. Congenital blaschkoid angiolymphoid hyperplasia with eosinophilia of the anogenital region. Am J Dermatopathol 2016;38:305–6.

13 Satpathy A, Moss C, Raafat F, Slator R. Spontaneous regression of a rare tumour in a child: angiolymphoid hyperplasia with eosinophilia of the hand: case report and review of the literature. Br J Plast Surg 2005;58:865–8.

14 Koizumi H, Okuyama R, Tagami H, Aiba S. Spontaneous regression of generalized angiolymphoid hyperplasia with eosinophilia in a 2-year-old boy. Acta Derm Venereol 2008;88:395–6.

15 Nishi M, Matsumoto K, Fujita T et al. Angiolymphoid hyperplasia with eosinophilia on penile skin in a 7-year-old child. J Pediatr Surg 2011;46:559–61.

16 **Jeon EK, Cho AY, Kim MY et al. Angiolymphoid hyperplasia with eosinophilia that was possibly induced by vaccination in a child. Ann Dermatol 2009;21:71–4.**

17 Korekawa A, Kaneko T, Hagiwara C et al. Angiolymphoid hyperplasia with eosinophilia in infancy. J Dermatol 2012;39:1052–4.

18 **Chou CY, Lee WR, Tseng J. Case of angiolymphoid hyperplasia with eosinophilia associated with scabies infestation. J Dermatol 2012;39:102–4.**

19 Azari AA, Kanavi MR, Lucarelli M et al. Angiolymphoid hyperplasia with eosinophilia of the orbit and ocular adnexa: Report of 5 cases. JAMA Ophthalmol 2014;132:633–6.

20 Ayachi K, Daoud R, Ben Youssef A et al. Angiolymphoid hyperplasia with eosinophilia. Rev Stomatol Chir Maxillofac Chir Orale 2013;114:331–3.

21 Shevchenko L, Aaberg T Jr, Grossniklaus HE. Conjunctival angiolymphoid hyperplasia with eosinophilia in a child. J Pediatr Ophthalmol Strabismus 2012;49:e66–9.

22 **Guinovart RM, Bassas-Vila J, Morell L, Ferrandiz C. Angiolymphoid hyperplasia with eosinophilia: A clinicopathologic study of 9 cases. Actas Dermosifiliogr 2014;105:e1–6.**

23 **Parimalam K, Thomas J. Angiolymphoid hyperplasia with eosinophilia associated with pregnancy – A rare report. Indian J Dermatol 2016;61:125.**

24 Al-Muharraqi MA, Faqi MK, Uddin F et al. Angiolymphoid hyperplasia with eosinophilia (epithelioid hemangioma) of the face: An unusual presentation. Int J Surg Case Rep 2011;2:258–60.

25 **Rascovan N, Bouchard SM, Grob JJ et al. Human polyomavirus-6 infecting lymph nodes of a patient with an angiolymphoid hyperplasia with eosinophilia or Kimura disease. Clin Infect Dis 2016;62:1419–21.**

26 San Nicolo M, Mayr D, Berghaus A. Angiolymphoid hyperplasia with eosinophilia of the external ear: case report and review of the literature. Eur Arch Otorhinolaryngol 2013;270:2775–7.

27 **Stewart N, Zagarella S, Mann S. Angiolymphoid hyperplasia with eosinophilia occurring after venipuncture trauma. J Dermatol 2013;40:393–5.**

28 Ahmad SM, Wani GM, Khursheed B, Qayoom S. Angiolymphoid hyperplasia with eosinophilia mimicking multiple cylindromas: A rare case report. Indian J Dermatol 2014;59:423.

29 Marcum CB, Zager JS, Belongie IP et al. Profound proliferating angiolymphoid hyperplasia with eosinophilia of pregnancy mimicking angiosarcoma. Cutis 2011;88:122–8.

30 Chen JF, Gao HW, Wu BY et al. Angiolymphoid hyperplasia with eosinophilia affecting the scrotum: a rare case report with molecular evidence of T-cell clonality. J Dermatol 2010;37:355–9.

31 **Manton RN, Itinteang T, Jong SD et al. Angiolymphoid hyperplasia with eosinophilia developing within a port wine stain. J Cutan Pathol 2016;43:53–6.**

32 Rahman A, Asad Shabbir SM, Tabassum S, Hafeez J. Auricular angiolymphoid hyperplasia with eosinophilia. J Coll Physicians Surg Pak 2011;21:623–5.

33 **Adler BL, Krausz AE, Minuti A et al. Epidemiology and treatment of angiolymphoid hyperplasia with eosinophilia (ALHE): A systematic review. J Am Acad Dermatol 2016;74:506–12.**

34 Chiu SC. An unusual case of angiolymphoid hyperplasia with eosinophilia of the nose. Ear Nose Throat J 2013;92:e10–11.

35 Singh P, Singh A. A rare case of angiolymphoid hyperplasia with eosinophilia in the submental region. J Oral Maxillofac Pathol 2013;17:311–14.

36 Ozkan BT, Eroglu CN, Cigerim L, Gunhan O. Angiolymphoid hyperplasia with eosinophilia in the angle region of the mandible. J Oral Maxillofac Pathol 2015;19:108.

37 **Padilla-Espana L, Fernandez-Morano T, Del Boz J, Funez- Liebana R. Angiolymphoid hyperplasia with eosinophilia: Analysis of 7 cases. Actas Dermosifiliogr 2013;104:353–5.**

38 Jung KE, Kim KM, Lee JY et al. Erythematous protruding skin lesion in the retroauricular area: A quiz. Acta Derm Venereol 2014;94:365–6.

39 Damle DK, Raotole SS, Belgaumkar VA, Mhaske CB. Angiolymphoid hyperplasia with eosinophilia on penis in HIV- positive patient: An unusual presentation. Indian J Dermatol Venereol Leprol 2013;79:109–11.

40 Parmar NV, Sandhu J, Kanwar AJ, Saikia UN. Angiolymphoid hyperplasia with eosinophilia of the infra-axillary region: report of a case. Dermatol Online J 2014;20:8.

41 Park J, Hwang SR, Song KH et al. Angiolymphoid hyperplasia with eosinophilia affecting the scrotum of a child. Eur J Dermatol 2013;23:423–4.

42 Kurihara Y, Inoue H, Kiryu H, Furue M. Epithelioid hemangioma (angiolymphoid hyperplasia with eosinophilia) in zosteriform distribution. Indian J Dermatol 2012;57:401–3.

43 Cunniffe G, Alonso T, Dinares C et al. Angiolymphoid hyperplasia with eosinophilia of the eyelid and orbit: the western cousin of Kimura's disease? Int Ophthalmol 2014;34:107–10.

44 Aggarwal A, Keluskar V. Epithelioid hemangioma (angiolymphoid hyperplasia with eosinophilia) in the oral mucosa. Indian J Dent Res 2012;23:271–4.

45 Ueda S, Goto H, Usui Y et al. Angiolymphoid hyperplasia with eosinophilia occurring in bilateral eyelids. BMC Ophthalmol 2013;13:38.

46 Bangal SV, Chitgopekar RP, Gupta AK, Karle R. Orbital extension of supraorbital angiolymphoid hyperplasia with eosinophilia. Australas Med J 2011;4:111–13.

47 Tirumalasetti N. Angiolymphoid hyperplasia with eosinophilia: A rare benign vascular tumor of breast. Indian J Pathol Microbiol 2013;56:405–7.

48 Das SK, Ghosh A, Banerjee N et al. Angiolymphoid hyperplasia with eosinophilia presenting with peri-ocular swelling. J Indian Med Assoc 2013;111:853–4.

49 Baker MS, Avery RB, Johnson CR, Allen RC. Methotrexate as an alternative treatment for orbital angiolymphoid hyperplasia with eosinophilia. Orbit 2012;31:324–6.

50 Tokoro S, Namiki T, Ueno M et al. Angiolymphoid hyperplasia with eosinophilia of the head arising within the aponeurosis. J Dermatol 2015;42:1190–1.

51 **Liu XK, Ren J, Wang XH et al. Angiolymphoid hyperplasia with eosinophilia and Kimura`s disease coexisting in the same patient: Evidence for a spectrum of disease. Australas J Dermatol 2012;53:e47–50.**

52 Horigome H, Sekijima T, Ohtsuka S, Shibasaki M. Life threatening coronary artery spasm in childhood Kimura`s disease. Heart 2000;84:e5.

53 Teraki Y, Katsuta M, Shiohara T. Lichen amyloidosis associated with Kimura's disease: successful treatment with cyclosporine. Dermatology 2002;204:133–5.
54 Danno K, Horio T, Miyachi Y et al. Coexistence of Kimura's disease and lichen amyloidosis in three patients. Arch Dermatol 1982;118:976–80.
55 Hamrick HJ, Jennette JC, LaForce CF. Kimura's disease: report of a pediatric case in the United States. J Allergy Clin Immunol 1984;73:561–6.
56 Jun R, Liu XK, Zeng K. Successful treatment of angiolymphoid hyperplasia with eosinophilia and Kimura's disease in the same patient with surgery. Dermatol Therapy 2014;27:36–8.
57 Chong WS, Thomas A, Coh CL. Kimura's disease and angiolymphoid hyperplasia with eosinophilia: two disease entity in the same patient: case report and review of the literature. Int J Dermatol 2006;45:139–45.
58 Reddy PK, Prasad AL, Sumathy TK et al. An overlap of angiolymphoid hyperplasia with eosinophilia and Kimura's disease: Successful treatment of skin lesions with cryotherapy. Indian J Dermatol 2015;60:216.
59 Hamaguchi Y, Fujimoto M, Matsushita Y et al. IgG4-related skin disease, a mimic of angiolymphoid hyperplasia with eosinophilia. Dermatol 2011;223:301–5.
60 Cole CM. Dermatopathology Diagnosis: Angiolymphoid hyperplasia with eosinophilia. Cutis 2013;92:110;117–18.
61 Rodriguez-Lomba E, Aviles-Izquierdo JA, Molina-Lopez I et al. Dermoscopic features in 2 cases of angiolymphoid hyperplasia with eosinophilia. J Am Acad Dermatol 2016;75:e19–21.
62 Lorente-Luna M, Alfageme-Roldan F, Suarez-Massa D, Jimenez-Blazquez E. Wooly pattern as a characteristic ultrasound finding in angiolymphoid hyperplasia with eosinophilia. Actas Dermosifiliogr 2014;105:718–20.
63 Okman JS, Bhatti TR, Jackson OA, Rubin AI. Angiolymphoid hyperplasia with eosinophilia: A previously unreported complication for ear piercing. Pediatr Dermatol 2014;31:738–41.
64 Gutte R, Doshi B, Khopkar U. Angiolymphoid hyperplasia with eosinophilia with follicular mucinosis. Indian J Dermatol 2013;58:159.
65 Grimwood R, Swinehart JM, Aeling JL. Angiolymphoid hyperplasia with eosinophilia. Arch Dermatol 1979;115:205–7.
66 Panicker VV, Dhramaratnam AD, Kuruvilla J. Angiolymphoid hyperplasia with eosinophilia. Indian Dermatol Online J 2012;3:80.
67 Tchernev G, Taneva T, Ananiev J et al. Angiolymphoid hyperplasia with eosinophilia-an incidental finding after surgical excision. Wien Med Wochenschr 2012;162:448–51.
68 Ali FR, Madan V. Facial angiolymphoid hyperplasia with eosinophilia: sustained remission following treatment with carbon dioxide laser. Clin Exp Dermatol 2016;41:96–8.
69 Rongioletti F, Cecchi F, Pastorino C, Scaparro M. Successful management of refractory angiolymphoid hyperplasia with eosinophilia with thalidomide. J Eur Acad Dermatol Venereol 2016; 30:527–9.
70 Gonzalez JA, Boixeda P, Diez MT et al. Angiolymphoid hyperplasia with eosinophilia treated with vascular laser. Lasers Med Sci 2011;26:285–90.
71 Fink CM, Maggio KL. Angiolymphoid hyperplasia with eosinophilia revisited: lack of durable response to intralesional interferon alfa-2a. Arch Dermatol 2011;147:507–8.
72 Lembo S, Balato A, Cirillo T, Balato N. A long-term follow- up of angiolymphoid hyperplasia with eosinophilia treated by corticosteroids: when a traditional therapy is still up-to-date. Case Rep Dermatol 2011;3:64–7.
73 Wang Y, Tu Y, Tao J, Li Y. Angiolymphoid hyperplasia with eosinophilia responsive to sclerotherapy. Dermatol Surg 2014;40:1042–3.
74 Nouchi A, Hickman G, Battistella M et al. Treatment of angiolymphoid hyperplasia with eosinophilia (ALHE) using topical tacrolimus: Two cases. Ann Dermatol Venereol 2015;142:360–6.
75 Chacon AH, Mercer J. Successful management of angiolymphoid hyperplasia with eosinophilia in a split-face trial of topical tacrolimus and timolol solution. G Ital Dermatol Venereol 2016;151:436–40.
76 Su YW, Wu XF. Angiolymphoid hyperplasia with eosinophilia treated with surgical excision and electrocoagulation forceps. Indian J Dermatol Venereol Leprol 2016;82:457–8.
77 Bazakas A, Solander S, Ladizinski B, Halvorson EG. Transarterial embolization followed by surgical excision of skin lesions as treatment for angiolymphoid hyperplasia with eosinophilia. J Am Acad Dermatol 2013;68:e48–9.
78 Lade NR, Banode P, Dhope N et al. Angiolymphoid hyperplasia with arterial ectasia and arteriovenous malformation: Response to intraarterial embolization. Indian J Dermatol Venereol Leprol 2016;82: 413–15.
79 Oguz O, Antonov M, Demirkesen C. Angiolymphoid hyperplasia with eosinophilia responding to interferon-alpha 2b. J Eur Acad Dermatol Venereol 2007;21:1277–8.
80 Singh S, Dayal M, Walia R et al. Intralesional radiofrequency ablation for nodular angiolymphoid hyperplasia on forehead: A minimally invasive approach. Indian J Dermatol Venereol 2014;80:419–21.
81 Isohisa T, Masuda K, Nakai N. Angiolymphoid hyperplasia with eosinophilia treated successfully with imiquimod. Int J Dermatol 2014;53:e43–4.
82 Horst C, Kapur N. Propranolol: a novel treatment for angiolymphoid hyperplasia with eosinophilia. Clin Exp Dermatol 2014;39:810–12.
83 Bito T, Kabashima R, Sugita K, Tokura Y. Angiolymphoid hyperplasia with eosinophilia on the leg successfully treated with T-helper cell 2 cytokine inhibitor suplatast tosilate. J Dermatol 2011;38:300–2.

CHAPTER 114
Fibromatoses

Jenna L. Streicher[1,2], *Moise L. Levy*[3] *& Albert C. Yan*[1,2]

[1] Section of Dermatology, Children's Hospital of Philadelphia, Philadelphia, PA, USA
[2] Departments of Pediatrics and Dermatology, Perelman School of Medicine at the University of Pennsylvania, Philadelphia, PA, USA
[3] Department of Pediatrics, Texas Children's Hospital, Baylor College of Medicine, Houston, TX and Department of Pediatrics, Dell Medical School/University of Texas and Pediatric Dermatology, Dell Children's Medical Center, Austin, TX, USA

Introduction, 1356
Lesions with a generally indolent course, 1357
Lesions with potential for a locally aggressive course, 1362

Abstract

The fibromatoses represent a heterogeneous collection of spindle cell tumours of the skin and soft tissues. These lesions have been described under a variety of different names, but all share a histology characterized principally by spindle cells. Depending on the specific fibromatosis, these tumours can be localized, multicentric or generalized; indolent or aggressive; occur solely in the skin or have visceral involvement; and may occur during infancy, childhood or adulthood. The variability in their presentation makes this a challenging group of disorders to characterize. This chapter will focus on an important subset of these tumours, the fibrous and myofibroblastic tumours of childhood.

Key points

- The principal fibromatoses can be divided into those with a generally indolent course and those with the potential for a locally aggressive course.
- Myofibromas that are solitary or multicentric (but not visceral) have a generally good prognosis with many lesions showing spontaneous regression. Visceral myofibromatosis, however, carries a guarded prognosis with significant morbidity and mortality.
- The fibromatoses with a more generally indolent course include myofibromas, fibromatosis colli, fibrous hamartoma of infancy, calcifying fibrous pseudotumour and nodular fasciitis.
- The fibromatoses with a greater potential for a more aggressive course include the infantile desmoid type, palmar–plantar type, gingival fibromatosis, infantile digital (inclusion body) fibromatosis, calcifying aponeurotic fibroma, giant cell fibroblastoma, dermatofibrosarcoma protuberans and infantile fibrosarcoma.
- Surgical approaches, where necessary, can be helpful when tumours can be removed in their entirety, but many of the more aggressive fibromatoses have a high rate of recurrence. Mohs micrographic surgical methods may provide higher rates of clearance in these cases. Systemic therapies targeted at underlying molecular mechanisms can be helpful in certain instances.

Introduction

In the first half of the twentieth century it was not unusual for doctors to collectively describe a great variety of reactive, hamartomatous, benign nonaggressive and benign locally aggressive lesions under the single encompassing classification of 'fibromatosis' [1]. Traditional attempts have been made to categorize these lesions on the basis of their anatomical location: namely, digital, palmar–plantar and generalized fibromatoses of childhood. Anatomical classifications, however, provide limited prognostic information and leave many entities without appropriate categories. Other classifications separate the diseases by those that correspond with similar lesions in adults and those that are peculiar to infancy and childhood [2]. Ultimately, until specific underlying genetic bases are elucidated, it may be best to consider these lesions on the basis of their biological behaviour: those that are relatively indolent lesions and those that often follow a more locally aggressive course (Box 114.1).

Box 114.1 Fibrous and myofibroblastic lesions of childhood

Those with a generally indolent course

- Myofibroma/myofibromatosis
- Fibromatosis colli
- Fibrous hamartoma of infancy
- Calcifying fibrous pseudotumour
- Nodular fasciitis

Those with potential for a locally aggressive course

- Infantile (desmoid-type) fibromatosis
- Palmar–plantar fibromatosis
- Gingival fibromatosis
- Digital (inclusion body) fibromatosis
- Calcifying aponeurotic fibroma
- Giant cell fibroblastoma and dermatofibrosarcoma protuberans
- Congenital/infantile fibrosarcoma

Harper's Textbook of Pediatric Dermatology, Fourth Edition. Edited by Peter Hoeger, Veronica Kinsler and Albert Yan.

References

1 Stout AP. Juvenile fibromatoses. Cancer 1954;7:953–78.
2 Thway K, Fisher C, Sebire NJ. Pediatric fibroblastic and myofibroblastic lesions. Adv Anat Pathol 2012;19:54–65.

Lesions with a generally indolent course

Myofibroma/myofibromatosis

Introduction/history. Myofibromas are benign mesenchymal tumours that are composed of cells having fibroblastic and myofibroblastic (smooth muscle) differentiation. Solitary lesions are called myofibromas, whereas multiple lesions are designated as myofibromatosis [1]. These tumours represent one of the most common benign fibrous tumours of infancy [2].

Epidemiology and pathogenesis. Solitary lesions are sporadic in most instances while patients with myofibromatosis have been reported with both autosomal dominant [3–6] and recessive patterns of inheritance [7,8]. Families with an autosomal dominant mode of inheritance have been found to have mutations in platelet-derived growth factor receptor-β (PDGFRB), which plays a role in early haematopoiesis and blood vessel formation and is known to promote growth of mesenchymal cells including blood vessels and smooth muscle [9,10]. A male predominance has been reported [6].

Clinical features and differential diagnosis. Myofibromas are usually first appreciated as a single (or, less often, multiple) subcutaneous or dermal nodule; these nodules may range in size from a few millimetres to 2 or 3 centimetres in their largest dimension. The nodules may be noted at birth or within the first few months; it is unusual for these lesions to develop after the first year or two (although examples of myofibromas in older children and adults have been reported) [6,11]. The more superficially located lesions often have a bluish hue and may have a vascularized surface appearance; deeply seated lesions may show little surface change. These lesions have a firm to rubbery quality, and present as painless masses.

Although the individual myofibromas themselves are not aggressive lesions, it is nevertheless important to distinguish those children with solitary lesions from those with multiple lesions. Three clinical patterns of disease are recognized: (i) solitary disease (often subcutaneous), which is a self-limiting process; (ii) multicentric disease, which involves the skin, subcutaneous tissues, muscles and bone, with a typical benign course and spontaneous resolution; and (iii) a generalized form which is defined by visceral involvement and poor prognosis.

Solitary myofibromas are the most common pattern, accounting for approximately half of cases. These frequently occur in the head/neck region and trunk [6]. Children with solitary lesions often see their lesions regress spontaneously (Fig. 114.1). In some cases, intrauterine regression has been observed.

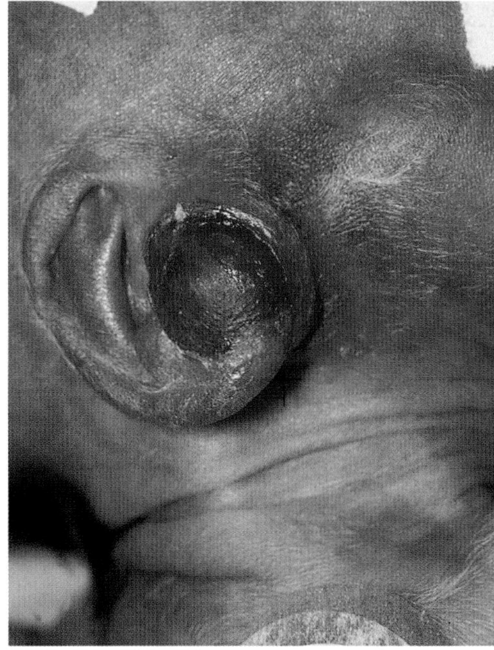

(a)

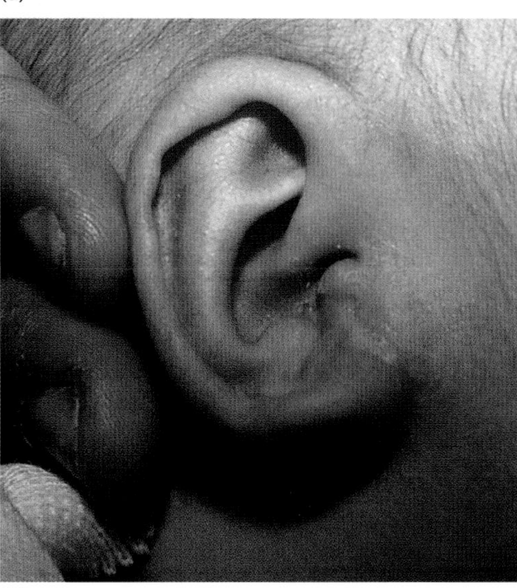

(b)

Fig. 114.1 (a) Firm erythematous tumour on the ear of a neonate typical of a myofibroma. (b) Same infant as in (a) at 6 months, with nearly complete spontaneous resolution of the myofibroma.

Patients with multicentric disease may develop lesions at a variety of sites, including the skin, subcutaneous tissue and muscle, accounting for approximately 98% of cases, and bones being involved in 50% of cases [6,12]. When bone involvement occurs, it is usually characterized by lytic lesions on skeletal radiography. These multifocal lesions may be quite numerous, ranging from a few dozen to perhaps 100 or more. Patients with multifocal disease often still have a good prognosis with most experiencing spontaneous resolution within the first 2 years of life [6]. If any complication does occur, it is usually a localized complication due to pressure-induced damage. Upon spontaneous resolution, the nodules may leave behind atrophic scars.

Patients with generalized myofibromatosis typically have severe systemic disease. Visceral involvement can involve the gastrointestinal tract, lungs, heart and endocrine organs [2,13]. Those children with visceral involvement may die of their disease, particularly as a result of pulmonary or gastrointestinal tract involvement. Most deaths occur within the first week of life or no later than 4 months. Paradoxically, the myofibromas do not themselves exhibit malignant behaviour, in the sense of growing uncontrollably or metastasizing; rather, it is the sheer volume of these lesions in the vital organs that interferes with their function and so may lead to death.

Clinically, the differential diagnosis includes any of a variety of tumours including neurofibroma, hyaline fibromatosis, vascular lesions such as congenital or infantile haemangioma, or sarcoma. Generalized forms without spontaneous regression show overlap with infantile systemic hyalinosis. Adequate biopsy material should distinguish these entities from myofibromatosis.

Pathology. One of the most characteristic features of a myofibroma on light microscopic examination is its architecture; there is a distinct zonation in its appearance (Fig. 114.2). Peripherally, myofibromas are marked by a proliferation of short bundles of spindle cells with a myoid appearance, i.e. plump nuclei and abundant pale cytoplasm, with cytoplasmic striations, which are frequently gathered into rounded aggregates. In the interior of these lesions, the spindle cells adopt a more fibrous appearance, i.e. they contain smaller, thinner nuclei with less cytoplasm and a more eosinophilic appearance overall (Fig. 114.3). The central region of the tumour is often marked by a proliferation of rather small round to oval cells with little cytoplasm. Centrally located round to oval cells are often arranged around prominent vascular spaces, in a pattern that is reminiscent of a haemangiopericytoma. This central region often develops changes of ischaemic necrosis [14]. It is not usually difficult to identify mitotic figures within this lesion; mitotic rates may approach one mitosis in each high-power field, particularly centrally. However, none of these mitoses is atypical. This degree of mitotic activity is not usually associated with the other fibrous/myofibroblastic lesions (with one exception, that of nodular fasciitis). No significant cytological atypia (of the degree seen in malignancies) will be appreciated within the cells of a myofibroma.

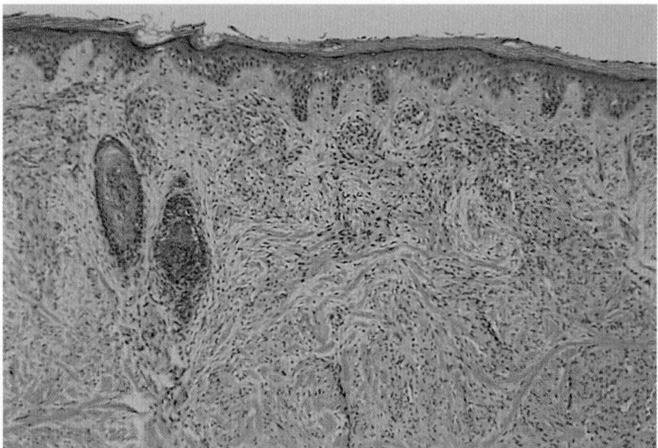

Fig. 114.2 The key characteristic of a myofibroma is its zonal architecture: the periphery of this lesion shows nodules of rounded to oval cells surrounding adnexal structures and approaching the epidermis.

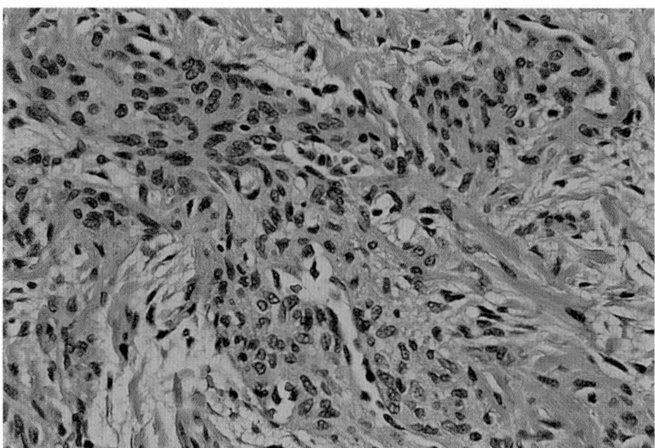

Fig. 114.3 At the periphery of a myofibroma the individual cells are characterized by eosinophilic cytoplasm, round to oval dark nuclei and a grouping into nodular aggregates.

These features are the same in solitary and multiple lesions and so light microscopic evaluation will not distinguish these two different clinical diagnoses on the basis of examining a single lesion. A myofibromatous nodule differs from the infiltrative fibromatoses discussed in following sections with regard to its borders; other fibromatoses have infiltrative borders, whereas the myofibromas are relatively well circumscribed (although not actually encapsulated) on both gross and microscopic examination. Moreover, true fibromatoses produce a degree of stromal collagen not seen in myofibromas. In keeping with their myoid appearance, myofibroma cells show focal actin and vimentin positivity by immunohistochemistry; these lesions are desmin negative and S100 protein negative [15].

Treatment. Ultimately, solitary myofibromas are best approached as benign, self-limiting lesions as the majority spontaneously regress over time. Involvement of the viscera is rare with a solitary myofibroma. Those children with multiple lesions are usually subjected to a biopsy for diagnosis and then undergo a full skin examination and consideration of imaging to determine the extent of disease. In patients with visceral involvement, a trial of systemic therapy may be necessary as fatality is reported in up to 75% of cases [2]. The combination of low-dose methotrexate and vinblastine has been reported to be helpful in the resolution of these lesions and may be considered in infants with extensive or life-threatening involvement [16].

References

1 Thway K, Fisher C, Sebire NJ. Pediatric fibroblastic and myofibroblastic lesions. Adv Anat Pathol 2012;19:54–65.

2 Wiswell TE, Davis J, Cunningham BE et al. Infantile myofibromatosis: the most common fibrous tumor of infancy. J Pediatr Surg 1988;23:315–18.

3 Jennings TA, Duray PH, Collins FS et al. Infantile myofibromatosis. Evidence for an autosomal-dominant disorder. Am J Surg Pathol 1984;8:529–38.
4 Ikediobi NI, Iyengar V, Hwang L et al. Infantile myofibromatosis: support for autosomal dominant inheritance. J Am Acad Dermatol 2003;49(2 Suppl Case Reports):S148–50.
5 Zand DJ, Huff D, Everman D et al. Autosomal dominant inheritance of infantile myofibromatosis. Am J Med Genet A 2004;126A: 261–6.
6 Mashiah J, Hadj-Rabia S, Dompmartin A et al. Infantile myofibromatosis: a series of 28 cases. J Am Acad Dermatol 2014;71:264–70.
7 Venencie PY, Bigel P, Desgruelles C et al. Infantile myofibromatosis. Report of two cases in one family. Br J Dermatol 1987;117:255–9.
8 Narchi H. Four half-siblings with infantile myofibromatosis: a case for autosomal-recessive inheritance. Clin Genet 2001;59:134–5.
9 Martignetti JA, Tian L, Li D et al. Mutations in PDGFRB cause autosomal-dominant infantile myofibromatosis. Am J Hum Genet 2013;92:1001–7.
10 Cheung YH, Gayden T, Campeau PM et al. A recurrent PDGFRB mutation causes familial infantile myofibromatosis. Am J Hum Genet 2013;92:996–1000.
11 Stanford D, Rogers M. Dermatological presentations of infantile myofibromatosis: a review of 27 cases. Australas J Dermatol 2000;41: 156–61.
12 Goldberg NS, Bauer BS, Kraus H et al. Infantile myofibromatosis: a review of clinicopathology with perspectives on new treatment choices. Pediatr Dermatol 1988;5:37–46.
13 Coffin CM, Neilson KA, Ingels S et al. Congenital generalized myofibromatosis: a disseminated angiocentric myofibromatosis. Pediatr Pathol Lab Med 1995;15:571–87.
14 Fukasawa Y, Ishikura H, Takada A et al. Massive apoptosis in infantile myofibromatosis. A putative mechanism of tumor regression. Am J Pathol 1994;144:480–5.
15 Hausbrandt PA, Leithner A, Beham A et al. A rare case of infantile myofibromatosis and review of literature. J Pediatr Orthop B 2010;19:122–6.
16 Azzam R, Abboud M, Muwakkit S et al. First-line therapy of generalized infantile myofibromatosis with low-dose vinblastine and methotrexate. Pediatr Blood Cancer 2009;52:308.

Fibromatosis colli

Introduction/history. Fibromatosis colli (synonyms: sternocleidomastoid tumour, congenital muscular fibromatosis, pseudotumour of infancy) is a benign soft tissue mass that originates from the sternocleidomastoid muscle. It is seen exclusively in newborn infants and often produces torticollis [1,2].

Epidemiology and pathogenesis. Fibromatosis colli is the most common neck mass that presents in the perinatal period and is reported to be more common in boys than girls [1]. The exact aetiology is unknown. Delivery trauma has been implicated in its pathogenesis; however, cases have developed following uncomplicated spontaneous vaginal delivery, suggesting that factors other than birth trauma may be involved. Another hypothesis is that these lesions develop due to poor venous flow to the area *in utero* or during delivery, which leads to oedema and muscle degeneration [3].

Clinical features and differential diagnosis. Fibromatosis colli usually presents clinically in one of two ways: as a palpable mass in the vicinity of the lower portion of the sternocleidomastoid muscle (typically within the first few weeks after birth), or as torticollis or wryneck. The lesion is not fixed to the overlying skin, but rather seems to be associated with the adjacent muscle tissue. After a period of growth spanning only a few months, these masses usually stabilize or even regress.

Other causes of torticollis may enter into the clinical differential diagnosis (e.g. infection, trauma later in life and muscular spasm, all of which may produce a tilting of the child's head to one side or another and so mimic fibromatosis colli). These are acquired lesions and so appear at a later age than fibromatosis colli.

Pathology. In its earliest phase of development, fibromatosis colli is marked by an infiltration of the skeletal muscle of the sternocleidomastoid muscle by a population of bland spindle cells, set in a myxoid background; neither cytological atypia nor mitotic activity is appreciable [2]. As the lesion ages, its stroma becomes more heavily collagenized.

Treatment. The diagnosis of fibromatosis colli can often be made based on the clinical presentation and natural history of the lesion with the help of radiological imaging as needed. Ultrasound has been shown to be helpful [4]. If tissue confirmation is needed, fine-needle aspiration can be used to make a definitive diagnosis [5].

Fibromatosis colli usually reaches its maximum growth within a few weeks of onset, stabilizes, and then often undergoes spontaneous regression. There have been lesions that have been reported to be progressive which could potentially lead to facial skull deformities due to traction of the muscle on facial anatomy [1]. In most cases, conservative management with physical therapy and massage is recommended [6]. Ultimately, surgical correction of any persisting deformity may be carried out in the minority of patients in whom such therapy is indicated [7,8].

References
1 Lowry KC, Estroff JA, Rahbar R. The presentation and management of fibromatosis colli. Ear Nose Throat J 2010;89:E4–8.
2 Coffin CM, Neilson KA, Ingels S et al. Congenital generalized myofibromatosis: a disseminated angiocentric myofibromatosis. Pediatr Pathol Lab Med 1995;15:571–87.
3 Ablin DS, Jain K, Howell L, West DC. Ultrasound and MR imaging of fibromatosis colli (sternomastoid tumor of infancy). Pediatr Radiol 1998;28:230–3.
4 Maddalozzo J, Goldenberg JD. Pseudotumor of infancy—the role of ultrasonography. Ear Nose Throat J 1996;75:248–54.
5 Sharma S, Mishra K, Khanna G. Fibromatosis colli in infants. A cytologic study of eight cases. Acta Cytol 2003;47:359–62.
6 Kumar V, Prabhu BV, Chattopadhayay A, Nagendhar MY. Bilateral sternocleidomastoid tumor of infancy. Int J Pediatr Otorhinolaryngol 2003;67:673–5.
7 Bredenkamp JK, Hoover LA, Berke GS, Shaw A. Congenital muscular torticollis. A spectrum of disease. Arch Otolaryngol Head Neck Surg 1990;116:212–16.
8 Cheng JC, Au AW. Infantile torticollis: a review of 624 cases. J Pediatr Orthop 1994;14:802–8.

Fibrous hamartoma of infancy

Introduction/history. Fibrous hamartoma of infancy was first described as a 'subdermal fibrous tumor of infancy' in 1956 by Reye [1]. He described six infants with tumours in the subcutaneous tissue that all had similar histological findings. The tumour was renamed fibrous hamartoma of infancy in 1965 by Enzinger [2].

Epidemiology and pathogenesis. Fibrous hamartoma of infancy is a benign mesenchymal tumour that often presents within in the first 2 years of life, with up to 23% of cases being congenital [3,4]. The aetiology of this tumour is controversial with no clear consensus whether the lesion represents a hamartoma or benign neoplasm. There have not been any significant syndromic associations with fibrous hamartoma of infancy, nor a familial predilection for the lesion [4]. As with many of the fibrous tumours seen in children, it is more commonly seen in boys compared to girls.

Clinical features and differential diagnosis. Fibrous hamartoma of infancy usually presents as a solitary, painless nodular or plaque-like mass that appears to be centred in the subcutaneous tissues or the deep dermis (Fig. 114.4). The lesion is neither fixed to the skin nor to underlying deep structures. Presentation as multiple lesions has occasionally been reported in the literature [3]. Hypertrichosis and hyperhidrosis of the overlying skin of these tumours have been reported [5–8]. Commonly affected areas include the upper extremity and axilla, the neck and the lower extremity and groin region (20% of cases arise in a genital location); the distribution therefore is central and not acral [3,4].

The clinical differential diagnosis includes infantile myofibromatosis, soft tissue sarcomas, juvenile hyaline fibromatosis, calcifying aponeurotic fibroma, lipoblastoma and fibrolipoma.

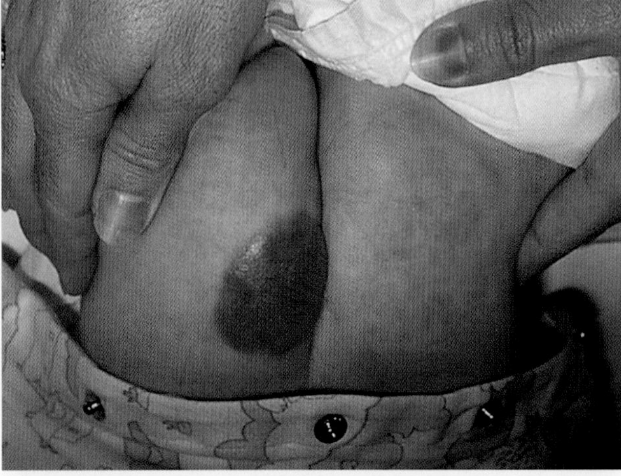

(a)

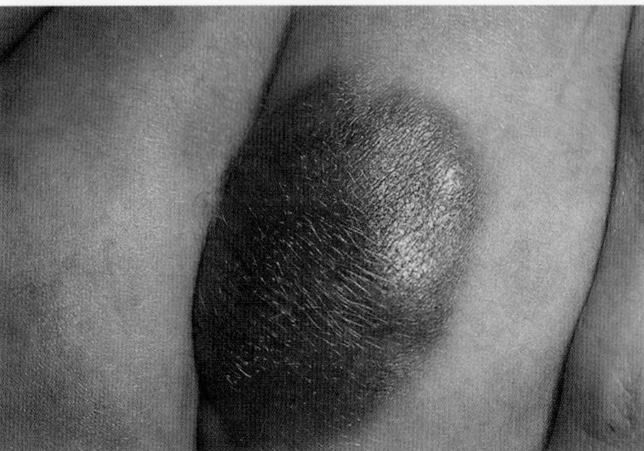

(b)

Fig. 114.4 (a and b) Fibrous hamartoma on the buttock of a 3-month-old girl.

Pathology. Fibrous hamartoma of infancy is classically a tripartite entity (referred to by some as an 'organoid' pattern); it contains areas of mature adipose tissue, bands of densely collagenized fibrous tissue and peculiar islands of immature cells that are disposed in a myxoid matrix (Fig. 114.5), all intimately admixed (Fig. 114.6) [4]. Although very occasional mitotic figures may be identified, they should not be prominent. The borders of these lesions may appear ill-defined on microscopic examination, blending into the host tissues owing to the similarity of the adipose tissue to normal tissue.

If the presence of the immature areas is not appreciated (either because of sampling or because they were simply overlooked) then fibrous hamartoma of infancy may be misinterpreted as a simple lipoma. The immature foci themselves may invite consideration of a malignant process; however, they are not marked by the same high rate of mitotic activity seen in malignant tumours. The spindled areas may resemble myoid or neural proliferations, but immunohistochemical studies will be of value in making this distinction (these fibrous areas in a fibrous

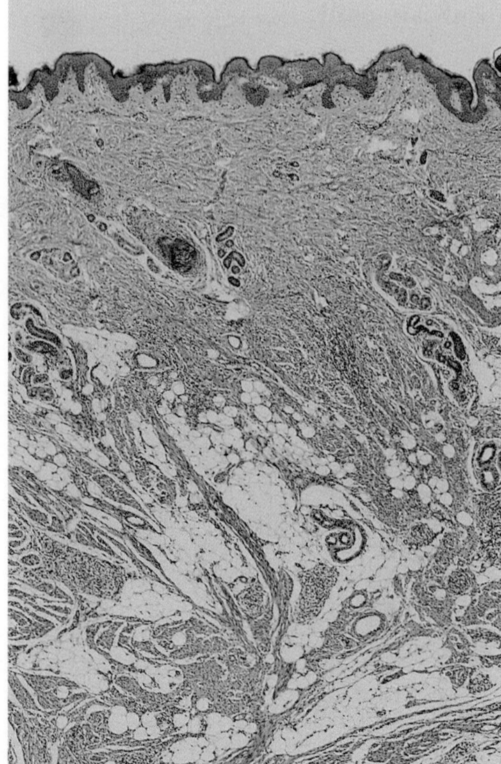

Fig. 114.5 Fibrous hamartoma of infancy comprises three components: mature adipose tissue, aggregates of primitive cells and bands of fibrous tissue.

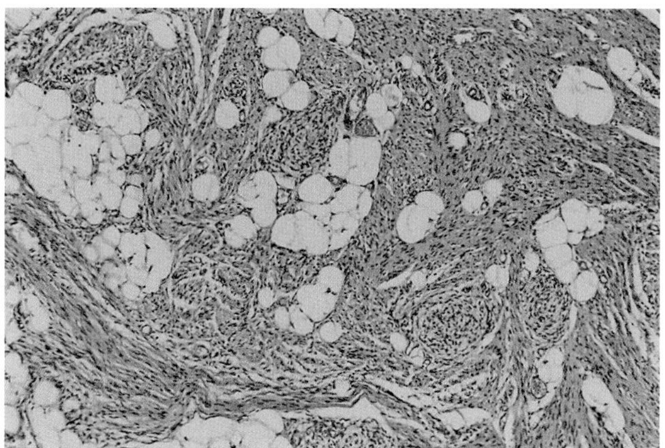

Fig. 114.6 The three components of fibrous hamartoma of infancy are intimately admixed.

hamartoma of infancy lack the desmin positivity of a smooth muscle tumour and they lack the S100 protein positivity of a neural lesion). Finally, when attention is focused upon the fibrous component of this lesion, confusion with infantile fibromatosis is possible; however, identification of the immature mesenchymal component should permit distinction between these two entities.

Treatment. Surgical excision of a fibrous hamartoma of infancy is recommended, as these lesions do not typically resolve spontaneously. In most instances, the lesions are cured by a complete local excision with only rare recurrence in less than 17% of cases [4,7]. If a putative fibrous hamartoma of infancy recurs after attempted complete surgical excision, the original diagnostic material should be reviewed to exclude the possibility of a malignancy or other more aggressive process.

References

1 Reye RD. A consideration of certain subdermal fibromatous tumours of infancy. J Pathol Bacteriol 1956;72:149–54.
2 Enzinger FM. Fibrous hamartoma of infancy. Cancer 1965;18:241–8.
3 Dickey GE, Sotelo-Avila C. Fibrous hamartoma of infancy: current review. Pediatr Dev Pathol 1999;2:236–43.
4 Saab ST, McClain CM, Coffin CM. Fibrous hamartoma of infancy: a clinicopathologic analysis of 60 cases. Am J Surg Pathol 2014;38: 394–401.
5 Melnick L, Berger EM, Elenitsas R et al. Fibrous hamartoma of infancy: a firm plaque presenting with hypertrichosis and hyperhidrosis. Pediatr Dermatol 2015;32:533–5.
6 Weinberger MS, Pransky SM, Krous HF. Fibrous hamartoma of infancy presenting as a perspiring neck mass. Int J Pediatr Otorhinolaryngol 1993;26:173–6.
7 Seguier-Lipszyc E, Hermann G, Kaplinski C, Lotan G. Fibrous hamartoma of infancy. J Pediatr Surg 2011;46:753–5.
8 Scott DM, Pena JR, Omura EF. Fibrous hamartoma of infancy. J Am Acad Dermatol1999;41:857–9.

Calcifying fibrous pseudotumour

Introduction/history. The calcifying fibrous pseudotumour is a rare benign tumour that was first reported as a 'childhood fibrous tumor with psammoma bodies' [1].

Epidemiology and pathogenesis. There is some debate as to its origin. Some authors have suggested that it is a true neoplasm, whereas others believe that it represents a late-stage ('burnt-out') inflammatory myofibroblastic tumour [2,3]. The typical patient is between 10 and 30 years of age. No sex predilection has been noted [4].

Clinical features and differential diagnosis. Calcifying fibrous pseudotumours may involve the subcutaneous tissues as well as deeper soft tissues. There are many reports of visceral involvement including the gastrointestinal tract (oropharynx, oesophagus, stomach, liver, spleen, intestine, omentum) [5–10], lungs [11], heart [12], mediastinum [13–15] retroperitoneum [16], adrenal gland [17], muscle [18], scrotum [19] and breast [20]. The majority of these lesions are located in the extremities. The lesions present as deep, slow-growing, painless nodules that may have associated systemic symptoms depending on their site of involvement.

Although clinical consideration might be given to a variety of fibrous proliferations (including desmoid-type fibromatosis, digital fibromatosis and nodular fasciitis), the calcifications are a distinctive feature whose presence, along with the distinctly low cellularity and relatively sharp circumscription from adjacent tissue, should suggest the diagnosis of calcifying fibrous pseudotumour.

Pathology. These lesions are reasonably well circumscribed, and better circumscribed, for example, than the desmoid-type fibromatoses discussed in this chapter. A sclerotic collagenous stroma is a dominant feature of calcifying fibrous pseudotumours on low-power microscopy; on closer scrutiny, widely scattered spindle cells are found distributed throughout this collagenous stroma. A minimal chronic inflammatory cell infiltrate may also be scattered throughout this stroma. The most characteristic microscopic feature of this lesion, however, is the presence of calcified bodies (psammomatous calcifications), which are found within the mass (either throughout the lesion or as only a focal finding).

Treatment. The calcifying fibrous pseudotumour has an excellent prognosis. It is a slowly growing mass that is usually successfully treated by surgical excision. Local recurrence is rare and may occur several years after the initial surgical excision [4].

References

1 Rosenthal NS, Abdul-Karim FW. Childhood fibrous tumor with psammoma bodies. Clinicopathologic features in two cases. Arch Pathol Lab Med 1988;112:798–800.
2 Hill KA, Gonzalez-Crussi F, Chou PM. Calcifying fibrous pseudotumor versus inflammatory myofibroblastic tumor: a histological and immunohistochemical comparison. Mod Pathol 2001;14:784–90.
3 Nascimento AF, Ruiz R, Hornick JL, Fletcher CD. Calcifying fibrous 'pseudotumor': clinicopathologic study of 15 cases and analysis of its relationship to inflammatory myofibroblastic tumor. Int J Surg Pathol 2002;10:189–96.
4 Fetsch JF, Montgomery EA, Meis JM. Calcifying fibrous pseudotumor. Am J Surg Pathol 1993;17:502–8.
5 Chatelain D, Lauzanne P, Yzet T et al. [Gastric calcifying fibrous pseudotumor, a rare mesenchymal tumor of the stomach]. Gastroenterol Clin Biol 2008;32:441–4.
6 Lewis CM, Bell DM, Lai SY. Pathology quiz case 2. Calcifying fibrous pseudotumor (CFT) of the oral cavity. Arch Otolaryngol Head Neck Surg 2010;136:841, 843–4.

7 Lee SW, Yeh HZ, Chang CS. Calcifying fibrous pseudotumor of the esophagus. J Chin Med Assoc 2010;73:599–601.
8 Liang HH, Chai CY, Lin YH et al. Jejunal and multiple mesenteric calcifying fibrous pseudotumor induced jejunojejunal intussusception. J Formos Med Assoc 2007;106:485–9.
9 Lee JC, Lien HC, Hsiao CH. Coexisting sclerosing angiomatoid nodular transformation of the spleen with multiple calcifying fibrous pseudotumors in a patient. J Formos Med Assoc 2007;106:234–9.
10 Medina AM, Alexis JB. A 27-year-old woman with incidental omental nodules. Calcifying fibrous pseudotumor of the omentum. Arch Pathol Lab Med 2006;130:563–4.
11 Suh JH, Shin OR, Kim YH. Multiple calcifying fibrous pseudotumor of the pleura. J Thorac Oncol 2008;3:1356–8.
12 Shimizu S, Funakoshi Y, Yoon HE et al. Small calcifying fibrous pseudotumor of the heart confined to the epicardium. Cardiovasc Pathol 2015;24:191–3.
13 Dissanayake SN, Hagen J, Fedenko A, Lee C. Calcifying fibrous pseudotumor of the posterior mediastinum with encapsulation of the thoracic duct. Ann Thorac Surg 2016;102:e39–40.
14 Chauhan KR, Shah HU, Trivedi PP, Shah MJ. Calcifying fibrous pseudotumor of the mediastinum: a rare case report. Indian J Pathol Microbiol 2014;57:155–6.
15 Chang JW, Kim JH, Maeng YH. Calcifying fibrous pseudotumor of the anterior mediastinum. Korean J Thorac Cardiovasc Surg 2011;44: 318–20.
16 Jaiswal SS, Agrawal A, Sahai K, Nair SK. Large retroperitoneal calcifying fibrous tumor. Med J Armed Forces India 2013;69:184–6.
17 Wu T, Zhu P, Duan X et al. Calcifying fibrous pseudotumor of the adrenal gland: A rare case report. Mol Clin Oncol 2016;5:252–4.
18 Shinohara N, Nagano S, Yokouchi M et al. Bilobular calcifying fibrous pseudotumor in soleus muscle: a case report. J Med Case Rep 201128;5:487.
19 Varghese RG, Toi PCh, Jacob SE et al. Calcifying pseudotumor of scrotum: a case report. Indian J Pathol Microbiol 2007;50:577–8.
20 Mangat A, Schiller C, Mengoni P et al. Calcifying fibrous pseudotumor of the breast. Breast J 2009;15:299–301.

Nodular fasciitis

Introduction/history. Nodular fasciitis is a reactive myofibroblastic proliferation. It has not usually been included in standard classification schemes of the fibromatoses of childhood, but its light microscopic appearance may overlap with that of the fibromatoses and so it is considered here [1–3]. It is often categorized as a pseudosarcoma, which is a group of benign fibroblastic–myofibroblastic tumours that simulate malignancy due to their rapid growth rate, histological appearance and clinical features [3].

Epidemiology and pathogenesis. Nodular fasciitis is most commonly seen in the second decade of life, but it can be seen in much younger children (<4% of cases occur in children younger than 10 years of age) [1]. It is more commonly seen in males. The lesion suggests a reactive proliferation on light microscopy, and so a suspicion persists that it might in some way be related to some inflammatory or traumatic stimulus. However, less than 15% of cases have a known history of preceding trauma [3].

Clinical features. This lesion typically presents as a subcutaneous mass. The overlying skin is movable. Nodular fasciitis is most often painless, although a minority of these lesions may be tender. Frequent sites of involvement include the head and neck region, arms or chest wall, but almost any site may give rise to this reactive process. Nodular fasciitis is, paradoxically, a more rapidly growing lesion than other potentially more aggressive processes. One distinctive paediatric form of nodular fasciitis is known as cranial fasciitis; this condition, largely restricted to infants in the first year of life, is distinguished by the presence of a rapidly growing scalp mass that may erode the outer table of the skull. Cranial fasciitis has the light microscopic attributes of nodular fasciitis and behaves as an altogether benign lesion despite its sometimes rapid growth. Some observers believe that cranial fasciitis may be related to birth trauma and so relegate it to the category of a reactive process [3].

Pathology. The essential light microscopic features include a loose proliferation of spindle cells set in a myxoid stroma, scattered foci of haemorrhage and scattered lymphocytes. Mitotic figures are often readily identifiable but are not, however, atypical appearing. Uncommonly, scattered multinucleated giant cells or even foci of ossification may be found within nodular fasciitis. Older lesions may lose some of their myxoid character and adopt a somewhat more collagenized appearance. Nodular fasciitis is reactive for vimentin and smooth muscle actin.

The spindle cells of nodular fasciitis lack either the cytoplasmic eosinophilia typical of a myofibroblastoma or the well-developed storiform architecture of a cutaneous fibrous histiocytoma. While the mitotic activity of nodular fasciitis may at first be disconcerting, it should be borne in mind that nodular fasciitis lacks the cytological atypia that is the hallmark of most true sarcomas.

Treatment. Nodular fasciitis is an entirely benign lesion. These lesions may regress spontaneously, and so recurrence after surgical excision is uncommon.

As is the case with myofibromas, a diagnostic biopsy is typically all the therapy that is required for the effective treatment of nodular fasciitis. However, excision of lesions is often sought by affected patients or parents.

References

1 Lu L, Lao IW, Liu X et al. Nodular fasciitis: a retrospective study of 272 cases from China with clinicopathologic and radiologic correlation. Ann Diagn Pathol 2015;19:180–5.
2 Pandian TK, Zeidan MM, Ibrahim KA et al. Nodular fasciitis in the pediatric population: a single center experience. J Pediatr Surg 2013;48:1486–9.
3 Coffin CM, Alaggio R. Fibroblastic and myofibroblastic tumors in children and adolescents. Pediatr Dev Pathol 2012;15(1 suppl):127–80.

Lesions with potential for a locally aggressive course

Infantile (desmoid-type) fibromatosis

Introduction/history. The locally recurring fibromatoses have traditionally been divided into two groups: the more superficially located lesions (considered under Palmar–plantar fibromatosis) and the deeply seated lesions (e.g. infantile fibromatosis). Infantile fibromatosis (synonym: deep fibromatosis) is a locally recurring lesion that, although not malignant, may be locally quite aggressive and infiltrate key regional structures including nerves and joints [1].

Epidemiology and pathogenesis. Infantile (desmoid-type) fibromatosis accounts for up to 60% of fibrous tumours in childhood [2,3]. Approximately 30% of these cases occur in children during the first year of life [2].

The aetiology of infantile desmoid-type fibromatosis is unclear. In the majority of cases, the lesions are sporadic tumours. However, in a minority of patients, desmoid fibromatosis represents an element of the presentation of Gardner syndrome (familial adenomatous polyposis) with autosomal dominant inheritance, which warrants genetic consultation and DNA analysis of the *APC* gene if the family history is positive for intestinal tumours [4]. Trauma or prior surgery can stimulate growth of desmoids in the setting of a patient having an *APC* gene mutation [2].

Clinical features and differential diagnosis. Infantile desmoid-type fibromatosis manifests as firm masses at any age from birth onwards. The lesions are usually painless. Owing to their rapid growth, patients will often promptly seek clinical evaluation. Untreated, infantile desmoid-type fibromatosis may grow to great proportions. In contrast with the true fibrosarcomas, however, infantile fibromatosis lacks the capacity for metastasis [1,5]. Although infantile desmoid-type fibromatosis may extend towards the superficial regions that fall within the province of the dermatologist, the epicentre of this lesion is rather deeply seated, associated with the muscle or fascia [5]. Among the favoured areas for the development of infantile fibromatosis are the shoulder girdle, head, neck and proximal lower extremity.

The most difficult disorder to distinguish from infantile desmoid-type fibromatosis is a true (high-grade) fibrosarcoma. Although the cellularity of a fibromatosis (developing in an older child) falls short of that of the usual (congenital) infantile fibrosarcoma, newborn infants with infantile desmoid-type fibromatosis may show a more cellular pattern than that seen in older patients, resembling a congenital fibrosarcoma. This distinction may be extremely difficult with only limited material for diagnosis.

Myofibromas, neural tumours, nodular fasciitis and dermatofibrosarcoma protuberans may also be considered in the differential diagnosis of infantile fibromatosis.

Pathology. Infantile desmoid-type fibromatosis comprises a rather homogeneous proliferation of bundles of spindle cells set in a collagenized stroma. Although widely scattered mitotic figures may be found, they are not a prominent feature of infantile fibromatosis. The individual nuclei are often characterized as 'bland', a reference to their lack of cytological atypia. In newborn infants, the cellularity of infantile fibromatosis is somewhat greater than that seen in older children or adults.

Treatment. Although infantile desmoid-type fibromatosis does not metastasize, it does show a stubborn tendency to persist and recur locally. In this regard, infantile fibromatosis is the most aggressive of the benign fibrous and myofibroblastic disorders considered here. In addition, infantile desmoid-type fibromatosis may entrap vital structures (including vascular, neural and articular structures) and so interfere with both the quality of life and the lifespan of the affected child.

The key to cure of infantile desmoid-type fibromatosis is complete surgical excision [5]. Both the extent of this disorder and infiltration of adjacent vital structures often conspire to frustrate the surgeon. More than half of these lesions recur after surgery [2]. In refractory or recurrent lesions, pharmacological treatments that have had some success include the combination of tamoxifen and celecoxib [6] and possibly tyrosine kinase inhibitors [7].

References

1 Keltz M, DiCostanzo D, Desai P, Cohen SR. Infantile (desmoid-type) fibromatosis. Pediatr Dermatol 1995;12:149–51.
2 Coffin CM, Alaggio R. Fibroblastic and myofibroblastic tumors in children and adolescents. Pediatr Dev Pathol 2012;15(1 suppl):127–80.
3 Roychoudhury A, Parkash H, Kumar S, Chopra P. Infantile desmoid fibromatosis of the submandibular region. J Oral Maxillofac Surg 2002;60:1198–202.
4 van der Luijt RB, Meera Khan P, Vasen HFet al. Germline mutations in the 3′ part of APC exon 15 do not result in truncated proteins and are associated with attenuated adenomatous polyposis coli. Hum Genet 1996;98:727–34.
5 Ruparelia MS, Dhariwal DK. Infantile fibromatosis: a case report and review of the literature. Br J Oral Maxillofac Surg 2011;49:e30–2.
6 Francis WP, Zippel D, Mack LA et al. Desmoids: a revelation in biology and treatment. Ann Surg Oncol 2009;16:1650–4.
7 Liegl B, Leithner A, Bauernhofer T et al. Immunohistochemical and mutational analysis of PDGF and PDGFR in desmoid tumours: is there a role for tyrosine kinase inhibitors in c-kit-negative desmoid tumours? Histopathology 2006;49:576–81.

Palmar–plantar fibromatosis

Introduction/history. Palmar–plantar fibromatosis (synonym: superficial fibromatosis) is a form of fibromatosis that is localized to the palms or soles, which, although more commonly found in older adults, may occasionally present in teenagers and young adults. In adults, plantar fibromatosis is sometimes known as Ledderhose disease, whereas palmar fibromatosis has been referred to as Dupuytren contracture. Although these eponyms do not usually evoke the image of a paediatric patient, they are nevertheless applicable to such lesions when they are diagnosed in the paediatric age group.

Epidemiology and pathogenesis. Palmar–plantar fibromatosis most commonly presents in late childhood and onwards with few cases reported before the age of 5 years [1]. For plantar involvement in childhood, a female predominance has been noted. It has been hypothesized that hormonal factors may play a role. From early adulthood onwards, Dupuytren contracture is more commonly seen in men until the sixth decade when female incidence then increases coinciding with menopause [1]. An autosomal dominant inheritance pattern has been observed. Knuckle pads, seizure disorders and keloids have been reported to be associated with palmar and plantar fibromatosis [1].

Clinical features and differential diagnosis. Palmar–plantar fibromatosis is a disease that is mostly seen in adults. Nevertheless, both plantar and palmar fibromatosis are occasionally encountered in children; plantar lesions are more commonly encountered in children than are palmar lesions. Palmar–plantar fibromatosis presents as a nodular or plaque-like thickening of the bottom of the foot or the palm of the hand. The lesions often involve adjacent tendinous structures which may result in flexion contractures of the digits. These secondary changes are seen less often in children than adults. Although the lesions are usually painless initially, the trauma of weightbearing with walking upon the plantar lesions often proves to be painful over time [1–3].

The differential diagnosis includes calcifying aponeurotic fibroma, desmoid fibromatosis, cellular dermatofibroma and fibrosarcoma.

Pathology. In their earliest stages, the lesions of palmar–plantar fibromatosis are marked by the combination of fascicular bands of spindle cells with nodular areas showing a distinctly increased cellularity. Cytological atypia is not seen. The mature lesions of palmar–plantar fibromatosis are quite similar to those of (the deeper situated) infantile fibromatosis, with fascicles of bland spindle cells set in a collagenous stroma.

Treatment. Palmar–plantar fibromatosis has a more favourable prognosis than infantile fibromatosis. It does often recur locally, but does not exhibit the insidious infiltrative growth pattern of infantile fibromatosis. As such, palmar–plantar fibromatosis does not pose the same risk of infiltration and compromise of adjacent vital structures as infantile fibromatosis.

Nonoperative intervention is considered first-line management as the infiltrative character often makes complete surgical excision technically difficult or impossible without the sacrifice of some degree of function. Triamcinolone acetonide injections [4], percutaneous collagenase [5] and radiation therapy [6] are alternatives to surgical management. For those patients with significant contractures, surgical intervention may be necessary. A high recurrence rate of 84% is noted after surgical excision with a 42% risk for multiple recurrences, probably due to the difficulty of complete surgical excision [1]. The recurrence typically occurs within the first 12 months after resection.

References

1 Fetsch JF, Laskin WB, Miettinen M. Palmar-plantar fibromatosis in children and preadolescents: a clinicopathologic study of 56 cases with newly recognized demographics and extended follow-up information. Am J Surg Pathol 2005;29:1095–105.

2 Sammarco GJ, Mangone PG. Classification and treatment of plantar fibromatosis. Foot Ankle Int 2000;21:563–9.

3 Jacob CI, Kumm RC. Benign anteromedial plantar nodules of childhood: a distinct form of plantar fibromatosis. Pediatr Dermatol 2000;17:472–4.

4 Ketchum LD, Donahue TK. The injection of nodules of Dupuytren's disease with triamcinolone acetonide. J Hand Surg Am 2000;25: 1157–62.

5 Gilpin D, Coleman S, Hall S et al. Injectable collagenase Clostridium histolyticum: a new nonsurgical treatment for Dupuytren's disease. J Hand Surg Am 2010;35:2027–38 e1.

6 Schuster J, Saraiya S, Tennyson N et al. Patient-reported outcomes after electron radiation treatment for early-stage palmar and plantar fibromatosis. Pract Radiat Oncol 2015;5:e651–8.

Gingival fibromatosis

Introduction/history. Gingival fibromatosis (synonyms: congenital idiopathic gingival fibromatosis, hereditary gingival hyperplasia, generalized hypertrophy of the gums, gingival elephantiasis) is a fibrous overgrowth of the gums that, in some patients, is associated with other conditions (including hypertrichosis, mental retardation and epilepsy) [1,2].

Epidemiology and pathogenesis. Patients with gingival fibromatosis may be divided into two groups: those whose disease is sporadic and those with an inherited condition (autosomal dominant or autosomal recessive). Those patients with inherited disease appear to be a heterogeneous group. A variety of different genetic syndromes have been associated with gingival fibromatosis including Zimmermann–Laband syndrome, Ramon syndrome and Klippel–Trenaunay–Weber syndrome [1,3–5]. A mutation in the son of sevenless-1 (SOS-1) gene has been suggested as a cause for nonsyndromic gingival fibromatosis [6]. Some have noted that many instances of gingival fibromatosis (which may develop at any age) have coincided with the development of dentition and so postulated a relationship between the eruption of teeth and the development of gingival fibromatosis. The enlargement of the gingiva is associated with increased deposition of extracellular matrix by fibroblasts, which has been hypothesized to occur due to increased signalling of transforming growth factor β1, a mediator of wound healing and tissue regeneration [7].

Clinical features and differential diagnosis. The gingival masses are slow-growing and painless, but symptomatic (in that they often interfere with eating and speaking). In patients with inherited disease, the process may be a solitary phenomenon or associated with other abnormalities (including hypertrichosis, epilepsy, mental retardation or skeletal abnormalities). The fibrous overgrowths of gingival fibromatosis may be restricted to only a portion of the gums or they may extensively involve both mandibular and maxillary regions and even extend to the adjacent palate.

Gingival fibromatosis is usually first biopsied for diagnosis. In general, the same differential diagnostic considerations discussed previously for infantile fibromatosis are applicable to gingival fibromatosis. Juvenile hyalinosis may involve the gums as well, but this condition usually exhibits cutaneous lesions, which helps in the clinical distinction between the two entities. Drug therapy (phenytoin, ciclosporin and calcium channel blockers) may produce gingival hypertrophy, as may chronic gingivitis or other reactive processes, all of which may produce lesions histologically similar to gingival fibromatosis. Gingival hypertrophy is also often observed in lysosomal storage disorders such as mucolipidoses and aspartylglucosaminuria.

Pathology. Gingival fibromatosis is marked by a densely collagenous stroma, and so to some extent histologically resembles juvenile hyalinosis: the stromal component predominates over the cellular component. In gingival fibromatosis, however, the stroma is a collagenous one (which contrasts with the homogeneous periodic acid–Schiff [PAS] positive hyalinized stroma of juvenile hyalinosis).

Treatment. The prognosis of gingival fibromatosis is most reminiscent of that of (superficial) palmar–plantar fibromatosis. Gingival fibromatosis is a benign fibrous proliferation that has a significant capacity for local recurrence. However, it lacks the more locally aggressive character of infantile (desmoid-type) fibromatosis, or the metastatic potential of a true fibrosarcoma.

Attempts at excision will be prompted by a desire to correct impairments in eating or speaking, which have been produced by the fibrous masses. Attempts at achieving a surgical cure are sometimes frustrated by recurrence of the disease. Interestingly, some smaller lesions have been treated by extraction of the adjacent erupting tooth, the presumed stimulus giving rise to the development of the fibrous overgrowth in the first place.

References

1 Ramnarayan BK, Sowmya K, Rema J. Management of idiopathic gingival fibromatosis: report of a case and literature review. Pediatr Dent 2011;33:431–6.
2 Thway K, Fisher C, Sebire NJ. Pediatric fibroblastic and myofibroblastic lesions. Adv Anat Pathol 2012;19:54–65.
3 Davalos IP, Brambila-Tapia AJ, Davalos NO et al. Wide clinical spectrum in Zimmermann-Laband syndrome. Genet Couns 2011;22:1–10.
4 Martins F, Ortega KL, Hiraoka C et al. Oral and dental abnormalities in Barber-Say syndrome. Am J Med Genet A 2010;152A:2569–73.
5 Suhanya J, Aggarwal C, Mohideen K et al. Cherubism combined with epilepsy, mental retardation and gingival fibromatosis (Ramon syndrome): a case report. Head Neck Pathol 2010;4:126–31.
6 Hart TC, Zhang Y, Gorry MC et al. A mutation in the SOS1 gene causes hereditary gingival fibromatosis type 1. Am J Hum Genet 2002;70: 943–54.
7 Wright HJ, Chapple IL, Matthews JB. TGF-beta isoforms and TGF-beta receptors in drug-induced and hereditary gingival overgrowth. J Oral Pathol Med 2001;30:281–9.

Infantile digital fibromatosis

Introduction/history. Infantile digital fibromatosis (synonyms: subdermal fibromatous tumour of infancy, infantile dermal fibromatosis, recurrent digital fibromatosis, inclusion body fibromatosis) is a fibrous proliferation of childhood that is marked both by its location (fingers and toes) and by its light microscopic appearance.

Epidemiology and pathogenesis. Infantile digital fibromatosis usually presents within the first year of life and may be present at the time of birth; rare cases in older children have been reported. It has no sex predilection. The pathogenesis of this disorder is unknown; however, it does not appear to be inherited. In some cases it has been associated with a past history of trauma [1,2].

Clinical features and differential diagnosis. Infantile digital fibromatosis presents on the fingers and toes; very few cases have been reported of lesions occurring in other areas. The affected digit is surmounted by a firm pink to flesh-coloured painless nodule (Fig. 114.7). The overlying

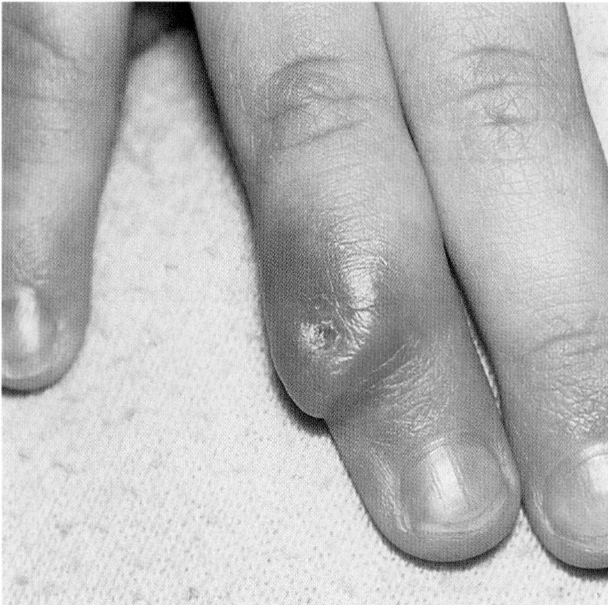

Fig. 114.7 Erythematous nodule over the lateral aspect of the fourth finger of this 3-year-old with digital fibromatosis.

skin is fixed to this lesion. The firm nodules are usually seen on the extensor sites of the affected digit. At first presentation they often appear rather small, in the order of 1 cm or less; they rarely reach more than 2 cm in greatest dimension. The nodules are either solitary or multiple, and sometimes are present on multiple digits of the hands and feet. The lesions are usually asymptomatic.

Other proliferative disorders should be considered, as discussed for infantile fibromatosis. Following attempts at surgical excision, recurrence may raise the possibility of a malignant process, but digital fibromatosis lacks the increased cellularity, high rate of mitotic activity and focal necrosis that are the hallmarks of a malignant process.

Pathology. On low-power examination, fascicles of spindle cells are found. These bundles of spindle cells fill the dermis and reach the dermoepidermal junction (Fig. 114.8). Cytological atypia is not a feature of this lesion. On low-power examination, digital fibromatosis bears a superficial resemblance to infantile fibromatosis (Fig. 114.9). On closer scrutiny, however, the most distinctive feature of digital fibromatosis is the presence of scattered cells possessing eosinophilic cytoplasmic inclusions on routine haematoxylin and eosin staining. These inclusions are typically juxtanuclear and may even indent the adjacent nucleus; they are phosphotungstic acid haematoxylin positive and Masson trichrome positive, but PAS negative. On ultrastructural examination, these cytoplasmic inclusion bodies prove to consist of an admixture of fibrillar and granular electron-dense material that probably represents densely packed actin microfilaments [3].

Treatment. Digital fibromatosis is a capricious disorder. Some children experience spontaneous regression of their lesions, whereas others (over 50% of the cases) see progression of their lesions with multiple recurrences despite

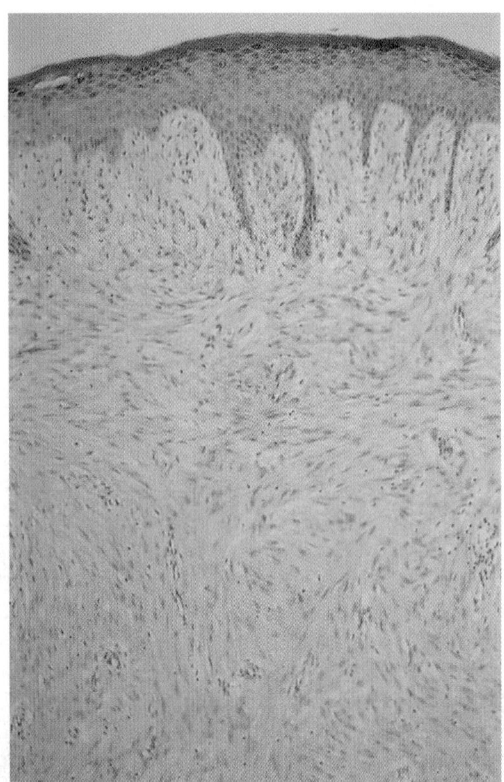

Fig. 114.8 Digital (inclusion body) fibromatosis fills the subcutis and dermis, approaching the dermoepidermal junction.

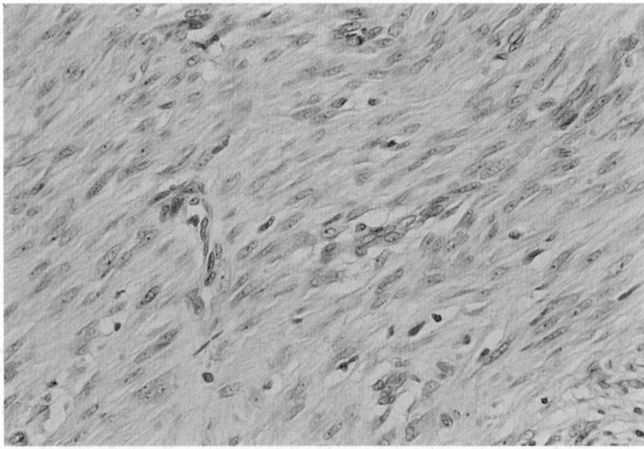

Fig. 114.9 Digital (inclusion body) fibromatosis resembles infantile fibromatosis in its fascicular arrangement of spindle cells, with one addition – eosinophilic cytoplasmic inclusions are found in most lesions (such inclusions are not characteristic of infantile or palmar–plantar fibromatosis).

attempts at surgical extirpation [4–6]. Digital fibromatosis is a process with a greater likelihood of local recurrence than some of the other more indolent fibromatoses. Digital fibromatosis, however, is less likely to infiltrate widely than infantile fibromatosis. After spontaneous regression, some deformity of the affected digit(s) may develop as a potential residual complication.

The unpredictable nature of this process prompts an understandable reluctance on the part of some treating clinicians to undertake extensive and potentially disfiguring excision of these lesions. Moreover, the knowledge that half to three quarters of lesions recur after attempted surgical excision is a further complicating factor. As some lesions will regress spontaneously, one reasonable approach in some patients (after biopsy confirmation of the nature of the process) may call for clinical observation and follow-up to monitor for changes in the lesion [7]. In some cases where the lesions make it difficult to wear shoes, debulking by shave technique has been helpful for two children we have cared for; recurrences, when they occurred, were slow to arise and eventually regressed without further intervention.

Clearly, the approach to a specific lesion in a particular patient will require individual tailoring. In progressive lesions, Mohs micrographic surgery is a surgical treatment option [8].

References

1 Miyamoto T, Mihara M, Hagari Y et al. Posttraumatic occurrence of infantile digital fibromatosis. A histologic and electron microscopic study. Arch Dermatol 1986;122:915–18.
2 Taylor HO, Gellis SE, Schmidt BA et al. Infantile digital fibromatosis. Ann Plast Surg 2008;61:472–6.
3 Mukai M, Torikata C, Iri H et al. Immunohistochemical identification of aggregated actin filaments in formalin-fixed, paraffin-embedded sections. I. A study of infantile digital fibromatosis by a new pretreatment. Am J Surg Pathol 1992;16:110–15.
4 Laskin WB, Miettinen M, Fetsch JF. Infantile digital fibroma/fibromatosis: a clinicopathologic and immunohistochemical study of 69 tumors from 57 patients with long-term follow-up. Am J Surg Pathol 2009;33:1–13.
5 Grenier N, Liang C, Capaldi L et al. A range of histologic findings in infantile digital fibromatosis. Pediatr Dermatol 2008;25:72–5.
6 Thway K, Fisher C, Sebire NJ. Pediatric fibroblastic and myofibroblastic lesions. Adv Anat Pathol 2012;19:54–65.
7 Niamba P, Leaute-Labreze C, Boralevi F et al. Further documentation of spontaneous regression of infantile digital fibromatosis. Pediatr Dermatol 2007;24:280–4.
8 Albertini JG, Welsch MJ, Conger LA et al. Infantile digital fibroma treated with mohs micrographic surgery. Dermatol Surg 2002;28: 959–61.

Calcifying aponeurotic fibroma

Introduction/history. First described by Keasbey in 1953, calcifying aponeurotic fibroma (synonyms: juvenile aponeurotic fibroma, calcifying fibroma) is a benign fibrous proliferation that most frequently occurs in childhood or adolescence and presents in the distal extremities [1].

Epidemiology and pathogenesis. The disease presents at any age, but most commonly in the first two decades of life (with a peak age incidence at about 10 years). The lesions are more common in males compared to females with a ratio of 2 : 1 [2]. It is not clear what stimulus gives rise to the development of calcifying aponeurotic fibroma. It is thought to be a sporadic event as no familial inheritance pattern has been identified. An *FN1–EGF* fusion gene resulting in epidermal growth factor expression has been found in a series of calcifying aponeurotic fibromas [3].

Clinical features and differential diagnosis. Calcifying aponeurotic fibromas present as slow-growing lesions that most commonly occur in the hands (palms or fingers).

Approximately 15% of the lesions occur on the feet in the ankle region or plantar surface [4]. Only rarely are other sites affected [2]. The lesions are often fixed to the overlying skin and present as a firm, mobile nodule. They may be painless or slightly tender on palpation. The lesions do not develop at the same rapid rate as infantile fibromatoses; rather, they may have been present for months to years before professional help is sought.

The differential diagnosis includes nodular fasciitis, fibrous hamartoma of infancy, infantile fibromatosis or fibrosarcoma.

Pathology

Histologically, calcifying aponeurotic fibroma shows a proliferation of spindle cells arranged in fascicles. This architecture overlaps with that of infantile fibromatosis and digital fibromatosis. Typical of calcifying aponeurotic fibroma is the focal development of cartilaginous and amorphous calcific deposits. The periphery of the lesion infiltrates the adjacent soft tissue.

Differential diagnosis

Infantile fibromatosis, palmar–plantar fibromatosis or fibrous hamartoma of infancy may be considered in the differential diagnosis; these lesions, however, lack calcification and chondroid foci. Fibrosarcoma should also be considered but will be distinguished by its greater cellularity and cytological atypia.

Treatment. In most cases, calcifying aponeurotic fibromas will stabilize over time or even regress. Their behaviour is similar to that of digital fibromatosis or infantile fibromatosis. Calcifying aponeurotic fibroma differs clinically from infantile fibromatosis in that it does not have the same propensity for extensive local infiltration with impairment of vital structures.

The initial therapy usually takes the form of an attempt at surgical excision. However, approximately half of the lesions so treated will recur. The incidence of local recurrence appears to be greater in the first 5 years of life than in older children [5]. This suggests that the proliferative process may undergo some sort of maturation with time. Indeed, some lesions (even recurrent ones) may become stable or even regress over time. Hence, some surgeons will elect to observe those lesions that recur after attempted excision and forgo attempts at re-excision unless unavoidable.

References

1 Keasbey LE. Juvenile aponeurotic fibroma (calcifying fibroma); a distinctive tumor arising in the palms and soles of young children. Cancer 1953;6:338–46.
2 Fetsch JF, Miettinen M. Calcifying aponeurotic fibroma: a clinicopathologic study of 22 cases arising in uncommon sites. Hum Pathol 1998;29:1504–10.
3 Puls F, Hofvander J, Magnusson L et al. FN1-EGF gene fusions are recurrent in calcifying aponeurotic fibroma. J Pathol 2016;238: 502–7.
4 Thway K, Fisher C, Sebire NJ. Pediatric fibroblastic and myofibroblastic lesions. Adv Anat Pathol 2012;19:54–65.
5 Allen PW, Enzinger FM. Juvenile aponeurotic fibroma. Cancer 1970;26:857–67.

Giant cell fibroblastoma and dermatofibrosarcoma protuberans

Introduction and history. Giant cell fibroblastoma and dermatofibrosarcoma protuberans (DFSP) both characteristically stain CD34 positive and are considered to be on a disease spectrum: giant cell fibroblastoma is more commonly seen in children, and DFSP more commonly in adolescents and adults. Reports exist of giant cell fibroblastomas that after excision are followed by recurrences that look like DFSPs, as well as reports of recurrent DFSPs that resemble giant cell fibroblastomas, and lesions that combine features of both entities [1–3]. These tumours are classified as fibrohistiocytic tumours of intermediate malignancy due to their low risk for metastasis; however, both lesions often recur if not completely excised.

Epidemiology and pathogenesis. Giant cell fibroblastoma usually presents in children younger than 5 years of age with a median age of 3 years [4]. It is most commonly seen in boys. The annual incidence of DFSP in the paediatric population has been estimated at 1 per 1 000 000 [5,6]. DFSP most commonly occurs in adults; however, when presenting in paediatric patients it most commonly presents between 7 and 16 years of age with a median age of 15 years [5]. Giant cell fibroblastoma and DFSP display identical molecular changes. Molecular studies have shown somatic (intratumoral) chromosomal abnormalities (either 17;22 translocations or ring chromosomes), leading to a fusion between exon 29 of the *COL1A1* gene and exon 2 of the *PDGFB* gene [7].

Clinical features and differential diagnosis. Giant cell fibroblastomas present as painless masses, centred in the dermis and subcutaneous region; their rate of growth is not as rapid as that of infantile fibromatosis or congenital/infantile fibrosarcoma. In contrast with some of the more distally located fibromatoses, giant cell fibroblastomas are most often centripetal lesions, preferring the back, thigh and chest. DFSP can have a heterogeneous presentation and is most commonly mistaken as a benign vascular malformation or hamartoma in the early stages. The tumour most commonly presents on the trunk and proximal extremities with very slow, progressive growth being characteristic of this lesion. DFSPs rarely metastasize and therefore do not require staging evaluation.

The clinical differential diagnosis includes a vascular malformation, fibrous hamartoma and infantile fibromatosis.

Pathology. Giant cell fibroblastoma comprises a proliferation of spindle cells as in other fibromatoses. There are, in addition, two other features of this disorder that are distinctive: the presence of cytological atypia and the presence of pseudo-vascular spaces. The cytologically atypical cells may be spindled or, more characteristically, large multinucleated giant cells. These multinucleated giant cells (sometimes described as having a 'floret-like' arrangement of their nuclei) are often found at the periphery of cleft-like or gaping spaces. However, these spaces are not actually lined by the endothelial cells and so are really only pseudo-vascular spaces.

The calcific bodies, coupled with the pseudo-vascular spaces, are a unique and specific feature that will serve to distinguish giant cell fibroblastoma from most other benign fibrous lesions. A more significant problem in light microscopic differential diagnosis may be presented by the pleomorphism of the component cells, a finding that quite naturally prompts consideration of a malignant process. However, the 'look-alike' sarcomas (such as malignant fibrous histiocytoma or liposarcoma) are exceedingly rare in children; moreover, their pleomorphism notwithstanding, the giant cell fibroblastomas do not exhibit the mitotic activity or necrotic foci that would support an interpretation of malignancy.

Treatment. More than half of these lesions recur after attempts at conventional surgical excision due to the infiltrating growth pattern, and so in this regard their behaviour is similar to that of other fibromatoses such as calcifying aponeurotic fibroma or infantile fibromatosis.

Giant cell fibroblastomas and DFSPs are best approached surgically, with complete wide local excision or preferably Mohs micrographic surgery, where available. When recurrences do occur, they are usually successfully treated by re-excision. For large DFSP tumours that are unable to be completely resected, imatinib mesylate, a tyrosine kinase inhibitor that has activity against PDGF, has been reported to be a possible therapeutic option [8–10].

References

1 Fletcher CD. Giant cell fibroblastoma of soft tissue: a clinicopathological and immunohistochemical study. Histopathology 1988;13:499–508.

2 Cherradi N, Malihy A, Benkiran L et al. [Giant cell fibroblastoma recurring as dermatofibrosarcoma. A pediatric case report]. Ann Pathol 2002;22:465–8.

3 Alguacil-Garcia A. Giant cell fibroblastoma recurring as dermatofibrosarcoma protuberans. Am J Surg Pathol 1991;15:798–801.

4 Goldblum JR, Folpe AL, Weiss SW et al. Enzinger and Weiss's Soft Tissue Tumors, 6th edn. Philadelphia, PA: Saunders/Elsevier, 2014:xiv, 1155.

5 Valdivielso-Ramos M, Torrelo A, Campos M et al. Pediatric dermatofibrosarcoma protuberans in Madrid, Spain: multi-institutional outcomes. Pediatr Dermatol 2014;31:676–82.

6 Kornik RI, Muchard LK, Teng JM. Dermatofibrosarcoma protuberans in children: an update on the diagnosis and treatment. Pediatr Dermatol 2012;29:707–13.

7 Simon MP, Pedeutour F, Sirvent N et al. Deregulation of the platelet-derived growth factor B-chain gene via fusion with collagen gene COL1A1 in dermatofibrosarcoma protuberans and giant-cell fibroblastoma. Nat Genet 1997;15:95–8.

8 Price VE, Fletcher JA, Zielenska M et al. Imatinib mesylate: an attractive alternative in young children with large, surgically challenging dermatofibrosarcoma protuberans. Pediatr Blood Cancer 2005;44:511–15.

9 Ugurel S, Mentzel T, Utikal J et al. Neoadjuvant imatinib in advanced primary or locally recurrent dermatofibrosarcoma protuberans: a multicenter phase II DeCOG trial with long-term follow-up. Clin Cancer Res 2014;20:499–510.

10 Gooskens SL, Oranje AP, van Adrichem LN et al. Imatinib mesylate for children with dermatofibrosarcoma protuberans (DFSP). Pediatr Blood Cancer 2010;55:369–73.

Congenital and infantile fibrosarcoma

Introduction. Congenital and infantile fibrosarcomas are rare tumours of low to intermediate malignant potential due to their ability for rapid growth and rare ability to metastasize [1]. Despite this, these tumours carry a favourable prognosis with a 94% 5-year survival [2].

Epidemiology and pathogenesis. There is a slight male predominance. Practically all of these lesions develop within the first 4 years of life, with most found between birth and 1 year. These tumours have been shown to contain a novel chromosomal translocation, t(12;15)(p13;q25), resulting in *ETV6–NTRK3* gene fusion and a number of chromosome polysomies [3]. This fusion protein results in ligand-independent chimeric tyrosine kinase activity leading to constitutive activation of Ras/MAPK and PI3K/ACT pathways [4]. Morphological, cytogenetic and biological evidence supports a relationship between congenital (infantile) fibrosarcoma and congenital mesoblastic nephroma (CMN). Also in CMN, *ETV6–NTRK3* fusion transcripts and/or *ETV6* region rearrangement have been consistently observed. It is likely that infantile fibrosarcoma and CMN represent a single neoplastic entity, arising in either renal or soft-tissue locations [5].

Clinical features and differential diagnosis. Two clinical patterns of disease have been identified: lesions present at birth (congenital fibrosarcoma) (Fig. 114.10) and those that develop later in life (infantile fibrosarcoma). Here, these two clinical patterns are considered together as a single entity, in view of the similarity of the course of the disease. Irrespective of whether the lesion is congenital or first noted later in life, these masses are painless, usually rather large at initial presentation and grow rapidly. These are often more distally located lesions; common sites of involvement include the extremity, head, trunk and pelvis [6].

The clinical differential includes a vascular malformation, congenital haemangioma, infantile haemangioma, infantile myofibroma, DFSP, desmoid fibromatosis and other sarcomas.

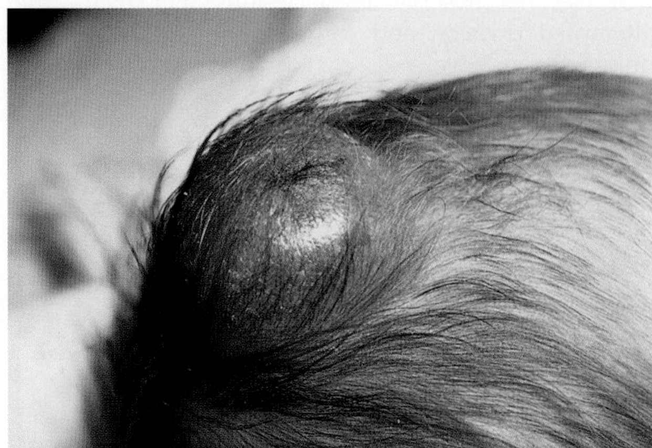

Fig. 114.10 Rapidly growing congenital infantile fibrosarcoma.

Pathology. The low-power appearance of a congenital/infantile fibrosarcoma is marked by an extremely cellular proliferation of hyperchromatic oval to spindle cells (Fig. 114.11). Mitotic figures are abundant (often more than one per high-power field); necrotic foci are often present and the individual tumour cells have pleomorphic nuclei (Fig. 114.12). Vasculature may be prominent and may in fact mimic, in some areas, a haemangiopericytic arrangement of the tumour cells. The spindle cells are typically arranged in fascicles that run at an angle to adjacent fascicles of tumour cells (described by some as a 'herringbone' pattern). Scattered chronic inflammatory cells may be present.

The high cellularity and mitotic activity of fibrosarcoma usually combine to suggest the diagnosis of malignancy on biopsy examination. Although clinically subject to confusion with fibromatosis, adequate biopsy material should permit distinction of fibrosarcoma from fibromatosis. With regard to other sarcomatous differential diagnostic considerations, the absence of rhabdomyoblastic differentiation (seen either by light microscopy or by desmin negativity on immunohistochemical study) serves to exclude rhabdomyosarcoma; a malignant haemangiopericytoma is both exceedingly rare in the first year of life and marked by a diffuse architectural arrangement into a pericytic pattern, not the focal change that may be seen in congenital/infantile fibrosarcoma.

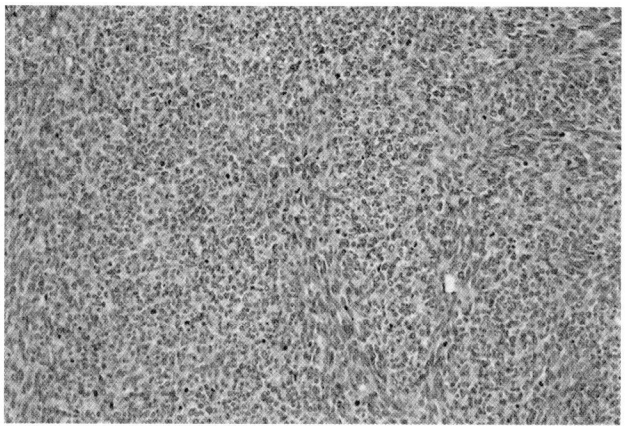

Fig. 114.11 The low-power appearance of congenital/infantile fibrosarcoma is marked by a population of closely packed hyperchromatic cells.

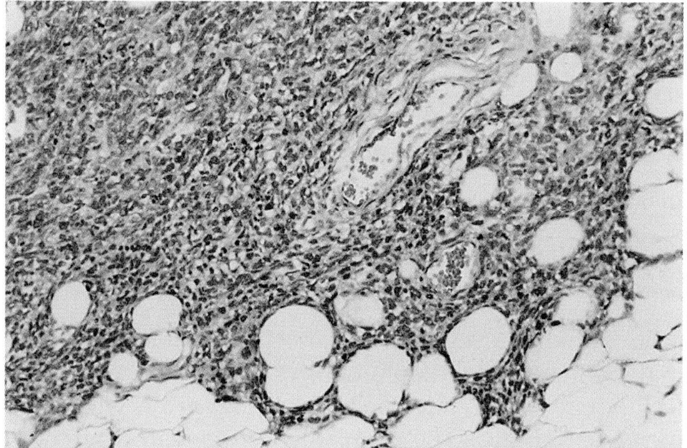

Fig. 114.12 The periphery of a congenital/infantile fibrosarcoma is an infiltrative one, with invasion and entrapment of adjacent structures by the advancing front of the tumour.

Treatment. Although the designation of any lesion as a sarcoma carries with it a powerful negative connotation, in the paediatric age group, the congenital/infantile fibrosarcomas are a decidedly more indolent group of lesions than the adult fibrosarcomas (lesions that have a similar light microscopic appearance to the paediatric lesions). When wide local excision successfully achieves tumour-free margins, this procedure may be curative. Indeed, such a good outcome is seen in the majority of cases; metastases can be anticipated in less than 10% of patients.

The best approach to treatment is a surgical one. Because complete surgical excision of the lesion is the goal of therapy, Mohs micrographic surgery is an attractive option. Although it is true that approximately half of these lesions recur after attempted surgical excision, the 5-year survival is still above 80% [7]. Some role may exist for the use of adjuvant chemotherapy in addition to surgery when resection alone is unfeasible [7,8].

Acknowledgements

We gratefully acknowledge the authors of the original chapter from the previous editions, Grazia Mancini, Arnold P. Oranje and Jan C. den Hollander, upon whose work this chapter is based.

References

1 van Grotel M, Blanco E, Sebire NJ et al. Distant metastatic spread of molecularly proven infantile fibrosarcoma of the chest in a 2-month-old girl: case report and review of literature. J Pediatr Hematol Oncol 2014;36:231–3.
2 Coffin CM, Jaszcz W, O'Shea PA, Dehner LP. So-called congenital-infantile fibrosarcoma: does it exist and what is it? Pediatr Pathol 1994;14:133–50.
3 Knezevich SR, McFadden DE, Tao W et al. A novel ETV6-NTRK3 gene fusion in congenital fibrosarcoma. Nat Genet 1998;18:184–7.
4 Tognon C, Garnett M, Kenward E et al. The chimeric protein tyrosine kinase ETV6-NTRK3 requires both Ras-Erk1/2 and PI3-kinase-Akt signaling for fibroblast transformation. Cancer Res 2001;61:8909–16.
5 Rubin BP, Chen CJ, Morgan TW et al. Congenital mesoblastic nephroma t(12;15) is associated with ETV6-NTRK3 gene fusion: cytogenetic and molecular relationship to congenital (infantile) fibrosarcoma. Am J Pathol 1998;153:1451–8.
6 Thway K, Fisher C, Sebire NJ. Pediatric fibroblastic and myofibroblastic lesions. Adv Anat Pathol 2012;19:54–65.
7 Parida L, Fernandez-Pineda I, Uffman JK et al. Clinical management of infantile fibrosarcoma: a retrospective single-institution review. Pediatr Surg Int 2013;29:703–8.
8 Orbach D, Rey A, Cecchetto G et al. Infantile fibrosarcoma: management based on the European experience. J Clin Oncol 2010;28:318–23.

CHAPTER 115
Carcinomas of the Skin

Karen Agnew
Starship Children's and Auckland City Hospitals, Auckland, New Zealand

Introduction, 1370
Basal cell carcinoma, 1370
Squamous cell carcinoma, 1373
Pilomatrix carcinoma, 1374
Sebaceous carcinoma, 1375
Merkel cell carcinoma, 1375

Abstract

Carcinomas of the skin are malignant epidermal tumours. They are rare in children, but can potentially be lethal. Basal cell carcinoma (basal cell epithelioma) develops from basal cells of the epidermis or its appendages, whereas squamous cell carcinoma (epidermoid carcinoma) originates from keratinocytes. The term nonmelanoma skin cancer is often used in reference to basal cell and squamous cell carcinomas. Nonmelanoma skin cancer in childhood generally arises in the context of predisposing risk factors such as chronic immunosuppression or an associated genetic condition. Both skin surveillance and photoprotective measures are important in the management of at-risk individuals. Merkel cell carcinoma, sebaceous carcinoma and pilomatrix carcinoma are further cutaneous malignances and are exceedingly rare in children. The diagnosis of a skin carcinoma is established histopathologically, and surgical excision is the treatment of choice for children with these malignancies.

Key points

- Carcinomas of the skin are malignant epidermal tumours and include basal cell carcinoma (BCC), squamous cell carcinoma (SCC), pilomatrix carcinoma, sebaceous carcinoma and Merkel cell carcinoma.
- Basal cell and squamous cell carcinomas are often referred to as nonmelanoma skin cancer.
- Childhood nonmelanoma skin cancer generally develops in individuals with predisposing risk factors such as chronic immunosuppression or an associated genetic condition.
- Although uncommon, the prevalence of childhood basal cell carcinoma is higher than that of squamous cell carcinoma. Pilomatrix carcinoma, sebaceous carcinoma and Merkel cell carcinoma are exceedingly rare in childhood.
- The diagnosis of a skin carcinoma is established by histopathological examination.
- Surgical excision is the treatment of choice for childhood carcinomas of the skin.

Introduction

Basal cell carcinoma (BCC), squamous cell carcinoma (SCC), pilomatrix carcinoma, sebaceous carcinoma and Merkel cell carcinoma are all epidermal malignant neoplasms. They are rare in children, but can cause significant morbidity and are potentially lethal.

BCC, also termed basal cell epithelioma, is a slow-growing low-risk malignancy that causes localized tissue destruction; metastases are very rare [1]. SCC, also termed epidermoid carcinoma, develops from keratinocytes. A small percentage of these tumours metastasize and this is usually locally or to the regional lymph nodes. BCC and SCC are often referred to as nonmelanoma skin cancer [2]. Childhood nonmelanoma skin cancer generally occurs in individuals with predisposing risk factors such as chronic immunosuppression or an associated genetic condition [3–5].

Pilomatrix carcinoma is a very rare malignant adnexal tumour with only a few reports in children [6–8]. Sebaceous carcinoma and Merkel cell carcinoma are also rare cutaneous malignancies [9–15]. The incidence is highest in the elderly population, however there are occasional reports of children developing these carcinomas [9,12,15,16].

Basal cell carcinoma

BCC, also known as basal cell epithelioma, is a cutaneous neoplasm arising from the basal cells of the epidermis or its appendages.

Epidemiology. BCC is the most common cutaneous malignancy and predominantly affects white-skinned individuals. The incidence is rising worldwide and increases with age. BCC prevalence is greatest in countries such as Australia, with high UV radiation exposure and ageing populations of people with Fitzpatrick skin types I and II [1,2]. These tumours are rare in children and generally occur when there are predisposing risk factors.

Harper's Textbook of Pediatric Dermatology, Fourth Edition. Edited by Peter Hoeger, Veronica Kinsler and Albert Yan.

There are recognized associated congenital and environmental risk factors for childhood BCC. The hereditary or congenital risk factors include basal cell naevus syndrome, oculocutaneous albinism, Bazex–Dupre–Christol syndrome, xeroderma pigmentosus, Rothmund–Thomson syndrome and naevus sebaceus [1,3–5,17,18]. Environmental or iatrogenic risk factors, including radiotherapy, chemotherapy and chronic immunosuppression such as that seen in solid organ transplantation, have all been reported in early-onset BCC [3,5,17,19,20].

In a study of 28 children and young adults in whom 182 nonmelanoma skin cancers were identified, 80% of these tumours were BCC. The remaining 6.5% and 13.5% of tumours were invasive SCC and SCC *in situ* respectively. Of the BCC, 43% developed in children who were under 10 years of age. Eighty four percent of individuals had Fitzpatrick skin type I or II and virtually all patients had associated risk factors. Predisposing conditions were identified in 50% of patients and environmental or iatrogenic risk factors in a further 46%. All patients with Fitzpatrick skin type III or greater had BCC associated with a predisposing condition and these were basal cell naevus syndrome, xeroderma pigmentosum and naevus sebaceus [3].

Children without congenital or iatrogenic risk factors have developed BCC, however this is rare [17,21]. Another study reviewed the literature and described 107 children with idiopathic BCC. In this cohort, the age range was from 2 to 18 years with a mean age of 11 years. Most children had white skin, however there were two Hispanic children and one child with black skin [17].

The established risk factors associated with childhood-onset BCC are presented in Table 115.1.

Pathogenesis. In the skin, as in any organ, there is a delicate balance between growth and differentiation of cells. Malignancy develops when a disturbance occurs resulting in increased cell division coupled with impaired differentiation. In BCC the tumour originates from the basal cells of the epidermis or its appendages.

Cancers arise as a result of cumulative DNA damage which generally occurs from the combination of carcinogen exposure and genetic vulnerability [22].

There are a number of well-recognized factors implicated in the pathogenesis of childhood-onset BCC. These include:

Carcinogens

Ultraviolet (UV) radiation or sun exposure is the primary carcinogen associated with the development of nonmelanoma skin cancer. It both damages DNA and has an immunosuppressive action on the skin. This can lead to malignancies when UV-induced DNA mutations occur in genes that regulate cell growth [22]. However, in children where cumulative UV radiation exposure is usually low, it tends to play a secondary role in the pathogenesis of nonmelanoma skin cancer.

Radiotherapy or ionizing radiation is another carcinogen that can cause DNA damage leading to malignancy. It is a risk factor for the development of BCC in children and adults [3,19,20].

Predisposing genodermatoses

A number of genetic mutations associated with nonmelanoma skin cancer have been identified and include:

Basal cell naevus syndrome (Gorlin–Goltz syndrome, Gorlin syndrome) has autosomal dominant inheritance and stems primarily from a mutation in the patched 1 gene (*PTCH1*) on chromosome 9q22-31 [4,5,22,23] (see Chapter 139). Spontaneous mutations occur in up to 50% of cases. *PTCH1* encodes a transmembrane glycoprotein, patched 1, which acts as a tumour suppressor in the Hedgehog signalling pathway, a pro-oncogenic pathway that stimulates growth. This syndrome is characterized by the clinical triad of BCC, odontogenic jaw keratocysts and cerebral calcification. BCC generally first develop in adolescence but have been known to occur as early as the first year of life [5,23].

Xeroderma pigmentosum (see Chapter 138) is a rare group of genetic disorders with autosomal recessive inheritance.

Table 115.1 Risk factors for childhood-onset nonmelanoma skin cancer

	Basal cell carcinoma (BCC)	Squamous cell carcinoma (SCC)
Ultraviolet radiation	Primary risk factor in fair-skinned individuals and adjuvant risk factor	Adjuvant risk factor
Radiotherapy	Risk factor	Reports in adults, however BCC is more common
Chronic iatrogenic immunosuppression	Risk factor but SCC is more common	Risk factor
Voriconazole following stem cell transplantation	No known association	Risk factor
Basal cell naevus syndrome	Risk factor and often multiple BCC	Not an established risk factor
Xeroderma pigmentosum	Risk factor	Risk factor
Oculocutaneous albinism	Risk factor	Risk factor
Epidermolysis bullosa	A few reports, however SCC more common	Risk factor particularly in severe generalized recessive dystrophic subtype
Rothmund–Thomson syndrome	Risk factor	Risk factor
Bazex–Dupre–Christol syndrome	Risk factor	Not an established risk factor
Fanconi anaemia	No known association	Risk factor and risk is compounded following stem cell transplantation
Naevus sebaceus	Risk factor	A few reports, however BCC more common

Patients with this rare condition have a mutation in one of the genes encoding proteins involved in the nucleotide excision repair pathway [4,5,22]. The role of this pathway is to remove damaged DNA, which in the skin is primarily UV-induced. Tumours arise when DNA damage in growth-regulating genes is not repaired.

Oculocutaneous albinism (see Chapter 124) is a group of genetic disorders in which affected individuals have complete or partial loss of pigmentation in their skin, hair and eyes [4,5]. The most common form is oculocutaneous albinism 1 where the pathological mutation is located in the tyrosinase gene. This gene encodes for the enzyme tyrosinase, which catalyses three steps in the melanin biosynthetic pathway, and the mutation results in a reduction of melanin within melanocytes [4,5]. Melanin is photoprotective and able to absorb UV photons that might otherwise damage DNA or cell membranes. Therefore the lack of melanin makes individuals more susceptible to cutaneous malignancies [22].

Immunosuppression

Prolonged immunosuppression is a recognized risk factor for childhood nonmelanoma skin cancer. It is presumed that dysplastic keratinocytes are not effectively identified and eradicated due to impaired immune surveillance resulting in uncontrolled growth of malignancies [3,5]. In children nonmelanoma skin cancer has been reported with iatrogenic immunosuppression in chronic graft-versus-host disease following haematopoietic stem cell transplantation, organ transplantation and chronic autoimmune conditions requiring prolonged immunosuppressive medication. As for adults, children with iatrogenic immunosuppression are more likely to develop SCC than BCC [3,24,25].

Clinical features and differential diagnosis. Clinical assessment including a thorough history and examination is essential for making an early diagnosis in children with cutaneous malignancies. A high index of suspicion is required for patients who have predisposing risk factors.

The clinical presentation for childhood BCC is similar to that seen in adults: tumours grow slowly and arise more commonly on the head. Children most often present with a nonhealing lesion that may bleed. On examination, BCC tumours are pink or pigmented with a characteristic pearly rolled periphery that can be accentuated on stretching the skin.

The clinicopathological variants of BCC are recognized in both childhood- and adult-onset malignancies. These variants include nodular (solid), micronodular, superficial, morphoeic (sclerosing), infiltrative, pigmented, adenocystic and basosquamous BCC [1,17]. The *nodular* or *micronodular variants* classically appear as a translucent pearly papule or nodule. These tumours are well defined and there is a tendency for central ulceration to develop after the lesion enlarges to a pivotal size. Dilated superficial capillaries are visible in the thin layer of epithelium covering the BCC. The *superficial basal cell carcinoma* predominantly arises on the trunk as a thin, well-defined plaque. These lesions may demonstrate central atrophy or scaling and display a thread-like raised edge. *Pigmented basal cell carcinoma* displays brown, red or black pigmentation within the tumour as a result of trapped melanin or altered blood composition. This pigmentation generally occurs in nodular, micronodular or superficial BCC. The *adenocystic variant* most commonly develops into a diffuse plaque with a rolled edge whereas the *infiltrative* and *morphoeic variants* both classically present as indurated scar-like plaques with ill-defined margins. *Basosquamous basal cell carcinoma* has histological features of both BCC and SCC, however clinically the lesions are more representative of SCC. There is some controversy over whether these lesions are a variant of SCC or BCC [22]. On very rare occasions BCC has been reported to metastasize.

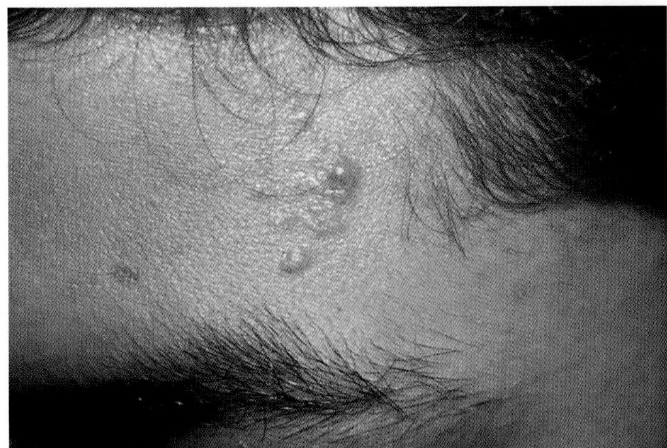

Fig. 115.1 Pigmented basal cell carcinoma (BCC) within a sebaceous naevus in a 10-year-old boy.

BCC is one of the tumours than can arise within a *sebaceous naevus* [3,18,22]. The BCC classically presents as a firm papule within the papillomatous naevus (Fig. 115.1).

A diagnosis of BCC can be made clinically, however it is confirmed on histopathological examination following incisional or excisional biopsy. The differential diagnosis for BCC includes amelanotic melanoma and adnexal lesions such as basaloid follicular hamartoma, trichoblastoma, trichofolliculoma and trichoepithelioma [17,21,26].

Histology findings. The histological features of a BCC vary with the different subtypes, however the unifying findings are of nests or islands of basaloid tumour cells in the dermis with peripheral palisading of nuclei at the margins of the cell nests (Fig. 115.2). The tumour cells have hyperchromatic nuclei with multiple mitoses and sparse cytoplasm. In superficial BCC the tumour cells are attached to the epidermis and confined to the papillary dermis. A morphoeic BCC has narrow strands of tumour cells embedded in a dense fibrous stroma [22].

Treatment. Surveillance and monitoring for nonmelanoma skin cancer is a fundamental component of management in individuals with recognized risk factors. High-risk individuals and their families require education, self-examination strategies and close observation to ensure early diagnoses are made.

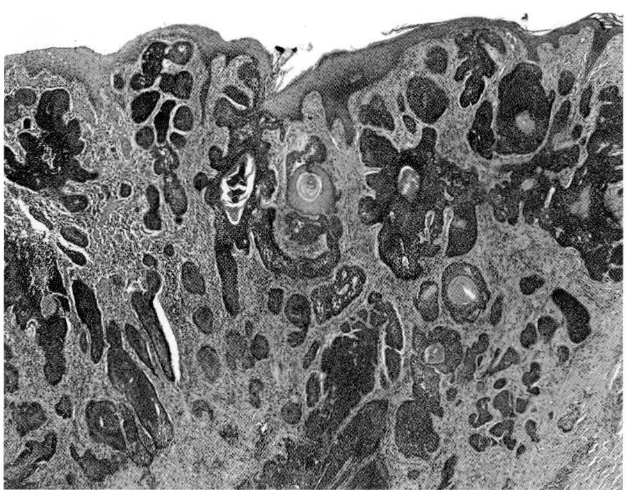

Fig. 115.2 Low-power light microscopy of a basal cell carcinoma demonstrating nests of basaloid cells within the dermis (haematoxylin and eosin). Source: Courtesy of Dr Patrick Emanuel, Auckland District Healthboard, New Zealand.

Surgical excision is the treatment of choice for BCC in childhood, and Mohs micrographic surgery has been successfully performed in selected cases [17,21]. Other potential treatment modalities include cryotherapy, curettage and electrodessication, photodynamic therapy and topical imiquimod [1,3,22]. Vismodegib is an orally administered inhibitor of the Hedgehog pathway and is therefore a therapeutic option for patients with basal cell naevus syndrome [23,27]. The safety and efficacy of both vismodegib and imiquimod have not been established in children.

Prevention. As UV radiation is the strongest recognized risk factor for BCC, photoprotective strategies are fundamental to prevention.

Photoprotective measures include sun avoidance, wearing sun-protective clothing and using sunscreens. Individuals, particularly children, should avoid sunbed use and not get sunburn. The intensity of the UV radiation varies considerably throughout the day with approximately two thirds of all UVB and half of UVA radiation reaching the earth between 10 a.m. and 4 p.m. [22,28].

Clothing offers good photoprotection and tends to absorb the spectrum of solar irradiation uniformly. Ultraviolet protection factor (UPF) for clothing is analogous to sun protection factor (SPF) for sunscreen and provides a measurement of the degree of photoprotection offered by a fabric. Fabrics with a tight weave, a dark colour and a heavy weight are more protective and have a higher UPF [22,28].

Sunscreens are topical preparations applied to the skin that attenuate UV radiation. They achieve this by reflecting and/or absorbing the UV radiation. The sunscreen needs to remain on the skin in sufficient quantity to be effective during sun exposure. Unfortunately sunscreen application is often inadequate; it should be applied liberally 30 minutes before sun exposure and reapplied after 2 hours or after swimming or sweating [28]. Broad-spectrum sunscreens are best as they protect against both UVB and UVA radiation. In New Zealand and Australia, where there are very high rates of skin cancer, the recommendation is for the use of a broad-spectrum SPF 50+ sunscreen.

Squamous cell carcinoma

SCC, also termed epidermoid carcinoma, is a malignant tumour originating from keratinocytes of the epidermis or its appendages.

Epidemiology. Cutaneous SCC represents approximately 20% of nonmelanoma skin cancer, and childhood SCC is rare with a lower incidence than that of childhood BCC [3,24]. This malignancy is virtually always described in children with predisposing risk factors; as with BCC, these can be congenital or environmental [3–5].

Congenital or hereditary risk factors include xeroderma pigmentosum. With this disorder of autosomal recessive inheritance, SCC or BCC appear at a median age of 8–9 years, in children who have not been protected from the sun [4]. The genodermatosis epidermolysis bullosa is associated with the development of mucocutaneous SCC and the risk increases with age [4,29,30]. These tumours are seen most often with severe generalized recessive dystrophic epidermolysis bullosa and are a leading cause of death in these patients. SCC has also been reported in children with other dystrophic subtypes and in junctional epidermolysis bullosa. Furthermore, SCC is the most common cutaneous malignancy in patients with oculocutaneous albinism [4,5,29,31]. Other hereditary conditions reported to have associated childhood SCC include Rothmund–Thomson syndrome, dyskeratosis congenita, Clericuzio-type poikiloderma with neutropenia, interferon-γ receptor 2 deficiency and Fanconi anaemia where the risk is compounded following haematopoietic stem cell transplantation [32–34].

Iatrogenic risk factors for childhood SCC are well recognized and include chronic immunosuppression as with organ transplantation, total body irradiation and the combination of haematopoietic stem cell transplantation or iatrogenic immunosuppression with voriconazole [3,24,25,35,36].

Risk factors associated with childhood-onset SCC are presented in Table 115.1.

Pathogenesis. The malignant cells in SCC are derived from the epidermal or appendageal keratinocytes. Carcinogens, predisposing genodermatoses and immunosuppression are also implicated in the pathogenesis of SCC as described in the section on BCC pathogenesis. Although BCC is the most common childhood nonmelanoma skin cancer, children with iatrogenic immunosuppression are more likely to develop SCC [3,24,25].

Epidermolysis bullosa (see Chapter 76) is a genodermatosis in which individuals with junctional and dystrophic subtypes are at increased risk of mucocutaneous SCC [4,29,30]. These tumours tend to arise on sites of chronic blistering and scarring. The mechanism by which SCC

Box 115.1 Established risk factors for carcinoma metastasis

Squamous cell carcinoma

Diameter of tumour >20 mm
Tumour depth >2 mm
Tumour invasion beyond subcutaneous fat
Poorly differentiated tumour
Perineural invasion
Host immunosuppression
Tumour location: temple, ear, lip, non-sun-exposed sites
Epidermolysis bullosa-associated
Tumour recurrence

Pilomatrix carcinoma

Tumour recurrence

develops in this group of skin fragility genodermatoses is not clearly understood [4,29].

Clinical features and differential diagnosis. SCC primarily develops on sun-exposed and photodamaged skin, therefore the face, lips, ears, scalp, dorsal hands and lower legs are common sites in adults [22,37]. These are also characteristic sites for SCC in immunocompromised children or those with hereditary conditions that make them susceptible to UV radiation carcinogenesis. However this does not apply to epidermolysis bullosa-associated SCC, which tend to develop at sites of chronic wounds and scarring [29].

Invasive SCC characteristically first present as an ill-defined firm indurated and often erythematous, tender lesion. The SCC is usually a scaly or crusted papule, plaque or nodule, however it may be ulcerated or verrucous [22,37]. Approximately 5% of SCC metastasize and this is predominantly to the regional lymph nodes [24]. A higher risk of metastasis is identified with tumours arising in non-sun-exposed sites and in areas of chronic inflammation or scars, as with epidermolysis bullosa. Other risk factors for metastasis include an immunosuppressed host, tumour diameter over 20 mm, tumour depth greater than 2 mm, perineural invasion, a poorly differentiated tumour, and temple, ear or lip lesion site [24,37,38]. The risk factors for carcinoma metastases are presented in Box 115.1.

Bowen disease is the most common form of *in situ SCC* and it presents as a thin scaly well-demarcated erythematous plaque [22,39].

The diagnosis of SCC is established by an incisional or excision biopsy [22,37,39]. The differential diagnosis includes keratoacanthoma, BCC, hyperkeratotic actinic keratosis and amelanotic melanoma.

Histology findings. Histopathologically, *invasive SCC* is characterized by dermal nests of atypical squamous epithelial cells arising from the epidermis. These tumour cells have large nuclei and abundant eosinophilic cytoplasm with varying degrees of keratinization. A greater degree of keratinization differentiation is associated with a more differentiated tumour [22]. With *SCC in situ* the malignancy is intraepidermal and therefore the abnormal keratinocytes are confined to the epidermis.

The histological report should include the histopathological pattern or subtype of SCC, degree of differentiation, level of dermal invasion, presence of perineural, vascular or lymphatic invasion and the tumour excision margins [37].

Treatment. As with BCC, surveillance and monitoring of individuals at high risk of SCC is important to ensure early identification of malignancies.

Surgical excision with or without margin control is the standard of care for *invasive SCC* [37]. The aim of therapy is to completely remove or destroy the primary tumour and any metastasis. Potential metastasis should be examined for and, if identified, in-transit metastases are usually treated with wide local excision and lymph node metastases with regional nodal dissection [37]. Wide local excision, ideally with a 2 cm margin, is considered the treatment of choice for primary epidermolysis bullosa-associated SCC as these tumours behave aggressively [29]. Patients with high-risk SCC and metastatic disease are best managed by a multidisciplinary team [37]. Both the American Joint Committee on Cancer and Brigham and Women's Hospital provide staging systems for cutaneous SCC [24,40]. The utility of sentinel lymph node biopsy for cutaneous SCC is not yet established [37,41].

In situ SCC can be treated with a variety of therapeutic modalities, however surgical excision with or without Mohs micrographic surgery is most commonly undertaken in children [3]. Other potential therapies include topical 5-fluorouracil, curettage with electrosurgery and photodynamic therapy [39].

Prevention. UV radiation is the strongest risk factor for development of SCC. As with BCC, photoprotective strategies are fundamental to prevention and are described previously in the section on BCC prevention. Chemoprophylaxis, such as oral retinoids, has a role in very high-risk adults who develop recurrent nonmelanoma skin cancer, however this is not an established treatment in children.

Pilomatrix carcinoma

Pilomatrix carcinoma originates from hair follicle matrix cells and is the malignant counterpart of pilomatricoma [6–8].

Epidemiology. Pilomatrix carcinoma is an extremely rare tumour. The youngest case was reported in a child 14 months of age, however the tumour characteristically develops in white middle- to older-aged individuals [7,42].

Pathogenesis. The pathogenesis of pilomatrix carcinoma is not clearly understood. There are reports describing malignant transformation of benign pilomatricoma into pilomatrix carcinoma, however de novo malignancies occur in the majority of cases [43].

Clinical features and differential diagnosis. Pilomatrix carcinomas generally present as firm asymptomatic dermal or subcutaneous lesions having a predilection for the head and neck. However they have been described at most body locations [6,7]. One study reported a range in tumour diameters from 0.5 to 20 cm with a median of 2.5 cm [7]. Pilomatrix carcinoma has a tendency for local recurrence and has the potential to metastasize. Metastases are most likely to develop at the same time as or after local recurrence (Box 115.1) and have been reported in the regional lymph nodes, lung, bone, other visceral organs and the brain [7]. A diagnosis is established histologically and usually following surgical excision. The foremost differential diagnosis is pilomatricoma.

Histology findings. Histological examination of a pilomatrix carcinoma reveals an asymmetrical, poorly circumscribed tumour originating in the dermis. The tumours are characterized by irregular basaloid cells with frequent atypical mitoses and eosinophilic anucleate shadow cells (Fig. 115.3). Foci of necrosis and a desmoplastic stroma are often described, and lymphovascular invasion has been reported [6,7].

Treatment. As this tumour is exceedingly rare there is no consensus on management other than the requirement for complete excision of the tumour. With its high recurrence rate, clinicians have opted for wide local excisions or Mohs micrographic surgery. There is not sufficient evidence available to determine adequate surgical margins for primary tumours or the best treatment approach for metastatic disease [7]. Furthermore, there is insufficient understanding of this malignancy to propose any preventative interventions.

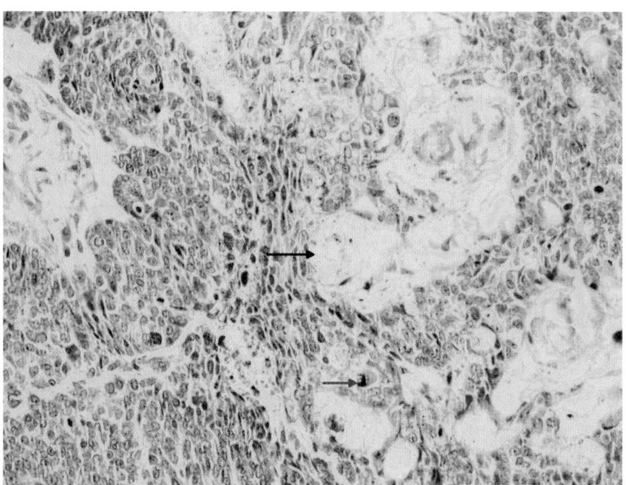

Fig. 115.3 High-power light microscopy of a pilomatrix carcinoma. The characteristic shadow cell is highlighted with the black arrow. The red arrow identifies an irregular basaloid cell with numerous mitoses (haematoxylin and eosin). Source: Courtesy of Dr Patrick Emanuel, Auckland District Healthboard, New Zealand.

Sebaceous carcinoma

Sebaceous carcinoma is an aggressive adnexal malignancy that arises from the epithelium of sebaceous glands [9,16].

Epidemiology. This is another rare tumour. The incidence appears to be rising, with highest rates seen in elderly individuals [10,11]. There have only been a few reported cases of sebaceous carcinoma in children [9,16].

Pathogenesis. The pathogenesis of sebaceous carcinoma in poorly understood. There is literature to support an association between this malignancy and the genodermatosis, Muir–Torre syndrome. This syndrome has not been reported in any childhood cases of sebaceous carcinoma. There are two cases of upper eyelid sebaceous carcinoma developing in children after radiation therapy [9,16].

Clinical features and differential diagnosis. Sebaceous carcinomas predominantly develop on the head and neck, with the periorbital region most frequently involved. The majority of paediatric presentations have arisen in periorbital skin [9,16]. This malignancy is often referred to as ocular or extraocular sebaceous carcinoma. The clinical presentation is of a painless enlarging firm papule, nodule, swelling or cyst-like lesion [9,16]. Sebaceous carcinoma has the potential to spread both regionally to tissue or lymph nodes as well as systemically to form distant metastases.

A diagnosis of sebaceous carcinoma is confirmed on histological examination. The differential diagnosis includes a chalazion, BCC, SCC, epidermal cyst, pilomatricoma and other adnexal tumours.

Histology. On histological examination, a sebaceous carcinoma presents as an asymmetrical dermal proliferation with varying degrees of differentiation. The majority of sebaceous carcinomas have a combination of sebaceous and basaloid cells arranged in irregular lobules. There may be pagetoid spread and extension into the epidermis. Lipid or periodic acid–Schiff (PAS) staining can assist with identifying glycogen, lipid and mucin, which is valuable in differentiating sebaceous carcinoma from other malignancies [9,16].

Treatment. Sebaceous carcinoma is treated surgically, usually with wide-margin excision. One child who suffered lymph node metastases also underwent a lymph node dissection with adjuvant radiotherapy and there was no reported disease recurrence [9,16].

Merkel cell carcinoma

Merkel cell carcinoma is an aggressive neuroendocrine skin cancer originating from the Merkel cell [12–14]. It is exceedingly rare in children, with approximately five cases reported in the literature, and is therefore not discussed in detail in this chapter [12,14,15]. Merkel cell carcinoma is most commonly seen in white-skinned elderly individuals and recognized risk factors include ultraviolet (UV) radiation, chronic immunosuppression and a number of haematological malignancies [12–16]. In addition, recent research has identified a polyomavirus to be associated with this carcinoma which was subsequently named the Merkel cell polyomavirus [13]. The characteristic clinical presentation is of a rapidly enlarging, painless, red or purple tumour and the diagnosis is often not suspected clinically. This malignancy has a high mortality rate and affected individuals can develop local recurrence, regional nodal metastases and distal metastases [12,14].

References

1 **Telfer NR, Colver GB, Morton CA. Guidelines for the management of basal cell carcinoma. Br J Dermatol 2008;159:35–48.**

2 Fransen M, Karahallos A, Sharma N et al. Non-melanoma skin cancer in Australia. Med J Aust 2012;197:565–8.

3 **Khosravi H, Schmidt B, Huang JT. Characteristics and outcomes of nonmelanoma skin cancer (NMSC) in children and young adults. J Am Acad Dermatol 2015;73:785–90.**

4 **Nikolaou V, Stratigos AJ, Tsao H. Hereditary nonmelanoma skin cancer. Semin Cutan Med Surg 2012;31:204–10.**

5 **Jaju PD, Ransohoff KJ, Yang JY, Sarin KY. Familial skin cancer syndromes. J Am Acad Dermatol 2016;74:437–51.**

6 **Sau P, Lupton GP, Graham JH. Pilomatrix carcinoma. Cancer 1993;71:2491–8.**

7 **Hermann JI, Allan A, Trapp KM, Morgan MB. Pilomatrix carcinoma: 13 new cases and review of the literature with emphasis on predictors of metastasis. J Am Acad Dermatol 2014;71:38–43.**

8 Yadia S, Randazzo CG, Malik S et al. Pilomatrix carcinoma of the thoracic spine: Case report and review of the literature. J Spinal Cord Med 2010;33:272–7.

9 **Omura NE, Collison DW, Perry AE, Myers LM. Sebaceous carcinoma in children. J Am Acad Dermatol 2002;47:950–3.**

10 Tripathi R, Chen Z, Li L, Bordeaux JS. Incidence and survival of sebaceous carcinoma in the United States. J Am Acad Dermatol 2016;75:1210–15.

11 Dasgupta T, Wilson LD, Yu JB. A retrospective review of 1349 cases of sebaceous carcinoma. Cancer 2009;115:158–65.

12 **Koksal Y, Toy H, Talim B et al. Merkel cell carcinoma in a child. J Pediatr Hematol Oncol 2009;31:359–61.**

13 Kaae J, Hansen A, Biggar R et al. Merkel cell carcinoma: incidence, mortality, and risk of other cancers. J Natl Cancer Inst 2010;102: 793–801.

14 Agelli M, Clegg LX. Epidemiology of primary Merkel cell carcinoma in the United States. J Am Acad Dermatol 2003;49:832–41.

15 Schmid CH, Beham A, Feichtinger J et al. Recurrent and subsequently metastasizing Merkel cell carcinoma in a 7-year-old girl. Histopathology 1992;20:437–43.

16 Mebazaa A, Boussofara L, Trabelsi A et al. Undifferentiated sebaceous carcinoma: an unusual childhood cancer. Pediatr Dermatol 2007; 24:501–4.

17 **Griffin JR, Cohen PR, Tschen JA et al. Basal cell carcinoma in childhood: Case report and literature review. J Am Acad Dermatol 2007;57:s97–102.**

18 Moody NM, Landau JM, Goldberg LH. Nevus sebaceous revisited. Pediatr Dermatol 2012;29:15–23.

19 **Watt TC, Inskip PD, Statton K et al. Radiation-related risk of basal cell carcinoma: a report from the Childhood Cancer Survivor Study. J Natl Cancer Inst 2012;104:1240–50.**

20 Unal S, Cetin M, Gumruk F. Basal cell carcinoma after treatment of childhood acute lymphoblastic leukaemia and concise review of the literature. Pediatr Dermatol 2015;32:e82–5.

21 Turan E, Yurt N, Yesilova Y, Turkcu G. Early-onset basal cell carcinoma. Turk J Pediatr 2013;55:354–6.

22 **Agnew KL, Bunker CB, Arron ST. Fast Facts: Skin Cancer, 2nd edn. Oxford: Health Press Ltd, 2013.**

23 **John AM, Schwartz RA. Basal cell naevus syndrome: an update on genetics and treatment. Br J Dermatol 2016;174:68–76.**

24 **Farasat S, Yu SS, Neel VA et al. A new American Joint Committee on Cancer staging system for cutaneous squamous cell carcinoma: creation and rationale for inclusion of tumor (T) characteristics. J Am Acad Dermatol 2011;64:1051–9.**

25 Wong JY, Kuzel P, Mullen J et al. Cutaneous squamous cell carcinoma in two pediatric lung transplant patients on prolonged voriconazole treatment. Pediatr Transplant 2014;18:E200–7.

26 Puente-Pablo N, Tardio JC, Najera L et al. Adnexal tumours in children clinically mimicking basal cell carcinoma. Eur J Pediat Dermatol 2015;25:7–11.

27 Sekulic A, Migden MR, Oro AE et al. Efficacy and safety of vismodegib in advanced basal-cell carcinoma. N Engl J Med 2012;366:2171–9.

28 **Kullavanijaya P, Lim HW. Photoprotection. J Am Acad Dermatol 2005;52:937–58.**

29 **Mellerio JE, Sobertson SJ, Bernardis C et al. Management of cutaneous squamous cell carcinoma in patients with epidermolysis bullosa: best clinical practice guidelines. Br J Dermatol 2016;174:56–67.**

30 Kawasaki H, Sawamura D, Iwao F et al. Squamous cell carcinoma developing in a 12-year-old boy with nonHallopeau-Siemens recessive dystrophic epidermolysis bullosa. Br J Dermatol 2003; 148:1047–50.

31 Luande J, Henschke CI, Mohammed N. The Tanzanian human albino skin. Natural history. Cancer 1985;55:1823–8.

32 Rodgers W, Ancliff P, Ponting CP et al. Squamous cell carcinoma in a child with Clericuzio-type poikiloderma with neutropenia. Br J Dermatol 2013;168:665–7.

33 Toyoda H, Ido M, Nakanishi K et al. Multiple cutaneous squamous cell carcinomas in a patient with interferon γ receptor 2 (IFNγR2) deficiency. J Med Genet 2010;47:631–4.

34 Rosenberg PS, Socie G, Alter BP, Gluckman E. Risk of head and neck squamous cell cancer and death in patients with Fanconi anemia who did and did not receive transplants. Blood 2005;105:67–73.

35 **Cowen EW, Nguyen JC, Miller DD et al. Chronic phototoxicity and aggressive squamous cell carcinoma of the skin in children and adults during treatment with voriconazole. J Am Acad Dermatol 2010;62:31–7.**

36 Sheu, J, Hawryluk EB, Guo D et al. Voriconazole phototoxicity in children: A retrospective review. J Am Acad Dermatol 2015;72:314–20.

37 **Motley RJ, Preston PW, Lawrence CM. Multi-professional guidelines for the management of the patient with primary cutaneous squamous cell carcinoma 2009. Available at: British Association of Dermatologists: http://www.bad.org.uk (accessed 10 February 2019).**

38 **Thompson AK, Kelley BF, Prokop LJ et al. Risk factors for cutaneous squamous cell carcinoma recurrence, metastasis, and disease-specific death: A systematic review and meta-analysis. JAMA Dermatol 2016;152:419–28.**

39 **Morton CA, Birnie AJ, Eedy DJ. British Association of Dermatologists' guidelines for the management of squamous cell carcinoma in situ (Bowen's disease) 2014. Br J Dermatol 2014;170:245–60.**

40 Karia PS, Jambusaria-Pahlajani A, Harrington DP et al. Evaluation of American Joint Committee on Cancer, International Union Against Cancer and Brigham and Women's Hospital tumor staging for cutaneous squamous cell carcinoma. J Clin Oncol 2014;32:327–34.

41 Navarrete-Dechent C, Veness MJ, Droppelmann N, Uribe P. High-risk cutaneous squamous cell carcinoma and the emerging role of sentinel lymph node biopsy: A literature review. J Am Acad Dermatol 2015;73:127–37.

42 Lui J, Li B, Fan Z et al. Pilomatrix carcinoma on the left side of the parotid region: A case report and review of the literature. Oncol Lett 2015;10:313–16.

43 Sassmannshausen J, Chaffins M. Pilomatrix carcinoma: A report of a case arising from a previously excised pilomatrixoma and a review of the literature. J Am Acad Dermatol 2001;44:358–61.

CHAPTER 116
Childhood Melanoma

Birgitta Schmidt[1] *& Elena B. Hawryluk*[2,3]

[1] Department of Pathology, Boston Children's Hospital, Harvard Medical School, Boston, MA, USA
[2] Department of Dermatology, Massachusetts General Hospital, Harvard Medical School, Boston, MA, USA
[3] Dermatology Program, Division of Allergy and Immunology, Department of Medicine, Boston Children's Hospital, Harvard Medical School, Boston, MA, USA

Abstract

Paediatric melanomas are rare, and their presentation is often challenging due to not only their rarity but also their distinct clinical features compared to those arising in adults. Lesions are diagnosed by histopathology, and although there are an increasing number of ancillary and genetic tests to better understand these challenging lesions, to date none has been proven as a gold standard for diagnosis of melanoma in paediatric skin lesions. Treatment of melanoma in children is primarily surgical, and there is debate in the literature regarding the utility of sentinel lymph node biopsy among borderline pigmented lesions. The overall prognosis among melanomas in childhood is better than in adolescents and adults.

Key points

- **Childhood melanoma is extremely rare, and most commonly presents in adolescence or is associated with giant congenital naevus or genetic disease.**
- **The presentation of melanoma among the paediatric population can differ significantly from adult melanomas, with higher frequency of amelanotic melanomas and suggested criteria for detection that differ from adult melanomas.**
- **Histopathology is the gold standard for diagnosis, although genetic testing holds promise for providing future diagnostic and/or therapeutic information.**

SECTION 24: NONVASCULAR SKIN TUMOURS

Brief introduction/history. Melanoma in childhood is exceedingly rare, and is distinguished from the historic term 'juvenile melanoma', used by Sophie Spitz in 1948 [1] to describe childhood melanocytic tumours with biopsy features of melanoma but banal clinical outcomes. The benign presentation is now termed a Spitz naevus; lesions with increasing atypical features are termed atypical Spitz tumours and can be particularly difficult to distinguish from Spitz melanomas. Although melanomas in children typically have a favourable clinical outcome relative to adult melanomas with similar histopathological features, it is important to respect the potential for aggressive behaviour, including metastasis and death.

Epidemiology and pathogenesis. Melanoma is extremely rare in children. The true incidence of cutaneous melanoma is unknown, and diagnosis is challenging based upon histological criteria, with discordance among even expert dermatopathologists. Melanoma in childhood can be difficult to distinguish from atypical Spitz tumours and other borderline pigmented tumours. It has been estimated that melanoma represents 1–4% of childhood malignancies [2,3].

The data available suggest that after puberty the incidence of melanoma starts to rise [3]. Incidence rates appeared to be increasing over the past few decades, but in 2015 Campbell and colleagues reported a decline in paediatric melanoma incidence in the USA [4], consistent with trends in Australia and Sweden where recent reductions in paediatric melanoma incidences have also been reported. Data from the Surveillance, Epidemiology, and End Results (SEER) registry suggest that in the USA there is a 5-year survival rate of 94% for children with melanoma [2].

Childhood melanoma may occur in the normal host but there are known predispositions: congenital melanocytic naevi (see Chapter 105), the atypical mole syndrome (see Chapter 105), and familial melanoma and other cancer family syndromes such as bilateral retinoblastoma and xeroderma pigmentosum (XP). There is also an increased risk of melanoma in childhood based upon immunosuppression, for example by medication, comorbid condition or transplantation [5]. Paediatric melanoma is usually postpubertal [6]. It may have a distinct presentation, genetic mutations, and clinical course in patients who present before puberty versus adolescence, in association with congenital naevi (including patients with neurocutaneous melanocytosis) versus spontaneous, and with melanomas that are amelanotic or have spitzoid features on histopathology. A similar risk factor profile is found among adolescent and adult patients with melanoma, including an abnormal naevus phenotype, positive family history of melanoma, red hair and freckling [7].

Harper's Textbook of Pediatric Dermatology, Fourth Edition. Edited by Peter Hoeger, Veronica Kinsler and Albert Yan.

Among patients with congenital naevi, the risk of development of malignant melanoma was studied by systematic review; this reported an overall incidence of melanoma of 0.7% (46 patients developed melanoma among 6571 patients with congenital naevi) [8]. The risk of melanoma increases with size of congenital naevus, with the highest risk among patients with large and giant congenital naevi; among 2578 patients with large and giant congenital naevi, there was a 2% incidence of melanoma [9], which is significantly higher than previously estimated incidences. Among patients with large and giant congenital naevi with melanomas, 14% presented viscerally and 55% were fatal [9].

A systematic analysis of the literature reporting fatal or metastatic melanomas described 178 cases associated with congenital naevi (112 cutaneous and 66 central nervous system [CNS]) with mean age at diagnosis of 5.8 years for cutaneous melanoma and 5.5 years for congenital naevus-associated central nervous system melanoma [10]. The majority of fatal/metastasizing melanomas developed in small and giant congenital naevi (vs. medium and large), and 53.9% of CNS melanomas developed in patients with multiple medium congenital naevi [10]. In contrast, among patients with fatal childhood melanoma in the absence of a congenital melanocytic naevus (n = 155), the mean age at diagnosis was 13.1 years (median 14 years). The mean Breslow index in this group was 8.5 mm for children aged 0–10 years and 3.7 mm for children aged 11–18 years [10].

The presentation of Spitz melanoma is more common among children than adolescents [11]. Spitz melanomas generally harbour kinase fusions, as do atypical Spitz tumours and Spitz naevi [12].

The atypical mole syndrome, also known as familial atypical multiple mole melanoma syndrome, is associated with genetic mutations of *CDKN2A* and elevated melanoma risk. However, many of these melanomas present after childhood. In one series, two out of 147 adolescent melanoma patients in a Queensland cohort had germline *CDKN2A* mutations [7], which approximates to the frequency in adult melanoma patients [13].

Xeroderma pigmentosum is a rare autosomal recessive condition that results from inherited mutation of nucleotide excision repair genes (see Chapter 138), and this condition has a number of subtypes with a range of severity. Severe xeroderma pigmentosum involves extreme photosensitivity, with freckling of the skin and the occurrence of multiple skin cancers, including melanoma, which can appear during the teen years. Melanoma susceptibility in these patients is associated with the *XPC* and *XPD* genes [14].

Melanoma may occur as a second malignancy in children predisposed to other malignancies, as a consequence of genetic predisposition or a treatment effect. Tumours may develop in an irradiation field, or after transplantation, which may involve irradiation and probably chronic immunosuppression. The role of chemotherapy in the induction of melanoma as a second malignancy is unclear. A study of 151 575 childhood cancer survivors reported that 0.14% of survivors developed a subsequent malignant melanoma, with risk factors including radiotherapy and the use of a combination of antimitotic and alkylating chemotherapies [15]. In other large studies, the time to development of melanoma as a subsequent neoplasm was a median of 21 years, with a range of 5.6–35.4 years, so often beyond the childhood period [16].

While the prognosis for a baby born to a woman diagnosed with a melanoma during pregnancy is usually excellent, there is rare dissemination of metastasis to the placenta or fetus in pregnant patients with stage IV disease. All reported cases of fetal metastasis have been accompanied by a microscopically examined placenta demonstrating metastatic disease with villous vascular invasion [17]. Among cases with placental metastases, an estimated 25% of the babies develop melanoma metastases [18].

Additional clinical presentations of melanoma during childhood include acral melanoma, ocular melanoma, and melanoma of unknown primary; at this time there are no distinguishing features of these subtypes compared to adults with these presentations.

Clinical features and differential diagnosis. The presentation of melanoma in children does not adhere to the conventional adult 'ABCDE' criteria: asymmetry, border irregularity, colour variegation, diameter greater than or equal to 6 mm, and evolution. A series of 70 children with melanoma identified that these criteria were lacking in 60% of melanomas in children under 11 years old, and 40% of adolescents [19]. The distinct presentation of paediatric melanomas prompted modified paediatric-specific ABCDE detection criteria, to include lesions that have the following characteristics: amelanotic, bleeding, bump, colour uniformity, de novo, any diameter, in addition to those lesions that are suspicious based upon adult criteria [19] (Fig. 116.1). Additional proposed detection criteria for paediatric melanomas include the 'CUP' criteria: lesions of colour pink/red, changing, ulceration, upward thickening, pyogenic granuloma-like lesions, and pop-up of new lesions [20]. Although melanoma in childhood is quite rare, a high index of suspicion is required, and complete excisional biopsy is important to assess atypical lesions. A retrospective study of childhood melanomas at one institution found that 66% that were originally diagnosed as benign melanocytic lesions exhibited changes in size, shape and colour [21], emphasizing the importance of monitoring paediatric lesions for bleeding and evolution.

Based on the clinical features of childhood melanoma, the differential diagnosis of childhood melanoma is broad. Among pigmented lesions, the differential includes common naevi, dysplastic naevi, Spitz naevi, atypical Spitz tumours and blue naevi. Among amelanotic lesions, the differential diagnosis includes warts, pyogenic granulomas, Spitz naevi and atypical Spitz tumours. Bleeding pyogenic granulomas and warts can present a particular challenge clinically, although both have characteristic findings on biopsy and histopathology is diagnostic.

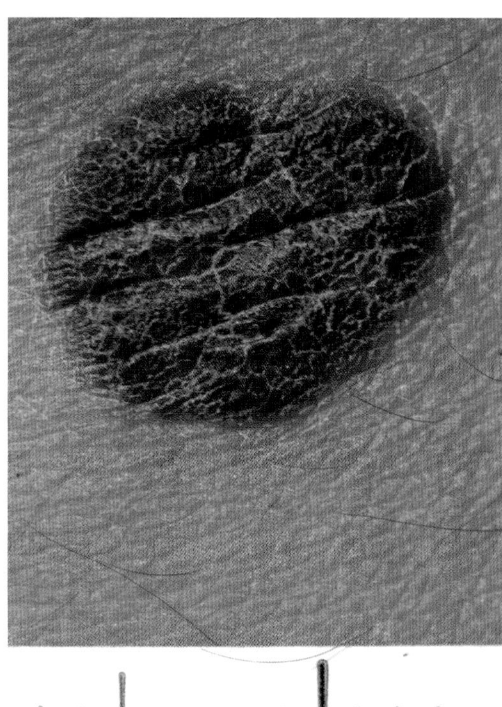

Fig. 116.1 A superficial spreading melanoma on the knee of a 3-year-old child. Source: Courtesy of Dr Newton-Bishop.

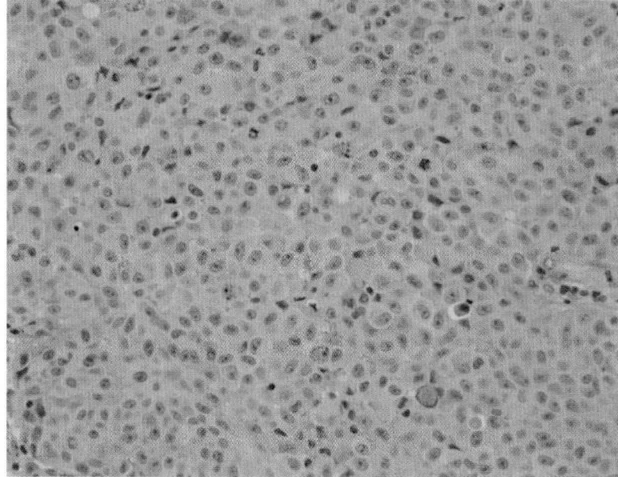

Fig. 116.2 Nodular malignant melanoma from the scalp arising in an 11-year-old girl.

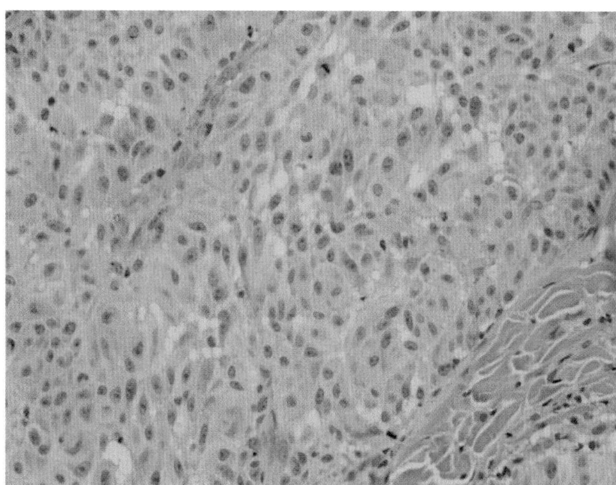

Fig. 116.3 Nodular malignant melanoma from the scalp arising in an 11-year-old girl, deeper tissue section.

In patients with congenital naevi, new growths within the lesions can also represent proliferative nodules or warts. Proliferative nodules have been shown to have atypical histopathology but more often arise from the dermis compared to melanomas arising within a congenital naevus. Further, proliferative nodules typically arise with multiple foci and, in contrast to melanomas, are infrequently ulcerated (14% of proliferative nodules vs. 100% of melanomas in one small cohort) [22].

Laboratory/histology findings. The pathological appearances of the majority of melanomas in childhood are usually those of superficial spreading or nodular melanomas [23] (Figs 116.2 and 116.3). It remains very challenging to distinguish so-called 'atypical Spitz' tumours from melanoma, and inclusion of these tumours in studies of paediatric melanoma may incorporate patients with a much better clinical outcome than patients with similar clinical stage conventional melanoma. Several studies to date have found no correlation between regional nodal involvement and aggressive disease outcome in atypical Spitz tumours [24]. In classic benign Spitz naevi (in contrast to melanoma), immunohistochemistry studies demonstrate diffuse positivity with MelanA and S100. HMB-45 usually only highlights the superficial portion of the lesion, and Ki-67 demonstrates a low proliferation index compared to malignant melanoma. P16 stain has shown characteristic staining in benign Spitz naevi and is negative in Spitz melanoma. Cytogenetic techniques demonstrate chromosome 11p amplifications in few Spitz naevi, and most exhibit a distinct mutation profile compared to common naevi and melanoma [25]. Crotty and colleagues reported the histological features they found to be most suggestive of melanoma: the presence of mitoses within 0.25 mm of the dermal margin, a dermal mitotic rate exceeding two per 1 mm^2, ulceration, surface exudate, large pigment granules and clear cell differentiation [23].

Cytogenetic approaches including comparative genomic hybridization (CGH) and fluorescence *in situ* hybridization (FISH) were initially thought to offer some promising insights to improve our understanding and diagnosis of paediatric pigmented lesions. Studies of atypical Spitz tumours of a range of clinical outcomes have demonstrated that homozygous 9p21 deletions are associated with clinically aggressive melanocytic tumours, from patients of all ages (including adults) [26], but subsequent data suggest that this is not as reliable a marker for aggressive behaviour and extranodal spread in the paediatric population [27,28]. A recent study reported that in more than 23 patients multiple copy number changes were seen on CGH and abnormal FISH assay, but only one patient in this group developed aggressive disease [29]. This and other recent studies found promising data that *TERTp* mutation may indicate aggressive behaviour [29]. Kinase fusions have been identified among benign Spitz naevi, borderline tumours and Spitz melanomas [12]. At this time, studies of cytogenetic approaches utilize largely adult tumours, and further studies are necessary to support the use of these techniques in clinical decision-making for paediatric pigmented lesions.

Treatment and prevention. The primary treatment of childhood melanoma is the same as for adult melanoma: surgical management is the first-line treatment with wide local excision to the deep fascia, and a margin depending on the thickness of melanoma and anatomical site.

A sentinel lymph node biopsy allows the identification of micrometastases and staging of melanoma in the regional lymph node basin. This technique is widely used in the management of adult invasive melanomas, for tumours over 1 mm in depth and/or those exhibiting high-risk histopathological features. Although the procedure has been performed in children, its use is controversial for childhood melanoma based upon data that suggest a higher rate of positivity in younger patients, and lack of correlation with an aggressive clinical course [30]. For atypical Spitz tumours or lesions not clearly defined as melanoma, a sentinel lymph node biopsy is not recommended, as results do not correlate with prognosis. If a sentinel lymph node biopsy is positive for melanoma, the option of observation with ultrasonography versus completion lymph node dissection is discussed, based on adult data indicating that the immediate completion lymph node dissection does not increase melanoma-specific survival [31].

For patients at higher risk for metastatic disease, adjuvant therapy is considered to improve disease-free and overall survival. Interferon alfa has been associated with prolonged disease-free and overall survival in a meta-analysis of 14 randomized trials, encompassing over 8000 patients [32]. High-dose interferon alfa is tolerated by paediatric patients [33,34]. Tumour genetic profiling may indicate *BRAF* mutation status and relevance of therapies directed at the MEK-signalling pathway. Clinical trials of immunotherapy and targeted therapies are underway in paediatric patients.

The cornerstone of melanoma prevention is modification of external risk factors, principally ultraviolet exposure. Childhood is a vital time period to establish sun-protection behaviours that can modify melanoma risk. For example, there is an increase in melanoma risk by 80% associated with sustaining five or more blistering sunburns during youth [35], and just one indoor tanning exposure is also associated with increased melanoma risk [36]. Conversely, regular sunscreen use (SPF 15 or higher) was associated with a 50% reduction in melanoma risk. Sun-protection counselling is most vital in patients with a high intrinsic melanoma risk (family history of melanoma, high-risk naevus phenotype, or red hair and freckles), and should be tailored to Fitzpatrick skin phenotype, with the goal of sunburn avoidance.

SECTION 24: NONVASCULAR SKIN TUMOURS

References

1 Spitz S. Melanomas of childhood. Am J Pathol 1948;24:591–609.
2 Austin MT, Xing Y, Hayes-Jordan AA et al. Melanoma incidence rises for children and adolescents: an epidemiologic review of pediatric melanoma in the United States. J Pediatr Surg 2013; 48:2207–13.
3 Strouse JJ, Fears TR, Tucker MA, Wayne AS. Pediatric melanoma: risk factor and survival analysis of the surveillance, epidemiology and end results database. J Clin Oncol 2005;23:4735–41.
4 Campbell LB, Kreicher KL, Gittleman HR et al. Melanoma incidence in children and adolescents: decreasing trends in the United States. J Pediatr 2015;166:1505–13.
5 Baker KS, DeFor TE, Burns LJ et al. New malignancies after blood or marrow stem-cell transplantation in children and adults: incidence and risk factors. J Clin Oncol 2003;21:1352–8.
6 Schmid-Wendtner MH, Berking C, Baumert J et al. Cutaneous melanoma in childhood and adolescence: an analysis of 36 patients. J Am Acad Dermatol 2002;46:874–9.
7 Youl P, Aitken J, Hayward N et al. Melanoma in adolescents: a case-control study of risk factors in Queensland, Australia. Int J Cancer 2002;98:92–8.
8 Krengel S, Hauschild A, Schafer T. Melanoma risk in congenital melanocytic naevi: a systematic review. Br J Dermatol 2006;155:1–8.
9 Vourc'h-Jourdain M, Martin L, Barbarot S; aRED. Large congenital melanocytic nevi: therapeutic management and melanoma risk: a systematic review. J Am Acad Dermatol 2013;68:493–8.e1–14.
10 Neuhold JC, Friesenhahn J, Gerdes N, Krengel S. Case reports of fatal or metastasizing melanoma in children and adolescents: a systematic analysis of the literature. Pediatr Dermatol 2015;32:13–22.
11 Bartenstein, DW, Kelleher CM, Friedmann AM et al. Contrasting features of childhood and adolescent melanomas. Pediatr Dermatol 2018;35:354–360.
12 Wiesner T, He J, Yelensky R et al. Kinase fusions are frequent in Spitz tumours and spitzoid melanomas. Nat Commun 2014;5:3116.
13 Begg CB, Orlow I, Hummer AJ et al.; Genes Environment and Melanoma Study Group. Lifetime risk of melanoma in CDKN2A mutation carriers in a population-based sample. J Natl Cancer Inst 2005;97:1507–15.
14 Paszkowska-Szczur K, Scott RJ, Serrano-Fernandez P et al. Xeroderma pigmentosum genes and melanoma risk. Int J Cancer 2013; 133:1094–100.
15 Braam KI, Overbeek A, Kaspers GJ et al. Malignant melanoma as second malignant neoplasm in long-term childhood cancer survivors: a systematic review. Pediatr Blood Cancer 2012;58:665–74.
16 Pappo AS, Armstrong GT, Liu W et al. Melanoma as a subsequent neoplasm in adult survivors of childhood cancer: a report from the childhood cancer survivor study. Pediatr Blood Cancer 2013;60:461–6.
17 Driscoll MS, Grant-Kels JM. Hormones, nevi, and melanoma: an approach to the patient. J Am Acad Dermatol 2007;57:919–31; quiz 932–6.
18 Baergen RN, Johnson D, Moore T, Benirschke K. Maternal melanoma metastatic to the placenta: a case report and review of the literature. Arch Pathol Lab Med 1997;121:508–11.
19 Cordoro KM, Gupta D, Frieden IJ et al. Pediatric melanoma: results of a large cohort study and proposal for modified ABCD detection criteria for children. J Am Acad Dermatol 2013;68:913–25.
20 Silverberg NB, McCuaig CC. Melanoma in childhood: changing our mind-set. Cutis 2013;92:217–18.
21 Mitkov M, Chrest M, Diehl NN et al. Pediatric melanomas often mimic benign skin lesions: A retrospective study. J Am Acad Dermatol 2016;75:706–11.
22 Yelamos O, Arva NC, Obregon R et al. A comparative study of proliferative nodules and lethal melanomas in congenital nevi from children. Am J Surg Pathol 2015;39:405–15.
23 Crotty KA, McCarthy SW, Palmer AA et al. Malignant melanoma in childhood: a clinicopathologic study of 13 cases and comparison with Spitz nevi. World J Surg 1992;16:179–85.
24 Lallas A, Kyrgidis A, Ferrara G et al. Atypical Spitz tumours and sentinel lymph node biopsy: a systematic review. Lancet Oncol 2014;15:e178–83.
25 Luo S, Sepehr A, Tsao H. Spitz nevi and other Spitzoid lesions part I. Background and diagnoses. J Am Acad Dermatol 2011;65:1073–84.
26 Gerami P, Scolyer RA, Xu X et al. Risk assessment for atypical spitzoid melanocytic neoplasms using FISH to identify chromosomal copy number aberrations. Am J Surg Pathol 2013;37:676–84.
27 Lu C, Zhang J, Nagahawatte P et al. The genomic landscape of childhood and adolescent melanoma. J Invest Dermatol 2015; 135:816–23.

28 **Massi D, Tomasini C, Senetta R et al. Atypical Spitz tumors in patients younger than 18 years. J Am Acad Dermatol 2015;72:37–46.**
29 Lee S, Barnhill RL, Dummer R et al. TERT promoter mutations are predictive of aggressive clinical behavior in patients with spitzoid melanocytic neoplasms. Sci Rep 2015;5:11200.
30 Howman-Giles R, Shaw HM, Scolyer RA et al. Sentinel lymph node biopsy in pediatric and adolescent cutaneous melanoma patients. Ann Surg Oncol 2010;17:138–43.
31 Faries, MB, Thompson JF, Cochran AJ et al. Completion dissection or observation for sentinel-node metastasis in melanoma. N Engl J Med 2017;376:2211–22.
32 Mocellin S, Pasquali S, Rossi CR, Nitti D. Interferon alpha adjuvant therapy in patients with high-risk melanoma: a systematic review and meta-analysis. J Natl Cancer Inst 2010;102:493–501.
33 Chao MM, Schwartz JL, Wechsler DS et al. High-risk surgically resected pediatric melanoma and adjuvant interferon therapy. Pediatr Blood Cancer 2005;44:441–8.
34 Navid F, Furman WL, Fleming M et al. The feasibility of adjuvant interferon alpha-2b in children with high-risk melanoma. Cancer 2005;103:780–7.
35 Wu S, Han J, Laden F, Qureshi AA. Long-term ultraviolet flux, other potential risk factors, and skin cancer risk: a cohort study. Cancer Epidemiol Biomarkers Prev 2014;23:1080–9.
36 Boniol M, Autier P, Boyle P, Gandini S. Cutaneous melanoma attributable to sunbed use: systematic review and meta-analysis. BMJ 2012;345:e4757.

CHAPTER 117
Other Malignant Skin Tumours

Andrea Bettina Cervini, Marcela Bocian, María Marta Bujan & Paola Stefano
Dermatology Department, Hospital de Pediatría 'Prof. Dr. Juan P. Garrahan', Buenos Aires, Argentina

Introduction, 1382
Rhabdomyosarcoma, 1382
Other soft tissue sarcomas, 1385
Malignant tumours of neural crest and germ cell origin, 1395
Papillary intralymphatic angioendothelioma, 1397

Abstract

Malignant tumours may arise from any of the normal structures that comprise the skin and its appendages. Moreover, the skin is frequently the site of metastases of internal malignancies and provides clues for prompt diagnosis of these processes in affected patients. Malignant soft tissue masses in children include the soft tissue sarcomas (STS) and other tumours of neural crest, germ cell or vascular origin.

STS in children and adolescents are rare, constituting about 8% of all cancer cases. Furthermore, they may have clinical and imaging features that overlap with more common benign and reactive processes. Rhabdomyosarcoma is the most common paediatric STS and accounts for more than 50%; the rest are included in the group of non-rhabdomyosarcoma soft tissue sarcomas (NRSTS). These tumours usually present as a painless enlarging mass or with symptoms of compression and/or infiltration of adjacent organs or structures. Many of them have characteristic chromosomal abnormalities.

Treatment of paediatric STS and other malignant tumours often involves surgery, chemotherapy and radiation (as needed) and the outcome depends on whether wide local excision with negative margins is possible.

Key points

- Soft tissue sarcomas (STS) and other malignant skin tumours are relatively rare in children and present as painless masses.
- STS have many differential diagnoses as their clinical and imaging features overlap with benign tumours, reactive processes and other malignant tumours.
- Rhabdomyosarcoma (RMS) is the most common STS in children under 15 years old.
- Infantile fibrosarcoma is the second most common STS (after RMS) in children under 1 year of age.
- Many STS and other malignant tumours of soft tissue have characteristic chromosomal abnormalities.
- The treatment of sarcomas comprises a multimodal approach that includes surgery, chemotherapy and/or radiation therapy.
- Infantile choriocarcinoma is a very rare tumour that develops in the first 6 months of life. It is a complication of gestational choriocarcinoma.
- Neuroblastoma is the most common extracranial malignant tumour of children under 4 years of age.
- Dermatofibrosarcoma protuberans (DFSP) is a rare cutaneous tumour of fibrohistiocytic origin characterized by intermediate malignancy and locally aggressive growth with frequent local recurrence but rare distant metastases.

Introduction

Malignant tumours are rarely seen in infancy but they deserve careful attention as they can lead to significant morbidity and mortality. Accurate and early diagnosis can result in a good prognosis, as better therapeutic options have improved the ominous outcomes that were observed in the past.

Malignant tumours may arise from any of the normal structures that comprise the skin and its appendages. Moreover, the skin is frequently the site of metastasis of internal malignancies and provides clues for prompt diagnosis of these processes in affected patients. Dermatologists and paediatricians must consider these malignant skin tumours in their differential diagnoses. This chapter provides the relevant information for accurate diagnosis and discusses the main types of therapy, from a multidisciplinary approach.

Rhabdomyosarcoma

Definition and epidemiology. Rhabdomyosarcoma (RMS) is a primary malignancy in children and adolescents that arises from embryonic mesenchymal striated precursor muscle. It is the most common soft tissue sarcoma (STS) of childhood and adolescence and represents 7–8% of all malignant tumours of childhood. Around 65% of the

Harper's Textbook of Pediatric Dermatology, Fourth Edition. Edited by Peter Hoeger, Veronica Kinsler and Albert Yan.

cases appear in children under 6 years of age. The ratio of males to females is 1.3–1.5 : 1. Primary cutaneous presentation is extremely unusual. Cutaneous metastasis of RMS, although rare, may be the first manifestation of the disease. Approximately 15% of children with RMS present with metastatic disease and their prognosis has not improved significantly over the last 15 years, despite changes in therapy [1,2].

Aetiology and pathogenesis. Most cases of RMS occur sporadically with no recognized predisposing factor. For patients with embryonal tumours, high birthweight and large size for gestational age are associated with an increased incidence of RMS. Genetic conditions associated with RMS include Li–Fraumeni cancer susceptibility syndrome (with germline *p53* mutations), pleuropulmonary blastoma (with *DICER1* mutations), neurofibromatosis type I, Costello syndrome (with germline *HRAS* mutations), Beckwith–Wiedemann syndrome (with which Wilms tumour and hepatoblastoma are more commonly associated) and Noonan syndrome.

RMS in paediatric patients is predominantly of the alveolar or embryonal histological subtypes.

Alveolar RMS often has chromosomal translocations resulting in fusions between either the *PAX3* gene on chromosome 2 (t(2; 13) (q35; q14)) or the *PAX7* gene on chromosome 1 (t(1; 13) (p36; q14)) and the *FOXO1* gene on chromosome 13. Translocations involving the *PAX3* gene occur in approximately 59% of alveolar RMS cases, while the *PAX7* gene appears to be involved in about 19% of cases. Around 22% of cases with alveolar histology have no detectable PAX gene translocation.

PAX–FOXO1 fusion status appears to be relevant to clinical outcome. Fusion-positive alveolar RMS has a more aggressive course than fusion-negative disease, and more frequently has metastases at presentation and a poorer event-free survival. Fusion-negative alveolar RMS may have a clinical course similar to that of embryonal RMS. Alveolar RMS associated with *PAX7–FOXO1* fusions, with or without metastases, appears to occur in patients at a younger age, and may be associated with longer event-free survival rates than those associated with *PAX3–FOXO1* gene rearrangements. In addition to *FOXO1* rearrangements, alveolar tumours are characterized by a lower mutational burden than fusion-negative tumours, with fewer genes having recurring mutations. *BCOR* and *PIK3CA* mutations and amplification of *MYCN*, *MIR17HG* and *CDK4* have also been described [1–7].

Embryonal RMS do not carry *PAX–FOXO1* fusions, but often show loss of heterozygosity at 11p15 and gains on chromosome 8 [6].

Rearrangement of the *NCOA2* (nuclear receptor coactivator 2) gene has been identified in paediatric cases of spindle cell RMS, but not in adult cases. In older children and adults with spindle cell/sclerosing RMS, a specific *MYOD1* mutation (p.L122R) has been observed in a large proportion of patients. The presence of the *MYOD1* mutation is associated with an increased risk of treatment failure [7].

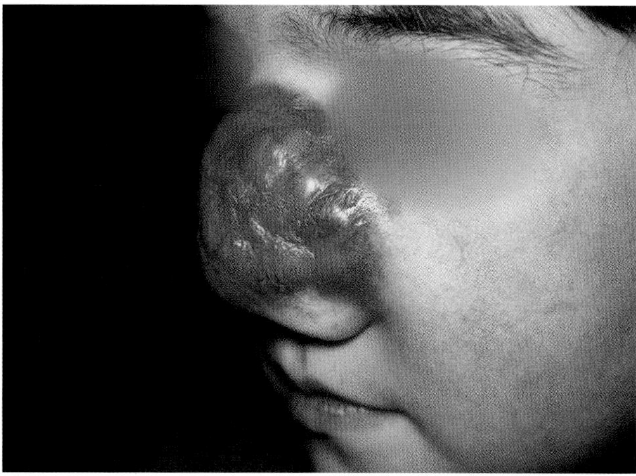

Fig. 117.1 Primary cutaneous rhabdomyosarcoma: bright red solid tumour infiltrating the nasal skin tissue.

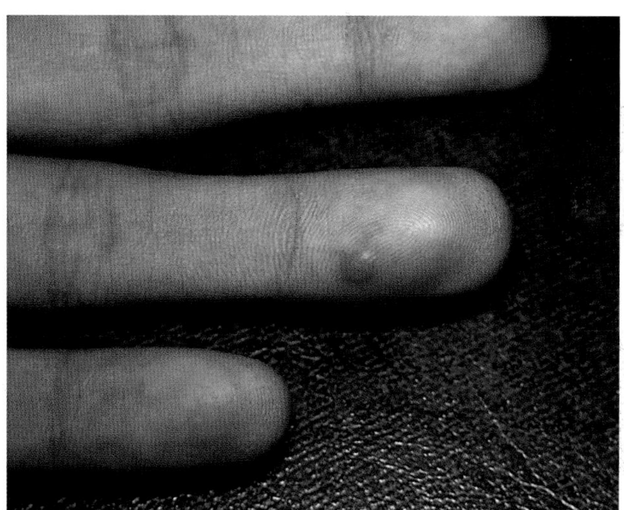

Fig. 117.2 Recurrent metastatic rhabdomyosarcoma presenting as a small firm purple nodule.

Clinical features. The clinical presentation of RMS will depend on the site of origin of the primary tumour, the age of the patient and the presence or absence of metastatic disease. The majority of symptoms will be related to compression of local structures and occasionally mild pain. There are no classic paraneoplastic syndromes associated with RMS. The most common sites in children are the head and neck region and the genitourinary tract, with only 20% involving the extremities (Figs 117.1 and 117.2).

The disease can arise at any site and in any tissue in the body except bone. Primary cutaneous RMS develops mainly on the face as subcutaneous or protruding exophytic masses. Orbital tumours produce proptosis and occasionally ophthalmoplegia. Those arising from parameningeal sites often produce nasal, ear or sinus obstruction with or without a mucopurulent or sanguineous discharge. Parameningeal tumours may extend into the cranium with resultant cranial nerve palsy and meningeal symptoms. When RMS is located on the trunk or

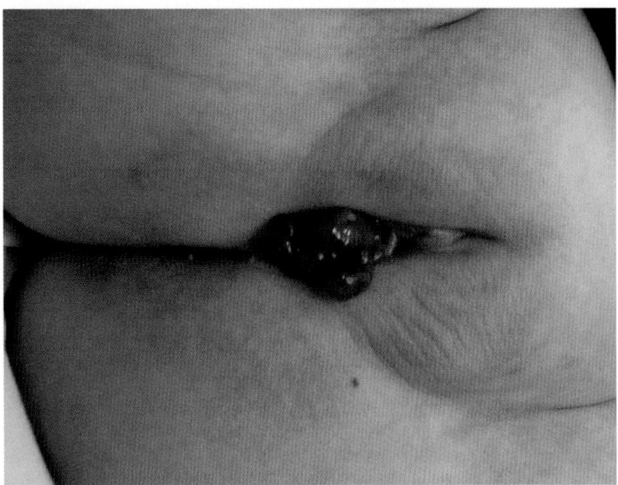

Fig. 117.3 Botryoid rhabdomyosarcoma in a 2-year-old girl.

limbs it is usually first noticed as a haematoma following trauma. The swelling persists or increases, and malignancy must be suspected. Vaginal tumours tend to occur in very young girls and present with a mass or vaginal bleeding and discharge (Fig. 117.3). Congenital alveolar RMS is a rare variant, characterized by multiple cutaneous metastases and aggressive behaviour leading to early death [1,5].

Pathology. RMS belongs to the group of 'small round cell tumours'. Its myogenic origin can be ascertained by immunohistochemical studies positive for muscle: actin, myogenin, desmin, vimentin, Myo D and Myo F4. There are four major histological subtypes:

- Embryonal: the most common form in children.
  - Botryoid: a variant of the embryonal type in which tumour cells and an oedematous stroma protrude into a body cavity (e.g. vagina, ear, nasopharynx).
- Alveolar: consists of cleft-like spaces between solid sheets of small cells resembling alveoli.
- Spindle cell/sclerosing rhabdomyosarcoma: composed of spindle-shaped, polygonal or round tumour cells with minimal cytoplasm embedded within a densely sclerotic stroma; dyshesion between tumour cells may result in a pseudovesicular growth pattern.
- Pleomorphic: this variant is present during adult life. It is rare in childhood and may also go by the name of anaplastic RMS [1,2,6,7].

Diagnosis. The diagnosis of RMS is usually made by direct open biopsy. There are no helpful serum markers.

Patients with RMS require a complete work-up before definitive surgery: history/physical examination (height and weight); measuring of the lesion (physical or imaging); complete blood count, bone marrow biopsy and aspirate; chest X-ray; magnetic resonance imaging (MRI) or computed tomography (CT) of primary site; CT of chest; bone scan; cerebral spinal fluid cytology (for parameningeal lesions); and electrocardiogram (ECG) or echocardiogram (selective) [1].

Differential diagnosis. Depending on the clinical appearance, RMS must be differentiated from haemolymphangioma, haemangioma, neuroblastoma, other soft tissue sarcomas and haematoma [2].

Treatment. The treatment is based on clinical staging according to primary tumour location, disease extension and molecular biology.

In group I tumours (localized disease) complete surgical excision is followed by chemotherapy. In group II (total gross resection with evidence of regional spread) and group III tumours (incomplete resection with gross residual disease) surgery is followed by local irradiation and multiple chemotherapy. In group IV tumours (distant metastatic disease present at onset), systemic chemotherapy and irradiation are the best choices of treatment [1,2,8].

Prognosis. Rapid diagnosis and recognition of RMS aids long-term survival. Currently, localized RMS has an overall survival of 70%. In contrast, the overall survival is generally less than 30% for patients with metastases at the time of diagnosis. Depending on the age of the patient at the time of diagnosis, the histological type and the primary location, the tumour is classified into low, medium or high risk. Indicators of a poor prognosis are age (under 1 or over 10 years of age), the alveolar histological type, size larger than 5 cm and primary location in the limbs [1,2,9]. Fusion-negative alveolar RMS have a better prognosis than fusion-positive tumours. However, among the fusion-positive alveolar RMS, preliminary data indicate that the type of chromosomal fusion may also predict outcome, with *PAX7–FOX01*-positive tumours having a more favourable overall survival than *PAX3–FOX01*-positive ones [10].

The prognosis of spindle cell RMS in adults is worse than in children, and recent insights into the genetics of this tumour suggest that there may be underlying genetic differences between paediatric and adult cases.

References

1 **Hayes-Jordan A, Andrassy R. Rhabdomyosarcoma in children. Curr Opin Pediatr 2009;21:373–8.**

2 Lanoel A, Fain A, Cervini AB et al. Rhabdomyosarcoma with cutaneous presentation. Eur J Pediatr Dermatol 2009;19:8–14.

3 Lampe AK, Seymour G, Thompson PW et al. Familial neurofibromatosis microdeletion syndrome complicated by rhabdomyosarcoma. Arch Dis Child 2002;87:444–5.

4 Hoang MP, Sinkre P, Albores-Saavedra J. Rhabdomyosarcoma arising in a congenital melanocytic nevus. Am J Dermatopathol 2002;24:26–9.

5 Grundy R, Anderson J, Gaze M et al. Congenital alveolar rhabdomyosarcoma: clinical and molecular distinction from alveolar rhabdomyosarcoma in older children. Cancer 2001;91:606–12.

6 **Fletcher C, Unni K, Mertens F (eds). World Health Organization Classification of Tumours. Pathology and Genetics of Tumours of Soft Tissue and Bone, 3rd edn. Lyon, France: IARC Press, 2002.**

7 **Doyle LA. Sarcoma classification: An update based on the 2013 World Health Organization Classification of Tumours of Soft Tissue and Bone. Cancer 2014;120:1763–74.**

8 Arndt CA, Hawkins DS, Meyer WH et al. Comparison of results of a pilot study of alternating vincristine/doxorubicin/cyclophosphamide and etoposide/ ifosfamide with IRS-IV in intermediate risk rhabdomyosarcoma: a report from the Children's Oncology Group. Pediatr Blood Cancer 2008;50:33–6.

9 Meza JL, Anderson J, Pappo AS, Meyer WH; Children's Oncology Group. Analysis of prognostic factors in patients with nonmetastatic rhabdomyosarcoma treated on intergroup rhabdomyosarcoma studies III and IV: The Children's Oncology Group. J Clin Oncol 2006;24:3844–51.
10 Skapek SX, Anderson J, Barr FG et al. PAX-FOXO1 fusion status drives unfavourable outcome for children with rhabdomyosarcoma: A children's oncology group report. Pediatr Blood Cancer 2013;60:1411–17.

Other soft tissue sarcomas

The non-RMS soft tissue sarcomas include tumours of different origins which are extremely rare in childhood. They can occur as primary tumours of the skin or be metastatic from other locations. Depending on the tissue type involved, it is possible to observe the following:

- liposarcoma
- fibrosarcoma
- epithelioid sarcoma
- angiosarcoma
- cutaneous Ewing sarcoma
- synovial sarcoma
- alveolar soft part sarcoma
- leiomyosarcoma
- dermatofibrosarcoma protuberans
- haemangiopericytoma/solitary fibrous tumour.

Liposarcoma

Definition and epidemiology. Liposarcoma is a rare malignant soft tissue tumour derived from the primitive mesenchymal tissue that undergoes adipose differentiation; it was first described by Virchow in 1890 [1].

Liposarcoma is predominantly a disease of adulthood and commonly occurs between 40 and 60 years of age. It is rare in paediatric patients, representing about 2–5% of all childhood soft tissue sarcomas, with a peak incidence occurring in the second decade of life [2].

In 2013, the World Health Organization (WHO) described four different histopathological subtypes of liposarcoma: atypical lipomatous tumour (previously known as well-differentiated liposarcoma), dedifferentiated liposarcoma, myxoid liposarcoma and pleomorphic liposarcoma [3]. These four main subgroups are characterized by distinctive morphologies, as well as unique genetic findings. In the paediatric population, myxoid liposarcoma is the most common subtype.

Aetiology and pathogenesis. Myxoid liposarcoma is characterized by two main karyotypic aberrations: more than 95% of cases carry a specific translocation t(12; 16)(q13;p11), which fuses the *DDIT3* (CHOP) gene on 12q13 with the *FUS* (TLS) gene on 16p11; the latter plays an important role in oncogenesis. Approximately, 5% of myxoid liposarcomas harbour a t(12;22)(q13;q12), which fuses *DDIT3* with *EWSR1* on 22q12.

Atypical lipomatous tumour (previously well-differentiated liposarcoma) has giant and ring chromosomes that are derived from chromosome 12 and can result in amplification of the 12q13–15 region [4].

Another common finding is amplification of the *MDM2* gene in well-differentiated and dedifferentiated liposarcomas. However, these histopathological subtypes are extremely rare in younger patients.

Amplifications of *MDM2* and alterations of *TP53* have been found in approximately 30–40% of pleomorphic liposarcomas [5].

Clinical features. Clinically, cutaneous liposarcoma appears as a painless, slowly growing, dome-shaped or polypoid mass, and measures between 1 and 20 cm. The majority of patients have tumours bigger than 5 cm at initial presentation (73%) [6]. Tumours limited to the dermis or subcutis can recur, but they do not metastasize or cause the patient's death.

The prognosis depends on the location, degree of differentiation and histopathological subtype. Myxoid liposarcoma usually occurs in extremities (71%) and has an excellent prognosis. Pleomorphic liposarcoma occurs in axial sites (57%) but can also arise in the retroperitoneum and/or in other viscera [7].

Pathology. Microscopically, well-differentiated liposarcoma is composed of a variable percentage of mature adipose tissue, transected by irregular fibrous bands containing enlarged, hyperchromatic stromal cells and occasional lipoblasts.

Myxoid liposarcoma resembles immature fat tissue and can be histologically indistinguishable from a lipoblastoma. Small and uniformly bland spindle cells are set in a myxoid matrix with plexiform vessels.

Pleomorphic liposarcoma is the least common subtype; it exhibits an extreme degree of nuclear pleomorphism and resembles a malignant fibrous histiocytoma.

Dedifferentiated liposarcoma is a biphasic tumour comprised of areas of well-differentiated liposarcoma/atypical lipomatous tumour and areas of nonlipogenic sarcoma [8,9].

Differential diagnosis. The differential diagnosis of liposarcoma is the lipoblastoma, which occurs more frequently in childhood (90% in children younger than 3 years old). Histologically, lipoblastoma consists of fat cells in a spectrum of maturation arranged in a lobulated pattern and separated by loose fibrous connective tissue. Peripherally, spindle-shaped tumour cells can be found. These histological features may also show a striking similarity to myxoid liposarcoma [2,9].

Treatment. As in other soft tissue sarcomas, wide local excision remains the preferred approach for local control of primary disease. It is not uncommon for liposarcomas to have a multinodular growth pattern and extend into muscle and fascial planes. Excision needs to be carefully planned using MRI and X-ray information. Adjuvant radiation therapy is effective at controlling microscopic residual disease after surgical resection. Myxoid tumours are radiosensitive, and preoperative, intraoperative and/or postoperative radiotherapy has been effective when complete resection is not possible. The use of chemotherapy for treatment of liposarcoma is controversial in paediatric patients [5].

References

1 Dadone B, Refae S, Lemarié-Delaunay C et al. Molecular cytogenetics of paediatric adipocytic tumours. Cancer Genet 2015;208:469–81.
2 Marcio F, Filho J, Temer Cursino S et al. Liposarcoma periorbital em paciente pediátrico: relato de caso. Arch Bras Oftalmol 2013;76:244–6.
3 Fletcher CDM, Bridge JA, Hogendoorn PCW et al. WHO classification of Tumours of Soft Tissue and Bone, 4th edn. Lyon, France: IARC Press, 2013.
4 Dei Tos A. Liposarcomas: diagnostic pitfalls and new insights. Histopathology 2014;64:38–52.
5 Huh WW, Yuen C, Mensell M et al. Liposarcoma in children and young adults: a multi-institutional experience. Pediatr Blood Cancer 2011;57:1142–6.
6 Kaddu S, Kohler S. Muscle, adipose and cartilage neoplasms. In: Bolognia JL, Jorizzo JL, Schaffer JV (eds) Dermatology, 3rd edn. Edinburgh: Mosby Elsevier, 2012:1979–91.
7 Buehler D, Marburger T, Billings S. Primary subcutaneous myxoid liposarcoma: a clinicopathologic review of three cases with molecular confirmation and discussion of the differential diagnosis. J Cutan Pathol 2014;41:907–15.
8 Boland J, Folpe A. The impact of advances in molecular genetics on the classification and diagnosis of liposarcoma. Diagn Histopathol 2012;17:348–54.
9 Goldblum JR, Folpe AL, Weiss SW. Liposarcoma. In: Weiss SW (ed.) Enzinger and Weiss's Soft Tissue Tumours, 6th edn. Philadelphia: Mosby Elsevier, 2014:484–93.

Fibrosarcoma

Definition and epidemiology. Infantile fibrosarcoma is a rare soft tissue sarcoma arising at birth or in early infancy. It comprises less than 1% of all childhood tumours and approximately 10% of all sarcomas. Congenital infantile fibrosarcoma is defined as a tumour occurring within 3 months after birth and is the most common soft tissue sarcoma in children younger than 1 year old.

Currently, the WHO Classification includes infantile fibrosarcoma as a tumour of intermediate malignancy (rarely metastasizing) [1]. It is a borderline malignancy and has a more favourable prognosis than its adult counterpart. Infantile fibrosarcomas frequently recur locally but they have a relatively good prognosis and only rarely metastasize, the lung being the preferential site [2,3].

Clinical features. The tumour arises in the extremities in 70% of cases, where it forms a hard irregular mass covered by normal, erythematous or purplish skin. The infantile form primarily affects the distal extremities, especially the ankle, foot and hand, followed by the head and neck and then the trunk [4]. As it increases in size, ulceration and bleeding appear on the surface [3,5].

Pathology. Fibrosarcoma is a tumour that presents many difficulties for histological diagnosis. The pattern of spindle-shaped cells, with a tendency to be arranged in fascicles or interlacing bands (herringbone pattern), is strongly suggestive of the diagnosis. Mitotic figures are common. Immunohistochemically, the tumour is made up of spindle cells that stain for vimentin and variable smooth muscle actin (SMA) and is negative for other lineage markers (pancytokeratin, epithelial membrane antigen [EMA], desmin, HHF35, myogenin, MYOD1, CD34 and S100 protein) [6,7].

Cytogenetic studies of infantile fibrosarcomas have shown characteristic trisomies of chromosomes 8, 11, 17 and 20. The *ETV6*–neurotropic tyrosine receptor kinase 3 (*NTRK3*) gene fusion is unique to congenital infantile fibrosarcoma as a result of the translocation t(12,15)(p13;q25) and can be used to confirm the diagnosis [8]. Although *ETV6–NTRK3* is a specific transcript, it is not always observed and diagnosis is sometimes difficult [9]. This chromosomal translocation and fusion protein are characteristic of infantile fibrosarcoma, but also occur in congenital mesoblastic nephroma and in some leukaemias and breast cancers. However, it has not been found in adult fibrosarcoma [2–5,8,9].

Differential diagnosis. Infantile fibrosarcoma is often mistaken for haemangioma and other infantile vascular tumours. Other differential diagnoses include congenital fibromatosis, myofibromatosis, desmoid tumour, haemangiopericytoma and rhabdomyosarcoma [3,4,10].

Treatment. Standard treatment of infantile fibrosarcoma has been primarily surgical, with wide local excision. Histologically, free margins are the goal, without additional radiation and chemotherapy. However, a number of factors can make primary complete resection difficult, such as the tendency of these tumours to surround and invade neurovascular bundles and replace muscle groups. Moreover, bleeding and coagulopathy can accompany the tumour.

Because of the low potential for distant metastasis and the high long-term survival rates, limb-sparing procedures should be attempted in all cases.

Infantile fibrosarcomas can be chemosensitive. Several chemotherapy approaches have been used as a preoperative adjuvant treatment to decrease the mass of the tumour before resection and in management of unresectable cases [2–5,9]. However, because of the rarity of infantile fibrosarcoma and the young age of affected infants, treatment guidelines are not strictly defined [9,10].

Prognosis. Infantile fibrosarcoma has an excellent prognosis with an 80–90% overall survival rate at 5 years, in contrast to the poorer prognosis in adolescent/adult fibrosarcoma [10]. There is a local recurrence rate of 17–40% following resection with low capacity for metastasis [11,12].

References

1 Doyle L. Sarcoma classification: an update based on the 2013 World Health Organization Classification of Tumours of Soft Tissue and Bone. Cancer 2014;120:1763–74.
2 DeComas AM, Heinrich SD, Craver R. Infantile fibrosarcoma successfully treated with chemotherapy, with occurrence of calcifying aponeurotic fibroma and pleomorphic/spindled celled lipoma at the site 12 years later. J Pediatr Hematol Oncol 2009;31:448–52.
3 Gülhan B, Küpeli S, Yalçin B et al. An unusual presentation of infantile fibrosarcoma in a male newborn. Am J Perinatol 2009;26:331–3.
4 Yan AC, Chamlin SL, Liang MG et al. Congenital infantile fibrosarcoma: a masquerader of ulcerated haemangioma. Pediatr Dermatol 2006;23:330–4.

5 Russell H, Hicks MJ, Bertuch AA et al. Infantile fibrosarcoma: clinical and histologic responses to cytotoxic chemotherapy. Pediatr Blood Cancer 2009;53:23–7.
6 Bellfield EJ, Beets-Shay L. Congenital infantile fibrosarcoma of the lip. Pediatr Dermatol 2014;31:88–9.
7 Tannenbaum-Dvir S, Glade Bender JL, Church AJ et al. Characterization of a novel fusion gene EML4-NTRK3 in a case of recurrent congenital fibrosarcoma. Cold Spring Harb Mol Cas Stud 2015;1:a000471.
8 Kerl K, Nowacki M, Leuschner I. Infantile fibrosarcoma – an important differential diagnosis of congenital vascular tumours. Pediatr Hematol Oncol 2012;29:545–8.
9 Yanagisawa R, Noguchi M, Fujita K et al. Preoperative treatment with pazopanib in a case of chemotherapy-resistant infantile fibrosarcoma. Pediatr Blood Cancer 2016;63:348–51.
10 Thacker MM. Malignant soft tissue tumours in children. Orthop Clin North Am 2013;44:657–67.
11 Farmackis SG, Herman TE, Siegel MJ. Congenital infantile fibrosarcoma. J Perinatol 2014;34:329–30.
12 Hayes-Jordan A. Recent advances in non-rhabdomyosarcoma soft-tissue sarcomas. Semin Pediatr Surg 2012;21:61–7.

Epithelioid sarcoma

Definition and epidemiology. Epithelioid sarcoma (ES) was first described by Enzinger in 1970 [1–4]. It is a rare soft tissue sarcoma, representing less than 1% of soft tissue sarcomas. It usually presents itself as a subcutaneous or deep dermal mass, most often involving the distal extremities of adolescents and young adults, with a median age of 26 years [1,2,5–7]. The tumour is approximately twice as common in males as it is in females [2].

Aetiology and pathogenesis. The origin of ES remains controversial. An analysis of the immunohistochemical pattern of both epithelial and mesenchymal markers led to the conclusion that ES is a mesenchymal tumour capable of partial epithelial transformation [4].

Cytogenetic studies of ES show principally nonspecific chromosomal gain and loss. However, loss of 22q11, the location of the *SMARCB1* gene, has been reported in few cases [2,6].

Clinical features. Two different categories of epithelioid sarcoma are described in the literature: 'classical or distal', and 'proximal' type [3].

Classic ES is often present as a small, indurated, sometimes ulcerated nodule which usually affects distal extremities of adolescents and young adults [2,4]. It most commonly involves the hands and fingers, followed by the wrists, lower arms, legs and knees, but may occur in any location. Involvement of tendons and aponeuroses is common but not invariably present. On some occasions, it has been present for several weeks or longer before coming to clinical attention.

Proximal-type ES tends to occur in older adults, most often involving the deep soft tissues of the perineum, genital region and pelvis. It typically presents as much larger masses than classic ES [2]. This variant differs from the classic form of ES in that it frequently occurs in older patients, in a proximal/axial often deep location, and it is more aggressive [1,6].

ES recurs in over 70% of cases and nearly 50% metastasize even after wide excision. The tumour metastasizes through lymphatic and blood vessels to regional lymph nodes, skin, lungs, heart, pleura, liver, pericardium, bone and soft tissue of other parts of the body. The lungs are the most common site of distant metastases [2–6].

Pathology. Histologically, the classic or distal variant consists of a subcutaneous or deeper nodular proliferation of rounded to plump cells with abundant eosinophilic cytoplasm palisading around areas of necrosis; such a pattern is termed 'pseudogranulomatous' (proliferation of cells around a necrotic zone) [1,5]. The proximal variant is characterized by a proliferation of epithelioid cells with rhabdoid features in the absence of a granuloma-like pattern [4,6].

Both variants of ES exhibit immunohistochemical reactivity for cytokeratin 5/6 (CK) and EMA and vimentin. S100 and CD31 are negative, while desmin and CD34 are positive in some cases [1–6].

Differential diagnosis. Clinically, classic ES should be considered in the differential diagnosis of chronic nodules, erythema nodosum, haematomas, infectious nodules, etc. [5,8]. Proximal ES of the genital area could be misdiagnosed as a benign lesion such as infectious granuloma, Bartholin cyst, fibroma, lipoma, dermoid cyst, fibrous histiocytoma, viral wart or squamous cell carcinoma [3].

Histopathological differential diagnoses include, among others, granuloma annulare, necrobiosis lipoidica, fibrous histiocytoma, nodular fasciitis, melanoma, clear-cell sarcoma of the tendon and aponeurosis, metastatic carcinoma, angiosarcoma, synovial sarcoma, epithelioid haemangioendothelioma, epithelioid leiomyosarcoma and malignant extrarenal rhabdoid tumour of the soft tissue [1,4,5].

Treatment. Surgery is the gold standard method of treatment [3,4]. Adequate treatment requires radical excision with extensive lymph node dissection. Any benefit of radiotherapy and/or chemotherapy in preventing recurrence or for palliative treatment has not been demonstrated and it is controversial [3,4].

Older age, male sex, proximal or axial location, deep location, tumour size, mitotic figures, necrosis, vascular invasion, tumour haemorrhage, local recurrence, nodal metastases and the extent of surgery were identified as adverse prognostic factors [2,4].

References

1 Santos LM, Nogueira L, Matsuo CY et al. Proximal-type epithelioid sarcoma – case report. An Bras Dermatol 2013;88:444–7.
2 Folpe A. Selected topics in the pathology of epithelioid soft tissue tumors. Mod Pathol 2014;27: 64–79.
3 Patrizi L, Corrado G, Saltari M et al. Vulvar "proximal-type" epithelioid sarcoma: report of a case and review of the literature. Diagn Pathol 2013;8:122.
4 Al-Salam S, Al Ashari M. Epithelioid sarcoma in a child presenting as a submandibular mass. Afr Health Sci 2010;10:400–4.
5 Akpinar F, Dervis E, Demirkesen C et al. Epithelioid sarcoma of the extremities. Indian J Dermatol Venereol Leprol 2014;80:168–70.
6 Lynch MC, Graber EM, Johnson TS et al. Epithelioid sarcoma resembling benign fibrous histiocytoma. Cutis 2015;95:83–6.

SECTION 24: NONVASCULAR SKIN TUMOURS

7 Hernández-Bel P, Marín S, Soler S et al. Epithelioid sarcoma: report of 3 cases. Cutis 2014;93:8–9.
8 Niimi R, Matsumine A, Kusuzaki K et al. Soft-tissue sarcoma mimicking large haematoma: a report of two cases and review of the literature. J Orthop Surg 2006;14:90–5.

Angiosarcoma

Definition and epidemiology. Angiosarcoma is a rare malignant neoplasm, comprising only 1% of all soft tissue sarcomas [1–3]. It is an aggressive malignant tumour of endothelial cells of vascular or lymphatic origin [4–7].

Cutaneous angiosarcoma is the most common presentation of this malignancy with one third of angiosarcomas occurring in the skin. This is typically a tumour of older individuals, with a median age of 70–75 years, having a predilection for the scalp and central area of the face [2,3,8]. Angiosarcoma has a higher incidence among Caucasians and males [3,4,9].

Aetiology and pathogenesis. The aetiology of cutaneous angiosarcoma is unclear and no comprehensive studies of molecular changes in angiosarcoma have been published.

Angiosarcoma may be related to previous exposure to chemicals (vinyl chloride, thorium dioxide, arsenic, radium and anabolic steroids), ionizing radiation, vascular insufficiency, chronic lymphoedema, sunlight and trauma [2–4,6–9]. In many cases, however, the exact cause is unknown [2].

Clinical features. Although the tumour can occur in any location, the most common sites are the scalp and face [1–3,9,10]. The initial presentation can be subtle, often resembling a bruise or a raised purplish-red papule. With increasing tumour size, tissue infiltration, oedema, ulceration and haemorrhage can develop. Deeper soft tissue and visceral lesions present as an expanding painful mass. The lesions can reach sizes of 20 cm or more [2,3,7–9]. The neoplasm tends to invade tissue more widely, expanding with gradual centrifugal infiltration. Angiosarcoma is a rapidly progressing tumour that can spread not only to nearby lymph nodes, but also metastasize through the blood to the lungs, liver, bone and other locations. As angiosarcoma is an extremely aggressive lesion, most patients present with locally advanced disease, regional lymph node involvement or distant metastases at the time of initial diagnosis, all of which are associated with a poor prognosis [2–4,7,8]. Late local and distant recurrences are possible years after local control, and most patients ultimately die secondary to disseminated disease [8].

Pathology. Angiosarcoma can show a wide spectrum of histological differentiation, from a well-differentiated neoplasm with anastomosing vascular channels lined by atypical endothelial cells with low mitotic activity to poorly differentiated tumours without prominent vasoformative activity, composed of solid sheets of epithelial-like or spindle cells [2–4,9].

Immunohistochemical markers include von Willebrand factor, CD34, CD31, *Ulex europaeus* agglutinin 1, vascular endothelial growth factor (VEGF) and factor VIII antigen [2–4,7,8].

Differential diagnosis. The clinical differential diagnoses include pyogenic granuloma, haemangioma, haemangioendothelioma, Kaposi sarcoma, squamous cell carcinoma and haematoma [2,3].

Treatment. Angiosarcoma tends to be aggressive and its prognosis is very poor, with a 5-year survival rate of only 12–33% [2–4,7,10].

Important prognostic factors are: extent of primary tumour, tumour size over 5 cm, the presence of cutaneous satellite lesions, resection status, histological tumour differentiation and metastases [1–5].

Treatment options vary depending on medical findings such as the presence of metastases and the patient's condition. The treatment of choice for cutaneous angiosarcoma is surgical excision followed by external beam radiotherapy [1,2,4,5,7–10]. Despite aggressive locoregional therapy, many patients progress to disseminated disease. If surgical excision is not possible, no standard treatment is documented. Palliative chemotherapy and radiotherapy, alone or combined, have been used with varying results [9]. Emerging data suggest a role for targeted therapy with agents directed at the VEGF receptor, including bevacizumab and the broad-spectrum tyrosine kinase inhibitor sorafenib [7,8].

References

1 Guadagnolo BA, Zagars GK, Araujo D et al. Outcomes after definitive treatment for cutaneous angiosarcoma of the face and scalp. Head Neck 2011;33:661–7.
2 Tenjarla S, Sheils LA, Kwiatkowski TM et al. Cutaneous angiosarcoma of the foot: a case report and review of the literature. Case Rep Oncol Med 2014;2014:1–5.
3 Fomete B, Samaila M, Edaigbini S et al. Primary oral soft tissue angiosarcoma of the cheek: a case report and literature review. J Korean Assoc Oral Maxillofac Surg 2015;41:273–7.
4 Huang X, Sun S. Primary eyelid angiosarcoma in a Chinese patient. Int J Clin Exp Pathol 2015;8:8636–8.
5 Gründahl JE, Hallermann C, Schulze HJ et al. Cutaneous angiosarcoma of head and neck: a new predictive score of locoregional metastasis. Transl Oncol 2015;8:169–75.
6 Olson MT, Puttgen KB, Westra WH. Angiosarcoma arising from the tongue of an 11-year-old girl with xeroderma pigmentosum. Head Neck Pathol 2012;6:255–7.
7 Young RJ, Brown NJ, Reed MW et al. Angiosarcoma. Lancet Oncol 2010;11:983–91.
8 Dossett LA, Harrington M, Cruse CW et al. Cutaneous angiosarcoma. Curr Probl Cancer 2015;39:258–63.
9 Shetty M, Bhat R, Kodan P. Cutaneous angiosarcoma – a rare case report in Indian female! J Clin Diagn Res 2015;9:12–13.
10 Kulyapina A, Salmeron Escobar JI. Infraorbital cutaneous angiosarcoma: successful surgical management applying Mitek anchorage system. J Cutan Aesthet Surg 2015;8:179–81.

Cutaneous Ewing sarcoma

Definition and epidemiology. Cutaneous Ewing sarcoma is a rare tumour that belongs to the Ewing sarcoma family of tumours (ESFT) because they share histological and cytogenetic features. Angervall and Enzinger reported the first large series of 39 soft tissue Ewing sarcomas in 1975 [1]. The last review of cutaneous Ewing sarcoma was in 2015. The median age at diagnosis in this review was 21.5 years (range 2–77 years) and most occurred in females (F : M 1.9 : 1). Tumours were mainly located on the extremities (48.5%), followed by the trunk (39%) [2].

Aetiology and pathogenesis. The Ewing sarcoma breakpoint region 1 gene (*EWSR1*) on chromosome 22q12 is ubiquitously expressed in human cells but the function of its encoded protein has not yet been elucidated. Rearrangements involving *EWSR1* were first described in Ewing sarcoma/peripheral neuroectodermal tumours (PNET) and are now seen in a variety of soft tissue tumours. Most Ewing sarcoma cases involve fusion with the *FLI1* gene, with a minority involving *ERG* and rarely *ETV1*, *ETV4* and *FEV* genes amongst others. Cutaneous primary presentation of Ewing sarcoma is rare and most cases present the classic translocation t(11;22)(q24;q12) *EWSR1–FLI1* [3]. This specific genetic abnormality can be routinely demonstrated by reverse transcription polymerase chain reaction (RT-PCR) or fluorescence *in situ* hybridization (FISH).

Clinical features. Cutaneous Ewing sarcoma is a superficial mass, usually small at diagnosis (median tumour size 4 cm; range 1–13 cm), of soft consistency, freely mobile and sometimes painful. Cutaneous Ewing sarcoma seems to behave as a less aggressive tumour than primary bone Ewing sarcoma. The presence of metastases is very rare [4].

Diagnosis. The diagnosis of Ewing sarcoma /PNET is based on histology, immunohistochemistry (with a strong membranous positivity for CD99) and molecular cytogenetic testing (FISH and/or RT-PCR) [5].

The presence of metastases should be explored at diagnosis, by local MRI, thoracic CT scan, bone scintigraphy, bone marrow investigation and if possible fluorodeoxyglucose positron emission tomography (FDG-PET) scan or whole-body MRI to enhance the detection of bone and soft tissue metastases [6]. Local MRI can show multiple masses confined to the subcutaneous and cutaneous areas, having nonspecific signals of low to intermediate intensity in T1-weighted images and intermediate to high signal intensity in T2-weighted images. The tumours enhance heterogeneously and may show no enhanced areas of haemorrhage or necrosis on contrast-enhanced images. These images are nonspecific [7].

A sentinel node biopsy is justified routinely in patients with cutaneous Ewing sarcoma because they have a higher rate of regional node involvement [8].

Pathology. Ewing sarcoma tumours comprise small round cells with round hyperchromatic nuclei and a single nucleolus. The cytoplasm is poorly defined with clear colouration and regular vacuoles resulting from intracellular deposits of glycogen. Most of the cells express CD99 [4]. The tumour is located in the middle dermis, deep dermis or superficial subcutaneous tissue but may involve the dermal papilla.

Molecular diagnosis of Ewing sarcoma is crucial nowadays, as new entities are being described in *EWS–ETS*-negative Ewing sarcoma, such as *BCOR–CCNB3* (Ewing-like) sarcoma and *CIC–DUX4* sarcomas. The latter subtype is more frequently metastatic Ewing sarcoma [2].

Differential diagnosis. The superficial location of cutaneous Ewing sarcoma might facilitate detection but the tumour can be confused with a lipoma or other soft tissue tumour. Histologically, the differential diagnosis includes other neoplasms composed of small round cells, both primary and metastatic tumours. The former may include Merkel cell carcinoma, eccrine spiradenoma, lymphoma, clear cell sarcoma, rhabdomyosarcoma, malignant rhabdoid tumour, malignant primitive neuroectodermal tumour, myoepithelial carcinoma, angiomatoid fibrous histiocytoma, poorly differentiated adnexal tumour and granulocytic sarcoma. The latter may derive from osseous Ewing sarcoma, large cell neuroendocrine carcinoma, small cell lung carcinoma and neuroblastoma [4].

The diagnosis of Ewing sarcoma/PNET is based on histology and immunohistochemical (with a strong membranous positivity for CD99) and molecular cytogenetic (FISH and/or RT-PCR) studies.

Treatment. The primary treatment is surgical resection, associated or not with chemotherapy and/or radiotherapy, depending on the size and location of the tumour. Radiotherapy is used when there are still positive margins after surgical resection. The cutaneous disease presents a slow course and an apparently favourable prognosis, with a 10-year survival rate of 91% [6,9], when compared to osseous or soft tissue Ewing sarcoma, which has a worse prognosis.

References

1 Angervall L, Enzinger FM. Extraskeletal neoplasm resembling Ewing's sarcoma. Cancer 1975;36:240–51.

2 Di Giannatale A, Frezza A, Le Deley A et al. Primary cutaneous and subcutaneous Ewing sarcoma. Pediatr Blood Cancer 2015;62: 1555–61.

3 Sabb J, Nicoll K, Santos L. Primary cutaneous Ewing's sarcoma. Pathology 2015;47:S114.

4 Oliveira Filho J, Tebet ACF, Oliveira ARFM et al. Primary cutaneous Ewing sarcoma – case report. An Bras Dermatol 2014;89:501–3.

5 Terrier-Lacombe M, Guillou L, Chibon F et al. Superficial primitive Ewing's sarcoma: a clinicopathologic and molecular cytogenetic analysis of 14 cases. Mod Pathol 2009;22:87–94.

6 Furth C, Amthauer H, Denecke T et al. Impact of whole-body MRI and FDG-PET on staging and assessment of therapy response in a patient with Ewing sarcoma. Pediatr Blood Cancer 2006;47:607–11.

7 Delaplace M, Lhommet C, Pinieux G et al. Primary cutaneous Ewing sarcoma. Br J Dermatol 2012;166:721–6.

8 Applebaum MA, Goldsby R, Neuhaus J et al. Clinical features and outcomes in patients with Ewing sarcoma and regional lymph node involvement. Pediatr Blood Cancer 2012;59:617–20.

9 Collier A, Simpson L, Monteleone P. Cutaneous Ewing sarcoma report of 2 cases and literature. Review of presentation, treatment, and outcome of 76 other reported cases. J Pediatr Hematol Oncol 2011;33:631–4.

Synovial sarcoma

Definition and epidemiology. Synovial sarcoma (SS) is a mesenchymal neoplasm with partial epithelial differentiation that accounts for approximately 5–10% of all soft tissue sarcomas [1–3]. It is reported to be the most frequent non-rhabdomyosarcoma soft tissue sarcoma encountered in adolescents and young adults (15–20% of cases) [2,3]. Although the incidence rate of synovial sarcoma peaks in the third decade of life, 30% of tumours occur in patients younger than 20 years of age [1,3,4].

There is a slight male preponderance, with a male: female ratio of approximately 1.2:1; there is no racial or ethnic predilection [3,5].

Aetiology and pathogenesis. In more than 90% of cases, synovial sarcomas contain the characteristic translocation t(X;18)(p11.2;q11.2) [1,3,5] that fuses the *SYT* gene from chromosome 18 with the *SSX1* (approximately two thirds of cases), *SSX2* (approximately one third of cases) or *SSX4* gene (rare cases) from the X chromosome [2–7].

A strong association has been reported between fusion type and morphology, with the majority of *SYT–SSX2* tumours showing a monophasic phenotype, whereas almost all biphasic tumours have a *SYT–SSX1* rearrangement [4].

Clinical features. Synovial sarcoma can arise in any location but is most often located in the extremities, hence its historical name. However, despite its tendency to arise near joints, its origin is not related to synovial tissue [7]. The most common primary site of synovial sarcoma is the extremities, with the lower extremity being most often affected, accounting for almost 70% of cases [3,5]. After the extremities, the head and neck region is the next most frequent site, representing approximately 5% of cases. Rare locations include trunk, mediastinum, lumbar spine, heart, abdomen and retroperitoneum [3,5].

Synovial sarcoma usually appears as a palpable, slowly growing, large juxta-articular mass, which is associated with local pain and tenderness in more than half of the cases. Symptoms may also vary depending on the specific location of the disease; constitutional symptoms are rare. Synovial sarcoma has an average time to diagnosis of 2–4 years, but lesions may remain without diagnosis as long as 20 years. This gradual onset often causes a delay in diagnosis [1,3,5,6].

Metastases occur in 50–70% of cases and are mainly located in the lungs and pleura (which are also known sites for primary synovial sarcoma), followed by regional lymph nodes and bones [3,5].

Pathology. Histologically, synovial sarcomas do not resemble synovial structures. However, owing to the similarity between synovial sarcoma tumour cells and primitive synoviocytes, the term synovial sarcoma was introduced. In fact, synovial sarcomas derive from multipotent stem cells that are capable of differentiating into mesenchymal and/or epithelial structures [5]. Histologically, synovial sarcomas are divided into three subtypes: biphasic (20–30%), monophasic (50–60%) and poorly differentiated (15–25%). The biphasic subtype typically demonstrates epithelioid cells arranged in whorls or primitive gland-like structures along with the presence of spindle-shaped cells. Monophasic synovial sarcomas are entirely composed of spindle cells. A poorly differentiated subtype is often composed of small blue round cells and has high mitotic activity [5,6]. Although synovial sarcoma can be graded according to mitotic index, necrosis and tumour differentiation, it should always be considered a high-grade sarcoma [3–7]. Immunostaining is positive for keratin and EMA in most cases [6].

Differential diagnosis. Clinically, the differential diagnosis of synovial sarcoma is with other non-rhabdomyosarcoma soft tissue sarcomas, which usually present with a palpable growing mass. Histologically, the differential diagnosis is wide and varies according to the specific morphological pattern. Carcinosarcoma or sarcomatoid carcinoma can be particularly difficult to distinguish from synovial sarcoma, and monophasic epithelial synovial sarcoma may be confused with well-differentiated adenocarcinoma [3].

Treatment. Similar to the treatment of other soft tissue sarcomas, local control is primarily achieved by adequate surgical excision. The role of adjuvant radiation therapy and chemotherapy remains controversial, as their influence on local control and overall survival is still unclear [1,5]. Chemotherapy as a primary treatment modality is mainly reserved for patients with metastatic disease [5].

Prognostic factors in synovial sarcoma remain a controversial topic. Tumour stage, male sex, tumours on the trunk, large tumour size (the main important prognostic factor), metastases at the time of diagnosis and higher-grade histology have all been associated with an adverse outcome [1,3,4].

Synovial sarcoma is associated with local recurrence and distant metastases. It is generally considered a high-grade, aggressive sarcoma, with 5- and 10-year survival rates from 56% to 76%, and from 45% to 63%, respectively [1,3–5,7]. Because local recurrences and metastatic disease in synovial sarcoma patients occur rather late, even after 5–10 years, these patients should be followed for years [3,5].

References

1 Speth BM, Krieg AH, Kaelin A et al. Synovial sarcoma in patients under 20 years of age: a multicenter study with a minimum follow-up of 10 years. J Child Orthop 2011;5: 335–42.
2 Bozzi F, Ferrari A, Negri T et al. Molecular characterization of synovial sarcoma in children and adolescents: Evidence of AKT activation. Transl Oncol 2008;1):95–101.
3 Thway K, Fisher C. Synovial sarcoma: defining features and diagnostic evolution. Ann Diagn Pathol 2014;18:369–80.
4 Kerouanton A, Jimenez I, Cellier C et al. Synovial sarcoma in children and adolescents. J Pediatr Hematol Oncol 2014;36:257–62.
5 Hass RJ, Bonenkamp JJ, Flucke UE et al. Synovial sarcoma of the abdominal wall: Imaging findings and review of the literature. J Radiol Case Rep 2015;9:24–30.
6 Silverstein D, Klein P. Large monophasic synovial sarcoma: a case report and review of the literature. Cutis 2014;93:13–16.
7 Vlenterie M, Jones RL, van der Graaf WT. Synovial sarcoma diagnosis and management in the era of targeted therapies. Curr Opin Oncol 2015;27:316–22.

Alveolar soft part sarcoma

Definition and epidemiology. Alveolar soft part sarcoma (ASPS) is a rare soft tissue neoplasm accounting for less than 1% of all soft tissue sarcomas [1–4]. Clinically, this disease primarily occurs in young patients, with a peak incidence age of 15–35 years. It is more common in females than in males with a 2 : 1 ratio [4–6].

Aetiology and pathogenesis. The pathogenesis of ASPS is unknown and there is some controversy over this. The tumour is characterized by a specific chromosomal alteration, der(17)t(X:17)(p11:q25), resulting in the fusion of the *TFE3* transcription factor gene (from Xp11) with alveolar soft part sarcoma critical region 1 (*ASPSCR1*) at 17q25 [1,6–9]. The detection of the fusion transcript (*ASPSCR1–TFE3*) by real-time PCR and FISH for *TFE3* rearrangement are considered accurate methods for diagnosis [2,3,9].

Clinical features. In adults, ASPS tends to involve the deep soft tissues of the limb, particularly in the thigh or buttock. In children and infants, ASPS has a predilection for the head and neck region, with the tongue and orbit being the most common sites. Other organs such as genital area, breasts, mediastinum, bladder and retroperitoneum are reported in all age groups [3,4,6,7,9,10].

The natural history of ASPS is of a slow-growing painless mass at the time of presentation. The neoplasm is often indolent and may therefore be present for years before medical attention is sought. Patients may have advanced metastatic disease in the brain, bones and lungs. Metastases can also occur long after resection of the primary tumour, after long disease-free intervals, even if there is no local recurrence [2–4,8–10].

Pathology. Histologically, ASPS is characterized by aggregates of large polyhedral or round mesenchymal cells, containing an abundant eosinophilic to clear granular cytoplasm and separated by capillary-sized vascular channels and connective tissue. The loss of intercellular cohesion, with neoplastic cells adhering only to the fibrovascular septa, results in a 'pseudo'-alveolar pattern [2,3,7,9,10].

On immunohistochemistry, the tumour cells are typically negative for epithelial markers (i.e. EMA and cytokeratins), chromogranin A, synaptophysin, S100, HMB45, and Melan-A. Desmin may be positive in around 50% of cases, and nonspecific markers such as neurone-specific enolase and vimentin may be positive in 30–50% [2,3].

Differential diagnosis. ASPS may be clinically misinterpreted as a benign or developmental lesion such as a haemangioma, lymphangioma or arteriovenous malformation [3,10].

ASPS can be differentiated from other histologically similar malignant neoplasms by its cytological uniformity, lack of nuclear atypia and paucity of mitotic figures. The differential diagnoses of ASPS include granular cell tumour, paraganglioma, metastatic renal cell carcinoma, melanoma, alveolar rhabdomyosarcoma and ectopic lingual thyroid [3,4,7,10].

Treatment. The traditional treatments for ASPS consist of surgery and radiotherapy. The role of adjuvant chemotherapy in ASPS remains uncertain. However, in advanced cases, chemotherapy may be considered as a treatment option [3,7,10].

Recently, more evidence has appeared for the use of antiangiogenic agents in the treatment of this tumour. Given the highly vascular nature of ASPS, antiangiogenic agents such as bevacizumab, sunitinib and cediranib have shown promise in small series and clinical trials for the treatment of primary and metastatic disease [2,3,10].

Despite being a slow-growing tumour with an asymptomatic course, ASPS demonstrates a disproportionate frequency of distant metastases even at the early stages of disease. Local recurrence occurs in 20–30% of cases. Prognosis is largely dependent on the initial presentation (localized versus metastatic disease), tumour size and age. Primary tumours measuring less than 5 cm and those occurring in patients in the first and second decades of life demonstrate a more favourable clinical course. The 5-year survival rate of children, adolescents and adults younger than 25 years old with ASPS is reportedly 83%. However, because of the propensity for late metastases, survival rates decline steadily [3,4,7].

References

1 **Wang H, Jacobson A, Harmon DC et al. Prognostic factors in alveolar soft part sarcoma: A SEER analysis. J Surg Oncol 2016;113:581–6.**
2 Mullins BT, Hackman T. Adult alveolar soft part sarcoma of the head and neck: a report of two cases and literature review. Case Rep Oncol Med 2014;2014ID:597291.
3 Argyris PP, Reed RC, Manivel JC et al. Oral alveolar soft part sarcoma in childhood and adolescence: report of two cases and review of literature. Head Neck Pathol 2013;7:40–9.
4 Jaber OI, Kirby PA. Alveolar soft part sarcoma. Arch Pathol Lab Med 2015;139:1459–62.
5 Chen Z, Sun C, Sheng W et al. Alveolar soft-part sarcoma in the left forearm with cardiac metastasis: A case report and literature review. Oncol Lett 2016;11:81–4.
6 Qiao PF, Shen LH, Gao Y et al. Alveolar soft part sarcoma: clinicopathological analysis and imaging results. Oncol Lett 2015;10:2777–807.
7 Knossos G, Chlorides P, Petropoulos I et al. Alveolar soft part sarcoma of the tongue in a 3-year-old boy: a case report. J Med Case Rep 2010;4:130.
8 Zany PL, Hurter A, Deleon R et al. Alveolar soft-part sarcoma in the sacrum: a case report and review of the literature. Skeletal Radiol 2014;43:115–20.
9 Wang HW, Dai W, Qin XJ et al. A new clinical manifestation for cheek alveolar soft-part sarcoma: a case report and review of the literature. J Oral Maxillofac Surg 2014;72:817–22.
10 **Cho YJ, Kim JY. Alveolar soft part sarcoma: clinical presentation, treatment and outcome in a series of 19 patients. Clin Orthop Surg 2014;6:80–6.**

Leiomyosarcoma

Definition and epidemiology. Cutaneous leiomyosarcoma is a malignant neoplasm showing pure smooth muscle differentiation. It is a rare tumour, comprising only 4–6.5% of soft tissue sarcomas [1].

SECTION 24: NONVASCULAR SKIN TUMOURS

It may occur in patients of either sex and at any age but is most common in men between the fifth and seventh decades. Children rarely develop these tumours and there is conflicting evidence as to whether leiomyosarcomas in children have a better prognosis.

Cutaneous leiomyosarcoma belongs to a subgroup of leiomyosarcoma tumours that arise from the arrector pili muscle in the dermis and secondarily invade the subcutis. Because of their superficial location and limited clinical stage, they have an excellent prognosis. Leiomyosarcomas located exclusively in the subcutis arise in many instances from vessels and, therefore, have much in common with soft tissue leiomyosarcomas with respect to their prognosis and risk of metastasis.

Aetiology and pathogenesis. Karyotypes of soft tissue leiomyosarcomas are usually highly complex with genomic instability and are often associated with defects in *TP53* or sometimes *FANCA* and *ATM* genes [2]. The most frequent alterations reported are the loss of chromosomes rather than the gain.

These are smooth muscle tumours with uncertain malignant potential that occur in immunocompromised patients with greater frequency than in the general population. Most Epstein–Barr virus smooth muscle tumours occur in children and, interestingly, develop in organs not traditionally considered preferred sites for leiomyosarcomas (soft tissue, liver, lung, spleen, dura). The diagnosis can be confirmed by *in situ* hybridization of Epstein–Barr virus early RNA (also known as EBER) [3].

Clinical features. Cutaneous and subcutaneous leiomyosarcomas classically present as a solitary, firm, skin-coloured to red-brown nodule or plaque [3]. They are usually less than 2 cm at presentation and frequently cause changes in the overlying skin, such as discolouration and ulceration. Sometimes the tumours are painful or become ulcerated [1].

Typically leiomyosarcomas present on the scalp and hair-bearing surfaces and lower extremities; the presence of multiple lesions should always raise the question of metastatic disease from a previously resected or occult leiomyosarcoma of retroperitoneal or deep soft tissue origin.

The prognosis for cutaneous leiomyosarcoma is usually excellent, whereas those involving the subcutis metastasize in approximately 30–40% of cases.

Pathology. Histologically, cutaneous leiomyosarcomas have characteristic interlacing bundles of packed spindle cells with elongated, round-ended nuclei. In contrast, in the subcutis subtype the tumours appear more circumscribed because they compress the surrounding tissue, creating a pseudocapsule. Most superficial leiomyosarcomas resemble retroperitoneal leiomyosarcomas in general organization. Haemorrhage, necrosis, hyalinization and myxoid changes, which are probably a reflection of the smaller size of these lesions, are rarely encountered. Giant cells may be present but, as in retroperitoneal tumours, it is uncommon to encounter a tumour with them. Mitotic figures, including atypical forms, are easily identified in these tumours. Immunophenotypic studies with antibodies to SMA, desmin and calponin represent the standard of diagnosis. A small number of cutaneous leiomyosarcomas contain cytokeratins [3,4].

The histopathological features of leiomyosarcomas span a morphological spectrum: whereas the well differentiated demonstrate an overlap with leiomyomas, poorly differentiated lesions closely resemble atypical fibroxanthomas or 'malignant fibrous histiocytomas' [1].

Differential diagnosis. Because the clinical features are not unique, the differential diagnoses include a number of tumours that can be present as a solitary firm nodule or plaque such as dermatofibrosarcoma protuberans or other soft tissue sarcomas, epidermoid inclusion cyst and, less often, panniculitis [1].

Treatment. Primary wide surgical resection with a median margin of 1 cm allows a high percentage of secure complete resection. Local recurrence implies increased risk of eventual metastases because there is a distinct tendency for recurrent lesions to be larger and to involve deeper structures. Mohs surgery has recently been used in the treatment of this tumour with a recurrence rate of 14% [5].

References

1 Kaddu S, Kohler S. Muscle, adipose and cartilage neoplasms. In: Bolognia JL, Jorizzo JL, Schaffer JV (eds) Dermatology, 3rd edn. Edinburgh: Mosby Elsevier, 2012:1979–91.

2 Fletcher CDM, Bridge JA, Hogendoorn PCW et al. WHO Classification of Tumours of Soft Tissue and Bone, 4th edn. Lyon, France: IARC Press, 2013.

3 Goldblum J, Folpe A, Weiss S. Leiomyosarcoma. In: Enzinger and Weiss's Soft Tissue Tumors, 6th edn. Philadelphia: Saunders Elsevier, 2014:549–68.

4 Calonje E, Langar H. Connective tissue tumours. In: Calonje E, Dip R, Brenn T et al (eds) McKee's Pathology of the Skin, 4th edn. Philadelphia: Saunders Elsevier, 2011:1588–1768.

5 Winchester D, Hocker T, Brewer J et al. Leiomyosarcoma of the skin: clinical, histopathologic, and prognostic factors that influence outcomes. J Am Acad Dermatol 2014;71:919–25.

Dermatofibrosarcoma protuberans

Definition and epidemiology. Dermatofibrosarcoma protuberans (DFSP), first described by Darier, Ferrand and Hoffman, is a rare cutaneous tumour of fibrohistiocytic origin characterized by intermediate malignancy and locally aggressive growth with frequent local recurrence after treatment, but rare distant metastases with an estimated rate of 3.4–4.7%. The lungs are the most frequent site of metastases, while lymph nodes are rarely involved. DFSP is typically diagnosed in young to middle-aged adults; only 6% of cases occur in paediatric patients [1,2]. In a review published in 2010, Gooskens et al. analysed reports of 166 cases in children, of which 38 were congenital cases [3].

Aetiology and pathogenesis. The mechanism by which DFSP arises is unknown. Trauma has been considered a possible aetiological factor, especially in childhood. Specific cytogenetic abnormalities have been found in the majority of cases of DFSP. A supernumerary ring chromosome containing sequences derived from chromosome 17 and 22 is the most consistent detectable cytogenetic change in adults. Reciprocal translocation t(17;22)(q22,q13) has been the most frequent (90%) abnormality in paediatric patients. Both of these rearrangements combine *PDGFB* (chromosome 22) and *COL1A1* (chromosome 17) and could lead to increased production of platelet-derived growth factor (PDGFB). It seems that autocrine PDGF-receptor stimulation contributes to neoplastic growth of these cells. Fusion of the *COL1A1* gene with the *PDGFB* gene has also been detected in metastatic lesions of DFSP [1,4].

In congenital cases, chromosomal abnormalities occur *in utero*, although the mechanism driving the change is not known. No epidemiological data have enabled identification of any predisposing or environmental risk factor for the development of DFSP during gestation [3].

Clinical features. DFSP presents initially in childhood as a bluish discolouration or as a small and firm nodule or plaque. The early-stage plaque can present different variants: an indurated flat plaque; a morphoea-like depressed sclerotic plaque; or an anetoderma-like depressed soft plaque. After a variable period of time, one or more nodules develop over the plaque. The colour ranges from brown to bluish-red, with a blue or red discolouration of the surrounding skin (Fig. 117.4).

DFSP is usually asymptomatic and grows slowly. Lesion size normally ranges from 1 to 5 cm. It tends to increase in dimension over the years and becomes larger if not treated.

DFSP can occur in any part of the body, most often on the trunk, the proximal extremities and the head and neck region. However, in childhood the tumour seems to prefer the acral areas (back and legs) [2,4]. Congenital DFSP lesions are also more frequently located on the trunk and proximal aspect of the limbs [3]. In such lesions, an atrophic variant is frequently encountered. In this variant, depressed plaques with a sclerotic appearance tend to remain flat. Also common among congenital tumours are anetodermic variants in the form of depressed plaques with a soft consistency.

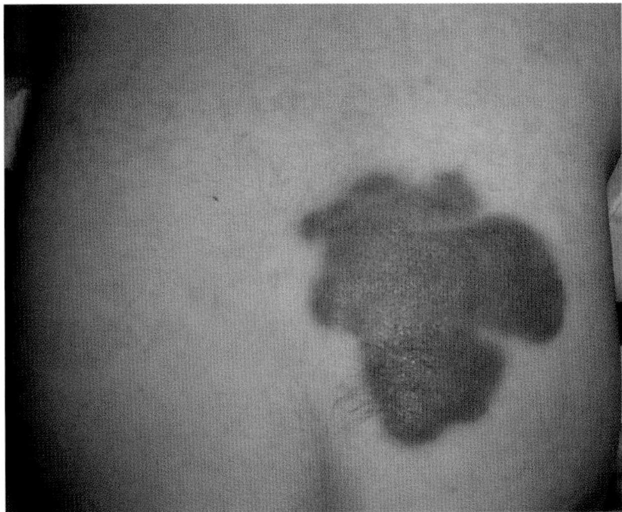

Fig. 117.4 Dermatofibrosarcoma protuberans: erythematous plaque on the thigh of a boy.

Pathology. Histologically, the tumour is composed predominantly of spindle-shaped fibrohistiocytic cells arranged in short fascicles that interweave [1]. Mitotic figures are rare in most tumours. DFSP is very often histologically indistinguishable from a low-grade fibrosarcoma or cellular fibroma occurring in the skin.

The fibrosarcomatous variant of DFSP represents an uncommon form. Histologically, the lesions show areas of typical low-grade DFSP adjacent to fibrosarcomatous areas.

Positive immunostaining for CD34 and vimentin and negative immunostaining for S100, factor XIIIa, desmin and SMA can confirm a diagnosis of DFSP [1,5]. Dermatofibroma, unlike DFSP, stains negative for CD34, while tenascin and factor XIIIa stains are positive. There are new markers proposed to differentiate dermatofibroma and DFSP: apolipoprotein D is positive in DFSP and negative in dermatofibroma, and stromelysin 342 and CD163 are positive in dermatofibroma and negative in DFSP.

An alternative method for confirming the diagnosis of DFPS is staining for PDGF receptor β (PDGFRB), thereby demonstrating overexpression of this molecule on the surface of tumour cells, although the usefulness of this approach has yet to be demonstrated [3].

Differential diagnosis. Unfortunately, DFSP in children may be misdiagnosed, often as a vascular tumour or malformation, morphoea, atrophoderma, atrophic scar and lipoatrophy, keloid and hypertrophic scars. However, it differs in the histological and immunohistochemical features. The distinction between DFSP and dermatofibroma is sometimes difficult, but immunostaining allows differentiation between these tumours [4–6].

Treatment. The treatment of choice is wide local excision with a margin of 1.5–3 cm, including the underlying fascia. Mohs micrographic surgery has been used but this technique may not be suitable for large lesions or for children due to the duration of the surgery. DFSP is a radiosensitive tumour. Radiotherapy can be considered as complementary to surgery in cases of resection with compromised margins.

Recent findings regarding the role of PDGFb and its receptor in the pathogenesis of DFSP have led investigators to target PDFG receptors as a novel treatment strategy for DFSP. In recently published results, imatinib mesylate, a protein tyrosine kinase inhibitor, has shown clinical activity against localized and metastatic DFSP tumours containing the t(17;22) translocation. Imatinib mesylate has recently been approved by the US Food and Drug Administration (FDA) for the treatment of unresectable, recurrent and/or metastatic DFSP CD34-positive tumours in adult patients. As tumours lacking the t(17;22) translocation may not respond to imatinib, molecular analysis with cytogenetics may be useful before initiating imatinib therapy [2,4,7,8].

In recurrences, whenever possible, tumours should be resected. Radiation therapy, if not given previously, or imatinib mesylate should be considered if surgery is not possible, or if additional resection would lead to unacceptable functional or cosmetic outcomes.

In the rare event of metastatic disease, consideration should be given to clinical trials, imatinib mesylate, chemotherapy, radiation therapy or repeat resection [2,4,7,8].

References

1 Patel KU, Szabo SS, Hernández VS et al. Dermatofibrosarcoma protuberans COL1A1-PDGFB fusion is identified in virtually all developed multiplex reverse transcription polymerase chain reaction and fluorescence *in situ* hybridization assays. Hum Pathol 2008;39:184–93.
2 Gerlini G, Mariotti G, Urso C et al. Dermatofibrosarcoma protuberans in childhood: two case reports and review of the literature. Pediatr Hematol Oncol 2008;25:559–66.
3 **Valdivielso-Ramos M, Hernanz JM. Dermatofibrosarcoma protuberans in childhood. Actas Dermosifiliogr 2012;103:863–73.**
4 **Jafarian F, McCuaig C, Kokta V et al. Dermatofibrosarcoma protuberans in childhood and adolescence: report of eight patients. Pediatr Dermatol 2008;25:317–25.**
5 Marque M, Bessis D, Pedetour F et al. Medallion-like dermal dendrocyte hamartoma: the main diagnostic pitfall is congenital atrophic dermatofibrosarcoma. Br J Dermatol 2009;160:190–3.
6 Mori T, Misago N, Yamamoto O et al. Expression of nestin in dermatofibrosarcoma protuberans in comparison to dermatofibroma. J Dermatol 2008;35:419–25.
7 Bague S, Folpe AL. Dermatofibrosarcoma protuberans presenting as a subcutaneous mass: a clinicopathological study of 15 cases with exclusive or near-exclusive subcutaneous involvement. Am J Dermatopathol 2008;30:327–32.
8 Miller SJ, Alam M, Andersen JS et al. NCCN Clinical Practice Guidelines, NCCN Guidelines in oncology for dermatofibrosarcoma protuberans. JNCCN 2012;10:312–18.

Haemangiopericytoma/solitary fibrous tumour

Definition. Haemangiopericytoma (HPC) is an unusual vascular soft tissue tumour. In the most recent World Health Organization (WHO) classification of soft tissue sarcomas, the concept of HPC as a vascular pericyte derived tumour was abandoned in favour of a fibroblastic cell origin, thus placing HPC more closely with solitary fibrous tumour (SFT). It is much more common in adults; only 5–10% of these tumours occur in the paediatric population. When it develops in childhood, HPC is considered a heterogeneous entity that comprises two distinct clinical forms: adult HPC/SFT and infantile HPC. Infantile HPC, occurring during the first year of life, is characterized by a more benign course with responsiveness to chemotherapy and even tendency to spontaneous regression. In contrast, the behaviour of HPC in adolescence does not appear to differ from that of adult HPC. Approximately 15–20% of HPC/SFT present a more aggressive behaviour leading to development of local recurrences or distant metastases despite surgery [1,2].

Aetiology and pathogenesis. Even when the aetiology is not well understood, studies have indicated that genetic alterations may have a role in the formation of all soft tissue sarcomas. Although many different chromosomal rearrangements have been reported, it is clear that involvement of chromosome 12 is a frequent finding in HPC specimens. Specifically, translocations seem to be most common, with a breakpoint at 12q13–15 reported in multiple cases including the paediatric population. Only two inversions have been reported, involving an X chromosome, and chromosome 12 [inv (12)(q14q24)]. Both specimens with inversions belonged to adult patients [2].

Clinical features. Soft tissue HPC is a firm, painless, slowly expanding mass that is often nodular and well localized. The skin overlying the mass does not have any discolouration or redness to indicate its vascular origin because the capillaries are emptied of blood by compression of massive numbers of pericytes surrounding them. The adult form is most common in the lower extremities but also occurs in thorax, pelvis, retroperitoneum, orbit and other sites. Paediatric HPC particularly affects the limbs [1,3].

Pathology. The infantile type, although histologically identical to the adult type, has a more benign clinical course. The reasons for this difference in the natural history of HPC are not well understood. Histologically, distinctive features of infantile HPC include immature cytology, multilobulated growth pattern, focal necrosis and mitotic activity in varying degrees. Capillaries are arranged in bands surrounded by cells with oval or spindle-shaped nuclei in a network of reticulum fibres. Additionally, some patients have a focal second tumour cell component consisting of spindle-shaped myofibroblastic cells forming fascicles and micronodules. Classically, immunohistochemical studies show expression of muscle-specific actin, SMA, tropomyosin and CD34 and are negative for desmin and h-caldesmon. However, this classic expression of markers is only present in 10–20% of HPC, with the majority expressing nonspecific patterns [1,3]. The morphological criteria suggested by Enzinger and Smith are used to distinguish a malignant from a benign tumour. These criteria are: large size (>5 cm), increased mitotic rate (four or more per 10 high-power fields), high degree of cellularity, immature and pleomorphic tumour cells, foci of haemorrhage and necrosis.

Differential diagnosis. The differential diagnosis of infantile HPC includes infantile haemangioma, infantile myofibromatosis, leukaemia cutis, neuroblastoma, Langerhans cell histiocytosis, kaposiform haemangioendothelioma, tufted angioma, pyogenic granuloma, fibrosarcoma, glomus tumour, rhabdomyosarcoma, reticulosarcoma and angiosarcoma.

Treatment. Surgical excision is the definitive therapy for HPC. Chemotherapy has been proved to be useful in a neoadjuvant setting for initially unresectable lesions and in cases where only a partial resection was possible or in the presence of metastases. Some centres use adjuvant therapy to reduce the risk of local recurrence. The value of the adjuvant therapy is difficult to assess because of the rarity of these tumours. Chemotherapeutic regimens have included the use of vincristine, actinomycin D, cyclophosphamide, methotrexate, doxorubicin, prednisone and dacarbazine. The role of radiation therapy alone is controversial. The rich vascular characteristics of HPC/SFT have been long recognized, and this observation has prompted the use of interferon alfa in a few cases of advanced disease based on the well-known antiangiogenic properties of the drug. Targeted therapy against the VEGF pathway and other pathways involved in angiogenesis may provide a novel, exciting approach to treatment. Combination therapy with temozolomide and bevacizumab appears to provide clinical benefit with a low rate of major toxicities. Future prospective studies with other antiangiogenic agents are necessary to investigate the biological mechanisms and the efficacy of these targeted agents in advanced tumours. Infantile HPC is characterized by a better clinical behaviour, with documented chemotherapy responsiveness and spontaneous regression, and requires a more conservative surgical approach [1,3–5].

References

1 **Parka MS, Araujo DM. New insights into the hemangiopericytoma/solitary fibrous tumour spectrum of tumours. Curr Opin Oncol 2009;21:327–31.**

2 Fletcher CD. The evolving classification of soft tissue tumours: an update based on the new WHO Classification. Histopathology 2006;48:3–12.

3 Gowans LK, Bentz ML, DeSantes KB et al. Successful treatment of an infant with constitutional chromosomal abnormality and hemangiopericytoma with chemotherapy alone. J Pediatr Hematol Oncol 2007;29:409–11.

4 Lackner H, Urban C, Dornbusch HJ et al. Interferon alfa-2a in recurrent metastatic hemangiopericytoma. Med Pediatr Oncol 2003;40:192–4.

5 **Perez EC, Brady CA, Luther W. Unusual non-epithelial tumours of the head and neck. In: Perez and Brady's Principles and Practice of Radiation Oncology, 5th edn. Lippincott Williams & Wilkins, 2008:235–48.**

Malignant tumours of neural crest and germ cell origin

Neuroblastoma

Definition and epidemiology. Neuroblastoma arises from the primitive neural crest cells that migrate during embryogenesis, and therefore can occur anywhere along the sympathetic ganglia. Thus, its clinical presentation includes a wide spectrum of symptoms depending on tumour location [1]. It is the most common extracranial malignant tumour of childhood. The incidence of neuroblastoma is 10.5 per million children under 15 years of age per year with over 650 new cases identified in North America annually. The incidence peak in children is under 4 years of age, with an average age of 19 months [2].

Aetiology and pathogenesis. Neuroblastoma is genetically and biologically heterogeneous, with numerous structural chromosomal abnormalities and allelic changes described. *MYCN*, the most critical oncogene, is amplified in approximately 20% of neuroblastomas, is an oncogenic driver and is one of the most powerful molecular markers of unfavourable prognosis [2]. There are several chromosomal gains and losses described: deletion of 1p36 (35% of neuroblastomas), deletion of 11q, gain of 17q, and others [3].

The large majority of neuroblastomas arise sporadically, however a small subset arise within families. *ALK* mutations appear in the majority of familial neuroblastomas with an autosomal dominant pattern with incomplete penetrance; 6% of familial neuroblastoma is associated with germline heterozygous *PHOX2B* mutations.

Clinical features. The most common presentation is a hard, smooth, non-tender abdominal mass. Cutaneous features, seen in 2.6% of all patients and 32% of newborn infants with this disorder, may at times be the first clinical manifestation of the disease.

Skin lesions consist of highly characteristic firm, non-tender, slightly blue or bluish-grey metastatic nodules that, because of release of catecholamines, tend to blanch and develop a surrounding halo of erythema within 2–3 minutes after being palpated, stroked or rubbed (Fig. 117.5). Blanching lasts for about 1 hour followed by a refractory period. Other manifestations include 'racoon eyes' (periorbital ecchymoses resulting from orbital metastases) and heterochromia of the iris (the result of involvement of the sympathetic innervation of the iris) [4–6].

Neuroblastoma staging is transitioning from the surgical–pathological International Neuroblastoma Staging System (INSS) to the more recently defined International Neuroblastoma Risk Group Staging System (INRGSS) [5,7].

The INRGSS uses radiological features to distinguish locoregional tumours that do not involve local structures (INRGSS L1) from locally invasive tumours (INRGSS L2) exhibiting image-defined risk factors. Stages M and MS refer to tumours that are widely metastatic, or children less than 18 months who have metastasis in skin, liver or bone marrow, respectively.

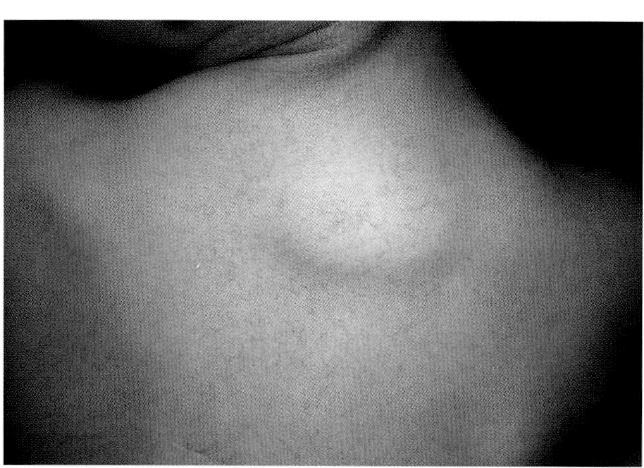

Fig. 117.5 Soft tumour on the back of a girl with neuroblastoma.

Laboratory studies and images. Most children affected by neuroblastoma have elevated levels of catecholamines and their metabolites (vanillylmandelic acid and homovanillic acid) in the urine. Their measurement is useful both for diagnosis and for the search for residual tumour after surgical treatment. Serum ferritin, lactic dehydrogenase and neurone-specific enolase levels have a special importance as prognostic factors [1,5,6].

Staging of neuroblastoma requires radiological studies and bone marrow aspiration and biopsy to determine the extent of local disease and distant spread. If there are skin lesions, their biopsy can help to diagnose and determine prognostic factors. Nuclear medicine scans performed with radionucleotides such as ^{131}I-metaiodobenzylguanidine (MIBG) may be more accurate and sensitive in the detection of extraosseous as well as osseous disease.

When tumour material is obtained, it should be submitted for determination of DNA content (tumour cell ploidy), detection of *MYCN* genomic amplification and cytogenetic analysis, and preserved for additional genomic evaluation [8].

Pathology. Cutaneous metastases of neuroblastoma are characterized by well-circumscribed nodules within the dermis and subcutaneous fat, formed by neoplastic cells that vary according to the degree of neural differentiation.

The more undifferentiated forms produce small blue round cells (neuroblasts). The cells have round dark nuclei with scant cytoplasm, and they are embedded in a fibrillary stroma. However, well-differentiated ganglion cells and Schwann cells are the only infiltrating cells in the so-called ganglioneuroma.

Immunohistochemistry of the tumour depends on the degree of differentiation. The more undifferentiated cells are identified by neurofilament proteins, synaptophysin and neurone-specific enolase markers. The S100 protein marks only the well-differentiated ganglioneuroblastoma cells [4–6].

Differential diagnosis. Skin lesions of neuroblastoma should be distinguished from other sarcomatous tumours such as rhabdomyosarcoma, and histiocytic tumours such as congenital self-healing reticulohistiocytosis. In the newborn period, blueberry muffin lesions, vascular tumours, cutaneous lesions of leukaemia and cysts may sometimes be confused with cutaneous lesions of neuroblastoma. Their characteristic blanching phenomenon as a result of catecholamine release following palpation or rubbing is strongly suggestive of the diagnosis.

Treatment. Great progress has been made in relating tumour genetic abnormalities to tumour behaviour and to clinical outcome; indeed, neuroblastoma provides a paradigm for the clinical importance of tumour genetic abnormalities. Knowledge of *MYCN* status is increasingly used in treatment decisions for individual children.

Tumours that are detected only on prenatal ultrasonography or postnatal neuroblastoma screening characteristically undergo spontaneous regression or maturation and require little or no treatment.

According to staging, age and biological factors, treatment can vary from observation, to surgery alone, to more aggressive treatments such as chemotherapy and/or immunotherapy [9,10].

References

1 Bowen KA, Chung DH. Recent advances in neuroblastoma. Curr Opin Pediatr 2009;21:350–6.

2 Park JR, Bagatell R, London WB et al; COG Neuroblastoma Committee. Children's Oncology Group's 2013 blueprint for research: neuroblastoma. Pediatr Blood Cancer 2013;60:985–93.

3 Park JR, Eggert A, Caron H. Neuroblastoma: biology, prognosis and treatment. Hematol Oncol Clin North Am 2011;24:65–86.

4 Lukens JN. Neuroblastoma in the neonate. Semin Perinatol 1999;23:263–73.

5 Brodeur GM, Pritchard J, Berthold F et al. Revisions of the international criteria for neuroblastoma diagnosis, staging, and response to treatment. J Clin Oncol 1993;11:1466–77.

6 Shimada H, Ambros IM, Dehner LP et al. The International Neuroblastoma. Pathology Classification (the Shimada system). Cancer 1999;86:364–72.

7 Monclair T, Brodeur GM, Ambros PF et al. The International Neuroblastoma Risk Group (INRG) staging system: An INRG Task Force report. J Clin Oncol 2009;27:298–303.

8 Dome J, Rodríguez-Galindo C, Spunt S et al. Pediatric solid tumors. In: Niederhuber J, Armitage J, Doroshow J et al (eds) Abeloff's Clinical Oncology, 5th edn. Philadelphia: Elsevier Saunders, 2014:1819–25.

9 Strother DR, London WB, Schmidt ML et al. Outcome after surgery alone or with restricted use of chemotherapy for patients with low-risk neuroblastoma: results of Children's Oncology Group study P9641. J Clin Oncol 2012;30:1842–8.

10 Baker DL, Schmidt ML, Cohn SL et al. Outcome after reduced chemotherapy for intermediate-risk neuroblastoma. N Engl J Med 2010;14:1313–23.

Choriocarcinoma

Definition and epidemiology. Choriocarcinomas are aggressive malignancies that may be separated into two groups: nongestational choriocarcinoma, which typically arises from the gonadal organs, but may also occur in extragonadal primary sites; and gestational choriocarcinoma, which is derived from any form of previously normal or abnormal pregnancy, such as a hydatidiform mole, spontaneous abortion or ectopic pregnancy. Infantile choriocarcinoma is a very rare tumour and is a complication of a gestational choriocarcinoma. It may occur between 0 and 6 months of age, and fewer than 30 cases have been described in the literature. NGCO is mostly seen in childhood and adolescence and can occur at any age and in any gender. Both types of choriocarcinoma are quite different in their genetic origin, immunogenicity, sensitivity to chemotherapy and prognosis [1–4].

History. Choriocarcinoma can occur in both gonadal and extragonadal sites. Ovarian choriocarcinoma can develop before puberty; testicular and mediastinal tumours are observed only in patients who have reached puberty. Very few cases of choriocarcinoma arising in the placenta and occurring simultaneously in mother and child have been described [3].

Aetiology and pathogenesis. Choriocarcinomas, as well as other germ cell tumours, originate from pluripotent germ cells of the fetal yolk sac. The result of extraembryonic differentiation can be either yolk sac carcinoma (from the yolk sac cells) or choriocarcinoma (from trophoblastic cells) [1–3].

Clinical features. Typical early symptoms are anaemia, failure to thrive, hepatomegaly, haemoptysis or respiratory failure. The tumour affects more than one organ in most cases; organs involved are liver, lung, brain or skin (10%). Cutaneous manifestations of choriocarcinoma are metastatic nodules, subcutaneous masses or multiple angiomatoid tumours, usually in midline sites, covered by normal skin. Gynaecomastia and precocious puberty may occur as the result of the secretion of large quantities of human chorionic gonadotrophin (hCG). Other symptoms depend on the site of the primary tumour and present themselves when compression of the organs is significant [3–6].

Laboratory studies. High serum levels of hCG are the main feature. Monitoring serum levels is useful, not only for diagnosis but also for the control of treatment. Microsatellite polymorphism analysis allows the distinction between both types of choriocarcinoma and can also be used to identify the causative pregnancy of gestational choriocarcinoma [1].

Pathology. Microscopically, the tumour exhibits a biphasic pattern with a central core of mononuclear cytotrophoblast surrounded by a peripheral rim of multinucleated syncytiotrophoblast. The viable and better preserved tumour cells are found mainly at the lesion periphery while extensive haemorrhage and necrosis are frequent in the central part of the lesion. The trophoblasts of choriocarcinoma show marked cytological atypia, and immunohistochemical biomarkers such as hCG, inhibin-α and human placental lactogen (hPL) confirm the diagnosis [1–5].

Differential diagnosis. The symptoms of abnormal vaginal bleeding and elevated hCG levels often lead to an incorrect diagnosis of ectopic pregnancy, threatened or incomplete abortion, cervical polyp or other types of malignancy. When external masses are the main lesion, the differential diagnoses include meningocoele, rhabdomyosarcoma, lipoma and/or haemangioma [2,3].

Treatment. The primary treatment is conservative surgery combined with multiple multiagent chemotherapy regimens, including MAC (methotrexate, actinomycin-D and cyclophosphamide) and CHAMOCA (cyclophosphamide, hydroxycarbamide, doxorubicin, actinomycin D, methotrexate, melphalan and vincristine). Currently, the most commonly used alternatives to the aforementioned multiagent chemotherapy regimens are EMA-CO (etoposide, methotrexate, actinomycin-D, cyclophosphamide and vincristine) and fluorouracil-based chemotherapy regimens [6].

Prognosis. The prognosis depends on the extent of the disease at diagnosis and on the primary site: extragonadal tumours and cutaneous metastases have a poor prognosis. Since maternal choriocarcinoma is associated with a risk of infantile choriocarcinoma in subsequent pregnancies, current guidelines suggest that women with such a history should be checked for β-hCG at the sixth and tenth weeks of every pregnancy.

References

1 Zhao J, Xiang Y, Wan XR et al. Molecular genetics analyses of choriocarcinoma. Placenta 2009;30:816–20.
2 Alkassar M, Gottschling S, Krenn T et al. Metastatic choriocarcinoma in a 17-year old boy. Klin Padiatr 2009;221:179.
3 Kong B, Tian YJ, Zhu WW et al. A pure nongestational ovarian choriocarcinoma in a 10-year-old girl: case report and literature review. J Obstet Gynaecol Res 2009;35: 574–8.
4 Isaacs H Jr. Cutaneous metastases in neonates: a review. Pediatr Dermatol 2011;28:85–93.
5 Brooks T, Nolting L. Cutaneous manifestation of metastatic infantile choriocarcinoma. Case Rep Pediatr 2014;2014:104652.
6 Blair S. Management of a 13-Year-Old Girl with Stage IV Metastatic Choriocarcinoma. Oncopedia#126. Available at: https://www.cure4kids.org/ums/oncopedia (12/14/2009).

Papillary intralymphatic angioendothelioma

Definition. Papillary intralymphatic angioendothelioma (PILA), originally termed endovascular papillary angioendothelioma, or Dabska tumour, is a locally aggressive, rarely metastasizing vascular lesion characterized by lymphatic- or vascular-like channels and papillary endothelial proliferation. The tumour is extremely rare and often affects the skin and subcutaneous tissues of the adult and paediatric populations. PILA is seen in both the male and female sexes uniformly. There is no known ethnic or racial preference [1–5].

Clinical features. PILA has no apparent predilection for any anatomical site. The head and extremities are commonly affected (but in many of the reports tumours are in the dermis and subcutaneous tissues of head, neck and extremities). Only a few cases of this tumour have been described in deeper locations, including spleen, tongue, testis and bone. Clinically, PILA presents as a slowly growing asymptomatic cutaneous or soft tissue nodule or tumour that is violaceous, pink or bluish-black. It usually comes to medical attention when significantly large in size (cases of reported PILA have ranged in size from 1 to 40 cm). Superficial PILA may look like capillary vascular malformations or red-blue or violet-coloured scars [1–5].

Pathology. The lesions are composed of multiple delicate interconnecting vascular channels with formation of papillae that project into the lumen, lined by atypical plump endothelial cells. Some of the papillae contain a hyalinized core. The vascular channels are also lined by plump cuboidal endothelial cells with a focal hobnail or 'match-head' appearance. In some areas, endothelial cells form solid-appearing aggregates with vessel lumens. A variable number of lymphocytes are seen within and around the vascular channels. Mitotic figures are rare. Immunohistochemically, vascular endothelial markers such as von Willebrand factor, CD34, CD31 and Fli-1 are commonly positive, which helps to identify and diagnose the tumour as a type of vascular neoplasm. Moreover, the presence of podoplanin (D2-40) and vascular endothelial growth factor receptor-3 (VEGFR3) has also been confirmed by immunohistochemical markers. These are highly specific lymphatic endothelial markers and suggest that the tumour is more similar to a tumour of lymphatic origin. However, the absence of D2-40 and CD34 in tumour cells has been found in several previously reported cases [1–5].

Differential diagnosis. Since this is an uncommon tumour, differential diagnosis with other more aggressive vascular tumour subtypes, such as angiosarcoma, is essential. In newborns kaposiform haemangioendothelioma should be considered.

Treatment. Wide local excision is the treatment of choice. However, PILA can be locally invasive with a potential to metastasize. Long-term follow-up should be performed to detect locoregional recurrence [5].

Acknowledgements

We would like to thank Dr Jéssica López Marti, Dr Walter Cacciavillano and Dr Adriana Rosé for their scientific contributions and Ms Mariana Tardío for her assistance with the English correction of this chapter.

References

1 Schwartz RA, Dabski C, Dabska M. The Dabska tumor: a thirty-year retrospect. Dermatology 2000;201:1–5.
2 Bhatia A, Nada R, Kumar Y, Menon P. Dabska tumor (endovascular papillary angioendothelioma) of testis: a case report with brief review of literature. Diagn Pathol 2006;1:12.
3 **Bin L, Yang L, Xiao-Ying T et al. Unusual multifocal intraosseous papillary intralymphatic angioendothelioma (Dabska tumor) of facial bones: a case report and review of literature. Diagn Pathol 2013;8:160.**
4 Fanberg-Smith JC. Papillary intralymphatic angioendothelioma. In: Fletcher CDM, Bridge JA, Hogendoorn PCW, Mertens F (eds) World Health Organization Classification of Tumours of Soft Tissue and Bone, 4th edn. Lyon, France: IARC Press, 2013:148–9.
5 **Neves RI, Stevenson J, Hancey MJ et al. Endovascular papillary angioendothelioma (Dabska tumour): underrecognized malignant tumor in childhood. J Pediatr Surg 2011;46:e25–8.**

CHAPTER 118
Vascular Malformations

Laurence M. Boon[1,2] *& Miikka Vikkula*[2]

[1] Centre for Vascular Anomalies, Division of Plastic Surgery, Cliniques Universitaires Saint Luc, University of Louvain, Brussels, Belgium
[2] Human Molecular Genetics, de Duve Institute, University of Louvain, Brussels, Belgium

Classification, 1399 | Fast-flow vascular malformations, 1399 | Slow-flow vascular malformations, 1405

Abstract

Vascular malformations are caused by developmental errors that occur *in utero*. They can be localized or diffuse and occur in any body part, including the viscera. Some are inconsequential, whereas others cause cosmetic problems, functional disability or threaten life. Clinical features permit diagnosis in about 90% of superficial vascular malformations in paediatric patients. Radiological imaging is rarely necessary for diagnosis; it is needed to delineate the malformation, detect an associated anomaly and determine therapy. Interdisciplinary collaboration is necessary not only for diagnosis, but also for treatment. Mutations have been found in several familial and, more recently, in sporadic types of vascular malformations. This offers hope for new forms of treatment.

Classification

In 1996, the International Society for the Study of Vascular Anomalies (ISSVA) approved and further developed a classification based on clinical, radiological, histopathological and haemodynamic characteristics: tumours and malformations [1–5] (www.issva.org). The most common tumour is haemangioma of infancy, a lesion that grows rapidly in neonatal life, involutes in childhood and never arises in an adolescent or an adult [6]. In contrast, vascular malformations are composed of malformed vessels without endothelial cell proliferation unless perturbed, and never regress. They can be divided into two groups, based on rheology and channel morphology (Table 118.1): fast-flow and slow-flow. There are also complex/combined vascular malformations; any combination is possible and many are known as eponymous syndromes [7,8]. They are present at birth but some become obvious later. Some vascular malformations are stable and others expand.

Fast-flow vascular malformations

Key points

- **Localized or extensive arteriovenous malformations (AVM) or syndromic AVM (Parkes Weber syndrome, Bonnet–Dechaume–Blanc or Wyburn–Mason syndrome, Cobb syndrome) or inherited AVM (hereditary haemorrhagic telangiectasia, capillary malformation-AVM).**
- **Histologically characterized by direct communications between arteries and veins.**
- **Can cause pain, distortion, bleeding and congestive heart failure.**
- **Need a multidisciplinary approach.**

Brief introduction. Fast-flow vascular malformations are rare. However, they can be the most devastating vascular anomalies. Most fast-flow cutaneous vascular anomalies are arteriovenous malformations (AVM). In skin, in contrast with the brain, a single, direct arteriovenous fistula (AVF) is almost always post-traumatic. AVM is composed of an epicentre, the nidus, consisting of arterial feeders, enlarged veins and micro- and macrofistulas. They are present at birth or they become evident in childhood [9]. They never regress.

Epidemiology. AVM is a rare, usually sporadic, fast-flow vascular malformation, with no sex preponderance. The exact incidence is unknown. Hereditary haemorrhagic telangiectasia (HHT) and capillary malformation-arteriovenous malformation (CM-AVM) are both autosomal inherited disorders with an estimated prevalence of 1 in 5000 individuals [10–17].

Pathogenesis. *Sporadic AVMs* can be caused by somatic activating MAP2K1 (MEK1) mutations (extracranial AVMs) [18] or somatic activating K-RAS mutations (brain AVMs) (S Nikolaev et al., ASHG 2016 abstract PgmNr 717/F). These lead to activation of the RAS-MAPK signalling pathway, similar to RASA1 mutations causing CM-AVM [17,19].

HHT is caused by alterations in the transforming growth factor-β (TGF-β) signalling pathway. Five types have been described: HHT1 and HHT2 being the most common. The genes most commonly implicated are *endoglin* (*ENG;* HHT1) and *ALK-1* (*ALK1;* HHT2); other genes (*SMAD4* [*JPHT*] and *HGF9* [*HHT5*]) are less frequently involved [20–23]. Endoglin and ALK-1 are type III and type I TGF-β

Harper's Textbook of Pediatric Dermatology, Fourth Edition. Edited by Peter Hoeger, Veronica Kinsler and Albert Yan.

Table 118.1 The 2014 updated International Society for the Study of Vascular Anomalies classification of vascular anomalies.

Vascular tumours			Vascular malformations	
Benign	**Locally aggressive**	**Malignant**	**Simple**	**Combined**
Infantile haemangioma	Kaposiform haemangioendothelioma	Angiosarcoma	Capillary malformation (C)	CVM, CLM
Congenital haemangioma	Retiform haemangioendothelioma	Epitheloid haemangioendothelioma	Lymphatic malformation (LM)	LVM, CLVM
Tufted haemangioma	PILA, Dabska tumor		Venous malformation (VM)	CAVM
Spindle-cell haemangioma	Composite hemanigoendothioma		Arteriovenous malformation (AVM)	CLAVM
Epithelioid haemangioma	Kaposi sarcoma		Arteriovenous fistula	
Pyogenic granuloma				

receptors, and both are well expressed on vascular endothelial cells. Loss of function of this signalling concomitantly increases PI3K-AKT signalling [24].

CM-AVM1 is caused by loss-of-function mutations in *RASA1*, a GTPase regulating RAS activit>y [14,19]. It converts the active GTP-bound RAS into its inactive GDP-bound form [25]. The high intrafamilial phenotypic variability is explained by the necessity of a somatic second-hit mutation to occur [15,26]. *CM-AVM2* is caused by loss-of-function mutation in EPHB4, an endothelial cell receptor on venous vessels [17]. The ligand, EPHRINB2, in contrast to EPHB4, is expressed on arterial endothelial cells. This bidirectional ligand-receptor system is important for arteriovenous identity and separation. EPHB4 signals using p120RASGAP, and the loss of function of either gene causes increased RAS-MAPK signalling [17,19,27–30].

AVM can also be caused by loss-of-function mutation in *PTEN*, a tumour suppressor gene, as seen in patients with PTEN hamartoma tumour syndrome (PHTS) (OMIM #158350 and 153480) [31]. PTEN regulates PI3K-AKT activity, which is moreover regulated at least by the HHT receptor complex (see previously). Loss of function of one of the partners of this complex or of PTEN itself leads to activation of PI3K [31–34].

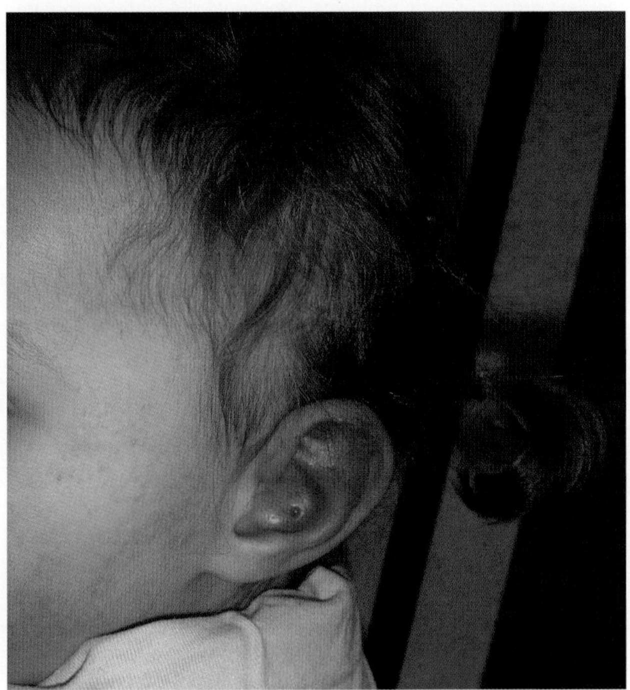

Fig. 118.1 Ear arteriovenous malformation in an infant: the ear is red, infiltrated, warm and throbbing on palpation.

Clinical features.

Localized or extensive AVM

AVM is often mistaken in childhood for haemangioma or port-wine stain (Figs 118.1 and 118.2). In a series of 200 consecutive cases, 40% (68 cases) of AVMs were visible at birth, 24.7% (42 cases) became evident during childhood, 10% (17 cases) at puberty and only 25.3% (43 patients) in adulthood [9].

Puberty and trauma can trigger expansion as fast-flow becomes clinically evident [35]. A purple colour and a mass develop. Other local signs include warmth, a thrill, a bruit and pulses of increased amplitude (Schobinger Stage I). The most common location is head and neck (70%) [9]. As an AVM worsens, draining veins become prominent, tortuous and distended (Schobinger Stage II) (see Fig. 118.1). Wherever the site of an AVM, the eventual consequences are darkening of skin colour, spontaneous and/or recurrent ulceration, pain and intermittent bleeding (Schobinger Stage III) [9,36,37]. These changes can occur in childhood, and haemorrhage can be life threatening. A facial AVM localized to the skin and/or bones (ethmoid, maxilla or mandible) can cause asymmetrical hypertrophy and gingival bleeding [37]. A nasal AVM can cause epistaxis. AVM in a digit gradually causes ischaemic cutaneous changes and shortening of the nail and distal phalanx. Pseudo-Kaposi sarcomatous cutaneous changes occur in association with AVM in the lower limb [38], but rarely before adolescence. Cardiac failure can be the end-stage of a large AVM (Schobinger Stage IV).

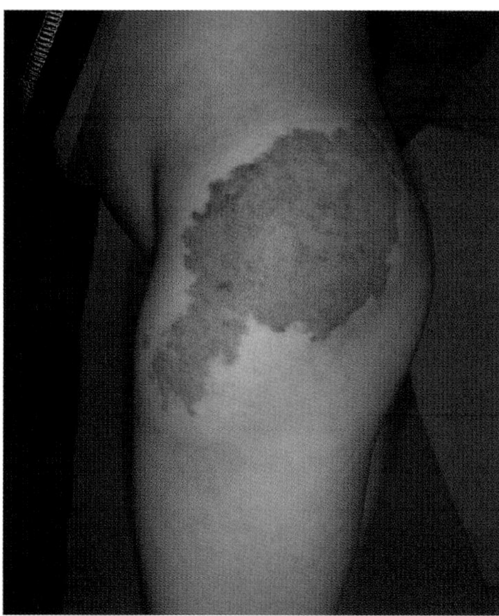

Fig. 118.2 Flank arteriovenous malformation in a 6-year-old child initially diagnosed as infantile haemangioma.

Parkes Weber syndrome (OMIM 608354 and 618196)

Parkes Weber syndrome is an eponym used for multiple capillary–arteriolovenular malformations (CAVM) with soft tissue and skeletal hypertrophy of the affected limb. Usually the lower extremity is involved, sometimes the upper limb [39]. It can also be part of the CM-AVM phenotype (see later).

Cutaneous warmth and bruit are present as a result of the numerous arteriovenous (AV) microfistulas along the affected limb, particularly near the joints. Leg length is measured clinically during infancy. Bony overgrowth may reach excess length of more than 5 cm. Common other complications during puberty or later are bony lesions, pathological fractures, painful skin ulceration, distal pseudo-Kaposi sarcoma skin changes, high cardiac output and congestive heart failure. Associated lymphoedema can also occur and causes major disability [39].

Bonnet–Dechaume–Blanc and Wyburn–Mason syndromes

These eponyms denote AVM in centrofacial and/or hemifacial skin, the eye and the mesodiencephalon [40–42]. Retinal involvement defines Bonnet–Dechaume–Blanc syndrome, also known as Wyburn–Mason syndrome, although it is not universal. Brégeat syndrome has no retinal or choroidal AVM, but exhibits vascular anomalies in the conjunctiva. The skin lesions are red, warm and thick, rarely following a trigeminal distribution (as in Sturge–Weber syndrome). Ipsilateral retinal, optic nerve, chiasma, optic pathway, basal ganglia and cerebral AVMs can be present. The jaws, nose and mouth are sometimes involved. AVM is present at birth and progressively worsens. Epistaxis, exophthalmos and hemianopia may occur. Some patients manifest a variety of neurological symptoms, including intracranial haemorrhage from the brain AVM, as well as mental changes.

Cobb syndrome

This sporadic syndrome is composed of cutaneous AVM, masquerading as capillary malformation, and spinal cord AVMs in the same metamere. The spinal cord AVM is either (i) intramedullary or perimedullary and fed by spinal cord arteries or (ii) dural and fed by radicular meningeal arteries [43]. AVM in the vertebrae and paraspinal muscles can also occur in the same metamere. Patients are at risk for local complications such as limb hypertrophy and ulceration. Neurological complications, often beginning in childhood, include pain, sensory disturbance and neurogenic bladder and bowel; motor symptoms (monoplegia, paraplegia or quadriplegia) depend on the location and extent of the lesion. We could postulate that Cobb syndrome is part of the CM-AVM phenotype; however, it is not known if these patients have distant multiple CMs [44].

Hereditary haemorrhagic telangiectasia

HHT manifests as the combination of the following triad: multiple cutaneous and mucosal telangiectasias, chronic epistaxis and familial history [45]. The diagnosis is clinical, in accordance with the Curaçao criteria (Tables 118.2 and 118.3). The estimated frequency of manifestations in HHT patients is: spontaneous, recurrent epistaxis (90%), skin telangiectasia (75%), hepatic or pulmonary AVMs (30%), and gastrointestinal bleeding (15%) [48].

Telangiectases are punctate, linear, stellate or nodular, and occur on the cheeks, nose, lips, tongue and other oral mucous membranes, and fingers (Fig. 118.3). Recurrent epistaxis, the most frequent symptom of HHT, occurs in 90% of patients and usually develops during late adolescence. Gastrointestinal bleeding, occuring in 10–40% of patients, begins in adulthood [49]. Symptoms may include abdominal pain, jaundice, symptoms of high-output cardiac failure, and bleeding from oesophageal varices [50].

AVMs located in the liver, brain or spinal cord, and/or lungs, manifest in 30% of cases [48]. Pulmonary AVMs affect about 50% of HHT, especially in HHT1. These patients can exhibit dyspnoea or haemoptysis, and can die from massive haemoptysis or haemothorax. Pulmonary AVMs place one-half of these patients at risk

Table 118.2 Hereditary haemorrhagic telangiectasia (HHT) subtypes.

	HHT1	HHT2	JPHT
Relative frequency	49%	49%	2%
Chromosome	9q34	12q	18q
Gene	Endoglin	Activin receptor-like kinase 1	SMAD4
Telangiectasias	80%	80%	80%?
Epistaxis	90%	90%	90%?
CNS AVM	9–16%	0–6%	
Liver AVM	44–66%	58–83%	
Pulmonary AVM	46–76%	5–48%	

AVM, arteriovenous malformation; CNS, central nervous system; HHT, hereditary haemorrhagic telangiecstasia; JPHT, juvenile polyposis hereditary hemorrhagic telangiectasia.

Source: Adapted from Bayrak-Toydemir et al. (2006) [46] and Shovlin et al. (2010) [47].

Table 118.3 Curaçao criteria for hereditary haemorrhagic telangiectasia.

Curaçao criteria	%	Diagnosis	Potential complications
1) Nosebleeds Spontaneous, recurrent	90	Evident	***Anaemia; massive acute haemorrhage***
2) Telangiectasia Lips; oral cavity, finger tip, nose	80	Evident	***Cosmetic, haemorrhage***
3) Visceral lesions, ***such as*** ***a) Gastrointestinal telangiectasia*** (with or without bleeding)	15–30	Endoscopy *(upper/lower)*	***Haemorrhage*** (chronic) ***Anaemia***
b) Pulmonary AVMs	50	CT scan C-Echo (CXR)	***Most asymptopmatic*** ***Right-to-left shunt:*** Hypoxaemia +/- dyspnoea; Stroke/TIA* Brain abscess Migraine Decompression illness ***Haemorrhage*** Haemoptysis Haemothorax *rare except specific circumstances*
c) Cerebral vascular malformations AV fistulae (AVF) Macro (nidus-type) AVM Micro AVM (<1cm) Capillary telangiectasia *Other forms can occur*	10–20	*MRI scan Angiography*	***Haemorrhage*** *depends on type:* AVF > macro > micro ≥ tel. For AVM (–0.5% per annum, lower than general population) ***Headache*** ***Epilepsy*** ***High output cardiac failure*** *(Paediatric cases)*
d) Hepatic vascular malformations Hepatic artery to hepatic vein Hepatic artery to portal vein Portal vein to hepatic vein	30–70	*Doppler US CT +/- invasive*	***Most (>90%) asymptomatic*** ***Hepatic AVMs:*** High cardiac output ± failure Post capillary pulm. hyp. ***Hepato-portal VMs:*** Portal hypertension + sequelae ***Porto-venous VMs:*** Biliary ischaemia
e) Spinal AVMs	<1%	*Spinal MRI*	***Haemorrhage;*** Paraplegia (acute, subacute or progressive) ***SOL*** +/- ***steal***: Pain, asymmetric growth progressive myelopathy in adults
4) FAMILY HISTORY: Affected first degree relative			

AVF, arteriovenous fistulae; AVM, arteriovenous malformation; CT, computed tomography; MRI, magnetic resonance imaging; TIA, transient ischaemic attack; US, ultrasound.
Source: Adapted from Shovlin et al. (2010) [47]. Reproduced with permission of Elsevier.

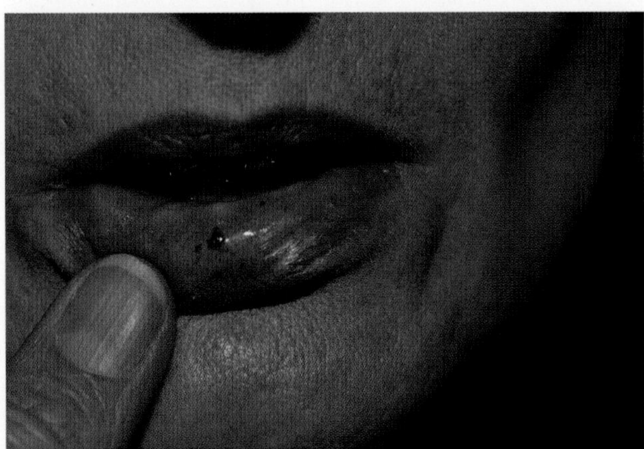

Fig. 118.3 Mucosal lip telangiectases of hereditary haemorrhagic telangiectasia.

for neurological complications from septic emboli, with brain abscesses. As a result of pulmonary AV shunting, a defect in the bacterial filtering function of the pulmonary circulation allows bacteria to enter the systemic circulation. Infection in a lung AVF can also result in bacteraemia.

Central nervous system AVM in HHT can cause acute headache and spinal cord or intracerebral haemorrhage, sometimes leading to significant cognitive and motor impairment [48]. Nasal, gastric or colonic endoscopy localizes bleeding sites [51].

CM-AVM

CM-AVM is characterized by multiple small pinkish-red, slightly tan round-to-oval CMs and familial history [13,14,52]. Telangiectasias seem more common in CM-AVM2. Some CMs are present at birth, whereas others

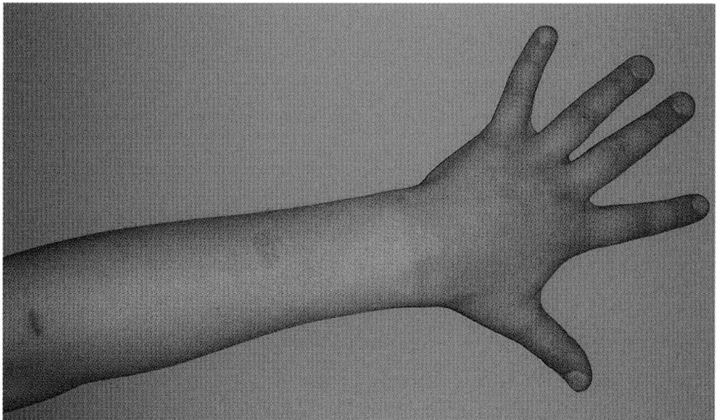

Fig. 118.4 Capillary malformations of capillary malformation-arteriovenous malformation: the lesion is pinkish-greyish with a pale halo.

appear later, but remain asymptomatic throughout life. Their size varies from a few millimetres to several centimetres in diameter. They often have a pale halo and an increased flow by hand-held Doppler examination (Fig. 118.4). There is a large inter- and intrafamilial phenotypic variability. AVM is present in 23% and 13% of CM-AVM1 and CM-AVM2 patients. Vein of Galen aneurysmal malformation, spinal and intracranial AVF represent 80% of AVM of CM-AVM2 [13,16,17,19,44]. They are often symptomatic at birth or in early childhood. In contrast to HHT, visceral AVMs are rare; extracranial lesions noticeably affect skin, subcutis and sometimes muscles and bones, and are located in the head and neck region. Parkes Weber syndrome associated with distant cutaneous CMs is also part of the phenotype [14,15].

PHTS

Previously known as Bannayan–Riley–Ruvalcaba syndrome (BRRS) and Cowden syndrome. These patients typically have the triad: macrocephaly, multiple lipomas and AVMs. Other symptoms include penile freckling, multiple developmental venous anomalies in the brain, and an increased risk of malignancy. The vascular malformations are often multifocal (57%) and musculoskeletal, and associated with ectopic fat deposition and disruption of the normal tissular architecture. Other vascular anomalies, such as capillary, venous or lymphatic malformations can also be part of the phenotype [53,54].

Differential diagnosis. In an infant or child, AVM must be distinguished from CM and infantile haemangioma (Figs 118.1 and 118.2). Ultrasonography and colour Doppler demonstrate that haemangiomas have equatorial feeding arteries, peripheral veins, variable echogenicity and fast-flow, but no true arteriovenous (AV) shunting. Hereditary benign telangiectasia (HBT) which is not associated with AVM, is the main differential diagnosis with CM-AVM.

A few other dermatological lesions, uncommon in the paediatric patient, mimic AVM. Epithelioid haemangio-endothelioma usually occurs on the distal extremity as a purple and locally aggressive lesion [55]. Lupus erythematosus tumidus or sarcoidosis on the ear or nose, and Melkersson–Rosenthal syndrome of the lip can masquerade as AVM. The pseudo-Kaposi sarcomatous changes, developing unilaterally in a severe AVM of the leg, are easily differentiated from true Kaposi sarcoma. Dabska tumour, in childhood, can simulate an AVM, when located in the ear (Fig. 118.5).

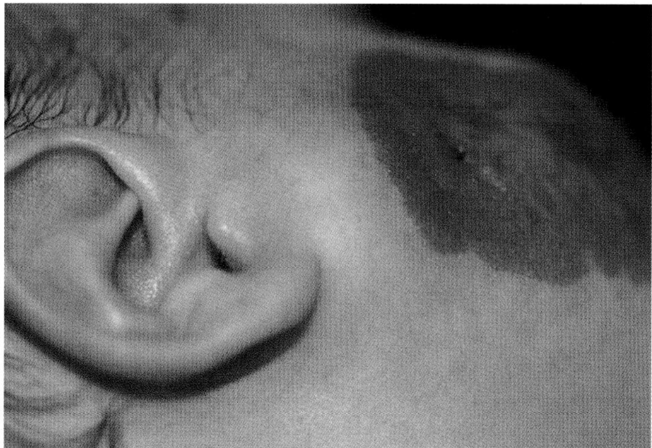

Fig. 118.5 Dabska tumour mimicking arteriovenous malformation in a 5-month-old girl. This lesion was slightly warm but no pulsatile artery was palpated.

Laboratory and histology findings. Radiological investigation is recommended whenever AVM is suspected clinically [36,56]. A number of techniques define the nature and extent of the lesion.

- *Ultrasonography combined with grey-scale and colour Doppler*: An AVM is heterogeneously echogenic and exhibits low-resistance, high-velocity arterial flow and pulsatile venous flow [36]. Vessels are tortuous. In contrast to infantile haemangioma, there is no mass. Pulsed Doppler measures the arterial output (of carotid, axillary or femoral arteries) compared with the uninvolved side and allows serial evaluation in a noninvasive fashion.
- *Computed tomography* (CT) with contrast cannot definitely differentiate between haemangioma, venous malformation (VM) and AVM. A three-dimensional angioscan may be useful to analyse the feeding and draining vessels portraying the AVM, especially in childhood.
- *Magnetic resonance imaging* (MRI) is the best imaging study to define the extent of an AVM. Flow-voids correspond to fast-flow vessels, in all sequences with gadolinium (spin-echo T1- and T2-weighted sequences) except gradient-echo (in which sequence-increased signal is present in vascular spaces).
- *Magnetic resonance angiography* (MRA) portrays the anomalous vascular network. It can replace arteriography for follow-up of AVM.
- *Arteriography* depicts the angio-architecture of an AVM, especially prior to embolization. In early childhood Parkes Weber syndrome, arteriography may show only diffuse hypervascularity of the limb, and AV fistulas become obvious later in life.
- Scaniometry is performed after the age of 2 years in all patients with Parkes Weber syndrome. If abnormal, it is repeated yearly.

Genetic testing should be performed in patients with multifocal CMs (CM-AVM1 and 2) or telangiectasia (HHT1/2/5 or *JPHT*) and AVM as well as in patients with AVM and associated macrocephaly (PTEN). It will enable genetic counselling, and further imaging for eventual undetected malformations and/or cancer [57]. This molecular diagnosis is recommended in newborns, because lethal cerebral haemorrhage from undiagnosed AVMs has been reported in such families [48]. Investigations in families with HHT can detect asymptomatic, unruptured intracranial AVMs [48,58–61]. Treatment guidelines must balance the lifetime risk for bleeding against surgical morbidity and mortality. The incidence of cerebrovascular anomalies, including microAVMs and cerebral telangiectasia, was considered to be 20%.

Histologically, an AVM is usually poorly delineated and consists of distorted arteries and veins with irregularly thickened fibromuscular walls, discontinuous elastic network, direct communications representing arteriovenous shunting, stromal fibrosis and a variable admixture of capillaries.

Treatment and prevention.

Prevention

AVM is the most unpredictable of all vascular malformations. Usually AVM remains quiescent in childhood, but tends to enlarge in time, and cause local destruction. A large AVM, usually in a limb, can cause congestive heart failure, but rarely in childhood. Once the initial diagnostic work-up is completed, the child should have periodic clinical evaluation and serial Doppler and/or MRI and MRA should be performed.

Failure to recognize its true nature can lead to dangerous mismanagement and complications. Partial excision and ligation of arterial feeders usually trigger AVM expansion, especially during puberty. Mismanagement of a limb AVM can lead to gangrene, necessitating amputation [13,62].

Treatment

In the paediatric age group, AVM is often clinically inconspicuous, but every AVM is potentially dangerous. Embolic and/or surgical treatment of a quiescent AVM is controversial. An AVM was usually not treated in its quiescent stage. However, recent study showed that surgical resection of stage I AVM is associated with a lower recurrence rate [35]. The management of an AVM should be multidisciplinary, modest about predicting outcome, and should never overestimate therapeutic possibility. The only acceptable surgical stratagem is complete resection [37,62–64]. Partial excision leads to transient improvement, but the AVM inevitably re-expands over time. Proximal ligation or embolization of arterial feeding vessels is contraindicated; after a period of transient benefit, vascular recruitment occurs, as neighbouring arteries supply the nidus. Furthermore, arterial ligation prevents access to the nidus at a time when therapeutic embolization becomes necessary [65,66].

A conservative approach is usually taken for patients with Parkes Weber syndrome. Management is fundamentally conservative. Elastic compression stockings provide relief of pain caused by venous engorgement. In the presence of leg length discrepancy, an adapted shoe-lift prevents compensatory tilting of the pelvis. In cases of increased vascularization of the growth zone, embolization of the knee cartilage artery may retard excess growth. Stapling epiphyseodesis can, in our experience, stimulate the AVM of this syndrome. In contrast, percutaneous epiphyseodesis is less aggressive. Lengthening of the normal leg is another option when the predicted final height of the child is poor; however, lengthening of a normal extremity has complications, and the risk/benefit ratio must be carefully considered.

Patients with anaemia require iron replacement and, occasionally, blood transfusion. In patients with HHT and pulmonary AVMs, antibacterial prophylaxis is recommended for dental, respiratory, gastrointestinal or genitourinary procedures that place the patient at risk for bacteraemia. A pharmacological approach using marimastat, a matrix metalloproteinase inhibitor, was successfully used to treat an extensive AVM of the arm that caused rapid progressive bony destruction in a young girl despite ethanol embolization. The treatment, performed over a 9-year period, resulted in improvement of the AV shunts and regrowth of bones. No adverse effects were reported [67]. Other antiangiogenic medications have also been effectively used to stop acute bleeding and epistaxis, such as thalidomide and bevacizumab [68,69].

Superselective arterial embolization

The most common embolic materials are liquid (ethanol, isobutylcyanoacrylate), particles (Ivalon) or implantable devices (coils, microspheres). Embolization alone as a palliative treatment is only indicated for complicated AVM (e.g. in case of ulceration or haemorrhage), when surgical excision will be disfiguring or mutilating. Embolization of an AVM, unlike embolization of a single direct AVF, is rarely 'curative'. The aim of the treatment is to occlude the shunts with a permanent or an irritating material, such as histoacryl glue or coils, or ethanol; particles are not indicated. The site of injection of the embolic agent must be as close as possible to the nidus. Proximal occlusion causes secondary refilling of the nidus through collateral arteries. In patients with maxillary or mandibular AVM, embolization should be performed prior to dental extraction, to minimize haemorrhage. Microcatheter guidewire systems, as used in interventional neuroradiology, permit a superselective approach to the nidus [70]. Direct puncture of the nidus, in association with local arterial and venous compression, is necessary when arteries are tortuous, or in patients who have previously had arterial ligation.

Surgical resection

Arterial embolization is usually performed prior to resection [70–72], to occlude the nidus and minimize bleeding during the procedure. It does not affect the margins of resection. Usually, the AVM and the overlying skin are widely excised. Microsurgical free-flap transfer may be necessary for reconstruction [71]. Cutaneous expansion, prior to embolization and resection, is an alternative surgical strategy. The overlying skin can be saved only if normal; vascular-stained skin left in place often leads to recurrence. Lytic bony lesions, for example in the mandible, can cause life-threatening haemorrhage requiring endovascular management [73], sometimes followed by resection. AVM in the distal extremity often recurs after technically successful embolization and a symptom-free interval [74,75]. Because AVM is so difficult to eradicate, the word 'control' rather than 'cure' should be used and patients must be followed for many years.

Treatment of orbital and/or intraspinal cord AVM is a challenge because of the anatomical and haemorrhagic characteristics of AVM in this location [42]. Neurosurgical procedures, consisting of complete removal of the nidus, are not always feasible. Neuroendovascular treatment is an alternative to surgical resection.

Other therapeutic modalities

Electrodesiccation and/or laser (Nd:YAG, diode, carbon dioxide or pulsed dye lasers) can be useful to stop bleeding of HHT cutaneous and mucosal lesions. In contrast to sporadic CM, pulsed-dye laser is rarely effective in CM of CM-AVM.

Slow-flow vascular malformations

Venous anomalies

Key points

- **Most common referrals to multidisciplinary centres for vascular anomalies.**
- **Bluish in colour, solitary or multifocal, localized or extensive.**
- **Compressible on palpation, presence of phleboliths is pathognomonic.**
- **Fifty percent have localized intravascular coagulopathy with elevated D-dimer level and normal-to-low fibrinogen level.**
- **Can be inherited as an autosomal dominant pattern: cutaneomucosal venous malformation fewer than 1% and glomuvenous malformation 5%.**
- **Can be part of a syndrome, such as Klippel–Trenaunay, blue rubber bleb naevus or Maffucci syndrome.**

Brief introduction. VMs involve the collecting side of the vascular network. Most lesions are sporadic and unifocal (VM, 93%); 1% are multifocal. VMs can be localized or extensive and may be located in the head and neck (the most common location), extremities and/or trunk. VMs occur in skin, mucous membranes, various soft tissues and viscera, and even bones. The lesions are present at birth, or they become clinically evident later [76–78]. VMs are mainly isolated, but can be part of complex vascular disorders, such as the Klippel–Trenaunay, Maffucci and blue rubber bleb naevus (BRBN) syndromes [2,79,80].

Epidemiology and pathogenesis. The exact incidence is unknown, but is estimated at 1:5–10 000, because VMs are the most common vascular malformations referred to multidisciplinary centres specializing in vascular anomalies [80]. Mainly sporadic, familial forms occur and include cutaneomucosal venous malformation (VMCM, <1%) and glomuvenous malformation (GVM, 5%) [81–83]. They both have an age-dependent variation in penetrance, which reaches its maximum by 20 years of age (87% for VMCM and 92.7% for GVM) [84]. Large VMCMs and GVMs are present at birth. However, 17% of affected individuals develop new small lesions over time [85]. Maffucci syndrome occurs sporadically, without gender predilection. Cerebral cavernous malformation is another inherited form of mixed malformation containing both capillary and venous vessel malformation [77,86,87].

Pathogenesis. Germline mutations in the gene encoding the angiopoietin receptor, *TIE2/TEK* (chromosome 9 p), have been identified in VMCM families [25,83,88,89]. These mutations have been shown to cause ligand-independent hyperphosphorylation of TIE2 and alteration of the downstream signalling specificity of this vascular endothelium-specific receptor tyrosine kinase [25,83,90]. A somatic second-hit was identified in two VMCM tissues. One causes a local loss of the protective wild-type allele, whereas the other is a second-hit on the allele carrying the germline mutation. This suggests paradominant inheritance [81,91,92]. These mutations activate the PI3K/AKT signalling pathway in endothelial cells [93,94].

GVMs are caused by loss-of-function mutations in *glomulin* (chromosome 1p21–p22), causing dysregulation of vascular smooth muscle cell differentiation [84,95,96]. A common five-nucleotide deletion is present in 40% of the patients [97]. In addition, a somatic second-hit is required for lesions to form, leading to complete loss of function of glomulin. The most common second-hit is acquired uniparental isodisomy that leads to homozygosity of the inherited mutation [98,99]. This explains the variable expressivity regarding penetrance, extent of the lesions, and number of lesions within family members [97,100]. So far, a mutation in glomulin has been found in almost all GVM families tested, demonstrating locus homogeneity [97,101,102].

Sporadic VMs are also caused by genetic mutations. In 60%, the cause is a somatic activating mutation in *TIE2* [91]. The most common one is L914F. The somatic mutations differ from the inherited VMCM mutations; L914F has never been seen as a germline change, suggesting its effects are too strong in the germline and are probably lethal [88,91,93,94]. Another 20% of sporadically occurring VMs are caused by somatic mutations in the *PIK3CA* gene [103]. Like the *TIE2* mutations, they have an activating effect. Both activate the PI3K/AKT signalling pathway, underscoring the importance of this signalling pathway in the pathogenesis of VMs [103,104].

Sporadically occurring multifocal venous malformation is also caused by *TIE2* mutations. These patients often have two *TIE2* mutations. Most frequently, a R915C mutation is present as a mosaic change in blood, and a somatic Y897C mutation occurs on top of it on the same allele [92].

BRBN is also caused by somatic mutations in *TIE2* [92]. The most common is a T1105N-T1106P double mutation. The same double mutations can be identified with equal allele frequencies in distinct, distally located lesions of the same BRBN patient. This suggests that separate lesions are formed by endothelial cells that originate from a single common site [92].

Maffucci syndrome, in contrast to Ollier disease, is not caused by *PTHR1* mutations [105]. Rather, somatic mutations are seen in isocitrate dehydrogenases genes 1 or 2 (IDH1 and 2) [106,107].

Cerebral 'cavernous' malformations (CCMs) have been mapped to three chromosomal loci: CCM1 to 7 q, CCM2 to 7 p and CCM3 to 3 p (Table 118.4). CCM1 patients demonstrated loss-of-function mutations of *KRIT1* (Krev1 interaction trapped 1) [86,109,110], CCM2 in malcavernin and CCM3 in PDCD10. The three molecules interact in an intracellular signalling pathway [111,112].

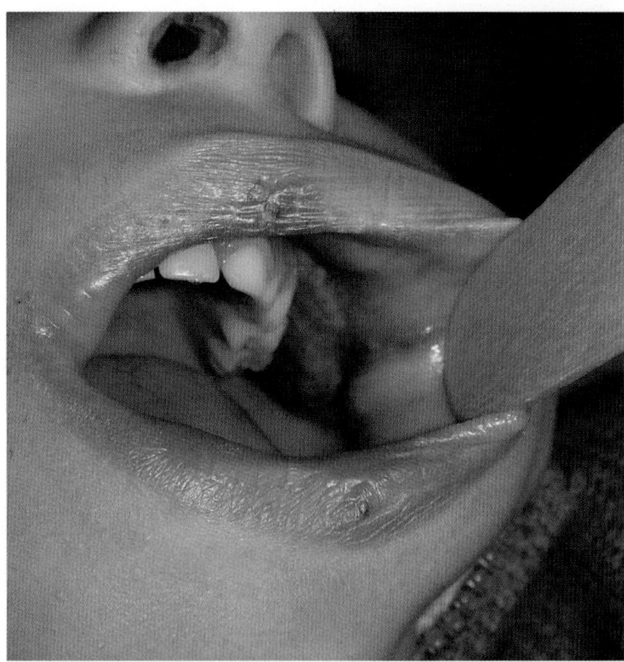

Fig. 118.6 Intrabuccal venous malformation causing dental malalignment.

Clinical features.

Localized or extensive venous malformations

Ectatic venous channels within the dermis give the lesions their characteristic blue colour. VMs swell with exertion and when the region is dependent. Deformation of involved tissues slowly worsens. Skin temperature is normal. There is no thrill or bruit. Depending on the size and site of their lesion, patients complain of swelling, pain or a burning sensation. Increased stiffness and pain upon awakening are frequent as well as painful thrombosis and phleboliths [80,113].

Head and neck VMs are usually unilateral; bilateral involvement occurs rarely. Owing to a mass effect, VMs can cause facial asymmetry, progressive distortion of features, dental malalignment and malocclusion (Fig. 118.6). Intraorbital VM varies in size, depending on head position. Enophthalmia can occur when the patient is standing, and minor exophthalmia when lying supine, but vision is not altered. Optic nerve compression rarely results from a VM in the orbital apex. Mucosal oral VMs involve the tongue, cheek or palate; they can extend to the parotid, parapharyngeal and laryngeal areas. VM in the oropharynx rarely impairs speech, but pharyngeal and laryngeal VMs can cause difficulties in swallowing, airway compromise and obstructive sleep apnoea.

A pure VM in an extremity commonly invades muscles and joints (Fig. 118.7) [85,114,115]. Distal upper or lower limb VMs cause enlarged blue fingers or toes with sagging skin. VM affecting an entire upper or lower limb and adjacent trunk causes increased limb girth, but length discrepancy is uncommon. Haemarthrosis is particularly troublesome in children with VM-associated chronic localized intravascular coagulopathy (LIC), mimicking haemarthrosis seen in haemophilia, and leading to degenerative joint disease and destructive cartilage/bone changes. Symptoms abate with bed rest but, if not treated,

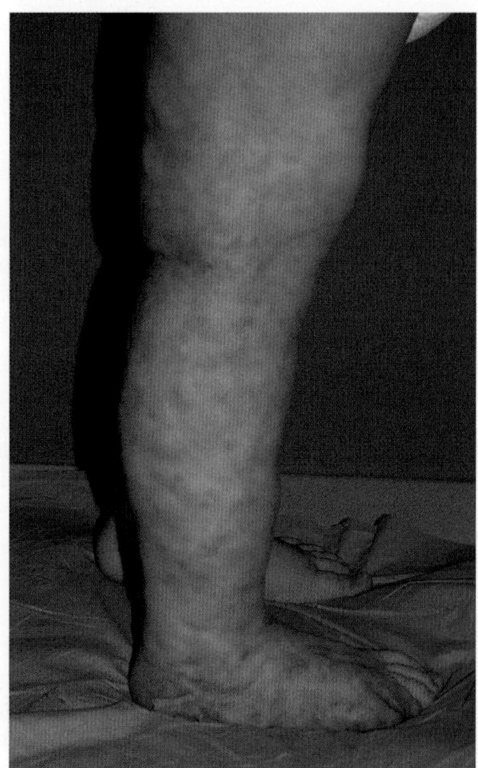

Fig. 118.7 Extensive venous malformation of lower extremity involving skin, subcutis, muscle and joint and associated with severe localized intravascular coagulopathy.

Table 118.4 Cerebral cavernous malformations (CCMs)

	CCM1	CCM2	CCM3
Relative frequency	53–65%	20%	10–16%
Chromosome	7q	7p	3q
Gene	*KRIT1*	*MGC4607* (malcavernin)	*PDCD10*

Source: Data from Akers et al. (2017) [108].

this ends in flexion deformity and ankylosis of the joint [114]. These lesions are often mislabelled in the literature as bony, intramuscular or synovial 'haemangioma' or 'cavernous haemangioma' [116].

Genitalia, in both males and females, are commonly involved when there is lower extremity VM. VM slowly worsens in childhood and adolescence, and phleboliths develop. Amyotrophy is a common, early finding in a child with extensive limb VM; slight limb undergrowth is common. Slight overgrowth can also occur, but never to the extent seen in Klippel–Trenaunay syndrome. Weakening of the bony shaft caused by intraosseous VM may result in pathological fracture after minimal trauma [114].

Blue rubber bleb naevus syndrome of Bean (OMIM 112200)

Bean named this VM disorder the *blue rubber bleb naevus syndrome*. Lesions are cutaneous and visceral. Familial examples (with autosomal dominant inheritance) are rare or nonexistent (obvious confusion exists in the literature with the familial VMCM). Cutaneous lesions consist of blue, soft nodules, which occasionally aggregate into large masses. There are small, colourless, dome-shaped, nipple-like lesions ('rubber bleb'), often associated with one large, so called 'dominant VM' (Fig. 118.8) [92]. The visceral vascular anomalies predominantly affect the gastrointestinal system. They are sessile (submucosal) or polypoid and visualized by endoscopy. Lesions are found throughout the gastrointestinal tract (oesophagus, stomach, small and large bowel) and in the mesentery, and may cause recurrent intestinal bleeding. Other visceral locations include the oral cavity, nasopharynx, anus, genitalia, bladder, brain, spinal cord, liver, spleen, lungs, bones and skeletal muscles [117].

Syndromic venous malformation Maffucci syndrome (OMIM 166000)

Maffucci syndrome was described in 1881. It combines spindle cell haemangioendotheliomas, which clinically mimic VMs, and enchondromas. Lesions are small or large, disseminated or localized, and some are segmental. Congenital cutaneous and bony lesions are rare (one-quarter of cases). More commonly, the lesions appear throughout childhood and adulthood [118–121].

Metaphyseal and diaphyseal enchondromas are considered similar to those seen in Ollier disease. The lesions, as seen on radiographs, are round or ovoid, well-demarcated radiolucent masses. They result from an abnormal development of cartilage into bone. Skeletal deformity and pathological fracture are common. Deformity of the hands is caused by both cutaneous and skeletal lesions. Secondary dwarfism may develop because of shortening and deformity of long leg bones. The hands are involved in 89% of patients, the fingers in 88% of cases, the toes in 61% and the long bones of the limbs in 30–40%. Cranial and pelvic bones are rarely affected. Various neurological defects and ocular complications (proptosis) occur with cranial lesions. The reported incidence of malignant transformation in enchondromas is 30%.

Vascular lesions in Maffucci syndrome consist of blue, exophytic nodules that can be emptied by manual compression. Phleboliths may develop.

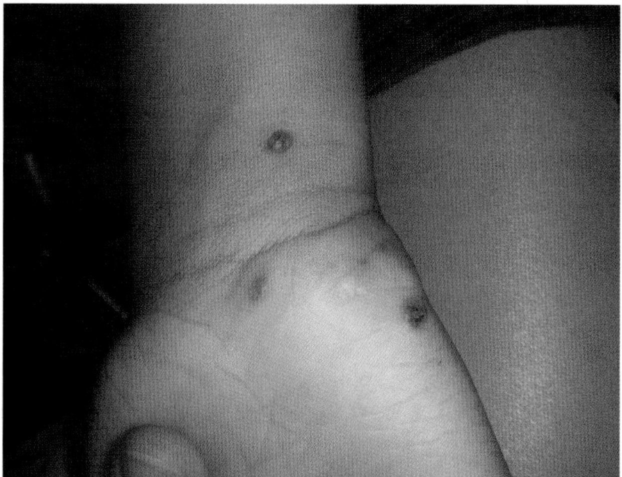

Fig. 118.8 Dome-shaped, nipple-like venous malformation lesion typical of blue rubber bleb nevus phenotype.

Venous malformation, multiple cutaneous and mucosal (VMCM) (OMIM #600195)

This autosomal dominant syndrome is characterized by multiple, small, dome-shaped VMs, although large venous anomalies can also be seen [25,83,85,88]. The cutaneous lesions are slightly similar to those seen in Bean syndrome (see previously), but they have no rubbery consistency and only rarely involve the gastrointestinal tract.

GVM (OMIM #138000)

This disorder is inherited in autosomal dominant fashion. Multiple, blue or purple, macular to papular and nodular dermal vascular lesions are isolated or grouped in a plaque-like segmental distribution (Fig.118.9) [85,100]. They occur anywhere on the skin, including the face. Congenital regional forms are difficult to diagnose because they appear more pink than blue, and are somewhat atrophic [100]. Thickening progressively develops later in life and the colour changes to deep blue. The lesions progress during childhood and adolescence and become tender with cold or manual compression. Some

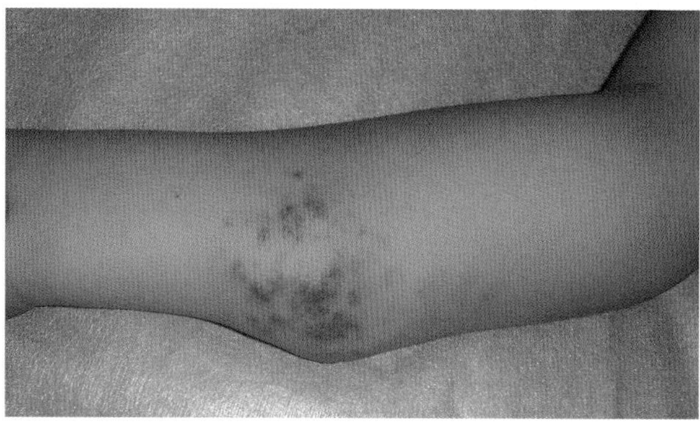

Fig. 118.9 Foream glomuvenous malformation.

SECTION 25: VASCULAR TUMOURS

individuals in a given family have few lesions, whereas other members can exhibit hundreds of lesions.

Familial cerebral 'cavernous' malformation (OMIM #116860)

This disorder is characterized by multiple cerebral and occasional retinal VMs. Symptoms include headache, epilepsy and abrupt intracranial haemorrhage, with a risk of sudden death [110]. Some CCM1 patients were associated with a peculiar cutaneous vascular malformation called 'hyperkeratotic cutaneous capillary–venous malformation' (HCCVM). This phenotype is characterized by cutaneous capillarovenous patches of hyperkeratotic purple papules overlying a bluish infiltration of the dermis [77,78,86,87,110]. In rare instances, cutaneous bluish or dark purple nodules or papules ('nodular VMs'), reminiscent of lesions seen in BRBN syndrome, have been associated with CCM1.

Differential diagnosis. A blue VM can be confused with the naevus of Ota or of Ito. Sinus pericranii, with abnormal cerebral venous drainage through a bony cranial defect, from or to the intracranial area, mimics a VM of the forehead or scalp. A dilated vein at the base of the nose is common in newborns, but prominent veins in the frontonasal area are occasionally caused by collateral cerebral venous circulation through the cavernous sinus, superior ophthalmic vein, angular vein and facial vein, as a result of a vein of Galen aneurysmal malformation. A deep cephalic VM and an intramuscular limb VM that has atypical MRI findings require a biopsy to rule out sarcoma or neurofibroma. VM deeply located in the neck area should be differentiated from various types of congenital cysts (thyroglossal duct, bronchogenic cyst, etc.). It is important to differentiate between extremity VMs and a complex/combined limb vascular malformation (see later).

Cerebral developmental venous anomaly (DVA) consists of dilated intramedullary veins converging into a large draining vein. This vessel enters either the superficial or the deep system. DVA is an uncommon pathway of cerebral drainage, occurring in 0.05–0.5% of the general population. By contrast, 20% of patients with extensive head and neck VMs have DVA [122], usually consisting of ectatic and dilated veins converging into the drainage system of the deep brain. In contrast with cerebral cavernous malformation, opacification of DVA appears in the venous phase, as do normal veins. CT and MRI with MRA image DVAs. These are usually asymptomatic. Some patients develop headaches, but intracerebral haemorrhage, seizures and neurological deficits do not occur.

Laboratory and histology findings. Venous malformations exhibit a continuous cycle of thrombosis and thrombolysis, causing the formation of phleboliths (Fig. 118.10). A *coagulation profile*, with platelet count, fibrinogen and D-dimer levels, should be obtained in any child with VM [80,114,123–125], because chronic LIC is pathognomonic of VM, in an otherwise healthy patient [124]. Severe LIC is often associated with large size deep involvement of underlying tissues and presence of phleboliths, and is rare in cervicofacial VMs [123–127]. Deep venous thrombosis is uncommon and pulmonary embolism is extremely rare.

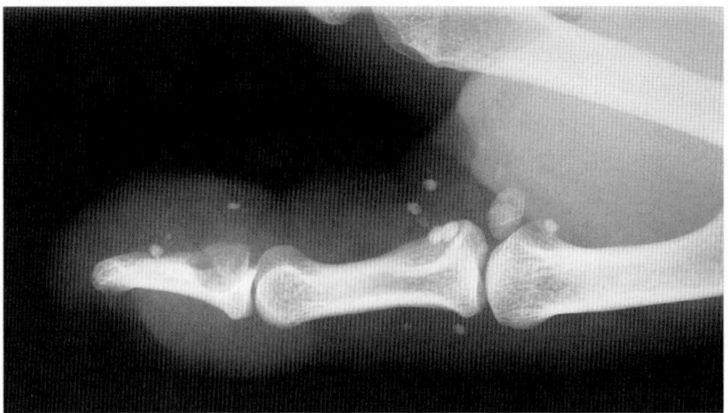

Fig. 118.10 Phleboliths seen on plain radiograph in a hand venous malformation.

A number of events, such as operation, sclerotherapy, prolonged immobilization, menstruation and pregnancy, can trigger the conversion of LIC to disseminated intravascular coagulopathy, with per- and postoperative bleeding related to consumption of fibrinogen and clotting factors.

This consumptive coagulopathy (very high D-dimer level with normal-to-low fibrinogen level) is completely different from the Kasabach–Merritt phenomenon (KMP), which is a profound thrombocytopenic coagulopathy, often associated with anaemia, low fibrinogen and variable elevation of D-dimers, and associated with aggressive vascular tumours of infancy (kaposiform haemangioendothelioma and tufted angioma) [128,129]. Confusion still exists in the literature; many patients with the VM-associated LIC are mislabelled as having 'haemangioma' and 'KMP', resulting in mismanagement.

Radiological imaging is necessary because a VM is often much more extensive than clinically anticipated. Plain radiography reveals phleboliths as early as the age of 2 years. These round calcifications are pathognomonic of slow venous flow and caused by intralesional thrombosis (Fig. 118.10). Radiographs show bony distortion in facial VMs, and bony thinning or periosteal reaction in limb VMs. The latter can mimic osteoid osteoma [117]. Ultrasonography and grey-scale and colour Doppler display the angioarchitecture and can confirm the diagnosis. VM is compressible with the probe. Most typically, a heterogeneous echogenicity and an ill-defined hypoechoic lacunar pattern are noted; arterial structures are not detected. Endoscopic evaluation is indicated in patients with chronic anaemia and multiple small VMs located on the palms and/or soles to confirm the diagnosis of BRBN.

MRI, with spin-echo (SE) T1-and T2-weighted sequences, is the best noninvasive radiological modality to delineate a VM. On SE T2-weighted sequences, VM is made up of well-delineated, often lobulated venous pouches giving a hypersignal. Three-dimensional reconstruction is particularly useful in demonstrating the involved structures [130,131]. In the case of a knee VM, MRI plus CT provides useful information, and eliminates the need for arthrography before treatment.

Phlebography shows a racemose complex of abnormal veins in limb VMs, but not the anatomical location and size of the lesion. Its usefulness is limited in comparison with Doppler and MRI. It should be done before sclerotherapy to ensure the absence of large draining veins. Arteriography is useless and need not to be performed. Venography obtained by direct contrast injection shows a well-demarcated dermal vascular anomaly; draining veins are not seen.

Genetic testing should be performed in patients with multiple venous anomalies. This would refine diagnosis and give the basis for precise genetic counselling. It will also delineate options for more targeted molecular treatment in the near future.

Histology findings. Venous malformations are composed of ectatic, poorly defined channels, interconnecting to form a complex network that permeates normal tissues. Some lesions contain only distorted, enlarged venous channels (erroneously labelled as 'cavernous haemangioma'). Other lesions consist of a spongy combination of ectatic venous channels intermingled with capillaries. The lining endothelium is flat and quiescent. Walls are thin and irregularly lined by a discontinuous layer of smooth muscle cells, positive for smooth muscle α-actin [25]. Thrombosis and calcifications (phleboliths) are frequent. The abnormal venous network drains to adjacent veins, many of which are varicose and lack valves.

GVMs differ from VMs by the presence in the vessel media of more or less developed clusters of α-actin-positive 'glomus' cells lining venous-like spaces [132]. Ultrastructurally, these smooth muscle cells are in contact with nonmyelinated nerve fibres. CCMs consist of thin-walled, capillary-like vessels that create lace-like structures [77,78].

Treatment and prevention. Venous malformations always expand, albeit slowly.

Medical treatment consists of iron replacement therapy and blood transfusion to control anaemia, especially in BRBN patients [133,134]. Elastic stockings provide comfort by reducing the venous pressure in an extremity [80]. In contrast, this will increase pain in GVM patients. Low molecular weight heparin (100 anti-Xa/kg/day) is usually given to patients with biological signs of LIC, 24 h before and for another 5–10 days after surgical and/or sclerotherapy procedures to minimize haemorrhagic risk [123,125,135,136]. The same treatment is given to patients with a painful episode of local thrombosis. In this circumstance, the duration of treatment is usually 2 weeks [80,123,137].

Targeted molecular therapies are becoming an additional possibility. As the PI3K-AKT signalling pathway is activated in the majority of VM forms, it has become the target to test small molecular inhibitors. Rapamycin was promising in a preclinical VM-mouse model trial [138], and in a Phase II clinical trial for difficult-to-treat extensive VMs [138,139]. Patients had almost complete relief from pain and symptoms, reduced coagulopathy, diminished functional restraint and increased self-perceived quality of life. Side-effects included mucositis, mild headache, fatigue and diarrhoea. A multicentric European study (VASE; NCT 02638389) is ongoing in order to determine which subtypes of VMs are best suited for rapamycin. Rapamycin should not be considered as treatment for small, localized and asymptomatic slow-flow vascular malformations that respond to standard of care. Bleeding in BRBN seems to respond fast, and it can stop within 24 hours if rapamycin is taken [140].

The best treatment for VM is *percutaneous intralesional sclerotherapy* [70,141–145]. Procedures are performed with real-time fluoroscopic control, and under general anaesthesia with careful monitoring. Local compression or intralesional coil injection is sometimes used to prevent passage into the systemic circulation. Absolute ethanol, the most efficient sclerosing agent, has been replaced by other agents because of frequent local and systemic complications. Local complications include inflammation, oedema, blistering, necrosis, chronic drainage and scarring, and temporary or permanent nerve deficit. Systemic complications, such as renal or pulmonary toxicity, myocardial depression and even cardiac arrest and death, have been reported [146,147]. Sodium tetradecyl-sulphate or lauromacrogol 400 injections, given with local anaesthesia or no anaesthesia, are effective for small VMs and cause fewer local side-effects. An acrylic glue is sometimes used preoperatively. Detergent sclerosants have been used as microfoam forms, using air bubbles or carbon dioxide to increase the volume and surface contact with endothelium [148,149]; however, neurological complications have been reported in 2% of patients [150]. More recently, a modified radio-opaque ethanol sclerosing agent has been developed which traps the ethanol within a mesh of ethylcellulose in order to increase its viscosity [151–153]. This decreases the amount of ethanol given and the frequency of possible complications.

Surgical resection is often performed after sclerotherapy to reduce recurrence risk [79]. If VM in the thigh or calf impairs function or causes severe pain, the involved muscle can be excised. Synovial knee VM creates recurrent episodes of haemarthrosis in active children as early as 6 years of age. Excision of the VM embedded in the synovia is possible and, after physical therapy, the child often recovers with pain-free joint mobility and normal function [114,154,155]. Aggressive surgical resection of all gastrointestinal VM lesions of BRBN can eliminate chronic bleeding often seen in these patients [156].

Lymphatic malformation

Key points

- **Less frequent than VM.**
- **Can be micro-, macro- or combined micro–macrocystic lymphatic malformation.**
- **Infection is the most common complication.**
- **Can be diagnosed *in utero* as early as the late first trimester of pregnancy.**
- **Always sporadic, except primary lymphoedema that is often inherited as an autosomal dominant pattern.**

Brief introduction. Lymphatic malformation (LM) consists of vesicles or pouches filled with lymphatic fluid. Microcystic LMs diffusely involve soft tissues and even bones. Macrocystic LM forms large translucent masses under normal skin. Combined micro–macrocystic forms often exist. LMs expand in the presence of regional inflammation or intralesional bleeding. Most LMs manifest during infancy or childhood. Ultrasonography detects intrauterine macrocystic LMs ('cystic hygroma') as early as the late first trimester of pregnancy [157,158].

Epidemiology and pathogenesis. The exact incidence of LM is unknown. Primary lymphoedema is inherited as an automosal pattern in 20% of cases. It can be isolated or part of a syndrome, such as in Turner and Noonan syndromes [159].

LMs are caused by mosaic/somatic mutations in PIK3CA. They activate the PI3K/AKT/mTor signalling pathway [160–162].

Primary lymphoedema is another lymphatic pathology. Over 20 genes have been identified to be mutated in various forms of primary lymphoedema [163]. Milroy disease is caused by inherited loss-of-function mutations in vascular endothelial growth factor receptor 3 (VEGFR3) [164–167], whereas lymphoedema distichiasis is caused by loss-of-function mutations in the *FOXC2* transcription factor [168]. Lymphoedema associated with microcephaly, with or without chorioretinopathy or developmental delay (MCLMR) is caused by dominantly inherited mutations in *KIF11* [169,170]. Hypotrichosis-lymphoedema-telangiectasia (HLT) that has an autosomal dominant or recessive pattern of inheritance, is caused by mutations in *SOX18* [166]. Hennekam syndrome is an autosomal recessive generalized lymphatic dysplasia, which is characterized by intestinal lymphangiectasia with severe and progressive lymphoedema of the limbs, genitalia and face, and severe mental retardation (OMIM #235510) [171]. It is caused by mutations in *CCBE1* (collagen and calcium-binding EGF domains 1) [172,173]. Lymphoedema is associated with haematological malignancies in Emberger syndrome caused by *GATA2* mutations [174]. In about 35–40% of familial primary lymphoedema patients, a germline mutation can be identified [163,175].

In patients with Gorham Stout syndrome, the increased osteoclastic formation, with increased osteoclastic activity and bone resorption, has been linked to increased sensitivity of osteoclast precursors to humoral osteoclastogenic factors such as macrophage-colony stimulating factor (M-CSF), interleukin 1 (IL-1), IL-6 and tumour necrosis factor α (TNF-α) [176].

Clinical features.

Macro- and/or microcystic LM

LM is rarely a localized lesion; it usually involves a large area of skin, mucosa, underlying soft tissues and bones [177–182]. Microcystic LM (lymphangioma circumscriptum) is a plaque-like lesion involving skin or mucosa. Clear and colourless or blood-filled dark-red vesicles overlie an area of diffuse swelling (Fig. 118.11). Other lesions present with intermittent red-brown dermal infiltration, flat-topped papules or slight hypertrichosis. Recurrent cellulitis and ecchymoses are common. Local redness and warmth will appear and the lesion will become painful.

In macrocystic LM (old term 'cystic hygroma') there are soft multilobular masses with slight bluish discoloration of the skin. Macrocystic LMs suddenly enlarge in response to nose, throat or dental infection, or to intralesional bleeding (Fig. 118.12).

LM in the cheek, forehead and orbit, frequently micro–macrocystic, causes facial asymmetry and distortion of features. Bony overgrowth occurs, commonly in the mandible, manifesting as class III malocclusion. Eyelid and intraorbital LMs produce orbital enlargement, ocular dystopia, exophthalmia, occlusion of the visual axis and amblyopia. Sudden orbital proptosis and possible visual loss result from bleeding within cysts. Bulky LM of the

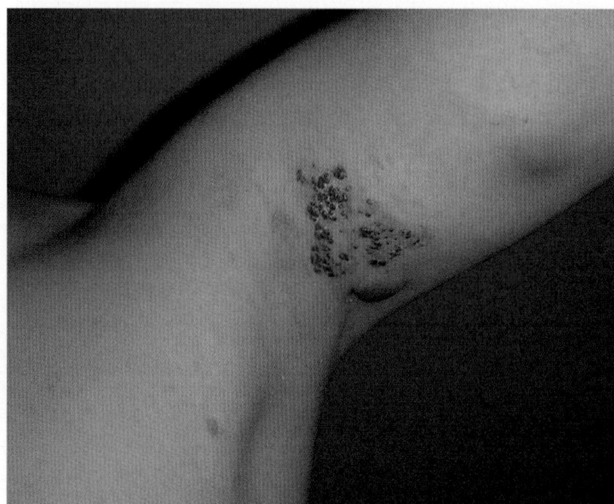

Fig. 118.11 Macro-microcystic lymphatic malformation in the axilla, with intralesional bleeding.

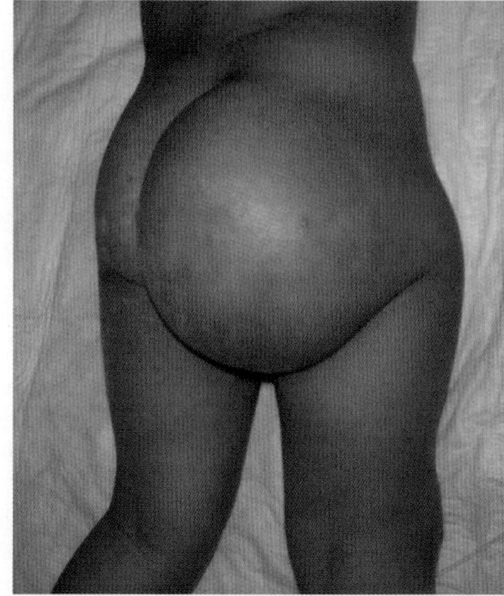

Fig. 118.12 Macrocystic lymphatic malformation of the buttock, with local infection.

tongue impairs speech; patients develop swelling of the tongue with infected bleeding vesicles, halitosis, aggressive caries and premature tooth loss. In the cervicofacial region, a diffuse LM can result in airway obstruction, necessitating tracheostomy [183,184]. Cervical and axillary LM can invade the thorax, causing chylothorax and pericardial effusion, as well as compression [184]. These complications can be lethal.

Localized angiokeratomas

Angiokeratomas circumscriptum are small, red to purple, keratotic papules. Lesions are localized, segmental or diffuse and are present from birth. They are often located on an extremity. Bleeding and irritation occur.

The terms angiokeratoma corporis circumscriptum or Fabry type II disease have been used to describe patients with localized hyperkeratotic lesions. Angioma serpiginosum of Hutchinson refers to patients with multiple small lesions with minimal hyperkeratosis, in a disseminated distribution; additional angiokeratomas develop over years. In angiokeratoma corporis diffusum, hundreds of small lesions develop over a large area of skin. In the Fordyce form, angiokeratomas develop on the scrotum. The Mibelli type, beginning during childhood, is characterized by angiokeratomas on the fingers [5].

Lymphoedema

Lymphoedema is characterized by swelling of the affected body part, usually a lower extremity, and caused by accumulation of lymphatic fluid into the extracellular space because of intrinsic lymphatic dysfunction. Various phenotypes exist depending on the age of onset, location and associated anomalies [163,173]. Milroy disease is suspected in the presence of swelling of the dorsum of the feet with familial history of congenital lymphoedema [185]. Other features can be associated with congenital lymphoedema, such as hydrocele (37% of males), prominent veins (23%), upslanting toenails (14%), papillomatosis (10%), or urethral abnormalities in males (4%). The most common complication is cellulitis. More rarely, pleural effusion, even *in utero*, hydrops fetalis, and chylous ascites can be observed [163,186,187].

Generalized lymphatic anomalies

In this rare syndrome, LMs are extensive and can invade any organ, such as bone, mediastinum, pericardium, pleura, or even gastrointestinal tract [188].

Gorham–Staout syndrome

Gorham–Stout syndrome ('vanishing bone disease') is another rare lymphatic anomaly that is more aggressive than generalized lymphatic anomalies. It is characterized by progressive demineralization and destruction of bones, which are replaced by lymphatic vessels and capillaries [189,190]. Depending on the location, this syndrome manifests as bone pain, muscular atrophy, fractures, pleural effusion, ascites and cerebrospinal fluid rhinorrhea. It is lethal in 16% of cases.

Differential diagnosis. Any mass under normal skin in an infant can be LM. The differential diagnosis includes deep haemangioma, teratoma, VM and haemangiopericytoma. Infantile fibrosarcoma and intramuscular alveolar rhabdomyosarcoma must be ruled out in an infant with a bulky mass under normal skin. These tumours are sometimes of soft consistency and cystic appearance on CT or MRI, and mimic LM; one-third is present at birth, and they grow to considerable size and metastasize [191]. Infantile rhabdomyosarcoma may present as an infiltrated pink plaque with firm pseudovesicles. Because lesions vary in volume because of the high content of blood vessels and lymphatic clefts, Kimura disease infiltrating the parotid and submaxillary gland under normal skin can be mistaken for macrocystic LM.

Microcystic LM, infiltrating large areas of skin, with intralesional bleeding, mimics the bruises of the Gardner–Diamond syndrome. Acquired lymphangiectasia of the vulva following resection and radiotherapy for genital cancer and lymphangiectasia in association with Crohn disease are indiscernible from microcystic vulvar LM [192]. Benign lymphangio-endothelioma presents as a brownish, slowly growing, cutaneous plaque with intermittent bruising in the extremities, trunk or face. It is composed of anastomosing dilated empty vascular channels in the superficial and deep dermis, and probably fits in the spectrum of LMs [193,194]. Acral microcystic LM with haematic vesicles must be differentiated from APACHE syndrome (acral pseudolymphomatous angiokeratoma of children), characterized by acquired, persistent painless, unilateral vascular papules on distal regions of the foot or hand [195]. Sinusoidal 'haemangioma' is a misnomer for a capillary dermal vascular anomaly occurring in childhood [196]. It presents as firm nodules or plaques mimicking LM. Interconnected, thin-lined, blood-filled, very large channels are in a striking lobular architecture, with pseudopapillary patterns.

Laboratory findings. When clinical diagnosis is equivocal, radiological imaging is needed. Useful techniques are ultrasonography (cysts are anechoic or hypoechoic and homogeneous), CT (cysts are hypodense), MRI (cystic spaces are hypointense on T1 sequence, hyperintense on T2 and show fluid–fluid levels if there is intracystic bleeding), direct puncture (liquid is analysed) and contrast injection.

Radiographically, radiolucency of the affected bones has a 'licked stick of candy' appearance.

Genetic counselling is essential in congenital lymphoedema, whether it is syndromic or not.

Histology findings. Microcystic LMs consist of dilated endothelium-lined, thin-walled and bloodless lymph capillaries and spaces that fill the dermis. Nodular collections of lymphocytes are often seen in the surrounding connective stroma. A dilated lymphatic vessel enlarging a dermal papilla creates a vesicle [132]. Blood within the anomalous spaces indicates either recent haemorrhage or a combined lymphatic–capillary malformation. Mural thrombi occur.

In macrocystic LMs, large cisterns do not communicate directly with the general lymphatic system. The vessel walls are of variable thickness, with both striated and smooth muscle elements. In combined macro–microcystic LMs, abnormal lymphatics connect deep cisterns to the superficial dermis in a complex meandering network. On electron microscopy, the basement membranes are either fragmented or well formed [197]. Endothelial cells express lymphatic markers such as VEGFR3, podoplanin and M2A oncofetal antigen [198].

Angiokeratomas consist of ectatic capillaries, which fill the dermal papilla. Marked acanthosis and hyperkeratosis are present. Endothelial cells lining the abnormal capillaries stain for factor VIII-related antigen.

Treatment and prevention.

Prevention

The child with diffuse LM can develop sepsis, which is unresponsive to antibiotics. Pelvic LM manifests with vulvar lymphangiectasia and vaginal chylous discharge, even before puberty. Abdominal LM with involvement of the gastrointestinal tract causes a protein-losing enteropathy and hypoalbuminaemia [199]. Transient inflammatory swelling usually improves with nonsteroidal anti-inflammatory drugs or corticosteroids, and antibiotics. Careful dental hygiene, tartar removal, and control of caries are important in the management of intrabuccal LMs. Bacterial infection within an LM sometimes necessitates intravenous administration of antibiotics; rarely is incision and drainage helpful.

Treatment

Macrocysts are treated with aspiration of the fluid, followed by percutaneous, image-guided, intralesional injection of sclerofibrosing agents. A number of substances have been used to produce an inflammation with subsequent shrinkage of the cysts. These include Ethibloc®, pure ethanol, bleomycin, dextrose, sodium morrhuate, sodium tetradecyl, OK-432 (a killed strain of group A *Streptococcus pyogenes*, also known as Picibanil®), tetracycline or doxycycline and bleomycin [200–204]. Side-effects are fever, erythema and oedema, and possible fistula with leakage. Partial regression, leaving a residual LM, may require excision.

Like sclerotherapy, surgical resection of the LM offers potential cure. Anatomical restrictions and difficulty in clearly separating normal from involved tissues can result in unsatisfactory outcome, incomplete excision and sacrifice of normal structures. The preferred operative strategy is to exstirpate the LM in a single region in one procedure. Staged excisions or cutaneous expansion are necessary for large lesions. Complications include fistula, infection, scarring and recurrences. Partial resection may facilitate the occurrence of multiple cutaneous or mucosal lymphatic vesicles, along and around the scar, causing intermittent lymph leakage, bleeding and infection. Orthodontic management is frequently needed in late childhood.

Nd:YAG laser photocoagulation, with or without continuous ice-cube surface cooling, or interstitial Nd:YAG laser, and diode laser photocoagulation have been used in the treatment of cutaneous and mucosal LM vesicles [205].

In extensive LM with lymphoedema in the limbs, medical management includes a pneumatic compression device, compressive bandaging and elastic support stockings. Multifocal extensive visceral LM, often labelled 'lymphangiectasia', has a poor prognosis and outcome [206]. Treatment with various pharmacological agents, including IFN-α, corticosteroids, vincristine and a few biotherapeutical trials, has usually failed. When there is a coexisting coagulopathy, protracted treatment with a low molecular weight heparin is necessary. There is one report of improved gastrointestinal symptoms with tranexamic acid [207]. *Rapamycin* has been effectively used in extensive lymphatic anomalies. Its efficacy is based on targeting the common pathogenic cause: activated PI3K-AKT-mTOR signalling because of activating PIK3CA mutations [208–211]. Patients had almost complete cessation of lymphatic leakage, infection, and reduced volume of the malformation on MRI. However, like for VMs, rapamycin should not be considered as treatment for small, localized and asymptomatic slow-flow vascular malformations that respond to standard care.

Capillary malformation

Key points

- Incidence of 0.3%.
- Pinkish red to purple in colour. Tend to darken and thicken with time.
- Can be part of a syndrome, such as Sturge–Weber or Klippel–Trenaunay syndrome.
- Can be part of inherited CM-AVM or PHTS.

Brief introduction.

Port-wine stain is a macular capillary malformation (CM) that is present at birth and persists throughout life. In most cases, CM is a cosmetic problem. It can also be an indicator of a more complex vascular disorder, such as Sturge–Weber syndrome (SWS) (see syndromic section), or CM-AVM (see AVM section) [13–16,19,212–214].

Epidemiology and pathogenesis.

CM has a prevalence of 0.3% [215]. There is no sex preponderance.

Sporadic CMs as well as SWS, can be caused by somatic activating GNAQ or GNAQ mutations [216]. The most common one is Arg183Gln. The mutations seem to have a weak activating effect eventually on both the RAS-MAPK and the PI3K-AKT pathways [18,216]. The mutations most likely exert their effects within the vascular endothelial cells [18].

Clinical features.

Localized or extensive capillary malformation ('port-wine stain')

Capillary malformation is characterized by a pinkish-red to deep purple homogeneous stain involving the skin, the subcutis and sometimes the mucosa. Lesions can be localized or extensive, and may occur on the face, trunk or limbs. Facial CM involves one or more of the so-called trigeminal areas (V1, V2, V3) and is unilateral or bilateral. A CM located on an extremity can remain unchanged throughout life, or it may be the first sign of a complex/combined vascular malformation. CM can present in a scattered distribution over the entire body, often associated with hemihypertrophy. This entity is called diffuse capillary malformation with overgrowth (DCMO) and is characterized by a reticulated ill-defined CM [217] (Dompmartin et al., in preparation). The lesions do not follow the lines of Blaschko. Areas of 'naevus anaemicus', composed of vessels with adrenergic tone, may be intermingled with the CM (Fig. 118.13). Acquired CM is not as uncommon as usually thought; trauma is considered the major cause [218].

CMs of CM-AVM (see AVM section)

These inherited CMs are multifocal and small in diameter. Most are present at birth but some appear later in life. They often manifest as round-to-oval lesions with a pale halo [19,219]. Sometimes they can be present as beer spots [17].

Occult spinal dysraphism and midline capillary malformations

Cutaneous hallmarks for occult spinal dysraphism (OSD) are common in the lumbosacral area but also occur at the dorsal and cervical level [220]. They include lipoma, hairy patch, skin dimple, dermal sinus, faun tail and vascular birthmark (haemangioma and CM). CM alone is seldom a clue for OSD. Most children with indicators of OSD have two or more cutaneous markers [221].

Midline occipital CM can be associated with dysraphism in the skull (meningocoele, encephalocoele), and the distinction between this CM and the common occipital and nuchal red 'naevus simplex' (the 'stork bite') is sometimes difficult. An association between scalp membranous aplasia cutis and neural tube closure defects or intracranial vascular malformation has been reported [222].

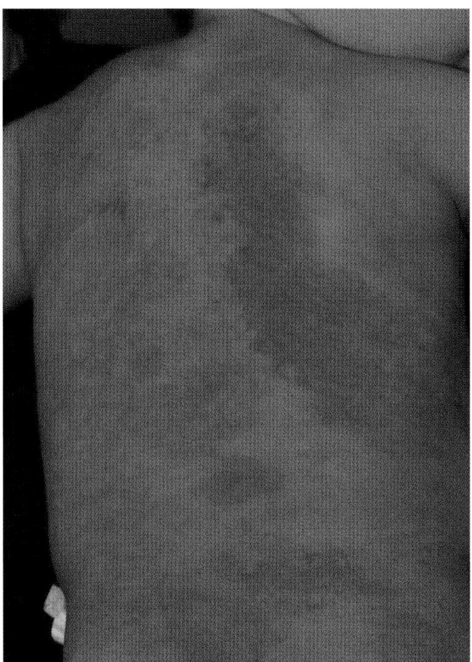

Fig. 118.13 Diffuse capillary malformation with overgrowth: extensive scattered capillary malformation with overgrowth.

Differential diagnosis. In infants, CM must be differentiated from a salmon patch (also known as naevus flammeus neonatorum – 'stork bite' when it occurs on the nucha and 'angel kiss' when it occurs on the forehead). These macules occur in about 50% of neonates on the nape of the neck, glabella, eyelid, nose and upper lip. They tend to fade in the facial region, and may persist in the occipital skin [223].

Early facial haemangiomas, including those in the 'beard' area and those associated with PHACES (posterior fossa anomalies, haemangioma, arterial defects, coarctation of aortic arch and cardiac defects, eye defects, scolioses; see Chapter 119) syndrome, may mimic CM. However, rapid thickening of the lesion indicates that it is actually a form of haemangioma.

In childhood, AVM often mimics CM. Both can develop multiple pyogenic granulomas. If there is concern about the possibility of AVM, Doppler evaluation is mandatory.

Tufted angioma (also known as angioblastoma of Nakagawa) is a benign vascular tumour appearing most often during childhood. It is considered as a minor form of Kaposiform haemangioendothelioma as it is less often associated with Kasabach– Merritt phenomenon. It grows slowly and usually stabilizes. Tender red or brownish patches, sometimes studded with red papules, grow on the neck, upper chest, shoulders or limbs [224–227]. Histologically, the collection of tightly packed capillaries, pericytes and endothelial cells, dispersed in the dermis in a 'cannonball' distribution, with semilunar bloodless clefts lining the tufts, is entirely different from a CM. Eccrine angiomatous hamartoma can also present as an erythematous irregularly stained area of skin but with localized hypertrichosis and intermittent hyperhidrosis.

Laboratory and histology findings. Usually no complementary exams are mandatory in patients with CMs. Exceptions arise in the presence of a CM in the frontopalpebral area (see SWS in syndromic section), in the midline to exclude OSD and on the lower extremity. Ultrasonography of a patient with midline CM and another axial sign can be performed as a screening test in infants less than 6 months of age. However, MRI is mandatory to exclude spinal dysraphism [220]. Scaniometry needs to be performed around the age of 6 years for every CM on the lower extremity to exclude asymmetric overgrowth. In addition, during an annual orthopaedic consultation, the need and timing for the medical or surgical correction of leg length is evaluated.

Genetic testing should be performed in patients with multiple CM.

Histologically, capillary malformation comprises regular, ectatic, thin-walled capillary to venular-sized channels, located in the papillary and upper reticular dermis. In adults, fibrosis around vessels and progressive vascular dilation develop [132].

Treatment and prevention.
Prognosis
CM usually grows in proportion to the rest of the body. The lesions are bright red at birth. During the first weeks they fade slightly, as the haemoglobin level of the newborn decreases. Then the red hue stabilizes. Facial CMs are prone to hyperplastic skin changes. Evenly thickened skin, purple nodules and pyogenic granulomas develop by adolescence [227–229]. This can mimic AVM.

Hyperplastic changes very rarely occur in trunk or extremity CM. Facial CM can also be associated with progressive hyperplasia of underlying soft and hard tissues. Lips and gums as well as alveolar bone enlarge in areas of vascular staining. Periodontal disease, bleeding and dental hygiene problems are common (Fig. 118.14). Overgrowth of the maxilla or mandible leads to skeletal asymmetry, occlusal tilt and open-bite deformity.

Increased limb girth can present at birth in children with a CM covering an entire limb; this asymmetry is stable and, unlike Klippel–Trenaunay syndrome, persists without progression until the child is fully grown. When the child has atopic dermatitis, psoriasis or acne, lesions are worse in the area of CM, a finding known as the Meyerson phenomenon [230].

Treatment
Pulsed dye laser is used to treat CM [231–236]. Laser therapy is more effective in lesions on the face and trunk than in those involving the distal extremity. A successful result is defined as fading of the CM, with little or no textural change. In a comparative study, the pulsed dye laser was found to be superior to the continuous-wave dye laser with the Hexascan robotized device in 45% of patients (with less hyper-or hypopigmentation), whereas the continuous-wave tunable dye laser was considered superior in 15% [232]. There was no appreciable difference in the remaining 40% of patients. There was no difference in the results obtained with a late (adult) treatment compared with pulsed dye laser treatment performed during childhood [233]. Nevertheless, for psychological reasons, most authors suggest early treatment [234]. Commonly, clearing of the stain progresses from the periphery [235]. There is a possibility of recurrence after cessation of laser treatment [236]. Soft tissue hypertrophy does not respond to laser and requires surgical correction. Skin grafting rarely provides identical colour and texture of skin, and a border effect is noticable. Contour resection for labial hypertrophy, orthodontic management for correction of the open bite and orthognathic correction can be required. Careful dental care and oral hygiene are important if there is gingival involvement. If epulis develops, electrodesiccation is curative.

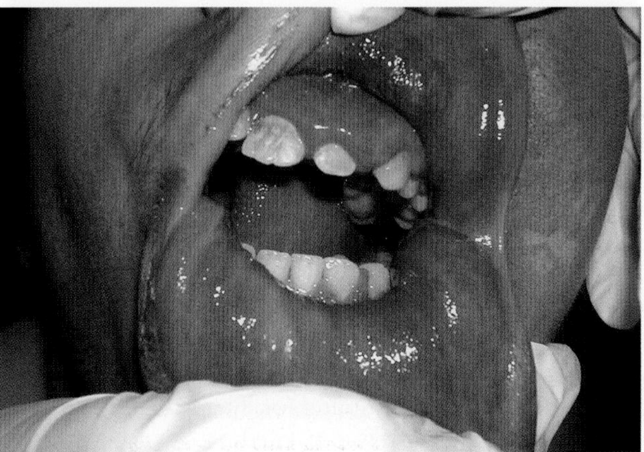

Fig. 118.14 Facial capillary malformation with lip, gums and alveolar bone enlargement.

Syndromic vascular anomalies

Key points

- **Incidence unknown.**
- **Mainly sporadic because of somatic mutations.**
- **Associate vascular malformations (often a CM) with other anomalies.**

Brief introduction. These syndromes associate CM with other anomalies such as pigmented naevi in phacomatosis pigmentovascularis (PPV). Overgrowth is a common feature. They are often called using eponyms, such Klippel–Trenaunay syndrome (KTS), or more recently acronyms such as CLOVES, CLAPO and PROS [237,238].

Epidemiology and pathogenesis. The incidence of these disorders is unknown except for SWS that occurs in 1 in 50 000 births. The syndromic forms are usually not inherited.

Described in 1947, Happle hypothesized the concept of 'twin spots' to explain the sporadic phenotype of PPV, which is more frequent in Asians and Africans [239]. This has not yet been demonstrated. SWS, like some sporadic CMs, is caused by somatic activating GNAQ or GNA11 mutations [216] (see CM section).

KTS, CLOVES and M-CAP are caused by mosaic/somatic mutations in PIK3CA. They activate the PI3K/AKT/mTor signalling pathway [160–162,240]. Their similar genotype suggests that they are part of a spectrum of a single phenotype that has recently been named PROS (PIK3CA related overgrowth syndrome) [240,241].

Clinical features.
PPV
PPV combines CM with pigmented naevi and is categorized into five variants (Box 118.1). Each category is cutaneous

Box 118.1 The various types of phacomatosis pigmentovascularis A and B

Cutaneous (A)

Type 1A = CM (naevus flammeus) + naevus pigmentosus and verrucosus
Type 2A = CM + aberrant Mongolian spots + naevus anaemicus
Type 3A = CM + naevus spilus (or giant speckled lentiginous naevus) + naevus anaemicus
Type 4A = CM + aberrant Mongolian spots + naevus spilus + naevus anaemicus
Type 5A = CMTC + aberrant Mongolian spots

Syndromic (B)

Types 1B, 2B, 3B, 4B = same as above plus either SWS or KTS, Ota naevus, etc.

CM, capillary malformation; CMTC, cutis marmorata telangiectatica congenita; KTS, Klippel–Trenaunay syndrome; SWS, Sturge–Weber syndrome.

(type A) or cutaneous and syndromic (type B). Related syndromes in type B include SWS, KTS and/or naevus of Ota [242,243].

According to the publication of Fernandez-Guarino and colleagues, 222 cases of PPV have been published (from 1947 to 2007), most of them being sporadic types observed in Japan, Mexico or Argentina [244]. The most common PPVs are type IIb (45%), followed by IIa (30%). The rest are much less frequent. In 2005, Happle revisited this classification and described four groups: phacomatosis cesioflammea, which associates blue spots to naevus flammeus; phacomatosis spilorosea with coexistence of naevus spilus and a pale-pink naevus; and phacomatosis cesiomarmorata, the association of a blue spot with cutis marmorata telangiectatica congenita. The fourth group is composed of unclassifiable PPV [245].

SWS

Children with SWS may have multifocal CMs, but always with involvement of the V1 skin [246]. Soft tissue overgrowth is more frequent than in nonsyndromic CM [227,247]. A leptomeningeal capillary–venular vascular anomaly, as in SWS, can rarely occur in the absence of facial CM. Impairment of the meningeal microvasculature affects the normal development of the brain [248]. Anomalies in the affected hemisphere are visible on MRI soon after birth [249]. In the presence of leptomeningeal involvement, patients usually develop contralateral seizures, neurological deficits and hemiparesis or hemiplegia. These neurological complications are seen before the age of 2 years in a majority of patients. It is noteworthy that about 10% of infants with V1 CM have only the neurological signs and symptoms of SWS. In addition, in children with SWS, developmental milestones can be delayed. Ocular anomalies include increase in the ipsilateral choroidal vascularity, glaucoma, retinal detachment and blindness.

KTS (OMIM 149000)

KTS has been used for CM in complex/combined slow-flow vascular malformations, including capillary venous malformation (CVM) and capillary lymphaticovenous malformation (CLVM) with progressive limb overgrowth [225,250]. Capillary malformations, dilated veins, occasional lymphangiectases and a more or less pronounced overgrowth in limb girth and length characterize this complex/combined vascular malformation of the extremities. Lower and upper extremities are affected, and truncal involvement commonly occurs.

Capillary malformation in this syndrome is often located on the anterolateral aspect of the thigh, in a geographical pattern, commonly in association with an embryonic lateral marginal vein. Lymphatic vesicles, clear or haemorrhagic, are sometimes present in the area of CM. There are no arteriovenous fistulas; thus, pulsations and bruit are absent. The involved vessels show evidence of inadequate venous return on ultrasonographic evaluation. Some patients have anomalous deep veins (agenesis, aplasia or duplication). Significant limb overgrowth, present since birth, causes severe disability. Vascular lesions may involve the limb and the adjacent trunk, and may be superficial or deep: KTS in the lower extremity may include genitourinary and intestinal lesions. Bleeding or protein-losing enteropathy from these lesions can be difficult to control. They can present with intermittent pain, caused by thrombotic events in some part of the anomalous venous network or in a deep vein.

CLOVES (OMIM 612918)

This newly recognized entity includes congenital lipomatous overgrowth, vascular malformations, epidermal naevi and scoliosis (CLOVES), as well as hemimegalencephaly, dysgenesis of the corpus callosum, neuronal migration defects, and the consequent seizures [237,251]. Limb overgrowth is minor at birth, but aggravates during infancy.

CLAPO syndrome (OMIM #613089)

This rare sporadic syndrome is characterized by capillary malformation of the lower lip, LM of the cervicofacial area and asymmetry and partial/generalized overgrowth [238].

Differential diagnosis. Differential diagnosis with other overgrowth syndromes with complex vascular anomalies (OSCVA) can be problematic [252,253]. These syndromes differ from pure limb VM, CM with congenital limb hypertrophy, regional glomuvenous malformation, BRBN and Maffucci syndrome. CLVM can be associated with SWS, and with PPV.

Laboratory findings. Patients with frontopalpebral CM must undergo brain MRI or CT and ophthalmological examination (visual evaluation, fundoscopic examination and eye pressure measurement) soon after birth. The latter should be repeated twice a year until puberty [254–257]. MRI T1-weighted sequences and gadolinium injection detect the leptomeningeal vascular anomaly, ipsilateral to the CM in SWS patients. Typically, but not always, it is located in the occipital brain. Other early features are an asymmetrically enlarged ipsilateral choroid plexus and, in infants younger than 6 months, accelerated myelination of the abnormal hemisphere. In advanced SWS, CT scans reveal dense calcifications moulding the convolutions. Both CT and MRI demonstrate cerebral atrophy, enlarged subarachnoid spaces and pachygyric cortical changes. DVAs are sometimes associated. Single photon emission computed tomography (SPECT), which determines regional cerebral blood flow, and positron emission tomography (PET), which determines local cerebral glucose metabolism, are useful tools for monitoring the activity of central nervous system disease. Local decreased cerebral blood flow and decreased cerebral glucose metabolism both correlate with anatomical involvement, as seen on CT or MRI. In early SWS, before the first seizures, SPECT and PET can detect hyperperfusion and hypermetabolic activity respectively. Thereafter, hypoperfusion and postnatal cerebral atrophy develop with the epileptic degradation, hypoxia, cortex venous stasis, venous thrombosis and calcifications. New sequences of dynamic contrast bolus magnetic resonance perfusion imaging are easier to perform than PET or SPECT scans. They give new insights on early vascular signs of SWS, showing often pronounced perfusion defect in the cerebral and/or cerebellar hemispheres, in children who still have normal neurological function. MR perfusion deficits match with the areas of gadolinium enhancement that correspond to leptomeningeal disease [258]. A neonatal neuroimaging work-up with CT and MRI may not demonstrate the pial vascular anomaly and should be repeated after 6–12 months in an at-risk infant.

A coagulation profile is mandatory in all syndromic malformations, except in patients with SWS or PPV, because they can have a chronic LIC [124,259]. This biological phenomenon is associated with high D-dimer levels and low fibrinogen, while platelet counts are usually only moderately lowered. This LIC carries the risk of thrombus migration and life-threatening pulmonary thromboembolism [259].

Children with overgrowth syndromes are evaluated annually. Leg length is evaluated clinically during infancy. After the age of 2 years, leg length is measured radiologically and, if abnormal, this is repeated yearly. Ultrasonography and grey-scale and colour Doppler evaluation of limb arterial and venous vessels should be performed when the child is 3 or 4 years old. Plain radiography detects skeletal changes. Phlebography is rarely indicated but is sometimes performed before surgical removal of varicose veins. It is replaced by the less invasive fast three-dimensional MRI venography (3D-MRV). Indications for lymphoscintigraphy are rare. In contrast to patients with pure extremity VMs, muscles and joints are rarely involved in PPV or KTS. MRI and MRA are sometimes useful to detect arterial feeders or draining veins penetrating muscles and bones.

Histology findings. Histologically, the anomalous veins seen in KTS have deformed, insufficient or absent valves. Venous fibromuscular anomalies are the most consistent mural finding. Some of the veins (such as the marginal vein in the thigh) might represent persistent embryonic veins [132].

Treatment and prevention.

Prognosis

The outlook in these syndromes depends on the extent and severity of this complex vascular anomaly, and on the bulk of the associated overgrowth. Children with extensive CVM and CLVM of the limbs and trunk (KTS) and associated vascular abnormalities in the abdomen or chest can develop haematuria, intestinal and vaginal bleeding, protein-losing enteropathy or haemothorax. These patients often have severe LIC and are at risk of chronic thromboembolic pulmonary hypertension and even life-threatening pulmonary embolism, but the incidence of this phenomenon is unknown [123,259].

Treatment

SWS

The development of seizures in patients with SWS, which may result in a permanent neurological deficit, or sudden corneal clouding, which indicates acute glaucoma, are near medical emergencies. Prompt pharmacological treatment of epilepsy prevents brain hypoxia, resultant neuronal death and psychomotor deterioration [260]. Pulsed dye laser therapy for the CM is possible after control of seizure activity. Surgical treatment may be necessary for severe glaucoma. Hemispherectomy, localized lobectomy or callosotomy usually provides dramatic control of epilepsy with marked improvement of quality of life, and these procedures can halt the progression of motor and cognitive deterioration in children unresponsive to pharmacological treatment [261]. Management of labial and gingival hypertrophy and occlusal anomalies may be indicated.

PROS

Recent evidence suggests that oral therapy with an inhibitor of PIK3CA gene activity (alpelisib) can lead to reduction of overgrowth [262]. Management of the coagulopathy when present in an overgrowth syndrome will prevent repeated thrombotic episodes and reduce the risk of pulmonary emboli, which could lead to chronic pulmonary arterial hypertension. It requires low molecular weight heparin (usually enoxaparin), which can also be used as a preventive therapeutic strategy before surgical procedures to avoid excess per- and/or postoperative bleeding. If the lower extremity is affected, elastic compression stockings provide relief from pain caused by venous engorgement. They are recommended after grey-scale and colour Doppler evaluation, confirming the malfunction of deep veins. Compressive bandaging or stockings and frequent massage minimize lymphoedema. Varicose veins rarely require surgical treatment during childhood. Multiple surgical procedures, performed by an experienced surgeon, are needed to obtain satisfactory and lasting results. Some reports of the long-term benefit of resection appear to be overenthusiastic [263]. Some patients will benefit from surgical resection of their symptomatic varicose veins, after careful evaluation of the venous anatomy in the KTS limb, and, in particular, verification of the presence of a patent deep venous system. Endovascular radiofrequency ablation of the KT veins, and sometimes of the great saphenous veins, has been more recently used in KTS as a safe therapy and is less damaging than stripping or intravenous laser [264,265].

In gross limb hypertrophy, staged surgical contour resection can be considered. These extensive procedures, albeit successful in the short term, often cause severe fibrosis and pedal lymphoedema. In rare instances, amputation (digits, forefoot or distal limb) is needed to permit the wearing of shoes and ambulation.

In the presence of leg length discrepancy, an adapted shoe-lift should be provided to prevent compensatory tilting of the pelvis. In cases of significant leg length discrepancy, epiphysiodesis (surgical epiphyseal arrest with stapling) is indicated. This procedure is performed when the child is approximately 11–13 years old, depending on the growth curve.

Bleeding from haemolymphatic vesicles on the thigh is a common problem. Diathermal coagulation, Nd:YAG laser coagulation, sclerotherapy, limited excision or skin grafting for resurfacing are recommended. It is sometimes possible to excise the entire area and perform primary closure after tissue expansion of the normal adjacent skin. Haemorrhage from visceral involvement, intestinal bleeding, haematuria or vaginal bleeding may require surgical management. Leg ulcers, infection, cellulitis and thrombophlebitis need specific medical treatment.

Telangiectases

Key points

- **Can be isolated or part of a syndrome.**
- **Incidence is unknown.**
- **Sporadic or inherited.**

Brief introduction. Telangiectasia denotes fine irregular red or purple lines, punctate macules, minute papules or stellate. They can be isolated or part of a syndrome. Although they are usually sporadic, they can also be inherited as an autosomal dominant trait, such as in HBT or in HHT (see AVM section) [46,266].

Epidemiology and pathogenesis. The incidence is unknown except for ataxia telangiectasia (AT). AT is a complex neurovascular disorder of autosomal recessive inheritance, occurring in approximately 1 in 40 000 live births. In contrast to cutis marmorata telangiectatica congenita (CMTC), unilateral naevoid telangiectasia (UNT) has a female predilection. It rarely presents before puberty and tends to worsen with pregnancy. Divry-van Bogaert syndrome is a rare disorder, sporadic or familial, affecting mostly males.

Pathogenesis. UNT been associated with elevated levels of oestrogen and progesterone receptors in involved skin [267]. Rare families of CMTC have been reported [268–272]. Mosaic PIK3CA mutations have been identified in megalencephaly-capillary malformation patients [273].

Adams Oliver syndrome can be inherited as an autosomal dominant or recessive trait. When dominant, it is caused by mutations in the *ARHGAP31*, *DLL4*, *NOTCH1*, or *RBPJ* gene. When recessive, it is caused by mutations in the *DOCK6* or *EOGT* gene.

AT is the result of a mutation in the *ATM* gene, which has been localized to chromosome 11q22–23 [274]. This mutation causes an impaired repair of ultraviolet-induced DNA damage of skin fibroblasts [275].

Clinical features.

Localized telangiectatic vascular malformation

UNT occurs in a systematized unilateral pattern. Individual telangiectasia is sometimes surrounded by a white or 'anaemic' halo. HBT is characterized by cutaneous and labial telangiectasias [266]. Generalized essential telangiectasia is another vascular syndrome described sporadically in adult females. In contrast to Rendu–Osler–Weber disease, visceral haemorrhage does not occur in UNT, HBT and generalized essential telangiectasia (see previously).

Syndromic angiokeratomas (angiokeratoma corporis diffusum and lysosomal storage disorders)

Angiokeratomas may be an indicator of Fabry disease or other disorders of lysosomal storage. These are discussed in Chapter 152.

CMTC (van Lohuizen syndrome)

CMTC consists of reticulated, purple bands, in a livedoid pattern, with intermingled telangiectases. Linear skin atrophy, located in the purple streaks over the joints, can ulcerate in infancy, and result in scarring. Lesions of CMTC fade over a period of years, but rarely disappear completely [272]. Persistence into adulthood results in a subtle or obvious network of purplish discolouration. Venous-like channels are commonly observed over the joints and dorsum of the hands, and may rarely occur in a diffuse network. Chronic ulcers can occur. Diffuse CMTC is rare: 1 in 22 cases in one series [276]. The localized form is the most common, occurring in 65% of a series of 85 patients [271]. Hypotrophy of the involved limb (mainly in girth) is a common finding. This change is present at birth and does not progress during the growth of the child. A constellation of other associated findings has been reported. Literature reviews [268,277] suggest that the frequency of association between CMTC and other anomalies has been overestimated, most likely because of reporting bias. Reports coming from a single department indicate lower numbers of associated anomalies, including other types of vascular malformation, glaucoma, cerebral malformation, epilepsy, mental retardation, cardiac defect, urinary or genital anomaly [269–271,276].

Adams–Oliver syndrome

This consists of lesions described as cutis marmorata or CMTC, aplasia cutis congenita in the scalp, with or without an underlying bony defect, and terminal transverse limb defects [278].

AT (Louis–Bar syndrome) (OMIM #208900)

Multiple telangiectases begin to develop around 3 years of age and are seen most commonly on the bulbar conjunctiva, near the canthus. Other locations include the face, neck and dorsum of the hand and foot. UV light hypersensitivity and premature photoageing, with associated freckling and loss of cutaneous fat, occur. Premature greying of the hair also occurs. Cerebellar ataxia typically begins during the second year of life. Dysarthric speech, choreo-athetosis, myoclonic jerks and impaired intelligence also develop during childhood.

Recurrent sinobronchopulmonary infections, secondary to combined immune deficiency, occur in about 80% of patients. Granulomatous skin lesions, in areas of ulceration and atrophy, have been reported [279]. Endocrinological dysfunction includes insulin-resistant diabetes, gonadal insufficiency and growth retardation. Both humoral and cellular immunodeficiency occur in AT.

There is an increased incidence of neoplasia. By adolescence, lymphoma and leukaemia are the main causes of death (10–15%). A variety of carcinomas, particularly breast cancer, occur in patients with AT. AT heterozygotes, estimated to make up 0.5–1.5% of the population, are also at increased risk of cancer.

SECTION 25: VASCULAR TUMOURS

Divry–van Bogaert syndrome

Most patients with this rare syndrome develop livedo reticularis or cutis marmorata during childhood. Neurological manifestations result from noncalcifying leptomeningeal 'angiomatosis'. These symptoms begin during adolescence; ischaemic attacks and seizures lead to progressive dementia, and pseudo-bulbar and extrapyramidal symptoms.

At present, it is unclear whether the nonfamilial form of Divry–van Bogaert syndrome, originally described in 1946, is identical to Sneddon syndrome, a brain vasculopathy described later, responsible for seizures, dementia and other neurological deficits, and associated in about half of the cases with antiphospholipid antibodies. In both conditions, MRI and arteriogram of the brain reveal similar anomalies (stenosis, collateral circulation and, rarely, moya-moya pattern).

Differential diagnosis. In an infant, the telangiectatic sequelae of neonatal lupus erythematosus are primarily located in sun-exposed areas. Anti-Ro (SSA), anti-La (SSB) and/or anti-U1 RNP antibodies can be detected in the sera of mothers and infants. The mothers have symptoms of connective tissue disease or are asymptomatic. Telangiectasia macularis eruptiva perstans, a mastocytosis, is uncommon in childhood. The terminology 'acquired naevoid telangiectasia' has been used for telangiectasia developing in a segmental distribution in the setting of collagen vascular diseases, such as lupus erythematosus and scleroderma [280]. The vascular papules of 'glomeruloid haemangioma' in POEMS syndrome (polyneuropathy, organomegaly, endocrinopathy, M protein, skin changes) are histologically distinct.

CMTC must be differentiated from livedo reticularis, or cutis marmorata physiological in neonates. Persistent livedo can be found in primary antiphospholipid syndrome and Sneddon syndrome. 'Generalized phlebectasia' is a misnomer for CMTC: this term should be reserved for the rare Bockenheimer syndrome. A syndrome that is probably distinct has been labelled 'cutis marmorata and macrocephaly'. These infants have a generalized reticulate CM, evenly distributed over the head and body. They lack the atrophic areas of classic CMTC and have a high risk of postnatal growth failure, and of associated vascular, neurological and ocular anomalies, including cardiac arrhythmia and sudden infant death [272,281,282].

Laboratory and histology findings. In patients with AT, MRI is useful to demonstrate cerebellar atrophy, a constant (although nonspecific) finding. Patients have decreased or absent serum immunoglobulin A (IgA), decreased serum IgG2, lymphopenia, decreased counts of CD4 lymphocytes and high levels of α-fetoprotein and carcinoembryonic antigen.

Treatment. Pulsed dye laser is the treatment of choice for these telangiectasias. In CMTC, there is a risk of scarring [283].

Affected homozygotes and carriers of AT have an acute sensitivity to ionizing radiation and radiomimetic drugs, and experience unexpected severe reactions to these therapeutic regimens. *ATM* mutation in females with breast cancer places them at risk of severe radiotherapy-induced late side-effects; it has been suggested that a reduced dosage of radiation should be delivered in their therapeutic regimen [284]. The discovery of *ATM*, the single gene responsible for AT, makes it possible to detect carriers. Antibiotic therapy and physical therapy prevent bronchiectasis. There is no treatment for the progressive cerebellar ataxia.

References

1 Mulliken JB, Glowacki J. Hemangiomas and vascular malformations in infants and children: a classification based on endothelial characteristics. Plast Reconstr Surg 1982;69:412–22.

2 Boon LM, Vikkula M. Molecular genetics of vascular malformations. In: Mulliken JB (ed.) Vascular Anomalies: Hemangiomas and Malformations, 2nd edn. Oxford: Oxford University Press, 2013:327–75.

3 Enjolras O, Riché MC, Mulliken JB, Merland J. Atlas des Hémangiomes et Malformations Vasculaires Superficielles. Paris: McGraw-Hill, 1990.

4 Takahashi K, Mulliken JB, Kozakewich HP et al. Cellular markers that distinguish the phases of hemangioma during infancy and childhood. J Clin Invest 1994;93:2357–64.

5 Wassef M, Blei F, Adams D et al. Vascular Anomalies Classification: Recommendations From the International Society for the Study of Vascular Anomalies. Pediatrics 2015;136:203–14.

6 Esterly NB. Cutaneous hemangiomas, vascular stains and malformations, and associated syndromes. Curr Probl Pediatr 1996;26:3–39.

7 Enjolras O, Mulliken JB. The current management of vascular birthmarks. Pediatr Dermatol 1993;10:311–3.
8 Enjolras O, Mulliken JB. Vascular tumors and vascular malformations (new issues). Adv Dermatol 1997;13:375–423.
9 Enjolras O, Logeart I, Gelbert F et al. [Arteriovenous malformations: a study of 200 cases]. Ann Dermatol Venereol 2000;127:17–22.
10 Abdalla SA, Letarte M. Hereditary haemorrhagic telangiectasia: current views on genetics and mechanisms of disease. J Med Genet 2006;43:97–110.
11 Shovlin CL, Sodhi V, McCarthy A et al. Estimates of maternal risks of pregnancy for women with hereditary haemorrhagic telangiectasia (Osler-Weber-Rendu syndrome): suggested approach for obstetric services. Br J Obstet Gynaecol 2008;115:1108–15.
12 Hosman AE, Devlin HL, Silva BM, Shovlin CL. Specific cancer rates may differ in patients with hereditary haemorrhagic telangiectasia compared to controls. Orphanet J Rare Dis 2013;8:195.
13 Boon LM, Mulliken JB, Vikkula M. RASA1: variable phenotype with capillary and arteriovenous malformations. Curr Opin Genet Dev 2005;15:265–9.
14 Revencu N, Boon LM, Mulliken JB et al. Parkes Weber syndrome, vein of Galen aneurysmal malformation, and other fast-flow vascular anomalies are caused by RASA1 mutations. Hum Mutat 2008;29:959–65.
15 Revencu N, Boon LM, Mendola A et al. RASA1 mutations and associated phenotypes in 68 families with capillary malformation-arteriovenous malformation. Hum Mutat 2013;34:1632–41.
16 Revencu N, Boon LM, Mulliken JB, Vikkula M. RASA1 and capillary malformation-arteriovenous malformation. In: Erickson RP, Wynshaw-Boris A (eds) Inborn Errors of Development Molecular Basis of Clinical Disorders of Morphogenesis. New York: Oxford University Press, 2016: 1423–8.
17 Amyere M, Revencu N, Helaers R et al. Germline loss-of-function mutations in EPHB4 cause a second form of capillary malformation–arteriovenous malformation (CM-AVM2) deregulating RAS-MAPK signaling. Circulation 2017;136:1037–48.
18 Couto JA, Huang AY, Konczyk DJ et al. Somatic MAP2K1 mutations are associated with extracranial arteriovenous malformation. Am J Hum Genet 2017;100:546–54.
19 Eerola I, Boon LM, Mulliken JB et al. Capillary malformation-arteriovenous malformation, a new clinical and genetic disorder caused by RASA1 mutations. Am J Hum Genet 2003;73:1240–9.
20 Johnson DW, Berg JN, Baldwin MA et al. Mutations in the activin receptor-like kinase 1 gene in hereditary haemorrhagic telangiectasia type 2. Nat Genet 1996;13:189–95.
21 McAllister KA, Grogg KM, Johnson DW et al. Endoglin, a TGF-beta binding protein of endothelial cells, is the gene for hereditary haemorrhagic telangiectasia type 1. Nat Genet 1994;8:345–51.
22 Gallione CJ, Repetto GM, Legius E et al. A combined syndrome of juvenile polyposis and hereditary haemorrhagic telangiectasia associated with mutations in MADH4 (SMAD4). Lancet 2004;363(9412):852–9.
23 Wooderchak-Donahue WL, McDonald J, O'Fallon B et al. BMP9 mutations cause a vascular-anomaly syndrome with phenotypic overlap with hereditary hemorrhagic telangiectasia. Am J Hum Genet 2013;93:530–7.
24 Ola R, Dubrac A, Han J et al. PI3 kinase inhibition improves vascular malformations in mouse models of hereditary haemorrhagic telangiectasia. Nat Commun 2016;7:13650.
25 Vikkula M, Boon LM, Carraway KL, 3rd, et al. Vascular dysmorphogenesis caused by an activating mutation in the receptor tyrosine kinase TIE2. Cell 1996;87:1181–90.
26 Macmurdo CF, Wooderchak-Donahue W, Bayrak-Toydemir P et al. RASA1 somatic mutation and variable expressivity in capillary malformation/arteriovenous malformation (CM/AVM) syndrome. Am J Med Genet A 2016;170:1450–4.
27 van der Geer P, Henkemeyer M, Jacks T, Pawson T. Aberrant Ras regulation and reduced p190 tyrosine phosphorylation in cells lacking p120-Gap. Mol Cell Biol 1997;17:1840–7.
28 Henkemeyer M, Rossi DJ, Holmyard DP et al. Vascular system defects and neuronal apoptosis in mice lacking ras GTPase-activating protein. Nature 1995;377(6551):695–701.
29 Kawasaki J, Aegerter S, Fevurly RD et al. RASA1 functions in EPHB4 signaling pathway to suppress endothelial mTORC1 activity. J Clin Invest 2014;124:2774–84.
30 Xiao Z, Carrasco R, Kinneer K et al. EphB4 promotes or suppresses Ras/MEK/ERK pathway in a context-dependent manner: implications for EphB4 as a cancer target. Cancer Biol Ther 2012;13:630–7.
31 Zhou XP, Marsh DJ, Hampel H et al. Germline and germline mosaic PTEN mutations associated with a Proteus-like syndrome of hemihypertrophy, lower limb asymmetry, arteriovenous malformations and lipomatosis. Hum Mol Genet 2000;9:765–8.
32 Marsh DJ, Dahia PL, Zheng Z et al. Germline mutations in PTEN are present in Bannayan-Zonana syndrome. Nat Genet 1997;16:333–4.
33 Marsh DJ, Kum JB, Lunetta KL et al. PTEN mutation spectrum and genotype-phenotype correlations in Bannayan-Riley-Ruvalcaba syndrome suggest a single entity with Cowden syndrome. Hum Mol Genet 1999;8:1461–72.
34 Celebi JT, Wanner M, Ping XL et al. Association of splicing defects in PTEN leading to exon skipping or partial intron retention in Cowden syndrome. Hum Genet 2000;107:234–8.
35 Liu AS, Mulliken JB, Zurakowski D et al. Extracranial arteriovenous malformations: natural progression and recurrence after treatment. Plast Reconstr Surg 2010;125:1185–94.
36 Paltiel HJ, Burrows PE, Kozakewich HP et al. Soft-tissue vascular anomalies: utility of US for diagnosis. Radiology 2000;214:747–54.
37 Kohout MP, Hansen M, Pribaz JJ, Mulliken JB. Arteriovenous malformations of the head and neck: natural history and management. Plast Reconstr Surg 1998;102:643–54.
38 Larralde M, Gonzalez V, Marietti R et al. Pseudo-Kaposi sarcoma with arteriovenous malformation. Pediatr Dermatol 2001;18: 325–7.
39 Enjolras O, Chapot R, Merland JJ. Vascular anomalies and the growth of limbs: a review. J Pediatr Orthop B 2004;13:349–57.
40 Brégeat P. Brégeat syndrome. In: Vinken PJ, Bruyn GW (eds) Handbook of Clinical Neurology: The Phakomatoses. Amsterdam: North Holland Publishers, 1975:474–9.
41 Bhattacharya JJ, Luo CB, Suh DC et al. Wyburn–Mason or Bonnet–Dechaume–Blanc as cerebrofacial arteriovenous metameric syndromes (CAMS). A new concept and a new classification. Intervent Neuroradiol 2001;7:5–17.
42 Jiarakongmun P, Alvarez A, Rodesch G, Lasjaunias P. Clinical course and angioarchitecture of cerebrofacial arteriovenous metameric syndromes: three demonstrative cases and literature review. Intervent Neuroradiol 2002;8:251–64.
43 Hodes JE, Merland JJ, Casasco A et al. Spinal vascular malformations: endovascular therapy. Neurosurg Clin N Am 1994;5:497–509.
44 Thiex R, Mulliken JB, Revencu N et al. A novel association between RASA1 mutations and spinal arteriovenous anomalies. Am J Neuroradiol 2010;31:775–9.
45 Letteboer TG, Mager HJ, Snijder RJ et al. Genotype-phenotype relationship for localization and age distribution of telangiectases in hereditary hemorrhagic telangiectasia. Am J Med Genet A 2008;146A:2733–9.
46 Bayrak-Toydemir P, McDonald J, Markewitz B et al. Genotype–phenotype correlation in hereditary haemorrhagic telangiectasia: mutations and manifestations. Am J Med Genet Part A 2006;140:463.
47 Shovlin, CL. Hereditary haemorrhagic telangiectasia: pathophysiology, diagnosis and treatment. Blood Review 2010;24:203–19. Bayrak-Toydemir P, McDonald J, Markewitz B et al. Genotype–phenotype correlation in hereditary haemorrhagic telangiectasia: mutations and manifestations. Am J Med Genet Part A 2006;140:463.
48 Morgan T, McDonald J, Anderson C et al. Intracranial hemorrhage in infants and children with hereditary hemorrhagic telangiectasia (Osler–Weber–Rendu syndrome). Pediatrics 2002;109:E12.
49 Ference BA, Shannon TM, White RI, Jr et al. Life-threatening pulmonary hemorrhage with pulmonary arteriovenous malformations and hereditary hemorrhagic telangiectasia. Chest 1994;106:1387–90.
50 Govani FS, Shovlin CL. Hereditary haemorrhagic telangiectasia: a clinical and scientific review. Eur J Hum Genet 2009;17:860–71.
51 Sabba C, Pasculli G, Lenato GM et al. Hereditary hemorrhagic telangiectasia: clinical features in ENG and ALK1 mutation carriers. J Thromb Haemost 2007;5:1149–57.
52 Eerola I, Boon LM, Watanabe S et al. Locus for susceptibility for familial capillary malformation ('port-wine stain') maps to 5q. Eur J Hum Genet 2002;10:375–80.
53 Cohen MM, Jr. Vasculogenesis, angiogenesis, hemangiomas, and vascular malformations. Am J Med Genet 2002;108:265–74.
54 Tan WH, Baris HN, Burrows PE et al. The spectrum of vascular anomalies in patients with PTEN mutations: implications for diagnosis and management. J Med Genet 2007;44:594–602.
55 Roudier-Pujol C, Enjolras O, Lacronique J et al. [Multifocal epithelioid hemangioendothelioma with partial remission after interferon alfa-2a treatment]. Ann Dermatol Venereol 1994;121:898–904.

56 Burrows PE, Laor T, Paltiel H, Robertson RL. Diagnostic imaging in the evaluation of vascular birthmarks. Dermatol Clin 1998;16:455–88.

57 Haneen S, Johanna H, Ulrich G et al. Mutation analysis of 'Endoglin' and 'Activin receptor-like kinase' genes in German patients with hereditary hemorrhagic telangiectasia and the value of rapid genotyping using an allele-specific PCR-technique. BMC Medical Genetics 2009;10:53.

58 ter Berg JW, Dippel DW, Habbema JD et al. Unruptured intracranial arteriovenous malformations with hereditary haemorrhagic telangiectasia. Neurosurgical treatment or not? Acta Neurochirurgica 1993; 121(1–2):34–42.

59 Kadoya C, Momota Y, Ikegami Y et al. Central nervous system arteriovenous malformations with hereditary hemorrhagic telangiectasia: report of a family with three cases. Surg Neurol 1994;42:234–9.

60 Matsubara S, Mandzia JL, ter Brugge K et al. Angiographic and clinical characteristics of patients with cerebral arteriovenous malformations associated with hereditary hemorrhagic telangiectasia. Am J Neuroradiol 2000;21:1016–20.

61 Maher CO, Piepgras DG, Brown RD, Jr et al. Cerebrovascular manifestations in 321 cases of hereditary hemorrhagic telangiectasia. Stroke 2001;32:877–82.

62 McClinton MA. Tumors and aneurysms of the upper extremity. Hand Clinics 1993;9:151–69.

63 Enjolras O, Borsik M, Herbreteau D, Merland JJ. [Management of arteriovenous malformations]. Ann Dermatol Venereol 1994;121:59–64.

64 Wu JK, Bisdorff A, Gelbert F et al. Auricular arteriovenous malformation: evaluation, management, and outcome. Plast Reconstr Surg 2005;115:985–95.

65 Coldwell DM, Stokes KR, Yakes WF. Embolotherapy: agents, clinical applications, and techniques. Radiographics 1994;14:623–43; quiz 45–6.

66 Yakes WF, Rossi P, Odink H. How I do it. Arteriovenous malformation management. Cardiovasc Intervent Radiol 1996;19:65–71.

67 Burrows PE, Mulliken JB, Fishman SJ et al. Pharmacological treatment of a diffuse arteriovenous malformation of the upper extremity in a child. J Craniofac Surg 2009;20 Suppl 1:597–602.

68 Dupuis-Girod S, Ginon I, Saurin JC et al. Bevacizumab in patients with hereditary hemorrhagic telangiectasia and severe hepatic vascular malformations and high cardiac output. JAMA 2012;307:948–55.

69 Lebrin F, Srun S, Raymond K et al. Thalidomide stimulates vessel maturation and reduces epistaxis in individuals with hereditary hemorrhagic telangiectasia. Nat Med 2010;16:420–8.

70 Burrows PE, Fellows KE. Techniques for management of pediatric vascular anomalies. In: Cope C (ed) Current Techniques in Interventional Radiology. 2. Philadelphia: Current Medicine, 1995:12–27.

71 Dompmartin A, Labbe D, Barrellier MT, Theron J. Use of a regulating flap in the treatment of a large arteriovenous malformation of the scalp. Br J Plast Surg 1998;51:561–3.

72 Enjolras O, Deffrennes D, Borsik M et al. [Vascular 'tumors' and the rules of their surgical management]. Ann Chir Plast Esthet 1998;43: 455–89.

73 Benndorf G, Campi A, Hell B et al. Endovascular management of a bleeding mandibular arteriovenous malformation by transfemoral venous embolization with NBCA. Am J Neuroradiol 2001;22:359–62.

74 Sofocleous CT, Rosen RJ, Raskin K et al. Congenital vascular malformations in the hand and forearm. J Endovasc Ther 2001;8:484–94.

75 White RI, Jr., Pollak J, Persing J et al. Long-term outcome of embolotherapy and surgery for high-flow extremity arteriovenous malformations. J Vasc Interv Radiol 2000;11:1285–95.

76 Eerola I, McIntyre B, Vikkula M. Identification of eight novel 5′-exons in cerebral capillary malformation gene-1 (CCM1) encoding KRIT1. Biochim Biophys Acta 2001;1517:464–7.

77 Sirvente J, Enjolras O, Wassef M et al. Frequency and phenotypes of cutaneous vascular malformations in a consecutive series of 417 patients with familial cerebral cavernous malformations. J Eur Acad Dermatol Venereol 2009;23:1066–72.

78 Toll A, Parera E, Gimenez-Arnau AM, Pou A et al. Cutaneous venous malformations in familial cerebral cavernomatosis caused by KRIT1 gene mutations. Dermatology 2009;218:307–13.

79 Boon LM, Vanwijck R. [Medical and surgical treatment of venous malformations]. Ann Chir Plast Esthet 2006;51(4–5):403–11.

80 Dompmartin A, Vikkula M, Boon LM. Venous malformation: update on aetiopathogenesis, diagnosis and management. Phlebology 2010;25:224–35.

81 Limaye N, Boon LM, Vikkula M. From germline towards somatic mutations in the pathophysiology of vascular anomalies. Hum Mol Genet 2009;18(R1):R65–74.

82 Brouillard P, Vikkula M. Genetic causes of vascular malformations. Hum Mol Genet 2007;16 Spec No. 2:R140–9.

83 Wouters V, Limaye N, Uebelhoer M et al. Hereditary cutaneomucosal venous malformations are caused by TIE2 mutations with widely variable hyper-phosphorylating effects. Eur J Hum Genet 2010;18:414–20.

84 Brouillard P, Boon LM, Mulliken JB et al. Mutations in a novel factor, glomulin, are responsible for glomuvenous malformations ('glomangiomas'). Am J Hum Genet 2002;70:866–74.

85 Boon LM, Mulliken JB, Enjolras O, Vikkula M. Glomuvenous malformation (glomangioma) and venous malformation: distinct clinicopathologic and genetic entities. Arch Dermatol 2004;140:971–6.

86 Eerola I, Plate KH, Spiegel R et al. KRIT1 is mutated in hyperkeratotic cutaneous capillary-venous malformation associated with cerebral capillary malformation. Hum Mol Genet 2000;9:1351–5.

87 Labauge P, Enjolras O, Bonerandi JJ et al. An association between autosomal dominant cerebral cavernomas and a distinctive hyperkeratotic cutaneous vascular malformation in 4 families. Ann Neurol 1999;45:250–4.

88 Boon LM, Mulliken JB, Vikkula M et al. Assignment of a locus for dominantly inherited venous malformations to chromosome 9p. Human Mol Genet 1994;3:1583–7.

89 Gallione CJ, Pasyk KA, Boon LM et al. A gene for familial venous malformations maps to chromosome 9p in a second large kindred. J Med Genet 1995;32:197–9.

90 Korpelainen EI, Karkkainen M, Gunji Y et al. Endothelial receptor tyrosine kinases activate the STAT signaling pathway: mutant Tie-2 causing venous malformations signals a distinct STAT activation response. Oncogene 1999;18:1–8.

91 Limaye N, Wouters V, Uebelhoer M et al. Somatic mutations in angiopoietin receptor gene TEK cause solitary and multiple sporadic venous malformations. Nat Genet 2009;41:118–24.

92 Soblet J, Kangas J, Natynki M et al. Blue rubber bleb nevus (BRBN) syndrome is caused by somatic TEK (TIE2) mutations. J Invest Dermatol 2017;137:207–16.

93 Uebelhoer M, Natynki M, Kangas J et al. Venous malformation-causative TIE2 mutations mediate an AKT-dependent decrease in PDGFB. Hum Mol Genet 2013;22:3438–48.

94 Nätynki M, Kangas J, Miinalainen I et al. Common and specific effects of TIE2 mutations causing venous malformations. Hum Mol Genet 2015;24:6374–89.

95 Boon LM, Brouillard P, Irrthum A et al. A gene for inherited cutaneous venous anomalies ('glomangiomas') localizes to chromosome 1p21-22. Am J Hum Genet 1999;65:125–33.

96 Irrthum A, Brouillard P, Enjolras O et al. Linkage disequilibrium narrows locus for venous malformation with glomus cells (VMGLOM) to a single 1.48 Mbp YAC. Eur J Hum Genet 2001;9:34–8.

97 Brouillard P, Ghassibe M, Penington A et al. Four common glomulin mutations cause two thirds of glomuvenous malformations ('familial glomangiomas'): evidence for a founder effect. J Med Genet 2005;42:e13.

98 Brouillard P, Boon LM, Mulliken JB et al. Mutations in novel factor, glomulin, are responsible for glomuvenous malformations ('glomangiomas'). Am J Hum Genet 2002;70:866–74.

99 Amyere M, Aerts V, Brouillard P et al. Somatic uniparental isodisomy explains multifocality of glomuvenous malformations. Am J Hum Genet 2013;92:188–96.

100 Mallory SB, Enjolras O, Boon LM et al. Congenital plaque-type glomuvenous malformations presenting in childhood. Arch Dermatol 2006;142:892–6.

101 Brouillard P, Enjolras O, Boon LM, Vikkula M. Glomulin and glomuvenous malformation. In: Epstein CJ, Erickson RP, Wynshaw-Boris A (eds) Inborn Errors of Development, 2nd edn. New York: Oxford University Press, 2008:1561–5.

102 Brouillard P, Boon LM, Revencu N et al. Genotypes and phenotypes of 162 families with a glomulin mutation. Mol Syndromol 2013;4:157–64.

103 Limaye N, Kangas J, Mendola A et al. Somatic activating PIK3CA mutations cause venous malformation. Am J Hum Genet 2015;97:914–21.

104 Boscolo E, Kang K-T, Limaye N et al. Venous malformation: from causative mutations to murine model and targeted therapy. J Clin Invest 2015;125:3491–504.

105 Couvineau A, Wouters V, Bertrand G et al. PTHR1 mutations associated with Ollier disease result in receptor loss of function. Hum Mol Genet 2008;17:2766–75.

106 Pansuriya TC, van Eijk R, d'Adamo P et al. Somatic mosaic IDH1 and IDH2 mutations are associated with enchondroma and spindle cell hemangioma in Ollier disease and Maffucci syndrome. Nat Genet 2011;43:1256–61.

107 Amyere M, Dompmartin A, Wouters V et al. Common somatic alterations identified in maffucci syndrome by molecular karyotyping. Mol Syndromol 2014;5:259–67.

108 Akers A, Al-Shahi Salman R, Awad IA et al. Synopsis of Guidelines for the Clinical Management of Cerebral Cavernous Malformations: Consensus Recommendations based on systematic literature review by the Angioma Alliance Scientific Advisory Board Clinical Experts Panel. Neurosurgery 2017;80:665–80.

109 Laberge-le Couteulx S, Jung HH, Labauge P et al. Truncating mutations in CCM1, encoding KRIT1, cause hereditary cavernous angiomas. Nat Genet 1999;23:189–93.

110 Revencu N, Vikkula M. Cerebral cavernous malformation: new molecular and clinical insights. J Med Genet 2006;43:716–21.

111 Liquori CL, Berg MJ, Squitieri F et al. Deletions in CCM2 are a common cause of cerebral cavernous malformations. Am J Hum Genet 2007;80:69–75.

112 Bergametti F, Denier C, Labauge P et al. Mutations within the programmed cell death 10 gene cause cerebral cavernous malformations. Am J Hum Genet 2005;76:42–51.

113 Boon L, Mulliken J, Enjolras O, Vikkula M. Glomuvenous malformation (glomangioma): distinct clinicopathologic and genetic entity. Arch Dermatol 2004;140:971–6.

114 Enjolras O, Ciabrini D, Mazoyer E et al. Extensive pure venous malformations in the upper or lower limb: a review of 27 cases. J Am Acad Dermatol 1997;36(2 Pt 1):219–25.

115 Hein KD, Mulliken JB, Kozakewich HP et al. Venous malformations of skeletal muscle. Plast Reconstr Surg 2002;110:1625–35.

116 Schajowicz F, Rebecchini AC, Bosch-Mayol G. Intracortical haemangioma simulating osteoid osteoma. J Bone Joint Surg Br 1979;61:94–5.

117 Ballieux F, Boon LM, Vikkula M. Blue bleb rubber nevus syndrome. Handb Clin Neurol 2015;132:223–30.

118 Weiss SW, Enzinger FM. Spindle cell hemangioendothelioma. A low-grade angiosarcoma resembling a cavernous hemangioma and Kaposi's sarcoma. Am J Surg Pathol 1986;10:521–30.

119 Johnson TE, Nasr AM, Nalbandian RM, Cappelen-Smith J. Enchondromatosis and hemangioma (Maffucci's syndrome) with orbital involvement. Am J Ophthalmol 1990;110:153–9.

120 Kaplan RP, Wang JT, Amron DM, Kaplan L. Maffucci's syndrome: two case reports with a literature review. J Am Acad Dermatol 1993;29:894–9.

121 Enjolras O, Wassef M, Merland JJ. [Maffucci syndrome: a false venous malformation? A case with hemangioendothelioma with fusiform cells]. Ann Dermatol Venereol 1998;125:512–5.

122 Boukobza M, Enjolras O, Guichard JP et al. Cerebral developmental venous anomalies associated with head and neck venous malformations. Am J Neuroradiol 1996;17:987–94.

123 Dompmartin A, Acher A, Thibon P et al. Association of localized intravascular coagulopathy with venous malformations. Arch Dermatol 2008;144:873–7.

124 Dompmartin A, Thibon P, Vikkula M, Boon LM. Oral contraceptive and D-Dimer level, a reply. Arch Dermatol 2009;145:210–1.

125 Mazoyer E, Enjolras O, Laurian C et al. Coagulation abnormalities associated with extensive venous malformations of the limbs: differentiation from Kasabach-Merritt syndrome. Clin Lab Haematol 2002;24:243–51.

126 Garzon MC, Huang JT, Enjolras O, Frieden IJ. Vascular malformations: Part I. J Am Acad Dermatol 2007;56:353–70; quiz 71–4.

127 Garzon MC, Huang JT, Enjolras O, Frieden IJ. Vascular malformations. Part II: associated syndromes. J Am Acad Dermatol 2007;56:541–64.

128 Enjolras O, Wassef M, Mazoyer E et al. Infants with Kasabach-Merritt syndrome do not have 'true' hemangiomas. J Pediatr 1997;130:631–40.

129 Sarkar M, Mulliken JB, Kozakewich HP et al.Thrombocytopenic coagulopathy (Kasabach–Merritt phenomenon) is associated with Kaposiform hemangioendothelioma and not with common infantile hemangioma. Plast Reconstr Surg 1997;100:1377–86.

130 Konez D, Burrows PE, Mulliken JB. Cervicofacial venous malformations. MRI features and interventional strategies. Intervent Neuroradiol 2002;8:227–34.

131 Trop I, Dubois J, Guibaud L et al. Soft-tissue venous malformations in pediatric and young adult patients: diagnosis with Doppler US. Radiology 1999;212:841–5.

132 Wassef M, Vanwijck R, Clapuyt P et al. [Vascular tumours and malformations, classification, pathology and imaging]. Ann Chir Plast Esthet 2006;51:263–81.

133 Goraya JS, Marwaha RK, Vatve M, Trehan A. Blue rubber bleb nevus syndrome: a cause for recurrent episodic severe anemia. Pediatr Hematol Oncol 1998;15:261–4.

134 Ertem D, Acar Y, Kotiloglu E et al. Blue rubber bleb nevus syndrome. Pediatrics 2001;107:418–20.

135 Mazoyer E, Enjolras O, Bisdorff A et al. Coagulation disorders in patients with venous malformation of the limbs and trunk: a case series of 118 patients. Arch Dermatol 2008;144:861–7.

136 Hermans C, Dessomme B, Lambert C, Deneys V. [Venous malformations and coagulopathy]. Ann Chir Plast Esthet 2006;51:388–93.

137 Dompmartin A, Ballieux F, Thibon P et al. Elevated D-dimer level in the differential diagnosis of venous malformations. Arch Dermatol 2009;145:1239–44.

138 Boscolo E, Limaye N, Huang L et al. Rapamycin improves TIE2-mutated venous malformation in murine model and human subjects. J Clin Invest 2015;125:3491–504.

139 Hammer J, Seront E, Dupont S et al. Rapamycin as treatment for complex vascular anomalies. submitted.

140 Yuksekkaya H, Ozbek O, Keser M, Toy H. Blue rubber bleb nevus syndrome: successful treatment with sirolimus. Pediatrics 2012;129: e1080–4.

141 Dubois JM, Sebag GH, De Prost Y et al. Soft-tissue venous malformations in children: percutaneous sclerotherapy with Ethibloc. Radiology 1991;180:195–8.

142 Herbreteau D, Riche MC, Enjolras O et al. [Venous vascular malformations and their treatment with Ethibloc]. Journal des maladies vasculaires 1992;17:50–3.

143 Suh JS, Shin KH, Na JB et al. Venous malformations: sclerotherapy with a mixture of ethanol and lipiodol. Cardiovasc Intervent Radiol 1997;20:268–73.

144 Berenguer B, Burrows PE, Zurakowski D, Mulliken JB. Sclerotherapy of craniofacial venous malformations: complications and results. Plast Reconstr Surg 1999;104:1–11; discussion 2–5.

145 Hammer FD, Boon LM, Mathurin P, Vanwijck RR. Ethanol sclerotherapy of venous malformations: evaluation of systemic ethanol contamination. J Vasc Interv Radiol 2001;12:595–600.

146 Mason KP, Michna E, Zurakowski D et al. Serum ethanol levels in children and adults after ethanol embolization or sclerotherapy for vascular anomalies. Radiology 2000;217:127–32.

147 Chapot R, Laurent A, Enjolras O et al. Fatal cardiovascular collapse during ethanol sclerotherapy of a venous malformation. Intervent Neuroradiol 2002;8:321–4.

148 Cabrera J, Cabrera J, Jr., Garcia-Olmedo MA, Redondo P. Treatment of venous malformations with sclerosant in microfoam form. Arch Dermatol 2003;139:1409–16.

149 Li L, Feng J, Zeng XQ, Li YH. Fluoroscopy-guided foam sclerotherapy with sodium morrhuate for peripheral venous malformations: Preliminary experience. J Vasc Surg 2009;49:961–7.

150 Forlee MV, Grouden M, Moore DJ, Shanik G. Stroke after varicose vein foam injection sclerotherapy. J Vasc Surg 2006;43:162–4.

151 Dompmartin A, Labbe D, Theron J et al. [The use of an alcohol gel of ethyl cellulose in the treatment of venous malformations]. Rev Stomatol Chir Maxillofac 2000;101:30–2.

152 Dompmartin A, Blaizot X, Théron J et al. Radio-opaque ethylcellulose-ethanol is a safe and efficient sclerosing agent for venous malformations. Eur Radiol 2011;21:2647–56.

153 Sannier K, Dompmartin A, Théron J et al. A new sclerosing agent in the treatment of venous malformations. Study on 23 cases. Interven Radiol 2004;10:113–27.

154 Boon LM, Bataille AC, Bernier V et al. [Medical treatment of juvenile hemangiomas]. Ann Chir Plast Esthet 2006;51:310–20.

155 Pireau N, Boon LM, Poilvache P, Docquier PL. Surgical treatment of intra-articular knee venous malformations: when and how? J Pediatr Orthop 2016;36:316–22.

156 Fishman SJ, Smithers CJ, Folkman J et al. Blue rubber bleb nevus syndrome: surgical eradication of gastrointestinal bleeding. Ann Surg 2005;241:523–8.

157 Gallagher PG, Mahoney MJ, Gosche JR. Cystic hygroma in the fetus and newborn. Sem Perinatol 1999;23:341–56.

158 Tanriverdi HA, Hendrik HJ, Ertan AK et al. Hygroma colli cysticum: prenatal diagnosis and prognosis. Am J Perinatol 2001;18:415–20.

159 Sybert VP, McCauley E. Turner's syndrome. New Engl J Med 2004;351:1227–38.

160 Osborn AJ, Dickie P, Neilson DE et al. Activating PIK3CA alleles and lymphangiogenic phenotype of lymphatic endothelial cells isolated from lymphatic malformations. Hum Mol Genet 2015;24:926–38.
161 Boscolo E, Coma S, Luks VL et al. AKT hyper-phosphorylation associated with PI3K mutations in lymphatic endothelial cells from a patient with lymphatic malformation. Angiogenesis 2015;18:151–62.
162 Luks VL, Kamitaki N, Vivero MP et al. Lymphatic and other vascular malformative/overgrowth disorders are caused by somatic mutations in PIK3CA. J Pediatr 2015;166:1048–54 e1–5.
163 Brouillard P, Boon L, Vikkula M. Genetics of lymphatic anomalies. J Clin Invest 2014;124:898–904.
164 Irrthum A, Karkkainen MJ, Devriendt K et al. Congenital hereditary lymphedema caused by a mutation that inactivates VEGFR3 tyrosine kinase. Am J Hum Genet 2000;67:295–301.
165 Evans AL, Bell R, Brice G et al. Identification of eight novel VEGFR-3 mutations in families with primary congenital lymphoedema. J Med Genet 2003;40:697–703.
166 Irrthum A, Devriendt K, Chitayat D et al. Mutations in the transcription factor gene SOX18 underlie recessive and dominant forms of hypotrichosis-lymphedema-telangiectasia. Am J Hum Genet 2003; 72:1470–8.
167 Ghalamkarpour A, Holnthoner W, Saharinen P et al. Recessive primary congenital lymphoedema caused by a VEGFR3 mutation. J Med Genet 2009;46:399–404.
168 Mansour S, Brice GW, Jeffery S, Mortimer P. Lymphedema-distichiasis syndrome. In: Pagon RA, Adam MP, Ardinger HH et al. (eds) GeneReviews(R). Seattle, WA, 1993.
169 Ostergaard P, Simpson MA, Mendola A et al. Mutations in KIF11 cause autosomal-dominant microcephaly variably associated with congenital lymphedema and chorioretinopathy. Am J Hum Genet 2012;90:356–62.
170 Schlogel MJ, Mendola A, Fastre E et al. No evidence of locus heterogeneity in familial microcephaly with or without chorioretinopathy, lymphedema, or mental retardation syndrome. Orphanet J Rare Dis 2015;10:52.
171 Hennekam RC, Geerdink RA, Hamel BC et al. Autosomal recessive intestinal lymphangiectasia and lymphedema, with facial anomalies and mental retardation. Am J Med Genet 1989;34:593–600.
172 Alders M, Hogan BM, Gjini E et al. Mutations in CCBE1 cause generalized lymph vessel dysplasia in humans. Nat Genet 2009;41:1272–4.
173 Connell F, Kalidas K, Ostergaard P et al. Linkage and sequence analysis indicate that CCBE1 is mutated in recessively inherited generalised lymphatic dysplasia. Hum Genet 2010;127:231–41.
174 Ostergaard P, Simpson MA, Connell FC et al. Mutations in GATA2 cause primary lymphedema associated with a predisposition to acute myeloid leukemia (Emberger syndrome). Nat Genet 2011;43:929–31.
175 Mendola A, Schlogel MJ, Ghalamkarpour A et al. Mutations in the VEGFR3 signaling pathway explain 36% of familial lymphedema. Mol Syndromol 2013;4:257–66.
176 Hirayama T, Sabokbar A, Itonaga I et al. Cellular and humoral mechanisms of osteoclast formation and bone resorption in Gorham-Stout disease. J Pathol 2001;195:624–30.
177 Gomez CS, Calonje E, Ferrar DW et al. Lymphangiomatosis of the limbs. Clinicopathologic analysis of a series with a good prognosis. Am J Surg Pathol 1995;19:125–33.
178 Boyd JB, Mulliken JB, Kaban LB et al. Skeletal changes associated with vascular malformations. Plast Reconstr Surg 1984;74:789–97.
179 Harris GJ, Sakol PJ, Bonavolonta G, De Conciliis C. An analysis of thirty cases of orbital lymphangioma. Pathophysiologic considerations and management recommendations. Ophthalmology 1990;97: 1583–92.
180 Alqahtani A, Nguyen LT, Flageole H et al. 25 years' experience with lymphangiomas in children. J Pediatr Surg 1999;34:1164–8.
181 Orvidas LJ, Kasperbauer JL. Pediatric lymphangiomas of the head and neck. Ann Otol Rhinol Laryngol 2000;109:411–21.
182 Padwa BL, Hayward PG, Ferraro NF, Mulliken JB. Cervicofacial lymphatic malformation: clinical course, surgical intervention, and pathogenesis of skeletal hypertrophy. Plast Reconstr Surg 1995;95:951–60.
183 Hartl DM, Roger G, Denoyelle F et al. Extensive lymphangioma presenting with upper airway obstruction. Arch Otolaryngol–Head & Neck Surg 2000;126:1378–82.
184 Konez O, Vyas PK, Goyal M. Disseminated lymphangiomatosis presenting with massive chylothorax. Pediatr Radiol 2000;30:35–7.
185 Brice G, Child AH, Evans A et al. Milroy disease and the VEGFR-3 mutation phenotype. J Med Genet 2005;42:98–102.
186 Ghalamkarpour A, Morlot S, Raas-Rothschild A et al. Hereditary lymphedema type I associated with VEGFR3 mutation: the first de novo case and atypical presentations. Clin Genet 2006;70:330–5.
187 Daniel-Spiegel E, Ghalamkarpour A, Spiegel R et al. Hydrops fetalis: an unusual prenatal presentation of hereditary congenital lymphedema. Prenat Diagn 2005;25:1015–8.
188 Lala S, Mulliken JB, Alomari AI et al. Gorham-Stout disease and generalized lymphatic anomaly – clinical, radiologic, and histologic differentiation. Skeletal Radiol 2013;42:917–24.
189 Gorham LW, Stout AP. Massive osteolysis (acute spontaneous absorption of bone, phantom bone, disappearing bone); its relation to hemangiomatosis. J Bone Joint Surg Am 1955;37–A:985–1004.
190 Moller G, Priemel M, Amling M et al. The Gorham–Stout syndrome (Gorham's massive osteolysis). A report of six cases with histopathological findings. J Bone Joint Surg Br 1999;81:501–6.
191 Hayward PG, Orgill DP, Mulliken JB, Perez-Atayde AR. Congenital fibrosarcoma masquerading as lymphatic malformation: report of two cases. J Pediatr Surg 1995;30:84–8.
192 Jappe U, Zimmermann T, Kahle B, Petzoldt D. Lymphangioma circumscriptum of the vulva following surgical and radiological therapy of cervical cancer. Sex Trans Dis 2002;29:533–5.
193 Jones EW, Winkelmann RK, Zachary CB, Reda AM. Benign lymphangioendothelioma. J Am Acad Dermatol 1990;23:229–35.
194 Guillou L, Fletcher CD. Benign lymphangioendothelioma (acquired progressive lymphangioma): a lesion not to be confused with well-differentiated angiosarcoma and patch stage Kaposi's sarcoma: clinicopathologic analysis of a series. Am J Surg Pathol 2000;24:1047–57.
195 Kaddu S, Cerroni L, Pilatti A et al. Acral pseudolymphomatous angiokeratoma. A variant of the cutaneous pseudolymphomas. Am J Dermatopathol 1994;16:130–3.
196 Calonje E, Fletcher CD. Sinusoidal hemangioma. A distinctive benign vascular neoplasm within the group of cavernous hemangiomas. Am J Surg Pathol 1991;15:1130–5.
197 Herron GS, Rouse RV, Kosek JC et al. Benign lymphangioendothelioma. J Am Acad Dermatol 1994;31:362–8.
198 Mentzel T, Kutzner H. [Tumors of the lymphatic vessel of the skin and soft tissue]. Der Pathologe 2002;23:118–27.
199 Gimeno Aranguez M, Colomar Palmer P, Gonzalez Mediero I, Ollero Caprani JM. [The clinical and morphological aspects of childhood lymphangiomas: a review of 145 cases]. Anales espanoles de pediatria 1996;45:25–8.
200 Ogita S, Tsuto T, Deguchi E, Tokiwa K et al. OK-432 therapy for unresectable lymphangiomas in children. J Pediatr Surg 1991;26: 263–8; discussion 8–70.
201 Dubois J, Garel L, Abela A et al. Lymphangiomas in children: percutaneous sclerotherapy with an alcoholic solution of zein. Radiology 1997;204:651–4.
202 Luzzatto C, Midrio P, Tchaprassian Z, Guglielmi M. Sclerosing treatment of lymphangiomas with OK-432. Arch Dis Childhood 2000;82: 316–8.
203 Sainsbury DC, Kessell G, Fall AJ et al. Intralesional bleomycin injection treatment for vascular birthmarks: a 5-year experience at a single United Kingdom unit. Plast Reconstr Surg 2011;127:2031–44.
204 Chaudry G, Guevara CJ, Rialon KL et al. Safety and efficacy of bleomycin sclerotherapy for microcystic lymphatic malformation. Cardiovasc Intervent Radiol 2014;37:1476–81.
205 Leboulanger N, Roger G, Caze A et al. Utility of radiofrequency ablation for haemorrhagic lingual lymphangioma. Int J Pediatr Otorhinolaryngol 2008;72:953–8.
206 Bruder E, Perez-Atayde AR, Jundt G et al. Vascular lesions of bone in children, adolescents, and young adults. A clinicopathologic reappraisal and application of the ISSVA classification. Virchows Arch 2009;454:161–79.
207 MacLean JE, Cohen E, Weinstein M. Primary intestinal and thoracic lymphangiectasia: a response to antiplasmin therapy. Pediatrics 2002;109:1177–80.
208 Hammill AM, Wentzel M, Gupta A et al. Sirolimus for the treatment of complicated vascular anomalies in children. Pediatr Blood Cancer 2011;57:1018–24.
209 Adams DM, Trenor CC, 3rd, Hammill AM et al. Efficacy and safety of sirolimus in the treatment of complicated vascular anomalies. Pediatrics 2016;137:1–10.
210 Mizuno T, Fukuda T, Emoto C et al. Developmental pharmacokinetics of sirolimus: Implications for precision dosing in neonates

and infants with complicated vascular anomalies. Pediatr Blood Cancer 2017;64:epub 2017 Feb 16.

211 **Hammer J, Seront E, Duez S et al. Sirolimus treatment for extensive slow-flow vascular malformations: a monocentric prospective phase-II study. Orphanet J Rare Dis 2018;13:191.**

212 Sturge WA. A case of partial epilepsy apparently due to a lesion of one of the motor centers of the brain. Trans Clin Soc London 1879;12:112.

213 Parkes W. Right-sided hemihypertrophy resulting from right-sided congenital spastic hemiplegia with a morbid condition of the left side of the brain revealed by radiogram. J Neurol Neurosurg Psychiatry 1922;37:301–11.

214 **Thomas-Sohl KA, Vaslow DF, Maria BL. Sturge-Weber syndrome: a review. Pediatr Neurol 2004;30:303–10.**

215 Jacobs AH, Walton RG. The incidence of birthmarks in the neonate. Pediatrics 1976;58:218–22.

216 **Shirley MD, Tang H, Gallione CJ et al. Sturge–Weber syndrome and port-wine stains caused by somatic mutation in GNAQ. New Engl J Med 2013;368:1971–9.**

217 **Lee MS, Liang MG, Mulliken JB. Diffuse capillary malformation with overgrowth: a clinical subtype of vascular anomalies with hypertrophy. J Am Acad Dermatol 2013;69:589–94.**

218 Adams BB, Lucky AW. Acquired port-wine stains and antecedent trauma: case report and review of the literature. Arch Dermatol 2000;136:897–9.

219 Larralde M, Abad ME, Luna PC, Hoffner MV. Capillary malformation-arteriovenous malformation: a clinical review of 45 patients. Int J Dermatol 2014;53:458–61.

220 **Enjolras O, Boukobza M, Jdid R. Cervical occult spinal dysraphism: MRI findings and the value of a vascular birthmark. Pediatr Dermatol 1995;12:256–9.**

221 Tavafoghi V, Ghandchi A, Hambrick GW, Jr., Udverhelyi GB. Cutaneous signs of spinal dysraphism. Report of a patient with a tail-like lipoma and review of 200 cases in the literature. Arch Dermatol 1978;114:573–7.

222 Drolet B, Prendiville J, Golden J et al. 'Membranous aplasia cutis' with hair collars. Congenital absence of skin or neuroectodermal defect? Arch Dermatol 1995;131:1427–31.

223 Leung AK, Telmesani AM. Salmon patches in Caucasian children. Pediatr Dermatol 1989;6:185–7.

224 Jones EW, Orkin M. Tufted angioma (angioblastoma). A benign progressive angioma, not to be confused with Kaposi's sarcoma or low-grade angiosarcoma. J Am Acad Dermatol 1989;20:214–25.

225 Tsang WY, Chan JK, Fletcher CD. Recently characterized vascular tumours of skin and soft tissues. Histopathology 1991;19:489–501.

226 Catteau B, Enjolras O, Delaporte E et al. [Sclerosing tufted angioma. Apropos of 4 cases involving lower limbs]. Ann Dermatol Venereol 1998;125:682–7.

227 Klapman MH, Yao JF. Thickening and nodules in port-wine stains. J Am Acad Dermatol 2001;44:300–2.

228 del Pozo J, Fonseca E. Port-wine stain nodules in the adult: report of 20 cases treated by CO2 laser vaporization. Dermatol Surg 2001;27:699–702.

229 Valeyrie L, Lebrun-Vignes B, Descamps V et al. Pyogenic granuloma within port-wine stains: an alarming clinical presentation. Eur J Dermatol 2002;12:373–5.

230 Hofer T. Meyerson phenomenon within a nevus flammeus. The different eczematous reactions within port-wine stains. Dermatology 2002;205:180–3.

231 **Ashinoff R, Geronemus RG. Flashlamp-pumped pulsed dye laser for port-wine stains in infancy: earlier versus later treatment. J Am Acad Dermatol 1991;24:467–72.**

232 Dover JS, Geronemus R, Stern RS et al. Dye laser treatment of port-wine stains: comparison of the continuous-wave dye laser with a robotized scanning device and the pulsed dye laser. J Am Acad Dermatol 1995;32:237–40.

233 **van der Horst CM, Koster PH, de Borgie CA et al. Effect of the timing of treatment of port-wine stains with the flash-lamp-pumped pulsed-dye laser. N Engl J Med 1998;338:1028–33.**

234 Troilius A, Wrangsjo B, Ljunggren B. Potential psychological benefits from early treatment of port-wine stains in children. Br J Dermatol 1998;139:59–65.

235 Namba Y, Mae O, Ao M. The treatment of port wine stains with a dye laser: a study of 644 patients. Scand J Plast Reconstr Surg Hand Surg 2001;35:197–202.

236 **Michel S, Landthaler M, Hohenleutner U. Recurrence of port-wine stains after treatment with the flashlamp-pumped pulsed dye laser. Br J Dermatol 2000;143:1230–4.**

237 **Sapp JC, Turner JT, van de Kamp JM et al. Newly delineated syndrome of congenital lipomatous overgrowth, vascular malformations, and epidermal nevi (CLOVE syndrome) in seven patients. Am J Med Genet A 2007;143A:2944–58.**

238 Lopez-Gutierrez JC, Lapunzina P. Capillary malformation of the lower lip, lymphatic malformation of the face and neck, asymmetry and partial/generalized overgrowth (CLAPO): report of six cases of a new syndrome/association. Am J Med Genet A 2008;146A:2583–8.

239 Happle R. Mosaicism in human skin. Understanding the patterns and mechanisms. Arch Dermatol 1993;129:1460–70.

240 **Keppler-Noreuil KM, Rios JJ, Parker VE et al. PIK3CA-related overgrowth spectrum (PROS): diagnostic and testing eligibility criteria, differential diagnosis, and evaluation. Am J Med Genet A 2015;167A:287–95.**

241 **Martinez-Lopez A, Blasco-Morente G, Perez-Lopez I et al. CLOVES syndrome: review of a PIK3CA-related overgrowth spectrum (PROS). Clin Genet 2017;91:14–21.**

242 Ruiz-Maldonado R, Tamayo L, Laterza AM et al. Phacomatosis pigmentovascularis: a new syndrome? Report of four cases. Pediatr Dermatol 1987;4:189–96.

243 Hagiwara K, Uezato H, Nonaka S. Phacomatosis pigmentovascularis type IIb associated with Sturge–Weber syndrome and pyogenic granuloma. J Dermatol 1998;25:721–9.

244 Fernandez-Guarino M, Boixeda P, de Las Heras E et al. Phakomatosis pigmentovascularis: clinical findings in 15 patients and review of the literature. J Am Acad Dermatol 2008;58:88–93.

245 Happle R. Phacomatosis pigmentovascularis revisited and reclassified. Arch Dermatol 2005;141:385–8.

246 **Enjolras O, Riche MC, Merland JJ. Facial port-wine stains and Sturge–Weber syndrome. Pediatrics 1985;76:48–51.**

247 Greene AK, Taber SF, Ball KL et al. Sturge–Weber syndrome: soft-tissue and skeletal overgrowth. J Craniofac Surg 2009;20 Suppl 1: 617–21.

248 Portilla P, Husson B, Lasjaunias P, Landrieu P. Sturge–Weber disease with repercussion on the prenatal development of the cerebral hemisphere. Am J Neuroradiol 2002;23:490–2.

249 Jacoby CG, Yuh WT, Afifi AK et al. Accelerated myelination in early Sturge–Weber syndrome demonstrated by MR imaging. J Comput Assist Tomogr 1987;11:226–31.

250 Capraro PA, Fisher J, Hammond DC, Grossman JA. Klippel–Trenaunay syndrome. Plast Reconstr Surg 2002;109:2052–60; quiz 61–2.

251 Gucev ZS, Tasic V, Jancevska A et al. Congenital lipomatous overgrowth, vascular malformations, and epidermal nevi (CLOVE) syndrome: CNS malformations and seizures may be a component of this disorder. Am J Med Genet A 2008;146A:2688–90.

252 Cohen MM, Jr. Proteus syndrome: an update. Am J Med Genet C Semin Med Genet 2005;137C:38–52.

253 Turner JT, Cohen MM, Jr., Biesecker LG. Reassessment of the Proteus syndrome literature: application of diagnostic criteria to published cases. Am J Med Genet A 2004;130A:111–22.

254 Adamsbaum C, Pinton F, Rolland Y et al. Accelerated myelination in early Sturge–Weber syndrome: MRI-SPECT correlations. Pediatr Radiol 1996;26:759–62.

255 Boukobza M, Enjolras O, Cambra M, Merland J. [Sturge–Weber syndrome. The current neuroradiologic data]. J Radiol 2000;81:765–71.

256 Pinton F, Chiron C, Enjolras O et al. Early single photon emission computed tomography in Sturge–Weber syndrome. J Neurol Neurosurg Psychiatry 1997;63:616–21.

257 Chugani HT, Mazziotta JC, Phelps ME. Sturge–Weber syndrome: a study of cerebral glucose utilization with positron emission tomography. J Pediatr 1989;114:244–53.

258 Evans AL, Widjaja E, Connolly DJ, Griffiths PD. Cerebral perfusion abnormalities in children with Sturge–Weber syndrome shown by dynamic contrast bolus magnetic resonance perfusion imaging. Pediatrics 2006;117:2119–25.

259 Huiras EE, Barnes CJ, Eichenfield LF et al. Pulmonary thromboembolism associated with Klippel–Trenaunay syndrome. Pediatrics 2005;116:e596–600.

260 Ville D, Enjolras O, Chiron C, Dulac O. Prophylactic antiepileptic treatment in Sturge–Weber disease. Seizure 2002;11:145–50.

261 Tuxhorn IE, Pannek HW. Epilepsy surgery in bilateral Sturge–Weber syndrome. Pediatr Neurol 2002;26:394–7.

262 Venot Q, Blanc T, Rabia SH. Targeted therapy in patients with PIK3CA-related overgrowth syndrome. Nature 2018;558:540–6

263 Baraldini V, Coletti M, Cipolat L et al. Early surgical management of Klippel–Trenaunay syndrome in childhood can prevent long-term haemodynamic effects of distal venous hypertension. J Pediatr Surg 2002;37:232–5.
264 Noel AA, Gloviczki P, Cherry KJ, Jr et al. Surgical treatment of venous malformations in Klippel–Trenaunay syndrome. J Vasc Surg 2000;32:840–7.
265 Frasier K, Giangola G, Rosen R, Ginat DT. Endovascular radiofrequency ablation: a novel treatment of venous insufficiency in Klippel–Trenaunay patients. J Vasc Surg 2008;47:1339–45.
266 Gold MH, Eramo L, Prendiville JS. Hereditary benign telangiectasia. Pediatr Dermatol 1989;6:194–7.
267 Uhlin SR, McCarty KS, Jr. Unilateral nevoid telangiectatic syndrome. The role of estrogen and progesterone receptors. Arch Dermatol 1983;119:226–8.
268 Pehr K, Moroz B. Cutis marmorata telangiectatica congenita: long-term follow-up, review of the literature, and report of a case in conjunction with congenital hypothyroidism. Pediatr Dermatol 1993;10:6–11.
269 Devillers AC, de Waard-van der Spek FB, Oranje AP. Cutis marmorata telangiectatica congenita: clinical features in 35 cases. Arch Dermatol 1999;135:34–8.
270 Gerritsen MJ, Steijlen PM, Brunner HG, Rieu P. Cutis marmorata telangiectatica congenita: report of 18 cases. Br J Dermatol 2000; 142:366–9.
271 Amitai DB, Fichman S, Merlob P et al. Cutis marmorata telangiectatica congenita: clinical findings in 85 patients. Pediatr Dermatol 2000;17:100–4.
272 Enjolras O. [Cutis marmorata telangiectatica congenita]. Ann Dermatol Venereol 2001;128:161–6.
273 Riviere JB, Mirzaa GM, O'Roak BJ et al. De novo germline and postzygotic mutations in AKT3, PIK3R2 and PIK3CA cause a spectrum of related megalencephaly syndromes. Nat Genet 2012;44:934–40.
274 Savitsky K, Bar-Shira A, Gilad S et al. A single ataxia telangiectasia gene with a product similar to PI-3 kinase. Science 1995; 268(5218):1749–53.
275 Hannan MA, Hellani A, Al-Khodairy FM et al. Deficiency in the repair of UV-induced DNA damage in human skin fibroblasts compromised for the ATM gene. Carcinogenesis 2002;23:1617–24.
276 Picascia DD, Esterly NB. Cutis marmorata telangiectatica congenita: report of 22 cases. J Am Acad Dermatol 1989;20:1098–104.
277 Gelmetti C, Schianchi R, Ermacora E. [Cutis marmorata telangiectatica congenita. 4 new cases and review of the literature]. Ann Dermatol Venereol 1987;114:1517–28.
278 Bork K, Pfeifle J. Multifocal aplasia cutis congenita, distal limb hemimelia, and cutis marmorata telangiectatica in a patient with Adams–Oliver syndrome. Br J Dermatol 1992;127:160–3.
279 Paller AS, Massey RB, Curtis MA et al. Cutaneous granulomatous lesions in patients with ataxia-telangiectasia. J Pediatr 1991;119: 917–22.
280 Wollina U, Barta U, Uhlemann C, Oelzner P. Acquired nevoid telangiectasia. Dermatology 2001;203:24–6.
281 Clayton-Smith J, Kerr B, Brunner H et al. Macrocephaly with cutis marmorata, haemangioma and syndactyly – a distinctive overgrowth syndrome. Clin Dysmorphol 1997;6:291–302.
282 Yano S, Watanabe Y. Association of arrhythmia and sudden death in macrocephaly–cutis marmorata telangiectatica congenita syndrome. Am J Med Genet 2001;102:149–52.
283 Mazereeuw-Hautier J, Carel-Caneppele S, Bonafe JL. Cutis marmorata telangiectatica congenita: report of two persistent cases. Pediatr Dermatol 2002;19:506–9.
284 Iannuzzi CM, Atencio DP, Green S, et al. ATM mutations in female breast cancer patients predict for an increase in radiation-induced late effects. Int J Rad Oncol Biol Phys 2002;52:606–13.

CHAPTER 119

Infantile Haemangiomas

Anna L. Bruckner[1], *Ilona J. Frieden*[2] *& Julie Powell*[3]

[1] University of Colorado School of Medicine, and Division of Dermatology, Children's Hospital Colorado, Aurora, CO, USA
[2] Division of Pediatric Dermatology, San Francisco School of Medicine, University of California, San Francisco, CA, USA
[3] Division of Dermatology, Department of Pediatrics, CHU Sainte-Justine, University of Montreal, QC, Canada

Abstract

Infantile haemangiomas (IH) are the most frequent vascular tumours of infancy, affecting about 5% of infants during the first year of life. They are characterized by an early proliferative phase followed by a plateau and spontaneous gradual involution. Their pathogenesis is still not clearly understood but appears to be triggered by hypoxia caused by maternal and/or fetal events. Although resolution occurs in the majority of cases, morbidity includes potential life and function compromise, ulceration and scarring as well as permanent disfigurement. Segmental IH carry a higher risk of complications and poorer prognosis than focal lesions. PHACE and LUMBAR syndromes are associated with segmental IH. Early recognition of potential complications allows for timely intervention and better outcome. Oral beta-blockers have revolutionized the treatment of complicated IH with excellent efficacy and good safety profile. They have replaced oral corticosteroids as first-line treatment.

Key points

- **Infantile haemangiomas (IH) are the most common vascular tumour of infancy.**
- **The pathogenesis of IH is still poorly understood but hypoxia is likely a key factor.**
- **IH have a characteristic life cycle with early proliferation followed by gradual involution.**
- **The diagnosis of IH is usually clinical but Doppler sonography may be a good screening tool.**
- **Early recognition of potential complications is essential for timely therapy and optimal outcome.**
- **Segmental IH should prompt further investigation for associated anomalies (PHACE syndrome, LUMBAR syndrome).**
- **Segmental IH are more frequently complicated than focal IH and require early treatment.**
- **Beta-blockers are now first-line treatment for complicated IH, with high efficacy and a good safety profile.**

Introduction. Infantile haemangiomas (IH) are the most common benign tumours of infancy but precise diagnosis has long been confounded by the lack of standardized nomenclature and confusion with other types of vascular lesions. Mulliken and Glowacki [1] clarified our thinking about vascular birthmarks by proposing a classification system based on biological characteristics that was modified and accepted by the International Society for the Study of Vascular Anomalies (ISSVA) in 1996 and updated in 2014 [2]. Vascular anomalies can be classified as either vascular tumours (proliferative lesions) or malformations (structural anomalies representing morphogenetic errors of developing blood vessels and lymphatics) (see Table 119.1). This dichotomy is not absolutely exclusive, because uncommon examples of coexisting tumours and malformations have been reported [3], yet its simplicity and elegance allow for a more accurate diagnosis, predictable prognosis and rational choice of therapy in the vast majority of cases.

Infantile haemangiomas are unique neoplasms that proliferate in infancy and eventually involute spontaneously in childhood. They do not occur in older children or adults. The terms 'infantile haemangioma' or 'haemangioma of infancy' are typically limited to vascular tumours arising in the first few weeks of life that display a period of active growth, in the vast majority of cases, followed by a period of apparent inactivity and subsequent involution. The diagnosis is usually made clinically but when histological confirmation is needed, these tumours stain positively for the glucose transporter protein, GLUT1 [4]. For the sake of simplicity, the term 'haemangioma' in this chapter will refer to such lesions unless otherwise specified.

Epidemiology and pathogenesis. Infantile haemangiomas are identified in approximately 1–2.5% of newborns [5–8] and although an incidence of 10% in the first year of life has been typically quoted [8], a better estimate is 4–5% [9,10]. They are more common in White non-Hispanic infants [11] and females are more frequently affected than males, with a sex ratio ranging from 2:1 to 3:1. Infants with IH are more likely to be born prematurely, to be the product of multiple gestation and to have mothers older than 30 years [11]. Low birthweight (less than 2500 g) is an independent risk factor associated with IH [12]. Preterm infants are more likely than term infants to have multiple tumours and the sex ratio is less skewed toward females

Harper's Textbook of Pediatric Dermatology, Fourth Edition. Edited by Peter Hoeger, Veronica Kinsler and Albert Yan.

Table 119.1 Classification of vascular anomalies

Vascular tumours	Vascular malformations
Benign Infantile haemangioma Congenital haemangioma: Rapidly involuting (RICH), Partially involuting (PICH), Non-involuting (NICH) Tufted angioma Pyogenic granuloma	Simple, low-flow malformations: VM, LM, CM Simple, fast-flow malformations: AM, AVF, AVM
Locally aggressive Kaposiform haemangioendothelioma Other	**Complex–combined vascular malformations:** Low-flow: CVM, CLM, CLVM, LVM Fast-flow: CAVM, CLAVM

A, arterial; AVF, arteriovenous fistula; C, capillary; L, lymphatic; M, malformation; V, venous.

[13,14]. Contrary to prior observations, newer prospective studies do not support chorionic villus sampling as a major risk factor [12,13]. Although most haemangiomas occur sporadically, presumed autosomal dominant transmission of these tumours, with and without vascular malformations, has been documented in six kindreds [15]. Superficial haemangiomas are the most common subtype, constituting approximately 50–60% of cases, whereas deep haemangiomas constitute about 15% and combined superficial and deep lesions 25–35%.

The *pathogenesis* of haemangiomas is still not completely understood; there is not yet a unifying mechanism that accounts for all aspects of the haemangioma phenotype nor a known single event that leads to haemangioma development. However, the patterns found in segmental haemangiomas suggest that the stage for at least some haemangiomas is set as early as 4–6 weeks of gestation, via a developmental error [16]. IH only occur in humans, and adequate animal or laboratory models have been difficult to develop. Several recently published articles comprehensively review proposed theories regarding IH pathogenesis [17–20].

While previous work suggested that IH arise because of aberrations in angiogenesis, recent investigations show that IH are the result of dysregulation in both vasculogenesis and angiogenensis [21,22]. It is speculated that hypoxia is likely the triggering signal, leading to an increase in angiogenic factors such as vascular endothelial growth factor (VEGF) via the HIFα pathway. VEGF overexpression then leads CD133+ stem cells to proliferate and differentiate into endothelial progenitor cells [23].

Implantation into immunodeficient mice of CD133+ cells isolated from IH gives rise to GLUT1+ vessels that later diminish and are replaced by adipocytes [24]. While not a perfect replica of IH growth, this model merits attention and additional study.

The recognition that a glucose transporter protein, GLUT1, is expressed in all stages of haemangioma maturation helped spur hypotheses on the pathogenesis of IH [4]. GLUT1 expression is absent in normal cutaneous vasculature but is found in placental blood vessels as well as in other so-called barrier tissues such as the blood–brain barrier. This, together with other immunohistochemical markers shared by IH and human placenta (see Histopathology, later), led to speculation that these tumours are of placental origin from either embolized placental cells or invading angioblasts that have differentiated towards a placental phenotype [25]. IH are unlikely to be placental emboli because they lack a villous architecture and do not express known placental trophoblastic markers [26]. Furthermore, it was determined that haemangioma endothelial cells are of fetal, not maternal origin [27].

Histopathology. Biopsies of both superficial and deep haemangiomas reveal relatively uniform vessel morphology [28]. In the proliferative stage, haemangiomas comprise syncytial aggregates of plump endothelial cells and pericytes, some of which form lumina and others solid cords. As involution progresses, the endothelial cells flatten and the vascular channels become more ectatic, producing large, thin-walled vessels. Islands of fatty tissue and fibrous strands gradually replace the tumour cells, giving the lesion a lobular architecture. Fully involuted IH contain few capillary-like feeding vessels and draining veins with flattened endothelium in a stroma of fatty and fibrous tissue, collagen and reticulin fibres. GLUT1 is expressed throughout these phases.

In addition to endothelial cells, haemangiomas contain pericytes, fibroblasts, interstitial cells and mast cells. An abundance of mast cells has been reported in both proliferating and involuting tumours but the significance of this finding is unclear [29].

Not surprisingly, immunohistochemical studies show that haemangiomas express many of the same markers as mature endothelial cells, such as alkaline phosphatase, factor VIII antigen, CD31, von Willebrand factor and urokinase [29]. These cellular markers have also defined distinctions between IH and vascular malformations as well as differences in the varying stages of haemangioma evolution. In the phase of rapid growth, haemangioma endothelia express large amounts of proliferating cell nuclear antigen, type IV collagenase, VEGF and E-selectin [30,31]. In contrast, elevated expression of TIMP-1 is a specific marker for the involution phase [30]. Use of these markers in biopsy tissue could conceivably provide a means for staging haemangiomas.

Positive immunohistochemical staining for GLUT1 confirms the diagnosis of haemangioma and helps differentiate it from other vascular tumours such as tufted angioma, pyogenic granuloma and congenital haemangioma as well as vascular malformations [4]. In addition to GLUT1, haemangiomas also show intense immunoreactivity for the placenta-associated vascular antigens FcγRII, merosin and LeY [25].

Clinical features. Infantile haemangiomas show considerable variation in appearance depending on their size, anatomical location, depth and stage of evolution (Figs 119.1–119.3). Approximately one-third to one-half

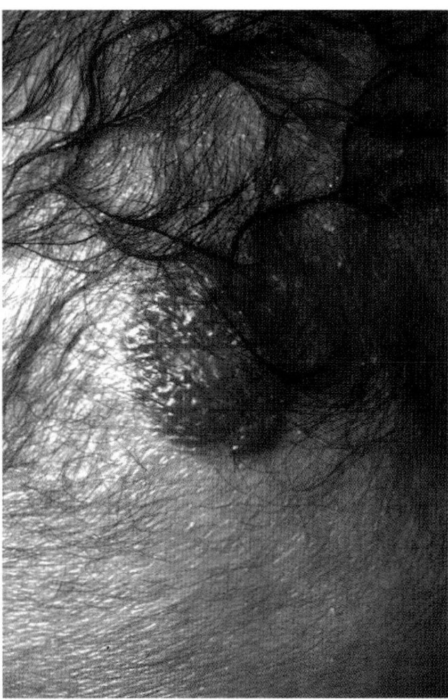

Fig. 119.1 Superficial haemangioma.

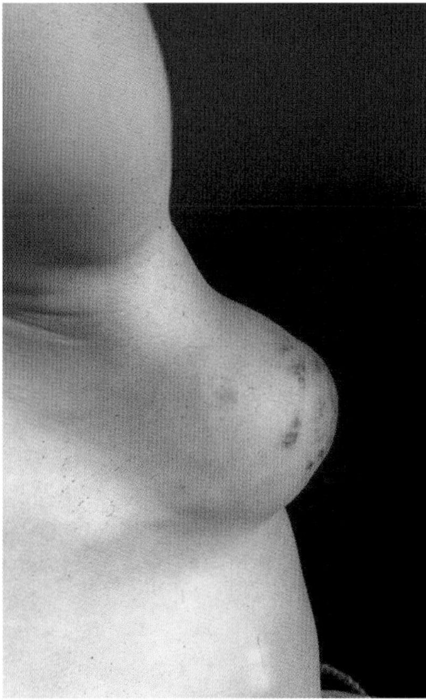

Fig. 119.2 Deep haemangioma.

are present at birth in some premonitory form and the remainder usually become evident during the first month of life. The precursor lesions often appear as a blanched macule, an erythematous or telangiectatic patch with or without a pale halo, a closely packed cluster of bright-red papules, or a blue-tinged bruise-like area (Fig. 119.4) [3,4]. Precursor lesions are sometimes confused with port-wine stains or a 'scratch' or 'bruise' attributed to perinatal or postnatal trauma.

Haemangiomas can be superficial, deep or mixed and all three types of lesions undergo the same natural history. Superficial haemangiomas (formerly called

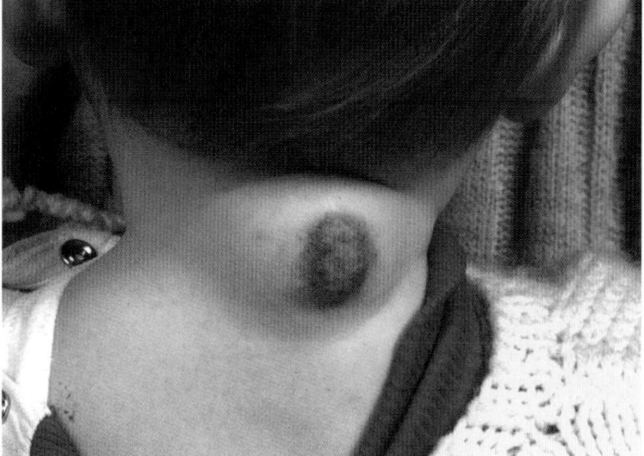

Fig. 119.3 Superficial and deep (mixed) haemangioma.

'capillary' or 'strawberry' haemangiomas) are vivid red or scarlet, sharply circumscribed plaques or nodules, whereas deep haemangiomas (formerly called 'cavernous') are skin-coloured or bluish purple and less well circumscribed. Mixed haemangiomas combine the features of both superficial and deep tumours. Focal lesions confined to a relatively small area of the body are 'localized' (Fig. 119.5), whereas larger, plaque-like tumours that are distributed in a developmental region or territory have been termed 'segmental' (Fig. 119.6) [32]. IH can also be defined by their stage of maturation and are referred to as nascent, proliferative, involuting or involuted.

Infantile haemangiomas are not randomly distributed. They show a clear predilection for the head and neck region with tumours at these sites constituting at least 50% of lesions in some series [33]. On the face, the midline and ocular axis are preferentially involved [34]. The majority of facial IH are focal tumours and a minority, so-called segmental haemangiomas, affect a broader, geographic region [32]. Four distinct segments that correspond to facial development units have been identified (Fig. 119.7) [16]. Segmental IH are more likely to be associated with complications and/or structural anomalies (see Associations, later) [32].

Virtually all IH undergo a proliferative phase followed by a period of stabilization and then gradual involution. IH tend to 'mark out' their area early on. Subsequent changes in size correlate with increases in volume, with 80% of proliferation being completed by 5 months of age [35,36]. A minority of haemangiomas, particularly those with segmental morphology, a deep component and often those affecting the parotid gland, may continue to enlarge slowly for months to years longer [37].

Signs of involution are clinically apparent in most IH at 1 year of age [35]. The first perceptible change is loss of the brilliant red colour, which is replaced by a more dull red colour in superficial haemangiomas. As this process continues, the colour becomes grey or milky-white, first centrally, then peripherally and as involution progresses the haemangioma begins to flatten and soften, gradually losing volume. Unfortunately, an exact timetable for regression of a particular lesion cannot be predicted but

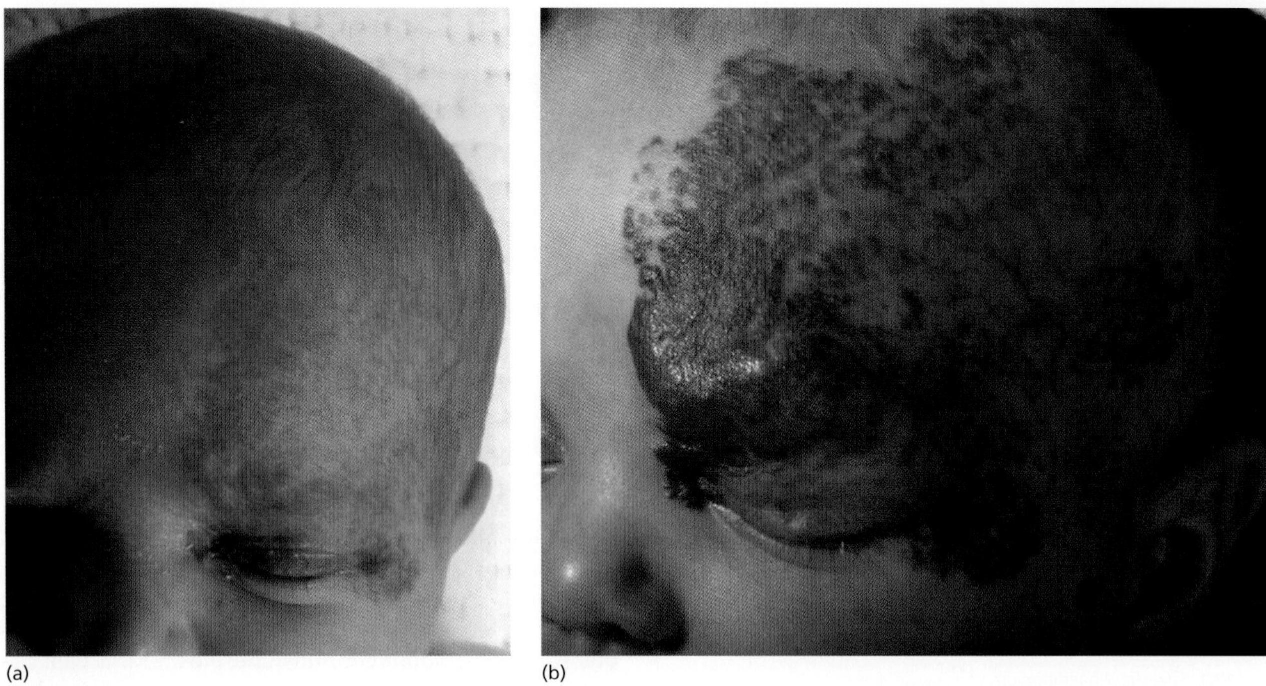

Fig. 119.4 (a) Large precursor lesion on the face, mimicking a port-wine stain. (b) Same lesion at one month of age.

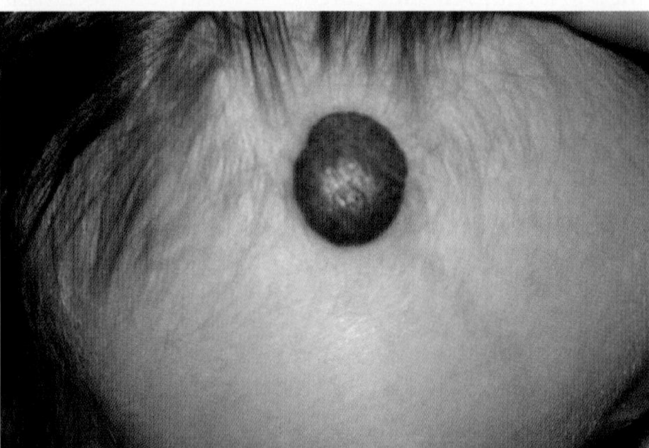

Fig. 119.5 Focal haemangioma on the forehead.

involution is typically slower than the proliferative phase. The time and rate of involution do not necessarily correlate with the sex of the child, or with the location, age of onset or type of haemangioma, but very small lesions do tend to complete involution sooner than very large ones.

Prognosis

Although the outcomes of haemangiomas are excellent in the majority of cases, the wide heterogeneity of the condition mandates that prognosis be assessed individually based on location, extent and any associated complications. All haemangiomas involute but usally at a slower rate than their growth. Approximately 50–60% will have completed involution by 5 years of age, 70–75% by 7 years of age and upwards of 90% by 9 years of age. However, involution does not correspond with complete disappearance of the lesion: precise figures regarding the percentage of children left with permanent skin changes from IH are lacking. These changes can be minor and trivial but in some patients they are severe and life-altering. Our best estimate is that at least 20% of children will have residual skin changes if untreated, including pallor, anetoderma, altered skin texture or overlying telangiectasia. IH may also destroy hair follicles, resulting in partial alopecia, but many lesions of the scalp resolve without this sequela. More significant changes, such as redundant skin and fibrofatty residuum, may occur if the tumour had a predominantly exophytic dermal component, especially if it

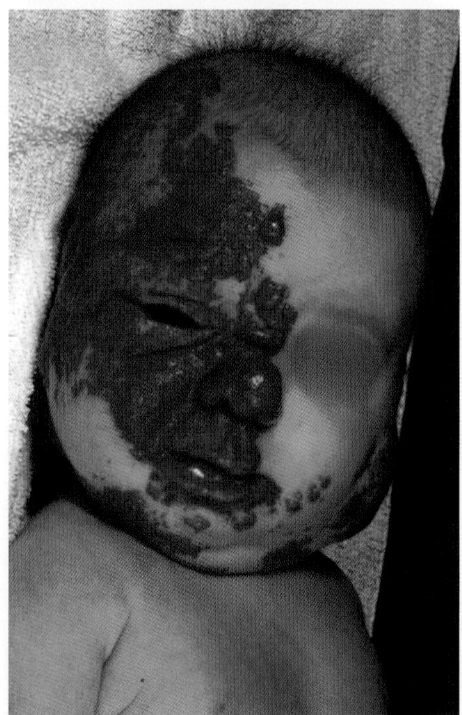

Fig. 119.6 Segmental facial haemangioma.

shows steep borders from the surrounding skin [38]. Ulceration resolves with variable scarring.

Complications. While the majority of IH are localized and pose no immediate or long-term threat, a significant minority develop complications. Haggstrom and colleagues [39] noted that 24% of patients with IH referred to tertiary paediatric dermatology centres had complications.

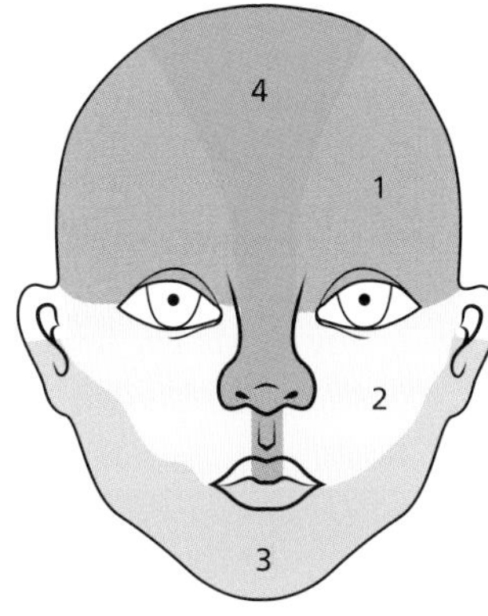

Fig. 119.7 Facial segments of infantile haemangioma. Source: Haggstrom et al. (2006) [16]. Copyright© 2006 by the AAP. Reproduced with permission of the American Academy of Pediatrics.

Large size, segmental morphology and facial and perineal location are associated with an increased likelihood of complications [39]. Early recognition of potentially problematic lesions, coupled with prompt intervention, is essential to minimize future problems.

Ulceration is the most common complication, occurring in approximately 15% of haemangiomas [40] (Figs 119.8–119.10). Characteristics associated with ulceration are large size, segmental morphology, superficial or mixed subtype and location on the lower lip, neck, or perineal area [40–42]. Ulceration typically occurs during rapid proliferation, with a median age of 4 months, and infants with ulcerated IH are likely to be referred to a specialist at a younger age [41]. Ulceration can cause considerable pain, particularly when the lips, genitalia, perirectal area or flexures are involved. It results in scar formation, causing variable disfigurement and, in some locations, functional impairment. Intervention is indicated to control pain, hasten re-epithelialization and prevent infection, No single treatment modality is uniformly effective and usually several modalities need to be used concurrently [43], making evaluation of each individual approach difficult. Treatment options include local wound care, barrier creams or occlusive dressings, topical or systemic antibiotics if infection is present, pulsed dye laser (PDL)

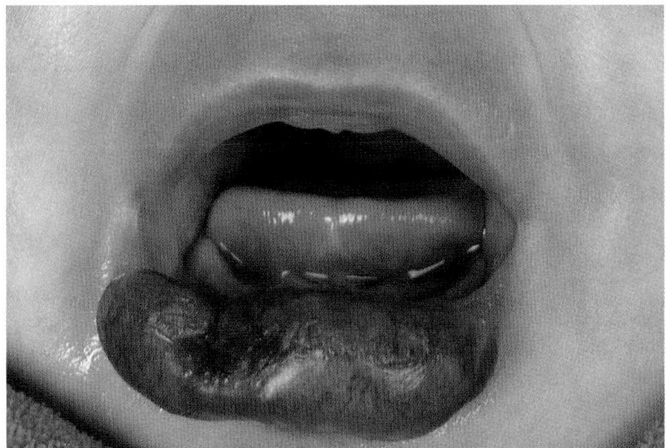

Fig. 119.8 Ulcerated haemangioma of the lower lip, a frequent site.

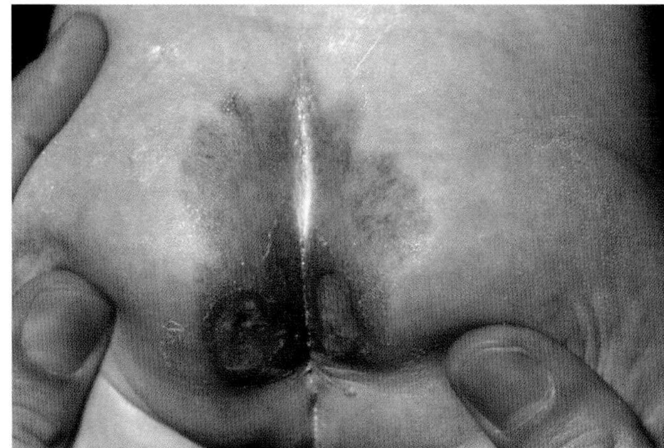

Fig. 119.10 Ulcerated segmental lumbosacral haemangioma.

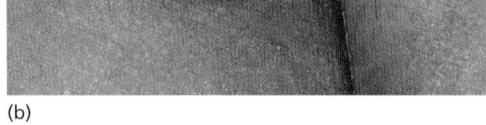

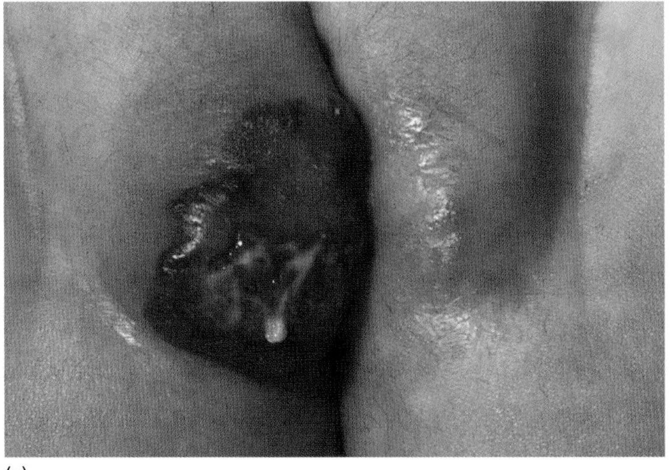

(a)

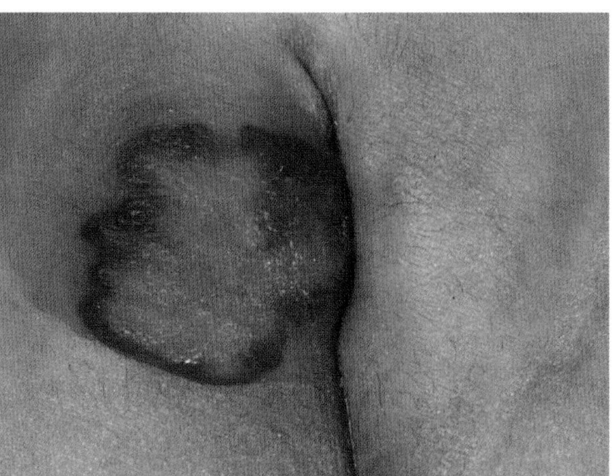

(b)

Fig. 119.9 (a) Ulcerated haemangioma on the buttock. (b) Residual scar after healing.

[44,45], and pain relief [46]. Recent studies have shown oral propranolol appears very promising in this setting [47,48]. Although topical timolol has been used successfully for ulcerated IHs [49], caution is advised because of increased absorption and the risk of toxicity. Rarely, surgical excision can be considered for refractory cases.

With rare exceptions, bleeding from an eroded or traumatized haemangioma in the absence of a coagulopathy is usually insignificant and responds to direct pressure. In the event of uncontrolled or persistent bleeding, the infant should be taken to an emergency room for haematological evaluation and additional therapeutic measures.

Ophthalmological complications occur in up to 80% of patients with untreated periocular haemangiomas (Fig. 119.11) [50–52]. The most common complication is anisometropia which can occur because of obstruction of the visual axis (caused by ptosis or mass effect), compression or displacement of the globe leading to asymmetrical refractive errors, or caused by strabismus. Abnormal visual input during the critical period when normal vision is required for visual development can result in permanent amblyopia. Periocular IH smaller than 1 cm in size are less likely to cause complications. Tumour location also seems to be an important predictor of amblyopia, with lesions affecting the nasal third of the eyelid associated with the highest risk. Other less common complications of periocular IH include proptosis and exophthalmos which are signs of deeper orbital involvement. Orbital involvement can cause compression of the optic nerve in rare cases. It is mandatory that patients with periocular haemangiomas undergo an ophthalmological assessment early in their course and periodically thereafter in order to detect and treat visual impairment.

Sequelae from *airway haemangiomas* are among the most alarming of all potential complications. Sites of involvement include both supra- and subglottic mucosa but subglottic location is most associated with airway compromise. Infants with subglottic disease typically present at between 6 and 12 weeks of age with noisy breathing, hoarse cry, inspiratory or biphasic stridor and, if severe, cyanosis [53,54]. Approximately 50% of these infants have IH elsewhere on the body, with the segmental mandibular and neck ('beard') area being strongly associated with symptomatic airway disease (Fig. 119.12) [53]. The airway haemangiomas themselves are most often segmental but can be more focal [54]. Definitive diagnosis is made by direct laryngoscopy. Treatment modalities have ranged from corticosteroids (intralesional or systemic) to laser ablation and surgical excision [55] but propranolol has dramatically changed the outcome of these patients [56–58]. The need for tracheostomy is nowadays just about nonexistent in these infants. Extrinsic compression from very large, bulky cervicofacial haemangiomas can rarely result in feeding difficulties or sleep apnoea.

Cardiac failure is a rare complication most often associated with hepatic haemangiomas (see Hepatic haemangiomas, see later) and occasionally with very large haemangiomas at other sites [59].

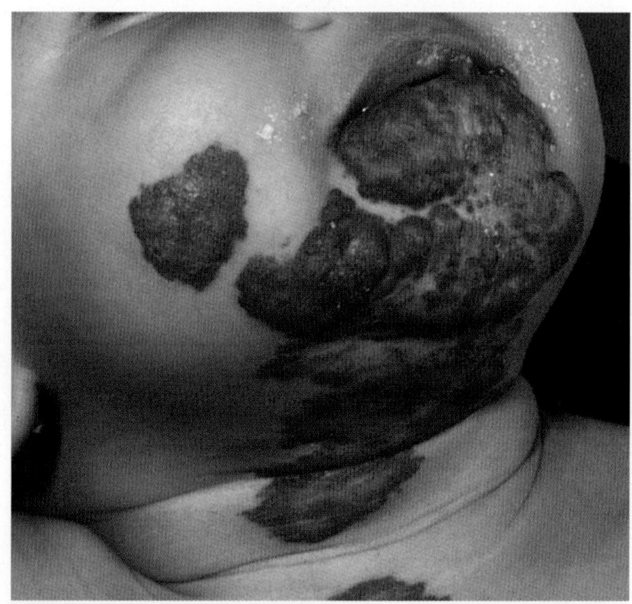

Fig. 119.12 Segmental haemangioma of the 'beard area' at high risk of airway involvement.

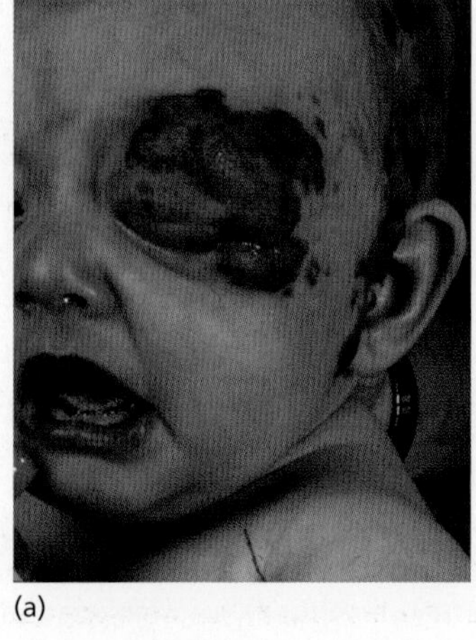

(a)

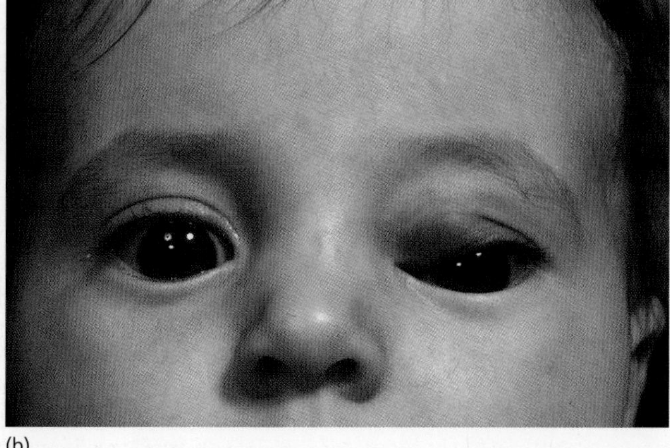

(b)

Fig. 119.11 (a) Periocular haemangioma requiring urgent ophthalmological evaluation and treatment. (b) Deep periocular haemangioma located nasally. Although nonobstructive, this haemangioma can also cause permanent amblyopia if untreated.

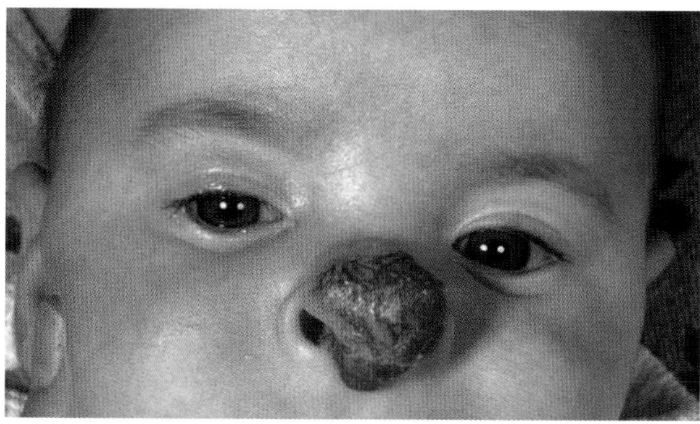

Fig. 119.13 Typical Cyrano nose, a haemangioma of the nasal tip.

Disfigurement, particularly from extensive and rapidly expanding IH of the head and neck, can be a serious problem and is an important reason for intervention. Certain locations are particularly prone to leaving permanent skin changes that can be problematic, particularly from a psychosocial standpoint [60,61]. Central face involvement is more problematic than the lateral face. Haemangiomas of the nasal tip (Cyrano nose, Fig. 119.13) are a case in point as they can significantly distort the nasal contour, causing permanent nasal deformity as well as tremendous distress and embarrassment to the child and family. The lips are another central facial site where even relatively small haemangiomas can leave permanent scarring. Large IH of the breast area in girls are also of concern. Early intervention with systemic agents, intralesional steroids or surgery may help to minimize disfigurement and psychosocial distress [62].

Differential diagnosis. Although numerous conditions can mimic haemangiomas [63–65], the diagnosis is usually made easily on the basis of the history and clinical findings. In a minority of cases, however, the true nature of the lesion may be in question and arriving at the correct diagnosis is critical, particularly when complications arise or if surgery is contemplated.

Haemangiomas may be mistaken for other types of birthmarks or neoplasms, depending on their stage of development. Nascent lesions may be confused with naevus anaemicus or naevus depigmentosus, capillary malformations or traumatic injury (a scratch or bruise). Superficial haemangiomas may resemble other vascular tumours such as pyogenic granulomas, congenital haemangiomas, tufted angiomas, kaposiform haemangioendotheliomas or haemangiopericytomas. Deeper tumours may mimic dermoid cysts, nasal gliomas, infantile myofibromatosis, lipomas, plexiform neurofibromas, neuroblastomas or other soft tissue sarcomas. Perhaps the greatest difficulty lies in the distinction from vascular malformations (either venous or lymphatic).

The correct diagnosis relies upon the typical natural history of the condition, particularly absence at birth or a premonitory mark followed by a period of rapid growth during the first month of life. IH are rarely present at birth as a fully formed soft tissue mass. They typically complete growth by 1 year of age, although there are some exceptions. The appearance of vascularity, particularly telangiectasias, should not be assumed to be definitive for IH because many rapidly expanding tumours, such as rhabdomyosarcoma, may also have overlying telangiectasias. Similarly, the imaging findings of high vascular flow should not be considered diagnostic, but the specific characteristics of IH have been well described in the radiology literature (see discussion later). Multifocal vascular appearing lesions are often assumed to represent IH and the term 'disseminated neonatal hemangiomatosis' has been applied to this clinical scenario, particularly when visceral involvement is present. However, a number of other conditions including multifocal lymphangioendotheliomatosis and pyogenic granuloma-like growths can resemble multiple haemangiomas. Biopsy of these lesions for analysis with GLUT1 staining may be needed to help differentiate these conditions from multifocal IH [63].

Imaging studies

Radiological evaluation can be helpful in confirming the diagnosis of haemangioma as well as delineating the extent of disease or associated structural anomalies (as in the case of PHACE syndrome). Doppler sonography has the advantage of being accessible, minimally invasive and inexpensive, making it a good screening modality to help differentiate IH from malformations or other tumours. The combination of high vessel density and high peak arterial Doppler shifts is a specific finding for proliferating IH [66]. Unfortunately, the value of this examination can be dependent on the experience of the radiologist and the extent of the tumour is not well defined. Ultrasonography is also valuable as a screening modality for liver haemangiomas. Computed tomography (CT) or magnetic resonance imaging (MRI) scans better delineate the extent of lesions and MRI with gadolinium enhancement is regarded as the best single technique to evaluate vascular anomalies [67–69]. CT scans and MRI show haemangiomas as well-circumscribed, lobulated masses with feeding and draining vessels at the centre and periphery and, on MRI, flow voids are observed on spin-echo images and enhancement with gadolinium is diffuse [67,68]. Angiography is rarely required for diagnostic purposes but is useful in the differentiation of arteriovenous malformation from IH or if embolization is contemplated for symptomatic high-flow lesions. On angiograms, haemangiomas appear as well-circumscribed masses with intense persistent tissue staining, a well-organized lobular pattern and a recognizable pattern of feeder vessels and draining veins [69]. Radiological studies should not be viewed as a substitute for a diagnostic biopsy, particularly in cases where a malignant tumour is a possible diagnosis. MR angiography (MRA) is needed to evaluate patients at risk for PHACE syndrome adequately (see discussion later).

Associations

The vascular lesions of several malformation syndromes have been mistakenly categorized as haemangiomas [70]. Although vascular malformations are more likely to be associated with structural anomalies, true IH are rarely the cardinal feature of genetic syndromes, except those described below.

PHACE syndrome

In 1996, Frieden and colleagues [71] reviewed 41 published cases of facial haemangiomas with associated anomalies such as coarctation of the aorta, midline ventral defects and central nervous system abnormalities and proposed the acronym PHACE (Posterior fossa malformations, Haemangioma, Arterial anomalies, Coarctation of the aorta and cardiac defects, Eye abnormalities, Sternal defects) (OMIM #606519) to unify the varying features of this syndrome (Fig. 119.14). Nearly 90% of affected infants are female, a much higher prevalence than the 2:1 to 5:1 ratio reported for common haemangiomas [71,72]. Consensus criteria for diagnosis have been proposed [73] and recently updated [74] (see Table 119.2).

A large segmental haemangioma, usually on the face, is the hallmark of the syndrome. In a prospective study of 108 infants with a large facial haemangioma, 31% were found to have PHACE syndrome [75]. Cerebrovascular anomalies are the most common extracutaneous manifestation, affecting mainly major arteries of the head and neck and include dysplasia, narrowing, aberrant course and persistence of fetal vasculature [76]. The arteriopathy is usually ipsilateral to the haemangioma. Structural brain anomalies include unilateral cerebellar hypoplasia, Dandy–Walker malformation or variants and less commonly cortical developmental anomalies. Neurological defects such as seizure disorder and developmental delay (language and gross motor especially) can be associated with these central nervous system abnormalities [77–79]. Acute ischaemic stroke may occur in the context of aplasia, hypoplasia, or occlusion of a major cerebral artery, especially when more than one vessel is involved or if there is coarctation of the aorta [79]. The most common cardiac anomalies are coarctation of the aorta and aberrant subclavian artery [80]. Eye anomalies include 'morning-glory' disc anomaly, persistent fetal vasculature, peripapillary staphyloma, microphthalmia and optic nerve hypoplasia, increased vascularity, microphthalmia and congenital cataracts [74,81]. Ventral developmental defects include sternal clefting and supraumbilical raphe. Hearing loss [82] and dental anomalies [83] have recently been described.

PHACE syndrome is uncommon but not rare and it is at least as common – if not more common – than Sturge–Weber syndrome from which it needs to be differentiated. Up to one-third of patients with large facial haemangiomas will be found to have PHACE syndrome when studied thoroughly. Those with haemangiomas affecting the frontotemporal or mandibular regions or affecting multiple facial segments are most likely to be affected [72]. At-risk patients should be examined thoroughly for signs and symptoms of PHACE syndrome and if possible, evaluation should include careful cardiac evaluation with echocardiogram, MRI/MRA imaging of the brain and neck and aortic arch, ophthalmological evaluation, serum thyroid studies and careful periodic developmental and neurological assessments as well as hearing screening and early dental examination [74]. Patients with PHACE syndrome may also have brain haemangiomas but these rarely seem to cause symptoms and limited data suggest that they, like their cutaneous counterparts, involute spontaneously [84]. Airway haemangiomas also occur with some frequency especially in association with IH in the mandibular and neck area ('beard IH'). Endocrine abnormalities such as hypothyroidism and pituitary abnormalities resulting in growth hormone deficiency are occasionally found [84,85].

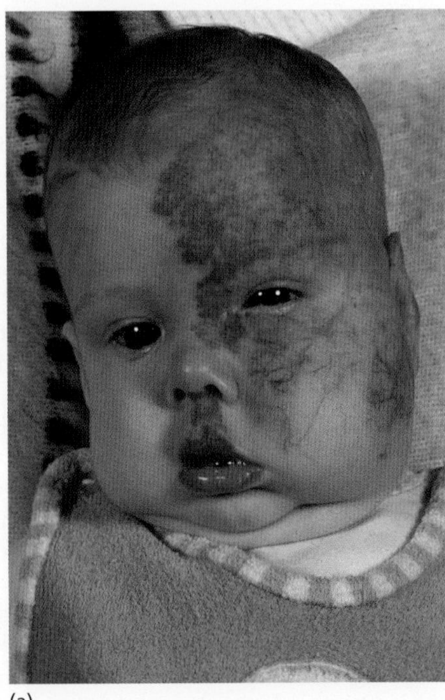
(a)

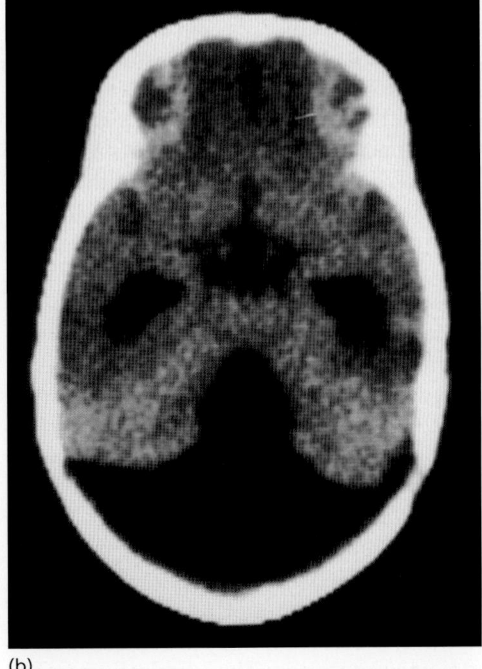
(b)

Fig. 119.14 (a) PHACE syndrome. This infant had a large segmental reticulated facial haemangima associated with Dandy–Walker anomaly (b).

SECTION 25: VASCULAR TUMOURS

Table 119.2 Diagnostic criteria (revised): PHACE syndrome

Definite PHACE		
Haemangioma >5 cm in diameter of the head including scalp	Haemangioma of the neck, upper trunk or trunk and proximal upper extremity PLUS 2 major criteria	
PLUS 1 major criterion OR 2 minor criteria		
Possible PHACE		
Haemangioma >5 cm in diameter of the head including scalp PLUS	Haemangioma of the neck, upper trunk or trunk and proximal upper extremity PLUS	No haemangioma PLUS
1 minor criterion	1 major criterion OR 2 minor criteria	2 major criteria
Organ system	**Major criteria**	**Minor criteria**
Arterial anomalies	Anomaly of major cerebral or cervical arteries[a] Dysplasia[b] of the large cerebral arteries Arterial stenosis or occlusion with or without moyamoya collaterals Absence or moderate to severe hypoplasia of the large cerebral and cervical arteries Aberrant origin or course of the large cerebral or cervical arteries except common arch variants such as bovine arch Persistent carotid–vertebrobasilar anastomosis (proatlantal segmental, hypoglossal, otic, and/or trigeminal arteries)	Aneurysm of any of the cerebral arteries
Structural brain	Posterior fossa brain anomalies Dandy–Walker complex or unilateral/bilateral Other hypoplasia/dysplasia of the mid and/or hind brain	Midline brain anomalies Malformation of cortical development
Cardiovascular	Aortic arch anomalies Coarctation of aorta Dysplasia[a] Aneurysm Aberrant origin of the subclavian artery with or without a vascular ring	Ventricular septal defect Right aortic arch /double aortic arch Systemic venous anomalies
Ocular	Posterior segment abnormality. Persistent fetal vasculature. Persistent hyperplastic primary vitreous. Retinal vascular anomalies. Morning-glory disc anomaly. Optic nerve hypoplasia. Peripapillary staphyloma	Anterior segment abnormalities Microphthalmia Sclerocornea Coloboma Cataracts
Ventral/midline	Anomaly of the midline chest and abdomen -Sternal defect -Sternal pit -Sternal cleft -Supraumbilical raphe	Hypopituitarism Ectopic thyroid Midline sternal papule/ hamartoma

[a] Internal carotid artery, middle cerebral artery, anterior cerebral artery, posterior cerebral artery or vertebrobasilar system.
[b] Includes kinking, looping, tortuosity and/or dolichoectasia.
Source: Garzon et al. (2016) [75]. Reproduced with permission of Elsevier.

The origin of PHACE syndrome is not known but evidence points to abnormalities in neuroectodermal or arterial vascular development that occur early in gestation, possibly between 4 and 8 weeks, as being the likely primary event, leading to downstream effects on brain development and other target organs [86].

Lower body haemangiomas and structural malformations (PELVIS/SACRAL/LUMBAR syndrome)

A second constellation of structural malformations is associated with haemangiomas overlying the lumbosacral spine or a segmental haemangioma of the lower extremity and may be viewed as the lower-body equivalent of PHACE syndrome (Figs 119.15 and 119.16). Several acronyms have been proposed: PELVIS syndrome (Perineal haemangioma, External genitalia malformations, Lipomyelomeningocoele, Vesicorenal abnormalities, Imperforate anus and Skin tag) [87]; SACRAL syndrome (Spinal dysraphism, Anogenital anomalies, Cutaneous anomalies, Renal and urological anomalies, associated with Angioma of Lumbosacral localization) [88]: and finally LUMBAR syndrome (Lower body haemangioma, Urogenital anomalies/Ulceration, Myelopathy, Bony deformities, Anorectal malformations/Arterial anomalies, and Renal anomalies) [89]. The most common of these anomalies is tethered spinal cord, often accompanied by an occult lipomeningocoele but as noted, genitourinary and other anomalies can also be found. These include imperforate anus, abnormal external genitalia and renal anomalies. At-risk patients typically have

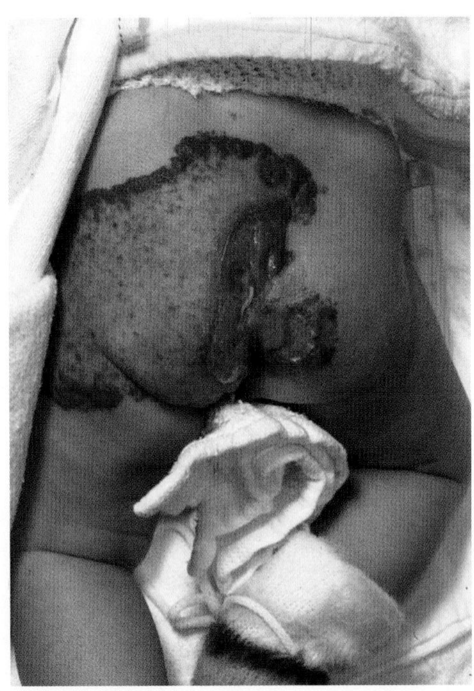

Fig. 119.15 LUMBAR syndrome. Infant with segmental lumbosacral haemangioma, imperforate anus and severe ulceration.

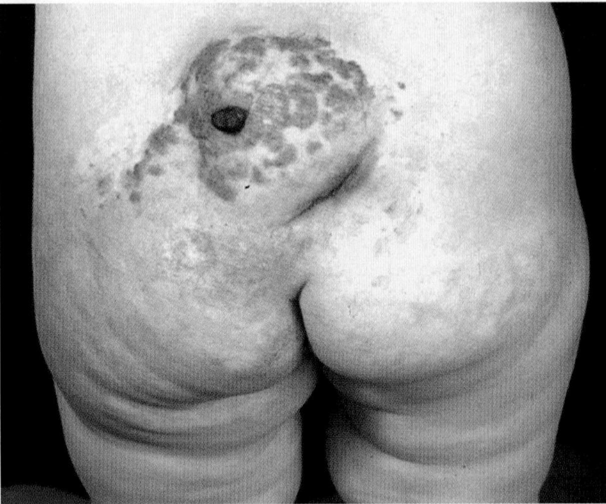

Fig. 119.16 LUMBAR syndrome. Lumbosacral mixed haemangioma associated with a cutaneous tag, extension into spinal canal and tethered cord.

large, plaque-like haemangiomas but the haemangioma may be nearly flat, with prominent ulceration and a reticular quality, as the most notable finding (Fig. 119.15) [39]. Infants with a haemangioma overlying the lumbosacral area or with a perianal haemangioma extending into the gluteal cleft should have MRI performed to evaluate for possible tethered spinal cord and occult spinal dysraphism. Other evaluations should be considered based on clinical findings [87–89].

Multifocal infantile haemangiomas

Multifocal haemangiomas may either be noted at birth or develop shortly thereafter [90], ranging from several to hundreds. They may vary in size from a few millimetres to centimetres in size but tend to be smaller, well localized and usually superficial in nature, appearing as dome-shaped, red papules or nodules (Fig. 119.17). The histological features of these tumours are identical to those of solitary haemangiomas and they may regress spontaneously as early as the first year of life and often involute completely by 2 years of age. Multiple cutaneous IH (arbitrarily established as five or more), are a potential marker for hepatic involvement [90] and an abdominal ultrasound is indicated. Although present in up to 16% of infants with more than five IH, the hepatic lesions usually are asymptomatic but can cause serious complications such as cardiac failure. A recent study showed that routine hepatic screening in infants with more than five cutaneous IH improved clinical outcomes, with a younger age of diagnosis and lower incidence of congestive heart failure, hypothyroidism and mortality than in those that were not screened [91]. Additional studies are not usually necessary if the clinical history and thorough physical examination are normal. Liver disease, if present, can range from completely asymptomatic (the most common outcome) to truly life-threatening [91]. Those that do become symptomatic usually do so within the first weeks to months of life. The classic triad for hepatic haemangiomatosis consists of hepatomegaly, varying numbers of cutaneous haemangiomas and high-output cardiac failure. Hepatic haemangiomas are classified as focal (27% cases), multifocal (57%) or diffuse (16%) [92,93]. The solitary localized form usually represents a rapidly involuting congenital haemangioma (RICH) and the multifocal or diffuse forms classic GLUT1 positive IH. Hypothyroidism

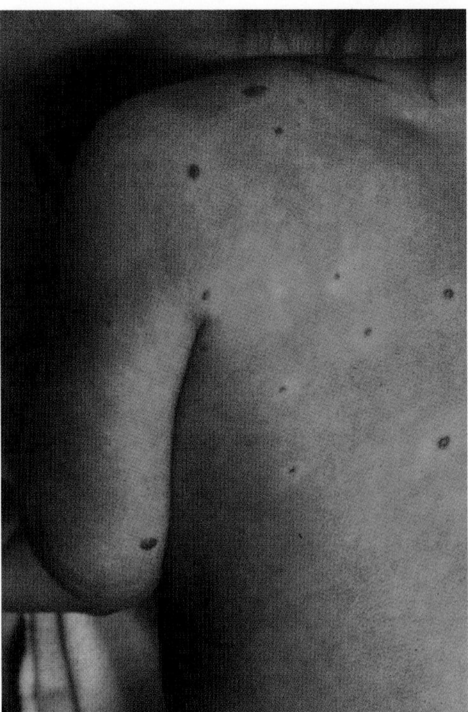

Fig. 119.17 Multifocal haemangiomatosis. This infant had hepatic involvement and high-output heart failure requiring aggressive systemic treatment and embolization (pre-propranolol era).

is a complication found mainly with diffuse or multifocal hepatic haemangiomas and is caused by increased iodothyronine deionidase [94]. Propranolol is now the most commonly used therapy for complicated hepatic IH [95,96].

Treatment. The approach to treatment of IH needs to be individualized as the spectrum of severity is very wide, making a 'one size fits all' approach difficult. In recent years, a better understanding of the growth features of IH, predictors of sequelae [97,98] and more effective and safe treatment options have somewhat changed our approach.

Most IH are small and tend to regress spontaneously without need for intervention. It is estimated that about 10% of IHs can cause complications and require treatment [97,99]. The major goals of management are: (i) preventing or reversing life- or function-threatening complications; (ii) preventing permanent disfigurement; (iii) minimizing psychosocial stress for the patient and family; (iv) avoiding aggressive and potentially scarring procedures; and (v) preventing or adequately treating ulceration to minimize scarring, infection and pain [100].

Infantile haemangiomas that are likely to require treatment are listed in Table 119.3. Clearly, those that are life or function threatening (see Complications, previously) need to be treated. Aptly named 'alarming haemangiomas', these tumours potentially represent approximately 10–20% of IH seen in referral centres [101]. Their rapid growth within the first weeks to months of infancy necessitates treatment with the goal of arresting growth, possibly hastening involution and preventing or minimizing further complications. Timely intervention early in the proliferative phase is crucial for optimal outcome. The decision of whether or not to treat less threatening IH can be more difficult. Factors such as the location, size and growth phase of the tumour need to be considered. The scarring produced by a large facial haemangioma, for instance, is more likely to result in visible disfigurement than a similar lesion on the torso. The child's cognitive and developmental status, especially in relation to social pressures, must also be considered. As a significant minority of school-aged children can have some residual tumour present, re-evaluation and discussion with the parents and child regarding treatment options should be undertaken prior to school entry.

Table 119.3 Haemangiomas likely to require treatment and their potential complications

Type of haemangioma	Potential complication
Subglottic (airway) with or without skin involvement	Airway occlusion
Ocular or periocular	Amblyopia
Large or multiple hepatic lesions	High-output cardiac failure
Diffuse hepatic	Abdominal compartment syndrome, hypothyroidism, cardiac failure
Large facial, perioral, perineal	Ulceration with subsequent scarring
Nasal, ear, lip, central face	Distortion of normal anatomy with disfigurement

Active non-intervention

As many IH are benign and self-limited, choosing not to treat can be the best approach. In such cases, 'active non-intervention' (also termed 'watchful waiting') rather than 'benign neglect' should be practised [97]. The anxiety associated with accepting the haemangioma, coping with an intrusive public and attaining perspective about the overall diagnosis can be great [61] and parents must be reassured that this choice is in the best interests of the child and will ultimately lead to the most satisfactory outcome. A proactive approach on the part of the physician may help to alleviate many of these anxieties. At the initial visit, the natural history of the tumour and a general sense of prognosis should be given. Photographs demonstrating the natural involution of IH can be helpful, as long as they are representative of the infant in question. The pros and cons of various treatment options should also be discussed. Visits at regular intervals to obtain measurements of the lesions as well as photographic documentation are also recommended. Often the changes associated with regression evolve slowly and the progress made over a fixed period of time is not easily appreciated without photographs. Simply asking the parents how they are coping with their child's haemangioma may also be comforting to families.

Propranolol

In 2008, Léauté-Labrèze and colleagues reported on the serendipitous discovery that propranolol appears to cause cessation of growth and shrinkage of IH [102]. The initial series of 11 infants was followed by a subsequent publication which included 32 patients given 2–3 mg/kg/day in two or three divided doses [103]. Since then, propranolol has rapidly become first-line treatment for complicated IHs, replacing oral corticosteroids (Fig. 119.18). Several randomized controlled trials [104–106] have confirmed the efficacy of propranolol at doses of 2–3 mg/kg/day for 6 months with complete or nearly complete regression in 60% of cases. In a recent meta-analysis of 1264 cases [107], the response rate of propranolol at a mean dose of 2.1 mg/kg/day was 98%. Observed side-effects are reversible and usually mild including sleep alteration (11%), acrocyanosis (5%), gastrointestinal symptoms (3%), asymptomatic transient hypotension, bronchospasm or bronchiolitis. More severe but rare occurrences of hypoglycaemia, bradycardia and symptomatic hypotension have been reported [107,108]. It is important to educate parents to temporarily discontinue treatment if the child is not feeding properly or has symptoms of bronchiolitis. Because propranolol is lipophilic and capable of crossing the blood–brain barrier, theoretical concerns have been raised regarding potential neurodevelopmental or cognitive, specifically memory, side-effects [109]. While some recent studies appear reassuring in that respect [110–112] others raise concerns about a (transient) gross motor delay [113]. Rebound growth can occur in up to 15–25% of cases at discontinuation of treatment [114,115]. Propranolol initation and treatment guidelines have been published by both European and American expert groups [99,116] but these recommendations are likely to evolve as more experience is reported. Propranolol

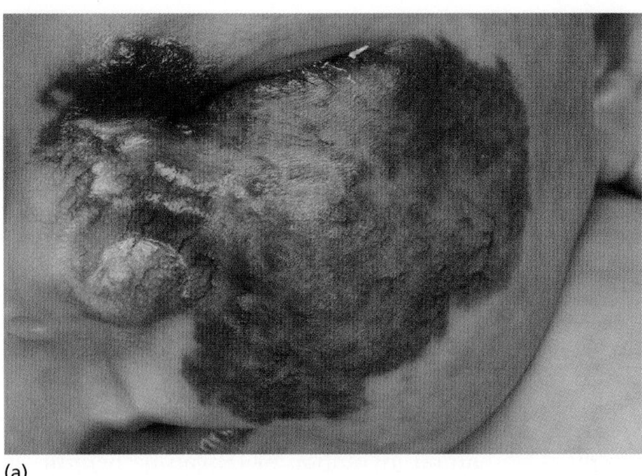
(a)

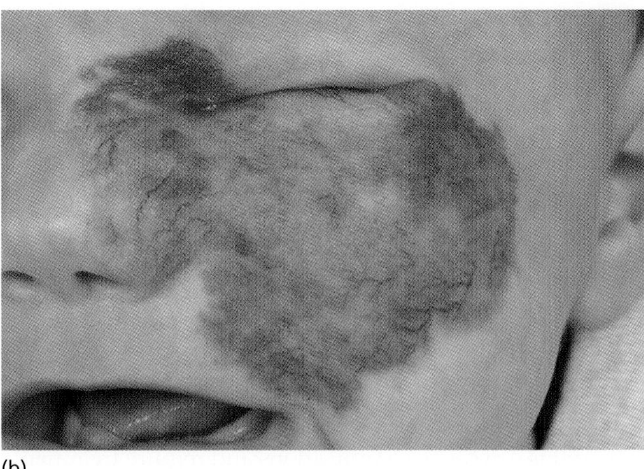
(b)

Fig. 119.18 Propranolol treatment. (a) Three-week-old infant with segmental proliferating haemangioma of the maxillary area. (b) After 1 month of propranolol, the lesion has flattened out.

is not absolutely contraindicated in PHACE syndrome but caution is warranted, especially if significant cerebral arterial anomalies and aortic coarctation are present [117].

Other beta blockers

Nadolol [118,119] and atenolol [120] have also been shown to be effective for the treatment of IH in several small studies. Because they are hydrophilic and do not cross the blood–brain barrier, they could theoretically be at lower risk of central nervous system adverse effects such as sleep disturbance and concerns for memory loss. Atenolol, a selective beta$_1$-blocker, is a good choice if respiratory side-effects are of concern.

Corticosteroids

Systemic corticosteroids were the gold-standard treatment for problematic IH for over 40 years [121] but have now been replaced by oral propranolol. They may still occasionally be considered in cases where propranolol is not well tolerated or ineffective. Prednisone or prednisolone, 2–3 mg/kg/day, is usually given as a single morning dose. Side-effects include irritability, insomnia, hypertension, gastrointestinal reflux, transient growth retardation, cushinoid facies and adrenal suppression. Compared with propranolol, prednisone has been shown in several studies to be less effective, with a slower onset of response and a higher rate of side-effects [122–124].

In an effort to avoid the side-effects associated with systemic corticosteroids, intralesional corticosteroids have been used to treat localized haemangiomas [125]. Commonly, triamcinolone 10 mg/mL at doses not exceeding 3 mg/kg per session is used and can be repeated at 4–8-week intervals if needed. This can be quite useful for growing localized haemangiomas of the lip and nasal tip. Caution should be used in the periocular region because of the risk of retinal arterial embolization causing blindness [126].

Other systemic therapies

Prior to the advent of propranolol, interferon-alpha and vincristine were occasionally used in severe corticosteroid-refractory IH. These have now been generally abandoned for IH because of their serious side-effects (spastic diplegia, peripheral neuropathy) and the high efficacy of propranolol.

Topical therapies

Given the success of propranolol in treating IH, *topical beta-blockers* have also been tried in clinical practice. Several recent studies [127,128] have shown that topical timolol 0.5% applied twice daily is useful in treating small, superficial, proliferating IH thus allowing avoidance of systemic treatment. Good indications for this treatment include small facial, eyelid and genital lesions. Little data is available on its absorption through the skin and caution should be used in treating ulcerated, mucosal or large lesions because of potential toxicity [129]. In the absence of randomized controlled studies, there is currently insufficient information regarding safety and comparative efficacy of topical timolol maleate for this indication [130].

Because of its antiangiogenic effects, *topical imiquimod* has been tried as a treatment for superficial IH [131]. Despite a recent report of equivalent efficacy to timolol gel [132], it unfortunately carries a high risk of skin irritation and potential ulceration, limiting its use.

The superpotent *topical corticosteroid* clobetasol propionate is another reasonable option for treatment of relatively flat superficial haemangiomas located in worrisome areas [133]. Risks include steroid atrophy, rosacea and systemic absorption.

Laser therapy

The use of lasers to treat haemangiomas is best divided into three separate indications: treatment of the proliferative phase, treatment of ulcerations and treatment of residual telangiectasias after involution has occurred.

PDL is an accepted treatment of haemangioma ulceration [134,135]. It is also widely accepted as a treatment for the residual erythema or telangiectasias that may remain after involution. Its role in treating proliferating haemangiomas is more controversial [136,137]. A subset of thin, superficial lesions may respond to laser treatments but because the depth of penetration of the PDL is only 1.2 mm, thicker tumours are not effectively treated, because the deeper component is not affected and may actually continue to proliferate. Moreover, the risk of scarring appears to be greater than that found in treating infants with port-wine stains. In addition, although uncommon, PDL therapy can result in persistent atrophic scarring or significant ulceration that heals with scarring [138]. Combining early PDL with oral propranolol [139] is advocated by some to achieve more rapid clearance. Combination of topical timolol and PDL is less convincing [140]. Fractional CO_2 laser resurfacing can be helpful in treating residual textural changes [137].

Surgery

In early infancy, excisional surgery may be considered for localized or pedunculated lesions that are virtually certain to resolve with permanent skin changes. Persistent bleeding or ulceration is another indication for surgery, if the lesion can be readily excised. Haemangiomas of the eyelid that do not respond to medical management could also be debulked or excised to minimize potential complications to the developing eye if medical treatment fails. Helpful guidelines for considering excision in early childhood include those where it appears that resection will be inevitable, if the scar will be the same whether performed as an infant or postponed, or if the scar can be easily hidden.

As children approach school age, the presence of a visible lesion may provoke teasing and embarrassment, leading to decreased self-esteem. It is appropriate to reconsider surgical or laser treatment of haemangioma residua or resultant skin changes at this age, with a goal of attaining as normal an appearance as possible. The risks of surgery and likely appearance of the surgical scar must be taken into account along with the potential for further involution and the child's concern about the haemangioma.

Embolization

Embolization is rarely indicated and is generally reserved for life-threatening haemangiomas that have not responded to medical management. Most lesions requiring this option are hepatic tumours causing severe congestive heart failure [141] and rare cases of severe bleeding. Consultation with both surgeons and interventional radiologists familiar with haemangiomas is imperative in this situation.

References

1 **Mulliken JB, Glowacki J. Hemangiomas and vascular malformations in infants and children: a classification based on endothelial cell characteristics. Plast Reconstr Surg 1982;12:412–20.**
2 **Wassef M, Blei F, Adams D et al. Vascular Anomalies Classification: Recommendations from the International Society for the Study of Vascular Anomalies. Pediatrics.2015;136:e203–14.**
3 Garzon MC, Enjolras O, Frieden IJ. Vascular tumors and vascular malformations: evidence for an association. J Am Acad Dermatol 2000;42:275–9.
4 **North PE, Waner M, Mizeracki A et al. Glut1: a newly discovered immunohistochemical marker for juvenile hemangiomas. Hum Pathol 2000;31:11–22.**
5 Hidano A, Nakajima S. Earliest features of the strawberry mark in the newborn. Br J Dermatol 1972;83:138–44.
6 Pratt AG. Birthmarks in infants. Arch Dermatol 1953;67:302–5.
7 Jacobs AH, Walton RG. The incidence of birthmarks in the neonate. Pediatrics 1976;58:218–22.
8 Jacobs AH. Strawberry hemangioma, natural history of the untreated lesion. Calif Med 1957;83:8–10.
9 **Kilcline C, Frieden IJ. Infantile hemangiomas: how common are they? A systematic review of the literature. Pediatr Dermatol 2008;25:168–73.**
10 **Munden A, Butschek R, Tom WL et al. Prospective study of infantile haemangiomas: incidence, clinical characteristics and association with placental anomalies. Br J Dermatol 2014;170:907–913.**
11 **Haggstrom AN, Drolet BA, Baselga E et al. Prospective study of infantile hemangiomas: demographic, prenatal and perinatal characteristics. J Pediatr 2007;150:291–4.**
12 **Drolet BA, Swanson EA, Frieden IJ. Infantile hemangiomas: an emerging health issue linked to an increased rate of low birth weight infants. J Pediatr 2008;153:712–15.**
13 **Garzon MC, Drolet BA, Baselga E et al. Comparison of infantile hemangiomas in preterm and term infants: a prospective study. Arch Dermatol 2008;144:1231–2.**
14 **Goelz R, Poets CF. Incidence and treatment of infantile haemangiomas in preterm infants. Arch Dis Child Fetal Neonatal Ed 2015;100: F85–91.**
15 **Blei F, Walter J, Orlow SJ et al. Familial segregation of hemangiomas and vascular malformations as an autosomal dominant trait. Arch Dermatol 1998;134:718–22.**
16 **Haggstrom AN, Lammer EJ, Schneider RA et al. Patterns of infantile hemangiomas: new clues to hemangioma pathogenesis and embryonic facial development. Pediatrics 2006;117:698–703.**
17 **Léauté-Labrèze C, Prey S, Ezzedine K. Infantile hemangioma: part 1. Pathophysiology, epidemiology, clinical features, life cycle and associated structural anomalies. J Eur Acad Dermatol Venereol 2011;25:1245–60.**
18 **Chen TS, Eichenfield LF, Fallon Friedlander S. Infantile hemangiomas:an update on pathogenesis and therapy. Pediatrics 2013;131:99–108.**
19 **Forbess Smith CJ, Fallon Friedlander S, Guma M et al. Infantile hemangiomas: an updated review on risk factors, pathogenesis and treatment. Birth Defects Res 2017;109:809–15.**
20 **Drolet B, Frieden IJ. Characteristics of infantile hemangiomas as clues to pathogenesis: does hypoxia connect the dots? Arch Dermatol 2010;146:1295–99.**
21 **Kleinman ME, Greives MR, Churgin SS et al. Hypoxia-induced mediators of stem/progenitor cell trafficking are increased in children with hemangioma. Arterioscler Thromb Vasc Biol 2007;27: 2664–70.**
22 **de Jong S, Itinteang T, Withers AH et al. Does hypoxia play a role in infantile hemangioma? Arch Dermatol Res 2016;308:219–27.**
23 Yu Y, Flint AF, Mulliken JB et al. Endothelial progenitor cells in infantile hemangioma. Blood 2004;103:1373–5.
24 **Khan ZA, Boscolo E, Picard A et al. Multipotential stem cells recapitulate human infantile hemangioma in immunodeficient mice. J Clin Invest 2008;118:2592–9.**
25 **North PE, Waner M, Mizeracki A et al. A unique microvascular phenotype shared by juvenile hemangiomas and human placenta. Arch Dermatol 2001;137:559–70.**
26 Bree AF, Siegfreid E, Sotelo-Avila C et al. Infantile hemangiomas: speculation on placental trophoblastic origin. Arch Dermatol 2001;137: 573–7.
27 **Pittman KM, Losken HW, Kleinman ME et al. No evidence for maternal-fetal microchimerism in infantile hemangioma: a molecular genetic investigation. J Invest Dermatol 2006;126:2533–8.**
28 **Mulliken JB, Young AG. Vascular Anomalies: Hemangiomas and Malformations, 2nd edn. New York:Oxford University Press, 2013.**
29 Tan ST, Velickovic M, Ruger BM et al. Cellular and extracellular markers of hemangioma. Plast Reconstr Surg 2000;106:529–38.
30 Takahashi K, Mulliken JB, Kosakewich HPW et al. Cellular markers that distinguish the phases of hemangioma during infancy and childhood. J Clin Invest 1994;93:2357–64.
31 Kraling BM, Razon MJ, Boon LM et al. E-Selectin is present in proliferating endothelial cells in human hemangiomas. Am J Pathol 1996; 148:1181–91.
32 **Chiller KG, Passaro D, Frieden IJ. Hemangiomas of infancy: clinical characteristics, morphologic subtypes and their relationship to race, ethnicity and sex. Arch Dermatol 2002;138:1567–76.**

33 Waner M, North PE, Scherer KA et al. The nonrandom distribution of facial hemangiomas. Arch Dermatol 2003;139:869–75.
34 Haggstrom AN, Baselga E, Chamlin SL et al. Localized infantile hemangiomas of the face and scalp: predilection for the midline and periorbital and perioral skin. Pediatr Dermatol 2018;35:774–9.
35 Chang LC, Haggstrom AN, Drolet BA et al. Growth characteristics of infantile hemangiomas: implications for management. Pediatrics 2008;122:360–7.
36 Tollefson MM, Frieden IJ. Early growth of infantile hemangiomas: what parents' photographs tell us. Pediatrics 2012;130:e314–20.
37 Brandling-Bennett HA, Metry DW, Baselga E et al. Infantile hemangiomas with unusually prolonged growth phase. Arch Dermatol 2008;144:1632–7.
38 Baselga E, Roe E, Coulie J et al. Risk factors for degree and type of sequelae after involution of untreated hemangiomas of infancy. JAMA Dermatol 2016;152:1239–43.
39 Haggstrom AN, Drolet BA, Baselga E et al. Prospective study of infantile hemangiomas: clinical characteristics predicting complications and treatment. Pediatrics 2006;118:882–7.
40 Chamlin S, Haggstrom A, Drolet B et al. Multicenter prospective study of ulcerated hemangiomas. J Pediatr 2007;151:684–9.
41 Hermans DJJ, Boezeman JBM, van de Kerkhof PCM et al. Differences between ulcerated and non-ulcerated hemangiomas, a retrospective study of 465 cases. Eur J Dermatol 2009;19:152–6.
42 Kim HJ, Colombo M, Frieden IJ. Ulcerated hemangiomas, clinical characteristics and response to therapy. J Am Acad Dermatol 2001;44:962–72.
43 McCuaig CC, Cohen L, Powell J et al. Therapy of ulcerated hemangiomas. J Cutan Med Surg 2013;17:233–42.
44 Morelli JG, Tan OT, Yohn JJ et al. Treatment of ulcerated hemangiomas in infancy. Arch Pediatr Adolesc Med 1994;148:1104–5.
45 David L, Malek M, Argenta L. Efficacy of pulse dye laser therapy for the treatment of ulcerated haemangiomas: a review of 78 patients. Br J Plast Surg 2003;56:317–27.
46 Yan A. Pain management for ulcerated hemangiomas. Pediatr Dermatol 2008;25:586–9.
47 Saint-Jean M, Léauté-Labrèze C, Mazereeuw-Hautier J et al. Propranolol for treatment of ulcerated infantile hemangiomas. J Am Acad Dermatol 2011;64:827–32.
48 Hermans DJ, van Beynum IM, Schultze Kool LJ et al. Propranolol, a very promising treatment for ulceration in infantile hemangiomas: a study of 20 cases with matched historical controls. J Am Acad Dermatol 2011;64:833–8.
49 Boos MD, Castelo-Soccio L. Experience with topical timolol maleate for the treatment of ulcerated infantile hemangiomas (IH). J Am Acad Dermatol 2016;7:567–70.
50 Ceisler EJ, Santos L, Blei F. Periocular hemangiomas: what every physician should know. Pediatr Dermatol 2004;21:1–9.
51 Schwartz SR, Blei F, Ceisler E et al. Risk factors for amblyopia in children with capillary hemangiomas of the eyelids and orbit. J AAPOS 2006;10:262–8.
52 Spence-Shishido AA, Good WV, Baselga E et al. Hemangiomas and the eye. Clin Dermatol 2015;33:170–8.
53 Orlow SJ, Isakoff MS, Blei F. Increased risk of symptomatic hemangiomas of the airway in association with cutaneous hemangiomas in a 'beard' distribution. J Pediatr 1997;131:643–6.
54 O TM, Alexander RE, Lando T et al. Segmental hemangiomas of the upper airway. Laryngoscope 2009;119:2242–7.
55 O-Lee TJ, Messner A. Subglottic hemangioma. Otolaryngol Clin North Am 2008;41:903–11.
56 Peridis S, Pilgrim G, Athanasopoulos I, Parpounas K. A meta-analysis of the effectiveness of propranololfor the treatment of infantile airway hemangiomas. Int J Pediatr Otorhinolaryngol 2011;75:455–60.
57 Denoyelle F, Leboulanger N, Enjolras O et al. Role of propranolol in the therapeutic strategy of infantile laryngotracheal hemangioma. Int J Pediatr Otorhinolaryngol 2009;73:1168–72.
58 Buckmiller L, Dyamenahalli U, Richter GT. Propranolol for airway hemangiomas: case report of novel treatment. Laryngoscope 2009;119: 2051–4.
59 Vaksman G, Rey C, Marache P et al. Severe congestive heart failure in newborns due to giant cutaneous hemangioma. Am J Cardiol 1987;60:392–4.
60 Dieterich-Miller C, Cohen B, Liggett J. Behavioral adjustment and self-concept of young children with hemangiomas. Pediatr Dermatol 1992;9:241–5.
61 Tanner JL, Dechert MP, Frieden IJ. Growing up with a facial hemangioma: parent and child coping and adaption. Pediatrics 1998;101:446–52.
62 Williams EF 3rd, Hochman M, Rodgers BJ et al. A psychological profile of children with hemangiomas and their families. Arch Facial Plast Surg 2003; 5:229–34.
63 Frieden IJ, Rogers M, Garzon MC. Conditions masquerading as infantile haemangioma: Part 1. Australas J Dermatol 2009;50:77–97.
64 Frieden IJ, Rogers M, Garzon MC. Conditions masquerading as infantile haemangioma: Part 2. Australas J Dermatol 2009;50:153–68.
65 Garzon MC, Weitz N, Powell J. Vascular anomalies: differential diagnosis and mimickers. Semin Cutan Med Surg 2016;35:170–6.
66 Dubois J, Patriquin HB, Garel L et al. Soft-tissue hemangiomas in infants and children: diagnosis using Doppler sonography. AJR 1998;171:247–52.
67 Dubois J, Garel L. Imaging and therapeutic approach of hemangiomas and vascular malformations in the pediatric age group. Pediatr Radiol 1999;29:879–93.
68 Konez O, Burrows PE. Magnetic resonance of vascular anomalies. Magn Reson Imaging Clin North Am 2002;10:363–88.
69 Burrows PE, Mulliken JB, Fellows KE et al. Childhood hemangiomas and vascular malformations: angiographic differentiation. AJR 1983;141: 483–8.
70 Hand JL, Frieden IJ. Vascular birthmarks of infancy: resolving nosologic confusion. Am J Med Genet 2002;108:257–64.
71 Frieden IJ, Reese V, Cohen D. PHACE syndrome, the association of posterior fossa brain malformations, hemangiomas, arterial anomalies, coarctation of the aorta and cardiac defects and eye abnormalities. Arch Dermatol 1996;132:307–11.
72 Metry DW, Garzon MC, Drolet BA et al. PHACE syndrome: current knowledge, future directions. Pediatr Dermatol 2009;26:381–98.
73 Metry D, Heyer G, Hess C et al. Consensus statement on diagnostic criteria for PHACE syndrome. Pediatrics 2009;124:1447–56.
74 Garzon MC, Epstein LG, Heyer GL et al. PHACE syndrome: consensus-derived diagnosis and care recommendations. J Pediatr 2016; 178:24–33.
75 Haggstrom AN, Garzon MC, Baselga E et al. Risk for PHACE syndrome in infants with large facial hemangiomas. Pediatrics 2010; 126:e418–26.
76 Hess CP1, Fullerton HJ, Metry DW et al. Cervical and intracranial arterial anomalies in 70 patients with PHACE syndrome. Am J Neuroradiol 2010;31:1980–6.
77 Tangtiphaiboontana J, Hess CP, Bayer M et al. Neurodevelopmental abnormalities in children with PHACE syndrome. J Child Neurol 2013;28:608–14.
78 Drolet BA, Dohil M, Golomb MR et al. Early stroke and cerebral vasculopathy in children with facial hemangiomas and PHACE association. Pediatrics 2006;117:959–64.
79 Siegel DH, Tefft KA, Kelly T, Johnson C et al. Stroke in children with posterior fossa brain malformations, hemangiomas, arterial anomalies, coarctation of the aorta and cardiac defects, and eye abnormalities (PHACE) syndrome: a systematic review of the literature. Stroke 2012;43(6):1672–4.
80 Bayer ML, Frommelt PC, Blei F et al. Congenital cardiac, aortic arch, and vascular bed anomalies in PHACE syndrome (from the International PHACE Syndrome Registry). Am J Cardiol 2013; 112:1948–52.
81 Spence-Shishido AA, Good WV, Baselga E, Frieden IJ. Hemangiomas and the eye. Clin Dermatol 2015;33:170–82.
82 Duffy KJ, Runge-Samuelson C, Bayer ML et al. Association of hearing loss with PHACE syndrome. Arch Dermatol 2010;146:1391–6
83 Chiu YE, Siegel DH, Drolet BA, Hodgson BD. Tooth enamel hypoplasia in PHACE syndrome. Pediatr Dermatol 2014;31:455–8.
84 Poindexter G, Metry DW, Barkovich AJ et al. PHACE syndrome with intracerebral hemangiomas, heterotopia and endocrine dysfunction. Pediatr Neurol 2007;36:402–6.
85 Carinci S, Tumini S, Consilvio NP et al. A case of congenital hypothyroidism in PHACE syndrome. J Pediatr Endocrinol Metab 2012;25:603–5.
86 Metry DW, Garzon MC, Drolet BA et al. PHACE syndrome: current knowledge, future directions. Pediatr Dermatol 2009;26:381–98.
87 Girard C, Bigorre M, Guillot B et al. PELVIS syndrome. Arch Dermatol 2006;142:884–8.
88 Stockman A, Boralevi F, Taïeb A et al. SACRAL syndrome: spinal dysraphism, anogenital, cutaneous, renal and urologic anomalies, associated with an angioma of lumbosacral localization. Dermatology 2007;214:40–5.
89 Iacobas I, Burrows PE, Frieden IJ et al. LUMBAR: association between cutaneous infantile hemangiomas of the lower body and regional congenital anomalies. J Pediatr 2010;157:795–801.
90 Horii KA, Drolet BA, Frieden IJ et al. Prospective study of the frequency of hepatic hemangiomas in infants with multiple cutaneous infantile hemangiomas. Pediatr Dermatol 2011;28:245–53.
91 Rialon KL, Murillo R, Fevurly RD et al. Impact of screening for hepatic hemangiomas in patients with multiple cutaneous infantile hemangiomas. Pediatr Dermatol 2015;32:808–12.

92 Christison-Lagay ER, Burrows PE, Alomari A et al. Hepatic hemangiomas: subtype classification and development of a clinical practice algorithm and registry. J Pediatr Surg 2007;42:62–7.
93 Kulungowski AM1, Alomari AI, Chawla A et al. Lessons from a liver hemangioma registry: subtype classification. J Pediatr Surg 2012;47:165–70.
94 Huang SA, Tu HM, Harney JW et al. Severe hypothyroidism caused by type 3 iodothyronine deiodinase in infantile hemangiomas. N Engl J Med 2000;343:185–9.
95 Mazereeuw-Hautier J, Hoeger PH, Benlahrech S et al. Efficacy of propranolol in hepatic infantile hemangiomas with diffuse neonatal hemangiomatosis. J Pediatr 2010;157:340–2.
96 Yeh I, Bruckner AL, Sanchez R, et al Diffuse infantile hepatic hemangiomas: a report of four cases successfully managed with medical therapy. Pediatr Dermatol 2011;28:267–75.
97 Frieden IJ. Which hemangiomas to treat: and how? Arch Dermatol 1997;133:1593–5.
98 Baselga E, Roe E, Coulie J et al. Risk factors for degree and type of sequelae after involution of untreated hemangiomas of infancy. JAMA Dermatol 2016;152:1239–43.
99 Hoeger PH, Harper JI, Baselga E et al. Treatment of infantile haemangiomas: recommendations of a European expert group. Eur J Pediatr 2015;174:855–65.
100 Frieden IJ, Eichenfield LF, Esterly NB et al. Guidelines of care for hemangiomas of infancy. J Am Acad Dermatol 1997;37:631–7.
101 Enjolras O, Riche MC, Merland JJ et al. Management of alarming hemangiomas in infancy: a review of 25 cases. Pediatrics 1990;85: 491–7.
102 Léauté-Labrèze C, Dumas de la Roque E, Hubiche T et al. Propranolol for severe hemangiomas of infancy. N Engl J Med 2008;358:2649–51.
103 Sans V, Dumas de la Roque E, Berge J et al. Propranolol for severe infantile hemangiomas: follow-up report. Pediatrics 2009;124:e423–31.
104 Léauté-Labrèze C, Hoeger P, Mazereeuw-Hautier J et al. A randomised, controlled trial of oral propranolol in infantile hemangioma. N Engl J Med 2015;372:735–46.
105 Léauté-Labrèze C, Dumas de la Roque E, Nacka F et al. Doubleblind randomized pilot trial evaluating the efiicacy of oral propranolol on infantile haemangiomas in onfants <4 months of age. Br J Dermatol 2013;169:181–3.
106 Hogeling M, Adams S, Wargon O. A randomized controlled trial of propranolol for infantile hemangiomas. Pediatrics 2011;128:e259–266.
107 Marqueling AL, Oza V, Frieden IJ et al. Propranolol and infantile hemangiomas four years later. Pediatr Dermatol 2013;30:182–191.
108 Wedgeworth E, Glover M, Irvine AD et al. Propranolol in the treatment of infantile haemangiomas: lessons from the European Propranolol In the Treatment of Complicated Haemangiomas (PITCH) Taskforce Survey. Br J Dermatol 2016;174:594–601.
109 Langley A, Pope E. Propranolol and central nervous system function: potential implications for pediatric patients with infantile hemangiomas. Br J Dermatol 2015;172:13–23.
110 Moyakine AV, Kerstjens JM, Spillekom-van Koulil S et al. Propranolol treatment of infantile hemangioma (IH) is not associated with developmental risk or growth impairment at age 4 years. J Am Acad Dermatol 2016;75:59–63.
111 Moyakine AV, Spillekom-van Koulil S, van der Vleuten CJM. Propranolol treatment of infantile hemangioma is not associated with psychological problems at 7 years of age. J Am Acad Dermatol 2017;77:105–8.
112 González-Llorente N, Del Olmo-Benito I, Muñoz-Ollero N et al. Study of cognitive function in children treated with propranolol for infantile hemangioma. Pediatr Dermatol 2017;34:554–8.
113 Mahon C, Heron G, Perkins D et al. Oral propranolol for infantile haemangioma may be associated with transient gross motor delay. Br J Dermatol 2018;178:1443–4.
114 Ahogo CK, Ezzedine K, Prey S et al. Factors associated with the relapse of infantile haemangiomas in children treated with oral propranolol. Br J Dermatol 2013;169:1252–6.
115 Shah SD, Baselga E, McCuaig C et al. Rebound growth of infantile hemangiomas after propranolol therapy. Pediatrics 2016;137: e20151754.
116 Drolet BA, Frommelt PC, Chamlin SL et al. Initiation and use of propranolol for infantile hemangioma: report of a consensus conference. Pediatrics 2013;131:128–40.
117 Metry D, Frieden IJ, Hess C et al. Propranolol use in PHACE syndrome with cervical and intracranial arterial anomalies: collective experience in 32 infants. Pediatr Dermatol 2013;30:71–89.
118 Pope E, Chakkittakandiyil A, Lara-Corrales I et al. Expanding the therapeutic repertoire of infantile hemangiomas: cohort-blinded study of oral nadolol compared with propranolol. Br J Dermatol 2013;168:222–4.
119 Bernabeu-Wittel J, Narvaez-Moreno B, de la Torre-Garcia JM et al. Oral nadolol for children with infantile hemangiomas and sleep disturbances with oral propranolol. Pediatr Dermatol 2015;32: 853–7.
120 Arbazua-Ataya A, Navarrete-Dechent CP, Heusser F et al. Atenolol vs propranolol for the treatment of infantile hemangiomas: a randomized controlled study. J Am Acad Dermatol 2014;70:1045–9.
121 Bennett ML, Fleischer AB Jr, Chamlin S et al. Oral corticosteroid use is effective for cutaneous hemangiomas:an evidence-based evaluation. Arch Dermatol 2001;137:1208–13.
122 Bertrand J, McCuaig C, Dubois J et al. Propranolol vs prednisone in the treatment of infantile hemangiomas: a retrospective comparative study. Pediatr Dermatol 2011;28:649–54.
123 Price CJ, Lattouf C, Baum B et al. Propranolol vs corticosteroids for infantile hemangiomas: a multicenter retrospective analysis. Arch Dermatol 2011;147;1371–6.
124 Malik MA, Menon P, Rao KL et al. Effect of propranolol vs prednisolone vs propranolol with prednisolone in the management of infantile hemangioma: a randomized controlled study. J Pediatr Surg 2013;48:2453–9.
125 Chen MT, Yeong EK, Horng SY. Intralesional corticosteroid therapy in proliferating head and neck hemangiomas: a review of 155 cases. J Pediatr Surg 2000;35:420–3.
126 Ruttum MS, Abrams GW, Harris GJ et al. Bilateral retinal embolization associated with intralesional corticosteroid injection for capillary hemangioma of infancy. J Pediatr Ophthalmol Strabismus 1993;30:4–7.
127 Püttgen K, Lucky A, Adams D et al. Topical timolol maleate treatment of infantile hemangiomas. Pediatrics 2016;138:pii: e20160355.
128 Chan H, McKay C, Adams S et al. RCT of timolol maleate gel for superficial infantile hemangiomas in 5-to 24-week-olds. Pediatrics 2013;131:e1739–47.
129 McMahon P, Oza V, Frieden IJ. Topical timolol for infantile hemangiomas:putting a note of caution in 'cautiously optimistic'. Pediatr Dermatol 2012;29:127–30.
130 Novoa M, Baselga E, Beltran S et al. Interventions for infantile haemangiomas of the skin. Cochrane Database Syst Rev 2018 Apr 18;4:CD006545. doi:10.1002/14651858.
131 McCuaig CC, Dubois J, Powell J et al. A phase II, open-label study of the efficacy and safety of imiquimod in the treatment of superficial and mixed infantile hemangioma. Pediatr Dermatol 2009; 26:203–12.
132 Qiu Y, Ma G, Yang J et al. Imiquimod 5% cream versus timolol 0.5% ophthalmic solution for treating superficial proliferating infantile haemangiomas: a retrospective study. Clin Exp Dermatol 2013;38:845–50.
133 Garzon MC, Lucky AW, Hawrot A et al. Ultrapotent topical corticosteroid treatment of hemangiomas of infancy. J Am Acad Dermatol 2005;52:281–6.
134 David L, Malek M, Argenta L. Efficacy of pulse dye laser therapy for the treatment of ulcerated haemangiomas: a review of 78 patients. Br J Plast Surg 2003;56:317–27.
135 Morelli JG, Tan OT, Yohn JJ et al. Treatment of ulcerated hemangiomas in infancy. Arch Pediatr Adolesc Med 1994;148:1104–5.
136 Batta K, Goodyear HM, Moss C et al. Randomised controlled study of early pulsed dye laser treatment of uncomplicated childhood haemangiomas: results of a 1 year analysis. Lancet 2002;360:521–7.
137 Brauer JA, Geronemus RG. Laser treatment in the management of infantile hemangiomas and capillary vascular malformations. Tech Vasc Interv Radiol 2013;16:51–4.
138 Witman PM, Wagner AM, Scherer K et al. Complications following pulsed dye laser treatment of superficial hemangiomas. Lasers Surg Med 2006;38:116–23.
139 Reddy KK, Blei F, Brauer JA et al. Retrospective study of the treatment of infantile hemangiomas using a combination of propranolol and pulsed dye laser. Dermatol Surg 2013;39:923–33.
140 Passeron T, Maza A, Fontas E et al. Treatment of port wine stains with pulsed dye laser and topical timolol: a multicenter randomized controlled trial. Br J Dermatol 2014;170:1350–3.
141 Hsi Dickie B, Fishman SJ, Azizkhan RG Hepatic vascular tumors. Semin Pediatr Surg 2014;23:168–72.

CHAPTER 120
Other Vascular Tumours

Ann M. Kulungowski[1], *Taizo A. Nakano*[1] *& Anna L. Bruckner*[2]

[1] University of Colorado School of Medicine, and Vascular Anomalies Center, Children's Hospital Colorado, Aurora, CO, USA
[2] University of Colorado School of Medicine, and Division of Dermatology, Children's Hospital Colorado, Aurora, CO, USA

Introduction, 1440
Benign vascular tumours, 1440
Locally aggressive or borderline vascular tumours, 1444
Malignant vascular tumours, 1448
Provisionally unclassified vascular anomalies, 1448

Abstract

This chapter reviews important vascular tumours in the paediatric population other than infantile haemangioma. Other than pyogenic granuloma, these growths are uncommon to quite rare. Congenital haemangioma present fully formed at birth and may rapidly involute thereafter, persist without change, or demonstrate an intermediate phenotype. Pyogenic granulomas are common, benign growths that typically require treatment because of their tendency to bleed. Tufted angioma and kaposiform haemangioendothelioma are locally invasive proliferations of endothelial and lymphatic cells that can be complicated by a serious coagulopathy called Kasabach–Merritt phenomenon. Malignant vascular tumours such as angiosarcoma are exceedingly rare and associated with underlying vascular anomalies or overgrowth, lymphoedema, or a history of radiation therapy. Multifocal lymphangioendotheliomatosis with thrombocytopenia and kaposiform lymphangioendotheliomatosis derive from lymphatic vessels and are associated with haematological abnormalities.

SECTION 25: VASCULAR TUMOURS

Introduction

The International Society for the Study of Vascular Anomalies classifies vascular tumours based on their malignant potential (see Table 120.1) [1]. Aside from infantile haemangioma and pyogenic granuloma, most of these tumours are rare. This chapter focuses on the tumours, other than infantile haemangioma, that present in infancy and childhood or have exceptional relevance in the paediatric population. In addition, two vascular anomalies that are considered 'provisionally unclassified' at this time, multifocal lymphangioendotheliomatosis with thrombocytopenia and kaposiform lymphangiomatosis, are included because they share features with tumours of lymphatic origin reviewed herein.

Benign vascular tumours

Key points

- **Congenital haemangiomas (CH) are uncommon vascular tumours that proliferate *in utero*.**
- **Three patterns of postnatal behavior occur: rapid involution, partial involution and noninvolution.**
- **Transient haematological changes can be associated with CH after birth.**
- **In most cases, treatment of CH in infancy is not needed. Persistent or residual tumour or atrophic skin may be excised in childhood.**

- **Pyogenic granuloma (PG, lobular capillary haemangioma) are common, acquired vascular proliferations that tend to bleed easily.**
- **In most cases, PG can be treated with shave removal and electrocautery with a low risk for recurrence and good aesthetic outcomes.**

Congenital haemangioma

Congenital haemangiomas (CH) are uncommon in comparison to infantile haemangiomas. They are benign vascular tumours that are observed *in utero* [2,3], present fully formed at birth, and do not exhibit postnatal proliferation. This natural history is distinct from that of infantile haemangiomas (see Chapter 119), which are either absent or present with a premonitory mark at birth, enlarge rapidly in the first few months, and involute slowly over years. CH occur equally between the genders. Their exact incidence is unknown.

There are three major subtypes of CH based upon their course after birth. Rapidly involuting congenital haemangioma (RICH) regresses in the first year of life, often by 14 months of age (Fig. 120.1) [4]. Noninvoluting congenital haemangioma (NICH) does not regress and grows proportionately with the child [5]. Partially involuting congenital haemangioma (PICH) regresses in the first 1–3 years after birth but fails to complete involution and persists as a noninvoluting-like CH (Fig. 120.2) [6].

Harper's Textbook of Pediatric Dermatology, Fourth Edition. Edited by Peter Hoeger, Veronica Kinsler and Albert Yan.

Ayturk and colleagues [7] recently identified somatic mutations that alter glutamic acid at amino acid 209 in *GNAQ* and *GNA11* in RICH and NICH specimens. This finding was confirmed by Funk and colleagues [8] who identified the same mutation in *GNA11* in an infant with an unusual phenotype of disseminated CH. *GNAQ* and *GNA11* encode the α-subunits of guanine nucleotide-binding proteins involved in transmembrane cell signalling. Activating mutations in *GNAQ* and *GNA11* lead to upregulation of the MAPK pathway, inducing changes in cellular morphology and growth [9]. However, other factors that are unknown at this time likely influence the postnatal course of CH.

Table 120.1 The International Society for the Study of Vascular Anomalies Classification of Vascular Tumours

Benign	Infantile haemangioma (see Chapter 119)
	Congenital haemangioma
	Rapidly involuting (RICH)
	Non-involuting (NICH)
	Partially involuting (PICH)
	Tufted angioma*
	Spindle-cell haemangioma
	Epithelioid haemangioma
	Pyogenic granuloma (lobular capillary haemangioma)
Locally progressive or borderline	**Kaposiform haemangioendothelioma**[a]
	Retiform haemangioendothelioma
	Papillary intralymphatic angioendothelioma (PILA), Dabska tumour
	Composite haemangioendothelioma
	Kaposi sarcoma
Malignant	**Angiosarcoma**
	Epithelioid haemangioendothelioma

Disorders in **bold** are discussed in this chapter.
[a] Tufted angioma and kaposiform haemangioendothelioma are considered by many experts to be variants on a spectrum.
Source: ISSVA Classification for Vascular Anomalies ©2018 International Society for the Study of Vascular Anomalies. Available at issva.org/classification. Licensed under a Creative Commons Attribution 4.0 International Licence.

CH are most often solitary tumours. Multifocal CH occur rarely [10] and a neonate with a large, symptomatic CH and numerous, small CH in a 'haemangiomatosis' pattern was recently described [8]. CH can occur concurrently with infantile haemangiomas [10,11]. Both RICH and NICH are warm on palpation [12]. RICH typically present on the head, neck, or extremities and range in size from small (a few centimetres) to large (>10 cm). While most lesions are focal, a segmental presentation may occur [13]. RICH may also occur in the liver as a focal hepatic haemangioma [14,15]. Morphology of RICH ranges from plaques covered with course telangiectasias to violaceous nodules or tumours that penetrate to the deeper dermis or subcutis with large draining peripheral veins. A halo-like rim of pallor is often observed in the skin bordering the tumour. A depression, ulceration or scar can be seen centrally. Ulceration can result in life-threatening haemorrhage. Transient thrombocytopenia (range 5000–62 000/μL) and coagulopathy can occur in the first weeks of life in some infants with RICH [16,17]. The thrombocytopenia and coagulopathy are not sustained or as severe as that seen in Kasabach–Merritt phenomenon. Most RICH start to involute days to weeks after birth, and involution is complete in 6–14 months, leaving redundant, atrophic, hypopigmented skin [3,12,18]. Some RICH undergo involution during fetal life and present with these findings at birth [19].

NICH and RICH share many features in common though there are subtle distinctions. NICH are encountered in the same anatomical locations as RICH. NICH are usually smaller, with an average diameter of 5 cm, and are round to ovoid plaques or nodules. NICH tend to be less exophytic than RICH. Telangiectasias may cover the surface, often with central or peripheral pallor (Fig. 120.3). NICH do not resolve spontaneously [5]. As differentiating RICH and NICH in a neonate based on morphology alone is challenging, observation for rapid involution over time is the most reliable distinguishing feature. The diagnosis of RICH versus NICH or PICH depends upon clinical history and is elucidated with time.

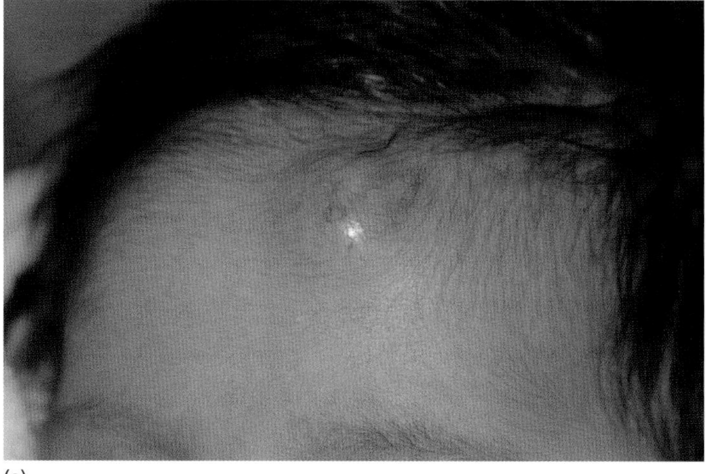
(a)

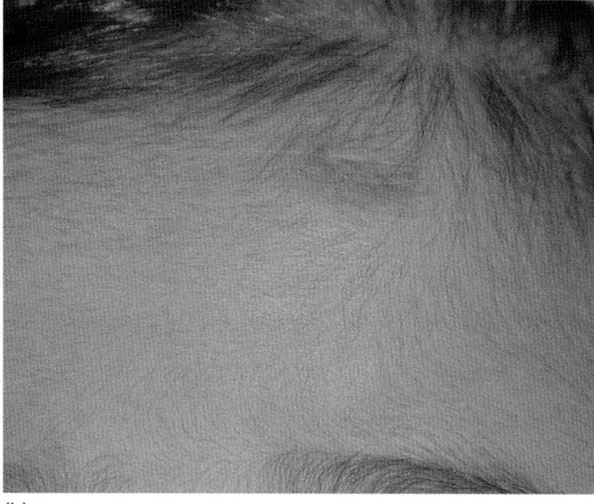
(b)

Fig. 120.1 A small rapidly involuting congenital haemangioma (RICH) on the forehead. (a) Lesion 2 months after birth and (b) at 11 months, where only subtle atrophy can be found.

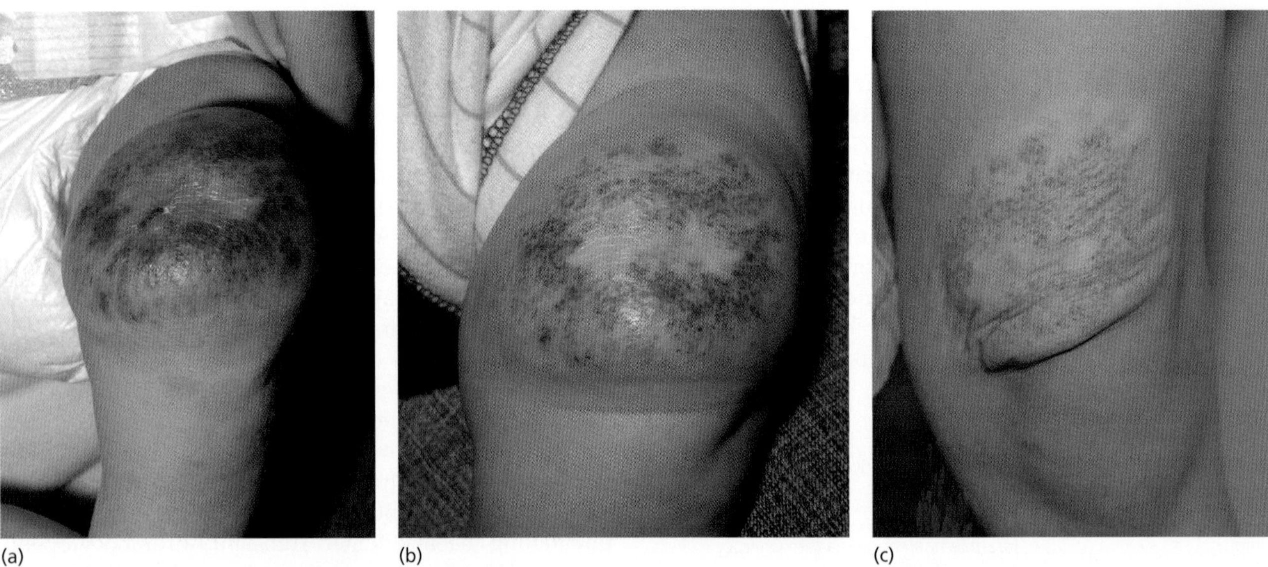

Fig. 120.2 The progression of a partially involuting congenital haemangioma (PICH) over time. (a) Protuberant red–violaceous tumour with peripheral pallor observed in a newborn. (b) The lesion is flatter 3 months after birth. (c) Residual vessels and pallor with atrophic, redundant skin seen at 4 years of age.

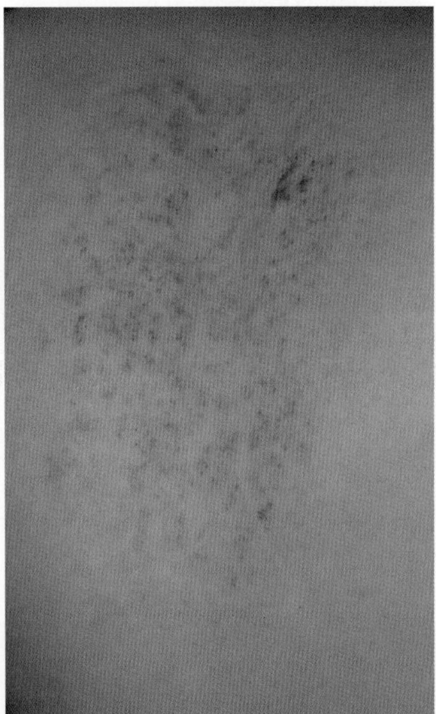

Fig. 120.3 Noninvoluting congenital haemangioma (NICH). The peripheral pallor and telangiectasias over the surface are typical.

CH exhibit unique histopathological findings that are distinct from infantile haemangiomas. RICH and NICH have similar histological appearances. The tumours are cellular lesions consisting of multiple well-defined lobules of proliferating capillaries separated by intervening bands of abnormal, dense fibrous tissue. Large dysplastic vessels surround the lobules. Focal thrombosis, calcifications and hemosiderin deposits are observed [4,5,11]. Glucose transporter-1 protein (GLUT-1) expression is lacking in CH [4]. Lobular areas stain with Wilms tumour-1 [20].

CH are commonly diagnosed by history and physical examination alone. Ultrasonography and magnetic resonance imaging (MRI) serve as adjuncts to clarify or confirm the diagnosis and delineate tumour extent and relation to adjacent structures. Ultrasonographic features of RICH and NICH include a solitary, heterogeneous, vascular mass with high vessel density. Occasional calcifications and varying degrees of shunting are also detected. MRI/angiography of RICH and NICH exhibit a vascular structure with flow voids, heterogenous enhancement, and hyperintensity on T2-weighted sequences [21]. CH can be detected antenatally with both ultrasonography and fetal MRI as they develop *in utero* [2,3,22].

The differential diagnosis of CH includes infantile fibrosarcoma, vascular malformations and other vascular tumours [12,23]. Biopsy is indicated in the face of diagnostic uncertainty and should be performed in a controlled environment because of bleeding risk. The periphery of the tumour should be included where the lobular architecture is preserved.

Management strategies for CH are based upon location, size and symptoms. Expectant management and anticipatory guidance are the mainstays. Large, ulcerated or bleeding tumours, especially RICH, may require surgical intervention to manage pain and prevent haemorrhage, especially when complicated by thrombocytopenia. There are no proven systemic medications for the treatment of CH. While propranolol and corticosteroids have been used, whether or not these treatments hasten the normal course of RICH is unclear. Pulsed dye laser may be used to ablate residual telangiectasias. Excision of redundant, atrophic skin is indicated postinvolution if disfigurement is present. Most NICH do not need treatment, but if causing pain, tissue distortion, or disfigurement, surgical excision is an option. Follow-up for congenital haemangiomas depends on the clinical course. In the face of complications, frequent visits are necessary.

Tufted angioma

Although the ISSVA classification categorizes tufted angioma as benign, many experts feel this tumour exists in the spectrum of kasposiform heamangioendothelioma, a tumour of intermediate malignant potential. Tufted angioma is fully discussed in the following section.

Spindle cell haemangioma

Although spindle cell haemangioma (SCH) is now recognized as a benign tumour, it was first described with malignant potential and termed spindle cell haemangioendothelioma [24]. A subsequent study of 78 cases determined this process is not malignant [25]. SCH is rare, and occurs in all ages, equally affecting females and males. It presents as a reddish-brown to blue nodule arising in the dermis or subcutaneous skin of the distal extremities. Solitary lesions can multiply within a focal area. SCH can be seen with other vascular tumours and malformations and are common in Maffucci syndrome which is characterized by venous malformations and enchondromas.

A hypothesis about the pathogenesis of SCH suggests an underlying malformation that is complicated by thrombosis and aberrant vascular remodelling. This concept is supported by histology of SCH which demonstrates two key features: thin-walled vessels with organizing thrombi and proliferations of spindle cells. The spindle cells express CD31, Prox-1 and are focally positive for D2-40, suggesting a possible lymphatic origin to the proliferative component of SCH [26]. Kurek and colleagues [27] recently identified somatic R132C mutations in *IDH1*, the same mutation in Mafucci syndrome, in 20 of 28 SCH specimens that were not associated with Maffucci syndrome.

Treatment for SCH has focused on excision when possible, although the recurrence rate is high.

Pyogenic granuloma (lobular capillary haemangioma)

Pyogenic granulomas (PG, also called lobular capillary haemangioma) are common, acquired, benign vascular neoplasms. The term pyogenic granuloma arose from the hypothesis that these tumours were a granulomatous response to an infectious agent and is clearly a misnomer. Lobular capillary haemangioma accurately describes the histological findings of these lesions, but the term PG persists in clinical practice and the medical literature. PG can occur at any age and are common in the paediatric population.

The pathogenesis of PG is not well understood. Trauma and an aberrant wound healing response may have a role. Lim and colleagues [28] found somatic activating mutations in *RAS* genes in a subset of PG specimens. Groesser and colleagues [29] identified *BRAF* c.1799T>A mutations in 8 of 10 PG associated with port wine stains and 3 of 25 sporadic PG specimens; other mutations in *BRAF*, *NRAS* and *KRAS* were also discovered. The role of this pathway in the pathogenesis of PG is also supported by the observation of PG as a cutaneous complication of *BRAF* inhibitors [30,31]. Blackwell and colleagues [32] hypothesize that PG may arise from primitive endothelial and interstitial cells based on their finding of embryonic stem cell markers in PG from 11 patients.

PG affect the skin and epithelial mucosa. The most common cutaneous locations are the head, neck and extremities, including the periungual area. The typical lesion is a bright red, friable papule that grows quickly and is prone to bleeding (Fig. 120.4a). A loosely adherent haemorrhagic crust may be seen. Thrombosed lesions appear brown to black. Lesions may be pedunculated or sessile and surrounded by an epithelial collarette. Most are solitary and less than 1 cm in size. Large, multiple or agminated presentations are reported. Other vascular anomalies – especially capillary malformations, burns and some medications (isotretinoin, others) – are associated with the development of PG.

The clinical diagnosis of PG is straightforward and based on the history and clinical characteristics of the lesion. The patient's age and underlying health risks should be taken into account when considering the differential diagnosis which includes infantile haemangioma,

SECTION 25: VASCULAR TUMOURS

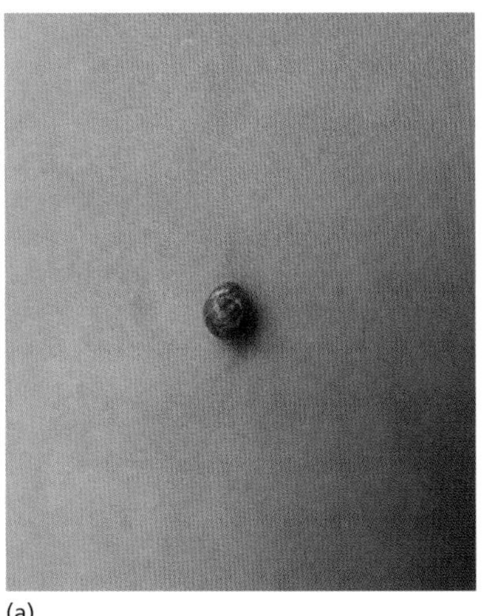

(a)

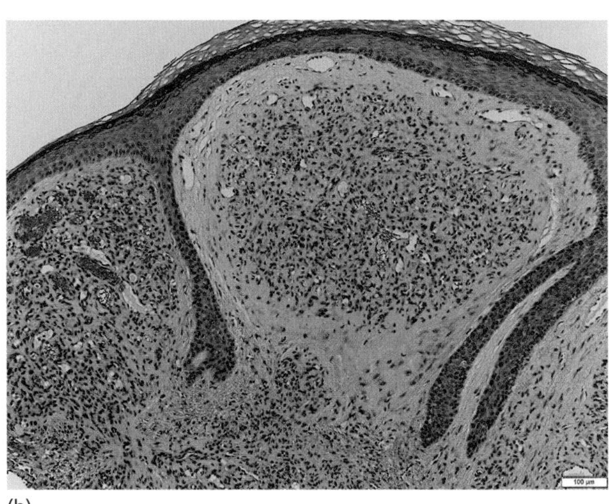

(b)

Fig. 120.4 Pyogenic granuloma (lobular capillary haemangioma). (a) Focal, bright red pedunculated papule. (b) Histology of PG shows lobular proliferations of capillary endothelial cells in the superficial dermis (×10). Source: Photomicrograph courtesy of Dr Lori Prok.

solitary angiokeratoma, Spitz nevus (particular for pink to red papules that have not bled), melanoma, eccrine poroma, Kaposi sarcoma and bacillary angiomatosis.

Histology of PG shows well-circumscribed proliferations of capillary endothelial cells that are arranged in lobules and separated by bands of fibrous stroma (Fig. 120.4b). An epithelial collarette, ulceration and inflammation are additional findings.

Although PG are benign, removal is typically recommended and performed on presentation to the physician because of the high likelihood of persistence and bleeding if not treated. The treatment of choice is shave removal (using a blade or curette) and electrocautery, which has a low risk for recurrence and good aesthetic outcomes [33]. Other procedural options include excision and pulsed dye laser ablation, although a single laser treatment is unlikely to resolve PG. Both imiquimod and timolol have also been reported as potential treatments for PG, although controlled studies are lacking.

Locally aggressive or borderline vascular tumours

Key points

- **Kaposiform haemangioendothelioma (KHE) and tufted angioma (TA) are considered to be varied clinical expressions on a spectrum of the same uncommon vascular proliferation.**
- **KHE tends to be deeper and more invasive, whereas TA is confined to the dermis.**
- **Both KHE and TA can be complicated by the Kasabach–Merritt phenomenon (KMP), a potentially life-threatening disorder characterized by severe thrombocytopenia, hypofibrinogenaemia, microangiopathic haemolytic anaemia, and consumptive coagulopathy.**
- **While corticosteroids and vincristine are considered the first-line treatment for KHE or TA complicated by KMP, a growing body of evidence also supports the use of sirolimus for these disorders.**

Kaposiform haemangioendothelioma and tufted angioma

Kaposiform haemangioendothelioma (KHE) and tufted angioma (TA) are two related vascular tumours of intermediate malignant potential that present in infancy and childhood. KHE and TA share histopathological features, consisting of the inappropriate proliferation of both endothelial and lymphatic cells, and are now considered to be varied clinical expressions on a spectrum of the same vascular anomaly. Rapid recognition of these lesions is critical given their common association with a life-threatening bleeding diathesis known as Kasabach–Merritt phenomenon (KMP). These aggressive and infiltrating lesions require a multidisciplinary approach to establish a timely diagnosis and coordinate a multimodal management plan.

Kaposiform haemangioendothelioma

KHE is a rare and locally aggressive vascular tumour of intermediate malignant potential named for its histopathological resemblance to Kaposi sarcoma. Although these lesions carry the potential for local infiltration through tissue plains and possible spread to local lymph nodes, they are not known to metastasize [34]. KHE do not undergo spontaneous involution and can demonstrate episodes of rapid growth associated with severe platelet and fibrinogen consumption and red cell destruction, referred to as KMP.

In a retrospective study of KHE, Croteau and colleagues estimated the incidence to be 0.7 cases per 100 000 children per year [35]. Males and females are equally affected with no identified ethnic prevalence.

KHE typically presents in early infancy, but congenital and adult onset has been described. The tumour appears as an intradermal or subcutaneous mass with overlying red–brown cutaneous discoloration or as violaceous plaques or nodules [36,37]. Common locations are the extremities and trunk; the retroperitoneal, cervicofacial, visceral and boney regions are less commonly affected [35,38]. Retroperitoneal and mediastinal disease may present in infants with symptoms such as haemothorax and ascites [39]. Cutaneous lesions can be associated with hypertrichosis and hyperhidrosis [37].

KHE can exhibit dramatic episodes of tumour growth in response to infectious, inflammatory and traumatic stimuli [40]. As the lesion expands, it infiltrates through local tissues, muscles and occasionally bone, which can greatly impair the structure and function of the affected area. These episodes of acute growth often correlate with the rapid consumption of platelets and fibrinogen and the destruction of red blood cells as part of a systemic bleeding diathesis, KMP, described in more detail later. Approximately 50–70% of cases are complicated by KMP [34,41]. In these cases, rapidly establishing a clinical diagnosis and promptly initiating a treatment plan is essential given the life-threatening nature of KMP.

Histological examination of KHE reveals infiltrating sheets and lobules of tightly packed, spindle-shaped endothelial cells with minimal atypia and infrequent mitoses. The infiltrating pattern forms crescentic vascular spaces that entrap erythrocytes and resembles the histology of Kaposi sarcoma [42,43]. Fibrin, microthrombi, red blood cell fragments and haemosiderin granules can be found within nodular collections of the spindle-shaped endothelial cells [34,36]. The immunophenotype is negative for GLUT-1 and human herpes virus 8 (HHV8), distinguishing KHE from infantile haemangioma and Kaposi sarcoma, respectively [34]. KHE stain diffusely positive for the endothelial markers CD31, CD34, and Friend Leukemia Integration 1 transcription factor (FLI1). Lymphatic channels may be seen at the periphery or deep to the tumour, and KHE stain positively for the lymphatic markers vascular endothelial growth factor receptor-3 (VEGFR-3) and D2-40, suggesting a lymphothelial origin, but the precise aetiology is unknown [44,45].

The differential diagnosis of KHE includes other vascular malformations and tumours, such as infantile haemangioma, CH, TA (see later), Kaposiform lymphangiomatosis (see later), infantile fibrosarcoma, rhabdomyosarcoma, venous malformations, glomuvenous malformations and subcutaneous fat necrosis of the newborn [17,46–49].

The prognosis of KHE varies, and poor outcomes can occur if the tumour compresses vital structures or is complicated by KMP and uncontrolled haemorrhage. Management of these tumours depends on their size, extent and presence or absence of coagulopathy. Small and intermediate-sized lesions may be excised or, if asymptomatic, monitored clinically. Therapies for more infiltrating lesions and those complicated by KMP are discussed later. Although aggressive interventions may reduce tumour morbidity and mortality, residual tissue fibrosis and/or lymphoedema may cause chronic impairment of local function [38].

Tufted angioma

TA, also known as angioblastoma of Nakagawa, is an uncommon and slower growing variant of KHE named for its characteristic histological pattern of tufts of endothelial cells that are typically confined to the dermis [50]. The aetiology of TA is basically unknown, but similar to KHE, TA may arise from an endothelial progenitor cell with both lymphatic and blood vessel characteristics.

TA may be present at birth but more often arises in infancy or childhood, although uncommon cases of adult onset are reported as well [46,51–54]. Most of these tumours have their onset before the age of 1 year. Boys and girls are equally affected with no identified ethnic prevalence. Lesions can occur at any site but are most commonly found on the torso or proximal extremities and vary in size from a few to 20 cm. In some cases, an extremity is circumferentially involved. Although usually solitary, rare multifocal cases occur [55]. The morphology may vary from that of a vascular stain with slight induration or nodularity (Fig. 120.5) to a discrete soft tissue tumour, the former being a more common presentation. The lesions may have a pink, red, violaceous or blue colour, and focal hypertrichosis and hyperhidrosis are noted in many patients. Intermittent tenderness is very common, even in the absence of KMP [54].

The clinical presentation of an indurated vascular stain with tenderness in an infant is relatively specific for either TA or KHE, but is occasionally seen in mixed vascular malformations. Although the diagnosis may be suspected clinically, confirmation requires a skin biopsy. The prognosis of TA is not well understood, and spontaneous resolution may occur [46,53]. Many tumours have a pattern of indolent growth, eventually reaching a maximum size in early childhood. Induration and apparent fibrosis can affect limb or joint function in some cases but, similar to KHE, malignant transformation has not been reported [56].

Histology of TA shows nodules of densely packed endothelial cells that are only partially canalized and are scattered throughout the dermis in a 'cannonball' pattern. The nodules are larger and more prominent in the mid and deep dermis (Fig. 120.6). At the periphery, the vessels may appear slit-like, reminiscent of Kaposi sarcoma. Similar to KHE, dilated lymphatic vessels are commonly seen at the periphery of the tufts in TA [51]. Additionally, TA and KHE share a comparable immunophenotype consisting of negative staining for GLUT-1 and HHV8 and positive staining for CD31, CD34 and lymphatic markers D2-40 and VEGFR-3 [50].

Treatment of TA depends on size, symptomatology and whether a coagulopathy is present. Observation without intervention may be a reasonable option in some cases. Small lesions can be excised surgically. There are no uniformly accepted pharmacological agents for treating TA, but anecdotal success has been reported with interferon-α, pulsed dye laser and sirolimus. Treatment of KMP is discussed in the next section.

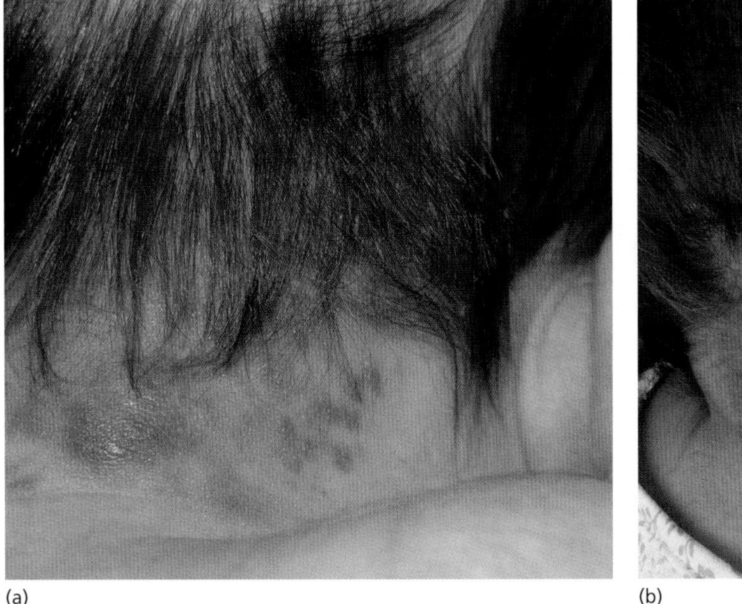
(a)

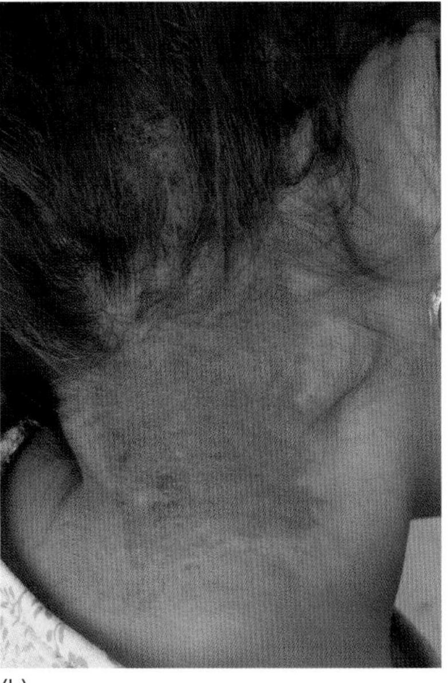
(b)

Fig. 120.5 Tufted angioma. (a) This infant presented with an uncomplicated, poorly defined reddish-blue plaque. (b) She returned a few years later complaining of persistence of the lesion and pain.

Kasabach–Merritt Phenomenon

KMP, originally described by Kasabach and Merritt in 1940, is a life-threatening bleeding diathesis associated with a rapidly enlarging KHE or TA. KMP consists of severe thrombocytopenia (platelets often <20 000/μL), hypofibrinogenaemia (often <1 g/L), microangiopathic haemolytic anaemia, and consumptive coagulopathy [57]. Although for decades KMP was widely accepted as a complication of infantile haemangiomas, it is now understood to be specific to KHE and TA [40,58]. The unique expansion of abnormal lymphoepithelial cells likely results in a prothrombotic intravascular microenvironment that manifests as KMP. Rare cases of similar bleeding diatheses have been reported in haemangiopericytomas and other lymphoepithelial neoplasms such as Kaposi sarcoma [59–61]. Fulminant KMP carries an associated mortality risk of 10–30%, often related to the development of uncontrolled haemorrhage, high-output cardiac failure and shock [62].

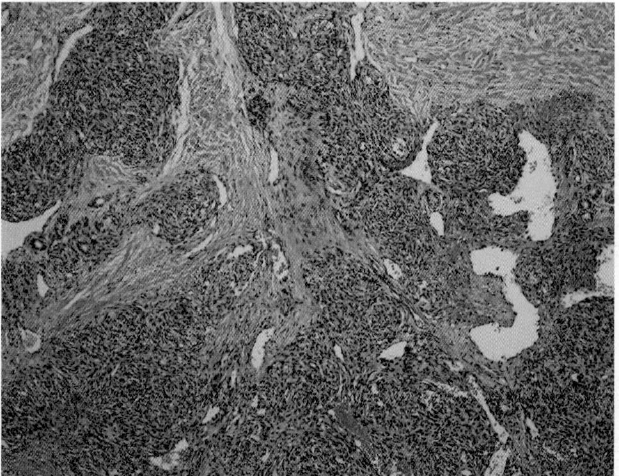

Fig. 120.6 Histology of tufted angioma demonstrates nodules of spindle-shaped endothelial cells in the mid to deep dermis (×10). Source: Photomicrograph courtesy of Dr Lori Prok.

KMP may occur at birth but more frequently presents in early infancy. It occurs equally in males and females, favours lesions of the extremities, trunk and retroperitoneum, and usually occurs in a solitary tumour that may be quite large [63]. As discussed previously, the associated tumours, KHE and TA, virtually never have a 'strawberry-like' appearance, but may have an overlying vascular pink, red, violaceous or red–brown stain. Clinical features suggesting the possibility of KMP are a violaceous, tender, rapidly enlarging, deep dermal and subcutaneous nodule or plaque. Additional clues are petechiae and ecchymoses surrounding the tumour (Fig. 120.7a). In many cases, the tumour enlarges rapidly, acquiring a woody consistency and haemorrhagic discoloration of the overlying skin, suggestive of cellulitis. The haemorrhagic lesions are restricted initially to the area of the tumour but subsequently become more widespread as the body is systemically depleted of platelets and fibrinogen.

When KHE or TA are suspected, haematological evaluation for KMP should be undertaken promptly. The most sensitive tests for detecting an associated coagulopathy are the platelet count and the fibrinogen level. Platelet counts may initially be only slightly decreased, but can drop as low as 3000–5000/μL as the tumour expands. A microangiopathic haemolytic anaemia, with evidence of fragmented red blood cells on peripheral blood smear, is often present [64,65]. D-dimers are frequently elevated. Prothrombin time (PT) and activated partial thromboplastin time (PTT) may be elevated but may be relatively less altered than the platelet count and fibrinogen level.

The thrombocytopenia of KMP has been attributed to sequestration and destruction of platelets within the expanding vascular mass [66]. Blood flow is markedly more turbulent and prone to stasis throughout the lesion.

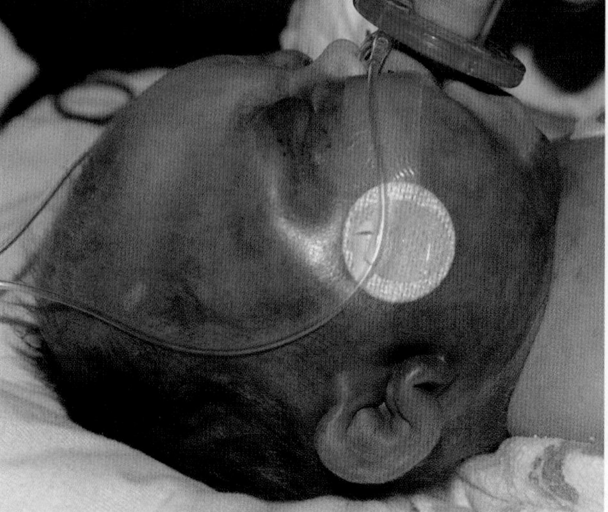

(a)

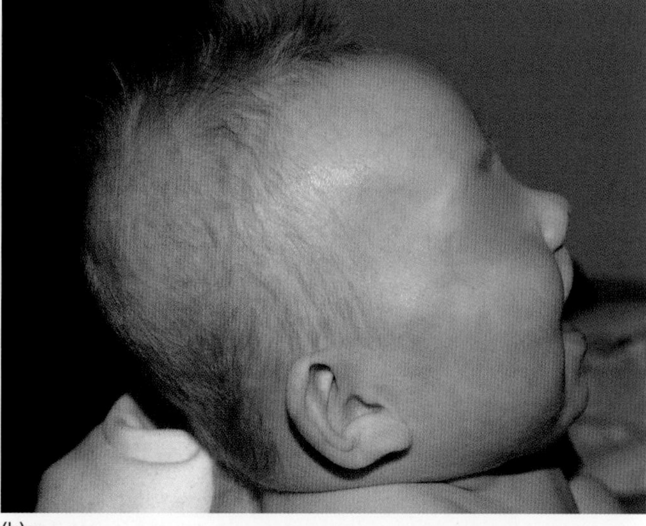

(b)

Fig. 120.7 Kasabach–Merritt phenomenon. (a) This infant had a large and poorly defined tumour involving the head and neck with associated thrombocytopenia and coagulopathy. Note the indurated swelling and cutaneous haemorrhage. (b) Treatment included supportive care, steroids and sirolimus, leading to an excellent outcome, shown here at 5 months of age.

The lymphoepithelial architecture likely contributes to a state of continuous hyperfibrinolysis; however, a clear mechanism for this has yet to be defined. KMP must be distinguished from the coagulopathy which can occur with CH, large venous and mixed venous–lymphatic malformations, and other vascular anomalies [67]. In contrast to KMP, the coagulopathy associated with venous malformations is characterized by localized intravascular coagulation (rather than platelet trapping) within the malformation, leading to consumption of clotting factors, elevated D-dimers, prolonged PT and PTT, with either normal or mildly decreased platelets [68].

The diagnosis of KMP is often established on the basis of the clinical presentation and the associated laboratory and imaging abnormalities. When the diagnosis of the underlying lesion is less clear, incisional biopsy for histological and immunohistochemical evaluation is recommended. Although tumour biopsy remains the gold standard to diagnose the primary lesion and exclude malignant tumours, the risk of severe bleeding in the setting of KMP may preclude this option.

MRI is helpful in delineating the extent and invasiveness of the underlying vascular tumour and may also help in the diagnosis of KMP. KHE and TA associated with KMP typically undergo periods of rapid growth and invade through multiple tissue planes, with cutaneous and subcutaneous thickening and oedema. KHE and TA enhance with gadolinium on T1-weighted MRI and are hyperintense on T2 MRI [69,70]. Lesions are less well circumscribed than infantile haemangiomas and peripheral haemorrhage may be evident. Intramuscular and bony involvement is more common, and superficial feeding and draining vessels are less common than with infantile haemangioma [71].

The majority of infants with KMP survive, but mortality is as high as 10–30% in some published series [63,66]. Less symptomatic patients recover with inconspicuous or mild cutaneous residua after the temporary crisis of platelet trapping and coagulopathy has resolved. However, a significant minority continue to have long-term or permanent sequelae with persistent residual tumour, residual fibrosis, and/or lymphoedema, which can affect muscle and joint function [38,60].

Therapeutic options

Management depends on the severity of the coagulopathy and severity of functional impairment. No single therapy is uniformly effective in all cases, but supportive and preventative care to maintain haemodynamic stability remains vital to patient survival. Young infants who are not yet ambulating usually tolerate mild to moderate thrombocytopenia relatively well and may be managed with close monitoring of their haematological status. However, patients with rapidly enlarging tumours and severe thrombocytopenia are at significant risk for systemic haemorrhagic complications and require aggressive intervention to rapidly reverse the coagulopathy.

Although platelet levels may dramatically fall, platelet transfusions can actually worsen the condition and should only be used if active bleeding is occurring or prior to operative procedures [72]. Cryoprecipitate and fresh-frozen plasma can be used to improve fibrinogen levels. Consider transfusion of cryoprecipitate with evidence of active bleeding, prior to surgical procedures, and prophylactically to maintain a fibrinogen level of more than 1 g/dL. Consider the transfusion of packed red blood cells for patients with symptomatic anaemia, including tachycardia, lethargy, and poor feeding. Heparin is ineffective for KMP and may actually worsen the condition.

Historically, KHE or TA with KMP were treated with complete surgical excision, which demonstrated some efficacy to resolve haematological abnormalities rapidly [73]. However, these large and infiltrative lesions can be aggravated by trauma, and procedures risk inducing more extensive haemorrhagic complications. Therefore, first-line intervention for KMP should be directed at inducing involution of the tumour using a variety of pharmacotherapeutic agents.

Although oral corticosteroids (prednisone or prednisolone) in doses of 2–5 mg/kg per day or intravenous corticosteroids (dexamethasone) in doses of 1.6 mg/kg per day have been effective at transiently maintaining an adequate platelet count and controlling tumour growth, they are frequently ineffective as monotherapy [64,74]. A response, measured as an increase in the platelet count and fibrinogen level, should be noticed within the first two weeks of initiating corticosteroid therapy [65]. Although corticosteroids are readily accessible and easy to administer, attempts should be made to reduce cumulative exposure in infants and children. In refractory cases, high-dose methylprednisolone (30 mg/kg bolus per day for three consecutive days) has been utilized with varying efficacy [64,75].

Vincristine is a potent agent to consider with rapidly expanding KHE or TA with KMP. Often dosed at 0.05 mg/kg per week, this antimitotic chemotherapeutic agent acts to inhibit endothelial growth and angiogenesis resulting in more rapid correction of hematological parameters [76–79]. The rapidity of response varies considerably, but in one case series of 15 infants, most responded to weekly treatments within 4 weeks, with an average of 12 weeks of therapy needed. Relapses may occur, requiring either additional medications or repeated courses of vincristine [77]. Recent consensus guidelines recommend the concurrent use of vincristine and corticosteroids as first-line pharmacotherapy in the treatment of KHE with KMP [73]. Of note, vincristine is a potent vesicant, and administration requires a central venous catheter. The degree of coagulopathy and clinical status of the patient should be considered to determine the safety of catheter placement.

An increasing body of literature has demonstrated the efficacy of sirolimus, also known as rapamycin, in the acute treatment of KHE or TA with KMP. Sirolimus, an inhibitor of the mammalian target of rapamycin (mTOR), inhibits lymphoepithelial cell proliferation and angiogenesis and has shown great efficacy to normalize platelet counts rapidly and induce tumour involution [80,81]. More commonly used as a mild immunosuppressant in post solid-organ transplant patients, the safety profile of sirolimus has been well documented, and its side-effects (including neutropenia, mucositis, poor wound healing and hypertriglyceridaemia) remain manageable. For the treatment of KHE or TA with KMP, sirolimus is now recognized as a standard adjuvant second-line therapy and, recently, has been used as a first-line intervention with encouraging results (Fig. 120.7b) [82].

Platelet sequestration within a KHE or TA, provokes an uncontrolled cycle of thrombosis and hyperfibrinolysis. The adjuvant use of antiplatelet agents such as aspirin and ticlopidine has previously been thought to reduce platelet adhesion and aggregation in KMP. Case reports demonstrate the use of low-dose aspirin to enhance reduction of bulk, improve colour and perilesional function [83]. However, it remains unclear if antiplatelet therapy could actually worsen the bleeding risk in patients with KMP, and initiating antiplatelet therapy up front has fallen out of standard practice. Antiplatelet therapy continues to be utilized in long-term maintenance management and in cases of KHE or TA without KMP.

Several historical adjuvant agents that have been administered with variable success include a combination of aspirin and dipyridamole, pentoxifylline, cyclophosphamide, and the antifibrinolytic agents tranexamic acid and ε-aminocaproic acid [84–87]. There remains little published data on the efficacy of these medications as mono- or multiagent therapy, likely secondary to the marked variability in protocols used and small cohorts of patients within each regimen. Large vessel tumour embolization can be considered in life-threatening lesions to control tumour size or as a preoperative treatment to diminish intraoperative bleeding [88]. Radiation therapy has also been advocated, but the long-term sequelae, including secondary malignancy and neuroendocrine dysfunction, make this modality a less acceptable choice which should be reserved for life-threatening disease if other treatments have failed [89,90]. Physical therapy may be necessary for patients with significant tumour residua or fibrosis. Compression garments may be helpful if residual lymphoedema is present.

Malignant vascular tumours

Angiosarcoma

Angiosarcoma is a rare, aggressive, malignant vascular neoplasm that typically affects adults. Cutaneous angiosarcoma is exceedingly rare in children. Reported cases are commonly associated with pre-existing conditions such as congenital hypertrophy, lymphoedema or prior radiation therapy [91]. Hepatic angiosarcoma is also quite rare but important to consider because of its strong association with infantile hepatic haemangiomas. In a recent series of eight patients, the mean age of presentation of hepatic angiosarcoma was 3 years, and seven had a history of hepatic haemangioma [92]. Cases of multifocal cutaneous haemangiomas with liver involvement and subsequent transformation to hepatic angiosarcoma are also reported [93,94]. The apparent recurrence (based on clinical symptoms or imaging findings) of hepatic vascular tumours after successful treatment should prompt evaluation for hepatic angiosarcoma. The overall prognosis is poor with liver transplant being the only modality linked to long-term survival.

Provisionally unclassified vascular anomalies

Key points

- **Multifocal lymphangioendotheliomatosis is a vascular disorder affecting the skin and gastrointestinal tract that is associated with variable thrombocytopenia.**
- **Kaposiform lymphangiomatosis exhibits features of both lymphatic neoplasia and malformation. It should be considered in patients with suspected KHE who also demonstrate a diffuse lymphatic disease pattern, bony lytic lesions or haemorrhagic effusions.**

Multifocal lymphangioendotheliomatosis (cutaneovisceral angiomatosis) with thrombocytopenia

Multifocal lymphangioendotheliomatosis (also known as cutaneovisceral angiomatosis) with thrombocytopenia (MLT/CAT) is a vascular disorder affecting various organs associated with fluctuating degrees of thrombocytopenia. Classically, the skin and gastrointestinal tract are involved [95,96]. Although cutaneous manifestations of MLT/CAT are present in most patients, a subgroup of patients may lack skin involvement [97].

The cutaneous lesions are present at birth and appear as multifocal, discrete, red–brown to burgundy papules, plaques and nodules, ranging in size from a few millimetres to several centimetres (Fig. 120.8a) [95,96]. A dominant large plaque is present in some patients. The number of lesions ranges from a few to hundreds. The trunk and extremities are more commonly involved. Gastrointestinal lesions present with haematemesis and/or melaena, usually early in infancy. The endoscopic appearance reveals several to numerous small vascular lesions of the mucosa of the gastrointestinal tract [95]. These lesions are usually slightly raised, 0.1–1 cm in size with indistinct margins and can ooze blood unprovoked [95]. Additional anatomical sites of involvement include lung, bone, liver, brain, bone, synovium and muscle. Pulmonary nodules often present with cough and/or haemoptysis. In the subpleural location, they appear as red and purple nodules by thoracoscopy. The course of lesions throughout the body can be progressive and increasing in number, static or regress with time [95,96].

Thrombocytopenia most commonly presents in the first month of life. It is usually sustained with an average platelet count of 50 000–100 000/μL. During disease exacerbations, infection or procedures, the platelet count may be <10 000/μL. Fibrinogen levels are normal and D-dimer levels are not detectable [95].

Histology of MLT/CAT reveals dilated thin-walled, blood-filled vascular channels and variable endothelial hyperplasia with most lesions displaying intraluminal

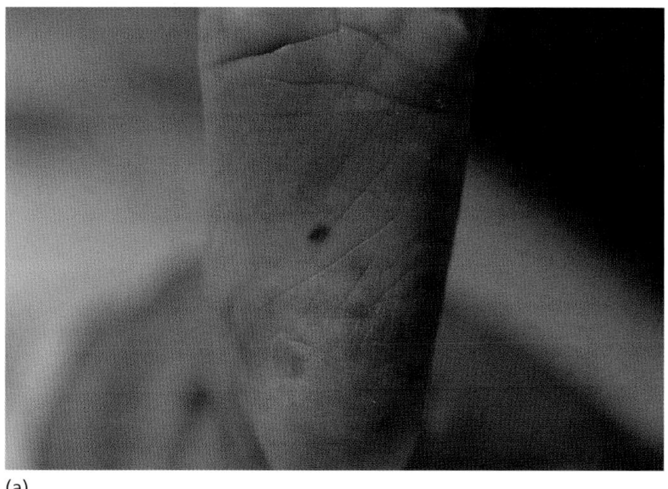
(a)

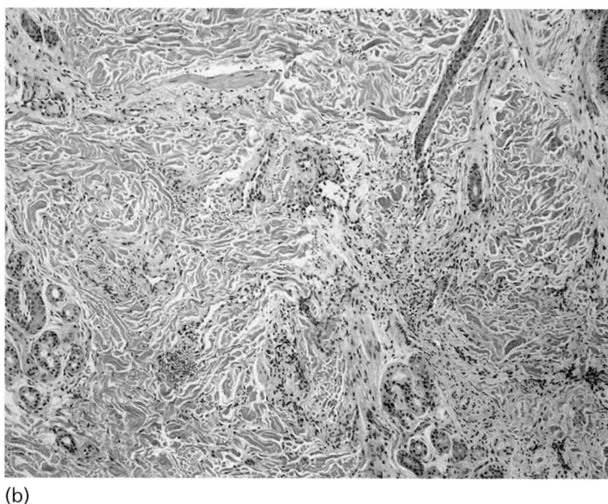
(b)

Fig. 120.8 Lymphangioendotheliomatosis. (a) This infant presented with a limited number of small, reddish-brown cutaneous papules and recurrent gastrointestinal bleeding and anaemia. (b) Histopathology showed small, ectatic, thin-walled vessels haphazardly scattered throughout the reticular dermis. The vessels are lined by hobnailed endothelium with focal intraluminal papillary projections. The endothelium was positive for lymphatic vessel endothelial hyaluronan receptor-1 and CD31 was negative for D2-40 (not shown). Source: Photomicrograph courtesy of Dr Soheil Sam Dadras.

papillary projections (Fig. 120.8b) [95,96]. The microvasculature appears dilated. The endothelial nuclei are elongated, round, crescentic or hobnailed. Immunostaining shows strong endothelial positivity for CD34 and lymphatic vessel endothelial hyaluronan receptor-1 (LYVE-1). GLUT-1 immunostaining is negative.

MRI and computed tomography are used to document the extent of disease in patients with MLT/CAT. MRI of the larger cutaneous lesions shows enhancement on T1 sequences and hyperintensity on T2 sequences [95]. Pulmonary nodules also exhibit enhancement. Lytic bone lesions can be seen with plain films.

Management of patients with MLT/CAT is supportive. Blood and platelets are administered for anaemia, bleeding and thrombocytopenia. Treatment strategies are not well established because of phenotypic variation and rarity of the disease. There is no clear pharmacological agent of choice. Corticosteroids, vincristine and interferon-alpha have all been tried [95,96]. Sirolimus has ameliorated blood and platelet transfusion requirements in some patients with CAT. In addition, some vascular lesions have resolved or partially responded to sirolimus, leading to clinical improvement in a small group of patients [98]. Bevacizumab ameliorated gastrointestinal bleeding for one patient [99].

MLT/CAT must be distinguished from other multifocal vascular diseases that affect the skin and viscera. These include multiple infantile haemangiomas, CH, and multifocal venous malformations (blue-rubber bleb nevus syndrome). Histological and immunohistochemical analysis of tissue biopsies is helpful when differentiating these lesions.

The clinical spectrum and course of MLT/CAT is wide, making its natural history and outcomes variable. For some patients, MLT/CAT may be lethal because of bleeding complications or intracranial hemorrhage [100]. In other cases, it is indolent or slowly progressive [95].

Kaposiform lymphangiomatosis

Kaposiform lymphangiomatosis (KLA) is a recently defined vascular anomaly that exhibits features of both lymphatic neoplasia and malformation. Although the primary lesion can aggressively infiltrate through local tissues, similar to KHE or TA, KLA shares more similarities with generalized lymphatic anomaly, including the diffuse proliferation of abnormal lymphatic vessels at multiple sites, often complicated by consumptive coagulopathy [49,101]. In the largest series reported to date, the most common presenting findings were respiratory symptoms, bleeding and subcutaneous mass, and thoracic cavity, bones and spleen are affected [49]. Individuals with intrathoracic KLA often demonstrate haemorrhagic pleural and/or pericardial effusions with a high risk for morbidity and mortality. Appropriate diagnosis requires physical examination, imaging, laboratory evaluation and, when possible, pathological biopsy analysis. The diagnosis of KLA should be considered in any patient with suspected KHE who also demonstrates a more diffuse and lymphatic disease pattern, bony lytic lesions or haemorrhagic effusions. While the study and treatment of KLA remains in its infancy, current approaches to management mimic the acute pharmacotherapy utilized to treat aggressive KHE, including corticosteroids, vincristine and sirolimus [82].

References

1 **ISSVA Classification of Vascular Anomalies. ©2018 International Society for the Study of Vascular Anomalies. Available at: issva.org/classification. Accessed December 14, 2018.**

2 Marler JJ, Fishman SJ, Upton J et al. Prenatal diagnosis of vascular anomalies. J Pediatr Surg 2002;37:318–26.

3 Boon LM, Enjolras O, Mulliken JB. Congenital hemangioma: evidence of accelerated involution. J Pediatr 1996;128:329–35.

4 **North PE, Waner M, James CA et al. Congenital nonprogressive hemangioma: a distinct clinicopathologic entity unlike infantile hemangioma. Arch Dermatol 2001;137:1607–20.**

5 **Enjolras O, Mulliken JB, Boon LM et al. Noninvoluting congenital hemangioma: a rare cutaneous vascular anomaly. Plast Reconstr Surg 2001;107:1647–54.**

6 Nasseri E, Piram M, McCuaig CC et al. Partially involuting congenital hemangiomas: a report of 8 cases and review of the literature. J Am Acad Dermatol 2014;70:75–9.

7 **Ayturk UM, Couto JA, Hann S et al. Somatic activating mutations in GNAQ and GNA11 are associated with congenital hemangioma. Am J Human Genet 2016;98:789–95.**

8 Funk T, Lim Y, Kulungowski AM et al. Symptomatic congenital hemangioma and congenital hemangiomatosis associated with a somatic activating mutation in GNA11. JAMA Dermatol 2016;152: 1015–20.

9 Lim YH, Bacchiocchi A, Qiu J et al. GNA14 somatic mutation causes congenital and sporadic vascular tumors by MAPK activation. Am J Human Genet 2016;99:443–50.

10 Mulliken JB, Bischoff J, Kozakewich HP. Multifocal rapidly involuting congenital hemangioma: a link to chorangioma. Am J Med Genet A. 2007;143A:3038–46.

11 Mulliken JB, Enjolras O. Congenital hemangiomas and infantile hemangioma: missing links. J Am Acad Dermatol 2004;50:875–82.

12 **Berenguer B, Mulliken JB, Enjolras O et al. Rapidly involuting congenital hemangioma: clinical and histopathologic features. Pediatr Dev Pathol 2003;6:495–510.**

13 Bonifazi E, Cutrone M. Unusually large patch-type noninvoluting congenital hemangioma of the shoulder: a report of two cases. Pediatr Dermatol 2015;32:710–3.

14 Christison-Lagay ER, Burrows PE, Alomari A et al. Hepatic hemangiomas: subtype classification and development of a clinical practice algorithm and registry. J Pediatr Surg 2007;42:62–7; discussion 7–8.

15 Kulungowski AM, Alomari AI, Chawla A et al. Lessons from a liver hemangioma registry: subtype classification. J Pediatr Surg 2012;47: 165–70.

16 Baselga E, Cordisco MR, Garzon M et al. Rapidly involuting congenital haemangioma associated with transient thrombocytopenia and coagulopathy: a case series. Br J Dermatol 2008;158:1363–70.

17 Rangwala S, Wysong A, Tollefson MM et al. Rapidly involuting congenital hemangioma associated with profound, transient thrombocytopenia. Pediatr Dermatol 2014;31:402–4.

18 Liang MG, Frieden IJ. Infantile and congenital hemangiomas. Semin Pediatr Surg 2014;23:162–7.

19 Maguiness S, Uihlein LC, Liang MG et al. Rapidly involuting congenital hemangioma with fetal involution. Pediatr Dermatol 2015;32: 321–6.

20 **Lee PW, Frieden IJ, Streicher JL et al. Characteristics of noninvoluting congenital hemangioma: a retrospective review. J Am Acad Dermatol 2014;70:899–903.**

21 Gorincour G, Kokta V, Rypens F et al. Imaging characteristics of two subtypes of congenital hemangiomas: rapidly involuting congenital hemangiomas and non-involuting congenital hemangiomas. Pediatr Radiol 2005;35:1178–85.

22 Elia D, Garel C, Enjolras O et al. Prenatal imaging findings in rapidly involuting congenital hemangioma of the skull. Ultrasound Obstet Gynecol 2008;31:572–5.

23 Boon LM, Fishman SJ, Lund DP, Mulliken JB. Congenital fibrosarcoma masquerading as congenital hemangioma: report of two cases. J Pediatr Surg 1995;30:1378–81.

24 Weiss SW, Enzinger FM. Spindle cell hemangioendothelioma. A low-grade angiosarcoma resembling a cavernous hemangioma and Kaposi's sarcoma. Am J Surg Pathol 1986;10:521–30.

25 **Perkins P, Weiss SW. Spindle cell hemangioendothelioma. An analysis of 78 cases with reassessment of its pathogenesis and biologic behavior. Am J Surg Pathol 1996;20:1196–204.**

26 Wang L, Gao T, Wang G. Expression of Prox1, D2-40, and WT1 in spindle cell hemangioma. J Cutan Pathol 2014;41:447–50.

27 Kurek KC, Pansuriya TC, van Ruler MA et al. R132C IDH1 mutations are found in spindle cell hemangiomas and not in other vascular tumors or malformations. Am J Pathol 2013;182:1494–500.

28 Lim YH, Douglas SR, Ko CJ et al. Somatic activating RAS mutations cause vascular tumors including pyogenic granuloma. J Invest Dermatol 2015;135:1698–700.

29 Groesser L, Peterhof E, Evert M et al. BRAF and RAS mutations in sporadic and secondary pyogenic granuloma. J Invest Dermatol 2016;136:481–6.

30 Sammut SJ, Tomson N, Corrie P. Pyogenic granuloma as a cutaneous adverse effect of vemurafenib. N Engl J Med. 2014;371:1265–7.

31 Henning B, Stieger P, Kamarachev J et al. Pyogenic granuloma in patients treated with selective BRAF inhibitors: another manifestation of paradoxical pathway activation. Melanoma Res 2016;26:304–7.

32 Blackwell MG, Itinteang T, Chibnall AM et al. Expression of embryonic stem cell markers in pyogenic granuloma. J Cutan Pathol 2016;43: 1096–101.

33 **Pagliai KA, Cohen BA. Pyogenic granuloma in children. Pediatr Dermatol 2004;21:10–3.**

34 Lyons LL, North PE, Mac-Moune Lai F et al. Kaposiform hemangioendothelioma: a study of 33 cases emphasizing its pathologic, immunophenotypic, and biologic uniqueness from juvenile hemangioma. Am J Surg Pathol 2004;28:559–68.

35 **Croteau SE, Liang MG, Kozakewich HP et al. Kaposiform hemangioendothelioma: atypical features and risks of Kasabach-Merritt phenomenon in 107 referrals. J Pediatr 2013;162:142–7.**

36 Zukerberg LR, Nickoloff BJ, Weiss SW. Kaposiform hemangioendothelioma of infancy and childhood. An aggressive neoplasm associated with Kasabach–Merritt syndrome and lymphangiomatosis. Am J Surg Pathol 1993;17:321–8.

37 Adams D, Frieden IJ. Tufted angioma, kaposifrom hemangioendothelioma, and the Kasabach–Merritt phernomenon. Up ToDate, Post TW (Ed), Up ToDate, Waltham, MA (accessed on December 14, 2018).

38 Enjolras O, Mulliken JB, Wassef M et al. Residual lesions after Kasabach–Merritt phenomenon in 41 patients. J Am Acad Dermatol 2000;42:225–35.

39 O'Regan GM, Irvine AD, Yao N et al. Mediastinal and neck kaposiform hemangioendothelioma: report of three cases. Pediatr Dermatol 2009;26:331–7.

40 **Enjolras O, Wassef M, Mazoyer E et al. Infants with Kasabach-Merritt syndrome do not have 'true' hemangiomas. J Pediatr 1997;130:631–40.**

41 Kelly M. Kasabach–Merritt phenomenon. Pediatr Clin North Am 2010;57:1085–9.

42 Le Huu AR, Jokinen CH, Rubin BP et al. Expression of prox1, lymphatic endothelial nuclear transcription factor, in Kaposiform hemangioendothelioma and tufted angioma. Am J Surg Pathol 2010;34: 1563–73.

43 Yuan SM, Hong ZJ, Chen HN et al. Kaposiform hemangioendothelioma complicated by Kasabach-Merritt phenomenon: ultrastructural observation and immunohistochemistry staining reveal the trapping of blood components. Ultrastruct Pathol 2013;37:452–5.

44 Debelenko LV, Perez-Atayde AR, Mulliken JB et al. D2-40 immunohistochemical analysis of pediatric vascular tumors reveals positivity in kaposiform hemangioendothelioma. Mod Pathol 2005;18:1454–60.

45 Folpe AL, Veikkola T, Valtola R, Weiss SW. Vascular endothelial growth factor receptor-3 (VEGFR-3): a marker of vascular tumors with presumed lymphatic differentiation, including Kaposi's sarcoma, kaposiform and Dabska-type hemangioendotheliomas, and a subset of angiosarcomas. Mod Pathol 2000;13:180–5.

46 Herron MD, Coffin CM, Vanderhooft SL. Tufted angiomas: variability of the clinical morphology. Pediatr Dermatol 2002;19:394–401.

47 Frieden IJ, Rogers M, Garzon MC. Conditions masquerading as infantile haemangioma: Part 2. Australas J Dermatol 2009;50:153–68; quiz 69–70.

48 Frieden IJ, Rogers M, Garzon MC. Conditions masquerading as infantile haemangioma: Part 1. Australas J Dermatol 2009;50:77–97; quiz 8.

49 Croteau SE, Kozakewich HP, Perez-Atayde AR et al. Kaposiform lymphangiomatosis: a distinct aggressive lymphatic anomaly. J Pediatr 2014;164:383–8.

50 Arai E, Kuramochi A, Tsuchida T et al. Usefulness of D2-40 immunohistochemistry for differentiation between kaposiform hemangioendothelioma and tufted angioma. J Cutan Pathol 2006;33:492–7.

51 Jones EW, Orkin M. Tufted angioma (angioblastoma). A benign progressive angioma, not to be confused with Kaposi's sarcoma or low-grade angiosarcoma. J Am Acad Dermatol 1989;20:214–25.

52 Satter EK, Graham BS, Gibbs NF. Congenital tufted angioma. Pediatr Dermatol 2002;19:445–7.

53 Browning J, Frieden I, Baselga E et al. Congenital, self-regressing tufted angioma. Arch Dermatol 2006;142:749–51.

54 Wong SN, Tay YK. Tufted angioma: a report of five cases. Pediatr Dermatol 2002;19:388–93.

55 Maronn M, Chamlin S, Metry D. Multifocal tufted angiomas in 2 infants. Arch Dermatol 2009;145:847–8.

56 Catteau B, Enjolras O, Delaporte E et al. Sclerosing tufted angioma. Apropos of 4 cases involving lower limbs. Ann Dermatol Venereol 1998;125:682–7.

57 Kasabach HH MK. Capillary hemangioma with extensive purpura: report of a case. Am J Dis Child 1940;59:1063.

58 Sarkar M, Mulliken JB, Kozakewich HP et al. Thrombocytopenic coagulopathy (Kasabach-Merritt phenomenon) is associated with Kaposiform hemangioendothelioma and not with common infantile hemangioma. Plast Reconstr Surg 1997;100:1377–86.

59 Chung KC, Weiss SW, Kuzon WM, Jr. Multifocal congenital hemangiopericytomas associated with Kasabach–Merritt syndrome. Br J Plast Surg 1995;48:240–2.

60 Mac-Moune Lai F, To KF, Choi PC et al. Kaposiform hemangioendothelioma: five patients with cutaneous lesion and long follow-up. Mod Pathol 2001;14:1087–92.

61 Sondel PM, Ritter MW, Wilson DG, Lieberman LM. Use of 111In platelet scans in the detection and treatment of Kasabach–Merritt syndrome. J Pediatr 1984;104:87–9.

62 Mulliken JB, Anupindi S, Ezekowitz RA, Mihm MC, Jr. Case records of the Massachusetts General Hospital. Weekly clinicopathological exercises. Case 13-2004. A newborn girl with a large cutaneous lesion, thrombocytopenia, and anemia. N Engl J Med. 2004;350:1764–75.

63 Maguiness S, Guenther L. Kasabach–Merritt syndrome. J Cutan Med Surg 2002;6:335–9.

64 Rodriguez V, Lee A, Witman PM, Anderson PA. Kasabach–Merritt phenomenon: case series and retrospective review of the Mayo clinic experience. J Pediatr Hematol Oncol 2009;31:522–6.

65 Ryan C, Price V, John P et al. Kasabach–Merritt phenomenon: a single centre experience. Eur J Haematol 2010;84:97–104.

66 Hall GW. Kasabach–Merritt syndrome: pathogenesis and management. Br J Haematol 2001;112:851–62.

67 Mazoyer E, Enjolras O, Laurian C et al. Coagulation abnormalities associated with extensive venous malformations of the limbs: differentiation from Kasabach–Merritt syndrome. Clin Lab Haematol 2002;24:243–51.

68 Dompmartin A, Acher A, Thibon P et al. Association of localized intravascular coagulopathy with venous malformations. Arch Dermatol 2008;144:873–7.

69 Gruman A, Liang MG, Mulliken JB et al. Kaposiform hemangioendothelioma without Kasabach–Merritt phenomenon. J Am Acad Dermatol 2005;52:616–22.

70 Fernandez Y, Bernabeu-Wittel M, Garcia-Morillo JS. Kaposiform hemangioendothelioma. Eur J Intern Med 2009;20:106–13.

71 Konez O, Burrows PE. Magnetic resonance of vascular anomalies. Magn Reson Imaging Clin N Am 2002;10:363–88, vii.

72 Phillips WG, Marsden JR. Kasabach–Merritt syndrome exacerbated by platelet transfusion. J R Soc Med 1993;86:231–2.

73 Drolet BA, Trenor CC, 3rd, Brandao LR et al. Consensus-derived practice standards plan for complicated Kaposiform hemangioendothelioma. J Pediatr 2013;163:285–91.

74 Esterly NB. Kasabach–Merritt syndrome in infants. J Am Acad Dermatol 1983;8:504–13.

75 Ozsoylu S. Megadose methylprednisolone for Kasabach–Merritt syndrome. Eur J Pediatr 2003;162:562; author reply 3–4.

76 Wang Z, Li K, Yao W et al. Steroid-resistant kaposiform hemangioendothelioma: a retrospective study of 37 patients treated with vincristine and long-term follow-up. Pediatr Blood Cancer 2015;62:577–80.

77 Haisley-Royster C, Enjolras O, Frieden IJ et al. Kasabach–Merritt phenomenon: a retrospective study of treatment with vincristine. J Pediatr Hematol Oncol 2002;24:459–62.

78 Fahrtash F, McCahon E, Arbuckle S. Successful treatment of kaposiform hemangioendothelioma and tufted angioma with vincristine. J Pediatr Hematol Oncol 2010;32:506–10.

79 Lopez V, Marti N, Pereda C et al. Successful management of Kaposiform hemangioendothelioma with Kasabach–Merritt phenomenon using vincristine and ticlopidine. Pediatr Dermatol 2009;26:365–6.

80 Kai L, Wang Z, Yao W et al. Sirolimus, a promising treatment for refractory Kaposiform hemangioendothelioma. J Cancer Res Clin Oncol 2014;140:471–6.

81 Jahnel J, Lackner H, Reiterer F et al. Kaposiform hemangioendothelioma with Kasabach–Merritt phenomenon: from vincristine to sirolimus. Klin Padiatr 2012;224:395–7.

82 Hammill AM, Wentzel M, Gupta A et al. Sirolimus for the treatment of complicated vascular anomalies in children. Pediatr Blood Cancer 2011;57:1018–24.

83 Javvaji S, Frieden IJ. Response of tufted angiomas to low-dose aspirin. Pediatr Dermatol 2013;30:124–7.

84 Koerper MA, Addiego JE, Jr., deLorimier AA et al.Use of aspirin and dipyridamole in children with platelet trapping syndromes. J Pediatr 1983;102:311–4.

85 de Prost Y, Teillac D, Bodemer C et al. Successful treatment of Kasabach–Merritt syndrome with pentoxifylline. J Am Acad Dermatol 1991;25:854–5.

86 Hurvitz CH, Alkalay AL, Sloninsky L et al. Cyclophosphamide therapy in life-threatening vascular tumors. J Pediatr 1986;109:360–3.

87 Warrell RP, Jr., Kempin SJ. Treatment of severe coagulopathy in the Kasabach–Merritt syndrome with aminocaproic acid and cryoprecipitate. N Engl J Med 1985;313:309–12.

88 Zhou SY, Li HB, Mao YM et al. Successful treatment of Kasabach–Merritt syndrome with transarterial embolization and corticosteroids. J Pediatr Surg 2013;48:673–6.

89 Leong E, Bydder S. Use of radiotherapy to treat life-threatening Kasabach–Merritt syndrome. J Med Imaging Radiat Oncol 2009;53: 87–91.

90 Kwok-Williams M, Perez Z, Squire R et al. Radiotherapy for life-threatening mediastinal hemangioma with Kasabach–Merritt syndrome. Pediatr Blood Cancer 2007;49:739–44.

91 Deyrup AT, Miettinen M, North PE et al. Pediatric cutaneous angiosarcomas: a clinicopathologic study of 10 cases. Am J Surg Pathol 2011;35:70–5.

92 Grassia KL, Peterman CM, Iacobas I et al. Clinical case series of pediatric hepatic angiosarcoma. Pediatr Blood Cancer 2017;64. Epub 2017, May 18.

93 Nord KM, Kandel J, Lefkowitch JH et al. Multiple cutaneous infantile hemangiomas associated with hepatic angiosarcoma: case report and review of the literature. Pediatrics 2006;118:e907–13.

94 Jeng MR, Fuh B, Blatt J et al. Malignant transformation of infantile hemangioma to angiosarcoma: response to chemotherapy with bevacizumab. Pediatr Blood Cancer 2014;61:2115–7.

95 Prasad V, Fishman SJ, Mulliken JB et al. Cutaneovisceral angiomatosis with thrombocytopenia. Pediatr Dev Pathol 2005;8:407–19.

96 North PE, Kahn T, Cordisco MR et al. Multifocal lymphangioendotheliomatosis with thrombocytopenia: a newly recognized clinicopathological entity. Arch Dermatol 2004;140:599–606.

97 Uller W, Kozakewich HP, Trenor CC et al. Cutaneovisceral angiomatosis with thrombocytopenia without cutaneous involvement. J Pediatr 2014;165:876.

98 Droitcourt C, Boccara O, Fraitag S et al. Multifocal lymphangioendotheliomatosis with thrombocytopenia: clinical features and response to Sirolimus. Pediatrics 2015;136:e517–22.

99 Kline RM, Buck LM. Bevacizumab treatment in multifocal lymphangioendotheliomatosis with thrombocytopenia. Pediatr Blood Cancer 2009;52:534–6.

100 Huang C, Rizk E, Iantosca M et al. Multifocal lymphangioendotheliomatosis with devastating intracranial hemorrhage. J Neurosurg Pediatr 2013;12:517–20.

101 Fernandes VM, Fargo JH, Saini S et al. Kaposiform lymphangiomatosis: unifying features of a heterogeneous disorder. Pediatr Blood Cancer 2015;62:901–4.

CHAPTER 121
Disorders of Lymphatics

Arin K. Greene & Jeremy A. Goss

Department of Plastic and Oral Surgery, Vascular Anomalies Center, Boston Children's Hospital, Harvard Medical School, MA, USA

Abstract

Lymphatic disorders are a group of congenital malformations that affect the lymphatic system. The lesions consist of: macrocystic/microcystic lymphatic malformation, primary lymphoedema, generalized lymphatic anomaly, Gorham–Stout disease, and overgrowth conditions associated with lymphatic malformations (CLOVES, Klippel–Trenaunay). Many lesions are caused by mutations in *PIK3CA*. Treatment is based on symptoms and the type of lymphatic disorder. Patients are typically best managed in an interdisciplinary centre focused on vascular anomalies.

Key points

- **First-line therapy for problematic macrocystic lymphatic malformations is sclerotherapy.**
- **Microcystic lymphatic malformations can be treated with resection, bleomycin, CO_2 laser or sirolimus.**
- **Definitive diagnosis of lymphoedema requires lymphoscintigraphy.**
- **Sirolimus can be used to treat problematic microcystic lymphatic malformations as well as generalized lymphatic anomaly and Gorham–Stout disease.**
- **Patients with lymphatic disorders usually are best managed in an interdisciplinary vascular anomalies centre.**

SECTION 25: VASCULAR TUMOURS

Introduction. Lymphatic malformations (LMs) are caused by genetic defects of lymphangiogenesis. There are several phenotypes of LM and most have a known mutation (Table 121.1). Although LMs are benign congenital lesions, they often do not present until childhood or adolescence and typically worsen during puberty. Morbidity is common because LMs can bleed, become infected, leak lymph fluid, obstruct vital structures and/or result in disfigurement and psychosocial distress. Phenotypes include macrocystic LM, microcystic LM, combined (macrocystic/microcystic) LM, primary lymphoedema, Gorham–Stout disease (GSD), generalized lymphatic anomaly (GLA) and LMs associated with syndromic overgrowth conditions (e.g. CLOVES [congenital lipomatosis overgrowth, vascular malformations, epidermal nevi and scoliosis] syndrome, Klippel–Trenaunay syndrome [KTS]). It is important to diagnose accurately the type of LM because each lesion has its own natural history and treatment. Patients with lymphatic disorders are usually best managed in an interdisciplinary centre focused on these diseases.

Aetiopathogenesis. Many theories exist concerning the origin of LMs: (i) disrupted lymph sacs arising in the sixth week of embryonic development; (ii) 'pinching off' of sprouting lymphatic channels from the principal lymphatic system causing abnormal collections of lymph fluid-filled spaces; (iii) aberrant budding from the lymphatic system with loss of connection to central lymph channels; or (iv) lymphatic tissues developing in anomalous locations. The cause of LM progression is also unknown. Possible mechanisms include disturbed angiogenesis, lymphangiogenesis, vasculogenesis or dilation of vascular spaces. Because lesions have a greater risk of enlargement during adolescence, pubertal hormones have been implicated in stimulating their growth [1,2]. Sporadic LMs (e.g. macrocystic, microcystic) as well as syndromes associated with LMs (CLOVES, KTS) are caused by a somatic mutation in the *PIK3CA* gene [3]. Multiple germline mutations are associated with primary (idiopathic) lymphoedema (e.g. *VEGFR3, FOXC2, SOX18, CCBE1, PTPN11/SOS1*) [4–9].

Clinical features.
Macrocystic LM
Solitary LM is characterized by the size of the malformed channels: microcystic, macrocystic or combined (macrocystic/microcystic). Although lesions are present at birth, small or deep LMs may not become evident until childhood or adolescence following enlargement. LMs are soft and compressible. Overlying skin typically appears normal but may also have a blue hue or pink–red discoloration and cutaneous vesicles. Facial lesions can lead to macroglossia, poor oral hygiene and dental caries. Periorbital LM causes reduction in vision (40%) and 7% of patients become blind in the affected eye [10].

Harper's Textbook of Pediatric Dermatology, Fourth Edition. Edited by Peter Hoeger, Veronica Kinsler and Albert Yan.

Table 121.1 Phenotypes of lymphatic disorders

Lesion	Mutation	Treatment options
Macrocystic lymphatic malformation	*PIK3CA*	Sclerotherapy Resection
Microcystic lymphatic malformation	*PIK3CA*	Resection Bleomycin injection Carbon dioxide laser Radiofrequency ablation Cutaneous cautery/ sclerotherapy Sirolimus
Combined lymphatic malformation(macrocystic and microcystic)	*PIK3CA*	Sclerotherapy Resection Bleomycin injection Carbon dioxide laser Radiofrequency ablation Cutaneous cautery/ sclerotherapy Sirolimus
Primary lymphoedema	*VEGFR3, FOXC2, SOX18, CCBE1*	Compression Liposuction
Gorham–Stout disease/ generalized lymphatic anomaly		Interferon and bisphosphonate Sirolimus
CLOVES	*PIK3CA*	Wilms tumour monitoring Resection of lipomatous lesions Treatment of vascular anomalies Orthopaedic intervention
Klippel–Trenaunay syndrome	*PIK3CA*	Leg-length monitoring Removal of embryonal veins Orthopaedic intervention Sclerotherapy Skin/subcutaneous resection

CLOVES, congenital lipomatosis overgrowth, vascular malformations, epidermal nevi and scoliosis.

Macrocystic LM is characterized by cysts large enough to be cannulated by a needle and treated with sclerotherapy (≥5mm) (Fig. 121.1). Lesions most commonly affect the neck or axilla.

Microcystic LM

Microcystic LM is defined by cysts <5mm which cannot be treated with sclerotherapy because they are too small to be cannulated by a needle (Fig. 121.2). Because they are unable to be managed by traditional sclerotherapy, microcystic disease has a worse prognosis than macrocystic LMs. Overlying skin typically is pink–red and studded with cutaneous vesicles which may leak lymph fluid (lymphorrhoea) and bleed.

Combined (macrocystic and microcystic) LM

In many cases, solitary LMs are not purely macrocystic or microcystic. Instead, lesions may contain both macro- and microcysts. A greater proportion of microcystic involvement portends a poorer prognosis.

Primary lymphoedema

Primary (idiopathic) lymphoedema affects 1/100000 persons [11] and results from aplasia or hypoplasia of the lymphatics (Fig. 121.3) [12]. The condition almost always affects the lower extremity and 50% have bilateral disease of the legs [13]. Rarely, isolated genital or upper extremity lymphoedema can occur. Boys typically present during infancy with bilateral lower extremity lymphoedema, and girls most commonly develop swelling of one leg during adolescence [13]. Adult-onset primary lymphoedema rarely can occur.

Many forms of primary lymphoedema have a familial/syndromic association (e.g. Milroy disease, Meige disease, lymphoedema–distichiasis, hypotrichosis–lymphoedema–telangiectasia syndrome, Aagenaes syndrome, Hennekam syndrome, Noonan syndrome, Turner syndrome). Milroy disease is defined by congenital lower extremity

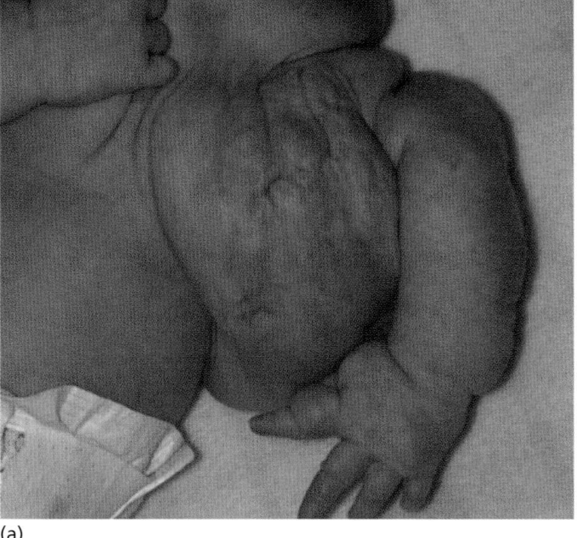
(a)

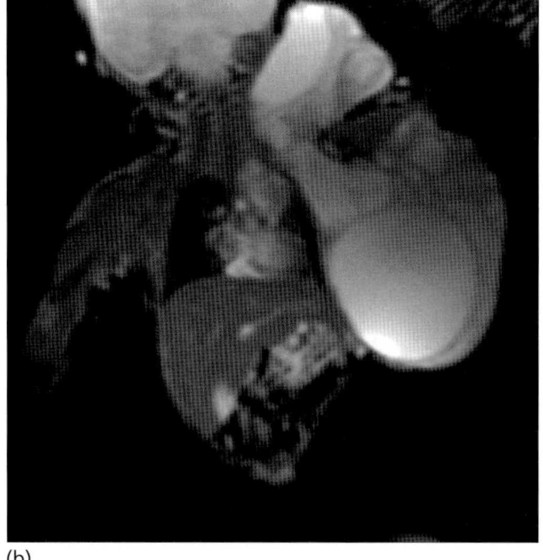
(b)

Fig. 121.1 Macrocystic lymphatic malformation. (a) This infant was born with a large lesion involving the axilla and chest. (b) Magnetic resonance image shows the large macrocysts.

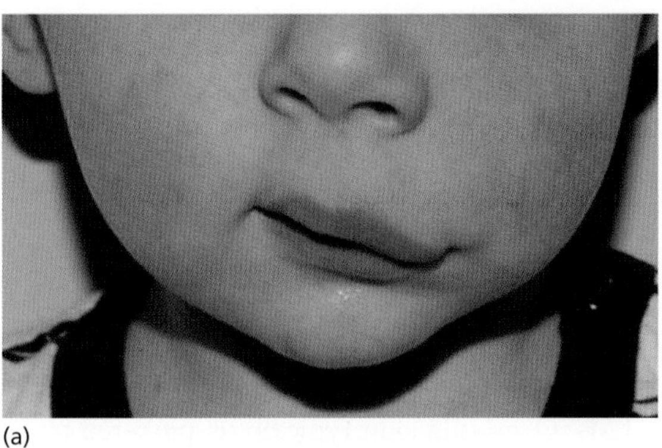
(a)

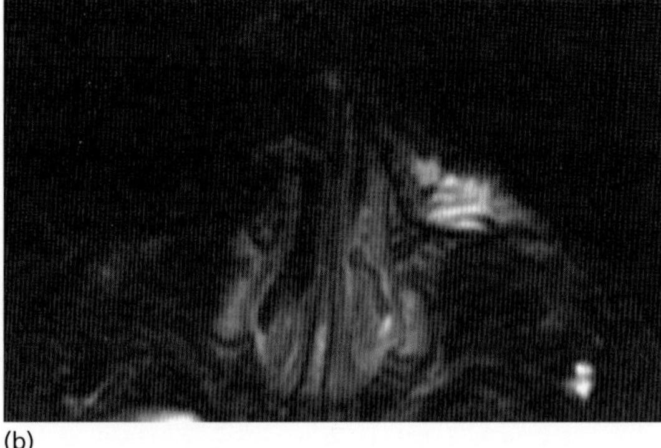
(b)

Fig. 121.2 Microcystic lymphatic malformation. (a) A young child was born with an enlarged lip and cheek. (b) Magnetic resonance image illustrates a microcystic lymphatic malformation involving the soft tissue.

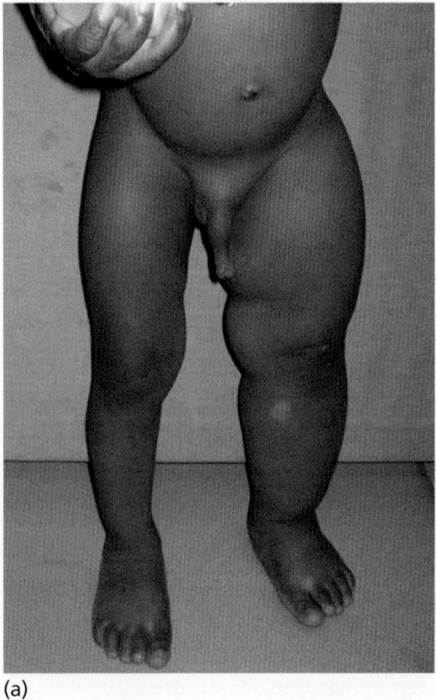
(a)

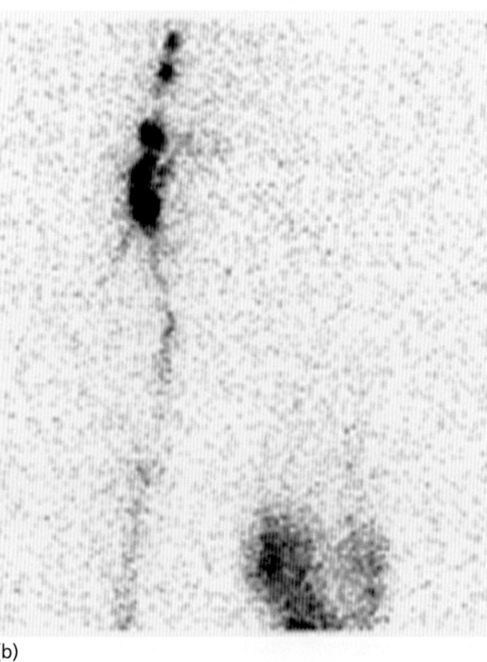
(b)

Fig. 121.3 Primary lymphoedema. (a) A child was noted to have an enlarged left lower extremity at birth. (b) Lymphoscintigraphy confirmed the diagnosis of lymphoedema by illustrating delayed transit of radiolabelled tracer to the inguinal nodes and dermal backflow of the affected leg.

lymphoedema (bilateral or unilateral) in patients with a family history of lymphoedema or a documented mutation in *VEGFR3* in the absence of a family history of the disease [14,15]. Meige disease refers to familial lymphoedema of the lower extremities presenting in adolescence. Patients with adolescent-onset lymphoedema without a family history of the disease should not be considered as having Meige disease as a mutation for this condition has not yet been identified [16,17]. Patients with lymphoedema–distichiasis inherited mutations in *FOXC2* and develop a second row of eyelashes, eyelid ptosis, and/or yellow nails in addition to lymphoedema [18]. Hypotrichosis–lymphoedema–telangiectasia is caused by dominant or recessively transmitted mutations in *SOX18* resulting in lymphoedema, sparse hair growth, and cutaneous telangiectasias [19]. Aagenaes syndrome or cholestasis lymphoedema syndrome is a rare cause of familial lymphoedema associated with intrahepatic cholestasis and lymphoedema of the lower extremities [20]. Hennekam syndrome is the result of a *CCBE1* mutation and is characterized by generalized lymphoedema with visceral involvement, developmental delay, flat faces, hypertelorism and a broad nasal bridge [21]. Patients with Noonan syndrome inherited dominant mutations in *PTPN11/SOS1* and have a 3% risk of developing lymphoedema along with intestinal lymphangiectasia and/or fetal hydrops [8,9,22]. Patients with Turner syndrome carry a 57% risk of developing lymphoedema and as many as 76% present with swelling in infancy [23].

Secondary lymphoedema is not a vascular anomaly and results from injury to lymphatic vessels or axillary/inguinal lymph nodes. The most common causes of secondary lymphoedema are: (i) radiation and/or lymphadenectomy for cancer treatment; (ii) a parasitic infection; (iii) obesity [24,25].

Over time, the diseased area increases in size because the interstitial lymphatic fluid stimulates subcutaneous fibrosis and production of adipose tissue [26,27].

Lymphoedema is a chronic condition that does not improve and slowly worsens. Lymphoedema progresses through four stages: *Stage 0* indicates a normal extremity clinically, but with abnormal lymph transport (i.e. illustrated by lymphoscintigraphy); *Stage 1* is early oedema which improves with limb elevation; *Stage 2* represents pitting oedema that does not resolve with elevation; *Stage 3* describes fibroadipose deposition and skin changes [28]. The severity of lymphoedema is categorized as mild (<20% increase in extremity volume), moderate (20–40%), or severe (>40%) [28].

The major morbidity of primary lymphoedema is lowered self-esteem because the overgrown extremity causes a deformity. Patients also have an increased risk of infection of the area. Difficulty using the extremity is rare. Patients typically have normal appearing skin although cutaneous problems such as bleeding from vesicles, hyperkeratosis and lymphorrhoea can occur. Lymphoedema is painless and ulceration is uncommon. Rarely, lymphangiosarcoma can occur.

GSD

GSD is a progressive, multifocal osteolytic lymphatic disorder (Fig. 121.4). The most common sites affected are the rib, cranium, clavicle and cervical spine. On average, seven bones are involved, and if multiple sites are affected they are contiguous. Over time bone resorption occurs which causes significant morbidity including pain and pathological fractures. The condition also has been called 'vanishing bone disease'. As many as 95% of lesions have an associated infiltrative soft tissue abnormality overlying the involved bone [15]. Forty-two percent of patients develop pleural effusions and 21% have splenic and/or hepatic lesions [29].

GLA

GLA is a multisystem disorder that involves noncontiguous areas. Eighty-five percent of patients have bony involvement and the mean number of affected bones is 30. Compared with GSD, GLA more often involves the appendicular skeleton (shoulders, pelvis, upper/lower extremities). The most commonly affected bones are rib, thoracic spine, humerus and femur. Fifty-six percent of patients have associated infiltrative soft tissue abnormalities adjacent to the bony lesions [29]. Fifty percent of patients have a macrocystic LM, 63% exhibit visceral (splenic or hepatic) lesions and 50% experience pleural effusions [29].

LM-associated overgrowth syndromes

CLOVES syndrome: CLOVES syndrome is a nonfamilial overgrowth syndrome caused by mutations in the *PIK3CA* gene (Fig. 121.5) [3]. Patients present with truncal lipomatous masses, a slow-flow vascular malformation (most commonly a capillary malformation overlying the lipomatous mass) and hand/foot anomalies (increased width, macrodactyly, first web-space 'sandal gap') [30]. Individuals also may have an arteriovenous malformation (28%), neurological impairment (50%) or scoliosis (33%) [30]. The lipomatous masses typically are painful and can infiltrate the retroperitoneum, mediastinum, paraspinal muscles and epidural space.

KTS: KTS is a capillary–lymphatic–venous malformation of an extremity that is associated with soft tissue and/or skeletal overgrowth (Fig. 121.6). The disease is caused by a mutation in PIK3CA [3]. Presentation varies greatly in KTS. Some patients experience slightly enlarged extremities with a capillary stain whereas others develop grotesquely enlarged limbs with malformed digits. KTS typically involves the lower extremity but the upper extremity and trunk can be affected. Upper extremity or truncal disease can affect the posterior mediastinum and retropleural space. The capillary malformation is distributed over the lateral side of the extremity, buttock, or thorax and is macular in the neonate but becomes studded with haemolymphatic vesicles later in life. Pelvic involvement can occur with KTS of a lower extremity; although usually asymptomatic, morbidity includes haematuria, bladder obstruction, cystitis and haematochezia. The lymphatic abnormalities are typically macrocystic in the pelvis and thighs and microcystic in the abdominal wall, buttock and distal limb.

Imaging and histopathology. Most LMs are diagnosed by history and physical examination. Small, superficial lesions do not require additional work-up. Large, deep LMs can be assessed with ultrasonography (US) or magnetic resonance imaging (MRI). Although US is not as

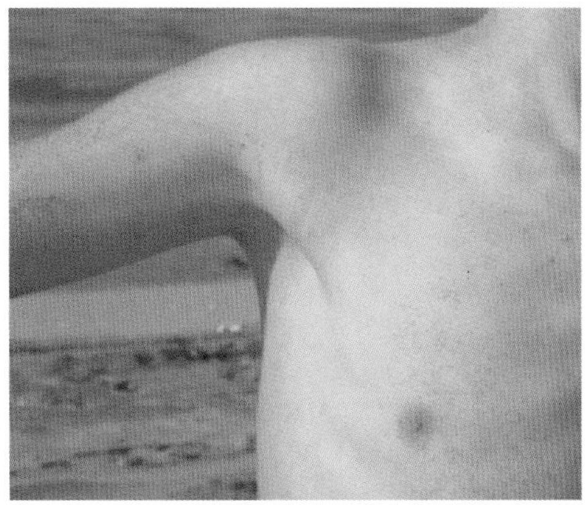
(a)

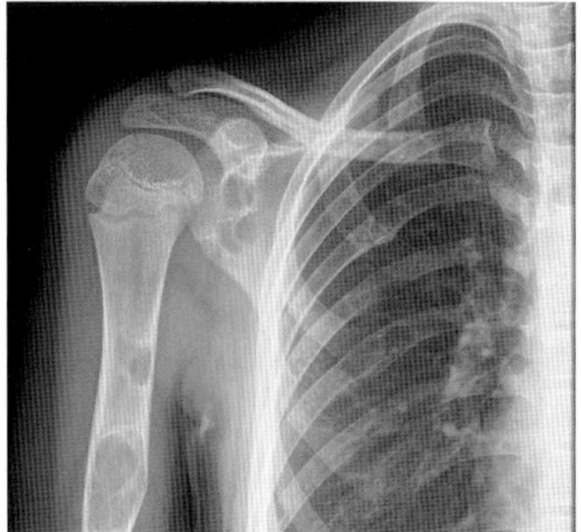
(b)

Fig. 121.4 (a) Generalized lymphatic anomaly. (b) A plain radiograph illustrates osteolytic lesions involving the humerus and scapula.

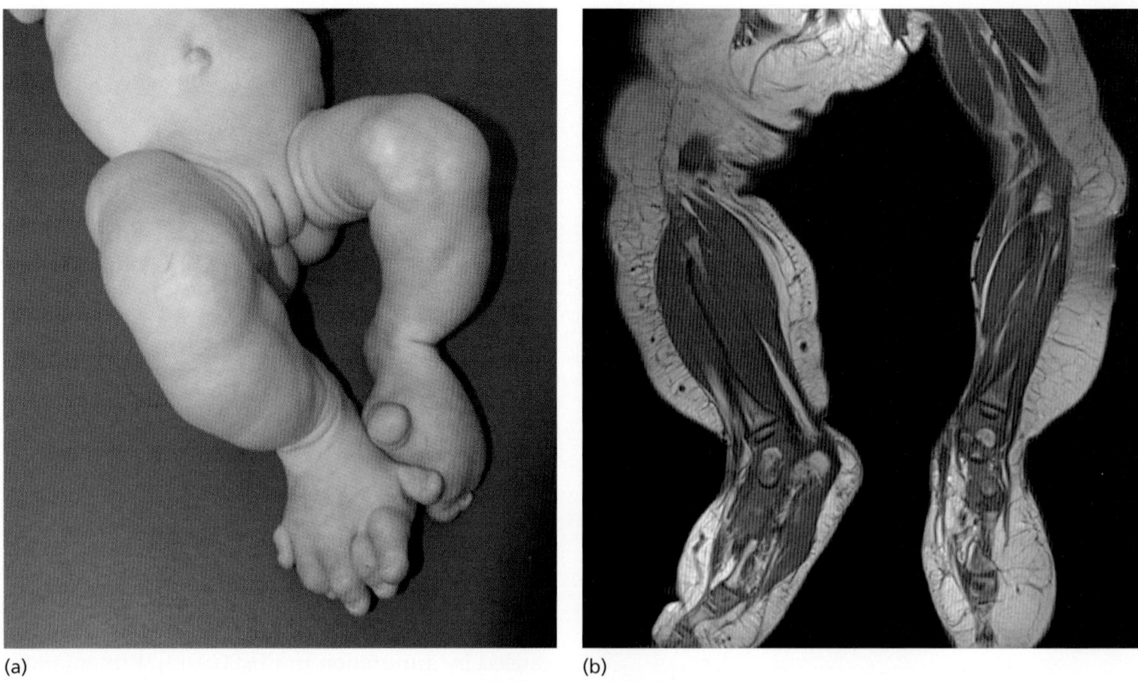

(a) (b)

Fig. 121.5 CLOVES (congenital lipomatosis overgrowth, vascular malformations, epidermal nevi and scoliosis) syndrome. (a) Young child with CLOVES syndrome. (b) Magnetic resonance image shows adipose overgrowth of the lower extremities.

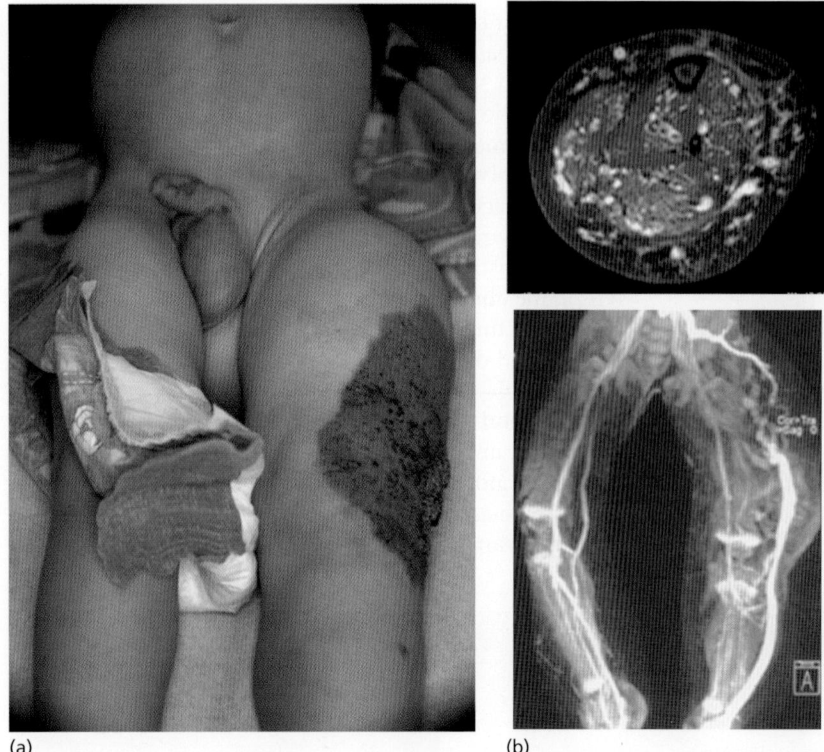

(a) (b)

Fig. 121.6 Klippel–Trenaunay syndrome. (a) The patient exhibits overgrowth of the left lower extremity with a cutaneous stain containing lymphatic vesicles. (b) Imaging shows venous and lymphatic malformations throughout all levels of the limb as well as a large lateral embryonic vein.

accurate as MRI, it can confirm the diagnosis and assess intralesional bleeding without requiring sedation in children. Macrocystic LM findings on US include anechoic cysts with septations, debris and/or fluid levels [31]. Microcystic LM exhibits poorly defined echogenic masses with diffuse involvement of adjacent tissues [31]. MRI assists in confirming the diagnosis, defining the extent of disease and planning treatment. Lesions appear hyperintense on T2-weighted images and do not show diffuse enhancement [31].

Lymphoscintigraphy is required to definitively diagnose lymphoedema. The test provides qualitative information (i.e. normal versus abnormal lymphatic function) and is 96% sensitive and 100% specific for lymphoedema [32]. Abnormal findings are delayed transit time of the radiolabelled protein to draining lymph nodes (>45 min), accumulation of tracer in cutaneous lymphatics (dermal backflow), asymmetric node uptake and/or formation of collateral lymphatic channels [33,34].

MRI is helpful in CLOVES and KTS to assess for phlebectasia or enlarged lower extremity embryonal veins which predispose patients to thromboembolic events. Individuals with CLOVES are at risk for developing Wilms tumour and require routine US examination every 3 months until age 7 [35]. In KTS, there is not an increased risk for Wilms tumour [36].

Histological confirmation of LM is rarely required. Findings include abnormally walled vascular spaces filled with many eosinophils and lymphocytes within a protein-rich fluid. D240, LYVE1, and PROX1 are lymph-specific markers which can be helpful in differentiating LMs from other vascular anomalies [37]. Compared with a solitary LM, GLA exhibits: (i) small channels, (ii) large lymphatic endothelial cells, (iii) endothelial hyperplasia, and (iv) an increased proliferation. In both GSD and GLA, histopathology reveals variably sized lymphatic channels in the medulla and cortex that are immunopositive for lymphatic markers. However, GLA exhibits greater bone formation, more marrow fibrosis and additional osteoclast/osteoblast activity compared with GSD. Histopathology is nonspecific in LM-associated overgrowth syndromes.

Management. Treatment of an LM is not mandatory. Intervention is reserved for lesions that lower self-esteem, cause pain, bleed or obstruct/destroy tissues. Resection and reconstruction should not leave a worse deformity than the LM. LMs causing significant symptoms require intervention regardless of the age of the patient. If possible, treatment should be delayed until at least 6 months of age because before this time the risks associated with anaesthesia are greater than for an adult. In addition, a young infant is less able to tolerate a procedure.

If it is likely that a patient will require a procedure to improve a deformity, intervention between 3 and 4 years of age is favorable. Because long-term memory and self-esteem begin to form at approximately 4 years of age, improving an LM prior to this time will treat the deformity before it causes psychosocial distress; the patient also may not remember the procedure. Another period to intervene is during late childhood/early adolescence when the child can communicate whether he/she would like to have a procedure. If a patient has a minor deformity or a large lesion that would require significant reconstruction, it is often best to wait until the child verbalizes the desire to be treated. If the lesion is minor, it may be possible to remove it using local anaesthesia by waiting until the patient is older. If the LM is significant, the process is facilitated for the family and surgeon if the child is a willing participant.

Macrocystic/combined LM

Macrocystic and combined LMs are managed with sclerotherapy because this technique is safer and more effective than resection (Fig. 121.7). Sclerotherapy involves the injection of an irritating substance into the lesion that causes fibrosis and shrinkage of the LM. The procedure is performed under general anaesthesia with ultrasound or fluoroscopy. Our centre prefers to inject doxycycline for LMs, but other types of sclerosants include ethanol, sodium tetradecyl sulfate and bleomycin. Asymptomatic macrocystic lesions generally should be treated because they are at risk for bleeding and infection. If a macrocyst has intralesional bleeding, then the LM can be converted to microcysts which are no longer amenable to sclerotherapy. Large, asymptomatic macrocystic LMs are treated prophylactically at 6 months of age before the lesion bleeds or becomes infected which would obviate future sclerotherapy. Sclerotherapy usually is performed at 6-week intervals until there are no cysts visible on post-treatment ultrasound that may be amenable to further injections.

Although sclerotherapy does not remove an LM, it effectively shrinks the lesion and improves symptoms. Usually the patient's symptoms are adequately alleviated and resection is unnecessary. If the individual continues to suffer morbidity following sclerotherapy, then exstirpation of the area is facilitated. Large lesions can leave behind redundant skin once they have been deflated using sclerotherapy which can be improved with resection. LMs may also have residual symptomatic microcystic disease following sclerotherapy that may necessitate excision.

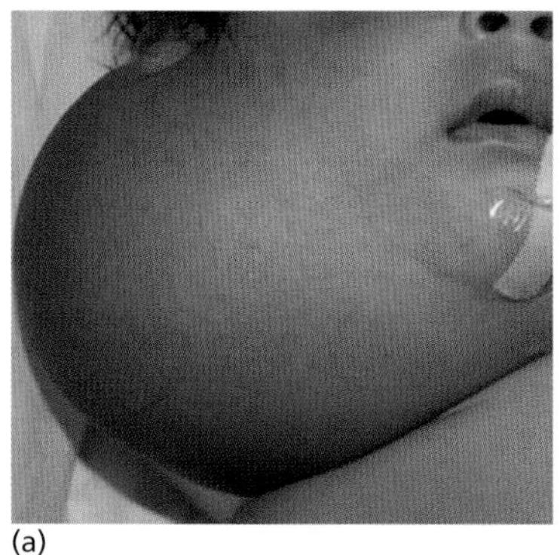
(a)

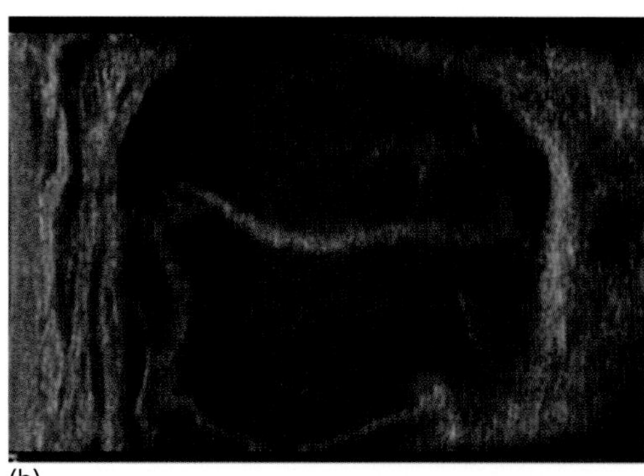
(b)

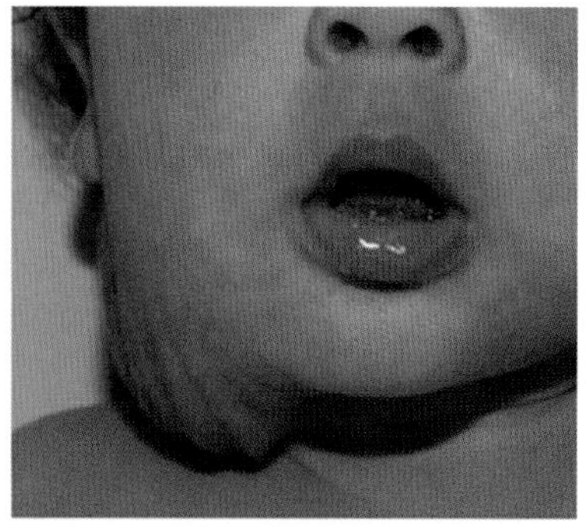
(c)

Fig. 121.7 Management of a macrocystic lymphatic malformation. (a) An infant was born with a large lesion involving the neck. (b) Ultrasound illustrates the large macrocysts. (c) He was managed with sclerotherapy which was much safer and more effective than attempting to resect the lesion. After sclerotherapy the cysts have been collapsed and the redundant skin can be excised.

Resection of a macrocystic LM is reserved for: (i) small lesions that may be completely removed for cure and (ii) symptomatic LMs that can no longer be managed with sclerotherapy (all the macrocysts have been treated). Generally, macrocystic/combined LMs should undergo sclerotherapy prior to resection because: (i) the lesion will be smaller; (ii) excision is facilitated because cysts are converted to fibrotic tissue; and (iii) peripheral vessels are permeated by the sclerosant which theoretically reduces the recurrence rate. Small lesions that can potentially be removed for cure do not require preoperative sclerotherapy.

Microcystic LM

Microcystic LM is more difficult to manage compared with macrocystic lesions. Microcystic LM usually involves the face and extremities. If the disease affects the integument, the patient may develop lymphatic vesicles which can bleed, become infected and cause lymphorrhoea. Asymptomatic microcystic LMs may be observed; intervention is reserved for problematic lesions. Generally, first-line therapy is resection (Figs 121.8 and 121.9). Localized LMs do not require preoperative imaging if only resection is planned. MRI is obtained prior to performing a resection of a large lesion to determine which surgical planes and anatomical structures are involved. Excision usually is subtotal because microcystic LMs often are diffuse and involve multiple tissue planes.

Lesions located in anatomically sensitive areas (e.g. face) should have minimal margins included in the resection. LM is not a malignancy and evidence does not show that a wide margin lowers the recurrence rate. The LM often involves a larger area than is appreciated clinically and radiographically. Intraoperatively, subcutaneous tissues can be cauterized at the periphery of the LM without removing skin. Cautery and fibrosis may destroy residual LM and reduce recurrence. If a lesion is in a non-sensitive area (e.g. abdomen) then larger margins can be taken as long as they don't complicate the exstirpation and reconstruction. Because most LMs are diffuse and involve multiple tissue planes, complete exstirpation rarely is possible. Instead, the goal usually is to alleviate symptoms and control the lesion. Despite subtotal and presumed 'complete' exstirpation, most LMs re-enlarge. Localized areas of skin involvement are best resected, but can recur along the scar. Larger regions of integument can be removed using serial excision. Wounds are reconstructed by letting them heal secondarily, mobilization of local tissues or skin grafts. Tissue expansion, regional muscle flaps, or free-flaps usually are not necessary. Patients and families are counselled that LM is likely to recur following resection and treatment may be needed in the future.

Diffuse lymphatic vesicles that are problematic to excise can be treated with carbon dioxide laser (Fig. 121.10). Alternatively, cutaneous vesicles can be managed with superficial sclerotherapy or cauterization. Intraoral lymphatic vesicles are best treated by radiofrequency ablation. This technique causes low-temperature tissue destruction which reduces damage to adjacent structures [38]. Compared with carbon dioxide laser there is less oedema, which is particularly favourable in the oral cavity because it minimizes the risk of airway obstruction.

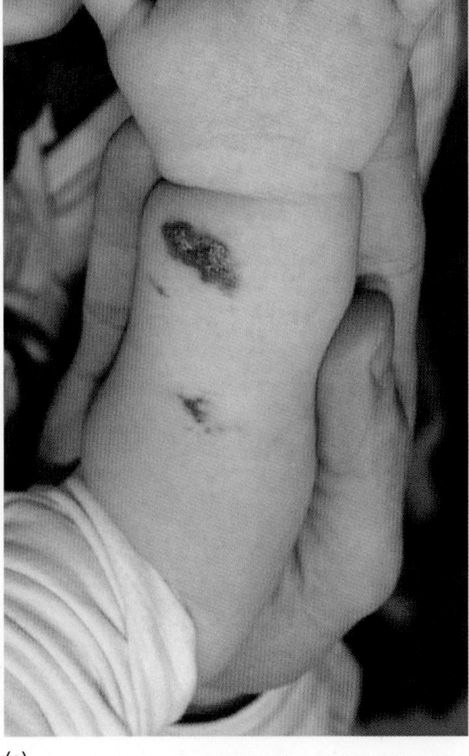
(a)

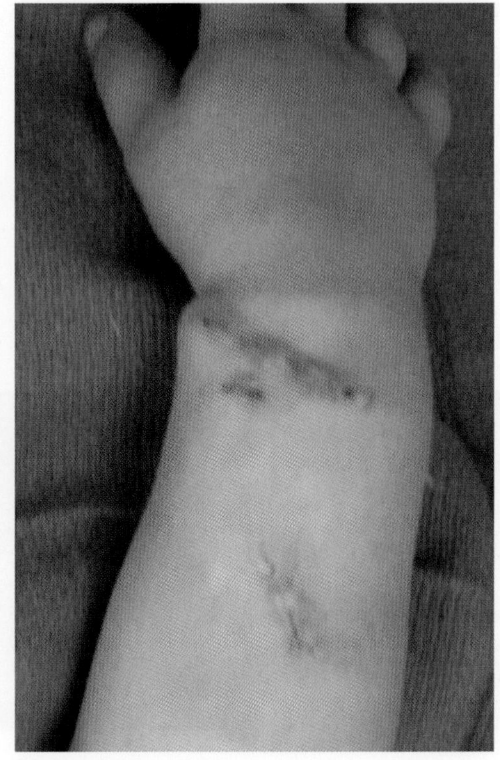
(b)

Fig. 121.8 Treatment of cutaneous microcystic lymphatic malformation by resection. (a) A child developed bleeding cutaneous lymphatic vesicles that were also causing a deformity. (b) Because the areas were localized, they were resected for potential cure.

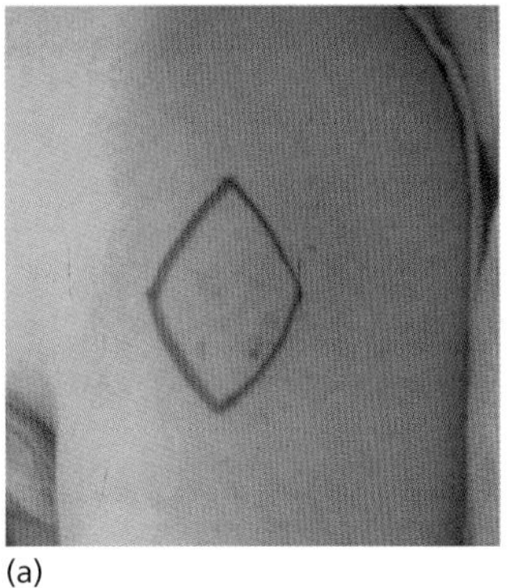

(a)

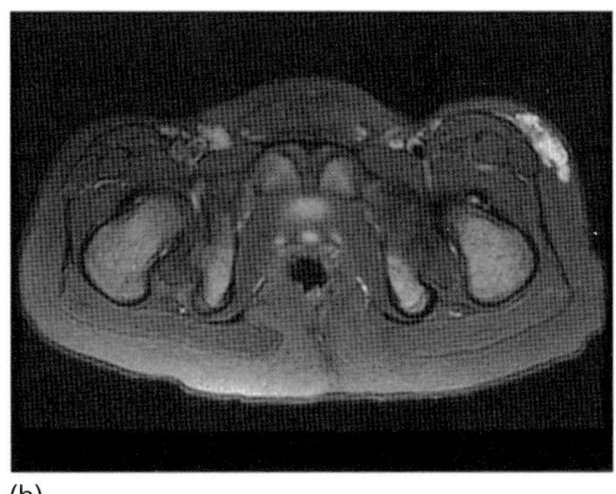

(b)

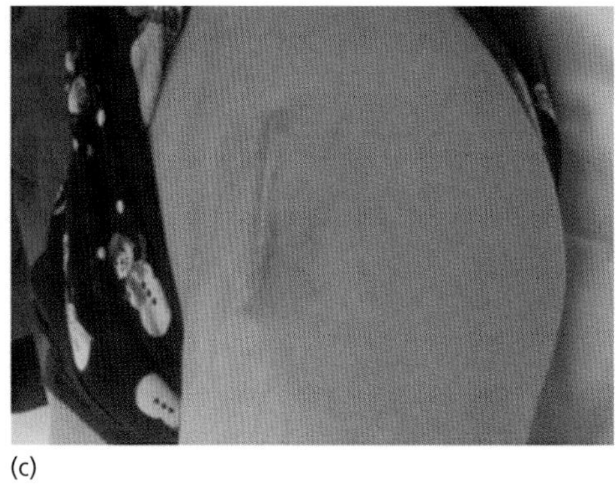

(c)

Fig. 121.9 Treatment of subcutaneous microcystic lymphatic malformation. (a) A child presented with a painful, enlarging lesion of the left leg. (b) Magnetic resonance image illustrates a primarily microcystic lymphatic malformation. (c) Because the lesion was localized, it was resected for potential cure.

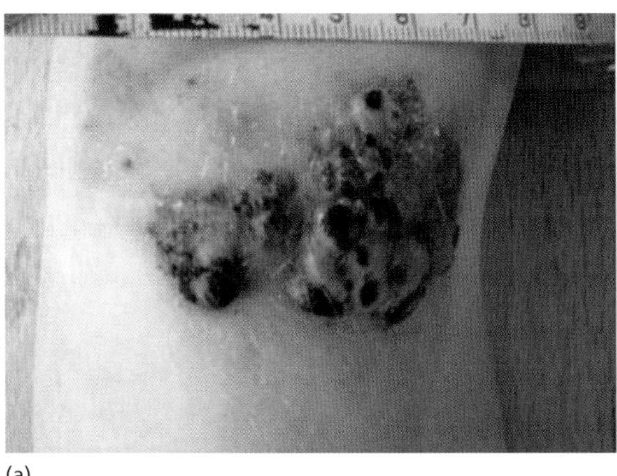

(a)

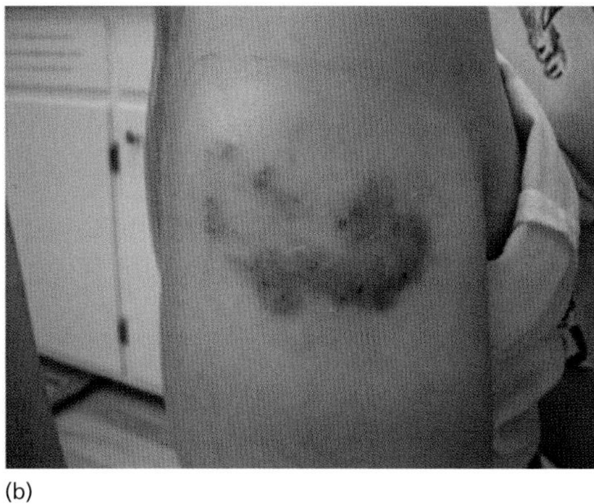

(b)

Fig. 121.10 Treatment of cutaneous microcystic lymphatic malformation by carbon dioxide laser. (a) An adolescent female presented with worsening bleeding from lymphatic vesicles involving her knee. Because the location was an unfavourable area for resection, she was treated with carbon dioxide laser to cause fibrosis of the area. (b) After treatment, bleeding from the vesicles resolved.

Other options to treat microcystic LMs are bleomycin sclerotherapy and oral sirolimus. Bleomycin can be diffusely injected throughout the tissues containing LM and most patients will have a 10–50% reduction in the size of the area and improvement in symptoms [39]. Bleomycin is useful for patients with symptomatic lesions that are in an unfavourable area for resection. The treatment may obviate the need for excision and a cutaneous scar. Individuals with diffuse, problematic microcystic LMs that have failed other interventions are candidates for oral sirolimus pharmacotherapy [40]. Our centre and others have had favourable outcomes using this medication; lesions exhibit reduced size, bleeding and lymphorrhoea. Sildenafil has been described for the treatment of LMs [41], but consistent results have not been achieved and the use of the drug is not well accepted. Our centre has not found efficacy with sildenafil and does not use it for the treatment of LMs.

Primary lymphoedema

Most patients with primary lymphoedema do not have significant morbidity. Patients are told to avoid incidental trauma to the affected area which is at higher risk for infection. Patients are advised to exercise the extremity and maintain a normal body mass index. Obesity can significantly worsen lymphoedema [42]. First-line therapy is compression of the area. Patients are prescribed a custom-fitted compression garment; young children wear commercially available tight stockings. Older children and adults may benefit from a pneumatic compression pump [43]. Complex decongestive therapy is another type of compression regimen but may be difficult in the paediatric age group. There are two categories of operation to treat lymphoedema. Excisional procedures remove subcutaneous fibroadipose tissue; the two most common types are suction-assisted lipectomy (liposuction) and staged skin/subcutaneous excision. Physiological operations attempt to improve lymphatic flow most often by lymphatic–venous anastomosis or vascularized lymph node transfer. Our preferred operative intervention for lymphoedema is liposuction because the technique gives consistent improvement and has minimal morbidity (Fig. 121.11) [44]. In addition, liposuction may improve the patient's underlying lymphatic function [45].

Physiological procedures do not predictably restore lymphatic flow and fail to remove excess subcutaneous adipose tissue. Lymphatic–venous anastomosis and vascularized lymph node transfer may have benefit for patients with early secondary lymphoedema from axillary or inguinal lymphadenectomy/radiation (before fibroadipose tissue has developed). Physiological procedures may be contraindicated in patients with primary

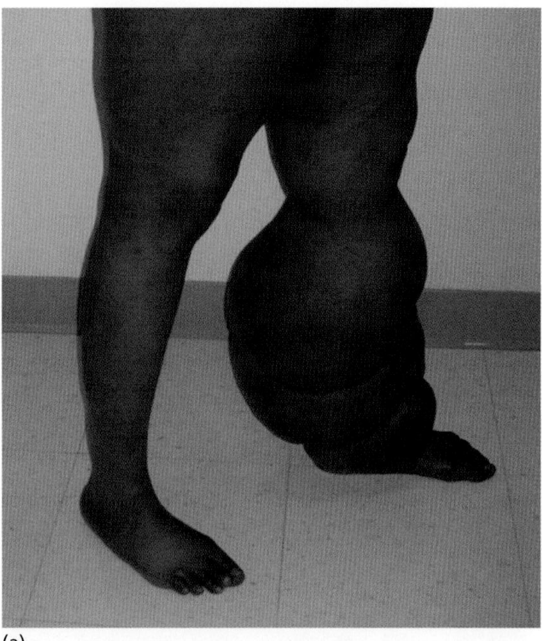
(a)

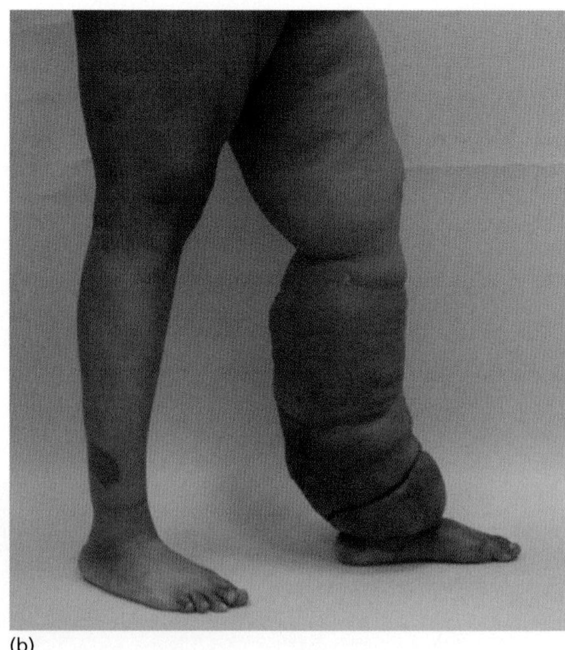
(b)

Fig. 121.11 Operative management of lymphoedema. (a) An adult female with adolescent-onset primary lymphoedema presented with continued enlargement of her left lower extremity. (b) She was treated with liposuction and the contour of her leg improved postoperatively.

disease because they have absent or hypoplastic lymphatics. Patients undergoing vascularized lymph node transfer also may develop donor-site lymphoedema at the site where the lymph nodes are harvested. This risk is higher in patients with primary lymphoedema who have an underlying anomaly of their lymphatic system.

Symptomatic patients who have failed conservative therapy undergo lymphoscintigraphy and MRI before proceeding with suction-assisted lipectomy [44]. Lymphoscintigraphy confirms the diagnosis of lymphoedema and determines the severity of lymphatic dysfunction. MRI documents subcutaneous fibroadipose overgrowth. Imaging of both extremities is necessary to compare the diseased limb with the contralateral side. If MRI shows that the arm or leg is primarily enlarged because of fluid, the patient is not a candidate for the excisional procedure and his/her compression regimen is maximized. It typically takes a few years following the onset of oedema for sufficient subcutaneous adipose tissue to be formed. If MRI illustrates significant subcutaneous adipose tissue then the patient may be improved with liposuction. Liposuction does not cure lymphoedema and patients are educated that they must continue their compression regimen postoperatively to slow recurrence. Penile/scrotal lymphoedema is not amenable to liposuction and requires staged skin/subcutaneous resection.

GSD/GLA

Our management for both diseases involves weekly subcutaneous interferon-alfa 2b injections (PEGylated interferon alfa-2b [Peg-Intron] 1.5μg/kg subcutaneously, weekly) and monthly intravenous bisphosphonates (zoledronate [Zometa] 0.05mg/kg intravenously, every other month). This treatment regimen helps to prevent progressive bone loss and improve bone remineralization. Oral sirolimus (0.8mg/m^2 per dose twice daily, with pharmacokinetic-guided target serum 12 h trough level of 7–13ng/mL) also is efficacious for these conditions [46]. Symptomatic areas of bone loss may require fracture stabilization and/or bone grafts.

LM-associated overgrowth syndromes

CLOVES: Patients are managed based on symptoms. Lipomatous masses can be resected but have a high recurrence rate. Paraspinal arteriovenous malformations or lipomatous lesions may require embolization or resection to protect the spinal cord. Lymphatic and venous malformations might necessitate sclerotherapy or resection. Capillary malformations can be treated with pulsed-dye laser. Patients may require orthopaedic intervention to correct a leg-length discrepancy or for amputations/soft-tissue debulking to fit shoes and facilitate ambulation. Also, individuals are monitored with serial ultrasounds for Wilms tumour. Recently, oral sildenafil has shown limited efficacy in a case report of a patient with *PIK3CA*-related overgrowth [46]. CLOVES is described in detail in Chapter 108.

KTS: Patients with large embryonal veins have these veins removed by sclerotherapy, coiling, or endovascular laser to prevent life-threatening thromboembolism. Individuals are followed for a leg-length discrepancy. If the discrepancy is >1.5cm, a shoe-lift for the shorter limb can prevent limping and scoliosis before an epiphysiodesis of the distal femoral growth plate is performed at approximately 11 years of age. Ray, midfoot, or Syme amputations may be required to allow the use of footwear. Patients are not at risk for Wilms tumour and thus do not require screening. Symptomatic venous and macrocystic LMs are managed with sclerotherapy.

Bleeding cutaneous microcystic LMs are treated with carbon dioxide laser or resection. Large areas may require skin graft reconstruction following excision. Circumferential leg overgrowth can be improved with staged skin and subcutaneous excision.

References

1 Kulungowski AM, Hassanein AH, Nosé V et al. Expression of androgen, estrogen, progesterone, and growth hormone receptors in vascular malformations. Plast Reconstr Surg 2012;129:919e–24e.
2 Hassanein AH, Mulliken JB, Fishman SJ et al. Lymphatic malformation: risk of progression during childhood and adolescence. J Craniofac Surg 2012;23:149–52.
3 Luks VL, Kamitaki N, Vivero MP et al. Lymphatic and other vascular malformative/overgrowth disorders are caused by somatic mutations in PIK3CA. J Pediatr 2015;166:1048–54.
4 Irrthum A, Karkkainen MJ, Devriendt K et al. Congenital hereditary lymphedema caused by a mutation that inactivates VEGFR3 tyrosine kinase. Am J Hum Genet 2000;67:295–301.
5 Fang J, Dagenais SL, Erickson RP, et al. Mutations in FOXC2 (MFH-1), a forkhead family transcription factor, are responsible for the hereditary lymphedema–distichiasis syndrome. Am J Hum Genet 2000;67:1382–8.
6 Irrthum A, Devriendt K, Chitayat D et al. Mutations in the transcription factor gene SOX18 underlie recessive and dominant forms of hypotrichosis–lymphedematelangiectasia. Am J Hum Genet 2003;72: 1470–8.
7 Alders M, Hogan BM, Gjini E et al. Mutations in CCBE1 cause generalized lymph vessel dysplasia in humans. Nat Genet 2009;41:1272–4.
8 Tartaglia M, Mehler EL, Goldberg R et al. Mutations in PTPN11, encoding the protein tyrosine phosphatase SHP-2, cause Noonan syndrome. Nat Genet 2001;29:465–8.
9 Roberts AE, Araki T, Swanson KD et al. Germline gain-of-function mutations in SOS1 cause Noonan syndrome. Nat Genet 2007;39:70–74.
10 Greene AK, Burrows PE, Smith L et al. Periorbital lymphatic malformation: clinical course and management in 42 patients. Plast Reconstr Surg 2005;115:22–30.
11 Smeltzer DM, Stickler GB, Schirger A. Primary lymphedemas in children and adolescents: a follow-up study and review. J Pediatr 1985;76:206–18.
12 Kinmonth JB, Taylor GW, Tracy GD, Marsh JD. Primary lymphoedema; clinical and lymphangiographic studies of a series of 107 patients in which the lower limbs were affected. Br J Surg 1957;45:1–9.
13 Schook CC, Mulliken JB, Fishman SJ et al. Primary lymphedema: clinical features and management in 138 pediatric patients. Plast Reconstr Surg 2011;127: 2419–31.
14 Ghalamkarpour A, Morlot S, Raas-Rothschild A et al. Hereditary lymphedema type I associated with VEGFR3 mutation: the first de novo case and atypical presentations. Clin Genet 2006;70:330–5.
15 Connell FC, Ostergaard P, Carver C et al. Analysis of the coding regions of VEGFR3 and VEGFRC in Milroy disease and other primary lymphoedemas. Hum Genet 2009;124:625–31.
16 Rezaie T, Ghoroghchian R, Bell R et al. Primary non-syndromic lymphoedema (Meige disease) is not caused by mutations in FOXC2. Eur J Hum Genet 2008;16:300–4.
17 Connell F, Brice G, Jeffery S et al. A new classification system for primary lymphatic dysplasias based on phenotype. Clin Genet 2010;77:438–52.
18 Fang J, Dagenais SL, Erickson RP et al. Mutations in FOXC2 (MFH-1), a forkhead family transcription factor, are responsible for the hereditary lymphedema–distichiasis syndrome. Am J Hum Genet 2000;67:1382–8.
19 Irrthum A, Devriendt K, Chitayat D et al. Mutations in the transcription factor gene SOX18 underlie recessive and dominant forms of hypotrichosis–lymphedema–telangiectasia. Am J Hum Genet 2003;72:1470–8.
20 Aagenaes O, Hagen van der CB, Refsum R. Hereditary recurrent intrahepatic cholestasis from birth. Arch Dis Child 1968;43:646–57.
21 Alders M, Hogan BM, Gjini E et al. Mutations in CCBE1 cause generalized lymph vessel dysplasia in humans. Nat Genet 2009;41:1272–4.
22 Shaw AC, Kalidas K, Crosby AH et al. The natural history of Noonan syndrome: a long-term follow-up study. Arch Dis Child 2007;92:128–32.
23 Welsh J, Todd M. Incidence and characteristics of lymphedema in Turner's syndrome. Lymphology 2006;39:152–3.
24 Maclellan RA, Couto RA, Sullivan JE et al. Management of primary and secondary lymphedema: analysis of 225 referrals to a center. Ann Plast Surg 2015;75:197–200.
25 Greene AK, Grant FD, Slavin SA. Lower-extremity lymphedema and elevated body-mass index. N Engl J Med 2012;366:2136–7.
26 Brorson H, Svensson H. Liposuction combined with controlled compression therapy reduces arm lymphedema more effectively than controlled compression therapy alone. Plast Reconstr Surg 1998;102:1058–67.
27 Brorson H, Ohlin K, Olsson G, Karlsson MK. Breast cancer-related chronic arm lymphedema is associated with excess adipose and muscle tissue. Lymphat Res Biol 2009;7:3–10.
28 International Society of Lymphology. The diagnosis and treatment of peripheral lymphedema: 2013 Consensus document of the international society of lymphology. Lymphology 2013;46:1–11.
29 Lala S, Mulliken JB, Alomari AI et al. Gorham-Stout disease and generalized lymphatic anomaly – clinical, radiologic, and histologic differentiation. Skeletal Radiol 2013;42:917–24.
30 Alomari AI. Characterization of a distinct syndrome that associates complex truncal overgrowth, vascular, and acral anomalies: a descriptive study of 18 cases of CLOVES syndrome. Clin Dysmorphol 2009;18:1–7.
31 Arnold R, Chaudry G. Diagnostic imaging of vascular anomalies. Clin Plast Surg 2011;38:21–9.
32 Hassanein AH, Maclellan RA, Grant FD, Greene AK. Diagnostic accuracy of lymphoscintigraphy for lymphedema and Analysis of false-negative tests. Plast Reconstr Surg Glob Open 2017;5:e1396.
33 Gloviczki P, Calcagno D, Schirger A et al. Noninvasive evaluation of the swollen extremity: experiences with 190 lymphoscintigraphic examinations. J Vasc Surg 1989;9:683–9.
34 Szuba A, Shin WS, Strauss HW, Rockson S. The third circulation: radionuclide lymphoscintigraphy in the evaluation of lymphedema. J Nucl Med 2003;44:43–57.
35 Peterman CM, Fevurly RD, Alomari AI et al. Sonographic screening for Wilms tumor in children with CLOVES syndrome. Pediatr Blood Cancer 2017;64. Epub 2017, June 19.
36 Greene AK, Kieran M, Burrows PE et al. Wilms tumor screening is unnecessary in Klippel–Trenaunay syndrome. Pediatrics 2004; 113:e326–9.
37 Gupta A, Kozakewich H. Histopathology of vascular anomalies. Clin Plast Surg 2011;38:31–44.
38 Grimmer JF, Mulliken JB, Burrows PE, Rahbar R. Radiofrequency ablation of microcystic lymphatic malformation in the oral cavity. Arch Otolaryngol Head Neck Surg 2006;132:1251–6.
39 Chaudry G, Guevara CJ, Rialon KL et al. Safety and efficacy of bleomycin sclerotherapy for microcystic lymphatic malformation. Cardiovasc Intervent Radiol 2014;37:1476–81.
40 Hammill AM, Wentzel M, Gupta A et al. Sirolimus for the treatment of complicated vascular anomalies in children. Pediatr Blood Cancer 2011;57:1018–24.
41 Tu JH, Tafoya E, Jeng M, Teng JM. Long-term follow-up of lymphatic malformations in children treated with sildenafil. Pediatr Dermatol 2017;34:559–65.
42 Greene AK, Grant F, Slavin SA, Maclellan RA. Obesity-induced lymphedema: clinical and lymphoscintigraphic features. Plast Reconstr Surg 2015;135:1715–9.
43 Maclellan RA, Greene AK. Lymphedema. Semin Pediatr Surg 2014;23:191–7.
44 Greene AK, Maclellan RA. Operative treatment of lymphedema using suction-assisted lipectomy. Ann Plast Surg 2016;77:337–40.
45 Greene AK, Voss SD, Maclellan RA. Liposuction for swelling in patients with lymphedema. N Engl J Med 2017;377:1788–9.
46 Adams DM, Trenor CC 3rd, Hammill AM et al. Efficacy and safety of sirolimus in the treatment of complicated vascular anomalies. Pediatrics 2016;137:e20153257.

CHAPTER 122

Inherited and Acquired Hyperpigmentation

Leslie Castelo-Soccio[1] *& Alexis Weymann Perlmutter*[2]

[1]Department of Pediatrics, Section of Pediatric Dermatology, University of Pennsylvania Perlman School of Medicine and Children's Hospital of Philadelphia, Philadelphia, PA, USA
[2]Department of Dermatology, Geisinger Medical Center, PA, USA

Introduction, 1463 | Acquired hyperpigmentation, 1463 | Inherited disorders of pigmentation, 1469

Abstract

Cutaneous hyperpigmentation can be congenital or acquired. Congenital hyperpigmentation is often related to gene changes and acquired as a result of skin inflammation, systemic diseases, environmental factors or medications. The vast majority of these disorders of hyperpigmentation are linked to alterations of the pigment melanin. This review will focus on the major acquired hyperpigmentation disorders and inherited/congenital pigmentation. Prominent aspects of diagnosis and therapy will be emphasized.

Key points

- Acquired pigmentation can be caused by infection, inflammation and inflammatory disorders, autoimmune disorders, medications, heavy metal toxicity, hormones and endocrinological disorders and nutritional abnormalities.
- Inherited disorders are due disorders in melanin production and transport, keratin and other inflammatory pathways and can be diffuse, localized or segmental.

Introduction

Pigmentary disorders have many etiologies and may present similarly in the clinical setting. Because treatment varies widely and is dependent on accurate diagnosis we present a review of common disorders of hyperpigmentation acquired and inherited to help make the diagnosis.

Acquired hyperpigmentation

Circumscribed hyperpigmentation

Infective causes of circumscribed hyperpigmentation

Cutaneous bacterial infections such as impetigo are common and may result in demarcated hyperpigmentation. Pityriasis versicolor (tinea versicolor) is another common condition that causes hyper- or hypopigmented macules and patches in a coalescing pattern on the trunk, neck and upper extremities. It is caused by overgrowth of a commensal skin organism of the *Malassezia* species, most commonly *M. globosa,* and next most commonly, *M. furfur*. This dimorphic fungus is difficult to grow and is best seen in a wet potassium hydroxide preparation, with the hyphae and clusters of spores appearing as the so-called 'spaghetti and meatballs' pattern. The hyperpigmentation appears to be caused by an increase in melanosome activity [1] or sequestering of melanosomes [2] as well as caused by inflammation. Dark-skinned patients with tinea versicolor are more likely to present with hypopigmented lesions rather than hyperpigmented lesions. These patients have an increased incidence of postinflammatory hyperpigmentation that may last for months despite adequate treatment of the mycotic infection and can be confused with inadequately treated tinea versicolor [2]. Several treponemal infections result in pigmentary change. *Treponema carateum* causes pinta, a disease of Central and South America. In the secondary stage, blue–grey papules and macules develop progressing to depigmentation in the later stage. *Treponema pallidum* (syphilis) may present with patches of hyperpigmentation on the upper trunk and neck (necklace of Venus), but because these areas are often superimposed with guttate leucoderma, they may also be regarded as acquired dyschromatosis.

Postinflammatory hyperpigmentation

Hyperpigmentation is a common result following an inflammatory insult to the skin and can occur at any age. Pigmentation occurs at the site of inflammation and is more pronounced in darkly pigmented skins or those who tan easily. Usually the process will resolve given time, but this may take months to years. Table 122.1 lists

Harper's Textbook of Pediatric Dermatology, Fourth Edition. Edited by Peter Hoeger, Veronica Kinsler and Albert Yan.

Table 122.1 Inflammatory disorders associated with hyperpigmentation

Inflammatory disease	Clinical clues (in addition to primary lesions)
Common	
Acne vulgaris	Head/neck region, upper trunk; <1 cm; perifollicular
Dermatitis	
Atopic	Atopic diathesis; face and forearms in infants then flexural areas; excoriations; atopic pleats; hyperpigmented transverse fold on nose; xerosis; hyperlinear palms
Lichen simplex chronicus	Common locations: neck, ankle, antecubital/popliteal fossae
Transient neonatal pustulosis	Newborns
Impetigo	Favours face
Insect bites	Favours exposed areas; usually <1 cm
Less common	
Irritant and allergic contact and photocontact dermatitis	Initial sites determined by aetiological agent and form of exposure; phytophotodermatitis discussed under 'Linear hyperpigmentation' in text
Pityriasis rosea	Favours trunk and proximal extremities; follows skin cleavage lines; oval-shaped
Psoriasis	Scalp/nail involvement; knees/elbows most common sites
Polymorphous light eruption	Face, extensor upper extremities and mid upper chest; often seasonal
Discoid lupus erythematosus	Face and conchal bowl; follicular plugging in latter; oral lesions; in scarred lesions, central hypopigmentation with rim of hyperpigmentation
Lichen planus	Wrists, presacral (Fig. 122.1); nail/oral involvement
Erythema dyschromicum perstans	Synonyms: ashy dermatosis; dermatosis cinecienta; face, neck, upper extremities, trunk (Fig. 122.2); round or oval in shape; long axis can follow skin cleavage lines similar to pityriasis rosea; possibly associated with HIV or trichuriasis; less commonly observed in fair-skinned individuals
Idiopathic eruptive macular pigmentation	Possibly separate entity from erythema dyschromicum perstans
Fixed drug eruption	Circular; perioral/genital common sites
Morbilliform drug eruption	Widespread; usually discrete lesions
Viral exanthem	Widespread; usually discrete lesions
Morphoea	Trunk or extremities; large-sized except in guttate variant; may be segmental
Atrophoderma of Parini and Pasini	Posterior trunk; large-sized; cliff sign (see Chapter 96)

common and unusual causes of inflammation that may occur in childhood and result in hyperpigmentation.

In addition, trauma such as friction or burns may result in hyperpigmentation.

Treatment. Initial treatment is to prevent further inflammation and depends on the underlying process. Sun protection may help to speed recovery in the authors' experience. Treatment of the pigmentation itself is often disappointing. Topical retinoids or hydroquinone may be tried, but care must be taken to protect surrounding normal skin and to avoid overtreatment resulting in hypopigmentation. Laser treatment, for example with Q-switched ruby or Q-switched Nd:YAG, has shown variable benefit, and hyperpigmentation is a real risk of treatment [3–5].

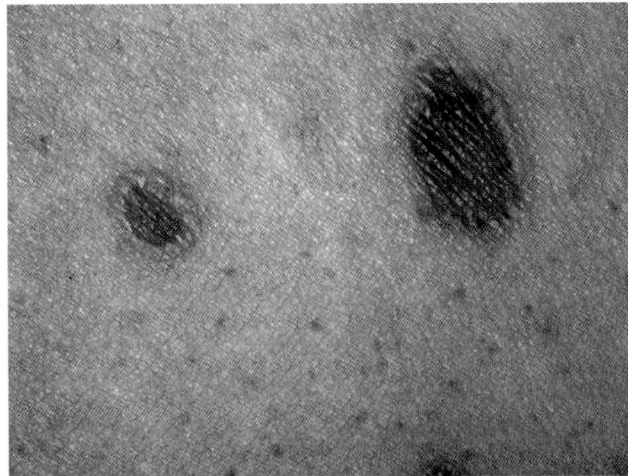

Fig. 122.1 Annular lichen planus with central postinflammatory hyperpigmentation.

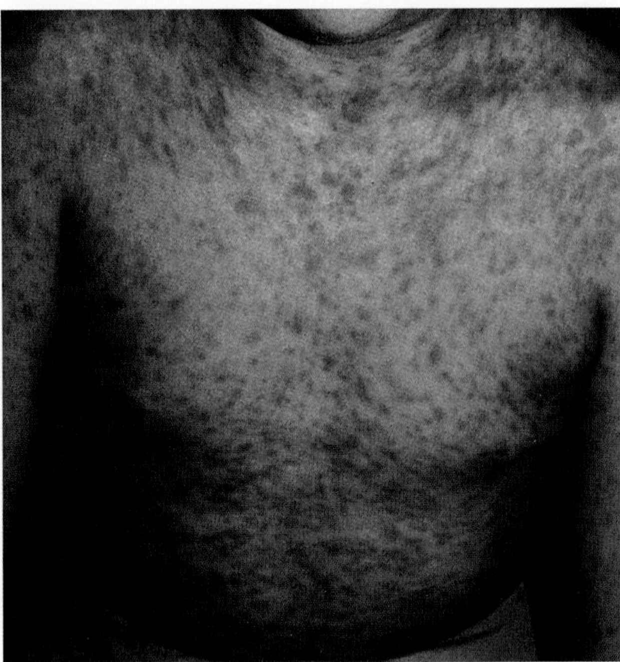

Fig. 122.2 Numerous oval-shaped grey–brown macules on the trunk of a child with erythema dyschromicum perstans. Source: Courtesy of the University Southern California residents' slide collection.

Drug-induced circumscribed hyperpigmentation

Drugs may affect the colour of the skin by altering melanin synthesis, through deposition of a drug-related material or as a result of postinflammatory changes. A wide and expanding range of drugs are implicated. The most commonly associated are minocycline, antimalarials, oral contraceptives, cytotoxic drugs and heavy metals.

Tetracyclines (except doxycycline) may potentially all cause hyperpigmentation [6]. Tetracycline is rarely

Table 122.2 Types of cutaneous pigmentation associated with minocycline

Pattern	Main clinical features
Type I	Blue–black macules at sites of scarring or inflammation, primarily acne scars
Type II	Blue–black, brown, or slate-grey pigmentation on healthy skin, predominantly ankles, shins and arms
Type III	Muddy-brown on healthy skin, generalized, symmetrical and accentuated at photoexposed sites

associated with blue-coloured osteomas [7]; however, most reports of hyperpigmentation are secondary to minocycline. Pigmentation with minocycline is thought to be secondary to deposition of a degradation product chelated to iron [8]. Because minocycline is a highly lipophilic drug, it has excellent tissue penetration, which may contribute to deposition in various tissues. Table 122.2 summarizes the types of cutaneous pigmentation associated with minocycline [9–14]. Pigmentation has been reported at many sites in addition to the skin, such as heart valves, sclerae, teeth, nails, mucous membranes, thyroid and breastmilk [6,11,13,14]. In the authors' experience, pigmentation in the skin usually resolves after months or years but may be permanent.

Chloroquine and hydroxychloroquine used in the treatment of malaria or connective tissue disease may result in a blue–black or brownish discoloration most often of the face, shins or hard palate, but also diffusely on the trunk and extremities. It may develop within 1 year of starting the medication. It can mimic the bruising [15]. It resolves upon cessation of the medication [16].

Bleomycin, an antibiotic used in the treatment of malignancy such as Hodgkin lymphoma, may produce diffuse or patchy pigmentation, which is often worse on extensor surfaces [17,18]. It may also produce a characteristic 'flagellate dermatitis' resulting in linear hyperpigmentation [19,20]. It has been postulated that secretion of chemotherapy agents onto the skin in sweat may explain hyperpigmentation at sites of tapes and ECG pads [21]. A number of other chemotherapy agents are associated with localized cutaneous hyperpigmentation including carmustine, 5-fluorouracil, dactinomycin, actinomycin-D, doxorubicin and thiotepa [22].

Heavy metals may affect pigmentation via systemic absorption or local contact. Argyria is a bluish-grey discoloration that may be localized or widespread and is caused by the deposition of silver in the skin. It may be caused by silver-containing medicines or by topical silver sulfadiazine [23]. Chrysiasis is a permanent bluish-grey discoloration caused by gold salts, such as intramuscular gold used in rheumatic diseases, and is limited to sites of sun exposure [24]. Arsenic is a carcinogen and a major pollutant in drinking water in many parts of the world. It may result in patchy bronze hyperpigmentation or hypopigmentation. Colour change can occur years following exposure [25].

Pigmentation caused by mastocytosis

In children cutaneous mastocytosis usually presents as either urticaria pigmentosa, solitary cutaneous mastocytoma or less commonly diffuse cutaneous mastocytosis. The prognosis is generally better in childhood mastocytosis than in adult disease [26]. The cause of pigmentation in these conditions is not yet fully understood. In adult forms mutations in *c-KIT* have been isolated and are believed to be the cause of mast cell proliferation [27,28]. In paediatric cases evidence for *c-KIT* mutation was less clear. However, recent evidence suggests that *c-KIT* mutations may be important in childhood mastocytosis, possibly via mosaicism [29]. c-KIT has an important role in melanocyte development and physiology, and loss-of-function mutations lead to depigmentation as in piebaldism (see Chapter 125), thus it is possible that activating mutations may influence pigmentation. This remains to be substantiated in the case of mastocytosis. Mastocytosis is reviewed in Chapter 92.

Erythema dyschromicum perstans

Erythema dyschromicum perstans (EDP), or ashy dermatosis, is an acquired disorder of unknown cause. Both sexes and all age ranges and races may be affected, though it is rare in children [30]. Clinical features are of asymptomatic ash-coloured (blue/brown–grey) macules, which slowly spread and leave long-lasting discoloration. In the early stages there may be a thin erythematous margin. It is most common on the trunk and limbs but may occur on the face also. Mucous membranes are spared. Lesions may be permanent but in children they may clear spontaneously [31]. There is no clearly effective treatment, though classically clofazimine and dapsone have been tried. Topical tacrolimus 0.1% ointment may be effective in some cases [32]. Narrow band UVB has also been reported as effective in one case report and anecdotally by others [33].

Periorbital hyperpigmentation

Periorbital hyperpigmentation affecting the skin of the upper and/or lower eyelids and adjacent areas is a descriptive term encompassing different clinical entities. Rarely this may be an inherited condition [34]. Periorbital hyperpigmentation has been reported in naevus of Ota [30], erythema dyschromicum perstans [35,36] and hyperthyroidism (Jellinek sign) [37]. Increased pigmentation of the lower eyelids is often seen in atopic individuals ('allergic shiners') and may be caused by congestion of the nasal and paranasal venous network [38] as a result of chronic allergic rhinitis. In those with atopic dermatitis this may be contributed to by scratching, resulting in postinflammatory hyperpigmentation [39]. Contact dermatitis may also result in postinflammatory hyperpigmentation [40].

Melasma

Melasma is an acquired condition presenting as patches of brown-to-black discoloration on the face. It is significantly more common in women than men [41,42]. Melasma is uncommon in childhood and early adolescence in most areas, although in parts of India, Pakistan and the Middle East the problem may develop before puberty [41]. It is more common in skin types V–VI [41] and in Hispanics [43]. Melasma may begin during pregnancy in many cases and is also known as 'the mask of pregnancy'. Hormonal influences may be important in its causation although in affected males this is not the case and ultraviolet exposure seems more significant [44]. Ultraviolet light may also play a significant role in its aetiology in females [44,45]. Hormone drugs such as the contraceptive pill can trigger the condition [46] as can antiseizure drugs, for example phenytoin [47]. Genetic predisposition is a further important causative factor [48]. The term chloasma (derived from a Greek word meaning to be green) is used interchangeably with melasma by many, although melasma is a more accurate description of the clinical findings, being derived from the Greek word for black [44].

Pathology. Melasma is usually divided histologically into one of three forms: a dermal form, an epidermal form and a mixed form [49]. In the epidermal form an increase in melanin is noted in the basal and suprabasal layers but may extend throughout the epidermis. In the dermal form macrophages laden with melanin are noted in the deep and superficial dermis [49]. Upregulation of various signalling pathways involved in melanogenesis are involved in the pathogenesis of melasma, including Wnt, KIT and melanocyte-stimulating hormone (MSH) [44].

Clinical features. Lesions consist of irregular, macular, brown-to-black patches. Three patterns of distribution predominate. These are centrofacial, malar and mandibular [41]. The centrofacial pattern occurs in around two-thirds of cases and includes forehead, nose, cheeks, upper lip and chin. The mandibular pattern occurs in about 15% of cases. The malar pattern is present in approximately 20% of cases [41]. Skin at other sun-exposed sites such as forearms may be involved regardless of facial pattern. Wood's lamp examination may indicate an epidermal (darker), dermal (no change), mixed involvement or indeterminate (lesions cannot be seen with Wood's lamp) pattern [41].

Prognosis. Once established, melasma may persist for a prolonged duration. After cessation of the oral contraceptive it may remain for more than 4 years [45,46]. Melasma of pregnancy usually resolves several months after delivery [47] but may recur in subsequent pregnancies. Melasma with dermal involvement is the most difficult pattern to manage, whilst the epidermal pattern tends to respond more favourably to treatment [47,50].

Differential diagnosis. Postinflammatory hyperpigmentation caused by cutaneous lupus, atopic dermatitis, contact dermatitis, photocontact or photosensitivity reactions may present with similar features but may have a history of an inflammatory phase. Actinic lichen planus may occur in childhood and can result in a similar facial appearance; the histology may differentiate it [51,52]. Where there is a history of hydroquinone use, particularly if melasma is deteriorating, exogenous ochronosis should be considered [53,54].

Treatment. Sun avoidance and regular use of a broad-spectrum sunscreen is a key part of management [55,56]. This may be difficult or unpopular. Any implicated drug such as an oral contraceptive or phenytoin should be stopped. Hydroquinone is the most commonly used agent [57] and may be used in monotherapy or in combination with a retinoid and/or a corticosteroid, so called triple-combination cream (TCC). TCC is more effective than hydroquinone alone at lightening melasma [58]. Azelaic acid 20% has also been demonstrated to be efficacious [57] and is more beneficial as a monotherapy than 2% hydroquinone alone [58]. Glycolic acid peels have shown some promise, alone or in combination with hydroquinone [58]. The Q-switched Nd:YAG is the most common laser used for treatment of melasma, though various laser regimens have been tried, including nonablative fractional lasers, with mixed results. Use of any laser to treat skin hyperpigmentation runs the risk of recurrence of the hyperpigmentation anomaly despite a temporary benefit, as well as development of postinflammatory hyperpigmentation [50]. Thus, a test spot should be utilized with any laser modality. Pretreatment with TCCs for 8 weeks before treatment with Q-switched ND:YAG laser may reduce the risk of postinflammatory hyperpigmentation and melasma recurrence [59].

Primary cutaneous localized amyloidosis

Amyloidosis is discussed further in Chapter 155 and is usually a condition beginning in adulthood. Two types have been associated with hyperpigmentation: macular amyloidosis and lichen amyloidosis. Macular amyloidosis usually presents on the upper back as poorly defined, brownish pigmented patches or linear rippling of the skin with closely aggregated greyish-brown macules [60]. Lichen amyloidosis appears as flesh- or brown-coloured papules, which may coalesce into plaques, and is more common on the legs or other extensor surfaces [61]. Amyloid is deposited in the papillary dermis in both conditions [62]. Both forms may be associated with pruritus and excoriation and there is ongoing debate as to the role of scratching in the causation of lichen amyloidosis [63,64]. The role of rubbing is becoming apparent in the aetiology of macular amyloidosis [60], and some prefer the term 'friction amyloidosis' in place of macular amyloidosis [65,66].

Notalgia paraesthetica [67], friction amyloidosis [65] and friction melanosis [68] have clinical similarities to macular amyloidosis. Macular amyloidosis and lichen amyloidosis are not associated with systemic deposition of amyloid. Lichen amyloidosis is reported in association with type 2A multiple endocrine neoplasia (Sipple syndrome) [69].

Diffuse hyperpigmentation

Endocrine and metabolic disorders

Increased pigmentation may be a feature of a number of endocrinopathies and may assist in diagnosis. Addison disease is the best-known example and consists of a diffuse brown pigmentation with accentuation at flexures, sites of trauma, buccal mucosa, lips, genitalia, areolae and palmar skin creases. It may be difficult to discern in darkly pigmented skin. The hyperpigmentation is a result of overproduction of adrenocorticotropic hormone (ACTH) by the pituitary because of failure of negative feedback. The structure of ACTH is closely related to MSH and both these substances stimulate melanocyte activity [70]. The aetiology of Addison disease in developed countries is predominantly autoimmune and it may occur alone or as part of an autoimmune polyglandular syndrome (type I), which often presents in childhood [70,71]. A similar pigmentary change may occur in Cushing disease and in Nelson syndrome [72].

Production of ectopic ACTH may result in hyperpigmentation and is associated with small cell lung cancer in adults. Ectopic ACTH is rare in children but has been reported in thymic carcinoid [73]. The hyperpigmentation that occurs in hyperthyroidism is often compared to Addison disease, but it is more variable, does not involve mucosal surfaces and tends to occur on shins, ankles, dorsal surfaces of the feet and nail beds [74].

It is the associated adrenal insufficiency in the very rare Siemerling–Creutzfeldt form of adrenoleucodystrophy that results in increased circulating levels of ACTH, which in turn causes hyperpigmentation [75]. A rare form of primary adrenal failure, familial ACTH unresponsiveness syndrome, presents with hyperpigmentation in childhood and may be associated with alacrima and achalasia [76]. Congenital adrenal hypoplasia is rare and hyperpigmentation usually develops slowly from several months of age. Extremely rarely, it may present in early infancy or at birth and pigmentation may be very dark [77].

In chronic renal failure, a diffuse brown pigmentation is common [78] and believed to be a result of failure of the kidney to excrete MSH [79]. Many patients with chronic hepatic disease have a degree of increased pigmentation, often a diffuse pattern. Haemochromatosis is an inherited iron storage disease and usually presents in adulthood; however, haemochromatosis type 2 (autosomal recessive) presents in childhood [80]. The iron deposits result in increased melanin [81]. Secondary haemochromatosis due, for example, to multiple blood transfusions, may also occur in childhood.

In adults with type I Gaucher disease, half of patients have diffuse brown or yellow–brown hyperpigmentation with easy tanning. There are no specific pigmentation patterns in type II (infantile) or type III (juvenile) Gaucher disease [82]. Porphyria cutanea tarda may present with pigmentation especially on photo-exposed sites, especially in sun-exposed sites; however, it usually presents in adults and is rare in children.

Drug-induced diffuse hyperpigmentation

The groups of drugs that can produce circumscribed hyperpigmentation can also cause diffuse pigmentary changes.

Minocycline usually results in local pigmentary change, but can produce a diffuse muddy-brown discoloration that is emphasized on sun-exposed areas [83]. Phototoxic reactions, such as with doxycycline, may precede generalized postinflammatory hyperpigmentation.

Chemotherapy drugs that may be used in the paediatric setting, such as cyclophosphamide, daunorubicin and hydroxyurea, may result in generalized hyperpigmentation [84].

Long-standing HIV infection can be associated with diffuse hyperpigmentation and therefore it can be difficult to assess the role of drugs especially in the context of polypharmacy. Azidothymidine (zidovudine) and emtricitabine have been reported to cause such reactions [85].

Dioxins may result in hyperpigmentation and porphyria cutanea tarda [86]. The heavy metals silver, bismuth and arsenic may cause a blue–grey pigmentation [87,88].

Hyperpigmentation resulting from nutritional abnormalities

Several vitamin deficiencies may result in increased cutaneous pigmentation. For example, folate deficiency can result in a greyish brown discoloration on sun-exposed areas [89]. Vitamin B_{12} deficiency may result in increased pigmentation in flexural areas, palms, soles and in the oral cavity [89]. Pigmentation results from an increase in tyrosinase activity secondary to the low vitamin B_{12} levels [89]. Deficiency in vitamin B_3 (niacin), results in pellagra. This has a variety of cutaneous manifestations including hyperpigmentation, following an erythematous dermatitis, on sun-exposed areas and around the neck (Casal's necklace) [90]. A shiny appearance of the skin is characteristic. The classic presentation of pellagra is of the three (or four) Ds – dermatitis, diarrhoea and dementia (and death if not treated). In up to one-third of cases the cutaneous signs alone may be present [90]. Protein-energy malnutrition in the form of kwashiorkor may result in hypo- or hyperpigmentation particularly at sites of trauma or pressure [91]. Carotenaemia results from excess intake of carotene-containing foods and manifests as yellow/orange discoloration of the skin, especially on palms, soles, forehead, chin, nasolabial grooves, anterior axillary skin folds and pressure areas. Sclerae and mucosal membranes are unaffected. It is usually seen in infants and results from excess consumption of foods such as carrot, squash, broccoli, apricots or egg yolk. It is a benign disorder and resolves upon reduction in carotene intake [92–94]. Other cutaneous and clinical manifestations of nutritional deficiency states are discussed in Chapter 71.

Autoimmune diseases

Autoimmune disease may result in adrenal failure and can present as hyperpigmentation (see Endocrine and metabolic disorders, previously). Systemic sclerosis can produce a variety of cutaneous manifestations including generalized hyperpigmentation, localized hyper- or hypopigmentation and a dyschromic appearance [95]. In POEMS syndrome (polyneuropathy, organomegalyendocrinopathy, M protein, skin changes), also known a Crow–Fukase syndrome, cutaneous changes include generalized hyperpigmentation, hypertrichosis and skin thickening [96,97]. It occurs mainly in the fifth and sixth decades, although there is a case report of an incomplete variant presenting in adolescence [98]. Hyper- and hypopigmented macules are reported as late-phase reactions adjacent to sclerodermatous changes in the toxic oil syndrome, caused by contaminated rapeseed oil, which affected large numbers of people in Spain in the 1980s [99].

Miscellaneous disorders of hyperpigmentation

In the neonatal period, a rare complication of cholestasis and phototherapy, bronze baby syndrome, results in a grey–brown discoloration. This condition of unknown aetiology usually resolves once phototherapy is stopped and cholestasis resolves [100]. Congenital adrenal hypoplasia may present with pigmentary change in neonates and was discussed earlier. An extremely rare condition, universal acquired melanosis (carbon baby syndrome), presents with generalized deep hyperpigmentation shortly after birth. Histology demonstrates a pattern of single melanosomes within keratinocytes, a pattern only seen normally in darkly pigmented skins [101,102].

Acropigmentation (acromelanosis or Spitzen pigment) presents with brown discoloration confined to the skin around nail beds and is not progressive [103]. Acromelanosis progressiva, another rare disorder, presents initially in a similar manner; however, pigmentation does not fade in adulthood and spreads to affect additional sites such as trunk and limbs [102]. Acquired facial pigmentation has also been described in young children without any preceding inflammation [104].

Diffuse hyperpigmentation has also been described in association with multifocal vascular sclerosis [103] and in a form of pseudoleprechaunism referred to as Patterson syndrome [105]. Additional clinical findings in this group of patients include cutis laxa, hirsutism, severe skeletal dysplasia and mental retardation.

Familial progressive hyperpigmentation (discussed later) and familial diffuse (or universal) melanosis are often regarded as causes of diffuse pigmentation. However, in the patients described by Wende and Baukus [106] and Pegum [107] there were 'zone-like' areas of varying intensity as well as multiple hypopigmented macules.

Linear hyperpigmentation

Pigmentary demarcation lines

Syn.

Voigt lines, Futcher lines, Ito lines

Pigmentary demarcation lines occur in all races however they are more commonly observed in those with deeply pigmented skin types. Five principal types are recognized:

1 Vertical line on the upper outer arm, which may extend into the pectoral region (with a number of variations in this locality);
2 Posteromedial portion of thigh, possibly extending to ankle;
3 A vertical or curved line in the pre- or parasternal area;
4 Vertical line pre- or paraspinal;
5 Bilateral markings on the chest from the mid-third of the clavicle to the periareolar skin.

Further subtypes affecting facial skin have been proposed [108,109]. The group A anterior pigmentation demarcation line has been referred to as Voigt's line [110]. This is derived from Voigt's boundary lines, which delineate the junction of dermatomes supplied by particular peripheral nerves [111]. Much of the work on pigmentary demarcation lines has been carried out in Japanese or African-American patients [112–114]. James *et al.* examined a mixed skin type group and found some kind of pigmentary demarcation line in 70% of black patients and in 6–14% of white patients [114].

Other causes of linear hyperpigmentation

Linear lesions on photo-exposed areas should suggest the possibility of phytophotodermatitis. This phototoxic reaction may be induced by contact with a number of plants such as giant hogweed, cow parsley, parsnip, lime and fig followed by sun exposure. The reaction begins with erythema and blisters and is followed by hyperpigmentation caused by melanin deposition [115]. Flagellate hyperpigmentation following administration of bleomycin in a number of conditions is reported [116]. Serpentine supravenous hyperpigmentation is reported overlying the vein used for injecting 5-fluorouracil and a variety of other antineoplastic agents [117].

Reticulated hyperpigmentation

There are a several acquired disorders presenting as reticular hyperpigmentation. These include erythema ab igne, which results in a net-like reticular pattern of postinflammatory hyperpigmentation following prolonged exposure to heat. Modern heat sources reported to have caused this eruption include heating pads, hot water bottles, laptops, cell phones and laptop batteries [118]. The atopic 'dirty neck' presents as a reticulate pattern affecting the anterolateral neck of individuals with atopic dermatitis and may demonstrate seasonal variation. This condition is reported in children as young as 5 years and also in adults [119,120]. Confluent and reticulated papillomatosis of Gougerot and Carteaud presents with asymptomatic hyperkeratotic pigmented papules, which coalesce to form plaques with a peripheral reticular pattern. Distribution is often on the upper anterior trunk. It occurs in all ages and is responsive to minocycline and a variety of other antibiotics [121]. Becker naevus may occasionally present with a cribriform pattern. Pruritus pigmentosa (Nagashima disease) is an acquired disorder of unknown cause that presents with outbreaks of pruritic papular lesions, which then resolve to leave reticular hyperpigmentation. It is mostly reported in Japanese women and may respond to minocycline [122].

There are a number of inherited disorders in which reticulate hyperpigmentation may be seen. Epidermolysis bullosa simplex with mottled pigmentation presents with mild acral blistering and a mottled, reticulated pigmentation at a variety of sites and may be associated with palmoplantar keratoderma [123,124]. It is associated with a mutation in keratin 5 [124]. There are a number of rare genetic disorders that have reticulated hyperpigmentation as a prominent feature. These will be discussed below. These include dyskeratosis congenita, Fanconi anaemia, Naegeli–Franceschetti–Jadassohn syndrome, dermatopathia pigmentosa reticularis, Dowling–Degos disease, X-linked reticulate pigmentary disorder and reticulate acropigmentation of Kitamura [125].

Inherited disorders of pigmentation

Variation in skin pigmentation is one of the most distinctive and socially significant human characteristics [126]. Differences in skin and hair colour are principally the result of differences in the melanin content of skin although additional elements including other pigments and skin thickness also determine shade variation in the skin [127].

Melanocytes are responsible for the synthesis of melanin, a complex quinone/indole-quinone-derived mixture of biopolymers [128]. Melanocytes migrate from the neural crest into the epidermis during the first trimester of gestation. They produce melanin within specialized vesicles known as melanosomes. Pigmentation differences arise from variation in the number, size, composition and distribution of melanosomes [129]. The major precursor of melanin is tyrosine. Tyrosinase catalyses the hydroxylation of tyrosine to DOPA (3,4, dihydroxy-phenylalanine). Once completely formed within melanocytes, melanosomes are transported along dendrites towards adjacent keratinocytes [130]. This process results from the concerted action of at least three proteins: the motor protein myosin Va, Rab27a, a member of the Rab GTPases family of proteins, and melanophilin [131]. The next step involves the extrusion of the melanosomes and their transfer into neighbouring keratinocytes, most probably through phagocytosis of released melanosomes by keratinocytes [132]. Activation of PAR-2 results in increased phagocytic activity of cultured keratinocytes toward isolated melanosomes [133].

After being transferred, melanosomes are translocated to the apical pole of the keratinocyte where they are best placed to absorb UV light and protect the nucleus from mutagenic damage. This trafficking process has been shown to require microtubule-associated motor proteins such as dynein [134] and cytoskeletal elements such as keratin and keratin-associated proteins [135]. Keratinocyte terminal differentiation is accompanied by concomitant degradation of melanosomes so that no melanosomes are normally visible in the very upper part of the epidermis.

In accordance with the biochemical complexity of the skin pigmentation process, more than 120 loci have been found to affect coat pigmentation in the mouse [135] and more than 100 inherited disorders of pigmentation have been described in humans, many of which have yet to be elucidated at the molecular level but an increasing number have a gene change identified (Table 122.3).

Patterned pigmentation occurs in a particular pattern on the skin. This can be an isolated finding or a signal of an underlying disorder with systemic manifestations. Happle described five types of patterned pigmentation: type 1a and 1b, narrow or thick bands respectively following lines of Blaschko; type 2, checkboard pattern; type 3, phylloid type or leaf pattern; and type 4, patchy pattern without midline separation [136].

Segmental pigmentary disorder (SegPD) is a term described by Hoegling and Frieden to describe a subset of patients with block-like and unilateral hypo- or hyperpigmentation who rarely have associated anomalies [137]. Large patches of hyperpigmentation in a unilateral distribution can be associated with McCune–Albright syndrome (polyostotic fibrous dysplasia with endocrinopathies including precocious puberty). This is caused by an activating mutation in the GNAS gene. The GNAS complex locus encodes the alpha-subunit of the stimulatory G protein (Gsα), a ubiquitous signalling protein mediating the actions of many hormones, neurotransmitters and paracrine/autocrine factors via generation of the second messenger cAMP [138].

Disorders of hyperpigmentation

Inherited disorders of pigmentation can be classified according to the pattern of pigmentation: diffuse, linear, reticulate and punctate. A full discussion of all inherited disorders of hyperpigmentation is beyond the scope of the present chapter. Punctate hyperpigmentation as seen in Peutz–Jeghers disease (Chapter 141) and Carney complex is discussed elsewhere (see Chapter 154).

Diffuse hyperpigmentation

Important metabolic disorders associated with diffuse hyperpigmentation include congenital adrenal hypoplasia, adrenal leucodystrophy, Wilson disease, porphyria cutanea tarda and haemochromatosis which are discussed in Chapter 154. Lysosomal storage disorders can also be accompanied by diffuse hyperpigmentation (e.g. Niemann–Pick disease, especially in sun-exposed areas, and Gaucher disease type I). Two disorders are discussed here below: familial progressive hyperpigmentation and familial primary cutaneous amyloidosis.

Familial progressive hyperpigmentation

Syn.
melanosis universalis hereditaria

This rare, autosomal dominant disorder is characterized by sharply demarcated and irregular skin and mucosal hyperpigmented patches which develop soon after birth and subsequently increase in size and number over time. There are no associated systemic anomalies. It is likely to be a heterogeneous genetic disease [139,140]. Histopathology demonstrates increased epidermal melanin, especially involving the stratum corneum [141]. A recent linkage analysis of an affected Chinese family demonstrated that a missense mutation on chromosome 12 which caused a mutant KIT ligand (KITL) had a gain-of-function effect on melanin synthesis in affected

Table 122.3 Inherited disorders of hyperpigmentation

Disease name	Inheritance	Gene	Locus	OMIM	Clinical features
Familial progressive hyperpigmentation	AD	KITL	12q	145250	Congenital sharply and irregular hyperpigmentary patches which increase in size and number with age
Primary cutaneous amyloidosis	AD	*OSMR*	5p13.1	105250	Chronic skin itching and multifocal hyperpigmentation
Incontinentia pigmenti	XLD	*IKBKG/ NEMO*	Xq28	308300	Pigmentation abnormalities consisted of whorls and streaks located over the trunk
Linear and whorled nevoid hypermelanosis	SO	Unknown	614323		Cardiovascular, neurological and musculoskeletal abnormalities
Dyskeratosis congenita					Reticulated pattern of hyperpigmentation, bone marrow dysplasia, haematological and epithelial malignancies
	XLR	*DKC1*	Xq28	305000	
	AD	*TERC*	5q21–3q28	127550	
	AD, AR	*TERT*	5p15.33	127550	
	AD, S	*TINF2*	14q12	127550	
	AR	*NOP10*	15q14	224230	
	AR	*NHP2*	22q13.2		
	AR	*TCAB1*	17p13.1		
Naegeli–Franceschetti–Jadassohn syndrome and dermatopathia pigmentosa reticularis	AD	*KRT14*	17q12–q21	161000/125595)	Complete absence of dermatoglyphics, a reticulate pattern of skin hyperpigmentation, palmoplantar keratoderma, abnormal sweating, dental anomalies and nail dystrophy
Dowling–Degos disease	AD	*KRT5*	12q12–q13	179850	Postpubertal reticulate hyperpigmentation of the flexures
Reticulate pigmentary disorder with systemic manifestations	XLD	POLA1	Xp22-p21	301220	Reticulate brown hyperpigmentation that follows the lines of Blashko in females and is generalized in males. Males also have neonatal colitis, neurological defects, hypohidrosis, dental anomalies, musculoskeletal defects and pulmonary complications
Reticulate acropigmentation of Kitamura	AD	ADAM10	15q21.3	615537	Hyperpigmented atrophic macules on the hand dorsa and pits on the palms and soles with abnormal dermatoglyphics

AD, autosomal dominant; AR, autosomal recessive; SO, somatic; XLD, X-linked dominant; XLR, X-linked recessive.

individuals [140]. KITL is a known regulator of melanocyte proliferation and melanin synthesis [142].

Familial primary cutaneous localized amyloidosis

This rare autosomal dominant form of cutaneous amyloidosis manifests with skin itching and macular or papular hyperpigmented lesions in an often multifocal distribution. It often presents in the second decade of life [143]. Familial primary cutaneous localized amyloidosis was found to result from impaired function of the oncostatin M-specific receptor β, which is part of the oncostatin M type II receptor and of the interleukin-31 receptor [144]. Recent evidence suggests that IL-31 plays a role in the pathophysiology of pruritus, which may help to elucidate the pathophysiology of non-familial cutaneous amyloidosis [143].

Linear hyperpigmentation

Incontinentia pigmenti

A thorough discussion of incontinentia pigmenti is presented in Chapter 136. This X-linked dominant disorder develops within the first month of life and involves four distinct stages of cutaneous morphology: vesicular, verrucous, hyperpigmentary and hypopigmentary. It results from mutations in the *IKBKG* gene [145]. The hyperpigmentation phase consists of striking whorls and 'marble cake' streaks following a Blaschko-linear distribution over the trunk and extremities. The pigmentation is most pronounced in the axilla or groin [146]. This phase lasts from just after the verrucous phase, often in infancy, until adolescence, and is highly characteristic of the disorder. There is melanin pigment incontinence on biopsy [146]. These lesions tend to fade by adulthood and usually evolve into hypopigmentary lesions.

Linear and whorled naevoid hypermelanosis (LWNH)

This disorder is now often grouped together with other pigment disorders as pigmentary mosaicism. Once gene causes are identified they are likely to be subdivided by gene change. In this sporadic disorder of hyperpigmentation resulting from genetic mosaicism, affected infants develop a swirled pattern of macular hyperpigmentation similar to that described above for the hyperpigmentary phase of incontinentia pigmenti. The absence of the prior vesicular and verrucous stages of incontinentia pigmenti help distinguish this as a distinct entity. In addition, skin biopsy of LWNH shows epidermal hypermelanosis without the incontinence of pigment seen in incontinentia pigmenti [147]. Associated systemic findings may include cardiovascular, neurological, ocular and musculoskeletal abnormalities [148], though a recent review suggests that serious extracutaneous anomalies are rarer than previously described because of a referral bias in the initial estimates [149]. A fuller discussion of this disorder is considered in Chapter 109.

Reticulate hyperpigmentation

Dyskeratosis congenita and Fanconi anaemia

Dyskeratosis congenita and Fanconi anaemia are fully discussed in Chapter 140. Dyskeratosis congenita is a multisystem disorder that features a reticulated pattern of hyperpigmentation predominantly on the neck, keratoderma, bullae, wrinkled skin on the extremities, nail dystrophy and premalignant oral leucokeratosis (Fig. 122.3a–c) [150]. Bone marrow dysplasia, and haematological and epithelial malignancies are frequent complications. Up to 90% of patients develop bone marrow failure, with the majority showing signs of failure by 30 years of age [151]. There is no treatment for this disorder. Abnormal skin pigmentation and nail changes usually manifest within the first decade, and as such, can be early indicators of disease. Dyskeratosis congenita can be inherited in an autosomal recessive, autosomal dominant or X-linked recessive fashion. The condition results from mutations critical to proper telomere function and maintenance [152]. To date, 10 causative genetic mutations have been identified [151].

A related disorder is autosomal recessive Fanconi anaemia, which is also associated with reticulated hyperpigmentation, café-au-lait spots, pancytopenia and an increased risk of neoplasia [153]. Change in pigmentation can often help corroborate the diagnosis especially in those without congenital malformations [154].

Naegeli–Franceschetti–Jadassohn syndrome and dermatopathia pigmentosa reticularis

These disorders are two closely related autosomal dominant ectodermal dysplasia syndromes that clinically share complete absence of dermatoglyphics, a reticulate pattern of skin hyperpigmentation mainly involving the trunk and face (Fig. 122.3d) palmoplantar keratoderma, abnormal sweating and other subtle developmental anomalies including plantar bullae in early childhood, alopecia, dental anomalies and nail dystrophy. These two syndromes have been shown to result from mutations affecting the region of the *KRT14* gene encoding the nonhelical head domain of keratin 14 [155]. These mutations were found to result in haploinsufficiency and to be associated with increased susceptibility of keratinocytes to proapoptotic stimuli [156]. Interestingly, mutations affecting other keratin 14 domains cause a completely different clinical phenotype – epidermolysis bullosa simplex [157] (see Chapter 76), which in some cases is also associated with mottled pigmentation [158].

Dowling–Degos disease, Galli-Galli disease and reticulate acropigmentation of Kitamura

Dowling–Degos disease (DDD) is an autosomal dominant disorder characterized by the presence of reticulate hyperpigmentation primarily of the flexures, and less so of the trunk, face and extremities (Fig. 122.3e), comedo-like lesions on the neck and pitted perioral acneiform scars [159]. Onset is usually postpubertal. No abnormalities of hair or nails are seen. Various mutations in the *KRT5* gene region have been demonstrated to cause this condition [159–161]. The fact that a mutation in *KRT5* causes epidermolysis bullosa simplex with mottled pigmentation suggests that keratin 5 has an important role in melanosome transport [162]. Galli-Galli disease, which clinically resembles DDD and features acantholysis on histology, is caused by a KRT5 mutation allelic to those seen in DDD [163]. Recently, mutations in POGLUT1 and POFUT1 have also been shown to underlie Dowling–Degos disease, with phenotypic correlation of a more diffuse distribution of pigmentary abnormalities in these genotypic variants [164,165]. These genes encode protein O-glucosyltransferase 1 and protein O-fucosyltransferase 1, respectively, both of which are part of the Notch signalling pathway. Reticulate acropigmentation of Kitamura (RAK) is characterized by the presence of hyperpigmented, atrophic macules on the dorsal hands and feet, pits on the palms and soles, and abnormal dermatoglyphics [166]. Onset is prepubertal, and in adulthood the hyperpigmented macules tend to spread to the trunk and proximal extremities. Because of clinical overlap between RAK and DDD, there has been debate as to whether these are overlapping entities. Recent research demonstrated that RAK is caused by loss-of-function mutations in *ADAM10*, clarifying RAK's distinctive genetic aetiology [167]. Of interest, ADAM10 is also a key part of the Notch signalling pathway, further emphasizing this pathway's role in pigmentation homeostasis [168].

X-linked reticulate pigmentary disorder

Reticulate, brown hyperpigmentation in this rare X-linked disease follows the lines of Blashko in female carriers and is generalized in affected males. Starting in infancy, affected males may also suffer from systemic complications including neonatal colitis, neurological defects, severe photophobia and pulmonary complications which can lead to early death [169]. Patients often have a characteristic dysmorphic facies with an upswept frontal hairline, hypohidrosis, hypodontia and onychodystrophy, leading a recent review to suggest this entity as a form of ectodermal dysplasia [170]. Histology reveals increased melanin epidermal content, pigment incontinence, dyskeratosis and amyloid in the papillary dermis [170].

Acknowledgement

The authors would like to thank Drs R.M. Ross Hearn, Eli Sprecher and Dov Hershkovitz for their contribution from the previous edition.

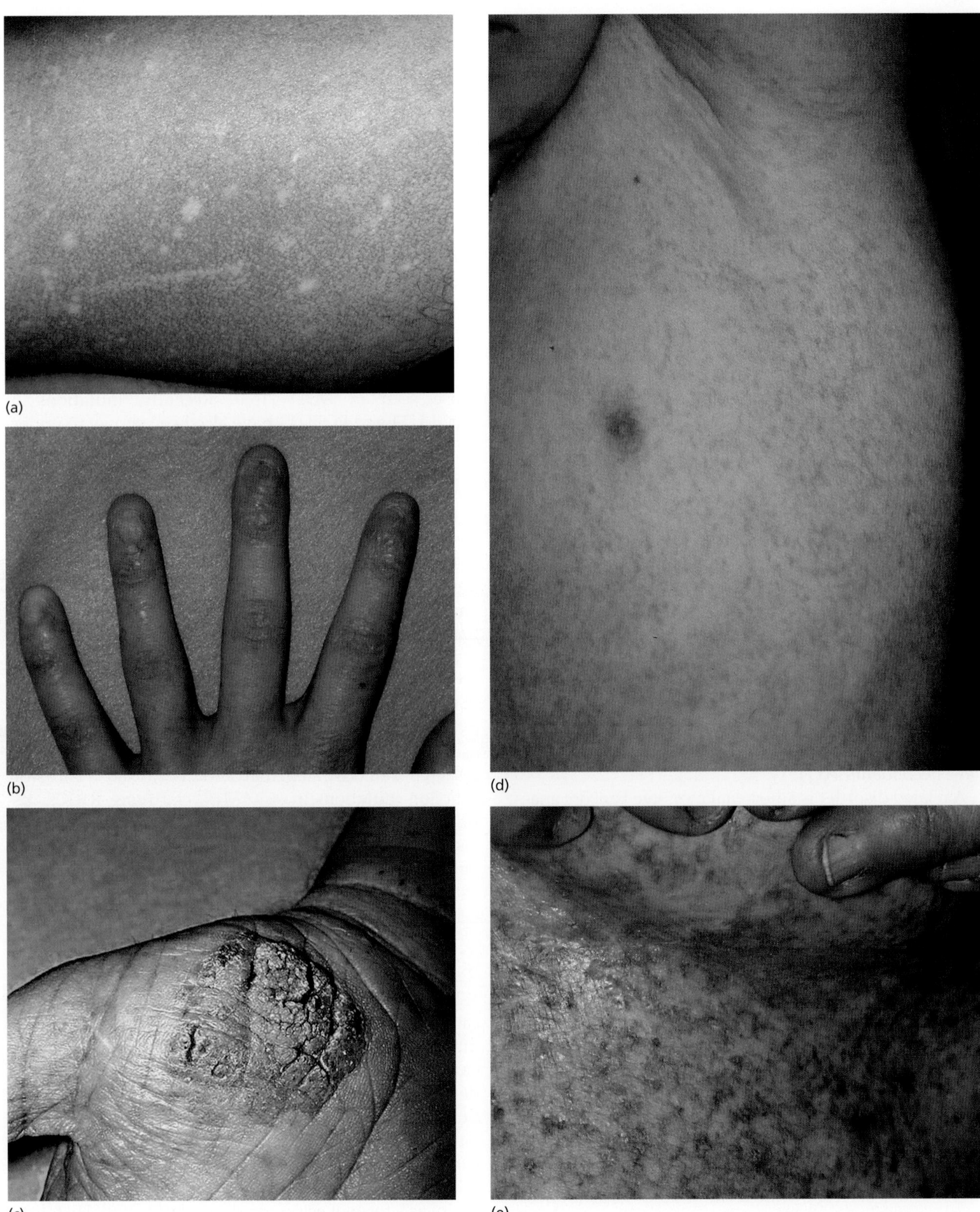

Fig. 122.3 Disorders of hyperpigmentation. (a) Reticulate pigmentation, (b) nail dystrophy and (c) squamous cell carcinoma in dyskeratosis congenita. (d) Reticulate hyperpigmentation in Naegeli–Franceschetti–Jadasshon syndrome. Source: Courtesy of Professor Gabriele Richard. (e) Flexural hyperpigmentation in Dowling–Degos syndrome.

References

1 Gupta AK, Bluhm R, Summerbell R. Pityriasis versicolor. J Eur Acad Dermatol Venereol 2002;16:19–33.
2 Kallini, JR, Riaz F, Khachemoune A. Tinea versicolor in dark-skinned individuals. Int J Dermatol 2014;53:137–41.
3 Arora, P, Sarkar, R, Garg, V, Arya, L. Laser treatment of melasma and post-inflammatory hyperpigmentation. J Cutan Aesth Surg 2012;5: 93–103.
4 Tse Y, Levine VJ, McClain SA, Ashinoff R. The removal of cutaneous pigmented lesions with the Q-switched ruby laser and the Q-switched neodymium:yttrium-aluminum-garnet laser. A comparative study. J Dermatol Surg Oncol 1994;20:795–800.
5 Omi, T, Yamashita, R, Kawana, S et al. Low fluence Q-switched ND-Yag laser toning and Q-switched ruby laser in the treatment of melasma: a comparative split face ultrastructural study. Laser Ther 2012;21:15–21.
6 Eisen D, Hakim MD. Minocycline-induced pigmentation. Incidence, prevention and management. Drug Safety 1998;18:431–40.
7 Walter JF, Macknet KD. Pigmentation of osteoma cutis caused by tetracycline. Arch Dermatol 1979;115:1087–8.
8 Okada N, Sato S, Sasou T et al. Characterization of pigmented granules in minocycline-induced cutaneous pigmentation: observations using fluorescence microscopy and high-performance liquid chromatography. Br J Dermatol 1993;129:403–7.
9 Goulden V, Glass D, Cunliffe WJ. Safety of long-term high-dose minocycline in the treatment of acne. Br J Dermatol 1996;134:693–5.
10 Fenske NA, Millns JL, Greer KE. Minocycline-induced pigmentation at sites of cutaneous inflammation. JAMA 1980;244:1103–6.
11 Fleming CJ, Hunt MJ, Salisbury EL et al. Minocycline-induced hyperpigmentation in leprosy. Br J Dermatol 1996;134:784–7.
12 Sabroe RA, Archer CB, Harlow D et al. Minocycline-induced discolouration of the sclerae. Br J Dermatol 1996;135:314–16.
13 Poliak SC, DiGiovanna JJ, Gross EG et al. Minocycline-associated tooth discoloration in young adults. JAMA 1985;254:2930–2.
14 Hunt MJ, Salisbury EL, Grace J, Armati R. Black breast milk due to minocycline therapy. Br J Dermatol 1996;134:943–4.
15 Cohen, Philip R. Hydroxychloroquine-associated hyperpigmentation mimicking elder abuse. Dermatol Ther 2013;3:203–10.
16 Tuffanelli D, Abraham RK, Dubois EI. Pigmentation from antimalarial therapy. Its possible relationship to the ocular lesions. Arch Dermatol 1963;88:419–26.
17 Cohen IS, Mosher MB, O'Keefe EJ et al. Cutaneous toxicity of bleomycin therapy. Arch Dermatol 1973;107:553–5.
18 Hendrix JD Jr, Greer KE. Cutaneous hyperpigmentation caused by systemic drugs. Int J Dermatol 1992;31:458–66.
19 Yamamoto T. Bleomycin and the skin. Br J Dermatol 2006;155:869–75.
20 Arseculeratne GB, Meiklejohn L, Mountain D et al. Bleomycin-induced 'flagellate dermatitis'. Arch Dermatol 2007;143:1461–2.
21 Singal R, Tunnessen WW Jr, Wiley JM, Hood AF. Discrete pigmentation after chemotherapy. Pediatr Dermatol 1991;8:231–5.
22 Alley E, Green R, Schuchter L. Cutaneous toxicities of cancer therapy. Curr Opin Oncol 2002;14:212–16.
23 Browning JC, Levy ML. Argyria attributed to silvadene application in a patient with dystrophic epidermolysis bullosa. Dermatol Online J 2008;14:9.
24 Smith RW, Leppard B, Barnett NL et al. Chrysiasis revisited: a clinical and pathological study. Br J Dermatol 1995;133:671–8.
25 Tchounwou PB, Patlolla AK, Centeno JA. Carcinogenic and systemic health effects associated with arsenic exposure—a critical review. Toxicol Pathol 2003;31:575–88.
26 Lange, M, Nedoszytko, B, Gorska, A et al. Mastocytosis in children and adults: clinical disease heterogeneity. Arch Med Sci 2010;8: 533–41.
27 Longley BJ Jr, Metcalfe DD, Tharp M et al. Activating and dominant inactivating c-KIT catalytic domain mutations in distinct clinical forms of human mastocytosis. Proc Natl Acad Sci U S A 1999;96:1609–14.
28 Longley BJ, Tyrrell L, Lu SZ et al. Somatic c-KIT activating mutation in urticaria pigmentosa and aggressive mastocytosis: establishment of clonality in a human mast cell neoplasm. Nat Genet 1996;12: 312–14.
29 Bodemer C, Hermine O, Palmerini F et al. Pediatric mastocytosis is a clonal disease associated with D816V and other activating c-KIT mutations. J Invest Dermatol 2010;130:804–15.
30 Schwartz RA. Erythema dyschromicum perstans: the continuing enigma of Cinderella or ashy dermatosis. Int J Dermatol 2004;43: 230–32.
31 Torrelo A, Zaballos P, Colmenero I et al. Erythema dyschromicum perstans in children: a report of 14 cases. J Eur Acad Dermatol Venereol 2005;19:422–6.
32 Mahajan VK, Chauhan PS, Mehta KS, Sharma AL. Erythema dyschromicum perstans: response to topical tacrolimus. Indian J Dermatol 2015;60:525.
33 Fabbrocini G, Cacciapuoti S, Izzo R et al. Efficacy of narrowband UVB phototherapy in erythema dyschromicum perstans treatment: case reports. Acta Dermatovenerol Croat 2015;23:63–5.
34 Goodman RM, Belcher RW. Periorbital hyperpigmentation. An overlooked genetic disorder of pigmentation. Arch Dermatol 1969;100: 169–74.
35 Kolde G, Schmollack KP, Sterry W. Periorbital hyperpigmentation. Bilateral nevus of Ota. Hautarzt 2001;52:460–3.
36 Sardana K, Rajpal M, Garg V, Mishra D. Periorbital hyperpigmentation mimicking fixed drug eruption: a rare presentation of erythema dyschromicum perstans in a paediatric patient. J Eur Acad Dermatol Venereol 2006;20:1381–3.
37 Ing EB, Buncic JR, Weiser BA et al. Periorbital hyperpigmentation and erythema dyschromicum perstans. Can J Ophthalmol 1992;27:353–5.
38 Woods A. The ocular changes of primary diffuse toxic goiter: a review. Medicine 1946;25:113–54.
39 Marks MB. Allergic shiners. Dark circles under the eyes in children. Clin Pediatr 1966;5:655–8.
40 Roh MR, Chung KY. Infraorbital dark circles: definition, causes, and treatment options. Dermatol Surg 2009;35:1163–71.
41 Handel, AC, Miot, LD, Miot, HA. Melasma: a clinical and epidemiological review. An Bras Dermatol 2014; 89:771–82.
42 Sarkar, R, Ailawadi, P, Gard, S. Melasma in men: a review of clinical, etiological and management issues. J Clin Aesthet Dermatol 2018;11:53–59
43 Cestari T, Arellano I, Hexsel D, Ortonne JP. Melasma in Latin America: options for therapy and treatment algorithm. J Eur Acad Dermatol Venereol 2009;23:760–72.
44 Lee, AY. Recent Progression in Melasma Pathogenesis. Pigment Cell Melanoma Res 2015;28:648–60.
45 Ortonne JP, Arellano I, Berneburg M et al. A global survey of the role of ultraviolet radiation and hormonal influences in the development of melasma. J Eur Acad Dermatol Venereol 2009;23:1254–62.
46 Resnik S. Melasma induced by oral contraceptive drugs. JAMA 1967;199:601–5.
47 Grimes PE. Melasma. Etiologic and therapeutic considerations. Arch Dermatol 1995;131:1453–7.
48 Holmo, NF, Ramos, GB, Salomao, H et al. Complex segregation analysis of facial melisma in Brazil: evidence for genetic suspectibility with dominant pattern of segregation. Arch Dermatol Res 2018;35:217–33.
49 Kwon,SH, Hwang, YJ, Lee, SK, Park, KC. Heterogeneous pathology of melasma and its clinical implications. Int J Mol Sci 2016;17:E824.
50 Gupta AK, Gover MD, Nouri K, Taylor S. The treatment of melasma: a review of clinical trials. J Am Acad Dermatol 2006;55:1048–65.
51 Aloi F, Solaroli C, Giovannini E. Actinic lichen planus simulating melasma. Dermatology 1997;195:69–70.
52 Dammak A, Masmoudi A, Boudaya S et al. [Childhood actinic lichen planus (6 cases)]. Archives de Pediatrie 2008;15:111–14.
53 Hull PR, Procter PR. The melanocyte: an essential link in hydroquinone-induced ochronosis. J Am Acad Dermatol 1990;22:529–31.
54 Tidman MJ, Horton JJ, MacDonald DM. Hydroquinone-induced ochronosis – light and electronmicroscopic features. Clin Exp Dermatol 1986;11:224–8.
55 Piamphongsant T. Treatment of melasma: a review with personal experience. Int J Dermatol 1998;37:897–903.
56 Jutley GS, Rajaratnam R, Halpern J et al. Systematic review of randomized controlled trials on interventions for melasma: an abridged Cochrane review. J Am Acad Dermatol 2014;70:369–73.
57 Balina LM, Graupe K. The treatment of melasma. 20% azelaic acid versus 4% hydroquinone cream. Int J Dermatol 1991;30:893–5.
58 Monheit GD, Dreher F. Comparison of skin lightening cream targeting melanogenesis on multiple levels to triple combination cream for melisma. J Drugs Dermatol 2013;12:2704.
59 Jeong SY, Shin JB, Yeo UC et al. Low-fluence Q switched neodymium-doped yttrium aluminum garnet laser for melasma with pre- or post-treatment triple combination cream. Dermatol Surg 2010;36:1–10.
60 Wang WJ. Clinical features of cutaneous amyloidoses. Clin Dermatol 1990;8:13–19.
61 Cho TH, Lee MH. A case of lichen amyloidosis accompanied by vesicles and dyschromia. Clin Exp Dermatol 2008;33:291–3.

62 Elder DE, Johnson B Jr, Murphy G (eds). Lever's Histopathology of the Skin, 11th edn. Philadelphia: Lippincott Williams & Wilkins, 2015.
63 Weyers W, Weyers I, Bonczkowitz M et al. Lichen amyloidosis: a consequence of scratching. J Am Acad Dermatol 1997;37:923–8.
64 Drago F, Rebora A. Lichen amyloidosis: a consequence of scratching? J Am Acad Dermatol 1999;41:501.
65 Wong CK, Lin CS. Friction amyloidosis. Int J Dermatol 1988;27: 302–7.
66 Venkataram MN, Bhushnurmath SR, Muirhead DE, Al-Suwaid AR. Frictional amyloidosis: a study of 10 cases. Australas J Dermatol 2001;42:176–9.
67 Weber PJ, Poulos EG. Notalgia paresthetica. Case reports and histologic appraisal. J Am Acad Dermatol 1988;18:25–30.
68 Al-Aboosi M, Abalkhail A, Kasim O et al. Friction melanosis: a clinical, histologic, and ultrastructural study in Jordanian patients. Int J Dermatol 2004;43:261–4.
69 Raue F, Frank-Raue K. Update on multiple endocrine neoplasia type 2. Fam Cancer 2010;Jan 20.
70 Nieman LK, Chanco Turner ML. Addison's disease. Clin Dermatol 2006;24:276–80.
71 Cutolo M, Autoimmune polyendocrine syndromes. Autoimmun Rev 2014;13:85–6.
72 Ahonen P, Myllarniemi S, Sipila I, Perheentupa J. Clinical variation of autoimmune polyendocrinopathy-candidiasis-ectodermal dystrophy (APECED) in a series of 68 patients. N Engl J Med 1990;322:1829–36.
73 Thomas CG Jr, Smith AT, Benson M, Griffith J. Nelson's syndrome after Cushing's disease in childhood: a continuing problem. Surgery 1984;96:1067–77.
74 Banba K, Tanaka N, Fujioka A, Tajima S. Hyperpigmentation caused by hyperthyroidism: difference from pigment from Addison's disease. Clin Exp Dermatol 1999;24:196–8.
75 Ropers HH, Burmeister P, von Petrykowski W, Schindera F. Leukodystrophy, skin hyperpigmentation, and adrenal atrophy: Siemerling–Creutzfeldt disease. Transmission through several generations in two families. Am J Hum Genet 1975;27:547–53.
76 Heinrichs C, Tsigos C, Deschepper J et al. Familial adrenocorticotropin unresponsiveness associated with alacrima and achalasia: biochemical and molecular studies in two siblings with clinical heterogeneity. Eur J Pediatr 1995;154:191–6.
77 Jones D, Kay M, Craigen W et al. Coal-black hyperpigmentation at birth in a child with congenital adrenal hypoplasia. J Am Acad Dermatol 1995;33:323–6.
78 Udayakumar P, Balasubramanian S, Ramalingam KS et al. Cutaneous manifestations in patients with chronic renal failure on hemodialysis. Indian J Dermatol Venereol 2006;72:119–25.
79 Smith AG, Shuster S, Thody AJ et al. Role of the kidney in regulating plasma immunoreactive beta-melanocyte-stimulating hormone. Br Med J 1976;i:874–6.
80 De Gobbi M, Roetto A, Piperno A et al. Natural history of juvenile haemochromatosis. Br J Haematol 2002;117:973–9.
81 Paller AS. Hurwitz Clinical Pediatric Dermatology, 5th edn. Philadelphia: Elsevier Saunders, 2015.
82 Goldblatt J, Beighton P. Cutaneous manifestations of Gaucher disease. Br J Dermatol 1984;111:331–4.
83 Eisen D, Hakim MD. Minocycline-induced pigmentation. Incidence, prevention and management. Drug Safety 1998;18:431–40.
84 Alley E, Green R, Schuchter L. Cutaneous toxicities of cancer therapy. Curr Opin Oncol 2002;14:212–16.
85 Borrás-Blasco J, Navarro-Ruiz A, Borrás C, Casterá E. Adverse cutaneous reactions associated with the newest antiretroviral drugs in patients with human immunodeficiency virus infection. J Antimicrob Chemother 2008;62:879–88.
86 Dunagin WG. Cutaneous signs of systemic toxicity due to dioxins and related chemicals. J Am Acad Dermatol 1984;10:688–700.
87 Granstein RD, Sober AJ. Drug and heavy metal-induced hyperpigmentation. J Am Acad Dermatol 1981;5:1–18.
88 Tchounwou PB, Patlolla AK, Centeno JA. Carcinogenic and systemic health effects associated with arsenic exposure – a critical review. Toxicol Pathol 2003;31:575–88.
89 Noppakun N, Swasdikul D. Reversible hyperpigmentation of skin and nails with white hair due to vitamin B12 deficiency. Arch Dermatol 1986;122:896–9.
90 MacDonald A, Forsyth A. Nutritional deficiencies and the skin. Clin Exp Dermatol 2005;30:388–90.
91 McLaren DS. Skin in protein energy malnutrition. Arch Dermatol 1987;123:1674–6a.
92 Burrows NP, Loo WJ. An orange-tinted baby!! Clin Exp Dermatol 2006;31:495–6.
93 McGowan R, Beattie J, Galloway P. Carotenaemia in children is common and benign: most can stay at home. Scot Med J 2004;49:82–4.
94 Karthik SV, Campbell-Davidson D, Isherwood D. Carotenemia in infancy and its association with prevalent feeding practices. Pediatr Dermatol 2006;23:571–3.
95 Burns T, Breathnach S, Cox N, Griffiths C (eds). Rook's Textbook of Dermatology. Oxford: Blackwell Publishing, 2004;Vol 3: Chapter 56.82.
96 Nakanishi T, Sobue I, Toyokura Y et al. The Crow–Fukase syndrome: a study of 102 cases in Japan. Neurology 1984;34:712–20.
97 Shelley WB, Shelley ED. The skin changes in the Crow-Fukase (POEMS) syndrome. Arch Dermatol 1987;123:85–7.
98 Marina S, Broshtilova V. POEMS in childhood. Pediatr Dermatol 2006;23:145–8.
99 Fonseca E. Skin manifestations of toxic syndrome due to denatured rapeseed oil. Actas Dermosifiliogr 2009;100:857–60.
100 Maisels MJ, McDonagh AF. Phototherapy for neonatal jaundice. N Engl J Med 2008;358:920–8.
101 Ruiz-Maldonado R, Tamayo L, Fernandez-Diez J. Universal acquired melanosis. The carbon baby. Arch Dermatol 1978;114:775–8.
102 Furuya T, Mishima Y. Progressive pigmentary disorder in Japanese child. Arch Dermatol 1962;86:412–8.
103 Bloom D. Acropigmentation in a child. Arch Dermatol Syphilol 1950;62:475.
104 Hernandez-Martin, A, Gilliam, ME, Baselga, E et al. Hyperpigmented macules on the face of young children: a series of 25 cases. J Am Acad Derm 2014;70:288–90.
105 David TJ, Webb BW, Gordon IR. The Patterson syndrome, leprechaunism, and pseudoleprechaunism. J Med Genet 1981;18:294–8.
106 Wende GW, Baukus HH. A hitherto undescribed generalized pigmentation of the skin appearing in infancy in brother and sister. J Cutan Dis 1919;37:685–701.
107 Pegum JS. Diffuse pigmentation in brothers. Proc R Soc Med 1955;48:179–80.
108 Malakar S, Dhar S. Pigmentary demarcation lines over the face. Dermatology 2000;200:85–6.
109 Somani VK, Razvi F, Sita VN. Pigmentary demarcation lines over the face. Indian J Dermatol Venereol Leprol 2004;70:336–41.
110 Ito K. The peculiar demarcation of pigmentation along the so-called Voigt's line among the Japanese. Dermatol Int 1965;4:45.
111 Millington PF, Wilkinson R (eds). Biological Structure and Function 9, Skin. Cambridge: Cambridge University Press, 1983:20.
112 Selmanowitz VJ, Krivo JM. Pigmentary demarcation lines. Comparison of Negroes with Japanese. Br J Dermatol 1975;93:371–7.
113 Miura O. On the demarcation lines of pigmentation observed among the Japanese, on inner sides of their extremities and on anterior and posterior sides of their medial regions. Tohoku J Exp Med 1951;54:135–40.
114 James WD, Carter JM, Rodman OG. Pigmentary demarcation lines: a population survey. J Am Acad Dermatol 1987;16:584–90.
115 Ferguson J, Dover JS (eds). Photodermatology. London: Manson, 2006:81–4.
116 Arseculeratne GB, Meiklejohn L, Mountain D et al. Bleomycin-induced 'flagellate dermatitis'. Arch Dermatol 2007;143:1461–2.
117 Geddes ER, Cohen PR. Antineoplastic agent-associated serpentine supravenous hyperpigmentation: superficial venous system hyperpigmentation following intravenous chemotherapy. South Med J 2010;103:231–5.
118 Riahi RR, Cohen PR. Laptop-induced erythema ab igne: report and review of literature. Dermatol Online J 2012;18:5.
119 Colver GB, Mortimer PS, Millard PR et al. The 'dirty neck'—a reticulate pigmentation in atopics. Clin Exp Dermatol 1987;12:14.
120 Humphreys F, Spencer J, McLaren K, Tidman MJ. An histological and ultrastructural study of the 'dirty neck' appearance in atopic eczema. Clin Exp Dermatol 1996;21:17–19.
121 Scheinfeld N. Confluent and reticulated papillomatosis: a review of the literature. Am J Clin Dermatol 2006;7:305–13.
122 Shannon JF, Weedon D, Sharkey MP. Prurigo pigmentosa. Australas J Dermatol 2006;47:289–90.
123 Andres C, Chen W, Hofmann H et al. Epidermolysis bullosa simplex with mottled pigmentation: a case report. Int J Dermatol 2009;48:753–4.
124 Irvine AD, Rugg EL, Lane EB et al. Molecular confirmation of the unique phenotype of epidermolysis bullosa simplex with mottled pigmentation. Br J Dermatol 2001;144:40–5.

125 Sardana K, Goel K, Chugh S. Reticulate pigmentary disorders. Indian J Dermatol Venereol Leprol 2013;79:17–29.

126 Slominski A, Tobin DJ, Shibahara S et al. Melanin pigmentation in mammalian skin and its hormonal regulation. Physiol Rev 2004;84:1155–228.

127 Abdel-Malek ZA, Scott MC, Furumura M et al. The melanocortin 1 receptor is the principal mediator of the effects of agouti signaling protein on mammalian melanocytes. J Cell Sci 2001;114:1019–24.

128 Rees JL. Genetics of hair and skin color. Annu Rev Genet 2003;37:67–90.

129 Lin JY, Fisher DE. Melanocyte biology and skin pigmentation. Nature 2007;445:843–50.

130 Boissy RE. Melanosome transfer to and translocation in the keratinocyte. Exp Dermatol 2003;12(suppl 2):5–12.

131 Hume AN, Ushakov DS, Tarafder AK et al. Rab27a and MyoVa are the primary Mlph interactors regulating melanosome transport in melanocytes. J Cell Sci 2007;120:3111–22.

132 Van Den Bossche K, Naeyaert JM, Lambert J. The quest for the mechanism of melanin transfer. Traffic 2006;7:769–78.

133 Seiberg M, Paine C, Sharlow E et al. Inhibition of melanosome transfer results in skin lightening. J Invest Dermatol 2000;115:162–7.

134 Betz RC, Planko L, Eigelshoven S et al. Loss-of-function mutations in the keratin 5 gene lead to Dowling-Degos disease. Am J Hum Genet 2006;78:510–19.

135 Planko L, Bohse K, Hohfeld J et al. Identification of a keratin associated protein with a putative role in vesicle transport. Eur J Cell Biol 2007;86:827–39.

136 Happle R. Mosaicism in human skin. Understanding the patterns and mechanisms. Arch Dermatol 1993;129:1460–70.

137 Hoegling, M, Frieden, I. Segmental pigmentation disorder. Br J Dermatol 2010;162:1337–41.

138 Turan, S, Bastepe, M. GNAS spectrum of disorders. Curr Osteoporos Rep 2015;13:146–58.

139 Hoekstra HE. Genetics, development and evolution of adaptive pigmentation in vertebrates. Heredity 2006;97:222–34.

140 Wang ZQ, Si L, Tang Q et al. Gain-of-function mutation of KIT ligand on melanin synthesis causes familial progressive hyperpigmentation. Am J Hum Genet 2009;84:672–7.

141 Ghonasgi S, Shah R, Meghana SM et al. Familial progressive hyperpigmentation: a case report. Case Rep Dent 2012;2012:840167.

142 Speeckaert R, Van Gele M, Speeckaert MM et al. The biology of hyperpigmentation syndromes. Pigment Cell Melanoma Res 2014;27:512–24.

143 Tanaka A, Lai-Cheong JE, van den Akker PC et al. The molecular skin pathology of familial primary localized cutaneous amyloidosis. Exp Dermatol 2010;19:416–23.

144 Arita K, South AP, Hans-Filho G et al. Oncostatin M receptor-beta mutations underlie familial primary localized cutaneous amyloidosis. Am J Hum Genet 2008;82:73–80.

145 Nelson DL. NEMO, NFkappaB signaling and incontinentia pigmenti. Curr Opin Genet Dev 2006;16:282–8.

146 Scheuerle AE, Ursini MV. Incontinentia Pigmenti. 1999 Jun 8 [Updated 2015 Feb 12]. In: Pagon RA, Adam MP, Ardinger HH et al. (eds) GeneReviews® [Internet]. Seattle (WA): University of Washington, Seattle;1993–2015

147 Maruani A, Khallouf R, Machet MC, Lorette G. Diffuse linear and whorled nevoid hypermelanosis in a newborn. J Pediatr 2012;160:171.

148 Hong SP, Ahn SY, Lee WS. Linear and whorled nevoid hypermelanosis: unique clinical presentations and their possible association with chromosomal abnormality inv(9). Arch Dermatol 2008;144:415–16.

149 Cohen, J, Shahrokh K, Cohen B. Analysis of 36 cases of Blaschkoid dyspigmentation: reading between the lines of Blaschko. Pediatr Dermatol 2014;31:471–6.

150 Ding YG, Zhu TS, Jiang W et al. Identification of a novel mutation and a de novo mutation in DKC1 in two Chinese pedigrees with Dyskeratosis congenita. J Invest Dermatol 2004;123:470–3.

151 García, M, Fernández S, Teruya-Feldstein J. The diagnosis and treatment of dyskeratosis congenita: a review. J Blood Med 2014;5:157.

152 Calado RT, Young NS. Telomere maintenance and human bone marrow failure. Blood 2008;111:4446–55.

153 Mathew CG. Fanconi anaemia genes and susceptibility to cancer. Oncogene 2006;25:5875–84.

154 Giampetro PF, Verlander PC, Davis JG, Auerbach AD. Diagnosis of Fanconi anemia in patients without congenital malformations: an international Fanconi Anemia Registry Study. Am J Med Genet 1997;68:58–61.

155 Lugassy J, Itin P, Ishida-Yamamoto A et al. Naegeli–Franceschetti–Jadassohn syndrome and dermatopathia pigmentosa reticularis: two allelic ectodermal dysplasias caused by dominant mutations in KRT14. Am J Hum Genet 2006;79:724–30

156 Lugassy J, McGrath JA, Itin P et al. KRT14 haploinsufficiency results in increased susceptibility of keratinocytes to TNF-alpha-induced apoptosis and causes Naegeli–Franceschetti–Jadassohn syndrome. J Invest Dermatol 2008;128:1517–24.

157 Hovnanian A, Pollack E, Hilal L et al. A missense mutation in the rod domain of keratin 14 associated with recessive epidermolysis bullosa simplex. Nat Genet 1993;3:327–32.

158 Harel A, Bergman R, Indelman M et al. Epidermolysis bullosa simplex with mottled pigmentation resulting from a recurrent mutation in KRT14. J Invest Dermatol 2006;126:1654–7.

159 Betz RC, Planko L, Eigelshoven S et al. Loss-of-function mutations in the keratin 5 gene lead to Dowling–Degos disease. Am J Hum Genet 2006;78:510–19.

160 Guo L, Luo X, Zhao A et al. A novel heterozygous nonsense mutation of keratin 5 in a Chinese family with Dowling-Degos disease. J Eur Acad Dermatol Venereol 2012;26:908–10.

161 Liao H, Zhao Y, Baty DU et al. A heterozygous frameshift mutation in the V1 domain of keratin 5 in a family with Dowling-Degos disease. J Invest Dermatol 2007;127:298–300.

162 Uttam J, Hutton E, Coulombe PA et al. The genetic basis of epidermolysis bullosa simplex with mottled pigmentation. Proc Natl Acad Sci USA 1996;93:9079–84.

163 Sprecher E, Indelman M, Khamaysi Z et al. Galli–Galli disease is an acantholytic variant of Dowling–Degos disease. Br J Dermatol 2007;156:572–4.

164 Basmanav FB, Oprisoreanu AM, Pasternack SM et al. Mutations in POGLUT1, encoding protein O-glucosyltransferase 1, cause autosomal-dominant Dowling-Degos disease. Am J Hum Genet 2014;94: 135–43.

165 Li M, Cheng R, Liang J et al. Mutations in POFUT1, encoding protein O-fucosyltransferase 1, cause generalized Dowling-Degos disease. Am J Hum Genet 2014;92:895–903.

166 Schnur RE, Heymann WR. Reticulate hyperpigmentation. Semin Cutan Med Surg 1997;16:72–80.

167 Kono M, Sugiura K, Suganuma M et al. Whole-exome sequencing identifies ADAM10 mutations as a cause of reticulate acropigmentation of Kitamura, a clinical entity distinct from Dowling-Degos disease. Hum Mol Genet 2013;22:3524–33.

168 Bozkulak EC, Weinmaster G. Selective use of ADAM10 and ADAM17 in activation of Notch1 signaling. Mol Cell Biol 2009;29:5679–95.

169 Jaeckle Santos LJ, Xing C, Barnes RB et al. Refined mapping of X-linked reticulate pigmentary disorder and sequencing of candidate genes. Hum Genet 2008;123:469–76.

170 Pezzani L, Brena M, Callea M et al. X-linked reticulate pigmentary disorder with systemic manifestations: a new family and review of the literature. Am J Med Genet Part A 2013;161A:1414–20.

CHAPTER 123
Vitiligo

Julien Seneschal[1], *Juliette Mazereeuw-Hautier*[2] *& Alain Taïeb*[1]

[1] Department of Dermatology and Paediatric Dermatology, Reference Center for Rare Skin Diseases, Hôpital Saint André, Bordeaux, France
[2] Department of Dermatology, Reference Center for Rare Skin Diseases, Larrey Hospital, Toulouse, France

Abstract

Vitiligo is a common inflammatory skin disease, characterized by the development of depigmented areas, with a worldwide prevalence estimated at 0.5–1% of the population. The exact prevalence in the paediatric age group remains unknown, although it is now assumed that vitiligo can begin very early in life. Vitiligo involves a complex combination of aetiological factors including genetic susceptibilities, mostly associated with components of the immune system and environmental triggers, leading to loss of melanocytes. The disease is disfiguring, with a major psychological impact on children and their parents. Management of vitiligo should take into account several factors, including extent of psychological impact, possible associations with other autoimmune diseases and the need to be associated with minimal side-effects.

Key points

- **Approximately 25% of vitiligo cases begin before the age of 10 years.**
- **Although vitiligo is not a life-threatening disease, it can be a life-altering disease.**
- **The most commonly reported autoimmune disease associated with vitiligo is thyroiditis, but an atopic background is also common in children**
- **Vitiligo is a microinflammatory disease, with little clinical evidence of inflammation. Early aggressive treatment is recommended to prevent rapid progression as well as maintenance treatment to stabilize the disease.**
- **Topical corticosteroids or topical tacrolimus (especially on face and neck) represent a first-line treatment for limited disease. Topical treatments yield better results when combined with ultraviolet light.**

Introduction. Vitiligo is an acquired disease characterized by the development of hypo- or depigmented areas of skin associated with substantial loss of functioning epidermal and/or hair follicle melanocytes. Vitiligo is a disorder that is usually generalized (vitiligo/nonsegmental vitiligo, NSV) (Fig. 123.1) or segmental (segmental vitiligo, SV) (Fig 123.2), focal, mixed (Fig. 123.3) or unclassifiable according to the revised international nomenclature [1]. Childhood vitiligo differs from adult onset vitiligo in several aspects, including a higher proportion of segmental cases, a higher prevalence of halo nevi and a higher proportion of cases with a family history of autoimmune diseases and atopic diathesis.

Aetiology and pathogenesis. In vitiligo there is a variable pattern of loss of melanocytes from the epidermis and follicular reservoir; this is most usually chronic and progressive, with periods of spontaneous remission. Vitiligo is a multifactorial disorder characterized histologically by a microinflammatory phase associated with melanocyte loss.

Genetic susceptibility

Most cases occur sporadically but about 15–20% of patients have one or more affected first-degree relatives. Familial aggregation of NSV follows a non-Mendelian pattern suggesting complex polygenic multifactorial inheritance. Genome-wide association studies have identified several susceptibility loci for generalized vitiligo, including the gene encoding tyrosinase, *TYR*. Tyrosinase is a melanocyte enzyme that catalyses melanin biosynthesis. However, in these studies, nearly all the susceptibility genes so far identified encode proteins associated with the immune system, supporting the hypothesis that vitiligo is linked to a dysregulation of the innate and the adaptative immune system. Several of these loci (e.g. *HLA* class I and II, *PTPN22*, *IL2R* α, *GZMB*, *FOXP3*, *BACH2*, *CD80* and *CCR6*) suggest a role for adaptive immunity. Other loci (e.g. *NLRP1*, *IFIH1* [*MDA5*], *TRIF*, *CASP7*, *XBP1* and *C1QTNF6*) point to components of the innate immune system. Some of them are shared with susceptibility to other autoimmune disorders, such as type 1 diabetes, thyroid disease and rheumatoid arthritis [2–6].

Harper's Textbook of Pediatric Dermatology, Fourth Edition. Edited by Peter Hoeger, Veronica Kinsler and Albert Yan.

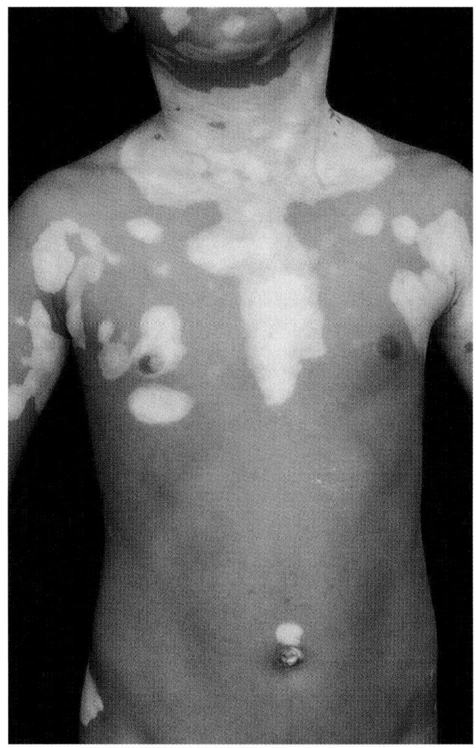

Fig. 123.1 Typical vitiligo in symmetrical patches on both sides of the body.

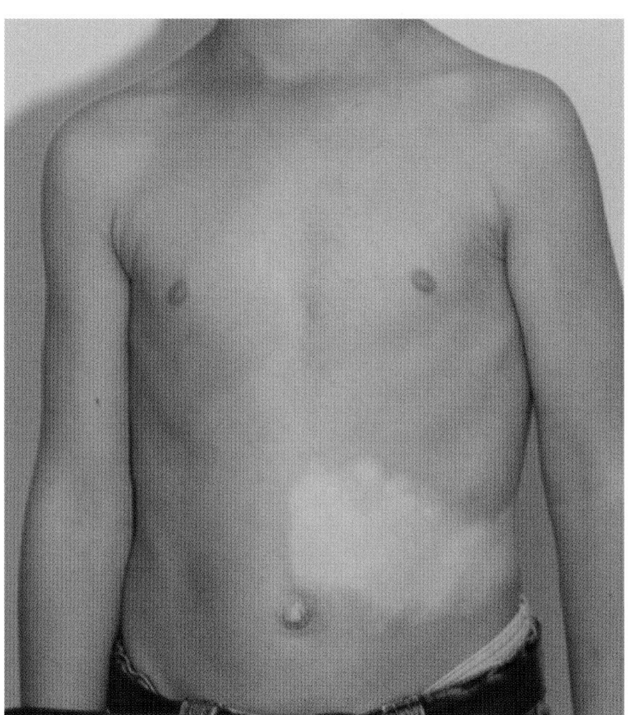

Fig. 123.2 Segmental vitiligo on the trunk.

Similar to other common chronic disorders, vitiligo may represent an interaction between inherited and environmental factors [7].

Melanocyte loss

Melanocyte loss is the classical hallmark of vitiligo. Multiple mechanisms have been suggested to be involved in melanocyte disappearance. However, the initiating

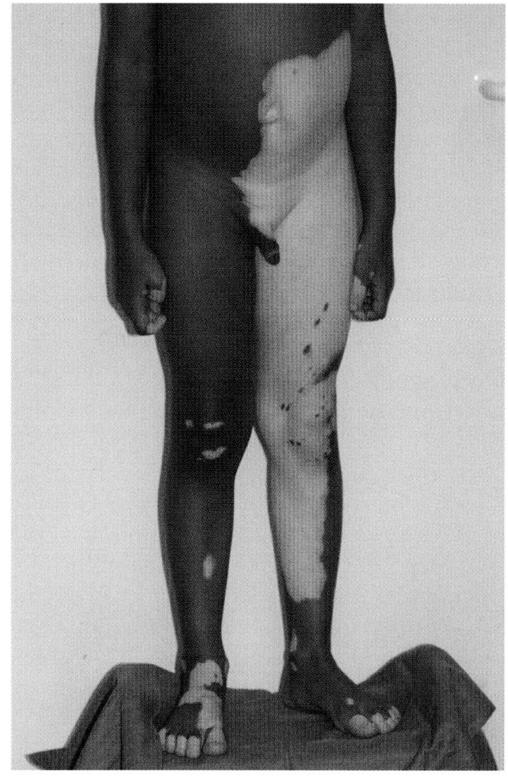

Fig. 123.3 Mixed vitiligo.

events and pathomechanisms leading to the loss of melanocytes remain largely unknown. Many studies support melanocyte-intrinsic abnormalities in vitiligo with increased levels of reactive oxygen species (ROS) leading to impaired melanocyte degeneration and/or proliferation, and activation of the innate and adaptive (cell-mediated or humoral immunity) responses. Therefore, melanocytes loss could result from the consequences of the immune response, apoptosis or decreased stability in the basement membrane zone [8,9].

The immune system

Increased levels of ROS can create a proinflammatory environment leading to the production of proinflammatory cytokines and the activation of the immune response. Chemicals known to trigger vitiligo (4-TBP and MBEH) induce the disruption of the folding machinery of the endoplasmic reticulum, leading to the accumulation of immature proteins and resulting in the activation of the unfolded protein response, XBP1 and the production of interleukin (IL)-6 and IL-8. ROS can also modulate the innate immune system through the activation of pathogen recognition receptors (PRRs). For example, in the cytosol, receptors involving the inflammasome formation have been linked to vitiligo. Increased expression of NLRP1 and IL-1β in perilesional skin of vitiligo has been shown to be associated with disease progression. Nucleic acid receptors have been also associated with vitiligo. For example, IFIH1 (MDA-5) is a cytosolic recognition receptor which recognizes dsRNA, and induces the production of type I interferon. Besides the role of these receptors, small molecules such as heat shock proteins have been shown to be elevated in vitiligo and activate PRRs. Stimulation of PRRs by various mechanisms induces the activation and recruitment of innate immune cells to promote adaptive immune responses. In vitiligo, various innate immune cells have been observed in perilesional or lesional skin such as natural killer cells, dendritic cells and more recently plasmacytoid dendritic cells. All these innate cells are important for the promotion of the adaptive immune response in particular via CD8+ T cells [10].

Other involved cells

Keratinocytes appear to be involved in vitiligo. Firstly, these cells can produce a number of soluble factors under the influence of environmental factors through activation of PRRs such as IL-1β, IL-6 and IL-8. Secondly, recent studies highlight a new role of keratinocytes in the pathogenesis of vitiligo. Keratinocytes were found to be the major producers of two chemokines ligands (CXCL9 and CXCL10) important for the recruitment of T cells into perilesional skin of vitiligo [11,12]. In addition, oxidative stress was found to induce expression of the chemokine ligand CXCL16 by keratinocytes leading to the recruitment of CD8+ T cells expressing CXCR6 [13].

Segmental vitiligo

The pathophysiology was formerly presumed to be different for segmental vitiligo, with limited influence of immune phenomena. Quite strikingly, the distribution of segmental vitiligo, at least in a subset of patients, suggests a developmental pattern usually associated with cutaneous mosaicism. However, biopsies taken in recent onset cases indicate also the presence of immune infiltrates as in common vitiligo [14].

Segmental vitiligo can be associated with nonsegmental vitiligo. It indicates a continuum between the two forms with shared predisposing genetic factors and a shared autoimmune-mediated process, including genes operating specifically in the skin. It also suggests, as in monogenic mosaic disorders, a mechanism of loss of heterozygosity for a dominant gene controlling part of the cutaneous phenotype [14].

Pathology. The clinical diagnosis of vitiligo is straightforward and a skin biopsy is usually not required. Histologically, melanocytes are completely absent in established lesions of vitiligo [15,16]. Immunohistochemical stains using antibodies to antigens on cells of neural crest derivation, or specific melanocyte antibodies such as antityrosinase or melan-A (A 103), can also confirm the absence of melanocytes [17].

In contrast, melanocytes are not absent in the sections from early lesions, but exhibit various cellular abnormalities including vacuolization, presence of dilated endoplasmic reticulum and granular deposits [18]. At the progressing border of active vitiligo macules, mononuclear cellular infiltrates are present, and there is indication of type I interferon production [11].

During repigmentation, especially when ultraviolet (UV)-induced, there is an influx of cells from the follicular reservoir of melanocytes [19,20]. This is confirmed by response to treatment: repigmentation is first visible principally around follicular orifices and depigmented lesions without hair follicles (glabrous skin) do not respond well to treatment [21]. However, repigmentation patterns in glabrous areas suggest alternative reservoirs [19,22].

Clinical features.

Prevalence and age of onset

The exact prevalence of vitiligo in the paediatric age group is unknown but the figure of approximately 25% of cases beginning before the age of 10 years obtained in a Danish study seems correct [20]. The mean age of onset in paediatric series varies between studies from 4 to 8 years [21], but very early onset, as young as 3 months, is acknowledged. Congenital vitiligo, however, is usually piebaldism misdiagnosed as vitiligo, and the existence of true 'congenital vitiligo' remains controversial. In fair-skinned individuals, vitiligo patches are usually detected only after the first exposure of the skin to sunlight, following the first summer of life.

Gender

In most reported paediatric series the majority of cases were girls, but this finding differs from population-based studies, which do not confirm a female sex predominance.

Race

All races can be affected. The prevalence probably varies according to geographic origin and seems to be higher in India than in other countries.

Morphology

The depigmented lesions are, as the name suggests, completely devoid of pigment and appear as milk white areas of skin (Fig. 123.4). Patches of vitiligo are made more visible by tanning of the surrounding skin or in dark skin. The use of a Wood's lamp is useful to delineate areas of involvement in fair-skinned children.

Psychological effects of vitiligo

Negative experiences from childhood vitiligo may influence adult life [23]. Although vitiligo is not a life-threatening disease, it can be a life-altering disease. Children are probably affected differently, depending on the location, extent and course of the disease, their age, individual capacities and social environment. It is important to assess as early as possible how the children themselves are coping with their disease, in order to make appropriate treatment plans.

Classification and distribution. Depigmented patches of vitiligo can occur anywhere on the body and no area is necessarily spared. The most commonly involved site is the head. In vitiligo/nonsegmental vitiligo, lesions are characteristically distributed in a remarkably symmetrical pattern involving both sides of the body. The most common location is the face, especially around the eyes,

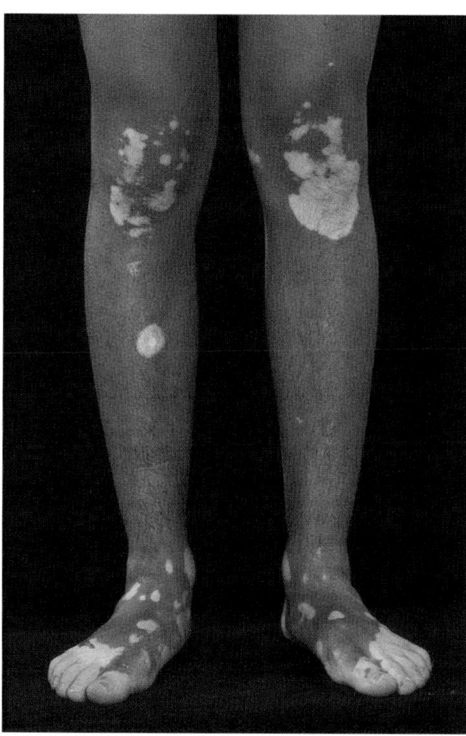

Fig. 123.4 Vitiligo on the lower legs and feet: ivory white symmetrical areas on the knees, ankles and feet.

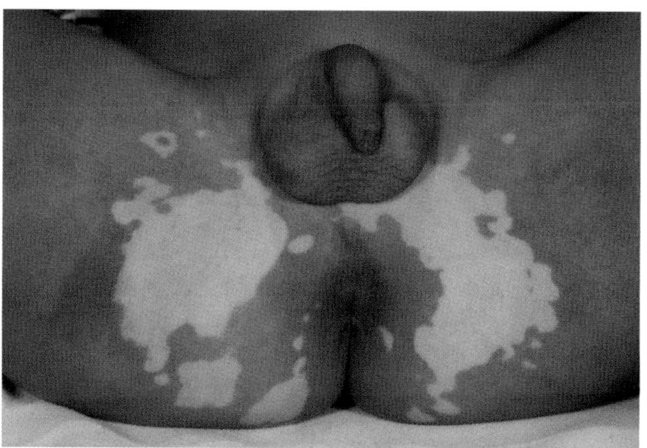

Fig. 123.5 Vitiligo presenting in infancy in the napkin area.

and neck, followed by the lower limbs, trunk and upper limbs. Involvement of the perineum, in particular the perianal and buttocks skin in contact with the nappy is common, suggesting Koebner's phenomenon (Fig. 123.5). The recently developed K-VSCOR, suggests a correlation between rapid spread and koebnerization [24]. Few studies have recorded the presence of the Koebner phenomenon in children with vitiligo. Handa and Dogra found evidence of koebnerization in 11.3% of children [25]. Examination of the hands and feet with a Wood's lamp confirms that these areas are commonly involved, including the palms, even in those with type 1 or 2 skin.

The skin and hair follicles on the scalp can also be involved, leading to poliosis (Fig. 123.6). In the literature, the prevalence of poliosis was found to be between 12.3% and 19.3%. Premature greying of the hair is sometimes

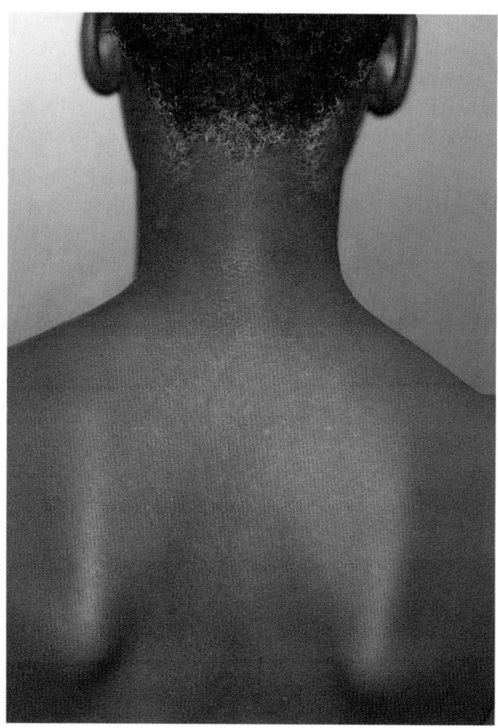

Fig. 123.6 Involvement of hair follicles (follicular vitiligo).

observed; Jaisankar and colleagues noted this finding in 4.4% of children [26]. There are a few individuals who develop totally white hair of the scalp, eyebrows and eyelashes. A follicular variant with preferential early hair involvement has recently been delineated [27]. An area rarely recognized to be affected by vitiligo is the oral cavity. The lips, buccal mucosa and gingiva can be involved but the incidence of involvement seems to be lower in children than in adults. The presence of halo naevi in a patient with segmental vitiligo may be a marker of risk for mixed vitiligo [28]. The significance of isolated halo naevi as a clinical marker of risk for vitiligo is frequently debated. A comparison to the general paediatric population is difficult because the prevalence of halo naevi in not well known, possibly around 1%. Prcic and colleagues [29] found that there are more halo naevi in children with vitiligo, compared with children without vitiligo (34% vs 3.3%). The prevalence of halo naevi in children with vitiligo varies widely according to series, from 2.5 to 34%, and based on personal experience some cases would have gone undetected without Wood's lamp examination. It is also unclear whether the prevalence of halo naevi in children with vitiligo is different from that found in adult vitiligo, but in general they are easier to detect, without skin ageing background. Vitiligo may develop within or around congenital naevi, and unusually on Becker's naevus. Halo naevi associated with non-segmental vitiligo was associated with an age of onset younger than 18 years [30].

Extension

The extent of involvement varies among patients. Handa and Dogra demonstrated that 96.4% of children have less than 20% of the body involved, and 89.7% have less than 5% of the body area involved [25]. Rarely, vitiligo can involve more than 90% of the body surface area (vitiligo universalis, Fig. 123.7).

Progression

It is important to determine the stage of disease progression in order to take the best therapeutic decision. Early or advancing lesions of vitiligo may be partially depigmented and have a freckled appearance or multishaded hue. In dark-skinned individuals this is termed trichrome vitiligo. In a few patients, an inflammatory border (oedematous, pruritic and erythematous) may be visible. Confetti-like lesions is a negative prognostic sign in patients with vitiligo, indicating rapidly progressing disease suggesting a more aggressive therapy for preventing rapid and potential permanent loss of pigmentation [31] (Figs 123.8 and 123.9). Evidence of recent Koebner's phenomenon is also an objective sign of progressive disease [25].

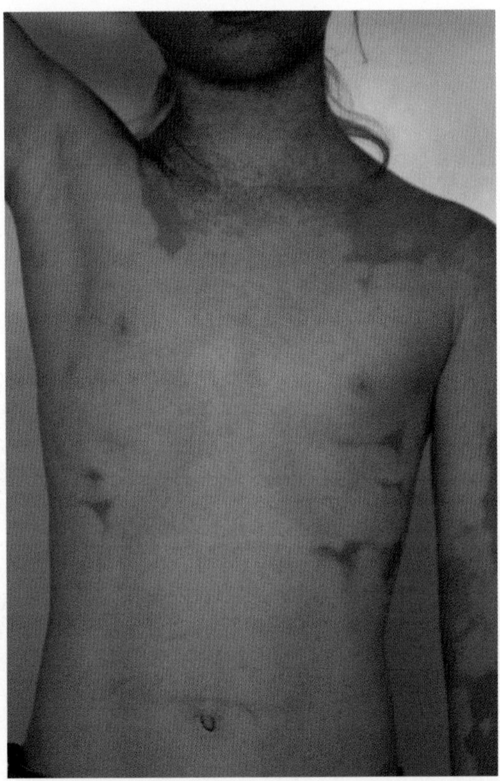

Fig. 123.7 Vitiligo universalis.

Repigmentation

Five repigmentation patterns have been described: perifollicular, marginal, diffuse, combined and, newly described, the medium spotted repigmentation pattern that occurs in sites with few or absent hair follicles such as palms and soles. Gan and colleagues demonstrated in a cohort of 109 paediatric patients that the combined pattern of repigmentation was the most frequently observed pattern in this population [22].

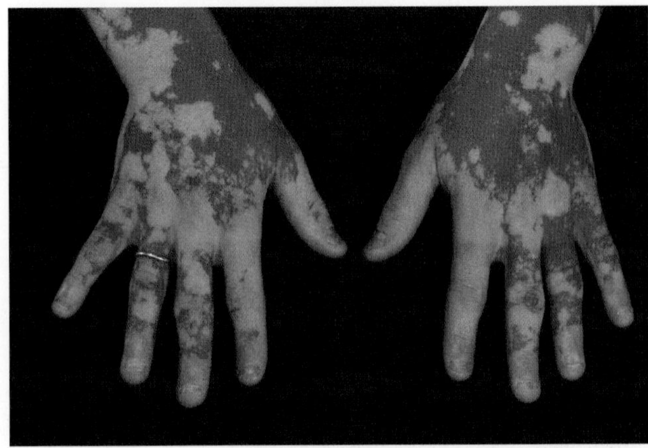

Fig. 123.8 Typical pattern of rapidly progressive vitiligo of the hands in an adolescent girl.

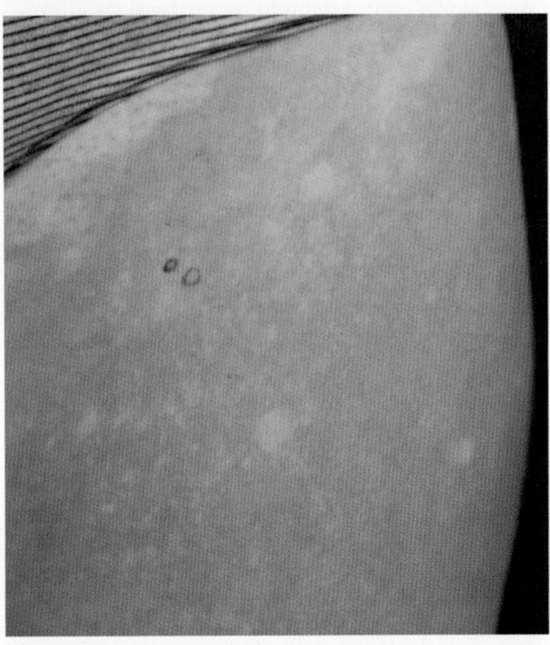

(a)

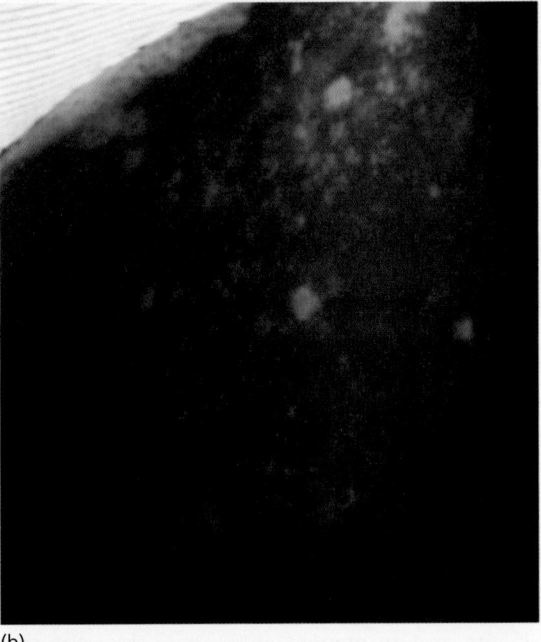

(b)

Fig. 123.9 Confetti-like lesions in patient with rapidly progressive disease. (a) Normal light. (b) Wood's lamp.

Associated skin conditions
Vitiligo can affect children with a history of atopic dermatitis. In a multivariate analysis of a prospective observational study, it was found that atopic dermatitis and an atopic diathesis is commonly found in children with vitiligo [32]. The location of the vitiligo may correspond to eczema lesions but not as a rule. In general, the two diseases follow a separate course in the same patient [32]. In another study including adults, the higher prevalence of atopic dermatitis with vitiligo was confirmed, and a history of atopic dermatitis was associated with more extensive disease [33]. In this situation, it is necessary to distinguish the depigmented areas of vitiligo from postinflammatory hypopigmentation or depigmentation secondary to eczema.

Associated diseases
Children suffering from vitiligo are generally healthy, but other autoimmune and allergic diseases can sometimes be associated. The most commonly reported autoimmune disease is thyroiditis. The prevalence of thyroid dysfunction in childhood vitiligo was found to vary from 0 to 14% among different studies [29,34–37]. Some authors have suggested that thyroid dysfunction increases with age. On the other hand, Kakourou and colleagues found no association between thyroid dysfunction and the following parameters: chronological age, age of onset, mean duration, clinical type of vitiligo, family history of autoimmunity/thyroid disorder or sex [38]. Ezzedine and colleagues showed that prepubertal onset of vitiligo was no more associated with thyroid disease than postpubertal onset [32].

The other autoimmune diseases reported in children with vitiligo include: alopecia areata, diabetes mellitus, Addison disease and autoimmune polyglandular syndrome. The prevalence of these other diseases seems to be very low (1.3–7.6% in total).

Antinuclear antibodies can be found in children with vitiligo. This probably represents the general autoimmune status of the child with vitiligo. One study [23] detected positive antinuclear antibodies in 4.8% of children, whereas two others recorded 0% antinuclear antibody positivity [24,26]. In clinical practice, there is no consensus for screening for associated autoimmunity, but it seems appropriate to perform routine thyroid screening in nonsegmental vitiligo, particularly if the child has a strong family history of autoimmune diseases. Some authors have suggested annual assessment of thyroid function [35], although there is little data to support this. The presence of antithyroid antibodies with normal thyroid function should trigger endocrinology follow-up. Other baseline tests could include: full blood count, fasting blood sugar and antinuclear antibodies.

Familial background
Based on a large study, children with vitiligo and a family history of vitiligo were more likely to have an earlier age of onset than those with no family history [39]. The family incidence for autoimmunity found in the different reported studies ranges from 3.3 to 27.3% [26,40,41]. A family history of dysimmunity is more frequently reported in children with vitiligo, as compared with adults with vitiligo [42]. A French multicentre study found a similar percentage of familial autoimmune diseases in children with SV and NSV [36].

A so far neglected finding has been the association of vitiligo with a familial atopic diathesis, a common finding at vitiligo pediatric clinics. This association has been confirmed in larger series [32,43] and genome-wide association studies have shown predisposing genes common to atopy and vitiligo such as thymic stromal lymphopoietin (TLSP) [44].

Segmental vitiligo
Unilateral lesions that do not cross the midline and may follow development lines are classified as segmental vitiligo. Segmental vitiligo is seen more frequently in children compared with adults [29,40]. The prevalence of segmental vitiligo among children varied among different reported case series and ranged from 4.6 to 32.5%. The most common involved site of vitiligo is the head. Mazereeuw-Hautier and colleagues compared the characteristics of segmental vitiligo with nonsegmental vitiligo [36]: thyroid abnormalities and a hyperpigmented rim around vitiligo lesions were observed only in nonsegmental vitiligo. In addition, more halo naevi were observed among children with nonsegmental vitiligo, compared with children with segmental vitiligo (20% vs 12%).

Differential diagnosis. If vitiligo is atypical, other disorders associated with hypopigmentation in children should be excluded. Vitiligo is an acquired and not a congenital disease, so the determination of the age of onset of the depigmented lesions is crucial. Furthermore, vitiligo is completely depigmented except in trichrome vitiligo or in the early stages of the disease.

The main differential diagnoses are postinflammatory hypopigmentation and naevus depigmentosus. Naevus depigmentosus is a single large hypopigmented or depigmented patch, with sometimes islands of normal skin that is usually present at birth but can be detected only later in infancy or early childhood; typically it does not progress. Wood's lamp examination does not enhance lesions as much as in vitiligo, which shows typically a marked fluorescent white reflection. If a biopsy is taken, melanocytes are present in naevus depigmentosus.

Other differential diagnoses include tinea versicolour, pityriasis alba, piebaldism, lichen sclerosus et atrophicus, tuberous sclerosis, scleroderma and systemic lupus erythematosus. Other causes of genetic hypomelanoses include Waardenburg syndrome, Menkes syndrome, Ziprkowski–Margolis syndrome, Griscelli syndrome and the various forms of albinism.

Tinea versicolor is characterized by hypopigmented patches that can resemble early vitiligo. However, differentiating features include lesions that are hypopigmented, not depigmented, with a fine scale on the surface, with poorly defined edges. The distribution of tinea versicolor is mainly the neck, chest and back. The diagnosis of tinea versicolor is confirmed by mycology of skin scrapings.

Pityriasis alba is another disorder of hypopigmentation. The lesions also have a fine scale with poorly defined edges and are typically located on the cheeks and upper portions of the arms or thighs in individuals who have atopic dermatitis. The association of pityriasis alba and vitiligo is common in children.

Piebaldism is a genetic disease, transmitted as an autosomal dominant trait, which is characterized by areas of depigmentation, often with hyperpigmented areas within the affected areas of skin. Involvement of the hair with a white forelock is common. The cutaneous manifestations are similar to vitiligo in many respects; however, the lesions are present at birth or visible soon after birth. They are stable in their size and location although the edges of the spots can change slightly with age with central and marginal repigmentation. The lesions are almost invariably located on the anterior surface of the body and have a typical pattern. A family history is usually present.

Ash leaf spots associated with tuberous sclerosis are hypopigmented macules that either are present at birth or develop during the neonatal period.

Albinism is a genetic disorder usually detectable at birth. It is not easily confused with vitiligo. Melanocytes are present but are unable to synthesize melanin. The entire body, the hair and the eyes are involved. The patient will have significant ocular abnormalities including nystagmus, strabismus and low visual acuity.

Two rare syndromes that include vitiligoid lesions as part of their clinical manifestations are the Vogt–Koyanagi–Harada syndrome (uveitis, meningitis, dysacousia, alopecia, poliosis and vitiligo) and Alezzandrini syndrome (segmental vitiligo associated with ipsilateral uveitis and loss of visual acuity in some).

Scleroderma is a disorder readily distinguished from vitiligo, but one that might exhibit postinflammatory hypopigmentation. The spots often have a confetti distribution.

Lupus erythematosus in various forms can also cause depigmentation. Leucoderma is most commonly observed in cutaneous (discoid) lupus. Lesions exhibit atrophy of all epidermal elements.

Mycosis fungoides, sarcoidosis, leprosy and syphilis are rarely encountered in children but can mimic vitiligo. A skin biopsy and appropriate specific tests are needed. Leprosy must be considered in the differential diagnosis of vitiligo in patients from endemic areas of the world.

Prognosis. Monitoring disease activity is essentially based on clinical observation and recording the spread of established areas of depigmentation or appearance of new areas. There are no blood tests that have been shown to be helpful in routine practice.

There is a lack of studies of the natural history and evolution of childhood vitiligo. Mazereeuw-Hautier and colleagues noted in 114 infants with vitiligo followed up for approximately 1 year, that vitiligo resolved in only 5.5% of the patients [36]. A retrospective case series of 208 children showed that patients with early-onset vitiligo (<3 years old) were more likely to develop greater than 10% body surface area involvement and new areas of depigmentation than children with late onset (3–18 years old). However, no significant differences in the incidence of repigmentation between the early- and the later-onset groups were observed suggesting similar responses to treatment [45]. Precipitating factors are often reported prior to the onset or spread of vitiligo, such as emotional or physical stress.

Treatment. Vitiligo is difficult to treat and no definitive cure is yet available [46,47]. There are minor differences in the management of childhood versus adult vitiligo due mostly because of feasibility and the aesthetic demand of treatment. The major difference is in the parent's behaviour and how they cope with the disease, especially in families with vitiligo. One important unsolved issue is the possible impact of early aggressive treatment on disease outcome in severe, rapidly progressive vitiligo in children. It is crucial to avoid undertreatment in vitiligo where early intervention is helpful to avoid a definitive loss of skin melanocytes.

Therapeutic efficacy varies greatly according to the modalities and the individual, and complete repigmentation is only rarely achieved. Treatment in vitiligo therefore aims to stabilize the depigmenting process and achieve some degree of repigmentation in the lesions. Repeated skin friction or pressure during disease flares can rapidly aggravate pigment cell loss. All therapies require sufficient time for melanocytes to proliferate and migrate into the depigmented skin, usually a minimum of 3 months, and thereafter the treatment must be continued. It is now well established that treatment must be started early to limit disease progression, and that combined therapy using topical or systemic anti-inflammatory drugs with phototherapy is the best option to achieve disease stabilization and repigmentation simultaneously [10].

Glabrous skin (skin without hair follicles) and hair-bearing skin in which the hair is white lack the follicular reservoir and therefore are unlikely to repigment following medical treatment. For this reason, it is important to determine if the hairs in the depigmented skin retain their colour or are white. Certain areas such as lips, nipples, genitals, eyelids and distal extremities are areas that are known to respond poorly to treatment. The response to treatment is better on light-exposed skin, in particular the face and especially around the eyes.

There are several options for the treatment of vitiligo, including topical and systemic drug intervention, phototherapy and surgical modalities. A child will not usually request treatment until around the age of 6, when entering primary school. However, earlier unformulated harm to self-image may remain undetected. As indicated before, early intervention is preferable, whatever the type of vitiligo, to limit disease extension. However, the benefits/risks of the treatment should be carefully considered, such as the time needed to apply topical treatment or, more importantly, if phototherapy is to be used.

Topical corticosteroids

Potent topical corticosteroids are the most commonly used treatment for limited vitiligo on extrafacial areas. Side-effects occur in 15–30% of cases [48], but can be avoided with discontinuous application schemes (e.g. 2 weeks/month).

Immunomodulatory drugs

Tacrolimus is an immunosuppressive/immunomodulatory drug; it is a topical preparation licensed for the treatment of atopic dermatitis but not currently licensed for the treatment of vitiligo. Studies performed in childhood vitiligo have reported some degree of repigmentation in more than 60% of cases [49,50]. In a study evaluating topical tacrolimus in 22 adults and 20 children, children had a better response than adult patients. A disease duration of 5 years or less correlated with better response [51]. This treatment is particularly useful on the face and neck, especially around the eyes, because it does not cause skin atrophy or affect intraocular pressure compared with the associated risk when using potent topical steroids. Ho and colleagues showed in a double-blind, randomized, placebo-controlled trial evaluating the use of topical tacrolimus (0.1%) vs clobetasol propionate (0.05%) similar benefits between the two regimens in childhood vitiligo. Facial lesions responded faster than nonfacial lesions [52].

Pimecrolimus was also studied in nonsegmental childhood vitiligo and seems to be effective alone or in combination with narrow-band ultraviolet B (NB-UVB) [53,54].

Indeed, several studies and reviews suggest that topical calcineurin inhibitors can enhance the efficacy of UV light therapy. In a recent systematic review and meta-analysis, topical tacrolimus in combination with an excimer light was more effective than an excimer lamp alone for localized lesions of vitiligo [55]. Another study evaluated the combination of topical tacrolimus with NB-UVB therapy in 20 children (4 to 14 years of age). Results on this small cohort showed better repigmentation in the combination group compared with UV light alone [56].

Phototherapy

The best results are observed when combining NB-UVB or excimer devices with topical corticosteroids and calcineurin inhibitors [56]. Commonly used phototherapy regimen are discussed below.

- **Photochemotherapy (PUVA; psoralen + ultraviolet A) and topical psoralens plus UVA (topical PUVA)** These treatments are not currently recommended options for reasons of safety, logistical complexity of visiting the hospital and the discipline of avoiding excess exposure to sunlight [56].
- **NB-UVB phototherapy TL-01 (311 nm)** This is now the standard of care in many countries. Treatment is usually administered twice a week. According to published studies, more than 75% of the involved skin areas repigmented in more than 50% of the children after 6–12 months of treatment [49,57,58]. Response to treatment correlates with localization of the lesions: the face and neck showed the best results, whereas the trunk and proximal extremities had moderate repigmentation. Acral sites, sites around bony prominences and those with lower hair follicle density hardly repigmented. This treatment had a positive effect on the quality of life in these children. Adverse effects were limited and transient. Long-term NB-UVB therapy carries lower risk for the development of skin cancer than PUVA therapy, although the risk is a factor in the decision of some clinicians to avoid treatment by this modality. In clinical practice, the problem is the availability of UVB near the patient's home, which has encouraged the development of supervised home phototherapy [59]. In children, if no response is observed after 6 months, further therapy should be discouraged, or the treatment limited to specific areas.
- **Excimer devices** The 308-nm xenon chloride excimer laser is targeted phototherapy with single-wavelength laser light. The degree of repigmentation after a relatively small number of treatments over a much shorter treatment time than with NB-UVB has shown very encouraging results. Cho and colleagues observed that in 30 children with 40 vitiligo patches 56.7% achieved an acceptable degree of repigmentation (>50%). The face and neck showed better results. The mean duration of the treatment was 7.7 months for the head and neck and 9.7 months for lower extremities [60]. Similar results have been observed with excimer lamps, mostly in adults. Another study suggests that calcipotriol combined with natural sunlight can be beneficial [61].

Systemic steroids

Systemic steroids can induce repigmentation in childhood vitiligo. In one study, 81 patients (adults and infants) with vitiligo were treated for 5 months. The patients took daily doses of oral prednisolone (0.3 mg/kg bodyweight) initially; the dosage was then reduced. Arrested progression of vitiligo and repigmentation were noted in 88% and 70% of patients respectively. The side-effects of treatment were minimal and did not affect the course of treatment [62]. Mini-pulses of oral systemic steroids, for example methylprednisolone 8 mg (<30 kg) or 16 mg (>30 kg), only at weekends, over 3–6 months, as used in adults, can stop disease progression efficiently in most cases, and for safety reasons is preferred to a continuous regimen.

Transplantation methods

Several methods of autologous transplantation of melanocytes have been developed to repigment small lesions that are stable (for at least 1–2 years) and those that are refractory to treatment (for at least 6–12 months) [63]. Patients with segmental or lip-tip (lips, hands, feet, fingers) vitiligo can be successfully treated with these transplantation methods with excellent long-term outcome. These methods are not indicated for children aged less than 12 years but can be considered later in adolescence. These procedures can be painful and can interfere with normal daily activities for a short time as the graft heals.

Photoprotection

Sun exposure can be beneficial and stimulate the growth and migration of melanocytes, but the family must be given advice on cautious sun exposure, making sure that the child is not put at risk of sunburn, which may trigger the Koebner phenomenon as well as increasing skin cancer risk. The authors advise a sunscreen with a high sun protection factor (SPF around 50 or higher) for strong sun exposure, and a sunscreen with a lower SPF (15–25) for mild to moderate sun exposure. Although vitiliginous skin has lost its pigment, it has not been shown that the skin is at high risk of sun-induced damage and skin cancer, as might be expected. Recent data are reassuring, indicating a tendency to better immune surveillance in patients with vitiligo [64,65].

Cosmetic camouflage

The use of cosmetic camouflage is not ideal in young children with vitiligo because it is easily removed during play, but for older children it can help psychologically, especially if the face is involved.

Choice of treatment

Any child with vitiligo should be evaluated for their perceptions regarding the cosmetic disfigurement and for the impact the vitiligo has on their interactions with other children. Similarly, parents should be questioned regarding their concern about the impact of the disease on their child's personal development. Especially in those with darker skin, vitiligo may cause more significant disfigurement that can lead to serious impairment of quality of life. Children and parents must be informed of all the available treatment options and their expected response and side-effect profiles. It is also important to inform the parents that the skin can repigment spontaneously and any of the treatments advised can take at least 2–3 months before an improvement may be noticed. Careful assessment of the risk/benefit ratio is necessary in children before embarking on treatment.

In the case of more limited vitiligo, topical corticosteroids represent a first-line treatment. Topical tacrolimus possibly represents another option, especially on the face and neck. Both treatments yield better results when combined with UV light (heliotherapy or home phototherapy are the best choices). When patients exhibit more generalized vitiligo, phototherapy may be considered. TL-01 (NB-UVB) is the first-choice phototherapy modality, especially if the child is less than 12 years old.

References

1 Ezzedine K, Lim HW, Suzuki T et al. Revised classification/nomenclature of vitiligo and related issues: the Vitiligo Global Issues Consensus Conference. Pigment Cell Melanoma Res 2012;25:E1–13.

2 Jin Y, Andersen G, Yorgov D et al. Genome-wide association studies of autoimmune vitiligo identify 23 new risk loci and highlight key pathways and regulatory variants. Nat Genet 2016;48:1418–24.

3 Jin Y, Andersen GH, Santorico SA, Spritz RA. Multiple functional variants of IFIH1, a gene involved in triggering innate immune responses, protect against vitiligo. J Invest Dermatol 2017;137:522–4.

4 Jin Y, Birlea SA, Fain PR et al. Genome-wide association analyses identify 13 new susceptibility loci for generalized vitiligo. Nat Genet 2012;44:676–80.

5 Jin Y, Birlea SA, Fain PR et al. Variant of TYR and autoimmunity susceptibility loci in generalized vitiligo. N Engl J Med 2010; 362:1686–97.

6 Jin Y, Birlea SA, Fain PR et al. Common variants in FOXP1 are associated with generalized vitiligo. Nat Genet 2010;42:576–8.

7 Manga P, Elbuluk N, Orlow SJ. Recent advances in understanding vitiligo. F1000Res 2016, September 6, 5.

8 Yildirim M, Baysal V, Inaloz HS et al. The role of oxidants and antioxidants in generalized vitiligo. J Dermatol 2003;30:104–8.

9 Picardo M, Bastonini E. A new view of vitiligo: looking at normal-appearing skin. J Invest Dermatol 2015;135:1713–14.

10 Boniface K, Seneschal J, Picardo M, Taïeb A. Vitiligo: focus on clinical aspects, immunopathogenesis, and therapy. Clin Rev Allergy Immunol 2018;54:52–67.

11 Bertolotti A, Boniface K, Vergier B et al. Type I interferon signature in the initiation of the immune response in vitiligo. Pigment Cell Melanoma Res 2014;27:398–407.

12 Richmond JM, Bangari DS, Essien KI et al. Keratinocyte-derived chemokines orchestrate T cell positioning in the epidermis during vitiligo and may serve as biomarkers of disease. J Invest Dermatol 2017;137:350–8.

13 Li S, Zhu G, Yang Y et al. Oxidative stress drives CD8+T cells skin trafficking in vitiligo via CXCL16 upregulation by activating the unfolded protein response in keratinocytes. J Allergy Clin Immunol 2017;140:177–89.

14 van Geel N, Mollet I, Brochez L et al. New insights in segmental vitiligo: case report and review of theories. Br J Dermatol 2012; 166:240–6.

15 Le Poole IC, van den Wijngaard RM, Westerhof W et al. Presence or absence of melanocytes in vitiligo lesions: an immunohistochemical investigation. J Invest Dermatol 1993;100:816–22.

16 Le Poole IC, Das PK. Microscopic changes in vitiligo. Clin Dermatol 1997;15:863–73.

17 Jungbluth AA, Iversen K, Coplan K et al. T311 – an anti-tyrosinase monoclonal antibody for the detection of melanocytic lesions in paraffin embedded tissues. Pathol Res Pract 2000;196:235–42.

18 Tobin DJ, Swanson NN, Pittelkow MR et al. Melanocytes are not absent in lesional skin of long duration vitiligo. J Pathol 2000; 191:407–16.

19 Gan EY, Eleftheriadou V, Esmat S et al. Repigmentation in vitiligo: position paper of the Vitiligo Global Issues Consensus Conference (VGICC). Pigment Cell Melanoma Res 2017;30:28–40.

20 Howitz J, Brodthagen H, Schwartz M, Thomsen K. Prevalence of vitiligo. Epidemiological survey on the Isle of Bornholm, Denmark. Arch Dermatol 1977; 113:47–52.

21 Mazereeuw-Hautier J, Taieb A. Vitiligo in childhood. Springer: Berlin, 2010:117–25.

22 Gan EY, Gahat T, Cario-Andre M et al. Clinical repigmentation patterns in paediatric vitiligo. Br J Dermatol 2016;175:555–60.

23 Linthorst Homan MW, de Korte J, Grootenhuis MA et al. Impact of childhood vitiligo on adult life. Br J Dermatol 2008;159:915–20.

24 Diallo A, Boniface K, Jouary T et al. Development and validation of the K-VSCOR for scoring Koebner's phenomenon in vitiligo/non-segmental vitiligo. Pigment Cell Melanoma Res 2013;26:402–7.

25 Handa S, Dogra S. Epidemiology of childhood vitiligo: a study of 625 patients from north India. Pediatr Dermatol 2003;20:207–10.

26 Jaisankar TJ, Baruah MC, Garg BR. Vitiligo in children. Int J Dermatol 1992; 31:621–3.

27 Gan EY, Cario-Andre M, Pain C et al. Follicular vitiligo: a report of 8 cases. J Am Acad Dermatol 2016;74:1178–84.

28 Ezzedine K, Diallo A, Leaute-Labreze C et al. Halo naevi and leukotrichia are strong predictors of the passage to mixed vitiligo in a subgroup of segmental vitiligo. Br J Dermatol 2012;166:539–44.

29 Prcic S, Duran V, Poljacki M. [Vitiligo in childhood]. Med Pregl 2002;55:475–80.

30 Ezzedine K, Diallo A, Leaute-Labreze C et al. Halo nevi association in nonsegmental vitiligo affects age at onset and depigmentation pattern. Arch Dermatol 2012;148:497–502.

31 Sosa JJ, Currimbhoy SD, Ukoha U et al. Confetti-like depigmentation: A potential sign of rapidly progressing vitiligo. J Am Acad Dermatol 2015;73:272–5.

32 Ezzedine K, Diallo A, Leaute-Labreze C et al. Pre- vs. post-pubertal onset of vitiligo: multivariate analysis indicates atopic diathesis association in pre-pubertal onset vitiligo. Br J Dermatol 2012;167:490–5.

33 Silverberg JI, Silverberg NB. Association between vitiligo and atopic disorders: a pilot study. JAMA Dermatol 2013;149:983–6.

34 Iacovelli P, Sinagra JL, Vidolin AP et al. Relevance of thyroiditis and of other autoimmune diseases in children with vitiligo. Dermatology 2005;210:26–30.

35 Kurtev A, Dourmishev AL. Thyroid function and autoimmunity in children and adolescents with vitiligo. J Eur Acad Dermatol Venereol 2004;18:109–11.

36 Mazereeuw-Hautier J, Bezio S, Mahe E et al. Segmental and nonsegmental childhood vitiligo has distinct clinical characteristics: a prospective observational study. J Am Acad Dermatol 2010;62:945–9.

37 Pagovich OE, Silverberg JI, Freilich E, Silverberg NB. Thyroid abnormalities in pediatric patients with vitiligo in New York City. Cutis 2008;81:463–6.

38 Kakourou R, Kanaka-Gantenbein C, Papadopoulou A. Increased prevalence of chronic autoimmune (Hashimoto's) thryoiditis in children and adolescents with vitiligo. J Am Acad Dermatol 2005; 53:220–3.

39 Pajvani U, Ahmad N, Wiley A et al. The relationship between family medical history and childhood vitiligo. J Am Acad Dermatol 2006;55:238–44.

40 Cho S, Kang HC, Hahm JH. Characteristics of vitiligo in Korean children. Pediatr Dermatol 2000;17:189–93.

41 Hu Z, Liu JB, Ma SS et al. Profile of childhood vitiligo in China: an analysis of 541 patients. Pediatr Dermatol 2006;23:114–16.

42 Halder RM. Childhood vitiligo. Clin Dermatol 1997;15:899–906.

43 Ezzedine K, Le Thuaut A, Jouary T et al. Latent class analysis of a series of 717 patients with vitiligo allows the identification of two clinical subtypes. Pigment Cell Melanoma Res 2014;27:134–9.

44 Birlea SA, Jin Y, Bennett DC et al. Comprehensive association analysis of candidate genes for generalized vitiligo supports XBP1, FOXP3, and TSLP. J Invest Dermatol 2011;131:371–81.

45 Mu EW, Cohen BE, Orlow SJ. Early-onset childhood vitiligo is associated with a more extensive and progressive course. J Am Acad Dermatol 2015;73:467–70.

46 Ezzedine K, Whitton M, Pinart M. Interventions for vitiligo. JAMA 2016;316:1708–9.

47 Whitton ME, Pinart M, Batchelor J et al. Interventions for vitiligo. Cochrane Database Syst Rev 2015:CD003263.

48 Kwinter J, Pelletier J, Khambalia A, Pope E. High-potency steroid use in children with vitiligo: a retrospective study. J Am Acad Dermatol 2007;56:236–41.

49 Kanwar AJ, Dogra S, Parsad D. Topical tacrolimus for treatment of childhood vitiligo in Asians. Clin Exp Dermatol 2004;29:589–92.

50 Silverberg NB, Lin P, Travis L et al. Tacrolimus ointment promotes repigmentation of vitiligo in children: a review of 57 cases. J Am Acad Dermatol 2004;51:760–6.

51 Udompataikul M, Boonsupthip P, Siriwattanagate R. Effectiveness of 0.1% topical tacrolimus in adult and children patients with vitiligo. J Dermatol 2011;38:536–40.

52 Ho N, Pope E, Weinstein M et al. A double-blind, randomized, placebo-controlled trial of topical tacrolimus 0.1% vs. clobetasol propionate 0.05% in childhood vitiligo. Br J Dermatol 2011;165:626–32.

53 Esfandiarpour I, Ekhlasi A, Farajzadeh S, Shamsadini S. The efficacy of pimecrolimus 1% cream plus narrow-band ultraviolet B in the treatment of vitiligo: a double-blind, placebo-controlled clinical trial. J Dermatolog Treat 2009;20:14–18.

54 Farajzadeh S, Daraei Z, Esfandiarpour I, Hosseini SH. The efficacy of pimecrolimus 1% cream combined with microdermabrasion in the treatment of nonsegmental childhood vitiligo: a randomized placebo-controlled study. Pediatr Dermatol 2009; 26:286–91.

55 Bae JM, Hong BY, Lee JH et al. The efficacy of 308-nm excimer laser/light (EL) and topical agent combination therapy versus EL monotherapy for vitiligo: a systematic review and meta-analysis of randomized controlled trials (RCTs). J Am Acad Dermatol 2016;74:907–15.

56 Dayal S, Sahu P, Gupta N. Treatment of childhood vitiligo using tacrolimus ointment with narrowband ultraviolet B phototherapy. Pediatr Dermatol 2016;33:646–51.

57 Brazzelli V, Prestinari F, Castello M et al. Useful treatment of vitiligo in 10 children with UV-B narrowband (311 nm). Pediatr Dermatol 2005;22:257–61.

58 Njoo MD, Bos JD, Westerhof W. Treatment of generalized vitiligo in children with narrow-band (TL-01) UVB radiation therapy. J Am Acad Dermatol 2000;42:245–53.

59 Eleftheriadou V, Ezzedine K. Portable home phototherapy for vitiligo. Clin Dermatol 2016;34:603–6.

60 Cho S, Zheng Z, Park YK, Roh MR. The 308-nm excimer laser: a promising device for the treatment of childhood vitiligo. Photodermatol Photoimmunol Photomed 2011; 27:24–9.

61 Parsad D, Saini R, Nagpal R. Calcipotriol in vitiligo: a preliminary study. Pediatr Dermatol 1999;16:317–20.

62 Kim SM, Lee HS, Hann SK. The efficacy of low-dose oral corticosteroids in the treatment of vitiligo patients. Int J Dermatol 1999;38: 546–50.

63 Mulekar SV, Isedeh P. Surgical interventions for vitiligo: an evidence-based review. Br J Dermatol 2013;169(Suppl 3):57–66.

64 Taieb A, Ezzedine K. Vitiligo: the white armour? Pigment Cell Melanoma Res 2013 Feb 8. doi: 10.1111/pcmr.12076.

65 Paradisi A, Tabolli S, Didona B et al. Markedly reduced incidence of melanoma and nonmelanoma skin cancer in a nonconcurrent cohort of 10,040 patients with vitiligo. J Am Acad Dermatol 2014;71:1110–16.

CHAPTER 124
Albinism

Fanny Morice-Picard & Alain Taïeb

Department of Dermatology and Paediatric Dermatology, Reference Center for Rare Skin Diseases, Hôpital Saint André, Bordeaux, France

Introduction, 1486
Oculocutaneous albinism (OMIM #606952), 1486
Hermansky–Pudlak syndrome (OMIM #203300), 1489
Chédiak–Higashi syndrome (OMIM #214500), 1489
Griscelli syndromes type I (OMIM #214450), type II (OMIM #607624) and type III (OMIM #609227), 1490
Cross syndrome (OMIM 257800), 1490

Abstract

Normal skin pigmentation is dependent upon efficient melanin synthesis and melanosome maturation within melanocytes, melanosome transfer to neighbouring keratinocytes and melanosome degradation concomitant with keratinocyte terminal differentiation. Several hundred genes are known to modulate the pigmentation type or pattern in skin, hairs/coat and eyes in mammals, during or after development, by acting directly or indirectly on the pigment cell lineage. Among these, oculocutaneous albinism is a rare genetic disorder characterized by generalized hypo- or depigmentation of the skin, hair and eye and by ophthalmological anomalies caused by a deficiency in melanin biosynthesis. Oculocutaneous albinism is a clinically and genetically heterogeneous disorder with a total of seven genes/loci so far identified. In addition, there are several syndromic forms of albinism, affecting the normal function of other organs, which can be grouped as Hermansky–Pudlak syndrome, Chédiak –Higashi syndrome and Griscelli–Prunieras syndrome. Management needs to be adapted to the severity of the presentation and an accurate diagnosis is important for planning the follow up in syndromic forms.

Key points

- Oculocutaneous albinism is a disorder of pigmentation associated with abnormal eye development.
- Pigment dilution is highly variable ranging from total absence of pigment to normal pigmentation.
- A high incidence of skin carcinoma is observed in sun-exposed patients in tropical countries.
- An accurate diagnosis of syndromic forms of albinism allows appropriate follow up.

Introduction

Normal skin pigmentation is dependent upon efficient melanin synthesis and melanosome maturation within melanocytes, melanosome transfer to neighbouring keratinocytes and melanosome degradation concomitant with keratinocyte terminal differentiation. Several hundred genes are known to modulate the pigmentation type or pattern in skin, hairs/coat, and eyes in mammals, during or after development, by acting directly or indirectly on the pigment cell lineage. Among these, oculocutaneous albinism (OCA) is a rare genetic disorder characterized by generalized hypo- or depigmentation of the skin, hair and eyes and by ophthalmological anomalies, caused by a deficiency in melanin biosynthesis [1]. The definition of OCA, initially based on clinical findings, has moved towards a molecular classification based upon the identification of causative genes (OCA1 to 7, Table 124.1). OCA is a genetically heterogeneous disorder. Initially, four types of OCA were known and recently three additional forms have been reported: *TYR*, responsible for OCA1, *OCA2* in OCA2, *TYRP1* in OCA3, *SLC45A2* in OCA4, *SLC24A5* in OCA6 and *C10orf11* in OCA7 [2–9]. OCA5 has been linked to locus 4q24 but the causative gene still remains to be identified.

In addition, there are several syndromic forms of albinism, affecting the normal function of other organs, which can be grouped as Hermansky–Pudlak syndrome (HPS1-9), Chédiak –Higashi syndrome (CHS1) and Griscelli–Prunieras syndrome (GPS) [10–12].

Oculocutaneous albinism (OMIM #606952)

Epidemiology and pathogenesis. OCA is the most frequent form of diffuse hypopigmentation worldwide with a prevalence estimated at around 1 in 20 000. The genetic

Harper's Textbook of Pediatric Dermatology, Fourth Edition. Edited by Peter Hoeger, Veronica Kinsler and Albert Yan.

Table 124.1 Summary of different types of albinism and associated genes

Albinism: defects in melanin synthesis			
OCA1A	AR	TYR	Absent skin and hair pigmentation, no ability to tan (OCA1A). Partial albinism, hair darkens with age (OCA1B)
OCA2	AR	OCA2	Prevalent in Blacks, blond to red–brown hair with age, ephelides
OCA3	AR	TYRP1	Rufous albinism in Blacks
OCA4	AR	SLC45A2	Similar to OCA1, more common in Japan
OCA5	AR	Unknown	One family described in Pakistan
OCA6	AR	SLC24A5/NCKX5	One family described from China and five from Europe
OCA7	AR	C10orf11	Faroe albinism
OA1	XLR	GPR143	Isolated ocular albinism
Defects in lysosomal biogenesis and transport, including melanosomes			
Hermansky-Pudlak syndrome			
HPS1	AR	HPS1	
HPS2	AR	AP3B1	
HPS3	AR	HPS3	
HPS4	AR	HPS4	Decreased pigmentation in eyes, hair and skin, easy bruising and bleeding tendency, lung interstitial fibrosis, granulomatous colitis
HPS5	AR	HPS5	
HPS6	AR	HPS6	
HPS7	AR	DTNBP1	
HPS8	AR	BLOC1S3	
HSP9	AR	BLOC1S6 (paladin)	
HSP10	AR	AP3D1	
Chediak-Higashi syndrome	AR	CHS1/LYST	Partial albinism (blond hair, fair skin) accompanied by immunodeficiency (pyogenic infections, haemophagocytic syndrome) and cerebellar syndrome
Griscelli syndrome			
GS1	AR	MYO5A	Silvery grey hair and fair skin, neurological defects
GS2	AR	RAB27A	Silvery grey hair and fair skin, immunological defects
GS3	AR	MLPH	Silvery grey hair and fair skin

prevalence varies considerably from one continent to another. OCA1 is the most frequent form worldwide. OCA2 is the most frequent form among African patients with a prevalence that reaches 1 in 1100 in some populations in western Africa.

OCA is caused by a deficiency of melanin biosynthesis but the melanocytes are normally distributed. The reduction in melanin production is responsible for the increased sensitivity to ultraviolet radiation and for the predisposition to skin cancer. The ophthalmological anomalies associated with albinism are not only a consequence of lack of melanin but also of a lack of L-DOPA, an intermediate early metabolite of the synthesis of melanin, which has been shown to be the only requirement to allow the retinal and visual development to proceed normally [13].

OCA1 is caused by mutations in *TYR*, encoding the tyrosinase gene [14]. Total lack of tyrosinase activity results in OCA type 1A whilst partial activity causes type 1B [15]. Some patients with type 1B OCA show variation in hair and skin pigmentation with dark hair being found in cooler areas of the body. This phenomenon has been related to the fact the underlying mutations in these cases are temperature sensitive. It has been shown that mutations in the mouse Tyr gene cause the Tyr protein to be retained in the endoplasmic reticulum, with subsequently early degradation.

OCA2 is caused by mutations in the *OCA2* gene, encoding the P protein, a transmembrane protein of importance for melanin biosynthesis and for the processing and transport of other melanosomal proteins such as tyrosinase [3]. It seems that OCA2 exerts at least some of its effects by maintaining an acidic pH in melanosomes.

Mutations in *TYRP1* are responsible for OCA3. The protein encoded by this gene catalyses the oxidation of DHICA monomers into eumelanin and serves also to stabilize tyrosinase. It is not required for pheomelanin production, explaining the accumulation of the latter in the skin and hair in OCA3 [4].

OCA4 is caused by mutations in *SLC45A2*, encoding the membrane-associated transporter protein (MATP), a membrane transporter in melanosomes [5]. OCA6 is caused by mutations in *SLC24A5*, the membrane-associated transporter protein (NCKX5). This protein is involved in correct maturation of melanosomes [8].

OCA7 is caused by mutations in C10orf11[6], thought from animal studies to be involved in melanocyte differentiation.

Clinical features. The pigmentation of the skin, hair and eyes is in general reduced but its degree varies with the type of albinism.

All types of OCA and ocular albinism have similar ocular findings, including various degrees of congenital nystagmus, hypopigmentation of the iris leading to iris translucency, reduced pigmentation of the retinal pigment epithelium, foveal hypoplasia, reduced visual acuity usually in the range 20/60–20/400 and refractive errors, and sometimes a degree of colour vision impairment [16].

Photophobia may be prominent. Iris translucency is demonstrable by slit lamp examination. A characteristic finding is misrouting of the optic nerves, consisting of an excessive crossing of the fibres in the optic chiasma, which can result in strabismus and reduced stereoscopic vision [17]. The abnormal crossing of fibres can be demonstrated by monocular visual evoked potential [18]. Absence of misrouting excludes the diagnosis of albinism.

Clinical variants: In the severe OCA1A form, there is a complete absence of pigmentation with white hair and pink skin (Fig. 124.1) [19]. There is no tendency to tan. Naevi are achromic. The visual impairment is severe with nystagmus, photophobia and errors of refraction.

In other types initially described as tyrosinase positive, pigmentation is highly variable and influenced by the phototype of the patient. Pigmentation can increase with age (Fig. 124.2). Patients develop dark brown freckles with age particularly in sun-exposed areas. Visual acuity may improve as patients get older and they may have less severe nystagmus.

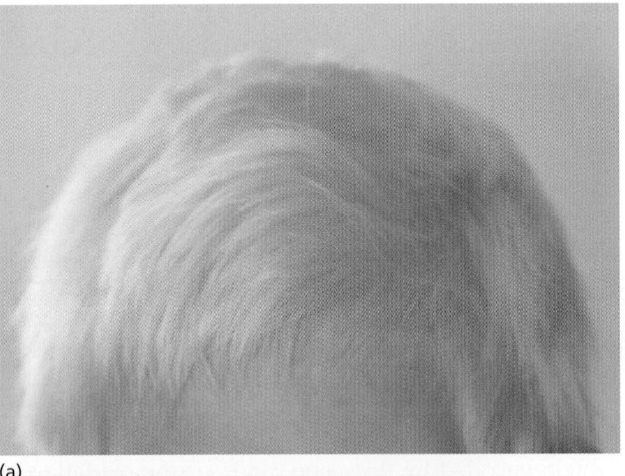

(a)

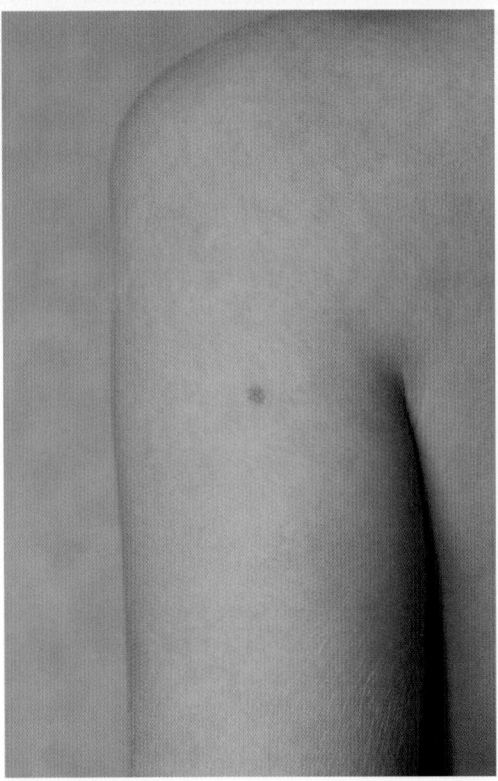

(b)

Fig. 124.1 Platinum white hair (a) and an achromic naevus (b) in a patient with oculocutaneous albinism type 1.

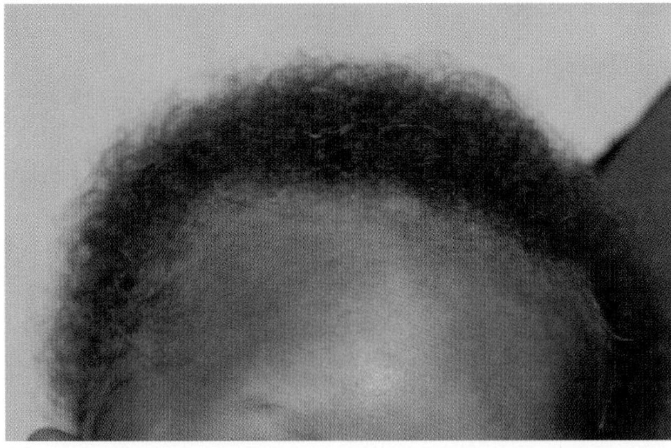

(a)

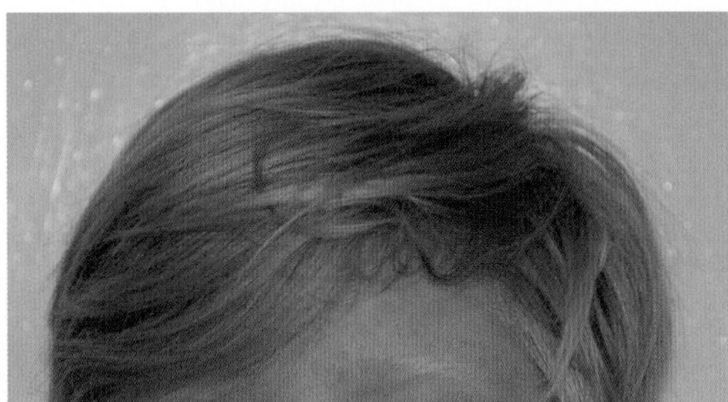

(b)

Fig. 124.2 Yellow hair in African (a) and White (b) patients with oculocutaneous albinism type 2.

Rufous albinism (OCA3) was originally described in African patients with *TYRP1* mutations, but recent molecular diagnoses indicate that it is not restricted to African populations [4,20,21].

Lifespan in patients with OCA is not limited and medical problems are generally not increased compared with those in the general population. Skin cancers may occur and regular skin checks should be offered. Development and intelligence are normal. Persons with OCA have normal fertility. The incidence of skin cancer is increased in patients with OCA, especially spinous cell carcinoma which is a cause of mortality in Africans with OCA2 [22]. Melanoma is less common [23].

Differential diagnosis. The presence of ocular albinism excludes a large number of diseases associated with pigment dilution. Diagnoses to be considered in the case of ocular and cutaneous hypopigmentation include histidinaemia, homocystinuria, phenylketonuria, as well as Cross and Tietz syndromes. OCA has to be distinguished from syndromic forms of OCA.

Laboratory findings. The diagnosis of OCA is based on clinical findings of hypopigmentation of the skin and hair. Ophthalmological examination should include an examination with optical-coherence-tomography of the retina showing the foveal hypoplasia [24,25]. Electrophysiological testing can demonstrate misrouting of the optic nerves, resulting in strabismus and impaired stereoscopic vision [26].

Electron microscopy examination of skin may show abnormal melanosome development in hair bulb melanocytes which progressed no further than stage II, indicating a lack of melanin [27]. Molecular diagnosis caused by the clinical overlap between the OCA subtypes is necessary in order to establish the gene defect and thus the OCA subtype. Molecular analysis of the OCA genes is available and will help to confirm the diagnosis and to give appropriate genetic counselling [21].

Treatment and prevention. No specific treatment is available. Sun protection is mandatory to avoid skin sunburns and skin cancers with a special emphasis in patients living in high ultraviolet risk environments. Early referral to an ophthalmologist is mandatory. Decreased visual acuity is usually managed with corrective lenses whereas strabismus requires eye patching or surgical correction. Dark glasses are important to protect the eyes and prevent photophobia [16]. L-DOPA, an intermediate product in the biosynthesis of melanin pigment, has been tried in albino patients without showing improvement in visual acuity [28]. Nitisinone, an FDA-approved inhibitor of tyrosine degradation, has been shown to improve pigmentation and potentially vision loss in albino mice [29].

Hermansky–Pudlak syndrome (OMIM #203300)

Epidemiology and pathogenesis. Hermansky–Pudlak syndrome is a rare type of OCA associated with a haemorrhagic diathesis [30,31]. About 250 cases have been reported, most of whom are from Puerto Rico or the south of the Netherlands. Here too, a molecular classification has now been universally accepted recognizing nine clinicogenetic subtypes of the disease (see Table 124.1). The disorder is rare except in Puerto Rico.

The disease results from abnormal biogenesis of lysosome-related organelles with impaired melanosome maturation and absent dense bodies in thrombocytes [31]. Hermansky–Pudlak syndrome is associated with mutations in 10 distinct genes: HPS1 (type 1) and HPS4 (type 4) encode components of the BLOC3 lysosomal complex, which is essential for the proper formation of lysosome-related organelles; AP3B1 (type 2) encodes a subunit of the AP3 complex, which is responsible for mediating protein sorting to lysosomes; HPS3 (type 3), HSP5 (type 5) and HSP6 (type 6) all encode components of BLOC2; and DTNBP1 (type 7), BLOC1S3 (type 8), BLOC1S6 (type 9) and AP3D1 (type 10) encode components of BLOC1 which are all required for proper melanosome maturation [32–40].

Clinical features. All subtypes of the syndrome share common clinical manifestations including decreased pigmentation in the eyes, hair and skin, easy bruising and bleeding tendency, interstitial pulmonary fibrosis and granulomatous colitis (Fig. 124.3) [31].

The complications of Hermansky–Pudlak syndrome are secondary to bleeding problems, pulmonary fibrosis and colitis. Prognosis is guarded with a life expectancy of 30–50 years.

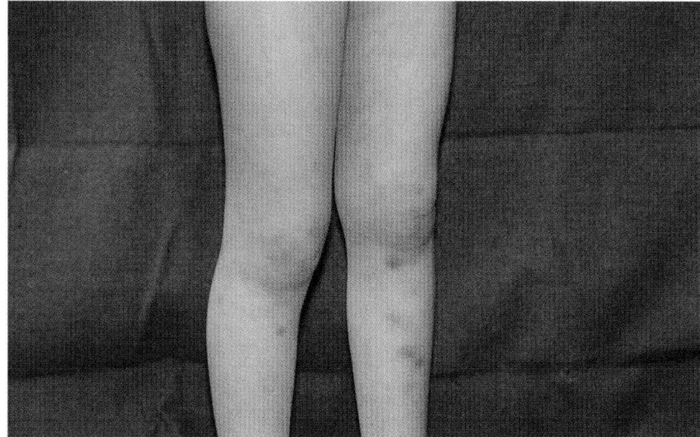

Fig. 124.3 Bruising in a 2-year-old patient with Hermansky-Pudlak syndrome type 4.

Laboratory findings. Absence of dense bodies on whole mount electron microscopy of platelets constitutes a standard diagnostic test. Moreover, upon stimulation of platelets, the dense bodies, which contain adenosine diphosphate, adenosine triphosphate, serotonin, calcium and phosphate, release their contents to attract other platelets, which can be tested to screen for Hermansky–Pudlak syndrome [10].

Treatment and prevention. No treatment is available. Protection of the skin from sunburn, and correction of refractive errors and use of low vision aids are required for the OCA. For detection and evaluation of lung fibrosis, pulmonary function tests should be performed on a regular basis in adulthood and computed tomography scans when necessary. Molecular analysis of the Hermansky–Pudlak syndrome genes helps to confirm the diagnosis and to give appropriate genetic counselling [10].

Chédiak–Higashi syndrome (OMIM #214500)

Epidemiology and pathogenesis. Chédiak–Higashi syndrome is a rare autosomal recessive disorder characterized by hypopigmentation of the skin and eye, immunodeficiency and possibly neurological symptoms [10].

The hereditary defect concerns membrane-bound organelles of various cell types and is caused by loss-of-function mutations in *CHS1* (LYST), a gene encoding a protein known as lysosomal trafficking regulator. The melanocytes contain giant pigment granules, which arise by autophagocytosis and fission of large melanosomes that show degradative changes within the cells [41]. Similar defects of granules and other organelles occur in white cells and platelets. Cytoplasmic inclusions are present in a variety of cells of neuroectodermal origin. The white cells are defective in combating infection and if children with this condition survive infancy, they usually die later from a malignant lymphoma.

Clinical features. The skin is fair, the retinae are pale and the irides translucent. The diagnosis of Chédiak–Higashi syndrome is suspected in individuals with clinical criteria for OCA combined with a significant history of pyogenic infections. Neutropenia is noted [42].

Neurological manifestations (e.g. progressive intellectual decline, cranial nerve palsies, decreased deep tendon reflexes, tremor and abnormal gait, seizures) can appear any time from childhood to early adulthood [43].

Attenuated forms have been described with genotype–phenotype correlation. Loss-of-function mutations are associated with the severe childhood-onset form [44]. The accelerated phase corresponding to a haemophagocytic lymphohistiocytosis, occurs in 85% of individuals at any age and can be fatal [42,43].

Laboratory findings. Peroxidase-positive giant inclusions seen in leukocytes is a first-line diagnostic test [44]. Light microscopy of hairs shows pigment clumping.

Treatment and prevention. The only curative treatment available for Chédiak–Higashi syndrome is bone marrow transplantation [45]. A case of complete remission after combination therapy with rituximab and ciclosporin has been reported [46].

Griscelli syndromes type I (OMIM #214450), type II (OMIM #607624) and type III (OMIM #609227)

Epidemiology and pathogenesis. Griscelli–Pruniéras syndrome is a rare autosomal recessive disorder that associates hypopigmentation and the presence of large clusters of pigment in the hair shaft, and the occurrence of either a primary neurological impairment or a severe immune disorder [47].

All genetic alterations associated with Griscelli–Pruniéras syndrome result in defective transport of melanosomes and consequently abnormal accumulation of melanosomes in melanocytes. Griscelli–Pruniéras syndrome type 1 results from mutations in *MYO5A*, encoding myosin 5a [48]. Type 2 disease results from mutations in the *RAB27A* gene whereas type 3 is caused by mutations in *MLPH* encoding melanophilin or by a specific genetic defect in *MYO5A* [12,49].

Clinical features. In 1978, Griscelli and Pruniéras described two patients with partial albinism of the hair and skin, frequent pyogenic infections and acute episodes of fever, hepatosplenomegaly, neutropenia and thrombocytopenia [47]. Dermatological findings included pigmentary abnormalities of the hair variably described as silvery grey, silvery, greyish-golden or dusty [9]. Neurological involvement is a prominent feature. In addition to pigmentary dilution, there is immune deficiency and the affected children are prone to recurrent pyogenic infection. There is hypogammaglobulinaemia and defective cell-mediated immunity with lymphohistiocytosis and haematophagocytosis. Patients with Griscelli–Pruniéras syndrome are predisposed to the occurrence of 'accelerated phases' similar to those encountered in Chédiak–Higashi syndrome [9].

Clinical variants. Patients with Griscelli–Pruniéras syndrome type 1 have primary central nervous system dysfunction, type 2 patients commonly develop haemophagocytic lymphohistiocytosis and type 3 patients have only partial albinism [12,48–50].

The differential diagnosis of the disease in the patient presenting with silvery hair includes primarily the Griscelli–Pruniéras, Chédiak–Higashi, and Elejalde syndromes. Elejalde syndrome is inherited in an autosomal recessive fashion and is characterized by pigment dilution, silvery grey hair and neurological defects [51]. Some authors suggest that the disease may in fact be identical to Griscelli-Pruniéras syndrome type 1.

Laboratory findings. Griscelli-Pruniéras syndrome is characterized by the presence of large clusters of pigment in the hair shaft [52].

Treatment and prevention. No specific treatment is available. Griscelli–Pruniéras syndrome has been successfully treated with bone marrow transplantation [53].

Cross syndrome (OMIM 257800)

Cross syndrome is one of the 'silvery hair' syndromes and is characterized by generalized hypopigmentation associated with ocular anomalies, mental and physical retardation, ataxia and spasticity [54].

About 10 cases of Cross syndrome have been described in Amish and Gipsy families and in South Africa. It is an autosomal recessive disorder [54,55]. The defective gene remains to be identified.

The pigmentary and ocular defects are manifest from birth. The hypopigmentation resembles albinism; blood tyrosine levels are normal and the light-coloured hair pigments poorly in tyrosine solution. The ocular defects include microphthalmos, a small opaque cornea and coarse nystagmus. Spasticity soon becomes evident, and physical and mental development is retarded [55].

References

1 Tomita Y, Suzuki T. Genetics of pigmentary disorders. Am J Med Genet C Semin Med Genet 15;131C:75–81.
2 Tomita Y, Takeda A, Okinaga S et al. Human oculocutaneous albinism caused by single base insertion in the tyrosinase gene. Biochem Biophys Res Commun 1989;164:990–6.
3 Rinchik EM, Bultman SJ, Horsthemke B et al. A gene for the mouse pink-eyed dilution locus and for human type II oculocutaneous albinism. Nature 1993;361(6407):72–6.
4 Manga P, Kromberg JG, Box NF et al. Rufous oculocutaneous albinism in southern African Blacks is caused by mutations in the TYRP1 gene. Am J Hum Genet 1997;61:1095–101.
5 Newton JM, Cohen-Barak O, Hagiwara N et al. Mutations in the human orthologue of the mouse underwhite gene (uw) underlie a new form of oculocutaneous albinism, OCA4. Am J Hum Genet 2001;69:981–8.
6 Grønskov K, Dooley CM, Østergaard E et al. Mutations in c10orf11, a melanocyte-differentiation gene, cause autosomal-recessive albinism. Am J Hum Genet 2013;92:415–21.

SECTION 26: DISORDERS OF PIGMENTATION

7 **Kausar T, Bhatti MA, Ali M et al. OCA5, a novel locus for non-syndromic oculocutaneous albinism, maps to chromosome 4q24. Clin Genet 2013;84:91–3.**

8 **Wei A-H, Zang D-J, Zhang Z et al. Exome sequencing identifies SLC24A5 as a candidate gene for nonsyndromic oculocutaneous albinism. J Invest Dermatol 2013;133:1834–40.**

9 **Morice-Picard F, Lasseaux E, François S et al. SLC24A5 mutations are associated with non-syndromic oculocutaneous albinism. J Invest Dermatol 2014;134:568–71.**

10 **Dotta L, Parolini S, Prandini A et al. Clinical, laboratory and molecular signs of immunodeficiency in patients with partial oculo-cutaneous albinism. Orphanet J Rare Dis 2013;8:168.**

11 Shiflett SL, Kaplan J, Ward DM. Chédiak-Higashi Syndrome: a rare disorder of lysosomes and lysosome related organelles. Pigment Cell Res 2002;15:251–7.

12 Ménasché G, Ho CH, Sanal O et al. Griscelli syndrome restricted to hypopigmentation results from a melanophilin defect (GS3) or a MYO5A F-exon deletion (GS1). J Clin Invest 2003;112:450–6.

13 Lavado A, Montoliu L. New animal models to study the role of tyrosinase in normal retinal development. Front Biosci 2006;11:743–52.

14 Tomita Y. Tyrosinase gene mutations causing oculocutaneous albinisms. J Invest Dermatol 1993;100(2 Suppl):186S–190S.

15 Oetting WS, King RA. Molecular basis of type I (tyrosinase-related) oculocutaneous albinism: mutations and polymorphisms of the human tyrosinase gene. Hum Mutat 1993;2:1–6.

16 **Summers CG. Albinism: classification, clinical characteristics, and recent findings. Optom Vis Sci 2009;86:659–62.**

17 Hoffmann MB, Lorenz B, Morland AB, Schmidtborn LC. Misrouting of the optic nerves in albinism: estimation of the extent with visual evoked potentials. Invest Ophthalmol Vis Sci 2005;46:3892–8.

18 Hoffmann MB, Lorenz B, Preising M, Seufert PS. Assessment of cortical visual field representations with multifocal VEPs in control subjects, patients with albinism, and female carriers of ocular albinism. Invest Ophthalmol Vis Sci 2006;47:3195–201.

19 Tanita M, Matsunaga J, Miyamura Y et al. Polymorphic sequences of the tyrosinase gene: allele analysis on 16 OCA1 patients in Japan indicate that three polymorphic sequences in the tyrosinase gene promoter could be powerful markers for indirect gene diagnosis. J Hum Genet 2002;47:1–6.

20 Rooryck C, Roudaut C, Robine E et al. Oculocutaneous albinism with TYRP1 gene mutations in a Caucasian patient. Pigment Cell Res 2006;19:239–42.

21 **Rooryck C, Morice-Picard F, Elçioglu NH et al. Molecular diagnosis of oculocutaneous albinism: new mutations in the OCA1-4 genes and practical aspects. Pigment Cell Melanoma Res 2008;21:583–7.**

22 Kiprono SK, Chaula BM, Beltraminelli H. Histological review of skin cancers in African Albinos: a 10-year retrospective review. BMC Cancer 2014;14:157.

23 Yakubu A, Mabogunje OA. Skin cancer in African albinos. Acta Oncol 1993;32:621–2.

24 McCafferty BK, Wilk MA, McAllister JT et al. clinical insights into foveal morphology in albinism. J Pediatr Ophthalmol Strabismus 2015;52:167–72.

25 Pakzad-Vaezi K, Keane P, Cardoso JN et al. Optical coherence tomography angiography of foveal hypoplasia. Br J Ophthalmol 2017; 101:985–8.

26 **Grønskov K, Ek J, Brondum-Nielsen K. Oculocutaneous albinism. Orphanet J Rare Dis 2007;2:43.**

27 **Summers CG, Connett JE, Holleschau AM et al. Does levodopa improve vision in albinism? Results of a randomized, controlled clinical trial. Clin Experiment Ophthalmol 2014;42:713–21.**

28 **Onojafe IF, Adams DR, Simeonov DR et al. Nitisinone improves eye and skin pigmentation defects in a mouse model of oculocutaneous albinism. J Clin Invest 2011;121:3914–23.**

29 Hermansky F, Pudlak P. Albinism associated with hemorrhagic diathesis and unusual pigmented reticular cells in the bone marrow: report of two cases with histochemical studies. Blood 1959;14:162–9.

30 Wei A-H, Li W. Hermansky-Pudlak syndrome: pigmentary and non-pigmentary defects and their pathogenesis. Pigment Cell Melanoma Res 2013;26:176–92.

31 Li W, Zhang Q, Oiso N et al. Hermansky-Pudlak syndrome type 7 (HPS-7) results from mutant dysbindin, a member of the biogenesis of lysosome-related organelles complex 1 (BLOC-1). Nat Genet 2003;35:84–9.

32 Morgan NV, Pasha S, Johnson CA et al. A germline mutation in BLOC1S3/reduced pigmentation causes a novel variant of Hermansky-Pudlak syndrome (HPS8). Am J Hum Genet 2006;78:160–6.

33 Cullinane AR, Curry JA, Golas G et al. A BLOC-1 mutation screen reveals a novel BLOC1S3 mutation in Hermansky-Pudlak Syndrome type 8. Pigment Cell Melanoma Res 2012;25:584–91.

34 Zhang Q, Zhao B, Li W et al. Ru2 and Ru encode mouse orthologs of the genes mutated in human Hermansky-Pudlak syndrome types 5 and 6. Nat Genet 2003;33:145–53.

35 Suzuki T, Li W, Zhang Q et al. Hermansky-Pudlak syndrome is caused by mutations in HPS4, the human homolog of the mouse light-ear gene. Nat Genet 2002;30:321–4.

36 Anikster Y, Huizing M, White J et al. Mutation of a new gene causes a unique form of Hermansky-Pudlak syndrome in a genetic isolate of central Puerto Rico. Nat Genet 2001;28:376–80.

37 Huizing M, Pederson B, Hess RA et al. Clinical and cellular characterisation of Hermansky-Pudlak syndrome type 6. J Med Genet 2009;46:803–10.

38 Oh J, Bailin T, Fukai K et al. Positional cloning of a gene for Hermansky-Pudlak syndrome, a disorder of cytoplasmic organelles. Nat Genet 1996;14:300–6.

39 Ammann S, Schulz A, Krägeloh-Mann I et al. Mutations in AP3D1 associated with immunodeficiency and seizures define a new type of Hermansky-Pudlak syndrome. Blood 2016;127:997–1006.

40 Durchfort N, Verhoef S, Vaughn MB et al. The enlarged lysosomes in beige j cells result from decreased lysosome fission and not increased lysosome fusion. Traffic 2012;13:108–19.

41 Ward DM, Shiflett SL, Kaplan J. Chédiak-Higashi syndrome: a clinical and molecular view of a rare lysosomal storage disorder. Curr Mol Med 2002;2:469–77.

42 Introne WJ, Westbroek W, Golas GA, Adams D. Chédiak-Higashi Syndrome. In: Pagon RA, Adam MP, Ardinger HH et al. (eds) GeneReviews(®) [Internet]. Seattle (WA): University of Washington, Seattle, 1993.

43 Karim MA, Suzuki K, Fukai K et al. Apparent genotype-phenotype correlation in childhood, adolescent, and adult Chédiak-Higashi syndrome. Am J Med Genet 2002;108:16–22.

44 Barak Y, Nir E. Chédiak-Higashi syndrome. Am J Pediatr Hematol Oncol 1987;9:42–55.

45 Eapen M, DeLaat CA, Baker KS et al. Hematopoietic cell transplantation for Chédiak-Higashi syndrome. Bone Marrow Transplant 2007;39:411–5.

46 Ogimi C, Tanaka R, Arai T et al. Rituximab and cyclosporine therapy for accelerated phase Chédiak-Higashi syndrome. Pediatr Blood Cancer 2011;57:677–80.

47 Griscelli C, Prunieras M. Pigment dilution and immunodeficiency: a new syndrome. Int J Dermatol 1978;17:788–91.

48 Pastural E, Barrat FJ, Dufourcq-Lagelouse R et al. Griscelli disease maps to chromosome 15q21 and is associated with mutations in the myosin-Va gene. Nat Genet 1997;16:289–92.

49 Ménasché G, Pastural E, Feldmann J et al. Mutations in RAB27A cause Griscelli syndrome associated with haemophagocytic syndrome. Nat Genet 2000;25:173–6.

50 Dotta L, Parolini S, Prandini A et al. Clinical, laboratory and molecular signs of immunodeficiency in patients with partial oculo-cutaneous albinism. Orphanet J Rare Dis 2013;8:168.

51 Lambert J, Vancoillie G, Naeyaert JM. Elejalde syndrome revisited. Arch Dermatol 2000;136:120–1.

52 Valente NYS, Machado MCMR, Boggio P et al. Polarized light microscopy of hair shafts aids in the differential diagnosis of Chédiak-Higashi and Griscelli-Prunieras syndromes. Clinics (Sao Paulo) 2006;61:327–32.

53 Patiroglu T, Akar HH, Unal E et al. Hematopoietic stem cell transplant for primary immunodeficiency diseases: a single-center experience. Exp Clin Transplant 2017;15:337–43.

54 Cross HE, McKusick VA, Breen W. A new oculocerebral syndrome with hypopigmentation. J Pediatr 1967;70:398–406.

55 Lerone M, Pessagno A, Taccone A et al. Oculocerebral syndrome with hypopigmentation (Cross syndrome): report of a new case. Clin Genet 1992;41:87–9.

CHAPTER 125
Disorders of Hypopigmentation

M.W. Bekkenk & A. Wolkerstorfer
Netherlands Institute for Pigment Disorders, Amsterdam University Medical Centers, Amsterdam, The Netherlands

General introduction, 1492 | Congenital hypopigmentation, 1492 | Acquired hypopigmentation, 1496

Abstract

Hypopigmentation of the skin is frequently encountered in childhood. Such a presentation can be either congenital or acquired, and generalized or more localized. Considering that hypopigmentation can be an early indication of serious (congenital) conditions, a medical history and thorough clinical examination, including Wood's light investigation, is important. In this chapter, the clinical diagnosis, aetiology and management of different types of congenital and acquired hypopigmentary disorders will be discussed.

Key points

- **Congenital hypopigmentation of the skin can be a sign of a multiorgan disorder, and special attention should be paid to vision, hearing and neurological symptoms.**
- **Solitary segmental localized hypopigmentation is rare and is generally a naevus depigmentosus with no systemic symptoms.**
- **Acquired hypopigmentation has a very diverse aetiology and is usually a symptom of an underlying skin disorder.**
- **The treatment of acquired hypopigmentation is to address the underlying skin disorder.**

General introduction

Hypopigmentation of the skin is observed frequently in paediatric patients. The presentation of hypopigmentation can be very diverse, from extensive congenital areas of depigmentation in piebaldism, to acquired mild and localized hypopigmentation in pityriasis alba. In addition, the implications of hypopigmentation can vary from a benign isolated skin condition to a key to the diagnosis of complex multisystem disorders. Distinction between depigmentation (total loss of pigment) and hypopigmentation (lighter skin compared with normal skin type, but some pigmentation remains) is important and usually straightforward. The use of a Wood's lamp makes distinction easier, especially in light colour skin types. In cases of extensive skin involvement it can be challenging to determine whether the lighter or darker skin is the normal colour. Hypopigmentation can be acquired or congenital, but not all hypopigmentation is clearly visible directly after birth. A segmental or Blaschkolinear distribution favours a congenital disorder, although there may be exceptions, as with segmental vitiligo. A comprehensive medical history and physical examination are generally sufficient for the diagnosis [1]. Key elements in the medical history are the age of onset (congenital or acquired), the clinical course of the lesions (stable, slowly progressive or exacerbations with remissions), the family history, subjective symptoms (itching, pain, anaesthesia) and associated symptoms from skin (abnormalities of hair, teeth and nails) or other organs (vision, hearing, skeletal, neurological). For an overview of hypopigmentation in children see Table 125.1 and for a flowchart on acquired localized hypopigmentation see Figure 125.1.

Reference

1 van Geel N, Speeckaert M, Chevolet I et al. Hypomelanoses in children. J Cutan Aesthet Surg 2013;6:65–72.

Congenital hypopigmentation

Introduction

There are several genodermatoses that show hypopigmentation of the skin: albinism (including the associated Hermansky–Pudlak, Chédiak–Higashi and Griscelli syndromes, see Chapter 124 for details), Waardenburg syndrome, Tietz albinism–deafness syndrome and piebaldism present with widespread (and generalized in albinism) hypo- to depigmentation at birth. In hypomelanosis of Ito (HI) and incontentia pigmenti (IP) there are areas of hypopigmentation that are often extensive, but the distribution is Blaschkolinear. In HI the hypopigmentation is present early, usually directly after birth, whereas

Harper's Textbook of Pediatric Dermatology, Fourth Edition. Edited by Peter Hoeger, Veronica Kinsler and Albert Yan.

Table 125.1 An overview of hypopigmentation in children

Early onset diffuse	Early onset localized	Acquired diffuse	Acquired localized
Albinism[a]	*Piebaldism* *Waardenburg syndrome* *Tietz syndrome*	*Malnutrition* Copper Selenium	*Vitiligo* Nonsegmental Segmental Vogt–Koyanagi–Harada[e]
Inborn metabolic disorders Phenylketonuria Homocysteinuria[b] Histadenaemia[b]	*Naevus depigmentosus/* hypopigmentary mosaicism *Naevus anaemicus* Tuberous sclerosis ('ash leaf' lesions)	Late (hypopigmented) stage of incontinentia pigmentii	*Postinflammatory* Eczema/pityriasis alba Pityriasis lichen chronica Lichen striatus Mycosis fungoides Other dermatitis Postinfection (lepra) Post-traumatic (nitrogen)
Genodermatoses Griscelli syndome[c] Menkes syndrome[c] EEC Syndrome[d]			*Lichen sclerosus/morphoea* *Bier spots*

[a] For subdivision see Chapter 124.
[b] First signs can also develop in older children.
[c] With neurological defects.
[d] With skeletal defects.
[e] Associated ear/eye/brain involvement.

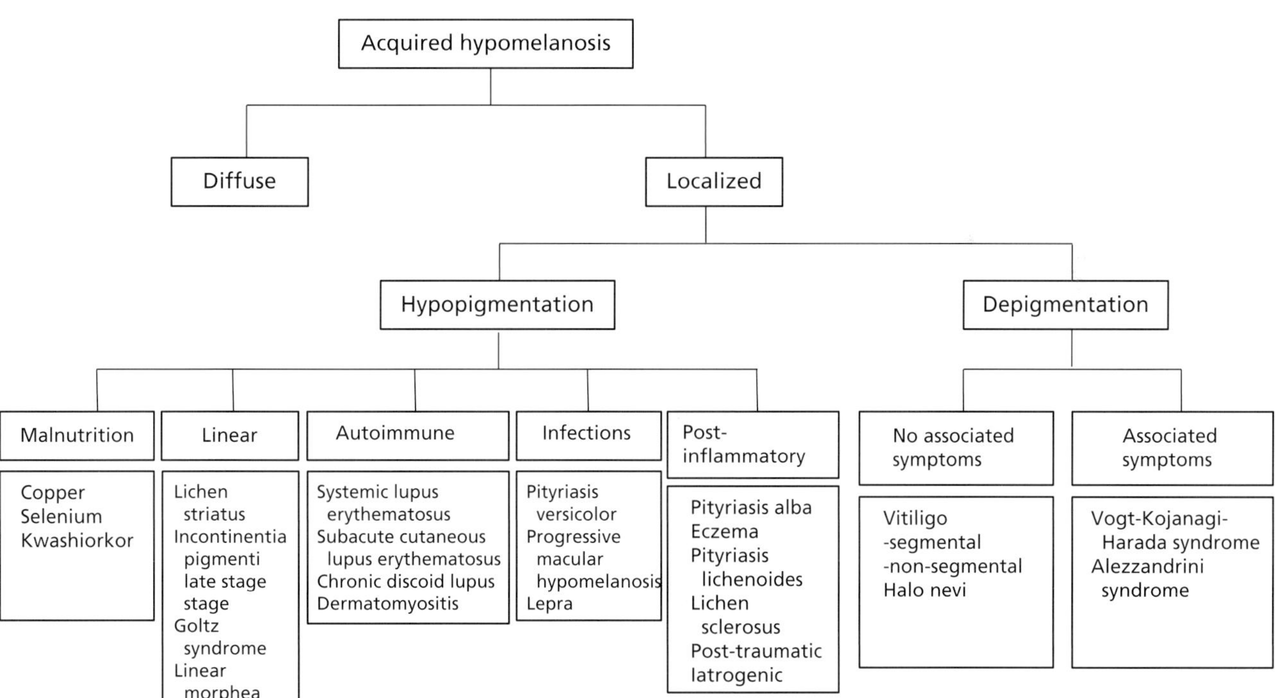

Fig. 125.1 Acquired localized hypopigmentation.

in IP hypopigmentation is a late sign (stage 4), following the vesicular, verrucous and hyperpigmented stages of this disorder. The hypopigmentation found in tuberous sclerosis (TS), the so-called 'ash-leaf macules', are an early indication for this genodermatosis. A naevus depigmentosus and anaemicus are mostly solitary, segmental and hypopigmented.

Piebaldism

Piebaldism is a rare autosomal dominant disorder caused by mutations in the *KIT* gene. Clinically it is characterized by a distinct type of symmetrical patchy depigmentation of the skin, often with areas of hyperpigmentation within and a characteristic midfrontal white forelock (Fig. 125.2). This disorder is present at birth and usually stable through life, unlike vitiligo.

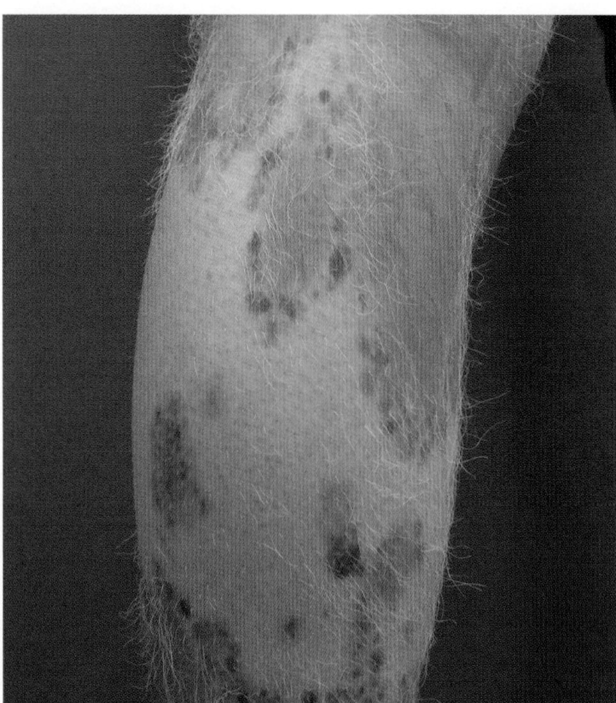

Fig. 125.2 Piebaldism. Sharply demarcated depigmentation on the leg with variably hyperpigmented macules along the border. Note the leucotrichia within the lesion.

Brief introduction and history. Piebaldism was already observed in early history with descriptions of persons with the striking skin and hair phenotype by Egyptians, Greek and Roman writers. Because of the dominant inheritance, the specific features were a specific family trait resulting in surnames such as Whitlock. The origin of the word is probably the medieval English word 'pied', indicating contrasting colours used in heraldry, but also in costumes of jesters and minstrels, such as the famous pied piper of Hamelin.

Epidemiology and pathogenesis. It is estimated that fewer than 1 in 20 000 children are born with piebaldism, with males and females equally affected [1]. The cause of piebaldism lies usually in the tyrosinase kinase domain of the KIT proto-oncogene, first described by Giebel and Spritz [2]. Several different mutations have been identified and can result in different phenotypes. The KIT gene encodes a tyrosinase kinase receptor involved in pigment cell development.

Clinical features and differential diagnosis. Anterior or ventral depigmentation centred on the midline, leading to a white forelock, central facial and anterior abdominal depigmentation, and presentation directly after birth [3,4] are the key features of piebaldism. The distribution of the irregular white patches are largely symmetrical. Involvement of the limbs is also common, centred on the elbows and knees. The extent of depigmentation is highly variable between individuals, but tends to be of similar severity within families. The depigmentation is usually stable, although rare cases with repigmentation [5] and progressive depigmentation [6] have been described in literature. In addition, patients frequently have islands of normal skin or darker than normal within the depigmented areas, and café-au-lait macules on top of normal skin, appearing as hyperpigmented macules. In patients with piebaldism there is no systemic involvement, and therefore it should be distinguished from Waardenburg syndrome. These patients show highly similar skin and hair features as piebaldism patients, but depending on the type of mutation also several other symptoms, most frequently sensory hearing loss [3,4,7]. Patients with vitiligo can show similar skin and hair depigmentation but can be easily distinguished from piebaldism patients by a good medical history. White skin and hair in patients with vitiligo are acquired and show a progressive rather than static course in life compared with piebaldism patients.

Laboratory and histology findings. Histology of the depigmented skin shows the absence or very sparse presence of melanocytes in the hypopigmented areas, whereas in the hyperpigmented areas the number of melanocytes is normal [1]. There should be no symptoms other than the skin disorders, but special attention should be paid to the presence of specific eye abnormalities, sensory hearing loss, bowel disorders, upper limb abnormalities and facial dysmorphic features. All these features can be present in Waardenburg syndrome (see later).

Treatment and prevention. Depigmented areas can be treated with surgical transplantation techniques. Minigrafting is an inexpensive and relatively simple and safe procedure that can be used with good results [8]. Split skin grafting is generally not feasible because of the large donor sites required for this technique. For the treatment of large areas as in piebaldism, the cultured or noncultured autologous cell suspension techniques are a possible option. Several autologous cell suspension techniques show promising results when applied on an ablative laser pretreated surface [9,10].

The risk of sunburn is elevated in individuals with piebaldism and ultraviolet protection is therefore advised. The subsequent risk of developing skin cancer is probably elevated in the hypopigmented areas, although no specific reports were found of skin cancer associated with piebaldism-related hypopigmented areas.

References

1 Agarwal S, Ojha A. Piebaldism: a brief report and review of the literature. Indian Dermatol Online J 2012;3:144–7.
2 Giebel LB, Spritz RA. Mutation of the KIT (mast/stem cell growth factor receptor) protooncogene in human piebaldism. Proc Natl Acad Sci 1991;88:8696–9.
3 Sundfor H. A pedigree of skin-spotting in man: 42 piebalds in a Norwegian family. J Hered 1939;30:67–77.
4 Thomas I, Kihiczak GG, Fox MD et al. Piebaldism: an update. Int J Derm 2004; 43:716–19.
5 Frances L, Betlloch I, Leiva-Salinas M, Silvestre JF. Spontaneous repigmentation in an infant with piebaldism. Int J Dermatol 2015;54:e244–6.
6 Kerkeni E, Boubaker S, Sfar S et al. Molecular characterization of piebaldism in a Tunisian family. Pathol Biol (Paris) 2015;63:113–6.
7 **Waardenburg PJ. A new syndrome combining developmental anomalies of the eyelids, eyebrows and nose root with pigmentary defects of the iris and head hair and with congenital deafness. Am J Hum Genet 1951;3:195–253.**

8 Komen L, Vrijman C, Prinsen CA et al. Optimising size and depth of punch grafts in autologous transplantation of vitiligo and piebaldism: a randomised controlled trial. J Dermatolog Treat 2017;28:86–91.
9 van Geel N, Wallaeys E, Goh BK et al. Long-term results of noncultured epidermal cellular grafting in vitiligo, halo naevi, piebaldism and naevus depigmentosus. Br J Dermatol 2010;163:1186–93.
10 Komen L, Vrijman C, Tjin EP et al.Autologous cell suspension transplantation using a cell extraction device in segmental vitiligo and piebaldism patients: a randomized controlled pilot study. J Am Acad Dermatol 2015;73:170–2.

Waardenburg syndrome

The skin manifestations in Waardenburg syndrome (WS) are undistinguishable from those in piebaldism, but apart from the pigmentation disorder other features are present depending on the mutation type. Sensorineural hearing loss and heterochromia irides are most frequently found, but upper limb abnormalities, bowel disorders and facial dysmorphic features may be present as well.

Brief introduction and history. The syndrome is named after Petrus Johannus Waardenburg, a Dutch ophthalmologist, who published a review on cases with a combination of skin and systemic features [1]. These cases showed eye abnormalities, deafness and pigment disorders. Different subtypes of this syndrome are acknowledged, classified by the different gene mutation (see Table 125.2 for details).

Epidemiology and pathogenesis. WS is rare and has an estimated incidence of 1 in 42 000 people [1]. An estimated 2–5% of people with sensory hearing loss are patients with WS and WS is the most common cause of congenital dominant syndromic hearing loss [2,3].

Mutations in different genes can result in WS and inheritance is usually autosomal dominant, although some rare cases have been described to be autosomal recessive. WS is caused by mutations of the *PAX3, MITF, WS2B, WS2C, SNAI2, EDNRB, EDN3* or *SOX10* gene; different mutations result in different phenotypes (see Table 125.2) [4,5].

Table 125.2 Subtypes of Waardenburg syndrome

Type	OMIM	Gene	Associated features[a]
WS1	193500	*PAX3*	Hypertelorism, prominent nasal root Dystopia canthorum Congenital hearing loss
WS2A	193510	*MITF*	Congenital hearing loss
WS2B	600193	*WS2B*	Heterochromia of the irises
WS2C	606662	*WS2C*	
WS2D	608890	*SNAI2*	
WS3	148820	*PAX3*	Upper limb abnormalities Dystopia canthorum Progressive hearing loss
WS4A	277580	*EDNRB*	Hirschsprung disease
WS4B	613265	*EDN3*	Congenital hearing loss
WS4C	613266	*SOX10*	

[a] All Waardenburg syndrome subtypes are characterized by pigmentary abnormalities of hair, iris and skin.
Type III is also known as Klein–Waardenburg syndrome and type IV is also known as Waardenburg–-Shah syndrome.
OMIM, Online Mendelian Inheritance of Man.

Clinical features and differential diagnosis. All WS patients have pigment disorders of the skin and hair (indistinguishable from piebaldism), with patchy depigmentations and a white forelock. Pigment disorders of the iris are often present, like heterochromia irides (irises of different colour) or brilliant blue eyes. Congenital sensorineural hearing loss is present and together with the prominent nasal root and increased intercanthal distance (dystopia canthorum) may suggest hypertelorism. Differentiation of the different subtypes of WS is mostly performed by genetic testing, but some clinical features are found in specific subgroups. In short, WS type 1 is distinguished by the presence of dystopia canthorum, whereas this feature is absent in WS type 2. Upper limb abnormalities are found only in WS type 3 and in WS type 4, also known as Waardenburg–Shah syndrome, Hirschsprung disease can be found [6,7].

Tietz albinism–deafness syndrome is closely related to WS2A, but the skin is totally depigmented (hence the term albinism), as in WS2A the *MITF* gene is mutated [8]

Laboratory and histology findings. An important test to perform is audiometry. If WS type 4 is suspected, evaluation of bowel transit time and a colon biopsy may be necessary. Genetic testing will result in definite diagnosis.

Treatment and prevention. There is no treatment for this syndrome; specific symptoms (like Hirschsprung's disease) can be treated as needed. The white patches on the skin can be treated as in piebaldism (see Piebaldism section for details).

References
1 Waardenburg PJ. A new syndrome combining developmental anomalies of the eyelids, eyebrows and nose root with pigmentary defects of the iris and head hair and with congenital deafness. Am J Hum Genet 1951;3:195–253.
2 Kochhar A, Hildebrand MS, Smith RJ. Clinical aspects of hereditary hearing loss. Genet Med 2007;9:393–408.
3 Zaman A, Capper R, Baddoo W. Waardenburg syndrome: more common than you think! Clin Otolaryngology 2015;40:44–8.
4 Zhang H, Chen H, Luo H et al. Functional analysis of Waardenburg syndrome-associated PAX3 and SOX10 mutations: report of a dominant-negative SOX10 mutation in Waardenburg syndrome type II. Hum Genet 2012;131:491–503.
5 Wollnik B, Tukel T, Uyguner O et al. Homozygous and heterozygous inheritance of PAX3 mutations causes different types of Waardenburg syndrome. Am J Med Genet A 2003;122A:42–5.
6 Horner ME, Abramson AK, Warren RB et al. The spectrum of oculocutaneous disease: part I. Infectious, inflammatory, and genetic causes of oculocutaneous disease. J Am Acad Dermatol 2014;70:795.e1–25.
7 Adam MP, Ardinger HH, Pagon RA et al. (eds). Waardenburg syndrome type 1. In: GeneReviews. Seattle (WA): University of Washington, 1993–2017.
8 Tietz W. A syndrome of deaf-mutism associated with albinism showing dominant autosomal inheritance. Am J Hum Genet 1962;15:259–64.

Localized congenital hypopigmentation

In HI there is extensive hypopigmentation along Blaschko lines; usually the term is reserved for patients with not only skin, but also organ (often cerebral) involvement [1,2]. HI is probably not a distinct entity [3,4] and skin symptoms may be part of the different state of the mosaicism [3].There is no good information on incidence, but estimates that between 1 in 1000 new patients in a paediatric neurological service and 1 in 10 000 patients in a children's hospital are diagnosed with HI [5] Usually HI occurs spontaneously, with parent–child inheritance rarely reported, but when it does occur, an autosomal dominant inheritance is suggested [6]. HI has been mapped to Xp11. HI and incontinentia pigmenti may represent allelic forms or a contiguous gene syndrome, with different genetic alterations in the Xp11 region showing HI or IP (or borderline) phenotypes [7]. The term linear naevoid hypomelanosis or segmental hypopigmentation is usually reserved for patients with only skin involvement; the delineation between patients with a (multifocal and segmental) naevus depigmentosus and HI is debatable. In young children with hypopigmentation along Blaschko lines, referral to a paediatrician is advised to exclude systemic involvement.

IP does not show hypopigmentation at first presentation (see Chapter 136 for details). Nevertheless, the clinical features of a later stage of IP can show an atrophic hypopigmented skin in Blaschko lines and can be mistaken for HI [3].

First presentation of TS is often the so-called 'ash leaf macules', that are present in the majority of TS patients [8,9]. Apart from these lesions, patients with TS usually have numerous symptoms of both skin and other organs, particularly the central nervous system.

A *naevus depigmentosus* is, despite its name, a localized and often segmental [10], *hypo*pigmentation present at birth or at an early age. It is probably a mosaic disorder, resulting in production of less or abnormal pigment (melanosomes) by a normal amount of melanocytes in the affected skin [11]. An association with systemic symptoms is rarely seen. Distinguishing a naevus anaemicus (NA) from a naevus depigmentosus can be difficult at first glance. Both present as a hypopigmented macule, but an NA is a vascular disorder and pigmentation is normal [12]. This can be appreciated by rubbing the lesion or when diascopy is performed, resulting in disappearance of the colour difference with the normal skin in an NA.

SECTION 26: DISORDERS OF PIGMENTATION

References

1 Ito M. Studies of melanin XI. Incontinentia pigmenti achromians: a singular case of nevus depigmentosus systematicus bilateralis. Tohoku Exper Med 1951;55(suppl):57–5

2 Jelinek JE, Bart RS, Schiff GM. Hypomelanosis of Ito ('incontinentia pigmenti achromians'): report of three cases and review of the literature. Arch Derm 1973;107: 596–601.

3 **Happle, R. Incontinentia pigmenti versus hypomelanosis of Ito: the whys and wherefores of a confusing issue (Letter). Am J Med Genet 1998;79: 64–5.**

4 Ruggieri, M. Familial hypomelanosis of Ito: implications for genetic counselling (Letter). Am J Med Genet 2000;95:82–4.

5 Pascual-Castroviejo I et al. Hypomelanosis of Ito. Neurological complications in 34 cases. Can J Neurol Sci 1988;15:124–9.

6 Klug H, Schreiber G, Hauschild R. [Incontinentia pigmenti achromicans (Ito syndrome). Cell morphological aspects.] Dermatol Monatschr 1982;168:680–5.

7 Koiffmann CP, de Souza DH, Diament A et al. Incontinentia pigmenti achromicans (hypomelanosis of Ito): further evidence of localization at Xp11. Am J Med Genet 1993;46:529–33.

8 Randle SC. Tuberous sclerosis complex: a review. Pediatr Ann 2017;46:e166–e171.

9 Cardis MA, DeKlotz CMC. Cutaneous manifestations of tuberous sclerosis complex and the paediatrician's role. Arch Dis Child 2017;102:858–63.

10 Lernia D. Segmental nevus depigmentosus: analysis of 20 patients. Pediatr Dermatol 1999;16:349–53.

11 Lee HS, Chun YS, Hann SK. Nevus depigmentosus: clinical features and histopathologic characteristics in 67 patients. J Am Acad Dermatol 1999;40:21–6.

12 Ahkami RN, Schwartz RA. Nevus anemicus. Dermatology 1999; 198:327–9.

Acquired hypopigmentation

Introduction

A wide range of conditions are associated with acquired hypopigmentation, including inflammatory, infectious and neoplastic disorders but also drug reactions, nutritional deficits and vitiligo. Individuals with darker skin are particularly prone to hypopigmentation following inflammation, infection or trauma of the skin, resulting in localized, patchy, hypopigmentation known as postinflammatory hypopigmentation.

Postinflammatory hypopigmentation is most commonly seen in patients with darker skin types and atopic dermatitis [1]. The clinical picture is variable, depending on the primary inflammatory disorder. The borders of the lesions are often blurred and the degree of hypopigmentation varies with both the age of the lesions and the degree of primary inflammation. However, sharply demarcated borders and mixed hypo- and hyperpigmentation can be present. These lesions are often a reason for concern and consultation with a doctor. In addition, concern about cosmetic appearance can be important [2]. However, at consultation it may be difficult to identify the underlying disorder because the patient may present at a late stage without any inflammation. A medical history should be taken in an attempt to identify an initial inflammatory stage, although sometimes the patients or parents do not remember any signs of inflammation. Moreover, postinflammatory hypopigmentation can evolve without any signs of inflammation, especially in darker skin types where erythema can easily be missed. In these cases, the clinical picture will often enable the diagnosis, but a skin biopsy may be necessary for the diagnosis and to rule out an ongoing inflammatory disease.

Pityriasis alba

Epidemiology. Pityriasis alba (PA) is a common hypopigmentary disorder occurring throughout the world in all ethnicities. The incidence ranges from 1.9 to 5.2% but is higher in populations with a darker skin type [3]. Although it may affect all age groups it is predominantly seen in children aged 3–16 years.

Clinical presentation. PA is characterized by spontaneous remissions and recurrences of hypopigmented macules with blurred borders (Fig. 125.3). Fine scaling is often present in the macules. Generally, the face is affected

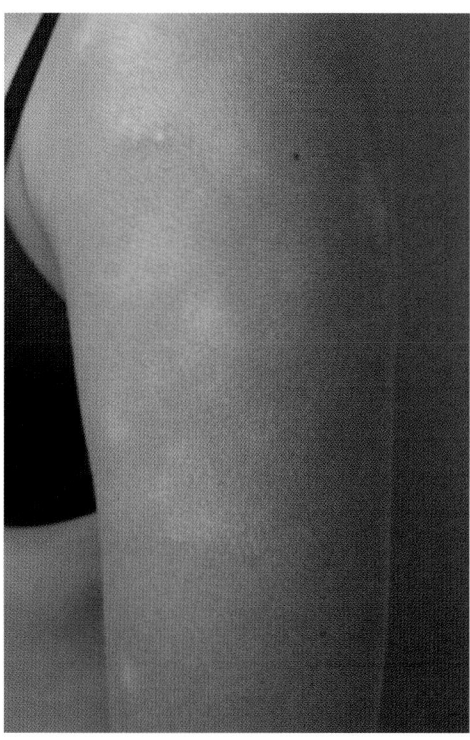

Fig. 125.3 Pityriasis alba. Hypopigmented macules with blurred borders on the left upper arm and shoulder.

followed by the extremities. Cases with disseminated lesions over the whole body are rare. Spontaneous resolution is the rule, although the hypopigmentation can remain for several years in some cases. Histopathology is rarely performed for the diagnosis of PA, but can show keratotic aggregates blocking hair follicles, sebaceous gland atrophy, irregular pigmentation of the basal layer and epidermal and follicular spongiosis. The number of melanocytes is usually normal.

Pathogenesis. Although the exact cause is unclear, it is regarded as a specific variant of atopic dermatitis with postinflammatory hypopigmentation. The strong link to atopic dermatitis is underlined by the fact that PA used to be one of the minor criteria for the diagnosis of atopic dermatitis according to the Hanifin and Raijka guidelines [3]. On the other hand, PA can be observed in children without any atopic signs.

Management. Similar to atopic dermatitis, the treatment of PA consists of skincare using emollients, avoidance of potential triggering factors, and in selected patients, topical anti-inflammatory treatment. Administration of emollient creams is considered helpful, especially when the lesions are scaling. Possible triggering factors, like sunlight, frequent bathing or use of exfoliating beauty treatments should be reduced [4]. Whether ultraviolet exposure really triggers the skin lesions or only makes them more visible is unclear. Topical corticosteroids are often prescribed although long-term use is limited because of the location. Topical tacrolimus and pimecrolimus are considered a safe and good option for long-term treatment [5].

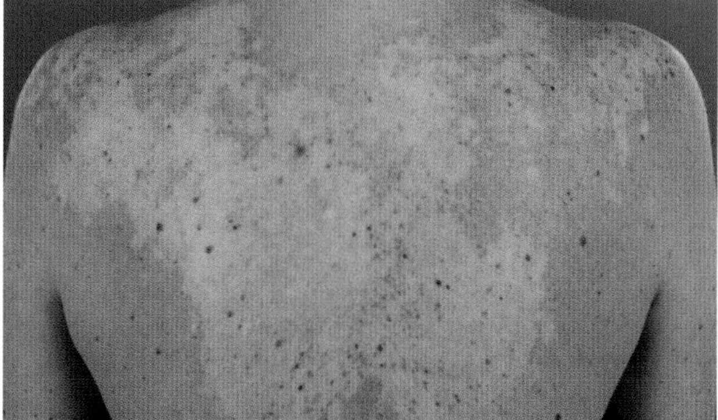

Fig. 125.4 Hypopigmentation in cutaneous lupus erythematosus. Multiple hypo- and depigmented macules with partly sharp and partly blurred demarcation. Note the persistence of the melanocytic naevi which differs from vitiligo.

Lichen sclerosus

When hypopigmentation is located in the anogenital area, lichen sclerosus can be suspected, although vitiligo and eczema are also often located in this region. When the inflammatory component is absent at consultation, vitiligo may be difficult to differentiate and a skin biopsy may be required. Although lichen sclerosus is rare at a young age, it is important to keep it in mind, because early diagnosis is important to prevent scarring and impaired function of the affected area [6]. Despite symptoms such as pruritus, dysuria, bleeding and constipation, the diagnostic delay in children is often long and sexual abuse incorrectly may be suspected. Treatment is similar to that in adults and involves long-term use of topical anti-inflammatory drugs.

Autoimmune disorders such as cutaneous lupus erythematosus, dermatomyositis and scleroderma are known to result in hypo- and hyperpigmentation (Fig. 125.4). Again, in children with darker skin types, the hypopigmentation can be the presenting symptom because the inflammatory component may no longer be visible.

Similarly, in pityriasis lichenoides chronica the inflammatory stage may be missed and the disease may present with extensive hypopigmentation and prominent facial involvement [7,8]. Hypopigmentation can also be the presenting symptom in superficial scaly dermatitis and small plaque parapsoriasis.

Mycosis fungoides

Epidemiology. In the differential diagnosis of hypopigmented macules, mycosis fungoides (MF) must also be considered. MF is the most frequent primary cutaneous lymphoma in childhood.

Clinical presentation. In children with darker skin types, hypopigmented MF has been reported to be the predominant clinical manifestation of MF [9]. The diagnosis in this variant of MF is commonly delayed because of a lack of specific clinical features [10]. Postinflammatory hypopigmentation or hypopigmented eczema may be diagnosed initially. Suspicion should arise when the patches are persistent and do not improve with conventional treatment. The presence of even a few papules or plaques should result in additional histopathological investigation. The management of MF is described in Chapter 88.

Other conditions associated with acquired hypopigmentation

Naevus anaemicus may be mistaken for a hypomelanotic lesion. In this condition the change in colour results from a localized reduction of perfusion whereas the melanin pigmentation is normal. The clinical distinction is easily made by using pressure on the edges, which will fade the lesion. Similarly, Bier spots result from localized reduction of skin perfusion leading to a marbled mottling pattern of the skin of the extremities.

Both segmental and nonsegmental *vitiligo* can be the cause of depigmentation in children. The diagnosis is straightforward in typical cases showing sharply demarcated depigmented macules on predilection sites. However, the diagnosis may be missed in progressive stages when blurred borders, pinpoint lesions and hypopigmentations instead of depigmentations are present. Well known but rare are syndromes where vitiligo is associated with ear and eye involvement (Vogt–Koyanagi–Harada syndrome and Alezzandrini syndrome) [11,12].

Hypochromic vitiligo was first described in 2015 [13]. Despite the name there are hardly any similarities with typical vitiligo. The lesions are hypopigmented instead of depigmented, less sharply demarcated, often located on the head and upper trunk, and tend to be unresponsive to any treatment used in vitiligo.

Any trauma, including that iatrogenically induced, for example cryotherapy, intralesional corticosteroids, laser treatment and vaccination, can result in localized hypopigmentation. Generally, the hypopigmentation will resolve spontaneously within 6–12 months.

Skin infections can also lead to hypopigmentation. Pityriasis versicolour is a common disorder with a characteristic distribution on the upper trunk and subtle scaling of the skin appearing after traction. However, the diagnosis may be more difficult in older lesions where scaling is absent and direct microscopic examination of a KOH (potassium hydroxide) preparation is negative. It is caused by a superficial *Malassezia furfur* (formerly known as *Pityrosporum ovale*) skin infection, which can result in both hypo- and hyperpigmentation. As in adults, topical antimycotic drugs are generally effective. The clinical features of progressive macular hypomelanosis can be somewhat similar, but the hypopigmented lesions are usually located more centrally on the trunk, do not scale and do not repigment spontaneously. When inspected with the Wood's lamp, orange–red follicular fluorescence can be observed because of the presence of Propionibacterium. It is hypothesized that this bacterium is the (indirect) cause of the hypopigmentation and therefore should be the target of treatment [14]. Accordingly, topical antiacne therapy has been proven to be effective (3 months treatment). Narrowband ultraviolet B is a therapeutic alternative. *Mycobacterium leprae* infection may result in hypopigmentation. In the tuberculoid form of the disease the lesions are anaesthetic. Secondary syphilis (*Leukoderma syphiliticum*) should not be forgotten as a possible cause of hypopigmentation in children. Viral infections can also lead to hypopigmentation; eruptive hypomelanosis is considered to be a specific type of viral exanthema presenting with disseminated hypopigmentation without a clear erythematous phase that can occur in children with darker skin types [15].

Kwashiorkor, a protein energy related *nutritional deficit* occurring in young children, may result in hypopigmentation especially around the mouth and on the legs; hyperpigmentation may develop on pressure sites. Desquamation of the skin and scalp hair loss and hair colour changes can also be present [16]. Selenium deficiency, a complication of long-term nutritional support, can result in pseudoalbinism, growth retardation and alopecia. These symptoms are reversible when adequate administration of selenite is given.

References

1 Vachiramon V, Thadanipon K. Postinflammatory hypopigmentation. Clin Exp Dermatol 2011;36:708–14.
2 Taylor A, Pawaskar M, Taylor SL et al. Prevalence of pigmentary disorders and their impact on quality of life: a prospective cohort study. J Cosmet Dermatol 2008;7:164–8.
3 Hanifin JM, Rajka G. Diagnostic features of atopic dermatitis. Acta Dermatol Venereol 1980;92:44–7.
4 Miazek N, Michalek I, Pawlowska-Kisiel M et al. Pityriasis alba – common disease, enigmatic entity: up-to-date review of the literature. Pediatr Dermatol 2015;32:786–91.
5 Rigopoulos D, Gregoriou S, Charissi C et al. Tacrolimus ointment 0.1% in pityriasis alba: an open-label, randomized, placebo-controlled study. Br J Dermatol 2006;155:152–5.
6 Nerantzoulis I, Grigoriadis T, Michala L. Genital lichen sclerosus in childhood and adolescence – a retrospective case series of 15 patients: early diagnosis is crucial to avoid long-term sequelae. Eur J Pediatr 2017;176:1429–32.
7 Clayton R, Warin A. Pityriasis lichenoides chronica presenting as hypopigmentation. Br J Dermatol 1979;100:297–302.
8 Lane TN, Parker SS. Pityriasis lichenoides chronica in black patients. Cutis 2010;85:125–9.
9 Rizzo FA, Vilar EG, Pantaleão L et al. Mycosis fungoides in children and adolescents: a report of six cases with predominantly hypopigmentation, along with a literature review. Dermatol Online J 2012;18:5.
10 Gameiro A, Gouveia M, Tellechea Ó, Moreno A. Childhood hypopigmented mycosis fungoides: a commonly delayed diagnosis. BMJ Case Rep 2014 Dec 23;2014.
11 Moorthy RS, Inomata H, Rao NA. Vogt–Koyanagi–Harada syndrome. Surv Ophthalmol 1995;39:265–92.
12 Casala AM, Alezzandrini AA. Vitiligo, poliosis unilateral con retinitis pigmentaria y hypoacusia. Arch Argent Dermatol 1959;9:449.
13 Ezzedine K, Mahé A, van Geel N et al. Hypochromic vitiligo: delineation of a new entity. Br J Dermatol 2015;172:716–21.
14 Relyveld GN, Westerhof W, Woudenberg J et al. Progressive macular hypomelanosis is associated with a putative Propionibacterium species. J Invest Dermatol 2010;130: 1182–4.
15 Chuh A, Bharatia P, Zawar V. Eruptive hypomelanosis in a young child as a 'paraviral exanthem'. Pediatr Dermatol 2016;33:e38–9.
16 Heilskov S, Vestergaard C, Babirekere E et al. Characterization and scoring of skin changes in severe acute malnutrition in children between 6 months and 5 years of age. J Eur Acad Dermatol Venereol 2015;29:2463–9.

CHAPTER 126
Dyschromatosis

Liat Samuelov & Eli Sprecher
Department of Dermatology, Tel-Aviv Sourasky Medical Center, Tel-Aviv, Israel

Introduction, 1499
Dyschromatosis symmetrica hereditaria, 1500
Dyschromatosis universalis hereditaria, 1502
Familial progressive hyperpigmentation and hypopigmentation, 1504
Cutis tricolor, 1505
Westerhof syndrome, 1506
Amyloidosis cutis dyschromica, 1507
Dyschromatosis ptychotropica, 1509
Other entities associated with dyschromia, 1509
Treatment, 1510

Abstract

Dyschromatoses refer to a group of pigmentary disorders characterized by both hypo- and hyperpigmented lesions. There are several causes of dyschromatosis including genodermatoses, inflammatory skin diseases, infections, drugs and environmental exposures or nutritional disorders. Genodermatoses account for most cases in the paediatric population, whereas in adults most conditions are acquired. Some conditions are confined to the skin whereas others may manifest with extracutaneous features. In contrast to inherited dyschromatoses in which no satisfactory treatment modality has been reported, prevention and treatment is possible in some of the acquired entities. This chapter summarizes the differential diagnosis and approach to diagnosis and management of both inherited and acquired dyschromatosis.

Key points

- Dyschromatosis symmetrica hereditaria, characterized by symmetrically distributed hypo- and hyperpigmented macules over the back of the hands and feet, is caused by mutations in the gene *ADAR1*. Hypomelanosis and a reduced number and density of dopa-positive melanocytes is evident in the hypopigmented areas. In contrast, dyschromatosis universalis hereditaria, caused by mutations in the gene *ABCB6*, features hypo- and hyperpigmented macules which are distributed over the entire skin surface and result from a defect in melanosome production or distribution (but not from abnormal melanocyte numbers).
- Familial progressive hyperpigmentation and hypopigmentation is an autosomal dominant disease caused by heterozygous mutations in the gene *KITLG* encoding KIT ligand that normally manifests at birth or early infancy. It is characterized by diffuse hyperpigmentation intermixed with confetti-like and ash leaf-like hypopigmented macules, café-au-lait spots and lentigines. Familial progressive hyperpigmentation, where hypopigmentation is absent, is allelic to familial progressive hyperpigmentation and hypopigmentation.
- Cutis tricolor refers to the coexistence of congenital hypo- and hyperpigmented lesions in close proximity to each other on a background of normal skin. Most cases are sporadic and the cause is unknown.
- Westerhof syndrome is characterized by multiple hereditary congenital hypopigmented and hyperpigmented macules which may be associated with retarded growth and mental deficiency.
- Amyloidosis cutis dyschromica is a rare type of primary cutaneous amyloidosis characterized by widely distributed hyperpigmentation admixed with hypopigmented macules which usually start before puberty. Unlike acquired amyloidosis cutis, there is little or no associated pruritus. Amyloid deposition is confined to the papillary dermis. Amyloidosis cutis dyschromica pathogenesis involves both genetic and environmental factors.
- Dyschromatosis ptychotropica appears during infancy and is characterized by reticular or mottled hypo- and hyperpigmented macules, mainly found in body folds (ptychotropism). It may be associated with neurological abnormalities.

Introduction

The dyschromatoses are a group of disorders characterized by hypo- and hyperpigmented macules giving the skin a mottled appearance. Genodermatoses account for most cases of dyschromatosis in the paediatric population as exemplified by dyschromatosis symmetrica hereditaria and dyschromatosis universalis hereditaria, caused by mutations in *ADAR1* and *ABCB6*, respectively. Both conditions are most commonly seen in Japan and China and are typically confined to the skin. Whereas dyschromatosis symmetrica hereditaria features symmetrically distributed hypo- and hyperpigmented macules over the back of the hands and feet, in DUS the lesions are distributed over the entire skin surface. Additional inherited entities are familial progressive hyper- and hypopigmentation caused by mutations in the gene *KITLG*, cutis tricolor, Westerhof syndrome, amyloidosis cutis dyschromica and dyschromatosis ptychotropica. Dyschromia is also a characteristic

Harper's Textbook of Pediatric Dermatology, Fourth Edition. Edited by Peter Hoeger, Veronica Kinsler and Albert Yan.

feature of several other genodermatoses including keratin disorders, ectodermal dysplasias and pigmentary dilution disorders. In contrast to the paediatric population, in adults most dyschromatoses are acquired in the context of inflammatory skin disorders, infections, drugs and chemical exposures [1–4]. The differential diagnosis of inherited and acquired dyschromatoses is listed in Table 126.1.

Dyschromatosis symmetrica hereditaria

History. Dyschromatosis symmetrica hereditaria (DSH; OMIM #127400), also known as reticulate acropigmentation of Dohi, was first described in 1910 by Toyama who reported a unique pigmentation pattern on the dorsal aspect of the distal extremities. Later on, Matsumoto termed the condition 'leucopathia punctata et reticularis' which was renamed DSH by Toyama in 1929 [1,5–7].

Table 126.1 Differential diagnosis of inherited and acquired dyschromatoses

Inherited disorders
Dyschromatosis symmetrica hereditaria
Dyschromatosis universalis hereditaria
Familial progressive hyperpigmentation and hypopigmentation
Cutis tricolor
Westerhof syndrome (hereditary congenital hypopigmented and hyperpigmented macules)
Amyloidosis cutis dyschromica
Dyschromatosis ptychotropica
Xeroderma pigmentosum
Dyskeratosis congenita
Rothmund–Thomson syndrome
Epidermolysis bullosa simplex with mottled pigmentation
Dowling–Degos disease and Galli-Galli disease
Naegeli–Franceschetti–Jadassohn syndrome
Dermatopathia pigmentosa reticularis syndrome
Chediak–Higashi syndrome
Griscelli syndrome
Ectodermal dysplasia with coexisting skin dyschromatosis
Wende–Bauckus syndrome
Ziprkowski–Margolis syndrome
Incontinenta pigmenti
Mismatch repair disorders
Acquired conditions
Inflammatory skin disorders
Cutaneous lupus erythematosus
Systemic sclerosis
Dermatomyositis
Infections
Secondary syphilis (syphilitic leucomelanoderma)
Pinta (tertiary)
Onchocerciasis
Drugs, chemical and physical agents
Chronic arsenic toxicity
Contact leucomelanosis (diphenylcyclopropenone, monobenzyl ether hydroquinone)
Drug-induced photoleucomelanodermatitis (afloqualone, thiazides or tetracyclines)
Psolaren ultraviolet A photochemotherapy
Betel leaf
Nutritional disorders
Kwashiorkor
Miscellaneous
Amyloidosis cutis dyschromica
Acquired brachial cutaneous dyschromatosis
Vagabond leucomelanoderma
Chronic radiation dermatitis
Poikiloderma

Epidemiology. DSH has been described predominantly in Japan and China but cases from Taiwan, Korea, Thailand, India, Europe and South America have also been reported [1,8–25]. The exact frequency of DSH is unknown because many cases remain unreported. The prevalence of DSH in Japan has been estimated to be 1.5 in 100 000 [26]. It has been speculated that the high prevalence of DSH in eastern Asia may reflect the fact that skin manifestations in White patients are inconspicuous and difficult to recognize [27].

Pathogenesis. DSH has a dominant pattern of inheritance with high penetrance. The disease is caused by mutations in the gene *ADAR1*, encoding adenosine deaminase acting on RNA1, also known as the double-stranded RNA specific adenosine deaminase (*DSRAD*) [25,26,28]. To date, over 100 mutations have been reported, the majority of which lie within the deaminase region of the protein. There is no clear genotype–phenotype correlation in patients with DSH because identical mutations may result in different clinical features and degrees of severity [24]. The *ADAR1* gene, ubiquitously expressed in human tissues, spans up to 40 kb, consists of 15 exons and encodes a 139 kDa protein [29,30]. ADAR1 mediates a post-transcriptional modification of the messenger RNA through a mechanism known as RNA editing during which adenosine is converted into inosine on double-stranded RNA following RNA transcription [31,32]. The gene produces interferon-inducible (p150) and constitutively expressed (p110) isoforms as a result of alternative splicing [33]. The p150 protein includes two Z-DNA-binding domains in its N-terminal region, three dsRNA-binding domains and a deaminase domain in the C-terminal region. The p110 isoform lacks one of the Z-DNA-binding domains which are considered to be important for antiviral response [34,35]. ADAR1 has been shown to be involved in several physiological processes including virus inactivation, neurotransmitter receptor activities, inhibition of apoptosis, regulation of cellular RNA interference efficacy and modulation of the innate antiviral response [36–41]. The latter is probably induced by the interferon-inducible isoform, p150. Elevated interferon levels induce upregulation of the p150 isoform in individuals with normal ADAR1 expression. Accordingly, viral encephalitis in a patient with DSH has been suggested to result from loss-of-function mutations in the ADAR1 p150 isoform which may be a risk factor for severe viral infections [42,43].

An epidermis-specific *Adar1* knockout mouse model resulted in epidermal necrosis and thickening of the stratum corneum, whereas *Adar1*-null knockout mice showed extensive apoptosis and embryonic lethality.

It has been postulated that impaired RNA editing during melanoblast migration from the neural crest causes their differentiation into hyper- and hypoactive melanocytes.

Thus, the most affected melanocytes are those which migrate farthest, to the hands and feet [26]. In addition, because the hypopigmented areas reveal decreased number of melanocytes with degenerative vacuolation indicating apoptosis, it was speculated that stress-induced apoptosis (e.g. viral infection) in melanocytes with *ADAR1* mutation results in hypopigmented lesions while remnant melanocytes in the bulge area of hair follicles migrate toward the epidermis to form hyperpigmented macules, leading to the classic appearance of DHS [5,40,44].

Although most cases are familial and dominant, some rare sporadic cases and a case of autosomal recessive inheritance have been reported [24,45,46]. In addition, DSH is allelic to Aicardi–Goutières syndrome, a genetic inflammatory disorder affecting the nervous system, caused by homozygous or compound heterozygous mutations in *ADAR1* (although two cases with heterozygous mutations have been reported). Recently, a case of DSH with neurological symptoms and brain calcification with compound heterozygous *ADAR1* mutations and a case of DSH with neurological symptoms and a heterozygous *ADAR1* mutation, have been reported. It has been shown that differences in editing efficiency as a result of heterozygous or homozygous mutations determine whether neurological abnormalities develop [27].

In addition to mutations in the gene *ADAR1*, heterozygous mutations in the tumour suppressor gene *SASHI*, encoding SAM and SH3 domain containing I, were identified in three families with clinical features reminiscent of DSH or resembling familial lentiginosis [47–49]. Homozygous mutations in the same gene were associated with dyschromatosis over the trunk, face and extremities, alopecia, palmoplantar keratoderma, teeth anomalies, onychodystrophy and recurrent squamous cell carcinoma in a consanguineous Moroccan family [50]. SASH1 has been shown to reduce E-cadherin expression (a known mediator of melanocyte–keratinocyte adhesion) which in turn increases cell motility and may alter melanin transfer [48,51]. Moreover, SASH1 has been reported to be involved in other cellular mechanisms including tumorigenesis, interaction with the actin cytoskeleton, cell migration and endothelial toll-like-receptor 4 (TLR4) signalling. In addition, SASH1 was identified as a regulator of ubiquitination of TNF receptor associated factor 6 (TRAF6), which in turn modulates the activity of nuclear factor kappa B (NF-kB) and has been implicated in the pathogenesis of hypohidrotic ectodermal dysplasia [52–56].

Clinical features. DSH appears during infancy or early childhood (before the age of six in approximately 70% of cases), although a case of adult-onset DSH at age 26 and a case of adolescence-onset have been reported [1,12,57]. DSH is characterized by asymptomatic hypo- and hyperpigmented macules of varying sizes (mostly pinpoint to pea-sized macules) distributed symmetrically on the dorsal aspect of the hands and feet (Fig. 126.1) that increase in size and number until adolescence and persist throughout life without any change in colour or distribution. The hypopigmented macules are followed by the appearance of hyperpigmented lesions within hypopigmented areas, with no evidence of any precedent event [58–60]. Darkening of skin lesions following sun exposure can occasionally occur [1,61]. Facial involvement consisting of small discrete freckle-like macules may be seen [61,62]. Skin lesions on the penis, heels, abdomen and chest have also been described [23,59,63,64]. The palms, soles and mucous membranes are usually spared.

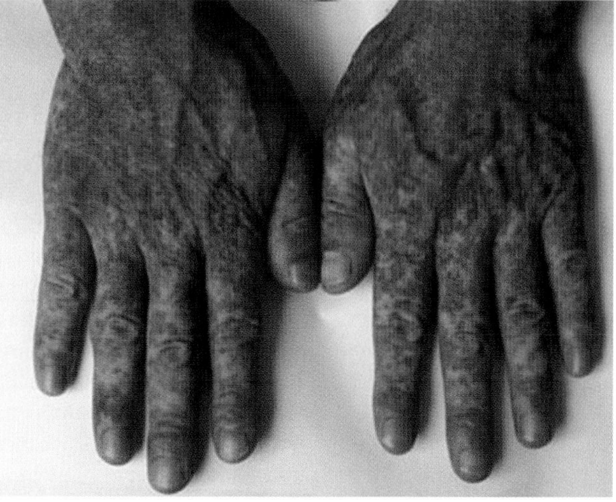

Fig. 126.1 Varying sizes of hypo- and hyperpigmented macules in a reticulate pattern over the dorsal hands in a patient with dischromatosis symmetrica hereditaria. Source: Sun et al. (2005) [28]. Reproduced with permission of John Wiley & Sons.

Dermoscopic features that were reported in DSH include 0.5–1.5 mm round pigmented spots showing a variety of pigmented appearances (reticulated hyperpigmented spots, diffuse pigmentation with hyperpigmented dots, reticulate pigmented spots, monotonous pigmented spots, reticulated hypopigmented spots and monotonous hypopigmented spots), connected to each other and producing oval hyperpigmented macules. In contrast, the hypopigmented lesions contain sparsely distributed and unconnected round pigmented spots [65].

Most cases are confined to the skin with no evidence of systemic manifestations. However, various associations have been reported including neurological abnormalities (mental deterioration, developmental regression, dystonia brain calcification), limb hypertrophy, dental root aplasia, aortic valve sclerosis, psoriasis and depression [39,58,59,66–69]. In addition, the appearance of DSH in conjunction with neurofibromatosis type 1 has been reported [70]. Moreover, a familial case with splice site *ADAR1* mutation associated with dental anomalies, longer thicker hypopigmented and hyperpigmented hair appearing on both hyper- and hypopigmented skin respectively, has been published [23]. In one study, in which a three-generation family with a single germline *ADAR1* mutation exhibited phenotypic variability, it was suggested that severe chilblains may aggravate the clinical phenotype of DSH [24].

Differential diagnosis. Given its quite restricted skin involvement, the main differential diagnosis for DSH is reticulate acropigmentation of Kitamura (RAK; OMIM #615537).

RAK is a rare autosomal dominant disease with high penetrance that has been shown to result from mutations in the gene *ADAM10* encoding a zinc metalloprotease [71,72]. The disease usually appears in the first or second decades of life and is characterized by slightly depressed angulated hyperpigmented lesions which appear over the dorsal surface of the hands and feet and progress towards the proximal extremities in conjunction with palmoplantar pits. There is no hypopigmentation and the face is usually uninvolved. Involved skin demonstrates epidermal atrophy with an increased number of basal melanocytes [72]. Characteristic dermoscopy findings are hyperpigmented macules forming a fine pigmented network and patchy brownish pigmented spots coinciding with the depressions seen on the palms and soles [73]. Vitiligo is another entity which should be taken into consideration. Although it lacks hyperpigmented macules, localized vitiligo involving the distal extremities in its early stages or in a state of repigmentation following treatment may share similar features with DSH. Other entities to be considered in the differential diagnosis are listed in Table 126.1.

Histopathology. Histopathological examination of skin lesions demonstrates significantly increased melanin content within basal keratinocytes of hyperpigmented macules whereas basal hypomelanosis is observed in the hypopigmented lesions. Moreover, reduced number and density of dopa-positive melanocytes is evident in the hypopigmented areas compared with control skin [58,74,75]. Electron microscopy analysis revealed the formation of cytoplasmic vacuoles and degenerative mitochondria in lesional skin suggesting an apoptotic process. Moreover, it was suggested that the process of melanosome transfer from melanocytes to adjacent keratinocytes is much activated compared with melanosome production resulting in small or immature, sparsely scattered melanosomes in melanocytes within the hyperpigmented areas, while numerous small melanosomes are aggregated within adjacent keratinocytes [58].

Dyschromatosis universalis hereditaria

History. Dyschromatosis universalis hereditaria (DUH) is a rare inherited disorder first described in Japan by Ichikawa and Hiraga in 1933 [76].

Epidemiology. Although most cases have been reported in Japan, it has also been described in China, Taiwan, Korea, Europe, South America, India and Africa. Both sexes are equally affected [8,77–90]. The exact prevalence of the disorder is unknown.

Pathogenesis. DUH is inherited in an autosomal dominant fashion with variable penetrance in most cases (DUH1/DUH3; OMIM 127500/#615402), although autosomal recessive inheritance (DUH2; OMIM 612715) and few sporadic cases have been reported [78,80,83,86,87,91,92].

Autosomal dominant DUH has been found to result in some cases from mutations in the *ABCB6* gene encoding ATP binding cassette subfamily B member 6 [93,94]. Mutations in *ABCB6* result in diverse disease phenotypes including DUH, ocular coloboma (a developmental defect of the eye caused by incomplete closure of the optic fissure), negative Lan blood type and dominant familial pseudohyperkalaemia [95–97]. *ABCB6* knockout mice do not show pigmentary abnormalities [98]. In contrast, *ABCB6* gene knockdown in the zebrafish model is associated with a significant lower number of pigmented melanocytes within the head region compared with control. This was partially rescued by coinjecting the mutant embryos with full length hABCB6 mRNA confirming the involvement of ABCB6 in the pigmentation process [93].

ABCB6 is ubiquitously expressed in tissues including the heart, skeletal muscles, fetal liver, melanocytes, melanoma cells but not in keratinocytes of the basal cell layer [93].

ABCB6 may contribute to pigment homeostasis in two different ways. Firstly, it is a transporter protein located in mitochondria, endoplasmic reticulum, Golgi apparatus, lysosomes and plasma membranes [99–101]. It functions as a porphyrin transporter and plays an important role in hemosynthesis and multidrug resistance. Moreover, it is also important for metal homeostasis (mainly that of copper) [100,102–105]. ABCB6 participates in the transport of enzymes required for normal melanogenesis in melanocytes. Copper is important for vertebrate pigmentation because it serves as a cofactor for tyrosinase [106,107]. Accordingly, it has been speculated that DUH-causing mutations in *ABCB6* result in abnormal melanin synthesis caused by disturbed copper homeostasis influencing tyrosinase activity. In line with this hypothesis, hyperpigmented lesions of DUH demonstrate increased RNA expression of *TYR* and *DCT*, encoding tyrosinase and dopachrome tautomerase respectively, compared with hypopigmented ones [91]. DUS is thus associated with a defect in melanosome production or distribution and not with abnormal melanocyte number [108].

Secondly, ABCB6 is present in exosomes which are vesicles secreted upon fusion of multivesicular bodies with the cell surface plasma membrane. This process is part of the melanosome transport machinery and many melanogenic proteins are sorted in exosomes (e.g. Pmel17/gp100, TYRP1 [tyrosinase-related protein 1], MART-1 [melanoma antigen recognized by T cells] and Rab27) [109–112]. In addition, wild type ABCB6 exhibits endosome-like distribution with subcellular localization in the dendrites of the mouse melanoma B16 cell line whereas mutant ABCB6 demonstrates retention in the Golgi body apparatus in those cells [94]. These findings suggest that ABCB6 plays an important role in melanosome transport and indicate that mutant ABCB6 may exert a dominant negative effect on melanogenesis through binding of mutant and wild-type ABCB6 transporters [100].

Clinical features. DUH tends to present during infancy or early childhood (80% appear before the age of 6 years) and approximately 20% manifest with dyspigmentation at birth, although adult-onset cases have been reported [2,79,91,113]. It is characterized by widespread, symmetrical and asymptomatic hypo- and hyperpigmented macules with irregular borders and varying sizes ranging from a few millimetres to several centimetres (Fig. 126.2). The lesions usually appear first over the extremities or trunk and slowly progress and increase their size within a few years to cover most of the body areas, mainly the extremities, trunk and abdomen. Stabilization of lesions may be seen prior to adolescence with persistent appearance throughout life with no seasonal variation or spontaneous regression [79]. A case of localized involvement with hypo- and hyperpigmented macules over the anterior neck in a 14-year-old girl has been described [114]. Although in most cases lesions tend to slowly progress over the years, some reports of abrupt onset have been described [115]. Facial involvement with hyperpigmented macules resembling ephelides occurs in 50% of cases. The mucous membranes, palms, soles, hair and nails (with dystrophy and pterygium formation) may seldom be affected [2,3,83,94,116]. A case of DUH with absent dermatoglyphics distal to the

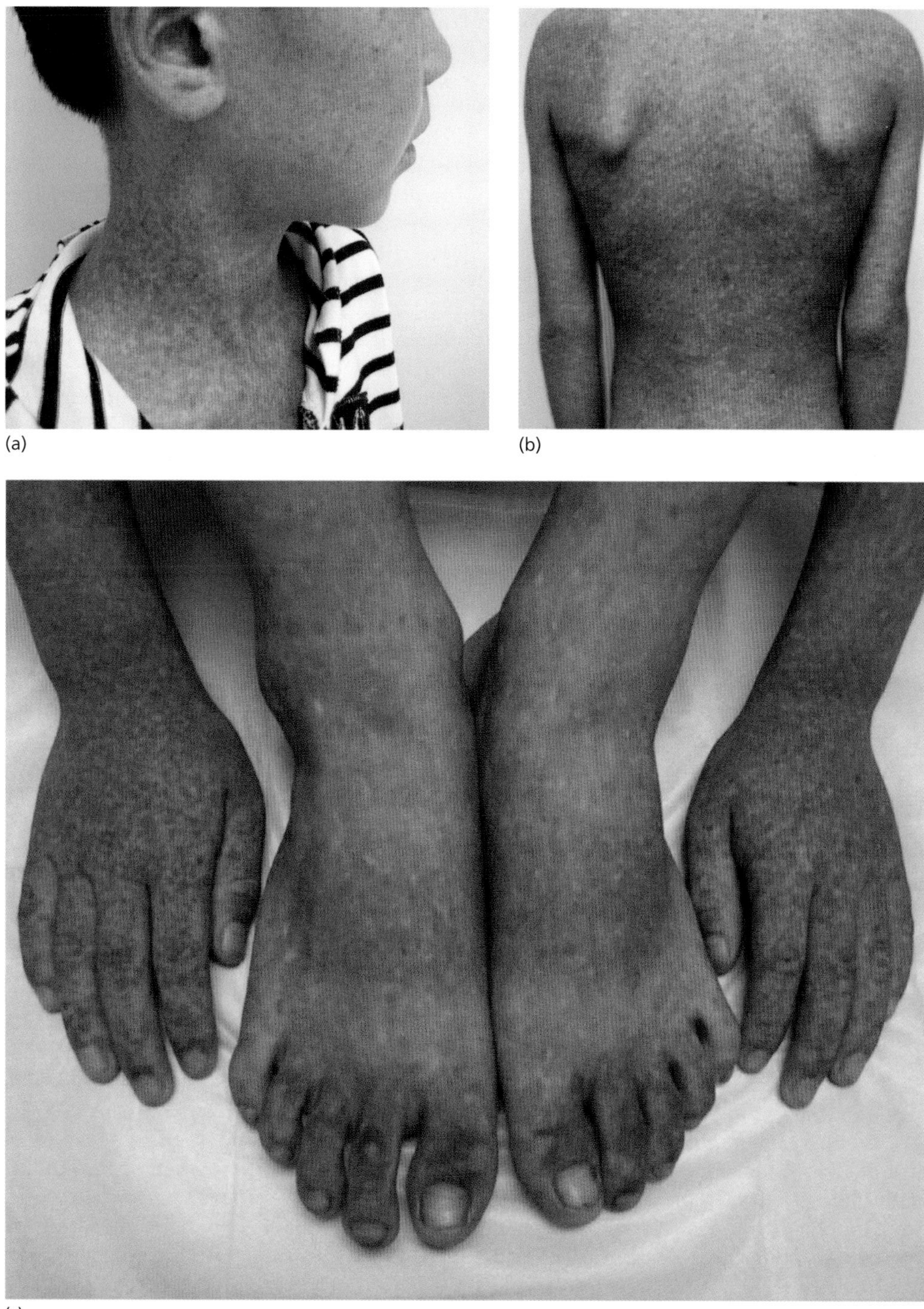

Fig. 126.2 Diffuse, symmetric distribution of hypo- and hyperpigmented macules in varying sizes and with a mottled appearance over the (a) face and neck, (b) trunk, and (c) the dorsal aspect of the hands and feet in a patient with dyschromatosis universalis hereditaria. Source: Zhang et al. (2013) [94]. Reproduced with permission of Elsevier.

distal creases has been reported [87]. Other dermatological abnormalities that have been reported with DUH in some cases include pruritus, dry skin with scaling, photosensitivity, solar elastosis, tuberous sclerosis (TS) and Dowling–Degos disease [87,117–119]. In most cases, disease manifestations are confined to the skin although systemic abnormalities have been reported in association with DUH including short stature, learning difficulties, mental retardation, insulin-dependent diabetes mellitus, haematological abnormalities, tryptophan metabolism abnormalities, renal failure, high-tone deafness and neurosensory hearing loss, ocular abnormalities and epilepsy [79,80,82,93,118,120,121].

Differential diagnosis. Several inherited disorders should be taken into consideration in the differential diagnosis of DUH including dyskeratosis congenita (DKC), Dowling-Degos disease (DDD), Naegeli-Franceschetti-Jadassohn (NFJ) syndrome, dermatopathia pigmentosa reticularis (DPR), epidermolysis bullosa simplex with mottled pigmentation (EBS-MP) and xeroderma pigmentosum (XP).

DKC is an inherited multisystem disease caused by defective telomere maintenance with a variable pattern of inheritance (X-linked recessive, autosomal dominant or autosomal recessive), and is characterized by a classic triad of reticulate hypo- and hyperpigmented macules mostly in sun exposed areas, nail dystrophy and oral leukoplakia in association with other dermatological (skin atrophy, telangiectasias, palmoplantar keratoderma, hyperhidrosis and alopecia) and systemic (pancytopenia, predisposition to malignancies and pulmonary fibrosis) manifestations [122].

DDD and its acantholytic form, Galli-Galli disease, is a rare autosomal dominant condition characterized by spotted and reticulate hyperpigmented macules in association with small brown hyperkeratotic papules affecting mainly the skin folds and pitted perioral scars. Lesions usually appear following puberty. Pruritus may be severe and lesions may be triggered by ultraviolet (UV) light, mechanical stress and sweating. DDD has been shown to be caused by mutations in *KRT5* encoding keratin 5, as well as (mostly in patients with generalized forms of DDD) in *POFUT1* or *POGLUT1*, encoding protein O-fucosyltransferase 1 and protein O-glucosyltransferase 1 respectively, which are involved in glycoprotein synthesis [123–126].

NFJ and DPR syndromes are allelic disorders caused by heterozygous nonsense or frameshift mutations in *KRT14*, encoding keratin 14, which result in increased keratinocytes apoptosis [127,128]. Whereas NFJ syndrome is characterized by reticulate hyperpigmentation mainly over the abdomen, perioral and periocular areas appearing during the first 2 years of life that tends to fade after adolescence in association with complete absence of dermatoglyphics, onychodystrophy, alopecia, palmoplantar hyperkeratosis, hypohidrosis and dental anomalies, DPR features a triad of reticulate hyperpigmentation mainly over the trunk, noncicatricial alopecia and onychodystrophy in association with other manifestations including abnormal sweating, keratosis pilaris, bullous keratoderma, ichthyosis and pigmentation of the mucosa and cornea [88,129,130].

EBS-MP is an autosomal dominant disorder caused by mutations in the gene *KRT5* encoding keratin 5. Most cases are associated with a missense mutation in the V1 domain of the protein which has been suggested to be important for melanosome transport. It is characterized by trauma-induced intraepidermal blisters accruing shortly after birth, palmoplantar hyperkeratosis, nail dystrophy and mottled pigmentation with reticulate hypo- and hyperpigmentation over the trunk and the extremities not related to areas of prior blister formation [131,132].

XP, a rare autosomal recessive disease with genetic heterogeneity involving genes encoding elements of importance for the nucleotide excision repair or the translation synthesis system (in XP-variant), is a multisystem disorder involving the skin, eyes and nervous system. XP is characterized by photosensitivity and the gradual development of erythema, xerosis, atrophy and freckle-like hyperpigmentation on sun exposed areas resulting in dyschromic changes and poikiloderma with gradual worsening during life and increased risk of nonmelanoma and melanoma skin cancer during the first decade of life [133].

Histopathology. The characteristic histopathological findings are increased melanin content in the basal layer and melanin incontinence in hyperpigmented lesions whereas hypopigmented lesions exhibit decreased melanin deposition in the basal layer [83]. Macromelanosome throughout the epidermis including the stratum corneum, lichenoid reaction in the papillary dermis and Civatte bodies have been reported [115,134,135].

Although electron microscopy demonstrated a comparable number of melanocytes in hypo- and hyperpigmented skin, numerous fully melanized melanosomes forming melanosome complexes are evident in melanocytes and keratinocytes of hyperchromic macules whereas significantly reduced melanosomes and empty immature melanosomes are seen in achromic lesions [79,91,108]. Accordingly, it was suggested that the main pathogenic process in DUH involves abnormal melanosome synthesis and maturation.

Familial progressive hyperpigmentation and hypopigmentation

History. Familial progressive hyperpigmentation and hypopigmentation (FPHH; OMIM #145250) is a rare inherited disorder first described in three families from south-east Germany in 2004 by Zanardo and colleagues [136].

Epidemiology. FPHH has only been described in a few families and a founder effect was suggested because several families sharing the same mutation have been shown to originate from a small area in south-east Germany [136,137]. FPHH has been described in Germany, Denmark and the USA [136,137]. A FPHH variant was reported in China [138].

Pathogenesis. FPHH is characterized by an autosomal dominant mode of inheritance with variable expression. The disease results from heterozygous mutations in the gene *KITLG* encoding KIT ligand (also known as the steel factor or mast cell growth factor/stem cell factor). In some families with FPHH, no mutations were identified in the *KITLG* gene [137], suggesting genetic heterogeneity.

Several mutations have been identified in an evolutionary conserved short amino-acid sequence (VTNN) located in the third β-strand of KITLG, that most likely result in gain-of-function, increasing KITLG affinity to its receptor c-Kit [137]. Following KITLG binding to the c-Kit receptor, oligomerization is triggered followed by initiation of signal transduction via the RAS/MAPK pathway to upregulate melanoblast proliferation [139,140]. Mutations in genes encoding proteins involved in this pathway also result in disorders featuring abnormal pigmentation including neurofibromatosis type 1 caused by loss-of-function mutations in *NF1,* encoding the RasGTPase neurofibromin, Legius syndrome resulting from gain-of-function mutations in *SPRED1*, encoding a RAS signalling pathway inhibitor, and piebaldism which results from dominant mutations in the gene encoding c-Kit [141–143]. One of the mutations identified in FPHH, c.107A > G, is a gain-of-function mutation previously reported in a single Chinese family with familial progressive hyperpigmentation (FPH; OMIM #145250), an autosomal dominant disorder characterized by progressive hyperpigmentation similar to that seen in FPHH, but without hypopigmented lesions [144]. Moreover, single-nucleotide polymorphisms in *KITLG* have been associated with hair colour in the Scottish population [145]. The relatively localized appearance of the lesions in FPHH and FPH may suggest the existence of an additional somatic second-hit mutation in the gene *KITLG* or in another gene involved in melanogenesis [137].

Clinical features. FPHH features are present at birth or early infancy. FPHH is characterized by progressive, diffuse, partly blotchy, hyperpigmentation, intermixed with scattered small confetti-like hypopigmented macules, larger hypopigmented areas resembling ash-leaf-like macules, café-au-lait spots and lentigines (Fig. 126.3). These features occur on the face, neck, trunk and extremities. The palms may be involved with hyperpigmented creases and lentigines. Hyperpigmented lesions may be accentuated following sun exposure. Lesions tend to increase in size and number with age.

A case associated with co-occurring classical vitiligo has been reported [136,137]. An FPHH variant also featuring multiple-band longitudinal melanonychia and mucosal brown pigmentation with no evidence of lentiginosis in association with mental retardation, epilepsy and recurrent infections has been described in China [138].

Differential diagnosis. Several disorders are included in the differential diagnosis, including Westerhof syndrome featuring widely distributed congenital hypo- and hyperpigmented macules that may be associated with retarded growth and mental deficiency [146] and FPH that lacks the component of hypopigmentation [144]. DUH should also be considered and the concurrent presence of hypo- and hyperpigmented macules may also resemble TS and neurofibromatosis type 1. FPHH should also be differentiated from Legius syndrome, characterized by familial cafe-au-lait spots and skin fold freckling, caused by mutations in *SPRED1* [147].

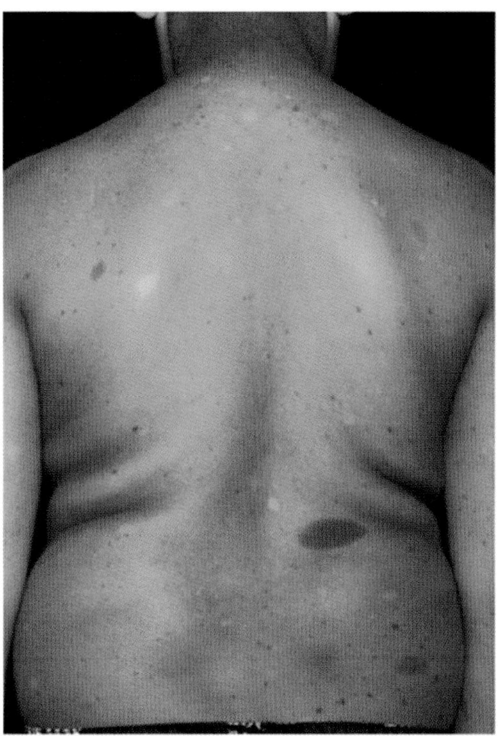

Fig. 126.3 Confluent hyperpigmentation with accentuation over the neck, with scattered café-au-lait macules, lentigines and small hypopigmented spots in a patient with familial progressive hyperpigmentation and hypopigmentation. Source: Amyere et al. (2011) [137]. Reproduced with permission of Elsevier.

Histopathology. At the histopathological level, FPHH features different degrees of hyperpigmentation and pigment incontinence in the basal layer of the epidermis in hyperpigmented lesions whereas hypopigmented macules display slight basal pigmentation with no evidence of dermal melanophages. Ultrastructural analysis reveals a varying content of regular melanosomes and melanosome complexes within keratinocytes [136].

Cutis tricolor

History. The term cutis tricolor was coined by Happle and colleagues in 1997 to describe the coexistence of congenital hypo- and hyperpigmented lesions in close proximity to each other on a background of normal skin. It is not yet clear if this is a distinct phenotype or a descriptive diagnosis which encompasses a variety of presentations of dyschromatosis.

Epidemiology. Cutis tricolor has been reported to date in several cases in Europe and it appears equally in both sexes [148–152]. Most cases are sporadic, although familial occurrence in two sisters has been reported [152].

Pathogenesis. The dichotomous pigmentary pattern seen in cutis tricolor was originally proposed to be caused by a theoretical 'twin spotting' phenomenon [149] by Rudolf Happle and colleagues. However, this theory in nonallelic form has now been disproved in a variety of mosaic conditions previously also proposed to be caused by twin spotting [153,154], and officially retracted by Happle [155]. Although allelic twin spotting has not yet been disproven by scientific evidence the burden of proof would now be to demonstrate it. Paradominant inheritance has been suggested in familial cases [152]. However, there is no evidence yet to support this, and simple postzygotic mosaicism is an equally feasible theory.

Clinical features. Skin manifestations in cutis tricolor appear at birth and have been described with various patterns, hence the term cutis tricolor may be a descriptive diagnosis encompassing different distinct disorders. The original description was of hypo- and hyperpigmented lesions in close proximity to each other on a background of normal skin that usually involve the trunk, extremities and neck. The various patterns of hypo- and hyperpigmented lesions are multiple well-demarcated small macules resembling café-au-lait spots or speckled lentiginous naevus, diffuse, spirally-shaped or streaky patches along the lines of Blaschko or in a segmental distribution [148–151], or in cutis tricolor 'parvimaculata' multiple, disseminated and much smaller café-au-lait macules and hypochromic spots (Fig. 126.4) [151,156]. A case associated with other dermatological findings including small congenital melanocytic naevus, multiple skin tags, periungual fibromas and dental abnormalities (small teeth, enamel pitting, conical shaped teeth) has been described [151].

Cutis tricolor may be associated with systemic conditions including facial dysmorphism (e.g. deep-set rotated ears, bulbous nose with anteverted or broad nostrils, prognathism), skeletal (e.g. kyphoscoliosis, pectus excavatum, leg length discrepancies, tibial bowing, clinodactyly), ophthalmological (e.g. strabismus, hyperopia and astigmatism), cardiac (ventricular septal defect) and neurological (e.g. mental retardation, delayed motor development, convulsions, white matter lesions, hypoplasia of the corpus callosum, oligodendroglioma brain tumour), abnormalities and ipsilateral breast hypoplasia [148–152].

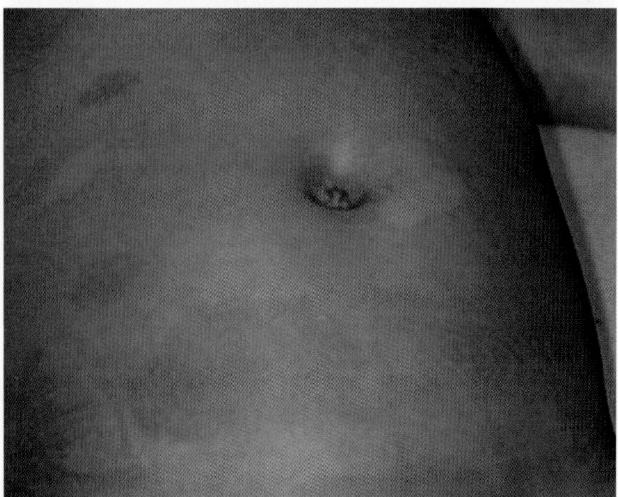

Fig. 126.4 Multiple hyper- and hypopigmented macules in close proximity on the abdomen in a patient with cutis tricolor parvimaculata. Source: del Carmen Boente et al. (2011) [156]. Reproduced with permission of John Wiley & Sons.

Differential diagnosis. The pigmentary pattern of cutis tricolor may give rise to other entities in the differential diagnosis. Narrow lesions distributed along the lines of Blaschko forming whorls, streaks and 'V'- or 'S'-shaped and linear arrangements may resemble hypomelanosis of Ito, incontinentia pigmenti or chromosomal mosaicism. Large asymmetric irregular pigmentary macules over the sacrum, buttocks and upper spine may resemble McCune–Albright syndrome, although this disorder does not feature hypopigmented lesions [157–162]. Inflammatory dermatoses with linear distribution including linear psoriasis, linear lichen planus and lichen striatus should also be ruled out. However, these entities have characteristic clinical and histopathological manifestations [163]. Other entities in the differential diagnosis are segmental neurofibromatosis, naevus depigmentosus or linear and whorled naevoid hypermelanosis [159,164,165]. The association of hypo- and hyperpigmented lesions with neurological abnormalities also exist in Westerhof syndrome. However, the latter is a hereditary disorder with an autosomal dominant mode of inheritance, in contrast to cutis tricolor which is mostly sporadic [146]. The case of cutis tricolor parvimaculata with multiple small hypo- and hyperpigmented lesions associated with periungual fibromas and enamel pitting is reminiscent of TS [151]. Patients with inv dup(15) syndrome manifest with multiple whorled, mottled or linear patterns of hypo- or hyperpigmented skin associated with facial dysmorphism and severe neurological and behavioural abnormalities. However, this entity is associated with an abnormal karyotype [166,167]. Lastly it is worth remembering mismatch repair disorders as a differential in dyschromatosis which has no clearly distinct pigmentary label (Fig. 126.5) [168].

Histopathology. Hypopigmented lesions show decreased basal melanin content and a decreased number of epidermal melanocytes whereas hyperpigmented lesions feature increased melanin content in the basal layer and/or pigmentary incontinence. Cytogenetic analysis of blood lymphocytes and dermal fibroblasts reveals normal karyotype with no evidence of mosaicism [150,152].

Westerhof syndrome

History. Westerhof syndrome (also known as hereditary congenital hypopigmented and hyperpigmented macules) was first described in 1978 by Westerhof and colleagues and is characterized by multiple hereditary congenital hypopigmented and hyperpigmented macules that may be associated with retarded growth and mental deficiency.

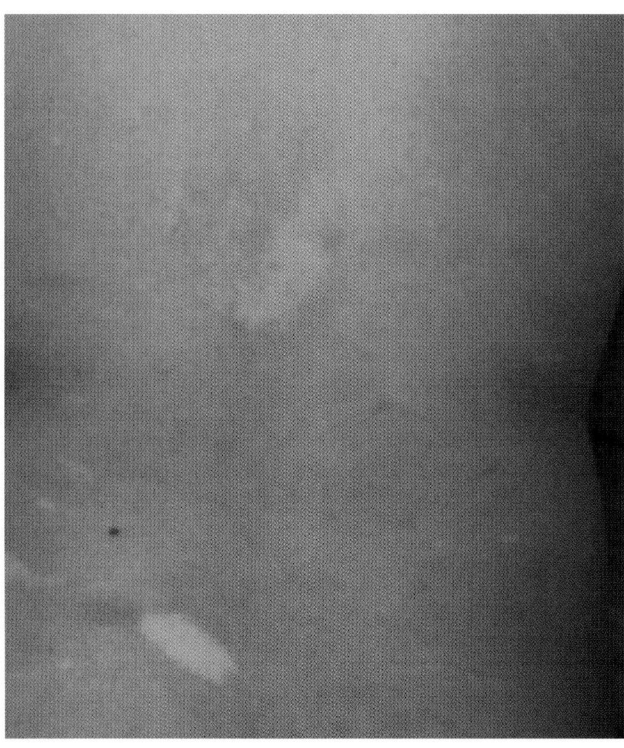

Fig. 126.5 Widespread hyperpigmented and hypopigmented macules in a patient with T-cell lymphoblastic lymphoma and homozygous truncating mutation in the mismatch repair gene MSH2. Source: Scott et al. (2007) [168]. Reproduced with permission from BMJ Publishing Group Ltd.

Epidemiology and pathogenesis. To date, Westerhof syndrome has been described in only two families with a suggested autosomal dominant or paradominant mode of inheritance [146,169]. It has been suggested that in contrast to cutis tricolor, the lack of strictly spatial proximity of the lesions in Westerhof syndrome is a result of lateralization movements of the trunk region in the embryo following the somatic recombination event [169]. However, this is theoretical only. With the expansion of the cutis tricolor phenotype it is possible that Westerhof syndrome will be included under this umbrella term, or more likely, that as the genetic basis of these overlapping phenotypes becomes clear we are able to regroup diseases, as in other areas of paediatric dermatology.

Clinical features. Multiple or solitary, 1–15 cm in diameter, well-defined asymmetric but nondermatome-confined hypopigmented and hyperpigmented macules appear at birth on any part of the body. Male patients tend to develop more lesions than females. Mucous membranes are spared. In one family, skin lesions were associated with retarded growth and mental deficiency whereas among two siblings from a second family retarded growth was evident in one whereas the second sibling was otherwise healthy. In general, growth retardation and low intelligence have been seen in male patients [146,169].

Differential diagnosis. The main differential diagnosis is TS and neurofibromatosis. However, no mutations in the genes *TSC1*, *TSC2* and *NF1* have been identified in patients with Westerhof syndrome [169] and although congenital hypopigmented macules are very common in TS, multiple congenital café-au-lait spots are not a frequent finding in this disorder [170].

Histopathology. Histopathological examination demonstrates a decreased number of epidermal melanocytes in the hypopigmented areas whereas an increased melanocyte number is observed in the dark macules [169]. Ultrastructurally, hypomelanotic skin showed small melanosomes within melanosome complexes in keratinocytes whereas hypermelanotic lesions revealed singly distributed large melanosomes in keratinocytes [146].

Amyloidosis cutis dyschromica

Introduction. Amyloidosis cutis dyschromica (ACD) is a rare distinct type of primary cutaneous amyloidosis which should be included in the differential diagnosis of childhood-onset dyschromatoses. It is characterized by the constellation of dotted, reticular or diffuse hyperpigmentation admixed with hypopigmented macules which usually appear before puberty. The disorder features no or little pruritus and is characterized by amyloid deposition confined to the papillary dermis on skin biopsy [171].

History. ACD was first described by Morishima in 1970 in a young female who had skin lesions suggestive of DUH in conjunction with lichenoid lesions involving her extremities, both containing amyloid deposition on histology [171]. In 1976, Eng and colleagues reported familial cases of ACD [172].

Epidemiology. To date, approximately 50 cases of ACD have been reported. Most patients were of east and south Asian ethnicity. A minority of cases was of White extraction. Moreover, the majority of cases displayed a positive family history [171–190]. In familial cases, the mean age at diagnosis was 30 years and males and females were equally affected. The rash usually develops before puberty (at around 6–10 years of age), although appearance shortly after birth has been described [174,177–179] and appearance after puberty was rarely noted [178]. Sporadic cases, which are significantly less common in ACD, are a little more frequent in females; the mean age at diagnosis was 40 years with disease onset at around 20 years on average [174]. The delayed diagnosis in both familial and sporadic cases is probably a result of the fact that the condition is asymptomatic with gradual and progressive pigmentary changes that mostly affect otherwise healthy patients with an originally darker complexion and subtle amyloid deposition on skin histology that can be easily missed in the early stages of the disease.

Pathogenesis. The aetiology of ACD is not clear and is probably multifactorial, including genetic and environmental factors. Familial cases are inherited in an autosomal dominant fashion with incomplete penetrance as males and females are equally affected and affected family members are not present in every generation [174]. However, autosomal recessive inheritance cannot be ruled out and cases of ACD following consanguineous marriages have been reported [175–178,182].

UV-B- and UV-C-induced damage to keratinocytes with hypersensitivity to UV-B and possible DNA repair defects are suggested to be the cause of this disease [171,178,185,187,188,191]. Destroyed keratinocytes undergo apoptosis as a result of abnormal DNA repair mechanisms and the released cytokeratin is phagocytosed by histiocytes and fibroblasts, leading to the formation and deposition of amyloid in the skin [182,192]. The epidermal origin of the amyloid was further validated by demonstrating its strong positivity to CK34βE12 and CK5/6 by immunohistochemical studies [178]. However, the fact that dyschromia did not show predilection to sun-exposed skin in all cases and displayed even milder involvement in those areas compared with the trunk argues against photosensitivity as a main aetiological factor [174,178].

It has been suggested that the dyschromia in ACD occurs as a result of the balance between epidermal pigment retention and dermal pigment deposition. Moreover, amyloid deposition in the papillary dermis may stretch the basement membrane with reduction of melanocyte density in the basal layer resulting in hypopigmentation [175].

Clinical features. ACD is characterized by widespread, symmetrical diffuse, macular or reticulate hyperpigmentation interspersed with well-defined mottled or spotty hypo- and depigmented macules of sizes varying from a few millimetres to a few centimetres (Fig. 126.6). Dyschromic lesions usually start on the trunk and gradually progress over years to the limbs, with widespread involvement of all the skin surface. More restricted involvement of distinct body sites has been described in several cases [185]. Scattered hyperpigmented keratotic papules or hypopigmented papules interspersed within the dyschromic lesions may be seen [178,180,182,185]. Facial involvement has been documented in 20% and 27% of familial and sporadic cases, respectively. Hair, nails, teeth and mucous membranes are normally spared. Palms and soles are not involved in most cases. Freckles, telangiectasias, atrophy and blisters have been rarely reported within ACD lesions [178,181,186,188]. Concurrent appearance of ACD with lichen, poikiloderma-like and bullous variants of primary cutaneous amyloidosis has been reported in one patient [189]. Pruritus may accompany skin lesions in approximately 20% of cases. In most cases there was no predilection to sun-exposed skin and no evidence of photosensitivity [174,177,181]. Spontaneous improvement or resolution have not been reported.

There are no reports of systemic amyloidosis in association with ACD. Although most cases are confined to the skin in otherwise healthy individuals, concomitant appearance of generalized morphoea, colon cancer and atypical Parkinsonism, with motor weakness and spasticity with no evidence of systemic amyloidosis, have been reported [178,179,186]. A case of ACD with a strong family history of vitiligo [175] and a single case of ACD associated with isolated secondary amyloidosis of lungs [172] have been reported.

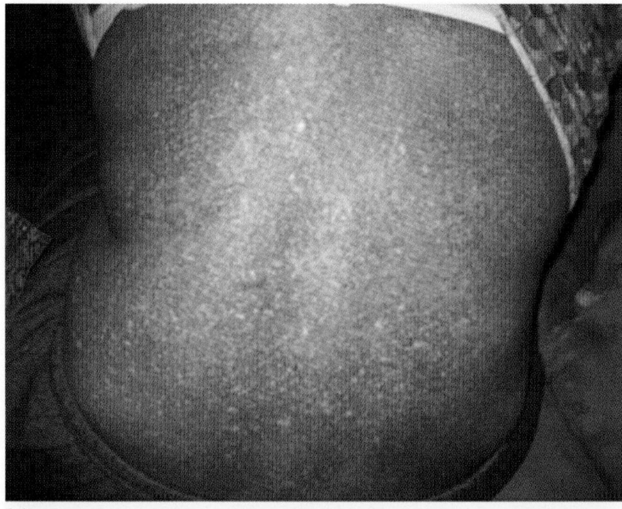

(a)

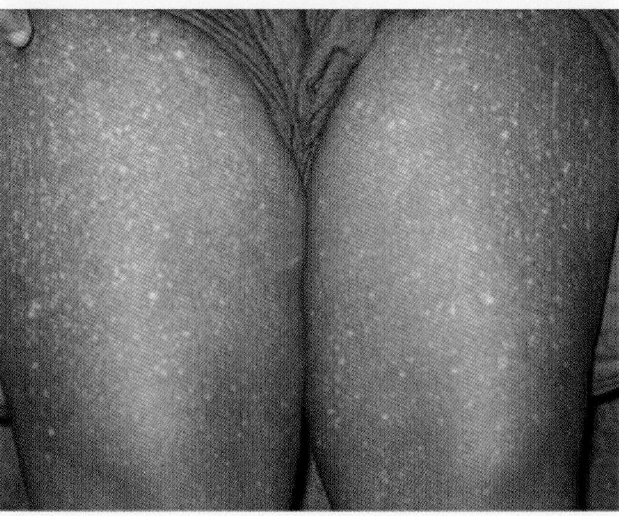

(b)

Fig. 126.6 Generalized hyperpigmentation with symmetric widespread distribution of hypopigmented macules over the (a) trunk and (b) thighs in a patient with amyloidosis cutis dyschromica. Source: Fernandes et al. (2011) [179]. Reproduced with permission of John Wiley & Sons.

Differential diagnosis. Clinically, ACD can be mistaken for DUH, generalized DDD, XP, DKC and poikiloderma. The amyloid deposition in the papillary dermis and the absence of other histological features facilitate the diagnosis of ACD. Moreover, ACD lacks the marked photosensitivity, premature actinic damage and the associated cutaneous malignancies seen in XP [174,182].

Other types of cutaneous amyloidosis and even other systemic diseases with cutaneous amyloid deposition should also be considered in the differential diagnosis [193]. Although lichen and macular amyloidosis exhibit cutaneous amyloid deposition in the papillary dermis which stains positive with anticytokeratin antibodies similar to ACD, lichen amyloidosis manifests with hyperkeratotic hyperpigmented papules on the extremities whereas macular amyloidosis is characterized by reticulated hyperpigmentation that tends to be limited to the upper back [194,195]. Poikiloderma-like cutaneous amyloidosis is a rare type of cutaneous amyloidosis that clinically resembles ACD. It is characterized by reticular hyper- and hypopigmentation, telangiectasias, atrophy, lichenoid papules and blisters, which appear in adult life, mostly involving the limbs, and may be associated with photosensitivity, short stature and keratoderma. Some authors considered ACD a subset of poikiloderma-like cutaneous amyloidosis [179,181,185,196–199]. In systemic amyloidosis, amyloid deposition, which demonstrates negative immunohistochemistry to cytokeratins, is much more extensive and involves the deeper dermis, the periappendageal and perivascular areas. Cutaneous amyloid deposition has also been described in various collagen vascular diseases (e.g. lupus erythematosus, dermatomyositis, morphea) [194,200–203].

Histopathology. Histopathological findings in both hypo- and hyperpigmented lesions consist of amorphous eosinophilic material within the papillary dermis with increased melanin in the basal layer and pigment incontinence in the papillary dermis. The amorphous eosinophilic material in the papillary dermis stains positive with Congo red and demonstrates an apple-green birefringence under polarized light [174]. A case in which the amyloid deposition extended beyond the papillary dermis towards the reticular dermis has been described [179]. Slightly widened dermal papillae, irregular elongation of rete ridges, a sparse lymphocytic infiltrate in the papillary dermis, basal vacuolar change and apoptotic bodies in the basal layer of the epidermis may be seen [176,180]. Immunohistochemistry with antibodies against high molecular weight cytokeratin show diffuse staining of the globules in the papillary dermis. Electron microscopy analysis displays randomly oriented, straight, non-branching thin fibrils characteristic of amyloid filaments [179,182]

Dyschromatosis ptychotropica

Dyschromatosis ptychotropica (DP) is a recently described entity characterized by irregular, small (2–4 mm in diameter) hypo- and hyperpigmented macules forming a reticular and mottled appearance that are initially noted over the neck (Fig. 126.7), axillae and inguinal region as the name of the disorder implies (ptychotropism = affinity to the body folds). Lesions appear during infancy but progress gradually to more extensive involvement including the trunk and the extremities but with pronounced affinity to body folds. The dermatological findings were associated with neurological abnormalities including nystagmus, developmental delay, microcephaly, epileptic encephalopathy, polyneuropathy, cerebellar, and supratentorial and optic atrophies suggesting the diagnosis of PEHO-like syndrome (progressive encephalopathy with oedema, hypsarrythmia, and optic atrophy; OMIM #260565) [204,205].

The differential diagnosis includes other neurocutaneous syndromes characterized by abnormal pigmentation and neurological abnormalities including incontinentia pigmenti, although those entities have distinct cutaneous

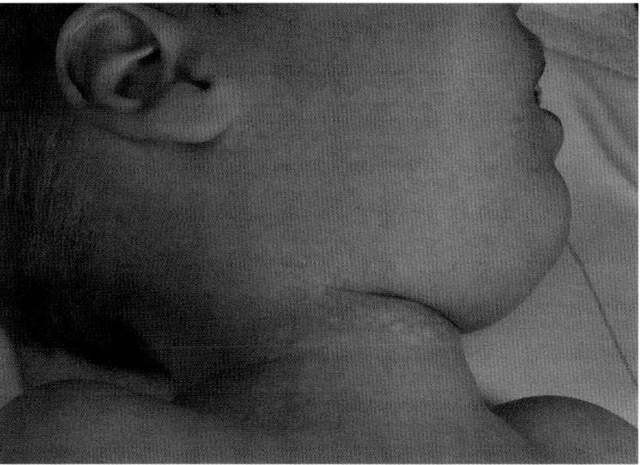

Fig. 126.7 Dyschromatosis ptychotropica manifests in a young child with irregular, small hypo- and hyperpigmented macules forming a reticular appearance over the neck. Source: Courtesy of Professor Rudolf Happle.

features. In addition, X-linked recessive hereditary macular bullous dystrophy (OMIM 302000), associated with mottled pigmentation, blistering, microcephaly and intellectual disabilities, should also be considered in the differential diagnosis [206,207]. Hypomelanosis of Ito is another entity characterized by both pigmentary and neurological defects, although it may be easily ruled out by its segmental distribution [208]. Large structural genomic aberrations were also reported to feature mottled hyperpigmentation, intellectual disability and epilepsy [166].

On histology, hyperpigmented lesions display marked pigmentation of the basal layer with a normal amount of active melanocytes containing a high number of fully melanized melanosomes demonstrated by ultrastructural analysis [204].

Other entities associated with dyschromia

A number of other inherited and acquired disorders may present with dyschromatosis as a main feature or as a part of constellation of manifestations (Table 126.1). Inherited disorders which should be considered in cases of childhood-onset dyschromatosis include pigment dilution disorders (Chediak–Higashi syndrome and Griscelli syndrome), keratin disorders (EBS-MP, DDD, NFJ and DPR syndromes), various types of ectodermal dysplasia with coexisting dyschromatosis, disorders of impaired DNA repair (e.g. XP), inherited poikilodermatous conditions (e.g. DKC, Rothmund–Thomson syndrome) and incontinenta pigmenti [122–126,129–132,209–216]. Acquired entities that may be associated with dyschromatosis are inflammatory skin disorders (cutaneous lupus erythematosus, systemic sclerosis, dermatomyositis), several types of infections (secondary syphilis and tertiary Pinta, onchocerciasis), nutritional disorders (Kwashiorkor), drugs, chemicals and environmental exposures (arsenic, contact leukomelanosis, drug-induced photoleucomelanodermatitis, photochemotherapy, betel leaf), chronic radiation dermatitis and poikiloderma [3,4]. An approach to the patient with inherited dyschromatoses is displayed in Fig. 126.8.

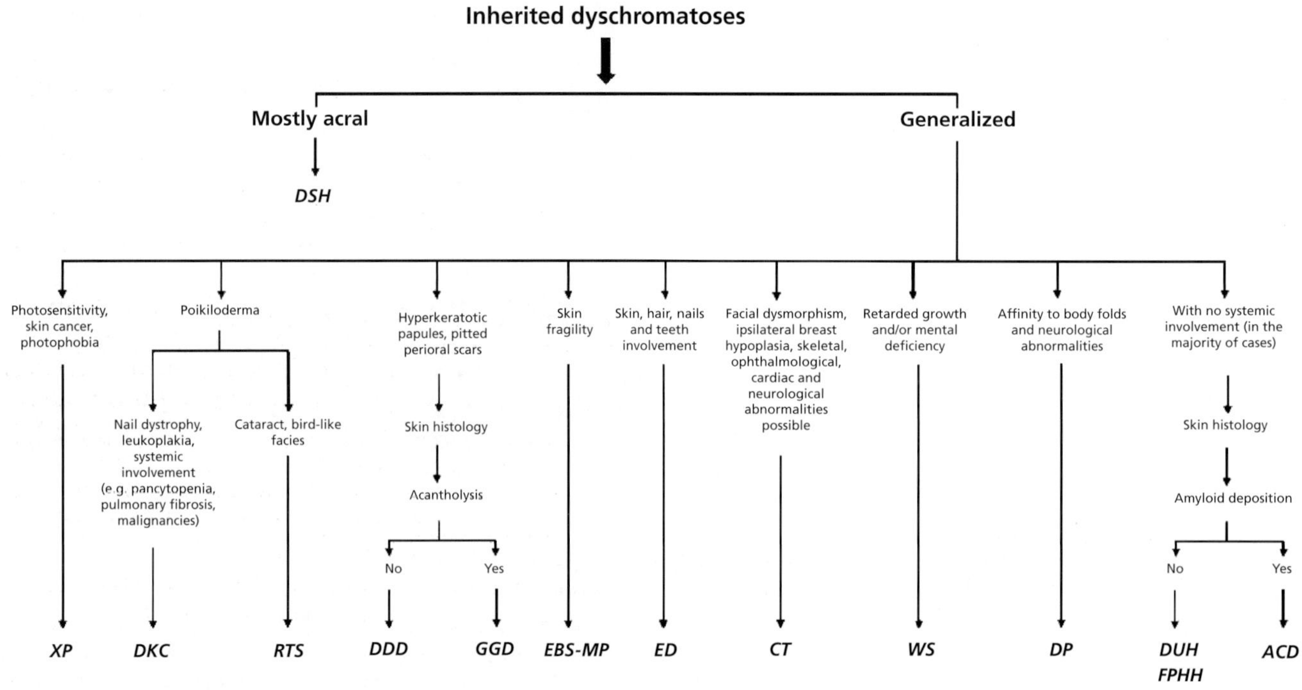

Fig. 126.8 An approach to the patient with inherited dyschromatosis. ACD, amyloidosis cutis dyschromica; CT, cutis tricolor; DDD, Dowling–Degos disease; DKC, dyskeratosis congenita; DP, dyschromatosis ptychotropica; DSH, dyschromatosis symmetrica hereditaria; DUH, dyschromatosis universalis hereditaria; EBS-MP, epidermolysis bullosa simplex with mottled pigmentation; ED, ectodermal dysplasia; FPHH, familial progressive hyperpigmentation and hypopigmentation; GGD, Galli-Galli disease; RTS, Rothmund–Thomson syndrome; WS, Westerhof syndrome; XP, xeroderma pigmentosum.

Treatment

In general, treatment options for most types of dyschromatoses are limited and there is no satisfactory or universal treatment modality that has been reported. In DSH, split-thickness autograft has been shown to improve appearance in some patients [217]. In addition, a 50-year-old man was successfully treated with 1-mm miniature punch grafting in the hypopigmented areas in combination with a 308-nm excimer light applied prior to punch grafting [218].

Dramatic improvement of facial and labial lentigines following treatment with Q-switched alexandrite laser in a 51-year-old woman with DUH has been reported [219].

In ACD, topical treatments (e.g. keratolytic agents, tazarotene) have been tried with variable response rates [177,178,180–183]. Antioxidant therapy (vitamin C, beta carotene, vitamin E, selenium, copper, manganese, zinc) resulted in minimal or no improvement. Oral acitretin may decrease the amount of apoptotic basal keratinocytes available for transformation into amyloid [220] and has been shown to lead to improvement in several cases [173,174,178,180,182,184,187]. Photoprotection, including sun avoidance and the use of broad-spectrum sunscreen, attenuates the contrast between hypo- and hyperpigmented areas, prevents lesions triggering (as in ACD) and is recommended in all cases. Camouflage with cosmetic makeup is the only treatment option in certain conditions.

References

1 Oyama M, Shimizu H, Ohata Y et al. Dyschromatosis symmetrica hereditaria (reticulate acropigmentation of Dohi): report of a Japanese family with the condition and a literature review of 185 cases. Br J Dermatol 1999;140:491–6.
2 Urabe K, Hori Y. Dyschromatosis. Semin Cutan Med Surg 1997; 16:81–5.
3 Vachiramon V, Thadanipon K, Chanprapaph K. Infancy- and childhood-onset dyschromatoses. Clin Exp Dermatol 2011;36:833–8, quiz 839.
4 Vachiramon V, Thadanipon K, Rattanakaemakorn P. Adult-onset dyschromatoses. Clin Exp Dermatol 2012;37:97–103.
5 Hayashi M, Suzuki T. Dyschromatosis symmetrica hereditaria. J Dermatol 2013;40:336–43.
6 Toyama I. An unknown disorder of hyperpigmentation. Jpn J Dermatol Urol 1910;10:644.
7 Toyama I. Dyschromatosis symmetrica hereditaria. Jpn J Dermatol 1929;27:95–6.
8 Gharpuray MB, Tolat SN, Patwardham SP. Dyschromatosis: its occurrence in two Indian families with unusual features. Int J Dermatol 1994;33:391–2.
9 Ostlere LS, Ratnavel RC, Lawlor F et al. Reticulate acropigmentation of Dohi. Clin Exp Dermatol 1995;20:477–9.
10 Fernandes NC, Andrade LR. [Case for diagnosis. Reticulate acropigmentation of Dohi]. An Bras Dermatol 2010;85:109–10.
11 Froes GC, Pereira LB, Rocha VB. [Case for diagnosis. Dyschromatosis symetrica hereditaria]. An Bras Dermatol 2009;84:425–7.
12 Gaiewski CB, Zuneda Serafini S, Werner B et al. Dyschromatosis symmetrica hereditaria of late onset? Case Rep Dermatol Med 2014; 2014:639537.
13 Muller CS, Tremezaygues L, Pfohler C et al. The spectrum of reticulate pigment disorders of the skin revisited. Eur J Dermatol 2012;22:596–604.
14 Lee YB, Lee SB, Kim SJ et al. A frameshift mutation in the ADAR gene in a Korean family with dyschromatosis symmetrica hereditaria. Eur J Dermatol 2014;24:693–5.
15 Namitha P, Sacchidanand S. Dyschromias: a series of five interesting cases from india. Ind J Dermatol 2015;60:636.
16 Bilen N, Akturk AS, Kawaguchi M et al. Dyschromatosis symmetrica hereditaria: a case report from Turkey, a new association and a novel gene mutation. J Dermatol 2012;39:857–8.
17 Chao SC, Lee JY, Sheu HM et al. A novel deletion mutation of the DSRAD gene in a Taiwanese patient with dyschromatosis symmetrica hereditaria. Br J Dermatol 2005;153:1064–6.
18 He PP, He CD, Cui Y et al. Refined localization of dyschromatosis symmetrica hereditaria gene to a 9.4-cM region at 1q21-22 and a literature review of 136 cases reported in China. Br J Dermatol 2004;150:633–9.

19 Hemanthkumar, Thappa DM. Dyschromatosis symmetrica hereditaria in an Indian family. J Dermatol 1999;26:544–5.
20 Liu Q, Liu W, Jiang L et al. Novel mutations of the RNA-specific adenosine deaminase gene (DSRAD) in Chinese families with dyschromatosis symmetrica hereditaria. J Invest Dermatol 2004;122:896–9.
21 Suzuki N, Suzuki T, Inagaki K et al. Ten novel mutations of the ADAR1 gene in Japanese patients with dyschromatosis symmetrica hereditaria. J Invest Dermatol 2007;127:309–11.
22 Murata I, Hayashi M, Hozumi Y et al. Mutation analyses of patients with dyschromatosis symmetrica hereditaria: five novel mutations of the ADAR1 gene. J Dermatol Sci 2010;58:218–20.
23 Kantaputra PN, Chinadet W, Ohazama A et al. Dyschromatosis symmetrica hereditaria with long hair on the forearms, hypo/hyperpigmented hair, and dental anomalies: report of a novel ADAR1 mutation. Am J Med Genet A 2012;158A:2258–65.
24 Zhang G, Shao M, Li Z et al. Genetic spectrum of dyschromatosis symmetrica hereditaria in Chinese patients including a novel nonstop mutation in ADAR1 gene. BMC Med Genet 2016;17:14.
25 Kawaguchi M, Hayashi M, Murata I et al. Eleven novel mutations of the ADAR1 gene in dyschromatosis symmetrica hereditaria. J Dermatol Sci 2012;66:244–5.
26 Miyamura Y, Suzuki T, Kono M et al. Mutations of the RNA-specific adenosine deaminase gene (DSRAD) are involved in dyschromatosis symmetrica hereditaria. Am J Hum Genet 2003;73:693–9.
27 Kono M, Matsumoto F, Suzuki Y et al. Dyschromatosis symmetrica hereditaria and Aicardi-Goutieres syndrome 6 are phenotypic variants caused by ADAR1 mutations. J Invest Dermatol 2016;136:875–8.
28 Sun XK, Xu AE, Chen JF et al. The double-RNA-specific adenosine deaminase (DSRAD) gene in dyschromatosis symmetrica hereditaria patients: two novel mutations and one previously described. Br J Dermatol 2005;153:342–5.
29 O'Connell MA, Krause S, Higuchi M et al. Cloning of cDNAs encoding mammalian double-stranded RNA-specific adenosine deaminase. Mol Cell Biol 1995;15:1389–97.
30 Wang Y, Zeng Y, Murray JM et al. Genomic organization and chromosomal location of the human dsRNA adenosine deaminase gene: the enzyme for glutamate-activated ion channel RNA editing. J Mol Biol 1995;254:184–95.
31 Bass BL. RNA editing by adenosine deaminases that act on RNA. Ann Rev Biochem 2002;71:817–46.
32 Kawakubo K, Samuel CE. Human RNA-specific adenosine deaminase (ADAR1) gene specifies transcripts that initiate from a constitutively active alternative promoter. Gene 2000;258:165–72.
33 Patterson JB, Samuel CE. Expression and regulation by interferon of a double-stranded-RNA-specific adenosine deaminase from human cells: evidence for two forms of the deaminase. Mol Cell Biol 1995; 15:5376–88.
34 Athanasiadis A. Zalpha-domains: at the intersection between RNA editing and innate immunity. Semin Cell Dev Biol 2012;23:275–80.
35 George CX, Gan Z, Liu Y et al. Adenosine deaminases acting on RNA, RNA editing, and interferon action. J Interferon Cytokine Res 2011;31:99–117.
36 Clerzius G, Gelinas JF, Daher A et al. ADAR1 interacts with PKR during human immunodeficiency virus infection of lymphocytes and contributes to viral replication. J Virol 2009; 83:10119–28.
37 Seeburg PH, Hartner J. Regulation of ion channel/neurotransmitter receptor function by RNA editing. Curr Opin Neurobiol 2003;13:279–83.
38 Taylor DR, Puig M, Darnell ME et al. New antiviral pathway that mediates hepatitis C virus replicon interferon sensitivity through ADAR1. J Virol 2005;79:6291–8.
39 Tojo K, Sekijima Y, Suzuki T et al. Dystonia, mental deterioration, and dyschromatosis symmetrica hereditaria in a family with ADAR1 mutation. Movement Dis 2006;21:1510–13.
40 Wang Q, Miyakoda M, Yang W et al. Stress-induced apoptosis associated with null mutation of ADAR1 RNA editing deaminase gene. J Biol Chem 2004;279:4952–61.
41 Yang W, Wang Q, Howell KL et al. ADAR1 RNA deaminase limits short interfering RNA efficacy in mammalian cells. J Biol Chem 2005; 280:3946–53.
42 Kono M, Akiyama M, Suganuma M et al. Dyschromatosis symmetrica hereditaria by ADAR1 mutations and viral encephalitis: a hidden link? Int J Dermatol 2013;52:1582–4.
43 Ward SV, George CX, Welch MJ et al. RNA editing enzyme adenosine deaminase is a restriction factor for controlling measles virus replication that also is required for embryogenesis. Proc Natl Acad Sci U S A 2011;108:331–6.
44 Sharma R, Wang Y, Zhou P et al. An essential role of RNA editing enzyme ADAR1 in mouse skin. J Dermatol Sci 2011;64:70–2.
45 Alfadley A, Al Ajlan A, Hainau B et al. Reticulate acropigmentation of Dohi: a case report of autosomal recessive inheritance. J Am Acad Dermatol 2000;43:113–17.
46 Consigli J, Zanni MS, Ragazzini L et al. Dyschromatosis symmetrica hereditaria: report of a sporadic case. Int J Dermatol 2010;49: 918–20.
47 Xing QH, Wang MT, Chen XD et al. A gene locus responsible for dyschromatosis symmetrica hereditaria (DSH) maps to chromosome 6q24.2-q25.2. Am J Hum Genet 2003;73:377–82.
48 Zhou D, Wei Z, Deng S et al. SASH1 regulates melanocyte transepithelial migration through a novel Galphas-SASH1-IQGAP1-E-Cadherin dependent pathway. Cell Signal 2013;25:1526–38.
49 Shellman YG, Lambert KA, Brauweiler A et al. SASH1 is involved in an autosomal dominant lentiginous phenotype. J Invest Dermatol 2015;135:3192–4.
50 Courcet JB, Elalaoui SC, Duplomb L et al. Autosomal-recessive SASH1 variants associated with a new genodermatosis with pigmentation defects, palmoplantar keratoderma and skin carcinoma. Eur J Hum Genet 2015;23:957–62.
51 Tang A, Eller MS, Hara M et al. E-cadherin is the major mediator of human melanocyte adhesion to keratinocytes in vitro. J Cell Sci 1994;107: 983–92.
52 Han Q, Yao F, Zhong C et al. TRAF6 promoted the metastasis of esophageal squamous cell carcinoma. Tumour Biol 2014;35:715–21.
53 Starczynowski DT, Lockwood WW, Delehouzee S et al. TRAF6 is an amplified oncogene bridging the RAS and NF-kappaB pathways in human lung cancer. J Clin Invest 2011;121:4095–105.
54 Fujikawa H, Farooq M, Fujimoto A et al. Functional studies for the TRAF6 mutation associated with hypohidrotic ectodermal dysplasia. Br J Dermatol 2013;168:629–33.
55 Wisniewski SA, Trzeciak WH. A rare heterozygous TRAF6 variant is associated with hypohidrotic ectodermal dysplasia. Br J Dermatol 2012;166:1353–6.
56 Dauphinee SM, Clayton A, Hussainkhel A et al. SASH1 is a scaffold molecule in endothelial TLR4 signaling. J Immunol 2013;191:892–901.
57 Liu Q, Jiang L, Liu WL et al. Two novel mutations and evidence for haploinsufficiency of the ADAR gene in dyschromatosis symmetrica hereditaria. Br J Dermatol 2006;154:636–42.
58 Kondo T, Suzuki T, Ito S et al. Dyschromatosis symmetrica hereditaria associated with neurological disorders. J Dermatol 2008;35:662–6.
59 Patrizi A, Manneschi V, Pini A et al. Dyschromatosis symmetrica hereditaria associated with idiopathic torsion dystonia. A case report. Acta Dermato-Venereol 1994;74:135–7.
60 Tomita Y, Suzuki T. Genetics of pigmentary disorders. Am J Med Genet C Semin Med Genet 2004;131C:75–81.
61 Hou Y, Chen J, Gao M et al. Five novel mutations of RNA-specific adenosine deaminase gene with dyschromatosis symmetrica hereditaria. Acta Dermato-Venereol 2007;87:18–21.
62 Suzuki N, Suzuki T, Inagaki K et al. Mutation analysis of the ADAR1 gene in dyschromatosis symmetrica hereditaria and genetic differentiation from both dyschromatosis universalis hereditaria and acropigmentatio reticularis. J Invest Dermatol 2005;124:1186–92.
63 Li M, Li C, Hua H et al. Identification of two novel mutations in Chinese patients with Dyschromatosis symmetrica hereditaria. Arch Dermatol Res 2005;297:196–200.
64 Mohana D, Verma U, Amar AJ et al. Reticulate acropigmentation of dohi: a case report with insight into genodermatoses with mottled pigmentation. Ind J Dermatol 2012;57:42–4.
65 Oiso N, Murata I, Hayashi M et al. Dermoscopic features in a case of dyschromatosis symmetrica hereditaria. J Dermatol 2011;38:91–93.
66 Kaliyadan F, Vinayan KP, Fernandes B et al. Acral dyschromatosis with developmental regression and dystonia in a seven-year-old child: dyschromatosis symmetrica hereditaria variant or a new syndrome? Ind J Dermatol Venereol Leprol 2009; 75: 412–414.
67 Dutta A, Ghosh SK, Mandal RK. Dyschromatosis symmetrica hereditaria with neurological abnormalities. Ind J Dermatol Venereol Leprol 2014;80:549–51.
68 Tojyo K, Hattori T, Sekijima Y et al. [A case of idiopathic brain calcification associated with dyschromatosis symmetrica hereditaria, aplasia of dental root, and aortic valve sclerosis]. Rinsho shinkeigaku = Clinical neurology 2001;41:299–305.
69 Luo S, Zheng Y, Ni H et al. Novel clinical and molecular findings in Chinese families with dyschromatosis symmetrica hereditaria. J Dermatol 2012;39:556–8.

70 Tan HH, Tay YK. Neurofibromatosis and reticulate acropigmentation of Dohi: a case report. Pediatr Dermatol 1997;14:296–8.
71 Kono M, Sugiura K, Suganuma M et al. Whole-exome sequencing identifies ADAM10 mutations as a cause of reticulate acropigmentation of Kitamura, a clinical entity distinct from Dowling-Degos disease. Hum Mol Genet 2013;22:3524–33.
72 Okamura K, Abe Y, Araki Y et al. Behavior of melanocytes and keratinocytes in reticulate acropigmentation of Kitamura. Pigment Cell Melanoma Res 2016;28:243–6.
73 Koguchi H, Ujiie H, Aoyagi S et al. Characteristic findings of handprint and dermoscopy in reticulate acropigmentation of Kitamura. Clin Exp Dermatol 2014;39:85–7.
74 Sheu HM, Yu HS. Dyschromatosis symmetrica hereditaria – a histochemical and ultrastructural study. Taiwan Yi Xue Hui Za Zhi 1985; 84:238–49.
75 Hata S, Yokomi I. Density of dopa-positive melanocytes in dyschromatosis symmetrica hereditaria. Dermatologica 1985;171:27–9.
76 Ichikawa T, Hiraga Y. A previously undescribed anomaly of pigmentation dyschromatosis universalis hereditaria. Jpn J Dermatol Urol 1933;34 360–4.
77 Merino de Paz N, Rodriguez-Martin M, Contreras Ferrer P et al. Photoletter to the editor: Dyschromatosis universalis hereditaria: an infrequently occurring entity in Europe. J Dermatol Case Rep 2012;6:96–7.
78 Yusuf SM, Mijinyawa MS, Maiyaki MB et al. Dyschromatosis universalis hereditaria in a young Nigerian female. Int J Dermatol 2009;48:749–50.
79 Al Hawsawi K, Al Aboud K, Ramesh V et al. Dyschromatosis universalis hereditaria: report of a case and review of the literature. Pediatr Dermatol 2002;19:523–6.
80 Bukhari IA, El-Harith EA, Stuhrmann M. Dyschromatosis universalis hereditaria as an autosomal recessive disease in five members of one family. J Eur Acad Dermatol Venereol 2006;20:628–9.
81 Kenani N, Ghariani N, Denguezli M et al. Dyschromatosis universalis hereditaria: two cases. Dermatol Online J 2008;14:16.
82 Nuber UA, Tinschert S, Mundlos S et al. Dyschromatosis universalis hereditaria: familial case and ultrastructural skin investigation. Am J Med Genet A 2004;125A:261–6.
83 Sethuraman G, Srinivas CR, D'Souza M et al. Dyschromatosis universalis hereditaria. Clin Exp Dermatol 2002;27:477–9.
84 Suenaga M. Genetical studies on skin diseases. VII. Dyschromatosis universalis hereditaria in 5 generations. Tohoku J Exp Med 1952; 55:373–6.
85 Udayashankar C, Nath AK. Dyschromatosis universalis hereditaria: a case report. Dermatol Online J 2011;17:2.
86 Kantharaj GR, Siddalingappa K, Chidambara MS. Dyschromatosis universalis: autosomal dominant pattern. Ind J Dermatol Venereol Leprol 2002;68:50–1.
87 Kumar S, Bhoyar P, Mahajan BB. A case of dyschromatosis universalis hereditaria with adermatoglyphia: a rare association. Indian Dermatol Online J 2015;6:105–9.
88 Rycroft RJ, Calnan CD, Allenby CF. Dermatopathia pigmentosa reticularis. Clin Exp Dermatol 1977;2:39–44.
89 Wang G, Li CY, Gao TW et al. Dyschromatosis universalis hereditaria: two cases in a Chinese family. Clin Exp Dermatol 2005;30:494–6.
90 Wu CY, Huang WH. Two Taiwanese siblings with dyschromatosis universalis hereditaria. Clin Exp Dermatol 2009;34:e666–9.
91 Gupta A, Sharma Y, Dash KN et al. Ultrastructural investigations in an autosomal recessively inherited case of dyschromatosis universalis hereditaria. Acta Dermatol Venereol 2015;95:738–40.
92 Kao CH, Yu HS, Ko SS. Dyschromatosis universalis hereditaria: report of a case. Taiwan Yi Xue Hui Za Zhi 1991;90:1205–10.
93 Lu C, Liu J, Liu F et al. Novel missense mutations of ABCB6 in two chinese families with dyschromatosis universalis hereditaria. J Dermatol Sci 2014;76:255–8.
94 Zhang C, Li D, Zhang J et al. Mutations in ABCB6 cause dyschromatosis universalis hereditaria. J Invest Dermatol 2013;133:2221–8.
95 Wang L, He F, Bu J et al. ABCB6 mutations cause ocular coloboma. Am J Hum Genet 2012; 90:40–8.
96 Andolfo I, Alper SL, Delaunay J et al. Missense mutations in the ABCB6 transporter cause dominant familial pseudohyperkalemia. Am J Hematol 2013;88:66–72.
97 Helias V, Saison C, Ballif BA et al. ABCB6 is dispensable for erythropoiesis and specifies the new blood group system Langereis. Nature Genet 2012;44:170–3.
98 Ulrich DL, Lynch J, Wang Y et al. ATP-dependent mitochondrial porphyrin importer ABCB6 protects against phenylhydrazine toxicity. J Biol Chem 2012;287:12679–90.
99 Heimerl S, Bosserhoff AK, Langmann T et al. Mapping ATP-binding cassette transporter gene expression profiles in melanocytes and melanoma cells. Melanoma Res 2007;17:265–73.
100 Krishnamurthy PC, Du G, Fukuda Y et al. Identification of a mammalian mitochondrial porphyrin transporter. Nature 2006;443:586–9.
101 Mitsuhashi N, Miki T, Senbongi H et al. MTABC3, a novel mitochondrial ATP-binding cassette protein involved in iron homeostasis. J Biol Chem 2000;275:17536–40.
102 Krishnamurthy P, Schuetz JD. The role of ABCG2 and ABCB6 in porphyrin metabolism and cell survival. Curr Pharm Biotech 2011;12: 647–55.
103 Krishnamurthy P, Xie T, Schuetz JD. The role of transporters in cellular heme and porphyrin homeostasis. Pharmacol Therapeut 2007; 114:345–58.
104 Jalil YA, Ritz V, Jakimenko A et al. Vesicular localization of the rat ATP-binding cassette half-transporter rAbcb6. Am J Physiol Cell Physiol 2008;294:C579–90.
105 Petris MJ, Strausak D, Mercer JF. The Menkes copper transporter is required for the activation of tyrosinase. Hum Mol Genet 2000; 9:2845–51.
106 Lutsenko S, Barnes NL, Bartee MY et al. Function and regulation of human copper-transporting ATPases. Physiol Rev 2007;87:1011–46.
107 Marks MS, Seabra MC. The melanosome: membrane dynamics in black and white. Nat Reviews Mol Cell Biol 2001;2:738–48.
108 Kim NS, Im S, Kim SC. Dyschromatosis universalis hereditaria: an electron microscopic examination. J Dermatol 1997;24:161–4.
109 Andre F, Schartz NE, Movassagh M et al. Malignant effusions and immunogenic tumour-derived exosomes. Lancet 2002;360:295–305.
110 Ostrowski M, Carmo NB, Krumeich S et al. Rab27a and Rab27b control different steps of the exosome secretion pathway. Nature Cell Biol 2010;12:19–30; suppl 11–13.
111 Simons M, Raposo G. Exosomes – vesicular carriers for intercellular communication. Curr Opin Cell Biol 2009;21:575–81.
112 Theos AC, Truschel ST, Tenza D et al. A lumenal domain-dependent pathway for sorting to intralumenal vesicles of multivesicular endosomes involved in organelle morphogenesis. Dev Cell 2006;10:343–54.
113 Kumar S, Mahajan BB, Singh R, Jr. Dyschromatosis universalis hereditaria: a rare entity. Dermatol Online J 2011;17:6.
114 Dhar S, Malakar S. Localized form of dyschromatosis universalis hereditaria in a 14-year-old girl. Pediatr Dermatol 1999;16:336.
115 Shi Y, Tan C. [Abrupt onset of dyschromatosis universalis hereditaria with macromelanosomes]. J German Soc Dermatol 2015; 13: 1028–1030.
116 Naveen KN, Dinesh US. Dyschromatosis universalis hereditaria with involvement of palms. Indian Dermatol Online J 2014;5:296–9.
117 Sandhu K, Saraswat A, Kanwar AJ. Dowling–Degos disease with dyschromatosis universalis hereditaria-like pigmentation in a family. J Eur Acad Dermatol Venereol 2004;18:702–4.
118 Shono S, Toda K. Universal dyschromatosis associated with photosensitivity and neurosensory hearing defect. Arch Dermatol 1990;126:1659–60.
119 Binitha MP, Thomas D, Asha LK. Tuberous sclerosis complex associated with dyschromatosis universalis hereditaria. Ind J Dermatol Venereol Leprol 2006;72:300–2.
120 Rojhirunsakool S, Vachiramon V. Dyschromatosis universalis hereditaria with renal failure. Case Rep Dermatol 2015;7:51–5.
121 Pirasath S, Sundaresan T, Tamilvannan T. Thrombocytopenia in dyschromatosis universalis hereditaria. Ceylon Medical J 2012;57:124–5.
122 Dokal I. Dyskeratosis congenita. Hematology/the Education Program of the American Society of Hematology. American Society of Hematology Education Program 2011: 480–6.
123 Li M, Cheng R, Liang J et al. Mutations in POFUT1, encoding protein O-fucosyltransferase 1, cause generalized Dowling–Degos disease. Am J Hum Genet 2013;92:895–903.
124 Pickup TL, Mutasim DF. Dowling–Degos disease presenting as hypopigmented macules. J Am Acad Dermatol 2011;64:1224–5.
125 Basmanav FB, Fritz G, Lestringant GG et al. Pathogenicity of POFUT1 in Dowling–Degos disease: additional mutations and clinical overlap with reticulate acropigmentation of kitamura. J Invest Dermatol 2015;135:615–18.
126 Basmanav FB, Oprisoreanu AM, Pasternack SM et al. Mutations in POGLUT1, encoding protein O-glucosyltransferase 1, cause autosomal-dominant Dowling–Degos disease. Am J Hum Genet 2014;94: 135–43.
127 Lugassy J, Itin P, Ishida-Yamamoto A et al. Naegeli–Franceschetti–Jadassohn syndrome and dermatopathia pigmentosa reticularis: two

allelic ectodermal dysplasias caused by dominant mutations in KRT14. Am J Hum Genet 2006;79:724–30.
128 Lugassy J, McGrath JA, Itin P et al. KRT14 haploinsufficiency results in increased susceptibility of keratinocytes to TNF-alpha-induced apoptosis and causes Naegeli–Franceschetti–Jadassohn syndrome. J Invest Dermatol 2008;128:1517–24.
129 Sparrow GP, Samman PD, Wells RS. Hyperpigmentation and hypohidrosis. (The Naegeli–Franceschetti–Jadassohn syndrome): report of a family and review of the literature. Clin Exp Dermatol 1976;1:127–40.
130 Itin PH, Lautenschlager S, Meyer R et al. Natural history of the Naegeli–Franceschetti–Jadassohn syndrome and further delineation of its clinical manifestations. J Am Acad Dermatol 1993;28:942–50.
131 Coleman R, Harper JI, Lake BD. Epidermolysis bullosa simplex with mottled pigmentation. Br J Dermatol 1993;128:679–85.
132 Uttam J, Hutton E, Coulombe PA et al. The genetic basis of epidermolysis bullosa simplex with mottled pigmentation. Proc Natl Acad Sci U S A 1996;93:9079–84.
133 Moriwaki S. Human DNA repair disorders in dermatology: a historical perspective, current concepts and new insight. J Dermatol Sci 2016;81:77–84.
134 Pranay T, Kumar AS, Chhabra S. Civatte bodies: a diagnostic clue. Ind J Dermatol 2013;58:327.
135 Sorensen RH, Werner KA, Kobayashi TT. Dyschromatosis universalis hereditaria with oral leukokeratosis–a case of mistaken identity and review of the literature. Pediatr Dermatol 2015;32:e283–287.
136 Zanardo L, Stolz W, Schmitz G et al. Progressive hyperpigmentation and generalized lentiginosis without associated systemic symptoms: a rare hereditary pigmentation disorder in south-east Germany. Acta Dermato-Venereol 2004;84:57–60.
137 Amyere M, Vogt T, Hoo J et al. KITLG mutations cause familial progressive hyper- and hypopigmentation. J Invest Dermatol 2011;131:1234–9.
138 Zhang RZ, Zhu WY. Familial progressive hypo- and hyperpigmentation: a variant case. Ind J Dermatol Venereol Leprol 2012;78:350–3.
139 Spritz RA. Molecular basis of human piebaldism. J Invest Dermatol 1994;103:137S–40S.
140 Steel KP, Davidson DR, Jackson IJ. TRP-2/DT, a new early melanoblast marker, shows that steel growth factor (c-kit ligand) is a survival factor. Development 1992;115:1111–19.
141 De Schepper S, Maertens O, Callens T et al. Somatic mutation analysis in NF1 cafe au lait spots reveals two NF1 hits in the melanocytes. J Invest Dermatol 2008;128:1050–3.
142 Spurlock G, Bennett E, Chuzhanova N et al. SPRED1 mutations (Legius syndrome): another clinically useful genotype for dissecting the neurofibromatosis type 1 phenotype. J Med Genet 2009;46:431–7.
143 Spritz RA, Giebel LB, Holmes SA. Dominant negative and loss of function mutations of the c-kit (mast/stem cell growth factor receptor) proto-oncogene in human piebaldism. Am J Hum Genet 1992;50:261–9.
144 Wang ZQ, Si L, Tang Q et al. Gain-of-function mutation of KIT ligand on melanin synthesis causes familial progressive hyperpigmentation. Am J Hum Genet 2009;84:672–7.
145 Mengel-From J, Wong TH, Morling N et al. Genetic determinants of hair and eye colours in the Scottish and Danish populations. BMC Genet 2009;10:88.
146 Westerhof W, Beemer FA, Cormane RH et al. Hereditary congenital hypopigmented and hyperpigmented macules. Arch Dermatol 1978;114:931–6.
147 Brems H, Pasmant E, Van Minkelen R et al. Review and update of SPRED1 mutations causing Legius syndrome. Human Mutat 2012;33:1538–46.
148 Ruggieri M, Iannetti P, Pavone L. Delineation of a newly recognized neurocutaneous malformation syndrome with 'cutis tricolor'. Am J Med Genet A 2003;120A:110–16.
149 Happle R, Barbi G, Eckert D et al. 'Cutis tricolor': congenital hyper- and hypopigmented macules associated with a sporadic multisystem birth defect: an unusual example of twin spotting? J Med Genet 1997;34:676–8.
150 Ruggieri M. Cutis tricolor: congenital hyper- and hypopigmented lesions in a background of normal skin with and without associated systemic features: further expansion of the phenotype. Eur J Pediatr 2000;159:745–9.
151 Larralde M, Happle R. Cutis tricolor parvimaculata: a distinct neurocutaneous syndrome? Dermatology 2005;211:149–51.
152 Baba M, Seckin D, Akcali C et al. Familial cutis tricolor: a possible example of paradominant inheritance. Eur J Dermatol 2003;13:343–5.
153 Groesser L, Herschberger E, Sagrera A et al. Phacomatosis pigmentokeratotica is caused by a postzygotic HRAS mutation in a multipotent progenitor cell. J Invest Dermatol 2013;133:1998–2003.
154 Thomas AC, Zeng Z, Riviere JB et al. Mosaic activating mutations in GNA11 and GNAQ are associated with phakomatosis pigmentovascularis and extensive dermal melanocytosis. J Invest Dermatol 2016;136:770–8.
155 Happle R. Mosaicism in Human Skin. Berlin: Springer, 2014.
156 del Carmen Boente M, Bazan C, Montanari D. Cutis tricolor parvimaculata in two patients with ring chromosome 15 syndrome. Pediatr Dermatol 2011;28:670–3.
157 Happle R. Mosaicism in human skin. Understanding the patterns and mechanisms. Arch Dermatol 1993;129:1460–70.
158 Paller AS. Pigmentary patterning as a clinical clue of genetic mosaicism. Arch Dermatol 1996;132:1234–5.
159 Bolognia JL, Orlow SJ, Glick SA. Lines of Blaschko. J Am Acad Dermatol 1994;31:157–90; quiz 190–52.
160 Ruggieri M, Pavone L. Hypomelanosis of Ito: clinical syndrome or just phenotype? J Chil Neurol 2000;15:635–44.
161 Happle R. An early drawing of Blaschko's lines. Br J Dermatol 1993;128:464.
162 Happle R. Transposable elements and the lines of Blaschko: a new perspective. Dermatology 2002;204:4–7.
163 Grosshans EM. Acquired blaschkolinear dermatoses. Am J Med Genet 1999;85:334–7.
164 Moss C, Green SH. What is segmental neurofibromatosis? Br J Dermatol 1994;130:106–10.
165 Zvulunov A, Esterly NB. Neurocutaneous syndromes associated with pigmentary skin lesions. J Am Acad Dermatol 1995;32:915–35; quiz 936–17.
166 Akahoshi K, Spritz RA, Fukai K et al. Mosaic supernumerary inv dup(15) chromosome with four copies of the P gene in a boy with pigmentary dysplasia. Am J Med Genet A 2004;126A:290–2.
167 Battaglia A, Gurrieri F, Bertini E et al. The inv dup(15) syndrome: a clinically recognizable syndrome with altered behavior, mental retardation, and epilepsy. Neurology 1997;48:1081–6.
168 Scott RH, Homfray T, Huxter NL et al. Familial T-cell non-Hodgkin lymphoma caused by biallelic MSH2 mutations. J Med Genet 2007;44:e83.
169 Velez A, Salido R, Amorrich-Campos V et al. Hereditary congenital hypopigmented and hyperpigmented macules (Westerhof syndrome) in two siblings. Br J Dermatol 2009;161:1399–400.
170 Jozwiak S, Schwartz RA, Janniger CK et al. Skin lesions in children with tuberous sclerosis complex: their prevalence, natural course, and diagnostic significance. Int J Dermatol 1998;37:911–17.
171 Morishima T. A clinical variety of localized cutaneous amyloidosis characterized by dyschromia (amyloidosis cutis dyschromica). Jpn J Dermatol Series B 1970;80:43–52.
172 Eng AM, Cogan L, Gunnar RM et al. Familial generalized dyschromic amyloidosis cutis. J Cutan Pathol 1976;3:102–8.
173 Hermawan M, Rihatmadja R, Sirait SP. Familial amyloidosis cutis dyschromica in three siblings: report from indonesia. Dermatol Rep 2014;6:5375.
174 Mahon C, Oliver F, Purvis D et al. Amyloidosis cutis dyschromia in two siblings and review of the epidemiology, clinical features and management in 48 cases. Australas J Dermatol 2016;57:307–11.
175 Verma S, Joshi R. Amyloidosis cutis dyschromica: a rare reticulate pigmentary dermatosis. Ind J Dermatol 2015;60:385–7.
176 Dehghani F, Ebrahimzadeh M, Moghimi M et al. Familial amyloidosis cutis dyschromica: a case report. Acta Med Iran 2014;52:163–5.
177 Kurian SS, Rai R, Madhukar ST. Amyloidosis cutis dyschromica. Indian Dermatol Online J 2013;4:344–6.
178 Qiao J, Fang H, Yao H. Amyloidosis cutis dyschromica. Orphanet J Rare Dis 2012;7:95.
179 Fernandes NF, Mercer SE, Kleinerman R et al. Amyloidosis cutis dyschromica associated with atypical Parkinsonism, spasticity and motor weakness in a Pakistani female. J Cutan Pathol 2011;38: 827–31.
180 Garg T, Chander R, Jabeen M et al. Amyloidosis cutis dyschromica: a rare pigmentary disorder. J Cutan Pathol 2011;38:823–6.
181 Yang W, Lin Y, Yang J et al. Amyloidosis cutis dyschromica in two female siblings: cases report. BMC Dermatol 2011;11:4.
182 Huang WH, Wu CY, Yu CP et al. Amyloidosis cutis dyschromica: four cases from two families. Int J Dermatol 2009;48:518–21.
183 Madarasingha NP, Satgurunathan K, De Silva MV. A rare type of primary cutaneous amyloidosis: amyloidosis cutis dyschromica. Int J Dermatol 2010;49:1416–18.

184 Ozcan A, Senol M, Aydin NE et al. Amyloidosis cutis dyschromica: a case treated with acitretin. J Dermatol 2005;32:474–7.
185 Choonhakarn C, Wittayachanyapong S. Familial amyloidosis cutis dyschromica: six cases from three families. J Dermatol 2002;29:439–42.
186 Morales Callaghan AM, Vila JB, Fraile HA et al. Amyloidosis cutis dyschromica in a patient with generalized morphoea. Br J Dermatol 2004;150:616–17.
187 Vijaikumar M, Thappa DM. Amyloidosis cutis dyschromica in two siblings. Clin Exp Dermatol 2001;26:674–6.
188 Moriwaki S, Nishigori C, Horiguchi Y et al. Amyloidosis cutis dyschromica. DNA repair reduction in the cellular response to UV light. Arch Dermatol 1992;128:966–70.
189 Chandran NS, Goh BK, Lee SS et al. Case of primary localized cutaneous amyloidosis with protean clinical manifestations: lichen, poikiloderma-like, dyschromic and bullous variants. J Dermatol 2011;38:1066–71.
190 Chuah SY, Chia HY, Tey HL. Acquired dyschromic patches. Int J Dermatol 2015;54:516–17.
191 Morishima T. Amyloidosis cutis dyschromica. Dermatol Clin 1981;3:627.
192 Chang YT, Wong CK, Chow KC et al. Apoptosis in primary cutaneous amyloidosis. Br J Dermatol 1999;140:210–15.
193 Schreml S, Szeimies RM, Vogt T et al. Cutaneous amyloidoses and systemic amyloidoses with cutaneous involvement. Eur J Dermatol 2010;20:152–60.
194 Taniguchi Y, Horino T, Terada Y. Cutaneous amyloidosis associated with amyopathic dermatomyositis. J Rheumatol 2009;36:1088–9.
195 Salim T, Shenoi SD, Balachandran C et al. Lichen amyloidosus: a study of clinical, histopathologic and immunofluorescence findings in 30 cases. Ind J Dermatol Venereol Leprol 2005;71:166–9.
196 Ho MH, Chong LY. Poikiloderma-like cutaneous amyloidosis in an ethnic Chinese girl. J Dermatol 1998;25:730–4.
197 Ogino A, Tanaka S. Poikiloderma-like cutaneous amyloidosis. Report of a case and review of the literature. Dermatologica 1977;155:301–9.
198 Unni M, Ankad B, Naidu V et al. A familial poikiloderma-like cutaneous amyloidosis. Ind J Dermatol 2014;59:633.
199 Zeng YP, Jin HZ, Fang K. Poikiloderma-like primary cutaneous amyloidosis confined to the calves in a Chinese man. J German Soc Dermatol 2012;10:663–4.
200 Aktas Yilmaz B, Duzgun N, Mete T et al. AA amyloidosis associated with systemic lupus erythematosus: impact on clinical course and outcome. Rheumatology Int 2008;28:367–70.
201 Li WM. Histopathology of primary cutaneous amyloidoses and systemic amyloidosis. Clin Dermatol 1990;8:30–5.
202 Ogiyama Y, Hayashi Y, Kou C et al. Cutaneous amyloidosis in patients with progressive systemic sclerosis. Cutis 1996;57:28–32.
203 Samuelov L, Arad U, Gat A et al. Diffuse scalp alopecia in a middle-aged patient. Clin Exp Dermatol 2013;38:936–9.
204 Helbig I, Folster-Holst R, Brasch J et al. Dyschromatosis ptychotropica: an unusual pigmentary disorder in a boy with epileptic encephalopathy and progressive atrophy of the central nervous system–a novel entity? Eur J Pediatr 2010;169:495–500.
205 Somer M. Diagnostic criteria and genetics of the PEHO syndrome. J Med Genet 1993;30:932–6.
206 Hassing JH, Doeglas HM. Dystrophia bullosa hereditaria, typus maculatus (Mendes da Costa-van der Valk): a rare genodermatosis [proceedings]. Br J Dermatol 1980;102:474–6.
207 Lungarotti MS, Martello C, Barboni G et al. X-linked mental retardation, microcephaly, and growth delay associated with hereditary bullous dystrophy macular type: report of a second family. Am J Med Genet 1994;51:598–601.
208 Ruiz-Maldonado R, Toussaint S, Tamayo L et al. Hypomelanosis of Ito: diagnostic criteria and report of 41 cases. Pediatr Dermatol 1992;9:1–10.
209 Berlin C. Congenital generalized melanoleucoderma associated with hypodontia, hypotrichosis, stunted growth and mental retardation occurring in two brothers and two sisters. Dermatologica 1961;123:227–43.
210 Chiba A, Miura T. A family with hypotrichosis associated with congenital hypoplasia of the thumb. Jinrui Idengaku Zasshi 1979; 24:111–17.
211 Lucky AW, Esterly NB, Tunnessen WW, Jr. Ectodermal dysplasia and abnormal thumbs. J Am Acad Dermatol 1980;2:379–84.
212 Siemens HW. Acromelanosis albo-punctata. Dermatologica 1964;128:86–7.
213 Winter RM, MacDermot KD, Hill FJ. Sparse hair, short stature, hypoplastic thumbs, single upper central incisor and abnormal skin pigmentation: a possible 'new' form of ectodermal dysplasia. Am J Med Genet 1988;29:209–16.
214 Dessinioti C, Stratigos AJ, Rigopoulos D et al. A review of genetic disorders of hypopigmentation: lessons learned from the biology of melanocytes. Exp Dermatol 2009; 18: 741–749.
215 Rufo M, Sierra J. [Neurocutaneous disorders with large dyschromia: incontinentia pigmenti, achromic nevus]. Revista de neurologia 1996;24:1060–7.
216 Ashley JR, Burgdorf WH. Incontinentia pigmenti: pigmentary changes independent of incontinence. J Cutan Pathol 1987; 14:248–50.
217 Taki T, Kozuka S, Izawa Y et al. Surgical treatment of speckled skin caused by dyschromatosis symmetrica hereditaria – case report. J Dermatol 1986;13:471–3.
218 Kawakami T, Otaguchi R, Kyoya M et al. Patient with dyschromatosis symmetrica hereditaria treated with miniature punch grafting, followed by excimer light therapy. J Dermatol 2013;40:771–2.
219 Nogita T, Mitsuhashi Y, Takeo C et al. Removal of facial and labial lentigines in dyschromatosis universalis hereditaria with a Q-switched alexandrite laser. J Am Acad Dermatol 2011;65:e61–3.
220 Haake AR, Polakowska RR. Cell death by apoptosis in epidermal biology. J Invest Dermatol 1993;101:107–12.

CHAPTER 127
Review of Keratin Disorders

Maurice A.M. van Steensel[1] *& Peter M. Steijlen*[2]

[1] Skin Research Institute of Singapore and Lee Kong Chian School of Medicine, Singapore
[2] Department of Dermatology, Maastricht University Medical Centre, The Netherlands

Introduction, 1515
Keratin biology, 1515
Disorders caused by keratin mutations, 1517
Conclusion, 1521

Abstract

This chapter deals with disorders caused by mutations in genes that code for epithelial keratins, which are intermediate filament proteins that make up much of the cytoskeleton in simple as well as multilayered epithelia. Keratins exist as obligate heterodimers, and the dimers in turn assemble into filaments that form the intermediate filament network. As such, keratins have a major role in maintaining structural integrity of cells and tissues, in addition to emerging functions in signal transduction. Mutations in epithelial keratins cause a plethora of disorders that mostly manifest in the skin, as well as in hair and nails. The phenotypes are quite variable and their impact on patients ranges from mild inconvenience to life-altering handicaps. Proper care for and counselling of the patients depends on accurate diagnosis, which is increasingly based on molecular genetics rather than subtleties of clinical appearance. To date there are no specific treatments for any keratin disorder, but this may soon change as insight into the underlying biology grows.

Key points

- Keratins are components of the cytoskeleton that contribute to maintaining cellular integrity in stratified as well as simple epithelia.
- Mutations in keratin genes give rise to a wide range of genetic disorders, most of which manifest in the skin with abnormal keratinization.
- Keratins have emerging functions in signal transduction, which might contribute to disease symptoms and represent possible therapeutic targets.

Introduction

In recent years, rapid progress has been made in our understanding of the molecular basis of many genetic skin diseases. Among these are several often distressing and sometimes even life-threatening disorders in which the process of keratinization is disturbed. Keratinization, defined as the process of stratum corneum formation, is a complex process and many molecules are involved in it. This chapter discusses epithelial keratins and disorders that result from mutations in them. There are still many gaps in our knowledge, but modern genetics and cell biology are increasing our insight into the function of keratins themselves, as well as the effects of keratin mutations.

To understand properly the effects of keratin mutations, some basic knowledge of keratin biology is necessary.

Keratin biology

The human genome codes for at least 54 different keratins. They belong to the family of intermediate filament (IF) proteins [1]. These evolutionarily conserved molecules are a major part of the cytoskeleton in many organisms and as such play an important role in maintaining the structural integrity of the cells and their surroundings, in addition to functions in signal transduction and metabolic control [2]. This overview is concerned with the so-called soft keratins that are found in multilayered and simple epithelia and the hard keratins that form the bulk of appendicular structures such as hairs and nails. Hard keratins differ from their soft counterparts by the number of cysteine residues they contain [3]. Having more, they can form more extensive cross-links between individual keratins and between filaments. This results in stiffer keratin intermediate filament (KIF) networks. There are 15 hard keratins in humans.

Like all other IF molecules, keratins have a central α-helical 'rod' domain, flanked by end domains that are specific to the type of keratin in question (Fig. 127.1) [4]. This basic structure is strongly conserved throughout evolution in all IF proteins, which suggests that it is essential to normal IF function.

Skin and hair/nail keratins are subdivided based on their end domains and their charge: type I acidic (soft keratins 10–21 and hard keratins 31–38) or type II basic/neutral (soft keratins 1–9 and hard keratins 81–86). The acidic keratins are coded for by a gene cluster on chromosome 17, the basic

SECTION 27: DISORDERS OF KERATIN AND KERATINIZATION

Harper's Textbook of Pediatric Dermatology, Fourth Edition. Edited by Peter Hoeger, Veronica Kinsler and Albert Yan.

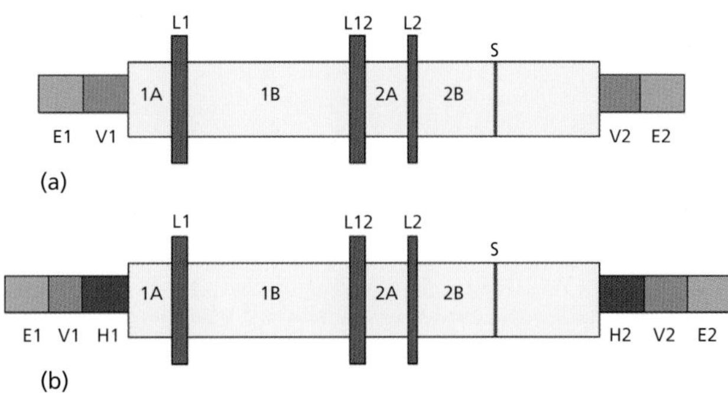

Fig. 127.1 Central α-helical rod domain. (a) Type I. (b) Type II.

ones by genes on chromosome 12. The two forms also differ slightly in their basic structure: type I keratins lack H1 and H2 domains [4].

Keratins exist as obligate heterodimers of type I and type II chains [5]. The association between the chains is thought to take place through the rod domain, which shows a motif of seven amino acids (the 'heptad motif'), thought to mediate the association of the helices. Short, strongly conserved sequences at the beginning and end of the rod domains, the helix initiation and helix termination motifs respectively, are essential for the initiation and proper termination of the dimerization process. Alterations in this motif perturb keratin function and are generally associated with severe skin disease. The keratin filaments aggregate into a network (Fig. 127.2), that interacts through specialized molecules called plakins with adhesion structures in the keratinocytes: desmosomes and hemidesmosomes [6,7]. Thus, the cytoskeleton of each cell is linked to its membrane and, via this membrane, to other cells. An increasing body of evidence suggests that keratins mediate interactions with various signalling pathways in the cell, implying the intermediate

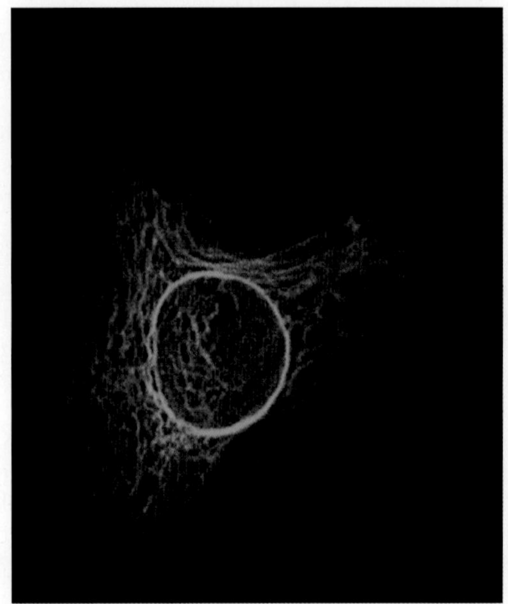

Fig. 127.2 HaCaT cell transfected with a green fluorescent protein-labelled keratin 1 construct. The intermediate filament network is clearly visible.

filament network in signal transduction. The recently uncovered connections between the inner nuclear lamina and cytoskeleton via the so-called LINC complex provide an excellent illustration [8]. It is increasingly recognized that such emerging, nonstructural functions of the keratins may contribute significantly to the clinical symptoms of keratin disorders [9].

During differentiation of the epidermal cells, the expression of keratins in the keratinocytes changes as the cells move upwards (Table 127.1). Basal keratinocytes express K5 and K14. Upon their maturation to spinous layer cells, K5 and K14 are downregulated and K1, K2e and K10 are expressed [10]. Nail and hair progenitor cells express mainly K6, K16 and K17. These keratins are also expressed in other regions in response to keratinocyte stress or injury. Because of this, they can also be found in the palms and soles. K6a and K16 are also expressed in mucosal epithelia. K9 is expressed in the palms and soles only [11]. Nonepidermal keratins are expressed in mucous membranes and two of these, K4 and K13, have been implicated in a disorder of the mucosa (see later).

As the keratinocytes reach the stratum granulosum, the expression of keratins ceases. Among the many proteins produced in the upper layer are loricrin and filaggrin [12]. These two are a major part of the so-called cornified envelope, an insoluble hydrophobic layer on the inner surface of the plasma membrane of the keratinocytes in the stratum corneum. This layer is made by cross-linking of the proteins mentioned, both to each other and to the KIF network. Several enzymes are involved in this process, mainly transglutaminases [12].

Keratins and other members of the IF family are involved in maintaining the structural integrity of the epidermis. Disruption of the IF network has been proposed to cause symptoms by decreasing resistance of the epidermis to mechanical stress. However, there is evidence that keratins (and other IF proteins) may have complex functions in cellular function, beyond their structural role in the cytoskeleton. For example, it has been shown that loss of K17 correlates with decreased Akt/mTOR signalling activity. Furthermore, two amino acids in K17 are required to relocalize the adaptor protein 14-3-3-σ from the nucleus to the cytoplasm [2]. These findings reveal a new role for the cytoskeleton in regulating cell growth and metabolism. More recently, it was discovered that K16 mutations in pachyonychia congenita can lead to oxidative stress, which can be corrected by agonists of the transcription factor NRF2,

Table 127.1 Differentiation-specific expression of keratins

Layer of epidermis	Expression of keratins
Stratum spinosum	
Upper	K2e
Lower	K1/K10, K6/K16, K4/K13, K9[a]
Stratum basale	K5/K14, K6b, K17

[a] Expression in palmoplantar skin only.

such as sulforaphane. Intriguingly, topical application of this small molecule (which is present in broccoli) ameliorated the phenotype in a mouse model of the disease [9].

Symptoms caused by keratin mutations may also be related to the affected cells' response to the presence of misfolded (mutant) keratin proteins. Meanwhile, the number of disorders caused by keratin mutations is growing and now includes liver and ocular disease, showing that keratins are also involved in the maintenance of simple epithelia (see, for example, reference [13]).

Disorders caused by keratin mutations

Known disorders caused by keratin mutations are listed in Table 127.2. These are discussed in this section. Note that several keratin diseases are grouped under other nosological headings and are discussed in more detail elsewhere. Therefore, this chapter will provide an overview of these disorders; for details the reader is referred to the appropriate chapters. Keratin gene mutations are catalogued in the Human Intermediate Filament database: www.interfil.org [14]. A note on terminology: keratin genes are indicated by '*KRT*', the proteins by 'K'.

Epidermolysis bullosa simplex (OMIM #131760, #131800, #131900, #615028, *KRT5/14, EXPH5*)

The inherited forms of epidermolysis bullosa (EB) have recently been reclassified and EB simplex (EBS) is no longer subdivided into three entities (Weber–Cockayne, Dowling–Meara and Koebner) [15]. Nowadays, EBS is considered as a single entity with variable expressivity, which is caused by mutations in *KRT5/14*. The term 'simplex' refers to the level of blistering. EB with mottled pigmentation can be caused by mutations in *KRT5/14* [16,17] and likewise is assigned to the EBS group. Recently, it was discovered that a recessive form of EBS can also be caused by mutations in the *EXPH5* gene, coding for a protein that is involved in vesicular transport [18]. Of note, there are some nonclassic forms of the disease with associated symptoms, described in Chapter 75. These must be distinguished because they have a different molecular background.

Table 127.2 Keratin disorders (see also Chapter 128)

Disorder (and subtypes)	Keratins affected
Epidermolysis bullosa, simplex type; Naegeli–Franceschetti–Jadassohn syndrome, dermatopathia pigmentosa reticularis	K5/14
Dowling–Degos disease[a]	K5
Epidermolytic ichthyosis (bullous congenital ichthyosiform erythroderma of Brocq)	K1/10
Epidermolytic epidermal naevus	K1/10 (mosaic)
Epidermolytic palmoplantar hyperkeratosis (Vörner)	K1/9
Superficial epidermolytic ichthyosis (ichthyosis bullosa Siemens)	K2e
Pachyonychia congenita	K6a/6b/16/17
Focal NEPPK	K6c, 16
White sponge naevus	K4/13
Cryptogenic liver cirrhosis	K8/18
Meesmann's corneal dystrophy	K3/12
Monilethrix	K83, 81, 86
Ectodermal dysplasia, 'pure' hair-nail type[a]	K74, 85
Pseudo-folliculitis barbae	K75

NEPPK, nonepidermolytic palmoplantar keratoderma.
[a] Phenocopies of these disorders are associated with nonkeratin genes (see respective sections in this chapter).

Both K5 and K14 are expressed in basal epidermal cells. Different mutations can give rise to phenotypes of varying severity; there are also strong environmental influences such as ambient heat and humidity. Disturbed intermediate filament network formation is considered as an essential component of EBS [19]. Interestingly, a few disorders formerly thought to be distinct are now known to be allelic to EBS. From a nosological point of view, one might argue that they should no longer be recognized as separate disease entities. However, their clinical appearance is sufficiently distinctive and of mnemonic value to retain them as separate categories. These are discussed below.

Naegeli–Franceschetti–Jadassohn syndrome and dermatopathia pigmentosa reticularis (OMIM #161000, #125595, *KRT14*)

These disorders are discussed under the same heading because their clinical features are highly similar, if not identical, and because they are allelic [20]. In the authors' opinion, they should probably be considered as manifestations of EBS. In their typical form, though, they are sufficiently distinct to be recognized as a defined phenotype.

Distinguishing symptoms of Naegeli–Franceschetti–Jadassohn syndrome (NFJS) are complete absence of dermatoglyphics (fingerprint lines), skin hyperpigmentation, palmoplantar keratoderma, reduced sweating, nail dystrophy and discoloured, yellow teeth that are lost early in life [21]. The hyperpigmentation is illustrated in Fig. 127.3. Dermatopathia pigmentosa reticularis (DPR) is characterized by the triad of nonscarring alopecia, onychodystrophy and reticular hyperpigmentation. It has been reported that in DPR the latter symptom is

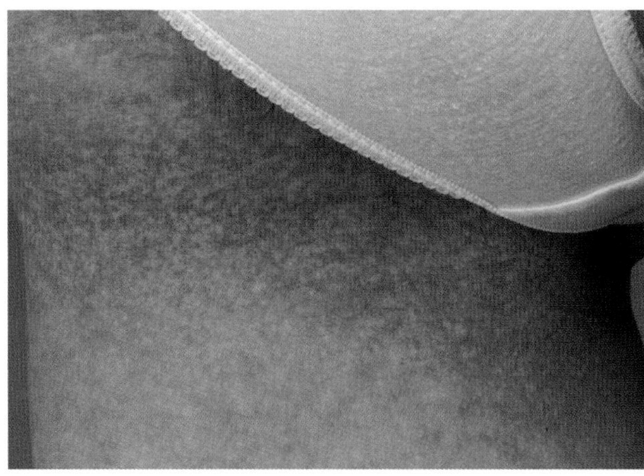

Fig. 127.3 Naegeli–Franceschetti–Jadassohn syndrome: inguinal reticular pigmentation.

persistent [22]. Blistering can also be present in DPR [23] but dental abnormalities are supposed to be absent. However, these differences are all anecdotal. The NFJS and DPR phenotypes are so similar that it is probably no longer useful to distinguish them.

In contrast with *KRT14* mutations affecting the central α-helical rod domain of K14, which are known to cause EBS, NFJS/DPR-associated mutations were found in a region of the gene encoding the nonhelical head (E1/V1) domain and are predicted to result in very early termination of translation [20]. It seems reasonable to assume from this that NFJS/DPR results from K14 haploinsufficiency. Apparently, K14 plays an important role during ontogenesis of dermatoglyphics and sweat glands. Among other functions, the N-terminal part of keratin molecules has been shown to protect against proapoptotic signals [24]. There is evidence for increased susceptibility to apoptosis induced by TNF-α in keratinocytes that are haploinsufficient for *KRT14*, suggesting that apoptosis is an important mechanism in the pathogenesis of NFJS/DPR [25]. The pathogenesis of the hyperpigmentation is not clear, but recent work on Dowling–Degos disease suggests involvement of cutaneous NOTCH signalling (see next section).

Dowling–Degos disease (OMIM #179850, *KRT5*)

Dowling–Degos disease (DDD) is a rare autosomal dominant disorder causing progressive reticular hyperpigmentation of skin folds and flexures to appear after puberty. The pigmentation is progressive and disfiguring. DDD is identical to Galli-Galli disease [26] and allelic to epidermolysis bullosa simplex with mottled pigmentation (EBS-MP, OMIM #131960). In contrast to EBS-MP, DDD is not associated with manifest blistering. It must be distinguished from the reticulate acropigmentations of Kitamura and Dohi (see also Chapter 122).

DDD is most often caused by heterozygous loss-of-function mutations in the *KRT5* gene, presumably leading to haploinsufficiency [27]. As in NFJS/DPR, the pathogenesis of the hyperpigmentation is not clear. However, it was recently discovered that a DDD phenotype can also be associated with loss-of-function mutations in the *POFUT1* or *POGLUT1* genes, which code for proteins that potentiate NOTCH signalling [28,29]. NOTCH is a receptor family that mediates interactions between neighbouring cells, and its activity is required for the maintenance of melanocyte precursors in the skin [30]. Thus, it is tempting to speculate that the pigmentation defect in DDD and related disorders is caused by defective melanocyte maintenance, consequent to defective NOTCH signalling. This notion is supported by the published observation that basal keratinocytes, which are affected in DDD, express the classic NOTCH ligand JAGGED2 [31]. Of note, this proposed mechanism also explains the pigmentary defects in EBS-MP and NFJS/DPR.

Epidermolytic ichthyoses (formerly: bullous congenital ichthyosiform erythroderma of Brocq and ichthyosis bullosa of Siemens, OMIM #113800 and #146800, *KRT1/10* and *KRT2e*)

In 2010, the ichthyoses were reclassified during the Ichthyosis Consensus Conference in Sorèze, France [15]. The entities formerly known as bullous congenital ichthyosiform erythroderma of Brocq (BCIE, OMIM #113800) and ichthyosis bullosa Siemens (IBS, OMIM #146800) have been grouped together as 'epidermolytic ichthyoses'. The disorders are rare. For clinical and mnemonic purposes, it is still useful to distinguish the two phenotypes.

BCIE is characterized by generalized blistering at birth, accompanied by varying erythroderma and the development later in life of hyperkeratosis that can be localized or generalized (Fig. 127.4).

Inheritance is autosomal dominant. Various mutations in K1 and K10 have been identified (www.interfil.org). These keratins are expressed mainly in the suprabasal layers of the epidermis, where the ultrastructural abnormalities of epidermolytic hyperkeratosis are found: clumping of intermediate filaments, vacuolation and

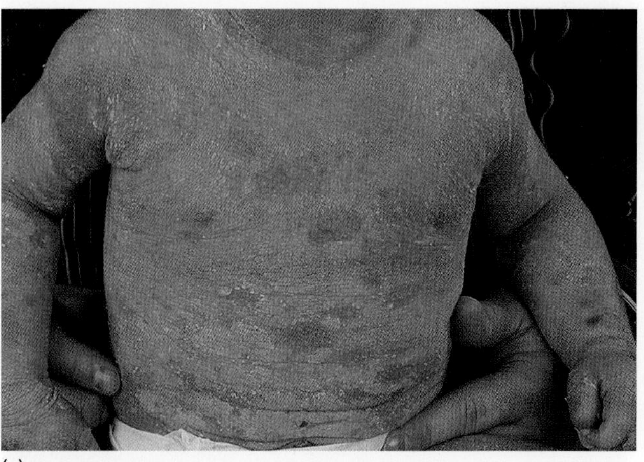

(a)

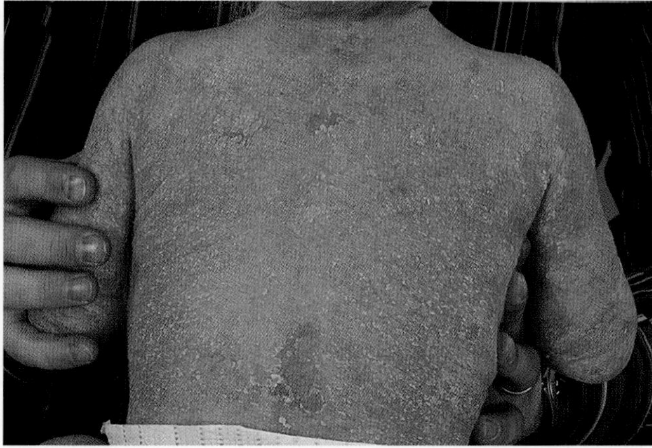

(b)

Fig. 127.4 Epidermolytic ichthyosis (BCIE Brocq) caused by a KRT10 mutation. (a) Generalized blistering at birth, evolving into (b) hyperkeratosis with erythroderma and superficial erosions.

hyperkeratosis. K1 mutations can cause palmoplantar keratoderma of varying severity. This symptom has also been observed in patients with K10 mutations [32] (see Chapter 128).

Mutations in K1 and K10 associated with severe BCIE are located at the beginning or end of the 1A rod domain, as in EBS [33]. Milder forms typically have mutations in the H1, L1 or L12 domain. However, pronounced phenotypic variation has been reported for mutations in the L12 domain, suggesting that the phenotype–genotype correlation might be less clear-cut than previously thought [34]. Symptoms can be so mild that they escape attention. It is interesting to note that in three different keratin disorders (BCIE, EBS and epidermolytic palmoplantar keratodermas, see later), the same residues are mutated in three different keratins (asparagine 160, arginine 162, methionine 156) [35]. This indicates the functional importance of the conserved heptad motif.

K10 mutations can also appear in a mosaic pattern in some individuals [36]. Mosaicism means that cells carrying a mutation are intermingled with normal cells in the same individual. K10 mutations in a mosaic give rise to an epidermolytic epidermal naevus (OMIM 113800), whereas the presence of the mutation in all cells gives rise to epidermolytic ichthyosis. Interestingly, mosaicism has never been described for K5/K14 mutations. The reason for this is not clear but it seems that in the hypothetical case of mosaicism for K5/K14 mutations, the blisters that result are healed by migration of normal stem cells expressing K5/K14. In the case of K10 mutations, there is no expression in stem cells; hence the mosaic state remains (D. Roop, personal communication). Meanwhile, mosaicism for K1 mutations has also been found [37]. Most recently, revertant mosaicism has been demonstrated for K10 mutations. Ichthyosis en confetti is a very rare condition in which patients develop round blanched macules formed by normal skin on an erythrodermic background. It was shown that the normal areas represent thousands of revertant clones of normal keratinocytes. The reversion was caused by loss of heterozygosity (on chromosome 17q) via mitotic recombination [38]. Predictably, a similar phenomenon has now been observed for *KRT1* [39]. BCIE and its manifestations do not generally respond well to retinoids (see also Chapter 129).

IBS (OMIM #146800) is a milder, superficial epidermolytic ichthyosis without erythroderma (Fig. 127.5). Hyperkeratosis is mild and located on the flexural areas as well as on the umbilical skin and shins. Erosions are caused by minor trauma. A very typical phenomenon is grey, scaling, almost flaky hyperkeratosis on the flexural

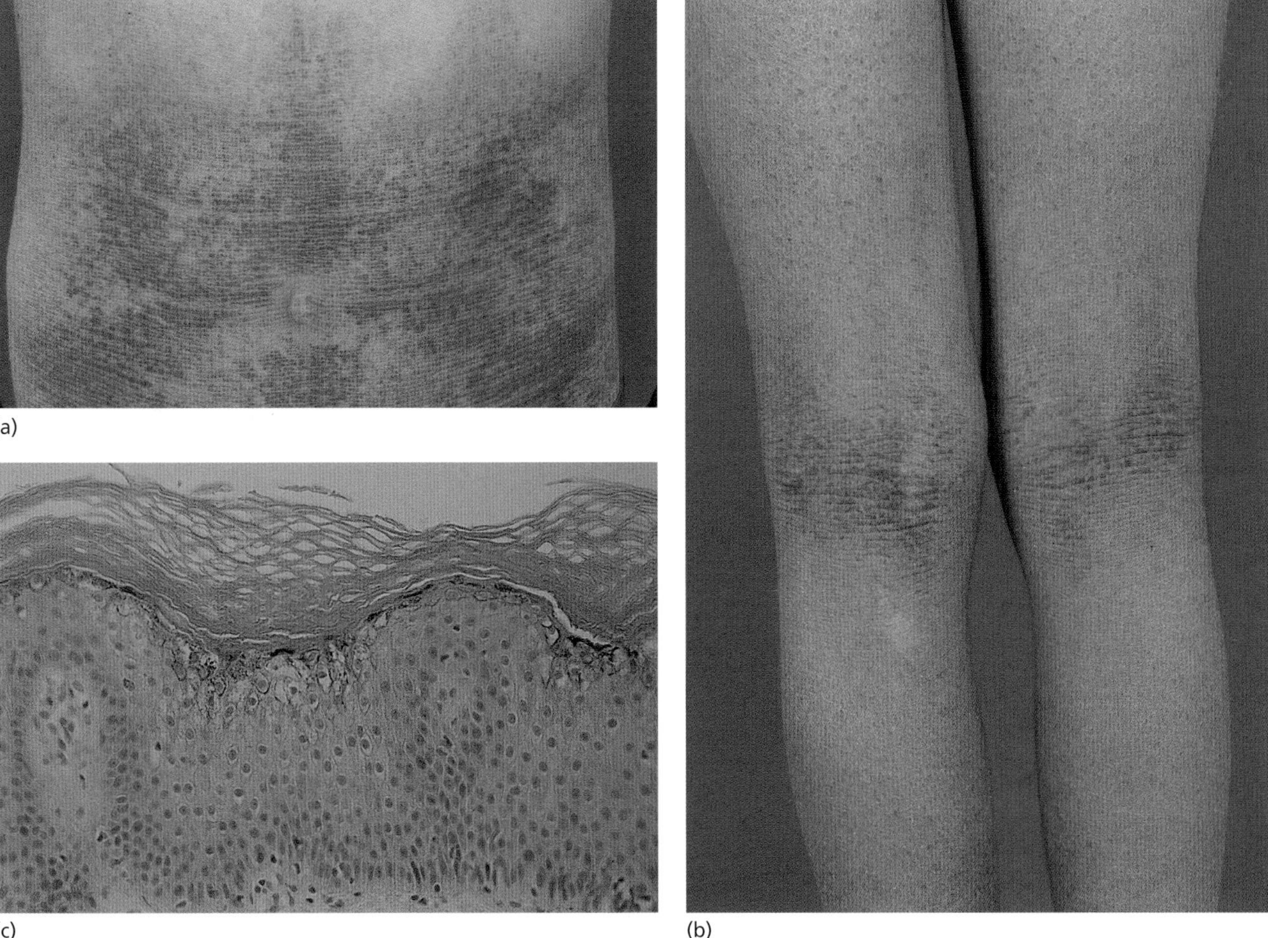

Fig. 127.5 Ichthyosis bullosa of Siemens. (a) Typical scaling in a boy. (b) Hyperkeratosis in flexural site of the knee. (c) Epidermolytic hyperkeratosis limited to the upper layers of the stratum spinosum.

surfaces known as 'moulting' or 'Mauserung' in German (Fig. 127.5b). Ultrastructural features in this disorder again are indicative of keratin mutations: KIF clumping and vacuolation, this time in the upper layers of the stratum spinosum. One of the keratins expressed in this layer, K2e, was found to harbour mutations [40]. Again, the mutations cluster within the conserved domains. The IBS phenotype responds well to low doses of acitretin (<0.5mg/kg).

Palmoplantar keratodermas

This is a heterogeneous group of disorders, all characterized by abnormal keratinization of the skin of palms and soles. Their classification is still mostly based on morphology and associated features. In recent years, the causative mutations of many palmoplantar keratodermas (PPKs) have been found. The PPKs, including those associated with mutations in keratin genes, are extensively discussed in Chapter 128. Here, it will suffice to say that mutations in the *KRT1* and *KRT9* genes can both cause a diffuse PPK, known as the Vörner or Unna–Thost type, whereas mutations in *KRT6a/b/c*, *16* and *17* cause pachyonychia congenita.

White sponge 'naevus' of Cannon (OMIM #193900, *KRT4*, *KRT13*)

This is a rare autosomal dominant disorder, characterized by the presence of thick white plaques in the mouth and occasionally on the mucosa of the oesophagus, nose, genitals and rectum. The pertinent differential diagnosis is with leucoplakia, lichen sclerosus, lichen planus and hereditary benign intraepithelial dyskeratosis (OMIM 127600 [41,42]). The latter disorder is distinguished by conjunctival lesions resembling pterygia. Microscopically, plaques show vacuolization of suprabasal cells in a manner similar to epidermolytic hyperkeratosis. The disorder is caused by heterozygous mutations in the *KRT4* and *KRT13* genes coding for the basic respectively acidic keratins K4 and K13 [43,44]. It will be no surprise that the mutations are in the beginning of the 1A domains. Of note, this disorder is not a true naevus. Naevi are the result of congenital or acquired genetic mosaicism [45]; white sponge 'naevus' is not.

Ectodermal dysplasia, 'pure' hair-nail types (OMIM #602032, *KRT85*; OMIM #614929, *KRT74*; OMIM #614931, *HOXC13*)

Several reports describe 'pure' hair-nail dysplasias that are not associated with other ectodermal abnormalities [46–48]. The extent of hair involvement is variable and both autosomal dominant and recessive inheritance patterns have been described. At least five different types, presumably with a different genetic background, may be distinguished. Currently, we know the causes of three types. In 2006, Naeem and colleagues described a consanguineous Pakistani pedigree in which four males and four females had universal alopecia and nail dystrophy present at birth. Affected individuals never developed axillary or pubic hair. The nails of all digits were dystrophic. Other ectodermal abnormalities were not present. Inheritance was autosomal recessive and homozygosity mapping indicated linkage to a cluster of type II hair keratins on chromosome 12. Subsequent sequencing of these candidate genes revealed homozygous missense mutations in the type II *KRT85* gene [49]. Subsequently, Shimomura and colleagues [50] reported that autosomal-dominant woolly hair (ADWH), a rare disorder characterized by poorly growing and tightly curled hair, can be caused by a heterozygous mutation, p.Asn148Lys, within the helix initiation motif of the inner root sheath-specific *KRT74* gene in all affected family members. The mutant K74 protein disrupts keratin intermediate filament formation in cultured cells, probably in a dominant-negative manner. Of interest, the authors sequenced the mouse *Krt71-74* genes in mice with a phenotype reminiscent of ADWH, Caracul-like 4. They identified a heterozygous mutation, p.Glu440Lys, not in *Krt74* but in the neighbouring gene, *Krt71*. *Krt71* mutations cause the Caracul and reduced coat phenotypes, which are characterized by a wavy coat [51]. Curly-coated dogs and cats have a coding SNP in their *Krt71* genes [52,53]. Thus, it seems plausible that at least KRT74, and possibly also KRT71, might influence normal hair texture in humans.

As discussed, it is evident that expression of keratins in hair and nails must be tightly regulated. How cells achieve such control is poorly understood. It has been reported that the homeobox transcription factor HOXC13 is involved [54]. In support of a key role for this protein in controlling the expression of hard keratins, its loss leads to a hair-nail dysplasia (OMIM #614931) [55].

Monilethrix (OMIM #158000, *KRT81*, *KRT83*, *KRT85*)

Monilethrix is an autosomal dominant disorder characterized by beaded hair that breaks easily. This is most obvious on the occiput. Alopecia may be a presenting manifestation, but the phenotype is quite variable and ranges from extensive scarring alopecia to slight fraying without overt hair loss (Fig. 127.6a). Follicular hyperkeratosis is quite commonly associated. The beading is strictly periodic and results from narrowing of the hair shaft every 0.7mm. Its origin is unknown. It is a useful sign for diagnosis and should be sought when monilethrix is suspected. Polarization microscopy is useful to assist visualization, but dermoscopy will often suffice [56] (Fig 127.6b).

Classically, the disease is caused by mutations in the type II (basic) hair keratin genes *KRT81*, *83* and *86* [33–35]. The three genes are clustered within a 40kb region on chromosome 12q13.13. This interesting arrangement, with *KRT86* in between *KRT81* and *KRT83* and oriented in the opposite direction, suggests that they may have arisen by duplication from a single ancestral hard keratin gene, which may have been *KRT86*. Most patients reported to date have mutations in either *KRT81* or *86*. Because keratins exist as obligate heterodimers, it is logical to assume that there exist forms of monilethrix caused by mutations in acidic hard keratins. These are yet to be reported. Of note, an autosomal recessive form of hypotrichosis resembling monilethrix is associated with homozygous loss-of-function mutations in the *DSG4* gene, which codes for the desmosomal cadherin DSG4 [57–59].

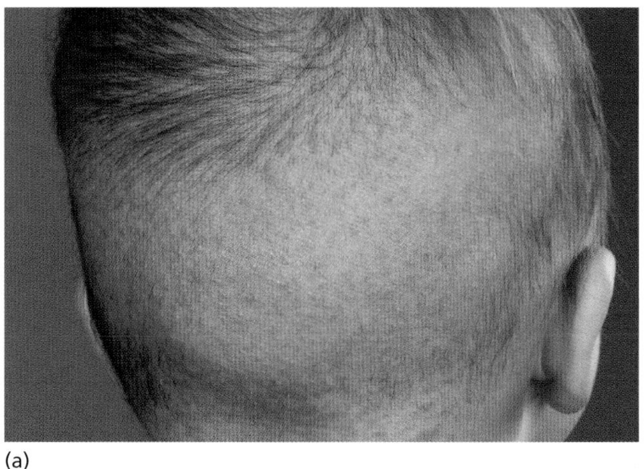

(a)

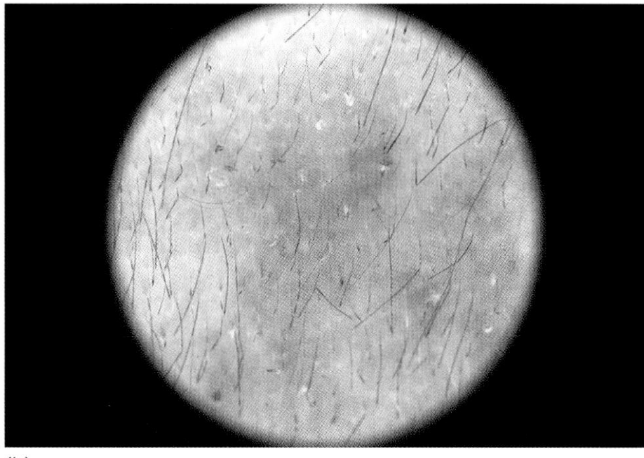

(b)

Fig. 127.6 Monilethrix. (a) Occipital hair loss with follicular hyperkeratosis. (b) Dermoscopy readily reveals the classic beading.

Pseudo-folliculitis barbae (OMIM 612318, *KRT75*)

Pseudo-folliculitis barbae, also known as pili incarnati or 'razor bumps', is a common disorder, in particular in persons with curly hair. Shaving against the grain, done to obtain a clean shave, is usually the precipitating factor. The short and sharp hairs produced by the razor penetrate the skin in an extra- or transfollicular manner. Ingrowing hairs cause a foreign body reaction and subsequent inflammation. The risk of developing pseudo-folliculitis is increased about fourfold in people carrying a polymorphism (A15T, alanine to threonine) in the companion-layer specific keratin K6hf, encoded by the gene *KRT75* [60].

Other diseases caused by keratin mutations

Keratins are expressed in a multitude of epithelia, including nonkeratinizing ones. Perhaps unsurprisingly, mutations in these keratins are also associated with disease. For example, cryptogenic and, in some cases, autoimmune cirrhosis of the liver can be associated with mutations in the *KRT8* or *KRT18* genes [61,62]. K8 mutations were later found to be associated with inflammatory bowel disease in some patients. The mutations were shown to be detrimental to K8/18 filament assembly [63]. Meesmann corneal dystrophy is an autosomal dominant disorder and characterized by fragility of the anterior corneal epithelium. It is caused by mutations in the type II keratin K3 or its partner, K12 [64].

The pace of discovery has slowed in the past few years, but still only 23 of the 54 known keratin genes are associated with a disease. It seems logical to assume that some of the remaining keratins will eventually be connected to epithelial disorders. These can be Mendelian but as for liver cirrhosis, the associations found may be risk factors. Several genome-wide association studies (GWAS) have found associations between genetic markers (SNPs) in the keratin loci and various disorders or traits (http://www.gwascentral.org/). The functional significance remains to be determined.

Conclusion

Given the present progress in our understanding of the basic biology of the keratin disorders, it can be expected that the near future will bring many more revelations. Disease classification is increasingly based on molecular data. Eponymous syndrome designations are disappearing and it is reasonable to expect that disorders thought to be distinct will prove to have the same molecular basis, and vice versa (see, for example, the expanding number of EBS variants). Patients increasingly benefit from our growing understanding of the mechanisms underlying their disease. For many disorders, prenatal diagnosis is possible. An accurate diagnosis is essential for reproductive counselling of patients and finding a mutation can confirm a clinical diagnosis.

Therapeutic interventions are still some way off, but progress is being made. In a patient with pachyonychia congenita, therapeutic gene silencing has been achieved by direct injection of therapeutic siRNA into a skin lesion [65]. Although this approach is not suitable for clinical use, the work did prove in principle that therapeutic gene modulation is feasible. The recently developed CRISPR/Cas9 technology promises therapeutic gene editing that could one day cure any genetic defect. Unfortunately, such interventions remain impractical for now. Skin penetration is still a major hurdle for large molecules, and systemic editing of gene defects is fraught with practical and ethical difficulties. As such, small molecule interventions directed towards cellular processes that are disrupted by mutant keratins may have a better chance of appearing in the clinic soon.

References

1 **McLean WHI, Irvine AD. Disorders of keratinisation: from rare to common genetic diseases of skin and other epithelial tissues. Ulster Med J 2007;76:72–82.**

2 **Kim S, Wong P, Coulombe PA. A keratin cytoskeletal protein regulates protein synthesis and epithelial cell growth. Nature 2006;441:362–5.**

3 Yu J, Yu DW, Checkla DM et al. Human hair keratins. J Invest Dermatol 1993;101:56S–59S.

4 Strelkov SV, Herrmann H, Aebi U. Molecular architecture of intermediate filaments. Bioessays 2003;25:243–51.

5 Herrmann H, Hesse M, Reichenzeller M et al. Functional complexity of intermediate filament cytoskeletons: from structure to assembly to gene ablation. Int Rev Cytol 2003;223:83–175.

6 **Hatzfeld M, Keil R, Magin TM. Desmosomes and Intermediate Filaments: Their Consequences for Tissue Mechanics. Cold Spring Harbor Perspectives in Biology 2017;9:a029157.**

7 Nahidiazar L, Kreft M, van den Broek B et al. The molecular architecture of hemidesmosomes, as revealed with super-resolution microscopy. J Cell Sci 2015;128:3714–9.

8 Janin A, Bauer D, Ratti F et al. Nuclear envelopathies: a complex LINC between nuclear envelope and pathology. Orphanet J Rare Dis 2017;12:147.

9 Kerns ML, Hakim JMC, Lu RG et al. Oxidative stress and dysfunctional NRF2 underlie pachyonychia congenita phenotypes. J Clin Invest 2016;126:2356–66.

10 Moll R, Divo M, Langbein L. The human keratins: biology and pathology. Histochem Cell Biol 2008;129:705–33.

11 Knapp AC, Franke WW, Heid H et al. Cytokeratin No. 9, an epidermal type I keratin characteristic of a special program of keratinocyte differentiation displaying body site specificity. J Cell Biol 1986;103:657–67.

12 Steinert PM, Marekov LN. The proteins elafin, filaggrin, keratin intermediate filaments, loricrin, and small proline-rich proteins 1 and 2 are isodipeptide cross-linked components of the human epidermal cornified cell envelope. J Biol Chem 1995;270:17702–11.

13 Ku N-O, Strnad P, Zhong B-H et al. Keratins let liver live: mutations predispose to liver disease and crosslinking generates Mallory-Denk bodies. Hepatology 2007;46:1639–49.

14 Szeverenyi I, Cassidy AJ, Chung CW et al. The Human Intermediate Filament Database: comprehensive information on a gene family involved in many human diseases. Hum Mutat 2008;29:351–60.

15 Fine J-D, Bruckner-Tuderman L, Eady RAJ et al. Inherited epidermolysis bullosa: updated recommendations on diagnosis and classification. J Am Acad Dermatol 2014;70:1103–26.

16 Uttam J, Hutton E, Coulombe PA et al. The genetic basis of epidermolysis bullosa simplex with mottled pigmentation. Proc Natl Acad Sci U S A 1996;93:9079–84.

17 Harel A, Bergman R, Indelman M, Sprecher E. Epidermolysis bullosa simplex with mottled pigmentation resulting from a recurrent mutation in KRT14. J Invest Dermatol 2006;126:1654–7.

18 McGrath JA, Stone KL, Begum R et al. Germline mutation in EXPH5 implicates the Rab27B effector protein Slac2-b in inherited skin fragility. Am J Hum Genet 2012;91:1115–21.

19 Sørensen CB, Andresen BS, Jensen UB et al. Functional testing of keratin 14 mutant proteins associated with the three major subtypes of epidermolysis bullosa simplex. Exp Dermatol 2003;12:472–9.

20 Lugassy J, Itin P, Ishida-Yamamoto A et al. Naegeli-Franceschetti-Jadassohn syndrome and dermatopathia pigmentosa reticularis: two allelic ectodermal dysplasias caused by dominant mutations in KRT14. Am J Hum Genet 2006;79:724–30.

21 Itin PH, Lautenschlager S, Meyer R et al. Natural history of the Naegeli-Franceschetti-Jadassohn syndrome and further delineation of its clinical manifestations. J Am Dermatol 1993;28:942–50.

22 Brar BK, Mehta V, Kubba A. Dermatopathia pigmentosa reticularis. Pediatr Dermatol 2007;24:566–70.

23 Bu TS, Kim YK, Whang KU. A case of dermatopathia pigmentosa reticularis. J Dermatol 1997;24:266–9.

24 Yoneda K, Furukawa T, Zheng Y-J et al. An autocrine/paracrine loop linking keratin 14 aggregates to tumor necrosis factor alpha-mediated cytotoxicity in a keratinocyte model of epidermolysis bullosa simplex. J Biol Chem 2004;279:7296–303.

25 Lugassy J, McGrath JA, Itin P et al. KRT14 haploinsufficiency results in increased susceptibility of keratinocytes to TNF-alpha-induced apoptosis and causes Naegeli-Franceschetti-Jadassohn syndrome. J Invest Dermatol 2008;128:1517–24.

26 Sprecher E, Indelman M, Khamaysi Z et al. Galli-Galli disease is an acantholytic variant of Dowling-Degos disease. Br J Dermatol 2007;156:572–4.

27 Betz RC, Planko L, Eigelshoven S et al. Loss-of-function mutations in the keratin 5 gene lead to Dowling-Degos disease. Am J Hum Genet 2006;78:510–9.

28 Li M, Cheng R, Liang J et al. Mutations in POFUT1, encoding protein O-fucosyltransferase 1, cause generalized Dowling-Degos disease. Am J Hum Genet 2013;92:895–903.

29 Basmanav FB, Oprisoreanu A-M, Pasternack SM et al. Mutations in POGLUT1, encoding protein O-glucosyltransferase 1, cause autosomal-dominant Dowling-Degos disease. Am J Hum Genet 2014;94:135–43.

30 Kumano K, Masuda S, Sata M et al. Both Notch1 and Notch2 contribute to the regulation of melanocyte homeostasis. Pigment Cell Melanoma Res 2008;21:70–8.

31 Moriyama M, Osawa M, Mak S-S et al. Notch signaling via Hes1 transcription factor maintains survival of melanoblasts and melanocyte stem cells. J Cell Biol 2006;173:333–9.

32 Morais P, Mota A, Baudrier T et al. Epidermolytic hyperkeratosis with palmoplantar keratoderma in a patient with KRT10 mutation. Eur J Dermatol 2009;19:333–6.

33 McLean WH, Eady RA, Dopping-Hepenstal PJ et al. Mutations in the rod 1A domain of keratins 1 and 10 in bullous congenital ichthyosiform erythroderma (BCIE). J Invest Dermatol 1994;102:24–30.

34 Nellen RGL, Nagtzaam IF, Hoogeboom AJM et al. Phenotypic variation in epidermolytic ichthyosis: clinical and functional evaluation of the novel p.(Met339Lys) mutation in the L12 domain of KRT1. Exp Dermatol 2015;24:883–5.

35 Rothnagel JA, Fisher MP, Axtell SM et al. A mutational hot spot in keratin 10 (KRT 10) in patients with epidermolytic hyperkeratosis. Hum Mol Genet 1993;2:2147–50.

36 Paller AS, Syder AJ, Chan YM et al. Genetic and clinical mosaicism in a type of epidermal nevus. N Engl J Med 1994;331:1408–15.

37 Tsubota A, Akiyama M, Sakai K et al. Keratin 1 gene mutation detected in epidermal nevus with epidermolytic hyperkeratosis. J Invest Dermatol 2007;127:1371–4.

38 Choate KA, Lu Y, Zhou J et al. Mitotic recombination in patients with ichthyosis causes reversion of dominant mutations in KRT10. Science 2010;330:94–7.

39 Choate KA, Lu Y, Zhou J et al. Frequent somatic reversion of KRT1 mutations in ichthyosis with confetti. J Clin Invest 2015;125:1703–7.

40 Rothnagel JA, Traupe H, Wojcik S et al. Mutations in the rod domain of keratin 2e in patients with ichthyosis bullosa of Siemens. Nature Genet 1994;7:485–90.

41 Scully C, Porter S. Orofacial disease: update for the dental clinical team: 3. White lesions. Dent Update 1999;26:123–9.

42 James WD, Lupton GP. Acquired dyskeratotic leukoplakia. Arch Dermatol 1988;124:117–20.

43 Rugg EL, McLean WH, Allison WE et al. A mutation in the mucosal keratin K4 is associated with oral white sponge nevus. Nature Genet 1995;11:450–2.

44 Richard G, De Laurenzi V, Didona B et al. Keratin 13 point mutation underlies the hereditary mucosal epithelial disorder white sponge nevus. Nature Genet 1995;11:453–5.

45 Happle R. What is a nevus? A proposed definition of a common medical term. Dermatology (Basel) 1995;191:1–5.

46 Pinheiro M, Freire-Maia N. Hair-nail dysplasia – a new pure autosomal dominant ectodermal dysplasia. Clin Genet 1992;41:296–8.

47 Barbareschi M, Cambiaghi S, Crupi AC, Tadini G. Family with 'pure' hair-nail ectodermal dysplasia. Am J Med Genet 1997;72:91–3.

48 Rasool M, Nawaz S, Azhar A et al. Autosomal recessive pure hair and nail ectodermal dysplasia linked to chromosome 12p11.1-q14.3 without KRTHB5 gene mutation. Eur J Dermatol 2010;20:443–6.

49 Naeem M, Wajid M, Lee K et al. A mutation in the hair matrix and cuticle keratin KRTHB5 gene causes ectodermal dysplasia of hair and nail type. J Med Genet 2006;43:274–9.

50 Shimomura Y, Wajid M, Petukhova L et al. Autosomal-dominant woolly hair resulting from disruption of keratin 74 (KRT74), a potential determinant of human hair texture. Am J Hum Genet 2010;86:632–8.

51 Kikkawa Y, Oyama A, Ishii R et al. A small deletion hotspot in the type II keratin gene mK6irs1/Krt2-6g on mouse chromosome 15, a candidate for causing the wavy hair of the caracul (Ca) mutation. Genetics 2003;165:721–33.

52 Cadieu E, Neff MW, Quignon P et al. Coat variation in the domestic dog is governed by variants in three genes. Science 2009;326:150–3.

53 Gandolfi B, Alhaddad H, Joslin SEK et al. A splice variant in KRT71 is associated with curly coat phenotype of Selkirk Rex cats. Sci Rep 2013;3:2000.

54 Jave-Suárez LF, Winter H, Langbein L et al. HOXC13 is involved in the regulation of human hair keratin gene expression. J Biol Chem 2002;277:3718–26.

55 Lin Z, Chen Q, Shi L et al. Loss-of-function mutations in HOXC13 cause pure hair and nail ectodermal dysplasia. Am J Hum Genet 2012;91:906–11.

56 Liu C-I, Hsu C-H. Rapid diagnosis of monilethrix using dermoscopy. Br J Dermatol 2008;159:741–3.

57 Zlotogorski A, Marek D, Horev L et al. An autosomal recessive form of monilethrix is caused by mutations in DSG4: clinical overlap with localized autosomal recessive hypotrichosis. J Invest Dermatol 2006;126:1292–6.

58 Schaffer JV, Bazzi H, Vitebsky A et al. Mutations in the desmoglein 4 gene underlie localized autosomal recessive hypotrichosis with monilethrix hairs and congenital scalp erosions. J Invest Dermatol 2006;126:1286–91.

59 Shimomura Y, Sakamoto F, Kariya N et al. Mutations in the desmoglein 4 gene are associated with monilethrix-like congenital hypotrichosis. J Invest Dermatol 2006;126:1281–5.
60 Winter H, Schissel D, Parry DAD et al. An unusual Ala12Thr polymorphism in the 1A alpha-helical segment of the companion layer-specific keratin K6hf: evidence for a risk factor in the etiology of the common hair disorder pseudofolliculitis barbae. J Invest Dermatol 2004;122:652–7.
61 Ku NO, Wright TL, Terrault NA et al. Mutation of human keratin 18 in association with cryptogenic cirrhosis. J Clin Invest 1997;99:19–23.
62 Ku NO, Gish R, Wright TL, Omary MB. Keratin 8 mutations in patients with cryptogenic liver disease. N Engl J Med 2001;344:1580–7.
63 Owens DW, Wilson NJ, Hill AJM et al. Human keratin 8 mutations that disturb filament assembly observed in inflammatory bowel disease patients. J Cell Sci 2004;117:1989–99.
64 Irvine AD, Corden LD, Swensson O et al. Mutations in cornea-specific keratin K3 or K12 genes cause Meesmann's corneal dystrophy. Nature Genet 1997;16:184–7.
65 Leachman SA, Hickerson RP, Schwartz ME et al. First-in-human mutation-targeted siRNA phase Ib trial of an inherited skin disorder. Mol Ther 2010;18:442–6.

CHAPTER 128

Mendelian Disorders of Cornification (MEDOC): The Keratodermas

Edel A. O'Toole

Department of Dermatology, Royal London Hospital, Barts Health NHS Trust and Centre for Cell Biology and Cutaneous Research, Barts and the London School of Medicine and Dentistry, London, UK

Introduction, 1524
History and clinical examination, 1525
Genetic diagnosis, 1525
Generic management, 1525
Diffuse hereditary palmoplantar keratodermas without associated features, 1525
Diffuse hereditary palmoplantar keratodermas with associated features, 1529
Focal hereditary palmoplantar keratodermas without associated features, 1537
Focal hereditary palmoplantar keratodermas with associated features, 1539
Papular hereditary palmoplantar keratodermas without associated features, 1545
Papular hereditary palmoplantar keratodermas with associated features, 1547
Palmoplantar keratodermas of uncertain identity, 1548

Abstract

This chapter focuses on the hereditary palmoplantar keratodermas (PPK), a heterogeneous group of disorders characterized by hyperkeratosis of palmoplantar skin. The PPKs can be divided into three groups according to the clinical pattern of the hyperkeratosis including diffuse, focal (which includes striate) and punctate PPK. Affected individuals may have a simple PPK without associated features, or a syndromic PPK with associated features, such as hearing loss, cardiomyopathy, hair, dentition or nail changes. In recent years, many causative genes of PPK have been identified, which has confirmed and/or altered the traditional clinical classification.

Key points

- The palmoplantar keratodermas (PPK) can be subdivided into three clinical patterns – diffuse, focal and punctate.
- The commonest PPK is diffuse epidermolytic PPK caused by *KRT9* mutations.
- Woolly hair and PPK may indicate the presence of desmosomal gene mutations causing cardiomyopathy. Associated hearing loss may suggest a mutation in connexin genes.
- For painful focal keratodermas, the current management includes paring down the calluses and appropriate footwear.
- Some PPKs are responsive to oral retinoids, but retinoids may increase skin fragility causing pain.
- Fungal superinfection is common and treatment can be beneficial.

Introduction

The palmoplantar keratodermas (PPKs) are a large and heterogeneous group of disorders characterized by excessive epidermal thickening of the palmoplantar skin. There are both hereditary and acquired forms. Examples of the latter category include psoriasis and pityriasis rubra pilaris.

Hereditary forms of PPK may occur as a sign of more generalized disorders, such as epidermolytic ichthyosis, autosomal recessive congenital ichthyosis, erythrokeratodermas and Darier disease. This chapter deals with the monogenic PPKs, with and without associated features. Among the former group, the PPK is one of the major findings and sometimes the hallmark of a congenital syndrome. Classification of the monogenic PPKs is often difficult because of inter- and intrafamilial variations, differences in nomenclature and the large number of reported cases.

Many authors have attempted to classify the hereditary forms [1–7]. In recent years, manifestations that were previously considered to be distinct entities have been shown to be variants of the same disease. Furthermore, the application of molecular biological techniques, such as mutation analysis of candidate genes and more recently exome sequencing, is increasingly leading to the reclassification of these diseases by showing that morphological distinctions made in the past often do not have a biological basis. The molecular classification is thus less complex than the clinical one. However, the clinical phenotype still guides the

Harper's Textbook of Pediatric Dermatology, Fourth Edition. Edited by Peter Hoeger, Veronica Kinsler and Albert Yan.

diagnostic process and mutation analysis is undertaken on the basis of the clinical diagnosis. The classification according to Greither still forms a useful starting point [3].

History and clinical examination

The most important features in the clinical classification of PPKs are the specific morphology and distribution of the hyperkeratosis or keratoderma (diffuse, focal, punctate/papular), the presence or absence of associated features (careful examination of the mucous membrane, nails, hair and the remainder of the skin is important) and the pattern of inheritance. It should always be kept in mind that the clinical features are often not fully expressed in early childhood. Additional criteria are the age at onset of the keratoderma, the severity of the disease process, association of fungal infection, response of the palmoplantar skin to water, associated hyperhidrosis and the histopathological findings. The author rarely biopsies children with PPK. However, a biopsy can be helpful in PPK to show epidermolysis, demonstrate loss of cell–cell adhesion suggestive of desmosomal disorders or to exclude inflammatory dermatoses.

Genetic diagnosis

For small genes such as keratins or connexins, if confident of the diagnosis, a single gene test, for example *KRT9* sequencing in diffuse epidermolytic PPK, is the most economical. However, next generation targeted sequencing panels are now becoming available for skin disorders and this is a good option if available locally. Pachyonychia Project (www.pachyonychia.org) currently offers a targeted panel of nine genes associated with focal keratoderma.

Generic management

Comfortable shoes and custom-made insoles are often helpful. In children with painful calluses, podiatry input to help with paring down calluses may be necessary. Sports socks that wick away moisture or Carnation silver socks can help if there is hyperhidrosis. Emollients to lubricate the skin and urea (up to 40%) to soften calluses also help. Some PPKs, for example Papillon–Lefevre are very responsive to oral retinoids. However, retinoids can also increase skin fragility which may be a problem in children with mutations in keratin genes, for example. In PPKs prone to fungal infection, a month of antifungal therapy every 6 months to a year can be useful.

An integrated approach is necessary for a correct diagnosis. The classification in this chapter is necessarily provisional and must be modified continually as new information becomes available. As a result, several entries have been updated and others removed since the last edition. New syndromes that have been described recently have been added. Note that disorders caused by deficiencies of desmosomal proteins, such as Naxos disease and Carvajal-Huerta syndrome (the cardiocutaneous diseases), can also be grouped with the palmoplantar keratoses. Because they are reviewed in another chapter (Chapter 134), these disorders will not be discussed further here.

The OMIM numbers accompanying several of the diseases refer to the online version of McKusick's Online Mendelian Inheritance in Man [8]. If the number is preceded by a '#', the causative gene defect is known.

References

1 Franceschetti A, Schnyder UW. Versuch einer klinisch-genetischen Klassifikation der hereditären Palmoplantarkeratosen unter Berücksichtigung assoziierter Symptome. Dermatologica 1960;120:154–78.
2 Schnyder UW, Klunker W. Erbliche verhornungsstörungen der Haut. In: Gottron HA, Schnyder UW (eds) Handbuch der Haut- und Geschlechtskrankeiten. Berlin: Springer, 1966:861–961.
3 Greither A. Erbliche Palmoplantarkeratosen. Hautarzt 1977;28: 395–403.
4 Voigtländer V, Schnyder UW. Palmoplantarkeratosen. In: Korting GW (ed.) Dermatologie in Praxis und Klinik. Stuttgart: Thieme Verlag, 1980:26–36.
5 Salamon T. An attempt at classification of inherited disorders of keratinization localized mainly, not exclusively on the palms and soles. Dermatol Monatsschr 1986;172:601–5.
6 **Lucker GPH, van de Kerkhof PCM, Steijlen PM. The hereditary palmoplantar keratoses: an updated review and classification. Br J Dermatol 1994;131:1–14.**
7 Stevens HP, Kelsell DP, Bryant SP et al. Linkage of an American pedigree with palmoplantar keratoderma and malignancy (palmo-plantar ectodermal dysplasia type III) to 17q24. Literature survey and proposed updated classification of the keratodermas. Arch Dermatol 1996;132:640–51.
8 OMIM. Online Mendelian Inheritance in Man: available via www.ncbi.nlm.nih.gov/omim/

Diffuse hereditary palmoplantar keratodermas without associated features

Diffuse epidermolytic palmoplantar keratoderma (OMIM #144200, *KRT9, KRT1*)

Syn.
- Palmoplantar keratoderma cum degeneratione granulosa Vörner
- Palmoplantar keratoderma type Thost
- Palmoplantar keratoderma type Unna
- Norbotten-type palmoplantar keratoderma

Brief introduction and history. In 1909, Vörner [1] described a diffuse PPK that was histologically characterized by epidermolytic hyperkeratosis (granular degeneration or epidermolysis). Küster and Becker [2] re-examined the family described by Thost clinically and histologically and demonstrated that the PPK in this family was identical to that described by Vörner. In fact, Vörner described the PPK of Unna and Thost. In 1994, Reis and colleagues [3] elucidated the cause of this disease by identifying mutations in the gene coding for keratin 9.

Epidemiology and pathogenesis. Diffuse epidermolytic PPK is the most common PPK. A prevalence of 4.4 per 100 000 was found in Northern Ireland [4]. It is an autosomal dominant disease and is most commonly caused by point mutations in the gene coding for keratin 9, which lies on chromosome 17q12–21 [3]. Keratin 1 (*KRT1*) gene mutations have also been described [4]. Both keratin 9 and keratin 1 are expressed in the suprabasal layer of the epidermis. Keratin 9 is expressed preferentially in palmoplantar skin [5].

Dominant pathogenic mutations in keratin disrupt intermediate filament assembly reducing the resilience of the cytoskeleton, leading to epidermolysis and hyperkeratosis [6]. Disruption of signalling pathways and endoplasmic reticulum stress are likely to contribute to the hyperkeratosis. The keratin 9 null mouse has both hyperkeratosis and impaired differentiation with induction of the stress-associated keratins, keratin 6 and 16 [7].

Clinical features (Fig. 128.1). The typical Vörner hyperkeratosis is diffuse, non-transgrediens keratoderma and has a brown-yellow colour with sometimes a greyish hue. Fissuring may be evident. There can be accentuation on areas subjected to stress, such as the Achilles tendon. There is usually a sharp demarcation and an erythematous edge. Sometimes there is pitted keratolysis, particularly on the feet. This may be indicative of a *Corynebacterium minutissimum* infection. Knuckle pads have been reported [8]. Onset is in infancy. Rarely, symptoms may appear in adulthood.

Differential diagnosis. PPK type Vörner can sometimes be differentiated from the other diffuse types of PPK by the histopathological characteristics of epidermolytic hyperkeratosis. Usually, associated features and the phenotype will suffice to establish the diagnosis, as well as examination of a parent. This can be difficult in the case of epidermolytic ichthyosis where some *KRT1* mutations can result in very mild or even absent blistering in friction areas, associated with a PPK that is indistinguishable from Vörner type. Considering that keratin 1 pairs with keratin 9 in palmoplantar skin, this is not suprising. Mutation analysis is required to establish the diagnosis in such cases.

Laboratory and histology findings. The author does not recommend biopsy for a clinically evident epidermolytic type PPK in a child. When in doubt as to the diagnosis, mutation analysis for *KRT9* can be performed. Occasionally a biopsy may be required and then epidermolytic changes should be specifically sought. It is characterized by perinuclear vacuolization, large keratohyaline granules, clumping of tonofilaments, cellular degeneration in spinous and granular cells and sometimes blister formation [9].

Treatment. Patients can be helped by the application of keratolytics such as salicylic acid (contraindicated in very young children), urea, lactic acid and propylene glycol in white soft paraffin, as a gel or an ointment. Occlusion under polyethylene (clingfilm) is often more beneficial. Topical retinoids have some effect but can cause irritation. Systemic retinoids such as acitretin are more effective, but can increase skin fragility [10]. Because of possible side-effects and teratogenicity, systemic retinoids should be prescribed only after serious consideration. Fungal and bacterial superinfections should be treated adequately, if necessary using systemic therapy. The majority of patients eventually discontinue their treatment because they have come to depend on the mechanical barrier that their hyperkeratosis provides. For the future, small inhibitory RNA therapy is a possibility [11].

References

1 Vörner H. Zur Kenntnis des Keratoma hereditarium palmare et plantare. Arch Derm Syph (Berlin) 1901;56:3–31.

2 Kuster W, Becker A. Indication for the identity of palmoplantar keratoderma type Unna–Thost with type Vorner. Thost's family revisited 110 years later. Acta Derm Venereol 1992;72:120–2.

3 **Reis A, Hennies HC, Langbein L et al. Keratin 9 gene mutations in epidermolytic palmoplantar keratoderma (EPPK). Nat Genet 1994;6:174–9.**

4 Smith F. The molecular genetics of keratin disorders. Am J Clin Dermatol 2003;4:347–64.

5 Langbein L, Heid HW, Moll I et al. Molecular characterization of the body site-specific human epidermal cytokeratin 9: cDNA cloning, amino

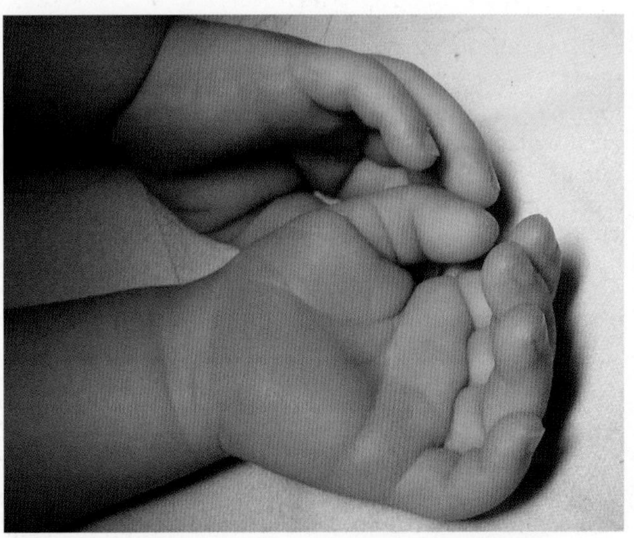
(a)

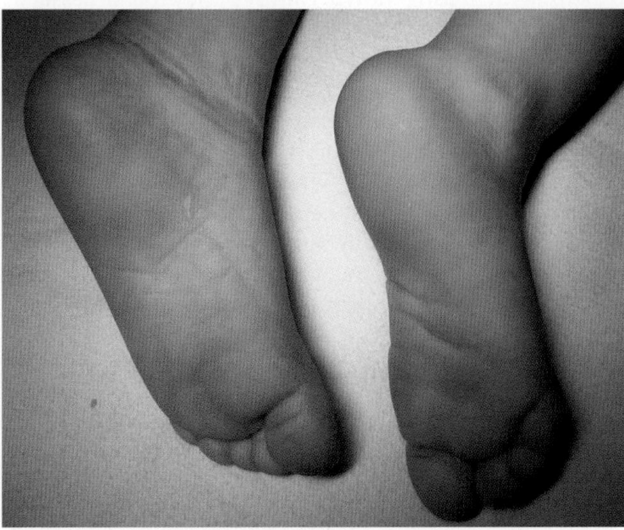
(b)

Fig. 128.1 Diffuse epidermolytic palmoplantar keratoderma in a child with *KRT9* mutation. (a) Palms and (b) soles.

acid sequence, and tissue specificity of gene expression. Differentiation 1994;55:164.
6 Magin TM, Vijayaraj P, Leube RE. Structural and regulatory functions of keratins. Exp Cell Res 2007;313:2021–32.
7 Fu DJ, Thomson C, Lunny DP et al. Keratin 9 is required for the structural integrity and terminal differentiation of the palmoplantar epidermis. J Invest Dermatol 2014;134:754–63.
8 Nogita T, Nakagawa H, Ishibashi Y. Hereditary epidermolytic palmoplantar keratoderma with knuckle pad-like lesions over the finger joints. Br J Dermatol 1991;125:496.
9 Navsaria HA, Swensson O, Ratnavel RC et al. Ultrastructural changes resulting from keratin-9 gene mutations in two families with epidermolytic palmoplantar keratoderma. J Invest Dermatol 1995;104:425–9.
10 Happle R, van de Kerkhof PC, Traupe H. Retinoids in disorders of keratinization: their use in adults. Dermatologica 1987;175(suppl 1): 107–24.
11 Leslie Pedrioli DM, Fu DJ, Gonzalez-Gonzalez E et al. Generic and personalized RNAi-based therapeutics for a dominant-negative epidermal fragility disorder. J Invest Dermatol 2012;132:1627–35.

Diffuse nonepidermolytic palmoplantar keratoderma

Introduction

Nonepidermolytic PPK usually refers to nonsyndromic forms of diffuse keratoderma that do not show epidermolysis in the upper spinous or granular layers histologically. At least three types can be distinguished: nonepidermolytic PPK type Bothnia, nonepidermolytic PPK type Nagashima and Mal de Meleda.

Nonepidermolytic PPK type Bothnia (OMIM #600231, *AQP5*)

Syn.
- Nonepidermolytic palmoplantar tylosis

Brief introduction and history. The original families described were from Bothnia in northern Sweden where there is a prevalence of 0.3–0.5% [1].

Epidemiology and pathogenesis. Using linkage analysis and exome sequencing in families from Sweden and the UK, this form of nonepidermolytic PPK (NEPPK) was shown to be caused by dominant missense mutation in the *AQP5* gene [2], which encodes the water channel protein, aquaporin 5. Aquaporins allow osmotic transport of water across cell membranes. In the skin, aquaporin 5 localizes to the plasma membrane of the keratinocytes in the granular layer of the epidermis. Mutations in *AQP5* cause the keratinocytes to have increased water uptake resulting in a white spongy appearance of palmar skin when patients immerse their hands in water. Palmar acetylated alpha-tubulin expression is increased in patient palmar skin compared with control, suggesting increased levels of microtubule stabilization in NEPPK palmar epidermis [2].

Clinical features. Typically, there is a smooth, waxy yellow hyperkeratosis affecting the palms and soles from infancy. There can be an erythematous margin, sometimes with a papular border. Hyperhidrosis is common with associated tinea superinfection which can cause a transgradiens, scaly erythema on the distal fingers (Fig. 128.2). The nails can be thickened and curved.

Differential diagnosis. The differential diagnosis will include mild Mal de Meleda keratoderma, diffuse epidermolytic PPK and aquagenic PPK. The persisting spongy appearance after immersion in water and the presence of tinea can be discriminating, but in early childhood it can be difficult to differentiate diffuse nonepidermolytic PPK (DNEPPK) from diffuse epidermolytic PPK (DEPPK). Examining an affected parent can be helpful.

Laboratory and histology findings. A skin biopsy will show acanthosis and hyperkeratosis without epidermolysis.

Treatment. Keratolytic measures can be helpful. Fungal infections should be treated with systemic therapy. Some patients benefit from 4 weeks of antifungal therapy annually. Topical macrolides may be helpful if there is pitted keratolysis. Low dose systemic retinoids can also help but are usually not necessary in children.

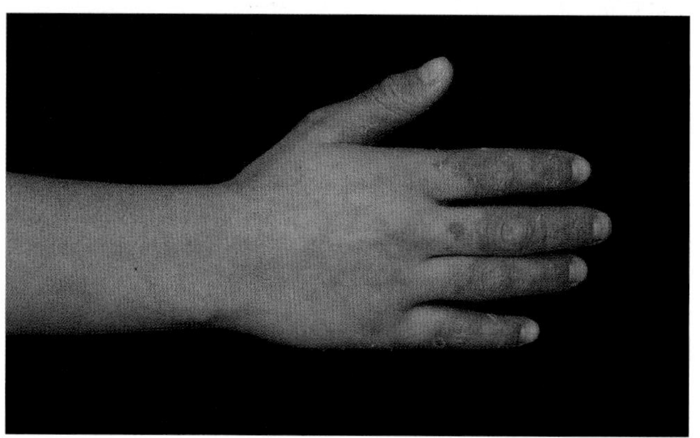
(a)

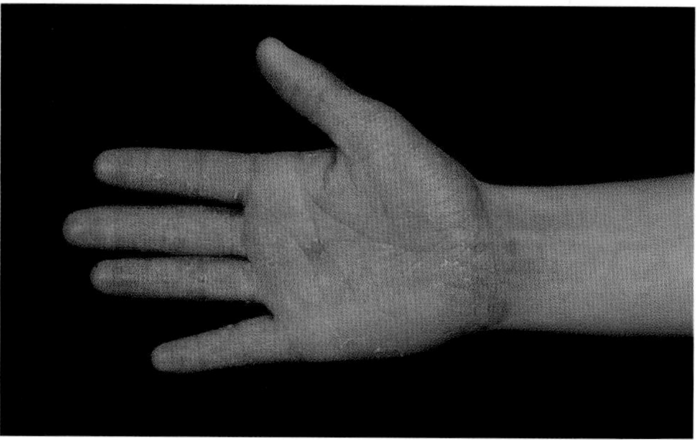
(b)

Fig. 128.2 Tinea infection in a 14-year-old girl with palmoplantar keratoderma Bothnia caused by an *AQ5* mutation. (a) Dorsum of hands and (b) palms.

References

1 Lind L, Lundström A, Hofer PA et al. The gene for diffuse palmoplantar keratoderma of the type found in northern Sweden is localized to chromosome 12q11-q13. Hum Mol Genet 1994;3:1789–93.

2 **Blaydon DC, Lind LK, Plagnol V et al. Mutations in *AQP5*, encoding a water-channel protein, cause autosomal-dominant diffuse nonepidermolytic palmoplantar keratoderma. Am J Hum Genet 2013;93:330–5.**

Nonepidermolytic PPK type Nagashima (OMIM #603357, *SERPINB7*)

Brief introduction and history. PPK Nagashima (PPKN) is an autosomal recessive PPK originally described in the Japanese literature by Nagashima in 1977 and subsequently in the English literature [1]. To date, it has only been described in Japanese and Chinese families [2–4].

Epidemiology and pathogenesis. The estimated prevalence of PPKN in the Japanese population is 1.2/10000 [2]. Whole exome sequencing in three unrelated Japanese patients with PPKN identified homozygous or compound heterozygous mutations in the *SERPINB7* gene in all three patients, which were confirmed by Sanger sequencing [2]. Analysis of *SERPINB7* in 10 additional unrelated Japanese individuals with PPKN revealed homozygosity or compound heterozygosity for the same mutations identified in the initial three patients. All of the patients carried the nonsense mutation R266X on at least one allele suggesting that this is a founder mutation causing PPKN in Asian populations [2–4].

Clinical features (Fig. 128.3). There is mild hyperkeratosis with a striking erythema extending onto the dorsum of the fingers, flexor aspect of the wrist and the dorsal surface of the feet. Hyperkeratosis on the ear lobes, elbows and knees has also been described. The palmar and plantar skin becomes white and spongy on immersion in water. Hyperhidrosis and dermatophyte infection are additional features.

Differential diagnosis. The differential diagnosis will include other nonepidermolytic PPKs, in particular PPK caused by mutations in *AQP5*, and the erythrokeratodermas.

Laboratory and histology findings. Biopsy of palmopantar skin shows acanthosis of the epidermis with orthokeratotic hyperkeratosis and hypergranulosis.

Treatment. Keratolytic measures and antifungal treatment (topical and/or systemic) can be helpful. If hyperhidrosis is a problem, anticholinergic medications can be tried in teenagers and young adults.

References

1 Kabashima K, Sakabe J, Yamada Y et al. 'Nagashima-type' keratosis as a novel entity in the palmoplantar keratoderma category. Arch Dermatol 2008;144:375–9.

2 **Kubo A, Shiohama A, Sasaki T et al. Mutations in *SERPINB7*, encoding a member of the serine protease inhibitor superfamily, cause Nagashima-type palmoplantar keratosis. Am J Hum Genet 2013;93: 945–56.**

3 Mizuno O, Nomura T, Suzuki S et al. Highly prevalent *SERPINB7* founder mutation causes pseudodominant inheritance pattern in Nagashima-type palmoplantar keratosis. Br J Dermatol 2014;171: 847–53.

4 Yin J. Xu G, Wang H et al. New and recurrent *SERPINB7* mutations in seven Chinese patients with Nagashima-type palmoplantar keratosis. J Invest Dermatol 2014;134:2269–72.

Mal de Meleda (OMIM #248300, *ARS*)

Syn.
- Meleda disease
- Mal de Mljet
- Keratosis extremitatum hereditaria transgrediens et progrediens
- Keratoderma palmoplantaris transgrediens

Brief introduction and history. This rare PPK was first described by Hovarka anad Ehlers in 1897 and further delineated by, among others, Brunner and Fuhrman in 1950 and Franceschetti and colleagues in 1972 [1–3]. The disorder takes its name from the Croatian island of Mljet (Meleda), where it is unusually frequent as a result of parental relatedness.

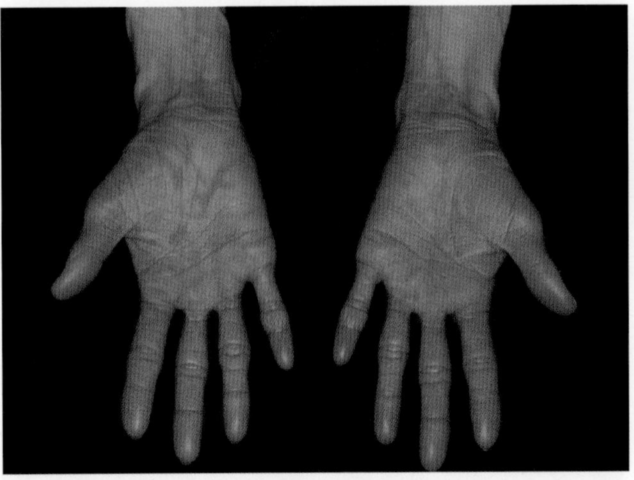
(a)

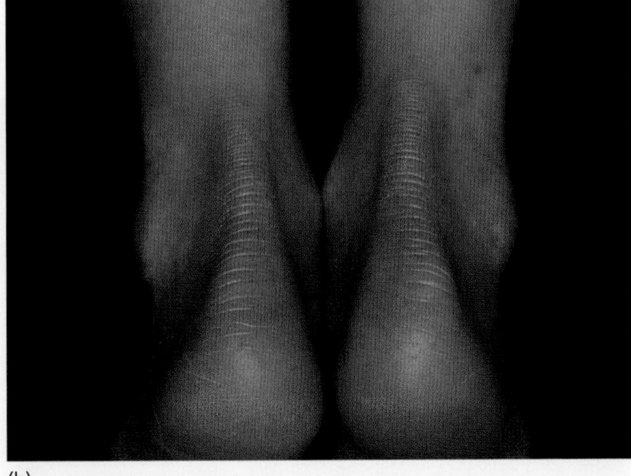
(b)

Fig. 128.3 Diffuse palmoplantar keratoderma Nagashima with (a) mild palmar keratoderma with striking erythema and (b) extension of plantar keratoderma onto the Achilles tendon. Source: Courtesy of Dr Akiharu Kubo, Keio University Hospital, Japan.

Epidemiology and pathogenesis. The inheritance is autosomal recessive. Fischer and colleagues [4] demonstrated that Mal de Meleda is associated with mutations in the *ARS* gene on chromosome 8q24.3 encoding the SLURP-1 (for secreted Ly6/uPAR-related protein-1) protein, a member of the Ly-6/uPAR protein family and homologous to snake venom and frog neurotoxins. The structure of the protein suggests that it may act as a neuromodulator in skin and SLURP-1 modulates the action of acetylcholine receptors present on keratinocytes [5,6]. It also has proapoptotic activity [6] and may play a role in regulating tumour necrosis factor (TNF)-α release by skin macrophages [5]. Involvement of acetylcholine signalling in the disorder is conceptually consistent with the hyperhidrosis. There is a founder effect in the Mediterranean basin with relatively few mutations, that is the mutation arose in a common ancestor of populations that later migrated and was maintained by inbreeding [4].

Clinical features. Mal de Meleda is characterized by a diffuse, thick, white to yellow, macerated-looking hyperkeratosis (Fig. 128.4) with a prominent transgredient erythematous border. The thick hyperkeratosis may lead to flexion contractures. The disease has its onset in early infancy and follows a progressive course with extension onto the dorsal surfaces. Constricting bands surrounding the digits are typical, resulting rarely in spontaneous amputation of the digits [7]. Concomitant lesions can be found at other sites, especially the elbows and knees [4]. Perioral erythema and hyperkeratosis may be present [8], resembling the clinical features of Olmsted's syndrome. Hyperhidrosis of the affected parts, with maceration, bacterial or fungal superinfection and the consequent stale odour, is pronounced. Examination with a Wood's lamp is recommended. Nail changes (koilonychia, nail thickening, subungual hyperkeratosis) can be present.

Differential diagnosis. It may be difficult to distinguish Mal de Meleda PPK from either Vörner or Olmsted PPK, in particular in very young children. Keratoderma of Gamborg–Nielsen mainly described in Scandinavia is now known to be also caused by mutations in ARS and thus is a milder variant of Mal de Meleda PPK [9].

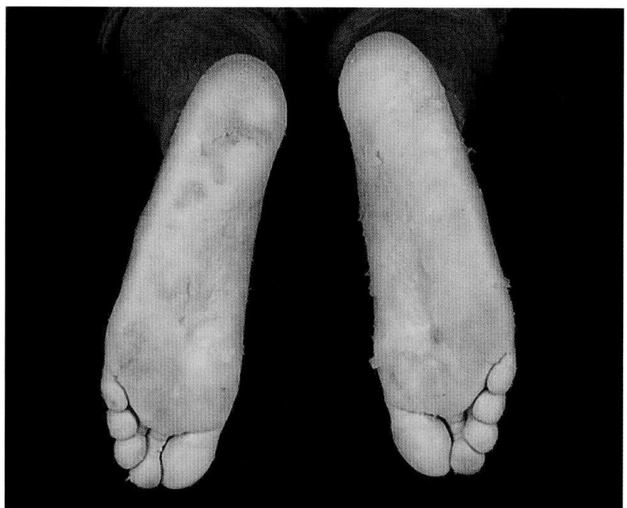

Fig. 128.4 Macerated diffuse keratoderma of Mal de Meleda.

Laboratory and histology findings. The histological findings include hyperkeratosis with some parakeratosis, prominence of the stratum lucidum and marked acanthosis. A prominent perivascular mononuclear infiltrate is often present.

Treatment. A good response to retinoids, including alitretinoin, has been reported [10,11], especially a reduction in the hyperkeratosis, but the erythema may become more prominent. Any bacterial or fungal superinfection should be treated, if possible with topical agents. The distinctive odour often improves after such interventions. The hyperhidrosis might result from alterations in acetylcholine signalling. Topical agents such as aluminium chloride may be useful.

References

1 Hovorka O, Ehlers E. Meledakrankheit. Arch Derm Syph 1896;34:51.
2 Brunner MJ, Fuhrman DL. Mal de Meleda. Report of a case and results of treatment with vitamin A. Arch Derm Syph 1950;61:820–3.
3 Franceschetti AT, Reinhart V, Schnyder UW. La maladie de Meleda. J Genet Hum 1972;20:267–96.
4 Fischer J, Bouadjar B, Heilig R et al. Mutations in the gene encoding SLURP-1 in Mal de Meleda. Hum Mol Genet 2001;10:875–80.
5 Chimienti F, Hogg RC, Plantard L et al. Identification of SLURP-1 as an epidermal neuromodulator explains the clinical phenotype of Mal de Meleda. Hum Mol Genet 2003;12:3017–24.
6 Arredondo J, Chernyavsky A, Webber R et al. Biological effects of SLURP-1 on human keratinocytes. J Invest Dermatol 2005;125:1236–41.
7 Degos MMR, Delort J, Charlas J. Ainhum avec kératodermie palmoplantaire. Bull Soc Fr Dermatol Syphiligr 1963;70:136–8.
8 Lestringant GG, Hadi SM, Qayed KI et al. Mal de Meleda: recessive transgressive palmoplantar keratoderma with three unusual facultative features. Dermatology 1992;184:78–82.
9 Zhao L, Vahlquist A, Virtanen M et al. Palmoplantar keratoderma of the Gamborg-Nielsen type is caused by mutations in the *SLURP1* gene and represents a variant of Mal de Meleda. Acta Derm Venereol 2014;94:707–10.
10 Van de Kerkhof PC, van Dooren-Greebe RJ, Steijlen PM. Acitretin in the treatment of Mal de Meleda. Br J Dermatol 1992;127:191–2.
11 Park HK, Kim EJ, Ko JY. Alitretinoin: treatment for refractory palmoplantar keratoderma. Br J Dermatol 2016;174:1143–4.

Diffuse hereditary palmoplantar keratodermas with associated features

Loricrin keratoderma (OMIM #604117, *LOR*)

Syn.
- Progressive symmetrical erythrokeratoderma
- Camisa variant of Vohwinkel syndrome

Brief introduction and history. This rare disorder was originally reported by Camisa and Rosana *et al.* as a variant of Vohwinkel syndrome [1]. They described a diffuse honeycomb keratoderma with annular constrictions around the digits, with mild ichthyosis. In true Vohwinkel syndrome there is hearing loss, but no ichthyosis. The first

LOR mutation defining this disorder as a separate entity was reported in 1996 by Maestrini *et al.* who likewise called this entity Vohwinkel syndrome [2]. Further confusion resulted from a report describing the finding of loricrin mutations in progressive symmetrical erythrokeratoderma, which is a manifestation of the erythrokeratodermas [3]. Loricrin mutations are therefore associated with a recognizable entity that we will refer to as 'loricrin keratoderma'.

Epidemiology and pathogenesis. Loricrin keratoderma is a rare autosomal dominant keratoderma with about 20 families reported in the literature. It is caused by insertion or deletion mutations in the *LOR* gene [2,4]. The commonest insertion results in extension of the loricrin peptide by 22 amino acids. The gene is in the epidermal differentiation complex on chromosome 1q21. Loricrin is a major component of the cornified envelope and contains three glycine-rich domains interspersed with glutamine-rich motifs. Thus, loricrin is thought to function as a major component of transglutaminase-formed cross-links in the cornified envelope [5]. The mutant protein is transported to the nucleus which is thought to interfere with regulation of formation of the cornified envelope [6]. Mice expressing a pathogenic loricrin mutation have generalized scaling, thickened footpads and autoamputation of the tail caused by a constricting band [7].

Clinical features. Loricrin keratoderma can rarely present as a collodion baby. It typically manifests in early childhood with nonmigratory erythematous sharply demarcated plaques of thickened skin over the extensor surfaces of large joints (Fig. 128.5). The associated PPK is usually diffuse, classically with a honeycomb pattern, transgrediens and can be quite erythematous. Pseudo-ainhum and extension onto the wrist and ankles can occur. Knuckle pads have also been reported [8]. Truncal ichthyosis is prominent in some patients. Importantly, hearing loss is absent.

Differential diagnosis. The disorder must be distinguished from Vohwinkel syndrome. The keratoderma in the latter is limited to the hands and feet and can show smooth palmoplantar hyperkeratosis. The major distinguishing feature is the hearing loss. Erythrokeratoderma variabilis can be a consideration but the migratory nature of hyperkeratotic plaques usually distinguishes this particular disorder. A rare disorder called KLICK syndrome (*vide infra*) can be potentially confused with loricrin keratoderma.

Laboratory and histology findings. Histological features include hypergranulosis, parakeratosis (retained nuclei in the stratum corneum), psoriasiform epidermal hyperplasia and a perivascular lymphocytic infitrate. Electron microscopy is more informative, showing intranuclear granules in upper granular layer cells and a conspicuous transitional cell layer. The cornified envelope is abnormal, containing lipid droplets and a lack of increase in thickness of cell envelopes [9].

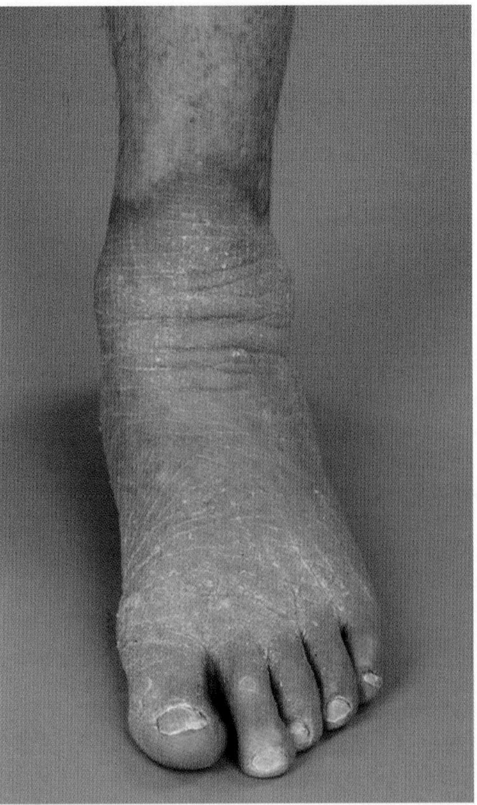

Fig. 128.5 Typical flexural erythema, thickening and scale of loricrin keratoderma.

Treatment. Topical keratinolytic agents are of limited use. Emollients can be helpful. It is worth trying topical vitamin D3 or retinoids but their effect in our experience is limited. Systemic retinoids can also be tried.

References

1 Camisa C, Rossana C. Variant of keratoderma hereditaria mutilans (Vohwinkel's syndrome). Treatment with orally administered isotretinoin. Arch Dermatol 1984;120:1323–8.

2 Maestrini E, Monaco AP, McGrath JA et al. A molecular defect in loricrin, the major component of the cornified cell envelope, underlies Vohwinkel's syndrome. Nat Genet 1996;13:70–7.

3 **Ishida-Yamamoto A, McGrath JA, Lam H et al. The molecular pathology of progressive symmetric erythrokeratoderma: a frameshift mutation in the loricrin gene and perturbations in the cornified cell envelope. Am J Hum Genet 1997;61:581–9.**

4 Kinsler VA, Drury S, Khan A et al. A novel microdeletion in *LOR* causing autosomal dominant loricrin keratoderma. Br J Dermatol 2015; 172:262–4.

5 Hitomi K. Transglutaminases in skin epidermis. Eur J Dermatol 2005; 15:313–19.

6 Ishida-Yamamoto A. Loricrin keratoderma: a novel disease entity characterized by nuclear accumulation of mutant loricrin. J Dermatol Sci 2003;31:3–8.

7 Koch PJ, de Viragh PA, Scharer E et al. Lessons from loricrin-deficient mice: compensatory mechanisms maintaining skin barrier function in the absence of a major cornified envelope protein. J Cell Biol 2000;151: 389–400.

8 Pohler E, Cunningham F, Sandilands A et al. Novel autosomal dominant mutation in loricrin presenting as prominent ichthyosis. Br J Dermatol 2015;173:1291–4.

9 Schmuth M, Fluhr JW, Crumrine DC et al. Structural and functional consequences of loricrin mutations in human loricrin keratoderma (Vohwinkel syndrome with ichthyosis). J Invest Dermatol 2004;122: 909–22.

Keratosis linearis with ichthyosis congenita and sclerosing keratoderma (KLICK) syndrome (OMIM #601952, 613386, *POMP*)

Brief introduction and history. In 1989, Pujol and colleagues described this rare entity in four Spanish siblings [1]. It was later further defined by Vahlquist and colleagues in an isolated case [2]. They coined the 'KLICK' acronym. A further case was reported from Holland [3].

Epidemiology/pathogenesis. Inheritance is autosomal recessive. All patients reported to date have the same causative mutation affecting the 5′ UTR of the *POMP* (proteasome maturation protein) gene on chromosome 13q [4]. POMP codes for a component of the proteasome which is the cellular machine for breaking down degraded, misfolded or otherwise nonfunctional proteins. In KLICK, proteasomal distribution in the upper epidermis is altered. As a result, protein breakdown is disturbed with resulting endoplasmic reticulum stress and hyperkeratosis.

Clinical features. The disorder typically presents with generalized erythroderma and fine scaling in early childhood. Erosions can also occur. Later, a diffuse PPK with constricting bands develops in addition to linear or starfish-shaped keratoderma affecting both flexor and extensor sides of large joints (Fig. 128.6). There are no other anomalies.

Differential diagnosis. The KLICK syndrome must be primarily distinguished from loricrin keratoderma. Clues to the diagnosis include PPK, which in KLICK is smooth without honeycombing, and the morphology of the flexural hyperkeratosis, which is typical.

Laboratory investigation and pathology. Palmoplantar skin histology is nonspecific showing orthohyperkeratosis and epithelial hyperplasia with hypergranulosis. Electron microscopy shows numerous large keratohyaline granules in superficial keratinocytes

Treatment. Topical emollients and keratolytics are not very effective. Acitretin can give satisfactory improvement of both the ichthyosis and the keratoderma [3].

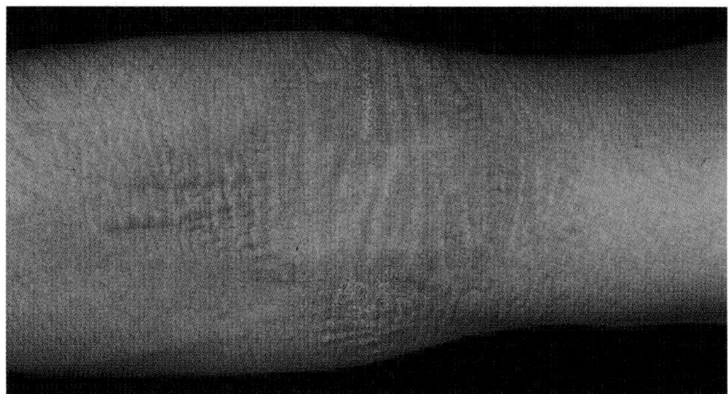

Fig. 128.6 Vertical, linear, flexural hyperkeratosis of KLICK syndrome.

References

1 Pujol RM, Moreno A, Alomar A et al. Congenital ichthyosiform dermatosis with linear keratotic flexural papules and sclerosing palmoplantar keratoderma. Arch Dermatol 1989;125:103–6.

2 Vahlquist A, Ponten F, Pettersson A. Keratosis linearis with ichthyosis congenita and sclerosing keratoderma (KLICK syndrome): a rare, autosomal recessive disorder of keratohyaline formation? Acta Derm Venereol 1997;77:225–7.

3 Van Steensel MA, van Geel M, Steijlen PM. A new type of erythrokeratoderma. Br J Dermatol 2005;152:155–8.

4 Dahlqvist J, Klar J, Tiwari N et al. A single-nucleotide deletion in the *POMP* 5′ UTR causes a transcriptional switch and altered epidermal proteasome distribution in KLICK genodermatosis. Am J Hum Genet 2010;86:596–603.

Palmoplantar keratoderma with scleroatrophy (Huriez syndrome) (OMIM 181600)

Brief introduction and history. This cancer-associated syndrome was first described by Huriez and colleagues [1,2] in two families resident in the north of France.

Epidemiology and pathogenesis. The condition is inherited in an autosomal dominant manner. There is a report of linkage to chromosome 4q23 [3]. There are several candidate genes in this region, but no pathogenic mutations have been identified to date. It is notable that a case of Huriez syndrome with 46, XX sex reversal has been published [4]. This was found to be caused by mutations in the *RSPO1* gene, coding for R-Spondin1, a member of the Wingless (Wnt) signalling family associated with malignancy and disturbance of epidermal and nail development [5].

Clinical features. The palmopantar findings are visible from the neonatal period. The PPK consists of discrete areas of hyperkeratosis with atrophy, diffusely covering especially the palmar skin. The plantar skin usually displays less severe involvement. Atrophic plaques may be found on the dorsa of the hands and fingers. The affected skin usually is erythematous. Sclerodactyly is present which is pseudosclerodermatous. Nail changes consist of aplasia, ridging and clubbing. Hypohidrosis is associated in half of the cases. The distinctive feature of this syndrome is the risk of development of squamous cell carcinoma on the affected skin, which may occur as early as the third or fourth decade.

Laboratory investigation and pathology. The epidermal Langerhans cells are virtually absent from the involved skin only [6]. There is compacting of dermal collagen with dilated vessels.

Treatment. Treatment with oral retinoids should be considered [7].

References

1 Huriez CL, Agache P, Bombart M et al. Epithéliomas spinocellulaires sur atrophie cutanée congénitale dans deux familles à morbidité canc éreuse élevée. Bull Soc Fr Dermatol Syphiligr 1963;70:24–8.

2 Huriez CL, Agache P, Souillart F et al. Scléroatrophie familiale des extrémités avec dégénérescence cellulaires multiples. Bull Soc Fr Dermatol Syphiligr 1963;70:743–4.

SECTION 27: DISORDERS OF KERATIN AND KERATINIZATION

3 Lee YA, Stevens HP, Delaporte E et al. A gene for an autosomal dominant scleroatrophic syndrome predisposing to skin cancer (Huriez syndrome) maps to chromosome 4q23. Am J Hum Genet 2000;66:326–30.
4 Vernole P, Terrinoni A, Didona B et al. An SRY-negative XX male with Huriez syndrome. Clin Genet 2000;57:61–6.
5 Parma P, Radi O, Vidal V et al. R-spondin1 is essential in sex determination, skin differentiation and malignancy. Nat Genet 2006; 38:1304–9.
6 Hamm H, Traupe H, Brocker EB et al. The scleroatrophic syndrome of Huriez: a cancer-prone genodermatosis. Br J Dermatol 1996;134:512–18.
7 Keratoderma with scleroatrophy of the extremities or sclerotylosis (Huriez syndrome): a reappraisal. Br J Dermatol 1995;133:409–16.

Palmoplantar hyperkeratosis with squamous cell carcinoma of skin and sex reversal (OMIM #610644, *RSPO1*)

Syn.

- Palmoplantar hyperkeratosis and true hermaphroditism

Brief introduction and history. This possibly unique entity was first reported as Huriez syndrome with 46, XX sex reversal [1, 2]. In 2005, four brothers from a consanguineous family, including the patient described by Guerriero and colleagues [2], were reported as having a 46, XX karyotype, with palmoplantar keratosis and predisposition to squamous cell carcinoma of the skin [3].

Epidemiology and pathogenesis. Homozygosity mapping in the individuals reported in 2005 led to the finding of a homozgous single-nucleotide insertion in the *RSPO1* gene coding for the protein R-Spondin1 [4]. The R-Spondin proteins potentiate Wnt signalling by binding to the Frizzled/LRP receptor complex [5]. 46, XX sex reversal is unusual and poorly understood. However, loss-of function *WNT4* mutations cause the SERKAL syndrome, a rare disorder which includes female sex reversal, explaining how loss of R-Spondin1 can cause this phenomenon [6]. The Wnt signalling pathway is further involved in dorsalventral polarization and determination of nail development (autosomal recessive anonychia, for example, is caused by absence of RSPO4 [7]). Furthermore, recent findings firmly imply Wnt signalling in skin carcinogenesis [8].

Clinical features. The cardinal feature is that of more or less complete sex reversal in a 46, XX individual with a Huriez-like PPK and abnormal nails. Patients presenting with Huriez-like keratoderma should be examined for signs of sex reversal and be offered karyotyping. The squamous cell carcinomas reported were moderately differentiated. Further abnormalities that have been reported include hypertriglyceridaemia, Leydig cell hyperplasia and loss of teeth in early adulthood caused by periodontitis.

Differential diagnosis. Huriez syndrome can be distinguished in males by a 46, XY karyotype. The PPK is quite similar but the sclerobrachydactyly that is so striking in Huriez is lacking. Odonto-onycho-dermal dysplasia is distinguished by abnormal tooth development and a much milder PPK.

Laboratory investigation and pathology. The only available description lists hyperkeratosis, vacuolar degeneration of keratinocytes in the upper stratum spinosum and a thickened granular layer with hypergranulosis [1].

Treatment. The sequelae of sex reversal and the squamous cell carcinomas will require a surgical approach. Topical emollients may be of benefit.

References

1 Vernole P, Terrinoni A, Didona B et al. An SRY-negative XX male with Huriez syndrome. Clin Genet 2000;57:61–6.
2 Guerriero C, Albanesi C, Girolomoni G et al. Huriez syndrome: case report with a detailed analysis of skin dendritic cells. Br J Dermatol 2000;143:1091–6.
3 Radi O, Parma P, Imbeaud S et al. XX sex reversal, palmoplantar keratoderma and predisposition to squamous cell carcinoma: genetic analysis in one family. Am J Med Genet A 2005;138A:241–6.
4 Parma P, Radi O, Vidal V et al. R-spondin1 is essential in sex determination, skin differentiation and malignancy. Nat Genet 2006; 38:1304–9.
5 Kim KA, Wagle M, Tran K et al. R-Spondin family members regulate the Wnt pathway by a common mechanism. Mol Biol Cell 2008;19: 2588–96.
6 Mandel H, Shemer R, Borochowitz ZU et al. SERKAL syndrome: an autosomal-recessive disorder caused by a loss-of-function mutation in *WNT4*. Am J Hum Genet 2008;82:39–47.
7 Blaydon DC, Ishii Y, O'Toole EA et al. The gene encoding R-spondin 4 (RSPO4), a secreted protein implicated in Wnt signaling, is mutated in inherited anonychia. Nat Genet 2006;38:1245–7.
8 Yang SH, Andl T, Grachtchouk V et al. Pathological responses to oncogenic Hedgehog signaling in skin are dependent on canonical Wnt/beta-catenin signaling. Nat Genet 2008;40:1130–5.

Odonto-onycho-dermal dysplasia spectrum (OODD, OMIM #257980, *WNT10A*)

Brief introduction and history. The first three families reported with this rare ectodermal dysplasia were Lebanese Muslim Shiites [1]. A few sporadic patients and another Lebanese family were subsequently reported [2,3]. It was recently shown that OODD is a manifestation of a phenotypic spectrum to which the Schöpf–Schulz–Passarge syndrome (SSPS) also belongs [4,5].

Epidemiology and pathogenesis. Using homozygosity mapping in three Lebanese Shiite families, Adaimy and colleagues assigned the disease locus to chromosome 2q35. They found the same homozygous nonsense mutation in the *WNT10A* gene in all three families (E233X) [6]. Heterozygous carriers have been noted to have features such as abnormally shaped teeth or mild nail dysplasia [7]. Nail specification, epidermal differentiation and tooth development all require WNT signalling [8].

Clinical features. The core phenotype consists of hypodontia with abnormal teeth, nail hypoplasia and a mild diffuse, erythematous palmoplantar hyperkeratosis with hyperhidrosis (Fig. 128.7). A smooth tongue has also been reported in some patients. Hypotrichosis may be present but is not a constant feature. Benign adnexal tumours,

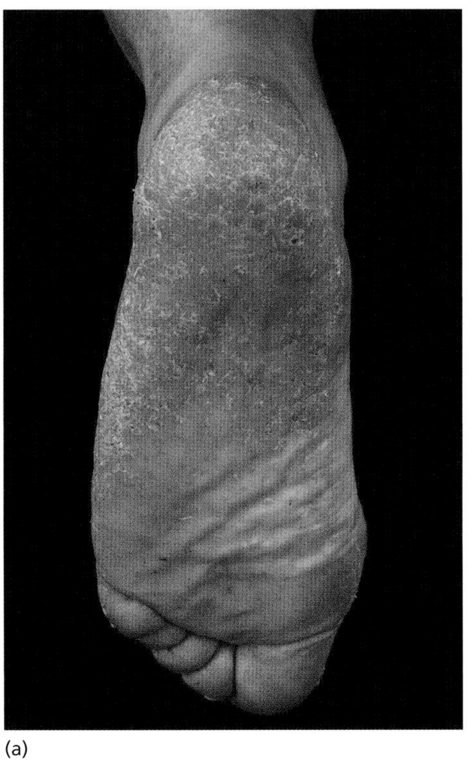
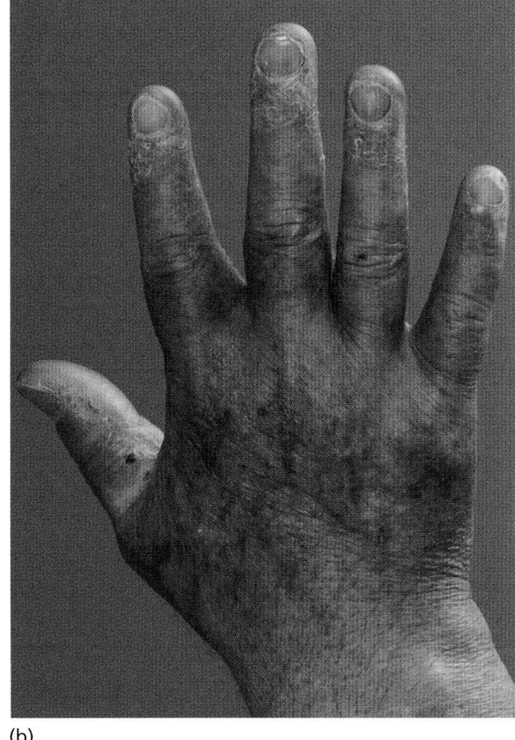

(a) (b)

Fig. 128.7 Keratoderma (a) and nail dystrophy (b) of odonto-onycho-dermal dysplasia.

including eccrine poroma, eyelid apocrine hydrocystoma and diffuse palmoplantar eccrine syringofibroadenomatosis have been reported in association with SSPS [9].

Differential diagnosis. Huriez syndrome can be distinguished by the sclerobrachydactyly and the absence of tooth abnormalities. The same applies to the PPK 46, XX sex reversal syndrome. The lack of a PPK and other distinctive phenotypic features in other ectodermal dysplasias usually readily differentiate them.

Laboratory investigation and pathology. Biopsy of palmoplantar skin in SSPS shows proliferation of anastomosing cords and strands of basaloid acrosyringeal cells, ductal differentiation and a mucinous fibrovascular stroma.

Treatment. The skin condition responds reasonably well to emollients with keratolytics and/or moisturisers containing urea. Benign tumours can be surgically treated if necessary. Bothersome eyelid cysts can be removed with an ablative laser (CO_2 or Er:YAG).

References

1 Fadhil M, Ghabra TA, Deeb M et al. Odontoonychodermal dysplasia: a previously apparently undescribed ectodermal dysplasia. Am J Med Genet 1983;14:335–46.
2 Arnold WP, Merkx MA, Steijlen PM. Variant of odontoonychodermal dysplasia? Am J Med Genet 1995;59:242–4.
3 Megarbane H, Haddad M, Delague V et al. Further delineation of the odonto-onycho-dermal dysplasia syndrome. Am J Med Genet A 2004;129A:193–7.
4 van Geel M, Gattas M, Kesler Y et al. Phenotypic variability associated with *WNT10A* nonsense mutations. Br J Dermatol 2010;162:1403–6.
5 **Bohring A, Stamm T, Spaich C et al. *WNT10A* mutations are a frequent cause of a broad spectrum of ectodermal dysplasias with sex-biased manifestation pattern in heterozygotes. Am J Hum Genet 2009;85:97–105.**
6 Adaimy L, Chouery E, Megarbane H et al. Mutation in *WNT10A* is associated with an autosomal recessive ectodermal dysplasia: the odonto-onycho-dermal dysplasia. Am J Hum Genet 2007;81:821–8.
7 Tardieu C, Jung S, Niederreither K et al. Dental and extra-oral clinical features in 41 patients with *WNT10A* gene mutations: a multicentric genotype-phenotype study. Clin Genet 2017;92:477–86.
8 Xu M, Horrell J, Snitow M et al. WNT10A mutation causes ectodermal dysplasia by impairing progenitor cell proliferation and KLF4-mediated differentiation. Nat Commun 2017;8:15397.
9 Castori M, Ruggieri S, Giannetti L et al. Schöpf-Schulz-Passarge syndrome: further delineation of the phenotype and genetic considerations. Acta Derm Venereol 2008;88:607–12.

Mutilating palmoplantar keratoderma with periorificial keratotic plaques (Olmsted syndrome) (OMIM #614594, 300918, *TRPV3, MTBSP2*)

Brief introduction and history. In 1927, Olmsted [1] described a congenital PPK that led to flexural deformities and spontaneous amputation of two digits. Since then, over 74 cases have been reported (reviewed in [2]).

Epidemiology and pathogenesis. This a rare keratoderma and most of the cases reported are sporadic. There are reports of autosomal recessive, autosomal dominant, semidominant and X-linked recessive inheritance [3–6]. In 2012, Lin and colleagues identified heterozygous missense mutations in the transient receptor potential vanilloid 3 (*TRPV3*) gene in five Chinese patients with autosomal dominant Olmsted syndrome [3]. Autosomal recessive mutations have also been reported in the same gene [4]. The protein encoded by *TRPV3* is a member of the TRP cation selective ion channels that are important in regulation of epidermal differentiation and skin barrier formation, itching and pain, skin inflammation and hair growth. Individuals with the X-linked recessive variant of Olmsted syndrome with severe alopecia and dystrophic nails have mutations in the *MTBSP2* gene, a zinc metalloprotease gene, that has also been associated with IFAP and keratosis follicularis spinulosa decalvans syndrome [6].

Clinical features. The syndrome usually manifests within the first 6 months of life and consists of a diffuse, sharply defined PPK with flexion deformities of the digits, leading to constriction or spontaneous amputation, periorificial keratoses and onychodystrophy. Periorificial plaques are common with warty hyperkeratosis and erythema in the perianal or perioral regions. Hyperkeratosis may also be present on the ears, nose or umbilicus. The course is relentlessly progressive, causing fingers and toes to disappear into a hyperkeratotic mass typical of Olmsted syndrome. Recent data suggest that the affected skin in Olmsted syndrome may be cancer prone as a number of patients have developed squamous cell carcinoma in affected skin [7]. Supporting this notion, a study provides clear evidence for hyperproliferation of basal keratinocytes in affected skin [8]. Several associated abnormalities have been reported, in particular hypotrichosis and alopecia, oral leukokeratosis, tooth anomalies, nail dystrophy and erythromelalgia [2,9]. Mutations in *TRPV3* can also cause a painful, inflammatory focal keratoderma (Fig. 128.8) with dystrophic nails [10].

Differential diagnosis. The principal genetic syndromes to be excluded in the differential diagnosis include pachyonchia congenita, Mal de Meleda and PPK of Vohwinkel. The perioral hyperkeratosis can mimic acrodermatitis enteropathica, which can be excluded by measuring the plasma zinc level.

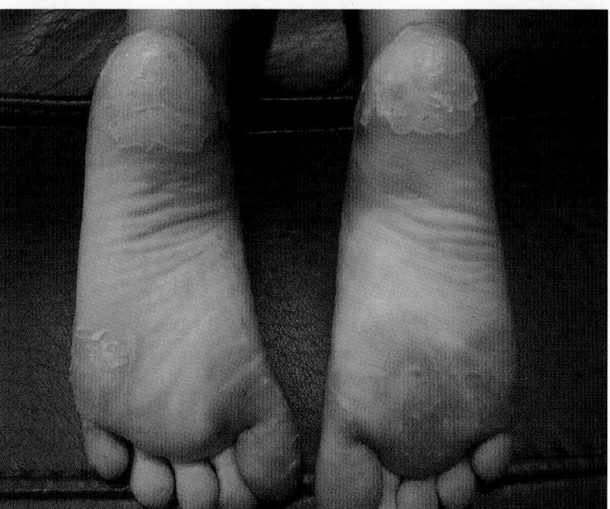

Fig. 128.8 Inflammatory focal keratoderma in a child caused by *TRYPV3* mutation.

SECTION 27: DISORDERS OF KERATIN AND KERATINIZATION

Laboratory and histology findings. Histology from the periorificial plaques shows psoriasiform hyperplasia, hyperkeratosis and parakeratosis with a perivascular inflammatory infiltrate containing some mast cells.

Treatment. Treatment is difficult. Variable improvement is seen with retinoids such as acitretin. Topical corticosteroids or tacrolimus may help relieve itching. In one female patient the epidermal growth factor (EGF) receptor inhibitor erlotinib led to a temporary thinning of the keratoderma and resolution of perioral plaques [11]. Mechanical removal, full-thickness excision of affected skin followed by grafting and systemic etretinate have been reported to be effective in individual cases [12].

References

1 Olmsted HC. Keratoderma palmaris et plantaris congenitalis. Am J Dis Child 1927;33:757–64.

2 Tao J, Huang CZ, Yu NW et al. Olmsted syndrome: a case report and review of literature. Int J Dermatol 2008;47:432–7.

3 Lin Z, Chen Q, Lee M et al. Exome sequencing reveals mutations in *TRPV3* as a cause of Olmsted syndrome. Am J Hum Genet 2012;90: 558–64.

4 Cao X, Wang H, Li Y et al. Semidominant Inheritance in Olmsted Syndrome. J Invest Dermatol 2016;136:1722–5.

5 Eytan O, Fuchs-Telem D, Mevorach B et al. Olmsted syndrome caused by a homozygous recessive mutation in *TRPV3*. J Invest Dermatol 2014;134:1752–4.

6 Haghighi A, Scott CA, Poon DS et al. A missense mutation in the *MBTPS2* gene underlies the X-linked form of Olmsted syndrome. J Invest Dermatol 2013;133:571–3.

7 Ogawa F, Udono M, Murota H et al. Olmsted syndrome with squamous cell carcinoma of extremities and adenocarcinoma of the lung: failure to detect loricrin gene mutation. Eur J Dermatol 2003; 13:524–8.

8 Requena L, Manzarbeitia F, Moreno C et al. Olmsted syndrome: report of a case with study of the cellular proliferation in keratoderma. Am J Dermatopathol 2001;23:514–20.

9 Duchatelet S, Pruvost S, de Veer S et al. A new *TRPV3* missense mutation in a patient with Olmsted syndrome and erythromelalgia. JAMA Dermatol 2014;150:303–6.

10 Wilson NJ, Cole C, Milstone LM et al. Expanding the phenotypic spectrum of Olmsted syndrome. J Invest Dermatol 2015;135:2879–83.

11 Kenner-Bell BM, Paller AS, Lacouture ME. Epidermal growth factor receptor inhibition with erlotinib for palmoplantar keratoderma. J Am Acad Dermatol 2010;63:e58–9.

12 Duchatelet S, Hovnanian A. Olmsted syndrome: clinical, molecular and therapeutic aspects. Orphanet J Rare Dis 2015;10:33.

Palmoplantar keratoderma with periodontitis (OMIM #245000, allelic disease: Haim–Munk syndrome #245010, *CTSC*)

Syn.

- Papillon–Lefèvre syndrome (PLS)
- Haim–Munk syndrome (HMS)

Brief introduction and history. In 1924, Papillon and Lefèvre reported PPK and severe dental anomalies in a brother and sister [1]. A very similar disorder, called HMS was described in a single family of Cochin Jews from South India [2]. Molecular analysis has shown that the disorders are allelic [3].

Epidemiology and pathogenesis. Both these conditions are caused by homozygous mutations in the *CTSC* gene encoding cathepsin C, a lysosomal protease expressed at high levels in polymorphonuclear leucocytes and macrophages [4]. In neutrophils, it has a crucial function in the activation of granule-derived serine proteases that are implicated in bacterial killing and activation of cytokines. This may explain the aggressive periodontitis, psoriasiform skin lesions and predisposition to systemic bacterial infections [5]. Absence of CTSC from osteoclasts [6] might be responsible for the acro-osteolysis seen in HMS but the underlying pathophysiology is not understood.

Clinical features. PLS is characterized by a diffuse transgredient PPK and periodontitis potentially causing premature loss of both deciduous (age 4 to 5 years) and permanent teeth (Fig. 128.9). In addition to the well-known palmoplantar hyperkeratosis, numerous PLS patients have erythematous plaques over the knees, elbows, interphalangeal joints and dorsum of the feet,

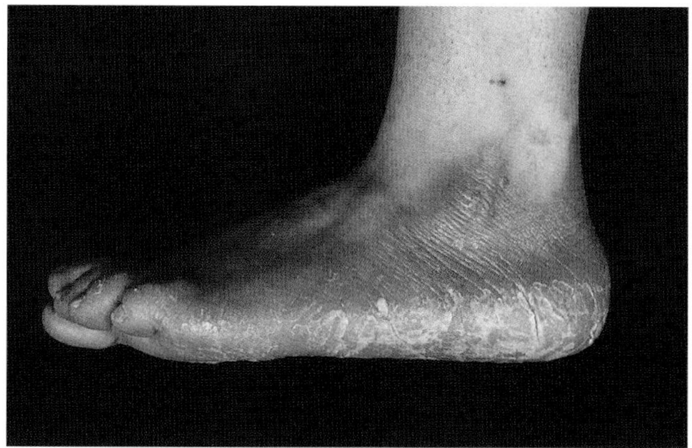

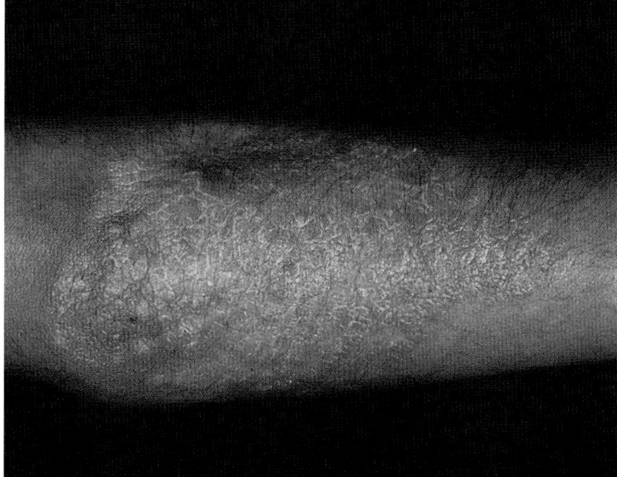

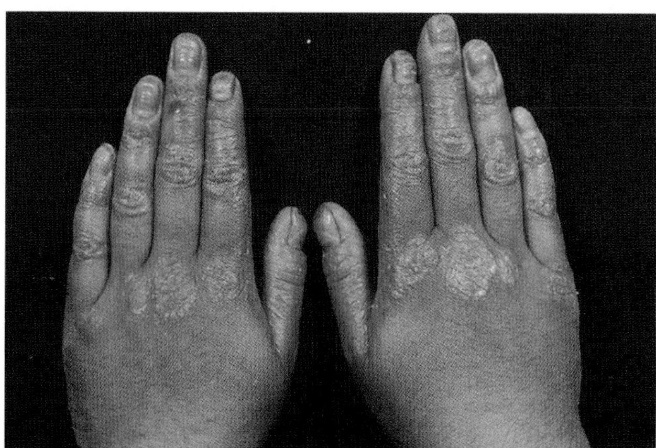

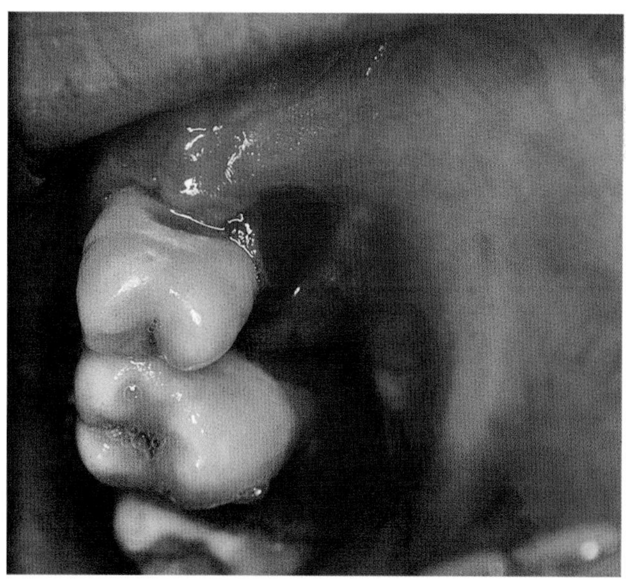

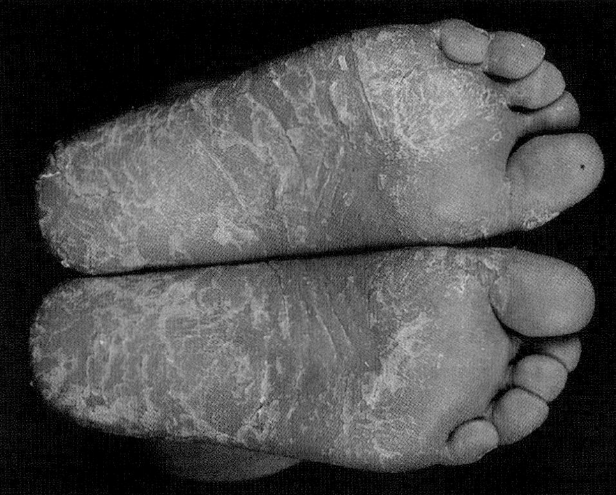

Fig. 128.9 Palmoplantar keratoderma with periodontitis (Papillon-Lefevre syndrome).

commonly misdiagnosed as psoriasis [7,8]. Redness and thickening of the palms and soles usually occur in the first years of life, together with the breakthrough of the deciduous teeth. A spontaneous improvement parallels the subsiding of the gingival inflammation after the loss of the permanent teeth [9]. Associated hyperhidrosis causes an unpleasant odour. An increased susceptibility to skin infections has been observed in about 20% of PLS patients [10]. Pyogenic liver abscesses are an increasingly recognized complication [11]. Affected individuals with HMS have archnodactyly, onychogryphosis and acro-osteolysis as well as the classic PLS features.

Differential diagnosis. Hypotrichosis–osteolysis–periodontitis–PPK syndrome (HOPP) does feature periodontitis but is distinguished by the unique pattern of PPK and the additional features of hypotrichosis, onychogryphosis and lingua plicata.

Laboratory and histology findings. Histopathological changes are nonspecific. Electron microscopic features include lipid-like vacuoles in the corneocytes and granulocytes, reductions in tonofilaments and irregular keratohyalin granules.

Treatment. Systemic retinoids appear to be effective in the treatment of hyperkeratosis and have been associated with improvement in periodontitis [10]. Professional oral hygiene and dental input are recommended from an early age [12]. In adults and children over 12, low-dose tetracyclines might be useful even in subtherapeutic doses for the treatment of periodontitis.

References

1 Papillon M, Lefèvre P. Deux cas de keratodermie palmaire et plantaire symmetrique familiale (Maladie devMeleda) chez le frere et la soeur. Coexistance dans les deux cas d'alterations dentaires graves. Societé Française de Dermatologie et de Syphiligraphie 1924;31:82.
2 Haim S, Munk J. Keratosis palmo-plantaris congenita, with periodontosis, arachnodactyly and a peculiar deformity of the terminal phalanges. Br J Dermatol 1965;77:42–54.
3 Hart TC, Hart PS, Michalec MD et al. Haim-Munk syndrome and Papillon–Lefevre syndrome are allelic mutations in cathepsin C. J Med Genet 2000;37:88–94.
4 **Toomes C, James J, Wood AJ et al. Loss-of-function mutations in the cathepsin C gene result in periodontal disease and palmoplantar keratosis. Nat Genet 1999;23:421–4.**
5 Roberts H, White P, Dias I et al. Characterization of neutrophil function in Papillon-Lefèvre syndrome. J Leukoc Biol 2016;100:433–44.
6 Goto T, Yamaza T, Tanaka T. Cathepsins in the osteoclast. J Electron Microsc (Tokyo) 2003;52:551–8.
7 **Ullbro C, Crossner CG, Nederfors T et al. Dermatologic and oral findings in a cohort of 47 patients with Papillon–Lefevre syndrome. J Am Acad Dermatol 2003;48:345–51.**
8 Tekin B, Yucelten D, Beleggia F et al. Papillon-Lefèvre syndrome: report of six patients and identification of a novel mutation. Int J Dermatol 2016; 55:898–902.
9 Posteraro AF. Papillon–Lefevre syndrome. J Ala Dent Assoc 1992;76: 16–19.
10 Bergman R, Friedman-Birnbaum R. Papillon–Lefevre syndrome: a study of the long-term clinical course of recurrent pyogenic infections and the effects of etretinate treatment. Br J Dermatol 1988;119:731–6.
11 Almuneef M, Al Khenaizan S, Al Ajaji S et al. Pyogenic liver abscess and Papillon–Lefevre syndrome: not a rare association. Pediatrics 2003;111:e85–8.
12 D'Angelo M, Margiotta V, Ammatuna P et al. Treatment of prepubertal periodontitis. A case report and discussion. J Clin Periodontol 1992;19:214–19.

Cerebral dysgenesis, neuropathy, ichthyosis and palmoplantar keratoderma syndrome (CEDNIK, OMIM #609528, *SNAP29*)

Brief introduction and history. Sprecher and colleagues reported this syndrome in seven individuals from two unrelated consanguineous Arab families in the north of Israel [1].

Epidemiology and pathogenesis. This rare disorder is caused by a homozygous mutation (currently 1 bp deletion or insertion reported) affecting the *SNAP29* gene on chromosome 22q12 [1]. The SNAP29 protein is a member of the SNARE (soluble N-ethylmaleimide-sensitive factor-attachment protein receptors) family which are essential proteins for fusion of cellular membranes. SNAREs localized on opposing membranes assemble to form a trans-SNARE complex which mediates fusion of transport vesicles in cells which is important for lipid and protein transport in keratinocytes and neuronal synapses. SNAP29 is also involved in autophagy, a cell death process which involves autodigestion of intracellular organelles [2,3]. Thus, SNAP29 mutations are expected to disrupt transport of lipid and proteins in the upper epidermis, thus causing a barrier defect and palmoplantar hyperkeratosis. A very similar disorder called MEDNIK syndrome (mental retardation, enteropathy, deafness, peripheral neuropathy, ichthyosis and keratoderma) features erythrokeratoderma variabilis-like skin changes and is caused by mutations in the gene coding for the adapter protein AP1S1, which is a subunit of the AP-1 protein complex regulating vesicle assembly and trafficking [4]. This is now known to be a disorder of copper metabolism as well as vesicular transport.

Clinical features. After a normal birth, affected infants develop failure to thrive, abnormal eye movements and poor head and body control over the first 4 months of life. Other features include progressive microcephaly, elongated facies, downward-slanting palpebral fissures, mild hypertelorism and a flat, broad nasal bridge. A diffuse PPK and ichthyosis appear before the age of 1 year. By then, major developmental delay is apparent. Other features include hypoplastic optic discs and sensorineural deafness. Magnetic resonance imaging shows defects of the corpus callosum, cortical dysplasia with polymicrogyria and pachygyria.

Differential diagnosis. The disorder must be distinguished from the closely related MEDNIK syndrome [4]. This disorder is differentiated by the erythrokeratoderma and the associated congenital diarrhoea. The differential diagnosis also includes the recently described autosomal recessive keratoderma ichthyosis and deafness (ARKID) syndrome also caused by a defect in cell transport (see next section).

Laboratory and histology findings. Skin biopsy in CEDNIK shows clear vesicles in the spinous, granular and stratum corneum layers, with retained glucosylceramides. This might suggest abnormal lamellar granule maturation. Patients with MEDNIK have increased aspartate transaminase/alanine transaminase, hyperbilrubinaemia, decreased serum copper and ceruloplasmin and increased serum very long chain fatty acids.

Treatment. General measures such as emollients and keratolytics are used for the ichthyosis and keratoderma. One MEDNIK patient with a homozygous *AP1S1* mutation showed an improvement of clinical signs and biochemical copper abnormalities on oral zinc acetate therapy [5].

References

1 **Sprecher E, Ishida-Yamamoto A, Mizrahi-Koren M et al. A mutation in *SNAP29*, coding for a SNARE protein involved in intracellular trafficking, causes a novel neurocutaneous syndrome characterized by cerebral dysgenesis, neuropathy, ichthyosis and palmoplantar keratoderma. Am J Hum Genet 2005;77:242–51.**

2 Su Q, Mochida S, Tian JH et al. SNAP-29: a general SNARE protein that inhibits SNARE disassembly and is implicated in synaptic transmission. Proc Natl Acad Sci U S A 2001;98:14038–43.

3 Pan PY, Cai Q, Lin L et al. SNAP-29-mediated modulation of synaptic transmission in cultured hippocampal neurons. J Biol Chem 2005;280:25769–79.

4 Montpetit A, Cote S, Brustein E et al. Disruption of AP1S1, causing a novel neurocutaneous syndrome, perturbs development of the skin and spinal cord. PLoS Genet 2008;4:e1000296.

5 Martinelli D, Travaglini L, Drouin CA et al. MEDNIK syndrome: a novel defect of copper metabolism treatable by zinc acetate therapy. Brain 2013;136:872–81.

Autosomal recessive keratoderma, ichthyosis and deafness (ARKID, no OMIM assigned yet, *VPS33B*)

Brief introduction and history. This is a recently described rare syndrome with PPK, ichthyosis and sensorineural deafness [1].

Epidemiology and pathogenesis. Three patients were reported with severe PPK associated with ichthyosis and sensorineural deafness. Biallelic mutations were found in *VPS33B*, encoding VPS33B, a Sec1/Munc18 family protein that interacts with Rab proteins and is involved in trafficking of the collagen-modifying enzyme lysyl hydroxylase 3 [1]. The epidermal ultrastructure of affected patients is similar to VPS33B-deficient mice with aberrant secretion of lamellar bodies. Mutations in *VPS33B* and VPS33B interacting protein, apical–basolateral polarity regulator (*VIPAR*) cause arthrogryposis–renal dysfunction–cholestasis (ARC) syndrome, which is usually fatal in early childhood [2].

Clinical features. Reported patients have a diffuse keratoderma with contractures and autoamputation, a mild ichthyosis which is worse on the limbs, sensorineural hearing loss and delayed psychomotor development. Neonatal hearing tests are usually normal, so the hearing loss is progressive.

Differential diagnosis. The differential diagnosis includes attenuated ARC syndrome (see previously) and other PPKs associated with deafness.

Laboratory and histology findings. Histology of affected skin from ARKID patients shows acanthosis with extensive orthohyperkeratosis, hypergranulosis, and elongation of rete ridges. Electron microscopy shows lamellar body entombment and inclusion of lipid bilayers within corneocytes.

References

1 Gruber R, Rogerson C, Windpassinger C et al. Autosomal Recessive Keratoderma-Ichthyosis-Deafness (ARKID) syndrome is caused by *VPS33B* mutations affecting rab protein interaction and collagen modification. J Invest Dermatol 2017;137:845–54.

2 Smith H, Galmes R, Gogolina E et al. Associations among genotype, clinical phenotype, and intracellular localization of trafficking proteins in ARC syndrome. Hum Mutat 2012;33:1656–-64.

Palmoplantar keratoderma, leukonychia and exuberant scalp hair (no OMIM assigned yet, *FAM83G*)

Brief introduction and history. Exome sequencing of two Pakistani siblings with PPK, leukonychia and exuberant scalp hair revealed a homozygous mutation in the *FAM83G* gene [1]. Although never reported in humans previously, mutations in this gene cause 'furry foot hyperkeratosis' in Kromfohrländer and Irish terrier dog breeds, a disease similar to the human phenotype with hyperkeratosis of the paws and a bushy coat [2].

Clinical features. Both siblings had a diffuse, verrucous hyperkeratosis of the soles, with a mild palmar keratoderma, leukonychia with dystrophy of the distal toe nails and curly hair with rapid growth requiring hair trimming every 3 weeks (Fig. 128.10).

References

1 **Maruthappu T, McGinty L, Blaydon DC et al. Recessive mutation in *FAM83G* associated with palmoplantar keratoderma and exuberant scalp hair. J Invest Dermatol 2018;138:984–7.**

2 Drögemüller M, Jagannathan V, Becker D et al. A mutation in the *FAM83G* gene in dogs with hereditary footpad hyperkeratosis (HFH). PLoS Genet 2014;10:e1004370.

Focal hereditary palmoplantar keratodermas without associated features

Striate palmoplantar keratoderma (OMIM 148700, 125647, 607654)

Syn.
- Keratosis palmoplantaris varians Siemens–Wachters
- Keratosis palmoplantaris areata et striata

Brief introduction and history. Originally, striata and areata types of PPK were described: in 1924 by Fuchs [1], in 1925 by Brünauer [2] and in 1929 by Siemens [3].

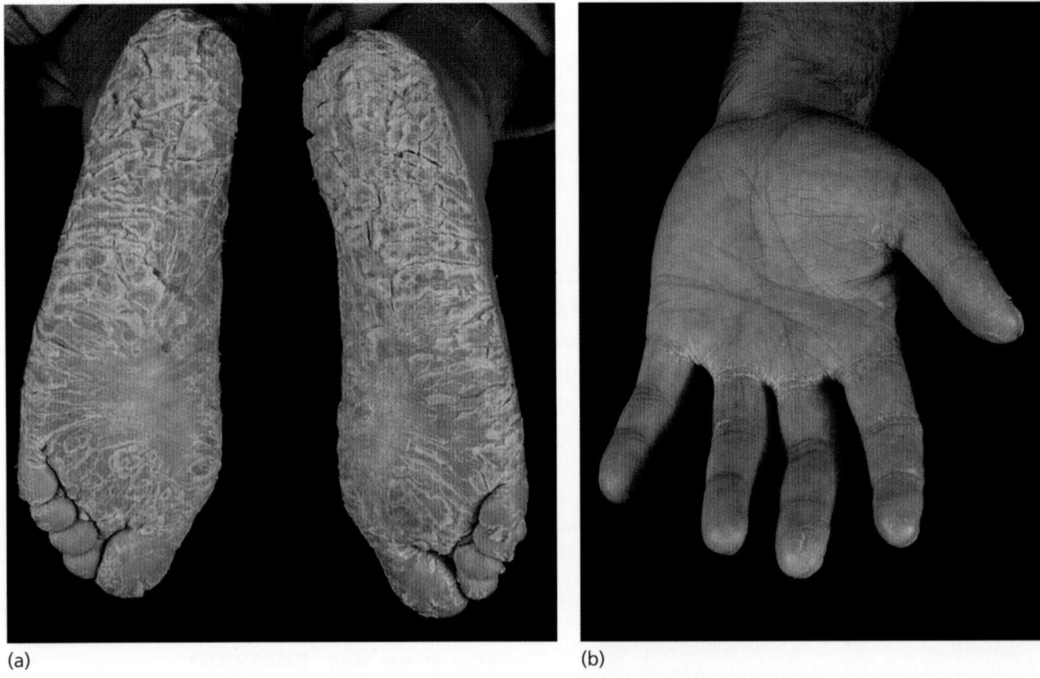

Fig. 128.10 (a) Verrucous plantar and (b) mild palmar keratoderma of patient with *FAM83G* mutation.

In 1963, Wachters demonstrated that both areata and striata types of keratosis occurred in one family. He considered both types as manifestations of the same disorder and proposed the term 'keratosis palmoplantaris varians' [4]. It is, however, possible to find only one subtype occurring in a family.

Epidemiology and pathogenesis. Molecular analysis has shown that the disorder has a heterogeneous genetic basis, but without a clear genotype–phenotype correlation. Heterozygous mutations in the gene coding for the desmosome component desmoglein 1 (DSG1) are associated with striate PPK type I (OMIM #148700) [5]. Heterozygous mutations in the *DSP1* gene coding for desmoplakin-1, a desmosome component, can also cause striate PPK, designated type II in this case [6]. Heterozygous and homozygous mutations in *DSP1* can cause striate keratoderma in association with woolly hair and cardiomyopathy (discussed in Chapter 134) [7]; complete homozygous loss of the desmoplakin tail results in lethal acantholytic epidermolysis bullosa [8]. Finally, striate PPK type III can be caused by a mutation in the keratin 1 gene (*KRT1*; OMIM #607654) [9]. Interestingly, the same mutation is associated with a severe form of epidermolytic ichthyosis formerly known as ichthyosis hystrix Curth–Macklin [10].

Clinical features. There is major variability between families and even members of the same family. Classically, patients with striate keratoderma have linear hyperatosis on the palmar aspects of the fingers (Fig. 128.11). However, focal, punctate or linear lesions may occur on the palms. Focal lesions may also occur in the first web space extending onto the thenar eminence. The plantar keratoderma is usually focal with calluses localized to the pressure points

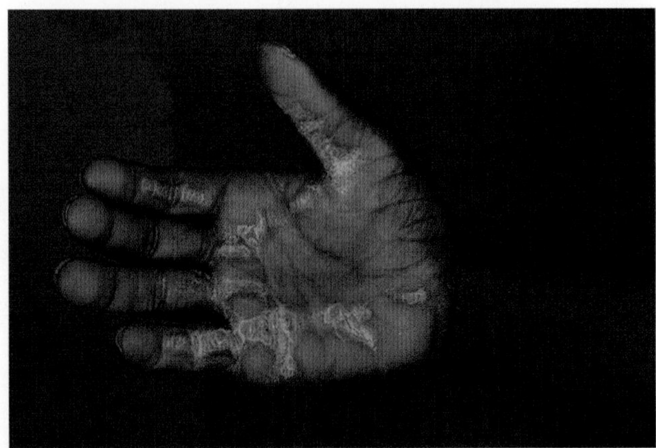

Fig. 128.11 Striate palmoplantar keratoderma caused by a *KRT1* mutation in a 12-year-old girl.

(Fig. 128.12) [11]. Diffuse and striate plantar keratoderma appearance have also been described [12]. Lesions appear on the soles in the first or second year of life. The palms are affected later in life and the hyperkeratosis is more severe in manual workers.

Differential diagnosis. Isolated striate PPK in children should be differentiated from pachyonychia congenita (PC) variants with focal keratoderma and mild nail changes usually caused by mutations in *KRT16* or *KRT6C*. Focal nonepidermolytic PPK caused by mutations in desmosomal component genes tends to be fissured rather than smooth and yellow as in PC. The plantar keratoderma is also less painful [12]. Carvajal/Naxos syndrome associated cardiomyopathy should be considered in patients with woolly/curly hair and dental anomalies (see Chapter 134). Two families have been described with autosomal recessive *palmoplantar striate keratoderma* with

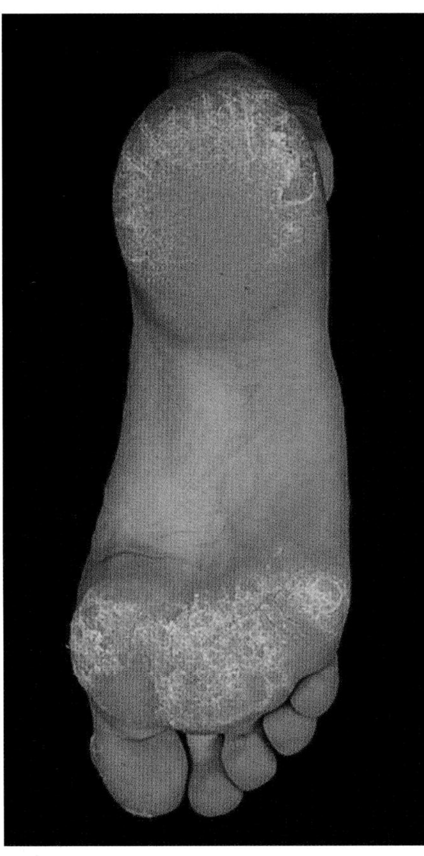

Fig. 128.12 Focal plantar palmoplantar keratoderma caused by *DSG1* mutation.

pseudo-ainhum of the fifth toe, woolly hair/hypotrichosis and leukonychia caused by mutations in *KANK2* (OMIM #616099), encoding a sequestering protein for steroid receptor coactivators [13].

Laboratory and histology findings. In patients with desmosomal mutations, skin biopsy shows loss of keratinocyte cell–cell adhesion or acantholysis in the epidermis because of the defective desmosomes. Electron microscopy may show small and/or disrupted desmosomes, or clumping of keratin filaments.

References

1 Fuchs H. Zur Kenntniss der herdweisen Keratosen an Händen und Füssen. Acta Derm Venereol (Stockh) 1924;5:11–58.

2 Brunauer SR. [Zur syptomatologie und histologie der kongenitalen dyskeratosen]. Dermatol Zschr 1925;42:6–26.

3 Siemens HW. Keratosis palmo-plantaris striata. Arch Derm Syph 1929;157:392–408.

4 Wachters DH. Over de verschillende morphologische vormen van de keratosis palmoplantaris, in het bijzonder over de 'keratosis palmoplantaris varians' Dermatology. Vol PhD. Leiden: State University Leiden, 1963.

5 **Rickman L, Simrak D, Stevens HP et al. N-terminal deletion in a desmosomal cadherin causes the autosomal dominant skin disease striate palmoplantar keratoderma. Hum Mol Genet 1999;8:971–6.**

6 **Armstrong DK, McKenna KE, Purkis PE et al. Haploinsufficiency of desmoplakin causes a striate subtype of palmoplantar keratoderma. Hum Mol Genet 1999;8:143–8.**

7 **Norgett EE, Hatsell SJ, Carvajal-Huerta L et al. Recessive mutation in desmoplakin disrupts desmoplakin-intermediate filament interactions and causes dilated cardiomyopathy, woolly hair and keratoderma. Hum Mol Genet 2000;9:2761–6.**

8 Jonkman MF, Pasmooij AM, Pasmans SG et al. Loss of desmoplakin tail causes lethal acantholytic epidermolysis bullosa. Am J Hum Genet 2005;77:653–60.

9 **Whittock NV, Smith FJ, Wan H et al. Frameshift mutation in the V2 domain of human keratin 1 results in striate palmoplantar keratoderma. J Invest Dermatol 2002;118:838–44.**

10 **Sprecher E, Ishida-Yamamoto A, Becker OM et al. Evidence for novel functions of the keratin tail emerging from a mutation causing ichthyosis hystrix. J Invest Dermatol 2001;116:511–19.**

11 Lucker GP, Steijlen PM. [Keratosis palmoplantaris varians et punctata. Clinical variability of a single genetic defect?] Hautarzt 1996; 47:858–9.

12 Lovgren ML, McAleer MA, Irvine AD et al. Mutations in desmoglein 1 cause diverse inherited palmoplantar keratoderma phenotypes: implications for genetic screening. Br J Dermatol 2017;176:1345–50.

13 Ramot Y, Molho-Pessach V, Meir T et al. Mutation in KANK2, encoding a sequestering protein for steroid receptor coactivators, causes keratoderma and woolly hair. J Med Genet 2014;51:388–94.

Focal hereditary palmoplantar keratodermas with associated features

Tylosis with oesophageal cancer (TOC, OMIM #148500, *RHBDF2*)

Syn.
- Tylosis
- Howell–Evans syndrome
- Palmoplantar keratoderma with oesophageal cancer
- Clarke–Howell–Evans–McConnell syndrome

Brief introduction and history. A family in whom six members developed an oesophageal carcinoma in two generations was reported in 1954 by Clarke and McConnell [1], and was subsequently described to have a PPK [2]. In 1958, Howell-Evans and colleagues further delineated the phenotype in both the families from Liverpool [3].

Epidemiology and pathogenesis. This is a rare disorder with a prevalence of less than one in a million [4]. The disease is inherited in an autosomal dominant fashion, with complete penetrance. Linkage mapping and targeted next generation sequencing revealed missense gain of function mutations in *RHBDF2* located on chromosome 17q25.1, which encodes an inactive rhomboid protein, iRhom2, that plays a role in epidermal growth factor receptor (EGFR) shedding [5,6]. iRhom2 regulates the trafficking and activation of ADAM17, a membrane-bound sheddase which is important for cleavage and release of TNFα and EGFR ligands [7]. As a consequence of increased ADAM17 activity, tylosis-derived keratinocytes show characteristics of 'constitutive wound healing' *in vitro* with upregulated shedding of ADAM17-dependent substrates such as EGF and TNFα, possibly underlying the propensity for oesophageal carcinoma.

Clinical features. Patients with tylosis have a focal keratoderma characterized by areas of yellowish thickened plaques restricted to areas of weight bearing and/or friction

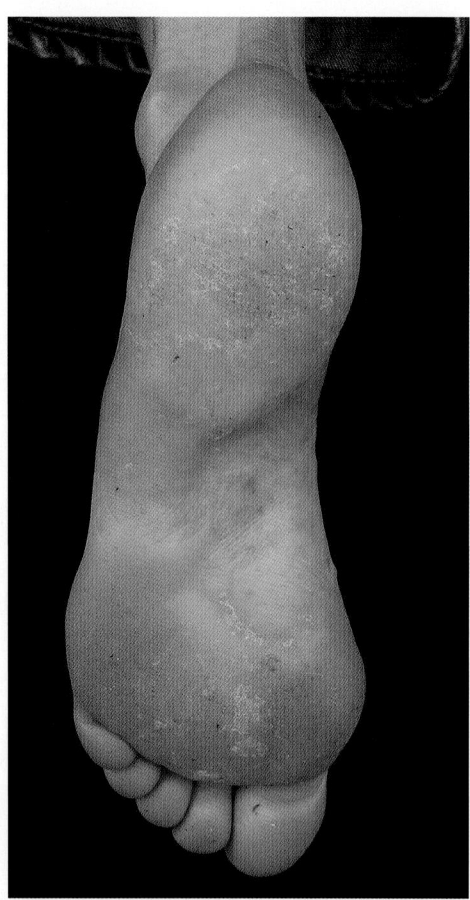

Fig. 128.13 Focal keratoderma of tylosis with oesophageal cancer.

on the palms and soles [8] (Fig. 128.13). The cutaneous features are completely penetrant and are usually evident by 7–8 years of age but can present as late as puberty [4]. Follicular hyperkeratosis is often seen. Oesophageal lesions present as small, white, polyploid lesions dotted throughout the oesophagus. The number and size of these varies between individuals but does not worsen with age or prior to the development of carcinomas. In addition, oral leukokeratosis has been described. Although the oral lesions are considered to be largely benign, two cases of squamous cancer of the oropharynx have been recorded [4]. A total of 21 out of 89 members of the Liverpool extended family had died of oesophageal cancer and 11 had died of other causes [9]. The risk of developing oesophageal cancer in the Liverpool family was calculated to be 95% at the age of 65.

Differential diagnosis. The main differential diagnosis is PC, in particular the variants associated with milder nail changes caused by mutations in *KRT16* or *KRT6C*. Patients with TOC usually have a family history of oesophageal cancer, but both TOC and PC have a focal keratoderma, follicular hyperkeratosis and oral leukokeratosis. The recent finding that iRhom2 binds to KRT16 provides a scientific basis for the clinical phenotypes [10].

Laboratory and histology findings. Histological features of the affected skin include acanthosis, hyperkeratosis and hypergranulosis without epidermolysis. Genetic testing for *RHBDF2* mutations is important to confirm the diagnosis.

Treatment. The management of the keratoderma is similar to other keratodermas. The key focus in patients with TOC is surveillance for early detection and treatment of oesophageal dysplasia from the early twenties onwards. A healthy diet, smoking cessation and alcohol restriction (known risk factors for oesophageal cancer) should also be encouraged.

References

1 Clarke CA, McConnell R. Six cases of carcinoma of the oesophagus occurring in one family. BMJ 1954;2:1137–8.
2 Clarke CA, Howel-Evans AW, McConnell RB. Carcinoma of the oesophagus associated with tylosis. BMJ 1957;1:945.
3 Howel-Evans W, McConnell R, Clarke CA et al. Carcinoma of the oesophagus with keratosis palmaris et plantaris (tylosis): a study of two families. Q J Med 1958;27:413–29.
4 Ellis A, Risk JM, Maruthappu T, Kelsell DP. Tylosis with oesophageal cancer: Diagnosis, management and molecular mechanisms. Orphanet J Rare Dis 2015;10:126.
5 **Blaydon DC, Etheridge SL, Risk JM et al. *RHBDF2* mutations are associated with tylosis, a familial esophageal cancer syndrome. Am J Hum Genet 2012;90:340–6.**
6 Saarinen S, Vahteristo P, Lehtonen R et al. Analysis of a Finnish family confirms RHBDF2 mutations as the underlying factor in tylosis with esophageal cancer. Fam Cancer 2012;11:525–8.
7 Brooke MA, Etheridge SL, Kaplan N et al. iRHOM2-dependent regulation of ADAM17 in cutaneous disease and epidermal barrier function. Hum Mol Genet 2014;23:4064–76.
8 Stevens HP, Kelsell DP, Bryant SP et al. Linkage of an American pedigree with palmoplantar keratoderma and malignancy (palmoplantar ectodermal dysplasia type III) to 17q24. Literature survey and proposed updated classification of the keratodermas. Arch Dermatol 1996;132:640–51.
9 **Ellis A, Field JK, Field EA et al. Tylosis associated with carcinoma of the oesophagus and oral leukoplakia in a large Liverpool family – a review of six generations. Eur J Cancer B Oral Oncol 1994;30B:102–12.**
10 **Maruthappu T, Chikh A, Fell B et al. Rhomboid family member 2 regulates cytoskeletal stress-associated Keratin 16. Nat Commun 2017;8:14174.**

Tyrosinaemia type II (OMIM #276600, *TAT*)

Syn.

- Richner–Hanhart syndrome
- Tyrosine transaminase deficiency

Brief introduction and history. This syndrome was first described by Richner in 1938 [1] and later, in 1947, by Hanhart [2].

Epidemiology and pathogenesis. Tyrosinaemia type II is a very rare disorder of tyrosine metabolism. Deficiency of the enzyme tyrosine aminotransferase (TAT), leading to increased serum levels of tyrosine and phenolic acid metabolites of tyrosine, is the biochemical basis for tyrosinaemia type II [3–5]. The *TAT* gene has been mapped to the long arm of chromososome 16 (16q22.1–q22.3) [6].

Clinical features. Early signs of eye disease are photophobia, pain, tearing and conjunctival erythema occurring in the first few months of life. Later, corneal epithelial opacities, superficial or deep dendritic ulceration, corneal neovascularization, and corneal scars and glaucoma occur. Hyperkeratosis following dermatoglyphics may be an early sign of the keratoderma [7]. The PPK is usually focal affecting weight-bearing areas often associated with hyperhidrosis [8]. It may begin as bullae and erosions that progress to painful, hyperkeratotic papules and plaques. Central nervous system involvement is variable, occurring in about 60% of patients, and can include intellectual deficit (mild to severe), behavioural problems, nystagmus, tremor, ataxia and convulsions.

Laboratory and histology findings. Increased tyrosine levels are found in blood and urine of affected individuals.

Treatment. The ocular and cutaneous signs respond well to the treatment which includes a low protein diet with tyrosine and phenylalanine-free supplements [8].

References

1 Richner H. Hornhautaffektionen bei Keratoma palmare et plantare hereditarium. Klin Monatsbl Augenheilkd 1938;100:580–8.
2 Hanhart E. Neue Sonderformen von Keratosis palmo-plantaris, u a eine regelmässig-dominante Form mit systematisierten Lipomen, ferner zwei einfach rezessive, mit Schwachsinn und z. T. mit Hornhautver änderungen des Auges (Ektodermalsyndrom). Dermatologica 1947;94:286–308.
3 Larrègue M, de Giacomoni PH, Bressieux JM et al. Syndrome de Richner–Hanhart ou tyrosinose oculo-cutanee. Ann Dermatol Vénéréol 1979;106:53–62.
4 Fellman JH, Vanbellinghen PJ, Jones RT et al. Soluble and mitochondrial forms of tyrosine aminotransferase. Relationship to human tyrosinaemia. Biochemistry 1969;8:615–22.
5 Goldsmith LA, Thorpe J, Roe CR. Hepatic enzymes of tyrosine metabolism in tyrosinaemia II. J Invest Dermatol 1979;73:530–2.
6 Natt E, Westphal E, Toth-Fejel SE et al. Inherited and de novo deletion of the tyrosine aminotransferase gene locus at 16q22.1–22.3 in a patient with tyrosinemia type II. Hum Genet 1987;77:352–8.
7 Rossi LC, Santagada F, Besagni F et al. Palmoplantar hyperkeratosis with a linear disposition along dermatoglyphics: a clue for an early diagnosis of tyrosinemia type II. G Ital Dermatol Venereol 2017; 152:182–3.
8 **Peña-Quintana L, Scherer G, Curbelo-Estévez ML et al. Tyrosinemia type II: mutation update, 11 novel mutations and description of 5 independent subjects with a novel founder mutation. Clin Genet 2017;92:306–317.**

Pachyonychia congenita (multiple OMIM #)

Syn.

- Jadassohn–Lewandowsky syndrome
- Jackson–Lawler syndrome
- PC1 and PC2
- Focal NEPPK

Brief introduction and history. PC is a heterogeneous group of diseases characterized by a painful focal keratoderma and nail dystrophy. It was originally described by Muller in 1904 [1] and Wilson in 1905 [2]. Jadassohn and Lewandowsky [3] reported in 1906 on the association with PPK and other ectodermal defects. Historically, PC was subdivided into type I (Jackson–Lawlor) and type II (Jadassohn–Lewandowsky) subgroups.

Epidemiology and pathogenesis. PC is inherited in an autosomal dominant manner. A recent reclassification identified five subtypes, PC-KRT6A, PC-KRT6B, PC-KRT6C, PC-KRT16 and PC-KRT17 [4]. Keratins 6 and 16 are present in the nailbed around nail progenitor cells; they are abundant in the suprabasal layers of palmoplantar skin, in mucosal epithelia, especially in the oral region and in hair follicles. Keratin 17 is highly expressed in the pilosebaceous unit, but has much less expression in palmoplantar skin and is undocumented in oral epithelium. Traumatic damage owing to a compromised keratin cytoskeleton leads to the distinct clinical features [4].

Clinical features. The focal plantar keratoderma usually presents during the first few years of life when a child starts weight bearing and walking [5] (Fig. 128.14). Blisters develop beneath the keratoderma resulting in intense pain. Pain usually becomes a problem over the age of 10 years. The blisters and plantar pain are more severe in summer. Excessive palmoplantar sweating is a problem for 50% of patients. The palmar keratoderma is less prominent with the exception of PC-KRT16 which can sometimes be striate [6,7].

Hypertrophic nail dystrophy, the predominant clinical feature of PC, is typically noted within the first few months of life, although it can present later (Fig. 128.14). The classic nail dystrophy appears to fall into two phenotypes: (i) nails that grow to full length and slant upwards caused by the prominent distal subungual hyperkeratosis; and (ii) nails that have a nail plate that terminates prematurely leaving a gently sloping distal region of hyperkeratosis [7]. Nail involvement can be complicated by paronychia and pus under the nails. Oral leukokeratosis (thickened white patches) is often present usually affecting the tongue and the buccal mucosa (Fig. 128.15). In babies, oral leukokeratosis can be misdiagnosed as *Candida albicans* and may cause difficulty in sucking [5].

Follicular keratoses, occur in areas of friction, usually the elbows, knees, buttocks and trunk (Fig. 128.15). These are usually visible by the age of 10 years. Cysts including widespread steatocystomas, epidermoid cysts, milia and vellus hair cysts occur in all PC subtypes and may increase in number at puberty [6,7]. Natal teeth are usually associated with pathogenic variants in *KRT17* and less commonly, *KRT6A* [5]. Primary and secondary dentition are normal.

Infants and young children with PC-KRT6A may experience ear pain. This manifests with difficult feeding as an infant and as severe pain anterior to the ear in children who can localize the problem usually when starting to eat or drink. The pathogenesis of this pain is unknown but it is hypothesized to be salivary gland related. Hoarseness in young children can be caused by laryngeal leukokeratosis in PC-KRT6A and rarely laryngeal involvement may cause life-threatening respiratory distress requiring intervention [8].

PC may present with a less severe presentation. The PC-KRT16 variant of PC may present with a painful focal keratoderma and dystrophy of a few nails, frequently

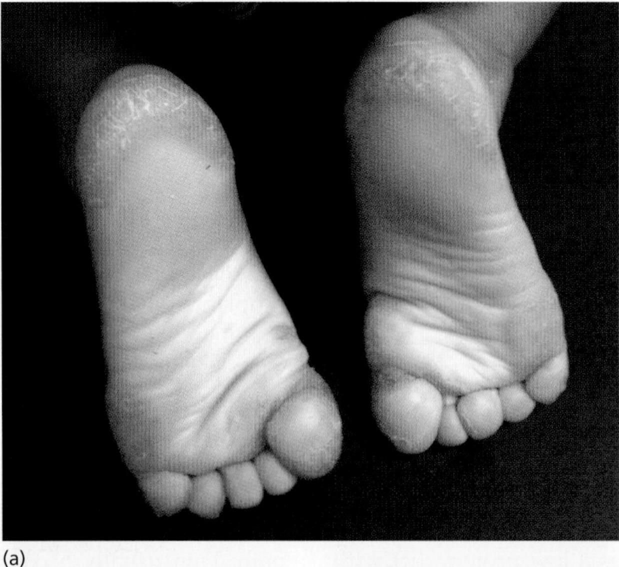

(a)

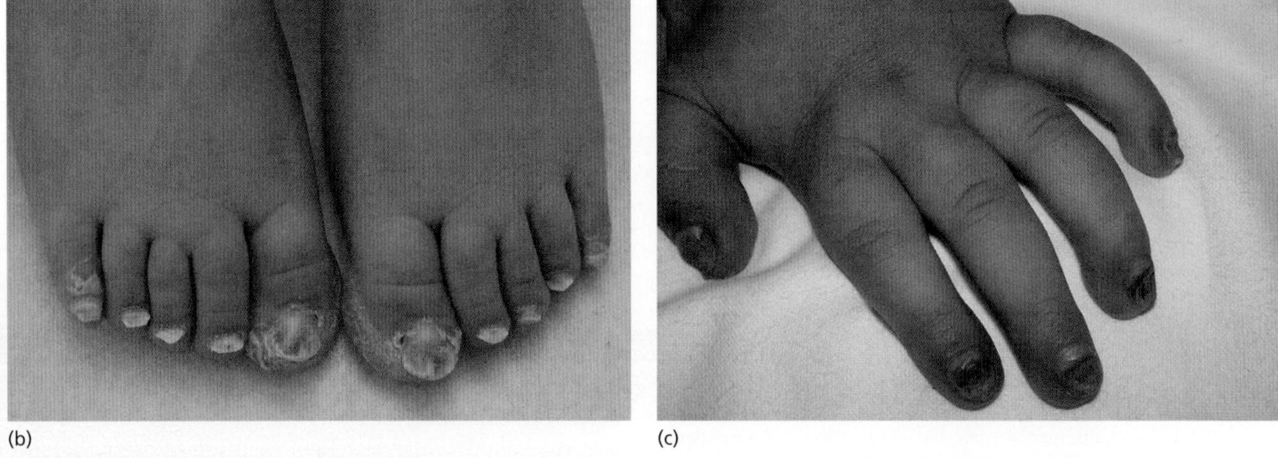

(b) (c)

Fig. 128.14 (a) Focal keratoderma and (b) nail dystrophy in a child with PC-KRT16 and (c) nail dystrophy in a child with PC-KRT17.

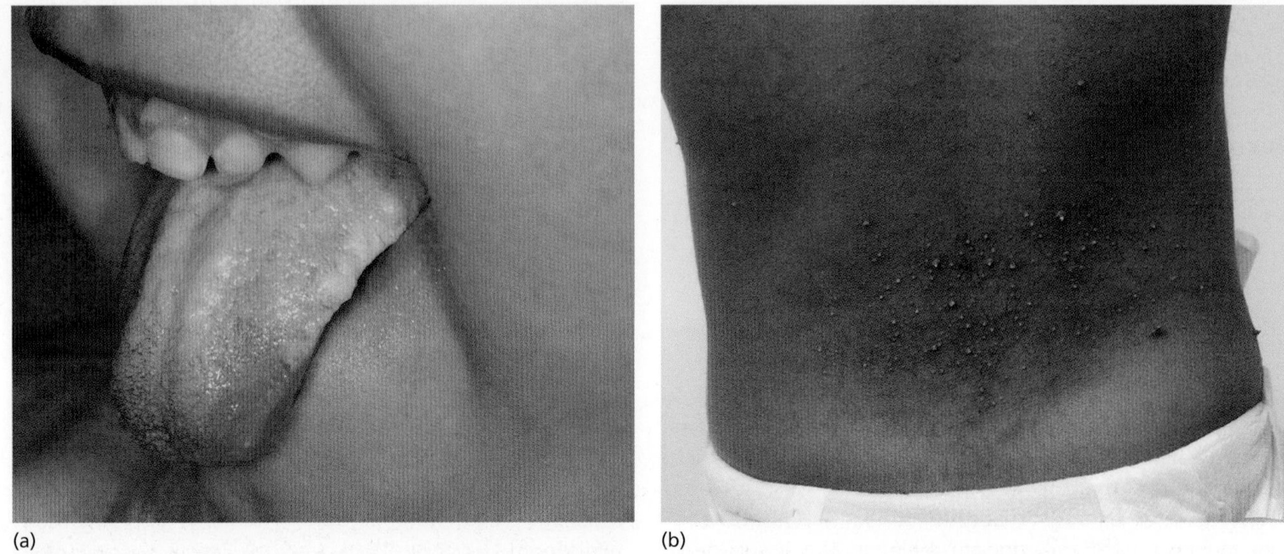

(a) (b)

Fig. 128.15 (a) Oral leukokeratosis and (b) follicular hyperkeratoses in children with PC-KRT6A.

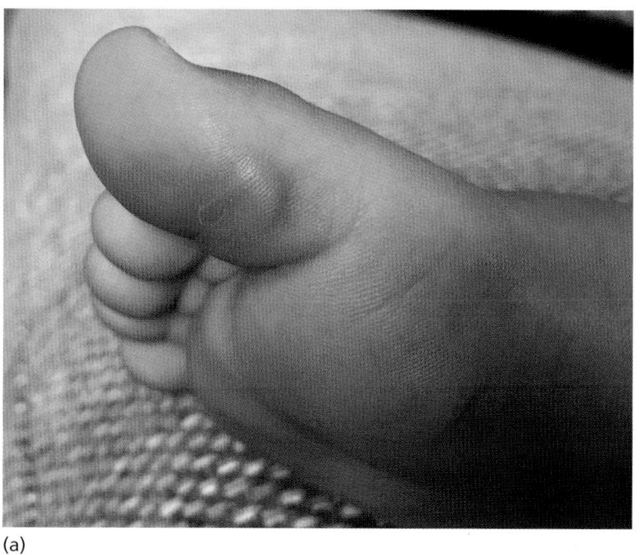
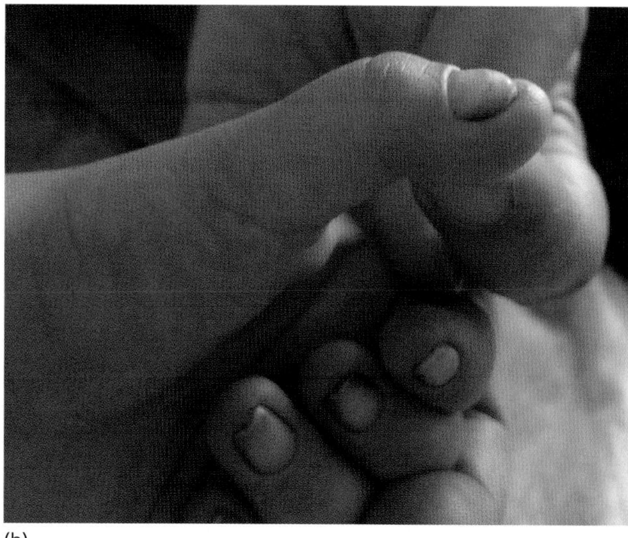

(a) (b)

Fig. 128.16 (a) Mild focal palmoplantar keratoderma in PC-KRT6C and (b) nail dystrophy in a patient with *FZD6* mutation (autosomal recessive nail dysplasia).

with visible splinter haemorrhages on the finger nails. The PC-KRT6C variant presents with a focal plantar keratoderma (Fig. 128.16) and mild nail dystrophy [9].

Differential diagnosis. PC should be differentiated from PPKs associated with oral leukokeratosis such as TOC. The differential diagnosis also includes focal keratoderma caused by *TRPV3* or *DSG1* mutations. Patients with *DSG1* muations generally have less pain. The keratoderma and nail dystrophy of Clouston syndrome are usually associated with hypotrichosis or alopecia which points to this diagnosis. Connexin 26 mutations can also be associated with focal PPK but patients will also have sensorineural hearing loss. Mutations in *FZD6* (Frizzled 6) can also cause a recessive nail dysplasia (Fig. 128.16) [10].

Laboratory and histology findings. Histology from palmoplantar skin shows gross hyperkeratosis, acanthosis and patchy hypergranulosis. There is usually no epidermolysis.

Treatment. The main treatment currently used for PC management is paring or filing of the calluses. This is usually done by a podiatrist or a parent in childhood and eventually older children learn to do it themselves. Comfortable footwear and customized insoles are also helpful. Local keratolytic measures are helpful for a few patients, but if too stringent can increase pain. Reducing hyperhidrosis with botulin toxin can also help the plantar pain of PC [11]. Some patients benefit from systemic retinoids usually at low dose [12]. The International Pachyonychia Congenita Consortium (IPCC) has demonstrated benefit from reducing keratin expression with rapamycin and siRNA [13,14]. Oral rapamycin helped some patients but was stopped because of side-effects. Clinical trials are in progress using topical rapamycin. The siRNA technology requires further development for clinical delivery. Pachyonychia Project offers free mutation analysis and maintains a database of mutations and phenotypes, a patient forum and a lot of advice for affected families. It also maintains an internet forum where patients can share tips and tricks for dealing with their disorder. Physicians caring for patients with PC should get in touch with PC Project and also refer their patients to this organization.

References

1 Muller C. On the causes of congenital onychogryphosis. München Med Wchnschr 1904;49:2180–2.
2 Wilson AG. Three cases of hereditary hyperkeratosis of the nail bed. Br J Dermatol 1905;17:13–14.
3 Jadassohn J, Lewandowsky F. Pachyonychia congenita. In: Jacobs Ikonographia Dermatologica. Berlin: Urban and Schwarzenberg, 1906:29–31.
4 McLean WH, Hansen CD, Eliason MJ, Smith FJ. The phenotypic and molecular genetic features of pachyonychia congenita. J Invest Dermatol 2011;131:1015–7.
5 **Shah S, Boen M, Kenner-Bell B et al. Pachyonychia congenita in pediatric patients: natural history, features, and impact. JAMA Dermatol 2014;150:146–53.**
6 **Smith FJD, Hansen CD, Hull PR et al. Pachyonychia Congenita. 2006 Jan 27 [updated 2017 Nov 30]. In: Adam MP, Ardinger HH, Pagon RA et al. (eds) GeneReviews® [Internet]. Seattle (WA): University of Washington, Seattle; 1993-2017. Available from http://www.ncbi.nlm.nih.gov/books/NBK1280/**
7 Eliason MJ, Leachman SA, Feng BJ et al. A review of the clinical phenotype of 254 patients with genetically confirmed pachyonychia congenita. J Am Acad Dermatol 2012;67:680–6.
8 O'Kane AM, Jackson CP, Mahadevan M, Barber C. Laryngeal manifestations of pachyonychia congenita: a clinical case and discussion on management for the otolaryngologist. J Laryngol Otol 2017;131: S53–S56.
9 **Wilson NJ, Messenger AG, Leachman SA et al. Keratin K6c mutations cause focal palmoplantar keratoderma. J Invest Dermatol 2010;130:425–9.**
10 **Fröjmark AS, Schuster J, Sobol M et al. Mutations in Frizzled 6 cause isolated autosomal-recessive nail dysplasia. Am J Hum Genet 2011;88:852–60.**
11 **Swartling C, Karlqvist M, Hymnelius K et al. Botulinum toxin in the treatment of sweat-worsened foot problems in patients with epidermolysis bullosa simplex and pachyonychia congenita. Br J Dermatol 2010;163:1072–6.**
12 Gruber R, Edlinger M, Kaspar RL et al. An appraisal of oral retinoids in the treatment of pachyonychia congenita. J Am Acad Dermatol 2012;66:e193–9.

13 Leachman SA, Hickerson RP, Schwartz ME et al. First-in-human mutation-targeted siRNA phase Ib trial of an inherited skin disorder. Mol Ther 2010;18:442–6.
14 Hickerson RP, Leake D, Pho LN et al. Rapamycin selectively inhibits expression of an inducible keratin (K6a) in human keratinocytes and improves symptoms in pachyonychia congenita patients. J Dermatol Sci 2009;56:82–8.

Hypotrichosis–osteolysis–periodontitis–palmoplantar keratoderma syndrome (HOPP, OMIM 607658)

Brief introduction and history. The authors described this rare syndrome in 2002 and named it after the most obvious abnormalities [1]. A third case was later reported by Brun and van Steensel, defining HOPP as an entity [2].

Epidemiology and pathogenesis. This is unknown. The phenotype suggests that the syndrome is related to PLS and HMS but no mutations were found in cathepsins C, K and L by Sanger sequencing [1]. Inheritance is probably autosomal dominant because mother-to-daughter transmission has been observed.

Clinical features. The abnormalities found are quite similar to what is seen in PLS and HMS, with periodontitis, acro-osteolysis, onychogryphosis and psoriasis-like skin lesions as prominent symptoms.

Hypotrichosis–osteolysis–periodontitis–PPK syndrome is distinguished by a peculiar pitted keratoderma that on the hands tends to form a network-like pattern with unaffected skin between the 'meshes' of the net, which may be rather small. A progressive hypotrichosis occurs from about 6 years old onwards and also distinguishes HOPP. Pili annulati was observed in two out of three affected individuals. Lingua plicata also seems to be part of the phenotype and is seen at an early age.

Differential diagnosis. Hypotrichosis–osteolysis–periodontitis–PPK syndrome must be distinguished from PLS and HMS. The hypotrichosis and lingua plicata should allow distinction, as should the unique keratoderma.

Treatment. Acitretin has been used with satisfactory effect on PPK. Osteolysis may respond to methotrexate. Severe onychogryphosis may eventually necessitate ablation of the nails and should be treated adequately by a skilled manicurist. Professional care is required for the teeth and gingiva. The periodontitis might also respond to low-dose oral tetracyclines (≥12 years of age in UK; ≥8 years of age in Europe/USA).

References

1 Van Steensel M, van Geel M, Steijlen P. New syndrome of hypotrichosis, striate palmoplantar keratoderma, acro-osteolysis and periodontitis not due to mutations in cathepsin C. Br J Dermatol 2002;147: 575–81.
2 Brun AM, van Steensel MA. A third case of HOPP syndrome – confirmation of the phenotype. Br J Dermatol 2004;150:1032–3.

Palmoplantar keratoderma-deafness syndromes (multiple OMIM entries, *GJB2* and *GJB6*)

Brief introduction and history. A number of mostly focal PPKs with hearing loss are caused by mutations in the gap junction genes *GJB2* and *GJB6* [1]. These disorders were originally reported as unique syndromes under a variety of names, such as Bart–Pumphrey syndrome, Vohwinkel syndrome and Clouston syndrome. The phenotypes can show considerable overlap but are recognizably distinct and associated with a unique mutation that in recent years has been found for most of these disorders (reviewed in [2]).

Epidemiology and pathogenesis. Most of the PPK-deafness syndromes are caused by mutations in *GJB2* coding for connexin 26. They are summarized in Table 128.1. A recent report describes PPK in a KID-like phenotype caused by a *GJB6* mutation [3]. The latter gene is typically associated with Clouston syndrome (see later) but as its product, connexin 30, interacts with connexin 26, it is perhaps not surprising to find overlapping phenotypes. Connexins are part of gap junctions, intercellular channels that are conserved throughout evolution and ubiquitously present in the body. Connexin 26 (*GJB2)* is expressed in the cochlea where it may allow the recycling of cations

Table 128.1 Overview of all skin phenotypes and genotypes of the *GJB2* gene

Syndrome	OMIM	Mutation	Domain
Keratitis-ichthyosis - deafness (KID)-like	148210	p.Gly12Arg, p.Asn14Tyr, p.Ser17Phe, p.Gly45Glu, p.Asp50Ans, p.AspTyr	NT, E1
Hystrix-like ichthyosis-deafness (HID)	602540	p.Asp50Asn	E1
Hypotrichosis-deafness	No entry	p.Asn14Lys	NT
PPK-deafness	148350	p.Gly59Arg, p.Gly59Ala, p.Arg75Trp, p.Arg75Gln, p. Δ Glu42, p.Gly130Val, p.Ser183Phe	E1, E2, CL
Bart–Pumphrey syndrome	149200	p.Asn54His, p.Asn54Lys, p.Gly59Ser	E1
Vohwinkel-like PPK-deafness	No entry	p.His73Arg	E1
Vohwinkel	124500	p.Asp66His, p.Tyr65His	E1
Mucositis-deafness	No entry	p.Phe142Leu	TM3

NT, N-terminus; E1, E2, first and second extracellular loop respectively; CL, cytoplasmatic loop; TM3, third transmembrane domain.

SECTION 27: DISORDERS OF KERATIN AND KERATINIZATION

to endolymph. In skin, it is expressed in palmoplantar epidermis and the sweat glands [4]. Mutant connexins are known to impair the epidermal calcium gradient, interfere with other connexins and are associated with endoplasmic reticulum stress [5–7]. The genotype–phenotype correlation is not well understood although we know that particular phenotypes tend to be associated with particular protein domains (Table 128.1).

Clinical features. The cardinal features are PPK of varying severity and nature in addition to sensory deafness of likewise varying severity. A papular appearance is sometimes observed at the palmar edge in diffuse keratoderma (Fig. 128.17). In Vohwinkel syndrome, shiny, translucent papules arise in childhood and gradually become confluent. Classic 'starfish keratoses' occur over the knuckles and sometimes on extensor sites. Circumferential bands leading to pseudo-ainhum occur. In Bart–Pumphrey syndrome, nail abnormalities such as leukonychia can be associated, as can knuckle pads. The associated abnormalities and the nature of the PPK usually indicate the mutation, as outlined in Table 128.1. In any patient presenting with a PPK, hearing loss should be sought.

Differential diagnosis. Although mutations in *GJB6* usually do not cause hearing loss, there are reports of patients with aberrant phenotypes resembling *GJB2* associated disease, including sensory deafness. Therefore, if a patient with symptoms suggestive of *GJB2* mutations has no mutations in that gene, *GJB6* must be sequenced. Clouston syndrome should be suspected in any patient with nail (both thinning and thickening [8]) and hair abnormalities. A PPK is not mandatory for the diagnosis and can be very mild. A rare disorder caused by mutations in *GJA1*, oculo-dento-digital syndrome, will occasionally feature a mild PPK [9]. Oculo-dento-digital syndrome can be distinguished by its associated features. Mitochondrial DNA mutations can also cause a PPK with deafness and maternal inheritance may suggest this [10].

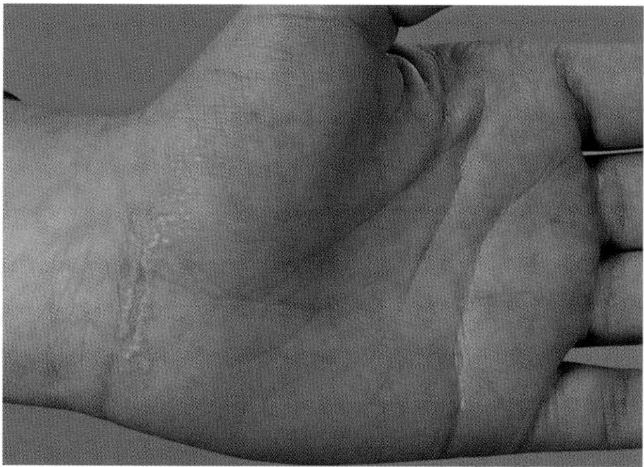

Fig. 128.17 One of the palmoplantar keratoderma-deafness disorders (mutation p.Ser183Phe in Cx26). Typical papular keratoderma that must be distinguished from acrokeratoelastoidosis.

Treatment. Retinoids are quite effective in Vohwinkel syndrome and may ameliorate the pseudo-ainhum. However, this symptom may eventually require surgical intervention. For the other phenotypes the effect of retinoids is mostly unknown. Topical keratolytic agents can be useful.

References

1 Van Steensel MA. Gap junction diseases of the skin. Am J Med Genet C Semin Med Genet 2004;131C:12–19.
2 Laird DW. Closing the gap on autosomal dominant connexin-26 and connexin-43 mutants linked to human disease. J Biol Chem 2008;283: 2997–3001.
3 Jan AY, Amin S, Ratajczak P et al. Genetic heterogeneity of KID syndrome: identification of a Cx30 gene (*GJB6*) mutation in a patient with KID syndrome and congenital atrichia. J Invest Dermatol 2004;122: 1108–13.
4 Skerrett IM, Di WL, Kasperek EM et al. Aberrant gating but a normal expression pattern, underlies the recessive phenotype of the deafness mutant Connexin26M34T. Faseb J 2004;18:860–2.
5 García IE, Bosen F, Mujica P et al. From hyperactive Connexin26 hemichannels to impairments in epidermal calcium gradient and permeability barrier in the keratitis-ichthyosis-deafness syndrome. J Invest Dermatol 2016;136:574–83.
6 Shuja Z, Li L, Gupta S et al. Connexin26 mutations causing palmoplantar keratoderma and deafness interact with Connexin43, modifying gap junction and hemichannel properties. J Invest Dermatol 2016;136:225–35.
7 Tattersall D, Scott CA, Gray C et al. EKV mutant connexin 31 associated cell death is mediated by ER stress. Hum Mol Genet 2009;18: 4734–45.
8 Van Steensel MA, Jonkman MF, van Geel M et al. Clouston syndrome can mimic pachyonychia congenita. J Invest Dermatol 2003;121:1035–8.
9 Van Steensel MA, Spruijt L, van der Burgt I et al. A 2-bp deletion in the *GJA1* gene is associated with oculo-dento-digital dysplasia with palmoplantar keratoderma. Am J Med Genet A 2005;132A:171–4.
10 Sevior KB, Hatamochi A, Stewart IA et al. Mitochondrial A7445G mutation in two pedigrees with palmoplantar keratoderma and deafness. Am J Med Genet 1998;75:179–85.

Papular hereditary palmoplantar keratodermas without associated features

Punctate palmoplantar keratoderma (OMIM #148600, 614936, *AAGAB*)

Syn.
- Palmoplantar keratderma punctate type 1 (PPKP1)
- Keratosis punctate palmoplantaris type Buschke–Fischer–Brauer

Brief introduction and history. This rare entity was first described by Buschke and Fischer in 1910 [1] and later confirmed as a hereditary disorder by Brauer in 1913 [2]. Several cases have since been described; Emmert and colleagues reported no less than 47 cases from 14 families [3].

Epidemiology and pathogenesis. Punctate PPK occurs in about 1 in 100 000 individuals and has autosomal dominant inheritance. This condition has been mapped to two chromosomal loci, 15q22, containing the *AAGAB* gene, and 8q24.13-8q24.21. Mutations in the *AAGAB* gene, which encodes the alpha- and gamma-adaptin-binding protein, p34, results in increased phosphorylation of the EGF receptor which drives keratinocyte proliferation [4]. The locus on 8q has been associated with one mutation in the *COL14A1* gene in a Chinese family [5].

Clinical features. Lesions generally develop after the age of 10 but lesions can start to appear from the teenage years up to the sixth decade. The clinical presentation is of numerous tiny keratotic papules, strictly limited to the volar aspects of the hands and feet [4–8] (Fig. 128.18). The papular keratoses progress slowly, becoming more warty and cause pain, particularly on the feet where they coalesce into focal plaques, in some patients. There is interfamilial and intrafamilial clinical variation [8]. Lesions are more florid in manual labourers. Most patients exhibit no associated features but an association with gastrointestinal malignancy has been reported in some families [9,10].

Differential diagnosis. In spiny keratoderma (also known as music box keratoderma, PPKP2, punctate porokeratotic keratoderma), the papules are tiny 1–2 mm prickly spines. Darier disease, Cowden syndrome, epidermodysplasia verruciformis and arsenic keratoses may all present with papules on the palms.

Laboratory and histology findings. Punctate lesions usually have compact acanthosis, hypergranulosis, hyperkeratosis and focal parakeratosis. Porokeratoses have a cornoid lamella.

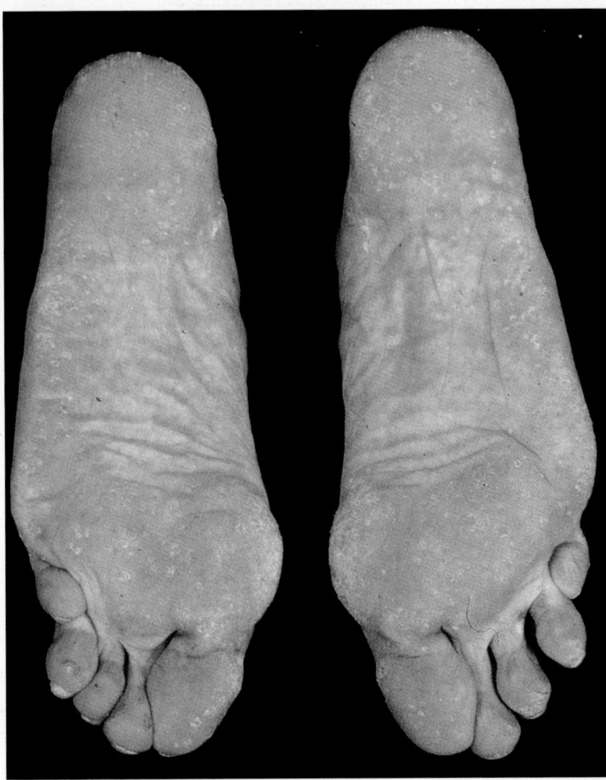

Fig. 128.18 Punctate keratoderma on the feet.

Treatment. Comfortable footwear is important. A pumice stone or similar device can be useful to reduce the hyperkeratosis. Oral retinoids are helpful in some patients and successful treatment with alitretinoin has recently been reported.

References

1 Buschke A, Fischer W. Keratodermia maculosa disseminata symmetrica palmaris et plantaris. In: Neisser A, Jacobi E (eds) Konographia Dermatologica 1. Berlin: Urban and Schwarzenberg, 1910:183–92.

2 Brauer A. Über eine besondere Form des hereditären Keratoms (Keratoma dissipatum hereditarium palmare et plantare). Arch Dermatol 1913;114:211–36.

3 Emmert S, Kuster W, Hennies HC et al. 47 patients in 14 families with the rare genodermatosis keratosis punctata palmoplantaris BuschkeFischer-Brauer. Eur J Dermatol 2003;13:16–20.

4 **Pohler E, Mamai O, Hirst J et al. Haploinsufficiency for *AAGAB* causes clinically heterogeneous forms of punctate palmoplantar keratoderma. Nat Genet 2012;44:1272–6.**

5 Guo BR, Zhang X, Chen G et al. Exome sequencing identifies a COL14A1 mutation in a large Chinese pedigree with punctate palmoplantar keratoderma. J Med Genet 2012;49:563–8.

6 Furniss M, Higgins CA, Martinez-Mir A et al. Identification of distinct mutations in *AAGAB* in families with type 1 punctate palmoplantar keratoderma. J Invest Dermatol 2014;134:1749–52.

7 Giehl KA, Herzinger T, Wolff H et al. Eight novel mutations confirm the role of AAGAB in punctate palmoplantar keratoderma type 1 (Buschke-Fischer-Brauer) and show broad phenotypic variability. Acta Derm Venereol 2016;96:468–72.

8 Eytan O, Sarig O, Israeli S et al. A novel splice-site mutation in the *AAGAB* gene segregates with hereditary punctate palmoplantar keratoderma and congenital dysplasia of the hip in a large family. Clin Exp Dermatol 2014;39:182–6.

9 Bennion SD, Patterson JW. Keratosis punctata palmaris et plantaris and adenocarcinoma of the colon. A possible familial association of punctate keratoderma and gastrointestinal malignancy. J Am Acad Dermatol 1984;10:587–91.

10 Stevens HP, Kelsell DP, Leigh IM et al. Punctate palmoplantar keratoderma and malignancy in a four-generation family. Br J Dermatol 1996;134:720–6.

Marginal papular keratoderma (OMIM 101850)

Syn.
- Palmoplantar keratderma punctate type 1 (PPKP3)
- Acrokeratoelastoidosis
- Focal acral hyperkeratosis

In 1953 and 1954, Costa described a clinical entity, which he called acrokeratoelastoidosis with fragmentation of dermal elastic fibres on skin biopsy [1,2]. Clinically, the disease is characterized by small, crateriform papules, extending along Wallace's line on the medial aspect of the foot, at the edge of the plantar skin or along the border of thenar or hypothenar eminences on the palms. The lesions usually become visible before the age of 10 but may occur later than this. Dowd described a similar clinical entity without the characteristic histology called focal acral hyperkeratosis, associated with knuckle pads and callosities at the flexor aspect of the wrist and extending onto the Achilles tendon in some patients [3]. Some patients also had plantar callosities. Inheritance seems to be autosomal dominant. The condition mainly occurs in individuals of African or Afro-Caribbean ethnicity (Fig. 128.19).

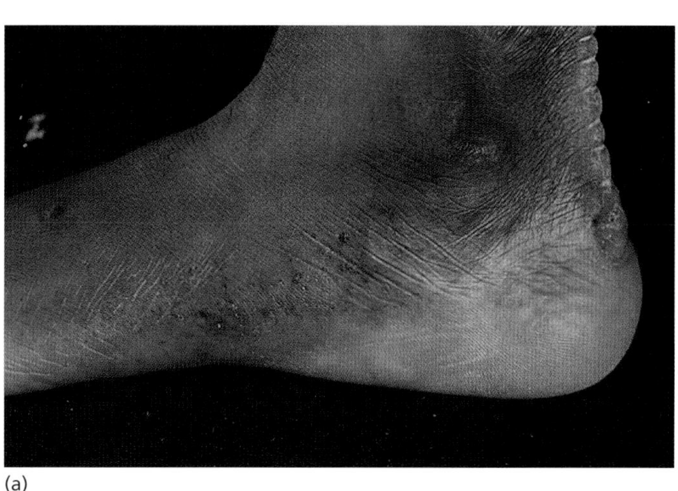
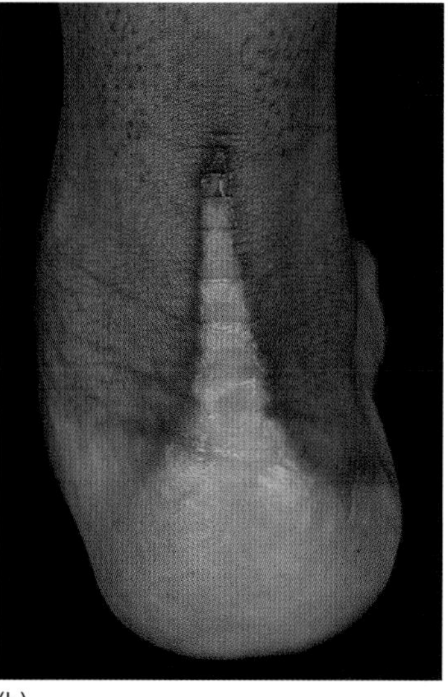

(a) (b)

Fig. 128.19 (a) Crateriform lesions on medial aspect of the foot and (b) hyperkeratosis of focal acral hyperkeratosis extending onto the Achilles tendon in a different patient.

References

1 Costa OG. Acrokeratoelastoidosis. AMA Arch Derm Syphilol 1954; 70:228–31.
2 Costa OG. Acrokeratoelastoidosis: a hitherto undescribed skin disease. Dermatologica 1953;107:164–8.
3 Dowd PM, Harman RR, Black MM. Focal acral hyperkeratosis. Br J Dermatol 1983;109:97–103.

Transient aquagenic keratoderma

Syn.
- Aquagenic reactive papulotranslucent keratoderma
- Aquagenic syringeal acrokeratoderma
- Aquagenic wrinkling of the palms

Brief introduction and history. This is a mild papular keratoderma which is triggered by contact with water or sweat.

Epidemiology and pathogenesis. Aquagenic wrinkling of the palms is classically associated in the literature with cystic fibrosis and is observed in about 10% of *CFTR* gene mutation carriers [1,2]. It has also been described in association with use of cyclo-oxygenase-2 inhibitors [3].

Clinical features. Affected individuals, most often young women, develop slightly itchy, whitish papular lesions on the palms associated with dilated acrosyringeal openings after exposure of the hands to water. Lesions subside a few minutes after drying the hands.

Treatment. Topical aluminium chloride or injection of botulinum toxin may help [4].

References

1 Weil B, Chaillou E, Troussier F et al. Aquagenic palmoplantar keratoderma in children with cystic fibrosis. Arch Pediatr 2013;20:1306–9.
2 Cabrol C, Bienvenu T, Ruaud L et al. Aquagenic palmoplantar keratoderma as a CFTR-related disorder. Acta Derm Venereol 2016;96:848–9.
3 Carder KR, Weston WL. Rofecoxib-induced instant aquagenic wrinkling of the palms. Pediatric Dermatology 2002;19:353–5.
4 Diba VC, Cormack GC, Burrows NP. Botulinum toxin is helpful in aquagenic palmoplantar keratoderma. Br J Dermatol 2005;152:394–5.

Papular hereditary palmoplantar keratodermas with associated features

Cole disease (OMIM #615522, *ENPP1*)

Brief introduction and history. In 1976, Cole reported a family in which six members over three generations had a generalized variegated pattern of hypopigmentation with palmoplantar punctate keratoses [1].

Epidemiology and pathogenesis. This is a very rare disorder with autosomal dominant and recessive inheritance. Ultrastructural examination of skin suggests defective melanosome transfer from melanocyte to keratinocyte. The dominant form is caused by missense mutations in the *ENPP1* gene (ectonucleotide pyrophosphatase/phosphodiesterase 1), encoding a cell surface protein that catalyses the hydrolysis of adenosine triphosphate to adenosine monophosphate generating extracellular pyrophosphate, which inhibits mineralization [2]. Recessive mutations in *ENPP1* have recently been reported with more extensive pigmentary change [3]. Cole disease mutations affect the somatomedin domain of ENPP1 which regulates insulin signalling. There is crosstalk with the EGF pathway making a possible link with isolated punctate PPK.

Clinical features. The disease presents during infancy with a punctate PPK and then affected children develop generalized well-demarcated hypopigmented macules most marked on the extremities. Some individuals with additional calcinosis cutis or tendon calcification have been reported.

References

1 Cole LA. Hypopigmentation with punctate keratosis of the palms and soles. Arch Derm 1976;112:998–1000.
2 Eytan O, Morice-Picard F, Sarig O et al. Cole disease results from mutations in *ENPP1*. Am J Hum Genet 2013;93:752–7.
3 Chourabi M, Liew MS, Lim S et al. *ENPP1* mutation causes recessive cole disease by altering melanogenesis. J Invest Dermatol 2018;138:291–300.

PLACK syndrome (OMIM #616295, *CAST*)

Brief introduction and history. This is a recently described syndrome encompassing peeling skin, leukonychia, acral keratoses, cheilitis and knuckle pads [1]. One of the described families was previously reported as autosomal recessive PC [2].

Epidemiology and pathogenesis. This is an autosomal recessive disorder and has been described in five individuals from four families so far [1,3]. It is caused by mutations in *CAST*, encoding calpastatin, a calpain that regulates keratinocyte cell–cell adhesion and apoptosis.

Clinical features. One of the first described cases presented at age 2 years with punctate keratoses on the palms and soles and also on the dorsum of the toes. Leukonychia and cheilitis of the lower lips was noted, as well as knuckle pads with hyperkeratotic micropapules and follicular hyperkeratosis on the extensor surface of the knees. At age 4 years, areas of peeling skin were observed particularly on the limbs. In the older patients described, generalized skin peeling was more prominent.

References

1 **Lin Z, Zhao J, Nitoiu D, Scott CA et al. Loss-of-function mutations in *CAST* cause peeling skin, leukonychia, acral punctate keratoses, cheilitis, and knuckle pads. Am J Hum Genet 2015;96:440–7.**
2 Haber RM, Rose TH. Identification of a *CAST* mutation in a cohort previously misdiagnosed as having autosomal recessive pachyonychia congenita. JAMA Dermatol 2015;151:1393–4.
3 Alkhalifah A, Chiaverini C, Del Giudice P et al. PLACK syndrome resulting from a new homozygous insertion mutation in *CAST*. J Dermatol Sci 2017;88:256–8.

Palmoplantar keratodermas of uncertain identity

There are several reports of patients suffering from PPKs that could not at the time of their publication be classified. These are listed in this section.

Palmoplantar keratoderma with clubbing of the fingers and toes and skeletal deformity (Bureau–Barrière–Thomas)

In 1959, Bureau, Barrière and Thomas described four members of one family who presented with a diffuse, symmetrical, nontransgredient palmoplantar keratosis, clubbing of the fingers and toes and skeletal changes consisting of bone hypertrophy and thinning of the cortex of long bones [1,2]. Hedstrand and colleagues [3] reported on two sisters of consanguineous parents, presenting with PPK starting in childhood, clubbing of fingers and toes and unusual skeletal changes in the terminal phalanges. Radiographic investigation revealed a peculiar deformity of the terminal phalanges. The distal end seemed splayed out and showed marginal effects suggesting atrophy [3]. In both families, the PPK was accompanied by a marked hyperhidrosis. A patient was described with PPK, drumstick finger, hypotrichosis, hypohidrosis and dental dysplasia [4].

References

1 Bureau Y, Horeau M, Barrière H et al. Deux observations de doigts en baguettes de tambors avec hyperkératose palmoplantaire et lésions osseuses. Bull Soc Fr Dermatol Syph 1958;65:328–30.
2 Bureau Y, Barrière H, Thomas M. Hippocratisme digital congénital avec hyperkératose palmo-plantaire et troubles osseux. Ann Derm Syph 1959;86:611–22.
3 Hedstrand H, Berglund G, Werner I. Keratodermia palmaris et plantaris with clubbing and skeletal deformity of the terminal phalanges of the hands and feet. Acta Derm Venereol (Stockh) 1972;52:278–80.
4 Koch HJ, Hübner U, Schaarschmidt E et al. Keratosis palmoplantaris mit Trommelschlegelfingern, Hypotrichose, Hypohidrose und Zahndysplasie. Hautarzt 1991;42:399–401.

Keratosis palmoplantaris papillomatosa et verrucosa Jakac–Wolf

In 1975, Jakac and Wolf described a clinically distinct keratoderma in four relatives of one family. Onset occurs between 2 and 6 years of age and is characterized by a verrucous–papillomatous aspect [1]. The PPK, accompanied by a violaceous red border, is nummular at onset and progresses to cover the entire surface of the palms and soles. The keratosis is sharply confined to the palms and soles. Fingers and toes have an atrophic skin and are contracted in flexion. Aberrant keratotic lesions may be present at the knees, lower arms and buttocks. Because of a profuse hyperhidrosis, which is a constant accompanying feature of the disease, and the pronounced papillomatosis, secondary infections may lead to periostitis and osteomyelitis. In one of the patients, gingivitis and periodontitis, leading to early loss of teeth, was observed. There is some resemblance to Mal de Meleda and PLS, suggesting a common pathogenetic mechanism.

Acknowledgements

The author would like to acknowledge Maurice van Steensel and Peter Steijlen, the authors of this chapter in the last edition, upon which this chapter was based. Thank you also to my patients, Pachyonychia Project and patients enrolled in the PC Registry for photographs.

Reference

1 Jakac D, Wolf A. Papillomatös-verruköse Form der palmo-plantaren Keratodermie kombiniert mit anderen Anomalien der Verhornung sowie dysplastischen Zahnveränderungen. Hautarzt 1975;26:25–9.

CHAPTER 129

Mendelian Disorders of Cornification (MEDOC): The Ichthyoses

Angela Hernández[1], Robert Gruber[2] & Vinzenz Oji[3]

[1] Department of Dermatology, Hospital Infantil del Niño Jesús, Madrid, Spain
[2] Department of Dermatology and Division of Human Genetics, Medical University of Innsbruck, Innsbruck, Austria
[3] Department of Dermatology, University Hospital Münster, Münster, Germany

Introduction, 1549
Nonsyndromic ichthyoses, 1551
Syndromic ichthyoses, 1576
Management of congenital ichthyoses, 1592

Abstract

The heterogeneous and large group of ichthyoses is highly relevant for neonatologists, paediatric dermatologists and paediatricians. The diseases are characterized by generalized hyperkeratosis and scaling. Nonsyndromic types of ichthyosis such as ichthyosis vulgaris, autosomal recessive congenital ichthyosis or keratinopathic ichthyosis can be distinguished from syndromic ichthyoses, e.g. Sjögren–Larsson or Chanarin–Dorfman syndrome. Management of the diseases is symptomatic and requires a multidisciplinary approach. This chapter follows the ichthyosis classification of Sorèze 2009 and discusses clinical findings, pathogenesis, genetics, as well as diagnostics and treatment options.

Key points

- The heterogeneous and large group of ichthyoses is highly relevant for neonatologists, paediatric dermatologists and paediatricians.
- Ichthyoses are characterized by generalized hyperkeratosis and scaling.
- Nonsyndromic types of ichthyosis, e.g. ichthyosis vulgaris, autosomal recessive congenital ichthyosis or keratinopathic ichthyosis, are distinguished from so-called syndromic ichthyoses, e.g. neuroichthyoses such as Sjögren–Larsson or Chanarin–Dorfman syndrome.
- Patients with congenital ichthyosis, e.g. born with collodion membranes, should be closely monitored for the disease course and examined for potential extracutaneous symptoms.
- Management of the diseases is symptomatic requiring a multidisciplinary approach. Specific aspects such as hypohidrosis and proneness for hyperthermia have to be considered for lifestyle recommendations.
- Patient organizations play an important role for coping with the disease.
- This chapter follows the ichthyosis classification of Sorèze 2009 and discusses clinical findings, pathogenesis, genetics, as well as diagnostics and treatment options. Of note, Netherton syndrome, erythrokeratodermia variabilis and acquired ichthyosis are discussed elsewhere in this book.

Introduction

History. The term 'ichthyosis' was first introduced more than 200 years ago by Robert Willan in his textbook on cutaneous diseases [1]. The literal translation 'scaly fish disease' (deriving from Greek 'Ιχθύς' = fish) certainly is embarrassing and should be avoided. As a technical term it is deeply entrenched in the medical literature and today refers to those Mendelian Disorders of Cornification (MeDOC) that share a conspicuous scaling, which is generalized and affects the whole integument [2,3].

Classification and nosology. In 2009 at the First Consensus Conference on Ichthyosis [4] it was agreed to differentiate between syndromic (Table 129.1a) and nonsyndromic (Table 129.1b) forms of ichthyoses. The onset of the diseases, i.e. the distinction between 'congenital onset' and 'non-congenital onset' [2,5], is no longer used as a major criterion. Definitely, almost all ichthyoses – with the prominent exception of Refsum disease – manifest at birth or in early childhood. Therefore, the heterogeneous and large group of ichthyoses (more than 36 entities) is highly relevant for neonatologists, paediatricians and paediatric dermatologists. From the diagnostic point of view, it is useful to distinguish between common and rare forms. Common ichthyoses include ichthyosis vulgaris (IV) and recessive X-linked ichthyosis (RXLI), keeping in mind that RXLI with a prevalence of 1 : 2000–3000 would formerly be considered a rare disease according to the criteria of the European Union [6]. Of note, there are entities that could be regarded either belonging to the ichthyoses or palmoplantar keratoderma (PPK) group. One such

Harper's Textbook of Pediatric Dermatology, Fourth Edition. Edited by Peter Hoeger, Veronica Kinsler and Albert Yan.

Table 129.1a Clinicogenetic classification of inherited ichthyoses: nonsyndromic forms

Disease	Mode of inheritance	Gene(s)
Common ichthyoses		
Ichthyosis vulgaris (IV) [146700]	Autosomal semidominant	*FLG*
Nonsyndromic recessive X-linked ichthyosis (RXLI) [308100]	XR	*STS*
Autosomal recessive congenital ichthyosis (ARCI)[a]		
Harlequin ichthyosis		
ARCI4B [242500]	AR	*ABCA12*
Lamellar ichthyosis (LI)/congenital ichthyosiform erythroderma (CIE)		
ARCI1 [242300]	AR	*TGM1*
ARCI2 [242100]		*ALOX12B*
ARCI3 [606545]		*ALOXE3*
ARCI4A [601277]		*ABCA12*
ARCI5 [604777]		*CYP4F22*
ARCI6 [612281]		*NIPAL4*
ARCI8 [613943]		*LIPN*[1]
ARCI9 [615023]		*CERS3*
ARCI10 [615024]		*PNPLA1*
Self-improving congenital ichtyosis (SICI)[b]		
ARCI1 [242300]	AR	*TGM1*
ARCI2 [242100]		*ALOX12B*
ARCI3 [606545]		*ALOXE3*
Bathing suit ichthyosis (BSI)		
ARCI1 [242300]	AR	*TGM1*
Keratinopathic ichthyosis (KPI)		
Epidermolytis ichthyosis (EI) [113800]	AD	*KRT1 / KRT10*
Superficial epidermolytic ichthyosis (SEI) [146800]	AD	*KRT2*
KPI variants		
Anular epidermolytic ichthyosis (AEI) [607602]	AD	*KRT1 / KRT10*
Ichthyosis Curth–Macklin (ICM) [146590]	AD	*KRT1*
Autosomal recessive epidermolytic ichthyosis (AREI) [113800]	AR	*KRT10*
Congenital reticular ichthyosiform erythroderma (CRIE) [609165][c]	AD	*KRT10 / KRT1*
Epidermolytic nevi [113800][d]	Somatic mutations	*KRT1 / KRT10*
Other nonsyndromic ichthyosis forms		
Loricrin keratoderma (LK) [604117]	AD	*LOR*
Erythrokeratodermia variabilis (EKV) [133200]	AD	*GJB3 / GJB4*
Peeling skin disease (PSD) [270300][e]	AR	*CDSN*
Exfoliative ichthyosis [607936][f]	AR	*CSTA*
Keratosis linearis-ichthyosis congenita keratoderma (KLICK) [601952]	AR	*POMP*

AD, autosomal dominant; AR, autosomal recessive.
[a] ARCI of late onset
[b] self-healing collodion baby (SHBC)
[c] ichthyosis with confetti (IWC), ichthyosis variegata
[d] may indicate a gonadal mosaicism, which can cause generalized EI in the offspring generation
[e] peeling skin syndrome (PSS) 1
[f] peeling skin syndrome (PSS) 4.
OMIM in [ ], http://www.ncbi.nlm.nih.gov/omim.
Source: Adapted from Oji et al. (2010). Revised nomenclature and classification of inherited ichthyoses: results of the First Ichthyosis Consensus Conference in Sorèze 2009. J Am Acad Dermatol 2010;63:607–41.

example is loricrin keratoderma [7] or keratosis linearis-ichthyosis congenita-keratoderma (KLICK) [8]. Still, for the clinician the distinction between ichthyosis and PPK is diagnostically valuable and helpful [9].

General pathophysiological aspects. In brief, ichthyoses are associated with abnormal differentiation and/or abnormal desquamation, e.g. showing impaired corneocyte shedding (retention hyperkeratosis) or accelerated keratinocyte production (epidermal hyperplasia/hyperproliferative hyperkeratosis). In many of the disorders, however, development of hyperkeratosis may be understood as a homeostatic repair response aimed at compensating for an abnormal epidermal barrier [3,4]. From a pathophysiological perspective it would be tempting to provide a classification based on molecular grounds, for instance unravelling keratinopathies related to mutations in keratin genes from diseases related to defects in lipid transport or cholesterol biosynthesis. However, the same class of genes may be associated with considerably different phenotypes, e.g. ranging from epidermolysis bullosa simplex to epidermolytic ichthyosis. Therefore, the present classification scheme is based upon clinicogenetic and morphological

Table 129.1b Clinicogenetic classification of inherited ichthyoses: syndromic forms

Disease		Mode of in heritance	Gene(s)
X-linked ichthyosis syndromes			
Syndromic recessive X-linked ichthyosis (RXLI)[a] [308100]		XR	*STS* (and others[a])
Ichthyosis follicularis alopecia photophobia (IFAP) Syndrome [308205]		XL	*MBTPS2*
Conradi–Hünermann–Happle syndrome (CDPX2) [302960]		XL	*EBP*
Autosomal ichthyosis syndrome/s with:			
Prominent hair abnormalities			
Netherton syndrome (NS) [256500]		AR	*SPINK5*
Ichthyosis hypotrichosis syndrome (IHS)[b] [602400]		AR	*ST14*
Neonatal ichthyosis-sclerosing cholangitis (NISCH)[c] [607626]		AR	*CLDN1*
Prominent neurological signs			
Refsum syndrome (HMSN4) [266500]		AR	*PHYH / PEX7*
Multiple sulphatase deficiency (MSD) [272200]		AR	*SUMF1*
Gaucher syndrome type 2 [230900]		AR	*GBA*
Sjögren–Larsson syndrome (SLS) [270200]		AR	*ALDH3A2*
Keratitis ichthyosis deafness (KID) syndrome [148210]		AD	*GJB2 (GJB6)*
Chanarin–Dorfman syndrome/neutral lipid storage disease (NLSD) with ichthyosis [275630]		AR	*ABHD5*
Trichothiodystrophy (TTD)			
TTD1	[601675]	AR	*ERCC2 / XPD*
TTD2	[616390]		*ERCC3 / XPB*
TTD3	[616395]		*GTF2H5 / TFIIH*
Cerebral dysgenesis-neuropathy-ichthyosis-palmoplantar keratoderma (CEDNIK) syndrome [609528]		AR	*SNAP29*
Mental retardation-enteropathy-deafness-neuropathy-ichthyosis-keratodermia (MEDNIK) syndrome [609313]		AR	*AP1S1*
Arthrogryposis-renal dysfunction-cholestasis (ARC) syndrome [208085]		AR	*VPS33B*
Ichthyosis, spastic quadriplegia, and mental retardation (ISQMR) [614457]		AR	*ELOVL4*
Other extracutaneous involvement			
Ichthyosis prematurity syndrome (IPS) [608649]		AR	*SLC27A4 (FATP4)*
Severe dermatitis-multiple allergies-metabolic wasting (SAM) syndrome [615508]		AR	*DSG1, DSP*

AD, autosomal dominant; AR, autosomal recessive; CDPX2, chondrodysplasia punctata type 2; HMSN4, hereditary motor and sensory neuropathy type 4.
[a] In the context of a contiguous gene syndrome
[b] clinical variant: congenital ichthyosis, follicular atrophoderma, hypotrichosis, and hypohidrosis syndrome
[c] also known as ichthyosis-hypotrichosis-sclerosing cholangitis (IHSC) syndrome.
OMIM in [ ], http://www.ncbi.nlm.nih.gov/omim.
Source: Adapted from Oji et al. (2010). Revised nomenclature and classification of inherited ichthyoses: results of the First Ichthyosis Consensus Conference in Sorèze 2009. J Am Acad Dermatol 2010;63:607–41.

features and the molecular pathology of the ichthyoses is discussed separately for each diagnosis.

Disclosure and acknowledgement

The present chapter for paediatric dermatology is in part based on our recent work for *Rook's Textbook of Dermatology* [10]. Therefore, the contribution of Prof. Dr Heiko Traupe (Münster, Germany) is gratefully acknowledged (refer to reference [10]).

References

1 **Willan R. On cutaneous diseases, Volume 1, Chapter 4, Ichthyosis. Barnard: London, 1808:197–212.**
2 Traupe H. The Ichthyoses. A Guide to Clinical Diagnosis, Genetic Counseling, and Therapy. Berlin: Springer-Verlag, 1989.
3 Elias PM, Williams ML, Crumrine D, Schmuth M. Ichthyoses, Clinical Biochemical, Pathogenic and Diagnostic Assessment. Basel: Karger Verlag, 2010.
4 **Oji V, Tadini G, Akiyama M et al. Revised nomenclature and classification of inherited ichthyoses: results of the First Ichthyosis Consensus Conference in Sorèze 2009. J Am Acad Dermatol 2010;63: 607–41.**
5 Oji V1, Traupe H. Ichthyoses: differential diagnosis and molecular genetics. Eur J Dermatol 2006;16:349–59.
6 Traupe H, Fischer J, Oji V. Nonsyndromic types of ichthyoses – an update. J Dtsch Dermatol Ges 2013;12:109–21.
7 Gedicke MM, Traupe H, Fischer B et al. Towards characterization of palmoplantar keratoderma cuased by gain-of-function mutation in loricrin: analysis of a family and review of the literature. Br J Dermatol 2006;154:167–171.
8 Pujol RM, Moreno A, Alomar A, De Moragas JM. Congenital ichthyosiform dermatosis with linear keratotic flexural papules and sclerosing palmoplantar keratoderma. Arch Dermatol 1989;125:103–6.
9 Peukert M. Über Ichthyosis. Eine Übersicht. Dermatol Z. Berlin 1844:171–204.
10 **Oji V, Metze D, Traupe H. Mendelian Disorders of Cornifcation (MeDOC). In: Griffiths C, Barker J, Bleiker T et al. (eds) Rook's Textbook of Dermatology, 9th edn. Chichester: John Wiley & Sons Ltd, 2016:65.1–75**

Nonsyndromic ichthyoses

Ichthyosis vulgaris

Epidemiology and pathogenesis. Ichthyosis vulgaris (IV; OMIM #146700) is the most prevalent disorder of cornification in humans. An incidence of up to 1 in 250 was reported [1,2]; however, recent studies suggest that up to

4% of northern Europeans and 3% of Asians show clinical evidence of IV [3–6]. There is no sex preference.

IV is caused by nonsense and frameshift mutations in exon 3 of the gene encoding profilaggrin (*FLG*), which is located within the epidermal differentiation complex on chromosome 1q21, resulting in a loss-of-function of the profilaggrin protein and thus a decrease in epidermal filaggrin expression [3,5,7]. The median prevalence of *FLG* mutations is 7.7% in Europe and 3% in Asia [8]. Although IV occurs in a variety of populations, the various *FLG* mutations are population-specific. In northern and central Europe two *FLG* mutations, c.1501C > T (p.Arg501Ter) and c.2282_2285delCAGT (p.Ser761CysfsTer36) are most frequent, accounting for approximately 80% of mutations in this population [5]. Severity of the IV phenotype appears to be dose dependent (semidominant mode of inheritance), with heterozygous *FLG* mutation carriers presenting mild clinical signs, whereas homozygous or compound heterozygous individuals exhibit a more severe scaling phenotype and a greater predisposition for early occurring and more intense atopic dermatitis [9]. Most individuals with a single *FLG* mutant allele only show dry skin, often with aggravation when exposed to a dry and cold climate, without knowing their underlying diagnosis.

The structural protein filaggrin, which represents the processed product of profilaggrin, is both a component of the cornified cell envelope and responsible for aggregating keratin filaments. Thereby it plays a major role in maintaining epidermal barrier function. Filaggrin breakdown products such as pyrrolidone-5-carboxylic acid serve as natural moisturizing factors contributing to a proper hydration level of the stratum corneum, and contribute to the acidic pH of the skin, which in turn is important for the activity of stratum corneum proteases involved in lipid synthesis and desquamation [10]. Therefore, *FLG* mutations lead to an impaired epidermal barrier with increased transepidermal water loss, xerosis and elevated skin surface pH in a dose-dependent fashion [11]. The increased skin surface pH likely contributes to both the scale retention and the deactivation of ceramide processing enzymes in IV. Reduced levels of trans-urocanic acid in IV have been correlated with increased levels of 25-OH vitamin D, because trans-urocanic acid shields against UVB radiation, which induces the vitamin D_3 production in the skin [12].

Clinical features. In contrast to many other forms of ichthyosis, IV is not present at birth, but usually manifests at 3 months of age or later within the first year of life [1,13]. Whereas heterozygous *FLG* mutation carriers show a mild phenotype that can be masked by maintaining proper topical treatment with moisturizers or become very discreet in the summer season because of increased humidity, homozygous and compound heterozygous individuals present a severe phenotype that tends to be more stable and chronic [6]. IV is characterized by generalized small fine white to light grey scaling, which is accentuated on the extensor surfaces of the extremities and the trunk, sparing the more hydrated axillae, groins and antecubital and popliteal fossae (Fig. 129.1). Scaling is most distinctive on the lower legs where scales can become coarse and polygonal. In contrast, the face often shows no scaling but only dry skin [1]. Scaling on the scalp is generally mild with scales attached centrally with peripheral peeling [14]. In Black and darker-skinned children, scales are hyperpigmented.

A crucial feature of IV is both hyperlinearity and marked creases of palms and soles (Fig. 129.1) and importantly this clinical sign is not changed by environmental factors. Palmoplantar hyperlinearity strongly correlates with a *FLG* mutation genotype; the positive and negative predictive value is 71% and 90% respectively [2]. Biallelic *FLG* mutation carriers show mild hyperkeratosis with

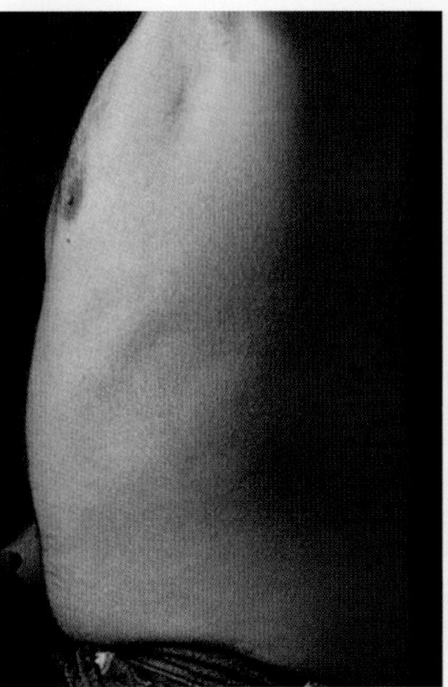

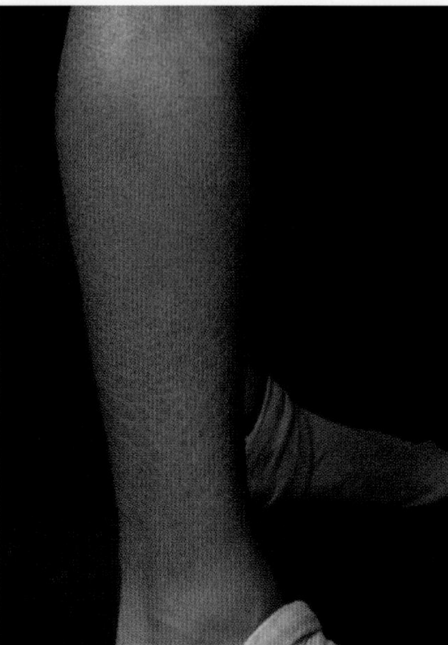

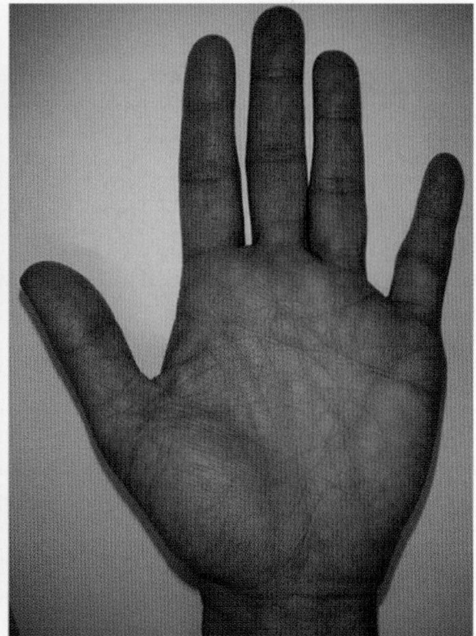

Fig. 129.1 Ichthyosis vulgaris with a generalized fine scaling phenotype, pronounced scaling of the lower limbs, and palmar hyperlinearity. Source: Courtesy of Dr R. Gruber, Innsbruck, Austria.

furrows and sometimes painful fissures of the heels. A further frequent feature of IV is keratosis pilaris, which is present in 100% of homozygous and 66% of heterozygous *FLG* mutation carriers. Thus, the absence of palmoplantar hyperlinearity as well as keratosis pilaris account for a negative predictive value for *FLG* mutations as high as 92% [2]. Subjective troubles include pruritus, xerosis and sensation of skin tightness, in particular in the winter season. Note a few patients with IV suffer from hypohidrosis and heat intolerance [15].

IV is frequently associated with the atopic triad of allergic rhinitis, asthma and atopic dermatitis. *FLG* mutations are the strongest genetic risk factor for developing atopic dermatitis. Concomitant atopic dermatitis occurs in up to 50% of IV patients, especially in those harbouring two *FLG* mutations, and dry inflamed skin can be the first clinical manifestation of IV, preceding the typical IV phenotype [4,5,15,16]. Overall, allergic rhinitis and asthma appear through the atopic march. Other than its association with atopy, IV shows no extracutaneous symptoms.

Differential diagnosis. In boys, clinical distinction from X-linked ichthyosis (XLI) may be difficult and sometimes biochemical or genetic testing is indicated to confirm the suspected diagnosis. However, XLI can often be differentiated clinically by larger, darker scales and an involvement of the neck and great flexures, absence of palmoplantar hyperlinearity and keratosis pilaris, a maternal history of delayed or prolonged labour pains, cryptorchidism and the mode of inheritance (males are affected) [17]. Autosomal recessive congenital ichthyosis (ARCI) caused by mutations in *ALOXE3*, *CERS3* or *PNPLA1*, which shows a mild phenotype can resemble IV clinically, but congenital manifestation and mode of inheritance (consanguinity) are clues for differentiation. In addition, mild forms of trichothiodystrophy can show a similar scaling phenotype to IV, but can have several extracutaneous manifestations (see later). Acquired ichthyosis, a nonheritable form of ichthyosis, can be distinguished by its onset during adulthood, a lacking family history, and the association with malnutrition, infections (leprosy), neoplasms (e.g. Hodgkin's lymphoma) and inflammatory disorders (e.g. sarcoidosis). Although palmoplantar hyperlinearity is characteristic of IV, it can also be present in Refsum disease and ARCI caused by mutations in *CYP4F22* and *CERS3*. Because IV is always a nonsyndromic ichthyosis, associated late-onset visual and neurological abnormalities point to Refsum disease.

Laboratory and histology findings. Largely, diagnosis of IV can be made clinically. Genetic testing is complementary but provides additional information about the genotype and is expedient for genetic counselling. Blood tests are unremarkable because there are no specific markers for IV. Most individuals with IV show elevated 25-OH vitamin D levels. However, this is not pathognomonic for IV [12].

Histological features of IV comprise orthohyperkeratosis or a basket weave pattern and depending on *FLG* genotype an attenuated or absent granular layer, because profilaggrin is the main component of the keratohyalin granules located within the stratum granulosum (Fig. 129.2). Ultrastructurally, heterozygous *FLG* mutation carriers exhibit a decrease in both size and number of F-type keratohyalin granules within the granular layer whereas in homozygous carriers there is a complete absence of these granules [11,18]. Further characteristics of filaggrin-depleted epidermis, assessed by electron microscopy, not only involve corneocyte defects (e.g. cytoskeletal abnormalities with intermediate filament retraction, impaired loading of lamellar body contents, attenuated cornified envelopes), but also abnormalities in the extracellular lipid matrix (e.g. inhomogeneous postsecretory dispersion and lipid bilayer organization) together with decreased tight junction expression and corneodesmosome degradation [11]. Particularly in biallelic *FLG* mutation carriers, sparse inflammatory infiltrates enriched in mast cells and increased expression of CD1a + dendritic

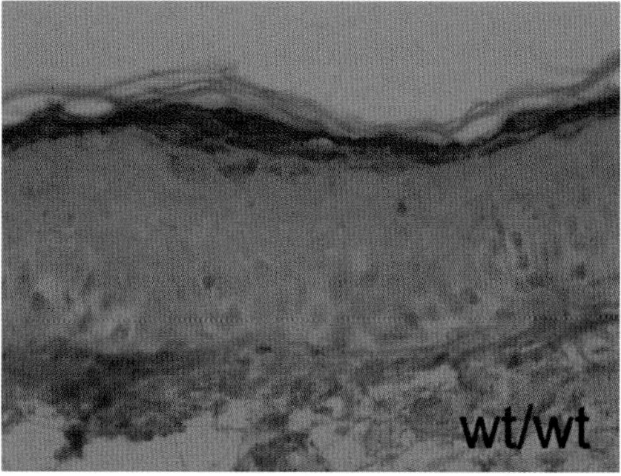

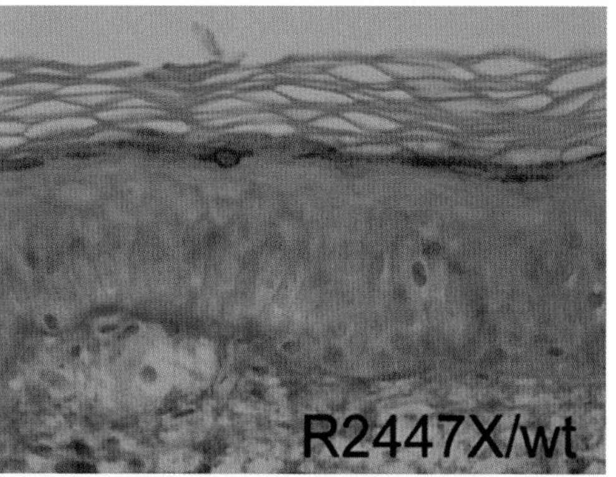

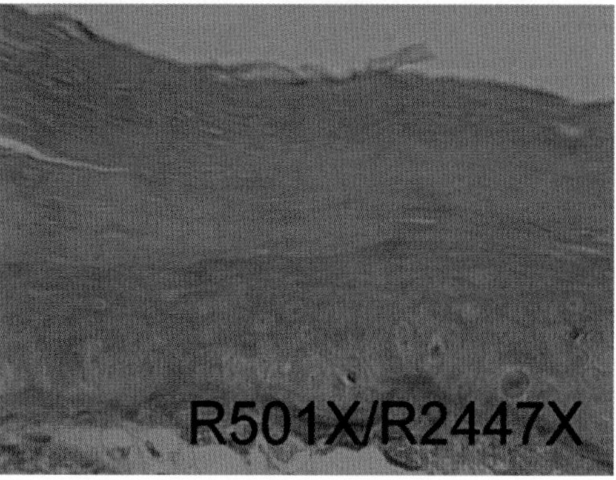

Fig. 129.2 Reduced or absent granular layer in heterozygous or compound heterozygous ichthyosis vulgaris. Source: Courtesy of Dr A. Hernandez-Martin, Madrid, Spain.

cells are detectable, suggesting sensitization in IV regardless of the existence of concomitant atopic dermatitis [11,15].

Treatment and prevention. Topical therapy is aimed at improving skin hydration as well as removal of excess scales, and should be applied frequently according to the phenotypical severity, for a lifelong period [19]. Oral retinoids are not recommended in IV. A variety of topical products, including emollients, keratolytics and epidermal proliferation modulators, have been proven to be effective. However, choice of treatment usually depends on the experience of parents and patients, and personal preferences.

Ointments and creams containing dexpanthenol, glycerol, ceramides, omega-3 fatty acids, low concentrations of salt, or urea <5% are favourable in maintaining skin softness and improving skin barrier function; however, because of irritation and a burning sensation, urea should not be used in children aged below 1 year [20,21]. Keratolytics such as urea 10–20%, and α-hydroxy, lactic, glycolic or salicylic acids are beneficial on body sites with stronger hornification, but use of salicylic acid should be avoided in small children and restricted to small body areas in older children to prevent salicylate toxicity. Topical retinoids are effective to decrease scaling in particular on the lower legs, but skin irritation limits their use. In children with concomitant atopic dermatitis, keratolytics and topical retinoids are often not well tolerated. When bathing, the addition of bath oils or synthetic detergents to the water and the subsequent application of ointments is recommended; however, some individuals with IV prefer showering. The incidence of developing atopic dermatitis in at risk neonates may be reduced by using an emollient therapy at least once daily after bathing [22].

For children with IV, having a cat in the home and tobacco smoke increase the risk of aggravating atopic dermatitis and asthma respectively and these triggers should be vigorously avoided. Moreover, individuals with IV should avoid nickel and other contact irritants as well as wet work, because they are more prone to contact sensitization and hand eczema [23,24].

References

1 **Wells RS, Kerr CB. Clinical features of autosomal dominant and sex-linked ichthyosis in an English population. Br Med J 1966:1(5493): 947–50.**
2 Brown SJ, Relton CL, Liao H et al. Filaggrin null mutations and childhood atopic eczema: a population-based case-control study. J Allergy Clin Immunol 2008;121:940–6 e943.
3 **Smith FJ, Irvine AD, Terron-Kwiatkowski A et al. Loss-of-function mutations in the gene encoding filaggrin cause ichthyosis vulgaris. Nat Genet 2006;38:337–42.**
4 **Palmer CN, Irvine AD, Terron-Kwiatkowski A et al. Common loss-of-function variants of the epidermal barrier protein filaggrin are a major predisposing factor for atopic dermatitis. Nat Genet 2006;38: 441–6.**
5 Sandilands A, Terron-Kwiatkowski A, Hull PR et al. Comprehensive analysis of the gene encoding filaggrin uncovers prevalent and rare mutations in ichthyosis vulgaris and atopic eczema. Nat Genet 2007;39:650–4.
6 Sinclair C, O'Toole EA, Paige D et al. Filaggrin mutations are associated with ichthyosis vulgaris in the Bangladeshi population. Br J Dermatol 2009;160:1113–15.
7 **Gruber R, Janecke AR, Fauth C et al. Filaggrin mutations p.R501X and c.2282del4 in ichthyosis vulgaris. Eur J Hum Genet 2007;15: 179–84.**
8 Thyssen JP, Godoy-Gijon E, Elias PM. Ichthyosis vulgaris: the filaggrin mutation disease. Br J Dermatol 2013;168:1155–66.
9 Irvine AD, McLean WH, Leung DY. Filaggrin mutations associated with skin and allergic diseases. N Engl J Med 2011;365:1315–27.
10 Kezic S, Kemperman PM, Koster ES et al. Loss-of-function mutations in the filaggrin gene lead to reduced level of natural moisturizing factor in the stratum corneum. J Invest Dermatol 2008;128:2117–19.
11 Gruber R, Elias PM, Crumrine D et al. Filaggrin genotype in ichthyosis vulgaris predicts abnormalities in epidermal structure and function. Am J Pathol 2011;178:2252–63.
12 Thyssen JP, Thuesen B, Huth C et al. Skin barrier abnormality caused by filaggrin (FLG) mutations is associated with increased serum 25-hydroxyvitamin D concentrations. J Allergy Clin Immunol 2012;130: 1204–7 e1202.
13 Ziprkowski L, Feinstein A. A survey of ichthyosis vulgaris in Israel. Br J Dermatol 1972;86:1–8.
14 Frost P, Van Scott EJ. Ichthyosiform dermatoses. Classification based on anatomic and biometric observations. Arch Dermatol 1966;94: 113–26.
15 Oji V, Seller N, Sandilands A, Gruber R et al. Ichthyosis vulgaris: novel FLG mutations in the German population and high presence of CD1a+ cells in the epidermis of the atopic subgroup. Br J Dermatol 2009;160:771–81.
16 Rodriguez E, Baurecht H, Herberich E et al. Meta-analysis of filaggrin polymorphisms in eczema and asthma: robust risk factors in atopic disease. J Allergy Clin Immunol 2009;123:1361–70 e1367.
17 Schmuth M, Martinz V, Janecke AR et al. Inherited ichthyoses/generalized Mendelian disorders of cornification. Eur J Hum Genet 2013;21:123–33.
18 Sybert VP, Dale BA, Holbrook KA. Ichthyosis vulgaris: identification of a defect in synthesis of filaggrin correlated with an absence of keratohyaline granules. J Invest Dermatol 1985;84:191–4.
19 Oji V, Traupe H. Ichthyosis: clinical manifestations and practical treatment options. Am J Clin Dermatol 2009;10:351–64.
20 Blanchet-Bardon C, Tadini G, Machado Matos M, Delarue A. Association of glycerol and paraffin in the treatment of ichthyosis in children: an international, multicentric, randomized, controlled, double-blind study. J Eur Acad Dermatol Venereol 2012;26:1014–19.
21 Vahlquist A, Ganemo A, Virtanen M. Congenital ichthyosis: an overview of current and emerging therapies. Acta Derm Venereol 2008;88:4–14.
22 Simpson EL, Berry TM, Brown PA, Hanifin JM. A pilot study of emollient therapy for the primary prevention of atopic dermatitis. J Am Acad Dermatol 2010;63:587–93.
23 Carlsen BC, Thyssen JP, Menne T et al. Association between filaggrin null mutations and concomitant atopic dermatitis and contact allergy. Clin Exp Dermatol 2011;36:467–72.
24 Novak N, Baurecht H, Schafer T et al. Loss-of-function mutations in the filaggrin gene and allergic contact sensitization to nickel. J Invest Dermatol 2008;128:1430–5.

Recessive X-linked ichthyosis

Definition. Recessive X-linked ichthyosis (RXLI; OMIM #308100), simply termed as X-linked ichthyosis (XLI) by geneticists, is a mild to moderate scaling disorder. It is the only type of ichthyosis that can be both syndromic and nonsyndromic, depending on the coexistence of extracutaneous manifestations.

Epidemiology and pathogenesis. RXLI is, after ichthyosis vulgaris (IV), the second most common form of ichthyosis. It has an overall prevalence of 1:3000 individuals [1]. RXLI is caused by mutations in the gene for steroid sulphatase (STS), a microsomal enzyme encoded in the distal short arm of the X chromosome (Xp22.3) responsible for the hydrolysis of the 3β-sulphate esters [2]. STS is expressed in the central nervous system, liver, adrenal cortex, placenta, gonads, skin and leukocytes. In the epidermis, the deficit STS results in a concentration of sulphate cholesterol in the stratum corneum 10 times higher than normal [3]. Accumulation of cholesterol sulphate in the epidermis inhibits proteases such as kallikrein 5 and kallikrein 7 that are pivotal for normal degradation of corneodesmosomes [4]. The subsequent increased intercellular cohesion delays desquamation and accounts for the retention hyperkeratosis. In the placenta, STS is responsible for dehydroepiandrosterone sulphate (DHEA-S) desconjugation within the oestrogen synthesis pathway [5]. Insufficient levels of oestrogen cause a slowing of labour secondary to insufficient dilation of the cervix and decreased response to oxytocin stimulation, which often determines prolonged labour, the need for caesarean section in female carriers and an increased risk of obstetric complications.

Clinical features. RXLI is characterized by the presence of large polygonal symmetrically distributed dark brown scales primarily located to the extensor surface of the limbs (Fig. 129.3). RXLI affects boys almost exclusively, whereas females are disease carriers and only exceptionally show clinical manifestations [6–9]. Although XLI appears very early in life, presentation as a collodion baby is uncommon. By the age of 2–6 months large, thick dark brown-to-yellow brown scales appear on the trunk, the extremities and the neck. This dark scaling on the lateral aspects of the neck and trunk give the characteristic appearance of a 'dirty look' (Fig. 129.3a). A substantial number of patients display a greyish fine desquamation that may be raise a differential diagnosis from IV or mild forms of ARCI. The antecubital and popliteal folds are usually involved but may as well be spared, whereas

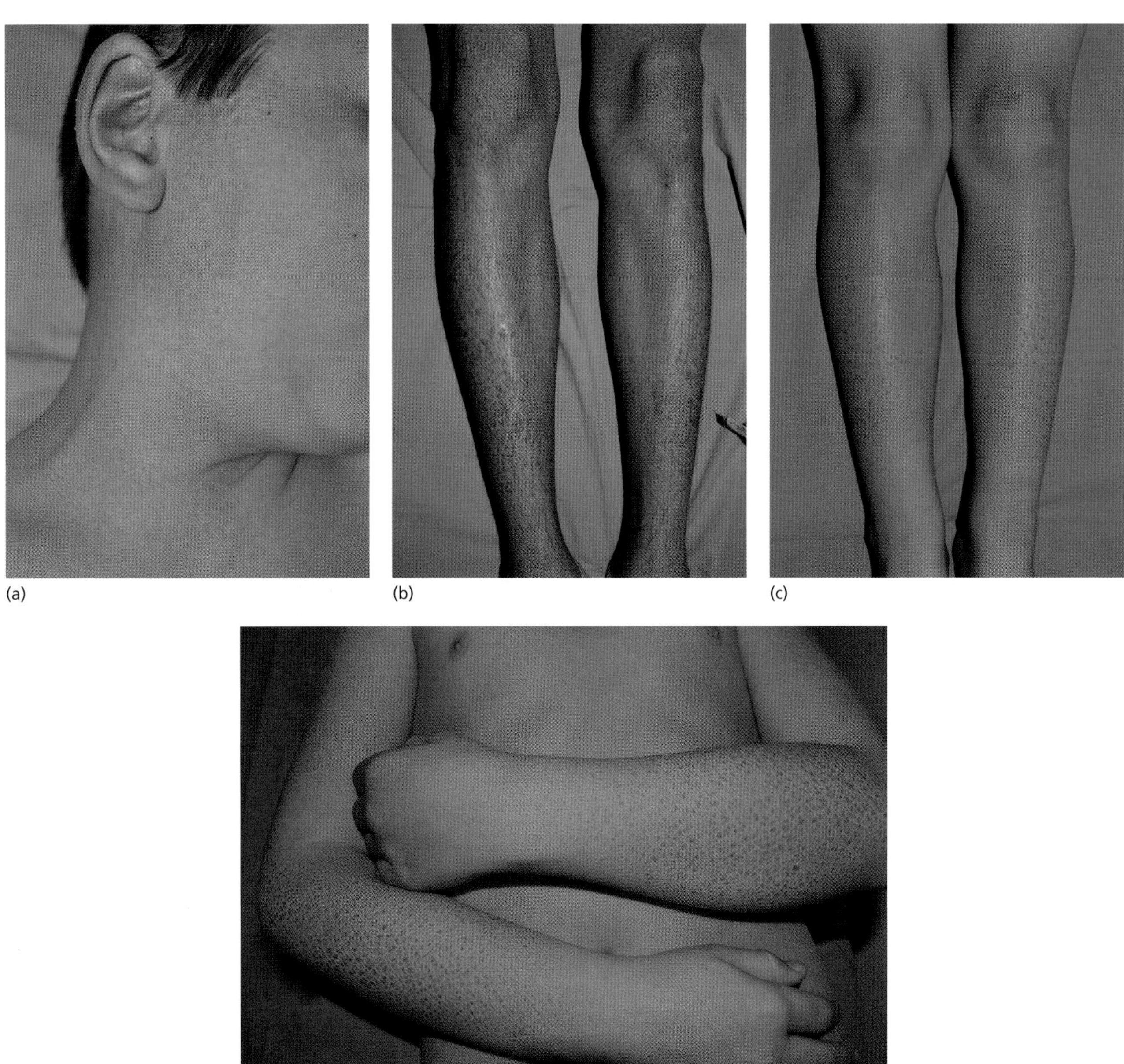

Fig. 129.3 (a) X-chromsomal recessive ichthyosis: 'dirty neck'. (b) Large scales of lower limbs. (c) Small scales of lower limbs and (d) upper limbs and trunk. Source: Rook's Textbook of Dermatology. Reproduced with permission of John Wiley & Sons.

palms and soles remain unaffected. Cephalic involvement is frequent, showing pre- and retro-auricular desquamation as well as a fine persistent scalp desquamation. Hair and nails are normal. Disease severity may be enhanced by concomitant filaggrin mutations [9], as well as by a further still unidentified modifier. Family anamnesis with affected males is very useful in making the diagnosis. The presence of an affected grandfather or uncles on the maternal side is consistent with the pattern of inheritance. Also, mothers of these boys frequently report birth complications relating to the enzyme defect in the placenta. Insufficient cervical dilatation is often found in pregnant women with placental sulphatase deficiency and may cause weakness of labour and a prolonged delivery, necessitating caesarean section or forceps delivery in around 30%.

Extracutaneous findings

Cryptorchidism is present in 5–20% of patients with RXLI [10], but it is also a relatively common finding in the general population. Diffuse corneal deposits that do not affect the visual acuity are present in about 50% of adult patients, but are infrequent in children [11]. Attention-deficit hyperactivity syndrome (ADHD) can be found in up to 40% and autism in around 25% of patients [12]. Of note, steroid sulphatase-deficient mice carrying a deletion of the *STS* gene exhibit behavioural abnormalities relevant to ADHD such as inattention and hyperactivity. Moreover, these mice display altered serotonergic function that may account for their abnormal behavior [13]. Nevertheless, patients with presumed *STS* gene mutations and ADHD have also been reported [12]. Other anecdotally reported associated findings include electroencephalographic abnormalities, pyloric hypertrophy, testicular cancer, hypogonadism, acute lymphoblastic leukaemia, congenital defect of the abdominal wall and dysthrophic epidermolysis bullosa [14,15].

Contiguity syndromes

Karyotypically normal subjects showing a deficit in STS can be classified in two different groups: nonsyndromic RXLI, where mucocutaneous findings are the only clinical manifestations, and syndromic RXLI, where patients show other associated phenotypic anomalies caused by broader chromosomal deletions. Deletions extending into adjacent genes may result in Kallman syndrome, short stature, the recessive form of X-linked chondrodysplasia punctata, brain abnormalities including mental retardation, unilateral polymicrogyria or retinitis pigmentosa [16,17].

Differential diagnosis. Although clinical diagnosis is relatively simple in most cases, genetic analysis is occasionally needed to reliably distinguish RXLI from other types of ichthyosis. In particular, patients with light grey scaling or with smaller than typical scales are often misdiagnosed with IV. Unlike IV, RXLI appears early in life and lacks palmoplantar hyperlinearity. Sparing of folds, pruritus, atopic eczema and asthma are also more frequent in IV. The absence of a granular layer on histology is diagnostic for bi-allelic IV, but when this finding is absent, histology is unspecific.

Laboratory, histology and genetic findings. Diagnosis of patients with RXLI is based on either demonstration of an STS deficiency or an *STS* gene abnormality. STS activity can be measured biochemically, e.g. in fibroblasts or in plasma. In addition, lipoprotein electrophoresis is a simple, but useful tool revealing increased mobility of beta lipoproteins. Analysis of cholesterol sulphate plasma levels by quantitative high-perfomance liquid chromatography (HPLC)/mass spectrometry is a very elegant method, but unfortunately currently available only for research purposes. Measurements of transepidermal water loss have revealed a clear-cut increase that is more pronounced than in IV patients, for example, whereas skin surface pH was not significantly altered [18]. Histology shows orthohyperkeratosis and a well-maintained, often thickened stratum granulosum. Ultrastructurally, a marked increase of persistent corneodesmosomes typical for retention hyperkeratosis can be seen. About 90% of cases show *STS* gene deletions which often (up to 25%) can be partial, whereas in 10%, point mutations are causal for RXLI [19]. Fluorescent *in situ* hybridization (FISH) allows rapid diagnosis in those cases that have large deletions, but will miss around 10% of cases. Next generation sequencing techniques can reveal small deletions as well as point mutations [20]. Absence of STS in affected male fetuses leads to low levels of maternal unconjugated oestriol [5], which may be noted on routine screening offered between 15 and 20 weeks of gestation [21]. However, although sensitive, an isolated low level of unconjugated oestriol (uE3) is not a specific marker for RXLI, because decreased uE3 can also be seen in other conditions such as fetal demise, trisomy 18 and 21, neural tube defects and Smith–Lemli–Opitz syndrome [22]. The identification of female carriers may be essential to prevent obstetric complications.

Treatment. RXLI patients benefit from the same therapeutic strategy that is applied for IV (see IV). Interestingly, treatment with moisturizers does not normalize the transepidermal water loss but rather tends to further increase it, whereas skin dryness does improve [18]. Similar to IV, most patients with RXLI improve during the warmer and more humid summer months. The need for systemic retinoids is exceptional, but may be considered in a low dosage during periods of increased disease expression [23,24].

References

1 **Craig WY, Roberson M, Palomaki GE et al. Prevalence of steroid sulfatase deficiency in California according to race and ethnicity. Prenatal Diagnosis 2010;30:893–8.**

2 Marinkovic-Ilsen A, Koppe JG, Jobsis AC, de Groot WP. Enzymatic basis of typical X-linked ichthyosis. Lancet 1978;2(8099):1097.

3 Elias PM, Williams ML, Choi EH, Feingold KR. Role of cholesterol sulfate in epidermal structure and function: lessons from X-linked ichthyosis. Biochim Biophys Acta 2014;1841:353–61.

4 **Elias PM, Crumrine D, Rassner U et al. Basis for abnormal desquamation and permeability barrier dysfunction in RXLI. J Invest Dermatol 2004;122:314–19.**
5 Bradshaw KD, Carr BR. Placental sulfatase deficiency: maternal and fetal expression of steroid sulfatase deficiency and X-linked ichthyosis. Obstet Gynecol Surv 1986;41:401–13.
6 Mevorah B, Frenk E, Muller CR, Ropers HH. X-linked recessive ichthyosis in three sisters: evidence for homozygosity. Br J Dermatol 1981;105:711–17.
7 Nagtzaam IF, Stegmann AP, Steijlen PM et al. Clinically manifest X-linked recessive ichthyosis in a female due to a homozygous interstitial 1.6-Mb deletion of Xp22.31. Br J Dermatol 2012;166:905–7.
8 Murtaza G, Siddiq S, Khan S et al. Molecular study of X-linked ichthyosis: report of a novel 2-bp insertion mutation in the STS and a very rare case of homozygous female patient. J Dermatol Sci 2014;74:165–7.
9 Ramesh R, Chen H, Kukula A et al. Exacerbation of X-linked ichthyosis phenotype in a female by inheritance of filaggrin and steroid sulfatase mutations. J Dermatol Sci 2011;64:159–62.
10 Traupe H, Fischer J, Oji V. Nonsyndromic types of ichthyoses – an update. J German Soc Dermatol 2014;12:109–21.
11 Fernandes NF, Janniger CK, Schwartz RA. X-linked ichthyosis: an oculocutaneous genodermatosis. J Am Acad Dermatol 2010;62: 480–5.
12 **Kent L, Emerton J, Bhadravathi V et al. X-linked ichthyosis (steroid sulfatase deficiency) is associated with increased risk of attention deficit hyperactivity disorder, autism and social communication deficits. J Med Genet 2008;45:519–24.**
13 Trent S, Cassano T, Bedse G et al. Altered serotonergic function may partially account for behavioral endophenotypes in steroid sulfatase-deficient mice. Neuropsychopharmacology 2012;37: 1267–74.
14 Hernandez-Martin A, Cuadrado-Corrales N, Ciria-Abad S et al. X-linked ichthyosis along with recessive dystrophic epidermolysis bullosa in the same patient. Dermatology 2010;221:113–16.
15 Hernandez-Martin A, Gonzalez-Sarmiento R, De Unamuno P. X-linked ichthyosis: an update. Br J Dermatol 1999;141:617–27.
16 Puri PK, Reddi DM, Spencer-Manzon M et al. Banding pattern on polarized hair microscopic examination and unilateral polymicrogyria in a patient with steroid sulfatase deficiency. Arch Dermatol 2012;148:73–8.
17 Ballabio A, Bardoni B, Carrozzo R et al. Contiguous gene syndromes due to deletions in the distal short arm of the human X chromosome. Proc Natl Acad Sci U S A 1989;86:10001–5.
18 Hoppe T, Winge MC, Bradley M et al. X-linked recessive ichthyosis: an impaired barrier function evokes limited gene responses before and after moisturizing treatments. Br J Dermatol 2012;167: 514–22.
19 Canueto J, Ciria S, Hernandez-Martin A et al. Analysis of the STS gene in 40 patients with recessive X-linked ichthyosis: a high frequency of partial deletions in a Spanish population. J Eur Acad Dermatol Venereol 2010;24:1226–9.
20 Ali RH, Mahmood S, Raza SI et al. Genetic analysis of Xp22.3 micro-deletions in seventeen families segregating isolated form of X-linked ichthyosis. J Dermatol Sci 2015;80:214–17.
21 Keren DF, Canick JA, Johnson MZ et al. Low maternal serum unconjugated estriol during prenatal screening as an indication of placental steroid sulfatase deficiency and X-linked ichthyosis. Am J Clin Pathol 1995;103:400–3.
22 Schoen E, Norem C, O'Keefe J et al. Maternal serum unconjugated estriol as a predictor for Smith-Lemli-Opitz syndrome and other fetal conditions. Obstet Gynecol 2003;102:167–72.
23 Bruckner-Tuderman L, Sigg C, Geiger JM, Gilardi S. Acitretin in the symptomatic therapy for severe recessive x-linked ichthyosis. Arch Dermatol 1988;124:529–32.
24 Pehamberger H, Neumann H, Holubar K. Oral treatment of ichthyosis with an aromatic retinoid. Br J Dermatol 1978;99:319–24.

Autosomal recessive congenital ichthyoses

Introduction. Autosomal recessive congenital ichthyoses (ARCI) is an 'umbrella' term that includes all nonsyndromic autosomal recessive congenital forms of ichthyosis without a tendency toward blistering [1]. Terms like lamellar ichthyosis or congenital ichthyosiform erythroderma describe extreme ends of the clinical spectrum, but are used in older textbooks as synonyms. The group includes harlequin ichthyosis, self-improving congenital ichthyosis, as well as transient manifestations, such as collodion baby [2,3].

Epidemiology and pathogenesis. Registry-based data from Spain [4] and Germany [5] show that the prevalence of ARCI in Europe is in the range of 1.6 : 100 000. ARCI is associated with mutations in several genes (Table 129.1a), which encode proteins involved in lipid transport, such as *ABCA12* [6], in lipid biosynthesis such as *CERS3* [7], in fatty acid metabolism, or have a role in assembling suprastructures such as the cornified envelope. A 'unified field theory' explaining how these various proteins interact with each other and result in a barrier defect and in hyperkeratosis has not yet been established, although it seems that further research on the role of ceramides, essential fatty acids, lipoxygenase enzymes and their hepoxilin products will significantly increase our functional understanding of the pathophysiology [8].

Genotype–phenotype correlations have been reported for some of these disorders. This is best illustrated by the *ABCA12* gene. Missense mutations in this gene cause either lamellar ichthyosis [9] or congenital ichthyosiform erythroderma [10], whereas nonsense or frameshift mutations result in life-threatening harlequin ichthyosis [6]. A combination of the two types of mutations results in an intermediate phenotype [11]. Similarly, bathing suit ichthyosis (BSI) has been associated with distinct temperature-sensitive mutations in *TGM1*About 10–20% of ARCI cases cannot be attributed to known genes [12].

References
1 **Oji V, Tadini G, Akiyama M et al. Revised nomenclature and classification of inherited ichthyoses: results of the First Ichthyosis Consensus Conference in Sorèze 2009. J Am Acad Dermatol 2010;63:607–41.**
2 **Vahlquist A, Bygum A, Gånemo A et al. Genotypic and clinical spectrum of self-improving collodion ichthyosis: ALOX12B, ALOXE3, and TGM1 mutations in Scandinavian patients. J Invest Dermatol 2010;130:438–43.**
3 Traupe H, Fischer J, Oji V. Nonsyndromic types of ichthyoses – an update. J Dtsch Dermatol Ges 2014;12:109–21
4 **Hernández-Martín A, Garcia-Doval I, Aranegui B et al. Prevalence of autosomal recessive congenital ichthyosis: a population-based study using the capture-recapture method in Spain. J Am Acad Dermatol 2012;67:240–4.**
5 **Hartz T, Hennies H, Oji V et al. The prevalence of autosomal recessive congenital ichthyosis and of transglutaminase-1 deficiency in Germany: Calculation of estimates using the three-source capture-recapture method. J Invest Dermatol 2013;133S:S91.**
6 Akiyama M, Sugiyama-Nakagiri Y, Sakai K et al. Mutations in lipid transporter ABCA12 in harlequin ichthyosis and functional recovery by corrective gene transfer. J Clin Invest 2005;115:1777–84.
7 Rabionet M, Gorgas K, Sandhoff R. Ceramide synthesis in the epidermis. Biochim Biophys Acta 2014;1841:422–34.
8 Muñoz-Garcia A, Thomas CP, Keeney DS, Zheng Y, Brash AR. The importance of the lipoxygenase-hepoxilin pathway in the mammalian epidermal barrier. Biochim Biophys Acta 2014;1841:401–8.
9 Lefévre C, Audebert S, Jobard F et al. Mutations in the transporter ABCA12 are associated with lamellar ichthyosis type 2. Hum Mol Genet 2003;12:2369–78.

10 Sakai K, Akiyama M, Yanagi T et al. ABCA12 is a major causative gene for non-bullous congenital ichthyosiform erythroderma. J Invest Dermatol 2009;129:2306–9.
11 Akiyama M, Sakai K, Sugiyama-Nakagiri Y et al. Compound heterozygous mutations including a de novo missense mutation in ABCA12 led to a case of harlequin ichthyosis with moderate clinical severity. J Invest Dermatol 2006 ;126:1518–23.
12 Fischer J. Autosomal recessive congenital ichthyosis. J Invest Dermatol 2009;129:1319–21.

Harlequin ichthyosis

Introduction. Harlequin ichthyosis (HI) is the most devastating type of ARCI. It is lethal in around 44% of cases [1].

Epidemiology and pathogenesis. Based on preliminary data from the Network for Ichthyoisis and Related Keratinization Disorders (NIRK) registry in Germany, the prevalence of HI is estimated to be in the range of 1 : 2 million. It appears to be roughly 10 times lower than transglutaminase-1 (TG1) deficient ARCI. Nonsense and/or frameshift mutations in the *ABCA12* gene cause lack of protein expression in HI [2–5]. ABCA12 transfers lipids such as glucosylceramides, which are essential for epidermal barrier formation, into lamellar bodies. It plays an essential role in the loading and formation of lamellar bodies that transport also proteases such as

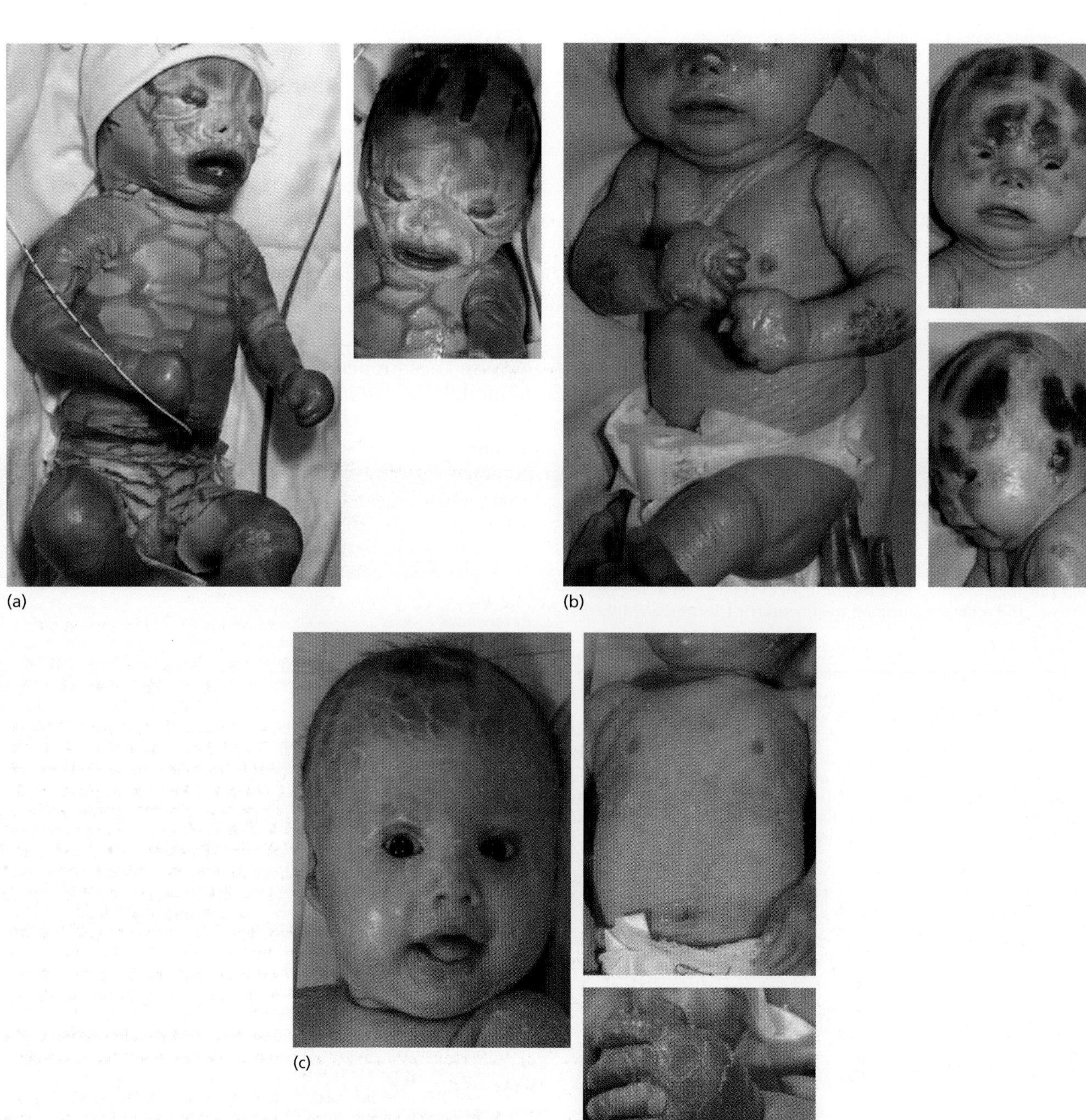

Fig. 129.4 Harlequin ichthyosis. (a) Neonate, (b) aged 6 weeks on retinoid therapy and (c) 6 months.

kallikrein 5, 7 and 14 and secrete these proteins into the intercellular space in the stratum corneum [6]. These proteases play an important role in desquamation by degrading corneodesmosomes [7], thus leading to a retention hyperkeratosis [8].

Clinical features. Neonates are born with armour-like skin (truncal plates with fissuring) (Fig. 129.4), which can considerably impair movement and the ability to drink and breath. Bilateral ectropion and eclabium are present and hyperkeratotic skin may result in ears lacking retroaural folds. Around 10% of children develop autoamputation of digits [1]. A major problem in early infancy is a proneness to infection of the skin, as well as other organs such as the lungs. Respiratory problems are the major cause of death in neonates [9]. In those children who survive the critical initial phase of the disease, the thickening of the stratum corneum improves somewhat and large, lamellar scales, accompanied by marked ichthyosiform erythroderma develop. In later life persistent ectropion is a frequent major problem, and often these patients have problems achieving and maintaining normal body weight despite high calorie supplementation. Vitamin D deficiency causing rickets and osteomalacia can occur [1].

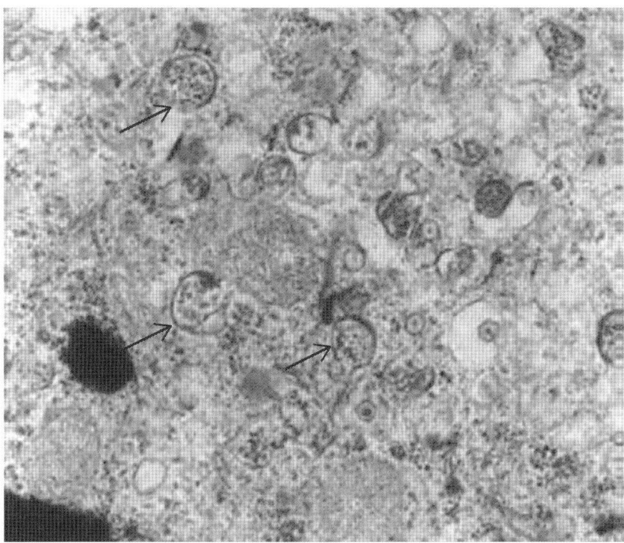

(a)

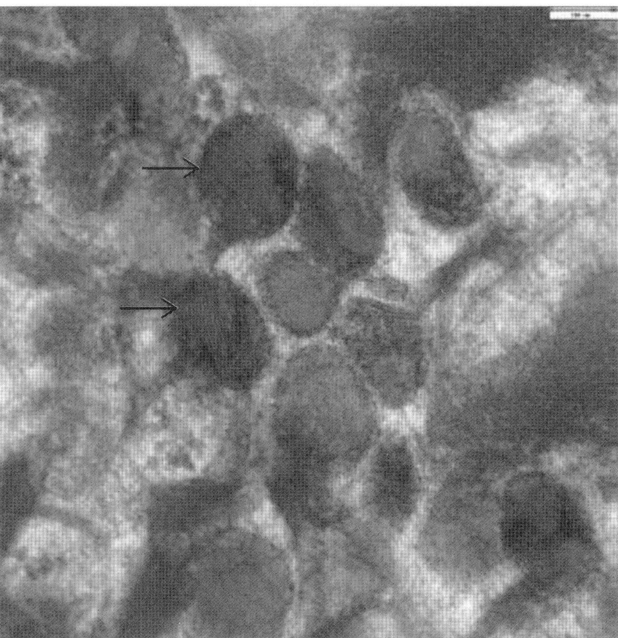

(b)

Fig. 129.5 Ultrastructural diagnosis of harlequin ichthyosis. (a) Abnormal lamellar bodies in *ABCA12* deficiency. (b) Morphology of normal lamellar bodies in granular layer cells with their diverse cargos: mostly lamellated, but also homogeneous areas (higher magnification). Source: Courtesy of Dr I. Hausser, Institute of Pathology, Heidelberg University Hospital, Heidelberg, Germany.

Histology and ultrastructure. HI has a striking histology showing an enormous thickness of the stratum corneum. There is parakeratosis and hypergranulosis, and nonpolar lipids are reduced, whereas expression of proteases like kallekrein 5 and cathepsin D are dramatically reduced [10]. Electron microscopy reveals numerous abnormal lamellar bodies in the stratum granulosum and accumulation of extruded irregular lamellar bodies as vesicular structures between the epidermal cornified cells. This defect of lamellar bodies is highly pathognomonic for HI (Fig. 129.5).

Treatment. Management requires an interdisciplinary approach – reviewed in [1] – and will be discussed in the section 'Management of collodion baby and harlequin ichthyosis'.

References

1 **Rajpopat S, Moss C, Mellerio J et al. Harlequin ichthyosis: a review of clinical and molecular findings in 45 cases. Arch Dermatol 2011;147:681–6.**

2 **Thomas AC, Cullup T, Norgett EE et al. ABCA12 is the major harlequin ichthyosis gene. J Invest Dermatol 2006;126:2408–13.**

3 **Akiyama M, Sugiyama-Nakagiri Y, Sakai K et al. Mutations in lipid transporter ABCA12 in harlequin ichthyosis and functional recovery by corrective gene transfer. J Clin Invest 2005;115: 1777–84.**

4 Akiyama M. ABCA12 mutations and autosomal recessive congenital ichthyosis: a review of genotype/phenotype correlations and of pathogenetic concepts. Hum Mutat 2010;31:1090–6.

5 Yamanaka Y, Akiyama M, Sugiyama-Nakagiri Y et al. Expression of the keratinocyte lipid transporter ABCA12 in developing and reconstituted human epidermis. Am J Pathol 2007;171:43–52.

6 Scott CA, Rajpopat S, Di WL. Harlequin ichthyosis: ABCA12 mutations underlie defective lipid transport, reduced protease regulation and skin-barrier dysfunction. Cell Tissue Res 2013;351:281–8.

7 **Caubet C, Jonca N, Brattsand M et al. Degradation of corneodesmosome proteins by two serine proteases of the kallikrein family, SCTE/KLK5/hK5 and SCCE/KLK7/hK7. J Invest Dermatol 2004;122: 1235–44.**

8 Thomas AC, Tattersall D, Norgett EE et al. Premature terminal differentiation and a reduction in specific proteases associated with loss of ABCA12 in Harlequin ichthyosis. Am J Pathol 2009;174:970–8.

9 Yanagi T, Akiyama M, Nishihara H et al. Harlequin ichthyosis model mouse reveals alveolar collapse and severe fetal skin barrier defects. Hum Mol Genet 2008;17:3075–83.

10 Milner ME, O'Guin WM, Holbrook KA, Dale BA. Abnormal lamellar granules in harlequin ichthyosis. J Invest Dermatol 1992;99:824–9.

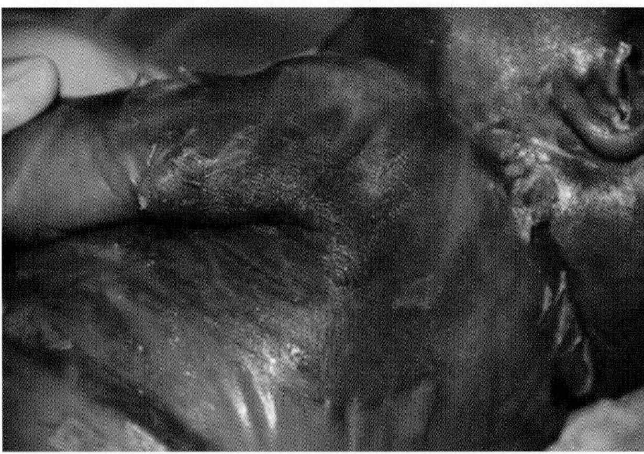

Fig. 129.6 Autosomal recessive congenital ichthyosis. Sheddding of collodion membranes after 1 week. Source: Rook's Textbook of Dermatology. Reproduced with permission of John Wiley & Sons.

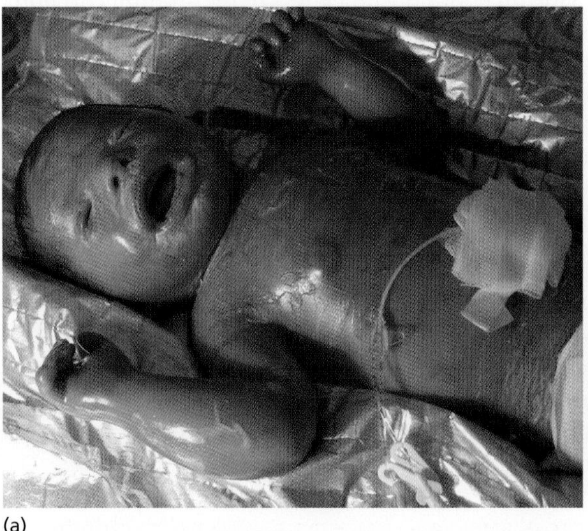

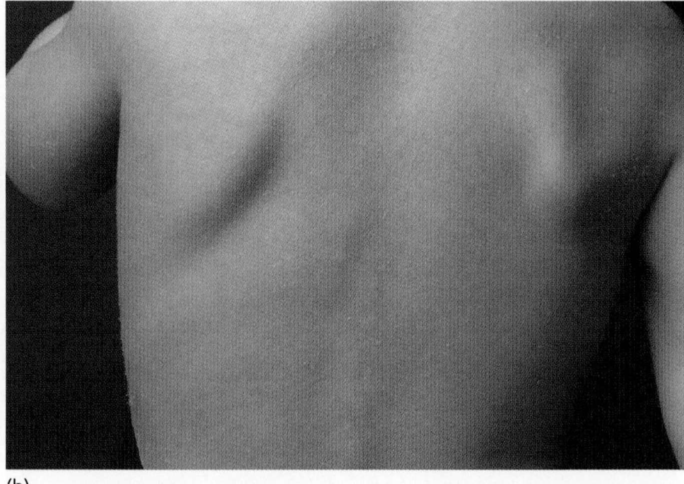

(a) (b)

Fig. 129.7 Self-improving congenital ichthyosis. (a) Collodion baby. (b) Mild ichthyosis at the age of 21 months. Source: Courtesy of the Department of Dermatology, University Hospital Münster, Münster, Germany.

Collodion baby and self-improving congenital ichthyosis

Definition. The term collodion baby describes a nonspecific transient condition in newborns. Lamellar ichthyosis typically presents at birth as 'collodion baby' [1], but the same is true for several syndromic types of congenital ichthyosis such as trichothiodystrophy or Gaucher syndrome type 2 (Table 129.1b).

Pathogenesis. Refer to lamellar ichthyosis (LI) and congenital ichthyosiform erythroderma (CIE), BSI or special forms of syndromic ichthyoses (see later).

Clinical features. The neonate is encased in a shiny parchment-like membrane (Fig. 129.6), which cracks within a few days after birth and usually peels off within the first 4 weeks of life. Initially the clinical presentation can be quite severe and often includes ectropion and everted lips of different degrees. Afterwards for a brief time healthy skin becomes visible. Collodion babies look similar at birth, but later on take different clinical courses. In around 80% of cases collodion baby is then followed by the onset of an ARCI subtype. The clinical presentations may evolve into BSI or into the phenotypes of LI, e.g. in severe TG1 deficiency, or CIE, e.g. in lipoxygenase deficiency. However, around 10–20 % of cases develop into self-improving congenital ichthyosis (SICI) [2] or self-healing collodion baby (SHCB) (Fig. 129.7) [3].

Differential diagnosis. Ichthyosis prematurity syndrome (IPS) is an important differential diagnosis of SICI and SHCB.

Treatment. Refer to the section 'Management of collodion baby and harlequin ichthyosis'.

References

1 Van Gysel D, Lijnen RL, Moekti SS et al. Collodion baby: a follow-up study of 17 cases. J Eur Acad Dermatol Venereol 2002;16:472–5.

2 Vahlquist A, Bygum A, Gånemo A et al. Genotypic and clinical spectrum of self-improving collodion ichthyosis: ALOX12B, ALOXE3, and TGM1 mutations in Scandinavian patients. J Invest Dermatol 2010;130:438–43.

3 Raghunath M, Hennies HC, Ahvazi B et al. Self-healing collodion baby: a dynamic phenotype explained by a particular transglutaminase-1 mutation. J Invest Dermatol 2003;120:224–8.

Bathing suit ichthyosis

Definition. Bathing suit icthyosis (BSI) is a peculiar type of ARCI first recognized in South African Bantu of the Nguni ethnic group [1]. Although children are born as collodion babies, they later develop a lamellar type of ichthyosis that spares the face and the extremities, and follows the distribution pattern of bathing suits.

Pathogenesis. BSI was found to be caused by peculiar missense mutations in *TGM1* that render the enzyme TG1 temperature sensitive [2,3]. Recombinant expression of the *TGM1* mutations in BSI showed that they exhibit a marked shift in temperature optimum from 37 °C to 31 °C [4]. Deficient activity of BSI mutants could be rescued and even reconstituted by decreasing the temperature to below 33 °C. All BSI mutations showed an activity above 10% at their temperature optimum at 31 °C and a dramatic decrease at 37 °C [4]. A few of these patients heal completely eventually and could also be regarded as examples of SICI [5–7].

Clinical features. The most striking aspect is the dynamic of the phenotype. Children are born as collodion babies involving the entire skin. Shedding of the collodion membrane is followed by development of large dark grey/brownish scales affecting the trunk and the scalp, but sparing the face and extremities (Fig. 129.8). Palms and soles are dry and diffusely mildly hyperkeratotic. Digital thermography validated a striking correlation between warmer body areas and presence of scaling in patients [2]. The disease tends to become worse in the summer months and to improve in winter [8]. Hypohydrosis that is often seen in ARCI may play a crucial role in local heat accumulation that results in additional reduction of TG1 activity [9]. In our experience, hyperkeratoses can develop in the ear canal affecting the ability to hear.

Laboratory, histology and ultrastructure findings. *In situ* assessment of TG1 activity reveals a deficiency only in affected skin, but sufficient activity in unaffected healthy appearing skin [2]. Likewise, ultrastructural analysis reveals a massively thickened stratum corneum displaying multiple cholesterol clefts which are typical for a TG1 deficiency, whereas stratum corneum is of normal thickness in healthy skin and shows no cholesterol clefts [2].

Treatment. Management corresponds to that of lamellar ichthyosis. In addition, special attention should be given to the ears and to removing keratotic material from the ear canal (see 'Special aspects of treatment').

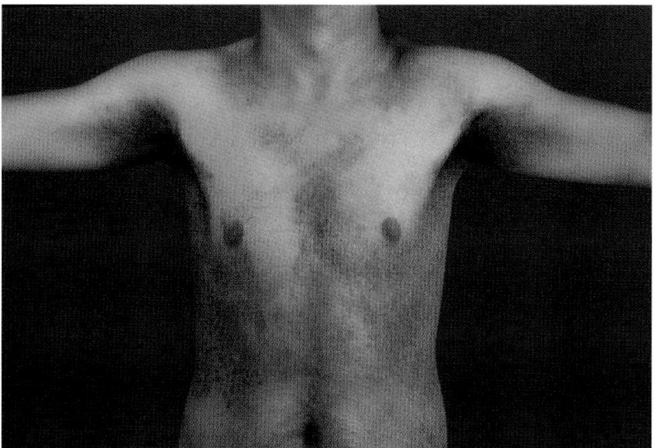

Fig. 129.8 Bathing suit ichthyosis affecting areas with high skin temperature. Source: Courtesy of the Department of Dermatology, University Hospital Münster, Münster, Germany.

References

1 **Jacyk WK. Bathing-suit ichthyosis. A peculiar phenotype of lamellar ichthyosis in South African blacks. Eur J Dermatol 2005;15:433–6.**
2 **Oji V, Hautier JM, Ahvazi B et al. Bathing suit ichthyosis is caused by transglutaminase-1 deficiency: evidence for a temperature-sensitive phenotype. Hum Mol Genet 2006;15:3083–97.**
3 Arita K, Jacyk WK, Wessagowit V et al. The South African 'bathing suit ichthyosis' is a form of lamellar ichthyosis caused by a homozygous missense mutation, p.R315L, in transglutaminase 1. J Invest Dermatol 2007;127:490–3.
4 Aufenvenne K, Oji V, Walker T et al. Transglutaminase-1 and bathing suit ichthyosis: molecular analysis of gene/environment interactions. J Invest Dermatol 2009;129:2068–71.
5 Trindade F, Fiadeiro T, Torrelo A et al. Bathing suit ichthyosis. Eur J Dermatol 2010;20:447–50.
6 Bourrat E, Blanchet-Bardon C, Derbois C et al. Specific TGM1 mutation profiles in bathing suit and self-improving collodion ichthyoses: phenotypic and genotypic data from 9 patients with dynamic phenotypes of autosomal recessive congenital ichthyosis. Arch Dermatol 2012;148:1191–5.
7 Hackett BC, Fitzgerald D, Watson RM et al. Genotype-phenotype correlations with TGM1: clustering of mutations in the bathing suit ichthyosis and self-healing collodion baby variants of lamellar ichthyosis. Br J Dermatol 2010;162:448–51.
8 Yamamoto M, Sakaguchi Y, Itoh M et al. Bathing suit ichthyosis with summer exacerbation: a temperature-sensitive case. Br J Dermatol 2012;166:672–4.
9 Washio K, Fukunaga A, Terai M et al. Hypohidrosis plays a crucial role in the vicious circle of bathing suit ichthyosis: a case with summer exacerbation. Acta Derm Venereol 2014;94:349–50.

Lamellar ichthyosis and congenital ichthyosiform erythroderma

Definition. When the term 'lamellar ichthyosis' (LI) was coined by the American dermatologist Frost [1] in the 1960s, it was used to denote a type of ARCI that is characterized by large, plate-like dark-brown hyperkeratoses covering the entire body (Fig. 129.9a). At the other end of the clinical spectrum, ARCI patients may present with very marked erythroderma, and mostly fine often whitish or grey scales. This is referred to as congenital ichthyosiform erythroderma CIE (Fig. 129.10).

Epidemiology and pathogenesis. Deficiency of TG1 as the most frequent cause of ARCI is responsible for 32% of ARCI cases in Germany, whereas in the USA it has been found in up to 55% of cases studied [2]. In Europe, mutations in *ALOX12B* account for 12% of ARCI, and *ALOXE3* mutations are responsible for a further 5% of cases. *NIPAL4* mutations account for 16% of ARCI and are thus a frequent cause. Around 8% of ARCI cases are caused by mutations in the *CYP4F22* gene [3,4]. The LI or CIE phenotype is not specific for a certain gene [5,6].

TG1 critically contributes to the assembly of the cornified envelope by catalysing calcium-dependent crosslinking of proteins, such as involucrin, loricrin, and proline-rich proteins, and by binding omega-hydroxy ceramides to proteins such as involucrin, thus connecting the corneocyte lipid envelope with the cornified envelope [7,8].

The epidermal lipoxygenases E3 and 12B act on adjacent steps in the hepoxilin pathway and are believed to play a role in the secretion of lamellar bodies so that mutations in the genes encoding these enzymes result in impaired secretion of lipids and formation of the intercellular lipids in the stratum corneum [9–11].

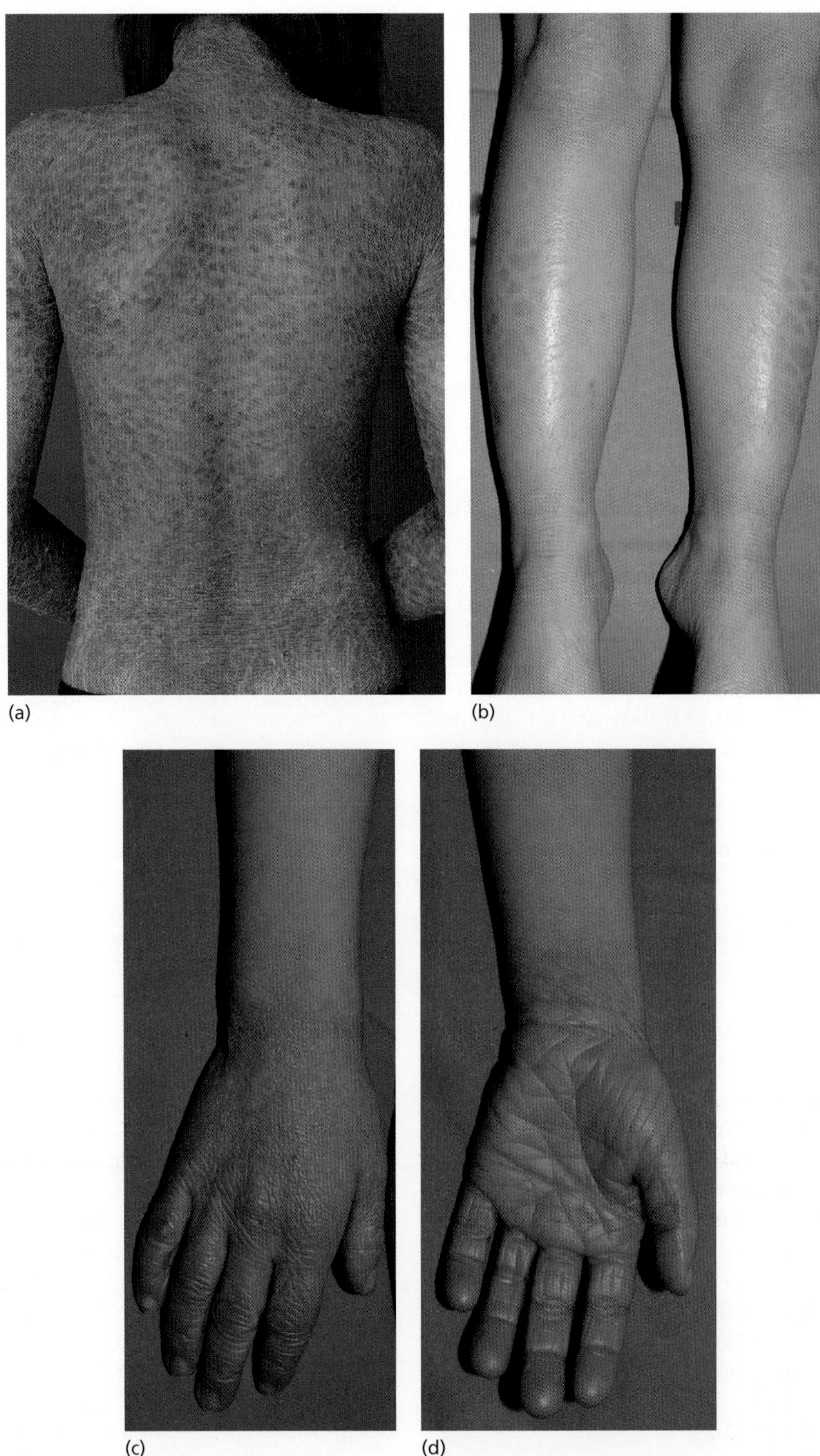

Fig. 129.9 Autosomal recessive congenital ichthyosis caused by transglutaminase 1 deficiency: classic lamellar scaling (a) and mild to moderate presentations when treated properly (b–d). Source: Courtesy of the Department of Dermatology, University Hospital Münster, Münster, Germany.

The *NIPAL4* gene encodes for the protein ichthyin. Patients with a *NIPAL4* mutation show a markedly increased expression of epidermal lipoxigenases and TG1 in their skin indicating a common metabolic pathway essential for skin barrier homeostasis [12,13]. Ichthyin appears to localize to desmosomes and keratins [14] and interacts with fatty acid transporter protein 4 [15], which is defective in IPS.

The gene *CYP4F22* encodes a cytochrome P450 polypeptide that is a homolog of a leukotriene B4 omega-hydroxylase. The actual function of this gene for the epidermal barrier has not been established, but it has been hypothesized that it participates in the hepoxilin pathway by catalysing the conversion of trioxilin A3 to 20 hydroxy-(R) trioxilin [16].

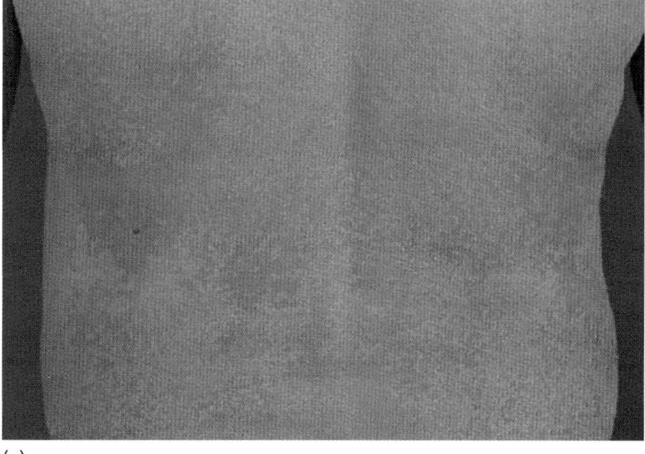
(a)

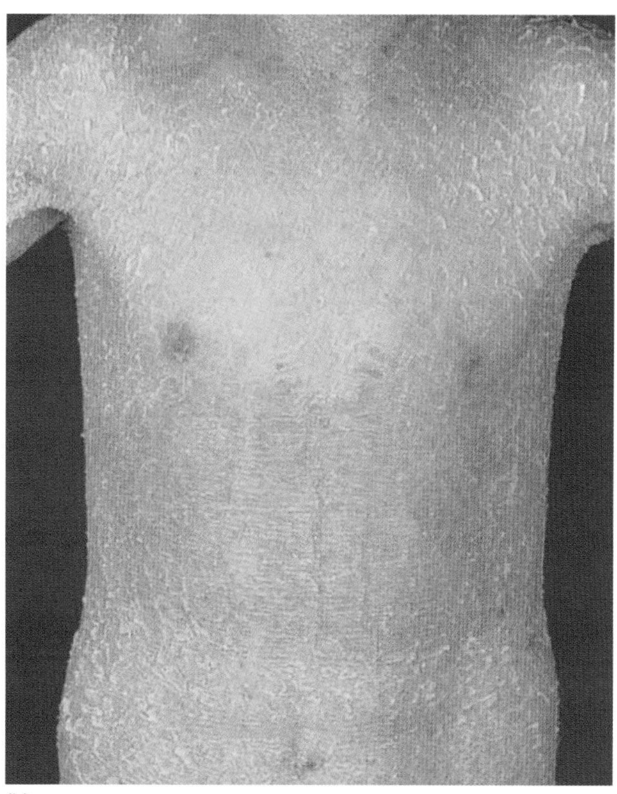
(b)

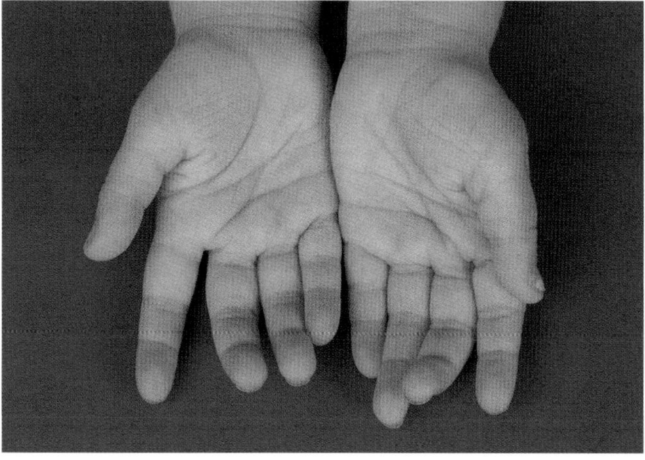
(c)

Fig. 129.10 Congenital ichthyosiform erythroderma. (a) Infancy. (b) Adulthood. (c) Palmoplantar hyperlinearity in *ALOXE3* mutations. Source: (a) and (b) courtesy of the Department of Dermatology, University Hospital Münster, Münster, Germany.

Mutations in the *CERS3* gene encoding ceramide synthase 3 are a rare cause of ARCI [17,18]. Inactivating mutations in this gene are associated with a loss of very long acyl chains from C26 up to C34 in terminally differentiating keratinocytes of affected patients and thus impair epidermal barrier formation.

LIPN encodes an acid lipase that is involved in triglyceride metabolism in mammals and is expressed exclusively in the epidermis. A 2 bp deletion in *LIPN* was found to be associated with a mild form of CIE showing diffuse ichthyosis on the legs [19].

PNPLA1 belongs to the patatin-like phospholipase family and is related to *PNPLA2*, which causes neutral lipid storage disease with myopathy but without ichthyosis. *PNPLA1* mutations may be associated with fine white scales, only mild erythroderma, palmoplantar keratoderma and a pseudosyndactyly of the second and third toes [20].

Clinical features. A definite genotype/phenotype relationship for LI and CIE has not yet been achieved, but in our experience there are clinical clues in ARCI that tend to be indicative for certain genes. The majority of patients with *TGM1* mutations presents with classical LI (Fig. 129.9) often showing ectropion or alopecia ichthyotica. There is no obvious erythroderma, but beneath the thick scales some erythema can be present. Ears are often deformed and small. As pointed out above, specific temperature sensitive mutations in *TGM1* are associated with BSI. Moreover, there are patients who initially present as collodion babies, progress to mild CIE and later on may develop a very mild or even absent scaling. This phenotype is referred to as SICI (Fig. 129.7) [6,21]. *TGM1* patients who carry premature termination codon mutations (e.g. nonsense or frameshift mutations) are more likely to report sweating abnormalities, such as hypohidrosis and overheating, than those who have missense mutations [2].

Neonates with lipoxygenase mutations are often born with a mild type of collodion membrane, which when shed reveals an underlying erythema and mild scaling in infancy (Fig. 129.10a), and in later life mostly present with the CIE phenotype (Fig. 129.10b), although some also present brownish scales (Fig. 129.11). Patients often progress to SICI [21]. Typically, they show striking palmoplantar hyperlinearity being reminiscent of IV (Fig. 129.10c) [10]. However, mild keratotic lichenifications of the elbow fossa or of the dorsum of the hands help to rule out this differential diagnosis. Patients with *ALOX12B* mutations

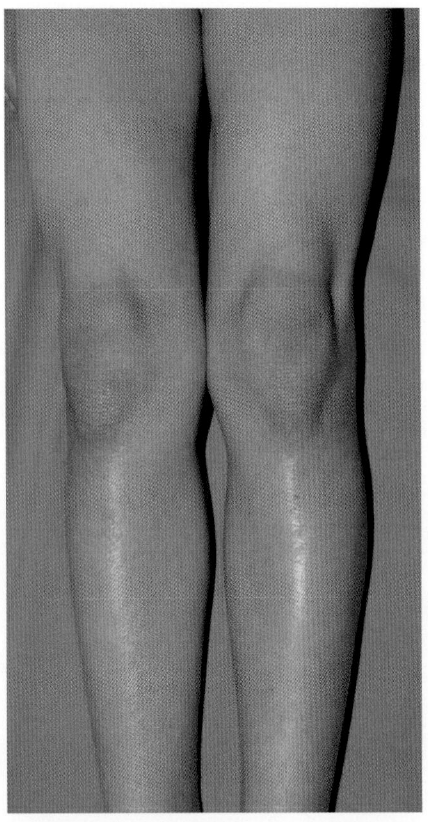

Fig. 129.11 Lipoxygenase deficiency. Source: Courtesy of Dr A. Hernandez-Martin, Madrid, Spain.

more often exhibit pronounced palmoplantar keratosis than those with *ALOXE3* mutations [10]. Many of these patients report reduced or completely absent sweating ability [22], and many complain of pruritus. Fungal superinfections are not unusual.

Patients with *NIPAL4* mutation often present with a CIE/LI overlapping phenotype, ectropion, clubbing of the nails and a pronounced and diffuse yellowish keratoderma on the palms and soles [23]. It often develops at the end of the first decade of life (Fig. 129.12) and may be reminiscent of classical PPKs such as a focal nonepidermolytic type.

Most patients with *CYP4F22* mutations present with a CIE or mild collodion baby phenotype [24] and may evolve into SICI (Fig. 129.13). As the children grow older, they develop whitish-grey scales which are more pronounced in the periumbilical region [16]. Palms and soles show pronounced hyperlinearity or even palmoplantar keratoderma.

Patients with mutations in *CERS3* are born as collodion babies and then progress to CIE often with improvement of the ichthyosis phenotype in the summer time. As in lipoxygenase deficiency, patients have marked plantar hyperlinearity (Fig. 129.14) and may experience pruritus and/or fungal infections [17].

LIPN mutations seem to cause a late onset form of ichthyosis (around the age of 5 years), so formally it is not a congenital ichthyosis [19].

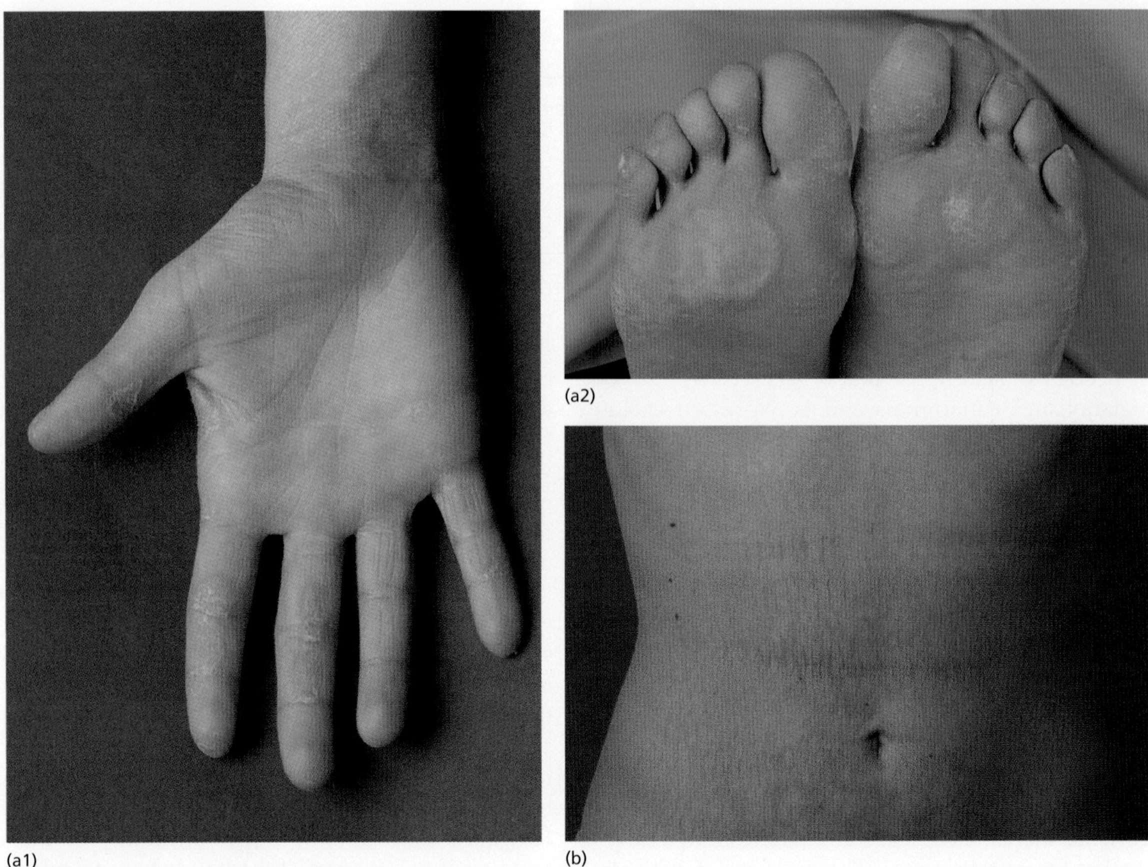

Fig. 129.12 Clinical phenotype of *NIPAL4* mutations. (a) Diffuse yellowish keratoderma on palms and soles. (b) Reticulate scaling on the trunk. Source: Courtesy of the Department of Dermatology, University Hospital Münster, Münster, Germany.

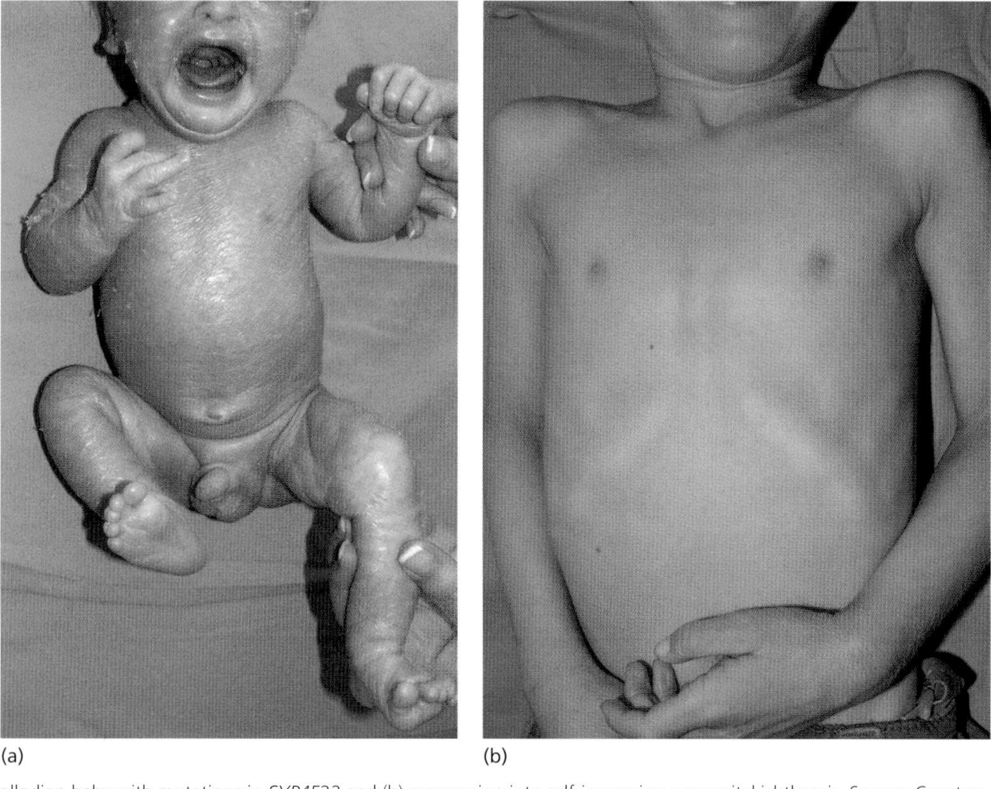

(a) (b)

Fig. 129.13 (a) Collodion baby with mutations in *SYP4F22* and (b) progression into self-improving congenital ichthyosis. Source: Courtesy of Dr A. Hernandez Martin, Madrid, Spain.

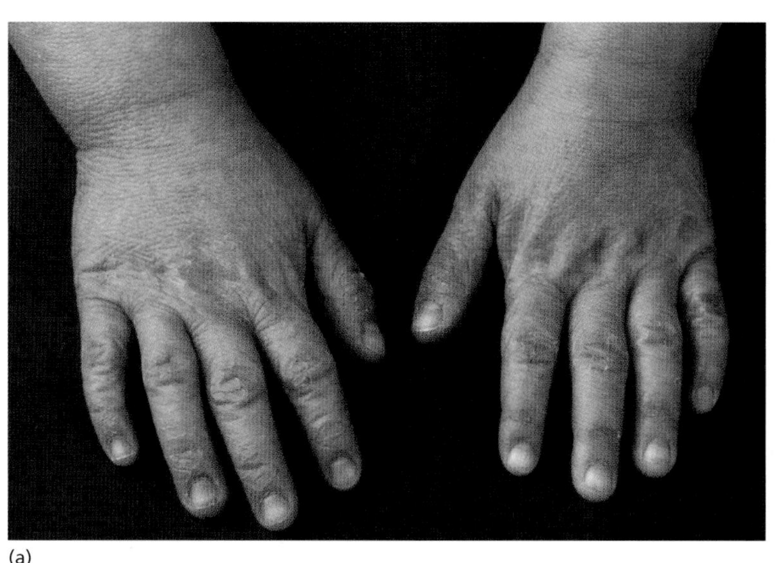

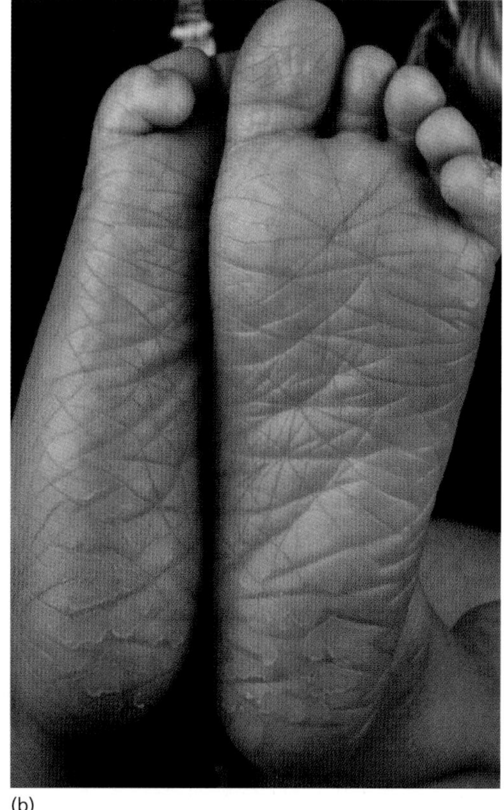

(a) (b)

Fig. 129.14 Palmoplantar keratoderma and lichenification in *CERS3* deficiency. Source: Courtesy of the Department of Dermatology, University Hospital Münster, Münster, Germany.

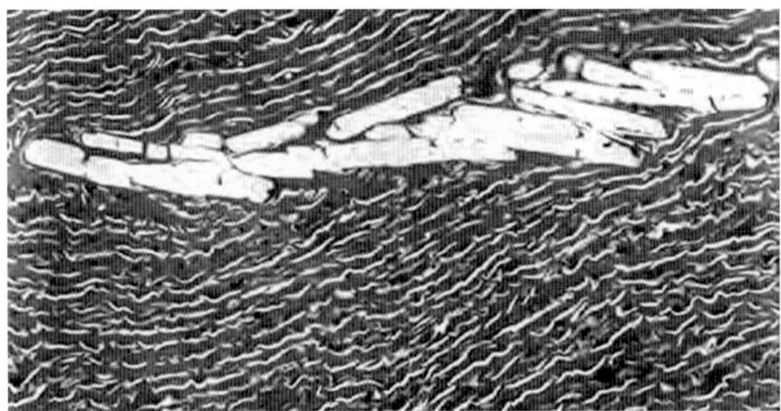

Fig. 129.15 Ultrastructure of transglutaminase-1 deficient skin with typical cholesterol clefts in the stratum corneum. Source: Courtesy of Dr I. Hausser, Institute of Pathology, Heidelberg University Hospital, Heidelberg, Germany.

Laboratory, histology, ultrastructure and genetic analyses. Diagnosis of TG1 deficiency can be made by sequencing [2,3,8] or by measuring *in situ* TG1 activity in cryostat sections [25]. Ultrastructural investigations reveal so-called cholesterol clefts in the stratum corneum (Fig. 129.15) [26]. NIPAL4 deficiency may correlate with the ultrastructure of abnormal lamellar bodies and elongated membranes in the stratum granulosum classified as ARCI electron microscope type III [27]. Biochemical measurements of lipoxygenase activity are feasible but available only in specialized research laboratories [28]. The same applies for ultrastructural methods with frozen sections or osmium tetroxide and ruthenium tetroxide postfixation that enable an advanced electron microscope diagnostic of all ARCI subtypes [29]. Direct sequencing is necessary for diagnosis of lipoxygenase deficiency and other ARCI subtypes (*CERS3, CYP4F2* or *LIPN*) that lack specific ultrastructural markers.

References

1 **Frost P, Weinstein GD, Van Scott EJ. The ichthyosiform dermatoses. II. Autoradiographic studies of epidermal proliferation. J Invest Dermatol 1966;47:561–7.**

2 Farasat S, Wei MH, Herman M, Liewehr DJ et al. Novel transglutaminase-1 mutations and genotype-phenotype investigations of 104 patients with autosomal recessive congenital ichthyosis in the USA. J Med Genet 2009;46:103–11.

3 **Fischer J. Autosomal recessive congenital ichthyosis. J Invest Dermatol 2009;129:1319–21.**

4 Eckl KM, de Juanes S, Kurtenbach J et al. Molecular analysis of 250 patients with autosomal recessive congenital ichthyosis: evidence for mutation hotspots in ALOXE3 and allelic heterogeneity in ALOX12B. J Invest Dermatol 2009;129:1421–8.

5 Hazell M, Marks R. Clinical, histologic, and cell kinetic discriminants between lamellar ichthyosis and nonbullous congenital ichthyosiform erythroderma. Arch Dermatol 1985;121:489–93.

6 Vahlquist A. Pleomorphic ichthyosis: proposed name for a heterogeneous group of congenital ichthyoses with phenotypic shifting and mild residual scaling. Acta Derm Venereol 2010;90:454–60.

7 Candi E, Schmidt R, Melino G. The cornified envelope: a model of cell death in the skin. Nat Rev Mol Cell Biol 2005;6:328–40.

8 **Huber M, Rettler I, Bernasconi K et al. Mutations of keratinocyte transglutaminase in lamellar ichthyosis. Science 1995;267:525–8.**

9 **Jobard F, Lefèvre C, Karaduman A et al. Lipoxygenase-3 (ALOXE3) and 12(R)-lipoxygenase (ALOX12B) are mutated in non-bullous congenital ichthyosiform erythroderma (NCIE) linked to chromosome 17p13.1. Hum Mol Genet 2002;11:107–13.**

10 Eckl KM, Krieg P, Küster W et al. Mutation spectrum and functional analysis of epidermis-type lipoxygenases in patients with autosomal recessive congenital ichthyosis. Hum Mutat 2005;26:351–61.

11 Akiyama M, Sakai K, Yanagi T et al. Partially disturbed lamellar granule secretion in mild congenital ichthyosiform erythroderma with ALOX12B mutations. Br J Dermatol 2010;163:201–4.

12 **Lefèvre C, Bouadjar B, Karaduman A et al. Mutations in ichthyin a new gene on chromosome 5q33 in a new form of autosomal recessive congenital ichthyosis. Hum Mol Genet 2004;13:2473–82.**

13 Li H, Loriè EP, Fischer J et al. The expression of epidermal lipoxygenases and transglutaminase-1 is perturbed by NIPAL4 mutations: indications of a common metabolic pathway essential for skin barrier homeostasis. J Invest Dermatol 2012;132:2368–75.

14 Dahlqvist J, Westermark GT, Vahlquist A, Dahl N. Ichthyin/NIPAL4 localizes to keratins and desmosomes in epidermis and Ichthyin mutations affect epidermal lipid metabolism. Arch Dermatol Res 2012;304:377–86.

15 Li H, Vahlquist A, Törmä H. Interactions between FATP4 and ichthyin in epidermal lipid processing may provide clues to the pathogenesis of autosomal recessive congenital ichthyosis. J Dermatol Sci 2013;69:195–201.

16 **Lefèvre C, Bouadjar B, Ferrand V et al. Mutations in a new cytochrome P450 gene in lamellar ichthyosis type 3. Hum Mol Genet 2006;15:767–76.**

17 **Eckl KM, Tidhar R, Thiele H et al. Impaired epidermal ceramide synthesis causes autosomal recessive congenital ichthyosis and reveals the importance of ceramide acyl chain length. J Invest Dermatol 2013;133:2202–11.**

18 Radner FP, Marrakchi S, Kirchmeier P et al. Mutations in CERS3 cause autosomal recessive congenital ichthyosis in humans. PLoS Genet 2013;9:e1003536

19 **Israeli S, Khamaysi Z, Fuchs-Telem D et al. A mutation in LIPN, encoding epidermal lipase N, causes a late-onset form of autosomal-recessive congenital ichthyosis. Am J Hum Genet 2011;88:482–7.**

20 **Grall A, Guaguère E, Planchais S et al. PNPLA1 mutations cause autosomal recessive congenital ichthyosis in golden retriever dogs and humans. Nat Genet 2012;44:140–7.**

21 **Vahlquist A, Bygum A, Gånemo A et al. Genotypic and clinical spectrum of self-improving collodion ichthyosis: ALOX12B, ALOXE3, and TGM1 mutations in Scandinavian patients. J Invest Dermatol 2010;130:438–43.**

22 Haenssle HA, Finkenrath A, Hausser I et al. Effective treatment of severe thermodysregulation by oral retinoids in a patient with recessive congenital lamellar ichthyosis. Clin Exp Dermatol 2008;33: 578–81.

23 Alavi A, Shahshahani MM, Klotzle B et al. Manifestation of diffuse yellowish keratoderma on the palms and soles in autosomal recessive congenital ichthyosis patients may be indicative of mutations in NIPAL4. J Dermatol 2012;39:375–81.

24 Sugiura K, Takeichi T, Tanahashi K et al. Lamellar ichthyosis in a collodion baby caused by CYP4F22 mutations in a non-consanguineous family outside the Mediterranean. J Dermatol Sci 2013;72:193–5.

25 Raghunath M, Hennies HC, Velten F et al. A novel in situ method for the detection of deficient transglutaminase activity in the skin. Arch Dermatol Res 1998;290:621–7.

26 Niemi KM, Kanerva L, Kuokkanen K. Recessive ichthyosis congenita type II. Arch Dermatol Res 1991;283:211–8.

27 Dahlqvist J, Klar J, Hausser I et al. Congenital ichthyosis: mutations in ichthyin are associated with specific structural abnormalities in the granular layer of epidermis. J Med Genet 2007;44:615–20.

28 Eckl KM, Krieg P, Küster W et al. Mutation spectrum and functional analysis of epidermis-type lipoxygenases in patients with autosomal recessive congenital ichthyosis. Hum Mutat 2005;26:351–61
29 Elias PM, Williams ML, Holleran WM et al. Pathogenesis of permeability barrier abnormalities in the ichthyoses: inherited disorders of lipid metabolism. J Lipid Res 2008;49:697–714.

Keratinopathic ichthyoses

Definition. Keratinopathic ichthyoses (KPI) comprise a group of severe hereditary cornification disorders which are caused by mutations in keratin genes (Tables 129.1a and 129.2). Germline mutations within *KRT1*, *KRT2* and *KRT10* result in generalized phenotypes characterized by age-related and ichthyosis-type specific erythroderma, blistering, ichthyosis and hyperkeratosis. In contrast, postzygotic mutations in *KRT1* and *KRT10* are the cause of epidermolytic naevi following the lines of Blaschko (see later) [1].

Epidemiology and pathogenesis. KPI are rare with a prevalence of approximately 1:350000 [2]. Epidermal keratins are structural proteins that combine to form heterodimers, e.g. *KRT1* and *KRT10*, which pair to tetramers and further aggregate to form keratin intermediate filament networks assembling the cytoskeleton of the keratinocyte and providing mechanical resilience. Within the keratinocyte, intermediate filament networks extend from the nucleus to the desmosomes or hemidesmosomes, thus attaching neighbouring cells [3]. Keratins are organized as central alpha-helical rod domains that are composed of alpha-helical coiled-coil domains (1A, 1B, 2A, 2B) interrupted by nonhelical linker segments, flanked by a N-terminal head and a C-terminal tail domain. Short sequence motifs at the beginning and the end of the rod domain are essential for the assembly of keratin intermediate filaments. Post-translational modifications including glycosylation and phosphorylation of keratins play an important role in protection of keratinocytes from injury [4].

The majority of reported mutations within the genes encoding suprabasal epidermal keratins, i.e. *KRT1*, *KRT2* and *KRT10*, are dominant missense mutations within the highly conserved ends of the rod domains, resulting in a dominant negative effect, i.e. the dominant mutation impairs the impact of the wildtype allele. The integration of mutated keratins into the keratin network disturbs the overall function and provokes the specific ultrastructural features with clumping of cytoplasmic keratins, the formation of perinuclear shells of aberrant keratin filaments, as well as the characteristic epidermolytic hyperkeratosis observed histologically (Fig. 129.16) [5]. These findings are most distinctive when individuals with KPI get exposed to environmental stress such as trauma, high temperature, fever or skin infections that are known triggers of disease aggravation. In this context, it was reported that oral retinoids can reduce the formation of keratin aggregates in heat stressed keratinocytes from a patient with epidermolytic ichthyosis caused by a *KRT10* mutation [6].

Interestingly, there is a functional link between *KRT1* and inflammation, because keratin aggregates can interact with activated MAP kinases, as well as chaperones such as Hsp70 and components of the ubiquitin–proteasome system [7]. In addition, *Krt1* knock-out mice show a high release of the proinflammatory IL-18, and transcriptome profiling revealed a *KRT1*-mediated gene expression signature similar to that of atopic dermatitis [8]. Further, mechanical stretching of *KRT10* mutant keratinocytes induces an increased release of TNF-α and CCL5. These findings could explain the pronounced inflammation phenotype existent in most KPI (Table 129.2).

Epidermolytic ichthyosis

Epidemiology and pathogenesis. Epidermolytic ichthyosis (EI; OMIM #113800), formerly termed epidermolytic hyperkeratosis or bullous congenital ichthyosiform erythroderma, is a severe congenital keratinization disorder with an incidence of approximately 1:200000 [9].

It is caused by mutations in both *KRT1* and *KRT10*, encoding the suprabasally expressed keratins 1 and 10 respectively. EI is predominantly inherited in a dominant mode, with up to 50% of the cases caused by *de novo* missense mutations, but some cases of autosomal recessive inheritance with nonsense mutations in *KRT10* and a case of semidominant inheritance with missense mutations in *KRT1* have been reported [9,10]. In severe forms of EI mutations are clustered predominantly within the highly conserved ends of the *KRT1* and *KRT10* rod domains. Mutations in milder cases of EI are often localized within less conserved regions, either within or outside the rod domain. Generally, mutations in *KRT1* and *KRT10* have a dominant negative effect resulting in an impairment of keratin intermediate filaments (see previously).

Whereas mutations in *KRT1* lead to severe palmoplantar keratoderma accompanying moderate EI, mutations in *KRT10* result in severe EI without or with only mild involvement of palms and soles [11]. These phenotypical differences can be explained by the fact that in palmoplantar epidermis, keratin 1 pairs solely with keratin 9, but in nonpalmoplantar epidermis, keratin 10 pairs only with keratin 2.

Clinical features. EI usually presents at birth with CIE as well as varying degrees of epidermal blisters, erosions and denuded skin areas (Fig. 129.17). Within the first weeks of life, blistering subsides and erosions are replaced by ichthyosis with white-brown moderate scaling and progressive hyperkeratosis with a predilection for friction areas and over joints. The basis for the shift in phenotype is thought to be the consequence of a postnatal adaption of the skin to the dryer surrounding conditions compared with the uterus, which stimulates epidermal proliferation. Whereas extensor surfaces show a characteristic cobblestone appearance, flexural surfaces present a keratotic lichenification with a rippled ridged or verrucous pattern (Figs 129.18 and 129.19).

In adolescents and adults hyperkeratosis is the main clinical feature. However, epidermal fragility with blisters

Table 129.2 Keratinopathic ichthyoses

	Epidermolytic ichthyosis (EI)	Superficial epidermolytic ichthyosis (SEI)	Congenital reticular ichthyosiform erythroderma (CRIE)	Ichthyosis Curth–Macklin (ICM)
OMIM	113800	146800	609165	146590
Also known as:	Epidermolytic hyperkeratosis (EHK), bullous CIE	Ichthyosis bullosa of Siemens	Ichthyosis with confetti (IWC), ichthyosis variegata	Ichthyosis hystrix Curth–Macklin
Mode of inheritance	AD (rarely AR in *KRT10*)	AD	AD	AD
Gene	*KRT1 or KRT10*	*KRT2*	*KRT10 or KRT1*	*KRT1*
Onset of phenotype	At birth	At birth	At or shortly after birth	Early childhood
Presentation of the baby	Severe CIE, erosions, denuded skin, blistering ('burned child')	CIE, localized superficial blistering, 'Mauserung (moulting effect)'	Severe CIE, palmoplantar keratoderma, no blistering	Striate or diffuse palmoplantar keratoderma, no blistering
Disease course	Within the first weeks, erosions are replaced by hyperkeratoses Annular type (AEI): mild form of EI with recurrent development of numerous annular, erythematous, scaly plaques	Within the first weeks, hyperkeratoses appear particularly over extensor sides of joints	In childhood (after third year) the characteristic skin-coloured confetti-like macules appear, which enlarge and increase in number (hundreds) with age, reticular pattern on the extremities	Progressive worsening of PPK and development of hyperkeratotic plaques over joints and/or hyperkeratotic papules on the trunk and extremities
Distribution of scaling	Generalized with predilection for friction areas and over joints	Friction areas and over joints	Generalized, later reticular pattern with nonscaling macules	Palms and soles, over large joints, rarely extremities and trunk
Characterization of scales	Adherent, moderate size, white-brown	Adherent, fine to moderate size, 'moulting effect'	Fine size, white-brown	Thick, spiky hyperkeratosis ('porcupine-quill-like'), yellow-brown
Erythroderma	Frequent	Initially, fades	Pronounced	Occasional
Palmoplantar keratoderma	*KRT1*: epidermolytic PPK *KRT10*: palms and soles are usually spared	Usually absent	Usually present	Massive PPK, deep, bleeding and painful fissures, flexural contractures, constriction bands
Hypohidrosis	Possible	Possible	Possible	None
Scalp abnormalities	Scaling, encasement of hair shafts	Rarely scaling	Scaling	None
Other skin findings	Pruritus, blisters after minor trauma, proneness to skin infections, malodour	Pruritus, become blisters after minor trauma (often in summer season)	Rarely pruritus, squamous cell carcinomas reported	Rarely pruritus, proneness to skin infections, malodour
Extracutaneous findings	Growth failure common, sometimes severe phenotypes	Growth failure possible	Growth failure common, sometimes severe phenotypes	Growth failure possible, gangrene and loss of digits ('pseudoainhum')
Histology and skin ultrastructure	EHK, aggregation and clumping of keratin filaments in SG and SS, accumulation and entombment of lamellar bodies, paucity of lamellar bilayers in SC	Superficial EHK, thickened keratin bundles, rarely keratin clumping, cytolysis in SG of affected body sites	Vacuolization or absence of SG, binuclear cells, perinuclear shells of keratin filaments, effete desmosomes, paucity of lamellar bilayers in SC	No epidermolysis or clumping of keratins, perinuclear shells of aberrant keratin filaments, defective organization of lamellar bilayers in SC

AD, autosomal dominant; AR, autosomal recessive; CIE, congenital ichthyosiform erythroderma; EHK, epidermolytic hyperkeratosis; PPK, palmoplantar keratoderma; SC, stratum corneum; SG, stratum granulosum; SS, stratum spinosum.

Source: Adapted from Oji et al. (2010). Revised nomenclature and classification of inherited ichthyoses: results of the First Ichthyosis Consensus Conference in Sorèze 2009. J Am Acad Dermatol 2010;63:607–41.

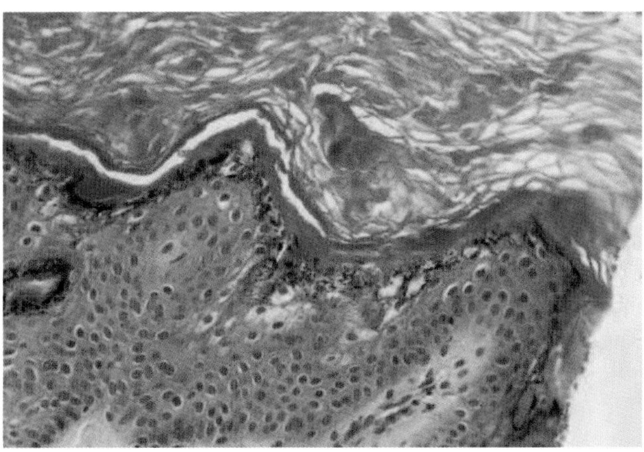

Fig. 129.16 Histological diagnosis of epidermolytic hyperkeratosis. Source: Reproduced from Oji et al. 2016 [10] with permission of John Wiley & Sons.

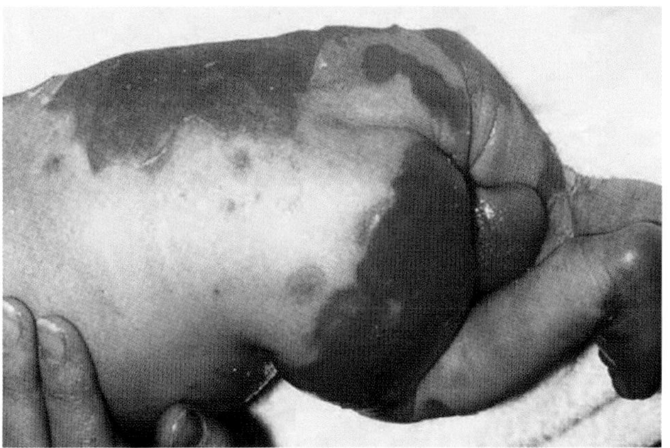

Fig. 129.17 Neonatal presentation of epidermolytic ichthyosis ('enfant brulé'). Source: Reproduced from Oji et al. 2016 [10] with permission of John Wiley & Sons.

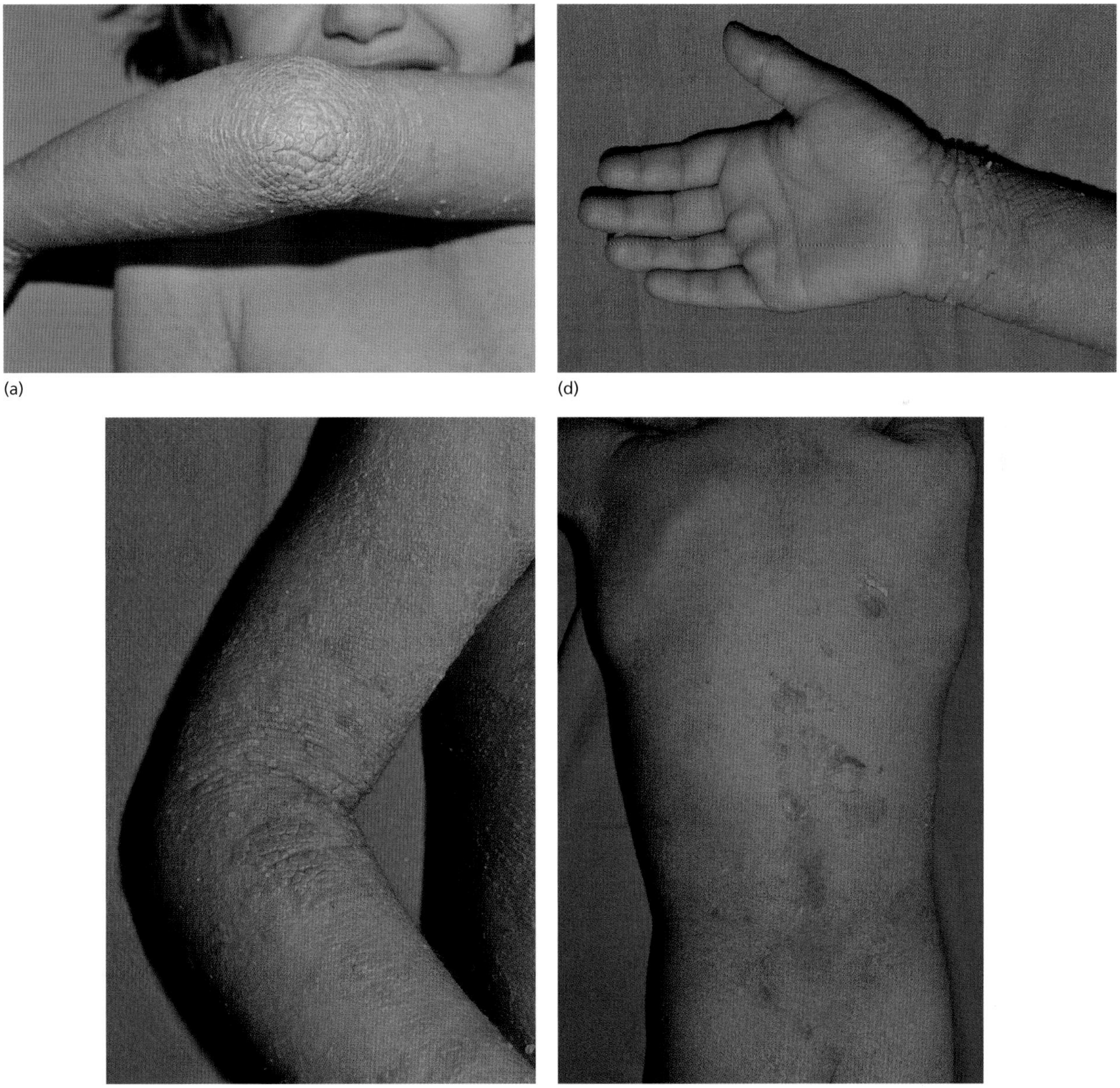

(a) (d)

(b) (c)

Fig. 129.18 Epidermolytic ichthyosis caused by *KRT10* mutation. (a,b) Pronounced hyperkeratosis over the joint area, (c) erosions on the trunk and (d) sparing of the palms. Source: Courtesy of Dr A. Hernandez-Martin, Madrid, Spain.

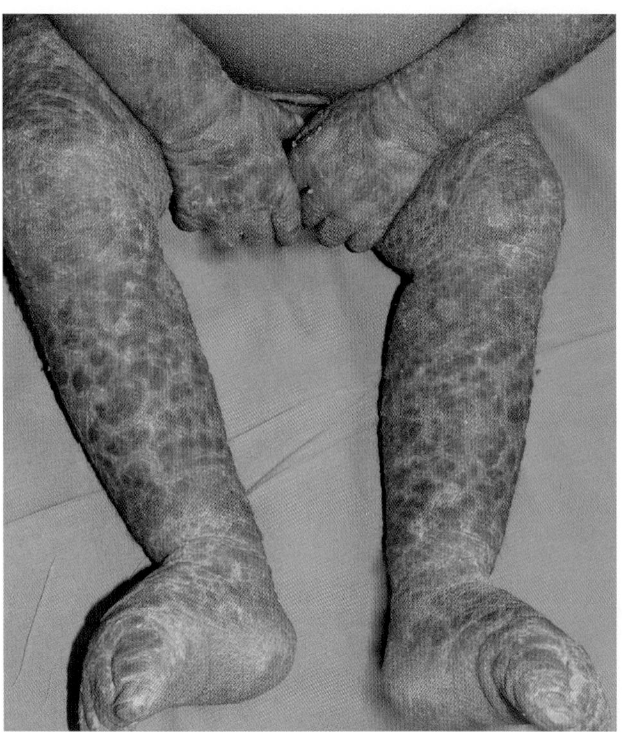

Fig. 129.19 Epidermolytic ichthyosis caused by *KRT1* mutation. Source: Courtesy of Dr A. Hernandez-Martin, Madrid, Spain.

and erosions remains at sites of minor trauma (Fig. 129.18c) or secondary skin infection, but also when patients suffer from fever or stay in a hot climate. On the knees and the lower legs patients sometimes exhibit spiny hyperkeratoses. Although a typical sign of superficial epidermolytic ichthyosis (see later), superficial skin peeling described as the Mauserung or moulting effect, is also present to some degree in EI. Palmoplantar keratoderma is a common feature of individuals with *KRT1* mutations, but predominantly missing in *KRT10* mutation carriers (Fig. 129.18d). The face is typically less involved than the remaining body and both ectropion and eclabion are not found. Scaling on the scalp is common with a nit-like covering of the hair shafts.

Concerning clinical features, the degree of phenotypical variability can be quite different amongst individuals with EI. Moreover, those with EI are prone to skin infections, in particular bacteria and fungi. Other ectodermal structures such as teeth, hair and nails as well as other organ systems are unaffected. Growth failure is common in children. Subjective troubles include pruritus and malodour caused by maceration of scales and bacterial overgrowth. Sometimes infants die from severe infection, but life expectancy is usually normal, although individuals with EI are often stigmatized and psychologically stressed.

Annular epidermolytic ichthyosis

Annular epidermolytic ichthyosis (AEI) is a mild very rare variant of EI, that shares a similar onset at birth, but later in life greatly improves and is characterized by recurrent flares of numerous annular, erythematous and scaly plaques, especially on the trunk and the extremities [11,12]. Exacerbations, or flare-ups, may occur during times of stress, i.e. high temperature in the summer, fever or pregnancy [13]. Between the flares, the skin appears normal except for palmoplantar hyperkeratoses in individuals with *KRT1* mutations. AEI is caused by distinct mutations outside the helix boundary regions of *KRT1* and *KRT10* [14].

Epidermolytic naevi (mosaic epidermolytic ichthyosis)

The mosaic form of EI exhibits unilateral or bilateral streaks of kyperkeratosis that follow the lines of Blaschko (Fig. 129.20) [1]. Sometimes, skin involvement can be extensive with severe hyperkeratoses characterized by protruding, porcupine-like spines. Epidermolytic naevi are caused by a postzygotic mutation in either *KRT1* or *KRT10* that occurs during embryogenesis. Importantly, if this mutation is also present in gonadal cells representing a germline mosaicism in the parent generation, it can potentially be transmitted to the offspring, resulting in a full blown generalized EI [1,15].

Differential diagnosis. The clinical distinction of mild EI from severe superficial epidermolytic ichthyosis is almost impossible and genetic testing is therefore necessary. In neonates, clinical distinction from epidermolysis bullosa, toxic epidermal necrolysis, severe herpes virus infections and the staphylococcal scalded skin syndrome can be difficult and requires a skin biopsy and/or cultures. Of note, careful skin inspection may reveal areas of fine scaling or beginning hyperkeratosis which argues for EI. Congenital

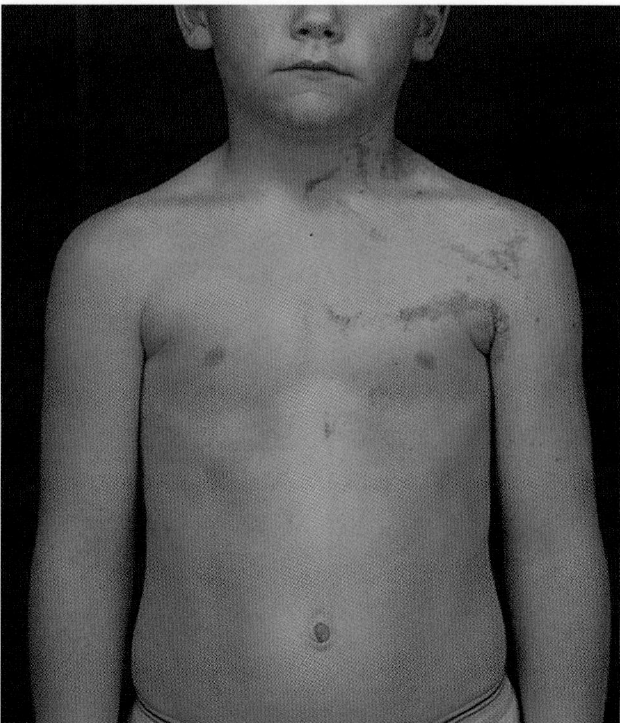

Fig. 129.20 Epidermolytic naevus caused by postzygotic mutations of *KRT1* or *KRT10* following the lines of Blaschko and indicating the risk of transmission of epidermolytic ichthyosis.

appearance of EI may resemble a severe combustion, explaining the term 'enfant brûlé (burned child)' used formerly in French literature. In addition, in girls, incontinentia pigmenti should be considered.

Laboratory, histology and genetic findings. Clinical diagnosis of EI in particular in neonates is difficult (see previously). However, because EI can be confirmed by histology, a skin biopsy is recommended in all newborns with this suspected diagnosis. Genetic testing provides additional information about the keratin genotype and is expedient for genetic counselling and prenatal diagnosis. Blood tests are unremarkable because there are no specific markers for EI.

Histologically, EI reveals the characteristic epidermolytic hyperkeratosis, i.e. marked hyperkeratosis and acanthosis with perinuclear vacuolar changes, cell lysis and coarse basophilic clumps in the granular and spinous layers (Fig. 129.16) [16]. Yet, an extensive degree of cytolysis leads to intraepidermal blister formation. Because the histological finding of epidermolytic hyperkeratosis can be less marked in AEI than in classical EI, it is crucial to take the skin biopsy from a site of maximal clinical involvement. The histology of epidermolytic naevi is identical to that of EI and the particular diagnosis can only be made with a clinical and histopathological correlation.

Specific ultrastructural features are clumping of cytoplasmic keratins, absent connection of keratin filaments to desmosomes, and formation of perinuclear shells of aberrant keratin filaments (see previously) [5]. In addition, the deficient cytoskeleton causes an accumulation of lamellar bodies at the cell periphery, an impaired secretion and a paucity of lamellar lipid bilayers within the extracellular spaces of the stratum corneum [17].

Treatment and prevention. Treatment is symptomatic and needs to be adapted concerning age and clinical issues of the patient. In the neonatal period, infants with EI require management in an intensive care nursery to prevent or treat mechanical trauma, dehydration, electrolyte imbalance, hypothermia, cutaneous superinfection and sepsis. In children and adults, topical therapy is important for removing or reducing hyperkeratosis (mechanical, keratolytics), softening the skin (emollients, humectants) and treating skin infections (antiseptics). Systemic antibiotics are often inevitable, but chronic preventive therapy is not recommended. Oral retinoids, preferably acitretin, can efficiently reduce hyperkeratosis, but they also increase epidermal fragility and blister formation. Therefore, low doses, e.g. acitretin 0.5 mg/kg body weight, and careful medical observation are advisable [18]. Interestingly, there is evidence for a correlation of keratin genotype and response to oral retinoids, i.e. individuals with a *KRT10* mutation respond much better than those with a *KRT1* mutation [19]. As skin fragility is increased, mechanical trauma must be avoided. Prenatal diagnosis can be performed when the underlying keratin mutation is known from affected family members [20].

Superficial epidermolytic ichthyosis

Epidemiology and pathogenesis. Superficial epidermolytic ichthyosis (SEI; OMIM #146800), formerly termed ichthyosis bullosa of Siemens, is a rare congenital ichthyosis, that represents a distinct entity. It is caused by dominant mutations in *KRT2*, encoding the suprabasally expressed keratin 2. The majority of mutations is located within the helix termination motif of the rod domain of *KRT2* [21,22].

Clinical features. The clinical presentation and symptoms resemble that of EI; however, the course of the disease is milder and hyperkeratoses are more localized. SEI usually presents at birth with mild CIE and blistering. During early childhood, erythroderma and blisters subside and grey- or brown-coloured hyperkeratotic and lichenified skin areas develop. Preferred sites are the extensor surfaces over joints, the axillary and periumbilical regions, the buttocks, as well as the dorsal aspects of hands and feet (Fig. 129.21). A characteristic phenotypical feature is superficial skin peeling with collarette-like borders, described as the Mauserung or moulting effect (Fig. 129.22). Palmoplantar keratoderma is absent in SEI.

Differential diagnosis. In neonates, it is similar to EI (see previously). In childhood, SEI can be distinguished from classic EI because it has a milder clinical appearance with more superficial skin shedding and missing erythema. Peeling skin syndromes can resemble the SEI phenotype. However, histologically they do not reveal epidermolytic hyperkeratosis.

Laboratory and histology findings. Findings are similar to that described in EI (see previously) but can be less pronounced. Thus, it is important to take the skin biopsy from a site of maximal clinical involvement such as the knees.

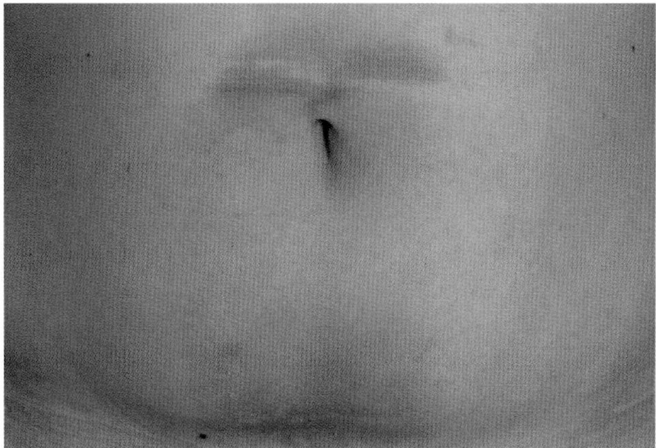

Fig. 129.21 Superficial epidermolytic ichthyosis. Involvement around the navel. Source: Courtesy of the Department of Dermatology, University Hospital Münster, Münster, Germany. Reproduced from Oji et al. 2016 with permission of John Wiley & Sons.

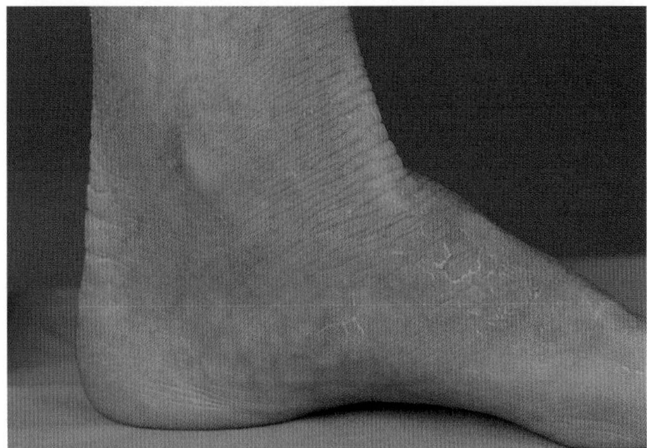

Fig. 129.22 Moulting ('Mauserung') phenomenon in superficial epidermolytic ichthyosis. Source: Courtesy of the Department of Dermatology, University Hospital Münster, Münster, Germany.

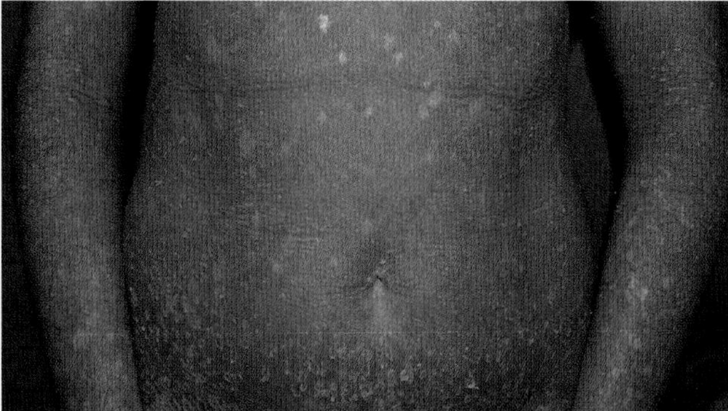

Fig. 129.23 Congenital reticular ichthyosiform erythroderma. Note pale, confetti-like spots representing localized spontaneous healing. Source: courtesy of Dr A. Hernandez-Martin, Madrid, Spain.

Treatment and prevention. Therapy is similar to that of EI (see previously). Low-dose oral retinoids, e.g. acitretin 0.1–0.5 mg/kg body weight, are very effective but should only be given to severe SEI cases.

Congenital reticular ichthyosiform erythroderma

Epidemiology and pathogenesis. Congenital reticular ichthyosiform erythroderma (CRIE; OMIM #609165), also termed ichthyosis with confetti (IWC), or formerly ichthyosis variegata, is a rare autosomal dominant keratinization disorder, characterized by the development of small, confetti-like islands of normal skin within an ichthyosiform erythroderma. It is mainly caused by heterozygous frameshift mutations in the C-terminal tail domain of *KRT10*, inserting an arginine-rich motif, which mislocalizes the mutant keratin 10 protein to the nucleolus. Recently, a *de novo* mutation in *KRT1* has also been reported as disease causing [23].

The genesis of the confetti spots can be explained by revertant mosaicism, i.e. localized spontaneous healing of the mutated keratin 10 based on mitotic recombination [24].

Clinical features. Infants are born with severe CIE and shortly after birth, mild palmoplantar keratoderma becomes apparent [25]. In later childhood (after the third year of life) the characteristic skin-coloured macules resembling confetti manifest, which slowly enlarge (up to 2 cm) and increase in number (hundreds) with age (Fig. 129.23). These spots of normal skin have a widespread, orderless distribution, and when appearing in high numbers can give the impression of a reticular pattern of the adjacent erythematous ichthyotic skin, which is mainly observed on the extremities. Palmoplantar keratoderma with orange to brown hyperkeratoses is usually present in CRIE. Generally, phenotypical expression varies within the individuals, because in adulthood some of them exhibit hundreds to thousands of confetti-like skin spots whereas others show much fewer numbers. Children with CRIE are prone to bacterial skin infections, are often severely ill, and growth failure is frequent.

Differential diagnosis. In neonates, it is similar to EI (see previously). With the development of confetti-like islands of normal skin, the disease becomes more distinctive. However, sometimes severe atopic dermatitis with pityriasis alba or postinflammatory pigmentary alterations can clinically mimic CRIE, and a skin biopsy can be advisable.

Laboratory, histology and genetic findings. Clinical diagnosis of CRIE is difficult in infants and a skin biopsy is recommended in all newborns with this suspected diagnosis (see previously). Genetic testing is expedient for genetic counselling and prenatal diagnosis. Blood tests are unspecific. Histology and ultrastructure are different from EI.

Histopathological findings include band-like parakeratosis, acanthosis, vacuolization or absence of the granular layer, as well as binuclear cells in the upper epidermis, sometimes associated with dermal amyloid deposition. Ultrastructural abnormalities comprise vacuolar degeneration of mitochondria, perinuclear shells formed from a network of fine filaments in the upper epidermis, effete desmosomes, and a paucity of lamellar bilayers in the stratum corneum.

Treatment and prevention. Therapy is similar to that of EI with a *KRT10* mutation (see previously). Treatment with low dose oral retinoids may result in an increase in the number and size of confetti-like macules [26].

Ichthyosis Curth Macklin

Epidemiology and pathogenesis. Ichthyosis Curth Macklin (ICM; OMIM 146590), also termed ichthyosis hystrix Curth Macklin, is a rare severe ichthyosis with autosomal dominant inheritance. It is caused by heterozygous deletion/insertion mutations in the C-terminal tail domain of *KRT1*, resulting in an abnormal keratin 1 protein with an aberrant tail domain in place of the naturally glycine loop motifs.

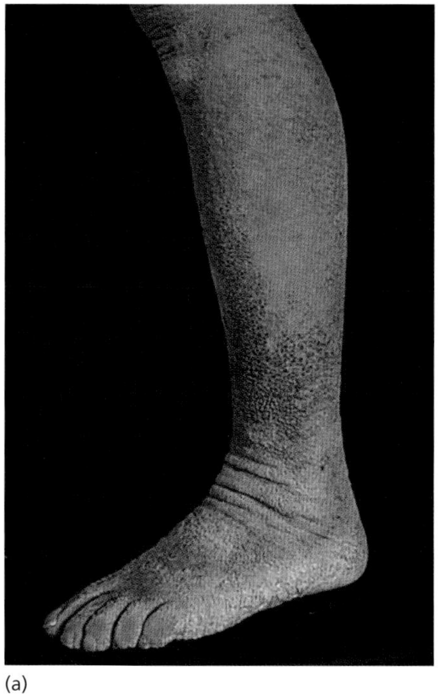

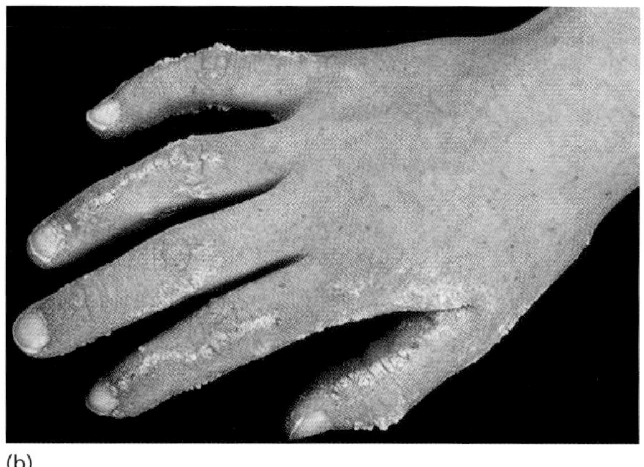

(a) (b)

Fig. 129.24 Epidermolytic ichthyosis with 'hystrix'-like presentation on (a) lower legs and (b) hand. (a) Source: Rook's Textbook of Dermatology. Reproduced with permission of John Wiley & Sons.

Clinical features. ICM becomes manifest in early childhood with striate or diffuse palmoplantar keratoderma. Importantly compared with EI, in ICM there is no blistering and epidermal fragility. The course of the disease is characterized by a progressive worsening of palmoplantar keratoderma and the development of massive cobblestone-like plaques with ridged surfaces over joints and/or hyperkeratotic papules on the trunk and extremities (Fig. 129.24a,b). The phenotypical expression often varies even within families, exhibiting a broad range from multiple localized hyperkeratotic plaques to generalized hystrix-like hyperkeratosis. Palmoplantar keratoderma can be massive, with deep, bleeding and painful fissures, as well as flexural contractures and mutilating circular constriction bands (pseudoainhum) [27]. Scales range from yellow-brown thick, spiky hyperkeratosis ('porcupine-quill-like') to dark excrescences. ICM is prone to skin infections and malodour caused by maceration of scales, and bacterial overgrowth can be pronounced. Growth failure is possible, but life expectancy is usually normal. Individuals with ICM are often stigmatized.

Differential diagnosis. Severe forms of EI can resemble ICM (see previously), however in the latter there is no blistering and skin fragility. Additionally, ultrastructural findings are different.

Laboratory, histology and genetic findings. Genetic testing is the basis for genetic counselling and prenatal diagnosis. Blood tests are unspecific as other organ systems are unaffected. Histology and ultrastructure are different from EI.

Histopathology is nonspecific and reveals orthokeratotic hyperkeratosis, acanthosis, church spire-like papillomatosis, hypergranulosis, as well as vacuolated or binuclear cells in the granular and spinous layers, but no epidermolysis. Ultrastructural abnormalities in the upper epidermis are diagnostic for ICM and comprise a failure in keratin intermediate filament bundling, often associated with perinuclear vacuolization, perinuclear shells of aberrant keratin filaments, and a defective organization of lamellar bilayers in the stratum corneum. However, there is no keratin clumping as in EI [27].

Treatment and prevention. Therapy is similar to that of EI (see previously), with a focus on reducing severe hyperkeratosis by both topical keratolytics and oral retinoids. Large-area application of salicylic acid in particular in children should be prohibited because of the risk of salicylate intoxication.

SECTION 27: DISORDERS OF KERATIN AND KERATINIZATION

References

1 **Paller AS, Syder AJ, Chan YM et al. Genetic and clinical mosaicism in a type of epidermal nevus. N Engl J Med 1994;21:1408–15.**
2 **Bygum A, Virtanen M, Brandrup F et al. Generalized and naevoid epidermolytic ichthyosis in Denmark: clinical and mutational findings. Acta Derm Venereol 2013:93:309–13.**
3 Uitto J, Richard G, McGrath JA. Diseases of epidermal keratins and their linker proteins. Exp Cell Res 2007;313:1995–2009.
4 Knobel M, O'Toole EA, Smith FJ. Keratins and skin disease. Cell Tissue Res 2015; 360:583–9.
5 **Anton-Lamprecht I. Ultrastructural identification of basic abnormalities as clues to genetic disorders of the epidermis. J Invest Dermatol 1994;103(5 Suppl):6S–12S.**
6 Li H, Torma H. Retinoids reduce formation of keratin aggregates in heat-stressed immortalized keratinocytes from an epidermolytic ichthyosis patient with a KRT10 mutation. Acta Derm Venereol 2013;93:44–9.

7 Chamcheu JC, Wood GS, Siddiqui IA et al. Progress towards genetic and pharmacological therapies for keratin genodermatoses: current perspective and future promise. Exp Dermatol 2012;21:481–9.

8 Roth W, Kumar V, Beer HD et al. Keratin 1 maintains skin integrity and participates in an inflammatory network in skin through interleukin-18. J Cell Sci 2012;125(Pt 22):5269–79.

9 Muller FB, Huber M, Kinaciyan T et al. A human keratin 10 knockout causes recessive epidermolytic hyperkeratosis. Hum Mol Genet 2006;15:1133–41.

10 Nousbeck J, Padalon-Brauch G, Fuchs-Telem D et al. Semidominant inheritance in epidermolytic ichthyosis. J Invest Dermatol 2013;133: 2626–8.

11 DiGiovanna JJ, Bale SJ. Clinical heterogeneity in epidermolytic hyperkeratosis. Arch Dermatol 1994;130:1026–35.

12 Joh GY, Traupe H, Metze D et al. A novel dinucleotide mutation in keratin 10 in the annular epidermolytic ichthyosis variant of bullous congenital ichthyosiform erythroderma. J Invest Dermatol 1997;108:357–61.

13 Sheth N, Greenblatt D, McGrath JA. New KRT10 gene mutation underlying the annular variant of bullous congenital ichthyosiform erythroderma with clinical worsening during pregnancy. Br J Dermatol 2007;157:602–4.

14 Irvine AD, McLean WH. Human keratin diseases: the increasing spectrum of disease and subtlety of the phenotype-genotype correlation. Br J Dermatol 1999;140:815–28.

15 Arin MJ, Oji V, Emmert S, Hausser I et al. Expanding the keratin mutation database: novel and recurrent mutations and genotype-phenotype correlations in 28 patients with epidermolytic ichthyosis. Br J Dermatol 2011;164:442–7.

16 Frost P, Van Scott EJ. Ichthyosiform dermatoses. Classification based on anatomic and biometric observations. Arch Dermatol 1966;94: 113–26.

17 Schmuth M, Yosipovitch G, Williams ML et al. Pathogenesis of the permeability barrier abnormality in epidermolytic hyperkeratosis. J Invest Dermatol 2001;117:837–47.

18 Lacour M, Mehta-Nikhar B, Atherton DJ, Harper JI. An appraisal of acitretin therapy in children with inherited disorders of keratinization. Br J Dermatol 1996;134:1023–9.

19 Virtanen M, Gedde-Dahl T, Jr., Mork NJ et al. Phenotypic/genotypic correlations in patients with epidermolytic hyperkeratosis and the effects of retinoid therapy on keratin expression. Acta Derm Venereol 2001;81:163–70.

20 Rothnagel JA, Lin MT, Longley MA et al. Prenatal diagnosis for keratin mutations to exclude transmission of epidermolytic hyperkeratosis. Prenat Diagn 1998;18:826–30.

21 Rothnagel JA, Traupe H, Wojcik S et al. Mutations in the rod domain of keratin 2e in patients with ichthyosis bullosa of Siemens. Nat Genet 1994;7:485–90.

22 Arin MJ. The molecular basis of human keratin disorders. Hum Genet 2009;125:355–73.

23 Choate KA, Lu Y, Zhou J et al. Frequent somatic reversion of KRT1 mutations in ichthyosis with confetti. J Clin Invest 2015;125:1703–7.

24 Choate KA, Lu Y, Zhou J et al. Mitotic recombination in patients with ichthyosis causes reversion of dominant mutations in KRT10. Science 2010;330(6000):94–7.

25 Spoerri I, Brena M, De Mesmaeker J et al. The phenotypic and genotypic spectra of ichthyosis with confetti plus novel genetic variation in the 3′ end of KRT10: from disease to a syndrome. JAMA Dermatol 2015;151:64–9.

26 Camenzind M, Harms M, Chavaz P, Saurat JH. [Confetti ichthyosis]. Ann Dermatol Venereol 1984;111:675–6.

27 Sprecher E, Ishida-Yamamoto A, Becker OM et al. Evidence for novel functions of the keratin tail emerging from a mutation causing ichthyosis hystrix. J Invest Dermatol 2001;116:511–19.

Other nonsyndromic ichthyosis forms

Exfoliative ichthyosis

Introduction. Exfoliative ichthyosis (according to OMIM 'peeling skin syndrome type 4', #607936) should be mentioned as an important differential diagnosis for ichthyoses such as SEI as well as certain PPKs or epidermolysis bullosa simplex.

Pathogenesis. Loss-of-function mutations in the *CSTA* gene encoding cystatin A are the cause of this autosomal recessive disease [1]. Cystatin A is a potent inhibitor of exogenous proteases, thus preventing epidermal barrier impairment.

Clinical features. The disease is characterized by pronounced palmoplantar keratoderma that tends to be sensitive to sweat and water exposure (Fig. 129.25). Of note, exfoliative ichthyosis affects the entire integument showing mild dry and scaly skin, and as such fulfils the criteria of a nonsyndromic form of congenital ichthyosis. Skin peeling may occur, easily elicited by moisture or minor trauma, and resemble the 'moulting' phenomenon in superficial epidermolytic ichthyosis [2].

Differential diagnosis. Palmoplantar keratoderma such as Mal de Meleda, superficial epidermolytic ichthyosis, epidermolysis bullosa simplex, CIEor acral peeling skin syndrome [3] are important differential diagnoses.

Laboratory and histology findings. Histology shows mild orthohyperkeratosis, a prominent granular layer, spongiosis in the spinous layer, but no signs of epidermolytic hyperkeratosis. Ultrastructural analysis reveals reduced cell–cell adhesion caused by intercellular oedema mainly in the spinous layer, normal appearing desmosomes, prominent keratin filaments within basal keratinocytes, reduced thickness of CEs, as well as impaired lamellar lipid bilayers caused by delayed processing of secreted LB contents [1,4]. The barrier abnormalities of exfoliative ichthyosis are reminiscent of, albeit less severe, Netherton syndrome, which results from a deficiency of the serine protease inhibitor LEKTI.

Treatment. Efficient symptomatic treatment options seem completely lacking, because local therapy tends to increase humidity associated sensibility.

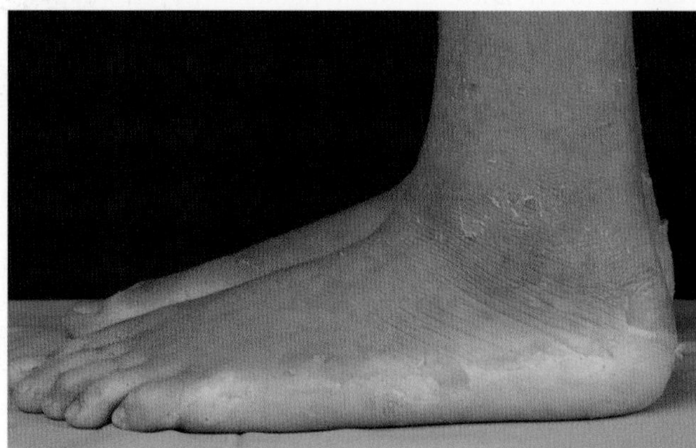

Fig. 129.25 Exfoliative ichthyosis with pronounced plantar keratoderma. Source: Courtesy of the Department of Dermatology, University Hospital Münster, Germany.

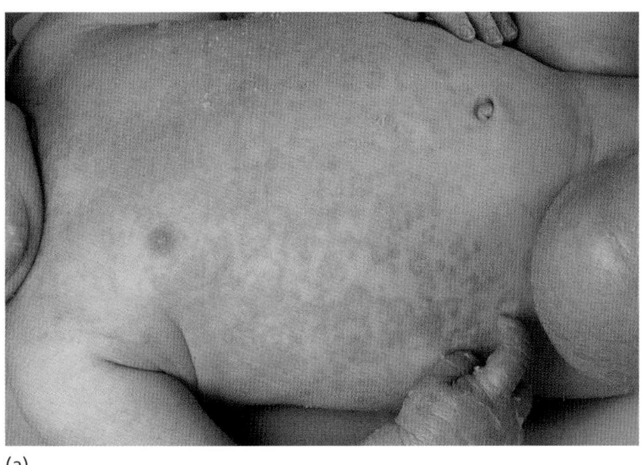
(a)

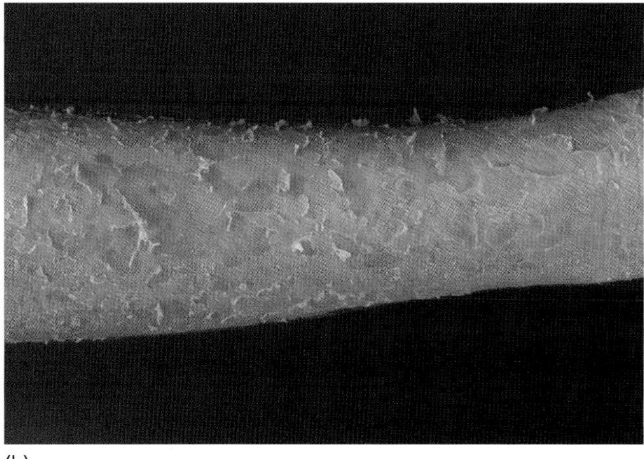
(b)

Fig. 129.26 Peeling skin disease type I. Source: Courtesy of the Department of Dermatology, University Hospital Münster, Germany.

Peeling skin disease

Definition. The term 'peeling skin syndrome' (PSS) was introduced by Levy and Goldsmith in 1982 [5]. Traupe differentiated PSS type A and B [6]. Inflammatory peeling skin disease (= PSS1; OMIM #270300) initially described by Wile in 1921 [7] refers to an ichthyosiform erythroderma characterized by lifelong patchy peeling of the skin with accompanying pruritus.

Pathogenesis. PSS1 is caused by autosomal recessive loss-of-function mutations in *CDSN* encoding corneodesmosin [8]. CDSN is a secreted protein expressed in cornified epithelia and hair follicles [9]. It is specific to corneodesmosomes, cell–cell junction structures responsible for the SC cohesion [10]. The essential role of CDSN for maintaining integrity of the epidermis and hair follicle is demonstrated in mice [11].

Clinical features. Inflammatory peeling skin disease presents at birth or a few days later [7,8]. Infants develop ichthyosiform erythroderma with skin abnormalities consisting of spontaneous patchy peeling affecting the entire skin (Fig. 129.26). Depending on mechnical stress, environmental factors, e.g. low humidity or temperature changes, patients experience recurrent episodes of peeling with severe pruritus. The presentation might be reminiscent of Netherton syndrome [12]. However, individuals do not show 'bamboo hairs' or hypotrichosis, and do not develop ichthyosis linearis circumflexa. The disease persists throughout life and is often accompanied by significant atopic manifestations.

Differential diagnosis. Hypotrichosis and failure to thrive seems unusual or less severe than in Netherton syndrome [8]. Peeling skin syndrome type A (PSS4) lacks skin inflammation and has a disease onset after the neonatal period [13,14]. Other exfoliative inflammatory phenotypes should be distinguished including SAM syndrome and exfoliative ichthyosis (see previously).

Laboratory and histology investigations. Histopathology reveals subcorneal splitting and/or enhanced detachment of corneocytes. Consequently, Netherton syndrome and PSS1 appear similar at the histological and ultrastructural level [15]. Immunostaining for corneodesmosin and LEKTI may help to distinguish between these two disorders [8].

Treatment. There is no effective treatment. Episodes of skin peeling are accompanied by severe and refractory pruritus. Allergies need to be prevented; tacalcitol cream [16], emollients with dexpanthenol and antiseptics or use of thermal water spray can be tried.

Erythrokeratoderma, loricrin keratoderma and KLICK

Comment

Erythrokeratoderma such as erythrokeratoderma variabilis shows a significant clinical overlap with several ichthyoses and has therefore been included into the list of hereditary ichthyoses [17]. This step is in accordance with the classification of KID (keratitis-ichthyosis-deafness) syndrome as an ichthyosis (refer to neuroichthyotic syndromes). Other forms of the erythrokeratoderma group are discussed elsewhere in this book (see Chapter 131). Similarly, loricrin keratoderma and keratosis linearis-ichthyosis congenita-keratoderma (KLICK) [18] which belong to the ichthyoses but show a pronounced palmoplantar phenotype are discussed under PPK (see Chapter 128).

References

1 **Blaydon DC, Nitoiu D, Eckl KM et al. Mutations in CSTA, encoding Cystatin A, underlie exfoliative ichthyosis and reveal a role for this protease inhibitor in cell-cell adhesion. Am J Hum Genet 2011;89:564–71.**

2 **Hatsell SJ, Stevens H, Jackson AP et al. An autosomal recessive exfoliative ichthyosis with linkage to chromosome 12q13. Br J Dermatol 2003;149:174–80.**

3 Moosbrugger-Martinz V, Jalili A, Schossig AS et al. Epidermal barrier abnormalities in exfoliative ichthyosis with a novel homozygous loss-of-function mutation in CSTA. Br J Dermatol 2015;172:1628–32.

4 Krunic AL, Stone KL, Simpson MA, McGrath JA. Acral peeling skin syndrome resulting from a homozygous nonsense mutation in the CSTA gene encoding cystatin A. Pediatr Dermatol 2013;30:e87–8.
5 **Levy SB, Goldsmith LA. The peeling skin syndrome. J Am Acad Dermatol 1982; 7:606–13.**
6 **Traupe H. Peeling-skin syndrome: clinical and morphological evidence for two types. In: Traupe H (ed.) The Ichthyoses: A Guide to Clinical Diagnosis, Genetic Counselling, and Therapy. Berlin; Springer, 1989:207–10.**
7 **Wile UJ. Familial study of three unusual cases of congenital ichthyosiform erythrodermia. Arch Dermatol Syph 1924;10:487–98.**
8 **Oji V, Eckl KM, Aufenvenne K et al. Loss of corneodesmosin leads to severe skin barrier defect, pruritus, and atopy: unraveling the peeling skin disease. Am J Hum Genet 2010;87:274–81**
9 Lundstrom A, Serre G, Haftek M, Egelrud T. Evidence for a role of corneodesmosin, a protein which may serve to modify desmosomes during cornification, in stratum corneum cell cohesion and desquamation. Arch Dermatol Res 1994;286:369–75.
10 Serre G, Mils V, Haftek M et al. Identification of late differentiation antigens of human cornified epithelia, expressed in re-organized desmosomes and bound to cross-linked envelope. J Invest Dermatol 1991;97:1061–72.
11 **Jonca N, Leclerc EA, Caubet C et al. Corneodesmosomes and corneodesmosin: from the stratum corneum cohesion to the pathophysiology of genodermatoses. Eur J Dermatol 2011;21:35–42.**
12 Farooq M, Kurban M, Abbas O et al. Netherton syndrome showing a large clinical overlap with generalized inflammatory peeling skin syndrome. Eur J Dermatol 2012; 22:412–3.
13 Fox H. Skin Shedding (keratolysis exfoliativa congenita): report of a case. Arch Dermatol 1921;3:202.
14 **Cabral RM, Kurban M, Wajid M et al. Whole-exome sequencing in a single proband reveals a mutation in the CHST8 gene in autosomal recessive peeling skin syndrome. Genomics 2012;99:202–8.**
15 **Komatsu N, Suga Y, Saijoh K et al. Elevated human tissue kallikrein levels in the stratum corneum and serum of peeling skin syndrome-type B patients suggests an over-desquamation of corneocytes. J Invest Dermatol 2006; 126:2338–42.**
16 Mizuno Y, Suga Y, Hasegawa T et al. A case of peeling skin syndrome successfully treated with topical calcipotriol. J Dermatol 2006;33: 430–2.
17 **Oji V, Tadini G, Akiyama M et al. Revised nomenclature and classification of inherited ichthyoses: results of the First Ichthyosis Consensus Conference in Sorèze 2009. J Am Acad Dermatol 2010;63:607–41.**
18 **Vahlquist A, Pontén F, Pettersson A. Keratosis linearis with ichthyosis congenita and sclerosing keratoderma (KLICK-syndrome): a rare, autosomal recessive disorder of keratohyaline formation? Acta Derm Venereol 1997;77:225–7.**

Syndromic ichthyoses

X-chromosomal ichthyosis syndromes

Conradi–Hünermann–Happle syndrome

Introduction. Conradi–Hünermann–Happle syndrome (X-linked dominant chondrodysplasia type II/CDPX2; OMIM #302960) is an ultra-rare X-linked dominant skin disorder that usually affects females and is lethal in males. Clinical hallmarks of the disease are a mosaic presentation of linear ichthyosis, chondrodysplasia punctata, asymmetrically shortened limbs, unilaterial, sometimes sectorial cataracts and short stature [1].

Pathogenesis. Mutations in the emopamil binding protein (EBP) encoding a delta8-delta7 sterol isomerase in the late stages of cholesterol biosynthesis were found to underlie CDPX2 in humans [2–4]. The genetic defect is associated with metabolic alterations in the serum, namely markedly elevated levels of 8-dehydrocholesterol and of cholest-8(9)-en-3b-ol that can help to identify somatic mosaicism even in clinically unaffected males. The process of X-inactivation underlies the Blaschkoid pattern of distribution of skin lesions. Mosaicism in the parent generation has been reported several times [4–6]. The syndrome is characterized by anticipation, namely worsening of disease severity in subsequent generations [7]. It is believed that the accumulation of 8-dehydrocholesterol and other cholesterol precursors interferes with sonic hedgehog signalling and thus explains the developmental abnormalities such as facial dysmorphism, chondrodysplasia punctata or kyphoscoliosis [8]. The ichthyosis phenotype is difficult to explain, but it has been shown that lamellar bodies lack their normal lamellar structure [9].

Clinical features. Affected babies are typically female, premature and born with either partial collodion membrane or generalized ichthyosiform erythroderma. Within the first year, generalized linear and swirling patterns of erythroderma and scaling, following the lines of Blaschko, are established (Fig. 129.27a). Intervening areas of skin are unaffected. Palmoplantar hyperkeratosis and nail dystrophy may occur. Recurrent infections especially in the flexures, can be troublesome, and scalp and eyebrow hair is sparse and lusterless. The ichthyosis improves in early childhood and the residual signs are often so subtle in adult life that an affected mother may be missed. Signs to be sought in older children and adults include swirls of fine scales, linear pigmentary change, patchy atrophy, follicular atrophoderma (Fig. 129.27b) mainly on the limbs and dorsal hands, and a striate cicatricial alopecia, all in a Blaschkoid pattern.

Other variable features include a rounded or asymmetrical facies with frontal bossing and hypertelorism, a broad flat nasal bridge, congenital asymmetric cataracts in 60% of patients, short stature, asymmetrical or, rarely, symmetrical shortening of limbs, kyphoscoliosis, supernumerary digits and other skeletal defects. Stippled calcification (asymmetric) of long-bone epiphyses is a characteristic but not universal radiological finding in the neonatal period, and usually resolves by adulthood. Neural hearing loss has been reported.

Differential diagnosis. Novel clinicogenetic entities caused by a hypomorphic mutation in *EBP*, have been described [10,11], and the term *MEND syndrome* (male *EBP* disorder with neurological defects) has been proposed [12]. MEND is inherited as an X-linked recessive trait with extreme behavioural symptoms, but female carriers of the hypomorphic EBP mutation seem to be unaffected [13]. The situation is reminiscent of CK syndrome (OMIM #300831), which is caused by hypomorphic temperature-sensitive mutations in *NSDHL* [14], whereas classic *NSDHL* mutations are associated with the X-linked dominant CHILD syndrome [15].

Treatment. Emollients are helpful in controlling ichthyosis and antimicrobial therapy may be needed for skin infections in infancy. The effect of retinoids is unknown and the need for treatment diminishes with age. Continued orthopaedic surveillance and appropriate procedures may

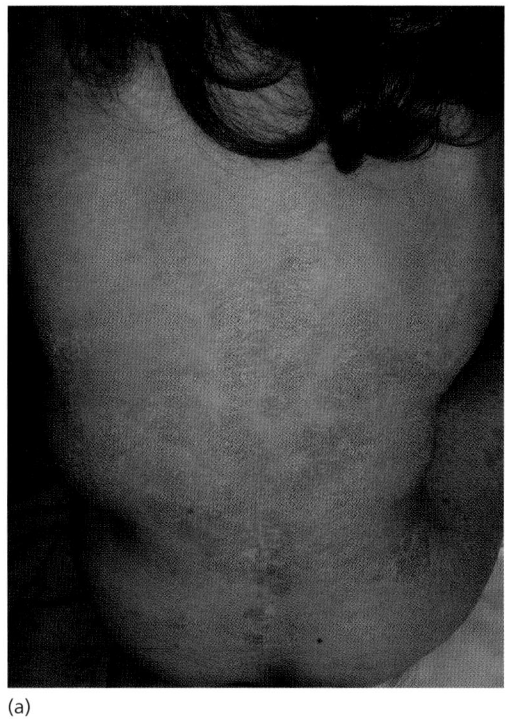

(a)

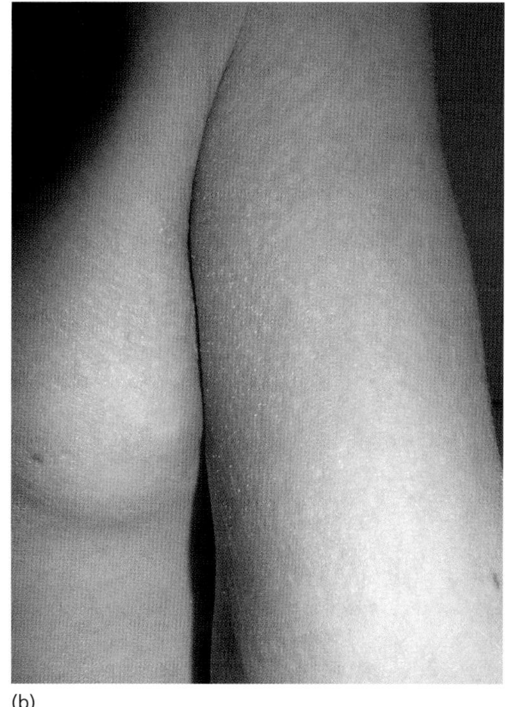

(b)

Fig. 129.27 Conradi–Hünermann–Happle syndrome. (a) Blaschko linear ichthyosis. and (b) follicular atrophoderma. Source: Courtesy of Dr A. Hernandez-Martin, Madrid, Spain.

be indicated for skeletal anomalies. Cataracts usually do not affect vision. The ichthyosis is probably caused by both cholesterol deficiency and accumulation of toxic sterol metabolites. Therefore, an approach similar to that used in treating hyperkeratosis in the metabolically related CHILD syndrome may be beneficial [16].

References

1 **Happle R, Phillips RJ, Roessner A, Jünemann G. Homologous genes for X-linked chondrodysplasia punctata in man and mouse. Hum Genet 1983;63:24–7.**

2 Derry JM, Gormally E, Means GD et al. Mutations in a delta 8-delta 7 sterol isomerase in the tattered mouse and X-linked dominant chondrodysplasia punctata. Nat Genet 1999;22:286–90.

3 **Braverman N, Lin P, Moebius FF et al. Mutations in the gene encoding 3 beta-hydroxysteroid-delta 8, delta 7-isomerase cause X-linked dominant Conradi-Hünermann syndrome. Nat Genet 1999;22:291–4.**

4 **Has C, Seedorf U, Kannenberg F et al. Gas chromatography-mass spectrometry and molecular genetic studies in families with the Conradi-Hünermann-Happle syndrome. J Invest Dermatol 2002;118:851–8.**

5 Hellenbroich Y, Grzeschik KH, Krapp M et al. Reduced penetrance in a family with X-linked dominant chondrodysplasia punctata. Eur J Med Genet 2007;50:392–8.

6 Morice-Picard F, Kostrzewa E, Wolf C et al. Evidence of postzygotic mosaicism in a transmitted form of Conradi-Hunermann-Happle syndrome associated with a novel EBP mutation. Arch Dermatol 2011;147:1073–6.

7 Traupe H, Müller D, Atherton D et al. Exclusion mapping of the X-linked dominant chondrodysplasia punctata/ichthyosis/cataract/short stature (Happle) syndrome: possible involvement of an unstable pre-mutation. Hum Genet 1992;89:659–65.

8 **Porter FD, Herman GE. Malformation syndromes caused by disorders of cholesterol synthesis. J Lipid Res 2011;52:6–34**

9 **Akiyama M, Sakai K, Hayasaka K et al. Conradi-Hünermann-Happle syndrome with abnormal lamellar granule contents. Br J Dermatol 2009;160:1335–7.**

10 Milunsky JM, Maher TA, Metzenberg AB. Molecular, biochemical, and phenotypic analysis of a hemizygous male with a severe atypical phenotype for X-linked dominant Conradi-Hunermann-Happle syndrome and a mutation in EBP. Am J Med Genet A 2003;116A:249–54.

11 Happle R. Hypomorphic alleles within the EBP gene cause a phenotype quite different from Conradi-Hünermann-Happle syndrome. Am J Med Genet A 2003;122A:279.

12 **Arnold AW, Bruckner-Tuderman L, Has C, Happle R. Conradi-Hünermann-Happle syndrome in males vs. MEND syndrome (male EBP disorder with neurological defects). Br J Dermatol 2012;166: 1309–13.**

13 **Hartill VL, Tysoe C, Manning N. An unusual phenotype of X-linked developmental delay and extreme behavioral difficulties associated with a mutation in the EBP gene. Am J Med Genet A 2014;164: 907–14.**

14 **McLarren KW, Severson TM, du Souich C et al. Hypomorphic temperature-sensitive alleles of NSDHL cause CK syndrome. Am J Hum Genet 2010;87:905–14.**

15 Bornholdt D, König A, Happle R et al. Mutational spectrum of NSDHL in CHILD syndrome. J Med Genet 2005;42:17.

16 **Paller AS1, van Steensel MA, Rodriguez-Martín M et al. Pathogenesis-based therapy reverses cutaneous abnormalities in an inherited disorder of distal cholesterol metabolism. J Invest Dermatol 2011;131:2242–8.**

Congenital hemidysplasia–ichthyosiform naevus-limb defect syndrome

Comment

Congenital hemidysplasia–ichthyosiform naevus-limb defect syndrome (CHILD) syndrome (OMIM #308050) is a very rare X-linked and, in males, lethal disorder of distal cholesterol biosynthesis featuring as a clinical hallmark the CHILD naevus [1]. In the initial report, the cutaneous phenotype was categorized as ichthyosis, but later the Happle group described it as an inflammatory naevus syndrome [2] (see Chapter 106).

References

1 **Happle R, Koch H, Lenz W. The CHILD syndrome. Congenital hemidysplasia with ichthyosiform erythroderma and limb defects. Eur J Pediatr 1980;134:27–33.**

2 **Happle R, Mittag H, Küster W. The CHILD nevus: a distinct skin disorder. Dermatology 1995;191:210–6.**

SECTION 27: DISORDERS OF KERATIN AND KERATINIZATION

Ichthyosis follicularis, with atrichia and photophobia syndrome

Introduction. Ichthyosis follicularis, with atrichia and photophobia (IFAP) syndrome (OMIM #308205) is a rare X-linked recessive trait featuring ichthyosis follicularis, atrichia, photophobia and severe retardation of growth and psychomotor development [1]. It has both clinical and molecular genetic overlap with two other disorders: BRESEK/BRESHEK syndrome with brain anomalies, retardation, ectodermal dysplasia, skeletal malformations, Hirschsprung disease, ear/eye anomalies, cleft palate/cryptorchidism, and kidney dysplasia/hypoplasia; and X-linked keratosis follicularis spinulosa decalvans (KFSDX; OMIM #308800).

Pathogenesis. X-inked inheritance [1] was firmly established by the observation of functional cutaneous mosaicism showing Blaschko-linear lesions reflecting lyonization in women heterozygous for IFAP syndrome [2]. Causative missense mutations were identified in the X-linked gene *MBTPS2* encoding membrane-bound transcription factor protease, site 2 [3]. Different and distinct mutations in the same gene are associated with keratosis follicularis spinulosa decalvans [4], BRESEK/BRESHEK syndrome [5,6] as well as an X-linked variant of Olmsted syndrome [7]. The transcription factor encoded by *MBTPS2* is a zinc metalloprotease essential for cholesterol homeostasis as well as endoplasmatic reticulum stress response [3,6]. Of note, only missense mutations and splice mutations partially affecting transcription [8] are known so far. It is most likely that total loss of *MBTPS2* is not tolerated in male embryos and a residual enzyme activity is required for survival [6].

Clinical features. The full-blown spectrum of IFAP syndrome is variable and seen only in males. All patients have the triad of follicular ichthyosis, congenital atrichia of the scalp (absence of hair), and photophobia. Children can be born as collodion babies and present with generalized follicular keratosis over the entire body including the scalp. It can improve markedly in early childhood. The most striking abnormality certainly is the congenital alopecia (atrichia) (Fig. 129.28). Superficial corneal ulceration and vascularization leads to progressive corneal scaring and underlies photophobia, the third cardinal feature [9]. Neurological features include mental retardation and seizures as well as olivo-cerebellar atrophy, malformation of the temporal lobes, mild inner cerebral atrophy and hypoplasia of the corpus callosum [10,11]. Female carriers can present with much milder symptoms such as cutaneous hyperkeratotic lesions that follow the lines of Blaschko, asymmetrical distribution of body hair or a Blaschko-linear presentation of hypohidrosis that can only be visualized by sweat testing [2,11].

Differential diagnosis. Hereditary mucoepithelial dysplasia featuring photophobia and keratosis pilaris could be misdiagnosed as IFAP syndrome [12].

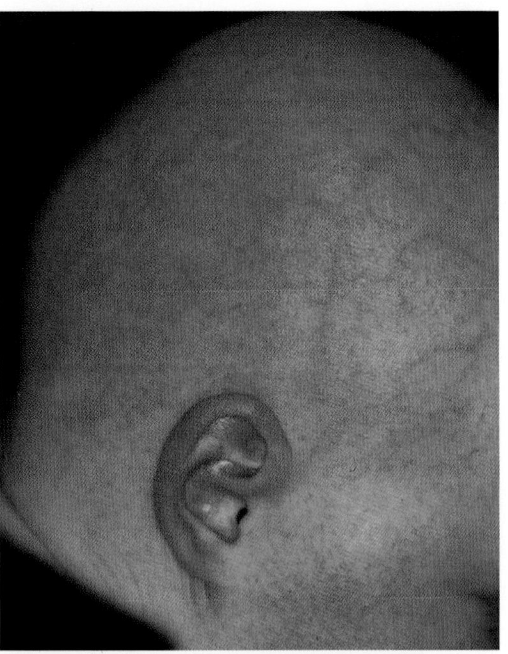

Fig. 129.28 Ichthyosis follicularis-alopecia-photophobia syndrome. Source: Courtesy of Dr A. S. Paller, Department of Dermatology and Pediatrics, Chicago, USA.

Treatment. A moderate response to low dose acitretin has been reported [13]. Emollients are helpful. Intensive lubrication of the ocular surface remains the mainstay of therapy for photophobia.

References

1 **Hamm H, Meinecke P, Traupe H. Further delineation of the ichthyosis follicularis, atrichia, and photophobia syndrome. Eur J Pediatr 1991;150:627–9.**

2 **König A, Happle R. Linear lesions reflecting lyonization in women heterozygous for IFAP syndrome (ichthyosis follicularis with atrichia and photophobia). Am J Med Genet 1999;85:365–8.**

3 **Oeffner F, Fischer G, Happle R et al. IFAP syndrome is caused by deficiency in MBTPS2, an intramembrane zinc metalloprotease essential for cholesterol homeostasis and ER stress response. Am J Hum Genet 2009;84:459–67.**

4 **Aten E, Brasz LC, Bornholdt D et al. Keratosis follicularis spinulosa decalvans is caused by mutations in MBTPS2. Hum Mutat 2010;31:1125–33.**

5 Naiki M, Mizuno S, Yamada K et al. MBTPS2 mutation causes BRESEK/BRESHECK syndrome. Am J Med Genet A 2012;158A: 97–102.

6 Bornholdt D, Atkinson TP, Bouadjar B et al. Genotype-phenotype correlations emerging from the identification of missense mutations in MBTPS2. Hum Mutat 2013;34:587–94.

7 Haghighi A, Scott CA, Poon DS et al. A missense mutation in the MBTPS2 gene underlies the X-linked form of Olmsted syndrome. J Invest Dermatol 2013;133:571–3.

8 Oeffner F, Martinez F, Schaffer J et al. Intronic mutations affecting splicing of MBTPS2 cause ichthyosis follicularis, alopecia and photophobia (IFAP) syndrome. Exp Dermatol 2011;20:447–9.

9 **Mégarbané H, Mégarbané A. Ichthyosis follicularis, alopecia, and photophobia (IFAP) syndrome. Orphanet J Rare Dis 2011;6:29.**

10 Bibas-Bonet H, Fauze R, Boente MC et al. IFAP syndrome 'plus' seizures, mental retardation, and callosal hypoplasia. Pediatr Neurol 2001;24:228–31.

11 Keyvani K, Paulus W, Traupe H et al. Ichthyosis follicularis, alopecia, and photophobia (IFAP) syndrome: clinical and neuropathological observations in a 33-year-old man. Am J Med Genet 1998;78:371–7.

12 Rothe MJ, Lucky AW. Are ichthyosis follicularis and hereditary mucoepithelial dystrophy related diseases. Pediatr Dermatol 1995;12:195.

13 Khandpur S, Bhat R, Ramam M. Ichthyosis follicularis, alopecia and photophobia (IFAP) syndrome treated with acitretin. J Eur Acad Dermatol Venereol 2005;19:759–62.

Netherton syndrome

Comment

(Comèl-)Netherton syndrome (OMIM #256500) is a specific genodermatosis characterized by premature desquamation and a thinner rather than thicker stratum corneum. Scaling and erythroderma as seen in the disease overlap with the clinical features of congenital ichthyoses. The disease has therefore been classified as syndromic ichthyosis. It is discussed separately in this book (see Chapter 132).

Differential diagnosis. Diseases such as hyper-IgE recurrent infection syndrome, atopic dermatitis, CIE, PSS type B (= peeling skin disease), Severe dermatitis-multiple allergies-metabolic wasting syndrome, trichothiodystrophy, neutral lipid storage disease with ichthyosis or erythrokeratoderma are important clinical differential diagnoses.

Severe dermatitis-multiple allergies-metabolic wasting syndrome

Epidemiology and pathogenesis. Severe dermatitis, multiple allergies, metabolic wasting syndrome (SAM syndrome; OMIM #615508) is an autosomal recessive or dominant disorder of cornification that has recently been recognized. It is very rare, with currently six families reported in the literature [1–5].

SAM syndrome is predominantly caused by biallelic loss-of-function mutations in *DSG1*, encoding desmoglein 1, that is a major constituent of desmosomes. In addition, one patient with SAM syndrome caused by a heterozygous *de novo* missense mutation in *DSP*, that encodes desmoplakin-assembling desmosomal plaques, has been reported. Desmosomes connect the cell surface to the keratin cytoskeleton and subsequently play an essential role in maintaining epidermal integrity. Thus, both *DSG1* and *DSP* mutations result in a loss of cell–cell adhesion and a severe barrier dysfunction. The position of the mutation within *DSG1* is suggested to play a role in the clinical presentation of SAM syndrome. However, a genotype–phenotype correlation cannot yet be made because the number of published cases is too low. Furthermore, it is likely that environmental factors or modifier genes account for the phenotypic variability.

Clinical features. SAM syndrome becomes manifest at birth or within the first weeks of life with CIE (see previously), patchy eczematous lesions, palmoplantar keratoderma and diffuse hypotrichosis (Fig. 129.29). During childhood, the palmoplantar keratoderma gradually grows thicker and extends to the dorsal aspects of palms and soles. In addition, hyperkeratotic plaques over the knees, elbows and the sacral region, as well as superficial skin erosions and a generalized itchy psoriasiform dermatitis develop. Severe skin infections with superficial pustulosis and a susceptibility to respiratory infections and sepsis (*Staphylococcus aureus*) are common. In addition, most infants show malabsorption and metabolic wasting with developmental delay and growth retardation. This is in part a consequence of multiple food allergies, but of note, in some children with SAM syndrome, food allergies are subtle.

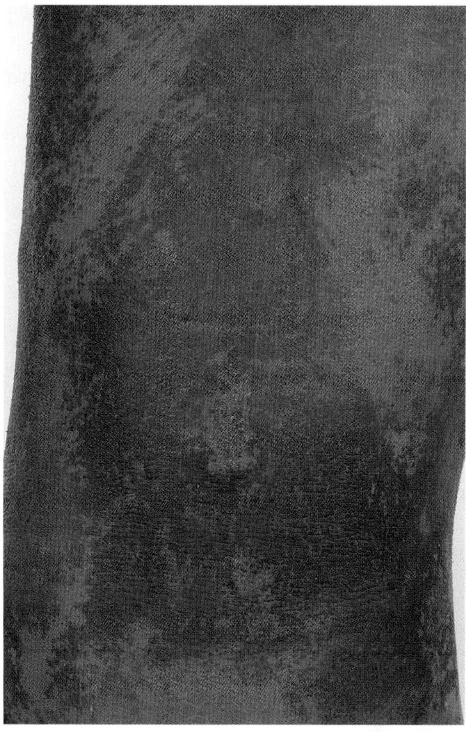

Fig. 129.29 Variant of SAM syndrome (severe dermatitis-multiple allergies-metabolic wasting syndrome) caused by *DSP* mutation. Patient made a local treatment with black tea and cream. Source: Courtesy of the University Hospital Münster, Münster, Germany

Additional reported features of SAM syndrome include collodion membrane, nail dystrophy, macrocephaly, nystagmus, photophobia, keratitis, hypodontia, eosinophilic esophagitis and ventricular septal defect.

Differential diagnosis. In neonates, clinical distinction from other disorders of cornification that present with CIE, including Netherton syndrome, neutral lipid storage disease with ichthyosis, Sjögren–Larsson syndrome and ARCI can be difficult. In addition, SAM syndrome with extensive superficial pustulosis can resemble infantile pustulosis, which is a rare cutaneous presentation for multiple dermatological conditions. The association of generalized eczema, elevated IgE plasma levels and skin infections is a characteristic finding not only of SAM syndrome, but also of atopic dermatitis and other genodermatoses such as hyper-IgE syndrome, Netherton syndrome, PSS type B, Omenn syndrome, Wiskott–Aldrich syndrome, prolidase deficiency and immune dysregulation, polyendocrinopathy, enteropathy, and X-linked (IPEX) syndrome. Because diagnosis is further complicated by the fact that the mentioned genodermatoses often share other clinical symptoms and laboratory findings, genetic testing is expedient in infants with suspected diagnosis of SAM syndrome.

Laboratory, histology and genetic findings. Blood tests exhibit persistent eosinophilia and increased IgE levels. Genetic testing is recommended for early differentiation of SAM syndrome. Light microscopy of the hair is unspecific.

Histopathological skin findings include psoriasiform dermatitis with alternating para- and orthohyperkeratosis, hypo- and hypergranulosis, as well as widespread acantholysis within the granular and spinous layers. Immunofluorescence analysis shows large accumulations of desmoglein 1 and desmoplakin, and striking reductions in both desmoglein 1 and keratin 10 staining.

Electron microscopy of individuals with SAM syndrome caused by *DSG1* mutations reveals a deficiency, as well as reduction or uneven distribution of desmosomes in the upper epidermis, leading to an expansion of intercellular spaces. In SAM syndrome, caused by a *DSP* mutation in the spinous layer, a striking dissociation between keratin intermediate filament bundles and desmosomes is detectable, and poorly formed desmosomal inner plaques that appear much less electron dense are also visible. Furthermore, the stratum corneum displays structural abnormalities, including marked attenuation of cornified envelopes, absence of corneodesmosomes, and an impairment in the postsecretory maturation and organization of secreted lamellar body contents.

Treatment and prevention. Neonates often require management in an intensive care unit to treat infections and failure to thrive. High calorific nutrition and a hypoallergenic diet are important. A percutaneous endoscopic gastrostomy tube can be necessary to provide essential supplemental feeding. Treatment of skin symptoms is dependent on the phenotypical severity and the age of the child. Topical therapy with emollients, corticosteroids, tacrolimus ointment and antiseptics is standard. Systemic acitretin (0.5 mg/kg/day) has been shown to be effective.

References

1 **Samuelov L, Sarig O, Harmon RM et al. Desmoglein 1 deficiency results in severe dermatitis, multiple allergies and metabolic wasting. Nat Genet 2013;45:1244–8.**

2 **McAleer MA, Pohler E, Smith FJ et al. Severe dermatitis, multiple allergies, and metabolic wasting syndrome caused by a novel mutation in the N-terminal plakin domain of desmoplakin. J Allergy Clin Immunol 2015;136:1268–76.**

3 Cheng R, Yan M, Ni C et al. Report of Chinese family with severe dermatitis, multiple allergies and metabolic wasting syndrome caused by novel homozygous desmoglein-1 gene mutation. J Dermatol 2016;43:1201–4.

4 Has C, Jakob T, He Y et al. Loss of desmoglein 1 associated with palmoplantar keratoderma, dermatitis and multiple allergies. Br J Dermatol 2015;172:257–61.

5 Schlipf NA, Vahlquist A, Teigen N et al. Whole-exome sequencing identifies novel autosomal recessive DSG1 mutations associated with mild SAM syndrome. Br J Dermatol 2016;174:444–8.

Neutral lipid storage disease with ichthyosis

Definition. Chanarin–Dorfman syndrome (neutral lipid storage disease with ichthyosis; NLSDI; OMIM #275630) is a rare type of syndromic ARCI featuring CIE and lipid droplets in various tissues.

Epidemiology and pathogenesis. Often patients originate from Mediterranean countries. NLSDI is caused by bi-allelic mutations in the *ABHD5* gene [1], that is widely expressed in tissues such as skin, muscle, liver, brain and lymphocytes [2,3]. The resultant acylceramide deficiency leads to lipid depositions in various organs [4]. It should not be confused with neutral lipid storage disease with myopathy – but without ichthyosis (NLSDM), which is caused by mutations in the *PNPLA2* gene [5]. Interestingly, common features of the diseases in noncutaneous tissues can be explained by the fact that the *ABHD5* gene product is a cofactor of adipose triglyceride lipase encoded by the *PNPLA2* gene [6].

Clinical features. The multisystem disorder initially manifests as congenital ichthyosis. Affected newborns are either collodion babies or erythrodermic [7–9]. Thereafter Chanarin–Dorfman syndrome resembles mild to moderate CIE with fine white scales (Fig. 129.30). The ichthyosis may improve with age. Pruritus and hypohidrosis have been described. Mild ectropion, flexural and neck lichenification, and palmoplantar hyperkeratosis are common.

Extracutaneous findings. Muscle involvement ranges from an asymptomatic or subclinical myopathy with elevated muscle enzymes in most patients to marked proximal myopathy in a few cases. Of note, hepatomegaly, abnormal liver enzymes and fatty infiltration of the liver are common. Cirrhosis can evolve rapidly, even in childhood. Spenomegaly and malabsorption, resulting from intestinal mucosal lipid deposition, are occasional features. Cataracts of the nuclear type (subcapsular) may be detected from infancy in over 50% of cases, but rarely affect vision. Nystagmus may occur. Short stature, retinal disease, nerve deafness, ataxia, microcephaly, spasticicity, neuropathy and developmental delay have been reported, but most patients are intellectually normal. Fetal renal complications occurred in an infant with NLSDI. Prognosis depends on the pattern and degree of organ involvement.

Laboratory findings. Diagnostics may involve an ultrastructural analysis of the skin, as well as liver parameters, and special haematology (Jordan's anomaly) (Fig. 129.30a) [7], ophthalmological and neurological assessment. In particular, the characteristic lipid inclusions have to be specifically looked for in both affected patients and possible gene carriers, because Jordans's anomaly is not detected by simple automated blood cell count. Liver biopsy is more sensitive than biochemical markers in detecting the degree of hepatic involvement. Finally, the disease should be confirmed by early molecular analysis.

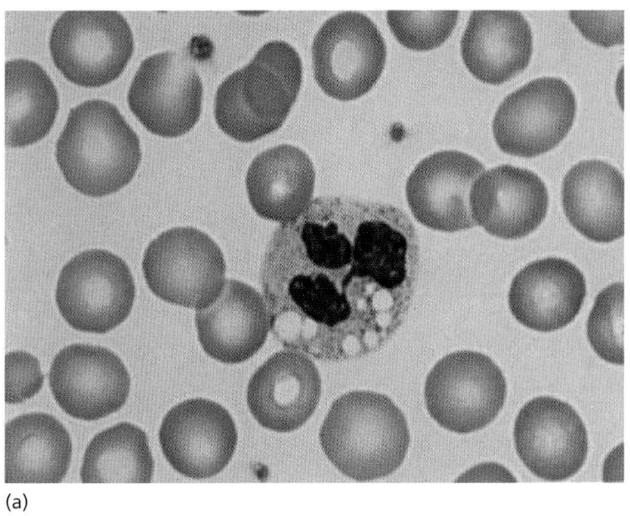
(a)

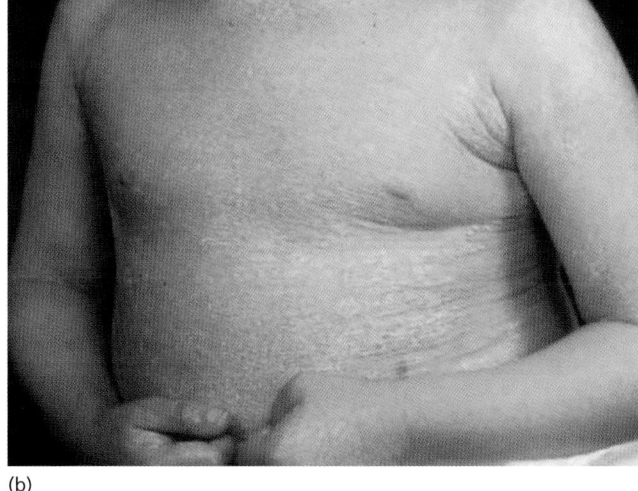
(b)

Fig. 129.30 Neutral lipid storage disease with ichthyosis. (a) Lipid vacuoles (Jordan's anomaly). (b) Ichthyosiform erythroderma. Source: Rook's Textbook of Dermatology. Reproduced with permission of John Wiley & Sons.

Treatment. Emollients are helpful and although liver function tests usually show abnormalities in these patients, administration of acitretin has been beneficial even in the presence of compromised liver function [10]. The effect of dietary approaches is doubtful [11].

References

1 **Lefèvre C, Jobard F, Caux F et al. Mutations in CGI-58, the gene encoding a new protein of the esterase/lipase/thioesterase subfamily, in Chanarin–Dorfman syndrome. Am J Hum Genet 2001;69:1002–12.**

2 **Badeloe S, van Geel M, Nagtzaam I et al. Chanarin–Dorfman syndrome caused by a novel splice site mutation in ABHD5 Br J Dermatol 2008;158:1378–80.**

3 Akiyama M, Sawamura D, Nomura Y et al. Truncation of CGI-58 protein causes malformation of lamellar granules resulting in ichthyosis in Dorfman–Chanarin syndrome. J Invest Dermatol 2003;121:1029–34.

4 Uchida Y, Cho Y, Moradian S et al. Neutral lipid storage leads to acylceramide deficiency, likely contributing to the pathogenesis of Dorfman–Chanarin syndrome. J Invest Dermatol 2010;130:2497–9.

5 Fischer J, Lefèvre C, Morava E et al. The gene encoding adipose triglyceride lipase (PNPLA2) is mutated in neutral lipid storage disease with myopathy. Nat Genet 2007;39:28–30.

6 Radner FP, Fischer J. The important role of epidermal triacylglycerol metabolism for maintenance of the skin permeability barrier function. Biochim Biophys Acta 2014;1841:409–15.

7 Wollenberg A, Geiger E, Schaller M, Wolff H. Dorfman–Chanarin syndrome in a Turkish kindred: conductor diagnosis requires analysis of multiple eosinophils. Acta Derm Venereol 2000;80:39–43.

8 Srebrnik A1, Tur E, Perluk C et al. Dorfman–Chanarin syndrome. A case report and a review. J Am Acad Dermatol 1987;17:801–8.

9 Peña-Penabad C, Almagro M, Martínez W et al. Dorfman–Chanarin syndrome (neutral lipid storage disease): new clinical features. Br J Dermatol 2001;144:430–2.

10 Israeli S, Pessach Y, Sarig O et al. Beneficial effect of acitretin in Chanarin–Dorfman syndrome. Clin Exp Dermatol 2012;37:31–3.

11 Judge MR, Atherton DJ, Salvayre R et al. Neutral lipid storage disease. Case report and lipid studies. Br J Dermatol 1994;130:507–10.

Ichthyoses with hair abnormalities, gastrointestinal or respiratory symptoms

Ichthyosis hypotrichosis syndrome

Definition. Ichthyosis hypotrichosis syndrome (OMIM #602400) presents at birth, without a collodion membrane (refer to Table 129.3). Two allelic variants have been described: (i) *autosomal recessive ichthyosis with hypotrichosis* features the ichthyosis and whole-body hypotrichosis, but no atrophoderma [1,2]; (ii) *congenital ichthyosis, follicular atrophoderma, hypotrichosis and hypohidrosis* refers to a very similar phenotype in addition associated with follicular atrophoderma (e.g. follicular pitting on dorsal aspects of hands and fingers) [3,4]. Both ichthyoses could be discussed as one nonsyndromic form, because its symptoms seem restricted to the skin and its appendages only.

Pathogenesis. The *ST14* gene [1,2] encodes matriptase, a novel key player of the epidermal protease network [5,6]. The transmembrane serine protease is an efficient activator of epidermal prokallikreins. Matriptase deficiency leads to a decrease of filaggrin processing [7] and may be seen as the functional counterpart to LEKTI deficiency, which leads to an increase of epidermal kallikrein activity [8]. Clinical heterogeneity may be caused by different types of *ST14* mutations [1,4,9,10]. The hair phenotype can be explained by the fact that matriptase is expressed in the cortex cells and shaft of the anagen hair [11].

Neonatal ichthyosis-sclerosing cholangitis

Pathogenesis. Neonatal ichthyosis-sclerosing cholangitis (NISCH) syndrome (OMIM #607626) belongs to the disorders of tight junctions and is caused by biallelic mutations in *CLDN1* encoding claudin-1 [12,13] (refer to Table 129.4). Claudin-1 is part of the epidermal tight junctions and is well expressed in cholangiocytes and hepatocytes [14]. Primary lack of claudin-1 leads to an increased paracellular permeability between epithelial cells explaining hypercholanaemia and epidermal barrier defect [12].

Clinical features. NISCH syndrome is characterized by scalp hypotrichosis with scarring alopecia and ichthyosis, and shows a primary sclerosing cholangitis of variable severity [15–17] (Fig. 129.31). Sclerosing cholangitis is a chronic condition characterized by inflammation and obliterative fibrosis of the intra- and extrahepatic bile

Table 129.3 Different neuroichthyotic syndromes

	Gaucher syndrome type 2	MEDNIK[a] syndrome	CEDNIK[b] syndrome	ARC[c] syndrome
OMIM	230900	609313	609528	208085
Mode of inheritance	AR	AR	AR	AR
Gene	*GBA*	*AP1S1*	*SNAP29*	*VPS33B*
Onset	At birth, or later	At birth or within first weeks of life	After 5–11 months	At birth, can sometimes be later
Initial clinical presentation	CIE or less frequently mild collodion membrane	Erythematous rashes, similar to EKV	Until up to one year of age, normal skin; thereafter LI type	Xerosis and scaling within a few days of birth
Disease course	Ranging from mild to moderate	Progressive	Fatal	Fatal
Distribution of scaling	Generalized	Generalized,	Generalized with sparing of skin folds	Generalized with sparing of skin folds
Scaling type	Fine or moderate; scaling may resolve after neonatal period	EKV-like	Coarse and large (plate-like)	Fine or platelike (extensor sites)
Scaling colour	White, grey or brown	EKV-like	Whitish	White or brownish
Erythema	Unusual	EKV-like	Absent	Absent
Palmoplantar involvement	-	Not specifically	Yes	Spared
Scalp abnormalities	-	Not specifically	Fine, sparse hair	Mild scarring alopecia
Other skin findings	-	Nail thickening, mucous membrane affected	None	Ectropion
Extracutaneous involvement	Hydrops fetalis; progressive neurological deterioration; hepatosplenomegaly, hypotonia, respiratory distress, arthrogryposis, facial anomalies	Congenital sensorineural deafness, peripheral neuropathy, psychomotor and growth retardation, chronic diarrhoea, mental retardation	Sensorineural deafness; cerebral dysgenesis; neuropathy; microcephaly; neurogenic muscle atrophy; optic nerve atrophy; cachexia	Arthrogryposis (wrist, knee or hip); intrahepatic bile duct hypoplasia with cholestasis; renal tubular degeneration; metabolic acidosis; abnormal platelet function; cerebral malformation
Risk of death	Death often by 2 years of age	Life-threatening congenital diarrhoea	Lethal within the first decade	Lethal within first year of life
Skin ultrastructure	Lamellar/nonlamellar phase separations in SC	Histology: hyperkeratosis with hypergranulosis	Impaired lipid loading onto LB and defective LB secretion	Defective LB secretion
Special analyses	Liver function tests; decreased beta-glucocerebrosidase activity (leukocytes); Gaucher cells (bone marrow); increased acid phosphatase (serum)	Elevation of VLCFAs (blood), treatable by zinc acetate therapy	Absent RAB protein on immunohistochemistry, MRI	Liver and renal biopsy

AR, autosomal recessive; CIE, congenital ichthyosiform erythroderma; EKV, erythrokeratodermia variabilis; IV, ichthyosis vulgairs; LB, lamellar body; LI, lamellar ichthysosis; SC, stratum corneum; VLCFA, very long-chain fatty acid.

[a] MEDNIK, mental retardation-enteropathy-deafness-neuropathy-ichthyosis-keratodermia (~erythrokeratodermia variabilis 3, Kamouraska type);

[b] CEDNIK, cerebral dysgenesis-neuropathy-ichthyosis-palmoplantar keratoderma

[c] ARC, Arthrogryposis-renal dysfunction-cholestasis.

Source: Adapted from Oji et al. (2010). Revised nomenclature and classification of inherited ichthyoses: results of the First Ichthyosis Consensus Conference in Sorèze 2009. J Am Acad Dermatol 2010;63:607–41.

Table 129.4 Examples of syndromic ichthyoses with hair abnormalities, gastrointestinal or respiratory symptoms

	Ichthyosis with hypotrichosis[a]	Neonatal ichthyosis-sclerosing cholangitis (NISCH)[b]	Ichthyosis prematurity syndrome (IPS)
OMIM	602400	607626	608649
Mode of inheritance	AR	AR	AR
Gene	*ST14*	*CLDN1*	*SLC27A4* (previously known as *FATP4*)
Onset	At birth	At birth (or shortly after)	At birth (polyhydramnion, prematurity, >6 weeks)
Initial clinical presentation	Lamellar ichthyosis, severe hypotrichosis, absent eyebrows and eyelashes	Mild scaling, neonatal jaundice with hepatomegaly, frontal alopecia in early childhood	Respiratory distress, generalized skin hyperkeratosis with focal accentuation on scalp, eyebrows
Disease course	Over time, scalp hair growth and appearance/colour may improve	Mild ichthyosis, liver involvement variable	Severe at birth, spontaneous improvement
Distribution of scaling	Generalized, including the scalp, face may be unaffected	Predominant on trunk	Focal accentuation (see above)
Scaling type	Coarse, plate-like, adherent	Fine to polygonal, thin	Caseous (vernix caseosa-like)
Scaling color	Brown to dark	Normal	Whitish
Erythema	Unusual	Unusual	Mild to moderate
Palmoplantar involvement	No	No	Yes, initially
Hypohidrosis	Yes	No	No
Scalp abnormalities	Hypotrichosis in youth, sparse, unruly hair in adolescence, recessing frontal hair line in adults	Major criterion: coarse thick hair, fronto-temporal scarring alopecia; hypotrichosis, curly/woolly hair	Extensive at birth
Other skin findings	Follicular atrophoderma	-	Follicular keratosis ('toad skin'), atopic eczema, asthma, eosinophilia
Extracutaneous involvement	Sparse and curly eyebrows, occasionally photophobia and pingueculum	Major criterion: sclerosing cholangitis or congenital paucity of bile ducts	Pulmonary involvement and asphyxia at birth, later on atopic asthma, eosinophilia and occasionally hyper IgE
Risk of death	Normal	Not observed, but theoretically possible from liver involvement	Perinatally potentially fatal because of respiratory asphyxia; otherwise normal
Skin ultrastructure	High presence of intact corneodesmosomes in the upper SC, residues of membranous structures in the SC	Splitting of desmosomal anchoring plaques in the SG	Deposits of trilamellar membranous curved lamellae in swollen corneocytes and perinuclearly in oedematous granular cells
Special analyses	Hair microscopy may reveal dysplastic hair, pili torti or pili bifurcati	Liver function tests, cholangiography, liver biopsy	Blood cell count (eosinophilia)

AR, autosomal recessive; SC, stratum corneum, SG, stratum granulosum.

[a] Allelic variant: congenital ichthyosis, follicular atrophoderma, hypotrichosis and hypohidrosis (IFAH)

[b] Also known as ichthyosis-hypotrichosis-sclerosing cholangitis or ILVASC syndrome.

Adapted from Oji et al. (2010). Revised nomenclature and classification of inherited ichthyoses: results of the First Ichthyosis Consensus Conference in Sorèze 2009. J Am Acad Dermatol 2010;63:607–41.

ducts. Hence, infantile jaundice and ichthyosis may be an important clinical symptom of the disease.

Laboratory findings. Early molecular analysis is recommended as pathognomonic histological and ultrastructural features have not been established so far [18].

Ichthyosis prematurity syndrome

Pathogenesis. Ichthyosis prematurity syndrome (IPS; OMIM #608649) is caused by biallelic mutations in *SLC27A4*, previously known as *FATP4* [19,20], encoding a fatty acid transporter and acyl coenzyme A synthetase expressed in the suprabasal layers of the epidermis [21] (refer to Table 129.3). Impaired function leads to a disturbance of the intercellular lipid bilayers of the stratum corneum [22]. Animal models suggest that *FATP4* might be more important for the generation of the epidermal barrier than for its maintenance, explaining the rapid self-improving character of the disease [23,24].

Clinical features. IPS is characterized by mild to moderate erythema and thick caseous scales predominantly on the scalp, neck, shoulders and back, as well as on the hands and feet. Affected neonates are often born between the 30th and 35th gestational week, and suffer from transient, potentially life-threatening asphyxia that is the result of reduced lung function and bronchial obstruction from keratin plugs [23,25,26]. Prenatal findings are a polyhydramnion with increased echogenic signals within the amniotic fluid [27]. In later life children are prone to pruritus and atopic manifestations [23].

Differential diagnosis. Neonatal erythroderma (Fig. 129.32a) evolves into a mild ichthyosis reminiscent of self-healing collodion baby [28] (Fig. 129.32b).

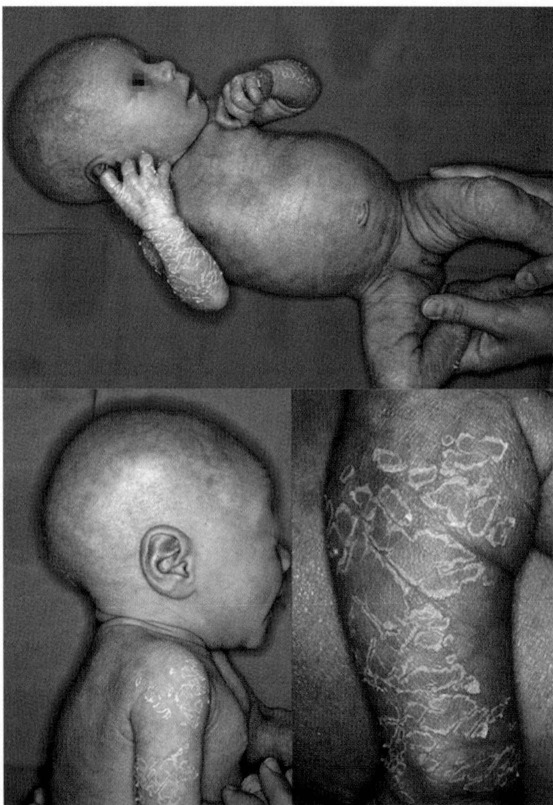

Fig. 129.31 Neonatal ichthyosis-sclerosing cholangitis-hypotrichosis syndrome.

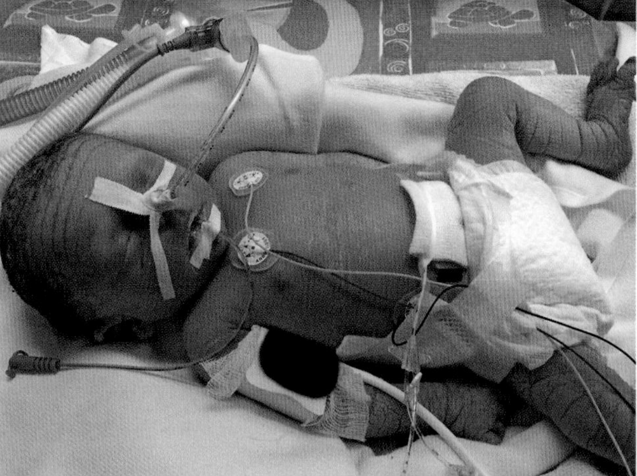

(a)

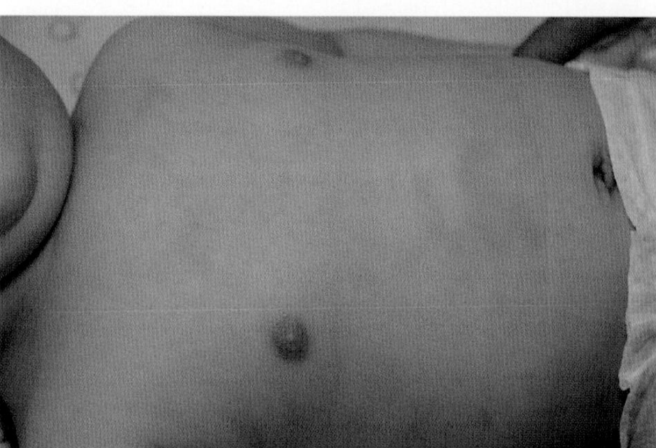

(b)

Fig. 129.32 Ichthyosis prematurity syndrome. (a) Neonatal presentation. (b) Same patient after 3 months. Note mild velvet-like skin texture. Source: Courtesy of the Department of Dermatology, University Hospital Münster, Germany.

Laboratory and ultrastructure findings. Apart from molecular diagnostics, ultrastructural analysis of the skin clearly distinguishes IPS from other ichthyoses [29].

Treatment and prevention. Infants with IPS require management in an intensive care nursery. Optimal treatment, i. e. adequate bronchial suction, if initiated early enough, and optimal perinatal care will avoid life-threatening hypoxaemia and/or complications such as infantile cerebral paresis [23]. Genetic counselling of the patient's parents is strongly recommended. Information about the risk of IPS and the danger of respiratory insufficiency at birth is important for subsequent pregnancies.

References

1 **Basel-Vanagaite L, Attia R, Ishida-Yamamoto A et al. Autosomal recessive ichthyosis with hypotrichosis caused by a mutation in ST14, encoding type II transmembrane serine protease matriptase. Am J Hum Genet 2007;80:467–77.**

2 Avrahami L, Maas S, Pasmanik-Chor M et al. Autosomal recessive ichthyosis with hypotrichosis syndrome: further delineation of the phenotype. Clin Genet 2008;74:47–53.

3 **Lestringant GG, Kuster W, Frossard PM, Happle R Congenital ichthyosis, follicular atrophoderma, hyotrichosis, and hypohidrosis: a new genodermatosis? Am J Med Genet 1998;75:186–9**

4 Alef T, Torres S, Hausser I et al. Ichthyosis, follicular atrophoderma, and hypotrichosis caused by mutations in ST14 is associated with impaired profilaggrin processing. J Invest Dermatol 2009;129:862–9.

5 Chen YW, Wang JK, Chou FP et al. Matriptase regulates proliferation and early, but not terminal, differentiation of human keratinocytes. J Invest Dermatol 2014;134:405–14.

6 Ishida-Yamamoto A, Igawa S. Genetic skin diseases related to desmosomes and corneodesmosomes. J Dermatol Sci 2014;74:99–105.

7 List K, Szabo R, Wertz PW et al. Loss of proteolytically processed filaggrin caused by epidermal deletion of Matriptase/MT-SP1. J Cell Biol 2003;163:901–10.

8 **Sales KU, Masedunskas A, Bey AL et al. Matriptase initiates activation of epidermal pro-kallikrein and disease onset in a mouse model of Netherton syndrome. Nat Genet 2010;42:676–83.**

9 Désilets A, Béliveau F, Vandal G et al. Mutation G827R in matriptase causing autosomal recessive ichthyosis with hypotrichosis yields an inactive protease. J Biol Chem 2008;283:10535–42.

10 Dereure O. [Recessive autosomal ichthyosis with hypotrichosis with mutation in the ST14 gene]. Ann Dermatol Venereol 2007;134:798.

11 List K, Currie B, Scharschmidt TC, el al. Autosomal ichthyosis with hypotrichosis syndrome displays low matriptase proteolytic activity and is phenocopied in ST14 hypomorphic mice. J Biol Chem 2007;282:36714–23.

12 **Hadj-Rabia S, Baala L, Vabres P et al. Claudin-1 gene mutations in neonatal sclerosing cholangitis associated with ichthyosis: a tight junction disease. Gastroenterology 2004;127:1386–90.**

13 **Nagtzaam IF, van Geel M, Driessen A et al. Bile duct paucity is part of the neonatal ichthyosis-sclerosing cholangitis phenotype. Br J Dermatol 2010;163:205–7.**

14 Morita K, Miyachi Y, Furuse M. Tight junctions in epidermis: from barrier to keratinization. Eur J Dermatol 2011;21:12–7.

15 Baala L, Hadj-Rabia S, Hamel-Teillac D et al. Homozygosity mapping of a locus for a novel syndromic ichthyosis to chromosome 3q27-q28. J Invest Derm 2002;119:70–6.

16 Feldmeyer L, Huber M, Fellmann F et al. Hohl D. Confirmation of the origin of NISCH syndrome. Hum Mutat 2006;27:408–10.

17 Shah I, Bhatnagar S. NISCH syndrome with hypothyroxinemia. Ann Hepatol 2010;9:299–301.
18 **Kirchmeier P, Sayar E, Hotz A et al. Novel mutation in the CLDN1 gene in a Turkish family with Neonatal Ichthyosis Sclerosing Cholangitis (NISCH) syndrome. Br J Dermatol 2014;170:976–8.**
19 **Klar J, Schweiger M, Zimmerman R et al. Mutations in the fatty acid transport protein 4 gene cause the ichthyosis prematurity syndrome. Am J Hum Genet 2009;85:248–53**
20 Inhoff O, Hausser I, Schneider SW et al. Ichthyosis prematurity syndrome caused by a novel fatty acid transport protein 4 gene mutation in a German infant. Arch Dermatol 2011;147:750–2.
21 Khnykin D, Miner JH, Jahnsen F. Role of fatty acid transporters in epidermis: implications for health and disease. Dermatoendocrinol 2011;3:53–61.
22 Lin MH, Khnykin D. Fatty acid transporters in skin development, function and disease. Biochim Biophys Acta 2014;1841:362–8.
23 **Khnykin D, Rønnevig J, Johnsson M et al. Ichthyosis prematurity syndrome: clinical evaluation of 17 families with a rare disorder of lipid metabolism. J Am Acad Dermatol 2012;66:606–16.**
24 Lin MH, Hsu FF, Miner JH. Requirement of fatty acid transport protein 4 for development, maturation, and function of sebaceous glands in a mouse model of ichthyosis prematurity syndrome. J Biol Chem 2013;288:3964–76.
25 Bygum A, Westermark P, Brandrup F. Ichthyosis prematurity syndrome: a well-defined congenital ichthyosis subtype. J Am Acad Dermatol 2008;59(Suppl):S71–4.
26 Dereksson K, Kjartansson S, Hjartardóttir H, Arngrimsson R. Ichthyosis prematurity syndrome with separation of fetal membranes and neonatal asphyxia. BMJ Case Rep 2012;2012.
27 **Blaas HG, Salvesen KÅ, Khnykin D et al. Prenatal sonographic assessment and perinatal course of ichthyosis prematurity syndrome. Ultrasound Obstet Gynecol 2012;39:473–7.**
28 Vahlquist A. Pleomorphic ichthyosis: proposed name for a heterogeneous group of congenital ichthyoses with phenotypic shifting and mild residual scaling. Acta Derm Venereol 2010;90:454–60.
29 **Anton-Lamprecht I. Diagnostic ultrastructural of non-neoplastic diseases. In: Papadimitriou J, Henderson DW, Spagnolo DV (eds) The skin. Edinburgh: Churchill and Livingstone, 1992:459–550.**

Neuroichthyotic syndromes

Sjögren–Larsson syndrome

Definition. Sjögren–Larsson syndrome (SLS; OMIM #270200) is a rare autosomal recessive neurocutaneous condition featuring congenital ichthyotic hyperkeratosis, spastic diplegia and mild to moderate mental retardation.

Epidemiology and pathogenesis. In the UK the prevalence is estimated to be 1 : 300 000 whereas in Sweden it is 1 : 100 000; in the Province of Västerbotten it is 1 : 10 000. Microsomal fatty aldehyde dehydrogenase (FALDH) deficiency underlies SLS [1]. FALDH encoded by the *ALDH3A2* gene catalyses oxidation of medium- and long-chain fatty aldehydes into fatty acids. Deficiency results in accumulation of fatty aldehydes and fatty alcohols in various tissues. LTB4 accumulation may explain the marked pruritus of the patients, who excrete large amounts of LTB4 in urine [2]. Oral zileuton, which inhibits LTB4 synthesis, may improve the pruritus, but has no effect on ichthyosis or neurological disease [3]. The pathogenesis of the ichthyosis has been linked to the hepoxilin pathway [4]. Neurological symptoms result from abnormal lipid composition of myelin. More than 72 *ALDH3A2* mutations have been reported in SLS [5,6].

Clinical features. Preterm birth is common and has been attributed to abnormal LTB4 inactivation [2]. Children are usually not born as collodion babies. At birth their skin may be erythematous and covered with horny material (similar to ichthyosis prematurity syndrome). Scaling develops within the first 3 month of life. Thereafter, a mild erythroderma persists and a variable degree of scaling develops (Fig. 129.33) consisting of diffuse peeling on the trunk and more pigmented, lamellar-type ichthyosis on the lower limbs. Keratotic lichenification is often seen around the flexures, neck and mid-abdomen. The face is usually spared. Severe and persistent pruritus is a notable feature of SLS, but skin infections are rare.

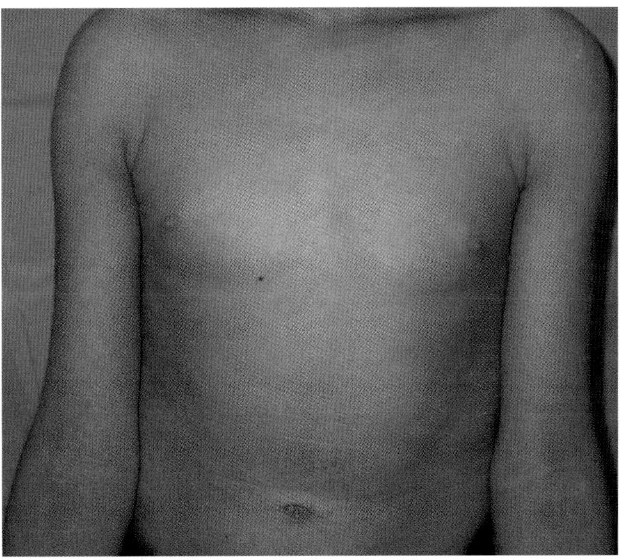

Fig. 129.33 Sjögren-Larsson syndrome. A 3-year-old girl with spastic diplegia. Source: Courtesy of Dr A. Hernandez-Martin, Madrid, Spain.

Extracutaneous symptoms

Neurological symptoms and signs appear during the first 2 years of life and consist of delay in reaching motor milestones caused by spastic diplegia or much less commonly, of spastic tetraplegia. Seizures may occur in up to 40% of patients. Delayed speech and dysarthria are common. Increased muscle tone leads to altered posture and movement, which predispose to contractures (ankles, knees, hips), kyphoscoliosis and dislocated hips. Distinctive ophthalmological findings are so-called glistening white dots surrounding the fovea that are caused by crystalline inclusions [7].

Differential diagnosis. Important differential diagnoses include ichthyosis prematurity syndrome, Netherton syndrome and congenital ichthyosiform erythroderma.

Laboratory findings. Histology and histochemistry may deliver unspecific hints for diagnosis. Increased fatty alcohols can be found in plasma; leukocytes may be checked for reduction in aldehyde dehydrogenase. However, early DNA analysis should be initiated. Clinical diagnostics requires a multidisciplinary approach. Patchy leukodystrophy and myelination defects have been reported on CT and MRI scanning studies.

Treatment and prevention. Dietary approaches with supplementation of medium-chain fatty acids have not been successful so far. Inhibition of LTB4 synthesis by zileuton may improve pruritus in some patients [3]. Retinoid therapy (etretinate, acitretin) has proven effective in relieving scaling and disabling keratotic lichenification, but less successful in controlling itching [8]. Intensive physiotherapy [9] and skills learning in early childhood clearly improve motor and social development in SLS. With early physiotherapy, most patients learn to walk unaided or with crutches in childhood. Bezafibrate, a lipid lowering agent, was shown to induce FALDH activity in fibroblasts in patients with residual enzyme activity, but clinical studies have not been carried out up to now [10].

References

1 **Rizzo WB, Dammann AL, Craft DA. Sjögren-Larsson syndrome. Impaired fatty alcohol oxidation in cultured fibroblasts due to deficient fatty alcohol:nicotinamide adenine dinucleotide oxidoreductase activity. J Clin Invest 1988;81:738–44.**

2 **Willemsen MA, Rotteveel JJ, de Jong JG et al. Defective metabolism of leukotriene B4 in the Sjögren–Larsson syndrome. J Neurol Sci 2001;183:61–7.**

3 Willemsen MA, Lutt MA, Steijlen PM et al. Clinical and biochemical effects of zileuton in patients with the Sjögren–Larsson syndrome. Eur J Pediatr 2001;160:711–7.

4 Rizzo WB. Sjögren–Larsson syndrome: molecular genetics and biochemical pathogenesis of fatty aldehyde dehydrogenase deficiency. Mol Genet Metab 2007;90:1–9.

5 De Laurenzi V, Rogers GR, Hamrock DJ et al. Sjögren–Larsson syndrome is caused by mutations in the fatty aldehyde dehydrogenase gene. Nat Genet 1996;12:52–7.

6 Rizzo WB, Carney G. Sjögren–Larsson syndrome: diversity of mutations and polymorphisms in the fatty aldehyde dehydrogenase gene (ALDH3A2). Hum Mutat 2005;26:1–10.

7 Fuijkschot J, Cruysberg JR, Willemsen MA et al. Subclinical changes in the juvenile crystalline macular dystrophy in Sjögren–Larsson syndrome detected by optical coherence tomography. Ophthalmology 2008;115:870–5.

8 **Gånemo A, Jagell S, Vahlquist A. Sjögren–larsson syndrome: a study of clinical symptoms and dermatological treatment in 34 Swedish patients. Acta Derm Venereol 2009;89:68–73.**

9 **Kathuria S, Arora S, Ramesh V. Sjögren–Larsson syndrome: importance of early diagnosis and aggressive physiotherapy. Dermatol Online J 2012;18:11.**

10 Gloerich J, Ijlst L, Wanders RJ, Ferdinandusse S. Bezafibrate induces FALDH in human fibroblasts; implications for Sjögren–Larsson syndrome. Mol Genet Metab 2006;89:111–15.

Keratitis ichthyosis deafness syndrome

Epidemiology and pathogenesis. Keratitis ichthyosis deafness syndrome (KID syndrome; OMIM #148210) is an autosomal dominant disorder of cornification overlapping with ectodermal dysplasia, that is characterized by progressive keratitis, erythrokeratoderma and congenital sensorineural hearing loss [1]. It is rare, with approximately 200 published cases, most of them arising sporadically.

KID syndrome is caused by heterozygous missense mutations in *GJB2*, encoding the gap junction protein connexin 26 [2]. Connexins are universal membrane proteins organizing intercellular channels that control a variety of cellular activities through the exchange of ions, metabolites and signalling molecules, which provides the basis of cell communication. Connexin 26 is expressed in both the inner ear and the skin. *GJB2* mutations result in a gain-of-function of mutated connexin 26, causing abnormal cell homeostasis and cell death. Because there is large phenotypical variability in KID syndrome, and both recurrent and rare mutations in *GJB2* have been reported, a phenotype–genotype correlation is currently not possible. In addition, equal *GJB2* mutations were detected for hystrix-like ichthyosis with deafness syndrome (HID syndrome), suggesting that these allelic diseases represent a single clinical entity [3].

Clinical features. KID syndrome manifests with transient erythroderma and sometimes mild scaling either at birth, or during infancy. Later on, most individuals develop symmetrically distributed erythrokeratoderma, i.e. well demarcated, erythematous hyperkeratotic plaques with rough, ridged or verrucous surface, and generalized xerotic skin (Fig. 129.34). Plaques are predominantly located on the extensor sites of the extremities and on the face. However, other body parts can also be affected to a less degree. Palmoplantar keratoderma is invariably present, typically presenting a leather-like grainy surface. Some individuals show diffuse thickening of the skin in the face, with a coarse-grained appearance, perioral radial furrows and cheilitis. Often, there is extensive scarring alopecia of the scalp and loss of eyelashes, eyebrows and body hair caused by follicular hyperkeratosis and atrophy. Dystrophic nails with or without leukonychia, and dental caries and malformed teeth are common. Heat intolerance rarely occurs in children. Additional mucocutaneous manifestations of KID syndrome are acne conglobata, dissecting cellulitis of the scalp and hidradenitis suppurativa, also known as follicular occlusion triad, as well as folliculitis, stomatitis with erythematous patches, and epidermoid and proliferating benign or malignant pilar tumours [4]. A serious complication of KID syndrome is the development of squamous cell carcinoma within hyperkeratotic lesions and oral mucosa, which can be detected in up to 20% of individuals at a median age of 20 years, but also in older children [5]. KID syndrome is prone to chronic mucocutaneous superinfections with

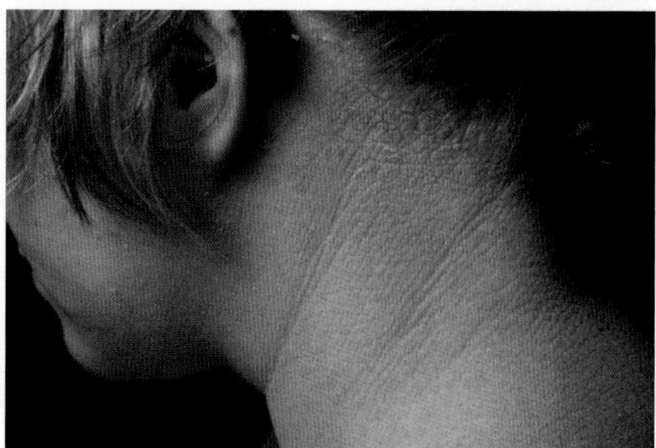

Fig. 129.34 Keratitis ichthyosis deafness syndrome. Source: Oji et al. (2009). Reproduced with permission of Elsevier.

bacteria (e.g. *Staphylococcus aureus*), fungi (e.g. *Candida* spp.) and viruses, and death in infancy from sepsis has been reported [6].

Almost all individuals with KID syndrome have ocular involvement, which manifests in early childhood with photophobia, tearing, conjunctivitis and blepharitis. With age, the latter become chronic and importantly vascularizing keratitis develops, which can lead to a progressive decline in visual acuity and even blindness in up to 75% of patients.

Congenital nonprogressive sensorineural hearing loss is noticeable by infancy in KID syndrome. It is generally bilateral and severe. However, unilateral or moderate hearing impairment has been reported. Neurological features such as cerebellar hypoplasia and anomaly of the fourth ventricle (Dandy–Walker malformation) are occasionally noted in KID syndrome. Individuals with KID syndrome are often stigmatized because of their appearance and body malodour.

Porokeratotic eccrine naevus

There is strong evidence that porokeratotic eccrine naevus (PEN) is a mosaic form of KID syndrome [7,8]. The amount of body involvement in PEN shows a high variability, ranging from a widespread distribution with linear spiky hyperkeratotic papules and plaques on the trunk, extremities and feet to more localized forms on the extremities, including the palms and soles. Histopathology features ortho- or parakeratotic plaques protruding from eccrine ducts. Postzygotic missense mutations in *GJB2* have been detected in skin samples, but not the blood of individuals with PEN. Importantly, individuals with PEN bear the possibility of a germline mosaicism, and thus the risk of transmitting systemic disease, resulting in a full-blown KID syndrome in their offspring. This situation is similar to mosaic epidermolytic ichthyosis (see previously).

Differential diagnosis. In children with classic KID syndrome, diagnosis is often straightforward and can be made on a clinical basis, without the need for further genetic testing. Compared to KID syndrome, HID syndrome shows a more severe skin phenotype, but a milder form of keratitis. However, nowadays these allelic diseases are thought to represent a single clinical entity.

The group of erythrokeratodermas (*GJB3*, *GJB4*) may resemble the skin features of KID syndrome, but it is not associated with keratitis and deafness. In children, both IFAP syndrome and keratosis follicularis spinulosa decalvans (KFSD) can present with keratitis and similar skin features to KID syndrome with prominent follicular keratoses, but they exhibit scarring alopecia and lack the hyperkeratotic plaques, palmoplantar keratoderma and hearing impairment. Additionally, they are X-linked and caused by mutations in *MBTPS2*. MEDNIK syndrome (*AP1S1*) and CEDNIK syndrome (*SNAP29*) share the symptom of deafness, however they include mental retardation, which is exceptional in KID syndrome.

Laboratory, histology and genetic findings. If possible, genetic testing is recommended, because it clearly differentiates from erythrokeratodermas and provides the basis for genetic counselling and prenatal diagnosis. Blood tests are nonspecific as other organ systems are unaffected. Histopathology is also nonspecific, including acanthosis, papillomatosis, basket-weave hyperkeratosis and follicular plugging, as well as vacuolization of cells in the granular layer.

Ocular involvement comprises centrally dyskeratotic, atrophic or absent corneal epithelium and/or absence of the Bowman's membrane. In the inner ear, the spiral organ is immature or atrophic.

Treatment and prevention. In infants and children topical therapy is essential for removing or reducing hyperkeratosis, softening the skin and treating cutaneous infections. Antiseptic baths and cleansers, intermittent antibiotic and antiviral therapy and prolonged systemic antifungal agents are usually required for the reduction of skin infections and malodour [9]. Skin debridement, excision and grafting of hyperkeratotic plaques may become necessary to reduce the potential for malignant transformation. Surveillance for the development of squamous cell carcinoma by examination of skin and mucous membranes is essential. Oral retinoids such as acitretin or alitretinoin can reduce hyperkeratosis, but should be used with caution because palmoplantar keratoderma does not often respond to treatment and ocular adverse effects may aggravate the keratitis and corneal neovascularization.

Starting in infants, routine ophthamological and audiological examinations are necessary to enable appropriate and early treatments. Ocular lesions are treated topically with lubricants, antibiotics, steroids or ciclosporin drops as indicated. Corneal transplants are often not successful because of revascularization [5]. Hearing aids, cochlear implants and speech correction are important to enable communication [10].

Trichothiodystrophy

Epidemiology and pathogenesis. Trichothiodystrophy (TTD; OMIM #601675 and 234050), also termed Tay syndrome, IBIDS (ichthyosis, brittle hair, infertility, developmental delay, short stature) syndrome, PIBIDS (photosensitivity + IBIDS) syndrome, or sulphur-deficient brittle hair syndrome, comprises a heterogeneous group of neurocutaneous disorders, variably affecting organs derived from the neuroectoderm, that have in common the finding of sulphur-deficient brittle short hair [11,12]. It is rare, with about 250 cases published in the literature. TTD is inherited in an autosomal recessive way, with the exception of one reported family, in which inheritance was presumed to be X-linked [13].

TTD can be subclassified into two major forms, i.e. TTD with and without photosensitivity, which occur in almost similar distribution. TTD with photosensitivity is caused by recessive mutations in *ERCC2/XPD* and less frequently *ERCC3/XPB*, both encoding the helicase subunits of transcription factor IIH (TFIIH). These genes are also mutated in individuals with xeroderma pigmentosum (XP). However, mutation type and gene loci are different. In fact, photosensitive TTD patients do not have a susceptibility to cancer, and otherwise XP patients do not display a sulphur content deficit in structural proteins. In addition, mutations in *GTF2H5*, encoding another subunit of TFIIH, have also been found in a subset of individuals with photosensitive TTD. The loss of functional TFIIH results in both a defect of DNA repair and suppressed transcription of genes that are expressed in differentiated cells of neuroectodermal tissues. In contrast, TTD without photosensitivity, which importantly also lacks the congenital ichthyosis and collodion baby phenotype, is caused by mutations in *MPLKIP* (former *C7ORF11*), encoding the protein TTDN1 involved in cytokinesis and mitosis.

Clinical features. TTD with photosensitivity typically presents at birth or in the neonatal period with ichthyosiform erythroderma, or sometimes as collodion baby [11,12]. Neonates often are small for gestational age with a low birth weight and require admission to a neonatal intensive care unit. Mothers carrying a child with TTD have a high risk for complications during pregnancy, e.g. HELLP (haemolysis, elevated liver enzyme levels, and low platelet levels) syndrome, and are considered as high-risk pregnancies [14]. Mostly, erythroderma resolves during infancy and is replaced by mild ichthyosis with fine scaling. However, sometimes ichthyosis can get severe with large brown scales (Fig. 129.35).

The pathognomonic feature of all TTD types is short, dry, brittle hair, mainly affecting the scalp hair, eyebrows and eyelashes, and also, but less pronounced, axillary and pubic hair. Broken hair or partial alopecia is typically seen on mechanically stressed areas on the scalp. The hair fragility is caused by abnormally low sulphur content. In addition, nail changes are common, comprising dystrophic nails, longitudinal ridging, splitting, discolouration and koilonychia.

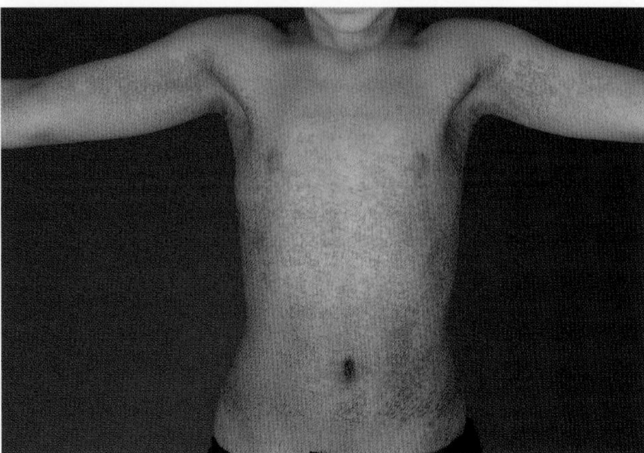

Fig. 129.35 Trichothiodystrophy with large brown scaling reminiscent of bathing suit ichthyosis. Source: Courtesy of the Department of Dermatology, University Hospital Münster, Germany.

Additional cutaneous symptoms in individuals with TTD are variable and include eczema, follicular keratosis, folliculitis, cheilitis, freckling, telangiectasia, poikiloderma, palmoplantar hyperkeratosis and digital flexion contractures, as well as pruritus and hypohidrosis. Photosensitivity and photophobia occur in most patients exhibiting TFIIH mutations, but this feature can improve with age. In children there is already a remarkable progeria-like facies caused by fat atrophy and hypoplastic aural cartilage.

Extracutaneous manifestations, which depend on the type of TTD, are congenital cataracts, osteosclerosis, dental anomalies, bone lesions, growth retardation with short stature, hypogonadism with infertility, and neurological symptoms such as mental retardation of varying degree, motor control impairment, spasticity, seizures and autism. A friendly, approachable disposition and affectionate behaviour are typical for individuals with TTD. Of notice, despite the DNA repair defect and in contrast to XP, an increased risk of malignancy is not regarded as a feature of photosensitive TTD. Moreover, recurrent (pulmonary) infections caused by severe immunodeficiency with chronic neutropenia are prevalent in TTD and early death from sepsis in children has been reported [12]. Of note, febrile infections can lead to a reversible aggravation of hair and skin phenotypes, with sudden hair loss and skin inflammation, but also to an impairment of neurological symptoms. This can be explained by a temperature-sensitive defect of transcription and DNA repair caused by thermoinstability of the TFIIH complex [15].

Prognosis is dependent on the severity of neurological manifestations and/or immunodeficiency, but in general life expectancy is reduced.

Differential diagnosis. In neonates, clinical distinction from Netherton syndrome, NLSDI (Chanarin–Dorfman syndrome), SLS and ARCI with a CIE phenotype can be difficult. However, the hair of these disorders does not reveal a tiger-tail pattern. Additionally, serum IgE levels are usually elevated in Netherton syndrome, whereas unremarkable in TTD. Cockayne syndrome shares a few symptoms with the photosensitive TTD, but shows no ichthyosis and no tiger-tail pattern of the hair. Other disorders that present with congenital hypotrichosis or alopecia, such as Menkes disease, can also be differentiated by microscopic hair analysis (see later). In children with TTD, both the fine scaling phenotype and the histology with a reduced granular layer can resemble IV (see previously); however, the latter is always nonsyndromic.

Laboratory, histology and genetic findings. Blood tests are unspecific. Genetic testing can be helpful for early differentiation of TTD with and without photosensitivity, and provides the basis for genetic counselling and prenatal diagnosis. Histopathological features are similar to those found in IV (see previously).

Investigation of hair is strongly recommended for the diagnosis of TTD. Amino acid analysis of hydrolysed hair demonstrates a low content of cysteine. On polarizing light microscopy, the presence of alternating light and dark bands within the hair shafts, the so-called 'tiger-tail pattern', is pathognomonic; however, it may be absent before the third year of life. Additional findings of hair analysis by light and electron microscopy include trichoschisis, an irregular surface and diameter, as well as an absent or severely damaged hair cuticle [12].

Treatment and prevention. Neonates require management in an intensive care unit to prevent or treat infections and failure to thrive. In childhood, treatment of ichthyosis is dependent on its severity, but topical therapy with emollients, humectants and at times antiseptics is invariably recommended. Oral retinoids can be used in severe cases of TTD, but the effect on ichthyosis is often disappointing. Mechanical trauma caused by hair treatment should be avoided to reduce further hair damage. In photosensitive TTD, strict sunscreen is essential.

References

1 **Skinner BA, Greist MC, Norins AL. The keratitis, ichthyosis, and deafness (KID) syndrome. Arch Dermatol 1981;117:285–89.**
2 **Richard G, Rouan F, Willoughby CE et al. Missense mutations in GJB2 encoding connexin-26 cause the ectodermal dysplasia keratitis-ichthyosis-deafness syndrome. Am J Hum Genet 2002;70: 1341–8.**
3 **van Geel M, van Steensel MA, Kuster W et al. HID and KID syndromes are associated with the same connexin 26 mutation. Br J Dermatol 2002;146:938–42.**
4 Mazereeuw-Hautier J, Bitoun E, Chevrant-Breton J et al. Keratitis-ichthyosis-deafness syndrome: disease expression and spectrum of connexin 26 (GJB2) mutations in 14 patients. Br J Dermatol 2007;156:1015–19.
5 Caceres-Rios H, Tamayo-Sanchez L, Duran-Mckinster C et al. Keratitis, ichthyosis, and deafness (KID syndrome): review of the literature and proposal of a new terminology. Pediatr Dermatol 1996;13:105–13.
6 Haruna K, Suga Y, Oizumi A, Mizuno Y et al. Severe form of keratitis-ichthyosis-deafness (KID) syndrome associated with septic complications. J Dermatol 2010;37:680–2.
7 Levinsohn JL, McNiff JM, Antaya RJ, Choate KA. A Somatic p.G45E GJB2 Mutation Causing Porokeratotic Eccrine Ostial and Dermal Duct Nevus. JAMA Dermatol 2015; 151:638–41.
8 Easton JA, Donnelly S, Kamps MA et al. Porokeratotic eccrine nevus may be caused by somatic connexin26 mutations. J Invest Dermatol 2012;132:2184–91.
9 **Coggshall K, Farsani T, Ruben B et al. Keratitis, ichthyosis, and deafness syndrome: a review of infectious and neoplastic complications. J Am Acad Dermatol 2013;69:127–34.**
10 **Smyth CM, Sinnathuray AR, Hughes AE, Toner JG. Cochlear implantation in keratitis-ichthyosis-deafness syndrome: 10-year follow-up of two patients. Cochlear Implants Int 2012;13:54–9.**
11 **Morice-Picard F, Cario-Andre M, Rezvani H et al. New clinico-genetic classification of trichothiodystrophy. Am J Med Genet A 2009;149A:2020–30.**
12 Faghri S, Tamura D, Kraemer KH, Digiovanna JJ. Trichothiodystrophy: a systematic review of 112 published cases characterises a wide spectrum of clinical manifestations. J Med Genet 2008;45(10):609–21.
13 Corbett MA, Dudding-Byth T, Crock PA et al. A novel X-linked trichothiodystrophy associated with a nonsense mutation in RNF113A. J Med Genet 2015;52:269–74.
14 **Tamura D, Khan SG, Merideth M et al. Effect of mutations in XPD(ERCC2) on pregnancy and prenatal development in mothers of patients with trichothiodystrophy or xeroderma pigmentosum. Eur J Hum Genet 2012;20(12):1308–10.**
15 Vermeulen W, Rademakers S, Jaspers NG et al. A temperature-sensitive disorder in basal transcription and DNA repair in humans. Nat Genet 2001;27:299–303.

Complex and ultra-rare neuroichthyotic syndromes

CEDNIK, MEDNIK, ARC, Gaucher disease type II, ISQMR, Stormorken syndrome (see Table 129.1b and Table 129.4)

Definitions. *Gaucher disease type II* represents a classic neuroichthyosis presenting at birth with a collodion membrane [1,2]. Diseases with poor prognosis when compared with other ichthyoses are the cerebral dysgenesis-neuropathy-ichthyosis-palmoplantar keratoderma (*CEDNIK*) syndrome [3–5], the arthrogryposis renal dysfunction cholestasis (*ARC*) syndrome [6–11], and the mental retardation-enteropathy-deafness-neuropathy-ichthyosis-keratodermia (*MEDNIK*) syndrome [12]. Ichthyosis, spastic quadriplegia and mental retardation (*ISQMR*) syndrome [13,14] has been regarded as an erythrokeratoderma with sensorineural deafness [15] – clinically reminiscent of KID syndrome. In a five generation Canadian pedigree, erythrokeratoderma appearing in infancy and clearing in later life was associated with late onset ataxia and neuropathy [16].

Patients with *Stormorken syndrome* [17] [OMIM #185070] may present with moderate thrombocytopenia, thrombocytopathia, muscle fatigue, asplenia, miosis, migraine, dyslexia and ichthyosis. The autosomal dominant disorder seems to belong to the group of channelopathies affecting calcium homeostasis in various tissues [18,19].

References

1 **Holleran WM, Ginns EI, Menon GK et al. Consequences of beta-glucocerebrosidase deficiency in epidermis. Ultrastructure and permeability barrier alterations in Gaucher disease. J Clin Invest 1994;93:1756–64.**
2 Tsuji S, Choudary PV, Martin BM et al. A mutation in the human glucocerebrosidase gene in neuronopathic Gaucher's disease. N Engl J Med 1987;316:570–5.
3 **Sprecher E, Ishida-Yamamoto A, Mizrahi-Koren M et al. A mutation in SNAP29, coding for a SNARE protein involved in intracellular trafficking, causes a novel neurocutaneous syndrome characterized by cerebral dysgenesis, neuropathy, ichthyosis, and palmoplantar keratoderma. Am J Hum Genet 2005;77:242–51.**
4 Fuchs-Telem D, Stewart H, Rapaport D et al. CEDNIK syndrome results from loss-of-function mutations in SNAP29. Br J Dermatol 2011;164:610–6.
5 Dereure O. [Differentiating between Mednik and Cednik syndromes]. Ann Dermatol Venereol 2009;136:850–1.
6 **Nezelof C, Martin G, Pruvost J. [A fatal syndrome associating a micromelic dwarfism, an ichthyosiform skin disorder and a severe combined immunologic deficiency. Report of a case and survey of the literature (author's transl)]. Ann Pediatr (Paris) 1979;26:309–14.**
7 **Gissen P, Johnson CA, Morgan NV et al. Mutations in VPS33B, encoding a regulator of SNARE-dependent membrane fusion, cause arthrogryposis-renal dysfunction-cholestasis (ARC) syndrome. Nat Genet 2004;36:400–4.**
8 Hershkovitz D, Mandel H, Ishida-Yamamoto A et al. Defective lamellar granule secretion in arthrogryposis, renal dysfunction, and cholestasis syndrome caused by a mutation in VPS33B. Arch Dermatol 2008;144:334–40.
9 Smith H, Galmes R, Gogolina E et al. Associations among genotype, clinical phenotype, and intracellular localization of trafficking proteins in ARC syndrome. Hum Mutat 2012;33:1656–64.
10 Jang JY, Kim KM, Kim GH et al. Clinical characteristics and VPS33B mutations in patients with ARC syndrome. J Pediatr Gastroenterol Nutr 2009;48:348–54.
11 **Dehghani SM, Bahador A, Nikeghbalian S et al. Liver transplant in a case of arthrogryposis-renal tubular dysfunction-cholestasis syndrome with severe intractable pruritus. Exp Clin Transplant 2013;11:290–2.**

SECTION 27: DISORDERS OF KERATIN AND KERATINIZATION

12 Montpetit A, Cote S, Burstein E et al. Disruption of AP1S1, causing a novel neurocutaneous syndrome, perturbs development of the skin and spinal cord. Proc Natl Acad Sci USA 2009;4:e1000296.
13 Aldahmesh MA, Mohamed JY, Alkuraya HS et al. Recessive mutations in ELOVL4 cause ichthyosis, intellectual disability, and spastic quadriplegia. Am J Hum Genet 2011;89:745–50.
14 Mir H, Raza SI, Touseef M et al. A novel recessive mutation in the gene ELOVL4 causes a neuro-ichthyotic disorder with variable expressivity. BMC Med Genet 2014; 26;15:25.
15 Giroux JM, Barbeau A. Erythrokeratodermia with ataxia. Arch Dermatol 1972;106:183–8.
16 Cadieux-Dion M, Turcotte-Gauthier M, Noreau A et al. Expanding the clinical phenotype associated with ELOVL4 mutation: study of a large French-Canadian family with autosomal dominant spinocerebellar ataxia and erythrokeratodermia. JAMA Neurol 2014;71:470–5.
17 Stormorken H, Sjaastad O, Langslet A et al. A new syndrome: thrombocytopathia, muscle fatigue, asplenia, miosis, migraine, dyslexia and ichthyosis. Clin Genet 1985;28: 367–74.
18 Misceo D, Holmgren A, Louch WE et al. A dominant STIM1 mutation causes Stormorken syndrome. Hum Mutat 2014;35:556–64.
19 Morin G, Bruechle NO, Singh AR et al. Gain-of-function mutation in STIM1 (p.R304W) is associated with Stormorken Syndrome. Hum Mutat 2014;35:1221–32.

Neu-Laxova syndrome

Definition. Neu-Laxova syndrome (NLS; OMIM #256520), also termed as phosphoglycerate dehydrogenase deficiency, is a lethal autosomal recessive malformation syndrome, in which the cutaneous features (congenital ichthyosis) have never been studied adequately. The tight skin described in several reports is reminiscent of restrictive dermopathy [1–3].

Pathogenesis. NLS is heterogeneous and inherited as an autosomal recessive trait. It is caused by mutations in the *PHGDH* gene that lead to phosphoglycerate dehydrogenase deficiency [4]. This enzyme is involved in the first and limiting step of L-serine biosynthesis. Two other enzymes of the L-serine biosynthesis pathway may be associated with NLS (*PSAT1* and *PSPH*) [5]. Histology of the skin reveals focal parakeratosis. No systematic analysis of the cutaneous phenotype with immunofluorescence studies or ultrastructure is available.

Clinical features. NLS is characterized by congenital ichthyosis, marked intrauterine growth retardation, microcephaly, short neck, central nervous system anomalies, limb deformities, hypoplastic lungs, oedema, and abnormal facial features including severe proptosis with ectropion, hypertelorism, micrognathia, flattened nose and malformed ears [1–3]. Prenatal ultrasound findings of marked ocular proptosis in a growth restricted, oedematous fetus are suggestive of the diagnosis [3,6].

Diffential diagnoses. Polyhydramion can also be seen in harlequin ichthyosis or IPS. From a dermatological point of view, restrictive dermopathy is the most relevant differential diagnosis. Similar to NLS it is characterized by intrauterine growth retardation, thin, tightly adherent, translucent skin, typical facial dysmorphology with a mouth forming an O, generalized joint contractures, fetal akinesia and polyhydramnion. Most cases are caused by mutations in the *ZMPSTE24* gene, whereas a few seem to be caused by mutations in *LMNA* [7,8].

Treatment and prevention. All reported cases have been lethal so far. Considering the metabolic basis of the disorder and similarity to other serine deficiency therapies, NLS might be a treatable condition when recognized and treated early [5,9]. A supplement therapy may be provided for pregnant women who previously had a child affected by NLS [4], which underscores the need for accurate diagnosis of neonates with congenital ichthyosis and a potential lethal course.

Coloboma-heart defect-ichthyosiform dermatosis-mental retardation-ear anomalies syndrome

Definition. Coloboma, heart defect, ichthyosiform dermatosis, mental retardation, ear anomalies (CHIME) syndrome (Zunich's neuroectodermal syndrome; OMIM #280000) is an exceedingly rare autosomal recessive neurocutaneous condition featuring coloboma, heart disease, ichthyosis, mental retardation and ear defects.

Pathogenesis. CHIME syndrome is a congenital disorder of glycosylation and is caused by mutations in the gene *PIGL*, which encodes the de-N-acetylase required for glycosyl phosphatidyl inisitol anchor formation [10]. *PIGL* is an enzyme localized in the endoplasmatic reticulum, that catalyses the second step of glycosyl phosphadidyl biosynthesis. Glycosylation is the biosynthetic process of adding glycans to proteins and lipids and is an important modification of secretory and membrane-bound proteins [11,12].

Clinical features. In 1983, Zunich and Kaye [13] reported a child with migratory CIE, retinal colobomas, neurological disease, fine sparse hair and dental abnormalities. Moreover, cases featuring cardiac abnormalities have been described [13–16]. Generalized pruritus, erythema and scaling develop within the first month, and figurate, red scaly and itchy patches migrate on the head and body from early childhood. Palm and soles are thickened; the scalp hair is fine, sparse and hypopigmented. Cranial defects, alopecia, hypertelorism, a broad nasal bridge, wide mouth, full lips and wide-spaced teeth contribute to a characteristic facial appearance. Neurological features include hearing loss, seizures, developmental delay and outbursts of violent behaviour. A 4-year-old with CHIME syndrome developed leukaemia. The disease is considered to be a cancer-prone genodermatosis [17].

Treatment. For the ichthyosis, emollients (moisturizers) have been recommended [15].

References

1 Neu RL, Kajii T, Gardner LI, Nagyfy SF. A lethal syndrome of microcephaly with multiple congenital anomalies in three siblings. Pediatrics 1971;47:610–2.
2 Laxova R, Ohara PT, Timothy JA. A further example of a lethal autosomal recessive condition in sibs. J Ment Defic Res 1972;16:139–43.
3 Manning MA, Cunniff CM, Colby CE et al. Neu-Laxova syndrome: detailed prenatal diagnostic and post-mortem findings and literature review. Am J Med Genet A 2004;125:240–9.

SECTION 27: DISORDERS OF KERATIN AND KERATINIZATION

4 Shaheen R, Rahbeeni Z, Alhashem A et al. Neu-Laxova syndrome, an inborn error of serine metabolism, is caused by mutations in PHGDH. Am J Hum Genet 2014;94:898–904.
5 Acuna-Hidalgo R, Schanze D, Kariminejad A et al. Neu-laxova syndrome is a heterogeneous metabolic disorder caused by defects in enzymes of the L-serine biosynthesis pathway. Am J Hum Genet 2014;95:285–93.
6 Shapiro I, Borochowitz Z, Degani S et al. Neu-Laxova syndrome: prenatal ultrasonographic diagnosis, clinical and pathological studies, and new manifestations. Am J Med Genet 1992;43:602–5.
7 Smigiel R, Jakubiak A, Esteves-Vieira V et al. Novel frameshifting mutations of the ZMPSTE24 gene in two siblings affected with restrictive dermopathy and review of the mutations described in the literature. Am J Med Genet A 2010;152A:447–52
8 Loucks C, Parboosingh JS, Chong JX et al. A shared founder mutation underlies restrictive dermopathy in Old Colony (Dutch-German) Mennonite and Hutterite patients in North America. Am J Med Genet A 2012;158A:1229–32.
9 **De Koning TJ. Treatment with amino acids in serine deficiency disorders. J Inherit Metab Dis 2006;29,347–51.**
10 **Ng BG, Hackmann K, Jones MA et al. Mutations in the glycosylphosphatidylinositol gene PIGL cause CHIME syndrome. Am J Hum Genet 2012;90:685–8.**
11 Jones MA, Ng BG, Bhide S et al. DDOST mutations identified by whole-exome sequencing are implicated in congenital disorders of glycosylation. Am J Hum Genet 2012;90:363–8.
12 Rymen D, Jaeken J. Skin manifestations in CDG. J Inherit Metab Dis 2014;36:699–708.
13 Zunich J, Kaye CI. New syndrome of congenital ichthyosis with neurologic abnormalities. Am J Med Genet 1983;15:331–3, 335.
14 Zunich J, Esterly NB, Holbrook KA, Kaye CI. Congenital migratory ichthyosiform dermatosis with neurologic and ophthalmologic abnormalities. Arch Dermatol 1985;121:1149–56.
15 Shashi V, Zunich J, Kelly TE, Fryburg JS. Neuroectodermal (CHIME) syndrome: an additional case with long term follow up of all reported cases. J Med Genet 1995;32:465–9.
16 **Tinschert S, Anton-Lamprecht I, Albrecht-Nebe H, Audring H. Zunich neuroectodermal syndrome: migratory ichthyosiform dermatosis, colobomas, and other abnormalities. Pediatr Dermatol 1996;13:363–71.**
17 **Schnur RE, Greenbaum BH, Heymann WR Acute lymphoblastic leukemia in a child with the CHIME neuroectodermal dysplasia syndrome. Am J Med Genet 1997;72:24–9.**

Ultra-rare neuroichthyotic syndromes with later disease presentations

Refsum disease

Definition. Refsum disease (RD; OMIM #266500), also known as heredopathia atactica polyneuritiformis, is an ultra-rare autosomal recessive neurocutaneous lipid storage disorder featuring deteriorating vision and hearing, ataxia, neuropathy and ichthyosis (of late onset) [1].

Pathogenesis. RD is caused by inactivating mutations in *PHYH* encoding a human phytanoyl-CoA hydroxylase, which is responsible for alpha oxidation of phytanic acid [2]. Biallelic mutations in *PEX7*, encoding peroxin 7, were found to cause an adult type of RD [3–5].

Clinical features. Age of onset usually is late childhood, but diagnosis may be delayed until early adult life. Ichthyosis with a fine scaling phenotype occurs in around 25% of RD patients and coincides with or postdates the onset of neurological signs. It resembles ichthyosis vulgaris or mild ichthyosiform erythroderma.

Extracutaneous findings

Progressive retinitis pigmentosa initially causes night blindness and later, failing vision and constricted visual fields. Neurological features develop in adolescence or in the early twenties. Anosmia and impaired taste is a frequent finding. Sensorineural deafness with tinnitus develops in more than 50%. A mixed sensorimotor polyneuropathy (type IV) with hypertrophic peripheral nerves and elevated cerebrospinal fluid protein are characteristic findings. Cerebellar ataxia causes increasing disability.

Differential diagnosis. From the dermatological point of view ichthyosis vulgaris (or RXLI) are important differential diagnoses, as well as nonhereditary acquired ichthyosis. Of note, accumulation of phytanic acid does not occur exclusively in RD, but can also be found in other diseases like Zellweger syndrome or hepatic peroxisome disorder with dysmorphic features, hepatomegaly, retinitis pigmentosa and hearing loss [5–7].

Laboratory and histology findings. Increased phytanic acid levels are found in the plasma. On histological examination basal cells may be vacuolated. Special lipid stains such as Oil-Red O stain will reveal numerous fat globules within the basal cell layer and other keratinocytes [8].

Treatment and prevention. Early diagnosis is the clue for proper management of these patients [9]. Exclusion of sources of chlorophyll in the diet is mandatory in the treatment of RD. The major dietary exclusions are green vegetables (phytanic acids) and animal fat (phytol). The aim of the dietary treatment is to reduce daily intake from the usual level of 50 mg/day to less than 5 mg/day. At the beginning lipid apheresis, i.e. extracorporeal elimination of lipoprotein–phytanic acid complexes, may be the treatment of choice [10], followed by a phytanic acid-poor diet [9]. Rapid weight loss should be avoided as it mobilizes tissue phytanic acid, which can lead to acute clinical manifestations.

Multiple sulphatase deficiency

Definition. Multiple sulphatase deficiency (MSD; multiple sulfatase deficiency; mucosulfatidosis; OMIM #272200) is an exceedingly rare, autosomal recessive lysosomal storage disorder.

Pathogenesis. All known sulphatases are deficient causing accumulation of glycosaminoglycans and sulphated lipids [11]. The underlying gene *SUMF1* encodes a protein which is responsible for post-translational modification of sulphatases and catalyses the conversion of a conserved cysteine within the catalytic domain of various sulphatases into a C-alpha formyl glycine [12].

Clinical features. The enzyme deficiency can present as a very severe neonatal MSD [13], as severe late-infantile MSD with onset in the first year of life, as mild late-infantile MSD with symptoms occurring between the age of 2 and 4 years, or as juvenile MSD presenting usually only a few of the symptoms such as mental retardation and ichthyosis. Hence, a mild ichthyosis and progressive neurological degeneration may evolve in the second or third year. The phenotype varies according to the reduction in the enzyme activity [14,15].

Extracutaneous findings
The disease is typically characterized by developmental delay, failure to thrive and features of mucopolysaccharidosis type I. A first neurological sign may be that children can no longer sit unsupported and lose their communication skills.

Treatment and prevention. No specific therapy is available. Children with predominant MPS II or MPS VI-like features may be candidates for enzyme replacement therapy.

References

1 **Kahlke W, Richterich R. Refsum's disease (herecopathia a tactica polyneuritiformis: an inborn error of lipid metabolism with storage of 3,7,11,15-tetramethyl hexadecanoic acid. II. Isolation and identivication of the storage product. Am J Med 1965;39:237–41.**

2 **Jansen GA, Hogenhout EM, Ferdinandusse S et al. Human phytanoyl-CoA hydroxylase: resolution of the gene structure and the molecular basis of Refsum's disease. Hum Mol Genet 2000;9:1195–200.**

3 van den Brink DM, Brites P, Haasjes J et al. Identification of PEX7 as the second gene involved in Refsum disease. Am J Hum Genet 2003;72:471–7.

4 **Horn MA, van den Brink DM, Wanders RJ et al. Phenotype of adult Refsum disease due to a defect in peroxin 7. Neurology 2007;68: 698–700.**

5 Jansen GA, Waterham HR, Wanders RJ. Molecular basis of Refsum disease: sequence variations in phytanoyl-CoA hydroxylase (PHYH) and the PTS2 receptor (PEX7). Hum Mutat. 2004;23:209–18.

6 Scotto JM, Hadchouel M, Odievre M et al. Infantile phytanic acid storage disease, a possible variant of Refsum's disease: three cases, including ultrastructural studies of the liver. J Inherit Metab Dis 1982;5:83–90.

7 **Poll-The BT, Saudubray JM, Ogier HA et al. Infantile Refsum disease: an inherited peroxisomal disorder. Comparison with Zellweger syndrome and neonatal adrenoleukodystrophy. Eur J Pediatr 1987;146:477–83.**

8 **Ramsay BC, Meeran K, Woodrow D et al. Cutaneous aspects of Refsum's disease. J R Soc Med 1991;84:559–60.**

9 **Kohlschütter A, Santer R, Lukacs Z et al. A child with night blindness: preventing serious symptoms of Refsum disease. J Child Neurol 2012;27:654–6.**

10 **Zolotov D, Wagner S, Kalb K et al. Long-term strategies for the treatment of Refsum's disease using therapeutic apheresis. J Clin Apher 2012;27:99–105.**

11 Artigalás OA, da Silva LR, Burin M et al. Multiple sulfatase deficiency: clinical report and description of two novel mutations in a Brazilian patient. Metab Brain Dis 2009;24:493–500.

12 **Dierks T, Dickmanns A, Preusser-Kunze A et al. Molecular basis for multiple sulfatase deficiency and mechanism for formylglycine generation of the human formylglycine-generating enzyme. Cell 2005;121:541–52.**

13 Busche A, Hennermann JB, Bürger F et al. Neonatal manifestation of multiple sulfatase deficiency. Eur J Pediatr 2009;168:969–73.

14 **Schlotawa L, Ennemann EC, Radhakrishnan K et al. SUMF1 mutations affecting stability and activity of formylglycine generating enzyme predict clinical outcome in multiple sulfatase deficiency. Eur J Hum Genet 2011;19:253–61.**

15 Loffeld A, Gray RG, Green SH et al. Mild ichthyosis in a 4-year-old boy with multiple sulphatase deficiency. Br J Dermatol 2002; 147:353–5.

Management of congenital ichthyoses

General aspects of therapy

Congenital ichthyoses (CI) are hereditary, noncurable diseases, in which currently only symptomatic relief can be provided. Their variable degrees of scaling, hyperkeratosis and erythema require different approaches. Ocular and ear complications are common in neonates and infants – in both syndromic and nonsyndromic ichthyoses; and children often suffer from pruritus, fissuring, sweating impairment (hypohidrosis) and superinfections that need individualized care. Although some types of CI may show spontaneous and seasonal variations, most patients will require daily therapy throughout life. In infancy and childhood almost all cases need to be managed with topical therapy/balneotherapy, whereas systemic treatment options – namely oral retinoids – are limited for most severe cases.

Since the ichthyoses are chronic life-long diseases, there is a need for well-tolerated, safe and effective treatments. However, the degree of scientific evidence on the benefits and risks of the available treatments is low. A recent systematic review of clinical studies for CI revealed only six randomized controlled trials (RCTs) that met the criteria of the methodology of the Cochrane collaboration [1]. However, the small number of patients included in the studies, the high risk of bias and the short follow up of patients require careful evaluation of the results. Similarly, there are no studies focused on long-term adverse effects, optimal management of particular forms of ichthyoses such as collodion baby, or about ocular and auditory complications, and consequently most recommendations in these guidelines are mainly based on the recommendations of experts and the experience of patients and caregivers. In 2016 the first EU consensus conference for the treatment of the ichthyoses was held in Toulouse, France. The therapy guideline report of the meeting has been published [2,3].

Topical treatment options

Topical therapy is aimed at restoring the epidermal barrier, facilitating desquamation and improving the overall cutaneous appearance. It is the mainstay of treatment in all types of CI, regardless of type and severity. A variety of topical products including emollients, topical keratolytics and epidermal proliferation modulators have been assayed with variable efficacy (Table 129.5) but, in practice, choice will depend on the experience and personal preferences of patients and clinicians. Also, local availability can vary depending on the country. The therapeutic outcome of topical therapy is largely limited by nonadherence, because treatments are not only time consuming and include greasy products, but often show disappointing results.

Emollients
Emollients include both moisturizers and lubricants. Moisturizers increase the ability of the stratum corneum to incorporate water whereas lubricants are occlusive substances with a high content of lipids that form a layer on the skin preventing water loss. Moisturizers are used in cream and contain mainly sodium chloride, urea and glycerol. Petrolatum and paraffin are common lubricating agents; however, although safe and inexpensive, they are

Table 129.5 Emollients and keratolytics commonly used for topical therapy of ichthyoses

Lubricating agents	Petrolatum/vaseline		
	Paraffin		
Hydrating agents	**Agent**	**Concentration (%)**	**Comment**
	Urea	<5	Better avoided during first year of life because of possible systemic absorption
	Lactic acid		Alternative to urea. Commercial preparations are often optimized by buffering
	Sodium chloride	3–10	In ointments often adverse effects (irritation/stinging), possible as bath additive
	Dexpanthenol	5–10	Supporting normal epidermal differentiation
	Macrogol 400	20–30	Moisturizer and keratolytic
	Propylene glycol	15–20	Moisturizer and keratolytic
	Vitamin E acetate	5	Moisturizer
	Glycerol	10–15	Moisturizer
Keratolytic agents	Urea	>5	Humectant and keratolytic
	Propyleneglycol	>20	
	α-hydroxy-acids (glycolic acid)		Critical/caution in children
Keratolytic agents with effects on the epidermal differentiation	Tretinoin, tazarotene, adapalene		Frequent stinging/risk of absorption and teratogenicity in women of childbearing age
	N-acetyl-cysteine		
	Calcipotriol, tacalcitol		High risk of systemic absorption, treat less than 10% of body surface
	Dexpanthenol		Supporting normal epidermal differentiation

Warning: salicylic acid might cause life-threatening poisoning in neonates and long-term toxicity in older patients.

greasy, may impair sweating and are cosmetically unacceptable for some patients. Among emollients, the association of 15% glycerol and paraffin 10% cream has been evaluated in a RCT showing good results in IV patients but no significant differences with respect to placebo in patients with RXLI and ARCI [4]. Emollients are usually safe and can be applied on all body surfaces. The frequency of application depends on the severity of the ichthyosis and the patient's choice, but most individuals need topical therapy at least twice a day.

Keratolytics

RCTs assessing keratolytic agents are also scarce and only include small numbers of patients of each ichthyosis type, preventing any recommendations for the best keratolytic agent. The keratolytic action of urea seems to rely on breakage of hydrogen bonds in the stratum corneum, loosening epidermal keratin, and increasing water-binding sites [5]. The beneficial effect of 10% urea lotion has been evaluated in two RCTs [6,7], showing better results than a urealess 5% lactic acid lotion [6] and the association of glycerol 15% and 10% paraffin cream [7]. Alpha-hydroxy-acids (AHAs) have also been evaluated in several studies [8–10]. One RCT, in which four different formulations with and without 5% lactic acid in patients with lamellar ichthyosis were compared, showed that formulas containing 5% lactic acid reduced scaling significantly but also increased erythema, interpreted as skin irritation. In particular, the combination of 5% lactic acid and 20% propylene glycol in a cream base was the preferred combination for 14 of 18 patients [9]. Salicylic acid (SA) is known to facilitate desquamation and to reduce the rate of keratinocyte proliferation. The potency and toxicity of SA formulations depend on their concentrations, but also on the vehicle (mineral oil or petrolatum vs solution) and the status of the epidermal barrier. In general, preparations for ichthyosis treatment contain concentrations lower than 5% of SA. Systemic toxicity or salicylism develops when blood concentrations of salicylates exceed 35 mg/dL and is characterized by nausea, vomiting, confusion, stupor, coma and finally death. Acidosis and hypoglycaemia in children and hyperglycaemia in adults may also occur. Several cases of salicylism in patients with ichthyosis have been reported, including some babies extensively treated with concentrations as low as 1% [11]. N-acetylcysteine (NAC) is a thiol derivative used as a mucolytic agent that inhibits both the keratinocyte and fibroblast proliferation by reversibly blocking the cell cycle in G1 phase [12]. Its effectiveness and tolerance has been reported in a series of five patients with lamellar ichthyosis [13] and a number of isolated case reports [14,15]. In the largest study, excellent results were observed with a water-in-oil emulsion of 10% NAC in combination with 5% urea topically applied twice daily [13]. No significant side-effects after a 4-year follow up were recorded except for mild and transient burning. An important disadvantage of NAC is the unpleasant sulphuric smell ('rotten eggs') that may be lessened by adding different fragrances [16]. Importantly, the compound needs buffering because the final formula may have a pH as low as 2; however, excessive buffering may inactivate NAC. The biologically active form of Vitamin D_3, 1-25 dihydroxyvitamin D_3, seems to improve disorders of cornification by modifying the epidermal growth factor. Vitamin D analogues include tacalcitol and calcipotriol. A RCT comparing calcipotriol and vehicle in several types of ichthyosis found that calcipotriol showed a higher reduction in skin roughness and scaling [17].

On the contrary, in a single-blind study of nine patients with different types of ichthyosis, tacalcitol did not show superiority over the vehicle [18]. It should be kept in mind that topical calcipotriol bears the risk of hypercalcaemia, and therefore a maximum quantity of 100 g per week in adults is recommended. Topical retinoids modulate keratinocyte proliferation and differentiation. Tazarotene is a third generation retinoid that has been evaluated in several types of ichthyosis in an open-label, nonrandomized trial [19]. Tazarotene gel (0.05%) was compared with a 10% urea lotion showing more favourable results in patients with IV and XLI but not in superficial epidermolytic ichthyosis. Nevertheless, skin irritation was observed in 25% of patients. Adapalene, another third generation retinoid, has recently been proved useful in a single case of a patient with epidermolytic ichthyosis [20].

Patient's age, ichthyosis type and severity as well as extent and location of the lesions must be taken into consideration before prescribing keratolytic agents. Children have a thinner skin and a higher skin surface area/body mass ratio, and therefore are at higher risk of systemic absorption. In particular, all kinds of keratolytics should be avoided in newborns and young infants, in particular salicylic acid. The frequency of application is variable and can be tapered depending on the clinical response. Side-effects are usually mild and include itching, burning sensation and irritation. In areas such as the face or the folds, less potent keratolytics are recommended to prevent irritation, and in areas of fissuring they should be avoided. Systemic toxicity caused by cutaneous absorption of salicylic and lactic acid is a rare but worrisome event.

Balneotherapy

Bathing helps to mechanically remove the scales and reduces discomfort. However, it is time-consuming, lasting approximately 30–60 minutes daily or twice daily. Additives such as salt, oil or sodium bicarbonate can be added to provide additional hydration and promote exfoliation. The mechanism behind the use of sodium bicarbonate is still unclear, but the addition of two handfuls of baking soda to a bath tub would raise the pH from 5.5 to 7.9 [21]. Normal desquamation requires the enzymatic dissolution of corneodesmosomes by serin proteases such as kallikrein 5 and kallikrein 7, which have an alkaline pH optima [22]. Interestingly, most fresh water or lake water has a pH of around 5, whereas ocean water, that many patients also report to be beneficial, usually has a pH above 8.1. Mild nonallergenic soaps and syndets are necessary to remove residual fat-soluble substances. After soaking the skin for around 20–30 minutes, a sponge, microfibre cloth, a silk glove or even a pumice stone can be used to rub the skin and facilitate mechanical scale removal. This can take additional 20–30 minutes. Drying with a towel and immediate application of large amounts of ointments onto the still 'hydrated' skin are beneficial to help retain hydration.

Bathing is also recommended for hygienic reasons. Antiseptics such as triclosan (contained in a number of soaps), chlorhexidine (dilution 5/1000–5/10000), octenidine 0.1%, polihexanide 0.1%, and potassium permanganate (dilution 1/10000) can be used to target bacterial colonization and infections. Also, diluted bleach baths (0.005%) may lessen microbial overgrowth and odour. Hydrotherapy with thermal water has proved useful in an open-label prospective study. Neither the composition nor the pH of the thermal water was specified, and wrapping with a thick layer of emollients was performed immediately after hydrotherapy [23].

Systemic treatment options

In children, systemic therapy is usually reserved for severe forms of ichthyosis that do not respond adequately to topical therapy. Because systemic therapy is a long-term, often life-long treatment, expected outcome and potential side-effects need to be discussed with the parents and caregivers before starting treatment.

Systemic retinoids (SR) are synthetic analogs of all-trans retinoic acid, a vitamin A derivative, that bind to retinoid acid receptors and retinoid X receptors regulating the transcription of genes involved in keratins, growth factors and cytokine expression [24]. In ichthyotic skin, oral retinoids seem to promote a reduction of hyperkeratosis, a tendency to normalization of keratinocyte proliferation and differentiation, and a lessening of coexisting inflammation. Different SR have been used in ichthyosis therapy, including etretinate (which is no longer available in most European countries), alitretinoin [25], acitretin and isotretinoin. Acitretin, a second-generation retinoid, is the first choice in treatment of ichthyoses because of numerous available literature. However, there are no studies comparing its efficacy and tolerability profile to isotretinoin.

SR improve scaling, hyperkeratosis, hair regrowth, hypohidrosis and ectropion. However, they tend to increase skin fragility and are only effective for as long as they are used. Although SR have been widely used, especially in ARCI and keratinopathic ichthyosis, there are no RCTs assessing the minimum starting age and optimal dose. In general, daily doses of up to 0.5 mg/kg adequately control the disease, but lower maintenance doses are often sufficient. SR have a slow turn-over in the body and the clinical effects last for days or even weeks; therefore, they can be administered once daily or even every second day, and interruption of therapy does not result immediately in clinical changes [26]. Thus, some patients may benefit from discontinuous therapy ('therapy holidays') particularly in warm weather for those with CIE. The clinical response is observed after 2–4 weeks after initiation of treatment. Although SR have numerous and feared potential side-effects, they are usually mild and reversible. Acute and chronic toxicities must be discussed before starting therapy. Acute mucocutaneous toxicity including xerosis, cheilitis, dry nose and conjunctiva irritation are common. Haematological abnormalities can be observed in liver enzymes, lipids and blood cell counts. Chronic toxicity mainly affects the skeletal system and consists of diffuse skeletal hyperostosis, that is, spurs and calcifications along the spine (usually the anterior spinal ligament) and at tendon and ligamentous insertions around joints [27]. Side-effects are usually mild and reversible except teratogenicity and bone changes.

Patients require a blood screen (blood cell count, biochemistry panel and human chorionic gonadotropin in female adolescents) before starting treatment and periodic follow up during therapy. Blood tests should be performed every 2–4 weeks at the beginning of treatment and every 3–6 months in long-term therapy, or more often if there are laboratory abnormalities or pregnancy issues. The optimal periodicity of skeletal survey is controversial in children. Baseline radiographs can be obtained but frequency of the follow up is not well established.

SR are teratogens and this issue requires thorough discussion and adequate contraception in female adolescents. SR are lipophilic drugs that are slowly eliminated from the body [28]; in particular, acitretin has the potential to persist in the body because of conversion to etretinate, and therefore pregnancy must be avoided for 3 years following acitretin therapy [29]. The shorter teratogenicity period of isotretinoin makes it a good therapeutic alternative for female adolescents [30]. Liarozole, an imidazole derivative belonging to retinoic acid metabolism blocking agents (RAMBAs), showed a shorter teratogenic period in pharmacokinetic studies [31], but an in-depth period of time to avoid its teratogenic effect has not been established. Liarozole was granted orphan drug status for congenital ichthyosis by the European Commission and the US Food and Drug Administration. Its development has now been discontinued, because it did not show significantly better results than acitretin in two RCTs [31,32].

Acitretin therapy noticeably improves the majority of patients with ARCI. Some patients with CIE may respond better to lower doses [33]. Whereas the effect of acitretin on ARCI phenotypes seems not to be related to the genetic abnormality, KPI show a clear correlation between the mutated keratin gene and the response to SR. In superficial KPI, caused by *KRT2* mutation, a silencing of this gene by retinoid therapy will be beneficial whereas in KPI caused by *KRT1* mutation downregulation of *KRT2* will be deleterious because wild-type keratin 2 partially compensates for mutated keratin 1 in the dimerization process with keratin 10. Therefore, the response to acitretin will be better in superficial KPI than in *KRT10* deficient KPI but still better than in KPI caused by *KRT1* deficiency [34]. In KPI, erythema and blistering are commonly exacerbated after starting SR therapy, particularly in hot and humid climates. To avoid this, starting with a low dose is recommended, followed by slowly increasing the dose.

SR have been used with some success in a few syndromic forms of CI including KID syndrome, SLS, ichthyosis follicularis, alopecia and photophobia (IFAP) syndrome, Chanarin–Dorfman syndrome, NISCH syndrome and Netherton syndrome. However, they should be used with caution in forms with liver involvement or biliary disease such as Chanarin–Dorfman syndrome or NISCH, and in CI with bone anomalies such as Conradi–Hünermann–Happle syndrome.

Special aspects of treatment

Therapy of the scalp

Scalp desquamation is a common issue in all types of ichthyosis. It ranges from fine scaling, such as in IV and RXLI, to adherent scales and thick crusts in severe types. Although early treatment of scalp desquamation is believed to help preventing cicatricial alopecia, no solid evidence exists supporting this theory. Mechanical removal of the scales with brushes and combs is advised to avoid excessive thickening of the scales and potential microbial super infection. In general, lotions, solutions and shampoos are more cosmetically acceptable than greasy products; however, in some instances, oil-in-water creams may be needed to remove thick adherent scales, with or without occlusion. Keratolytics may also be useful but attention must be paid to increased absorption through the scalp. Brushing and scalp care must be particularly careful in ichthyosis with brittle hair such as Netherton syndrome and trichothiodystrophy.

Ophthalmological aspects

Eye problems are common in all types of ichthyosis. Scales on the eyelashes, blepharoconjunctivitis, madarosis, lagophthalmos and ectropion may eventually lead to corneal damage [35–37]. The main goal of eye care is maintaining the ocular surface integrity, so careful prophylactic ocular lubrication is strongly recommended. In patients who require frequent eye drop administration, preservative-free topical medication is preferred [38,39]. In addition to ocular lubrication, room humidifiers may also improve the corneal hydration status. Intensive treatment with eyelid emollients and massage may improve eyelid retraction, ectropion and lagophthalmos. Although surgical techniques may be required in severe cases, therapy with topical retinoids, N-acetylcysteine and hyaluronic acid fillers have proved useful [40–42] and may prevent or postpone the need for surgery in cases with mild ectropion. Patients with chronic corneal involvement, persistent corneal epithelial defects or ectropion and eyelid retraction require specialized ophthalmic care and should be followed up regularly.

ENT

Hearing loss is another frequent finding in patients with CI. Excessive desquamation within the external auditory canal promotes ear plugging and predisposes to outer ear infections and conduction deafness [43]. Ear pruritus and ear pain are also important complaints in CI in all age groups [44]. Although the best topical therapy to remove ear plugs and the ideal periodicity of ENT follow ups remain to be elucidated, involvement of ENT specialists in the management of patients with CI is crucial to ensure the application of the best therapeutic and preventive measures [44,45].

Nutritional issues and growth

Impairment of the epidermal barrier and increased transepidermal water loss have been proven to play a central role in CI-associated growth failure [46]. Additionally, increased epidermal turnover, chronic skin inflammation and cutaneous protein losses, especially in CI patients with erythroderma, contribute to increased resting energy expenditure [47]. Therefore, although auxological outcomes in children with CI have not yet been studied in prospective clinical trials, close monitoring of weight and height gain at regular intervals is mandatory, particularly in neonates and infants with severe CI. As the child grows, follow up intervals can widen. Special attention should also be paid to signs of delayed puberty in older school children and adolescents. Vitamin D deficiency has been reported in up to 41% of children with CI [48], particularly in those with darker phenotypes and suffering from ARCI or KPI. Scale thickness, low sun exposure and low vitamin D intake have been the advocated causes. In one French study [49], ichthyosis severity, dark skin, and winter/spring seasons were identified as independent risk factors for vitamin D deficiency [50]. Also, the possible causative effect of SR in vitamin D deficiency rickets has been pointed out [51]. Recently, dramatic improvement of CI with vitamin D supplements has been reported [52], supporting the role of vitamin D as a regulator of genes involved in epidermal differentiation [53]. Consequently, regular monitoring for clinical, biochemical and hormonal parameters is strongly recommended as well as adequate vitamin D supplementation according to the degree of deficiency.

Lifestyle recommendations

Sweating impairment is a major problem in CI. Patients are at risk of overheating, heat exhaustion and heat stroke. Physical activity must be limited, particularly in warm and humid weather, and natural fibre clothing is preferred over synthetic fabrics. Children should stay in a fresh environment with air conditioning, fans or other cooling devices. Sun exposure has advantages and disadvantages; although it improves some types of ichthyosis (IV and RXLI) and may prevent rickets, it may worsen heat intolerance and sun protection may be difficult.

Psychosocial aspects

CI are characterized by visible clinical signs and distressing symptoms such as pruritus, pain or heat intolerance that can disturb a patient's personal well being and social relationships. In addition, topical treatment is time consuming and expensive, interfering with daily life and budget. It has been shown that CI not only impact negatively on the quality of life of both the patient and their relatives [49] but the economic impact of the disease is considerable when there is no possibility of reimbursement [54]. The ideal moment to offer specialized psychological support is not clear. New parents can be devastated in the early stages but may need some time to adapt before seeking psychological support. School children may need help to cope with bullying issues, as well as children transitioning to adolescence. Dermatologists responsible for the patients must address this issue and direct patients and caregivers to receive psychological support when needed.

Management of collodion baby and harlequin ichthyosis

Collodion baby as well as harlequin ichthyosis (HI) should be regarded as dermatological emergencies and require an interdisciplinary approach [55,56]. Infants suffering from these two conditions have a profoundly disturbed epidermal barrier which is associated with increased transepidermal water loss that may result in hypothermia and/or hypernatraemic dehydration [57,58]. Other problems include proneness to infection, ectropion, poor sucking, restricted pulmonary ventilation and occasionally digital vascular constriction [58,59]. Neonates should be transferred to a neonatal intensive care unit. Infants suffering from collodion baby should be placed in a high humidity incubator with close monitoring of body temperature. It is generally recommended to start with humidity levels in the range of 60–80%, and decrease levels every 3–4 days to reach normal humidity conditions until the children can be moved into an open crib. In our experience it is sufficient to use bland ointments, e.g. a dexpanthenol containing ointment two to four times a day. Occlusive products such as petrolatum or vaseline may ease skin infections and miliaria. Percutaneous absorption is very high and substances typically used in older children with ichthyosis, such as urea or lactic acid, should be avoided in the first year of life. In particular, *the use of salicylic acid is strictly forbidden*, because its use can result in metabolic acidosis within 72 hours even when used in very low concentrations [60,61]. Although their real value remains unproven, SR can be considered in HI. In the largest series published so far of 45 HI patients, 83% of babies who survived were given SR, whereas long-term survival was only 24% for those untreated [58]. However, there are also reports of survival without oral treatment, and for some authors 'a more active management approach overall' might have contributed to the apparent success of oral retinoids [62]. For further information on the nursing care of collodion baby and harlequin ichthyosis see Chapter 176.

Patient organizations and other resources

Patient organizations are nonprofit organizations that inform, educate and support patients and their families, often in collaboration with health professionals. They organize meetings where members can meet others in the same situation and share experiences, uncertainties and advice. Therefore, membership of a patient organization can be extremely helpful for patients and their families and should be recommended. There are active patient associations in many European countries. At the European level these national self-support groups have formed the European Network for Ichthyoses (ENI). In the USA the Foundation for Ichthyosis and related skin types (FIRST) has been active since 1981 and has the aim to educate, inspire and connect all those touched by ichthyosis and related disorders. Sources for general information on the disease are, for example, the homepage of the German network for ichthyoses (NIRK; www.netzwerk-ichthyose.de) or the network of FIRST (www.firstskinfoundation.org) (Table 129.6). Genetic analysis can be performed in expert centres throughout Europe; detailed information is provided at www.orpha.net. Finally, social media such as Facebook and Twitter allow easy and quick connection of worldwide patients, caregivers and all interested individuals in the field.

Table 129.6 Resources and further information

Patient organizations for ichthyoses	
Denmark	www.iktyosis.dkwww.iholiitto.fi/
Finland	www.anips.net/
France	www.ichthyose.dewww.ittiosi.it/
Germany	www.ictiosis.orgwww.ichthyose.chwww.ichthyosis.org.uk/
Italy	http://www.firstskinfoundation.org
Spain	
Switzerland	
UK	
USA	
Other databases and internet links	
Web site hosted at NCBI	www.genetests.orgwww.orpha.netwww.interfil.orghttp://www.awmf.org/en/ clinical-practice-guidelines.html
Portal for rare diseases and orphan drugs	
Human intermediated filament database	
German guidelines for ichthyoses	

Future directions

Nonsyndromic CI seem to be the ideal scenario for topical targeted therapy, because the genetic defect is limited to the skin and topical treatments easily hit the target. Liposomal technology has been used to introduce recombinant TGM1 into the TGM1-deficient keratinocytes in humanized skin models in mice [63]. The authors found not only normalization of histochemistry and ultrastructure after rhTG1-liposome treatment but also a dramatic improvement of the skin barrier. Topical therapy with cholesterol and lovastatin is another pathogenesis-based therapy that has been reported as successful in inherited disorders of distal cholesterol metabolism [64].

References

1 **Hernandez-Martin A, Aranegui B, Martin-Santiago A et al. A systematic review of clinical trials of treatments for the congenital ichthyoses, excluding ichthyosis vulgaris. J Am Acad Dermatol 2013;69:544–9.**

2 **Mazereeuw-Hautier J, Vahlquist A, Traupe H et al. Management of congenital ichthyoses: European guidelines of care, part one. Br J Dermatol 2019;180:272–81.**

3 **Mazereeuw-Hautier J, Hernández-Martín A, O'Toole EA et al. Management of congenital ichthyoses: European guidelines of care, part two. Br J Dermatol 2019;180:484–95.**

4 **Blanchet-Bardon C, Tadini G, Machado Matos M et al. Association of glycerol and paraffin in the treatment of ichthyosis in children: an international, multicentric, randomized, controlled, double-blind study. J Eur Acad Dermatol Venereol 2012;26:1014–9.**

5 Gloor M, Fluhr J, Lehmann L et al. Do urea/ammonium lactate combinations achieve better skin protection and hydration than either component alone? Skin Pharmacol Appl Skin Physiol 2002;15:35–43.

6 **Kuster W, Bohnsack K, Rippke F et al. Efficacy of urea therapy in children with ichthyosis. A multicenter randomized, placebo-controlled, double-blind, semilateral study. Dermatology 1998;196:217–22.**

7 Tadini G, Giustini S, Milani M. Efficacy of topical 10% urea-based lotion in patients with ichthyosis vulgaris: a two-center, randomized, controlled, single-blind, right-vs.-left study in comparison with standard glycerol-based emollient cream. Curr Med Res Opin 2011;27:2279–84.

8 Buxman M, Hickman J, Ragsdale W et al. Therapeutic activity of lactate 12% lotion in the treatment of ichthyosis. Active versus vehicle and active versus a petrolatum cream. J Am Acad Dermatol 1986;15:1253–8.

9 Gånemo A, Virtanen M, Vahlquist A. Improved topical treatment of lamellar ichthyosis: a double-blind study of four different cream formulations. Br J Dermatol 1999:1027–32.

10 Kempers S, Katz HI, Wildnauer R et al. An evaluation of the effect of an alpha hydroxy acid-blend skin cream in the cosmetic improvement of symptoms of moderate to severe xerosis, epidermolytic hyperkeratosis, and ichthyosis. Cutis 1998;61:347–50.

11 Madan RK, Levitt J. A review of toxicity from topical salicylic acid preparations. J Am Acad Dermatol 2014;70:788–92.

12 Redondo P, Bauza A. Topical N-acetylcysteine for lamellar ichthyosis. Lancet 1999;354:1880.

13 Bassotti A, Moreno S, Criado E. Successful treatment with topical N-acetylcysteine in urea in five children with congenital lamellar ichthyosis. Pediatr Dermatol 2011;28:451–5.

14 Gicquel JJ, Vabres P, Dighiero P. [Use of topical cutaneous N-acetylcysteine in the treatment of major bilateral ectropion in an infant with lamellar ichthyosis]. J Fr Ophthalmol 2005;28:412–5.

15 Sarici SU, Sahin M, Yurdakok M. Topical N-acetylcysteine treatment in neonatal ichthyosis. Turk J Pediatr 2003;45:245–7.

16 Davila-Seijo P, Florez A, Davila-Pousa C et al. Topical N-acetylcysteine for the treatment of lamellar ichthyosis: an improved formula. Pediatr Dermatol 2014;31:395–7.

17 Kragballe K, Steijlen PM, Ibsen HH et al. Efficacy, tolerability, and safety of calcipotriol ointment in disorders of keratinization. Results of a randomized, double-blind, vehicle-controlled, right/left comparative study. Arch Dermatol 1995;131:556–60.

18 Okano M. Assessment of the clinical effect of topical tacalcitol on ichthyoses with retentive hyperkeratosis. Dermatology 2001;202:116–8.

19 Hofmann B, Stege H, Ruzicka T et al. Effect of topical tazarotene in the treatment of congenital ichthyoses. Br J Dermatol 1999;141:642–6.

20 Ogawa M, Akiyama M. Successful topical adapalene treatment for the facial lesions of an adolescent case of epidermolytic ichthyosis. J Am Acad Dermatol 2014;71:e103–5.

21 Milstone LM. Scaly skin and bath pH: rediscovering baking soda. J Am Acad Dermatol 2010;62:885–6.

22 Brattsand M, Stefansson K, Lundh C et al. A proteolytic cascade of kallikreins in the stratum corneum. J Invest Dermatol 2005;124: 198–203.

23 Bodemer C, Bourrat E, Mazereeuw-Hautier J et al. Short- and medium-term efficacy of specific hydrotherapy in inherited ichthyosis. Br J Dermatol 2011;165:1087–94.

24 Torma H. Regulation of keratin expression by retinoids. Dermatoendocrinol 2011;3:136–40.

25 Ganemo A, Sommerlund M, Vahlquist A. Oral alitretinoin in congenital ichthyosis: a pilot study shows variable effects and a risk of central hypothyroidism. Acta Derm Venereol 2012;92:256–7.

26 **Vahlquist A, Ganemo A, Virtanen M. Congenital ichthyosis: an overview of current and emerging therapies. Acta Derm Venereol 2008;88:4–14.**

27 Digiovanna JJ, Mauro T, Milstone LM et al. Systemic retinoids in the management of ichthyoses and related skin types. Dermatol Ther 2013;26:26–38.

28 DiGiovanna JJ, Zech LA, Ruddel ME et al. Etretinate. Persistent serum levels after long-term therapy. Arch Dermatol 1989;125:246–51.

29 Lebwohl M, Drake L, Menter A et al. Consensus conference: acitretin in combination with UVB or PUVA in the treatment of psoriasis. J Am Acad Dermatol 2001;45:544–53.

30 Baden HP, Buxman MM, Weinstein GD et al. Treatment of ichthyosis with isotretinoin. J Am Acad Dermatol 1982;6:716–20.

31 **Verfaille CJ, Vanhoutte FP, Blanchet-Bardon C et al. Oral liarozole vs. acitretin in the treatment of ichthyosis: a phase II/III multicentre,**

double-blind, randomized, active-controlled study. Br J Dermatol 2007:965–73.

32 **Vahlquist A, Blockhuys S, Steijlen P et al. Oral liarozole in the treatment of patients with moderate/severe lamellar ichthyosis: results of a randomized, double-blind, multinational, placebo-controlled phase II/III trial. Br J Dermatol 2014;170:173–81.**

33 Steijlen PM, Van Dooren-Greebe RJ, Van de Kerkhof PC. Acitretin in the treatment of lamellar ichthyosis. Br J Dermatol 1994;130:211–4.

34 Virtanen M, Gedde-Dahl T, Jr., Mork NJ et al. Phenotypic/genotypic correlations in patients with epidermolytic hyperkeratosis and the effects of retinoid therapy on keratin expression. Acta Derm Venereol 2001;81:163–70.

35 Bhallil S, Chraibi F, Andalloussi IB et al. Optical coherence tomography aspect of crystalline macular dystrophy in Sjogren–Larsson syndrome. Int Ophthalmol 2012;32:495–8.

36 Singh AJ, Atkinson PL. Ocular manifestations of congenital lamellar ichthyosis. Eur J Ophthalmol 2005;15:118–22.

37 Jay B, Blach RK, Wells RS. Ocular manifestations of ichthyosis. Br J Ophthalmol 1968;52:217–26.

38 Huber-van der Velden KK, Thieme H, Eichhorn M. [Morphological alterations induced by preservatives in eye drops]. Ophthalmologe 2012;109:1077–81.

39 Messmer EM. [Preservatives in ophthalmology]. Ophthalmologe 2012;109:1064–70.

40 Craiglow BG, Choate KA, Milstone LM. Topical tazarotene for the treatment of ectropion in ichthyosis. JAMA Dermatol 2013;149: 598–600.

41 Deffenbacher B. Successful experimental treatment of congenital ichthyosis in an infant. BMJ Case Rep 2013;2013.

42 Litwin AS, Kalantzis G, Drimtzias E et al. Nonsurgical treatment of congenital ichthyosis cicatricial ectropion and eyelid retraction using Restylane hyaluronic acid. Br J Dermatol 2015;173:601–3.

43 Martin-Santiago A, Rodriguez-Pascual M, Knopfel N et al. Otologic manifestations of autosomal recessive congenital ichthyosis in children. Actas Dermosifiliogr 2015;106:733–9.

44 Huang JT, Mallon K, Hamill S et al. Frequency of ear symptoms and hearing loss in ichthyosis: a pilot survey study. Pediatr Dermatol 2014;31:276–80.

45 Hernandez-Martin A, Davila'Seijo P, Soria de Francisco JM et al. Fragmented health care delivery in ichthyosis. Actas Dermosifiliogr 2015;106:514–5.

46 Moskowitz DG, Fowler AJ, Heyman MB et al. Pathophysiologic basis for growth failure in children with ichthyosis: an evaluation of cutaneous ultrastructure, epidermal permeability barrier function, and energy expenditure. J Pediatr 2004;145:82–92.

47 Fowler AJ, Moskowitz DG, Wong A et al. Nutritional status and gastrointestinal structure and function in children with ichthyosis and growth failure. J Pediatr Gastroenterol Nutr 2004;38:164–9.

48 Sethuraman G, Sreenivas V, Yenamandra VK et al. Threshold levels of 25-hydroxyvitamin D and parathyroid hormone for impaired bone health in children with congenital ichthyosis and type IV and V skin. Br J Dermatol 2015;172:208–14.

49 Dreyfus I, Bourrat E, Maruani A et al. Factors associated with impaired quality of life in adult patients suffering from ichthyosis. Acta Derm Venereol 2014;94:344–6.

50 Frascari F, Dreyfus I, Rodriguez L et al. Prevalence and risk factors of vitamin D deficiency in inherited ichthyosis: a French prospective observational study performed in a reference center. Orphanet J Rare Dis 2014;9:127.

51 Neema S, Mukherjee S, Vasudevan B et al. Vitamin D deficiency after oral retinoid therapy for ichthyosis. Pediatr Dermatol 2015;32:e151–5.

52 Sethuraman G, Marwaha RK, Challa A et al. Vitamin D: a new promising therapy for congenital ichthyosis. Pediatrics 2016;137.

53 Lu J, Goldstein KM, Chen P et al. Transcriptional profiling of keratinocytes reveals a vitamin D-regulated epidermal differentiation network. J Invest Dermatol 2005;124:778–85.

54 Dreyfus I, Pauwels C, Bourrat E et al. Burden of inherited ichthyosis: a French national survey. Acta Derm Venereol 2015;95:326–8.

55 Prado R, Ellis LZ, Gamble R et al. Collodion baby: an update with a focus on practical management. J Am Acad Dermatol 2012;67: 1362–74.

56 Van Gysel D, Lijnen RL, Moekti SS et al. Collodion baby: a follow-up study of 17 cases. J Eur Acad Dermatol Venereol 2002;16:472–5.

57 Buyse L, Graves C, Marks R et al. Collodion baby dehydration: the danger of high transepidermal water loss. Br J Dermatol 1993;129:86–8.

58 Rajpopat S, Moss C, Mellerio J et al. Harlequin ichthyosis: a review of clinical and molecular findings in 45 cases. Arch Dermatol 2011;147:681–6.

59 Harvey HB, Shaw MG, Morrell DS. Perinatal management of harlequin ichthyosis: a case report and literature review. J Perinatol 2010;30:66–72.

60 Galea P, Goel KM. Salicylate poisoning in dermatological treatment. Arch Dis Child 1990;65:335.

61 Ward PS, Jones RD. Successful treatment of a harlequin fetus. Arch Dis Child 1989;64:1309–11.

62 Milstone LM, Choate KA. Improving outcomes for harlequin ichthyosis. J Am Acad Dermatol 2013;69:808–9.

63 Aufenvenne K, Larcher F, Hausser I et al. Topical enzyme-replacement therapy restores transglutaminase 1 activity and corrects architecture of transglutaminase-1-deficient skin grafts. Am J Hum Genet 2013;93:620–30.

64 Paller AS, van Steensel MA, Rodriguez-Martin M et al. Pathogenesis-based therapy reverses cutaneous abnormalities in an inherited disorder of distal cholesterol metabolism. J Invest Dermatol 2011; 131:2242–8.

CHAPTER 130
Keratosis Pilaris and Darier Disease

Flora B. de Waard-van der Spek[1] *& Arnold P. Oranje*[2]

[1] Department of Dermatology, Franciscus Gasthuis & Vlietland, Rotterdam/Schiedam, The Netherlands
[2] Kinderhuid.nl, Rotterdam, Hair Clinic, Breda and Dermicis Skin Clinic, Alkmaar, The Netherlands

Introduction, 1599 | Keratosis pilaris, 1599 | Darier disease, 1603

Abstract

Keratosis pilaris is a cutaneous abnormality associated with a variety of clinical entities and has been a source of historical confusion. Recently, keratosis pilaris has also been described as being induced by biologic drugs. Darier disease (DD) is an inherited keratinizing disorder that exhibits autosomal dominant inheritance with complete penetrance, but variable expression. DD is caused by the mutations of ATP2A2, which encodes an endoplasmic reticulum calcium pump, sarco/endoplasmic reticulum ATPase type 2 (SERCA2). DD often develops in childhood, persists through adolescence and causes small papules. Skin lesions are present predominantly in seborrhoeic areas such as the face, chest and back. Acral involvement is common, and children may have hand involvement before any other signs of the disease. Longitudinal red and white lines in the nail are an early sign of DD. There are no currently validated curative treatments available for keratosis pilaris and DD, with the majority of cases treated symptomatically or left untreated.

Key points

- **Keratosis pilaris is a cutaneous abnormality associated with a variety of clinical entities and has been a source of historical confusion.**
- **Whole exome sequencing identified low density lipoprotein receptor-related protein 1 (LRP1) as a pathogenic gene in autosomal recessive keratosis pilaris atrophicans.**
- **Keratosis follicularis spinulosa decalvans X-linked (KFSDX), and ichthyosis follicularis, alopecia and photophobia (IFAP) syndrome are probably related diseases (OMIM #308800).**
- **Darier disease (DD) is an inherited keratinizing disorder that exhibits autosomal dominant inheritance with complete penetrance, but variable expression.**
- **DD is caused by the mutations of ATP2A2, which encodes an endoplasmic reticulum calcium pump, sarco/endoplasmic reticulum ATPase type 2 (SERCA2).**
- **There are no currently validated curative treatments available for keratosis pilaris and DD.**

Introduction

Keratosis pilaris is a cutaneous abnormality associated with a variety of diseases. It is defined by the presence of keratotic plugging of hair follicles, surrounded by varying degrees of erythema. In the isolated form, keratosis pilaris is an essentially normal physiological finding. Lesions occur predominantly on the extensor surfaces of the arms and legs, but may also involve the face, buttocks and trunk. About 40% of children suffer from mild keratosis pilaris. Keratosis pilaris atrophicans occurs in a number of syndromes with different inheritance patterns. The differential diagnosis of keratosis pilaris includes Darier disease, also known as keratosis follicularis or Darier–White disease. Darier disease is an autosomal dominantly inherited genodermatosis, characterized by brown, keratotic papules of sizes varying from pin-head to millet seed which develop in seborrhoeic areas such as the forehead, central chest, back and scalp margins. The rough skin in keratosis pilaris is caused by follicular plugs of keratin. In Darier disease narrow intraepidermal clefts or lacunae containing acantholytic cells form above the basal cells. Dyskeratotic keratinocytes (corps ronds and grains), contain clumped cytokeratin filaments and cytoplasmic vacuoles.

Keratosis pilaris

Definition. Keratosis pilaris is a cutaneous abnormality associated with a variety of diseases. It is defined by the presence of keratotic plugging of hair follicles, surrounded by varying degrees of erythema. When keratosis pilaris is accompanied by atrophy, it is referred to as keratosis pilaris atrophicus [1,2].

History. The clinical entities of keratosis pilaris and keratosis pilaris atrophicus have been a source of historical confusion. This is the result of overlap among syndromes, the presence of intermediate forms and the

Harper's Textbook of Pediatric Dermatology, Fourth Edition. Edited by Peter Hoeger, Veronica Kinsler and Albert Yan.

existence of numerous synonyms in the dermatology and genetics literature [3].

Particularly confusing is the entity 'ichthyosis follicularis', a term coined by Lesser in 1885 [4,5]. Another disorder that, historically, has received much attention is keratosis follicularis spinulosa decalvans (also initially described as ichthyosis follicularis). This entity was first described in the Dutch literature by Lameris in 1905 and Rochat in 1906 in a Dutch–German family [6,7]. In 1925, Siemens investigated this same family clinically [8]. Van Osch and colleagues performed an update of the clinical study with the goal of performing a linkage study [9]. In 2010, Aten and colleagues detected and identified *MBTPS2* as the candidate gene carrying a c.1523A>G (p.Asn508Ser) missense mutation [10].

Aetiology and pathogenesis. In the isolated form, keratosis pilaris is essentially a normal physiological finding. About 40% of children suffer from mild keratosis pilaris. In a questionnaire study undertaken by Poskitt and Wilkinson, the mean age of improvement was 16 years [11]. Keratosis pilaris may also be seen in relation to malnutrition/nutritional deficiency, xerosis and ichthyosis vulgaris, and may be induced by biologic drugs [12,13].

Keratosis pilaris atrophicans occurs in a number of syndromes with different inheritance patterns: (i) keratosis pilaris atrophicans faciei; (ii) atrophoderma vermiculata; (iii) keratosis follicularis spinulosa decalvans; and (iv) folliculitis spinulosa decalvans [12,14].

Keratosis pilaris atrophicans faciei, or ulerythema ophryogenes, is inherited in an autosomal dominant fashion. Physical findings demonstrate follicular keratotic papules associated with alopecia and predominantly occur in the eyebrows. Genetic linkage studies have not yet been performed.

Atrophoderma vermiculata, also known as atrophoderma reticulata, acne vermoulante, folliculitis ulerythema reticulata, folliculitis ulerythematosa and honeycomb atrophy, is characterized by reticulate scarring on the cheeks. The disease is inherited as an autosomal recessive trait, and genetic linkage has not yet been performed.

Keratosis follicularis spinulosa decalvans (KFSD) has been extensively studied. Families have been described in Finland, Switzerland and the Netherlands. In all three family studies, pedigree analysis shows an X-linked inheritance pattern [9]. Nearly complete expression in women can be explained by skewed lyonization. Richard and Harth have described fully expressed keratosis follicularis spinulosa decalvans in a woman [15].

In a large Dutch family which descends from the cohort originally investigated by Lameris and Siemens, Oosterwijk and colleagues. localized the gene to Xp21.2 – p22.2 [9,16]. The gene locus has since been narrowed to Xp22.13–p22.2 [17] but in another German family, the same research team could not confirm these results and suggested the possibility of genetic heterogeneity [18]. Now the exact mutation is known: whole exome sequencing identified *LRP1* as a pathogenic gene in autosomal recessive keratosis pilaris atrophicans [10,13].

In the Dutch family with KFSDX mentioned above, described in detail by van Osch, Oranje and colleagues [9,12], Aten and colleagues [10] identified a mutation in the MBTPS2 gene [6,8,9,10]. The same mutation was found in not-related families from the UK and the USA [10]. In obligate female carriers, imbalances in allelic expression perfectly matched with skewed levels of X inactivation and with the clinical phenotype. The findings suggested that KFSDX and ichthyosis follicularis, alopecia and photophobia (IFAP) syndrome are related diseases (OMIM #308800).

Interestingly, KFSD has also been described with possible autosomal dominant inheritance and a slightly different clinical presentation [18,19].

Pathology. The histopathology is nonspecific and is generally not useful in diagnosis. The follicular orifice is distended by a keratin plug [20]. In keratosis pilaris, mild inflammation is present. In keratosis pilaris atrophicans, severe inflammation may occur in the early stages and in the late stages, atrophy of the epidermis is noted [9,20].

Clinical features.

Keratosis pilaris

Lesions occur predominantly on the extensor surfaces of the arms (Fig. 130.1) and legs, but may also involve the face, buttocks and trunk. Keratosis pilaris often improves in the summer months and flares in the winter. Clinical signs of atopy are observed in at least one-third of patients [2,11].

Keratosis pilaris is characterized by the presence of rough, follicular papules and varying degrees of erythema. Erythema may be particularly severe in children with extensive facial involvement (keratosis pilaris rubra faciei). A number of diseases are associated with keratosis pilaris (Box 130.1)

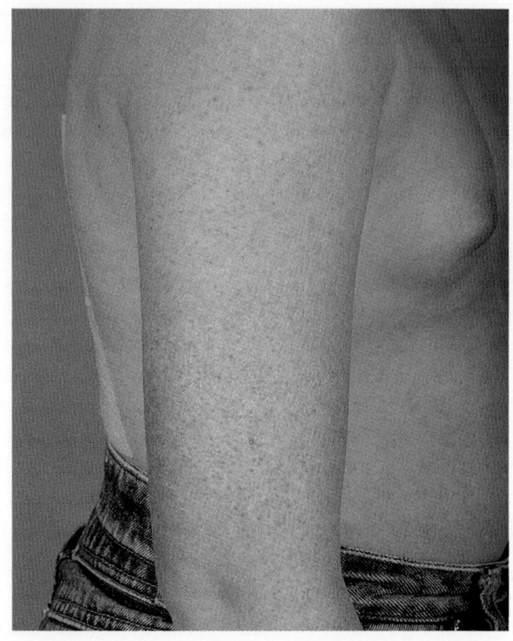

Fig. 130.1 Keratosis pilaris on the arms.

Box 130.1 Keratosis pilaris and keratosis pilaris atrophicans associated disorders and syndromes in childhood

Keratosis pilaris

- Physiological
- Atopic dermatitis
- Lichen spinulosa
- Ichthyosis vulgaris
- Other ichthyoses (Mevorah et al. [21])
- Renal insufficiency (Guillet et al. [22])
- Prolidase deficiency (Larrègue et al. [23])
- Down syndrome (Finn et al. [24])
- Monilethrix
- Fairbank syndrome (Marks [25])
- Keratosis pilaris follicularis non-atrophicans

Keratosis pilaris atrophicans

- Keratosis pilaris atrophicans faciei (ulerythema ophryogenes)
- Atrophoderma vermiculata
- Keratosis follicularis spinulosa decalvans
- Folliculitis spinulosa [12]
- Noonan syndrome (now called cardiofaciocutaneous syndrome) (Ward et al. [26])
- Woolly hair

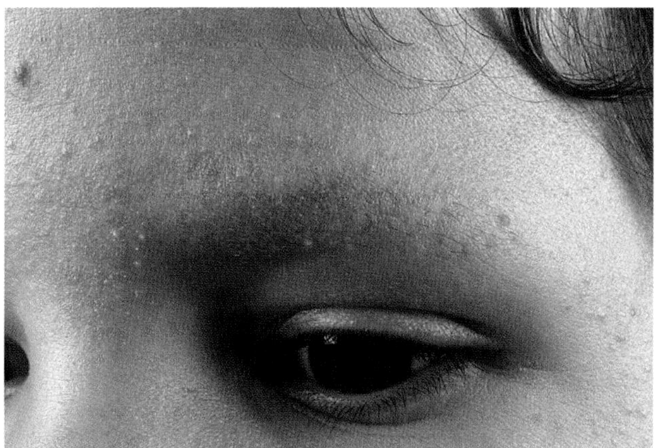

Fig. 130.2 Keratosis pilaris atrophicans faciei.

Keratosis pilaris atrophicans

Keratosis pilaris atrophicans faciei is characterized by redness and atrophic scarring of the eyebrows (Fig. 130.2). The symptoms are present at birth or begin during infancy. Typical keratosis pilaris is observed at other sites. Combinations of keratosis pilaris atrophicans faciei and Noonan syndrome or woolly hair have been described [27,28]. The association with Noonan syndrome has been designated as cardio-facio-cutaneous syndrome [26].

Atrophoderma vermiculata is characterized by symmetrical reticulate atrophy and scarring of the cheeks. Small pits with sharp edges give the skin a 'worm-eaten' appearance. Lesions are always limited to the face, and begin after the age of 5 years. Asymmetrical forms limited to one cheek have been described [29].

KFSD is a rare X-linked disease that affects both the skin (Fig. 130.3) and the eyes (Fig. 130.4). It is characterized by follicular hyperkeratosis of the skin and corneal dystrophy. Several families have been described, the largest one being of German–Dutch origin [9]. The follicular papules are associated with loss of hair, especially from the scalp, eyebrows

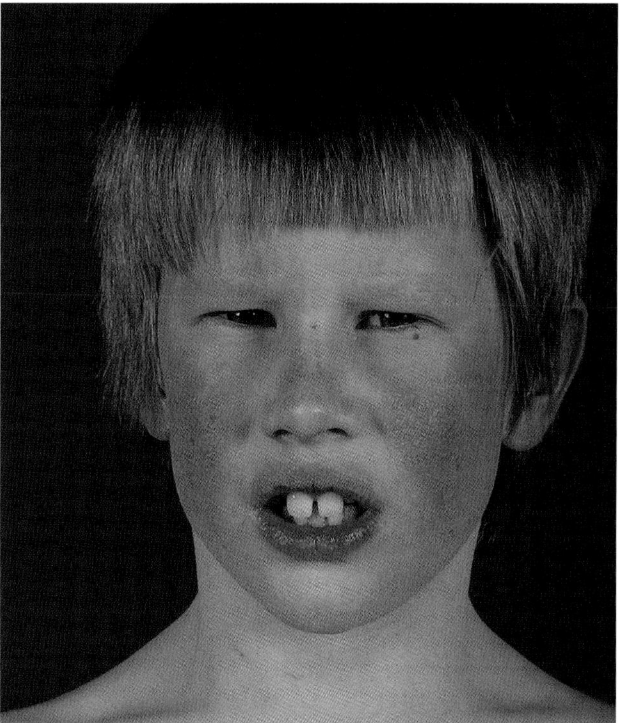

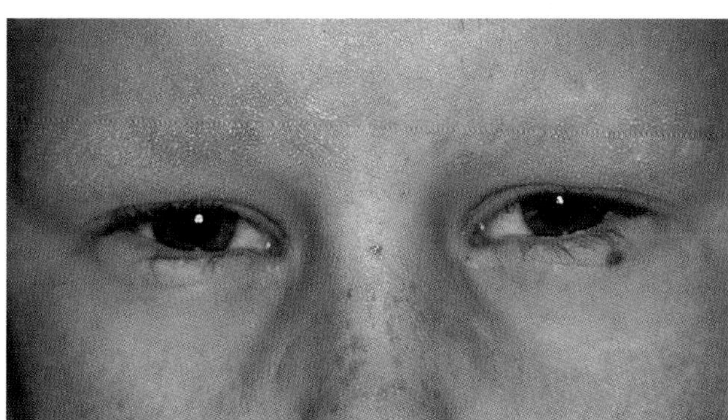

Fig. 130.3 Keratosis follicularis spinulosa decalvans in the face.

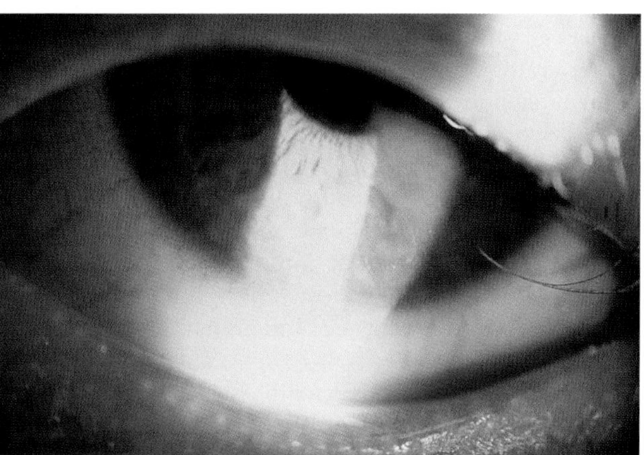

Fig. 130.4 Patchy corneal dystrophy in keratosis follicularis spinulosa decalvans.

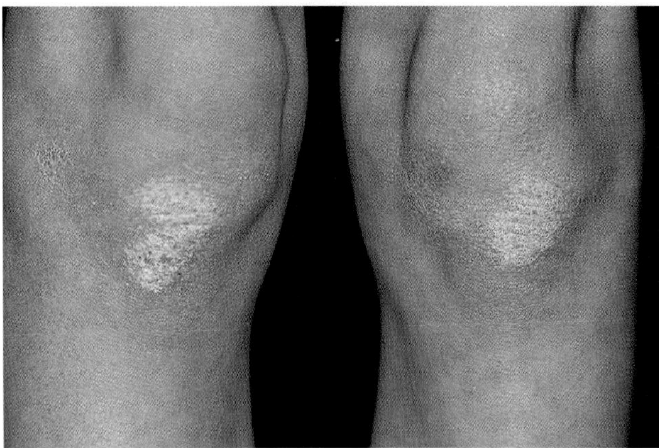

Fig. 130.5 Hyperkeratosis on the knees in keratosis follicularis spinulosa decalvans.

and eyelashes. Marked photophobia may result from the corneal dystrophy. Other prominent findings are scarring alopecia of the scalp and absence of the eyebrows and eyelashes. X-linked KFSD lacks severe inflammation. In our study of the largest known pedigree, hyperkeratosis of the knees (Fig. 130.5) and calcaneal region of the soles was noted, together with a high cuticle on the nails (Fig. 130.6) [9].

Symptoms are never present at birth and generally develop in early childhood. Complete spontaneous improvement often occurs at puberty [9]. Full expression of KFSD in a woman has been described [30]. An autosomal dominant variant has also been described. In these cases, the inflammation becomes worse in adulthood [31].

Of female carriers of X-linked KFSD, 50% are asymptomatic [9]. Symptomatic female carriers develop dry skin, minimal follicular hyperkeratosis and mild hyperkeratosis of the soles, but have no eye findings.

Phrynoderma

Nicholls observed hyperkeratotic folliculitis in some African labourers who suffered from vitamin A deficiency [32]. Keratosis pilaris-like eruption has been noted to occur after intestinal bypass [33]. Phrynoderma has not been described extensively in children.

Prognosis. Keratosis pilaris resolves completely in at least one-third of cases. Lesions involving the arms and legs are more likely to persist into adulthood than facial lesions. Most cases of keratosis pilaris atrophicans result in atrophy, without persistent inflammation [11,12].

Differential diagnosis. Normally, the diagnosis of keratosis pilaris is not difficult. Keratosis pilaris involving the face may mimic milia, miliaria and acne vulgaris. Other childhood causes of follicular keratoses include pityriasis rubra pilaris and Darier disease. Early cases of keratosis pilaris atrophicans faciei may be confused with the common form of keratosis pilaris, and late forms with seborrhoeic dermatitis. Atrophoderma vermiculata may be misdiagnosed as acne vulgaris or lupoid sycosis.

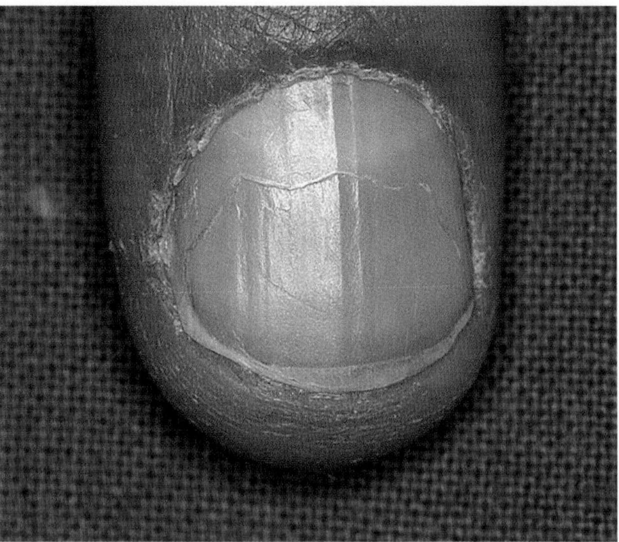

Fig. 130.6 A prominent cuticle of the nails in keratosis follicularis spinulosa decalvans (nonspecific sign).

Treatment. There is no effective therapy for keratosis pilaris. Emollients are rarely effective. Mild, temporary relief can be obtained with keratolytic agents, such as 10% urea. Response to all therapies (keratolytics, antibiotics, corticosteroids and retinoids) is limited.

Treatment with different lasers show limited results; a recent trial showed improvement in roughness but not in redness [34,35]

References

1 McKusick VA. Mendelian Inheritance in Man, 13th edn. Baltimore: Johns Hopkins University Press, 1995.
2 Rand RE, Arndt KA. Follicular syndromes with inflammation and atrophy. In: Fitzpatrick TB, Eisen AZ, Wolff K et al. (eds) Dermatology in General Medicine, 3rd edn. New York: McGraw Hill, 1979:717–21.
3 Touraine A. Essai de classification des keratoses congenitales. Ann Dermatol 1958;85:257–66.
4 Eramo LR, Burton Esterly N, Zieserl EJ et al. Ichthyosis follicularis with alopecia and photophobia. Arch Dermatol 1985;121:1167–74.
5 Lesser E. Ichthyosis follicularis. In: Eiemssen N (ed.) Handbook of Skin Diseases. New York: William Wood, 1885.
6 Lameris HJ. Ichthyosis follicularis. Ned Tijdschr Geneeskd (Dutch J Med) 1905;41:1524.
7 Rochat GF. Familiaire cornea degeneratie. Ned Tijdschr Geneeskd (Dutch J Med) 1906;42:515–18.
8 Siemens HW. Keratosis follicularis spinulosa decalvans. Arch Dermatol Syph 1926;151:384–7.
9 Van Osch LDM, Oranje AP, Keukens FM et al. Keratosis follicularis spinulosa decalvans. J Med Genet 1992;29:36–40.
10 Aten E, Brasz LC, Bornholdt D et al. keratosis follicularis spinulosa decalvans is caused by mutations in MBTPS2. Hum Mutat 2010; 31:1125–33.
11 Poskitt L, Wilkinson JD. Natural history of keratosis pilaris. Br J Dermatol 1994;130:711–13.
12 Oranje AP, van Osch LDM, Oosterwijk JC. Keratosis pilaris atrophicans. Arch Dermatol 1994;130:500–2.
13 Braunstein I, Gangadhar TC, Elenitsas R, Chu EY. Vemurafenib-induced interface dermatitis manifesting as radiation-recall and a keratosis pilaris-like eruption. J Cutan Pathol 2014;41:539–43.
14 Klar J, Schuster J, Khan TN et al. Whole exome sequencing identifies LRP1 as a pathogenic gene in autosomal recessive keratosis pilaris atrophicans. J Med Genet 2015;52:599–606.
15 Richard G, Harth W. Keratosis follicularis spinulosa decalvans. Therapie mit Isotretinoin und Etretinat im entzundlichen Stadium. Hautarzt 1993;44:529–34.

16 Oosterwijk JC, Nelen M, van Zandvoort PM et al. Linkage analysis of keratosis follicularis spinulosa decalvans, and regional assignment to human chromosome Xp21.2–p22.2. Am J Hum Genet 1992;50:801–7.
17 Oosterwijk JC, van der Wielen MJ, van de Vosse E et al. Refinement of the localisation of the X linked keratosis follicularis spinulosa decalvans (KFSD) gene in Xp22.13–p22.2. J Med Genet 1995;32:736–9.
18 Oosterwijk JC, Richard G, van der Wielen MJ et al. Molecular genetic analysis of two families with keratosis follicularis spinulosa decalvans: refinement of gene localisation and evidence for genetic heterogeneity. Hum Genet 1997;100:520–4.
19 Khumalo NP, Loo WJ, Hollowood K et al. Keratosis pilaris atrophicans in mother and daughter. J Eur Acad Dermatol Venereol 2002; 16:397–400.
20 Sallakachart P, Nakjang Y. Keratosis pilaris: a clinicohistopathologic study. J Med Assoc Thai 1987;70:386–9
21 Mevorah B, Marazzi A, Frenk E. The prevalence of accentuated palmoplantar marking and keratosis pilaris in atopic dermatitis, autosomal dominant ichthyosis and control dermatological patients. Br J Dermatol 1985;112:679–85
22 Guillet G, Sanciaume C, Hennunestre JP et al. Keratose pilaire generalis ée. Ann Dermatol Vénéréol 1982;109:1061–6.
23 Larrègue M, Charpentier C, Laidet B et al. Déficit en prolidase et en manganese. Ann Dermatol Vénéréol 1982;109:667–8.
24 Finn OA, Grant PW, McCallum DI et al. A singular dermatosis of Mongols. Arch Dermatol 1978;114:1493–4.
25 Marks R. Follicular hyperkeratosis and ocular abnormalities associated with Fairbank's syndrome. Br J Dermatol 1967;79:118–19.
26 Ward KA, Moss C, McKeown C. The cardio-facio-cutaneous syndrome: a manifestation of the Noonan syndrome? Br J Dermatol 1994;131:270–4.
27 Pierini DO, Pierini AM. Keratosis pilaris atrophicans faciei (ulerythema oophryogenes): a cutaneous marker of Noonan's syndrome. Br J Dermatol 1979;100:409–16.
28 Neild VS, Pegum JS, Wells RS. The association of keratosis pilaris atrophicans and woolly hair, with and without Noonan's syndrome. Br J Dermatol 1984;110:357–62.
29 Arrieta E, Milgram-Sternberg Y. Honeycomb atrophy on the right cheek. Arch Dermatol 1994;130:481–2.
30 Harth W, Richard G, Schubert H. Keratosis follicularis spinulosa decalvans: the complete syndrome in a female (in German). Z Hautkr 1992;67:1080–4.
31 Khumalo NP, Loo WJ, Hollowood K et al. Keratosis pilaris atrophicans in mother and daughter. J Eur Acad Dermatol Venereol 2002; 16:397–400.
32 Nicholls L. Phrynoderma: a condition due to vitamin deficiency. Ind Med Gazette 1933;68:681–7.
33 Barr RJ, Riley RJ. Bypass phynoderma. Arch Dermatol 1984;120: 919–21.
34 Ibrahim O, Khan M, Bolotin D et al. Treatment of keratosis pilaris with 810-nm diode laser. JAMA Dermatol 2015;151:187–91.
35 Lee SJ, Choi MJ, Zheng Z et al. Combination of 595-nm pulsed dye laser, long-pulsed 755-nm alexandrite laser, and microdermabrasion treatment for keratosis pilaris: retrospective analysis of 26 Korean patients J Cosmet Laser Ther 2013;15:150–4.

Darier disease

Definition and history. Darier disease (DD) is a rare keratinizing disorder with an autosomal dominant inheritance, first reported in 1889 in France by Darier and in the USA by White [1–6].

Epidemiology and pathogenesis. The prevalence of DD is reported to range from 1/30 000 to 100 000 [1–3]. This rare autosomal dominantly inherited skin disorder is caused by mutations in *ATP2A2*, which is expressed in both the skin and the brain and encodes for SERCA2 [7]. Inheritance is autosomal dominant with complete penetrance, but variable expression. Studies suggest a prevalence of around 1 in 30 000 in the UK [1,8]. *ATP2A2*, the defective gene in Darier disease, encodes the p-type cation pump, sarco/endoplasmic reticulum Ca^{2+}-ATPase isoform 2 (SERCA2), the pump that maintains intraluminal Ca^{2+} in the endoplasmic reticulum (ER) of keratinocytes [9].

The ER Ca^{2+} pool is required for intracellular signalling as well as for the correct folding, sorting and post-translational processing of proteins. Most mutations cause complete or partial loss of function of SERCA2 [6] and haploinsufficiency is the primary mechanism of dominant inheritance. A variety of mutations have been described but few correlations demonstrated between genotype and phenotype. Postzygotic mosaicism for *ATP2A2* mutations causes unilateral or 'segmental' DD [10]. Some cases of acrokeratosis verruciformis of Hopf can also be attributed to mutations in the Darier gene and might be better classified as a form of DD [11,12].

DD is characterized by loss of intercellular adhesion (acantholysis) and abnormal keratinization [13]. The pathogenesis of DD is incompletely understood, but one of the earliest changes is disruption of desmosomes, the adhesion junctions that mechanically couple keratinocytes. It seems likely that intracellular signalling is abnormal and that the depletion of the ER Ca^{2+} pool also destabilizes desmosomes by altering the folding of desmosomal proteins or their sorting and trafficking to the cell membrane. Reduced ER Ca^{2+} also enhances the influx of Ca^{2+} into the cytosol through plasma membrane channels and this may stimulate cell proliferation [14]. Alterations in the epidermal calcium gradient combined with activation of apoptosis appear to contribute to abnormal differentiation [15,16]. Savignac and colleagues (2014) illustrated that endoplasmic stress impairs the formation of both adherens junctions and desmosomes, and showed that ER Ca^{2+} signalling may control not only keratinocyte growth and differentiation, but also cell-to-cell adhesions [17].

External factors such as ultraviolet-B, heat and oral lithium may exacerbate disease by reducing transcription of *ATP2A2* and decreasing the already haploinsufficient SERCA2 protein to a critical level [18–20].

Clinical features. Expression of the disease varies, but males and females are affected with equal frequency. More than 60% of patients develop signs between the ages of 6 and 20, with onset peaking between the ages of 11 and 15. Congenital DD has been reported but is rare [21].

DD is characterized by brown, keratotic papules of sizes varying from pin-head to millet seed which develop in seborrhoeic areas such as the forehead, central chest, back and scalp margins [4]. More than 95% of patients have acral involvement and children may have hand involvement before any other signs of the disease. In one study, seven of 13 children had nail involvement, eight had palmar pits and 10 had acrokeratosis verruciformis. Only three of these children had the typical rash of DD [8].

The most specific acral sign of DD is a combination of longitudinal red and white lines extending from the base to the free edge of the nail plate. These may be associated with V-shaped notching of the free edge of the nail, subungual hyperkeratosis or splinter haemorrhages (Fig. 130.7). The nails are fragile so they break and split, but at first these changes may be attributed to nail biting. Most patients have pits or punctate keratotic papules on palms and soles. The fine palmar pits are easier to detect in children by using palm prints [8]. Children may develop haemorrhagic macules or blisters on the hands and feet, but these are uncommon [2]. Discrete flat-topped warty papules (acrokeratosis verruciformis) are an early sign on the backs of the hands and feet (Fig. 130.8). The skin-coloured papules are always bilateral.

The greasy, crusted papules in DD are flesh-coloured, yellow or brown (Fig. 130.9) but in pigmented skin, DD may present as hypopigmented macules and papules (Fig. 130.10) [22–24]. Papules appear on seborrhoeic areas of the trunk, the supraclavicular fossae, the sides of the neck, the forehead, the ears and the scalp. At first the lesions are discrete but later may coalesce into crusted, malodorous plaques. Itching is common but not invariable. Pain is unusual in uncomplicated disease. Most patients have some flexural involvement; occasionally this is severe.

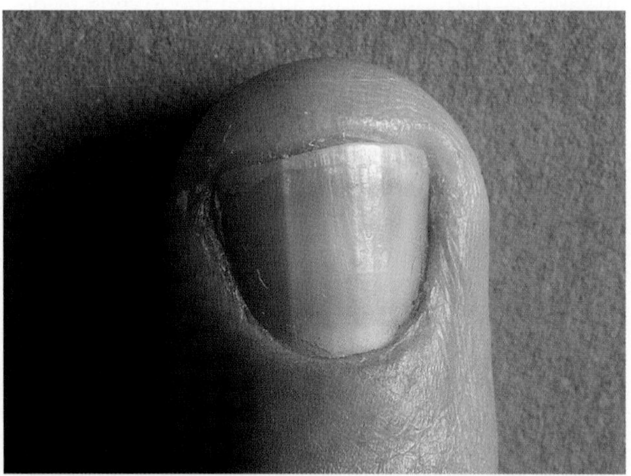

Fig. 130.7 Longitudinal red and white lines in the nail are an early sign of Darier disease. These may be associated with nail fragility, notching and splitting.

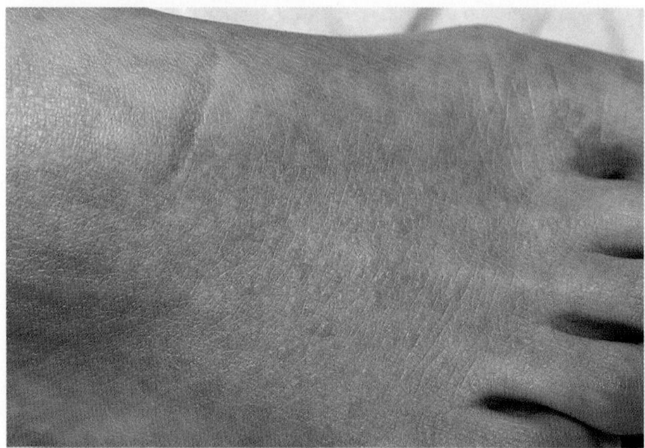

Fig. 130.8 Small flesh-coloured papules of acrokeratosis verruciformis are scattered over the dorsum of both feet in this patient with Darier disease.

Fig. 130.9 The crusted papules on the chest are yellowish-brown and rather greasy. Some are coalescing into plaques.

Fig. 130.10 Darier disease may present with hypopigmented lesions in children with pigmented skin. This child had typical hyperpigmented papules in addition to hypopigmented macules and papules.

The condition is usually mild in children, so the rash is often overlooked until summer, when symptoms and signs are exacerbated by heat or sweating. Lesions may develop 1–2 weeks after an episode of sunburn [25,26].

Mucosal involvement has been described in some patients, including salivary gland obstruction [27]. Papules or verrucous plaques develop on the palate, alveolar ridges, buccal mucosa or tongue (Fig. 130.11).

Children who are mosaic for the Darier mutation may present with localized disease [10,28–30]. Keratotic papules appear on one side of the body in streaks or whorls following Blaschko's lines. Palmar pits and nail changes may be present on the same side of the body. Heat, sweating and sunburn also aggravate segmental disease.

Complications. Patients are prone to widespread cutaneous infections, but no specific or consistent abnormality in immune function has been demonstrated [31]. Herpes simplex infection causes erythema, vesiculation, erosions, crusting and pain. The possibility of herpetic infection should be considered in any patient with a painful exacerbation, even if vesicles are not obvious. Infection with *Staphylococcus aureus* may also cause blisters. Secondary

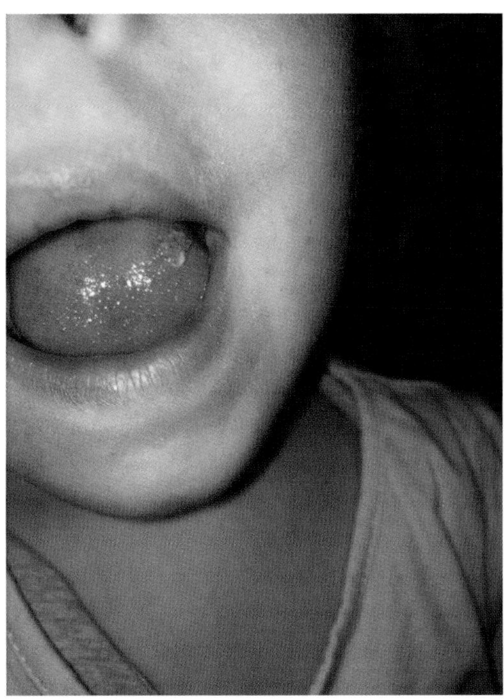

Fig. 130.11 Papilloma of the tongue in children could be an initiating symptom of Darier Disease. The differential diagnosis is HPV infection and lymphangioma.

bacterial overgrowth is common in the keratotic debris and may contribute to malodour.

Associated conditions. Bipolar affective disorder and mental impairment have been described in some patients, but the prevalence of these conditions in DD is low [2]. A gene that confers susceptibility to bipolar affective disorder may be present in the Darier region [32–34]. Lithium exacerbates DD and if possible should be avoided for the treatment of bipolar affective disorder in these patients [35,36].

Prognosis. DD is chronic and life-long, but severity is unpredictable and fluctuates. Some patients always have relatively mild disease, whereas in others the condition worsens inexorably. Occasionally patients do improve in old age [2].

Differential diagnosis.

Clinical

Crusted plaques on the trunk, flexural papules and scaling on the scalp may suggest seborrhoeic dermatitis. Comedones with keratotic papules on the face or chest may be misdiagnosed as acne. Acrokeratosis verruciformis may simulate plane warts. Solitary longitudinal red or white lines in the nails may indicate a subungual tumour.

Flexural DD may simulate Hailey–Hailey disease, but Hailey–Hailey disease usually presents in the third decade and is characterized by painful erosions without keratotic papules. Nails in Hailey–Hailey disease may also have longitudinal white lines, but are not fragile as they are in DD [37]. Palmar pits have also been described in Hailey–Hailey disease.

Benign forms of acanthosis nigricans may develop during childhood. Flexural skin is pigmented, thickened and papillomatous, but the soft tags differ from the warty papules of Darier disease. Confluent and reticulate papillomatosis presents around puberty, usually in girls. The flat, brown papules appear between the breasts and in the middle of the back, and gradually spread across the trunk. Although the distribution and colour may suggest Darier disease, the papules are not hyperkeratotic. Lesions of the tongue or palatum could be misdiagnosed as condylomata acuminata.

Histology findings

Histological features include separation between suprabasal epidermal cells (acantholysis) with proliferative 'budding' at the base of lesions and a distinctive dyskeratosis (Fig. 130.12). Narrow intraepidermal clefts or lacunae containing acantholytic cells form above the basal cells. Dyskeratotic keratinocytes, known as corps ronds and grains, contain clumped cytokeratin filaments and cytoplasmic vacuoles [38,39]. Corps ronds in the spinous and granular layers have a central homogeneous nucleus surrounded by a clear halo. Grains with elongated pyknotic nuclei surrounded by homogeneous dyskeratotic material are seen in or just below the horny layer.

Immunoelectron microscopy indicates that some desmosomal glycoproteins are quantitatively less concentrated in perilesional epidermis [40]. Lesional keratinocytes express keratins and extracellular matrix components characteristic of hyperproliferation [41,42]. Involucrin is also expressed prematurely [43]. In acantholytic cells, the extracellular domains of desmogleins are lost, whereas intracellular domains of desmogleins and desmosomal plaque proteins are distributed diffusely in the cytoplasm, where they may be trapped in tonofilament aggregates [40,44–47].

Acantholytic dyskeratosis is a feature of Hailey–Hailey disease, but acantholysis is more widespread and dyskeratosis less severe than in Darier disease. Acantholytic dyskeratosis is also seen in transient or persistent acantholytic

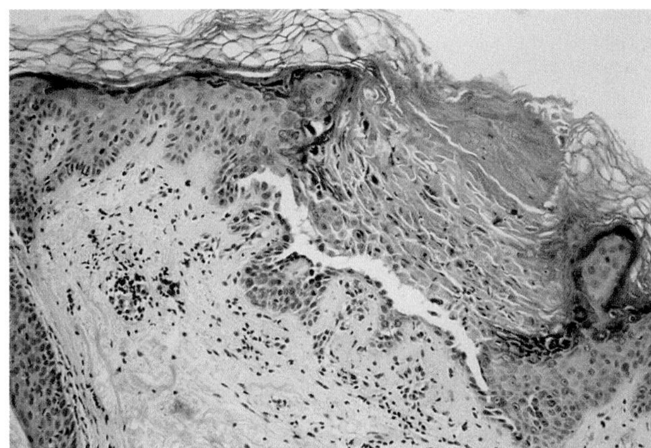

Fig. 130.12 The hyperkeratotic papule in this biopsy shows typical features of Darier disease. The suprabasal cleft contains acantholytic cells. Dyskeratotic cells are present in the granular layer and the horny plug (×200; stain H&E).

dermatosis (Grover disease) but this condition affects adults, not children. Localized perineal papules and plaques with acantholytic histology have been described in children and adults, but the relationship of this condition to DD is uncertain [48,49].

Treatment. There are no currently validated curative treatments available for Darier disease, with the majority of cases treated symptomatically [4]. Lifestyle advice is important in eliminating exacerbating factors such as high temperatures, high humidity, ultraviolet rays and mechanical irritation. [4]

Information, explanation and education are important issues in the care of children with DD and their families. Genetic counselling should be offered. Written information may be helpful for the family, as well as for schoolteachers or employers. Teenagers should be advised to avoid careers that will involve work in hot or sweaty conditions.

Children reluctant to reveal the affected skin or to participate in activities such as swimming will need psychological support, some of which may be provided by a paediatric-trained dermatology nurse or clinical psychologist. Older children may appreciate cosmetic camouflage, including artificial nails.

Treatment must be tailored to the child. Those with mild disease may not need specific treatment. Itching is the most troublesome symptom, but cool cotton clothing, sun avoidance and sun protection creams will reduce exacerbations in the summer. Emollients used as a soap substitute may reduce irritation and crusting. Emollients containing urea or lactic acid may reduce hyperkeratosis, but often sting. A mild or moderately potent topical corticosteroid may reduce irritation. Topical corticosteroids may be prescribed in combination with an antibiotic to reduce secondary infection in crusted plaques or malodorous flexural disease. Antiseptics may be helpful in the bath. Antiviral treatment with aciclovir should be considered in any child with a painful exacerbation in view of the possibility of a herpetic superinfection.

Retinoids, the vitamin A derivatives, are the most effective treatments for moderate to severe Darier disease. Topical retinoids reduce hyperkeratosis, but irritation limits efficacy. Adapalene cream or tazarotene gel may be better tolerated than isotretinoin gel or tretinoin cream [50–53,54]. Retinoids may be combined with mild topical corticosteroids to reduce inflammation.

The oral retinoids, acitretin and isotretinoin, are of value in severe Darier disease. Acitretin 0.6 mg/kg/day has been recommended for long-term treatment of inherited disorders of keratinization in children, but side-effects must be monitored carefully, particularly liver function [55,56]. Isotretinoin, 0.5–1 mg/kg/day, is not as effective in disorders of keratinization but is a more suitable choice than acitretin for teenage girls because of its comparatively short half-life. All oral retinoids are teratogenic. Pregnancy must be avoided during treatment and for 2 years after stopping acitretin (or etretinate) or for 1 month after stopping isotretinoin. Dose-related side-effects include mucosal dryness, nosebleeds, skin fragility, itching and elevated triglycerides, cholesterol and liver enzymes. Retinoids may cause skeletal hyperostosis and extraosseous calcification, but the long-term significance of these changes is not known.

Doxycycline may be an interesting treatment option in older children with DD, as mentioned in a case report in a 77-year-old patient with a 57-year history of DD. Mechanism of action may be caused by powerful metal chelation properties of tetracyclines. Tetracyclines bind divalent metal cations and circulate in blood plasma primarily as calcium and magnesium chelators. Chelated tetracyclines can act as ionophores capable of transporting bound calcium and magnesium through lipophilic phases. These lipophilic phases are present in cellular membranes, and so chelated tetracyclines may deliver ions into intracellular compartments [13].

Oral contraceptives have been recommended to treat females with DD [57] but this strategy has not been subjected to randomized controlled trials and no consistent relationship has been demonstrated to the menstrual cycle.

New insights and molecular knowledge may lead to new treatment modalities in the future. SERCA2 dysfunction in DD causes ER stress and impaired cell-to-cell adhesion strength. Treatment with miglustat, used for Gaucher disease, also acts to inhibit glucosylceramide synthetase, and may modulate the ceramide/sphingolipid pathway, playing a role in the pathogenesis of Darier disease. Miglustat acts as a chaperone, and allows adhesion molecules to escape from the ER stress-induced unfolded protein response. Because of this, the adhesion molecules will be able to reach the plasma membrane, and form adherens junctions and desmosomes. In summary, miglustat may facilitate redistribution of adhesion molecules to plasma membrane [17].

Acknowledgement

The authors are grateful to Susan M. Burge, dermatologist, for her work on the Darier Disease chapter in the previous edition.

References

1 **Tavadia S, Mortimer E, Munro CS. Genetic epidemiology of Darier's disease: a population study in the west of Scotland. Br J Dermatol 2002;146:107–9.**
2 Burge SM, Wilkinson JD. Darier–White disease: a review of the clinical features in 163 patients. J Am Acad Dermatol 1992;27:40–50.
3 Svendsen I, Alberchtsen B. The prevalence of dyskeratosis follicularis in Denmark. An investigation into heredity in 22 families. Acta Derm Venereol 1959;39:256–9.
4 Takagi A, Kamijo M, Ikeda S. Darier disease. Review article. J Dermatol 2016;43:275–9.
5 **White J. A case of keratosis (ichthyosis) follicularis. J Cutan Genito-Urin Dis 1889;7:201–9.**
6 Darier J. Psorospermose folliculaire vëgëtant. Ann Dermatol Syphilol 1889;10:597–612.
7 Green EK, Gordon-Smith K, Burge Susan M et al. Novel ATP2A2 mutations in a large sample of individuals with Darier disease. J Dermatol 2013;40:259–66.
8 Munro CS. The phenotype of Darier's disease: penetrance and expressivity in adults and children. Br J Dermatol 1992;127:126–30.
9 Hovnanian A. Darier's disease: from dyskeratosis to endoplasmic reticulum calcium ATPase deficiency. Biochem Biophys Res Commun 2004;322:1237–44.

SECTION 27: DISORDERS OF KERATIN AND KERATINIZATION

10 Sakuntabhai A, Dhitavat J, Burge S et al. Mosaicism for ATP2A2 mutations causes segmental Darier's disease. J Invest Dermatol 2000;115: 1144–7.

11 Macfarlane CS, McSween R, Sakuntabhai A et al. Acrokeratosis verruciformis of Hopf is caused by mutation in ATP2A2, the gene which is defective in Darier's disease. Br J Dermatol 2000;143:47.

12 Braun-Falco M, Fesq H, Ring J et al. Acrokeratosis verruciformis Hopf als minimal variante des M. Darier (Acrokeratosis verruciformis Hopf as a minimal manifestation of Darier's disease). H+G Zeitschrift fur Hautkrankheiten 2001;76:449–52.

13 Sfecci A, Orion C, Darrieux L et al. Extensive Darier disease successfully treated with doxycycline monotherapy. Case Rep Dermatol 2015;7:311–315.

14 Pani B, Singh BB. Darier's disease: a calcium-signaling perspective. Cell Mol Life Sci 2008;65:205–11.

15 Pasmatzi E, Badavanis G, Monastirli A et al. Reduced expression of the antiapoptotic proteins of Bcl-2 gene family in the lesional epidermis of patients with Darier's disease. J Cutan Pathol 2007;34:234–8.

16 Leinonen PT, Hagg PM, Peltonen S et al. Reevaluation of the normal epidermal calcium gradient, and analysis of calcium levels and ATP receptors in Hailey–Hailey and Darier epidermis. J Invest Dermatol 2009;129:1379–87.

17 Savignac M, Simon M, Edir A et al. SERCA2 dysfunction in Darier disease causes endoplasmic reticulum stress and impaired cell-to-cell adhesion strength: rescue by Miglustat. J Invest Dermatol 2014;134:1961–70.

18 Mayuzumi N, Ikeda S, Kawada H et al. Effects of ultraviolet B irradiation, proinflammatory cytokines and raised extracellular calcium concentration on the expression of ATP2A2 and ATP2C1. Br J Dermatol 2005;152:697–701.

19 Mayuzumi N, Ikeda S, Kawada H et al. Effects of drugs and anticytokine antibodies on expression of ATP2A2 and ATP2C1 in cultured normal human keratinocytes. Br J Dermatol 2005;152:920–4.

20 Sule N, Teszas A, Kalman E et al. Lithium suppresses epidermal SERCA2 and PMR1 levels in the rat. Pathol Oncol Res 2006;12:234–6.

21 Fong G, Capaldi L, Sweeney SM et al. Congenital Darier disease. J Am Acad Dermatol 2008;59:S50–1.

22 Berth-Jones J, Hutchinson PE. Darier's disease with peri-follicular depigmentation. Br J Dermatol 1989;120:827–30.

23 Ohtake N, Takano R, Saitoh A et al. Brown papules and leukoderma in Darier's disease: clinical and histological features. Dermatology 1994;188:157–9.

24 Peterson CM, Lesher JL Jr, Sangueza OP. A unique variant of Darier's disease. Int J Dermatol 2001;40:278–80.

25 Baba T, Yaoita H. UV radiation and keratosis follicularis. Arch Dermatol 1984;120:1484–7.

26 Hedblad MA, Nakatani T, Beitner H. Ultrastructural changes in Darier's disease induced by ultraviolet irradiation. Acta Dermato-Venereol 1991;71:108–12.

27 Macleod RI, Munro CS. The incidence and distribution of oral lesions in patients with Darier's disease. Br Dent J 1991;171:133–6.

28 Starink T, Woerdeman MJ. Unilateral systematized keratosis follicularis. A variant of Darier's disease or an epidermal naevus (acantholytic dyskeratotic epidermal naevus)? Br J Dermatol 1981;105:207–14.

29 Munro CS, Cox NH. An acantholytic dyskeratotic epidermal naevus with other features of Darier's disease on the same side of the body. Br J Dermatol 1992;127:168–71.

30 Itin PH, Buchner SA, Happle R. Segmental manifestation of Darier disease. What is the genetic background in type 1 and type 2 mosaic phenotypes? Dermatology 2000;200:254–7.

31 Patrizi A, Ricci G, Neri I et al. Immunological parameters in Darier's disease. Dermatologica 1989;178:138–40.

32 Jacobsen NJ, Franks EK, Elvidge G et al. Exclusion of the Darier's disease gene, ATP2A2, as a common susceptibility gene for bipolar disorder. Mol Psychiatry 2001;6:92–7.

33 Jones I, Jacobsen N, Green EK et al. Evidence for familial cosegregation of major affective disorder and genetic markers flanking the gene for Darier's disease. Mol Psychiatry 2002;7:424–7.

34 Green E, Elvidge G, Jacobsen N et al. Localization of bipolar susceptibility locus by molecular genetic analysis of the chromosome 12q23-q24 region in two pedigrees with bipolar disorder and Darier's disease. Am J Psychiatry 2005;162:35–42.

35 Clark R Jr, Hammer CJ, Patterson SD. A cutaneous disorder (Darier's disease) evidently exacerbated by lithium carbonate. Psychosomatics 1986;27:800–1.

36 Ehrt U, Brieger P. Comorbidity of keratosis follicularis (Darier's Disease) and bipolar affective disorder: an indication for valproate instead of lithium. Gen Hosp Psychiatry 2000;22:128–9.

37 Burge SM. Hailey–Hailey disease: the clinical features, response to treatment and prognosis. Br J Dermatol 1992;126:275–82.

38 Gottlieb S, Lutzner M. Darier's disease. An electron microscopic study. Arch Dermatol 1973;107:225–30.

39 Mesquita-Guimarïes J, Mesquita-Guimarïes I. Cellular differentiation in Darier's disease. Ultrastructural aspects. J Submicrosc Cytol 1984; 16:387–94.

40 Tada J, Hashimoto K. Ultrastructural localization of cell junctional components (desmoglein, plakoglobin, E-cadherin, and beta-catenin) in Hailey–Hailey disease, Darier's disease, and pemphigus vulgaris. J Cutan Pathol 1998;25:106–15.

41 Burge SM, Fenton DA, Dawber RPR et al. Darier's disease: an immunohistochemical study using monoclonal antibodies to human cytokeratins. Br J Dermatol 1988;118:629–40.

42 Steijlen PM, Maessen E, Kresse H et al. Expression of tenascin, biglycan and decorin in disorders of keratinization. Br J Dermatol 1994;130:564–8.

43 Kassar S, Charfeddine C, Zribi H et al. Immunohistological study of involucrin expression in Darier's disease skin. J Cutan Pathol 2008;35: 635–40.

44 Burge SM, Garrod DR. An immunohistological study of desmosomes in Darier's disease and Hailey–Hailey disease. Br J Dermatol 1991;124: 242–51.

45 Burge SM, Schomberg K. Adhesion molecules and related proteins in Darier's disease and Hailey–Hailey disease. Br J Dermatol 1992;127: 335–43.

46 Hashimoto K, Fujiwara K, Tada J et al. Desmosomal dissolution in Grover's disease, Hailey–Hailey's disease and Darier's disease. J Cutan Pathol 1995;22:488–501.

47 Hakuno M, Shimizu H, Akiyama M et al. Dissociation of intra- and extracellular domains of desmosomal cadherins and E-cadherin in Hailey–Hailey disease and Darier's disease. Br J Dermatol 2000;142: 702–11.

48 Salopek TG, Krol A, Jimbow K. Case report of Darier disease localized to the vulva in a 5-year-old girl. Pediatr Dermatol 1993;10:146–8.

49 Wong TY, Mihm MC Jr. Acantholytic dermatosis localized to genitalia and crural areas of male patients: a report of three cases. J Cutan Pathol 1994;21:27–32.

50 Burge SM, Buxton PK. Topical isotretinoin in Darier's disease. Br J Dermatol 1995;133:924–8.

51 English JC 3rd, Browne J, Halbach DP. Effective treatment of localized Darier's disease with adapalene 0.1% gel. Cutis 1999;63: 227–30.

52 Micali G, Nasca MR. Tazarotene gel in childhood Darier disease. Pediatr Dermatol 1999;16:243–4.

53 Cianchini G, Colonna L, Camaioni D et al. Acral Darier's disease successfully treated with adapalene. Acta Derm Venereol 2001;81:57–8.

54 Abe M, Inoue C, Yokoyama Y et al. Successful treatment of Darier's disease with adapalene gel. Pediatr Dermatol 2011;28:197–8.

55 Christophersen J, Geiger JM, Danneskiold Samsoe P et al. A double blind comparison of acitretin and etretinate in the treatment of Darier's disease. Acta Dermato-Venereol 1992;72:150–2.

56 Lacour M, Atherton DJ, Harper JI. An appraisal of acetretin treatment in children with inherited disorders of keratinisation. JEADV 1995;5(suppl 1): S109.

57 Oostenbrink JH, Cohen EB, Steijlen PM et al. Oral contraceptives in the treatment of Darier–White disease – a case report and review of the literature. Clin Exp Dermatol 1996;21:442–4.

CHAPTER 131
The Erythrokeratodermas

Juliette Mazereeuw-Hautier[1], *S. Leclerc-Mercier*[2] *& E. Bourrat*[3]

[1] Reference Center for Rare Skin Diseases, Dermatology Department, CHU Larrey, Toulouse, France
[2] Reference Center for Rare and Inherited Skin Diseases (MAGEC), Departments of Dermatology and Pathology, CHU Necker-Enfants Malades, Paris, France
[3] Reference Center for Inherited Skin Disease, Dermatology Department, CHU Saint Louis, Paris, France

Abstract

Erythrokeratoderma is a clinical term that refers to a group of inherited disorders with both clinical and genetic heterogeneity. Lesions usually start in infancy and are clinically characterized by localized and well demarcated erythematous and hyperkeratotic plaques, sometimes with a migratory nature. Lesions favour the extensor surface of the upper and lower extremities and they may involve palms and soles. Erythrokeratoderma is a genetic disease, often inherited as an autosomal dominant trait, caused by mutations in different genes including the connexin genes *GJB3*, *GJB4* and *GJA1*. Erythrokeratoderma in association with neurological anomalies and caused by *ELOVL4* has also been reported. Erythrokeratoderma must be clearly distinguished from other dermatoses with erythema and hyperkeratosis, either in a diffuse distribution, or restricted to palms and soles. Histopathological features are not specific but skin biopsy can sometimes be helpful. Symptomatic treatment includes local therapies with emollients, keratolytics or calcipotriol. Retinoids usually have a significant and prompt efficacy.

Key points

- **Erythrokeratoderma is characterized by localized, well demarcated and sometimes migratory, erythematous and hyperkeratotic plaques.**
- **Erythrokeratoderma is a genetic disease, often inherited as an autosomal dominant trait, caused by mutations in different genes including the connexin genes *GJB3*, *GJB4* and *GJA1*.**
- **Histopathological features are not specific but skin biopsy can sometimes be helpful.**
- **Symptomatic treatment includes local therapies with emollients, keratolytics or calcipotriol. Retinoids have a significant and prompt efficacy.**

Introduction and history. Erythrokeratoderma is a clinical term that refers to a group of inherited disorders characterized by localized and well-demarcated erythematous and hyperkeratotic plaques [1]. This definition clearly distinguishes erythrokeratoderma from other dermatoses with erythema and hyperkeratosis, either in a diffuse distribution, or restricted to palms and soles (palmoplantar keratodermas, PPK). Two major clinical types of erythrokeratodermas have initially been defined: erythrokeratoderma variabilis (EKV), a migratory form described by Mendes da Costa [2]; and progressive symmetric erythrokeratoderma (PSEK), a fixed form, first documented by Darier in 1911 [3] and later by Gottron in 1923 [4]. Later, following the report of EKV and PSEK within a single family [5] and the identification of the same gene mutation in patients with EKV [6] and PSEK [7], it was suggested that both forms of erythrokeratoderma were two clinical manifestations of the same disease, rather than two distinctive diseases. The designation 'erythrokeratoderma variabilis progressiva' (EKVP) was proposed to cover the diversity of clinical phenotypes of erythrokeratoderma [7].

Erythrokeratoderma annularis migrans or erythrokeratoderma en cocardes are old terms that can be found in the literature or textbooks.

Epidemiology and pathogenesis. EKVP is a rare skin disease whose prevalence can be estimated at around one in 2 000 000 people. Both sexes are equally affected.

EKVP is genetically heterogeneous and caused by mutations in different genes including the connexin genes. The connexins are proteins forming gap junctions. There are at least 10 different connexin proteins that are expressed in several organs, including the skin. Connexins are abundant in the epidermis and allow the transport and signalling between neighbouring cells.

In EKVP, causal mutations were found in the *GJB3* [7], *GJB4* [7] and *GJA1* [8] genes, encoding connexins 31, 30.3 and 43, respectively. These three connexin genes associated with EKVP are also linked to other clinical entities. Mutations in *GJB3* cause hearing loss, neuropathy and deafness [9]. Mutations in *GJA1* cause nonsyndromic deafness, oculo-dento-digital dysplasia, PPK and congenital alopecia [10,11].

The majority of EKVP cases follow an autosomal dominant mode of inheritance, but 40% of cases occur sporadically. Autosomal recessive inheritance has also been described and should be considered when providing genetic counselling, especially in consanguineous families.

Harper's Textbook of Pediatric Dermatology, Fourth Edition. Edited by Peter Hoeger, Veronica Kinsler and Albert Yan.

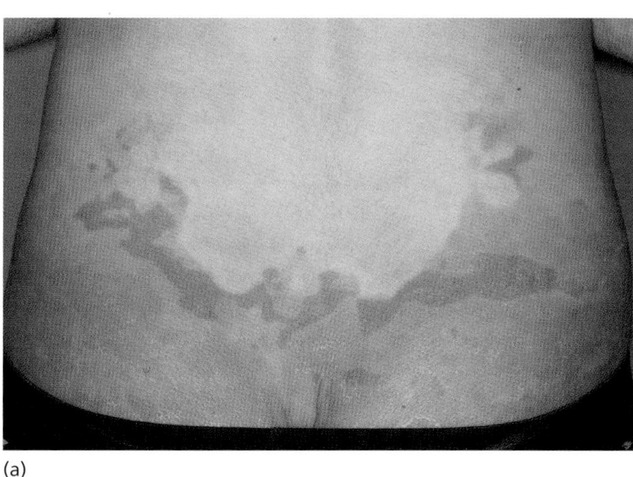

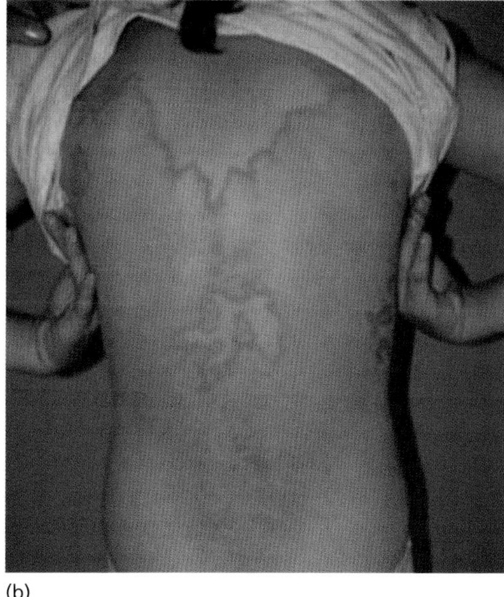

(a) (b)

Fig. 131.1 (a) and (b) Patients present with well-demarcated, erythematous and hyperkeratotic plaques with irregular and accentuated borders. Source: (b) courtesy of Dr E. Mahé.

Erythrokeratoderma in association with other anomalies and caused by other gene mutations have also been described. A heterozygote mutation in *ELOVL4* was identified in affected individuals from a family with autosomal dominant spinocerebellar ataxia and erythrokeratoderma [12]. The gene *ELOVL4* encodes a member of the elongase family, which is responsible for the elongation of very long-chain fatty acids. Patients presented with mild neurological and dermatological phenotype made of early-onset patches of erythema and hyperkeratosis. Mutations of this gene have also been reported in families with macular degeneration. Recently, homozygous mutations in *ELOVL4* were found in patients with ichthyosis, spastic paraplegia and severe neurodevelopmental defects [13].

Other genes are likely to be discovered in the future because some families with erythrokeratoderma (without associated anomalies) do not carry mutations in any of the genes discovered so far.

Clinical features. Erythrokeratoderma usually starts in the first months of life. Rarely, lesions may develop later, during late childhood or early adulthood. In some patients, erythema may be present at birth. The plaques tend to progress during childhood, with lesions stabilizing thereafter. Improvement in adulthood has rarely been reported.

Patients present with well-demarcated, erythematous and hyperkeratotic plaques with irregular and accentuated borders (Fig. 131.1). The severity of the lesions is variable. Lesions may be pigmented, especially if the skin is dark (Fig. 131.2). A fine scaling may be present. The lesions are arranged symmetrically and can occur at any site but favour the extensor surface of the upper and lower extremities, buttocks and face. The extension is variable: from localized to more widespread lesions. Minimal pruritus or a burning sensation may be noted. Considerable clinical overlap exists between PSEK and EKV, the main distinguishing feature being the presence of migratory erythema in patients with EKV. In this case, lesions migrate over time and last from hours to days. Erythema gyratum repens-like features, characterized by rapidly migrating figurate erythema 1–2 cm wide in an annular garland or spiral arrangement has been described in some patients [6,14]. The palms and soles are normal or exhibit PPK, usually in the form of a fine erythematous scaling

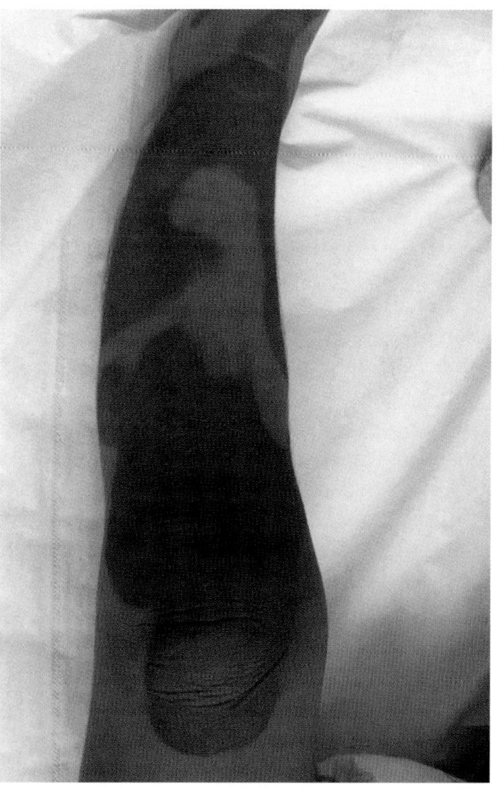

Fig. 131.2 Erythrokeratoderma presented as pigmented lesions in a child with dark skin. Source: Courtesy of Dr E. Mahé.

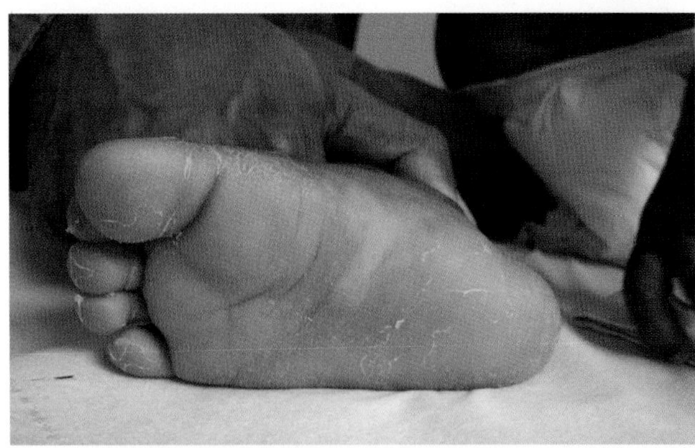

Fig. 131.3 Palms and soles exhibiting palmoplantar keratoderma in the form of a fine erythematous scaling. Source: Courtesy of Dr E. Mahé.

(Fig. 131.3). Patients carrying *GJA1* mutations may present with porcelain-white proximal nails [8]. Lesions are influenced by emotions, physical stressors such as temperature changes (lesions usually become worse in summer and improve in winter), friction or pressure, ultraviolet exposure and hormonal changes. A great variability of clinical features exists between different patients, patients from the same family, as well as in a single patient over time.

EKVP is not a life-threatening disease and general health is unaffected. Nevertheless, there is an impact on the patient's quality of life and it can be a social handicap because of the skin's appearance and symptoms.

Differential diagnosis.

Skin diseases with erythematous and hyperkeratotic lesions in a generalized distribution

Lesions in EKVP may be extensive but are not generalized and therefore should not be confused with other skin disorders such as inherited ichthyosis. The particular case of keratitis, ichthyosis and deafness (KID) syndrome (syndromic ichthyosis) caused by *CX26* mutations may be difficult to differentiate. Patients present with erythematous and hyperkeratotic lesions that are usually localized but are associated with diffuse hyperkeratosis. There are also associated anomalies such as PPK with leather-like appearance, keratitis, deafness and increased risk for squamous cell carcinomas.

Skin diseases with erythematous and hyperkeratotic lesions in a localized and well-demarcated pattern

EKVP must be distinguished from other skin diseases with erythematous and hyperkeratotic lesions in a localized and well-demarcated pattern. There are two types of situations, depending on the presence or absence of associated anomalies.

In case of associated anomalies, the diagnosis of MEDNIK (a unique syndrome characterized by mental retardation, enteropathy, deafness, peripheral neuropathy, ichthyosis, and keratodermia) caused by *AP1S1* mutations needs to be discussed [15].

If there are no associated anomalies, the differential diagnoses are as follows:

- Psoriasis may start in infancy and present with well-demarcated erythematous and hyperkeratotic plaques. Other members of the family may suffer from psoriasis;
- Pityriasis rubra pilaris is a papulo-squamous disorder phenotypically related to psoriasis. The disease has occasionally been shown to be inherited in an autosomal dominant fashion. All affected individuals show well-demarcated erythematous plaques coalescing into large areas interspersed with islands of normal skin, follicular papules or accentuation, PPK and a lack of psoriasis-associated nail changes. Histopathology of skin lesions showed alternating orthokeratosis and parakeratosis, acanthosis with broadening of the rete ridges, follicular plugging, lymphocytic infiltrate in the dermis and lack of neutrophils in the epidermis. Age of onset varied from 4 to 36 months of age. It was identified that pityriasis rubra pilaris was caused by heterozygous mutations in *CARD14*, a known activator of nuclear factor kappa B signalling, which has been implicated in other inflammatory disorders [16].
- Some variants of keratinopathic ichthyosis caused by mutations in the *KRT1* or *KRT10* genes may be confounded with EKVP, especially the annular form characterized by migratory erythematous plaques. Verrucous hyperkeratosis and PPK are also present in the Curth–Macklin form.
- Erythematous and hyperkeratotic lesions in a localized and well-demarcated pattern have been observed in a patient with KLICK syndrome. This patient also had a slight hyperkeratosis in a linear distribution on several folds and subtle digital constrictions bands [17].
- EKVP should also not be confused with hereditary PPKs that start in infancy. The differential diagnosis is easy when the lesions are strictly localized to palms and soles. Differential diagnosis is much more difficult if the lesions spread to the dorsal surfaces, posterior aspects of the forearms, anterior aspects of the legs, knees, elbows, the Achilles tendon or perioral areas. Nevertheless, contrarily to PPKs, palmoplantar lesions in EKVP are not at the foreground of the clinical features.
- Loricrine keratoderma, belonging to the group of PPK with ichthyosis, is an important differential diagnosis [18]. Loricrine keratoderma is caused by mutations in the loricrin gene. Skin lesions start at birth, sometimes presenting initially as a collodion baby [19,20] or later in infancy. The phenotype is heterogeneous and the severity is variable. Lesions can be generalized or located, closely resembling that of EKV. In case of localized lesions, the most distinctive, but inconstant feature, is the presence of a honeycomb PPK with digital constriction (pseudo-ainhum) (Fig. 131.4). Histology may help with the diagnosis (see below).

Laboratory and histology findings. The diagnosis of EKVP is based on the presence of characteristic clinical features. Histopathological features are not specific but skin biopsy can be helpful [21]. Stratum corneum is usually hyperorthokeratotic and sometimes parakeratotic. The epidermal acanthosis is irregular, with variably marked papillomatosis. A slight perivascular inflammatory infiltrate is observed in the dermis. There are some distinctive characteristics between PSEK and EKV. In EKV, the granular layer

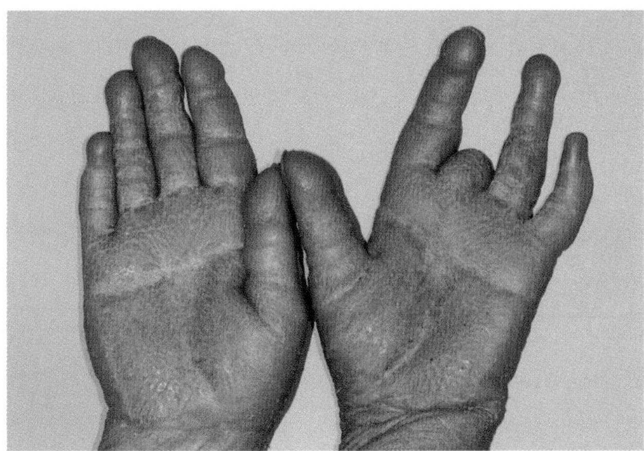

Fig. 131.4 Palmoplantar keratoderma with digital constriction (pseudo-ainhum) in a patient with loricrin keratoderma.

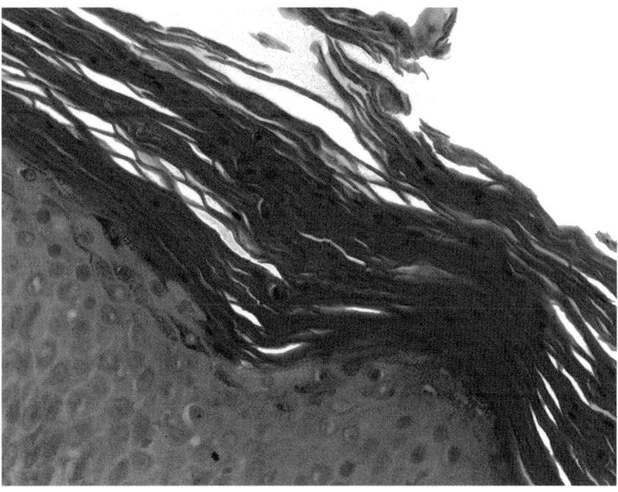

Fig. 131.5 Marked hyperkeratosis, dyskeratotic cell in the upper epidermis and aspect of 'remnant cells' in the stratum corneum (×400; stain H&E).

is present and appears normal. Electron microscopy was reported in different observations, revealing a diminished number of keratinosomes and perinuclear condensed keratin filaments. More specific aspects are seen in PSEK (Fig. 131.5) [22]. Parakeratosis is frequently present with big nuclei and sometimes an aspect of remnant cells. In the granular layer, cells can be vacuolated and basophilic granules can be observed. Dyskeratosis is not rare. Electron microscopy showed enlarged keratohyalin, large amounts of keratinosomes, and granular cells were described as having thin membrane structures and abnormal tubular structures. The horny layer can have more than 35 cells layers, with the presence of dyskeratotic cells and laminated inclusions.

Ichthyosis and loricrin keratoderma caused by loricrin mutations share some histological characteristics with EKVP. The epidermis is also psoriasiform with parakeratosis (which is reported as condensed crenelated basophilic nuclei). Electron microscopy shows intranuclear granules rich in loricrin in the stratum granulosum.

Treatment. There is no specific and curative treatment. Treatment is symptomatic and helps to reduce the thickness of the lesions and the redness to a lesser degree. Local therapies include emollients, topical keratolytics or calcipotriol (bioactive form of vitamin D_3) [23,24]. Oral therapies include low-dose acitretin or isotretinoin. If the patient is attempting a pregnancy, alitretin may also be used in the short term. Systemic retinoids must be used at low dose. Efficacy is usually very good and swift [25,26]. Some authors use retinoid plus psoralen and ultraviolet-A therapy [27]. Hopefully, novel therapies targeting connexin defects could be available in the future.

References

1 Ishida-Yamamoto A. Erythrokeratodermia variabilis et progressiva. J Dermatol 2016;43:280–5.
2 Mendes da Costa S. Erythrokeratodermia variabilis in a mother and a daughter. Acta Derm Venerol 1925;6:255–61.
3 Darier J. Erythro-keratodermie verruqueuse en nappes, symetrique et progressive. Bull Soc Fr Derm Syph 1911;22:252–64.
4 Gottron H. Congenital symmetrical progressive erythrokeratoderma. Arch Dermatol Syph 1923;7:416.
5 Macfarlane AW, Chapman SJ, Verbov JL. Is erythrokeratoderma one disorder? A clinical and ultrastructural study of two siblings. Br J Dermatol 1991;124:487–91.
6 Richard G, Brown N, Rouan F *et al.* Genetic heterogeneity in erythrokeratodermia variabilis: novel mutations in the connexin gene GJB4 (Cx30.3) and genotype-phenotype correlations. J Invest Derm 2003; 120:601–9.
7 Van Steensel MAM, Oranje AP, van der Schroeff JG et al. The missense mutation G12D in connexin30.3 can cause both erythrokeratodermia variabilis of Mendes da Costa and progressive symmetric erythrokeratodermia of Gottron. Am J Med Genet 2009;149:657–61.
8 Boyden LM, Craiglow BG, Zhou J et al. Dominant de novo mutations in GJA1 cause erythrokeratodermia variabilis et progressiva, without features of oculodentodigital dysplasia. J Invest Dermatol 2015;135: 1540–7.
9 Rabionet R, Gasparini P, Estivill X. Molecular genetics of hearing impairment due to mutations in gap junction genes encoding beta connexins. Hum Mutat 2000;16:190–202.
10 Duchatelet S, Hovnanian A. Erythrokeratodermia variabilis et progressive allelic to oculo-dento-digital dysplasia. J Invest Dermatol 2015;135:1475–8.
11 Wang H, Cao X, Lin Z et al. Exome sequencing reveals mutation in GJA1 as a cause of keratoderma-hypotrichosis-leukonychia totalis syndrome. Hum Mol Genet 2014;24:243–50.
12 Cadieux-Dion M, Turcotte-Gauthier M, Noreau A et al. Expanding the clinical phenotype associated with ELOVL4 mutation: study of a large French-Canadian family with autosomal dominant spinocerebellar ataxia and erythrokeratodermia. JAMA Neurol 2014;71:470–5.
13 Aldahmesh MA, Mohamed JY, Alkuraya HS et al. Recessive mutations in ELOVL4 cause ichthyosis, intellectual disability, and spastic quadriplegia. Am J Hum Genet 2011;89:745–50.
14 Macari F, Landau M, Cousin P et al. Mutation in the gene for connexin 30.3 in a family with erythrokeratodermia variabilis. Am J Hum Genet 2000;67:1296–301.
15 Montpetit A, Côté S, Brustein E et al. Disruption of AP1S1, causing a novel neurocutaneous syndrome, perturbs development of the skin and spinal cord. PLoS Genet 2008;4:12.
16 Fuchs-Telem D, Sarig O, van Steensel MA et al. Familial pityriasis rubra pilaris is caused by mutations in CARD14. Am J Hum Genet 2012;91:163–70.
17 Onnis G, Bourrat E, Jonca N et al. KLICK syndrome: an unusual phenotype. Br J Dermatol 2018;178:1445–6.
18 Ishida-Yamamoto A. Loricrin keratoderma: a novel disease entity characterized by nuclear accumulation of mutant loricrin. J Dermatol Sci 2003;31:3–8.
19 Yeh JM, Yang MH, Chao SC. Collodion baby and loricrin keratoderma: a case report and mutation analysis. Clin Exp Dermatol 2013;38:147–50.

20 Hotz A, Bourrat E, Hausser I et al. Two novel mutations in the LOR gene in three families with loricrin keratoderma. Br J Dermatol 2015;172:1158–62.
21 Metze D. Disorders of keratinisation. In: Calonje JE, Brenn T, Lazar A, McKee P (eds) McKee's Pathology of the Skin. Philadelphia: Saunders, 2011:71–3.
22 Niemi KM, Kanerva L. Histological and ultrastructural study of a family with erythrokeratodermia progressiva symmetrica. J Cutan Pathol 1993;20:242–9.
23 Bilgin I, Bozdağ KE, Uysal S, Ermete M. Progressive symmetrical erythrokeratoderma - response to topical calcipotriol. J Dermatol Case Rep 2011;21:50–2.
24 Tarikci N, Göncü EK, Yüksel T et al. Progressive symmetrical erythrokeratoderma on the face: a rare condition and successful treatment with calcipotriol. JAAD Case Rep 2016;4:70–1.
25 Singh N, Thappa DM. Erythrokeratoderma variabilis responding to low-dose isotretinoin. Pediatr Dermatol 2010;27:111–13.
26 Bilan P, Levy A, Sin C et al. Erythrokeratodermia variabilis. Ann Dermatol Venereol 2013;140:129–33.
27 Yüksek J, Sezer E, Köseoğlu D et al. Erythrokeratodermia variabilis: successful treatment with retinoid plus psoralen and ultraviolet A therapy. J Dermatol 2011;38:725–7.

CHAPTER 132
Netherton Syndrome

Wei-Li Di[1] *& John Harper*[1,2]

[1] Infection, Immunity and Inflammation Programme, Immunobiology Section, Institute of Child Health, University College London, London, UK
[2] Paediatric Dermatology, Great Ormond Street Hospital for Children NHS Trust, London, UK

Abstract

Netherton syndrome (NS) is an autosomal recessive disorder characterized by the triad of ichthyosiform erythroderma, a specific hair shaft defect known as trichorrhexis invaginata and atopic manifestations. The gene responsible for NS is *SPINK5* (serine protease inhibitor Kazal type 5) and is located on chromosome 5q32. It encodes for a protein called lymphoepithelial Kazal type-related inhibitor (LEKTI). LEKTI protein is a serine protease inhibitor localized in the uppermost spinous and granular layers of normal human epidermis. In patients with NS, deficient LEKTI expression causes increased serine proteases, in particular kallikreins KLK5 and 7, which severely compromises the structure and function of the skin barrier. Early infancy is often stormy and complicated by life-threatening events, which include hypernatraemic dehydration, hypothermia and sepsis. The severe cases usually persist as generalized erythroderma, whereas milder cases often evolve into characteristic ichthyosis linearis circumflexa. NS shares a number of clinical features with atopic dermatitis, as well as a high IgE. Treatment is based on protecting the skin barrier with the frequent application of ointment-based emollients as the mainstay of treatment. Topical steroids and calcineurin inhibitors are of limited value and best avoided, as there is increased percutaneous absorption, because of the poor skin barrier, with a high risk of systemic side-effects. Intravenous immunoglobulin has been shown to be of some benefit. Experimental new approaches to treatment include serine protease inhibitor targeted therapy and the potential for gene therapy.

Key points

- Netherton syndrome is potentially life-threatening in early infancy.
- The skin barrier is severely compromised caused by a lack of the serine protease inhibitor, LEKTI.
- Netherton syndrome shares a number of immunological and clinical features with atopic dermatitis.
- Prognosis is improved with better early supportive management.
- Exciting new experimental approaches to treatment are underway: serine protease inhibitor targeted therapy and the potential for gene therapy.

Introduction and history. Netherton syndrome (NS), also known as Comel–Netherton syndrome, is a rare autosomal recessive disorder characterized by the triad of ichthyosiform erythroderma, a specific hair shaft defect known as trichorrhexis invaginata and atopic manifestations. It was first described by Comel [1] in 1949 as a new type of congenital ichthyosis, when he wrote about a young woman with erythematous, serpiginous and migratory plaques that had a characteristic double-edged scale at the margin of the erythema, which he termed *ichthyosis linearis circumflexa* (ILC). In 1958, Netherton reported a case of a girl who presented at 4 years of age with congenital ichthyosiform erythroderma (CIE) associated with sparse brittle hair, which, on examination, revealed unique nodular fragile deformities that he called *bamboo hairs* [2]; some hairs also showed pili torti. This patient also had recurrent respiratory infections and later angioedema.

In 1961, Marshall and Brede [3] described a child with a similar clinical history. In 1964, Wilkinson and colleagues [4] proposed the eponym of *Netherton's disease* for this combination of congenital ichthyosis, bamboo hairs and atopy. They suggested naming the hair shaft abnormality as *trichorrhexis invaginata* for the ball-and-socket deformity noted on the hair [4]. Because an increasing number of NS cases were reported in the literature, Altman and Stroud [5] recognized the association of NS with specific skin changes called ILC and they suggested that these two were the same entity.

In 1974, Mevorah and colleagues [6] established the clinico-statistical relationship between NS and ILC. All cases of ILC in which the hair had been carefully examined showed trichorrhexis invaginata. The atopic manifestations occur in all patients.

Aetiology and pathogenesis. NS affects an estimated 1 in 200 000 babies [7] and accounts for up to 18% of congenital erythrodermas [8]. A high neonatal mortality rate and frequent misdiagnosis of this condition may result in underestimation of the true incidence. NS has an equal sex distribution although it was initially thought to have a female predominance [9]. Traupe [10] argued, however, that the higher incidence in females was usually seen in the mild ILC cases, whereas the most severe CIE that sometimes caused death at an early age affected more boys than girls. The condition appears to take a more severe course in males than in females [10,11]. NS has an autosomal recessive mode of transmission, occurring in

Harper's Textbook of Pediatric Dermatology, Fourth Edition. Edited by Peter Hoeger, Veronica Kinsler and Albert Yan.

offspring of unaffected parents, especially in consanguineous families, as well as in siblings [9,12].

The gene responsible for NS is known as *SPINK5* (serine protease inhibitor Kazal type 5) and is located on chromosome 5q32 [13,14]. The premessenger *SPINK5* has 34 exons and spans a region of 73.31 kb on the genome (NCBI: www.ncbi.nlm.nih.gov). The gene contains 38 different GT-AG introns, which flank the beginning and end of the majority of vertebrate exons. To date, more than 80 mutations in the *SPINK5* gene have been reported [7,13–39]. Except for exons 28 to 34, mutations are distributed in every exon and intron–exon boundary, with high mutation frequencies in exons 2 to 8 and exons 21 to 26. The mutations include nonsense mutations, splice-site mutations, small nucleotide deletions and insertions. All mutations cause either an immediate premature termination codon or a frameshift/premature termination codon in the encoding region, resulting in null or very low expression of the gene *SPINK5*, presumably via accelerated mRNA decay [7].

Patients with NS have two copies of the mutant *SPINK5* gene (homozygous). Three or four mutations in *SPINK5* in one patient have also been reported, but it is rare [40]. As a recessive condition, both parents of a patient are asymptomatic heterozygous carriers and the risk of recurrence based on the Mendelian principle is 25% for subsequent pregnancies [41]. There is, however, an exception to this based on uniparental disomy. This is a genetic situation in which a pair of chromosomes is inherited from only one parent [42]. There were studies showing maternal isodisomy of chromosome 5 in patients with NS [13,17]. Although the frequency of uniparental disomy is rare, this genetic situation should be considered when carrying out mutation screening and genetic counselling for NS.

The complete mRNA of *SPINK5* is 3648 bp long and encodes for a 1094-amino-acid protein, lymphoepithelial Kazal type-related inhibitor (LEKTI), which has a molecular weight of 124.1 kDa and isoelectric point (pI) of 7.7. The LEKTI protein is a serine protease inhibitor containing 15 Kazal-type related inhibitory domains. It is expressed in many tissues including the thymus, epithelial tissues, oral mucosa, tonsils, parathyroids and Bartholin glands [13,16,43]. Because patients with NS have a severe skin phenotype, the biological role of LEKTI in the skin and keratinocytes has been extensively investigated in the past decade. *In situ* hybridization and immunohistochemistry have indicated that the gene *SPINK5* and its encoded protein LEKTI are localized in the uppermost spinous and granular layers of normal human epidermis [13,44]. In keratinocytes, pro-LEKTI synthesized in cells is rapidly processed into proteolytic fragments and secreted into extracellular compartments. More than five secreted LEKTI fragments with heterogeneous molecular weights have been found in the epidermis and conditional culture medium [45,46]. *In vitro* studies have confirmed that full-size LEKTI and its fragments are able to inhibit various serine proteases such as plasmin, trypsin, elastase and tissue kallikreins (KLKs), in particular KLK5 and 7 [28,47–49]. KLK5 is one of the major serine proteases expressed in the uppermost layers of the epidermis. It has a typical serine protease catalytic domain and its major biological role in the epidermis is in desquamation by degrading the adhesive ectodomain of desmoglein I, which is one of the corneodesmosomal proteins, to maintain epidermal tissue integrity in the superficial layers. Activated KLK5 further activates other KLKs including KLK6, 7, 8, 11, 13 and 14, most of which can coordinate to destabilize corneodesmosomes, subsequently resulting in a proteolytic cascade in the skin [50,51]. The pathomechanism of the defective skin barrier caused by enhanced KLK5 activity in NS has been further demonstrated in transgenic KLK5 mice, in which cutaneous and systemic hallmarks of NS were reproduced [52].

The LEKTI protein controls the activity of KLK5 by forming an inhibitory complex with KLK5 in a pH-dependent manner [45]. Under acidic pH, which occurs in the upper epidermal layers in normal skin, the LEKTI–KLK5 inhibitory complex is dissociated to allow inhibitor-free KLK5 to degrade corneodesmosomes [53]. In patients with NS, deficient LEKTI expression causes increased inhibitor-free KLK5 in the epidermis, resulting in premature degradation of corneodesmosomes in the granular layer as well as in the lower stratum corneum, where an inflammatory cascade mediated by the protease-activated receptor (PAR2)–nuclear factor κB (NFκB) pathway can be activated and further impair skin barrier formation [53–56]. Understanding the pathophysiological pathway of loss of function of LEKTI in the epidermis has been further expanded by two studies: (i) apart from degrading corneodesmosomes, hyperactivated KLK5 mediated by deficient LEKTI expression can upregulate the epidermal protease elastase 2, resulting in excessive degradation of (pro-)filaggrin and alteration of intercorneocyte lipid formation in the skin barrier [57]; and (ii) once the LEKTI–KLK5 complex is dissociated, the inhibitor-free KLK5 is activated by matriptase, a transmembrane serine protease having the ability to undergo efficient autoactivation to initiate proteolytic cascades [53,58,59]. There are other studies indicating that LEKTI can also target caspase 1 [60] and caspase 14 [61], but the actual pathophysiological relationship needs to be further elucidated.

Because NS shares a number of clinical features with atopic dermatitis (AD), single nucleotide polymorphisms (SNPs) in *SPINK5* in atopic dermatitis individuals have been sought. Earlier studies showed that the c.1258G>A polymorphism in *SPINK5* resulting in the p.Glu420Lys substitution in LEKTI was significantly associated with atopy and atopic dermatitis [62–65]. Another study showed an association of *SPINK5* polymorphism with disease severity and food allergy in children with AD [66]. Although some genome-wide association studies carried out in French, German and Irish/English cases of AD showed no significant relationship between *SPINK5* Glu420Lys SNP and AD [67,68], a recent functional investigation has confirmed that the polymorphism Glu420Lys can cause abnormal proteolytic activity of LEKTI, suggesting that the SNP is associated with AD [69].

Pathology. A study of 80 skin biopsies from 67 patients with confirmed NS with either a negative LEKTI immunohistochemistry and/or molecular confirmation by identified mutation in SPINK5 revealed the most frequent histological finding was psoriasiform hyperplasia. Additional, less common, or previously unreported findings included compact parakeratosis with large nuclei, subcorneum or intracorneum splitting, presence of clear cells in the upper epidermis or stratum corneum, dyskeratosis, dermal infiltrate with neutrophils and/or eosinophils and dilated blood vessels in the superficial dermis [70]. Another feature is spongiosis, which is usually more pronounced in the lower epidermal cell layers.

Ultrastructural studies of the skin show evidence of inhibition of terminal differentiation of the keratinocytes and impaired cornification. On electron microscopy, cells in the outer nucleated layer appear in various stages of transition into corneocytes. The stratum corneum is less cohesive than normal with the corneocytes containing numerous intracellular lipid droplets, nuclear membrane and inclusions. There are decreased numbers of desmosomal connections and tonofilaments resulting in loosening of the stratum corneum [71,72].

The granular layer shows signs of suppressed or incomplete keratinization, indicated by low amounts of irregularly dispersed keratin filaments and a near complete absence of keratohyalin. Keratinocytes in the granular layer are not flattened, as occurs in normal skin, and contain numerous inclusion bodies [10,72–74], which is not reported in other ichthyoses [10]. The formation and discharge of epidermal lipids at the stratum corneum–granulosum interface, which provide the lamellar sheets important for epidermal barrier function, is also disturbed [75].

Lamellar body secretion also occurs into the extracellular spaces in four or more layers of the stratum granulosum and upper spinosum. The prematurely secreted lamellar body contents remain unprocessed. In some areas where the cornified envelope is present, elongated membrane sheets are evident, but fully processed mature lamellar membrane structures, as observed in normal skin, do not occur [71]. In the extracellular compartment of the lower stratum corneum, fusiform dilations are present containing foci of electron-dense material, which may disturb the transformation to mature lamellar membrane structures. These electron-dense materials create clefts in the mid to upper stratum corneum.

The defective skin barrier accounts for many of the clinical findings in NS, such as increased transepidermal water loss, hypernatraemic dehydration, susceptibility to skin infections and allergy.

Clinical features.

Presentation in infancy

NS usually presents within the first few days of life with a CIE (Fig. 132.1). The neonatal course is often stormy and complicated by life-threatening events. Neonatal hypernatraemia, hypothermia, seizures, diarrhoea and recurrent sepsis contribute to the high mortality and morbidity rate in the first year of life [75–79]. The condition tends to improve thereafter.

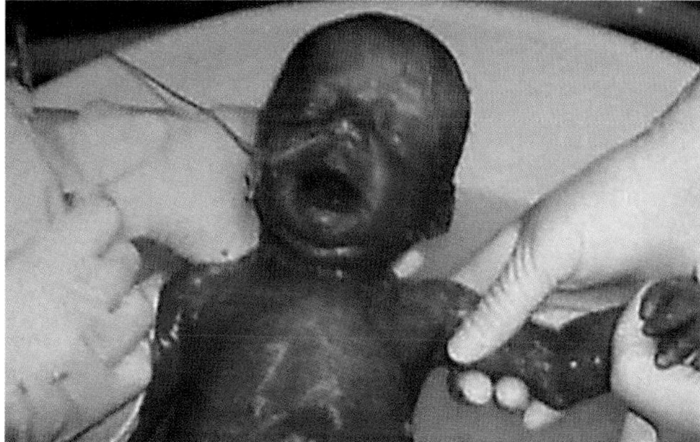

Fig. 132.1 Netherton syndrome presenting as congenital erythroderma.

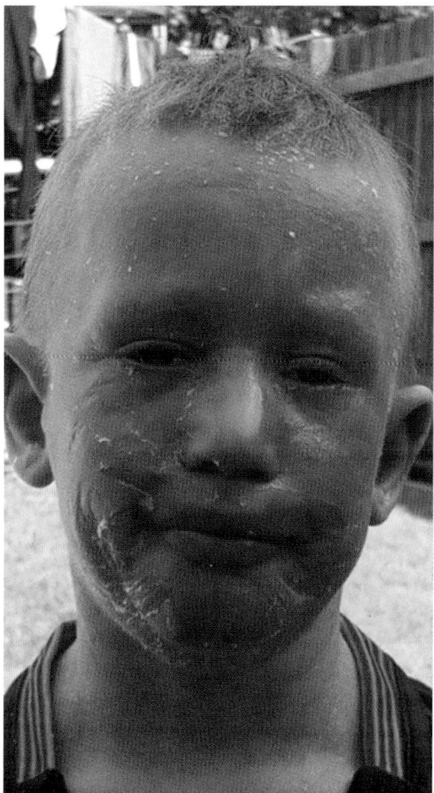

Fig. 132.2 Netherton syndrome: same boy as in Fig. 132.1, exhibiting the characteristic facial appearance and short hair.

Skin manifestations

Ichthyosiform erythroderma presents at or soon after birth and can range from mild patchy involvement to severe generalized ichthyosiform erythroderma. The severe cases usually persist as generalized erythroderma (Fig. 132.2), whereas milder cases often evolve into characteristic ILC (Fig. 132.3) on the trunk and limbs after 1–2 years [10,76,77,80]. ILC may be episodic, with flares lasting up to 2–3 weeks and then clearing for weeks and months at a time [77]. Patients with predominantly ILC have normal

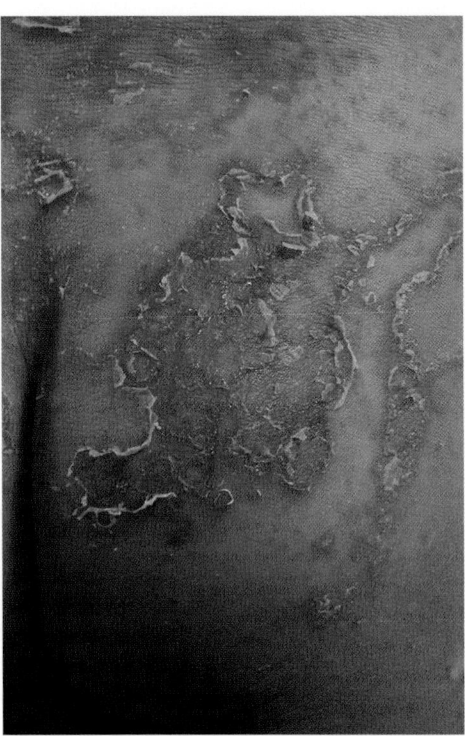

Fig. 132.3 Ichthyosis linearis circumflexia: erythematous, serpiginous and migratory plaques that have a characteristic double-edged scale at the margin of the erythema.

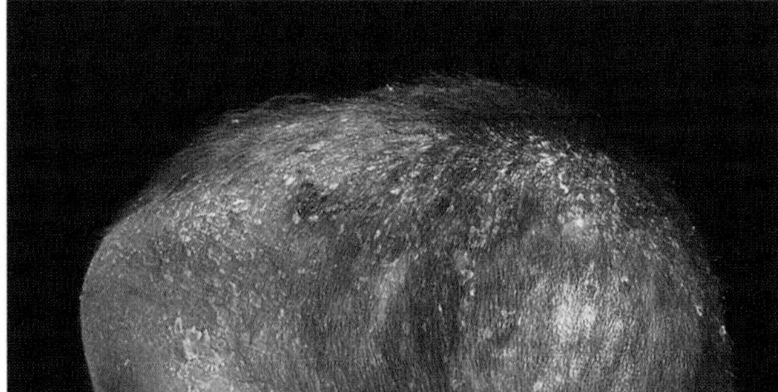

Fig. 132.4 Netherton syndrome: short broken hairs displaying a characteristic spiky appearance.

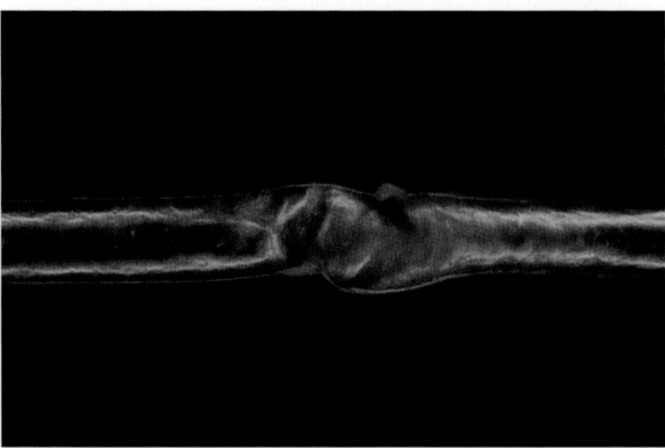

Fig. 132.5 Trichorrhexis invaginata: a ball-and-socket hair shaft deformity caused by the invagination of the distal hair shaft into the cup formed by the proximal hair shaft, pathognomonic for Netherton syndrome.

physical development in general, whereas those with persistent generalized erythroderma have a more severe course, with failure to thrive and life-threatening events occurring in early childhood [10,76,77]. Skin erosions with peeling of the skin, itchiness and redness can give rise to the misdiagnosis of peeling skin syndrome [10,81]. There is a tendency for spontaneous improvement with the transition from generalized erythroderma to patchy or episodic involvement. Despite the improvement, some patients remain severely affected with a fluctuating course throughout childhood and adult life [77].

Pruritus is a common feature in NS, causing irritability especially in infancy [7,77]. Other skin manifestations include lichenification similar to that seen in AD [11,77]. The palms and soles are normally spared but may appear hyperkeratotic [82]. Although the nails are usually unaffected, nail dystrophy, pterygia and loss of several fingernails have been reported [77].

Papillomatous skin lesions can present at various sites such as the groin, axillae, and genitoanal regions [83–85]. Squamous cell carcinoma has been reported on the dorsum of the hand, the upper arm and the vulva [86–88]. Krasagakis and colleagues [89] reported a case of early aggressive cutaneous neoplasia in an area of papillomatous lesions on sun-exposed skin and suggested that the underlying genetic defect may be the cause of the malignancy in these patients. Weber and colleagues [85] suggested that the nonmelanoma skin cancer in NS patients might be associated with EV-HPV (epidermodysplasia verruciformis-associated human papillomavirus)-type infection, similar to that seen in immunosuppressed transplant recipients.

Hair abnormalities

Hair growth is often sparse and delayed in NS patients. Individual hairs are short, dry, lustreless and brittle, growing a few centimetres before breaking and displaying a characteristic spiky appearance (Fig. 132.4) [77,90]. The hair abnormalities can affect all parts of the body, including scalp, eyebrow, eyelashes and body hair. The type of abnormalities seen include trichorrhexis invaginata, trichorrhexis nodosa and pili torti [3,4,90]. Trichorrhexis nodosa and pili torti can feature in various other medical conditions and syndromes ranging from hypothyroidism [91], Menkes hair disease [92], ectodermal dysplasia [93], mitochondrial disorders [94] to argininosuccinic aciduria [95].

Trichorrhexis invaginata, on the other hand, is considered to be pathognomonic for NS [80]. Trichorrhexis invaginata can be readily identified on light microscopy (including dermoscopy) wherein the so-called 'golf tee' or 'matchstick' structures can be identified, but the findings are best demonstrated on electron microscopy. It is a ball-and-socket hair shaft deformity caused by the invagination of the distal hair shaft into the cup formed by the proximal hair shaft (Fig. 132.5) [4]. In trichorrhexis invaginata, the invagination occurs at the site of a transient keratinizing defect of the hair cortex resulting from incomplete conversion of sulphydryl groups into the disulphide bonds in the protein of the cortical fibres. The incomplete conversion means fewer cross-linkages of the keratin structures, resulting in weak architectural structure of the cortical cells. This defect leads to cortical softness, which, when driven upwards by growing, is forced to fold around the more stable distal hair shaft forming the typical trichorrhexis invaginata deformity [90,96,97]. Trichorrhexis invaginata has been reported to be present in an 11-day-old infant [98] but is usually not obvious in early infancy. It may also be difficult to detect given the sparsity of hair in babies with NS, making it difficult to obtain adequate samples. Even when hairs are examined microscopically, not all of them will have the obvious abnormality required to make the diagnosis. Hair microscopy often has to be repeated on several occasions over a period of time before the diagnosis is made [99]. In some instances, only the proximal half of the invaginate node is seen under electron microscopy, representing the golf tee sign, which may be the only clue to the diagnosis of trichorrhexis invaginata [99]. Powell and colleagues [100] described an increased density of trichorrhexis invaginata in eyebrow hair compared with scalp hair (about 10 times) in patients with NS. Hence examination of both the eyebrow and scalp hair will increase the chances of making a positive diagnosis. In some cases of NS only vellus [101] or eyebrow hairs [5,96,102,103] are abnormal. Improvement of hair growth can occur during childhood [103,104] but although it may approach a normal-looking appearance the hair never returns completely to normal. There is currently no known treatment for trichorrhexis invaginata. If there is significant hair loss, a wig may need to be considered.

Pili torti and trichorrhexis nodosa are the two other most common hair abnormalities in NS. Trichorrhexis nodosa is a disorder of the hair shaft in which there is a distinctive response to injury. The hair is fragile and on examination regularly spaced pale node-like swellings are observed [104]. It may affect normal hair following injury or occur after minimal trauma in cases of inherent defects in keratin synthesis, leading to abnormally brittle hair. When the cuticle of the hair is absent, the hair cortex is exposed and its integrity is broken down. The hair can then split and fray into strands at the point of the break. Trichorrhexis nodosa may be localized or generalized to all hair [105,106]. Pili torti is the twisting of the hair fibre at focal points along its length. The hair cuticle is still intact but the twisting creates stress in the fibre, causing longitudinal fractures in the cuticle and internal hair cortex. This results in weak points in the hair fibre, which subsequently break [107,108].

Atopic manifestations and allergy

Atopy is a feature of all patients with NS [77,82]. Atopic dermatitis, asthma, urticaria, angioedema and allergic rhinitis occur in some form or other in patients with NS [7,77,82,109]. A positive family history of atopy is also frequently observed [77]. Some patients may even have concomitant presentation of several atopic features. Reaction to food allergens, particularly nuts, egg and milk, is common [9,82,106]. In some cases, the patients may have a delayed response as seen in atopic dermatitis [5,110,111] but more often anaphylactoid-type reactions with angioedema occur [7,77]. Positive skin tests or radioallergosorbent test (RAST) responses to allergens such as house dust mite, grass pollen and cat dander are frequent [9,77]. Peripheral eosinophilia is present in the blood and the IgE level is high, ranging from 400 to 15 000 IU/mL [9,77,82,103,112,113].

Immunological abnormalities and infections

Recurrent cutaneous, sinus and chest infections are frequent in NS patients [7,77]. It has been suggested that the recurrent infections are caused by an underlying immunodeficiency [10,86,114]. Greene and Muller [9] reported that 12 out of the 45 patients they reviewed had recurrent infections, with six having decreased serum IgG levels. Judge and colleagues [77] in 1994 reported that two NS patients had decreased IgG_2 subclasses, and two others who did not show clinically significant viral infections also had a reduced number of natural killer cells. However, most patients with NS have normal immunoglobulins apart from a high level of IgE.

Stryk and colleagues [115] reported selective antibody deficiency to bacterial polysaccharide antigens in three of their patients with NS, who had recurrent sinopulmonary infections. The study emphasized the importance of checking for functional antibody response to both protein and bacterial polysaccharide, and not simply relying on IgG subclass levels alone. In these patients, prophylactic antibody can usually control the rate of infection [116], but in some patients intravenous immunoglobulin therapy may be helpful in preventing infections. Serial immunological evaluation is important as the deficient antibody response may simply represent maturation delay.

Severe recurrent or chronic skin infections suffered by patients with NS include: bacterial infections such as *Staphylococcus aureus*, including meticillin-resistant *Staphylococcus aureus*; *Candida albicans* and viral infections (herpes simplex and human papillomavirus) [10,117]. Other infections such as conjunctivitis, otitis media and bacterial vaginosis [118] have also been reported [77,79,119]. Gross and colleagues [120] documented a case of vaccine-associated poliomyelitis. Some of these infections can lead to severe sepsis and in some cases life-threatening septicaemia, especially in early childhood, accounting for the high mortality seen in this age group [7,79,121]. Renner and colleagues [23] carried out an extensive immunological study in patients with NS and revealed reduced memory B-cells and defective response to vaccination with Pneumovax and bacteriophage phiX174. They also reported that patients with NS had a skewed T-helper 1 phenotype, elevated pro-inflammatory cytokine levels – interleukin (IL)-1β, IL-12, tumour necrosis factor α, granulocyte-macrophage colony-stimulating factor, IL-1 receptor antagonist – and decreased natural killer cell cytotoxicity although the absolute numbers of natural killer cells were normal or elevated in patients.

Growth and development

Failure to thrive is a major problem especially in the first year of life. This is attributed to a combination of a high catabolic rate and a defective skin barrier, leading to fluid loss and increased susceptibility to recurrent infections [77]. These children usually have chronic diarrhoea and malabsorption, which further exacerbates the failure to thrive. Jejunal biopsy has revealed villous atrophy in a significant proportion of patients: three out of five in the report by Pradeaux and colleagues [122] and 26% in the series by Bitoun and colleagues [7]. Nutritional support is a significant part of management from an early stage in order to maintain adequate growth and development. For most patients a hypoallergenic diet is advised, and for infants, especially those with diarrhoea and failure to thrive, Neocate®, an amino acid-based formula milk substitute, is recommended. The input of a dietitian is essential.

By the second year of life most children show improved weight gain, but some degree of growth retardation persists and those who are most severely affected in early infancy remain below the 25th centile [6,74,75,77,102,123]. Greig and Wishart [123] reviewed the growth of 34 patients with NS and found 12 to be less than the third percentile and two less than the tenth percentile. Short stature is characteristic of NS.

Neurodevelopment is usually normal in NS. Mild mental retardation has been reported in a minority of patients and may be a consequence of neonatal events, such as cerebral haemorrhage following hypernatraemic dehydration [77,82,124].

Other clinical features

Hypernatraemic dehydration and hypothermia are major causes of neonatal morbidity and mortality in NS [7,9,75,125]. These features are a consequence of the markedly increased transepidermal water loss [9,75] resulting from the impaired skin permeability barrier [71]. Intermittent aminoaciduria has been reported in NS patients, although no related specific renal problem has been identified [9].

Other features that have been described in patients with NS are: hydroureter; hypoplastic left heart; atresia of the pulmonary artery; hemihypertrophy; and acute bilateral renal thrombosis [6,75,126–128].

Diagnosis. Confirming the diagnosis of NS is often difficult in early infancy, in a baby who is usually very unwell with erythroderma and profound failure to thrive. The main important differential diagnosis is Omenn syndrome, but in practice a frequent misdiagnosis is atopic dermatitis. In this situation a significant clue is the lack of response to topical steroids, and indeed this is one situation that can rapidly lead to steroid toxicity and cushingoid features.

With the identification of the gene responsible for NS (*SPINK5*), DNA analysis for known mutations in NS is now possible and would assist in the diagnosis of these patients. A more rapid investigation is to look for the presence of LEKTI in the skin by immunohistochemistry using an antibody with a specific epitope for the LEKTI protein (C-terminus). Absence of LEKTI expression can be detected using this anti-LEKTI antibody (Fig. 132.6). Therefore, if LEKTI expression is absent or significantly decreased, when compared with normal skin as a control, this is strongly indicative of NS. The immunostaining test

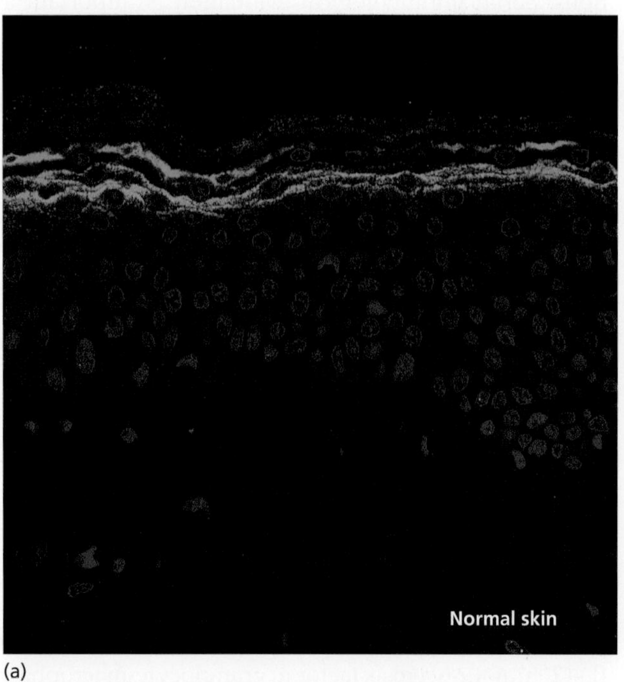

(a)

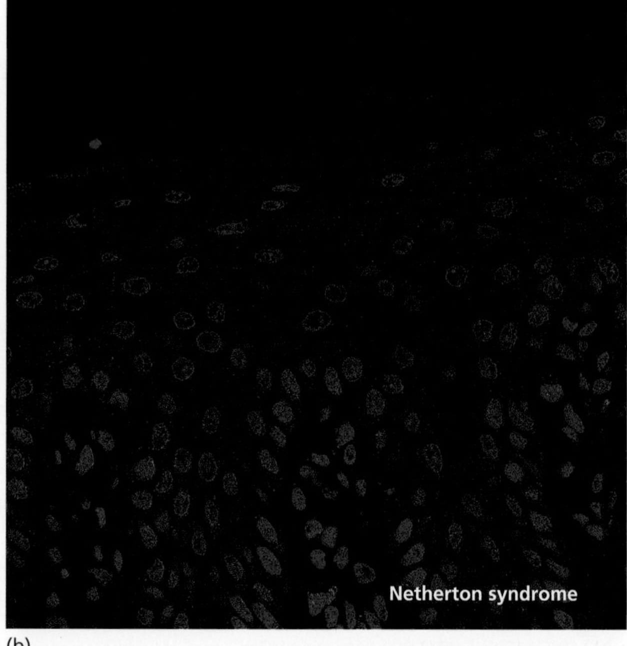

(b)

Fig. 132.6 Staining for LEKTI protein in (a) normal skin and (b) the skin of a patient with Netherton syndrome, using a polyclonal antibody. It shows almost complete absence of LEKTI in Netherton syndrome.

can be done on paraffin-embedded tissue and provides a result within 24 hours [129]. Other investigations should include: a routine haematological and biochemical profile; a full immunological screen to exclude an underlying immunodeficiency; total IgE and specific IgE to a panel of common atopic allergens; a skin biopsy; and microscopic examination of a sample of hair (either dermoscopically or using cut, not plucked hair for light microscopy or electron microscopy). Unfortunately, erythrodermic babies have little or no scalp hair and examination of eyebrow hair has been suggested [100]; however, trichorrhexis invaginata is rarely detectable at presentation. A presumptive diagnosis of NS is made and repeated hair samples need to be taken. Usually, trichorrhexis invaginata is confirmed from the age of about 6 months, but diagnosis can certainly take much longer, even several years. In the latter situation only a small proportion of hairs are affected and it is necessary to take samples from different sites on the scalp.

'Leiner disease' is an old term that was used for infants with erythroderma, sparse hair, diarrhoea and failure to thrive. Many of these babies have NS. In a clinical study by Glover and colleagues [130] of five patients with 'erythroderma, failure to thrive and diarrhoea', four developed clinical features consistent with NS. These infants are often subjected to extensive investigations for immunological, metabolic or nutritional deficiencies.

Treatment and prognosis. To date, there is no curative therapy for NS. Regular application of ointment-based emollients (such as a 50:50 mixture of white soft paraffin and liquid paraffin) is the mainstay of treatment. Topical steroids do not help in this condition and there is the risk of increased percutaneous absorption. This aspect is particularly relevant in infancy, because it can result in systemic side-effects and cushingoid features [77].

The use of topical calcineurin inhibitors, tacrolimus and pimecrolimus, for the treatment of the skin in NS is controversial. Allen and colleagues [131] reported significantly high blood levels of tacrolimus in three patients with NS who were treated with topical tacrolimus, caused by increased absorption through the skin. Bens and colleagues [132], on the other hand, described effective treatment with careful monitoring of blood levels.

Small and Cordoro reported two patients with NS mimicking pustular psoriasis who responded well to treatment with intravenous immunoglobulin [133]. Retinoid therapy is uncertain, with some groups reporting success [10] and others showing no real improvement [77]. In our experience, oral retinoid treatment (acitretin) has no therapeutic role and in some cases can make the skin worse, causing extensive skin erosions.

Other promising treatments that have been tried and reported to be beneficial, include omalizumab (anti-IgE) [134] and infliximab (anti-TNF) [135]; however, these are case reports with no formal clinical trials performed as yet. Evidence of increased expression of anti-IL-17/IL-23 among patients with NS has been reported [136] and raises the possibility of IL-17-targeting strategies.

Serine protease inhibitor targeted therapy

Improved understanding of the pathogenesis of NS has led to the development of novel therapies that target tissue KLKs, in particular KLK5. An *in vivo* study showed that KLK5 knock-out in newborn mice with LEKTI-deficiency rescued neonatal lethality, reverses the severe skin barrier defect, restores epidermal structure and prevents skin inflammation [137]. A case of NS was reported in whom there was markedly reduced skin exfoliation, hypertension, hypernatremia and alkalosis following treatment with an ointment containing sodium bicarbonate and 40% zinc oxide, a potent KLK5 inhibitor [138]. This has led to extensive investigations in this field and a growing list of KLK inhibitors has been reported in the past decade [139,140]. However, currently all are laboratory-based studies and no treatment trials have been published to date.

The potential for gene therapy

With the development of a high-efficiency gene transfer system, which has allowed delivery of foreign DNA into keratinocyte stem cells, and advances in culture techniques, which have allowed keratinocyte stem cells to be cultured as sheets of epithelium in laboratories and grafted back onto donors [141,142], gene-based therapy for patients with NS has been developed; patients' keratinocytes obtained from small skin biopsies are transduced with the wild-type *SPINK5* gene using a lentiviral vector system. Corrected cells are then cultured as epidermal sheets with the potential for this to be grafted back to patients. This therapeutic strategy has been examined in a human/murine chimeric model *in vivo* and results showed that skin grafts generated from transduced patients' cells with NS have a marked correction of epidermal architecture, even when relatively low numbers of LEKTI-expressing cells were present in the skin grafts [25]. Linking this result with the fact that LEKTI is a secreted protein, the genetically modified skin grafts may act as 'protein factories' secreting functional LEKTI to produce a generalized beneficial effect. This is especially feasible for small infants where relatively small gene-corrected skin sheets could provide significant clinical benefit. Based on preclinical results, a first-in-man *ex vivo* autologous skin graft gene therapy for NS has commenced. The aims are: determination of the feasibility and safety of lentivirus modified autologous epithelial sheets and assessment of whether SPINK5 gene transfer can mediate localized correction of skin architecture inside and outside of the graft [143]. The trial has been approved by the Gene Therapy Advisory Committee (GTAC) and Medicines and Healthcare products Regulatory Agency (MHRA) in the UK and registered with ClinicalTrials.gov (http://clinicaltrials.gov/number) under identifier number NCT01545323.

Prenatal diagnosis

Prenatal diagnosis for families with known mutations has been performed by two groups [73,98].

Prognosis

The mortality rate is high in the first year of life, especially in the neonatal period. Thereafter there is a tendency towards improvement, although NS remains a lifelong condition. The generalized skin condition and hair abnormality persist and the course is punctuated by acute exacerbations.

Acknowledgement

We wish to thank Christina Ong for her contribution to this chapter in the first two editions.

References

1 Comel M. Ichthyosis linearis circumflexa. Dermatologica 1949; 98:133–6.
2 Netherton EW. A unique case of trichorrhexis nodosa; bamboo hairs. AMA Arch Derm 1958;78:483–7.
3 Marshall J, Brede HD. Black piedra in a child with pili torti, bamboo hair and congenital ichthyosiform erythroderma. S Afr Med J 1961;35:221–5.
4 Wilkinson RD, Curtis Ch, Hawk WA. Netherton's disease; trichorrhexis invaginata (bamboo hair), congential ichthyosiform erythroderma and the atopic diathesis. A histopathologic study. Arch Dermatol 1964;89:46–54.
5 Altman J, Stroud J. Netherton's syndrome and ichthyosis linearis circumflexa. Arch Dermatol 1969;100:550–8.
6 Mevorah B, Frenk E, Brooke EM. Ichthyosis linearis circumflexa comel. A clinico-statistical approach to its relationship with Netherton's syndrome. Dermatologica 1974;149:201–9.
7 Bitoun E, Chavanas S, Irvine AD et al. Netherton syndrome: disease expression and spectrum of SPINK5 mutations in 21 families. J Invest Dermatol 2002;118:352–61.
8 Pruszkowski A, Bodemer C, Fraitag S et al. Neonatal and infantile erythrodermas: a retrospective study of 51 patients. Arch Dermatol 2000;136:875–80.
9 Greene SL, Muller SA. Netherton's syndrome. Report of a case and review of the literature. J Am Acad Dermatol 1985;13:329–37.
10 Traupe H. Guide to Clinical Diagnosis, Genetic Counselling, and Therapy. Berlin: Springer Verlag, 1985:168–78.
11 Dupre A, Bonafe JL, Carrere S. [Comel's linear circumflex ichthyosis and Netherton's syndrome. General conceptions based on study of 4 cases (author's transl.)]. Ann Dermatol Venereol 1978;105:49–54.
12 van Furth AM, Boontje RP, Louwers MJ et al. [Netherton's syndrome in two sisters]. Ned Tijdschr Geneeskd 2002;146:1087–90.
13 Chavanas S, Bodemer C, Rochat A et al. Mutations in SPINK5, encoding a serine protease inhibitor, cause Netherton syndrome. Nat Genet 2000;25:141–2.
14 Sprecher E, Chavanas S, DiGiovanna JJ et al. The spectrum of pathogenic mutations in SPINK5 in 19 families with Netherton syndrome: implications for mutation detection and first case of prenatal diagnosis. J Invest Dermatol 2001;117:179–87.
15 Chao SC, Tsai YM, Lee JY. A compound heterozygous mutation of the SPINK5 gene in a Taiwanese boy with Netherton syndrome. J Formos Med Assoc 2003;102:418–23.
16 Komatsu N, Takata M, Otsuki N et al. Elevated stratum corneum hydrolytic activity in Netherton syndrome suggests an inhibitory regulation of desquamation by SPINK5-derived peptides. J Invest Dermatol 2002;118:436–43.
17 Raghunath M, Tontsidou L, Oji V et al. SPINK5 and Netherton syndrome: novel mutations, demonstration of missing LEKTI, and differential expression of transglutaminases. J Invest Dermatol 2004;123:474–83.
18 Shimomura Y, Sato N, Kariya N et al. Netherton syndrome in two Japanese siblings with a novel mutation in the SPINK5 gene: immunohistochemical studies of LEKTI and other epidermal molecules. Br J Dermatol 2005;153:1026–30.
19 Kilic G, Guler N, Ones U et al. Netherton syndrome: report of identical twins presenting with severe atopic dermatitis. Eur J Pediatr 2006;165:594–7.
20 Mizuno Y, Suga Y, Muramatsu S et al. A Japanese infant with localized ichthyosis linearis circumflexa on the palms and soles harbouring a compound heterozygous mutation in the SPINK5 gene. Br J Dermatol 2005;153:661–3.
21 Mizuno Y, Suga Y, Haruna K et al. A case of a Japanese neonate with congenital ichthyosiform erythroderma diagnosed as Netherton syndrome. Clin Exp Dermatol 2006;31:677–80.
22 Zhao Y, Ma ZH, Yang Y et al. SPINK5 gene mutation and decreased LEKTI activity in three Chinese patients with Netherton's syndrome. Clin Exp Dermatol 2007;32:564–7.
23 Renner ED, Hartl D, Rylaarsdam S et al. Comel–Netherton syndrome defined as primary immunodeficiency. J Allergy Clin Immunol 2009;124:536–43.
24 Tuysuz B, Ojalvo D, Mat C et al. A new SPINK5 donor splice site mutation in siblings with Netherton syndrome. Acta Derm Venereol 2010;90:95–6.
25 Di WL, Larcher F, Senemova E et al. Ex-vivo gene therapy restores LEKTI activity and corrects the architecture of Netherton syndrome derived skin grafts. Mol Ther 2011;19:408–16.
26 Fong K, Akdeniz S, Isi H et al. New homozygous SPINK5 mutation, p.Gln333X, in a Turkish pedigree with Netherton syndrome. Clin Exp Dermatol 2011;36:412–15.
27 Roedl D, Oji V, Buters JT et al. rAAV2-mediated restoration of LEKTI in LEKTI-deficient cells from Netherton patients. J Dermatol Sci 2011;61:194–8.
28 Alpigiani MG, Salvati P, Schiaffino MC et al. A new SPINK5 mutation in a patient with Netherton syndrome: a case report. Pediatr Dermatol 2012;29:521–2.
29 Lacroix M, Lacaze-Buzy L, Furio L et al. Clinical expression and new SPINK5 splicing defects in Netherton syndrome: unmasking a frequent founder synonymous mutation and unconventional intronic mutations. J Invest Dermatol 2012;132:575–82.
30 Fortugno P, Grosso F, Zambruno G et al. A synonymous mutation in SPINK5 exon 11 causes Netherton syndrome by altering exonic splicing regulatory elements. J Hum Genet 2012;57:311–15.
31 Diociaiuti A, Castiglia D, Fortugno P et al. Lethal Netherton syndrome due to homozygous p.Arg371X mutation in SPINK5. Pediatr Dermatol 2013;30:e65–e67.
32 Konishi T, Tsuda T, Sakaguchi Y et al. Upregulation of interleukin-33 in the epidermis of two Japanese patients with Netherton syndrome. J Dermatol 2014;41:258–61.
33 Aydin BK, Bas F, Tamay Z et al. Netherton syndrome associated with growth hormone deficiency. Pediatr Dermatol 2014;31:90–4.
34 Israeli S, Sarig O, Garty BZ et al. Molecular analysis of a series of Israeli families with Comel-Netherton syndrome. Dermatology 2014;228:183–8.
35 Numata S, Teye K, Krol RP et al. A compound synonymous mutation c.474G>A with p.Arg578X mutation in SPINK5 causes splicing disorder and mild phenotype in Netherton syndrome. Exp Dermatol 2016;25:568–70.
36 Hannula-Jouppi K, Laasanen SL, Ilander M et al. Intrafamily and interfamilial phenotype variation and immature immunity in patients with Netherton Syndrome and Finnish SPINK5 Founder Mutation. JAMA Dermatol 2016;152:435–42.
37 Macknet CA, Morkos A, Job L et al. An infant with Netherton syndrome and persistent pulmonary hypertension requiring extracorporeal membrane oxygenation. Pediatr Dermatol 2008;25:368–72.
38 Numata S, Hamada T, Teye K et al. Complete maternal isodisomy of chromosome 5 in a Japanese patient with Netherton syndrome. J Invest Dermatol 2014;134:849–52.
39 Lin SP, Huang SY, Tu ME et al. Netherton syndrome: mutation analysis of two Taiwanese families. Arch Dermatol Res 2007;299:145–50.
40 Ilias C, Evgenia B, Aikaterini P et al. Netherton Syndrome in a Neonate with Possible Growth Hormone Deficiency and Transient Hyperaldosteronism. Case Rep Pediatr 2015;2015:818–961.
41 Fassihi H, Lu L, Wessagowit V et al. Complete maternal isodisomy of chromosome 3 in a child with recessive dystrophic epidermolysis bullosa but no other phenotypic abnormalities. J Invest Dermatol 2006;126:2039–43.
42 Zlotogora J. Parents of children with autosomal recessive diseases are not always carriers of the respective mutant alleles. Hum Genet 2004;114:521–6.
43 Magert HJ, Standker L, Kreutzmann P et al. LEKTI, a novel 15 domain type of human serine proteinase inhibitor. J Biol Chem 1999;274:21499–502.
44 Bitoun E, Micheloni A, Lamant L et al. LEKTI proteolytic processing in human primary keratinocytes, tissue distribution and defective expression in Netherton syndrome. Hum Mol Genet 2003; 12:2417–30.
45 Deraison C, Bonnart C, Lopez F et al. LEKTI fragments specifically inhibit KLK5, KLK7, and KLK14 and control desquamation through a pH-dependent interaction. Mol Biol Cell 2007;18:3607–19.

46 Jayakumar A, Kang Y, Henderson Y et al. Consequences of C-terminal domains and N-terminal signal peptide deletions on LEKTI secretion, stability, and subcellular distribution. Arch Biochem Biophys 2005; 435:89–102.

47 Egelrud T, Brattsand M, Kreutzmann P et al. hK5 and hK7, two serine proteinases abundant in human skin, are inhibited by LEKTI domain 6. Br J Dermatol 2005;153:1200–3.

48 Jayakumar A, Kang Y, Mitsudo K et al. Expression of LEKTI domains 6–9′ in the baculovirus expression system: recombinant LEKTI domains 6–9′ inhibit trypsin and subtilisin A. Protein Expr Purif 2004;35:93–101.

49 Mitsudo K, Jayakumar A, Henderson Y et al. Inhibition of serine proteinases plasmin, trypsin, subtilisin A, cathepsin G, and elastase by LEKTI: a kinetic analysis. Biochemistry 2003;42:3874–81.

50 Borgono CA, Michael IP, Komatsu N et al. A potential role for multiple tissue kallikrein serine proteases in epidermal desquamation. J Biol Chem 2007;282:3640–52.

51 Caubet C, Jonca N, Brattsand M et al. Degradation of corneodesmosome proteins by two serine proteases of the kallikrein family, SCTE/KLK5/hK5 and SCCE/KLK7/hK7. J Invest Dermatol 2004;122:1235–44.

52 **Furio L, de Veer S, Jaillet M et al. Transgenic kallikrein 5 mice reproduce major cutaneous and systemic hallmarks of Netherton syndrome. J Exp Med 2014;211:499–513.**

53 Sales KU, Masedunskas A, Bey AL et al. Matriptase initiates activation of epidermal pro-kallikrein and disease onset in a mouse model of Netherton syndrome. Nat Genet 2010;42:676–83.

54 Descargues P, Deraison C, Prost C et al. Corneodesmosomal cadherins are preferential targets of stratum corneum trypsin- and chymotrypsin-like hyperactivity in Netherton syndrome. J Invest Dermatol 2006;126:1622–32.

55 Hachem JP, Crumrine D, Fluhr J et al. pH directly regulates epidermal permeability barrier homeostasis, and stratum corneum integrity/cohesion. J Invest Dermatol 2003;121:345–53.

56 Briot A, Deraison C, Lacroix M et al. Kallikrein 5 induces atopic dermatitis-like lesions through PAR2-mediated thymic stromal lymphopoietin expression in Netherton syndrome. J Exp Med 2009;206:1135–47.

57 **Bonnart C, Deraison C, Lacroix M et al. Elastase 2 is expressed in human and mouse epidermis and impairs skin barrier function in Netherton syndrome through filaggrin and lipid misprocessing. J Clin Invest 2010;120:871–82.**

58 Netzel-Arnett S, Currie BM, Szabo R et al. Evidence for a matriptase prostasin proteolytic cascade regulating terminal epidermal differentiation. J Biol Chem 2006;281:32941–5.

59 Kilpatrick LM, Harris RL, Owen KA et al. Initiation of plasminogen activation on the surface of monocytes expressing the type II transmembrane serine protease matriptase. Blood 2006;108:2616–23.

60 Hosomi N, Fukai K, Nakanishi T et al. Caspase-1 activity of stratum corneum and serum interleukin-18 level are increased in patients with Netherton syndrome. Br J Dermatol 2008;159:744–6.

61 **Bennett K, Callard R, Heywood W et al. New role for LEKTI in skin barrier formation: label-free quantitative proteomic identification of caspase 14 as a novel target for the protease inhibitor LEKTI. J Proteome Res 2010;9:4289–94.**

62 Kabesch M, Carr D, Weiland SK, von Mutius E. Association between polymorphisms in serine protease inhibitor, kazal type 5 and asthma phenotypes in a large German population sample. Clin Exp Allergy 2004;34:340–5.

63 Kato A, Fukai K, Oiso N et al. Association of SPINK5 gene polymorphisms with atopic dermatitis in the Japanese population. Br J Dermatol 2003;148:665–9.

64 Nishio Y, Noguchi E, Shibasaki M et al. Association between polymorphisms in the SPINK5 gene and atopic dermatitis in the Japanese. Genes Immun 2003;4:515–17.

65 **Walley AJ, Chavanas S, Moffatt MF et al. Gene polymorphism in Netherton and common atopic disease. Nat Genet 2001;29:175–8.**

66 **Kusunoki T, Okafuji I, Yoshioka T et al. SPINK5 polymorphism is associated with disease severity and food allergy in children with atopic dermatitis. J Allergy Clin Immunol 2005;115:636–8.**

67 Hubiche T, Ged C, Benard A et al. Analysis of SPINK 5, KLK 7 and FLG genotypes in a French atopic dermatitis cohort. Acta Derm Venereol 2007;87:499–505.

68 Weidinger S, Baurecht H, Wagenpfeil S et al. Analysis of the individual and aggregate genetic contributions of previously identified serine peptidase inhibitor Kazal type 5 (SPINK5), kallikrein-related peptidase 7 (KLK7), and filaggrin (FLG) polymorphisms to eczema risk. J Allergy Clin Immunol 2008;122:560–8.

69 **Fortugno P, Furio L, Teson M et al. The 420K LEKTI variant alters LEKTI proteolytic activation and results in protease deregulation: implications for atopic dermatitis. Hum Mol Genet 2012; 21:4187–200.**

70 **Leclerc-Mercier S, Bodemer C, Furio L et al. Skin biopsy in Netherton syndrome: a histological review of a large series and new findings. Am J Dermatopathol 2016;38:83–91.**

71 Fartasch M, Williams ML, Elias PM. Altered lamellar body secretion and stratum corneum membrane structure in Netherton syndrome: differentiation from other infantile erythrodermas and pathogenic implications. Arch Dermatol 1999;135:823–32.

72 Frenk E, Mevorah B. Ichthyosis linearis circumflexa Comel with Trichorrhexis invaginata (Netherton's Syndrome): an ultrastructural study of the skin changes. Arch Dermatol Forsch 1972;245:42–9.

73 Muller FB, Hausser I, Berg D et al. Genetic analysis of a severe case of Netherton syndrome and application for prenatal testing. Br J Dermatol 2002;146:495–9.

74 Thorne EG, Zelickson AS, Mottaz JH et al. Netherton's syndrome: an electronmicroscopic study. Arch Dermatol Res 1975;253:177–83.

75 Jones SK, Thomason LM, Surbrugg SK, Weston WL. Neonatal hypernatraemia in two siblings with Netherton's syndrome. Br J Dermatol 1986;114:741–3.

76 Hausser I, Anton-Lamprecht I, Hartschuh W, Petzoldt D. Netherton's syndrome: ultrastructure of the active lesion under retinoid therapy. Arch Dermatol Res 1989;281:165–72.

77 Judge MR, Morgan G, Harper JI. A clinical and immunological study of Netherton's syndrome. Br J Dermatol 1994;131:615–21.

78 Smith DL, Smith JG, Wong SW, deShazo RD. Netherton's syndrome. Br J Dermatol 1995;133:153–4.

79 De WK, Ferster A, Sass U, Andre J et al. Netherton's syndrome: a severe neonatal disease. A case report. Dermatology 1996;192:400–2.

80 Plantin P, Delaire P, Guillet MH et al. [Netherton's syndrome. Current aspects. Apropos of 9 cases]. Ann Dermatol Venereol 1991;118:525–30.

81 Sardy M, Fay A, Karpati S, Horvath A. Comel–Netherton syndrome and peeling skin syndrome type B: overlapping syndromes or one entity? Int J Dermatol 2002;41:264–8.

82 Smith DL, Smith JG, Wong SW, deShazo RD. Netherton's syndrome: a syndrome of elevated IgE and characteristic skin and hair findings. J Allergy Clin Immunol 1995;95:116–23.

83 Folster-Holst R, Swensson O, Stockfleth E et al. Comel–Netherton syndrome complicated by papillomatous skin lesions containing human papillomaviruses 51 and 52 and plane warts containing human papillomavirus 16. Br J Dermatol 1999;140:1139–43.

84 Sedlacek V, Krenar J. [Symptomatology of Comel's linear circumflex ichthyosis (a case associated with genito-anal papillomatosis)]. Hautarzt 1971;22:390–7.

85 Weber F, Fuchs PG, Pfister HJ et al. Human papillomavirus infection in Netherton's syndrome. Br J Dermatol 2001;144:1044–9.

86 Hintner H, Jaschke E, Fritsch P. [Netherton syndrome: weakened immunity, generalized verrucosis and carcinogenesis]. Hautarzt 1980;31:428–32.

87 Kubler HC, Kuhn W, Rummel HH et al. [Development of cancer (vulvar cancer) in the Netherton syndrome (ichthyosis, hair anomalies, atopic diathesis)]. Geburtshilfe Frauenheilkd 1987;47:742–4.

88 Saghari S, Woolery-Lloyd H, Nouri K. Squamous cell carcinoma in a patient with Netherton's syndrome. Int J Dermatol 2002;41:415–16.

89 Krasagakis K, Ioannidou DJ, Stephanidou M et al. Early development of multiple epithelial neoplasms in Netherton syndrome. Dermatology 2003;207:182–4.

90 Stevanovic DV. Multiple defects of the hair shaft in Netherton's disease. Association with ichthyosis linearis circumflexa. Br J Dermatol 1969;81:851–7.

91 Lurie R, Hodak E, Ginzburg A, David M. Trichorrhexis nodosa: a manifestation of hypothyroidism. Cutis 1996;57:358–9.

92 Taylor CJ, Green SH. Menkes' syndrome (trichopoliodystrophy): use of scanning electron-microscope in diagnosis and carrier identification. Dev Med Child Neurol 1981;23:361–8.

93 Silengo M, Pietragalla A, Jarre L. Trichorrhexis nodosa and lip pits in autosomal dominant ectodermal dysplasia–central nervous system malformation syndrome. Am J Med Genet 1997;71:226–8.

94 Silengo M, Valenzise M, Spada M et al. Hair anomalies as a sign of mitochondrial disease. Eur J Pediatr 2003;162:459–61.

95 Shelley WB, Rawnsley HM. Aminogenic alopecia. Trans Assoc Am Physicians 1966;79:146–56.

96 Ito M, Ito K, Hashimoto K. Pathogenesis in trichorrhexis invaginata (bamboo hair). J Invest Dermatol 1984;83:1–6.

97 Taneda A, Ogawa H, Hashimoto K. The histochemical demonstration of protein-bound sulfhydryl groups and disulfide bonds in human hair by a new staining method (DACM staining). J Invest Dermatol 1980;75:365–9.
98 Bitoun E, Bodemer C, Amiel J et al. Prenatal diagnosis of a lethal form of Netherton syndrome by SPINK5 mutation analysis. Prenat Diagn 2002;22:121–6.
99 de Berker DA, Paige DG, Ferguson DJ, Dawber RP. Golf tee hairs in Netherton disease. Pediatr Dermatol 1995;12:7–11.
100 Powell J, Dawber RP, Ferguson DJ, Griffiths WA. Netherton's syndrome: increased likelihood of diagnosis by examining eyebrow hairs. Br J Dermatol 1999;141:544–6.
101 Menne T, Weisman K. Canestick lesion of vellus hair in Netherton's syndrome. Arch Dermatol 1985;121:451.
102 Adamson JE, Marten RH. Ichthyosis linearis circumflexa and Netherton's syndrome with idiopathic dwarfism. Proc R Soc Med 1973;66:624–5.
103 Caputo R, Vanotti P, Bertani E. Netherton's syndrome in two adult brothers. Arch Dermatol 1984;120:220–2.
104 Brodin MB, Porter PS. Nertherton's syndrome. Cutis 1980;26:185–8.
105 Dawber R, Comaish S. Scanning electron microscopy of normal and abnormal hair shafts. Arch Dermatol 1970;101:316–22.
106 Leonard JN, Gummer CL, Dawber RP. Generalized trichorrhexis nodosa. Br J Dermatol 1980;103:85–90.
107 Kurwa AR, Abdel-Aziz AH. Pili torti – congenital and acquired. Acta Derm Venereol 1973;53:385–92.
108 Selvaag E, Aas AM, Heide S. Structural hair shaft abnormalities in hypomelanosis of Ito and other ectodermal dysplasias. Acta Paediatr 2000;89:610–12.
109 Krafchik BR. What syndrome is this? Netherton syndrome. Pediatr Dermatol 1992;9:157–60.
110 Nikulin A, Salamon T. [The origin of the hair nodosities in Netherton's disease. (Polarization microscope studies)]. Z Haut Geschlechtskr 1969;44:1015–22.
111 Stankler L, Cochrane T. Netherton's disease in two sisters. Br J Dermatol 1967;79:187–96.
112 Gupta AK, Love P, Rasmussen JE. Hair abnormalities and a rash with a double-edged scale. Netherton's syndrome. Arch Dermatol 1986;122:1201,1203–4.
113 Kassis V, Nielsen JM, Klem-Thomsen H et al. Familial Netherton's disease. Cutis 1986;38:175–8.
114 Renz H, Brodie C, Bradley K et al. Enhancement of IgE production by anti-CD40 antibody in atopic dermatitis. J Allergy Clin Immunol 1994;93:658–68.
115 Stryk S, Siegfried EC, Knutsen AP. Selective antibody deficiency to bacterial polysaccharide antigens in patients with Netherton syndrome. Pediatr Dermatol 1999;16:19–22.
116 Knutsen AP. Chronic sinusitis in children. Pediatr Asthma Allerg Immunol 1997;11:147–69.
117 Arslanagic N, Arslanagic R. [Netherton syndrome with recurrent herpes of facial skin]. Medicinski Arhiv (Sarajevo) 2002;56:221–4.
118 Nicholls S, Patel HC, Jones M. Recurrent bacterial vaginosis and Netherton's syndrome. Int J STD AIDS 1999;10:202–3.
119 De WK, Ferster A, Sass U et al. Netherton's syndrome: a severe neonatal disease. A case report. Dermatology 1996;192:400–2.
120 Gross TP, Khurana RK, Higgins T et al. Vaccine associated poliomyelitis in a household contact with Netherton's syndrome receiving long-term steroid therapy. Am J Med 1987;83:797–800.
121 Hausser I, Anton-Lamprecht I. Severe congenital generalized exfoliative erythroderma in newborns and infants: a possible sign of Netherton syndrome. Pediatr Dermatol 1996;13:183–99.
122 Pradeaux L, Olives JP, Bonafe JL et al. [Digestive and nutritional manifestations of Netherton's syndrome]. Arch Fr Pediatr 1991;48:95–8.
123 Greig D, Wishart J. Growth abnormality in Netherton's syndrome. Australas J Dermatol 1982;23:27–31.
124 Stoll C, Alembik Y, Tchomakov D et al. Severe hypernatremic dehydration in an infant with Netherton syndrome. Genet Couns 2001;12:237–43.
125 Ergin H, Kilic I, Tekinalp G. Netherton's syndrome and neonatal hypernatremia. A case report. Turk J Pediatr 1997;39:409–13.
126 Pohl M, Zimmerhackl LB, Hausser I et al. Acute bilateral renal vein thrombosis complicating Netherton syndrome. Eur J Pediatr 1998;157:157–60.
127 Yerebakan O, Uguz A, Keser I et al. Netherton syndrome associated with idiopathic congenital hemihypertrophy. Pediatr Dermatol 2002;19:345–8.
128 Julius CE, Keeran M. Netherton's syndrome in a male. Arch Dermatol 1971;104:422–4.
129 Ong C, O'Toole EA, Ghali L et al. LEKTI demonstrable by immunohistochemistry of the skin: a potential diagnostic skin test for Netherton syndrome. Br J Dermatol 2004;151:1253–7.
130 Glover MT, Atherton DJ, Levinsky RJ. Syndrome of erythroderma, failure to thrive, and diarrhea in infancy: a manifestation of immunodeficiency. Pediatrics 1988;81:66–72.
131 Allen A, Siegfried E, Silverman R et al. Significant absorption of topical tacrolimus in 3 patients with Netherton syndrome. Arch Dermatol 2001;137:747–50.
132 Bens G, Boralevi F, Buzenet C, Taieb A. Topical treatment of Netherton's syndrome with tacrolimus ointment without significant systemic absorption. Br J Dermatol 2003;149:224–6.
133 Small AM, Cordoro KM. Netherton syndrome mimicking pustular psoriasis: clinical implications and response to intravenous immunoglobulin. Pediatr Dermatol 2016;33:e222–3.
134 Yalcin AD. A case of Netherton syndrome: successful treatment with omalizumab and pulse prednisolone and its effects on cytokines and immunoglobulin levels. Immunopharmacol Immunotoxicol 2016;38:162–6.
135 Fontao L, Laffitte E, Briot A et al. Infliximab infusions for Netherton syndrome: sustained clinical improvement correlates with a reduction of thymic stromal lymphopoietin levels in the skin. J Invest Dermatol 2011;131:1947–50.
136 Paller AS, Renert-Yuval Y, Suprun M et al. An IL-17-dominant immune profile is shared across the major orphan forms of ichthyosis, J Allergy Clin Immunol 2017;139:152–65.
137 Furio L, Pampalakis G, Michael IP et al. KLK5 Inactivation Reverses Cutaneous Hallmarks of Netherton Syndrome. PLoS Genet 2015;11(9):e1005389.
138 Tiryakioğlu NO, Önal Z, Saygili SK et al. Treatment of ichthyosis and hypernatremia in a patient with Netherton syndrome with a SPINK5 c.153delT mutation using kallikrein inhibiting ointment. Int J Dermatol 2017;56:106–8.
139 Prassas I, Eissa A, Poda G, Diamandis EP. Unleashing the therapeutic potential of human kallikrein-related serine proteases. Nat Rev Drug Discov 2015;14:183–202.
140 de Veer SJ, Swedberg JE, Brattsand M et al. Exploring the active site binding specificity of kallikrein-related peptidase 5 (KLK5) guides the design of new peptide substrates and inhibitors. Biol Chem 2016;397:1237–49.
141 Ferrari S, Pellegrini G, Matsui T et al. Towards a gene therapy clinical trial for epidermolysis bullosa. Rev Recent Clin Trials 2006;1:155–62.
142 Mavilio F, Pellegrini G, Ferrari S et al. Correction of junctional epidermolysis bullosa by transplantation of genetically modified epidermal stem cells. Nat Med 2006;12:1397–402.
143 Di WL, Mellerio JE, Bernadis C et al. Phase I study protocol for ex vivo lentiviral gene therapy for the inherited skin disease, Netherton syndrome. Hum Gene Ther Clin Dev 2013;24:182–90.

CHAPTER 133
Porokeratosis

Leslie Castelo-Soccio
University of Pennsylvania Perlman School of Medicine and Children's Hospital of Philadelphia, Philadelphia, PA, USA

Abstract

Porokeratoses are clonal disorders of keratinization. Risk factors include genetic inheritance, ultraviolet radiation and immunosuppression. Therapy is individualized and is based on size, location and number of lesions. Active nonintervention with regular follow up to monitor for malignant transformation is appropriate for many. For some, localized therapy with topical therapy such as steroids, antimetabolites, or retinoids are prescribed. Cryotherapy and excision, as well as laser therapy, are also utilized.

Key points

- **Porokeratoses are clonal disorders of keratinization.**
- **They can be localized or diffuse.**
- **Genetic inheritance, ultraviolet light therapy and immunosuppression are risk factors.**

Definition. Porokeratoses are a collection of clonal disorders of keratinization that share a histologically distinct hyperkeratotic ridge-like border called the cornoid lamella (Fig. 133.1). There are five common clinical variants: classic porokeratosis of Mibelli (PM), disseminated superficial actinic porokeratosis (DSAP), porokeratosis palmaris et plantaris disseminata (PPPD), linear porokeratosis and punctate porokeratosis [1–4]. There is also an additional disseminated variant known as disseminated superficial porokeratosis and lesser known variants such as porokeratosis ptychotropica, a pustular variant of DSAP, porokeratotic eccrine ostial and dermal duct nevus and genital/penoscrotal porokeratosis.

Aetiology. Several risk factors exist for porokeratosis including genetic inheritance, ultraviolet radiation (including electron beam, radiation therapy and artificial ultraviolet radiation) and immunosuppression [5–7]. Porokeratosis has been observed in patients with the human immunodeficiency virus (HIV) and lymphomas as well as patients on immunosuppressive medications for transplant or autoimmune diseases [8]. Most patients who develop porokeratosis have less pigmented skin, although porokeratosis can be seen in more darkly pigmented individuals [9]. The formation of nonmelanoma skin cancers including squamous cell carcinomas and basal cell carcinomas have been reported for all types of porokeratosis although linear porokeratosis and large lesions of long duration appear to have the greatest risk [10–13]. Reports of malignant transformation into skin tumours range from 7.5 to 11.6%. Instability in chromosome 3 has been associated with development of malignancy in cultured fibroblasts derived from porokeratosis lesions [5,14].

Online Mendelian Inheritance in Man lists nine types of porokeratosis. Changes in the mevalonate pathway and the gene *MVK* has been implicated in some causes of DSAP [15]. More recently three additional genes, *MVD, PMVK* and *FDPS* have also been identified as novel genes [15]. All four genes are involved in the mevalonate pathway. Previous microarray analysis from porokeratosis patients' lesional and nonlesional skin identified three candidate genes: *SART3, SSH1* and *ARPC3* (actin related protein 2/3 complex, subunit 3) which were upregulated in lesional skin. Keratin 6a was identified as a specific biomarker for porokeratotic keratinocytes because it was the most significantly upregulated gene in the nine patient samples. Keratin 6A, BB, 16, 17, S100A7 (S-100 calcium binding proteinA7/psoriasin), A8, A9, FABP5 (fatty acid binding protein 5, psoriasis-associated), GJB2 (gap junction protein beta 2/connexin 26) and SPRP1A (small proline-rich protein 1A) were previously shown upregulated in lesional compared with nonlesional skin [16,17].

The subtypes of porokeratosis arise at different time points in an individual's lifetime with linear porokeratosis and PPPD occurring at any time between birth and adulthood, whereas PM develops in childhood and DSAP typically occurs in the third or fourth decade of life. There are reports of multiple types of porokeratosis arising in a single patient [18].

Harper's Textbook of Pediatric Dermatology, Fourth Edition. Edited by Peter Hoeger, Veronica Kinsler and Albert Yan.

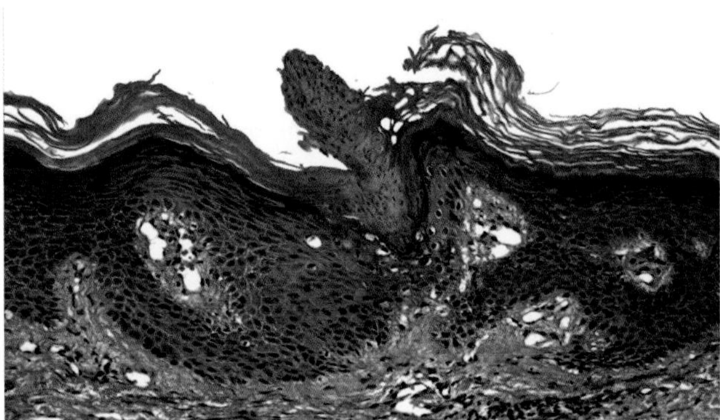

Fig. 133.1 Histology of porokeratosis. Haematoxylin and eosin stained image (×10) showing characteristic cornoid lamella. Source: Courtesy of Dr Adam Rubin.

Clinical variants.

Porokeratosis of Mibelli

This entity was first reported in 1889 by Vittorio Mibelli in a 21-year-old patient with an affected father and sibling, as multiple annular and gyrate plaques with central atrophy and elevated keratotic borders containing a longitudinal furrow [1]. Mibelli coined the term 'porokeratosis' to emphasize what he believed to be representative features of the lesion: abnormal keratinization and origination within the pores of sweat ducts. PM lesions are typically asymptomatic or very slightly itchy, light brown keratotic papules that develop in childhood. Although there is usually an autosomal dominant inheritance pattern, this entity can also be acquired. As the lesion progresses, papules slowly expand to form an annular plaque with a raised border and atrophic centre. These lesions may expand rapidly if the patient becomes immunosuppressed. There are reports of patients developing this entity after diagnosis of HIV [19]. Frequently there is a history of antecedent burn, radiation therapy or other trauma to the area where the lesion first appears [20]. For PM, the main differential diagnoses include guttate psoriasis and warts. There are rare reports of cutaneous T-cell lymphoma mimicking porokeratosis so this should be considered. Use of dermoscopy to identify the hyperkeratotic border has been proposed recently. Under dermoscopy a white peripheral rim, which corresponds to cornoid lamellae, is the essential pathognomonic feature for diagnosis [21].

Disseminated superficial actinic porokeratosis

Four years after Mibelli described porokeratosis, Respighi described the disseminated superficial variant. In 1967, Chernosky defined DSAP (also known as porokeratosis of Chernosky) as a distinct clinical entity characterized by small inconspicuous lesions occurring on sun-exposed areas in adults [22]. A subsequent detailed light microscopic analysis of 35 clinically varied cases was published by Reed and Leone in 1970 [23]. They observed that the majority of lesions were not associated with ostia of eccrine or pilosebaceous ducts, and asserted that the well-accepted term 'porokeratosis' was a misnomer. A more precise term was not proposed. This entity is composed of multiple small scaly brown keratotic papules with raised borders which occur on the extensor surfaces. Lesion numbers range from a few to several hundred but typically more than 50 lesions are present. They may be asymptomatic or slightly itchy. Half of patients note exacerbation of their lesions during the summer months. Facial lesions are uncommon and occur in less than 15% of patients. Most patients who develop DSAP are women in their fourth and fifth decades with an extensive history of ultraviolet radiation exposure (such as repeated tanning/tanning bed exposure or ultraviolet exposure from phototherapy) [24,25]. Immunosuppression also can trigger DSAP [24]. For DSAP the main differential diagnoses include psoriasis, stuccokeratoses, actinic keratoses, squamous cell carcinoma, warts and Darier disease.

In 2002, two loci for DSAP were mapped to 12q23.2–24.1 and 15q25.1–26.1 in two Chinese families and in 2004 an additional locus was mapped to chromosome 18p11.3 [26,27]. Since then *MVP* has been identified as a causal gene in patients with DSAP. In 2015, three additional genes in the mevalonate pathway have been identified as causal: *PMVK*, *MVD* and *FDPS*. The *SART3* gene has also been identified as a candidate gene from previous work. SLC17A9 mutations have also been reported in patients with DSAP [15].

In 2009, a new variant was described with neutrophilic pustules within the cornoid lamellae which corresponds to pustules on the outer rim clinically. This was the second report of porokeratosis with pustules [28].

Linear porokeratosis

This rarer subtype was historically described in 1974 by Rahbari as an entity distinct from PM [29]. These lesions typically occur in infancy or childhood and do not appear to be inherited. They are red–brown linear keratotic papules and annular plaques often in a Blaschkoid distribution (Fig. 133.2). Nail dystrophy has been associated with this disorder. Loss of heterozygosity may account for a higher risk of malignant degeneration within these lesions. These lesions may also have increased risk for p53 mutations [30]. For linear porokeratosis, the main differential diagnoses include linear verrucous epidermal naevus, lichen striatus, incontinentia pigmenti, linear lichen planus, linear psoriasis, linear Darier disease and warts.

Porokeratosis palmaris and plantaris disseminata

This is a variant originally described by Guss in 1971 [31]. These are small keratotic papules, which are sometimes itchy, on the palms and soles which occur during adolescence and early adulthood. These may become generalized and involve the trunk and extremities. The appearance is similar to DSAP except that the lesions are not limited to sun-exposed areas. Mucosal lesions have been noted occasionally. Squamous cell carcinomas are reported to develop within these lesions [24,32,33]. These lesions can be transmitted in an autosomal

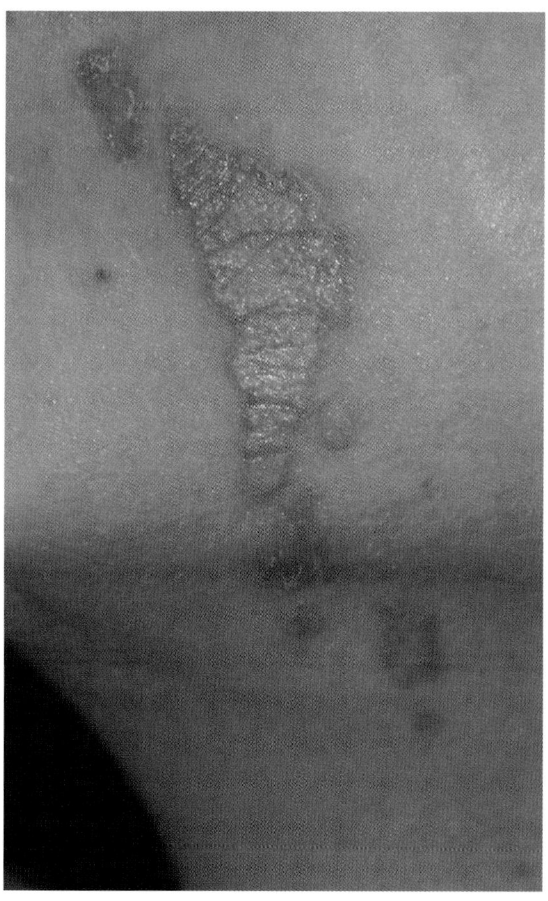

Fig. 133.2 Linear porokeratosis on the chin of a child. Source: Courtesy of Dr Albert Yan.

dominant mode or caused by immunosuppression. Sudden development of these lesions should prompt a search for internal malignancy. Differential diagnoses include palmo-plantar keratodermas, calluses and warts.

In 2003, a locus was located at chromosome 12q24.1–24.2 but no disease genes or mechanisms were identified [27]. Two candidate genes, *SSH1* and *SART3*, with uncertain significance were isolated from one screen. Flow cytometry of cells from lesional skin have shown abnormal DNA ploidy.

Punctate porokeratosis

Punctate porokeratosis is manifested by multiple small (0.2–1.0 cm) firm flesh-coloured hyperkeratotic papules on the palms and soles of adults. Papules are firmly attached at their bases. There is no inheritance pattern (although both sporadic and autosomal dominant forms have been reported) and usually these are associated with other forms of porokeratosis [34]. Clinically, these lesions resemble punctate porokeratotic keratoderma which is considered a sign of internal malignancy. Differential diagnoses include punctate, palmoplantar keratoderma (Buschke–Fischer disease), acrokeratoelastoidosis, punctate keratosis of palmar creases, focal acral hyperkeratosis, calluses and warts.

The aetiology of this disease is not certain. Lesions do not resolve spontaneously.

Porokeratosis ptychotropica

This lesser known variant is characterized by circumferential perianal plaques. These lesions have the typical cornoid lamella histology but with underlying amyloid deposition [35]. Differential diagnoses include inverse psoriasis, chronic contact or irritant dermatitis, acrodermatitis enteropathica, necrolytic migratory erythema, chronic intertrigo, Darier disease and Hailey–Hailey disease. These are sometimes associated with giant plaques.

Genital/penoscrotal porokeratosis

This variant has been considered a distinct form of porokeratosis that can be associated with diabetes, sexually transmitted disease (one report of a patient with condyloma acuminata and one with syphilis) [36] and in one case CD4/CD8 suppression in the absence of HIV infection [37]. Porokeratosis of the genital area is extremely rare. There does not appear to be a genetic inheritance pattern. Most lesions are confined to the genital area but some patients have involvement of the inguinal area and buttocks. Severe burning and itching has been associated. This entity is difficult to diagnose clinically at first and initial clinical impressions include atopic dermatitis, gumma, condylomata lata, extramammary Paget disease, granuloma annulare, warts and lichen simplex chronicus. Biopsy can assist in differentiation. It appears to progress rapidly initially but stabilizes quickly without further extension. The majority of cases reported were in men in their 20s. Malignant transformation has not been reported.

Diagnosis. Overall, appearance, age of onset and distribution categorize these lesions. Biopsy will show characteristic cornoid lamella and help rule out other diagnoses. Dermoscopic examination may be of diagnostic use [38]. Dermoscopy of disseminated porokeratosis shows a characteristic central scar-like area with a single or double 'white track' structure at the margin. The 'white track' corresponds to the cornoid lamella histologically.

Key management criteria. Treatment is individualized and based on size, location and number of lesions. For many patients observation for malignant degeneration, aggressive sun protection and emollients are all that is required. Active non-intervention should always be accompanied by anticipatory guidance for patients and caregivers, along with regular follow up to monitor for significant changes. High-quality close-up photographic images can be of value in this effort. If lesions are widespread or there is a concern for malignant degeneration, a number of surgical, topical and oral therapies can be utilized [39]. Overall, treatments are documented as single case reports and small case series and these include both topical agents like tacrolimus as well as systemic agents and light [40–45]. The majority of reports are for adult patients with DSAP. There are few case reports for use of these treatments in children [46,47]. The ideal treatment is pain-free, effective, safe and nonscarring.

As with any genodermatosis, a genetic history should be obtained and counselling should be provided. Parents of a child with PM should be examined for skin lesions. There is a 50% risk of disease in each child born to an affected individual. The inheritance pattern of linear porokeratosis is unclear. An autosomal pattern of transmission has been reported for other genodermatoses that present as somatic mosaics. CDAGs syndrome (craniosynostosis, anal anomalies, and porokeratosis) has been reported in four families [48]. No gene has been identified.

Topical therapies

Topical therapy is the most acceptable route for the majority of patients. However, long-term therapy is often required. Poor compliance will result in suboptimal results, and prolonged use of some medications (potent topical corticosteroids, calcipotriol) requires close follow up, paying special attention to problems associated with systemic absorption.

Topical 5-fluouracil (5-FU), an antimetabolite that inhibits DNA synthesis, can induce remission if it is used for at least 3–4 weeks and a brisk inflammatory response is achieved. This therapy is often combined with topical retinoids, salicylic acid or other keratolytics [40,45]. It is thought that topical retinoids decrease abnormal keratinization. Patients will develop extreme redness and irritation and should be warned about these effects.

Topical 5% imiquimod cream, an imidazoquinoline amine, has been used effectively for PM and may be beneficial for other types of porokeratosis including linear porokeratosis [43,49]. The precise mechanism is not known but appears to be related to induction of cytokines such as interferon-α (IFN-α), IFN-γ, tumour necrosis factor α and interleukin-12 which results in the promotion of cell-mediated immune responses. In these case reports and small case series, topical imiquimod (5%) is applied once per day, 5 days per week under occlusion for 2–4 months. Strong inflammatory reactions were noted but were decreased with either topical steroids or decreasing frequency of application. Good responses were noted but long-term follow up is needed to evaluate safety and efficacy. There is one report of a patient with disseminated porokeratosis palmaris and plantaris with a history of multiple basal cell carcinomas and squamous cell carcinomas treated with imiquimod to prevent malignancy. This patient used daily therapy for 6 months. No new carcinomas were noted in the 6-month period and clinically there was decreased scale and red–brown coloration of porokeratotic plaques [43].

There are no data on the efficacy of topical 5-FU for the treatment of paediatric porokeratoses. Case reports have documented the relative safety of extensively applied topical 5% 5-FU cream for up to 10 years in children with other problems [46,47]. A potential adverse effect is injury from inadvertent transfer to other sensitive tissues, such as the cornea. Systemic absorption in adults is estimated to be 6 mg following a daily application of 2 g, far below the 12 mg/kg/day for cancer chemotherapy, and toxic effects have not been reported. However, enhanced absorption is expected from eroded areas, and the increased ratio of body surface area to weight in small children puts them at higher risk for systemic toxicity.

Topical vitamin D_3 analogues can regulate keratinocyte differentiation and can be used in this disorder [50]. Daily topical calcipotriol or talcalcitol applied for 8 weeks to 5 months can be effective for DSAP. Caution is advised because these can potentially elevate serum calcium levels.

Topical retinoids and salicylic acid alone are third-line therapies and are more typically used in combination with topical chemotherapy [40]. Diclofenac topical gel has also been used for genital lesions and DSAP with mixed success. Diclofenac topical gel is a nonsteroidal anti-inflammatory which is thought to block prostaglandin production by inhibiting cyclo-oxygenase [51,52]. Patients who have used this therapy typically report a subjective improvement in lesions and overall skin texture. It may stabilize progression of disease, as documented in one case report of a patient with genital porokeratosis, and provide symptomatic relief. An open label study of 17 patients in which patients were enrolled for 12–24 weeks of twice daily topical treatment, a mean decrease of 4% in target area lesions after 12 weeks and a 12% decrease in 24 weeks was found. Half of the patients showed a decrease in progression of disease [51].

In a single case report in two patients with PM, cantharadin has been reported to be effective. It was applied under occlusion for 8 hours [53].

Surgical management

Cryotherapy is a first-line therapy for smaller lesions [54]. Lesions are typically treated for 30 seconds with a spray tip after keratotic borders are removed. The main drawback of cryotherapy is that it can be painful and lead to dyschromia and atrophy. Multiple treatments are often needed for complete resolution.

Surgical methods can also be used including electrodessication and curettage for small to medium lesions. Dermabrasion has been shown to be successful in one case. Surgery is needed for any lesions that have undergone malignant transformation. It is unclear if prophylactic excision reduces the incidence of malignant transformation. If a painful surgical approach is indicated, age-appropriate recommendations for control of pain and anxiety should be followed [39].

Oral therapies

Oral retinoids may reduce malignant degeneration in patients on immunosuppression. Both acitretin and etretinate have been shown to be effective in disseminated porokeratosis and PM [44,55,56]. Doses of 30 mg/day acitretin and 75 and 50 mg/day etretinate have been used in adults. Patients noticed improvement within 2–4 weeks. Recurrence has been observed after cessation of therapy. Low-dose isotretinoin (20 mg/day) has also been used for PPPD. Gradual recurrence is noted 3 months after treatment. The risks of these medications usually outweigh the benefits in children but may be warranted if there is concern for malignant degeneration in immunosuppressed children.

Laser and light therapies

Laser ablation using pulsed dye laser (one case report in linear porokeratosis), ND:YAG laser (one case report) [57], Q-switched ruby (two case reports in DSAP) [58] and CO_2 laser ablation (multiple case reports)[59] has been used but recurrence has also been observed after these therapies. These methods are destructive methods and can cause scarring. Overall, these case reports describe each therapy as moderately successful. Postoperative pain may be poorly tolerated, and traditional wound care, with frequent dressing changes, is not easily accomplished in young children.

Light therapy, most prominently photodynamic therapy, has been used successfully for DSAP and linear porokeratosis. Photodynamic therapy uses light to activate a photosensitizer in diseased skin leading to the formation of cytotoxic reactive oxygen species and selective cell damage. There are three case reports in adults with DSAP, one case series in adults with DSAP and one case report in a child with linear porokeratosis for efficacy of this therapy [41,42,60]. In these reports, patients were treated with methyl aminolevulinate hydrochloride cream, a sensitizer, for 2–3 hours under occlusion. The area was subsequently illuminated with red light for 9–16 minutes. Authors note good tolerance of the procedure and no need for anaesthesia. Two to four total sessions were performed in these cases with no recurrence noted up to 11 months after last treatment. One patient continued 5-FU during therapy and these authors felt this combination was more effective than either alone [60].

Close observation and education about strict sun protection is important. If familial inheritance is suspected, other family members should be screened. Screening for causes of immunosuppression including haematological malignancies and HIV is appropriate for PM, DSAP or sudden exacerbation of lesions.

References

1 Mibelli V. Porokeratosis. In: Morris MA (ed.) International Atlas of Rare Skin Diseases. Hamburg: Leopold Voss, 1889:8–10.
2 Schamroth JM, Zlotogorski A, Guead L. Porokeratosis of Mibelli: overview and review of the literature. Acta Derm Venereol 1997;77:207–13.
3 Kim C. Linear porokeratosis. Dermatol Online J 2005;11:22.
4 Lorenz GE, Ritter SE. Linear porokeratosis: a case report and review of the literature. Cutis 2008;81:479–83.
5 Scappaticci S, Lambiase S, Orecchia G, Fraccaro M. Clonal chromosome abnormalities with preferential involvement of chromosome 3 in patients with porokeratosis of Mibelli. Cancer Genet Cytogenet 1989;43:89–94.
6 Paller AS, Syder AJ, Yiu-Mo Chan BS. Genetic and clinical mosaicism in a type of epidermal nevus. N Engl J Med 1994;331:1408–15.
7 Xia K, Deng H, Xia JH et al. A novel locus (DSAP2) for disseminated superficial actinic porokeratosis maps to chromosome 15q25.1–26.1. Br J Dermatol 2002;147:650–4.
8 Diluvio L, Campione E, Paterno EJ et al. Acute onset disseminated superficial porokeratosis heralding diffuse large B-cell lymphoma. Eur J Dermatol 2008;18:349–50.
9 Doherty CB, Krathen RA, Smith-Zagone MJ, Hsu S. Disseminated superficial actinic porokeratosis in black skin. Int J Dermatol 2009;48:160–1.
10 Otsuka F, Someya T, Ishibashi Y. Porokeratosis and malignant skin tumors. Cancer Res Clin Oncol 1991;117:55–60.
11 Ninomiya Y, Urano Y, Yoshimoto K. P53 gene mutation analysis in porokeratosis and porokeratosis associated squamous cell carcinomas. J Dermatol Sci 1997;14:173–8.
12 Ma DL, Vano-Galvan S. Squamous cell carcinoma arising from giant porokeratosis. Dermatol Surg 2009;35:1999–2000.
13 James WD, Rodman OG. Squamous cell carcinoma arising in porokeratosis of Mibelli. Int J Dermatol 1986;25:389–91.
14 Happle R. Cancer proneness of linear porokeratosis may be explained by allelic loss. Dermatology 1997;195:20–5.
15 Leng Y, Yan L, Feng H et al. Mutations in Mevalonate pathway genes in patients with familial or sporadic porokeratosis. J Dermatol 2018;45:862–6.
16 Hivnor C, Williams N, Singh F et al. Gene expression profiling of porokeratosis demonstrates similarities to psoriasis. J Cutan Pathol 2004;31:657–64.
17 Zhang ZH, Wang ZM, Crosby ME et al. Reassessment of microarray expression data of porokeratossi by quantitative real time polymerase chain reaction. J Cutan Pathol 2002;37:371–5.
18 Bhaskar S, Jaiswal AK, Raj N et al. Porokeratosis – head to toe: an unusual presentation. Indian Dermatol Online J 2015;6:101–4.
19 Rodriguez EA, Jakubowicz S, Chinchilla DA et al. Porokeratosis of Mibelli and HIV infection. Int J Dermatol 1996;35:402–4.
20 Nova MP, Goldberg LJ, Mattison T, Halperin A. Porokeratosis arising in a burn scar. J Am Acad Dermatol 1991;25:354–6.
21 Pizzichetta MA, Canzonieri V, Massone C, Soyer HP. Clinical and dermscopic features of porokeratosis of Mibelli. Arch Dermatol 2009;141:91–2.
22 Chernosky, ME, Freeman, RG. Disseminated superficial actinic porokeratosis (DSAP). Arch Dermatol 1967;96:611–24.
23 Reed RJ, Leone P. Porokeratosis – a mutant clonal keratosis of the epidermis. I. Histogenesis. Arch Dermatol 1970;101:340–47.
24 Jung JY, Yeon JH, Ryu HS et al. Disseminated superficial porokeratosis developed by immunosuppression due to rheumatoid arthritis treatment. J Dermatol 2009;36:466–7.
25 Bencini PL, Tarantino A, Grimalt R et al. Porokeratosis and immunosuppression. Br J Dermatol 1995;132:74–8.
26 Wei S, Zhang TD, Zhou Y et al. Fine mapping of the disseminated superficial porokeratosis locus to a 2.7 Mb region at 18p11.3. Clin Exp Dermatol 2010;35:664–7.
27 Wei SC, Yang S, Li M et al. Identification of a locus for porokeratosis palmaris et plantaris disseminata to a 6.9-cM region at chromosome 12q24.1–24.2. Br J Dermatol 2003;149:261–7S.
28 Miller DD, Ruben BS. Pustular porokeratosis. J Cutan Pathol 2009;36:1191–2.
29 Rahbari H, Cordero AA, Mehregan AH. Linear porokeratosis: a distinctive clinical variant of porokeratosis of Mibelli. Arch Dermatol 1974;109:526–8.
30 Arranz-Salas I, Sanz-Trelles A, Bautista-Ojeda D. P53 alterations in porokeratosis. J Cutan Pathol 2003;30:455–8.
31 Guss, SB, Osbourn, RA, Lutzner, MA. Porokeratosis plantaris, palmaris et disseminate: a third type of porokeratosis. Arch Dermatol 1971;104:366–73.
32 Sasson M, Krain AD. Porokeratosis and cutaneous malignancy: a review. Dermatol Surg 1996;22:339–42.
33 Sherman V, Reed J, Hollowod K et al. Poromas and porokeratosis in patients treated for solid organ and haematological malignancies. Clin Exp Dermatol 2010;35:130–2.
34 Alikhan A, Burns T, Zargari O. Punctate porokeratotic keratoderma. Dermatol Online J 2010;16:13.
35 Tallon B, Blumental G, Bhawn J. Porokeratosis ptychotropica: a lesser known variant. Clin Exp Dermatol 2009;34:e895–7.
36 Chen TJ, Chou YC, Chen CH et al. Genital porokeratosis: a series of 10 patients and review of the literature. Br J Dermatol 2006; 155:325–9.
37 Benmously Mlika R, Kenani N, Badri T et al. Localized genital porokeratosis in a female patient with multiple myeloma. Eur Acad Dermatol Venereol 2008;23:584–5.
38 Delfino M, Argenziano G, Nino M. Dermscopy for the diagnosis of porokeratosis. J Eur Acad Dermatol Venereol 2004;18:194–5.
39 Martin-Clavijo A, Kanelleas A, Vlachou C et al. (eds). Treatment of Skin Disease: Comprehensive Therapeutic Strategies, 3rd edn. Philadelphia: Saunders Elsevier, 2010:584–6.
40 Danby W. Treatment of porokeratosis with fluorouracil and salicylic acid under occlusion. Dermatol Online J 2003;9:33.

41 Fernandez-Guarino M, Harto A, Perez-Garcia B et al. Photodynamic therapy in disseminated superficial actinic keratosis. J Euro Acad Dermatol Venereol 2009;23:176–7.
42 Garcia-Navarro X, Garces JR, Baselga E, Alomar A. Linear porokeratosis: excellent response to photodyamic therapy. Arch Dermatol 2009;145:526–7.
43 Jensen JM, Egberts F, Proksch E, Hauschild A. Disseminated porokeratosis palmaris and plantaris treated with imiquimod cream to prevent malignancy. Acta Derm Venereol 2005;85:550–1.
44 Hong JB, Hsiao CH, Chu CY. Systematized linear porokeratosis: a rare variant of diffuse porokeratosis with good response to systemic acitretin. J Am Acad Dermatol 2009;60:713–5.
45 Levitt J, Emer JJ, Emanuel PO. Treatment of porokeratosis of Mibelli with combined use of photodynamic therapy and fluorouracil cream. Arch Dermatol 2010;146:371–3.
46 Kwok, C, Gibbs, S, Bennett, C et al. Topical treatment for cutaneous warts. Cochrane Database Syst Rev 2012;12:CD00178.
47 Hamoudan, B, Jamila Z, Najet, R et al. Topical 5-fluorouracil to treat multiple or unresectable facial squamous cell carcinoma in xeroderma pigmentosum. J Am Acad Dermat 2001;44:1054.
48 Chouvery, E, Guissart, C, Megarbane, H et al. Craniosynostosis, anal anomalies and porokeratosis (CDAGS syndrome): case report and review. Eur J Med Genet 2013;56:674–7.
49 Agarwal S, Berth-Jones J. Porokeratosis of Mibelli: successful treatment with 5% imiquimod cream. Br J Dermatol 2002;146:331–4.
50 Bakardzhiev, I, Kavaklieva, S, Pehlivanov, G. Successful treatment of DSAP with calcipotriol. Int J Dermatol 2012;51:1139–42.
51 Varma SM, Cantrell W, Chen SC et al. Diclofenac sodium 3% gel as a potential treatment for disseminated actinic porokeratosis. J Eur Dermatol Venereol 2009;23:42–5.
52 Vlachou C, Kanelleas AI, Martin-Clavijo A, Berth-Jones J. Treatment of disseminated superficial actinic porokeratosis with topical diclofenac gel: a case series. Eur J Dermatol Venereol 2008; 22:1343–5.
53 Levitt, JO, Kelley, BR, Phelps, RG. Treatment of porokeratosis of Mibelli with cantharadin. J Am Acad Derm 2013; 69:e254–55.
54 Dereli T, Ozyurt S, Ozturk G. Porokertosis of Mibelli: successful treatment with cryosurgery. J Dermatol 2004;31:223–7.
55 McAllister RE, Estes SA, Yarbrough CL. Porokeratosis plantaris, palmaris et disseminata: report of a case and treatment with isotretinoin. J Am Acad Dermatol 1986;13:598–603.
56 Campbell JP, Voorhees JJ. Etretinate improves localized porokeratosis of Mibelli. Int J Dermatol 1985;24:261–3.
57 Liu HT. Treatment of lichen amyloidosis (LA) and disseminated superficial porokeratosis (DSP) with frequency-doubled Q-switched Nd-YAG laser. Dermatol Surg 2000;26:958–62.
58 Lolis MS, Marmur ES. Treatment of disseminated superficial actinic porokeratosis (DSAP) with the Q-switched ruby laser. J Cosmetic Laser Ther 2008;10:124–7.
59 Barnett JH. Linear porokeratosis: treatment with the carbon dioxide laser. J Am Acad Dermatol 1986;14:902–4.
60 Cavicchini S, Tourlaki A. Successful treatment of disseminated superficial actinic porokeratosis with methyl aminolevulinate–photodyamic therapy. J Dermatol Treat 2006;17:190–1.

CHAPTER 134
Ectodermal Dysplasias

Cathal O'Connor[1], *Yuka Asai*[2] *& Alan D. Irvine*[1]
[1] Paediatric Dermatology, Trinity College Dublin and Our Lady's Children's Hospital, Dublin, Ireland
[2] Division of Dermatology, Queen's University, Kingston, Ontario, Canada

Introduction, 1629
Ectodermal dysplasias caused by mutations in tumour necrosis factor like/NF-κB signalling pathways, 1669
Transcription factors and homeobox genes: major regulators of gene expression, 1677
Defects in the Wnt-β-catenin pathway, 1686
Defects in gap junction proteins, 1691
Disorders caused by mutations in structural and adhesive molecules, 1697
Management of ectodermal dysplasia: general overview, 1704

Abstract

The ectodermal dysplasias (EDs) encompass a complex and highly diverse group of heritable disorders that have developmental abnormalities of ectodermal appendages in common. Recent advances in molecular genetic testing have changed the paradigm of classification to correlate with underlying genotypes. EDs can be divided into defects in developmental regulation and epithelial–mesenchymal interaction, and defects in proteins of cytoskeleton or adhesion, which are involved in cell–cell communication as well as structural integrity. Management of EDs is multidisciplinary and specific to the ED involved.

Key points

- Ectodermal dysplasias (EDs) are a group of inherited disorders that have two or more of the following developmental abnormalities in common: skin, hair, teeth, nails, sweat glands and other ectodermal structures.
- Other structures derived from embryonic ectoderm include the mammary gland, thyroid gland, thymus, anterior pituitary, adrenal medulla, central nervous system, external ear, melanocytes, cornea, conjunctiva, lacrimal gland and lacrimal duct.
- Previous clinical classification systems distinguished EDs according to the presence or absence of affected tissues. The advent of molecular genetic testing has resulted in a shift to classification according to underlying genotype, and a deeper understanding of pathogenicity.
- Over 170 individual conditions have been described.
- Mutations in the NF-κB complex impair immune and stress responses, cell adhesion, and protection against apoptosis and inflammatory reactions, causing hypohidrotic ED with various patterns of inheritance, as well as ED associated with immunodeficiency and incontinentia pigmenti.
- Mutations in TP63 interfere with transcription factors and cause EDs associated with ectrodactyly, cleft palate, and ankyloblepharon.
- Defects in the Wnt-β-catenin pathway are particularly associated with impaired hair and tooth formation, causing odonto-onycho-dermal dysplasia syndrome, Schöpf–Schulz–Passarge syndrome, focal dermal hypoplasia, atrichia with papular lesions and alopecia universalis congenital.
- Mutations in gap junction proteins such as connexin affect cell–cell communication and cause Clouston syndrome, keratitis, ichthyosis and deafness syndrome, oculodentodigital dysplasia, Bart–Pumphrey syndrome, Vohwinkel syndrome and palmoplantar keratoderma associated with hearing loss.
- Mutations in epithelial structural proteins (cytokeratins) or adhesive molecules (desmosal components) disrupt integrity of ectodermal structures and cause conditions such as pachonychia congenital and McGrath syndrome.

Introduction

The ectodermal dysplasias (EDs) encompass a complex and highly diverse group of heritable disorders that have developmental abnormalities of ectodermal appendages in common. This chapter briefly discusses the historical clinical challenges in defining and classifying these conditions, and the impact of recent developments in molecular biology. A summary is presented of the great majority of reported EDs that have a cutaneous phenotype. A more detailed description of the more common disorders that present to dermatologists is also given. Online Mendelian Inheritance in Man numbers (OMIM) [1] are given where appropriate for ease of reference.

What is an ED?

More than 170 different conditions have been described under the umbrella term 'ectodermal dysplasia'. The history of the terminology throughout the literature is instructive. The first clinical cases with features of what would now be classified as ED were reported in the literature as early as 1792, when Danz reported two Jewish boys with congenital absence of hair and teeth [2]. However, the term 'ectodermal dysplasia' did not appear in the literature until coined by Weech in 1929 [3]. Prior to this report, a small series of patients with hypotrichosis, hypodontia, onychodysplasia and anhidrosis had been described under various names such as 'dystrophy of hair

Harper's Textbook of Pediatric Dermatology, Fourth Edition. Edited by Peter Hoeger, Veronica Kinsler and Albert Yan.

and nails', 'imperfect development of skin, hair and teeth' and 'congenital ectodermal defect'. The designation outlined by Weech specified three essential aspects of EDs:

1 Most of the disturbances must affect tissues of ectodermal origin;
2 These disturbances must be developmental;
3 Heredity plays a causal role.

Weech had in mind the X-linked anhidrotic form, Christ–Siemens–Touraine syndrome (CST), or hypohidrotic ED (HED; OMIM #305100) in males but noted that it had also been reported in females; he also noted that this pattern of involvement was occasionally inherited as a non-sex linked trait. Some authors and clinicians still used the term 'ectodermal dysplasia' specifically regarding CST syndrome and the autosomal dominant and recessive forms of HED. As more clinical reports of patients with similar but subtly distinct patterns of anomalies were recorded, the term 'ectodermal dysplasia' became extended to include many different genetic entities. To encapsulate this heterogeneity and the diversity of symptoms seen, Touraine proposed the term 'ectodermal polydysplasia' [4]. Attempts at more formal classification soon followed; initially conditions were classified as hidrotic or anhidrotic, but this simple classification failed to reflect the complexity of nail, hair and dental anomalies associated with the various forms of ED.

Currently, the most widely accepted and used definition of EDs is a group of inherited disorders that have in common developmental abnormalities of two or more of the following: skin, hair, teeth, nails, sweat glands and other ectodermal structures. Other structures derived from embryonic ectoderm include the mammary gland, thyroid gland, thymus, anterior pituitary, adrenal medulla, central nervous system, external ear, melanocytes, cornea, conjunctiva, lacrimal gland and lacrimal duct. These authors subscribe to this definition because the problems encountered by many patients and families are similar regardless of the specific subtype of ED; parents and children can benefit by being part of larger support networks exemplified by the Ectodermal Dysplasia Society (UK-based: www.ectodermaldysplasia.org) and the National Foundation for Ectodermal Dysplasias (US-based: www.nfed.org). This wide-ranging classification is also helpful in research, because several EDs are now known to have shared genetic mechanisms. Although the broader definition forms the basis for this chapter, many conditions that lie within this broad definition are often considered separately. For example, pachyonychia congenita, incontinentia pigmenti, dyskeratosis congenita and Goltz syndrome are all, by definition, EDs, but common practice has been to consider them as separate entities; these conditions are given in-depth coverage elsewhere.

Clinical classification of ED

Having accepted the broadest definition of an ED, a second challenge presented by this group of conditions is that of designing a meaningful and functional classification system. Until the end of the twentieth century, classification systems for EDs were, because of lack of molecular understanding, based on clinical features. Several authors addressed the issue of delineating nosological groups of conditions linked by shared phenotypic features. The most comprehensive accounts of clinical features and inheritance patterns of ED are to be found in the classic 1984 monograph by Freire-Maia and Pinheiro [5] and in subsequent publications [6]. Their classification designated conditions by groups depending on the presence of features in hair, nails, teeth or sweat glands, and assigned conditions to groups using a '1234 system' to collate conditions that involved the hair (1), teeth (2), nails (3) or sweat glands (4) to groups such as 1–2 or 1–2–3. This classification was a comprehensive attempt at ordering an unwieldy group of conditions but was difficult to use and grouped together intuitively disparate clinical entities such as Goltz syndrome and pachyonychia congenita. In common with any other classification of EDs based on clinical findings, this system is confounded by the subtleties of inheritance such as incomplete penetrance and variable expressivity of phenotype. This is especially true in the EDs, in which sweating is often not formally measured and teeth or nail anomalies may be subtle. A comprehensive contemporaneous consideration of the breadth of ED conditions in the tradition of Freire-Maia and Pinheiro is presented in Table 134.1.

EDs may also be divided into those with isolated involvement of hair, teeth and nails – 'pure' EDs – whereas those with abnormalities of other structures and organs are referred to as 'ectodermal dysplasia syndromes'. The construction of a practical, convenient classification of ED is made challenging because of the complex interplay between clinical presentation, mode of inheritance and the genes, proteins and molecular pathways involved.

Molecular basis and classification of ED

The last decade has seen several important insights into the molecular basis of several of the EDs. In some cases, the molecular data have confirmed clinical impressions; for example, Hay–Wells syndrome and ectrodactyly, ectodermal dysplasia, clefting (EEC) syndrome have ED and clefting of the palate and lip as common clinical features and these conditions are now known to be allelic. In a few conditions, a unifying molecular mechanism has been shown to underlie clinically very distinct conditions. In recognition of the recent advances in understanding the molecular mechanisms underlying these EDs, conditions that share molecular mechanisms are considered together below.

One important concept in ectodermal appendage morphogenesis that recurs throughout the EDs is an early dermal signal initiating morphogenesis, followed by an ectodermal signal to organize the mesenchyme, with a secondary dermal signal to coordinate growth and development of the epithelial appendage. For a recent summary, see Fuchs and colleagues [7]. The molecular mechanisms delineated to date in EDs can be considered under the broad categories of defects in the nuclear factor κB (NF-κB) signalling pathway, p63 transcription factor pathway, Wnt-β-catenin pathway, gap junctions

Table 134.1 Clinical characteristics of the EDs

Name (alternative names)	OMIM number/ primary ref	Inheritance	Phenotypic characteristics					Genetic basis and OMIM number
			Nails	Hair	Teeth	Sweat glands	Other	
Basan syndrome (ectodermal dysplasia, absent dermatoglyphic pattern, changes in nails, and simian crease); adermatoglyphia	129200 136000	AD	Fingernails attached distally to the hyponychium; rough in texture; horizontal and vertically grooved	Normal	Normal	Palmoplantar anhidrosis	**Skin:** at birth, multiple milia (on chin); several vesicular/bullous lesions (on fingers and soles); leather-like texture and callosities in adults; simian creases in some patients. May also have palmoplantar fissures and flexion contractures	*SMARCAD1* (612761)
Short-limb skeletal dysplasia with severe combined immunodeficiency	200900	AR?	Normal	Slow growing, in one family failed to grow after initial pelage	No data	No data	**Skin:** erythroderma; mild hyperkeratosis; generalized scaliness; ichthyosiform lesions; redundant, especially on the limbs, suggesting cutis laxa. Biopsy showed keratosis, fissuring of keratotic layer and thickening of granular layer **Other:** dyschondroplastic (short-limbed) dwarfism; lymphopenia; gammaglobulinaemia; prominent eosinophilia; hypoplastic thymus; microscopic alterations of thymus, spleen, lymph nodes, gastrointestinal tract, bones	NK
Ackerman syndrome (molar roots, pyramidal, with juvenile glaucoma and unusual upper lip)	200970	AR?	Horizontal ridging of the fingernails with distal onychoschizia	Scanty body hair; vellus hairs in the moustache and beard areas	Taurodontia, pyramidal or fused molar roots	Normal	**Skin:** indurated and hyperpigmented over the interphalangeal joints of the fingers **Face:** upper lip characterized by absence of 'Cupid's bow'; thickening and widening of the philtrum; ectropion of both lower lids **Other:** complete sensorineural hearing loss; juvenile glaucoma; syndactyly (third and fourth fingers); clinodactyly of the fifth finger	NK
Acrorenal field defect, ectodermal dysplasia, lipoatrophic diabetes (AREDYLD) syndrome	207780	AR	Normal	Scalp hypotrichosis, scant axillary and pubic hair; normal eyebrows and lashes	Two natal and four deciduous teeth with enamel dysplasia; absence of permanent teeth buds; anodontia by 11 years	Normal	**Skin:** hypoplastic and hypopigmented areolae; absence of DIP extension and flexion creases **Face:** prominent forehead and bridge of nose; slight mongoloid slant of palpebral fissures; short nasal septum with flat tip of nose; short upper lip; relatively flat philtrum; prominent chin with mandibular prognathism; posteriorly angulated auricles with broad intertragal incisure; hypoplastic tragus and small groove at antitragus	NK

(*Continued*)

Table 134.1 *Continued*

Name (alternative names)	OMIM number/ primary ref	Inheritance	Phenotypic characteristics					Genetic basis and OMIM number
			Nails	Hair	Teeth	Sweat glands	Other	
							Other: short stature; difficulty in grasping with left hand; limb abnormalities; lipoatrophic diabetes; hypoplasia of mammary gland; lumbar scoliosis; hyperostosis of cranial vault; cranial dysostosis; prominent subcutaneous leg veins; hypoplasia of the middle right major renal calyx and hypotonia of the right ureter	
Acro-dermato-ungual-lacrimal-tooth (ADULT) syndrome (allelic with EEC3, limb–mammary syndrome, AEC, Rapp–Hodgkin syndrome, split hand–foot malformation 4)	103285	AD	Finger- and toenail dysplasia	Frontal alopecia	Hypodontia; loss of permanent teeth	Normal	**Skin:** intensive freckling **Other:** lacrimal duct atresia; ectrodactyly, syndactyly; hypoplastic breasts and nipples	*TP63* (603273)
Alopecia–anosmia–deafness–hypogonadism syndrome (Johnson neuroectodermal syndrome)	147770	AD	Normal	Absent or sparse scalp hair, eyebrows and lashes, axillary and pubic hair	Carious, leading to extensive premature loss	Hypohidrosis	**Skin:** multiple café-au-lait spots **Other:** conductive hearing loss; protruding ears, hypogonadism; occasional congenital heart defects; cleft palate; choanal stenosis; anosmia or hyposmia; mental retardation; speech impairment; hypodontia; unilateral facial asymmetry or palsy; retro/micrognathia	NK
Alopecia–onychodysplasia–hypohidrosis	Freire-Maia and Pinheiro [5]	NK	Severely dystrophic (thick and yellow)	Absence of scalp and body hair; no eyebrows or lashes; virtually no body hair	Normal	Hypohidrosis with hyperthermia	**Skin:** thick, scaly skin in patches over most of the body (the scalp, soles and legs are more severely affected); eczema; scaly lesions with crusting and some open sores most pronounced around orifices **Other:** photophobia; horizontal nystagmus, legal blindness; short stature, low IQ; seizures; hypospadias; non-palpable testes	NK
Alopecia–onychodysplasia–hypohidrosis–deafness	Freire-Maia and Pinheiro [5]	NK	Normal fingernails; thick, slightly deformed toenails, with subungual hyperkeratosis; congenital anonychia	Extensive scalp hypotrichosis; absence of eyebrows	Normal	Hypohidrosis	**Skin:** hyperpigmented, dry and slightly rough, with hyperkeratosis of palms, soles knees and elbows; dermatoglyphs with extensive ridge dissociation **Face:** unusual, with prominent nose; slightly anteverted auricles with broad upper antihelical region; mongoloid palpebral slanting and narrow palpebral fissures **Other:** sensorineural deafness; bilateral ectropia; photophobia; short stature; pectus excavatum; retarded bone age	NK

Alopecia universalis congenita (ALUNC; generalized atrichia) (allelic with atrichia with papular lesions, OMIM 209500)	203655	AR	Normal	Complete alopecia of scalp, body hair, eyelashes, eyebrows variably affected	Normal	Normal		*HR* (602302)
Alopecia universalis–onychodystrophy–total vitiligo	Lerner [10]	AR?	Dystrophic fingernails and toenails with transverse ridging	Progressive loss of body and scalp hair, eyebrows and lashes	Normal	Hyperhidrosis	**Skin:** total vitiligo; skin becomes light and translucent and prone to sunburn	NK
Amelo onycho hypohidrotic dysplasia	104570	AD	Onycholysis with subungual hyperkeratosis	Normal	Hypocalcified–hypoplastic enamel	Hypohidrosis	**Skin:** generally xerotic with keratosis pilaris over the buttocks and extensor surfaces of the limbs; seborrhoeic dermatitis of scalp	NK
Ankyloblepharon–ectodermal defects–cleft lip and palate (AEC) syndrome (Hay–Wells syndrome) (allelic with EEC3, limb–mammary syndrome, ADULT syndrome, Rapp–Hodgkin syndrome, split hand–foot malformation 4)	106260	AD	Severe dystrophy	Hypotrichosis; absent or scanty eyebrows and lashes; coarse, wiry hair	Poorly formed and pointed; widely spaced; carious; severe hypodontia	Slight hypohidrosis; no hyperthermia	**Skin:** dry and smooth; palmoplantar hyperkeratosis with obliteration of dermatoglyphic patterns; occasional reticulate hyperpigmentation; supernumerary nipples; severe recurrent scalp pustulations **Face:** ankyloblepharon filiforme adnatum with partial fusion of eyelids at birth; broad nasal bridge; hypoplastic maxilla; auricular abnormalities; cleft lip/palate **Other:** lacrimal duct atresia; choana atresia; photophobia	*TP63* (603273)
Anonychia–onychodystrophy with brachydactyly type b and ectrodactyly (same as Cook syndrome? – see below)	106990	AD	Anonychia; onychodystrophy	Normal	Normal	Normal	**Limbs:** ectrodactyly; absent/hypoplastic metacarpals; absent/hypoplastic distal phalanges; hypoplastic metatarsals	NK
Anonychia with flexural pigmentation	106750	AD	Generalized absence on the fingers and toes; in a few instances rudimentary	Slow-growing and coarse scalp hair, thinning early in adult life	Highly carious	Mild hypohidrosis without hyperthermia	**Skin:** hypo- and hyperpigmentation, particularly in the groins, axillae and breasts; distortion of epidermal ridges on palms and soles; mild palmoplantar hyperkeratosis; increased palmar markings; distorted fingertip patterns; small macular telangiectasias in a few regions	NK
Arthrogryposis and ectodermal dysplasia (tricho oculodermovertebral syndrome; Alves syndrome)	601701	AR	Absence at birth; later normal length; tendency toward longitudinal breaks	Hypotrichosis of scalp (atrichia at birth) and body; scanty eyebrows and lashes	Enamel hypoplasia	Hypohidrosis	**Skin:** dry; tendency to excessive bruising and scarring after injuries and scratching **Other:** bilateral epicanthic folds; slight mongoloid slant; short stature; probable low-normal intelligence level; arthrogryposis of all joints; bilateral clinodactyly; slight bilateral syndactyly of second and third toes; diabetes mellitus	NK

(Continued)

Table 134.1 *Continued*

Name (alternative names)	OMIM number/ primary ref	Inheritance	Phenotypic characteristics					Genetic basis and OMIM number
			Nails	Hair	Teeth	Sweat glands	Other	
Atrichia with papular lesions (allelic with alopecia universalis congenita OMIM 203655)	209500	AR	Normal	Atrichia at birth, or hair present at birth with shedding shortly afterwards that is not replaced Alopecia may include eyebrows, eyelashes, axillary and pubic hair	Normal	Normal	**Skin:** skin-coloured cystic and papular lesions over the body, primarily on elbows and knees, and face	*HR* (602302)
Autoimmune polyendocrinopathy–candidiasis–ectodermal dystrophy (APECED) syndrome; autoimmune polyendocrinopathy syndrome, type 1	240300	AR	Thickened and dystrophic	Occasional alopecia areata	Hypoplastic enamel	Normal	**Other: o**ral candidiasis; autoimmune endocrinopathies (hypergonadotropic hypogonadism, insulin dependent diabetes mellitus, autoimmune thyroid diseases and pituitary defects); autoimmune or immunomediated gastrointestinal diseases (chronic atrophic gastritis, achalasia, pernicious anaemia and malabsorption); chronic active hepatitis; autoimmune skin diseases (vitiligo and alopecia); keratoconjunctivitis, immunological defects (cellular and humoral); asplenia and cholelithiasis	*AIRE* (607358)
Baisch syndrome	Baisch [11]	NK	Almost total absence of the finger- and toenails	Normal	Delayed eruption; absence of lateral incisors	Normal	**Limbs:** polydactyly with syndactyly in the hands (6/7 fingers); hypoplasia of the distal interphalangeal joints of fingers and toes; short and wide hands and feet; adduction of feet; delayed bone age	NK
Blepharocheilodontic syndrome (clefting, ectropion and conical teeth syndrome; Elschnig syndrome)	119580	AD	Normal	Distichiasis of eyelashes in some	Conical teeth, hypodontia	Normal	**Other:** cleft lip and palate; hypertelorism; ectropia; euryblepharon, lagophthalmia	*CDH1* (192090)
Book dysplasia (premolar aplasia, hyperhidrosis and canities prematura [PHC] syndrome)	112300	AD	Normal	Premature canities	Hypodontia of the premolar region	Palmoplantar hyperhidrosis	**Eyes:** blue irides	NK
Brachymetapody–anodontia–hypotrichosis–albinoidism (oculo-osteocutaneous syndrome; Tuomaala syndrome)	211370	AR	Normal	Poor hair growth, distichiasis	Congenital anodontia	Normal	**Skin:** albinoidism **Other:** multiple ocular abnormalities (strabismus, nystagmus, lenticular opacities, high-grade myopia); mandibular prognathism; short stature; short metacarpals/ metatarsals	NK

Camarena syndrome	Freire-Maia and Pinheiro [5]	NK	Dysplastic	Thin, hypopigmented, and very sparse; poor growth	Anodontia	Absence of sweat glands in the scalp; anhidrosis on face and scalp	**Skin:** thin and smooth; palmoplantar erythema; naevus vascularis on the right lid and above the nose; euhidrosis on the rest of the body; mild 'cara devieja' (old woman's face) **Other:** hypertelorism; abnormal auricles; micrognathia; microstomia; bilateral clinodactyly of the fifth fingers; high-arched palate	NK
Cardiofaciocutaneous syndrome	115150	AD	Normal or thin opalescent nails	Sparse, brittle, slow-growing curly hair; absence of eyebrows and eyelashes, sparse body hair	Normal	Normal	**Skin:** severe atopic dermatitis, patchy to severe ichthyosis; multiple palmar and plantar creases; hyperkeratosis (especially extensor surfaces); keratosis pilaris, ulerythema ophryogenes **Face:** coarse facial features, similar to Noonan's syndrome; relative macrocephaly; prominent forehead; bitemporal narrowing; shallow orbital ridges; prominent philtrum; posteriorly rotated ears; downslanting palpebral fissures; hypertelorism; exophthalmos; short upturned nose; depressed nasal bridge; submucous cleft palate; high-arched palate **Other:** postnatal short stature; hearing loss; nystagmus; strabismus; cardiac defects (atrial septal defects, pulmonic stenosis, hypertrophic cardiomyopathy); splenomegaly; hyperextensible fingers; mild to moderate mental retardation; seizures; hypotonia or hypertonia; hydrocephalus; cortical atrophy; frontal lobe hypoplasia; brain stem atrophy	*BRAF* (164757)
Carey syndrome	Freire-Maia and Pinheiro [5]	NK	Dystrophy from early childhood	Thin, hypopigmented and very sparse	Discoloration; microdontia; hypodontia	Decreased number of sweat pore openings	**Skin:** aplasia cutis congenita-like scalp defects **Other:** moderate conductive hearing loss; absence of tear ducts; displacement of the inner canthi; U-shaped mouth; flat nasal bridge; maxillary hypoplasia; incomplete two- to three-toe syndactyly; cleft palate	NK

(*Continued*)

Table 134.1 *Continued*

Name (alternative names)	OMIM number/ primary ref	Inheritance	Phenotypic characteristics					Genetic basis and OMIM number
			Nails	Hair	Teeth	Sweat glands	Other	
Cartilage–hair hypoplasia syndrome (metaphyseal chondrodysplasia, McKusick type)	250250	AR	Normal	Sparse eyebrows, eyelashes, beard, light-coloured hair, small calibre, fine hairs	Normal	Normal	**Other:** increased risk of malignancy (non-Hodgkin's, squamous cell carcinoma, basal cell carcinoma); immune defect (lymphopenia, neutropenia, severe varicella and herpes simplex virus); short-limbed dwarfism; mild scoliosis; short hands; limited elbow extension; malabsorption; Hirschsprung's disease; oesophageal atresia	*RMRP* (157660)
Carvajal syndrome (palmoplantar keratoderma with left ventricular cardiomyopathy and woolly hair)	605676	AR	Normal	Woolly hair at birth	Normal	Normal	**Skin:** striate palmoplantar keratoderma **Other:** dilated left ventricular cardiomyopathy; altered contractility	*DSP* (125647)
Cataract–alopecia–sclerodactyly syndrome; palmoplantar keratoderma and congenital alopecia	212360	AR	Normal	Total alopecia	Normal	Normal	**Skin:** sclerodactyly; hyperkeratosis **Other:** congenital bilateral cataracts; contractures, digits; pseudo-ainhum; patients from Rodrigues in the Indian Ocean	NK
Cataract, hypertrichosis, mental retardation (CAHMR) syndrome	211770	AR	Normal	Generalized congenital hypertrichosis (back, shoulders, face)	Normal	Normal	**Other:** mental retardation; congenital lamellar cataracts	NK
Cleft lip/palate–ectodermal dysplasia syndrome (CLEPD1; Zlotogora–Ogur syndrome) (allelic to Margarita Island ectodermal dysplasia, see below)	225060	AR	Subungual hyperkeratosis, sulci; transverse and longitudinal striae; irregularities of free margins; hallucal nails with absence of the lamina	Woolly, thin, coarse, opaque and short; pili torti	Hypodontia of upper lateral incisors; transverse striation; irregularities of the free margins	Normal; ? mild tendency to perspiration	**Face:** cleft lip; hypoplasia of the auricular lobes; flat nasal pyramid **Other:** cleft palate; malformation of the genitourinary system; absence or fusion of the last lumbar vertebra; syndactyly of second and third fingers, mental retardation	*NECTIN-1* (600644)
Conductive deafness, with ptosis and skeletal anomalies	221320	AR	Normal	Delayed hair growth	Dysplastic teeth	Normal	**Other:** conductive hearing loss from combined atresia of the external auditory canal and the middle ear space, complicated by chronic infection; ptosis; thin, pinched-nose facial appearance **Skeletal:** internal rotation of hips; dislocation of the radial heads; fifth finger clinodactyly	NK

Coffin–Siris syndrome (fifth digit syndrome)	135900	NK	Absent to hypoplastic fifth fingernails and toenails; other nails occasionally hypoplastic or absent	Sparse scalp hair; bushy eyebrows and lashes; hirsutism of limbs, forehead and back	Delayed eruption; microdontia	Normal	**Skin:** dermatoglyphic changes; simian crease **Other:** coarse face with thick lips, wide mouth and nose, anteverted nostrils and low nasal bridge; retardation of psychomotor and growth development; hypotonia; lax joints; clinodactyly of the fifth fingers; general absence of terminal phalanges of fifth fingers and toes; general aplasia or variable hypoplasia of middle and proximal phalanges of other fingers and toes; bilateral or unilateral dislocation of the radial heads; small or absent patella; frequent respiratory infections; umbilical and inguinal hernias; cleft palate; feeding problems in infancy; six lumbar vertebrae; short sternum; sternal anomalies; microcephaly; patent ductus arteriosus	*ARID1B* (614556)
Congenital hypotrichosis with juvenile macular dystrophy (HJMD)	601553	AR	Normal	Congenital hypotrichosis secondary to decreased ratio of terminal to vellus hairs; beading of hair shaft (flat shaft and pili torti); normal eyelashes/eyebrows	Normal	Normal	**Other:** not true macular dystrophy; pigmentary abnormalities extending beyond macula; progressive cone/rod dystrophy	*CDH3* (114021)
Congenital insensitivity to pain with anhidrosis (CIPA; familial dysautonomia, type II; hereditary sensory and autonomic neuropathy, type IV)	256800	AR	Normal	Hypotrichosis in areas of the scalp	Enamel aplasia	Hypohidrosis or anhidrosis with hyperthermia, normal sweat glands	**Skin:** dry; scars from self-inflicted bites may be present on the fingers and arms; chronic sores are common on the hands, feet and pressure points, such as the buttocks	*NTRK1* (191315)

(*Continued*)

Table 134.1 *Continued*

Name (alternative names)	OMIM number/ primary ref	Inheritance	Phenotypic characteristics					Genetic basis and OMIM number
			Nails	Hair	Teeth	Sweat glands	Other	
							Other: irregular lacrimation; mental retardation; fever; corneal ulcers; multiple fractures from trauma resulting in deformities; joint degeneration (Charcot joints); universal sensory loss; absence of pain perception and physiological responses to painful stimuli; impaired temperature and touch perception; diminished tendon reflexes; occasional encopresis and enuresis; ulceration of the mouth and scars from biting the tongue and lips	
Cook syndrome (same as anonychia–onychodystrophy with brachydactyly type b and ectrodactyly? – see above)	106995	AD	Congenital onychodystrophy; anonychia	Normal	Normal	Normal	**Skin:** prominent finger pads **Other:** fifth finger brachydactyly; digitalization of thumbs; absent/hypoplastic distal phalanges of hands and feet	NK
Corneodermato-osseous syndrome	122440	AD	Distal onycholysis	Normal	Soft teeth; early tooth decay	Normal	**Skin:** diffuse palmoplantar hyperkeratosis; erythematous scaly skin (knees, elbows, hands/feet); generalized erythroderma **Eyes:** corneal dystrophy; photophobia; burning/watering of eyes **Other:** brachydactyly; short distal phalanges; short stature; medullary narrowing of hand bones; premature birth	NK
Cranio-ectodermal syndrome (Levin syndrome I; Sensenbrenner syndrome)	218330	AR	Broad and short	Thin, sparse and slow-growing; abnormal structure	Microdontia; hypodontia; widely spaced; enamel hypoplasia; taurodontism	Normal	**Skin:** dimples over elbows and knees; bilateral hallucal creases; single flexion crease on each toe; bilateral single palmar creases, cutis laxa **Skeletal:** rhizomelic shortness (greatest in upper limbs); disproportionate shortness of the fibulae; pronounced shortness of middle and distal phalanges of toes and fingers; cutaneous syndactyly; clinodactyly; increased space between first and second toes; hallux valgus; dolichocephaly; generalized osteoporosis; highly arched palate; sagittal suture synostosis; short and narrow thorax; pectus excavatum	*IFT122* (606045)

							Other: hyperopia; myopia; nystagmus; retinal dystrophy; frontal bossing; epicanthal folds and anti-mongoloid slant; full cheeks; posteriorly angulated pinnae with hypoplastic antihelix; hypotelorism; broad nasal bridge; anteverted nares; everted lower lip; capillary naevus on the forehead; multiple oral frenula; nephronophthisis; hepatic fibrosis; congenital heart defects	
Curly hair–ankyloblepharon–nail dysplasia syndrome (CHAND syndrome)	214350	AR	Hypoplastic finger- and toenails	Curly	Normal	Normal	**Eyes:** fused eyelids at birth (ankyloblepharon) **Other:** bilateral lip pits (at commisures of mouth), inferiorly attached frenulum, inguinal hernia	*RIPK4* (605706)
Deafness and onychodystrophy (Robinson syndrome)	124480	AD	Absent, hypoplastic, fissured and dystrophic finger- and toenails	Normal	Coniform; hypodontia; delayed primary and secondary dentition	Normal	**Other:** syndactyly of toes; severe sensorineural hearing loss (high frequency)	*ATP6V1B2* (606939)
Deafness, onychodystrophy, osteodystrophy, mental retardation and seizures syndrome (DOOR syndrome)	220500	AR	Hypoplastic and dystrophic finger- and toenails; anonychia	Normal	Hypoplastic and discoloured; irregular placement	Normal	**Skin:** dermatoglyphic abnormalities (arched pattern) **Other:** congenital sensorineural deafness; apparently low-set ears; seizures and mental retardation; triphalangy of both thumbs and halluces; hypoplasia or aplasia of terminal phalanges of fingers and toes; occasional clinodactyly and camptodactyly; ↑ 2 oxo-gutarate associated with severe phenotype	*TBC1D24* (613577)
Dermatopathia pigmentosa reticularis (allelic with Naegeli–Franceschetti–Jadassohn syndrome)	125595	AD	Onychodystrophy	Alopecia, wiry hair	No dental anomalies	Hypohidrosis or hyperhidrosis	**Skin:** reticulate hyperpigmentation that persists throughout life (unlike Naegeli–Franceschetti–Jadassohn syndrome); adermatoglyhpia; palmoplantar hyperkeratosis; punctate hyperkeratosis of palms and soles. Rarely digital fibromatous thickening, acral non-scarring blisters	*KRT14* (148066)
Dermo-odonto-dysplasia	125640	AD	Dysplastic; brittle	Dry; slow-growing (scalp, moustache and beard); circumscribed area of alopecia; normal eyebrows and lashes; sparse axillary and pubic hair	Hypodontia; microdontia; persistence of deciduous teeth	Normal	**Skin:** dry and thin to variable degree (especially on palmoplantar regions); simian crease **Face:** left palpebral ptosis; prognathic mandible	NK

(Continued)

Table 134.1 *Continued*

Name (alternative names)	OMIM number/ primary ref	Inheritance	Phenotypic characteristics					Genetic basis and OMIM number
			Nails	Hair	Teeth	Sweat glands	Other	
Dermotrichic syndrome ?related to IFAP syndrome (308205) (see below)	Freire-Maia and Pinheiro [5]	XR	Dystrophic and hyperconvex fingernails	Generalized atrichia from birth	Normal	Hypohidrosis without hyperthermia	**Skin:** general ichthyosiform lesions, including palmoplantar area and scalp **Face:** prominent forehead; large ears; small nose with mildly low nasal bridge; blepharophimosis **Other:** severe psychomotor retardation; abnormal EEG; frequent apyretic seizures; short stature; hemivertebrae at the dorsolumbar region; congenital aganglionic megacolon; narrow arched palate; positive Benedict and glucose oxidase tests; discrete increase in tyrosinaemia; discrete anaemia; no ocular/respiratory disorders as in IFAP	NK
Dubowitz syndrome	223370	AR	Normal	Sparse scalp hair, sparse lateral eyebrows	Delayed eruption; caries	Normal	**Skin:** eczema **Face:** elongation of face with age; shallow supraorbital ridge; facial asymmetry; micrognathia; high, sloping forehead; prominent ears; short palpebral fissures; ptosis; blepharophimosis; microphthalmia; broad nasal tip; high-arched palate; submucous cleft palate; velopharyngeal insufficiency **Other:** intrauterine growth restriction; short stature; pilonidal dimples; spina bifida occulta; microcephaly; mild mental retardation with behaviour problems; high-pitched, hoarse voice; recurrent infections; hypogammaglobulinaemia; IgA deficiency; neoplasia including aplastic anaemia; acute lymphatic leukaemia, lymphoma and neuroblastoma; hypospadias; cryptorchidism; low cholesterol	NK

Dyskeratosis congenita, X-linked (Zinsser–Cole–Engman syndrome)	305000	XR	Dystrophy with late-onset paronychia occasionally leading to anonychia; hypoplasia	Hypotrichosis; loss of cilia owing to blepharitis and ectropion; absence of eyebrows and lashes; premature cavities	Poorly aligned; early carious degeneration	Generalized hyperhidrosis	**Skin:** hyper- and hypomelanosis, telangiectatic erythema; ulcers; dry desquamation; atrophy; hyperkeratotic plaques (palmoplantar and over joints); premalignant lesions; absent fingerprints; malignant leucoplakia on lips, mouth, anus, urethra and conjunctiva **Eyes:** blepharitis; ectropion of the lower lids; obliteration of the puncta lacrimalia; bullous conjunctivitis; continuous lacrimation **Other:** sharp facial features; occasional mental and growth retardation; Fanconi-like pancytopenia; frail skeletal structure; oesophageal dysfunction and/or diverticulum; atrophic lingual papillae; gingivitis; testicular atrophy	*DKC1* (300126)
Dyskeratosis congenita, autosomal dominant (Scoggins type)	127550	AD	Dystrophic	Hypotrichosis	Carious	Normal	**Skin:** hyper- and hypomelanosis; telangiectatic erythema; ulcers; dry desquamation; atrophy; hyperkeratotic plaques (palmoplantar and over joints); premalignant lesions; absence of fingerprints; premalignant leucoplakia on lips, mouth, anus, urethra and conjunctiva **Eyes:** blepharitis; ectropion of the lower lids; obliteration of the puncta lacrimalia; bullous conjunctivitis; continuous lacrimation **Other:** pulmonary fibrosis, hepatic fibrosis, ataxia; sharp facial features; occasional mental and growth retardation; Fanconi-like pancytopenia; frail skeletal structure; osteoporosis; genital anomalies; oesophageal dysfunction and/or diverticulum; atrophic lingual papillae; gingivitis	*TERC* (602322)
Dyskeratosis congenita (autosomal recessive)	224230	AR	Dystrophic, hypoplastic	Hypotrichosis, sparse hair and eyelashes	Carious	Normal	**Skin:** hyper- and hypomelanosis; periorbital telangiectatic erythema; ulcers; dry desquamation **Other:** pancytopenia; thrombocytopenia; small platelets; T-cell abnormalities; dystrophic fingers and toes	*NOLA3* (aka *NOP10*) (606471)

(Continued)

Table 134.1 *Continued*

Name (alternative names)	OMIM number/ primary ref	Inheritance	Phenotypic characteristics					Genetic basis and OMIM number
			Nails	Hair	Teeth	Sweat glands	Other	
Ectodermal dysplasia with short stature	616029 Petfor et al. [12]	AR	Dystrophy, hypoplasia	None	Delayed dentition, hypodontia, enamel hypoplasia	None	**Skin:** palmoplantar keratoderma **Other:** Short stature, oromucosal hyperpigmentation, sensorineural hearing loss, asthma, oesophageal strictures	*GRHL2* (608576)
Ectodermal defect with skeletal abnormalities	Wallace [13]	NK	Finger- and toenails poorly developed and foreshortened	Scalp hair is slightly coarse; very sparse axillary hair	Hypodontia; hypoplastic teeth	Normal	**Skin:** thin, fine and dry; fine, light, granular pigmentation; translucent appearance; rudimentary nipples **Face:** striking appearance; central portion is relatively underdeveloped; the cheeks, upper jaw and nose are sunken with the 'inverted, dish-shaped deformity' and somewhat prominent eyes **Other:** low intelligence; short metacarpals; some absorption of the terminal tufts of the distal phalanges; flexion anomalies of hands and feet; absence of breasts; narrow and highly arched palate	NK
Ectodermal dysplasia and neurosensory deafness (Mikaelian syndrome)	224800	AR	Normal	Coarse and brittle; hypotrichosis of scalp	Caries	Normal	**Skin:** hyperkeratotic; increased melanin in the basal layer **Other:** bilateral sensorineural loss; coarse facial features; arachnodactyly; contracture of fifth fingers; kyphoscoliosis	NK
Ectodermal dysplasia with natal teeth (Turnpenny type)	601345	AD	Normal	Thin scalp hair; scanty body hair	Oligodontia by late adolescence	Variable heat tolerance; no anhidrosis	**Skin:** flexural acanthosis nigricans	NK
Ectodermal dysplasia with palatal paralysis	Wesser and Vistnes [14]	NK	No data	Absence of frontal hair, eyebrows and lashes	Stunted and peg-shaped; enamel hypoplasia	Anhidrosis on face (absent sweat glands)	**Skin:** absence of sebaceous glands on the face **Other:** conductive loss; otitis; frontal bossing; depressed nasal bridge; highly arched palate; palatal paralysis; diminished sensation in the palate, posterior pharyngeal wall and tonsillar pillar area; abnormal and distorted speech with a marked nasal component	NK
Ectodermal dysplasia with severe mental retardation	Kirman [15]	NK	Almost absent from fingers and toes	Absent scalp (except for a small wisp in the centre of the head) and body hair	Normal	Hypohidrosis without hyperthermia	**Skin:** fine, thin and shiny with some desquamation over the hands, feet and the top of the head; absence of both nipples **Other:** blindness with bilateral cataract; abnormal ears; severe mental retardation; absence of menstruation; prepubertal vulva	NK

Ectodermal dysplasia with mental retardation and syndactyly	600906	NK	Severe onychogryposis	Short, abundant and stiff, sparse eyebrows	No data	Mild hypohidrosis	**Skin:** dry; large scalp defect **Other:** syndactyly involving the third and fourth fingers and the second and third toes; mild mental retardation; a peculiar face with large palpebral fissures, broad nasal bridge and constantly open mouth; abnormally modelled ears	NK
Ectodermal dysplasia with syndactyly	613573 Wiedemann et al. [16]	AR	Yellowish and partially thickened	Hypotrichosis; brittle scalp hair; pili torti; sparse eyebrows and lashes	Severe crown hypoplasia; delayed and atypical eruption of permanent teeth	Normal	**Skin:** dry with hyperkeratosis, especially at the distal third of the trunk, lower limbs and palmoplantar regions (axillae and elbow are normal); transverse crease on both palms **Other:** mild crowding of the lenses; discrete hypermetropia; syndactyly on both fingers and toes to variable degrees; lordosis; highly arched palate	*PVRL-4* (609607)
Ectodermal dysplasia with adrenal cyst (odonto-onycho hypohidrotic dysplasia with midline scalp defect)	129550	AD	Dystrophic fingernails	Alopecia cutis verticis	Delayed eruption; diastemata; minor shape alterations	Hypohidrosis	**Skin:** midline scalp defect (aplasia cutis vertices); hypoplastic areolae and nipples **Other:** breast hypoplasia (inability to lactate); hypertension of undetermined pathogenesis; large adrenal cyst	NK
Ectodermal dysplasia with distinctive facies and preaxial polydactyly of feet	129540	AD	Rounded nails	Scalp alopecia; body alopecia; sparse eyebrows; sparse eyelashes	Thin enamel; dental caries	Normal	**Other:** micrognathia; flat philtrum; malar hypoplasia; dystopia canthorum; flat nasal bridge; thin upper lip; thickened frenulum; fifth finger clinodactyly; preaxial polydactyly; duplicated halluces; duplicated first metatarsals; language delay	NK
Ectodermal dysplasia with ectrodactyly and macular dystrophy (EEM syndrome)	225280	AR	Dysplastic	Hypotrichosis or normal	Normal	Dental anomalies, small wide-spaced teeth	**Other:** ectrodactyly; syndactyly; cleft hand; macular dystrophy	*CDH3* (114021)
Ectodermal dysplasia 4; pure hair and nail type	602032	AR	Congenital onychodystrophy; micronychia; onycholysis; onychorrhexis	Brittle hair; temporal hypotrichosis	Normal	Normal	**Skin:** folliculitis decalvans of neck	*KRT85* (602767)
Ectrodactyly–ectodermal dysplasia-cleft lip/palate syndrome (EEC3)	604292	AD	Dysplastic, thin, pitted, brittle and striated	Hypotrichosis of scalp and body; fair and dry; scanty or absent eyebrows and lashes	Anodontia; hypodontia; microdontia; enamel hypoplasia; poorly formed; peg-shaped incisors	Occasional hypohidrosis without hypothermia	**Skin:** dry, translucent, palmoplantar hyperkeratosis; eczematous patches; pigmented naevi **Face:** cleft lip; broad nose; defective auricles; pointed chin; malar hypoplasia	*TP63* (603273)

(*Continued*)

Table 134.1 *Continued*

Name (alternative names)	OMIM number/ primary ref	Inheritance	Phenotypic characteristics					Genetic basis and OMIM number
			Nails	Hair	Teeth	Sweat glands	Other	
							Other: conductive hearing loss; tear duct anomaly or malfunction; speckled iris; photophobia; strabismus; blepharitis; clouding of the cornea; congenital adhesions between the eyelids; ectrodactyly; syndactyly; clinodactyly; cleft palate; renal abnormalities; rhinitis; respiratory infections; genital anomalies	
Ectrodactyly–ectodermal dysplasia-cleft lip/palate (EEC1) syndrome	129900	AD	Dysplastic, thin, pitted, brittle and striated	Sparse, brittle hair	Anodontia	Hypohidrosis uncommon	**Skin:** dry, translucent, palmoplantar hyperkeratosis; eczematous patches; pigmented naevi **Face:** cleft lip and/or palate; low-set, posteriorly rotated ears; lacrimal duct anomalies very common (atresia, non-canalization, hypoplasia, small punctum, dysfunction), leading to secondary keratitis **Other:** genitourinary abnormalities; large omphalocoele; anal atresia frequent; conductive hearing loss; distal limb defects (ectodactyly, polydactyly, syndactyly, tetramelic cleft hand and foot); recurrent upper respiratory, urogenital and eye infections, secondary to structural anomalies; growth hormone deficiency secondary to hypothalamic defect	*EEC1* (7q11.2-121.3)
Ectrodactyly and ectodermal dysplasia without cleft lip/palate (EEC without cleft lip/ palate)	129810	AD	Normal	Hypotrichosis	Abnormal dentition	Normal	**Other:** no clefting of the lip or palate, as seen in classic EEC syndrome; ectrodactyly ranges from almost normal presentation to tetramelic clefting of hands and feet	NK
Ellis–van Creveld syndrome (chondroectodermal dysplasia, mesoectodermal dysplasia) (see entry for Weyer acrofacial dysostosis later)	225500	AR	Dysplastic (brittle, furrowed and underdeveloped)	Thin, brittle and hypochromic; absent or scanty eyebrows and lashes	Natal teeth; precocious exfoliation; hypodontia; occasional hypoplastic enamel	Normal	**Skin:** eczema; petechiae are described in different patterns	*EVC* (604831); *EVC2* (607261)

							Other: occasional strabismus; cataract; coloboma of the iris; microphthalmia; exophthalmia; short-limbed dwarfism; bilateral postaxial polydactyly (generally of the hands); brachymetacarpia; thick and short bones of limbs; fusion of the hamate and capitate; club-foot; genu valga; syndactyly; occasionally mild mental retardation; congenital heart disease; respiratory difficulties; gingivolabial fusion; cleft palate; epispadias; hypospadias; hypoplastic genitalia **Face:** broad nose; occasional cleft lip; frontal bossing and hypertelorism	
Fischer syndrome (Fischer–Volavsek syndrome)	Fischer [17]	AD	Onychogryposis; onycholysis	Sparse scalp hair, eyebrows and lashes	Normal	Palmoplantar hyperhidrosis	**Skin:** occasional xeroderma; palmoplantar keratosis **Other:** eyelid oedema; occasional mental deficiency; clubbing of distal phalanges of the fingers and toes; syringomyelia; apathy	NK
Focal dermal hypoplasia syndrome (Goltz syndrome; Goltz–Gorlin syndrome)	305600	XD	Thin, spooned, narrow, grooved hypopigmented or absent	Hypotrichosis	Hypodontia; microdontia; enamel hypoplasia; delayed eruption; irregular placement; dental pitting	Hypohidrosis or hyperhidrosis	**Skin:** absence of skin from various parts at birth; areas of underdevelopment or thinness; linear hypo- or hyperpigmentation; telangiectasia; herniation of subcutaneous fat; multiple papillomas of mucous membranes of periorificial skin; follicular hyperkeratotic papules; angiofibromatous nodules around lips, vulva and anus; palmoplantar hyperkeratosis; occasional dermatoglyphic changes **Eyes:** colobomas; microphthalmia; irregularity of pupils; clouding of cornea or vitreous; blue sclerae; ectopia lentis **Face:** lip papillomas; malformed auricles; asymmetry and notching of the alae nasi; pointed chin; triangular face; hypertelorism **Other:** osteopathia striata; occasional hearing loss; mental retardation; epilepsy; short stature; syndactyly; polydactyly; hypoplasia of the external genitalia; umbilical and/or inguinal hernia; vertebral anomalies (scoliosis, spina bifida, etc.); highly arched palate; gum papillomas; small breasts	*PORCN* (300651)

(*Continued*)

Table 134.1 *Continued*

Name (alternative names)	OMIM number/ primary ref	Inheritance	Phenotypic characteristics					Genetic basis and OMIM number
			Nails	Hair	Teeth	Sweat glands	Other	
Focal facial dermal dysplasia, type I (FFDD type I, hereditary symmetrical aplastic naevi of temples, bitemporal aplasia cutis, Brauer syndrome) ? same as FFDD type II	136500	AD	Normal	Alopecia areata; generally sparse eyebrows and lashes or multiple rows of lashes on upper lids; normal to absent lashes on lower lids	Normal	Localized hypohidrosis (scarce to absent sweat glands in the focal lesions)	**Skin:** round, focal temporal lesions that have a smooth or wrinkled surface and may be hyperpigmented (usually bitemporal, can be unilateral); occasional multiple vertical linear depressions on the lower forehead; absence of sebaceous glands in the temporal lesions	NK
Focal facial dermal dysplasia, type II (FFDD type II, bitemporal forceps marks syndrome) ? same as FFDD type I	614973	AD	Normal	Alopecia areata; some have unruly scalp hair; generally sparse eyebrows and lashes or multiple rows of lashes on upper lids; normal to absent lashes on lower lids; upward slanting eyebrows	Normal	Localized hypohidrosis (scarce to absent sweat glands in the focal lesions)	**Skin:** round, focal temporal lesions that have a smooth or wrinkled surface and may be hypo- or hyperpigmented; occasional multiple vertical linear depressions on the lower forehead; absence of sebaceous glands in the temporal lesions **Eyes:** chronic bilateral blepharitis in a few cases **Face:** leonine appearance; wrinkles periorbitally; wide nasal bridge; fleshy nose with the tip bent down; bilateral epicanthic folds; developmental delay	NK
Focal facial dermal dysplasia, type III	227260	AR						*TWIST2* (607556)
Focal facial dermal dysplasia, type IV	614974	AR						*CYP26C1* (608428)
Fried tooth and nail syndrome (?same as Witkop syndrome 189500; see later)	Fried [18]	AR	Small, thin and slightly concave	Fine and short; scanty eyebrows	Hypodontia; peg-shaped teeth	Normal	**Face:** prominent lips and chin **Other:** branchial cyst on the left side of the neck	NK
Gingival fibromatosis and hypertrichosis (hypertrichosis terminalis, generalized, with or without gingival hyperplasia)	135400	AR	Normal	Generalized hypertrichosis; black and coarse (terminal hairs)	Widely spaced, dentition may be obscured by gingival fibromatosis	Normal	**Skin:** occasional pigmented naevi and hyperelasticity **Other:** occasional large ears, peculiar nose and coarse features; mental retardation; epilepsy; gingival fibromatosis; occasional hypoplastic breasts	Microdeletion or microduplication in 17q24.2-q24.3
Gingival fibromatosis–sparse hair–malposition of teeth	Jorgenson [19]	AR	No data	Excessively thick in childhood; begins to thin out during early teens; sparse later	Malpositioned and malformed; serrated incisors	No data	**Face:** coarse appearance; protruding lips (secondary to gingival fibromatosis); prognathic mandible; broad and flat nasal alae **Other:** alternating strabismus; rotating nystagmus; myopia; abnormal EEG; low IQ; large hands; broad and relatively short feet; highly arched palate	NK

Gorlin–Chaudhry–Moss syndrome (craniofacial dysostosis, hypertrichosis, hypoplasia of labia majora; dental and eye anomalies, patent ductus arteriosus, normal intelligence)	612289	AR?	No data	Hypertrichosis, coarse hair, low frontal hairline	Hypodontia; microdontia; some pulp chambers small or missing	Normal	**Face:** characteristic with 'dished out' appearance of middle face; ectropion of lower lid; antimongoloid slant; short stature **Other:** mild bilateral conductive hearing loss; hyperopia; microphthalmia; horizontal nystagmus; corneal ulcers; defective eyelid development; craniofacial dysostosis; patent ductus arteriosus; hypoplasia of labia majora; highly arched palate; mild umbilical hernia; short distal phalanges of fingers and toes	*SLC25A24* (608744)
Growth retardation–alopecia–pseudoanodontia–optic atrophy (GAPO)	230740	AR	Hyperconvexity on fingers and toes in two patients	Generalized atrichia	Failure of eruption (pseudoanodontia) of both primary and permanent dentition with absence of alveolar ridges	Normal	**Skin:** dry; fragile with inadequate wound healing (small, depressed scars); depigmented areas; unusual wrinkles; leather-like and thick on nape and upper back; abnormal dermatoglyphics **Face:** 'small' and 'characteristic'; asymmetrical; craniofacial dysostosis; micrognath a; protruding and thickened lips; protruding auricles; prominent supraorbital ridges; depressed nasal bridge; minor auricular malformations **Other:** sensorineural hypoacusia; optic atrophy; glaucoma; keratoconus; nystagmus; photophobia; dwarfism; occasional mental retardation; hypoplasia of mammary glands; pectus excavatum; umbilical hernia; delayed bone maturation through childhood and adolescence; respiratory infection	*ANTXR1* (606410)
Haim–Munk syndrome (keratosis palmoplantaris with periodontopathia and onychogryphosis, Cochin Jewish disorder) (allelic with Papillon–Lefèvre syndrome)	245010	AR	Onychogryphosis	Normal	Severe periodontitis with onset at young age, loss of teeth		**Skin;** palmoplantar keratoderma **Other:** arachnodactyly; acro-osteolysis	*CTSC* (602365)

(*Continued*)

Table 134.1 *Continued*

Name (alternative names)	OMIM number/ primary ref	Inheritance	Phenotypic characteristics					Genetic basis and OMIM number
			Nails	Hair	Teeth	Sweat glands	Other	
Hallerman–Streiff syndrome (Francois dyscephalic syndrome)	234100	AR Heterogeneity?	Normal	Thin and light; generalized or sutural alopecia of scalp	Natal; supernumerary; hypodontia; deciduous; premature caries; coniform teeth; hypoplastic enamel	Normal	**Skin:** cutaneous atrophy largely limited to the face and/or scalp; telangiectases; xerosis **Face:** characteristically bird-like; the head has an abnormal shape, usually brachycephalic or scaphocephaly with frontal and parietal bossing; micrognathia; microstomia with thin lips; apparently low-set ears; 'double chin'; beaked nose **Other:** bilateral microphthalmia; congenital cataract; congenital corectopia; occasional nystagmus; strabismus; blue sclerae; optic disc coloboma; various chorioretinal pigment alterations; occasional syndactyly; winging of the scapulae; proportionate short stature; intelligence ranges from normal to mental retardation; narrow and highly arched palate; delayed ossification of craniofacial sutures; microcephaly; cardiac defects; hypogenitalism; cryptorchidism; vertebral anomalies; funnel chest	NK
Hayden syndrome	Freire-Maia and Pinheiro [5]	NK	Severe pachyonychia (hands and feet)	No scalp hair, eyebrows or lashes; virtually no body hair	Normal	Severe hypohidrosis	**Skin:** follicular and plaque-like hyperkeratosis; ichthyosis-like hyperkeratosis on the shins; extremely severe palmoplantar hyperkeratosis to the point of almost complete stiffness of the fingers and toes; severe chronic scalp infection with many pustules **Other:** chronic external otitis leading to virtual deafness; severe chronic conjunctivitis leading to virtual blindness; saddle nose; narrow palpebral fissures	NK
Hereditary mucoepithelial dysplasia	158310	AD	Chronic monilial nail infection	Non-scarring alopecia	Gingival inflammation	Normal	**Skin:** flat red periorificial mucosal lesions; follicular keratosis **Other:** photophobia; nystagmus; keratoconjunctivitis; keratitis; pannus; cataracts; repeated pneumonia; fibrocystic lung disease; cor pulmonale; mucocutaneous candidiasis; diarrhoea in infancy; T- and B-cell abnormalities; abnormal Papanicolau smears; vulvovaginal erythema	NK

Hidrotic ectodermal dysplasia (Clouston syndrome, ED2)	129500	AD	Variable degrees of dystrophy; thickened and slightly discoloured; paronychia	Dry, fine, usually blond, slow-growing; ranging from hypotrichosis to complete alopecia; absent/scanty eyebrows and lashes	Occasional hypodontia, anodontia, widely spaced; natal teeth; caries	Normal	**Skin:** dry and rough; tendency towards scaliness; hyperpigmentation of some areas; thick cyskeratotic palms and soles **Other:** occasional strabismus, cataract and myopia; occasional mental deficiency and short stature; speech difficulties; tufting of terminal phalanges; clubbing of fingers; thickening of skull bones	*GJB6* (604418)
Hidrotic ectodermal dysplasia, Christianson–Fourie type	601375	AD	Dystrophic thickened nails; unattached distal half of nails	Short, thin, sparse, pale scalp hair; absent eyebrows; short, sparse eyelashes; sparse axillary and pubic hair	Normal	Normal	**Other:** episodic supraventricular tachycardia; bradycardia; skin normal	NK
Hypertrichosis and dental defects	Freire-Maia and Pinheiro [5]	AD	Normal	Generalized hypertrichosis (except on palms, soles and mucous membranes)	Occasional persistence of deciduous teeth, delayed eruption, hypodontia, anodontia	Normal		NK
Hypohidrotic ectodermal dysplasia-X-linked (ED1; Christ–Siemens–Touraine [CST] syndrome) (see Lelis syndrome 608290 later)	305100	XR	Generally normal; sometimes dystrophic or absent at birth and/or fragile and brittle with incomplete development and celonychia	Fine and dry; hypochromic; hypotrichosis of scalp and body; absent or scanty eyebrows and lashes; moustache and beard generally normal	Hypodontia; peg-shaped incisors and/or canines; persistence of deciduous teeth; delayed eruption; occasional anodontia	Hypohidrosis with or without hyperthermia; absent or decreased number of epidermal ridge sweat pores	**Skin:** thin, smooth and dry owing to hypoplastic or absent sebaceous glands; occasional pigmentation and dermatoglyphic changes; absent or supernumerary nipples and areolae **Face:** highly characteristic in persons who are severely affected (generally males) with thick and prominent lips, depressed nasal bridge (saddle nose), frontal bossing, hypoplasia of the maxilla, wrinkles beneath the eyes, or around the eyes, nose and mouth, and minor alterations of the auricles; the periorbital region is often more darkly pigmented than the rest of the body **Other:** occasional conductive hearing loss; photophobia; decreased function of the lacrimal glands; aplasia or hypoplasia of the lacrimal ducts; atrophic rhinitis; otitis media; decreased sense of taste and/or smell; atrophied mucous glands of the upper respiratory tract; respiratory difficulties; chronic pharyngitis and laryngitis; aplasia or hypoplasia of the mammary glands	*EDA* (300451)

(*Continued*)

Table 134.1 *Continued*

Name (alternative names)	OMIM number/ primary ref	Inheritance	Phenotypic characteristics					Genetic basis and OMIM number
			Nails	Hair	Teeth	Sweat glands	Other	
Ectodermal dysplasia 10A, hypohidrotic/hair/nail type, autosomal dominant; includes Jorgenson syndrome	129490	AD	Generally normal; sometimes hypoplastic	Sparse, fuzzy, lightly pigmented scalp hair; absent or scanty eyebrows, lashes and body hair	Hypodontia; anodontia; conical teeth; delayed eruption of teeth	Hypohidrosis with hyperthermia	**Skin:** smooth, thin, dry and hypoplastic; can be eczematous **Other:** photophobia; hypoplasia of lacrimal ducts; decreased function of the lacrimal glands; saddle nose; thick and protruding lips; frontal bossing and prominent auricles; chronic rhinitis, frequent respiratory infections	*EDAR* (604095)
Ectodermal dysplasia 10B, hypohidrotic/hair/tooth type, autosomal recessive	224900	AR	Generally normal; sometimes hypoplastic	Sparse, fuzzy, lightly pigmented scalp hair; absent or scanty eyebrows, lashes and body hair	Hypodontia; anodontia; conical teeth	Hypohidrosis with hyperthermia; hypoplastic eccrine sweat glands	**Skin:** smooth, thin, dry and hypoplastic; hyperpigmentation; rarely palmoplantar keratoderma **Other:** photophobia; periorbital wrinkling; hypoplasia of lacrimal ducts; decreased function of the lacrimal glands; saddle nose; thick and protruding lips; frontal bossing and prominent auricles; chronic rhinitis; frequent respiratory infections; absence of breasts	*EDAR* (604095)
Hypohidrotic ectodermal dysplasia (HED) with immune deficiency	300291	XR	Generally normal; sometimes hypoplastic	Sparse, fuzzy, lightly pigmented scalp hair; absent or scanty eyebrows, lashes and body hair	Hypodontia; anodontia; conical teeth	Hypohidrosis with hyperthermia	**Other:** milder ectodermal dysplasia features than classic HED; failure to thrive; recurrent infections of digestive tract; recurrent respiratory infections; dysgammaglobulinaemia; high morbidity/mortality	*IKBKG* (300248)
HED with immune deficiency, osteopetrosis and lymphoedema	300301	XR?	Generally normal; sometimes hypoplastic	Sparse, fuzzy, lightly pigmented scalp hair; absent or scanty eyebrows, lashes and body hair	Hypodontia; anodontia; conical teeth	Hypohidrosis with hyperthermia	**Other:** milder ectodermal dysplasia features than classic HED; failure to thrive; recurrent infections of digestive tract; recurrent respiratory infections; dysgammaglobulinaemia; osteopetrosis; generally more severe phenotype than 300291	*IKBKG* (300248)
HED with deafness	125050	AD	Generally normal; sometimes hypoplastic	Sparse, fuzzy, lightly pigmented scalp hair; absent or scanty eyebrows, lashes and body hair	Hypodontia; anodontia; conical teeth	Hypohidrosis with hyperthermia	**Other:** progressive hearing loss	NK
Hypohidrotic ectodermal dysplasia with hypothyroidism and ciliary dyskinesia (HEDH syndrome) (possibly a CGS with 225040; see later) (?same as ANOTHER syndrome)	225050	NK	Dystrophic, ridged finger- and toenails with a shrivelled appearance	Scanty and wispy scalp hair with a hard, hay-like consistency; scanty eyebrows and normal lashes	Normal	Hypohidrosis with hyperthermia; low number of sweat gland pores in the palms	**Skin:** poorly developed palmar dermal ridges; mottled brownish skin pigmentation of the trunk during the first months of life; urticaria pigmentosa like skin and mucosal pigmentation	NK

							Other: lacrimal ducts frequently blocked with resultant bilateral epiphora; frequent conjunctivitis; short stature; structural ciliary abnormalities of the respiratory tract; recurrent and severe upper and lower respiratory infections; severe cow's milk intolerance in infancy; elevated thyrotropin; decreased thyroid hormone production from early childhood; first degree hypothyroicism – no evidence of thyroid tissue shown by radiolabelled iodine studies	
Hypohidrotic ectodermal dysplasia with hypothyroidism and agenesis of the corpus callosum	225040	NK ?CGS	Dystrophic, ridged finger- and toenails with a shrivelled appearance	Scanty and wispy scalp hair	Normal, or microdontia, enamel defect	Hypohidrosis with hyperthermia	**Other:** severe mental retardation; agenesis of corpus callosum; primary hypothyroidism; absent normal thyroid and ectopic goitre on technetium-99 thyroid scintigram; respiratory tract and eye infections; hypoplastic maxilla; hypertelorism; protruding tongue	NK
Hypotrichosis and recurrent skin vesicles	613102	AR	Normal	Hairs present at birth, with regrowth after ritual shaving postnatally Increased hair loss at age 2–3 months, resulting in sparse and fragile scalp hair, eyebrows, eyelashes, axillary and body hair	Normal	Normal	**Skin:** vesicles, less than 1 cm in size, on scalp and skin, which burst and heal after 34 months with scarring	*DSC3* (600271)
Hypotrichosis–osteolysis–periodontitis–palmoplantar keratoderma syndrome (HOPP syndrome)	607658	AD	Onychogryphosis	Hypotrichosis; pili torti et annulati; congenital absence of eyebrows and lashes; ↓ hair follicles	Caries and periodontitis	Normal	**Skin:** severe, reticulate palmoplantar keratoderma with pits; nummular or striate palmoplantar keratoderma; acro osteolysis; psoriasis-like skin lesions; **Other:** lingua plicata, ventricular tachycardia	NK
Hypotrichosis simplex	146520	AD	Normal	Hair usually present at birth, but can have alopecia at birth; gradual hair loss beginning in first decade, complete hair loss by third decade; facial and body hair normal	Normal	Normal	No other findings	*CDSN*, (602593)

(*Continued*)

Table 134.1 *Continued*

Name (alternative names)	OMIM number/ primary ref	Inheritance	Phenotypic characteristics					Genetic basis and OMIM number
			Nails	Hair	Teeth	Sweat glands	Other	
Ichthyosis follicularis, atrichia and photophobia syndrome (IFAP syndrome); keratosis follicularis spinulosa decalvans	308205 308800	XR	Normal	Congenital atrichia	Enamel dysplasia	Hypohidrosis	**Skin:** ichthyosis follicularis **Other:** photophobia; short stature; mental retardation; seizures; congenital aganglionic megacolon; inguinal hernia; vertebral anomalies; renal anomalies; recurrent respiratory infections **Bresheck variant:** brain anomalies, retardation, ectodermal dysplasia, skeletal malformations, Hirschprung disease, ear/eye anomalies, cleft palate/cryptorchidism, kidney dysplasia/hypoplasia	*MBTPS2* (300294)
Immune dysfunction with T-cell inactivation due to calcium entry defect 1 and 2 (immunodeficiency 9 and 10)	612782 612783 McCarl et al. [20]	AR	Normal	Normal	Enamel hypoplasia	Anhydrosis	**Skin:** ichthyosis **Immunodeficiency:** Recurrent infections due to defective T-cell activation **Congenital myopathy**	*ORAI1* (610277) *STIM1* (605921)
Incontinentia pigmenti (familial male-lethal type IP, Bloch–Sulzberger syndrome)	308300	XD	Dystrophic in all or most of the fingers and toes in about one-tenth of cases	Scarring alopecia in one-third	Hypodontia; anodontia; peg-shaped; delayed eruption. Both deciduous and permanent teeth are affected	Normal	**Skin:** vesicular-bullous eruption in the neonatal period followed or accompanied by verrucous lesions and bizarre 'marble cake' pigmentation; pigmented macules may be present **Other:** occasional congenital hearing loss; ophthalmological alterations in about one-fifth of patients include blindness, strabismus, cataract, uveitis, retrolental fibroplasias, optic nerve atrophy, microphthalmia; occasional club-foot, cleft palate, microcephaly; about one-third of the cases present severe central nervous system anomalies: spastic tetraplegia, hemiplegia, diplegia; epilepsy; mental retardation; occasional short stature	*IKBKG* (300248)
Johanson–Blizzard syndrome	243800	AR	No data	Sparse, dry and fine or coarse; marked frontal upsweep	Oligodontia of both dentitions; peg-shaped teeth; absent permanent teeth	Normal	**Skin:** pale and smooth; café-au-lait spots on lower limbs and abdomen; patches of vitiligo on the lower back and abdomen; midline scalp defects (aplasia cutis congenita); tiny nipples with almost no areolae; transverse palmar creases	*UBR1* (605981)

							Other: exocrine pancreatic insufficiency; congenital sensorineural deafness; aplasia of the inferior puncta; strabismus; aplastic alae nasi, beak-like appearance to nose; variable mental retardation; occasional akinetic seizures; microcephaly; hypothyroidism; imperforate anus; genitourinary defects; failure to thrive/oedema; malabsorption; epiphyseal dysgenesis; dilated cardiomyopathy; nasolacrimocutaneous fistulae; highly arched palate; delayed bone age; hyperextensibility	
Keratitis, ichthyosis and deafness (KID) syndrome, incorporates hystrix-like ichthyosis with deafness (HID) syndrome 602540	148210	AD	Absence at birth; delayed development; leuconychia and thickening (most marked in the fingernails); destructive dystrophy	Hair loss varies from alopecia to fine, thin scalp hair; scanty or absent eyebrows and lashes; occasional trichorrhexis nodosa in some scalp hairs	Delayed eruption of deciduous teeth; brittleness; tendency to develop caries; unspecified defects	Hypohydrosis (with hypothermia)	**Skin:** ichthyosiform erythroderma with sebaceous dysfunction; furrowing around mouth and chin; erythematous hyperkeratotic plaques on elbows, knees and dorsa of hands and feet; marked thickening (leather-like consistency) of palms and soles; increased susceptibility to squamous cell carcinoma **Other:** congenital sensorineural deafness; vascularization of the cornea with pannus formation resulting in loss of vision; keratitis; occasional decreased tear production; photophobia; bilateral flexion contractures at knees and elbows with tight heel cords	*GJB2* (121011)
Keratosis palmoplantaris striata I (PPKS1)	148700	AD	Normal	Normal	Normal	Normal	**Skin:** linear palmoplantar keratoderma of the palms, may be more diffuse on the soles	*DSG1* (125670)
Keratosis palmoplantaris striata II (PPKS2)	612908	AD	Normal	Normal	Normal	Normal	**Skin:** linear palmoplantar keratoderma of the palms, may be more diffuse on the soles	*DSP* (125647)
Keratosis palmoplantaris striata III (PPKS3)	607654	AD	Normal	Normal	Normal	Normal	**Skin:** linear palmoplantar keratoderma of the palms, may be more diffuse on the soles	*KRT1* (139350)
Kirghizian dermato-osteolysis	221810	AR?	Some dystrophic fingernails	Normal	Hypodontia; abnormally shaped	Normal	**Skin:** multiple ulcerations on face, trunk and limbs, with healing of the more superficial ones and fistulous cicatrization of the deeper ones	NK

(*Continued*)

Table 134.1 *Continued*

Name (alternative names)	OMIM number/ primary ref	Inheritance	Phenotypic characteristics					Genetic basis and OMIM number
			Nails	Hair	Teeth	Sweat glands	Other	
							Other: recurrent keratitis with corneal scarring leading to visual impairment; acromegaloid enlargement of hands and feet; arthralgia; osteolysis around joints; claw hands; enlarged and deformed joints; short fingers; flexion contractures in some fingers	
Kohlschutter–Tonz syndrome (epilepsy, dementia and amelogenesis imperfecta)	226750	AR	Normal	Normal or coarse hair	Yellow owing to enamel hypoplasia	Hypohidrosis	**Skin:** scarce sebaceous glands and nerve fibres **Other:** myopia, progressive central nervous system degeneration with severe epileptiform seizures appearing between 11 months and 4 years of age; muscle spasticity; abnormal EEG; ventricular enlargement; broad thumbs and toes	*ROGDI* (614574)
Lelis syndrome (hypohidrotic ectodermal dysplasia with acanthosis nigricans) (? manifestation of X-linked HED 305100, see previously)	608290	AR?	Short and dystrophic	Generalized hypotrichosis; scalp hair is dry, fine, lustreless and slow growing; also scanty axillary, pubic hair; moustache/beard; eyebrows and lashes	Hypoplastic and carious	Hypohidrosis, small number of sweat glands (detected by biopsy)	**Skin:** dry; palmoplantar hyperkeratosis; hyperpigmented and hyperkeratotic skin with wrinkles, papillomas and a symptomatic acanthosis nigricans in the neck, axillae and genitofemoral regions; increased cornification and presence of follicular plugs on the 'normal' skin; unusual wrinkles around lips **Other:** plicate tongue with papillomatosis	*EDA* (300451)
Limb–mammary syndrome (allelic with EEC3, ADULT syndrome, AEC, Rapp–Hodgkin syndrome, split hand-foot malformation 4)	603543	AD	Nail dysplasia	Normal	Variable degrees of hypodontia	Hypohidrosis	**Other:** hypoplasia/aplasia of the mammary glands; cleft lip/palate +/− bifid uvula; lacrimal duct atresia; absence of uterus/ovaries	*TP63* (603273)
Localized autosomal recessive hypotrichosis, type 1 (LAH1); Hypotrichosis 6	607903	AR	Normal	Hypotrichosis, localized to scalp, chest, arms and legs; facial hair may be spared; eyebrows and eyelashes may be thinned, axillary and pubic hair usually normal Thin atrophic hair shafts that are unable to penetrate through the skin surface; swelling within the base of the hair shaft at precortical region	Normal	Normal	**Skin:** small papules on scalp may be seen due to ingrown hairs	*DSG4* (607892)

Localized autosomal recessive hypotrichosis, type 2 (LAH2); Hypotrichosis 7	604379	AR	Normal	Congenital hypotrichosis of scalp; any hairs present wiry and twisted; sparse or absent eyebrows and eyelashes; pubic and axillary hair affected, little body hair; in men, beard hair may be normal	Normal	Normal	**Skin:** follicular hyperkeratosis in two cases, possibly unrelated to alopecia	*LIPH* (607365)
Localized autosomal recessive hypotrichosis, type 3 (LAH3); hypotrichosis 8	278150	AR	Normal	Diffuse and progressive hair loss, beginning in childhood; sparse or absent scalp hair; sparse eyebrows and lashes, axillary and body hair; in men beard hair may be normal	Normal	Normal		*LPAR6* (609239)
Margarita Island ED (allelic to cleft lip/palate–ectodermal dysplasia syndrome [CLEPD1])	225060	AR	Dysplastic	Sparse, short scalp hair; sparse eyebrows	Hypodontia, especially upper lateral incisors	Normal	**Other:** cleft lip/palate; syndactyly of fingers; no mental retardation compared with CLEPD1	*NECTIN-1* (600644)
Marshall syndrome (allelic to Stickler syndrome [108300], but no ectodermal dysplasia in Stickler syndrome)	154780	AD	Normal	Sparse scalp hair and eyelashes in some families	Occasional hypodontia, microdontia, abnormalities of eruption and malposition	Occasional mild hypohidrosis	**Face:** characteristic, with congenital and persistently severe flat nasal bridge, anteversion of nostrils, malar hypoplasia, frontal bossing and sometimes hypertelorism; bifid uvula; large appearing eyeballs 2° to shallow orbit **Other:** occasional mental retardation; short to normal stature; hypoextensible joints; cranial and spondyloepiphyseal abnormalities; progressive congenital sensorineural deficit; myopia; fluid vitreous; congenital and juvenile cataracts with spontaneous and sudden maturation and absorption; calcification of falx cerebri and meninges	*COL11A1* (120280)
McGrath syndrome (ectodermal dysplasia–skin fragility syndrome)	604536	AR	Thickened and dystrophic	Short and sparse, some improvement with time	Normal	Hypohidrosis, some improvement with age	**Skin:** at birth, blistering and desquamation, especially on the face, limbs and buttocks; lifelong fragility, with trauma-induced tearing and blisters on the pressure points of the soles after prolonged standing or walking; plantar hyperkeratosis **Cardiomyopathy** associated with DSP mutation	*PKP1* (601975)

(*Continued*)

Table 134.1 *Continued*

Name (alternative names)	OMIM number/ primary ref	Inheritance	Phenotypic characteristics					Genetic basis and OMIM number
			Nails	Hair	Teeth	Sweat glands	Other	
Melanoleucoderma, infantilism, mental retardation, hypodontia, hypotrichosis	246500	AR	Normal	Dry and abundant scalp hair; sparse lateral eyebrows; normal eyelashes; axillary and pubic hair almost normal in women, absent in men	Delayed eruption of deciduous and permanent teeth; hypodontia	Mild palmoplantar hyperhidrosis	**Skin:** pale, thin, dry, smooth, pliable and feminine; generalized mottled dyschromia consisting of various shades of hyper- and hypopigmentation; aneto-poikiloderma-like lesions over the elbows, knees and proximal phalangeal articulations; pyoderma over the lower regions of the legs leading to atrophic scars; palmoplantar hyperkeratosis **Face:** typical 'family' face with flat saddle nose, thick lips with slight telangiectasia and deep furrows around the eyes and mouth **Other:** mental retardation; short stature; hyperextensibility of the fingers; slender legs; sexual underdevelopment in men (hypospadias, small penis and scrotum; atrophy of the testes; absence of secondary sexual characteristics)	NK
Mesomelic dwarfism–skeletal abnormalities–ectodermal dysplasia	Brunoni et al. [21]	NK	Hypoplastic toenails	Hypotrichosis	Dysmorphic; irregular eruption; malpositioned	Normal	**Skin:** extremely hypoplastic papillary dermal ridges; bilateral transitional palmar flexion creases **Face:** depressed nasal root; micrognathia; hypertelorism; antimongoloid palpebral slanting; epicanthal folds; long philtrum; thin lips **Limbs:** short forearms and hands; broad thumbs; brachymesophalangy; camptodactyly of both fifth fingers; short legs; flattened acetabular margins; broad halluces **Other:** esotropia; short stature; mild psychomotor retardation; brachycephaly; narrow and highly arched palate; retarded ossification of the anterior fontanelle with the presence of Wormian bones	NK
Monilethrix	158000	AD	Occasionally dystrophic	Brittle, beaded, highly variable degrees of alopecia	Normal	Normal	**Skin:** keratosis pilaris, especially over nape of neck	*KRT81 (602153)) KRT83 602765) or KRT86* (601928)

Naegeli–Franceschetti–Jadassohn syndrome (allelic with dermatopathia pigmentosa reticularis)	161000	AD	Normal; congenital malalignment of great toenails	Normal	Carious and yellowish spotted; early total loss of teeth	Hypohidrosis; discomfort in heat	**Skin:** reticular cutaneous pigmentation (appearing at age 2 and disappearing with age); diffuse palmoplantar hyperkeratosis; punctate keratoses; absent dermatoglyphics	*KRT14* (148066)
Naxos disease (palmoplantar keratoderma with arrhythmogenic right ventricular cardiomyopathy and woolly hair)	601214	AR	Normal	Dense, rough, bristly, woolly hair at birth; resembles steel wire, fragile hair	Normal	Normal	**Skin:** palmoplantar keratoderma, diffuse **Other:** arrhythmogenic right ventricular dysplasia and cardiomyopathy (abnormal electrocardiogram, cardiomegaly, ventricular tachycardia, sudden death)	*JUP* (173325)
Oculo-dentodigital dysplasia (ODDD) syndrome, autosomal dominant	164200	AD	Normal	Brittle, sparse and dry; slow growing	Generalized enamel hypoplasia; occasional hypodontia; microdontia and premature loss	Normal	**Eyes:** microcornea; microphthalmia with small orbits; reduced lid apertures; occasional findings: optic atrophy, synechiae, disc coloboma, persistence of papillary membrane, nystagmus, congenital cataract, glaucoma, strabismus and epicanthal folds **Limbs:** syndactyly and camptodactyly of the fourth and fifth fingers and of one or more toes; occasional ulnar clinodactyly of the fifth fingers and syndactyly of the third and fourth toes; hip dislocation; cubitus valgus **Other:** face characterized by a thin nose, prominent columella, hypoplastic alae and narrow nostrils; cleft lip; orbital hypotelorism; occasional micrognathia and mild pinna defects; microcephaly; cranial hyperostosis; cleft palate; osteopetrosis; occasional conductive impairment; spastic paraplegia; neurogenic bladder; ataxia; seizures; mild mental retardation	*GJA1* (121014)
Oculo-dentodigital dysplasia (ODDD) syndrome, autosomal recessive	257850	AR	Normal	Sparse fine hair, delayed onset of growth (2 years)	Malformed teeth; abnormal enamel; delayed eruption; hypoplastic teeth; chronic infection	Normal	**Eyes:** more severe ocular disease than the dominant form; prominent epicanthal folds; microphthalmia; microcornea; telecanthus; dysplastic iris; hyaloid system remnants; deep-set eyes; persistent pupillary membrane; cataract **Face:** long, narrow nose; hypoplastic nasal alae; micrognathia; markedly obtuse mandibular angle; mandibular overgrowth	*GJA1* (121014)

(*Continued*)

Table 134.1 *Continued*

Name (alternative names)	OMIM number/ primary ref	Inheritance	Phenotypic characteristics					Genetic basis and OMIM number
			Nails	Hair	Teeth	Sweat glands	Other	
							Limbs: syndactyly of fourth and fifth fingers; bilateral distal phalanx; clinodactyly of the fifth finger; soft tissue syndactyly of the second, third and fourth toes; widening of the long bones of the limbs; wide diaphyses **Other:** spinal cord compression at the base of the skull; calcification of the basal ganglia fontanelles; widely separated sutures; developmental delay	
Oculotrichodysplasia	257960	AR	Brittle finger- and toenails	Generalized hypotrichosis, sparse scalp, axillary and pubic hair; scanty eyelashes and sparse eyebrows in distal two-thirds	Hypodontia, carious with extensive extractions; small, pointed and widely spaced	Normal	**Skin:** dry and scaly **Other:** retinitis pigmentosa	NK
Odontomicronychial dysplasia	601319	AR	Short, thin, slow-growing nails	Normal	Precocious eruption and shedding of deciduous teeth; precocious eruption of secondary teeth with short rhomboid roots	Normal		NK
Odonto-onycho-dermal dysplasia	257980	AR	Dystrophic; small thin concave toenails; thin fingernails	Dry and sparse with thinning of eyebrows in some	Misshapen teeth; peg-shaped incisors; partial adontia; persistent deciduous teeth	Hyperhidrosis or normal sweating	**Skin:** thickening of the palms and soles; erythematous lesions of face; thickening of the palmar skin with painful chafing **Other:** mild mental deficiency, chronic irritative conjunctivitis secondary to short lashes; delayed psychomotor development; mild generalized hypotonia	*WNT10A* (606268)
Oligodontia-colorectal cancer syndrome	608615 Marvin et al. [22]	AD		Sparse hair and eyebrows	Oligodontia		**Colonic polyps and neoplasia** **Breast cancer**	*AXIN2* (604025)
Onychotrichodysplasia and neutropenia	258360	AR	Hypoplastic finger- and toenails; koilonychia; onychorrhexis	Congenitally absent; later dry, fine, lustreless, short, curly, sparse on scalp, eyebrows and lashes; trichorrhexis; absent axillae and pubic hair	Normal	Normal		NK

Orofaciodigital (OFD) syndrome type 1 (Papillon–Leage and Psaume syndrome)	311200	XD	Normal	Dryness and/or variable degree of alopecia (65%)	Absence of the lower lateral incisors (50%); malposition; occasional supernumerary canines and enamel hypoplasia	Normal	**Skin:** evanescent facial milia **Face:** broad nasal root; dystrophia canthorum; hypoplasia of alae nasi; median cleft of the upper lip; occasional short philtrum, frontal bossing; ear abnormalities **Limbs:** several types of malformations including brachydactyly, clinodactyly, syndactyly, polydactyly **Other:** occasional mental retardation (usually mild); agenesis of corpus callosum; dysarthria; gait disturbance; tremor; short stature; multiple hypertrophied lingual and labial frenula; lateral grooving of maxillary alveolar process; grooved ankyloglossia; cleft palate; hypoplasia of malar bone; hypoplasia of the base of the skull; renal abnormalities	*OFD1* (300170)
Pachyonychia congenita type 1 (Jadassohn–Lewandowsky type)	167200	AD	Severe wedge-shaped thickening	Usually normal	No natal teeth	Palmoplantar hyperhidrosis	**Skin:** focal palmoplantar keratoderma; verrucous lesions on the knees, elbows, buttocks, ankles and popliteal regions; follicular keratoses/keratosis pilaris **Other:** oral leucokeratosis; hoarseness	*KRT 16* (148067)
Pachyonychia congenita type 2 (Jackson–Lawler type)	167210	AD	Severe wedge-shaped thickening	Usually normal	Natal teeth	Palmoplantar hyperhidrosis	**Skin:** focal palmoplantar keratoderma; verrucous lesions on the knees, elbows, buttocks, ankles and popliteal regions; follicular keratoses/keratosis pilaris; multiple pilosebaceous cysts (steatocysts) with onset at puberty distinguish this form from PC type 1 **Other:** oral leucokeratosis; hoarseness	*KRT 17* (148069)
Pachyonychia congenita, autosomal recessive type	260130	AR	Thickened distorted nails, or prominent white nails	Normal	Normal	Hyperhidrosis	**Skin:** blistering at sites of friction; focal and punctate palmoplantar keratoderma; oral leukokeratoses; epidermal cysts; follicular keratotic papules on knees, elbows and buttocks	NK
Palmoplantar hyperkeratosis with congenital alopecia (alopecia congenita with keratosis palmoplantaris)	104100	AD	Short and dystrophic with onycholysis	Hypotrichosis to alopecia; absence of eyebrows and lashes; hypotrichosis of axillae and pubic regions	Normal	Normal	**Skin:** palmoplantar hyperkeratosis	*GJA1* (121014)

(*Continued*)

Table 134.1 *Continued*

Name (alternative names)	OMIM number/ primary ref	Inheritance	Phenotypic characteristics					Genetic basis and OMIM number
			Nails	Hair	Teeth	Sweat glands	Other	
Palmoplantar keratoderma with deafness	148350	AD	Normal	Normal	Normal	Normal	**Skin:** palmoplantar hyperkeratosis, progressive, onset mid-childhood **Other:** high-frequency sensorineural deafness, onset in early childhood	*GJB2* (121011)
Papillon–Lefèvre syndrome (keratosis palmoplantaris with periodontopathia) (allelic with Haim–Munk syndrome)	245000	AR	Occasionally dystrophic (spoon-shaped and striated; onychogryposis)	Occasionally thin and loose	Periodontal degeneration with consequent shedding of all teeth	Palmoplantar hyperhidrosis; occasional generalized hypohidrosis	**Skin:** hyperkeratosis of the palmar and plantar surfaces with a tendency towards fissuring and cracking; dry and dirty-appearing on the dorsal surface of the arms and the ventral surface of the legs; occasional eczema and erythema of the face as well as of the sacral and gluteal regions **Other:** severe gingivostomatitis; occasional intracranial calcifications; abnormal liver function; renal abnormalities; generalized osteoporosis; increased susceptibility to infections; liver abscess; ocular squamous neoplasia	*CTSC* (602365)
Pili torti and developmental delay	261990	AR	Normal	Pili torti	Normal	Normal	**Other:** growth and developmental delay; mild to moderate neurological abnormalities	NK
Pili torti and onychodysplasia (Beare type)	Beare [23]	AD	Short fragile and brittle	Initially normal, followed by hypotrichosis on the scalp, axillary and pubic areas; pili torti	Normal	Normal	**Skin:** normal, dry or greasy; slight atrophy on the top of the scalp **Other:** low IQ; severe mental retardation; 'irresponsible personality'	NK
Pili torti and onychodysplasia	Calzavara Pinton et al. [24]	AD	Distal nail dystrophy	Pilitorti of scalp, beard, pubic and axillary hair; absent eyebrows, eyelashes and body hair	Normal	Normal		NK
Pilodental dysplasia with refractive errors	262020	AR	Normal	Scalp hypotrichosis; pili annulati	Hypodontia; abnormally shaped teeth	Normal	**Other:** follicular hyperkeratosis of trunk and limbs; marked hyperopia; astigmatism	NK
Poikiloderma with neutropenia (Navajo poikiloderma; poikiloderma with neutropenia, Clericuzio type)	604173	AR	Thickened and dystrophic; subungual hyperkeratosis	Normal	Normal	Normal	**Skin:** eczematous rash at birth, becomes poikilodermatous over first 2 years of life **Other:** cyclical and noncyclical neutropenia; recurrent upper respiratory tract infections and chest infections; similarity to Rothmund–Thompson syndrome but no mutations in *RECQL4*	*USB1* (613276)

Polyposis, skin pigmentation, alopecia and fingernail changes (Cronkhite–Canada syndrome)	175500	?AD	Onychodystrophy	Alopecia	Normal	Normal	**Skin:** diffuse hyperpigmentation **Other:** cachexia; cataracts; xerostomia; glossitis; diminution of sense of taste; gastrointestinal hamartomatous polyps (stomach, small bowel, colon); gastrointestinal carcinoma; protein-losing enteropathy; malabsorption; haematochezia; clubbing of fingers; peripheral neuropathy; thromboembolism; hypocalcaemia; hypomagnesaemia; hypokalaemia	?Autoimmune mechanism
Rapp–Hodgkin syndrome (allelic with EEC3, limb–mammary syndrome, AEC, ADULT syndrome, split hand-foot malformation 4)	129400	AD	Small, narrow and dysplastic	Coarse and stiff on scalp; pili torti; absence or scarcity on scalp and body; sparse eyebrows and lashes	Conically shaped; short, square incisors and canines; hypoplastic enamel; extensive caries; hypodontia	Hypohidrosis; lower number of sweat glands	**Skin:** dry and coarse; thickened over the extensor surface of the elbows and knees; hypoplastic dermatoglyphics **Face:** cleft lip; hypoplastic maxilla; mild frontal prominence; microstomia; mildly depressed nasal bridge; prominent and malformed auricles **Other:** conductive loss (secondary to otitis media); chronic epiphora; corneal opacities; photophobia; atresia of puncta; ectropion; lacrimal papillae; short stature; occasional syndactyly	*TP63* (603273)
Rosselli–Gulienetti syndrome	225000	NK	Nail dysplasia	Hypotrichosis	Microdontia	Anhidrosis	**Skin:** tendency to desquamation with erythematous patches; popliteal and perineal pterygium (unlike CLEPD1 or Margarita Island ED; see above) **Face:** cleft lip and palate, aplasia or hypoplasia of thumb **Other:** genitourinary malformations, syndactyly	NK
Rothmund–Thomson syndrome	268400	AR	Frequently dystrophic	Hypotrichosis of scalp and body; eyebrows and lashes usually fall out during the first year of life and remain sparse or absent	Hypodontia; microdontia; supernumerary teeth; pronounced caries; delayed eruption	Normal	**Skin:** poikiloderma including atrophy, irregular pigmentation and telangiectasias beginning during the first 3–6 months; palmoplantar hyperkeratosis; sensitivity to sunlight; initial rash is red, elevated with oedematous patches appearing symmetrically on the cheeks, hands, forearms and buttocks and subsequently on the trunk and lower limbs; after a few years the active phase persists and a dry, scaling and atrophic skin develops with areas of hyperpigmentation, hypopigmentation and telangiectasia	*RECQL4* (603780)

(Continued)

Table 134.1 *Continued*

Name (alternative names)	OMIM number/ primary ref	Inheritance	Phenotypic characteristics					Genetic basis and OMIM number
			Nails	Hair	Teeth	Sweat glands	Other	
							Other: cataract, usually bilateral (onset between 3 and 6 years); occasionally degenerative lesions of the cornea; small hands and feet; short terminal phalanges; syndactyly: absence of metacarpals; rudimentary ulna and radius; increased risk of osteosarcoma; short stature; occasional mental retardation; hypogonadism; cryptorchidism; skull abnormalities; scoliosis	
Sabina brittle hair and mental deficiency syndrome (brittle hair and mental deficit) (?same as nonphotosensitive trichothiodystrophy, Pollitt syndrome, 234050)	211390	AR	Dystrophic (splitting and cracking proximally)	Dry, brittle, coarse, wiry in texture; reduced eyebrows and lashes; absence of axillary and pubic hair	No data	Normal	**Skin:** scalp hyperkeratosis on exposed areas **Other:** pigmentary retinopathy; unilateral congenital tortuosity of the retina vessels; pale optic discs and hyperopic astigmatism; maxillary hypoplasia; mental retardation; delayed bone age	NK
Scalp–ear–nipple syndrome (Finlay–Marks syndrome)	181270	AD	Brittle fingernails	Congenitally denuded areas on scalp; sparse axillary and secondary sexual hair	Widely spaced/missing teeth	Reduced apocrine secretion	**Skin:** scalp defects at birth, later become raised firm scalp nodules **Other:** small tragi; cupped and protruding ears; absent/rudimentary nipples; breast aplasia; partial third/fourth finger syndactyly; diabetes; colobomata; cataract; renal abnormalities	*KCTD1* (613420)
Schinzel–Giedion midface retraction syndrome	269150	AD	Narrow, deeply set, triangular and hyperconvex	Generalized hypertrichosis	Delayed eruption	No data	**Skin:** abundant on the neck; hypoplastic nipples; hypoplastic dermal ridges; simian creases **Face:** saddle nose with depressed root and short bridge; high/protruding forehead; orbital hypertelorism; small/malformed auricles; anteverted nostrils; midface hypoplasia; facial haemangiomata; alacrima; corneal hypoesthesia **Limbs:** mesomelic brachymelia; hypoplasia of distal phalanges in hands and feet; short metacarpals of thumbs; talipes	*SETBP1* (611060)

							Other: severe mental retardation; growth retardation; abnormal EEG and seizures; spasticity; recurrent apnoeic spells; multiple Wormian bones; wide cranial sutures and fontanelles; broad ribs, broad cortex and increased density of long tubular bones and vertebrae; hypoplastic/aplastic pubic bones; choanal stenosis; short and broad neck; genitourinary abnormalities (short penis with hypospadias, megaureter, megacalycosis)	
Schopf–Schulz–Passarge syndrome (cystic eyelids–palmoplantar keratosis–hypodontia–hypotrichosis)	224750	AR	Brittle with longitudinal and oblique furrows; onycholysis	Generalized hypotrichosis of scalp and body	Extensive hypodontia; persistence of deciduous teeth	Normal or hyperhidrosis	**Skin:** palmoplantar keratosis; telangiectatic facial skin; papules; multiple tumours with follicular differentiation **Other:** bilateral early senile cataract; arteriosclerotic fundi; myopia; cysts of eyelids developing late	*WNT10A* (606268)
Sener syndrome (frontonasal dysplasia and dilated Virchow–Robin spaces)	606156	NK	Dystrophic nails	Thin, coarse, brittle hair	Hypodontia; dental occlusion; natal teeth; irregular, pointed	Normal	**Face:** hypertelorism with a wide mouth, long, smooth philtrum and small posteriorly rotated ears **Other:** multiple cystic areas within the white matter radiating from the ventricles into oval lobes with sparing of the basal ganglia, brainstem and corpus callosum; mild developmental delay	NK
Sensorineural hearing loss, enamel hypoplasia and nail defects (Heimler syndrome)	234580	AR	Beau's lines (toenails); leuconychia (fingernails)	Normal	Generalized enamel hypoplasia; hypomineralized amelogenesis imperfecta	Normal	**Other:** severe, early-onset sensorineural hearing loss	*PEX1* (602136)
Skeletal anomalies–ectodermal dysplasia–growth and mental retardation	Schinzel [25]	NK	Hypoplastic toenails	Almost complete absence of body hair; a few curled hairs are present in the parieto-occipital and pubic regions	Normal	Normal	**Skin:** dry and hyperkeratotic with rhomboid type of scaling, especially on the lower legs; absence of flexion creases on thumbs; fifth fingers with single flexion creases **Face:** large, prominent nose; upslanting palpebral fissures; short upper lip; large, poorly formed ears **Other:** microbrachycephaly; multiple uni- or bilateral fusion of vertebral bodies in the lower thoracic and upper lumbar regions; multiple limb abnormalities; syndactyly; bone fusions	NK

(*Continued*)

Table 134.1 *Continued*

Name (alternative names)	OMIM number/ primary ref	Inheritance	Phenotypic characteristics					Genetic basis and OMIM number
			Nails	Hair	Teeth	Sweat glands	Other	
Skin fragility–woolly hair syndrome	607655	AR	Progressively worsening nail dystrophy	Woolly hair; generalized alopecia; sparse eyelashes and eyebrows	Abnormal teeth		**Skin:** fragile skin in the immediate newborn period, that decreases in severity; intraoral blisters with poor feeding; hyperkeratosis of palms and soles	*DSP* (125647)
Split hand-foot malformation (SHFM1)	183600	AD	Dysplastic, dystrophic, underdeveloped, absent	Sparse hair, alopecia	Oligodontia, abnormally shaped teeth		**Other:** lacrimal involvement, ectrodactyly, preaxial involvement of the upper extremities least common in SHFM1 (most common in SHFM3)	7q21.2-q21.3
Split hand-foot malformation 4	605289	AD	Underdeveloped, absent, dystrophic or dysplastic	Sparse hair, alopecia	Oligodontia, abnormally shaped teeth		**Skin:** freckling **Face:** lacrimal involvement **Other:** ectodermal features most common in SHFM4; SHFM3 has only dental and nail findings	*TP63* (603273)
Taurodontia, absent teeth and sparse hair (? same as Witkop syndrome, 189500; see later)	272980	AR	Slow-growing nails; thin, spoon-shaped nails	Sparse hair; slow-growing hair	Congenital hypodontia; taurodontia; lack of permanent lateral maxillary incisors	Normal		NK
Tetramelic deficiencies, ectodermal dysplasia, deformed ears and other abnormalities (odontotrichomelic syndrome)	273400	AR	Platonychia, mildly dysplastic toenails, hypoplastic?	Severe hypotrichosis of scalp and body	Hypodontia; microdontia; coniform teeth; persistence of deciduous teeth	Normal	**Skin:** hypoplastic nipples; hypoplastic or absent areolae; thin, dry and shiny; an unusual number of wrinkles are formed when patients smile or grimace; dermatoglyphic disturbances **Face:** protruding lips; enlarged nose; large, thin, prominent and deformed auricles; incomplete right cleft lip in one patient; esotropia; wide nasal root **Other:** bipartite right clavicle; short and distally curved left clavicle; coxa valga; steep femoral necks; synostosis of cuboid and lateral cuneiform bones; cutaneous syndactyly; EEG abnormalities; growth retardation; extensive tetramelic deficiencies; metabolic abnormalities; electrocardiogram abnormalities; mild mental retardation; short stature; microcephaly; constant tearing and repeated infections of the conjunctivae; atresia of the nasolacrimal ducts	NK

Thumb deformity and alopecia	188150	AD	Normal	Alopecia	Single central upper incisor	Normal	**Other:** hypoplastic thumbs; short stature; mental retardation; increased groin pigmentation with raindrop depigmentation	NK
Trichodental dysplasia	601453	AD	Normal	Slow-growing, fine and lustreless appearance; relatively thin shafts with a slight beading effect; scanty or absent distal eyebrows and sparse eyelashes	Hypodontia; peg-shaped teeth; shell teeth (thin dentin, large pulp chamber), missing teeth; retained deciduous teeth	No data	**Other:** one case of microcephaly and mental retardation	NK
Trichodento-osseous syndrome	190320	AD	Flat, thickened, misshapen and striated; brittle	Dry, thick, tough with short curls, often straightens in childhood; balding may occur with age in men	Thin enamel; small, widely spaced teeth; teeth pits; taurodontism; periapical abscesses	Normal	**Face:** occasional frontal bossing **Other:** occasional clinodactyly; some of the calvaria sutures show evidence of premature fusion leading to mild to moderate dolichocephaly	*DLX3* (600525)
Tricho-odonto-onychial dysplasia (tricho odonto-onychial dysplasia with amastia)	129510	AR?	Variable degree of dystrophy of finger- and toenails; brittle nails	Alopecia totalis; sparse eyebrows and eyelashes	Enamel hypoplasia in both dentitions; secondary anodontia; delayed eruption	Normal	**Skin:** increased number of pigmented naevi; extranumerary nipples; keratotic actinic lesions; crusts, ephelides in the scalp; mild palmoplantar hyperkeratosis; dermatoglyphic alterations; irregular hyperpigmentation of the back **Other:** one patient had a mixed mild hearing deficit on the left; short stature; amastia, athelia	NK
Tricho-odonto-onycho dermal syndrome	Pinheiro et al. [26]	NK	Severely dystrophic or absent finger and toenails	Parieto-occipital hypotrichosis; aplasia cutis congenita; sparse eyelashes; sparse and irregular eyebrows	Hypodontia; persistence of deciduous teeth; enamel hypoplasia; delayed eruption	Normal	**Skin:** dry with hypochromic, atrophic and poikiloderma like spots; irregular areolae; wrinkled back of hands; palmar keratosis; dermatoglyphic alterations; aplasia cutis congenita of the scalp **Face:** long philtrum; microstomia with thin lips; hyperpigmented eyelids and periorbital regions **Limbs:** bilateral clinodactyly; syndactyly; hypoplastic thumb; pronounced manus cava; hypoplastic distal and middle phalanges of both second fingers; absent middle phalanges of all toes **Other:** mild asymmetry of the skull; congenital hypertrophy of the frenum linguae	NK

(*Continued*)

Table 134.1 *Continued*

Name (alternative names)	OMIM number/ primary ref	Inheritance	Phenotypic characteristics					Genetic basis and OMIM number
			Nails	Hair	Teeth	Sweat glands	Other	
Tricho-odonto-onychial dysplasia with bone deficiency	275450	?AR	Dystrophic	Severe hypotrichosis; peripheral fringe of hair on the temporal and occipital regions; dry, brittle, sparse hair	Enamel hypoplasia; secondary anodontia	Normal	**Skin:** supernumerary nipples; naevus pigmentosus; mild palmoplantar keratoderma **Other:** bone deficiency in the frontoparietal region **Skin:** fine textured	NK
Tricho-onycho-dental (TOD) dysplasia	Koshiba et al. [27]	AD	Thin with longitudinal striations and cracks	Scanty, fine, curled; sparse eyebrows and lashes	Taurodontic molars; hypoplastic–hypomature enamel; hypodontia	Hypohidrosis with hyperthermia		NK
Trichorhinophalangeal syndrome types I and III	190350, 190351	AD	Occasional thin, short, with long longitudinal grooves; flattened, koilonychia-like and normal in colour; racket thumbnails	Fine, usually blond and sparse (especially in the frontotemporal areas); sparse or absent eyebrows	Occasional supernumerary incisors; microdontia; poorly aligned	Normal	**Other:** pear-shaped nose; long and wide philtrum; large, prominent ears; occasional exotropia and photophobia; short stature; increased susceptibility to upper respiratory tract infections; narrow palate; scoliosis; lordosis or kyphosis; pectus carinatum **Limbs:** brachymesophalangy; brachymetacarpy; brachymetatarsy; peripheral dysostosis with type 12 cone-shaped epiphyses at some of the middle phalanges of the hands (the joints are thickened); ulnar and radial deviation of the fingers; occasional clinodactyly; winged scapulae; coxa valga; Perthes-like abnormalities (type III: severe brachydactyly, short metacarpals, severe short stature) Pubertal delay, gynaecomastia	*TRSPS1* (604386)
Trichorhinophalangeal syndrome type II (Langer–Giedion syndrome)	150230	AD	Occasional thin, short, with long longitudinal grooves; flattened, koilonychia-like and normal in colour; racket thumbnails	Fine, usually blond and sparse (especially in the frontotemporal areas); sparse or absent eyebrows	Occasional supernumerary incisors; microdontia; poorly aligned	Normal	As above for trichorhinophalangeal syndrome types I and III, plus multiple cartilaginous exostoses; mental retardation is common, seizures	Microdeletion of 8q42.11 to 8q24.13 (includes *TRPS1*, *RAD21* and *EXT1*)

Trichothiodystropy 4, nonphotosensitive (Pollitt syndrome, trichothiodystrophy neurocutaneous syndrome) (?same as Sabina brittle hair and mental deficiency syndrome 211390; see earlier)	234050	AR	Hypoplastic nails; spoon-shaped nails	Trichorrhexis nodosa; short, woolly hair; stubby eyebrow hair	No data	Normal	**Skin:** ichthyotic skin, flexural eczema; photosensitivity **Other:** mental retardation; hypotonia; titubation; spastic diplegia; extensor plantar reflexes; absent deep tendon reflexes; partial agenesis of the corpus callosum; central nuclear cataracts; jerky ocular pursuit movements; growth retardation; microcephaly; receding chin; protruding ears	*MPLKIP* (609188)
Ulnar mammary syndrome (Schinzel syndrome, ulnar mammary syndrome of Pallister)	181450	AD	Normal	Sparse axillary hair; scant lateral eyebrows	Ectopic upper canines; hypodontia	Axillary apocrine gland hypoplasia	**Other:** delayed growth; obesity; subglottic stenosis; hypoplastic scapula; hypoplastic clavicle; breast hypoplasia; nipple hypoplasia; anal atresia or stenosis; pyloric stenosis; small penis; delayed puberty; shawl scrotum; imperforate hymen **Limbs:** hypoplastic/absent/deformed ulna; hypoplastic/absent/deformed radius; hypoplastic humerus; absent third, fourth and fifth ulnar rays; postaxial polydactyly; short fourth and fifth toes	*TBX3* (601621)
Uncombable hair, retinal pigmentary dystrophy, dental anomalies and brachydactyly (Bork syndrome)	191482	AD	Normal	Uncombable hair; pili canaliculi; congenital hypotrichosis	Oligodontia; supernumerary inferior lateral incisors; microdontia	Normal	**Other:** juvenile cataracts; retinal pigmentary dystrophy; brachymetacarpy; mild mental retardation	NK
Walbaum–Dehane–Schlemmer syndrome	Walbaum et al. [28]	AR	Normal	Initially thin and blond; alopecia later; hypotrichosis of body hair	Hypodontia; supernumerary teeth; microdontia; malposition	Normal	**Skin:** abnormal dermatoglyphics **Face:** swollen, with flat nasal bridge and enlarged tip of nose **Other:** mild gingival hypertrophy; growth retardation	NK
Witkop syndrome (tooth and nail syndrome) (?same as taurodontia, absent teeth and sparse hair (272980); see earlier: ?Fried tooth and nail syndrome included)	189500	AD	Koilonychia; longitudinal ridging; nail pits; seen in childhood; toenails more affected than fingernails	Fine scalp hair, normal eyelashes and eyebrows	Partial or total anodontia; permanent teeth fail to erupt; absent maxillary canines, mandibular incisors, second molars	Normal	**Other:** lower lip eversion; polycystic ovaries	*MSX1* (142983)
Weyer acrofacial dysostosis (acrodental dysostosis of Weyer, Curry–Hall syndrome) (?milder AD form of Ellis–van Creveld [225500] *ibid*)	193530	AD	Hypoplastic/dysplastic	Normal	Incisors abnormal in shape and number; single central incisor; conical	Normal	**Other:** short stature; postaxial polydactyly; short limbs; acrofacial dysostosis; abnormal mandible; hypotelorism; prominent ear antihelices	*EVC* (607261) *EVC2* (604831)

(*Continued*)

Table 134.1 *Continued*

Name (alternative names)	OMIM number/ primary ref	Inheritance	Phenotypic characteristics					Genetic basis and OMIM number
			Nails	Hair	Teeth	Sweat glands	Other	
Woolly hair, hypotrichosis, everted lower lip and outstanding ears (Salamon syndrome)	278200	AD	Highly dystrophic; brittle; ungues plicatae; toenails more severely affected; onycholysis	General hypotrichosis of scalp and body hair; woolly hair	Extensive hypodontia (rudimentary permanent teeth); persistence of deciduous teeth	Normal	**Skin:** palmoplantar keratosis; telangiectatic facial skin; papules; multiple tumours with follicular differentiation **Other:** bilateral early senile cataract; arteriosclerotic fundi; myopia; eyelid cysts; everted lower lip; protruding ears	NK
Xeroderma–talipes–enamel defect (XTE syndrome)	Moynahan [29]	NK	Deformed on fingers +/– toes	Coarse and dry; slow growing; hypotrichosis; no lashes on lower lids	Poorly formed; yellow enamel	Hypohidrosis	**Skin:** generally dry, scaling with numerous bullae on face and limbs; scanty hair follicles **Other:** photophobia; hypoplasia of the ocular puncta leading to epiphora and blepharitis; EEG alterations; mild mental retardation; bilateral club foot; cleft palate	NK
X-linked tooth agenesis	313500	XD	Normal	Normal	Congenital absence of central and lateral incisors, also canine teeth, but maxillary and permanent molars unaffected	Normal		*EDA* (300451)
Zanier–Roubicek syndrome (?same as AD HED, 129490)	Zanier and Roubicek [30]	AD	Occasionally brittle	Hypotrichosis; normal eyebrows and lashes	Hypodontia; conical teeth; early loss of deciduous teeth	Hypohidrosis, often severe hyperthermia in infancy	**Skin:** smooth and dry **Other:** reduced lacrimation; normal or slightly reduced stature; hypoplasia of the mammary glands	NK

AD, autosomal dominant; AR, autosomal recessive; CGS, contiguous gene syndrome; EEG, electroencephalogram; NK, not known; OMIM, Online Mendelian Inheritance in Man; XD, X-linked dominant; XR, X-linked recessive.

and structural/adhesive molecules. Based on these pathophysiological mechanisms, EDs can also be sorted into two broad categories: Group 1, indicating defects in developmental regulation and epithelial–mesenchymal interaction, and Group 2, indicating defects in proteins of cytoskeleton or adhesion, which are involved in cell–cell communication as well as structural integrity [8,9].

References

1 **Online Mendelian Inheritance in Man, OMIM™. McKusick–Nathans Institute for Genetic Medicine, Johns Hopkins University and National Center for Biotechnology Information, National Library of Medicine, Bethesda, MD. www.ncbi.nlm.gov/omim/**
2 Danz DFG. Sechste Bemerkung. Von Menschen ohne Haare und Zahne. Stark Arch Geburtch Frauenz Neugeb Kinderkr 1792;4:684.
3 **Weech A. Hereditary ectodermal dysplasia (congenital ectodermal defect). A report of two cases. Am J Dis Child 1929;37:766–90.**
4 Touraine A. L'anidrose hereditaires avec hypotrichose et anodontie (polydysplasie ectodermique héréditaire). Presse Méd 1936;44:145–9.
5 **Freire-Maia N, Pinheiro M. Ectodermal Dysplasias: A Clinical and Genetic Study. New York: Alan R. Liss, 1984.**
6 **Pinheiro M, Freire-Maia N. Ectodermal dysplasias: a clinical classification and a causal review. Am J Med Genet 1994;53:153–62.**
7 **Fuchs E, Merrill BJ, Jamora C et al. At the roots of a never-ending cycle. Dev Cell 2001;1:13–25.**
8 **Priolo, M, Laganà C. Ectodermal dysplasias: a new clinical-genetic classification. J Med Genet 2001;38:579–85.**
9 **Priolo M. Ectodermal dysplasias: an overview and update of clinical and molecular-functional mechanisms. Am J Med Genet A 2009;149A:2003–13.**
10 Lerner AB. Three unusual pigmentary syndromes. Arch Dermatol 1961;83:151–9.
11 Baisch A. Anonychia congenita, Kombiniert mit Polydaktykie and verzogertem abnormen Zahndurchbruch. Dtsch Z Chir 1931;232:450–7.
12 Petfor G, Nanda A, Howden J et al. Mutations in GRHL2 result in an autosomal-recessive ectodermal dysplasia syndrome. Am J Hum Genet. 2014;95:308–14.
13 Wallace HJ. Ectodermal defect with skeletal abnormalities. Proc C Soc Med Edinb 1958;51:707–8.
14 Wesser DW, Vistnes LM. Congenital ectodermal dysplasia, anhidrotic, with palatal paralysis and associated chromosome abnormality. Plast Reconstr Surg 1969;8:396–8.
15 Kirman BH. Idiocy and ectodermal dysplasia. Br J Dermatol 1955;67:303–7.
16 Wiedemann HR, Grosse FR, Dibbern H. Caracteristicas das Sindromes em Pediatria. Atlas de Diagnostico Diferencial. São Paulo: Editoria Manole, 1978.
17 Fischer H. Familiar hereditares Vorkommen von Keratoma palamare et plantare, Nagelverandergungen, Haaranomalien und Verdickung der Endglieder der Finger und Zehen in 5 Generationen (die Beziehungen dieser Veranderungen zur inneren Sekretion). Dermatol Zeitschr 1921;32:114–42.
18 Fried K. Autosomal recessive hydrotic ectodermal dysplasia. J Med Genet 1977;14:137–9.
19 Jorgenson RJ. Gingival fibromatosis. Birth Defects 1971;VII:278–80.
20 McCarl C-A, Picard C, Khalil S, et al. ORAI1 deficiency and lack of store-operated Ca^{2+} entry cause immunodeficiency, myopathy and ectodermal dysplasia. J Allergy Clin Immunol 2009;124:1311–18.
21 Brunoni D, Lederman H, Ferrari S et al. Uma sindrome malformativa com nanismo mesomelico, malformacoes esqueleticas, displasia ectodermica e facies tipica. Cienc Cult 1982;34:694.
22 Marvin ML et al. AXIN2-associated autosomal dominant ectodermal dysplasia and neoplastic syndrome. Am J Med Genet A. 2011; 155A:898–902.
23 Beare JM. Congenital pilar defect showing features of pili torti. Br J Dermatol 1952;64:366–72.
24 Calzavara-Pinton P, Carlino A, Benetti A et al. Pili torti and onychodysplasia. Report of a previously undescribed hidrotic ectodermal dysplasia. Dermatologica 1991;182:184–7.
25 Schinzel A. A case of multiple skeletal anomalies, ectodermal dysplasia, and severe growth and mental retardation. Helv Paediatr Acta 1980;35:243–51.
26 Pinheiro M, Pereira LC, Freire-Maia N. A previously undescribed condition: tricho-odonto-onycho-dermal syndrome. A review of the tricho-odonto-onychial subgroup of ectodermal dysplasias. Br J Dermatol 1981;105:371–82.
27 Koshiba H, Kimura O, Nakata M et al. Clinical, genetic, and histologic features of the trichoonychodental (TOD) syndrome. Oral Surg Oral Med Oral Pathol 1978;46:376–85.
28 Walbaum R, Dehaene P, Schlemmer H. Dysplasie ectodermique: une forme autosomique recessive? Arch Fr Pediatr 1971;28:435–42.
29 Moynahan EJ. XTE syndrome (xeroderma, talipes and enamel defect): a new heredo-familial syndrome. Proc Roy Soc Med Lond 1970;63:1–2.
30 Zanier JM, Roubicek MM. Hypohidrotic ectodermal dysplasia with autosomal dominant transmission. Fifth International Congress on Human Genetics, Mexico, 1976: Communication 273.

Ectodermal dysplasias caused by mutations in tumour necrosis factor like/NF-κB signalling pathways

Overview of molecular pathways

The transcription factor NF-κB regulates the expression of multiple genes with functions in controlling the immune and stress responses, cell adhesion, protection against apoptosis and inflammatory reactions [1,2]. NF-κB is composed of homo- or heterodimers of five proteins belonging to the Rel family (p50, p52, c-rel, relA and relB). NF-κB is usually maintained in an inactive state within the cytoplasm by association with inhibitory proteins of the IB (IκB) family: IBα, IBβ and IBε. IB molecules are phosphorylated on two critical serine residues in response to multiple stimuli such as cytokines, various stress signals and viral and bacterial infections. An increasing number of signals that initiate this phosphorylation are identified year-on-year, but the best studied signals include the tumour necrosis factors (TNFs), lipopolysaccharides (LPS) and interleukin 1 (IL-1). Phosphorylation at these sites allows IB molecules to be recognized by a ubiquitination complex; following polyubiquitation, IBs are degraded by proteasomes, thus freeing free NF-κB to enter the nucleus and activate target genes [3].

The kinase that phosphorylates IB has been designated IKK (for IκB kinase) and has been shown to consist of two catalytic subunits (IKKα/IKK1, now known as CHUK, and IKKβ/IKK2, now known as IKBKB) and a third component IKKγ (now known as IKBKG, previously known as NEMO – NF-κB essential modulator) that provides a structural and regulatory function to the complex. Cell lines lacking IKBKG are unable to activate NF-κB in response to most stimuli [4]. Extensive work with mouse models has confirmed the centrality of the NF-κB pathway in apoptosis and inflammatory and immune functions [5]. Complete absence of NF-κB leads to prenatal death owing to massive TNF-induced liver apoptosis, and more subtle knockouts that alter NF-κB activity all lead to immune defects. CHUK is also an important suppressor of skin cancer [6].

The elucidation of the NF-κB pathway has recently generated much interest in the EDs, and defects at various levels have been identified in several EDs [7]. In many cases, these predominantly phenotype-driven, mouse–human comparison studies have yielded significant

Table 134.2 Genotype–phenotype correlation in disorders due to mutations in the NF-κB signalling pathway

Gene	Human disease (OMIM number; abbreviation)
EDAR	Autosomal dominant hypohidrotic ectodermal dysplasia (129490) and autosomal recessive hypohidrotic ectodermal dysplasia recessive (224900)
EDA	X-linked hypohidrotic ectodermal dysplasia (305100)
EDARADD	Autosomal recessive hypohidrotic ectodermal dysplasia (614941) and autosomal dominant hypohidrotic ectodermal dysplasia (614940)
TRAF6	Familial osteoporosis (611739)
IKBKG (amorphic mutations)	Incontinentia pigmenti (308300; IP)
IKBKG (hypomorphic mutations)	Hypohidrotic ectodermal dysplasia with immune deficiency (300291; ED-ID)
IKBKG (stop codons)	Anhidrotic ectodermal dysplasia with immunodeficiency, osteopetrosis and lymphoedema (300301; OL-EDA-ID)
NFKBIA (hypermorphic dominant mutations)	Autosomal dominant ectodermal dysplasia with a severe and unique T-cell immunodeficiency (612132; EDA-ID)
IRAK1 (amorphic mutations)	None yet identified; ?lupus susceptibility

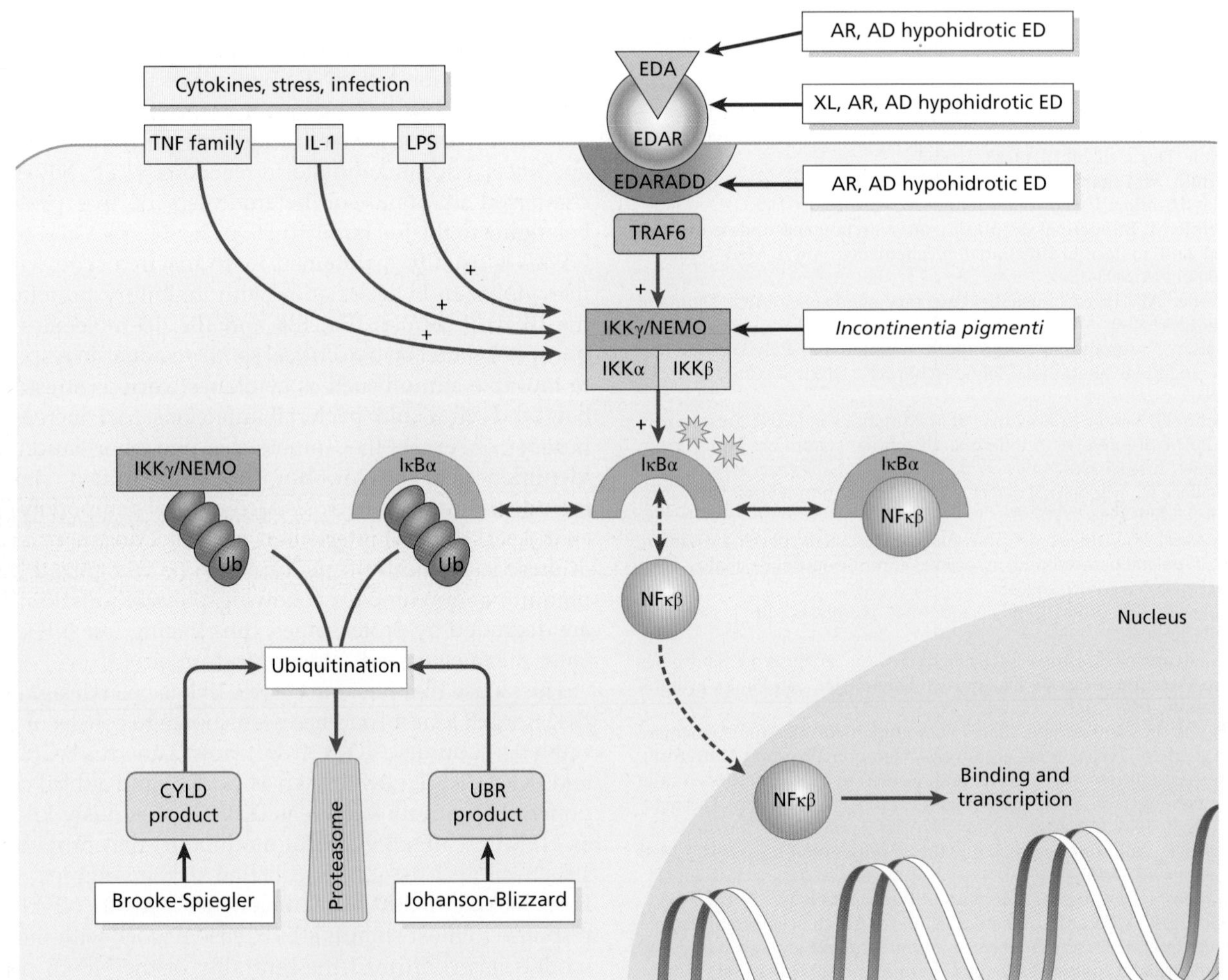

Fig. 134.1 Schematic of NF-κB pathway. EDA binds to EDAR, which interacts with EDARADD. Downstream signalling from this complex, as well as input from cytokines and other stressors, leads to activation of the IKK (inhibitor κ B kinase) complex via TRAF 6 and other signalling molecules. When activated, the IKK complex, which is made up of three subunits (α, β and γ), phosphorylates IκB α (inhibitor κ B α), which results in its targeting for ubiquitination and degradation. This causes the release of NF-κB, allowing it to enter the nucleus, bind to transcriptional elements, and cause upregulation of NF-κB mediated gene targets. AD, autosomal dominant; AR, autosomal recessive; ED, ectodermal dysplasia; EDAR, ectodysplasin A; EDARADD, EDAR-associated death domain; IL-1, interleukin 1; LPS, lipopolysaccharides; TNF, tumour necrosis factor; Ub, ubiquitin; XL, X-linked.

new insights in molecular pathways (Table 134.2) [1]. One of the best characterized pathways in NF-κB activation is the ectodysplasin pathway, an upstream activator (Fig. 134.1). Since 1997, defects in this pathway have been demonstrated in the X-linked, autosomal dominant and recessive subtypes of HED. Subsequently, mutations in downstream components have been shown to underlie familial incontinentia pigmenti and HED associated with immunodeficiency and/or osteopetrosis and HED associated with T cell immune deficiency.

The X-linked HED gene, *EDA*, which maps to Xq12–13.1 and is also mutated in the mouse orthologue *tabby* [8], was first described in 1996 [9]. Canine and bovine models for X-linked HED have mutations in the similar genes [10–12]. *EDA* encodes two isoforms of a transmembrane protein, ectodysplasin-A (EDA), that has homology to the TNF family. The extracellular domain of EDA has a collagen-like repeat and a furin cleavage site, unique in TNF proteins. Cleavage is necessary to enable solubility and functionality of EDA. The two longest iso forms, EDA-A1 and EDA-A2, bind to two different receptors: EDA-A1 binds to the EDAR protein and EDA-A2 binds to another X-linked receptor, XEDAR [13]. Mutations have been identified in all domains of EDA in patients with HED; many of these mutations are thought to affect solubility or cleavage of EDA, rendering it non-unctional [14]. Mutations in the EDA Gly-X-Y domain are thought to prevent bundling of EDAR trimers but do not appear to affect EDA–EDAR binding. EDA mutations are also responsible for X-linked hypodontia (OMIM 313500), a condition notable for the congenital absence of incisors but not molars [15].

The physiological role of EDA in hair follicle morphogenesis was reinforced by the isolation of the gene for autosomal dominant/recessive HED. Patients with autosomal dominant or recessive HED are phenotypically identical to those with X-linked HED. The mutated gene, previously named *downless* (*DL*) after the mouse homologue, encodes a member of the tumour necrosis factor receptor (TNFR) superfamily which functions as an ectodysplasin receptor (EDAR) [16]. Loss-of-function mutations throughout *EDAR* have been reported in autosomal recessive HED and dominant negative mutations have been reported in autosomal dominant HED within the death domain of this transmembrane protein [17].

The EDA–EDAR pathway was further refined when the molecular basis of a third mouse homologue was identified. The *crinkled* mouse (*cr*) is a spontaneous mouse mutant with an identical phenotype to *downless* and *tabby*. Using positional cloning techniques, the causative gene was identified in an adapter protein (EDAR-associated death domain, termed Edaradd) for the EDA–EDAR complex [18]. The same group also identified mutations in a family with autosomal recessive HED [18]. The Edaradd death domain interacts with the intracellular death domain of EDAR, linking it to downstream signals leading to NF-κB activation [18]. Edaradd associates with TNFR-associated factor (TRAF) 1, 2 and 3. The gene encoding the Edaradd protein, *EDARRADD*, may be mutated in both autosomal recessive and dominant HED [19,20].

NF-κB activation by the EDAR pathway is *IKBKG* dependent [21], and the relevance of this interaction to human EDs became clear when loss-of function mutations were identified in the *IKBKG* gene (*NEMO*) in incontinentia pigmenti [22]. This discovery was followed by identification of less critical mutations in *IKBKG* in several male patients with an unusual phenotype of HED associated with immune deficiency (EDA-ID) [21,23,24]. Mutations in the coding region are associated with the EDA-ID phenotype, and specific mutations in the stop codon of *IKBKG* cause a more severe syndrome of osteopetrosis and/or lymphoedema associated with EDA-ID [21]. *IKBKG* C-terminal deletion mutations are associated with inflammatory skin and intestinal disease in addition to ED with anhidrosis and immunodeficiency [25]. TNF blockade has been shown to be useful in these patients [26].

Recently, two other EDAR-related members of the TNFR superfamily, X-linked ectodysplasin-A2 receptor (XEDAR) [13] and TNFR superfamily member 19 (TNFRSF19), also known as TROY or TAJ (toxicity and JNK inducer) [27,28], have been reported. Signals from each of these receptors were shown to activate NF-κB, providing further candidate genes and candidate signalling systems for human HED. TRAF-6 is a cytoplasmic adapter protein that links signals from members of the TNFR superfamily to activation of transcription factors such as NF-κB through IKK activation. TRAF-6 –/– mice display HED, revealing yet more complexity to these signalling systems [29]. It is likely that several of these genes will, in time, be shown to have relevance in human HED.

Regulatory modulators of the NF-κB system may also prove relevant to ED in the future; recently mutations in a gene encoding a protein involved in deubiquitinization of inhibitor proteins has been found in familial cylindromatosis (Brooke–Spiegler syndrome, OMIM #605041), and its allelic disorders, familial cylindromatosis (OMIM #132700) and multiple familial trichoepitheliomas (OMIM #601606). Mutations in the cylindromatosis gene (*CYLD*) are associated with these disorders, and this protein has an important role in negative regulation of the NF-κB pathway, because it deubiquitinates multiple NF-κB regulators, including *TRAF2*, *TRAF6* and *IKGKB* [30–34]. Johanson–Blizzard syndrome, another ED, is caused by mutations in *UBR1*, which encodes ubiquitin-protein ligase E3 component N-recognin, a protein that binds to a destabilizing N-terminal residue of a substrate protein and participates in the formation of a substrate-linked multiubiquitin chain [35].

X-linked, autosomal dominant and recessive HED

The phenotypic appearances of the X-linked (OMIM #305100), autosomal recessive (OMIM 606603) and autosomal dominant types (OMIM #129490) are identical.

Definition. X-linked HED is the most common of the EDs and is characterized by hypotrichosis, hypodontia, hypohidrosis and distinctive facial features. Autosomal recessive HED is clinically identical to X-linked HED and females are as severely affected as males.

History. X-linked HED was first described in 1848 by Thurnam [36]. In 1921, Thadani [37] determined that it was an X-linked disorder and later reported that female carriers manifest varying signs of the condition.

Pathology. The epidermis is thin, with effacement of rete ridges. The striking finding is absent or sparse eccrine glands and ducts in affected males (Fig. 134.2) [38,39]. Hair follicles and sebaceous glands are variably reduced in number and may appear rudimentary [38–40]. Apocrine glands may be absent, sparse or even normal. The nasal mucosa demonstrates almost complete loss of ciliated cells [41]. Mucous glands of the upper respiratory tract may be sparse or absent [38]. Mucus-secreting glands in the duodenum may also be absent [39]. Light and scanning electron microscopic findings of hair shaft abnormalities are variable and include longitudinal clefts or grooves and transverse fissuring. The bulb of the hair shaft is dystrophic in some individuals [42]. Radiographs of the mandible reveal dental hypoplasia or aplasia [38,43].

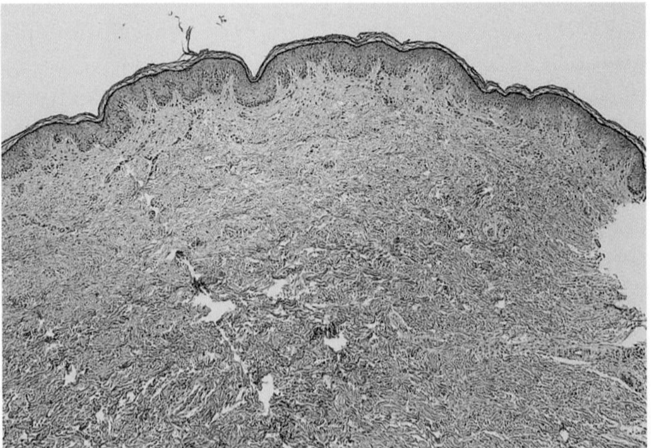

Fig. 134.2 Skin biopsy from the trunk of an affected male with X-linked hypohidrotic ectodermal dysplasia. Note the absence of hair follicles, sebaceous glands and eccrine glands (haematoxylin and eosin; ×10).

Clinical features.

Hair

The scalp hair is sparse, fine and lightly pigmented, and grows slowly (Fig. 134.3). Eyebrows are scanty or absent; sometimes just the outer two-thirds are missing. The eyelashes may be normal, sparse or completely absent. Secondary sexual hair in the beard, pubic and axillary regions is variably present and may be normal. Hair on the torso and extremities is usually absent [38,40,44,45]. Approximately 70% of obligate female carriers of X-linked HED describe their hair as being sparse or fine [44].

Teeth

Dental abnormalities vary from complete absence of teeth to sparse, abnormally shaped teeth. Studies reveal a mean of 24 missing teeth, out of a total of 28, in affected males [44,46]. Dentition is delayed and the erupted teeth tend to be small and widely spaced, and are frequently conical or peg-shaped. Both deciduous and permanent teeth are affected. The alveolar ridges are hypoplastic (Fig. 134.4), which gives rise to full, everted lips [43,47]. About 80% of obligate female carriers of X-linked HED have distinct dental abnormalities, including absent permanent teeth and small or peg-shaped teeth (Fig. 134.5) [44]. Oligodontia in the primary dentition is an important clinical predictor of EDA mutation in females [48]. Furthermore, antenatal ultrasonographic detection of tooth germ has recently been shown to be a reliable indicator of prenatal diagnosis in XLHED between 18 and 28 weeks of gestation [49].

Nails

The nails are normal in most individuals. Thin, brittle nail plates with longitudinal ridges have been described in some individuals.

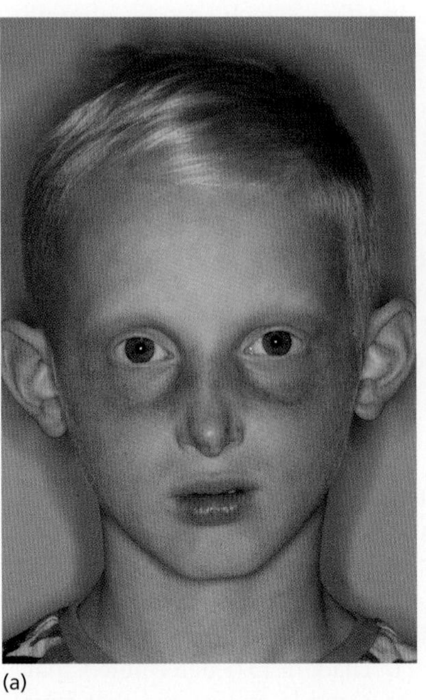

(a)

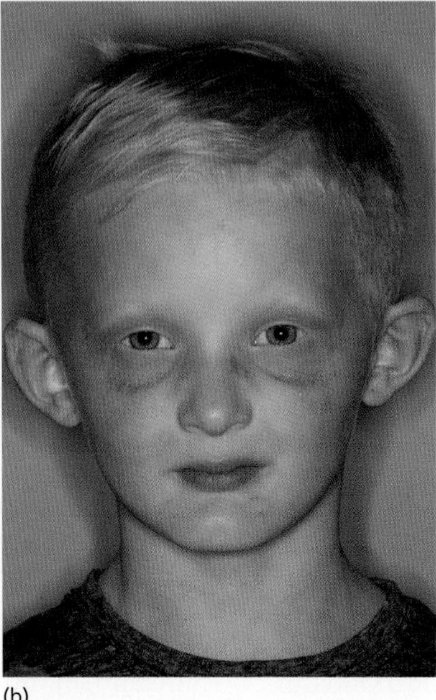

(b)

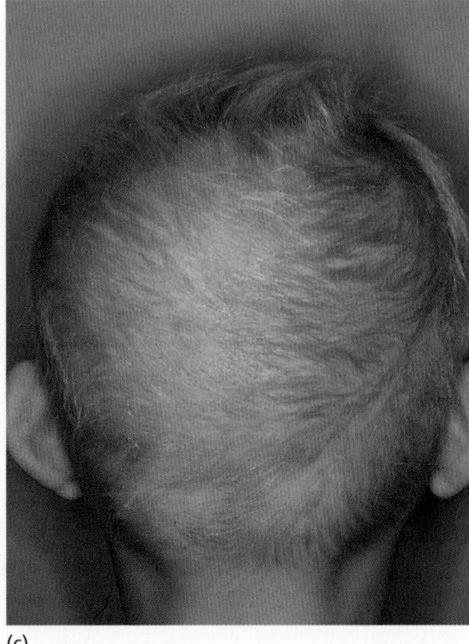

(c)

Fig. 134.3 Two young brothers with X-linked hypohidrotic ectodermal dysplasia. The hair is fine, lightly pigmented and sparse. There is a periocular dermatitis secondary to swimming goggles.

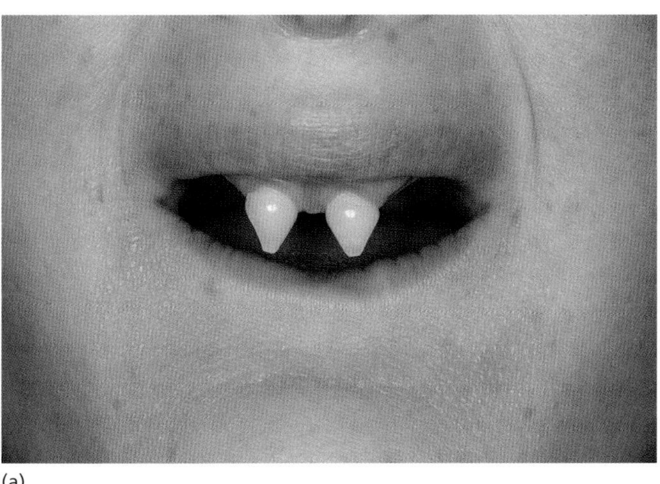

(a)

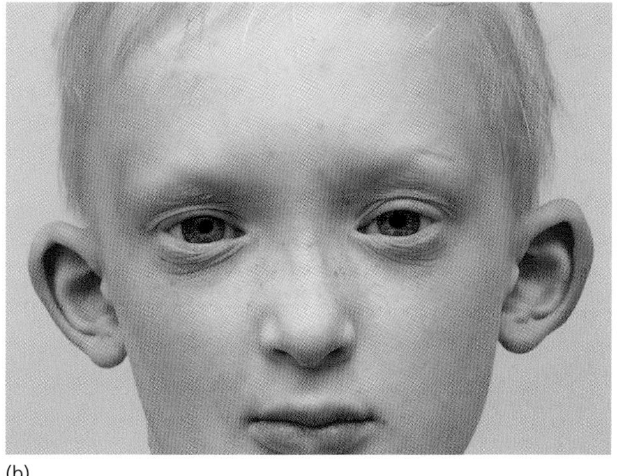

(b)

Fig. 134.4 Hypoplastic aveolar ridges and peg-shaped teeth, with perioral and periocular wrinkling in an affected male with X-linked hypohidrotic ectodermal dysplasia.

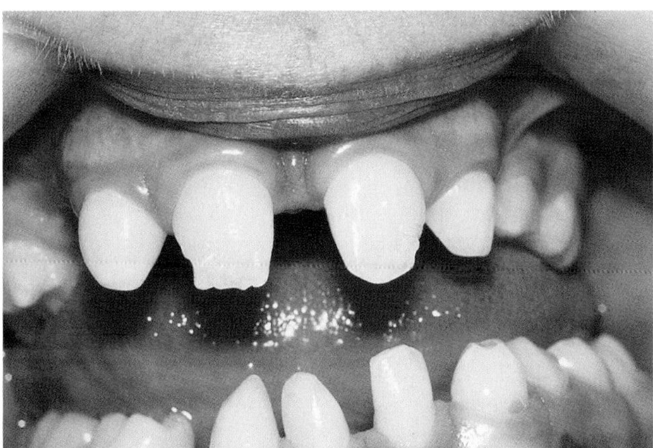

Fig. 134.5 This female heterozygous for X-linked hypohidrotic ectodermal dysplasia exhibits abnormally shaped and absent permanent teeth. Source: Courtesy of Dr Virginia Sybert.

Sweat glands

Sweating is severely diminished or absent owing to a paucity or absence of eccrine glands. The ability to thermoregulate by evaporative cooling is inadequate and hyperthermia can occur with physical exertion or in a warm environment. This is particularly problematic in infants and young children, who may experience recurrent bouts of fever as high as 42 °C. Heat intolerance does occur in older children and adults, but they learn to control their body temperature by drinking cold liquids, wetting their skin or clothing and seeking out cool surroundings [40]. About 25% of heterozygote females experience heat intolerance, and almost half notice that their ability to sweat is reduced [44]. The hypohidrotic areas of skin in carrier females of X-linked HED occur in defined linear patterns corresponding to the lines of Blaschko [50]. Diminished apocrine sweating in affected individuals is not problematic.

Skin

At birth, affected males may demonstrate marked scaling or peeling of their skin that may be mistaken for a collodion membrane [51]. In children and adults, the skin is fine, smooth and dry. Periorbital hyperpigmentation and fine wrinkling around the eyes are characteristic features of the disorder. Eczema is common and is prominent in flexural areas [45,52]. Small milia-like papules may be found on the face [40,53].

Other ectodermal structures

Diminished or absent salivary glands and mucous glands of the nose, mouth and ears cause numerous otolaryngological complications including nasal obstruction caused by thick, foetid nasal discharge and adherent nasal crusts, sinusitis, recurrent upper respiratory tract infections, feeding problems in infancy, xerostomia, hoarse voice and impacted cerumen [40,52–54]. Diminished production of tear film from the lacrimal glands may cause dry eyes, photophobia and corneal damage [53,55]. A third of affected males have abnormalities of the nipples including absent, simple or accessory nipples [44,56]. Female carriers may also be affected with marked breast asymmetry, inadequate breast milk production, athelia or amastia. Pituitary and adrenal insufficiency have been reported [52], as have ovarian teratomas [57].

Craniofacial features

The facies are distinctive with relative frontal bossing, concave midface, saddle nose and everted lips [38,40,43]. A third of affected males have ears that are described as simple or satyr [44]. The distinctive facial features may not be obvious at birth but become more noticeable with age (Figs 134.6 and 134.7).

Other clinical features

Diminished or absent mucous glands of the tracheal, bronchial, oesophageal, gastric and colonic mucosa cause problems with recurrent bronchitis, pneumonia, dysphagia and gastro-oesophageal reflux and constipation [44,51,53]. Reactive airways associated with wheezing are a common problem [44]. There is no convincing evidence for thyroid or parathyroid abnormalities, nor for a primary immune deficiency associated with X-linked HED [44].

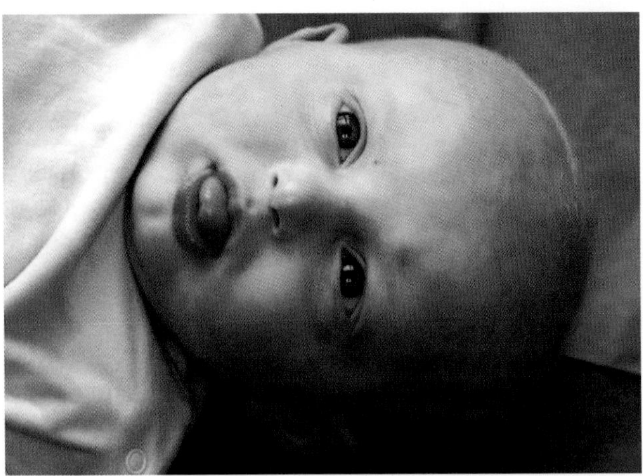

Fig. 134.6 The facial features of X-linked hypohidrotic ectodermal dysplasia. may not be obvious at birth but become more pronounced over time.

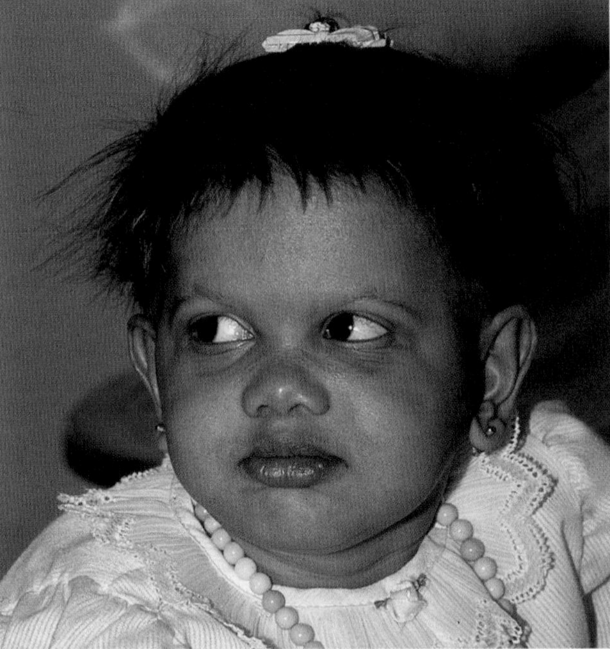

Fig. 134.7 This female exhibits a concave midface, saddle nose and everted lips. Source: Courtesy of Dr Virginia Sybert.

Prognosis. Failure to thrive occurs in up to 40% of affected males [44]. Height and weight are compromised in early childhood but appear to normalize with time. Mortality in infancy and early childhood is historically 25%, primarily owing to hyperthermia, failure to thrive and respiratory infections [44]. Febrile seizures can occur with hyperpyrexia [44,52]. Speech problems may exist because of hypodontia, nasal obstruction and impacted cerumen [52,54].

Differential diagnosis. Affected infants with scaling skin may be misdiagnosed as collodion babies with lamellar ichthyosis. The saddle nose and abnormal teeth have caused diagnostic confusion with congenital syphilis [40,53]. Once the characteristic facies and lack of sweating are evident, there are very few disorders to consider in the differential diagnosis. HED with hypothyroidism displays hypohidrosis with hyperthermia and hypotrichosis but the teeth are normal, the nails are significantly dystrophic and the skin has mottled-brown areas of pigmentation [58]. Fried tooth and nail syndrome manifests as hypotrichosis, hypodontia and prominent everted lips, but sweating is normal [58]. Basan syndrome is characterized by hypotrichosis, hypodontia and hypohidrosis but also by severe nail dystrophy and congenital absence of dermatoglyphics [44]. It has recently been proposed to be part of a spectrum with autosomal dominant adermatoglyphia [59], because both phenotypes have been found to be caused by mutations in *SMARCAD1* [60–62].

For the purposes of genetic counselling and reproductive planning, it is possible to perform DNA-based molecular genetic diagnosis in selected patients. This can help to conclusively distinguish between X-linked and autosomal forms where there is no family history to indicate the mode of inheritance.

Treatment. A multidisciplinary approach to the management of these individuals is advocated [58]. Early diagnosis is crucial to avoid life-threatening complications in infancy, for planning long-term management and to define recurrent risks for families [63]. Female carriers may be detected in most cases by careful clinical examination for patchy distribution of scalp and body hair, sweat pores and hypodontia [52]. DNA-based molecular diagnosis in affected families can detect female carriers of X-linked HED with considerable accuracy. DNA-based prenatal diagnosis is also possible in families at risk for the disorder.

Prevention of hyperthermia is critical. This is done by avoiding heat and physical overexertion, cooling the body with wet clothing and cool drinks, and by airconditioning home and school environments. Early dental restoration with bonding, overdentures or implants is imperative [54,64,65]. Nasal crusting and discharge can be managed with saline nose drops and a home humidifier. Consumption of large amounts of liquids or the use of artificial saliva preparations minimizes dry mouth and swallowing difficulties [66]. Dry eyes may be treated with artificial tears. The daily use of lubricating drops facilitates the removal of impacted earwax. Pulmonary difficulties are managed by avoidance of smoky, dusty environments, adequate humidification and the use of chest physiotherapy and antibiotics when appropriate [67]. Topical minoxidil has been used to treat congenital alopecia [68].

Studies on animal models of X-linked HED suggest the possibility of more targeted therapies for this condition in the future, although currently no such therapies are available. Previously, *in utero* administration of recombinant EDA was found to permanently correct the phenotype of newborn affected mice [69]. More recently, postnatal intravenous administration of soluble recombinant EDA to affected dogs resulted in normalization of adult teeth, improved ability to sweat, restoration of normal lacrimation, and decreased respiratory infection, caused by improved mucociliary clearance from correction of glandular deficit in the trachea and bronchi [70,71]. Initial postnatal human treatment studies using synthetic ectodysplasin-A1 failed to produce a response [72]. Dramatically, however, recent protein replacement therapy delivered intra-amniotically to two pregnancies (three fetuses) has demonstrated what appears to be complete phenotypic rescue at a follow up time of 14–22 months of age [73].

Hypohidrotic ED with immunodeficiency (OMIM #300291); HED with immunodeficiency with osteopetrosis and lymphoedema (OMIM #300301)

Both these conditions are caused by mutations in the *IKBKG* gene, formerly known as *NEMO*. The observation of unusually severe recurrent infections in a small subset of patients with otherwise typical HED features led to the suggestion that there may be a specific syndrome of HED and immunodeficiency (EDA–ID). The EDA–ID syndrome was first reported in a boy with miliary tuberculosis [74]. The second reported patient had recurrent life-threatening infections caused by *Pseudomonas aeruginosa*, *Mycobacterium avium* and cytomegalovirus [75]. A third child had a milder phenotype with repeated infections caused by *Staphylococcus aureus* and *Streptococcus pneumoniae* [76]. Three siblings from a different kindred had recurrent severe infections with *S. pneumoniae*, with impaired response to polysaccharide antigens [77]. Disseminated bacillus Calmette–Guérin infection has also been described [78,79]. All these patients were male, suggesting X-linked inheritance. Further cases have extended our knowledge of the phenotype, and severe life-threatening or recurrent bacterial infections have been reported in the lower respiratory tract, skin, soft tissues, bones and gastrointestinal tract, as well as meningitis and septicaemia in early childhood.

Overall, the causative pathogens have most often been Gram-positive bacteria (*S. pneumoniae* and *S. aureus*) followed by Gram-negative bacteria (*Pseudomonas* spp. and *Haemophilus influenzae*) and mycobacteria. Most patients have severe hypogammaglobulinaemia with low serum IgG levels and varied levels of other immunoglobulin isotypes (IgA, IgM and IgE) [4]. Some patients have massively elevated IgM levels [21,23,80], and an impaired antibody response to polysaccharides is the most consistent feature of this condition [4]. Impaired natural killer (NK) cell activity is reported in some, but not all, patients with EDA–ID [81,82]; the degree and range of immunological abnormalities seen may relate to the type of *NEMO* mutation involved. Treatment of one such case with allogenic transplantation of umbilical cord blood resulted in the resolution of the eczematous eruption, although it is not clear if the defect in cellular immunity also resolved [83]. Immune thrombocytopaenic purpura has also been described [84].

One patient has been described with a wide range of abnormalities associated with a duplication at Xq28, which includes the *IKBKG* gene. This patient's phenotype overlapped with different *IKBKG*-associated phenotypes, including HED, incontinentia pigmenti, immunodeficiency, recurrent isolated invasive pneumococcal disease and anhidrotic ED with immunodeficiency, osteopetrosis and lymphoedema. In addition, she also had macrocephaly, peripheral neuropathy, gastroparesis and various benign tumors, but no intellectual disability [85].

Autosomal dominant anhidrotic ED with T cell immunodeficiency (OMIM #612132)

The importance of these pathways was further emphasized when a mutation was identified in a 7-year-old boy with autosomal dominant anhidrotic ED and T cell immunodeficiency. A 94G-T transversion resulting in a serine 32 to isoleucine (S32I) change was found in the *IκBα* gene (inhibitor of kappa light chain gene enhancer in B cells alpha), now known as *NFKBIA* (nuclear factor of kappa light chain gene enhancer in B cell inhibitor alpha) [86]. Ser32 is a key phospho-acceptor site of *NFKBIA*, and is conserved in the other two IκB proteins. The mutation appeared to be a *de novo* event. The patient was born to unrelated parents. From 2 months of age he had chronic diarrhoea, recurrent bronchopneumonitis, hepatosplenomegaly and failure to thrive. A diagnosis of ED with immunodeficiency was made at the age of 3 years based on dry rough skin, moderately sparse scalp hair and conical teeth. The patient had no other overt developmental defects. This patient was treated with a successful bone marrow transplant, although occasional immunoglobulin substitution was required post transplant [87]. Three other cases, including one female, have been described with similar immunodeficiency, presenting with recurrent infections, abnormal teeth, coarse, wrinkled or dry skin and, in some, thin hair and recessed hairline [88–90]. Noninfectious inflammation can also be a presenting feature [91]. A heterozygous S32I mutation in *NFKBIA* in mice has been shown to be associated with defective lymphoid organogenesis, decreased *NFKBIA* phosphorylation and degradation, and impaired contact hypersensitivity and B-cell function [92].

Familial incontinentia pigmenti (incontinentia pigmenti type 2; OMIM #)

Please see Chapter 136 for a full discussion of this condition.

References

1 Ghosh S, May MJ, Kopp EB. NF-kappa B and Rel proteins: evolutionarily conserved mediators of immune responses. Annu Rev Immunol 1998;16:225–60.
2 Kaufman CK, Fuchs E. It's got you covered. NF-kappaB in the epidermis. J Cell Biol 2000;149:999–1004.
3 Karin M, Ben-Neriah Y. Phosphorylation meets ubiquitination. The control of NF-[kappa]B activity. Annu Rev Immunol 2000;18:621–63.
4 Smahi A, Courtois G, Rabia SH et al. The NF-kappaB signalling pathway in human diseases: from incontinentia pigmenti to ectodermal dysplasias and immune-deficiency syndromes. Hum Mol Genet 2002;11:2371–5.
5 Gerondakis S, Grossmann M, Nakamura Y et al. Genetic approaches in mice to understand Rel/NF-kappaB and IkappaB function: transgenics and knockouts. Oncogene 1999;18:6888–95.
6 Descargues P, Sil AK, Karin M. IKKalpha, a critical regulator of epidermal differentiation and a suppressor of skin cancer. EMBO J 2008;27:2639–47.

7 **Trzeciak WH, Koczorowski R. Molecular basis of hypohidrotic ectodermal dysplasia: an update. J Appl Genet 2016;57:51–61.**
8 Ferguson BM, Brockdorff N, Formstone E et al. Cloning of Tabby, the murine homolog of the human EDA gene: evidence for a membraneassociated protein with a short collagenous domain. Hum Mol Genet 1997;6:1589–94.
9 **Kere J, Srivastava AK, Montonen O et al. X-linked anhidrotic (hypohidrotic) ectodermal dysplasia is caused by mutation in a novel transmembrane protein. Nat Genet 1996;13:409–16.**
10 Drogemuller C, Distl O, Leeb T. Partial deletion of the bovine ED1 gene causes anhidrotic ectodermal dysplasia in cattle. Genome Res 2001;11:1699–705.
11 Drogemuller C, Peters M, Pohlenz J et al. A single point mutation within the ED1 gene disrupts correct splicing at two different splice sites and leads to anhidrotic ectodermal dysplasia in cattle. J Mol Med 2002;80:319–23.
12 Casal ML, Scheidt JL, Rhodes JL et al. Mutation identification in a canine model of X-linked ectodermal dysplasia. Mamm Genome 2005;16:524–31.
13 Yan M, Wang LC, Hymowitz SG et al. Two-amino acid molecular switch in an epithelial morphogen that regulates binding to two distinct receptors. Science 2000;290:523–7.
14 Chen Y, Molloy SS, Thomas L et al. Mutations within a furin consensus sequence block proteolytic release of ectodysplasin-A and cause X-linked hypohidrotic ectodermal dysplasia. Proc Natl Acad Sci USA 2001;98:7218–23.
15 Han D, Gong Y, Wu H et al. Novel EDA mutation resulting in X-linked non-syndromic hypodontia and the pattern of EDA-associated isolated tooth agenesis. Eur J Med Genet 2008;51:536–46.
16 Barsh G. Of ancient tales and hairless tails. Nat Genet 1999;22:315–16.
17 Headon DJ, Overbeek PA. Involvement of a novel TNF receptor homologue in hair follicle induction. Nat Genet 1999;22:370–4.
18 Headon DJ, Emmal SA, Ferguson BM et al. Gene defect in ectodermal dysplasia implicates a death domain adapter in development. Nature 2001;414:913–16.
19 Bal E, Baala L, Cluzeau C et al. Autosomal dominant anhidrotic ectodermal dysplasias at the EDARADD locus. Hum Mutat 2007;28:703–9.
20 Monreal AW, Ferguson BM, Headon DJ et al. Mutations in the human homologue of mouse dl cause autosomal recessive and dominant hypohidrotic ectodermal dysplasia. Nat Genet 1999;22:366–9.
21 Doffinger R, Smahi A, Bessia C et al. X-linked anhidrotic ectodermal dysplasia with immunodeficiency is caused by impaired NF-kappaB signaling. Nat Genet 2001;27:277–85.
22 Smahi A, Courtois G, Vabres P et al. Genomic rearrangement in NEMO impairs NF-kappaB activation and is a cause of incontinentia pigmenti. The International Incontinentia Pigmenti (IP) Consortium. Nature 2000;405:466–72.
23 Zonana J, Elder ME, Schneider LC et al. A novel X-linked disorder of immune deficiency and hypohidrotic ectodermal dysplasia is allelic to incontinentia pigmenti and due to mutations in IKK-gamma (NEMO). Am J Hum Genet 2000;67:1555–62.
24 Fusco F, Pescatore A, Conte AI et al. EDA-ID and IP, two faces of the same coin: how the same IKBKG/NEMO mutation affecting the NF-κB pathway can cause immunodeficiency and/or inflammation. Int Rev Immunol. 2015;34:445–59.
25 Zilberman-Rudenko J. Recruitment of A20 by the C-terminal domain of NEMO suppresses NF-κB activation and autoinflammatory disease. Proc Natl Acad Sci U S A. 2016;113:1612–7.
26 Mizukami T, Obara M, Nishikomori R et al. Successful treatment with infliximab for inflammatory colitis in a patient with X-linked anhidrotic ectodermal dysplasia with immunodeficiency. J Clin Immunol 2012;32:39–49.
27 Kojima T, Morikawa Y, Copeland NG et al. TROY, a newly identified member of the tumor necrosis factor receptor superfamily, exhibits a homology with Edar and is expressed in embryonic skin and hair follicles. J Biol Chem 2000;275:20742–7.
28 Eby MT, Jasmin A, Kumar A et al. TAJ, a novel member of the tumor necrosis factor receptor family, activates the c-Jun N-terminal kinase pathway and mediates caspase-independent cell death. J Biol Chem 2000;275:15336–42.
29 Naito A, Yoshida H, Nishioka E et al. TRAF6-deficient mice display hypohidrotic ectodermal dysplasia. Proc Natl Acad Sci U S A 2002; 99:8766–71.
30 Blake PW, Toro JR. Update of cylindromatosis gene (CYLD) mutations in Brooke–Spiegler syndrome: novel insights into the role of deubiquitination in cell signaling. Hum Mutat 2009;30:1025–36.
31 Trompouki E, Hatzivassiliou E, Tsichritzis T et al. CYLD is a deubiquitinating enzyme that negatively regulates NF-kappaB activation by TNFR family members. Nature 2003;424(6950):793–6.
32 Kovalenko A, Chable-Bessia C, Cantarella G et al. The tumour suppressor CYLD negatively regulates NF-kappaB signalling by deubiquitination. Nature 2003;424(6950):801–5.
33 Brummelkamp TR, Nijman SM, Dirac AM et al. Loss of the cylindromatosis tumour suppressor inhibits apoptosis by activating NF-kappaB. Nature 2003;424(6950):797–801.
34 Hutti JE, Shen RR, Abbott DW et al. Phosphorylation of the tumor suppressor CYLD by the breast cancer oncogene IKK-epsilon promotes cell transformation. Molec Cell 2009;34:461–72.
35 Zenker M, Mayerle J, Lerch MM et al. Deficiency of UBR1, a ubiquitin ligase of the N-end rule pathway, causes pancreatic dysfunction, malformations and mental retardation (Johanson–Blizzard syndrome). Nat Genet 2005;37:1345–50.
36 Thurnam J. Two cases in which the skin, hair and teeth were very imperfectly developed. Med Chir Trans 1848;31:71–82.
37 Thadani KI. A toothless type of man. J Hered 1921;12:87–8.
38 Clouston H. The major forms of hereditary ectodermal dysplasia (with an autopsy and biopsies on the anhydrotic type). Can Med Assoc J 1939;40:1–7.
39 Arnold ML, Rauskolb R, Anton-Lamprecht I et al. Prenatal diagnosis of anhidrotic ectodermal dysplasia. Prenat Diagn 1984;4:85–98.
40 Weech A. Hereditary ectodermal dysplasia (congenital ectodermal defect). A report of two cases. Am J Dis Child 1929;37:766–90.
41 Baer ST, Coulson IH, Elliman D. Anhidrotic ectodermal dysplasia: an ENT presentation in infancy. J Laryngol Otol 1988;102:458–9.
42 Micali G, Cook B, Blekys I et al. Structural hair abnormalities in ectodermal dysplasia. Pediatr Dermatol 1990;7:27–32.
43 Vierucci S, Baccetti T, Tollaro I. Dental and craniofacial findings in hypohidrotic ectodermal dysplasia during the primary dentition phase. J Clin Pediatr Dent 1994;18:291–7.
44 Clarke A, Phillips DI, Brown R et al. Clinical aspects of X-linked hypohidrotic ectodermal dysplasia. Arch Dis Child 1987;62:989–96.
45 Reed WB, Lopez DA, Landing B. Clinical spectrum of anhidrotic ectodermal dysplasia. Arch Dermatol 1970;102:134–43.
46 Crawford PJ, Aldred MJ, Clarke A. Clinical and radiographic dental findings in X linked hypohidrotic ectodermal dysplasia. J Med Genet 1991;28:181–5.
47 Clauss F, Manière MC, Obry F et al. Dento-craniofacial phenotypes and underlying molecular mechanisms in hypohidrotic ectodermal dysplasia (HED): a review. J Dent Res 2008;87:1089–99.
48 Levin LS. Dental and oral abnormalities in selected ectodermal dysplasia syndromes. Birth Defects Orig Artic Series 1988;24:205–27.
49 Hammersen J, Wohlfart S, Goecke TW et al. Reliability of prenatal detection of X-linked hypohidrotic ectodermal dysplasia by tooth germ sonography. Prenat Diagn 2018: doi: 10.1002/pd.5384.
50 Happle R, Frosch PJ. Manifestation of the lines of Blaschko in women heterozygous for X-linked hypohidrotic ectodermal dysplasia. Clin Genet 1985;27:468–71.
51 Executive and Scientific Advisory Boards of the National Foundation for Ectodermal Dysplasias, Mascoutah, Illinois. Scaling skin in the neonate: a clue to the early diagnosis of X-linked hypohidrotic ectodermal dysplasia (Christ–Siemens–Touraine syndrome). J Pediatr 1989;114:600–2.
52 Clarke A. Hypohidrotic ectodermal dysplasia. J Med Genet 1987; 24:659–63.
53 Butterworth T, Ladda R. Clinical Genodermatology. Westpoint, CT: Praeger, 1981:208–17.
54 Coston GN, Salinas CF. Speech characteristics in patients with hypohidrotic ectodermal dysplasia. Birth Defects Orig Artic Series 1988;24:229–34.
55 Wright JT, Finley WH. X-linked recessive hypohidrotic ectodermal dysplasia. Manifestations and management. Ala J Med Sci 1986;23:84–7.
56 Soderholm AL, Kaitila I. Expression of X-linked hypohidrotic ectodermal dysplasia in six males and in their mothers. Clin Genet 1985;28:136–44.
57 Wohlfart S, Soder S, Smahi A, Schneider H. A novel missense mutation in the gene EDARADD associated with an unusual phenotype of hypohidrotic ectodermal dysplasia. Am J Med Genet A 2016;170:249–53.

58 Freire-Maia N, Pinheiro M. Ectodermal Dysplasias: A Clinical and Genetic Study. New York: Alan R. Liss, 1984.
59 Valentin MN, Solomon BD, Richard G et al. Basan gets a new fingerprint: mutations in the skin-specific isoform of SMARCAD1 cause ectodermal dysplasia syndromes with adermatoglyphia. Am J Med Genet A 2018;176:2451–5.
60 Marks KC, Banks WR, 3rd, Cunningham D et al. Analysis of two candidate genes for Basan syndrome. Am J Med Genet A 2014;164A:1188–91.
61 Li M, Wang J, Li Z et al. Genome-wide linkage analysis and whole-genome sequencing identify a recurrent SMARCAD1 variant in a unique Chinese family with Basan syndrome. Eur J Hum Genet 2016;24:1367–70.
62 Nousbeck J, Burger B, Fuchs-Telem D et al. A mutation in a skin-specific isoform of SMARCAD1 causes autosomal-dominant adermatoglyphia. AmJ Human Genet 2011;89:302–7.
63 Sybert VP. Early diagnosis in the ectodermal dysplasias. Birth Defects Orig Artic Series 1988;24:277–8.
64 Nowak AJ. Dental treatment for patients with ectodermal dysplasias. Birth Defects Orig Artic Series 1988;24:243–52.
65 Guckes AD, Brahim JS, McCarthy GR et al. Using endosseous dental implants for patients with ectodermal dysplasia. J Am Dent Assoc 1991;122:59–62.
66 Myer CM 3rd. The role of an otolaryngologist in the care of ectodermal dysplasia. Pediatr Dermatol 1987;4:34–5.
67 Myer CM 3rd. Otolaryngologic manifestations of the ectodermal dysplasias – clinical note. Int J Pediatr Otorhinolaryngol 1986;11:307–10.
68 Lee HE, Chang IK, Im M et al. Topical minoxidil treatment for congenital alopecia in hypohidrotic ectodermal dysplasia. J Am Acad Dermatol 2013;68:e139–40.
69 Gaide O, Schneider P. Permanent correction of an inherited ectodermal dysplasia with recombinant EDA. Nat Med 2003;9:614–18.
70 Casal ML, Lewis JR, Mauldin EA et al. Significant correction of disease after postnatal administration of recombinant ectodysplasin A in canine X-linked ectodermal dysplasia. Am J Hum Genet 2007;81:1050–6.
71 Mauldin EA, Gaide O, Schneider P et al Neonatal treatment with recombinant ectodysplasin prevents respiratory disease in dogs with X-linked ectodermal dysplasia. Am J Med Genet A 2009;149A:2045–9.
72 Huttner K. Future developments in XLHED treatment approaches. Am J Med Genet A 2014;164A:2433–6.
73 Schneider H, Faschingbauer F, Schuepbach-Mallepell S et al. Prenatal correction of X-linked hypohidrotic ectodermal dysplasia. New Engl J Med 2018;378:1604–10.
74 Frix CD 3rd, Bronson DM. Acute miliary tuberculosis in a child with anhidrotic ectodermal dysplasia. Pediatr Dermatol 1986;3:464–7.
75 Sitton JE, Reimund EL. Extramedullary hematopoiesis of the cranial dura and anhidrotic ectodermal dysplasia. Neuropediatrics 1992; 23:108–10.
76 Abinun M, Spickett G, Appleton AL et al. Anhidrotic ectodermal dysplasia associated with specific antibody deficiency. Eur J Pediatr 1996;155:146–7.
77 Schweizer P, Kalhoff H, Horneff G et al. Polysaccharide specific humoral immunodeficiency in ectodermal dysplasia. Case report of a boy with two affected brothers. Klin Padiatr 1999;211:459–61.
78 Imamura M, Kawai T, Okada S et al. Disseminated BCG infection mimicking metastatic nasopharyngeal carcinoma in an immunodeficient child with a novel hypomorphic NEMO mutation. J Clin Immunol 2011;31:802–10.
79 Karaca NE, Aksu G, Ulusoy E et al. Disseminated BCG, infectious disease, and hyperferritinemia in a patient with a novel nemo mutation. J Investig Allergol Clin Immunol 2016;26:268–71.
80 Jain A, Ma CA, Liu S et al. Specific missense mutations in NEMO result in hyper-IgM syndrome with hypohydrotic ectodermal dysplasia. Nat Immunol 2001;2:223–8.
81 Orange JS, Brodeur SR, Jain A et al. Deficient natural killer cell cytotoxicity in patients with IKK-gamma/NEMO mutations. J Clin Invest 2002;109:1501–9.
82 Dupuis-Girod S, Corradini N, Hadj-Rabia S et al. Osteopetrosis, lymphedema, anhidrotic ectodermal dysplasia, and immunodeficiency in a boy and incontinentia pigmenti in his mother. Pediatrics 2002;109:e97.
83 Minakawa S, Takeda H, Nakano H et al. Successful umbilical cord blood transplantation for intractable eczematous eruption in hypohidrotic ectodermal dysplasia with immunodeficiency. Clin Exp Dermatol 2009;34:e441–2.
84 Ramirez-Alejo N, Alcantara-Montiel JC, Yamazaki-Nakashimada M et al. Novel hypomorphic mutation in IKBKG impairs NEMO-ubiquitylation causing ectodermal dysplasia, immunodeficiency, incontinentia pigmenti, and immune thrombocytopenic purpura. Clin Immunol 2015;160:163–71.
85 Van Asbeck E, Ramalingam A, Dvorak C et al. Duplication at Xq28 involving IKBKG is associated with progressive macrocephaly, recurrent infections, ectodermal dysplasia, benign tumors, and neuropathy. Clin Dysmorphol 2014;23:77–82.
86 Courtois G, Smahi A, Reichenbach J et al. A hypermorphic IκBα mutation is associated with autosomal dominant anhidrotic ectodermal dysplasia and t-cell immunodeficiency. J Clin Invest 2003;112:1108–15.
87 Dupuis-Girod S, Cancrini C, Le Deist F et al. Successful allogeneic hemopoietic stem cell transplantation in a child who had anhidrotic ectodermal dysplasia with immunodeficiency. Pediatrics 2006;118: 205–11.
88 Janssen R, van Wengen A, Hoeve MA et al. The same I-kappa-B-alpha mutation in two related individuals leads to completely different clinical symptoms. J Exp Med 2004;200:559–68.
89 Lopez-Granados E, Keenan JE, Kinney MC et al. A novel mutation in NFKBIA/IKBA results in a degradation-resistant N-truncated protein and is associated with ectodermal dysplasia with immunodeficiency. Hum Mutat 2008;29:861–8.
90 McDonald DR, Mooster JL, Reddy M et al. Heterozygous N-terminal deletion of I-kappa-B-alpha results in functional nuclear factor kappa-B haploinsufficiency, ectodermal dysplasia, and immune deficiency. J Allergy Clin Immunol 2007;120:900–7.
91 Yoshioka T, Nishikomori R, Hara J et al. Autosomal dominant anhidrotic ectodermal dysplasia with immunodeficiency caused by a novel NFKBIA mutation, p.Ser36Tyr, presents with mild ectodermal dysplasia and non-infectious systemic inflammation. J Clin Immunol 2013;33:1165–74.
92 Mooster JL, Le Bras S, Massaad MJ et al. Defective lymphoid organogenesis underlies the immune deficiency caused by a heterozygous S32I mutation in IκBα. J Exp Med 2015;212:185–202.

Transcription factors and homeobox genes: major regulators of gene expression

TP63-related phenotypes: overview of molecular pathway

The *TP53 etc* gene family is a key regulator of the cell cycle and is mutated in more than 50% of human cancers. *TP63* and *TP73* are recently discovered [1–5], related genes that share high amino acid identity with *TP53*. The role of *TP63* and *TP73* in human cancers has been extensively studied, but neither molecule is believed to play a significant role in tumorigenesis. Both *TP63* and *TP73* are distinct from *TP53* in that they each have a C-terminal protein–protein interacting motif (sterile α motif – SAM domain) that is not present in *TP53*. The *TP63* and *TP73* genes also differ from *TP53* in that they can each encode several different isoforms by utilizing two different transcription initiation sites (for review see [6]). The expression of *TP63* is more restricted than the ubiquitous nature of *TP53* expression and is restricted to the embryonic ectoderm and the basal regenerative layers of epithelial tissues in adults (skin, cervix, tongue, oesophagus, mammary glands, prostate and urothelium [5]). *p63 −/−* mice die at birth and have truncation of limbs (especially the forelimbs, with complete absence of phalanges and carpals) and absence of ectodermal derivatives including the epidermis and appendages (whiskers, hair, etc.), the prostate, lacrimal, breast and urothelial tissues [7,8].

Limb defects are best explained by a failure of the apical ectodermal ridge to develop [8].

Autosomal dominant mutations in the human *p63* gene, *TP63*, have now been identified in six distinct human phenotypes, all of which have ED as a key feature. Some genotype–phenotype correlation is possible in that there is clustering of mutations in some of the phenotypes to specific sites of the *p63* molecule (for review see [6]). *TP63* mutations account for most cases of EEC syndrome. In an authoritative paper, van Bokhoven and colleagues [9] were able to demonstrate mutations in 40 out of 43 families with EEC; all but one of these mutations were sited within the DNA-binding domain, and five amino acid residues accounted for 75% of all mutations [9]. In ankyloblepharon-ectodermal dysplasia-clefting syndrome (AEC syndrome, also known as Hay–Wells syndrome), in which the limb abnormalities are absent or minimal, mutations have been exclusively detected within the SAM domain and are associated with complex gain-of-function as well as loss- and change-of-function effects [9]. In limb–mammary syndrome (LMS), *TP63* frameshift mutations leading to truncations of p63 protein have been reported in exon 13 in two unrelated patients [9] and an N-terminal mutation was found in a further family [6]. Mutations in acro-dermato-ungual-lacrimal-tooth syndrome (ADULT syndrome) have yielded interesting insights in that the first mutation was identified in exon 3′, which is only expressed in the transactivating isotypes of *p63* and causes an amino acid substitution outside the DNA-binding domain [10]. A subsequent report has demonstrated a mutation that confers significant transactivation activity on ΔN-p63γ, an otherwise inert isoform of *p63* [6]. Nonsyndromic split hand–split foot syndrome (SHFM) is a genetically heterogeneous group of conditions, but some cases (possibly around 10%) are attributable to *p63* mutations [9]. Some of these mutations seem specific for SHFM, but others underlie both EEC and SHFM [6]. It is therefore understandable that of the six known types of SHFM, ED features are most commonly seen in SHFM4, which shares the same gene as EEC, whereas SHFM3, which maps to 10q24, has only dental and nail findings [11].

The *TP63* gene product can act as an activator or a repressor, and mutations in the 5′ end of *TP63* in AEC and Rapp–Hodgkin syndrome show loss of activator function, and even dominant-negative activity [12,13]. While clustering of mutations is determined in part by the characteristics of the mutated residue, whether it is a CpG site, etc., the degree of clustering in this group of conditions suggests that each condition has a specific pathogenetic mechanism. This site specificity also presumably suggests that the p63 protein has several functions, each with a specific site, and that each of these functions can be disturbed in isolation from the others. However, overlapping phenotypes are not uncommon and further elucidation of *TP63* may shed light on the role of this protein and its downstream pathway [14,15]. One target of p63 is *PERP* (p53 effector related to PMP22), a gene that has an effect on cell–cell adhesion and is a potential tumour suppressor gene [16, 17]. PERP levels may vary in patients with the same *TP63* mutation; therefore, modifier genes and other proteins are likely to be involved in the phenotypic expression of *TP63* mutations [18]. A functional link has been established between fibroblast growth factor and p63 in the expansion of epithelial progenitor cells to provide mechanistic insights into the pathogenesis of AEC syndrome [19]. IKKα (now known as CHUK), discussed above, is a direct transcriptional target of ΔNp63α [20,21]. A mouse model may shed further light on the role of p63 in ED [22].

AEC syndrome (Hay–Wells syndrome; OMIM #106260)

Definition. AEC syndrome is characterized by cleft lip/palate, severe scalp erosions and abnormalities of the epidermal appendages including hypotrichosis, hypodontia, absent or dystrophic nails and mild hypohidrosis. One distinctive feature is ankyloblepharon filiforme adnatum, which is partial-thickness fusion of the eyelid margins. Recently, mutations in *TP63* have also been identified in Rapp–Hodgkin syndrome (OMIM #129400) (Fig. 134.8) [23], demonstrating that this disorder is allelic with AEC syndrome. Clinical distinction between these two disorders is probably not warranted. The same mutation can cause marked phenotypic variability, underscoring the clinical heterogeneity of the condition [24].

History. In 1976, Hay and Wells described seven patients from four families with an inherited disorder characterized by congenital filiform fusion of the eyelids, dysplasia of the epidermal appendages and cleft lip/palate. Five of these original seven patients had ankyloblepharon filiforme adnatum and one had small nodules removed from her eyelids as a child, presumably remnants of spontaneously lysed ankyloblepharon [25].

Pathology. Hair shafts are thin and atrophic, and show various defects, including fractures of the cuticle, bent shafts, trichoclasis, trichorrhexis nodosa, pili canaliculi, pili annulati, pili triangulati and pili torti, none of which is specific for the disorder [26,27]. Dyspigmentation of the hair is relatively common, with pigment variation both between and within hairs; pigment may be normal, clumped or nearly absent [27].

Skin biopsy of involved scalp tissue shows a thin granular layer and stratum corneum [28]. Biopsies from clinically 'normal' skin show mild hyperkeratosis and papillomatosis, epidermal atrophy and pigment incontinence, as well as a prominent superficial perivascular plexus with minimal to mild perivascular lymphocyte infiltrates [27]. Hair follicles are reduced in size and arrector pili muscles appear hypertrophic [28]. Sweat stimulation tests reveal a patchy loss of sweat glands over most of the body [25].

Clinical features.

Hair

Scalp hair is wiry, coarse and sparse; alopecia is common. The eyebrows and eyelashes are almost always short, brittle and sparse or absent. Body, pubic and

SECTION 28: FOCAL OR GENERALIZED HYPOPLASIA

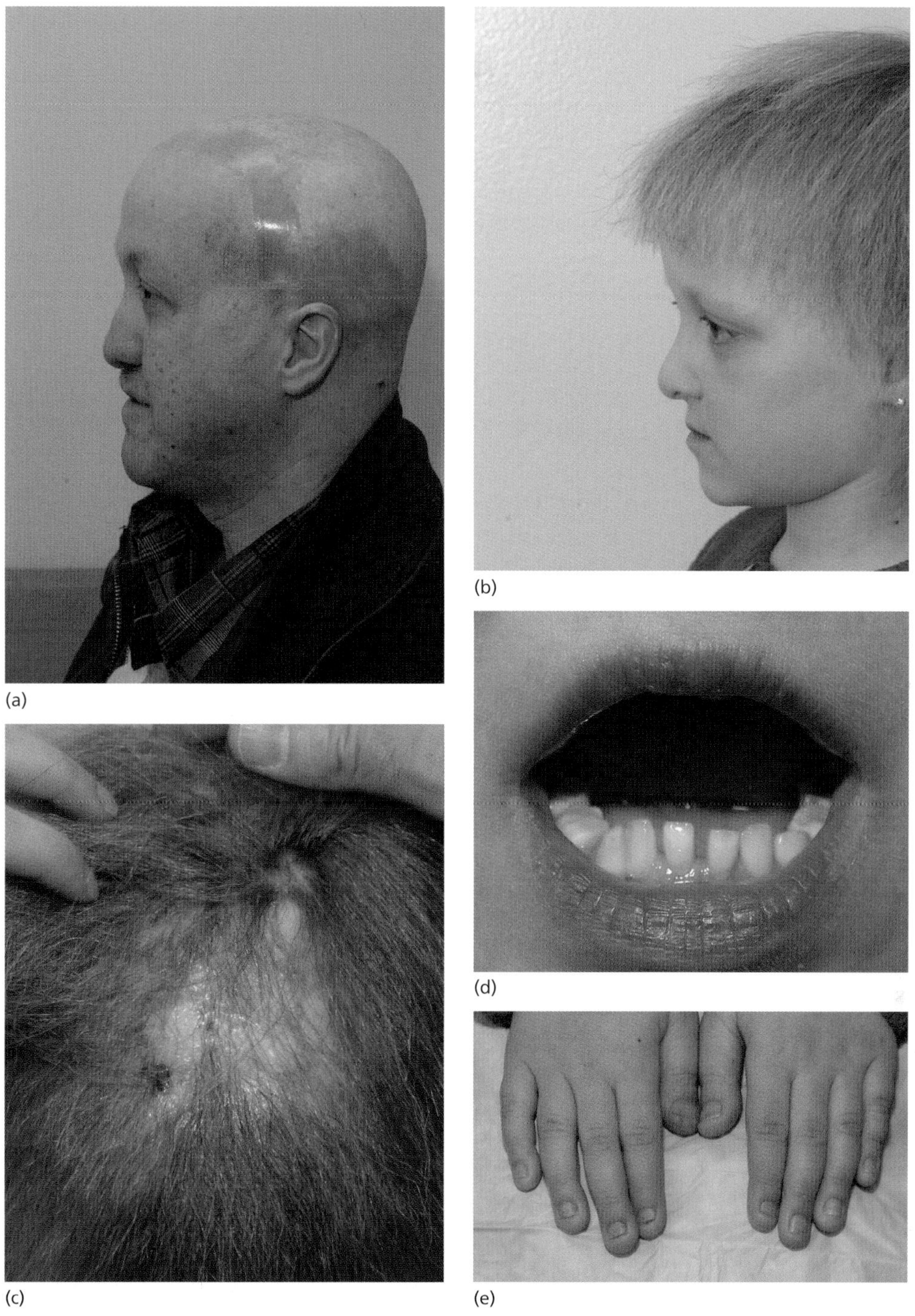

Fig. 134.8 (a, b) A father and daughter with Rapp–Hodgkin syndrome (AEC). Both have history of cleft palate. Note the typical facies (high forehead, hypoplastic maxilla and thin upper lip) and brittle, wiry hair in childhood, which can progress to alopecia in adulthood. The father was previously wearing a hairpiece. (c) Scalp dermatitis with alopecia seen in Rapp–Hodgkin syndrome (AEC). (d, e) Hypodontia and nail dysplasia in Rapp–Hodgkin syndrome (AEC). Source: Courtesy of Dr Jean Bernard.

axillary hair may be sparse or absent [25,26,28]. Some may also display scarring alopecia or 'spun-glass' uncombable hair [30].

Teeth

Hypodontia is common. Those teeth that are present are frequently small, conical and discoloured with white or yellow spots secondary to enamel hypoplasia [25,26,29,31,32]. Maxillary and mandibular first molars are the most likely of the permanent teeth to be present, whereas maxillary incisors and canines tend to be absent, probably caused by the alveolar cleft defect [32].

Nails

Nail abnormalities are variable even within an individual and include distal hypoplasia and thickened, hyperconvex plates. Complete absence of nails is a frequent finding [25]. Chronic paronychia has been reported [26].

Sweat glands

Decreased sweat production and heat intolerance is described by a significant number of individuals but hyperpyrexia is not a problem [29,30]. Sweat pores are reduced in a number in affected individuals [25]. A recent genotype-phenotype study of sweating in AEC and EEC has proposed that only certain genotypes are associated with decreased sweating [33], but this is yet to be confirmed in other studies.

Skin

At birth, over three-quarters of affected newborns have red, eroded, peeling skin like a collodion membrane (Fig. 134.9) [29] or may present with erythroderma [34]. Erosions are most prominent over the scalp [30]. These symptoms resolve over the first few weeks and the underlying skin is dry (Fig. 134.10). Erosions may heal with residual scarring, in a cribriform, reticulate, stellate or punctate pattern [30]. Over two-thirds of individuals have chronic problems with severe recurrent scalp erosions and scalp infections, which are a major feature of AEC syndrome (Fig. 134.11) [29]. Palmoplantar keratoderma was reported in four of the original seven patients described by Hays and Wells [25]. It is not a common finding in affected children but may be more pronounced in adults. Both hypopigmentation and hyperpigmentation can occur, commonly in a reticulate pattern in intertriginous areas; this may progress with age [30].

Other ectodermal structures

Ankyloblepharon filiforme adnatum (strands of epithelial tissue between the eyelids) are a cardinal feature of the disorder but are noted in only 70% of patients (Fig. 134.12) [25,26,29]. The strands may lyse spontaneously and may be difficult to detect. Lacrimal duct atresia or obstruction occurs in over half of affected individuals [29]. Supernumerary nipples may be present [26,29]. Nutritional issues are common, which are not

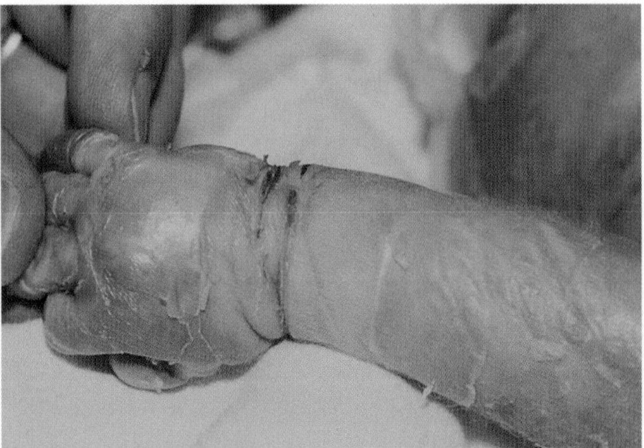

Fig. 134.9 Peeling, red, parchment-like skin in a newborn with AEC syndrome. Source: Courtesy of Dr Virginia Sybert.

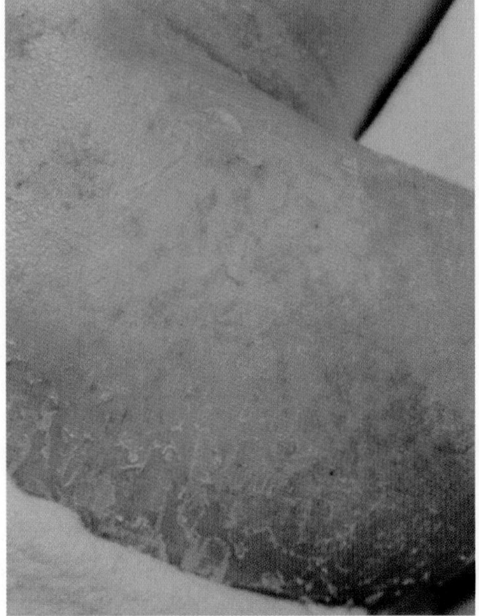

Fig. 134.10 The parchment skin resolves over the first few weeks of life and the underlying skin is dry as seen in this 1-month-old baby with AEC syndrome.

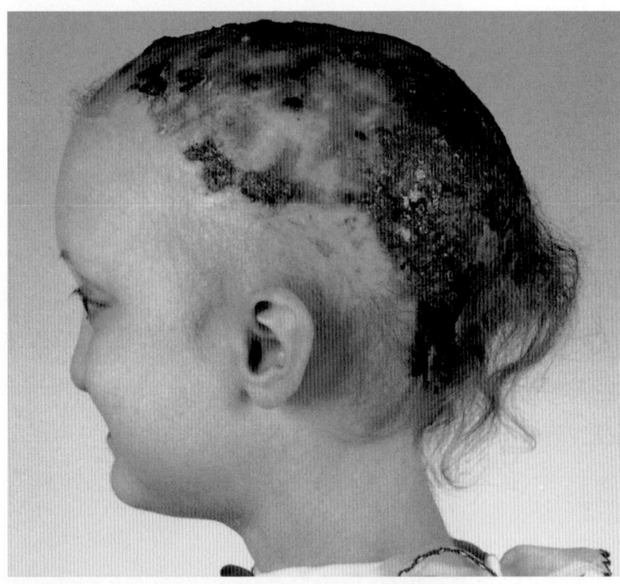

Fig. 134.11 Severe scalp erosions and extensive granulation tissue in a 5-year-old girl with AEC syndrome. Source: Courtesy of Dr Virginia Sybert and Dr Mark Stephan.

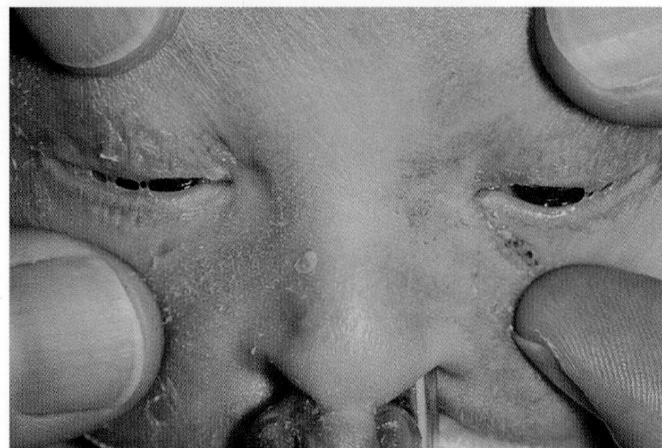

Fig. 134.12 Ankyloblepharon filiforme adnatum (strands of epithelial tissue between the eyelids) in a newborn with AEC syndrome. Source: Courtesy of Dr Virginia Sybert

specifically related to cleft palate and lip. One-quarter of patients require gastrostomy placement, and nutritional supplements at some point in time are required in two-thirds of patients. Low birthweight is common, although birth length is unaffected. Weight issues resolve with time, but AEC patients have significantly lower height-for-age than the reference population [35].

Craniofacial features

Typical craniofacial features include a broadened nasal bridge and maxillary hypoplasia [36]. The ears may be small and low-set with deformities of the auricle [29]. The ear canals may be webbed and abnormally shaped [26]. Cleft lip is a variable feature but cleft palate is seen in most individuals [25–29].

Other abnormalities

Other features seen occasionally in AEC syndrome include cutaneous syndactyly of the second and third toes, genitourinary abnormalities, hypospadias, micropenis, and vaginal dryness and erosions [29].

Prognosis. Abnormalities of the external ear canals and palate frequently cause problems with chronic otitis

Differential diagnosis. Curly hair–ankyloblepharon–nail dysplasia syndrome (CHANDS) is a rare autosomal recessive ED with curly, kinky hair, hypoplastic nails and the defining feature of ankyloblepharon. It can be distinguished from AEC by absence of cleft palate and lack of typical craniofacial features [37,38]. In the newborn period, the eroded, peeling skin seen in AEC syndrome may be mistaken for epidermolysis bullosa [39].

Treatment. Emollients are appropriate for the collodion-like membrane in the newborn. Neonates with AEC often have extremely fragile skin and they should be handled with extreme care. Neonatal intensive care nursing protocols such as those used for neonates with epidermolysis bullosa should be used. The ankyloblepharon filiforme adnatum may require surgical correction or may lyse spontaneously. The lacrimal duct atresia may be surgically correctable [40]. The scalp requires aggressive wound care and treatment with topical or systemic antibiotics as warranted [29]. Potent topical steroids may be of use [40]. Other abnormalities, such as cleft lip/palate, hypospadias and the maxillary hypoplasia, may be surgically corrected [41]. Teeth preservation and restoration are imperative [32].

EEC (OMIM 129900)

Definition. The main features of the EEC syndrome are ectrodactyly (spilt hand or foot deformity), cleft lip/palate, tear duct anomalies and abnormalities of the epidermal appendages including hypotrichosis, hypodontia, dystrophic nails and occasional hypohidrosis.

History. The association of ectrodactyly, cleft lip/palate and ED was initially described by Rüdiger and colleagues [43], who recognized that this combination of defects represents a specific syndrome, termed EEC syndrome. Over 150 cases have subsequently been described [28].

Pathology. Radiographs of hand or foot deformities show missing or hypoplastic metacarpals and metatarsals [44]. Scanning electron microscopic studies of hair shafts of affected individuals show longitudinal grooves, distorted bulbs and cuticular defects [45, 46]. These findings can be seen in a number of other EDs and are not specific to EEC syndrome.

Clinical features.

Hair

The scalp hair is fine and sparse, light-coloured and may be wiry in texture. Eyebrows and eyelashes are short, thin and sparse. Axillary, pubic and body hair may also be affected [43–45,47].

Teeth

Teeth may be small, abnormally shaped or missing [43–44,47]. Premature loss of secondary teeth is common, presumably owing to multiple caries from enamel hypoplasia.

Nails

The nail plates may be dystrophic, hypoplastic or completely absent even when there are no bony defects of the involved digit [47,48].

Sweat glands

Sweating is usually normal but heat intolerance is noted by a few individuals [44,47,49].

Skin

Dry skin and hyperkeratosis, particularly of the lower extremities, are reported in some individuals [50,51]. Scalp dermatitis is seen rarely [45,51]. Naevoid hypermelanosis has been described [52].

Other ectodermal structures

Atresia or hypoplasia of the lacrimal duct is seen in over 90% of affected individuals [28,50,53]. Secretions from the lacrimal gland may be diminished [53]. Nipple anomalies are reported in a few individuals [50].

Craniofacial features

The nose may be broad, the chin pointed, and there may be minor variable ear anomalies, but the facies are not distinct. Cleft palate with or without cleft lip occurs in three-quarters of affected individuals and is a major feature of this disorder [50]. Choanal atresia has been reported [54], as has holoprosencephaly [55].

Other abnormalities

Ectrodactyly (lobster claw deformity) is a major feature of this disorder and occurs in over 90% of affected individuals (Fig. 134.13). About three-quarters of individuals with ectrodactyly have both hand and foot involvement [50]. Structural abnormalities of the genitourinary tract occur in about one-third of individuals,

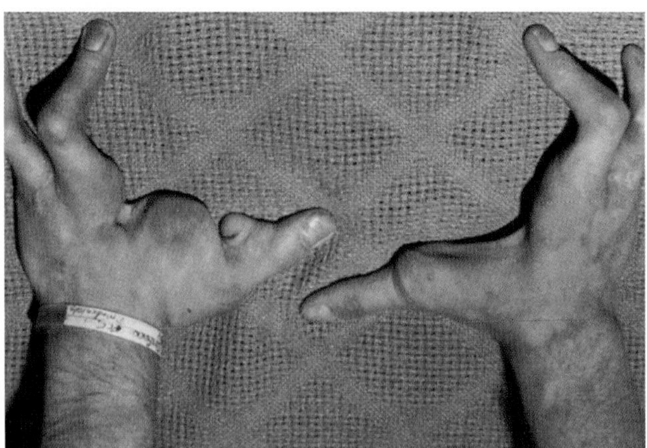

Fig. 134.13 Ectrodactyly of the hands in a young man with EEC syndrome. Source: Courtesy of Dr Virginia Sybert.

including cryptorchidism, hypospadias, hydronephrosis and hydroureters, renal agenesis, and duplication of the kidneys and collecting system [50]; the most common structural finding is megaureter [56,57]. Urinary abnormalities may be more common in those cases of EEC with an Arg227Gln *TP63* mutation [58]. Abnormalities of the external genitalia and genitourinary tract have also been described [59].The acronym EECUT represents ectrodactyly, ED, clefting, urinary tract abnormalities and thymic abnormalities [60].

Intellectual disability is a variable and uncommon feature of the disorder, occurring in fewer than 10% of affected individuals [50], and may be limited to those with chromosomal deletions as part of a contiguous gene syndrome. Hearing loss occurs in about 15% of individuals [50]. It is uncertain whether this is primary or secondary to recurrent otitis media. Isolated growth hormone deficiency has been reported in one individual [61]. Endocrine anomalies such as hypogonadotropic hypogonadism, thyroid stimulating hormone and prolactin deficiency have also been reported [62]. Tetralogy of Fallot has been reported [63], as have cases of concomitant Hodgkin, non-Hodgkin and B-cell lymphoma in EEC [62,64–65].

Prognosis. A significant number of affected individuals experience excessive tearing, conjunctivitis and blepharitis as a result of lacrimal duct hypoplasia. Photophobia and corneal ulcers as well as corneal scarring and perforation may occur as a result of lacrimal gland hypoplasia [54]. Blindness has been described [66]. Recurrent urinary tract infections, both symptomatic and asymptomatic, may be a problem in individuals with genitourinary anomalies [57].

Differential diagnosis. A few other EDs involve limb abnormalities and cleft palate/lip. Although clefting is not a constant feature, odontotrichomelic syndrome may be differentiated by severe tetramelic reductions and autosomal recessive mode of inheritance [28]. Other rare syndromes, such as Martinez syndrome, Zlotogora–Ogur syndrome and Rosselli–Gulienetti syndrome, can be differentiated from EEC by specific limb abnormalities and mode of inheritance (see Table 134.1).

Treatment. Treatment involves surgical correction of the cleft lip/palate, lacrimal duct and limb defects and genitourinary abnormalities as indicated. DNA-based prenatal diagnosis is available for families in which the gene defect is known. Mutant p63 has been corrected *in vitro* using siRNA-mediated allele specific silencing to restore defective stem cell function [67].

ADULT (OMIM #103285)

ADULT syndrome is a rare condition distinguished from EEC syndrome by an absence of facial clefting. Patients have, in addition, excessive freckling and exfoliative dermatitis of the digits [68]. Other features, such as hyperextensibility of the distal interphalangeal joints, bilateral duplicate thumbs, bifid toenails, genitourinary defects and conductive hearing loss, have also been described [69].

LMS (OMIM #603543)

This previously unrecognized autosomal dominant syndrome was described in a Dutch family with a constellation of features that had not previously been reported. The major features were a combination of hand and foot anomalies and mammary gland aplasia/hypoplasia. The skin and hair were normal in all affected individuals but some had lacrimal duct atresia, nail dysplasia, hypohidrosis, hypodontia or cleft palate [6]. LMS is distinguished from EEC syndrome by the consistent finding of mammary anomalies in LMS (infrequent in EEC) and the much more frequent finding of skin, nail and tooth anomalies in EEC syndrome. The clefting in LMS is of the palate only whereas in EEC syndrome the lip and palate are affected [6].

Nonsyndromic SHFM (OMIM #183600)

This condition has no dermatological features and is not discussed in detail here.

Defects in transcription factors other than *p63*

In addition to the *p63* pathway, several other EDs have now been attributed to defects in transcription factors that control the expression of several target genes important in ectodermal morphogenesis. In many cases, positional cloning studies have yielded the primary mutation but the detailed molecular signalling pathways have yet to be delineated. Ellis–van Creveld syndrome is a recessive ED that is characterized by a skeletal dysplasia with short limbs, short ribs, postaxial polydactyly and congenital heart defects [70]. Mutations in the *EVC* and *EVC2* genes have been identified in this syndrome [71,72] and these proteins, although not fully characterized, are most likely transcription factors, given the hypothetical structural characteristics (nuclear localization, two DNA-binding domains, leucine-rich zipper domain). The products of these two genes are thought to function coordinately in cardiac development [73]. Mutations in these genes may also cause Weyer acrofacial dysostosis (OMIM #193530), an autosomal dominant allelic disorder [71]. Witkop syndrome (OMIM #189500) is an autosomal dominant ED with primary manifestation in the teeth (taurodontia, partial or complete anodontia) and nails (koilonychia, longitudinal ridging and nail pits) [74]. Recently, mutations have been identified in the *MSX1* gene, a member of the homeobox gene family and an important regulator of transcription [74].

Of the EDs more likely to be seen by a paediatric dermatologist, trichodento-osseous (TDO) syndrome and trichorhinophalangeal syndrome (TRPS) have both been attributed to mutations in transcription factors. The causative gene for TDO is *DLX3* [75], a homeodomain transcription factor that is developmentally expressed in many structures derived from epithelial–mesenchymal interactions such as teeth, hair follicle and limb buds [76]. Mutations in this gene were previously thought to cause amelogenesis imperfecta (type IV) [77]; however, this condition is now thought to simply be an attenuated phenotype of TDO [78].

The *TRPS1* gene underlies TRPS types I and III [79,80] and a microdeletion syndrome (8q42.11-8q24.1), which includes *TRPS1* and *EXT1*, underlies TRPS type II [81,82]. Computer analysis of the protein encoded by *TRPS1* suggests that it is a novel transcription factor with an unusual composition of nine putative zinc-finger motifs of four different types [83]. All the mutations in *TRPS1* probably act as loss-of-function mutations, meaning that haploinsufficiency is the likely mechanism in TRPS. TDO and TRPS are discussed in detail below.

TDO syndrome (OMIM #190320)

Definition. TDO syndrome is a well-defined ED manifesting in kinky hair, hypoplasia of tooth enamel and asymptomatic sclerotic bone changes.

History. Lichtenstein and colleagues [84] defined the features of this disorder in 107 individuals and proposed the name TDO syndrome. Robinson and Miller [85] were the first authors to describe this syndrome, but they did not detect bone involvement as part of the disorder. Some authors argue that the clinical manifestations observed in some families are sufficiently varied to suggest genetic heterogeneity and classify TDO syndrome into three subtypes that differ primarily by the degree of bone involvement [86,87]. Variable expression of a single gene seems a more plausible explanation for other authors [88].

Pathology. On dental radiographs, unerupted teeth and taurodontia (increased size of the tooth pulp chamber) are found [89]. Scanning electron microscopic analysis of affected teeth shows pits and depressions in the tooth enamel, uniformly thin tooth enamel and an abnormal collagenous membrane around the open apices [90]. Radiographs of the skull reveal sclerosis and sometimes thickening of the calvarium. The long bones may also be sclerotic [88].

Clinical features [82,85,86,88].

Hair

At birth, the scalp hair is thick and kinky or curly; it may straighten in later life. The eyelashes may also be curly.

Teeth

Teeth abnormalities are present in all patients and include pitted, hypoplastic enamel with brownish-yellow discoloration of both primary and permanent teeth, and taurodontia. Tooth eruption may be delayed and abscesses are common. Multiple dental caries occur and lead to early loss of teeth.

Nails

Fingernails are thin and brittle and peel readily. Toenails may be thickened or normal.

Sweat glands

Sweating abnormalities are not found in this disorder.

Skin

The skin is normal and other ectodermal structures are normal.

Craniofacial features

There is frontal bossing, the jaw is square and the head is elongated. Partial premature fusion of the cranial sutures occurs in three-quarters of affected individuals. The bones of the skull are radiographically dense and may be thick. This is not problematic for the patient and may be found incidentally when radiographs of the skull are obtained for unrelated reasons.

Other abnormalities

Clinodactyly is rarely seen.

Prognosis. Affected individuals are healthy but lose most of their teeth by the age of 30 years [84].

Differential diagnosis. Curly hair and nail dysplasia is also seen in CHANDS syndrome (curly hair, ankylo blepharon and nail dysplasia), but ankyloblepharon makes this disorder distinct. Tooth and nail syndrome lacks kinky or curly hair.

Treatment. This includes appropriate dental restoration [91].

TRPS type I (OMIM #190350); TRPS type II (Langer–Giedion syndrome; OMIM #150230); TRPS type III (Sugio–Kajii syndrome; OMIM #190531)

Definition. TRPS is characterized by sparse scalp hair, bulbous pear-shaped nose, small teeth with dental malocclusion, thin nails, coneshaped epiphyses, short stature and occasional skeletal abnormalities.

Clinical features [92,93].

Hair

The hair is usually fine, blond and sparse; the most prominently affected areas are the frontotemporal areas. The eyebrows are sparse or absent.

Teeth

Dental abnormalities are frequent, with supernumerary incisors, microdontia and poorly aligned teeth.

Nails

The nails are occasionally thin and short, with long longitudinal grooves. They can be flattened, koilonychia-like and normal in colour. 'Racket' thumbnails have been described.

Sweat glands and skin

There are no abnormalities of sweat glands or skin.

Other ectodermal structures

There is occasional exotropia and photophobia.

Craniofacial features

Many patients have a characteristic facies with a pear-shaped nose, a long and wide philtrum and large, prominent ears. A narrow palate is often noted.

Other features

Short stature is common and a wide range of skeletal abnormalities have been described, including brachymesophalangy, brachymetacarpy, brachymetatarsy and peripheral dysostosis with type 12 cone-shaped epiphyses at some of the middle phalanges of the hands. Joints are often thickened, ulnar and radial deviation of the fingers is seen and there are occasional abnormalities such as clinodactyly, winged scapulae and coxa valga. Perthes-like abnormalities have been reported in a few cases [94]. Chest wall deformities such as pectus carinatum, lordosis or kyphoscoliosis are occasional features.

Type II TRPS shares many characteristics with types I and III but is more significantly associated with intellectual disability. In addition, there are multiple cutaneous exostoses and marked redundant or loose skin and more marked joint laxity. Type III TRPS differs from TRPS I by the presence of severe brachydactyly, owing to short metacarpals, and more severe short stature [95,96]. There is an emerging genotype–phenotype correlation in that mutations in the GATA DNA-binding zinc finger seem to predict a type III phenotype, whereas mutations elsewhere are associated with TRPS I [80].

EGFR-related ectodermal dysplasia-like disease

Recently, loss-of-function mutations in gene *EGFR* encoding the epidermal growth factor receptor have been described in association with cutaneous erosions, dry scale and alopecia, with subsequent papules and pustules in the skin, recurrent cutaneous and pulmonary infections, and death in early childhood [97]. These were noted to be similar to the cutaneous side effects seen with EGFR inhibitors [97]. Other similar patients have since been reported [98,99].

SECTION 28: FOCAL OR GENERALIZED HYPOPLASIA

References

1 **Jost CA, Marin MC, Kaelin WG Jr. p73 is a simian [correction of human] p53-related protein that can induce apoptosis. Nature 1997;389:191–4.**

2 Kaghad M, Bonnet H, Yang A et al. Monoallelically expressed gene related to p53 at 1p36, a region frequently deleted in neuroblastoma and other human cancers. Cell 1997;90:809–19.

3 Osada M, Ohba M, Kawahara C et al. Cloning and functional analysis of human p51, which structurally and functionally resembles p53. Nat Med 1998;4:839–43.

4 Senoo M, Seki N, Ohira M et al. A second p53-related protein, p73L, with high homology to p73. Biochem Biophys Res Commun 1998;248:603–7.

5 **Yang A, Kaghad M, Wang Y et al. p63, a p53 homolog at 3q27–29, encodes multiple products with transactivating, death-inducing, and dominant-negative activities. Mol Cell 1998;2:305–16.**

6 **Brunner HG, Hamel BC, van Bokhoven H. P63 Gene mutations and human developmental syndromes. Am J Med Genet 2002;112:284–90.**

7 **Mills AA, Zheng B, Wang X-J et al. p63 is a p53 homolog required for limb and epidermal morphogenesis. Nature 1999;398:708–13.**

8 **Yang A, Schweizer R, Sun D et al. p63 is essential for regenerative proliferation in limb, craniofacial and epithelial development. Nature 1999;398:7147–8.**

9 Van Bokhoven H, Hamel BC, Bamshad M et al. p63 Gene mutations in EEC syndrome, limb–mammary syndrome, and isolated split hand-split foot malformation suggest a genotype-phenotype correlation. Am J Hum Genet 2001;69:481–92.

10 Amiel J, Bougeard G, Francannet C et al. TP63 gene mutation in ADULT syndrome. Eur J Hum Genet 2001;9:642–5.

11 Elliott AM, Evans JA. Genotype-phenotype correlations in mapped split hand foot malformation (SHFM) patients. Am J Med Genet A 2006;140:1419–27.

12 Rinne T, Bolat E, Meijer R et al. Spectrum of p63 mutations in a selected patient cohort affected with ankyloblepharon-ectodermal defects-cleft lip/palate syndrome (AEC). Am J Med Genet A 2009;149A:1948–51.

13 Rinne T, Clements SE, Lamme E et al. A novel translation re-initiation mechanism for the p63 gene revealed by amino-terminal truncating mutations in Rapp–Hodgkin/Hay–Wells-like syndromes. Hum Mol Genet 2008;17:1968–77.

14 Chiu YE, Drolet BA, Duffy KJ et al. A case of ankyloblepharon, ectodermal dysplasia, and cleft lip/palate syndrome with ectrodactyly: are the p63 syndromes distinct after all? Pediatr Dermatol 2011;28;15–19.

15 Slavotinek AM, Tanaka J, Winder A et al. Acro-dermato-ungual lacrimal-tooth (ADULT) syndrome: report of a child with phenotypic overlap with ulnar-mammary syndrome and a new mutation in TP63. Am J Med Genet A 2005;138A:146–9.

16 Hildebrandt T, Preiherr J, Tarbe N et al. Identification of THW, a putative new tumor suppressor gene. Anticancer Res 2000;20:2801–10.

17 Ihrie RA, Marques MR, Nguyen BT et al. Perp is a p63-regulated gene essential for epithelial integrity. Cell 2005;120:843–56.

18 Beaudry VG, Pathak N, Koster MI et al. PERP regulation by TP63 mutants provides insight into AEC pathogenesis. Am J Med Genet A 2009;149A:1952–7.

19 Ferone G, Thomason HA, Antonini D et al. Mutant p63 causes defective expansion of ectodermal progenitor cells and impaired FGF signalling in AEC syndrome. EMBO Mol Med 2012;4:192–205.

20 Koster MI, Dai D, Marinari B et al. p63 induces key target genes required for epidermal morphogenesis. Proc Natl Acad Sci USA 2007;104:3255–60.

21 Marinari B, Ballaro C, Koster MI et al. IKKalpha is a p63 transcriptional target involved in the pathogenesis of ectodermal dysplasias. J Invest Dermatol 2009;129:60–9.

22 Koster MI, Marinari B, Payne AS et al. DeltaNp63 knockdown mice: a mouse model for AEC syndrome. Am J Med Genet A 2009;149A:1942–7.

23 Chan I, McGrath JA, Kivirikko S. Rapp–Hodgkin syndrome and the tail of p63. Clin Exp Dermatol 2005;30:183–6.

24 Eiesenkraft A, Pode-Shakked B, Goldstein N et al. Clinical variability in a family with an ectodermal dysplasia syndrome and a nonsense mutation in the TP63 gene. Fetal Pediatr Pathol 2015;34:400–6.

25 Hay RJ, Wells RS. The syndrome of ankyloblepharon, ectodermal defects and cleft lip and palate: an autosomal dominant condition. Br J Dermatol 1976;94:277–89.

26 Greene SL, Michels VV, Doyle JA. Variable expression in ankyloblepharon-ectodermal defects-cleft lip and palate syndrome. Am J Med Genet 1987;27:207–12.

27 Dishop MK, Bree AF, Hicks MJ. Pathologic changes of skin and hair in ankyloblepharon-ectodermal defects-cleft lip/palate (AEC) syndrome. Am J Med Genet A 2009;149A:1935–41.

28 Fosko SW, Stenn KS, Bolognia JL. Ectodermal dysplasias associated with clefting: significance of scalp dermatitis. J Am Acad Dermatol 1992;27:249–56.

29 Vanderhooft SL, Stephan MJ, Sybert VP. Severe skin erosions and scalp infections in AEC syndrome. Pediatr Dermatol 1993;10: 334–40.

30 Julapalli MR, Scher RK, Sybert VP et al. Dermatologic findings of ankyloblepharon-ectodermal defects-cleft lip/palate (AEC) syndrome. Am J Med Genet A 2009;149A:1900–6.

31 Rule DC, Shaw MJ. The dental management of patients with ankyloblepharon (AEC) syndrome. Br Dent J 1988;164:215–18.

32 Farrington F, Lausten L. Oral findings in ankyloblepharon-ectodermal dysplasia-cleft lip/palate (AEC) syndrome. Am J Med Genet A 2009;149A:1907–9.

33 Ferstl P, Wohlfart S, Schneider H. Sweating ability of patients with p63-associated syndromes. Eur J Pediatr 2018; 177: 1727–31.

34 Yoo J, Beck DR, Fabre E et al. Ankyloblepharon-ectodermal dysplasia clefting (AEC) syndrome with neonatal erythroderma: report of two cases. Int J Dermatol 2007;46:1196–7.

35 Motil KJ, Fete TJ. Growth, nutritional, and gastrointestinal aspects of ankyloblepharon-ectodermal defect-cleft lip and/or palate (AEC) syndrome. Am J Med Genet A 2009;149A:1922–5.

36 Bronshtein M, Gershoni-Baruch R. Prenatal transvaginal diagnosis of the ectrodactyly, ectodermal dysplasia, cleft palate (EEC) syndrome. Prenat Diagn 1993;13:519–22.

37 Baughman FA Jr. CHANDS: the curly hair–ankyloblepharon–nail dysplasia syndrome. Birth Defects Orig Artic Series 1971;7:100–2.

38 Toriello HV, Lindstrom JA, Waterman DF et al. Re-evaluation of CHANDS. J Med Genet 1979;16:316–17.

39 Taieb A, Legrain V, Surleve-Bazeille JE et al. Generalized epidermolysis bullosa with congenital synechiae, associated malformations and unusual ultrastructure: a new entity? Dermatologica 1988;176: 76–82.

40 Hicks C, Pitts J, Rose GE. Lacrimal surgery in patients with congenital cranial or facial anomalies. Eye 1994;8:583–91.

41 Satoh K, Tosa Y, Ohtsuka S et al. Ankyloblepharon, ectodermal dysplasia, cleft lip and palate (AEC) syndrome: surgical corrections with an 18-year follow-up including maxillary osteotomy. Plast Reconstr Surg 1994;93:590–4.

42 Theiler M, Frieden IJ. High-potency topical steroids: an effective therapy for chronic scalp inflammation in rapp-hodgkin ectodermal dysplasia. Pediatr Dermatol 2016;33:84–7.

43 Rüdiger RA, Haase W, Passarge E. Association of ectrodactyly, ectodermal dysplasia, and cleft lip–palate. Am J Dis Child 1970;120:160–3.

44 Bixler D, Spivack J, Bennett J et al. The ectrodactyly–ectodermal dysplasia–clefting (EEC) syndrome. Report of 2 cases and review of the literature. Clin Genet 1972;3:43–51.

45 Trueb RM, Bruckner-Tuderman L, Wyss M et al. Scalp dermatitis, distinctive hair abnormalities and atopic disease in the ectrodactyly–ectodermal dysplasia–clefting syndrome. Br J Dermatol 1995;132:621–5.

46 Micali G, Cook B, Blekys I et al. Structural hair abnormalities in ectodermal dysplasia. Pediatr Dermatol 1990;7:27–32.

47 Kuster W, Majewski F, Meinecke P. EEC syndrome without ectrodactyly? Report of 8 cases. Clin Genet 1985;28:130–5.

48 Rosenmann A, Shapira T, Cohen MM. Ectrodactyly, ectodermal dysplasia and cleft palate (EEC syndrome). Report of a family and review of the literature. Clin Genet 1976;9:347–53.

49 Richieri-Costa A, de Vilhena-Moraes SA, Ferrareto I et al. Ectodermal dysplasia/ectrodactyly in monozygotic female twins. Report of a case-review and comments on the ectodermal dysplasia/ectrodactyly (cleft lip/palate) syndromes. Rev Brasil Genet 1986;9:349–74.

50 Rodini ES, Richieri-Costa A. EEC syndrome. Report on 20 new patients: clinical and genetic considerations. Am J Med Genet 1990;37:42–53.

51 Trueb RM, Bruckner-Tuderman L, Burg G. Ectrodactyly-ectodermal dysplasia–clefting syndrome with scalp dermatitis. J Am Acad Dermatol 1993;29:505–6.

52 Pratsou P, Defty CL, Ozoemena L et al. Limited ectrodactyly, ectodermal dysplasia and cleft lip-palate syndrome with a p63 mutation, associated with linear and whorled naevoid hypermelanosis. Clin Exp Dermatol 2014;39:266–8.

53 McNab AA, Potts MJ, Welham RA. The EEC syndrome and its ocular manifestations. Br J Ophthalmol 1989;73:261–4.

54 Christodoulou J, McDougall PN, Sheffield LJ. Choanal atresia as a feature of ectrodactyly–ectodermal dysplasia–clefting (EEC) syndrome. J Med Genet 1989;26:586–9.

55 Metwalley Kalli KA, Fargalley HS. Holoprosencephaly in an Egyptian baby with ectrodactyly-ectodermal dysplasia-cleft syndrome: a case report. J Med Case Rep 2012;24:35.

56 Nardi AC, Ferreira U, Netto NR Jr et al. Urinary tract involvement in EEC syndrome: a clinical study in 25 Brazilian patients. Am J Med Genet 1992;44:803–6.

57 Rollnick BR, Hoo JJ. Genitourinary anomalies are a component manifestation in the ectodermal dysplasia, ectrodactyly, cleft lip/palate (EEC) syndrome. Am J Med Genet 1988;29:131–6.

58 Maclean K, Holme SA, Gilmour E et al. EEC syndrome, Arg227Gln TP63 mutation and micturition difficulties: is there a genotypepheno-type correlation? Am J Med Genet A 2007;143A:1114–19.

59 Hyder Z, Beale V, O'Connor R et al. Genitourinary malformations: an under-recognized feature of ectrodactyly, ectodermal dysplasia and cleft lip/palate syndrome. Clin Dysmorphol 2017;26:78–82.

60 Giampietro PF et al. Novel mutation in TP63 associated with ectrodactyly ectodermal dysplasia and clefting syndrome and T cell lymphopenia. Am J Med Genet A 2013;161A:1432–5.

61 Knudtzon J, Aarskog D. Growth hormone deficiency associated with the ectrodactyly–ectodermal dysplasia–clefting syndrome and isolated absent septum pellucidum. Pediatrics 1987;79:410–12.

62 Gershoni-Baruch R, Goldscher D, Hochberg Z. Ectrodactyly ectodermal dysplasia-clefting syndrome and hypothalamo-pituitary insufficiency. Am J Med Genet 1997;68:168–72.

63 Sharma D, Kumar C, Bhalerao S et al. Ectrodactyly, ectodermal dysplasia, cleft lip, and palate (EEC syndrome) with tetralogy of Fallot: a very rare combination. Front Pediatr 2015;16:51.

64 Balci S, Engiz O, Okten G et al. A 19-year follow-up of a patient with type 3 ectrodactyly-ectodermal dysplasia-clefting syndrome who developed non-Hodgkin lymphoma. Oral Surg Oral Med Oral Pathol Oral Radiol Endod 2009;108:e91–5.

65 Akahoshi K, Sakazume S, Kosaki K et al. EEC syndrome type 3 with a heterozygous germline mutation in the P63 gene and B cell lymphoma. Am J Med Genet A 2003;120A:370–3.

66 Rosenberg JB, Butrus S, Bazemore MG et al. Ectrodactyly-ectodermal dysplasia-clefting syndrome causing blindness in a child. J AAPOS 2011;15:80–2.

67 Barbaro V, Nasti AA, Del Vecchio C et al. Correction of mutant p63 in EEC syndrome using siRNA mediated allele specific silencing restores defective stem cell function. Stem Cells 2016;34:1588–600.

68 Propping P, Zerres K. ADULT syndrome: an autosomal-dominant disorder with pigment anomalies, ectrodactyly, nail dysplasia, and hypodontia. Am J Med Genet 1993;45:642–8.

69 Reisler TT, Patton MA, Meagher PPJ. Further phenotypic and genetic variation in ADULT syndrome. Am J Med Genet A 2006; 140A:2495–500.

70 Ellis RWB, van Creveld S. A syndrome characterized by ectodermal dysplasia, polydactyly, chondrodysplasia and congenital morbus cordis: report of three cases. Arch Dis Child 1940;15:65–84.

71 Ruiz-Perez VL, Ide SE, Strom TM et al. Mutations in a new gene in Ellis–van Creveld syndrome and Weyer's acrodental dysostosis. Nat Genet 2000;24:283–6.

72 Galdzicka M, Patnala S, Hirshman MG et al. A new gene, EVC2, is mutated in Ellis–van Creveld syndrome. Mol Genet Metab 2002;77:291–5.

73 Sund KL, Roelker S, Ramachandran V et al. Analysis of Ellis van Creveld syndrome gene products: implications for cardiovascular development and disease. Hum Mol Genet 2009;18:1813–24.

74 Jumlongras D, Bei M, Stimson JM et al. A nonsense mutation in MSX1 causes Witkop syndrome. Am J Hum Genet 2001;69:67–74.

75 Price JA, Bowden DW, Wright JT et al. Identification of a mutation in DLX3 associated with tricho-dento-osseous (TDO) syndrome. Hum Mol Genet 1998;7:563–9.

76 Robinson GW, Mahon KA. Differential and overlapping expression domains of Dlx-2 and Dlx-3 suggest distinct roles for Distal-less homeobox genes in craniofacial development. Mech Dev 1994;48:199–215.

77 Dong J, Amor D, Aldred MJ et al. DLX3 mutation associated with autosomal dominant amelogenesis imperfecta with taurodontism. Am J Med Genet 2005;133A:138–41.
78 Wright JT, Hong SP, Simmons D et al. DLX3 c.561_562delCT mutation causes attenuated phenotype of tricho-dento-osseous syndrome. Am J Med Genet 2008;146A:343–9.
79 Momeni P, Glockner G, Schmidt O et al. Mutations in a new gene, encoding a zinc-finger protein, cause tricho–rhino–phalangeal syndrome type I. Nat Genet 2000;24:71–4.
80 Ludecke HJ, Schaper J, Meinecke P et al. Genotypic and phenotypic spectrum in tricho-rhino-phalangeal syndrome types I and III. Am J Hum Genet 2001;68:81–91.
81 Ludecke HJ, Wagner MJ, Nardmann J et al. Molecular dissection of a contiguous gene syndrome: localization of the genes involved in the Langer–Giedion syndrome. Hum Mol Genet 1995;4:31–6.
82 Hou J, Parrish J, Ludecke HJ et al. A 4-megabase YAC contig that spans the Langer–Giedion syndrome region on human chromosome 8q24.1: use in refining the location of the trichorhinophalangeal syndrome and multiple exostoses genes (TRPS1 and EXT1). Genomics 1995;29:87–97.
83 Dai KS, Liew CC. Characterization of a novel gene encoding zinc finger domains identified from expressed sequence tags (ESTs) of a human heart cDNA database. J Mol Cell Cardiol 1998;30:2365–75.
84 Lichtenstein J, Warson R, Jorgenson R et al. The tricho-dento-osseous (TDO) syndrome. Am J Hum Genet 1972;24:569–82.
85 Robinson GC, Miller JR. Hereditary enamel hypoplasia: its association with characteristic hair structure. Pediatrics 1966;37:498–502.
86 Freire-Maia N, Pinheiro M. Ectodermal Dysplasias: A Clinical and Genetic Study. New York: Alan R. Liss, 1984.
87 Shapiro SD, Quattromani FL, Jorgenson RJ et al. Tricho-dento-osseous syndrome: heterogeneity or clinical variability. Am J Med Genet 1983;16:225–36.
88 Quattromani F, Shapiro SD, Young RS et al. Clinical heterogeneity in the tricho-dento-osseous syndrome. Hum Genet 1983;64:116–21.
89 Levin LS. Dental and oral abnormalities in selected ectodermal dysplasia syndromes. Birth Defects Orig Artic Series 1988;24:205–27.
90 Melnick M, Shields ED, El-Kafrawy AH. Tricho-dento-osseous syndrome: a scanning electron microscopic analysis. Clin Genet 1977;12:17–27.
91 Sclar AG, Kannikal J, Ferreira CF et al. Treatment planning and surgical considerations in implant therapy for patients with agenesis, oligodontia, and ectodermal dysplasia: review and case presentation. J Oral Maxillofac Surg 2009;67(11 Suppl):2–12.
92 Giedion A, Burdea M, Fruchter Z et al. Autosomal dominant transmission of the tricho-rhino-phalangeal syndrome. Report of 4 unrelated families, review of 60 cases. Helv Paediatr Acta 1973;28:249–59.
93 Beals RK. Tricho-rhino-phalangeal dysplasia. Report of a kindred. J Bone Joint Surg Am 1973;55:821–6.
94 Sugiura Y. Tricho-rhino-phalangeal syndrome associated with Perthes disease-like bone change and spondylolisthesis. Jinrui Idengaku Zasshi 1978;23:23–30.
95 Sugio Y, Kajii T. Ruvalacaba syndrome: autosomal dominant inheritance. Am J Med Genet 1984;19:741–53.
96 Niikawa N, Kamei T. The Sugio–Kajii syndrome, proposed tricho rhino-phalangeal syndrome type III. Am J Med Genet 1986; 24:759–60.
97 Campbell P, Morton PE, Takeichi T et al. Epithelial inflammation resulting from an inherited loss-of-function mutation in EGFR. J Invest Dermatol 2014;134:2570–8.
98 Ganetzky R, Finn E, Bagchi A et al. EGFR mutations cause a lethal syndrome of epithelial dysfunction with progeroid features. Mol Genet Genomic Med 2015;3:452–8.
99 Hayashi S, Yokoi T, Hatano C et al. Biallelic mutations of EGFR in a compound heterozygous state cause ectodermal dysplasia with severe skin defects and gastrointestinal dysfunction. Hum Genome Var 2018;5:11.

Defects in the Wnt-β-catenin pathway

The Wnt-β-catenin pathway is highly conserved and seen in all species from invertebrates to humans. It plays a prominent role in embryogenesis and carcinogenesis. The term 'Wnt' is the result of a combination between 'wingless', also known as Wg, the identified gene in *Drosophila melanogaster*, and the homologous 'int', the murine mammary tumour virus integration site. There are at least 19 *WNT* genes in humans that are involved in a variety of developmental and regulatory processes, including the decision between self-renewal and differentiation [1]. They are also notably involved in hair and tooth formation [2–5]. Recently, *WNT10A* missense mutations have been associated with both odonto-onycho-dermal dysplasia syndrome (OMIM #257980) and Schöpf–Schulz–Passarge (SSP) syndrome (OMIM #224750) [6–8]. This is understandable because one kindred exhibited both conditions among its family members [8]. Focal dermal hypoplasia, also known as Goltz syndrome (OMIM #305600), is caused by mutations in the *PORCN* gene [9,10]. The product of this gene is homologous to *Porc*, which encodes an *O*-acyltransferase enzyme in the endoplasmic reticulum, responsible for modification of Wg in *Drosophila*. Due to the conservation of this pathway throughout evolution, it is likely that the product of *PORCN* performs a similar function for Wnt [9].

In the canonical Wnt-β-catenin pathway, the downstream effector is β-catenin, whose concentrations are altered when Wnt interacts with Frizzled, a transmembrane protein, and the LRP5/6 receptor (Fig. 134.14). In the absence of Wnt signalling, β-catenin is free in the cytoplasm and is rapidly bound by a 'destruction complex', followed by polyubiquitination and degradation. With Wnt binding, a downstream cascade leads to stabilization of β-catenin, allowing it to enter the nucleus and activate its target genes [11]. Mutations in the gene *Hairless* (*HR*) have been discovered in two conditions that feature hair loss: atrichia with papular lesions (OMIM #209500) [12] and alopecia universalis congenita (OMIM #203655) [13]. The HR protein is involved in the regulation of gene expression during the hair cycle, specifically by controlling Wnt signalling through its actions as a repressor of a Wnt inhibitor, Wise; thus HR increases the amount of Wnt signalling, allowing for proper regrowth of hair at the beginning of the hair cycle [14]. Wnt signalling is also involved in myriad other processes, including tooth and limb formation, myogenesis and neural development [15].

Multiple developmental signalling pathways, of which the Wnt-β-catenin pathway is one, have complex and interconnected relationships. A patient with vitamin D-resistant rickets caused by a compound heterozygote mutation in the vitamin D receptor gene (*VDR*) had an identical phenotype to atrichia with papular lesions (APL), suggesting its importance in the hair growth cycle [16]. Wnt is repressed by Notch signalling, another important and highly conserved protein in cell regulation. The *p63* signalling pathway, discussed above, inhibits Notch, and Notch in turn represses *p63* [17].

Odonto-onycho-dermal dysplasia syndrome (OMIM #257980)

Definition. The main features of odonto-onycho-dermal dysplasia (OODD) syndrome include hypotrichosis, hypodontia and nail dystrophy. Other characteristics that may be observed include hyperhidrosis, palmoplantar keratoderma (PPK) and loss of lingual papillae, resulting

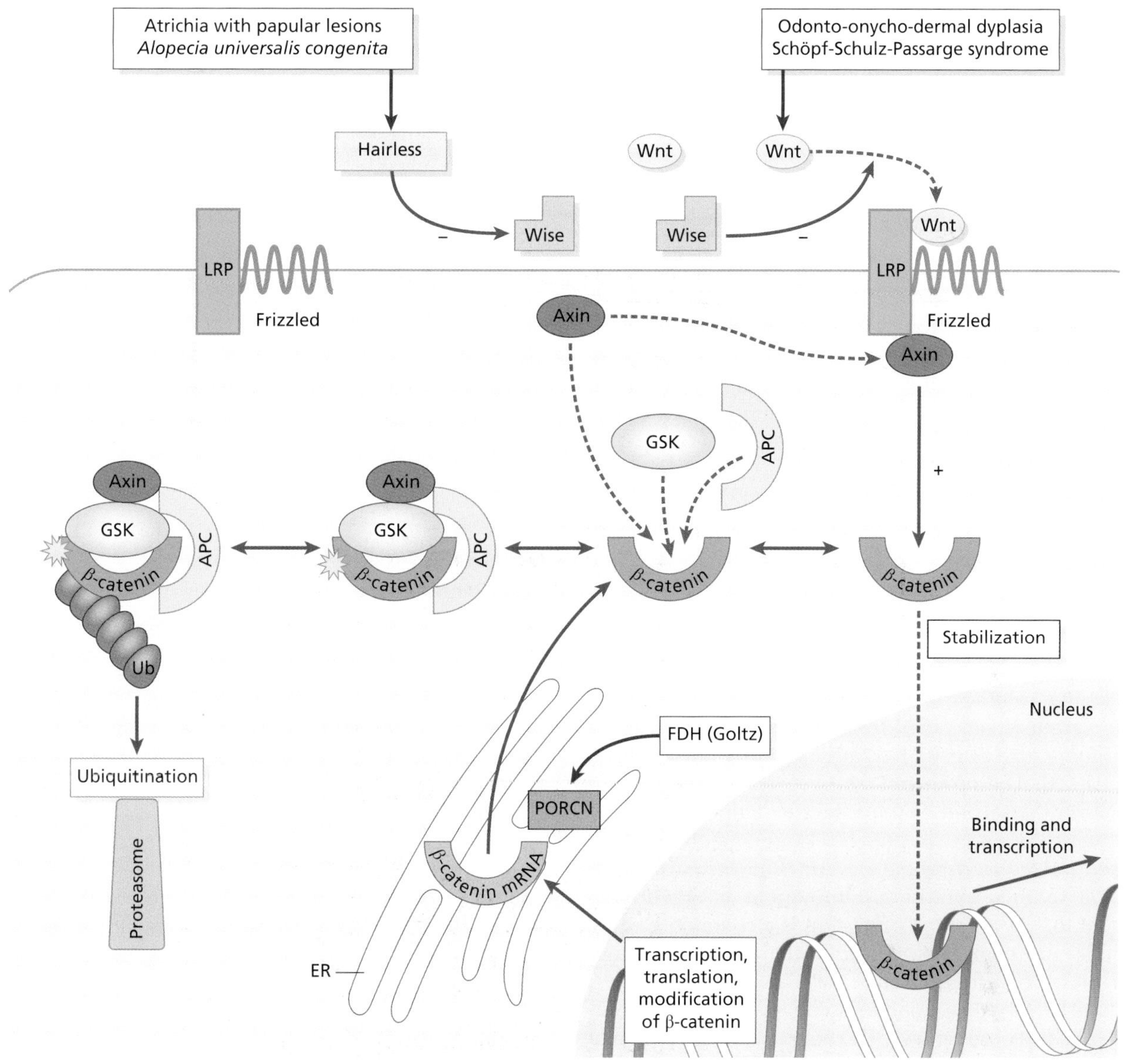

Fig. 134.14 Overview of the Wnt-related pathways and their role in human ectodermal dysplasias. Wnt binding to Frizzled and LRP causes stabilization of β-catenin, resulting in its translocation to the nucleus, where it binds to DNA and causes transcription of β-catenin upregulated genes. Wnt binding to Frizzled is impaired by Wise, whereas Wise is inhibited by the Hairless gene product. β-catenin is usually held inactive by binding of the APC destruction complex. APC, along with Axin, binds β-catenin, allowing it to be phosphorylated by GSK. Phosphorylation results in ubiquitination of β-catenin and its targeting for destruction. APC, adenomatosis polyposis coli protein; ER, endoplasmic reticulum; FDH, focal dermal hypoplasia; GSK, glycogen synthase kinase 3 β; PORCN, *PORCN* gene product; Ub, ubiquitin.

in a smooth tongue. Patients may also exhibit mild intellectual disability and recurrent infection.

History. OODD was initially reported by Fried in 1977 in boy and girl cousins who were products of consanguineous marriages. They were described as having a similar presentation to Witkop syndrome, with partial adontia, conical teeth and nail dystrophy [18]. The disease was further characterized in a large Lebanese Muslim [7,19–21] and Pakistani kindred [6]. This condition is autosomal recessive; sporadic cases have been reported [22].

Pathology. Histology of the hyperkeratotic plantar skin shows mild epidermal acanthosis with hypergranulosis, orthokeratosis and hyperkeratosis [7,21]. A mild perivascular infiltrate in the papillary dermis may also be present [21]. Sweat glands are decreased in number and poorly developed [8,21]. The erythematous plaques of the face show an atrophic epidermis with basophilic collagen degeneration of the upper dermis [19]. Irregular hairs with longitudinal depressions are observed on scanning electron microscopy [21], at the bottom of which are cuticular cells with a longitudinal striated aspect [7].

Clinical features.

Hair

Hypotrichosis is common, and lack of hair may be congenital [6,20,21], but hair may be normal at birth [21]. Both scalp and body hair may be affected [6]. Hair that is present is often dry, thin and sparse [7,23], or has a coarse texture [21]. Eyebrows and eyelashes may be thinned [6,7,19,22,23].

Teeth
Severe oligodontia is nearly always present [7]; congenital absence of secondary dentition is often seen [6,21]. Deciduous teeth may be widely spaced and malformed [7,19,21]. If permanent teeth are absent, some deciduous teeth may be retained into adulthood [6]. Misshapen teeth, including conical and bifid incisors, and five-cusped molars have been described [19,21,23]

Nails
Nails may be congenitally absent [21,23]. Nail dystrophy may or may not be present; toenails are more commonly affected than fingernails [7,19,21–23]. Nails are thin, concave and may exhibit longitudinal ridging or central grooved dystrophy [7,21,23]. Thickening, tenting and onycholysis have also been described [23].

Sweat glands
Hyperhidrosis of the palms and soles is commonly reported, although not in all cases [7,19,21,23]. Hypohidrosis and heat intolerance are less commonly reported [6,8].

Skin
Thickening of the palms and soles is common, and hyperkeratosis can range from mild to severe, causing symptoms such as pain, laceration or impaired dexterity [6–8,21–23]. The onset can be as early as 3–4 years or appear in the second or third decade. Palmar erythema is a very common finding [7,21]. A smooth tongue, caused by reduced fungiform and filiform papillae, is notable for this condition, although it is not always present [6,7,21]. Diffusely dry skin is a common finding [6–8,21]. Erythematous, telangiectatic atrophic plaques in a malar distribution have been described in select patients [19,24]; these tend to become worse in the summer [19,23]. Those with OODD may have keratosis pilaris and follicular hyperkeratosis on the body [6,21,24], and recurrent folliculitis has been described [7]. Some photographs of these erythematous malar plaques bring to mind keratosis pilaris atrophicans rubra faciei (ulerythema ophryogenes), especially when considering the presence of keratosis pilaris.

Other ectodermal structures
Patients with this condition may have chronic irritative conjunctivitis secondary to short lashes [23] and a few have also reported photophobia [8,23]. One case of seizures associated with this condition has been reported [22].

Craniofacial features
There are no characteristic craniofacial features.

Other abnormalities
Mild mental deficiency has been described [22], recurrent cutaneous dermatophytosis [21] and folliculitis [7].

Prognosis. The nail and skin dystrophies can become more pronounced over time. Physical development and lifespan are unaffected. It is unknown if this condition has a risk of skin cancer, as in the allelic condition of SSP.

Differential diagnosis. The allelic SSP syndrome is in the differential for this condition. A lack of eyelid cysts is not discriminatory in children because they present later on in life. If present, a smooth tongue may also help to make the diagnosis. The facial eruption may bring to mind keratitis, ichthyosis deafness syndrome (KID), discussed later, but the quality of PPKand lack of deafness would delineate OODD from KID syndrome.

Treatment. Treatment is symptomatic. Suggested treatments have included topical keratolytic agents and physical debridement with warm water soaks and pumice stone [24]. Emollients are suggested for dry skin. It is unclear if topical corticosteroids improve the facial eruption associated with this syndrome [24].

SSP syndrome (OMIM #224750)

Definition. The main features of SSP syndrome (SSPS) include hypodontia, persistence of deciduous teeth, generalized hypotrichosis of both scalp and body, and normal sweating. Eyelid cysts are helpful in the diagnosis but may not always be present. Age of onset of symptoms may vary greatly. These patients have a risk of benign and malignant skin tumours.

History. The condition was described by Schöpf in 1971 [25]. SSPS generally exhibits autosomal recessive inheritance; other reported forms of inheritance include one German kindred with autosomal dominant inheritance, and one case of possible uniparental isodisomy for a recessive trait [26,27].

Pathology. Eccrine syringofibroadenoma is characteristic of SSPS. This is a rare tumour that presents with anastomosing cords of pale-staining epithelial cells, extending from the epidermis into the papillary dermis, with focal luminal formation. The cords of cells are surrounded by an oedematous stroma containing dilated capillaries. Rarely, this tumour may become malignant [28]. The pale epithelial cells are negative for SMA, S100 and CAM5.2, with weak to intermediate staining for EMA. CEA is positive only at the inner border of ductal structures. In areas of malignant degeneration, more intense staining of EMA is seen, with weak CAM5.2 positivity. CEA, EMA and CAM5.2 are all strongly positive in ductal areas [28].

Biopsy of the eyelid cysts characteristic in this condition show intradermal papillary cystic stuctures composed of two layers of cells – a cuboidal inner lining of cells and an outer myoepithelial layer. These findings are consistent with apocrine hidrocystomas [29].

Clinical features.
Hair
Hair loss is common, although not always present, and may affect the scalp and body [8,27,28]. Sparse eyelashes

and eyebrows have also been described [27,28]. Hair may be thin or fine [27]. Pili torti has also been associated with this syndrome [30]. Despite the many findings, hair may also be normal [29].

Teeth
Extensive hypodontia is common in this condition. Primary teeth may be abnormal, lost early or retained, and permanent teeth may be missing completely or have partial development [8,25,27,28,31]. Tooth abnormalities include conical and widely spaced teeth [28,29].

Nails
Both fingernail and toenail dystrophy are seen [8,27,28]. Nails may be fragile and brittle or exhibit furrowing or onycholysis [25,29,32]. Splitting, koilonychia and pterygium unguis have also been described [31]. Longitudinal narrowing of the fingernails and complete absence of the fingernails have also been noted in this condition [33].

Sweat glands
Sweating is usually normal but hyperhidrosis is not uncommon [8,31,34]. Tumours and cysts of eccrine origin are common; this will be discussed further later.

Skin
The PPK in Schöpf's original description began at approximately the age 12 years [25]; other cases became symptomatic in their twenties and thirties [20,28,33]. The palmar and plantar findings include erythematous hyperkeratosis, scaling hyperkeratosis and a lace-like network of erythema and scale [28]. Findings may also include dyshidrotic blistering of glabrous skin and hyperkeratosis of the dorsal hands [8]. These may be symptomatic caused by thickening or fissuring.

Multiple eccrine tumours are noted, specifically eccrine poroma and eccrine syringofibroadenoma [28, 4]. Eccrine syringofibroadenoma can present as PPK in a mosaic pattern [35]. Benign adnexal tumours, such as tumour of the follicular infundibulum, and poroma with follicular differentiation have also been reportedly associated with this condition [36]. Malignant skin tumours have also been described, suggesting an elevated risk of skin cancer in these patients requiring increased vigilance. Some of these are common tumours, such as basal cell and squamous cell carcinomas [26,28,29,37]; others are neoplastic counterparts to eccrine tumours, such as malignant degeneration of eccrine syringofibroadenoma, and porocarcinoma [8,28].

Eyelid cysts present as milky or translucent papules located mostly along the lash border; they are bilateral and symmetrically distributed. These apocrine hidrocystomas were originally thought to originate from the glands of Moll [29], but others suggest they are ectopic remnants of fetal apocrine glands [38]. Milia on the face have also been described in a few cases [29,31]. Telangiectatic rosacea has also been reported [31].

Other ectodermal structures
Photophobia has been described [29], similar to cases of OODD. Optic atrophy and hypoplastic nipples were reported in one case [31]. Vaginal dryness and decreased salivary gland secretion have also been described [32].

Craniofacial features
There are generally no characteristic craniofacial features, although a 'curious bird-like facies' has been described in one kindred [33].

Other abnormalities
Breast cancer and hypernephroma have been described in patients with this condition [28,33].

Prognosis. Patients may present during childhood [25], or during their second and third decades [20,28,29,33]. Eyelid cysts can become symptomatic much later, after the age of 50 and into the seventies [25,27,28]. As many features may have late presentation in the fifth and sixth decades, counselling younger patients or their parents on prognosis may be difficult; a milder presentation at a younger age does not necessarily predict lack of lifetime symptoms.

Differential diagnosis. The main differential for this condition is OODD, as both present with severe oligodontia, hypotrichosis, PPK and nail dystrophy. Patients with both of these conditions may also display hyperhidrosis. Significant differences between the two conditions include the presence of eyelid cysts and eccrine tumours in SSPS, and the smooth tongue caused by loss of lingual papillae in OODD.

Treatment. Apocrine hidrocystomas of the eyelid can present significant cosmetic impairment, and simple excision of eyelid cysts is rarely adequate. Radical excision of the anterior lamella may result in sustained improvement [32]. Treatment of hyperkeratosis involves keratolytic therapy. For lesions unresponsive to treatment, a biopsy may be warranted. Unresponsive lesions may in fact be eccrine tumours, and clinicians must remain vigilant for cutaneous malignancies.

Focal dermal hypoplasia (FDH; Goltz syndrome; OMIM #305600)

Definition. The main features of Goltz syndrome include linear, streaked blaschkoid arrangements of markedly thinned dermis, resulting in fat herniation. Skin is dry and involvement of other ectodermal structures may be present, such as sparse hair, hypodontia, notched incisors and dysplastic or absent nails [39]. Ophthalmological abnormalities are common, as is cleft palate. This is an X-linked dominant condition caused by mutations in the *PORCN* gene [8,9]; cases may also be sporadic [39]. The majority (90%) of affected patients are female, and severity may be affected by lyonization in females and by somatic mosaicism in males [40,41].

Please see Chapter 135 for a full discussion of this condition.

Atrichia with papular lesions (OMIM #209500); alopecia universalis congenita (OMIM #203655)

Definition. These two syndromes are probably the same or a continuum of the same disease, the main feature of which is diffuse hair loss. In atrichia with papular lesions (APL), this hair loss can be accompanied by skin-coloured papules, which are not present in alopecia universalis congenita. They are both autosomal recessive conditions, caused by mutations in the *Hairless* gene (*HR*), a co-repressor in the Wnt signalling pathway (see previously) [12,13].

History. In 1952 Tillman reported two families with congenital alopecia [42]. This condition was further characterized in a large Pakistani kindred [43], in which the gene for alopecia universalis congenita was eventually mapped and identified [13,44].

Pathology. Skin biopsy of the area of alopecia shows an unremarkable epidermis and a dermis containing hair follicles without hair [43]. Aborted follicles are seen, with only well-developed infundibula but no hair shaft or other parts of the hair follicle. The papular lesions contain small keratinous cysts surrounded by normal sebaceous glands and pilar muscle; these cysts are lined by epithelial cells similar to those that line the mid and lower portions of the hair follicle [45].

Clinical features.

Hair

Patients may present with a history of atrichia at birth or, more commonly, with a history of normal hair present at birth that is shed normally but is not replaced; this may occur between 3 and 24 months of age [43,45]. Alopecia may be complete and include eyebrows, eyelashes, axillary and pubic hair [43], but sparse eyelashes and eyebrows may be present in some cases [45].

Teeth, nails, sweat glands and other ectodermal structures

Teeth, nails and sweat glands are normal. No other ectodermal abnormalities have been reported [43,45]. Intelligence is normal [43].

Skin

In APL, patients may present with skin-coloured to white cystic and/or papular lesions, similar to milia, ranging in size from 1 to 3 mm. These papules are primarily seen over the elbows and knees but can be present elsewhere on the body, including thighs and buttocks; if other sites are involved, the face is a common location [45].

Prognosis. As this is a defect in the hair growth cycle, hair loss does not grow back. The condition does not affect patient lifespan.

Differential diagnosis. The differential diagnosis of this condition includes autoimmune-induced alopecia totalis and universalis, and localized autosomal recessive hypotrichosis. These conditions should be distinguishable upon history, except for cases of APL or alopecia universalis congenita that present with congenital hair loss – these may be more difficult to distinguish from localized autosomal recessive hypotrichosis. Biopsy showing an inflammatory infiltrate would differentiate autoimmune alopecia from APL and alopecia universalis congenita.

Treatment. There is currently no specific treatment for this condition. Treatment involves wigs or hats for cosmesis.

References

1 **Staal FJ, Tiago CL. Wnt signaling in hematopoiesis: crucial factors for self-renewal, proliferation, and cell fate decisions. J Cell Biochem 2010;109:844–9.**

2 **Wang J, Shackleford GM. Murine Wnt10a and Wnt10b: cloning and expression in developing limbs, face and skin of embryos and in adults. Oncogene 1996;13:1537–44.**

3 Dassule HR, McMahon AP. Analysis of epithelial-mesenchymal interactions in the initial morphogenesis of the mammalian tooth. Dev Biol 1998;202:215–27.

4 **Millar SE, Willert K, Salinas PC et al. WNT signaling in the control of hair growth and structure. Dev Biol 1999;207:133–49.**

5 Andl T, Reddy ST, Gaddapara T et al. WNT signals are required for the initiation of hair follicle development. Dev Cell 2002;2:643–53.

6 **Nawaz S, Klar J, Wajid M et al. WNT10A missense mutation associated with a complete odonto-onycho-dermal dysplasia syndrome. Eur J Hum Genet 2009;17(12):1600–5.**

7 **Adaimy L, Chouery E, Mégarbané H et al. Mutation in WNT10A is associated with an autosomal recessive ectodermal dysplasia: the odonto-onycho-dermal dysplasia. Am J Hum Genet 2007;81:821–8.**

8 **Bohring A, Stamm T, Spaich C et al. WNT10A mutations are a frequent cause of a broad spectrum of ectodermal dysplasias with sexbiased manifestation pattern in heterozygotes. Am J Hum Genet 2009;85:97–105.**

9 **Grzeschik KH, Bornholdt D, Oeffner F et al. Deficiency of PORCN, a regulator of Wnt signaling, is associated with focal dermal hypoplasia. Nat Genet 2007;39:833–5.**

10 Wang X, Sutton VR, Peraza-Llanes JO et al. Mutations in X-linked PORCN, a putative regulator of Wnt signaling, cause focal dermal hypoplasia. Nat Genet 2007;39:836–8.

11 Cadigan KM, Peifer M. Wnt signaling from development to disease: insights from model systems. Cold Spring Harb Perspect Biol 2009;1:a002881.

12 Ahmad W, Irvine AD, Lam H et al. A missense mutation in the zinc finger domain of the human hairless gene underlies congenital atrichia in a family of Irish travelers. Am J Hum Genet 1998;63:984–91.

13 **Ahmad W, Haque MF, Brancolini V et al. Alopecia universalis associated with a mutation in the human hairless gene. Science 1998;279:720–4.**

14 Thompson CC, Sisk JM, Beaudoin GM. Hairless and wnt signaling: allies in epithelial stem cell differentiation. Cell Cycle 2006;5:1913–17.

15 Clements SE. Importance of PORCN and Wnt signaling pathways in embryogenesis. Am J Med Genet A 2009;149A:2050–1.

16 Miller J, Djabali K, Chen T et al. Atrichia caused by mutations in the vitamin D receptor gene is a phenocopy of generalized atrichia caused by mutations in the hairless gene. J Invest Dermatol 2001;117:612–17.

17 Okuyama R, Tagami H, Aiba S. Notch signaling: its role in epidermal homeostasis and in the pathogenesis of skin diseases. J Dermatol Sci 2008;49:187–94.

18 Fried K. Autosomal recessive hydrotic ectodermal dysplasia. J Med Genet 1977;14:137–9.
19 Fadhil M, Ghabra TA, Deeb M et al. Odontoonychodermal dysplasia: a previously apparently undescribed ectodermal dysplasia. Am J Med Genet 1983;14:335–46.
20 Mégarbané A, Noujeim Z, Fabre M et al. New form of hidrotic ectodermal dysplasia in a Lebanese family. Am J Med Genet 1998;75:196–9.
21 Mégarbané H, Haddad M, Delague V et al. Further delineation of the odonto-onycho-dermal dysplasia syndrome. Am J Med Genet 2004;129A:193–7.
22 Arnold WP, Merkx MA, Steijlen PM. Variant of odontoonychodermal dysplasia? Am J Med Genet 1995;59:242–4.
23 Zirbel GM, Ruttum MS, Post AC et al. Odonto-onycho-dermal dysplasia. Br J Dermatol 1995;133:797–800.
24 Adams BB. Odonto-onycho-dermal dysplasia syndrome. J Am Acad Dermatol 2007;57:732–3.
25 Schöpf E, Schulz HJ, Passarge E. Syndrome of cystic eyelids, palmo-plantar keratosis, hypodontia and hypotrichosis as a possible autosomal recessive trait. Birth Defects Orig Artic Ser 1971;VII:219–21.
26 Küster W, Hammerstein W. Das Schöpf-Syndrom. Hautarzt 1992; 43:763–6.
27 Craigen WJ, Levy ML, Lewis RA. Schöpf-Schulz-Passarge syndrome with an unusual pattern of inheritance. Am J Med Genet 1997;71:186–8.
28 Starink TM. Eccrine syringofibroadenoma: multiple lesions representing a new cutaneous marker of the Schöpf syndrome, and solitary nonhereditary tumors. J Am Acad Dermatol 1997; 36:569–76.
29 Font RL, Stone MS, Schanzer MC et al. Apocrine hidrocystomas of the lids, hypodontia, palmarplantar hyperkeratosis, and onychodystrophy: a new variant of ectodermal dysplasia. Arch Ophthalmol 1986;104:1811–13.
30 Szepetiuk G, Vanhooteghem O, Muller G et al. Schöpf-Schulz-Passarge syndrome with pili torti: a new association? Eur J Dermatol 2009;19:517–18.
31 Castori M, Ruggieri S, Giannetti L et al. Schöpf-Schulz-Passarge syndrome: further delineation of the phenotype and genetic considerations. Acta Derm Venereol 2008;88:607–12.
32 Maillaiah U, Dickinson J. Photo essay: bilateral multiple eyelid apocrine hidrocystomas and ectodermal dysplasia. Arch Ophthalmol 2001;119:1866–7.
33 Monk BE, Pieris S, Soni V. Schöpf-Schulz-Passarge syndrome. Br J Dermatol 1992;127:33–5.
34 Nordin H, Mansson T, Svensson A. Familial occurrence of eccrine tumours in a family with ectodermal dysplasia. Acta Dermatol Venereol 1988;68:523–30.
35 Hampton PJ, Angus B, Carmichael AJ. A case of Schöpf-Schulz-Passarge syndrome. Clin Exp Dermatol 2005;30:528–30.
36 Verplancke P, Driessen L, Wynants P et al. The Schöpf-Schulz-Passarge syndrome. Dermatology 1998;196:463–6.
37 Perret C. Schöpf syndrome. Br J Dermatol 1989;120:131–2.
38 Alessi E, Gianotti R, Coggi A. Multiple apocrine hidrocystomas of the eyelids. Br J Dermatol 1997;137:642–5.
39 Leoyklang P, Suphapeetiporn K, Wananukul S et al. Three novel mutations in the PORCN gene underlying focal dermal hypoplasia. Clin Genet 2008;73:373–9.
40 Maas SM, Lombardi MP, van Essen AJ et al. Phenotype and genotype in 17 patients with Goltz-Gorlin syndrome. J Med Genet 2009; 46:716–20.
41 Harmsen MB, Azzarello-Burri S, García González MM et al. Goltz Gorlin (focal dermal hypoplasia) and the microphthalmia with linear skin defects (MLS) syndrome: no evidence of genetic overlap. Eur J Hum Genet 2009;17:1207–15.
42 Tillman WG. Alopecia congenita: report of two families. BMJ 1952;2:428.
43 Ahmad M, Abbas H, Haque S. Alopecia universalis as a single abnormality in an inbred Pakistani kindred. Am J Med Genet 1993;46:369–71.
44 Nöthen MM, Cichon S, Vogt IR et al. A gene for universal congenital alopecia maps to chromosome 8p21–22. Am J Hum Genet 1998; 62:386–90.
45 Sprecher E, Bergman R, Szargel R et al. Atrichia with papular lesions maps to 8p in the region containing the human hairless gene. Am J Med Genet 1998;80:546–50.

Defects in gap junction proteins

Gap junctions facilitate efficient cell–cell communication between all cells in multicellular organisms. This system facilitates a synchronized cellular response to a variety of intercellular signals by regulating the direct passage of low molecular weight metabolites (<1000 Da) and ions between the cytoplasm of adjacent cells [1]. In humans, gap junction channels are formed by a polygenic family of 20 different connexin proteins with a predicted molecular mass of 25–62 kDa. Six connexin units oligomerize to rosette-like hemichannels (connexins) that dock end to end with an apposing cell. Connexins are integral membrane proteins that couple with four α-helical transmembrane domains, two rigid extracellular domains that couple with those of a partner connexin, and three cytoplasmic portions of variable length and sequence that determine connexin specificity and selective channel properties. Gap junction channels may be composed of two similar hemichannels formed by the same type of connexin (homotypic) or two distinct hemichannels, each formed by a different connexin protein (heterotypic) (Fig. 134.15). In addition, each connexin could be assembled from different connexin subunits (heterotypic heterochannels). Each combination of connexins has different qualities of permeability, and this is probably highly significant in terms of function.

Most cell types express more than one type of connexin, but the skin and inner ear have a particularly large number of gap junctions and utilize up to 10 of the 20 different connexin proteins. In the skin, connexins appear to have

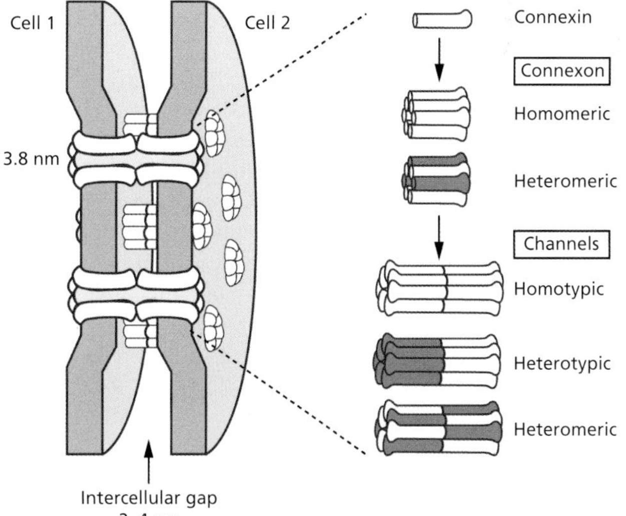

Fig. 134.15 Model of a gap junctional plaque and organization of connexion channels. Six connexin units oligomerize to form a connexon, which is homomeric if the connexins are of the same type or heteromeric if there are different connexins. Connexins of opposing cells dock in the intercellular gap to form a complete connexin channel. These channels are homotypic if both connexons are of the same type, heterotypic if homomeric connexons are of different types and heteromeric if both connexons are heteromeric. Source: Richard G. (2000) [5]. Reproduced with permission of John Wiley & Sons.

SECTION 28: FOCAL OR GENERALIZED HYPOPLASIA

a role in the coordination of keratinocyte growth and differentiation [2]. Connexin genes may be classified in three major groups (*GJA*, *GJB* and *GJC*) based on sequence homology.

Mutations in connexin genes result in hereditary peripheral neuropathy, complex conotruncal heart malformations, autosomal dominant forms of cataract and hearing loss. The first connexin mutations associated with skin disease were identified in *GJB3*, encoding Cx31, leading to erythrokeratodermia variabilis [3]. Mutations associated with distinct skin phenotypes were subsequently identified in three additional genes, *GJB3*, *GJB4* and *GJB6*, encoding the β-connexins Cx26, Cx30.3 and Cx30 respectively [4,5]. Most of these connexins are also expressed in the inner ear, and the relationship between epidermal disease and deafness is complex – three out of the four autosomal dominant connexin mutations that are associated with epidermal disease are also associated with hearing loss.

In 1996, Clouston syndrome was linked to chromosome 13q11–q12.1 [6], and subsequent studies have shown genetic homogeneity to this locus [7–9]. Mutations in *GJB6* encoding the connexin Cx30 were identified in all available kindreds [10]. Several dominant-negative mutations have now been identified within the amino terminus and transmembrane domains of Cx30. Mutations in *GJB6* had previously been identified in a small family with dominant nonsyndromic hearing loss [11], emphasizing the complexity and diversity of phenotypes caused by dominant acting connexin mutations. Mutations may result in reduced protein stability or increased expression leading to cell death [12].

Several dominant-negative mutations have been reported within the first extracellular loop and in the cytoplasmic amino terminus of the closely related Cx26 in patients with the KID syndrome [13]. A D50N mutation in Cx26 is particularly common, and has been associated with a phenotype resembling both KID and Clouston syndromes [14]. Mutations in Cx26 had previously been documented in patients with the mutilating keratoderma Vohwinkel syndrome (see later). To emphasize the overlap in genotype–phenotype correlation in the connexin disorders, patients carrying identical mutations in Cx30 (V37E) have been shown to have classic Clouston syndrome [15] and a KID syndrome-like phenotype [16].

The role of connexins in EDs was further expanded with the identification of mutations in the α-connexin gene, *GJA1*, encoding Cx43, in oculodentodigital dysplasia [17].

Clouston syndrome (hidrotic ED; OMIM #129500)

Definition. Hidrotic ED is an autosomal dominant ED defined by generalized hypotrichosis, dystrophic nails and hyperkeratosis of the palms and soles.

History. This distinct ED is named after Clouston, a doctor in Quebec, Canada, who defined much of what we know about the disorder [18,19]. Several reports describe a large kindred originally from France, who then migrated to Canada, the USA and Scotland [18–22]. Five generations of a large Malaysian-Chinese kindred have also been reported [23].

Pathology. Various abnormal physical properties of the hair shaft have been found, including low disulphide bonded protein content, increased water content, altered birefringence in polarized light, reduced elastic modulus and reduced tensile strength. The hair shaft is abnormally shaped; it may be twisted, small, have longitudinal grooves and be square in cross-section. The pigment may be absent [24]. Cells of the cuticle are atrophic or even absent near the tips of the hair shafts though relatively normal near the base. The cortex of the hair shaft is more fibrillar, coarser and more disorganized than normal hair shafts [24]. Hair follicles in skin biopsies are reduced in number and, when present, may appear dystrophic, with thickened connective tissue sheaths surrounding them [25]. Sebaceous glands are sparse and apocrine glands are sparse or absent. Eccrine glands are normal in number; in one affected individual, a single, rather than a double, layer of eccrine ductal cells was present [25]. Skin biopsy of the palmoplantar thickening shows acanthosis, orthohyperkeratosis and hypergranulosis [25].

Clinical features.

Hair

Scalp hair is sparse, fine, brittle, pale in colour and slow growing. Hair loss may become more pronounced over time and total alopecia can occur (Fig. 134.16a). The eyebrows and eyelashes are thin or absent. Body, pubic and axillary hairs are also affected.

Teeth

The teeth are normal but caries are common.

Nails

Nail dystrophy is characteristic of HED but can be variable. Generally, the nail plate is short, thick, slow growing and discoloured (Fig. 134.17). The nail plate may be completely absent (Fig. 134.16b). Frequent infections of the nailfolds can occur.

Sweat glands

Sweating is normal in affected individuals.

Skin

The skin tends to be dry and rough; it is unclear how this is related to the paucity of sebaceous glands described in some affected individuals. Diffuse, stippled palmar and plantar hyperkeratosis is a frequent finding (Fig. 134.16c), and can be severe. It may extend onto the dorsum of the hands and feet, and fissuring can occur. The skin may also be thickened over the knees, elbows, joints of the fingers and knuckles. Localized hyperpigmentation of the skin is a striking finding and may be found over the knuckles, elbows, axillae, areolae and bony prominences. In the original kindred, cutaneous carcinomas of the nail bed

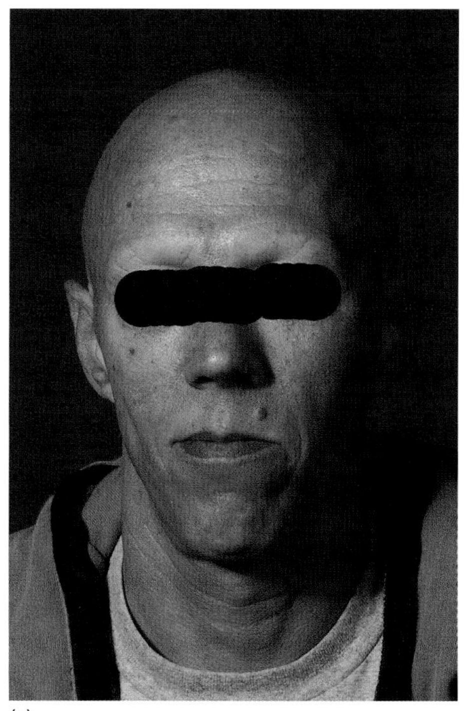
(a)

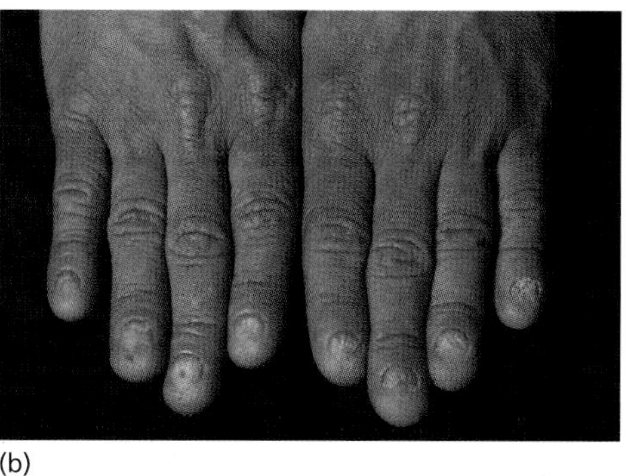
(b)

(c)

Fig. 134.16 (a) Alopecia in a patient with hypohidrotic ectodermal dysplasia (HED). This patient is a descendent of the original family described by Clouston. (b) Dystrophic/absent nails in a patient with HED. (c) Palmoplantar keratoderma in a patient with HED. Source: Courtesy of Dr Audrey Lovett.

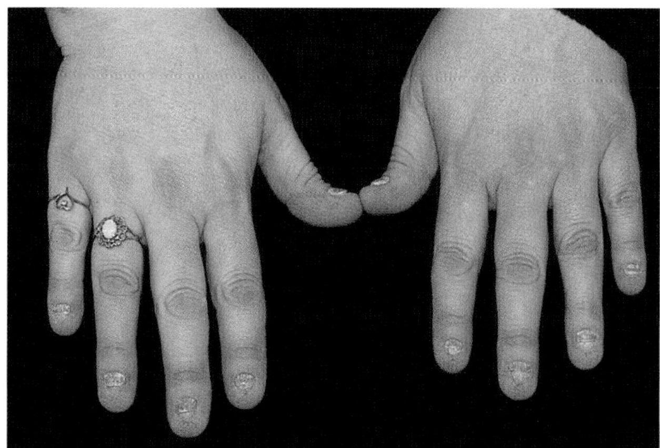

Fig. 134.17 The nail plates are thick, short and discoloured in this individual with hidrotic ectodermal dysplasia.

and palmar tissue were observed in several affected individuals [18,19]. Squamous cell carcinomas, most often subungual, have been reported, as well as one case of subungual melanoma that metastasized [26–28].

Other ectodermal structures

Various eye abnormalities have been described, including conjunctivitis, strabismus and congenital cataract. In one family, five affected individuals developed bilateral premature cataracts [29]. Oral leucoplakia has been described in a number of families [30,31]. Diffuse eccrine poromatosis was reported in one patient [32]. Sensorineural hearing loss has rarely been reported.

Craniofacial features

There are no characteristic craniofacial features. Thickened skull bones have been described.

Other features

Tufting of the terminal phalanges was described in Clouston's original report [18].

Prognosis. The nail and skin dystrophies can become more pronounced over time. Physical development and lifespan are unaffected.

Differential diagnosis. Pachyonychia congenita shares the features of palmoplantar hyperkeratosis, oral leucoplakia and thickened, discoloured nails but the hair is usually normal and the teeth erupt prematurely [31,33]. Individuals with Coffin–Siris syndrome have sparse hair and absent or hypoplastic nails, most notably the fifth fingernail and toenail. They lack the palmoplantar hyperkeratosis, their facial features are characteristic and they have associated mental retardation [30].

Treatment. Nail ablation may sometimes be necessary, emollients for hyperkeratosis sometimes helpful and artificial hairpieces useful in some individuals. Similar to KID syndrome, nonhealing, painful or treatment-resistant lesions should be biopsied to rule out squamous cell carcinoma.

KID syndrome (OMIM 242150)

Definition. The constellation of vascularizing keratitis, ichthyosiform hyperkeratosis and neurosensory deafness is the characteristic feature of KID syndrome. This was probably first reported as early as 1915 [34], with the acronym being coined relatively recently, in 1981 [35]. There is a broad clinical spectrum of manifestations.

Pathology. Biopsy of skin shows nonspecific acanthosis with papillomatosis and basketweave hyperkeratosis. Hair follicles may be atrophic.

Clinical features.

Hair

Alopecia occurs overall in 80% of patients, ranging from minimal loss of eyebrows or eyelashes to total scalp alopecia; in 25% of patients, the alopecia is congenital. An additional 17% of patients have sparse, fine hair without frank alopecia.

Teeth

These show no abnormalities.

Nails

Nails are dystrophic in the majority of patients.

Sweat glands

Sweating may be decreased or absent.

Skin

Patients with KID syndrome are usually born with erythematous or erythrokeratodermatous skin that is mildly scaling; in 7% of patients these skin features develop during the first 4 weeks of life [36]. The sharply demarcated, erythematous plaques are symmetrically distributed on the face and extremities. The characteristic thick, leathery skin with tiny stippled papules develops during the first year of life, particularly during the first 3 months. Well-defined verrucous hyperkeratotic plaques develop in 90% of patients, often localized to the face and limbs. Diffuse palmoplantar hyperkeratosis with a stippled or leathery pattern also occurs in almost all patients; occasionally knuckle pads are noted. After puberty, follicular occlusion syndrome, occasionally with severe acne, may develop, with severe sinuses in the axillae, groin and perianal region. Maternal mosaicism presenting as bilateral blaschkoid, hyperkeratotic, hyperpigmented, linear lesions has been reported [37]. KID can also be inherited from the same mosaic mutations in a parent who has linear porokeratotic eccrine and ostial dermal duct naevus [38].

Other ectodermal structures

Ophthalmological features are progressive and most commonly develop in childhood or early adolescence, although photophobia from birth has been described. The keratoconjunctivitis sicca with corneal vascularization leads to pannus formation and markedly decreased visual acuity. Severity of ocular disease may vary regardless of age. Other symptoms include corneal epithelial defects, thickened and keratinized lids, trichiasis, and presumed limbal insufficiency in one patient. While some patients may be maintained with conservative management, such as close follow up and artificial tears, some may require extensive surgery [39].

Craniofacial features

There are no characteristic cranio-ectodermal features.

Other features

The hearing loss is neurosensory, congenital and nonprogressive. It can be detected in the neonate by brainstem-evoked auditory potential testing. Approximately 45% of patients have recurrent infections, especially bacterial and candidal infections of the skin, auditory canals and eyes. Some patients have shown evidence of immunodeficiency, with moderate increases in IgE levels, defective chemotaxis and absent lymphocyte proliferative responses to *Candida albicans* [40]. Squamous cell carcinoma of the skin and of the tongue has been described in more than 10% of patients, and may occur during childhood. One such case of tongue neoplasm was fatal; the p.Ser17Phe mutation may have a more severe phenotype and could be at higher risk for tongue carcinoma [41]. Malignant pilar tumours, resulting in metastases and death, can also be seen in this condition, and care must be taken to remove tumours at an early stage to prevent poor outcome [42].

Prognosis. Ophthalmological manifestations are progressive; the hearing loss is generally felt not to change with time, but in the authors' experience progressive hearing loss may occur. Vigilance is required for development of squamous carcinoma and pilar tumours. A fatal form of the disease, caused by a G45E mutation, has been described [43].

Differential diagnosis. The stippled PPK and alopecia are reminiscent of Clouston syndrome.

Treatment. Therapy is supportive. Corneal transplants have been successfully performed to treat corneal vascularization. Cochlear implants [44] have been used to treat the hearing loss, but the sustainability of these in persons with such abnormally healing skin has yet to be proven. Oral fluconazole treatment for recalcitrant fungating candidiasis resulted in complete resolution and remission for at least a year [45].

Vohwinkel syndrome (OMIM #124500); PPK associated with hearing loss (OMIM #148350)

Vohwinkel syndrome (VS) is an autosomal dominant mutilating keratoderma characterized by extensive PPK with a distinct 'honeycomb' pattern and constrictions (pseudoainhum) that may lead to amputation of distal digits. In some cases, distinctive hyperkeratotic 'starfish'-like plaques are present over the knuckles. In addition to the epidermal changes, sensorineural deafness is a common accompanying feature and considerable variation has been reported in the penetrance of these characteristics in several families [46–49]. A specific mutation, D66H in the *GJB2* gene (encoding Cx26), has been shown to underlie VS in two families [50]. A variant form of VS that does not present with deafness, mutilating keratoderma with ichthyosis (OMIM #604117), is caused by mutation in the gene for loricrin and is not discussed in this section (please see Chapter 128 for further details). Further genotype–phenotype correlation has emerged as more heterozygous mutations are discovered in families with PPK and deafness. A missense mutation (G59A) in *GJB2* was identified in one family with autosomal dominant PPK and high-frequency hearing loss (classified as OMIM #148350) [51] and a 3 bp deletion has been identified in a further family with deafness and keratoderma. Another mutation, R75W, has been reported as underlying a VS-like phenotype in an Egyptian family [52], whereas the same mutation in another family was associated with hearing loss and a very mild diffuse PPK [53]. A clinically similar condition presenting with progressive sensorineural hearing loss and PPK, with maternal inheritance, is caused by a mitochondrial point mutation in the *MTTS1* gene, encoding mitochondrial transfer RNA for serine [54–57].

Bart–Pumphrey syndrome (OMIM #149200)

The Bart–Pumphrey syndrome [58,59] (knuckle pads, leuconychia and deafness) shares many characteristics with VS and mutations have been found in the first extracellular loop of Cx26 [60].

Oculodentodigital dysplasia (oculodento-osseous dysplasia; OMIM #164200)

Definition. Oculodentodigital dysplasia is characterized by sparse hair, enamel hypoplasia, camptodactyly and characteristic facies with small eyes. The majority of cases display dominant inheritance with variable expressivity although an autosomal recessive form caused by mutations in the same gene, *GJA1*, has been reported [17,61]. Some cases of Hallerman–Streiff syndrome (Francois dyscephalic syndrome; OMIM 234100), are caused by mutations in the same gene [62].

History. The syndrome was originally described by Lohmann in 1920 and more fully defined by Gorlin and colleagues in 1963 [63].

Pathology. Radiographs show shortening of the fifth finger, with a cube-shaped hypoplastic middle phalanx. Despite a normal clinical appearance, radiographs of the feet show hypoplasia or absence of the middle phalanx of one or more toes. Radiographs of the teeth show generalized enamel hypoplasia.

Clinical features [63–68].

Hair

The scalp hair is dry, lustreless and slow growing and can be sparse. The eyebrows and eyelashes may be sparse or absent.

Teeth

All teeth exhibit severe hypoplasia of the enamel. The teeth are friable, small, prone to caries and yellowish in colour. Both primary and secondary teeth are affected.

Nails

Nails are normal, as are the sweat glands and skin.

Other ectodermal structures

Individuals may have microcornea, microphthalmia or both. Variable iris abnormalities have been described.

Craniofacial features

The facies are distinctive, with small palpebral fissures, a long slender nose, hypoplastic alae nasi and prominent columella. Ocular hypertelorism and epicanthal folds are seen in some individuals. The mandible may be large and broad. Minor ear anomalies have been described, such as thin pinnae and bifid ear lobes. Cleft palate has been described in several individuals.

Other abnormalities

Bony anomalies are seen in almost every individual and include hyperostoses of the calvarium, small paranasal sinuses, broad, thick clavicles and ribs, and abnormal trabeculation of the long bones. The most frequent skeletal abnormality is absence of the middle phalanx of the fifth finger. Camptodactyly of the fourth and fifth fingers occurs in over 80% of individuals and syndactyly of the fourth and fifth fingers and toes may be present but is not a constant feature.

Prognosis. Rare neurological abnormalities have been described owing to spinal cord compression from severe cranial hyperostosis [68]. Despite the associated eye abnormalities, vision is usually normal. Glaucoma is reported in 10–15% of affected individuals [67]. Conductive hearing loss may occur possibly as a result of deformity of the bony ossicles.

Differential diagnosis. Microphthalmos is described in a number of other syndromes but none with the characteristic facies and hair and teeth abnormalities seen in oculodentodigital dysplasia.

Treatment. Syndactyly may require surgical correction.

References

1 Pitts JD. The discovery of metabolic co-operation. Bioessays 1998;20:1047–51.

2 **Choudhry R, Pitts JD, Hodgins MB. Changing patterns of gap junctional intercellular communication and connexin distribution in mouse epidermis and hair follicles during embryonic development. Dev Dyn 1997;210:417–30.**

3 **Richard G, Smith LE, Bailey RA et al. Mutations in the human connexin gene GJB3 cause erythrokeratodermia variabilis. Nat Genet 1998;20:366–9.**

4 **Kelsell DPWL, Houseman MJ. Connexin mutations in skin disease and hearing loss. Am J Hum Genet 2001;68:559–68.**

5 **Richard G. Connexins: a connection with the skin. Exp Dermatol 2000;9:77–96.**

6 Kibar Z, Der Kaloustian VM, Brais B et al. The gene responsible for Clouston hidrotic ectodermal dysplasia maps to the pericentromeric region of chromosome 13q. Hum Mol Genet 1996;5:543–7.

7 Radhakrishna U, Blouin JL, Mehenni H et al. The gene for autosomal dominant hidrotic ectodermal dysplasia (Clouston syndrome) in a large Indian family maps to the 13q11–q12.1 pericentromeric region. Am J Med Genet 1997;71:80–6.

8 Taylor TD, Hayflick SJ, McKinnon W et al. Confirmation of linkage of Clouston syndrome (hidrotic ectodermal dysplasia) to 13q11–q12.1 with evidence for multiple independent mutations. J Invest Dermatol 1998;111:83–5.
9 Kibar Z, Dube MP, Powell J et al. Clouston hidrotic ectodermal dysplasia (HED): genetic homogeneity, presence of a founder effect in the French Canadian population and fine genetic mapping. Eur J Hum Genet 2000;8:372–80.
10 Lamartine J, Munhoz Essenfelder G, Kibar Z et al. Mutations in GJB6 cause hidrotic ectodermal dysplasia. Nat Genet 2000; 26:142–4.
11 Grifa A, Wagner CA, d'Ambrosio L et al. Mutations in GJB6 cause nonsyndromic autosomal dominant deafness at DFNA3 locus. Nat Genet 1999;23:16–18.
12 Terrinoni A, Codispoti A, Serra V et al. Connexin 26 (GJB2) mutations as a cause of the KID syndrome with hearing loss, Biochem Biophys Res Commun 2010;395:25–30.
13 Richard G, Rouan F, Willoughby CE et al. Missense mutations in GJB2 encoding connexin-26 cause the ectodermal dysplasia keratitis–ichthyosis–deafness syndrome. Am J Hum Genet 2002;70: 341–8.
14 Markova TG, Brazhkina NB, Bliznech EA et al. Phenotype in a patient with p.D50N mutation in GJB2 gene resembles both KID and Clouston syndromes. Int J Pediatr Otorhinolaryngol. 2016;81:10–14.
15 Smith FJD, Morely SM, McLean WH. A novel connexin 30 mutation in Clouston syndrome. J Invest Dermatol 2002;118:530–2.
16 Jan AY, Amin S, Ratajczak P et al. Genetic heterogeneity of KID syndrome: identification of a Cx30 gene (GJB6) mutation in a patient with KID syndrome and congenital atrichia. J Invest Dermatol 2004;122:1108–13.
17 Paznekas WA, Boyadjiev SA, Shapiro RE et al. Connexin 43 (GJA1) mutations cause the pleiotropic phenotype of oculodentodigital dysplasia. Am J Hum Genet 2003;72:408–18.
18 Clouston H. A hereditary ectodermal dystrophy. Can Med Assoc J 1929;21:18–31.
19 Clouston H. The major forms of hereditary ectodermal dysplasia (with an autopsy and biopsies on the anhydrotic type). Can Med Assoc J 1939;40:1–7.
20 Joachim H. Hereditary dystrophy of the hair and nails in six generations. Ann Intern Med 1936;10:400–2.
21 Wilkey WD, Stevenson GH. A family with inherited ectodermal dystrophy. Can Med Assoc J 1945;53:226–30.
22 Williams M, Fraser FC. Hydrotic ectodermal dysplasia – Clouston's family revisited. Can Med Assoc J 1967;96:36–8.
23 Rajagopalan K, Tay CH. Hidrotic ectodermal dysplasia: study of a large Chinese pedigree. Arch Dermatol 1977;113:481–5.
24 Escobar V, Goldblatt LI, Bixler D et al. Clouston syndrome: an ultrastructural study. Clin Genet 1983;24:140–6.
25 Pierard GE, van Neste D, Letot B. Hidrotic ectodermal dysplasia. Dermatologica 1979;158:168–74.
26 Campbell CJ, Keokarn T. Squamous-cell carcinoma of the nail bed in epidermal dysplasia. J Bone Joint Surg Am 1966;48:92–9.
27 Mauro JA, Maslyn R, Stein AA. Squamous-cell carcinoma of nail bed in hereditary ectodermal dysplasia. N Y State J Med 1972;72:1065–6.
28 Parhizkar N, Jones VE, McClay EF et al. Metastatic melanoma in a patient with Clouston syndrome successfully treated with isolated hyperthermic limb perfusion. J Cutan Med Surg 2003;7:43–6.
29 Hazen PG, Zamora I, Bruner WE et al. Premature cataracts in a family with hidrotic ectodermal dysplasia. Arch Dermatol 1980;116:1385–7.
30 Levin LS. Dental and oral abnormalities in selected ectodermal dysplasia syndromes. Birth Defects Orig Artic Ser 1988;24:205–27.
31 George DI Jr, Escobar VH. Oral findings of Clouston's syndrome (hidrotic ectodermal dysplasia). Oral Surg Oral Med Oral Pathol 1984;57:258–62.
32 Wilkinson RD, Schopflocher P, Rozenfeld M. Hidrotic ectodermal dysplasia with diffuse eccrine poromatosis. Arch Dermatol 1977; 113:472–6.
33 Freire-Maia N, Pinheiro M. Ectodermal Dysplasias: A Clinical and Genetic Study. New York: Alan R. Liss, 1984.
34 Burns FS. A case of generalized congenital keratoderma with unusual involvement of the eyes, ears and nasal and buccal mucous membranes. J Cutan Dis 1915;33:255–60.
35 Skinner BA, Greist MC, Norins AL. The keratitis, ichthyosis, and deafness (KID) syndrome. Arch Dermatol 1981;117:285–9.
36 Caceres-Rios H, Tamayo-Sanchez L, Duran-Mckinster C et al. Keratitis, ichthyosis, and deafness (KID syndrome): review of the literature and proposal of a new terminology. Pediatr Dermatol 1996;13:105–13.
37 Titeux M, Mendonça V, Décha A et al. Keratitis-ichthyosis-deafness syndrome caused by GJB2 maternal mosaicism. J Invest Dermatol 2009;129:776–9.
38 Easton JA, Donnelly S, Kamps MAF et al. Porokeratotic eccrine nevus may be caused by somatic connexin26 mutations. J Invest Dermatol 2012;132:2184–91.
39 Messmer EM, Kenyon KR, Rittinger O et al. Ocular manifestations of keratitis-ichthyosis-deafness (KID) syndrome. Ophthalmology 2005;112:e1–6.
40 Harms M, Gilardi S, Levy PM et al. KID syndrome (keratitis, ichthyosis, and deafness) and chronic mucocutaneous candidiasis: case report and review of the literature. Pediatr Dermatol 1984;2:1–7.
41 Mazereeuw-Hautier J, Bitoun E, Chevrant-Breton J et al. Keratitis ichthyosis-deafness syndrome: disease expression and spectrum of connexin 26 (GJB2) mutations in 14 patients. Br J Dermatol 2007;156:1015–19.
42 Nyquist GG, Mumm C, Grau R et al. Malignant proliferating pilar tumors arising in KID syndrome: a report of two patients. Am J Med Genet A 2007;143:734–41.
43 Janecke AR, Hennies HC, Günther B et al. GJB2 mutations in keratitis ichthyosis-deafness syndrome including its fatal form. Am J Med Genet A 2005;133A:128–31.
44 Hampton SM, Toner JG, Small J. Cochlear implant extrusion in a child with keratitis, ichthyosis and deafness syndrome. J Laryngol Otol 1997;111:465–7.
45 Shiraishi S, Murakami S, Miki Y. Oral fluconazole treatment of fungating candidiasis in the keratitis, ichthyosis and deafness (KID) syndrome. Br J Dermatol 1994;131:904–7.
46 Fitzgerald DA, Verbov JL. Hereditary palmoplantar keratoderma with deafness. Br J Dermatol 1996;134:939–42.
47 Crosby EF, Vidurrizaga RH. Knuckle pads, leukonychia, deafness, and keratosis palmoplantaris: report of a family. Johns Hopkins Med J 1976;139(Suppl):90–2.
48 Hatamochi A, Nakagawa S, Ueki H et al. Diffuse palmoplantar keratoderma with deafness. Arch Dermatol 1982;118:605–7.
49 Sharland M, Bleach NR, Goberdhan PD et al. Autosomal dominant palmoplantar hyperkeratosis and sensorineural deafness in three generations. J Med Genet 1992;29:50–2.
50 Kelsell DP, Wilgoss AL, Richard G et al. Connexin mutations associated with palmoplantar keratoderma and profound deafness in a single family. Eur J Hum Genet 2000;8:141–4.
51 Heathcote K, Syrris P, Carter ND et al. A connexin 26 mutation causes a syndrome of sensorineural hearing loss and palmoplantar hyperkeratosis (MIM 148350). J Med Genet 2000;37:50–1.
52 Richard G, White TW, Smith LE et al. Functional defects of Cx26 resulting from a heterozygous missense mutation in a family with dominant deaf-mutism and palmoplantar keratoderma. Hum Genet 1998;103:393–9.
53 Loffeld A, Kelsell DP, Moss C. Palmoplantar keratoderma and sensorineural deafness in an 8-year old boy: a case report. Br J Dermatol 2000;143(Suppl. 57):38.
54 Reid FM, Vernham GA, Jacobs HT. Complete mtDNA sequence of a patient in a maternal pedigree with sensorineural deafness. Hum Mol Genet 1994;3:1435–6.
55 Fischel-Ghodsian N, Prezant TR, Fournier P et al. Mitochondrial mutation associated with nonsyndromic deafness. Am J Otolaryngol 1995;16:403–8.
56 Hatamochi A, Nakagawa S, Ueki H et al. Diffuse palmoplantar keratoderma with deafness. Arch Dermatol 1982;118:605–7.
57 Martin L, Toutain A, Guillen C et al. Inherited palmoplantar keratoderma and sensorineural deafness associated with A7445G point mutation in the mitochondrial genome. Br J Dermatol 2000;143:876–83.
58 Bart RS, Pumphrey RE. Knuckle pads, leukonychia and deafness. A dominantly inherited syndrome. N Engl J Med 1967;276:202–7.
59 Ramer JC, Vasily DB, Ladda RL. Familial leuconychia, knuckle pads, hearing loss, and palmoplantar hyperkeratosis: an additional family with Bart–Pumphrey syndrome. J Med Genet 1994;31:68–71.
60 Richard G, Brown N, Ishida-Yamamoto A et al. Expanding the phenotypic spectrum of Cx26 disorders: Bart–Pumphrey syndrome is caused by a novel missense mutation in GJB2. J Invest Dermatol 2004;123:856–63.
61 Richardson RJ, Joss S, Tomkin S et al. A nonsense mutation in the first transmembrane domain of connexin 43 underlies autosomal recessive oculodentodigital syndrome. J Med Genet 2006;43:e37.
62 Pizzuti A, Flex E, Mingarelli R et al. A homozygous GJA1 gene mutation causes a Hallermann-Streiff/ODDD spectrum phenotype. Hum Mutat 2004;23:286.

63 Gorlin RJ, Meskin LH, St Geme JW. Oculodentodigital dysplasia. J Pediatr 1963;63:69–75.
64 Reisner SH, Kott E, Bornstein B et al. Oculodentodigital dysplasia. Am J Dis Child 1969;118:600–7.
65 Eidelman E, Chosack A, Wagner ML. Orodigitofacial dysostosis and oculodentodigital dysplasia. Two distinct syndromes with some similarities. Oral Surg Oral Med Oral Pathol 1967;23:311–19.
66 Gillespie FD. A hereditary syndrome: 'dysplasia oculodentodigitalis'. Arch Ophthalmol 1964;71:187–92.
67 Judisch GF, Martin-Casals A, Hanson JW et al. Oculodentodigital dysplasia. Four new reports and a literature review. Arch Ophthalmol 1979;97:878–84.
68 Beighton P, Hamersma H, Raad M. Oculodento-osseous dysplasia: heterogeneity or variable expression? Clin Genet 1979;16:169–77.

Disorders caused by mutations in structural and adhesive molecules

A number of EDs are caused by mutations in epithelial structural proteins (cytokeratins) or adhesive molecules (desmosomal components).

Cytokeratins: overview of basic biology

The cytoplasm of animal cells is structured by scaffolding composed of actin microfilaments, microtubules and intermediate filaments. Intermediate filaments are so named because their 7–10nm diameter is intermediate between that of microfilaments such as actin (6nm) and microtubules such as tubulin (23nm). The intermediate filaments have long been presumed to have a predominantly structural function, a role that was clarified when human epithelial fragility syndromes became attributed to mutations within epidermal keratin genes (type I and II intermediate filament proteins). Keratins are expressed specifically in the cytoplasm of epithelial cells, where they form a dense meshwork of 10nm filaments [1]. More than 30 cytokeratins and trichocyte keratins ('hard' or hair/nail keratins) have been identified to date, and it is thought that several more remain to be discovered. Keratins are expressed as obligate heterodimers of type I/type II pairs in a tissue- and differentiation-specific fashion [2]. Keratins form type I–type II heterodimers [3,4], whereas type III intermediate filaments such as desmin and vimentin form homopolymers.

Keratins were initially characterized by immunohistochemical techniques that allowed their subclassification into some 30 different types [5]. It was soon recognized that these keratins were coexpressed in pairs that showed great tissue specificity [6,7]. Variations in the head and tail domains largely account for differences between the individual keratin proteins within each type and may account for functional fine tuning between the different keratin pairs. K8 (type II) and K18 (type I), thought to be the oldest keratin pair in evolutionary terms [8,9], form the first embryonic keratins expressed in the oocyte and preimplantation blastocyst. The genes for K8 and K18 are, uniquely for keratin pairs, located on the same chromosome, chromosome 12. The genes encoding other human keratin pairs are spatially separated in two compact gene-dense clusters on chromosomes 12q (type II keratins) and 17q (type I keratins) [1].

The tissue-specific distribution of keratins can be exemplified by the keratin expression profile of the interfollicular epidermis. Keratin 5 (type II) and K14 (type I) are the primary keratins of basal cells in the many types of stratifying squamous epithelia. Throughout the suprabasal keratinocytes of the epidermis, *K5* and *K14* gene expression is downregulated and replaced by *K10* and *K1* expression. From the upper spinous layer outwards, an additional type II keratin, K2e, is also expressed. The reason for the many tissue-specific keratins is unknown but it may involve qualitative requirements for cytoskeleton in differing epithelia and tissue-specific interactive functions that may reside in the head and tail domains. Type II keratins are almost always expressed before their type I partner in differentiating epithelia [10], possibly reflecting a differential stringency in the gene regulation of type I and type II keratins [11].

Since 1991, mutations in several keratin genes have been found to cause a variety of human diseases affecting the epidermis and other epithelial structures. Epidermolysis bullosa simplex was the first keratin disease to be identified, with mutations in both the *K5* and *K14* genes rendering basal epidermal keratinocytes less resilient to trauma and resulting in skin fragility [12–14]. The site and type of amino acid substitution within the keratin protein correlate to a degree with phenotypic severity in this disorder. Since mutations were identified in the basal cell keratins, the total number of keratin genes associated with diseases has risen, and now includes not only hereditary skin disease, but also gastrointestinal and ocular diseases (for review see [15,16]). Pseudofolliculitis barbae (OMIM #612318) is a common condition that is most often seen in African–American males that has recently been shown in association with a polymorphism in the keratin 75 gene, also known as hair follicle keratin 6 [17]. White sponge naevus, an autosomal dominant condition of oral leucokeratosis, is caused by mutations in keratin 3 and 14, and Dowling–Degos disease is caused by mutations in keratin 5 [18–20]. Keratin-related diseases tend to manifest when there is mechanical disturbance, such as friction in palmoplantar keratoderma or shaving against the grain of hair growth in pseudofolliculitis barbae [15]. Many of the keratin disorders, such as epidermolysis bullosa and ichthyoses, are discussed elsewhere in this book.

A complete, regularly updated catalogue of human intermediate filament mutations and their associated phenotype may be accessed at www.interfil.org. Descriptions of specific EDs associated with mutations in human keratin genes follow.

Monilethrix (OMIM #158000)

Monilethrix is an autosomal dominant disorder characterized by varying degrees of alopecia and beaded hairs with an alternating structure of elliptical nodes which represent normal hair shafts and constrictions, known as internodes. Affected hairs show an increased susceptibility to fracturing and weathering. The alopecia shows marked interindividual variation, even between members of the same family, a feature common to most keratin disorders. There may be associated nail abnormalities. The first mutations in a human hair shaft, keratin 86 (trichocyte keratin hHb6), were reported in two families in 1997 [21], as well as mutations in another type II hair keratin, keratin 81 (hHb1) [22], a protein that is coexpressed with hHb6 in cortical trichocytes of the hair shaft. More recently, a mutation in the human hair keratin 83 gene (*hHb3*) was reported in monilethrix [23]. Interestingly, mutations in the gene encoding desmoglein 4 (*DSG4*) have also been found in monilethrix [24].

ED, 'pure' hair-nail type (OMIM #602032)

This ED is significant for lack of involvement of teeth, sweating, skin and nonectodermal structures. Both autosomal dominant and autosomal recessive forms have been described [25–28]. In 2006, a mutation in the highly conserved head domain of the hair matrix and cuticle keratin 85 (*KRT85*; also known as *KRTHB5*) was discovered in a consanguineous Pakistani family with ED [28]. Affected individuals were homozygous for a 233G-A transition in exon 1 of the *KRT85* gene, resulting in an arginine-to-histidine substitution. This family showed autosomal recessive inheritance of total alopecia and congenital nail dystrophy. Nails were small and malformed. Scalp and body hair were absent since birth, including absence of eyebrows and eyelashes, and pubic and axillary hair never developed. Heterozygous individuals had normal hair and nails [28]. The presence of *KRT85* mutations was confirmed in other families with pure hair-nail ED [29]. Homozygosity for a *KRT74* missense variant has also been associated with this type [30]. Other autosomal recessive reports describe pili torti, with broken hairs of scalp, beard, axillary and pubic hair, as well as lack of eyebrows, eyelashes and other body hair. These findings were accompanied by distal onychodysplasia [27]. More recently, homozygous loss-of-function mutations in gene *HOXC13* have been described as a cause of pure hair and nail ED [31].

Autosomal dominant cases of pure hair and nail ED have variable phenotype. Thin, fragile, straight, slow-growing and sparse hair is described over the scalp and body. Severity ranges from complete alopecia of the scalp and body hair, excepting only eyelashes, to mild thinning of scalp hair [26]. Onychodystrophy in this family was mild, with only short, fragile, spoon-shaped nails. The fingernails were more severely affected than the toenails. Others report temporal hypotrichosis, associated with folliculitis decalvans of the neck, and onychodystrophy with micronychia, onychorrhexis and triangular nails [25]. A sporadic case has been reported, which demonstrated nail dystrophy, trichorrhexis nodosa and hypotrichosis that was responsive to 5% minoxidil [32].

Pachyonychia congenita; focal nonepidermolytic PPK; steatocystoma multiplex (OMIM #167200, #167210, #184500 and #600962)

Pachyonychia congenita (PC) describes a group of inherited EDs whose most prominent clinical feature is hypertrophic nail dystrophy. Two main clinical variants of PC are generally recognized: PC-1 (Jadassohn–Lewandowsky syndrome; OMIM #167200) [33] and PC-2 (Jackson–Lawlor syndrome; OMIM #167210) [34]. In PC-1, pachyonychia is accompanied by severe focal PPK and also by features such as angular cheilosis, follicular keratosis, hoarseness and oral leucokeratosis that are not fully penetrant. The PC-2 form is also associated with focal PPK and follicular keratoses but is most readily distinguished by the presence of multiple steatocysts, which appear at puberty. Children with PC-2 may have curly hair. Natal teeth appear to be associated only with the PC-2 form, but this phenotype is also not fully penetrant. Mutations have been identified in differentiation-specific keratins, which are expressed in the particular epithelia affected in each type of PC. Genetic linkage analysis in a large PC-2 family from Glasgow indicated a type I keratin defect [35]. The mutation in this family was later found to be a point mutation in the 1A domain of *KRT17* [35]. PC-1 results from similar mutations in *KRT16* [36]. Another group identified the first mutation in *KRT6A*, the expression partner of *KRT16*, also giving rise to PC-1 [37]. *KRT17* mutations have since been shown to be consistently associated with the PC-2 phenotype [38,39], and a mutation in its expression partner, *KRT6B*, was reported in a PC-2 family [40].

Intra- and interfamilial phenotypic variation has been observed in families carrying mutations in the *KRT16* or *KRT17* genes. *KRT16* mutations can present as focal keratoderma without nail changes or other features of PC-1 [41]. Similarly, *KRT17* mutations have been found in families presenting with steatocystoma multiplex without abnormalities of nails or other ectodermal structures [38,42]. The reason for these phenotypical differences is not clear but appears to be unrelated to the specific genetic mutation and is therefore thought to be caused by the action of additional unknown modifying genes [42]. Recently, a case of late-onset PC-1 was attributed to a novel missense mutation in *KRT6* [43], reinforcing the considerable clinical heterogeneity in this condition. In addition, a mosaic mutation in *KRT16* was shown to underlie a unilateral palmoplantar naevus [44]. A recessive form of PC (OMIM 260130) has been described, but its genetic basis is unknown.

Naegeli–Franceschetti–Jadassohn syndrome (OMIM #161000 dermatopathia pigmentosa reticularis (OMIM #125595)

Both Naegeli–Franceschetti–Jadassohn syndrome (NFJS) and dermatopathia pigmentosa reticularis (DPR) have been associated with mutations in the gene encoding keratin 14 (*KRT14*) [45–47], which may cause increased susceptibility of keratinocytes to apoptosis [48]. NFJS is an autosomal dominant condition, which presents with reticulate pigmentation that begins in the first few years of life. There is also accompanying hypohidrosis, diffuse or punctate PPK and tooth anomalies [49]. Some may also have bullae on the hands and feet at birth, which subsequently resolve. A lack of dermatoglyphs is a singular finding, although it may also be present in several other disorders, including Basan's syndrome and DPR. NFJS may present with tooth enamel defects, with yellow and spotted teeth, caries and early loss of teeth. It also has congenital malalignment of great toenails [49]. In NFJS, the reticulate cutaneous pigmentation disappears with age, decreasing in intensity during the mid-teens and fading almost completely toward the sixth decade of life [49]. Hypohidrosis remains a problem throughout life.

Dermatopathia pigmentosa reticularis is also autosomal dominant in inheritance [50] and similarly presents with onychodystrophy, variable presentation of alopecia and reticulate pigmentation. Hair may be wiry in texture. The other clinical aspects seen in NFJS of palmoplantar keratoderma, adermatoglyphia and nonscarring acral blisters may also be observed in DPR [47,51]. Although NFJS and DPR have many similarities and are probably a spectrum of the same disease, the key difference is the duration of the reticulate pigmentation. While pigmentation fades with time in NFJS, it remains the same in DPR. Patients with DPR appear to lack the tooth involvement seen in NFJS. Digital fibromatous thickening has also been reported in DPR [47]. Patients with DPR may exhibit both hypo- and hyperhidrosis.

The differential diagnosis of these conditions includes other genodermatoses with reticulate hyperpigmentation, especially dyskeratosis congenita and incontinentia pigmenti [52]. See Chapter 139 for further information. The lack of eye findings, X-linked inheritance, malignant leucoplakia and other symptoms should help distinguish these conditions from NFJS and DPR. The PPK and dental anomalies are not present in incontinentia pigmenti, and lack of dermatoglyphs should aid in making the diagnosis of NFJS and DPR. Dowling–Degos disease, caused by a mutation in the keratin 5 gene, also presents with similar reticulate pigmentation, but lacks the hair and nail changes. Pachyonychia congenita may also be considered in the differential diagnosis.

Keratosis palmoplantaris striata type III (PPKS3; OMIM #607654)

This PPK features linear keratosis of the volar surfaces of the hands with more diffuse keratoderma of the feet. It is an autosomal dominant condition, caused by a mutation in keratin 1 [53]. Lesions develop on the palms and soles during early childhood. There is no involvement of hair, nails or nonpalmoplantar skin. Keratosis palmoplantaris striata types I and II are caused by mutations in the desmoglein 1 and desmoplakin genes, respectively, and are discussed below.

Uncombable hair syndrome (UHS 1 OMIM #191480, UHS2 OMIM #617251, UHS3 OMIM #617252)

Uncombable hair syndrome is a rare condition of hair shaft abnormality characterized by silver, blonde, or straw-coloured hair, which tends to improve with age, and is not associated with any other ectodermal features. Recently homozygous or compound heterozygous mutations in three genes have been identified as causative of this phenotype, *TGM3*, *PADI3*, and *TCHH* [54].

Desmosomes: overview of basic biology

Desmosome junctions are present in large numbers in all tissues that experience mechanical stress and are thought to have a primarily structural function (for review see [55,56]). Desmosomes show both tissue- and differentiation-specific expression in epithelia, and their composition changes as cells move towards the surface of stratified squamous epithelia [57,58]. In epithelial tissues, including the skin, they anchor keratin intermediate filaments to the cell membrane; tissue-specific desmosomes perform similar roles in the heart, meningeal cells and follicular dendritic cells of lymph nodes.

Desmosomes are largely formed from proteins encoded by three gene superfamilies: the plakins, which include desmoplakin, plectin and the cell envelope proteins periplakin and envoplakin; the armadillo family proteins including plakoglobin and plakophilins 1–4; and the desmosomal cadherins, which are subdivided into desmogleins 1–4 and desmocollins 1–3 (Fig. 134.18). The structure and combination of components of a desmosome will depend on its localization within a stratified epithelial sheet, because desmosomal components are expressed in a stratification-specific pattern.

Understanding of desmosomes has been, to some extent, based on analogy with the adherens junction–microfilament arrangement. Briefly, intermediate filaments are tethered to the membrane through a linear complex: desmogleins and desmocollins associate with plakoglobin, which in turn binds to desmoplakin, which links intermediate filaments to the membrane. In addition to their well-appreciated structural role, desmosomes may also function as signalling centres. For example, *in vitro* and *in vivo* research indicates that a decrease of plakophilin 2 results in decreased cell surface expression of connexin 43 [59,60].

The role of desmosome protein targets in autoimmune blistering skin disease has long been recognized; more recently, mutations in desmosomal constituent proteins were shown to underlie several single gene disorders. Many of these conditions have abnormal keratinization as a key feature, and are discussed below, whereas others present only in the heart, with cardiomyopathy and sudden death. Mutations in the plakophilin 2 (*PKP2*), plakoglobin (*PG*), desmoplakin (*DSP*), desmoglein 2 (*DSG2*) and desmocollin 2 (*DSC2*) genes have been found in arrhythmogenic right ventricular cardiomyopathy and dysplasia. This is understandable, because considerable tensile strength is required in both skin and heart and the signalling role of desmosomal proteins would explain the abnormal development. Phenotypical variation can be explained by differential desmosomal protein expression both between and within tissue types.

Ectodermal dysplasia/skin fragility syndrome (McGrath syndrome; OMIM #604536)

A recessive skin fragility syndrome has been attributed to homozygous mutations in the *PKP1* gene encoding the accessory desmosomal plaque protein plakophilin 1 [61]. This usually hypohidrotic form of ED is characterized by skin fragility, nail dystrophy and sparse hair. In the first few years of life, patients develop hyperkeratotic plaques on the limbs and palmoplantar keratoderma; a reduced ability to sweat is also noted. Light microscopy of the

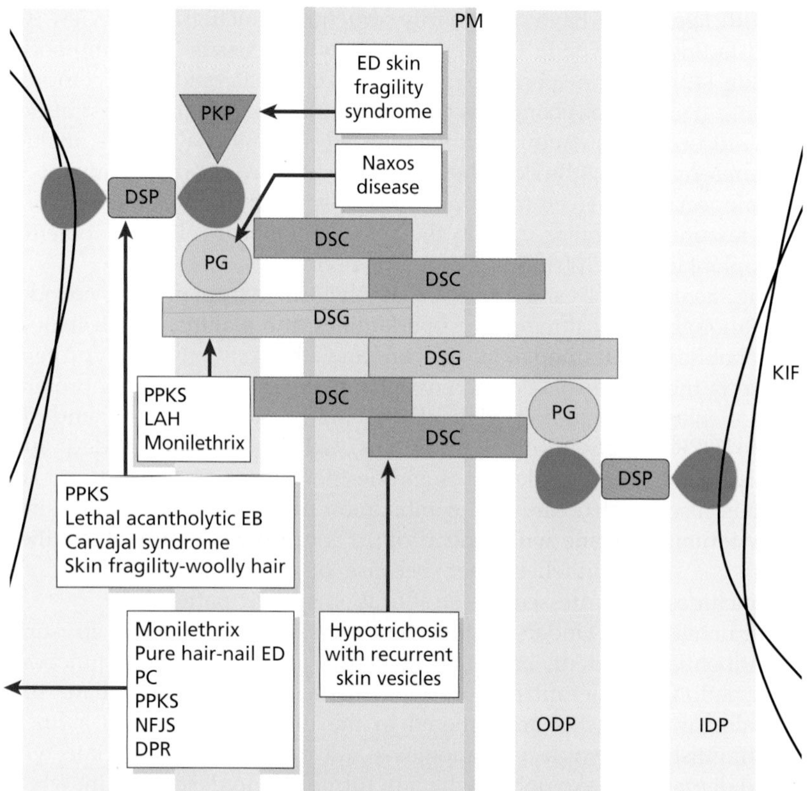

Fig. 134.18 Structure and components of desmosomes and some associated genodermatoses. DPR, dermatopathia pigmentosa reticularis; DSC, desmocollin; DSG, desmoglein; DSP, desmoplakin; ED, ectodermal dysplasia; IDP, inner dense plaque; KIF, keratin intermediate filaments; LAH, localized autosomal recessive hypotrichosis; NFJS, Naegeli-Franceschetti-Jadassohn syndrome; ODP, outer dense plaque; PC, pachyonychia congenita; PG, plakoglobin; PKP, plakophilin; PM, plasma membrane; PPKS, palmoplantar keratoderma, striate. Source: Adapted from Getsios et al. (2004) [54] by permission from Macmillan Publishers Ltd.

skin reveals thickening of the epidermis and extensive widening of keratinocyte intercellular spaces, extending from the first suprabasal layer upward. Plakophilin 1 plays an important role in the recruitment of desmosomal proteins and the stabilization of desmosomes [62]. Electron microscopy shows a loss of keratinocyte–keratinocyte adhesion, and desmosomes, particularly in the lower suprabasal layers, are small and reduced in number. Immunostaining for plakophilin 1 in the skin is negative [61]. Several families and sporadic cases have now been reported [63–68].

Plakophilin 1 is an entirely intracellular protein and has a role in binding desmosomes to the cytoskeleton of keratinocytes; this connection is effected through binding to the intracellular component of desmosomal cadherins, especially desmocollin 1. As a member of the armadillo protein family, plakophilin shares about 25% sequence homology with the other members such as β-catenin, and it is likely that plakophilin also has a role in signal transduction. Plakophilin is preferentially expressed in the spinous layer of the epidermis and in the outer root sheath of hair follicles [69], but is not expressed in cardiac muscle and, accordingly, excepting one case of patent foramen ovale, no cardiac pathology is associated with this condition [70]. Recently, a mutation in the gene encoding desmoplakin (*DSP*) was found to cause a phenotype similar to ED-skin fragility syndrome, associated with early-onset cardiomyopathy. This is understandable, because *DSP* is expressed in cardiac tissue, whereas *PKP1* is not [71].

Naxos disease (PPK with arrhythmogenic right ventricular cardiomyopathy and woolly hair; OMIM #601214)

This autosomal recessive condition was first described in four families on the Greek island of Naxos [72]. Mutations in the *JUP* gene, encoding the desmosomal component plakoglobin, have been shown to underlie this condition [73]. Patients present with a diffuse PPK that appears between 6 and 12 months of age. Hair is rough, dull and bristly in texture and resembles steel wire. The cardiac abnormalities are the most significant part of the phenotype and are commonly known as arrhythmogenic ventricular cardiomyopathy (ARVC) or dysplasia. In a study of 26 affected subjects, 92% showed ECG abnormalities, 92% ventricular arrhythmias, 100% right ventricular structural alterations and 27% left ventricular involvement. During follow up, 16 (62%) developed structural progression, 12 (46%) arrhythmic events and seven (27%) heart failure. The annual disease-related and sudden death mortality rates were 3% and 2.3% respectively [74]. Heterozygotes have a slightly increased rate of echocardiographic abnormalities but are otherwise normal. Short fingers and curved nails were also noted in the original description [72].

A two base-pair (TG) deletion at the 3′ end of the gene results in a frameshift and premature truncation of the C-terminus of plakoglobin in Naxos disease [73] whereas the amino terminus of the protein is affected in the *JUP* mutations causing ARVC with no skin findings [75]. The different areas of protein defect and thus protein function may explain the phenotypical variation caused by mutations in the same protein, and the genetic heterogeneity of ARVC.

In this chapter, we refer to Naxos disease as being the full complement of skin and heart findings. This is in comparison with much of the cardiology literature, which may refer to all types of ARVC or dysplasia related to all desmosomal proteins, both with or without skin findings, as Naxos disease. The genetic heterogeneity of ARVC is further underscored by the recent discovery of an Arabic family with a Naxos-like syndrome, who lacked mutations in multiple desmosomal genes [76]. Regardless of classification, evaluation and follow up by a cardiologist are necessary. If required, possible interventions include implantation of an automatic cardioverter defibrillator for prevention of sudden cardiac death, antiarrhythmic drugs for prevention of ventricular tachycardia, and treatment of congestive heart failure. Heart transplantation may be considered in end-stage disease [77]. Treatment of PPK with physical debridement or topical keratolytics is recommended if symptomatic.

Carvajal syndrome (PPK with left ventricular cardiomyopathy and woolly hair; OMIM #605676); skin-fragility–woolly hair syndrome (OMIM #607655); keratosis palmoplantaris striata type II (PPKS2; OMIM #612908)

Carvajal syndrome was first described by Carvajal-Huerta in Ecuador in 1998 [78]. These patients were found to have woolly hair at birth, PPK and cardiac abnormalities, similar to Naxos disease, and are considered by some to have a variant of Naxos disease. However, the original report describes a left ventricular rather than right-sided cardiomyopathy, and a striate epidermolytic PPK rather than diffuse. Keratoses of the palms and soles begin to appear at approximately 10 months of age and are striate, starting at the wrists and extending down the ventral fingers. Patients also have follicular keratoses on the elbows and knees or scattered across the abdomen and lower limbs, and fingernail clubbing. Transient pruritic vesicles and blisters and psoriasiform keratosis were also described [78]. Management is similar to that discussed above for Naxos disease.

This condition is caused by a mutation in the gene coding for desmoplakin, *DSP* [79]. Desmoplakin is one of the main components of desmosomes, and has two splice variants [80]. *DSP* mutations have also been reported in striate PPK [81,82], as well as skin fragility and woolly hair [83]. A lethal acantholytic form of epidermolysis bullosa has also been described with *DSP* mutations [84,85], indicating that the C-terminus and rod domain of the desmoplakin protein are required for function of the inner dense plaque of desmosomes. This variable clinical presentation sheds light on the function of the desmoplakin protein. Haploinsufficiency of desmoplakin leads to striate PPK alone [81].

Loss of the type I splice variant results in right ventricular cardiomyopathy with woolly hair and epidermolytic PPK [86]. While desmoplakin is necessary for life, disturbance in the rod domain and C terminus causes lethal acantholytic EB [84,85]. Similarly, acantholysis is seen in a reported 'Naxos-like syndrome', which presents with arrhythmogenic right ventricular dysplasia, woolly hair, dry skin and vesicular acral lesions which show acantholysis on biopsy [87]. This presentation was caused by a C-terminal mutation in desmoplakin, close to the binding sites of the keratin filaments. Compound heterozygosity of nonsense and missense mutations results in skin fragility–woolly hair syndrome [83], and a *DSP* mutation has been found to cause a phenotype similar to ED-skin fragility syndrome [71].

Keratosis palmoplantaris striata type I (PPKS3; OMIM #148700)

This type of striate PPK is clinically similar to types II and III, with linear keratoderma of the volar surfaces of the hands and feet, inherited in autosomal dominant fashion. It is caused by mutations in the desmoglein 1 gene (*DSG1*), which affects the highly conserved extracellular region, leading to a null mutation or a truncated protein [88,89]. This type of PPK may be histologically differentiated from other types by widening of the intercellular spaces and disadhesion of keratinocytes in the suprabasal epidermis [90].

Localized autosomal recessive hypotrichosis, type 1 (OMIM #607903)

Localized autosomal recessive hypotrichosis, type 1 (LAH1) is an autosomal recessive condition caused by mutations in *DSG4*, which encodes desmoglein 4 [91], and in which mutations are also a rare cause of monilethrix [92]. LAH is characterized by hypotrichosis of the scalp and body hair. Facial hair may be spared, although eyebrows and eyelashes are usually thin. Axillary and pubic hair is generally normal. Small papules on the scalp, similar to ingrown hairs, are visible and show abnormal hair follicles and shafts that are unable to penetrate the dermis, and are coiled up as a result [91]. Follicular keratoses have been reported, but may be an incidental finding [93]. Comedo-like structures, reminiscent of follicles, may be present on biopsy [94]. Teeth, sweating and hearing are normal [95]. However, phenotype can vary greatly, even within the same kindred [96].

Two other clinically similar forms, localized autosomal recessive hypotrichosis type 2 (LAH2; OMIM #604379) and type 3 (LAH3; OMIM #278150) are known. LAH2 is caused by mutations in lipase (*LIPH*), thought to be involved in cell proliferation [97,98]. *P2RY5* encodes a G protein-coupled receptor, probably involved in cell signalling, which is the cause of LAH3 [94,99,100].

Hypotrichosis and recurrent skin vesicles (OMIM #613102)

This autosomal recessive condition was described in a consanguineous Afghan pedigree in 2009 [101]. Hairs are present at birth and regrow after ritual shaving. At approximately 2–3 months of age, however, increased hair loss is noted, resulting in sparse and fragile scalp hair, eyebrows and eyelashes. Axillary and body hair are also affected. Although teeth, nails and sweating appear normal, vesicles less than 1 cm in size are apparent on the scalp and skin. These burst then heal over 3–4 months. Homozygous nonsense mutations of the desmocollin 3 gene (*DSC3*) have been found in affected individuals [101].

Hypotrichosis simplex of the scalp (OMIM #146520)

Hypotrichosis simplex of the scalp was first described by Toribio and Quiñones in 1974 [102]. In this autosomal dominant condition, hair is usually normal at birth, with a progressive loss with age, although some may have absence of hair at birth [103]. Hair thinning generally begins in the first decade of life, with complete hair loss by the third decade [102–105]. Eyebrows and lashes, beard, axillary and pubic hair are normal. No other tooth, nail or other ectodermal structures are affected. This condition was mapped to 6p21 [104] and nonsense mutations in the gene encoding corneodesmosin (*CDSN*) were found shortly thereafter [106]. Corneodesmosin is a skin barrier protein most notably studied as a candidate gene for psoriasis. It plays a role in terminal differentiation and the epidermal barrier as well as hair regulation [107], although its function is yet to be fully elucidated. Recently, biallelic mutations in gene *LSS* encoding lanosterol synthase have also been found to cause hypotrichosis simplex [108].

Other molecules involved in cell-to-cell adhesion: hypotrichosis with juvenile macular degeneration (OMIM #601553)

Hypotrichosis with juvenile macular dystrophy (HJMD) is an autosomal recessive condition described in the Druze, a Muslim minority population living in northern Israel. Affected individuals are born with apparently normal hair but develop alopecia of the scalp at around 3 months. There is partial regrowth during puberty. The second feature is progressive macular degeneration with slight peripheral retinal dystrophy. A frameshift mutation leading to a premature stop codon and a missense mutation in the *CDH3* gene encoding P-cadherin, have been identified in affected families [109,110]. The exact mechanism by which these mutations cause HJMD is not clear, but classic cadherins have a role in maintaining cell–cell adhesion through Ca^2-dependent homophilic interactions. Another similar condition, ED, ectrodactyly, muscular dystrophy syndrome (EEM syndrome; OMIM #225280) is also caused by mutations in *CDH3* [111].

Desmosomes, integrins and cadherins are not the sole molecules involved in cell adhesion; poliovirus receptor-like 1 (*PVRL1*) codes for nectin 1, a transmembrane cell–cell adhesion molecule that is part of the NAP cell adhesion system. A mutation in the gene encoding this protein causes cleft-lip-palate-ED syndrome (OMIM #225060) [112].

SECTION 28: FOCAL OR GENERALIZED HYPOPLASIA

References

1 **Quinlan RA, Hutchison CJ, Lane EB. Intermediate filaments. In: Sheterline P (ed.) Protein Profiles. London: Academic Press, 1994.**

2 **Lane EB. Keratins. In: Royce PM, Steinmann B (eds) Connective Tissue and its Heritable Disorders. Molecular, Genetic and Medical Aspects. New York: Wiley-Liss, 1993:237–47.**

3 Hatzfeld M, Weber K. The coiled coil of in vitro assembled keratin filaments is a heterodimer of type I and II keratins: use of sitespecific mutagenesis and recombinant protein expression. J Cell Biol 1990;110:1199–210.

4 Steinert PM. The two-chain coiled-coil molecule of native epidermal keratin intermediate filaments is a type I-type II heterodimer. J Biol Chem 1990;265:8766–74.

5 **Moll R, Franke WW, Schiller DL et al. The catalog of human cytokeratins: patterns of expression in normal epithelia, tumors and cultured cells. Cell 1982;31:11–24.**

6 Fuchs E, Green H. Changes in keratin gene expression during terminal differentiation of the keratinocyte. Cell 1980;19:1033–42.

7 Sun T-T, Eichner R, Schermer A et al. Classification, Expression and Possible Mechanisms of Evolution of Mammalian Epithelial Keratins: A Unifying Model. Cold Spring Harbor Laboratory, NY: Cold Spring Harbor Laboratory Press, 1984.

8 Oshima RG, Howe WE, Klier G et al. Intermediate filament protein synthesis in preimplantation murine embryos. Dev Biol 1983; 99:447–55.

9 Waseem A, Alexander CM, Steel JB et al. Embryonic simple epithelial keratins 8 and 18: chromosomal location emphasizes difference from other keratin pairs. New Biol 1990;2:464–78.

10 Roop DR, Huitfeldt H, Kilkenny A et al. Regulated expression of differentiation-associated keratins in cultured epidermal cells detected by monospecific antibodies to unique peptides of mouse epidermal keratins. Differentiation 1987;35:143–50.

11 Stasiak PC, Purkis PE, Leigh IM et al. Keratin 19: predicted amino acid sequence and broad tissue distribution suggest it evolved from keratinocyte keratins. J Invest Dermatol 1989;92:707–16.

12 **Bonifas JM, Rothman AL, Epstein EH Jr. Epidermolysis bullosa simplex: evidence in two families for keratin gene abnormalities. Science 1991;254:1202–5.**

13 Coulombe PA, Hutton ME, Letai A et al. Point mutations in human keratin 14 genes of epidermolysis bullosa simplex patients: genetic and functional analyses. Cell 1991;66:1301–11.

14 Lane EB, Rugg EL, Navsaria H et al. A mutation in the conserved helix termination peptide of keratin 5 in hereditary skin blistering. Nature 1992;356:244–6.

15 Irvine AD, McLean WH. Human keratin diseases: the increasing spectrum of disease and subtlety of the phenotype-genotype correlation. Br J Dermatol 1999;140:815–28.

16 **Arin MJ. The molecular basis of human keratin disorders. Hum Genet 2009;125:355–73.**

17 Winter H, Schissel D, Parry DA et al. An unusual ala12thr polymorphism in the 1A alpha-helical segment of the companion layerspecific keratin K6hf: evidence for a risk factor in the etiology of the common hair disorder pseudofolliculitis barbae. J Invest Dermatol 2004;122:652–7.

18 Richard G, de Laurenzi V, Didona B et al. Keratin 13 point mutation underlies the hereditary mucosal epithelia disorder white sponge nevus. Nat Genet 1995;11:453–5.

19 Rugg EL, McLean WH, Allison WE et al. A mutation in the mucosal keratin K4 is associated with oral white sponge nevus. Nat Genet 1995;11:450–2.

20 **Betz RC, Planko L, Eigelshoven S et al. Loss-of-function mutations in the keratin 5 gene lead to Dowling–Degos disease. Am J Hum Genet 2006;78:510–19.**

21 **Winter H, Rogers MA, Langbein L et al. Mutations in the hair cortex keratin hHb6 cause the inherited hair disease monilethrix. Nat Genet 1997;16:372–4.**

22 Winter H, Labrèze C, Chapalain V et al. A variable monilethrix phenotype associated with a novel mutation, Glu402Lys, in the helix termination motif of the type II hair keratin hHb1. J Invest Dermatol 1998;111:169–72.

23 Van Steensel MA, Steijlen PM, Bladergroen RS et al. A missense mutation in the type II hair keratin hHb3 is associated with monilethrix. J Med Genet 2005;42:e19.

24 Zlotogorski A, Marek D, Horev L et al. An autosomal recessive form of monilethrix is caused by mutations in DSG4: clinical overlap with localized autosomal recessive hypotrichosis. J Invest Dermatol 2006;126:1292–6.

25 Barbareschi M, Cambiaghi S, Crupi AC et al. Family with 'pure' hair-nail ectodermal dysplasia. Am J Med Genet 1997;72:91–3.

26 **Pinheiro M, Freire-Maia N. Hair-nail dysplasia – a new pure autosomal dominant ectodermal dysplasia. Clin Genet 1992;41:296–8.**

27 Calzavara-Pinton P, Carlino A, Benetti A et al. Pili torti and onychodysplasia: report of a previously undescribed hidrotic ectodermal dysplasia. Dermatologica 1991;182:184–7.

28 Naeem M, Wajid M, Lee K et al. A mutation in the hair matrix and cuticle keratin KRTHB5 gene causes ectodermal dysplasia of hair and nail type (letter). J Med Genet 2006;43:274–9.

29 Shimomura Y, Wajid M, Kurban M et al. Mutations in the keratin 85 (KRT85/hHb5) gene underlie pure hair and nail ectodermal dysplasia. J Invest Dermatol 2010;130:892–5.

30 Raykova D et al. Autosomal recessive transmission of a rare KRT74 variant causes hair and nail ectodermal dysplasia: allelism with dominant woolly hair/hypotrichosis. PLoS One 2014;9:e93607.

31 Lin Z, Chen Q, Shi L et al. Loss-of-function mutations in HOXC13 cause pure hair and nail ectodermal dysplasia. Am J Human Genet 2012;91:906–11.

32 Harrison S, Sinclair R. Hypotrichosis and nail dysplasia: a novel hidrotic ectodermal dysplasia. Australas J Dermatol 2004;45:103–5.

33 Jadassohn J, Lewandowsky F. Pachyonychia congenita. In: Jacobs Ikonographia Dermatologica. Berlin: Urban and Schwarzenberg, 1906: 29.

34 Jackson ADM, Lawler SD. Pachyonychia congenita: a report of six cases in one family. Ann Eugen 1951;16:142–6.

35 Munro CS, Carter S, Bryce S et al. A gene for pachyonychia congenita is closely linked to the keratin gene cluster on 17q12–q21. J Med Genet 1994;31:675–8.

36 McLean WH, Rugg EL, Lunny DP et al. Keratin 16 and keratin 17 mutations cause pachyonychia congenita. Nat Genet 1995;9:273–8.

37 Bowden PE, Haley JL, Kansky A et al. Mutation of a type II keratin gene (K6a) in pachyonychia congenita. Nat Genet 1995;10:363–5.

38 Smith FJD, Corden LD, Rugg EL et al. Mutations in keratin-17 cause steatocystoma multiplex. J Invest Dermatol 1996;106:225.

39 Smith FJ, Corden LD, Rugg EL et al. Missense mutations in keratin 17 cause either pachyonychia congenita type 2 or a phenotype resembling steatocystoma multiplex. J Invest Dermatol 1997;108:220–3.

40 Smith FJ, Jonkman MF, van Goor H et al. A mutation in human keratin K6b produces a phenocopy of the K17 disorder pachyonychia congenita type 2. Hum Mol Genet 1998;7:1143–8.

41 Shamsher MK, Navsaria HA, Stevens HP et al. Novel mutations in keratin 16 gene underlie focal non-epidermolytic palmoplantar keratoderma (NEPPK) in two families. Hum Mol Genet 1995;4:1875–81.

42 Covello SP, Smith FJ, Sillevis Smitt JH et al. Keratin 17 mutations cause either steatocystoma multiplex or pachyonychia congenita type 2. Br J Dermatol 1998;139:475–80.

43 Connors JB, Rahil AK, Smith FJ et al. Delayed-onset pachyonychia congenita associated with a novel mutation in the central 2B domain of keratin 16. Br J Dermatol 2001;144:1058–62.

44 Terrinoni A, Puddu P, Didona B et al. A mutation in the V1 domain of K16 is responsible for unilateral palmoplantar verrucous nevus. J Invest Dermatol 2000;114:1136–40.

45 Lugassy J, Itin P, Ishida-Yamamoto A et al. Naegeli–Franceschetti–Jadassohn syndrome and dermatopathia pigmentosa reticularis: two allelic ectodermal dysplasias caused by dominant mutations in KRT14. Am J Hum Genet 2006;79:724–30.

46 Van Steensel MA, Lemmink HH. A missense mutation in KRT14 causing a dermatopathia pigmentosa reticularis/Naegeli–Franceschetti–Jadassohn phenotype. J Eur Acad Dermatol Venereol 2010;24:1116–17.

47 Goh BK, Common JE, Gan WH et al. A case of dermatopathia pigmentosa reticularis with wiry scalp hair and digital fibromatosis resulting from a recurrent KRT14 mutation. Clin Exp Dermatol 2009;34:340–3.

48 Lugassy J, McGrath JA, Itin P et al. KRT14 haploinsufficiency results in increased susceptibility of keratinocytes to TNF-alpha-induced apoptosis and causes Naegeli–Franceschetti–Jadassohn syndrome. J Invest Dermatol 2008;128:1517–24.

49 Itin PH, Lautenschlager S, Meyer R et al. Natural history of the Naegeli–Franceschetti–Jadassohn syndrome and further delineation of its clinical manifestations. J Am Acad Dermatol 1993;28:942–50.

50 Heimer WL, Brauner G, James WD. Dermatopathia pigmentosa reticularis: a report of a family demonstrating autosomal dominant inheritance. J Am Acad Dermatol 1992;26:298–301.

51 Brar BK, Mehta V, Kubba A. Dermatopathia pigmentosa reticularis. Pediatr Dermatol 2007;24:566–70.

52 Itin PH, Lautenschlager S. Genodermatosis with reticulate, patchy and mottled pigmentation of the neck – a clue to rare dermatologic disorders. Dermatology 1998;197:281–90.

53 Whittock NV, Smith FJ, Wan H et al. Frameshift mutation in the V2 domain of human keratin 1 results in striate palmoplantar keratoderma. J Invest Dermatol 2002;118:838–44.

54 FB UB, Cau L, Tafazzoli A et al. Mutations in three genes encoding proteins involved in hair shaft formation cause uncombable hair syndrome. Am J Human Genet 2016;99:1292–304.

55 Green KJ, Gaudry CA. Are desmosomes more than tethers for intermediate filaments? Nat Rev Mol Cell Biol 2000;1:208–16.

56 Getsios S, Huen AC, Green KJ. Working out the strength and flexibility of desmosomes. Nat Rev Mol Cell Biol 2004;5:271–81.

57 Schmidt A, Heid HW, Schafer S et al. Desmosomes and cytoskeletal architecture in epithelial differentiation: cell type-specific plaque components and intermediate filament anchorage. Eur J Cell Biol 1994;65:229–45.

58 Kowalczyk AP, Bornslaeger EA, Norvell SM et al. Desmosomes: intercellular adhesive junctions specialized for attachment of intermediate filaments. Int Rev Cytol 1999;185:237–302.

59 Oxford EM, Musa H, Maass K et al. Connexin43 remodeling caused by inhibition of plakophilin-2 expression in cardiac cells. Circ Res 2007;101:703–11.

60 Fidler LM, Wilson GJ, Liu F et al. Abnormal connexin43 in arrhythmogenic right ventricular cardiomyopathy caused by plakophilin-2 mutations. J Cell Mol Med 2009;13:4219–28.

61 McGrath JA, McMillan JR, Shemanko CS et al. Mutations in the plakophilin 1 gene can result in ectodermal dysplasia/skin fragility syndrome. Nat Genet 1997;17:240–4.

62 McMillan JR, Haftek M, Akiyama M et al. Alterations in desmosome size and number coincide with the loss of keratinocyte cohesion in skin with homozygous and heterozygous defects in the desmosomal protein plakophilin 1. J Invest Dermatol 2003;121:96–103.

63 McGrath JA, Hoeger PH, Christiano AM et al. Skin fragility and hypohidrotic ectodermal dysplasia resulting from ablation of plakophilin 1. Br J Dermatol 1999;140:297–307.

64 Whittock NV, Haftek M, Angoulvant N et al. Genomic amplification of the human plakophilin 1 gene and detection of a new mutation in ectodermal dysplasia/skin fragility syndrome. J Invest Dermatol 2000;115:368–74.

65 Hamada T, South AP, Mitsuhashi Y et al. Genotype-phenotype correlation in skin fragility-ectodermal dysplasia syndrome resulting from mutations in plakophilin 1. Exp Dermatol 2002;11:107–14.

66 Sprecher E, Molho-Pessach V, Ingber A et al. Homozygous splice site mutations in PKP1 result in loss of epidermal plakophilin 1 expression and underlie ectodermal dysplasia/skin fragility syndrome in two consanguineous families. J Invest Dermatol 2004;122:647–51.

67 Zheng R, Bu DF, Zhu XJ. Compound heterozygosity for new splice site mutations in the plakophilin 1 gene (PKP1) in a Chinese case of ectodermal dysplasia-skin fragility syndrome. Acta Dermatol Venereol 2005;85:394–9.

68 Ersoy-Evans S, Erkin G, Fassihi H et al. Ectodermal dysplasia-skin fragility syndrome resulting from a new homozygous mutation, 888delC, in the desmosomal protein plakophilin 1. J Am Acad Dermatol 2006;55:157–61.

69 Moll I, Kurzen H, Langbein L et al. The distribution of the desmosomal protein, plakophilin 1 in human skin and skin tumours. J Invest Dermatol 1997;108:139–46.

70 McGrath JA, Mellerio JE. Ectodermal dysplasia-skin fragility syndrome. Dermatol Clin 2010;28:125–9.

71 Tanaka A, Lai-Cheong JE, Café ME et al. Novel truncating mutations in PKP1 and DSP cause similar skin phenotypes in two Brazilian families. Br J Dermatol 2009;160:692–7.

72 Protonotarios N, Tsatsopoulou A, Patsourakos P et al. Cardiac abnormalities in familial palmoplantar keratosis. Br Heart J 1986; 56:321–6.

73 McKoy G, Protonotarios N, Crosby A et al. Identification of a deletion in plakoglobin in arrhythmogenic right ventricular cardiomyopathy with palmoplantar keratoderma and woolly hair (Naxos disease). Lancet 2000;355:2119–24.

74 Protonotarios N, Tsatsopoulou A, Anastasakis A et al. Genotype phenotype assessment in autosomal recessive arrhythmogenic right ventricular cardiomyopathy (Naxos disease) caused by a deletion in plakoglobin. J Am Coll Cardiol 2001;38:1477–84.

75 Asimaki A, Syrris P, Wichter T et al. A novel dominant mutation in plakoglobin causes arrhythmogenic right ventricular cardiomyopathy. Am J Hum Genet 2007;81:964–73.

76 Djabali K, Martinez-Mir A, Horev L et al. Evidence for extensive locus heterogeneity in Naxos disease. J Invest Dermatol 2002; 118:557–60.

77 Protonotarios N, Tsatsopoulou A. Naxos disease: cardiocutaneous syndrome due to cell adhesion defect. Orphanet J Rare Dis 2006;1:4.

78 Carvajal-Huerta L. Epidermolytic palmoplantar keratoderma with woolly hair and dilated cardiomyopathy. J Am Acad Dermatol 1998;39:418–21.

79 Norgett EE, Hatsell SJ, Carvajal-Huerta L et al. Recessive mutation in desmoplakin disrupts desmoplakin-intermediate filament interactions and causes dilated cardiomyopathy, woolly hair and keratoderma. Hum Mol Genet 2000;9:2761–6.
80 Green KJ, Parry DA, Steinert PM et al. Structure of the human desmoplakins. Implications for function in the desmosomal plaque. J Biol Chem 1990;265:2603–12.
81 Armstrong DK, McKenna KE, Purkis PE et al. Haploinsufficiency of desmoplakin causes a striate subtype of palmoplantar keratoderma. Hum Mol Genet 1999;8:143–8.
82 Wan H, Dopping-Hepenstal PJ, Gratian MJ et al. Striate palmoplantar keratoderma arising from desmoplakin and desmoglein 1 mutations is associated with contrasting perturbations of desmosomes and the keratin filament network. Br J Dermatol 2004;150:878–91.
83 Whittock NV, Wan H, Morley SM et al. Compound heterozygosity for non-sense and mis-sense mutations in desmoplakin underlies skin fragility/woolly hair syndrome. J Invest Dermatol 2002; 118:232–8.
84 Jonkman MF, Pasmooij AM, Pasmans SG et al. Loss of desmoplakin tail causes lethal acantholytic epidermolysis bullosa. Am J Hum Genet 2005;77:653–60.
85 Bolling MC, Veenstra MJ, Jonkman MF et al. Lethal acantholytic epidermolysis bullosa due to a novel homozygous deletion in DSP: expanding the phenotype and implications for desmoplakin function in skin and heart. Br J Dermatol 2010; 162:1388–94.
86 Uzumcu A, Norgett EE, Dindar A et al. Loss of desmoplakin isoform I causes early onset cardiomyopathy and heart failure in a Naxoslike syndrome. J Med Genet 2006;43:e5.
87 Alcalai R, Metzger S, Rosenheck S et al. A recessive mutation in desmoplakin causes arrhythmogenic right ventricular dysplasia, skin disorder, and woolly hair. J Am Coll Cardiol 2003;42:319–27.
88 Rickman L, Simrak D, Stevens HP et al. N-terminal deletion in a desmosomal cadherin causes the autosomal dominant skin disease striate palmoplantar keratoderma. Hum Mol Genet 1999;8:971–6.
89 Hunt DM, Rickman L, Whittock NV et al. Spectrum of dominant mutations in the desmosomal cadherin desmoglein 1, causing the skin disease striate palmoplantar keratoderma. Eur J Hum Genet 2001;9:197–203.
90 Bergman R, Hershkovitz D, Fuchs D et al. Disadhesion of epidermal keratinocytes: a histologic clue to palmoplantar keratodermas caused by DSG1 mutations. J Am Acad Dermatol 2010;62:107–13.
91 Kljuic A, Bazzi H, Sundberg JP et al. Desmoglein 4 in hair follicle differentiation and epidermal adhesion: evidence from inherited hypotrichosis and acquired pemphigus vulgaris. Cell 2003;113:249–60.
92 Zlotogorski A, Marek D, Horev L et al. An autosomal recessive form of monilethrix is caused by mutations in DSG4: clinical overlap with localized autosomal recessive hypotrichosis. J Invest Dermatol 2006;126:1292–6.
93 Rogaev EI, Zinchenko RA, Dvoryachikov G et al. Total hypotrichosis: genetic form of alopecia not linked to hairless gene. Lancet 1999;354(9184):1097–8.
94 Azeem Z, Jelani M, Naz G et al. Novel mutations in G proteincoupled receptor gene (P2RY5) in families with autosomal recessive hypotrichosis (LAH3). Hum Genet 2008;123:515–19.
95 Wali A, Chishti MS, Ayub M et al. Localization of a novel autosomal recessive hypotrichosis locus (LAH3) to chromosome 13q14.11-q21.32. Clin Genet 2007;72:23–9.
96 Wajid M, Bazzi H, Rockey J et al. Localized autosomal recessive hypotrichosis due to a frameshift mutation in the desmoglein 4 gene exhibits extensive phenotypic variability within a Pakistani family. J Invest Dermatol 2007;127:1779–82.
97 Kazantseva A, Goltsov A, Zinchenko R et al. Human hair growth deficiency is linked to a genetic defect in the phospholipase gene LIPH. Science 2006;314(5801):982–5.
98 Ali G, Chishti MS, Raza SI et al. A mutation in the lipase H (LIPH) gene underlie autosomal recessive hypotrichosis. Hum Genet 2007;121(3–4):319–25.
99 Pasternack SM, von Kügelgen I, Aboud KA et al. G protein-coupled receptor P2Y5 and its ligand LPA are involved in maintenance of human hair growth. Nat Genet 2008;40:329–34.
100 Shimomura Y, Wajid M, Ishii Y et al. Disruption of P2RY5, an orphan G protein-coupled receptor, underlies autosomal recessive woolly hair. Nat Genet 2008;40:335–9.
101 Ayub M, Basit S, Jelani M et al. A homozygous nonsense mutation in the human desmocollin-3 (DSC3) gene underlies hereditary hypotrichosis and recurrent skin vesicles. Am J Hum Genet 2009; 85:515–20.
102 Toribio J, Quiñones PA. Hereditary hypotrichosis simplex of the scalp. Evidence for autosomal dominant inheritance. Br J Dermatol 1974;91:687–96.
103 Hess RO, Uno H. Hereditary hypotrichosis of the scalp. Am J Med Genet 1991;39:125–9.
104 Betz RC, Lee YA, Bygum A et al. A gene for hypotrichosis simplex of the scalp maps to chromosome 6p21.3. Am J Hum Genet 2000;66:1979–83.
105 Kohn G, Metzker A. Hereditary hypotrichosis simplex of the scalp. Clin Genet 1987;32:120–4.
106 Levy-Nissenbaum E, Betz RC, Frydman M et al. Hypotrichosis simplex of the scalp is associated with nonsense mutations in CDSN encoding corneodesmosin. Nat Genet 2003;34:151–3.
107 Matsumoto M, Zhou Y, Matsuo S et al. Targeted deletion of the murine corneodesmosin gene delineates its essential role in skin and hair physiology. Proc Natl Acad Sci U S A 2008;105:6720–4.
108 Romano MT, Tafazzoli A, Mattern M et al. Bi-allelic mutations in LSS, encoding lanosterol synthase, cause autosomal-recessive hypotrichosis simplex. Am J Human Genet 2018;103:777–85.
109 Sprecher E, Bergman R, Richard G et al. Hypotrichosis with juvenile macular dystrophy is caused by a mutation in CDH3, encoding P-cadherin. Nat Genet 2001;29:134–6.
110 Indelman M, Bergman R, Lurie R et al. A missense mutation in CDH3, encoding P-cadherin, causes hypotrichosis with juvenile macular dystrophy. J Invest Dermatol 2002;119:1210–13.
111 Kjaer KW, Hansen L, Schwabe GC et al. Distinct CDH3 mutations cause ectodermal dysplasia, ectrodactyly, macular dystrophy (EEM syndrome). J Med Genet 2005;42:292–8.
112 Suzuki K, Hu D, Bustos T et al. Mutations of PVRL1, encoding a cell-cell adhesion molecule/herpesvirus receptor, in cleft lip/palateectodermal dysplasia. Nat Genet 2000;25:427–30.

Management of ectodermal dysplasia: general overview

Treatment of ED is relatively condition specific and a multidisciplinary approach is generally necessary. Dependent upon the type of ED, the variety of professionals involved may include dermatologists, paediatricians, immunologists, audiologists, ophthalmologists and geneticists as well as multiple surgical specialties including otorhinolaryngologists, plastic surgeons and orthopaedic surgeons. Additional expertise of occupational and physiotherapists, and prostheticians may be required.

Dental restoration is a common issue, because patients with ED can have significant orofacial dysfunction [1]. Hypodontia can cause considerable social impairment and involvement of oral specialists is necessary for retention and maintenance of any existing dentition, to maximize range of foods tolerated and to improve speech, aesthetics and patient self- and social acceptance [2]. Considerations of age, skeletal growth status, as well as location and number of missing teeth all affect the type and timing of restoration; restorations may include removable dentures, orthodontic treatment, composite build-ups, implants, surgery or a combination of treatments (Table 134.3). These decisions may require the involvement of multiple dental specialists, including dentists, orthodontists, periodontists, oral maxillofacial surgeons and prosthodontists [3]. If present, xerostomia and the resultant elevated risk of caries may also need to be managed [4].

Ectodermal dysplasias may cause significant psychosocial impairment [5,6]. As well as patient support organizations, involvement of procurers and fitters of wigs, as well as chiropodists or podiatrists for management of

Table 134.3 Expected approximate age at which dentition is radiologically and clinically apparent

Teeth		Radiograph	Oral cavity
Primary	Incisors	Birth	6–9 months
	Canines	Birth	18 months
	First molars	Birth	12 months
	Second molars	Birth	24 months
Permanent	Central incisors	6 months	6–8 years
	Lateral incisors	9–12 months	7–9 years
	Canines – mandibular	6 months	9–10 years
	Canines – maxillary	6 months	11–12 years
	Premolars	2–3 years	10–12 years
	First molars	Birth	6 years
	Second molars	4 years	11–13 years

Source: Adapted from Nunn et al. (2003) [2] with permission from Macmillan Publishers Ltd

associated palmoplantar or nail findings may ease both physical and social discomfort of affected children.

Genetic testing of ED syndromes has expanded significantly in recent times. Testing for rarer syndromes through research labs may also be obtainable. As the availability of genetic testing is rapidly increasing, please consult www.genetests.org for the most up to date listing of tests. Before offering a genetic test, clinicians should ascertain the goal of such testing. Clinical utility of the test, with regard to patient care, screening of family members or prenatal diagnosis, should be considered, as well as how long it will take for the result to become available, which may range between months to years [7].

Despite some promising studies in animal models for X-linked hypohidrotic ED, gene therapy and protein targeted treatments for ED are currently not available [8].

Specific management issues particular to individual ectodermal subtypes are discussed separately above.

Acknowledgement

The authors would like to acknowledge the original contribution made by Dr Julie Francis to this chapter in the previous editions of this book.

References

1 Bergendal B, McAllister A, Stecksen-Blicks C. Orofacial dysfunction in ectodermal dysplasias measured using the Nordic Orofacial Test-Screening protocol. Acta Odontol Scand 2009;67:377–81.

2 Nunn JH, Carter NE, Gillgrass TJ et al. The interdisciplinary management of hypodontia: background and role of paediatric dentistry. Br Dent J 2003;194:245–51.

3 Sclar AG, Kannikal J, Ferreira CF et al. Treatment planning and surgical considerations in implant therapy for patients with agenesis, oligodontia, and ectodermal dysplasia: review and case presentation. J Oral Maxillofac Surg 2009;67(11 Suppl):2–12.

4 Gill DS, Jones S, Hobkirk J et al. Counselling patients with hypodontia. Dent Update 2008;35:344–6, 348–50, 352.

5 Lane MM, Dalton WT 3rd, Sherman SA et al. Psychosocial functioning and quality of life in children and families affected by AEC syndrome. Am J Med Genet A 2009;149A:1926–34.

6 Hummel P, Guddack S. Psychosocial stress and adaptive functioning in children and adolescents suffering from hypohidrotic ectodermal dysplasia. Pediatr Dermatol 1997;14:180–5.

7 Bale SJ, Mitchell AG. Genetic testing in ectodermal dysplasia: availability, clinical utility, and the nuts and bolts of ordering a genetic test. Am J Med Genet A 2009;149A:2052–6.

8 Gaide O. Gene therapy and protein therapy of ectodermal dysplasias: a perspective. Am J Med Genet A 2009;149A:2042–4.

CHAPTER 135

Focal Dermal Hypoplasia

Bret L. Bostwick[1], *Ignatia B. Van den Veyver*[1,2] *& V. Reid Sutton*[1]

[1]Department of Molecular and Human Genetics, Baylor College of Medicine, Houston, TX, USA
[2]Department of Obstetrics and Gynecology, Baylor College of Medicine, Houston, TX, USA

Abstract

Focal dermal hypoplasia (aka Goltz syndrome) is an ectodermal dysplasia primarily involving the skin, skeleton and eyes. The hallmarks of the congenital cutaneous manifestations are atrophic and hypoplastic areas of skin, nodular fat herniation in the dermis, linear pigmentary changes and cutis aplasia. Limb malformations include ectrodactyly, oligodactyly and syndactyly, whereas ocular anomalies include anophthalmia, microphthalmia, iris colobomas and chorioretinal colobomas. Ninety per cent of individuals with focal dermal hypoplasia are females, because this X-linked condition is lethal in hemizygous males and only mosaic males survive. Although clinical diagnosis can be made through recognition of classic ectodermal findings and characteristic limb findings, molecular genetic testing of *PORCN* is recommended to confirm the diagnosis.

Key points

- **Focal dermal hypoplasia primarily affects skin, skeleton and eyes.**
- **Classic skin findings include atrophic patches of skin, linear hypo/hyperpigmentation, nodular fat herniation and cutis aplasia.**
- **Characteristic limb malformations include ectrodactyly, oligodactyly and syndactyly.**
- **Ocular anomalies include anophthalmia, microphthalmia and iris or chorioretinal colobomas.**
- **X-linked condition affecting mostly females because of lethality in hemizygous males.**
- **Caused by variants in *PORCN*, detectable by sequencing and deletion testing.**

Syn.
Goltz syndrome, Goltz–Gorlin syndrome

Epidemiology and pathogenesis. Focal dermal hypoplasia (FDH) is a rare developmental disorder of which several hundred cases have been described in the literature [1–3] but the exact prevalence is unknown. Considering the high degree of variability in the phenotype, mildly affected individuals may be unrecognized, whereas the most severe cases may not be compatible with neonatal survival. About 90% are females and 10% are males, consistent with X-linked dominant inheritance. Surviving males with FDH are mosaic. Ninety-five per cent of affected female cases are sporadic and 5% are familial, but 100% of males with FDH are sporadic, which is expected because of the mosaic nature of the mutation in these cases [1,3,4]. Women with FDH have a higher incidence of pregnancy loss, presumably of hemizygous affected males [5].

Genetics

FDH is an X-linked dominant disorder that affects predominantly females; all males with FDH have been demonstrated to have somatic mosaicism [5]. Such males have never been shown to transmit FDH to their sons, but can have severely affected daughters [1,4].

In 2007, it was demonstrated that variants in *PORCN* cause FDH [4,6]. *PORCN* is currently the only known gene to cause FDH. To date, nearly 70 different single nucleotide variants are known [4,6–10]. *PORCN*, the human homologue of the fruit fly (*Drosophila melanogaster*) Porcupine gene, is located on the X chromosome in Xp11.2 and encodes a transmembrane endoplasmic reticulum protein [11]. Most of the information regarding the function of human Porcupine is derived from studies in fruit flies and mice, where it has been shown to be essential for processing and secretion of Wnt proteins [12–16]. The Wnt proteins are a highly conserved family of proteins that function as morphogens during embryonic development and organ differentiation. In the canonical Wnt signalling pathway, Wnt proteins are secreted from Wnt-producing cells and interact with receptors and coreceptors on the target cells to activate an intracellular signalling cascade that is crucial for cell differentiation, proliferation and organogenesis. Whether all Wnt proteins require Porcupine, whether other protein families require Porcupine for their secretion from the endoplasmic reticulum, and whether Wnt protein secretion from the endoplasmic reticulum is Porcupine's only function are currently unresolved questions. Nevertheless, many of the phenotypic features of FDH can be explained by defective function of one or more Wnt proteins [4].

Harper's Textbook of Pediatric Dermatology, Fourth Edition. Edited by Peter Hoeger, Veronica Kinsler and Albert Yan.

Several new mouse models [14–16] have been developed that will be helpful in further understanding the normal function of Porcupine and investigating potential new therapeutic approaches. Inactivation of *Porcn* in mouse embryos results in early embryonic lethality, revealing a critical role for normal development of the ectoderm and mesenchymal-derived structures during gastrulation [14,15]. Conditional inactivation of *Porcn* causes alopecia caused by lack of hair follicle development [14] and accompanying skeletal limb defects are reminiscent of those seen in humans with FDH [14,15]. The ability of these mouse models to recapitulate features of the human phenotype is encouraging, because it suggests a reliable animal model for investigating potential therapies for the features of FDH that can progress postnatally, including papillomatosis, nodular fat herniation and skin defects.

PORCN is a gene that undergoes X inactivation, a process that inactivates most genes on one of a female's two X chromosomes to assure equal dosage of X-chromosome genes between males and females. X inactivation initiates early in embryonic development, and the choice of which X (maternally inherited or paternally inherited) is inactivated is random. However, once the choice is made in a particular cell, it is clonally propagated to all its daughter cells during cell division. This results in specific mosaic patterns of cells with either the maternal or paternal X inactive. Mosaicism caused by X inactivation is thought to be responsible for the linear pattern of the skin lesions in FDH, following the lines of Blaschko, as well as the osteopathia striata [17] and the asymmetrical distribution of defects [18].

Figure 135.1 shows the distribution of FDH-causing pathogenic variants along the *PORCN* gene. All types of variants have been described and all areas of the gene can be affected but some 'hot-spots' seem to exist [7,8,19]. In addition to smaller single nucleotide variants, larger genomic deletions that encompass *PORCN*, as well as neighbouring genes, have also been identified in up to 20% of sporadic and familial cases [7]. Smaller deletions of one or more exons of the *PORCN* gene [7,8] are also known. Deletions and a subset of single nucleotide variants are often associated with extremely skewed X chromosome inactivation, presumably preferentially inactivating the mutant X chromosome [4,6,19]. Genetic testing by sequencing of the *PORCN* gene or by testing for chromosomal deletions that include *PORCN* is now clinically available and can aid in the confirmation of the diagnosis. Limited studies have shown that at least 80% of individuals with a well-characterized clinical diagnosis of FDH have an identifiable pathogenic variant in *PORCN* or a deletion of this gene [4,7,9]. It is currently unclear whether others carry as yet unidentifiable variants in *PORCN* that affect its function, whether there are other genes that can cause FDH, or whether they represent atypical cases of different aetiology. Hence, although molecular testing is important to confirm FDH, it remains a clinical and pathological diagnosis in some cases that cannot be molecularly confirmed.

With the discovery that pathogenic variants in a major regulator in *PORCN* are the cause of FDH, these observations of developmental abnormalities of proliferation and differentiation involving various components of the skin are probably the result of faulty ectomesodermal Wnt signalling, which is important for normal specification of components of skin and appendages. Disrupted Wnt signalling, involving different Wnt proteins, is also the likely explanation for the defects observed in other organs and the skeleton.

Clinical features. FDH is a multisystem disorder primarily involving skin, skeletal system, eyes and face (Box 135.1). Most individuals have multiple classic skin lesions and limb malformations, thus these findings are used in the clinical diagnostic criteria [20]. Combined ectomesodermal defects are thought to be the basis of the observed abnormalities. There is extreme variability in severity, including within families with several affected individuals [1]. Findings are often asymmetrical and follow patterns consistent with mosaicism, such as the distribution of skin lesions along the lines of Blaschko [18], reflecting X inactivation patterns in females and somatic mosaicism in males with the disorder (see Genetics) [4,18].

Skin

Skin involvement is usually the key presenting feature, together with skeletal findings, that supports a clinical diagnosis of FDH and is thus present in nearly all reported cases [2]. However, mildly affected or unaffected carriers may not have skin lesions [5] and the phenotypic spectrum of the condition will probably expand now that the genetic defect has been identified and more individuals with atypical presentations are being tested [4,6,7] as well as the increased use of untargeted genomic testing.

The typical skin lesions in FDH usually present at birth, but can show progression and changes into adulthood [21]. The first types of lesions are streaky areas of linear hypoplastic-appearing skin with telangiectasia and hyper- or hypopigmentation. These can be found on any part of the body, but typically involve the thighs, buttocks and trunk and may be limited or affect very large areas of the body (Figs 135.2 and 135.3) [1]. These striate lesions may be pink, brown, pale to flesh-coloured and can be slightly raised or depressed. They are often asymmetrical and follow the distribution of fine lines of Blaschko [18]. Occasionally, there is an initial inflammatory phase at birth with oedematous, blistered, eroded, crusted or scaling erythematous lesions that is sometimes confused with incontinentia pigmenti [1] but evolves by 5–6 months of age into the more typical lesions [22]. Atrophic lesions or atrophy-like cutaneous depressions comprise depressed areas of skin that can be pink, red, brown, grey and white and striate, elliptical, round, oval, reticulate or cribriform. The lipomatous lesions are very characteristic and present as soft pinkish-yellow to brown nodules that can be present from birth or appear later and increase in size and number during childhood [23]. Similar to the striate lesions, they can occur anywhere but are more common on the torso and the limbs, particularly in the popliteal

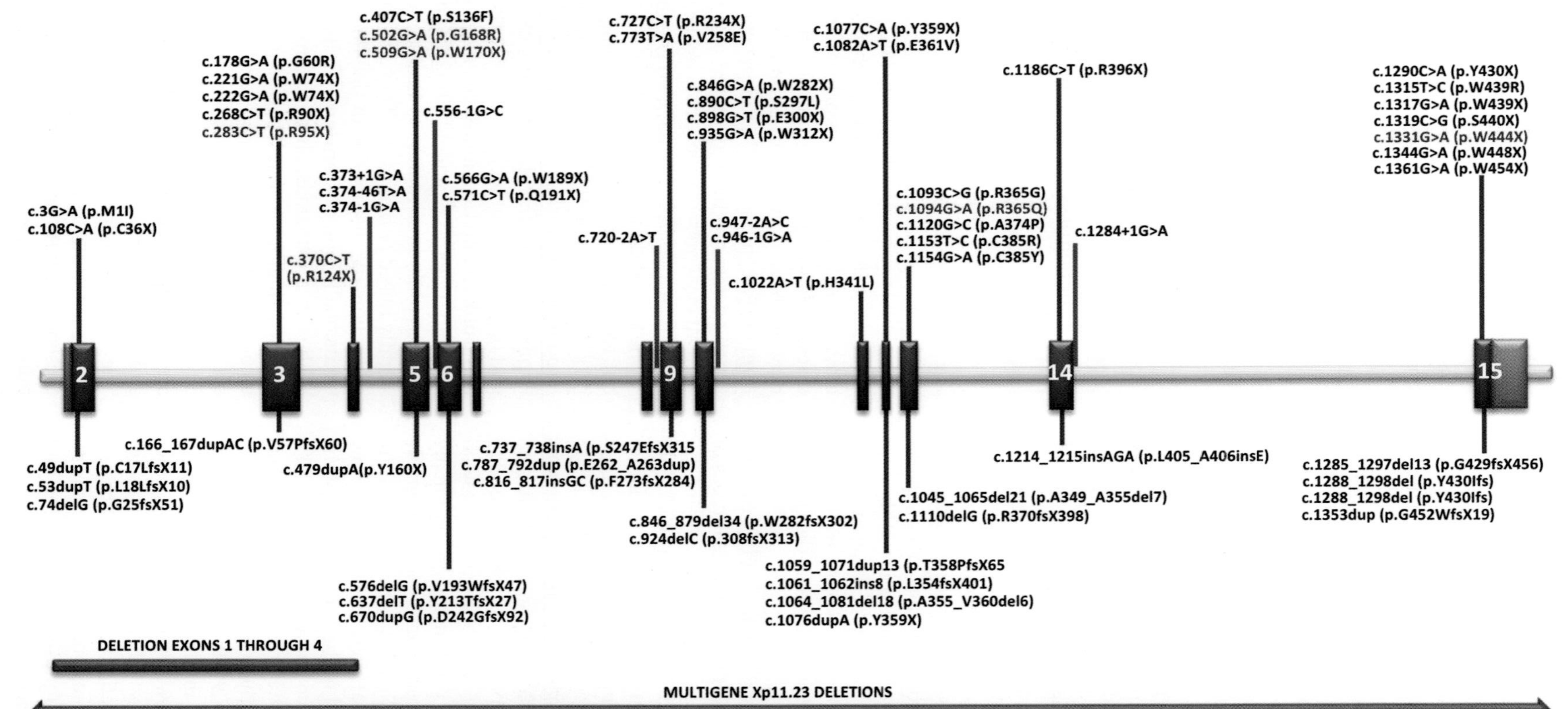

Fig. 135.1 *PORCN* gene diagram with examples of pathogenic variants found in focal dermal hypoplasia. The yellow line represents the genomic region. Coding exons are in blue, noncoding 3′ and 5′ untranslated regions of exons 2 and 15 respectively are in orange. Red lines point to coding-exon variants; green lines point to intronic variants, affecting splicing. Missense, nonsense and splice-site variants are above the gene diagram and frame-shift variants and deletions are below it. The purple lines represent examples of larger genomic deletions that have been described. Red text indicates examples of variants observed repeatedly in unrelated affected individuals ('mutation hot-spots').

Box 135.1 Clinical diagnosis and features of focal dermal hypoplasia

Clinical diagnosis

- Three of more characteristic skin findings *and* ≥1 characteristic limb malformation [20]

Main features (~ % prevalence when available from [20])

Skin
- Streaky linear dermal atrophy or atrophic lesions (94%)
- Lipomatous lesions (ectopic fat nodules) (67%)
- Linear hypo- or hyperpigmentation (100%)
- Papillomas (verrucoid) (67%)
- Telangiectasias (79%)
- Atrophy-like cutaneous depressions
- Hypopigmented poikiloderma
- Aplasia cutis congenita

Skeleton
- Hand ectrodactyly (lobster claw deformity) (44%)
- Foot ectrodactyly (split-foot deformity) (61%)
- Hand syndactyly (67%)
- Foot syndactyly (67%)
- Transverse limb reduction defects (17%)
- Long bone reduction (78%)
- Polydactyly
- Absence or hypoplasia of digits
- Osteopathia striata of long bones
- Scoliosis
- Spina bifida occulta
- Diastasis pubis
- Deformities of ribs and clavicles
- Osteoporosis
- Cystic lesions, tumours of bone
- Joint hyperlaxity

Face
- Notching of alae nasi (61%)
- Asymmetry (50%)
- Abnormal ear morphology (44%)
- Pointed chin
- Maxillary hypoplasia
- Broad nasal tip with narrow bridge
- Facial clefts, tongue clefts
- Notching of alveolar ridge
- Thin protruding ears

Eyes
- Chorioretinal colobomata (61%)
- Colobomata of the iris (50%)
- Microphthalmia (44%)
- Anophthalmia (11%)
- Microcornea
- Ectopia lentis
- Aniridia
- Corneal clouding
- Cataracts
- Optic atrophy

Teeth
- Enamel hypoplasia with or without discoloration (78% [27])
- Vertical enamel grooving (68% [27])
- Peg-shaped teeth (52% [27])
- Irregular spacing, malocclusion (15% [27])
- Hypodontia and anodontia
- Delayed eruption
- Notched incisors
- Ridged teeth

Other
- Nail hypoplasia or dystrophy (67%)
- Nail ridging (89%)
- Alopecia, sparse hair, brittle hair or wiry hair (67%)
- Genital labial hypoplasia (94% of females)
- Anonychia
- Grooving and spooning of nails
- Orophayngeal, laryngeal and oesophageal papillomas
- Intestinal malrotation
- Diaphragmatic hernia
- Kidney defects
- Bicornuate uterus, asymmetric labia
- Cardiac defects
- Mental deficiency in 15%
- CNS anomalies are rare
- Agenesis of corpus callosum
- Mild growth retardation
- Normal lifespan

and cubital fossae. These fat nodules were initially referred to as 'fat herniations' [1]; however, it has not been established that they embryologically represent true herniations of the subcutaneous adipose tissue, rather than localized dysplasia of the dermis [21]. Telangiectasias and hypo- or hyperpigmentation can accompany the atrophic, striate and lipomatous lesions. Aplasia cutis congenita, in which one or a few large or multiple smaller areas of the epidermis are not developed, probably owing to absence of the underlying dermis, can be found in some individuals [1,24]. Generalized skin dryness associated with pruritus, photosensitivity [5], sweat abnormalities [25], apocrine gland anomalies [26], hypoplastic dermatoglyphics on the digits and hypothenar eminence [25] and palmar hyperkeratosis, hypohidrosis and hyperhidrosis have all been reported.

Papillomas

These can appear at any time on the skin and mucous membranes, but are rarely present at birth. They are most common at the transition from mucosal epithelium to cutaneous epithelium, as around the lips and eyes and on vulvar, perianal and perineal areas where they can be confused with condylomata acuminata. They have also been reported at other sites including the oesophagus and larynx where they may result in breathing and swallowing difficulties [28,29].

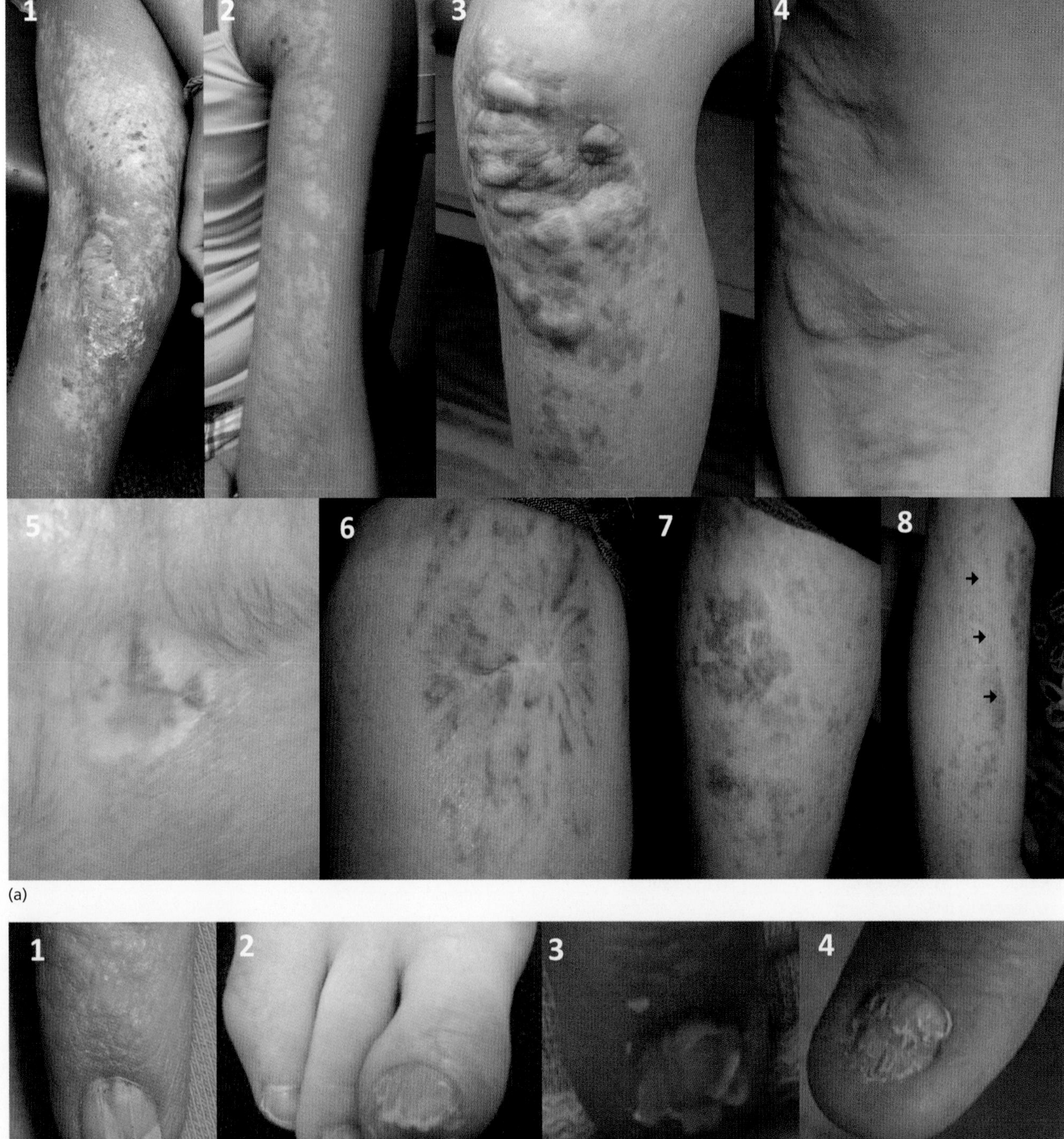

Fig. 135.2 (a) Dermatological manifestations of FDH: (1,2) skin aplasia and hypopigmented areas of poikiloderma; (3) nodular fat herniation; (4) skin atrophy and fat herniation; (5) cutis aplasia of scalp; (6,7,8) Hypo-/hyper-pigmentation following Blaschkolinear distribution (black arrows in 8). (b) Nail manifestations of FDH. (1) longitudinal linear ridging and onycholysis; (2,3,4) dysplastic nails. Source: Bostwick et al. 2016 [20]. Reproduced with permission of John Wiley & Sons.

Recurrence after excision has been observed and they can occasionally take on giant proportions [30].

Skeletal system

Individuals with FDH have typical skeletal findings that are asymmetrical and variable, with predominant involvement of hands and feet in 70% of cases [1]. These include syndactyly, polydactyly, ectrodactyly and absence or hypoplasia of digits. Lobster claw deformity (split hand or split foot with syndactyly and absence of rays) is a major distinct feature of this condition [5] (see Figs 135.3 and 135.4). In rare cases, the hands or feet and part of long

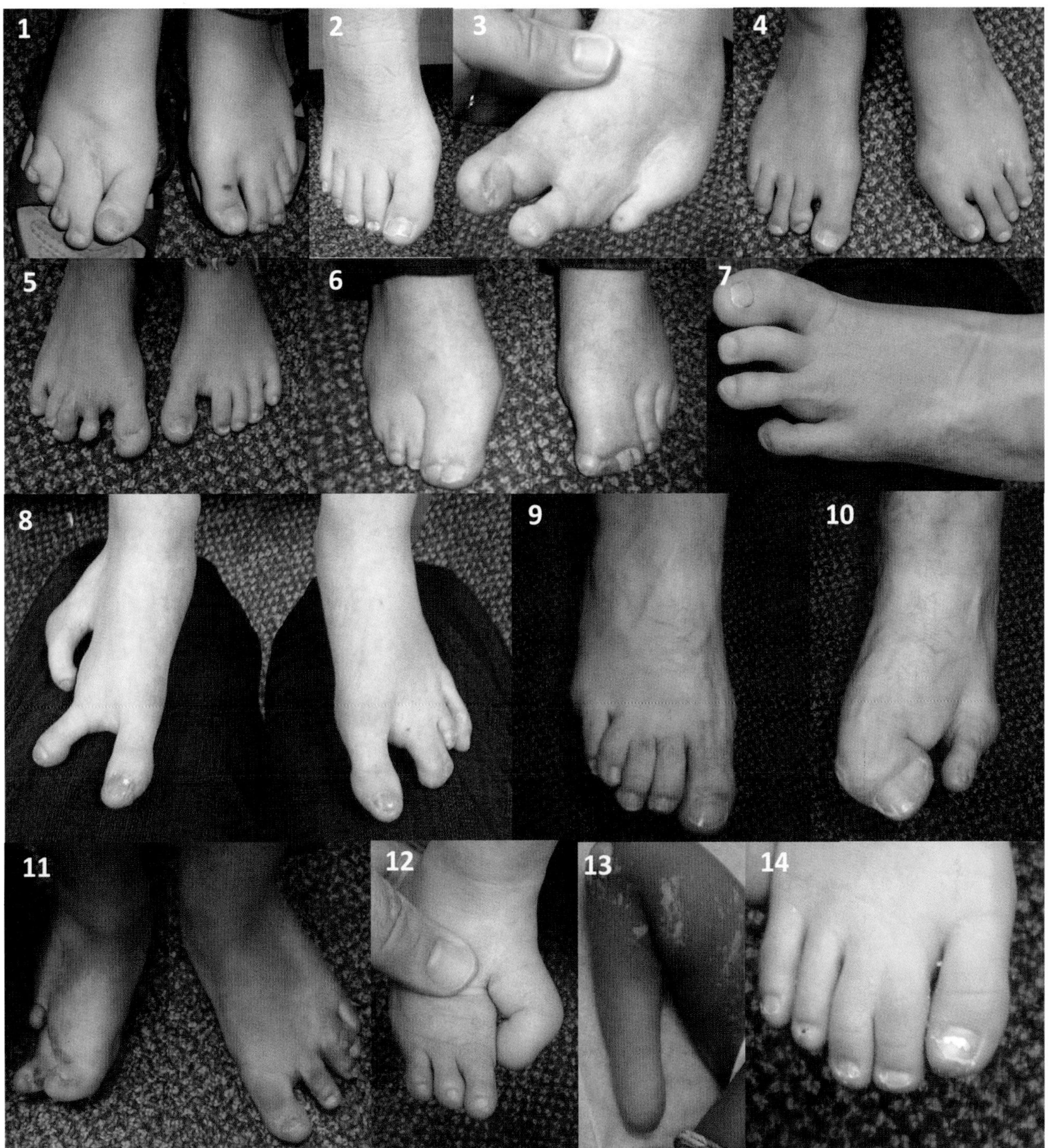

Fig. 135.3 Foot deformities in FDH: (1) syndactyly and clefting; (2) mild sandal gap deformity; (3) oligodactyly and clefting; (4) left foot 4–5 syndactyly and small 3–4 cleft representing subtle ectrodactyly; (5) sandal-gap, dysplastic phalanges; (6) syndactyly and ectrodactyly bilaterally; (7) split-foot deformity (ectrodactyly) and oligodactyly; (8) bilateral median and paramedian ectrodactyly; (9,10) demonstrates asymmetric limb involvement in an individual; (10,11,12) ectrodactyly; (13) complete transverse limb defect; (14) subtle 2–3 toe syndactyly. Source: Bostwick et al. 2016 [20]. Reproduced with permission of John Wiley & Sons.

bones may be missing in an asymmetrical pattern. Scoliosis occurs in 15–20% of cases and asymmetry in the size and shape of the face, trunk or limbs in 30% of cases [5]. In 20% of cases, there is osteopathia striata, which are longitudinal linear striations in the metaphyses of long bones seen on radiography [1,17]. It is highly characteristic of FDH but has also been seen in other disorders. A separate X-linked dominant condition, osteopathia striata with cranial sclerosis, was hypothesized to be allelic with FDH but recently, variants in the *WTX* gene in Xp have been shown to be responsible for this disorder, establishing it as distinct from FDH [31].

Other findings include spina bifida occulta, diastasis pubis [25,32], joint hyperlaxity, deformities of ribs and clavicles, split sternum, reduction in bone density, osteoporosis, fibrous dysplasia of the bone, cystic lesions and

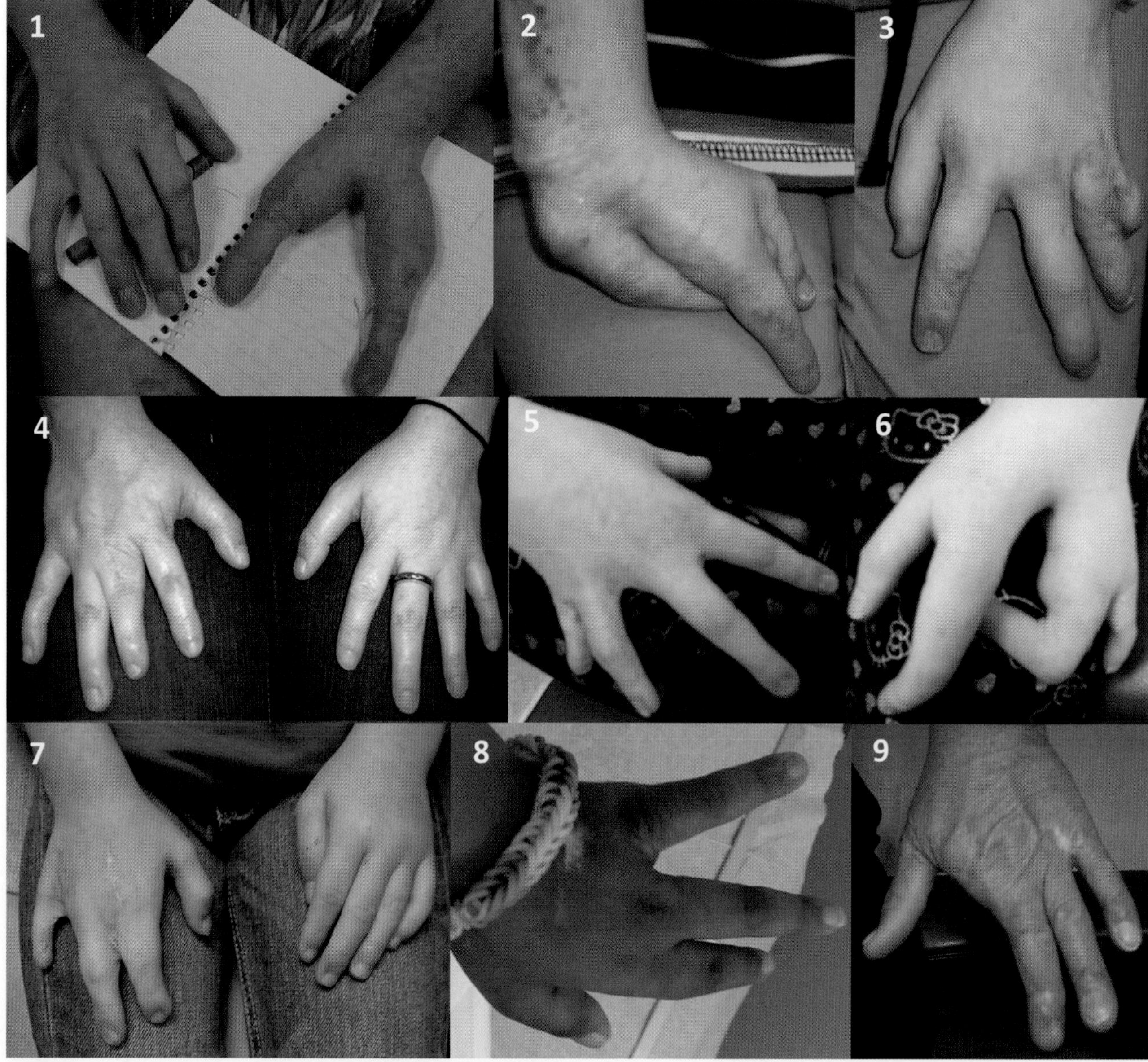

Fig. 135.4 Hand deformities in FDH: (1) marked ectrodactyly (median cleft of the left hand). Note variability in limb manifestations; (2,3) right ectrodactyly/oligodactyly and left syndactyly with dysplastic digits; (4) right 2/3 syndactyly/bachydactyly; (5,6) bilateral ectrodactyly with left hand median cleft; (7) right ectrodactyly after surgical repair and hypoplastic 5th finger; (8,9) ectrodactyly and oligodactyly. Source: Bostwick et al. 2016 [20]. Reproduced with permission of John Wiley & Sons.

expanding lesions including giant cell tumours of bone [33] and osteochondroma in one case [34].

Face

Individuals with FDH may have facial asymmetry, a pointed chin, maxillary hypoplasia, broad nasal tip with a narrow bridge and sometimes notching of the alae nasi. Papillomas of the lips, perioral fissures, leukokeratosis, gum hyperplasia, notching of the alveolar ridge, bifid or notched uvula and tongue clefts have been reported in several individuals. Cleft lip and cleft and high-arched palate are present in a few per cent and some severe cases have complex extensive facial clefts [24]. The ears are often thin and protruding and can be low-set, asymmetrical, small or deformed with poor development of cartilage, and auricular appendages, cholesteatoma and hearing deficit can be present.

Teeth

Approximately 40% of people with FDH have dental abnormalities [5,25]. Findings include typical longitudinal grooving of teeth, taurodontia, enamel defects with caries, anodontia, hypoplastic or dysplastic teeth, delayed eruption, irregular spacing, malocclusion and notched incisors [27].

Hair

The hair in FDH is often sparse and brittle. Localized areas of absent scalp and pubic hair have been reported [5,25].

Eyes
In 20–40% of reported cases there is significant eye involvement [1,5,35], mostly chorioretinal colobomas [36] but microphthalmia, microcornea and ectopia lentis are also frequently present. In addition, anophthalmia, papillomas of the eyelids, aniridia, heterochromia, microcornea, corneal clouding, keratoconus, cataracts, optic atrophy [2], retinal neovascularization and vitreous haemorrhage [37], irregularity of pupils and lacrimal duct abnormalities and cysts [2,26] have also been reported. These can be associated with strabismus or nystagmus, or result in blindness or significant visual handicap in some individuals [5] (see Fig 135.5).

Nails
Dystrophy, atrophy, anonychia, grooving (see Fig. 135.2) and spooning of both fingernails and toenails is very frequently present [5,25].

Gynecological
Hypoplasia of the labia minora is common in females, whereas vulvar papillomas along with breast or nipple asymmetry are less commonly seen [38].

Other rarer features
There can be respiratory and digestive tract abnormalities, including duodenal atresia, intestinal malrotation [39], anterior placement of the anus [32,39], anal stenosis [40], omphalocoele [5], and inguinal, diaphragmatic [41], epigastric and hiatus hernias. In the genitourinary tract, renal agenesis [24], hypoplastic kidney [40], horseshoe kidney [25,40,42], cystic renal dysplasia [5] and hydronephrosis [39,40] have all been reported. In addition, a bicornuate uterus, asymmetrical labia and vaginal canal were reported in one individual [40]. Cardiovascular system abnormalities associated with FDH include mediastinal dextroposition, patent ductus arteriosus [39], total anomalous pulmonary venous return, truncus arteriosus with truncal origin of hypoplastic pulmonary arteries, cardiac ventricular septal defect and hypoplasia of the lungs and pulmonary veins [24,40]. Recurrent tonsillitis, respiratory infections, conjunctivitis, urinary tract infections and otitis media have been observed [5]. However, no immunological deficiency has been reported and these infections are probably related to predisposing underlying structural defects of these organ systems. Rare cases with absent nipples are also reported.

Central nervous system
About 15% of individuals with FDH have intellectual disability of varying severity, which may be overestimated because of sensory deprivation and difficulty assessing mental function in more severely affected individuals who may have combined hearing and vision loss [5]. Agenesis of the corpus callosum [43], meningomyelocoele, hydrocephalus, Arnold–Chiari malformation [44], gyral abnormalities and absent cerebellar vermis [40] have been reported. However, overall, CNS anomalies are uncommon in FDH and there is no clear increased incidence of seizures.

Growth and lifespan
Growth retardation *in utero* and mild short stature have been described, but poorly characterized. The lifespan is normal in the majority of cases [1].

Histopathology. The histological changes of some skin lesions are characteristic and, prior to identification of the causative gene, had been studied extensively in search for

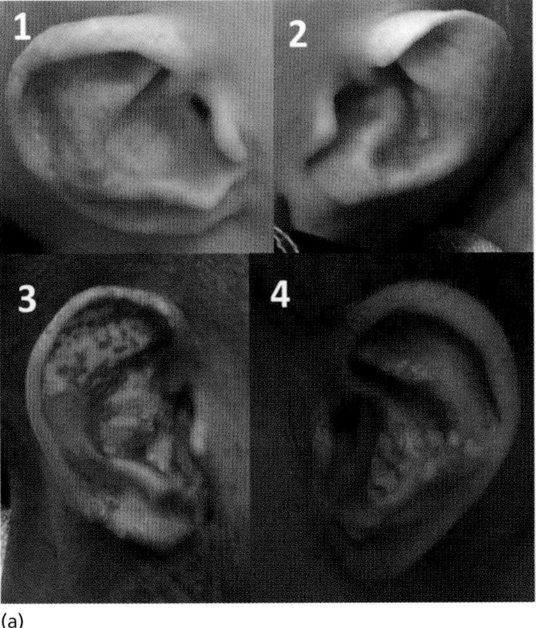

(a)

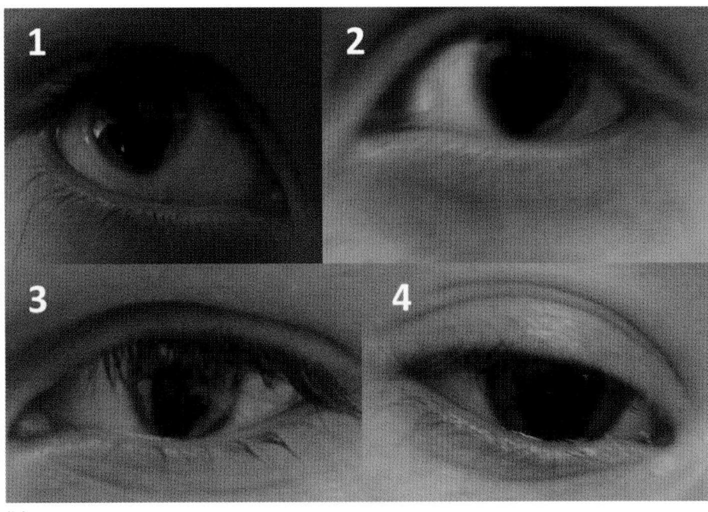

(b)

Fig. 135.5 (a) Ear abnormalities in FDH: (1) absent crus of helix and auricular hypoplasia; (2) hypoplastic helix and scapha (note generalized thinning of the auricle); (3) hypoplastic crus and hypopigmented poikiloderma; (4) hypopigmented antitragus. (b) Ocular manifestations in FDH: (1,2,3,4) varying severity of iris colobomas. Source: Bostwick et al. 2016 [20]. Reproduced with permission of John Wiley & Sons.

clues for the pathogenesis of the disorder. These histopathological abnormalities can now be reinterpreted in the context of *PORCN* function and Wnt signalling. Goltz and colleagues initially concluded that the observed lipomatous lesions resulted from fat herniation through a congenital dermal defect and proposed the name 'focal dermal hypoplasia' [2]. However, based on observations that suggest that there is rather a local proliferation of heterotopic fat tissue in the dermis, Ishibashi and Kurihara [36] proposed the term 'dermal dysplasia' instead. Howell and Freeman [21] also provided evidence in a longitudinal analysis of lesions in a few individuals over time that the ectopic adipose tissue was naevoid and resulted from a dysplasia within the dermis, rather than herniation of subcutaneous fat. This is consistent with the presence of immature adipocytes in an electron microscopic study of the skin lesions, which suggests adipose tissue proliferation [45,46]. In addition to abnormal adipocyte development, incomplete tropocollagen–precollagen fibres, paucity of collagen within the dermis and increased ground substance suggest a primary connective tissue disturbance, along with the adipocyte abnormalities [45,46]. This may be secondary to abnormalities in the fibroblasts which show decreased organelles, abnormal Golgi and endoplasmic reticulum. Uitto and colleagues [47] demonstrated *in vitro* that the synthesis of collagen by individual fibroblasts was normal but that they had a reduced proliferative capacity. On the other hand, Sato and colleagues [48] did not find any abnormal growth kinetics in fibroblasts, or abnormal collagen, but demonstrated decreased accumulation of hyaluronic acid.

Atrophic, striate and lipomatous lesions

The hallmark features of the typical atrophic, striate and lipomatous lesions of FDH syndrome are the diminished thickness of the dermis with evidence for defective collagen formation [25], widened blood vessels in the papillary dermis and islands of mature adipose tissue deposits scattered within the reticular and papillary dermis [25] that are thought to initiate around these capillaries [21], but can be restricted initially to the reticular dermis. It has been suggested that the lipomatous lesions represent different degrees of the same process [21]. The combination of increased papillary dermal blood vessels, decreased thickness of dermis and adipocytes high in the dermis are felt to strongly suggest a diagnosis of FDH [49].

In early-stage skin lesions, the epidermis is usually normal. The papillary dermis shows increased numbers of small blood vessels and sometimes a perivascular lymphohistiocytic infiltrate [26,45]. The dermis is thinned, with attenuated collagen fibres. The elastic tissue can be increased or decreased [46]. Adipocytes or adipocyte-like cells can be found in small deposits 3–4 cells thick around blood vessels in the dermis, but not in continuity with the subcutaneous fat layer. These aggregates tend to enlarge and result in fat nodule formation. When large lobulated fat masses have developed in later stages, the relationship with blood vessels can be lost. The fat masses can be separated from the epidermis by only a few collagen fibres [25,46]; there is usually a layer of dermal connective tissues beneath the fat nodules, separating them from the subcutaneous layer. Atrophic lesions have a paucity of appendages [46]. Hyperpigmented areas can be associated with epidermal acanthosis and papillomatosis and increased melanin pigment in the epidermal basal layer [45].

Electron microscopy reveals loosely arranged collagen bundles composed of scattered abnormally formed and orientated fibres [45,46]. Elastic fibres are scarce but of normal morphology, but the fibroblasts in affected areas appear more oval, larger and have reduced organelle content with vacuoles, and irregular thickening below the nuclear lamina [45,46]. In these cells, the Golgi is enlarged and the rough endoplasmic reticulum cisternae are dilated and contain amorphous material [47]. Both mature, uniloculated and immature, multiloculated adipocytes can be found in the dermal fat nodules [45,46].

Congenital aplasia

Absence of epidermis and sometimes dermis is observed in the lesions of congenital aplasia. The subcutaneous fat may be deficient. On the scalp, sometimes only the appendages fail to develop.

Inflammatory lesions

The inflammatory lesions [22] with marked oedema in the papillary dermis, perivascular lymphocytic infiltration, increased numbers of fibroblasts and clusters of lipocytes at the mid-dermis occur in some individuals at birth and diminish with time. It has been suggested that these histological findings represent a transitional phase and may contribute to the process of fat deposition.

Papillomas

The papillomas consist of a fibrovascular stalk covered by a layer of acanthotic stratified squamous epithelium. Hyperkeratosis and parakeratosis are often present [25]. A case of a papilloma with lymphocytic infiltration has been reported [50].

Differential diagnosis.

Incontinentia pigmenti

Incontinentia pigmenti is an X-linked disorder that affects the skin, eyes, hair, teeth and central nervous system. The characteristic skin manifestations evolve through a stage of vesiculation followed by verrucous lesions, pigmentation and atrophy following the lines of Blaschko. Skin biopsy is characteristic and has no dermal underdevelopment. Eye abnormalities may also be present, but they involve the posterior chamber. *NEMO* is the only known gene associated with incontinentia pigmenti [51].

Rothmund–Thomson syndrome

Rothmund–Thomson syndrome is an autosomal recessive disorder that affects the skin, eyes, hair and skeletal system. Typically, the skin is not affected at birth. The rash usually presents as erythema, swelling and blistering of the face at 3–6 months of age, later spreading to the buttocks and extremities. Over months to years, the rash evolves into the chronic pattern of reticulated hypo- and hyperpigmentation, punctate atrophy and telangiectases, collectively known as poikiloderma [52]. Short stature, skeletal dysplasia, juvenile cataract, sparse hair, hypogonadism and midface hypoplasia are other features. Papillomas of the genital and anal region are common. The intelligence of those affected is usually normal. *RECQL4* is the only known gene associated with Rothmund–Thomson syndrome [53].

Microphthalmia with linear skin defects

Microphthalmia with linear skin defects is an X-linked dominant disorder in which eye and CNS anomalies and linear skin lesions on the head and neck are observed that show mild overlap with those of FDH [54]. Heart and skeletal anomalies can also occur but are uncommon. Although originally proposed to be allelic with FDH, Microphthalmia with linear skin defects is now known to be caused by deletions and single nucleotide variants in the *HCCS* gene [55].

Naevus lipomatosus cutaneous superficialis (Hoffmann–Zurhelle)

Naevus lipomatosus cutaneous superficialis usually presents in early adulthood as grouped soft yellow or flesh-coloured nodules, often localized on the lower trunk, buttocks and hips. Histologically, there are fat cells around blood vessels in the mid- and upper dermis, similar to the lesions of FDH, but the extreme thinning of the dermis is usually absent and there are no anomalies of eyes and other connective tissues.

Anetoderma

Anetoderma is characterized by damage of elastic tissue, resulting in skin laxity and herniation, but is not present at birth. The histology shows fragmented, shortened or absent elastic fibres in some lesions.

Angioma serpiginosum with oesophageal papillomatosis

This condition is characterized by linearly grouped lesions with capillary ectasias in the papillary dermis, present from birth. This rash resembles purpura and patterns can follow the lines of Blaschko. A family with this condition in which the gene mapped to Xp11.3–Xq12 was described to have a deletion encompassing *PORCN*, which suggested that this condition is allelic to FDH [56]. However, it was subsequently argued that this was a family segregating a mild form of FDH and that the diagnosis of angioma serpiginosum was incorrect [57].

Treatment. A multidisciplinary approach, including dermatology, ophthalmology, otorhinolaryngology, and orthopaedic and plastic surgery services, is required, as well as other specialties relevant to the individual medical problems.

Skin lesions are not only a cosmetic concern, but they can also become painful, pruritic or infected resulting in disease morbidity. For areas with significant dermal aplasia, the use of occlusive dressings and potentially topical antibiotics may help prevent secondary infections. Some individuals report that moisturizers help in managing erosive lesions that become painful or pruritic. Pulsed dye laser and photodynamic therapy can aid in managing excessive granulation tissue [58,59]. The combination of curettage and photodynamic therapy has also been used to treat refractory exophytic granulation tissue [60].

Papillomatous lesions can be excised or treated with cautery or cryotherapy but can recur. Laser therapy is the method of choice for laryngeal papillomas, which can be hypopharyngeal, tonsillar or tracheal. Skarzynski and Podskarbi-Fayette treated one individual with FDH with a CO_2 laser for papillomatous lesions on her face and neck. They reported a good aesthetic result without recurrence at a 6-month follow up examination after a second stage of laser was given [61]. Oesophageal papillomatosis can cause swallowing dysfunction and has been treated with both endoscopic removal [62], as well as balloon-assisted radiofrequency ablation [63].

Prior to general anaesthesia, an otolaryngologist should be consulted for evaluation of tonsillar or pharyngeal papillomas that could complicate endotracheal intubation. The papillomas may be friable and prone to bleeding; when papillomas are present, the airway must be handled as gently as possible and fibreoptic bronchoscopy for intubation rather than direct laryngoscopy may be employed [64]. Since the size and location of airway papillomas can change significantly over time, the otolaryngology evaluation should be within a few months of the scheduled procedure.

Dental care with special attention to caries development, orthopaedic consultation and treatment of musculoskeletal problems, ophthalmology and audiology evaluation and treatment are all important for the supportive care of individuals with FDH.

Acknowledgements

We thank the families who participate in our research on Goltz syndrome.

References

1 Goltz RW. Focal dermal hypoplasia syndrome. An update. Arch Dermatol 1992;128:1108–11.
2 Goltz RW, Peterson WC, Gorlin RJ, Ravits AG. Focal dermal hypoplasia. Arch Dermatol 1962;86:708–17.
3 Bostwick BL, Van den Veyver IB, Sutton VR. Focal dermal hypoplasia. In: GeneReviews at GeneTests: Medical Genetics Information Resource. Available at www.genetests.org.
4 Wang X, Reid Sutton V, Omar Peraza-Llanes J et al. Mutations in X-linked PORCN, a putative regulator of Wnt signaling, cause focal dermal hypoplasia. Nat Genet 2007;39:836–8.
5 Temple IK, MacDowall P, Baraitser M, Atherton DJ. Focal dermal hypoplasia (Goltz syndrome). J Med Genet 1990;27:180–7.
6 Grzeschik KH, Bornholdt D, Oeffner F et al. Deficiency of PORCN, a regulator of Wnt signaling, is associated with focal dermal hypoplasia. Nat Genet 2007;39:833–5.
7 Fernandes PH, Wen S, Sutton VR et al. PORCN mutations and variants identified in patients with focal dermal hypoplasia through diagnostic gene sequencing. Genet Test Mol Biomarkers 2010;14:709–13.
8 Bornholdt D, Oeffner F, Konig A et al. PORCN mutations in focal dermal hypoplasia: coping with lethality. Hum Mutat 2009;30:E618–28.
9 Clements SE, Mellerio JE, Holden ST et al. PORCN gene mutations and the protean nature of focal dermal hypoplasia. Br J Dermatol 2009;160:1103–9.

SECTION 28: FOCAL OR GENERALIZED HYPOPLASIA

10 Lombardi MP, Bulk S, Celli J et al. Mutation update for the PORCN gene. Hum Mutat 2011:32:723–8.
11 Kadowaki T, Wilder E, Klingensmith J et al. The segment polarity gene porcupine encodes a putative multitransmembrane protein involved in Wingless processing. Genes Dev 1996;10:3116–28.
12 Takada R, Satomi Y, Kurata T et al. Monounsaturated fatty acid modification of Wnt protein: its role in Wnt secretion. Dev Cell 2006;11:791–801.
13 Willert K, Brown JD, Danenberg E et al. Wnt proteins are lipid modified and can act as stem cell growth factors. Nature 2003;423: 448–52.
14 Liu W, Shaver TM, Balasa A et al. Deletion of Porcn in mice leads to multiple developmental defects and models human focal dermal hypoplasia (Goltz syndrome). PLoS One. 2012;7(3).
15 Barrott JJ, Cash GM, Smith AP et al. Deletion of mouse Porcn blocks Wnt ligand secretion and reveals an ectodermal etiology of human focal dermal hypoplasia/Goltz syndrome. Proc Natl Acad Sci U S A 2011;108:12752–7.
16 Biechele S, Adissu HA, Cox BJ, Rossant J. Zygotic Porcn paternal allele deletion in mice to model human focal dermal hypoplasia. PLoS One 2013:8(11).
17 Larregue M, Maroteaux P, Michel Y, Faure C. [Osteopathia striata, radiological manifestation of focal dermal hypoplasia.] Ann Radiol (Paris) 1972;15:287–95.
18 Happle R. The lines of Blaschko: a developmental pattern visualizing functional X- chromosome mosaicism. Curr Probl Dermatol 1987;17:5–18.
19 Maas SM, Lombardi PM, van Essen AJ et al. Phenotype and genotype in 17 patients with Goltz–Gorlin syndrome. J Med Genet 2009;46: 716–20.
20 Bostwick B, Fang P, Patel A, Sutton VR. Phenotypic and molecular characterization of focal dermal hypoplasia in 18 individuals. Am J Med Genet Part C Semin Med Genet 2016;172C:9–20.
21 Howell JB, Freeman RG. Cutaneous defects of focal dermal hypoplasia: an ectomesodermal dysplasia syndrome. J Cutan Pathol 1989;16:237–58.
22 Mann M, Weintraub R, Hashimoto K. Focal dermal hypoplasia with an initial inflammatory phase. Pediatr Dermatol 1990;7:278–82.
23 Bree AF, Grange DK, Hicks MJ, Goltz RW. Dermatologic findings of focal dermal hypoplasia (Goltz syndrome). Am J Med Genet C Semin Med Genet 2016;172C:44–51.
24 Han XY, Wu SS, Conway DH et al. Truncus arteriosus and other lethal internal anomalies in Goltz syndrome. Am J Med Genet 2000; 90:45–8.
25 Goltz RW, Henderson RR, Hitch JM, Ott JE. Focal dermal hypoplasia syndrome. A review of the literature and report of two cases. Arch Dermatol 1970;101:1–11.
26 Buchner SA, Itin P. Focal dermal hypoplasia syndrome in a male patient. Report of a case and histologic and immunohistochemical studies. Arch Dermatol 1992;128:1078–82.
27 Wright JT, Puranik CP, Farrington F. Oral phenotype and variation in focal dermal hypoplasia. Am J Med Genet C Semin Med Genet 2016;172C:52–8.
28 Brinson RR, Schuman BM, Mills LR et al. Multiple squamous papillomas of the esophagus associated with Goltz syndrome. Am J Gastroenterol 1987;82:1177–9.
29 Gordjani N, Herdeg S, Ross UH et al. Focal dermal hypoplasia (Goltz–Gorlin syndrome) associated with obstructive papillomatosis of the larynx and hypopharynx. Eur J Dermatol 1999;9:618–20.
30 Kore-Eda S, Yoneda K, Ohtani T et al. Focal dermal hypoplasia (Goltz syndrome) associated with multiple giant papillomas. Br J Dermatol 1995;133:997–9.
31 Jenkins ZA, van Kogelenberg M, Morgan T et al. Germline mutations in WTX cause a sclerosing skeletal dysplasia but do not predispose to tumorigenesis. Nat Genet 2009;41:95–100.
32 Hancock S, Pryde P, Fong C et al. Probable identity of Goltz syndrome and Van Allen-Myhre syndrome: evidence from phenotypic evolution. Am J Med Genet 2002;110:370–9.
33 D'Alise MD, Timmons CF, Swift DM. Focal dermal hypoplasia (Goltz syndrome) with vertebral solid aneurysmal bone cyst variant. A case report. Pediatr Neurosurg 1996;24:151–4.
34 Cox NH, Paterson WD. Osteochondroma of humerus in focal dermal hypoplasia (Goltz) syndrome. Clin Exp Dermatol 1991;16:283–4.
35 Gisseman JD, Herce HH. Ophthalmologic manifestations of focal dermal hypoplasia (Goltz syndrome): a case series of 18 patients. Am J Med Genet C Semin Med Genet 2016;172C:59–63.
36 Ishibashi A, Kurihara Y. Goltz's syndrome: focal dermal dysplasia syndrome (focal dermal hypoplasia): report of a case and on its etiology and pathogenesis. Dermatologica 1972;144:156–67.
37 Dunlop AA, Harper JI, Hamilton AM. Retinal neovascularisation in Goltz syndrome (focal dermal hypoplasia). Br J Ophthalmol 1999;83:1094.
38 Adeyemi-Fowode OA, Mansouri R, Dietrich JE. Gynecologic findings in Goltz syndrome: a case series. Am J Med Genet C Semin Med Genet 2016;172C:64–6.
39 Irvine AD, Stewart FJ, Bingham EA et al. Focal dermal hypoplasia (Goltz syndrome) associated with intestinal malrotation and mediastinal dextroposition. Am J Med Genet 1996;62:213–15.
40 Kilmer SL, Grix AW Jr, Isseroff RR. Focal dermal hypoplasia: four cases with widely varying presentations. J Am Acad Dermatol 1993;28:839–43.
41 Kunze J, Heyne K, Wiedemann HR. Diaphragmatic hernia in a female newborn with focal dermal hypoplasia and marked asymmetric malformations (Goltz–Gorlin syndrome). Eur J Pediatr 1979;131:213–18.
42 Toro-Sola MA, Kistenmacher ML, Punnett HH, DiGeorge AM. Focal dermal hypoplasia syndrome in a male. Clin Genet 1975;7:325–7.
43 Baughman FA Jr, Worcester DD. Agenesis of the corpus callosum in a case of focal dermal hypoplasia. Mt Sinai J Med 1970;37:702–9.
44 Almeida L, Anyane-Yeboa K, Grossman M, Rosen T. Myelomeningocele, Arnold–Chiari anomaly and hydrocephalus in focal dermal hypoplasia. Am J Med Genet 1988;30:917–23.
45 Del Carmen Boente M, Asial RA, Winik BC. Focal dermal hypoplasia: ultrastructural abnormalities of the connective tissue. J Cutan Pathol 2007;34:181–7.
46 Tsuji T. Focal dermal hypoplasia syndrome. An electron microscopical study of the skin lesions. J Cutan Pathol 1982;9:271–81.
47 Uitto J, Bauer EA, Santa-Cruz DJ et al. Focal dermal hypoplasia: abnormal growth characteristics of skin fibroblasts in culture. J Invest Dermatol 1980;75:170–5.
48 Sato M, Ishikawa O, Yokoyama Y et al. Focal dermal hypoplasia (Goltz syndrome): a decreased accumulation of hyaluronic acid in three-dimensional culture. Acta Derm Venereol 1996;76:365–7.
49 Ko CJ, Antaya RJ, Zubek A et al. Revisiting histopathologic findings in Goltz syndrome. J Cutan Pathol 2016;43:418–21.
50 Rosen SA, Bocklage T, Clericuzio CL. Mucocutaneous squamous papilloma with reactive lymphoid hyperplasia in two patients with focal dermal hypoplasia. Pediatr Dev Pathol 2005;8:250–2.
51 Aradhya S, Woffendin H, Jakins T et al. A recurrent deletion in the ubiquitously expressed NEMO (IKK-gamma) gene accounts for the vast majority of incontinentia pigmenti mutations. Hum Mol Genet 2001;10:2171–9.
52 Wang LL, Levy ML, Lewis RA et al. Clinical manifestations in a cohort of 41 Rothmund–Thomson syndrome patients. Am J Med Genet 2001;102:11–17.
53 Siitonen HA, Sotkasiira J, Biervliet M et al. The mutation spectrum in RECQL4 diseases. Eur J Hum Genet 2009;17:151–8.
54 Van den Veyver IB. Microphthalmia with linear skin defects (MLS), Aicardi, and Goltz syndromes: are they related X-linked dominant male-lethal disorders? Cytogenet Genome Res 2002;99:289–96.
55 Wimplinger I, Morleo M, Rosenberger G et al. Mutations of the mitochondrial holocytochrome c-type synthase in X-linked dominant microphthalmia with linear skin defects syndrome. Am J Hum Genet 2006;79:878–89.
56 Houge G, Oeffner F, Grzeschik KH. An Xp11.23 deletion containing PORCN may also cause angioma serpiginosum, a cosmetic skin disease associated with extreme skewing of X-inactivation. Eur J Hum Genet 2008;16:1027–8.
57 Happle R. Angioma serpiginosum is not caused by PORCN mutations. Eur J Hum Genet 2009;17:881–2; author reply 2.
58 Alster TS, Wilson F. Focal dermal hypoplasia (Goltz's syndrome). Treatment of cutaneous lesions with the 585-nm flashlamp-pumped pulsed dye laser. Arch Dermatol 1995;131:143–4.
59 Liu J, Hsu PT, VanderWielen BA, Teng JM. Treatment of recalcitrant excessive granulation tissue with photodynamic therapy in an eight-year-old patient with focal dermal hypoplasia syndrome. Pediatr Dermatol 2012;29:324–6.
60 Mallipeddi R, Chaudhry SI, Darley CR, Kurwa HA. A case of focal dermal hypoplasia (Goltz) syndrome with exophytic granulation tissue treated by curettage and photodynamic therapy. Clin Exp Dermatol 2006;31:228–31.
61 Skarzynski H, Podskarbi-Fayette R. Treatment of otorhinolaryngo-logical manifestations of three rare genetic syndromes: branchiooculo-facial

SECTION 28: FOCAL OR GENERALIZED HYPOPLASIA

(BOF), ectrodactyly ectodermal dysplasia clefting (EEC) and focal dermal hypoplasia (Goltz syndrome). Int J Pediatr Otorhinolaryngol 2009;73:143–51.

62 Kashyap P, Sweetser S, Farrugia G. Esophageal papillomas and skin abnormalities. Focal dermal hypoplasia (Goltz syndrome) manifesting with esophageal papillomatosis. Gastroenterology 2011;140:784.

63 Bertani H, Mirante VG, Caruso A et al. Successful treatment of diffuse esophageal papillomatosis with balloon-assisted radiofrequency ablation in a patient with Goltz syndrome. Endoscopy 2014;46: E404–5.

64 Rhee KY, Baek RM, Ahn KJ. Airway management in a patient with focal dermal hypoplasia. Anesth Analg 2006;103:1342.

CHAPTER 136
Incontinentia Pigmenti

Elizabeth A. Jones & Dian Donnai

Manchester Centre for Genomic Medicine, St Mary's Hospital, Manchester University NHS Foundation Trust and Division of Evolution and Genomic Sciences, Faculty of Biology Medicine and Health, University of Manchester, Manchester, UK

Abstract

Incontinentia pigmenti is a multisystem disorder affecting predominantly females. It is characterized by distinct cutaneous features which classically occur in four stages in the distribution of Blaschko lines: vesicular, verrucous, hyperpigmented and atrophic. These stages often occur in a temporal sequence but all stages do not necessarily occur and several stages may overlap. Additional abnormalities that commonly occur include: dental anomalies such as hypodontia or abnormally shaped teeth, peripheral neovascularization of retina and neurodevelopmental abnormalities. Incontinentia pigmenti is an X-linked dominant disorder caused by mutations in the *IKBKG* gene (previously known as the *NEMO* gene). In the majority of affected women, a recurrent deletion in the *IKBKG* gene is responsible and molecular diagnosis is available. Knowledge of this multisystem disorder and early diagnosis is important for clinical management, particularly because of the risk of neovascularization of retina which can result in visual loss if not detected in time.

Key points

- **Incontinentia pigmenti is a neonatal onset, multisystem disorder.**
- **Incontinentia pigmenti has four distinct cutaneous phases: vesicular, verrucous, hyperpigmented and atrophic.**
- **Dental anomalies are common, such as hypodontia or abnormally shaped teeth.**
- **Peripheral neovascularization of the retina can lead to visual loss and requires early proactive screening.**
- **Neurodevelopmental abnormalities include seizures and intellectual disability.**
- **Incontinentia pigmenti is an X-linked dominant disorder caused by mutations in the *IKBKG* gene.**

Introduction. Incontinentia pigmenti (IP) is a multisystem disorder with characteristic skin manifestations affecting predominantly females. It was probably first described in 1906 by Garrod [1], although Bardach [2], Bloch [3], Siemens [4] and Sulzberger [5] defined the condition further. IP is characterized by cutaneous features which classically occur in four stages in the distribution of Blaschko lines: vesicular, verrucous, hyperpigmented, and atrophic. These stages often occur in a temporal sequence but all stages do not necessarily occur and several stages may overlap. IP and pigmentary mosaicism (hypomelanosis of Ito, incontinentia pigmenti achromians) are often confused in the older literature but it is important that they are distinguished from each other because they have different aetiologies, clinical effects and implications for genetic counselling. The clinical similarities of IP and pigmentary mosaicism are caused by the distribution of skin lesions in Blaschko lines. Individuals with IP often have dental abnormalities and may also have visual loss secondary to neovascularization of the retina and neurodevelopmental problems. IP is an X-linked dominant single-gene disorder whereas pigmentary mosiacism is the dermatological phenotype associated with various types of genetic mosaicism. The causative gene for IP was mapped in 1989 to Xq28 [6] and identified as the *NEMO* gene (now the *IKBKG* gene) in 2000 [7].

Epidemiology and pathogenesis. In 1976, Carney [8] reviewed the literature and, from published reports and his personal series, derived risk figures for cutaneous and noncutaneous features. However, this analysis is of a group of patients that has been ascertained in a biased way (by publication) and may also be aetiologically heterogeneous. Not all the published reports contained sufficient information to be sure that the individuals reported had classic IP and some may be examples of pigmentary mosaicism. A review of clinical features from the literature and from a large study was published in 1993 [9], and subsequently several reviews and series of male cases have been published [10–14]. These studies have elucidated data on the frequency of the different features of IP. The cutaneous manifestations are universal, affecting 100% of individuals, whereas 43.5% have dental anomalies, 30% central nervous system (CNS) defects and 30% ophthalmic complications [14]. Prevalence at birth is estimated to be 1.2 per 100 000 [15].

Harper's Textbook of Pediatric Dermatology, Fourth Edition. Edited by Peter Hoeger, Veronica Kinsler and Albert Yan.

Review of pedigrees with IP is compatible with X-linked dominant inheritance, with lethality usually occurring in affected males. This mode of inheritance is supported by the high female:male ratio, female–female transmission and by the increased incidence of miscarriage. In a study of familial IP [9], 53 out of 111 patients were adult females who had been pregnant at least once. They had a total of 158 pregnancies; 40 (25%) ended in miscarriage, 32 produced normal males, 56 affected females and 30 normal females.

The most convincing evidence of X-linkage came from close linkage of IP to markers in the subchromosomal band Xq28 [6]. In 2000 an international consortium found a recurrent deletion mutation in 80% of index cases in the *IKBKG* gene (inhibitor of kappa polypeptide gene enhancer in B cells kinase gamma) – previously known as the *NEMO* gene (nuclear factor κB, essential modulator) which encodes the regulatory subunit of the inhibitor of κB kinase (IKK) complex [7]. NEMO is central to many immune, inflammatory and apoptotic pathways in the cell and required for the activation of the transcription factor NF-κB. Cells in which the active X carries the mutated gene are more liable to undergo cell death. Curtis and colleagues [16] reported skewed X inactivation in affected females, with preferential inactivation of the IP X chromosome. X-inactivation is thought to be the major contributory factor to the wide phenotypic variability in affected females even within the same family. In males, extensive cellular apoptosis usually results in early fetal lethality [17,18]. However, IP has been reported in liveborn males. In such cases, the male may have Klinefelter syndrome (47, XXY) [19,20] or somatic mosaicism [21,22]. Father-to-daughter transmission has been reported [22–24].

In female patients with IP the *IKBKG* gene mutation is always heterozygous and can either preserve a residual NF-κB activation (hypomorphic mutation) or completely abolish it (amorphic mutation) [25]. The recurrent *IKBKG* gene mutation results from a complex rearrangement that deletes exons 4–10 of the gene. Males with hypomorphic *IKBKG* mutations have a milder, clinically distinct anhydrotic ectodermal dysplasia-immunodeficiency syndrome (known as X-linked hypohidrotic ectodermal dysplasia and immunodeficiency, HED-ID), though interestingly, their mothers may show signs of classic IP [26–30].

Clinical features.

Skin

The cutaneous manifestations of IP are diagnostic where these arise in the classic order, or once sufficient numbers of stages have been seen; however, their absence does not entirely exclude the diagnosis, especially in first-degree female relatives of classic patients who have several noncutaneous features. Classically, the dermatological features are described in four stages, but all stages do not necessarily occur; they may arise out of order, and several stages may overlap. The cutaneous features occur in the pattern of fine and whorled Blaschko lines, that is, circumferential around the trunk, forming a V pattern over the spine, stopping in the midline anteriorly and in linear streaks over the shoulders and hips and down the limbs. There may be a stage that precedes stage 1, the vesicular stage. We have observed so-called erythema toxicum neonatorum distributed in Blaschko lines, which lasted 24 hours before the occurrence of typical vesicles at the age of 48 hours in the affected daughter of an affected mother.

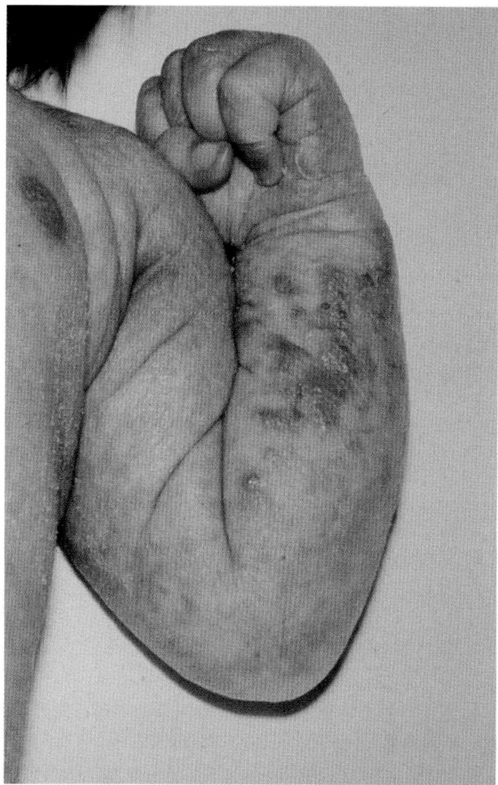

Fig. 136.1 Female, aged 3 weeks, showing the characteristic stage 1 vesicular rash on the left arm.

Stage 1: The first stage is characterized by vesicles often preceded by localized erythema, which occur anywhere on the body but usually sparing the face. The lesions of the first stage develop within the first few weeks after birth, often within the first week. A linear distribution along the limbs and circumferentially around the trunk is classic, although not always so well defined (Fig. 136.1). Crops of blisters may occur in the groin and axillary regions and on the vertex of the scalp. Each crop of blisters clears within weeks and may be replaced by new crops at the same or different sites. In general, the vesicles clear within the first 6 months of life, although they may recur during acute febrile illness in childhood. These later eruptions are less severe and more short-lived than those that appear in the neonatal period.

Stage 2: The so-called verrucous lesions were observed in just over one-third of the 111 patients reported by Landy and Donnai [9]. These lesions were often short-lived and trivial compared with the initial vesicular eruption and therefore might have been underreported. In the patients in whom there was a positive history, the lesions had appeared by 2 months and all had cleared by 3 years. The lesions were predominantly seen on the distal limbs, especially the digits and ankles (Fig. 136.2).

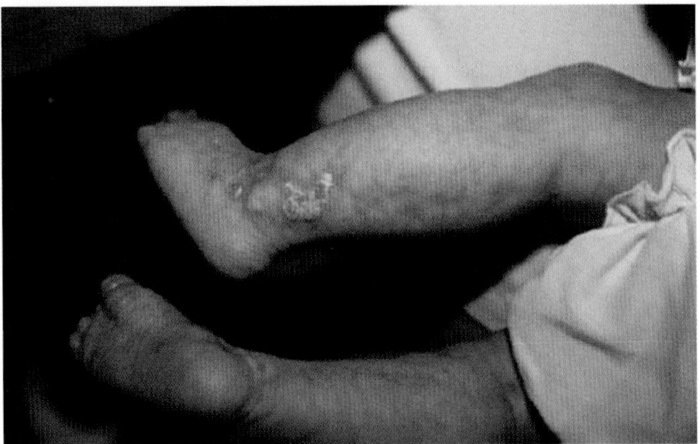

Fig. 136.2 Female, aged 6 months, demonstrating stage 2 verrucous phase of incontinentia pigmenti.

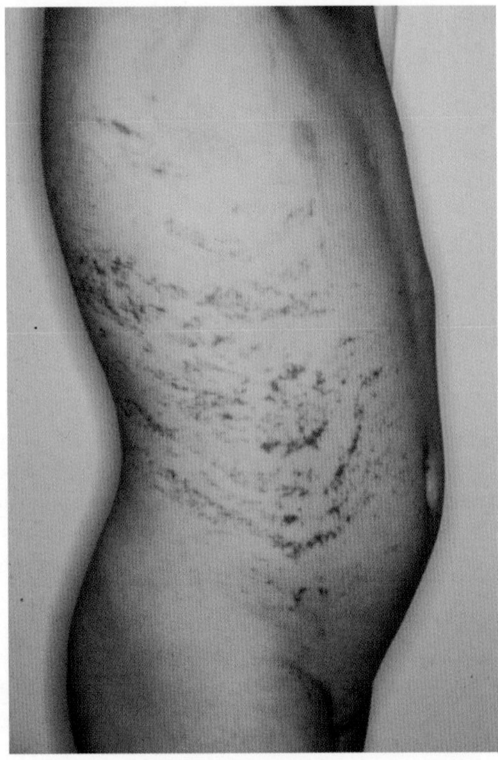

Fig. 136.3 Female, aged 4 years, demonstrating stage 3 widespread pigmentation in the distribution of Blaschko lines over the torso.

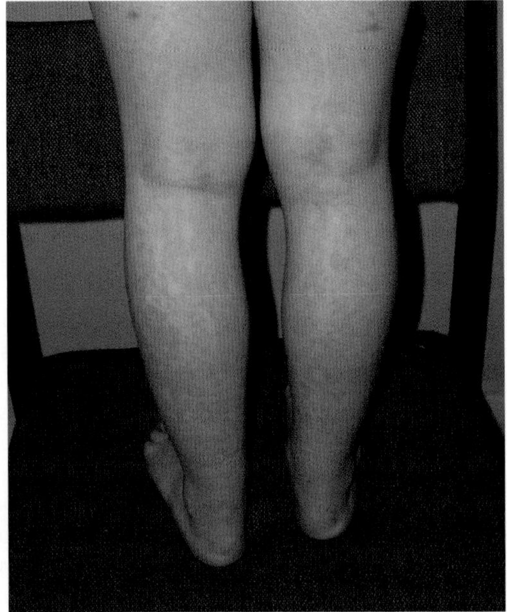

Fig. 136.4 Female, aged 7 years, demonstrating the stage 4 atrophic phase of incontinentia pigmenti in a linear distribution over the back of both legs.

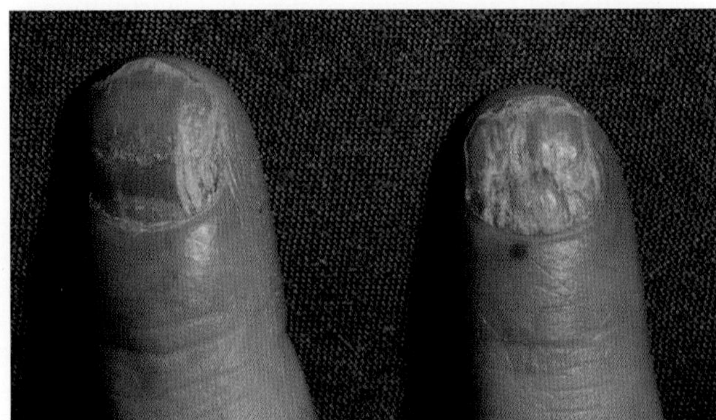

Fig. 136.5 Nails of female with incontinentia pigmenti illustrating the nail dystrophy.

They did not necessarily appear in the same areas as the vesicles. The crusting lesions that develop at the vertex following blistering at that site may be similar to the verrucous lesions but these tended to persist and to be followed by an area of alopecia.

Stage 3: This is the stage that gives its name to the condition but its presence and extent are very variable. It can range from small streaks of pigmentation in the groin to more extensive lesions, especially following Blaschko lines around the trunk (Fig. 136.3). The distribution, however, is not necessarily classically Blaschkolinear, and is classically referred to as 'Chinese Figurate' in appearance. The nipples are frequently involved in the increased pigmentation and the axillae and groins are invariably affected in patients with pigmentation elsewhere. The pigmentation has usually appeared by 6 months but, occasionally, not until 2–3 years, and occasionally it precedes all other stages. By 10 years, the lesions have faded in about 25% of cases and in the majority these pigmented lesions disappear by the age of 16 years.

Stage 4: This is the so-called atrophic phase classically seen in affected adult females. However, in the series reported by Landy and Donnai [9], these pale linear lesions were observed in many girls under the age of 10 years, concurrent with hyperpigmented or even vesicular and verrucous lesions. The atrophic lesions are less frequently observed on the trunk and are more often seen on the posterior aspect of the upper and lower legs (Fig. 136.4) and over the shoulders and upper arms. It is not clear that these follow Blaschko lines.

Nails

Nail dystrophy is frequent, occurring in approximately 40% of affected individuals (Fig. 136.5). The range of manifestations is wide, from mild ridging or pitting to severe nail dystrophy resembling onychomycosis.

Nail dystrophy may be a transient phenomenon. Subungual keratotic lesions have been described [31,32]. The histology of these lesions corresponds to that seen in the verrucous cutaneous lesions of stage 2, showing hyperkeratosis, acanthosis, papillomatosis and focal dermal dyskeratosis.

Hair

Although hair abnormalities are common (26%), it is rare for affected females to have major cosmetic problems. Alopecia, especially at the vertex and usually after blistering or verrucous lesions at this site, is common. Hair is often described as sparse early in childhood and later in life as lustreless, wiry and coarse.

Teeth

Dental abnormalities are common, occurring in over 40% of cases. Either, or both, deciduous and permanent dentition may be affected and abnormalities include hypodontia, delayed eruption, impaction and malformation of the crowns, especially conical forms and accessory cusps [32]. Deciduous teeth may be retained into adult life (Fig. 136.6). Dental features can be of diagnostic value in adult females and, if present in adult first-degree female relatives of an affected case, they should stimulate a search for other signs such as atrophic skin lesions or hair anomalies.

Eyes

The incidence of ocular abnormalities in IP is high and may approach 40%. The characteristic lesion of ocular IP involves anomalies of the developing retinal vessels and the underlying pigmented cells [33,34]. Areas of retinal ischaemia promote new vessel proliferation with subsequent bleeding and fibrosis, a process with similarities to those found in retinopathy of prematurity. Signs of this process are present in many IP patients but the process is generally limited and progression to gross intraocular scarring with severe visual loss occurs in only 10% of patients. When this does occur, it is usually only in one eye.

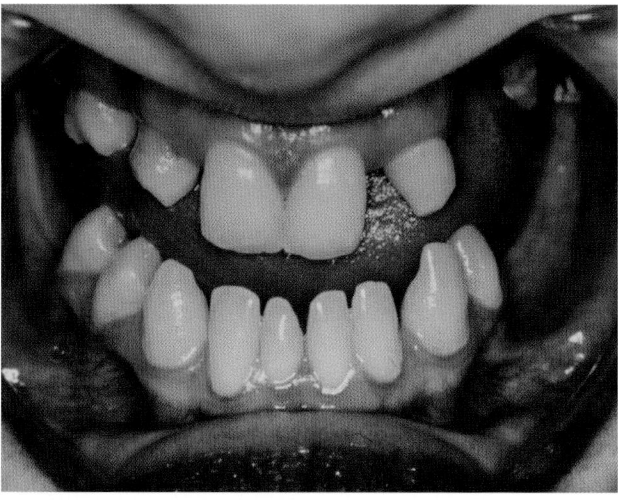

Fig. 136.6 Teeth of adult female with incontinentia pigmenti, demonstrating hypodontia and missing upper incisors.

When visual loss occurs in younger patients (some as early as the first couple of weeks), it is usually caused by tractional retinal detachment secondary to contraction of fibrovascular tissue, whereas in older patients it is caused by rhegmatogenous detachment related to holes in atrophic, avascular retina [35]. Strabismus occurs in almost one-third of patients, often in association with refractive errors. Occasionally microphthalmos, cataract and optic atrophy are seen. Despite the high frequency of ophthalmic complications, over 90% of patients have normal vision.

Neurological signs

Although Carney's review [8] found a high frequency of neurological abnormalities, the group of patients reviewed may have been biased towards those with a neurological presentation, and possibly also aetiologically heterogeneous. The study by Landy and Donnai [9], in which strict diagnostic criteria were applied, suggest a considerably lower incidence of CNS abnormalities and this is concordant with Fusco and colleague's recent series [14]. In Donnai and Landy's series [9] 14% of patients had seizures, 8% had transient seizures without associated intellectual disability and only 6% of patients had persistent seizures. In this group, the seizures developed before 12 weeks of age, often in the first week of life, and were associated with a degree of intellectual disability. Around 10% of the 111 patients studied had intellectual disability, although in only one-third of these was it classed as severe. The incidence of intellectual disability in familial cases is 3% compared with 15% in the sporadic cases studied.

In Fusco and colleague's series [14], 97 out of 308 had CNS defects (31.5%) and of these 39 had seizures and 29 had intellectual impairment. Minic and colleagues [36] published a systematic review of CNS anomalies in IP and again these were present in 30%. In 58% of those affected, the age of first neurological manifestation was in the first week and 88% had presented in the first year of life. The most frequent CNS anomalies were seizures, motor impairment, intellectual impairment and microcephaly. Severe neurological problems are uncommon but Wolf and colleagues [37], Loh and colleagues [38] and Maingay-de Groof and colleagues [39] have reported cases with proven *IKBKG* mutations that presented with neonatal encephalopathy and extensive cerebral infarction with major developmental problems. However, Bryant and Rutledge [40] reported a child with significant white matter abnormalities but with no neurological problems.

Breasts

Breast anomalies have rarely been reported in patients with IP but in the series by Landy and Donnai [9], breast anomalies occurred in 10% of cases. One woman had unilateral breast and nipple aplasia whereas 10 others had supernumerary nipples.

Other signs

Although there have been reports of IP patients with recurrent infections, suggesting that immunodeficiency might be a factor, this does not seem to be a common

Table 136.1 Diagnostic criteria for incontinentia pigmenti. For a clinical diagnosis of incontinentia pigmenti two major criteria or one major criterion and at least one minor criterion should be present.

Major criteria	Minor criteria
Typical incontinentia pigmenti cutaneous stages distributed along Blaschko lines:	Dental anomalies
Vesiculo-bullous stage	Peripheral neovascularization of retina
Verrucous stage	Central nervous system abnormalities
Hyperpigmented stage	Abnormal hair
Atrophic/hypopigmented stage	Abnormal nails
Confirmed pathogenic mutation in *IKBKG* gene	Breast or nipple hypoplasia
	Multiple miscarriages of male fetuses

problem. Anomalies of the palate including a high arched palate, cleft lip and cleft palate have been reported to occur in association with IP [36]. Pulmonary hypertension is a rare complication of IP [41,42].

Diagnostic criteria. Any condition with skin manifestations in Blaschko lines may be confused with IP and so strict diagnostic criteria are crucial. Diagnostic criteria for IP were initially suggested by Landy and Donnai [9] and later updated by Minic and colleagues [43]. The skin manifestations represent major criteria with the other features making up the minor criteria. With the increased availability of diagnostic testing a confirmed pathogenic mutation in the *IKBKG* gene can also be included as a major diagnostic criterion (Table 136.1).

Differential diagnosis.

Pigmentary mosaicism (hypomelanosis of Ito, incontinentia pigmenti achromians)

This heterogeneous group of mosaic conditions should be considered in any 'atypical' or severely affected sporadic case of IP particularly in the absence of a clear history of a vesicular or verrucous phase (see Chapter 109),

X-autosome translocation

A similar but clinically distinct disorder has been observed in several females with X-autosome translocations involving a possible locus at Xp11. At first, this was thought to indicate the genetic locus for familial IP. Confusingly the disorder associated with X-autosome translocations was sometimes referred to as IP1 and the familial form as IP2. In the reported women with X-autosome translocations with a breakpoint at Xp11, the early stage 1 and 2 lesions of classic IP are not observed; rather, whorled pigmentation or hypopigmentation is seen from early on. As a group, these individuals have more severe developmental problems. Molecular studies by Hatchwell and colleagues [44] have demonstrated random X inactivation in uncultured fibroblasts, lending support to the hypothesis that the phenotype is a manifestation of mosaicism, with some cells being functionally disomic for a portion of the X chromosome rather than the effects being caused by disruption of a single genetic locus.

Goltz focal dermal hypoplasia

This condition with lesions in Blaschko lines is sometimes confused with IP and has the same X-linked dominant mode of inheritance. However, the skin lesions are quite distinct, consisting of focal absence of the dermis in the distribution of Blaschko lines, with multiple papillomas of mucous membranes as well as linear hyper- and hypopigmentation. Skeletal abnormalities, including limb reduction defects and major eye abnormalities, such as microphthalmia and anophthalmia, are common. This disorder is caused by mutations in the *PORCN* gene, a regulator of Wnt signalling [45,46].

X-linked dominant chondrodysplasia punctata

The early phases of skin manifestations in this condition are ichthyosiform erythroderma and these can sometimes be mistaken for the verrucous phase of IP. The hyperkeratotic phase is followed by linear scarring with follicular pitting. Alopecia is sometimes a major problem, as are skeletal abnormalities and cataracts. Mutations have been found in the *EBP* (emopamil-binding protein) gene which codes for an enzyme catalysing a key step in the formation of cholesterol and vitamin D [47].

Laboratory findings.

Histology

In the early vesicular cutaneous stage of IP, there is massive infiltration of eosinophils into the epidermis. There is also marked peripheral blood eosinophilia. In stage I of the lesions, eosinophilic spongiosis is usually present on skin biopsy.

Genetic testing

Genetic testing of the *IKBKG* gene is available. Approximately 75% of individuals who meet clinical diagnostic criteria will have the common exon 4-10 deletion mutation; 22% will have point mutations; and 4% Xq28 rearrangements [14]. In those in whom a mutation in the *IKBKG* gene cannot be found, somatic mosaicism should be considered. If possible, genetic testing should be performed using DNA extracted from an affected area of skin to look for a somatic *IKBKG* gene mutation. In males with clinical features of IP, chromosomal analysis should be undertaken as well to look for sex chromosome abnormalities.

Prenatal diagnosis is available and can be offered to women with an increased chance of having a child with IP if the causative mutation is known.

Medical surveillance and treatment. During the neonatal period and when blisters are present, it is important to guard against infection and keep the lesions as dry as possible. There is no effective treatment to hasten resolution of any of the phases of IP.

The ocular abnormalities can occur early and lead to significant visual loss and so there should be lifelong regular screening for retinal abnormalities. If the diagnosis of IP is made in the newborn period, an ophthalmic evaluation should take place before discharge from hospital and be repeated regularly (at least monthly) in the first 4 months. This may require general anaesthesia to ensure adequate retinal examination. Newborn examination may be normal but rapid progression of the vascular abnormalities can occur in the first weeks of life. Examinations should then be repeated 3 monthly until 1 year of age and six monthly until 3 years of age. A fluorescein angiogram is a useful investigation. The risk of retinal detachment decreases after 3 years of age and so follow-up interval can be increased to 12 months, but surveillance should be lifelong. Adult patients or parents of children with IP should be educated to be aware of the symptoms of retinal detachment. Interventions to promote regression of neovascular changes may include laser photocoagulation or cryotherapy of the nonperfused retina.

All patients with IP should have regular dental reviews and receive education regarding oral health. If dental abnormalities are detected, referral to a specialist dental team should be considered.

Patients with IP should all have an initial neurological examination. If there is a history of seizures an EEG may be useful. Standard antiepileptic therapies should be prescribed for seizure control but phenobarbitone may be less effective in infantile seizures. Cranial imaging studies should be considered in those with seizures or other neurological signs and magnetic resonance imaging with the combined use of diffusion-weighted imaging and susceptibility-weighted imaging has been shown to be useful [48]. Standard supportive therapies should be offered to individuals with intellectual impairment.

Genetic counselling to individuals with IP and parents of a child with IP should be offered. Examination of first-degree female relatives and/or genetic testing if the causative mutation is known should be offered.

References

1 Garrod AE. Peculiar pigmentation of the skin of an infant. Trans Clin Soc Lond 1906;39:216.

2 Bardach M. Systematisierte Naevusbildungen bei einem eineiigen Zwillingspaar. Z Kinderheilkd 1925;39:542–50.

3 Bloch B. Eigentumliche, bischer nicht beschriebene Pigmentaffektion (incontinentia pigmenti). Schweiz Med Wochenschr 1926;7:404–5.

4 Siemens HW. Die Melanosis corii degenerativa eine neue Pigmentdermatose. Arch Dermatol Syph (Berl) 1929;157:382–91.

5 Sulzberger MB. Uber eine bischer nicht beschriebene congenitale Pigmentanomalie (IP). Arch Dermatol Syph (Berl) 1928;154:19–32.

6 Sefiani A, Abel L, Heuertz S et al. The gene for incontinentia pigmenti is assigned to Xq28. Genomics 1989;4:427–9.

7 Smahi A, Courtois G, Vabres P et al. Genomic rearrangement in NEMO impairs NF-B activation and is a cause of incontinentia pigmenti. Nature 2000;405:466–72

8 Carney RG. Incontinentia pigmenti: a world statistical analysis. Arch Dermatol 1976;112:535–42.

9 Landy SJ, Donnai D. Incontinentia pigmenti (Bloch–Sulzberger syndrome). J Med Genet 1993;30:53–9.

10 Sheuerle AE. Male cases of incontinentia pigmenti: case report and review. Am J Med Genet 1998;77:201–18.

11 Pacheco TR, Levy M, Collyer JC et al. Incontinentia pigmenti in male patients. J Am Acad Dermatol 2006;55:251–5.

12 Ardelean D, Pope E Incontinentia pigmenti in boys: a series and review of the literature. Pediatr Dermatol 2007;23:523–7.

13 Fusco F, Fimiani G, Tadini G et al. Clinical diagnosis of incontinentia pigmenti in a cohort of male patients. J Am Acad Dermatol 2007;56:264–7.

14 Fusco F, Paciolla M, Conte, MI et al. Incontinentia pigmenti: report on data from 2000 to 2013. Orphanet J Rare Dis 2014;9:93.

15 Orphanet Report Series, Prevalence and incidence of rare diseases, June 2018 – http://www.orpha.net/orphacom/cahiers/docs/GB/Prevalence_of_rare_diseases_by_alphabetical_list.pdf

16 Curtis ARJ, Lindsay S, Boye E et al. A study of X chromosome activity in two incontinentia pigmenti families with probable linkage to Xq28. Eur J Hum Genet 1994;2:51–8.

17 Courtois G, Smahi A, Israël A. NEMO/IKK gamma: linking NF-kappa B to human disease Trends Mol Med. 2001;7(10):427–30.

18 Nelson DL. NEMO, NFkappaB signaling and incontinentia pigmenti. Curr Opin Genet Dev 2006;16:282–8.

19 Ormerod AD, White MI, McKay E et al. Incontinentia pigmenti in a boy with Klinefelter's syndrome. J Med Genet 1987;24:439–41.

20 Garcia-Dorado J, de Unamo P, Fernandez-Lopez E et al. Incontinentia pigmenti: XXY male with family history. Clin Genet 1990;38:128–38.

21 Kenwrick S, Woffendin H, Jakins T et al. Survival of male patients with incontinentia pigmenti carrying a lethal mutation can be explained by somatic mosaicism or Klinefelter syndrome. Am J Hum Genet 2001;69:1210–7.

22 Rashidghamat E, Hsu CK, Nanda A et al. Incontinentia pigmenti in a father and daughter. B J Derm 2016;175:1059–60.

23 Sommer AM, Liu PH. Incontinentia pigmenti in a father and his daughter. Am Med Genet 1984;17:655–9.

24 Emery MM, Siegfried EC, Stone MS et al. Incontinentia pigmenti: transmission from father to daughter. J Am Acad Dermatol 1993;29:368–72.

25 Fusco F, Pescatore A, Conte MI et al. EDA-ID and IP, Two faces of the same coin: how the same IKBKG/NEMO mutation affecting the NF-κB pathway can cause immunodeficientcy and/or inflammation. Int Rev Immunol 2015;34:445–59.

26 Smahi A, Courtois G, Rabia SH et al. The NF kappaB signalling pathway in human diseases: from incontinentia pigmenti to ectodermal dysplasias and immune-deficiency syndromes. Hum Mol Genet 2002;11:2371–5.

27 Zonana J, Elder ME, Schneider LC et al. A novel X-linked disorder of immune deficiency and hypohidrotic ectodermal dysplasia is allelic to incontinentia pigmenti and due to mutations in IKK-(NEMO). Am J Hum Genet 2000; 67:1555–62.

28 Mansour S, Woffendin H, Mitton S et al. Incontinentia pigmenti in a surviving male is accompanied by hypohidrotic ectodermal dysplasia and recurrent infection. Am J Med Genet 2001;99:172–7.

29 Aradhya S, Courtois G, Rajkovic A et al. Atypical forms of incontinentia pigmenti in males result from mutations of a cytosine tract in exon 10 of NEMO (IKK). Am J Hum Genet 2001;68:765–71.

30 Dupuis-Girod S, Corradini N, Hadj-Rabia S et al. Osteopetrosis, lymphedema, anhydrotic ectodermal dysplasia and immunodeficiency in a boy and incontinentia pigmenti in his mother. Pediatrics 2002;109:e97.

31 Simmons DA, Kegel MF, Scher RK et al. Subungual tumours in incontinentia pigmenti. Arch Dermatol 1986;122:1431–4.

32 Mascaro JM, Palon J, Vires P et al. Painful subungual keratotic tumours in incontinentia pigmenti. J Am Acad Dermatol 1985;13:913–18.

33 Goldberg MF, Custis PH. Retinal and other manifestations of incontinentia pigmenti (Bloch–Sulzberger syndrome). Ophthalmology 1993;100:1645–54.

34 Francois J. Incontinentia pigmenti and retinal changes. Br J Ophthalmol 1984;68:19–25.

35 Chen CJ, Han IC, Tian J et al Extended follow-up of treated and untreated retinopathy in incontinentia pigmenti. JAMA Ophthalmol 2015;133:542–8.

36 Minic S, Trpinac D, Obradovic M Systematic review of central nervous system anomalies in incontinentia pigmenti. Orphanet J Rare Dis 2013;8:25.

37 Wolf NI, Kramer N, Harting I et al. Diffuse cortical necrosis in a neonate with incontinentia pigmenti and an encephalitis-like presentation. Am J Neuroradiol 2005;26:1580–2.

38 Loh NR, Jadresic LP, Whitelaw A. A genetic cause for neonatal encephalopathy: incontinentia with NEMO mutation. Acta Paediatr 2008;97:379–81.

39 Maingay-de Groof F, Lequin MH, Roofhooft DW et al Extensive cerebral infarction in the newborn due to incontinentia pigmenti. Eur J Paediatr Neurol 2008;12:284–9.
40 Bryant SA, Rutledge SL. Abnormal white matter in a neurologically intact child with incontinentia pigmenti. Pediatr Neurol 2007;36:199–201.
41 Alshenqiti A, Nashabat M, AlGhoraibi H et al. Pulmonary hypertension and vasculopathy in incontinentia pigmenti: a case report. Ther Clin Risk Manag 2017;13:629–34.
42 Godambe S, McNamara P, Rajguru M, Hellman J. Unusual neonatal presentation of incontinentia pigmenti with persistent pulmonary hypertension of the newborn: a case report. J Perinatol 2005;25:289–92.
43 Minic S, Trpinac D, Obradovic M. Incontinentia pigmenti diagnostic criteria update. Clin Genet 2014;85:536–42.
44 Hatchwell E, Robinson D, Crolla JA et al. X inactivation analysis in a female with hypomelanosis of Ito associated with a balanced X;17 translocation: evidence for functional disomy of Xp. J Med Genet 1996;33:216–20.
45 Grzeschik KH, Bornholdt D, Oeffner F et al. Deficiency of PORCN, a regulator of Wnt signaling, is associated with focal dermal hypoplasia. Nat Genet 2007;39: 833–5.
46 Wang X, Sutton VR, Peraza-Llanes JO et al. Mutations in X-linked PORCN, a putative regulator of Wnt signaling, cause focal dermal hypoplasia. Nat Genet 2007;39: 836–8.
47 Derry JMJ, Gormally E, Means GD et al. Mutations in a delta8-delta7 sterol isomerase in the tattered mouse and X-linked dominant chondrodysplasia punctata. Nat Genet 1999;22:286–90.
48 Salamon AS, Lichtenbelt K, Cowan F et al. Clinical presentation and spectrum of neuroimaging findings in newborn infants with incontinentia pigmenti. Dev Med Child Neurol 2016;58: 1076–84.

CHAPTER 137
Premature Ageing Syndromes

Helga V. Toriello[1] *& Caleb P. Bupp*[2]

[1]Department of Pediatrics/Human Development, Michigan State University College of Human Medicine, Grand Rapids, MI, USA
[2]Spectrum Health Genetics, Grand Rapids, MI, USA

Conditions with true premature ageing, 1725
Conditions with skin atrophy/lipoatrophy, 1729
Conditions in which individuals appear aged, 1735
Conditions with skin laxity, 1738

Abstract

Key diseases in this group include Hutchinson–Gilford progeria, Werner syndrome, Cockayne syndrome, and the mandibuloacral dysplasias. The causes of a prematurely aged phenotype are heterogeneous. In general, true premature ageing, thin skin with local or generalized lipoatrophy, cutis laxa or skin hyperextensibility, or simply an older appearance than would be expected for the person's age can all lead to what is considered a prematurely aged phenotype. However, classical key clinical features which should be recognized are appearance of the skin (thin, excessively wrinkled or easily sunburned?), altered growth patterns, and the presence of additional manifestations. The heterogeneity of disease is because of differences in underlying mechanisms, primarily genetic variations. The diagnostic and genetic features of the prematurely aged phenotypes are reviewed, with emphasis on differential diagnosis.

Key points

- Premature ageing syndromes are heterogeneous, including diagnoses such as Hutchinson–Gilford progeria, mandibuloacral dysplasias, and numerous rare conditions.
- Key clinical features of premature ageing are alterations in skin appearance, diminished growth, and additional phenotypic manifestations. Underlying disease mechanisms can be an accelerated ageing process, lipodystrophy, or skin laxity.
- Prognosis is dependent on the underlying cause.
- Most, if not all have a genetic basis and diagnosis is based on the component manifestations and identification of the causative mutation.

Conditions with true premature ageing

Hutchinson–Gilford progeria syndrome

Syn.
Progeria

Brief introduction and history. Hutchinson–Gilford progeria syndrome (HGPS) is characterized by the rapid appearance of ageing with development of characteristic facial features, alopecia and what are usually adult-onset medical conditions in childhood. This condition is initially marked by failure to thrive, and lifespan is typically markedly reduced. A general rule of thumb is that in one calendar year, HGPS individuals age one clinical decade [1].

Hutchinson [2] first described this condition in 1886; 11 years later Gilford [3] reported a similar patient. Since then, over 130 cases have been reported [4]. The causative gene, *LMNA*, was discovered in 2003 by two groups [5,6]. The function of *LMNA* as it relates to cellular ageing has prompted much interest and study regarding potentially harnessing and altering the ageing process.

Epidemiology and pathogenesis. Best estimates of incidence are 1 in 4–8 million, and there may be a slightly increased male:female sex ratio [4]. With most early cases being reported sporadically and linked based on similar phenotypic features, the underlying cause of HGPS first remained unclear. A seminal review article from DeBusk in 1972 looked at 60 cases from across the globe [7]. The discovery of the causative gene proved autosomal dominant inheritance. The *LMNA* gene was identified by two groups using differing lines of inquiry. One group used noted lipodystrophy phenotype similarities to mandibulo-acral dysostosis and used autozygosity mapping to target chromosome 1q21 where *LMNA* is located. The other group utilized areas of homozygosity and the detection of two patients with uniparental disomy of 1q to identify *LMNA* as a candidate gene [8,9].

LMNA produces the protein Lamin A, a member of the lamin family of intermediate filaments. They are located in the nuclei of eukaryotes and help with strength, shape and anchoring other proteins. B-type lamins are expressed in all cells but A-type lamins are only in differentiated cells. There are four isoforms caused by alternate mRNA splicing. Initially, Lamin A exists as prelamin A, which has a C-terminal tail that is seen in farnesylated proteins. Prelamin A is altered after translation by addition of a farnesyl group then altering of the amino acid tail in multiple steps. A zinc metalloproteinase *ZMPSTE24* is involved in this process, and cases of atypical HGPS are possibly caused by mutations in that gene. After farnesylation, Lamin A can be utilized in the inner nuclear membrane [4].

In almost all cases of classic HGPS a p.G608G (c.1824C>T) mutation takes place in exon 11 of *LMNA*. This does not change the amino acid, but it does create a cryptic splice site that causes the elimination of 150 nucleotides. This alters the ability of prelamin A to be farnesylated and prelamin A is not turned into Lamin A, instead ending up altered and termed Progerin [3]. It is likely that the presence of Progerin, not the absence of Lamin A, is the cause of the HGPS phenotype. This has been demonstrated *in vitro* by the inability of Lamin A addition to counteract the presence of Progerin [10]. The pathogenic function of Progerin is not entirely understood and has led to much thought regarding treatment for HGPS and understanding of the ageing process in general. It may function in enhanced DNA damage and defective repair or altered cell proliferation and ageing [11]. Other mutations in the *LMNA* gene have been reported more rarely to cause HGPS in classic and nonclassic form. Also, there are probably other causative genes associated with this condition. There may be a paternal age effect for *LMNA* mutations [4].

Pathology. Early reports of abnormal findings on histology include a superabundant network of thick and irregular elastin fibres in the reticular dermis [12], epidermal atrophy and hyaline fibrosis of the dermis with loss of appendages [13] and capillary dilation in the dermis [14]. More recently, however, Mazereeuw-Hautier and colleagues [15] only noted a mild increase in the number of elastic fibres in three children with p.G608G mutations. It is therefore possible that the previously reported alterations might have been seen in children with either atypical forms of HGS or related conditions, or that there is variability in histopathological changes.

Clinical features (Figs 137.1 and 137.2). The most common clinical features of classic HGPS are failure to thrive resulting in marked short stature, premature hair loss, scleroderma leading to skin atrophy, lipodystrophy, decreased joint mobility and characteristic facies. Pregnancy is typically unremarkable and infants have a normal appearance at birth other than slightly reduced birthweight and size. Growth parameters plummet to below the third centile (weight worse than height) in the first year of life. Osteolysis takes place in membranous bones such as the distal phalanges (causing the skin over the phalanges to be red and swollen along with dystrophic nails), clavicle (causing narrowing at the shoulders),

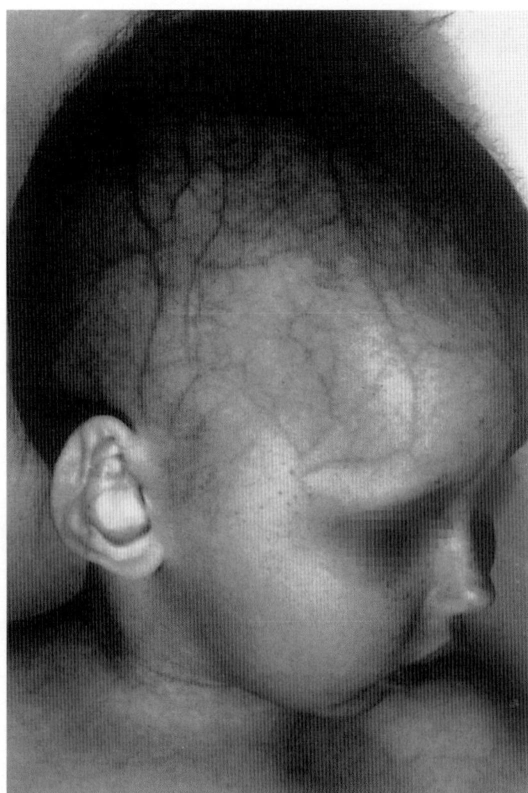

Fig. 137.1 Progeria: there is loss of hair with prominent scalp veins, micrognathia and abnormal ears. Source: Reproduced courtesy of Professor D.J. Gawkrodger and Butterworth Heinemann.

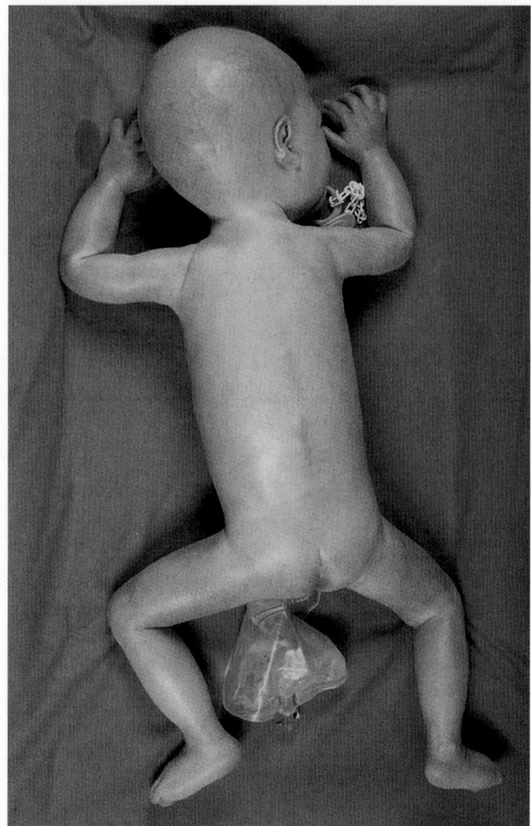

Fig. 137.2 Progeria: typical posture. Source: Courtesy of Professor Arnold P. Oranje.

mandible (causing retrognathia), viscerocranium (causing teeth crowding) and neurocranium (causing a wide, open fontanelle and preserving head size secondary to normal brain growth giving the face a smaller appearance). Lipodystrophy develops and contributes to the skin appearing more translucent and the presence of visible veins. It typically spares the abdomen giving a 'pear shaped' appearance. A vein seen across the nasal bridge is a characteristic sign of HGPS. Transient sclerodermatous skin develops in the first couple years of life then improves without treatment resulting in thin, dry, atrophic skin on which dyspigmentation and early solar lentigines can appear on the neck and upper thorax. With similar timing, hair initially develops but falls out by age two, along with eyelashes and eyebrows. Decreased joint mobility eventually causes a shuffling gait and 'horse riding stance' when standing, along with winging of the scapulae. Muscle bulk is decreased and joints can become painful, but these are not because of developing skin problems. Individuals with HGPS have a high-pitched voice, increased dental decay despite good hygiene, delayed tooth eruption and dental crowding. Cataracts, hearing loss, increased infections, and secondary sexual development are not typically seen. Development and intellect are normal [4,16].

Cardiovascular features are most closely linked to morbidity and mortality. There are not increased cardiovascular abnormalities at birth and blood pressure is normal. There is a gradual development of hypertension, dyspnoea with exertion, fatigue and heart enlargement over the first years of life. Blood vessels have little intima and media resulting in a small diameter, and smooth muscle cells are lost. Myocardial cells hypertrophy and valve leaflets thicken. All these processes lead to vascular problems, strokes, atherosclerosis and myocardial infarction. The average age of stroke is nine years and death is 14.6 years, most often secondary to myocardial infarction [4,17]. The clinical features of HGPS are well detailed in a review of this condition [4].

HGPS is an excellent example of a segmental or organ-restricted ageing syndrome because there is no neurocognitive decline and no major increased cancer risk. Multiple organs such as the liver, kidney, lung, gastrointestinal tract, bone marrow and brain are essentially spared [18].

Prognosis. The average age for diagnosis of HGPS is 2.9 years [4]. There is no curative treatment for HGPS, but medications such as statins and bisphosphonates can be given. Clinical trials of attempts to inhibit farnesylation of progerin have shown some promise. Other proposed methods for treatment include antisense oligonucleotides, and there are mouse models for HGPS used in research [9,16]. Surveillance and management guidelines have been suggested [19]. Reported lifespan ranges from 6 to 20 years [16].

Differential diagnosis. Atypical HGPS is notable for similar findings but with later onset, slower progression and slightly longer lifespan. Osteolysis is more severe [3]. Many of these cases are caused by nonclassic mutations in *LMNA* and others may be attributed to other related or modifying genes [4,16]. Werner syndrome can appear similar but has later onset, cataracts and increased cancer risk [20]. Many other disorders that share similarities in clinical presentation are discussed within this chapter.

References

1 Pollex RL, Hegele RA. Hutchinson–Gilford progeria syndrome. Clin Genet 2004; 66:375–81

2 Hutchinson J. Congenital absence of hair and mammary glands with atrophic condition of skin and its appendages. Med Chir Trans 1886;69:473–7.

3 Gilford H. On a condition of mixed premature and immature development. Med Chir Trans 1897;80:17–45.

4 Hennekam RCM. Hutchinson–Gilford progeria syndrome: review of the phenotype. Am J Med Genet A 2006;140A:2603–24.

5 Eriksson M, Brown WT, Gordon LB et al. Recurrent de novo point mutations in lamin A cause Hutchinson–Gilford progeria syndrome. Nature 2003;423:293–8.

6 De Sandre-Giovannoli A, Bernard R, Cau P et al. Lamin a truncation in Hutchinson–Gilford progeria. Science 2003;300:2055.

7 DeBusk FL. The Hutchinson–Gilford progeria syndrome. J Pediatr 1972;80:697–724.

8 Novelli G, Muchir A, Sangiuolo F et al. Mandibuloacral dysplasia is caused by a mutation in LMNA-encoding lamin A/C. Am J Hum Genet 2003; 71:426–431.

9 Eriksson M, Brown WT, Gordon LB et al. Recurrent de novo point mutations in lamin A cause Hutchinson–Gilford Progeria syndrome. Nature 2003;423:293–8.

10 Scaffidi P, Misteli T. Reversal of the cellular phenotype in the premature aging disease Hutchinson–Gilford progeria syndrome. Nat Med 2005;11:440–5.

11 Burtner CR, Kennedy BK. Progeria syndromes and ageing: what is the connection? Nat Rev Mol Cell Biol 2010;11:567–78.

12 Colige A, Roujeau JC, de la Rocque F et al. Abnormal gene expression in skin fibroblasts from a Hutchinson–Gilford patient. Lab Invest 1991;64:799–806.

13 Beauregard S, Gilchrest BA. Syndromes of premature ageing. Dermatol Clin 1987;5:109–21.

14 Erdem N, Gunes AT, Avci O et al. A case of Hutchinson–Gilford progeria syndrome mimicking scleroderma in early infancy. Dermatology 1994;188:318–21.

15 Mazereeuw-Hautier J, Wilson LC, Mohammed S et al. Hutchinson–Gilford progeria syndrome: clinical findings in three patients carrying the G608G mutation in LMNA and review of the literature. Br J Dermatol 2007;156:1308–14.

16 Gordon LB, Brown WT, Collins FS. (Updated January 8, 2015). Hutchinson–Gilford Progeria Syndrome. In: *GeneReviews* at GeneTests Medical Genetics Information Resource (database online). Copyright, University of Washington, Seattle. 1997-2013. Available at http://www.genetests.org (accessed 11 December 2018).

17 Gordon LB, Massaro J, D'Agostino RB Sr et al. Impact of farnesylation inhibitors on survival in Hutchinson–Gilford progeria syndrome. Circulation 2014;130:27–34.

18 Kieran MW, Gordon L, Kleinman M. New approaches to progeria. Pediatrics 2007;120;834–41.

19 Progeria Research Foundation. The Progeria Handbook: A Guide for Families & Health Care Providers of Children with Progeria. http://www.progeriaresearch.org/assets/files/PRFhandbook_0410.pdf (accessed 11 December 2016).

20 Yu CE, Oshima J, Fu YH et al. Positional closing of the Werner's syndrome gene. Science 1996;272:258–62.

Werner syndrome

Brief introduction and history. Werner syndrome (WS) is a teenage and adult-onset premature ageing syndrome with the four cardinal features of bilateral ocular cataracts, premature greying and thinning of scalp hair, short stature and characteristic skin findings. The first decade of life is normal with symptoms developing during the teenage years or twenties. An unusual cancer predisposition accompanies WS.

Werner, in a 1904 doctoral thesis, first described this condition in four siblings, emphasizing their scleroderma-like skin and cataracts [1]. Since then there have been over 200 patients reported. An international patient registry and mutation database is available [2].

Epidemiology and pathogenesis. The *RECQL2* gene is located at chromosome 8p12, and homozygous and compound heterozygous loss of function mutations in this gene are known to cause WS [3]. It codes for a DNA helicase protein which plays a role in DNA repair, homologous recombination, replication, and helps with telomere maintenance [4]. The pathogenesis of WS as it pertains to ageing likely reflects the multiple roles of the gene and accumulation of cellular dysfunction [5,6]. There have been over 70 mutations reported of varying types, including deletions, duplications and intronic changes. The most common point mutation, c.1105C>T, is present in 20–25% of individuals [7,8]. There have been some genotype–phenotype associations noted, with specific genotypes predictive of the resulting cancer phenotype. WS is inherited as an autosomal recessive condition and carriers are asymptomatic. Prevalence is highest in Japan at 1:20 000–40 000 with a likely founder mutation effect. Estimates of prevalence in the USA approach 1:200 000 [4,9,10].

Pathology. Gawkrodger and colleagues [11] described skin biopsy findings in one patient. Significant findings included hyalinization of dermal collagen but no epidermal atrophy or loss of appendages. Electron microscopic evaluation demonstrated accumulation of amorphous material between normal collagen bundles.

Clinical features. Individuals with WS typically have no uncommon health concerns throughout the first decade of life. The first diagnostic clue may be delayed pubertal growth. Adult height will be at a lower growth centile than in childhood. Beginning between late teenage years and the early thirties, individuals develop scalp hair loss and greying, cataracts and scleroderma-like skin changes. Limbs are thin with fat deposition in the trunk, and the face has a pinched appearance (sometimes termed 'bird-like'). Osteoporosis develops in the long bones, not as typically in the vertebrae, and deep, chronic ulceration begins at the ankles and elbows. Osteolytic lesions can develop in the distal joints of the fingers. The voice is often high-pitched. Hypogonadism and quickly declining fertility take place, but childbearing is possible. There is a high risk for type 2 diabetes mellitus, as well as arteriosclerosis (particularly of the arterioles) and myocardial infarction. Higher rates of dementia are not reported [9,10].

The cancer risk in WS merits specific mention as the type, site and frequency of tumours are unusual [12]. Higher rates of thyroid neoplasm, soft tissue sarcoma, melanoma and osteosarcoma are present, and the risk of cancer has been estimated at 44% [2,9]. Sarcoma is more likely to be of epithelial origin, melanoma is more of an acral lentigenous type unrelated to sun exposure and osteosarcoma is present more in lower extremities [10]. Risk of leukaemia might also be elevated [12]. The nature of the *RECQL2* gene function, coupled with DNA damaging effects of cancer treatment, may relate to the increased risk for multiple cancers affecting one WS individual [10].

Treatment and prognosis. Patients with WS have a shortened lifespan, with an average life expectancy of 54 years [13]. The most common causes of death are cancer and myocardial infarction. Screening and surveillance are recommended for diabetes, hyperlipidemia, cataracts and cancer. Patients should be counselled to maintain a healthy lifestyle. Treatment is otherwise symptomatic [9]. Potential avenues for treatment focus on remediating the loss of *RECQL2* gene function at the biochemical and cellular level, but no active clinical trials are currently in place [14,15].

Differential diagnosis. About 10% of clinically diagnosed WS patients do not have a *RECQL2* mutation identified [7,8,9]. Among these, approximately 15% were found to have *LMNA* mutations [16]. *LMNA* is associated with HGPS. These mutations in *LMNA* were missense mutations or are suggested to be weak activators of the cryptic splice site that is the hallmark of classic HGPS [17]. Clinical presentation is onset of cancer at a younger age and faster progression. Classic HGPS has a much earlier onset than WS. Mandibuloacral dysplasia, also caused by *LMNA* mutations, has short stature and some similar facial features, but it does not have cataracts, a finding in nearly 100% of WS [10]. Some cancer-specific similarities can be seen in Rothmund–Thomson syndrome and Bloom syndrome, which interestingly have genetic causes in other helicase genes. Their cancer onset is typically younger than WS [12]. Individual components of WS can each generate a differential diagnosis list, but the combination is rather unique to WS.

References

1 Werner CWO. Uber Kataract in Verbindung mit Sklerodermie. Thesis. Kiel, Germany: Schmidt and Klauning, 1904.

2 University of Washington. Werner Syndrome. http://www.wernersyndrome.org/ (accessed 11 December 2018).

3 Yu CE, Oshima J, Fu YH et al. Positional closing of the Werner's syndrome gene. Science 1996;272:258–62.

4 Bohr VA. Deficient DNA repair in the human progeroid disorder, Werner syndrome. Mutat Res 2005;577:252–9.

5 Rossi ML, Ghosh ML, Bohr VA. Roles of Werner syndrome protein in protection of genome integrity. DNA Repair (Amst) 2010;9:331–44.

6 Bohr A. Rising from the RecQ-age: the role of human RecQ helicases in genome maintenance. Trends Biochem Sci 2008;33:609–20.

7 Matsumoto T, Imamura O, Yamabe Y, et al. Mutation and haplotype analyses of the Werner's syndrome gene based on its genomic structure: genetic epidemiology in the Japanese population. Hum Genet 1997;100:123–30.

8 Friedrich et al. WRN mutations in Werner syndrome patients: genomic rearrangements, unusual intronic mutations and ethnic-specific alteration. Hum Genet 2010;128:103–11.

9 Oshima J, Martin GM, Hisama FM (Updated January 27, 2014). Werner Syndrome. In: GeneReviews at GeneTests Medical Genetics Information Resource (database online). Copyright, University of Washington, Seattle. 1997–2013. Available at http://www.genetests.org. (accessed 11 December 2018).

10 **Muftuoglu M, Oshima J, von Kobbe C et al. The clinical characteristics of Werner syndrome: molecular and biochemical diagnosis. Hum Genet 2008; 124:369–77.**
11 Gawkrodger DJ, Priestley GC, Vijayalaxmi Ross JA et al. Werner's syndrome. Biochemical and cytogenetic studies. Arch Dermatol 1985;121:636–41.
12 Lauper JM, Krause A, Vaughan TL et al. Spectrum and risk of neoplasia in Werner syndrome: a systematic review. PLOS ONE 2013;e59709:1–8.
13 Huang S, Lee L, Hanson NB et al. Hum Mutat 2006;27:558–67.
14 Kudlow BA, Kennedy BK, Monnat RJ. Werner and Hutchinson–Gilford progeria syndromes: mechanistic basis of human progeroid diseases. Nat Rev Mol Cell Biol 2007;8:394–404.
15 US National Institutes of Health. http://clinicaltrials.gov/ (accessed 11 December 2018).
16 Chen L, Lee L, Kudlow BA et al. LMNA mutations in atypical Werner's syndrome. Lancet 2003;362:440–5.
17 Oshima J, Hisama FM. Search and insights into novel genetic alterations leading to classical and atypical Werner syndrome. Gerontology 2014;60:239–46.

Cockayne syndrome (see Chapter 138)

Cockayne syndrome (CS) is a heterogeneous condition, which has been separated into CSA and CSB based on the gene involved, as well as into types I, II and III based on clinical severity. The classic form (termed CS type I) is characterized by postnatal growth deficiency and microcephaly, cataracts, pigmentary retinopathy, skin photosensitivity, hearing loss and intellectual disability. A severe form (CS type II) has been described and includes prenatal growth deficiency and earlier onset of symptoms. CS type II has clinical and molecular overlap with the cerebro-oculofacial syndrome. A mild form (CS type III) has also been described and includes normal growth and intelligence. Causative genes are *ERCC8* and *ERCC6*, mutations in which cause CSA and CSB respectively. Mutations in *ERCC5* may also cause the severe CS phenotype, as well as other overlapping disorders [1–3].

References

1 Drury S, Boustred C, Tekman M et al. A novel homozygous ERCC5 truncating mutation in a family with prenatal arthrogryposis – further evidence of genotype-phenotype correlation. Am J Med Genet Part A 2014;164A:1777–83.
2 Laugel V, Dalloz C, Tobias ES, et al. Cerebro-oculo-facio-skeletal syndrome: three additional cases with CSB mutations, new diagnostic criteria and an approach to investigation. J Med Genet 2008; 45:564–71.
3 Wilson BT, Stark Z, Sutton RE et al. The Cockayne syndrome natural history (CoSyNH) study: clinical findings in 102 individuals and recommendations for care. Genet Med 2015;18:483–93.

Rothmund–Thomson syndrome (see Chapter 140)

Rothmund–Thomson syndrome (RTS) is an inherited disorder whose phenotype includes early childhood-onset poikiloderma, with occasional occurrence of cataracts and skeletal anomalies. An increased risk of malignancy is one of the manifestations. RTS is genetically heterogeneous, with mutations in *ReCQL4* not identified in all patients [1]. RTS also overlaps clinically with Baller–Gerold and RAPADILINO syndromes, with the cause of all three phenotypes attributable to *ReCQL4* mutations [2–5], and with Clericuzio-type poikiloderma with neutropenia, caused by mutation in *USB1* [1]

References

1 Suter AA, Itin P, Heinimann K et al. Rothmund–Thomson syndrome: novel pathogenic mutations and frequencies of variants in the RECQL4 and USB1 (C16orf57) gene. Mol Genet Genomic Med 2016;24:359–66.
2 Kitao S, Shimamoto A, Goto M et al. Mutations in RECQL4 cause a subset of cases of Rothmund–Thomson syndrome. Nat Genet 1999;22:82–4.
3 Siitonen H, Sotkasiira J, Biervliet M et al. The mutation spectrum in RECQL4 diseases. Europ J Hum Genet 2009;17:151–8.
4 Van Maldergem L, Siitonen HA, Jalkh N et al. Revisiting the craniosynostosis-radial ray hypoplasia association: Baller-Gerold syndrome caused by mutations in the RECQL4 gene. J Med Genet 2006; 43:149–52.
5 Piard J, Aral B, Vabres P et al. Search for ReCQL4 mutations in 39 patients genotyped for suspected Rothmund–Thomson /Baller-Gerold syndromes. Clin Genet 2015;87:244–51.

Dyskeratosis congenita (see Chapter 140)

Dyskeratosis congenita is a heterogeneous condition characterized by skin and nail manifestations, oral leukoplakia, premature greying, tooth loss, osteoporosis and increased frequency of malignancy.

Conditions with skin atrophy/ lipoatrophy

Wiedemann–Rautenstrauch syndrome

Syn.
Neonatal progeroid syndrome

Brief introduction and history. Wiedemann–Rautenstrauch syndrome (WRS) is a premature ageing syndrome characterized by intrauterine growth retardation, short stature, typical facial appearance, natal teeth, lipoatrophy and paradoxical caudal fat accumulation. WRS was first described by Rautenstrauch & Snigula [1] in 1977, who reported two sisters with a progeria-like syndrome. Wiedemann [2] described two additional patients 2 years later; Devos and colleagues [3] suggested the acronym WRS.

Epidemiology and pathogenesis. Over 30 patients have been described to date [4].

This is almost certainly an autosomal recessive trait in that both affected siblings and parental consanguinity have been described [1,3,5–7]. The basic genetic defect is unknown, although Beavan and colleagues [8] described deficient decorin expression in one patient originally described by Rautenstrauch & Snigula [1]. Decorin is a small proteoglycan that may interact with collagen I and II to influence the rate of fibril formation. However, the authors did not consider a decorin deficiency to be the primary defect because decorin expression returned to normal levels in adolescence in that patient. Mazzarello and colleagues [9] described reduced thymidine kinase activity in skin fibroblasts, suggesting a DNA metabolism defect. Mutations in *LMNA*, *ZMPSTE24* and *ERCC8* have been sought, but not found [7,10,11]. Therefore, the cause of WRS remains elusive, but with the increasing use of exome sequencing to identify causative genes, it is likely the relevant gene will be identified.

Clinical features. Affected individuals have intrauterine growth retardation with failure to thrive and short stature. The progeroid appearance is apparent at birth, with the phenotype consisting of a pseudo-hydrocephaloid appearance (although the occipitofrontal circumference is within normal limits), sparse hair, prominent scalp veins, widened anterior fontanelles and malar hypoplasia. One to four natal teeth are almost always present, with these teeth lost and subsequent dentition delayed. Skin is dry, thin and wrinkled. Hands and feet appear large. Generalized lipoatrophy is present, although paradoxical caudal fat accumulation occurs during childhood. One child also had fat accumulation in the axillae and on the proximal portion of the digits [12]. Feeding difficulties are common. Over time, the nose appears beaked. Cognitive impairment is usually present, with mild to severe degrees of impairment reported. Joint contractures, cardiac defects, hydronephrosis and congenital hearing loss are occasional manifestations. Ocular anomalies are an under-reported manifestation, but a range of ocular anomalies, including microphthalmia, are being increasingly recognized [4,7]. Some patients have been reported to have elevated insulin and triglyceride levels [13], but this is not a consistent manifestation [14,15]. The oldest patient described was 17 years old at the time of the report [16], and the mean age of survival is 7 months [16]. As noted above, cognitive impairment may be present, ranging from mild to severe.

Differential diagnosis. Natal teeth are present in Hallerman–Streiff, Ellis–van Creveld and Ullrich Fremerez–Dohna syndromes. Progeroid facial appearance at birth can occur in Hallermann–Streiff, Berardinelli–Seip, Bamatter and DeBarsy syndromes. Paradoxical caudal fat accumulation occurs in congenital disorders of glycosylation. One child thought to have WRS was subsequently found to have somatic mosaicism for triploidy and tetraploidy, so a skin biopsy for karyotyping should be considered, particularly when unusual manifestations such as cardiac defects and syndactyly of the fingers are present [17]. The syndrome described by Petty and colleagues [18] should be distinguished from WRS.

Laboratory and histology findings. Brain examination by Martin and colleagues [19] on the patient described by Devos and colleagues [3] showed a sudanophilic leucodystrophy with tigroid streaks. Hagadorn and colleagues [20] did not find this in their patient and suggested that heterogeneity may exist. Ulrich and colleagues [21] described absence of mature myelin in their patient's brain. They also suggested that WRS may be heterogeneous, neuropathologically and probably genetically. Arboleda and colleagues [7] reported autopsy findings in one child and described the skull bones as consisting of cartilaginous tissue surrounded by unossified fibrous tissue. Jager and colleagues [22] described deficiency of osteoblast regeneration capacity *in vitro*. Skin biopsy from one patient demonstrated only marked hypoplasia of dermis [12]. Proliferation rate of fibroblasts was one-half of that of normal control patients.

Treatment and prevention. Treatment is supportive.

References

1 Rautenstrauch T, Snigula F. Progeria: a cell culture study and clinical report of familial inheritance. Eur J Pediatr 1977;124:101–11.
2 Wiedemann HR. An unidentified neonatal progeroid syndrome: follow up report. Eur J Pediatr 1979;130:65–70.
3 Devos EA, Leroy JG, Fryns JP et al. The Wiedemann–Rautenstrauch or neonatal progeroid syndrome: report of a patient with consanguineous parents. Eur J Pediatr 1981;136:245–8.
4 Barkley MR, O'Hagan SB. Ophthalmic manifestations in a case of Wiedemann-Rautenstrauch syndrome. J AAPOS 2015;19:559–61.
5 Castincyra G, Panal M, Presas HL et al. Two sibs with Wiedemann–Rautenstrauch syndrome: possibilities of prenatal diagnosis by ultrasound. J Med Genet 1992;29:434–6.
6 Pivnick EK, Angle B, Kaufman RA et al. Neonatal progeroid (Wiedemann–Rautenstrauch) syndrome: report of five new cases and review. Am J Med Genet 2000;90:131–40.
7 Arboleda G, Morales LC, Quintero L et al. Neonatal progeroid syndrome (Wiedemann-Rautenstrauch syndrome): report of three affected sibs. Am J Med Genet Part A 2011;155:1712–15.
8 Beavan LA, Quentin-Hoffmann E, Schonherr E et al. Deficient expression of decorin in infantile progeroid patients. J Biol Chem 1993;268:9856–62.
9 Mazzarello P, Verri A, Mondello C et al. Enzymes of DNA metabolism in a patient with Wiedemann–Rautenstrauch progeroid syndrome. Ann NY Acad Sci 1992;663:440–1.
10 Cao H, Hegele RA. LMNA is mutated in Hutchinson–Gilford progeria (MIM 176670) but not in Wiedemann–Rautenstrauch progeroid syndrome (MIM 264090). J Hum Genet 2003;48:271–4.
11 Hou J-W. Natural course of neonatal progeroid syndrome. Pediatr Neonatol 2009;50:102–9.
12 Rudin C, Thommen L, Fliegel C et al. The neonatal pseudohydrocephalic progeroid syndrome (Wiedemann–Rautenstrauch). Eur J Pediatr 1988;147:433–8.
13 Dinleyici EC, Tekin N, Dinleyici M et al. Clinical and laboratory findings of two newborns with Wiedemann–Rautenstrauch syndrome: additional features, evaluation of bone turnover and review of the literature. J Pediatr Endocrinol Metab 2008;21:591–6.
14 O'Neill B, Simha V, Kotha V et al. Body fat distribution and metabolic variables in patients with neonatal progeroid syndrome. Am J Med Genet 2007;143A:1421–30.
15 Kiraz A, Ozen S, Tubas F et al. Wiedemann-Rautenstrauch syndrome: report of a variant case. Am J Med Genet Part A 2012;158A:1434–6.
16 Arboleda H, Arboleda G. Follow-up study of Wiedemann–Rautenstrauch syndrome: long-term survival and comparison with Rautenstrauch's patient 'G'. Birth Defects Res A 2005;73:562–8.
17 Karteszi J, Kosztolanhi G, Czako M et al. Transient progeroid phenotype and lipodystrophy in mosaic polypoidy. Clin Dysmorph 2006;15:29–31.
18 Petty EM, Laxova R, Wiedemann HR. Previously unrecognized congenital progeroid disorder. Am J Med Genet 1990;35:383–7.
19 Martin JJ, Ceuterick CM, Leroy JG et al. The Wiedemann–Rautenstrauch or neonatal progeroid syndrome. Neuropathological study of a case. Neuropediatrics 1984;15:43–8.
20 Hagadorn JI, Wilson WG, Hogge WA et al. Neonatal progeroid syndrome: more than one disease? Am J Med Genet 1990;35:91–4.
21 Ulrich J, Rudin C, Bubl R et al. The neonatal progeroid syndrome (Wiedemann–Rautenstrauch) and its relationship to Pelizaeus–Merzbacher's disease. Neuropath Appl Neurobiol 1995;21:116–20.
22 Jager M, Thorey F, Westhoff B, et al. In vitro osteogenic differentiation is affected in Wiedemann-Rautenstrauch (WRS). In Vivo 2005;19:831–6.

DeBarsy syndrome

Brief introduction and history. DeBarsy syndrome (DBS) phenotype consists of progeroid appearance, growth retardation and intellectual disability, cutis laxa, corneal clouding and athetoid movements. DeBarsy and colleagues [1] described the combination of prenatal growth retardation, skin laxity, minor craniofacial anomalies, cloudy corneae, large anterior fontanelle with delayed closure, and athetoid movements in a single girl in 1968. Since then, over 25 patients have been described, including three as unknown cases [2–12]. Some of the cases reported as having DBS, however, probably have a distinct condition [3,8].

Epidemiology and pathogenesis. DBS is a rare, genetically heterogeneous condition, with both autosomal recessive and autosomal dominant forms described [13–15]. The autosomal recessive forms are caused by biallelic mutations in either *PYCR1* or *ALDH18A1*, encoding pyrroline-5-carboxylate reductase 1 and pyrroline-5-carboxylate synthase, respectively. Both genes are involved in the mitochondrial proline cycle. The autosomal dominant form is caused by heterozygous mutations in *ALDH18A1*. To date, all patients with the autosomal dominant form have had *de novo* mutations.

Clinical features. Children with DBS generally have intrauterine growth retardation and subsequent slow growth. Corneal clouding or cataracts are virtually universal and the facial phenotype is described as progeroid. Specifically, these children have a prominent forehead, small nose with upturned nares and thin lips. The eyes usually appear deeply set. The ears are described as large and dysplastic, with a relatively unfolded helix. Hypotonia is a virtually constant finding, as is mild cutis laxa and thin wrinkled skin, particularly of the extremities. Small joints are often hyperflexible and hip dislocation or club foot occur frequently. Athetoid movements had initially been described as a common manifestation of DBS, but more recently it has been found these movements occur in less than half of those affected [14]. Cognitive impairment is present, being severe in almost half [12], and no child was reported to have normal development. There is also some evidence for genotype–phenotype correlation, in that individuals with *ALDH18A1* mutations are more likely to have cataracts/corneal clouding and hypotonia, and those with *PYCR1* mutations are more likely to suffer easy bruising [14,15].

Lifespan is unknown, because most patients were reported as infants. The oldest reported individual was 24 years old at the time of the report and did not have any life-threatening health problems [3]. However, it has been questioned whether this individual and his siblings have DBS, particularly because they have a different facial phenotype, had normal birthweights, and had hyper- and hypopigmented skin patches, which are not seen in other individuals with DBS [12].

Differential diagnosis. Apparently some children with DBS are initially diagnosed as having WRS, but the presence of natal teeth and caudal fat accumulation in WRS should distinguish between the two. The other premature ageing syndromes should also be considered in the differential diagnosis [13].

Laboratory and histology findings. Skin biopsy performed by DeBarsy and colleagues [1] demonstrated normal epidermis, but thinner than normal dermis. The collagen fibres were described as having few fasciculations and elastic fibres were thin, short and decreased in number. Karnes and colleagues [11] and Skidmore and colleagues [13] described decreased elastic fibres. Karnes and colleagues [11] also described the skin biopsy changes over time. In the neonatal period, their patient had hyperkeratosis and papillomatosis of the epidermis, with a deficiency of elastic fibres. At 10 months, the epidermis was normal and the dermis thin. The adnexal structures were located at the dermoepidermal junction instead of their usual location. Elastic fibres remained decreased in number and size.

Electron microscopy demonstrated variability in the collagen bundle size, as well as an increased microfibrillar component of elastin and thinning of the amorphous component of elastin. The elastic fibres were described as appearing 'moth-eaten' [11,13].

Treatment. No specific treatment is known.

References

1 DeBarsy AM, Moens E, Dierckx L. Dwarfisms, oligophrenia and degeneration of the elastic tissue in skin and cornea: a new syndrome? Helv Pediatr Acta 1968;23:305–13.
2 Schierenberg M, Donne W, Schiafone P et al. De Barsy–Moens–Dierckx-Syndrom: ein ungewohnlicher Verlauf bei einem Fruhgeborenen. Klin Padiatr 1994;206:444–6.
3 Kunze J, Majewski F, Montgomery P et al. DeBarsy syndrome: an autosomal recessive, progeroid syndrome. Eur J Pediatr 1985; 144:348–54.
4 Stanton RP, Rao N, Scott CI. Orthopaedic manifestations in De Barsy syndrome. J Pediatr Orthop 1994;14:60–2.
5 Harrod MJ, Keele D, Stevenson RE. The De Barsy syndrome. Proc Greenwood Genet Cent 1984;3:134.
6 Hoefnagel D, Pomeroy J, Wurster D et al. Congenital athetosis, mental deficiency, dwarfism, and laxity of skin and ligaments. Helv Pediatr Acta 1971;26:397–402.
7 Burck U. De Barsy-Syndrom: eine weitere Beobachtung. Klin Padiatr 1974;186:441–4.
8 Riebel T. DeBarsy–Moens–Dierckx-Syndrom: Beobachtung bei Geschwistern. Mschr Kinderheilk 1976;124:96–8.
9 Siedel H, Stengel-Rutkowski S, Schimanek P et al. Non-chromosomal dysmorphic syndromes (MCA/MR syndromes). 1. Similar abnormal phenotype in two mentally retarded brothers. Dysmorph Clin Genet 1987;1:101–8.
10 Saul R (ed.). Unknown case (R.F.W.). Proc Greenwood Genet Cent 1983;2:70–1.
11 Karnes PS, Shamban AT, Olsen DR et al. De Barsy syndrome: report of a case, literature review, and elastic gene expression studies of the skin. Am J Med Genet 1992;42:29–34.
12 Kivuva EC, Parker MJ, Cohen MC et al. De Barsy syndrome: a review of the phenotype. Clin Dysmorphol 2008;17:99–207.
13 Skidmore DL, Chitayat D, Morgan T et al. Further expansion of the phenotypic spectrum associated with mutations in ALDH18A1, encoding Δ^1-pyrroline-5-carboxylate synthase (P5CS). Am J Med Genet Part A 2011;155:1848–56.
14 Zampatti S, Castori M, Fischer B et al. De Barsy syndrome: a genetically heterogeneous autosomal recessive cutis laxa syndrome related to P5CS and PYCR1 dysfunction. Am J Med Genet Part A 2012;158A:927–31.
15 Fischer-Zirnsak B, Escande-Beillard N, Ganesh J et al. Recurrent de novo mutations affecting residue Arg138 of pyrroline-5-carboxylate synthase cause a progeroid form of autosomal dominant cutis laxa. Am J Hum Genet 2015;97:483–92.

Acrometageria

Brief introduction and history. This is a presumed spectrum of phenotypes that encompasses *acrogeria*, which primarily affects the hands and feet, and *metageria*, which involves the limbs as well as other structures. This entity is clearly heterogeneous.

Gottron [1] first described a progeroid syndrome that primarily affected the skin of the hands and feet. Since then, over 50 cases have been described. In 1974, Gilkes and colleagues [2] described two patients with phenotypes similar to but believed to be distinct from acrogeria and HGPS or WS. In 1992 Greally and colleagues [3] described a boy with features of both acrogeria and metageria, and hypothesized that acrogeria and metageria are part of the phenotypic spectrum of a single disease entity. They suggested *acrometageria* as the name for this condition. It is now clear that this is a group of similar, but genetically distinct, conditions.

Epidemiology and pathogenesis. Although most affected individuals are the only family members affected, Kaufman and colleagues [4] described a pedigree consistent with autosomal dominant inheritance, in which one individual clinically had metageria and two others had acrogeria. The other cases therefore could represent *de novo* mutations. Although a defect in collagen III synthesis was suggested by Pope and colleagues [5] and Bouillie and colleagues [6], Bruckner-Tuderman and colleagues [7] and Blaszczyk and colleagues [8] did not find abnormal collagen III levels. It is likely that acrometageria is heterogeneous and that some patients with collagen III deficiency (which also causes Ehlers–Danlos IV) have an acrogeroid phenotype [9,10]. Hunzelmann and colleagues [11] described deficiency of type I collagen in a man with metageria and his sister with acrogeria. Hadj-Rabia and colleagues [12] described a man with acrogeria who had a pathogenic mutation in *LMNA*.

Clinical features. Clinical manifestations in patients with acrogeria were reviewed by Meurer and colleagues [13] and Greally and colleagues [3] and are essentially limited to the skin and skeleton. Cutaneous findings include: skin atrophy of the extremities, particularly the hands and feet; atrophic nose tip; hyperpigmentation; dystrophic and thickened nails; hypertrophic scars; and in rare cases other cutaneous manifestations (e.g. psoriasis, scleroderma). Skeletal changes are minor and are most often limited to short limbs. Other described changes include osteoporosis, acro-osteolysis and hypermobile joints [14].

The described cutaneous changes in metageria are more severe, and the phenotype also includes metabolic and cardiovascular changes. Skin manifestations include more severe atrophy affecting the limbs, thin scalp hair and generalized limb lipoatrophy. Metabolic disturbances are primarily limited to early-onset diabetes; cardiovascular changes consist of premature atherosclerosis. The facial phenotype includes beaked nose and prominent eyes.

In general, the lifespan is dependent on the severity of the diabetes and atherosclerosis, if present. Intellect appears unimpaired, although the patient of Greally and colleagues [3] was moderately cognitively impaired.

Differential diagnosis. WS and DBS must be included in the differential diagnosis but can be distinguished by age of onset in the case of WS and phenotypic differences in the case of DBS. Rezai-Delui and colleagues [15] described acrogeria occurring in an autosomal recessive pattern in a family; it is likely that the affected individuals actually have mandibuloacral dysplasia.

Laboratory and histology findings. Meurer and colleagues [13] examined the skin in a man diagnosed with acrogeria. Subcutaneous fat was diminished, dermal papillae were flattened and there was orthokeratotic hyperkeratosis. Collagen fibre number was decreased, whereas elastin fibres were increased, although they were fragmented in appearance. The granular endoplasmic reticulum was dilated, so cells appeared vacuolized. In the vacuoles, as well as extracellular areas, pseudo-elastin was present. Bruckner-Tuderman and colleagues [7] also examined the skin from a patient with acrogeria, but noted differences between biopsy sites. These differences included reduced thickness of the dermis and more collagen bundle abnormalities in the foot specimen compared with the axilla specimen. A third report of skin biopsy results did not note any abnormalities in a specimen taken from the buttock [3]. Tajima and colleagues [16] described late-onset focal dermal elastosis in a patient, and Hadj-Rabia and colleagues [12] described epidermal hyperplasia and disorganization of collagen bundles in a skin biopsy taken from the right arm.

Treatment. Diabetes and atherosclerosis should be treated.

References

1 Gottron H. Familiare akrogerie. Arch Dermatol Syph 1941;181:571–83.
2 Gilkes JJH, Sharvill DE, Wells RS. The premature ageing syndromes. Reports of eight cases and description of a new entity named metageria. Br J Dermatol 1974;91:243–62.
3 Greally JM, Boon LY, Lenkey SG et al. Acrometageria: a spectrum of 'premature ageing' syndromes. Am J Med Genet 1992;44:334–9.
4 Kaufman I, Thiele B, Mahrle G. Simultaneous occurrence of metageria and Gottron's acrogeria in one family. Z Hautkr 1985;60:975–84.
5 Pope FM, Nicholls AC, Jones PM et al. EDS IV (acrogeria): new autosomal dominant and recessive types. J Roy Soc Med 1980;73:180–6.
6 Bouillie MC, Venencie PY, Thomine E et al. Syndrome d'Ehlers–Danlos type IV à type d'Acrogerie. Ann Dermatol Vénéréol 1986;113:1077–85.
7 Bruckner-Tuderman L, Vogel A, Schnyder UW. Fibroblasts of an acrogeria patient produce normal amounts of type I and III collagen. Dermatology 1987;174:157–65.
8 Blaszczyk M, DePaepe A, Nuytinck L et al. Acrogeria of the Gottron type in a mother and son. Eur J Dermatol 2000;10:36–40.
9 Pope FM, Narcisi P, Nicholls AC et al. Col3A1 mutations cause variable clinical phenotypes including acrogeria and vascular rupture. Br J Dermatol 1996;135:163–81.
10 Jansen T, DePaepe A, Luytinck N et al. Col3A1 mutation leading to acrogeria (Gottron type). Br J Dermatol 2000;142:177–99.
11 Hunzelmann N, Ueberham U, Eckes B et al. Transforming growth factor-α reverses deficient expression of type(1) collagen in cultured fibroblasts of a patient with metageria. Biochim Biophys Acta 1997; 1360:64–70.
12 Hadj-Rabia S, Mashiah J, Roll P et al. A new lamin A mutation associated with acrogeria syndrome. J Invest Dermatol 2014; 134:2274–7.
13 Meurer A, Lohmoller G, Keller C. Gottron's acrogeria and sarcoidosis. Clin Invest 1993;71:387–91.
14 Ho A, White SJ, Rasmussen JE. Skeletal abnormalities of acrogeria, a progeroid syndrome. Skel Radiol 1987;16:463–8.
15 Rezai-Delui H, Lotfi N, Mamoori G et al. Hereditary Gottron's acrogeria with recessive transmission: a report of four cases in one family. Pediatr Radiol 1999;29:124–30.
16 Tajima S, Inazumi T, Kobayashi T. A case of acrogeria associated with late-onset focal dermal elastosis. Dermatology 1996;192:264–8.

Mandibuloacral dysplasia

Brief introduction and history. Mandibuloacral dysplasia (MAD) is characterized by the combination of growth failure, progressive osteolytic skeletal changes and skin abnormalities. Lipodystrophy can also occur.

Cavallazzi and colleagues [1] first described this condition as an atypical form of cleidocranial dysostosis. Young and colleagues [2] termed this condition mandibuloacral dysplasia (MAD). Danks and colleagues [3] recognized that the patient of Cavallazzi and colleagues [1] had MAD. Since then, numerous cases have been reported, and it is now recognized that two forms, MADA and MADB, exist. MADA is far more common than is MADB.

Epidemiology and pathogenesis. The condition is inherited as an autosomal recessive trait and can be caused by mutations in *LMNA* or *ZMPSTE24* [4–9], causing MAD type A (MADA) and MADB respectively [9].

Clinical features. In the more typical cases of MADA, age of onset is between 3 and 14 years, with facial and digital changes occurring first. Those with MADB have an earlier onset of symptoms, with manifestations present in early infancy [10]. The phenotype consists of short stature, thin, hyperpigmented skin, partial alopecia, prominent eyes, beaked nose, tooth loss, micrognathia, short fingers and, on radiography, evidence of bone resorption of the clavicles and distal phalanges. In areas of alopecia, prominent scalp veins are present. The skin is described as sclerodermoid in areas, and fingernails and toenails can be dystrophic or absent. Lipodystrophy can affect only extremities or trunk, face and extremities [9,11]. Those with MADB tend to have most of the manifestations by 5 years of age, including total resorption of the clavicles. Atherosclerosis, hypertension, and renal disease occur during early childhood in these individuals [12]. Some individuals with MADB develop subcutaneous and vascular calcifications, with the subcutaneous lumps ultimately extruding through the skin [3,12,13]. One individual also had areas of subcutaneous tissue necrosis and, at the age of 27 years, had a tracheostomy for airway management and a kidney transplant for renal failure secondary to focal sclerosis [13].

Finally, there exists a group of patients who have some manifestations of MAD but are missing cardinal findings and have atypical manifestations. For example, some of the patients described by Friedenberg and colleagues [14] had normal stature, hearing loss and hepatomegaly.

There is evidence that genotype–phenotype correlation might exist. For example, those with *ZMPSTE24* mutations (but not those with *LMNA* mutations) tend to have premature greying of the hair and renal disease. In individuals with *LMNA* mutations, those with the common R527H/R527H genotype have hyperinsulinaemia and hypertriglyceridaemia, whereas those with A529V/A529V genotype do not [5].

Lifespan appears to be close to normal for individuals with a more typical presentation of MAD, although there are reports of early death in some patients. Intellect is unimpaired in either form.

Differential diagnosis. The most important condition to distinguish is cleidocranial dysostosis, where no skin changes occur and the bony manifestations are present at birth. Pycnodysostosis should also be considered in the differential diagnosis but, as in cleidocranial dysostosis, no skin changes occur. There have also been descriptions of individuals with the diagnosis of HGPS but in whom MAD is suspected to be the correct diagnosis [15,16].

Laboratory and histology findings. Skin biopsy results described by Welsh [17] included moderate homogenization of the dermis and mild elastosis. Zina and colleagues [18] noted loss of rete pegs, but normal dermis and well-developed elastic fibres. Al-Haggar and colleagues [19] described ultrastructural skin changes in patients with MADA and in their heterozygous mothers. The patients' skin showed numerous abnormalities, including epidermal cells with disturbed desmosomes which were separated by vacuoles of different sizes. The dermis showed collagen bundle depletion and abnormal fibroblasts. The heterozygous mothers had some minor abnormalities noted on their biopsies, and the authors suggested that these women be followed for possible development of skin atrophy and signs of premature ageing.

Treatment. Treatment is supportive.

References

1 Cavallazzi C, Cremoncini R, Quadri A. Si du caso di disostosi clediocranica. Rev Clin Pediatr 1960;65:313–26.

2 Young LW, Radebaugh JF, Rubin P et al. New syndrome manifested by mandibular hypoplasia, acroosteolysis, stiff joints and cutaneous atrophy (mandibulo-acral dysplasia) in two unrelated boys. BDOAS 1971;7:291–7.

3 Danks DM, Mayne V, Wettenhall HNB et al. Craniomandibular dermatodysostosis. BDOAS 1974;x:99–105.

4 Shen JJ, Brown CA, Lupski JR et al. Mandibuloacral dysplasia caused by homozygosity for the R527H mutation in lamin A/C. J Med Genet 2003;40:854–7.

5 Garg A, Cogulu O, Ozkinay F et al. A novel homozygous Ala529Val LMNA mutation in Turkish patients with mandibuloacral dysplasia. J Clin Endocrinol Metab 2005;90:5259–64.

6 Agarwal AK, Zhou XJ, Hall RK et al. Focal segmental glomerulosclerosis in patients with mandibuloaral dysplasia owing to ZMPSTE24 deficiency. J Invest Med 2006;54:208–13.

7 Lombardi F, Gullott F, Columbaro M et al. Compound heterozygosity for mutations in LMNA in a patient with a myopathic and lipodystrophic mandibuloacral dysplasia type A phenotype. J Clin Endocrinol Metab 2007;92:4467–71.

8 Kosho T, Takahashi J, Momose T et al. Mandibuloacral dysplasia and a novel LMNA mutation in a woman with severe progressive skeletal changes. Am J Med Genet 2007;143A:2598–603.

9 Garavelli L, d'Apice MR, Rivieri F et al. Mandibuloacral dysplasia type A in childhood. Am J Med Genet 2009;149A:2258–64.

10 Kwan JM. Mandibuloacral dysplasia type B in an infant: a rare progeroid genodermatosis. JAMA Dermatol 2015;151:561–2.

11 Simha V, Garg A. Body fat distribution and metabolic erangements in patients with familial partial lipodystrophy associated with mandibuloacral dysplasia. J Clin Endocrinol Metab 2002;87:776–85.

12 Ben Yaou R, Navarro C, Quijano-Roy S, et al. Type B mandibuloacral dysplasia with congenital myopathy due to homozygous ZMPSTE24 missense mutation. Eur J Hum Genet 2011;19:647–54.

13 Schrander-Stumpel C, Spaepen A, Fryns J-C et al. A severe case of mandibuloacral dysplasia in a girl. Am J Med Genet 1992;43:877–81.

14 Friedenberg GR, Cutler DL, Jones MC et al. Severe insulin resistance and diabetes mellitus in mandibuloacral dysplasia. Am J Dis Child 1992;146:93–9.
15 Liang L, Zhang H, Gu X. Homozygous LMNA mutation R527C in atypical Hutchinson–Gilford progeria syndrome: evidence for autosomal recessive inheritance. Acta Paediatr 2009;98:1365–7.
16 Ramesh V, Jain RK. Progeria in two brothers. Aust J Dermatol 1987;28:33–5.
17 Welsh O. Study of a family with a new progeroid syndrome. BDOAS 1975;xi:25–38.
18 Zina AM, Cravario A, Bundino S. Familial mandibuloacral dysplasia. Br J Dermatol 1981;105:719–23.
19 Al-Haggar M, Shams A, Madej-Pilarczyk A et al. Ultrastructural skin changes in Egyptian mandibuloacral dysplasia patients with p.Arg527Leu LMNA mutation in their asymptomatic heterozygotic mothers. J Clin Pathol 2013; 66:1000–4.

Megarbane–Loiselet neonatal progeroid syndrome

Brief introduction and history. This condition is characterized by neonatal progeroid phenotype, joint contractures, thumb adduction, inguinal herniae and early death.

Megarbane & Loiselet [1] described siblings with a 'new' progeroid syndrome. Jukkola and colleagues [2] described a child who probably had the same condition.

Epidemiology and pathogenesis. Inheritance is probably autosomal recessive. The basic gene defect is unknown.

Clinical features. Affected individuals have: pre- and postnatal growth retardation; a characteristic face with hypertelorism, pinched nose, small mouth and micrognathia; sparse hair; thin skin on the face and scalp; prominent occiput; cataracts; adduction of the thumb; inguinal herniae; and talipes. Both joint contractures [1] and joint hyperextensibility were described [2]. Cardiac defects are also a common manifestation. The lifespan is less than 1 year and death may be related to associated cardiac defects.

Differential diagnosis. This condition most closely resembles Wiedemann–Rautenstrauch, DeBarsy and Hallermann–Streiff syndromes, but the course of the condition and severity of manifestations should distinguish this from the others.

Laboratory and histology findings. The patient of Jukkola and colleagues [2] demonstrated insufficient production of types I and III procollagens.

References

1 Megarbane A, Loiselet J. Clinical manifestation of a severe neonatal progeroid syndrome. Clin Genet 1997;51:200–4.
2 Jukkola A, Kauppila S, Risteli L et al. New lethal disease involving type I and III collagen defect resembling geroderma osteodysplatica, De Barsy syndrome, and Ehlers–Danlos IV. J Med Genet 1998;35:513–18.

Penttinen progeroid disorder

This entity has only been described in three patients. Manifestations include postnatal onset, progeroid appearance, skeletal findings and skin lesions resembling juvenile hyaline fibromatosis [1,2]. Inheritance of this condition is unknown, as is the basic gene defect.

Progeroid features develop in infancy/early childhood. The earliest manifestations appear to be premaxillary and maxillary retrusion with proptosis and broad thumbs and halluces. The skin is described as being slightly dry and translucent and joint hypermobility is present. Over time, keloid-like nodular lesions develop on the dorsa of the hands and feet as well as on the buttocks. Scalp hair becomes sparse and acro-osteolysis develops. The oldest described patient died at age 20 years of respiratory insufficiency. Ocular pterygia and corneal clouding, hearing loss and craniosynostosis have also been described. Growth and intellectual function were normal in all three patients. In addition, Haugen and Bertelsen [3] described a family with similar, albeit milder manifestations, which could be the same entity.

Other progeroid conditions (e.g. MADA, MADB, etc.) should be ruled out. Skin biopsy in one patient demonstrated similarities to juvenile hyaline fibromatosis, but differed in that staining with periodic acid-Schiff and Alcian blue was only faintly positive [1].

References

1 Pentinnen M, Niemi K-M, Vinkka-Puhakka H et al. New progeroid disorder. Am J Med Genet 1997;69:182–7.
2 Zufferey F, Hadj-Rubia S, De Sandre-Giovannoli A et al. Acro-osteolysis, keloid like-lesions, distinctive facial features, and overgrowth: two newly recognized patients with premature aging syndrome, Penttinen type. Am J Med Genet Part A 2012;161A:1786–91.
3 Haugen OH, Bertelsen T. A new hereditary conjunctivo-corneal dystrophy associated with dermal keloid formation. Report of a family. Acta Ophthalmol Scand 1998;76:461–5.

Lenz–Majewski syndrome

Brief introduction and history. The Lenz–Majewski syndrome (LMS) is a rare disorder of progeroid appearance, facial and limb defects and skeletal anomalies, first recognized by Lenz & Majewski [1] as a distinct entity. It had been described previously by Braham [2] and MacPherson [3] in patients diagnosed with craniodiaphyseal or diaphyseal dysplasia. Robinow and colleagues [4] suggested the eponym. Others have also reported patients [5–13].

Epidemiology and pathogenesis. This is an autosomal dominant trait, caused by heterozygous gain-of-function mutations in *PTDSS1* [12].

Clinical features. Affected individuals have: pre- and postnatal growth retardation; a characteristic face with relative macrocephaly, frontal bossing, midface hypoplasia, hypertelorism, short nose, long philtrum, thin upper lip and large posteriorly rotated ears; dental enamel hypoplasia; short hands and feet with marked cutaneous syndactyly; and loose, atrophic skin with prominent venous patterns. Moderate to severe intellectual disability is present and sensorineural hearing loss can also occur. Skeletal manifestations include progressive sclerosis of the skull base and vertebrae, bone remodelling in tubular bones, various synostoses, and rib and vertebral anomalies. The lifespan is unknown, although the patient described by Lenz & Majewski [1] was alive at 30 years and the subject of a more recent report [9].

Differential diagnosis. The conditions that need to be considered in the differential diagnosis, radiographically, include craniometaphyseal dysplasia, diaphyseal dysplasia and craniodiaphyseal dysplasia. However, other phenotypic manifestations should distinguish among these.

Laboratory and histology findings. Hood and colleagues [8] described the absence of elastin fibres in a child who was reported to have a new syndrome but who was later recognized to have LMS. The infant girl reported by Whyte and colleagues [14] had hyperphosphoserinuria on urine amino acid analysis.

Treatment. Treatment is supportive.

References

1 Lenz WD, Majewski F. A generalized disorder of the connective tissues with progeria, choanal atresia, symphalangism, hypoplasia of the dentine, and craniodiaphyseal hypostosis. BDOAS 1974;x:133–6.
2 Braham RL. Multiple congenital abnormalities with diaphyseal dysplasia (Camurati–Engelmann's syndrome). Oral Surg 1969;27:20–6.
3 MacPherson RI. Craniodiaphyseal dysplasia, a disease or group of diseases. J Can Assoc Radiol 1974;25:22–3.
4 Robinow M, Johanson AJ, Smith T. The Lenz–Majewski hyperostotic dwarfism. J Pediatr 1977;91:417–21.
5 Gorlin RJ, Whitley CB. Lenz–Majewski syndrome. Radiology 1983;149:129–31.
6 Chrzanowska KH, Fryns J-P, Krajewska-Walasek M et al. Skeletal dysplasia syndrome with progeroid appearance, characteristic facial and limb anomalies, multiple synostoses, and distinct skeletal changes: a variant example of the Lenz–Majewski syndrome. Am J Med Genet 1989;32:470–4.
7 Saraiva JM. Dysgenesis of corpus callosum in Lenz–Majewski hyperostotic dwarfism. Am J Med Genet 2000;91:198–200.
8 Hood OJ, Lockhart LH, Hughes TE. Cutis laxa with craniofacial, limb, genital, and brain defects. J Clin Dysmorph 1984;2:23–6.
9 Majewski F. Lenz–Majewski hyperostotic dwarfism: re-examination of the original patient. Am J Med Genet 2000;93:335–8.
10 Dateki S, Kondoh T, Nishimura G et al. A Japanese patient with a mild Lenz–Majewski syndrome. J Hum Genet 2007;52:686–9.
11 Wattanasirichaigoon D, Visudtibhan A, Jaovisidha S et al. Expanding the phenotypic spectrum of Lenz–Majewski syndrome: facial palsy, cleft palate and hydrocephalus. Clin Dysmorphol 2004;13:137–42.
12 Sousa SB, Jenkins D, Chanudet E et al. Gain-of-function mutations in the phosphatidylserine synthase 1 (PTDSS1) gene cause Lenz-Majewski syndrome. Nat Genet 2014;46:70–8.
13 Mizuguchi K, Miyazaki O, Nishimura G et al. Craniovertebral junction stenosis in Lenz-Majewski syndrome. Pediatr Radiol 2015;45:1567–70.
14 Whyte MP, Blythe A, McAlister WH et al. Lenz-Majewski hyperostotic dwarfism with hyperphosphoserinuria from a novel mutation in PTDSS1 encoding phosphatidylserine synthase 1. J Bone Miner Res 2015;30:606–14.

Conditions in which individuals appear aged

Mulvihill–Smith syndrome

Brief introduction and history. This is a rare syndrome in which short stature, minor craniofacial anomalies, postnatal onset naevi and immunodeficiency occur. The Mulvihill–Smith syndrome (MSS) was described in 1975 [1] by the two authors after whom this condition is named, although Shepard [2] is now recognized as having published the first description of this rare syndrome. Elliott reported on the same patient in 1975 [3]. Since then, descriptions of several other definite patients [4–13] and one possible patient [14] have been published.

Epidemiology and pathogenesis. The cause of this condition is unknown; all reported individuals have been the only such affected family member. The patient reported by Ohashi and colleagues [14] was born to consanguineous parents; if this individual does indeed have MSS, then the possibility that this is an autosomal recessive condition exists.

Clinical features. MSS is characterized by low birthweight and subsequent short stature in almost all patients. Microcephaly is another common manifestation. The face is distinctive, with relative lack of subcutaneous fat, broad forehead, malar flattening, small and pointed chin and prominent ears. The voice is often highly pitched; hypodontia and irregular teeth are common. Most have sensorineural hearing loss.

The most characteristic finding is the pigmented naevi, which occur on all parts of the body. However, age at appearance of the naevi is variable, with the naevi noted in the patient of Bartsch and colleagues [6] at the age of 1 year, in the patient of Baraitser and colleagues [5] at the age of 5–6 years and in the patient of Ohashi and colleagues [14] at the age of 25 years. Additional skin manifestations include normal subcutaneous fat distribution on the trunk and limbs, dryness and increased hirsutism. Immunodeficiency and recurrent infections have been reported often, with T cell dysfunction and decreased levels of immunoglobulins A (IgA) and G (IgG) noted. Advanced bone age was reported in two patients [5,8]. So-called 'dry eye disease' was reported in one adult with MSS [10]. Intellectual disability is an inconstant finding, ranging from severe to mild in those with this manifestation. Lifespan is unknown, although several patients were adults at the time of the reports. Cognitive decline during adulthood might be an additional manifestation [9]. An increased risk of tumour development is also likely, given that four patients [6,8,9,12] developed tumours while in their late teens or twenties.

Differential diagnosis. Other progeroid syndromes, such as WS, need to be ruled out, although definitive diagnosis is difficult prior to the appearance of the naevi. The LEOPARD syndrome includes lentigines and short stature in the phenotype (plus electrocardiogram abnormalities, ocular hypertelorism, pulmonary stenosis, abnormalities of the genitalia and deafness), but can be distinguished by the characteristic facial appearance in MSS.

Laboratory and histology findings. De Silva and colleagues [7] described skin biopsy findings in their patient, and noted that fibroblast growth in culture was slow, with small size and large numbers of inclusions found. Primary cilia were absent.

Treatment. None is known, other than for infections when they occur.

References

1 Mulvihill JJ, Smith DW. Another disorder with prenatal shortness of stature and premature ageing. BDOAS 1975;xi:368–71.
2 Shepard MK. An unidentified syndrome with abnormality of skin and hair. BDOAS 1971;vii:353–4.
3 Elliott DE. Undiagnosed syndrome of psychomotor retardation, low birthweight dwarfism, skeletal, dental, dermal and genital anomalies. BDOAS 1975;xi:364–7.
4 Wong W, Cohen MM, Miller M et al. Case report for syndrome identification. Cleft Palate J 1979;16:286–90.
5 Baraitser M, Insley J, Winter RM. A recognisable short stature syndrome with premature ageing and pigmented naevi. J Med Genet 1986;25:53–6.
6 Bartsch O, Tympner K-D, Schwinger E et al. Mulvihill–Smith syndrome: case report and review. J Med Genet 1994;31:707–11.
7 De Silva DC, Wheatley DN, Herriot R et al. Mulvihill–Smith progeria like syndrome. A further report with delineation of phenotype, immunologic deficits, and novel observation of fibroblast abnormalities. Am J Med Genet 1997;69:56–64.
8 Ferri R, Lanuzza G, Cosentino FI et al. Agrypnia excitata in a patient with progeroid short stature and pigmented Nevi (Mulvihill–Smith syndrome). J Sleep Res 2005;14:463–70.
9 Yagihashi T, Kato M, Izumi K et al. Case report: adult phnotype of Mulvihill–Smith syndrome. Am J Med Genet 2009;149A:496–500.
10 Ibrahim OM, Takefumi Y, Dogru M et al. Ocular complications in Mulvihill-Smith syndrome. Eye (Lond) 2010;24:1123–4.
11 Fuhler-Stiller M, Tronnier M. Suspicious pigmented tumor in Mulvihill-Smith syndrome. J Dtsch Dermatol Ges 2011;9:308–11.
12 Stevic M, Simic D, Milojevic I. Anesthesia in a child with Mulvihill-Smith syndrome. J Anesth 2014;28:313.
13 Breinis P, Alves FG, Alves CAE, et al. The eleventh reported case of Mulvihill-Smith syndrome in the literature. BMC Neurol 2014;14:4.
14 Ohashi H, Tsukahara M, Murano I et al. Premature ageing and immunodeficiency: Mulvihill–Smith syndrome? Am J Med Genet 1993;45:597–600.

Lenaerts syndrome

Brief introduction and history. This is a rare hereditary syndrome that includes premature ageing, joint dislocations and minor craniofacial anomalies among the phenotypical manifestations. Only one family has been described, by Lenaerts and colleagues in 1994 [1].

Epidemiology and pathogenesis. This condition is probably inherited as an autosomal dominant trait, although X-linked dominant inheritance cannot be excluded. The basic genetic defect is unknown.

Clinical features. Full expression of this condition is characterized by: short stature; sparse hair and blue sclerae; thin nose; thin lips; joint anomalies, including large joint hyperlaxity; subluxation of the interphalangeal joints of the hands and feet, and talipes equinovarus; carpal synostosis; and thin skin with lower extremity livedo reticularis. Documented panhypogammaglobulinaemia developed during adulthood in the proposita, but may have affected others in the family as well. Lifespan and intellectual functioning appear to be normal.

Differential diagnosis. This condition most closely resembles Larsen syndrome with regard to joint dislocations but can be distinguished by the additional skin and immune system findings.

Laboratory and histology findings. None were reported.

Treatment. Antibiotics for infections or intravenous provision of γ-globulin may be indicated.

Reference

1 Lenaerts J, Fryns JP, Westhovens R et al. A familial syndrome of dwarfism, bilateral club feet, premature ageing and progressive panhypogammaglobulinemia. J Rheumatol 1994;21:961–3.

MDPL syndrome

Brief introduction and history. Shastry and colleagues [1] described seven patients with *m*andibular hypoplasia, *d*eafness, *p*rogeroid features and *l*ipodystrophy, and proposed that these individuals had a previously undescribed syndrome which they named MDP. The condition was later termed MDPL, which is an acronym for the cardinal manifestations [2]. Since the initial report, other patients have been reported [3–5].

Epidemiology and pathogenesis. MDPL syndrome is caused by heterozygous mutation in the polymerase delta 1 (*POLD1*) gene.

Clinical features. MDPL is characterized by childhood onset lipodystrophy, dysmorphic facial appearance and development of sensorineural hearing loss. Facial features include prominent eyes, beaked nose, mandibular hypoplasia and crowded teeth. Hypogonadism is common in males whereas females exhibit lack of breast development. The skin is described as sclerodermatous. Notably, sparse hair, clavicular hypoplasia or acro-osteolysis do not occur, and lifespan and intellect appear not to be significantly affected.

Differential diagnosis. Mandibuloacral dysplasia and WS should be considered in the differential diagnosis.

Laboratory and histology findings. Adult patients can have a number of metabolic disturbances, including abnormal glucose metabolism, liver function tests and lipid profiles, although these findings are not universal [2,4].

Treatment. Treatment is supportive, with treatment of metabolic disturbances indicated.

References

1 Shastry S, Simha V, Godbole K et al. A novel syndrome of mandibular hypoplasia, deafness, and progeroid features associated with lipodystrophy, undescended testes, and male hypogonadism. J Clin Endocrinol Metab 2010;95:E192–E197.
2 Pelosini C, Martinelli S, Ceccarini G et al. Identification of a novel mutation in the polymerase delta 1 (POLD1) gene in a lipodystrophic patient affected by mandibular hypoplasia, deafness, progeroid features (MDPL) syndrome. J Metabol 2014;63:1385–9.
3 Weedon MN, Ellard S, Prindle MH et al. An in-frame deletion at the polymerase active site of POLD1 causes a multisystem disorder with lipodystrophy. Nat Genet 2013;45:947–50.
4 Lessel D, Hisama FM, Szakszon K et al. POLD1 germline mutations in patients initially diagnosed with Werner syndrome. Hum Mutat 2015;36:1070–9.
5 Reinier F, Zoledziewska M, Hanna D et al. Mandibular hypoplasia, deafness, progeroid features and lipodystrophy (MDPL) syndrome in the context of inherited lipodystrophies. J Metabol 2015;64:1530–40.

Marfanoid progeria–lipodystrophy syndrome

Brief introduction and history. Grauel-Neumann and colleagues [1] described an adult patient with some manifestations of Marfan syndrome, but also with a progeroid facial appearance and lipodystrophy. Since then, other patients have been reported [2–7].

Epidemiology and pathogenesis. The cause of this condition is mutation in exon 64 (the terminal exon) of *FBN1*, the gene associated with classic Marfan syndrome.

Clinical features. Affected individuals have low birthweight and a generalized lipodystrophy at birth. The lack of facial fat leads to a prematurely aged appearance. Marfan syndrome-associated manifestations variably occur, and include arachnodactyly, joint contractures, severe myopia, lens dislocation, aortic root dilatation and mitral valve prolapse. Cognitive function is normal. The skin is described as thin with easy bruising [5,6]. Prognosis is unknown; the oldest reported patient was 27 years at the time of the report [1].

Differential diagnosis. Neonatal Marfan syndrome, caused by mutations in exons 24–32 [8] and Wiedemann–Rautenstrauch syndrome should be considered in the differential diagnosis.

Laboratory and histology findings. Glucose metabolism is normal, with no evidence of insulin resistance or diabetes.

Treatment. Treatment is supportive, with routine screening of vision and cardiac status indicated.

References

1 Graul-Neumann LM, Kienitz T, Robinson PN et al. Marfan syndrome with neonatal progeroid syndrome-like lipodystrophy associated with a novel frameshift mutation at the 3′ terminus of the FBN-1 gene. Am J Med Genet Part A 2010;152A:2749–55.
2 Goldblatt J, Hyatt J, Edwards C et al. Further evidence for a marfanoid syndrome with neonatal progeroid features and severe generalized lipodystrophy due to frameshift mutations near the 3′ end of the FBN1 gene. Am J Med Genet Part A 2011;155A:717–20.
3 Horn D, Robinson PN. Progeroid facial features and lipodystrophy associated with a novel splice site mutation in the final intron of the FBN1 gene. Am J Med Genet Part A 2011;155A:721–4.
4 Takenouchi T, Hida M, Sakamoto Y et al. Severe congenital lipodystrophy and a progeroid appearance: mutation in the penultimate exon of FBN1 causing a recognizable phenotype. Am J Med Genet Part A 2013;161:3057–62.
5 Jacquinet A, Verloes A, Callewaert B et al. Neonatal progeroid variant of Marfan syndrome with congenital lipodystrophy results from mutations at the 3′ end of FBN1 gene. Eur J Med Genet 2014;57:230–4.
6 Garg A, Xing C. De novo heterozygous FBN1 mutations in the extreme C-terminal region cause progeroid fibrillinopathy. Am J Med Genet Part A 2014;164A:1341–5.
7 Passarge E, Robinson PN, Graul-Neumann LM. Marfanoid-progeroid-lipodystrophy syndrome: a newly recognized fibrillinopathy. Eur J Hum Genet 2016;24:1244–7.
8 Maeda J, Kosaki K, Shiono J et al. Variable severity of cardiovascular phenotypes in patients with an early-onset form of Marfan syndrome harboring FBN1 mutations in exons 24-32. Heart Vessels 2016;31:1717–23.

CAV1-associated lipodystrophy

Brief introduction and history. This condition is characterized by neonatal-onset lipodystrophy, mottled skin, pulmonary hypertension and failure to thrive. To date only three patients have been reported [1,2].

Epidemiology and pathogenesis. This condition is caused by heterozygous mutation in *CAV1*, which encodes caveolin 1, an integral membrane protein.

Clinical features. Two of the reported children were known to have prenatal-onset pulmonary effusions, which resolved prior to or soon after birth. These children were also noted at birth to have mottled skin, described as cutis marmorata, and decreased subcutaneous fat. Two of the children were reported to need feeding assistance using G-tubes. The facial features were described as consisting of a triangular face with small lips and/or small mouth. The anterior fontanelle remained open for at least the first few years of life. Scalp hair is thin, and lipodystrophy affects most of the body, with sparing only of the buttocks. Cognitive development was normal. The oldest reported patient was 7 years at the time of the report.

Differential diagnosis. Other congenital lipodystrophies and the congenital disorders of glycosylation should be considered in the differential diagnosis.

Laboratory and histology findings. Lipid metabolism appears to be abnormal, in that low HDL and high triglycerides were present in one or more patient.

Treatment. Treatment is supportive. It is unknown whether treatment with statins is indicated.

References

1 Schrauwen I, Szelinger S, Siniard AL et al. A frame-shift mutation in CAV1 is associated with a severe neonatal progeroid and lipodystrophy syndrome. PLOS ONE 2015; published online.
2 Garg A, Kircher M, del Campo M et al. Whole exome sequencing identifies de novo heterozygous CAV1 mutations associated with a novel neonatal onset lipodystrophy syndrome. Am J Med Genet Part A 2015;167A:1796–806.

Nestor–Guillermo syndrome

Brief introduction and history. Cabanillas and colleagues [1] described two unrelated males with a phenotype reminiscent of, but distinct from, that of mandibuloacral dysplasia or HGPS. The syndrome is named after these two original patients. As of early 2016, there have been no other reported patients.

Epidemiology and pathogenesis. Nestor–Guillermo syndrome is an autosomal recessive condition, and is caused by biallelic mutation in the barrier-to-autointegration factor 1 (*BANF1*) gene [2,3].

SECTION 28: FOCAL OR GENERALIZED HYPOPLASIA

Clinical features. Both individuals had a normal phenotype until the age of 2 years. From this age onwards, loss of subcutaneous fat, finger joint stiffness, and mandibular and clavicular bone resorption began to occur. By adulthood, mandibular, maxillary and clavicular osteolysis was severe, with complete resorption noted. The skin is described as thin, dry and atrophic, with areas of hyperpigmentation. Cognition is normal, although growth is impaired.

Differential diagnosis. Mandibuloacral dysplasia type A and HGPS most resemble this condition.

Laboratory and histology findings. Neither patient had any metabolic complications. Skeletal densitometry identified severe osteoporosis in one.

Treatment. Treatment is supportive.

References

1 Cabanillas R, Cadinanos J, Villameytide JAF et al. Nestor-Guillermo progeria syndrome: a novel premature aging condition with early onset and chronic development caused by BANF1 mutations. Am J Med Genet Part A 2011; 155:2617–25.
2 Paquet N, Box JK, Ashton NW et al. Nestor-Guillermo progeria syndrome: a biochemical insight into barrier-to-Autointegration factor 1, alanine 12 threonine mutation. BMC Mol Biol 2014;15:27.
3 Puente XS, Quesada V, Osorio et al. Exome sequencing and functional analysis identifies BANF1 mutation as the cause of a hereditary progeroid syndrome. Am J Hum Genet 2011;88:650–6.

Petty syndrome

Brief introduction and history. Petty and colleagues [1] described two unrelated patients with a progeroid phenotype that overlapped with that of Wiedemann–Rautenstrauch syndrome and HGPS, but which was felt to be distinct from these two. It has been pointed out by others [2,3] that this might be the same condition as that described by Fontaine and colleagues [4]. Additional patients with what might be a single condition (i.e. the Petty and Fontaine–Farriaux syndromes) have been described [5–9].

Epidemiology and pathogenesis. The molecular basis is unknown, but this is presumed to be an autosomal dominant trait attributable to a *de novo* mutation based on the lack of family history in any of the reported individuals.

Clinical features. Patients are small at birth and have several dysmorphic features. The cranial sutures are wide and the skull poorly ossified. The hair pattern is unusual and appears to have a disorganized growth pattern. Lipodystrophy is also present and skin is loose and wrinkled. Distal digital and nail dysplasia also occur. All children have also had umbilical hernias and most have had craniosynostosis, whereas other manifestations such as abdominal muscle hypoplasia, genital anomalies, central nervous system anomalies or heart defects are more variable. Most individuals do not have cognitive impairment.

Differential diagnosis. Mandibuloacral dysplasia type B and Wiedemann–Rautenstrauch syndrome as well as some of the rarer progeroid syndromes should be considered in the differential.

Laboratory and histology findings. None were reported.

References

1 Petty EM, Laxova R, Wiedemann HR. Previously unrecognized congenital progeroid disorder. Am J Med Genet 1990;35:383–7.
2 Castori M, Silvestri E, Pedace L et al. Fontaine-Farriaux syndrome: a recognizable craniosynostosis syndrome with nail, skeletal, abdominal, and central nervous system anomalies. Am J Med Genet Part A 2009;149A:2193–9.
3 Braddock SR, Ardinger HH, Yang CS et al. Petty syndrome and Fontaine-Farriaux syndrome: delineation of a single syndrome. Am J Med Genet Part A 2010;152A:1718–23.
4 Fontaine G, Farriaux JP, Blanckaert D et al. Un nouveau syndrome polymalformatif complexe. J Genet Hum 1977;25:109–19.
5 Wiedemann HR. Newly recognized congenital progeroid syndrome. Am J Med Genet 1992;42:857.
6 Delgado-Luengo WN, Petty EM, Solis-Anez E et al. Further phenotypical delineation and confirmation of a rare syndrome of premature aging. Am J Med Genet Part A 2009;149A:2200–5.
7 Priolo M, De Toni T, Baffico M et al. Fontaine-Farriaux craniosynostosis: second report in the literature. Am J Med Genet 2001;100:214–18.
8 Faivre L, Khau Van Kien P, Madinier-Chappat N et al. Can Hutchinson-Gilford progeria syndrome be a neonatal condition? Am J Med Genet 1999;87:450.
9 Rodriguez JI, Perez-Alonso P, Funes R et al. Am J Med Genet 1999;82:242–8.

Conditions with skin laxity

Cutis laxa (see Chapter 94)

Cutis laxa is a connective tissue disorder marked by inelastic skin that often hangs loose from the body. Other organs can be affected and hernias often develop. Forms are divided based on inheritance pattern as autosomal dominant (*ELN*, *FBLN5* mutations), autosomal recessive (*EFEMP2*, *ATP6V0A2*, *FBLN5*) or X-linked (*ATP7A*) [1,2]. Alibert [3] is attributed with the first description of autosomal recessive cutis laxa, which was published in 1833. Rossbach [4] described the first instance of autosomal dominant cutis laxa in 1884.

Recessive forms have more severe phenotypes including levels of developmental delay, seizures and movement problems. The X-linked form is also termed occipital horn syndrome and is considered part of the Menkes syndrome spectrum, a disorder of copper metabolism. Some forms of cutis laxa that were thought to be separate entities are now included in the molecular classification. This includes cutis laxa with intellectual disability and wrinkly skin syndrome, which are now known to be forms of autosomal recessive cutis laxa type IIa caused by mutations in the *ATP6V0A2* gene. These both can have aged appearance along with growth retardation, ligamentous laxity, joint dislocation, craniofacial anomalies and developmental delay (cutis laxa with intellectual disability) or wrinkled skin on the hands, feet and abdomen, multiple skeletal anomalies, microcephaly and intellectual disability (wrinkly skin syndrome).

References

1 Mohamed M et al. Cutix laxa. Adv Exp Med Biol 2014;802:161–84.
2 Genetics Home Reference. Cutis laxa. https://ghr.nlm.nih.gov/condition/cutis-laxa (accessed 11 December 2018).
3 Alibert JL. Histoire d'un berger des environs de Gisore (dermatose hypermorphe). Monogr Dermatol 1833;2:719.
4 Rossbach MJ. Ein merkwurdiger Fall von greisenhafter Veranderung der allgemeinen Korperdecke bei einem achtzehnjahrigen Jungling. Dtsch Arch Klin Med 1884;36:197–203.

Macrocephaly, alopecia, cutis laxa and scoliosis (MACS syndrome)

Only described in four consanguineous families, some heterogeneity is present beyond the original family's features [1].

The condition is autosomal recessive with mutations found in *RIN2*, which is involved in Rab5 interaction, which affects endosomal trafficking [1,2].

Light microscopy on skin biopsies revealed sparse elastic fibres, with a complete absence of oxytalin fibres in the upper dermis. [1]. Other studies have shown abnormal collagen fibril morphology with fibroblasts having dilated endoplasmic reticulum and abnormal Golgi apparatus [2]. Golgi had swollen cisternae and vacuole accumulation [3].

The most consistent features appear to be facial coarsening, scoliosis, thin/sparse hair (not necessarily alopecia), joint hypermobility, easy bruising and skin hyperextensibility (not cutis laxa-like skin relaxation). Droopiness of the cheeks appears to be related to soft tissue swelling [2]. Macrocephaly does not appear to be a key feature. With most of the findings included in the acronym name not consistently found, *RIN2* syndrome may be a more proper name for this condition [3,4].

Lifespan is unknown. Differential diagnosis includes other forms of cutis laxa and Ehlers–Danlos syndrome (EDS), Costello syndrome, and GAPO (growth retardation, alopecia, pseudoanodontia and optic atrophy), caused by *ANTXR1* mutations [5].

References

1 Basel-Vanagatte L, Sarig O, Hershkovitz D et al. RIN2 deficiency results in macrocephaly, alopecia, cutis laxa, and scoliosis: MACS syndrome. Am J Hum Genet 2009;85:254–63.
2 Syx D, Malfait F, Van Laer L. The RIN2 syndrome: a new autosomal recessive connective tissue disorder caused by deficiency of Ras and Rab interactor 2 (RIN2). Hum Genet 2010;128:79–88.
3 Albrecht B, de Brouwer AP, Lefeber DJ. MACS Syndrome: a combined collagen and elastin disorder due to abnormal Golgi trafficking. Am J Med Genet Part A 2010;152A:2916–8.
4 Aslanger AD, Altunoglu U, Aslanger E. Newly described clinical features in two siblings with MACS syndrome and a novel mutation in RIN2. Am J Med Genet Part A 2014;164A:484–9.
5 Stranecky V, Hoischen A, Hartmannova H, et al. Mutations in ANTXR1 cause GAPO syndrome. Am J Hum Genet 2013;92:792–9.

Geroderma osteodysplastica

Definition. Geroderma osteodysplastica (GO) is a rare autosomal recessive condition marked by lax, wrinkled skin, joint hypermobility and characteristic aged-looking face [1].

History. Credit for the first description and naming goes to Bamatter and colleagues [2]. They identified five affected siblings and used the term 'Walt Disney dwarfs' because of the similar facial features. Initially a clinical diagnosis, there has been significant overlap with other conditions such as cutis laxa and wrinkly skin syndrome. The molecular basis has clarified this somewhat but led to other areas of difficulty with reclassification. Review of the literature for cases reported prior to gene identification is especially challenging.

Aetiology and pathogenesis. Hennies and colleagues identified *SCYL1BP1* as the causative gene for GO in 2008 [3]. Highest expression levels were in osteoblasts and skin. The protein product was noted to be involved in Golgi apparatus function. Since renamed *GORAB*, the specific function of the gene is not entirely clear. It interacts with Ras-like GTPase RAB6 which helps with transport processes [1,4]. Causative mutations in *GORAB* cause loss-of-function [3]. With molecular diagnosis replacing clinical diagnoses of the past, some individuals with clinical GO have been found to have *PYCR1* mutations [5]. *PYCR1* is causative of autosomal recessive cutis laxa, types IIB and IIIB. There are some clinical differences between the *GORAB* and *PCYR1* genotypes, so molecular diagnosis should be used to give the most accurate diagnosis.

Pathology. Skin biopsy findings reported by Hunter [6] included nonspecific fragmentation of elastic fibres.

Clinical features. The classic facial features include oblique furrowing from the lateral border of the supraorbital ridge along the scalp hairline superolaterally up to the outer canthus inferomedially. This causes the upper eyelid to appear full [1]. The face appears long and triangular with larger ears that protrude [5]. Malar hypoplasia and lax facial skin contribute to the aged appearance [4]. The main other areas of skin laxity are the dorsum of the hands and feet [5]. Mandibular frenulum has been reported to be consistently absent or hypoplastic [1]. Skeletal findings include joint hypermobility and varying degrees of osteoporosis, which can lead to fractures or growth problems [1,3,4]. GO is considered a segmental progeroid disorder.

Treatment and prognosis. Treatment is mainly symptomatic. Facial and dental surgery may be required [7], and bone density issues can be addressed appropriately [8]. Adults with GO have been reported in the literature, and there does not appear to be any clear data supporting significant risks for morbidity and mortality [9].

Differential diagnosis. GO should be differentiated from autosomal recessive cutis laxa caused by *PYCR1* by the presence of intellectual disability associated with the latter. Osteopenia is also seen more often in GO [5]. Wrinkly skin syndrome (now molecularly found to be another subtype of autosomal recessive cutis laxa) should also be considered [9]. In infancy and childhood, there may be some similarities to EDS and HGPS [10]. The initial clinical classification of GO followed by relabelling after the molecular cause was identified illustrates the challenges present in differentiating GO from other similar conditions.

References

1 Al-Dosari M, Alkuraya FS. A Novel Missense Mutatino in SCYL1BP1 produces geroderma osteodysplastica phenotype indistinguishable from that caused by nullimorphic mutations. Am J Med Genet Part A 149A:2093–8.
2 Bamatter F, Franschetti A, Klein D et al. Gerodermie osteodysplastique hereditaire. Un noveau biotype de la progeria. Confin Neurol 1949;9:397.
3 **Hennies HC, Kornak U, Zhang H et al. Geroderma osteodysplastica is caused by mutations in SCYL1BP1, a Rab-6 intercting golgin. Nat Genet 2008;40:1410–12.**
4 Egerer J, Emmerich D, Fischer-Zirnsak B. GORAB missense mutations disrupt RAB6 and ARF5 binding and golgi targeting. J Invest Dermatol 2015;135:2368–76.
5 Yildirim Y, Tolun A, Tuysuz B. The phenotype caused by PYCR1 mutations corresponds to geroderma osteodysplasticum rather than autosomal recessive cutis laxa type 2. Am J Med Genet Part A 2011;155:134–40.
6 Hunter AGW, Martsolf JT, Baker CG. Geroderma osteodysplastica: report of two affected families. Hum Genet 1978;40:311–24.
7 Lustmann J, Nahlieli O, Harary D et al. Geroderma osteodysplastica: report on two patients and surgical correction of facial deformity. Am J Med Genet 1993;47:261–7.
8 Noordam C, Funke S, Knoers NV et al. Decreased bone density and treatment in patients with autosomal recessive cutis laxa. Acta Paediatrica 2009;98:490–4.
9 Rajab A, Kornak U, Budde BS. Geroderma osteodysplasticum hereditaria and wrinkly skin syndrome in 22 patients from Oman. Am J Med Genet Part A 2008; 146A:965–76.
10 Sommer A. Photo essay – geroderma osteodysplastica. Am J Med Genet Part C 2007;145C:291–2.

Costello syndrome (see Chapter 144)

Definition. Costello syndrome is a multiple congenital anomaly syndrome characterized by the combination of postnatal onset poor growth, relative macrocephaly, typical facial appearance, developmental delay and nasal papillomas. The skin exhibits cutis laxa, and the palmar and plantar creases are deep [1].

History. Two children were first described in 1971 and again in 1977 by Costello [2,3]. Subsequently, other examples have been reported in the literature [4–8]. There is debate as to whether children described by Borochowitz and colleagues [9,14] had Costello syndrome or a distinct entity. Resolution of this issue is important, because the two conditions probably have different modes of inheritance. Johnson and colleagues [15], Philip & Sigaudy [16] and Quezada & Gripp [1] provide good reviews.

Aetiology and pathogenesis. The cause of Costello syndrome is a heterozygous mutation in *HRAS*, which is virtually always *de novo*. This gene is in the MAPK signalling pathway. The most common mutation is p.G12S and is present in 84% of cases [17]. Other mutations are associated with slight variations in the phenotype [18] or more severe manifestations and early lethality [19].

Pathology. Skin biopsy has usually demonstrated normal elastic tissue, although Hatamochi and colleagues [20] and Torrelo and colleagues [21] both described abnormal elastic fibres in skin biopsies.

Clinical features. Because of postnatal failure to thrive, the head looks too large for the body, leading to the appearance of relative macrocephaly. Ectodermal defects include: slow-growing brittle hair, which tends to become curly and soft; slow-growing nails; lax skin, particularly on the hands and feet, with deep palmar and plantar creases; papillomas that occur not only in the perinasal region, but also in other areas (e.g. perianal, perioral); and development of pigmented naevi and acanthosis nigricans. The voice is often hoarse. Cardiovascular abnormalities include congenital heart defects (most commonly pulmonary valve stenosis), hypertrophic cardiomyopathy and arrhythmia (often atrial tachycardia) [17]. Diagnosis is difficult in the newborn period, because many of the manifestations do not develop until later. However, Digilio and colleagues [22] pointed out that neonatal macrosomia (often with hydrops) with subsequent failure to thrive, hypotonia, coarse facial appearance, and hyperpigmented, loose skin on the hands and feet should raise the suspicion of Costello syndrome. Prenatal findings that might suggest Costello syndrome include polyhydramnios, fetal overgrowth, relative macrocephaly and fetal atrial tachycardia [23,24].

Prognosis. Developmental delay and cognitive impairment are common, with a mean IQ score of 57 (range 30–87) reported [25]. Lifespan is unknown, but cardiac defects or cardiomyopathy, when present, may affect this. In addition, there is a 10–15% risk for the development of malignant tumours, particularly rhabdomyosarcoma, neuroblastoma and transitional cell carcinoma of the bladder [1,26]. Among these, rhabdomyosarcoma is by far the most common. The possibility of sudden worsening requires lifetime cardiac surveillance [17].

Differential diagnosis. There are several similarities to the Noonan and cardiofaciocutaneous syndromes, but phenotypical differences should distinguish among them. Some children initially identified as having cutis laxa with intellectual disability were subsequently diagnosed with Costello syndrome [27]. Larger size and hypoglycaemia might also suggest Simpson–Golabi–Behmel or Beckwith–Wiedemann syndromes [19].

Treatment. Nutritional support does not alleviate growth failure, although studies on use of growth hormone indicate that growth hormone supplementation led to increased growth velocity [28]. Orthopaedic intervention may be necessary for valgus deformities or hip dislocation. There is also work under way to evaluate several drugs that target various elements of the Ras pathway [28,29]. Some clinical trials for RASopathies have already begun with more likely to follow [20].

References

1 **Quezada E, Gripp KW. Costello syndrome and related disorders. Curr Opinion Pediatr 2007;19:636–44.**
2 Costello JM. A new syndrome. NZ Med J 1971;74:397.
3 Costello JM. A new syndrome: mental subnormality and nasal papillomata. Aust Pediatr J 1977;13:114–18.

4 Der Kaloustian VM, Noroz B, McIntosh N et al. Costello syndrome. Am J Med Genet 1991;41:69–73.
5 Martin RA, Jones KL. Delineation of Costello syndrome. Am J Med Genet 1991;41:346–9.
6 Say B, Gucsavas M, Morgan H et al. The Costello syndrome. Am J Med Genet 1993;47:163–5.
7 Teebi AS, Shabaani IS. Further delineation of Costello syndrome. Am J Med Genet 1993;47:166–8.
8 Zampino G, Mastroiacovo P, Ricci R et al. Costello syndrome: further clinical delineation, natural history, genetic definition, and nosology. Am J Med Genet 1993;47:176–83.
9 Borochowitz Z, Pavone L, Mazor G et al. New multiple congenital anomalies: mental retardation syndrome (MCA/MR) with facio-cutaneous-skeletal involvement. Am J Med Genet 1992;42:678–85.
10 Philip N, Mancini J. Costello syndrome and facio–cutaneous–skeletal syndrome. Am J Med Genet 1993;47:176–83.
11 Martin RA, Jones KL. Facio–cutaneous–skeletal syndrome is the Costello syndrome. Am J Med Genet 1993;47:169.
12 Der Kaloustian VM. Not a new MCA/MR syndrome but probably Costello syndrome? Am J Med Genet 1993;47:170–1.
13 Teebi AS. Costello or facio–cutaneous–skeletal syndrome? Am J Med Genet 1993;47:172.
14 Borochowitz Z, Pavone L, Mazor G et al. Facio–cutaneous–skeletal syndrome. Am J Med Genet 1993;47:173.
15 Johnson JP, Golabi M, Norton ME et al. Costello syndrome: phenotype, natural history, and differential diagnosis, and possible cause. J Pediatr 1998;133:441–8.
16 Philip N, Sigaudy S. Costello syndrome. J Med Genet 1998;35: 238–40.
17 Lin AE, Alexander ME, Colan SD et al. Clinical, pathological, and molecular analysis of cardiovascular abnormalities in Costello syndrome: A Ras/MAPK pathway syndrome. Am J Med Genet Part A 2011;155:486–507.
18 Gripp KW, Hopkins E, Sol-Church K et al. Phenotypic analysis of individuals with Costello syndrome due to HRAS p.G13C. Am J Med Genet Part A 2011;155:706–16.
19 Lo IF, Brewer C, Shannon N et al. Severe neonatal manifestations of Costello syndrome. J Med Genet 2008;45:167–71.
20 Hatamochi A, Nagayama H, Kuroda K et al. Costello syndrome with decreased gene expression of elastin in cultured dermal fibroblasts. Dermatology 2000;201:366–9.
21 Torrelo A, Lopez-Avila A, Mediero IG et al. Costello syndrome. J Am Acad Dermatol 1995;32:904–7.
22 Digilio MC, Sarkozy A, Capolino R et al. Costello syndrome: clinical diagnosis in the first year of life. Eur J Pediatr 2008;167:621–8.
23 Smith LP, Podraza J, Proud VK. Polyhydramnios, fetal overgrowth, and macrocephaly: prenatal ultrasound findings of Costello syndrome. Am J Med Genet Part A 2009;149A:779–84.
24 Lin AE, O'Brien B, Demmer LA et al. Prenatal features of Costello syndrome: ultrasonographic findings and atrial tachycardia. Prenat Diagnosis 2009;29:682–90.
25 Axelrad ME, Nicholson L, Stabley DL et al. Longitudinal assessment of cognitive characteristics in Costello syndrome. Am J Med Genet 2007;143A:3185–93.
26 Sigaudy S, Vittu G, David A et al. Costello syndrome: report of six patients including one with an embryonal rhabdomyosarcoma. Eur J Pediatr 2000;159:139–42.
27 Davies SJ, Hughes HE. Costello syndrome: natural history and differential diagnosis of cutis laxa. J Med Genet 1994;31:486–9.
28 Rauen KA, Hefner E, Carrillo K et al. Molecular aspects, clinical aspects and possible treatment modalities for Costello syndrome: proceedings from the 1st international Costello syndrome research symposium 2007. Am J Med Genet 2008;146A:1205–17.
29 Rauen KA, Banerjee A, Bishop WR. Costello and Cardio-facio-cutaneous syndrome: moving toward clinical trials in RASopathies. Am J Med Genet Part C 2011;157:136–46.

Ehlers–Danlos, progeroid type

Definition. This condition classically involves features of EDS-like hypermobility and loose skin with the addition of aged appearance, developmental delay and other musculoskeletal findings. Original clinical diagnoses giving way to molecular clarification has broadened and shifted the phenotype somewhat.

History. First reports come from Hernandez and colleagues in 1981, 1986 and 1987 [1–3]. None of these patients has ever had molecular testing at a later time. Kresse and colleagues described a similar patient and suggested a biochemical basis for a progeroid-like condition [4]. Since the molecular aetiology was described, several other patients have been reported with varying features despite having proven genetic mutations, calling into question the true clinical nature of this entity and wonderment as to whether the Hernandez cases should be included or separated out.

Aetiology and pathogenesis. Almeida and colleagues and Okajima and colleagues separately reported *B4GALT7* as the causative gene in 1999 [5,6]. Skin fibroblasts from the Kresse patient had been previously shown to incompletely convert the core protein of the small proteodermatan sulfate to mature glycosaminoglycan chain-bearing proteoglycan [4]. This was then shown to be secondary to deficiency of galactosyltransferase I, the protein product of *B4GALT7* [5]. Inherited as autosomal recessive, homozygous mutations and compound heterozygous mutations have both been noted, most often in the catalytic domain of the enzyme [5–7]. Affected individuals had enzyme levels at approximately 5% of the normal level and carriers were nearly 50% [6]. *B4GALT7* is differentially expressed in rodent growth plates, perhaps relating to the short stature seen clinically in humans [8]. Mutations in *B3GALT6* have been found in cases with similar phenotype but no *B4GALT7* mutation [9]. This has been classified in the Online Mendelian Inheritance of Man as EDS-progeroid type 2, suggesting genetic heterogeneity for EDS-progeroid type.

Pathology. A skin biopsy was performed on one Hernandez patient and it did not demonstrate epidermal or dermal defects at the light microscopic level. Using electron microscopy, there was slight distension of intracellular spaces in the epidermal spinous layer and fragmentation of elastic fibres [3]. Little other pathology information is available with most investigations focusing on molecular and biochemical aspects of this condition.

Clinical features. The classic description should be seen in the context of clinical reports and classification giving way to molecular testing. The syndromic features of the first cases included mild intellectual disability, cryptorchidism, curly/fine hair, scant eyebrows/eyelashes and wrinkled facies, in addition to more common features of EDS such as skin hyperextensibility, joint hypermobility, easy bruising, pectus excavatum, winged scapula and papiraceous scarring [1–3]. Developmental delay and progeroid features were not cardinal features of later reported patients, especially among those with proven molecular diagnoses. This has suggested either a wider phenotype spectrum, perhaps because of differing effects of various mutation types and locations in *B4GALT7*, or improper classification of the initial Hernandez cases. Some have even advocated for the removal of the term 'progeroid' in the description [8].

In addition to flexibility and extensibility EDS features, short stature, forearm abnormalities like radioulnar synostosis, and bowing of the legs appear to be the most consistent features associated with *B4GALT7* mutations [8]. For *B3GALT6*, short stature, hypotonia, bone fragility, kyphoscoliosis and progressive contractures are key features in addition to more traditional EDS findings [9,10].

Treatment and prognosis. Treatment is mainly supportive based on symptoms. Based on cases reported, lifespan appears generally normal.

Differential diagnosis. The possibility of this diagnosis being a form of Noonan syndrome was raised in early reports [3]. HGPS has diminished subcutaneous fat and alopecia. Severe intellectual disability and neurological problems may suggest DBS and hearing loss and photosensitivity may suggest CS [4].

References

1 Hernandez A, Aguirre-Negrete MG, Ramirez-Soltero S et al. A distinct variant of the Ehlers–Danlos syndrome. Clin Genet 1979;16:335–9.
2 Hernandez A, Aguirre-Negrete MG, Liparoli JC et al. Third case of a distinct variant of the Ehlers–Danlos syndrome. Clin Genet 1981;20:222–4.
3 Hernandez A, Aguirre-Negrete MG, Gonzalez-Flores S et al. Ehlers–Danlos features with progeroid facies and mild mental retardation. Clin Genet 1986;30:456–61.
4 Kresse H, Rosthoj S, Quentin E et al. Glycosaminoglycan-free small proteoglycan core protein is secreted by fibroblasts from a patient with a syndrome resembling progeroid. Am J Hum Genet 1987;41:436–53.
5 Almeida R, Levery SB, Mandel U. Cloning and expression of a proteoglycan UDP-galactose:β-xylose β1,4-galactosyltransferase I. J Biol Chem 1999;274:26165–171.
6 Okajima T, Fukumoto S, Furukawa K et al. Molecular basis for the progeroid variant of Ehlers–Danlos syndrome. J Biol Chem 1999; 274:28841–4.
7 Faiyaz-Ul-Haque M, Zaidi SHE, Al-Ali M et al. A novel missense mutation in the galactosyltransferase-I (B4GALT7) gene in a family exhibiting facioskeletal anomalies and Ehlers–Danlos syndrome resembling the progeroid type. Am J Med Genet 2004;128A:39–45.
8 Guo MH, Stoler J, Lui J. Redefining the progeroid form of Ehlers-Danlos syndrome: report of the fourth patient with B4GALT7 deficiency and review of the literature. Am J Med Genet Part A 2013;161A:2519–27.
9 Nakajima M, Mizumoto S, Miyake N et al. Mutations in B3GALT6, which encodes a glycosaminoglycan linker region enzyme, cause a spectrum of skeletal and connective tissue disorders. Am J Human Genet 2013;92:927–34.
10 Byers PH, Murray ML. Ehlers-Danlos syndrome: a showcase of conditions that lead to understanding matrix biology. Matrix Biology 2014;33:10–15.

CHAPTER 138
Xeroderma Pigmentosum and Related Diseases

Steffen Schubert[1] *& Steffen Emmert*[2]

[1]Department of Dermatology, Venereology and Allergology, University Medical Centre Göttingen, Göttingen, Germany
[2]Clinic for Dermatology and Venereology, University Medical Centre Rostock, Rostock, Germany

Cellular DNA repair systems, 1743
Nucleotide excision repair, 1744
Nucleotide excision repair defective syndromes, 1748
Disease susceptibility in heterozygous carriers of defective DNA repair genes, 1765
Senescence, 1766
Mitochondrial repair, 1767
Novel therapeutic strategies/DNA repair creams, 1768

Abstract

Nucleotide excision repair (NER) is the most versatile DNA repair system in humans. NER can repair a variety of bulky DNA damage including ultraviolet light-induced DNA damage. The consequences of defective NER factors are demonstrated by the three most common but still rare autosomal recessive NER defective syndromes: xeroderma pigmentosum (XP), Cockayne syndrome (CS), and trichothiodystrophy (TTD). XP patients show severe sun sensitivity, freckling in sun exposed skin and develop skin cancers already during childhood. CS patients exhibit sun sensitivity, severe neurological abnormalities and cachectic dwarfism. Clinical features of TTD patients include sun sensitivity, ichthyosis and short brittle sulphur-deficient hair. In contrast to XP patients, CS and TTD patients are not prone to ultraviolet light-induced skin cancers (melanoma, squamous and basal cell carcinomas). Because the genotype–phenotype correlations are complex, these syndromes can serve as disease models for skin cancer development, neurodegeneration and epidermal cell differentiation, potentially leading to new prevention and therapeutic strategies.

Key points

- **The DNA repair defective disorders xeroderma pigmentosum (XP), Cockayne syndrome (CS), and trichothiodystrophy (TTD) are autosomal recessive diseases.**
- **In XP, key symptoms include sun sensitivity and freckling as well as early skin cancer development.**
- **The prevalence is approximately 1:1 million of the population.**
- **Polygeneity of a phenotype exists, that is, defects in different genes can lead to the same phenotype.**
- **Polypheneity of a gene exists, that is, different mutations in the same gene can lead to different phenotypes.**
- **Genotype–phenotype correlations are complicated because of involvement of XP genes in several essential pathways like DNA repair, transcription, transactivation of nuclear receptors and epigenetic remodelling.**
- **The DNA repair defective disorders are primarily diagnosed on the clinical level.**
- **Functional cell test systems as well as genetic testing affirm the diagnosis.**
- **The nucleotide excision repair system protects against the development of skin cancer in the normal population for around 50 to 60 years.**
- **Variations in DNA repair capacity (gene variations) can influence the skin cancer risk and cancer treatment prospects in a negative as well as a positive way.**
- **Beside nucleotide excision repair, error-free translesional synthesis contributes to maintenance of the genomic pool after ultraviolet radiation.**

Cellular DNA repair systems

The genome of prokaryotes and eukaryotes is permanently exposed to endogenous or exogenous cellular DNA-damaging substances. Cells contain evolutionarily conserved mechanisms to protect themselves against such damage [1–3]. To counteract these toxic effects, the genomic integrity is secured by more than 130 DNA repair enzymes [4]. The total genome is constantly scanned by DNA repair enzymes which detect and remove DNA damage like strand breaks, crosslinks, mismatches or dimers as well as damage to single nucleotides [5–7]. The ultraviolet (UV) portion of sunlight is one of the most common and relevant exogenous toxic agents to DNA. In living organisms, the excision of DNA damage, double-strand break DNA repair via homologous or nonhomologous recombination, as well as direct reversion of DNA damage are the most important DNA repair mechanisms. Within excision repair, three different mechanisms can be distinguished: nucleotide excision repair (NER), mismatch repair (MMR) and base excision repair (BER). If DNA damage persists despite action of these repair mechanisms, specific types of DNA damage can be bypassed by special DNA polymerases (translesional synthesis) [3,4,8].

Harper's Textbook of Pediatric Dermatology, Fourth Edition. Edited by Peter Hoeger, Veronica Kinsler and Albert Yan.

Direct reversion

A good example of DNA damage repair via direct reversion is the bacterial enzyme photolyase, which only exists in prokaryotes. Two different photolyases are known that can specifically separate cyclobutane pyrimidine dimers or pyrimidine-6,4-pyrimidone photoproduct dimers, the two most relevant UV-induced DNA lesions, into their original monomeric state, respectively. If the enzyme photolyase is bound to the dimer, it needs to be photoreactivated by irradiation with visible light (300–500 nm) [9]. In eukaryotes, the photolyase gene has most probably converged evolutionary to blue light receptors in order to control the circadian clock [10].

Translesional synthesis

It has been shown that, despite multiple DNA damage, a cell can continue to proliferate. The existence of polymerases that can bypass specific DNA lesions can partly explain this phenomenon. This process is called translesional synthesis [8,11]. Polymerase eta is one of the best studied polymerases. It was identified in 1999 and is able to bypass TT cyclobutane pyrimidine dimers in an error-free manner [12]. The consequence of a functional loss of polymerase eta is demonstrated by xeroderma pigmentosum variant (XPV) patients. These patients accumulate DNA UV signature mutations because of the alternative use of more error-prone polymerases but display a normal nucleotide excision repair capacity. It is most interesting that the loss of polymerase eta function in XPV patients leads to the same clinical xeroderma pigmentosum (XP) symptoms found in other XP patients with defective nucleotide excision repair [13]. Those patients accumulate DNA mutations caused by defects in NER of UV-induced DNA photoproducts because they have a defect in one of the seven major NER-associated XP genes, *XPA* to *XPG*, which correspond to the complementation groups A–G [14].

Excision repair

Regarding the elimination of UV-induced DNA damage, the NER and BER pathways are the most relevant DNA repair systems in humans. BER eliminates (UVA-induced) oxidative DNA adducts and NER is capable of eliminating UVB-induced photoproducts. The process of BER excises and replaces a single oxidatively damaged nucleotide [3,4,15]. Falsely paired bases or small DNA loops that occur during DNA slippage at microsatellites during replication are eliminated by a third DNA repair system, the mismatch repair system [16,17].

Multistep cancer theory

In general, for complete transformation of a cell into a tumour cell, multiple different gene mutations are necessary. Spontaneous DNA mutations have been shown to occur at a frequency too low to solely account for human cancer development, for example because of the large proportion of noncoding (intron) sequences in the genome [18]. However, if a mutation leads to inactivation of a gene that is involved in the maintenance of genomic stability, a 'mutator phenotype' is established, leading to an increased cellular mutation rate and accelerated malignant transformation. Inherited diseases with DNA repair defects are classic models for this multistep cancer theory. In the normal population, spontaneous DNA repair gene mutations may also accelerate cancer development but at a much greater latency compared with the inherited DNA repair defective disorders [18]. With respect to UV-induced skin cancer, this suggests that more subtle changes in NER as compared with patients with XP may determine whether an individual develops skin cancer in their seventh or eighth decade [19].

References

1 **Bauer NC, Corbett AH, Doetsch PW. The current state of eukaryotic DNA base damage and repair. Nucleic Acids Res 2015;43: 10083–101.**
2 Pan MR, Li K, Lin SY et al. Connecting the dots: from DNA damage and repair to aging. Int J Mol Sci 2016;17:pii:E685.
3 Lindahl T, Wood RD. Quality control by DNA repair. Science 1999;286:1897–905.
4 Wood RD, Mitchell M, Sgouros J et al. Human DNA repair genes. Science 2001;291:1284–9.
5 Lee AJ, Warshaw DM, Wallace SS. Insights into the glycosylase search for damage from single-molecule fluorescence microscopy. DNA Repair (Amst) 2014;20:23–31.
6 Shell SM, Hawkins EK, Tsai MS et al. Xeroderma pigmentosum complementation group C protein (XPC) serves as a general sensor of damaged DNA. DNA Repair (Amst) 2013;12:947–53.
7 Sancar A, Lindsey-Boltz LA, Unsal-Kacmaz K et al. Molecular mechanisms of mammalian DNA repair and the DNA damage checkpoints. Annu Rev Biochem 2004;73:39–85.
8 Goodman MF, Woodgate R. Translesion DNA polymerases. Cold Spring Harb Perspect Biol 2013;5:a010363.
9 Liu Z, Wang L, Zhong D. Dynamics and mechanisms of DNA repair by photolyase. Phys Chem Chem Phys 2015;17:11933–49.
10 Thompson CL, Sancar A. Photolyase/cryptochrome blue-light photoreceptors use photon energy to repair DNA and reset the circadian clock. Oncogene 2002;21:9043–56.
11 Lehmann AR. Replication of damaged DNA by translesion synthesis in human cells. FEBS Lett 2005;579:873–6.
12 Yuasa M, Masutani C, Eki T et al. Genomic structure, chromosomal localization and identification of mutations in the xeroderma pigmentosum variant (XPV) gene. Oncogene 2000;19:4721–8.
13 Inui H, Oh KS, Nadem C et al. Xeroderma pigmentosum-variant patients from America, Europe, and Asia. J Invest Dermatol 2008;128: 2055–68.
14 Schärer OD. Nucleotide excision repair in eukaryotes. Cold Spring Harb Perspect Biol 2013;5:a012609.
15 Carter RJ, Parsons JL. Base excision repair, a pathway regulated by posttranslational modifications. Mol Cell Biol 2016;36:1426–37.
16 Groothuizen FS, Sixma TK. The conserved molecular machinery in DNA mismatch repair enzyme structures. DNA Repair (Amst) 2016;38:14–23.
17 Marti TM, Kunz C, Fleck O. DNA mismatch repair and mutation avoidance pathways. J Cell Physiol 2002;191:28–41.
18 Hoeijmakers JH. Genome maintenance mechanisms for preventing cancer. Nature 2001;411:366–74.
19 Kraemer KH, Rünger TM. Genome stability, DNA repair and cancer. In: Wolff K, Goldsmith LA, Katz SI et al. (eds) Fitzpatrick's Dermatology in General Medicine. McGraw-Hill: New York, 2008: 977–86.

Nucleotide excision repair

A wide variety of different forms of DNA damage is eliminated by NER. NER processes bulky DNA damage that leads to a distortion of the DNA helix including UV-induced DNA photoproducts [1,2].

UV-induced DNA damage

When UV light is absorbed by skin, many effects are noted [3]. Pigmentation occurs as well as immunosuppression. More importantly, light energy may be directly absorbed by cellular DNA that leads to the formation of photoproducts which interfere with the normal processes of DNA replication and transcription. Alternatively, light energy may be absorbed by photosensitizers in the cytosol, leading to the formation of free radicals and other reactive oxygen species which then indirectly lead to the formation of DNA adducts such as oxidative DNA damage, e.g. 8-hydroxyguanine. The type of adducts formed depends on the wavelengths of photons absorbed. Longer wavelengths (320–400 nm) cannot be absorbed by the DNA molecule directly and therefore produce predominantly free radicals. Shorter wavelengths (280–320 nm) are more energetic and produce DNA photoproducts by direct action.

The UVB portion in sunlight predominantly induces two types of DNA photoproducts: pyrimidine-6,4-pyrimidone photoproducts (6-4PP) and cyclobutanepyrimidine dimers (CPD). 6-4PP are repaired five times faster by the NER pathway than CPD. Polycyclic aromatic hydrocarbons, which can be found in tobacco smoke as well as DNA crosslinking agents, induce other substrates of NER. Such crosslinking agents include chemotherapeutics such as cisplatin [4].

Nucleotide excision repair pathway

The nucleotide excision repair mechanism is the most critical system for repairing DNA adducts created by UV radiation. NER consists of a multistep process [1,5,6]. At least 30 proteins are involved in this process in a defined manner. At first, the DNA damage is recognized (I), then demarcated (II), followed by strand incision up- and downstream of the DNA lesion (III). After that, the DNA lesion containing oligonucleotide is removed (IV) and the gap is filled with a newly synthesized oligonucleotide by DNA polymerases using the complementary strand as a template (V) (Fig. 138.1). All seven XP genes identified so far, *XPA* to *XPG*, are critically involved in this process. Multiple organisms of different hierarchies utilize the NER principle. Interestingly, only three proteins are needed to perform NER in *Escherichia coli* [7]. This may demonstrate the astonishing evolution and specialization of this important DNA repair mechanism to maintain genomic integrity.

I Damage recognition

Cellular DNA damage can be sensed and located in two ways (see Fig. 138.1) [8]. The *global genome repair* (GGR) subpathway operates in a genome-wide manner but in a rather slow fashion. Here, the XPC-HR23B-Centrin 2 heterotrimeric complex binds to the damage and initiates

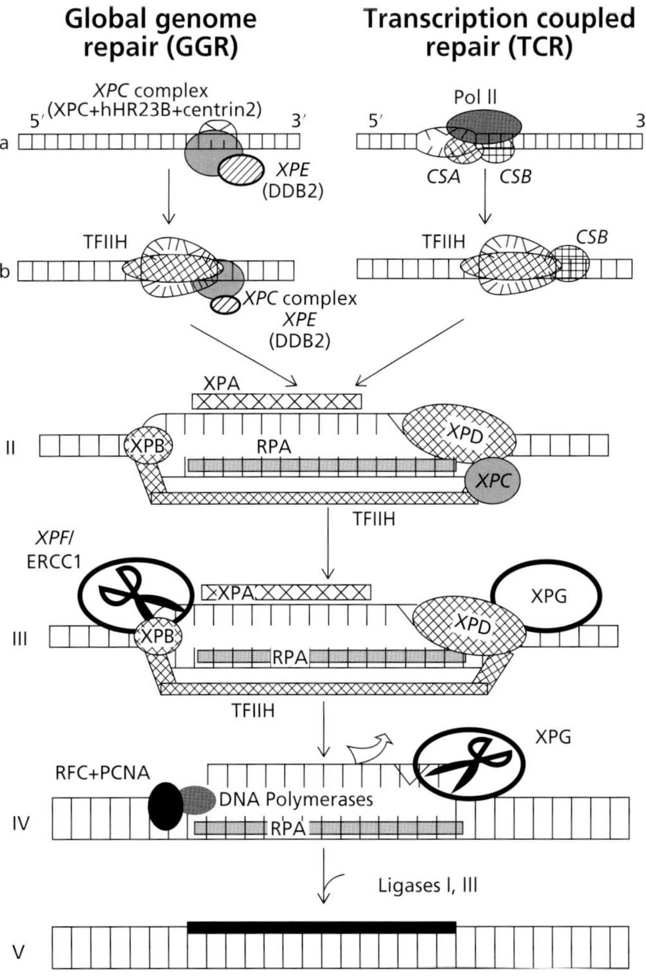

Fig. 138.1 The nucleotide excision repair (NER) pathway. (Ia) In the global genome *XPC* and *XPE* recognize DNA damages and initiate the NER cascade (GGR). In actively transcribed genes, the stalled polymerase II in concert with *CSA* and *CSB* are thought to initiate the NER cascade (TCR). (Ib) XPB and XPD are components of the 10 units containing multiprotein complex TFIIH that is subsequently recruited to the damage and to demarcate the damage. (II) TFIIH facilitates unwinding of the DNA double helix around the lesion and XPA and RPA are stabilizing the open complex. (III) *XPF* is the first endonuclease that cuts the damage-containing DNA strand upstream of a lesion. (IV) A damage-containing oligonucleotide (24-32 nts) is released after recruitment of DNA polymerases (δ, ε or κ) and the second cleavage by XPG. (V) The resulting gap is filled by DNA polymerases using the complementary DNA strand as a template and DNA ligases I or III, which finally close the nick. Abbreviations: hHR23B, human homolog of Rad23b; PCNA, proliferating cell nuclear antigen; Pol II, RNA Polymerase II; RFC, replication factor C; RPA, replication protein A; TFIIH, basal transcription factor IIH; RFC, replication factor C. Source: Leibeling et al. 2006 [2]. Reproduced with permission of Springer Nature.

further repair steps. The XPC protein is functionally the major component of this complex and acts as a thermodynamic sensor of base pair disruptions and mediator for subsequent recruitment steps [9,10]. Another damage sensor in GGR is the UV-damaged DNA-binding protein (UV-DDB) consisting of the DDB1 and DDB2 subunits. DDB2 corresponds to the *XPE* gene product. DDB has a higher binding affinity and specificity for certain types of DNA lesion with minor DNA-backbone bending (like cyclobutane pyrimidine dimers) and enhances XPC's affinity by ubiquitination [11,12]. Patients with *XPC* gene mutations usually develop a classic XP phenotype with skin cancer proneness but no neurological abnormalities. This may be because of the retained transcription coupled repair activity in XPC patients [6].

The stalled RNA polymerase II mediates damage recognition in actively transcribed genes [13]. This second NER subpathway is called *transcription coupled repair* (TCR). TCR acts much faster than GGR (see Fig. 138.1). XPC and DDB proteins are dispensable in the TCR subpathway. Patients belonging to the XPC and XPE complementation groups therefore have normal TCR capabilities. In contrast, normal GGR accompanied by a deficiency in TCR are hallmarks of Cockayne syndrome (CS) patients (*CSA* or *CSB* gene defective, respectively). The exact functions of the *CSA* and *CSB* gene products still remain to be elucidated. CS proteins CSA and CSB may be involved in this recognition process but are not essential for transcription. CSB binds to DNA–RNA–RNA polymerase II complexes, and the resulting quaternary complexes are able to recruit transcription factor IIH (TFIIH), thus initiating the NER complex. CSA has been shown to bind to the p44 subunit of TFIIH as well as ubiquitin ligase complexes [14,15]. CSB binds to CSA, XPA, XPB, XPG and the p34 subunit of TFIIH [16,17]. In general, the CS proteins may support the polymerase II complex to allow its temporary removal and may play a general role in the processing of stalled polymerases during transcription in nuclei and mitochondria. This general role in facilitating transcription may be one reason for the severe neurological abnormalities in some CS patients, whereas there are usually no neurological abnormalities in XPC or XPE patients [18].

II Damage demarcation

The DNA double helix has to be unwound around the damage to be accessible for excision repair. This is accomplished by the multifunctional basal TFIIH complex. TFIIH consists of 10 subunits including the XPB, XPD, and TTD-A proteins. ATPase activity of the XPB protein and the 5′-3′helicase activity of the XPD protein are essential for NER [19]. Furthermore, XPD was shown to fulfil a major role during damage demarcation while it gets stuck at the lesion and ensures correct positioning of TFIIH [20,21]. Trichothiodystrophy (TTD)-A was identified in 2004 and is the smallest component of TFIIH (8 kDa). If TTD-A is mutated, the autosomal recessive disease trichothiodystrophy results (see later). Furthermore, mouse model studies identified TTD-A as an important

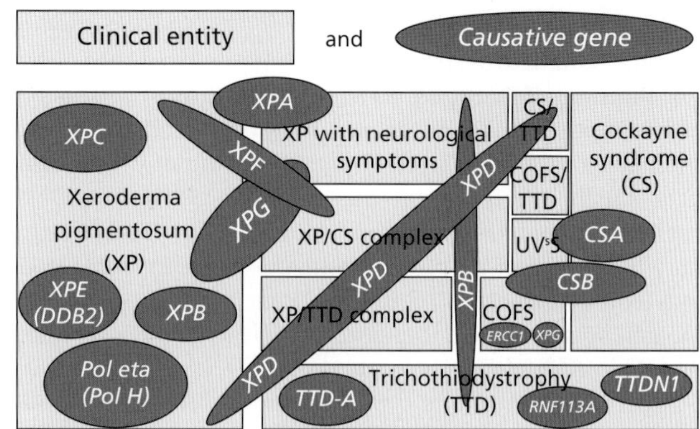

Fig. 138.2 Ten clinical entities (rectangles) based on 14 defective genes (ovals) demonstrate the complex genotype–phenotype interactions. Different mutations at different locations within the same gene can result in different clinical entities. Conversely, mutations in different genes may cause the same clinical entity. COFS, cerebro-oculo-facial-skeletal syndrome; UVSS, UV sensitive syndrome. Source: Modified from Kraemer and Rünger 2008 [5].

component for embryonic development, basal transcription as well as NER [22,23]. RNA polymerase II also utilizes TFIIH to initiate transcription at promoter sites. Thus, at least two different functions of TFIIH can be discerned, namely basal transcription and NER. The great phenotypic heterogeneity of defects in the *XPD* and *XPB* genes may be explained by this dual function of TFIIH (Fig. 138.2). Either NER or basal transcription or both may be disabled, depending on the type and location of the mutation within the respective gene. This can lead to clinical phenotypes that represent combinations of XP, TTD or even CS. The activity of TFIIH and stabilization of the 'DNA bubble' around the damage is supported by the ssDNA binding protein replication protein A (RPA) (see Fig. 138.1). The XPA protein is recruited to the site of DNA damage later than TFIIH and complexes with RPA. XPA in conjunction with RPA monitors DNA bending and unwinding, verifies the damage-specific localization of repair complexes and establishes the preincision complex rather than recognizes DNA damage [24]. However, the exact role of the XPA-RPA complex is not well understood. XPA patients usually are defective in GGR as well as in TCR which can explain the preponderance of XP with neurological symptoms, if *XPA* is mutated (see Fig. 138.2) [25].

III Incision of the damaged DNA strand

The heterodimer XPF/ERCC1 and XPG, two endonucleases, are recruited to form the incision complex [26]. First, the DNA strand upstream of the lesion is cleaved by ERCC1-XPF and, after a molecular switch, XPG cleaves downstream of the lesion (see Fig. 138.1) in order to release a damage-containing oligonucleotide [27]. This so called 'cut-patch-cut-patch' mechanism ensures correct positioning of all components at any time in order to avoid unwanted unspecific cuts. XPG is described as the eleventh subunit of TFIIH with a structural scaffold-function during NER and basal transcription [28].

The connection between XPG and TFIIH is especially important to anchor the cdk-activating kinase (CAK) and the seven subunit core TFIIH complexes for catalysation of basal transcription with implications for the XP/CS complex phenotype. Hence, mutated XPG proteins identified in XPG patients failed to stably connect to TFIIH (XPD) and lead to neurological symptoms in XPG/CS combined phenotypes [29].

IV Removal of the DNA damage-containing oligonucleotide

At any time, an oligonucleotide of 24–32 nucleotides in size is excised by the sequential processes described above. In addition, the DNA damage is always located 5–6 nucleotides upstream of the 3′ end of the excised oligonucleotide. After excision, ssDNA fragments are further degraded to even smaller stretches (3–4 nts-long oligomers) [30,31]. It is not known yet if the oligonucleotide is simply degraded after transport into the cytoplasm or if it subsequently induces UV-protective cell functions. Small oligonucleotides with specific sequences have been demonstrated to induce DNA repair as well as melanogenesis without UV exposure of the cells [32]. Furthermore, TFIIH-bound complexes were found in UV-irradiated nuclei only if DNA repair synthesis and ligation are carried out properly [33]. Otherwise, UV photoproduct removal is decreased and RPA-oligonucleotide complexes are accumulating. This indicates a regulatory role of excision fragment processing for appropriate termination of NER events.

V Gap filling

The excision process results in a single-stranded gap which is filled by a newly synthesized oligonucleotide using the complementary strand as a template [34]. This DNA repair synthesis involves DNA polymerases δ, ε, or κ, and depends on proliferating cell nuclear antigen (PCNA) and replication factor C (RFC). Reconstitution of *in vitro* repair synthesis was successfully accomplished using purified PCNA, RFC and either polymerase δ or polymerase ε. The very last step of NER consists of 3′ strand rejoining by DNA ligase I or III [1].

Normal repair of UV-damaged DNA requires the integrity of all the gene products mentioned above. Mutations in *XPA–XPG* and polymerase eta (XPV) are responsible for the clinical phenotype of xeroderma pigmentosum. Mutations in *CSA* and *CSB* are responsible for the clinical phenotype of Cockayne syndrome. The clinical disease trichothiodystrophy results from mutations in *TTD-A*, *XPD* and *XPB*. Some nonphotosensitive TTD patients have been identified who have a mutation in *TTDN1*, a gene involved in cell cycle maintenance [35], or in the X-chromosomally encoded gene *RNF113A* (see Fig. 138.2) [36, 37].

References

1 **Schärer OD. Nucleotide excision repair in eukaryotes. Cold Spring Harb Perspect Biol 2013;5:a012609.**
2 Leibeling D, Laspe P, Emmert S. Nucleotide excision repair and cancer. J Mol Histol 2006;37:225–38.
3 Matsumura Y, Ananthaswamy HN. Toxic effects of ultraviolet radiation on the skin. Toxicol Appl Pharmacol 2004;195:298–308.
4 Wood RD. Mammalian nucleotide excision repair proteins and interstrand crosslink repair. Environ Mol Mutagen 2010;51:520–6.
5 Kraemer KH, Rünger TM. Genome stability, DNA repair and cancer. In: Wolff K, Goldsmith LA, Katz SI et al. (eds) Fitzpatrick's Dermatology in General Medicine. McGraw-Hill: New York, 2008:977–86.
6 Thoms KM, Kuschal C, Emmert S. Lessons learned from DNA repair defective syndromes. Exp Dermatol 2007;16:532–44.
7 Kisker C, Kuper J, Van Houten B. Prokaryotic nucleotide excision repair. Cold Spring Harb Perspect Biol 2013;5:a012591.
8 Hanawalt PC. Subpathways of nucleotide excision repair and their regulation. Oncogene 2002;21:8949–56.
9 Shell SM, Hawkins EK, Tsai MS et al. Xeroderma pigmentosum complementation group C protein (XPC) serves as a general sensor of damaged DNA. DNA Repair (Amst) 2013;12:947–53.
10 Sugasawa K, Akagi J, Nishi R et al. Two-step recognition of DNA damage for mammalian nucleotide excision repair: directional binding of the XPC complex and DNA strand scanning. Mol Cell 2009;36:642–53.
11 Sugasawa K. UV-DDB: a molecular machine linking DNA repair with ubiquitination. DNA Repair (Amst) 2009;8:969–72.
12 Puumalainen MR, Ruthemann P, Min JH et al. Xeroderma pigmentosum group C sensor: unprecedented recognition strategy and tight spatiotemporal regulation. Cell Mol Life Sci 2016;73:547–66.
13 Brueckner F, Cramer P. DNA photodamage recognition by RNA polymerase II. FEBS Lett 2007;581:2757–60.
14 Angers S, Li T, Yi X et al. Molecular architecture and assembly of the DDB1-CUL4A ubiquitin ligase machinery. Nature 2006;443:590–3.
15 Fischer ES, Scrima A, Bohm K et al. The molecular basis of CRL4DDB2/CSA ubiquitin ligase architecture, targeting, and activation. Cell 2011;147:1024–39.
16 Aamann MD, Muftuoglu M, Bohr VA et al. Multiple interaction partners for Cockayne syndrome proteins: implications for genome and transcriptome maintenance. Mech Ageing Dev 2013;134:212–24.
17 Velez-Cruz R, Egly JM. Cockayne syndrome group B (CSB) protein: at the crossroads of transcriptional networks. Mech Ageing Dev 2013;134:234–42.
18 Jaarsma D, van der Pluijm I, van der Horst GT et al. Cockayne syndrome pathogenesis: lessons from mouse models. Mech Ageing Dev 2013;134:180–95.
19 Oksenych V, Bernardes de Jesus B, Zhovmer A et al. Molecular insights into the recruitment of TFIIH to sites of DNA damage. EMBO J 2009;28:2971–80.
20 Mathieu N, Kaczmarek N, Naegeli H. Strand- and site-specific DNA lesion demarcation by the xeroderma pigmentosum group D helicase. Proc Natl Acad Sci U S A 2010;107:17545–50.
21 Mathieu N, Kaczmarek N, Ruthemann P et al. DNA quality control by a lesion sensor pocket of the xeroderma pigmentosum group D helicase subunit of TFIIH. Curr Biol 2013;23:204–12.
22 Theil AF, Hoeijmakers JH, Vermeulen W. TTDA: big impact of a small protein. Exp Cell Res 2014;329:61–8.
23 Theil AF, Nonnekens J, Steurer B et al. Disruption of TTDA results in complete nucleotide excision repair deficiency and embryonic lethality. PLoS Genet 2013;9:e1003431.
24 Fadda E. Role of the XPA protein in the NER pathway: a perspective on the function of structural disorder in macromolecular assembly. Comput Struct Biotechnol J 2016;14:78–85.
25 Emmert S. Xeroderma pigmentosum, Cockayne syndrome, Trichothiodystrophy – defects in DNA repair and carcinogenesis. In: Allgayer H, Rehder H, Fulda S (eds) Hereditary Tumors. Weinheim: Wiley-VCH2009:421–39.
26 Fagbemi AF, Orelli B, Schärer OD. Regulation of endonuclease activity in human nucleotide excision repair. DNA Repair (Amst) 2011;10:722–9.
27 Staresincic L, Fagbemi AF, Enzlin JH et al. Coordination of dual incision and repair synthesis in human nucleotide excision repair. EMBO J 2009;28:1111–20.
28 Ito S, Kuraoka I, Chymkowitch P et al. XPG stabilizes TFIIH, allowing transactivation of nuclear receptors: implications for Cockayne syndrome in XP-G/CS patients. Mol Cell 2007;26:231–43.
29 Schäfer A, Schubert S, Gratchev A et al. Characterization of three XPG-defective patients identifies three missense mutations that impair repair and transcription. J Invest Dermatol 2013;133:1841–9.

30 Kemp MG, Reardon JT, Lindsey-Boltz LA et al. Mechanism of release and fate of excised oligonucleotides during nucleotide excision repair. J Biol Chem 2012;287:22889–99.
31 Kemp MG, Sancar A. DNA excision repair: where do all the dimers go? Cell Cycle 2012;11:2997–3002.
32 Eller MS, Asarch A, Gilchrest BA. Photoprotection in human skin—a multifaceted SOS response. Photochem Photobiol 2008;84:339–49.
33 Kemp MG, Gaddameedhi S, Choi JH et al. DNA repair synthesis and ligation affect the processing of excised oligonucleotides generated by human nucleotide excision repair. J Biol Chem 2014;289:26574–83.
34 Lehmann AR. DNA polymerases and repair synthesis in NER in human cells. DNA Repair (Amst) 2011;10:730–3.
35 Zhang Y, Tian Y, Chen Q et al. TTDN1 is a Plk1-interacting protein involved in maintenance of cell cycle integrity. Cell Mol Life Sci 2007;64:632–40.
36 Rünger TM, DiGiovanna JJ, Kraemer KH. Hereditary diseases of genome instability and DNA repair. In: Wolff K, Goldsmith LA, Katz SI et al. (eds) Fitzpatrick's Dermatology in General Medicine. McGraw-Hill: New York, 2008:1311–25.
37 Corbett MA, Dudding-Byth T, Crock PA et al. A novel X-linked trichothiodystrophy associated with a nonsense mutation in RNF113A. J Med Genet 2015;52:269–74.

Nucleotide excision repair defective syndromes

As discussed previously, it is evident that cancer development is a multistep process. The process of tumour initiation is started if, for example, UV-induced DNA damage is not properly repaired. In terms of skin cancer development, the incomplete repair of UVB-induced pyrimidine dimers by the NER machinery prevails here. The clinical consequences of defective NER compounds are vividly demonstrated by three major, but still rare, autosomal recessive inherited model diseases: XP, CS and the photosensitive form of TTD (Table 138.1) [1]. Increased sun sensitivity and freckling in sun-exposed skin areas are clinical symptoms shared by all three clinical entities. However, XP patients differ from CS and TTD patients with respect to their risk of a skin cancer [2–5] (Table 138.2). The genotype–phenotype correlations are quite complex. In total, 10 distinct clinical entities and 14 causative genes have been distinguished to date (see Fig. 138.2). Different mutations in one gene can give rise to more than one clinical entity (variable expression) and conversely, each clinical entity can arise from mutations in more than one gene (genetic heterogeneity).

Xeroderma pigmentosum

History. Moritz Kaposi described the first patient with 'dry skin (xeroderma) and hyperpigmentations' in 1863 [6]. This entity was finally named xeroderma pigmentosum in 1882 [7]. However, it was another 100 years before the pathogenic defect of XP was identified. Cleaver found in 1968 that cells from XP patients were defective in nucleotide excision repair [8]. Normal cells repair UV-induced pyrimidine dimers by excising these dimers and replacing the gap in the DNA strand with newly synthesized DNA. DNA replication is normally restricted to the S phase of the cell cycle. Nucleotide excision repair, however, can occur at any time during the cell cycle. This phenomenon was called 'unscheduled' repair synthesis. The repair defect of XP cells was thus identified by showing that XP cells have decreased rates of unscheduled DNA synthesis. Eventually, it was shown by Epstein and colleagues in 1970 that all cell types in XP patients exhibit the excision repair defect including epidermal cells, fibroblasts, conjunctival cells, corneal cells and lymphocytes [4,9,10].

In 1972, de Weerd-Kastelein and colleagues fused together fibroblasts from different patients with XP to form heteropolykaryons (multinucleated cells containing nuclei from the two different strains) [11]. They were able to demonstrate correction of the excision repair defect in these heteropolykaryons, suggesting that different genetic defects could produce one similar phenotypic disease. Groups of patients whose cells failed to complement each other in culture were placed within a single complementation group. In this manner, seven complementation groups of XP have been identified and are designated A–G. Again, it took more than two decades until the genetic basis of these complementation groups began to unravel. Today, the seven complementation groups, XPA to XPG, correspond to seven distinct XP genes, *XPA-XPG* [4,12,13].

Epidemiology and pathogenesis. The rare autosomal recessive inherited genetic disease XP occurs worldwide. Patients have been reported in all ethnic groups and skin types. An examination of the literature demonstrated that 830 XP cases were reported from the first case in 1863 until 1982 [14]. In Japan, 91 cases were published, 210 cases in Europe, 49 cases in Egypt and 241 cases in the USA. The incidence of XP in the USA and Europe is lower than 1:1 million [4,15]. Because of less mobile and more isolated populations, the incidence of XP is 10 times higher in northern Africa and Japan. Both sexes are affected equally. Consanguinity of the parents was present in about 30% of all cases [14].

If the patient carries homozygous, compound heterozygous or hemizygous mutations in one of the genes causing XP, clinical XP symptoms occur. Heterozygous carriers of XP mutations are regarded as 'healthy' to date. Notably, the frequency of such clinically normal individuals who are heterozygous carriers of an XP gene mutation is much higher (1:500) than XP patients (1:1 000 000). However, whether individuals heterozygous for a mutation in an XP gene are at increased risk of an UV-induced skin malignancy is not well understood. Of note, heterozygous 'healthy' carriers of a defective XPC allele displayed reduced *XPC* mRNA levels to an intermediate state (~60%) between healthy controls (100%) and XPC patients (~20%) [16]. However, this gene dose effect only holds true for XPC patients. The only study to date of cancer risk in XP heterozygotes was published in 1979, before the XP genes were cloned [17]. This study was conducted on the pedigrees of XP families. The authors found that proposed carriers of one mutated XP allele have an elevated incidence of skin cancer. The National Cancer Institute (NCI, USA) is currently performing a clinical study to determine the cancer risk in carriers of a gene defect for xeroderma pigmentosum (NCT00046189).

Clinical features. First XP symptoms (see Table 138.2) occur at a median age of 1–2 years [14]. Severe sun sensitivity is usually the first symptom that becomes apparent.

Table 138.1 Nucleotide excision repair defective syndromes: clinical hallmarks and affected genes

Syndrome	Benign (skin) symptoms	Malignant (skin) symptoms	Affected gene
Xeroderma pigmentosum (XP) XP-A (OMIM 278700) XP-B (OMIM 610651) XP-C (OMIM 278720) XP-D (OMIM 278730) XP-E (OMIM 278740) XP-F (OMIM 278760) XP-G (OMIM 278780) XPV (OMIM 278750)	Sunburns, hyper- and hypopigmentation, atrophy, telangiectasias in sun-exposed skin regions (poikiloderma), xerosis, neurological symptoms	Basal cell carcinomas, squamous cell carcinomas, cutaneous melanomas (UV-induced skin tumours) in childhood, internal tumours, CNS tumours	*XPA* (OMIM 611153) *XPB* (OMIM 133510) *XPC* (OMIM 278720) *XPD* (OMIM 126340) *DDB1* (OMIM 600045) *DDB2* (OMIM 600811) *XPF* (OMIM 133520) *XPG* (OMIM 133530) *Pol H* (OMIM 603968)
XP plus neurological symptoms	Same as XP plus loss of deep tendon reflexes, sensorineural deafness, progressive neurological degeneration, primary neurodegeneration	Same as XP	*XPA* (OMIM 611153) *XPB* (OMIM 133510) *XPC* (OMIM 278720) *XPD* (OMIM 126340) *XPG* (OMIM 133530) *XPF* (OMIM 133520)
Cockayne syndrome (CS) CSA (OMIM 216400) CSB (OMIM 133540)	Sunburns, growth retardation, bird-like face (deep-set eyes, prominent nose, loss of subcutaneous tissue), retinitis pigmentosa, caries, progressive neurological and psychomotoric impairment, brain calcifications, primary demyelination	No increased (skin) cancer risk	*CSA* (OMIM 609412) *CSB* (OMIM 609413)
XP/CS complex	XP symptoms plus CS symptoms	XP-associated cancers, especially basal cell carcinomas, squamous cell carcinomas	*XPB* (OMIM 133510) *XPD* (OMIM 126340) *XPF* (OMIM 133520) *XPG* (OMIM 133530)
Photosensitive form of trichothiodystrophy (TTD) OMIM 601675 OMIM 616395 OMIM 616390	Sunburns, erythema, ichthyosis-like skin changes, nail and other neuroectodermal dysplasias, short, brittle sulphur-deficient hair (tiger-tail sign), congenital cataracts, mental retardation with outgoing personality, recurrent infections	No increased (skin) cancer risk	*TTD-A* (OMIM 608780) *XPB* (OMIM 133510) *XPD* (OMIM 126340)
Nonphotosensitive form of trichothiodystrophy (TTD) OMIM 234050	Same as photosensitive form of trichothiodystrophy except sunburns and sun sensitivity	No increased (skin) cancer risk	*TTDN1* (OMIM 609188) *RNF113A* (OMIM 300951)
XP/TTD complex	XP symptoms plus TTD symptoms	XP-associated cancers	*XPD* (OMIM 126340)
Cerebro-oculo-facio-skeletal (COFS) syndrome OMIM 610756 OMIM 214150 OMIM 616570 OMIM 610758	Microcephaly, cerebral atrophy, severe mental retardation, joint contractures, postnatal growth deficiency, cataracts, microcornea, optic atrophy	No increased (skin) cancer risk	*XPD* (OMIM 126340) *XPG* (OMIM 133530) *CSB* (OMIM 609413) *ERCC1* (OMIM 126380)
XFE progeroid syndrome (XFEPS) OMIM 610965	Dwarfism, cachexia and microcephaly, sun-sensitivity, mild learning disabilities, bird-like facies, scoliosis, hearing loss and visual impairment	No increased (skin) cancer risk	*XPF (OMIM 133520)*
De Sanctis-Cacchione syndrome OMIM 278800	Xeroderma pigmentosum, mental deficiency, progressive neurological deterioration, dwarfism and gonadal hypoplasia, defects in oculomotor system	Same as XP, acute lymphatic leukaemia	*CSB* (OMIM 609413)
UV sensitive syndrome (UV^{s}S) OMIM 600630 OMIM 614621 OMIM 614640	Photosensitivity	No increased (skin) cancer risk	*CSA* (OMIM 609412) *CSB* (OMIM 609413)

OMIM, Online Mendelian Inheritance in Man.

Table 138.2 Clinical features of nucleotide excision repair defective syndromes

Clinical feature	Phenotype				
	XP	**XP plus neurological abnormalities**	**CS (±XP)**	**TTD (±XP)**	**COFS**
Sun-sensitivity	Yes	Yes, severe	Yes	Yes/no	Yes, in some
Freckling	Yes	Yes			
Skin cancer (NM[a] and M[b])	Yes	Yes		No	
Photophobia	Yes	Yes	Yes	Yes/no	
Conjunctival growths	Yes	Yes			
Cancer (anterior eye portion)	Yes	Yes		No	
Congenital cataracts			Yes	Yes	
Pigmentary retinal degeneration			Yes		
Sensorineural deafness		Yes	Yes		
Ataxia		Yes, in some	Yes		
Progressive cognitive impairment		Yes	Yes	Yes, in some	Yes
Developmental delay		Yes	Yes	Yes	
Primary neuronal degeneration		Yes			
Loss of subcutaneous tissue			Yes		
Dwarfism/growth deficiencies		Yes, in some	Yes	Yes, in some	Yes
Brain calcification			Yes	Yes, in some	
Demyelinating neuropathy			Yes	Yes, in some	
Ichthyosis				Yes	
Brittle hair				Yes	
Brittle nails				Yes	
Tiger-tail hair				Yes	
Sulphur-deficient hair				Yes	
Dental abnormalities/caries				Yes, in some	
Facial dysmorphism			Yes	Yes	Yes, in some
Infections				Yes	
Hypertrichosis					Yes
Skeletal abnormalities				Yes, in some	Yes
microcephaly/craniofacial abnormalities					Yes
Increased mortality	Yes, in some	Yes, in some	Yes	Yes	Yes

COFS, cerebro-oculo-facio-skeletal syndrome; CS, Cockayne syndrome; TTD, trichothiodystrophy; XP, xeroderma pigmentosum.
[a] Non-melanoma skin cancer (basal and squamous cell carcinoma).
[b] Melanoma skin cancer.
Source: Adapted from Emmert 2009 [22]. Reproduced with permission of John Wiley & Sons.

However, approximately one-half of XP patients tan normally without excessive burning. In the other half, severe sunburn with blisters may develop after a very short sun exposure, even through window glass. The severe skin burning reaches a maximum after 24 hours and then resolves within the next 4–6 days, lasting longer than in normal healthy individuals. Infants may be misdiagnosed as being scalded; doctors may then initiate investigations concerning child abuse. In later stages of infancy, pigmentary changes in sun-exposed skin develop. Poikiloderma becomes apparent, including telangiectasia and atrophic hyper- as well as hypopigmentation (Fig. 138.3). This is a sign of premature skin ageing, because poikiloderma normally develops after chronic sun exposure over decades. The poikilodermic skin changes are usually sharply demarcated from sun-protected skin.

Later on, in early childhood, the first skin cancers appear that include all common UV-induced skin cancers such as basal and squamous cell carcinoma, and cutaneous melanoma (see Fig. 138.3). Basal cell carcinomas and squamous cell carcinomas of the face, head and neck account for 80% of all cutaneous malignancies in the USA. In patients with XP, 97% arise on these sun-exposed sites. The risk of developing a cutaneous malignancy, including melanoma, under 20 years of age is increased 1000-fold in XP patients and is characterized by a typical UV mutation pattern predominantly in the PTEN gene [18]. In a retrospective study of more than 830 XP patients, the median age of first skin cancer development was assessed as 8 years. In contrast, the median age of first skin cancer development in the normal White population is about 60 years [4,19,20]. There is no method or marker to predict the severity of the disease. The age of onset of symptoms is no marker for disease progression, nor is the progression predictable within family members [21].

Ocular manifestations

XP patients also suffer from UV damage to the sun-exposed portions of the eyes, as the repair defect is present in all cells of the body. Photophobia, conjunctivitis, keratitis, pterygium (see Fig. 138.3) and neoplasia of the eyelids and conjunctivae may develop. The posterior

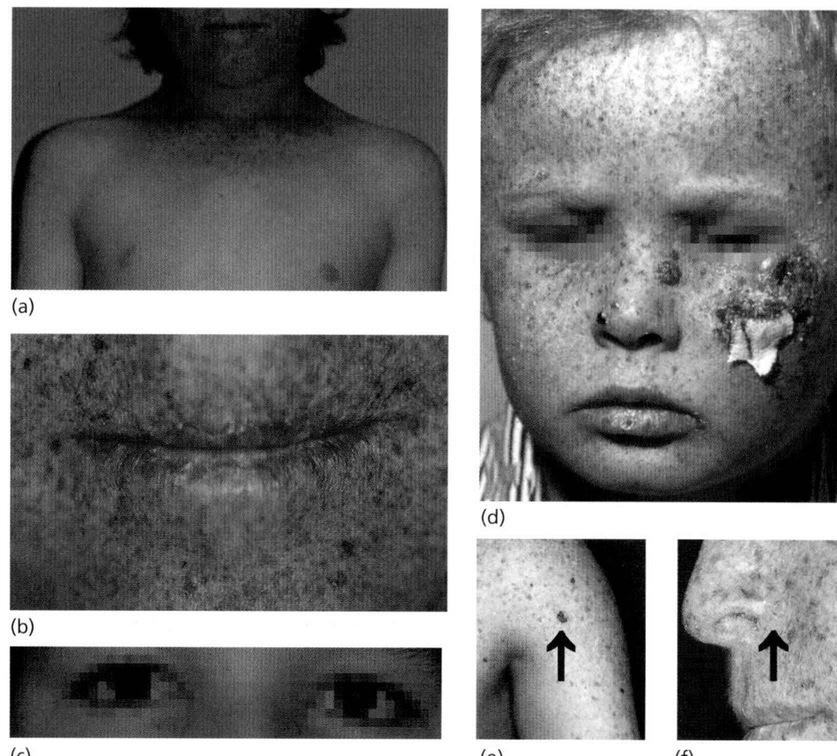

Fig. 138.3 Clinical symptoms of xeroderma pigmentosum (XP). (a) Skin changes sharply demarcated to sun-exposed skin. (b) Typical poikilodermic aspect of XP skin changes including the lips (atrophic dry skin with hyper- and hypopigmentations and telangiectasias). (c) Involvement of the anterior eyes (pterygium). (d) Child with classic XP symptoms and large squamous cell carcinoma on the left cheek. (e) Melanoma on XP skin (arrow). (f) Basal cell carcinoma on XP skin (arrow). Source: Emmert 2009 [22]. Reproduced with permission of John Wiley & Sons.

portions of the eye, such as the retina, are usually unaffected because only visible light (400–800 nm) reaches the retina and UV light is absorbed by anterior portions of the eye. Therefore, XP patients may want to wear UV-protective glasses with side shields. The cornea can be moisturized with methyl cellulose eye drops. Patients with corneal opacity from severe keratitis may benefit from corneal transplantations but there is a risk of graft rejection caused by neovascularization. In addition, atrophic rash, telangiectasia and neoplasia at the tip of the tongue reflect relevant sun exposure to that area [4,23].

Neurological symptoms

XP patients may additionally develop neurological symptoms in about 25% of cases (see Fig. 138.2) [24]. There is great variability in the onset and severity of these neurological symptoms, but all share a progressive character (see Table 138.2). The onset may be in early infancy or delayed until puberty and the neurological abnormalities may be mild or severe. Reduction or losses of deep tendon reflexes, followed by progressive deafness, are normally the first neurological symptoms. Then, mental deterioration with disabilities in speaking, hearing, walking and balance may follow.

Neurological deficiency in XP was first reported by DeSanctis & Cacchione in 1932 [25]. The patients described were three severely affected Italian brothers with intellectual impairment, microcephaly, delayed motor development, sensorineural deafness, peripheral neuropathy and, finally, dementia, beginning at 2 years of age. Patients with DeSanctis–Cacchione syndrome have XP and severe neurological progressive deficiencies, including choreoathetosis, Achilles tendon shortening resulting from eventual quadriparesis and immature sexual development. In clinical practice, testing of deep tendon reflexes and routine audiometry can usually serve as a screen for XP-associated neurological abnormalities. In cases where there is clinical evidence of early neurological abnormalities, a brain magnetic resonance imaging (MRI) scan may show enlarged ventricles. The pathological correlate of the neurological symptoms is a primary axonal degeneration with loss of neurons, particularly in the cerebrum and cerebellum (see Table 138.2). XP patients with defects in the *XPA* and the TFIIH-associated genes *XPB*, *XPD* or *XPG* are mostly affected with additional neurological abnormalities. The molecular basis for this differs between the groups. In the case of *XPA* one possible explanation would be that they are caused by an accumulation of endogenously caused, for example oxidative, DNA damage or defective apoptosis to which nonproliferating neurons would be most susceptible and start to degrade [26,27]. It was found that some XP genes are also involved in BER of oxidative DNA damage [28]. In parallel, there are indications that some oxidative DNA damage is repaired via the NER system. TFIIH and its associated genes are also involved in transcription. Transcriptional deficiencies may therefore constitute another cause of neurological abnormalities.

Internal neoplasias

The risk of development of internal neoplasia may also be increased in XP patients (see Table 138.1). It has been estimated that the overall risk of noncutaneous malignancy is increased approximately 10–20-fold. Primary brain tumours, sarcomas, leukaemia and lung cancers have been reported in XP patients [22]. Benzo[a]pyrene derivates induce DNA damage that is repaired by NER. Thus, tobacco smoke may be regarded as 'internal sun' for XP patients [4,29]. It is recommended that XP patients refrain from smoking and that parents should protect children with XP from being exposed to second-hand smoke. XP may also be associated with metabolic diseases. In 1998, an XP patient with a splice site mutation within the *XPC* gene was reported, who suffered from hypoglycinaemia [30]. This may comprise a new syndrome analogous to the XP/CS complex syndrome (see later).

The development of skin cancer, progressive neurological symptoms and resulting complications drastically reduces the life expectancy of XP patients, who die 30 years earlier than healthy individuals on average. It has been estimated that the probability of a 40-year life expectancy for XP patients is about 70% [14].

Histopathology. The histological features of XP patients are similar to the features of severe sun damage. Hyperkeratosis, atrophy of the epidermis and irregular elongation or atrophy of the rete ridges can be found. Irregular hyperpigmentation of the basal layer, either with or without an increase in the number of melanocytes, is often present. Hypopigmented macules in between show decreased numbers of melanocytes. A nonspecific chronic inflammatory infiltrate may be present in the upper dermis. In addition, typical histologies of UV-induced malignant skin tumours may be seen, including cutaneous melanoma, basal cell and squamous cell carcinoma, and keratoacanthoma. Taken together, the histological features resemble sun-damaged aged skin but are nonspecific for XP.

Differential diagnoses. The diagnosis of XP should be established as early as possible to implement UV-protective measures. Photosensitivity, often expressed as crying on exposure to sunlight in an infant, and sunburn comprise early signs. Such symptoms may also be found in differential diagnoses such as erythropoietic protoporphyria, erythropoietic porphyria, polymorphous light eruption, Rothmund–Thomson syndrome and Hartnup or Bloom syndrome (Box 138.1). Drug-induced photosensitivity or severe sunburn may also result in such symptoms. Biopsies and examination of the urine, stool and blood for porphyrins should be performed to help with clarification of these differential diagnoses. As pigmentation is noted, other differential diseases may come to mind. These include urticaria pigmentosa, dyskeratosis congenita, radiodermatitis, Carney complex or other premature ageing syndromes such as progeria. The occurrence of malignancies may resemble basal cell naevus syndrome or familial atypical multiple mole–melanoma (FAMMM) syndrome (see Box 138.1).

Laboratory tests. In addition to the clinical hallmarks of sun sensitivity, freckling and increased risk of skin cancer, XP may be diagnosed by further laboratory tests [31,32].

Box 138.1 Potential differential diagnoses of nucleotide excision repair defective syndromes

Xeroderma pigmentosum	Numerous ephelids on nontypical localizations, e.g. lips
	Polymorphous light eruption
	Drug-induced photosensitivity
	Hydroa vacciniforme
	Subacute cutaneous lupus erythematosus
	Erythropoietic porphyria
	Urticaria pigmentosa
	Basal cell naevus syndrome (Gorlin–Goltz syndrome)
	FAMMM syndrome (familial melanoma and multiple melanoma)
	Dyskeratosis congenita
	LEOPARD syndrome
	Hartnup disease
	Progeria (Werner syndrome)
	Rothmund–Thomson syndrome
	Bloom syndrome (congenital teleangiectatic erythema)
	Carney complex
Cockayne syndrome	Chromosomal abnormalities
	Hallermann–Streiff syndrome
	Russell–Silver syndrome
	Brachmann–deLange syndrome
	Dubowitz syndrome
	Tyrosinaemia
	Leucodystrophies
	Peroxisomal disorders
Trichothio-dystrophy	Ectodermal dysplasias
	Clouston ectodermal dysplasia
	Ichthyoses

These include functional assessment of cellular repair capacity and genetic tests (mutational analysis). Cell lines from XP patients can be established either from blood (virus-transformed lymphoblastoid cell lines) or from a skin punch biopsy (primary fibroblasts). Such cultured cells grow normally when not exposed to damaging agents. However, after UV irradiation, the population growth or the colony-forming ability is reduced to a greater extent than normal. Cells from XPV patients show this phenomenon only in the presence of caffeine, as it reverses the cell cycle to S-phase where translesion polymerases are acting predominantly, which is a hallmark for XPV cells [12]. The cellular NER capacity can be measured with a host cell reactivation assay. Here, UV-damaged plasmids encoding for reporter genes (e.g. luciferases) are brought into the patient cells. In every form of XP cell tested, there is a deficiency in the ability to repair the plasmids to a functionally active state compared with normal cells. Such functional tests may be followed by genetic investigations on the base sequence, mRNA and protein level. In general, XP cells have a normal karyotype without excessive chromosome breakage or increased sister chromatid exchange. If a mutation is known in an affected family, prenatal diagnosis by amniocentesis in future pregnancies is possible using cells from amniotic fluid.

Treatment and prevention. The treatment of XP patients consists of three main steps: making the diagnosis as early as possible, rigorous sun protection and regular skin examination with treatment of all premalignant and malignant skin changes. Sun protection includes, for example, very strict sun avoidance and wearing of protective clothing, UV-absorbing glasses and a long hairstyle [33]. Special suits have been developed that completely block UV but consist of light fabrics. Patients should adopt a lifestyle to minimize UV exposure and use sunscreens with high sun protection factor (SPF) ratings daily (best SPF 50+). Some families use UV meters to measure the UV levels in their environment. Such measures should be paralleled by careful and frequent skin examinations for early skin cancer detection. Ideally, a family member should be instructed in the recognition of cutaneous neoplasms. A complete (digital) photo documentation of the entire skin surface with additional close-ups (e.g. by digital epiluminescence microscopy) of lesions is often useful in detecting new lesions. A dermatologist should examine patients at short intervals (every 3–6 months).

The most common premalignant skin lesions are actinic keratoses. These can be treated with the common treatment modalities listed in treatment guidelines, including cryotherapy, curettage or topical 5-fluorouracil. For the treatment of larger skin areas, topical use of imiquimod is also feasible. Caution is recommended, however, in the use of photodynamic therapy or other light- or laser-based therapies, because an abnormal response cannot be excluded in XP patients. Therapeutic dermabrasion or dermatome shaving has been applied to remove the more UV-damaged superficial skin layers and to allow repopulation of these layers by more UV-shielded cells from hair follicles or glands. That this is a valid hypothesis is demonstrated by patients who received a larger skin graft to the face. The graft taken from sun-protected areas like the buttocks or upper thighs is often more resistant to the development of skin cancers for many years than the surrounding ungrafted skin [34].

If skin cancer occurs, it should be treated according to guidelines, with surgical excision being first choice as it is for patients who do not have XP. Because XP patients may need hundreds of surgical excisions on their face over a lifetime, removal of undamaged skin should be minimized. This may be accomplished by Mohs micrographic surgery. Interestingly, most XP patients are not abnormally sensitive to therapeutic X-rays and respond normally to full doses of therapeutic X-radiation for treatment of inoperable neoplasms. However, because some XP patient cells show hypersensitivity to X-rays, it may be prudent to test for clinical X-ray hypersensitivity with an initial low dose. XP patients should not smoke or be exposed to second-hand smoke, because tobacco smoke (indeed benzo[a]pyrenes) produces DNA lesions that are repaired by the NER system [35].

High-dose oral isotretinoin can significantly reduce the frequency of skin cancers at least in some XP patients. Because of its side-effects (hepatic, hyperlipidaemic, teratogenic, calcification of ligaments and tendons, premature closure of the epiphyses), this treatment may be reserved for XP patients who are actively developing large numbers of new skin cancers. However, after cessation of isotretinoin the skin cancer frequency may recur. The topical use of T4 endonuclease V, a prokaryotic DNA repair enzyme that initiates repair of UV-induced CPDs by direct removal, has been shown to reduce the rate of skin cancers (actinic keratoses and basal cell carcinomas) in patients with XP [36]. To deliver the agent, T4 endonuclease V is encapsulated in a liposomal lotion. This treatment on a daily basis is well tolerated and no side-effects have been reported so far. However, it is still subject to research and has not been approved for clinical use. In general, follow up and treatment of XP patients should be performed by an interdisciplinary team of experts because multiple organ systems can be involved (dermatologist, ophthalmologist, ear, nose and throat specialist, geneticist, etc.) [31].

Complementation groups

Four clinical entities can be distinguished in patients with XP symptoms: XP, XP with neurological abnormalities, and XP/CS or XP/TTD combined symptoms (see Fig. 138.2). Besides classification according to the presented clinical phenotype, XP patients can also be classified according to their mutated gene. Seven XP complementation groups, XPA to XPG, can be discerned according to this genotypic classification (Table 138.3). XP patients with neurological symptoms typically fall into complementation groups XPA, XPB, XPD or XPG. Between groups as well as within a single group, there

Table 138.3 Characteristics of the seven xeroderma pigmentosum (XP) complementation groups and XP variant

Complementation group	Frequency (%)	Skin cancer	Neurological involvement	Cellular repair capability (%)	Defective gene	Chromosome
XPA	30	++	+++	<10	*XPA*	9q22.3
XPB	0.5	+	+	3~7	*XPB/ERCC3*	2q21
XPC	27	++	+	10~20	*XPC*	3p25
XPD	15	++	+++	25~50	*XPD/ERCC2*	19q13.2-q13.3
XPE	1	+	-	40~50	*XPE-DDB2*	11p12-p11
XPF	2	+	-	10~20	*XPF/ERCCC4*	16p13.3
XPG	1	+	++	<5; 25	*XPG/ERCC5*	13q33
Variant	23.5	+	-	100	*Pol H*	6p21.1-p12

can be great variability in the severity of symptoms [4,37,38]. This variability depends on the special type and location of the respective XP gene mutation and the extent to which one or more XP gene functions are disrupted. These complex genotype–phenotype relations relate to the roles of DNA repair genes in transcription and other chromatin-associated functions [39–42].

Complementation group A

XP patients in this group represent the second largest group worldwide. Patients are reported from Japan, the USA, Europe and the Middle East. Often, severe XP symptoms are seen in this group with an early age of onset. Additional (late onset) neurological symptoms are common, although subsets of patients within this group have been reported to develop minimal or no neurological abnormalities at all. XPA patients are totally deficient in NER.

The *XPA* gene has been identified on chromosome 9q22. It contains 273 amino acids and binds specifically to damaged DNA via a zinc-binding domain in the C-terminal region [43]. Although this protein was originally hypothesized to be responsible for the recognition of damaged DNA, recent studies have demonstrated that it is rather involved in damage verification and recruitment of other NER subunits such as RPA and TFIIH (see Fig. 138.1). Many mutations have been identified within the *XPA* gene. Most result in protein truncations, although missense mutations in the zinc finger domain of the protein that produce a severe phenotype have also been identified. More mildly affected patients have been identified with mutations in the final exon 6, indicating that the function of that portion of the protein is less critical. These studies revealed a relationship between the genotype and the resulting phenotype. Patients with the most severe disease symptoms appear to have truncating mutations in both alleles of the *XPA* gene and no detectable XPA protein expression. Patients with additional minimal neurological symptoms have splice-site mutations that permit a small amount of normal *XPA* mRNA to be made. In the Japanese population, *XPA* gene mutations are the most common cause of XP. About 85% of patients have the same mutation in the splice acceptor site of intron 3. Because of the isolated island situation, this mutation, which results in a truncated protein lacking the C-terminal half, is regarded as a founder mutation. This founder mutation enables rapid genetic testing of Japanese XP patients using restriction fragment length polymorphism (RFLP) techniques. The estimated frequency of heterozygous carriers of this mutation in Japan is about 1% (1:100).

Complementation group B

Only very few patients have been reported with this complementation group worldwide [12,44]. Five patients had the combined features of XP and CS. Stigmata of CS with typical ocular and neurological findings were noted. In another family, two siblings exhibited XP without any CS symptoms. Surprisingly, in a single patient, a defect in the *XPB* gene resulted in a trichothiodystrophy phenotype.

The gene for this protein has been localized to chromosome 2q21. It encodes a 782-amino acid 3′–5′ helicase with DNA-dependent ATPase activity. The clinical spectrum of disease can best be explained on the basis of the multiple functions of the XPB protein. The XPB helicase function is dispensable for NER, but DNA binding, allowing binding of the TFIIH complex for excision repair, and its ATPase activity are essential for the process [45]. It also functions in transcription initiation by unwinding or opening the promoter region to allow DNA synthesis to occur. The hypothesis is that, if the mutation in *XPB* affects only NER, a XP phenotype results. If the transcription function of the protein is affected, CS or TTD are developed. The low number of families carrying mutations in this gene suggests that the transcriptional role of XPB as part of the TFIIH complex is vital for life, and mutations of this function are usually not tolerated.

Complementation group C

This represents the most common group worldwide and is particularly common in the USA, Europe, the Maghreb region and the Middle East [46–49]. It has rarely been found in Japan. Patients in complementation group C suffer from XP with skin and ocular involvement but without neurological abnormalities. A history of severe sun sensitivity is not typical in XPC patients. They are normally diagnosed with the appearance of severe freckling or skin cancer in childhood. Skin and ocular findings are moderately severe, but neurological disease is very rarely seen. Robbins reported a single patient in this group with very mild, late-onset neurological deficiencies [50]. Repair of actively transcribed genes (TCR) in patients of this group is usually normal. This may account for the clinical findings reported without neurological symptoms.

The gene product of *XPC* is a 92 kDa polypeptide located on chromosome 3. The heterotrimeric complex of XPC with hHR23B and Centrin 2 is involved in detection of DNA damage as the initiation step in NER. This protein is only involved in repair of UV-damaged DNA that is not undergoing transcription. Mutations in most cases result in protein truncations leading to undetectable levels of *XPC* mRNA, most probably caused by involvement of XPC in several cellular functions beside NER [51,52].

Complementation group D

Approximately 20% of cases of XP account for this complementation group. This gene product is unique, however, because mutations in this gene result in seven different clinical entities (see Fig. 138.2) [53,54]. Patients may develop XP without neurological symptoms or XP with late onset of neurological symptoms. Neurological abnormalities can be quite severe; however, the onset is later in life, typically in the teens or early twenties. Other patients may exhibit the combined symptoms of XP and CS (XP/CS complex – see later). Yet other patients with *XPD* gene mutations developed TTD symptoms and two patients were reported with combined symptoms of XP and TTD (XP/TTD complex – see later). A CS/TTD complex case was also reported. Finally, *XPD* gene mutations may also result in cerebro-oculo-facio-skeletal (COFS/TTD) syndrome (see later).

The gene maps to chromosome 19q13 encoding a 760-amino acid 5′–3′ helicase that is also a component of the TFIIH complex. The helicase is believed to be involved in the 3′ unwinding of the DNA in the vicinity of an existing damaged base [55]. Furthermore, XPD was shown to be the major factor for DNA damage demarcation, verification as well as correct positioning of TFIIH during NER reactions [56,57]. The dual role of XPD in transcription initiation, as well as DNA repair, may help explain the broader spectrum of clinical symptoms in patients with defects in the *XPD* gene. These phenotypes can be explained, at least in part, by the site of the mutation in the *XPD* gene. Patients with XPD or XPD/CS complex have mutations within one of the highly conserved helicase domains. Most of the mutations (75%) in patients with *XPD* are localized to one site: arg683 [37]. The reduced function of the helicase repair activity accounts for the severity of the clinical syndrome. Patients whose causative mutations are in the DNA/RNA helicase regions that cluster at the C-terminus of the protein have TTD, which is predominantly a transcription disorder producing proteins that interfere with the ability of XPD to interact with other parts of the TFIIH complex or TFIIH interaction partners and destabilize the complex. This hypothesis does not adequately explain how different phenotypes can occur from different changes of the same or adjacent amino acids. For example, two XP patients, one with mild features, are described with a mutation at arg601. Mutation of the adjacent amino acid gly602 produces a severe phenotype of XP/CS. Another possible explanation for this phenotypic variability may relate to the gene dosage. If the mutated XPD protein is unstable in the TFIIH complex, there may be reduced levels of the complex and therefore reduced transcription capability. Severe reduction in transcription capability could produce a severe phenotype, if even a single amino acid difference resulted in a less stable protein product [53]. However, like in complementation group B, complete loss of XPD would be deleterious for life.

Complementation group E

Clinically, patients in this group have one of the least severe forms of XP. Cutaneous findings are mild and there are no neurological abnormalities. Cases have been reported from Europe and Japan, and heterogeneity is present in both clinical presentation and laboratory studies. Cells from these patients have an NER level ranging from 40 to 60% of normal cells and only slight UV sensitivity. Some patients who were thought to have the variant form of XP turned out to belong to the XPE complementation group after gene sequencing.

The XPE complementation group results from defects in a dimeric protein that has two subunits of 127 kDa (*DDB1*), localizing to chromosome 11q12–q13, and 48 kDa (*DDB2*), localizing to chromosome 11p12–p11. The XPE protein is specifically involved in lesion detection during global genome repair of CPDs via Cullin 4 dependent ubiquitination of XPC and DDB2 [58]. It has no role in TCR. The *DDB2* gene is inducible by UV irradiation and the induction is dependent on p53 [59].

Complementation group F

The XPF complementation group is rare, with the majority of patients originating in Japan and a few patients reported from Europe. Cells from patients in group F are more photosensitive than those from group E patients but only a few skin tumours have been noted clinically. No neurological deficits are reported in most patients, although some patients were reported with adult onset of severe neurodegeneration, the XFE progeroid syndrome and even Fanconi anaemia [60–62].

The gene for XPF is located on chromosome 16p13.3 and encodes a structure-specific endonuclease (ERCC4) of 916 amino acids. This protein associates with the ERCC1 protein to a heterodimeric complex and functions to incise DNA upstream of the UV-damaged site before XPG incises downstream. Mutations in *ERCC1* have recently been identified in one patient as the cause of COFS, implying that this protein, along with the XPF protein, is essential for viability and probably has a second function, in addition to its role in NER [63]. The yeast homologues of these proteins are essential for recombination between short repeats and it is likely that these proteins have a similar function. Null mutations are not compatible with life [64].

Complementation group G

Fewer than 30 patients in complementation group G have been reported from Europe, Japan as well as North- and South America [65–67]. Patients in this group are clinically heterogeneous. The clinical spectrum ranges from XP symptoms that are very mild with little sun sensitivity to several European and US patients who had severe symptoms with the additional stigmata of CS. XPG/CS complex presents as a much more severe phenotype than that seen in XPB/CS patients. Neurological disease was present in patients with XP/CS complex and the clinical picture was of CS, as well as XP neurological disease.

XPG is located on chromosome 13q33 and encodes an 1186-amino acid structure-specific endonuclease that incises DNA downstream of the UV-damaged site. Although few patients have been identified within this complementation group, the clinical spectrum of patient severity is wide. Milder affected patients with this defect have missense mutations that reduce the nuclease activity. More severely affected patients have mutations that result in XPG proteins unable to stably interact with TFIIH and in a XP/CS complex phenotype caused by destabilization of TFIIH and subsequent failure during basal transcription [39,66]. Furthermore, the severity of clinical disease in patients with mutations of *XPG* compared with patients with *XPA* mutations supports the hypothesis that XPG has a second function. XPG has been shown to stimulate the binding of hNth1 to DNA [68].

This protein is a DNA glycosylase that cleaves oxidatively damaged DNA bases in terms of BER. Mutations that result in interaction deficiencies of the XPG protein with TFIIH compounds abolish all functions of XPG and lead to CS symptoms, whereas missense mutations can abolish nuclease activity during NER, responsible for XP phenotype, while leaving BER functions or basal transcription intact.

Variant form of XP

In addition to the seven complementation groups, a variant form of XP (XPV) exists. Despite having a normal NER capability, these patients develop the same clinical symptoms as other XP patients with defective NER [69]. Cutaneous and ocular abnormalities may also range from severe to mild. XPV patients usually do not develop additional neurological symptoms. However, severely affected patients have been reported. One-third of all patients with XP are of the variant type. Patients have been identified from Europe and the USA. It represents the most common form of XP seen in Japan. Unlike the complementation groups of XP, patients with the variant form of XP have normal NER and normal levels of unscheduled DNA synthesis after UV exposure. However, a slower rate of recovery following UV light injury is observed, especially in the presence of caffeine. Cells are less viable and show more marked mutagenesis than normal cells after UV injury. UV-irradiated cells produce newly synthesized DNA of a reduced molecular weight and demonstrate a delay in the production of intact high molecular weight DNA strands following UV injury.

POLH was identified in 1999 as the disease causing gene of XPV. *POLH* is a homologue of the yeast *RAD30* gene. This polymerase is involved in translesional synthesis and has the capability to specifically bypass UV-induced CPD photoproducts in a less error-prone manner. It is localized to chromosome 6p21–p12. When NER fails to remove UV-damaged DNA, translesion synthesis allows for generation of daughter-strand DNA, despite the presence of pre-existing UV damage in the parental DNA strands. XPV patients are deficient in the ability to bypass a single thymine dimer by error-free synthesis of two adenines. Most mutations result in frameshifts and premature termination of the protein, but inactivating missense mutations have also been reported [32].

Cockayne syndrome

History. Cockayne first reported this syndrome in 1936 [70]. He described a phenotype including the hallmarks of cachectic dwarfism, hearing disability and retinal atrophy [4,64]. The two siblings described by Cockayne presented with cachectic dwarfism, progressive mental retardation, an erythematous dermatitis and an odd facial appearance in which loss of subcutaneous fat resulted in a 'wizened' look with typical 'bird-headed' facies and prominent ears. Further details on these patients that Cockayne reported in 1946 included loss of vision associated with an unusual pigmentary degeneration of the retina and progressive hearing loss [71]. In 1950 Neil and Dingwall described two siblings with similar clinical features [72]. Subsequently, CS has been reported in over 180 patients. Because of the dermatological similarities recognized in some patients with XP and CS, the discovery of defective DNA repair in XP in 1968 resulted in a search for an underlying defect in DNA repair in CS after a breakthrough discovery in this field [8]. Although the usual assays of DNA excision repair were found to be normal, it was soon discovered that CS cells were delayed in recovery of DNA and RNA synthesis following UV irradiation [73].

Epidemiology and pathogenesis. CS is a very rare disease caused by a deficiency in the transcription-coupled subpathway of NER and is inherited in an autosomal recessive manner. Like XP patients, CS patients experience increased sun sensitivity. However, in contrast to XP patients, CS patients do not exhibit an increased skin cancer risk [5]. CS affects males and females with almost equal frequency. Most reported patients have been White or Japanese. Black patients have been reported, as well as patients from Argentina, India, Saudi Arabia and Iraq. Parental consanguinity has been reported in many cases. However, parents of affected children, obligate heterozygotes, are asymptomatic.

Clinical features. The clinical features of the multisystem disorder CS are quite heterogeneous and can vary considerably in their severity [74]. Classic CS symptoms include growth retardation (dwarfism), neurological and psychomotor impairment with mental retardation, skin sensitivity to sunlight (with or without xerosis), progressive ophthalmological disorders including cataracts or retinitis pigmentosa, deafness, dental caries and a characteristic facies including a thin face, flat cheeks and prominent tapering nose (bird-like face). CS patients exhibit cutaneous photosensitivity, but are not prone to skin cancer [5] (see Table 138.2). Also commonly noted are microcephaly and calcifications of the basal ganglia or elsewhere in the central nervous system (Fig. 138.4).

The neurological impairment of CS patients correlates to a primary demyelinization of neurons. This contrasts with the primary neuronal degeneration found in XP patients. Beside other explanations (see later), one reason for this difference could be that the specific inability of CS cells to repair cyclobutane-pyrimidine dimers in actively transcribed genes may result in repeated injury to myelin-producing cells, which is not fully repaired. Myelin-producing cells eventually die from this damage. Mature neurons lack the ability to divide and have reduced transcription. This may explain the progressive neurological damage that occurs in patients with CS. The exact nature of the damage that occurs in these cells and the reason why damage occurs in such a specific anatomical location are not understood and most are probably because of a highly complex interplay between several functions of CS proteins in cellular integrity [75]. Early hallmarks for a clinical diagnosis of CS include cachectic dwarfism and neurological disabilities. This leads to premature death at

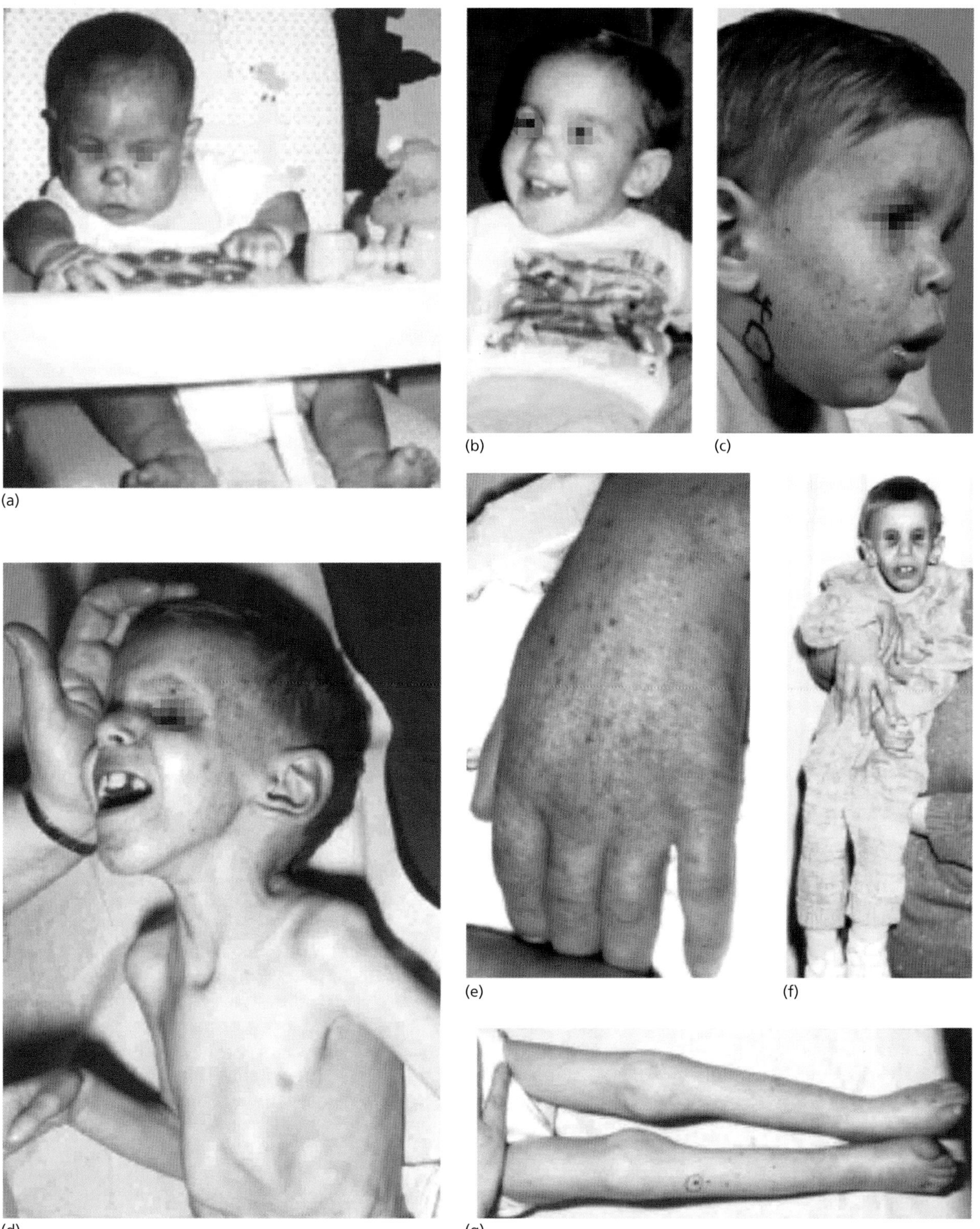

Fig. 138.4 (a) Patient with xeroderma pigmentosum (XP)/Cockayne syndrome (CS) complex at age 4 months after he developed severe sunburn in March, the first sign of illness. Note the sharp change in redness on his lower legs where his socks blocked some sunlight. (b) Normal fullness of the face at age 1 year. (c) Age 1.5 years. Characteristic skin lesions of XP: freckling and hypopigmented macules of skin and lips. A benign pedunculated lesion is circled. (d) Age 6 years. Typical appearance of CS with deep-set eyes, prominent ears and profound cachexia with posturing of the hand. (e) Age 6 years. Pigmentary changes and wrinkling of the dorsum of the hand showing signs of premature ageing. (f) Age 6 years. Signs of advanced CS with profound weakness of dorsiflexion of the hand. Note small size in comparison with the mother who is holding him. (g) Profound wasting and contractures of the legs with distal cyanosis and permanently upgoing toes. Source: Lindenbaum et al. 2001 [77]. Reproduced with permission from Elsevier/European Paediatric Neurology Society.

a mean age of 12 years. Nance & Berry [76] published a clinical review of 140 CS patients in 1992 and suggested three clinical CS categories: CSI, a classic form including most CS patients; CSII, a severe form with early onset and rapid progression; CSIII, a mild form with late onset and slow progression of symptoms.

CSI becomes apparent after the first year of life, with severe growth failure and neurodevelopmental dysfunction. These two hallmarks, together with one or more of the following features, generally allow the clinical diagnosis: progressive retinitis pigmentosa or cataracts, sensorineural hearing loss or dental caries (see Table 138.2). As a consequence of the deficiency in the transcription-coupled subpathway of NER, classic CS patients are sun sensitive. In about 75% of CS patients, such hyperkeratotic erythemas in sun-exposed skin that may resolve leaving poikiloderma (hyperpigmentations, skin atrophy, telangiectasias) are often first symptoms in the second year of life. Appearance and development in the first year of life are often normal.

A second early sign is growth failure. This comprises height, weight and head circumference. Height and weight measurements below the fifth percentile by 2 years of age are the rule. A small encephalon can be radiologically documented. Delayed psychomotor development as indicated by delayed milestones for speech and ambulation is usually the earliest neurological abnormality. Neurological examinations typically reveal cerebellar abnormalities. Tremor, incoordination and dysarthric speech are common findings. Leg spasticity, ataxia and contractures of the hips, knees and ankles lead to progressive gait disorder. About 5–10% of the patients experience seizures later in life. X-ray of the skull and computed tomography (CT) show calcification of the basal ganglia and other brain structures. MRI shows mild ventricular enlargement and delay in myelination of the cerebrum and cerebellum (white matter abnormalities). Auditory or visual evoked potentials are further tests that show abnormalities.

Severe cognitive impairment is common. In more mildly affected CS patients, progressive deterioration is expected in teenage years. Eye problems are also common in CS patients. Pigmentary degeneration of the retina leading to a 'salt and pepper' retinal change is a hallmark of CS and the most frequent ophthalmological complication. Other common eye problems include cataracts, optic nerve atrophy and optic disc pallor. Less common are iris hypoplasia and microphthalmos which, together with cataracts, indicate severe CS and poor prognosis. Progressive sensorineural hearing loss may not manifest until the teenage years, but is seen in most patients caused by loss of auditory neurons. Dental caries are a major problem for CS patients. Renal abnormalities with decreased creatinine clearance and hypertension have been reported in CS patients. Reproductive development is also retarded. Undescended testes occur in 30% of male CS patients.

These features lead to a typical appearance. Because of the microcephaly and small oral cavity, the ears as well as the teeth appear prominent. Hands and limbs are disproportionately large in contrast to the smaller trunk. Kyphosis and contractures and a bird-like face caused by loss of subcutaneous fat tissue define the CS habitus (see Fig. 138.4).

CSII, a severe form of CS with early onset and rapid progression, has been reported in over 20 patients. Most patients die of cachexia at 6 or 7 years of age. A low birthweight is common. However, there is only little growth after birth and often progressive loss of subcutaneous tissue, leading to a total bodyweight not exceeding 8 kg. Cachectic dwarfism, progeric features and progressive spasticity are noted after the first year of life. Neurological development is absent. In 30% of cases structural abnormalities of the eye and early or congenital cataracts are present. Cutaneous symptoms, and dental and auditory complications are less commonly noted.

CSIII comprises a mild form with late onset and slow progression of symptoms. Such patients exhibit some CS features but lack one of the hallmarks of abnormal growth and mental retardation. Patients may have normal intelligence, growth and reproductive capacity.

Many of the clinical features of CS are reminiscent of normal ageing, such as systemic growth failure, neurological degeneration and cataracts. Although the process of normal ageing is not well understood, it has been suggested that the gradual accumulation of damaged DNA that has not been removed during the cellular lifetime contributes to the process of normal ageing. Because the CS proteins are involved in transcription-coupled NER but also in transcription (via interaction with TFIIH) and in the base excision of oxidative DNA damage (especially repair of oxidative DNA damage in actively transcribed genes), these and several other functions of this protein can provide an explanation for the multisystem manifestations of CS and some of the phenotypic diversity accounting for some of the clinical symptoms that mimic normal senescence [78–81].

Histopathology. Histology of the skin of patients with CS is nonspecific. Facial erythema caused by sun sensitivity histologically appears as nonspecific dermatitis. The synthesis of collagen fibres was assessed in the skin of CS patients and found to be normal. One report 25 years ago found abnormally small eccrine glands for age in the skin of CS patients, but this has not been verified in larger studies [64]. Neuropathological features of CS are more distinct. There is multifocal, patchy or diffuse demyelination in the central and peripheral nervous system and cerebral as well as cerebellar atrophy. In addition, dilated ventricles may be found. Calcifications in the basal ganglia and in the cortex of the cerebrum and cerebellum are typical features. Widespread demyelination and neuronal loss, especially in the cerebellum, comprise the hallmarks of CS neuropathology. Reduced nerve conduction velocity, sensorineural hearing loss and changes in muscle innervation (hyperreflexia) are signs of peripheral nerve defects [64].

Differential diagnoses. The hallmarks of CS include short stature and/or failure to thrive with developmental delay. In younger infants and children, the typical CS symptoms may not have fully developed, whereas in older patients the differential considerations are usually limited (see Box 138.1). Therefore, it is necessary, particularly in infants, to perform a complete examination of the skin, eyes, ears, teeth, skeletal system and neurological function. Limb and trunk contractures and the cachectic facial appearance (bird-like face) are not typically identifiable in the first several years of life. Profound growth failure usually suggests a chromosomal abnormality or a genetic syndrome such as Hallermann–Streiff, Russell–Silver, Brachmann–deLange, Dubowitz or others. The onset of growth failure after birth without physical anomalies makes chromosomal abnormalities less likely.

Skeletal dysplasias can be ruled out with routine X-ray examination. Endocrine and metabolic testing is indicated and feeding history is helpful to exclude gastrointestinal problems. Photosensitivity, a facial rash and dry or atrophic hair suggest XP, TTD or Bloom syndrome, dyskeratosis congenita, the premature ageing syndromes such as progeria, Werner syndrome, Rothmund–Thompson syndrome or tyrosinaemia. Appropriate diagnostic tests can look for chromosome breakage, DNA repair in fibroblasts or other diagnostic features. If neurological deterioration exists or even seizures, an MRI of the brain will show primary involvement of the white matter and possibly the presence of brain calcifications. None of the leucodystrophies causes severe growth failure. Intracranial calcifications might suggest congenital infections or disorders of calcium or phosphate metabolism, but these should be easily eliminated by examination of other organ systems. Finally, the presence of retinitis pigmentosum with neurological abnormalities might be seen in peroxisomal disorders and mitochondrial encephalomyopathy with ragged-red fibres. These conditions lack the growth, cutaneous and dental findings of CS. Corroborative tests in cases where the diagnosis is uncertain would include a CT or MRI of the brain, auditory or visual evoked potentials, electromyogram (EMG) or nerve conduction velocity (NCV), audiometry, and the analysis of the sensitivity of fibroblasts to UV light in combination with other assays of DNA metabolism [82].

Clinical and laboratory tests. Clinical laboratory testing often shows sensorineural deafness, an abnormal neuropathic EMG and slow motor NCV. Height and weight are usually below the third percentile for the age. Bone age is normal. There may be abnormalities on electroencephalogram. X-ray examination of the head can show thickened skull and microcephaly. CT scans of the brain can detect normal-pressure hydrocephalus or calcifications of the basal ganglia and other brain structures. MRI of the brain typically shows atrophy and demyelination of the cerebrum and cerebellum at older age.

Chromosome karyotype and sister chromatid exchange frequency is normal in patients with CS. Cultured fibroblasts and lymphocytes from all patients with CS are hypersensitive to UV irradiation, for example as assessed by their colony-forming ability. As in XP cells, CS cells exhibit reduced host cell reactivation of UV-damaged reporter plasmids but to a lesser extent compared with XP. Recovery of RNA synthesis is delayed following UV injury. This reflects a defective repair of actively transcribed genes. Transcriptionally active genes are normally repaired at a faster rate than are inactive genes in the global genome. In addition, it has been demonstrated that CS cells are not able to repair cyclobutane-pyrimidine dimers in actively transcribed DNA. 6-4PP are repaired normally. However, they only account for approximately 25% of UV-derived lesions in the human genome [83,84]. The UV cancer resistance in CS may relate, in part, to the ability of cells from these patients to repair 6-4PP in actively transcribed genes normally, a function that is absent in patients with XP [85].

Treatment and prevention. Unfortunately, CS patients can only be treated symptomatically and in a supportive way. There is currently no specific or causal treatment for CS available. Because most patients experience sun sensitivity and burn easily, photo protective measures as described for XP patients are advisable. The molecular reason for the cachectic dwarfism is still unknown. The cachexia and loss of subcutaneous tissue can usually not be fully compensated by enhanced nutritive uptake and are progressive. In individuals who have problems with eating and drinking caused by additional severe neurological impairment, the placement of a gastric tube may be beneficial. There is no treatment to avoid the short stature. Routine patient follow up may include assessment of neurological symptoms, social, auditory and visual function. MRI examinations of the brain can indicate intracranial calcifications. Appropriate services should be provided for the various symptoms. Symptoms such as hypertension, tooth decay or hearing loss can be specifically addressed. To prevent development and progression of contractures, early intervention with physical therapy is mandatory. Exercise and physical therapy to compensate for deteriorating neurological function are also important. In an affected family, prenatal diagnosis using fetal amniocytes is possible and has been performed based on the delay in recovery of post-UV RNA synthesis and the increased cell death following UV radiation. Because life expectancy is short and growth is poor we would recommend paediatric services with experienced clinicians for coordination of care.

Complementation groups and molecular basis

CS patients may be categorized according to their defective gene in addition to their clinical phenotypical categorization. Two complementation groups have been identified: CS complementation group A (CSA), corresponding with a smaller group of patients with later onset and less severe disease, and CS complementation group B (CSB) comprising the largest number of patients (~80%) with a severe infantile form of the disease leading to early death (see Table 138.1) [86,87]. Cells from CS patients exhibit genomic hypermutability, chromosomal instability after UV irradiation and defective processing of UV-induced DNA damage, for example reduced unscheduled DNA or RNA synthesis [88]. Both CS genes are involved in TCR of active genes (see Fig. 138.1).

A defect in transcription beyond bulky DNA damage, including UV-induced DNA photoproducts, may be present in CS cells. CS symptoms may also result as a consequence of defective repair of endogenous oxidative DNA damage in actively transcribed genes [81]. However, there is an ongoing debate about the importance of defective cellular processes other than DNA repair for the neurological symptoms in CS patients. The involvement of CS proteins in basal transcription [79], RNA polymerase I transcription (rRNA) [78] as well as mitochondrial functions [80] are discussed.

CSA, also named *ERCC8*, is located on chromosome 5 and encodes a 396-amino acid protein that is involved in the coupling between transcription and repair. CSA has been shown to bind to the p44 subunit of TFIIH, a component of the CSB–/RNA PolII complex that stalls at damaged sites in transcriptionally active DNA [89]. If cells have mutations in *CSA*, they cannot ubiquitinate RNA polymerase II after UV exposure nor remove the transcription complex stalled at a damaged site by, for example, degradation of CSB [90,91]. *CSB*, also named *ERCC6*, is located on chromosome 10q11 and encodes a 1493-amino acid protein with helicase motifs. Like *CSA*, it is involved in the coupling between repair and transcription. *CSB* has a nucleotide binding site, multiple interaction partners in a brought variety of cellular processes and acts as a DNA-dependent ATPase [92]. One proposed model is that CS proteins, by binding to DNA, chromatin and the TFIIH complex, allow a conformational change in the complex that switches the complex from transcriptional mode to NER mode, and then, after damage repair is complete, back to transcriptional mode to restore RNA synthesis [22,93].

XP/CS complex

The identification of patients who exhibit both XP and CS symptoms simultaneously paved the way for the establishment of this separate clinical entity: XP/CS complex. Robbins [50] recognized these patients as having a distinct clinical phenotype (see Table 138.2). XP/CS complex patients exhibit defects in their mental and physical development, dwarfism, bird-like facies and severe neurological and psychomotor disabilities (CS symptoms) as well as sun sensitivity of their skin and an increased skin cancer risk (XP symptoms) (see Fig. 138.4) [77,94,95]. XP/CS complex patients may have other features of CS including pigmentary retinal degeneration, calcification of the basal ganglia, normal-pressure hydrocephalus and, in contrast to XP with neurological symptoms, hyperreflexia. These patients are distinguishable, clinically, from XP patients with the DeSanctis–Cacchione syndrome because they lack the typical neurological features of primary neuronal degeneration. The underlying causes of the neurological symptoms here are demyelination and cerebellar dysfunction.

Worldwide, fewer than 30 patients with XP/CS complex have been described. Genotyping of these patients revealed that they had no mutations in either the *CSA* or *CSB* genes. However, mutations were found in the *XPB*, *XPD* and *XPG* genes (see Fig. 138.2, Table 138.1) [3]. Recently, a patient with XP/CS features as well Fanconi anaemia symptoms was identified with mutations in the *XPF* gene [60]. Thus, certain mutations in XP genes can lead to XP plus additional CS symptoms.

The location of the mutation correlates to some degree with the clinical phenotypes in XP/CS complex patients. Mutations that affect the helicase domain of XPD or the ATPase domain of XPB result in XP phenotypes, because unwinding of the DNA cannot occur and is essential to repair. Similarly, patients whose *XPG* mutation affects the endonuclease activity have XP. Patients whose mutation abolishes the scaffold function of XPG during transcription develop the clinical picture of XP plus CS [96]. The hypothesis is that in XP/CS complex patients, at least two different XP gene functions are affected. One function relates to a disturbed NER and the other one to a deficiency in transcription or repair of other DNA lesions like oxidative DNA damage.

Trichothiodystrophy

History. Price and colleagues introduced the term 'trichothiodystrophy' in 1980 [97]. TTD comprises the third major NER defective syndrome and is also inherited in an autosomal recessive fashion. The first reported cases of TTD appeared a decade before when Pollitt and colleagues described patients with trichorrhexis nodosa, low sulphur content of hair and associated mental and physical retardation. Two years later, Brown and colleagues reported a case of trichoschisis with the typical pattern of sulphur-deficient hair seen on polarized light microscopy. Tay reported three patients with ichthyosiform erythroderma, hair shaft abnormalities, and mental and growth retardation. Other authors have since reported cases of Tay syndrome with TTD [82].

In TTD, as in CS, a variety of neurological and psychomotor developmental defects may occur. Retrospectively, several syndromes can now be encompassed under the broad term TTD, including Pollitt syndrome, Tay syndrome, Sabinas syndrome, Marinesco–Sjögren syndrome and ONMR (onychotrichodysplasia, neutropenia, mental retardation) [98]. PIBIDS represents yet another specific constellation of TTD symptoms. The genetic basis of TTD was initially studied in PIBIDS patients [99]. PIBIDS summarizes the symptoms photosensitivity, ichthyosis, brittle hair and nails, intellectual impairment, decreased fertility and short stature [100].

Clinical features. Trichothiodystrophy is a rare autosomal recessive inherited disease characterized by sulphur-deficient brittle hair and a variety of neuroectodermal symptoms (Figs 138.5 and 138.6) [101]. Of note, TTD patients, especially children, have a very sociable, outgoing personality. More severely affected individuals exhibit a typical dysmorphic facies with protruding ears, deep-set eyes, micrognathia and head elongation (fronto-occipital) as well as a raspy voice. In addition, other tissues of ectodermal or neuroectodermal origin may be

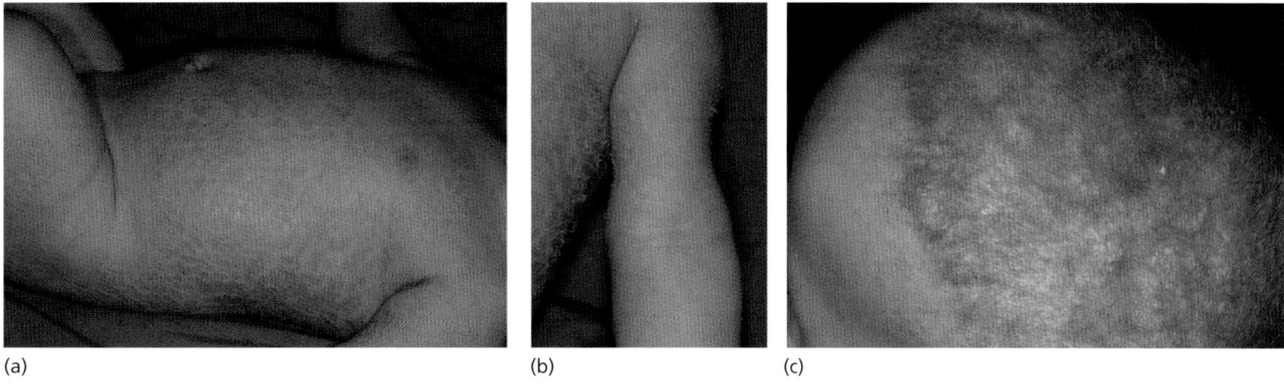

Fig. 138.5 Clinical features of trichothiodystrophy in a young boy showing dry, scaly skin on the trunk and dorsal extremities sparing the flexures at eight weeks (a, b) and short, brittle hair at two years of age (c). Source: Brauns et al. 2016 [103]. Reproduced with permission of Wiley-VCH.

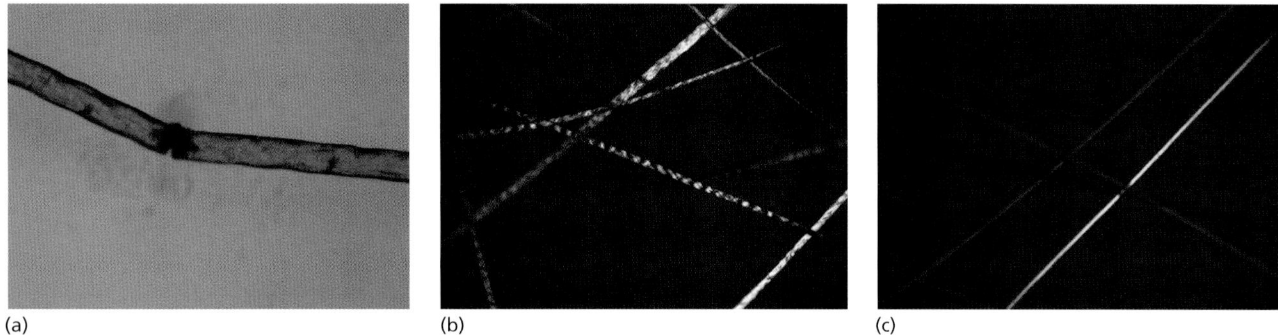

Fig. 138.6 Tiger tail hair of trichothiodystrophy in a 2-year-old boy. Light microscopy revealed trichoschisis (a; magnification ×10) and polarizing microscopy showed alternating dark and light bands of hair shafts ('tiger-tail' banding) (b) compared with hair shafts of a healthy person (c; magnification ×5). Source: Brauns et al. 2016 [103]. Reproduced with permission of Wiley-VCH.

dystrophic in great variability. Classic TTD skin symptoms are increased sun sensitivity, ichthyotic skin changes, nail changes and erythemas (see Table 138.2). An increased sun sensitivity on exposed skin is the hallmark of about half of all TTD patients. A cellular repair defect of UV-induced photoproducts is mirrored by this photosensitivity. However, this defect does not translate into either an increased skin cancer risk or poikiloderma (hyperpigmentation, atrophy, telangiectasias) as in XP patients [100,102]. Collodion baby, generalized ichthyosis, erythroderma and eczema are common cutaneous findings (Fig. 138.5). Nail dystrophies include longitudinal ridging and splitting, and koilonychia. Dental abnormalities including enamel hypoplasia, caries and a high-arched palate can be found. Eye abnormalities include cataracts as well as conjunctivitis, epicanthal folds and photophobia. Neurological findings include nystagmus, intention tremor, spasticity and ataxia. Mental and growth retardation (osteosclerosis) as well as reduced fertility comprise other typical TTD symptoms. Finally, there are recurrent infections in TTD patients. Chronic neutropenia with monocytosis and disturbed intracellular killing during phagocytosis has been reported. The prognosis of TTD depends on the severity of the neuroectodermal symptoms. There is a spectrum ranging from early death caused by infections to mild symptoms with normal intelligence and a normal lifespan.

Hair phenotype

All patients with TTD have clinically abnormal hair on the scalp, eyelashes and eyebrows. Hairs are brittle, unruly, of variable lengths, easily broken, sparse and dry (Fig. 138.5). Hypotrichosis, patchy scalp alopecia, scarce eyebrows and eyelashes, and sparse axillary and pubic hair are typical. Other body hair may be scant or absent. Hair colour does not seem to be affected. Intermittent hair loss may occur with periodic cyclicity or during infection (temperature dependent instability of the mutated protein). Hair shaft stability is normally conferred by sulphur-rich hair matrix proteins. Changes in elasticity of the hair shaft lead to hair breakage in TTD patients. The sulphur deficiency leads to a typical tiger tail pattern of the hair that can be seen under a polarizing microscope (see Fig. 138.6). However, tiger-tail hair is not diagnostic for TTD because it can be found in other circumstances. Changes of the amino acid content of the hair caused by the lack of sulphur-rich hair matrix proteins can also be identified. The amounts of the amino acids cysteine, proline, threonine and serine are greatly reduced. In contrast, a relative increase in methionine, phenylalanine, alanine, leucine, lysine and aspartic acid can be found in mice [104]. Quantification of the hair sulphur content is regarded as a diagnostic test. Scanning electron microscopy showed severe cuticular and secondary cortical degeneration, trichorrhexis nodosa formation and trichoschisis.

Transmission electron microscopy identified a quantitative decrease in sulphur protein resulting in cuticular weathering and weakness of the hair shaft [100,102]. In addition, patients have hair shaft abnormalities including trichoschisis, trichorrhexis nodosa and ribboning.

Differential diagnoses. The differential diagnosis of TTD includes the spectrum of ectodermal dysplasias (ED) because abnormalities in ectodermal structures are a common feature in TTD patients (see Box 138.1). EDs comprise a large and heterogeneous group of disorders characterized by abnormal development or growth of tissues and structures that originate from the outer embryonal layer, the ectoderm. An inherited skin defect is classified as an ED when two or more of the following structures are affected: skin, hair, teeth, nails or sweat glands. Also, conditions that combine a defect in one of those structures with an anomaly of another ectodermal structure are referred to as ED. Besides various combinations of ectodermal defects, ED patients can also manifest other congenital abnormalities, such as orofacial clefting, limb malformations, diminished immune defence, hearing impairment, renal abnormalities or mental retardation, which are subsequently termed ED syndromes [100,105]. Currently about 170 different ED conditions have been described. Nail and teeth abnormalities which are often found in TTD patients overlap with ED syndromes. The reduced sulphur content of the hair helps to distinguish TTD from ED. However, although an increasing number of EDs have been linked to specific gene mutations, the majority of ED syndromes, predominantly the rare conditions, remain unsolved. However, these syndromes may represent different closely related genetic alterations that regulate keratinization in hair, nails, etc. For example, the ED genes *EDA*, *EDAR*, *EDARADD*, *IKBKG* and *NFKBIA* all converge on NF-κB signalling [106].

It should be noted that not all patients with reduced sulphur content of the hair suffer from TTD. Ichthyosis patients may also have cysteine or other amino acid deficiencies in their hair. Patients with hidrotic ectodermal dysplasia have been reported with cysteine content of hydrolysed hair in the 25% range. Nutrition can influence the sulphur content of hair, too, with normalization after treatment of the nutritional deficiency. In addition, many products used in the hair industry, such as cold-waving lotions, hair bleaching solutions and synthetic organic hair dyes, can change the cysteine content of hair. Similarly, the pattern of trichoschisis and alternating bands of light and dark under polarizing microscopy (tiger-tail hair) has been described in patients with other genetic hair abnormalities who do not have low sulphur content [102].

Laboratory tests. All patients with congenitally brittle hair should undergo sulphur analysis of hair to look for TTD. Evaluation of clipped hairs under light, polarized, scanning electron, or transmission electron microscopy can aid in establishing the diagnosis. Neurological and developmental assessments as well as eye examinations may be performed. MRI of the brain can demonstrate demyelination. Prophylactic antibiotics may be needed in cases of recurrent infections and patients can profit from rehabilitation medicine support. In photosensitive TTD patients cell survival measurements after UV irradiation and other DNA repair assays may be helpful as well as base sequencing analysis of possibly affected genes (see later). Prenatal diagnosis may be considered for the more severe and potentially lethal phenotypes. For patients with reduced DNA repair, prenatal diagnosis can be accomplished by measuring DNA repair in trophoblasts or amniotic cells. Microscopic analysis of fetal hairs has also been performed [82].

Treatment. As in CS, there is no specific treatment in TTD patients (see previously). Patient care is symptomatic. Sun protection is recommended in sun-sensitive individuals. The ichthyotic skin problems can be treated with moisturizing ointments. There is also not much that can be done for the sulphur-deficient short brittle hair. Traumas and mechanical or environmental stresses should be avoided. A hair cut is rarely necessary; trimming of some hairs is usually sufficient. Oral uptake of biotin does not improve the hair condition.

Genetic classification

A genetic classification of TTD patients developed eventually as it did in XP and CS patients. Photosensitive, repair-deficient TTD cells were used for genetic testing because a suitable functional screening test was and still is lacking for the other half of nonphotosensitive TTD cells. Four genes causing TTD have been identified so far: ~60% of all photosensitive TTD patients exhibited mutations in the *XPD* gene [102]; in two patients a mutation in the *XPB* gene was detected (see Fig. 138.2) [107]. *XPD* and *XPB* are both subunits of the TFIIH complex and essential for basal transcription (see Fig. 138.1). One TTD patient was identified who had no XP gene defect but a TFIIH defect [108]. The putative gene was named *TTD-A* (TTD complementation group A) and was recently identified as the human *TFB5* orthologue of yeast and tenth subunit of TFIIH (see Figs 138.1 and 138.2) [109,110]. TFIIH is a high molecular weight protein complex with dual function in NER as well as initiation of RNA polymerase II transcription. TTD cells have reduced amounts of TFIIH. Because TTD is thought to be a transcriptional disease, studies in mouse models demonstrated that the impairment of basal transcription of some specific genes may account for the wide range of clinical symptoms except photosensitivity which may be a consequence of the disruption in the DNA repair function of TFIIH [111]. Reduced amounts of TFIIH may prevent transcription of important genes in terminally differentiated cells like keratinocytes or neurones that cannot synthesize TFIIH de novo, resulting in brittle hair and nails or demyelination [112]. Some nonphotosensitive TTD patients have been identified with a mutation in the so-called *TTDN1* gene, a gene of still unknown function [113] and a different mechanism of disease than in TTD-A patients is suspected [114]. Very recently, a new gene, named *RNF113A*,

SECTION 29: DISEASES PREDISPOSING TO MALIGNANCY

involved in nonphotosensitive TTD pathogenesis was identified in two patients [115].

XP/TTD complex

XP/CS complex was initially identified as an independent clinical entity by careful patient examinations. In the case of XP/TTD, genetics suggested the existence of a XP/TTD complex phenotype. The *XPD* gene was mutated in patients with the photosensitive form of TTD. An overview of *XPD* mutations revealed that they either led to XP or TTD symptoms or were null mutations, depending on their location in *XPD* [53]. This implied that TTD results as a consequence of an *XPD*-triggered deficiency in basal transcription and that XP is caused by a defect in NER. Thus, investigators looked specifically for individuals carrying compound heterozygous *XPD* mutations (one mutation leading to XP and the other to TTD). Such patients should present a XP/TTD complex phenotype. Two patients, XP189MA and XP38BR, confirmed this hypothesis [116].

Cerebro-oculo-facio-skeletal syndrome

COFS syndrome is a very rare autosomal recessive condition. It was initially described in French–Indian families within the genetically isolated Manitoba Aboriginal population which has a high frequency of consanguineous marriages [117]. Although initially reported as early as 1971 by Lowry and colleagues, COFS syndrome was delineated by Pena & Shokeir in 1974 as an autosomal recessive progressive brain and eye disorder leading to microcephaly with cerebral atrophy, hypoplasia of the corpus callosum, hypotonia, severe mental retardation, cataracts, microcornea, optic atrophy, progressive joint contractures and postnatal growth deficiency [118]. Some symptoms appear quite similar to CS, for example progressive demyelination with brain calcification or cataracts. But COFS syndrome eye defects (e.g. microcornea) appear to be more severe than those associated with CS and in contrast to CS, cutaneous photosensitivity is not always noted in COFS patients (see Table 138.2). Meira and colleagues demonstrated that COFS cells showed features indistinguishable from those observed in classic CS and identified a mutation in the *CSB* gene causally related to COFS [119]. Furthermore, mutations in the *XPG* gene as well as the *XPD* gene and the *ERCC1* gene were identified in COFS patients (see Fig. 138.2) [63,118].

UV-sensitive syndrome, COFS/TTD and CS/TTD

Because different mutations at different locations within the same gene can lead to different clinical entities it is understandable that 'combined' clinical entities have been described where patients are compound heterozygous for two mutations that each cause different clinical symptoms. With potential implications for oxidative and energy metabolism, patients that exhibit combined symptoms of COFS and TTD (COFS/TTD) as well as CS together with TTD symptoms have been discovered [120]. Yet another distinct clinical entity is the UV-sensitive syndrome (UVSS) first described in 1994 [121]. Patients with this rare syndrome exhibit mild photosensitivity without pigmentary skin abnormalities or apparent defects in the central nervous system. Their growth, mental development, and lifespan are normal and there appears to be no increased cancer risk. Disease-causing defects in the *CSA* [122] or *CSB* genes [123] have been described. UVSS patient cells have the same transcription defects as CS cells. Because neurological symptoms are absent in UVSS patients, the CS genes obviously have functions related to UV sensitivity as well as central nervous functions. The latter may include processing of oxidative DNA damage [122].

References

1 **Kraemer KH, Patronas NJ, Schiffmann R et al. Xeroderma pigmentosum, trichothiodystrophy and Cockayne syndrome: a complex genotype-phenotype relationship. Neuroscience 2007;145:1388–96.**
2 Moriwaki S. Human DNA repair disorders in dermatology: a historical perspective, current concepts and new insight. J Dermatol Sci 2016;81:77–84.
3 Rapin I. Disorders of nucleotide excision repair. Handb Clin Neurol 2013;113:1637–50.
4 Bootsma D, Kraemer KH, Cleaver JE et al. Nucleotide excision repair syndromes: xeroderma pigmentosum, Cockayne syndrome, and trichothiodystrophy. In: Vogelstein B, Kinzler KW (eds) The Genetic Basis of Human Cancer. McGraw-Hill: New York, 2002:211–37.
5 de Boer J, Hoeijmakers JH. Nucleotide excision repair and human syndromes. Carcinogenesis 2000;21:453–60.
6 Moriz Kaposi (1837–1902 – Disciple of Von Hebra). JAMA 1964; 187:227–8.
7 Emmert S, Leibeling D, Rünger TM. Syndromes with genetic instability: model diseases for (skin) cancerogenesis. J Dtsch Dermatol Ges 2006;4:721–31.
8 Cleaver JE. Defective repair replication of DNA in xeroderma pigmentosum. Nature 1968;218:652–6.
9 Epstein JH, Fukuyama K, Fye K. Effects of ultraviolet radiation on the mitotic cycle and DNA, RNA and protein synthesis in mammalian epidermis in vivo. Photochem Photobiol 1970;12:57–65.
10 Epstein JH, Fukuyama K, Reed WB et al. Defect in DNA synthesis in skin of patients with xeroderma pigmentosum demonstrated in vivo. Science 1970;168:1477–8.
11 De Weerd-Kastelein EA, Keijzer W, Bootsma D. Genetic heterogeneity of xeroderma pigmentosum demonstrated by somatic cell hybridization. Nat New Biol 1972;238:80–3.
12 Schubert S, Lehmann J, Kalfon L et al. Clinical utility gene card for: Xeroderma pigmentosum. Eur J Hum Genet 2014;22.
13 Leibeling D, Laspe P, Emmert S. Nucleotide excision repair and cancer. J Mol Histol 2006;37:225–38.
14 Kraemer KH, Lee MM, Scotto J. Xeroderma pigmentosum. Cutaneous, ocular, and neurologic abnormalities in 830 published cases. Arch Dermatol 1987;123:241–50.
15 Kleijer WJ, Laugel V, Berneburg M et al. Incidence of DNA repair deficiency disorders in western Europe: xeroderma pigmentosum, Cockayne syndrome and trichothiodystrophy. DNA Repair (Amst) 2008;7:744–50.
16 Khan SG, Oh KS, Shahlavi T et al. Reduced XPC DNA repair gene mRNA levels in clinically normal parents of xeroderma pigmentosum patients. Carcinogenesis 2006;27:84–94.
17 Swift M, Chase C. Cancer in families with xeroderma pigmentosum. J Natl Cancer Inst 1979;62:1415–21.
18 Masaki T, Wang Y, DiGiovanna JJ et al. High frequency of PTEN mutations in nevi and melanomas from xeroderma pigmentosum patients. Pigment Cell Melanoma Res 2014;27:454–64.
19 Kraemer KH, Slor H. Xeroderma pigmentosum. Clin Dermatol 1985;3:33–69.
20 Seebode C, Lehmann J, Emmert S. Photocarcinogenesis and skin cancer prevention strategies. Anticancer Res 2016;36:1371–8.
21 Kraemer KH, Sander M, Bohr VA. New areas of focus at workshop on human diseases involving DNA repair deficiency and premature aging. Mech Ageing Dev 2007;128:229–35.
22 Emmert S. Xeroderma pigmentosum, Cockayne syndrome, trichothiodystrophy – defects in DNA repair and carcinogenesis. In: Allgayer H, Rehder H, Fulda S (eds) Hereditary Tumors. Weinheim: Wiley-VCH2009:421–39.

23 DiGiovanna JJ, Kraemer KH. Shining a light on xeroderma pigmentosum. J Invest Dermatol 2012;132:785–96.
24 Bradford PT, Goldstein AM, Tamura D et al. Cancer and neurologic degeneration in xeroderma pigmentosum: long term follow-up characterises the role of DNA repair. J Med Genet 2011;48:168–76.
25 Muramoto O, Mukoyama M, Nonaka I et al. [De Sanctis-Cacchione syndrome: a report of a case and a review of the literature (author's transl)]. Rinsho Shinkeigaku 1981;21:986–92.
26 Fu L, Xu X, Ren R et al. Modeling xeroderma pigmentosum associated neurological pathologies with patients-derived iPSCs. Protein Cell 2016;7:210–21.
27 Viana LM, Seyyedi M, Brewer CC et al. Histopathology of the inner ear in patients with xeroderma pigmentosum and neurologic degeneration. Otol Neurotol 2013;34:1230–6.
28 Melis JP, van Steeg H, Luijten M. Oxidative DNA damage and nucleotide excision repair. Antioxid Redox Signal 2013;18:2409–19.
29 Lagerqvist A, Hakansson D, Lundin C et al. DNA repair and replication influence the number of mutations per adduct of polycyclic aromatic hydrocarbons in mammalian cells. DNA Repair (Amst) 2011;10:877–86.
30 Khan SG, Levy HL, Legerski R et al. Xeroderma pigmentosum group C splice mutation associated with autism and hypoglycinemia. J Invest Dermatol 1998;111:791–6.
31 Lehmann J, Schubert S, Emmert S. Xeroderma pigmentosum: diagnostic procedures, interdisciplinary patient care, and novel therapeutic approaches. J Dtsch Dermatol Ges 2014;12:867–72.
32 Inui H, Oh KS, Nadem C et al. Xeroderma pigmentosum-variant patients from America, Europe, and Asia. J Invest Dermatol 2008;128:2055–68.
33 Tamura D, DiGiovanna JJ, Khan SG et al. Living with xeroderma pigmentosum: comprehensive photoprotection for highly photosensitive patients. Photodermatol Photoimmunol Photomed 2014;30:146–52.
34 Sharquie KE, Ibrahim GA. Is the skin graft immune against new malignancy? J Saudi Soci Dermatol Dermatol Surg 2011;15:73–5.
35 Hess MT, Gunz D, Luneva N et al. Base pair conformation-dependent excision of benzo[a]pyrene diol epoxide-guanine adducts by human nucleotide excision repair enzymes. Mol Cell Biol 1997;17:7069–76.
36 Cafardi JA, Elmets CA. T4 endonuclease V: review and application to dermatology. Expert Opin Biol Ther 2008;8:829–38.
37 Feltes BC, Bonatto D. Overview of xeroderma pigmentosum proteins architecture, mutations and post-translational modifications. Mutat Res Rev Mutat Res 2015;763:306–20.
38 van Steeg H, Kraemer KH. Xeroderma pigmentosum and the role of UV-induced DNA damage in skin cancer. Mol Med Today 1999; 5:86–94.
39 Ito S, Kuraoka I, Chymkowitch P et al. XPG stabilizes TFIIH, allowing transactivation of nuclear receptors: implications for Cockayne syndrome in XP-G/CS patients. Mol Cell 2007;26:231–43.
40 Singh A, Compe E, Le May N et al. TFIIH subunit alterations causing xeroderma pigmentosum and trichothiodystrophy specifically disturb several steps during transcription. Am J Hum Genet 2015; 96:194–207.
41 Ziani S, Nagy Z, Alekseev S et al. Sequential and ordered assembly of a large DNA repair complex on undamaged chromatin. J Cell Biol 2014;206:589–98.
42 Le May N, Fradin D, Iltis I et al. XPG and XPF endonucleases trigger chromatin looping and DNA demethylation for accurate expression of activated genes. Mol Cell 2012;47:622–32.
43 Sugitani N, Sivley RM, Perry KE et al. XPA: a key scaffold for human nucleotide excision repair. DNA Repair (Amst) 2016;44:123–5.
44 Oh KS, Khan SG, Jaspers NG et al. Phenotypic heterogeneity in the XPB DNA helicase gene (ERCC3): xeroderma pigmentosum without and with Cockayne syndrome. Hum Mutat 2006;27:1092–103.
45 Compe E, Egly JM. TFIIH: when transcription met DNA repair. Nat Rev Mol Cell Biol 2012;13:343–54.
46 Ben Rekaya M, Messaoud O, Talmoudi F et al. High frequency of the V548A fs X572 XPC mutation in Tunisia: implication for molecular diagnosis. J Hum Genet 2009;54:426–9.
47 Chavanne F, Broughton BC, Pietra D et al. Mutations in the XPC gene in families with xeroderma pigmentosum and consequences at the cell, protein, and transcript levels. Cancer Res 2000;60:1974–82.
48 Schäfer A, Hofmann L, Gratchev A et al. Molecular genetic analysis of 16 XP-C patients from Germany: environmental factors predominately contribute to phenotype variations. Exp Dermatol 2013;22:24–9.
49 Soufir N, Ged C, Bourillon A et al. A prevalent mutation with founder effect in xeroderma pigmentosum group C from north Africa. J Invest Dermatol 2010;130:1537–42.
50 Robbins JH. Xeroderma pigmentosum. Defective DNA repair causes skin cancer and neurodegeneration. JAMA 1988;260:384–8.
51 Fong YW, Inouye C, Yamaguchi T et al. A DNA repair complex functions as an Oct4/Sox2 coactivator in embryonic stem cells. Cell 2011;147:120–31.
52 Le May N, Egly JM, Coin F. True lies: the double life of the nucleotide excision repair factors in transcription and DNA repair. J Nucleic Acids 2010;2010:1–10.
53 Lehmann AR. The xeroderma pigmentosum group D (XPD) gene: one gene, two functions, three diseases. Genes Dev 2001;15:15–23.
54 Liu H, Rudolf J, Johnson KA et al. Structure of the DNA repair helicase XPD. Cell 2008;133:801–12.
55 Kuper J, Braun C, Elias A et al. In TFIIH, XPD helicase is exclusively devoted to DNA repair. PLoS Biol 2014;12:e1001954.
56 Mathieu N, Kaczmarek N, Ruthemann P et al. DNA quality control by a lesion sensor pocket of the xeroderma pigmentosum group D helicase subunit of TFIIH. Curr Biol 2013;23:204–12.
57 Spies M. DNA repair: trust but verify. Curr Biol 2013;23:R115–7.
58 Matsumoto S, Fischer ES, Yasuda T et al. Functional regulation of the DNA damage-recognition factor DDB2 by ubiquitination and interaction with xeroderma pigmentosum group C protein. Nucleic Acids Res 2015;43:1700–13.
59 Bennett D, Itoh T. The XPE gene of xeroderma pigmentosum, its product and biological roles. Adv Exp Med Biol 2008;637:57–64.
60 Kashiyama K, Nakazawa Y, Pilz DT et al. Malfunction of nuclease ERCC1-XPF results in diverse clinical manifestations and causes Cockayne syndrome, xeroderma pigmentosum, and Fanconi anemia. Am J Hum Genet 2013;92:807–19.
61 Bogliolo M, Schuster B, Stoepker C et al. Mutations in ERCC4, encoding the DNA-repair endonuclease XPF, cause Fanconi anemia. Am J Hum Genet 2013;92:800–6.
62 Niedernhofer LJ, Garinis GA, Raams A et al. A new progeroid syndrome reveals that genotoxic stress suppresses the somatotroph axis. Nature 2006;444:1038–43.
63 Jaspers NG, Raams A, Silengo MC et al. First reported patient with human ERCC1 deficiency has cerebro-oculo-facio-skeletal syndrome with a mild defect in nucleotide excision repair and severe developmental failure. Am J Hum Genet 2007;80:457–66.
64 Kraemer KH, Rünger TM. Genome stability, DNA repair and cancer. In: Wolff K, Goldsmith LA, Katz SI et al. (eds) Fitzpatrick's Dermatology in General Medicine. McGraw-Hill: New York, 2008:977–86.
65 Lehmann J, Schubert S, Schäfer A et al. An unusual mutation in the XPG gene leads to an internal in-frame deletion and a XP/CS complex phenotype. Br J Dermatol 2014;171:903–5.
66 Schäfer A, Schubert S, Gratchev A et al. Characterization of three XPG-defective patients identifies three missense mutations that impair repair and transcription. J Invest Dermatol 2013;133:1841–9.
67 Soltys DT, Rocha CR, Lerner LK et al. Novel XPG (ERCC5) mutations affect DNA repair and cell survival after ultraviolet but not oxidative stress. Hum Mutat 2013;34:481–9.
68 Klungland A, Hoss M, Gunz D et al. Base excision repair of oxidative DNA damage activated by XPG protein. Mol Cell 1999;3:33–42.
69 Gratchev A, Strein P, Utikal J et al. Molecular genetics of Xeroderma pigmentosum variant. Exp Dermatol 2003;12:529–36.
70 Cockayne EA. Dwarfism with retinal atrophy and deafness. Arch Dis Child 1936;11:1–8.
71 Cockayne EA. Dwarfism with retinal atrophy and deafness. Arch Dis Child 1946;21:52–4.
72 Neill CA, Dingwall MM. A syndrome resembling progeria: a review of two cases. Arch Dis Child 1950;25:213–23.
73 Lehmann AR, Thompson AF, Harcourt SA et al. Cockayne's syndrome: correlation of clinical features with cellular sensitivity of RNA synthesis to UV irradiation. J Med Genet 1993;30:679–82.
74 Wilson BT, Stark Z, Sutton RE et al. The Cockayne Syndrome Natural History (CoSyNH) study: clinical findings in 102 individuals and recommendations for care. Genet Med 2016;18:483–93.
75 Wilson DM, 3rd, Bohr VA. Special issue on the segmental progeria Cockayne syndrome. Mech Ageing Dev 2013;134:159–60.
76 Nance MA, Berry SA. Cockayne syndrome: review of 140 cases. Am J Med Genet 1992;42:68–84.
77 Lindenbaum Y, Dickson D, Rosenbaum P et al. Xeroderma pigmentosum/cockayne syndrome complex: first neuropathological study and review of eight other cases. Eur J Paediatr Neurol 2001;5:225–42.
78 Brooks PJ. Blinded by the UV light: how the focus on transcription-coupled NER has distracted from understanding the mechanisms of Cockayne syndrome neurologic disease. DNA Repair (Amst) 2013;12:656–71.

79 Velez-Cruz R, Egly JM. Cockayne syndrome group B (CSB) protein: at the crossroads of transcriptional networks. Mech Ageing Dev 2013;134:234–42.
80 Scheibye-Knudsen M, Croteau DL, Bohr VA. Mitochondrial deficiency in Cockayne syndrome. Mech Ageing Dev 2013;134:275–83.
81 D'Errico M, Pascucci B, Iorio E et al. The role of CSA and CSB protein in the oxidative stress response. Mech Ageing Dev 2013;134:261–9.
82 Wagner AM. Xeroderma pigmentosum, Cockayne's syndrome and trichothiodystrophy. In: Harper J, Oranje A, Prose N (eds) Textbook of Pediatric Dermatology. Wiley-Blackwell: Weinheim, 2006:1557–82.
83 Rastogi RP, Richa, Kumar A et al. Molecular mechanisms of ultraviolet radiation-induced DNA damage and repair. J Nucleic Acids 2010;2010:592980.
84 Yokoyama H, Mizutani R, Satow Y et al. Structure of the DNA (6-4) photoproduct dTT(6-4)TT in complex with the 64M-2 antibody Fab fragment implies increased antibody-binding affinity by the flanking nucleotides. Acta Crystallogr D Biol Crystallogr 2012;68:232–8.
85 Thoms KM, Kuschal C, Emmert S. Lessons learned from DNA repair defective syndromes. Exp Dermatol 2007;16:532–44.
86 Lehmann AR. Three complementation groups in Cockayne syndrome. Mutat Res 1982;106:347–56.
87 Miyauchi H, Horio T, Akaeda T et al. Cockayne syndrome in two adult siblings. J Am Acad Dermatol 1994;30:329–35.
88 Mallery DL, Tanganelli B, Colella S et al. Molecular analysis of mutations in the CSB (ERCC6) gene in patients with Cockayne syndrome. Am J Hum Genet 1998;62:77–85.
89 Saijo M, Hirai T, Ogawa A et al. Functional TFIIH is required for UV-induced translocation of CSA to the nuclear matrix. Mol Cell Biol 2007;27:2538–47.
90 Fischer ES, Scrima A, Bohm K et al. The molecular basis of CRL4DDB2/CSA ubiquitin ligase architecture, targeting, and activation. Cell 2011;147:1024–39.
91 Groisman R, Kuraoka I, Chevallier O et al. CSA-dependent degradation of CSB by the ubiquitin-proteasome pathway establishes a link between complementation factors of the Cockayne syndrome. Genes Dev 2006;20:1429–34.
92 Aamann MD, Muftuoglu M, Bohr VA et al. Multiple interaction partners for Cockayne syndrome proteins: implications for genome and transcriptome maintenance. Mech Ageing Dev 2013;134: 212–24.
93 Beerens N, Hoeijmakers JH, Kanaar R et al. The CSB protein actively wraps DNA. J Biol Chem 2005;280:4722–9.
94 Emmert S, Slor H, Busch DB et al. Relationship of neurologic degeneration to genotype in three xeroderma pigmentosum group G patients. J Invest Dermatol 2002;118:972–82.
95 Rapin I, Lindenbaum Y, Dickson DW et al. Cockayne syndrome and xeroderma pigmentosum. Neurology 2000;55:1442–9.
96 Arab HH, Wani G, Ray A et al. Dissociation of CAK from core TFIIH reveals a functional link between XP-G/CS and the TFIIH disassembly state. PLoS One 2010;5:e11007.
97 Price VH, Odom RB, Ward WH et al. Trichothiodystrophy: sulfur-deficient brittle hair as a marker for a neuroectodermal symptom complex. Arch Dermatol 1980;116:1375–84.
98 Lambert WC, Gagna CE, Lambert MW. Trichothiodystrophy: photosensitive, TTD-P, TTD, Tay syndrome. Adv Exp Med Biol 2010;685:106–10.
99 Stefanini M, Lagomarsini P, Arlett CF et al. Xeroderma pigmentosum (complementation group D) mutation is present in patients affected by trichothiodystrophy with photosensitivity. Hum Genet 1986;74:107–12.
100 Itin PH, Sarasin A, Pittelkow MR. Trichothiodystrophy: update on the sulfur-deficient brittle hair syndromes. J Am Acad Dermatol 2001; 44:891–920; quiz 1–4.
101 Stefanini M, Botta E, Lanzafame M et al. Trichothiodystrophy: from basic mechanisms to clinical implications. DNA Repair (Amst) 2010;9:2–10.
102 Faghri S, Tamura D, Kraemer KH et al. Trichothiodystrophy: a systematic review of 112 published cases characterises a wide spectrum of clinical manifestations. J Med Genet 2008;45:609–21.
103 Brauns B, Schubert S, Lehmann J et al. Photosensitive form of trichothiodystrophy associated with a novel mutation in the XPD gene. Photodermatol Photoimmunol Photomed 2016;32:110–2.
104 Van Neste DJ, Gillespie JM, Marshall RC et al. Morphological and biochemical characteristics of trichothiodystrophy-variant hair are maintained after grafting of scalp specimens on to nude mice. Br J Dermatol 1993;128:384–7.
105 Priolo M, Silengo M, Lerone M et al. Ectodermal dysplasias: not only 'skin' deep. Clin Genet 2000;58:415–30.
106 Cui CY, Schlessinger D. EDA signaling and skin appendage development. Cell Cycle 2006;5:2477–83.
107 Weeda G, Eveno E, Donker I et al. A mutation in the XPB/ERCC3 DNA repair transcription gene, associated with trichothiodystrophy. Am J Hum Genet 1997;60:320–9.
108 Stefanini M, Vermeulen W, Weeda G et al. A new nucleotide-excision-repair gene associated with the disorder trichothiodystrophy. Am J Hum Genet 1993;53:817–21.
109 Giglia-Mari G, Coin F, Ranish JA et al. A new, tenth subunit of TFIIH is responsible for the DNA repair syndrome trichothiodystrophy group A. Nat Genet 2004;36:714–9.
110 Lehmann AR, Bootsma D, Clarkson SG et al. Nomenclature of human DNA repair genes. Mutat Res 1994;315:41–2.
111 Marteijn JA, Lans H, Vermeulen W et al. Understanding nucleotide excision repair and its roles in cancer and ageing. Nat Rev Mol Cell Biol 2014;15:465–81.
112 Theil AF, Hoeijmakers JH, Vermeulen W. TTDA: big impact of a small protein. Exp Cell Res 2014;329:61–8.
113 Botta E, Offman J, Nardo T et al. Mutations in the C7orf11 (TTDN1) gene in six nonphotosensitive trichothiodystrophy patients: no obvious genotype-phenotype relationships. Hum Mutat 2007;28:92–6.
114 Heller ER, Khan SG, Kuschal C et al. Mutations in the TTDN1 gene are associated with a distinct trichothiodystrophy phenotype. J Invest Dermatol 2015;135:734–41.
115 Corbett MA, Dudding-Byth T, Crock PA et al. A novel X-linked trichothiodystrophy associated with a nonsense mutation in RNF113A. J Med Genet 2015;52:269–74.
116 Broughton BC, Berneburg M, Fawcett H et al. Two individuals with features of both xeroderma pigmentosum and trichothiodystrophy highlight the complexity of the clinical outcomes of mutations in the XPD gene. Hum Mol Genet 2001;10:2539–47.
117 Graham JM, Jr., Hennekam R, Dobyns WB et al. MICRO syndrome: an entity distinct from COFS syndrome. Am J Med Genet A 2004;128A:235–45.
118 Graham JM, Jr., Anyane-Yeboa K, Raams A et al. Cerebro-oculo-facio-skeletal syndrome with a nucleotide excision-repair defect and a mutated XPD gene, with prenatal diagnosis in a triplet pregnancy. Am J Hum Genet 2001;69:291–300.
119 Meira LB, Graham JM, Jr., Greenberg CR et al. Manitoba aboriginal kindred with original cerebro-oculo- facio-skeletal syndrome has a mutation in the Cockayne syndrome group B (CSB) gene. Am J Hum Genet 2000;66:1221–8.
120 Hosseini M, Ezzedine K, Taieb A et al. Oxidative and energy metabolism as potential clues for clinical heterogeneity in nucleotide excision repair disorders. J Invest Dermatol 2015;135:341–51.
121 Itoh T, Ono T, Yamaizumi M. A new UV-sensitive syndrome not belonging to any complementation groups of xeroderma pigmentosum or Cockayne syndrome: siblings showing biochemical characteristics of Cockayne syndrome without typical clinical manifestations. Mutat Res 1994;314:233–48.
122 Nardo T, Oneda R, Spivak G et al. A UV-sensitive syndrome patient with a specific CSA mutation reveals separable roles for CSA in response to UV and oxidative DNA damage. Proc Natl Acad Sci U S A 2009;106:6209–14.
123 Horibata K, Iwamoto Y, Kuraoka I et al. Complete absence of Cockayne syndrome group B gene product gives rise to UV-sensitive syndrome but not Cockayne syndrome. Proc Natl Acad Sci U S A 2004;101:15410–5.

Disease susceptibility in heterozygous carriers of defective DNA repair genes

Heterozygous carriers of XP mutations are regarded as 'healthy'. However, in the western world the frequency of such clinically normal individuals (1:500) within the general population is much higher than XP patients (1:1 000 000). Whether individuals who are heterozygous for a mutation in an XP gene are at increased risk of developing a malignancy later in life is unknown. The only study to date of cancer risk in XP heterozygotes was published in 1979, long before the XP genes were cloned [1].

The study was conducted on the pedigrees of XP families. The authors suggested that carriers of one mutated XP allele have an elevated incidence of skin cancer. In addition, and in contrast to humans, mice with a homozygous knockout of the *XPC* gene have a markedly increased susceptibility to UV induction of skin cancer. *XPC* heterozygous mice have an increased cancer susceptibility after prolonged UV exposure [2]. Since 2002 the National Cancer Institute (USA) has been conducting a clinical trial to determine the cancer risk in carriers of mutations in XP genes (NCT00046189).

In the human population, the identification of heterozygous XP gene carriers in early phases of life is hampered by the lack of an easy-to-apply, reliable and high-throughput test system. Recently, at least for XPC, the level of XPC mRNA reduction was correlated with the number of defective XPC alleles [3]. Heterozygous XPC gene mutation carriers exhibit approximately 66% and homozygous diseased XPC patients exhibit maximally 33% of normal XPC mRNA expression. Thus, XPC mRNA levels may be evaluated as a marker of cancer susceptibility in carriers of mutations in the XPC gene who may then be thoroughly protected from UV exposure and followed by a dermatologist during life [4]. Of note, in other human diseases with defects in DNA repair enzymes involved in different repair pathways, heterozygotes do develop late-onset disease symptoms. For example, relatives of ataxia telangiectasia (AT) patients (obligate AT carriers) are more likely to develop breast cancer at an early age. About 1% of the general population are AT carriers [5]. Colorectal cancer is reported to be 2.76 times more likely in carriers of a *BLM* mutation (the gene for Bloom syndrome) compared with disease-free controls in the population of Ashkenazi Jews [6]. The observation that carriers of a single defective BLM allele are cancer prone is supported by results from analyses of a transgenic mouse model [7].

References

1 **Swift M, Chase C. Cancer in families with xeroderma pigmentosum. J Natl Cancer Inst 1979;62:1415–21.**

2 Thoms KM, Kuschal C, Emmert S. Lessons learned from DNA repair defective syndromes. Exp Dermatol 2007;16:532–44.

3 Schäfer A, Hofmann L, Gratchev A et al. Molecular genetic analysis of 16 XP-C patients from Germany: environmental factors predominately contribute to phenotype variations. Exp Dermatol 2013;22:24–9.

4 Khan SG, Oh KS, Shahlavi T et al. Reduced XPC DNA repair gene mRNA levels in clinically normal parents of xeroderma pigmentosum patients. Carcinogenesis 2006;27:84–94.

5 Athma P, Rappaport R, Swift M. Molecular genotyping shows that ataxia-telangiectasia heterozygotes are predisposed to breast cancer. Cancer Genet Cytogenet 1996;92:130–4.

6 Gruber SB, Ellis NA, Scott KK et al. BLM heterozygosity and the risk of colorectal cancer. Science 2002;297:2013.

7 Goss KH, Risinger MA, Kordich JJ et al. Enhanced tumor formation in mice heterozygous for Blm mutation. Science 2002;297:2051–3.

Senescence

Two types of cellular senescence are described in the literature: replicative senescence caused by telomeres shortening [1] and stress-induced senescence [2], which involves DNA damage and/or the overexpression of oncogenes. Cortopassi & Wang were the first to show a positive correlation between the lifespan of fibroblasts of several different species from mouse to human and their DNA repair capacity [3]. Hart & Setlow showed that the rate of nucleotide excision repair capacity is proportional to the logarithm of the lifespan [4]. Furthermore, the involvement of DNA damage response in senescence was clearly demonstrated by *p53*-dependent senescence [5] as well as a $p16^{Ink4a}$-dependent ageing process [6]. DNA repair and transcription deficiency were related to premature ageing in mice. The loss of proliferative capacity defines cellular senescence. Senescence-associated DNA damage foci mediate the signalling for permanent growth arrest in the vicinity of different DNA lesions. The two kinases, 'ataxia telangiectasia mutated' (ATM) and 'ataxia telangiectasia and Rad3 related' (ATR), are such DNA damage response factors mediating senescence. *ATM* as well as *ATR* deficiency lead to accelerated ageing [7] and stem cell loss [8] in mice, respectively. Both enzymes play a critical role in early signal transmission after DNA damage. Interestingly, accelerated skin ageing can result from the combination of psoralens plus UVA (PUVA) irradiation commonly used for the treatment of different skin disorders. Interstrand cross-links are induced by PUVA treatment, leading to stalled replication forks which are repaired in dependency of the NER machinery [9] and by themselves activate the *ATR* kinase. Premature cellular senescence in human dermal fibroblasts is also induced by PUVA. This depends on *ATR* which is essential to induce and maintain the senescent cellular phenotype [10]. Additionally, the DNA damage response cascade involves manifold secondary protein modifications with implications for senescence and ageing. Ubiquitin-Spezific Protease 3 (USP3) deubiquitinates histones and is involved in maintenance of the haematopoietic stem cell reservoir as well as chromosomal stability and ageing in mice [11]. N-terminal RCC1 methyltransferase 1 (NRMT1) was shown to be involved in methylation of DNA damage binding protein 2 (DDB2) during NER [12] with implications for premature ageing in mice [13]. Under increased oxidative stress the presence of DDB2 is more important for controlled cellular senescence than DDB2 secondary protein modifications [14]. The accumulation of reactive oxygen species is important for the induction of premature senescence as well as posttranslational modifications like glycation, which enhances the insolubility of proteins [15]. Accumulation of oxidized glycated proteins ('glycoxidation') is known to be involved in Alzheimer's disease [16]. Further involvement of NER factors in the ageing process is demonstrated by the phenotype of CS as well as TTD patients (see previously). The factors associated with basal transcription, like CS-proteins or TTDA, were shown to be especially essential for normal ageing and senescence in mutant mice, thereby mimicking phenotypes observed in humans [17]. Nevertheless, accumulation of DNA damage, hence genome instability, can be regarded as the initial trigger from cellular senescence to systemic (normal or pathological) ageing. As a first step, senescence exhausts the pool progenitor cells or stem cells, which leads to decline of tissue homeostasis and to progress in organ ageing [18,19].

Secondly, senescence induces tissue degeneration especially in neural cells which leads a disturbed endocrine/exocrine system followed by unbalanced hormone depletion and accelerated organ ageing, as is demonstrated by, for example, CS patients (see previously). The third consequence of senescence is chronic inflammation, found in aged mice as well as in aged individuals, for example by monitoring proinflammatory factors like interleukin-6 levels [20,21]. Taken together, these developments on a cellular level will trigger changes in the immune response and in the vascular system and finally lead to mitochondrial dysfunction (see later), intercellular malfunctions in communication and nutrition sensing, and finally organ/tissue ageing [17,22].

References

1 **Campisi J. Senescent cells, tumor suppression, and organismal aging: good citizens, bad neighbors. Cell 2005;120:513–22.**
2 Courtois-Cox S, Jones SL, Cichowski K. Many roads lead to oncogene-induced senescence. Oncogene 2008;27:2801–9.
3 Cortopassi GA, Wang E. There is substantial agreement among interspecies estimates of DNA repair activity. Mech Ageing Dev 1996;91:211–8.
4 Hart RW, Setlow RB. Correlation between deoxyribonucleic acid excision -repair and life-span in a number of mammalian species. Proc Natl Acad Sci U S A 1974:2169–73.
5 Tyner SD, Venkatachalam S, Choi J et al. p53 mutant mice that display early ageing-associated phenotypes. Nature 2002;415:45–53.
6 Baker DJ, Wijshake T, Tchkonia T et al. Clearance of p16Ink4a-positive senescent cells delays ageing-associated disorders. Nature 2011; 479:232–6.
7 Wong KK, Maser RS, Bachoo RM et al. Telomere dysfunction and Atm deficiency compromises organ homeostasis and accelerates ageing. Nature 2003;421:643–8.
8 Ruzankina Y, Pinzon-Guzman C, Asare A et al. Deletion of the developmentally essential gene ATR in adult mice leads to age-related phenotypes and stem cell loss. Cell Stem Cell 2007;1:113–26.
9 Moldovan GL, D'Andrea AD. How the fanconi anemia pathway guards the genome. Annu Rev Genet 2009;43:223–49.
10 Thoms KM, Kuschal C, Emmert S. Lessons learned from DNA repair defective syndromes. Exp Dermatol 2007;16:532–44.
11 Lancini C, van den Berk PC, Vissers JH et al. Tight regulation of ubiquitin-mediated DNA damage response by USP3 preserves the functional integrity of hematopoietic stem cells. J Exp Med 2014;211:1759–77.
12 Cai Q, Fu L, Wang Z et al. alpha-N-methylation of damaged DNA-binding protein 2 (DDB2) and its function in nucleotide excision repair. J Biol Chem 2014;289:16046–56.
13 Bonsignore LA, Tooley JG, Van Hoose PM et al. NRMT1 knockout mice exhibit phenotypes associated with impaired DNA repair and premature aging. Mech Ageing Dev 2015;146–148:42–52.
14 Roy N, Stoyanova T, Dominguez-Brauer C et al. DDB2, an essential mediator of premature senescence. Mol Cell Biol 2010;30:2681–92.
15 Soskic V, Groebe K, Schrattenholz A. Nonenzymatic posttranslational protein modifications in ageing. Exp Gerontol 2008;43:247–57.
16 Gella A, Durany N. Oxidative stress in Alzheimer disease. Cell Adh Migr 2009;3:88–93.
17 Vermeij WP, Hoeijmakers JH, Pothof J. Genome Integrity in Aging: Human Syndromes, Mouse Models, and Therapeutic Options. Annu Rev Pharmacol Toxicol 2016;56:427–45.
18 Goodell MA, Rando TA. Stem cells and healthy aging. Science 2015;350:1199–204.
19 Lee HW, Blasco MA, Gottlieb GJ et al. Essential role of mouse telomerase in highly proliferative organs. Nature 1998;392:569–74.
20 Starr ME, Evers BM, Saito H. Age-associated increase in cytokine production during systemic inflammation: adipose tissue as a major source of IL-6. J Gerontol A Biol Sci Med Sci 2009;64:723–30.
21 Maggio M, Guralnik JM, Longo DL et al. Interleukin-6 in aging and chronic disease: a magnificent pathway. J Gerontol A Biol Sci Med Sci 2006;61:575–84.
22 Pan MR, Li K, Lin SY et al. Connecting the dots: from DNA damage and repair to aging. Int J Mol Sci 2016;17:p.ii: E685.

Mitochondrial repair

In the past, most studies focused on nuclear DNA repair. A growing body of evidence is developing to suggest that even repair of mitochondrial DNA is connected with diseases. Mitochondrial DNA (mtDNA) damage may result in congenital disorders, ageing, photoaging and carcinogenesis [1]. The main function of mitochondria is the generation of energy for the cell. This is accomplished by the respiratory chain which is located at the inner mitochondrial membrane. The mitochondrial DNA exists in about 4–10 copies per mitochondrion and comprises a 16559 bp double-stranded circular molecule. Congenital disorders like Kearns–Sayre syndrome, Alzheimer disease and diabetes in addition to ageing are associated with a common 4977 bp deletion in the mitochondrial genome, which was also found in hair samples in an age-dependent manner [2]. Several mechanisms similar to nuclear DNA repair exist for the repair of mtDNA damage. The best characterized mechanism in mitochondria is BER of oxidative DNA damage. In addition, MMR activities, repair of DNA double-strand breaks (DSBR) as well as NER have been demonstrated in purified human mitochondria [3]. In comparison to 6-4PPs, the elimination of UV-induced CPDs was very much slower in mtDNA [4]. However, there is a reduced repair capacity of 8-oxoguanine in mitochondrial extracts of *CSB*-deficient cells [5]. The *CSB* protein is a component of the basal transcription machinery and NER. Homozygous knock-in mice expressing a proof reading-deficient polymerase γ, which is involved in all repair processes of mitochondria, exhibit an ageing phenotype characterized by progeroid symptoms such as weight loss, kyphosis, osteoporosis, alopecia and subcutaneous fat reduction [6]. Recent findings correlated the interplay between the occurrence of DNA breaks in mtDNA, cellular NAD^+/NADH levels, mitochondrial maintenance and neuronal degeneration [7]. NAD^+ is the rate-limiting substrate for the epigenetic regulator Sirtuin 1 (SIRT1) and poly(ADP-ribose)-polymerase 1 (PARP1), initiator of PARylation, both with comparable K_m values [8–10]. Hence, both enzymes compete for the same substrate with nearly the same affinity. PARP1 detects DNA breaks and initiates a DNA repair cascade by flagging these sites through generation of PAR. SIRT1 is a major deacetylase in nuclei and mitochondria with a variety of substrates. Several animal models for ageing and DNA repair diseases (nematodes, mice) and human cells (e.g. CS cells, XPA patient cells) showed persisting hyperactivation of PAR and low SIRT1 activity, which, for example, deacetylates XPA during NER [7,8,11,12]. This imbalance is furthermore associated with the pathogenesis of certain diseases like Alzheimer disease or Parkinson disease. However, NAD^+ level is crucial for this tightly regulated interplay and is consumed by cells during normal and accelerated ageing, which leads to acetyl coenzyme A (acetyl-CoA) production [13]. Interestingly, acetyl-CoA is increased by fasting or ketogenic diets, which were also found to increase lifespan (healthspan) in, for example, worms, mice and humans [14]. Taken together, PARylation is an important process for maintenance of mtDNA integrity, but persisting PAR activation inhibits necessary epigenetic remodelling activities of SIRT1 and leads to mitochondrial dysfunction, which is a major feature of ageing and neurodegenerative diseases like XP with neurological symptoms or Cockayne syndrome [7,15,16].

References

1 Thoms KM, Kuschal C, Emmert S. Lessons learned from DNA repair defective syndromes. Exp Dermatol 2007;16:532–44.
2 Zheng Y, Luo X, Zhu J et al. Mitochondrial DNA 4977 bp deletion is a common phenomenon in hair and increases with age. Bosn J Basic Med Sci 2012;12:187–92.
3 Fang EF, Scheibye-Knudsen M, Chua KF et al. Nuclear DNA damage signalling to mitochondria in ageing. Nat Rev Mol Cell Biol 2016;17:308–21.
4 Lee MH, Wang L, Chang ZF. The contribution of mitochondrial thymidylate synthesis in preventing the nuclear genome stress. Nucleic Acids Res 2014;42:4972–84.
5 Stevnsner T, Nyaga S, de Souza-Pinto NC et al. Mitochondrial repair of 8-oxoguanine is deficient in Cockayne syndrome group B. Oncogene 2002;21:8675–82.
6 Kujoth GC, Bradshaw PC, Haroon S et al. The role of mitochondrial DNA mutations in mammalian aging. PLoS Genet 2007;3:e24.
7 Fang EF, Scheibye-Knudsen M, Brace LE et al. Defective mitophagy in XPA via PARP-1 hyperactivation and NAD(+)/SIRT1 reduction. Cell 2014;157:882–96.
8 Canto C, Menzies KJ, Auwerx J. NAD(+) Metabolism and the Control of Energy Homeostasis: A Balancing Act between Mitochondria and the Nucleus. Cell Metab 2015;22:31–53.
9 Gibson BA, Kraus WL. New insights into the molecular and cellular functions of poly(ADP-ribose) and PARPs. Nat Rev Mol Cell Biol 2012;13:411–24.
10 Rodgers JT, Lerin C, Haas W et al. Nutrient control of glucose homeostasis through a complex of PGC-1alpha and SIRT1. Nature 2005;434:113–8.
11 Mouchiroud L, Houtkooper RH, Moullan N et al. The NAD(+)/sirtuin pathway modulates longevity through activation of mitochondrial UPR and FOXO signaling. Cell 2013;154:430–41.
12 Fan W, Luo J. SIRT1 regulates UV-induced DNA repair through deacetylating XPA. Mol Cell 2010;39:247–58.
13 Ross JM, Oberg J, Brene S et al. High brain lactate is a hallmark of aging and caused by a shift in the lactate dehydrogenase A/B ratio. Proc Natl Acad Sci U S A 2010;107:20087–92.
14 Longo VD, Mattson MP. Fasting: molecular mechanisms and clinical applications. Cell Metab 2014;19:181–92.
15 Scheibye-Knudsen M, Mitchell SJ, Fang EF et al. A high-fat diet and NAD(+) activate Sirt1 to rescue premature aging in cockayne syndrome. Cell Metab 2014;20:840–55.
16 Scheibye-Knudsen M, Ramamoorthy M, Sykora P et al. Cockayne syndrome group B protein prevents the accumulation of damaged mitochondria by promoting mitochondrial autophagy. J Exp Med 2012;209:855–69.

Novel therapeutic strategies/DNA repair creams

Studying NER-defective syndromes may lead to the development of new therapeutic approaches. For example, a delivery system has been studied over the last decade that utilizes the packaging of repair enzymes into liposomes that can be applied to the skin as a hydrogel lotion on a regular basis. Any repair enzyme at a defined concentration and frequency could be delivered with this technique to epidermal skin cells. This offers a new dimension in topical dermatotherapy. The efficacy of a T4 endonuclease liposomal therapy was investigated in 30 XP patients in a first prospective pilot study [1]. In XP patients who applied the repair cream, 68% and 30% reductions in the development of actinic keratoses and basal cell cancers, respectively, were documented. This demonstrates that improved DNA repair inhibits tumour promotion as well as tumour progression. The efficacy of this treatment in skin cancer prevention in renal transplant patients is currently under investigation [2]. Stege and colleagues investigated the efficacy of the liposomal encapsulated repair enzyme photolyase in DNA damage reversion [3]. The enzyme specifically binds to cyclobutane-pyrimidine dimers and can separate the dimer into the original monomers (direct reversion, only in prokaryotes). This treatment reduced the content of cyclobutane-pyrimidine dimers in the UVB-irradiated skin of 19 healthy volunteers by up to 45%. In addition, the extent of UVB-induced skin erythema was reduced.

More recently, topical antibiotics have been applied to attempt to facilitate 'read-through' of stop codon mutations. *In vitro*, Kuschal and colleagues could show that, for example, gentamycin can overcome stop codon mutations in the XPC gene resulting in the expression of some wildtype full length XPC mRNA, and enhanced cellular DNA repair [4]. Thus, application of antibiotic creams could be beneficial in XP patients harbouring stop codon mutations in postponing skin cancer development. However, a clinical trial to approve such a treatment approach is needed [5].

Thus, clinical and molecular studies of DNA repair defective syndromes may have great implications for the normal population and lead to novel approaches for disease prevention, genetic susceptibility testing, disease diagnostics and more individualized therapeutic strategies.

Acknowledgement

Steffen Emmert is supported by the European Union (EU grant number ESF/14-BM-A55), the Deutsche Forschungsgemeinschaft, the Deutsche Krebshilfe e.V., the Damp Foundation, the Niedersächsische Krebsgesellschaft e.V., the Heinz und Heide Dürr Stiftung, the Wilhelm Sander Stiftung, the Claudia von Schilling Foundation for Breast Cancer Research, and the Bundesministerium für Wirtschaft und Technologie.

References

1 Yarosh D, Klein J, O'Connor A et al. Effect of topically applied T4 endonuclease V in liposomes on skin cancer in xeroderma pigmentosum: a randomised study. Xeroderma Pigmentosum Study Group. Lancet 2001;357:926–9.
2 Yarosh DB. DNA repair, immunosuppression, and skin cancer. Cutis 2004;74(5 Suppl):10–3.
3 Stege H, Roza L, Vink AA et al. Enzyme plus light therapy to repair DNA damage in ultraviolet-B-irradiated human skin. Proc Natl Acad Sci U S A 2000;97:1790–5.
4 Kuschal C, DiGiovanna JJ, Khan SG et al. Repair of UV photolesions in xeroderma pigmentosum group C cells induced by translational readthrough of premature termination codons. Proc Natl Acad Sci U S A 2013;110:19483–8.
5 Lehmann J, Schubert S, Emmert S. Xeroderma pigmentosum: diagnostic procedures, interdisciplinary patient care, and novel therapeutic approaches. J Dtsch Dermatol Ges 2014;12:867–72.

CHAPTER 139

Gorlin (Naevoid Basal Cell Carcinoma) Syndrome

Kai Ren Ong[1] *& Peter A. Farndon*[2]

[1]West Midlands Regional Clinical Genetics Service, Birmingham Women's Hospital, Birmingham, UK
[2]University of Birmingham, Birmingham, UK

Abstract

Gorlin syndrome is a rare inherited genodermatosis characterized by the development of multiple basal cell carcinomas (BCCs), odontogenic keratocysts in the mandible and maxilla, and other dermatological and nondermatological features. Palmar pits and ectopic calcification of the falx cerebri are also major diagnostic features. Typical facial characteristics and macrocephaly are common. Intellectual development is affected only in a small minority and lifespan is not usually shortened. Wide phenotypic variability is seen both between and within families. Skin type and sun exposure influences the development of BCCs. Gorlin syndrome is inherited in an autosomal dominant manner and is associated with mutations in the *PTCH1* and *SUFU* genes. Mutation analysis of these genes is an important diagnostic test. The mainstay of treatment is surgical enucleation of odontogenic keratocysts and surgical or medical treatment of BCCs, with the avoidance of radiotherapy which raises the risk of BCCs in the radiation field.

Key points

- **Gorlin syndrome is a rare inherited genodermatosis characterized by the development of multiple basal cell carcinomas (BCCs), odontogenic keratocysts in the mandible and maxilla, and other dermatological and nondermatological features.**
- **Palmar pits and ectopic calcification of the falx cerebri are also major diagnostic features.**
- **Typical facial characteristics and macrocephaly are common. Intellectual development is affected only in a small minority and lifespan is not usually shortened.**
- **Wide phenotypic variability is seen both between and within families.**
- **Skin type and sun exposure influences the development of BCCs.**
- **Gorlin syndrome is inherited in an autosomal dominant manner and is associated with mutations in the *PTCH1* and *SUFU* genes. Mutation analysis of these genes is an important diagnostic test.**
- **The mainstay of treatment is surgical enucleation of odontogenic keratocysts and surgical or medical treatment of BCCs, with the avoidance of radiotherapy which raises the risk of BCCs in the radiation field.**

Definition. The three main components of the Gorlin syndrome (naevoid basal cell carcinoma or NBCC syndrome) are multiple basal cell carcinomas (BCCs), recurrent jaw cysts and nonprogressive skeletal anomalies. Other hallmarks are palmar and plantar pits, ectopic calcification and an increased incidence of congenital malformations. It is a fully penetrant autosomal dominant disorder with extremely variable expression, both within and between families. Not only does the variability manifest itself in the presence or absence of a particular feature, but also in its severity.

Adult patients with the Gorlin syndrome may present to any specialty, because there are over 100 recognized features. In the absence of a family history, most children are diag-nosed because of jaw cysts, a (usually unexpected) histological diagnosis of BCC in a biopsied skin lesion or skeletal anomalies found on radiographs taken for other medical reasons. Occasionally, a child may present with hundreds of 'naevi' but it is unusual for aggressive BCCs to be the presenting feature in childhood [1].

Another common name for the syndrome is basal cell naevus syndrome but this name is inappropriate because, histologically, the naevi are BCCs rather than naevi, although not all behave aggressively. It has also been suggested that it be known as the NBCC syndrome, although 10% of adults do not develop BCCs. Rather than focus on one feature of the condition, it may be better to use the eponymous title of Gorlin syndrome, in recognition of Professor Robert Gorlin's contributions, especially because parents and patients prefer not to have a condition that contains the word 'carcinoma'.

History. Skeletal signs of the syndrome have been found in Egyptian mummies, presumed to be father and son [2]. The first reported cases appear to be those of Jarisch and White in 1894 [3,4].

The term 'basal cell naevus' was coined by Nomland [5] when he reported an unusual case of invasive BCC of the face that occurred in adult life from congenital pigmented basal cell tumours. Clinically, the tumours resembled melanocytic naevi; microscopically the cells

Harper's Textbook of Pediatric Dermatology, Fourth Edition. Edited by Peter Hoeger, Veronica Kinsler and Albert Yan.

were 'like dark staining basal cells'. Thus, the name 'naevus of basal cells' was used.

Gorlin and Goltz's description of two patients and review of the literature in 1960 [6] drew the condition to wide attention. However, Howell and Caro in the dermatological literature in 1959 [7] had attempted to correlate the clinical features of the unusual tumours in the syndrome with the interpretations that then prevailed and introduced the term 'basal cell naevus syndrome'. For many years, clinicians had puzzled over rare cases of multiple tumours that, histologically, seemed to be epithelioma adenoides cysticum, but clinically behaved like rodent ulcers. Some believed that the tumours were unique, whereas others believed that they were epithelioma adenoides cysticum transformed into rodent ulcers. Howell and Caro proposed that the tumours were a unique type of BCC that was capable of aggressive behaviour in adults, and which was associated with developmental anomalies. They pointed out that the harmless clinical appearance of the tumours, especially in childhood, contrasted strikingly with the microscopic appearance and destructive behaviour of tumours in adulthood. They also felt that although ionizing radiation was curative, its use was not prudent because of the multiplicity of tumours and the concern over new ones erupting in the irradiated area. Mason and colleagues [8] proposed the term 'naevoid basal cell carcinoma syndrome' because of the confusion over the term 'naevus'.

Gorlin presented extensive reviews of the syndrome in 1987 [9] and 1995 [10], combining information from a personal series of patients and a review of 216 papers.

Aetiology and pathogenesis. A population-based study in north-west England in 1991 gave a minimum prevalence of 1 in 55 600 [11]; the latest figures from that continuing study are 1 in 30 827 prevalence and birth incidence 1 in 18 976 [12]. A study in Australia gave a minimum prevalence of 1 in 164 000 [13].

Rahbari and Mehregan [14] reported a group of 59 children under the age of 19 years with a histologically proven BCC; 10 had a BCC that had developed in a preexisting naevus sebaceous. Of the others, 13 (26%) had features of Gorlin syndrome. Two other children were developing a second BCC but they had no signs of the syndrome on radiograph or examination.

The syndrome is an autosomal dominant condition, each child of a parent with the condition having a probability of 1 in 2 that he or she will inherit Gorlin syndrome.

A new mutation rate of up to 40% has been suggested [15] and a paternal age effect reported [16]. The new mutation rate obtained from the literature may be an overestimate because not all parents were thoroughly investigated and the intrafamilial expression is variable. The authors know of several families whose child was considered to have a new mutation until careful examination confirmed that one of the parents had the syndrome, albeit with very mild features.

Gorlin syndrome is associated with the *patched (PTCH1)* gene which is located at 9q22.3 [17–19]. There had been no evidence of genetic heterogeneity until the publication of a single Chinese family with a missense mutation in *PTCH2* which segregated with the condition [20], and a further case report of a 13-year-old girl with a frameshift mutation and characteristic clinical features [21]. *PTCH2* is highly homologous to *PTCH1* and is located on 1p32.1–32.2 [22]. No mutations were found in 11 sporadic and 11 familial NBCC patients in whom PTCH screening by single strand conformational polymorphism had been negative and the role of *PTCH2* remains to be fully elucidated. Clinical testing is initially focused on *PTCH1*.

Mutations in the *SUFU* gene have also been found in patients with features of Gorlin syndrome. The first mutation reported was a splice-site mutation in a child who was diagnosed with a medulloblastoma at 8 months. Both father and son had macrocephaly and pits; the father at age 37 had falx calcification [23]. Further mutations have been found in families with features of Gorlin syndrome and medulloblastoma, suggesting a particularly high frequency of medulloblastoma associated with *SUFU* mutations compared with *PTCH1* mutations [24].

The patched gene and the hedgehog signalling pathway
The *PTCH1* gene was isolated by positional cloning in 1996 [25,26]. PTCH is a component of the hedgehog signalling pathway, a pathway that is particularly critical in cellular growth and differentiation during embryonic development. Inherited or sporadic mutations in genes in this pathway have been implicated in a number of human birth defects and adult cancers [27–29].

Spectrum of mutations. The human *PTCH1* gene has 23 exons covering 62 kb of genomic DNA. It encodes an integral membrane protein of 1500 amino acids with 12 transmembrane regions and two extracellular loops that are required for binding with the extracellular protein, Sonic Hedgehog (SHH) (Fig. 139.1). When SHH is absent, PTCH suppresses the activation of smoothened (SMO), a 7-span transmembrane protein, resulting in repression of transcription of downstream genes (Fig. 139.2a). In normal tissues, human PTCH has three transcripts that are differentially regulated, encoding proteins that confer different levels of inhibition [30].

When extracellular SHH binds to PTCH, the inhibition of SMO is released, activating the signalling pathway and transcription of downstream target genes (Fig. 139.2b).

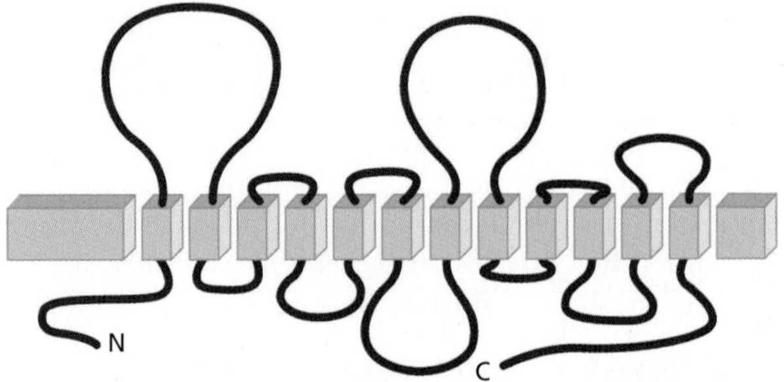

Fig. 139.1 Predicted human PTCH protein structure. PATCHED encodes a 12-pass transmembrane glycoprotein with two large extracellular domains and a smaller intracellular domain. C, carboxyl terminus; N, amino terminus.

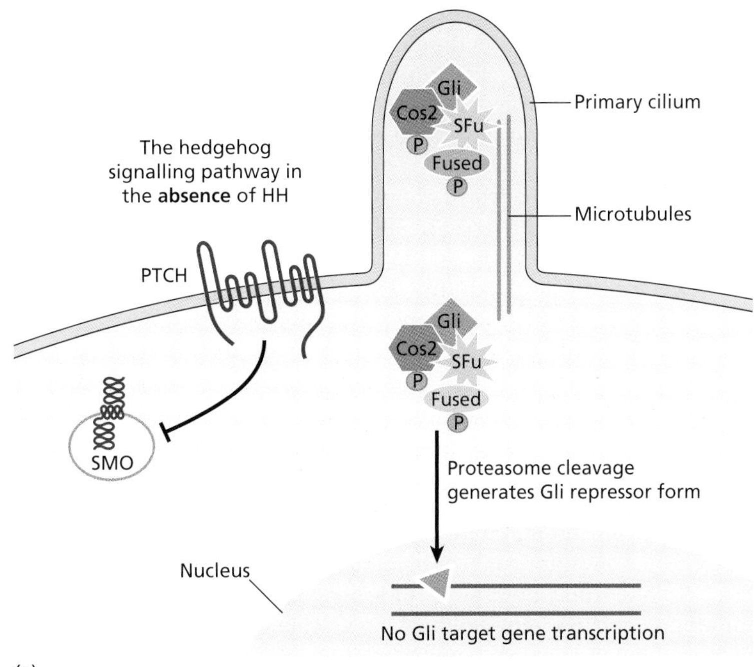

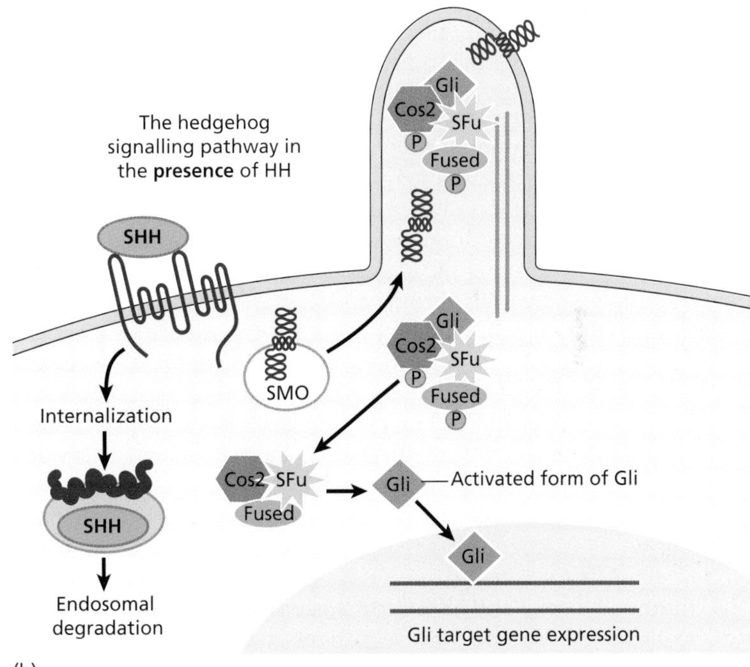

Fig. 139.2 The HH–PTCH–SMO pathway (a postulated view incorporating information from *Drosophila*, mouse and human). (a) In cells not exposed to HH, PTCH blocks SMO from entering the primary cilium and becoming activated. The activation of Gli (part of a tetrameric complex at the microtubules) is inhibited. (b) In the presence of hedgehog, the inhibition of SMO by PTCH is released and SMO migrates from intracellular endosomes to the cell membrane of the cilium. SMO is activated in the cilium and activates a signal transduction cascade resulting in mature active Gli being released from the tetrameric complex to promote transcription of target genes. The patched/hedgehog complex is internalized and degraded or destabilized.

GLi is colocalized with the SUFU protein, which inhibits the transcriptional activating function of GLi. Mutations in the *SUFU* gene abrogate this effect.

The SHH–PTCH–GLi pathway appears to be sensitive to the levels of its various proteins. Any mutation or polymorphism in one or more of the genes may affect the amount of functional protein, so affecting the activation or repression of downstream genes. A wide range of variation in transcription could therefore result from different levels of activity of PTCH. There is experimental evidence for this: complete inactivation of one allele (resulting in 50% patched activity) leads to the features of Gorlin syndrome in mice [31] and *PTCH* missense alleles produce active proteins but with reduced activities [32]. That the pathway is dosage sensitive may explain the spectrum of clinical presentation, as seen between and within families in Gorlin syndrome.

The jaw cysts and BCCs in Gorlin syndrome are associated, however, with a different mechanism – loss of function of the usual *PTCH1* allele [33,34], thereby releasing the cell from the remaining control of the SHH–PTCH–GLi pathway exerted by that allele. In fact, inactivation of PTCH or oncogenic activation of SMO occurs in almost all nonsyndromic BCCs as well, suggesting that dysregulation of SHH signalling is a prerequisite for BCC formation [29].

A wide spectrum of *PTCH1* mutations has been found in patients with Gorlin syndrome [35]. The mutations are spread throughout the whole coding region, with no apparent clustering.

Mutations are detected in about 75% of patients who meet the diagnostic criteria [36,37]. The authors' experience is that the detection rate is lowest in people who are the first affected individual in their family, most probably because of somatic mosaicism. The mutation may often be more easily detected if an affected child is tested. For patients in whom there is a clinical suspicion of mosaicism, detecting the same *PTCH1* mutation in several tumours but not in lymphocyte DNA may confirm this.

The frequency of classes of mutations in *PTCH1*, obtained from the literature [25,26,37–41] and the DNA Diagnostic Laboratory at Birmingham Women's Hospital, UK, is 65% truncating, 16% missense, 13% splice site mutations and 6% intragenic or large-scale deletions or rearrangements.

There appears to be no genotype–phenotype correlation with truncating mutations [41]. It is not possible to make predictions about clinical severity for developmental and neoplastic features associated with specific mutations because of the likely modifying effects of other genes and environmental factors.

PTCH1 germline mutations have not been associated with any other heritable syndromes, but somatic mutations have been found in a range of sporadically occurring tumours including those observed in Gorlin syndrome: nonsyndromic BCC, skin trichoepithelioma, medulloblastoma, ovarian fibroma and keratocysts.

Missense mutations of *PTCH1* have been reported in 5% of unrelated probands with holoprosencephaly [42]. The authors hypothesized that the missense mutations would lead to enhanced PTCH repressive activity on the hedgehog signalling pathway, unlike the mechanism in NBCC in which the pathway is activated.

Pathology.

Histology of BCCs

The childhood 'naevi' and NBCCs are histologically identical to BCCs. About one-third of patients have two or more types of NBCCs, including superficial, multicentric, solid, cystic, adenoid and lattice-like [43]. NBCCs are more commonly associated with melanin pigmentation and foci of calcification than nonsyndromic BCCs, but otherwise cannot be distinguished [8,44].

Histology of jaw cysts

The histological features of jaw cysts are characteristic [45]. The cysts are lined by a parakeratotic stratified squamous epithelium, which is usually about 5–8 cell layers thick and without rete ridges. Rarely, the form of keratinization is orthokeratotic. The basal layer is well defined with regularly orientated palisaded cells. Satellite cysts, epithelial rests and proliferating dental lamina are sometimes seen in the cyst capsules.

Palmar and plantar pits

The pits appear to be caused by premature desquamation of horny cells along the intercellular spaces, but are not caused by degeneration of the horny cells themselves. Light microscopy reveals a lack of keratinization of pit tissue and a proliferation of basaloid cells in irregular rete ridges [46].

Electron microscopy [47] showed that the epithelium at the base of the pits consists of keratinocytes containing poorly developed tonofibrils. Discharge of cementsomes from the horny cells was incomplete, which the authors suggested was perhaps caused by a shortened transit time of keratinocytes.

Scanning electron microscopy [46] showed the stratum corneum overlying the epithelium at the bases of the pits to be thin, irregular and containing large defects. The stratum corneum at the margins of the pits was thicker, more compact and more adherent. The pit walls descended from a gently rounded top to a point of sharp transition between pit epithelium and normal epithelium.

Response to radiation. As some patients respond to therapeutic irradiation by later developing crops of BCCs in the treated area, *in vitro* studies of cellular radiation hypersensitivity have been undertaken, with conflicting results. It appears, however, that the cancer susceptibility is neither caused by nor manifested as chromosome instability, or that increased cell killing is a major effect of the gene.

Little and colleagues [48] demonstrated a moderate degree of radiation hypersensitivity in one family member whereas the remaining affected and nonaffected individuals from the same family responded normally. They suggested that isolated cases of *in vitro* radiation hypersensitivity might not relate to the underlying genetic disorder. It seems likely that the response to radiation may be affected by other genes of major effect, and their delineation by comparing family members with the syndrome would be useful research.

There is supporting evidence in an animal model for the adverse effects of radiation. With age, mice heterozygous for an inactivating *PTCH* mutation spontaneously developed BCC-like tumours [49]. However, the BCCs were of far greater number and size in mice that had received ultraviolet irradiation. A single dose of ionizing radiation markedly enhanced development of BCCs [49].

Ultraviolet radiation

Circumstantial evidence that exposure to sunlight may be deleterious comes from population studies: 14% of cases in a north-west England study [11] developed a BCC before the age of 20 years, compared with 47% in Australia (G. Trench, personal communication).

Laboratory experiments with ultraviolet (UV) radiation, however, have been inconclusive. Fibroblasts have been found to have no differences in sensitivity [50] following ultraviolet C (UVC), whereas others were more sensitive to UVC [51].

The majority of experiments have been conducted with UVC radiation (254 nm), but epidemiological and clinical studies indicate that UVB radiation (280–320 nm) in sunlight is responsible for the induction of most skin cancers in humans.

Gorlin syndrome fibroblasts have been shown to be hypersensitive to killing by UVB but not UVC radiation [52,53] compared with skin fibroblasts from normal individuals. This was not caused by a defect in the excision repair of pyrimidine dimers [53].

Clinical features and natural history. The major features of the syndrome which present in childhood are shown in Table 139.1, compiled from a review of the literature and from the clinical experience of one of the authors (P.F.) of over 200 patients, many of whom have been followed for more than 15 years Some features are described in more detail below. Several large studies all give similar results [11,13,54,55].

Developmental history

In a series of 25 children of pre- or school-age 62% had an operative delivery [56]. The average birthweight was 4.1 kg and head circumference was 38 cm, both greatly increased when compared with siblings. Walking was delayed until an average of 18 months; siblings walked at 12–13 months. Several children had investigations for hydrocephalus because of striking macrocephaly – the head circumference was grossly above the 97th centile but growth continued parallel with the centile lines. Many children initially have a motor delay, but appear to catch up. All children known to the authors have attended mainstream school, with a few needing additional help.

In the literature, 'mental retardation' has been reported in about 3% [57]. In the population study in the northwest of England, there were no cases of moderate or severe mental retardation in 84 cases [11], apart from treated cases of medulloblastoma. About 6% of patients in that study required prolonged anticonvulsant therapy for grand mal seizures.

Build

Patients tend to be tall [58]. Their heights are usually above the 97th centile, often in marked contrast with unaffected siblings. Some patients exhibit a marfanoid build [59].

Shape and size of cranium

One of the most striking features is the increased head size present from birth. All children and adults in a series of 75 [56] had a head circumference on or above the 97th centile and above the corresponding centile line for height. The head gives the appearance of being long in the anteroposterior (AP) plane, with a prominent and low occiput.

Facial appearance

About 70% of patients have the characteristic facies but there is intrafamilial variation [56]. Figures 139.3 and 139.4 show children and an adult with the syndrome. Frontal, temporal and biparietal bossing in 80% give a prominent appearance to the upper part of the face, and patients

Table 139.1 Frequency of features in childhood Gorlin syndrome by organ system

Features	%
Skin	
Milia	42
Meibomian cysts	6
Epidermal cysts	44
Skin tags	6
Palmar pits	
<10 years	65
<15 years	80
Plantar pits	49
'Naevi'[a] <20 years	53
Basal cell carcinomas[b]	
<20 years	14
>20 years	73
>40 years	92
Jaw cysts	
10 years	13
20 years	51
>40 years	79–90
Misshapen/missing teeth	30
Skeletal	
High arched palate	6
Sloping shoulders	61
Sprengel shoulder	46
Pectus excavatum	20
Thoracic scoliosis	47
Short fourth metacarpal	26
Short terminal phalanx thumbs	9
Stiff thumbs	6
Polydactyly	8
Occipitofrontal head circumference	97
Operative delivery	62
Facial features	
Bossing	79
'Typical face'	70
Prognathism	46
Eyebrows arched	28
Palpebral fissures downslanting	30
Upslanting	13
Eye anomalies	30
Strabismus	19
Cataracts	4
Cleft lip and palate	7
Other features	
Mental retardation	?3
Epilepsy	6
Medulloblastoma	5
Ovarian fibroma	24 women
Undescended testes	6 males
Inguinal hernia	17 males
Cardiac fibroma	2.5
X-ray findings	
Cervical/thoracic vertebral anomalies	60
Rib anomalies	70
Calcification: falx <15 years	40
Diaphragm sella (20 years)	100

[a]This term is used to refer to the 'naevi' as seen in Fig. 139.7. They usually remain static but the histology is that of a basal cell carcinoma.
[b]This term is used to refer to lesions which behave clinically like an aggressive basal cell carcinoma.

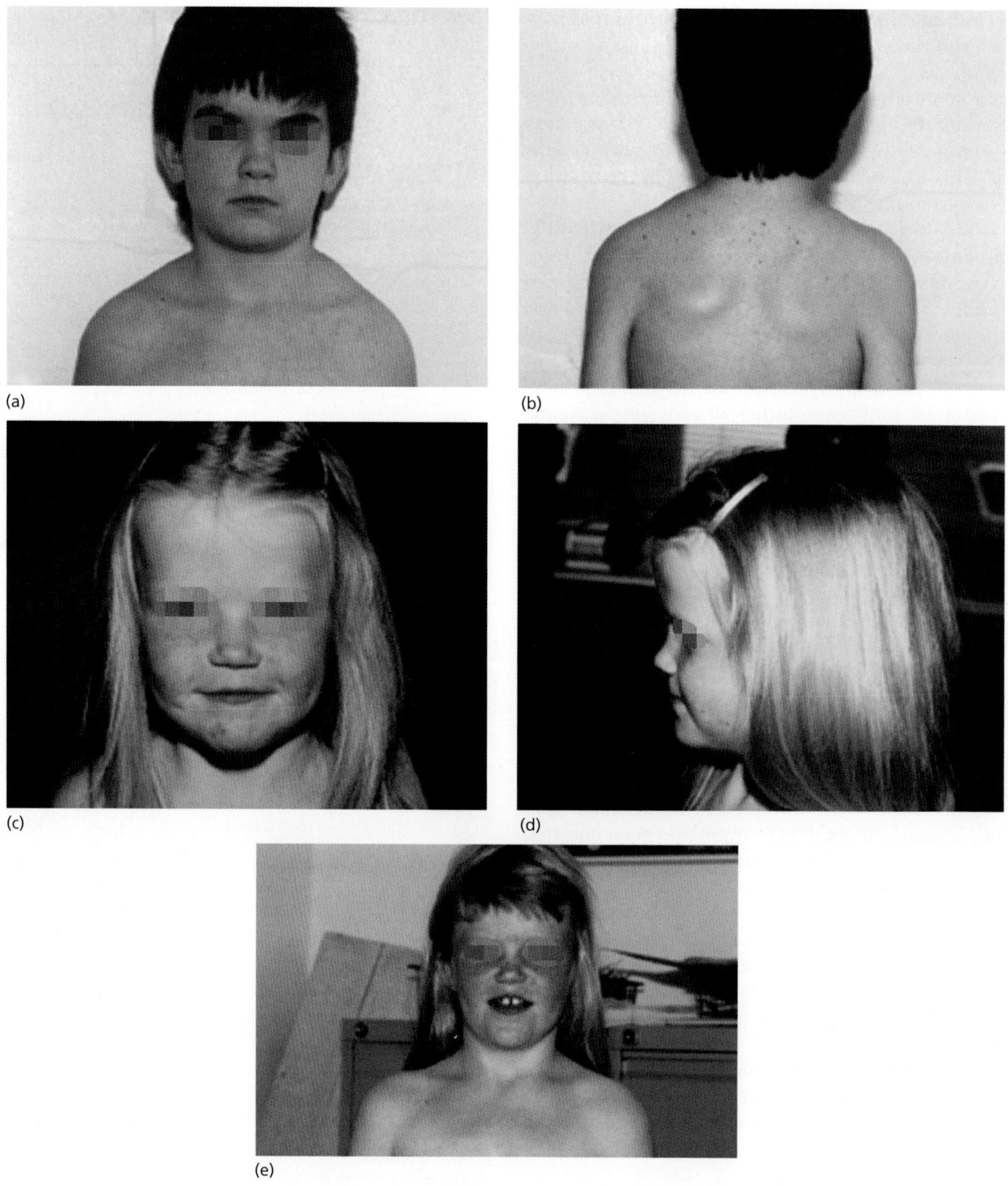

Fig. 139.3 Two children with Gorlin syndrome showing the degree of variation in facial appearance, frontal bossing and sloping of the shoulders. Sprengel shoulder is also shown (b).

often adopt hairstyles that disguise the bossing. There is often facial asymmetry. Some patients have well-developed supraorbital ridges, giving the eyes a sunken appearance. The eyebrows are often heavy, fused and arched. There is a broad nasal root and hypertelorism. The inner canthal, interpupillary and outer canthal distances are all generally above the 97th centile but appear to be in proportion with the head circumference. The mandible is long and often prominent with the lower lip protruding in front of the upper. There is a well-established association with cleft lip/palate, which occurs in 5–6% [9,11].

It can be very helpful to compare a person's facial appearance with siblings because there is usually a striking difference in the facial gestalt between unaffected and affected siblings.

Of patients reported in the literature, 10–25% have ophthalmic abnormalities including congenital blindness caused by corneal opacity, congenital glaucoma, coloboma of the iris, choroid or optic nerve, convergent or divergent strabismus, nystagmus, cataracts and microphthalmia, ptosis, proptosis, medullated nerve fibres and retinal hamartomas [58,60].

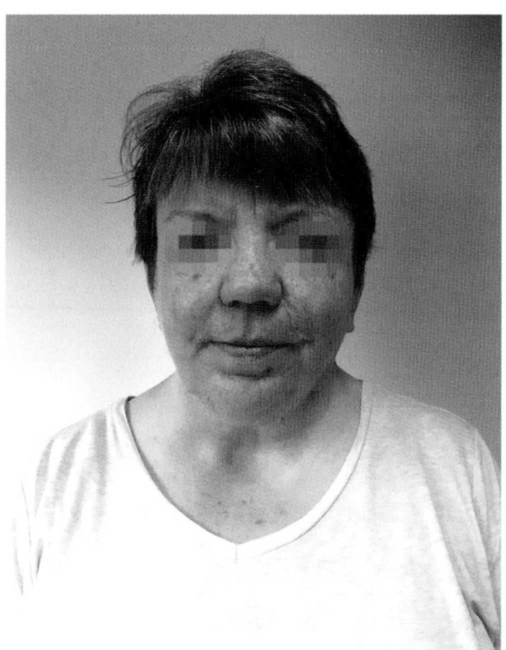

Fig. 139.4 An adult patient with Gorlin syndrome showing many of the facial features associated with the syndrome – arched eyebrows, downslanting palpebral fissures and sloping shoulders. Frontal bossing is disguised by the cut of the hair.

Small keratin-filled cysts (milia) are found on the face in 30% of cases, most commonly in the infraorbital areas, but they can also occur on the forehead. Meibomian cysts on the corneal surface of the eyelids can cause great distress because they repeatedly discharge material. 'Skin tags' are especially common around the neck; like the naevi, histology reveals the typical features of a BCC, but the skin tags do not generally change in size or shape.

Jaw cysts

Thirteen percent of 80 people with the syndrome developed a jaw cyst by the age of 10 years and 51% by the age of 20 years, the majority occurring after the seventh year although the youngest affected person presented with jaw swelling at 5 years old [56]. The peak incidence was in the third decade, about 10 years earlier than isolated odontogenic keratocysts [56]. Gorlin reported that 10% of individuals over the age of 40 with Gorlin syndrome had not developed signs or symptoms of cysts [9].

The mandible is involved far more frequently than the maxilla, with keratocysts occurring most usually at the angle of the mandible (Fig. 139.5).

Patients can be remarkably free of symptoms until cysts reach a large size, especially when the ascending ramus is involved. Presentation can be with swelling and/or pain of the jaw, pus discharging into the oral cavity or displaced, impacted or loose teeth.

Misshapen teeth, missing teeth and a susceptibility to caries are more common in patients than in unaffected relatives.

Chest and trunk

Epidermoid cysts may occur on the limbs and trunk in over 50% of cases and are usually 1–2 cm in diameter [61].

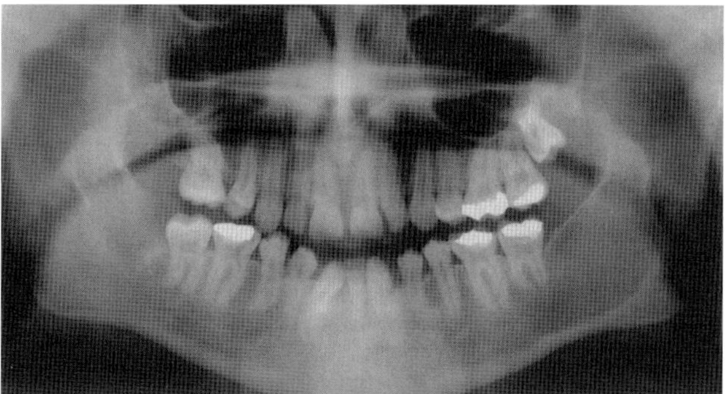

Fig. 139.5 An orthopantogram of a 17-year-old male showing a large cyst in the angle and ramus of the left mandible.

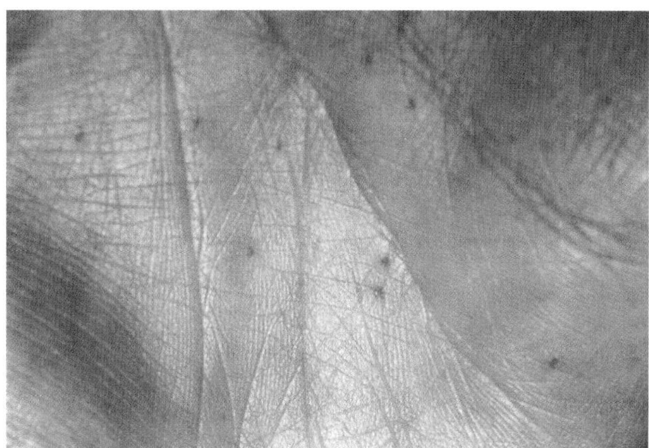

Fig. 139.6 Palmar pits.

Rib anomalies may give an unusual shape to the chest, including a characteristic downward sloping of the shoulders (see Fig. 139.3). The rib anomalies together with kyphoscoliosis may cause pectus deformity in about 13–30% of patients [56,62,63]. Sprengel deformity has been found in some surveys to be as common as 18% particularly if diagnosis is made in a child [64]. Inguinal hernia was noted in 6 of 36 (17%) males by one of the authors (P.F.) [56].

Hands and feet

The distinctive pits found on the palms and soles appear to be pathognomonic [65]. They increase in number with age, are permanent and, when found in a child, are a strong diagnostic indicator. They may vary from only a few to over a hundred. BCCs have very rarely arisen in the base of the pits. Palmar pits were present in 65% of people by the age of 10 years, in 80% by the age of 15 years and in 85% over the age of 20 years [56].

The pits are small (1–2 mm), often asymmetrical, shallow depressions, with the colour of the base being white, flesh-coloured or pale pink (Fig. 139.6). They are found more commonly on the palms (77%) than on the soles (50%). Pits can also appear independently on the sides of the fingers, when they are tiny, bright-red pinpricks.

Although the pits will be easier to see in children who have been playing in a dirty environment, they should be differentiated from palmar lesions caused by excoriation of dirt under the skin. In most patients the pits can be better visualized if the hands are soaked in warm water for about 10 minutes.

Thumb anomalies (short terminal phalanges and/or small stiff thumbs) occur in about 10% [56]. Pre- or post-axial polydactyly of hands or feet was found in 6 of 74 cases (8%) [56]. The fourth metacarpal is short in 15–45% of patients [64], but is not a good diagnostic sign as it is found in about 10% of the normal population [66]. Hallux valgus can be severe, requiring operation [56].

Naevi and BCCs

As 'naevi' and the BCCs found in the syndrome are histologically identical, they can both be classified as NBCCs. Clinically, however, the 'naevi' often develop first and behave differently from the BCCs, which can appear to arise from naevi. For the purposes of the clinical description that follows, it is helpful to treat 'naevi' and 'NBCCs' as though they are separate entities.

Naevi. Naevi affect 53% of patients less than 20 years old, rising to 74% over the age of 20 years. Ordinary naevus cell naevi occur in about 4% of unaffected relatives but are present from birth, whereas affected family members report that the naevi tend to appear in crops, their numbers increasing with time [56]. Naevi also appear as individual lesions. A patient may develop no naevi, a few or many hundreds. The naevi are flesh-coloured, reddish-brown or pearly (Fig. 139.7). Some grow rapidly for a few days to a few weeks, but then most remain static.

Naevoid BCCs. BCCs can arise in any area of the skin, affecting the face, neck and upper trunk in preference to the abdomen, lower trunk and extremities. The areas around the eyes, nose, malar regions and upper lip are the most frequently affected sites on the face. Usually only a few become aggressive, when they are locally invasive and behave like ordinary BCCs. Evidence of aggressive transformation of an individual lesion includes, as expected, an increase in size, ulceration, bleeding or crusting. Some patients can develop aggressive BCCs without first developing naevi. It is rare for metastasis to occur [9].

Aggressive BCCs are unusual before puberty. In a series of 80 individuals, 20% of those aged 15 years had received treatment for one or more NBCC, 45% of those aged 20 years, 70% of those aged 25 years, 80% of those aged 40 years and 92% of those aged 45 years [53].

Skeletal radiographs

Musculoskeletal features may be readily apparent on clinical examination. X-ray investigation may be helpful when the syndrome is suspected. In a series of 82 individuals, bifid ribs were present in 26%, anteriorly splayed, fused or misshapen ribs in 16%, and partially missing or hypoplastic ribs were found in 6% (Fig. 139.8) [62]. The third and fourth ribs are most frequently involved. Bifid ribs are found in about 0.6% of the normal population [67].

Abnormalities of the cervical or thoracic vertebrae are helpful diagnostic signs, being found in about 49% [63]

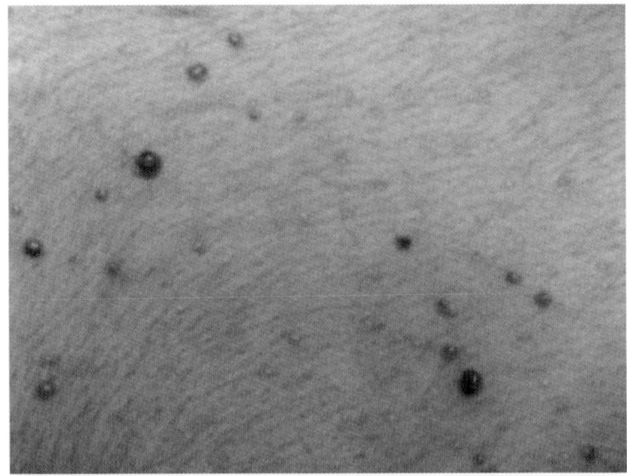

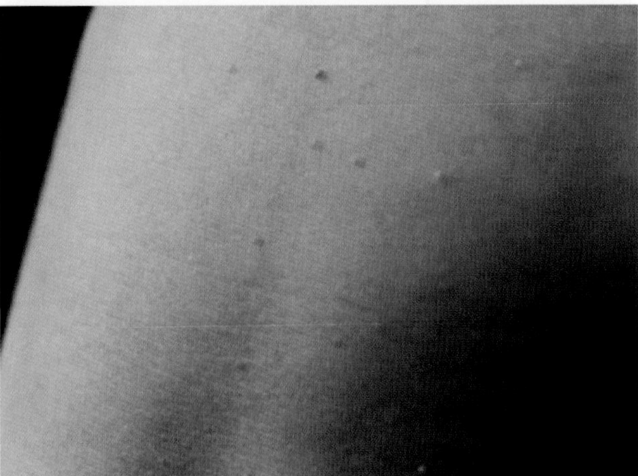

Fig. 139.7 Naevi. Note variation in size and appearance, some being reddish-brown, skin-coloured or translucent.

(Fig. 139.9). C6, C7, T2 and T1 are most frequently involved. Spina bifida occulta of the cervical vertebrae, or malformations at the occipitovertebral junction, are common [63]. In addition to lack of fusion of the cervical or upper thoracic vertebrae, fusion or lack of segmentation has been documented in about 40% [9]. A defective medial portion of the scapula is occasionally found [9].

As rib and spine anomalies are present at birth, they are helpful diagnostic signs.

Small pseudo-cystic lytic bone lesions, most often in the phalanges, metapodial and carpal and tarsal bones, may be found in up to 35% patients [58,68]. There may be just one or two lesions or they may involve almost the entire bone. The long bones, pelvis and calvarium may also be affected. Histologically, these bone radiolucencies are hamartomas composed of fibrous connective tissue, nerves and vessels [69].

Ectopic calcification

Calcification of the falx cerebri is a very useful diagnostic sign. It can appear very early in life, is often strikingly apparent from late childhood and its degree progresses with age. It was present in 40% of patients aged less than 15 years and 95% by age 25 years [56]. Falx calcification first appears as a faint line in the upper falx on plain X-ray

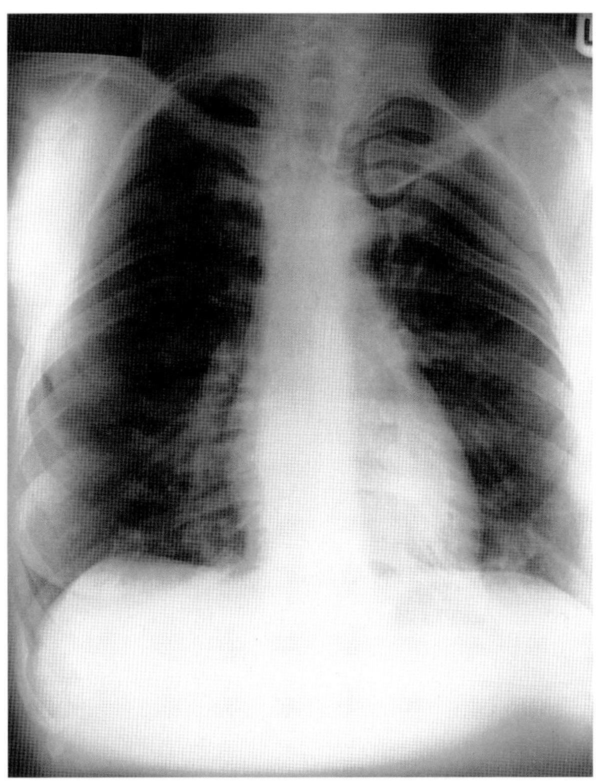

Fig. 139.8 Chest radiograph showing upper vertebral anomalies, variation in thickness of ribs and bifid ribs. The sloping left shoulder is caused by the rib anomalies.

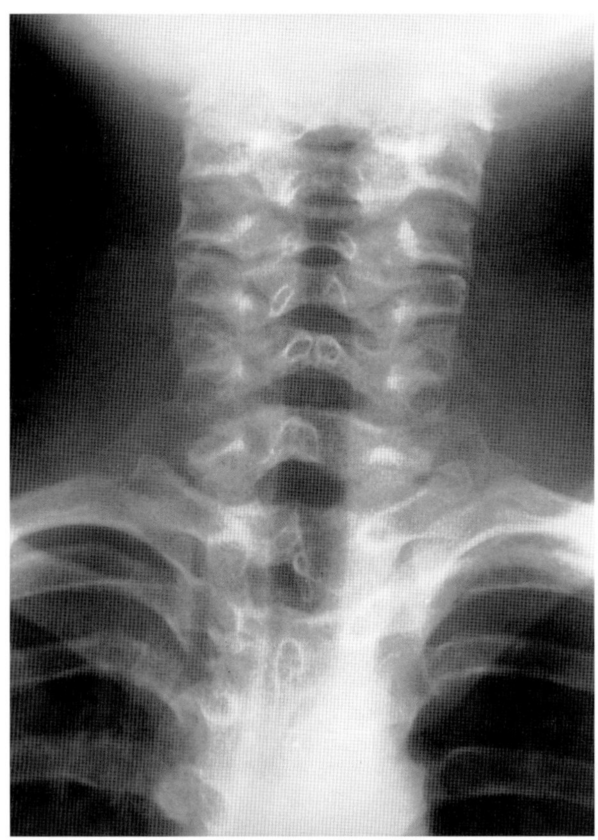

Fig. 139.9 Cervical and upper thoracic spine radiograph of a 10-year-old girl showing spina bifida occulta of C2–T3. The spinous processes of T1 and T2 are fused.

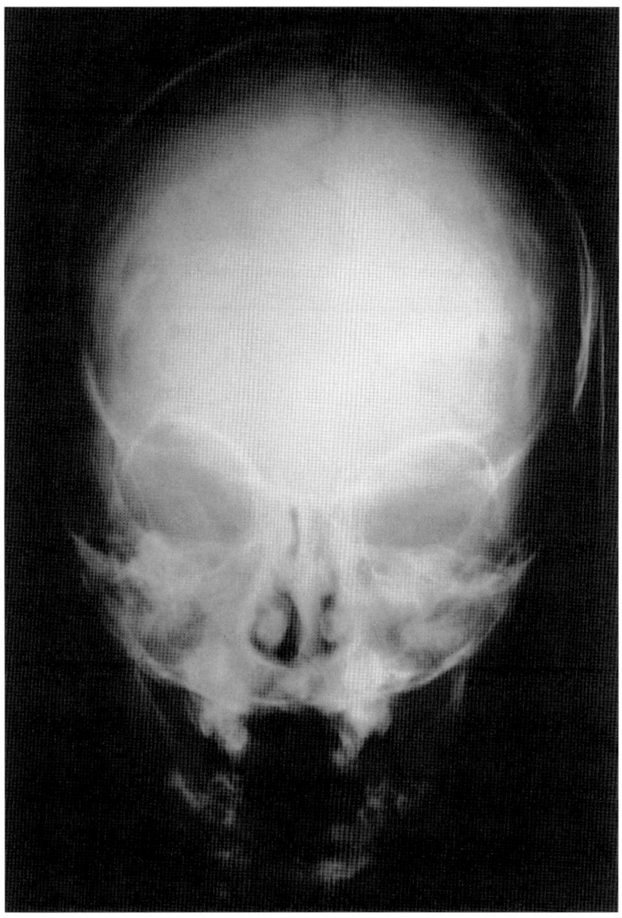

Fig. 139.10 Falx calcification. Skull radiograph of 2-year-old boy: a fine line of calcification is just visible in the upper falx.

films of the skull (Fig. 139.10), the faint line becoming more prominent and giving the appearance of several individual sheets of calcification (Fig. 139.11). In some patients it can be very florid, up to 1 cm wide. It has a characteristic lamellar appearance (Fig. 139.12), in comparison with the single sheet of calcification found in 7% of the normal older population [70].

Calcification of the falx in a child should strongly raise the possibility of Gorlin syndrome as a diagnosis. A normal variant of the skull, a prominent frontal crest, can simulate falx calcification on the AP skull film, and should be considered if the calcification appears to be a single line beginning inferiorly.

Ectopic calcification also occurs in other membranes: the tentorium cerebelli (20%), petroclinoid ligaments (15%) [62], dura, pia and choroid plexus.

Calcification of the diaphragma sellae causing the appearance of bridging of the sella turcica (Fig. 139.13) is another useful early diagnostic sign, found in 60–80% of cases, compared with 4% of the normal population in later life [9,56]. In one study, intracranial calcification was present in 100% of 43 individuals by the age of 20 years [56].

Calcification may also occur subcutaneously in apparently otherwise normal skin of the fingers and scalp [71].

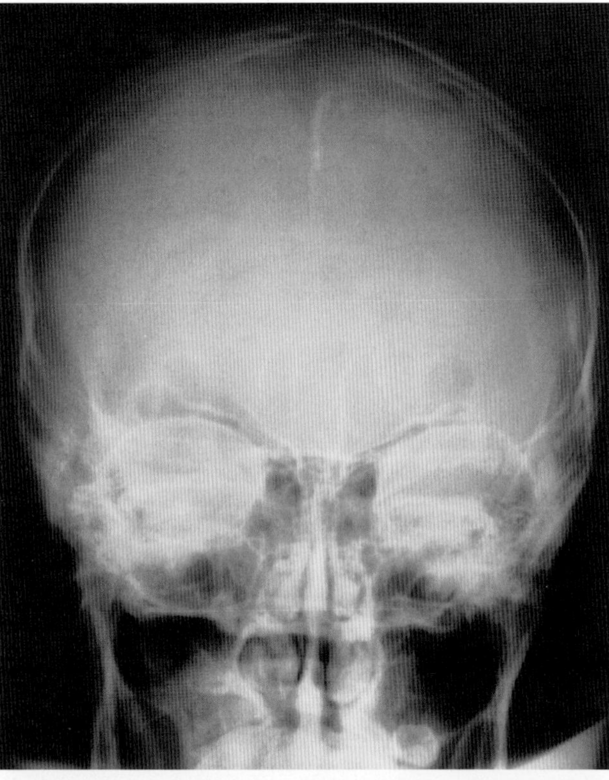

Fig. 139.11 Skull radiograph of an 18-year-old man showing upper falx calcification in plaques.

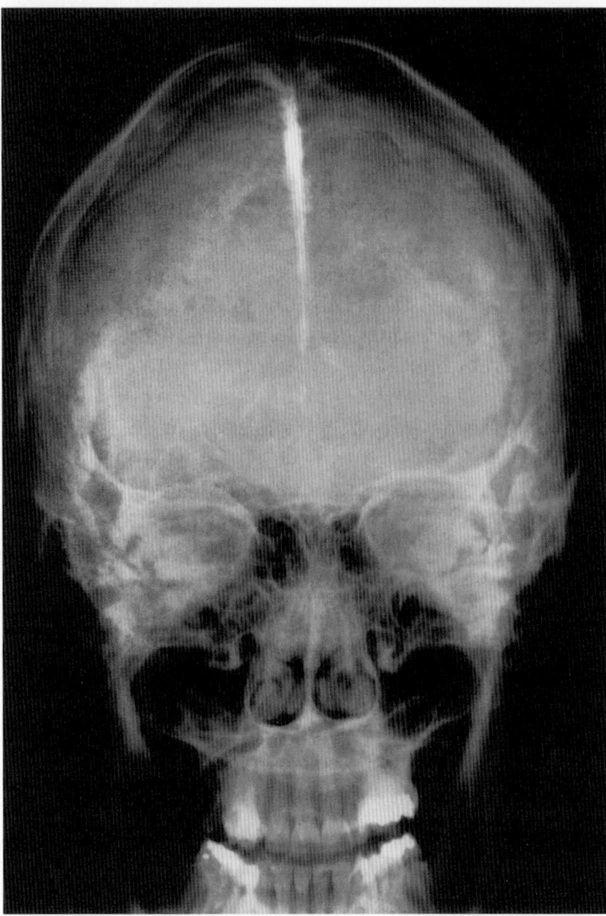

Fig. 139.12 Falx calcification. Skull radiograph of a 24-year-old woman showing florid falx calcification, extending inferiorly.

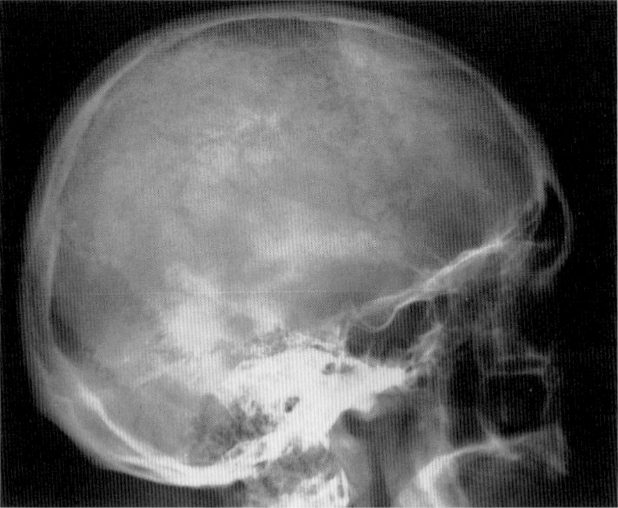

Fig. 139.13 Skull radiograph of a 44-year-old man showing bridged sella and characteristic 'low' occiput.

Central nervous system

Medulloblastoma (now often called primitive neuroectodermal tumour, PNET) is a well-recognized complication of the syndrome, occurring in approximately 5% of patients. Conversely, Gorlin syndrome is found in about 3% of children with medulloblastoma, and in 10% of those under the age of 2 years [72,73]. The average age of presentation in Gorlin syndrome is 2 years, about 5 years before the average age of presentation in children with isolated medulloblastoma. Patients with medulloblastoma associated with Gorlin syndrome are likely to have long-term survival, perhaps associated with the desmoplastic nature of the lesion, but there is a high chance that craniospinal irradiation will result in hundreds of BCCs appearing in the irradiated field [74–77]. There is an additional concern that there may be an increased risk of other second cancers in the radiation field [78].

One study [24] of individuals without mutations in *PTCH1*, found mutations in *SUFU* in three families which fulfilled diagnostic criteria for Gorlin syndrome, although none had jaw cysts. Each family included a single case of medulloblastoma. Of individuals in whom a *PTCH1* mutation had been detected, only two (1.7%) developed medulloblastoma. The authors pointed out that their findings of <2% risk in *PTCH1* mutation-positive individuals, with a risk up to 20 times higher in *SUFU* mutation-positive individuals could suggest that brain magnetic resonance imaging surveillance is justified in children with *SUFU*-related, but not *PTCH1*-related, Gorlin syndrome.

Meningioma, glioblastoma multiforme and craniopharyngioma have also been described in adults.

Cardiovascular system

In the north-west England population study, cardiac fibroma was found in 2.5% [11]. One child died at 3 months of age from multiple cardiac fibromas, whereas another case has been followed for over 20 years with a single 2 cm cardiac fibroma in the interventricular septum, which has remained unchanged. Long-term prognosis is generally good, but resection may be necessary.

The incidence in childhood of an isolated cardiac fibroma is between 0.027% and 0.08%, affecting most frequently the interventricular septum.

Mesentery
Just as cysts of the skin and jaws are integral parts of the syndrome, so are chylous or lymphatic cysts of the mesentery, but these are rare. They may present, if large, as painless movable masses in the upper abdomen or rarely may cause symptoms of obstruction. In most cases, however, they are discovered at laparotomy or on radiography if calcified.

Genitourinary system
Calcified ovarian fibromas have been reported in 25–50% of women with the syndrome [11] and may be mistaken for calcified uterine fibroids, especially if they overlap medially. They do not seem to reduce fertility but may undergo torsion. There is no evidence to suggest that they should be removed prophylactically.

Kidney malformations (horseshoe kidney, unilateral renal agenesis, renal cysts) have been described in isolated case reports but it is not known if their frequency is increased.

Neoplasia in other organs
Tumours in many other organs have been reported but rarely affect children. They include renal fibroma, melanoma, leiomyoma, rhabdomyosarcoma, adrenal cortical adenoma, seminoma, fibroadenoma of the breast, thyroid adenoma, carcinoma of the bladder, Hodgkin disease and chronic leukaemia. There does not appear to be a single particular neoplasm occurring at a frequency that would warrant selective screening.

Diagnosis. Diagnosis in a child with a 50% probability of having inherited the condition may not be easy because of the extreme variation in expression, both within and between families. Some children may have only rib anomalies, whereas others have the 'typical face' without other signs. Mutation analysis may be helpful for presymptomatic diagnosis.

For apparently isolated cases, detailed examination and X-ray investigation of the parents should be undertaken before concluding that a child's condition is the result of a new mutation. If a parent has no physical signs, no pertinent history and normal radiology, it is unlikely that he or she has Gorlin syndrome. If the mutation is known, DNA analysis will be helpful.

Confident diagnosis is obviously vital for subsequent surveillance for complications such as BCCs and jaw cysts, and for giving genetic information. Clinically, it relies on a detailed family history, and physical and X-ray examinations.

Family history
The family history may help to confirm the diagnosis in cases of doubt, although the variability of the condition may give seemingly disparate features in family members.

Physical examination
Particularly helpful are skeletal anomalies, typical facies, 'naevi', and palmar and plantar pits. The most valuable measurement is the head circumference. Measurements should also include height, inner and outer canthal and interpupillary distances. The head circumference should be plotted on a chart that takes height into account [79].

Radiography and imaging investigations
Radiograph signs may aid diagnosis in those who have equivocal physical signs. Radiographs should include the following:
1 Skull: AP;
2 Skull: lateral;
3 Panoramic views of the jaws (orthopantogram), as plain films may miss lesions;
4 Chest radiograph;
5 Cervical and thoracic spine: AP and lateral; and
6 Hands (for pseudocysts).

Ultrasound examinations for ovarian and cardiac fibromas may be helpful according to age.

Diagnostic criteria
Diagnostic criteria are given in Box 139.1, based on the most frequent and/or specific features of the syndrome [11]. These criteria were based on examination of family cases in England, a land not noted for excessive sunlight. The numbers of BCCs in adults accepted as a major diagnostic criterion may need to be increased in countries where there is high UV radiation exposure. The statement of the first International Colloquium on Basal Cell Nevus Syndrome words this criterion more loosely: 'BCC prior to 20 years old or excessive numbers of BCCs out of

Box 139.1 Diagnostic criteria for NBCC syndrome

Major criteria

1. Multiple (>2*) BCCs or one under the age of 30 years or >10 basal cell naevi
2. Odontogenic keratocyst (proven on histology) or polyostotic bone cyst
3. Palmar or plantar pits (three or more)
4. Ectopic calcification: lamellar or early (<20 years) falx calcification
5. First degree relative with NBCC syndrome

Minor criteria

1. Congenital skeletal anomaly: bifid, fused, splayed or missing rib or fused vertebrae
2. Occipitofrontal head circumference >97th centile with bossing
3. Cardiac or ovarian fibroma
4. Medulloblastoma
5. Lymphomesenteric cysts
6. Congenital malformation: cleft lip and/or palate, polydactyly, eye anomaly (cataract, coloboma, microphthalmia)

A diagnosis can be made when two major or one major and two minor criteria are fulfilled. If a first-degree relative is affected, the presence of one major or two minor criteria is diagnostic.
*Note that the numbers of BCC given were based on a study carried out in England; the numbers of BCC for diagnosis will be inappropriate for sunnier climes.

proportion to prior sun exposure and skin type' [36]. The colloquium also considered making medulloblastoma a major criterion as recognition as such may lead to earlier diagnosis.

Confirmation of diagnosis by mutation analysis

The definitive diagnostic test is to demonstrate a mutation in the *PTCH1* gene. In some children, clinical examination may not be conclusive because of age-dependent features of the syndrome. Mutation analysis for the familial mutation can be justified to institute surveillance and sun protection precautions. The demand for prenatal diagnosis has been low.

Identifying a pathogenic mutation (nonsense, frameshift, deletion/insertion, splice site) in *PTCH1* will of course confirm a clinical diagnosis. Because of technical limitations, a negative mutation screen cannot rule out NBCC but in an individual falling short of clinical diagnostic criteria will at least be partially reassuring, as long as a comprehensive analysis has been performed and the patient does not have mosaicism. It may be difficult to interpret the significance of missense mutations in an isolated patient falling short of diagnostic criteria.

Mutation detection appears to be less sensitive in the first affected individual in a family because a proportion of patients have somatic mosaicism.

Prognosis. Because of the variability, presumably because of the other genes in a dosage-sensitive pathway, members of a sibship may be affected to different degrees. There is no evidence that children are more severely affected than their parents, although jaw cysts and BCCs may be detected earlier through surveillance and may give the impression that these features have occurred at an earlier age [56]. The skeletal signs are nonprogressive and are not consistent between family members. Of adults with the syndrome, up to 10% develop neither jaw cysts nor BCCs [9,56]. A child in whom the diagnosis is made on histological examination of an isolated lesion will not necessarily develop a large number of BCCs later.

The authors have the clinical impression that some families seem especially prone to develop BCCs – occurring at a younger age and in greater number – than other families, in which members develop relatively few BCCs and perhaps much later in life. This may be caused by either the presence of background modifying genetic factors or shared environmental exposures. A study of 125 individuals with *PTCH1* mutations found DNA variants (in the *MC1R* gene and the *TERT-CLPTM1L* locus) were significantly associated with an earlier age of BCC onset [80]. The congenital malformations, however, generally do not follow a family-specific pattern: usually only one member is affected.

Differential diagnosis. Several rare conditions may need to be considered when an individual presents with only some, or very mild, features of Gorlin syndrome.

Somatic mosaicism for a *PTCH* mutation could explain the unilateral distribution of multiple BCCs, comedones and epidermoid cysts [81]. Occasional families show an autosomal dominant pattern of multiple BCCs but no other features of Gorlin syndrome; *PTCH* mutation analysis is likely to be negative [82] and *SUFU* analysis should be considered [83].

Differential diagnosis of the palmar pitting is porokeratosis of Mantoux [65], which is a rare form of nonhereditary papular keratosis of the hands and feet, with a few lesions occasionally sprinkled over the ankles. The lesions are changeable and usually disappear with time. The depressions are always found on the summit of the papillary excrescences, resembling an enlarged sudoriferous pore. Older lesions show a blackish vegetation with a finely lobulated or mulberry-like surface at the bottom of the depression, which is eventually shed, leaving a small depression with a slightly raised margin and a red base. The material resembles a cornified comedone. The characteristic lesion is a translucent papule that erupts in recurring crops over months or years.

A family with trichoepitheliomas, milia and cylindromas presenting in the second and third decades and inherited as an autosomal dominant was reported by Rasmussen [84]. The milia were miniature trichoepitheliomas and appeared only in sun-exposed areas. Cylindromatosis [85] (turban tumour syndrome) demonstrates considerable variation in the extent of distribution and age of onset within families, and may be the same condition.

Multiple BCCs, follicular atrophoderma on the dorsum of hands and feet, decreased sweating and hypotrichosis are features of Bazex syndrome [86]. The pitting on the backs of the hands is reminiscent of orange peel and quite unlike the pits of Gorlin syndrome.

The inheritance pattern is either autosomal or X-linked dominant.

A dominantly inherited condition similar to Bazex syndrome was reported in a single family [87]. Rombo syndrome is characterized by vermiculate atrophoderma, milia, hypotrichosis, trichoepitheliomas, BCCs and peripheral vasodilation with cyanosis. The skin is normal until later childhood; BCCs develop later and there is no reduction in sweating.

A single family with another autosomal or X-linked dominant syndrome of hypotrichosis, BCCs, milia and excessive sweating was reported by Oley and colleagues [88].

In Cowden syndrome (multiple hamartoma syndrome) [89], mucocutaneous changes develop in the second decade, consisting of multiple facial papules, both smooth and keratotic, concentrated around the orifices, and generally associated with hair follicles. Numerous small hyperkeratotic and verrucous growths are found on the dorsal aspect of the hands and feet, and round translucent palmoplantar keratoses are also common. Similar lesions, including verrucous papules, occur on the oral mucosa. Multiple skin tags are also frequent. Most patients have a broad forehead and a large head circumference. Adenomas occur in the thyroid; gastrointestinal polyps occur in 60% and there is an increased incidence of breast cancer.

Arsenic exposure may cause multiple BCCs.

Patients with Gorlin syndrome may have café-au-lait patches but they number less than the six required for the diagnosis of neurofibromatosis type 1 (NF1), nor is axillary freckling present. In fact, physical appearances of some patients with NF1 and Gorlin syndrome are very similar.

Pseudo-hypoparathyroidism may be considered because of ectopic calcification and short fourth metacarpals.

Cardiac fibromas are also found in tuberous sclerosis and Beckwith–Wiedemann syndrome.

Surveillance and prophylaxis. It is recommended that families are offered regular screening and that one clinician monitors and coordinates the overall programme [11]. Predictive testing by DNA analysis may be justified to identify family members for surveillance.

The following recommendations are based on clinical experience from a population study of 84 cases followed for 10 years [11].

During pregnancy

Ultrasound scans may be offered during pregnancy to detect cardiac tumours and developmental malformations, which may require early decisions about neonatal surgery, and to detect an extremely enlarged head that may necessitate operative delivery.

Neonatal

A detailed neonatal examination may confirm the physical signs of a large head, cleft palate or eye anomaly. X-rays may confirm bifid ribs or vertebral abnormalities. An echocardiogram is best performed early as at least two cases have presented before 3 months of age with fibromas.

Childhood

Six-monthly neurological examination may detect a deficit indicative of a medulloblastoma (primitive neuroectodermal tumour). Routine scanning with computed tomography (CT) or excessive use of X-rays is not recommended because of concerns about inducing skin malignancies. (Information from molecular analysis in one study has suggested that scanning may best be targeted to children with a mutation in *SUFU* [24].) At 3 years the clinical examinations could be reduced to annually until 7 years, after which a medulloblastoma is very unlikely. Although these examinations are of low sensitivity and specificity a parent should contact a specialist department if suspicious symptoms develop. Magnetic resonance imaging has been suggested annually until the age of 8 years [36] but because this may require general anaesthetic, it may not be justified in children with *PTCH1*-related Gorlin syndrome because the risk is around 2% [37].

Baseline ophthalmological examination and routine hearing, vision and developmental surveillance programmes are recommended.

Annual dental screening should commence as soon as tolerated, usually including a panoramic radiograph of the jaw. Orthopantograms are justified because of complications of untreated jaw cysts.

At least annual to 4-monthly examination of the skin from puberty is recommended but because a lesion may suddenly become aggressive, the patient needs open access to the specialist taking responsibility for treatment of the skin. It is especially important to offer early treatment for lesions of the eyelids, nose, ears and scalp. Patients must be warned to inspect all areas of the body – BCCs have been reported on the vulva and the mucosa of the anal sphincter.

Exposure to sunlight

As sunlight may be one of the environmental agents promoting the appearance of BCCs [90], sun protection precautions should be strongly recommended, including the wearing of a wide-brimmed hat to offer some protection to the areas around the eyes.

Treatment.

Skin

Alarm can be generated particularly in childhood when a skin tag or naevus is shown on histology to be a BCC. This may result in a feeling that immediate treatment is required for all other skin lesions present, and indeed, some authors do urge treatment for all such lesions. Other authors reserve treatment for lesions that show signs that they are active. As many naevi remain quiescent for long periods, they may not need to be removed but kept under frequent review. The authors' practice is to have a lower threshold for local treatment for individual lesions occurring around the eyes, nose, mouth and ears.

The most suitable form of treatment may vary depending on the type, size and site of an NBCC and patients may best be managed by a multidisciplinary treatment team able to access a wide range of treatment modalities. Surgical excision, cryotherapy, curettage and diathermy, topical 5-fluorouracil, Mohs microsurgery [91], carbon dioxide laser vaporization [92] and photodynamic therapy have all been used. Systemic retinoids are also used in some centres.

The priorities are to ensure complete eradication of aggressive BCCs and to preserve normal tissue to prevent disfigurement. A few patients (usually adults) have hundreds of aggressive BCCs and treatment may seem overwhelming and hopeless. A great deal of support may therefore be required, not least to encourage attendance at follow up clinics and to accept early treatment. There are active patient support groups in the UK and USA.

Local treatment. Topical 5-fluorouracil appears effective for superficial multicentric BCCs without follicular involvement but should not be used for deeply invasive BCCs. Topical 5-fluorouracil was used successfully in a 30-year-old man with multiple progressive superficial and nodular BCCs and Gorlin syndrome [93]. Superficial BCCs were cleared but nodular BCCs required surgical excision or photodynamic therapy. The main side-effects were pain and infection. Systemic levels of 5-fluorouracil were undetectable.

Topical imiquimod also appears effective for superficial BCCs but some people find the local inflammatory response difficult to tolerate [94–97] and new lesions appear on cessation of therapy [97].

The management of a girl who had inherited Gorlin syndrome from her father was reported after being treated for 10 years with a combination of topical tretinoin and 5-fluorouracil [98]. At 25 months of age, she had several red papules and numerous naevocellular and milia-like lesions confirmed on biopsy to be BCCs. After invasive BCCs had been removed, the other lesions were treated with twice-daily total body application of 0.1% tretinoin cream followed by 5% 5-fluorouracil cream. Lesions around the eyes were treated with 5-fluorouracil alone twice daily. The hundreds of tumours disappeared after initiation of the combined therapy; most of the remaining tumours did not grow. The patient was examined every 3 months and lesions that demonstrated signs of growth or appeared to be deeply invasive were managed by shave excision and curettage. Development appeared normal and she showed neither clinical nor laboratory evidence of toxicity. However, a study of tazarotene, a topical retinoid, demonstrated a very poor response in patients with Gorlin syndrome both in terms of prevention of new BCCs and treatment of existing lesions [99].

Treatment by radiation. The traditional approach is that radiotherapy should be avoided because of clinical evidence that new lesions can appear in the irradiated field; radiosensitive patients may develop more long-term complications from the treatment than from the original BCCs [100,101]. It may be that some families are not as radiosensitive as others, but until laboratory tests can detect these, the recommendation is that radiotherapy is avoided for all families.

Children who received craniospinal irradiation as part of the treatment for a medulloblastoma [74–77] or Hodgkin disease [102] have developed thousands of BCCs in the irradiated area (Fig. 139.14). The BCCs often develop within an extremely short latent period of 6 months to 3 years. This is earlier than, and in a distribution different from, other affected family members [101]. NBCC patients treated for eczema by irradiation to the hands have developed multiple BCCs on the palms.

Increased skin pigmentation may be protective against UV, but not ionizing, radiation as an African–American boy treated with craniospinal irradiation for a medulloblastoma developed numerous BCCs in the irradiated area [103].

One adult patient has been reported where radiotherapy was used as treatment for a 4.0 × 4.5 cm treatment-refractory BCC in a nasolabial fold leading to complete regression with no secondary malignancy after 57 months follow up. The authors suggest that whilst surgery and topical therapies should remain the first-line treatments, radiotherapy may not necessarily be excluded in adults for those lesions which are treatment-refractory or poorly located. Because higher susceptibility to secondary malignancy after ionizing radiation is age dependent, they do not recommend radiotherapy for BCCs in children [104].

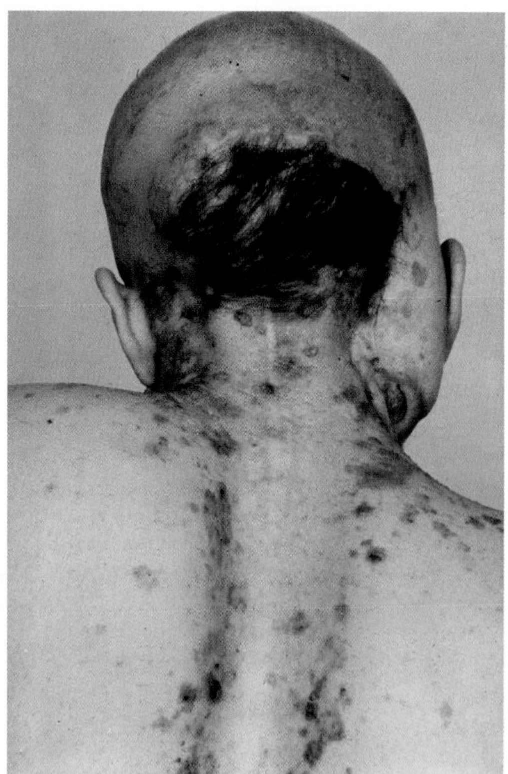

Fig. 139.14 Multiple basal cell carcinomas arising in the field irradiated some years previously as part of treatment for a medulloblastoma.

Systemic retinoids. Oral synthetic retinoids (etretinate, isotretinoin and 13-cis-retinoic acid) have been reported to prevent the development of new tumours, inhibit the growth of existing tumours and cause the regression of superficially invasive BCCs. However, high doses are required and recurrence occurs on cessation of treatment. In two reports [105,106], etretinate at a dose of 1 mg/kg per day resulted in regression of 76% and 83% of lesions for 5 months, respectively, but new lesions appeared in both adult patients within 3 months of treatment being discontinued. Less aggressive surgery was required in a 63-year-old woman, who received treatment with oral etretinate, initially at 1 mg/ kg per day [107]. Isotretinoin at 0.4 mg/kg per day prevented the formation of the majority of new BCCs and reduced the rate of growth of existing lesions in twin 26-year-old men who had hundreds of lesions [108]. The protective effect was lost following dose reduction to 0.2 mg/kg per day.

In a series of reports, Peck and colleagues [109] followed the progress of 12 adult patients with multiple BCCs, five of whom had Gorlin syndrome. Oral isotretinoin was given at 1 mg/kg per day increasing to an average maximum dose of 4.6 mg/kg per day for an average of 8 months. Approximately 8% of 270 selected BCCs underwent complete clinical and histological remission; 20% of tumours showed partial and a further 44% minimal regression. Five patients withdrew because of the side-effects associated with retinoids. The dose of isotretinoin was reduced to 0.25–1.5 mg/kg per day in the seven remaining patients. Partial regression of tumours was shown in only one patient.

A study of the chemopreventive potential of retinoids gave disappointing results in 981 adult patients with a previous history of two or more BCCs. Low-dose isotretinoin (10 mg/day) administered for 36 months did not significantly reduce the rate of development of new tumours [110].

There is significant toxicity associated with prolonged retinoid use. As well as potential teratogenicity, there are side-effects such as chelitis, pruritus, peeling of the palms and soles, eczema and diffuse idiopathic skeletal hyperostosis [111], dictating that retinoids should be used in carefully controlled circumstances. Their long-term role in the management of Gorlin syndrome is uncertain until synthetic retinoids become available that demonstrate reduced toxicity while maintaining an antineoplastic effect. At the time of writing, no trials are known to be taking place.

Photodynamic therapy. Photodynamic therapy (PDT) is proving to be a valuable treatment modality for patients with Gorlin syndrome. Original studies involved systemic administration of a photosensitizer followed by exposure of the target area to light, but topical treatments are now being used. In 1984, Tse and colleagues [112] treated 40 BCCs in which conventional treatments had failed or were no longer possible by systemic PDT in three adult patients with Gorlin syndrome, with 82.5% complete and 17.5% partial clinical response. There was a 10.8% recurrence rate.

Complete clinical BCC response rate was high (93%) in 796 nodular and superficial lesions in 20 adults with 1 mg/kg systemic Photofrin®; the results in three children were less satisfactory, with a poorer response and scarring [113]. Systemic PDT is therefore not recommended for prepubertal children. A subsequent study reported on the treatment of 2041 BCCs in 77 adult patients [114]. A major disadvantage of Photofrin® is that it can produce a generalized photosensitivity for 4–8 weeks.

Topical treatment has been reported using 5-aminolaevulinic acid (ALA) or methyl aminolaevulinate (MAL) [115,116]. Three children with 12–25% of their body surface areas affected by BCCs were treated with topical ALA PDT. Two children had hundreds of BCCs in the radiation field following treatment for medulloblastoma and one had clinical signs compatible with Gorlin syndrome and had more than 500 basaloid follicular hamartomas. The patients had excellent cosmetic results without scarring and 85–98% overall clearance rates [117]. This approach appears to be especially useful in such cases where there are thousands of superficial BCCs in children.

PDT gave local control rates of 56% at 12 months for 138 lesions treated in 33 (adult) patients with the syndrome. Ultrasound was used to measure the lesion thickness in order to determine optimum treatment. Lesions measuring <2 mm thick were generally treated using a topical photosensitizer, thicker lesions being treated with systemic photosensitizers and interstitial optical fibres [115]. A consensus recommendation in 2014 considered topical MAL-PDT safe in patients with Gorlin syndrome and of similar efficacy to that used in patients with sporadic BCC [118].

Small molecule inactivators of SMO. These include the drug vismodegib, which acts by inhibiting SMO and preventing the activation of downstream transcriptional pathways. A large phase II trial [119] demonstrated a clinically useful response in adult patients with inoperable locally advanced or metastatic BCCs. Based on this, the drug received FDA approval in 2012. In patients with Gorlin syndrome, and large numbers of BCCs, vismodegib reduced the rate of development of BCCs requiring surgical treatment and reduced the size of existing carcinomas [120]. Vismodegib may also be effective in reducing the size and tumour burden of odontogenic keratocysts [121].

Jaw cysts

As proliferating dental lamina and satellite cysts may occur in the fibrous wall of the primary cyst cavity, marsupialization is successful only if no satellite cysts are left behind. Small single lesions with regular spherical outlines can usually be completely enucleated provided that access is good. For the large multilocular lesions, excision and immediate bone grafting is the treatment of choice at the first operation [122].

The odontogenic keratocyst has a tendency to recur after surgical treatment, with reported rates varying up to 62%. New cysts may form from satellite cysts associated with the original or from the dental lamina.

References

1 **Rayner CR Towers JF Wilson JS. What is Gorlin's syndrome? Diagnosis and management of the basal cell naevus syndrome based on a study of 37 patients. Br J Plast Surg 1977;30:62–7.**
2 Satinoff MI, Wells C. Multiple basal cell naevus syndrome in ancient Egypt. Med Hist 1969;13:294–6.
3 Jarisch W. Zur Lehre con den Hautgeschwulsten. Arch Dermatol Syph 1894;28:162–222.
4 White JC. Multiple benign cystic epitheliomas. J Cutan Genitourin Dis 1894;12:477–84.
5 Nomland R. Multiple basal cell epitheliomas originating from congenital pigmented basal cell nevi. Arch Dermatol Syph 1932;25:1002–8.
6 **Gorlin RJ, Goltz RW. Multiple nevoid basal-cell epithelioma, jaw cysts and bifid rib: a syndrome. N Engl J Med 1960;262:908–12.**
7 Howell JB, Caro MR. The basal cell nevus: its relationship to multiple cutaneous cancers and associated anomalies of development. Arch Dermatol 1959;79:67–80.
8 Mason JK, Helwig EB, Graham JH. Pathology of the nevoid basal cell carcinoma syndrome. Arch Pathol 1965;79:401–8.
9 **Gorlin RJ. Nevoid basal-cell carcinoma syndrome. Medicine 1987;66:96–113.**
10 **Gorlin RJ. Nevoid basal cell carcinoma syndrome. Dermatol Clin 1995;13:113–25.**
11 **Evans DGR, Ladusans EJ, Rimmer S et al. Complications of the naevoid basal cell carcinoma syndrome: results of a population based study. J Med Genet 1993;30:460–4.**
12 Evans DG, Howard E, Giblin C et al. Birth incidence and prevalence of tumour prone syndromes: estimates from a UK genetic family register service. Am J Med Genet 2010;15(152A):327–32.
13 Shanley S, Ratcliffe J, Hockey A et al. Nevoid basal cell carcinoma syndrome: review of 118 affected individuals. Am J Med Genet 1994;50:282–90.
14 Rahbari H, Mehregan AH. Basal cell epithelioma (carcinoma) in children and teenagers. Cancer 1982;49:350–3.
15 Jones KL, Smith DW, Harvey MA et al. Older paternal age and fresh gene mutation: data on additional disorders. J Pediatr 1975;86:84–8.

16 **Gorlin RJ. Multiple nevoid basal cell carcinoma syndrome. In: Gorlin RJ, Cohen MM, Levin LS (eds) Syndromes of the Head and Neck, 3rd edn. Oxford: Oxford University Press, 1990:372–80.**

17 **Farndon PA, del Mastro RD, Evans DGR et al. Location of gene for Gorlin syndrome. Lancet 1992;339:581–2.**

18 Reis A, Kuster W, Gebel E et al. Localisation of the gene for the naevoid basal cell carcinoma syndrome. Lancet 1992;339:617.

19 Gailani MR, Bale SJ, Leffell DJ et al. Developmental defects in Gorlin syndrome related to a putative tumor suppressor gene on chromosome 9. Cell 1992;69:111–17.

20 Fan Z, Li J, Du J et al. A missense mutation in PTCH2 underlies dominantly inherited NBCCS in a Chinese family. J Med Genet 2008;45:303–8.

21 Fujii K, Ohashi H, Suzuki M et al. Frameshift mutation in the PTCH2 gene can cause nevoid basal cell carcinoma syndrome. Fam Cancer 2013;12:611–14.

22 Smyth I, Narang MA, Evans T et al. Isolation and characterisation of human Patched 2 (PTCH2), a putative tumour suppressor gene in basal cell carcinoma and medulloblastoma on chromosome 1p32. Hum Mol Genet 1999;8:291–7.

23 Pastorino L, Ghiorzo P, Nasti S et al. Identification of a SUFU germline mutation in a family with Gorlin syndrome. Am J Med Genet A 2009;149A(7):1539–43

24 Smith MJ, Beetz C, Williams SG et al. Germline mutations in SUFU cause Gorlin syndrome-associated childhood medulloblastoma and redefine the risk associated with PTCH1 mutations. J Clin Oncol 2014;32:4155–61.

25 **Hahn H, Wicking C, Zaphiropoulos PG et al. Mutations of the human homolog of Drosophila patched in the nevoid basal cell carcinoma syndrome. Cell 1996;85:841–51.**

26 Johnson RL, Rothman AL, Xie J et al. Human homolog of patched, a candidate gene for the basal cell nevus syndrome. Science 1996; 272:1668–71.

27 **Villavicencio EH, Walterhouse DO, Iannaccone PM. The Sonic Hedgehog-patched-Gli pathway in human development and disease. Am J Hum Genet 2000;67:1047–54.**

28 Bale AE, Yu K-P. The hedgehog pathway and basal cell carcinomas. Hum Mol Genet 2001;10:757–62.

29 Epstein EH. Basal cell carcinomas: attack of the hedgehog. Nature Rev Cancer 2008;8:743–754.

30 Kogerman P, Krause D, Rahnama F et al. Alternative first exons of PTCH1 are differentially regulated in vivo and may confer different functions of the PTCH1 protein. Oncogene 2002;21:6007–16.

31 Goodrich LV, Milenkovic L, Higgins KM et al. Altered neural cell fates and medulloblastoma in mouse patched mutants. Science 1997;277:1109–13.

32 Bailey EC, Milenkovic L, Scott MP et al. Several PATCHED1 missense mutations display activity in patched-1 deficient fibroblasts. J Biol Chem 2002;37:33632–40.

33 Bonifas JM, Bare JW, Kerschmann RL et al. Parental origin of chromosome 9q22.3–q31 lost in basal cell carcinomas from basal cell nevus syndrome patients. Hum Mol Genet 1994;3:447–8.

34 Levanat S, Gorlin RJ, Fallet S et al. A two-hit model for developmental defects in Gorlin syndrome. Nature Genet 1996;12:85–7.

35 **Lindstrom E, Shimokawa T, Toftgard R, Zaphiropoulos PG. PTCH mutations: distribution and analyses. Hum Mutat 2006 27:215–19.**

36 **Bree AF, Shah MR, BCNS Colloquium Group. Consensus statement from the first international colloquium on basal cell nevus syndrome (BCNS). Am J Med Genet A 2011; 155A(9):2091–7.**

37 **Evans DGR, Farndon PA. Nevoid Basal Cell Carcinoma Syndrome. Gene Reviews [Internet]. University of Washington, Seattle, WA, USA. 1993–2019, 2018. https://www.ncbi.nlm.nih.gov/books/NBK1151/**

38 Aszterbaum M, Rothman A, Johnson RL et al. Identification of mutations in the human PATCHED gene in sporadic basal cell carcinomas and in patients with the basal cell nevus syndrome. J Invest Dermatol 1998;110:885–8.

39 Lench NJ, Telford EAR, High AS et al. Characterisation of human patched germ line mutations in naevoid basal cell carcinoma syndrome. Hum Genet 1997;100:497–502.

40 Wicking C, Gillies S, Smyth I et al. De novo mutations of the patched gene in nevoid basal cell carcinoma syndrome help to define the clinical phenotype. Am J Med Genet 1997;73:304–7.

41 Wicking C, Shanley S, Smyth I et al. Most germ-line mutations in the nevoid basal cell carcinoma syndrome lead to a premature termination of the PATCHED protein, and no genotype-phenotype correlations are evident. Am J Hum Genet 1997;60:21–6.

42 Ming JE, Kaupas ME, Roessler E et al. Mutations in PATCHED-1, the receptor for SONIC HEDGEHOG, are associated with holoprosencephaly. Hum Genet 2002;110:297–301.

43 Gorlin RJ, Vickers RA, Klein E et al. The multiple basal cell nevi syndrome. Cancer 1965;18:89–104.

44 Graham JH, Mason JK et al. Differentiation of nevoid basal cell carcinoma from epithelioma adenoids cysticum. J Invest Derm 1965;33:197–200.

45 Ahlfors E, Larsson A, Sjogren S. The odontogenic keratocyst: a benign cystic tumor? J Oral Maxillofac Surg 1984;42:10–19.

46 Howell JB, Freeman RG. Structure and significance of the pits with their tumors in the nevoid basal cell carcinoma syndrome. J Am Acad Dermatol 1980;2:224–38.

47 Hashimoto K, Howell JB, Yamanishi Y et al. Electron microscope studies of palmar and plantar pits of nevoid basal cell epithelioma. J Invest Dermatol 1972;59:380–93.

48 Little JB, Nichols WW, Troilo P et al. Radiation sensitivity of cell strains from families with genetic disorders predisposing to radiation-induced cancer. Cancer Res 1989;49:4705–14.

49 Aszterbaum MA, Epstein J, Oro A. A mouse model of human basal cell carcinoma: ultraviolet and gamma radiation enhance basal cell carcinoma growth in patched heterozygote knock-out mice. Nature Med 1999;5:1285–91.

50 Lehmann AR, Kirk-Bell S, Arlett CF et al. Repair of UV light damage in a variety of human fibroblast cell strains. Cancer Res 1977;37:904–10.

51 Nagawaswa F, Little FF, Burke MJ et al. Study of basal cell nevus fibroblasts after treatment with DNA damaging agents. Basic Life Sci 1984;29B:775–85.

52 Ananthaswamy HN, Applegate LA, Goldberg LH et al. Skin fibroblasts from basal cell nevus patients are hypersensitive to killing by solar UVB radiation. Photochem Photobiol 1989;49:60S.

53 Applegate LA, Goldberg LH, Ley RD et al. Hypersensitivity of skin fibroblasts from basal cell nevus syndrome patients to killing by ultraviolet B but not by ultraviolet C radiation. Cancer Res 1990;50:637–41.

54 **Kimonis VE, Goldstein AM, Pastakia B et al. Clinical manifestations in 105 persons with nevoid basal cell carcinoma syndrome. Am J Med Genet 1997;69:299–308.**

55 **Lo Muzio L, Nocini PF, Savoia A et al. Nevoid basal cell carcinoma syndrome: clinical findings in 37 Italian affected individuals. Clin Genet 1999;55:34–40.**

56 **Farndon PA. The Gorlin (naevoid basal cell carcinoma) syndrome: a clinical and genetic study. MD Thesis King's College London School of Medicine and Dentistry, University of London. 1995.**

57 Gorlin RH, Sedano HO The multiple nevoid basal cell carcinoma syndrome revisited. Birth Defects, Original Article series, 1971;7:140–8.

58 **Gorlin R. Nevoid basal cell carcinoma (Gorlin) syndrome. Genet Med 2004; 6:530–9.**

59 Boyer BE Martin MM Marfan's syndrome: report of a case manifesting a giant bone cyst of the mandible and multiple (110) basal cell carcinomata. Plast Reconst Surg 1958;22:257–63.

60 Chen JJ, Sartori J, Aakau V et al. Review of ocular manifestations of nevoid basal cell carcinoma syndrome: what an ophthalmologist needs to know. Middle East Afr J Ophthalmol 2015;22:421–7.

61 Leppard BJ. Skin cysts in the basal cell naevus syndrome. Clin Exp Dermatol 1983;:603–12.

62 Kimonis VE, Mehta SG, DiGiovanna JJ et al. Radiological features in 82 patients with nevoid basal cell carcinoma (NBCC or Gorlin) syndrome. Genet Med 2004;6: 495–502.

63 Ratcliffe JF, Shanley S, Chenevix-Trench G. The prevalence of cervical and thoracic congenital skeletal abnormalities in basal cell naevus syndrome; a review of cervical and chest radiographs in 80 patients with BCNS. Br J Radiol 1995;68(810):596–9.

64 Kimonis VE, Singh KE, Zhong R et al. Clinical and radiological features in young individuals with nevoid basal cell carcinoma syndrome. Genet Med 2013;15:79–83.

65 Howell JB, Mehregan AH. Pursuit of the pits in the nevoid basal cell carcinoma syndrome. Arch Dermatol 1970;102:586–97.

66 Bloom RA The metacarpal sign. Br J Radiol 1970;43:133–5.

67 Etter LE. Osseous abnormalities of the thoracic cage seen in 40,000 consecutive chest photoroentograms. Am J Roentgenol 1944;51:359–63.

68 Dunnick NR, Head GL, Peck GL, Yoder FW. Nevoid basal cell carcinoma syndrome: radiographic manifestations including cystlike lesions of the phalanges. Radiology 1978;127:331–4.

69 Miller RF Cooper RR Nevoid basal cell carcinoma syndrome. Histogenesis of skeletal lesions. Clin Orthoped Rel Res 1972;89:246–52.

70 Dyke CG. Indirect signs of brain tumour as noted in routine roentgen examinations. Am J Roentgenol 1930;23:598–606.
71 Murphy KJ. Subcutaneous calcification in the naevoid basal cell carcinoma syndrome. Clin Radiol 1969;20:287–93.
72 Evans DGR, Farndon PA, Burnell LD et al. The incidence of Gorlin syndrome in 173 consecutive cases of medulloblastoma. Br J Cancer 1991;64:959–61.
73 Cowan R, Hoban P, Kelsey A et al. The gene for the naevoid basal cell carcinoma syndrome acts as a tumour-suppressor gene in medulloblastoma. Br J Cancer 1997;76:141–5.
74 Walter AW, Pivnick EK, Bale AE. Complications of the nevoid basal cell carcinoma syndrome: a case report. J Pediatr Hematol Oncol 1997;19:258–62.
75 O'Malley S, Weitman D, Olding M et al. Multiple neoplasms following craniospinal irradiation for medulloblastoma in a patient with nevoid basal cell carcinoma syndrome. J Neurosurg 1997;86:286–8.
76 Atahan IL, Vildiz F, Ozyar E et al. Basal cell carcinomas developing in a case of medulloblastoma associated with Gorlin's syndrome. Pediatr Hematol Oncol 1998;15:187–91.
77 Evans DGR, Birch J, Orton C. Brain tumours and the occurrence of severe invasive basal cell carcinomas in first degree relatives with Gorlin syndrome. Br J Neurosurg 1991;5:643–6.
78 Goldstein AM, Yuen J, Tucker MA. Second cancers after medulloblastoma: population-based results from the United States and Sweden. Cancer Causes Control 1997;8:865–71.
79 Bushby KMD, Cole T, Matthews JNS et al. Centiles for adult head circumference. Arch Dis Child 1992;67:1286–7.
80 Yasar B, Byers HJ, Smith MJ et al. Common variants modify the age of onset for basal cell carcinomas in Gorlin syndrome. Eur J Hum Genet 2015;23:708–10.
81 Bleiberg J, Brodkin RH. Linear unilateral basal cell nevus with comedones. Arch Dermatol 1969;100:187–90.
82 Klein RD, Dykas DJ, Bale AE. Clinical testing for the nevoid basal cell carcinoma syndrome in a DNA diagnostic laboratory. Genet Med 2005;7:611–19.
83 Schulman JM, Oh DH, Sanborn JZ et al. Multiple hereditary infundibulocystic basal cell carcinoma syndrome associated with a germline SUFU mutation. JAMA Dermatol 2016:152:323–7.
84 Rasmussen JE. A syndrome of trichoepitheliomas, milia and cylindromas. Arch Dermatol 1975;111:610–14.
85 Welch JP, Wells RS, Kerr CB. Ancell–Spiegler cylindromas (turban tumours) and Brooke–Fordyce trichoepitheliomas: evidence for a single genetic entity. J Med Genet 1968;5:29–35.
86 Viksnins P, Berlin A. Follicular atrophoderma and basal cell carcinomas: the Basex syndrome. Arch Dermatol 1977;113:948–51.
87 Michaelsson G, Olsson E, Westermark P. The Rombo syndrome. Acta Dermatol Venereol 1981;61:497–503.
88 Oley CA, Sharpe H, Chenevix-Trench G. Basal cell carcinomas, coarse sparse hair, and milia. Am J Med Genet 1992;43:799–804.
89 Starink TM, van der Veen JPW, Arwert F et al. The Cowden syndrome: a clinical and genetic study in 21 patients. Clin Genet 1986;29:222–33.
90 Goldstein AM, Bale SJ, Peck GL et al. Sun exposure and basal cell carcinomas in the nevoid basal cell carcinoma syndrome. J Am Acad Dermatol 1993;29:34–41.
91 Mohs FE, Jones DL, Koranda FC. Microscopically controlled surgery for carcinomas in patients with nevoid basal cell carcinoma syndrome. Arch Dermatol 1980;116:777–9.
92 Kopera D, Cerroni L, Fink-Puches R et al. Different treatment modalities for the management of a patient with nevoid basal cell carcinoma syndrome. J Am Acad Dermatol 1996;34:937–9.
93 van Ruth S, Jansman FGA and Sanders CJ. Total body topical 5-fluorouracil for extensive non-melanoma skin cancer. Pharm World Sci 2006;28:159–62.
94 Kagy MK, Amonette R. The use of imiquimod 5% cream for the treatment of superficial basal cell carcinomas in a basal cell nevus syndrome patient. Dermatol Surg 2000;26:577–8.
95 Stockfleth E, Ulrich C, Hauschild A et al. Successful treatment of basal cell carcinomas in a nevoid basal cell carcinoma syndrome with topical 5% imiquimod. Eur J Dermatol 2002;12:569–72.
96 Alessi SS, Sanches JA, de Oliveira WR et al. Treatment of cutaneous tumors with topical 5% imiquimod cream. Clinics (Sao Paulo) 2009;64:961–6.
97 Quist SR, Franke I, Helmdach M et al. Complete basal cell carcinoma remission with imiquimod in a patient with naevoid basal cell carcinoma syndrome and associated basal cell carcinoma of the scalp and invasive ductal breast cancer. J Am Acad Dermatol 2011;64:611–3.
98 Strange PR, Lang PG Jr. Long-term management of basal cell nevus syndrome with topical tretinoin and 5-fluorouracil. J Am Acad Dermatol 1992;27:842–5.
99 Tang JY, Chiou AS, Mackay-Wiggan JM et al. Tazarotene: randomized, double-blind, vehicle-controlled and open-label concurrent trials for basal cell carcinoma prevention and therapy in patients with basal cell nevus syndrome. Cancer Prev Res (Phila) 2014;7:292–9.
100 Southwick GJ, Schwartz RA. The basal cell nevus syndrome: disasters occurring among a series of 36 patients. Cancer 1979;44:2294–305.
101 Strong LC. Genetic and environmental interactions. Cancer 1977;40:1861–6.
102 Zvulunov A, Strother D, Zirbel G. Nevoid basal cell carcinoma syndrome: report of a case with associated Hodgkin's disease. J Pediatr Hematol Oncol 1995;17:66–70.
103 Korczak JF, Brahim JS, DiGiovanna JJ et al. Nevoid basal cell carcinoma syndrome with medulloblastoma in an African–American boy: a rare case illustrating gene–environment interaction. Am J Med Genet 1997;69:309–14.
104 Baker S, Joseph K, Tai P. Radiotherapy in Gorlin Syndrome: can it be safe and effective in adult patients? J Cut Med Surg 2016;20:159–62.
105 Cristofolini M, Zumiani G, Scappni P et al. Aromatic retinoid in chemoprevention of the progression of nevoid basal cell carcinoma syndrome. J Dermatol Surg Oncol 1984;10:778–81.
106 Hodak E, Ginzburg A, David M et al. Etretinate treatment of the nevoid basal cell carcinoma syndrome. Int J Dermatol 1987;26:606–9.
107 Sanchez-Conejo-Mir J, Camacho F. Nevoid basal cell carcinoma syndrome: combined etretinate and surgical treatment. J Dermatol Surg Oncol 1989;15:868–71.
108 Goldberg LH, Hsu SH, Alcalay J. Effectiveness of isotretinoin in preventing the appearance of basal cell carcinomas in basal cell nevus syndrome. J Am Acad Dermatol 1989;21:144–5.
109 Peck GL, DiGiovanna JJ, Sarnoff DS et al. Treatment and prevention of basal cell carcinoma with oral isotretinoin. J Am Acad Dermatol 1988;19:176–85.
110 Tangrea JA, Edwards BK, Taylor PR et al. Long-term therapy with low-dose isotretinoin for prevention of basal cell carcinoma: a multicenter clinical trial. J Natl Cancer Inst 1992;84:328–32.
111 Theiler R, Hubscher E, Wagenhauser FJ et al. Diffuse idiopathic skeletal hyperostosis (DISH) and pseudocoxarthritis following long-term etretinate therapy. Schweiz Med Wochenschr 1993;123:649–53.
112 Tse DT, Kersten RC, Anderson RL. Hematoporphyrin derivative photoradiation therapy in managing nevoid basal cell carcinoma syndrome. A preliminary report. Arch Ophthalmol 1984;102:990–4.
113 Zeitouni NC, Shieh S, Oseroff AR. Laser and photodynamic therapy in the management of cutaneous malignancies. Clin Dermatol 2001;19:328–39.
114 Oseroff AR, Blumenson LR, Wilson BD et al. A dose ranging study of photodynamic therapy with porfimer sodium (Photofrin) for treatment of basal cell carcinoma. Lasers Surg Med 2006;38:417–26.
115 Loncaster J, Swindell R, Slevin F et al. Efficacy of photodynamic therapy as a treatment for Gorlin syndrome-related basal cell carcinomas. Clin Oncol (R Coll Radiol) 2009;21:502–8.
116 Gilchrest BA, Brightman LA, Thiele JJ, Wasserman DI. Photodynamic therapy for patients with basal cell nevus syndrome. Dermatol Surg 2009;35:1576–81.
117 Oseroff AR, Shieh S, Frawley NP et al. Treatment of diffuse basal cell carcinomas and basaloid follicular harmatomas in nevoid basal cell carcinoma syndrome by wide-area 5-aminolevulinic acid photodynamic therapy. Arch Dermatol 2005;141:60–7.
118 Basset-Seguin N, Bissonnette R, Girard C et al. Consensus recommendations for the treatment of basal cell carcinomas in Gorlin syndrome with topical methylaminolaevulinate-photodynamic therapy. J Eur Acad Dermatol Venereol 2014;28:626–32.
119 Sekulic A, Migden M, Oro A et al. Efficacy and safety of vismodegib in advanced basal-cell carcinomas. New Engl J Med 2012; 366:2171–9.
120 Tang JY, Mackay-Wiggan JM, Aszterbaum M et al. Inhibiting the Hedgehog pathway in patients with the basal-cell nevus syndrome. N Engl J Med 2012;366:2180–8.
121 Ally MS, Tang JY, Joseph T et al. The use of vismodegib to shrink keratocystic odontogenic tumours in basal cell nevus syndrome patients. JAMA Dermatol 2014;150:542–5.
122 Posnick JC, Clokie CML, Goldstein JA. Maxillofacial considerations for diagnosis and treatment in Gorlin's syndrome: access osteotomies for cyst removal and orthognathic surgery. Ann Plast Surg 1994;35:512–18.

CHAPTER 140

Rothmund–Thomson Syndrome, Bloom Syndrome, Dyskeratosis Congenita, Fanconi Anaemia and Poikiloderma with Neutropenia

Lisa L. Wang[1] *& Moise L. Levy*[1,2]

[1]Department of Pediatrics, Texas Children's Hospital, Baylor College of Medicine, Houston, TX, USA
[2]Department of Pediatrics, Dell Medical School/University of Texas and Dell Children's Medical Center, Austin, TX, USA

Rothmund–Thomson syndrome, 1786
Bloom syndrome, 1791
Dyskeratosis congenita, 1793
Fanconi anaemia, 1796
Poikiloderma with neutropenia, 1798

Abstract

There are several genetic disorders with prominent skin findings which predispose affected individuals to malignancies or bone marrow failure states. Some of these, such as Rothmund–Thomson syndrome, Bloom syndrome and Clericuzio-type poikiloderma with neutropenia have known pathogenic variants in single genes and are all inherited in an autosomal recessive manner. Other disorders, including dyskeratosis congenita and Fanconi anaemia, are associated with pathogenic variants in multiple genes and can have more than one inheritance pattern. Although there are many overlapping phenotypes among these disorders, including skin pigmentation changes, hair and nail defects, small stature, involvement of the skeletal and haematopoietic systems, and cancer predisposition, there are also distinct differences in the clinical manifestations which may be a reflection of the specific molecular defects underlying each disorder. Key features regarding the pathogenesis and clinical findings in these inherited syndromes will be described in this chapter.

Key points

- Keys clinical features of Rothmund–Thomson syndrome include poikiloderma, hyperkeratosis, small stature, sparse hair, abnormal teeth and nails, and skeletal abnormalities.
- Rothmund–Thomson syndrome patients with pathogenic variants in the *RECQL4* gene are at increased risk for developing osteosarcoma.
- Bloom syndrome is caused by pathogenic variants in the *BLM* gene which is in the same family of *RECQ* helicase genes as *RECQL4*.
- Bloom syndrome patients are prone to all cancers seen in the general population but at a much earlier age and at higher frequency.
- Dyskeratosis congenita is a telomere biology disorder that is caused by pathogenic variants in over 10 genes all involved in proper telomere maintenance and function.
- The 'classic triad' of dyskeratosis congenita includes irregular pigmentation, nail dystrophy and oral leukoplakia. Patients are at increased risk for bone marrow failure as well as cancers such as squamous cell carcinoma of the head and neck.
- Fanconi anaemia is caused by pathogenic variants in over 15 genes involved in DNA crosslink repair.
- Individuals affected by Fanconi anaemia can have congenital malformations, such as radial ray defects with missing thumbs, renal abnormalities and pigmentation defects, and they are at increased risk of bone marrow failure and solid malignancies such as head and neck, oesophagus, breast and brain cancers.
- Poikiloderma with neutropenia, Clericuzio-type, is caused by pathogenic variants in the *USB1* gene which is important for RNA splicing.
- Patients with poikiloderma with neutropenia have poikiloderma affecting their whole body, thickened nails and frequent sinopulmonary infections, and they can go on to develop haematological disorders such as myelodysplastic syndrome and acute leukaemia.

Rothmund–Thomson syndrome

Introduction and history. Rothmund–Thomson syndrome (RTS; OMIM #268400) is a rare autosomal recessive genetic disorder characterized by poikiloderma affecting mainly the face and extremities. Other clinical features are more heterogeneous and include small stature, sparse hair, cataract, gastrointestinal disturbance and bone abnormalities. Patients have an increased risk of developing squamous and basal cell carcinomas of the skin and, in particular, osteosarcoma of the bone.

In 1868, Auguste Rothmund, a German ophthalmologist, reported from an isolated Bavarian village several related individuals with poikiloderma, often associated with rapidly progressive, bilateral juvenile cataracts [1].

Harper's Textbook of Pediatric Dermatology, Fourth Edition. Edited by Peter Hoeger, Veronica Kinsler and Albert Yan.

In 1923, Sydney Thomson, a British dermatologist, reported three similar patients with a 'hitherto undescribed familial disease', which he subsequently named 'poikiloderma congenitale' [2]. His patients did not have the cataracts described by Rothmund, but instead had prominent skeletal defects. Subsequently, William Taylor, a dermatologist in the USA coined the eponym 'Rothmund–Thomson syndrome' to unite the disorders described separately by Rothmund and Thomson [3]. By 1992, over 200 cases of RTS had been reported in the world literature [4] with a total of 260 cases by 2008 [5].

Epidemiology and pathogenesis. RTS is inherited in an autosomal recessive pattern and is caused by germline pathogenic variants in the *RECQL4* gene at chromosome locus 8q24.3 in approximately two-thirds of cases, suggesting presence of genetic heterogeneity [6,7]. *RECQL4* is a member of the highly conserved RECQ DNA helicase family that share sequence homology in the helicase domain. RECQ helicases are able to unwind duplex DNA to provide single-stranded templates for replication, repair, recombination and transcription [8,9]. In humans there are five such *RECQ* genes, and germline mutations in three of them – *BLM*, *WRN*, and *RECQL4* – give rise to disorders that share overlapping features of growth deficiency, premature aging and significant predisposition to malignancy, namely Bloom syndrome, Werner syndrome, and RTS, respectively [10–12]. RECQL4 is a multifunctional protein that has been implicated in several cellular processes, including DNA replication [13,14], DNA damage repair, including homologous recombination [15], nonhomologous end-joining [16], nucleotide excision repair [17] and base excision repair [18, 19], maintenance of telomeres [20,21] and of mitochondrial DNA integrity [22–25]. Genetically engineered mouse models of RTS demonstrate that Recql4 plays an important role in normal haematopoiesis [26] and bone development [27,28].

Clinical features. The characteristic poikiloderma of RTS develops usually between 3 and 6 months of age [12,29]. It appears first on the cheeks as erythema and, by the end of the first year, it usually spreads to the extensor surfaces of the arms and legs and may or may not involve the buttocks. Lesions may also appear on the pinnae of the ears (Fig. 140.1). The trunk, abdomen and back tend to be spared. Initially during the acute phase, the affected areas appear inflamed and occasionally blistered, but after a few weeks or months the inflammation settles into the chronic phase of poikiloderma, consisting of hyper- and hypopigmentation, punctate atrophy and telangiectases. Areas of normal skin within the affected areas may produce a reticulate pattern (Fig. 140.2).

Transient photosensitivity has been reported in early childhood based on the typical distribution of inflammatory lesions on the face and backs of the hands, but this is not supported as an aetiological trigger by the occurrence of poikiloderma on the buttocks (Fig. 140.3). Some patients report 'heat sensitivity' which may also be misinterpreted as photosensitivity. Studies in the laboratory have been conflicting regarding sensitivity to ultraviolet (UV) radiation due in part to the various different assays used to assess UV sensitivity [30,31]. One study using primary fibroblasts from RTS patients showed that RTS fibroblasts did not have increased sensitivity to UV radiation compared with controls [32].

Sparse hair affecting particularly the scalp, eyebrows and eyelashes is commonly reported. Patients may have

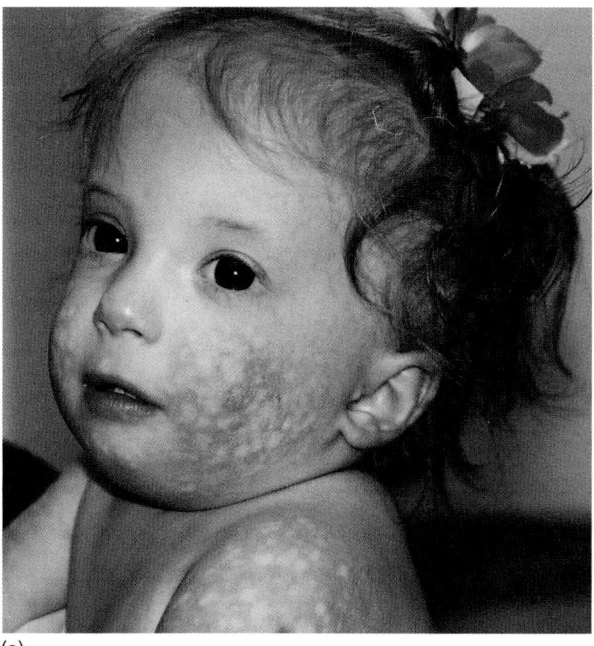
(a)

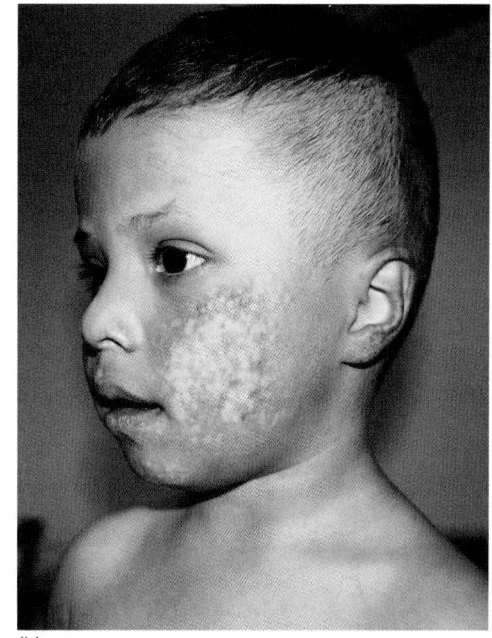
(b)

Fig. 140.1 Classic poikiloderma of the face in (a) a 1-year-old female and (b) a 4-year-old male with Rothmund–Thomson syndrome. Note involvement of the pinnae of the ears.

different combinations of sparseness (e.g. normal scalp hair but sparse eyelashes and/or eyebrows, or vice versa), and some have complete alopecia (Fig. 140.4). Body hair may also be reduced. The nails are usually slow growing and hypotrophic. Keratoses are commonly found on the extremities of older children and adults, often around the joints of the fingers or knee, and may be particularly severe on the heels (Fig. 140.5) [29]. A variety of dental anomalies has been reported such as short root anomaly, delayed or ectopic eruption of teeth, or rudimentary or hypoplastic teeth [33,34]; however, none of these findings is characteristic.

The reported incidence of juvenile cataracts has decreased over time, being 50% in Vennos and colleagues [4] 1992 review and only 6% in the series by Wang and colleagues in 2001 [12]. This is likely caused by genetic heterogeneity. Patients with *RECQL4* pathogenic variants do not typically develop cataracts; most cases of cataracts have been in those individuals lacking *RECQL4* pathogenic variants (likely the 'Rothmund phenotype'). Cataracts usually occur in all affected members of a sibship, and are generally of rapid onset, bilateral and of the subcapsular type; 73% develop before the age of 6 years [4]. A variety of other ocular abnormalities has been reported occasionally, including corneal atrophy, blue sclerae and iris dysgenesis [35,36].

Skeletal dysplasia is an important feature of RTS [12,37]. Proportional small stature is common and may be severe. Approximately 75% of patients demonstrated a significant skeletal abnormality on skeletal survey in a cohort

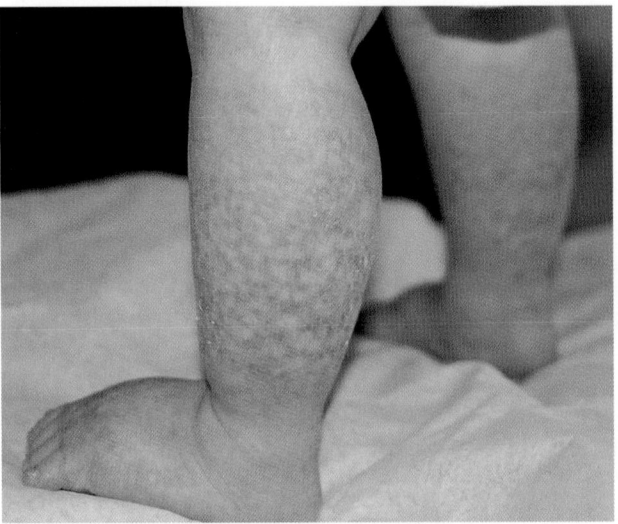

Fig. 140.2 Chronic poikiloderma on the lower extremities.

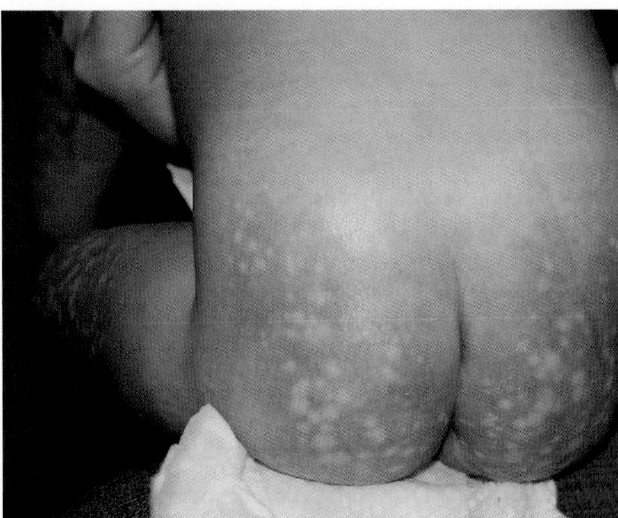

Fig. 140.3 Poikiloderma involving the buttocks in Rothmund–Thomson syndrome as well as the extremities with relative sparing of the back.

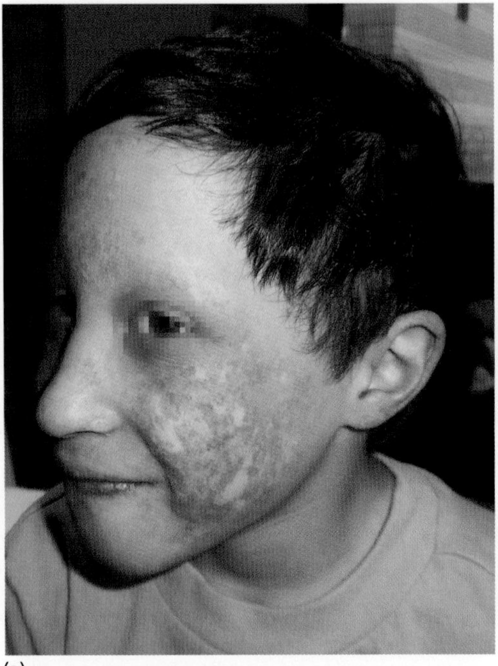

(a)

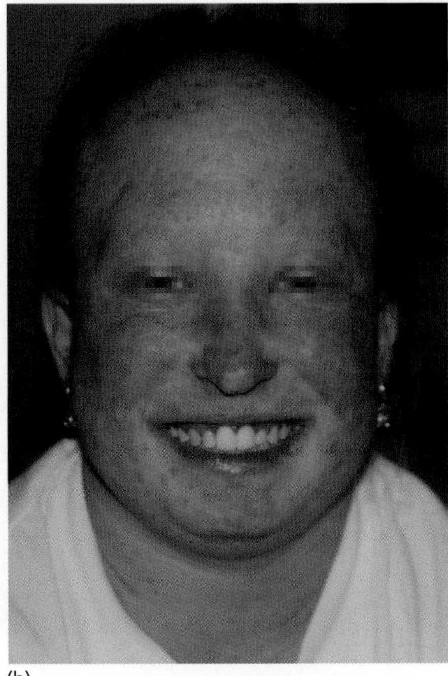

(b)

Fig. 140.4 Rothmund–Thomson syndrome patients with absent eyelashes and eyebrows with (a) normal and (b) sparse scalp hair.

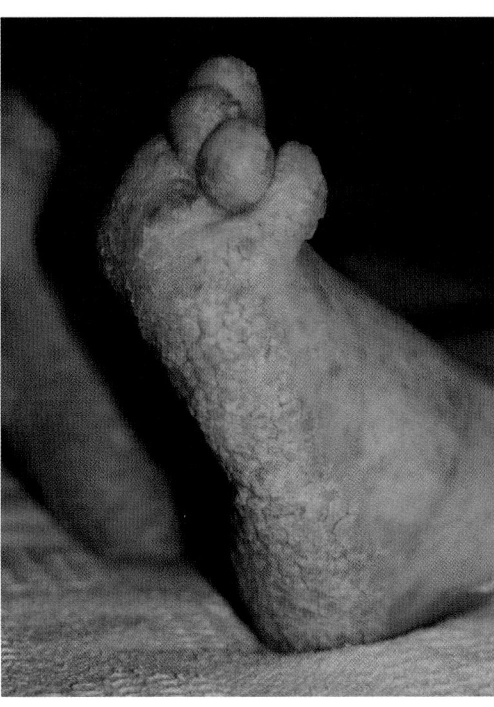

Fig. 140.5 Severe hyperkeratosis on the soles of the feet of a 19-year-old female with Rothmund–Thomson syndrome.

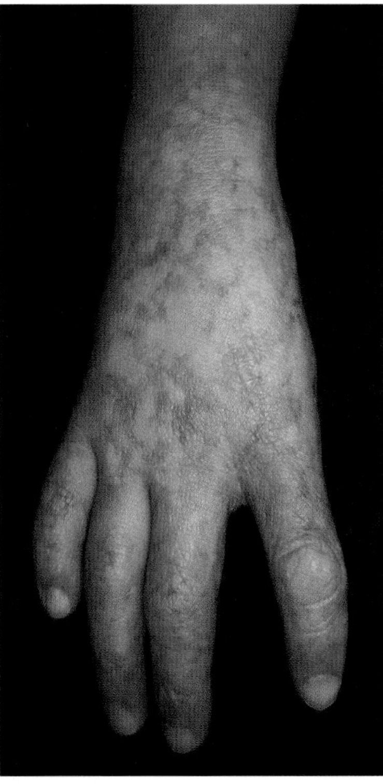

Fig. 140.6 Thumb aplasia in an 8-year-old male with Rothmund–Thomson syndrome.

study of 28 RTS patients. These findings included abnormal metaphyseal trabeculation, brachymesophalangy, thumb aplasia or hypoplasia (Fig. 140.6), osteopenia, dislocation of the radial head, radial aplasia or hypoplasia, and patellar ossification defects [37]. Genotype–phenotype analysis showed a significant positive correlation between those individuals with confirmed *RECQL4* pathogenic variants and the presence of skeletal abnormalities.

RTS is a cancer predisposition syndrome and patients have a very high risk of developing osteosarcoma, which is a primary malignant tumour that arises in bone, usually in the distal metaphyses of long bones. In a cohort of patients with RTS, the prevalence of osteosarcoma was 30% [12]. The median age at diagnosis of 11 years was younger than that seen in the general population. Families with more than one sibling with RTS and osteosarcoma have been described [12,38]. Presence of pathogenic variants in *RECQL4* has been shown to be significantly correlated with the risk of developing osteosarcoma [6,39].

Individuals with RTS are also at increased risk of developing skin cancer, most commonly basal cell and squamous cell carcinomas [4], although melanoma has also been described [40–42]. The prevalence of skin cancers in individuals with RTS is estimated from the literature to be 5%. Skin cancer can occur at any age, although it often arises earlier than in the general population. The mean age for epithelial tumours has been estimated at 34.4 years [5]. Piquero-Casals and colleagues [43] reported on a consanguineous Brazilian family with classic features of RTS including poikiloderma and bilateral cataracts. All three affected siblings developed cutaneous squamous cell carcinoma in adulthood (age 35–48 years). The cancers occurred on non-sun-exposed surfaces. Other forms of cancer that have been described in individuals with RTS include squamous cell carcinoma of the oropharynx, myelodysplasia and leukaemia [44–49].

Patients with RTS are generally of normal intelligence with no neurological problems, although delayed speech and delay in reaching childhood milestones have been reported [12]. Life expectancy in the absence of death from cancer appears to be normal in the authors' experience, although further natural history study is needed.

Differential diagnosis. Radial hypoplasia in a child too young to have developed the characteristic skin changes may be misdiagnosed as Fanconi syndrome or Holt–Oram syndrome [50]. The initial inflammation on the face or light-exposed areas may be mistaken for eczema or photosensitivity. Vesiculation at the onset of poikiloderma may suggest Weary–Kindler syndrome. The facial rash, with telangiectases, and pigmentation changes along with small stature may mimic Bloom syndrome. Patients with Clericuzio-type poikiloderma with neutropenia (PN) also have chronic poikiloderma, although the location of onset and pattern of spread is different from RTS, because it tends to start peripherally in PN and spread centrally to involve the trunk, abdomen and back [51–53]. Patients with PN also tend to have very thick nails and normal hair, unlike patients with RTS. Pathogenic variants in the *USB1* gene are causative of PN [54]. There are two other allelic disorders in which *RECQL4* pathogenic variants have been identified: RAPADILINO syndrome (OMIM

266280), and Baller–Gerold syndrome (BGS) (OMIM 218600) [55,56]. The name RAPADILINO is an acronym for a series of clinical features seen in patients with this disorder: radial ray defects (RA), patellae hypoplasia/aplasia and cleft or high arched palate (PA), diarrhoea in infancy and dislocated joints (DI), small stature (LI, little size), and long slender nose and normal intelligence (NO). Most of these findings overlap with RTS except for the poikiloderma. RAPADILINO patients also have an increased risk of developing lymphoma and osteosarcoma [7]. BGS is characterized primarily by radial ray defects and craniosynostosis, and lymphoma has been reported in a single BGS patient [57].

Laboratory and histology findings. Patients with a clinical diagnosis of RTS should undergo screening of the *RECQL4* gene for pathogenic variants. Early on by pathology, the affected skin is oedematous, with a perivascular lymphocytic infiltrate. Later, the poikilodermatous skin shows hyperkeratosis, epidermal atrophy with dyskeratotic cells, dilation of the superficial vessels in the papillary dermis, pigmentary incontinence, basal cell vacuolization, fragmentation of elastic tissue and loss of appendages. The keratoses display dysplastic and Bowenoid changes [58]. Several patients have been reported with various karyotypic abnormalities, including mosaic trisomies of chromosomes 2, 7, 8 and 15 as well as mosaicism for complex karyotypes [12,59–63].

Treatment and prevention. Treatment is largely symptomatic. Patients should employ sensible sun protection to prevent skin cancers and should monitor skin for lesions with unusual colour or texture. Retinoids may improve the hyperkeratoses [64]. Pulsed dye laser therapy may be helpful cosmetically for the telangiectatic portion of the rash [65]. Patients should undergo an ophthalmological evaluation to screen for cataracts. Skeletal surveys are recommended to define underlying bone defects and serve as a baseline in case of bone symptoms suggestive of osteosarcoma. RTS patients who develop osteosarcoma should be treated using standard chemotherapy protocols, with dose modifications based on individual patient toxicities [66]. There are currently no formal screening guidelines for osteosarcoma other than counselling and increased awareness.

References

1 Rothmund A. Uber Kataract in Verbindung mit einer eigentumliche Haut Degenerationen. Arch Ophthal 1868;14:159–82.
2 Thomson MS. Poikiloderma congenitale. Br J Dermatol 1936;48:221.
3 Taylor WB. Rothmund's syndrome; Thomson's syndrome; congenital poikiloderma with or without juvenile cataracts. AMA Arch Derm 1957;75:236–44.
4 Vennos EM, Collins M, James WD. Rothmund–Thomson syndrome: review of the world literature. J Am Acad Dermatol 1992;27:750–62.
5 Stinco G, Governatori G, Mattighello P et al. Multiple cutaneous neoplasms in a patient with Rothmund–Thomson syndrome: case report and published work review. J Dermatol 2008;35:154–61.
6 Wang LL, Gannavarapu A, Kozinetz CA et al. Association between osteosarcoma and deleterious mutations in the RECQL4 gene in Rothmund–Thomson syndrome. J Natl Cancer Inst 2003;95:669–74.
7 Siitonen HA, Sotkasiira J, Biervliet M et al. The mutation spectrum in RECQL4 diseases. Eur J Hum Genet 2009;17:151–8.
8 Chu WK, Hickson ID. RecQ helicases: multifunctional genome caretakers. Nat Rev Cancer 2009;9:644–54.
9 Croteau DL, Popuri V, Opresko PL et al. Human RecQ helicases in DNA repair, recombination, and replication. Annu Rev Biochem 2014;83:519–52.
10 de Renty C, Ellis NA. Bloom's syndrome: why not premature aging? A comparison of the BLM and WRN helicases. Ageing Res Rev 2016;S1568–1637(16)30089–7.
11 Monnat RJ Jr. '...Rewritten in the skin': clues to skin biology and aging from inherited disease. J Invest Dermatol 2015;135:1484–90.
12 Wang LL, Levy ML, Lewis RA et al. Clinical manifestations in a cohort of 41 Rothmund–Thomson syndrome patients. Am J Med Genet 2001;102:11–17.
13 Sangrithi MN, Bernal JA, Madine M et al. Initiation of DNA replication requires the RECQL4 protein mutated in Rothmund-Thomson syndrome. Cell 2005;121:887–98.
14 Matsuno K, Kumano M, Kubota Y et al. The N-terminal noncatalytic region of Xenopus RecQ4 is required for chromatin binding of DNA polymerase alpha in the initiation of DNA replication. Mol Cell Biol 2006;26:4843–52.
15 Petkovic M, Dietschy T, Freire R et al. The human Rothmund-Thomson syndrome gene product, RECQL4, localizes to distinct nuclear foci that coincide with proteins involved in the maintenance of genome stability. J Cell Sci 2005;118:4261–9.
16 Shamanna RA, Singh DK, Lu H et al. RECQ helicase RECQL4 participates in non-homologous end joining and interacts with the Ku complex. Carcinogenesis 2014;35:2415–24.
17 Fan W, Luo J. RecQ4 facilitates UV light-induced DNA damage repair through interaction with nucleotide excision repair factor xeroderma pigmentosum group A (XPA). J Biol Chem 2008;283:29037–44.
18 Woo LL, Futami K, Shimamoto A et al. The Rothmund-Thomson gene product RECQL4 localizes to the nucleolus in response to oxidative stress. Exp Cell Res 2006;312:3443–57.
19 Schurman SH, Hedayati M, Wang Z et al. Direct and indirect roles of RECQL4 in modulating base excision repair capacity. Hum Mol Genet 2009;18:3470–83.
20 Ghosh AK, Rossi ML, Singh DK et al. RECQL4, the protein mutated in Rothmund-Thomson syndrome, functions in telomere maintenance. J Biol Chem 2012;287:196–209.
21 Ferrarelli LK, Popuri V, Ghosh AK et al. The RECQL4 protein, deficient in Rothmund-Thomson syndrome is active on telomeric D-loops containing DNA metabolism blocking lesions. DNA Repair (Amst) 2013;12:518–28.
22 Croteau DL, Rossi ML, Canugovi C et al. RECQL4 localizes to mitochondria and preserves mitochondrial DNA integrity. Aging Cell 2012;11:456–66.
23 De S, Kumari J, Mudgal R et al. RECQL4 is essential for the transport of p53 to mitochondria in normal human cells in the absence of exogenous stress. J Cell Sci 2012;125:2509–22.
24 Gupta S, De S, Srivastava V et al. RECQL4 and p53 potentiate the activity of polymerase γ and maintain the integrity of the human mitochondrial genome. Carcinogenesis 2014;35:34–45.
25 Kumari J, Hussain M, De S et al. Mitochondrial functions of RECQL4 are required for the prevention of aerobic glycolysis-dependent cell invasion. J Cell Sci 2016;129:1312–8.
26 Smeets MF, DeLuca E, Wall M et al. The Rothmund-Thomson syndrome helicase RECQL4 is essential for hematopoiesis. J Clin Invest 2014;124:3551–65.
27 Lu L, Harutyunyan K, Jin W et al. recql4 regulates p53 function in vivo during skeletogenesis. J Bone Miner Res 2015;30:1077–89.
28 Ng AJ, Walia MK, Smeets MF et al. The DNA helicase recql4 is required for normal osteoblast expansion and osteosarcoma formation. PLoS Genet 2015;11:e1005160.
29 Wang LL, Plon SE. Rothmund-Thomson Syndrome. In: Pagon RA, Adam MP, Ardinger HH et al. editors. GeneReviews® [Internet]. Seattle (WA): University of Washington, Seattle; 1993–2016 [updated 2016 Aug 11].
30 Smith PJ, Paterson MC. Enhanced radiosensitivity and defective DNA repair in cultured fibroblasts derived from Rothmund–Thomson patients. Mutat Res 1982;94:213–28.
31 Shinya A, Nishigori C, Moriwaki S et al. A case of Rothmund–Thomson syndrome with reduced DNA repair capacity. Arch Dermatol 1993;129:332–6.
32 Jin W, Liu H, Zhang Y et al. Sensitivity of RECQL4-deficient fibroblasts from Rothmund–Thomson syndrome patients to genotoxic agents. Hum Genet 2008;123:643–53.

33 Roinioti TD, Stefanopoulos PK. Short root anomaly associated with Rothmund-Thomson syndrome. Oral Surg Oral Med Oral Pathol Oral Radiol Endod 2007;103:e19–22.
34 Haytaç MC, Oztunç H, Mete UO, Kaya M. Rothmund-Thomson syndrome: a case report. Oral Surg Oral Med Oral Pathol Oral Radiol Endod 2002;94:479–84.
35 Moss C. Rothmund–Thomson syndrome: a report of two patients and a review of the literature. Br J Dermatol 1990;122:821–9.
36 Mak RK, Griffiths WA, Mellerio JE. An unusual patient with Rothmund–Thomson syndrome, porokeratosis and bilateral iris dysgenesis. Clin Exp Dermatol 2006;31:401–3.
37 Mehollin-Ray AR, Kozinetz CA, Schlesinger AE et al. Radiographic abnormalities in Rothmund–Thomson syndrome and genotype–phenotype correlation with RECQL4 mutation status. AJR 2008; 191:W62–6.
38 Lindor NM, Furuichi Y, Kitao S et al. Rothmund-Thomson syndrome due to RECQ4 helicase mutations: report and clinical and molecular comparisons with Bloom syndrome and Werner syndrome. Am J Med Genet 2000;90:223–8.
39 Lu L, Jin W, Liu H et al. RECQ DNA helicases and osteosarcoma. Adv Exp Med Biol 2014;804:129–45.
40 Howell SM, Bray DW. Amelanotic melanoma in a patient with Rothmund–Thomson syndrome. Arch Dermatol 2008;144:416–7.
41 Simon T, Kohlhase J, Wilhelm C et al. Multiple malignant diseases in a patient with RECQL4 mutations: case report and literature review. Am J Med Genet A 2010;152A:1575–9
42 Jaju PD, Ransohoff KJ, Tang JY et al. Familial skin cancer syndromes. J Am Acad Dermatol 2016;74:437–51
43 Piquero-Casals J, Okubo AY, Nico MM. Rothmund–Thomson syndrome in three siblings and development of cutaneous squamous cell carcinoma. Pediatr Dermatol 2002;19:312–6.
44 Borg MF, Olver IN, Hill MP. Rothmund-Thomson syndrome and tolerance of chemoradiotherapy. Australas Radiol 1998;42:216–8.
45 Rizzari C, Bacchiocchi D, Rovelli A et al. Myelodysplastic syndrome in a child with Rothmund-Thomson syndrome: a case report. J Pediatr Hematol Oncol 1996;18:96–7.
46 Ilhan I, Arikan Ü, Büyükpamukçu M. Myelodysplatic syndrome and RTS. Pediatr Hematol Oncol 1996;13:197.
47 Pianigiani E, de Aloe G, Andreassi A et al. Rothmund–Thomson syndrome (Thomson type) and myelodysplasia. Pediatr Dermatol 2001;18:422–5.
48 Narayan S, Fleming C, Trainer AH, Craig JA. Rothmund-Thomson syndrome with myelodysplasia. Pediatr Dermatol 2001;18:210–2.
49 Porter WM, Hardman CM, Abdalla SH et al. Haematological disease in siblings with Rothmund-Thomson syndrome. Clin Exp Dermatol 1999;24:452–4.
50 Moss C, Bacon CJ, Mueller RF. 'Isolated' radial ray defect may be due to Rothmund–Thomson syndrome. Clin Genet 1990;38:318–9.
51 Wang LL, Gannavarapu A, Clericuzio CL et al. Absence of RECQL4 mutations in poikiloderma with neutropenia in Navajo and non-Navajo patients. Am J Med Genet A 2003;118A:299–301.
52 Van Hove JL, Jaeken J, Proesmans M et al. Clericuzio type poikiloderma with neutropenia is distinct from Rothmund-Thomson syndrome. Am J Med Genet A 2005;132A:152–8.
53 Clericuzio C, Harutyunyan K, Jin W et al. Identification of a novel C16orf57 mutation in Athabaskan patients with poikiloderma with neutropenia. Am J Med Genet A 2011;155A:337–42.
54 Hilcenko C, Simpson PJ, Finch AJ et al. Aberrant 3′ oligoadenylation of spliceosomal U6 small nuclear RNA in poikiloderma with neutropenia. Blood 2013;121:1028–38
55 Siitonen HA, Kopra O, Kääriäinen H et al. Molecular defect of RAPADILINO syndrome expands the phenotype spectrum of RECQL diseases. Hum Mol Genet 2003;12:2837–44
56 Van Maldergem L, Siitonen HA, Jalkh N et al. Revisiting the craniosynostosis-radial ray hypoplasia association: Baller-Gerold syndrome caused by mutations in the RECQL4 gene. J Med Genet 2006;43:148–52.
57 Debeljak M, Zver A, Jazbec J. A patient with Baller-Gerold syndrome and midline NK/T lymphoma. Am J Med Genet A 2009; 149A:755–9.
58 Shuttleworth D, Marks R. Epidermal dysplasia and skeletal deformity in congenital poikiloderma (Rothmund-Thomson syndrome). Br J Dermatol 1987;117:377–84.
59 Orstavik KH, McFadden N, Hagelsteen J et al. Instability of lymphocyte chromosomes in a girl with Rothmund-Thomson syndrome. J Med Genet 1994;31:570–2.
60 Der Kaloustian V, McGill JJ, Vekemans M et al. Clonal lines of aneuploid cells in Rothmund-Thomson syndrome. Am J Med Genet 1990;37:336–9.
61 Ying KL, Oizumi J, Curry CJ. Rothmund-Thomson syndrome associated with trisomy 8 mosaicism. J Med Genet 1990;27:258–60.
62 Lindor NM, Devries EM, Michels et al. Rothmund-Thomson syndrome in siblings: evidence for acquired in vivo mosaicism. Clin Genet 1996;49:124–9.
63 Miozzo M, Castorina P, Riva P et al. Chromosomal instability in fibroblasts and mesenchymal tumors from 2 sibs with Rothmund-Thomson syndrome. Int J Cancer 1998;77:504–10.
64 Shuttleworth D, Marks R. Congenital poikiloderma: treatment with etretinate. Br J Dermatol 1988;118:729–30.
65 Potozkin JR, Geronemus RG. Treatment of the poikilodermatous component of the Rothmund-Thomson syndrome with the flashlamp-pumped pulsed dye laser: a case report. Pediatr Dermatol 1991;8:162–5.
66 Hicks MJ, Roth JR, Kozinetz CA et al. Clinicopathologic features of osteosarcoma in patients with Rothmund–Thomson syndrome. J Clin Oncol 2007;25:370–5.

Bloom syndrome

Introduction and history. Bloom syndrome (BS; OMIM #210900) is a rare genetic disorder characterized by small stature, immunodeficiency, erythematous telangiectatic facial rash and other pigmentary abnormalities, and a significant predisposition for multiple types of cancers. David Bloom, a New York City dermatologist, first described this syndrome in 1954 [1], and he subsequently contributed cases [2] to the Bloom Syndrome Registry established by James German in the early 1960s [3].

Epidemiology and pathogenesis. BS is inherited in an autosomal recessive fashion. It is relatively less rare in the Ashkenazi Jewish population compared with the general population, likely caused by a founder effect, but it has been described in all races. In the BS Registry as of 2016, 72 of the 265 persons (27%) were of Ashekenazi Jewish ancestry [4]. The first cellular abnormalities identified in BD were increased sensitivity to UV light [5] and increased sister chromatid exchange (SCE) [6]. SCEs are the result of crossover events during repair via homologous recombination of damaged replication forks and are characteristic of BS cells. Other chromosomal aberrations are also present, including chromatid gaps and breaks, formation of quadriradial chromosomes and telomere associations [7].

In 1995, Ellis and colleagues [8] identified the BS gene as *RECQL2* (known as *BLM*) localized to 15q26.1. Homozygous or compound heterozygous pathogenic variants are causative of the disorder. *BLM* encodes a DNA helicase which unwinds complementary double strands and belongs to the conserved family of RECQ helicases that also includes genes associated with Werner syndrome (*WRN*) and RTS (*RECQL4*). These proteins are important for maintaining genomic stability [9]. In a 2007 report from the BS Registry [10], 64 different mutations were identified in 125 of 134 patients. These mutations all result in inactivation of the BLM protein either by premature termination of protein translation or by missense mutations that abrogate its helicase activity [7]. BLM is a multifunctional protein which plays a role in several cellular processes including homologous recombination

(DNA repair), DNA replication (stabilization and repair of stalled replication forks), sister chromatid segregation during normal mitosis and maintenance of telomeres [7].

Clinical features. Affected individuals show both pre- and postnatal growth deficiency [11]. The body proportions are normal apart from a slightly disproportionately small head. Patients have sparse subcutaneous fat and a characteristic facies with a narrow profile, underdeveloped malar and lower mandibular areas with resulting prominence of the nose and ears, and somewhat beaked nose [4]. Patients often have a high-pitched voice. Growth hormone levels are reported as normal.

The rash of BS usually appears on the face as erythema during the first or second years of life after sun exposure. It typically involves the cheeks and nose ('butterfly rash') but may involve other areas of the face (Fig. 140.7), as well as the forearms and hands. There may be a telangiectatic component to the rash. Vesiculation and fissure formation may also occur especially around the mouth. The severity of the rash is quite variable among different persons with BS. Often the rash becomes less severe with age and sometimes it can disappear completely. Café-au-lait spots are increased in BS; these are often associated with contiguous hypopigmented areas [4,7] (Fig. 140.8). Infants and children with BS have been described to have poor feeding and general lack of interest in food. Severe gastro-intestinal reflux has been described and may account for the increase in pneumonia and otitis media seen in BS. Immunodeficiency has been reported as a feature of BS with reduced levels of plasma immunoglobulins (IgA and IgM) and abnormal delayed hypersensitivity reaction, although this has not been fully delineated [12]. Diabetes mellitus resembling Type 2 adult-onset diabetes mellitus [13] occurs at an earlier age in BS patients (18% in BS Registry, median age 27 years), and chronic obstructive pulmonary disease, including chronic bronchitis and bronchiectasis, is also a known complication. Infertility is impaired in BS; males are infertile (azoospermia or severe oligospermia), whereas females are fertile and enter menarche at the normal age, but have premature cessation of menstruation. Intelligence appears to be normal overall, although some patients have minor learning disabilities [4].

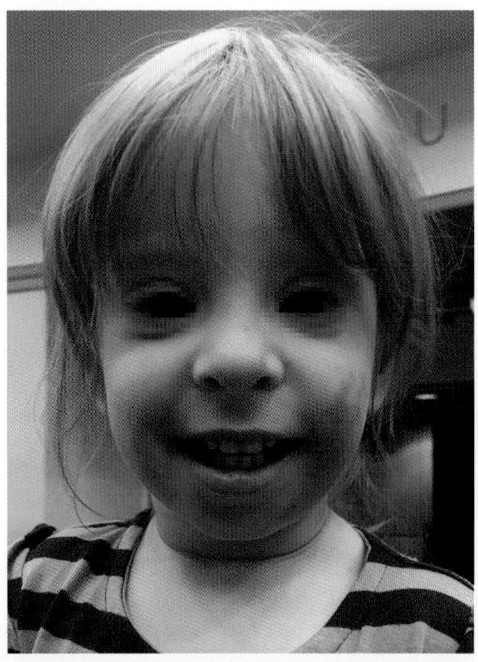

Fig. 140.7 Facial erythema in a 2-year-old girl with Bloom syndrome.

Cancer is the most frequent medical complication of BS and the most common cause of death. The spectrum of cancers reflects that of the general population, but the cancers arise at a much earlier age and at a higher frequency in BS patients. These include the major epithelial cancers such as lung, colorectal, breast, skin, genitourinary tract and oesophageal carcinomas, of which colorectal cancer is the most common in BS. Haematological malignancies including lymphomas, acute lymphoblastic leukaemia and acute myelogenous leukaemia are common, as is myelodysplasia. Rare paediatric tumours such as Wilm's tumour, retinoblastoma and osteosarcoma also occur. Shi and colleagues demonstrated through analysis of incidence ratios that persons with BS are 99 times more

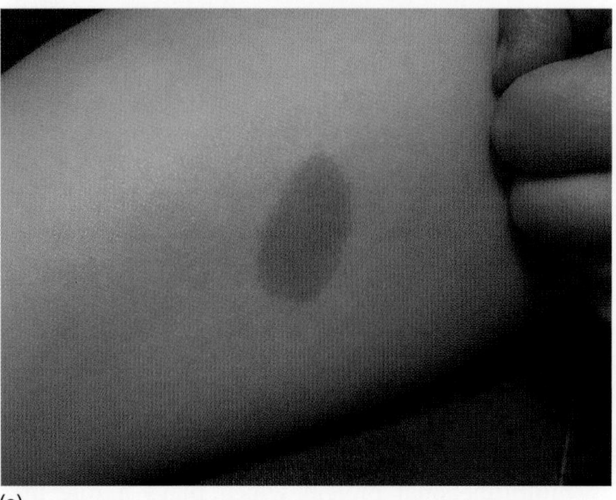

(a)

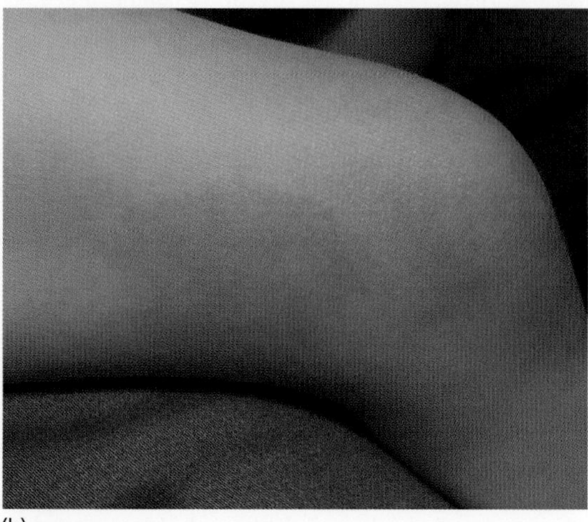

(b)

Fig. 140.8 Café-au-lait spots on the (a) left thigh and (b) right thigh in a child with Bloom syndrome.

likely to be diagnosed with any cancer compared with the general population (95% confidence interval 83–117) [7,14]. Life expectancy is reduced caused by the increased incidence and earlier age of malignancy, as well as other serious complications such as chronic obstructive pulmonary disease and diabetes mellitus.

Differential diagnosis. The symmetrical small stature and facial telangiectasia may be confused with RTS, but RTS patients have more prominent poikiloderma, hyperkeratosis, sparse hair, skeletal defects and they are uniquely and highly predisposed to osteosarcoma. Café-au-lait macules with immunodeficiency are also seen in Fanconi anaemia, as well as small stature and increased incidence of bone marrow failure and hematological malignancies. Patients with Fanconi anaemia often have thumb and forearm abnormalities which is more similar to RTS than BS. However, the increased SCE rate and molecular analysis of the *BLM* gene provide specific diagnostic tests for BS.

Laboratory and histology findings. Increased SCEs, usually a mean of 40–100 per metaphase versus fewer than 10 in controls, are pathognomonic of BS. These are demonstrated in cultured cells (lymphocytes, fibroblasts, fetal cells) allowed to proliferate in a medium containing 5′bromo-2′-deoxyuridine (BrdU). Molecular genetic testing identifying biallelic pathogenic variants in the *BLM* gene establishes a diagnosis. Plasma levels of immunoglobulins may be reduced [12,15]. The histology of the affected skin is nonspecific showing epidermal atrophy, telangiectasia and a mild perivascular inflammatory infiltrate. An interface pattern by histopathology, as in lupus erythematosus, is commonly seen [16].

Treatment and prevention. Treatment is geared toward the clinical manifestations. Laser therapy to areas of telangiectasia may improve cosmesis. Standard chemotherapy and/or radiation regimens for treatment of cancer typically require dose reduction given the hypersensitivity of BS patients to DNA damaging agents. Affected individuals should avoid carcinogens such as smoking, ultraviolet and ionizing radiation and should routinely use sunscreen protection. Regular screening tests for cancers in the general population, such as colonoscopy, mammogram and cervical pap smear, should be started earlier and at more frequent intervals [4,17].

References

1 Bloom D. Congenital telangiectatic erythema resembling lupus erythematosus in dwarfs; probably a syndrome entity. AMA Am J Dis Child 1954;88:754–8.

2 Bloom D. The syndrome of congenital telangiectatic erythema and stunted growth. J Pediatr 1966;68:103–13.

3 German J, Passarge E. Bloom's syndrome. XII. Report from the Registry for 1987. Clin Genet 1989;35:57–69

4 Sanz MM, German J, Cunniff C. Bloom's syndrome. In: Pagon RA, Adam MP, Ardinger HH (eds) GeneReviews® [Internet]. Seattle (WA): University of Washington, Seattle; 1993–2016. 2006 Mar 22 [updated 2016 Apr 7].

5 Gianneli F, Benson PF, Pawsey SA et al. Ultraviolet light sensitivity and delayed DNA chain maturation in Bloom's syndrome fibroblasts. Nature 1977;265:466–9.

6 Dicken CH, Dewald G, Gordon H. Sister chromatid exchanges in Bloom's syndrome. Arch Dermatol 1978;114:755–60.

7 de Renty C, Ellis NA. Bloom's syndrome: why not premature aging? A comparison of the BLM and WRN helicases. Ageing Res Rev 2016:S1568–1637(16)30089–7.

8 Ellis NA, Groden J, Ye TZ et al. The Bloom's syndrome gene product is homologous to RecQ helicases. Cell 1995;83:655–66.

9 Croteau DL, Popuri V, Opresko PL et al. Human RecQ helicases in DNA repair, recombination, and replication. Annu Rev Biochem 2014;83:519–52.

10 German J, Sanz MM, Ciocci S et al. Syndrome-causing mutations of the BLM gene in persons in the Bloom's Syndrome Registry. Hum Mutat 2007;28:743–53.

11 Keller C, Keller KR, Shew SB et al. Growth deficiency and malnutrition in Bloom syndrome. J Pediatr 1999;134:472–9.

12 Babbe H, McMenamin J, Hobeika E et al. Genomic instability resulting from Blm deficiency compromises development, maintenance, and function of the B cell lineage. J Immunol 2009;182:347–60.

13 Diaz A, Vogiatzi MG, Sanz MM, German J. Evaluation of short stature, carbohydrate metabolism and other endocrinopathies in Bloom's syndrome. Horm Res 2006;66:111–17.

14 Shi W, Zauber A, Sanz M et al. Analysis of the markedly increased incidence of cancer in individuals with Bloom's syndrome (Abstract). In: 56th Annual Meeting of the American Society of Human Genetics, New Orleans, 2006.

15 Kondo N, Ozawa T, Kato Y et al. Reduced secreted mu mRNA synthesis in selective IgM deficiency of Bloom syndrome. Clin Exp Immunol 1992;88:35–40.

16 McGowan J, Maize J, Cook J. Lupus-like histopathology in Bloom syndrome: Reexamining the clinical and histopathologic implications of photosensitivity. Am J Dermatopathol 2009;31:786–91

17 Thomas ER, Shanley S, Walker L et al. Surveillance and treatment of malignancy in Bloom syndrome. Clin Oncol (R Coll Radiol) 2008;20:375–9.

Dyskeratosis congenita

Introduction and history. Dyskeratosis congenita (DC) is a telomere biology disorder characterized by a classic triad of reticulated skin pigmentation, dystrophic nails and oral leucoplakia. Other prominent features include progressive bone marrow failure, increased risk for myelodysplastic syndrome and haematological malignancies, as well as epithelial tumours and pulmonary fibrosis.

The disorder was first described by Zinsser in 1906 [1] and later recognized as a clinical entity by Engman in 1926 [2] and Cole and colleagues in 1930 [3,4]. About 200 cases had been reported in the literature by 1995 [5], and more than 500 by 2009 [6]. Much information about the clinical features of DC has been gleaned from the DC Registry, which was founded in 1995 at the Hammersmith Hospital in London, UK, later relocating to the Royal London Hospital in 2006 [7]. A second registry was established as part of the larger International Bone Marrow Failure Syndrome Registry at the National Cancer Institute of the National Institutes of Health (NIH) in the USA and began accruing patients in 2002 for a prospective cohort study of DC [7]. There has been intense research interest in DC in the last few decades given the role of known causative genes in normal telomere biology and their potential roles in normal ageing and contribution to idiopathic forms of haematological disorders and pulmonary fibrosis.

There are two severe variants of DC that have additional findings not present in the classic form: Hoyeraal Hreidarsson syndrome which is characterized by cerebellar hypoplasia [4,8], and Revesz syndrome

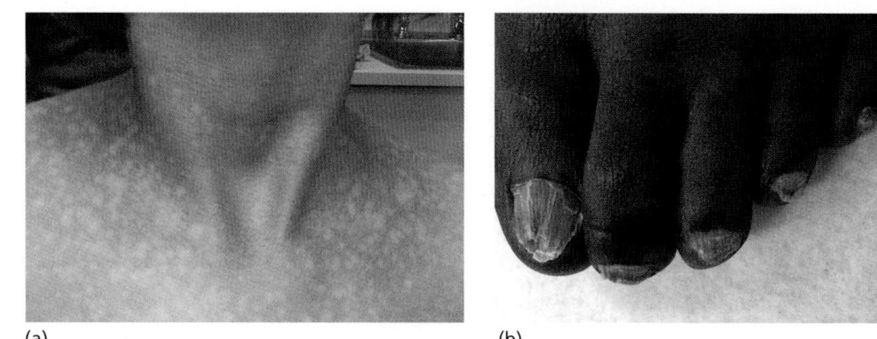
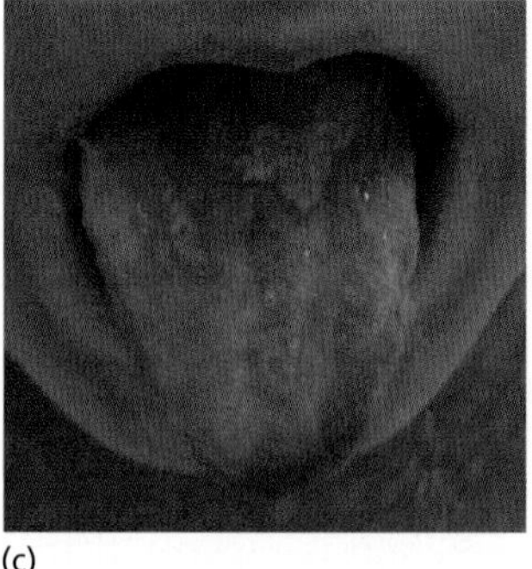

(a) (b) (c)

Fig. 140.9 Classic triad of dyskeratosis congenita consisting of (a) reticulated pigmentation changes, (b) nail dystrophy and (c) oral leukoplakia of the tongue. Source: Photos courtesy of Dr Alison A. Bertuch, Baylor College of Medicine, Houston, TX, USA.

which is associated with bilateral exudative retinopathy and intracranial calcifications [9]. Patients with all forms of DC have abnormally short telomeres for their age [10].

Epidemiology and pathogenesis. It was known from the many cases in the literature that DC could be inherited in three forms: as an X-linked, autosomal dominant or autosomal recessive trait. The key development in understanding the pathology of DC came in 1986 with the cloning of the gene responsible for the X-linked form of the disorder, *DKC1* [11] at Xq28, which encodes a protein called dyskerin. This nucleolar protein is associated with complexes that are involved in the synthesis of ribosomal RNA, but in addition in higher vertebrates it associates with telomerase RNA (TERC) which is important for the assembly and function of the telomerase enzyme and thus the synthesis of telomere repeats at the ends of chromosomes [12]. Since then, many more telomere biology genes have been identified as causative of DC. In addition to *DKC1* (OMIM #300126), which is the only known gene responsible for the X-linked form and which is responsible for the majority of cases of DC, there are 10 other known DC genes all involved in telomere biology. These include *TERC* (OMIM #602322) and *TINF2* (OMIM #604319) (autosomal dominant forms), *ACD* (OMIM #609377), *RTEL1* (OMIM #6608833), and *TERT* (OMIM #187270) (autosomal dominant or recessive forms) and *CTC1* (OMIM #613129), *NHP2* (OMIM #606470), *NOP10* (OMIM #606471), *PARN* (OMIM #604212), and *WRAP53* (OMIM #612661) (autosomal recessive forms). Patients with the severe variant Hoyeraal–Hreidarsson syndrome can have pathogenic variants in *DKC1*, *TERT*, *TINF2*, *RTEL1*, *ACD* and *PARN* [10,13,14]. Revesz syndrome has been shown to be caused by pathogenic variants in *TINF2* [15]. All causative pathogenic variants are in genes that are important for telomerase activity or assembly or in telomere integrity. Overall, approximately 70% of individuals who meet the clinical diagnostic criteria for DC will have pathogenic variants in the 11 aforementioned genes, the most common of which are *DKC1* and *TINF2* [10].

Clinical features. Not all patients with DC will have the classic triad of irregular pigmentation, nail dystrophy and oral leukoplakia (Fig, 140.9), but may have one or two of the classic features plus other suggestive physical findings, such as alopecia, abnormal eyelashes, premature grey hair, epiphora or blepharitis, periodontal disease, small stature, microcephaly, osteoporosis, urethral stenosis and hypogonadism [15]. Other severe associated conditions include pulmonary fibrosis, progressive bone marrow failure, myelodysplastic syndrome, acute myelogenous leukaemia or other solid tumours, usually squamous cell carcinoma of the head and neck region or anogenital adenocarcinoma. The diagnosis can be challenging because the onset of clinical findings, including the classic triad, is quite variable. Some patients may present with bone marrow failure in the absence of other clinical features.

The characteristic skin abnormality consists of reticulated hyperpigmentation affecting the flexural areas, particularly the neck, axillae and the inner upper thighs. The affected skin may show features of poikiloderma (pigmentation, telangiectasia and atrophy). The palms and soles sometimes show hyperhidrosis, loss of dermatoglyphics or keratoderma [16].

Nail dystrophy may be congenital but usually appears in childhood, with longitudinal ridging and progressive atrophic changes, including koilonychias. The dysplastic nail features may worsen with time until the nails are barely visible. Teeth may be missing or poorly formed, with thin enamel, early decay and periodontitis, but more commonly there is decreased root to crown ratio and taurodontism (enlarged pulp chambers of the teeth) [17].

Leucoplakia can affect any of the peripheral mucosal surfaces but most commonly presents in the mouth. This change is reported in 65% of patients and most commonly affects the tongue, but can also involve the buccal mucosa, palate and gingiva [17]. It may present as a large plaque on the tongue, small patches or a lacy network, often associated with papillary atrophy seen as a smooth red patch on the tongue. Oral leucoplakia appears later in childhood than the pigmentation and nail dystrophy. Development of squamous carcinoma is not uncommon. The same mucosal abnormality may be responsible for oesophageal [18] and urethral stenosis [19]. Severe gingival inflammation has also been reported [20].

Bone marrow failure develops in about 85% of patients and usually presents in the second to third decades, although it can occur any time from early childhood up to the seventh decade of life [21]. Patients may present with one affected lineage (often thrombocytopenia) and then progress to involve all three haematopoietic lineages. As mentioned earlier, bone marrow failure can be the first sign of DC and distinguishing it from other causes of bone marrow failure such as acquired aplastic anaemia is important because the management, prognosis, surveillance and counselling differ substantially between the two groups [15].

Alter and colleagues reviewed the cancer incidence in DC through a literature review of 500 published case reports in addition to the 50 DC patients enrolled in the National Cancer Institute's International Bone Marrow Failure Syndrome Registry [5]. Among both groups, the cumulative incidence of cancer was 40–50% by age 50 years. Patients with DC have an 11-fold increased risk of malignancy compared with the general population, the most common tumours being head and neck squamous carcinomas, followed by skin and anorectal cancer [5,15].

Pulmonary fibrosis and other pulmonary diseases have been described in about 20% of individuals with DC [15,22]. Approximately 16% of patients display premature greying or loss of hair [22]. Gastrointestinal involvement including liver disease, peptic ulceration and enteropathy has also been reported in about 7% of DC patients [15]. Bone abnormalities such as osteoporosis or avascular necrosis of the hip or shoulders has also been described in about 5% of patients [10,22]. Occasional ophthalmological features include blepharitis, conjunctivitis, lachrymal duct obstruction presenting as epiphora, ectropion with eyelash abnormalities and retinal vasculopathy [23,24].

The main causes of death in individuals with DC are bone marrow failure (60–70%), pulmonary complications (10–15%) and malignancy (10%) [21].

Differential diagnosis. Several other disorders that have cancer predisposition and features of poikiloderma are considered in the differential diagnosis, including RTS, in which the affected skin also shows mottled pigmentation. RTS can usually be distinguished by the earlier onset of poikiloderma, and its distribution initially on the cheeks and later on the extensor surfaces of the arms and legs, rarely affecting the trunk. Patients can also have small stature and sparse hair. The skin changes of Clericuzio-type PN are similar with areas of mottled hyper- and hypopigmentation, and these patients have severe neutropenia. They can also have transient anaemia and thrombocytopenia. Both RTS and PN patients can have dysplastic nails; usually thin and malformed in RTS and thickened in PN. Abnormal pigmentation also occurs in Fanconi anaemia (which may be haematologically indistinguishable from dyskeratosis congenita) but usually takes the form of café-au-lait macules. BD also shows patchy dyspigmentation, café-au-lait spots, telangiectasia and chromosomal instability but, more specifically, increased sister chromatid exchange. Genetic testing for pathogenic variants in causative genes for these disorders is available to help distinguish the diagnosis.

Laboratory and histology findings. Leukocyte telomere length testing by multicolour flow-fluorescent *in situ* hybridization (FISH) should be performed in an individual suspected of having DC. Patients with DC demonstrate telomere lengths less than the first percentile for age in lymphocytes. Molecular genetic testing of the DC genes to look for pathogenic variants should be performed to establish the diagnosis [10]. Other studies that may be performed based on the individual clinical presentation and course of disease include a complete blood count, bone marrow aspiration and biopsy, and liver and pulmonary function tests. Histology of pigmented skin shows nonspecific changes including epidermal atrophy, a mild chronic inflammatory infiltrate, dilated capillaries and pigment-laden macrophages in the upper dermis.

Treatment and prevention. Monitoring recommended by the 2008 NIH workshop should include yearly or twice-yearly complete blood count and annual bone marrow examination, pulmonary function tests, liver function tests and dermatological and oral examinations for malignancy [7,10]. Patients should be urged to avoid carcinogens such as sun exposure (ultraviolet light) and smoking, and to engage early with healthcare services regarding monitoring for common malignancies (e.g. breast, cervix, prostate, bowel) [25]. Leucoplakia should be documented, biopsied and closely monitored, and areas showing clinical or histological dysplasia should be excised. Etretinate has been reported to cause regression in leucoplakia of the mouth [26], and retinoids might theoretically defer malignant degeneration. Haematopoietic cell transplantation is the only curative treatment for severe bone marrow failure, myelodysplastic syndrome or leukaemia in DC. Treatment for malignancy should be tailored to the specific type of cancer. Management of pulmonary fibrosis is mainly supportive, although lung transplantation may be considered for severe cases.

References

1 Zinsser F. Atrophia Cutis Reticularis cum Pigmentations, Dystrophia Unguium et Leukoplakis oris (Poikioodermia atrophicans vascularis Jacobi.). Ikonographia Dermatologica 1910;5:219–23.
2 Engman MFS. A unique case of reticular pigmentation of the skin with atrophy. Arch Dermatol Syphiligraphie 1926;13:685–7.
3 Cole HN, Rauschkolb JC, Toomey J. Dyskeratosis congenita with pigmentation, dystrophia unguis and leukokeratosis oris. Arch Dermatol Syphiligraphie 1930;21:71–95.
4 Walne AJ, Dokal I. Dyskeratosis congenita: a historical perspective. Mech Ageing Dev 2008;129:48–59.
5 Alter BP, Giri N, Savage SA, Rosenberg PS. Cancer in dyskeratosis congenita. Blood 2009;113:6549–57.
6 Kirwan M, Dokal I. Dyskeratosis congenita: a genetic disorder of many faces. Clin Genet 2008;73:103–12.
7 Savage SA, Dokal I, Armanios M et al. Dyskeratosis congenita: the first NIH clinical research workshop. Pediatr Blood Cancer 2009;53:520–3.
8 Hoyeraal HM, Lamvik J, Moe PJ. Congenital hypoplastic thrombocytopenia and cerebral malformations in two brothers. Acta Paediatr Scand 1970;59:185–91.
9 Revesz T, Fletcher S, al-Gazali LI et al. Bilateral retinopathy, aplastic anaemia, and central nervous system abnormalities: a new syndrome? J Med Genet 1992;29:673–5.

10 **Savage S. Dyskeratosis congenita. In: Pagon RA, Adam MP, Ardinger HH et al. (eds) GeneReviews® [Internet]. Seattle (WA): University of Washington, Seattle; 1993–2016. 2009 Nov 12 [updated 2016 May 26].**

11 Heiss NS, Knight SW, Vulliamy TJ et al. X-linked dyskeratosis congenita is caused by mutations in a highly conserved gene with putative nucleolar functions. Nat Genet 1998;19:32–8.

12 **Mason PJ, Bessler M. The genetics of dyskeratosis congenita. Cancer Genet 2011;204:635–45.**

13 Savage SA, Vulliamy T. The genetics of dyskeratosis congenita. In: Savage SA, Cook EF (eds) Dyskeratosis Congenita and Telomere Biology Disorders: Diagnosis and Management Guidelines, 1st edn. Dyskeratosis Congenita Outreach, Inc., 2015: 68–81. Available online at: www.dcoutreach.org

14 Burris AM, Ballew BJ, Kentosh JB et al. Hoyeraal-Hreidarsson syndrome due to PARN mutations: fourteen years of follow-up. Pediatr Neurol 2016;56:62–8.

15 **Savage SA, Bertuch AA. The genetics and clinical manifestations of telomere biology disorders. Genet Med 2010;12:753–64.**

16 Nambudiri VE, Cowen EW. Dermatologic manifestations in dyskeratosis congenita. In: Savage SA, Cook EF (eds) Dyskeratosis congenita and telomere biology disorders: diagnosis and management guidelines, 1st edn. Dyskeratosis Congenita Outreach, Inc., 2015:182–96. Available online at: www.dcoutreach.org

17 Atkinson JC, Harvey KE, Domingo DL et al. Oral and dental phenotype of dyskeratosis congenita. Oral Dis 2008;14:419–27.

18 Sawant P, Chopda NM, Desai DC et al. Dyskeratosis congenita with esophageal stricture and dermatological manifestations. Endoscopy 1994;26:711–2.

19 Kirwan M, Dokal I. Dyskeratosis congenita: a genetic disorder of many faces. Clin Genet 2008;73:103–12.

20 Lourenço SV, Boggio PA, Fezzi FA et al. Dyskeratosis congenita – report of a case with emphasis on gingival aspects. Pediatr Dermatol 2009;26:176–9.

21 Dokal I. Dyskeratosis congenita. Hematol Am Soc Hematol Educ Program 2011;2011:480–6.

22 Marrone A, Walne A, Dokal I. Dyskeratosis congenita: telomerase, telomeres and anticipation. Curr Opin Genet Dev 2005;15:249–57.

23 Nazir S, Sayani N, Phillips PH. Retinal hemorrhages in a patient with dyskeratosis congenita. J AAPOS 2008;12:415–17.

24 Teixeira LF, Shields CL, Marr B et al. Bilateral retinal vasculopathy in a patient with dyskeratosis congenita. Arch Ophthalmol 2008;126:134–5.

25 Alter BP, Savage SA. Cancer in dyskeratosis congenita. In: Savage SA, Cook EF (eds) Dyskeratosis Congenita and Telomere Biology Disorders: Diagnosis and Management Guidelines, 1st edn. Dyskeratosis Congenita Outreach, Inc., 2015:318–32. Available online at: www.dcoutreach.org

26 Koch HF. Effect of retinoids on precancerous lesions of the oral cavity. In: Orfanos CE, Braun-Falco O, Farber EM et al. (eds) Retinoids. Advances in Basic Research and Therapy. Berlin: Springer-Verlag, 1981:307–12.

Fanconi anaemia

Introduction and history. Fanconi anaemia (FA) is a rare inherited disorder characterized by bone marrow failure, radial ray hypoplasia, abnormal pigmentation, increased risk of malignancy, and less commonly renal, cardiac and central nervous system anomalies. The disorder was first described by the Swiss paediatrician Guido Fanconi in 1927 in three brothers who had pancytopenia, short stature, hypogonadism and abnormal pigmentation [1]. Forty years later spontaneous chromosome breakage was recognized as a significant abnormality in this condition. By 2008, over 1000 North American patients had been enrolled in the International Fanconi Anaemia Registry which was established at the Rockefeller University in 1982 [2].

Epidemiology and pathogenesis. Increased sensitivity to crosslinking agents such as mitomycin C and diepoxybutane resulting in increased chromosomal breakage is a hallmark of cells from FA patients [2,3]. Through complementation analysis using cell fusion and correction of crosslinker hypersensitivity [4], several 'complementation groups' have been defined and their associated genes identified. There are currently 16 genes known to be involved in crosslink repair that are associated with FA complementation groups: *FANCA* (OMIM# 607139), *FANCB* (OMIM# 300515), *FANCC* (OMIM# 613899), *FANCD1* (OMIM# 605724)/*BRCA2* (OMIM# 600185), *FANCD2* (OMIM# 613984), *FANCE* (OMIM# 613976), *FANCF* (OMIM# 613897), *FANCG* (OMIM# 602956), *FANCI* (OMIM# 611360), *FANCJ* (OMIM# 609054)/*BRIP1* (OMIM# 605882), *FANCL* (OMIM# 608111), *FANCM* (OMIM# 609644), *FANCN* (OMIM# 610832)/ *PALB2* (OMIM# 610355), *FANCO* (OMIM# 613390)/ *RAD51C* (OMIM# 179617), *FANCP* (OMIM# 613951)/ *SLX4* (OMIM# 613278), *FANCQ* (OMIM# 615272)/*ERCC4* (OMIM# 133520) [5]. The latter three have been less well characterized because there have been fewer individuals diagnosed with FA who carry pathogenic variants in those genes [6]. The products of these FA genes function together to coordinate multiple processes involved in the repair of interstrand crosslinks. Eight of them (FANCA, FANCB, FANCC, FANCE, FANCF, FANCG, FANCL and FANCM) along with FAAP100 and FAAP24 are part of the nuclear core complex which has E3 ubiquitin ligase activity [6]. FA defects are inherited in an autosomal recessive manner for all groups except FANCB which is X-linked. The majority of FA patients are accounted for by complementation groups A (~65%), C (~15%), and G (~10%) [5]. Three of the genes, *FANCD1/BRCA2*, FANC*J/BRIP1* and FANC*N/PALBB2* and *FANCO* have also been associated with an increased risk of breast and other cancers in heterozygous carriers in the general population [5].

FA affects approximately 1 in 100000 live births and is inherited in an autosomal recessive manner for all groups except the *FANCB* group which is X-linked [5]. Somatic mosaicism is not uncommon, caused by either new mutation or spontaneous reversion of an inherited mutation [3,7]. Cells from heterozygous carriers have not been shown to have increased sensitivity to DNA crosslinking agents [2].

Clinical features. The phenotype of FA is extremely variable, even within families and between monozygotic twins [2]. Somatic mosaicism is one of many genetic and epigenetic factors complicating phenotype–genotype correlation. The main clinical characteristics of FA can be grouped in physical malformations, haematological abnormalities with progressive bone marrow failure and cancer susceptibility.

Two-thirds of children have congenital malformations, which involve multiple systems and organs, including the skeletal system, skin, ears, heart, kidneys, genitourinary system and central nervous system. About 40% of patients have short stature, often linked to hormonal deficiencies [2]. Prominent skeletal anomalies include radial ray defects and patients can have both unilateral and bilateral thumb defects, such as absent or hypoplastic, bifid, rudimentary or low set thumbs (seen in 35% of patients). A wide variety of other skeletal anomalies affecting the limbs, spine and skull have also been described. Bony abnormalities of the middle ear and canal can lead to hearing loss in about 10%. Congenital heart defects may include patient ductus arteriosus, septal defects, coarctation of the aorta and truncus arteriosus in about 6% of patients. Renal abnormalities including horseshoe, ectopic and hypoplastic kidneys are found in 20% of patients. Males can have reduced fertility caused by hypo- or azoospermia as well as hypospadias, undescended or absent testes and females have been described to have uterine malformations or malposition and small ovaries. Central nervous system abnormalities are not common but can include absent corpus callosum, small pituitary, cerebellar hypoplasia and hydrocephalus [6,8].

With regard to dermatological manifestations, the majority (about 64%) of patients show pigmentary anomalies, which become more apparent with time. Pigmentary changes may precede the haematological manifestations [2]. Most often patients have hyperpigmentation distributed proximally and in the flexures, as well as café-au-lait spots. Macules of lighter and darker pigmentation may be superimposed on this background. Oral pigmentation may be seen as well [9]. These dermatological features may be the sole presenting features in the early stages of FA.

Analysis of International Fanconi Anaemia Registry data revealed that haematological abnormalities develop in almost all patients at a median age of 7 years (birth to 41 years) and bone marrow failure in 90% by 40 years [10]. Thrombocytopenia associated with macrocytosis often preceded onset of anaemia or neutropenia [6]. Haemoglobin F may be elevated. Bone marrow cellularity is decreased, and cytogenetic abnormalities become increasingly common with age. A review of 1300 published cases revealed that leukaemia (usually acute myelogenous) occurred in 9% and myelodysplastic syndrome in 7% of patients [11].

Patients with FA also have a higher incidence of solid malignancies, with an estimated cumulative risk of 76% by the age of 45 years [11]. Malignancy precedes the diagnosis of Fanconi anaemia in 25% of cases. Review of patients in both the German FA Registry [12] and the National Institutes of Health Bone Marrow Failure Registry [13] showed significantly elevated ratios of observed to expected cancers of the head and neck, oesophagus, vulva, breast and brain. Heterozygote carriers have no general increase in cancer susceptibility, with the possible exception of *FANCC* mutation carriers who may have an increased susceptibility to breast cancer [14].

The median estimated survival for FA patients is 24 years [10]. There is a 98% risk of developing haematological abnormalities, and an 81% risk of dying from them, by 40 years of age [2]. The risks of developing bone marrow failure, haematological and nonhaematological malignancy by 40 years are, respectively, 90%, 33% and 28% [10]. Patients with fewer congenital anomalies are seemingly paradoxically at higher risk of malignancy [7].

Differential diagnosis. The progressive marrow aplasia and generalized hyperpigmentation seen in FA patients may be confused with dyskeratosis congenita. Another disorder characterized by haematological abnormalities and skin dyspigmentation PN [15]. Severe neutropenia is most prominent in PN, but patients can also have transient anaemia and thrombocytopenia as well as abnormal bone marrow findings. PN patients have more classic poikiloderma, similar to patients with RTS. Similar to patients with FA, RTS patients can present with radial ray defects and other skeletal abnormalities prior to the development of the poikiloderma [16,17]. Patients diagnosed with Baller–Gerold syndrome and VACTERL (vertebral anomalies, anal atresia, cardiac anomalies, tracheo-esophageal fistula, renal and radial anomalies) have also been reclassified as FA once the haematological abnormality appeared [2].

Laboratory and histology findings. Patients with FA demonstrate increased sensitivity to crosslinking agents with increased chromosome breaks on diepoxybutane testing. Mutation testing should be performed to confirm the diagnosis and the specific subtype of FA. Blood counts and bone marrow studies should be performed after consultation with a haematologist. Other laboratory testing should be performed based on the specific clinical features present in the patient.

Treatment and prevention. Haematopoietic stem cell transplantation is the only curative treatment for the haematological manifestations of FA [6]. Ideally this should occur prior to the development of myelodysplastic syndrome or leukaemia and before multiple transfusions have been administered [18]. FA patients require reduced doses of chemotherapy and radiation preparative regimens because of their increased sensitivity to cytotoxic agents [6]. Survival rates have improved with the use of fludarabine-based regimens for both matched related and alternative donors and improvement in graft-versus-host disease. Current survival rates after allogenic matched sibling donor transplant for children younger than 10 years exceeds 85% and is approximately 65% for children and adults combined [19–21]. Transplant is not without complications including an increased risk of developing post-transplant solid tumours, particularly squamous cell carcinomas of the oral cavity [6,22].

Androgens such as oxymethalone have been used to improve blood counts and may be useful in increasing counts in up to 50% of patients. This effect is earliest and least transient for red blood cells compared with platelets and white blood cells. Resistance to therapy may develop over time and patients must be monitored for liver toxicities that include elevated liver enzymes, cholestasis, peliosis hepatis and hepatic tumours [8,23]. Growth factors such as granulocyte colony-stimulating factor can improve the neutrophil count in some patients, but should be used with caution and its use should be preceded and monitored by bone marrow aspirate and biopsy to look for clonal bone marrow cytogenetic abnormalities [6].

Patients with FA should in general avoid toxic agents that could enhance risk of malignancy such as excessive radiation, smoking and alcohol. In addition, transfusion of blood products should be minimized if possible for potential future haematopoietic stem cell transplant.

References

1 Fanconi G. Familiare infantile pernizosaaritige anamie (pernizioeses Blutbild und Konstitution). Jahrbuch Kinderheild 1927;117:257–80.

2 Auerbach AD. Fanconi anemia and its diagnosis. Mutat Res 2009;668:4–10.

3 Tischkowitz MD, Hodgson SV. Fanconi anaemia. J Med Genet. 2003;40:1–10.

4 Chandra S, Levran O, Jurickova I et al. A rapid method for retrovirus-mediated identification of complementation groups in Fanconi anemia patients. Mol Ther 2005;12:976–84.

5 Auerbach AD. Diagnosis of Fanconi anemia by diepoxybutane analysis. Curr Protoc Hum Genet 2015;85:8.7.1–17.

6 Alter BP, Kupfer G. Fanconi Anemia. In: Pagon RA, Adam MP, Ardinger HH et al. (eds) GeneReviews® [Internet]. Seattle (WA): University of Washington, Seattle; 1993–2016. 2002 Feb 14 [updated 2013 Feb 7].

7 Neveling K, Endt D, Hoehn H, Schindler D. Genotype–phenotype correlations in Fanconi anemia. Mutat Res 2009;668:73–91.

8 Shimamura A, Alter BP. Pathophysiology and management of inherited bone marrow failure syndromes. Blood Rev 2010;24:101–22.

9 Karalis A, Tischkowitz M, Millington GWM. Dermatological manifestations of inherited cancer syndromes in children. Br J Dermatol 2011;164:245–56.

10 Kutler DI, Singh B, Satagopan J et al. A 20-year perspective on the International Fanconi Anemia Registry (IFAR). Blood 2003; 101:1249–56.

11 Alter BP. Cancer in Fanconi anemia, 1927–2001. Cancer 2003;97:425–40.

12 Rosenberg PS, Alter BP, Ebell W. Cancer risks in Fanconi anemia: findings from the German Fanconi Anemia Registry. Haematologica 2008;93:511–17.

13 Alter BP, Giri N, Savage SA et al. Malignancies and survival patterns in the National Cancer Institute inherited bone marrow failure syndromes cohort study. Br J Haematol 2010;150:179–88.

14 Berwick M, Satagopan JM, Ben-Porat L et al. Genetic heterogeneity among Fanconi anemia heterozygotes and risk of cancer. Cancer Res 2007;67:9591–6.

15 Clericuzio C, Harutyunyan K, Jin W et al. Identification of a novel C16orf57 mutation in Athabaskan patients with Poikiloderma with Neutropenia. Am J Med Genet A 2011;155A:337–42.

16 Moss C, Bacon CJ, Mueller RF. 'Isolated' radial ray defect may be due to Rothmund–Thomson syndrome. Clin Genet 1990;38:318–19.

17 Wang LL, Levy ML, Lewis RA et al. Clinical manifestations in a cohort of 41 Rothmund-Thomson syndrome patients. Am J Med Genet 2001;102:11–7.

18 MacMillan ML, Wagner JE. Haematopoeitic cell transplantation for Fanconi anaemia – when and how? Br J Haematol 2010;149:14–21.

19 Wagner J. Hematopoietic stem cell transplantation. In: Frohnmayer D, Frohnmayer L, Guinan E et al. (eds) Fanconi Anemia: Guidelines for Diagnosis and Management, 4th edn. Fanconi Anemia Research Fund, 2014:219–43. Available at: www.fanconi.org

20 MacMillan ML, Hughes MR, Agarwal S, Daley GQ. Cellular therapy for Fanconi anemia: the past, present, and future. Biol Blood Marrow Transplant 2011;17(1 Suppl):S109–14.

21 Smetsers SE, Smiers FJ, Bresters D et al. Four decades of stem cell transplantation for Fanconi anaemia in the Netherlands. Br J Haematol 2016;174:952–61.

22 Bonfim C, Ribeiro L, Nichele S et al. Long-term survival, organ function, and malignancy after hematopoietic stem cell transplantation for Fanconi anemia. Biol Blood Marrow Transplant 2016;22:1257–63.

23 Paustian L, Chao MM, Hanenberg H et al. Androgen therapy in Fanconi anemia: a retrospective analysis of 30 years in Germany. Pediatr Hematol Oncol 2016;33:5–12.

Poikiloderma with neutropenia

Introduction and history. PN, Clericuzio-type (OMIM #604173) was first described as 'immune deficient poikiloderma' by Clericuzio and colleagues [1] in 14 patients of Native American Navajo descent. Because it was identified in this population, it was later referred to as 'Navajo poikiloderma' [2]. This condition is one of several genetic disorders enriched in the Southwestern Athabaskan Native American populations, which comprises both Navajo and Apache groups [3]. Subsequently, in 2003 the disorder was identified in patients who were not of Navajo descent; therefore, it was renamed 'poikiloderma with neutropenia' to reflect its cardinal features [4]. In 2005, van Hove and colleagues described a Turkish family with PN, and he proposed renaming the disorder Clericuzio-type PN [5]. PN is characterized primarily by widespread postinflammatory poikiloderma, severe neutropenia, pachyonychia (thickened nails), palmar–plantar hyperkeratosis, recurrent sinopulmonary infections and chronic lung disease. Some patients can develop myelodysplastic syndrome or malignancies such as leukaemia or skin cancer [6].

Epidemiology and pathogenesis. PN is inherited in an autosomal recessive fashion. To date over 40 individuals with poikiloderma with neutropenia have been reported. The prevalence is unknown. In 2010, Volpi and colleagues [7] identified *C16orf57* (NM_024598.2) located on chromosome 16q21 as a causative gene in PN in a large inbred Italian family. This was confirmed in a Moroccan family [8] and in another European family [9]. In 2011, Clericuzio and colleagues examined a larger contemporary cohort of 11 PN patients to determine the prevalence and spectrum of *C16orf57* pathogenic variants in PN patients of both Athabaskan and non-Athabaskan descent. All patients were found to have *C16orf57* pathogenic variants, and all Athabaskan patients had a common mutation (c.496delA) which was not detected in the non-Athabaskan patients [10]. The *C16orf57* (*USB1*) gene encodes a protein called USB1(Mpn1) which plays a crucial role in the stability of spliceosomal U6 small nuclear RNA (snRNA) which is essential for RNA splicing by protecting it from exosome damage [11–13].

Pathogenic allelic variants. Approximately 20 pathogenic variants have been published that distribute from exon 2 to exon 6 containing splice sites. Pathogenic variant types include deletion, splice-site, nonsense and missense variants [14,15]. A genotype-ethnic origin correlation hypothesis was suggested by Colombo and colleagues and strengthened by a following study [16,17], whereby three frequent recurrent pathogenic variants were considered to be associated with European, Native American and North African origins, respectively. The most common pathogenic variant reported to date, c.531delA, has been detected in nine Caucasian PN patients, four of whom were from unrelated Turkish families [6,16,17]. The second most common pathogenic variant, c.496delA, has been identified in five PN patients from Athabaskan ancestry [10]. The third most common pathogenic variant, c.179delC, has been detected in four North African PN patients [6,8,16].

Clinical features. The papular, erythematous rash of PN begins between birth and age 18 months usually on the

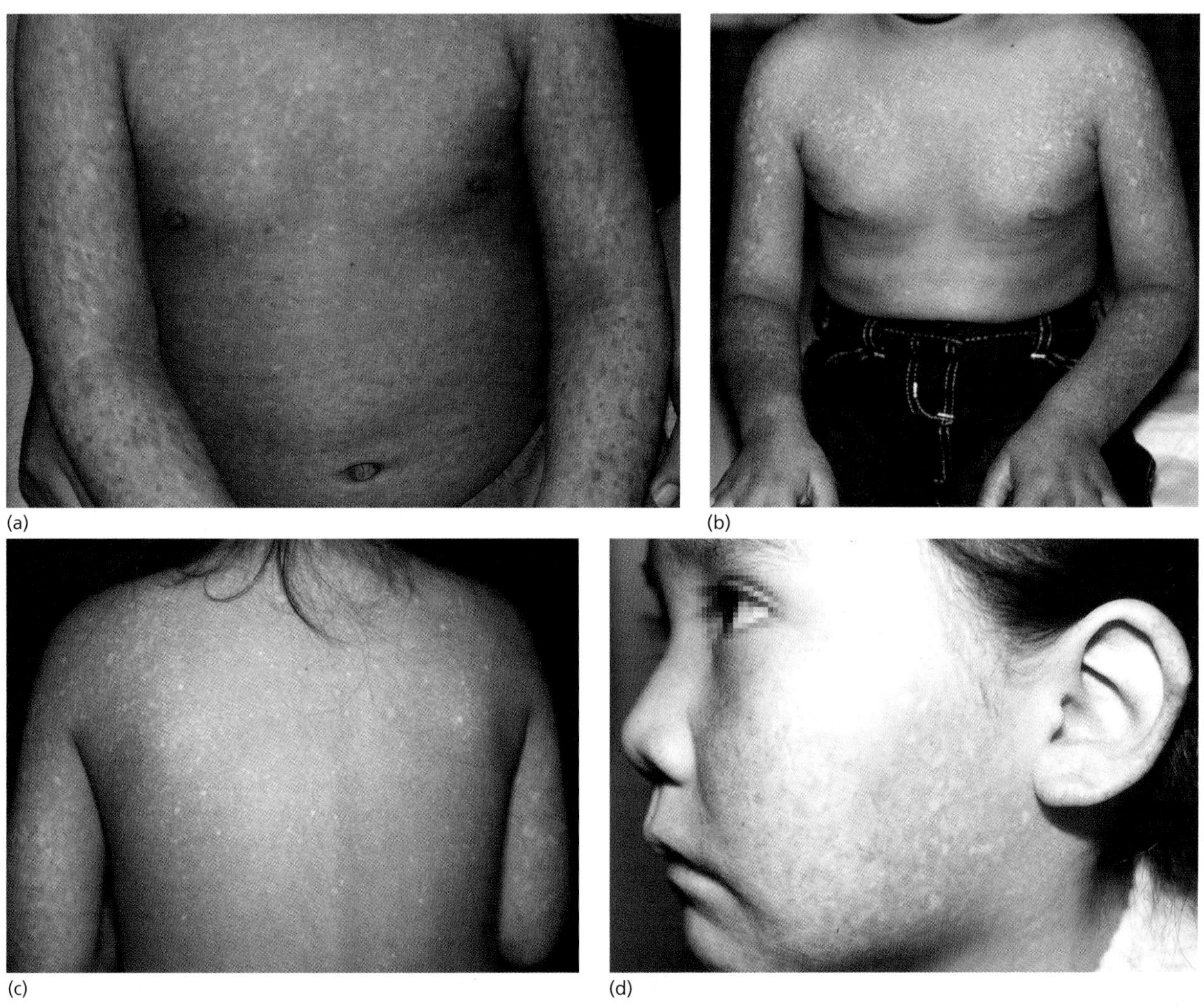

Fig. 140.10 Characteristic poikiloderma involving the (a,b) extremities and torso, (c) back and (d) face in individuals with poikiloderma with neutropenia. Source: Photos courtesy of Dr Carol Clericuzio, University of New Mexico, Albuquerque, NM, USA.

extremities and extends centrally to the trunk, back and face [9,16], although it has also been described as starting on the face [18]. It has a prominent postinflammatory, eczematous appearance early on. These changes eventually evolve into poikiloderma, characterized by hypo- and hyperpigmentation, telangiectasia and atrophy (Fig. 140.10). Poikiloderma persists throughout life. Palmoplantar hyperkeratosis is observed in about half the patients. Calcinosis cutis has been described in patients with PN. The deposits are usually asymptomatic, but may be painful if they cause eruptions on the knees and elbows and are frequently diffuse [10,19]. Pachyonychia and nail dystrophy/thickening of the toenails are common and can be quite severe (Fig. 140.11). Anonychia and subungual hyperkeratosis can also occur [16]. Dry, thin and sparse hair (including eyebrows and eyelashes) has been reported although is not common [16,20]. Squamous cell carcinoma of the skin has been reported in two affected individuals [6,21]. Dental abnormalities may be present including caries and missing teeth caused by neutropenia-associated gingivitis and poor dental hygiene [17].

Neutropenia and infections are a significant problem in PN patients. Moderate to severe noncyclic neutropenia is typically observed in the first year of life and is usually accompanied by recurrent infections. Respiratory infections are common; however, more severe infections can include meningitis, sepsis, bronchiectasis, sinusitis, otitis media and dermal ulcers [1,4,16]. Other haematological abnormalities include transient leucopenia usually during infection, transient anaemia and transient thrombocytopenia. Bone marrow studies may reveal hypocellularity and myelodysplasia [20,22]. Defective oxidative burst has been reported in some patients studied early on by a variety of assays, but this needs to be reevaluated with more standardized testing, such as the use of dihydrorhodamine to measure the neutrophil respiratory burst measured by flow cytometry. Polyclonal hypergammaglobulinaemia has been observed rarely [22].

Bone marrow failure manifested as myelodysplastic syndrome and acute myeloid leukaemia has been reported in several affected individuals, including a few patients who were previously diagnosed with other conditions [7,6,10,16,18,23,24].

Other features that have been described in PN include skeletal abnormalities, such as osteopenia and osteoporosis with fractures, and dysplasia of the fingers and toes [16]. Craniofacial dysmorphic features have been commonly described including midfacial hypoplasia,

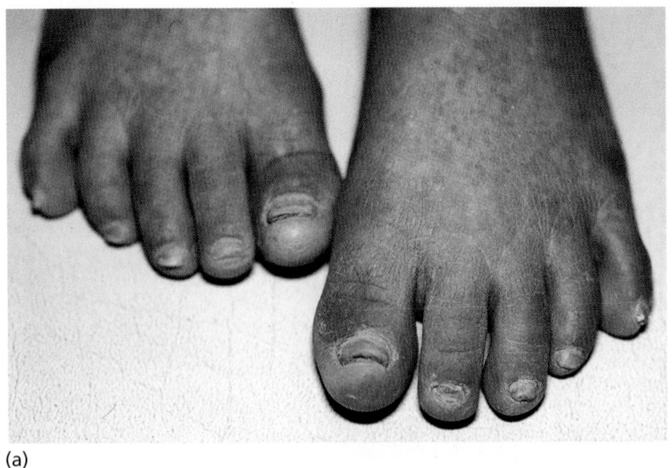
(a)

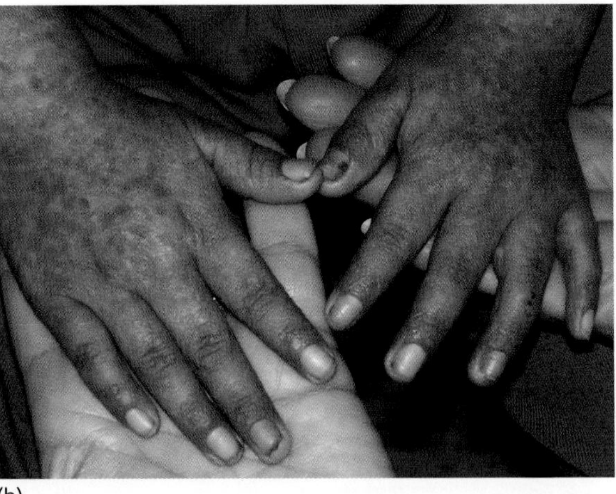
(b)

Fig. 140.11 Dystrophic (a) toenails and (b) fingernails in individuals with poikiloderma with neutropenia. Source: Photos courtesy of Dr Carol Clericuzio, University of New Mexico, Albuquerque, NM, USA.

hypertelorism, small or saddle nose with depressed nasal bridge [16–18]. Splenomegaly and less often hepatomegaly have been reported in roughly one-third of affected individuals [9]. In the absence of malignancy, the lifespan appears normal. However, the data are limited by the small number of reported individuals.

Differential diagnosis. RTS and DC should be considered (see previously).

Rothmund–Thomson syndrome (RTS) is an autosomal recessive genodermatosis characterized by poikiloderma; sparse hair, eyelashes, and/or eyebrows; small stature; skeletal, dental, and nail abnormalities; cataracts; and an increased risk for cancer, especially osteosarcoma and skin cancers. RTS is caused in two-thirds of cases by pathogenic variants in *RECQL4* [25]. The pattern of spread of the poikiloderma is an important distinctive feature for RTS. Poikiloderma in RTS tends to start in the face and then spreads towards the extremities, usually sparing the trunk, abdomen and back. This is in contrast to poikiloderma with neutropenia which usually starts peripherally and spreads centrally to the trunk and face. Other distinguishing features are permanent neutropenia (observed in PN but not RTS) and radial ray abnormalities (observed in RTS but not PN).

Dyskeratosis congenita (DC) is also considered an inherited poikiloderma and is characterized by a classic triad of dysplastic nails, lacy reticular pigmentation of the upper chest and/or neck, and oral leukoplakia. DC, a telomere biology disorder [26], differs from PN by the presence of oral leukoplakia and absence of isolated neutropenia. Individuals with DC have an increased risk for bone marrow failure and skin cancers similar to PN. Mutation of one of eleven 11 genes has been associated with DC. Listed by inheritance pattern, they include: autosomal recessive (*CTC1, NHP2, NOP10, PARN, WRAP53*), autosomal dominant (*TERC, TINF2*), autosomal recessive/dominant (*ACD, RTEL1, TERT*) and X-linked recessive (*DKC1*) [27].

Laboratory and histology findings. Complete blood count in patients with PN will demonstrate neutropenia. Elevated lactate dehydrogenase (and sometimes ferritin) levels, are seen almost universally and are of unknown aetiology [9,18,20]. Bone marrow aspirate and biopsy should be performed if there is depression of a second cell line. These may show decreased maturation of the neutrophil lineage with decreased numbers of neutrophil precursors. They may also show central eosinophilia and lymphocytosis, as well as increased numbers of immature cells with no abnormal clonality [5,18,22]. Skin biopsies demonstrate characteristic histological features of poikiloderma which can include hyperkeratosis, epidermal atrophy, basal cell vacuolization, melanin incontinence and dilated vessels.

Treatment and prevention. Treatment is largely symptomatic. Retinoids may improve the appearance of the hyperkeratoses. Antibiotics should be employed for infected skin ulcers and debridement of those that are slow to heal. Other infections should be treated with appropriate antibiotic and supportive therapies. If patients develop bone marrow failure and leukaemia, they should undergo standard treatment. Protection of skin from excessive sun exposure by use of sunscreens containing both UVA and UVB should be employed. Patients should avoid contact with other sick individuals because of risk of infection from neutropenia. It is not clear that granulocyte colony stimulating factor is useful on a chronic basis, but may be helpful during acute infections [20].

Surveillance should include close monitoring for lung infections. Regular skin examination should be performed because of the increased risk of infectious ulcers and possibly squamous cell carcinoma. Annual complete blood count is recommended. Biannual dental examination should be performed because of the high incidence of gingivitis and caries.

Acknowledgements

The authors thank Professor Celia Moss, Department of Dermatology, Birmingham Children's Hospital, Birmingham, UK, for her contribution to this chapter in previous editions. We also wish to acknowledge all the patients and families worldwide for their participation.

References

1 Clericuzio C, Hoyme HE, Aase JM. Immune deficient poikiloderma: a new genodermatosis. Am J Hum Genet 1991;49:A661.

2 Erickson RP. Southwestern Athabaskan (Navajo and Apache) genetic diseases. Genet Med 1999;1:151–7.

3 Erickson RP. Autosomal recessive diseases among the Athabaskans of the southwestern United States: recent advances and implications for the future. Am J Med Genet Part A 2009;149A:2602–11.

4 Wang LL, Gannavarapu A, Clericuzio CL et al. Absence of RECQL4 mutations in poikiloderma with neutropenia in Navajo and non-Navajo patients. Am J Med Genet A 2003;118A:299–301.

5 Van Hove JL, Jaeken J, Proesmans M et al. Clericuzio type poikiloderma with neutropenia is distinct from Rothmund-Thomson syndrome. Am J Med Genet A 2005;132A:152–8.

6 Walne AJ, Vulliamy T, Beswick R et al. Mutations in C16orf57 and normal-length telomeres unify a subset of patients with dyskeratosis congenita, poikiloderma with neutropenia and Rothmund-Thomson syndrome. Hum Mol Genet 2010;19:4453–61.

7 Volpi L, Roversi G, Colombo EA et al. Targeted next-generation sequencing appoints c16orf57 as clericuzio-type poikiloderma with neutropenia gene. Am J Hum Genet 2010;86:72–6.

8 Tanaka A, Morice-Picard F, Lacombe D. Identification of a homozygous deletion mutation in C16orf57 in a family with Clericuzio-type poikiloderma with neutropenia. Am J Med Genet A 2010;152A:1347–8.

9 Arnold AW, Itin PH, Pigors M et al. Poikiloderma with neutropenia: a novel C16orf57 mutation and clinical diagnostic criteria. Br J Dermatol 2010;163:866–9.

10 Clericuzio C, Harutyunyan K, Jin W et al. Identification of a novel C16orf57 mutation in Athabaskan patients with poikiloderma with neutropenia. Am J Med Genet A 2011;155A:337–42.

11 Hilcenko C, Simpson PJ, Finch AJ et al. Aberrant 3′ oligoadenylation of spliceosomal U6 small nuclear RNA in poikiloderma with neutropenia. Blood 2013;121:1028–38

12 Mroczek S, Krwawicz J, Kutner J et al. C16orf57, a gene mutated in poikiloderma with neutropenia, encodes a putative phosphodiesterase responsible for the U6 snRNA3′ end modification. Genes Dev 2012;26:1911–25.

13 Shchepachev V, Wischnewski H, Missiaglia E et al. Mpn1, mutated in poikiloderma with neutropenia protein 1, is a conserved 3′-to-5′ RNA exonuclease processing U6 small nuclear RNA. Cell Rep 2012;2:855–65.

14 Larizza L, Negri G, Colombo EA et al. Clinical utility gene card for: poikiloderma with neutropenia. Eur J Hum Genet 2013;21(10).

15 Suter AA, Itin P, Heinimann K et al. Rothmund-Thomson Syndrome: novel pathogenic mutations and frequencies of variants in the RECQL4 and USB1 (C16orf57) gene. Mol Genet Genomic Med 2016;4:359–66.

16 Colombo EA, Bazan JF, Negri G et al. Novel C16orf57 mutations in patients with poikiloderma with neutropenia: bioinformatic analysis of the protein and predicted effects of all reported mutations. Orphanet J Rare Dis 2012;7:7.

17 Koparir A, Gezdirici A, Koparir E et al. Poikiloderma with neutropenia: genotype-ethnic origin correlation, expanding phenotype and literature review. Am J Med Genet A 2014;164A:2535–40.

18 Concolino D, Roversi G, Muzzi GL et al. Clericuzio-type poikiloderma with neutropenia syndrome in three sibs with mutations in the C16orf57 gene: delineation of the phenotype. Am J Med Genet A 2010;152A:2588–94.

19 Chantorn R, Shwayder T. Poikiloderma with neutropenia: report of three cases including one with calcinosis cutis. Pediatr Dermatol 2012;29:463–72.

20 Farruggia P, Indaco S, Dufour C et al. Poikiloderma with neutropenia: a case report and review of the literature. J Pediatr Hematol Oncol 2014;36:297–300

21 Rodgers W, Ancliff P, Ponting CP et al. Squamous cell carcinoma in a child with Clericuzio-type poikiloderma with neutropenia. Br J Dermatol 2013;168:665–7.

22 Mostefai R, Morice-Picard F, Boralevi F et al. Poikiloderma with neutropenia, Clericuzio type, in a family from Morocco. Am J Med Genet A 2008;146A:2762–9.

23 Pianigiani E, De Aloe G, Andreassi A et al. Rothmund-Thomson syndrome (Thomson-type) and myelodysplasia. Pediatr Dermatol 2001;18:422–5.

24 Porter WM, Hardman CM, Abdalla SH et al. Haematological disease in siblings with Rothmund-Thomson syndrome. Clin Exp Dermatol 1999;24:452–4.

25 Wang LL, Gannavarapu A, Kozinetz CA et al. Association between osteosarcoma and deleterious mutations in the RECQL4 gene in Rothmund–Thomson syndrome. J Natl Cancer Inst 2003;95:669–74.

26 Mason PJ, Bessler M. The genetics of dyskeratosis congenita. Cancer Genet 2011;204:635–45.

27 Savage SA. Dyskeratosis congenita. In: Pagon RA, Adam MP, Ardinger HH et al. (eds) GeneReviews. Seattle, WA: University of Washington, Seattle (updated 26 May 2016).

CHAPTER 141

Other Genetic Disorders Predisposing to Malignancy

Julie V. Schaffer

Division of Pediatric and Adolescent Dermatology, Hackensack University Medical Center, Hackensack, NJ, USA

Bazex–Dupré–Christol syndrome, 1802
Beckwith–Wiedemann syndrome, 1807
Birt–Hogg–Dubé syndrome, 1808
Brooke–Spiegler syndrome, multiple familial trichoepitheliomas and familial cylindromatosis, 1810
Epidermodysplasia verruciformis, 1811
Gardner syndrome, 1812
Hereditary leiomyomatosis and renal cell cancer syndrome, 1813
Muir–Torre and constitutional mismatch repair deficiency syndromes, 1815
Peutz–Jeghers syndrome, 1816
PTEN hamartoma-tumour syndrome, 1818

Abstract

This chapter reviews selected genodermatoses associated with a predisposition to malignancies of the skin and/or extracutaneous tissues. Recognition of the characteristic mucocutaneous manifestations of these disorders facilitates diagnosis and cancer surveillance. Disorders reviewed in detail herein include epidermodysplasia verruciformis and the following syndromes: Bazex–Dupré–Christol, Birt–Hogg–Dubé, Brooke–Spiegler, Gardner, hereditary leiomyomatosis and renal cell cancer, Muir–Torre, Peutz–Jeghers and PTEN hamartoma-tumour.

Introduction

Hereditary cancer syndromes that affect the skin can be divided into the following groups: (i) disorders that predispose patients to mucocutaneous malignancies (Table 141.1); (ii) disorders that predispose patients to mucocutaneous and extracutaneous malignancies (Table 141.2); and (iii) disorders that have cutaneous stigmata and predispose patients to extracutaneous malignancies (Table 141.3). Selected genodermatoses with malignant potential are discussed in this chapter, and others are presented elsewhere in this book.

Bazex–Dupré–Christol syndrome

Key points

- **X-linked semidominant disorder featuring follicular atrophoderma, hypotrichosis, multiple milia and hypohidrosis.**
- **Patients are predisposed to the development of basal cell carcinomas.**

Introduction. The Bazex–Dupré–Christol syndrome (BDCS) is characterized by follicular atrophoderma, hypotrichosis, multiple milia, hypohidrosis and early development of basal cell carcinomas (BCCs) [1,2].

Pathogenesis. BDCS is inherited in an X-linked semidominant manner, with more severe manifestations in male patients and milder findings in female patients. It was recently found to be caused by mutations in the *ACTRT1* gene encoding actin-related protein T1, which inhibits GLI1 expression; loss of ACTRT1 function in BDCS patients leads to activation of the Hedgehog pathway [3].

Clinical features. (Fig. 141.1). The congenital hypotrichosis of BDCS is diffuse in boys, whereas abnormal hairs are admixed with normal hairs in girls [4–6]. The eyebrows as well as scalp hairs may be affected and hair shaft abnormalities can include trichorrhexis nodosa and twisted hairs mimicking pili torti. Numerous milia are often present in infancy and childhood. The milia have a predilection for the face but may also occur on the scalp, trunk and extremities. Follicular atrophoderma can be evident at birth or appear during childhood. It primarily affects the dorsal aspects of the hands, feet, elbows and knees; the lower back and face are occasionally

SECTION 29: DISEASES PREDISPOSING TO MALIGNANCY

Harper's Textbook of Pediatric Dermatology, Fourth Edition. Edited by Peter Hoeger, Veronica Kinsler and Albert Yan.

Table 141.1 Hereditary disorders associated with mucocutaneous malignancies. Diseases in bold text are covered in this chapter

Disorder	Tumour susceptibility	Mode of inheritance	Gene product	Gene symbol
Albinism, oculocutaneous (see Chapter 124)	SCC, BCC, melanoma	AR	Tyrosinase (OCA1) P protein (pink-eye dilution homologue; OCA2) Tyrosinase-related protein 1 (OCA3) Solute carrier family: 45 member 2 (OCA4) and 24 member 5 (OCA6) Leucine-rich melanocyte differentiation associated (OCA7)	*TYR* *OCA2* *TYRP1* *SLC45A2* *SLC24A5* *LRMDA*
Bazex–Dupré–Christol syndrome	BCC	XR	Actin-related protein T1	*ACTRT1*
Epidermodysplasia verruciformis	SCC	AR	Transmembrane channel-like 6	*TMC6*
		AR	Transmembrane channel-like 8	*TMC8*
Epidermolysis bullosa, particularly recessive dystrophic (see Chapter 76)	SCC, melanoma	AR	Collagen VII, α1 chain	*COL7A1*
KID (keratitis–ichthyosis–deafness) syndrome (see Chapter 129)	SCC (mucocutaneous), malignant proliferating pilar tumours	AD	Connexin 26 (gap junction protein β2)	*GJB2*
Multiple self-healing squamous epitheliomas (Ferguson–Smith syndrome)	SCC (self-healing/ keratoacanthoma-like)	AD	Transforming growth factor-β receptor 1	*TGFBR1*
Palmoplantar keratoderma with cutaneous SCC and sex reversal (see Chapter 128)	SCC	AR	R-spondin 1	*RSPO1*
Pigmentation defects, palmoplantar keratoderma, and cutaneous SCC	SCC	AR	SAM and SH3 domain-containing 1	*SASH1*
Porokeratosis: disseminated superficial (actinic) ± linear (see Chapter 133)	SCC (highest risk for linear lesions)	AD ± type 2 mosaicism	Mevalonate kinase, phosphomevalonate kinase, other enzymes in the mevalonate pathway, solute carrier family 17 member 9	*MVK, PMVK, MVD, FDPS, SLC17A9*

AD, autosomal dominant; AR, autosomal recessive; BCC, basal cell carcinoma; SCC, squamous cell carcinoma, XR, X-linked recessive.

involved. Exaggerated follicular or pseudofollicular funnels ('ice-pick' marks) represent deep, wide ostia rather than true atrophy. Approximately half of BDCS patients have hypohidrosis, which is frequently limited to the head.

Multiple BCCs usually begin to arise on the face during the second or third decade of life [4–6]. They often present as hyperpigmented papules that resemble melanocytic naevi but can exhibit locally aggressive behaviour. Basal cell naevi and multiple trichoepitheliomas on the face or in the genital area have also been described [7,8].

Differential diagnosis. BDCS should be distinguished from the autosomal dominant naevoid BCC syndrome (Gorlin syndrome), which is caused by defects in the *PTCH* gene and features palmoplantar pits, odontogenic keratocysts of the jaws, calcification of the falx cerebri and skeletal abnormalities as well as early-onset BCCs (see Chapter 139). Rombo syndrome, like BDCS, manifests with hypotrichosis, milia, follicular atrophoderma and BCCs. However, Rombo syndrome can be differentiated by an autosomal dominant inheritance pattern, cyanotic acral erythema and follicular atrophoderma affecting primarily the face (atrophoderma vermiculatum) rather than the extremities.

The findings of BDCS also overlap with those of basaloid follicular hamartoma syndrome, an autosomal dominant condition that presents with hypotrichosis, milia, comedone-like lesions, palmoplantar pits and skin-coloured to hyperpigmented papules (basal cell naevi) favouring the head and neck but not follicular atrophoderma or true BCCs. In Happle–Tinschert syndrome and the related Curry–Jones syndrome caused by mosaic gain-of-function smoothened (*SMO*) mutations, linear/segmental basaloid follicular hamartomas or BCCs are variably accompanied by atrophoderma, hypo-/hypertrichosis, and hypo-/hyperpigmentation; skeletal, dental and cerebral anomalies may also be present [9]. Of note, acrokeratosis paraneoplastica is also referred to as Bazex syndrome but represents a completely different disorder characterized by acral hyperkeratotic plaques in association with carcinomas of the upper aerodigestive tract.

Table 141.2 Hereditary skin disorders associated with mucocutaneous and extracutaneous malignancies. Muir–Torre syndrome, which can present with keratoacanthomas and sebaceous carcinomas in addition to internal malignancies, is included in Table 141.3 to allow juxtaposition with the constitutional mismatch repair deficiency syndrome. Diseases in bold text are covered in this chapter. Other conditions associated with mucocutaneous and/or extracutaneous malignancies include multiple primary immunodeficiency syndromes (see Chapter 156), certain ichthyoses and some mosaic conditions presenting with epidermal and/or melanocytic naevi.

Disorder	Tumour susceptibility	Mode of inheritance	Gene or gene product	Gene symbol
Ataxia–telangiectasia (see Chapter 155)	Lymphoma, leukaemia, gastric carcinoma, BCC	AR	Ataxia–telangiectasia mutated	*ATM*
Brooke–Spiegler syndrome, multiple familial trichoepitheliomas and familial cylindromatosis	BCC, cylindrocarcinoma, spiradenocarcinoma, salivary gland adenocarcinoma (all rare)	AD	CYLD (deubiquitinating enzyme)	*CYLD*
Cartilage–hair hypoplasia (see Chapters 134, 155 and 159)	Non-Hodgkin's lymphoma, BCC	AR	RNA component of mitochondrial RNA-processing endoribonuclease	*RMRP*
Dyskeratosis congenita (see Chapter 140)	SCC (mucosal), lymphoma, leukaemia	XR	Dyskerin	*DKC1*
			Nucleolar protein family A member 3	*NOLA3*
		AD	TERF1-interacting nuclear factor 2	*TINF2*
		AD	Telomerase RNA component	*TERC*
		AD, AR	Telomerase reverse transcriptase	*TERT*
		AD, AR	Regulator of telomere elongation helicase 1	*RTEL1*
		AR	Conserved telomere maintenance component 1	*CTC1*
		AR	Telomerase Cajal body protein 1	*WRAP53 (TCAB1)*
		AR	NHP2 or NOP10 ribonucleoproteins	*NHP2, NOP10*
		AR	Poly(A)-specific ribonuclease	*PARN*
		AD, AR	TINF-interacting protein 1	*ACD (TINT1)*
Familial atypical mole–malignant melanoma (FAMMM) syndrome	Melanoma; pancreatic cancer, astrocytoma (rare; with particular *CDKN2A* mutations)	AD	Cyclin-dependent kinase inhibitor 2A	*CDKN2A*
		AD	Cyclin-dependent kinase 4	*CDK4*
BAP1 tumour predisposition syndrome	Melanoma (cutaneous, uveal); BCC; mesothelioma, renal cell carcinoma	AD	BRCA1-associated protein 1	*BAP1*
Gorlin (naevoid basal cell carcinoma) syndrome (see Chapter 139)	BCC, medulloblastoma, glioblastoma, fibrosarcoma	AD	Patched homologue 1	*PTCH1*
Huriez syndrome (sclerotylosis) (see Chapter 128)	SCC (mucocutaneous), gastrointestinal carcinoma (rare)	AD		(4q23)
Neurofibromatosis 1 (see Chapter 142)	Malignant peripheral nerve sheath tumour, glioma (most often optic), other CNS tumours, pheochromocytoma, juvenile myelomonocytic leukaemia, rhabdomyosarcoma, duodenal carcinoid, gastrointestinal stromal tumour, breast cancer	AD	Neurofibromin 1	*NF1*
Rothmund–Thomson syndrome (see Chapter 140)	Osteosarcoma, SCC, BCC	AR	RecQ protein-like 4	*RECQL4*
Xeroderma pigmentosa (see Chapter 138)	BCC, SCC, melanoma; various internal malignancies (later in life)	AR	XPA	*XPA*
			ERCC3 (XPB)	*ERCC3*
			XPC	*XPC*
			ERCC2 (XPD)	*ERCC2*
			DDB2 (XPE)	*DDB2*
			ERCC4 (XPF)	*ERCC4*
			ERCC5 (XPG)	*ERCC5*
			DNA polymerase-η	*POLH*

AD, autosomal dominant; AR, autosomal recessive; BCC, basal cell carcinoma; DDB2, DNA damage-binding protein 2; ERCC, excision repair cross-complementing; SCC, squamous cell carcinoma; XR, X-linked recessive.

References

1 Bazex A, Dupré A, Christol B. Genodermatose complexe de type indetermine associant une hypotrichose, un état atrophodermique généralisé et des degenerescences cutanées multiples (epitheliomas basocellulaires). Bull Soc Fr Dermat Syph 1964;71:206.

2 **Viksnins P, Berlin A. Follicular atrophoderma and basal cell carcinomas. The Bazex syndrome. Arch Dermatol 1977;113:948–51.**

3 **Bal E, Park HS, Belaid-Choucair Z et al. Mutations in ACTRT1 and its enhancer RNA elements lead to aberrant activation of Hedgehog signaling in inherited and sporadic basal cell carcinomas. Nat Med 2017;23:1226–33.**

SECTION 29: DISEASES PREDISPOSING TO MALIGNANCY

Table 141.3 Hereditary skin disorders associated with extracutaneous malignancies. Diseases in bold text are covered in this chapter

Disorder	Tumour susceptibility	Typical skin findings	Mode of inheritance	Gene product	Gene symbol(s)
Beckwith–Wiedemann syndrome	Hepatoblastoma, Wilms tumour, adrenocortical carcinoma, rhabdomyosarcoma	Glabellar vascular stain, earlobe grooves, posterior helical depressions	Sporadic > AD	Cyclin-dependent kinase inhibitor 1C and other products of imprinted genes at 11p15.5	11p15.5: *CDKN1C*, *KCNQ1OT1*, *IGF2*
Birt–Hogg–Dubé syndrome	Renal cell carcinoma	Fibrofolliculomas, trichodiscomas, acrochordons	AD	Folliculin	*FLCN*
Bloom syndrome (see Chapter 140)	Leukaemia, lymphoma, GI carcinoma	Photosensitivity, malar erythema and telangiectasias, CALM, hypopigmented macules	AR	Bloom's syndrome RecQ helicase-like 3	*BLM (RECQL3)*
Fanconi syndrome (see Chapter 140)	Leukaemia, hepatic carcinoma, SCC (head/neck)	Hyperpigmentation (favouring flexures) ± hypopigmented macules; CALM	AR >> XR	Products of at least 13 complementation group genes	13 complementation group genes
Familial mastocytosis + gastrointestinal stromal tumours (GIST)	Malignant GIST	Mastocytomas	AD	KIT proto-oncogene	*KIT*
Gardner syndrome	Colorectal carcinoma, other internal malignancies, fibrosarcomas (rare)	Epidermoid cysts, pilomatricomas, fibromas, desmoid tumour, lipomas	AD	Adenomatous polyposis coli	*APC*
Howel–Evans syndrome (tylosis–oesophageal cancer) (see Chapter 128)	Oesophageal carcinoma	Palmoplantar keratoderma	AD	Rhomboid 5 homologue 2	*RHBDF2*
Leiomyomatosis, cutaneous and uterine (Reed syndrome)	Renal cell carcinoma, leiomyosarcoma (rare)	Leiomyomas	AD	Fumarate hydratase	*FH*
Muir–Torre syndrome	Colorectal and genitourinary carcinomas, other internal malignancies	Sebaceous neoplasms (occasionally carcinoma), keratoacanthomas	AD AD AD	MutS homologue 2 (mismatch repair enzyme) MutS homologue 6 (mismatch repair enzyme) MutL homologue 1 (mismatch repair enzyme)	*MSH2* *MSH6* *MLH1*
Constitutional mismatch repair deficiency syndrome	CNS, haematological and gastrointestinal malignancies	CALM, lentigines, neurofibromas, hypopigmented macules	AR AR AR AR	MutS homologue 2 MutS homologue 6 MutL homologue 1 Postmeiotic segregation increased 2 (mismatch repair enzyme)	*MSH2* *MSH6* *MLH1* *PMS2*
Maffucci syndrome (see Chapter 118)	Chondrosarcoma	Venous/lymphatic malformations, spindle cell haemangio-endothelioma	Mosaic	Isocitrate dehydrogenase 1	*IDH1*
Multiple endocrine neoplasia (MEN) 1A (see Chapter 154)	Pituitary adenoma, parathyroid adenoma, pancreatic adenoma/carcinoma, foregut carcinoid	Angiofibromas, collagenomas, lipomas, hypopigmented macules, gingival papules	AD	Menin	*MEN1*
MEN2A (see Chapter 154)	Parathyroid adenoma, medullary thyroid carcinoma, pheochromocytoma	Lichen/macular amyloidosis	AD	Ret proto-oncogene (cysteine-rich extracellular domain)	*RET*
MEN2B (see Chapter 154)	Medullary thyroid carcinoma, pheochromocytoma	Mucosal neuromas	AD	Ret proto-oncogene (esp. Met918Thr)	*RET*
Peutz–Jeghers syndrome	GI, breast and ovarian malignancies	Lentigines (oral, perificial, acral)	AD	Serine-threonine kinase 11	*STK11 (LKB1)*
Tuberous sclerosis (see Chapter 143)	Astrocytoma, renal cell carcinoma	Hypopigmented macules, angiofibromas, periungual and gingival fibromas, connective tissue naevi	AD	Hamartin Tuberin	*TSC1* *TSC2*

(*Continued*)

Table 141.3 *Continued*

Disorder	Tumour susceptibility	Typical skin findings	Mode of inheritance	Gene product	Gene symbol(s)
Von Hippel–Lindau disease	Renal cell carcinoma, haemangioblastoma, pheochromocytoma	Capillary malformations	AR	Von Hippel–Lindau	*VHL*
Werner syndrome (see Chapter 137)	Soft-tissue sarcoma, osteosarcoma; possibly thyroid cancer and melanoma in Japanese patients	Atrophic or sclerodermoid skin, mottled hyperpigmentation, keratoses and ulcers over pressure points, subcutaneous calcification	AR	Werner syndrome, RecQ helicase-like 2	*WRN (RECQL2)*
Wiskott–Aldrich syndrome (see Chapter 156)	Lymphoma, leukaemia	Eczematous dermatitis, petechiae/purpura	XR	Wiskott–Aldrich protein	*WASP*
Bannayan–Riley–Ruvalcaba syndrome[a]	Thyroid, breast and endometrial carcinomas	Pigmented genital macules, vascular anomalies, lipomas	AD	Phosphatase and tensin homologue	*PTEN*
Cowden syndrome[a]		Trichilemmomas, acral keratoses, sclerotic fibromas	AD		
SOLAMEN syndrome[a] ('Proteus-like' syndrome)		Segmental overgrowth, lipomatosis, arteriovenous malformation, epidermal naevus	AD + type 2 mosaicism		
Disorders with increased RAS-extracellular signal-regulated kinase (ERK) signalling (see also neurofibromatosis 1 above)					
Cardiofaciocutaneous syndrome[b]	Leukaemia (very low risk)	Keratosis pilaris, ichthyosiform dermatitis, curly/woolly hair	AD	B-Raf serine/threonine kinase Mitogen-activated protein kinase kinase 1 Mitogen-activated protein kinase kinase 2 K-Ras GTPase	*BRAF* *MAP2K1 (MEK1)* *MAP2K2 (MEK2)* *KRAS*
Costello syndrome[b] (see Chapter 137)	Rhabdomyosarcoma, neuroblastoma	Acanthosis nigricans, lax acral skin, deep palmoplantar creases, periorificial papillomas, curly/woolly hair	AD	H-Ras GTPase	*HRAS*
Noonan syndrome with multiple lentigines (LEOPARD syndrome)	Leukaemia (very low risk)	Lentigines, café-noir macules	AD	Protein tyrosine phosphatase, nonreceptor type 11 Raf-1 serine/threonine kinase B-Raf serine/threonine kinase Mitogen-activated protein kinase kinase 1	*PTPN11* *RAF1* *BRAF* *MAP2K1*
Noonan syndrome[b]	Leukaemia, neuroblastoma, rhabdomyosarcoma (low risk)	Keratosis pilaris, curly/woolly hair, CALM, melanocytic naevi	AD	Protein tyrosine phosphatase, non-receptor type 11 Son of sevenless homologue 1 (guanine nucleotide exchange factor) Raf-1 serine/threonine kinase Ras-like without CAAX 1 K-Ras GTPase	*PTPN11* *SOS1* *RAF1* *RIT1* *KRAS*

AD, autosomal dominant; AR, autosomal recessive; CALM, café-au-lait macules; CNS, central nervous system; GI, gastointestinal; LEOPARD, lentigines, ECG changes, ocular hypertelorism, pulmonary stenosis, abnormal genitalia, retardation of growth, deafness; XR, X-linked recessive; SOLOMEN, segmental overgrowth, lipomatosis, arteriovenous malformation, epidermal naevus.

[a] The findings of Bannayan–Riley–Ruvalcaba, Cowden and SOLOMEN syndromes overlap.

[b] Distal phalangeal transverse creases, especially on the volar thumbs, represent an additional feature.

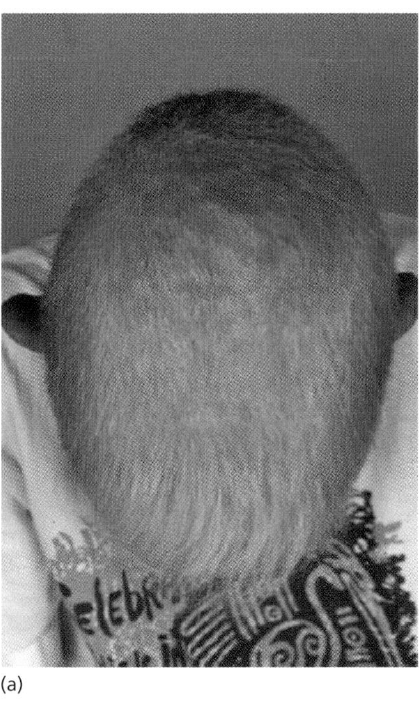

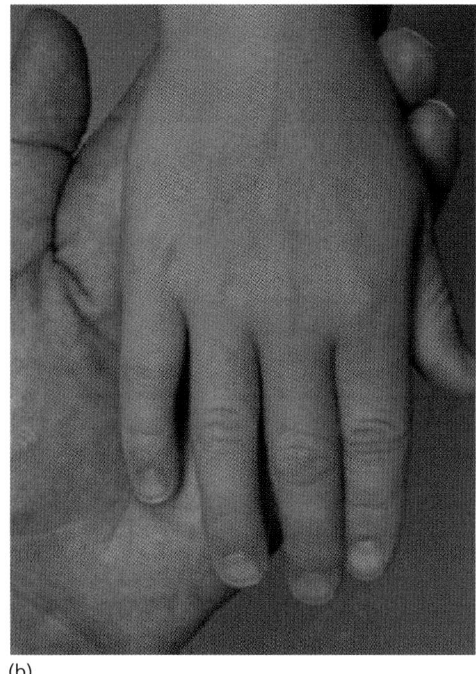

Fig. 141.1 Bazex–Dupré–Christol syndrome: (a) hypotrichosis and (b) follicular atrophoderma. Source: Courtesy of Professor Arnold Oranje.

4 **Goeteyn M, Geerts ML, Kint A et al. The Bazex–Dupré–Christol syndrome. Arch Dermatol 1994;130:337–42.**
5 Kidd A, Carson L, Gregory DW et al. A Scottish family with Bazex–Dupré–Christol syndrome: follicular atrophoderma, hypotrichosis and basal cell carcinoma. J Med Genet 1996;33:493–7.
6 Torrelo A, Sprecher E, Mediero IG et al. What syndrome is this? The Bazex–Dupré–Christol syndrome. Pediatr Dermatol 2006;23:286–90.
7 Yung A, Newton-Bishop JA. A case of Bazex–Dupré–Christol syndrome associated with multiple genital trichoepitheliomas. Br J Dermatol 2005;153:682–4.
8 **Castori M, Castiglia D, Passarelli F et al. Bazex–Dupré–Christol syndrome: an ectodermal dysplasia with skin appendage neoplasms. Eur J Med Genet 2009;52:250–5.**
9 **Twigg SR, Hufnagel RB, Miller KA. A recurrent mosaic mutation in SMO, encoding the hedgehog signal transducer smoothened, is the major cause of Curry-Jones syndrome. Am J Med Genet 2016;98:1256–65.**

Beckwith–Wiedemann syndrome

Syn.
Exomphalos-macroglossia-gigantism syndrome

Key points

- **Overgrowth disorder caused by genetic and epigenetic alterations of imprinted genes on chromosome 11p15.**
- **Characterized by hemihyperplasia, organomegaly, omphalocele and cutaneous findings including earlobe grooves, posterior helical depressions and a prominent glabellar naevus simplex.**
- **Increased risk of malignancies including hepatoblastoma and Wilms tumour.**

Introduction. Beckwith–Wiedemann syndrome (BWS) is characterized by visceral and somatic overgrowth, omphalocoele and increased risk of early childhood malignancies [1,2].

Pathogenesis. BWS can result from a variety of genetic or epigenetic alterations that affect a cluster of imprinted growth regulatory genes on chromosome 11p15.5 [3,4]. Imprinted genes are normally expressed preferentially or exclusively from either the paternal or maternal allele. The molecular aetiologies of BWS include: (i) loss-of-methylation of imprinting centre 2 (IC2) on the maternal chromosome (~50% of patients), resulting in expression of both alleles of *KCNQ1OT1*, which encodes an antisense RNA that down-regulates cyclin-dependent kinase inhibitor 1C (*CDKN1C*) gene expression; (ii) rare heterozygous loss-of-function mutations in the maternal *CDKN1C* gene; (3) gain-of-methylation of imprinting centre 1 (IC1) on the maternal chromosome, resulting in expression of both alleles of the insulin-like growth factor 2 (*IGF2*) gene and reduced expression of the oncosuppressor *H19* gene [5]; and (iv) uniparental disomy that replaces the maternal alleles of all these genes with a second paternal copy [4,6,7]. BWS usually occurs sporadically, although autosomal dominant inheritance with preferential maternal transmission accounts for approximately 15% of cases [6,7].

Clinical features. The characteristic cutaneous manifestations of BWS are anterior earlobe grooves and circular depressions on the posterior helical rim [6,7]. A prominent glabellar naevus simplex is another common finding. Extracutaneous features include macroglossia, midline umbilical wall defects (e.g. omphalocoele, umbilical hernia), organomegaly (e.g. liver, spleen, pancreas, kidneys, adrenal glands), and neonatal hypoglycaemia caused by increased insulin production. Somatic overgrowth can be prenatal and/or postnatal in nature and may result in gigantism or hemihyperplasia. Children with BWS have an increased risk of developing hepatoblastoma, Wilms tumour, rhabdomyosarcoma, adrenocortical carcinoma and neuroblastoma; overall, malignancy occurs in approximately 10% of patients during the first decade of life [7,8]. In patients with underlying IC2 loss-of-methylation, overall malignancy risk is lower and does not generally include Wilms tumour [8].

Treatment. Surveillance for malignancy includes serial abdominal ultrasounds and serum α-fetoprotein measurement, typically every 3 months until 8 and 4 years of age, respectively [9]. However, recently proposed guidelines recommend monitoring protocols based on the (epi) genetic aetiology, with less surveillance for patients with IC2 loss-of-methylation [8,10].

References

1 Wiedemann HR. Complexe malformatif familial avec hernie ombilicale et macroglossie: un 'syndrome nouveau'? J Genet Hum 1964; 13:223–32.
2 Beckwith JB. Macroglossia, omphalocele, adrenal cytomegaly, gigantism, and hyperplastic visceromegaly. Birth Defects 1969; v:188–96.
3 Koufos A, Grundy P, Morgan K et al. Familial Wiedemann–Beckwith syndrome and a second Wilms' tumor locus both map to 11p15.5. Am J Hum Genet 1989;44:711–19.
4 Weksberg R, Smith AC, Squire J et al. Beckwith–Wiedemann syndrome demonstrates a role for epigenetic control of normal development. Hum Mol Genet 2003;12:R61–R68.
5 Weksberg R, Shen DR, Fei Y-L et al. Disruption of insulin-like growth factor 2 imprinting in Beckwith–Wiedemann syndrome. Nat Genet 1993;5:143–50.
6 Weksberg R, Shuman C, Smith AC. Beckwith–Wiedemann syndrome. Am J Med Genet 2005;137C:12–23.
7 Weksberg R, Shuman C, Beckwith JB. Beckwith–Wiedemann syndrome. Eur J Hum Genet 2010;18:8–14.
8 Mussa A, Molinatto C, Baldassarre G et al. Cancer risk in Beckwith-Wiedemann syndrome: a systematic review and meta-analysis outlining a novel (epi)genotype specific histotype targeted screening protocol. J Pediatr 2016;176:142–9.
9 Zarate YA, Mena R, Martin et al. Experience with hemihyperplasia and Beckwith–Wiedemann syndrome surveillance protocol. Am J Med Genet 2009;149A:1691–7.
10 Maas SM, Vansenne F, Kadouch DJ et al. Phenotype, cancer risk, and surveillance in Beckwith-Wiedemann syndrome depending on molecular genetic subgroups. Am J Med Genet A 2016; 170:2248–60.

Birt–Hogg–Dubé syndrome

Key points

- **Autosomal dominant disorder caused by mutations in the folliculin gene (*FLCN*).**
- **Triad of fibrofolliculomas, trichodiscomas and acrochordons together with an increased risk of renal tumours and spontaneous pneumothoraces.**

Introduction. Birt–Hogg–Dubé syndrome (BHDS) is an autosomal dominant genodermatosis that features a classic triad of skin lesions – fibrofolliculomas, trichodiscomas and acrochordons – together with an increased risk of renal tumours and spontaneous pneumothoraces [1].

Pathogenesis. BHDS is caused by heterozygous loss-of-function mutations in the folliculin (*FLCN*) tumour suppressor gene [2]. Approximately 150 mutations in the *FLCN* gene have been identified, with almost all producing a truncated protein and approximately half involving insertion or deletion of a cytosine in a 'hot spot' hypermutable polycytosine tract in exon 11 [3–6]. Mutations in orthologous *bhd* genes underlie hereditary renal cancer in the Nihon rat and hereditary multifocal renal cystadenocarcinoma and nodular dermatofibrosis in the German shepherd dog. A high frequency of somatic inactivation of the germline wild-type *FLCN*/*bhd* allele has been noted in renal tumours from affected humans and rats.

The folliculin protein is expressed in the kidney, lung and skin. It associates with folliculin-interacting proteins, FNIP1 and FNIP2 [7,8]. FNIP1 binds to the AMP-activated protein kinase, a key energy sensing molecule that acts as a negative regulator of the mammalian target of rapamycin (mTOR) signalling pathway that stimulates cellular growth and survival (Fig. 141.2). Recent studies found that folliculin regulates an alternate mTOR pathway that controls browning of adipose tissue [9]. The exact relationships between folliculin and mTOR activity remain to be determined [8].

Pathology. In fibrofolliculomas, anastomosing strands of infundibular epithelium radiate from a distorted central follicle that is surrounded by a delicate fibromyxoid stroma. In trichodiscomas, the latter mesenchymal component predominates.

Clinical features. During the third or fourth decade of life, individuals with BHDS typically begin to develop multiple fibrofolliculomas, which affect more than 85% of patients, and (less often) trichodiscomas [5]. Both of these entities present as small, firm, whitish papules on the face, neck and upper trunk (Fig. 141.3). Angiofibromas and perifollicular fibromas, folliculocentric lesions otherwise similar to angiofibromas, have been described in patients with BHDS and are thought to exist on a spectrum with fibrofolliculomas [10–12]. Soft, skin-coloured, acrochordon-like papules in flexural sites represent another finding in BHDS. Mucosal fibromas and additional mesenchymal skin lesions such as perivascular fibromas, collagenomas, focal cutaneous mucinosis, angiomatous nodules and lipomas are also occasionally observed [3–5,9,13]. Cutaneous neoplasms that have been rarely reported in patients with BHDS include trichoblastoma, BCC, leiomyoma, leiomyosarcoma and dermatofibrosarcoma protuberans.

Individuals with BHDS have increased risk of developing renal tumours, particularly hybrid oncocytic and chromophobe renal carcinomas, which may be bilateral or multifocal. These tumours affect as many as a third of patients and develop at ages ranging from 20 to 70 years [3–5]. Recurrent spontaneous pneumothoraces are a frequent manifestation in BHDS; although most common in young adults, they have been reported in adolescents and

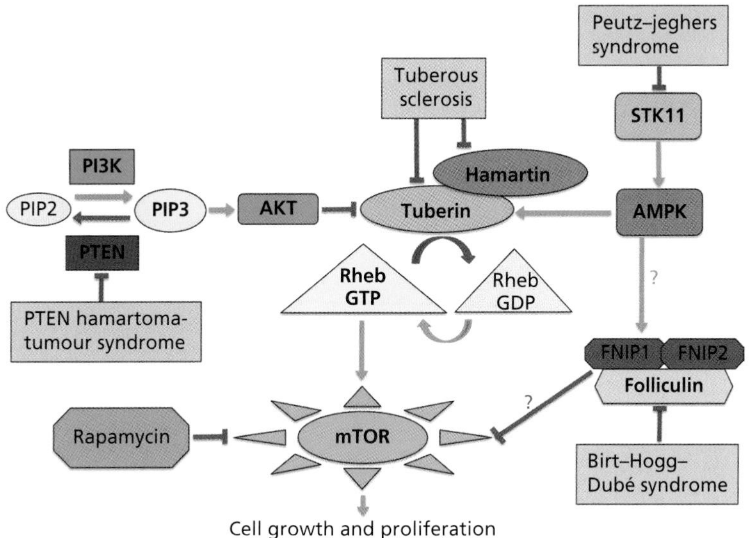

Fig. 141.2 Mammalian target of rapamycin (mTOR) signalling in cancer-prone genodermatoses. The PTEN protein negatively regulates the PI3K/AKT pathway, which inhibits the GTPase activating-protein tuberin. Decreased tuberin activity leads to increased mTOR signalling and resultant cell growth. During periods of nutrient depletion (high AMP/low ATP), serine-threonine kinase 11 (STK11) promotes AMP-activated protein kinase (AMPK)-mediated activation of tuberin, which results in decreased mTOR signalling and less protein synthesis. Folliculin and folliculin-interacting protein 1 (FNIP1) form a complex with and are phosphorylated by AMPK, and mTOR activation (potentially via the AKT pathway) has been observed in renal tumors from Birt-Hogg-Dubé syndrome patients and (in some studies) folliculin-deficient mice. Increased mTOR signalling therefore contributes to the development of tumours in genodermatoses characterized by defects in PTEN, tuberin, STK11 or folliculin proteins. AMP, adenosine monophosphate; ATP, adenosine triphosphate; GDP, guanosine diphosphate; GTP, guanosine triphosphate; PIP2, phosphatidylinositol diphosphate; PIP3, phosphatidylinositol triphosphate; PTEN, phosphatase and tensin homologue deleted on chromosome 10.

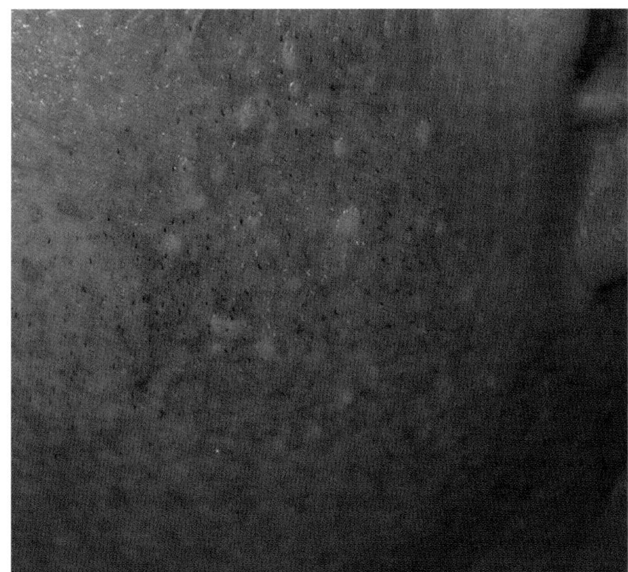

Fig. 141.3 Birt–Hogg–Dubé syndrome: multiple fibrofolliculomas presenting as whitish papules on the cheek.

children as young as 7 years [14]. Lung cysts are evident via computed tomographic scanning in more than 85% of adults with BHDS [5]. Patients with BHDS may also be predisposed to the development of renal cysts and parotid oncocytomas. Lastly, although colonic polyps and carcinomas were described as central features of the related and perhaps overlapping Hornstein–Knickerberg syndrome, which also manifests with perifollicular fibromas, an increased incidence of colonic neoplasia has not been consistently observed in large series of patients with BHDS [3–5].

Differential diagnosis. BHDS shares several mucocutaneous features with tuberous sclerosis, which also involves dysregulation of the mTOR pathway (see Fig. 141.2) and multiple endocrine neoplasia type 1A, including facial angiofibromas, collagenomas and mucosal fibromas. Renal tumours and cystic lung disease represent additional overlapping manifestations of tuberous sclerosis and BHDS.

Treatment. Recognition of the cutaneous manifestations of BHDS is important in order to facilitate early diagnosis of associated renal tumours and cystic lung disease.

References

1 **Birt AR, Hogg GR, Dubé WJ. Hereditary multiple fibrofolliculomas with trichodiscomas and acrochordons. Arch Dermatol 1977; 113:1674–7.**

2 **Nickerson ML, Warren MB, Toro JR et al. Mutations in a novel gene lead to kidney tumors, lung wall defects, and benign tumors of the hair follicle in patients with the Birt-Hogg-Dubé syndrome. Cancer Cell 2002;2:157–64.**

3 **Schmidt LS, Nickerson ML, Warren MB et al. Germline BHD-mutation spectrum and phenotype analysis of a large cohort of families with Birt-Hogg-Dubé syndrome. Am J Hum Genet 2005;76:1023–33.**

4 Leter EM, Koopmans AK, Gille JJ et al. Birt-Hogg-Dubé syndrome: clinical and genetic studies of 20 families. J Invest Dermatol 2008; 128:45–9.

5 **Toro JR, Wei MH, Glenn GM et al. BHD mutations, clinical and molecular genetic investigations of Birt-Hogg-Dubé syndrome: a new series of 50 families and a review of published reports. J Med Genet 2008;45:321–31.**

6 **Schmidt LS, Linehan WM. Molecular genetics and clinical features of Birt-Hogg-Dubé syndrome. Nat Rev Urol 2015;12:558–69.**

7 Baba M, Hong SB, Sharma N et al. Folliculin encoded by the BHD gene interacts with a binding protein, FNIP1, and AMPK, and is involved in AMPK and mTOR signaling. Proc Natl Acad Sci USA 2006;103: 15552–7.

8 **Hartman TR, Nicolas E, Klein-Szanto A et al. The role of the Birt Hogg-Dubé protein in mTOR activation and renal tumorigenesis. Oncogene 2009;28:1594–604.**
9 Wada S, Neinast M, Jang C et al. The tumor suppressor FLCN mediates an alternate mTOR pathway to regulate browning of adipose tissue. Genes Dev 2016;30:2551–64.
10 Schaffer JV, Gohara MA, McNiff JM et al. Multiple facial angiofibromas: a cutaneous manifestation of Birt-Hogg-Dubé syndrome. J Am Acad Dermatol 2005;53:S108–S111.
11 **Misago N, Kimura T, Narisawa Y. Fibrofolliculoma/trichodiscoma and fibrous papule (perifollicular fibroma/angiofibroma): a revaluation of the histopathological and immunohistochemical features. J Cutan Pathol 2009;36:943–51.**
12 Shvartsbeyn M, Mason AR, Bosenberg MW, Ko CJ. Perifollicular fibroma in Birt-Hogg-Dubé syndrome: an association revisited. J Cutan Pathol 2012;39:675–9.
13 Nikolaidou C, Moscarella E, Longo C et al. Multiple angiomatous nodules: a novel skin tumor in Birt-Hogg-Dubé syndrome. J Cutan Pathol 2016;43:1197–202.
14 Bessis D, Giraud S, Richard S. A novel familial germline mutation in the initiator codon of the BHD gene in a patient with Birt-Hogg-Dubé syndrome. Br J Dermatol 2006;155:1067–9.

Brooke-Spiegler syndrome, multiple familial trichoepitheliomas and familial cylindromatosis

Key points

- **Overlapping autosomal dominant disorders caused by mutations in the CYLD tumour suppressor gene.**
- **Characterized by a predisposition for the development of trichoepitheliomas, cylindromas and/or spiradenomas.**

Introduction. Brooke–Spiegler syndrome (BSS), multiple familial trichoepitheliomas (MFT; epithelioma adenoides cysticum of Brooke) and familial cylindromatosis (FC) are overlapping, allelic autosomal dominant disorders characterized by a predisposition for the development of trichoepitheliomas, cylindromas and/or spiradenomas.

Pathogenesis. BSS, FMT and FC are caused by heterozygous loss-of-function mutations in the *CYLD* tumour suppressor gene [1–3]. These are typically truncating lesions or (less often) missense mutations affecting the ubiquitin-specific protease domain. Although the clinical findings and severity vary among kindreds with the same mutation and even within families [2,3], missense mutations are more likely to be associated with MFT [4]. The adnexal tumours that develop in affected individuals usually have somatic inactivation of the germline wildtype *CYLD* allele. The CYLD protein functions as a deubiquitinating enzyme that is relatively specific for lysine 63-linked ubiquitin chains. It negatively regulates the nuclear factor-κB (NF-κB) and c-Jun N-terminal kinase (JNK) pathways that promote cell survival and proliferation [5].

Clinical features. BSS, MFT and FC exist on a spectrum and manifest between late childhood and early adulthood with progressive development of characteristic adnexal neoplasms [2,3]. Trichoepitheliomas and cylindromas occur together in BSS (sometimes along with spiradenomas), whereas trichoepitheliomas and cylindromas predominate in MFT and FC, respectively. Trichoepitheliomas are firm skin-coloured papulonodules with a predilection for the central face, especially the nose and melolabial folds (Fig. 141.4). Cylindromas present as slowly growing nodules that favour the scalp, referred to as 'turban tumours' in their fulminant form. Spiradenomas are less common and classically develop on the trunk and extremities as paroxysmally painful nodules with a slightly bluish hue. Syringomas have also been reported in individuals with BSS.

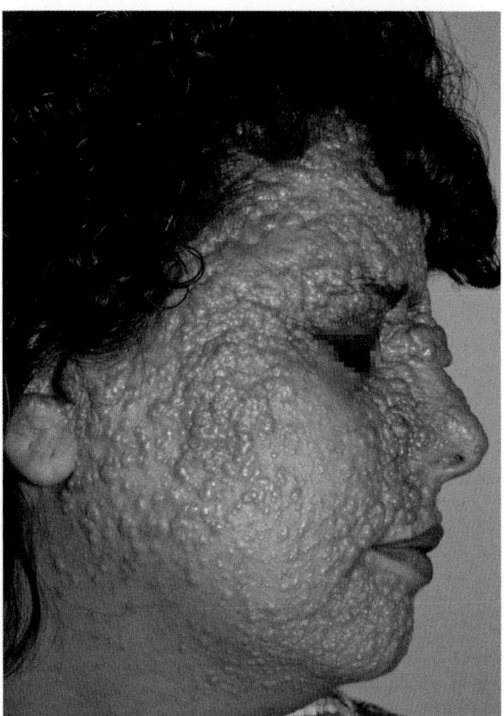

Fig. 141.4 Multiple familial trichoepitheliomas: numerous facial tumours.

Cylindrocarcinomas and spiradenocarcinomas occasionally arise in patients with BSS-spectrum disorders and tend to behave aggressively, with destructive local growth and metastases [3,6]. BCCs have been noted to originate in continuity with trichoepitheliomas in BSS/MFT patients, and adenocarcinomas as well as adenomas of the parotid and other salivary glands have also been observed [3].

Histological findings. Trichoepitheliomas, cylindromas and spiradenomas are tumours with follicular-apocrine differentiation [3]. Trichoepitheliomas feature small clusters or cribriform cords of basaloid cells with follicular germinative differentiation surrounded by dense fibrocytic stroma as well as small keratinizing cystic spaces with superficial follicular differentiation. Cylindromas, spiradenomas and spiradenocylindromas (hybrid tumours with features of both lesions) have apocrine lineage but are less obviously differentiated. Cylindromas display a 'jigsaw puzzle' pattern of angulated nests of basaloid cells enveloped by dense eosinophilic basement membrane material, whereas spiradenomas have larger, rounded nests composed of trabeculae with peripheral basaloid cells.

Treatment. Surgical excision, electrosurgical techniques and other ablative modalities (e.g. carbon dioxide or erbium:YAG laser treatment) can be used to control tumour burden [7,8]. Use of tumour necrosis factor-α inhibitors and aspirin to decrease the NF-κB signalling that is augmented in these disorders has also been described [8], and a topical tropomycin receptor kinase inhibitor is under investigation [9].

References

1 Bignell GR, Warren W, Seal S et al. Identification of the familial cylindromatosis tumour-suppressor gene. Nat Genet 2000;25:160–5.

2 Saggar S, Chernoff KA, Lodha S et al. CYLD mutations in familial skin appendage tumours. J Med Genet 2008;45:298–302.

3 Blake PW, Toro JR. Update of cylindromatosis gene (CYLD) mutations in Brooke-Spiegler syndrome: novel insights into the role of deubiquitination in cell signaling. Hum Mutat 2009;30:1025–36.

4 Nagy N, Farkas K, Kemeny L, Szell M. Phenotype-genotype correlations for clinical variants caused by CYLD mutations. Eur J Med Genet 2015;58:271–8.

5 Courtois G. Tumor suppressor CYLD: negative regulation of NF-κB signaling and more. Cell Mol Life Sci 2008;65:1123–32.

6 Kazakov DV, Zelger B, Rutten A et al. Morphologic diversity of malignant neoplasms arising in preexisting spiradenoma, cylindroma, and spiradenocylindroma based on the study of 24 cases, sporadic or occurring in the setting of Brooke-Spiegler syndrome. Am J Surg Pathol 2009;33:705–19.

7 Rajan N, Trainer AH, Burn J et al. Familial cylindromatosis and Brooke-Spiegler syndrome: a review of current therapeutic approaches and the surgical challenges posed by two affected families. Dermatol Surg 2009;35:845–52.

8 Fisher GH, Geronemus RG. Treatment of multiple familial trichoepitheliomas with a combination of aspirin and a neutralizing antibody to tumor necrosis factor alpha: a case report and hypothesis of mechanism. Arch Dermatol 2006;142:782–3.

9 Tropomyosin receptor antagonism in cylindromatosis (TRAC), an early phase trial of a topical tropomyosin kinase inhibitor as a treatment for inherited CYLD defective skin tumours: study protocol for a randomized controlled trial. Trials 2017;18:111.

Epidermodysplasia verruciformis

Key points

- **Autosomal recessive condition characterized by susceptibility to infections with β-genus human papillomavirus types caused by mutations in the transmembrane channel-like 6 or 8 gene (*TMC6* and *TMC8*).**
- **Affected individuals develop skin lesions resembling flat warts or tinea versicolor as well as squamous cell carcinomas.**

Introduction. Epidermodysplasia verruciformis (EDV) is an autosomal recessive condition characterized by genetic susceptibility to cutaneous infections with a particular group of human papillomavirus (HPV) types and the development of squamous cell carcinomas (SCCs) in affected skin.

Pathogenesis. Patients with EDV are prone to infection with the β genus of HPV, which includes types 5, 8, 9, 12, 14, 15, 17, 19–25, 36–38, 46, 47, 49, 50 and others [1–3]. These HPV types are ubiquitous but generally do not cause clinical lesions in immunocompetent individuals. EDV patients are usually infected by multiple β-HPV types, and infections with other HPV types such as 3 and 10 can also occur. Particular HPV types may be associated with distinct skin lesion morphologies within an affected individual. HPV types 5 and 8 are most often detected in the SCCs that develop in EBV patients.

EDV is caused by biallelic loss-of-function mutations in either of two adjacent genes located on chromosome 17q25: transmembrane channel-like 6 (*TMC6*; previously *EVER1*) and transmembrane channel-like 8 (*TMC8*; previously *EVER2*) [4]. *TMC6* and *TMC8* encode integral membrane proteins in the endoplasmic reticulum. These proteins form a complex with the zinc transporter 1 (ZnT1), which has a role in regulation of intracellular zinc distribution [4]. The ZnT1-TMC6/8 complex is thought to inhibit zinc influx to nucleoli and downregulate transcription factors stimulated by zinc and keratinocytes from EDV patients have an increased replication rate [3,5]. The HPV E5 protein, which is present in HPV types that are typically pathogenic but not in β-HPV types, inhibits ZnT1-TMC6/8 function. This may explain how the *TMC6/8* defect that underlies EDV enables β-HPV types to cause clinical disease.

Clinical features. EDV typically presents during childhood with widespread, polymorphic skin lesions [1–3,6]. Hyperpigmented or hypopigmented to pinkish flat-topped papules that resemble flat warts favour the face and dorsal hands (Fig. 141.5). Larger red-brown to pink-tan

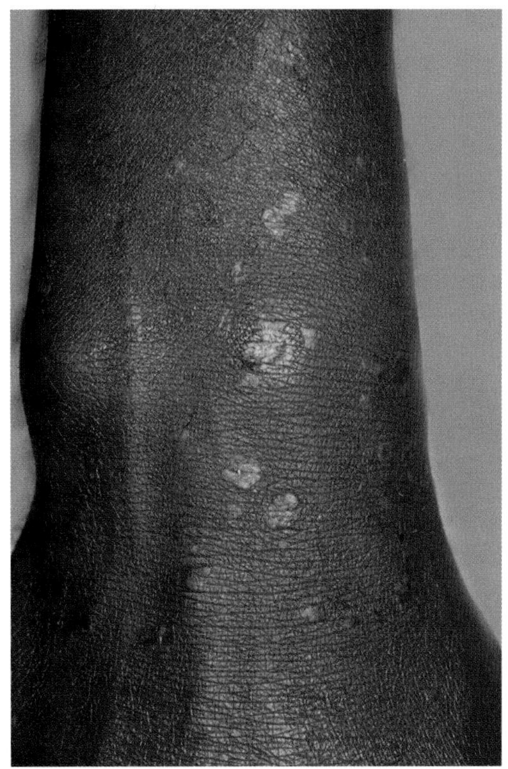

Fig. 141.5 Epidermodysplasia verruciformis: hypopigmented flat-topped papules on the dorsal wrist.

SECTION 29: DISEASES PREDISPOSING TO MALIGNANCY

or hypopigmented macules and thin scaly plaques reminiscent of tinea versicolor have a predilection for the neck, trunk and proximal extremities. Thicker scaly plaques may also appear, especially on the extensor surfaces and distal extremities.

SCCs, *in situ* or invasive, develop in approximately half of patients and usually affect chronically sun-exposed sites. The SCCs often begin to arise during the third or fourth decade of life but can occur in affected adolescents [6]. Deafness was described in two otherwise healthy teenage siblings with classic EDV skin lesions [7], which is interesting considering that mutations in other genes in the transmembrane channel-like family cause hearing loss.

Differential diagnosis. EDV-like manifestations have been reported in patients with a variety of primary immunodeficiency syndromes, including those caused by deficiencies in coronin 1A, serine/threonine kinase 4 (STK4/MST1), LCK tyrosine kinase, RhoH GTPase and dedicator of cytokinesis 8 (DOCK8) [8]. Other immunosuppressed patients, such as those with solid organ transplants or human immunodeficiency virus infection, can also develop extensive warts caused by infection with β-HPV types as well as standard pathogenic HPV types.

Histological findings. Benign skin lesions of EDV classically display large keratinocytes with pale blue-grey cytoplasm and occasional perinuclear halos. Keratohyaline granules with variable shapes and sizes may also be observed [9]. However, histological evaluation cannot reliably distinguish EDV lesions from ordinary flat warts.

Treatment. EDV patients should practise diligent sun protection and avoidance. The warty lesions tend to be resistant to treatment, although improvement has been described with use of oral retinoids, sometimes in conjunction with interferon-α, and photodynamic therapy with topical 5-aminolaevulinic acid [1,10]. Lesions with rapid growth or other features suggestive of SCC should be biopsied.

References

1 **Gewirtzman A, Bartlett B, Tyring S. Epidermodysplasia verruciformis and human papilloma virus. Curr Opin Infect Dis 2008;21:141–6.**

2 **Burger B, Itin PH. Epidermodysplasia verruciformis. Curr Probl Dermatol 2014;45:123–31.**

3 Lazarczyk M, Cassonnet P, Pons C et al. The EVER proteins as a natural barrier against papillomaviruses: a new insight into the pathogenesis of human papillomavirus infections. Microbiol Molec Biol Rev 2009;73:348–70.

4 Ramoz N, Rueda L-A, Bouadjar B et al. Mutations in two adjacent novel genes are associated with epidermodysplasia verruciformis. Nat Genet 2002;32:487–9.

5 Lazarczyk M, Pons C, Mendoza J et al. Regulation of cellular zinc balance as a potential mechanism of EVER-mediated protection against pathogenesis by cutaneous oncogenic human papillomaviruses. J Exp Med 2008;205:35–42.

6 **Gul U, Kilic A, Gonul M et al. Clinical aspects of epidermodysplasia verruciformis and review of the literature. Int J Dermatol 2007; 46:1069–72.**

7 Al Rubaie S, Breuer J, Inshasi J et al. Epidermodysplasia verruciformis with neurological manifestations. Int J Dermatol 1998;37:766–71.

8 Li SL, Duo LN, Wang HJ et al. Identification of LCK mutation in a family with atypical epidermodysplasia verruciformis with T-cell defects and virus-induced squamous cell carcinoma. Br J Dermatol 2016;175:1204–9.

9 **Nuovo G, Ishag M. The histologic spectrum of epidermodysplasia verruciformis. Am J Surg Pathol 2000;24:1400–6.**

10 Rallis E, Papatheodorou G, Bimpakis E et al. Systemic low-dose isotretinoin maintains remission status in epidermodysplasia verruciformis. J Eur Acad Dermatol Venerol 2008;22:523–5.

Gardner syndrome

Key points

- **Autosomal dominant condition caused by mutations in the fumarate hydratase (*FH*) tumour suppressor gene.**
- **Characterized by leiomyomas of the skin and uterus as well as an increased risk of renal cell cancer.**

Introduction. Gardner syndrome is an autosomal dominant condition that features epidermoid cysts, fibrous tumours, osteomas, intestinal polyposis and early-onset colorectal carcinoma [1]. It is considered to represent a phenotypic variant of familial adenomatous polyposis (FAP) with prominent extraintestinal manifestations.

Pathogenesis. Both Gardner syndrome and isolated FAP are caused by heterozygous loss-of-function mutations in the adenomatous polyposis coli (*APC*) tumour suppressor gene [2]. Some studies have found that mutations in certain regions of the *APC* gene are associated with a higher frequency of particular extraintestinal manifestations [3,4], although there is considerable phenotypic variability among individuals with the same mutation and even within affected families. The APC protein downregulates β-catenin, which has important functions in cell adhesion and development.

Clinical features. Epidermoid cysts typically begin to appear between ages 4 and 10 years but can be congenital. They may become numerous and are located on the head, neck and extremities more often than the trunk. Multiple pilomatricomas have also been reported [5,6]. The spectrum of fibrous tumours in Gardner syndrome includes fibromas (cutaneous, subcutaneous or mesenteric), desmoid tumours (classically within abdominal incisional scars) and occasionally fibrosarcomas [7,8]. Leiomyomas and lipomas may develop in the skin and subcutis as well as in extracutaneous sites.

Osteomas affect the majority of patients with Gardner syndrome and have a predilection for the maxilla, mandible and sphenoid bones, although they can also occur in other bones of the skull and in long bones [7,9]. Osteomas typically develop around puberty and may present as a slowly enlarging mass or require radiographic studies for detection. Dental anomalies can include supernumerary teeth, unerupted teeth and odontomas. Congenital hypertrophy of the retinal pigment epithelium (CHRPE) is frequent in patients with Gardner syndrome and can represent a useful clue to the diagnosis in young children who have not yet developed other manifestations [10].

Polyps of the colon, small intestine and stomach typically begin to arise during the second decade of life and are evident in at least half of patients by age 20 years [9]. They are frequently asymptomatic and intussusception is not a feature. Without intervention, colorectal carcinoma inevitably develops, usually before age 40 years [9]. Patients are also predisposed to other malignancies including duodenal and pancreatic carcinoma, hepatoblastoma (especially during the first 5 years of life), papillary thyroid carcinoma (with a 100-fold increased incidence in affected women) and medulloblastoma [7,9,11].

Differential diagnosis. A tendency to epidermoid cyst formation may be inherited as an isolated abnormality. The presence of multiple epidermoid cysts in a child is an indication for obtaining a detailed family history, an ophthalmological evaluation for CHRPE and radiological examination of the skull. Analysis of the *APC* gene can confirm the diagnosis. Of note, mutations in the *MUTYH* base excision repair gene can cause an autosomal recessive form of colorectal adenomatous polyposis that occasionally presents with pilomatricomas, desmoid tumours, sebaceous neoplasms (see below), osteomas or CHRPE.

Histological findings. Although the cutaneous cysts of Gardner syndrome are usually indistinguishable from ordinary epidermoid cysts, pilomatricoma-like changes are evident in a subset of lesions [5].

Treatment. Early recognition of Gardner syndrome allows affected children and adolescents to be monitored by a gastroenterologist, typically with annual colonoscopy or flexible sigmoidoscopy beginning at 10–12 years of age, and enables prophylactic colectomy to be performed prior to malignant transformation of polyps [8]. Because of the increased risk of hepatoblastoma, abdominal ultrasound and measurement of serum α-fetoprotein levels every 3–6 months during the first 5 years of life have been recommended by some experts [7,12]. Additional surveillance includes annual thyroid examination beginning in the late teenage years and periodic oesophagogastroduodenoscopy beginning in the third decade of life. Genetic counselling is crucial, and family members should be evaluated for extraintestinal and intestinal signs of the disorder.

References

1 Gardner EJ, Richards RC. Multiple cutaneous and subcutaneous lesions occurring simultaneously with hereditary polyposis and osteomatosis. Am J Hum Genet 1953;5:139–47.

2 Groden J, Thliveris A, Samowitz W et al. Identification and characterization of the familial adenomatous polyposis coli gene. Cell 1991;66:589–600.

3 Wallis YL, Morton DG, McKeown CM et al. Molecular analysis of the APC gene in 205 families: extended genotype-phenotype correlations in FAP and evidence for the role of APC amino acid changes in colorectal cancer predisposition. J Med Genet 1999;36:14–20.

4 Bisgaard ML, Bulow S. Familial adenomatous polyposis (FAP): genotype correlation to FAP phenotype with osteomas and sebaceous cysts. Am J Med Genet 2006;140A:200–4.

5 Cooper PH, Fechner RE. Pilomatricoma-like changes in the epidermal cysts of Gardner's syndrome. J Am Acad Dermatol 1983;8:639–44.

6 Pujol RM, Casanova JM, Egido R et al. Multiple familial pilomatricomas: a cutaneous marker for Gardner syndrome? Pediatr Dermatol 1995;12:331–5.

7 Green EJ, Roos A, Muntinghe FL et al. Extra-intestinal manifestations of familial adenomatous polyposis. Ann Surg Oncol 2008;15:2439–50.

8 van Geel MJ, Wijnen M, Hoppenreijs EP et al. Hypertrophic left calf and multiple flesh-coloured subcutaneous tumours in a 5-year-old girl: Gardner-associated fibroma. Acta Derm Venereol 2014; 94:619–22.

9 Galiatsatos P, Foulkes WD. Familial adenomatous polyposis. Am J Gastroenterol 2006;101:385–98.

10 Traboulsi EI, Krush AJ, Gardner EJ et al. Prevalence and importance of pigmented ocular fundus lesions in Gardner's syndrome. N Engl J Med 1987;316:661–7.

11 Giardiello FM, Petersen GM, Bresinger JD et al. Hepatoblastoma and APC gene mutation in familial adenomatous polyposis. Gut 1996; 39:867–9.

12 Aretz S, Koch A, Uhlhaas S et al. Should children at risk for familial adenomatous polyposis be screened for hepatoblastoma and children with apparently sporadic hepatoblastoma be screened for APC germline mutations? Pediatr Blood Cancer 2006;47:811–18.

Hereditary leiomyomatosis and renal cell cancer syndrome

Syn.
Leiomyomatosis cutis et uteri, multiple cutaneous and uterine leiomyomatosis syndrome, Reed syndrome

Key points

- **Autosomal dominant phenotypic variant of familial adenomatous polyposis.**
- **Features epidermoid cysts, fibrous tumours, osteomas, intestinal polyposis and early-onset colorectal carcinoma.**

Introduction. Hereditary leiomyomatosis and renal cell cancer (HLRCC) syndrome is an autosomal dominant condition characterized by leiomyomas of the skin and uterus as well as an increased risk of renal cell cancer (RCC).

Pathogenesis. HLRCC syndrome is caused by mutations in the fumarate hydratase (*FH*) tumour suppressor gene, which encodes a Krebs cycle (tricarboxylic acid cycle) enzyme [1–4]. The heterozygous germline *FH* mutations that underlie HLRCC syndrome are most often missense but occasionally truncating and the latter may have a stronger association with RCC [4]. Leiomyomas and other tumours that develop in association with HLRCC syndrome almost always have a 'second hit' that results in loss of the germline wild-type *FH* allele [5].

Inactivation of *FH* leads to accumulation of fumarate, which inhibits a hydroxylase enzyme that normally functions together with the von Hippel–Lindau protein to target hypoxia inducible factor (HIF) for proteasomal degradation [6]. As a result, HIF accumulates and stimulates increased transcription of genes encoding proteins that promote cellular growth and angiogenesis, including platelet-derived growth factor (PDGF), vascular endothelial growth factor (VEGF) and transforming growth factor-α (TGF-α). This provides the rationale for using drugs that disrupt PDGF and VEGF signalling (e.g. bevacizumab, sorafenib, sunitinib) in the treatment of HLRCC-related malignancies.

Clinical features. Cutaneous (pilar) leiomyomas affect more than 75% of HLRCC patients and are usually the first manifestation of the disorder. Onset is typically during the second to fourth decades of life (mean ~25 years), with lesions developing as early as 9 years of age [7]. In female patients, cutaneous leiomyomas become apparent a median of 7 years prior to the diagnosis of uterine leiomyomas [7].

The skin lesions present as red-brown to pink-tan, firm dermal papules or nodules that may be scattered in a disseminated fashion but are often clustered or segmental in distribution (Fig. 141.6), which is thought to reflect a postzygotic 'second hit' in the *FH* gene during embryonic development, i.e. type 2 mosaicism in an autosomal dominant skin condition [8,9]. Cutaneous leiomyomas typically measure 2 mm to 2 cm in diameter and favour the trunk and extremities. Most patients report lesional pain precipitated by a cold environment, minor trauma or palpation [7]. Cutaneous leiomyosarcomas have been reported in a few HLRCC patients; metastasis of these lesions has not been described [2,3,10].

Multiple uterine leiomyomas (fibroids) occur in almost all affected women, with an eightfold increased risk compared with the general population [11]. The fibroids develop in younger women (mean ~30 years) than in the general population (mean ~40 years), and surgical intervention (myomyectomy or hysterectomy) is often required [11]. Uterine leiomyosarcoma was described in one of Reed's original patients and in as many as 15% of young women from Finnish kindreds; however, it has not been reported in North American families with HLRCC [12].

RCC develops in approximately 15% of patients with multiple cutaneous and uterine leiomyoma and is usually unilateral [2,13,14]. Although the median age at diagnosis is 40–45 years, RCC arising during adolescence has been described in HLRCC kindreds [7,13]. The RCCs have traditionally been categorized as primarily papillary type 2, tubulocystic, or collecting duct tumours that behave aggressively, with a 5-year mortality rate of up to 70% [15]. However, the 2016 WHO classification of urinary system tumours includes a new entity termed HLRCC-associated RCC with papillary architecture [16]. Wilms tumour has also reported in a 2-year-old child with HLRCC [17].

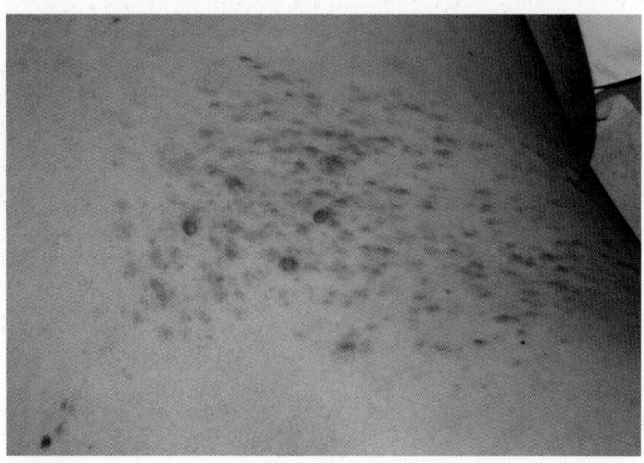

Fig. 141.6 Familial leiomyomatosis: segmental distribution of cutaneous leiomyomas.

Other potential manifestations of HLRCC include renal cysts, bladder carcinoma, ovarian neoplasms (e.g. mucinous cystadenoma), testicular neoplasms (e.g. Leydig cell tumours) and pheochromocytoma/paraganglioma.

Differential diagnosis. The clinical appearance of a cutaneous leiomyoma may resemble that of a dermatofibroma, schwannoma, neurofibroma (typically softer upon palpation) or adnexal neoplasm. Clustered lesions and pain associated with cold or light touch represent clues to the diagnosis, which can be confirmed via skin biopsy.

Patients diagnosed with a cutaneous leiomyoma should be examined for the presence of other lesions and questioned about a personal or family history of cutaneous leiomyomas, uterine fibroids, early hysterectomy and renal cancer. If additional features of HLRCC are identified in the patient or family members, genetic counselling and analysis of the *FH* gene should be offered. Almost 90% of patients who present with multiple cutaneous leiomyomas have an underlying germline *FH* mutation and can therefore be diagnosed as having HLRCC [7].

Pathology. The cutaneous leiomyomas of HLRCC originate from arrector pili muscles and are characterized by intersecting dermal bundles of well-differentiated smooth muscle cells. These myocytes are fusiform in shape and have abundant eosinophilic cytoplasm, central elongated nuclei with blunt ends (cigar-shaped) and perinuclear vacuolization [18]. Smooth muscle differentiation can be confirmed with a trichrome stain (where muscle appears red) or immunohistochemical staining for smooth muscle actin or desmin. Cutaneous leiomyomas associated with HLRCC demonstrate characteristic immunohistochemical staining for 2-succinocysteine caused by aberrant protein succination as well as variable loss of fumarate hydratase expression [19,20].

Hereditary leiomyomatosis and renal cell cancer-associated RCCs (papillary type II and collecting duct; see later) have characteristic histological features including abundant cytoplasm, large nuclei and prominent eosinophilic nucleoli with a clear halo [13].

Treatment. Patients with HLRCC should be monitored for the development of RCC with yearly magnetic resonance imaging (MRI) of the abdomen as well as complete skin and gynecological examinations [9,13,21].

References

1 **Tomlinson IP, Alam NA, Rowan AJ, Multiple Leiomyoma Consortium. Germline mutations in FH predispose to dominantly inherited uterine fibroids, skin leiomyomata and papillary renal cell cancer. Nat Genet 2002;30:406–10.**

2 **Toro JR, Nickerson ML, Wei MH et al. Mutations in the fumarate hydratase gene cause hereditary leiomyomatosis and renal cell cancer in families in North America. Am J Hum Genet 2003; 73:95–106.**

3 Wei MH, Toure O, Glenn GM et al. Novel mutations in FH and expansion of the spectrum of phenotypes expressed in families with hereditary leiomyomatosis and renal cell cancer. J Med Genet 2006;43:18–27.

4 Bayley JP, Launonen V, Tomlinson IP. The FH mutation database: an online database of fumarate hydratase mutations involved in the MCUL (HLRCC) tumor syndrome and congenital fumarase deficiency. BMC Med Genet 2008;9:20.

5 Alam NA, Rowan AJ, Wortham NC et al. Genetic and functional analyses of FH mutations in multiple cutaneous and uterine leiomyomatosis, hereditary leiomyomatosis and renal cancer, and fumarate hydratase deficiency. Hum Mol Genet 2003; 12:1241–52.

6 Ratcliffe PJ. Fumarate hydratase deficiency and cancer: activation of hypoxia signaling? Cancer Cell 2007;11:303–5.

7 **Alam NA, Barclay E, Rowan AJ et al. Clinical features of multiple cutaneous and uterine leiomyomatosis: an underdiagnosed tumor syndrome. Arch Dermatol 2005;141:199–206.**

8 Badeloe S, van Geel M, van Steensel MA et al. Diffuse and segmental variants of cutaneous leiomyomatosis: novel mutations in the fumarate hydratase gene and review of the literature. Exp Dermatol 2006;15:735–41.

9 **Patel VM, Handler MZ, Schwartz RA, Lambert C. Hereditary leiomyomatosis and renal cell cancer syndrome: an update and review. J Am Acad Dermatol 2017;77:149–58.**

10 **Muller M, Ferlicot S, Guillaud-Bataille M et al. Reassessing the clinical spectrum associated with hereditary leiomyomatosis and renal cell carcinoma syndrome in French FH mutation carriers. Clin Genet 2017;92:606–15.**

11 Stewart L, Glenn GM, Stratton P et al. Association of germline mutations in the fumarate hydratase gene and uterine fibroids in women with hereditary leiomyomatosis and renal cell cancer. Arch Dermatol 2008;144:1584–92.

12 Lehtonen HJ, Kiuru M, Ylisaukko-Oja SK et al. Increased risk of cancer in patients with fumarate hydratase germline mutation. J Med Genet 2006;43:523–6.

13 **Menko FH, Maher ER, Schmidt LS et al. Hereditary leiomyomatosis and renal cell cancer (HLRCC): renal cancer risk, surveillance and treatment. Fam Cancer 2014;13:637–44.**

14 Alam NA, Olpin S, Leigh IM. Fumarate hydratase mutations and predisposition to cutaneous leiomyomas, uterine leiomyomas and renal cancer. Br J Dermatol 2005;153:11–17.

15 Grubb RL, Franks ME, Toro J et al. Hereditary leiomyomatosis and renal cell cancer: a syndrome associated with an aggressive form of inherited renal cancer. J Urol 2005;177:2074–80.

16 Moch H, Cubilla AL, Humphrey PA et al. The 2016 WHO classification of tumours of the urinary system and male genital organs—part A: renal, penile, and testicular tumours. Eur Urol 2016; 70:93–105.

17 Badeloe S, van Spaendonck-Zwarts KY, van Steensel MA et al. Wilms tumour as a possible early manifestation of hereditary leiomyomatosis and renal cell cancer? Br J Dermatol 2009;160:707–9.

18 **Buelow B, Cohen J, Nagymanyoki Z et al. Immunohistochemistry for 2-succinocysteine (2SC) and fumarate hydratase (FH) in cutaneous leiomyomas may aid in identification of patients with HLRCC (hereditary leiomyomatosis and renal cell sarcinoma syndrome). Am J Surg Pathol 2016;40:982–8.**

19 Carter CS, Skala SL, Chinnaiyan AM et al. Immunohistochemical characterization of fumarate hydratase (FH) and succinate dehydrogenase (SDH) in cutaneous leiomyomas for detection of familial cancer syndromes. Am J Surg Pathol 2017;41:801–9.

20 Merino MJ, Torres-Cabala C, Pinto P et al. The morphologic spectrum of kidney tumors in hereditary leiomyomatosis and renal cell carcinoma (HLRCC) syndrome. Am J Surg Pathol 2007; 31:1578–85.

21 Rothman A, Glenn G, Choyke L et al. Multiple painful cutaneous nodules and renal mass. J Am Acad Dermatol 2009;55:683–6.

Muir–Torre and constitutional mismatch repair deficiency syndromes

Key points

- **Muir–Torre syndrome is an autosomal dominant phenotypic variant of Lynch syndrome characterized by adult onset of sebaceous neoplasms, keratoacanthomas and internal malignancies, especially gastrointestinal and genitourinary carcinomas.**
- **Constitutional mismatch repair deficiency syndrome is an allelic autosomal recessive disorder that features childhood onset of cutaneous findings similar to those of neurofibromatosis type 1 together with brain tumours and haematological malignancies.**

Introduction. Muir–Torre syndrome (MTS) is an autosomal dominant condition characterized by adult onset of sebaceous neoplasms, keratoacanthomas and internal malignancies; it is considered to represent a subtype of Lynch syndrome (hereditary nonpolyposis colorectal cancer syndrome) [1]. Constitutional mismatch repair deficiency syndrome (CMRDS or childhood cancer syndrome) is an allelic autosomal recessive disorder that features childhood onset of cutaneous findings similar to those of neurofibromatosis type 1 (NF1) together with brain tumours and haematological malignancies [2].

Pathogenesis. MTS is caused by heterozygous loss-of-function germline mutations in a mismatch repair gene, most often *MSH2* and occasionally *MLH1* or *MSH6* [1,3]. The tumours that arise in patients with MTS typically have a somatic 'second-hit' mutation in the other copy of the affected mismatch repair gene, which abolishes function of that protein. CMRDS patients have loss-of-function germline mutations in both copies of a mismatch repair gene such as *MLH1*, *MSH2*, *MSH6* or *PMS2* [2,4–6].

Defective mismatch repair protein function leads to accumulation of single nucleotide base pair mismatches and small insertion-deletion loops during DNA replication. This impairs maintenance of genomic integrity and results in a predisposition to tumour formation. The tumours that develop are characterized by microsatellite instability, which refers to increased variability in the lengths of repetitive 'microsatellite' sequences dispersed throughout the genome that are particularly prone to replication errors [1,2].

Clinical features. Patients with MTS present at a mean age of approximately 50 years with sebaceous neoplasms (adenomas > sebaceomas and carcinomas) of the head, neck and trunk [7,8]. Keratoacanthomas, sometimes with sebaceous differentiation, also develop in a quarter of patients. Colorectal carcinomas, often occurring at or proximal to the splenic flexure, and genitourinary carcinomas account for more than 50% and approximately 25% of associated cancers, respectively. These malignancies typically present a decade earlier (mean 50 years) and have a less aggressive course than their sporadic counterparts [7]. Almost half of patients develop more than one internal malignancy.

Patients with CMRDS syndrome usually present during early childhood with multiple café-au-lait macules (CALMs) [2,9]. Axillary freckling, hypopigmented macules and (less often) neurofibromas are evident in some affected children; extensive dermal melanocytosis has also been described. Haematological malignancies, most often non-Hodgkin lymphoma and acute lymphoblastic leukaemia, develop at a mean age of 5 years, brain tumours (primarily glioblastomas) occur at a mean age of 8 years and colorectal carcinoma arises at a mean age of 16 years, considerably earlier than in Lynch syndrome. Other malignancies such as rhabdomyosarcoma, neuroblastoma and Wilms tumour have also been reported in young children with CMRDS [2,10].

Differential diagnosis. Sebaceous adenomas and carcinomas as well as colorectal carcinomas and other malignancies have been described in patients with autosomal recessive colorectal adenomatous polyposis caused by mutations in the *MUTYH* base excision repair gene [11]. Patients with multiple self-healing squamous epithelioma of Ferguson-Smith, an autosomal dominant condition caused by transforming growth factor-β receptor 1 (*TGFB1*) mutations, present with keratoacanthoma-like tumours that tend to regress spontaneously within 6 months with residual scarring; affected individuals do not have an increased risk of internal malignancies. The time of onset varies from childhood to late adulthood (mean age = ~25 years), and the lesions favour chronically sun-exposed sites [12].

The cutaneous findings of CMRDS overlap with those of NF1 and a subset of CMRDS patients meets clinical criteria for diagnosis of NF1 (Chapter 142). The CALMs of CMRDS tend to be more irregular in pigmentation, configuration and size than those of NF1 and are more likely to be accompanied by hypopigmented macules [2]. CMRDS should be considered in the differential diagnosis for children with multiple CALMs, especially when associated with a malignancy that is not linked to NF1.

Histological findings. Immunohistochemical staining demonstrating a lack of expression of MSH2, MLH1, MSH6 and/or PMS2 may be utilized as a marker of MTS-associated neoplasms [13,14]. The MSH2 and MSH6 proteins form a heterodimer, so loss of one can lead to the absence of the other. However, reduced staining is sometimes observed in sporadic sebaceous neoplasms, especially in immunocompromised patients, and staining is occasionally normal in lesions from patients with a mismatch repair gene mutation [15,16]. In addition, lesional tissue from MTS-associated neoplasms often demonstrates microsatellite instability, which can be identified with polymerase chain reaction-based techniques [13,14].

Treatment. Recognition of the cutaneous findings of MTS and CMRDS, with confirmation via analysis of tumours for loss of a mismatch repair protein and microsatellite instability, can facilitate early diagnosis and treatment of associated malignancies in patients and their family members [17]. Long-term aspirin therapy may decrease the risk of colorectal carcinoma in patients with Lynch syndrome.

References

1 **Ponti G, Ponz de Leon M. Muir–Torre syndrome. Lancet Oncol 2005;6:980–7.**
2 **Wimmer K, Etzler J. Constitutional mismatch repair-deficiency syndrome: have we so far seen only the tip of an iceberg? Hum Genet 2008;124:105–22.**
3 Mangold E, Rahner N, Friedrichs N et al. MSH6 mutation in Muir–Torre syndrome: could this be a rare finding? Br J Dermatol 2007;156:158–62.
4 Ricciardone MD, Ozçelik T, Cevher B et al. Human MLH1 deficiency predisposes to hematological malignancy and neurofibromatosis type 1. Cancer Res 1999;59:290–3.
5 Wang Q, Lasset C, Desseigne F et al. Neurofibromatosis and early onset of cancers in hMLH1-deficient children. Cancer Res 1999;59:294–7.
6 **Poley JW, Wagner A, Hoogmans MM et al. Biallelic germline mutations of mismatch-repair genes: a possible cause for multiple pediatric malignancies. Cancer 2007;109:2349–56.**
7 **Cohen PR, Kohn SR, Kurzrock R. Association of sebaceous gland and internal malignancy: the Muir–Torre syndrome. Am J Med 1991;90:606–13.**
8 Singh RS, Grayson W, Redston M et al. Site and tumor type predicts DNA mismatch repair status in cutaneous sebaceous neoplasia. Am J Surg Pathol 2008;32:936–42.
9 **Wimmer K, Kratz CP, Vasen HF et al. Diagnostic criteria for constitutional mismatch repair deficiency syndrome: suggestions of the European consortium 'care for CMMRD' (C4CMMRD) J Med Genet 2014;51:355–65.**
10 Kratz CP, Holter S, Etzler J et al. Rhabdomyosarcoma in patients with constitutional mismatch-repair-deficiency syndrome. J Med Genet 2009;46:418–20.
11 Vogt S, Jones N, Christian D et al. Expanded extracolonic tumor spectrum in MUTYH-associated polyposis. Gastroenterology 2009;137:1976–85.
12 Goudie DR, D'Alessandro M, Merriman B et al. Multiple self-healing squamous epithelioma is caused by a disease-specific spectrum of mutations in TGFBR1. Nat Genet 2011;43:365–9.
13 **Ponti G, Losi L, di Gregorio C et al. Identification of Muir–Torre syndrome among patients with sebaceous tumors and keratoacanthomas: role of clinical features, microsatellite instability and immunohistochemistry. Cancer 2005;103:1018–25.**
14 **Abbas O, Mahalingam M. Cutaneous sebaceous neoplasms as markers of Muir–Torre syndrome: a diagnostic algorithm. J Cutan Pathol 2009;36:613–19.**
15 **Everett JN, Raymond VM, Dandapani M. Screening for germline mismatch repair mutations following diagnosis of sebaceous neoplasm. JAMA Dermatol 2014;150:1315–21.**
16 **Kim RH, Nagler AR, Meehan SA. Universal immunohistochemical screening of sebaceous neoplasms for Muir-Torre syndrome: putting the cart before the horse? J Am Acad Dermatol 2016;75:1078–9.**
17 **Giardiello FM, Allen JI, Axilbund JE et al. Guidelines on genetic evaluation and management of Lynch syndrome: a consensus statement by the US Multi-Society Task Force on Colorectal Cancer. Dis Colon Rectum 2014;57:1025–48.**

Peutz–Jeghers syndrome

Syn.
Periorificial lentiginosis

Key points

- **Autosomal dominant disorder caused by mutations in the serine/threonine kinase 11 (*STK11*) tumour suppressor gene.**
- **Characterized by periorificial and acral mucocutaneous lentigines, gastrointestinal hamartomatous polyps and an increased incidence of internal malignancies.**

Introduction. Peutz–Jeghers syndrome (PJS) is an autosomal dominant disorder characterized by mucocutaneous lentigines with a predilection for periorificial sites, gastrointestinal hamartomatous polyps, and an increased incidence of internal malignancies [1,2].

Pathogenesis. PJS is caused by heterozygous loss-of-function mutations in the serine/threonine kinase 11 (*STK11*; also known as *LKB1*) tumour suppressor gene [3]. Some studies have found that truncating *STK11* mutations are associated with the development of more gastrointestinal polyps and malignancies [4,5], and variants affecting the protein kinase domain XI may increase the risk of dysplastic gastrointestinal polyps [6]. The STK11 protein activates adenosine monophosphate-activated protein kinase (AMPK) and thereby stimulates activation of the tuberous sclerosis complex 2 (*TSC2*) gene product tuberin, which inhibits the mTOR pathway that promotes cellular growth and survival [7]. PJS is therefore characterized by increased mTOR signalling, and the mTOR inhibitor sirolimus (rapamycin) has been shown to reduce gastrointestinal polyp burden in the $lkb1^{+/-}$ mouse model of PJS [8].

Clinical features. The brown-to-black hyperpigmented macules of PJS, which represent lentigo simplex or mucosal melanotic macules, usually develop by early childhood [9,10]. The cutaneous lentigines typically measure 1–5 mm in diameter and favour perioral (Fig. 141.7), periorbital and other periorificial regions (e.g. around the nares or anus) as well as the hands (especially the fingers) and feet. The lips (vermilion and mucosal) and buccal mucosa are commonly affected, and additional mucosal sites may include the gingiva, palate and tongue. Lesions on the skin and vermilion lip tend to fade after puberty, but those in mucosal areas usually persist. Longitudinal melanonychia is sometimes observed.

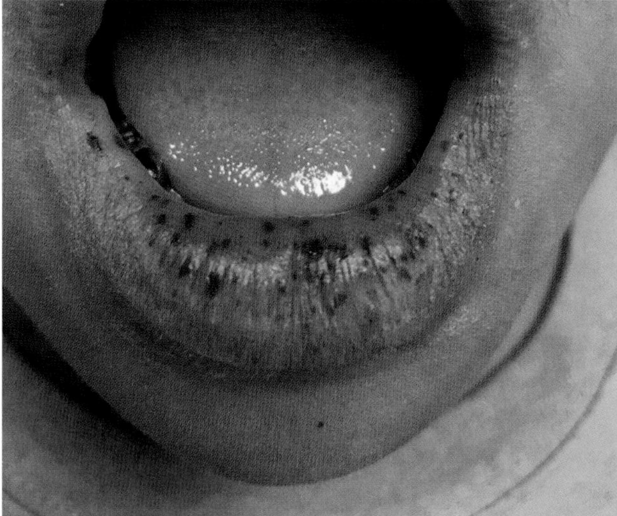

Fig. 141.7 Peutz–Jeghers syndrome: pigmented macules on the lip. Source: Courtesy of Joyce Teng, MD, PhD.

The hamartomatous polyps of PJS have a predilection for the small intestine but can occur anywhere in the gastrointestinal tract. The majority of patients have clinical manifestations such as abdominal pain, bleeding (often leading to anaemia), intussusception and other forms of bowel obstruction during childhood [8,9]. Nasal polyposis has also been described in PJS patients. Girls with PJS occasionally develop benign ovarian sex cord tumours with annular tubules, which can manifest with precocious puberty or abnormal menstrual bleeding and boys may present with gynaecomastia caused by aromatase production by large cell calcifying Sertoli cell tumours of the testes [11].

PJS patients have a 10–15-fold increase in the overall risk of cancer, with onset at younger ages than in the general population [12,13]. Predisposition to breast, colorectal, small intestinal, gastric, pancreatic, lung, ovarian, endometrial and cervical (adenoma malignum) malignancies has been documented [14,15].

Treatment. Patients with PJS should undergo periodic endoscopy beginning by age 10 years, with removal of large or otherwise troublesome polyps. Surveillance for extraintestinal as well as intestinal malignancies is required, and published protocols provide recommendations for types, starting ages and frequencies of procedures [8,9,16].

References

1 Peutz JL. Very remarkable case of familial polyposis of mucous membrane of intestinal tract and nasopharynx accompanied by peculiar pigmentations of skin and mucous membrane. Ned Maandschr Geneeskd 1921;10:134.

2 Jeghers H, McKusick BA, Katz KH. Generalised intestinal polyposis and melanin spots of the oral mucosa, lips and digits. N Engl J Med 1949;241:1031.

3 **Hemminki A, Markie D, Tomlinson I et al. A serine/threonine kinase gene defective in Peutz–Jeghers syndrome. Nature 1998; 391:184–7.**

4 Amos CI, Keitheri-Cheteri MB, Sabripour M et al. Genotype–phenotype correlations in Peutz–Jeghers syndrome. J Med Genet 2004; 41:327–33.

5 Salloch H, Reinacher-Schick A, Schulmann K et al. Truncating mutations in Peutz–Jeghers syndrome are associated with more polyps, surgical interventions and cancers. Int J Colorectal Dis 2010; 25:97–107.

6 Wang Z, Wu B, Mosig RA et al. STK11 domain XI mutations: candidate genetic drivers leading to the development of dysplastic polyps in Peutz-Jeghers syndrome. Hum Mutat 2014;35:851–8.

7 Shaw RJ, Kosmatka M, Bardeesy N et al. The tumor suppressor LKB1 kinase directly activates AMP-activated kinase and regulates apoptosis in response to energy stress. Proc Natl Acad Sci USA 2004; 101:3329–35.

8 Shakelford DB, Vasquez DS, Corbeil J et al. mTOR and HIF-1-mediated tumor metabolism in an LKB1 mouse model of Peutz–Jeghers syndrome. Proc Natl Acad Sci USA 2009;106:11137–42.

9 McGarrity TJ, Aos C. Peutz–Jeghers syndrome: clinicopathology and molecular alterations. Cell Mol Life Sci 2006;63:2135–44.

10 **Giardiello FM, Trimbath JD. Peutz–Jeghers syndrome and management recommendations. Clin Gastroenterol Hepatol 2006;4:408–15.**

11 Winterfield L, Schultz J, Stratakis CA et al. Gynecomastia and mucosal lentigines in an 8-year-old boy. J Am Acad Dermatol 2005;53:660–2.

12 Boardman LA, Thibodeau SN, Schaid DJ et al. Increased risk for cancer in patients with the Peutz–Jeghers syndrome. Ann Intern Med 1998;128:896–9.

13 Lim W, Hearle N, Shah B et al. Further observations on LKB1/STK11 status and cancer risk in Peutz–Jeghers syndrome. Br J Cancer 2003;89:308–13.

14 Lim W, Olschwang S, Keller JJ et al. Relative frequency and morphology of cancers in STK11 mutation carriers. Gastroenterology 2004; 126:1788–94.

15 **Hearle N, Schumacher V, Menko FH et al. Frequency and spectrum of cancers in the Peutz–Jeghers syndrome. Clin Cancer Res 2006; 12:3209–15.**

16 **Syngal S, Brand RE, Church JM et al. Clinical guideline: genetic testing and management of hereditary gastrointestinal cancer syndromes. Am J Gastroenterol 2015;110:223–62.**

PTEN hamartoma-tumour syndrome

Syn.

Bannayan–Riley–Ruvalcaba syndrome, Bannayan–Zonana syndrome, Cowden disease, Cowden syndrome, linear Cowden naevus, multiple hamartoma syndrome, Proteus-like syndrome, Riley–Smith syndrome, Ruvalcaba–Myhre–Smith syndrome, SOLAMEN syndrome

Key points

- **Spectrum of autosomal dominant disorders featuring macrocephaly, hamartomas and tumors (benign and malignant) caused by mutations in the *PTEN* tumour suppressor gene.**
- **Bannayan–Riley–Ruvalcaba syndrome is characterized by pigmented macules of the genitalia, lipomas and fast-flow vascular malformations that present at birth or during childhood.**
- **Cowden syndrome characterized by trichilemmomas, acral keratoses and sclerotic fibromas that typically develop in adolescence or early adulthood.**

Introduction. PTEN hamartoma-tumour syndrome (PHTS) is a multisystem disorder that features hamartomatous overgrowth of tissues with ectodermal, mesodermal and endodermal origin. Two overlapping autosomal dominant genodermatoses included within the spectrum of PHTS are: (i) Bannayan–Riley–Ruvalcaba syndrome (BRRS) characterized by pigmented macules of the genitalia, lipomas and fast-flow vascular malformations that present at birth or during childhood; and (ii) Cowden syndrome characterized by trichilemmomas, acral keratoses and sclerotic fibromas that typically develop in adolescence or early adulthood [1–3]. Macrocephaly and an increased incidence of benign and malignant neoplasms of the thyroid gland, breast and uterus represent additional manifestations of PHTS.

Pathogenesis. PHTS is caused by heterozygous loss-of-function germline mutations in the *PTEN* (phosphatase and tensin homolog) tumour suppressor gene [4,5]. One important function of the PTEN lipid phosphatase is to negatively regulate the phosphatidylinositol 3-kinase (PI3K)/AKT pathway that inhibits the tuberin tumour suppressor protein and thereby stimulates the mTOR pathway of increased cellular growth and survival [2,3].

Most studies have failed to correlate particular germline *PTEN* mutations with specific phenotypic characteristics [6–8]. Although large deletions are more often found in BRRS, identical mutations have been described in patients with BRRS and Cowden syndrome phenotypes. Clinical features vary considerably within PHTS kindreds, and BRRS and Cowden syndrome phenotypes can be observed in different members of the same family or even in the same individual, sometimes with diagnosis of BRRS as a young child and then meeting Cowden syndrome criteria later in life. It has been suggested that BRRS and Cowden syndrome represent a single condition with variable expressivity, with BRRS features having onset earlier in life than Cowden syndrome features. In PHTS patients with congenital manifestations in a mosaic distribution, e.g. epidermal naevi and segmental vascular anomalies, the presence of a postzygotic 'second hit' (presumably arising during embryogenesis) that results in loss of the germline wildtype *PTEN* allele in lesional tissue (type 2 mosaicism) has been documented [9,10].

Clinical features (Fig. 141.8). The classic skin findings of BRRS are usually apparent at birth or during early childhood. Pigmented genital macules favour the glans penis and vulva. Vascular anomalies tend to be multifocal lesions with fast-flow channels, intramuscular involvement and associated ectopic fat [11]. They have variable capillary, venous and lymphatic components and are sometimes associated with regional soft tissue and bony overgrowth. Separate lipomatous tumours may also be observed, and testicular lipomatosis is common in men with PHTS. Additional mucocutaneous findings in children with PHTS can include nonepidermolytic verrucous epidermal naevi and facial, acral and mucosal neuromas [12].

In contrast, the mucocutaneous hallmarks of Cowden syndrome typically develop during the second or third decade of life, although they are occasionally evident in younger children [13–15]. Trichilemmomas present as skin-coloured to yellowish-tan, verrucous or keratotic papules that favour the nose, periorificial face, ears and neck. Other papillomatous papules resembling warts or skin tags are also common in these locations. Punctate palmoplantar keratoses, which appear as translucent yellowish papules with or without a central depression, have been described in affected children as young as 3 years of age [16]. In addition, acral keratoses resembling flat warts may be seen on the dorsal aspects of the hands and feet, wrists and ankles, and extensor surfaces of the forearms and lower legs. Cutaneous sclerotic fibromas manifest as skin-coloured to white, smooth-surfaced, dome-shaped, firm papules. Mucosal papules, which may represent sclerotic fibromas or (less often) glycogenic acanthosis [17], can occur anywhere in the oral cavity, including the lips, tongue, buccal mucosa and gingiva; multiple lesions frequently lead to a cobblestone-like appearance.

Macrocephaly affects ≥80% of patients with PHTS, and neurological manifestations such as developmental delay, autism and seizures are occasionally observed [18,19]. Intracranial developmental venous anomalies are a common MRI finding in PHTS patients. Lhermitte–Duclos disease, a hamartomatous dysplastic gangliocytoma of the cerebellum, affects a small minority of patients with PHTS but (particularly when present in adults) is relatively specific for the condition. Craniofacial

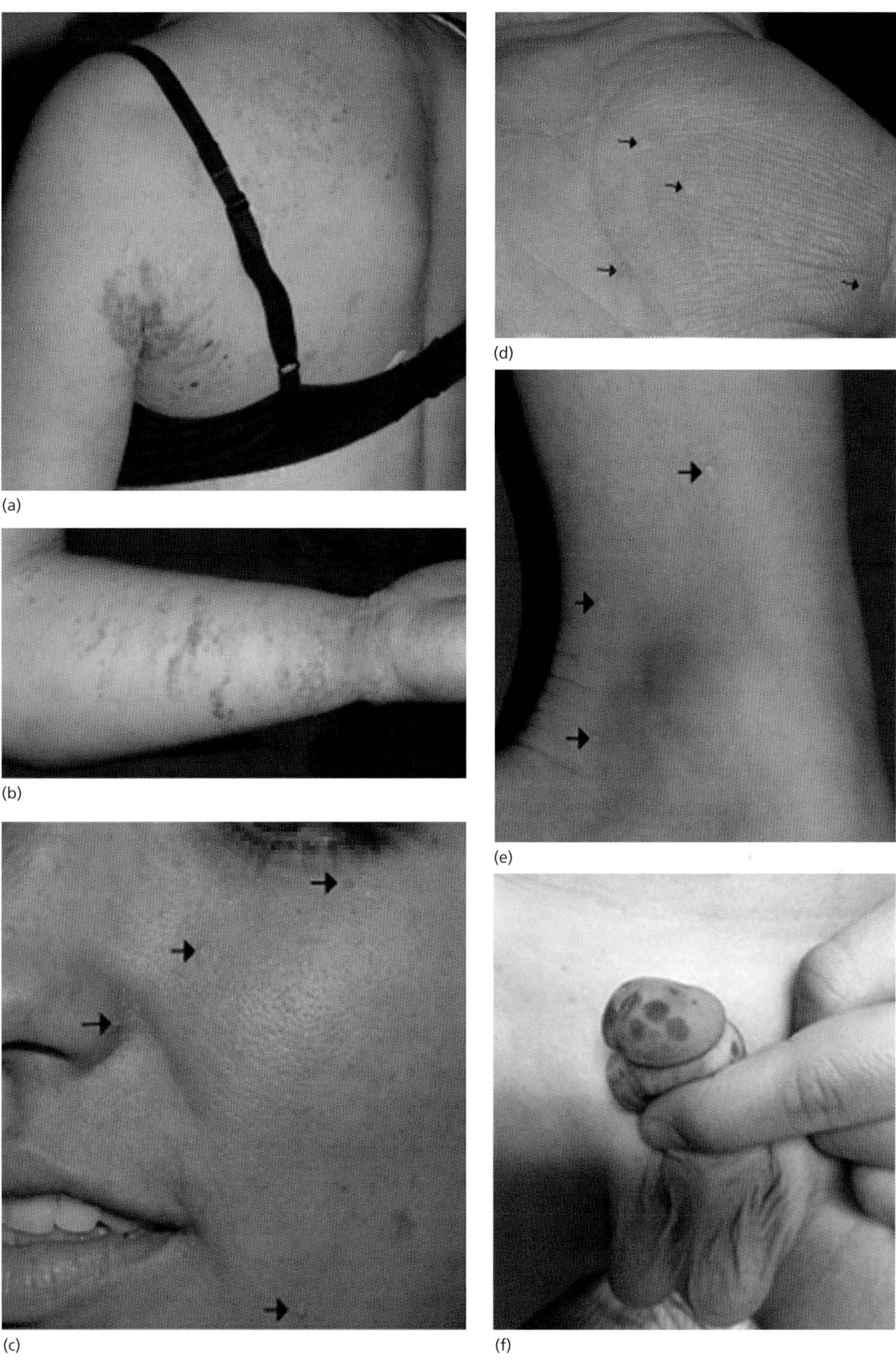

Fig. 141.8 PTEN hamartoma-tumour syndrome: (a, b) vascular malformation with arteriovenous and lymphatic components associated with overgrowth of the affected arm; (c) facial trichilemmomas; (d, e) acral keratoses; (f) pigmented macules on the glans penis.

and skeletal abnormalities may include adenoid facies, a high-arched palate, scoliosis, pectus excavatum, joint hyperextensibility and digital anomalies. Neonatal macrosomia, hypotonia and lipoid storage myopathy represent early extracutaneous findings in a small subset of patients.

Individuals with PHTS are at increased risk for the development of benign and malignant neoplasms of the thyroid, breast and uterus [2,3,20,21]. Thyroid cancer (follicular > papillary) affects 10–30% of patients, including children as young as 7 years of age. Breast cancer occurs in up to 85% of affected women at a mean age of approximately 40 years, whereas endometrial carcinoma develops in 15–30% of women at a somewhat older mean age. Although the majority of children and adults with PHTS have hamartomatous gastrointestinal polyps, colon cancer occurs in ≤10% of affected individuals. The lifetime risk of renal cell carcinoma is as high as 30%, and PHTS patients may also have an increased risk of cutaneous melanoma [2].

Differential diagnosis. The most recent diagnostic criteria for Cowden syndrome are provided in Table 141.4 [2]. A scoring system incorporating age and clinical findings has also been developed to estimate a patient's risk of having a *PTEN* mutation [21]. Despite their designation as 'pathognomonic' in the Cowden syndrome criteria, a combination of facial papules, oral mucosal papules and acral (including palmoplantar) keratoses can be observed in patients with Darier disease. Facial papules (e.g. angiofibromas and fibrofolliculomas) and gingival fibromas also occur together in tuberous sclerosis and BHDS. However, these conditions can usually be easily differentiated from Cowden syndrome by their distinct clinical and histological features.

Table 141.4 Clinical diagnostic criteria for the PTEN hamartoma tumour syndrome

Major criteria
- Any of the following mucocutaneous lesions:
  - Trichilemmomas (≥3, at least one biopsy-proven)
  - Acral keratoses (≥3 papules or palmoplantar pits)
  - Mucocutaneous neuromas
  - Oral papillomas, particularly on tongue and gingiva (≥3, biopsy-proven or dermatologist-diagnosed)
- Pigmented macules on the glans penis
- Macrocephaly (>97th percentile; for adults, 58 cm in women, 60 cm in men)
- Lhermitte-Duclos disease (in an adult)
- Breast cancer
- Endometrial cancer (epithelial)
- Thyroid cancer (follicular)
- Multiple gastrointestinal hamartomas or ganglioneuromas (≥3; excluding hyperplastic polyps)

Minor criteria
- Vascular anomalies (including intracranial developmental venous anomalies)
- Lipomas (≥3)
- Testicular lipomatosis
- Autism spectrum disorder
- Intellectual disability (IQ ≤ 75)
- Thyroid cancer (papillary or follicular variant of papillary)
- Thyroid structural lesions (e.g. adenoma, nodules, goiter)
- Renal cell carcinoma
- Colon cancer
- Esophageal glycogenic acanthosis

Operational diagnosis in an individual:
3 major criteria including macrocephaly, Lhermitte-Duclos disease or gastrointestinal hamartomas *or*
2 major criteria + 3 minor criteria
Operational diagnosis when a family member meets diagnostic criteria or has a PTEN *mutation:*
2 major criteria *or* 1 major + 2 minor criteria *or* 3 minor criteria
Source: Adapted from the National Comprehensive Cancer Network 2017 (www.nccn.org/professionals/physician_gls/PDF/genetics_screening.pdf) and reference [2].

The PHTS spectrum includes the type 2 mosaic SOLAMEN syndrome, which features segmental overgrowth, lipomatosis, arteriovenous malformations, and epidermal naevi. Proteus syndrome is caused by postzygotic *AKT1* mutations and has similar findings; however, it differs in its relentlessly progressive course, disproportionate overgrowth, highly characteristic cerebriform connective tissue naevi, and completely mosaic distribution of lesions (e.g. no disseminated/nonsegmental gastrointestinal polyposis as observed in PHTS). Postzygotic mutations in *PIK3CA* (phosphatidylinositol-4,5-biphosphate 3-kinase catalytic subunit α) that activate the PI3K/AKT pathway present with an overgrowth spectrum including CLOVES – congenital lipomatous overgrowth, vascular anomalies, epidermal naevi, scoliosis/skeletal abnormalities – and megalencephaly–capillary malformation syndromes.

Cowden syndrome-like disorders featuring predisposition to the same malignancies can result from heterozygous germline mutations in the *SDHB/C/D* genes, which encode subunits of mitochondrial succinate dehydrogenase, and germline epigenetic alteration in the *KLLN* gene, which encodes a p53-regulated DNA replication inhibitor. However, these conditions typically lack mucocutaneous manifestations. A Cowden syndrome-like phenotype has also been reported in patients with germline mutations in *PIK3CA* or *AKT1*; cutaneous findings such as trichilemmomas and lipomas were noted in a few affected individuals [22].

Pathology. Histological examination of trichilemmomas reveals lobular proliferations of pale keratinocytes with peripheral palisading surrounded by a prominent eosinophilic basement membrane [23,24]. The surface of trichilemmomas often demonstrates papillomatosis and hyperkeratosis. Papules on the face, neck and extremities of PHTS patients can also have histological features of verrucae or acrochordons and acral keratoses may resemble acrokeratosis verruciformis. Cutaneous and mucosal sclerotic fibromas are hypocellular lesions composed of short, thick, parallel collagen bundles arranged in plywood-like whorls embedded in abundant mucin [23,24].

Treatment. All patients with PHTS, including individuals with a known germline *PTEN* mutation and those with Cowden syndrome, should undergo surveillance for associated malignancies [2,19]. Current guidelines recommend a yearly comprehensive physical examination beginning at age 18 years and a yearly thyroid ultrasound. Women should have twice yearly clinical breast examinations beginning at age 25 years plus yearly mammography and breast MRI beginning at age 30–35 years. Prophylactic mastectomy can be considered on an individual basis. Periodic colonoscopy beginning at age

35 years is also recommended, as well as consideration of surveillance for endometrial and renal cancer, especially for patients with a family history of these malignancies. The mTOR inhibitor sirolimus (rapamycin) has been reported to decrease the growth of benign and malignant tumours in a few patients with PHTS and in pten-deficient mice [19,25,26].

References

1 Lloyd KM, Dennis M. Cowden's disease: a possible new symptom complex with multiple system involvement. Ann Intern Med 1963;58:136–42.

2 Pilarski R, Burt R, Kohlman W et al. Cowden syndrome and the PTEN hamartoma tumor syndrome: systematic review and revised diagnostic criteria. J Natl Cancer Inst 2013;105:1607–16.

3 Blumenthal GM, Dennis PA. PTEN hamartoma tumor syndromes. Eur J Hum Genet 2008;16:1289–300.

4 Liaw D, Marsh DJ, Li J et al. Germline mutations of the PTEN gene in Cowden disease, an inherited breast and thyroid cancer syndrome. Nat Genet 1997;16:64–7.

5 Marsh DJ, Dahia PL, Zheng Z et al. Germline mutations in PTEN are present in Bannayan–Zonana syndrome. Nat Genet 1997; 16:333–4.

6 Marsh DJ, Kum JB, Lunetta KL et al. PTEN mutation spectrum and genotype-phenotype correlations in Bannayan–Riley–Ruvalcaba syndrome suggest a single entity with Cowden syndrome. Hum Mol Genet 1999;8:1461–72.

7 Pilarski R, Eng C. Will the real Cowden syndrome please stand up (again)? Expanding mutational and clinical spectra of the PTEN hamartoma tumour syndrome. J Med Genet 2004;41:323–6.

8 Lachlan KL, Lucassen AM, Bunyan D et al. Cowden syndrome and Bannayan–Riley–Ruvalcaba syndrome represent on condition with variable expression and age-related penetrance: results of a clinical study of PTEN mutation carriers. J Med Genet 2007;44:579–85.

9 Caux F, Plauchu H, Chibon F et al. Segmental overgrowth, lipomatosis, arteriovenous malformation and epidermal nevus (SOLAMEN) syndrome is related to mosaic PTEN nullizygosity. Eur J Hum Genet 2007;15:767–73.

10 Happle R. Linear Cowden nevus: a new distinct epidermal nevus. Eur J Dermatol 2007;17:133–6.

11 Tan WH, Baris HN, Burrows PE et al. The spectrum of vascular anomalies in patients with PTEN mutations: implications for diagnosis and management. J Med Genet 2007;44:594–602.

12 Schaffer JV, Kamino H, Witkiewicz A et al. Mucocutaneous neuromas: an underrecognized manifestation of PTEN hamartoma-tumor syndrome. Arch Dermatol 2006;142:625–32.

13 Salem OS, Steck WD. Cowden's disease (multiple hamartoma and neoplasia syndrome). J Am Acad Dermatol 1983;8:686–96.

14 Starink TM. Cowden's disease: analysis of 14 new cases. J Am Acad Dermatol 1984;11:1127–41.

15 Starink TM, van der Veen JPW, Arwert F et al. The Cowden syndrome: a clinical and genetic study in 21 patients. Clin Genet 1986;29:222–33.

16 Ferran M, Bussaglia E, Matias-Guiu X et al. Bilateral and symmetrical palmoplantar punctuate keratoses in childhood: a possible clinical clue for an early diagnosis of PTEN hamartoma-tumour syndrome. Clin Exp Dermatol 2009;34:e28–e30.

17 Nishizawa A, Satoh T, Watanabe R et al. Cowden syndrome: a novel mutation and overlooked glycogenic acanthosis in gingiva. Br J Dermatol 2009;160:1116–8.

18 Lynch NE, Lynch SA, McMenamin J et al. Bannayan–Riley–Ruvalcaba syndrome: a cause of extreme macrocephaly and neurodevelopmental delay. Arch Dis Child 2009;94:553–4.

19 Hobert JA, Eng C. PTEN hamartoma tumor syndrome: an overview. Genet Med 2009;11:687–94.

20 Bubien V, Bonnet F, Brouste V et al. High cumulative risks of cancer in patients with PTEN hamartoma-tumour syndrome. J Med Genet 2013;50:255–63.

21 Tan M-H, Mester J, Peterson C et al. A clinical scoring system for selection of patients for PTEN mutation testing is proposed on the basis of a prospective study of 3042 probands. Am J Hum Genet 2011;88:42–56.

22 Orloff MS, He X, Peterson C et al. Germline PIK3CA and AKT1 mutations in Cowden and Cowden-like syndromes. Am J Hum Genet 2013;92:76–80.

23 Brownstein MH, Mehregan AM, Bikowski B et al. The dermatopathology of Cowden's syndrome. Br J Dermatol 1979;100:667–73.

24 Starink TM, Meijer CJLM, Brownstein MH. The cutaneous pathology of Cowden's disease: new findings. J Cutan Pathol 1985;12:83–93.

25 Squarize CH, Castilho RM, Gutkind JS. Chemoprevention and treatment of experimental Cowden's disease by mTOR inhibition with rapamycin. Cancer Res 2008;68:7066–72.

26 Schmid GL, Kässner F, Uhlig HH et al. Sirolimus treatment of severe PTEN hamartoma tumor syndrome: case report and in vitro studies. Pediatr Res 2014;75:527–34.

CHAPTER 142
The Neurofibromatoses

Amy Theos[1], *Kevin P. Boyd*[2] *& Bruce R. Korf*[3]

[1] Department of Dermatology, University of Alabama at Birmingham, Birmingham, AL, USA
[2] University of Alabama at Birmingham, Birmingham, AL, USA
[3] Department of Genetics, University of Alabama at Birmingham, Birmingham, AL, USA

Neurofibromatosis type 1, 1823
Segmental or mosaic neurofibromatosis type 1, 1831
Neurofibromatosis type 2, 1832

Abstract

The neurofibromatoses encompass three distinct inherited disorders: neurofibromatosis type 1 (NF1), neurofibromatosis type 2 (NF2) and schwannomatosis. These disorders share the propensity to develop multiple benign tumours of the peripheral and/or central nervous system, but are distinguished by specific clinical features, distinct genetic mutations, natural history and management. In this chapter, NF1 is reviewed in detail and the others are discussed briefly, with emphasis on how they may present to the paediatric dermatologist.

Key points

- The neurofibromatoses include three distinct genetic disorders: neurofibromatosis type 1 (NF1), neurofibromatosis type 2 (NF2) and schwannomatosis.
- NF1 has an estimated prevalence of 1 in 3000 and is the most likely to present to a dermatologist.
- NF1 is caused by mutations in the *NF1* gene, which encodes for neurofibromin, a tumour suppressor protein.
- The most common cutaneous features of NF1 are multiple (≥6) café-au-lait macules, (CALMs) skinfold freckling and neurofibromas.
- Patients presenting with six or more CALMs should be considered to have NF1 until proven otherwise.
- NF1 can involve any organ system: skeletal dysplasias, scoliosis, Lisch nodules, optic pathway gliomas and learning disabilities occur frequently in patients with NF1.
- CALMs with skinfold freckling, once thought to be pathognomonic for NF1, also occur in Legius syndrome. Patients with Legius syndrome do not develop other features of NF1 including neurofibromas, malignant peripheral nerve sheath tumours, Lisch nodules or optic pathway gliomas.
- Molecular genetic testing is available for NF1 and is useful for diagnostic confirmation.
- Segmental NF1 describes patients with characteristic features of NF1 (usually cutaneous)–localized to a body region(s) and is caused by postzygotic mosaicism of the *NF1* gene.
- NF2 is an autosomal dominant disorder caused by mutations in the *NF2* gene, which encodes for merlin, a tumour suppressor protein.
- Patients with NF2 typically have fewer than five CALMs, lack skinfold freckling and develop cutaneous schwannomas, not neurofibromas.
- NF2 phenotype is more restricted than NF1 with disease features being limited to the central nervous system and eye. Bilateral vestibular schwannomas are the hallmark of NF2.
- A few CALMs, cutaneous tumours and ocular abnormalities (cataracts, ambylopia) are the earliest findings in children with NF2.
- Molecular genetic testing is available for NF2 and is important for diagnostic confirmation, prediction of disease severity and screening at-risk family members.
- Ideally, patients with NF1 or NF2 should be managed in a multidisciplinary clinic.

Neurofibromatosis type 1

Neurofibromatosis type 1 (NF1), formerly known as von Recklinghausen disease, is an autosomal dominant, multisystem disorder affecting approximately 1 in 3000. Approximately half of affected individuals have a *de novo* mutation. NF1 is caused by mutations in the *NF1* gene that encodes for neurofibromin, a tumour suppressor protein. Cutaneous features, including multiple CALMs, axillary and inguinal freckling, and neurofibromas, are prevalent in NF1. Multiple CALMs are often the earliest diagnostic finding in NF1. Other cutaneous features that occur at a higher frequency in NF1 include juvenile xanthogranulomas, naevus anaemicus, and glomus tumours. Common extracutaneous findings in NF1 are Lisch nodules, optic pathway glioma, skeletal dysplasias and intellectual disabilities. Individuals also have an increased risk of malignancy, especially malignant peripheral nerve sheath tumour, leukaemia, and rhabdomyosarcoma. Thus, dermatologists play a critical role in the recognition and early diagnosis of patients with NF1.

Epidemiology and pathogenesis.

Epidemiology

NF1 is one of the most common autosomal dominant disorders, with an estimated prevalence of 1 in 3000

Harper's Textbook of Pediatric Dermatology, Fourth Edition. Edited by Peter Hoeger, Veronica Kinsler and Albert Yan.

Table 142.1 The neurofibromatoses

	NF1	NF2	Schwannomatosis
Incidence	1 in 3000	1 in 33 000	1 in 50 000
Cutaneous features	Café-au-lait macules, skinfold freckling, neurofibromas	Café-au-lait macules (< NF1), no freckling, schwannomas	Subcutaneous schwannomas
Inheritance	Autosomal dominant	Autosomal dominant	Autosomal dominant (15%)
Gene/chromosome	*NF1*/17q11.2	*NF2*/22q12.2	*SMARCB1*/22q11.23 LZTR1/22q11.21
Protein	Neurofibromin	Merlin	Chromatin remodelling complex

NF1, neurofibromatosis type 1; NF2, neurofibromatosis type 2.

(Table 142.1) [1]. The incidence has been reported to be between 1 in 2500 to 1 in 4000 [2]. NF1 affects all racial groups with no apparent predilection among any one particular group, although most epidemiological studies have involved mainly populations of European descent [3].

Genetics of NF1

NF1 is inherited as an autosomal dominant trait. Approximately half of affected individuals have a *de novo* mutation and therefore have no family history of NF1. Penetrance approaches 100% by the age of 20, but expression is extremely variable, even within families [4]. This point is important for genetic counselling, because an individual with mild clinical findings can have a child with a more severe phenotype, or vice versa.

NF1 gene and neurofibromin

The *NF1* gene was mapped to chromosome 17 by linkage analysis in 1987 and cloned in 1990 [5–9]. The gene is large, spanning 350 kb of genomic DNA, encoding an RNA of 11–13 kb and has 60 exons [10]. The *NF1* gene encodes a protein called neurofibromin, which contains 2818 amino acids and has an estimated molecular mass of 220 kDa [11]. Neurofibromin contains several functional domains. The most well characterized is the GRD domain (GAP-related domain). GAP proteins convert RAS from its active GTP-bound form to its inactive GDP-bound form, thus suppressing cell proliferation. The presence of this domain supports a tumour suppressor function for the NF1 gene. Other domains include CSRD (cysteine/serine rich domain), Sec14-PH module (Sec14 and pleckstrin homology domain) and CTD (C-terminal domain). These other less well-characterized domains suggest that in addition to the tumour suppressive function, neurofibromin acts as a large scaffold to interface with multiple proteins to coordinate signalling events central to normal neuronal development [12].

The cutaneous manifestations of NF1 have been shown to result from mutational events in accordance with Knudson's two-hit hypothesis of tumour formation, further evidence to support the tumour suppressor function of neurofibromin. Several studies have shown that cutaneous neurofibromas develop only after both copies of the *NF1* gene are lost [13–15]. Notably, it is only a subpopulation of Schwann cells that harbour the somatic (second-hit) mutation and not the other tumour cells (e.g. fibroblasts, mast cells), suggesting that the Schwann cell is the tumour cell of the neurofibroma [16]. It is hypothesized that the subpopulations of Schwann cells with two mutated *NF1* alleles secrete growth factors with subsequent recruitment and proliferation of other cells [17]. The somatic mutations in neurofibromas are distinct from the germline (first-hit) mutation and different for each neurofibroma [16]. CALMs have also been shown to result from loss of both *NF1* alleles in one study. DeSchepper and colleagues found second-hit *NF1* mutations in melanocytes cultured from CALMs; second-hit mutations were not present in fibroblasts, keratinocytes or melanocytes from uninvolved skin [18].

The large size of the gene and the lack of mutational hotspots have made mutation analysis challenging. Messiaen and colleagues developed a comprehensive multistep detection protocol that is able to identify mutations in greater than 95% of patients (both familial and sporadic) who fulfil NIH criteria [19]. Pathogenic mutations have been found in most of the 60 exons and comprise a wide diversity of mutation types, including complete gene deletions, chromosome rearrangements, smaller deletions or insertions, stop mutations, amino acid substitutions and splicing mutations. Indeed, most mutations result in absent or nonfunctional protein [20].

Clinical features.

Diagnostic criteria

The National Institutes of Health (NIH) Consensus Development Conference on Neurofibromatosis published clinical diagnostic criteria for NF1 in 1988, which were reaffirmed unchanged in 1997 (Box 142.1) [21,22]. A diagnosis of NF1 can be confidently made after thorough clinical and ophthalmological examination in an individual when at least two of the features (excluding CALMs and skinfold freckling only) listed in Box 142.1 are present.

These criteria have been shown to be both highly sensitive and specific for adults with NF1, but are less sensitive in children, particularly children under 8 years old, because of the fact that the number of clinical features increases with age. Forty-six percent of sporadic NF1 cases fail to meet NIH diagnostic criteria by 1 year of age, but 95% of these children meet criteria by 8 years of age, and all do so by 20 years old [23]. The usual order of appearance of these features is multiple café-au-lait spots,

Box 142.1 NIH diagnostic criteria for neurofibromatosis type 1 (two are required for diagnosis)

1. Six or more café-au-lait macules (>5 mm prepuberty, >15 mm postpuberty)
2. Two or more neurofibromas of any type, or one or more plexiform neurofibromas
3. Freckling in the axillae or groin
4. Optic pathway glioma
5. Two or more Lisch nodules
6. Dysplasia of the sphenoid; dysplasia or thinning of long bone cortex
7. First degree relative with NF1

Table 142.2 Typical age of onset and frequency of common clinical features in NF1 [23]

Clinical feature	Age of onset (years)	Frequency (%)
≥6 café-au-lait macules	Birth to 2	>99
Skinfold freckling	3–5	90
Lisch nodules	10	85
≥2 neurofibromas	16–20	>99

axillary or inguinal freckling, Lisch nodules and neurofibromas. Characteristic osseous lesions are generally apparent within the first year and symptomatic optic gliomas are often diagnosed by the age of 4. Table 142.2 summarizes the characteristic age of onset of the diagnostic criteria.

Dermatological features

Three of the seven diagnostic criteria involve the skin; thus dermatologists play an important and often early role in the recognition and diagnosis of NF1. The major cutaneous features, café-au-lait spots, skinfold freckling and neurofibromas, will be reviewed in detail. Other cutaneous signs that have been reported to occur at an increased frequency in patients with NF1 will be briefly reviewed.

CALMs

CALMs are discrete, uniformly pigmented brown patches of varying sizes (Fig. 142.1). One to three CALMs are common in the population at large, occurring in up to 36% of children, but greater than three CALMs are significantly less common, occurring in only 0.3% of the general population and often indicate an underlying disorder, most commonly NF1 [24]. Crowe & Schull established six CALMs larger than 1.5 cm as being useful in distinguishing those individuals with multiple CALMS and NF1 [25]. A prospective study evaluating the diagnostic outcome of multiple CALMs followed 41 children with at least six CALMs and 30 (73%) developed other signs of NF1 (24/41) or segmental NF1 (6/41) [26].

CALMs are the earliest manifestation of NF1 and are present in essentially 100% of children with NF1. Conservatively, 80% of children with NF1 will manifest with multiple CALMs by the age of 1 year old [27]. If a child has not developed at least six CALMs by the age of 4 years old, they are unlikely to do so [23]. CALMs continue to appear during childhood, but stop appearing or may disappear in adulthood. The spots vary in diameter from 0.5 to 50 cm or more, but are usually less than 10 cm. The pigmentation is usually several shades darker than the surrounding skin and in children with very pale complexions they are best seen under ultraviolet light. CALMs with a typical morphology (distinct smooth edges and homogeneous pigmentation) versus an atypical morphology (indistinct or irregular borders or nonhomogeneous pigmentation) have been shown to have predictive value in the diagnosis of patients with NF1 [28]. A retrospective study found that 47% of children presenting with more than six typical CALMs were eventually diagnosed with NF1 versus 5% of children presenting with atypical CALMs.

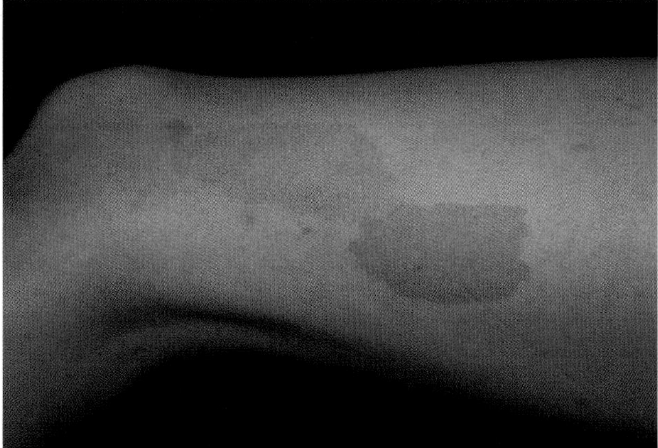

Fig. 142.1 Multiple cafe-au-lait macules in a child with NF1. Source: Boyd et al. 2009 [85]. Reproduced with permission of Elsevier.

Skinfold freckling

Skinfold freckling (Crowe's sign) presents as multiple (>3) 1–3 mm tan macules in the axillae and inguinal folds (Fig. 142.2). Skinfold freckling is uncommon in infants and typically becomes evident around the age of 3 years old, reaching a prevalence of 90% by the age of 7 years old [23]. In children with multiple CALMs and no family history of NF1, the appearance of skinfold freckling is typically the next diagnostic feature to appear. Skinfold freckling was once thought to be pathognomonic for NF1, but is now known to occur in Legius syndrome. In addition to the axillae and inguinal folds, freckling can occur around the neck, in the inframammary region, in other skin folds and occasionally is a generalized finding in adult patients.

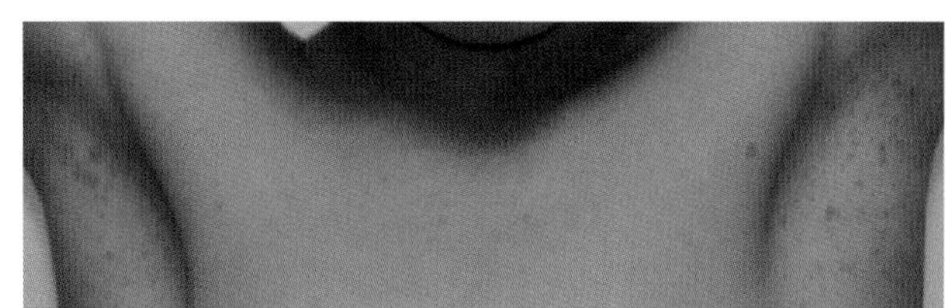

Fig. 142.2 Axillary freckling. Source: Boyd et al. 2009 [85]. Reproduced with permission of Elsevier.

Neurofibromas

Neurofibromas are benign tumours of the nerve sheath, which can occur at any point along any peripheral nerve, from the spinal roots to the cutaneous free nerve endings. Neurofibromas can be broadly classified as focal (localized to a single site on a nerve) or 'plexiform'. Dermatologists will most frequently encounter focal cutaneous and subcutaneous neurofibromas and superficial plexiform neurofibromas (PNFs).

Cutaneous neurofibromas are generally first noticed in adolescence and continue to increase in size and number throughout adulthood. Younger children may have neurofibromas that appear as subtle cutaneous swellings that are best seen with side lighting. Almost all adults with NF1 will develop cutaneous neurofibromas [27]. The number an individual will ultimately develop is unpredictable, even among family members, and can range from a few to thousands of lesions. Women with NF1 often report an increase in size and number of neurofibromas during pregnancy. Cutaneous neurofibromas appear as soft, dome-shaped, flesh-coloured to slightly hyperpigmented papules or nodules or as more subtle bluish lesions that barely project above the skin surface (Fig. 142.3). When pressed, the tumours tend to invaginate into the subcutaneous tissue, a sign called buttonholing [25]. Cutaneous neurofibromas do not have a risk of malignant degeneration, but have a negative impact on quality of life because of disfigurement from the visibility and sheer number of lesions [29]. Cutaneous neurofibromas can be pruritic and occasionally, especially if large and pedunculated, infarct, which can present with pain and swelling.

Subcutaneous neurofibromas are less prevalent than cutaneous neurofibromas and arise along peripheral nerves under the skin. These lesions present as well-defined, ovoid, firm subcutaneous nodules, best appreciated with palpation. Subcutaneous neurofibromas are often painful and can cause neurological symptoms, such as paraesthesia or weakness. While the risk of malignancy in these tumours is low, it is important to recognize individuals with multiple subcutaneous tumours because they are more likely to have internal spinal or PNFs, which are at a higher risk for peripheral neuropathy and malignant change [30,31]. The presence of multiple subcutaneous neurofibromas has also been reported to be associated with a higher mortality rate [32].

PNFs are neurofibromas that develop along the length of the nerve and involve multiple nerve fascicles and even multiple branches of nerves. The term 'plexiform' arises from the histopathological appearance and implies a network-like growth of neurofibroma involving multiple nerve fascicles. PNFs may be superficial and visible on examination, or deep and apparent only with imaging. Superficial PNFs are usually noticed early in life. A population study in Wales found that 27% of individuals with NF1 had a plexiform neurofibroma apparent on examination and up to 44% have a plexiform neurofibroma apparent with imaging [27,33]. When they are superficial, there is often associated overlying hyperpigmentation, hypertrichosis, and/or increased vascular markings (similar in appearance to a capillary malformation) (Fig. 142.4). The skin appears thickened and there are palpable cord-like masses, often likened to a 'bag of worms'. Overlying irregular hyperpigmentation is sometimes the earliest clue to an underlying plexiform neurofibroma and can appear before the skin thickens. PNFs can be associated with soft tissue overgrowth leading to massive hypertrophy and disfigurement. When PNFs involve the face they can cause facial asymmetry and there is often associated dysplasia of the greater wing of the sphenoid [34]. Unlike cutaneous neurofibromas, there is a risk of PNFs transforming into a malignant peripheral nerve sheath tumour (MPNST). The estimated lifetime risk of MPNST in individuals with NF1 is 8–13% [35]. Unrelenting pain, sudden growth or increased firmness in a previously stable plexiform neurofibroma are all signs suggestive of malignant transformation and should be evaluated. Positron emission tomography (PET) and PET computed tomography has been shown to be useful for evaluating malignant transformation in symptomatic PNFs [36].

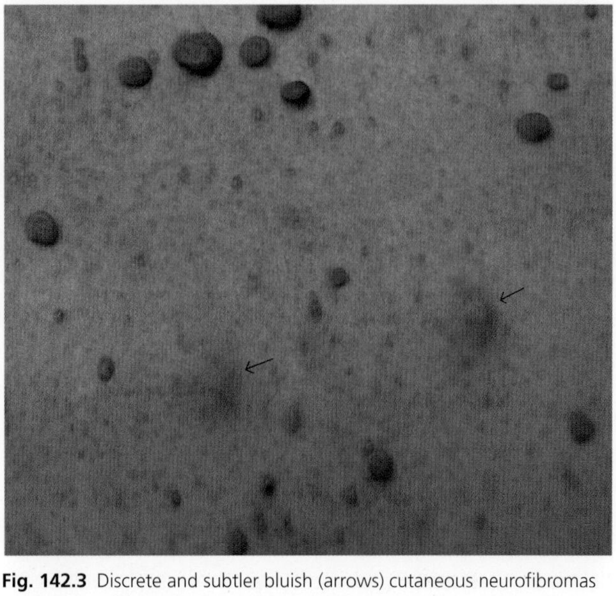

Fig. 142.3 Discrete and subtler bluish (arrows) cutaneous neurofibromas in a patient with NF1.

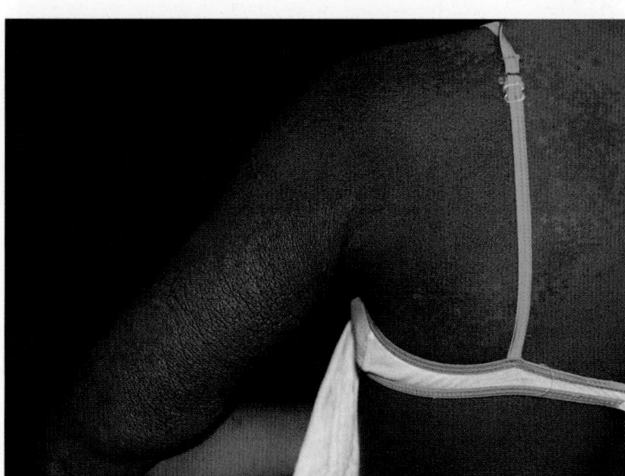

Fig. 142.4 Plexiform neurofibroma with characteristic overlying hyperpigmentation.

Other dermatological features

Juvenile xanthogranulomas (JXGs) occur at an increased frequency in the NF1 population with an estimated prevalence in children of 4–10% [37–39]. They are most frequent before the age of 2 with a tendency to regress over time. JXGs in patients with NF1 present as solitary or multiple (commonly) yellow-brown papules or nodules that have a predilection for the scalp, face and groin [40]. The association of JXGs, NF1 and the development of juvenile myelomonocytic leukaemia has been reported but the exact frequency is a source of debate [41–45]. Routine haematological screening in patients with NF1 and JXGs is currently not recommended, but clinicians should be aware of the possibility of juvenile myelomonocytic leukaemia and be vigilant for its presenting features (hepatosplenomegaly, lymphadenopathy, pallor, petechiae).

Naevus anaemicus (NA) has an estimated prevalence of 50% in patients with NF1 and, along with multiple CALMs, may be a useful clinical feature for the early diagnosis of NF1 [40]. NA appears as a pale patch with polylobulated borders caused by sustained vasoconstriction, which fails to develop reactive erythema with rubbing or heat (Fig. 142.5). The association of NA with NF1 was first reported in 1915, but only recently systematically evaluated. Two prospective studies identified NA in 50% of patients with definitive NF1 [39,46]. NA was most frequent in patients under18 years of age, multiple, present on the anterior chest and neck, and less than 10 cm in size. NA was not seen at high frequency in patients with segmental NF1 or other genodermatoses characterized by multiple CALMs. NA may be an early and specific finding in patients with NF1 and its presence should be purposefully evaluated in any patient with suspected NF1.

Generalized hyperpigmentation has been noted in individuals with NF1 compared with their unaffected siblings or parents [47]. Interestingly, the involved body regions of patients with segmental NF1 often have a background of hyperpigmentation. Although the cause of the generalized hyperpigmentation has not been studied, it is interesting to theorize that it is caused by a single mutation of the *NF1* gene, whereas CALMS are caused by loss of both alleles.

Glomus tumours are part of the tumour spectrum of NF1 [48–50]. NF1-associated glomus tumours are typically subungual and are more likely to be multifocal. These tumours exhibit biallelic inactivation of the *NF1* gene and loss of neurofibromin immunoreactivity [49,50]. Patients with subungual glomus tumours present with severe paroxysmal pain localized to one or more fingers and cold intolerance. It is important to recognize the increased risk of glomus tumours in NF1 patients because surgical removal of the tumour eliminates the pain.

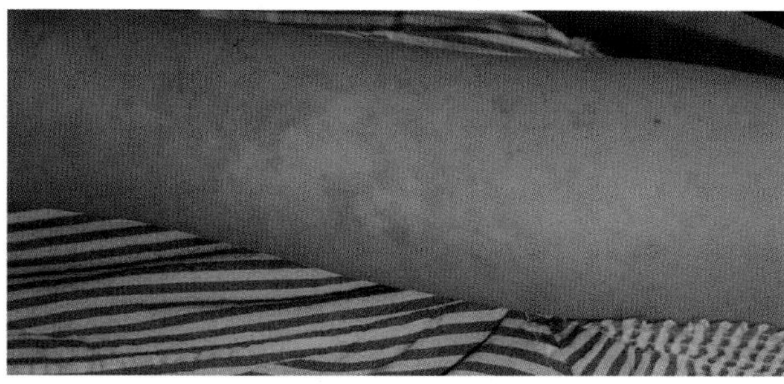

Fig. 142.5 Naevus anaemicus on the arm of a child with NF1.

Nondermatological features

NF1 can involve any organ system. Reported noncutaneous manifestations are summarized in Table 142.3. The noncutaneous features that comprise the diagnostic criteria, those that may be recognized during physical examination and learning disabilities are reviewed.

Orthopaedic

Orthopaedic manifestations are frequent and include mildly short stature, skeletal dysplasia, scoliosis and more recently recognized osteopenia/osteoporosis. Sphenoid wing or long bone dysplasias are the most distinctive bony lesions in NF1. Approximately 14% of patients with NF1 fulfil this diagnostic criterion, which is usually evident by the age of 1 year [23]. Long bone dysplasia should be suspected clinically when an infant or child presents with anterolateral bowing of the lower leg or, less commonly, the distal arm. These children are at an increased risk for fractures, which often fail to heal normally and can lead to pseudo-arthrosis. Contrary to the wording of the NIH criteria, thinning of the long bone cortex is uncommon and the characteristic radiographic finding is cortical thickening with medullary canal narrowing [51]. Sphenoid wing dysplasia presents as facial asymmetry with either enophthalmos or proptosis, depending on whether there is associated orbital plexiform neurofibroma. If physical examination does not suggest a bony abnormality, routine radiographs are not recommended. Scoliosis is also common, with an incidence of 10–25% [52]. Although the dermatologist's role is limited, periodic screening of children and adolescents is simple and if evidence of scoliosis is found, referral to orthopaedics is warranted.

Ophthalmological

Lisch nodules (iris hamartomas) are 1–2 mm smooth dome-shaped lesions on the iris [53]. They can occasionally be detected on general examination as yellow-brown lesions, but are best viewed and distinguished from iris naevi with slit-lamp examination. Lisch nodules are innocuous, but are useful for diagnostic confirmation of NF1. They generally appear later than CALMs and skinfold freckling and are found in approximately 40% of children under 6 years old, 85% of children under 18 years old and 93% of adults [54,55].

Optic pathway gliomas (OPGs) are classified as low-grade pilocytic astrocytomas of the optic nerve, optic chiasm, hypothalamus or optic tracts. OPGs are estimated to occur in 15% of children [56]; one-third to one-half of these cause clinical symptoms, such as decreased visual acuity, diminished visual fields, proptosis or precocious puberty [57]. OPGs are slow to progress and many never require intervention. Symptomatic OPGs usually manifest by the age of 6 years, but there are an increasing number of reports of late-onset or late-progressive OPGs [58]. The 1997 OPG Task Force determined there was not enough

Table 142.3 Noncutaneous manifestations and typical period of presentation

	Congenital/ infancy	Early childhood	Late childhood	Adolescence	Adult
Skeletal					
Scoliosis			X (severe)	X	
Dysplasia of the long bone/sphenoid	X				
Macrocephaly	X				
Prominent brow		X			
Short stature		X			
Pectus excavatum	X				
Pseudoarthrosis (esp. of tibia)	X	X			
Neurological/psychological					
Headaches			X	X	
Learning disabilities/attention deficit hyperactivity disorder (ADHD		X	X		
Astrocytoma		X			X
Seizures		X			
Ophthalmological					
Lisch nodules			X		
Optic glioma		X			
Cardiovascular					
Hypertension			X		X
Vascular dysplasia				X	
Endocrine					
Precocious puberty		X	X		
Carcinoid tumour					X
Pheochromocytoma			X		X
Gastrointestinal					
Gastrointestinal stromal tumors (GIST)					X
Associated malignancies					
Juvenile myelomonocytic leukaemia (JMML)		X			
Malignant peripheral nerve sheath tumour (MPNST)					X
Rhabdomyosarcoma		X			

evidence to recommend routine neuroimaging in asymptomatic children. Instead, children with known or suspected NF1 should have yearly ophthalmological assessments until at least 7 years of age and then at less frequent intervals from 8 to 25 years [59].

Learning disabilities

Learning disabilities are the most common complication in children with NF1. The reported frequency of learning disability ranges between 30 and 69% [60]. Several studies have shown a consistent shift to the left of IQ, but it is within 1 SD of the population mean; mental retardation (IQ <70) is uncommon [61–64]. Learning problems in children with NF1 can be global learning deficits (with associated lowered IQ) or specific learning deficits, with a normal IQ, but lower than expected academic achievement. Children with NF1 have particular difficulties with visuospatial orientation, receptive and expressive language skills, and gross and fine motor coordination [65] The learning problems are compounded by an increased prevalence of attention deficit hyperactivity disorder (ADHD); 46 of 93 patients in one series satisfied the criteria for ADHD [66].

Differential diagnosis. The diagnosis of NF1 is generally straightforward when one follows the NIH diagnostic criteria. As discussed above, the clinical features of NF1 are age-dependent and a definitive diagnosis may not always be possible in a young child without a family history of NF1. A child with six or more CALMs should be followed as if they have NF1, because other disease features usually become apparent by the age of 8 years. This statement is supported by two recent studies evaluating the predictive value of multiple CALMs as the initial presentation of NF1 in young children [28,67]. Nunley and colleagues found that 34 of 59 (58%) children presenting with six or more CALMs eventually met diagnostic criteria for NF1 [28]. Yao and colleagues diagnosed NF1 in 13 of 19 (68%) Chinese children with six or more CALMs using diagnostic criteria and molecular testing [67]. The most common conditions misdiagnosed as NF1 are other forms of neurofibromatosis, particularly NF2, which is reviewed later in this chapter.

An important entity to distinguish from NF1 is Legius syndrome, initially named NF1-like syndrome [68]. Individuals with Legius syndrome present with multiple CALMs with or without skinfold freckling, indistinguishable from

NF1. However, other NF1-associated features including Lisch nodules, neurofibromas, OPGs, bone lesions and MPNST are notably absent [69]. This syndrome is autosomal dominant and the responsible gene is *SPRED1*, which maps to chromosome 15 and encodes a protein that downregulates the RAS-mitogen activated protein kinase pathway. Learning disabilities, ADHD, macrocephaly and Noonan-like features are commonly reported in children with Legius syndrome. Molecular genetic testing is necessary for confirmation of this diagnosis. It is estimated that 1–4% of persons with multiple CALMs and a presumptive diagnosis of NF1 have Legius syndrome [70].

Multiple (more than five) CALMs are extremely rare in conditions other than NF1. Syndromes associated with multiple CALMs include multiple familial CALMs, Jaffe–Campanacci syndrome, constitutional mismatch repair deficiency syndrome and ring chromosome syndromes [24,71,72]. Other conditions associated with abnormal skin pigmentation and confused with NF1 include McCune–Albright syndrome, Noonan syndrome with multiple lentigines (formerly known as LEOPARD syndrome), Bannayan–Riley–Ruvalcaba syndrome and urticaria pigmentosa [71]. These syndromes generally have other distinguishing features that permit differentiation from NF1 (Table 142.4). Syndromes with multiple cutaneous or subcutaneous tumours without pigmentary features that can be misdiagnosed as NF1 include multiple lipomatosis syndromes, PTEN-hamartoma tumour syndrome, multiple endocrine neoplasia type 2b and Proteus syndrome.

Laboratory and histology findings.

Molecular Genetic Testing

Molecular testing for NF1 is available and is a useful adjunct when the diagnosis is in doubt. A comprehensive screening approach described by Messiaen and colleagues identified the *NF1* gene mutations in 95% of individuals fulfilling NIH diagnostic criteria [19]. Molecular testing is not indicated for the routine care of patients with NF1, because it will likely not alter management, but can be helpful in individuals suspected of having NF1 (e.g. a young child with more than five CALMs and unaffected parents, a child or families with CALMs and freckling only [to distinguish from Legius syndrome], segmental forms) or when prenatal or preimplantation genetic diagnosis is desired. It is important to counsel the patient that although useful for diagnostic confirmation, a positive test will generally not predict severity or outcome. Genetic testing is also available for Legius syndrome, as well as many of the other syndromes that can be confused with NF1. Recently, targeted next-generation sequencing (NGS) has been shown to be a more cost effective, rapid method for simultaneously identifying *NF1* and *SPRED1* mutations [73]. This method identified 100% of mutations in 30 patients with a molecular diagnosis of NF1. Subsequently, targeted NGS was performed in 279 patients with a clinical diagnosis of NF1 and an *NF1* or *SPRED1* alteration was found in 88% and 4% of patients, respectively.

Genotype–phenotype correlations have been difficult to establish because of the complexity of both the phenotype and the gene, but there are three of interest to dermatologists. Individuals with total loss of the *NF1* gene, along with flanking genes, have a more severe phenotype. This 1.5 Mb microdeletion occurs in 5% of patients with NF1 [74]. These patients have a greater neurofibroma burden with earlier onset of neurofibromas, more severe cognitive impairment, large hands and feet, dysmorphic facial features and a higher lifetime risk of developing MPNSTs [75–78]. A more recently identified 3 bp inframe deletion in exon 17 of the *NF1* gene has been reported to

Table 142.4 Key features and genetic defect of disorders associated with hyperpigmented macules or patches

Disorder	Key distinguishing features	Genetics
Neurofibromatosis 1	≥6 CALMs, skinfold freckling, Lisch nodules, neurofibromas	Autosomal dominant; *NF1*
Neurofibromatosis 2	Few CALMs, schwannomas, CNS tumours, cataracts	Autosomal dominant; *NF2*
Legius syndrome	Multiple CALMs, skinfold freckling, learning disability, no neurofibromas	Autosomal dominant; *SPRED1*
Multiple familial CALMs	Multiple CALMs only	Autosomal dominant; unknown
Jaffe–Campanacci syndrome	Multiple CALMs (typically ≥6), multiple nonossifying fibromas of long bones, mandibular giant cell lesions, no neurofibromas	Unknown; need to exclude *NF1* mutation
Constitutional mismatch repair deficiency syndrome	Multiple CALMs, freckling, haematological, GI, CNS malignancies, FHx HNPCC	Autosomal recessive; *MLH1, MSH2, MSH6, PMS2*
Ring chromosome syndrome	CALMs, hypopigmented macules, microcephaly, delay, facial dysmorphism	Sporadic; multiple chromosomes
McCune–Albright syndrome	Polyostotic fibrous dysplasia, increased endocrine activity; large CALMs with jagged edges classically respecting the midline	Mosaic; *GNAS*
Noonan syndrome with multiple lentigines (LEOPARD)	Café 'noir' (darker colour) spots, lentigines, ocular hypertelorism, genital abnormalities, deafness	Autosomal dominant; *PTPN11* (90%); *RAF1* (< 5%); *BRAF, MAP2K1*
Bannayan–Riley–Ruvalcaba syndrome	Hyperpigmented macules on penis, multiple lipomas, intestinal polyposis, haemangiomas	Autosomal dominant; *PTEN*
Urticaria pigmentosa	Darier's sign (urtication following stroking of lesion), larger number of hyperpigmented lesions, eventual resolution	Activating mutation in *c-kit*

CALMs, café-au-lait macules; CNS, central nervous system; GI, gastrointestinal; HNPCC, hereditary nonpolyposis colorectal cancer.

result in a milder phenotype. Individuals with this mutation have typical pigmentary features of NF1, but few, if any, cutaneous neurofibromas, no obvious external PNFs and appear to have a lower incidence of serious complications [79]. Lastly, patients carrying *NF1* missense mutations affecting p.Arg1809 also demonstrate a decreased frequency of NF1-associated benign and malignant tumours, including cutaneous and PNFs. However, these patients have a higher incidence of Noonan syndrome features, including Noonan-like facial features, short stature, pulmonic stenosis and learning disabilities [80]. It is likely that additional genotype–phenotype correlations will emerge as more carefully phenotyped patients are studied.

Histology findings

Only the histological features of CALMs, neurofibromas and PNFs will be reviewed. For other tumours that occur, the underlying pathology is usually the same as when they occur in isolation [81].

CALMs

Microscopically, CALMs present as focal hyperpigmentation in the basal layer of an otherwise normal epidermis; axillary freckles show a similar appearance. There is an increase in dopa-positive melanocytes, which show an increased number of melanin macroglobules [82]. Melanocytes with melanin macroglobules are also found, though in much lower numbers, throughout the skin of NF1 patients. Macroglobules are not specific to NF1 and are an occasional finding in normal individuals and other disorders including McCune–Albright syndrome, LEOPARD syndrome and xeroderma pigmentosum [83].

Neurofibromas

Histologically, they are indistinguishable from neurofibromas occurring as isolated lesions in the general population. Dermal neurofibromas are well circumscribed but not encapsulated, and although they arise from the terminal branches of cutaneous nerves, the nerve of origin is not usually obvious. Conversely, subcutaneous neurofibromas develop on major peripheral nerves, are more sharply demarcated and have an apparent capsule of perineural cells. The fibres of the nerve of origin pass through subcutaneous neurofibromas and are not stretched over their surface as is seen in schwannomas [84].

Microscopically, both dermal and subcutaneous neurofibromas are spindle cell tumours originating from peripheral nerve sheaths [85,86]. They are composed of five cell types including Schwann cells, neurons, fibroblasts, perineurial and mast cells. Common features include the formation of collagen fibres and myxoid degeneration. Mitotic activity is low. The tumour is not locally invasive. Cutaneous neurofibromas are not thought to have the potential for sarcomatous degeneration.

PNFs

PNFs are classically thought to always occur in association with NF1 but they can occasionally be seen as isolated lesions in otherwise healthy individuals and presumably they then represent somatic mosaicism. PNFs can be discrete nodular tumours developing on a nerve root or diffuse tumours associated with hypertrophy of surrounding connective tissue and other structures [86]. The tumour cells are embedded in an abundant extracellular myxoid matrix, which often contains mast cells. PNFs are locally invasive, growing within and along the nerve, enlarging nerve fascicles and elongating each fascicle. In the early stages of the lesion, hypercellular fascicles are found. As the lesion develops, there is an increase in the number of Schwann cells and/or perineurial cells. A few residual axons that have not been destroyed by the tumour can be found. As the lesion grows, the fascicle can become either hypocellular and myxomatous or even more cellular; the two pathologies can be found side by side in a single lesion. PNFs have the potential for malignant degeneration into sarcomas [85,86].

Management of NF1. The mainstay of care in NF1 is anticipatory guidance, surveillance for complications and genetic counselling. Annual evaluations (or more often, if indicated) should be performed in all patients with NF1 or suspected NF1. Specialized neurofibromatosis clinics offer coordinated care and follow up by a multidisciplinary group of physicians. The dermatologist's role is primarily diagnosing and differentiating NF1 from other conditions based on thorough skin examination, recognizing potential complications that may present to the dermatologist and managing cutaneous manifestations, primarily neurofibromas. History should focus on symptoms associated with NF1, including assessment of developmental milestones, growth problems, pain, visual complaints, headaches, seizures, weakness, learning disabilities and family history. Skin evaluation should include documentation of number and morphology of CALMs, skin fold freckling, cutaneous neurofibromas and PNFs. Evaluation should also look for the presence of facial asymmetry, ptosis or proptosis, bony abnormalities (anterolateral bowing of the leg or arm, scoliosis), presence of NA, JXGs or subcutaneous neurofibromas, and signs of precocious puberty. Routine evaluations should include yearly ophthalmological evaluations in children under the age of 8 years, developmental assessment and, if indicated, neuropsychiatric testing in children approaching school age, and documentation of growth parameters (height, weight, head circumference) and blood pressure. Routine screening with cranial computed tomography or magnetic resonance imaging in asymptomatic individuals is not recommended [87]. A consensus statement published by clinicians of the United Kingdom Neurofibromatosis Association in 2007 details the present strategies for diagnosing, monitoring and managing complications of NF1 and would serve as an excellent reference for any clinician evaluating a patient with suspected NF1 [88].

Genetic counselling is important and individuals with NF1 need to be aware that there is a 50% chance of having a child with NF1 with each conception. As discussed above, NF1 is a highly variable disorder and the risk of serious complications in offspring with NF1 is unpredictable.

Parents of a child with NF1 who have a normal skin and eye examination have a very low risk of having another child with NF1, barring the rare possibility of gonadal mosaicism in one of the parents. The estimate of recurrence in a subsequent sibling arising from gonadal mosaicism is usually estimated at 1–2%.

There is no medical treatment currently available to prevent or reverse the complications of NF1. Cutaneous neurofibromas can be removed surgically or, if small, by laser ablation or electrocautery. PNFs can be debulked, but complete removal is usually not possible and regrowth is common. Clinical trials are underway exploring the efficacy of new treatments that target pathogenetic pathways in NF1. Malignant tumours are usually treated with a combination of surgery, radiation and chemotherapy.

Segmental or mosaic neurofibromatosis type 1

Segmental NF1 is the term used to describe patients with the typical features of NF1 (usually cutaneous) localized to one or more body region(s). Segmental NF1 was initially referred to as neurofibromatosis type 5 by the Riccardi classification scheme; however, we now know that segmental NF1 is not a distinct variant of neurofibromatosis and this term should be abandoned. In 2001 Ruggieri and Huson proposed the term mosaic NF1 and subdivided this into three types: (1) mosaic generalized NF1 – to describe patients with generalized disease (shown to often have a mild NF1 phenotype) but who are found to be somatic mosaics on mutation analysis; (2) mosaic localized/segmental NF1 – to describe patients with disease features limited to one or a few body segments; (3) pure gonadal mosaicism – to describe patients with no clinical or molecular findings of NF1 in somatic tissue who have more than one affected child with generalized NF1 [89].

Epidemiology and pathogenesis.

Epidemiology

The reported prevalence is 1 in 36 000, but this is probably an underestimation because many mild cases never come to medical attention or go undiagnosed [89].

Pathogenesis

Somatic mosaicism of the *NF1* gene as the likely cause of segmental NF1 was suggested in 1952 and confirmed at the molecular level in 2000 [90]. Tinschert and colleagues demonstrated a microdeletion of the *NF1* gene in a percentage of cultured fibroblasts from a CALM in a patient with segmental NF1 [90]. This mutation was not present in fibroblasts from uninvolved skin or peripheral blood leukocytes. More recently, Maertens and colleagues were able to detect mutations in both *NF1* alleles (representing first hit and second hit mutations) from cultured Schwann cells and melanocytes from neurofibromas and CALMS, respectively, in two patients with mosaic NF1 [91]. Again, *NF1* mutations were not identified in normal skin or blood. The phenotypic features of segmental NF1 depend on the timing of the postconceptional *NF1* mutation and the embryonic cell line(s) involved. Mutations early on in embryogenesis lead to generalized disease, whereas mutations occurring later give rise to disease in a more localized distribution. Generalized disease from somatic mosaicism can be difficult to differentiate from nonmosaic NF1, but a clue on cutaneous examination is the presence of sharply demarcated areas of normal skin (Fig. 142.6) [92].

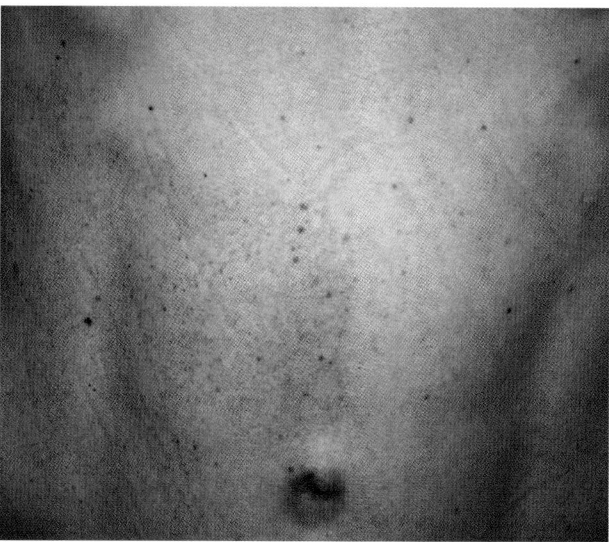

Fig. 142.6 Hyperpigmentation and freckling well demarcated from the normal skin in a patient with generalized mosaic NF1.

Clinical features. Cutaneous manifestations are the prominent and often only feature in patients with segmental NF1. CALMs with or without skinfold freckling, neurofibromas (cutaneous, subcutaneous or plexiform) or a combination of both are possible. The extent of involvement can range from a narrow strip to one quadrant or half of the body, but can also include more than one segment on both sides of the midline, either in a symmetrical or asymmetrical arrangement [89]. Interestingly, in patients with pigmentary features there is often background hyperpigmentation of the entire affected segment, suggesting that the *NF1* gene has an effect on global skin pigmentation [91]. Similar to nonmosaic NF1, CALMs, freckling and PNFs appear in childhood and neurofibromas in adolescence and adulthood. Not all patients with pigmentary changes develop neurofibromas. Patients with solitary PNFs presumably also have a form of segmental NF1. The clinical features and natural history of such lesions appear to be the same as when they occur as a complication of the generalized disease.

Noncutaneous findings and associated complications in segmental NF1 are rare, with a prevalence of around 5% [89]. Sporadic case reports of visceral neurofibromas, skeletal abnormalities (sphenoid wing dysplasia, tibial pseudoarthrosis), unilateral Lisch nodules, optic pathway gliomas and malignant peripheral nerve sheath tumours occurring in segmental NF1 exist [93–95].

The majority of reported cases of segmental NF1 have no family history of NF1. There are, however, several instances of individuals with segmental NF1 having children with generalized nonmosaic NF1, presumably from gonadal mosaicism [96,97]. Consoli and colleagues confirmed the occurrence of gonosomal mosaicism in segmental NF1 [98]. A recent review of the literature and an earlier large case series found that 2.5% and 6.4%, respectively, of patients with segmental NF1 had offspring with NF1 and all but one case occurred in the group with only pigmentary changes [99,89]. The exact risk of transmission is not known, but data extrapolated from animal work suggests the risk is proportional to the percentage of body area involved [89]. It is important to note that risk does not correlate with involvement of skin overlying the genitalia [99].

Differential diagnosis. The differential diagnosis of localized segmental NF1 includes segmental pigmentation disorder, McCune–Albright syndrome (see Table 142.4), speckled lentiginous naevus and agminated or partial unilateral lentiginosis. Segmental pigmentation disorder presents as block-like hyperpigmented patches that closely resemble CALMS but lack multiple smaller CALMs, freckling and neurofibromas within the hyperpigmentation [100]. Speckled lentiginous naevus contains multiple melanocytic naevi within a background patch of CALM-like pigmentation. Patrial unilateral lentiginosis consists of clustered unilateral lentigines on normal skin and has been found, in some patients, to coexist with CALMs, skinfold freckling, Lisch nodules and/or neurofibromas in the same segmental distribution [101]. Partial unilateral lentiginosis may represent a forme fruste of segmental NF1. Mosaic Legius syndrome should also be considered in the differential diagnosis of segmental NF1. This can present identical to segmental NF1 with multiple CALMs within a large hyperpigmented patch and identification of a mutation in *SPRED1* is necessary to confirm diagnosis [102].

Treatment and prevention. There are no specific management recommendations for segmental NF1. Patients should be advised they do not have generalized NF1; the risk of specific complications depends on the extent of mosaicism, clinical lesion(s) present and body areas affected, but is significantly lower than in patients with NF1. Those considering children need to be aware of the potential risk of transmission of NF1 to offspring. As mentioned above, it is possible to detect low-level *NF1* mutations in cells cultured from biopsies of specific cutaneous lesions (Schwann cells for neurofibromas and/or melanocytes for pigmentary lesions) in patients with segmental NF1. Identification of the *NF1* mutation can provide a useful molecular marker in the prenatal and presymptomatic diagnostic setting [92].

Neurofibromatosis type 2

Neurofibromatosis type 2 (NF2) is a genetic disorder clinically and molecularly distinct from NF1. The clinical overlap arises because CALMs and peripheral nerve tumours occur in both conditions. In NF2, CALMs are not as numerous and the nerve tumours are almost always schwannomas, not neurofibromas. Additionally, skinfold freckling is not a feature of NF2. NF2 is generally an adult-onset disease; CALMs, cutaneous tumours and ocular abnormalities (cataracts, strabismus, ambylopia) are the most common findings to occur in childhood [103].

Epidemiology and pathogenesis. NF2 is much less common than NF1, with an estimated incidence of 1:33 000 and a disease prevalence of 1 in 60 000 [104]. NF2 is caused by mutations in the *NF2* gene. It is inherited as an autosomal dominant trait. Approximately half of all patients will have a family history of NF2; the other half represent *de novo* mutations. Furthermore, mutation studies have indicated that more than one-third of these *de novo* cases of NF2 are mosaic, with the mutation detected only in tumour material [105].

The *NF2* gene was provisionally localized to chromosome 22 through studies showing loss of heterozygosity in vestibular schwannomas in 1986 [106]. This was confirmed by linkage studies the following year [107]. The identification of germline deletions in NF2 patients in the critical area of chromosome 22q11.2 facilitated the cloning of the disease gene in 1993 [108,109]. The *NF2* gene is a tumour suppressor gene that encodes for a protein named Merlin (moezin/ezrin/radixin-like protein), although others prefer the name schwannomin [106,109].

Merlin is expressed at high levels in large numbers of tissues during embryonic development. In adult tissue, significant expression is detected in Schwann cells, meningeal cells, the lens and nerves compatible with the development of the major disease features in these tissues. Within the cell, Merlin appears to localize in cell membranes at sites involved in cell–cell contact and motility. The protein interactions and exact mechanism that underlie Merlin's role as a tumour suppressor are gradually being elucidated [110–112].

Clinical features.

NIH diagnostic criteria

The initial NIH diagnostic criteria for NF2 proved too narrow for routine clinical use and modifications have been suggested to enable earlier diagnosis in patients without bilateral vestibular schwannomas or a family history of NF2 [113–116]. According to the modified criteria, NF2 can be diagnosed in individuals with any *one* of the following sets of manifestations:

- Bilateral vestibular schwannomas
- A first-degree relative with NF2 *and* unilateral vestibular schwannoma *or* any two of the following: meningioma, schwannoma, glioma, neurofibroma, posterior subcapsular lenticular opacities
- Unilateral vestibular schwannomas *and* any two of the following: meningioma, schwannomas, glioma, neurofibroma, posterior subcapsular lenticular opacities
- Multiple meningiomas *and* unilateral vestibular schwannomas *or* any two of the following: schwannoma, glioma, neurofibroma, posterior subcapsular lenticular opacities.

Dermatological features

A small but significant number of NF2 patients seek a dermatological consultation prior to the onset of symptoms from their neurological tumours. Those with more florid skin involvement are occasionally misdiagnosed as having NF1 prior to the development of the more characteristic NF2 tumours. Skin tumours and CALMs may be the presenting symptoms in some children and earlier diagnosis has been shown to improve survival [103,117]. The main cutaneous features, CALMs and peripheral nerve tumours will be reviewed.

CALMs

CALMs are more frequent in patients with NF2 compared with the general population. Forty-three percent of patients in the study of Evans and colleagues had between one and six spots, 39% had three or fewer spots, 3% had four spots and only 1% had six spots [115]. It is therefore only very occasional NF2 cases that have sufficient CALMs to satisfy the NF1 diagnostic criterion. Patients with NF2 do not develop skinfold freckling.

Peripheral nerve tumours

These occur less consistently and in much smaller numbers than in NF1. In the study of Evans and colleagues, 68% of patients had peripheral nerve tumours, which varied in number from one to 27 [115]. Clinically, there are three types of peripheral nerve tumours in NF2–NF2 plaques, peripheral nerve schwannomas, and NF1-like cutaneous lesions–although histologically they are all usually schwannomas.

NF2 plaques are the most frequent cutaneous lesions in NF2 and occurred in 48% of patients in the study by Evans and colleagues [115]. They are discrete, well circumscribed, slightly raised cutaneous lesions, usually less than 2 cm in diameter. Their surface is rough, may be slightly pigmented and often contains excess hair (Fig. 142.7). The age at which these lesions develop has not been formally studied, but they probably develop in early childhood.

Peripheral nerve schwannomas cannot be distinguished clinically from the subcutaneous neurofibromas seen in NF1. They present as firm, deep, spherical nodules that develop on the larger peripheral nerves. The nerve is often thickened at either end of the tumour and a number of nodular tumours may develop in one particular part of the same nerve. In the study of Evans and colleagues, 43% of patients had these lesions [115]. Histological examination is necessary to differentiate this tumour from a neurofibroma.

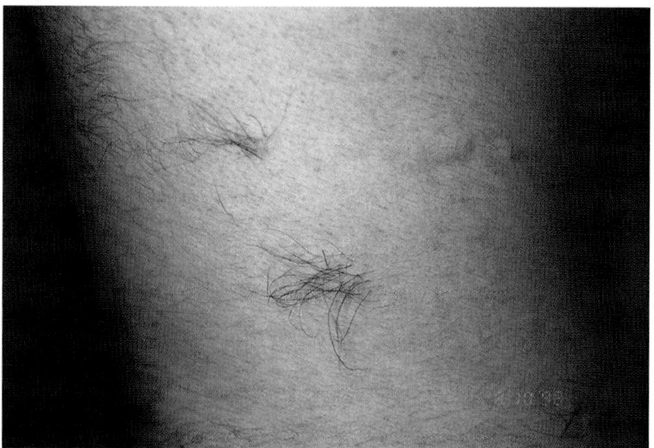

Fig. 142.7 NF2 plaque with prominent hypertrichosis.

NF1-like cutaneous lesions are the least common type of peripheral nerve tumour and appear similar to the dermal neurofibromas seen in NF1. They occurred in 27% of patients in the study by Evans and colleagues, but were much fewer in number than would normally be seen in an adult with NF1 [115].

Non-dermatological features

The phenotype of NF2 is much more restricted than NF1 with the symptomatic disease features being limited to the nervous system (including the eye). The key feature of NF2 is bilateral vestibular schwannomas. This term is preferred to the older name of acoustic neuromas because the lesions are histologically schwannomas and arise on the vestibular branch of the eighth cranial nerve. Bilateral vestibular schwannomas develop in 85–92% of individuals with NF2 [115,118]. The most common initial symptoms are unilateral hearing loss, with or without associated vertigo and/or tinnitus. The tumours usually become symptomatic in early adult life (average age 22.6 years, range 2–52 years) [115]. Patients with a unilateral vestibular schwannoma at presentation are much more likely to have mosaic disease [119]. Other neurological tumours that may develop are meningiomas, gliomas, spinal root schwannomas, astrocytomas and ependymomas.

Posterior subcapsular or cortical cataracts are the most common ophthalmological manifestation in NF2 and are often apparent in childhood. These lesions are usually asymptomatic but are useful for diagnostic confirmation of NF2. Cataracts were present in 81% of the patients in the series of Parry and colleagues: 72.4% had posterior subcapsular cataracts, 41.4% had cortical cataracts and 32.8% had both types [118]. The lesions only caused significant visual disturbances in 2 out of 47 individuals. Other ocular lesions seen at a much lower frequency are retinal hamartomas, epiretinal membranes, optic disc gliomas and optic nerve sheath meningiomas.

Differential diagnosis. NF2 should be distinguished from the other neurofibromatoses, NF1 and schwannomatosis. As discussed above, NF2 can be mistaken for NF1 because of the presence of CALMs and schwannomas, which can be mistaken for neurofibromas. Schwannomatosis is characterized by the formation of multiple, often painful, central and peripheral schwannomas and lack of vestibular and ocular involvement. Recently, schwannomatosis has been linked to mutations in *SMARCB1* and LZTR1, both tumour suppressor genes [120–122].

Genetic testing. The diagnosis of NF2 is based on clinical criteria, but molecular genetic testing can be a useful test for early diagnostic confirmation, screening at-risk family members and predicting disease severity. Early diagnosis of NF2 through genetic testing facilitates appropriate screening with MRI and brainstem auditory evoked response and improves outcome. Therefore, presymptomatic genetic testing is an integral part of the management of NF2 families [123]. Genotype–phenotype correlations have been well established for NF2. Nonsense or frameshift mutations resulting in a truncated protein cause more severe disease, with more tumours developing at a younger age and increased mortality [124]. Missense mutations and large deletions are associated with milder disease [125].

The mutation detection rate is 93% in nonfounder familial cases and 70% in sporadic cases [126]. Lower rates have been found in other studies probably because of the inclusion of more mildly affected patients. Approximately 25–30% of sporadic cases are caused by somatic mosaicism and a mutation will not be identified in blood lymphocytes [127,128]. Molecular genetic testing of tumour tissue in these individuals can be useful.

Pathology. Of the tumours that can occur in NF2, only the schwannoma is likely to present to the dermatologist for diagnosis and hence is the only one discussed here. Schwannomas are histologically distinct from neurofibromas, although terminology can be confusing as schwannomas are sometimes referred to as neurinomas, neurilemmomas or neuromas. In addition, occasional tumours from patients with both NF1 and NF2 can have mixed histology with schwannomatous and neurofibromatous components [86].

Macroscopically, the surface of schwannomas is usually firm and the tissue has a white or yellowish colour. The nerve of origin can often be identified in the capsule of the tumour [86,129]. Microscopically, fusiform cells predominate within a fibrous capsule. Many schwannomas show a biphasic histopathological growth pattern. One architecture, designated Antoni type A, consists of interwoven fascicles of elongated cells with conspicuous spindle-shaped nuclei that often exhibit palisading and contribute to the formation of Verocay bodies. Occasionally, the spindle cells form whirls resembling those found in meningiomas or isolated wavy fascicles similar to those occurring in neurofibromas [130]. The other architecture, Antoni type B, consists of a reticular, microcystic appearance, lower cellularity and regressive changes, including fatty degeneration and accumulation of macrophages. Immunohistochemical reactivity can be useful in distinguishing schwannomas from other spindle cell neoplasms [86]. The calcium-binding protein S100 is strongly expressed in both normal and neoplastic Schwann cells.

Treatment and prevention. The diagnosis of NF2 should be considered in patients with cutaneous schwannomas and CALMs or in patients with a family history of NF2. The management of patients with NF2 is outside the scope of dermatologists. Any patient with suspected or definitive NF2 should be referred to a physician with expertise in NF2 for further evaluation, management and genetic counselling.

Acknowledgement

The authors acknowledge that material has been used from the chapter in the second edition entitled The Neurofibromatoses, written by Susan M. Huson and Martino Ruggieri.

References

1 Lammert M, Friedman JM, Kluwe L et al. Prevalence of neurofibromatosis 1 in German children at elementary school enrollment. Arch Dermatol 2005;141:71–4.
2 Poyhonen M, Kytola S, Leisti J. Epidemiology of neurofibromatosis type 1 (NF1) in northern Finland. J Med Genet 2000;37:632–6.
3 Friedman JM. Epidemiology of neurofibromatosis type 1. Am J Med Genet 1999;89:1–6.
4 Easton DF, Ponder MA, Huson SM et al. An analysis of variation in expression of neurofibromatosis (NF) type 1 (NF1): evidence for modifying genes. Am J Hum Genet 1993;53:305–13.
5 Barker D, Wright E, Nguyen K et al. Gene for von Recklinghausen neurofibromatosis is in the pericentromeric region of chromosome 17. Science 1987;236:1100–2.
6 Seizinger BR, Rouleau GA, Ozelius LJ et al. Genetic linkage of von Recklinghausen neurofibromatosis to the nerve growth factor receptor gene. Cell 1987;49:589–94.
7 Cawthon RM, Weiss R, Xu GF et al. A major segment of the neurofibromatosis type 1 gene: cDNA sequence, genomic structure, and point mutations. Cell 1990;62:193–201.
8 Viskochil D, Bucherg AM, Xu G et al. Deletions and a translocation interrupt a cloned gene at the neurofibromatosis type 1 locus. Cell 1990;62:18–192
9 Wallace MR, Marchuk DA, Andersen LB et al. Type 1 neurofibromatosis gene: identification of a large transcript disrupted in three NF1 patients. Science 1990;249:181–6.
10 Viskochil D. Genetics of neurofibromatosis 1 and the NF1 gene. J Child Neurol 2002;17:562–70.
11 Marchuk DA, Saulino AM, Tavakkoi R et al. cDNA cloning of the type 1 neurofibromatosis gene: complete sequence of the NF1 gene product. Genomics 1991;11:931–40.
12 Rad E, Tee AR. Neurofibromatosis type 1: fundamental insights into cell signalling and cancer. Semin Cell Dev Biol 2016;52:39–46.
13 Serra E, Puig S, Otero D et al. Confirmation of a double-hit model for the NF1 gene in benign neurofibromas. Am J Hum Genet 1997;61:512–9.
14 Kluwe L, Friedrich R, Mautner VF. Loss of NF1 allele in Schwann cells but not in fibroblasts derived from an NF1-associated neurofibroma. Genes Chromosomes Cancer 1999;24:283–5.
15 Serra E, Rosenbaum T, Winner U et al. Schwann cells harbor the somatic NF1 mutation in neurofibromas: evidence of two different Schwann cell populations. Hum Mol Genet 2000;9:3055–64.
16 Maertens O, Brems H, Vandesompele J et al. Comprehensive NF1 screening on cultured Schwann cells from neurofibromas. Hum Mutat 2006;27:1030–40.
17 Yang FC, Ingram DA, Chen S et al. Nf1-dependent tumors require a microenvironment containing Nf1+/- and c-kit dependent bone marrow. Cell 2008;135:437–48.
18 De Schepper S, Maertens O, Callens T et al. Somatic mutation analysis in NF1 café au lait spots reveals two NF1 hits in melanocytes. J Invest Dermatol 2008;128:1050–3.
19 Messiaen LM, Callens T, Mortier G et al. Exhaustive mutation analysis of the NF1 gene allows identification of 95% of mutations and reveals a high frequency of unusual splicing defects. Hum Mutat 2000;15:541–55.
20 Theos A, Korf BR. Pathophysiology of neurofibromatosis type 1. Ann Intern Med 2006;144:842–9.
21 National Institutes of Health Consensus Development Conference. Neurofibromatosis: Conference statement. Arch Neurol 1988;45:575–8.
22 Gutmann DH, Aylsworth A, Carey JC, et al. The diagnostic evaluation and multidisciplinary management of neurofibromatosis 1 and neurofibromatosis 2. JAMA 1997;278:51–7.
23 DaBella K, Szudek J, Friedman JM. Use of the National Institutes of Health criteria for diagnosis of neurofibromatosis 1 in children. Pediatrics 2000;105:608–14.
24 Landau M, Krafchik BR. The diagnostic value of café-au-lait macules. J Am Acad Dermatol 1999;40:877–90.
25 Crowe FW, Schull WJ, Neel JV. A Clinical, Pathological and Genetic Study of Multiple Neurofibromatosis. Springfield, IL: C Thomas, 1956.

26 **Korf BR. Diagnostic outcome in children with multiple café au lait spots. Pediatrics 1992;90:924–7.**
27 Huson SM, Harper PS, Compston DA. Von Recklinghausen neurofibromatosis. A clinical and population study in south-east Wales. Brain 1988;111:1355–81.
28 Nunley KS, Gao F, Albers AC et al. Predictive value of café au lait macules at initial consultation in the diagnosis of neurofibromatosis type 1. Arch Dermatol 2009;145:883–7.
29 **Wolkenstein P, Zeller J, Revuz J et al. Quality-of-life impairment in neurofibromatosis type 1: a cross-sectional study of 128 cases. Arch Dermatol 2001;137:1421–5.**
30 Tucker T, Wolkenstein P, Revuz J et al. Association between benign and malignant peripheral nerve sheath tumors in NF1. Neurology 2005;65:205–11.
31 Sbidian E, Bastuji-Garin S, Valeyrie-Allanore L et al. At-risk phenotype of neurofibromatosis-1 patients: a multicentre case-control study. Orphanet J Rare Dis 2011;6:51.
32 Khosrotehrani K, Bastuji-Garin S, Riccardi VM et al. Subcutaneous neurofibromas are associated with mortality in neurofibromatosis 1: a cohort study of 703 patients. Am J Med Genet 2005;132A:49–53.
33 Tonsgard JH, Kwak SM, Short MP et al. CT imaging in adults with neurofibromatosis-1: frequent asymptomatic plexiform lesions. Neurology 1998;50:1755–60.
34 Korf BR. Plexiform neurofibromas. Am J Med Genet 1999;89:31–7.
35 **Evans DG, Baser ME, McGaughran J et al. Malignant peripheral nerve sheath tumours in neurofibromatosis 1. J Med Genet 2002;39:311–4.**
36 Ferner RE, Golding JF, Smith M et al. [18F]2-fluoro-2-deoxy-D-glucose positron emission tomography (FDG PET) as a diagnostic tool for neurofibromatosis 1 (NF1) associated malignant peripheral nerve sheath tumors (MPNSTs): a long-term clinical study. Ann Oncol 2008;19:90–394.
37 Cambiaghi S, Restano L, Caputo R. Juvenile xanthogranuloma associated with neurofibromatosis 1: 14 patients without evidence of hematologic malignancies. Pediatr Dermatol 2004;21:97–101.
38 Sbidian E, Hadj-Rabia S, Riccardi VM et al. Clinical characteristics predicting internal neurofibromas in 357 children with neurofibromatosis-1: results from a cross-sectional study. Orphanet J Rare Dis 2012;7:62.
39 **Hernandez-Martin A, Garcia-Martinez FJ, Duat A et al. Nevus anemicus: a distinctive cutaneous finding in neurofibromatosis type 1. Pediatr Dermatol 2015;32:342–7.**
40 **Ferrari F, Masurel A, Olivier-Faivre et al. Juvenile xanthogranuloma and nevus anemicus in the diagnosis of neurofibromatosis type 1. JAMA Dermatol 2014;150:42–6.**
41 Morier P, Merot Y, Paccaud D et al. Juvenile chronic granulocytic leukemia, juvenile xanthogranulomas, and neurofibromatosis. Case report and review of the literature. J Am Acad Dermatol 1990; 22:962–5.
42 **Zvulunov A, Barak Y, Metzker A. Juvenile xanthogranulomas, neurofibromatosis, and juvenile chronic myelogenous leukemia. World statistical analysis. Arch Dermatol 1995;131:904–8.**
43 Shin HT, Harris MB, Orlow SJ. Juvenile myelomonocytic leukemia presenting with features of hemophagocytic lymphohistiocytosis in association with neurofibromatosis and juvenile xanthogranulomas. J Pediatr Hematol Oncol 2004;26:591–5.
44 Gutmann DH, Gurney JG, Shannon KM. Juvenile xanthogranuloma, neurofibromatosis 1, and juvenile chronic myeloid leukemia. Arch Dermatol 1996;132:1390–1.
45 Burgdorf WH, Zelger B. JXG, NF1, and JMML: alphabet soup or a clinical issue. Pediatr Dermatol 2004;21:174–6.
46 Marque M, Roubertie A, Jaussent A et al. Nevus anemicus in neurofibromatosis type 1: a potential new diagnostic criterion. J Am Acad Dermatol 2013;69:768–75.
47 **Riccardi VM, Eichner JE. Neurofibromatosis: Phenotype, Natural History, and Pathogenesis. Baltimore, MD: Johns Hopkins University Press, 1986.**
48 Sawada S, Honda M, Kamide R et al. Three cases of subungual glomus tumors with von Recklinghausen neurofibromatosis. J Am Acad Dermatol 1995;32:277–8.
49 Kumar MG, Emnett RJ, Bayliss SJ et al. Glomus tumors in individuals with neurofibromatosis type 1. J Am Acad Dermatol 2014;71:44–8.
50 **Brems J, Park C, Maertens O et al. Glomus tumors in neurofibromatosis type 1: genetic, functional, and clinical evidence of a novel association. Cancer Res 2009;69:7393–401.**
51 Stevenson DA, Viskochil DH, Schorry EK et al. The use of anterolateral bowing of the lower leg in the diagnostic criteria for neurofibromatosis type 1. Genet Med 2007;9:409–12.
52 Alwan S, Tredwell SJ, Friedman JM. Is osseous dysplasia a primary feature of neurofibromatosis 1 (NF1)? Clin Genet 2005;67:378–90.
53 Savar A, Cestari CM. Neurofibromatosis type 1: genetics and clinical manifestations. Semin Ophthalmol 2008;23:45–51.
54 Flueler U, Boltshauser E, Kilchhofer A. Iris hamartomata as diagnostic criterion in neurofibromatosis. Neuropediatrics 1986;17:183–5.
55 Huson S, Jones D, Beck L. Ophthalmic manifestations of neurofibromatosis. Br J Ophthalmol 1987;71:235–8.
56 Listernick R, Charrow J, Greenwald M, Mets M et al. Natural history of optic pathway tumors in children with neurofibromatosis type 1: a longitudinal study. J Pediatr 1994;125:63–6.
57 King A, Listernick R, Charrow J et al. Optic pathway gliomas in neurofibromatosis type 1: the effect of presenting symptoms on outcome. Am J Med Genet 2003;122A:95–9.
58 Listernick R, Ferner RE, Piersall L et al Late-onset optic pathway tumors in children with neurofibromatosis 1. Neurology 2004;63: 1944–6.
59 **Listernick R, Ferner Re, Liu GT et al. Optic pathway gliomas in neurofibromatosis-1: controversies and recommendations. Ann Neurol 2007;61:189–98.**
60 Hyman SL, Arthur Shores E, North KN. Learning disabilities in children with neurofibromatosis type 1: subtypes, cognitive profile, and attention-deficit-hyperactivity disorder. Dev Med Child Neurol 2006;48:973–7.
61 Hofman KJ, Harris EL, Bryan RN et al. Neurofibromatosis type 1: the cognitive phenotype. J Pediatr 1994;124:S1–S8.
62 Legius E, Descheemaeker MJ, Spaepen A et al. Neurofibromatosis type 1 in childhood: a study of the neuropsychological profile in 45 children. Genet Couns 1994;5:51–60.
63 North K, Joy P, Yuille D et al. Specific learning disability in children with neurofibromatosis type 1: significance of MRI abnormalities. Neurology 1994;44:878–83.
64 Ferner RE, Hughes RA, Weinman J. Intellectual impairment in neurofibromatosis 1. J Neurol Sci 1996;138:125–33.
65 North K, Hyman S, Barton B. Cognitive deficits in neurofibromatosis 1. J Child Neurol 2002;17:605–12.
66 Mautner VF, Kluwe L, Thakker SD et al. Treatment of ADHD in neurofibromatosis type 1. Dev Med Child Neurol 2002;44:164–70.
67 Yao R, Wang L, Yu Y et al. Diagnostic value of multiple café-au-lait macules for neurofibromatosis 1 in Chinese children. J Dermatol 2016;43:537–42.
68 **Brems H, Chmara M, Sahbatou M et al. Germline loss-of-function mutations in SPRED1 cause a neurofibromatosis 1-like phenotype. Nat Genet 2007;39:1120–6.**
69 Brems H, Legius E. Legius syndrome, an update. Molecular pathology of mutations in SPRED1. Keio J Med. 2013;62:107–12.
70 Messiaen L, Yao S, Brems H et al. Clinical and mutational spectrum of neurofibromatosis type 1-like syndrome. JAMA 2009;302:2111–18.
71 **Shah KN. The diagnostic and clinical significance of café-au-lait macules. Pediatr Clin North Am 2010;57:1131–53.**
72 Stewart DR, Brems H, Gomes AG et al. Jaffe-Campanacci syndrome, revisited: detailed clinical and molecular analyses determine whether patients have neurofibromatosis type 1, coincidental manifestations, or a distinct disorder. Genet Med 2014;16:448–59.
73 Pasmant E, Parfait B, Luscan A et al. Neurofibromatosis type 1 molecular diagnosis: what can NGS do for you when you have a large gene with loss of function mutations? Eur J Hum Genet 2015;23:596–601.
74 Kluwe L, Siebert R, Gesk S et al. Screening 500 unselected neurofibromatosis 1 patients for deletions of the NF1 gene. Hum Mutat 2004;23:111–16.
75 Leppig KA, Kaplan P, Viskochil D et al. Familial neurofibromatosis 1 microdeletions: cosegregation with distinct facial phenotype and early onset of cutaneous neurofibromas. Am J Med Genet 1997; 73:197–204.
76 Kayes LM, Burke W, Riccardi VM et al. Deletions spanning the neurofibromatosis 1 gene: identification and phenotype of five patients. Am J Hum Genet 1994;54:424–36.
77 Descheemaeker MJ, Roelandts K, De Raedt T et al. Intelligence in individuals with a neurofibromatosis type 1 microdeletion. Am J Med Genet 2004;131A:325–6.
78 De Raedt T, Brems J, Wolkenstein P et al. Elevated risk for MPNST in NF1 microdeletion patients. Am J Hum Genet 2003;72:1288–92.
79 Upadhyaya M, Huson SM, Davies M et al. An absence of cutaneous neurofibromas associated with a 3-bp inframe deletion in exon 17 of the NF1 gene (c2970-2972 delAAT): evidence of a clinically significant NF1 genotype-phenotype correlation. Am J Hum Genet 2007; 80:140–51.

80 Rojnueangnit K, Xie J, Gomes A et al. High incidence of Noonan syndrome features including short stature and pulmonic stenosis in patients carrying NF1 missense mutations affecting p.Arg1809: Genotype-phenotype correlation. Hum Mutat 2015;36:1052–63.
81 Enzinger FM, Weiss SW. Soft Tissue Tumours, 2nd edn. St Louis, MO: C.V. Mosby, 1998.
82 De Schepper S, Boucneau J, Vander Haeghen Y et al. Café-au-lait spots in neurofibromatosis type 1 and in healthy control individuals: hyperpigmentation of a different kind? Arch Dermatol Res 2006;297:439–49.
83 Martuza RL, Philippe I, Fitzpatrick TB et al. Melanin macroglobules as a cellular marker of neurofibromatosis: a quantitative study. J Invest Dermatol 1985;85:347–50.
84 Fitzpatrick TB, Martuza RL. Clinical diagnosis of von Recklinghausen's neurofibromatosis. Ann NY Acad Sci 1986;486:383–5.
85 Harkin JC, Reed RJ. Tumors of the peripheral nervous system. In: Atlas for Tumor Pathology, 2nd series, fascicle 3. Washington, DC: Armed Forces Institute of Pathology, 1969:67–106.
86 Wiestler OD, Radner J. Pathology of neurofibromatosis 1 and 2. In: Huson SM, Hughes RAC (eds) The Neurofibromatoses: A Pathogenetic and Clinical Overview. London: Chapman & Hall, 1994:135–59.
87 Boyd KP, Korf BR, Theos A. Neurofibromatosis type 1. J Am Acad Dermatol 2009;61:1–14.
88 Ferner RE, Huson SM, Thomas N et al. Guidelines for the diagnosis and management of individuals with neurofibromatosis 1. J Med Genet 2007;44:81–8.
89 Ruggieri M, Huson SM. The clinical and diagnostic implications of mosaicism in the neurofibromatoses. Neurology 2001;56:1433–43.
90 Tinschert S, Naumann I, Stegmann E et al. Segmental neurofibromatoss is caused by somatic mutation of the neurofibromatosis type 1 (NF1) gene. Eur J Hum Genet 2000;8:455–9.
91 Maertens O, De Schepper S, Vandesompele J et al. Molecular dissection of isolated disease features in mosaic neurofibromatosis type 1. Am J Hum Genet 2007;81:243–51.
92 Vandenbroucke I, van Doorn R, Callens T et al. Genetic and clinical mosaicism in a patient with neurofibromatosis type 1. Hum Genet 2004;114:284–90.
93 Listernick R, Mancini AM, Charrow J. Segmental neurofibromatosis in childhood. Am J Med Genet 2003;121A:132–5.
94 Ruggieri M, Pavone P, Polizzi A et al. Ophthalmological manifestations in segmental neurofibromatosis type 1. Br J Ophthalmol 2004;88:1429–33.
95 Schwarz J, Belzberg AJ. Malignant peripheral nerve sheath tumors in the setting of segmental neurofibromatosis. Case report. J Neurosurg 2000;92:342–6.
96 Moss C, Green SH. What is segmental neurofibromatosis? Br J Dermatol 1994;130:106–10.
97 Poyhonen M. A clinical assessment of neurofibromatosis type 1 (NF1) and segmental NF in Northern Finland. J Med Genet 2000;37:E43.
98 Consoli C, Moss C, Green S et al. Gonosomal mosaicism for a nonsense mutation (R1947X) in the NF1 gene in segmental neurofibromatosis type 1. J Invest Dermatol 2005;125:463–6.
99 Garcia-Romero MT, Parkin P, Lara Corrales I. Mosaic neurofibromatosis type 1: a systematic review. Pediatr Dermatol 2016;33:9–17.
100 Hogeling M, Frieden IJ. Segmental pigmentation disorder. Br J Dermatol 2010;162:1337–41.
101 Chen W, Fan PC, Happle R. Partial unilateral lentiginosis with ipsilateral Lisch nodules and axillary freckling. Dermatology 2014; 209:228–9.
102 Jobling RK, Lara-Corrales I, Hsiao MC et al. Mosaicism for a SPRED1 deletion revealed in a patient with clinically suspected mosaic NF. Br J Dermatol 2017;176:1077–8.
103 Ruggieri M, Iannetti P, Polizzi A et al. Earliest clinical manifestations and natural history of neurofibromatosis type 2 (NF2) in childhood: a study of 24 patients. Neuropediatrics 2005;36:21–34.
104 Evans DG, Howard E, Giblin C et al. Birth incidence and prevalence of tumor-prone syndromes: estimates from a UK family genetic register service. Am J Med Genet 2010;77:163–70.
105 Evans DG, Ramsden RT, Shenton et al. Mosaicism in neurofibromatosis type 2: an update of risk based on uni/bilaterality of vesibular schwannoma at presentation and sensitive mutation analysis including multiple ligation-dependent probe amplification. J Med Genet 2007;44:424–8.
106 Seizinger BR, Martuza RL, Gusella JF. Loss of genes on chromosome 22 in tumourigenesis of human acoustic neuroma. Nature 1986;322:644–7.
107 Rouleau GA, Seizinger BR, Ozelius LG et al. Genetic linkage analysis of bilateral acoustic neurofibromatosis to a DNA marker on chromosome 22. Nature 1987;329:246–8.
108 Rouleau GA, Merel P, Lutchman M et al. Alteration in a new gene encoding a putative membrane organizing protein causes neurofibromatosis type 2. Nature 1993;363:515–21.
109 Trofatter JA, MacCollin MM, Rutter JL et al. A novel moesin-, ezrin-, radixin-like gene is a candidate for the neurofibromatosis 2 tumour suppressor. Cell 1993;75:826.
110 Baser ME, Evans DGR, Gutmann DH. Neurofibromatosis 2. Curr Opin Neurol 2003;16: 27–33.
111 Uhlmann EJ, Gutmann DH. Tumour suppressor gene regulation of cell growth: recent insights into neurofibromatosis 1 and 2 gene function. Cell Biochem Biophys 2001;34:61–71.
112 Sun C-X, Robb VA, Gutmann DH. Protein 4.1 tumour suppressors: getting a FERM grip on growth regulation. J Cell Sci 2002;115: 3991–4000.
113 National Institutes of Health Consensus Development Conference. Neurofibromatosis: conference statement. Arch Neurol 1988; 45:575–8.
114 Gutmann DH, Aylsworth A, Carey JC et al. The diagnostic evaluation and multidisciplinary management of neurofibromatosis 1 and neurofibromatosis 2. JAMA 1997;278:51–7.
115 Evans DG, Huson SM, Donnai D et al. A clinical study of type 2 neurofibromatosis Q J Med 1992;84:603–18.
116 Baser ME, Friedman JM, Wallace AJ et al. Evaluation of clinical diagnostic criteria for neurofibromatosis 2. Neurology 2002;59:1759–65.
117 Baser ME, Friedman JM, Aeschliman D et al. Predictors of the risk of mortality in neurofibromatosis 2. Am J Hum Genet 2002;71:715–23.
118 Parry DM, Eldridge R, Kaiser-Kupfer MI et al. Neurofibromatosis (NF2): clinical characteristics of 63 affected individuals and clinical evidence for heterogeneity. Am J Med Genet 1994;52:450–61.
119 Evans DG, Ramsden RT, Shenton A et al. Mosaicism in neurofibromatosis type 2: an update of risk based on uni/bilaterality of vestibular schwannoma at presentation and sensitive mutation analysis including multiple ligation-dependent probe amplification. J Med Genet 2007;44:424–8.
120 MacCollin M, Willet C, Heinrich B et al. Familial schwannomatosis: Exclusion of the NF2 locus as the germline event. Neurology 2003;60:1968–974.
121 Boyd C, Smith MJ, Kluwe L et al. Alterations in the SMARCB1 (INI1) tumor suppressor gene in familial schwannomatosis. Clin Genet 2008;74:358–66.
122 Piotrowski A, Xie J, Liu YF et al. Germline loss-of-function mutations in LZTR1 predispose to an inherited disorder of multiple schwannomas. Nat Genet 2014;46:182–7.
123 Evans DG. Neurofibromatosis type 2 (NF2): a clinical and molecular review. Orphanet J Rare Dis 2009;4:16.
124 Hexter A, Jones A, Joe H et al. Clinical and molecular predictors of mortality in neurofibromatosis 2: a UK national analysis of 1192 patients. J Med Genet 2015;52:699–705.
125 Selvanathan SK, Shenton A, Ferner R et al. Further genotype—phenotype correlations in neurofibromatosis 2. Clin Genet 2010; 77:163–70.
126 Evans DG. Neurofibromatosis 2 [Bilateral acoustic neurofibromatosis, central neurofibromatosis, NF2, NF type 2]. Genet Med 2009; 11:599–610.
127 Kluwe L, Mautner V, Heinrich B et al. Molecular study of frequency of mosaicism in neurofibromatosis 2 patients with bilateral vestibular schwannomas. J Med Genet 2003;40:109–14.
128 Moyhuddin A, Baser ME, Watson C et al. Somatic mosaicism in neurofibromatosis 2: prevalence and risk of disease transmission to offspring. J Med Genet 2003;40:459–63.
129 Bouldin TW. Nerve biopsy. In: Garcia JH, Escalona-Zapata J, Sandbank U et al. (eds) Diagnostic Neuropathology, Vol II. New York: Macmillan, 1990:175–92.
130 Kleihues P, Burger PC, Scheithauer BW. Histological Typing of Tumours of the Central Nervous System, 2nd edn. Berlin: Springer-Verlag, 1993.

CHAPTER 143
Tuberous Sclerosis Complex

Francis J. DiMario Jr

University of Connecticut School of Medicine, Farmington, CT, USA and Department of Pediatrics and Tuberous Sclerosis Clinic, Division of Pediatric Neurology, Connecticut Children's Medical Center, Hartford, CT, USA

Abstract

Tuberous sclerosis complex (TSC) is an autosomal dominant, multisystem neurocutaneous disorder characterized by cellular hyperplasia and tissue dysplasia. Population studies estimate prevalence between 1 in 6000–9000 in the USA to 1 in 38 000 elsewhere. Both genders are equally affected and TSC is found in all ethnicities, totalling 2 million people worldwide. Substantial progress in understanding the genetics and pathophysiology of TSC has been made. Mutations in two genetic loci are known to cause TSC: *TSC1* located on chromosome 9q34; and *TSC2* found on chromosome 16p13. Significant genetic and phenotypic variation occurs among individuals harbouring pathogenic mutations. TSC occurs spontaneously in an estimated 65–75% of affected individuals. Up to 15% of affected individuals have no detectable mutation. Translational research trials have been successful in utilizing drug inhibitors of the mammalian (mechanistic) target of rapamycin (mTOR), a key regulator of cell signalling, to ameliorate the effects of TSC.

Key points

- **Hypomelanotic skin macules in patients with epilepsy and/or autism are important diagnostic clues of tuberous sclerosis complex (TSC).**
- **Prenatal cardiac rhabdomyomas may be the initial diagnostic presentation of TSC.**
- **Infantile spasms are often the initial epileptic manifestation of TSC.**
- **Multiple organ tissue hamartomas are a hallmark of TSC.**
- **An uninhibited mechanistic target of rapamycin (mTOR) pathway leads to unregulated cell function that characterizes the molecular basis of TSC.**
- **The treatment of renal angiomyolipomas, lymphangioleiomyomatosis of the lung and brain subependymal giant cell astrocytomas with mTOR inhibitors and of facial angiofibromas with topical mTOR inhibitors has been demonstrated to be effective in reducing lesion size and improving function in clinical trials.**

Introduction. Tuberous sclerosis complex (TSC) is an autosomal dominant neurocutaneous multisystem disorder with an estimated population prevalence of between 1 in 6000–9000 in the USA to 1 in 38 elsewhere [1–3]. TSC is characterized by cellular hyperplasia, tissue dysplasia and multiple organ hamartomas [1,4]. Significant research efforts into the genetic and pathophysiological mechanisms of TSC have resulted in our current understanding and new treatment options. We have now identified two known genetic loci: *TSC1* found on chromosome 9q34 and *TSC2* on chromosome 16p13 [5,6]. As in most disorders with an autosomal dominant inheritance pattern, there is a high spontaneous mutation rate approaching 65–75% and up to 10–15% of affected individuals with no mutation identified with significant variation among those with similar pathogenic mutations [7–10]. Mutations in either gene produces TSC with similar manifestations although mutations in *TSC2* have been found to produce slightly more severe clinical manifestations such as more hypomelanotic macules and learning disabilities; and more frequent neurological and ophthalmological symptoms, renal cysts and ungual fibromas in males [7,9]. The genetic mutations have a direct consequence on the clinical manifestations as a result of an uninhibited mechanistic target of rapamycin (mTOR) pathway, which serves to regulate cell signalling [11].

Over the course of several international consensus conferences, the diagnostic criteria for TSC have been agreed upon and regularly updated. The most current diagnostic requirements are listed in Table 143.1 [12].

Historical perspective. The clinical identification of TSC begins with a brief necropsy description from von Recklinghausen in 1862 who described heart 'myomata' and brain 'scleroses' [13]. The initial neuropathology of tuberous sclerosis was carefully described by the French neurologist Bourneville in 1880 [14]. He coined the term 'tubereuse' when describing the potato-like firmness of the gyral protrusions identified during a postmortem examination of the brain from a girl who died of status epilepticus (Fig. 143.1) [14]. She had suffered with epilepsy, mental retardation and was also described to have had small kidney tumors and a facial rash. Pringle later referred to this rash as adenoma sebaceum in 1890 [15]. Between the years 1880 and 1900 Bourneville and colleagues described 10 additional deceased patients with brain and kidney lesions, referring to the condition as tuberous sclerosis [16]. In 1905, Perusini noted the

Harper's Textbook of Pediatric Dermatology, Fourth Edition. Edited by Peter Hoeger, Veronica Kinsler and Albert Yan.

Table 143.1 Diagnostic criteria according to the International Tuberous Sclerosis Complex Consensus Conference [12]

Definite diagnosis Two major features or one major feature with more than two minor features or presence of a TSC1 or TSC2 mutation of confirmed pathogenicity[1]

Possible diagnosis Either one major feature or more than two minor features

Major criteria

Skin

- Hypomelanotic macules ($n > 3$, at least 5 mm diameter)
- Angiofibromas ($n > 3$) or fibrous cephalic plaque
- Ungual fibromas ($n > 2$)
- Shagreen patch

Central nervous system

- Cortical dysplasias (includes tubers and cerebral white matter radial migration lines)
- Subependymal nodules
- Subependymal giant cell astrocytoma

Heart

- Cardiac rhabdomyoma

Lungs

- Lymphangioleiomyomatosis[2]

Kidney

- Angiomyolipomas ($n > 2$)[2]

Eyes

- Multiple retinal hamartomas

Minor criteria

Skin/oral cavity

- 'Confetti' skin lesions
- Dental enamel pits ($n > 3$)
- Intraoral fibromas ($n > 2$)

Kidney

- Multiple renal cysts

Eyes

- Retinal achromic patch

Other organs

- Nonrenal hamartomas

Genetics Identification of either a TSC1 or TSC2 pathogenic[1] mutation in DNA from normal tissue is sufficient to make a definite diagnosis

[1] A pathogenic mutation is defined as a mutation that clearly inactivates the function of the TSC1 or TSC2 proteins, prevents protein synthesis or is a missense mutation whose effect on protein function has been established by functional assessment (www.lovd.nl/TSC1, www.lovd.nl/TSC2).

[2] A combination of the two major clinical features (lymphangioleiomyomatosis and angiomyolipomas) without other features does not meet criteria for a definite diagnosis.

Source: Adapted from Northrup and Krueger 2013 [12]. Reproduced with permission of Elsevier.

association of brain, kidney, cardiac and skin manifestations in additional deceased patients identified with tuberous sclerosis [17]. However, it was not until 1908 when Heinrich Vogt diagnosed a living patient with tuberous sclerosis on the basis of his classic triad: mental retardation, seizures and the facial skin rash called adenoma sebaceum, now more appropriately termed facial angiofibroma [18]. Berg identified the familial autosomal dominant inheritance in a 1913 report of a family with affected members spanning three generations [19]. It was in 1920 that van der Hoeve described retinal lesions that he called retinal 'phacomas' (the Greek word *phakos* means spot) and also noted that 'phacomas' occurred in the intestine, bone and thyroid [20]. Critchley and Earl identified the importance of hypomelanotic skin macules (white ash leaf patches) in 1932 [21].

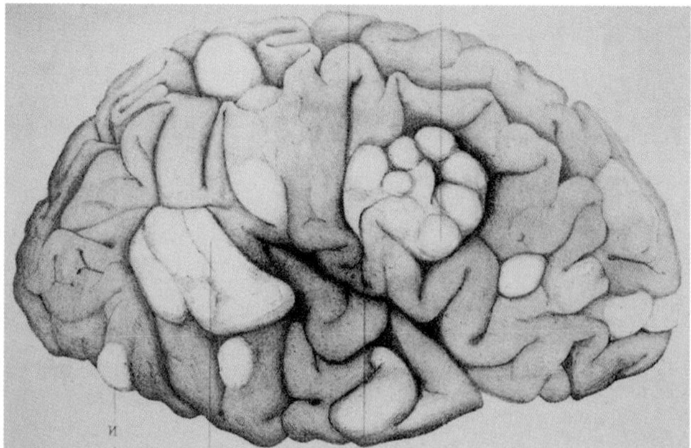

Fig. 143.1 A copy of one of the original illustrations from Bourneville's paper in 1880, showing 'tuber-like' growths with areas of sclerosis, hence the term TSC. Source: [14].

Epidemiology. Early epidemiological studies of TSC were based upon evolving diagnostic criteria and variable sampling methods that impacted sample ascertainment and biased results. Identifying affected subjects has become more standardized with international diagnostic consensus criteria (Table 143.1) and will undoubtedly improve further as the availability of better genetic testing proliferates.

Initial prevalence estimates in 1935, extrapolated from the number of affected individuals in psychiatric institutions, suggested a figure of 1 in 30 000 [22]. However, a number of prevalence studies from around the world have been undertaken since then (Table 143.2), most suggesting an overall prevalence of 1 in 27 000–39 000 for all ages [2,3,23–32] with an apparently higher prevalence in young children of 1 in 10 000–15 000. There is a paucity of data from Eastern countries. However, there have been estimates of 1 in 31 000–95 000 from Japan and Taiwan [3,30]. The higher estimates are supported by a long-term study in Minnesota, USA that suggested a figure of 1 in 9000–10 000 for a whole population [2]. Because intellectually normal children with TSC may not come to medical attention, the birth incidence may be as high as 1 in 7000 [32]. Using capture–recapture techniques, a prevalence of 8.8 cases per 100 000 (1 in 11 364) was obtained in the UK but this has since been revised downwards to 3.8 per 100 000 (1 in 26 315) after a second ascertainment of the population [24,25].

Pathogenesis. The search for a genetic aetiology for TSC reached an important milestone in 1987 when the *TSC1* gene was linked to the ABO blood group on chromosome 9q34 [33]. It would take another 10 years to identify the *TSC1* gene and its gene product *hamartin* [4]. During this interval, investigators in 1992 uncovered a second genetic locus that caused TSC on chromosome 16p13, which was adjacent to the gene for autosomal dominant polycystic kidney disease (ADPKD) [34]. The *TSC2* locus and its gene product *tuberin* were characterized shortly

Table 143.2 Epidemiology of tuberous sclerosis complex

Area and year	Prevalence (per 100 000)	Incidence	Case numbers	Reference
Japan, 1979	1:31 000 (3.22)	NA	52	30
Rochester, MN, USA, 1950–1982	1:9434 (10.6)	0.56:100 000	8	2
Scotland, UK, 1983	1:38 168 (2.62)	NA	1 family	28
Oxford, UK, 1984		NA	68	23
<65 years old	1:29 990 (3.34)			
<30 years old	1:21 500 (4.65)			
<5 years old	1:15 400 (6.49)			
Olmsted County, MN, USA, 1950–1989	1:16 667(6)	0.28	12	31
Sweden, 1994	1:12 900 (7.75)	NA	32	29
Wessex, UK, 1996	1:26 315 (3.8)	NA	131	24,25
	1:11 364 (8.8)		300 estimated	
Northern Ireland, 2006, 1956	1:24 956 (4.00)	NA	73	26,27
	1:142 857 (0.7)		31	
Taiwan, 2009	1:95 136 (1.051)	NA	208	3
<6 years old	1:14 608 (6.845)		50	
<12 years old	1:18 851 (5.305)		115	
<18 years old	1:24 617 (4.062)		150	
<30 years old	1:37 415 (2.673)		191	

NA, not available.

thereafter [35]. Both genetic loci may produce a similar phenotypic expression of TSC (genetic heterogeneity). Those individuals with a *TSC2* mutation generally have more severe clinical manifestations when compared with individuals harbouring *TSC1* gene mutations. These individuals often have more: hypomelanotic macules, learning disabilities, neurological and ophthalmological signs, renal cysts and ungual fibromas (in males) [7]. The genetic heterogeneity is made more complex by phenotypic heterogeneity and variable clinical expression among family members despite having the same genetic mutation [6]. It is the *TSC2* gene, however, which accounts for as much as 80–90% of the clinical cases with an identified genetic mutation [5–7]. None-the-less, there remains nearly 15% of affected individuals with no detectable mutation [10]. This group of patients has generally milder clinical manifestations with a lower incidence of neurological symptoms and signs and neuroimaging abnormalities yet concurrent renal and lung findings that suggest a possible mosaicism with *TSC2* and perhaps a unique pathogenesis [10].

The Tuberous Sclerosis Complex Variation Database of small mutations, small and large deletions, and rearrangements for both genes has compiled over 600 different mutations [7]. The majority of *TSC1* gene mutations are small deletions that result in nonsense or frameshifts, which lead to protein truncation [5–7]. In comparison, the majority of *TSC2* gene mutations involve missense mutations (25–32%) and large deletions/rearrangements (12–17%) [5–7]. The *TSC2* gene mutations are the most common overall whether found in familial cases (~65%) or in sporadic cases (~75%) resulting in a ratio of TSC2:TSC1 of almost 2:1 in familial cases and 3.5:1 in sporadic cases. However, when mutations in the *TSC1* gene are identified they are twice as likely in familial cases as in sporadic cases.

When an individual is born with a germline mutation of one allele of either *TSC1* or *TSC2* then it will be found in all cells. It is the additional loss of the second allele in somatic tissue or the end organ that will result in an organ lesion. The loss of the second allele results in no function at all in the *TSC1* or *TSC2* gene within the affected cells. This is referred to as a loss of heterozygosity and is consistent with Knudson's model of a two-hit tumour suppressor gene [36]. Analyses of multiple TSC organ hamartomas have demonstrated loss of heterozygosity including: cardiac rhabdomyomas, subependymal giant cell astrocytomas, renal angiomyolipomas, lung lymphangioleiomyomatosis cells, angiofibromas and a few cerebral cortical tubers [37–39].

Pathophysiology. The pathology of TSC hamartomas is consistent across tissues. The histological hallmarks include cellular hyperplasia and tissue dysplasia and are directly attributed to poorly regulated cell growth, cell proliferation and autophagy mechanisms. After the discovery of the *TSC1* and *TSC2* genes their respective protein products, TSC1 (hamartin) and TSC2 (tuberin), were subjected to extensive functional study in order to identify their sequential targets and critical signalling pathways (Fig. 143.2). These studies were initially informed through work on the fruit fly, *Drosophila melanogaster* [40]. The TSC gene proteins, hamartin and tuberin, together with a third protein, TBC1D7, form the TSC protein complex [41]. Normally, TSC2 is inactivated by protein kinase B (AKT) that leads to mTOR activation. The TSC protein complex interfaces with a number of other intracellular processes but most importantly serves as a critical negative regulator of mTOR complex 1 (mTORC1), a kinase that is pivotal to initiating many cell functions in response to growth factors, amino acids and nutrients [42–45]. The Ras homolog enriched in brain

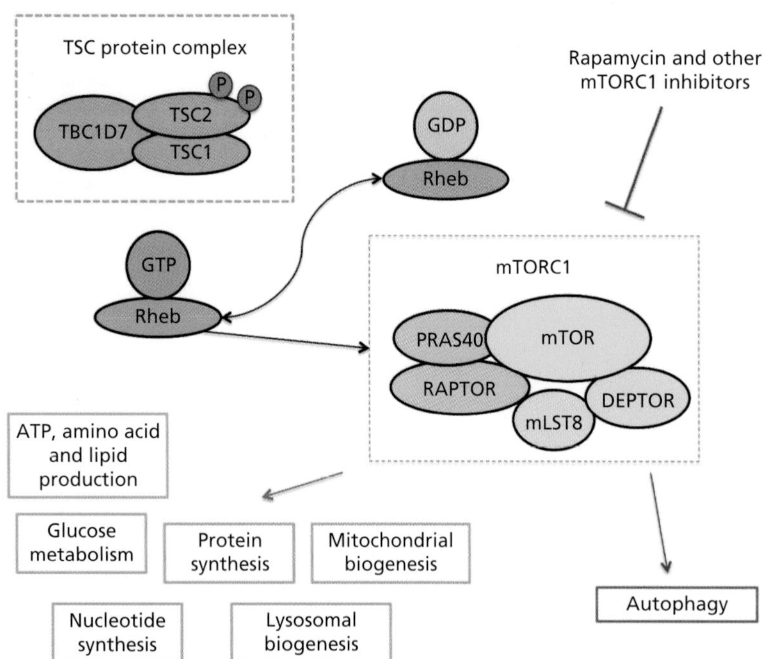

Fig. 143.2 Tuberous sclerosis complex (TSC) protein complex and mTOR signalling. Source: DiMario et al. 2015 [51]. Reproduced with permission of Elsevier.

(Rheb) is a specific GTPase downstream of the TSC protein complex that functionally links TSC1-TSC2 to mTORC1 (Fig. 143.2). TSC1-TSC2 complex functions as a GTPase activating protein (GAP) for Rheb and stimulates the conversion of Rheb-GTP to a GDP-bound state thereby inactivating Rheb signalling and thus removing its stimulatory effect on mTORC1. As a logical result, any loss-of-function mutation in either *TSC1* or *TSC2* will lead to enhanced Rheb-GTP signalling and mTORC1 activation. This sequence and interruption of cellular control constitutes the molecular basis of TSC.

When in its active state, mTORC1 phosphorylates the translational regulators eukaryotic translation initiation factor 4E-binding protein-1 (4E-BP1) and S6 kinase-1 (S6K1), which in turn stimulate protein synthesis, regulate anabolic pathways, and lead to cell hyperplasia and proliferation. Active mTORC1 directly stimulates the biosynthesis of ribosomes, lipid biogenesis, glucose metabolism, nucleotide synthesis, mitochondrial and lysosomal biogenesis, ATP and amino acid production and serves as a negative regulator for autophagy [45,46].

As a consequence to our understanding of these pathways was the recognition that there existed compounds, which could manipulate them in response to directed drug therapy. The mTORC1 complex can be bound to and its activity blocked by the macrolide antibiotic rapamycin and other related compounds [47–51]. These agents effectively restore control of the cellular signalling pathways lost with mutations in either *TSC1* or *TSC2*.

Diagnostic approach. The diagnosis of TSC is made by careful clinical examination, especially of the skin, nails, teeth and eyes. Selective organ imaging and genetic testing are utilized to support or confirm a clinical diagnosis in index cases [1,4,12]. These investigations can be valuable to determine the extent of organ involvement at that point in time. When investigations are pursued in parents these results can help refine recurrence risks.

As an autosomal dominant disorder TSC has full penetrance and a spontaneous mutation rate approaching 65–75% [7,10]. Still, there are up to 10–15% of affected individuals who have no mutation identified in either the *TSC1* or *TSC2* gene when tested [7,10]. An affected individual carries a 50% risk of passing the disease on to each prospective progeny. The apparently healthy parents of a child with clinical TSC who have no diagnostic signs of TSC, although it is unlikely they are gene mutation carriers, should be offered confirmatory testing. This can be accomplished through genetic testing especially when a *TSC* gene alteration is found in their child or through detailed dermatological and ophthalmological clinical examination, followed by cranial and renal imaging if no gene alteration is identified. When genetic testing identifies a *TSC1* or *TSC2* pathogenic gene mutation this supersedes clinical criteria [12]. When a diagnosis is made the anticipated severity of TSC cannot be predicted for an individual or extrapolated from affected family members [6]. However, when genetic testing is obtained, those individuals with a *TSC2* gene mutation in comparison to a *TSC1* gene mutation may be anticipated to have more severe clinical manifestations [7].

Despite the characteristic clinical features of TSC there are no specific symptoms unique to TSC. Importantly, the recognition of several common clinical presentations associated with TSC should prompt further consideration of this diagnosis. First and foremost is identification of a family member with TSC. If a patient under evaluation has any first-degree relative (i.e. a parent or sibling) diagnosed with TSC then there is up to a 50% risk for them to have the disorder. Multiple siblings can be affected in the absence of a definitive diagnosis in either parent when there exists gonadal mosaicism in one of the parents [1,4,12]. This condition occurs when the gonads and their affected gametes is the only organ affected with the TSC mutation. Gonadal mosaicism allows the potential for multiple affected offspring from a parent who is otherwise normal and apparently unaffected. The recurrence risk for all clinically unaffected parents with an affected child is estimated to be less than 2% from the potential of underlying gonadal mosaicism [1,4,12].

The diagnosis of TSC should be considered when patients are identified with certain clinical hallmarks (Table 143.1). Equally important are clinical scenarios through which patients with TSC commonly come to medical attention. These presentations include prenatal identification of fetal cardiac rhabdomyomas, postnatal identification of hypomelanotic skin macules, the development of seizures especially infantile spasms and an evaluation for autism with or without cognitive impairment. These specific clinical encounters carry a high potential for the individual to carry an underlying diagnosis of TSC and warrant a heightened clinical suspicion for it.

Among infants born with cardiac rhabdomyomas, whether single or multiple, 80% or more are ultimately diagnosed with TSC. Identification of these cardiac lesions has been as early as 22 weeks' gestation [52]. These lesions are most often located within the ventricular septum rather than within the walls or atria [1,4,12]. Most patients have an average of three lesions, 3–25 mm in size, but isolated lesions still harbour diagnostic significance.

Hypomelanotic macules are identifiable in 90–95% of TSC affected individuals. The ash leaf spot, although characteristic, is not diagnostic. This has a pyramidal shape with a rounded bottom and pointed end. The use of an ultraviolet light (Wood's lamp) may enhance the visualization of these macules but most can be seen under ambient light [1,4,12].

The development of epilepsy occurs in up to 80–90% of patients with TSC over the course of a lifetime. With the possible exception of pure absence epilepsy, all seizure types may develop. Childhood is the most common time of epilepsy onset with infantile spasms as the presenting feature in one third of these children [1,4,12].

Patients with TSC can be affected with a wide range of behavioural problems. Prominent among those problems are the autism spectrum disorders (ASD) that can be identified in 40–50% of patients with TSC [1,53]. Concurrent cognitive impairment exists in 75% of patients affected with ASD and there is an additional 75–100% prevalence of concurrent epilepsy [1,53].

Clinical features.

Differential diagnosis

The diagnosis of TSC can be straightforward for individuals experienced in the identification of the common hallmark skin manifestations. There are other disorders with similar dermatological findings that can be mistaken for TSC, however (Table 143.3). These other genodermatoses are also genetically inherited multisystem skin disorders that may have additional malignant associations. The multiple endocrine neoplasia type-1 syndrome (MEN-1) is important because patients also exhibit facial angiofibromas in common with the more prevalent TSC [54]. The MEN syndromes manifest a concurrence of tumours involving the parathyroid glands, the anterior pituitary and the pancreatic islet cells. MEN-1 and MEN-2 are the result of autosomal dominant inheritance of the tumour suppressor gene *MEN-1* and the proto-onco gene *RET*, respectively [54].

Table 143.3 Differential diagnostic considerations of tuberous sclerosis complex [54,55,119]

Genodermatoses	Cutaneous manifestations	Gene
Birt–Hogg–Dube syndrome	Fibrofolliculoma Trichodiscoma Acrochordoma Angiofibroma	*BHD (FLCN)*
Muir–Torre syndrome	Sebaceous adenoma	*MLH-1*
Brook–Spiegler syndrome	Cylindroma Trichoepithelioma Spiradenoma	*CYLD-1*
Cowden syndrome	Tricholemmoma	*PTEN*
Gardener syndrome	Epidermal cysts Fibromas	*APC*
Multiple endocrine neoplasia syndrome type-1	Angiofibromas	*MEN-1*
Neurofibromatosis type-2	Angiofibromas	*NF-2*

The most pertinent to consider in a differential, however, is the Birt–Hogg–Dubé syndrome (BHDS). This is a rare autosomal dominant disorder first described in 1977. There are several skin lesions found on the face of patients affected with BHDS: fibrofolliculoma, trichodiscoma and acrochordons, which resemble the angiofibromas of TSC [55]. These, however, develop at a much later age than the angiofibromas of TSC and can be distinguished on skin biopsy. Similar to TSC, these patients may also have renal tumours: chromophobe/oncocytic renal carcinomas, chromophobe renal carcinoma, clear cell carcinomas and oncocytomas [55]. An additional overlapping feature of BHDS with TSC is the possible development of lung cysts and pneumothorax. BHDS is caused by the tumour suppressor gene *BHD (FLCN)* [55]. The *BHD* gene also interacts with the mTOR signalling pathway [55].

Dermatological findings

The earliest skin manifestations of TSC are the hypomelanotic macules followed later by cephalic plaques and shagreen patches. Hypomelanotic macules (*major criterion*) may be visible at birth or become apparent over the first several months of life. Despite the name, these are often amelanotic macules. These should be ≥5 mm and individuals should have at least three in number to be considered clinically significant from a diagnostic standpoint (Fig. 143.3a). More numerous smaller macules are referred as confetti lesions (minor criteria) and most often identified over the calves of adults (Fig. 143.3b), although they can be present in infants. When hair follicles are contained within the macule the hair also appears hypomelanotic and is referred to as

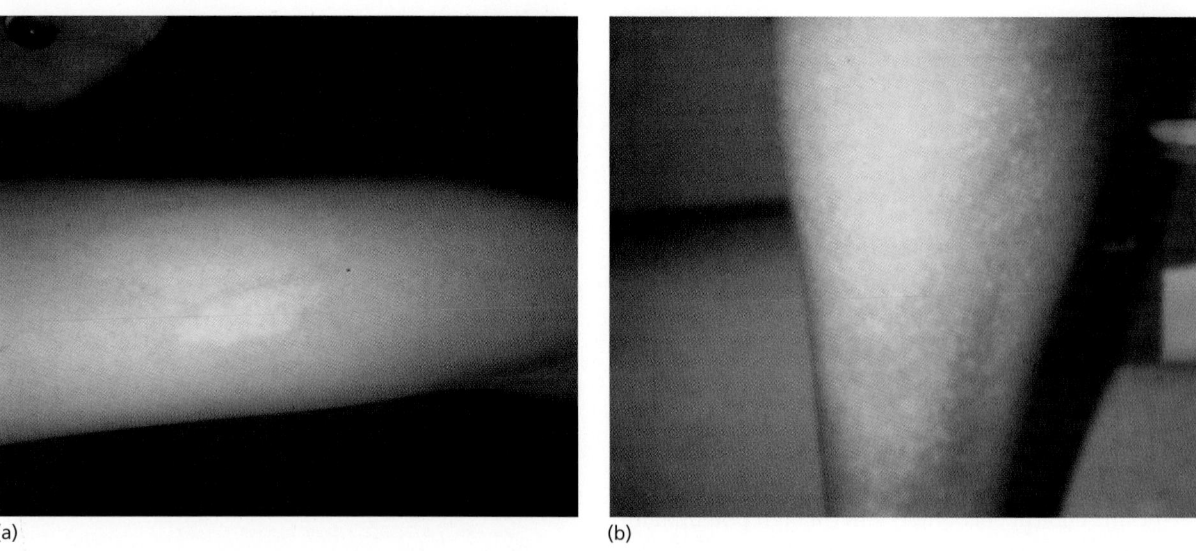

Fig. 143.3 (a) Hypomelanotic macules. The larger macule with a rounded base and pointed end is an ash leaf. (b) Confetti lesions over the lower leg. Source: DiMario et al. 2015 [51]. Reproduced with permission of Elsevier.

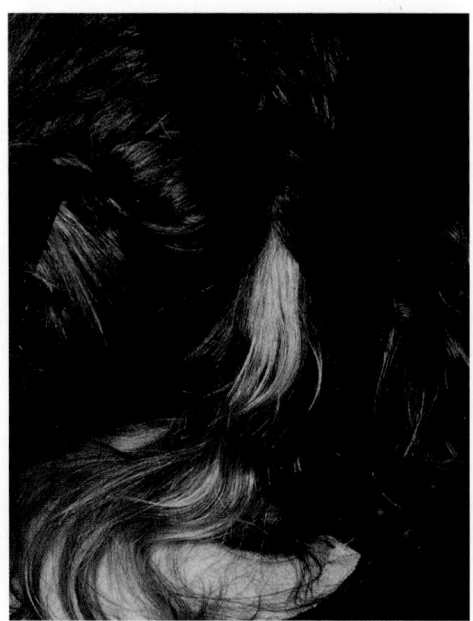

Fig. 143.4 Poliosis shown in the scalp. Source: Photo courtesy Dr A.J. Green.

poliosis (Fig. 143.4). These macules can produce single isolated hairs or patches. Over 90% of TSC patients will have hypomelanotic macules. Although the vast majority of hypomelanotic macules are identifiable in ambient light, the use of UV light can assist (Fig. 143.5). Larger macules with a rounded base and pointed end have the appearance of an ash leaf (Fig. 143.3a). These have no additional significance and count as one single hypomelanotic macule. Early biopsy and later iontophoresis studies have demonstrated abnormal sudomotor function with reduced sweat volume and aberrant sympathetic innervation within them [56]. Histologically, these lesions have normal numbers of melanocytes but absent melanosomes. These features have no clinical significance.

Cephalic plaques (*major criterion*) formerly called forehead plaques are found in about 10% of TSC patients. These may be present at birth and be identified anywhere over the scalp. These are most commonly seen over the forehead although larger lesions can be found over the vertexes (Fig. 143.6). The early appearance of these plaques resembles a capillary haemangioma but they gradually become firm, raised and waxy to touch. The initial erythematous colour deepens to yellow-brown. They are slow to evolve but enlarge and harden with fibrous tissue and often calcify by adulthood. Cephalic plaques and angiofibromas carry equivalence in diagnostic utility and are considered a single criterion whether or not one or both are present in an individual simultaneously.

Angiofibromas (*major criterion*) are initially small ruddy areas of the skin (Fig. 143.7). These often appear as small flushed areas on the face when in the sun or after exertion but are rarely obvious before the age of 2 years. Typical lesions are bilateral, symmetrically appearing erythematous papules or nodules usually located over the nasolabial folds, cheeks and chin. They rarely affect the forehead, scalp or upper lip but can be present elsewhere over the skin surface. They are present in about 80–85% of patients over the age of 4 years and can occasionally arise for the first time in adult life. These are not unique to TSC and individuals need more than three lesions to contribute as a diagnostic finding (Tables 143.1 and 143.3). The histological features of angiofibroma with characteristic giant cells on biopsy are also found in forehead plaques, shagreen patches and ungual fibromas. Skin tags, or molluscum fibrosum pendulum, are common especially around the neck, but do not contribute to the diagnosis of TSC.

Shagreen patches (*major criterion*) are easily overlooked in childhood and generally become apparent in late childhood and early adolescence. They can be elongated over several to many centimetres or occur in multiple millimetre nummular patches. Their initial puckered appearance evolves into a raised, thickened, palpable 'orange peel' surface to the dermis. The typical location is along the

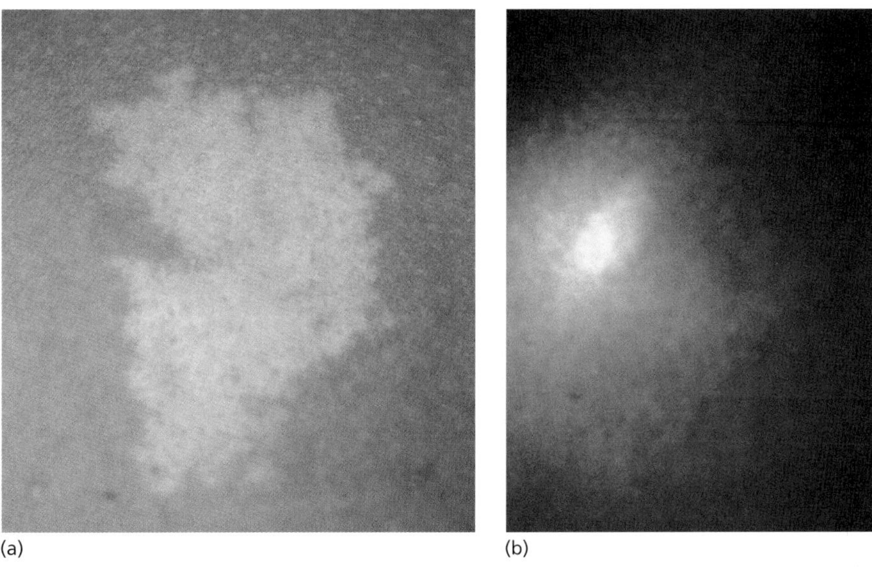

Fig. 143.5 (a) Hypomelanotic macule in ambient and (b) UV light. Irregular macules are not commonly seen in TSC. Source: Photo courtesy Dr A.J. Green.

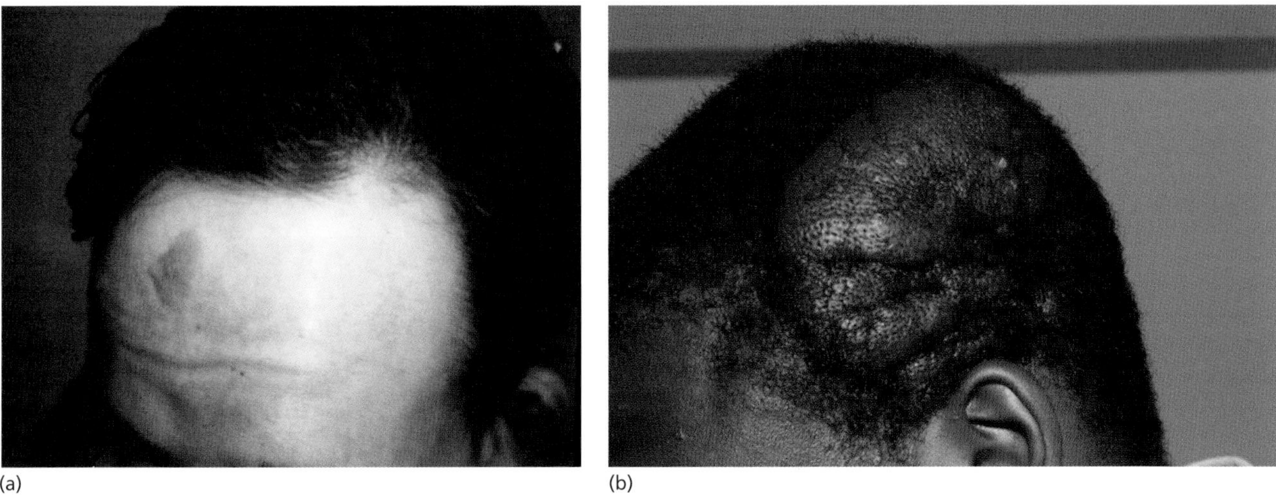

Fig. 143.6 Cephalic plaques. (a) The forehead is a common location. (b) Cephalic plaques can be seen elsewhere. This is a large cephalic plaque over the vertex in tuberous sclerosis complex. Source: DiMario et al. 2015 [51]. Reproduced with permission of Elsevier.

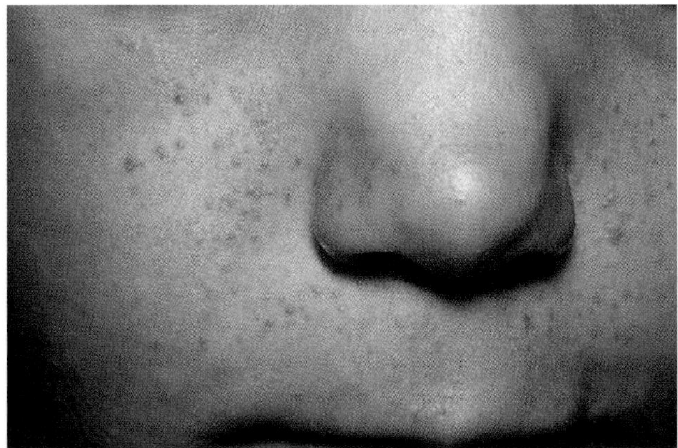

Fig. 143.7 Facial angiofibromas. Source: Photo courtesy Dr A.J. Green.

flanks in the lumbar region, up the back and occasionally at the top of the thigh (Fig. 143.8). Histologically, these are angiofibromas and are asymptomatic apart from their cosmetic appearance and are found in about 15–20% of individuals with TSC.

Ungual fibromas (*major criterion*) are generally adjacent to the nail but can be underneath it. About 15–20% of individuals with TSC will develop them. These are more often found on the toes rather than fingers and in females more than males. A longitudinal groove extending along the nail may the only indication of its presence. When evident adjacent to the nail these may feel fleshy or firm but can occasionally be identified underneath the nail also (Fig. 143.9). Histologically, these too are angiofibromas. These develop over time and are uncommon in the first decade; they can initially appear in later adulthood. Intraoral fibromas (*minor criterion*) can be identified along the gum lines in about 40–50% of TSC affected individuals. These are papular, fleshy outgrowths extruding from between the teeth. They can be a source of bleeding and if large enough may disrupt tooth alignment (Fig. 143.10). Two fibromas, whether ungual or intraoral, are required to contribute as a diagnostic sign.

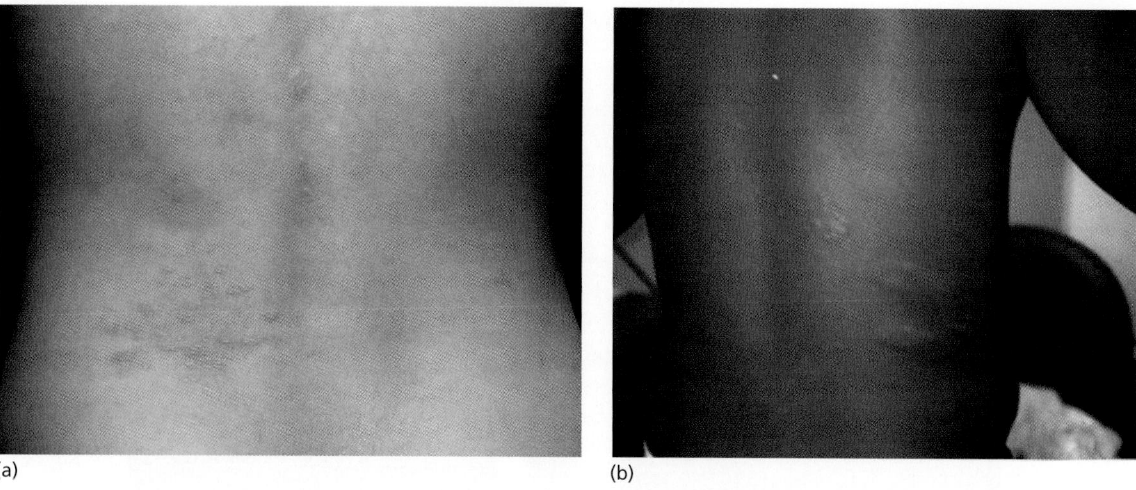

Fig. 143.8 Examples of shagreen patches. (a) A typical site with multiple small areas of affected skin called satellite lesions. Source: Photo courtesy Dr A.J. Green. (b) Larger flank lesion. Source: DiMario et al. 2015 [51]. Reproduced with permission of Elsevier.

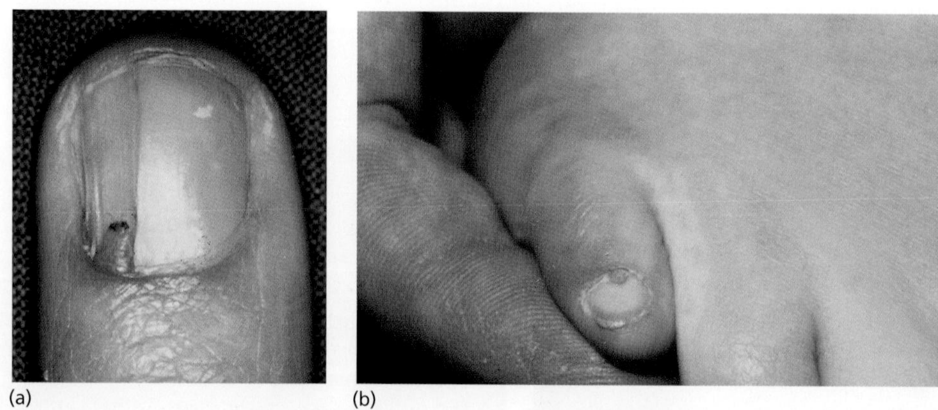

Fig. 143.9 (a) This ungual fibroma has caused a groove to develop in the finger nail. (b) This toe ungual fibroma was found in a boy of 3.5 years.

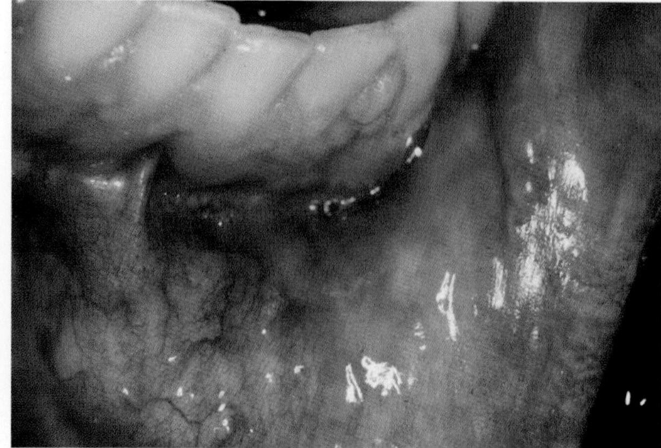

Fig. 143.10 A gum fibroma is visible next to the canine tooth. Source: Photo courtesy Dr A.J. Green.

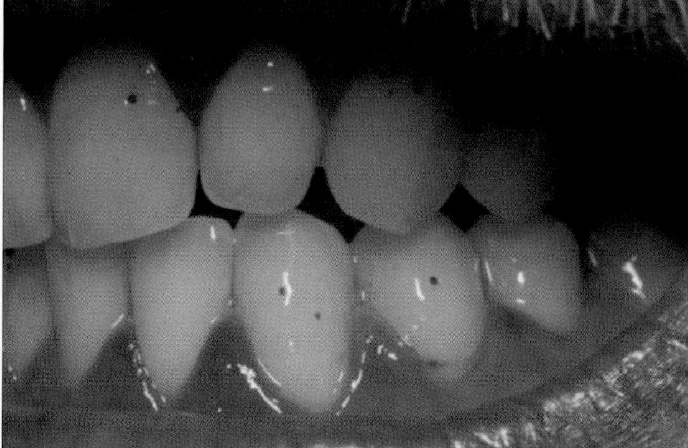

Fig. 143.11 Dental enamel pitting. Source: Courtesy Dr G. Mlynarczyk.

Dental enamel pitting (*minor criterion*) is a feature of TSC that virtually all patients develop in their permanent teeth [57]. These can be readily identified with a dental disclosing solution (Fig. 143.11). These can predispose to caries that may be prevented by using fluorides and applying sealants. These are also seen in persons unaffected with TSC. However, to contribute to a diagnosis of TSC there must be more than three pits present.

Neurological findings

The impact of TSC is probably most profoundly seen in its effects on the nervous system. Epilepsy is the presenting symptom of TSC in over 65–75% of patients. Up to 80–90% of all TSC patients develop epilepsy over their lifetimes. All seizure types (localization-related and generalized seizures) are encountered, with the exception of pure absence epilepsy. Of those with seizures, two-thirds will have seizure onset in the first year of life and 10% will occur in later childhood. Only 4% of TSC patients develop new onset seizures in adulthood [58]. A particularly devastating seizure type identified in up to 15–20% of those presenting with childhood epilepsy are infantile spasms (IS). These are massive myoclonic seizures where infants flex at the waist with arms extended in a repeated series. Commonly, IS manifest upon arousal from or entry into sleep. The typical EEG pattern of hypsarrhythmia, an extremely high amplitude and chaotic pattern, is often absent at onset only to develop over time [59,60].

Neurocognitive impairments span a multitude of effects from deficits in attention, multistep reasoning, learning disabilities and behavioural problems, to frank and profound intellectual disabilities and autism. While a gamut of additional sleep disturbances and psychiatric manifestations of all types and with variable degrees of severity are common, none are necessarily universal. In fact, the distribution of cognitive functioning in individuals with TSC is bimodal. There are 60–70% who fall within a normal full-scale IQ range but with a lower than the general population mean and a remaining 30–40% with profound disability and IQ scores of 40 or less [61,62]. These individuals require lifelong supervision for activities of daily living yet despite often having little or no language have full functional mobility. As noted previously, ASD are identified in up to 50% of patients with TSC [1,53]. Concurrent cognitive impairment exists in 75% of these patients with an additional near 100% prevalence of concurrent epilepsy [1,53]. Many of these features can be screened for using the TSC-associated neuropsychiatric disorders (TAND) checklist [63].

Among the key contributors to neurological dysfunction in TSC are the histological hallmarks cellular hyperplasia and tissue dysplasia identifiable within the central nervous system. These lesions are directly attributed to poorly regulated cell growth, cell proliferation and autophagy mechanisms, and manifest as cortical dysplasia, subependymal nodules and subependymal giant cell astrocytomas.

Cortical dysplasia (*major criterion*) is the preferred term that incorporates lesions individually identifiable as tubers and cerebral white matter migration lines (Fig. 143.12). Multiple areas of cortical dysplasia serve as a single diagnostic criterion however. These regions of disorganized cortical development can be localized from a few millimetres to centimetres of the cortex to as large as an entire cerebral lobe and are identified in up to 80–90% of TSC patients [1,58]. Tubers are developmental abnormalities histologically characterized by a loss of the normal six-layered cortical structure with the presence of dysmorphic neurons and giant astrocytes [64]. These are somewhat poorly demarcated in their full extent at the grey–white junction stretching medially from the cortex

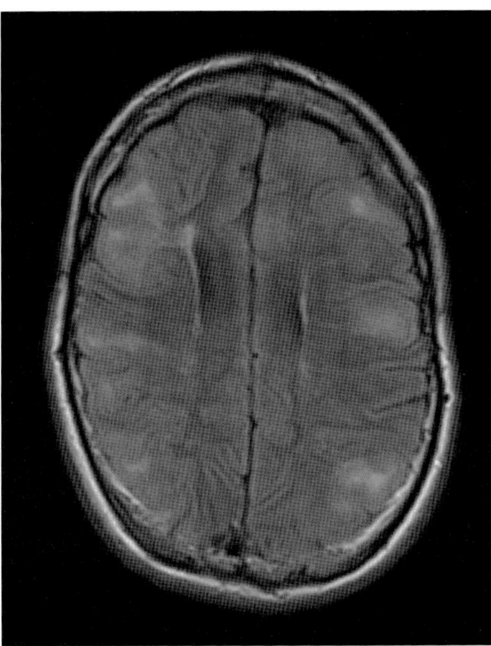

Fig. 143.12 Cortical dysplasias (tubers and migration lines on brain magnetic resonance imaging FLAIR sequence).

into the white matter on neuroimaging. They are typically multiple and equally distributed throughout all lobes but less frequently identified within the cerebellum and brainstem. They remain throughout a patient's life yet can become cystic in appearance on magnetic resonance imaging (MRI). There is recent evidence to suggest a more dynamic evolution of the tuber and the perituber tissue on a microstructural level using MRI diffusion tensor imaging (DTI) [65]. Identification of dysplasia with computed tomography (CT) scanning is less sensitive than with MRI. Hypodense and thickened cortical regions with or without accompanying calcification can be seen with CT whereas the different imaging sequences of MRI allow both correlative hyper- and hypointense thickened cortical regions on T2/FLAIR sequences to appear more readily. Migration lines themselves are identified exclusively with MRI as a fine linear hyperintense streak extending from the ventricular region peripherally toward the cortex. These are histologically comprised of displaced giant astrocytes.

Subependymal nodules (SEN) (*major criterion*) are also composed of dysmorphic neurons and giant astrocytes with varying foci of calcification positioned adjacent to and along the periphery of the ventricular walls. Histologically these are also comprised of a mixed lineage of astrocytes. SENs are clearly evident with either CT or MRI imaging modalities (Fig. 143.13). In contrast to other regions of dysplasia, SENs more frequently exhibit calcification. While most SENs remain fairly static in size there are some that enlarge over time. This growth is biologically more likely to occur when the SEN is located within the frontal periventricular regions than elsewhere, but not exclusively so.

Subependymal giant cell astrocytomas (SEGA) (*major criterion*) are comprised of dysmorphic neurons, proliferating astrocytes and giant astrocytes just as the other

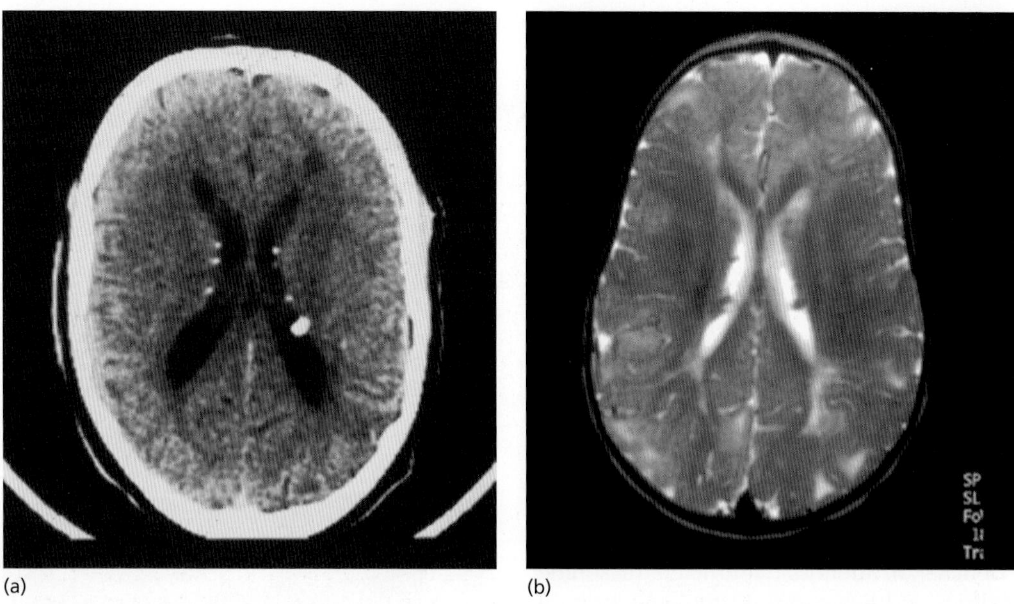

Fig. 143.13 (a) Subependymal nodules (SEN) on cranial computed scan shows multiple calcified subependymal nodules. (b) Similar slice from same patient on T2-weighted brain magnetic resonance imaging axial image shows SEN and cortical dysplasia (tubers and migration lines). Source: DiMario et al. 2015 [51]. Reproduced with permission of Elsevier.

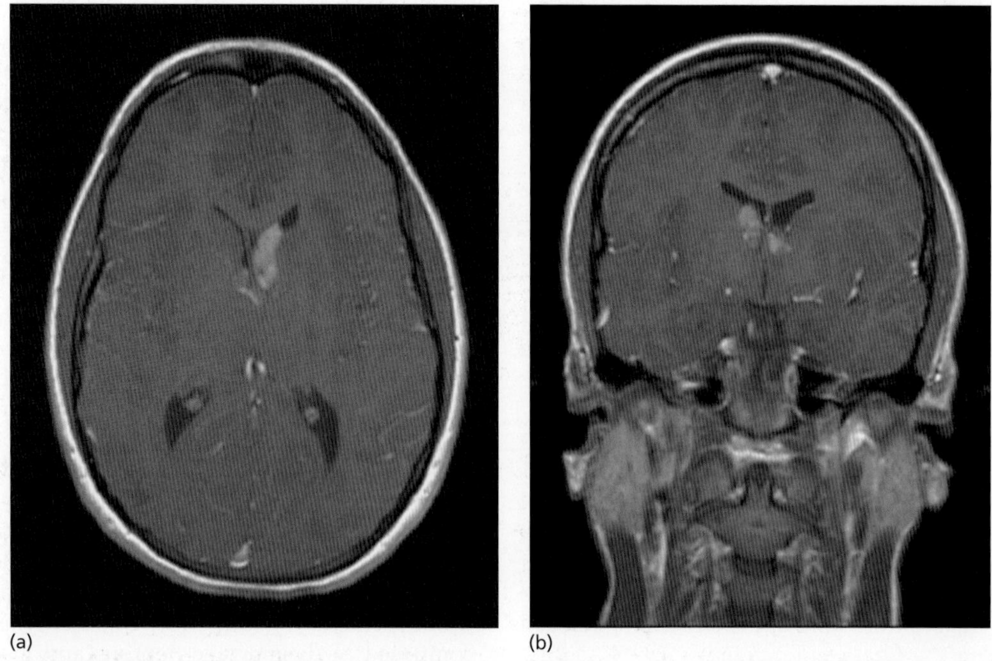

Fig. 143.14 T1-weighted contrast enhanced brain magnetic resonance imaging images. (a) Axial and (b) coronal planes show bilateral subependymal giant cell astrocytomas adjacent to the foramen of Monro.

dysplastic central nervous system lesions found in TSC. These are histologically equivalent to and emanate from SENs but are biologically more active. They have a predilection to occur within the frontal subventricular zone in and around the foramen of Monro (Fig. 143.14). As a consequence to their nonmalignant but hyperplastic growth, there is a risk of cerebrospinal fluid pathway occlusion and potential invasion into the adjacent hypothalamus and optic chiasm [1,12]. Approximately 10–15% of TSC patients develop these lesions, which unlike SEN and the cortical dysplasia of TSC, clearly develop and evolve over time [1,58]. Their peak identification is in late childhood and during the second decade of life, with growth rates plateauing in adulthood [66].

Ophthalmological findings

Multiple (more than one) retinal hamartomas (*major criterion*) are present in 20–25% of TSC affected individuals [1,58]. These are comprised histologically of astrocyte hyperplasia similar to other areas of cortical dysplasia. Most commonly these have the appearance on direct ophthalmoscopy of a flat, smooth, translucent salmon-coloured oval-shaped

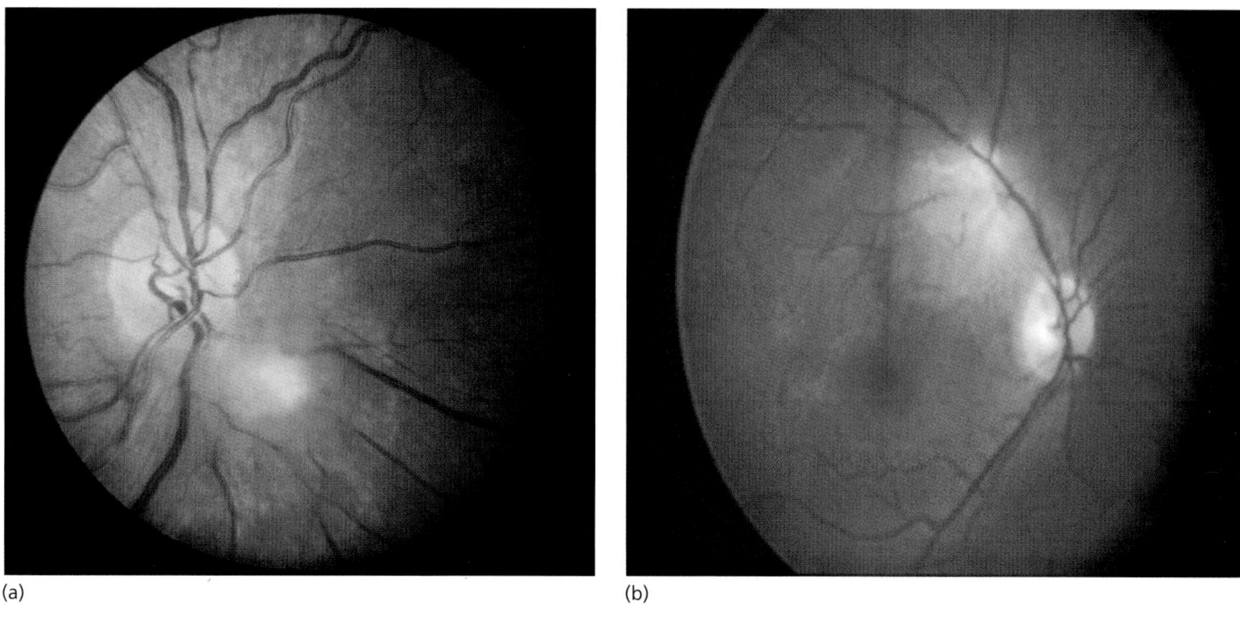

Fig. 143.15 Retinal photographs. (a) A partially translucent and partially calcified retinal hamartoma. (b) A retinal achromic patch.

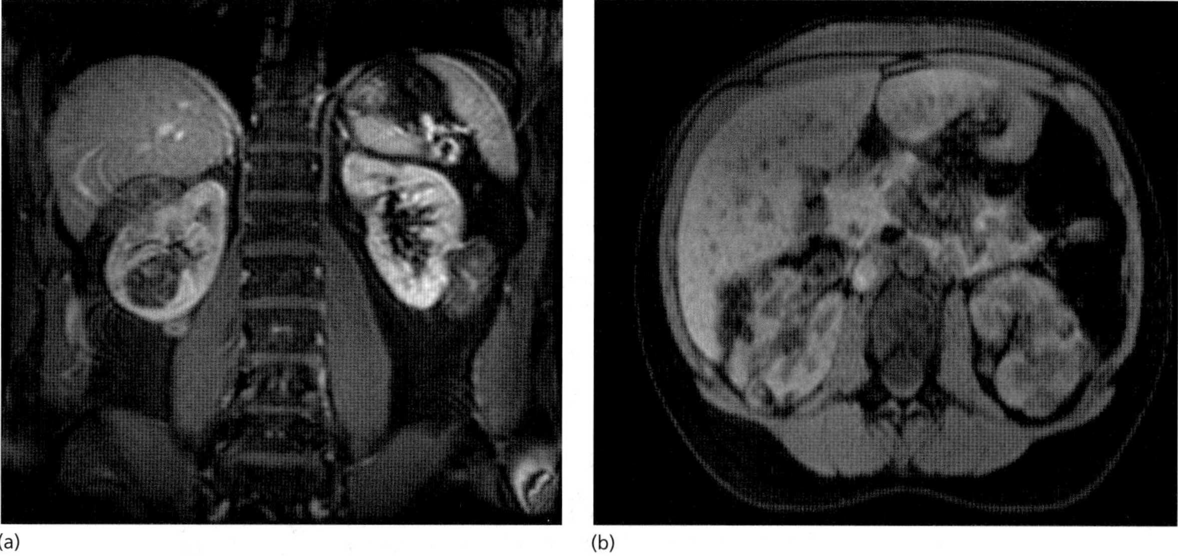

Fig. 143.16 Renal angiomyolipomas. (a) Bilateral intrarenal and exophytic low intensity tumours on magnetic resonance imaging (MRI). (b) Bilateral intrarenal tumours with scattered low intensity small cysts on MRI.

lesion in the superficial layer (Fig. 143.15a). Alternatively, they can be raised, nodular, opaque and calcified, resembling tapioca. Combinations of these two appearances can variably occur [67]. These lesions do not grow but they can become calcified over time. New lesions do not develop over a lifetime. There is rarely any visual impairment associated with them except when they develop directly over the optic nerve or invade the macula. A retinal achromic patch (*minor criterion*) is even less often identified (Fig. 143.15b). These are small areas on the retina or along retinal vessels where there is no pigment.

Renal findings

TSC-associated renal disease is identified in up to 55% of young children and increases in prevalence to about 70–80% by adolescence [68]. Lesions identified within the kidney include angiomyolipomas and multiple cysts (Fig. 143.16). Angiomyolipomas (two or more) is a *major diagnostic criterion*. However, these are not specific to the kidney and may be found in other organs such as the liver, pancreas, spleen and gonads [12,69]. Angiomyolipomas are benign tumours composed of vascular, smooth muscle and adipose tissue, and occur in 55–80% of TSC patients. They are one of a family of tumours, which exhibit perivascular epithelioid cell differentiation and express melanocytic protein, which suggests a neural crest lineage of origin. As such these may arise from multiple sites. These lesions generally contain adipose tissue but 'fat poor' lesions are also identified in TSC. In the kidney, these fat poor lesions are difficult to differentiate from oncocytomas and renal cell carcinomas. Renal biopsy may be necessary to confirm a diagnosis, however; angiomyolipoma tissue is often difficult to interpret histologically and has the appearance of renal carcinoma. Staining with HMB-45 or melanin A antibody confirms angiomyolipoma because these are negative in renal carcinoma.

The renal lesions are a significant source of morbidity and mortality for patients with TSC [70,71]. Renal angiomyolipomas have a high risk of haemorrhage from the development of micro- and macroaneurysms that are prone to rupture [70]. The risk of haemorrhage is proportional to the size of the aneurysm with greatest risk assigned to those larger than 5 mm [70]. Renal angiomyolipomas may grow to impinge upon normal renal parenchyma inducing chronic renal damage and hypertension. The growth rate of these lesions is slow in prepubertal children such that lesions 4 cm or larger in size are found only after puberty. Serial imaging (MRI preferred) is required on an annual or semiannual basis once a lesion is identified, primarily to assess size and evaluate for aneurysm development.

Renal cystic disease (*minor criterion*) occurs in over 40–45% of TSC patients. These are bilateral in over 60% with most having fewer than five in number and a mean diameter of 2 cm in size [7,72]. Cysts range from microcystic size to grossly enlarged polycystic kidneys when associated with the contiguous *PKD1* gene deletion adjacent to *TSC2* on chromosome 16p13. Fortunately, this has been identified in only about 1–2% of TSC patients (Fig. 143.17) [7,72]. Histologically, the cysts are lined with a hyperplastic eosinophilic epithelium that is thought to be pathognomonic. Enlarging cysts may disrupt kidney function to the point of renal failure in TSC affected individuals [71].

Cardiac findings

Cardiac rhabdomyomas (*major criterion*) are the primary lesion identified within the heart of patients with TSC. These are benign tumours identified in up to 50–60% of patients with TSC [73,74]. Conversely, patients with cardiac rhabdomyomas have a 70–80% estimated risk of having TSC [73,74]. This risk is highest with multiple lesions compared with single ones (Fig. 143.18a). However, the cardiac lesion may be the earliest identified sign of TSC. Prenatal diagnosis of cardiac rhabdomyomas in the late second and early third trimester is usual [73,74]. Even a single lesion requires further evaluation for TSC. These arise predominantly from the ventricular septum but can be located in the atria and within the nonseptal walls. The lesions may vary in size, commonly 3–25 mm and are rarely larger. Fetal hydrops and outflow obstruction may occur but are rare [75]. Theoretical consideration for embolic disease exists when lesions are adjacent to cardiac valves. However in reality, this is not a clinical consequence. Cardiac arrhythmias including atrial and ventricular arrhythmia and the Wolff–Parkinson–White syndrome (WPWS) are the more common complications of rhabdomyomas and warrant surveillance.

Histologically, the rhabdomyomas contain hypertrophied spindle cells, which are structurally similar to Purkinje cells. When lesions are located within the atrioventricular junction they can function as accessory conduction

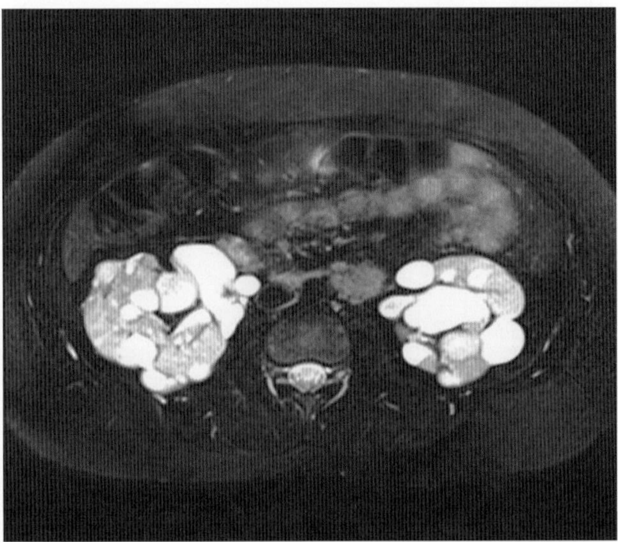

Fig. 143.17 Multicystic kidneys in *TSC2* associated with *PKD1* gene deletion syndrome.

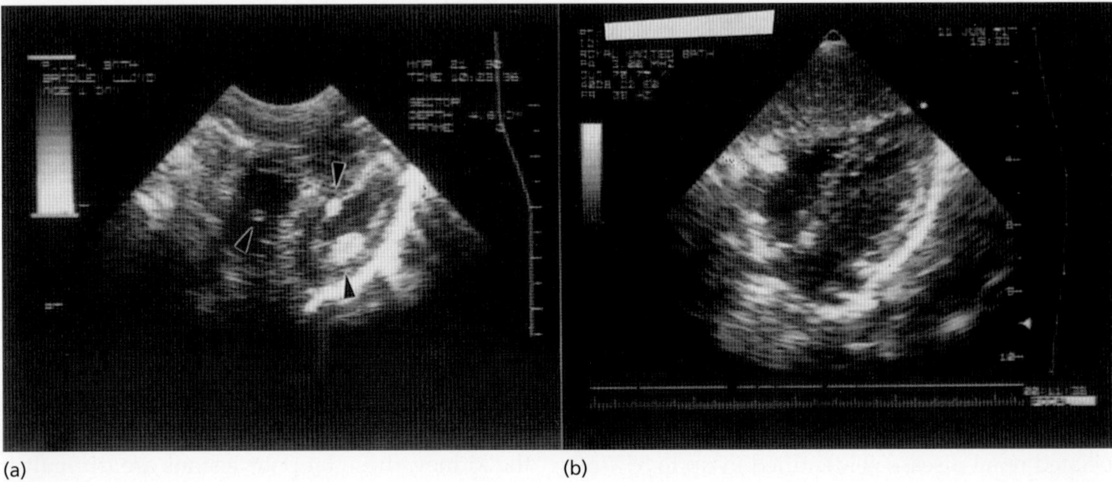

(a) (b)

Fig. 143.18 These two echocardiograms were taken 6 weeks apart. (a) At birth, three rhabdomyomas were present but they are no longer visible at (b) 6 weeks of age. Source: Courtesy Dr A.J. Green.

pathways. The incidence of WPWS has been noted to be about 1.5% in patients with TSC compared with 0.15% in the general population [76,77]. Since after birth these cells no longer divide, the tumour regresses and with this can be resolution of the arrhythmia. Most cardiac lesions spontaneously regress within early childhood (Fig. 143.18). At birth, if an infant has a normal electrocardiogram (ECG) and no cardiac compromise from rhabdomyomas then in the author's experience cardiac problems should not develop in later life.

Pulmonary findings

The most common pulmonary manifestation of TSC is lymphangioleiomyomatosis (*major criterion*) (aka lymphangiomyomatosis or LAM) [78]. It is the third leading cause of death in patients with TSC [71]. This is typically identified in women during childbearing age, but not exclusively [78]. Most identified TSC-LAM patients are asymptomatic when radiographic screening with high-resolution, non-contrast CT scanning (HRCT) reveals cystic changes (Fig. 143.19) [78]. HRCT scanning demonstrates bilateral symmetrical, thin-walled cysts of variable numbers ranging in size from 1 to 50 mm in diameter [78,79]. There may be accompanying hilar and mediastinal adenopathy, nodular densities and thoracic duct dilatation. The incidence of TSC-LAM has been estimated at 30–40% with some estimates as high as 80% when accounting for screening at later ages [12,79]. This complication occurs nearly exclusively in females but upwards of 10% of asymptomatic males with TSC has also been found to have cystic changes on radiographs [80,81].

The natural history of TSC-LAM is not well characterized. However, symptoms often develop by the age of 30–40 years. Patients with moderate cystic changes suffer from progressive exertional dyspnoea and pneumothorax complicated by haemoptysis and ultimately respiratory insufficiency and failure [78]. LAM also occurs spontaneously in the absence of TSC and is designated as S-LAM. Patients with S-LAM are more likely to develop lymphatic complications such as chylous effusion or chylous ascites. Importantly, 30–60% of S-LAM patients have associated renal angiomyolipomas, compared with over 90% of TSC-LAM patients [78,79]. They do not have concurrent dermatological or neurological findings, however. The most recent consensus panel emphasized the need to differentiate S-LAM and TSC-LAM: 'When angiomyolipomas and LAM are both present in a patient with suspected TSC, together they constitute only one major criterion' [12].

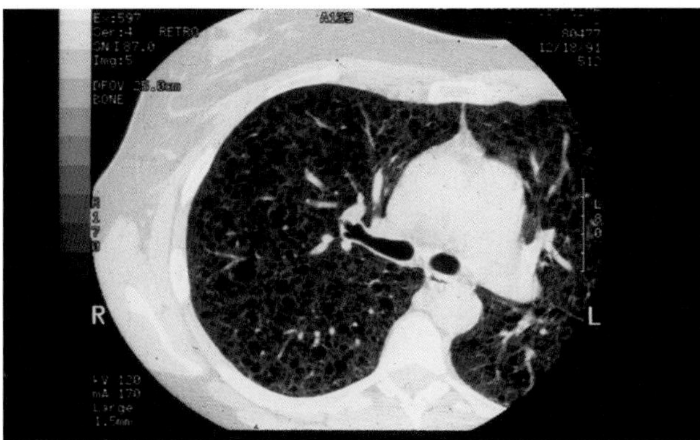

Fig. 143.19 Pulmonary lymphangiomyomatosis on high resolution computed tomography.

An important corollary to the association of patients with angiomyolipoma and S-LAM has been the hypothesis that LAM is a consequence of a benign metastasis. This proposes that benign cells with TSC1 or TSC2 mutations metastasize to the lungs via lymphatic channels or through haematogenous spread from renal angiomyolipomas or from uterine angioleiomyolipoma to seed LAM in the lungs. There are several lines of evidence to support the benign metastasis hypothesis including: (i) LAM cells within lymphadenopathy, lymph ducts and pleural effusions [82]; (ii) LAM cells with LOH for *TSC2* in blood [83]; and (iii) LAM recurs after lung transplantation with LAM cells derived from the recipient's own renal angiomyolipomas [84].

Another potential avenue of therapeutic research stems from the discovery that one of the high mobility group (HMG) of proteins, HMGA2, has been shown to play a major role in aberrant cell proliferation in several benign tumours including: lipomas, uterine leiomyomas, endometrial polyps, adenomas of the salivary gland and pulmonary chondroid hamartomas [85]. HMGA2 was also found in lung tissue samples from 21 patients with LAM and not from normal adult lung or other proliferative interstitial lung diseases, suggesting that HMGA2 in LAM represents aberrant gene activation not just from cellular proliferation [85]. *In vivo* transgenic mice studies found that HMGA2 in smooth muscle cells caused proliferation of these cells in the lung surrounding epithelial cells thus similarly leading to abnormal proliferation and LAM [85]. These results suggest that HMGA2 may also play a central role in the pathogenesis of LAM and is another potential therapeutic candidate. Whether there is a more direct role for this gene, *HMGA2*, in renal angiomyolipomas and TSC pathogenesis awaits further study.

Multifocal micronodular pneumocyte hyperplasia (MMPH) is another but nonspecific pulmonary finding seen in TSC patients. It is suggested by the radiographic identification of small nodular densities scattered throughout the lung fields [86]. These are composed of benign alveolar type II cells that stain with cytokeratin and surfactant proteins A and B, but not with HMB-45. MMPH has no known prognostic or physiological consequences [86].

Nonrenal hamartoma

There are other hamartomatous lesions identified within several organs. They occur in low frequencies and generally without clinical consequence aside from radiographic or clinical identification. Each are considered a minor criterion when encountered. These include: thyroid papillary adenoma, angiomyolipoma/fibroadenoma in the pituitary gland, pancreas or gonads, and hamartomatous rectal polyps [87,88]. Liver and adrenal angiomyolipomas (10–25%) are included as a major criterion under angiomyolipomas previously [12,88].

Skeletal findings
Bony changes on radiographs include cysts, periosteal new bone formation and areas of sclerosis but these are neither considered among the diagnostic criteria for TSC nor clinically important to identify.

Treatment.

Epilepsy
There has been a burgeoning interest in the care of patients with TSC. This is supported by the growing number of TSC specialist clinics worldwide and the increase in translational and clinical trials currently underway and recently published. The discovery of the genetic cause for TSC directly led to our understanding of the mTORC pathway and the pathophysiological basis of the manifestations for TSC. These new insights have propelled further research and hastened the discovery of successful treatment paradigms. A comprehensive review of all treatment approaches required for this multisystem disease would be beyond the scope of this chapter but may be found elsewhere [1,89,90]. A review of some key treatment issues and novel approaches will be highlighted later.

Updated recommendations for the surveillance and management of TSC manifestations have been recently published (Table 143.4) [91]. These undergo revisions periodically when sufficient new data become available to warrant such revision. Nevertheless, because TSC is uniquely manifest in each individual, these general approaches always require individualization depending upon the clinical circumstances and patient wishes.

Epilepsy is an important and often disabling symptom of TSC. Early recognition and effective treatment is thought to improve cognitive development and minimize the detrimental effects it has on quality of life. Approaches to treatment mostly remain in concert with epilepsy treatment of non-TSC patients. These include antiepileptic drug therapy, corticosteroids and adrenocorticotropic hormones, vagus nerve stimulation, ketogenic diet and cortical surgical resection. Antiepileptic drugs are the first-line and mainstay of treatment. All therapeutic interventions are judicially utilized in order to maximize benefit and minimize adverse effects particularly when polytherapies are needed.

TSC-associated infantile spasms (TSC-IS) and focal seizures in infancy present a need for special interventions. TSC-IS occur in 30–40% of TSC patients. This seizure type and an earlier onset portend a worse developmental outcome and greater likelihood for intractable epilepsy. A number of studies have demonstrated a high responsiveness rate for TSC-IS of almost 95% with use of vigabatrin and 35–45% responsiveness for focal seizures in infancy [92,93]. This has prompted international guidelines to advocate for the early institution of vigabatrin in these circumstances [93,94]. Vigabatrin has a mechanism of action that elevates gamma-aminobutyric acid (GABA) levels in the brain and also binds to mTOR. Taurine deficiency coupled with elevated GABA levels in the retina produce the retinal toxicity and explains the resultant irreversible concentric visual field loss identified in 30–40% of treated adult patients [92,95]. Despite identification using visual

Table 143.4 Surveillance and management recommendations for newly diagnosed or suspected tuberous sclerosis complex [91]

Organ system or specialty area	Recommendations
Genetics	• Obtain three-generation family history to assess for additional family members at risk of TSC • Offer genetic testing for family counselling or when TSC diagnosis is in question but cannot be clinically confirmed
Brain	• Perform MRI of the brain to assess for the presence of tubers, subependymal nodules, migrational defects, and subependymal giant cell astrocytoma • Evaluate for TAND • During infancy, educate parents to recognize infantile spasms, even if none have occurred at time of first diagnosis • Obtain baseline routine EEG. If abnormal, especially if features of TAND are also present, follow-up with a 24-hour video EEG to assess for subclinical seizure activity
Kidney	• Obtain MRI of the abdomen to assess for the presence of angiomyolipoma and renal cysts • Screen for hypertension by obtaining an accurate blood pressure • Evaluate renal function by determination of glomerular filtration rate
Lung	• Perform baseline pulmonary function testing (pulmonary function testing and 6-minute walk test) and high-resolution chest computed tomography, even if asymptomatic, in patients at risk of developing lymphangioleiomyomatosis, typically females 18 years or older. Adult males, if symptomatic, should also undergo testing • Provide counsel on smoking risks and oestrogen use in adolescent and adult females
Skin	• Perform a detailed clinical dermatological inspection/examination
Teeth	• Perform a detailed clinical dental inspection/examination
Heart	• Consider fetal echocardiography to detect individuals with high risk of heart failure after delivery when rhabdomyomas are identified via prenatal ultrasound • Obtain an ECG in paediatric patients, especially if younger than 3 years of age • Obtain an ECG in all ages to assess for underlying conduction defects
Eye	• Perform a complete ophthalmological evaluation, including dilated fundoscopy

ECG, electrocardiogram; EEG, electroencephalogram; MRI, magnetic resonance imaging; TAND, TSC-associated neuropsychiatric disorder; TSC, tuberous sclerosis complex.
Source: Krueger and Northrup 2013 [91]. Reproduced with permission of Elsevier.

field perimetry testing there is almost no functional impact and most patients are unaware of their deficit. Supplementation with taurine has minimized this toxicity [95]. The superior responsiveness of TSC-IS over the alternative standard therapy with steroids or adrenocorticotropic hormones injections may be in part caused by its interaction with the mTOR pathway.

The use of mTOR inhibitors for epilepsy has become a focus of clinical trial research. Enhanced mTOR activity is provoked by the excitatory neurotransmitter glutamate, which in turn promotes increased glutamate receptor and potassium channel synthesis and density, altered neuronal dendritic morphology and affects neuronal firing patterns among other effects [96]. These have detrimental effects on memory and learning in mice models of epilepsy. These effects have been abated in these models after treatment with the mTOR inhibitors everolimus and rapamycin (also called sirolimus) [97]. Human multicentre randomized clinical trials have also been underway [98]. Initial prospective open-labelled series had shown reductions in both seizure frequency and duration of 50–70% in a majority of participants treated with everolimus [99]. Currently, a larger scale multicentre, randomized double-blind, placebo-controlled trial in 366 TSC patients with refractory epilepsy has shown efficacy, with reduction in seizure frequency compared with placebo of 29% in the low trough dose and 39% in the high trough dose over 12 weeks [99].

Evaluation for epilepsy surgery in TSC patients is also a suitable intervention for many who are refractory to medical therapy. With appropriate evaluation there is a good likelihood of identifying a primary tuber and surrounding zone that initiates a majority of seizure activity [93,94]. Surgical interruption of epileptic circuits despite multifocal epileptic activity can be beneficial. Multiple cortical resections at one surgery or a staged procedure can be planned. In a recent meta-analysis of 13 studies, compiling the outcomes for 229 TSC patients, the overall rate of postoperative seizure freedom was 59%. Factors predicting better outcomes and a higher rate of seizure freedom were seizure onset later than 1 year of age, unilateral epileptic discharges and lobectomy [100].

SEGA

The development of SEGA in 10–15% of patients with TSC represents a significant disease burden. The typical location of SEGA near the foramen of Monro either unilaterally or bilaterally, has the potential to ultimately produce cerebrospinal fluid obstruction with progressive enlargement. Continued tumour expansion may invade adjacent brain parenchyma compromising the basal ganglia, hypothalamus, thalamus, optic chiasm and optic tracts. These tumours may also continue to grow without symptoms, however, and attain a large size before coming to clinical attention. For this reason, screening neuroimaging is recommended every 1–3 years until 25 years of age depending upon symptoms and findings.

The standard therapeutic approach to management involves surgical resection. Total resection is important because residual tumour ultimately produces recurrence in the same region. Although the majority of SEGAs are surgically resectable, some lesions invade adjacent brain parenchyma early and are less amenable to a complete surgical resection. If there are signs of aggressive growth, or complicating imaging features such as hypothalamic involvement, significant surrounding oedema or an atypical location, then an alternative intervention may be necessary.

An initial pilot treatment trial in five TSC patients using the mTOR inhibitor rapamycin demonstrated reduction in SEGA volume in all patients [101]. This was followed by an open label study of 28 TSC patients with rapamycin, where 32% of 28 patients (9 of 28) had more than 50% SEGA volume reduction at 6 months that persisted through 1 year of treatment [102]. The Exist-1 multicentre, randomized, double-blind, placebo-controlled phase-3 trial using the mTOR inhibitor everolimus with dose titration to a trough level of 5–15 ng/mL, culminated in a sustained volume reduction of more than 50% SEGA at 4 years in 58% of 111 patients (64 of 111) from baseline [103]. Only 7.8% of patients (5 of 111) experienced SEGA growth progression despite treatment. Everolimus now has US Food and Drug Administration (FDA) and European Medicines Agency (EMEA) approval for use in patients who cannot be curatively resected. The overall frequency of side effects have been acceptably low with an incidence of Grade 3–4 adverse effects of less than 4–9%. These include noninfectious pneumonitis, minor infections, angioedema, oral ulceration, acne, increased serum lipids, hyperglycaemia, elevated liver enzymes, lowered blood and platelet counts and rare renal failure [103]. The majority of the adverse effects can be managed with everolimus dose modification and other symptomatic treatment interventions.

Renal angiomyolipomas

The high prevalence of TSC-associated renal disease deserves careful delineation and clinical surveillance. The majority of renal disease exhibited in the 70–80% of patients so afflicted is caused by the development of angiomyolipomas [68]. These are typically multiple and often too numerous to count within an individual kidney, vary in size with a mean of 2.1 cm diameter and are bilaterally present in over 89% of patients [104]. In spite of angiomyolipomas being benign tumours, their progressive growth rate and vascular composition predisposes them to cause the potentially life-threatening complications of renal failure, haemorrhage and malignancy. Fortunately, these outcomes are not common and most patients are asymptomatic. The symptoms of flank or abdominal pain, haematuria, abdominal distension or mass, pernicious vomiting and progressive loss in renal function may herald more ominous complications. The risk of haemorrhage is greatest when individual lesions are more than 4 cm in size and or are accompanied by enlarging aneurysms measuring more than 5 mm in the feeding artery. The estimated frequency of bleeding approaches 25–50% over a lifetime with 20% of those individuals presenting in shock [104,105].

The use of selective arterial embolization is a first-line therapy for symptomatic patients with angiomyolipoma lesions more than 4 cm in diameter, active haemorrhage or in those individuals with asymptomatic lesions more than 8 cm in diameter [105,106]. This procedure results in angioinfarction of the tumour mass that enables preservation of the surrounding unaffected renal parenchyma. A total of 524 patient outcomes were reported in a recent meta-analysis of transarterial embolization for angiomyolipoma [106]. There was a high technical success rate reported at 93.3% associated with a low retreatment rate of 20.9% overall [106]. Lesions underwent a mean reduction in size of 3.4 cm (38.3% reduction in size) over a mean follow-up of 39 months [106]. There was 0% mortality reported but a high rate of postembolization adverse effects of 42.8%. The majority (35.9%) of adverse effects resulted from the self-limited postembolization syndrome, which is an inflammatory response that results in the constellation of symptoms: fever, nausea, vomiting and pain within the first 72 hours after the procedure [106]. Renal sparing treatment approaches are optimal and necessary because of the anticipated progressive growth of angiomyolipoma tumours and the continued accrual of renal compromise from them. Nephrectomy, partial or otherwise, should be considered as a last option or if there is a high suspicion for malignancy [105].

The clinical use of mTOR inhibitors for the management of large angiomyolipomas was prompted by the need for better interventional strategies. Initial case reports using rapamycin to inhibit tumour growth demonstrated tumour size reduction, bleeding control and preserved renal function in patients with TSC and angiomyolipoma and also for patients treated for LAM who had angiomyolipoma [107–111]. These initial reports have been followed by large scale, randomized, double-blind, placebo-controlled multicentre trials using both rapamycin and everolimus [112–114]. In a study of 36 patients with TSC or TSC-LAM using rapamycin, the overall response rate was 44.4% (16 of 36) with a partial response and 47.2% (17 of 36) with stable disease [112]. The mean decrease in kidney tumour size was 29.9% at 1 year [112]. There were three drug-related grade 3 adverse events: lymphopenia, headache and weight gain. Importantly, renal angiomyolipomas regrew when rapamycin was discontinued but response persisted when treatment was continued. There was the observation of SEGA regression, liver angiomyolipoma reduction, subjective improvement in facial angiofibromas in 57% and stable lung function in women with TSC-LAM ($n = 15$). Serum vascular endothelial growth factor D (VEGF-D) levels were elevated at baseline and decreased with rapamycin treatment and were identified as a correlative biomarker [112].

The more recent multicentre, randomized, double-blind, placebo-controlled, phase-3 EXIST-2 trial (everolimus for angiomyolipoma associated with TSC or sporadic lymphangioleiomyomatosis), enrolled 118 TSC patients with at least one renal lesion measuring 3 cm or more to receive 10 mg daily of everolimus or placebo. The angiomyolipoma response rate of a 50% or more reduction in the size of the largest target lesion was achieved at 6 months in 42% (33 of 79) for the everolimus group and 0% (0 of 39) for placebo. The most common adverse events in the everolimus group were stomatitis (48%), nasopharyngitis (24%) and acne-like skin lesions (22%) [113]. In the subsequent extension phase of this trial the response rate in 107 patients at a median exposure of 28.9 months was 54% [114]. The proportion of patients who demonstrated size reduction in lesions increased over time such that angiomyolipoma reductions of 30% or more and 50% or more reached 81.6% (62 of 76) and 64.5% (49 of 76), respectively, by 96 weeks [114]. Renal bleeding was not observed in patients treated with everolimus [114].

Pulmonary LAM

TSC-LAM is an insidiously progressive disorder that initially manifests symptoms of exertional dyspnea and pneumothorax in women of child-bearing age. This presentation has a profound impact upon their quality of life by virtue of influencing family planning decisions, air travel implications, escalation in healthcare needs and limitations upon physical activity. An estimated 30–40% of women with TSC and an additional five persons per million sporadically are affected [78,115].

The destruction of lung tissue with associated cystic cavitation is induced by the invasion of hyperproliferative smooth-muscle cells that express two lymphangiogenic growth factors: VEGF-C and VEGF-D [116]. High-resolution noncontrast chest CT scans for screening and in follow-up after diagnosis is coupled with oximetry at rest and with exertion. Bronchodilator therapy may be effective at symptom control and improvement in hypoxaemia for patients with reversible airway obstruction to maintain oxygen saturations greater than 90% [78,117]. The need for mechanical or chemical pleurodesis at the first onset of pneumothorax is also indicated [78]. Pulmonary function measures such as forced expiratory volume in one second (FEV_1), can show an inexorable yearly decline at a rate of up to 75–118 mL per year despite the use of progesterone [117,118]. When FEV_1 declines to less than 30% of predicted or there is disabling dyspnoea and hypoxaemia, lung transplantation may be considered.

The responsiveness of LAM to mTOR inhibitor therapy was observed during preclinical studies and suggested with observations made during early trials designed for the treatment of angiomyolipomas in TSC patients and lymphangioleiomyomatosis [110–112]. A subsequent large scale international, multicentre, randomized, placebo-controlled study using rapamycin for 1 year in 89 eligible LAM patients demonstrated a significant reduction in the rate of decline in the FEV_1 measure [115]. The enrollees had a mean FEV_1 measured at 48% predicted at enrolment. There was only a 1 mL ± 2 mL per month decline observed in the rapamycin treated group (n=43) compared with a 12 mL ± 2 mL per month decline in the placebo group [115]. This amounted to an 11% (153 mL) absolute difference between groups at 1 year [115]. This degree of improvement in FEV_1 is perceived by patients and deemed clinically meaningful. Nonetheless, there was no significant difference between groups on the 6-minute walk test. Improvements in quality of life and other functional performance measures paralleled reduction in VEGF-D levels [115]. There was a concomitant corresponding decline in lung function between groups with discontinuation of the study treatment without any observed rebound rapid decline [115].

Facial angiofibromas

Angiofibromas can be identified on the skin in patients with several genetic disorders but are the hallmark of TSC [54,119]. Facial angiofibromas appear in 80–85% of TSC patients and are a major diagnostic criterion. These lesions are hamartoma, just as many of the associated lesions of TSC, with a proliferation of fibroblasts and dilated blood vessels surrounded by collagen fibres and giant cells. Epidermal hyperkeratosis and melanocytic hyperplasia can also be identified on skin biopsies [120]. After the initial papular erythematous eruption develops many can undergo coalescence into plaques. Larger lesions located internally or subcutaneously are uncommon (see Fig. 143.7). Aside from the obvious cosmetic appearance these lesions can be prone to excoriation and bleeding from minor trauma and shaving. This is particularly of true of the larger papules. The majority of treatments described for facial angiofibromas are based primarily upon case reports and small series experience with limited rigorous evidence of response. These treatment modalities fall under three main categories: physical treatments, laser treatments and medical treatments (Table 143.5).

Physical treatments are often painful and should be considered invasive with general anaesthesia required in most instances. Although many patients will experience good results the potential for hypertrophic scarring, altered skin pigmentation and infection can occur as complications. Often repeated treatments are needed over time because of the recurrence and regrowth of treated skin areas. Cryotherapy does not require anaesthesia but may need multiple treatments for adequate results. Dermabrasion is the technique most often utilized, especially for large lesions. This involves 'shaving' the skin surface under anaesthesia and has had generally good outcomes in the short term [121]. Extensive areas of dermabrasion have been coupled with cultured epithelial autografts to re-epithelialize the skin surface [122]. The grafts need to be protected so as to ensure survival, which limits the applicability of this technique. This would not be a good option for children or cognitively impaired individuals.

Table 143.5 Treatment modalities for facial angiofibromas [120]

Modality
Physical treatments
Radiofrequency ablation
Cryotherapy
Electrocoagulation
Dermabrasion
Laser treatments
Argon
Potassium-titanyl-phosphate
Copper vapour
Carbon dioxide
Pulsed dye laser
Medical treatments
Tranilast (N-3,4-dimethoxycinnamoyl-anthranilic acid)
Podophyllotoxin
Timolol 0.5% gel
Rapamycin ointments

Laser treatments have become the primary treatment intervention for facial angiofibromas in many circumstances. This technique also often requires general anaesthesia but can be accomplished in serial sessions using topical anaesthetics as well. There are various types of lasers available. The carbon dioxide (CO_2) lasers are capable of treating larger, particularly nodular and deeper fibrous lesions effectively. However, the risk of hypertrophic scarring has been high 53.8% [123]. Despite the initial good results after treatment, lesions commonly recur over several years. The pulsed dye laser (PDL) has become the better laser option for the less nodular but erythematous angiofibromas. The PDL utilizes the photocoagulation properties of the laser to maximally ablate vascular components of the lesion [123]. As a result there is reduction in the erythema but minimal effect upon the fibrous component. Combination approaches may be needed in circumstances where both nodular and erythematous angiofibromas are present.

Up until now, medical treatments have been limited and anecdotal. However, with recent research there are more options to complement the physical and laser therapies described above. Several topical and oral agents have been reported for use in TSC angiofibroma treatment. Tranilast is a compound with antiallergic properties used to prevent keloid and hypertrophic scarring [124]. Early effectiveness for facial angiofibromas and ungual fibromas has been reported in a limited number of TSC patients [125]. Podophyllotoxin (25% solution), a topically applied agent for warts, has also been reported with successful use in a patient with TSC facial angiofibromas [126]. Similarly, a single TSC patient has been reported with good responsiveness to twice daily topical application of the β-blocker, timolol 0.5% gel, prior to combination therapy with PDL and CO_2 laser treatment [127]. The reduction in erythema was marked in comparison to facial regions not treated with the gel beforehand despite the use of PDL [127]. The study of oral mTOR inhibitors (rapamycin and everolimus) for SEGA, renal angiomyolipomas and LAM have all yielded observations that suggested facial angiofibromas are also responsive to the systemic effects of these agents [50,102,103,112,113,128]. However, the use of an oral and systemic mTOR inhibitor solely for a dermatological lesion is not an approved indication for this treatment approach. Alternatively, topically applied but not commercially prepared or approved mTOR inhibitor preparations for this use have become more applicable and evidenced based. An extensive review of the literature reporting topical mTOR inhibitors used for TSC facial angiofibromas and hypomelanotic macules has summarized data to date [129]. The most commonly used formulations were crushed tablets of rapamycin compounded with oil or water-based ointment at concentrations ranging from 0.003 to 1% (0.1 to

Table 143.6 Internet resources for patients and professionals

Tuberous Sclerosis Complex International: http://www.tscinternational.org
Tuberous Sclerosis Association UK: http://www.tuberous-sclerosis.org
Tuberous Sclerosis Alliance: http://www.tsalliance.org
Tuberous Sclerosis Canada: http://www.tscanada.ca
OrphaNet: http://www.orpha.net
Autism Society: http://www.autism-society.org
The LAM Foundation: https://www.thelamfoundation.org/
TSC1 & *TSC2* database site: http://chromium.lovd.nl/LOVD2/TSC

Table 143.7 Research opportunities

Priorities moving forward
1. Understanding phenotypic heterogeneity in tuberous sclerosis complex (TSC)
2. Gaining a deeper knowledge of TSC signalling pathways and the cellular consequences of TSC deficiency
3. Improving TSC disease models
4. Developing clinical biomarkers for TSC
5. Facilitating therapeutics and clinical trials research

Source: Adapted from [131] (https://www.ninds.nih.gov/Disorders/All-Disorders/Tuberous-Sclerosis-Information-Page4).

0.2% most common) with observation times ranging from 6 weeks to 30 months [129]. There has been only one randomized, double-blind controlled trial of topical rapamycin. This trial administered very low dose concentrations ranging from 0.003% to 0.015% in comparison with other reports [130]. Overall, there was subjective responsiveness of angiofibromas in almost all treated patients. Children younger than 10 years seem to benefit most and patients with lesions that elevate more than 3–4 mm benefit least [129,130]. There were limitations in outcome methods, however, because most were self-reports and there were few with right–left face comparison or serial photographic analysis. A few studies also found some reduction in the hypomelanotic macule size [129]. There were no significant systemic or local adverse effects.

Moving forward. The Tuberous Sclerosis international organization along with affiliated National TSC Associations worldwide aim to increase knowledge, promote research and provide support and resources for the TSC community (Table 143.6). Additional research efforts are currently underway in the important areas of neurocognition and behaviour, the extension of our understanding of the TSC signalling pathways, further exploration of animal models of TSC, an expansion of our current treatment approaches and the development of novel therapies. The identification and implementation of effective preventative strategies against the development of TSC-associated complications will be a priority. Table 143.7 contains the outline of the recommendations from the 2015 Strategic Planning Conference.

References

1 **Kwiatkowsi D, Whittemore V, Thiele E (eds). Tuberous Sclerosis Complex: Genes, Clinical Features, and Therapeutics. Weinheim: Wiley-Blackwell, 2010.**

2 Wiederholt WC, Gomez MR, Kurland LT. Incidence and prevalence of tuberous sclerosis in Rochester, Minnesota, 1950 through 1982. Neurology 1985;35:600–3.

3 Hong C-H, Darling TN, Lee C-H. Prevalence of tuberous sclerosis complex in Taiwan: a national population-based study. Neuroepidemiology 2009;33:335–41

4 Hyman MH, Whittemore VH. National Institutes of Health consensus conference: tuberous sclerosis complex. Arch Neurol 2000;57:662–5.

5 **European Chromosome 16 Tuberous Sclerosis Consortium. Identification and characterization of the tuberous sclerosis gene on chromosome 16. Cell 1993;75:1305–15.**

6 **van Slegtenhorst M, de Hoogt R, Hermans C et al. Identification of the tuberous sclerosis gene TSC1 on chromosome 9q34. Science 1997;277:805–8.**

7 **Dabora SL, Joswiak S, Franz DN et al. Mutational analysis in a cohort of 224 tuberous sclerosis patients indicates increased severity of TSC2, compared to TSC1, disease in multiple organs. Am J Hum Genet 2001;68:64–80.**

8 **Cheadle J, Reeve M, Samson J et al. Molecular genetic advances in tuberous sclerosis. Hum Genet 2000;62:345–57.**

9 **Au KS, Williams AT, Roach ES et al. Genotype/phenotype correlation in 325 individuals referred for a diagnosis of tuberous sclerosis complex in the United States. Genet Med 2007;9:88–100.**

10 Camposano SE, Greenberg E, Kwaitkowski DJ, Thiele EA. Distinct clinical characteristics of tuberous sclerosis complex patients with no mutation identified. Ann Hum Genet 2009;73:141–6.

11 **Tee AR, Fingar DC, Manning BD et al. Tuberous sclerosis complex-1 and -2 gene products function together to inhibit mammalian target of rapamycin (mTOR)-mediated downstream signaling. Proc Natl Acad Sci USA 2002;99:13571–6.**

12 **Northrup, H, Krueger, DA, on behalf of the International Tuberous Sclerosis Complex Consensus Group. Tuberous Sclerosis Complex Diagnostic Criteria Update: Recommendations of the 2012 International Tuberous Sclerosis Complex Consensus Conference. Pediatr Neurol 2013;49:243–54.**

13 von Recklinghausen F. Ein Herz von einem Neugeborenen welches mehrere Theil nach aussen, Theils nach den hohlen prominirende Tumoren (Myomen) trug. Verh Ges Geburtsh 25 Marz. Monatsschr Geburtskd 1862;20:1–2.

14 Bourneville DM. Sclerose tubereuse des circonvolutions cerebrales: idiotie et epilepsie hemiplegique. Arch Neurol (Paris) 1880;1:81–91.

15 Pringle JJ. A case of congenital adenoma sebaceum. Br J Dermatol 1890;2:1–14.

16 Bourneville DM, Brissaud E. Idiotie et epilepsie symptomatiques de sclerose tubereuse ou hypertrophique. Arch Neurol (Paris) 1900;10:29–39.

17 Perusini G. Uber einen Fall von Sclerosis tuberosa hypertropica. Monatsschr Psychiatr Neurol 1905;17:69–255.

18 Vogt H. Zur diagnostik der tuberosen Skelrose. Z Erforsch Behandl Jugendl Schwachsinns 1908;2:1–12.

19 Berg H. Vererbung der tuberosen Sklerose durch zweibzw. Drei Generationen. Z Ges Neurol Psychiatr 1913;19:528–39.

20 Van der Hoeve J. Eye symptoms in tuberous sclerosis of the brain. Trans Ophthalmol Soc UK 1920;40:329–34.

21 Critchley M, Earl CJC. Tuberous sclerosis and allied conditions. Brain 1932;55:311–46.

22 Gunther M, Penrose LS. The genetics of epiloia. J Genet 1935;31:413–30.

23 Hunt A, Lindenbaum RH. Tuberous sclerosis: a new estimate of prevalence within the Oxford region. J Med Genet 1984;21:272–7.

24 Webb DW, Fryer AE, Osborne JP. Morbidity associated with tuberous sclerosis: a population study. Dev Med Child Neurol 1996;38:146–55.

25 O'Callaghan FJ, Shiell AW, Osborne JP, Martyn CN. Prevalence of tuberous sclerosis estimated by capture-recapture analysis. Lancet 1998;351:1490.

26 Devlin LA, Shepherd CH, Crawford H, Morrison PJ. Tuberous sclerosis complex: clinical features, diagnosis, and prevalence within Northern Ireland. Dev Med Child Neurol 2006;48:495–9.

27 Fisher OD, Stevenson AC. Frequency of epiloia in Northern Ireland. Br J Prev Soc Med 1956;10:134–5.

28 Umapathy D, Johnston AW. Tuberous sclerosis: prevalence in the Grampian region of Scotland. J Ment Defic Res 1989;33:349–55.

29 Ahlsen G, Gillberg IC, Lindblom R, Gillberg C. Tuberous sclerosis in western Sweden. A population study of cases with early childhood onset. Arch Neurol 1994;51:76–81.

30 Ohno K, Takeshita K, Arima M. Frequency of tuberous sclerosis in Sanin district (Japan) and birth weight of patients with tuberous sclerosis. Brain Dev 1981;3:57–64.

31 Shepherd CW, Beard CM, Gomez MR et al. Tuberous sclerosis complex in Olmsted County, Minnesota 1950–1989. Arch Neurol 1991;48:400–1.

32 Webb DW, Fryer AE, Osborne JP. On the incidence of fits and mental retardation in tuberous sclerosis. J Med Genet 1991;28:395–7.

33 Fryer AE, Chalmers A, Connor JM et al. Evidence that the gene for tuberous sclerosis is on chromosome 9. Lancet 1987;i:659–61.

34 Kandt RS, Haines JL, Smith M et al. Linkage of an important gene locus for tuberous sclerosis to a chromosome 16 marker for polycystic kidney disease. Nature Genet 1992;2:37–41.

35 European Chromosome 16 Tuberous Sclerosis Consortium. Identification and characterization of the tuberous sclerosis gene on chromosome 16. Cell 1993;75:1305–15.

36 Knudson AG Jr. Mutation and cancer: statistical study of retinoblastoma. Proc Natl Acad Sci USA 1971;68:820–3.

37 Chan JA, Zhang H, Roberts PS et al. Pathogenesis of tuberous sclerosis subependymal giant cell astrocytomas: biallelic inactivation of TSC1 or TSC2 leads to mTOR activation. J Neuropathol Exp Neurol 2004;63:1236–42.

38 Henske EP, Scheithauer BW, Short MP et al. Allelic loss is frequent in tuberous sclerosis kidney lesions but rare in brain lesions. Am J Hum Genet 1996;59:400–6.

39 Niida Y, Stemmer-Rachamimov AO, Logrip M et al. Survey of somatic mutations in tuberous sclerosis complex (TSC) hamartomas suggests different genetic mechanisms for pathogenesis of TSC lesions. Am J Hum Genet 2001;69:493–503.

40 Potter CJ, Pedraza LG, Xu T. Akt regulates growth by directly phosphorylating Tsc2. Nature Cell Biol 2002;4:658–65.

41 Inoki K, Li Y, Zhu T et al. TSC2 is phosphorylated and inhibited by Akt and suppresses mTOR signaling. Nature Cell Biol 2002;4:648–57.

42 Mannaa M, Kramer S, Boschmann M, Gollasch M. mTOR and regulation of energy homeostasis in humans. [Review]. J Mol Med 2013;91:1167–75.

43 Laplante M, Sabatini DM. mTOR signaling in growth control and disease. Cell 2012;149:274–93.

44 Lipton JO, Sahin M. The neurology of mTOR. Neuron 2014;84:275–91.

45 Ebrahimi-Fakhari D, Wahlster L, Hoffmann GF et al. Emerging role of autophagy in pediatric neurodegenerative and neurometabolic diseases. Pediatr Res 2014;75:217–26.

46 Brown EJ, Albers MW, Shin TB et al. A mammalian protein targeted by G1-arresting rapamycin-receptor complex. Nature 1994;369:756–8.

47 Sabers CJ, Martin MM, Brunn GJ et al. Isolation of a protein target of the FKBP12-rapamycin complex in mammalian cells. J Biol Chem 1995;270:815–22.

48 Sahin M. Targeted treatment trials for tuberous sclerosis and autism: no longer a dream. Curr Opin Neurobiol 2012;22:895–901.

49 Julich K, Sahin M. Mechanism-based treatment in tuberous sclerosis complex. Pediatr Neurol 2014;50:290–6.

50 Kohrman MH. Emerging treatments in the management of tuberous sclerosis complex. Pediatr Neurol 2012;46:267–75.

51 DiMario FJ, Sahin M, Ebrahimi-Fakhari D. Tuberous sclerosis complex. Pediatr Clin N Am 2015;62:633–48.

52 Park SH, Pepkowitz SH, Kerfoot C et al. Tuberous sclerosis in a 20-week gestation fetus: immunohistochemical study. Acta Neuropathol (Berl) 1997;94:180–6.

53 De Vries P, Humphrey A, McCartney D et al. TSC Behaviour Consensus Panel. Consensus clinical guidelines for the assessment of cognitive and behavioural problems in tuberous sclerosis. Eur Child Adolesc Psychiatry 2005;14:183–90.

54 Vidal A, Iglesias MJ, Fernández B et al. Cutaneous lesions associated to multiple endocrine neoplasia syndrome type 1. J Eur Acad Derm Ven 2008;22:835–8.

55 Spring P, Fellman F, Giraud S et al. Syndrome of Birt-Hogg-Dube', a histological pitfall with similarities to tuberous sclerosis: a report of three cases. Am J Dermatolopathol 2013;35:241–5.

56 Chudnow RS, Wolfe GI, Sparagana SP et al. Abnormal sudomotor function in the hypomelanotic macules of tuberous sclerosis complex. J Child Neurol 2000;15:529–32.

57 Mlynarczyk G. Enamel pitting: a common symptom of tuberous sclerosis. Oral Surg Oral Med Oral Pathol 1991;71:63–7.

58 Webb DW, Fryer AE, Osborne JP. Morbidity associated with tuberous sclerosis: a population study. Dev Med Child Neurol 1996;38:146–55.

59 Curatolo P, Verdecchia M, Bombardieri R. Tuberous sclerosis complex: a review of neurological aspects. Eur J Paediatr Neurol 2002;6:15–23.

60 Theile E. Managing epilepsy in tuberous sclerosis complex. J Child Neurol 2004;19:680–6.

61 Prather P, de Vries P. Behavioral and cognitive aspects of tuberous sclerosis complex. J Child Neurol 2004;19:666–74.

62 Pulsifer M, Winterkorn E, Theile E. Psychological profile of adults with tuberous sclerosis complex. Epilepsy Behav 2007;10:402–6.

63 de Vries PJ, Whittemore VH, Leclezio L et al. Tuberous sclerosis associated neuropsychiatric disorders (TAND) and TAND checklist. Pediatr Neurol 2015;52:25–35.

64 Mizuguchi M, Takashima S. Neuropathology of tuberous sclerosis. Brain Dev 2001;23:508–15.

65 Peters J, Prohl AK, Tomas-Fernandez XK et al. Tubers are neither static nor discrete. Neurology 2015;85:1536–45.

66 Goh S. Subependymal giant cell tumors in tuberous sclerosis complex. Neurology 2004;63:1457–61.

67 Robertson DM. Ophthalmic manifestations of tuberous sclerosis. Ann N Y Acad Sci 1991;615:17–25.

68 McCullough DL, ScottR Jr, Seybold HM. Renal angiomyolipoma (hamartoma): a review of the literature and case report of 7 cases. J Urol 1971;105:32–44.

69 Fricke BL, Donnelly LF, Casper KA, Bissler JJ. Frequency and imaging appearance of hepatic angiomyolipomas in pediatric and adult patients with tuberous sclerosis. Am J Roentgenol 2004;182:1027–30.

70 Bissler J, Kingswood J. Renal angiomyolipomata. Kidney Int 2004;66:924–34.

71 Shepherd C, Gomez M, Lie J, Crowson C. Causes of death in patients with tuberous sclerosis. Mayo Clin Proc 1991;66:792–6.

72 Brook-Carter P, Peral B, Ward C et al. Deletion of the TSC2 and PKD1 genes associated with severe infantile polycystic kidney disease a contiguous gene syndrome. Nat Genet 1994;8:328–32.

73 Harding CO, Pagon RA. Incidence of tuberous sclerosis in patients with cardiac rhabdomyoma. Am J Med Genet 1990;37:443–6.

74 Tworetzky W, McElhinney DB, Margossian R et al. Association between cardiac tumors and tuberous sclerosis in the fetus and neonate. Am J Cardiol 2003;92:487–9.

75 Black M, Kadlez M, Smallhorn J, Freedom R. Cardiac rhabdomyomas and obstructive left heart disease: histologically but not functionally benign. Ann Thorac Surg 1998;65:1388–90.

76 Freedom RM, Lee KJ, MacDonald C, Taylor G. Selected aspects of cardiac tumors in infancy and childhood. Pediatr Cardiol 2000;21:299–316.

77 Mas C, Penny DJ, Menahem S. Pre-excitation syndrome secondary to cardiac rhabdomyomas in tuberous sclerosis. J Paediatr Child Health 2000,36:84–6.

78 McCormack F, Henske E. Lymphangioleiomyomatosis and pulmonary disease in TSC. In: Kwiatkowsi D, Whittemore V, Thiele E (eds) Tuberous Sclerosis Complex: Genes, Clinical Features, and Therapeutics. Weinheim: Wiley-Blackwell, 2010.

79 Cudzilo C, Szczesniak R, Brody A et al. Lymphangioleiomyomatosis screening in women with tuberous sclerosis. Chest 2013;144:578–85.

80 McCormack FX, Moss J. S-LAM in a man? Am J Respir Crit Care Med 2007;176:3–5.

81 Adriaensen ME, Schaefer-Prokop CM, Duyndam DA et al. Radiological evidence of lymphangioleiomyomatosis in female and male patients with tuberous sclerosis complex. Clin Radiol 2011;66:625–8.

82 Kumasaka T, Seyama K, Mitani K. Lymphangiogenesis-mediated shedding of LAM cell clusters as a mechanism for dissemination in lymphangioleiomyomatosis. Am J Surg Pathol 2005;29:1356–66

83 Crooks DM, Pacheco-Rodriguez G, DeCastro RM. Molecular and genetic analysis of disseminated neoplastic cells in lymphangioleiomyomatosis. Proc Natl Ac Sci USA 2004;101:17462–7.

84 Karbowniczek M, Astrinidis A, Balsara BR et al. Recurrent lymphangiomyomatosis after transplantation: Genetic analyses reveal a metastatic mechanism. Am J Respir Crit Care Med 2003;167:976–82.

85 D'Armiento J, Imai K, Schiltz J et al. Identification of the benign mesenchymal tumor gene HMGA2 in lymphangiomyomatosis. Cancer Res 2007;67:1902–9.

86 Kobashi Y, Sugiu T, Mouri K et al. Clinicopathological analysis of multifocal micronodular pneumocyte hyperplasia associated with tuberous sclerosis in Japan. Respirology 2008;13:1076–81.

87 O'Callaghan F, Osborne J. Endocrine, gastrointestinal, hepatic, and lymphatic manifestations of tuberous sclerosis complex. In: Kwiatkowski D, Whittemore V, Thiele E (eds) Tuberous Sclerosis Complex: Genes, Clinical Features, and Therapeutics. Weinheim: Wiley-Blackwell, 2010:369–85.

88 Nakhleh RE. Angiomyolipoma of the liver. Pathol Case Rev 2009;14:47–9.

89 DiMario FJ. Tuberous sclerosis complex. e-Pocrates online. Point of Care Monograph. Br Med J, July 2008. Updated July 2015.

90 Curatolo P, Maria BL. Tuberous sclerosis complex. In: Dulac O, Lassonde M, Sarnat HB (eds) Pediatric Neurology Part I: Chapter 38, Handbook of Clinical Neurology. New York: Elsevier, 2013.

91 Krueger DA, Northrup H, on behalf of the International Tuberous Sclerosis Complex Consensus Group. Tuberous Sclerosis Complex Surveillance and Management: Recommendations of the 2012 International Tuberous Sclerosis Complex Consensus Conference. Pediatr Neurol 2013;49:255–65.

92 Hancock E, Osborne J. Vigabatrin in the treatment of infantile spasms in tuberous sclerosis: literature review. J Child Neurol 1999;14:71–4.

93 Curatolo P, Jozwiak S, Nabbout R et al. Management of epilepsy associated with tuberous sclerosis complex (TSC): clinical recommendations. Eur J Paediatr Neurol 2012;16:582–6.

94 Thiele E. Managing epilepsy in tuberous sclerosis complex. J Child Neurol 2004;19:680–6.

95 Fecarotta C, Sergott RC. Viagabatrin-associated visual field loss. Int Ophthal Clin 2012;52:87–94.

96 Wong M. Mammilian target of rapamycin (mTOR) inhibition as a potential antiepileptogenic therapy: from tuberous sclerosis to common acquired epilepsies. Epilepsia 2009;51:27–36.

97 Zeng LH, Rensing NR, Wong M. The mammilian target of rapamycin signaling pathway mediates epileptogenesis in a model of temporal lobe epilepsy. J Neurosci 2009;29:6964–72.

98 Curatolo P. Mechanistic target of rapamycin (mTOR) in tuberous sclerosis complex-associated epilepsy. Pediatr Neurol 2015;52:281–9.

99 French JA, Lawson JA, Yapici Z et al. Adjunctive everolimus therapy for the treatment of refractory seizures associated with tuberous sclerosis complex: results from a randomized, placebo-controlled, phase 3 trial. Presented at American Academy of Neurology meeting, April 15–21, 2016. Vancouver, BC, Canada.

100 Zhang K, Hu WH, Zhang C et al. Predictors of seizure freedom after surgical management of tuberous sclerosis complex: a systematic review and meta-analysis. [Review]. Epilepsy Res 2013;105:377–83.

101 Franz DN, Leonard J, Tudor C et al. Rapamycin causes regression of astrocytomas in tuberous sclerosis complex. Ann Neurol 2006;59:490–8.

102 Kruger DA, Care MM, Holland K et al. Everolimus for subependymal giant-cell astrocytomas in tuberous sclerosis. N Eng J Med 2010;363:1801–11.

103 Franz DN, Belousova E, Sparagna S et al. Efficacy and safety of everolimus for subependymal giant cell astrocytomas associated with tuberous sclerosis complex (EXIST-1): a multicentre, randomized, placebo-controlled phase 3 trial. Lancet 2013;381:125–32.

104 Casper KA, Donnelly LF, Chen B, Bissler JJ. Tuberous sclerosis complex: renal imaging finding. Radiol 2002;225:451–6.

105 Kessler OJ, Gillon G, Neuman M et al. Management of renal angiomyolipomas: analysis of 15 cases. Eur Urol 1998;33:572–5.

106 Murray TE, Doyle F, Lee M. Transarterial embolization of angiomyolipoma: a systematic review. J Urol 2015;194:635–9.

107 Wienecke R, Fackler I, Linsenmaier U et al. Antitumoral activity of rapamycin in renal angiomyolipoma associated with tuberous sclerosis complex. Am J Kidney Dis 2006;48:27–9.

108 Peces R, Peces C, Cuesta-Lopez E et al. Low-dose rapamycin reduces kidney volume angiomyolipomas and prevents the loss of renal function in a patient with tuberous sclerosis complex. Nephrol Dial Transplant 2010;25:3787–91.

109 Krischock L, Beach R, Taylor J. Sirolimus and tuberous-associated renal angiomyolipomas. Arch Dis Child 2010;95:391–2

110 Davies DM, Johnson SR, Tattersfield AE et al. Sirolimus therapy in tuberous sclerosis or sporadic lymphangioleiomyomatosis. N Engl J Med 2008;358:200–3.

111 Bissler JJ, McCormack FX, Young LR et al. Sirolimus for angiomyolipoma in tuberous sclerosis complex or lymphangioleiomyomatosis. N Engl J Med 2008;358:140–51.

112 Dabora SL, Franz DN, Ashwal S et al. Multicenter phase 2 trial of sirolimus for tuberous sclerosis: Kidney angiomyolipomas and other tumors regress and VEGF- D levels decrease. PLoS ONE 2011;6: e23379.

113 Bissler JJ, Kingswood JC, Radzikowska E et al. Everolimus for angiomyolipoma associated with tuberous sclerosis complex or sporadic lymphangioleiomyomatosis (EXIT-2): a multicenter, randomized, double-blind, placebo-controlled trial. Lancet 2013;381:817–24.

114 Bissler JJ, Kingswood JC, Radzikowska E et al. Everolimus for angiomyolipoma associated with tuberous sclerosis complex or sporadic lymphangioleiomyomatosis: extension of a randomized controlled trial. Neph Dial Transpl 2016;31:111–19.

115 McCormack FX, Inoue Y, Moss J et al. Efficacy and safety of sirolimus in lymphangioleiomyomatosis. New Engl J Med 2011;364:1595–606.

116 Kumasaka T, Seyama K, Mitani K et al. Lymphangiogenesis in lymphangioleiomyomatosis: its implication in the progression of lymphangioleimyomatosis. Am J Surg Pathol 2004;28:1007–16.

117 Taveira-DaSilva A, Hedin C, Stylianou MP et al. Reversible airflow obstruction, proliferation of abnormal smooth muscle cells, and impairment of gas exchange as predictors of outcome in lymphangioleiomyomatosis. Am J Resp Crit Care 2001;164:1072–6.

118 Taveira-DaSilva A, Hedin C et al. Decline in lung function in patients with lymphangioleiomyomatosis treated with or without progesterone. Chest 2004;126:1867–74.

119 Jaffe AT, Heymann WR, Schnur RE. Clustered angiofibromas on the ear of a patient with Neurofibromatosis type 2. Arch Dermatol 1998;134:760–1.

120 Salido-Vallejo R, Garnacho-Saucedo G, Moreno-Gimenez JC. Current options for the treatment of facial angiofibromas. [Review]. Actas Dermo-Sifiliograficas 2014;105:558–68.

121 El-Musa KA, Shehadi RS, Shehadi S. Extensive facial adenoma sebaceum: successful treatment with mechanical dermabrasion: case report. Br J Plast Surg 2005;58:1143–7.

122 Hori K, Soejima K, Nozaki M et al. Treatment of facial angiofibromas of tuberous sclerosis using cultured epithelial autografts. Ann Plast Surg 2006;57:415–17.

123 Papadavid E, Markey A, Bellaney G, Walker NP. Carbon dioxide and pulsed dye laser treatment of angiofibromas in 29 patients with tuberous sclerosis. Br J Dermatol 2002;147:337–42.

124 Rogosnitzky M, Danks R, Kardash E. Therapeutic potential of tranilast, an anti-allergy drug, in proliferative disorders. Anti-cancer Res 2012;32:2471–8.

125 Wang L, Gao L, Abe T, Mizoguchi M. Effects of tranilast on angiofibromas of tuberous sclerosis. Pediatr Int 1999;41:701–3.

126 Turkmen M, Ertam I, Unal I, Dereli T. Facial angiofibromas of tuberous sclerosis: successful treatment with podophyllin. J Eur Acad Dermatol Venereol 2009;23:713–14.

127 Krakowski AC, Nguyen TA. Inhibition of angiofibromas in a tuberous sclerosis patient using topical timolol 0.5% Gel. Pediatr 2015;136:e709–13.

128 Nathan N, Wang J-A, Li S et al. Improvement of tuberous sclerosis complex (TSC) skin tumors during long-term treatment with oral sirolimus. J Am Acad Dermatol 2015;73:802–8.

129 Jozwiak S, Sadowski K, Kotluska K, Schwartz RA. Topical use of mammalian target of rapamycin (mTOR) inhibitors in tuberous sclerosis complex-A comprehensive review of the literature. Pediatr Neurol 2016;61:1–7.

130 Koenig MK, Hebert AA, Roberson J et al. Topical rapamycin therapy to alleviate the cutaneous manifestations of tuberous sclerosis complex: a double-blind, randomized, controlled trial to evaluate the safety and efficacy of topically applied rapamycin. Drugs R D 2012;12:121–6.

131 Sahin M, Henske EP, Brendan D. Manning BD et al. Advances and future directions for tuberous sclerosis complex research: recommendations from the 2015 strategic planning conference. Pediatr Neurol 2016;60:1–12.

CHAPTER 144
Other RASopathies

Fanny Morice-Picard
Pediatric Dermatology Unit and Department of Dermatology, Reference Centre for Rare Disorders of Skin, Bordeaux Children Hospital, CHU de Bordeaux, France

Introduction, 1857
Noonan syndrome, 1857
Noonan syndrome with multiple lentigines, 1859
Cardiofaciocutaneous syndrome, 1860
Costello syndrome, 1861

Abstract

Constitutional overactivation at various levels of the Ras/MAPK pathway is responsible for overlapping syndromes, comprising characteristic facial features, cardiac defects, cutaneous abnormalities, growth deficit, neurocognitive delay and predisposition to malignancies. Each syndrome also exhibits unique features that probably reflect genotype-related specific biological effects. Cutaneous findings are important because they may guide diagnosis and help to distinguish the different RASopathies one from the other.

Key points

- **RASopathies are characterized by a recognizable phenotype including typical craniofacial anomalies, congenital heart defects, short stature, variable cognitive deficits and skeletal anomalies.**
- **Molecular characterization of the patients presenting with RASopathies is useful and determines the follow-up and prognosis of the disease.**
- **Patients with Costello syndrome have an increased risk of developing malignancies which requires following of the recommendations for monitoring.**
- **Knowledge of the skin abnormalities observed in RASopathies is important and may help to guide clinical diagnosis.**

Introduction

The Ras/MAPK pathway has been implicated in several developmental syndromes with cutaneous manifestations in addition to neurofibromatosis 1 (NF1). The RASopathies constitute a group of human genetic syndromes that are caused by germline mutations in genes which encode components of the Ras/MAPK pathway [1]. The main RASopathies include: Noonan syndrome, Noonan syndrome with multiple lentigines (LEOPARD syndrome: lentigines-ophthalmological anomalies-atrial defect-deafness), cardiofaciocutaneous syndrome and Costello syndrome.

Noonan syndrome, Costello syndrome and cardiofaciocutaneous syndrome have overlapping findings such as similar facial features, cardiac defects and learning disabilities [2]. Prior to identification of the causative genes for the different RASopathies, the clinical diagnosis was challenging. Recent advances in molecular diagnosis have helped to make the distinction between the different Ras-related disorders (Table 144.1).

RAS-GTPases are ubiquitous small molecules that act as central molecular switches by cycling between an active GTP-bound and an inactive GDP-bound form [3]. Through association with RAF, GTP-bound RAS initiates an activation cascade of MAPKs (Fig. 144.1). The Ras/MAPK pathway is characterized by several isoforms of RAS, RAF, MEK and ERK (extracellular signal-regulated kinase) encoded by different genes. Somatic mutations in many genes encoding key proteins on the MAPK pathway, including *RAS* and *RAF* genes, are among the most common genetic alterations observed in a variety of malignancies [4]. Mutations described in cancers are often considered to cause overactivation of Ras/MAPK signalling [3,4].

Noonan syndrome

Definition, history and aetiology. Noonan syndrome (NS, OMIM #163950) is the eponymous name for the disorder described by the paediatric cardiologist Jacqueline Noonan in 1960 [5]. It is one of the most common genetic disorders with an autosomal dominant mode of inheritance and affects approximately 1 in 1000–2000 newborns. Many individuals with NS have a *de novo* pathogenic variant. NS is a genetically heterogeneous and currently mutations in *PTPN11, SOS1, KRAS, NRAS, RAF1, BRAF,*

Harper's Textbook of Pediatric Dermatology, Fourth Edition. Edited by Peter Hoeger, Veronica Kinsler and Albert Yan.

Table 144.1 Summary of RASopathies

Syndrome	Gene	Skin phenotype	Other
Costello	*HRAS*	Papilloma	Dysmorphic craniofacial features, congenital heart defects, failure to thrive with short stature, developmental delay, predisposition to cancer
Noonan	*PTPN11* *KRAS* *NRAS* *RAF1* *BRAF* *SHOC2* *CBL* *RIT1* *SOS1* *MAP2K1* *PPP1CB*	Lymphoedema, naevi, café-au-lait spots, follicular keratosis, thick and curly hair	Craniofacial dysmorphic features, congenital heart defects, short stature, undescended testicles, ophthalmological abnormalities, bleeding disorders, normal to mild neurocognitive delay, predisposition to cancer
Cardiofaciocutaneous	*BRAF* *MAP2K1* *MAP2K2* *KRAS*	Follicular keratosis, ulerythema ophryogenes, multiple naevi,	Craniofacial dysmorphic features, congenital heart defects, failure to thrive with short stature, ophthalmological abnormalities and developmental hypotonia
LEOPARD	*PTPN11* *RAF1*	Same as Noonan syndrome but may develop multiple skin lentigines as individuals get older	Congenital heart defects, short stature

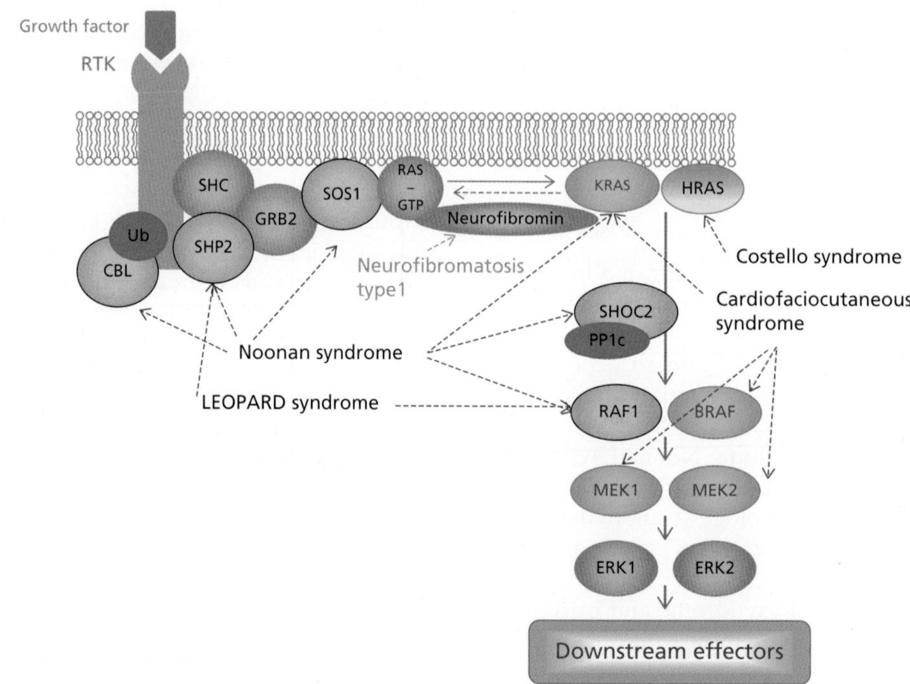

Fig. 144.1 The Ras/MAPK signal transduction pathway. Disorders related to the different components of the pathway are indicated and include neurofibromatosis type 1 (NF1), Noonan syndrome, LEOPARD syndrome, Costello syndrome and cardiofaciocutaneous syndrome.

SHOC2, MAP2K1/MEK1, CBL, RIT1 and *PPP1CB* have been causally associated with this disease or to the related conditions, including LEOPARD syndrome (OMIM #151100), Noonan-like syndrome with loose anagen hair (NS/LAH, OMIM #607721), and '*CBL* mutation-associated' syndrome [6–16].

Missense mutations in *PTPN11* (OMIM 176876), a gene encoding the nonreceptor protein tyrosine phosphatase SHP-2, which contains two Src homology 2 (SH2) domains, cause NS and account for 50% of the cases in different series [6,16,17]. All *PTPN11* missense mutations cluster in interacting portions of the amino N-SH2 domain and the phosphotyrosine phosphatase domains, which are involved in switching the protein between its inactive and active conformations. An energetics-based structural analysis of two N-SH2 mutants indicates that in these mutants there may be a significant shift of the equilibrium favouring the active conformation. This implies that they are gain-of-function changes and that the pathogenesis of NS arises from excessive SHP-2 activity [6].

Clinical features. NS is characterized by typical facial features, proportionate short stature and congenital heart disease associated with skin anomalies [18].

Cutaneous features

Lymphatic vessel dysplasia, hypoplasia or aplasia are common findings in NS. They lead to generalized lymphoedema, peripheral lymphoedema, pulmonary lymphangiectasia or intestinal lymphangiectasia. Lymphoedema of limbs is most common, which usually disappears during childhood. Varying degrees of oedema or hydrops are present during intrauterine life [19,20].

Abnormalities of pigmentation in NS include pigmented naevi, cafe-au-lait spots and lentigines. Ulerythema ophryogenes (keratosis pilaris atrophicans faciei) may lead to a lack of eyebrows. NS is also often accompanied by keratosis pilaris on the upper arms [16]. Approximately one-third of the patients have thick curly hair. Some may have thin sparse hair [16].

Other features

Facial features mainly include high forehead, ocular hypertelorism, down-slanting palpebral fissures, epicanthic folds, ptosis, low-set posteriorly rotated ears and short neck. Length at birth is usually normal. Postnatal growth failure is often obvious from the first year of life. Mean height then follows the third centile from age 2–4 years until puberty [21]. Congenital heart disease, including pulmonary valve stenosis, occurs in more than half of individuals [22]. Mild intellectual disability is observed in a quarter of NS patients.

NS associated with a germline pathogenic variant in *PTPN11* have a predisposition to juvenile myelomonocytic leukaemia, an unusual childhood leukaemia [23]. Individuals with NS are at an eightfold greater risk of developing a childhood cancer than are those without NS [24].

Other findings can include broad neck, unusual chest shape with superior pectus carinatum and inferior pectus excavatum, cryptorchidism, varied coagulation defects and ocular abnormalities [18].

Clinical variants

NS/LAH. Subjects with NS/LAH (OMIM #607721) show easily pluckable, sparse, thin, slow-growing hair in the anagen phase, but lacking an inner and outer root sheath. Loose anagen hair can be confirmed by microscopic examination of plucked hairs. Patients with NS/LAH may present with hairless and darkly pigmented skin with eczema or ichthyosis, and a tendency to pruritus. Ectodermal anomalies also include sparse eyebrows and dystrophic nails. Cardiac anomalies are observed in the majority of cases. NS/LAH appears to be genetically homogeneous. All affected individuals described so far share the same c.4A>G missense change (p.Ser2Gly) in *SHOC2* [8,25].

Noonan syndrome-like disorder with or without juvenile myelomonocytic leukaemia (OMIM #613563). Germline heterozygous pathogenic variants in *CBL* underlie a variable phenotype with features overlapping NS [13]. This condition is characterized by a relatively high frequency of neurological features, a predisposition to juvenile myelomonocytic leukaemia, and low prevalence of cardiac defects, reduced growth and cryptorchidism [26].

Diagnosis. Diagnosis of NS is based on clinical grounds by observation of key features. Diagnostic criteria developed by van der Burgt in 1997 were published in 2007 [18]. Affected individuals usually have normal chromosome studies. However, rare cases of copy number changes are described as causal. Molecular genetic testing identifies a pathogenic variant in *PTPN11* in around half of affected individuals, *SOS1* in approximately 13%, *RAF1* and *RIT1* each in 5%, and *KRAS* in fewer than 5% [27]. *NRAS*, *BRAF* and *MAP2K1* have been reported to cause NS in fewer than 1% of cases. Several additional genes associated with a Noonan-syndrome-like phenotype in fewer than 10 individuals have been identified.

Treatment. Treatment is symptomatic. Cardiovascular anomalies in NS are usually treated as in the general population. Some studies suggested that lovastatin or MEK inhibitors may be useful for treating the cognitive deficits in NS [28]. Treatment for serious bleeding is guided by knowledge of the specific factor deficiency or platelet aggregation anomaly. Growth hormone treatment increases growth velocity [21]. Bleeding disorders may require appropriate treatment and follow-up, as may hearing problems. Follow-up of the patients is based on a monitoring of anomalies found in any system, including cardiovascular abnormalities. Despite the apparent increased incidence of haematological and solid tumour malignancies, no surveillance strategies have been evaluated or recommended. Clinical management guidelines provide details of recommended baseline investigations and age-specific management [29].

Noonan syndrome with multiple lentigines

Definition, history and aetiology. Noonan syndrome with multiple lentigines (NSML) or LEOPARD syndrome (OMIM #151100) is an autosomal dominant trait that overlaps clinically with NS. The acronymic name refers to the major features: Lentigines, ECG conduction abnormalities, Ocular hypertelorism, Pulmonic stenosis, Abnormal genitalia, Retardation of growth, and sensorineural Deafness. NSML is caused by a restricted spectrum of heterozygous mutations in *PTPN11* [30]. LEOPARD syndrome has also been rarely causally linked to mutations in RAF1 or BRAF [11,12]. The most common NSML-associated *PTPN11* mutations affect amino acids in the catalytic PTP domain, which results in reduced SHP2 catalytic activity *in vitro*, causing a loss of function [31].

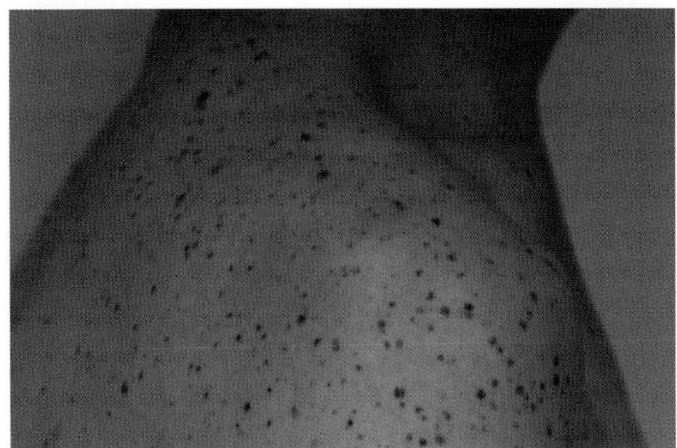

Fig. 144.2 Lentigines in Noonan syndrome with multiple lentigines.

Clinical features. The cardinal features of NSML consist of lentigines, hypertrophic cardiomyopathy, short stature and pectus deformity. Characteristic facial features include widely spaced eyes and ptosis. Multiple lentigines present as dispersed flat, black–brown macules, mostly on the face, neck and upper part of the trunk with sparing of the mucosa (Fig. 144.2). In general, lentigines do not appear until the age of 4–5 years but then increase to the thousands by puberty [32]. Some individuals with NSML do not exhibit lentigines. Café-au-lait macules are also observed in up to 70–80% of affected individuals [32]. Skin hyperelasticity has also been described.

Other features

Approximately 85% of affected individuals have heart defects, including hypertrophic cardiomyopathy (typically appearing during infancy and sometimes progressive) and pulmonary valve stenosis. Postnatal growth retardation resulting in short stature occurs in less than half of patients. Sensorineural hearing deficits are often present. A mild intellectual disability might be observed.

Diagnosis. The diagnosis of NSML is established either by clinical findings or, if clinical findings are insufficient, by identification of a heterozygous pathogenic variant in one of four genes (*PTPN11*, *RAF1*, *BRAF* and *MAP2K1*) by molecular genetic testing [30].

Treatment. Treatment of cardiovascular anomalies and cryptorchidism is the same as in the general population. Treatment of hearing loss includes hearing aids, enrolment in an educational programme for the hearing impaired and consideration of cochlear implantation. Developmental disability is managed by early occupational therapy, physical therapy and speech therapy as needed.

Cardiofaciocutaneous syndrome

Definition, history and aetiology. CFCS (OMIM #115150) is a rare, multiple congenital anomaly disorder characterized by distinctive craniofacial features, congenital heart defects, psychomotor delay, failure to thrive and abnormalities of the skin and hair.

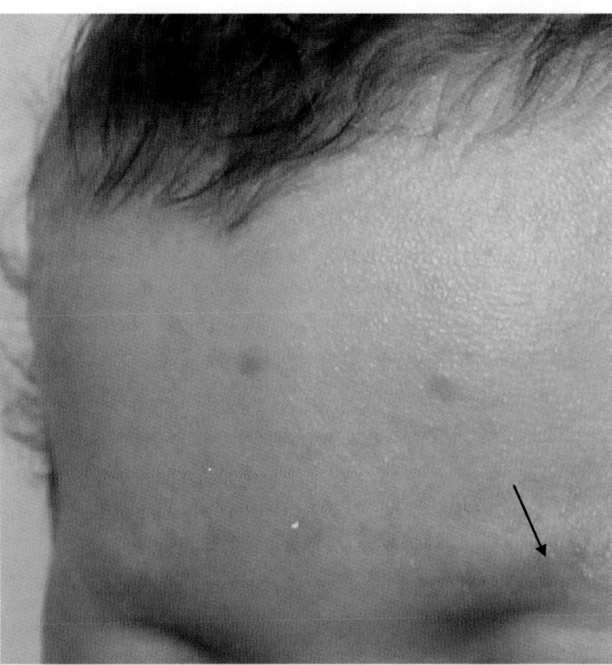

Fig. 144.3 Ulerythema ophryogene in a patient with cardiofaciocutaneous syndrome.

The syndrome was first described in 1986 by Reynolds and colleagues, in eight children [33]. CFCS is a heterogeneous autosomal dominant disorder caused by mutations either in *BRAF*, *MEK1* or *MEK2* encoding proteins of the RAF/MAPK pathway downstream of RAS [3]. Most affected individuals have CFCS as the result of a *de novo* pathogenic variant. Prenatal testing for pregnancies at risk is possible if the *BRAF, MAP2K1, MAP2K, or KRAS* pathogenic variant has been identified in the proband.

Clinical features. CFCS is characterized by cardiac abnormalities, distinctive craniofacial appearance and skin abnormalities [34].

Cutaneous features are mainly characterized by xerosis, keratosis pilaris and ulerythema (Fig. 144.3) [35,36]. Palmoplantar hyperkeratosis is observed. Patients have a high number of melanocytic naevi and café-au-lait spots. The hair is typically sparse, curly, fine or thick, woolly or brittle; eyelashes and eyebrows may be absent or sparse. Nails may be dystrophic or fast growing.

Cardiac anomalies are variable and include pulmonic stenosis and other valve dysplasias, septal defects, hypertrophic cardiomyopathy and rhythm disturbance [37]. These defects may be identified at birth or diagnosed later. Hypertrophic cardiomyopathy may be progressive.

Facial features mainly include high forehead, relative macrocephaly, bitemporal narrowing, ocular hypertelorism, downslanting palpebral fissures, epicanthal folds, ptosis, short nose with depressed bridge and anteverted nares, ear lobe creases, low-set ears that may be posteriorly rotated, deep philtrum and cupid's bow configuration of the upper lip [33,34]. The face is generally broader and coarser than in NS but not as coarse as in Costello syndrome.

Variable neurological abnormalities and cognitive delay are seen in all affected individuals.

The risk for malignancies in CFCS is not fully established. Acute lymphoblastic leukaemia has been reported in some individuals [38].

Diagnosis. Diagnosis is based on clinical findings and molecular genetic testing. The four genes known to be associated with CFCS are: *BRAF* (~75%), *MAP2K1* and *MAP2K2* (~25%) and *KRAS* (<2%) [39].

Treatment. A multidisciplinary approach is necessary. Management of cardiac defects and arrhythmias is as in the general population. Periodic echocardiogram (hypertrophic cardiomyopathy) and electrocardiogram (rhythm disturbances) are required.

For skin conditions, increased ambient humidity or hydrating lotions for xerosis and pruritus are important. A follow-up of melanocytic lesions is recommended.

Feeding problems may require increased caloric intake, a nasogastric tube or gastrostomy. Management of growth hormone deficiency and ocular abnormalities is routine. Management of seizures may require polytherapy. Occupational therapy, physical therapy and speech therapy may be needed. Consensus medical management guidelines have been published [40].

Costello syndrome

Definition, history and aetiology. Costello syndrome (CS; OMIM #218040) is the eponymous name for the disorder originally described in 1971 and further delineated in 1977 [41]. CS is one of the rarest RASopathies [3] and has a distinctive phenotype. Costello syndrome is an autosomal dominant disorder caused by germline mutations in the *HRAS* gene [42]. *HRAS* is an oncogene and aberrant activation of its gene product caused by missense mutations is seen in sporadic tumours. Similarly, increased activation of the abnormal gene product occurs caused by the germline mutations in CS. CS is mostly caused by a *de novo* pathogenic variant [43].

Clinical features. CS is characterized by prenatal overgrowth followed by severe failure to thrive, distinctive coarse facial features, developmental delay, short stature, cardiac defects, and musculoskeletal and skin abnormalities.

Cutaneous features include loose, soft skin with deep palmar and plantar creases, increased pigmentation, papillomata of the face and perianal region (typically absent in infancy but may appear in childhood; diagnosis must be confirmed in doubtful cases), premature aging, hair loss and curly or sparse fine hair (Fig. 144.4).

Diffuse hypotonia and joint laxity is associated with ulnar deviation of the wrists and fingers, and tight Achilles tendons.

Neurological anomalies consist of electrophysiological and structural disorders including ventricular dilatation, brain atrophy, Chiari malformation and syringomyelia [44]. Screening, including cerebral magnetic resonance imaging and an electroencephalogram, should be proposed after a diagnosis of Costello syndrome.

Cardiac involvement includes hypertrophic cardiomyopathy and arrhythmia. Individuals with Costello syndrome have an increased risk for malignant tumours including rhabdomyosarcoma and neuroblastoma in young children and transitional cell carcinoma of the bladder in adolescents and young adults [45].

Diagnosis. Diagnosis of CS is based on clinical findings and is confirmed by molecular genetic testing. Sequence analysis of *HRAS*, the only gene currently known to be associated with CS, detects pathogenic missense variants in 80–90% of individuals with the clinical diagnosis [43]. The clinical diagnosis should be reconsidered if an *HRAS* pathogenic variant is not identified, and other syndromes of the Ras/MAPK pathway should be considered as alternative diagnoses.

Management.

Treatment of manifestations

Treatment is symptomatic and depends on initial complications presented by the patients [45,46]. Most infants require nasogastric or gastrostomy feeding for failure to

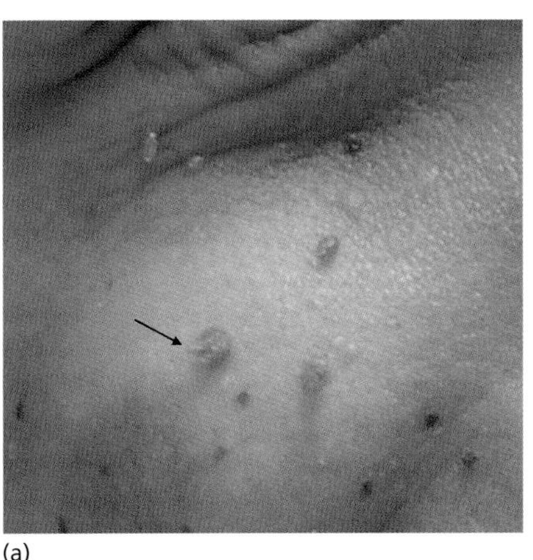

(a)

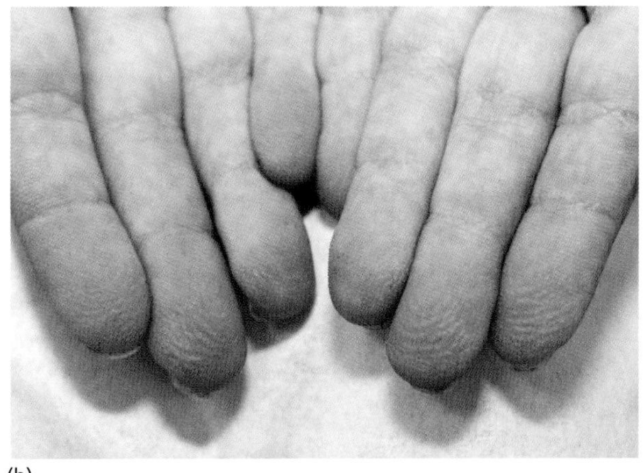

(b)

Fig. 144.4 (a) Papillomatosis and (b) pachydermatoglyphia with stippled dermatoglyphs on the fingertips in Costello syndrome.

thrive. Treatment of cardiac manifestations and malignancy is routine [47]. Orthopaedic manifestations require early bracing and physical therapy; tight Achilles tendons may require surgical tendon lengthening. Recurrent facial papillomata may require routine removal with dry ice.

Surveillance

Patients should be monitored for neonatal hypoglycaemia. Echocardiography with an electrocardiogram performed at diagnosis should be followed up by a cardiologist who is aware of the spectrum of cardiac disease and its natural history. Abdominal and pelvic ultrasound examinations to screen for rhabdomyosarcoma and neuroblastoma may be performed every 3–6 months until the age of 8–10 years. Annual urinalysis for evidence of haematuria to screen for bladder cancer should begin at the age of 10 years [48].

References

1 Tidyman WE, Lee HS, Rauen KA. Skeletal muscle pathology in Costello and cardio-facio-cutaneous syndromes: developmental consequences of germline Ras/MAPK activation on myogenesis. Am J Med Genet C Semin Med Genet 2011;157C:104–14.

2 Nava C, Hanna N, Michot C et al. Cardio-facio-cutaneous and Noonan syndromes due to mutations in the RAS/MAPK signalling pathway: genotype-phenotype relationships and overlap with Costello syndrome. J Med Genet 2007;44:763–71.

3 Aoki Y, Niihori T, Inoue S, Matsubara Y. Recent advances in RASopathies. J Hum Genet 2016;61:33–9.

4 Halaban R, Krauthammer M. RASopathy gene mutations in melanoma. J Invest Dermatol 2016;136:1755–9.

5 Noonan JA. Hypertelorism with Turner phenotype. A new syndrome with associated congenital heart disease. Am J Dis Child 1968;116:373–80.

6 Tartaglia M, Mehler EL, Goldberg R et al. Mutations in PTPN11, encoding the protein tyrosine phosphatase SHP-2, cause Noonan syndrome. Nat Genet 2001;29:465–8.

7 Tartaglia M, Pennacchio LA, Zhao C et al. Gain-of-function SOS1 mutations cause a distinctive form of Noonan syndrome. Nat Genet 2007;39:75–9.

8 Cordeddu V, Di Schiavi E, Pennacchio LA et al. Mutation of SHOC2 promotes aberrant protein N-myristoylation and causes Noonan-like syndrome with loose anagen hair. Nat Genet 2009;41:1022–6.

9 Carta C, Pantaleoni F, Bocchinfuso G et al. Germline missense mutations affecting KRAS Isoform B are associated with a severe Noonan syndrome phenotype. Am J Hum Genet 2006;79:129–35.

10 Cirstea IC, Kutsche K, Dvorsky R et al. A restricted spectrum of NRAS mutations causes Noonan syndrome. Nat Genet 2010;42:27–9.

11 Pandit B, Sarkozy A, Pennacchio LA et al. Gain-of-function RAF1 mutations cause Noonan and LEOPARD syndromes with hypertrophic cardiomyopathy. Nat Genet2007;39:1007–12.

12 Sarkozy A, Carta C, Moretti S et al. Germline BRAF mutations in Noonan, LEOPARD, and cardiofaciocutaneous syndromes: molecular diversity and associated phenotypic spectrum. Hum Mutat 2009;30:695–702.

13 Martinelli S, De Luca A, Stellacci E et al. Heterozygous germline mutations in the CBL tumor-suppressor gene cause a Noonan syndrome-like phenotype. Am J Hum Genet 2010;87:250–7.

14 Aoki Y, Niihori T, Banjo T et al. Gain-of-function mutations in RIT1 cause Noonan syndrome, a RAS/MAPK pathway syndrome. Am J Hum Genet 2013;93:173–80.

15 Gripp KW, Aldinger KA, Bennett JT et al. A novel rasopathy caused by recurrent de novo missense mutations in PPP1CB closely resembles Noonan syndrome with loose anagen hair. Am J Med Genet A 2016;170:2237–47.

16 Jongmans M, Sistermans EA, Rikken A et al. Genotypic and phenotypic characterization of Noonan syndrome: new data and review of the literature. Am J Med Genet A 2005;134A:165–70.

17 Chen J-L, Zhu X, Zhao T-L et al. Rare copy number variations containing genes involved in RASopathies: deletion of SHOC2 and duplication of PTPN11. Mol Cytogenet 2014;7:28.

18 van der Burgt I. Noonan syndrome. Orphanet J Rare Dis 2007;2:4.

19 Gandhi SV, Howarth ES, Krarup KC, Konje JC. Noonan syndrome presenting with transient cystic hygroma. J Obstet Gynaecol 2004;24:183–4.

20 Sharland M, Burch M, McKenna WM, Paton MA. A clinical study of Noonan syndrome. Arch Dis Child 1992;67:178–83.

21 Şıklar Z, Genens M, Poyrazoğlu Ş et al. The growth characteristics of patients with Noonan syndrome: results of the 3 years of growth hormone treatment: a nationwide multicenter study. J Clin Res Pediatr Endocrinol 2016;8:305–12.

22 Sarkozy A, Conti E, Seripa D et al. Correlation between PTPN11 gene mutations and congenital heart defects in Noonan and LEOPARD syndromes. J Med Genet 2003;40:704–8.

23 Jongmans MCJ, van der Burgt I, Hoogerbrugge PM et al. Cancer risk in patients with Noonan syndrome carrying a PTPN11 mutation. Eur J Hum Genet 2011;19:870–4.

24 Kratz CP, Franke L, Peters H et al. Cancer spectrum and frequency among children with Noonan, Costello, and cardio-facio-cutaneous syndromes. Br J Cancer 2015;112:1392–7.

25 Hannig V, Jeoung M, Jang ER et al. A novel SHOC2 variant in rasopathy. Hum Mutat 2014;35:1290–4.

26 Martinelli S, Stellacci E, Pannone L et al. Molecular diversity and associated phenotypic spectrum of germline CBL mutations. Hum Mutat 2015;36:787–96.

27 Bezniakow N, Gos M, Obersztyn E. The RASopathies as an example of RAS/MAPK pathway disturbances - clinical presentation and molecular pathogenesis of selected syndromes. Dev Period Med 2014;18:285–96.

28 Lee Y-S, Ehninger D, Zhou M et al. Mechanism and treatment for learning and memory deficits in mouse models of Noonan syndrome. Nat Neurosci 2014;17:1736–43.

29 Romano AA, Allanson JE, Dahlgren J et al. Noonan syndrome: clinical features, diagnosis, and management guidelines. Pediatrics 2010;126:746–59.

30 Digilio MC, Conti E, Sarkozy A et al. Grouping of multiple-lentigines/LEOPARD and Noonan syndromes on the PTPN11 gene. Am J Hum Genet 2002;71:389–94.

31 Kontaridis MI, Swanson KD, David FS et al. PTPN11 (Shp2) mutations in LEOPARD syndrome have dominant negative, not activating, effects. J Biol Chem 2006;281:6785–92.

32 Digilio MC, Sarkozy A, de Zorzi A et al. LEOPARD syndrome: clinical diagnosis in the first year of life. Am J Med Genet A 2006;140:740–6.

33 Reynolds JF, Neri G, Herrmann JP et al. New multiple congenital anomalies/mental retardation syndrome with cardio-facio-cutaneous involvement--the CFC syndrome. Am J Med Genet 1986;25:413–27.

34 Narumi Y, Aoki Y, Niihori T et al. Molecular and clinical characterization of cardio-facio-cutaneous (CFC) syndrome: overlapping clinical manifestations with Costello syndrome. Am J Med Genet A 2007;144A:799–807.

35 Siegel DH, Mann JA, Krol AL, Rauen KA. Dermatological phenotype in Costello syndrome: consequences of Ras dysregulation in development. Br J Dermatol 2012;166:601–7.

36 Morice-Picard F, Ezzedine K, Delrue M-A et al. Cutaneous manifestations in Costello and cardiofaciocutaneous syndrome: report of 18 cases and literature review. Pediatr Dermatol 2013;30:665–73.

37 Narumi Y, Aoki Y, Niihori T et al. Molecular and clinical characterization of cardio-facio-cutaneous (CFC) syndrome: overlapping clinical manifestations with Costello syndrome. Am J Med Genet A 2007;144A:799–807.

38 Makita Y, Narumi Y, Yoshida M et al. Leukemia in cardio-facio-cutaneous (CFC) syndrome: a patient with a germline mutation in BRAF proto-oncogene. J Pediatr Hematol Oncol 2007;29:287–90.

39 Rauen KA. Cardiofaciocutaneous syndrome. In: Pagon RA, Adam MP, Ardinger HH et al. (eds) GeneReviews® [Internet]. Seattle (WA): University of Washington, Seattle, 1993.

40 Pierpont MEM, Magoulas PL, Adi S et al. Cardio-facio-cutaneous syndrome: clinical features, diagnosis, and management guidelines. Pediatrics 2014;134:e1149–1162.

41 Costello JM. A new syndrome: mental subnormality and nasal papillomata. Aust Paediatr J 1977;13:114–8.

42 Aoki Y, Niihori T, Kawame H et al. Germline mutations in HRAS proto-oncogene cause Costello syndrome. Nat Genet 2005;37:1038–40.

43 Gripp KW, Lin AE, Stabley DL et al. HRAS mutation analysis in Costello syndrome: genotype and phenotype correlation. Am J Med Genet A 2006;140(1):1–7.

44 Delrue M-A, Chateil J-F, Arveiler B, Lacombe D. Costello syndrome and neurological abnormalities. Am J Med Genet A 2003;123A:301–5.

45 Korf B, Ahmadian R, Allanson J et al. The third international meeting on genetic disorders in the RAS/MAPK pathway: towards a therapeutic approach. Am J Med Genet A 2015;167A:1741–6.

46 **Gripp KW, Lin AE. Costello syndrome. In: Pagon RA, Adam MP, Ardinger HH et al. (eds) GeneReviews® [Internet]. Seattle (WA): University of Washington, Seattle, 1993.**

47 Lin AE, Grossfeld PD, Hamilton RM et al. Further delineation of cardiac abnormalities in Costello syndrome. Am J Med Genet 2002;111:115–29.

48 Gripp KW. Tumor predisposition in Costello syndrome. Am J Med Genet C Semin Med Genet 2005;137C:72–7.

CHAPTER 145
Cutaneous Vasculitis

Joyce C. Chang[1] *& Pamela F. Weiss*[1,2]

[1] Division of Rheumatology, The Children's Hospital of Philadelphia, Philadelphia, USA
[2] Center for Clinical Epidemiology and Biostatistics, University of Pennsylvania, Philadelphia, PA, USA

Introduction, 1865
Leukocytoclastic vasculitis, 1866
Pigmented purpuras, 1876
Cutaneous polyarteritis nodosa, 1879
Systemic diseases with secondary cutaneous vasculitis, 1882

Abstract

Vasculitis is an inflammatory process that causes destruction of blood vessel walls with subsequent haemorrhage and ischaemia. Cutaneous vasculitis can be seen in a heterogeneous group of disorders, both as a primary phenomenon and secondary to underlying systemic disease, infection or drug exposure. Palpable purpura is the most common manifestation; infiltrated erythema, nodules, ulcerations and peripheral gangrene are also seen. Leukocytoclastic vasculitis involving dermal small vessels is the most frequent histopathological finding and is typically associated with immune complex deposition. This chapter focuses on select diseases associated with cutaneous vasculitis in children, including Henoch–Schönlein Purpura, acute haemorrhagic oedema of infancy, urticarial vasculitis, erythema elevatum diutinum and cutaneous polyarteritis nodosa. The pigmented purpuras will also be discussed although they do not represent true vasculitis. Systemic vasculitis and autoimmune diseases can present with vasculitic skin lesions, therefore knowledge of their distinguishing features is crucial to making the diagnosis.

Key points

- **Cutaneous vasculitis can be limited to the skin or associated with systemic disease.**
- **Leukocytoclastic vasculitis refers to neutrophilic infiltration of small vessel walls with fibrinoid necrosis, typically associated with immune complex deposition. It is the histopathological correlate of most vasculitic skin lesions seen in childhood.**
- **Henoch–Schönlein purpura is the most common vasculitis of childhood.**
- **There is a close association between hypocomplementemic urticarial vasculitis and systemic lupus erythematosus.**
- **Erythema elevatum diutinum is extremely rare in children and often associated with underlying infection or systemic disease.**
- **Cutaneous polyarteritis nodosa is a skin-limited form of systemic polyarteritis nodosa with an overall benign prognosis.**
- **The differential diagnosis of cutaneous vasculitis is broad and includes primary cutaneous vasculitis, infections, drug reactions, systemic vasculitis, as well as connective tissue diseases.**

Introduction

Cutaneous vasculitis is a heterogeneous group of diseases characterized pathologically by inflammation and cell-mediated destruction of blood vessel walls, leading to ischaemia, haemorrhage and subsequent damage to surrounding tissues. Clinically these are manifested by purpuric macules or infiltrated erythema in the setting of superficial vessel involvement, palpable purpura or superficial ulcers with deeper dermal involvement, and deep ulcers, nodules or pits with dermal and subcutaneous involvement. Whereas primary cutaneous vasculitis is limited to the skin, secondary cutaneous vasculitis is frequently associated with underlying autoimmune or inflammatory disease, which can have prominent systemic symptoms and multiorgan involvement. Depending on the aetiology, the skin manifestations may have either a self-limited, relapsing and remitting, or chronic course [1]. The pathogenesis also varies among different types of vasculitis, and as a result, the treatment varies widely based on aetiology.

The classification of vasculitis in children has been particularly challenging. The most widely used classification system is the Chapel Hill Consensus Conference (CHCC) nomenclature, which is based on pathological criteria and categorizes diseases by size of the most commonly affected arteries, but is only validated in adults and has poor predictive value for use in individual patients [2,3]. In 2008, the European League against Rheumatism (EULAR), the Pediatric Rheumatology International Trials Organization (PRINTO), and the Paediatric Rheumatology European Society (PRES) proposed and validated revised classification criteria for a subset of childhood vasculitis syndromes that was demonstrated

Harper's Textbook of Pediatric Dermatology, Fourth Edition. Edited by Peter Hoeger, Veronica Kinsler and Albert Yan.

Table 145.1 Histological classification of cutaneous vasculitis

Small vessel vasculitis
Neutrophilic (leukocytoclastic)
Henoch–Schönlein purpura
Acute infantile haemorrhagic oedema
Urticarial vasculitis
Hypersensitivity vasculitis
Erythema elevatum diutinum
Lymphocytic
Rickettsial and viral infections
Arthropod bites
Mixed small and medium vessel vasculitis
Neutrophilic with immune-complex deposition
Cryoglobulinaemia
Connective tissue disease associated vasculitis
ANCA-associated, pauci-immune
Granulomatosis with polyangiitis (Wegener's)
Microscopic polyangiitis
Eosinophilic granulomatosis with polyangiitis (Churg–Strauss syndrome)
Miscellaneous
Septic vasculitis
Behçet's disease
Medium muscular vessel vasculitis
Neutrophilic
Polyarteritis nodosa (systemic and cutaneous)
Nodular vasculitis (erythema induratum)

Source: Adapted from Carlson JA, Chen K-R. 2006 [6].

to have high sensitivity and specificity [4]. Unfortunately, neither the CHCC nor the EULAR/PRINTO/PRES classification systems are easily applied to cutaneous vasculitis, particularly if cutaneous findings are the first manifestation of a systemic disease. Thus, some authors have proposed classification of cutaneous vasculitis using a combination of vessel size, histopathological findings and laboratory studies (Table 145.1) [5,6].

This chapter will focus on select vasculitides more commonly encountered in paediatric patients, the largest of which are the small vessel leukocytoclastic vasculitides, including Henoch–Schönlein purpura, acute haemorrhagic oedema of infancy, urticarial vasculitis and erythema elevatum diutinum. There will also be a brief discussion on pigmented purpuras although they are not considered to be true vasculitis. Cutaneous polyarteritis nodosa will be discussed as an example of primary medium vessel vasculitis. Lastly, there is a brief review of cutaneous findings associated with systemic vasculitis and connective tissue diseases. Infectious causes of vasculitis and drug-induced reactions are discussed elsewhere.

Leukocytoclastic vasculitis

Leukocytoclastic vasculitis is a descriptive term that refers to the histological presence of neutrophilic infiltration into vessel walls, resulting fibrinoid necrosis and granulocytic debris (leukocytoclasis) (Fig. 145.1) [7]. Clinically, the most frequent manifestation of leukocytoclastic vasculitis is palpable purpura. Pathologically it is associated with immune complex deposition and can be seen in a wide variety of diseases, including Henoch–Schönlein purpura, urticarial vasculitis, hypersensitivity vasculitis, systemic autoimmune diseases or infection (Box 145.1). Leukocytoclastic vasculitis can also be observed incidentally in association with several mimics of vasculitis, such as neutrophilic dermatoses and primary vasculopathies. Lastly, it can be a rare presentation of malignancy, either as a paraneoplastic process or from direct invasion of dermal blood vessels by leukaemic cells.

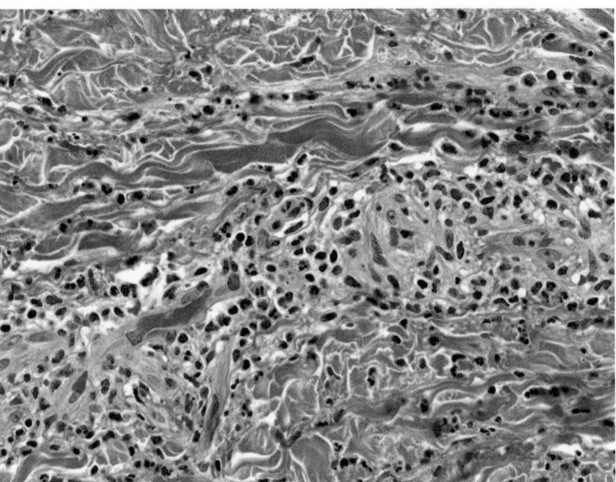

Fig. 145.1 Histological appearance of leukocytoclastic vasculitis. Note the predominantly neutrophilic infiltrate, fibrinoid degeneration and nuclear debris (leukocytoclasis). Source: Courtesy of Portia Krieger, MD, Children's Hospital of Philadelphia, PA, USA.

Box 145.1 Conditions associated with leukocytoclastic vasculitis

Henoch–Schönlein purpura
Acute haemorrhagic oedema of infancy
Urticarial vasculitis
Hypersensitivity vasculitis
Erythema elevatum diutinum
Mixed cryoglobulinaemia
Antineutrophil cytoplasmic antibody-associated (ANCA) vasculitis
Cutaneous polyarteritis nodosa
Goodpasture syndrome
Collagen–vascular disorders
Relapsing polychondritis
Inflammatory bowel disease
Infectious endocarditis
Viral infections (hepatitis, HIV)
Antiphospholipid antibody syndrome
Degos disease
Sweet syndrome
CANDLE (chronic atypical neutrophilic dermatosis with lipodystrophy and elevated temperature)
Febrile ulceronecrotic Mucha–Habermann disease
Leukaemia/Lymphoma

Henoch-Schönlein purpura

History and definition. The first case of Henoch–Schönlein purpura (HSP) was reported in the literature in 1801 by William Heberden, who described a 5-year-old boy with concurrent abdominal pain, vomiting, melaena, arthralgia, haematuria and a purpuric rash [8]. In 1837,

Table 145.2 EULAR/PRINTO/PRES classification criteria for Henoch–Schönlein Purpura (2010)

Criterion	Definition
Purpura (mandatory)	Purpura or petechiae, with lower limb predominance[1], not related to thrombocytopenia
And at least one of the following:	
Abdominal pain	Diffuse, acute, colicky abdominal pain. May include intussusception and gastrointestinal bleeding
Histopathology	Leukocytoclastic vasculitis with predominant IgA deposit or proliferative glomerulonephritis with predominant IgA deposit
Arthritis or arthralgias	Arthritis: acute joint swelling or pain with limitation in motion Arthralgia: acute joint pain without swelling or limitation in motion
Renal involvement	Proteinuria: >0.3 g/24 h or urine protein/creatinine ratio >30 mmoL/mg Haematuria: >5 red blood cells/HPF or red blood cell casts in urine sediment

[1] For purpura with an atypical distribution, demonstration of IgA deposit on biopsy is required.

EULAR, European League against Rheumatism; HPF, high-power field; PRINTO, Pediatric Rheumatology International Trials Organization; PRES, Paediatric Rheumatology European Society.

Source: Adapted from Ozen et al. 2010 [4]. Reproduced with permission of BMJ Publishing Group Ltd.

Johann Schönlein named the triad of arthralgia, abnormal urinary sediment and purpuric rash, peliosis rheumatica. Then in 1874, Schönlein's former scholar Eduard Henoch described the association of purpuric rash, abdominal pain, joint pain, bloody diarrhoea and proteinuria, which years later became known as Henoch–Schönlein purpura [9]. More recently HSP has been classified under the CHCC nomenclature as IgA vasculitis, defined as IgA-predominant immune complex deposition in small vessels, often involving skin, the gastrointestinal tract and joints, and sometimes causing glomerulonephritis that resembles IgA nephropathy [3]. Formal classification criteria for HSP in children were validated in 2010 by EULAR/PRINTO/PRES and have a diagnostic sensitivity of up to 100% and specificity of 87% (Table 145.2) [4].

Epidemiology. HSP is the most common vasculitis of childhood, accounting for at least half of all vasculitis cases and upwards of 90% of cutaneous vasculitis [10,11]. The annual incidence ranges from 6 to 26 per 100 000, with higher rates reported in Caucasian and Asian children than in African or African-American populations. The majority of cases occur in patients under the age of 10, with a peak incidence at ages 4–6 [12–14]. Unlike other vasculitides, there is a slight male predominance at a 1.2–1.8:1 ratio. A characteristic seasonality with a predilection for late autumn and winter has been observed across multiple epidemiological studies, suggesting that infectious triggers may play a role [12,14–16].

Pathogenesis. Although the pathogenesis is still poorly understood, the histological finding of IgA immune complex deposition in blood vessel walls and renal mesangium suggests that IgA plays a pivotal role in the pathophysiology. A dysregulated IgA-mediated immune response to some antigenic trigger may result in IgA immune complex deposition, activation of the alternative complement cascade and subsequent small vessel damage [17]. Immune complexes in HSP have consistently been shown to contain only the IgA_1 subtype of IgA antibodies [18]. Furthermore, patients with HSP nephritis have higher serum levels of poorly galactosylated IgA_1 [19]. Thus, it has been proposed that antiglycan IgG or IgA antibodies triggered by infection recognize poorly galactosylated IgA_1, resulting in immune complex formation and mesangial deposition [20,21]. Local complement activation by IgA_1 immune complexes and mesangial cell activation and proliferation are also thought to have important pathophysiological roles in glomerular injury [17]. Genes controlling IgA galactosylation, IgA synthesis and abnormal mesangial cell activation may confer susceptibility to disease, but the specific genes are unknown.

Several potential triggers have been proposed, including infection, medications and vaccines. Preceding infections, especially upper respiratory tract infections, are the most commonly implicated, which is consistent with the observed peak incidence in winter. Evidence of concomitant or recent beta-haemolytic streptococcal infection has been documented in 20–50% of patients with HSP [21–23]. Other reported associations include *Bartonella henselae* [24], *Staphylococcus aureus* [16,25], *Helicobacter pylori* [26,27], *Mycoplasma pneumonia* [28,29], as well as various viral infections, including parvovirus B19, coxsackievirus and hepatitis B [21,30], although the significance of these associations are unclear. Specific medications that have been implicated as potential triggers in adults include clarithromycin [31], nonsteroidal anti-inflammatory drugs (NSAIDs), TNF inhibitors [32–34] and vaccines [35], again suggesting that an antigenic exposure is important in the pathogenesis of this disease. Cases attributed to vaccines, however, have been refuted in large population-based studies and more recently by a systematic review [36,37].

Clinical features.

Cutaneous findings

Palpable purpura in the setting of a normal platelet count is characteristic of HSP (Fig. 145.2a). By definition, purpura is present in 100% of cases, and it is the presenting sign in nearly three-quarters of cases [14,38]. The classic distribution is in dependent areas, particularly the legs and buttocks, as well as areas exposed to pressure, such as sock lines or underneath blood pressure cuffs (Fig. 145.2b and 145.2c). The arms, trunk, face and area behind the ears may also be involved. Lesions range from petechiae to large coalescent ecchymoses. Occasionally the purpura develops a targetoid appearance mimicking erythema multiforme [14]. Rarely, there are haemorrhagic bullae that ulcerate and result in scarring [39]. All of the purpura variants may be preceded by a blanching, nonpruritic urticarial or maculopapular rash [40]. As the purpuric lesions heal they often turn brown or rust-coloured and

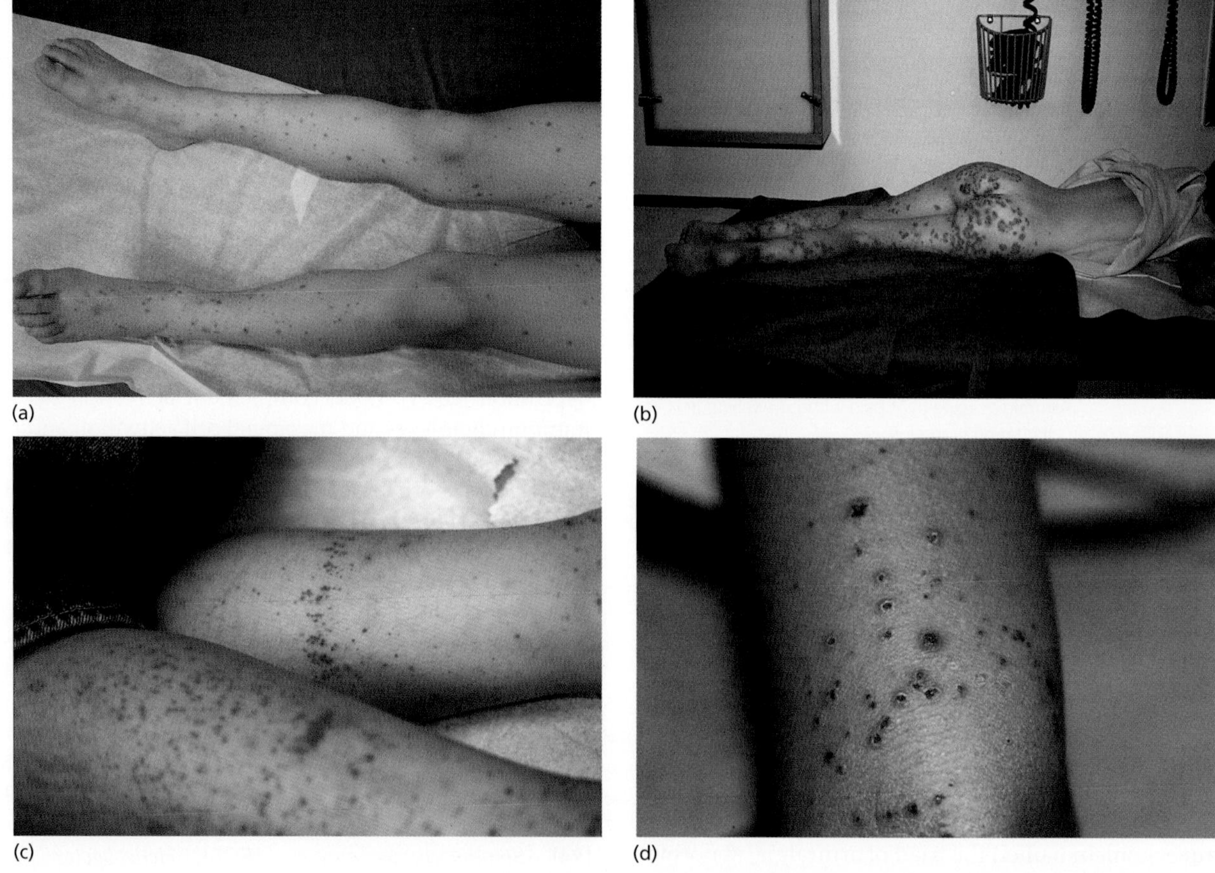

Fig. 145.2 (a) Palpable purpura on the lower extremities in a patient with Henoch–Schönlein purpura (HSP). (b) Classic distribution of HSP lesions over the legs and buttocks. Note the targetoid appearance of some purpura. (c) Petechiae appear under the sock line of a child with HSP. (d) Older HSP lesions can develop necrotic centres and scab over. Sources: (a) Courtesy of Lehn Weaver, MD; (b–d) Courtesy of David Sherry, MD, Children's Hospital of Philadelphia, PA, USA.

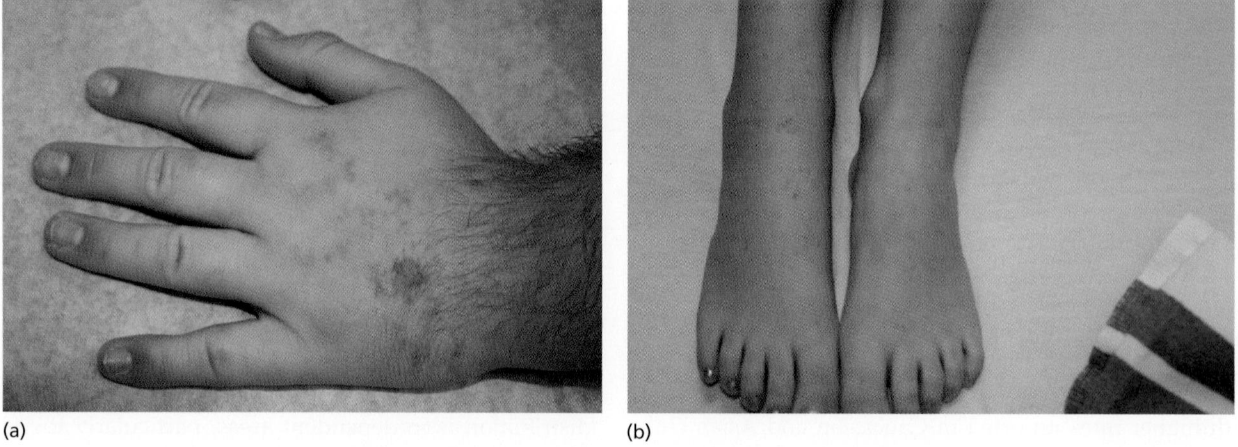

Fig. 145.3 (a) Soft tissue swelling is most prominent over the dorsum of the hand and proximal phalanges of this 8 year-old male with Henoch–Schönlein purpura. (b) Foot swelling and ankle pain was the presenting symptom of this 10 year-old female who subsequently developed purpura consistent with Henoch–Schönlein purpura. Sources: (a) Courtesy of Lehn Weaver, MD; (b) Courtesy of Sabrina Gmuca, MD and David Sherry, MD, Children's Hospital of Philadelphia, PA, USA.

scab over prior to resolving completely (Fig. 145.2d). Subcutaneous oedema, particularly over the dorsum of hands and feet, can be a prominent feature (Fig. 145.3). Scrotal and facial oedema are also seen, especially in infants and young children [9].

Gastrointestinal manifestations

Gastrointestinal involvement affects 50–75% of children with HSP and can precede the appearance of purpura by up to 2 weeks [22]. Symptoms include abdominal pain, vomiting and intestinal bleeding (ranging from occult blood to gross haematochezia). Ileo-ileal intussusception is a well-recognized complication that develops from lead-point formation after mural injury and occurs in 1–5% of cases. Other less common gastrointestinal manifestations that can occur include protein-losing enteropathy, pancreatitis, bowel ischaemia or perforation [40–42].

Arthritis and arthralgia

Joint pain or swelling affects up to 75% of children. Large joints such as the knees and ankles are predominantly affected. The arthritis is typically oligoarticular (less than four joints), nondestructive and self-limited. In 15–25% of cases joint manifestations precede the purpura [41,43].

Renal involvement

Renal involvement in HSP can lead to chronic morbidity and mortality and significantly impacts the long-term prognosis. Thirty to 50% of patients develop renal disease manifested by microscopic haematuria or proteinuria from glomerular injury. Less common presentations include hypertension, nephritic or nephrotic syndrome, and rarely renal failure. In contrast to gastrointestinal manifestations, renal disease almost never precedes the onset of purpura. Longitudinal studies of HSP nephritis have shown that renal involvement develops within the first 6 weeks in 91% of cases, and within 6 months in 97% of cases [20]. End-stage renal disease (ESRD) is a rare but serious complication of HSP.

Other manifestations

Low-grade fever and malaise are common nonspecific constitutional complaints that affect up to 50% of children [44]. In males, scrotal oedema or pain is not infrequent and true orchitis can also be seen [22]. Other rare manifestations of HSP include neurological complications, including seizures, central nervous system vasculitis and neuropathy, as well as ocular and pulmonary involvement [9].

Differential diagnosis. The differential diagnosis may include disseminated intravascular coagulation, sepsis, idiopathic thrombocytopenic purpura, thrombotic thrombocytopenic purpura, systemic lupus erythematosus or other systemic vasculitides, many of which can have both cutaneous and renal involvement. Detailed attention to the history, physical examination and laboratory findings often distinguish these other diseases from HSP.

Laboratory findings. Laboratory findings are nondiagnostic and generally correspond with mild systemic inflammation. Notably, the platelet count is normal or elevated, and the presence of thrombocytopenia should point toward a different diagnosis. There can be a moderate leukocytosis and inflammatory markers are usually normal or mildly elevated. A normocytic anaemia may be present secondary to gastrointestinal bleeding and fecal occult blood tests can be positive even in the absence of abdominal symptoms [38]. Urinalysis shows varying degrees of haematuria with or without proteinuria and red blood cell casts. Hypoalbuminaemia may also be seen in association with significant proteinuria. Complement levels are usually normal [45]. One study found IgA antineutrophil cytoplasmic antibodies (ANCA) in a large percentage of HSP patients compared with healthy controls and disease controls with other types of leukocytoclastic vasculitis [46]. The significance of IgA ANCA in the pathogenesis of HSP remains to be determined.

Imaging studies are not routinely indicated for patients with HSP. However, abdominal ultrasound is a useful, noninvasive test for evaluation of possible intussusception in children presenting with severe abdominal pain.

Histology. HSP is characterized pathologically by leukocytoclastic vasculitis with perivascular IgA deposition. In most cases, skin biopsy is not needed to diagnose HSP. However, punch biopsies of early lesions can be helpful to confirm the diagnosis in atypical or severe cases, particularly when there is prominent systemic inflammation, which is found in other types of systemic vasculitis. Classic histological findings of leukocytoclastic vasculitis include primarily neutrophilic transmural infiltrates, associated fibrinoid necrosis, granulocytic debris and extravasated erythrocytes. In HSP skin lesions, the dermal capillaries and postcapillary venules of the superficial dermis are most commonly involved. Direct immunofluorescence shows predominant IgA deposition, with some C3, fibrin and IgM [47]. However, if biopsies are taken from the centre of older necrotic lesions, immunostaining can be misleadingly negative for IgA [48].

Renal biopsies are generally undertaken for severe presentations such as nephritic or nephrotic syndrome and acute renal failure. Renal pathology shows an endocapillary proliferative glomerulonephritis that ranges from focal segmental to severe crescenteric disease [49]. Mesangial deposits composed primarily of IgA are characteristic, although IgG, C3, fibrin and properdin are frequently also present [50].

Treatment and prognosis. Supportive measures remain the mainstay of treatment for the majority of children with HSP. Acetaminophen and NSAIDs are most commonly used to provide symptomatic relief for abdominal or joint pain. Cutaneous manifestations rarely require treatment, although oral prednisone provides rapid symptom relief and may be indicated for haemorrhagic bullous lesions [51].

The use of systemic corticosteroids for the treatment of HSP remains controversial, as it has not been shown to prevent the development of persistent renal disease [52]. However, several studies suggest that early corticosteroid use is beneficial for symptomatic relief of joint and gastrointestinal symptoms, as well as for preventing gastrointestinal comorbidities in hospitalized patients [53–55]. Rapid corticosteroid tapers should be avoided, because they may precipitate rebound symptoms [55]. For patients with severe renal involvement, immunosuppression with intravenous methylprednisolone, cyclosporine, azathioprine and cyclophosphamide have been tried with variable success [56–60]. A few studies have suggested that plasmapheresis used early in the disease course is beneficial [61,62]. Despite the lack of evidence-based recommendations for immunosuppressive therapies, most experts believe that early treatment is still necessary for severe HSP nephritis [17]. Further investigation is needed to guide choice of therapy.

HSP typically resolves spontaneously within 4–6 weeks and the majority of patients carry an excellent long-term prognosis. A third of patients will have recurrence of disease, but recurrences are typically shorter and milder in duration and are more common in patients with nephritis [22]. It is recommended that providers check urinalysis and blood pressure weekly during the acute phase of disease and monthly for 6 months after initial presentation to screen for late-onset or persistent renal disease. Patients with documented nephritis may need to be followed more frequently and for longer. An estimated 1–2% of patients with HSP nephritis progress to ESRD, with a higher proportion (up to 44%) of those patients having nephritic or nephrotic syndrome at onset of disease [63,64]. Thus far there are no interventions known to decrease the risk of ESRD.

Acute haemorrhagic oedema of infancy

History. Acute haemorrhagic oedema of infancy (AHEI) is a benign leukocytoclastic vasculitis of infancy that overlaps in many ways with HSP but has distinct clinical and histological features. AHEI is also known as 'infantile Henoch–Schönlein purpura', cockade purpura and oedema, and Finkelstein–Seidlmayer syndrome. The names can be somewhat misleading, because AHEI is neither truly haemorrhagic nor is it simply an infantile version of HSP. The condition was first described in 1913 by Irving Snow [65]. Later, it was reported in Germany by Hubert Seidlmayer (1939) and Heinrich Finkelstein (1956) for whom the disease was named [66,67]. While long recognized as a distinct clinical entity in European countries, AHEI has only existed as a separate entity in the English language literature since the 1990s. There is continued debate about whether it is a variant of HSP or a distinct clinicopathological entity, with more emphasis on the latter [68,69].

Epidemiology. AHEI typically affects infants aged 4 months to 2 years, with a 2:1 predilection for males. Between 66 and 75% of patients have an infectious prodrome or preceding vaccination [70,71]. Similarly to HSP, there likely is a peak incidence in winter that corresponds with preceding infectious triggers. However, no epidemiological studies have been undertaken to prove this hypothesis [72].

Pathogenesis. The histological finding of leukocytoclastic vasculitis implicates immune complex deposition and neutrophil recruitment in the pathogenesis of AHEI. Direct immunofluorescence reveals a predominance of IgM (80%), although IgA (30%), IgE (30%) and IgG (20%) can also be seen. The presence of C3 and C1q in the immune deposits of involved skin also suggests that activation of the classical complement pathway plays an important role in the development of lesions [68]. The predilection for the face in infants, as opposed to the lower legs as seen with most leukocytoclastic vasculitis in children or adults, may be secondary to their more often prone position as well as proportionally larger head size corresponding to an increased blood supply [73].

A recent upper respiratory tract infection is the most commonly reported trigger [72]. Other purported infectious triggers include cytomegalovirus [71], rotavirus [74], herpes simplex [75], pneumococcal bacteraemia [76], and *Escherichia coli* urinary tract infection [77]. Fewer than 10% of cases occur following vaccination [72,78]. Although many of the reported cases of AHEI include a history of recent exposure to acetaminophen, NSAIDs or antibiotics, re-exposure to these medications did not result in recurrence of disease, arguing against a drug-induced pathogenesis [72].

Clinical features. AHEI is classically described as a triad of acute onset purpuric rash, oedema and low-grade fever in an otherwise well-looking infant. The cutaneous findings are dramatic in appearance and rapidity of onset, mimicking the purpura of HSP [79]. Despite the alarming nature of the rash, the overall appearance of wellness in the infant helps distinguish AHEI from other more serious diseases [71]. Fever is generally mild (less than 38.5 °C) [70].

The cutaneous eruption in AHEI occurs abruptly over the course of 24–48 hours, classically in a 'cockade' or targetoid pattern of ecchymotic, red to purple purpuric macules distributed symmetrically over the face, ears, lower extremities, upper extremities and perianal region, in that order of frequency (Fig. 145.4). Individual lesions are 1– 5 cm in size with surrounding indurated oedema

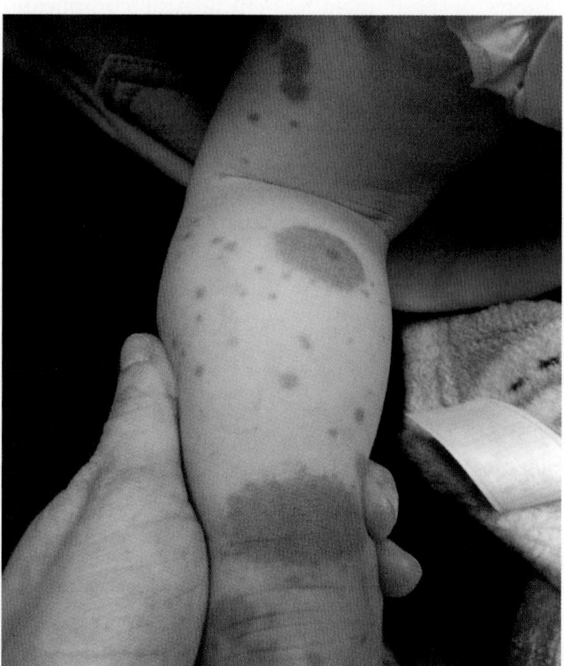

Fig. 145.4 Purpura and large coalescent ecchymoses on the upper extremities of an infant with acute haemorrhagic oedema of infancy. Source: Courtesy of Patrick McMahon, MD and Leslie Castelo-Soccio, MD, Children's Hospital of Philadelphia, PA, USA.

and can remain discrete or coalesce. Although the oedematous lesions may be tender, pruritus is typically absent [78]. Mucous membrane involvement is very uncommon but can include conjunctival injection or oral petechiae [70,71]. During the course of illness there can be between one to four crops of new lesions [80].

The inflammatory oedema of AHEI is nonpitting and can be both painful and extensive, often involving the face and ears. Scrotal swelling is sometimes also seen in boys (Fig. 145.5). In contrast to HSP, AHEI is typically confined to the skin, and additional systemic symptoms such as arthralgia, renal involvement, gastrointestinal bleeding and intussusception are exceedingly rare [70]. In the few reported cases of renal involvement, disease was mild and transient [81].

Krause and colleagues proposed a set of four clinical criteria for the diagnosis of AHEI: (i) age < 2 years old; (ii) purpuric or ecchymotic skin lesions, with oedema of the face, auricles and extremities, with or without mucosal involvement; (iii) lack of systemic or visceral involvement; and (iv) spontaneous recovery within a few days or weeks [69].

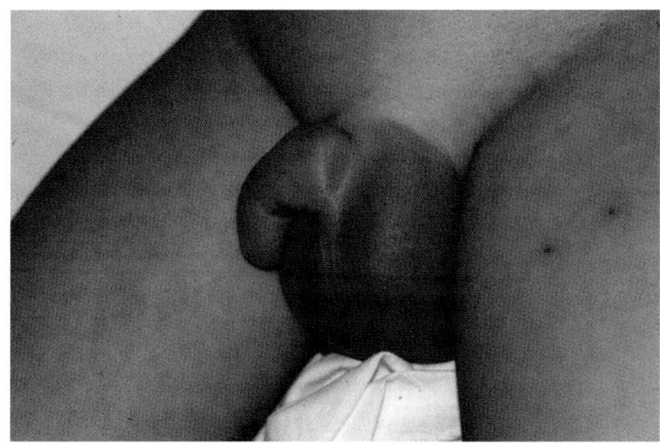

Fig. 145.5 Scrotal swelling can be a prominent feature of both Henoch–Schönlein purpura and acute haemorrhagic oedema of infancy. Source: Courtesy of David Sherry, MD, Children's Hospital of Philadelphia, PA, USA.

Differential diagnosis. The main differential diagnosis for AHEI is HSP if considered as separate entities. Table 145.3 details differences that help distinguish the two diseases. The targetoid appearance of the lesions in AHEI can also be confused with erythema multiforme. In contrast to erythema multiforme, however, AHEI lesions are more ecchymotic and mucous membrane involvement is rare. Other differential diagnoses include nonaccidental trauma, sepsis, meningococcemia, purpura fulminans, urticarial and drug-induced vasculitis, Kawasaki disease, Sweet syndrome, Gianotti–Crosti disease and Wells syndrome.

Laboratory findings. There are no diagnostic laboratory findings in AHEI. Inflammatory markers are normal or slightly elevated. A mild leukocytosis or thrombocytosis can also be seen. Liver function tests are usually normal but can in rare cases be slightly elevated, consistent with mild systemic inflammation. Urinalysis and creatinine are almost always normal [72,78]. Serum complement levels are also usually normal and in contrast to HSP there is no isolated increase in serum IgA [80]. One case report demonstrated transiently low C4, C1q and CH50, supporting the hypothesis that complement activation occurs via the classical pathway [81]. Antinuclear antibodies and antineutrophil cytoplasmic autoantibodies are absent [78].

Histology. Histological examination typically demonstrates an intense leukocytoclastic vasculitis involving the capillaries and postcapillary venules of the upper and mid-dermis. Fibrinoid necrosis and red blood cell extravasation are frequently present. Perivascular deposits are composed predominantly of fibrinogen, IgM (80%) and C3, with only 25–30% of cases also staining positive for IgA [68,70]. The additional presence of C1q deposition also distinguishes AHEI from HSP, supporting a different pathological mechanism [68].

Table 145.3 Comparison of typical findings in acute haemorrhagic oedema of infancy (AHEI) and Henoch–Schönlein purpura (HSP)

	AHEI	HSP
Clinical characteristics		
Age	4–24 months	Peaks at 4–6 years, rarely seen under 2 years
Gender	Male predominance 2:1	Slight male predominance
Purpura	Cockade pattern of ecchymoses	Petechiae, palpable purpura
Distribution	Face/ears > lower extremities > upper extremities	Lower legs and buttocks
Oedema	Frequent and extensive	+/–
Visceral involvement	Rare	Frequent
Duration	1–3 weeks	4 weeks
Recurrence	–	33%
Chronic renal disease	–	+/–
Histopathology		
Leukocytoclastic vasculitis	+	+
IgA deposits	+/– (2 of 3 negative)	+
C1q deposits	+	–
Fibrinoid necrosis	+	+/–

Treatment and prognosis. Because AHEI is a self-limited disease, no specific treatment is indicated. Supportive care directed toward symptomatic relief is generally adequate. The prognosis is excellent, and spontaneous resolution is almost always seen within 1–3 weeks with no known long-term complications. Unlike HSP, patients do not need monitoring for renal disease following the illness. Although rare recurrences have been described, in a review of 300 cases, no true recurrences were seen [70].

Urticarial vasculitis

History and definition. Urticarial vasculitis is a clinicopathological entity characterized by the clinical presentation of urticarial lesions with histopathological evidence of leukocytoclastic vasculitis. Unlike true urticaria, individual lesions persist for more than 24 hours and often resolve with postinflammatory hyperpigmentation, representative of blood vessel damage. However, the precise definition of urticarial vasculitis varies in the literature, especially with respect to the extent of blood vessel damage required for histopathological diagnosis [82].

Urticarial vasculitis is usually divided into normocomplementemic (NUV) and hypocomplementemic urticarial vasculitis (HUV), which may represent a spectrum of disease with HUV having more systemic features [82–84]. HUV is also known as anti-C1q vasculitis based on the 2012 Revised Chapel Hill Consensus Conference nomenclature [3]. Most cases are primary or idiopathic, but they can be associated with underlying systemic illness, including connective tissue diseases, infections, drug hypersensitivities and malignancy. HUV in particular is closely associated with systemic lupus erythematosus (SLE) [85].

Hypocomplementemic urticarial vasculitis syndrome (HUVS) is a rare but severe form of HUV with prominent systemic features, including renal, joint, ocular and gastrointestinal manifestations that was first described in adults by McDuffie and colleagues in 1972 [86]. Rare cases of HUVS have also been reported in children, most of which are associated with severe renal involvement [87–94]. Some authors believe that HUV and HUVS represent a continuum of disease severity, with HUVS being characterized by more systemic involvement, whereas others view HUVS as a distinct entity. However, the precise relationship between HUV and HUVS is not well defined, and nomenclature varies in the literature [85,95,96].

Epidemiology. Overall urticarial vasculitis is a rare cause of chronic and recurrent urticaria among children [87,88]. Of adults with chronic urticaria, approximately 10% may have urticarial vasculitis [85]. Up to two-thirds of urticarial vasculitis cases occur in women [83,97]. Although a slight female predominance has been observed in NUV, HUV is almost exclusively seen in females. The mean age of onset is approximately 40 years of age [95,97,98]. However, it can occur in the paediatric population, with the youngest reported case in a 2-month-old infant [99].

Pathogenesis. Urticarial vasculitis is recognized as a type III hypersensitivity reaction, in which immune complex deposition and complement activation play important roles, although the exact mechanism is not well understood. IgG autoantibodies against the collagen-like region of C1q in addition to decreased serum C1q levels have been found in nearly 100% of HUVS patients, 35–60% of SLE patients and in much smaller percentages of patients with other connective tissues diseases such as rheumatoid arthritis, Sjögren syndrome and scleroderma [100,101]. While it is not known whether anti-C1q antibodies are pathological, it has been proposed that immune complexes containing C1q-C1q antibody precipitins deposit within vessel walls and activate the classical pathway of the complement system, generating C3a/C5a anaphylotoxins and inducing mast cell degranulation. Mast cell activation is thought to drive the urticaria and angioedema that characterizes the early stages of disease [96]. Subsequent release of proinflammatory mediators lead to increased vascular permeability and recruitment of eosinophils and neutrophils with resulting vessel damage [102,103]. The exact mechanism may differ in various types of urticarial vasculitis.

Infectious triggers have been implicated in some cases, but much less commonly than in other types of cutaneous vasculitis. In one study, paediatric cases were often preceded by upper respiratory tract infections [104]. Lyme disease was implicated in a single paediatric case [105]. In adults, associations with HIV, syphilis, hepatitis, various drug exposures and physical stimuli, including exercise, cold exposure and ultraviolet light have all been described [82]. Numerous cases have also occurred in the setting of various malignancies, suggestive of a paraneoplastic phenomenon [104,106].

The hypocomplementemic forms of urticarial vasculitis have been closely associated with connective tissues diseases, especially SLE and Sjögren syndrome [82]. In one adult study, as many as half of the patients with HUV had SLE [98]. There have also been several paediatric cases of HUV described in association with SLE, as either manifestations of disease flare or as the presenting sign prior to development of positive antinuclear and antidouble-stranded DNA (anti-dsDNA) antibodies [89,107,108]. As such, HUV may in some cases represent either a minor form of SLE or lupus in evolution [98]. The high percentage of SLE patients with anti-C1q antibodies also suggests that SLE and HUV may share a similar pathogenetic basis. However, different binding specificities of the anti-C1q antibodies have been demonstrated in these two diseases and may account for the difference in clinical outcomes [102]. Lastly, the reported occurrence of urticarial vasculitis in a set of twins and two separate groups of siblings suggests there could be a genetic component to the disease [89,109,110]. Reported cases of HUV associated with hereditary C3 deficiency and C3 nephritic factor represent specific examples where underlying immune dysregulation results in a predisposition toward disease [111,112].

Other forms of urticarial vasculitis are associated with specific diseases, including AHA syndrome (arthritis, hives and angioedema) [113], Schnitzler syndrome, a

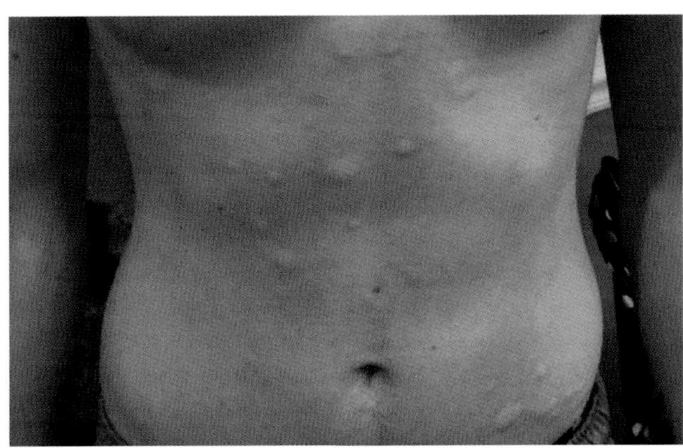

Fig. 145.6 Early pruritic wheals in a teenage male with urticarial vasculitis are indistinguishable from classic urticaria.

monoclonal IgM gammopathy with chronic urticaria [114] and Cogan's syndrome, a chronic inflammatory disorder characterized by interstitial keratitis, sensorineural hearing loss and systemic vasculitis [115,116].

Clinical manifestations. Urticarial vasculitis typically presents with raised, erythematous wheals that initially may be indistinguishable from urticaria in appearance (Fig. 145.6). However, in contrast to true urticaria which is transient, wheals in urticarial vasculitis are fixed, lasting at least 24 hours, and resolve with bruising or hyperpigmentation, presumably caused by extravasation of blood cells [97,117]. Dermascopy may reveal evidence of purpura, which helps distinguish urticarial vasculitis from true urticaria [118]. Less common cutaneous manifestations include palpable purpura, livedo reticularis, or rarely, erythema multiforme-like lesions [95,119,120]. The wheals in urticarial vasculitis can be pruritic but are more often painful or burning [97]. They are also usually much less responsive to antihistamines than true urticaria [95].

HUV is more commonly associated with systemic symptoms, including fever, angioedema (40–50% of cases), arthralgias (up to 75% of cases) and nonspecific gastrointestinal symptoms such as abdominal pain, diarrhoea, or vomiting [83,95,97]. Hypocomplementemic urticarial vasculitis syndrome is the most severe form, characterized by multiorgan involvement and the presence of anti-C1q antibodies. Associated findings may include glomerulonephritis, arthritis, uveitis, episcleritis, pulmonary haemorrhage, obstructive pulmonary disease, hepatosplenomegaly, serositis, central nervous system involvement and Raynaud's phenomenon [83,96]. Renal disease can develop up to 10 years after the onset of cutaneous manifestations [94].

Schwartz and colleagues developed diagnostic criteria for HUVS in 1982, which requires the presence of two major criteria (chronic urticaria and hypocomplementaemia) with at least two of six minor criteria (Table 145.4) [121]. HUVS is generally considered to be a distinct autoimmune disease and as such the diagnosis requires exclusion of other diseases such as SLE. While an elevated antinuclear antibody (ANA) titre is one of the exclusion criteria in the original Schwartz criteria, given the

Table 145.4 Diagnostic criteria for hypocomplementemic urticarial vasculitis syndrome

Two mandatory criteria:	
	Chronic urticarial exanthema (>6 months)
	Hypocomplementemia
And at least two of six minor criteria:	
	Leukocytoclastic vasculitis
	Arthralgia or arthritis
	Uveitis or episcleritis
	Glomerulonephritis
	Abdominal pain
	Positive anti-C1q antibody

Exclusion criteria[1]: Systemic lupus erythematosus, cryoglobulinaemia, hereditary complement or C1 esterase inhibitor deficiency, positive anti-dsDNA or hepatitis B antigen

[1] Elevated antinuclear antibody (ANA) titre was one of the original exclusion criteria but is not included here given the frequency of positive ANAs with negative double-stranded DNA (dsDNA) in urticarial vasculitis.
Source: Adapted from Schwartz et al. 1982 [121].

frequency of positive ANAs seen in urticarial vasculitis, subsequent authors have proposed that the ANA can be positive as long as anti-dsDNA and anti-Smith antibodies are negative [96,122].

Differential diagnosis. Urticarial vasculitis needs to be distinguished from urticaria multiforme, serum sickness, other types of cutaneous vasculitis and autoinflammatory diseases. Urticaria multiforme often presents with acral oedema and intense polycyclic urticarial lesions with dusky, ecchymotic-appearing centres that resolve within hours, and thus are not representative of true ecchymoses [123]. Furthermore, the wheals in urticaria multiforme classically coalesce into serpiginous lesions or giant urticaria rather than remaining discrete wheals as in urticarial vasculitis [85]. Serum sickness is somewhat more difficult to distinguish from urticarial vasculitis, because the presence of fever, arthralgias, hypocomplementaemia and urticarial rashes that resolve with bruising is seen in both conditions. However, serum sickness is an acute, self-limited condition [123].

For patients with multiorgan involvement, HSP and ANCA-associated vasculitis should be considered in the differential, although hypocomplementaemia is not characteristic of either disease, and each is distinguished by characteristic histopathological findings [124]. Autoinflammatory diseases in children also frequently present with urticarial lesions in the setting of systemic symptoms such as fever, arthralgia and abdominal pain. Hyperimmunoglobulinaemia D with periodic fever syndrome (hyper IgD syndrome) is an example wherein the urticarial lesions have histopathological features of mild vasculitis. The cryopyrin-associated periodic fever syndromes, namely familial cold autoinflammatory syndrome, Muckle–Wells syndrome and neonatal-onset multisystem inflammatory disease (NOMID), are also frequently characterized by recurrent urticarial lesions. However, biopsy features are more consistent with true urticaria than vasculitis [125].

Laboratory and imaging findings. Serum complement levels, including C1q, C3, C4 and CH50, are low in HUV, indicating activation of the classical complement pathway. C1 esterase inhibitor should be normal, distinguishing urticarial vasculitis from hereditary angioedema [95,97]. The erythrocyte sedimentation rate (ESR) is elevated in a third of cases [83]. ANA titres are often positive, but anti-dsDNA and anti-Smith are usually absent, except in cases where HUV is a manifestation of SLE [96].

Patients with HUVS characteristically have extremely low serum levels of C1q, in addition to markedly decreased C3 and C4. The degree of hypocomplementaemia seems to correlate with the severity of disease [96]. Anti-C1q antibodies are present in 90–100% of adults with HUVS, but it is not a specific finding [100]. In several paediatric cases that otherwise met clinical criteria for HUVS, anti-C1q antibodies were not always present [87,110].

In cases where multiorgan involvement is suspected, additional testing should be considered, including chest radiography, pulmonary function tests, abdominal ultrasonography, echocardiography and slit-lamp examination. Microscopic urinalysis, urine protein quantification and serum creatinine should be performed to screen for renal involvement, and significant proteinuria, haematuria or acute kidney injury may warrant renal biopsy [96].

Histology. Urticarial vasculitis is characterized by the classic appearance of a necrotizing leukocytoclastic vasculitis involving postcapillary venules of the superficial and mid-dermis. Skin biopsies are best performed on early lesions and multiple biopsies may be needed to make the diagnosis [126]. Evidence of vascular damage, including fragmented nuclei (leukocytoclasis), fibrinoid deposits and perivascular dermal haemorrhage are commonly seen, although there is no consensus on which features are required for diagnosis [82]. The inflammatory infiltrate is predominantly neutrophilic as expected with leukocytoclastic vasculitis. However, lymphocyte-predominant infiltrates have been described in a minority of cases, which may represent later stages of inflammation [33,103]. In addition to perivascular infiltrates, dermal neutrophilia is present in nearly half of cases. Other findings characteristic of urticaria are also observed, including dermal oedema and tissue eosinophilia [83]. In a timed experiment with exercise-induced urticarial vasculitis, eosinophils were the first inflammatory cells present, followed by an influx of neutrophils [103].

Direct immunofluorescence reveals IgG, C3 and C1q deposition both perivascularly and along the basement membrane [83]. This pattern of immune deposition is also seen in SLE and is not specific to urticarial vasculitis [82]. Similarly, renal biopsy findings may appear indistinguishable from lupus nephritis [102].

Treatment and prognosis. Although antihistamines and NSAIDs are traditionally considered first-line therapy for isolated cutaneous involvement, they are generally not effective. Other first-line agents frequently used in adults for mild disease include plaquenil, dapsone, colchicine and corticosteroids. For relapsing or refractory disease, a wide variety of immunosuppressive agents have been used, including azathioprine, cyclosporine, methotrexate, mycophenolate mofetil (MMF) and cyclophosphamide [104,117,127]. In a recent descriptive study of 57 patients, azathioprine, MMF and cyclophosphamide all had similar efficacy and were more effective than methotrexate. In the same study, rituximab achieved the highest response rates (75%) compared with corticosteroids and conventional immunosuppressive agents [95]. Rituximab has also been reported to be very effective for SLE-associated HUV [128]. More recently, omalizumab (anti-IgE monoclonal antibody) has been tried in several cases of refractory urticarial vasculitis with good success and tolerability [129]. Intravenous immunoglobulin (IVIG), plasmapheresis and biologic therapies including anakinra (IL-1 receptor antagonist), canakinumab (monoclonal anti–IL-1β antibody) and tocilizumab (monoclonal anti-IL-6 antibody) remain potential alternative options [123,130–134].

In the majority of paediatric cases reported in the literature, corticosteroids have been used with variable success [91,94], either as monotherapy or in combination with conventional immunosuppressive agents, including mycophenolate, dapsone, cyclosporine and azathioprine. Cyclophosphamide has also been used for severe renal disease and pulmonary hemorrhage [90,92]. IVIG was found to be effective in one paediatric case of HUV associated with SLE [135].

All forms of urticarial vasculitis tend to have a chronic or recurrent course, although idiopathic urticarial vasculitis with isolated cutaneous involvement often resolves over time and has the best prognosis. Despite the potential severity and frequency of systemic involvement, outcomes of urticarial vasculitis in adult studies are generally good, without significant increases in mortality [95,104]. In the few paediatric cases that have been described, outcomes are also generally good [87,88,92,93]. However, a few cases with severe renal involvement progressed to ESRD despite treatment with immunosuppressive therapy [89,90,94]. Some patients initially diagnosed with idiopathic HUV progressed to meet criteria for SLE, so it is recommended that patients be followed closely for association with SLE [84].

Erythema elevatum diutinum

History and definition. Erythema elevatum diutinum (EED) is a rare, localized cutaneous small vessel leukocytoclastic vasculitis characterized by a chronic course with progressive fibrosis. It was first described as persistent, raised, purple plaques occurring in middle-aged men by Hutchinson in 1888 [136]. One year later, Bury reported the first female case in a 12-year-old with significant disfigurement of her hands [137]. In 1894, Radcliff-Crocker and Williams described a 6-year-old female with similar cutaneous findings and concluded that their case, along with Hutchinson and Bury's, should be described as a single entity which they named erythema elevatum diutinum

[138]. Historically, cases occurring in young women with underlying rheumatic disease were considered the 'Bury type' of EED, whereas cases in middle-aged men were considered the 'Hutchinson type' [139]. However, these distinctions are no longer relevant because they are considered the same entity regardless of the underlying cause [139].

In the 1930s, the name 'extracellular cholesterolosis' was applied to persistent red-orange plaques and nodules that appeared to contain cholesterol deposits. Later studies showed that the lipid deposits were actually intracellular and this finding is now considered a chronic form of EED [140].

Epidemiology. EED is extremely rare. It most commonly presents in the fourth to sixth decade, although it can occur at any age and does not appear to have any racial predilection [141]. Only a few cases have been reported in children, with the youngest being 2 months of age [142–145]. The disease presents earlier in patients with HIV and in those with underlying rheumatic or haematological conditions. Numerous reports have demonstrated an association between EED and hypergammaglobulinaemia, particularly IgA paraproteinaemia [146]. Systemic autoimmune diseases associated with EED include coeliac disease [143], Crohn's disease [147,148], SLE [149] and rheumatoid arthritis [150,151]. Chronic infections [149,152,153] and malignancy, including multiple myeloma, myelodysplasia [151] and a single case of lymphoma [154], have also been reported. There was one report of EED in a juvenile idiopathic arthritis patient being treated with abatacept, and the authors surmise that the underlying arthritis rather than the drug exposure triggered the development of EED [145].

Pathogenesis. Immune complex deposition caused by an unknown chronic antigenic trigger is thought to be central to the pathogenesis of EED. It has been hypothesized that repeated immune complex deposition in postcapillary venules, complement activation and incomplete resolution of inflammation leads to the persistent fibrotic response and cholesterol deposition that characterizes EED [139,155].

In cases associated with IgA gammopathy, some authors postulate that high levels of IgA activate the alternative complement pathway and contribute to the pathogenesis of dermal vessel damage. However, the pathogenic role of IgA has not been proven, and the association with IgA gammopathy may represent an epiphenomenon [156]. The association with chronic infectious triggers and connective tissue diseases also support an immune complex-driven pathogenesis. There have been 19 cases of EED reported in patients with HIV [141]. It is possible that HIV infection itself triggers immune complex deposition or that other concomitant infections act as antigenic stimuli [157]. In support of the latter, recurrent flares of EED were temporally associated with episodes of respiratory infections in this population [158].

Lastly, activation of cytokines such as IL-8 may have a role in the initiation of EED through selective recruitment of neutrophils to tissue sites [159].

Clinical manifestations. EED is characterized by firm, red-brown or violaceous papules, plaques and nodules, which persist chronically and often coalesce or gradually enlarge. Lesions can also blister or ulcerate [151]. Chronic nodules often acquire more of a pink–yellow tinge, indicative of intracellular lipid deposits [160]. Lesions are symmetrically distributed over the extensor surfaces of extremities, preferentially overlying joints and tendons of the fingers, hands, elbows, ankles and knees (Fig. 145.7) [161]. Rarely the trunk, retroauricular scalp, palms or soles are involved [160]. Without treatment, lesions can either persist chronically or resolve spontaneously, sometimes leaving postinflammatory hypo- or hyperpigmentation [162]. Although EED is typically asymptomatic, early lesions can be pruritic, painful or burning [136,160]. Established lesions may become tender to palpation. Occasionally constitutional symptoms or arthralgias are also present [138].

Differential diagnosis. The differential diagnosis of EED includes granuloma annulare, granuloma faciale, pyoderma gangrenosum and neutrophilic dermatoses (Sweet syndrome), which can be differentiated from EED histopathologically. In HIV patients in particular, EED needs to be distinguished from Kaposi sarcoma and bacillary angiomatosis [163].

Laboratory findings. There are no diagnostic laboratory findings in EED. It is advisable to look for evidence of past streptococcal infection, HIV, hepatitis, syphilis or underlying autoimmune disease within the appropriate clinical context. Given the strong association with IgA gammopathies, routine immunoelectrophoresis has been recommended by some authors [151]. In one study, all patients with EED had a positive IgA ANCA, which could potentially serve as a marker of disease but needs further characterization [164].

Histology. A histological spectrum of leukocytoclastic vasculitis to vessel occlusion and dermal fibrosis is seen in EED [162]. Initially, neutrophilic perivascular infiltrates, leukocytoclasis and fibrinoid deposits resemble early changes of leukocytoclastic vasculitis. Early papillary oedema can be observed and clinically relates to pseudovesiculation [146]. Vessel occlusion can also occur, which in rare cases causes ischaemia and necrosis of the epidermis [162]. During later stages, an increasing number of histiocytes along with rare eosinophils surround vessel walls. Chronic dermal injury leads to well-circumscribed areas of concentric or storiform dermal fibrosis, associated with granulation and spindle cell proliferation [141,165,166]. Direct immunofluorescence can reveal perivascular deposition of complement, IgA, IgG, IgM and fibrin, which is nonspecific [24].

With chronic lesions, lipid-laden histiocytes are seen throughout the dermis. Electron microscopy reveals exclusively intracellular lipid deposits in histiocytes, epidermal keratinocytes, mast cells and lymphocytes. As such, the terminology 'extracellular cholesterolosis' is a misnomer and no longer used [167].

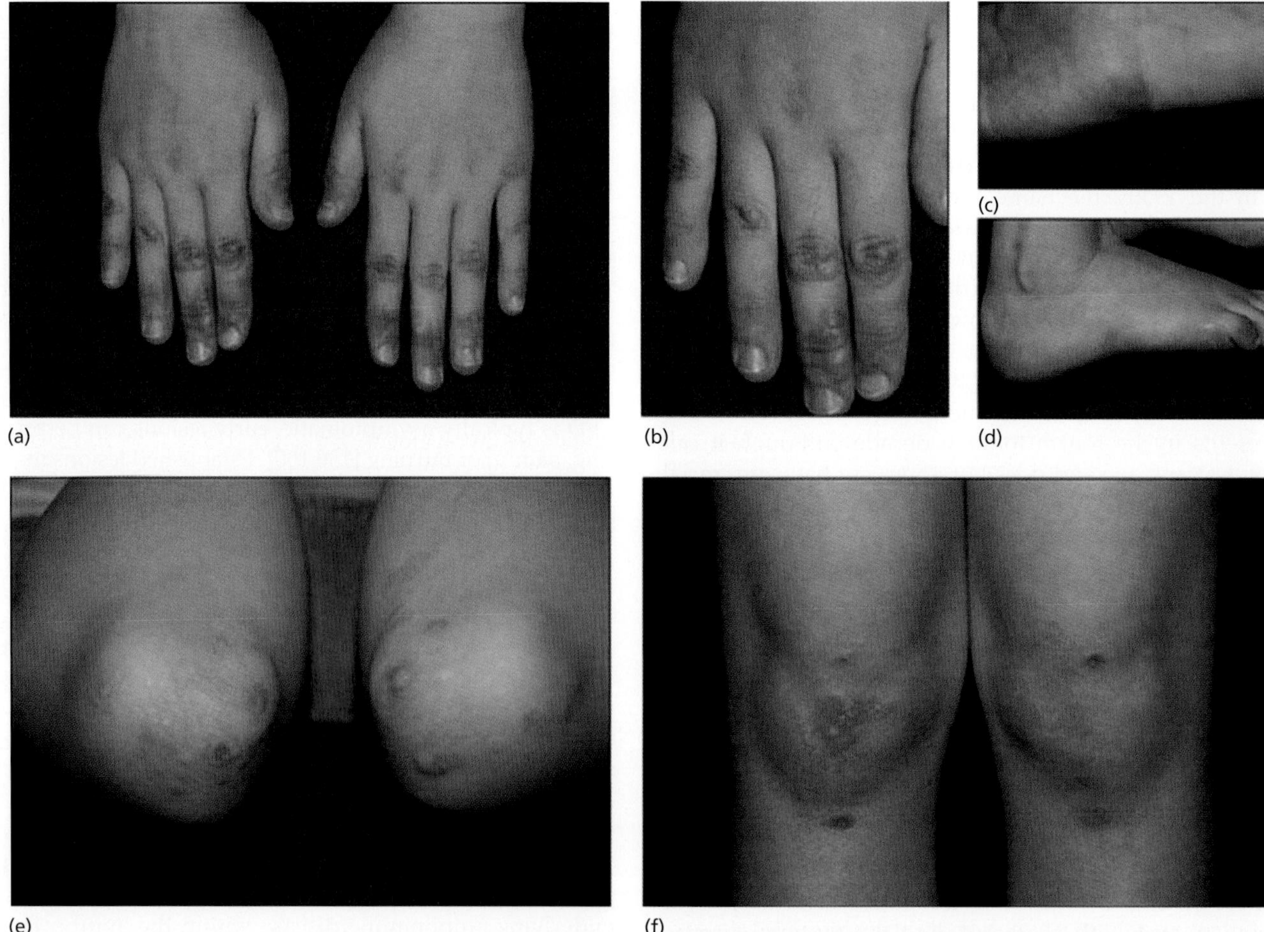

Fig. 145.7 (a) Multiple erythematous to flesh-coloured papules and nodules on the extensor surfaces of the hands of a child with erythema elevatum diutinum. (b) Closer view of the right hand. (c) Involvement of the wrist, (d) right foot, (e) extensor surfaces of the elbows and (f) knees. Source: Kim G-W et al. 2011 [161]. Reprinted with permission of Korean Dermatological Society. Copyright 2011 Korean Dermatological Association. http://anndermatol.org

Treatment and prognosis. Emphasis is placed on treatment of the underlying cause if there is one, because successful treatment of the associated infection or systemic disease often results in simultaneous resolution of the EED [143,149,168,169]. Otherwise, the first-line agent most commonly used for early EED lesions is oral dapsone, which was effective as monotherapy in up to 80% of cases [141]. However, relapse after therapy is common [152] and dapsone has no clinical effect on nodular lesions that are already in the chronic fibrotic stage [170]. Topical dapsone was also observed to improve early lesions but was not as effective as oral dapsone in achieving resolution [171].

Other therapies that have been tried with variable success include antibiotics (tetracyclines, sulphonamides, macrolides) [153], niacinamide [172], corticosteroids [173], intralesional corticosteroid injections [174], colchicine [175] and methotrexate [141,156]. For treatment of EED associated with IgA paraproteinaemia, there are reports of success with plasmapheresis [176]. Lastly, surgical excision can be considered for localized disease that is either in the chronic fibrotic stage or not amenable to medical therapy [174,177].

The overall prognosis is tied to the underlying cause. EED typically evolves over the course of 5–10 years and can spontaneously remit. There is no excess mortality. However, the cosmetic disfigurement can cause significant morbidity [178].

Pigmented purpuras

Overview

The pigmented purpuras are a group of benign dermatoses characterized clinically by petechiae and purpura on a brown, red or yellow base and histologically by capillaritis. Fibrinoid destruction of the vessel walls is absent, therefore the pigmented purpuras are classified as noninflammatory purpura without true vasculitis, or purpura simplex [179]. They are discussed along with the cutaneous vasculitides, given their clinical similarities. This family of dermatoses includes progressive pigmented purpuric dermatosis (Schamberg disease), pigmented purpuric lichenoid dermatosis of Gougerot and Blum, purpura annularis telangiectoides (Majocchi disease), lichen aureus and itching purpura (eczematoid-like purpura of Doucas and Kapetanakis) [180].

The pigmented purpuras are primarily seen in middle-aged adults, but paediatric cases have been reported in all types except for pigmented purpuric lichenoid dermatosis. Lesions are symmetrically distributed on the legs, suggesting a gravitational role. Although each variant has distinct morphological patterns, they are histopathologically indistinguishable and may represent different clinical features of the same disease [180,181]. Histological findings include lymphohistiocytic perivascular infiltrates in the papillary dermis and endothelial cell swelling. Red blood cell extravasation and haemosiderin-laden macrophages result in the characteristic pigmentary changes. The aetiology of these disorders is unclear, although an abnormal cell-mediated immune response has been implicated in the pathogenesis [181]. They all have a chronic persistent or recurrent course and present a therapeutic challenge.

Schamberg disease

History. Schamberg disease is the prototype of the pigmented purpuras. It was first described by Schamberg in 1901 in a 15-year-old male with red–brown oval patches on his lower legs bordered by punctate 'cayenne pepper' spots, which Schamberg termed progressive pigmentary disease [182]. It is also known as progressive pigmented purpura and progressive pigmentary dermatosis.

Epidemiology. Schamberg disease is by far the most common of the pigmented purpuras as well as the most common variant seen in children [183,184]. It typically presents later in adolescence or adulthood but can occur at any age, with the youngest reported case occurring in a 1-year-old child [185]. There is a male predominance [184].

Aetiology. Although the precise aetiology of pigmented purpura is largely unknown, cell-mediated immunity in the context of a delayed type hypersensitivity reaction is thought to be the underlying pathogenic mechanism [181,186]. Drug exposures such as acetaminophen, aspirin, carbamols and meprobamate have occasionally been implicated in cases of pigmented purpura, particularly with Schamberg disease in children [184,187,188]. Other triggers, including local contact allergens, wool clothing and exercise have also been described [180]. Most cases, however, appear to be idiopathic. Immunohistochemistry reveals perivascular infiltrates primarily comprised of CD4+ T lymphocytes in close contact with dendritic cells, supporting a cell-mediated immune mechanism similar to that of delayed hypersensitivity reactions [189]. Activation of Langerhans cells is also thought to play an important role [186]. In addition, modulated expression of cell adhesion molecules has been observed, suggesting a mechanism for lymphocyte recruitment and interaction with dermal endothelial cells and Langerhans cells [190]. Upregulation of E-selectins on endothelial cells also stimulates cytokines such as tumour necrosis factor alpha (TNF-α) [184]. Increased capillary hydrostatic pressure in dependent areas explains the predominantly lower limb involvement, whereas capillary dilation and fragility are thought to contribute to red blood cell extravasation [191].

Clinical manifestations. Patients classically present with pretibial reddish-brown macules of varying size that contain a sprinkling of petechiae concentrated near the periphery, commonly referred to as 'cayenne pepper' spots. Macules are slowly progressive and may enlarge or extend proximally. Older lesions coalesce into irregular plaques with an orange or darker brown pigmentation from haemosiderin deposition (Fig. 145.8) [180,184]. The lesions are usually distributed symmetrically over the lower limbs with a slow ascending progression, although unilateral involvement can occur [192]. The trunk and upper limbs are less commonly involved [185]. Patients are typically asymptomatic, although mild pruritus can occur [180]. The differential diagnosis includes HSP, coagulopathies, infection, thrombocytopenic purpura, traumatic ecchymoses, cryoglobulinaemia, and hypersensitivity reactions. In contrast to HSP and other forms of leukocytoclastic vasculitis, the lesions seen with Schamberg disease are never palpable and develop very slowly. There are also rare case reports of young males with pigmented purpura-like eruptions evolving to cutaneous T-cell lymphoma, which should be considered in the differential [193].

Laboratory findings. Laboratory studies are notably normal, including platelet count and coagulation studies. Other normal investigations, such as urinalysis, serum creatinine, erythrocyte sedimentation rate, cryoglobulins,

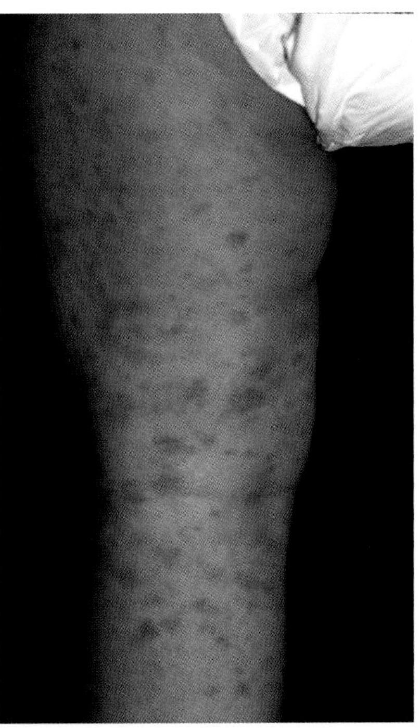

Fig. 145.8 Pigmented purpura on the lower extremities of a young toddler. Source: Courtesy of Patrick McMahon, MD and Leslie Castelo-Soccio, MD, Children's Hospital of Philadelphia, PA, USA.

antinuclear antibodies and liver enzymes also help distinguish Schamberg disease from other causes of purpura [185,188,192].

Histology. As with all pigmented purpuras, skin biopsy demonstrates a lymphohistiocytic perivascular infiltrate of superficial small vessels in the papillary dermis with endothelial cell swelling and luminal narrowing. Capillary dilation, red blood cell extravasation and haemosiderin-laden macrophages are typically seen in varying degrees. Despite the presence of inflammation and haemorrhage, fibrinoid necrosis is notably absent [194].

Treatment and prognosis. The pigmented purpuras as a whole have a chronic, persistent course. Lesions may regress spontaneously over months to years, but recurrences are also common [180]. No effective treatments have been established for Schamberg disease [185]. For the majority of patients, no treatment is necessary other than time and reassurance. Antihistamines and topical steroids can be used for symptomatic relief of pruritus [179]. Lesions are responsive to systemic corticosteroids but almost always recur after withdrawal of the medication [195]. In most cases systemic steroids are not indicated in children, given the benign nature of the condition and significant toxicity associated with chronic steroid use. Other therapies reported in the literature with variable success include ascorbic acid plus rutoside [196], cyclosporine [197], pentoxifylline [198] and griseofulvin [199]. Ultraviolet therapy remains the most promising treatment modality. There have been several reports of success with psoralen plus ultraviolet A (PUVA) [200,201] and narrowband ultraviolet B therapy in both adults and children [202,203]. However, PUVA should generally be avoided in children because of its carcinogenic potential.

Majocchi disease

Clinical overview. Majocchi disease, also known as purpura annularis telangiectoides, was first described by Majocchi in 1896 [204]. It is the single variant of pigmented purpura that presents primarily in adolescents or younger adults, and it is also the only variant more common in females. The disease is characterized clinically by annular macules with peripheral telangiectasias localized symmetrically over the lower extremities. Like Schamberg disease, lesions may extend proximally to involve the trunk and upper extremities. The purpura progress through three stages, beginning as punctate telangiectatic macules that gradually enlarge into erythematous annular patches with a peripheral rim of cayenne pepper petechiae. As each macule expands, the centre fades into a golden-brown colour, giving it the annular configuration. In the final stage, centres may become slightly atrophic [179,180,205]. The patches range from a few centimetres up to 20 cm in size. Lesions are either asymptomatic or mildly pruritic [206].

Treatment and prognosis. As with Schamberg disease, the course is chronic, often recurring and remitting over months to years [179,180]. There is no standard effective treatment. In addition to the aforementioned therapies for pigmented purpura, colchicine and methotrexate have been tried in single case reports of Majocchi disease [205,207].

Lichen aureus/lichen purpuricus

Clinical overview. Lichen aureus is a rare, distinct form of pigmented purpura that is localized, persistent and differs histologically from other subtypes [208]. It was first described by Marten in 1958 under the terminology 'lichen purpuricus' [209] and was later named lichen aureus to highlight the golden colour of the lesions. There is a predilection for younger patients; children comprise up to 17% of cases [210]. Lichen aureus is characterized clinically by localized, grouped lichenoid papules with a distinctive golden rust colour, distributed asymmetrically over the lower extremities (Fig. 145.9) [211]. The lesions can range in colour from yellow to copper and sometimes purple with scattered petechiae. Papules may coalesce into single or multiple well-demarcated plaques up to 20 cm in size. In contrast to Schamberg disease, lesions in lichen aureus are more often asymmetric or unilateral [208,212]. Occasionally a segmental or dermatomal distribution is seen [213,214].

Histology. Histologically, lichen aureus is distinguished from other subtypes of pigmented purpura by a normal epidermis and the presence of a dense band-like lymphohistiocytic infiltrate in the papillary dermis, often with marked accumulation of haemosiderin-laden macrophages [208]. The infiltrate is sometimes separated from the epidermal layer by a Grenz zone of normal collagen and closely resembles the histopathology of mycosis fungoides [215].

Treatment and prognosis. Lesions often persist unchanged for many years but occasionally spontaneously regress [205]. In one small cohort of children, the disease regressed without treatment on average over 2–4 years [210]. Topical steroids are occasionally beneficial [216] and topical calcineurin inhibitors have also been tried [217,218]. More recently, success with PUVA and pulsed-dye laser has been reported in adults [219,220].

Itching purpura

Clinical overview. Itching purpura, also known as eczematoid-like purpura of Doucas and Kapetanakis, is thought to be a more generalized and pruritic variant of Schamberg disease. It occurs primarily in middle-aged men and is characterized clinically by intensely pruritic reddish papules with mild scaling, localized to the lower legs. Lesions often extend proximally to the thighs, trunk and upper extremities. Lichenification from chronic scratching can be seen [184]. As with Schamberg disease, drug exposures and contact allergens have been implicated in the pathogenesis of disease [180].

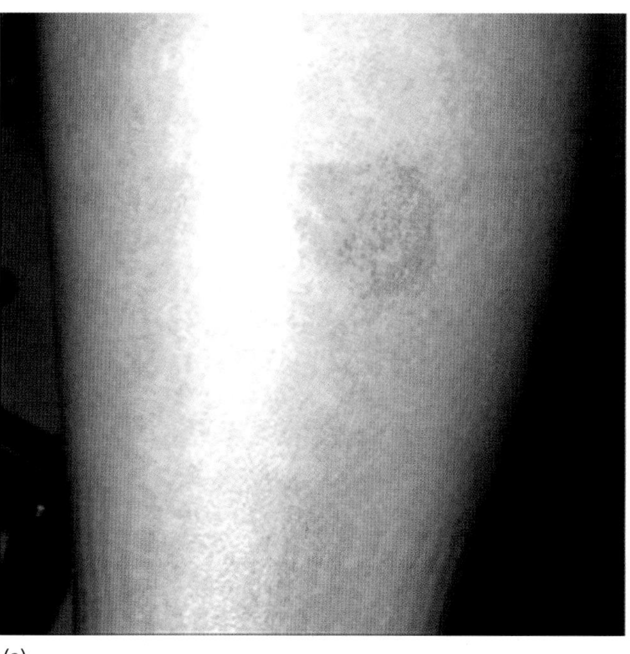

(a)

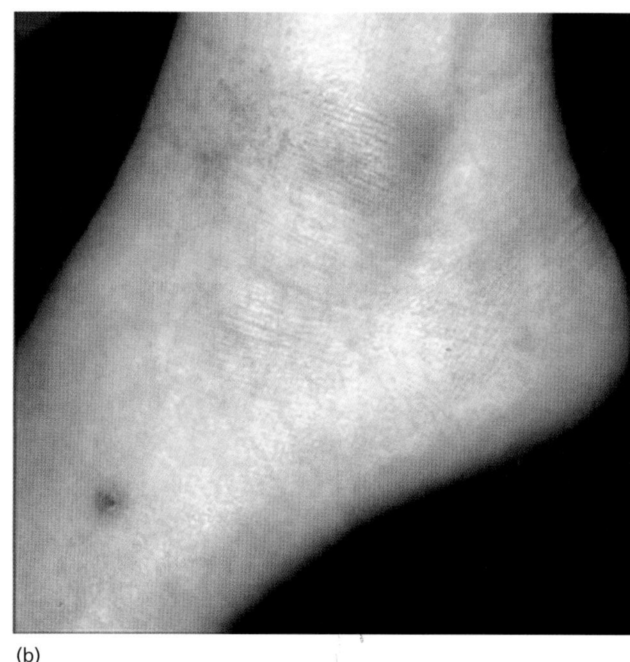

(b)

Fig. 145.9 (a) Golden-brown patches on the calf and (b) over the lateral malleolus in an 8-year-old female with lichen aureus. Source: Kim MJ et al. 2009 [211]. Reprinted with permission of Korean Dermatological Society. Source: Copyright 2009 Korean Dermatological Association. http://anndermatol.org

Treatment and prognosis. Lesions often spontaneously resolve over a period of months to years, but numerous recurrences are common [184]. Pruritus is managed with topical steroids and antihistamines.

Cutaneous polyarteritis nodosa

History. Systemic polyarteritis nodosa (PAN) is a necrotizing vasculitis of small and medium-sized arteries characterized by tissue necrosis and multiorgan involvement. Cutaneous PAN was first described in 1931 by Lindberg as a limited form of PAN that primarily involves the skin [221]. In contrast to systemic PAN, cutaneous PAN is a benign condition that does not affect other major organs. There has been some debate about whether cutaneous PAN can progress to systemic PAN. However, studies suggest they are distinct clinical entities on a continuum of disease and that there is no systemic transformation [222]. In children, PAN has some distinct characteristics and is often referred to as 'juvenile PAN', which can also be divided into cutaneous and systemic subtypes [223,224].

Epidemiology. PAN is a rare vasculitis in childhood and accounts for up to 5.6% of all vasculitides [225]. Its mean age of onset is 9 years old and has equal prevalence in both sexes. Cutaneous PAN comprises approximately one-third of juvenile PAN cases [226]. Fewer than 150 paediatric cases have been reported in the literature, with no apparent age or gender predilection [84,227].

Pathogenesis. The precise aetiology of cutaneous PAN is unknown, but is presumed to be immune complex-mediated given the presence of IgM and C3 deposition within affected arterial walls [228]. There is often a history of a preceding trigger, including streptococcal pharyngitis, viral illness, insect sting, vaccine or medication exposure; these exposures may serve as an antigenic trigger for immune complex formation. Group A streptococcal infection is the most commonly reported infectious association, as evidenced by elevated antistreptolysin (ASO) titres or positive throat cultures in up to 86% of cases [227], and has been implicated in the pathogenesis of disease in both adults and children [229–232]. ASO titres correlate with disease flares in a subset of patients, and long-term disease control with penicillin prophylaxis has been demonstrated, supporting a causal role for streptococcal infection [233]. Although hepatitis B infection is a well-known cause of PAN in adults, this association is rarely seen in children because of widespread vaccination practices [226].

Clinical manifestations. Cutaneous PAN has several clinical presentations including painful subcutaneous nodules, livedo reticularis and cutaneous ulcerations. Lesions can rarely be complicated by skin necrosis and peripheral gangrene. Petechiae, purpura and nonspecific maculopapular rashes can also be seen, but are not as helpful diagnostically unless skin biopsy confirms a necrotizing medium vessel vasculitis.

Cutaneous nodules

Most commonly, cutaneous PAN presents with painful, erythematous or violaceous subcutaneous nodules distributed over the distal lower extremities (Fig. 145.10) [232,234]. Individual nodules are small, often easier to palpate than to visualize, and may coalesce into larger areas of induration [224,232]. They often start over the malleoli and can extend proximally to include the thighs, buttocks or upper extremities [235]. The nodular manifestation is caused by involvement of small to medium vessels in the lower dermis and subcutaneous fat, as opposed to purpura, which typically represents small vessel vasculitis that is limited to the upper dermis [224].

Livedo reticularis

Livedo reticularis is another characteristic finding that may occur either alone or with subcutaneous nodules [232]. Livedo reticularis is characterized as a persistent violaceous, red or cyanotic net-like discolouration of the skin involving a wide area (Fig. 145.11a and 145.11b). The pattern can contain either regular unbroken circles (livedo reticularis), or irregular broken circles lesions (livedo racemosa) with pale centres, and does not resolve with rewarming [224]. This definition implies a pathological process and is distinct from physiological livedo reticularis (cutis marmorata), which is responsive to ambient temperature. Some authors argue that the term livedo racemosa is a more accurate description of the finding in PAN [224,236]. The characteristic mottled appearance results from microvascular thrombi and dilation of venules, which can be seen in association with many other diseases, including SLE, antiphospholipid antibody syndrome and rheumatoid arthritis.

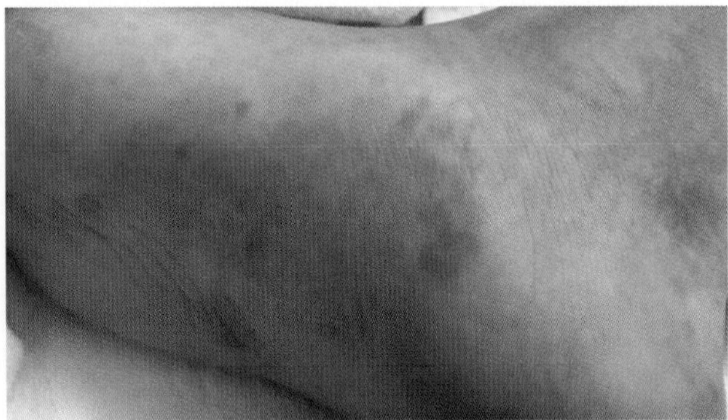

Fig. 145.10 Painful subcutaneous nodules on the foot of a 12-year-old male with polyarteritis nodosa.

Livedo reticularis must be distinguished from livedoid vasculopathy (LV), which is an occlusive microvascular disorder characterized by thrombosis and hyalinization of vessel walls, most often associated with an underlying hypercoagulable state [237]. LV presents with painful retiform purpura on the distal lower extremities that eventually ulcerate and heal with stellate atrophic porcelain-white scars (atrophie blanche) bordered by telangiectasias and haemosiderin deposition [238]. Although the appearance can be difficult to differentiate from cutaneous PAN, LV is not a true vasculitis. It is characterized histologically by intraluminal thrombi and prominent hyalinization of dermal vessel walls. In contrast to livedo reticularis, perivascular inflammation is mostly absent. Laboratory work-up should focus on excluding underlying connective tissue diseases, infections associated with cryoglobulinaemia and prothrombotic risk factors, such as lupus anticoagulants, antiphospholipid antibodies, Factor V Leiden, proteins C and S deficiencies and prothrombin gene mutations [239]. Treatment rests on anticoagulation rather than anti-inflammatory agents, although recent studies suggest intravenous immunoglobulin therapy may also be effective [237,240].

Cutaneous ulcerations and ischaemic injury

Other less common manifestations of cutaneous PAN that result from ischaemic injury include superficial and deep ulcerations, necrotic patches and peripheral gangrene [226]. Subcutaneous nodules and livedo can progress to ulceration. A 'star-burst pattern' of irregular livedo surrounding an ulcer is highly suggestive of cutaneous PAN [241,242]. The ulcers heal with porcelain-white, stellate, atrophic scarring, referred to as atrophie blanche [224]. Younger children are at higher risk for

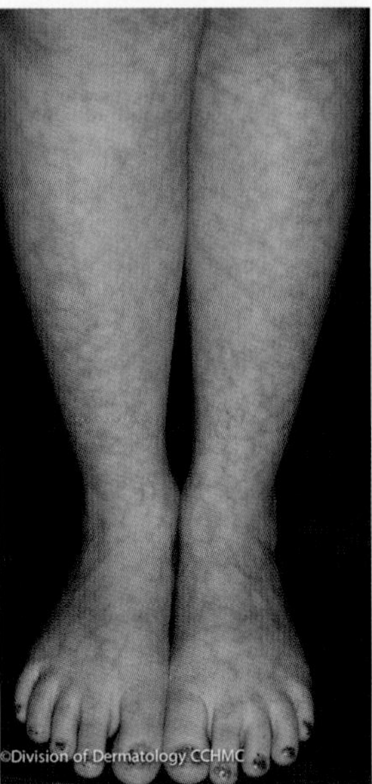

(a)

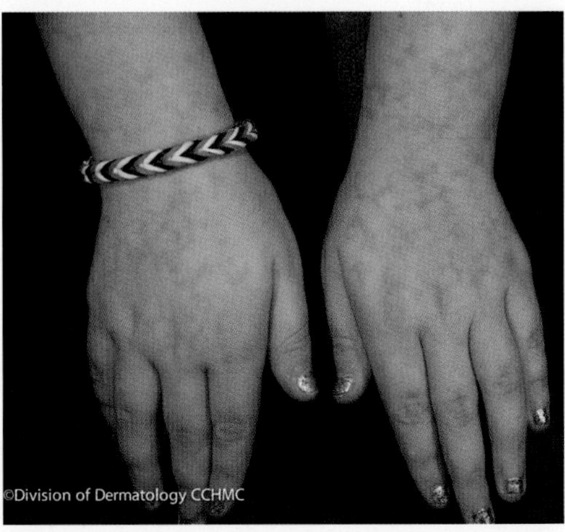

(b)

Fig. 145.11 (a) Livedo reticularis is most commonly observed on the lower limbs. (b) Hand involvement can also be seen. Source: Courtesy of Kara Shah, MD, Cincinnati Children's Hospital Medical Center, OH, USA.

Table 145.5 Comparison of systemic vasculitides

	Common cutaneous manifestations	Systemic features	Laboratory findings	Histopathology
Small vessel vasculitis, immune complex-mediated				
HSP	Palpable purpura	Glomerulonephritis Arthritis/arthralgia Gastrointestinal bleeding	Haematuria, proteinuria	Small vessel LCV; +IgA
Pauci-immune small vessel vasculitis				
GPA (Wegener)	Palpable purpura Oral/nasal ulcerations (septal perforation)	Upper respiratory (sinusitis, subglottic stenosis) Pulmonary (haemorrhage, cavitary lesions) Glomerulonephritis	c-ANCA/PR3	Small vessel necrotizing vasculitis or LCV, + granulomas
MPA	Palpable purpura	Pulmonary haemorrhage Glomerulonephritis	p-ANCA/MPO > c-ANCA/PR3	Small and medium vessel necrotizing vasculitis
EGPA (Churg–Strauss)	Painful subcutaneous nodules	Asthma Allergy Eosinophilic pneumonia Mononeuritis	p-ANCA/MPO, high serum IgE Eosinophilia	Small and medium vessel LCV or necrotizing vasculitis, + granulomas, + eosinophilia
Mixed small–medium vessel vasculitis				
Behçet disease	Oral and genital ulcerations Pathergy Erythema nodosum Papulopustular lesions	Ocular (uveitis, retinal vasculitis) Gastrointestinal ulcers Neurological Thrombophlebitisk		Affects arteries and veins of all sizes; septal panniculitis
Predominantly medium vessel vasculitis				
Kawasaki disease	Maculopapular rash Strawberry tongue Conjunctival injection Desquamation of hands and feet	Coronary artery aneurysms Cervical lymphadenopathy	Elevated ESR/CRP Elevated WBC/plt Sterile pyuria	Medium vessel necrotizing vasculitis
PAN	Cutaneous nodules, livedo reticularis, ulcerations, peripheral gangrene	Renal/hypertension Muscle pain Peripheral neuropathy	Elevated ESR/CRP ElevatedWBC/plt (ANCA negative)	Medium or small artery necrotizing vasculitis

ANCA, antineutrophil cytoplasmic antibodies (c-, cytoplasmic; p-, perinuclear); CRP, C-reactive protein; EGPA, eosinophilic granulomatosis with polyangiitis; ESR, erythrocyte sedimentation rate; GPA, granulomatosis with polyangiitis; HSP, Henoch–Schönlein purpura; LCV, leukocytoclastic vasculitis; MPA, microscopic polyangiitis; MPO, myeloperoxidase; plt, platelet count; PR3, antiproteinase 3; WBC, white blood cell count.

serious complications from ischaemic injury, including peripheral gangrene and digital autoamputation [230].

Extracutaneous manifestations

Although by definition cutaneous PAN is a skin-limited form of disease, it has been recognized that up to two-thirds of patients have extracutaneous manifestations, including peripheral neuropathy, myalgia and arthralgia/arthritis in areas adjacent to active skin disease. Constitutional symptoms such as fever, malaise and weight loss may also be present in the absence of visceral involvement [222,226,230]. The skin findings and corresponding histological features in systemic PAN and cutaneous PAN are identical. Localized myalgia and neuropathy may also be present in children with cutaneous PAN [222]. Neuropathy, in particular, is more commonly seen in association with recalcitrant ulcerative disease [232].

Differential diagnosis. Cutaneous PAN must first be distinguished from systemic PAN. Evidence of systemic involvement can include, but is not limited to, hypertension, renal failure, abdominal pain, liver injury, medium vessel aneurysms, central nervous symptoms and peripheral neuropathy or myalgias not adjacent to cutaneous lesions. Lower extremity cutaneous nodules in PAN may be confused with erythema nodosum, which is characterized histologically by septal panniculitis as opposed to the periarteriolar panniculitis described in cutaneous PAN [243,244]. Lastly, other types of vasculitis, both primary and secondary, should be considered in the differential (Table 145.5).

Laboratory findings. Inflammatory markers, including ESR and C-reactive protein (CRP) are almost always elevated, though to higher degrees in the systemic than the cutaneous form [226,245]. Other nonspecific signs of inflammation, including leukocytosis, thrombocytosis or mild anaemia may also be present. Routine testing for evidence of past streptococcal infection, including ASO and DNAse B titres, is recommended [229]. The remaining laboratory work-up should focus on excluding systemic diseases, which may include a comprehensive metabolic panel, urinalysis, ANA, ANCA, antiphospholipid antibodies and hypercoagulability work-up.

Histology. Wedge or excisional biopsies of both cutaneous nodules and livedo reticularis reveal a necrotizing nongranulomatous vasculitis of small to medium arterioles and arteries with microvascular thrombus in the lower dermis to subcutaneous fat [224]. Early stages of inflammation are characterized by fibrinoid degradation of the arterial wall and a predominantly neutrophilic infiltrate with some eosinophils [241,242]. Leukocytoclasia and erythrocyte extravasation may be present [224]. Direct immunofluorescence sometimes reveals IgM and C3 deposits [228,234,246]. In later stages, a predominantly lymphohistiocytic infiltrate is seen, with intimal proliferation and thrombosis of the artery, leading to infarction and ulceration. Healed end-stage disease is then characterized by perivascular fibroblastic proliferation [247]. For late-stage cutaneous ulcerations, multiple deep or full thickness biopsies at the edges of the ulceration may be needed to obtain conclusive evidence of necrotizing vasculitis.

Treatment and prognosis. NSAIDs may be used for mild disease. However, most patients require at least one course of systemic corticosteroids [244]. For refractory or recurrent disease, steroid-sparing agents have been used with success including colchicine, dapsone, methotrexate, mycophenolate mofetil, azathioprine, cyclophosphamide and IVIG [227,229,230,248,249]. There have been no controlled studies to guide the choice of immunosuppressive therapy. The efficacy of TNF-α inhibition in a number of systemic vasculitides suggests that TNF-α inhibitors may also be useful for refractory cutaneous PAN [250–252]. In the setting of acute distal extremity necrosis, prompt initiation of systemic vasodilators (nifedipine, sildenafil, pentoxifylline, bosentan) and anticoagulants (aspirin, heparin) in addition to systemic steroids is warranted for reperfusion and tissue salvage [249,253]. For patients with evidence of recent streptococcal infection, antibiotic treatment followed by long-term penicillin prophylaxis is recommended [226,229,233,244].

Overall, cutaneous PAN has a relatively benign course, characterized by periodic exacerbations and remissions that may persist for many years. Serious complications, however, such as digital necrosis and autoamputation can occur, especially in young children [141,230]. While evolution to systemic PAN is extremely rare, careful follow up with attention to systemic involvement is recommended [227].

Systemic diseases with secondary cutaneous vasculitis

ANCA-associated vasculitis

The antineutrophil cytoplasmic antibody (ANCA)-associated vasculitides (AAV) are a group of disorders characterized by necrotizing small vessel vasculitis with few or no immune complex deposits in the vessel walls [254]. Patients with AAV have autoantibodies against granular contents of neutrophils, which may either stain in a cytoplasmic (c-ANCA) or perinuclear (p-ANCA) pattern by indirect immunofluorescence after fixation, corresponding to the presence of antiproteinase 3 (PR3) and myeloperoxidase (MPO) antibodies respectively. The AAVs include granulomatosis with polyangiitis, microscopic polyangiitis and eosinophilic granulomatosis with polyangiitis.

Each type of AAV has distinctive characteristics as outlined in Table 145.5. Usually other associated systemic findings will help distinguish the diseases. However, skin lesions can in rare cases precede systemic involvement by months to years [6,255]. Cutaneous findings of AAV may include palpable purpura, urticarial lesions and painful subcutaneous nodules. Cutaneous findings should improve with treatment of the systemic disease, which usually involves a combination of steroids and a cytotoxic agent, such as cyclophosphamide or rituximab.

Granulomatosis with polyangiitis

Previously known as Wegener's granulomatosis, granulomatosis with polyangiitis (GPA) is characterized by necrotizing granulomatous inflammation of the upper and lower respiratory tract and kidneys. Skin involvement occurs in approximately 50% of patients [256,257], but is the initial presenting sign in only 8–9% of cases [255,256]. Cutaneous findings are variable and include palpable purpura, naso-oral ulcers, petechiae, subcutaneous nodules, erythematous patches, vasculitic papules, acneiform lesions, urticaria, necrotic ulcers and pyoderma gangrenosum-like ulcerations, of which palpable purpura is the most common [255–260]. With the exception of septal perforation from nasal ulcers, no single lesion is specific for GPA [4].

Skin biopsies reveal leukocytoclastic vasculitis, granulomatous vasculitis with lymphohistiocytic infiltrates or focal granular necrosis and fibrinoid degeneration preceding development of palisading granulomatous dermatitis [255,260]. Leukocytoclastic vasculitis is the most common histological correlate to palpable purpura in GPA. In contrast, acneiform lesions are typically characterized by a granulomatous folliculitis and subcutaneous nodules display an erythema nodosum-like septal panniculitis. Concurrent biopsies at multiple sites may be needed to confirm the presence of granulomatous inflammation [261]. Approximately 80–90% of GPA patients with cutaneous involvement have a positive c-ANCA [255,260,261]. In the few patients with negative ANCA serologies, biopsy can be particularly useful diagnostically.

Microscopic polyangiitis

Microscopic polyangiitis (MPA) is a systemic necrotizing small vessel vasculitis without granulomas. MPA manifests with a rapidly progressive necrotizing glomerulonephritis with or without pulmonary capillaritis, constituting a pulmonary–renal syndrome similar to that of GPA or Goodpasture's syndrome. Extrarenal manifestations are common and may include skin, joint, gastrointestinal, ocular and central nervous system involvement [262]. Skin disease is observed in 30–60% of patients and is the initial presenting sign in up to 15–30% of cases [263–265]. Palpable purpura over the lower extremities is the most common skin manifestation, followed by livedo reticularis, subcutaneous nodules, urticaria, ulcerations and necrosis [262,263]. Vesicles and splinter haemorrhages have also been reported in children [266]. Palpable purpura and subcutaneous nodules can be seen with either MPA or PAN, and histological features of the lesions cannot be used to differentiate the diseases [263]. Approximately 75–90% of MPA patients are ANCA positive, of which the majority are MPO and p-ANCA positive [254,262,264].

Histologically, the cutaneous lesions of MPA are characterized by leukocytoclastic vasculitis in small dermal vessels [267]. Intense inflammatory infiltrates characterize deeper dermal and subcutaneous involvement, but granulomatous inflammation is notably absent [266].

Eosinophilic granulomatosis with polyangiitis

Eosinophilic granulomatosis with polyangiitis (EGPA), also known as Churg–Strauss syndrome and allergic granulomatosis, is characterized by asthma, allergy, eosinophilia and systemic vasculitis. It is the rarest of the AAVs in children, comprising fewer than 2% of cases in one series [268]. Persistent asthma is a cardinal feature of disease, and along with other atopic diatheses such as allergic rhinitis, usually precedes the onset of other symptoms by many years. The second phase of disease is characterized by a marked peripheral and tissue eosinophilia. Systemic vasculitis is not seen until the third and final phase of the disease. Cutaneous findings, peripheral neuropathy (mononeuritis multiplex) and cardiomyopathy can also be seen [269,270]. While EGPA is classically associated with a positive p-ANCA and MPO, only 30–40% of adult patients are positive [271,272], and the percentage is even lower in children [273,274].

In addition to lower extremity palpable purpura, EGPA also presents with ecchymoses, haemorrhagic bullae, ulcerations, digital ischaemia, urticarial papules and painful subcutaneous nodules. The nodules are often located on the scalp and extensor surfaces of joints, such as the elbows, which are similar to those seen in PAN [6,275]. Cutaneous findings associated with mononeuritis multiplex can, in rare cases, be the only initial manifestation of vasculitis, in which case biopsy is particularly helpful [276]. Histologically, EGPA is characterized by a small vessel eosinophil-rich neutrophilic vasculitis, dermal eosinophilia and 'red granulomas' comprised of palisading granulomatous dermatitis [6]. While extravascular eosinophilia is almost always present, granulomas may not be seen without larger tissue samples [274].

Medium vessel vasculitis

Kawasaki Disease

Kawasaki disease (KD), the second most common systemic vasculitis in children [13], is an acute, self-limited small to medium vessel vasculitis with a predilection for coronary artery involvement. The classic mucocutaneous findings and systemic features are discussed in detail elsewhere. Although KD is a systemic vasculitis, the classic polymorphic skin eruptions are characterized by nonspecific inflammation; true cutaneous vasculitis associated with KD is extremely rare. Reports of cutaneous vasculitis have been limited to infants or very young children who developed purpura, peripheral gangrene or necrotic lesions during the course of disease [277–279]. Biopsy of a purpuric lesion in one case showed a pauci-immune small vessel vasculitis with mild leukocytoclasia, red blood cell extravasation and intravascular thrombi [277].

Systemic PAN

Systemic PAN is the third most common systemic vasculitis of childhood, after HSP and KD [225]. The cutaneous findings are clinically and histopathologically identical to that of cutaneous PAN [224]. However, the multiorgan involvement in systemic PAN causes significant complications if left untreated. The lungs are typically spared, which helps to distinguish PAN from AAV. Coronary artery aneurysms are more common in the juvenile form of disease [247] and can masquerade as atypical KD. Angiography in these cases is particularly helpful, as other evidence of aneurysmal dilation or stenosis in medium-sized arteries is virtually pathognomonic of PAN [4].

Collagen vascular diseases

In contrast to the primary vasculitides, where the primary pathology involves blood vessels, secondary cutaneous vasculitis occurs as a complication of an underlying disease process, most commonly systemic autoimmune disease. SLE, mixed connective tissue disease and Sjögren syndrome are examples of collagen vascular diseases seen in the paediatric population that are associated with cutaneous manifestations of secondary systemic vasculitis.

SLE

As with adult SLE, the disease process in paediatric onset SLE is characterized broadly by a systemic vasculopathy. True lupus vasculitis is less common and presents most often with cutaneous small vessel vasculitis, although medium vessel and visceral vasculitis can also occur [280–282]. Skin findings include erythematous to violaceous nonblanching punctate lesions on the fingertips or palms, palpable purpura, ischaemic or ulcerated lesions, erythematous papules, urticarial lesions and nodules (Fig. 145.12a and 145.12b). The lower extremities are most commonly involved, followed by the hands and face [280,283]. As with cutaneous PAN, severe cutaneous lupus vasculitis can result in peripheral neuropathy from underlying sensory nerve injury [284]. Livedo reticularis is less common in childhood-onset than in adult-onset SLE [283,285] and is associated with the presence of lupus vasculitis and antiphospholipid antibodies [236].

On biopsy, leukocytoclastic small vessel vasculitis is the most frequent finding, followed by necrotizing or lymphocytic vasculitis [280,283]. Whenever vasculitis is suspected or diagnosed, laboratory testing for antiphospholipid antibody syndrome (APS) is strongly recommended. Thrombotic lesions in APS appear clinically similar to vasculitic lesions, particularly in the fingertips. It is critical to distinguish them, because APS warrants anticoagulation rather than increased immunosuppression [280,286]. Lupus vasculitis and APS can also occur concomitantly, compounding the risk of vascular insufficiency and infarction [287]. In addition to vasculitis, petechiae and purpura can be seen in the setting of other

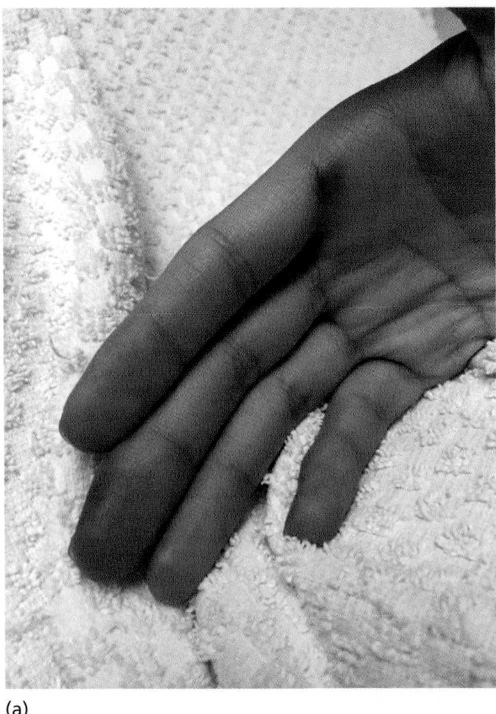

(a)

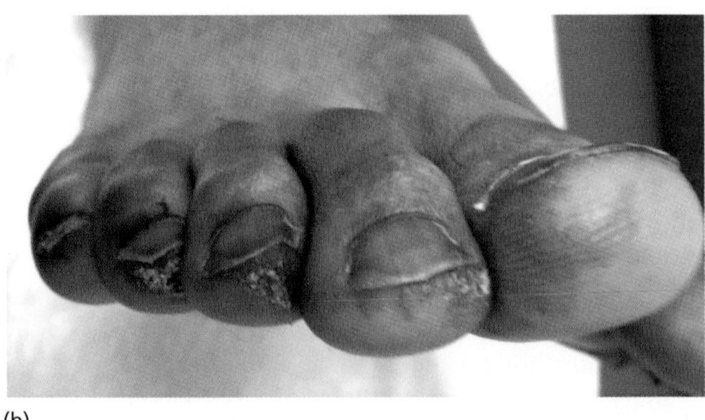

(b)

Fig. 145.12 (a) Nonblanching, painful, red nodule on the palm of a patient with lupus vasculitis. Note also the indurated erythema of the third finger with a dusky centre. (b) Chronic ulcerations of the toes (and fingers) are the primary manifestation of lupus vasculitis in this teenager.

nonvasculitic complications of lupus, including immune-mediated thrombocytopenia, thrombotic thrombocytopenic purpura or infection.

Mixed connective tissue disease

Mixed connective tissue disease (MCTD) is an overlap syndrome characterized clinically by features from two or more connective tissue diseases, including SLE, juvenile arthritis, dermatomyositis or systemic sclerosis. Serologically it is classically associated with a high titre of antiribonucleoprotein antibodies [288]. Clinically, the same cutaneous manifestations of lupus can also be seen in MCTD, including vasculitis [289]. However, vasculopathy predominates over vasculitis and is enhanced in the setting of sclerodermatous features and dermatomyositis. Raynaud phenomenon occurs in 85% of children at onset of disease and is a risk factor for severe digital pitting or ulcerations that can either mimic vasculitic lesions or enhance progression of digital infarction when coexistent with vasculitis [290].

Sjögren syndrome

Sjögren syndrome is a systemic autoimmune disease with chronic lymphocytic inflammation of the exocrine glands, classically leading to dry eyes and dry mouth (sicca symptoms). The disease is frequently associated with anti-Sjögren syndrome A (SSA) or anti-Sjögren syndrome B (SSB) autoantibodies and may occur as a primary disorder or secondarily in association with other autoimmune diseases like SLE. In children, Sjögren syndrome is rare and often presents differently than in adults. Parotitis is the initial presenting sign in 50–70% of children, whereas sicca symptoms are relatively uncommon [291,292]. Extraglandular manifestations can occur, including fatigue, arthritis, pulmonary disease, nephritis, peripheral neuropathy, Raynaud phenomenon and cutaneous vasculitis. Vasculitic lesions manifest as palpable purpura, petechiae, urticarial lesions or erythematous maculopapules. Histological examination typically reveals a non-IgA leukocytoclastic vasculitis in both adults and children, but adults are more likely to also fulfil criteria for urticarial or cryoglobulinemic vasculitis [292–294].

References

1 Chen K-R, Carlson JA. Clinical approach to cutaneous vasculitis. Am J Clin Dermatol 2008;9:71–92.

2 Carlson JA, Ng BT, Chen K-R. Cutaneous vasculitis update: diagnostic criteria, classification, epidemiology, etiology, pathogenesis, evaluation and prognosis. Am J Dermatopathol 2005;27:504–28.

3 Jennette JC, Falk RJ, Bacon PA et al. 2012 revised International Chapel Hill Consensus Conference Nomenclature of Vasculitides. Arthritis Rheum 2013;65:1–11.

4 Ozen S, Pistorio A, Iusan SM et al. EULAR/PRINTO/PRES criteria for Henoch-Schönlein purpura, childhood polyarteritis nodosa, childhood Wegener granulomatosis and childhood Takayasu arteritis: Ankara 2008. Part II: Final classification criteria. Ann Rheum Dis 2010;69:798–806.

5 Kawakami T. New algorithm (KAWAKAMI algorithm) to diagnose primary cutaneous vasculitis. J Dermatol 2010;37:113–24.

6 Carlson JA, Chen K-R. Cutaneous vasculitis update: small vessel neutrophilic vasculitis syndromes. Am J Dermatopathol 2006;28:486–506.

7 Carlson JA. The histological assessment of cutaneous vasculitis. Histopathology 2010;56:3–23.

8 Heberden W. Commentarii di morborium historia et curatione. London: Payne, 1801. In: Reprinted as Commentaries on the history and cure of disease. Birmingham, AL. The classics of Medicine Library, Division of Griphon Editions, Ltd, 1982:395–7.

9 Petty RE, Laxer RM, Lindsley CB, Wedderburn LR. Leukocytoclastic vasculitis: Henoch-Schönlein purpura and hypersensitivity vasculitis. In: Textbook of Pediatric Rheumatology, 7th edn, 2016:452–61.

10 Bowyer S, Roettcher P. Pediatric rheumatology clinic populations in the United States: results of a 3 year survey. Pediatric Rheumatology Database Research Group. J Rheumatol 1996;23:1968–74.

11 Blanco R,tínez-Taboada VM, Rodríguez-Valverde V et al. Cutaneous vasculitis in children and adults. Associated diseases and etiologic factors in 303 patients. Medicine (Baltimore) 1998;77:403–18.

12 Piram M, Mahr A. Epidemiology of immunoglobulin A vasculitis (Henoch-Schönlein): current state of knowledge. Curr Opin Rheumatol 2013;25:171–8.

13 Gardner-Medwin JMM, Dolezalova P, Cummins C et al. Incidence of Henoch-Schönlein purpura, Kawasaki disease, and rare vasculitides in children of different ethnic origins. Lancet 2002;360(9341): 1197–202.

14 Trapani S, Micheli A, Grisolia F et al. Henoch Schonlein purpura in childhood: epidemiological and clinical analysis of 150 cases over a 5-year period and review of literature. Semin Arthritis Rheum 2005;35:143–53.

15 Atkinson SR, Barker DJ. Seasonal distribution of Henoch-Schönlein purpura. Br J Prev Soc Med 1976;30:22–5.

16 Weiss PF, Klink AJ, Luan X et al. Temporal association of Streptococcus, Staphylococcus, and parainfluenza pediatric hospitalizations and hospitalized cases of Henoch-Schönlein purpura. J Rheumatol 2010;37:2587–94.

17 Davin J-C. Henoch-Schonlein purpura nephritis: pathophysiology, treatment, and future strategy. Clin J Am Soc Nephrol 2011;6:679–89.

18 Conley ME, Cooper MD, Michael AF. Selective deposition of immunoglobulin A1 in immunoglobulin A nephropathy, anaphylactoid purpura nephritis, and systemic lupus erythematosus. J Clin Invest 1980;66:1432–6.

19 Saulsbury FT. Henoch-Schönlein purpura. Curr Opin Rheumatol 2001;13:35–40.

20 Lau KK, Suzuki Hak J, Wyatt RJ. Pathogenesis of Henoch-Schönlein purpura nephritis. Pediatr Nephrol 2010;25:19–26.

21 Yang Y-H, Chuang Y-H, Wang L-C et al. The immunobiology of Henoch-Schönlein purpura. Autoimmun Rev 2008;7:179–84.

22 Saulsbury FT. Henoch-Schönlein purpura in children. Report of 100 patients and review of the literature. Medicine (Baltimore) 1999;78:395–409.

23 Schmitt R, Carlsson F, Mörgelin M et al. Tissue deposits of IgA-binding streptococcal M proteins in IgA nephropathy and Henoch-Schonlein purpura. Am J Pathol 2010;176:608–18.

24 Ayoub EM, McBride J, Schmiederer M et al. Role of Bartonella henselae in the etiology of Henoch-Schönlein purpura. Pediatr Infect Dis J 2002;21:28–31.

25 Satoskar AA, Molenda M, Scipio P et al. Henoch-Schönlein purpura-like presentation in IgA-dominant Staphylococcus infection - associated glomerulonephritis - a diagnostic pitfall. Clin Nephrol 2013;79:302–12.

26 Cai H-B, Li Y-B, Zhao H, Zhou S-M, Zhao X-D. [Prognostic analysis of children with Henoch-Schonlein purpura treated by Helicobacter pylori eradication therapy]. Zhongguo Dang Dai Er Ke Za Zhi Chin J Contemp Pediatr 2014;16:234–7.

27 Reinauer S, Megahed M, Goerz G et al. Schönlein-Henoch purpura associated with gastric Helicobacter pylori infection. J Am Acad Dermatol 1995;33:876–9.

28 Hu P, Guan Y, Lu L. Henoch-Schönlein purpura triggered by Mycoplasma pneumoniae in a female infant. Kaohsiung J Med Sci 2015;31:163–4.

29 Lim CSH, Lim S-L. Henoch-Schönlein purpura associated with Mycoplasma pneumoniae infection. Cutis 2011;87:273–6.

30 Saulsbury FT. Epidemiology of Henoch-Schönlein purpura. Cleve Clin J Med 2002;69 Suppl 2:SII87–9.

31 Borrás-Blasco J, Enriquez R, Amoros F et al. Henoch-Schönlein purpura associated with clarithromycin. Case report and review of literature. Int J Clin Pharmacol Ther 2003;41:213–6.

32 Asahina A, Ohshima N, Nakayama H et al. Henoch-Schönlein purpura in a patient with rheumatoid arthritis receiving etanercept. Eur J Dermatol 2010;20:521–2.

33 Lee A, Kasama R, Evangelisto A et al. Henoch-Schönlein purpura after etanercept therapy for psoriasis. J Clin Rheumatol Pract Rep Rheum Musculoskelet Dis 2006;12:249–51.

34 Rolle AS, Zimmermann B, Poon SH. Etanercept-induced Henoch-Schönlein purpura in a patient with ankylosing spondylitis. J Clin Rheumatol Pract Rep Rheum Musculoskelet Dis 2013;19:90–3.

35 Lambert EM, Liebling A, Glusac E, Antaya RJ. Henoch-Schonlein purpura following a meningococcal vaccine. Pediatrics 2003;112:e491.

36 Goodman MJ, Nordin JD, Belongia EA et al. Henoch-Schölein purpura and polysaccharide meningococcal vaccine. Pediatrics 2010;126:e325–9.

37 Bonetto C, Trotta F, Felicetti P et al. Vasculitis as an adverse event following immunization - systematic literature review. Vaccine 2015;34:6641–51.

38 Jauhola O, Ronkainen J, Koskimies O et al. Clinical course of extrarenal symptoms in Henoch-Schonlein purpura: a 6-month prospective study. Arch Dis Child 2010;95:871–6.

39 Trapani S, Iotti P, Resti M et al. Severe hemorrhagic bullous lesions in Henoch Schonlein purpura: three pediatric cases and review of the literature. Rheumatol Int 2010;30:1355–9.

40 Tizard EJ, Hamilton-Ayres MJJ. Henoch Schonlein purpura. Arch Dis Child Educ Pract Ed 2008;93:1–8.

41 González LM, Niger CK, Schwartz RA. Pediatric Henoch-Schönlein purpura. Int J Dermatol 2009;48:1157–65.

42 Robson WL, Leung AK. Henoch-Schönlein purpura. Adv Pediatr 1994;41:163–94.

43 Jithpratuck W, Elshenawy Y, Saleh H et al. The clinical implications of adult-onset Henoch-Schonelin purpura. Clin Mol Allergy 2011;9:9.

44 Rostoker G. Schönlein-Henoch purpura in children and adults: diagnosis, pathophysiology and management. BioDrugs Clin Immunother Biopharm Gene Ther 2001;15:99–138.

45 Garcia-Fuentes M, Tin A, Chantler C, Williams DG. Serum complement components in Henoch-Schönlein purpura. Arch Dis Child 1978;53:417–9.

46 Ozaltin F, Bakkaloglu A, Ozen S et al. The significance of IgA class of antineutrophil cytoplasmic antibodies (ANCA) in childhood Henoch-Schönlein purpura. Clin Rheumatol 2004;23:426–9.

47 Giangiacomo J, Tsai CC. Dermal and glomerular deposition of IgA in anaphylactoid purpura. Am J Dis Child 1977;131:981–3.

48 Shin JI, Kim JH, Lee JS. The diagnostic value of IgA deposition in Henoch-Schönlein purpura. Pediatr Dermatol 2008;25:140–1; author reply 141.

49 Vogler C, Eliason SC, Wood EG. Glomerular membranopathy in children with IgA nephropathy and Henoch Schönlein purpura. Pediatr Dev Pathol Off J Soc Pediatr Pathol Paediatr Pathol Soc 1999;2:227–35.

50 Levy M, Broyer M, Arsan A et al. Anaphylactoid purpura nephritis in childhood: natural history and immunopathology. Adv Nephrol Necker Hosp 1976;6:183–228.

51 den Boer SL, Pasmans SGMA, Wulffraat NM et al. Bullous lesions in Henoch Schönlein Purpura as indication to start systemic prednisone. Acta Paediatr Oslo Nor 2010;99:781–3.

52 Dudley J, Smith G, Llewelyn-Edwards A et al. Randomised, double-blind, placebo-controlled trial to determine whether steroids reduce the incidence and severity of nephropathy in Henoch-Schonlein Purpura (HSP). Arch Dis Child 2013;98:756–63.

53 Jauhola O, Ronkainen J, Koskimies O et al. Renal manifestations of Henoch-Schonlein purpura in a 6-month prospective study of 223 children. Arch Dis Child 2010;95:877–82.

54 Weiss PF, Feinstein JA, Luan X et al. Effects of corticosteroid on Henoch-Schönlein purpura: a systematic review. Pediatrics 2007;120: 1079–87.

55 Weiss PF, Klink AJ, Localio R et al. Corticosteroids may improve clinical outcomes during hospitalization for Henoch-Schönlein purpura. Pediatrics 2010;126:674–81.

56 Niaudet P, Habib R. Methylprednisolone pulse therapy in the treatment of severe forms of Schönlein-Henoch purpura nephritis. Pediatr Nephrol Berl Ger 1998;12:238–43.

57 Jauhola O, Ronkainen J, Autio-Harmainen H et al. Cyclosporine A vs methylprednisolone for Henoch-Schönlein nephritis: a randomized trial. Pediatr Nephrol 2011;26:2159–66.

58 Bergstein J, Leiser J, Andreoli SP. Response of crescentic Henoch-Schoenlein purpura nephritis to corticosteroid and azathioprine therapy. Clin Nephrol 1998;49:9–14.

59 Flynn JT, Smoyer WE, Bunchman TE et al. Treatment of Henoch-Schönlein purpura glomerulonephritis in children with high-dose corticosteroids plus oral cyclophosphamide. Am J Nephrol 2001;21:128–33.

60 Tarshish P, Bernstein J, Edelmann CM. Henoch-Schönlein purpura nephritis: course of disease and efficacy of cyclophosphamide. Pediatr Nephrol 2004;19:51–6.

61 Hattori M, Ito K, Konomoto T et al. Plasmapheresis as the sole therapy for rapidly progressive Henoch-Schönlein purpura nephritis in children. Am J Kidney Dis Off J Natl Kidney Found 1999;33:427–33.

62 Shenoy M, Ognjanovic MV, Coulthard MG. Treating severe Henoch-Schönlein and IgA nephritis with plasmapheresis alone. Pediatr Nephrol 2007;22:1167–71.

63 Narchi H. Risk of long term renal impairment and duration of follow up recommended for Henoch-Schonlein purpura with normal or minimal urinary findings: a systematic review. Arch Dis Child 2005;90:916–20.

64 Goldstein AR, White RH, Akuse R et al. Long-term follow-up of childhood Henoch-Schönlein nephritis. Lancet 1992;339(8788):280–2.

65 Snow IM. Purpura, urticaria and angioneurotic edema of the hands and feet in a nursing baby. J Am Med Assoc 1913;61:18.

66 Seidlmayer H. Die frühinfantile, postinfektiöse Kokarden-Purpura. Z Für Kinderheilkd 1939;61:217–55.

67 Rosenstern I. Heinrich Finkelstein, 1865–1942. J Pediatr 1956;49: 499–503.

68 Saraclar Y, Tinaztepe K, Adalioğlu G et al. Acute hemorrhagic edema of infancy (AHEI) – a variant of Henoch-Schönlein purpura or a distinct clinical entity? J Allergy Clin Immunol 1990;86(4 Pt 1): 473–83.

69 Krause I, Lazarov A, Rachmel A et al. Acute haemorrhagic oedema of infancy, a benign variant of leucocytoclastic vasculitis. Acta Paediatr Oslo Nor 1996;85:114–7.

70 Fiore E, Rizzi M, Ragazzi M et al. Acute hemorrhagic edema of young children (cockade purpura and edema): a case series and systematic review. J Am Acad Dermatol 2008;59:684–95.

71 Savino F, Lupica MM, Tarasco V et al. Acute hemorrhagic edema of infancy: a troubling cutaneous presentation with a self-limiting course. Pediatr Dermatol 2013;30:e149–52.

72 Fiore E, Rizzi M, Simonetti GD et al. Acute hemorrhagic edema of young children: a concise narrative review. Eur J Pediatr 2011;170:1507–11.

73 Amitai Y, Gillis D, Wasserman D et al. Henoch-Schönlein purpura in infants. Pediatrics 1993;92:865–7.

74 Di Lernia V, Lombardi M, Lo Scocco G. Infantile acute hemorrhagic edema and rotavirus infection. Pediatr Dermatol 2004;21:548–50.

75 Garty BZ, Pollak U, Scheuerman Ocus N et al. Acute hemorrhagic edema of infancy associated with herpes simplex type 1 stomatitis. Pediatr Dermatol 2006;23:361–4.

76 Morrison RR, Saulsbury FT. Acute hemorrhagic edema of infancy associated with pneumococcal bacteremia. Pediatr Infect Dis J 1999;18:832–3.

77 Breda L, Franchini Szetti V, Chiarelli F. Escherichia coli urinary infection as a cause of acute hemorrhagic edema in infancy. Pediatr Dermatol 2015;32:e309–11.

78 Ferrarini A, Benetti C, Camozzi P et al. Acute hemorrhagic edema of young children: a prospective case series. Eur J Pediatr 2016;175:557–61.

79 Crowe MA, Jonas PP. Acute hemorrhagic edema of infancy. Cutis 1998;62:65–6.

80 Legrain V, Lejean S, Taïeb A et al. Infantile acute hemorrhagic edema of the skin: study of ten cases. J Am Acad Dermatol 1991;24:17–22.

81 Watanabe T, Sato Y. Renal involvement and hypocomplementemia in a patient with acute hemorrhagic edema of infancy. Pediatr Nephrol 2007;22:1979–81.

82 Davis MDP, Brewer JD. Urticarial vasculitis and hypocomplementemic urticarial vasculitis syndrome. Immunol Allergy Clin North Am 2004;24:183–213, vi.

83 Mehregan DR, Hall MJ, Gibson LE. Urticarial vasculitis: a histopathologic and clinical review of 72 cases. J Am Acad Dermatol 1992;26:441–8.

84 Ting TV. Diagnosis and management of cutaneous vasculitis in children. Pediatr Clin North Am 2014;61:321–46.

85 Wisnieski JJ. Urticarial vasculitis. Curr Opin Rheumatol 2000;12:24–31.

86 McDuffie FC, Sams WM, Maldonado JE et al. Hypocomplementemia with cutaneous vasculitis and arthritis. Possible immune complex syndrome. Mayo Clin Proc 1973;48:340–8.

87 Cadnapaphornchai MA, Saulsbury FT, Norwood VF. Hypocomplementemic urticarial vasculitis: report of a pediatric case. Pediatr Nephrol 2000;14:328–31.

88 Al Mosawi ZSA, Al Hermi BEA. Hypocomplementemic urticarial vasculitis syndrome in an 8-year-old boy: a case report and review of literature. Oman Med J 2013;28:275–7.

89 Ozçakar ZB, Yalçınkaya F, Altugan FS et al. Hypocomplementemic urticarial vasculitis syndrome in three siblings. Rheumatol Int 2013;33:763–6.

90 Pasini A, Bracaglia C, Aceti A et al. Renal involvement in hypocomplementaemic urticarial vasculitis syndrome: a report of three paediatric cases. Rheumatology 2014;53:1409–13.

91 Geha RS, Akl KF. Skin lesions, angioedema, eosinophilia, and hypocomplementemia. J Pediatr 1976;89:724–7.

92 Martini A, Ravelli A, Albani S et al. Hypocomplementemic urticarial vasculitis syndrome with severe systemic manifestations. J Pediatr 1994;124:742–4.

93 Renard M, Wouters C, Proesmans W. Rapidly progressive glomerulonephritis in a boy with hypocomplementaemic urticarial vasculitis. Eur J Pediatr 1998;157:243–5.

94 Waldo FB, Leist PA, Strife CF et al. Atypical hypocomplementemic vasculitis syndrome in a child. J Pediatr 1985;106:745–50.

95 Jachiet M, Flageul B, Deroux A et al. The clinical spectrum and therapeutic management of hypocomplementemic urticarial vasculitis: data from a French nationwide study of fifty-seven patients. Arthritis Rheumatol 2015;67:527–34.

96 Grotz W, Baba HA, Becker JU et al. Hypocomplementemic urticarial vasculitis syndrome: an interdisciplinary challenge. Dtsch Ärztebl Int 2009;106:756–63.

97 Sanchez NP, Winkelmann RK, Schroeter AL et al. The clinical and histopathologic spectrums of urticarial vasculitis: study of forty cases. J Am Acad Dermatol 1982;7:599–605.

98 Davis MD, Daoud MS, Kirby B et al. Clinicopathologic correlation of hypocomplementemic and normocomplementemic urticarial vasculitis. J Am Acad Dermatol 1998;38:899–905.

99 Koch PE, Lazova R, Rosen JR et al. Urticarial vasculitis in an infant. Cutis 2008;81:49–52.

100 Wisnieski JJ, Jones SM. IgG autoantibody to the collagen-like region of Clq in hypocomplementemic urticarial vasculitis syndrome, systemic lupus erythematosus, and 6 other musculoskeletal or rheumatic diseases. J Rheumatol 1992;19:884–8.

101 Chang S, Carr W. Urticarial vasculitis. Allergy Asthma Proc Off J Reg State Allergy Soc 2007;28:97–100.

102 Jara LJ, Navarro C, Medina G et al. Hypocomplementemic urticarial vasculitis syndrome. Curr Rheumatol Rep 2009;11:410–5.

103 Kano Y, Orihara M, Shiohara T. Cellular and molecular dynamics in exercise-induced urticarial vasculitis lesions. Arch Dermatol 1998;134:62–7.

104 Loricera J, Calvo-Río V, Mata C et al. Urticarial vasculitis in northern Spain: clinical study of 21 cases. Medicine (Baltimore) 2014;93:53–60.

105 Olson JC, Esterly NB. Urticarial vasculitis and Lyme disease. J Am Acad Dermatol 1990;22:1114–6.

106 Kulthanan K, Cheepsomsong M, Jiamton S. Urticarial vasculitis: etiologies and clinical course. Asian Pac J Allergy Immunol 2009;27:95–102.

107 DeAmicis T, Mofid MZ, Cohen B et al. Hypocomplementemic urticarial vasculitis: report of a 12-year-old girl with systemic lupus erythematosus. J Am Acad Dermatol 2002;47(5 Suppl):S273–4.

108 Soylu A, Kavukçu S, Uzuner N et al. Systemic lupus erythematosus presenting with normocomplementemic urticarial vasculitis in a 4-year-old girl. Pediatr Int 2001;43:420–2.

109 Wisnieski JJ, Emancipator SN, Korman NJ et al. Hypocomplementemic urticarial vasculitis syndrome in identical twins. Arthritis Rheum 1994;37:1105–11.

110 Al Riyami BMS, Al Kaabi JK, Elagib EM et al. Subclinical pulmonary haemorrhage causing a restrictive lung defect in three siblings with a unique urticarial vasculitis syndrome. Clin Rheumatol 2003;22:309–13.

111 McLean RH, Weinstein A, Chapitis J et al. Familial partial deficiency of the third component of complement (C3) and the hypocomplementemic cutaneous vasculitis syndrome. Am J Med 1980;68: 549–58.

112 Carmichael AJ, Marsden JR. Urticarial vasculitis: a presentation of C3 nephritic factor. Br J Dermatol 1993;128:589.

113 McNeil DJ, Kinsella TD, Crawford AM et al. The AHA syndrome: arthritis, hives and angioedema. Rheumatol Int 1987;7:277–9.

114 Eiling E, Möller M, Kreiselmaier I et al. Schnitzler syndrome: treatment failure to rituximab but response to anakinra. J Am Acad Dermatol 2007;57:361–4.

115 St Clair EW, McCallum RM. Cogan's syndrome. Curr Opin Rheumatol 1999;11:47–52.

116 Ochonisky S, Chosidow O, Kuentz M et al. Cogan's syndrome. An unusual etiology of urticarial vasculitis. Dermatologica 1991;183:218–20.

117 Venzor J, Lee WL, Huston DP. Urticarial vasculitis. Clin Rev Allergy Immunol 2002;23:201–16.
118 Vázquez-López F, Fueyo A, Sánchez-Martín J et al. Dermoscopy for the screening of common urticaria and urticaria vasculitis. Arch Dermatol 2008;144:568.
119 Oishi M, Takano M, Miyachi K et al. A case of unusual SLE related syndrome characterized by erythema multiforme, angioneurotic edema, marked hypocomplementemia, and Clq precipitins of the low molecular weight type. Int Arch Allergy Appl Immunol 1976;50:463–72.
120 Gammon WR, Wheeler CE. Urticarial vasculitis: report of a case and review of the literature. Arch Dermatol 1979;115:76–80.
121 Schwartz HR, McDuffie FC, Black LF et al. Hypocomplementemic urticarial vasculitis: association with chronic obstructive pulmonary disease. Mayo Clin Proc 1982;57:231–8.
122 Wisnieski JJ, Baer AN, Christensen J et al. Hypocomplementemic urticarial vasculitis syndrome. Clinical and serologic findings in 18 patients. Medicine (Baltimore) 1995;74:24–41.
123 Shah D, Rowbottom AW, Thomas CL et al. Hypocomplementaemic urticarial vasculitis associated with non-Hodgkin lymphoma and treatment with intravenous immunoglobulin. Br J Dermatol 2007;157:392–3.
124 Chimenti MS, Ballanti E, Triggianese P et al. Vasculitides and the complement system: a comprehensive review. Clin Rev Allergy Immunol 2015;49:333–46.
125 Farasat S, Aksentijevich I, Toro JR. Autoinflammatory diseases: clinical and genetic advances. Arch Dermatol 2008;144:392–402.
126 Black AK. Urticarial vasculitis. Clin Dermatol 1999;17:565–9.
127 Worm M, Sterry W, Kolde G. Mycophenolate mofetil is effective for maintenance therapy of hypocomplementaemic urticarial vasculitis. Br J Dermatol 2000;143:1324.
128 Saigal K, Valencia IC, Cohen J et al. Hypocomplementemic urticarial vasculitis with angioedema, a rare presentation of systemic lupus erythematosus: rapid response to rituximab. J Am Acad Dermatol 2003;49(5 Suppl):S283–5.
129 Ghazanfar MN, Thomsen SF. Omalizumab for urticarial vasculitis: case report and review of the literature. Case Rep Dermatol Med 2015;2015:576893.
130 Staubach-Renz P, von Stebut E, Bräuninger W et al. [Hypocomplementemic urticarial vasculitis syndrome. Successful therapy with intravenous immunoglobulins]. Hautarzt Z Für Dermatol Venerol Verwandte Geb 2007;58:693–7.
131 Kartal O, Gulec M, Caliskaner Z et al. Plasmapheresis in a patient with 'refractory' urticarial vasculitis. Allergy Asthma Immunol Res 2012;4:245–7.
132 Botsios C, Sfriso P, Punzi L et al. Non-complementaemic urticarial vasculitis: successful treatment with the IL-1 receptor antagonist, anakinra. Scand J Rheumatol 2007;36:236–7.
133 Krause K, Mahamed A, Weller K et al. Efficacy and safety of canakinumab in urticarial vasculitis: an open-label study. J Allergy Clin Immunol 2013;132:751–4.e5.
134 Makol A, Gibson LE, Michet CJ. Successful use of interleukin 6 antagonist tocilizumab in a patient with refractory cutaneous lupus and urticarial vasculitis. J Clin Rheumatol Pract Rep Rheum Musculoskelet Dis 2012;18:92–5.
135 Yamazaki-Nakashimada MA, Duran-McKinster C, Ramírez-Vargas N et al. Intravenous immunoglobulin therapy for hypocomplementemic urticarial vasculitis associated with systemic lupus erythematosus in a child. Pediatr Dermatol 2009;26:445–7.
136 Hutchinson J. On two remarkable cases of symmetrical purple congestion of the skin in patches, with induration. Br J Dermatol 1888:10–5.
137 Bury J. A case of erythema with remarkable nodular thickening and induration of the skin associated with intermittent albuminuria. Ill Med News 1889:145–9.
138 Radcliff-Crocker H, Williams C. Erythema elevatum diutinum. Br J Dermatol 1894:1–9.
139 Haber H. Erythema elevatum diutinum. Br J Dermatol 1955;67:121–45.
140 Wolff HH, Maciejewski W, Scherer R. [Erythema elevatum diutinum. I. Electron microscopy of a case with extracellular cholesterosis (author's transl)]. Arch Dermatol Res 1978;261:7–16.
141 Momen SE, Jorizzo J, Al-Niaimi F. Erythema elevatum diutinum: a review of presentation and treatment. J Eur Acad Dermatol Venereol 2014;28:1594–602.
142 Tomasini C, Seia Z, Dapavo P et al. Infantile erythema elevatum diutinum: report of a vesiculo-bullous case. Eur J Dermatol 2006;16:683–6.
143 Rodriguez-Serna M, Fortea JM, Perez A et al. Erythema elevatum diutinum associated with celiac disease: response to a gluten-free diet. Pediatr Dermatol 1993;10:125–8.
144 Golmia A, Grinblat B, Finger E et al. The development of erythema elevatum diutinum in a patient with juvenile idiopathic arthritis under treatment with abatacept. Clin Rheumatol 2008;27:105–6.
145 Hernández-Cano N, De Lucas R, Lázaro TE et al. Erythema elevatum diutinum after liver transplantation: disappearance of the lesions associated with a reduction in cyclosporin dosage. Pediatr Dermatol 1998;15:411–2.
146 Wilkinson SM, English JS, Smith NP et al. Erythema elevatum diutinum: a clinicopathological study. Clin Exp Dermatol 1992;17:87–93.
147 Walker KD, Badame AJ. Erythema elevatum diutinum in a patient with Crohn's disease. J Am Acad Dermatol 1990;22:948–52.
148 Orteu CH, McGregor JM, Whittaker SJ et al. Erythema elevatum diutinum and Crohn disease: a common pathogenic role for measles virus? Arch Dermatol 1996;132:1523–5.
149 Woody CM, Lane JE, Davis LS. Erythema elevatum diutinum in the setting of connective tissue disease and chronic bacterial infection. J Clin Rheumatol Pract Rep Rheum Musculoskelet Dis 2005;11:98–104.
150 Nakajima H, Ikeda M, Yamamoto Y et al. Erythema elevatum diutinum complicated by rheumatoid arthritis. J Dermatol 1999;26:452–6.
151 Yiannias JA, el-Azhary RA, Gibson LE. Erythema elevatum diutinum: a clinical and histopathologic study of 13 patients. J Am Acad Dermatol 1992;26:38–44.
152 Katz SI, Gallin JI, Hertz KC et al. Erythema elevatum diutinum: skin and systemic manifestations, immunologic studies, and successful treatment with dapsone. Medicine (Baltimore) 1977;56:443–55.
153 Muratori S, Carrera C, Gorani A et al. Erythema elevatum diutinum and HIV infection: a report of five cases. Br J Dermatol 1999;141:335–8.
154 Futei Y, Konohana I. A case of erythema elevatum diutinum associated with B-cell lymphoma: a rare distribution involving palms, soles and nails. Br J Dermatol 2000;142:116–9.
155 Gibson LE, Su WP. Cutaneous vasculitis. Rheum Dis Clin North Am 1990;16:309–24.
156 Chowdhury MMU, Inaloz HS, Motley RJ et al. Erythema elevatum diutinum and IgA paraproteinaemia: 'a preclinical iceberg.' Int J Dermatol 2002;41:368–70.
157 Martín JI, Dronda F, Chaves F. Erythema elevatum diutinum, a clinical entity to be considered in patients infected with HIV-1. Clin Exp Dermatol 2001;26:725–6.
158 Cockerell CJ. Noninfectious inflammatory skin diseases in HIV-infected individuals. Dermatol Clin 1991;9:531–41.
159 Grabbe J, Haas N, Möller A et al. Erythema elevatum diutinum – evidence for disease-dependent leucocyte alterations and response to dapsone. Br J Dermatol 2000;143:415–20.
160 Gibson LE, el-Azhary RA. Erythema elevatum diutinum. Clin Dermatol 2000;18:295–9.
161 Kim G-W, Park H-J, Kim H-S et al. Dapsone hypersensitivity syndrome that occurred during treatment of pediatric patient with erythema elevatum diutinum. Ann Dermatol 2011;23(Suppl 3):S290–95.
162 Wahl CE, Bouldin MB, Gibson LE. Erythema elevatum diutinum: clinical, histopathologic, and immunohistochemical characteristics of six patients. Am J Dermatopathol 2005;27:397–400.
163 Revenga F, Vera A, Muñoz A et al. Erythema elevatum diutinum and AIDS: are they related? Clin Exp Dermatol 1997;22:250–1.
164 Ayoub N, Charuel J-L, Diemert M-C et al. Antineutrophil cytoplasmic antibodies of IgA class in neutrophilic dermatoses with emphasis on erythema elevatum diutinum. Arch Dermatol 2004;140:931–6.
165 Porneuf M, Duterque M, Sotto A et al. Unusual erythema elevatum diutinum with fibrohistiocytic proliferation. Br J Dermatol 1996;134:1131–4.
166 High WA, Hoang MP, Stevens K et al. Late-stage nodular erythema elevatum diutinum. J Am Acad Dermatol 2003;49:764–7.
167 Kanitakis J, Cozzani E, Lyonnet S et al. Ultrastructural study of chronic lesions of erythema elevatum diutinum: 'extracellular cholesterosis' is a misnomer. J Am Acad Dermatol 1993;29:363–7.
168 Marie I, Courville P, Levesque H. Erythema elevatum diutinum associated with dermatomyositis. J Am Acad Dermatol 2011;64:1000–1.
169 Fort SL, Rodman OG. Erythema elevatum diutinum. Response to dapsone. Arch Dermatol 1977;113:819–22.
170 Di Giacomo TB, Marinho RT, Nico MMS. Erythema elevatum diutinum presenting with a giant annular pattern. Int J Dermatol 2009;48:290–2.
171 Frieling GW, Williams NL, Lim SJM et al. Novel use of topical dapsone 5% gel for erythema elevatum diutinum: safer and effective. J Drugs Dermatol 2013;12:481–4.

172 Kohler IK, Lorincz AL. Erythema elevatum diutinum treated with niacinamide and tetracycline. Arch Dermatol 1980;116:693–5.
173 Delgado J, Gómez-Cerezo J, Sigüenza M et al. Relapsing polychondritis and erythema elevatum diutinum: an unusual association refractory to dapsone. J Rheumatol 2001;28:634–5.
174 Zacaron LH, Gonçalves JC de F, Curty VMA et al. Clinical and surgical therapeutic approach in erithema elevatum diutinum – case report. An Bras Dermatol 2013;88(6 Suppl 1):15–8.
175 Henriksson R, Hofer PA, Hörnqvist R. Erythema elevatum diutinum – a case successfully treated with colchicine. Clin Exp Dermatol 1989;14:451–3.
176 Chow RK, Benny WB, Coupe RL et al. Erythema elevatum diutinum associated with IgA paraproteinemia successfully controlled with intermittent plasma exchange. Arch Dermatol 1996;132:1360–4.
177 Rinard JR, Mahabir RC, Greene JF et al. Successful surgical treatment of advanced erythema elevatum diutinum. Can J Plast Surg 2010;18:28–30.
178 Mat C, Yurdakul S, Tüzüner N et al. Small vessel vasculitis and vasculitis confined to skin. Baillières Clin Rheumatol 1997;11:237–57.
179 Newton RC, Raimer SS. Pigmented purpuric eruptions. Dermatol Clin 1985;3:165–9.
180 Sardana K, Sarkar R, Sehgal VN. Pigmented purpuric dermatoses: an overview. Int J Dermatol 2004;43:482–8.
181 Smoller BR, Kamel OW. Pigmented purpuric eruptions: immunopathologic studies supportive of a common immunophenotype. J Cutan Pathol 1991;18:423–7.
182 Schamberg J. A peculiar progressive pigmentary disease of the skin. Br J Dermatol 1901;13:1–5.
183 Sharma L, Gupta S. Clinicoepidemiological study of pigmented purpuric dermatoses. Indian Dermatol Online J 2012;3:17–20.
184 Tristani-Firouzi P, Meadows KP, Vanderhooft S. Pigmented purpuric eruptions of childhood: a series of cases and review of literature. Pediatr Dermatol 2001;18:299–304.
185 Torrelo A, Requena C, Mediero IG et al. Schamberg's purpura in children: a review of 13 cases. J Am Acad Dermatol 2003;48:31–3.
186 Aiba S, Tagami H. Immunohistologic studies in Schamberg's disease. Evidence for cellular immune reaction in lesional skin. Arch Dermatol 1988;124:1058–62.
187 Abeck D, Gross GE, Kuwert C et al. Acetaminophen-induced progressive pigmentary purpura (Schamberg's disease). J Am Acad Dermatol 1992;27:123–4.
188 Draelos ZK, Hansen RC. Schamberg's purpura in children: case study and literature review. Clin Pediatr 1987;26:659–61.
189 Ghersetich I, Lotti T, Bacci S et al. Cell infiltrate in progressive pigmented purpura (Schamberg's disease): immunophenotype, adhesion receptors, and intercellular relationships. Int J Dermatol 1995;34:846–50.
190 von den Driesch P, Simon M. Cellular adhesion antigen modulation in purpura pigmentosa chronica. J Am Acad Dermatol 1994;30: 193–200.
191 Baselga E, Drolet BA, Esterly NB. Purpura in infants and children. J Am Acad Dermatol 1997;37:673–705; quiz 706–7.
192 Hersh CS, Shwayder TA. Unilateral progressive pigmentary purpura (Schamberg's disease) in a 15-year-old boy. J Am Acad Dermatol 1991;24:651.
193 Barnhill RL, Braverman IM. Progression of pigmented purpura-like eruptions to mycosis fungoides: report of three cases. J Am Acad Dermatol 1988;19:25–31.
194 Ratnam KV, Su WP, Peters MS. Purpura simplex (inflammatory purpura without vasculitis): a clinicopathologic study of 174 cases. J Am Acad Dermatol 1991;25:642–7.
195 Carpentieri U, Gustavson LP, Grim CB et al. Purpura and Schamberg's disease. South Med J 1978;71:1168–70.
196 Schober SM, Peitsch WK, Bonsmann G et al. Early treatment with rutoside and ascorbic acid is highly effective for progressive pigmented purpuric dermatosis. J Dtsch Dermatol Ges J Ger Soc Dermatol 2014;12:1112–9.
197 Okada K, Ishikawa O, Miyachi Y. Purpura pigmentosa chronica successfully treated with oral cyclosporin A. Br J Dermatol 1996;134:180–1.
198 Kano Y, Hirayama K, Orihara M et al. Successful treatment of Schamberg's disease with pentoxifylline. J Am Acad Dermatol 1997;36:827–30.
199 Tamaki K, Yasaka N, Osada A et al. Successful treatment of pigmented purpuric dermatosis with griseofulvin. Br J Dermatol 1995;132:159–60.
200 Seckin D, Yazici Z, Senol A et al. A case of Schamberg's disease responding dramatically to PUVA treatment. Photodermatol Photoimmunol Photomed 2008;24:95–6.
201 Milea M, Dimov H-A, Cribier B. [Generalized Schamberg's disease treated with PUVA in a child]. Ann Dermatol Vénéréologie 2007;134:378–80.
202 Fathy H, Abdelgaber S. Treatment of pigmented purpuric dermatoses with narrow-band UVB: a report of six cases. J Eur Acad Dermatol Venereol 2011;25:603–6.
203 Can B, Turkoglu Z, Kavala M et al. Successful treatment of generalized childhood Schamberg's disease with narrowband ultraviolet B therapy. Photodermatol Photoimmunol Photomed 2011;27:216–8.
204 Majocchi D. Sopra una dermatosi telangiectode non ancora descritla: purpura annularis. Ital Mal Ven 1896;31:263–4.
205 Hoesly FJ, Huerter CJ, Shehan JM. Purpura annularis telangiectodes of Majocchi: case report and review of the literature. Int J Dermatol 2009;48:1129–33.
206 Miller K, Fischer M, Kamino H et al. Purpura annularis telangiectoides. Dermatol Online J 2012;18:5.
207 Pandhi R, Jain R, Radotra BD et al. Purpura annularis telangiectoides with vasculitic ulcers treated with colchicine. Int J Dermatol 2002;41:388–9.
208 Price ML, Jones EW, Calnan CD et al. Lichen aureus: a localized persistent form of pigmented purpuric dermatitis. Br J Dermatol 1985;112:307–14.
209 Marten R. Case for diagnosis. Trans St Johns Hosp Dermatolo Soc 1958;112:307–14.
210 Gelmetti C, Cerri D, Grimalt R. Lichen aureus in childhood. Pediatr Dermatol 1991;8:280–3.
211 Kim MJ, Kim BY, Park KC, Youn SW. A case of childhood lichen aureus. Ann Dermatol 2009;21:393–5.
212 Kahana M, Levy A, Schewach-Millet M et al. Lichen aureus occurring in childhood. Int J Dermatol 1985;24:666–7.
213 Zhao Y-K, Luo D-Q, Sarkar R et al. Segmental lichen aureus in a young woman with spontaneous improvement. J Dtsch Dermatol Ges 2014;12:260–2.
214 Moche J, Glassman S, Modi D et al. Segmental lichen aureus: a report of two cases treated with methylprednisolone aceponate. Australas J Dermatol 2011;52:e15–8.
215 Fink-Puches R, Wolf P, Kerl H et al. Lichen aureus: clinicopathologic features, natural history, and relationship to mycosis fungoides. Arch Dermatol 2008;144:1169–73.
216 Rudolph RI. Lichen aureus. J Am Acad Dermatol 1983;8:722–4.
217 Hazan C, Fangman B, Cohen D. Lichen aureus. Dermatol Online J 2007;13:23.
218 Murota H, Katayama I. Lichen aureus responding to topical tacrolimus treatment. J Dermatol 2011;38:823–5.
219 Ling TC, Goulden V, Goodfield MJD. PUVA therapy in lichen aureus. J Am Acad Dermatol 2001;45:145–6.
220 Hong D, Chang I-K, Lee Y et al. Treatment of segmental lichen aureus with a pulsed-dye laser: new treatment options for lichen aureus. Eur J Dermatol 2013;23:891–2.
221 Lindberg K. Ein beitrag zur kenntnis der periarteritis nodosa. Acta Med Scand 1931;76:183.
222 Nakamura T, Kanazawa N, Ikeda T et al. Cutaneous polyarteritis nodosa: revisiting its definition and diagnostic criteria. Arch Dermatol Res 2009;301:117–21.
223 Ozen S. Juvenile polyarteritis: is it a different disease? J Rheumatol 2004;31:831–2.
224 Kawakami T. A review of pediatric vasculitis with a focus on juvenile polyarteritis nodosa. Am J Clin Dermatol 2012;13:389–98.
225 Ozen S, Bakkaloglu A, Dusunsel R et al. Childhood vasculitides in Turkey: a nationwide survey. Clin Rheumatol 2007;26:196–200.
226 Ozen S, Anton J, Arisoy N et al. Juvenile polyarteritis: results of a multicenter survey of 110 children. J Pediatr 2004;145:517–22.
227 Bansal N-K, Houghton KM. Cutaneous polyarteritis nodosa in childhood: a case report and review of the literature. Arthritis 2010;2010:687547.
228 Diaz-Perez JL, Schroeter AL, Winkelmann RK. Cutaneous periarteritis nodosa: immunofluorescence studies. Arch Dermatol 1980;116: 56–8.
229 Fathalla BM, Miller L, Brady S et al. Cutaneous polyarteritis nodosa in children. J Am Acad Dermatol 2005;53:724–8.
230 Kumar L, Thapa BR, Sarkar B et al. Benign cutaneous polyarteritis nodosa in children below 10 years of age – a clinical experience. Ann Rheum Dis 1995;54:134–6.

231 David J, Ansell BM, Woo P. Polyarteritis nodosa associated with streptococcus. Arch Dis Child 1993;69:685–8.

232 Daoud MS, Hutton KP, Gibson LE. Cutaneous periarteritis nodosa: a clinicopathological study of 79 cases. Br J Dermatol 1997;136:706–13.

233 Tonnelier JM, Ansart S, Tilly-Gentric A et al. Juvenile relapsing periarteritis nodosa and streptococcal infection. J Bone Spine 2000;67:346–8.

234 Bauzá A, España A, Idoate M. Cutaneous polyarteritis nodosa. Br J Dermatol 2002;146:694–9.

235 Marzano AV, Vezzoli P, Berti E. Skin involvement in cutaneous and systemic vasculitis. Autoimmun Rev 2013;12:467–76.

236 Uthman IW, Khamashta MA. Livedo racemosa: a striking dermatological sign for the antiphospholipid syndrome. J Rheumatol 2006;33:2379–82.

237 Kerk N, Goerge T. Livedoid vasculopathy – current aspects of diagnosis and treatment of cutaneous infarction. J Dtsch Dermatol Ges 2013;11:407–10.

238 Dabiri G, Damstetter E, Chang Y et al. Coagulation disorders and their cutaneous presentations: diagnostic work-up and treatment. J Am Acad Dermatol 2016;74:795–804.

239 Alavi A, Hafner J, Dutz JP et al. Livedoid vasculopathy: an in-depth analysis using a modified Delphi approach. J Am Acad Dermatol 2013;69:1033–42.

240 Monshi B, Posch C, Vujic I et al. Efficacy of intravenous immunoglobulins in livedoid vasculopathy: long-term follow-up of 11 patients. J Am Acad Dermatol 2014;71:738–44.

241 Diaz-Perez JL. Cutaneous periarteritis nodosa. Arch Dermatol 1974 1;110:407.

242 Morgan AJ, Schwartz RA. Cutaneous polyarteritis nodosa: a comprehensive review. Int J Dermatol 2010;49:750–6.

243 Shiau CJ, Abi Daoud MS, Wong SM et al. Lymphocytic panniculitis: an algorithmic approach to lymphocytes in subcutaneous tissue. J Clin Pathol 2015;68:954–62.

244 Díaz-Pérez JL, De Lagrán ZM, Díaz-Ramón JL et al. Cutaneous polyarteritis nodosa. Semin Cutan Med Surg 2007;26:77–86.

245 Jelusic M, Vikic-Topic M, Batinic D et al. Polyarteritis nodosa in Croatian children: a retrospective study over the last 20 years. Rheumatol Int 2013;33:3087–90.

246 Kawakami T, Yamazaki M, Mizoguchi M et al. High titer of antiphosphatidylserine-prothrombin complex antibodies in patients with cutaneous polyarteritis nodosa. Arthritis Rheum 2007 15;57:1507–13.

247 Fauci AS, Haynes B, Katz P. The spectrum of vasculitis: clinical, pathologic, immunologic and therapeutic considerations. Ann Intern Med 1978;89:660–76.

248 Gedalia A, Correa H, Kaiser M et al. Case report: steroid sparing effect of intravenous gamma globulin in a child with necrotizing vasculitis. Am J Med Sci 1995;309:226–8.

249 Williams VL, Guirola R, Flemming K et al. Distal extremity necrosis as a manifestation of cutaneous polyarteritis nodosa: case report and review of the acute management of a pediatric patient. Pediatr Dermatol 2012;29:473–8.

250 Valor L, Monteagudo I, de la Torre I et al. Young male patient diagnosed with cutaneous polyarteritis nodosa successfully treated with etanercept. Mod Rheumatol 2014;24:688–9.

251 Feinstein J, Arroyo R. Successful treatment of childhood onset refractory polyarteritis nodosa with tumor necrosis factor alpha blockade. J Clin Rheumatol Pract Rep Rheum Musculoskelet Dis 2005;11:219–22.

252 Eleftheriou D, Melo M, Marks SD et al. Biologic therapy in primary systemic vasculitis of the young. Rheumatology (Oxford) 2009;48:978–86.

253 González-Fernández MA, García-Consuegra J. Polyarteritis nodosa resistant to conventional treatment in a pediatric patient. Ann Pharmacother 2007;41:885–90.

254 McKinney EF, Willcocks LC, Broecker V et al. The immunopathology of ANCA-associated vasculitis. Semin Immunopathol 2014;36:461–78.

255 Wright AC, Gibson LE, Davis DMR. Cutaneous manifestations of pediatric granulomatosis with polyangiitis: a clinicopathologic and immunopathologic analysis. J Am Acad Dermatol 2015;72:859–67.

256 Rottem M, Fauci AS, Hallahan CW et al. Wegener granulomatosis in children and adolescents: clinical presentation and outcome. J Pediatr 1993;122:26–31.

257 Belostotsky VM, Shah V, Dillon MJ. Clinical features in 17 paediatric patients with Wegener granulomatosis. Pediatr Nephrol 2002;17: 754–61.

258 Brazzelli V, Vassallo C, Baldini F et al. Wegener granulomatosis in a child: cutaneous findings as the presenting signs. Pediatr Dermatol 1999;16:277–80.

259 Nasir N, Ali SA, Mehmood Riaz HM. Cutaneous ulcers as initial presentation of localized granulomatosis with polyangiitis: a case report and review of the literature. Case Rep Rheumatol 2015;2015:517025.

260 Daoud MS, Gibson LE, DeRemee RA et al. Cutaneous Wegener's granulomatosis: clinical, histopathologic, and immunopathologic features of thirty patients. J Am Acad Dermatol 1994;31:605–12.

261 Comfere NI, Macaron NC, Gibson LE. Cutaneous manifestations of Wegener's granulomatosis: a clinicopathologic study of 17 patients and correlation to antineutrophil cytoplasmic antibody status. J Cutan Pathol 2007;34:739–47.

262 Sun L, Wang H, Jiang X et al. Clinical and pathological features of microscopic polyangiitis in 20 children. J Rheumatol 2014;41: 1712–9.

263 Kluger N, Pagnoux C, Guillevin L et al. Comparison of cutaneous manifestations in systemic polyarteritis nodosa and microscopic polyangiitis. Br J Dermatol 2008;159:615–20.

264 Guillevin L, Durand-Gasselin B, Cevallos R et al. Microscopic polyangiitis: clinical and laboratory findings in eighty-five patients. Arthritis Rheum 1999;42:421–30.

265 Chung SA, Seo P. Microscopic polyangiitis. Rheum Dis Clin N Am 2010;36:545–58.

266 Peñas PF, Porras JI, Fraga J et al. Microscopic polyangiitis. A systemic vasculitis with a positive P-ANCA. Br J Dermatol 1996;134:542–7.

267 Yamada Y, Kitagawa C, Kamioka I et al. A case of microscopic polyangiitis with skin manifestations in a seven-year-old girl. Dermatol Online J 2013;19:19624.

268 Cabral DA, Uribe AG, Benseler S et al. Classification, presentation, and initial treatment of Wegener's granulomatosis in childhood. Arthritis Rheum 2009;60:3413–24.

269 Iudici M, Puéchal X, Pagnoux C et al. Brief report: childhood-onset systemic necrotizing vasculitides: long-term data from the French Vasculitis Study Group Registry. Arthritis Rheumatol 2015;67:1959–65.

270 Guillevin L, Cohen P, Gayraud M et al. Churg-Strauss syndrome. Clinical study and long-term follow-up of 96 patients. Medicine (Baltimore) 1999;78:26–37.

271 Sablé-Fourtassou R, Cohen P, Mahr A et al. Antineutrophil cytoplasmic antibodies and the Churg-Strauss syndrome. Ann Intern Med 2005;143:632–8.

272 Comarmond C, Pagnoux C, Khellaf M et al. Eosinophilic granulomatosis with polyangiitis (Churg-Strauss): clinical characteristics and long-term followup of the 383 patients enrolled in the French Vasculitis Study Group cohort. Arthritis Rheum 2013;65:270–81.

273 Gendelman S, Zeft A, Spalding SJ. Childhood-onset eosinophilic granulomatosis with polyangiitis (formerly Churg-Strauss syndrome): a contemporary single-center cohort. J Rheumatol 2013;40:929–35.

274 Zwerina J, Eger G, Englbrecht M et al. Churg-Strauss syndrome in childhood: a systematic literature review and clinical comparison with adult patients. Semin Arthritis Rheum 2009;39:108–15.

275 Davis MD, Daoud MS, McEvoy MT et al. Cutaneous manifestations of Churg-Strauss syndrome: a clinicopathologic correlation. J Am Acad Dermatol 1997;37:199–203.

276 Kawakami T, Soma Y, Kawasaki K et al. Initial cutaneous manifestations consistent with mononeuropathy multiplex in Churg-Strauss syndrome. Arch Dermatol 2005;141:873–8.

277 Gomez-Moyano E, Vera Casaño A, Camacho J et al. Kawasaki disease complicated by cutaneous vasculitis and peripheral gangrene. J Am Acad Dermatol 2011;64:e74–5.

278 Durall AL, Phillips JR, Weisse ME et al. Infantile Kawasaki disease and peripheral gangrene. J Pediatr 2006;149:131–3.

279 Kourda M, Bouaziz A, Tougourti MN. [Necrotic lesions of the face in Kawasaki disease]. Arch Pédiatrie Organe Off Sociéte Fr Pédiatrie 2010;17:1667–9.

280 Ramos-Casals M, Nardi N, Lagrutta M et al. Vasculitis in systemic lupus erythematosus: prevalence and clinical characteristics in 670 patients. Medicine (Baltimore) 2006;85:95–104.

281 Medina F, Ayala A, Jara LJ et al. Acute abdomen in systemic lupus erythematosus: the importance of early laparotomy. Am J Med 1997;103:100–5.

282 Drenkard C, Villa AR, Reyes E et al. Vasculitis in systemic lupus erythematosus. Lupus 1997;6:235–42.

283 Chiewchengchol D, Murphy R, Edwards SW et al. Mucocutaneous manifestations in juvenile-onset systemic lupus erythematosus: a review of literature. Pediatr Rheumatol 2015;13:1.
284 Tseng M-T, Hsieh S-C, Shun C-T et al. Skin denervation and cutaneous vasculitis in systemic lupus erythematosus. Brain J Neurol 2006;129:977–85.
285 Font J, Cervera R, Espinosa G et al. Systemic lupus erythematosus (SLE) in childhood: analysis of clinical and immunological findings in 34 patients and comparison with SLE characteristics in adults. Ann Rheum Dis 1998;57:456–9.
286 Bouaziz JD, Barete S, Le Pelletier F et al. Cutaneous lesions of the digits in systemic lupus erythematosus: 50 cases. Lupus 2007;16:163–7.
287 Tomizawa K, Sato-Matsumura KC, Kajii N. The coexistence of cutaneous vasculitis and thrombosis in childhood-onset systemic lupus erythematosus with antiphospholipid antibodies. Br J Dermatol 2003;149:439–41.
288 Amigues JM, Cantagrel A, Abbal M et al. Comparative study of 4 diagnosis criteria sets for mixed connective tissue disease in patients with anti-RNP antibodies. Autoimmunity Group of the Hospitals of Toulouse. J Rheumatol 1996;23:2055–62.
289 Magro CM, Crowson AN, Regauer S. Mixed connective tissue disease. A clinical, histologic, and immunofluorescence study of eight cases. Am J Dermatopathol 1997;19:206–13.
290 Petty RE, Laxer RM, Lindsley CB et al. Mixed and undifferentiated connective tissue disease. In: Textbook of Pediatric Rheumatology, 7th edn, 2016:418–26.
291 Stiller M, Golder W, Döring E et al. Primary and secondary Sjögren's syndrome in children – a comparative study. Clin Oral Investig 2000;4:176–82.
292 Civilibal M, Canpolat N, Yurt A et al. A child with primary Sjögren syndrome and a review of the literature. Clin Pediatr 2007;46:738–42.
293 Singer NG, Tomanova-Soltys I, Lowe R. Sjögren's syndrome in childhood. Curr Rheumatol Rep 2008;10:147–55.
294 Ramos-Casals M, Anaya J-M, García-Carrasco M et al. Cutaneous vasculitis in primary Sjögren syndrome: classification and clinical significance of 52 patients. Medicine (Baltimore) 2004;83:96–106.

CHAPTER 146
Purpura Fulminans

Michael Levin[1], *Brian Eley*[2] *& Saul N. Faust*[3]

[1]Imperial College London, London, UK
[2]University of Cape Town, South Africa
[3]University of Southampton and University Hospital Southampton NHS Foundation Trust, Southampton, UK

Abstract

Purpura fulminans is a very rare complication of infection, autoimmunity, drugs or snake bite. Identification of the specific cause in individual cases is important because specific treatment options are available based on the underlying pathophysiology. In the emergency situation, supportive medical and surgical treatments are similar regardless of cause.

Key points

- **The causes of purpura fulminans include congenital absence of protein C or protein S, bacterial and viral infection, autoimmune diseases, vasculitis and drugs.**
- **Distinction between the different forms of purpura fulminans is made on the basis of the clinical, epidemiological and laboratory features.**
- **Treatment should be supportive and directed at the cause.**
- **Prognosis is variable but surgical intervention should be delayed because it may be possible to retain functionally useful limbs and digits even when the initial appearance suggests extensive ischaemia.**

Definition. Purpura fulminans is a descriptive term used to describe a heterogeneous group of disorders characterized by rapidly progressive purpuric lesions, which may develop into extensive areas of skin necrosis and peripheral gangrene (Fig. 146.1a). The disorder is associated with laboratory evidence of consumptive coagulopathy. The histopathological features are of widespread thrombosis of the dermal capillaries and venules with haemorrhagic infarction of the surrounding tissues. The condition is often fatal and survivors may suffer loss of digits, limbs or areas of skin [1,2].

History. The term purpura fulminans was first introduced by Henoch in 1887 [3]. Since then an extensive literature on the disorder has been published, containing clear descriptions of the clinical features of the disorder and its histopathology [1–4]. The term purpura fulminans is now accepted as applying to patients with a devastating illness associated with extensive areas of purpura [2,3]. Despite the large number of cases reported in the literature, the cause of the disorder has remained unclear and a confusing, and often conflicting, array of different theories have been presented on its aetiology and pathogenesis. A large number of different processes have been reported to initiate purpura fulminans, including bacterial and viral infection [4], autoimmune diseases [5], vasculitis and a number of drugs [6]. Several disease mechanisms have been proposed to explain the central features of the disorder, the widespread thrombosis within dermal blood vessels. These including endothelial injury, primary activation of coagulation pathways, impaired anticoagulation mechanisms or activation of platelets [2,4,6]. Not surprisingly in view of the confusion surrounding the aetiology and the pathogenesis, the literature also contains conflicting recommendations as to treatment. Faced with a progressive and life-threatening illness of unclear aetiology, clinicians have utilized a wide variety of experimental or unproven treatments for the disorder. These include clotting factor replacement [7], anticoagulation [8], antiplatelet agents, glucocorticosteroids and immunosuppression [4], plasmapharesis or whole blood exchange [9], hyperbaric oxygen [10] and fibrinolytic agents [11].

Recognition that congenital deficiencies of protein C or S are associated with purpura fulminans [12,13], has highlighted the importance of the protein C pathway in the aetiology of the disorder. More recently, reports of purpura fulminans associated with acquired deficiency of protein C or S, either occurring during fulminant sepsis [14,15], or resulting from autoimmune processes [16], have highlighted the importance of primary thrombotic processes in the initiation of the disorder. The reports published in the past few years have not only provided a clearer understanding of the pathogenesis of the disorder, but also increasingly allow purpura fulminans to be understood as a syndrome that can result from several distinct disease processes.

Harper's Textbook of Pediatric Dermatology, Fourth Edition. Edited by Peter Hoeger, Veronica Kinsler and Albert Yan.

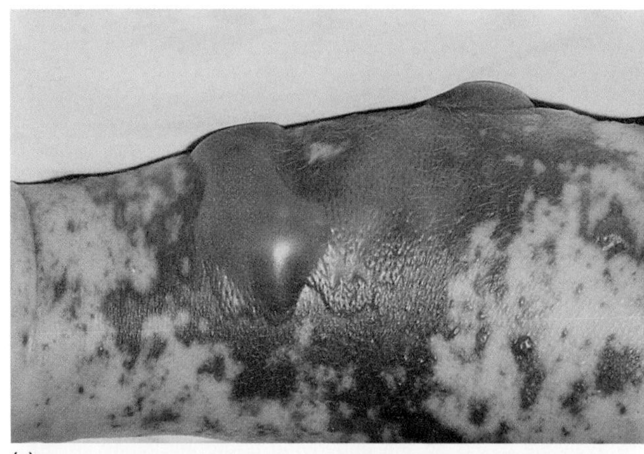
(a)

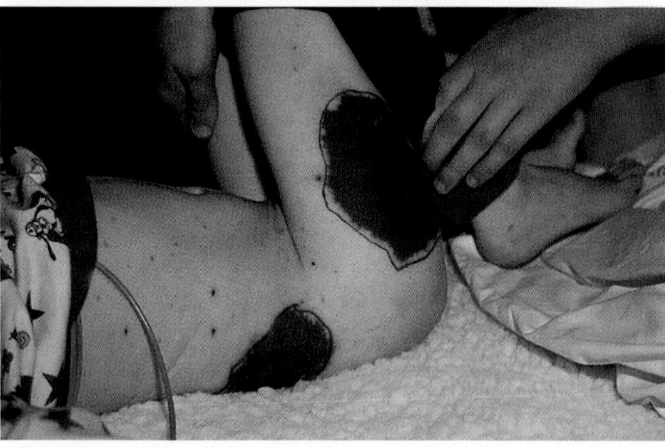
(b)

Fig. 146.1 (a) Acute infectious purpura fulminans due to meningococcal sepsis. Sharply demarcated areas of purpura are seen with bullous formation in the overlying skin. (b) Postinfectious purpura fulminans. Large areas of purpura are seen sharply demarcated from the surrounding tissues. Healing varicella vesicles are visible elsewhere on the body.

Classification of purpura fulminans based on aetiology and pathogenesis. As with many other clinical disorders that were initially defined simply by description of the major clinical and histopathological features, it is now apparent that purpura fulminans is not a single disease, but a common clinical and histopathological manifestation of a number of distinct disease processes. Thus, the major clinical feature (extensive purpura) is the result of a single histopathological process [17,18] (dermal vascular thrombosis and haemorrhagic infarction of the surrounding tissues). These clinical and histopathological features may be caused by a wide range of different disease processes involving the blood vessel wall, platelets or prothrombotic or antithrombotic pathways. Effective treatment of individual patients depends on identification of the underlying aetiological and pathophysiological mechanism, and the introduction of specific treatments to correct the disordered physiological process.

In this chapter a classification of purpura fulminans is proposed, which enables patients presenting with purpura fulminans to be classified into one of eight groups on the basis of clinical and epidemiological criteria and laboratory findings (Table 146.1). Each of these groups has a distinct aetiology and pathogenesis. Treatment recommendations are based on the current understanding of the pathophysiological mechanisms.

Acute infectious purpura fulminans

Purpura fulminans occurring in the context of acute bacterial sepsis is the most common form of the disorder. A variety of different bacteria have been associated with purpura fulminans, including *Staphylococcus aureus* [19], groups A and B β-haemolytic streptococci [20,21], *Streptococcus pneumoniae* [22], *Haemophilus influenzae* [23], *H. aegyptius* [24] and *Pseudomonas aeruginosa* [25]. Although purpura fulminans can be seen as an occasional complication of any of these bacterial infections, it occurs so commonly in the context of *Neisseria meningitidis* infection that its presence is considered a cardinal feature of meningococcal septicaemia [11,26,27]. Purpura fulminans associated with acute bacterial sepsis occurs in all age groups but is most common in children. Patients with purpura fulminans associated with acute bacterial infection such as meningococcaemia invariably present with the features of systemic infection and the majority will have evidence of shock [26,28–30]. The presenting features are often high fever, shivering, muscle aches, vomiting and abdominal pain. A particularly common presenting feature of children with severe purpura fulminans in the context of sepsis is intense limb pain, which may be an early sign of venous thrombosis. As the disease progresses, confusion, impaired consciousness, laboured breathing and other signs of systemic underperfusion become more apparent. Signs of shock are usually present including tachycardia, prolonged capillary refill, a wide gap between central and peripheral temperature, oliguria and elevated respiratory rate. Hypotension ultimately occurs once compensatory vasoconstrictive mechanisms are unable to maintain blood pressure in the face of severe shock. The disorder is frequently associated with multiorgan failure, but with recent advances in the early recognition and aggressive treatment of the disease, childhood mortality rates of 20–40% have been reduced to below 5% in countries where modern paediatric intensive care is available [26,27,31,32].

The pathophysiology of sepsis associated with purpura fulminans is complex (see Chapter 38 on meningococcaemia). Bacteria or their toxins (principally lipopolysaccharide in the case of Gram-negative organisms) trigger an intense inflammatory process, with activation of neutrophils, macrophages, complement and the clotting cascade [29,33]. Recently, meningococci have been shown in a mouse model to interact with CD147 and the β_2-adrenoceptor at the apical surface of endothelial cells mediated by bacterial type IV pili which may explain the initial endothelial injury [34,35] Endothelial injury mediated by bacterial toxins directly or secondary to host inflammatory factors, such as tumour necrosis factor (TNF), interleukin-1 (IL-1), reactive oxygen intermediates or proteolytic enzymes, results in disruption of the endothelium and loss of antithrombotic mechanisms [33]. Endotoxin induces upregulation of adhesion molecules

Table 146.1 Classification of purpura fulminans based on aetiology and pathogenesis

Clinical subgroup	Aetiology	Clinical features	Laboratory features	Pathophysiology	Medical therapy	Outcome
Acute infectious purpura fulminans	*Neisseria meningitidis* *Streptococcus pneumoniae*	Any age Acute febrile illness	Coagulopathy Positive blood culture	Circulatory insufficiency Endothelial dysfunction	*General*: Antimicrobial therapy	Mortality rate 20–40% May require skin grafting, amputation of digits or limbs
	Haemophilus influenzae	Hypotension	Other evidence of specific infections	Coagulation activation	Treatment of shock	Long-term orthopaedic problems including disrupted bone growth
	Staphylococcus aureus β-haemolytic streptococci Other bacteria	Multiorgan failure		Platelet activation Anticoagulant dysfunction Fibrinolytic dysfunction	Support of multiorgan failure *Specific*: ? Heparin	
	Rickettsiae *Candida albicans*				*Experimental*: AT III, protein C concentrates Fibrinolytic agents	
Postinfectious purpura fulminans	Varicella Group A β-haemolytic streptococci Other viruses, e.g. rubella	Usually young children Biphasic illness Initial febrile illness Sudden onset of purpura fulminans Haemodynamically stable	Coagulopathy Specific factor deficiency	Acquired protein S or C deficiency Autoantibody mediated ?Other mechanisms	FFP Heparin ± fibrinolytics *Speculative*: Factor concentrates Plasmapheresis Gamma globulin	Self-limiting Mortality rate 15–20% Surgical intervention may be necessary
Congenital protein C or S deficiency	Homozygous or compound heterozygous genetic defects	Usually early neonatal period	Coagulopathy	Inherited protein C or S deficiency	*Immediate*:	Lifelong deficiency
		Spontaneous onset of purpura fulminans Haemodynamically stable	Specific factor depletion Specific deficiency in family members		FFP or factor concentrate Heparin	Fatal if untreated Neurological and ophthalmic sequelae are common
		Family history of thromboembolism			*Prophylaxis*:	
					Anticoagulation: warfarin ± protein C concentrate	Continuous risk of recurrence Surgical intervention may be necessary
Acquired protein C or S deficiency associated with drugs or disease	Coumarin drugs Cholestasis	Any age Predisposing factors: drugs, interventions, hepatic or renal disease	Coagulopathy Specific factor depletion	Acquired protein C or S dysfunction or depletion	FFP or protein C concentrate Heparin	Usually self-limiting Surgical intervention may be necessary
	Renal dialysis Nephrotic syndrome Bone marrow transplantation				Address underlying cause	

(Continued)

Table 146.1 *Continued*

Clinical subgroup	Aetiology	Clinical features	Laboratory features	Pathophysiology	Medical therapy	Outcome
Antiphospholipid antibody syndrome	Autoimmunity	Usually older children and adults ± underlying SLE	Prolonged APTT ± slightly prolonged PT	Haemostatic dysregulation: multiple autoantibody mediated mechanisms identified	*Immediate:*	Fulminant variant is frequently fatal
			Lupus anticoagulant		Anticoagulation Fibrinolytics	Long-term prophylaxis is required to prevent recurrences
			Antiphospholipid antibodies		Immunosuppression	Surgical intervention may be necessary
					Plasmapheresis *Prophylaxis:* Anticoagulation: warfarin antiplatelet therapy	
Vasculitic disorders	Polyarteritis Henoch–Schönlein purpura	Fever Multiorgan involvement	Acute-phase response Leucocytosis	Vasculitic damage to blood vessel wall	Immunosuppression steroids Cyclophosphamide ± anticoagulation	Significant mortality Prognosis depends on response to underlying disease
	Other systemic vasculitides	Vasculitic rash Arthritis	Organ dysfunction		Antiplatelet agents	
Platelet-mediated purpura fulminans	Heparin therapy	Usually subcutaneous heparin Purpura fulminans at injection site	± Thrombocytopenia	Antibody-mediated platelet aggregation	Discontinue heparin therapy ± cyclo oxygenase inhibitors	Self-limiting Surgical intervention may be necessary
Toxins/poisons	Spider bites Snake bites	History of envenomation Purpura maximum at site of bite	Coagulopathy	Toxic damage to blood vessels Activation of coagulation	Specific antitoxins Supportive treatment	Self limiting Surgical intervention may be required

APTT, activated partial thromboplastin time; AT III, antithrombin III; FFP, fresh-frozen plasma; PT, plasma thromboplastin; SLE, systemic lupus erythematosus.

on the endothelial surface, which facilitate the attachment of neutrophils to the endothelial surface [33,36]. Upregulation of endothelial procoagulant activities, including tissue factor, occurs [37]. Neutrophils, activated by endotoxin, induce loss of the anticoagulant glycosaminoglycans, heparin sulphate and chondroitin sulphate from the endothelial surface [38], downregulation of prostacyclin production [39] and a defect in the activation of antithrombin by the endothelium [40].

The normal regulatory systems preventing uncontrolled coagulation are disturbed. Acquired deficiencies of tissue factor pathway inhibitor [41], antithrombin and proteins C and S [14,15,18,42,43] are caused by the profound capillary leak, together with consumption by the thrombotic processes. Reduced thrombomodulin and endothelial protein C receptor expression on the endothelium cause a defect of protein C activation in the dermal vessels [18]. The fibrinolytic system is also impaired, caused by elevation of plasminogen activator inhibitor 1 (PAI-1), the physiological inhibitor of tissue plasminogen activator (t-PA). In sepsis, elevated PAI-1 has been correlated with the development of shock, renal impairment and mortality [44]. In meningococcaemia, an increased in PAI-1 has been associated with death [45]. Variation in the PAI-1 gene does not affect the probability of an individual contracting meningococcal disease, but instead influences whether that person will develop septic shock or die from the disease [46,47].

The intravascular thrombosis seen in infectious purpura fulminans is therefore caused by a combination of sluggish vascular circulation caused by shock and platelet degranulation leading to local vasoconstriction [33], together with upregulation of procoagulant pathways and downregulation of anticoagulation regulatory pathways [33,48].

Postinfectious purpura fulminans

In contrast to purpura fulminans occurring as a complication of acute bacterial sepsis, 'idiopathic' or 'postinfectious purpura fulminans' characteristically occurs 1–3 weeks after an acute infectious process [4]. The disorder is more common in young children, and varicella and streptococcal infections are the most common antecedents [4], although a variety of other childhood illnesses have been reported to precede the disorder [1,4,16]. The disorder follows a biphasic course. After appearing to recover from an otherwise uncomplicated childhood illness, affected patients suddenly develop extensive areas of purpura, principally affecting the buttocks and lower limbs (Fig. 146.1b). Patients are usually afebrile and, except for areas of skin infarction or peripheral gangrene, are well perfused and normotensive. The disease may progress rapidly to cause extensive areas of skin necrosis and gangrene of the limbs or digits. Thromboembolic complications of internal organs may subsequently occur. Thrombosis of large vessels may lead to pulmonary emboli and embolization or thrombosis within the kidneys, brain, heart or other organs [16,49].

Affected patients have laboratory evidence of disseminated intravascular coagulation, with prolongation of prothrombin time, partial thromboplastin time and thrombin time, hypofibrinogenaemia and elevation of fibrin degradation products.

A wide range of different theories on the aetiology of the disorder have been presented. Although it is possible that the purpura fulminans following varicella may be mediated by a different process from that occurring in the context of streptococcal infections or other viral infections [4,6], there is now clear evidence that an acquired deficiency of protein S [49,50], induced by autoantibodies against protein S, is a consistent feature of the disorder [16]. In 1993, D'Angelo and colleagues reported a single case of thromboembolic disease occurring in a child who had recently had varicella [51]. The patient had an acquired deficiency of protein S caused by autoantibodies directed against protein S. Although their patient did not have purpura fulminans, or any cutaneous manifestations of thrombosis, their report led the authors to search for the presence of autoantibodies in similar patients with postvaricella purpura fulminans. In five consecutive children presenting with purpura fulminans following varicella or other viral infections, the authors documented severe acquired protein S deficiency caused by immunoglobulin G (IgG) or IgM autoantibodies directed against protein S, and this now appears to be the common mechanism underlying postinfectious purpura fulminans [16]. Varicella or other bacterial or viral infections may trigger the production of an autoantibody, which crossreacts with the protein S. Because no known varicella proteins exist with similar structure to that of protein S, it is likely that the antibody is directed against a neoantigen exposed during the varicella infection. The antibodies appear to increase the clearance of protein S, perhaps by rapid removal of the protein S antibody complex, through binding to Fc receptors on the reticuloendothelial system. The enhanced clearance of protein S not only explains the low levels of protein S present at the time of admission, but also explains the difficulties which may be found in restoring protein S levels to normal even following the infusion of large volumes of plasma. Levels of the anti-protein S autoantibodies decline spontaneously within 1–6 weeks after the onset of the disease [16] (Fig. 146.2). Because IgG responses would normally be expected to be long lasting, the rapid disappearance of the antibody from the circulation may suggest involvement of an anti-idiotype response. Anticardiolipin antibodies are present in some of the patients with postvaricella purpura fulminans, including those with antiprotein S antibodies. Low titres of IgM and IgG anticardiolipin antibodies are detected in some of the patients with antiprotein S antibodies, and may be implicated in the pathogenesis, but it is not yet clear whether this represents a crossreaction or the production of two distinct sorts of crossreacting antibodies [16,52]. It is also possible that autoantibodies directed against protein C may cause a similar picture in some cases.

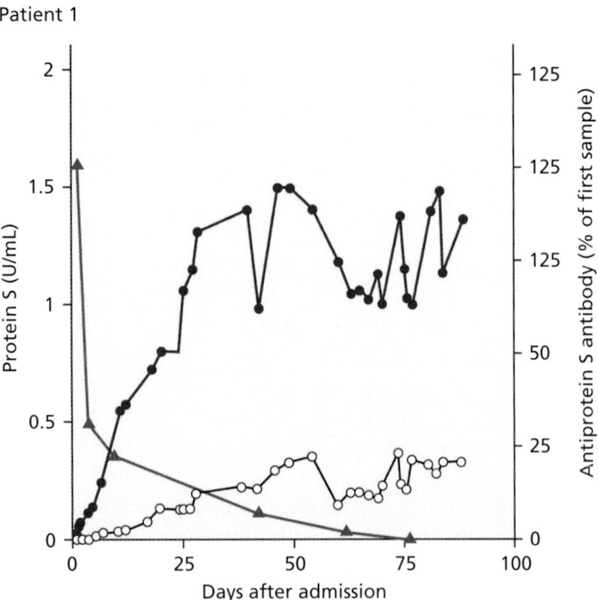

Fig. 146.2 Postinfectious purpura fulminans following varicella. The time courses of changes in protein S level are shown following admission of a child with purpura fulminans. On admission both free protein S (○) and total protein S (●) levels were undetectable. Levels of antiprotein S antibodies were markedly increased (▲). Over the next 4 weeks, antiprotein S antibody levels progressively declined, with a concurrent rise in both free and total protein S.

Congenital purpura fulminans caused by defects in the protein C or S pathway

Children with congenital protein C and S deficiency may present in the neonatal period with thrombosis of major organs including the brain with or without the cutaneous manifestations of purpura fulminans [12,53]. Severely affected patients have either homozygous protein C or S deficiency, or are functionally homozygous caused by compound heterozygous states. The cutaneous features of purpura fulminans may occur spontaneously either in the neonatal period or within the first months of life. In some cases, cutaneous or internal organ thrombosis occurs spontaneously but, in other cases, a precipitating infectious or inflammatory insult appears to trigger the disease. Unlike those patients with acute infectious purpura fulminans, those with congenital protein C or S deficiency are often haemodynamically stable and afebrile at the time of presentation unless an infection has precipitated the onset of purpura. A family history of thromboembolism is common as the heterozygous carriers of the disorder are at increased risk of thromboembolism. Any child presenting in the neonatal period or early months of life with purpura fulminans or thromboembolism should be suspected as having protein C or S deficiency and should be investigated appropriately [12,13,53–55].

Acquired protein C or S deficiency caused by drugs or specific diseases

Purpura fulminans has increasingly been recognized in patients treated with drugs such as coumarin derivatives, which suppress production of protein C and S, in addition to the production of the vitamin K-dependent clotting factors [6]. Patients heterozygous for deficiency of protein C or S appear to be at risk [56–58]. Acquired protein C and S deficiency may also occur in patients with cholestatic hepatic disease [59], the nephrotic syndrome, peritoneal dialysis [60] and bone marrow transplantation [61]. The clinical features in this subgroup include the use of drugs which affect protein C or S production, or the presence of underlying predisposing diseases. In the case of coumarin drug usage, patients developing purpura fulminans appear to have a more rapid decline in levels of protein C and S than the desired depletion of the vitamin K-dependent procoagulant factors. Patients heterozygous for protein C or S deficiency are at risk of this complication. Patients with the nephrotic syndrome have increased urinary clearance of protein C and S as part of the generalized proteinuria. Impaired production of protein C and S or increased clearance underlie the association of depletion of these proteins with hepatic disease or dialysis.

Purpura fulminans associated with the antiphospholipid antibody syndrome

Purpura fulminans may occur in patients with systemic autoimmune disease such as systemic lupus erythematosus (SLE) [62], polyarteritis nodosa or Henoch–Schönlein purpura [63]. It may also occur as a component of the antiphospholipid antibody syndrome [64,65] (Fig. 146.3). The clinical features of patients presenting with purpura fulminans in the context of these systemic disorders are usually dominated by those of the systemic illness. Patients with SLE or polyarteritis nodosa may have a prolonged febrile illness with evidence of multiorgan involvement including arthritis, nephritis, central nervous

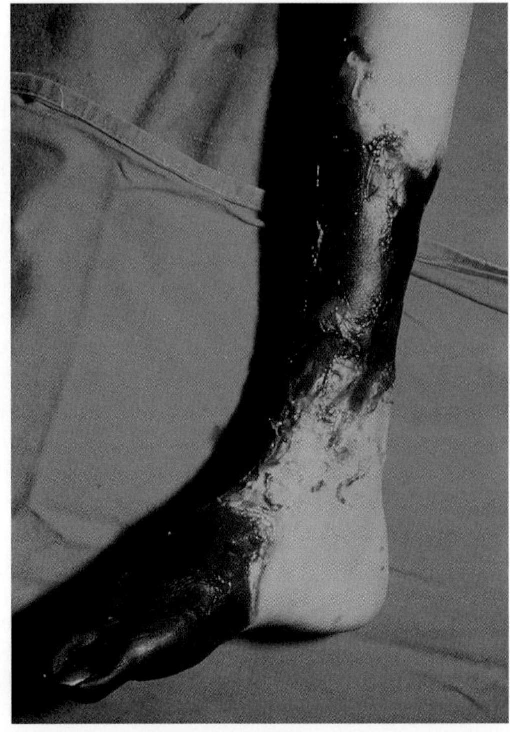

Fig. 146.3 Purpura fulminans and peripheral gangrene in a child with systemic lupus erythematosus and antiphospholipid antibodies.

system disease or pneumonitis [66,67]. Occasionally, patients with antiphospholipid antibodies may have no underlying systemic illness and may present acutely with either purpura fulminans or major organ thrombosis [64,65]. Laboratory features include an acute inflammatory response, with elevation of the erythrocyte sedimentation rate. Neutrophil leucocytosis and elevation of C-reactive protein are common in the acute vasculitides, whereas paradoxical depression of C-reactive protein, neutropenia and thrombocytopenia may occur in SLE. Antiphospholipid antibodies may occur in association with other markers of SLE, including anti-DNA antibodies, antibodies to extractable nuclear antigens, and low C3 and C4. A number of antibody-mediated mechanisms initiating thrombosis have been identified in patients with antiphospholipid antibodies, including inhibition of protein C activation by thrombomodulin, inhibition of the anticoagulant action of activated protein C and interference with antithrombin 3 binding to endothelial glycosaminoglycans [64,65]. Platelet activation may also occur. Non-antibody-mediated mechanisms may also be involved, including acute vasculitic damage to the vessel wall mediated by neutrophils and the lymphocytes or other inflammatory cells. Patients with systemic vasculitis may have evidence of antineutrophil cytoplasmic antibodies.

Platelet-mediated purpura fulminans occurring during heparin therapy

Heparin-induced skin necrosis, caused by antibody-mediated platelet aggregation, occurs primarily after subcutaneous administration of heparin, usually at the injection site [68,69]. Platelet-mediated mechanisms have also been proposed to explain purpura fulminans occurring in the course of thrombotic thrombocytopenic purpura [70], or paroxysmal nocturnal haemoglobinuria [71]. Diagnosis of platelet-mediated purpura fulminans is usually suggested by its occurrence in the context of heparin treatment or in patients with thrombocytopenic purpura. The disease is usually self-limiting once heparin therapy is discontinued but treatment with alternative anticoagulant agents such as coumarin derivatives, or the use of platelet inhibitors such as nonsteroidal anti-inflammatory agents or prostacyclin, may be required in severe cases.

Purpura fulminans following bites or envenomation

Purpura fulminans may occur after a number of toxic insults including snake bites or spider bites (see Chapter 61). Activation of coagulation and endothelial injury appear to be the underlying mechanisms. The purpura is usually present locally around the site of the toxin inoculation but, in severe cases, extensive areas of purpura may be apparent.

Pathology. Although purpura fulminans may be caused by a variety of distinct disease processes, the histopathological findings are common to all patients with the disorder. The hallmark of the disease is thrombotic occlusion of dermal vessels [2,4,6,17]. In mild cases the process is confined to the dermal capillaries and venules. In more severe cases thrombosis extends into the deeper tissues involving larger vessels and, in the most severely affected patients, thrombotic occlusion of the major veins draining entire limbs may also occur (Fig. 146.4). Veins and small venules are distended and occluded by fibrin thrombi and large aggregates of red cells. Haemorrhage into the surrounding tissues occurs resulting in oedema and the appearance of extravascular red blood cells [17].

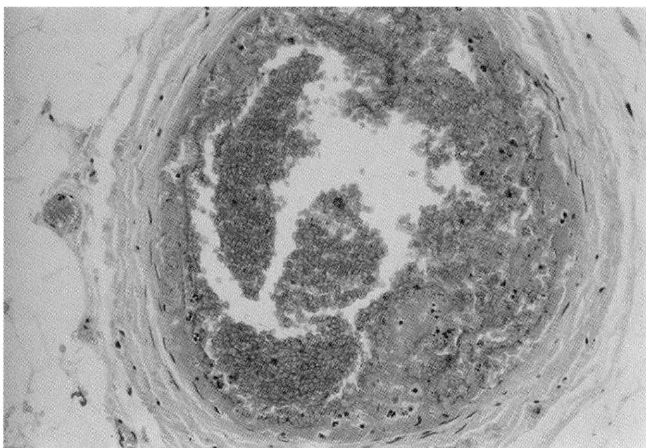

Fig. 146.4 Histology of purpura fulminans. Thrombosis within the saphenous vein is visible in a child who required below-knee amputation following meningococcal sepsis. The lumen of the vein is occluded by fibrin/thrombus. No inflammatory infiltrate was visible in the vessel wall.

The intravascular thrombosis affecting capillaries, veins and venules frequently occurs without any evidence of underlying vasculitis or inflammatory cell-induced disruption of the vessel wall. This is particularly true of postinfectious purpura fulminans, which is primarily a thrombotic process. In contrast, in patients with purpura fulminans associated with meningococcal sepsis or in vasculitis-associated purpura fulminans, there may be evidence of vasculitis surrounding areas of venous thrombosis [2,18]. Even in patients with purpura fulminans associated with meningococcaemia, venous thrombosis may occur without any evidence of inflammatory cell infiltrate into the vessel wall [26]. Areas of vasculitis may be interspersed between areas of thrombosis without evidence of underlying vessel wall inflammation.

Clinical features. The major presenting symptoms and clinical signs in purpura fulminans differ amongst clinical subgroups as described in Table 146.1, and largely depend on the different aetiological processes. For example, the presenting features of patients with acute infectious purpura fulminans associated with meningococcal sepsis are dominated by the features of sepsis and septic shock. Similarly, patients with purpura fulminans associated with SLE or vasculitic disease will present with features of the underlying disorder. In this section, those clinical features which are common to all patients with purpura fulminans are discussed.

The first cutaneous sign of purpura fulminans is usually the appearance of erythematous or purplish sharply defined skin lesions (Fig. 146.5a). These are most common on the periphery but may occur elsewhere on the body

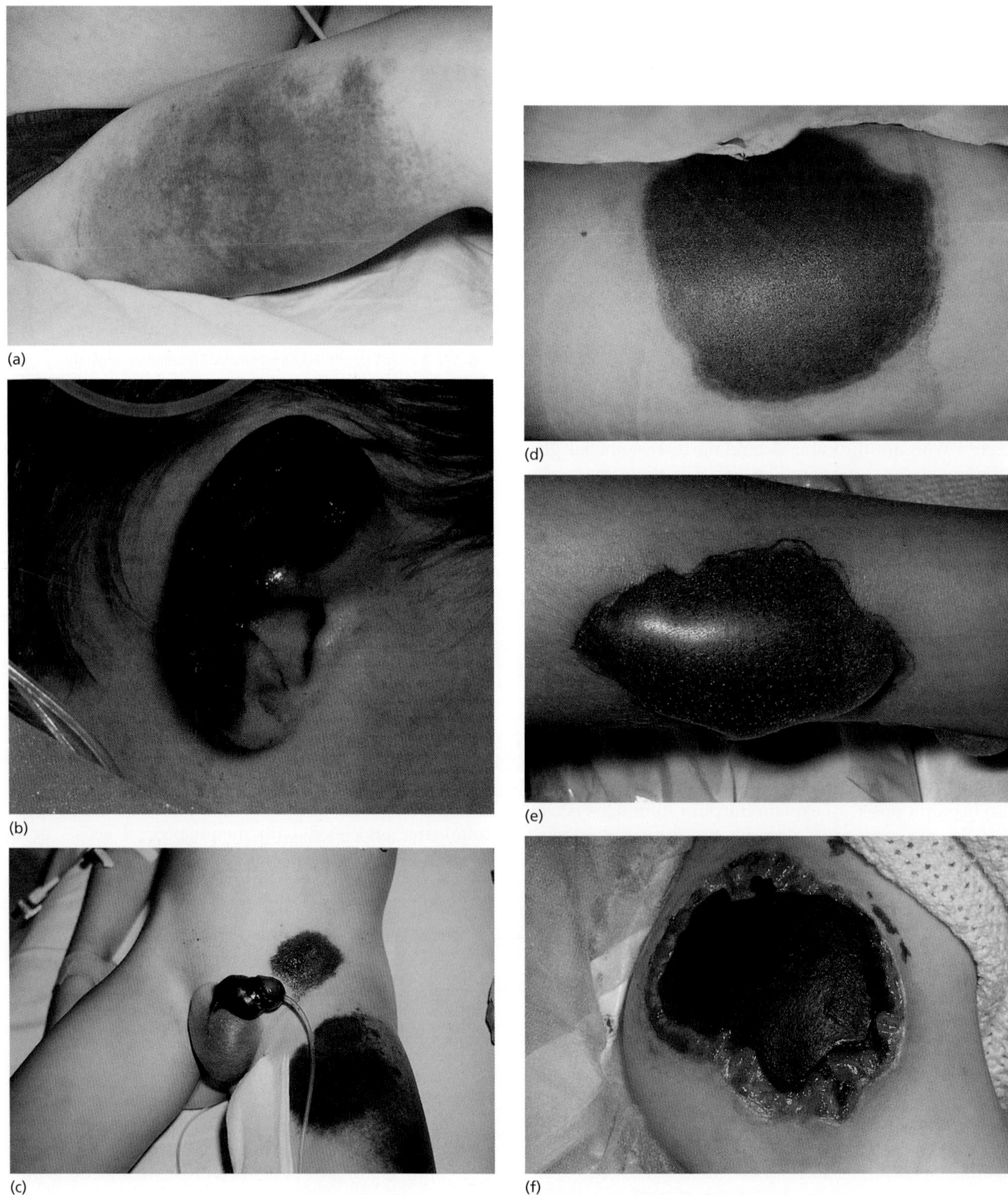

Fig. 146.5 (a) Early lesions of purpura fulminans. The child presenting with postinfectious purpura fulminans with early erythematous discoloration is seen with a small area of blue–black bruising in the centre of the lesion. (b,c) Purpura involving the earlobes and penis in a child with postvaricella purpura fulminans (composite). (d) Later lesions in postinfectious purpura fulminans. A sharply demarcated area of purpura is seen separated from surrounding skin by an area of erythema. (e) Haemorrhagic bullous lesions. A large blood-filled bullous area in a child with postinfectious purpura fulminans. (f) Late lesions of postinfectious purpura fulminans. Granulation tissue surrounds a deep area of skin necrosis on the buttock of a child with postvaricella purpura fulminans.

and frequently involve the tips of the nose, ears and penis (Fig. 146.5b,c). Within a few hours, the initial lesions may progress to sharply defined bruises ranging in size from a few centimetres to large confluent areas that may affect entire limbs. With time, the lesions become black in colour indicating infarction of the affected area of skin (Fig. 146.5d). Haemorrhagic bullae or vesicles may be seen in some cases, with the accumulation of haemorrhagic oedema fluid round the thrombosed vessels (Fig. 146.5e). In patients with progressive disease, lesions at different stages of evolution may be visible at the same time. Early lesions with erythema and bluish discoloration may coexist with blackened areas of infarcted skin. Well-established lesions frequently have a zone of erythema surrounding the blue–black area of cutaneous infarction (Fig. 146.5d,f).

In patients with circumferential lesions of limbs, or those who develop major vein thrombosis, signs of peripheral ischaemia of whole limbs or multiple limbs may become apparent (Fig. 146.6). Loss or diminution of pulses in the affected limbs, poor capillary refill, pallor and reduced temperature are signs of impending gangrene. In severely affected cases, the disorder may progress to critical ischaemia of entire limbs within a few hours of onset of the disease.

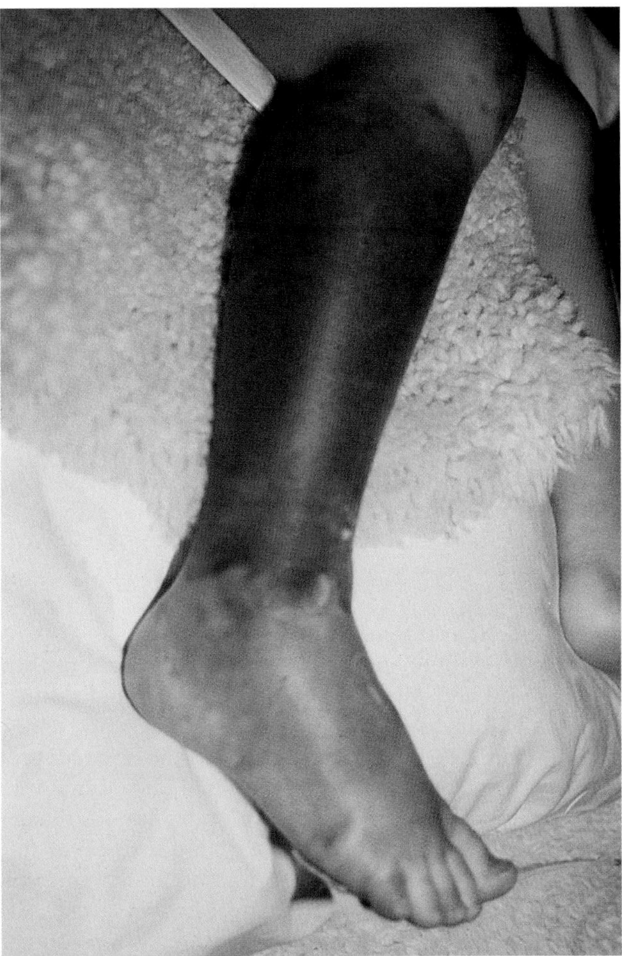

(a)

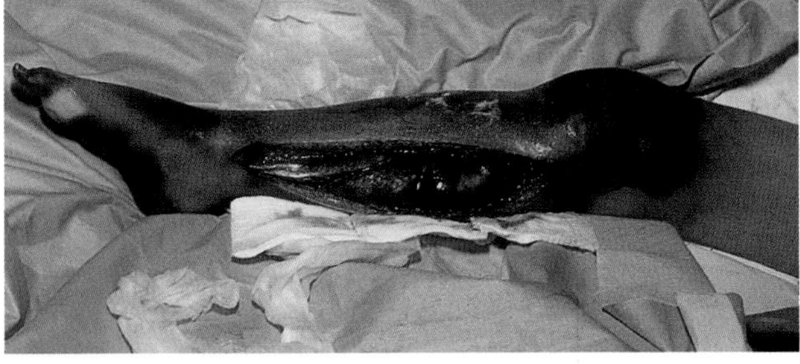

(b)

Fig. 146.6 (a) Circumferential areas of purpura in a child with postvaricella purpura fulminans. The foot is pale and pulses were not present. (b) Following fasciotomy, the muscles of the calf can be seen to be black and discoloured. Amputation of the leg below the knee was required.

In the days and weeks following the onset of the disease, areas of purpura become sharply demarcated from the surrounding tissues. Whatever the cause of the purpura fulminans, once the underlying disease process has been treated and progression of the disease halted (by treatment of sepsis in the case of meningococcaemia or following the administration of anticoagulants in the case of postinfectious purpura fulminans), the areas of cutaneous purpura persist, surrounded by uninvolved areas of skin which may be warm and well perfused. Where the thrombotic process has extended into the deep tissues, necrosis of the overlying skin will occur. The skin will initially become blackened and mummified. Thrombosed veins are often seen as black lines within the parchment-like dried and thickened skin. With time, the thrombosed and blackened dead skin sloughs off, revealing underlying healthy granulation tissue (Fig. 146.5f). In superficial lesions, blistering or bullous formation may occur but once the surface has been removed or fallen off viable skin may regrow without the need for skin grafting. The underlying depth of the lesions may be difficult to estimate early in the process and some patients may show dramatic recoveries without scarring, even when there have been extensive areas of apparent skin necrosis. In contrast, patients with deep and extensive lesions will require skin grafting and plastic surgery to cover extensive areas of skin loss, and may be left severely scarred by the disorder (Fig. 146.7).

Prognosis. Purpura fulminans remains a devastating condition that carries a significant mortality and may cause considerable long-term disability in severe cases. The prognosis of the disorder is largely dependent on the underlying condition (Table 146.1). For patients presenting with purpura fulminans as a component of meningococcal septicaemia or other forms of sepsis, the prognosis is largely that of the underlying disorder. With earlier disease recognition and modern aggressive intensive care, a higher proportion of patients with septic shock are now surviving and mortality rates for patients with meningococcal sepsis may now be as low as 5% [27,31,72]. However, with improvements in the survival rates for patients with severe sepsis, many patients who previously may have died of shock and multiorgan failure are now surviving but being left with the consequences of severe purpura fulminans, including ischaemia of whole limbs or digits and loss of extensive areas of skin [73–76]. Recently, a large study from the Netherlands showed the incidence of long-term skin scarring to be 48% and orthopaedic sequelae to be 14% in children surviving meningococcal sepsis. Although the severity of these sequelae varied, children with more severe scarring or who had suffered orthopaedic sequelae were demonstrated to have had more severe disease [77].

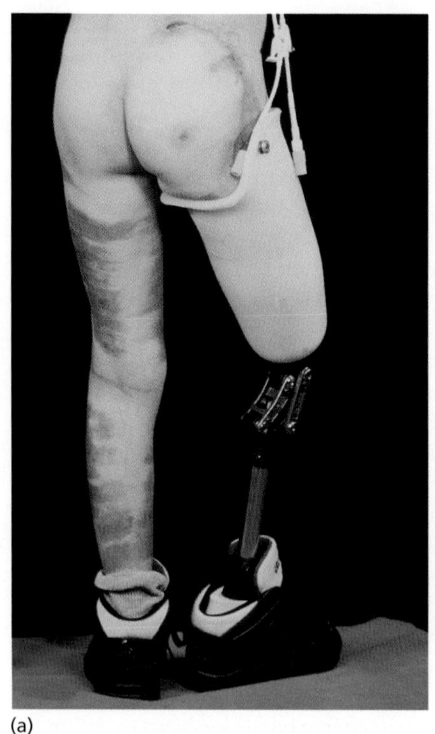

(a)

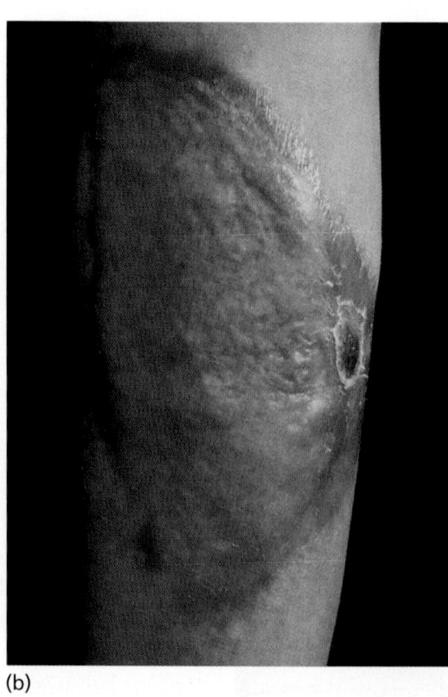

(b)

Fig. 146.7 (a,b) Consequences of postinfectious purpura fulminans. The same patient as in Fig. 146.6. Amputation of the lower leg was required and extensive scarring is seen in other areas.

For the other forms of purpura fulminans, including postinfectious purpura fulminans, the prognosis has improved as a result of a better understanding of the disease. Reports in the literature of patients with postinfectious purpura fulminans suggested mortality rates of 20–30% [1,4]. With early anticoagulation, and judicious use of fibrinolytic agents, the prognosis has undoubtedly improved, and the majority of patients in whom the diagnosis is made and appropriate treatment administered should now survive. Clearly, those patients in whom the true nature of the illness is not appreciated, and appropriate treatment withheld, continue to have a poor prognosis. Children with congenital protein C and S deficiency continue to have a poor prognosis. Affected children are at life-long risk of major vessel thrombosis, thrombosis of major organs and of recurrence of purpura. The availability of protein C concentrates [78,79] has dramatically improved the prognosis for children with this deficiency, but the requirement for life-long replacement therapy, continual vascular access with the attendant risks of infection and large vessel thrombosis, and the risk of neurological and ophthalmic thrombosis result in these disorders having an uncertain prognosis. Therefore, liver transplantation has been considered in some cases.

Specific treatment for individual subgroups. Effective treatment of individual patients depends on identification of the underlying aetiological and pathophysiological mechanisms, and the introduction of specific treatments to correct the disordered physiological process. Previously, a large number of different therapeutic modalities have been offered to individual patients without a clear understanding of the underlying physiological process. The clinicopathological classification proposed in this chapter now enables patients presenting with purpura fulminans to be assigned at the time of presentation to one of the distinct clinical subgroups, based on the history and the presenting features. Treatment can therefore be administered that is specifically designed to correct the pathophysiological derangement underlying each of the subgroups.

Acute infectious purpura fulminans

The major component of treatment for children with septic shock and purpura fulminans is directed against treatment of the underlying systemic infection and shock [28–30]. Patients should be admitted to a paediatric intensive care unit as soon as possible after diagnosis. Those presenting with shock and purpura fulminans should receive broad-spectrum antibiotics to cover not only *N. meningitidis*, but also the less common organisms associated with purpura fulminans such as *S. pneumoniae*, *P. aeruginosa* and staphylococcal and streptococcal infection. A combination of third-generation cephalosporin and consideration of the need for an antipseudomonal agent such as an aminoglycoside would be appropriate.

The main goal of treatment is to improve peripheral and organ perfusion by aggressive treatment of shock. The infusion of large volumes of colloid to correct hypovolaemia, inotropes to improve myocardial output and elective ventilation are indicated. Meticulous attention to fluid and electrolyte balance and the use of renal replacement therapies are often required. The treatment of shock in meningococcal septicaemia has been described in detail elsewhere [28,30].

Specific treatments of the purpura fulminans and the ischaemia of limbs and digits are increasingly used, but there have been few controlled trials to date. Fresh frozen plasma (FFP) infusions are required to correct the severe deficiencies of coagulation factors and to reduce the risk of haemorrhage associated with hypofibrinogenaemia. Despite theoretical concerns that the complement components present in FFP may accentuate the inflammatory process [80,81], FFP is indicated to correct hypofibrinogenaemia and specific clotting factor deficiency, and to reduce the risk of haemorrhage [33,82]. Prostacyclin has been used to try to reverse some vasoconstriction where impending gangrene is seen in a 'glove and stocking' distribution. However, there is no clinical trial supporting its use and, when used in large doses, this agent may cause further hypotension [33,39]. Heparin has also been suggested in the past as a logical treatment in disseminated intravascular coagulation [83,84]. However, limited clinical trials have not shown a benefit for routine heparin therapy in sepsis [85] and it is not recommended as standard therapy except as an adjunct to haemofiltration required for renal replacement.

A large number of other modalities of treatment are theoretically attractive based on the growing understanding of the pathophysiology of the disorder. As a result of uncontrolled series, some have suggested administration of concentrates of protein C [86,87] and antithrombin [88] may be beneficial in the face of the depletion of these anticoagulant proteins that have been documented in this disorder [14,15]. It is clear, however, that it is not possible at present to predict which patients who have been administered protein C concentrate will be able to activate the drug [18,87]. Even where activated protein C is detectable in the plasma, there is evidence of an activation defect in the dermal vascular endothelium and a theoretical risk that unactivated protein C in excess may displace activated protein C at the endothelial protein C receptor and thus worsen dermal vessel thrombosis [18,89]. A phase 3 trial of recombinant activated protein C was shown to reduce the mortality in adult sepsis [90], but the phase 3 trial in childhood sepsis has recently been stopped caused by futility and some safety concerns. Activated protein C was withdrawn from adult use in 2011 due to lack of efficacy [91]. Although the use of antithrombin to restore circulating levels was suggested by animal data and some human series [92–94], a placebo-controlled trial of this agent in adult sepsis showed no survival benefit of using the drug, together with an increased risk of bleeding where administered with heparin [95].

There have been a number of case reports of the use of t-PA in patients with critical limb ischaemia [96,97], and the use of t-PA to treat severe meningococcaemia has a sound theoretical basis [44–47]. However, in a retrospective European study of 62 children with meningococcal disease treated with t-PA, 8% suffered serious intracerebral bleeding and its use cannot now be recommended [98].

Many clinicians who are faced with a devastating illness and the prospect of limb loss and death in young children feel justified in attempting to utilize experimental treatments in an uncontrolled way. The potential beneficial effects of anticoagulant or fibrinolytic agents must be balanced against the potential risk of haemorrhage around venepuncture sites, or into the gastrointestinal, respiratory or central nervous systems. The experience in evaluating t-PA in severe meningococcal disease highlights the need to avoid such strategies and to participate in multicentre trials. The authors' own policy is to use plasma to replace clotting factors and fibrinogen, or cryoprecipitate, in patients resistant to the multiple doses of FFP. Patients are currently offered entry to the phase 3 randomized placebo-controlled trial of activated protein C. The role of fasciotomy [76] is discussed below.

Postinfectious purpura fulminans

With the recognition that the pathophysiology of postinfectious purpura fulminans involves acquired deficiency of protein S, and that the disorder is primarily a disorder of venous thrombosis, treatment has become much clearer [16,49]. Immediate heparinization should be undertaken in any patient presenting with purpura fulminans following varicella. In patients with severe evidence of disseminated intravascular coagulation, heparinization should be started concurrently with infusions of large volumes of FFP. Correction of hypofibrinogenaemia and replacement of clotting factors will usually enable full heparinization to be achieved without major risk of haemorrhage. Heparinization is achieved by immediate administration of 100 units/kg of heparin, followed by a constant infusion of 25 units/kg/h. Patients with purpura fulminans are frequently heparin resistant and much larger doses may be required to achieve anticoagulation. In most patients, heparin alone will be adequate to prevent progression of the disease. However, in patients with critical limb ischaemia or impending infarction of large areas of the body or with evidence of thromboembolism, t-PA may be considered in addition to anticoagulation [47]. Our most frequent regime would be to administer FFP on a daily basis (10–20 mL/kg) and to administer heparin continually, initially by the intravenous route and then switch to low molecular weight heparins to complete therapy [99,100]. Heparinization is generally indicated until levels of protein S return to normal 2–6 weeks after the onset of the disease [11].

Infection is a common precipitant of purpura fulminans and may also be a complication occurring in patients with large areas of skin damage. Appropriate antibiotics should be given until the underlying aetiology has been established and until the sepsis has been excluded.

Although immunosuppression, or plasmapheresis, would theoretically hasten the reduction in plasma levels of anti-protein S antibodies, these treatments are generally not indicated. The antibody levels decline spontaneously within a few weeks and it is dubious whether immunosuppression with steroids, or plasmapheresis would result in a decline of the levels much more rapidly. In addition, there are significant complications of central venous access that may be required in order to undertake plasmapheresis. In the presence of purpura fulminans and protein S deficiency, major vessel thrombosis including intracardiac thrombosis formation may occur and central venous cannulation should be avoided if at all possible.

Purpura fulminans associated with the antiphospholipid syndrome or systemic vasculitides

Patients presenting with purpura fulminans in the context of SLE or a systemic vasculitic illness present a complex management problem, because the pathophysiology of the disorder is less clear than in the case of postinfectious purpura fulminans. A combination of platelet-mediated thrombosis, defects in antithrombotic mechanisms including the protein C pathway and damage to the vessel wall by the vasculitic process is common. Immediate therapy for a patient developing critical ischaemia of limbs or large areas of purpura should involve initiating anticoagulation with heparin. In those patients with evidence of arterial occlusion, prostacyclin can be considered in addition. Correction of specific clotting factor deficiencies and hypofibrinogenaemia by infusion of FFP may also be necessary.

Treatment of the underlying disease and the vasculitic process could also be initiated with corticosteroids such as methylprednisolone and, for those patients with progressive and fulminant disease and evidence of multiorgan involvement, the addition of potent immunosuppressant agents such as cyclophosphamide or azothioprin may also be required. Plasmapheresis may be beneficial for patients with rapidly progressive multiorgan involvement [66].

The long-term treatment of patients with the antiphospholipid syndrome involves maintenance treatment of underlying SLE with steroids and immunosuppressive agents, and the use of oral anticoagulants. Immunosuppressive treatment may not be effective in removing antiphospholipid antibodies, and long-term oral anticoagulation with warfarin has been shown to reduce the risk of venous thrombosis [67].

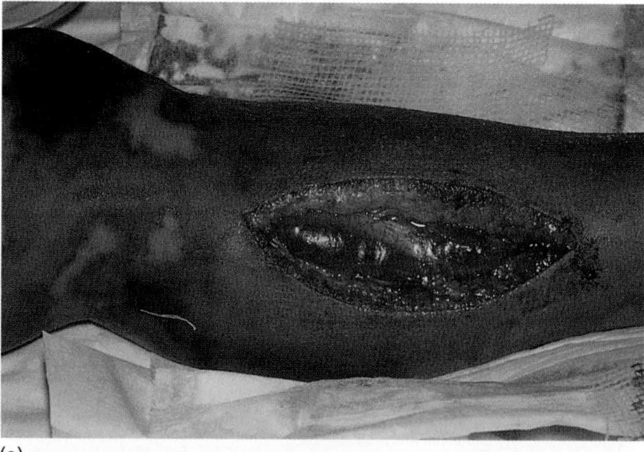

(a)

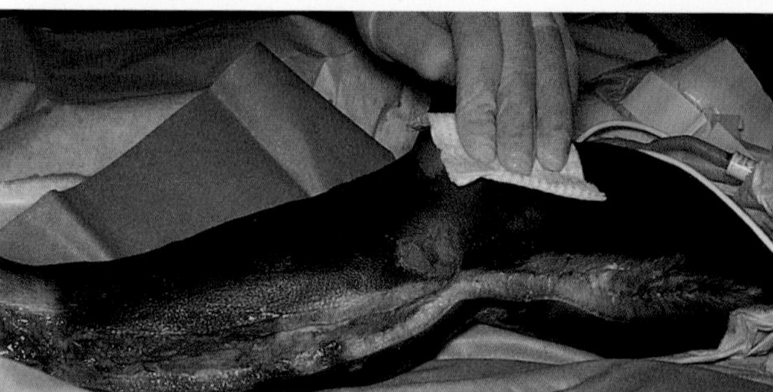

(b)

Fig. 146.8 (a) Purpura fulminans in meningococcal infection. A child with extensive purpura of both lower legs following meningococcal sepsis. Despite extensive cutaneous purpura, the muscles exposed by fasciotomy are viable. The oedematous muscle can be seen bulging through the incision site. (b) Meningococcal sepsis. A child with severe purpura fulminans and ischaemia of both lower legs is shown. Despite devitalized appearance of the skin and tissue exposed at fasciotomy, the child survived without loss of limbs, but required extensive skin grafting.

Surgical, orthopaedic and other aspects of treatment

Patients with extensive purpura fulminans and ischaemia of the limbs or digits require interdisciplinary treatment involving doctors, haematologists and a variety of surgical specialities. Meticulous nursing care and emotional support to the child and family are required throughout the illness.

Surgical intervention other than fasciotomy is rarely required during the early phases of extensive cutaneous purpura, and debridement and skin grafting to large purpuric areas should be delayed until complete demarcation of the infarcted areas of skin from the surrounding tissues has occurred, and the underlying disease process has been controlled [75,76,101–103].

In children with fulminant meningococcal shock who have a capillary leak syndrome, marked swelling and oedema of the limbs and other tissues may occur extremely rapidly. Compression of the arterial and venous blood supply to the periphery may develop in a period of only a few hours in children who are requiring large volumes of colloid replacement. Careful watch should be kept on the state of perfusion of the periphery in all such patients. Constriction of the blood supply may be further accentuated by plasters and tapes which have been used to secure intravenous cannulae. Because the tissues swell, adhesive tapes may produce circumferential constriction of the blood supply and contribute to the peripheral ischaemia.

For patients developing critical ischaemia of limbs or digits, early surgical opinion should be obtained and the compartment pressures measured. Fasciotomies may be required [104] if there is evidence of compression of the arteries or veins by the oedematous tissues (Fig. 146.8a). The venous thrombosis often results in the development of extensive tissue oedema and a compartment syndrome. Although there is a risk of bleeding at the site of the fasciotomy, particularly in patients who are treated with anticoagulation, those patients with evidence of vascular compression by the oedematous tissues may have a rapid improvement in perfusion of the limbs following the fasciotomy. If fasciotomies are required, they should be sufficiently extensive to release any possible constrictions to the major veins or arteries.

Decisions as to the timing and need for skin grafting or amputations should be taken after close interdisciplinary discussion between the paediatric intensive care specialists, and orthopaedic, plastic or vascular surgeons.

Surgical intervention to remove necrotic skin or amputate limbs or digits is generally not indicated during the acute phase of the disease for several reasons.

First, in patients with shock, multiorgan failure and severe coagulopathy, major surgical procedures are hazardous, and there will be major risks of bleeding. Second, clear demarcation between viable and dead tissue is extremely difficult in the early days of the illness. The area of skin blackening visible externally does not give an accurate indication of the condition of the underlying tissue. Because the disease process in all forms of purpura fulminans begins with thrombosis of the dermal vessels, patients may have large areas of blackened and infarcted skin, yet have underlying viable tissues (Fig. 146.8a). Even in patients who have evidence of blackening of muscle beds visible at the time of fasciotomy, the muscle infarction may only extend to the superficial visible areas of muscle, with viable tissues being left in deeper layers. The child shown in Fig. 146.8b, who appeared to have bilateral ischaemia of both lower limbs, has survived after extensive skin grafting with lower limbs intact. Although amputation may enable earlier discharge from hospital than is possible with a prolonged period of skin grafting, it may be possible to retain functionally useful limbs and digits even when the initial appearance suggests extensive ischaemia. Because purpura fulminans has generally resulted from venous infarction, the ischaemic tissues are seldom in contact with the general circulation, and most patients will not develop serious myoglobinuria or other evidence of systemic illness as a consequence of the gangrenous tissues.

For these reasons, amputations and skin grafting should be delayed for several days or weeks after the acute onset of the illness. In the case of children with fulminant meningococcal sepsis, stabilization of the child's condition and recovery from multiorgan failure should be allowed to take place before major surgical interventions are undertaken [105]. Secondary infection in the devitalized tissues does remain a significant risk. Virtually all patients who have large areas of necrotic skin and ischaemic tissues will have persistent fever, neutrophil leucocytosis and elevation of acute phase proteins. It may be difficult to distinguish fever and an inflammatory response because of the dead tissues from the effects of secondary infection in the devitalized tissues. If there is evidence of ongoing sepsis or persistent inflammatory state, earlier debridement should be considered.

Differential diagnosis. In children presenting with extensive areas of purpura leading to infarction of areas of the skin or digits, the diagnosis of purpura fulminans is usually obvious, and the major difficulties are therefore in the recognition of the individual disease processes which can lead to purpura fulminans. A number of other conditions may be associated with extensive areas of bruising. These would include subcutaneous bleeding in patients with primary haemostatic defects such as clotting factor deficiencies, anticoagulant overdose or thrombocytopenic disorders. However, in these primary bleeding disorders, although extensive subcutaneous bleeding may occur, infarction of areas of the skin, which is typical of purpura fulminans, does not occur.

The distinction between the different forms of purpura fulminans is made on the basis of the clinical, epidemiological and laboratory features outlined in Table 146.1

References

1 Hjort PF, Rapaport SI, Jorgensen L. Purpura fulminans: report of a case successfully treated with heparin and hydrocortisone: review of 50 cases from the literature. Scand J Haematol 1964;1:169–92.

2 Adcock DM, Hicks MJ. Dermatopathology of skin necrosis associated with purpura fulminans. Semin Thromb Hemost 1990;16:283–92.

3 Henoch E. Ueber Purpura fulminans. Berl Klin Wochenschr 1887:8–10.

4 Francis RB, Jr. Acquired purpura fulminans. Semin Thromb Hemost 1990;16:310–25.

5 Dodd HJ, Sarkany I, O'Shaughnessy D. Widespread cutaneous necrosis associated with the lupus anticoagulant. Clin Exp Dermatol 1985;10:581–6.

6 Adcock DM, Brozna J, Marlar RA. Proposed classification and pathologic mechanisms of purpura fulminans and skin necrosis. Semin Thromb Hemost 1990;16:333–40.

7 Branson HE, Katz J. A structured approach to the management of purpura fulminans. J Natl Med Assoc 1983;75:821–5.

8 Hatterley PG. Purpura fulminans: complete recovery with intravenously administered heparin. Am J Dis Child 1970;120:467–71.

9 Daeschner CW, 3rd, Carpentieri U. Purpura fulminans. Tex Med 1981;77:62–4.

10 Dudgeon DL, Kellogg DR, Gilchrist GS et al. Purpura fulminans. Arch Surg 1971;103:351–8.

11 Nadel S, Levin M, Habibi P. Treatment of meningococcal disease in childhood. In: Cartwright K (ed.) Meningococcal Disease. Chichester: John Wiley & Sons Ltd, 1995:207–43.

12 Marlar RA, Neumann A. Neonatal purpura fulminans due to homozygous protein C or protein S deficiencies. Semin Thromb Hemost 1990;16:299–309.

13 Dreyfus M, Magny JF, Bridey F et al. Treatment of homozygous protein C deficiency and neonatal purpura fulminans with a purified protein C concentrate. N Eng J Med 1991;325:1565–8.

14 Fourrier F, Lestavel P, Chopin C et al. Meningococcemia and purpura fulminans in adults: acute deficiencies of proteins C and S and early treatment with antithrombin III concentrates. Int Care Med 1990;16:121–4.

15 Powars D, Larsen R, Johnson J et al. Epidemic meningococcemia and purpura fulminans with induced protein C deficiency. Clin Infect Dis 1993;17:254–61.

16 Levin M, Eley BS, Louis J et al. Postinfectious purpura fulminans caused by an autoantibody directed against protein S. J Pediatrics 1995;127:355–63.

17 Sotto MN, Langer B, Hoshino-Shimizu S et al. Pathogenesis of cutaneous lesions in acute meningococcemia in humans: light, immunofluorescent, and electron microscopic studies of skin biopsy specimens. J Infect Dis 1976;133:506–14.

18 Faust SN, Levin M, Harrison OB et al. Dysfunction of endothelial protein C activation in severe meningococcal sepsis. N Engl J Med 2001;345:408–16.

19 Shennan AT. Purpura necrotica as a complication of ventriculoatrial shunts in hydrocephalus. Arch Dis Child 1972;47:821–3.

20 Issacman SH, Heroman WM, Lightsey AL. Purpura fulminans following late-onset group B beta-hemolytic streptococcal sepsis. Am J Dis Child 1984;138:915–6.

21 Canale ST, Ikard ST. The orthopaedic implications of purpura fulminans. J Bone Joint Surg Am 1984;66:764–9.

22 Johansen K, Hansen ST, Jr. Symmetrical peripheral gangrene (purpura fulminans) complicating pneumococcal sepsis. Am J Surg 1993;165:642–5.

23 Santamaria JP, Kenney S, Stiles AD. Purpura fulminans associated with Haemophilus influenzae type B infection. N C Med J 1985; 46:516–7.

24 Brazilian Purpuric Fever Study Group. Haemophilus aegyptius bacteraemia in Brazilian purpuric fever. Brazilian Purpuric Fever Study Group. Lancet 1987;2(8562):761–3.

25 Schafer J, Ambrus M, Morvay L et al. [Repeated attack of purpura fulminans associated with Pseudomonas pyocyanea septicemia]. Orv Hetil 1972;113:1608–11.

26 Toews WH, Bass JW. Skin manifestations of meningococcal infection; an immediate indicator of prognosis. Am J Dis Child 1974;127:173–6.
27 Wong VK, Hitchcock W, Mason WH. Meningococcal infections in children: a review of 100 cases. Pediatr Infect Dis J 1989;8:224–7.
28 Pollard AJ, Britto J, Nadel S et al. Emergency management of meningococcal disease. Arch Dis Child 1999;80:290–6.
29 Pathan N, Faust SN, Levin M. Pathophysiology of meningococcal meningitis and septicaemia. Arch Dis Child 2003;88:601–7.
30 Welch SB, Nadel S. Treatment of meningococcal infection. Arch Dis Child 2003;88:608–14.
31 Booy R, Habibi P, Nadel S et al. Reduction in case fatality rate from meningococcal disease associated with improved healthcare delivery. Arch Dis Child 2001;85:386–90.
32 Thorburn K, Baines P, Thomson A et al. Mortality in severe meningococcal disease. Arch Dis Child 2001;85:382–5.
33 Faust SN, Heyderman RS, Levin M. Disseminated intravascular coagulation and purpura fulminans secondary to infection. Baillieres Best Pract Res Clin Haematol 2000;13:179–97.
34 Coureuil M, Bourdoulous S, Marullo S et al. Invasive meningococcal disease: a disease of the endothelial cells. Trends Mol Med 2014; 20:571–8.
35 Lecuyer H, Borgel D, Nassif X et al. Pathogenesis of meningococcal purpura fulminans. Pathog Dis 2017;75.
36 Dixon GL, Heyderman RS, Kotovicz K et al. Endothelial adhesion molecule expression and its inhibition by recombinant bactericidal/permeability-increasing protein are influenced by the capsulation and lipooligosaccharide structure of Neisseria meningitidis. Infect Immun 1999;67:5626–33.
37 Heyderman RS, Klein NJ, Daramola OA et al. Induction of human endothelial tissue factor expression by Neisseria meningitidis: the influence of bacterial killing and adherence to the endothelium. Microb Pathog 1997;22:265–74.
38 Klein NJ, Shennan GI, Heyderman RS et al. Alteration in glycosaminoglycan metabolism and surface charge on human umbilical vein endothelial cells induced by cytokines, endotoxin and neutrophils. J Cell Sci 1992;102:821–32.
39 Heyderman RS, Klein NJ, Shennan GI et al. Deficiency of prostacyclin production in meningococcal shock. Arch Dis Child 1991;66:1296–9.
40 Heyderman RS, Klein NJ, Shennan GI et al. Reduction of the anticoagulant activity of glycosaminoglycans on the surface of the vascular endothelium by endotoxin and neutrophils: evaluation by an amidolytic assay. Thromb Res 1992;67:677–85.
41 Eling M, Stephens AC, Oragui EE et al. Tissue factor pathway inhibitor (TFPI) levels in the plasma and urine of children with meningococcal disease. Thromb Haemost 2001;85:240–4.
42 Esmon CT, Taylor FB, Jr, Snow TR. Inflammation and coagulation: linked processes potentially regulated through a common pathway mediated by protein C. Thromb Haemost 1991;66:160–5.
43 Leclerc F, Hazelzet J, Jude B et al. Protein C and S deficiency in severe infectious purpura of children: a collaborative study of 40 cases. Intensive Care Med 1992;18:202–5.
44 Brandtzaeg P, Joo GB, Brusletto B et al. Plasminogen activator inhibitor 1 and 2, alpha-2-antiplasmin, plasminogen, and endotoxin levels in systemic meningococcal disease. Thromb Res 1990;57:271–8.
45 Kornelisse RF, Hazelzet JA, Savelkoul HF et al. The relationship between plasminogen activator inhibitor-1 and proinflammatory and counterinflammatory mediators in children with meningococcal septic shock. J Infect Dis 1996;173:1148–56.
46 Westendorp RG, Hottenga JJ, Slagboom PE. Variation in plasminogen-activator-inhibitor-1 gene and risk of meningococcal septic shock. Lancet 1999;354(9178):561–3.
47 Hermans PW, Hibberd ML, Booy R et al. 4G/5G promoter polymorphism in the plasminogen-activator-inhibitor-1 gene and outcome of meningococcal disease. Meningococcal Research Group. Lancet 1999;354(9178):556–60.
48 Brandtzaeg P, Sandset PM, Joo GB et al. The quantitative association of plasma endotoxin, antithrombin, protein C, extrinsic pathway inhibitor and fibrinopeptide A in systemic meningococcal disease. Thromb Res 1989;55:459–70.
49 Nguyen P, Reynaud J, Pouzol P et al. Varicella and thrombotic complications associated with transient protein C and protein S deficiencies in children. Eur J Pediatr 1994;153:646–9.
50 Phillips WG, Marsden JR, Hill FG. Purpura fulminans due to protein S deficiency following chickenpox. Br J Dermatol 1992;127:30–2.
51 D'Angelo A, Della Valle P, Crippa L et al. Brief report: autoimmune protein S deficiency in a boy with severe thromboembolic disease. N Engl J Med 1993;328:1753–7.
52 Manco-Johnson MJ, Nuss R, Key N et al. Lupus anticoagulant and protein S deficiency in children with postvaricella purpura fulminans or thrombosis. J Pediatr 1996;128:319–23.
53 Marlar RA, Montgomery RR, Broekmans AW. Diagnosis and treatment of homozygous protein C deficiency. Report of the Working Party on Homozygous Protein C Deficiency of the Subcommittee on Protein C and Protein S, International Committee on Thrombosis and Haemostasis. J Pediatr 1989;114:528–34.
54 Millar DS, Allgrove J, Rodeck C et al. A homozygous deletion/insertion mutation in the protein C (PROC) gene causing neonatal Purpura fulminans: prenatal diagnosis in an at-risk pregnancy. Blood Coagul Fibrinol 1994;5:647–9.
55 Marlar RA, Sills RH, Groncy PK et al. Protein C survival during replacement therapy in homozygous protein C deficiency. Am J Hematol 1992;41:24–31.
56 McGehee WG, Klotz TA, Epstein DJ et al. Coumarin necrosis associated with hereditary protein C deficiency. Ann Intern Med 1984; 101:59–60.
57 Teepe RG, Broekmans AW, Vermeer BJ et al. Recurrent coumarin-induced skin necrosis in a patient with an acquired functional protein C deficiency. Arch Dermatol 1986;122:1408–12.
58 Friedman KD, Marlar RA, Houston JG et al. Warfarin induced skin necrosis in a patient with protein S deficiency. Blood 1986;68(Supp; 1): 333a (abstract).
59 Michiels JJ, Bertina RM. Thrombo-haemorrhagic skin necrosis due to rapid development of severe vitamin K deficiency associated with cholestasis. Thromb Haemost 1987:413 (abstract).
60 Kant KS, Glueck HI, Coots MC et al. Protein S deficiency and skin necrosis associated with continuous ambulatory peritoneal dialysis. Am J Kidney Dis 1992;19:264–71.
61 Gordon BG, Haire WD, Patton DF et al. Thrombotic complications of BMT: association with protein C deficiency. Bone Marrow Transplant 1993;11:61–5.
62 Jindal BK, Martin MF, Gayner A. Gangrene developing after minor surgery in a patient with undiagnosed systemic lupus erythematosus and lupus anticoagulant. Ann Rheum Dis 1983;42:347–9.
63 Kisker CT, Glueck H, Kauder E. Anaphylactoid purpura progressing to gangrene and its treatment with heparin. J Pediatr 1968; 73:748–51.
64 Stephens CJ. The antiphospholipid syndrome. Clinical correlations, cutaneous features, mechanism of thrombosis and treatment of patients with the lupus anticoagulant and anticardiolipin antibodies. Br J Dermatol 1991;125:199–210.
65 Key NS. Toward an understanding of the pathophysiologic mechanism of thrombosis in the antiphospholipid antibody syndrome. J Lab Clin Med 1995;125:16–7.
66 Asherson RA. The catastrophic antiphospholipid syndrome. J Rheumatol 1992;19:508–12.
67 Khamashta MA, Cuadrado MJ, Mujic F et al. The management of thrombosis in the antiphospholipid-antibody syndrome. N Engl J Med 1995;332:993–7.
68 White PW, Sadd JR, Nensel RE. Thrombotic complications of heparin therapy: including six cases of heparin-induced skin necrosis. Ann Surg 1979;190:595–608.
69 Warkentin TE, Levine MN, Hirsh J et al. Heparin-induced thrombocytopenia in patients treated with low-molecular-weight heparin or unfractionated heparin. N Engl J Med 1995;332:1330–5.
70 Luttengs WF. Skin necrosis in a patient with thrombotic thrombocytopenic purpura. Ann Intern Med 1957:1207–13.
71 Rietschel RL, Lewis CW, Simmons RA et al. Skin lesions in paroxysmal nocturnal hemoglobinuria. Arch Dermatol 1978;114:560–3.
72 Levin M, Quint PA, Goldstein B et al. Recombinant bactericidal/permeability-increasing protein (rBPI21) as adjunctive treatment for children with severe meningococcal sepsis: a randomised trial. rBPI21 Meningococcal Sepsis Study Group. Lancet 2000;356(9234):961–7.
73 Genoff MC, Hoffer MM, Achauer B et al. Extremity amputations in meningococcemia-induced purpura fulminans. Plast Reconstr Surg 1992;89:878–81.
74 Erickson L, De Wals P. Complications and sequelae of meningococcal disease in Quebec, Canada, 1990–1994. Clin Infect Dis 1998; 26:1159–64.

75 Huang DB, Price M, Pokorny J et al. Reconstructive surgery in children after meningococcal purpura fulminans. J Pediatr Surg 1999;34:595–601.

76 Hunt DM. The orthopaedic management of purpura fulminans in meningococcal disease in children. Care Critical Ill 2001;17:118–20.

77 Buysse CM, Oranje AP, Zuidema E et al. Long-term skin scarring and orthopaedic sequelae in survivors of meningococcal septic shock. Arch Dis Child 2009;94:381–6.

78 Muller FM, Ehrenthal W, Hafner G et al. Purpura fulminans in severe congenital protein C deficiency: monitoring of treatment with protein C concentrate. Eur J Pediatr 1996;155:20–5.

79 Dreyfus M, Masterson M, David M et al. Replacement therapy with a monoclonal antibody purified protein C concentrate in newborns with severe congenital protein C deficiency. Semin Thromb Hemost 1995;21:371–81.

80 Lehner PJ, Davies KA, Walport MJ et al. Meningococcal septicaemia in a C6-deficient patient and effects of plasma transfusion on lipopolysaccharide release. Lancet. 1992;340(8832):1379–81.

81 Busund R, Straume B, Revhaug A. Fatal course in severe meningococcemia: clinical predictors and effect of transfusion therapy. Crit Care Med 1993;21:1699–705.

82 de Jonge E, Levi M, Stoutenbeek CP et al. Current drug treatment strategies for disseminated intravascular coagulation. Drugs 1998; 55:767–77.

83 Kuppermann N, Inkelis SH, Saladino R. The role of heparin in the prevention of extremity and digit necrosis in meningococcal purpura fulminans. Pediatr Infect Dis J 1994;13:867–73.

84 Feinstein DI. Diagnosis and management of disseminated intravascular coagulation: the role of heparin therapy. Blood 1982;60:284–7.

85 Ockelford P. Heparin 1986. Indications and effective use. Drugs 1986;31:81–92.

86 White B, Livingstone W, Murphy C et al. An open-label study of the role of adjuvant hemostatic support with protein C replacement therapy in purpura fulminans-associated meningococcemia. Blood 2000;96:3719–24.

87 De Kleijn ED, De Groot R, Hack CE et al. Activation of protein C following infusion of protein C concentrate in children with severe meningococcal sepsis and purpura fulminans: a randomized, double-blinded, placebo-controlled, dose-finding study. Crit Care Med 2003;31:1839–47.

88 Balk R, Emerson T, Fourrier F et al. Therapeutic use of antithrombin concentrate in sepsis. Semin Thromb Hemost 1998;24:183–94.

89 Bernard G, Artigas A, Dellinger P et al. Clinical expert round table discussion (session 3) at the Margaux Conference on Critical Illness: the role of activated protein C in severe sepsis. Crit Care Med 2001;29(7 Suppl):S75–7.

90 Bernard GR, Vincent JL, Laterre PF et al. Efficacy and safety of recombinant human activated protein C for severe sepsis. N Engl J Med 2001;344:699–709.

91 Poole D, Bertolini G, Garattini S Withdrawal of 'Xigris' from the market: old and new lessons. J Epidemiol Commun Health 2012; 66:571–2.

92 Giudici D, Baudo F, Palareti G et al. Antithrombin replacement in patients with sepsis and septic shock. Haematologica 1999;84:452–60.

93 Emerson TE, Jr. Antithrombin III replacement in animal models of acquired antithrombin III deficiency. Blood Coagul Fibrinolysis 1994;5 Suppl 1:S37–45;discussion S59–64.

94 Taylor FB Jr, Emerson TE Jr, Jordan R et al. Antithrombin-III prevents the lethal effects of Escherichia coli infusion in baboons. Circ Shock 1988;26:227–35.

95 Warren BL, Eid A, Singer P et al. Caring for the critically ill patient. High-dose antithrombin III in severe sepsis: a randomized controlled trial. JAMA 2001;286:1869–78.

96 Zenz W, Muntean W, Gallistl S et al. Recombinant tissue plasminogen activator treatment in two infants with fulminant meningococcemia. Pediatrics 1995;96:44–8.

97 Nadel S, De Munter C, Britto J et al. Recombinant tissue plasminogen activator restores perfusion in meningococcal purpura fulminans [letter; comment]. Crit Care Med 1998;26:971–2; discussion 2–3.

98 Zenz W, Zoehrer B, Levin M et al. Use of recombinant tissue plasminogen activator in children with meningococcal purpura fulminans: a retrospective study. Crit Care Med 2004;32:1777–80.

99 Albisetti M, Andrew M. Low molecular weight heparin in children. Eur J Pediatr 2002;161:71–7.

100 Dix D, Andrew M, Marzinotto V et al. The use of low molecular weight heparin in pediatric patients: a prospective cohort study. J Pediatr 2000;136:439–45.

101 Arevalo JM, Lorente JA, Fonseca R. Surgical treatment of extensive skin necrosis secondary to purpura fulminans in a patient with meningococcal sepsis. Burns 1998;24:272–4.

102 Harris NJ, Gosh M. Skin and extremity loss in meningococcal septicaemia treated in a burn unit. Burns 1994;20:471–2.

103 Hudson DA, Goddard EA, Millar KN. The management of skin infarction after meningococcal septicaemia in children. Br J Plast Surg 1993;46:243–6.

104 Fitton AR, Dickson WA, Shortland G et al. Peripheral gangrene associated with fulminating meningococcal septicaemia. Is early escharotomy indicated? J Hand Surg (Br) 1997;22:408–10.

105 Morris ME, Maijub JG, Walker SK et al. Meningococcal sepsis and purpura fulminans: the surgical perspective. Postgrad Med J 2013;89(1052):340–5.

CHAPTER 147
Kawasaki Disease

Wynnis L. Tom[1,2] *& Jane C. Burns*[2]

[1]Department of Dermatology, Rady Children's Hospital and the University of California, San Diego, CA, USA
[2]Department of Pediatrics, Rady Children's Hospital and the University of California, San Diego, CA, USA

Abstract

Kawasaki disease (KD) is an acute systemic inflammatory illness with vasculitis that predominantly affects infants and young children. It is characterized by fever and five cardinal clinical features, although incomplete cases are not uncommon. KD results in cardiovascular complications in about 25% of untreated cases and is the leading cause of acquired heart disease in children in developed countries. Late adverse events occurring in those with coronary abnormalities make accurate diagnosis, treatment and continued monitoring critical. While significant advances have been made in characterizing factors influencing disease susceptibility and response to therapies, the underlying aetiology of KD remains unknown.

Key points

- **Kawasaki disease (KD) is an acute systemic inflammatory illness that predominantly affects infants and young children.**
- **The underlying aetiology of KD remains unknown, but epidemiological data suggest that it is caused by one or more widely distributed infectious agents or antigens triggering an abnormal immune response in a small subset of genetically susceptible individuals.**
- **The diagnosis is established by the presence of fever and five principal clinical features (changes in peripheral extremities, polymorphous skin eruption, bilateral conjunctival injection, changes in lips and oral cavity, and acute nonpurulent cervical adenopathy). Incomplete cases are not uncommon and it is important to recognize and treat them promptly.**
- **Medium-size vessel vasculitis, with a significant predilection for the coronary arteries, is the hallmark of KD. Coronary aneurysms may lead to myocardial infarction, arrhythmia or death during the inflammatory illness, with the potential for cardiac events later in adulthood if changes persist.**
- **At present, the most effective treatment in the acute stage is intravenous immunoglobulin (IVIG) plus aspirin, with a second dose of IVIG, infliximab, corticosteroids and cyclosporine being options if the response is inadequate. Clinical trials are ongoing, assessing the utility of the interleukin-1 signalling pathway blockade.**

Brief introduction and history. Kawasaki disease (KD) is an acute systemic inflammatory illness with vasculitis that predominantly affects infants and young children. The highest incidence is in Japan but KD occurs worldwide, having been observed on all continents and in all ethnic groups. Although originally believed to be a benign illness, KD is now known to result in cardiovascular complications in about 25% of untreated cases; sequelae range from asymptomatic coronary artery dilation or aneurysm to giant coronary artery aneurysms with thrombosis, myocardial infarction and sudden death. KD is the leading cause of acquired heart disease in children in developed countries.

Since the disease was first reported in 1967, significant advances have been made in its clinical, pathological and epidemiological characterization. However, the aetiology remains unknown. The recognition of late adverse events in those with coronary abnormalities makes accurate diagnosis, treatment and continued monitoring critical.

Epidemiology. KD predominantly affects young children, with peak incidence at 6–12 months of age in Japan and at 1.5–2 years of age in the USA and European countries [1]. Nearly 80% of all cases occur between 6 months and 5 years of age. The rarity in the first few months of life and after early childhood suggests that transplacental antibodies from the mother may protect the neonate from disease and that widespread immunity develops over time. Males are more often affected (1.4:1) [1,2].

Asian children, especially those of Japanese, Korean and Taiwanese descent, have the highest incidence of KD (respective rates of 265, 217 and 83 per 100 000 children under 5 years of age) [3–5]. In the USA, African-Americans and Hispanics show intermediate incidence and Caucasians have the lowest rate of illness (22.5 per 100 000 children under 5 years of age) [6]. The increased frequency of KD in children of Asian descent holds true even for those living a western lifestyle after migration to other countries, supporting a genetic predisposition for the disease. Cases occur year-round, but there are mini-epidemics and a seasonal peak of KD during the winter and spring months and again in mid-summer [2,7]. The incidence continues to gradually rise in Japan and other east Asian countries, but appears to be at a plateau in other developed countries such as the USA and the UK [8]. Rates of disease have increased more rapidly in

Harper's Textbook of Pediatric Dermatology, Fourth Edition. Edited by Peter Hoeger, Veronica Kinsler and Albert Yan.

developing countries such as India, although this may stem from increased recognition [2,9].

Person-to-person transmission appears unlikely as secondary cases rarely occur in the same household, school or daycare facility. The recurrence rate is 2–4% and is highest within the first 12 months after the first episode [10]. The fatality rate is estimated at 0.01%, based on the latest national survey in Japan [3].

Pathogenesis and theories of aetiology. The disease is characterized by marked activation of the innate immune system, with increased serum levels of proinflammatory cytokines such as tumour necrosis factor-α (TNF-α), interleukin (IL)-1, and IL-6 during the acute febrile phase [11]. Neutrophils are the predominant inflammatory cell type in the peripheral blood but in affected tissues, early infiltration by neutrophils is followed by CD8+ T cells, macrophages and plasma cells [11–13]. Three linked vasculopathic processes are described that disrupt the normal architecture of the vascular wall and result in aneurysm formation acutely and stenotic lesions after months to years [14]. Myocarditis has been noted in virtually all right ventricular biopsies during the acute phase of the illness, while myocardial fibrosis has been a common finding at autopsy decades after the acute illness [15,16]. Secretion of IL-10 by expanding populations of regulatory T cells and tolerogenic myeloid dendritic cells is associated with resolution of inflammation [17]. Oligoclonal IgA plasma cells have been found infiltrating the coronary arteries, pancreas, kidney and upper respiratory tract [1,11].

What causes KD remains an enigma, but epidemiological data suggest that it is caused by one or more widely distributed infectious agents or antigens triggering an abnormal immune response in a small subset of genetically susceptible individuals.

A genetic influence has been long suspected given that a parent of a child with KD is twice as likely to have had a personal history of KD; siblings of affected children have 10–20 times increased likelihood of disease development. In addition, Asian children have high rates of disease independent of geographic location [18]. As with other inflammatory illnesses, KD is genetically complex, with multiple genes contributing to overall disease susceptibility and outcome [19]. Genetic variation in the transforming growth factor (TGF)-β signalling pathway has shown consistent association with both susceptibility to KD and aneurysm formation [20,21]. The influence of polymorphisms in calcium signalling pathway genes including *inositol 1,4,5-triphosphate 3-kinase C (ITPKC)*, *ORAI calcium release-activated calcium modulator 1 (ORAI1)*, and *solute carrier family 8 member A1 (SLC8A1)* have been validated across different populations [22–24] and represent an intriguing therapeutic target because these pathways all converge on phosphorylation of the nuclear factor of activated T-cells (NFAT) transcription factor, the site of action of cyclosporine. Genome-wide association studies have identified single nucleotide variants in *caspase-3 (CASP3)*, *B lymphocyte kinase* (*BLK*), *CD40* and *Fc fragment of IgG low affinity IIa receptor* (*FCGR2A*) that influence KD susceptibility [25,26]. The first family-based analysis of whole genome sequence revealed an influence of variants in Toll-like receptor 6 on KD susceptibility [27].

Despite the seasonality, temporal clustering of cases and usually self-limited course suggestive of an infectious aetiology, no clear agent or environmental trigger has been found. KD shares many clinical features with scarlet fever and toxic shock syndrome, diseases known to be mediated by bacterial toxins, but toxin-producing bacteria have not been identified and the clinical illness does not respond to antibiotics [28–30]. In a search for a viral causative agent, Rowley et al. used synthetic antibodies derived from cloned IgA sequences from plasma cells in acute KD arterial tissue and demonstrated an antigen in the cytoplasm of bronchial epithelial cells and a subset of macrophages [31]. Light and electron microscopic studies localized the antigen to intracytoplasmic inclusion bodies consistent with aggregates of viral proteins and nucleic acids. This suggests a conventional antigen from an unidentified RNA virus potentially playing an important role in KD aetiology. Recent epidemiological data suggests that the trigger for KD may be carried by large-scale tropospheric winds, with provinces in northeastern China serving as a source for the seasonal clustering and annual epidemic of cases in Japan, Hawaii and southern California [32]. Investigations are ongoing for agent(s) that may have a respiratory portal of entry and tropism for vascular tissue.

Clinical features and diagnosis. The diagnosis of KD is established by the presence of fever and five principal clinical features. The most widely used criteria (established by the American Heart Association [AHA]) require fever of at least 5 days and at least four of the five other clinical findings, although diagnosis and treatment can occur before day 5 of fever if four clinical criteria are present or if coronary artery dilation is documented by echocardiography (Box 147.1) [33]. The duration of fever is usually 1–3 weeks in untreated patients. The fever responds poorly to antipyretics, but subsides rapidly in the majority of patients following treatment with intravenous immunoglobulin (IVIG) [34].

Box 147.1 Diagnostic criteria for Kawasaki disease

- Fever persisting for at least 5 days AND
- Changes in peripheral extremities:
  - Initial stage: reddening of palms and soles, indurative oedema
  - Convalescent stage: membranous desquamation from fingertips
- Polymorphous exanthem
- Bilateral conjunctival injection
- Changes in the lips and oral cavity: reddening of lips with fissuring, strawberry tongue, diffuse injection of oral and pharyngeal mucosa
- Acute non-opurulent cervical lymphadenopathy

Fever and at least four of five principal symptoms should be satisfied for the diagnosis of classic KD. However, patients with fewer than four of the principal symptoms can be diagnosed as having KD when coronary artery dilation or aneurysm is recognized by two-dimensional echocardiography or when patients meet laboratory criteria outlined in the American Heart Association algorithm (see [33] and Box 147.2).

1. Changes in peripheral extremities

The findings on the hands and feet in KD are distinctive. Within the first week after fever onset, erythema of the palms and soles (Fig. 147.1) and/or indurative oedema of the dorsum of the hands and feet (Fig. 147.2) occur. There may be a fusiform swelling of the digits with frank arthritis of the proximal interphalangeal joints and associated tenderness can be severe enough to limit walking or use of the hands [35]. After the fever subsides, the erythema and swelling disappear in most cases. About 10–15 days after the onset of illness, there is desquamation of the skin between the nails and the tips of the fingers and toes (Fig. 147.3), after which the peeling spreads proximally, often in large thick pieces (Fig. 147.4). While desquamation in this pattern is extremely characteristic of KD, it is only noted in two-thirds of patients [36].

2. Polymorphous skin eruption

During the first week after the onset of fever, an exanthem usually appears on the trunk and/or proximal extremities (Fig. 147.5). Perineal involvement is common (about two-thirds of cases), ranging from confluent macules to a plaque-type erythema (Fig. 147.6). Perineal and perianal

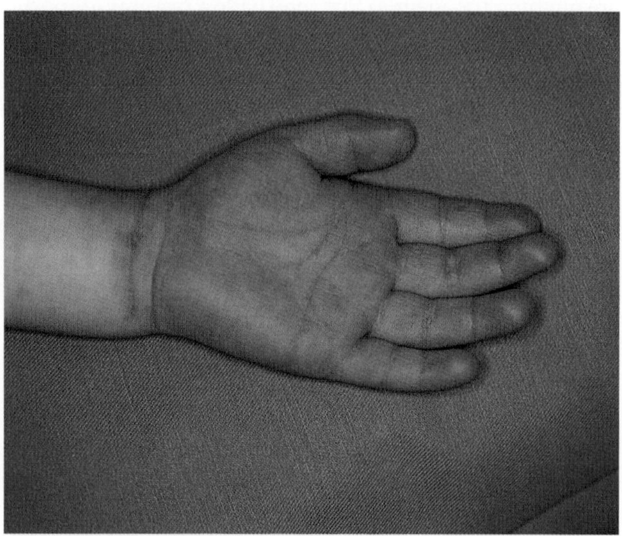

Fig. 147.1 Palmar erythema.

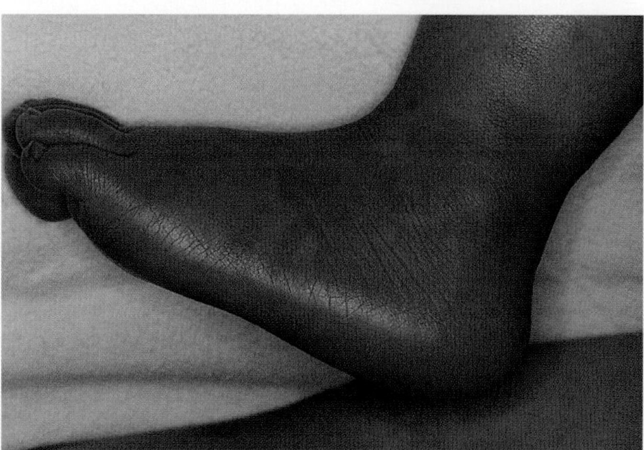

Fig. 147.2 Erythema and oedema of the foot.

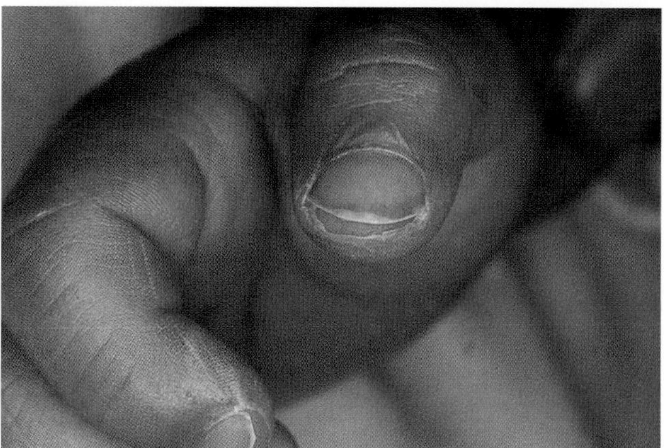

Fig. 147.3 Desquamation beginning at the fingertips.

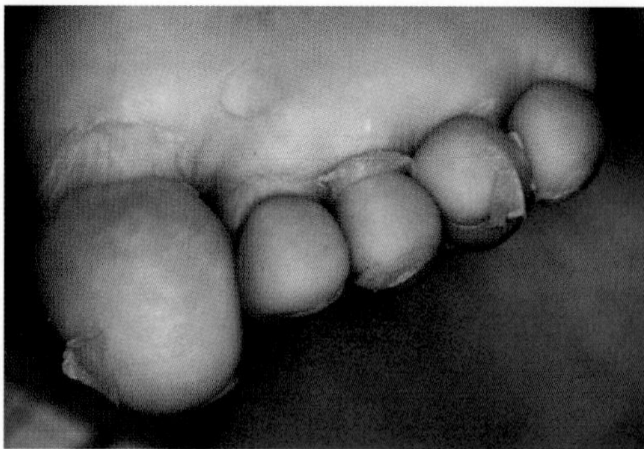

Fig. 147.4 Desquamation continues proximally, often in large thick pieces.

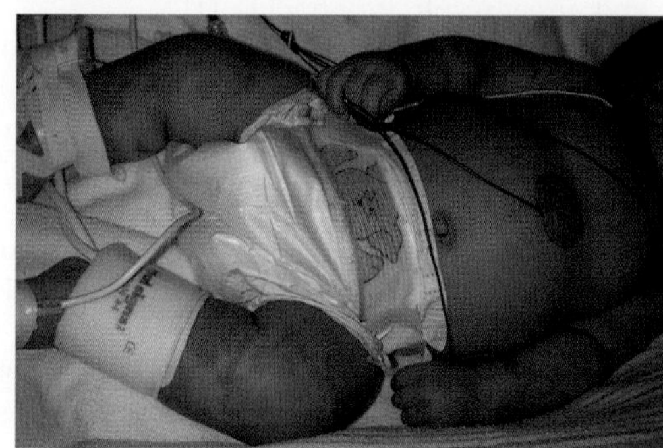

Fig. 147.5 The exanthem seen with KD is polymorphous and not specific to the disorder.

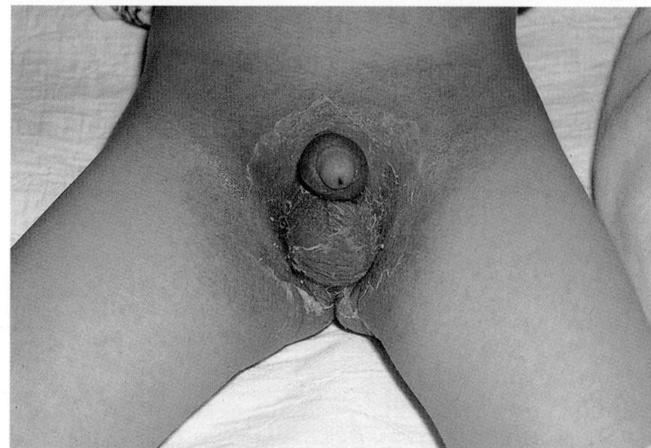

Fig. 147.6 Erythema, oedema, and desquamation at the groin and perineum.

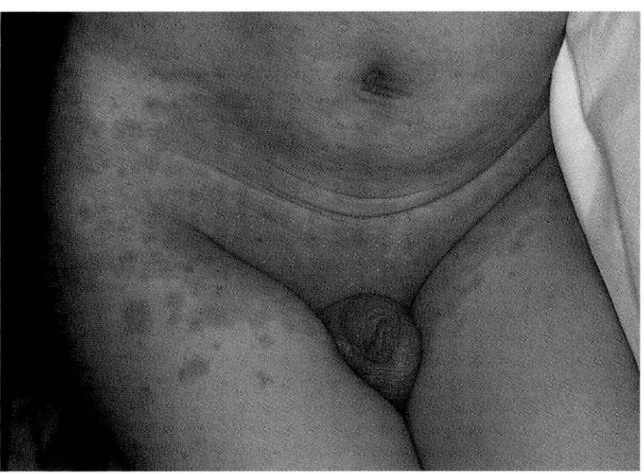

Fig. 147.7 Diffuse erythema with small pustules.

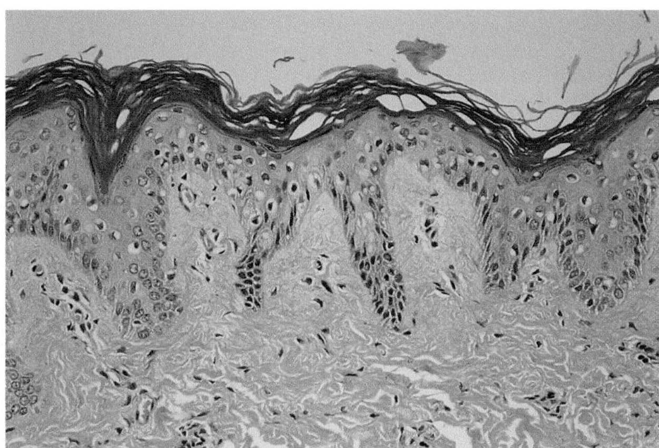

Fig. 147.8 Skin histology from an erythematous patch of the exanthem, showing a sparse perivascular mononuclear cell infiltrate in the papillary dermis.

desquamation may occur during the acute febrile phase and precedes the desquamation on the hands and feet. The more generalized eruption can be of many forms: an urticarial eruption with large erythematous plaques, a scarlatiniform or morbilliform rash, or in rare cases, erythema multiforme-like lesions with central clearing or targetoid lesions. Each lesion becomes increasingly large and often lesions coalesce. Vesicles or bullae are not seen; however, about 5% of patients show 0.5–1 mm, aseptic micropustules on the knees, buttocks or extensor surfaces (Fig. 147.7) [37]. Histologically, the lesions have nonspecific findings that include marked oedema of dermal papillae, focal intercellular oedema of the basal cell layer and very slight perivascular infiltration of mononuclear cells in the papillary dermis, with the dilation of small vessels (Fig. 147.8) [38]. Notably, small vessel vasculitis is not seen and skin biopsies are only useful in eliminating other diagnoses.

3. Bilateral conjunctival injection

Within 2–4 days of disease onset, injection of the ocular conjunctiva develops (Fig. 147.9). It is nonpurulent and often shows limbic sparing [39]. Each dilated capillary is clearly seen. Conjunctival biopsy reveals no inflammatory response so the term 'conjunctivitis' is not appropriate [40]. Careful slit-lamp examination early in the course of the disease may reveal anterior uveitis. The conjunctival injection usually subsides with IVIG treatment but sometimes continues for more than a few weeks. Anterior uveitis follows a similar course and has few sequelae in KD, unlike with many other inflammatory causes of uveitis [41].

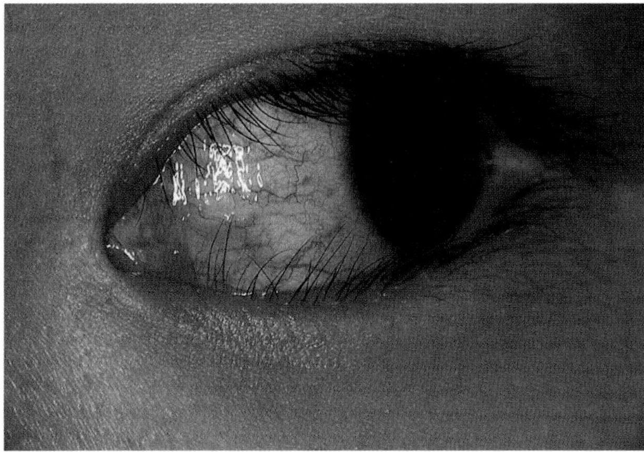

Fig. 147.9 Conjunctival injection in KD, which is nonexudative. Perilimbal sparing, signifying absence of oedema and inflammation in the conjunctiva, is apparent as a white halo around the iris.

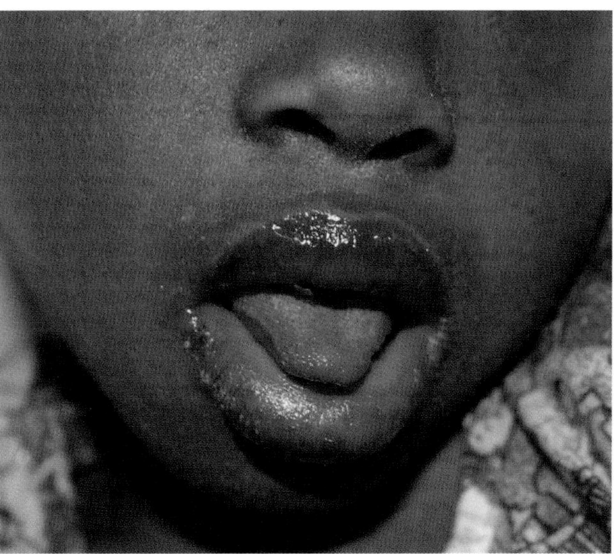

Fig. 147.10 Dryness, erosion and crusting of the mucosal lips.

4. Changes in lips and oral cavity

Changes in the lips and oral cavity are characterized by redness, dryness, fissuring, peeling and bleeding of the lips, diffuse erythema of the oropharyngeal mucosa and strawberry tongue without pseudomembrane formation (Figs 147.10 and 147.11). Aphthae and ulcerations of the oral mucosa are not seen. Redness of the lips may often continue for 2–3 weeks after the disappearance of other symptoms. Bilateral injection of the eyes together with the changes in the lips combine to give the characteristic appearance of KD and can be an important aid to diagnosis (Fig. 147.12).

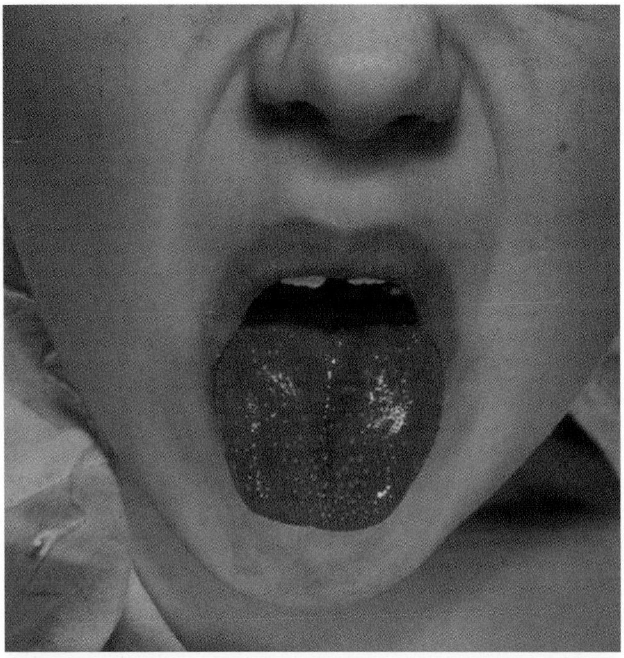

Fig. 147.11 Strawberry tongue with apparent fungiform papillae, but no pseudomembrane.

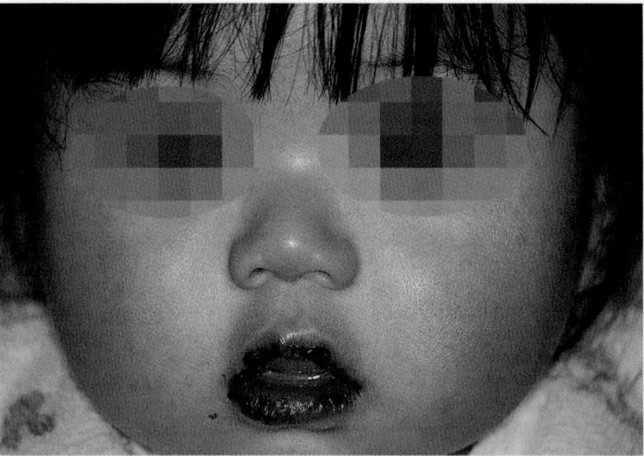

Fig. 147.12 Typical appearance of acute KD: redness, dryness and bleeding of the lips with bilateral conjunctival injection. Source: Courtesy of the Kawasaki Disease Foundation.

5. Acute nonpurulent cervical adenopathy

Approximately one-third of patients develop a single firm, nonfluctuant and painful mass, ranging from 1.5 to 5 cm in diameter (Fig. 147.13). Involvement occasionally may be bilateral and be misdiagnosed as mumps. In some older patients, a cervical lymph node mass with fever is the initial clinical presentation and may delay diagnosis because antibiotic treatment is given for presumed bacterial lymphadenitis. Imaging of the lymph node mass by ultrasound or computed tomography reveals a classic 'cluster of grapes' appearance in KD, in contrast to a predominant, large hypoechoic node in the case of bacterial infection [42]. Retropharyngeal phlegmon and oedema can also be associated with this presentation of KD. Hoarseness with swelling of the vocal folds has also been reported [43].

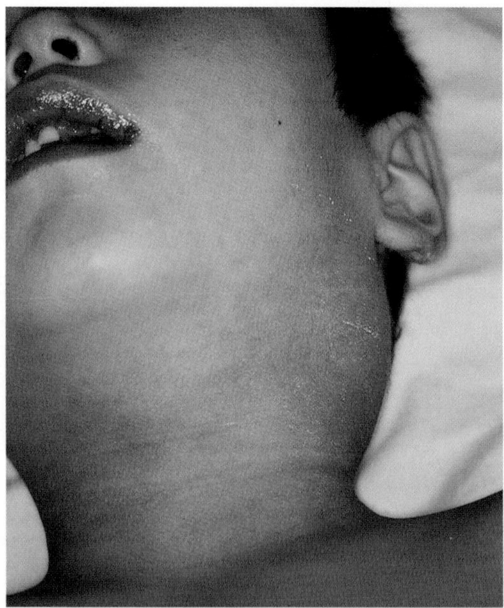

Fig. 147.13 Cervical lymph node mass with overlying erythema. Imaging of this mass would show a cluster of enlarged nodes.

In addition to these classic findings, the child with KD appears ill and is often very irritable, much more than with other febrile illnesses. About one-third, however, present with lethargy instead. Nuchal rigidity and aseptic meningitis can occur, with the CSF showing mild mixed cell pleocytosis but normal glucose and protein [44]. Less frequently, patients develop transient unilateral facial palsy or high-frequency sensorineural hearing loss [45,46]. Urethritis and sterile pyuria occur in 33–79% of patients [47]. Gastrointestinal findings include diarrhoea, vomiting and abdominal pain. In addition, hepatic enlargement, acute distension of the gallbladder, jaundice and transient elevation in the serum transaminases and γ-glutamyltranspeptidase may be seen [48,49]. Diffuse arthralgias that involve multiple small and large joints can occur early in the illness. Later, arthralgias and arthritis are more common in the large weight-bearing joints [50].

The clinical course of KD is generally divided into three phases. The acute phase lasts 7–14 days and is characterized by fever, the mucocutaneous changes and other acute signs of illness described previously. Coronary artery dilation or aneurysms and myocarditis may be apparent by echocardiography. In addition, a macrophage activation syndrome may rarely be evident [51]. The subacute phase (day 10–25) begins when fever and other acute signs have abated, but irritability, anorexia, arthralgias and conjunctival injection may persist. It is in this phase that desquamation and thrombocytosis occur. The risk of sudden death in those who have developed aneurysms is highest during this period. The convalescent phase begins around day 20 when all clinical signs of illness have disappeared and continues until the erythrocyte sedimentation rate (ESR) and C-reactive protein (CRP) return to normal, approximately 6–8 weeks after the onset of illness. In patients with previously normal echocardiograms, development of aneurysms does not occur after week 8 of the illness [33]. However, for those who do develop cardiovascular abnormalities, a fourth chronic phase of lifetime significance may be identified, where there is risk for complications extending into adulthood.

Other cutaneous findings

A unique feature of KD is acute inflammation at the site of prior bacillus Calmette–Guérin (BCG) vaccination. This may be localized erythema, peeling/crusting or even a bullous lesion that can become an ulcer [52–54]. The reaction may be secondary to crossreactivity between specific epitopes of mycobacterial and human heat shock proteins [53]. Studies from Taiwan suggest a significant association between reactivation of inflammation at the BCG vaccination site and a functional polymorphism in *ITPKC* gene that modulates T-cell activation [55,56].

The subacute and convalescent phases of KD may be complicated by the first episode of atopic dermatitis in patients with no previous history of this condition. Frequently, there is a family history of atopic dermatitis and/or personal history of other atopic conditions. It has been postulated that the intense activation of the immune system associated with acute KD precipitates the first appearance of this chronic skin condition in a genetically susceptible host [57,58].

Psoriasiform eruptions have been described in all three phases of KD [59,60]. This includes plaque, guttate and pustular lesions, with some being more crusted (Fig. 147.14) and others having finer scale than classic psoriasis. In one retrospective study of 476 children with KD, nine (1.9%) were affected, similar to the rate of psoriasis expected in the general adult population but higher than that in the general paediatric population [59]. Two of the children had a family history of psoriasis. A recent case-control study noted that diaper lesions were less prevalent among KD cases compared with psoriasis controls [60]. A more refractory case of KD showed psoriasiform papules and plaques on the extensor extremities along with crusted hyperkeratotic papules at the tips of the digits following treatment with IVIG, aspirin, methlyprednisolone and infliximab [61]. It is unclear if this may have any relationship to therapy or if the eruption could have been modulated given treatment with infliximab, a chimeric antibody also used to treat psoriasis. Also unclear is whether the co-occurrence of psoriasiform lesions and KD reflects activation of latent psoriasis in genetically predisposed individuals or a common aetiological agent for both KD and psoriasis. The psoriasiform eruption usually lasts several weeks to months and thus far, no cases associated with KD have been reported to become chronic psoriasis [59–62]. Having this eruption also does not appear to portend worse coronary outcomes [60].

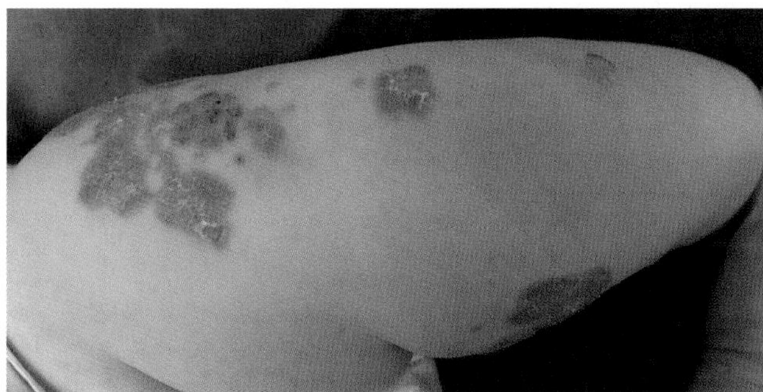

Fig. 147.14 Psoriasiform eruption that developed during the subacute phase.

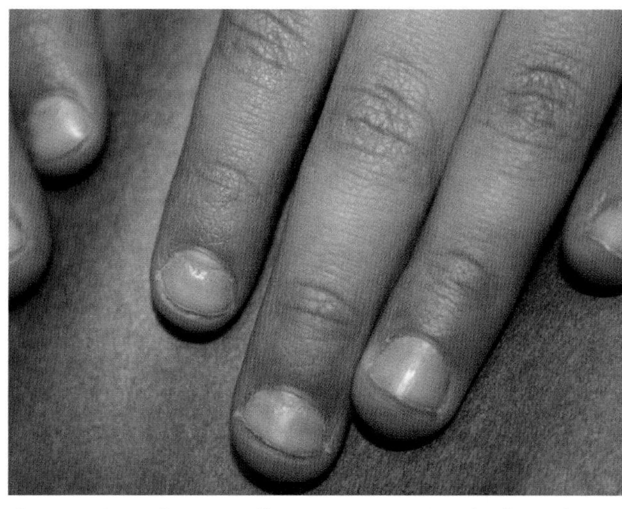

Fig. 147.15 Beau lines caused by temporary cessation of nail growth.

Rarely, Raynaud phenomenon leading to distal ischaemia and even gangrene of the fingers and toes may occur during the acute phase of the illness [63]. Nearly all cases have involved infants younger than 9 months of age and most had incomplete clinical criteria for KD [64–66]. Some case reports have documented the successful treatment of this complication with administration of prostaglandin E1, which suggests that the mechanism is vasospasm and not peripheral vasculitis [63,67].

Because of the prolonged high fever and systemic inflammation of KD, telogen effluvium can be noted weeks to months later. Beau lines (Fig. 147.15) and even shedding of the nails may also occur. In up to 10% of cases, recurrent peeling of the skin can occur for several years after KD, usually following minor upper respiratory tract infections [68].

Differential diagnosis. The differential diagnosis of KD includes scarlet fever, toxic shock syndrome, staphylococcal scalded skin syndrome, viral infections such as measles and adenovirus infection, Rocky Mountain spotted fever, drug eruptions, erythema multiforme and Stevens–Johnson syndrome. With the advent of PCR-based viral diagnostics, caution must be exercised not to reject the diagnosis of KD in the setting of a compatible clinical picture plus a positive PCR viral diagnosis, because infection with a variety of viruses may coexist with acute KD [69]. A KD-like syndrome has also been observed in adults infected with the human immunodeficiency virus [70,71]. Although the presentation of adenovirus infection can be quite similar to KD, it tends to have more prominent respiratory tract symptoms, a purulent conjunctivitis, and a rash without perineal accentuation [72]. The specific injury pattern on the tongue (strawberry tongue) is similar in scarlet fever and toxic shock syndrome, but occurs much less commonly in KD (about 50% of cases). Strawberry tongue is not seen in viral illnesses. Staphylococcal scalded skin syndrome shows radial crusting/furrowing periorally and a positive Nikolsky sign. Erythema multiforme and Stevens–Johnson syndrome have diffuse oral and/or labial erosions with haemorrhagic crusts.

Laboratory findings. There are no specific or diagnostic laboratory findings in KD, although values compatible with acute inflammation may support the diagnosis [33]. A moderate to marked leukocytosis (20 000–30 000 cells/mm^3) with a left shift, elevation of the ESR and positive CRP are common [13]. Thrombocytosis (greater than 450 000/mm^3) is noted in 50% of patients on presentation. The platelet count increases in virtually all patients in the subacute phase, peaking at about 3 weeks, but may persist for several months in some cases. A low platelet count may suggest low-grade intravascular consumption with depletion of the fibrinolytic system and an elevated D-dimer level. Sterile pyuria with mononuclear cells is frequently noted in the acute phase in KD and almost always disappears in the convalescent phase [47]. Other reported abnormalities include a normocytic, normochromic anaemia, mild to moderate elevations in serum transaminases, bilirubin, γ-glutamyl transpeptidase levels and hypoalbuminaemia. Hyponatraemia may occur in association with the development of inappropriate antidiuretic hormone secretion (SIADH) [73].

Incomplete cases. Patients with incomplete clinical signs, for whom the above diagnostic criteria are not met, may still develop coronary artery involvement and are often quite challenging for clinicians. About 15–20% of cases fall into this category [33]. Of the major criteria, cervical lymphadenopathy is the least common finding and occurs in only 30–50% of KD patients in the USA and 60–70% in Japan [74]. Those younger than 6 months of age or older than 5 years of age are more likely to have incomplete forms of KD and a higher rate of coronary artery aneurysms [75]. Newer data in infants younger than 6 months suggests that even with appropriate treatment administered within the first 10 days after fever onset, the rate of coronary artery aneurysms is greater than 20% [76].

In a patient with fever of unknown origin, a diagnosis of KD should always be considered. In such patients, especially infants and small children, fingertip desquamation, even in the absence of the other principal symptoms, is a strong indicator of KD [36]. Mild conjunctival injection may also be the only finding other than fever. Thus, prolonged fever in combination with any one of the principal symptoms should suggest KD and lead to prompt laboratory investigation, consideration for therapy and careful investigation by echocardiography for coronary complications. For those younger than 6 months of age, the AHA guidelines recommend echocardiography if there is fever of at least 7 days, laboratory evidence of systemic inflammation and no other explanation for the illness, even if no other clinical criteria are present [33].

Box 147.2 Summary of algorithm to aid early detection of incomplete Kawasaki disease (American Heart Association and American Academy of Pediatrics)

When fever plus two or three of the clinical criteria are present for 5 days or more, and patient characteristics suggest possible KD, a CRP and ESR should be obtained.

1. If CRP is <3 mg/dL and ESR is <40 mm/h, the patient may be followed daily and reassessed. If after the fever resolves, there is typical peeling at the distal fingers and toes, an echocardiogram should be performed.
2. If CRP is ≥3 mg/dL and/or ESR is ≥40 mm/h, supplemental laboratory studies should be performed, including albumin, complete blood cell count, alanine aminotransferase (ALT) and urinalysis (for pyuria).
   Abnormal findings include the following:
   Albumin <3 g/dL
   Anaemia for age
   Elevated ALT level
   Platelets >450 000/mm^3 after 7 days
   WBC count >15 000/mm^3
   Urinary white blood cell count of >10 cells per high-power field

a. If three or more supplemental laboratory criteria are met, a diagnosis of KD can be made. The child should have an echocardiogram and be treated.
b. If fewer than three supplemental laboratory criteria are present, cardiac echocardiogram should be performed. If negative but fever persists, a repeat echocardiogram may be performed. If the echocardiogram is negative and the fever abates, KD is unlikely. If the echocardiogram is positive, the child is treated for KD.

The AHA and American Academy of Pediatrics have published an algorithm to help in the early detection of incomplete KD (Box 147.2) [33]. It is based on expert consensus and uses commonly available laboratory tests and echocardiography, when indicated. Use is recommended in all children with unexplained fever for 5 or more days associated with two or three of the principal clinical features of KD. A multicentre, retrospective study on the use of this algorithm in 195 patients with KD and coronary artery aneurysms found that 190 (97%) would have received IVIG treatment at presentation and an additional two would have entered the algorithm and received IVIG at follow-up monitoring [77]. In a 2-year prospective study of German children under 5 years of age, 58% of the 64 incomplete KD cases were diagnosed based on echocardiographic findings and 42% based on laboratory criteria alone [78].

Cardiovascular and other complications. All children with suspected KD should undergo two-dimensional echocardiography to evaluate myocardial function and measure the internal diameter of the coronary arteries normalized for body surface area and expressed as standard deviations from the mean (Z scores) [33]. Follow up for patients with normal initial echocardiograms should include a repeat echocardiogram at 10–14 days after treatment [33].

Acute inflammation of medium-sized elastic arteries with a significant predilection for the coronary arteries is

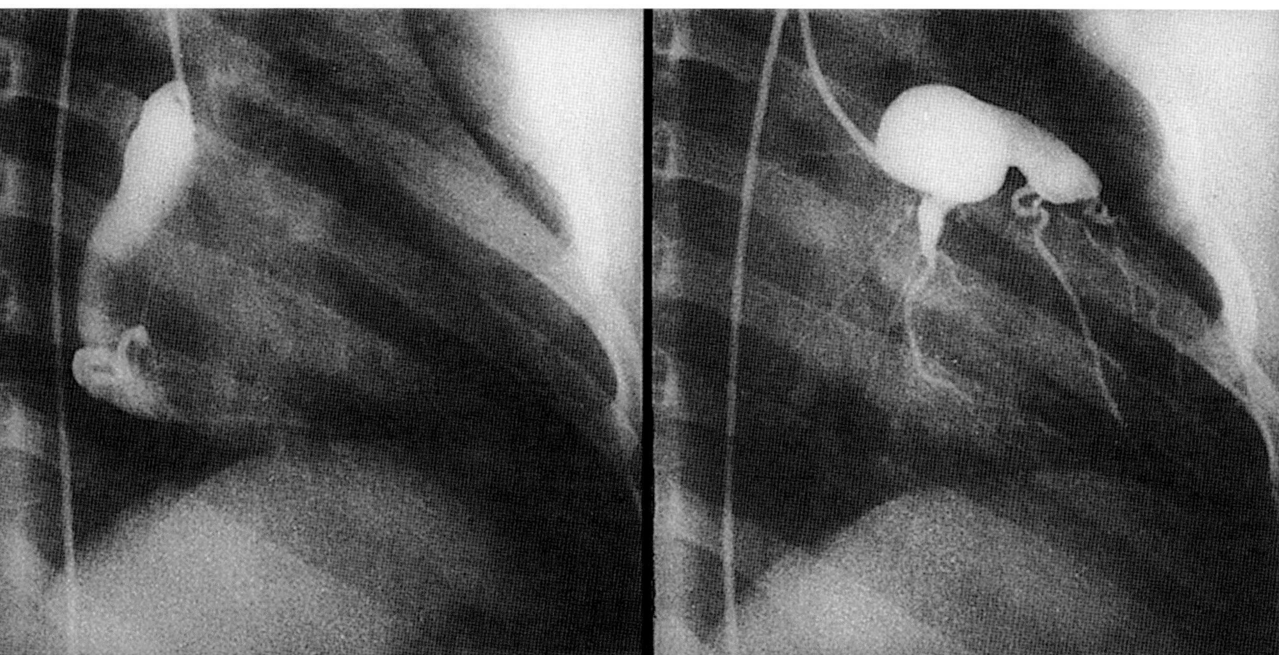

Fig. 147.16 Right and left giant coronary aneurysms.

the hallmark of KD. Coronary artery aneurysms may lead to myocardial infarction, arrhythmia or death. Risk factors for developing cardiac sequelae include male gender, age younger than 1 year or over 5 years, CRP greater than 100 mg/L, white blood count greater than 30 × 10^9/L, low platelet count, low serum albumin and sodium, and treatment after 6 days of illness [79–82].

Myocarditis can be associated with tachycardia in excess of the fever and occasionally is associated with reduced left ventricular ejection fraction. A KD shock syndrome related to inappropriate peripheral vascular resistance (warm shock), alone or in combination with decreased left ventricular contractility, was noted in 13 of 187 (7%) children with KD over a 4-year period [83]. Patients were more often female, had more severe laboratory markers of inflammation, and had impaired systolic and diastolic function. Diastolic dysfunction is common and aortic root dilation occurs in 15% of patients [84]. Electrocardiographic changes may include arrhythmia, prolonged PR interval or nonspecific ST- and T-wave changes. Rarely, there may be severe arrhythmia leading to cardiac arrest. Valvulitis with mitral and/or aortic regurgitation may also occur.

Coronary artery dilation by transthoracic echocardiography may be transient, with regression within the first 30 days after onset of KD. Progression to aneurysms occurs in 5–7% of patients despite treatment with IVIG within the first 10 days after fever onset [85,86]. Medium (5–8 mm internal diameter or Z score 5–9) and giant (>8 mm or Z score >10, see Fig. 147.16) aneurysms carry a high risk of thrombosis and need systemic anticoagulation [33,81]. Rarely, giant aneurysms may rupture within the first few months after KD, with fatal consequences.

Remodelling and fibrosis of affected coronary arteries can lead to stenosis, particularly with giant aneurysms.

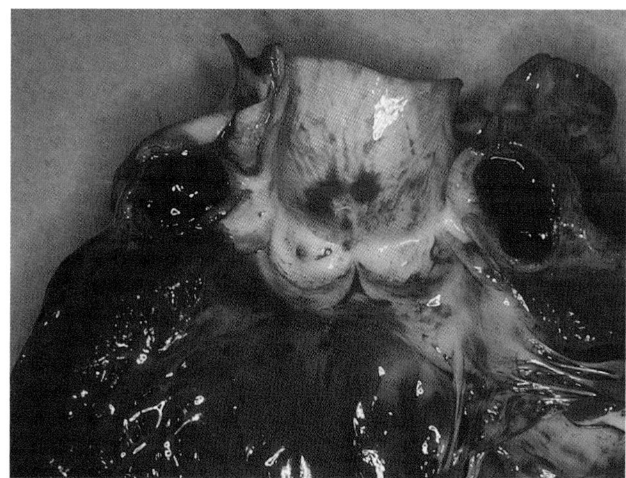

Fig. 147.17 Autopsy of the heart. Coronary artery aneurysms with thrombosis.

Stenoses often progress over time and lead to significant coronary obstruction and myocardial ischaemia. Myocardial infarction caused by thrombotic occlusion in an aneurysmal, stenotic coronary artery (Fig. 147.17) is the principal cause of death from KD and the highest risk of infarction is in the first year after onset of the disease. Over time, coronary occlusion in KD may be followed by the development of recanalized vessels and collateral flow [87]. Based on long-term studies from Japan, approximately 75% of patients who develop aneurysms during the acute phase will develop ischaemic symptoms and require cardiovascular interventions [88]. Inflammation of the coronary arteries is the most clinically significant aspect of the illness, but other medium-sized extraparenchymal arteries (e.g. brachial, iliac, mesenteric, abdominal aortic, etc.) can be involved [89].

Treatment and management. The management of KD is aimed at reducing systemic and cardiac/coronary inflammation to prevent aneurysm, thrombosis and myocardial infarction. All patients should be hospitalized during the acute febrile stage of illness. At present, the most effective treatment in the acute stage is IVIG (2g/kg) plus aspirin (30–80mg/kg/day divided every 6 hours). This combination has been shown to reduce fever and the rate of coronary lesion development to 3–5% [85]. Despite its demonstrated efficacy, the mechanism of action of IVIG is still under study. Current mechanisms include the stimulation and expansion of Fc-specific natural regulatory T cells and tolerogenic myeloid dendritic cells [17,90]. What is clear is a rapid and profound downregulation of inflammation, with improvement in clinical signs and cardiac contractility apparent within the first 12 hours after starting the infusion [91]. Aspirin has important anti-inflammatory effects at high doses and antiplatelet activity at low doses, but by itself it does not appear to decrease the frequency of development of coronary abnormalities [92].

Approximately 75–80% of patients treated with IVIG and aspirin respond promptly with defervescence within 36 hours of completing the IVIG infusion. However, 10–20% have persistent fever and inflammatory signs or only transient improvement and are termed IVIG-resistant [33,93]. Treatment for this group of patients differs between centres, with some administering a second infusion of IVIG and others treating with corticosteroids or infliximab, a chimeric mouse–human monoclonal antibody that binds soluble and membrane-bound TNF-α. A small, prospective pilot study found that treatment of IVIG-resistant patients with infliximab (5mg/kg) led to shorter fever duration, fewer days of hospitalization and a more rapid fall in inflammatory markers compared with patients treated with a second infusion of IVIG, but the study was not powered to see a difference in coronary artery Z scores [94]. A Phase III, randomized, double-blind, placebo-controlled trial studied the addition of infliximab to IVIG as a primary treatment for KD [95]. The use of infliximab did not reduce initial treatment resistance but did shorten fever duration, decreased the time to normalization of inflammatory markers (CRP, ESR), and was associated with a larger decrease in the Z score of the left anterior descending coronary artery. Additional studies are needed to clarify the role of TNF-α inhibition as adjunctive therapy for acute KD.

In contrast to other vasculitides, which usually respond to systemic corticosteroids, their benefit in KD is inconclusive. Two meta-analyses found benefit but there was great variability in the studies included [96,97]. A multicentre, randomized, double-blind, placebo-controlled trial of pulse steroids did not find this advantageous and this regimen has been largely abandoned in favour of the Japanese RAISE protocol that treats high risk patients with 4–6 weeks of oral methylprednisolone (2mg/kg/day) [98,99].

Cyclosporine A, a calcineurin inhibitor that targets the calcium/NFAT signalling pathway, has also been used for refractory disease. In a retrospective review of 19 patients given cyclosporine (4mg/kg/day) for 14 days, 14 of 19 patients became afebrile within 5 days [100]. Significantly lower serum inflammatory cytokines have been noted [100,101]. A randomized trial of the efficacy and safety of immunoglobulin plus cyclosporine in high risk KD patients based on a scoring system used in Japan (KAICA trial) has completed enrolment and is under analysis [102]. Methotrexate, cyclophosphamide and plasmapheresis are other agents used in some cases of refractory KD. Recently, great interest in the IL-1 signalling pathway has led to three international trials of IL-1 blockade with either anakinra (blocks both IL-1a and b) or canikinumab (Il-1b only) [103]. Interest in this approach was stimulated by the observation of high transcript levels for IL-1 pathway genes in the whole blood of acute KD patients [104].

Long-term management depends on the degree of cardiovascular risk based on coronary artery status [33]. Those with no coronary abnormalities at any time do not need aspirin or other antiplatelet medications beyond 2–3 months after the onset of disease. For patients with transient dilation resolved by 6–8 weeks, aspirin should be continued until the echocardiogram normalizes. If there are isolated small and medium aneurysms, low-dose aspirin should be continued at least until regression. Ibuprofen should be avoided in children with coronary aneurysms because it antagonizes the irreversible platelet inhibition that is induced by aspirin. For children who develop aneurysms with a Z score ≥10, systemic anticoagulation is recommended and the AHA guidelines should be followed [33].

Pharmacotherapy with antiplatelet agents, vasodilators, calcium channel blockers, β-blockers and/or angiotensin receptor blockers may be needed in those with ischaemic heart disease and myocardial infarction [81]. Catheter intervention with percutaneous transluminal rotational ablation, coronary angioplasty and stent implantation have all been used for the management of coronary stenosis caused by KD, with some patients requiring coronary artery bypass grafting [105]. Cardiac transplantation has been performed in a small number of patients with severe myocardial dysfunction, ventricular arrhythmias and coronary arterial lesions for which interventional catheterization or coronary artery bypass procedures were not feasible [106].

Prognosis. Early diagnosis and treatment are the key to good outcomes in KD. If diagnosis is delayed until 10 or more days after onset, treatment with IVIG and aspirin is still recommended if inflammatory markers are elevated, but the ability to prevent cardiovascular sequelae is less certain [33].

The only longitudinal angiographic study of KD to date was conducted in Japan prior to the institution of IVIG therapy [107]. Among 594 Japanese KD patients assessed 10–21 years later, 48% showed regression, 24% had persistent aneurysms without stenosis and 19% had stenosis in a coronary aneurysm. Eleven experienced myocardial infarction and there were five deaths. Those with giant aneurysms had the worst prognosis, with nearly all late deaths occurring in this subgroup. Other patient series have reported new dilated or expanding lesions in 3% of patients with coronary artery lesions from 2 to 19 years after disease onset, vascular calcifications becoming significant 5 or more years after the illness, and late-onset congestive heart failure in a subset of patients [105,108–110].

The mortality rate from KD has declined with the advent of IVIG therapy and most patients without coronary artery changes are considered to have good prognosis [82]. Prospective, longitudinal studies of the growing population of adults who had childhood KD are essential to assess the long-term outcomes.

References

1 Yim D, Curtis N, Cheung M et al. Update on Kawasaki disease: epidemiology, aetiology and pathogenesis. J Paediatr Child Health 2013;49:704–8.

2 Singh S, Vignesh P, Burgner D. The epidemiology of Kawasaki disease: a global update. Arch Dis Child 2015;100:1084–8.

3 Makino N, Nakamura Y, Yashiro M et al. Descriptive epidemiology of Kawasaki disease in Japan, 2011–2012: from the results of the 22nd nationwide survey. J Epidemiol 2015;25:239–45.

4 Ha S, Seo GH, Kim KY et al. Epidemiologic study on Kawasaki disease in Korea, 2007–2014: based on health insurance review and assessment service claims. J Korean Med Sci 2016;31:1445–9.

5 Lin MC, Lai MS, Jan SL et al. Epidemiologic features of Kawasaki disease in acute stages in Taiwan, 1997–2010: effect of different case definitions in claims data analysis. J Chin Med Assoc 2015;78:121–6.

6 Callinan LS, Holman RC, Vugia DJ et al. Kawasaki disease hospitalization rate among children younger than 5 years in California, 2003–2010. Pediatr Infect Dis J 2014;33:781–3.

7 Burns JC, Herzog L, Fabri O et al. Seasonality of Kawasaki disease: a global perspective. PLoS One 2013;8:e74529.

8 Uehara R, Belay ED. Epidemiology of Kawasaki disease in Asia, Europe, and the United States. J Epidemiol 2012;22:79–85.

9 Kushner HI, Bastian JF, Turner CL et al. The two emergencies of Kawasaki syndrome and the implications for the developing world. Pediatr Infect Dis J 2008;27:377–83.

10 Maddox RA, Holman RC, Uehara R et al. Recurrent Kawasaki disease: USA and Japan. Pediatr Int 2015;57:1116–20.

11 Shulman ST, Rowley AH. Kawasaki disease: insights into pathogenesis and approaches to treatment. Nat Rev Rheumatol 2015;11:475–82.

12 Brown TJ, Crawford SE, Cornwall ML et al. CD8 T lymphocytes and macrophages infiltrate coronary artery aneurysms in acute Kawasaki disease. J Infect Dis 2001; 184:940–3.

13 Tremoulet AH, Jain S, Chandrasekar D et al. Evolution of laboratory values in patients with Kawasaki disease. Pediatr Infect Dis J 2011;30:1022–6.

14 Orenstein JM, Shulman ST, Fox LM et al. Three linked vasculopathic processes characterize Kawasaki disease: a light and transmission electron microscopic study. PLoS One 2012;7:e38998.

15 Shimizu C, Sood A, Lau HD et al. Cardiovascular pathology in 2 young adults with sudden, unexpected death due to coronary aneurysms from Kawasaki disease in childhood. Cardiovasc Pathol 2015;24:310–6.

16 Yonesaka S, Nakada T, Sunagawa Y et al. Endomyocardial biopsy in children with Kawasaki disease. Acta Paediatr Jpn 1989;31:706–11.

17 Burns JC, Song Y, Bujold M et al. Immune-monitoring in Kawasaki disease patients treated with infliximab and intravenous immunoglobulin. Clin Exp Immunol 2013;174:337–44.

18 Uehara R, Yashiro M, Nakamura Y et al. Kawasaki disease in parents and children. Acta Paediatr 2003;92:694–7.

19 Onouchi Y. Genetics of Kawasaki disease: what we know and don't know. Circ J 2012;76:1581–6.

20 Shimizu C, Jain S, Davila S et al. Transforming growth factor-beta signaling pathway in patients with Kawasaki disease. Circ Cardiovasc Genet 2011;4:16–25.

21 Shimizu C, Oharaseki T, Takahashi K et al. The role of TGF-beta and myofibroblasts in the arteritis of Kawasaki disease. Hum Pathol 2013;44:189–98.

22 Onouchi Y, Fukazawa R, Yamamura K et al. Variations in ORAI1 gene associated with Kawasaki Disease. PLoS One 2016;11:e0145486.

23 Shimizu C, Eleftherohorinou H, Wright VJ et al. Genetic variation in the SLC8A1 calcium signaling pathway is associated with susceptibility to Kawasaki disease and coronary artery abnormalities. Circ Cardiovasc Genet 2016;9:559–68.

24 Alphonse MP, Duong TT, Shumitzu C et al. Inositol-triphosphate 3-kinase C mediates inflammasome activation and treatment response in Kawasaki disease. J Immunol 2016;197:3481–9.

25 Kim KY, Kim DS. Recent advances in Kawasaki disease. Yonsei Med J 2016;57:15–21.

26 Burgner D, Davila S, Breunis WB et al. A genome-wide association study identifies novel and functionally related susceptibility Loci for Kawasaki disease. PLoS Genet 2009;5:e1000319.

27 Kim J, Shimizu C, Kingsmore SF et al. Whole genome sequencing of an African American family highlights toll like receptor 6 variants in Kawasaki disease susceptibility. PLoS One 2017;12:e0170977.

28 Leung DY, Meissner HC, Shulman ST et al. Prevalence of superantigen-secreting bacteria in patients with Kawasaki disease. J Pediatr 2002;140:742–6.

29 Rowley AH, Shulman ST. New developments in the search for the etiologic agent of Kawasaki disease. Curr Opin Pediatr 2007;19:71–4.

30 Matsubara K, Fukaya T. The role of superantigens of group A Streptococcus and Staphylococcus aureus in Kawasaki disease. Curr Opin Infect Dis 2007;20:298–303.

31 Rowley AH, Baker SC, Orenstein JM et al. Searching for the cause of Kawasaki disease--cytoplasmic inclusion bodies provide new insight. Nat Rev Microbiol 2008;6:394–401.

32 Rodo X, Curcoll R, Robinson M et al. Tropospheric winds from northeastern China carry the etiologic agent of Kawasaki disease from its source to Japan. Proc Natl Acad Sci U S A 2014;111: 7952–7.

33 Newburger JW, Takahashi M, Gerber MA et al. Diagnosis, treatment, and long-term management of Kawasaki disease: a statement for health professionals from the Committee on Rheumatic Fever, Endocarditis, and Kawasaki Disease, Council on Cardiovascular Disease in the Young, American Heart Association. Pediatrics 2004;114:1708–33.

34 Durongpisitkul K, Gururaj VJ, Park JM et al. The prevention of coronary artery aneurysm in Kawasaki disease: a meta-analysis on the efficacy of aspirin and immunoglobulin treatment. Pediatrics 1995;96:1057–61.

35 Yun SH, Yang NR, Park SA. Associated symptoms of kawasaki disease. Korean Circ J 2011;41:394–8.

36 Wang S, Best BM, Burns JC. Periungual desquamation in patients with Kawasaki disease. Pediatr Infect Dis J 2009;28:538–9.

37 Kimura T, Miyazawa H, Watanabe K et al. Small pustules in Kawasaki disease. A clinicopathological study of four patients. Am J Dermatopathol 1988;10:218–23.

38 Sugawara T. [Immunopathology of skin lesions in Kawasaki disease]. Arerugi 1991;40:476–82.

39 Smith LB, Newburger JW, Burns JC. Kawasaki syndrome and the eye. Pediatr Infect Dis J 1989;8:116–8.

40 Burns JC, Wright JD, Newburger JW et al. Conjunctival biopsy in patients with Kawasaki disease. Pediatr Pathol Lab Med 1995;15:547–53.

41 Burns JC, Joffe L, Sargent RA et al. Anterior uveitis associated with Kawasaki syndrome. Pediatr Infect Dis 1985;4:258–61.

42 Kanegaye JT, Van Cott E, Tremoulet AH et al. Lymph-node-first presentation of Kawasaki disease compared with bacterial cervical adenitis and typical Kawasaki disease. J Pediatr 2013;162:1259–63.

43 Leuin SC, Shanbhag S, Lago D et al. Hoarseness as a presenting sign in children with Kawasaki disease. Pediatr Infect Dis J 2013;32:1392–4.

44 Dengler LD, Capparelli EV, Bastian JF et al. Cerebrospinal fluid profile in patients with acute Kawasaki disease. Pediatr Infect Dis J 1998;17:478–81.

45 Knott PD, Orloff LA, Harris JP et al. Sensorineural hearing loss and Kawasaki disease: a prospective study. Am J Otolaryngol 2001;22:343–8.

46 Terasawa K, Ichinose E, Matsuishi T et al. Neurological complications in Kawasaki disease. Brain Dev 1983;5:371–4.

47 Shike H, Kanegaye JT, Best BM et al. Pyuria associated with acute Kawasaki disease and fever from other causes. Pediatr Infect Dis J 2009;28:440–3.

48 Eladawy M, Dominguez SR, Anderson MS et al. Abnormal liver panel in acute kawasaki disease. Pediatr Infect Dis J 2011;30:141–4.

49 Baker AL, Lu M, Minich LL et al. Associated symptoms in the ten days before diagnosis of Kawasaki disease. J Pediatr 2009;154:592–5.

50 Hicks RV, Melish ME. Kawasaki syndrome. Pediatr Clin North Am 1986;33:1151–75.

51 Palazzi DL, McClain KL, Kaplan SL. Hemophagocytic syndrome after Kawasaki disease. Pediatr Infect Dis J 2003;22:663–6.

52 Antony D, Jessy PL. Involvement of BCG scar in Kawasaki disease. Indian Pediatr 2005;42:83–4.

53 Chalmers D, Corban JG, Moore PP. BCG site inflammation: a useful diagnostic sign in incomplete Kawasaki disease. J Paediatr Child Health 2008;44:525–6.

54 Kuniyuki S, Asada M. An ulcerated lesion at the BCG vaccination site during the course of Kawasaki disease. J Am Acad Dermatol 1997;37:303–4.

55 Lin MT, Wang JK, Yeh JI et al. Clinical implication of the C Allele of the ITPKC Gene SNP rs28493229 in Kawasaki disease: association with disease susceptibility and BCG scar reactivation. Pediatr Infect Dis J 2011;30:148–52.

56 Onouchi Y, Gunji T, Burns JC et al. ITPKC functional polymorphism associated with Kawasaki disease susceptibility and formation of coronary artery aneurysms. Nat Genet 2008;40:35–42.

57 Brosius CL, Newburger JW, Burns JC et al. Increased prevalence of atopic dermatitis in Kawasaki disease. Pediatr Infect Dis J 1988;7:863–6.

58 Burns JC, Shimizu C, Shike H et al. Family-based association analysis implicates IL-4 in susceptibility to Kawasaki disease. Genes Immun 2005;6:438–44.

59 Eberhard BA, Sundel RP, Newburger JW et al. Psoriatic eruption in Kawasaki disease. J Pediatr 2000;137:578–80.

60 Haddock ES, Calame A, Shimizu C et al. Psoriasiform eruptions during Kawasaki disease (KD): a distinct phenotype. J Am Acad Dermatol 2016;75:69–76.

61 Kishimoto S, Muneuchi J, Takahashi Y et al. Psoriasiform skin lesion and supprative acrodermatitis associated with Kawasaki disease followed by the treatment with infliximab: a case report. Acta Paediatr 2010;99:1102–4.

62 Liao YC, Lee JY. Psoriasis in a 3-month-old infant with Kawasaki disease. Dermatol Online J 2009;15:10.

63 Dogan OF, Kara A, Devrim I et al. Peripheral gangrene associated with Kawasaki disease and successful management using prostacycline analogue: a case report. Heart Surg Forum 2007;10:E70–2.

64 Durall AL, Phillips JR, Weisse ME et al. Infantile Kawasaki disease and peripheral gangrene. J Pediatr 2006;149:131–3.

65 Kim NY, Choi DY, Jung MJ et al. A case of refractory Kawasaki disease complicated by peripheral ischemia. Pediatr Cardiol 2008;29:1110–4.

66 Chang JS, Lin JS, Peng CT et al. Kawasaki disease complicated by peripheral gangrene. Pediatr Cardiol 1999;20:139–42.

67 Westphalen MA, McGrath MA, Kelly W et al. Kawasaki disease with severe peripheral ischemia: treatment with prostaglandin E1 infusion. J Pediatr 1988;112:431–3.

68 Michie C, Kinsler V, Tulloh R et al. Recurrent skin peeling following Kawasaki disease. Arch Dis Child 2000;83:353–5.

69 Song E, Kajon AE, Wang H et al. Clinical and virologic characteristics may aid distinction of acute adenovirus disease from Kawasaki disease with incidental adenovirus detection. J Pediatr 2016;170:325–30.

70 Stankovic K, Miailhes P, Bessis D et al. Kawasaki-like syndromes in HIV-infected adults. J Infect 2007;55:488–94.

71 Blanchard JN, Powell HC, Freeman WR et al. Recurrent Kawasaki disease-like syndrome in a patient with acquired immunodeficiency syndrome. Clin Infect Dis 2003;36:105–11.

72 Barone SR, Pontrelli LR, Krilov LR. The differentiation of classic Kawasaki disease, atypical Kawasaki disease, and acute adenoviral infection: use of clinical features and a rapid direct fluorescent antigen test. Arch Pediatr Adolesc Med 2000; 154:453–6.

73 Shin JI, Kim JH, Lee JS et al. Kawasaki disease and hyponatremia. Pediatr Nephrol 2006;21:1490–1; author reply 1492.

74 Rowley AH. Incomplete (atypical) Kawasaki disease. Pediatr Infect Dis J 2002; 21:563–5.

75 Burns JC, Wiggins JW Jr, Toews WH et al. Clinical spectrum of Kawasaki disease in infants younger than 6 months of age. J Pediatr 1986;109:759–63.

76 Salgado A, Ashouri N, Berry K et al. High risk of coronary artery aneurysms in infants younger than 6 months with Kawasaki disease despite timely treatment. J Pediatr 2017;185:112–16.

77 Yellen ES, Gauvreau K, Takahashi M et al. Performance of 2004 American Heart Association recommendations for treatment of Kawasaki disease. Pediatrics 2010; 125:e234–41.

78 Jakob A, Whelan J, Kordecki M et al. Kawasaki disease in Germany: a prospective, population-based study adjusted for underreporting. Pediatr Infect Dis J 2016;35:129–34.

79 Honkanen VE, McCrindle BW, Laxer RM et al. Clinical relevance of the risk factors for coronary artery inflammation in Kawasaki disease. Pediatr Cardiol 2003; 24:122–6.

80 Nakamura Y, Yashiro M, Uehara R et al. Use of laboratory data to identify risk factors of giant coronary aneurysms due to Kawasaki disease. Pediatr Int 2004; 46:33–8.

81 Guidelines for diagnosis and management of cardiovascular sequelae in Kawasaki disease (JCS 2013). Digest version. Circ J 2014;78:2521–62.

82 Newburger JW, Takahashi M, Burns JC. Kawasaki Disease. J Am Coll Cardiol 2016;67:1738–49.

83 Kanegaye JT, Wilder MS, Molkara D et al. Recognition of a Kawasaki disease shock syndrome. Pediatrics 2009;123:e783–9.

84 Ravekes WJ, Colan SD, Gauvreau K et al. Aortic root dilation in Kawasaki disease. Am J Cardiol 2001;87:919–22.

85 Newburger JW, Takahashi M, Beiser AS et al. A single intravenous infusion of gamma globulin as compared with four infusions in the treatment of acute Kawasaki syndrome. N Engl J Med 1991;324:1633–9.

86 Ogata S, Tremoulet AH, Sato Y et al. Coronary artery outcomes among children with Kawasaki disease in the United States and Japan. Int J Cardiol 2013;168:3825–8.

87 Senzaki H. Long-term outcome of Kawasaki disease. Circulation 2008;118:2763–72.

88 Tsuda E, Hamaoka K, Suzuki H et al. A survey of the 3-decade outcome for patients with giant aneurysms caused by Kawasaki disease. Am Heart J 2014;167:249–58.

89 Hoshino S, Tsuda E, Yamada O, Characteristics and fate of systemic artery aneurysm after Kawasaki Disease. J Pediatr 2015;167: 108–12.

90 Burns JC, Touma R, Song Y et al. Fine specificities of natural regulatory T cells after IVIG therapy in patients with Kawasaki disease. Autoimmunity 2015;48:181–8.

91 Newburger JW, Sanders SP, Burns JC et al. Left ventricular contractility and function in Kawasaki syndrome. Effect of intravenous gamma-globulin. Circulation 1989;79:1237–46.

92 Terai M, Shulman ST. Prevalence of coronary artery abnormalities in Kawasaki disease is highly dependent on gamma globulin dose but independent of salicylate dose. J Pediatr 1997;131:888–93.

93 Tremoulet AH, Best BM, Song S et al. Resistance to intravenous immunoglobulin in children with Kawasaki disease. J Pediatr 2008;153:117–21.

94 Youn Y, Kim J, Hong YM et al. Infliximab as the first retreatment in patients with Kawasaki disease resistant to initial intravenous immunoglobulin. Pediatr Infect Dis J 2016;35:457–9.

95 Tremoulet AH, Jain S, Jaggi P et al. Infliximab for intensification of primary therapy for Kawasaki disease: a phase 3 randomised, double-blind, placebo-controlled trial. Lancet 2014;383(9930):1731–8.

96 Athappan G, Gale S, Ponniah T. Corticosteroid therapy for primary treatment of Kawasaki disease – weight of evidence: a meta-analysis and systematic review of the literature. Cardiovasc J Afr 2009;20: 233–6.

97 Wardle AJ, Connolly GM, Seager MJ et al. Corticosteroids for the treatment of Kawasaki disease in children. Cochrane Database Syst Rev 2017 Jan 27;1:CD011188.

98 Newburger JW, Sleeper LA, McCrindle BW et al. Randomized trial of pulsed corticosteroid therapy for primary treatment of Kawasaki disease. N Engl J Med 2007;356:663–75.

99 Kobayashi T, Saji T, Otani T et al. Efficacy of immunoglobulin plus prednisolone for prevention of coronary artery abnormalities in severe Kawasaki disease (RAISE study): a randomised, open-label, blinded-endpoints trial. Lancet 2012:379(9826):1613–20.

100 Hamada H, Suzuki H, Abe J et al. Inflammatory cytokine profiles during Cyclosporin treatment for immunoglobulin-resistant Kawasaki disease. Cytokine, 2012;60:681–5.

101 Tremoulet AH, Pancoast P, Franco A et al. Calcineurin inhibitor treatment of intravenous immunoglobulin-resistant Kawasaki disease. J Pediatr 2012;161:506–512.

102 Aoyagi R, Hamada H, Sato Y et al. Study protocol for a phase III multicentre, randomised, open-label, blinded-end point trial to evaluate the efficacy and safety of immunoglobulin plus cyclosporin A in patients with severe Kawasaki disease (KAICA Trial). BMJ Open 2015;5:e009562.

103 Burns JC, Kone-Paut I, Kuijpers T et al. Found in translation: international initiatives pursuing interleukin-1 blockade for treatment of acute Kawasaki Disease. Arthritis Rheumatol 2016;69:268–76.

104 Hoang LT, Shimizu C, Ling L et al. Global gene expression profiling identifies new therapeutic targets in acute Kawasaki disease. Genome Med 2014;6:541.

105 Gordon JB, Daniels LB, Kahn AM et al. The spectrum of cardiovascular lesions requiring intervention in adults after Kawasaki disease. JACC Cardiovasc Interv 2016;9:687–96.

106 Checchia PA, Pahl E, Shaddy RE et al. Cardiac transplantation for Kawasaki disease. Pediatrics 1997;100:695–9.

107 Kato H, Sugimura T, Akagi T et al. Long-term consequences of Kawasaki disease. A 10- to 21-year follow-up study of 594 patients. Circulation 1996;94:1379–85.

108 Arnold R, Goebel B, Ulmer HE et al. An exercise tissue Doppler and strain rate imaging study of diastolic myocardial dysfunction after Kawasaki syndrome in childhood. Cardiol Young 2007;17:478–86.

109 Tsuda E, Kamiya T, Ono Y et al. Dilated coronary arterial lesions in the late period after Kawasaki disease. Heart, 2005;91:177–82.

110 Kahn AM, Budoff MJ, Daniels LB et al. Usefulness of calcium scoring as a screening examination in patients with a history of Kawasaki disease. Am J Cardiol 2017;119:967–71.

CHAPTER 148

Polyarteritis Nodosa, Granulomatosis with Polyangiitis and Microscopic Polyangiitis

Paul A. Brogan

University College London, Institute of Child Health and Great Ormond Street Hospital NHS Foundation Trust, London, UK

Polyarteritis nodosa, 1918
Granulomatosis with polyangiitis (formerly Wegener granulomatosis), 1924
Microscopic polyangiitis, 1931

Abstract

Primary systemic vasculitides of the young are relatively rare diseases, but are associated with significant morbidity and mortality, particularly if there is diagnostic delay. This chapter provides an overview of polyarteritis nodosa (PAN), and two of the more commonly encountered antineutrophil cytoplasmic antibodies-associated vasculitides: granulomatosis with polyangiitis (GPA, formerly Wegener granulomatosis) and microscopic polyangiitis (MPA, formerly microscopic polyarteritis). Significant advances in the field of vasculitis research include the development of classification criteria for PAN and GPA in children, recent discovery of the contribution of genetic mutations causing monogenic forms of PAN and a growing evidence base for treatment, albeit mainly in trials involving adults, but with considerable relevance to paediatric practice.

Key points

- **Polyarteritis nodosa (PAN) is a rare medium vessel vasculitis affecting children and adults.**
- **Recently, recessive mutations in *ADA2* have been shown to cause a monogenic form of PAN, caused by deficiency of adenosine deaminase type 2, with important diagnostic and therapeutic implications.**
- **There has never been a randomized controlled trial of treatment for children with PAN, an important unmet need.**
- **Granulomatosis with polyangiitis and microscopic polyangiitis are two of the more commonly encountered antineutrophil cytoplasmic antibodies-associated vasculitides (AAV).**
- **The pathogenesis of AAV is beginning to be unravelled, with important genetic contributions now described in the context of genome-wide association studies, and a better understanding of the role of aberrant innate and adaptive immunity including neutrophils, the alternative complement pathway, B lymphocyte and T lymphocyte dysregulation.**
- **There is a growing evidence base from adult trials for the treatment of AAV, with important implications for paediatric practice.**

Polyarteritis nodosa

Introduction and history. Classic (macroscopic) polyarteritis nodosa (PAN) predominantly affects medium-sized arteries, and should be differentiated from the small vessel antineutrophil cytoplasmic antibodies (ANCA)-associated vasculitis microscopic polyangiitis (MPA), which is now classified separately from PAN but was historically referred to as 'microscopic PAN'. Thus, for the purposes of this chapter, MPA and PAN will be described separately.

PAN was first described in 1866 by Kussmaul and Maier in the autopsy of a 27-year-old man who had proteinuria, myalgia, neuritis and abdominal pain. It is a disease predominantly of small- and medium-sized muscular arteries with aneurysmal dilation, especially at arterial branching points. Although it is rare, PAN does occur in childhood [1–4]. PAN may present as multisystem disease, but there is also a group of patients in whom the cutaneous manifestations predominate and in whom the prognosis is considerably better [5–7].

Epidemiology and classification criteria. In adults from Europe and the USA, the estimated annual incidence of PAN is 2–9/million [8]. Although comparatively rare in childhood, it is the most common form of systemic vasculitis after Henoch–Schönlein purpura and Kawasaki disease [9]. However, the epidemiological data are difficult to interpret because the incidence in various reports differs widely dependent on which criteria are used to classify patients into the PAN category. New criteria for the classification of PAN in children have recently been described (Box 148.1) [10], which may facilitate more accurate epidemiological studies in the future. Sensitivity

Harper's Textbook of Pediatric Dermatology, Fourth Edition. Edited by Peter Hoeger, Veronica Kinsler and Albert Yan.

Box 148.1 Criteria for the classification of polyarteritis nodosa in children [10]

Histopathological evidence of necrotizing vasculitis in medium or small arteries or angiographic abnormality (aneurysm, stenosis or occlusion) as a mandatory criterion plus one of the following five:

- skin involvement (see later)
- myalgia or muscle tenderness
- hypertension
- peripheral neuropathy
- renal involvement

and specificity of these new criteria were 73% and 100% respectively [10]. It should be noted, however, that recent genetic advances have led to the discovery of an important monogenic form of polyarteritis nodosa called deficiency of adenosine deaminase type 2 (DADA2; see below). Thus, some patients who were previously considered as having PAN are now known to have this monogenic disease, making the diagnosis of true PAN even rarer and casting some doubt on the validity of historical epidemiological paediatric data for this very rare disease. In adults, the majority of cases present between the ages of 25 and 50 years; the peak age of onset in children is 9–10 years of age [2,4]. In children, males and females are equally affected; however, PAN in adults occurs more commonly in males [2,4,11].

Pathogenesis. Genetic predisposing factors may make individuals vulnerable to develop PAN [12]. An association of childhood PAN with mutations in the familial Mediterranean fever (*MEFV*) gene has been shown in Turkish children [13]. This suggests that at least in certain populations where *MEFV* mutations are frequent, these mutations may be acting as one of the susceptibility factors for PAN [13]. Mutations in the *ADA2* (formerly *CECR1*) gene encoding adenosine deaminase 2 (ADA2), have been recently described in two reports of patients with symptoms suggestive of PAN and whose disease met all existing classification criteria for PAN, thus defining the rare entity of monogenic PAN [13–15]. Positive family history, livedo racemosa and haemorrhagic stroke were common in this form of the disease [13–15]. Although data are currently limited, ADA2 deficiency almost certainly accounts for the vast minority of patients with PAN [16]. Another recently described autoinflammatory disease with distinct vascular and pulmonary involvement resembling polyarteritis nodosa is caused by mutations in the gene *TMEM173*, encoding stimulator of interferon genes protein (STING), a major regulator of interferon signalling and is referred to as STING-associated vasculopathy with onset in infancy (SAVI) [17,18].

Regarding environmental triggers, the association with a previous streptococcal infection is well documented, particularly in those with cutaneous involvement [6,19,20]. The association between PAN and hepatitis B is well recognized in adults but is uncommon in children. Other infectious links include parvovirus B19 and cytomegalovirus in PAN patients compared with control populations [21,22]. HIV has also been implicated [23], and PAN-like illnesses in adults have additionally been reported in association with cancers and haematological malignancies [24], although this association is rare in children. An immune complex mechanism has been suggested and the finding of immune complexes persisting throughout months of active disease is consistent with this. In terms of pathogenetic mechanisms, it seems likely that the immunological processes involved are similar to those in other systemic vasculitides and include immune complexes, complement, possibly autoantibodies, cell adhesion molecules, cytokines, growth factors, chemokines, neutrophils and T cells [9].

There is some evidence that autoantibodies to vascular endothelial cells may be involved, again implicating an immunopathogenetic mechanism in vasculitis [25]. There has been evidence to support the role of superantigens in PAN with alterations in the T-cell Vβ repertoire in children with primary vasculitis [26].

Clinical features. Nonspecific constitutional manifestations such as malaise, fever, weight loss and musculoskeletal features such as arthralgia and myalgia as well as skin manifestations are common presenting features [2,4]. In children, various systems are involved in PAN with the skin, the musculoskeletal system, the kidneys and the gastrointestinal tract most prominently affected; cardiac, neurological and respiratory manifestations occur less frequently [2,4]. In the largest multicentre series describing 110 children with PAN (63 had systemic PAN) cutaneous lesions developed in 92 and 71.4% had myalgia [4]. Hypertension was described in 43 and 11.1% had impaired renal function during disease course [4]. One-third of patients had central nervous system (CNS) involvement [4]. Cardiac and pulmonary involvement was reported in 14 and 11%, respectively [4]. In a systematic retrospective study of 348 adult patients with PAN, the most frequent findings were general symptoms (93.1%) such as fever (63.8%), weight loss (69.5%), myalgia (58.6%) and arthralgia (48.9%), neurological manifestations (79%), urological and renal manifestations (50.6%), skin involvement (49.7%) and gastrointestinal manifestations (37.9%) [27].

The cutaneous features described in the most recent international classification exercise for PAN in children [10] occurred commonly and are defined in Box 148.2. Others have reported similar cutaneous manifestations, including erythematous subcutaneous nodules (Fig. 148.1) and livedo reticularis, to be common. In addition, ulcerated lesions, haemorrhage, bullae, urticaria and petechial lesions have been documented in other series [6,7,28,29].

In a report of 10 children with cutaneous PAN, clinical features included fever in all patients, peripheral gangrene in eight, livedo reticularis in four, ulceration, nodules and vesicobullous lesions alone or in combination in 10, black necrotic patches over limbs and trunk in three, and arthralgia and swelling of large joints in seven [5]. Abdominal pain has been reported to be a presenting feature of 'cutaneous PAN' but the subsequent

Box 148.2 Cutaneous features of polyarteritis nodosa defined in the 2010 classification criteria [10]

- *Livedo reticularis:* purplish reticular pattern usually irregularly distributed around subcutaneous fat lobules, often more prominent with cooling
- *Skin nodules:* tender subcutaneous nodules
- *Superficial skin infarctions:* superficial skin ulcers (involving skin and superficial subcutaneous tissue) or other minor ischaemic changes (nailbed infarctions, splint haemorrhages, digital pulp necrosis)
- *Deep skin infarctions:* deep skin ulcers (involving deep subcutaneous tissue and underlying structures), digital phalanx or other peripheral tissue (nose and ear tips) necrosis/gangrene

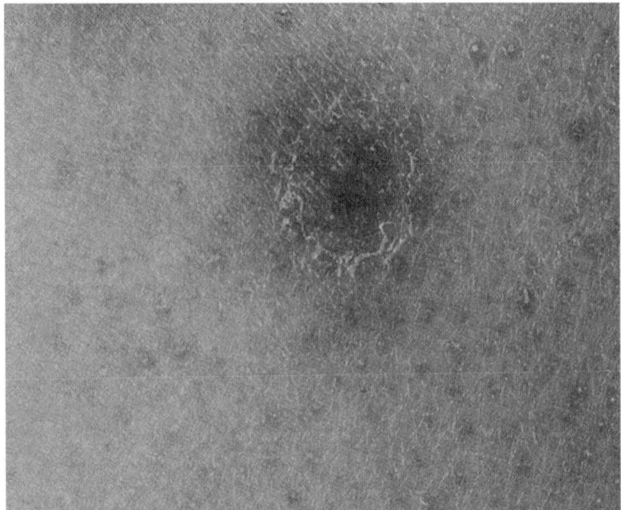

Fig. 148.1 Subcutaneous nodule in polyarteritis nodosa.

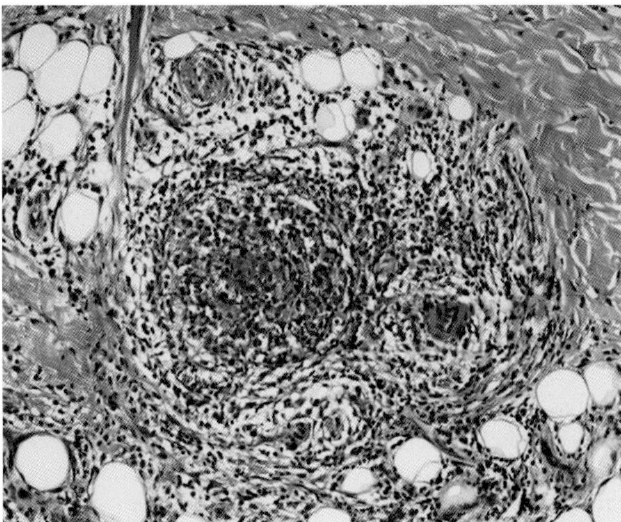

Fig. 148.2 Skin biopsy demonstrating fibrinoid necrosis of blood vessels in polyarteritis nodosa. Source: Dillon et al. 2010 [12]. Reproduced with permission from Springer.

development of anterior uveitis too may suggest an overlap with the more systemic form, although the outcome may be favourable [30]. Bauzá and colleagues [31] also described abdominal pain as a feature of cutaneous PAN. Figures 148.1–5 illustrate some of the aforementioned cutaneous features of PAN. Table 148.1 compares clinical features observed in two paediatric series.

Differential diagnoses for PAN. Differential diagnoses for PAN are summarized in Box 148.3.

Laboratory and histological findings. Laboratory work-up usually reveals leucocytosis and thrombocytosis along with elevated acute phase reactants. ANCAs are typically negative [2,4]. Positive hepatitis B serology is unusual in childhood PAN [4]. Furthermore, if the vasculitis is related to hepatitis B infection, it should now be classified under 'vasculitis associated with probable aetiology' according to the Chapel Hill Consensus Criteria (CHCC 2012) [32]. The renal findings reflect the involvement of the medium-sized arteries before the glomerular capillaries, such as the lobar and arcuate arteries [2,4]. Thus, varying amounts of proteinuria and mild haematuria may be present [2,4]. Necrotizing vasculitis of these arteries can result in the luminal arterial changes observed

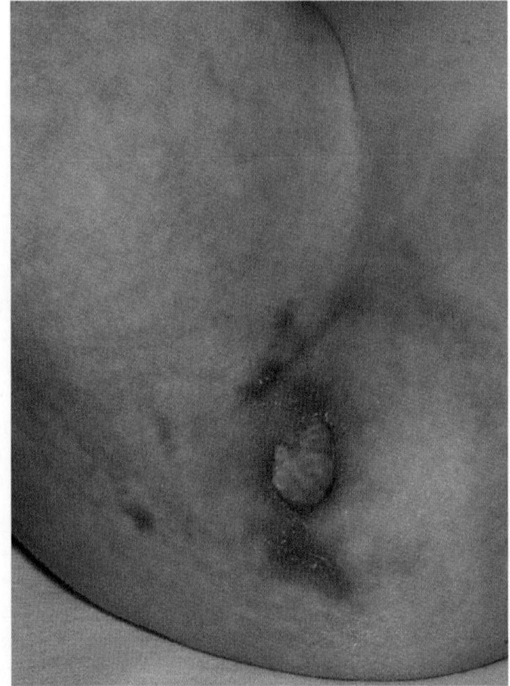

Fig. 148.3 Necrotizing lesion of the buttock in polyarteritis nodosa.

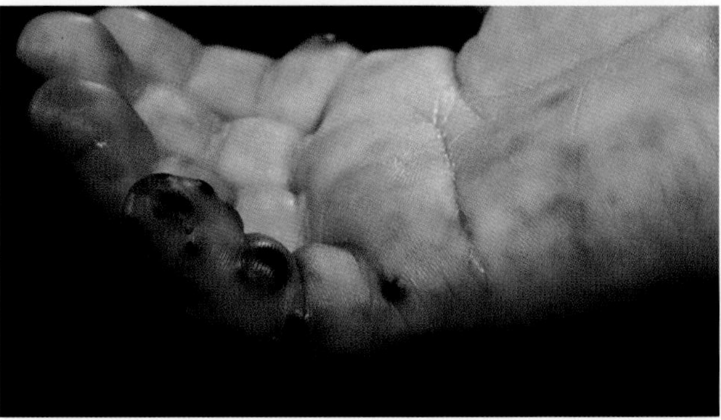

Fig. 148.4 Necrotizing vasculitis of the digits in polyarteritis nodosa.

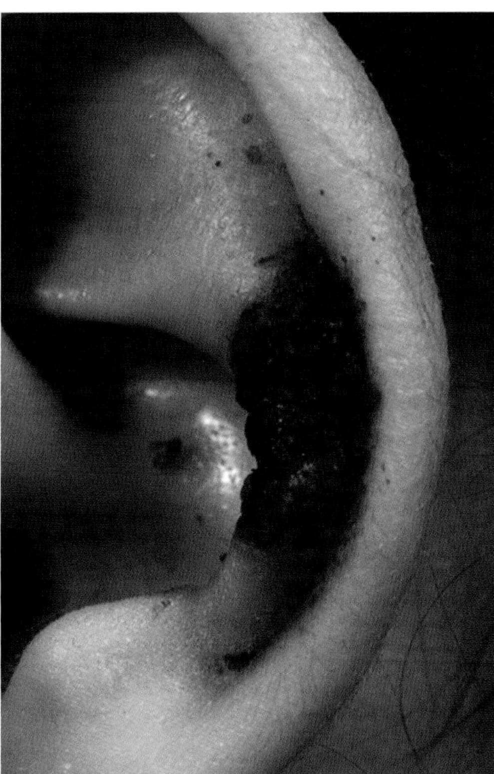

Fig. 148.5 Necrotizing vasculitic lesions of the pinna in polyarteritis nodosa.

using arteriography [2,4]. Although the classical arteriographic finding is aneurysmal dilatation, other luminal changes that may also suggest vasculitis in children include beaded tortuosity, abrupt cut-offs, tapering stenosis of smaller order vessels and pruning of the peripheral renal arterial tree [2,4]. Similar changes are also observed in adults. Because of the smaller calibre of the arteries typically involved in PAN, the gold standard for radiological diagnosis is conventional catheter digital subtraction. An important caveat is that the monogenic disease DADA2 produces identical changes on angiography to those typically associated with systemic PAN (Fig. 148.6). Hepatic and mesenteric catheter angiography, although invasive, can also be an extremely useful investigation in the demonstration of arteritis, often showing discrete aneurysms [33] (Fig. 148.7).

Macroscopic renal disease may be indicated on a technetium-99m dimercaptosuccinic acid (DMSA) scan (Fig. 148.6), which shows patchy areas of decreased uptake [34], but again is not specific for the differentiation of PAN from DADA2.

The classic pathological lesion is an inflammatory vasculitis of predominantly medium-sized vessels with fibrinoid necrosis of the media and cellular infiltration. There may be evidence of aneurysmal dilation and arterial thromboses [12]. Biopsies of affected organs, particularly the skin, may reveal a typical histological appearance. However, the absence of these changes does not exclude the diagnosis of PAN because the patchy nature of the disease may result in the pathological area being missed [1,35].

Table 148.1 Clinical features of polyarteritis nodosa

Clinical feature	Percentage of patients (total n = 31) affected [3]	Percentage of patients (total n = 110) affected [4]
Fever	65	51
Skin lesions (including livedo reticularis, maculopapular purpuric lesions, gangrene, nodules, digital infarction)	81	75
Myalgia, arthralgia	81	71
Gastrointestinal (abdominal pain/haemorrhage)	61	17
Neurological (including numbness, paraesthesia, polyneuropathy, encephalitis, hemiparesis, ptosis, fits)	48	15
Hypertension	65	15
Nephrological (including proteinuria/haematuria/ rapidly progressive nephritis)	65	12
Cardiological (including pericarditis, arrhythmias, cardiac failure, myocardial infarction)	16	4
Pulmonary (including pulmonary infiltrates, pleural effusion, haemoptysis)	10	2
Anaemia	32	
Acute-phase reactants (including raised ESR, CRP, leucocytosis)	90	
HBsAg	10	8
Male sex	70	49

CRP, C-reactive protein; ESR, erythrocyte sedimentation rate; HBsAg, hepatitis B surface antigen.

Box 148.3 Differential diagnoses for polyarteritis nodosa

- *Other primary vasculitides:* HSP, GPA, MPA, KD
- *Autoimmune or autoinflammatory diseases:*
  JIA – particularly the systemic form
  JDM
  SLE
  Undifferentiated connective tissue disease
  Sarcoidosis
  Behçet disease
- *Infections:*
  Bacterial, particularly streptococcal infections and subacute bacterial endocarditis.
  Viral – many: specifically look for hepatitis B/C, CMV, EBV, parvovirus B19 and consider HIV.
- *Malignancy:* lymphoma, leukaemia and other malignancies can mimic PAN.
- *DADA2:* cardinal clinical features are livedo racemosa, lacunar stroke, and systemic inflammation.

CMV, cytomegalovirus; DADA2, deficiency of adenosine deaminase type 2; EBV, Epstein–Barr virus; GPA, granulomatosis with polyangiitis; HIV, human immunodeficiency virus; HSP, Henoch–Schönlein purpura; JDM, juvenile dermatomyositis; JIA, juvenile idiopathic arthritis; KD, Kawasaki disease; MPA, microscopic polyangiitis; PAN, polyarteritis nodosa; SLE, systemic lupus erythematosus.

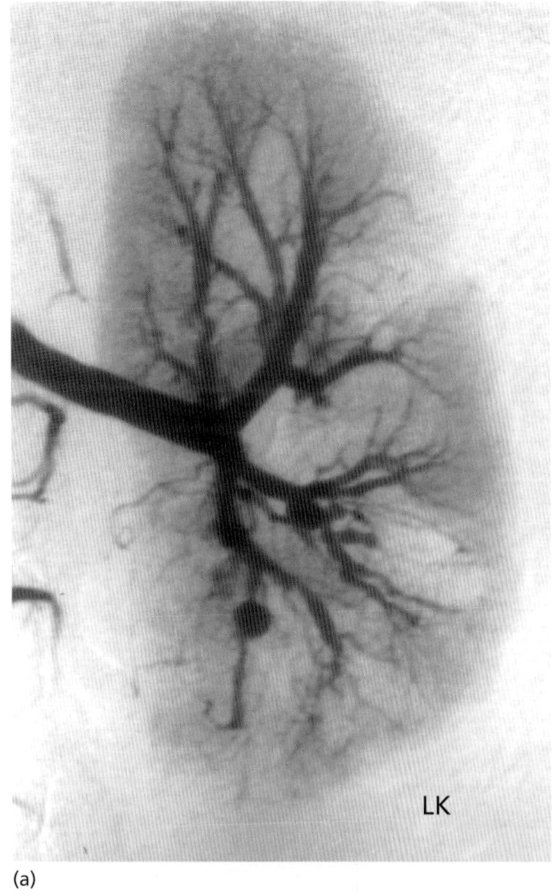

(a)

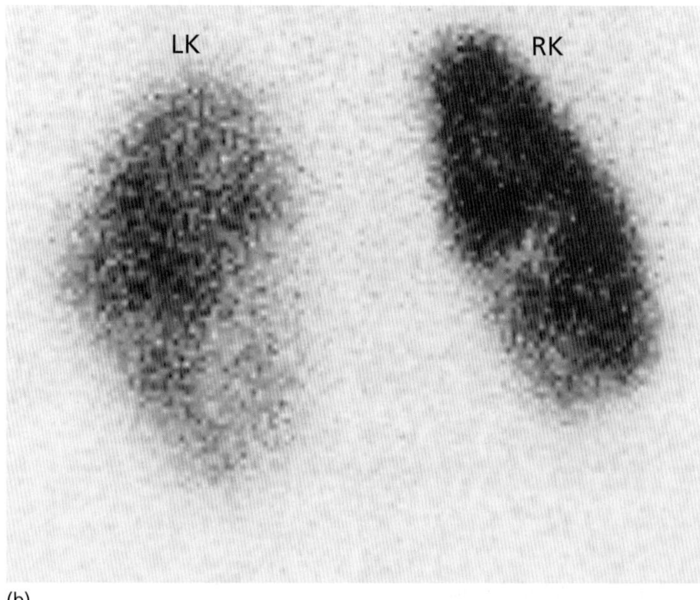

(b)

Fig. 148.6 (a) Left renal angiogram demonstrating multiple aneurysms in a child previously considered to have polyarteritis nodosa; subsequent genetic testing revealed the true diagnosis of DADA2 (deficiency of adenosine deaminase type 2). (b) DMSA (dimercaptosuccinic acid) scan from the same patient demonstrating defects of isotope uptake consistent with renal scarring. LK, left kidney; RK, right kidney. Source: Dillon et al. 2010 [12]. Reproduced with permission from Springer.

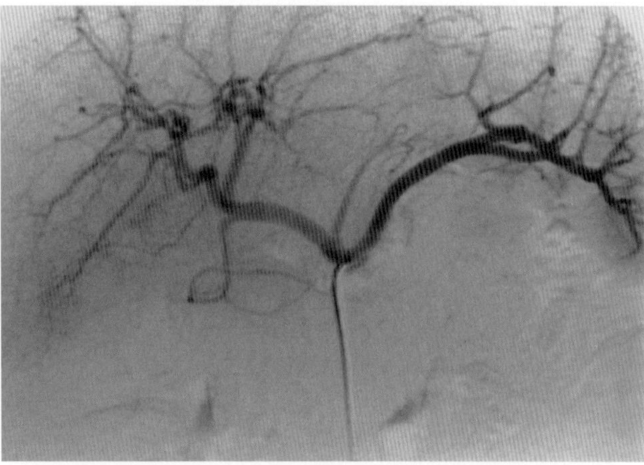

Fig. 148.7 Coeliac/hepatic angiogram demonstrating aneurysms in polyarteritis nodosa.

Treatment and prognosis. The treatment of PAN should be tailored to the extent of systemic involvement. In pure cutaneous PAN, corticosteroids alone or even anti-inflammatory drugs may suffice, whereas some also require more potent immunosuppression [5–7].

Treatment to induce remission of systemic PAN typically involves high doses of corticosteroids and intravenous cyclophosphamide (typically given monthly at a dose of 500–750 mg/m^2); once remission is achieved, maintenance therapy with low-dose corticosteroid and azathioprine is frequently used [2,4]. Long-term maintenance therapy with immunosuppressives may be necessary, but it is usually possible to discontinue treatment after 18 months to 3 years. Recently, successful treatment with biological agents such as infliximab or rituximab has been reported in refractory cases [36]. However, treatment of PAN in children is based mainly on trial data involving adult patients and there has never been a randomized controlled trial of treatment for children with PAN (see later). Plasma exchange could play a role in severe cases [37]. Children with PAN have better outcomes when compared with adults and a possibility of permanent remission can be anticipated in children with PAN [2,4]. The mortality rate was reported as 1–4% in children in recent studies [2,4]. The mortality rate was 24.6% in 349 adult PAN patients registered in the French Vasculitis Study Group database [38]. In a recent randomized trial involving 118 adult patients with MPA and PAN without poor prognostic factors, the 5- and 8-year overall survival rates were 93 and 86%, respectively, with no difference between MPA and PAN [39]. Poor prognostic factors in adults with PAN associated with higher 5-year mortality were as follows: age older than 65 years, cardiac symptoms, gastrointestinal involvement and renal insufficiency [11]. The worst outcome was significantly correlated with renal and neurological involvement in a cohort of 52 children with PAN [40]; in another recent paediatric series, severe gastrointestinal disease was associated with an increased risk of relapse of systemic PAN [2]. More recently, successful treatment with biological agents such as anti-TNFα or rituximab has been reported, particularly for relapsing cases. Anti-TNFα is particularly efficacious for the monogenic form of PAN, DADA2 [16], and in the opinion of this author this should be considered before cyclophosphamide, because for DADA2 patients the latter treatment is not successful [16]. In hepatitis B-associated PAN, interferon-α has been reported to be of benefit [41].

PAN, unlike some other vasculitides such as *granulomatosis with polyangiitis*, appears to be a condition in which permanent remission can be achieved. Relapses can occur but in spite of these, a real possibility of 'cure' can be anticipated. However, if treatment is delayed or inadequate, life-threatening complications can occur caused by the vasculitic process and, after treatment has commenced, similarly severe complications, especially infective, can arise as a sequel to the immunosuppressive drugs used [2,42,43]. In comparison to the almost 100% mortality seen in the presteroid era, mortality rates are currently remarkably low, with a mortality rate of 1–4% [2,4]. Late morbidity can occur years after childhood PAN from chronic vascular injury resulting in premature atherosclerosis [2]. This remains a cause for concern and an area of ongoing active research.

References

1 Blau EB, Morris RF, Yunis EJ. Polyarteritis nodosa in older children. Pediatrics 1977;60:227–34.

2 Eleftheriou D, Dillon MJ, Tullus K et al. Systemic polyarteritis nodosa in the young: a single-center experience over thirty-two years. Arthritis Rheum 2013;65:2476–85.

3 Ozen S, Besbas N, Saatci U et al. Diagnostic criteria for polyarteritis nodosa in childhood. J Pediatr 1992;120(2 Pt 1):206–9.

4 Ozen S, Anton J, Arisoy N et al. Juvenile polyarteritis: results of a multicenter survey of 110 children. J Pediatr 2004;145:517–22.

5 Kumar L, Thapa BR, Sarkar B et al. Benign cutaneous polyarteritis nodosa in children below 10 years of age – a clinical experience. Ann Rheum Dis 1995;54:134–6.

6 Sheth AP, Olson JC, Esterly NB. Cutaneous polyarteritis nodosa of childhood. J Am Acad Dermatol 1994;31:561–6.

7 Siberry GK, Cohen BA, Johnson B. Cutaneous polyarteritis nodosa. Reports of two cases in children and review of the literature. Arch Dermatol 1994;130:884–9.

8 Watts RA, Scott DG. Epidemiology of vasculitis. In: Ball R, Bridges SL, Jr (eds) Vasculitis, 2nd edn. Oxford: Oxford University Press, 2008:7–21.

9 Eleftheriou D, Batu ED, Ozen S, Brogan PA. Vasculitis in children. Nephrology Dialysis Transplantation 2015;30(suppl 1):i94–i103.

10 Ozen S, Pistorio A, Iusan SM et al. EULAR/PRINTO/PRES criteria for Henoch-Schonlein purpura, childhood polyarteritis nodosa, childhood Wegener granulomatosis and childhood Takayasu arteritis: Ankara 2008. Part II: Final classification criteria. Ann Rheum Dis 2010;69:798–806.

11 Guillevin L, Lhote F, Gayraud M et al. Prognostic factors in polyarteritis nodosa and Churg-Strauss syndrome. A prospective study in 342 patients. Medicine (Baltimore) 1996;75:17–28.

12 Dillon MJ, Eleftheriou D, Brogan PA. Medium-size-vessel vasculitis. Pediatr Nephrol 2010;25:1641–52.

13 Yalcinkaya F, Ozcakar ZB, Kasapcopur O et al. Prevalence of the MEFV gene mutations in childhood polyarteritis nodosa. J Pediatr 2007;151:675–8.

14 Navon Elkan P, Pierce SB, Segel R et al. Mutant adenosine deaminase 2 in a polyarteritis nodosa vasculopathy. N Engl J Med 2014;370:921–31.

15 Zhou Q, Yang D, Ombrello AK et al. Early-onset stroke and vasculopathy associated with mutations in ADA2. N Engl J Med 2014;370:911–20.

16 Nanthapisal S, Murphy C, Omoyinmi E et al. Deficiency of adenosine deaminase type 2 (DADA2): a description of phenotype and genotype in 15 cases. Arthritis Rheumatol 2016;68:2314–22.

17 Liu Y, Jesus AA, Marrero B et al. Activated STING in a vascular and pulmonary syndrome. N Engl J Med 2014;371:507–18.

18 Omoyinmi E, Melo GS, Nanthapisal S et al. Stimulator of interferon genes-associated vasculitis of infancy. Arthritis Rheumatol 2015;67:808.

19 David J, Ansell BM, Woo P. Polyarteritis nodosa associated with streptococcus. Arch Dis Child 1993;69:685–8.

20 Fink CW. The role of the streptococcus in poststreptococcal reactive arthritis and childhood polyarteritis nodosa. J Rheumatol Suppl 1991;29:14–20.

21 Finkel TH, Torok TJ, Ferguson PJ et al. Chronic parvovirus B19 infection and systemic necrotising vasculitis: opportunistic infection or aetiological agent? Lancet 1994;343(8908):1255–8.

22 Golden MP, Hammer SM, Wanke CA, Albrecht MA. Cytomegalovirus vasculitis. Case reports and review of the literature. Medicine (Baltimore) 1994;73:246–55.

23 Pagnoux C, Cohen P, Guillevin L. Vasculitides secondary to infections. Clin Exp Rheumatol 2006;24(2 Suppl 41):S71–S81.

24 Fain O, Hamidou M, Cacoub P et al. Vasculitides associated with malignancies: analysis of sixty patients. Arthritis Rheum 2007;57:1483–80.

25 Brasile L, Kremer JM, Clarke JL, Cerilli J. Identification of an autoantibody to vascular endothelial cell-specific antigens in patients with systemic vasculitis. Am J Med 1989;87:74–80.

26 Brogan PA, Shah V, Bagga A et al. T cell Vbeta repertoires in childhood vasculitides. Clin Exp Immunol 2003;131:517–27.

27 Pagnoux C, Seror R, Henegar C et al. Clinical features and outcomes in 348 patients with polyarteritis nodosa: a systematic retrospective study of patients diagnosed between 1963 and 2005 and entered into the French Vasculitis Study Group Database. Arthritis Rheum 2010;62:616–26.

28 Chen KR. Cutaneous polyarteritis nodosa: a clinical and histopathological study of 20 cases. J Dermatol 1989;16:429–42.

29 Verbov J. Cutaneous polyarteritis nodosa in a young child. Arch Dis Child 1980;55:569–72.

30 Falcini F, Lionetti P, Simonini G et al. Severe abdominal involvement as the initial manifestation of cutaneous polyarteritis nodosa in a young girl. Clin Exp Rheumatol 2001;19:349–51.

31 Bauza A, Espana A, Idoate M. Cutaneous polyarteritis nodosa. Br J Dermatol 2002;146:694–9.

32 Jennette JC, Falk RJ, Bacon PA et al. 2012 revised International Chapel Hill Consensus Conference Nomenclature of Vasculitides. Arthritis Rheum 2013;65:1–11.

33 Brogan PA, Davies R, Gordon I, Dillon MJ. Renal angiography in children with polyarteritis nodosa. Pediatr Nephrol 2002;17:277–83.

34 Dillon MJ. Childhood vasculitis. Lupus 1998;7:259–65.

35 Reimold EW, Weinberg AG, Fink CW, Battles ND. Polyarteritis in children. Am J Dis Child 1976;130:534–41.

36 Eleftheriou D, Melo M, Marks SD et al. Biologic therapy in primary systemic vasculitis of the young. Rheumatology (Oxford) 2009;48:978–86.

37 Wright E, Dillon MJ, Tullus K. Childhood vasculitis and plasma exchange. Eur J Pediatr 2007;166:145–51.

38 Guillevin LC, Pagnoux C, Seror R et al. The Five-Factor Score revisited: assessment of prognoses of systemic necrotizing vasculitides based on the French Vasculitis Study Group (FVSG) cohort. Medicine 2011;90:19–27.

39 Samson M, Puéchal X, Devilliers H et al. Long-term outcomes of 118 patients with eosinophilic granulomatosis with polyangiitis (Churg-Strauss syndrome) enrolled in two prospective trials. J Autoimmun 2013;43:60–9.

40 Falcini F, La Torre F, Martini G et al. Predictors of outcome in juvenile polyarteritis nodosa: a multi-center study. Clin Exp Rheumatol 2011;29:430–1.

41 Duzova A, Bakkaloglu A, Yuce A et al. Successful treatment of polyarteritis nodosa with interferon alpha in a nine-month old girl. Eur J Pediatr 2001;160:519–20.
42 Brogan PA, Dillon MJ. The use of immunosuppressive and cytotoxic drugs in non-malignant disease. Arch Dis Child 2000;83:259–64.
43 Gayraud M, Guillevin L, Le Toumelin P et al. Long-term followup of polyarteritis nodosa, microscopic polyangiitis, and Churg-Strauss syndrome: analysis of four prospective trials including 278 patients. French Vasculitis Study Group. Arthritis Rheum 2001;44:666–75.

Granulomatosis with polyangiitis (formerly Wegener granulomatosis)

Introduction and history. ANCA-associated vasculitides (AAV) comprise granulomatosis with polyangiitis (GPA) (previously WG, but hereafter only referred to as GPA), microscopic polyangiitis (MPA), eosinophilic granulomatous polyangiitis (EGPA; previously Churg–Strauss syndrome) and single organ disease including renal-limited vasculitis [1]. ANCA, autoantibodies to neutrophil constituents, in particular proteinase 3 (PR3) and myeloperoxidase (MPO) are considered central to the pathogenesis of this autoimmune disease [2,3]. GPA is associated with granulomatous inflammation involving the respiratory tract (Fig. 148.8), with necrotizing vasculitis affecting small- to medium-sized vessels (e.g. capillaries, venules, arterioles and arteries), typically with cytoplasmic (c-) ANCA positivity (Fig. 148.9). Necrotizing glomerulonephritis is common [4] and is an important determinant of prognosis. Although rare, AAV do occur in childhood and are associated with significant morbidity and mortality, especially if diagnosis is delayed [2]. The classification criteria for GPA in children are summarized below [5]. There are no classification criteria in children for MPA or EGPA; consequently, these diseases are referred to using CHCC 2012 definitions [6].

Although the earliest reports of GPA were first described by McBride in 1897 as mid-facial granuloma syndrome, the full description of GPA is attributed to Friedrich Wegener in 1936, based on three similar autopsy cases. Nearly 20 years later, Godman and Churg named it the 'Wegener triad' [7]. It is a multisystem disease affecting the ears, nose, larynx, eyes, lungs, kidneys, heart, joints, skin and CNS [8].

Paediatric classification for GPA requires the presence of three of the following six criteria:

- renal involvement (proteinuria or haematuria or red blood cell casts)

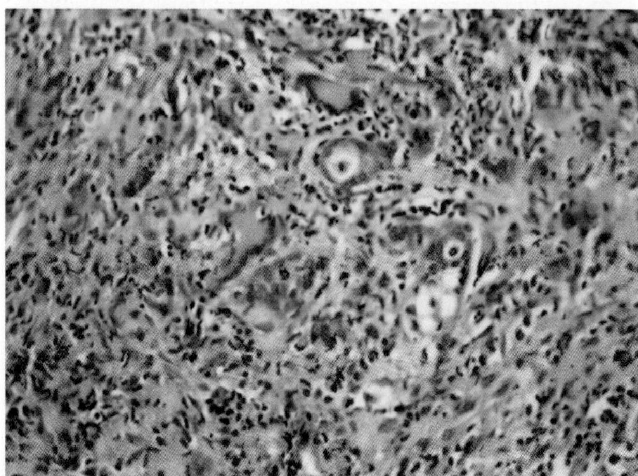

Fig. 148.8 Nasal biopsy of granulomatosis with polyangiitis: granulomatous inflammation with giant cells and generalized destructive acute inflammation involving nasal mucous glands.

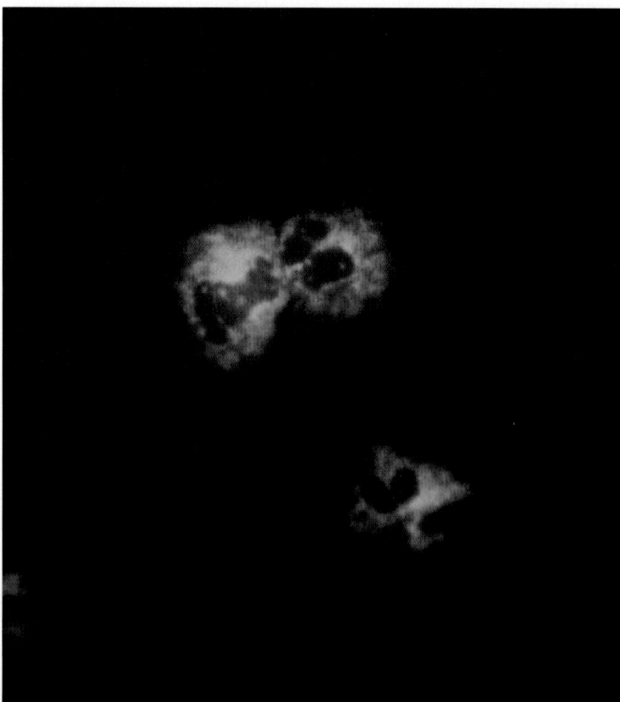

(a)

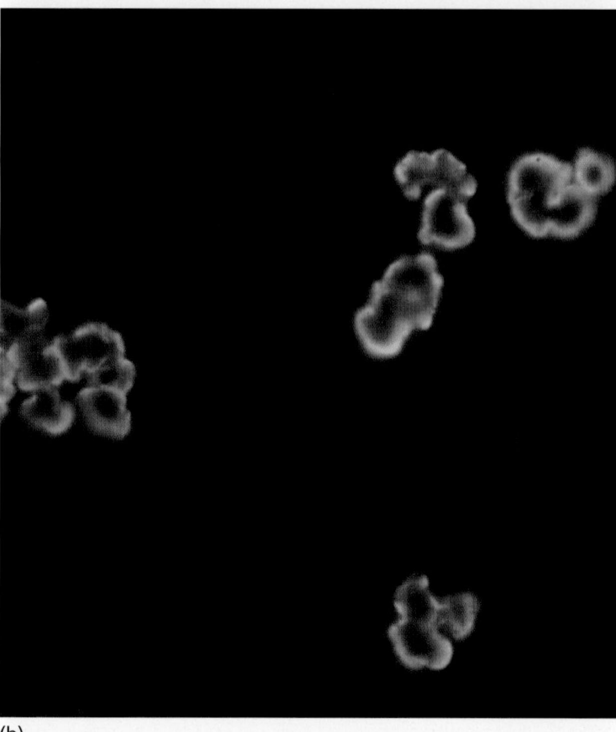

(b)

Fig. 148.9 Immunofluorescence pattern of (a) c-ANCA (cytoplasmic antineutrophil cytoplasmic antibodies and (b) p-ANCA (perinuclear antineutrophil cytoplasmic antibodies).

- positive histopathology (granulomatous inflammation within the wall of an artery or in the perivascular or extravascular area)
- upper airway involvement (nasal discharge or septum perforation, sinus inflammation)
- laryngo-tracheo-bronchial involvement (subglottic, tracheal or bronchial stenosis)
- pulmonary involvement (chest X-ray or computed tomography scan)
- ANCA positivity (by immunofluorescence, or enzyme-linked immunosorbent assay [ELISA] revealing PR3-ANCA or MPO-ANCA).

Sensitivity and specificity of the European League against Rheumatism/Pediatric Rheumatology International Trials Organization/Paediatric Rheumatology European Society (EULAR/PRINTO/PRES) criteria are 93% and 99% respectively for the differentiation of GPA from other forms of vasculitis in the young [5].

Epidemiology of GPA. The overall incidence of GPA is 0.8–1.2/100 000 population [9,10]. Regional differences have been described, with higher incidences in Norway and parts of the UK compared with Spain or Japan [11,12]. GPA is predominantly a disease of adults, usually 40–50-year-olds, with a male-to-female ratio of 1.6:1 [12,13]. However, although the epidemiology for GPA in children is poorly described, the disease does occur in the paediatric population, and of the AAV occurring in the young, GPA is seen most frequently [1]. In the paediatric population the disease tends to occur in the second decade and with a female preponderance [2,14–16].

Pathogenesis of AAV (GPA and MPA). The pathogenesis of AAV is an area of very active research, and the reader is referred to a recent in-depth review [17]. Clinical and experimental data strongly suggest a role for autoimmune responses to PR3 and MPO in disease development. The most accepted model of pathogenesis suggests that ANCA activate cytokine-primed neutrophils within the microvasculature, leading to bystander damage to endothelial cells themselves and rapid escalation of inflammation with recruitment of mononuclear cells [18,19]. Evidence for a pathogenic role of MPO-ANCA in AAV additionally comes from animal models for MPO-ANCA-associated vasculitis. Xiao and colleagues immunized mice deficient for MPO with mouse MPO and transferred splenocytes from these immunized mice into immunodeficient or normal mice [20]. The recipient mice developed pauci-immune necrotizing glomerulonephritis and haemorrhagic pulmonary capillaritis, similar to the clinical manifestations and the histopathology of MPO-ANCA-associated vasculitis [20]. In addition, transfer of IgG alone from MPO-immunized mice resulted in pauci-immune focal necrotizing glomerulonephritis in the recipient, demonstrating the pathogenic potential of anti-MPO antibodies [20]. In humans, transplacental transfer of MPO ANCA has been reported to cause a pulmonary–renal syndrome in a newborn, providing the best evidence of direct pathogenicity caused by ANCA [21]. Pathogenicity of anti-PR3 antibodies is perhaps less well-established, with no definitive animal model of anti-PR3 ANCA disease [22].

Genome-wide association studies (GWAS) emphasize that genetic risk factors predispose individuals to form either MPO ANCA or PR3 ANCA, rather than determine the clinical phenotype per se: patients with PR3 ANCA associated with HLA-DP, SERPINA1 (encoding alpha-1 antitrypsin), PRTN3 (encoding PR3) and Semaphorin 6A; in contrast patients with MPO ANCA associated mainly with HLA DQ polymorphisms [23,24].

Infectious episodes may trigger relapses of AAV [25]. Further studies of upper airway involvement in GPA showed good responses to treatment with trimethoprim/sulfamethoxazole [26]. Long-term studies demonstrated that chronic nasal carriage of *Staphylococcus aureus* is a major risk factor for relapse in GPA in conjunction with persistence of ANCA, and maintenance treatment with trimethoprim/sulfamethoxazole reduced the occurrence of relapses by 60% in patients with GPA [26]. Possible mechanisms whereby *S. aureus* could result in flares of GPA include superantigen production and T and B cell activation, direct tropism of *S. aureus* for endothelial cells with binding and internalization of the organism by endothelial cells, or by priming of neutrophils [25,27,28].

Whilst there are still many unanswered questions about why individuals develop ANCA in the first instance, in addition to clues provided by GWAS, it is suggested that dysregulation of neutrophil extracellular trap (NET) formation may contribute to the generation of autoimmunity and the formation of ANCA in some individuals, a proposal that is supported by animal data [29]. NETs may induce endothelial cell death, and thus may participate in vascular damage in patients with AAV [30]. An important role of B cells in AAV pathogenesis is underscored by recent positive experience in clinical trials of targeting B-cells therapeutically (see later). B cells may play a role in AAV by participating both in ANCA generation, and ANCA immune response regulation. T cells are also undoubtedly important in the pathogenesis of AAV and have been targeted in therapeutic trials [31]. Other important immunological pathways include the alternative complement pathway. In particular, the importance of C5 activation is emerging and may represent a novel therapeutic target for AAV [17].

Thus, the pathogenesis of AAV is complex and involves dysregulation of both innate and adaptive immune responses. Neutrophils remain as central players in the pathogenesis of AAV, both as a target of ANCA and as downstream mediators of endothelial damage. In particular, dysregulation of NET formation and activation of the imperative complement pathway are emerging as important components of AAV pathogenesis.

Clinical features of GPA. From a clinical perspective it may be useful to think of GPA as having two forms: a predominantly granulomatous form with mainly localized disease with a chronic course, and a florid, 'true' acute small vessel vasculitic form characterized by severe pulmonary haemorrhage and/or rapidly progressive vasculitis or other severe vasculitic manifestation [1]. These two broad pathogenic processes may coexist or present sequentially in individual paediatric/adult patients alike. In a series of 17 children with GPA, the frequency of different system involvement was respiratory 87%, renal 53%, ear, nose and throat 35%, musculoskeletal 53%, eyes 53%, nervous system 12% and skin 53% [2]. Another paediatric series of GPA reported an even higher frequency of renal involvement with 22 of 25 cases having glomerulonephritis at first presentation, and only 1 of 11 patients who had renal impairment in that series recovered renal function with therapy [14].

Cabral and colleagues described 65 children with GPA reporting renal involvement in up to 75.4% of cases [15]. Dialysis was necessary in seven patients (10.8%) and end-stage renal disease was present in a single patient of that series [15]. In adult patients, data suggest that 73.5% of adults with GPA have histological evidence of glomerulonephritis [32]. Of note, renal involvement in GPA is accrued with increasing age, which could account in part for the variation in reported renal involvement in paediatric GPA.

Similar distribution of symptoms and organ involvement was noted in the cases submitted for the validation exercise of the EULAR/PRES/PRINTO paediatric vasculitis classification criteria [33]. Comparing the paediatric and adult cohorts, whereas organ involvement, signs and symptoms are similar, there are differences in their frequencies at disease presentation. In general, adult patients have lower frequencies of constitutional symptoms (fever, weight loss), certain ear, nose and throat features (oral/nasal ulceration, chronic or recurrent otitis media/aural discharge), respiratory (tracheal/endobronchial stenosis, obstruction, haemoptysis/alveolar haemorrhage) and renal (haematuria or red blood cells casts) involvement; and a higher frequency of conductive hearing loss than children [4,33].

Chondritis of the nose results in the typical saddle nose deformity (Fig. 148.10) [34]. Sinuses are often affected, ranging from mucosal thickening to pansinusitis and bone destruction. Oral features include jaw pain, gingival hyperplasia and palatal ulceration. Subglottic stenosis is the most commonly affected area in the tracheobronchial tree in children, affecting up to 48% of children (Fig. 148.11) [2,16]. In a child with stridor, laryngoscopy with biopsies of any lesions in the airway may be helpful diagnostically. Pulmonary involvement may be asymptomatic. Single or multiple nodular masses with or without cavitation may be seen, as can focal (Fig. 148.12) or diffuse infiltrates [35].

Clinical manifestations relating to renal involvement include hypertension, haematuria and/or proteinuria, nephritic and nephrotic syndrome, and in some cases a rapidly progressive nephritis with acute renal failure [1]. Coronary arteritis, myocardial infarction, granulomatous valvulitis of the aortic or mitral valves [36], pericarditis or pancarditis are all rare complications, but are important to recognize early.

Skin disease may present as erythema, urticarial lesions, petechiae, purpura, ulcerative lesions, pyoderma gangrenosum and necrotic lesions (Fig. 148.13). In both paediatric and adult series, skin disease is reported in approximately 50% [2,8,16]. In one large series of 244 adults, 30 (14%) were found to have skin involvement and detailed clinical, histopathological and c-ANCA findings were reported [37]. Initial presentation with skin disease is less common, occurring in 8.6–13% of cases [16,38,39]. No single lesion is pathognomonic and lesions must be considered together with other findings. One case report described a child presenting with nodular

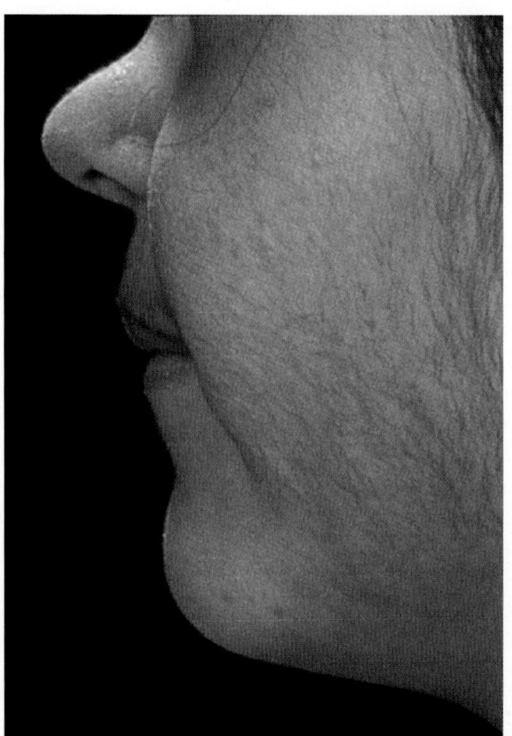

Fig. 148.10 Chondritis of the nasal bridge resulting in 'saddle nose' deformity in granulomatosis with polyangiitis.

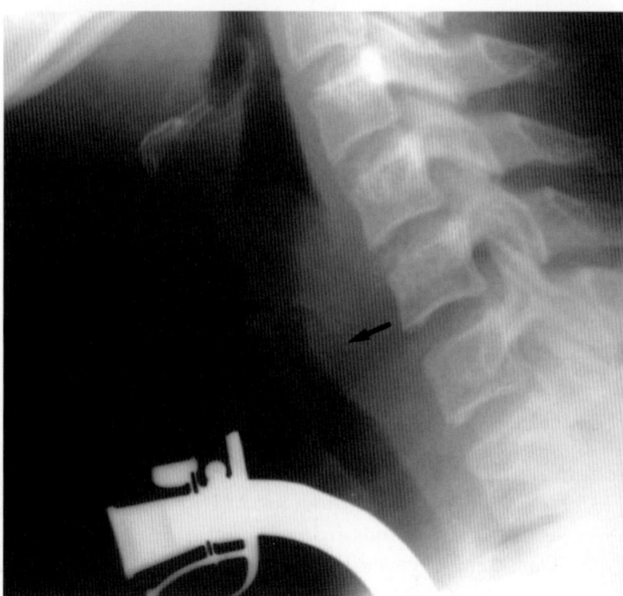

Fig. 148.11 Radiograph of narrowing of the subglottic region in granulomatosis with polyangiitis, necessitating tracheostomy.

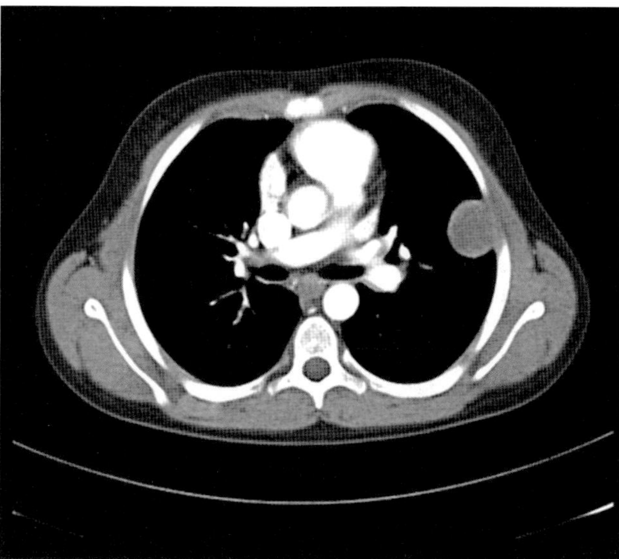

Fig. 148.12 Pulmonary nodule in a child with granulomatosis with polyangiitis. Source: Brogan et al. 2010 [1]. Reproduced with permission from Springer.

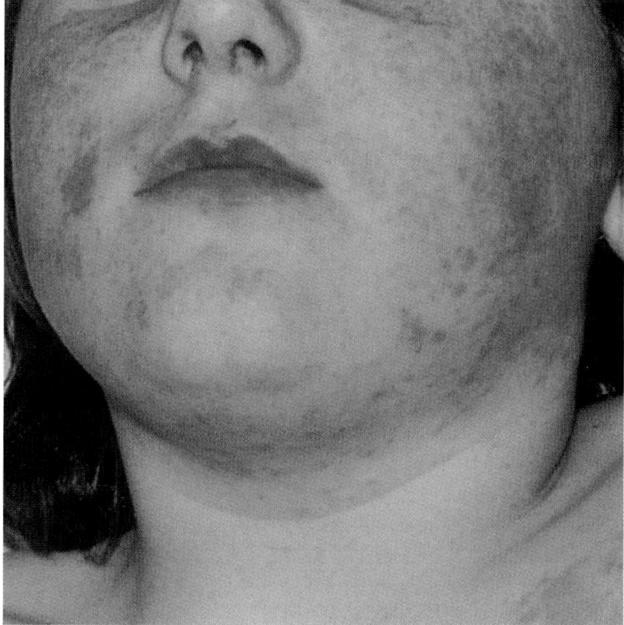

Fig. 148.13 Vasculitic rash of the face in granulomatosis with polyangiitis.

and necrotic acneiform lesions predominantly on her forehead, which then progressed to ulcers on the arms and buttocks [38], but at presentation other features of GPA were also identified.

Migratory arthralgias may affect several joints and symmetrical polyarthritis can occur, but destructive arthritis is rare. Neurological involvement may result in cranial nerve palsies, mononeuritis multiplex, symmetrical peripheral neuropathy, cerebral infarction (Fig. 148.14) and transverse myelitis. Ophthalmological disease, causing conjunctivitis, episcleritis, corneoscleral ulcers, uveitis, vasculitis of the retina, optic neuritis and central artery occlusion, is documented. Unilateral or bilateral proptosis may be caused by granulomatous pseudotumours of the orbit [40,41] (Fig. 148.15). Gastrointestinal symptoms are rare although vasculitic ischaemia may

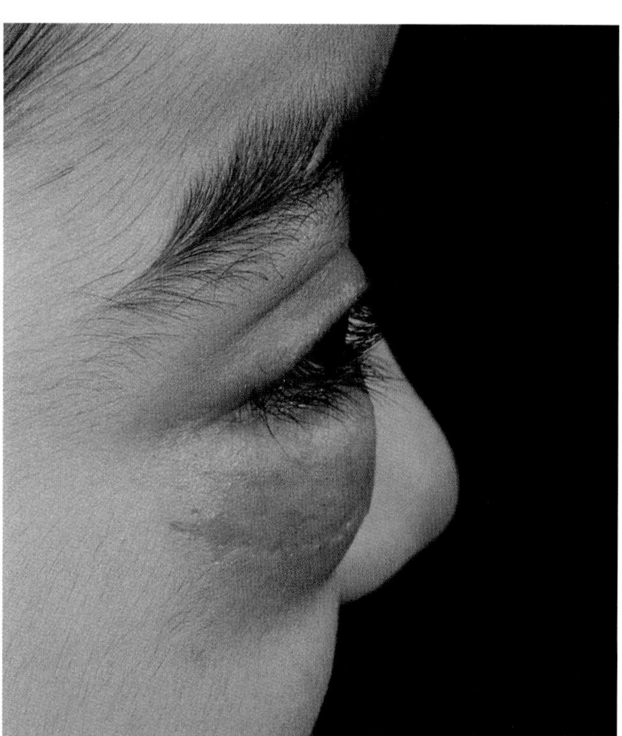

Fig. 148.15 Proptosis caused by granulomatous pseudotumour of the orbit in granulomatosis with polyangiitis.

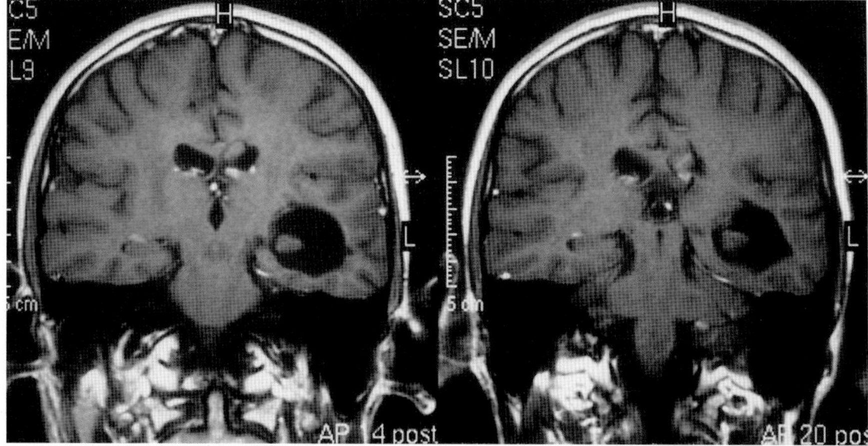

Fig. 148.14 Magnetic resonance image of brain cystic dilation following necrotic haemorrhagic cerebral vasculitis in granulomatosis with polyangiitis.

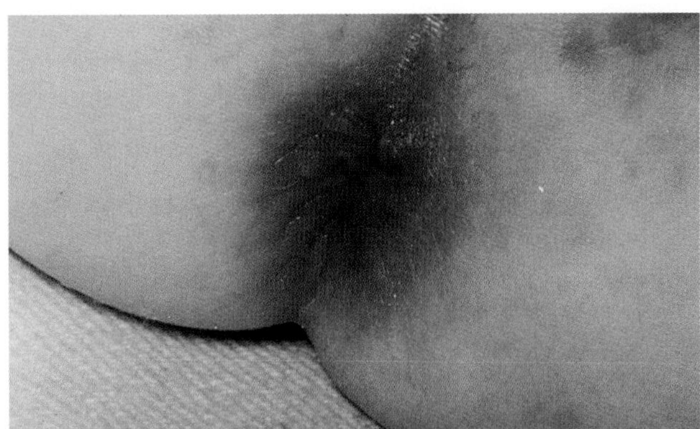

Fig. 148.16 Necrotizing vasculitic involvement of the anus and rectum in granulomatosis with polyangiitis.

result in bowel perforation, and necrotizing vasculitic involvement of the anus and rectum has been seen (Fig. 148.16).

A limited form of GPA also exists, in which the pathological findings are confined to the respiratory tract. Subglottic stenosis is a feature of GPA that has been reported in the absence of other clinical markers but in association with ANCA, demonstrating the benefit of a laboratory marker that allows early diagnosis and intervention with appropriate treatment [42]. A comparison of the clinical findings in children and adults is shown in Table 148.2

Differential diagnoses for GPA in children. Important differential diagnoses are summarized in Box 148.4.

Laboratory and histological findings of AAV. Davies and colleagues in 1982 [43] described antibodies directed against antigenic determinants in the neutrophil cytoplasm of patients with segmental necrotizing glomerulonephritis, the first description of ANCA linked to glomerulonephritis. Methodological improvements for the detection of ANCA have resulted in increased sensitivity and specificity. Both indirect immunofluorescence (IIF) and ELISA are used for routine diagnostic purposes. Typically, GPA is associated with a cytoplasmic staining pattern of ANCA on IIF, and ELISA reveals specificity against proteinase 3 (PR3-ANCA). However, perinuclear ANCA (p-ANCA) with specificity directed against myeloperoxidase (MPO-ANCA) can also be found in patients with GPA (Fig. 148.9). MPA and renal-limited AAV are typically associated with p-ANCA on IIF and MPO-ANCA on ELISA. Lastly, it should always be remembered that ANCA-negative forms of GPA, MPA, renal-limited vasculitis and EGPA are well described in children, although with improved sensitivity of modern ANCA assays, clinicians should consider the differential diagnosis carefully for patients with suspected 'ANCA negative' AAV.

The presence of ANCA (especially c-ANCA) has been found by some authors to be highly specific for GPA, with up to 91% sensitivity and 98% specificity during active disease being reported in adults [44]. In children, there is

Box 148.4 Differential diagnoses for granulomatosis with polyangiitis

- *Other primary vasculitides:* EGPA,HSP, MPA, PAN
- *Primary and postinfectious glomerulonephritides:* e.g. membranoproliferative or membranous glomerulonephritis, poststreptococcal glomerulonephritis
- *Autoimmune, autoinflammatory disease and primary immunodeficiency:* SLE, sarcoidosis, Blau syndrome, relapsing polychondritis, pyoderma gangrenosum, antiglomerular basement membrane disease, chronic granulomatous disease, TAP1 deficiency.
- *Infections:* mycobacterial infection, subacute bacterial endocarditis, *Pneumocystis jiroveci* pneumonia, bacterial pneumonia, fungal pneumonia.
- *Malignancy:* lymphoma, leukaemia, neuroblastoma, rhabdomyosarcoma of the orbit, histiocytic disorders and other malignancies can mimic GPA.
- *Miscellaneous:* cocaine, levamisole

EGPA, eosinophilic granulomatous polyangiitis; GPA, granulomatosis with polyangiitis; HSP, Henoch–Schönlein purpura; MPA, microscopic polyangiitis; PAN, polyarteritis nodosa; SLE, systemic lupus erythematosus.

Table 148.2 Comparison of features of granulomatosis with polyangiitis in children and adults

Feature	Akikusa et al. (2007) [14] *n* = 25 children Affected percentage	Rottem et al. (1993) [16] *n* = 23 children Affected percentage	Belostotsky et al. (2002) [2] *n* = 17 children Affected percentage	Fauci et al. (1983) [8] *n* = 85 adults Affected percentage
Renal	88	61	53	85
ENT (total)	96	91	58	–
Sinusitis	56	83	–	91
Nasal disease	60	65	–	64
Lung	84	74	87	94
Eye disease	60	48	53	58
Joints	44	78	53	67
Skin	48	52	53	45
CNS disease	8	17	12	22
Heart	–	9	–	12

ENT, ear, nose and throat; CNS, central nervous system.

also evidence to show a significant association with ANCA. In one report, 10 out of 12 paediatric GPA patients had ANCA detected on ELISA, compared with 7/12 on IIF [45]. In subsequent reports, ANCA positivity was found in 59–95% [2,14]. It is likely that this range of ANCA positivity in children with GPA reflects differences in age, variation in disease severity and methodological differences in laboratory detection of ANCA between these two series. Whilst early reports by van der Woude and colleagues [46] demonstrated the presence of these antibodies in adults with GPA and correlated their presence with disease activity, more recent studies have questioned the usefulness of measuring ANCA to monitor disease activity [47].

Whilst the diagnostic value of ANCA is without question important, ANCA for the longitudinal monitoring of disease activity is probably unreliable for many patients with GPA [47], although it can be used in some individuals for this purpose (Fig. 148.17). The reasons for this are not fully understood, but are likely to include methodological limitations of ANCA detection (including epitope specificity), the partial dissociation of ANCA levels and disease activity associated with immunosuppressive therapy, and the as yet undefined complexity in the exact role of ANCA in the pathogenesis of GPA [48].

Other commonly observed nonspecific findings include a mild normochromic normocytic anaemia together with a leucocytosis and thrombocytosis. The erythrocyte sedimentation rate (ESR) and C-reactive protein (CRP) are frequently elevated. Raised immunoglobulins (polyclonal IgG) may also support the diagnosis, although this finding is not specific. Laboratory manifestations relating to renal involvement include dipstick haematuria and proteinuria, a raised protein

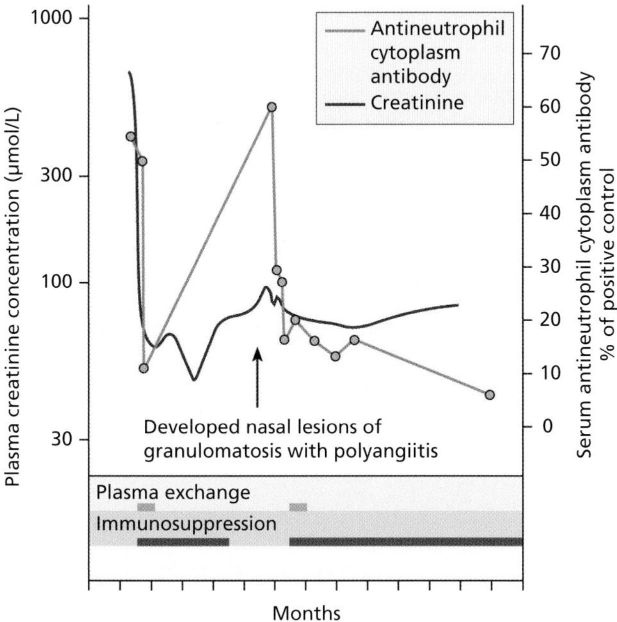

Fig. 148.17 Antineutrophil cytoplasmic antibodies (ANCA) relating to disease activity in a child with granulomatosis with polyangiitis. Whilst this case broadly reflects disease activity, overall ANCA are a poor biomarker for disease activity (see text).

creatinine ratio, raised serum creatinine and other associated laboratory features of renal failure.

Radiological findings. In addition to the haematological and immunological investigations discussed above, radiology can be of diagnostic benefit in GPA. Chest radiograph/CT may demonstrate pulmonary infiltrates or discrete nodular and/or cavitating lesions; sinus radiographs/CT may be abnormal, and neck views may demonstrate subglottic stenosis [1,35]. Increasingly, magnetic resonance imaging has a role for imaging in GPA, including of orbital lesions, of the airway and of the CNS [49].

Histological findings. GPA is a necrotizing granulomatous vasculitis, predominantly affecting small vessels, which are infiltrated with polymorphonuclear leucocytes followed by mononuclear cells. Granulomas are particularly seen in the upper and lower airways (Fig. 148.8), although there may be an absence of the classic granulomatous histological changes, with the only abnormality being chronic inflammation. Renal lesions are variable: a focal and segmental glomerulonephritis is most commonly found, although a diffuse proliferative glomerulonephritis with crescents is seen in those with a rapidly progressive clinical course and marked renal functional decline. Granulomas are often absent in renal biopsies. Skin biopsies may give supportive evidence for the diagnosis of GPA. In a report of GPA in a 10-year-old child, the finding of leucocytoclastic vasculitis with organizing thrombi in the dermis, and panniculitis in the absence of granulomatous changes was typical of changes that are consistent with but not absolutely diagnostic of GPA [50].

Treatment of GPA and MPA. Renal morbidity and mortality are a major concern in the AAV, hence therapy aimed at preservation of renal function is a recurring theme for the treatment of AAV in adults and children [51]. Treatment for paediatric AAV is broadly similar to the approach in adults, with corticosteroids, cyclophosphamide (usually 6–10 intravenous doses at 500–1000 mg/m^2 [maximum 1.2 g] per dose given 3–4 times weekly), and in select patients plasma exchange (particularly for pulmonary capillaritis and/or rapidly progressive glomerulonephritis – 'pulmonary–renal syndrome') routinely employed to induce remission [51]. Intravenous pulsed cyclophosphamide is increasingly favoured over oral continuous cyclophosphamide in adults and children, because of reduced cumulative dose and less neutropenic sepsis in adult patients, albeit without good paediatric evidence [52]. This is followed by low-dose corticosteroids and azathioprine (1.5–3 mg/kg/day; maximum 200 mg/day) to maintain remission [53]. Antiplatelet doses of aspirin (1–5 mg/kg/day; typically 37.5–75 mg/day) are empirically employed on the basis of the increased risk of thrombosis associated with the disease process [54]. Methotrexate may have a role for induction of remission in patients with limited GPA but is less commonly used as an induction agent in children with AAV [55]. Cotrimoxazole is commonly added for the treatment of

GPA, particularly in those with upper respiratory tract involvement, serving both as prophylaxis against opportunistic infection and as a possible disease-modifying agent to reduce the frequency of upper respiratory tract relapses [26]. Recommendations regarding duration of maintenance therapy are based on adult trial data, suggesting that the strongest predictor of relapse is withdrawal of therapy, and hence maintenance therapy is usually continued for 2–3 years, sometimes longer [56]. Because the use of cyclophosphamide may contribute to the burden of disease with infection being particularly common, and because disease relapses occur in 50% of the patients with AAV as drugs are reduced or withdrawn, newer immunosuppressive agents and immunomodulatory strategies are being explored in both adults and children. Treatments currently undergoing evaluation in clinical trials in children include mycophenolate mofetil (MMF) and rituximab [51]. Rituximab has already been reported to be effective at inducing remission in adults with AAV [57,58]; the recently published MYCYC trial suggests efficacy and safety of MMF in adults and children with AAV, although relapses might be higher than with cyclophosphamide [59].

Prognosis. Despite therapeutic advances over the past 10 years, the AAV are still associated with high disease-related morbidity and mortality in the young [2,14,15]. Irreversible end organ injury including renal failure, aggressive respiratory involvement and therapy-related complications such as sepsis are of particular concern [2,14,15]. Organ injury that accrues in the prediagnostic phase of the disease is unfortunately still relatively common, because AAV are rare in children and hence diagnosis is unfortunately often delayed [2,14,15]. The mortality for paediatric GPA from one recent paediatric series was 12% over a 17-year period [2]. Another paediatric series of GPA reported 40% chronic renal impairment at 33 months follow up despite therapy [14]. For MPA in children, mortality during paediatric follow up is reportedly between 0 and 14% (see later) [60]. In adults, absence of renal involvement in AAV is associated with a 95% 5-year survival rate, compared with 70% survival in individuals with renal disease, with an overall better renal prognosis for those with PR3-ANCA compared with MPO-ANCA [9,61].

References

1 Brogan P, Eleftheriou D, Dillon M. Small vessel vasculitis. Pediatr Nephrol 2010;25:1025–35.

2 Belostotsky VM, Shah V, Dillon MJ. Clinical features in 17 paediatric patients with Wegener granulomatosis. Pediatr Nephrol 2002; 17:754–61.

3 Ruperto N, Ozen S, Pistorio A et al. EULAR/PRINTO/PRES criteria for Henoch-Schonlein purpura, childhood polyarteritis nodosa, childhood Wegener granulomatosis and childhood Takayasu arteritis: Ankara 2008. Part I: Overall methodology and clinical characterisation. Ann Rheum Dis 2010;69:790–7.

4 Eleftheriou D, Batu ED, Ozen S, Brogan PA. Vasculitis in children. Nephrology Dialysis Transplantation 2015;30(suppl 1):i94–i103.

5 Ozen S, Pistorio A, Iusan SM et al. EULAR/PRINTO/PRES criteria for Henoch-Schonlein purpura, childhood polyarteritis nodosa, childhood Wegener granulomatosis and childhood Takayasu arteritis: Ankara 2008. Part II: Final classification criteria. Ann Rheum Dis 2010;69:798–806.

6 Jennette JC, Falk RJ, Bacon PA et al. 2012 revised International Chapel Hill Consensus Conference Nomenclature of Vasculitides. Arthritis Rheum 2013;65:1–11.

7 Godman GC, Churg J. Wegener's granulomatosis: pathology and review of the literature. AMA Arch Pathol 1954;58:533–53.

8 Fauci AS, Haynes BF, Katz P, Wolff SM. Wegener's granulomatosis: prospective clinical and therapeutic experience with 85 patients for 21 years. Ann Intern Med 1983;98:76–85.

9 Mohammad AJ, Jacobsson LT, Westman KW et al. Incidence and survival rates in Wegener's granulomatosis, microscopic polyangiitis, Churg–Strauss syndrome and polyarteritis nodosa. Rheumatology 2009;48:1560–5.

10 Ntatsaki E, Watts RA, Scott DG. Epidemiology of ANCA-associated vasculitis. Rheum Dis Clin North Am 2010;36:447–61.

11 Fujimoto S, Watts RA, Kobayashi S et al. Comparison of the epidemiology of anti-neutrophil cytoplasmic antibody-associated vasculitis between Japan and the UK. Rheumatology (Oxford) 2011;50:1916–20.

12 Watts RA, Gonzalez-Gay MA, Lane SE et al. Geoepidemiology of systemic vasculitis: comparison of the incidence in two regions of Europe. Ann Rheum Dis 2001;60:170–2.

13 Koldingsnes W, Nossent H. Epidemiology of Wegener's granulomatosis in northern Norway. Arthritis Rheum 2000;43:2481–7.

14 Akikusa JD, Schneider R, Harvey EA et al. Clinical features and outcome of pediatric Wegener's granulomatosis. Arthritis Rheum 2007;57:837–44.

15 Cabral DA, Uribe ArG, Benseler S et al. Classification, presentation, and initial treatment of Wegener's granulomatosis in childhood. Arthritis Rheum 2009;60:3413–24.

16 Rottem M, Fauci AS, Hallahan CW et al. Wegener granulomatosis in children and adolescents: clinical presentation and outcome. J Pediatr 1993;122:26–31.

17 Jarrot PA, Kaplanski G. Pathogenesis of ANCA-associated vasculitis: an update. Autoimmun Rev 2016;15:704–13.

18 Hong Y, Eleftheriou D, Hussain AA et al. Anti-neutrophil cytoplasmic antibodies stimulate release of neutrophil microparticles. J Am Soc Nephrol 2012;23:49–62.

19 Hong Y, Eleftheriou D, Klein NJ, Brogan PA. Impaired function of endothelial progenitor cells in children with primary systemic vasculitis. Arthritis Res Ther 2015;17:292.

20 Xiao H, Heeringa P, Hu P et al. Antineutrophil cytoplasmic autoantibodies specific for myeloperoxidase cause glomerulonephritis and vasculitis in mice. J Clin Invest 2002;110:955–63.

21 Schlieben DJ, Korbet SM, Kimura RE et al. Pulmonary-renal syndrome in a newborn with placental transmission of ANCAs. Am J Kidney Dis 2005;45:758–61.

22 Salama AD, Little MA. Animal models of antineutrophil cytoplasm antibody-associated vasculitis. Curr Opin Rheumatol 2012;24:1–7.

23 Lyons PA, Rayner TF, Trivedi S et al. Genetically distinct subsets within ANCA-associated vasculitis. N Engl J Med 2012;367:214–23.

24 Xie G, Roshandel D, Sherva R et al. Association of granulomatosis with polyangiitis (Wegener's) with HLA-DPB1*04 and SEMA6A gene variants: evidence from genome-wide analysis. Arthritis Rheum 2013;65:2457–68.

25 Cohen Tervaert JW, Stegeman CA, Manson WL et al. Staphylococcus aureus superantigens: a risk factor for disease reactivation in Wegener's granulomatosis. FASEB J 1998;12:A488.

26 Stegeman CA, Tervaert JW, de Jong PE, Kallenberg CG. Trimethoprim-sulfamethoxazole (co-trimoxazole) for the prevention of relapses of Wegener's granulomatosis. Dutch Co-Trimoxazole Wegener Study Group. N Engl J Med 1996;335:16–20.

27 Cohen Tervaert JW, Popa ER, Bos NA. The role of superantigens in vasculitis. Curr Opin Rheumatol 1999;11:24–33.

28 Cohen Tervaert JW. Infections in primary vasculitides. Cleve Clin J Med 2002;69 Supplement 2:SII–24–SII–26.

29 Sangaletti S, Tripodo C, Chiodoni C et al. Neutrophil extracellular traps mediate transfer of cytoplasmic neutrophil antigens to myeloid dendritic cells toward ANCA induction and associated autoimmunity. Blood 2012;120:3007–18.

30 Saffarzadeh M, Juenemann C, Queisser MA et al. Neutrophil extracellular traps directly induce epithelial and endothelial cell death: a predominant role of histones. PLoS One 2012;7:e32366.

31 Walsh M, Chaudhry A, Jayne D. Long-term follow-up of relapsing/refractory anti-neutrophil cytoplasm antibody associated vasculitis treated with the lymphocyte depleting antibody alemtuzumab (CAMPATH-1H). Ann Rheum Dis 2008;67:1322–7.

32 Hilhorst M, Wilde B, van Paassen P et al. Improved outcome in anti-neutrophil cytoplasmic antibody (ANCA)-associated glomerulonephritis: a 30-year follow-up study. Nephrol Dialys Transplant 2013;28:373–9.

33 Bohm M, Fernandez MIG, Ozen S et al. Clinical features of childhood granulomatosis with polyangiitis (Wegener's granulomatosis). Pediatr Rheum 2014;12:1–5.

34 Orlowski JP, Clough JD, Dyment PG. Wegener's granulomatosis in the pediatric age group. Pediatrics 1978;61:83–90.

35 Wadsworth DT, Siegel MJ, Day DL. Wegener's granulomatosis in children: chest radiographic manifestations. Am J Roentgenol 1994;163:901–4.

36 Varnier GC, Sebire N, Christov G et al. Granulomatosis with polyangiitis mimicking infective endocarditis in an adolescent male. Clin Rheumatol 2016;35:2369–72.

37 Daoud MS, Gibson LE, DeRemee RA et al. Cutaneous Wegener's granulomatosis: clinical, histopathologic, and immunopathologic features of thirty patients. J Am Acad Dermatol 1994;31:605–12.

38 Brazzelli V, Vassallo C, Baldini F et al. Wegener granulomatosis in a child: cutaneous findings as the presenting signs. Pediatr Dermatol 1999;16:277–80.

39 Chyu JY, Hagstrom WJ, Soltani K et al. Wegener's granulomatosis in childhood: cutaneous manifestations as the presenting signs. J Am Acad Dermatol 1984;10:341–6.

40 Haynes BF, Fishman ML, Fauci AS, Wolff SM. The ocular manifestations of Wegener's granulomatosis. Fifteen years experience and review of the literature. Am J Med 1977;63:131–41.

41 Sacks RD, Stock EL, Crawford SE et al. Scleritis and Wegener's granulomatosis in children. Am J Ophthalmol 1991;111:430–3.

42 Hoare TJ, Jayne D, Rhys EP et al. Wegener's granulomatosis, subglottic stenosis and antineutrophil cytoplasm antibodies. J Laryngol Otol 1989;103:1187–91.

43 Davies DJ, Moran JE, Niall JF, Ryan GB. Segmental necrotising glomerulonephritis with antineutrophil antibody: possible arbovirus aetiology? Br Med J (Clin Res Ed) 1982;285(6342):606.

44 Rao JK, Weinberger M, Oddone EZ et al. The role of antineutrophil cytoplasmic antibody (c-ANCA) testing in the diagnosis of Wegener granulomatosis. A literature review and meta-analysis. Ann Intern Med 1995;123:925–32.

45 Wong SN, Shah V, Dillon MJ. Antineutrophil cytoplasmic antibodies in Wegener's granulomatosis. Arch Dis Child 1998;79:246–50.

46 van der Woude FJ, Rasmussen N, Lobatto S et al. Autoantibodies against neutrophils and monocytes: tool for diagnosis and marker of disease activity in Wegener's granulomatosis. Lancet 1985 ;1(8426):425–9.

47 Finkielman JD, Merkel PA, Schroeder D et al. Antiproteinase 3 antineutrophil cytoplasmic antibodies and disease activity in Wegener granulomatosis. Ann Intern Med 2007;148:611–9.

48 Jayne D. Review article: progress of treatment in ANCA-associated vasculitis. Nephrology (Carlton) 2009;14:42–8.

49 Iglesias E, Eleftheriou D, Mankad K et al. Microscopic polyangiitis presenting with hemorrhagic stroke. J Child Neurol 2014;29:NP1–NP4.

50 Stein SL, Miller LC, Konnikov N. Wegener's granulomatosis: case report and literature review. Pediatr Dermatol 1998;15:352–6.

51 Eleftheriou D, Brogan PA. Therapeutic advances in the treatment of vasculitis. Pediatr Rheumatol Online J 2016;14:26.

52 Harper L, Morgan MD, Walsh M et al. Pulse versus daily oral cyclophosphamide for induction of remission in ANCA-associated vasculitis: long-term follow-up. Ann Rheum Dis 2012;71:955–60.

53 Hiemstra TF, Walsh M, Mahr A et al. Mycophenolate mofetil vs azathioprine for remission maintenance in antineutrophil cytoplasmic antibody-associated vasculitis: a randomized controlled trial. JAMA 2010;304:2381–8.

54 Merkel PA, Lo GH, Holbrook JT et al. Brief communication: high incidence of venous thrombotic events among patients with Wegener granulomatosis: the Wegener's Clinical Occurrence of Thrombosis (WeCLOT) Study. Ann Intern Med 2005;142:620–6.

55 de Groot K, Rasmussen N, Bacon PA et al. Randomized trial of cyclophosphamide versus methotrexate for induction of remission in early systemic antineutrophil cytoplasmic antibody-associated vasculitis. Arthritis Rheum 2005;52:2461–9.

56 Mukhtyar C, Guillevin L, Cid MC et al. EULAR recommendations for the management of primary small and medium vessel vasculitis. Ann Rheum Dis 2009;68:310–7.

57 Jones RB, Cohen Tervaert JW, Hauser T et al. Rituximab versus cyclophosphamide in ANCA-associated renal vasculitis. N Engl J Med 2010;363:211–20.

58 Stone JH, Merkel PA, Spiera R et al. Rituximab versus cyclophosphamide for ANCA-associated vasculitis. N Engl J Med 2010; 363:221–32.

59 Jones RB, Hiemstra TF, Ballarin J et al. Mycophenolate mofetil versus cyclophosphamide for remission induction in ANCA-associated vasculitis: a randomised, non-inferiority trial. Ann Rheum Dis 2019;78:399–405.

60 Ozen S, Anton J, Arisoy N et al. Juvenile polyarteritis: results of a multicenter survey of 110 children. J Pediatr 2004;145:517–22.

61 Mohammad AJ, Segelmark M. A population-based study showing better renal prognosis for proteinase 3 antineutrophil cytoplasmic antibody (ANCA)-associated nephritis versus myeloperoxidase ANCA-associated nephritis. J Rheumatol 2014;41:1366–73.

Microscopic polyangiitis

Introduction. Microscopic polyangiitis (MPA, formerly microscopic polyarteritis) is one of the AAV, and differs from classic PAN by the presence of extensive glomerular and pulmonary involvement, and is defined as a necrotizing vasculitis with few or no immune deposits, predominantly affecting small vessels (i.e. capillaries, venules or arterioles), although arteritis of the small and medium-sized arteries may be present [1]. Necrotizing glomerulonephritis is very common and pulmonary capillaritis may occur, usually in the context of pulmonary–renal syndrome. Clinically, it can be difficult to distinguish from GPA and often presents with rapidly progressive pauci-immune glomerulonephritis [2] in association with p-ANCA and MPO-ANCA positivity [1].

Renal-limited AAV describes those with rapidly progressive glomerulonephritis, often with ANCA positivity (usually MPO-ANCA) but without other organ involvement, and probably represents a forme fruste MPA.

Epidemiology. Epidemiological data are limited because the disease is very rare and because it was originally considered as a form of PAN. It is now considered with the other AAVs as discussed above. The estimated incidence in the UK is 3.6 cases per million [3]. In a survey study in the USA and Canada, paediatric rheumatologists recognized MPA as frequently as PAN, and about half as frequently as GPA [4]. The average age of onset in adults is 50 years with a male to female ratio of between 1.0 and 1.8:1. There are very few paediatric data, but published reports suggest an average age of onset between 9 and 12 years, with a slight female preponderance [5,6].

Pathogenesis. This is described in more detail previously (see section on GPA). Unlike GPA there is less of an association with infectious triggers; drug triggers may include exposure to propylthiouracil [7], hydralazine [8]; or levamisole (which may contaminate cocaine, therefore may be an issue for illicit drug abusers) [9].

Clinical features and differential diagnosis. The typical clinical manifestations are rapidly progressive glomerulonephritis and alveolar haemorrhage. Other possible symptoms resemble those encountered in polyarteritis nodosa (see previously). In adults, 75–80% of patients have p-ANCA/MPO-ANCA. Renal limited forms are described in children and adults. The main differential diagnosis is GPA, although consideration should be given to other causes of 'pulmonary renal syndrome' including systemic lupus erythematosus, antiglomerular basement membrane disease and other forms of glomerulonephritis.

Cutaneous manifestations include purpura and vasculitic ulcers, collectively affecting 58–100% of paediatric patients. Other cutaneous lesions such as petechiae, livedo reticularis, urticaria and erythema are observed [10,11].

Whilst the pulmonary and renal manifestations of MPA are often emphasized in reviews, it should be remembered that MPA can affect any organ in the body: CNS vasculitis may present with convulsions and severe headaches [12], ocular features include episcleritis, scleritis and conjunctivitis, and vasculitis of the gut with severe gastrointestinal haemorrhage are worthy of particular emphasis.

Laboratory and histological findings. As for GPA, nonspecific laboratory parameters of systemic inflammation are frequently observed: increased ESR and CRP, anaemia, thrombocytosis and hypoalbuminaemia (particularly in the context of rapidly progressive glomerulonephritis). MPO-ANCA/p-ANCA are typical in MPA, although some patients with MPA have PR3-ANCA. It is important to monitor renal function carefully, and also urinary protein excretion from an early morning urine sample (to avoid orthostatic proteinuria). Twenty-four hour urine protein excretion is often difficult to obtain accurately; a urine albumin creatinine ratio usually suffices to quantify proteinuria accurately. During the course of the disease, the relationship between ANCA positivity and disease activity is questionable (see previously). Pauci-immune immune necrotizing vasculitis including necrotizing glomerulonephritis are typical of MPA and is usually indistinguishable from GPA. Granulomatous inflammation is absent and if present may suggest the diagnosis of GPA.

Treatment and prognosis. The treatment of MPA is similar to that previously described for GPA, with corticosteroids and cyclophosphamide used for the induction of remission, followed by maintenance of remission with azathioprine. Plasma exchange should be considered for those with rapidly progressive glomerulonephritis and or pulmonary capillaritis [13]. Newer agents, including mycophenolate mofetil and rituximab, are also increasingly used in children and adults [14], both as induction of remission agents and as maintenance agents [15,16]. In adults, it has recently been suggested that patients with MPO-ANCA positivity may have less relapses than those associated with PR3-ANCA; the latter group may respond particularly well to rituximab rather than cyclophosphamide [15,16].

For MPA in children, mortality during paediatric follow up is reportedly 0–14% [14]. Two of seven children reported by Peco-Antic and colleagues [6] progressed to end-stage renal disease; one developed chronic renal failure and four normalized renal function. A selected population of 31 children with necrotizing pauci-immune glomerulonephritis and positive ANCA from Japan reported by Hattori and colleagues suggested a poor renal prognosis despite therapy [5]. In that series, at 43 months' follow up, 29% developed end-stage renal failure, 19.4% had reduced renal function and only 48.4% had normal renal function. Using these data, the authors suggested overall 75% renal survival at 39 months, compared with the poor renal prognosis of MPA in adults.

References

1. **Jennette JC, Falk RJ, Bacon PA et al. 2012 revised International Chapel Hill Consensus Conference Nomenclature of Vasculitides. Arthritis Rheum 2013;65:1–11.**
2. **van der Woude FJ, Rasmussen N, Lobatto S et al. Autoantibodies against neutrophils and monocytes: tool for diagnosis and marker of disease activity in Wegener's granulomatosis. Lancet 1985 23;1(8426):425–9.**
3. **Lyons PA, Rayner TF, Trivedi S et al. Genetically distinct subsets within ANCA-associated vasculitis. N Engl J Med 2012;367:214–23.**
4. Wilkinson NM, Page J, Uribe AG et al. Establishment of a pilot pediatric registry for chronic vasculitis is both essential and feasible: a Childhood Arthritis and Rheumatology Alliance (CARRA) survey. J Rheumatol 2007;34:224–6.
5. Hattori M, Kurayama H, Koitabashi Y. Antineutrophil cytoplasmic autoantibody-associated glomerulonephritis in children. J Am Soc Nephrol 2001;12:1493–500.
6. **Peco-Antic A, Bonaci-Nikolic B, Basta-Jovanovic G et al. Childhood microscopic polyangiitis associated with MPO-ANCA. Pediatr Nephrol 2006;21:46–53.**
7. Slot MC, Links TP, Stegeman CA, Tervaert JW. Occurrence of antineutrophil cytoplasmic antibodies and associated vasculitis in patients with hyperthyroidism treated with antithyroid drugs: a long-term followup study. Arthritis Rheum 2005 15;53:108–13.
8. Dobre M, Wish J, Negrea L. Hydralazine-induced ANCA-positive pauci-immune glomerulonephritis: a case report and literature review. Ren Fail 2009;31:745–8.
9. **McGrath MM, Isakova T, Rennke HG et al. Contaminated cocaine and antineutrophil cytoplasmic antibody-associated disease. Clin J Am Soc Nephrol 2011;6:2799–805.**
10. Kawakami T, Soma Y, Saito C et al. Cutaneous manifestations in patients with microscopic polyangiitis: two case reports and a minireview. Acta Derm Venereol 2006;86:144–7.
11. **Seishima M, Oyama Z, Oda M. Skin eruptions associated with microscopic polyangiitis. Eur J Dermatol 2004;14:255–8.**
12. Iglesias E, Eleftheriou D, Mankad K et al. Microscopic polyangiitis presenting with hemorrhagic stroke. J Child Neurol 2014; 29:NP1–NP4.
13. **Wright E, Dillon MJ, Tullus K. Childhood vasculitis and plasma exchange. Eur J Pediatr 2007;166:145–51.**
14. **Eleftheriou D, Brogan PA. Therapeutic advances in the treatment of vasculitis. Pediatr Rheumatol Online J 2016;14:26.**
15. **Yates M, Watts RA, Bajema IM et al. EULAR/ERA-EDTA recommendations for the management of ANCA-associated vasculitis. Ann Rheum Dis 2016;75:1583–94.**
16. **Schirmer JH, Wright MN, Herrmann K et al. Myeloperoxidase-ANCA associated Granulomatosis with polyangiitis is a clinically distinct subset within ANCA-associated vasculitis. Arthritis Rheumatol 2016;68:2953–63.**

CHAPTER 149

Juvenile Idiopathic Arthritis, Systemic Lupus Erythematosus and Juvenile Dermatomyositis

Elena Moraitis[1,2] *& Despina Eleftheriou*[1,2,3]

[1] Infection, Inflammation and Rheumatology Section, UCL Institute of Child Health, London, UK
[2] Paediatric Rheumatology Department, Great Ormond Street Hospital for Children NHS Foundation Trust, London, UK
[3] Arthritis Research UK Centre for Adolescent Rheumatology, University College London, UK

Juvenile idiopathic arthritis, 1933 | Systemic lupus erythematosus, 1940 | Juvenile dermatomyositis, 1945

Abstract

In this chapter we provide an overview of the clinical symptoms, laboratory findings and treatment for the following inflammatory diseases: juvenile idiopathic arthritis (JIA), juvenile systemic lupus erythematosus (JSLE) and juvenile dermatomyositis (JDM). For all these inflammatory conditions, the pathogenesis is likely to involve complex interactions between host susceptibility, infectious agents and other environmental triggers. Importantly, an understanding of these pathogenetic mechanisms has resulted in improved therapies and outcomes for the majority of patients affected by these diseases. The JIA clinical presentation can be classified into subtypes according to the number of joints involved (oligoarticular, polyarticular) and the presence of other symptoms such as psoriasis (psoriatic arthritis), enthesitis (for enthesitis-related arthritis) and systemic symptoms (fever, rashes for systemic JIA). The major new revolution in the management of JIA has been the advent of biologic therapies, developed to block specific targets of the inflammatory response. JSLE is an autoimmune disease characterized by a variety of clinical manifestations and a wide profile of autoantibodies. Cutaneous manifestations may include facial erythema (butterfly rash, discoid rash, Raynaud phenomenon, alopecia, photosensitivity and oral or nasopharyngeal ulceration). The severity spectrum of SLE is wide, and specific treatment should be individualized and take into consideration the extent and severity of the disease. JDM is considered an immune-mediated vasculopathy which presents characteristically with typical skin rashes (Gottron papules, heliotrope rash) and proximal muscle weakness, but can involve other organs. Calcinosis is a severe complication of JDM that is often extremely challenging to treat.

Key points

- **Juvenile idiopathic arthritis (JIA) is classified into systemic JIA, oligoarticular JIA, rheumatoid factor (RF)–negative polyarticular JIA, RF-positive polyarticular JIA, psoriatic arthritis, enthesitis-related arthritis and undifferentiated arthritis.**
- **Systemic JIA can be complicated by macrophage activation syndrome, a fatal complication caused by uncontrolled inflammation.**
- **Biologic therapies have revolutionized the outcome for JIA.**
- **Juvenile systemic lupus erythematosus is an autoimmune disease characterized by a variety of clinical manifestations and a wide profile of autoantibodies.**
- **The severity spectrum of systemic lupus erythematosus is wide, and specific treatment should be individualized and take into consideration the extent and severity of the disease.**
- **Juvenile dermatomyositis (JDM) is considered an immune-mediated vasculopathy which presents characteristically with typical skin rashes (gottron papules, heliotrope rash) and proximal muscle weakness, but can involve other organs.**
- **Calcinosis is a severe complication of JDM that is often extremely challenging to treat.**

Juvenile idiopathic arthritis

Introduction. Juvenile idiopathic arthritis (JIA) encompasses a heterogeneous group of diseases presenting with arthritis of unknown aetiology which persists longer than 6 weeks and affects children younger than 16 years of age [1]. The diagnosis of JIA requires exclusion of other conditions with similar presentation listed in Box 149.1.

Epidemiology, classification and pathogenesis. JIA is the most common rheumatic disease of childhood that on occasions is associated with significant disability caused by the effect of chronic arthritis on a growing skeleton, with either growth retardation or overgrowth of the involved joint. The annual incidence of the disease has been reported to be 2–20 cases per 100 000 population and the prevalence that of 16–150 cases per 100 000 population

Harper's Textbook of Pediatric Dermatology, Fourth Edition. Edited by Peter Hoeger, Veronica Kinsler and Albert Yan.

Box 149.1 Differential diagnosis of juvenile idiopathic arthritis

- Infection
- Other inflammatory and noninflammatory connective tissue diseases
- Leukaemia and other malignancies, e.g. neuroblastoma
- Haemoglobinopathies
- Genetic metabolic diseases, e.g. Hurler syndrome
- Chondrodysplasias
- Autoinflammatory syndromes

Source: Adapted from Ravelli A, Martini A. Juvenile idiopathic arthritis. Lancet 2007;369:767–78.

[2], with a yearly incidence in the UK of 10 cases per 100 000 population [3].

The International League of Associations for Rheumatology (ILAR) expert committee proposed a classification system for JIA with an aim to group the heterogenous disorders included under the JIA definition into mutually exclusive homogenous categories [1]. This classification has not only enabled a more consistent and directed clinical care, but also helped with research on pathogenesis, epidemiology, outcome studies and therapeutic trials. The term JIA was adopted instead of juvenile chronic arthritis or juvenile rheumatoid arthritis, which were previously used in Europe and North America, respectively. Based on the number of affected joints and other clinical features during the first 6 months of disease, the ILAR classification recognizes seven clinical subtypes: systemic onset JIA, oligoarticular JIA, rheumatoid factor (RF)-negative polyarticular JIA, RF-positive polyarticular JIA, psoriatic arthritis, enthesitis-related arthritis (ERA), and undifferentiated arthritis (Box 149.2) [1]. This classification system is currently being revised to account for our increased knowledge in the genetics and pathogenesis of JIA as well as the significant clinical heterogeneity in certain subtypes such as RF-positive polyarticular JIA and psoriatic arthritis.

The pathogenesis of JIA is still poorly understood, but seems to reflect the combination of complex genetic traits and unknown environmental triggers. Infections and vaccinations have been suggested as potential triggers in genetically susceptible individuals. However, this hypothesis lacks supporting evidence. Twin and family studies suggest a substantial role for genetic factors in the predisposition to JIA [4–6]. Utilizing a variety of techniques including candidate gene studies, the use of genotyping arrays such as Immunochip, and genome-wide association studies (GWAS), both human leukocyte antigen (HLA) and non-HLA susceptibility loci associated with JIA have been described [6–9]. Several of these polymorphisms (e.g. HLA class II, PTPN22, STAT4) are shared with other common autoimmune conditions; other novel polymorphisms that have been identified may be unique to JIA [8,10,11]. Associations with oligoarticular and RF-negative polyarticular JIA are the best characterized. A strong association between HLA DRB1:11:03/04 and DRB1:08:01, and a protective effect of DRB1:15:01 have been described; HLA DPB1:02:01 has also been associated with oligoarticular and RF-negative

Box 149.2 International League of Associations for Rheumatology (ILAR) classification of juvenile idiopathic arthritis subtypes [1]

Oligoarthritis

Arthritis of four or fewer joints within the first 6 months

- Persistent – affecting not more than four joints throughout the disease process
- Extended – extending to affect more than four joints after the first 6 months

Polyarthritis

Arthritis of five or more joints within the first 6 months

- RF positive – subdivided according to the presence of RF
- RF negative

Systemic arthritis

Arthritis with or preceded by quotidian (daily) fever for at least 3 days, accompanied by one or more of:

- Evanescent skin rash
- Lymphadenopathy
- Hepatomegaly and/or splenomegaly conditions
- Serositis

(Mandatory exclusion of infection and malignancy; arthritis may not present early in the course)

Psoriatic arthritis

Arthritis and psoriasis or arthritis with at least two of:

- Dactylitis
- Nail pitting or onycholysis
- Psoriasis in first-degree relative

Enthesitis-related arthritis

Arthritis and enthesitis or arthritis or enthesitis with two of:

- Sacroiliac joint tenderness of inflammatory lumbosacral pain
- HLA-B27 antigen
- Onset after 6 years in a male
- Acute (symptomatic anterior uveitis)
- History of HLA-B27-associated disease in a first-degree relative

Undifferentiated arthritis

Arthritis that fulfils the criteria in no or more than two of the above categories

HLA, human leukocyte antigen; RF, rheumatic factor.

polyarticular JIA [10,12]. Besides PTPN22, STAT4 and PTPN2 variants, IL2, IL2RA, IL2RB, as well as IL6 and IL6R loci also harbour variants associated with oligoarticular and RF-negative polyarticular JIA [11]. RF-positive polyarticular JIA is associated with many of the shared epitope encoding HLA DRB1 alleles, as well as PTPN22, STAT4 and TNFAIP3 variants [11]. ERA is associated with HLA B27 [10,11]. Most other associations between JIA categories and HLA or non-HLA variants need confirmation. The formation of International Consortia to ascertain and analyse large cohorts of JIA categories, validation of reported findings in independent cohorts, and functional studies will further enhance our understanding of the genetic underpinnings of JIA.

Systemic onset JIA is a distinct disease which shares similarities with the autoinflammatory diseases more than the classic autoimmune diseases, a fact reflected by the prominent systemic features besides arthritis and absence of autoantibodies [13]. Recent studies have provided insight into the pathogenesis of systemic onset JIA, showing that abnormalities of the innate immune response are contributing to the pathogenesis of the disease [14–17]; more specific, systemic onset JIA is characterized by overproduction of interleukin (IL)-6 and IL-18 [15,17] and a unique IL-1 signature [14], which has led to successful treatment with IL-6 or IL-1 blockade [18,19]. A recent study used meta-analysis of directly observed and imputed SNP genotypes and imputed classic HLA types, and identified HLA-DRB1*11 and variants of the MHC class II as bona fide susceptibility loci with effects on sJIA risk that transcended geographically defined strata thus solidifying the relationship between the class II HLA region and sJIA, implicating adaptive immune molecules in the pathogenesis of sJIA [20].

In terms of immunohistological characteristics of the synovial inflammation in JIA, studies have revealed that the synovium shows a pronounced hyperplasia of the lining layer and a cell infiltrate that includes mononuclear cells, T cells, B cells, macrophages, dendritic cells and plasma cells [21,22]. Growing evidence suggests that regulatory T (Treg) cells, a subpopulation of T cells known to suppress immune responses, and also T-helper (Th)17 cells are increased in number in the synovial fluid of patients with JIA, supporting their role in the pathogenesis of the disease [23]. T-helper (Th)17 cells, highly proinflammatory cells, have been shown in a higher number in the synovial fluid from patients with extended oligoarticular JIA, the more severe form of JIA, compared with other JIA subgroups, and the balance between IL-17+ T cells and Treg cells could be critical to the disease outcome [23]. Analyses of the proportions of synovial lymphocytes, levels of CCL5, and differential gene expression of synovial fluid from patients with JIA have also yielded potential biomarkers to predict the likelihood of extension of oligoarticular JIA to a more severe disease phenotype [24]. In addition, several studies have assessed blood and synovial cytokine concentrations in children with the various subsets of JIA with inconsistent reported results [13]. The therapeutic effect of antitumour necrosis factor (TNF) therapies in many patients, however, supports an important pathogenic role for TNF-α.

Clinical features.

sJIA

This form accounts for approximately 10% of cases of JIA [2]. The disease typically affects young children, even as young as the age of 1 year; however, the majority of studies indicate no definite peak age at onset of systemic arthritis [25]. The male:female ratio is approximately the same [26]. The diagnosis of sJIA is commonly based on the presence of fevers for more than 2 weeks, with a quotidian pattern for at least three consecutive days, accompanied by at least one of the following: an evanescent skin rash, generalized lymphadenopathy, serositis or hepatosplenomegaly [25]. By the time the diagnosis is made, children with sJIA may often be very unwell, with prominent systemic features, fatigue, significant articular pain and weight loss. The onset of the disease is typically one of recurrent high fevers of at least 39 °C, often occurring at the same time of day, usually late afternoon or evening, and in between the temperature returns to baseline. An evanescent macular rash, which often shows target lesions, is associated with the fever; the rash is characteristically described as 'salmon pink', but it is not rare that the rash is discretely erythematous. Sometimes the rash can be urticarial and itchiness is often described by the child (Fig. 149.1). The rash usually occurs on the limbs and the cheeks, but can be all over the body and there is marked dermographism (Fig. 149.2). Although it could be mistaken for a drug reaction or viral exanthem, what clearly distinguishes the rash of sJIA is that it is evanescent. At presentation, there can also be associated hepatosplenomegaly, generalized lymphadenopathy, serositis, cardiac complications such as pericardial effusion and pericarditis, and/or myocarditis, which can compromise cardiac function [27]. Very often, serositis has been mistaken for an acute abdomen. Typically, arthritis occurs after the onset of fever and polyarthritis becomes prominent when the fever fades away (Fig. 149.3) [28]. The most devastating complication of sJIA is macrophage activation syndrome (MAS), which is associated with significant morbidity. If it is not recognized and treated early and aggressively it can often lead to death. MAS is characterized by activation of T cells and macrophages, leading to an excessive systemic inflammatory response [25]. MAS is characterized by unremitting fever, lymphadenopathy, hepatosplenomegaly, hepatic dysfunction, mucosal bleeding, encephalopathy, or in severe cases multiorgan failure and shock [29]. The bone marrow aspirate reveals haemophagocytosis but not in all cases [29]. The laboratory investigations indicate the diagnosis showing low/falling/unexpectedly normal platelet or white blood cells counts, hyperferritinaemia, coagulation abnormalities, elevated AST (aspartate aminotransferase), ALT (alanine aminotransferase), GGT (gamma-glutamyl transpeptidase), bilirubin and LDH (lactate dehydrogenase), low/falling/unexpected normal fibrinogen, low or falling ESR (erythrocyte sedimentation rate) in the context of active inflammatory disease or high CRP (C-reactive protein), low serum sodium, elevated plasma

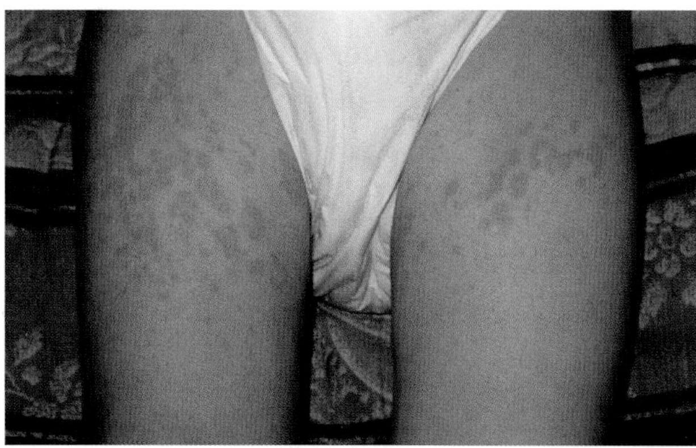

Fig. 149.1 A typical rash of systemic juvenile idiopathic arthritis.

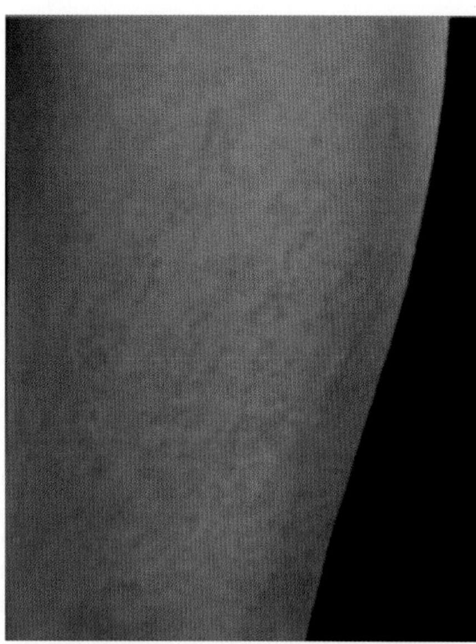

Fig. 149.2 Dermographism in a child with systemic juvenile idiopathic arthritis.

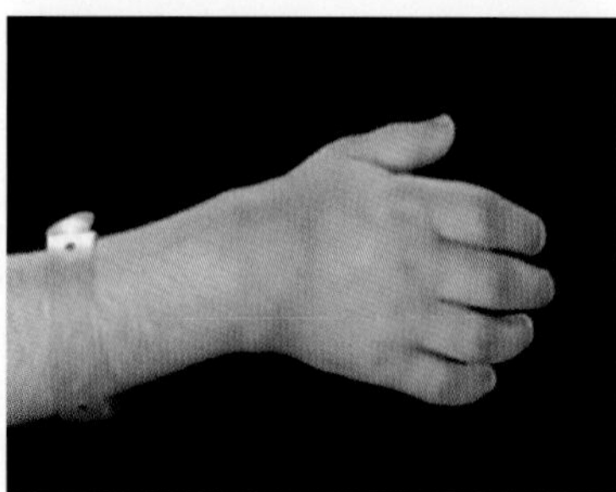

Fig. 149.3 The joints of the wrist and hand of a child with long standing systemic juvenile idiopathic arthritis. The wrist joint, distal interphalangeal joints and metacarpophalangeal joints are swollen, and deformities are noted.

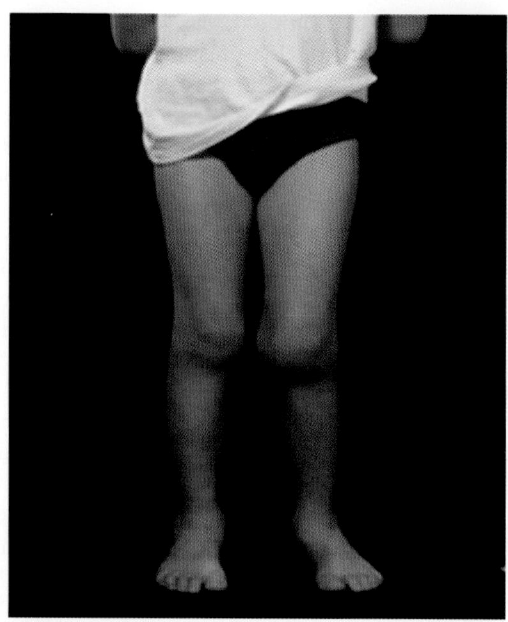

Fig. 149.4 Monoarthritis of the left knee in a child with oligoarticular juvenile idiopathic arthritis

d-dimers and soluble CD25. Classification criteria for MAS associated with sJIA have been recently developed and published by an international expert group [30]; a patient with known or suspected sJIA is classified as having MAS based on raised ferritin higher than 684 ng/mL and two of the following: platelet count ≤181 × 10^9/L, AST >48/litre, triglycerides >156 mg/dL, fibrinogen ≤360 mg/dL [30]. From the 1950s to the 1960s, amyloidosis was the major complication and the main cause of death in this disease. Approximately 10% of sJIA patients develop this complication [31,32]. Interestingly, polymorphisms in perforin or *UNC13D* genes have been shown to increase susceptibility to MAS in sJIA patients [33,34].

Oligoarthritis

This is the most common form of JIA in children, comprising approximately 50–60% of all JIA cases [2]. Sufferers have four or fewer joints involved at onset (Fig. 149.4) [1]. Approximately 20% of these children have more joints involved in the next year or so (classified as extended oligoarthritis) [1,2]. The rest of the group has a better prognosis and the condition is called 'persistent oligoarthritis' [1]. Anterior uveitis has been found associated with this form, in particular in younger children, typically girls around the age of 2–3 years in Europe and North America, with a positive antinuclear antibody (ANA) as an associated marker [35, 36]. This is not seen in other ethnic groups, such as Costa Ricans, Orientals and African black people [35,36]. Typically, the course of persistent oligoarthritis is mild and remits within 2–3 years. The course of uveitis is independent of arthritis and can continue into adulthood. The extended oligoarthritis patients have a more prolonged disease course, similar to the form or polyarthritis.

Polyarthritis, rheumatoid factor negative

This group is heterogenous, with one subgroup of patients with onset of the disease at a young age and similarities to oligoarthritis patients, in that they are often associated with uveitis and are positive for ANA [2]. A second subgroup presents at a school age, is ANA negative and shares similarities to the adult rheumatoid arthritis [2].

Polyarthritis, rheumatoid factor positive

This is a small group of polyarthritis patients with symptoms that resemble adult rheumatoid arthritis in presentation, affecting mainly preteen and teenage girls [2,37]. Young-onset polyarthritis patients are rarely rheumatoid factor positive and these patients often convert, in later years, to RF-negative polyarthritis.

Enthesitis-related arthritis

This group is characterized by the presence of enthesitis and arthritis affecting, predominantly, the lower limb joints in boys of preteen years [1,38]. The distribution of the arthritis is usually asymmetrical at onset and HLA-B27 is often positive in the Caucasian population [38,39]. A proportion of patients develop sacroiliitis at puberty and becomes true ankylosing spondylitis in late teenage and adulthood [39].

Psoriatic arthritis

The distinguishing features of this group are the characteristic pattern of joint involvement, dactylitis, asymmetrical involvement of large and small joints and the presence of psoriasis, either in the patient or a first-degree relative [39,40].

Differential diagnosis. The differential diagnosis of oligoarticular JIA includes septic arthritis, reactive arthritis, foreign body synovitis, pigmented villonodular synovitis, arterial–venous malformation, trauma or haemophilia. Polyarthritis needs to be differentiated from conditions such as infection, inflammatory bowel disease, lymphoma, leukaemia or viral synovitis lasting longer than 6 weeks. Box 149.1 summarizes the differential diagnosis of juvenile idiopathic arthritis.

The diagnosis of sJIA is a clinical diagnosis and based on excluding other conditions which can have a similar presentation. Especially at onset when the child can have systemic features but no arthritis, the diagnosis may be difficult and it is very important to rule out infections, other systemic inflammatory conditions or malignancy. Box 149.3 summarizes the differential diagnosis of sJIA.

Laboratory findings. Polyarthritis may be associated with elevated acute phase reactants and mild anaemia of chronic disease. The ANA are positive in up to 40% and the RF is positive or negative [43]. Oligoarthritis is usually associated with a normal or only mildly elevated ESR and sometimes positive ANA. The laboratory findings of sJIA reflect the ongoing systemic inflammatory response, with high white cell count, thrombocytosis, elevated ESR and CRP, moderately elevated ferritin, fibrinogen and complement, and anaemia. Myeloid-related proteins 8 and 14 (MRP-8/MRP-14) have been suggested as useful biomarkers in distinguishing between sJIA and infections or other conditions presenting with systemic inflammation [44].

Box 149.3 Differential diagnosis of systemic juvenile idiopathic arthritis [25,41,42]

1. Infections
   - Bacterial endocarditis
   - Acute rheumatic fever
   - Cat scratch disease *(Bartonella)*
   - Lyme disease *(Borrelia burgdorferi)*
   - Brucellosis, mycoplasma
2. Other rheumatic and inflammatory conditions
   - Systemic lupus erythematosus
   - Polyarteritis nodosa
   - Kawasaki disease
   - Serum sickness
   - Sarcoidosis
   - Castleman disease
3. Autoinflammatory conditions including NLRC4 mutation
   - Mevalonate kinase deficiency (mevalonic aciduria and hyperimmunoglobulin D syndrome)
   - Rheumatic fever
   - TNF receptor-associated periodic syndrome (TRAPS)
   - Muckle–Wells syndrome
   - Chronic infantile neurological cutaneous and articular syndrome (CINCA)
4. Malignancy
5. Inflammatory bowel disease
6. Primary haemophagocytic lymphohistiocytosis

Treatment and prevention. In terms of management, it is imperative to control the disease early and as quickly as possible to prevent cumulative side-effects and complications from the disease process. Until recently, the management of JIA relied on nonsteroidal anti-inflammatory drugs, corticosteroids and methotrexate.

The era of biologic therapies

The major new revolution in the management of JIA has been the advent of biologic therapies, developed to block specific targets of the inflammatory response. Used successfully in patients failing conventional disease-modifying antirheumatic drugs (DMARD), their benefit has a led to a shift in the paradigm of therapy for JIA [2]. Table 149.1 summarizes the biologic agents currently used to treat JIA in children. Etanercept (soluble TNF p75 receptor fusion protein) has become an established part of managing JIA based on double-blind controlled trials of its efficacy in treating the disease [45–49]. Other agents include infliximab (chimeric human/mouse monoclonal antibody that binds to soluble TNF-α), adalimumab (humanized immunoglobulin G1 monoclonal antibody that binds to TNF-α) and abatacept (soluble fully human fusion protein of cytotoxic T lymphocyte antigen 4, CTLA-4). Tocilizumab, anakinra and canakinumab are other biologic therapies for sJIA.

The drug management of polyarticular JIA is with methotrexate, given as a single weekly dose of 15 mg/m^2, often as a subcutaneous injection owing to better absorption profiles [37]. About 30% fail to respond to methotrexate and anti-TNF agents (etanercept, infliximab) are added. There is strong evidence to support the efficacy and safety of biologic agents over the short-term in juvenile arthritis with polyarticular course, with randomized clinical trials for etanercept, infliximab, adalimumab, abatacept and anakinra in polyarticular JIA, and one each looking at etanercept or infliximab as first-line therapies [50]. Long-term data is available for etanercept, but for other treatments it is sparse [46,48,49].

Sulphasalazine has been shown to be efficacious in enthesitis-related arthritis, but not long lasting, whereas methotrexate is effective in all ages. Anti-TNF therapy is effective in those who fail to respond completely to methotrexate [45].

As mentioned earlier in this chapter, novel therapies targeting key pathogenic molecules in sJIA have been explored in recent years, and biologic agents that inhibit IL-1 and IL-6 have already changed the approach to the treatment of sJIA. Two phase II and two phase III clinical trials of the use of tocilizumab, a humanized recombinant anti-IL-6 receptor antibody, in patients with sJIA have shown that tocilizumab is effective, and improved symptoms and laboratory markers [18,51–55]. Furthermore, anakinra, an IL-1 receptor antagonist, has

Table 149.1 Biologic agents used for the treatment of juvenile idiopathic arthritis

Biologic agent	Mode of action	Route of administration	Indication	Studies
Abatacept	Humanized selective T-cell costimulatory modulator	IV infusion	Polyarticular-JIA; JIA- associated uveitis	[57,58]
Adalimumab	Humanized soluble anti-TNF monoclonal antibody	SC	Polyarticular-JI, JIA-associated uveitis, systemic vasculitis	[59,60]
Anakinra	Humanized anti-IL-1 receptor antagonist	SC	SJIA	[18,61]
Canakinumab	Human anti-IL-1b monoclonal antibody	SC	SJIA	[51]
Etanercept	Human TNF receptor p75 Fc fusion protein	SC	Polyarticular-JIA, ERA, PsA, extended oligo JIA	[45,46,47,48,62,63]
Infliximab	Chimeric human–murine anti-TNF IgG1 monoclonal antibody	IV infusion	Polyarticular-JIA, JIA associated uveitis, PsA, ERA	[64,65,66]
Rituximab	Chimeric anti-CD20 monoclonal antibody	IV infusion	SJIA, refractory polyarticular JIA,	[67,68]
Tocilizumab	Humanized recombinant anti-IL-6 receptor monoclonal antibody	IV infusion	SJIA, refractory polyarticular-JIA	[51–55,68,69]
Certolizumab	Polyethylene glycolated Fab fragment of a humanized anti-TNF-α antibody	SC	Polyarticular-JIA	[65,70]
Golimumab	Humanized monoclonal anti-TNF-α antibody	SC	Refractory polyarticular JIA	[65,70]

ERA, enthesitis-related arthritis; IV, intravenous; JIA, juvenile idiopathic arthritis; PsA, psoriatic arthritis; SC, subcutaneous; SJIA, systemic juvenile idiopathic arthritis; TNF, tumour necrosis factor.

been shown to be effective in some patients with sJIA, resulting in resolution of systemic and articular symptoms [18]. Other IL-1 antagonists such as the fully human anti-IL-1β antibody canakinumab have shown convincing benefits in placebo-controlled clinical trial [56].

Other treatment and management

Physiotherapy has a major role in maintaining joint function and muscle tone during the active disease stage. This includes weight-bearing exercises because it has been shown that, if the child is not weight bearing and has hip disease, the acetabulae do not develop normally [71]. Intra-articular steroid therapy has been a major advance in recent years and early intervention with intra-articular steroids would be highly desirable, especially in joints such as the hip. If there are radiological changes already in the hip joint affecting the bones, intra-articular steroids could accelerate avascular necrosis. When physiotherapy and exercise fail to prevent deformity of the joints, surgical release of muscle spasm and later joint replacement therapy are all options in further management. Splinting of joints in positions of function is vital during the acute disease phase. Involvement of a podiatrist in correcting hindfoot deformity is important for normal growth of the tibia to prevent tibial torsion as well as abnormal development of the forefoot. A multidisciplinary team approach, including psychosocial input, is critical to maintain the child's development and quality of life.

References

1 **Petty RE, Southwood TR, Manners P et al. and International League of Associations for Rheumatology. International League of Associations for Rheumatology classification of juvenile idiopathic arthritis: second revision, Edmonton, 2001. J Rheumatol 2004;31;390–2**

2 **Ravelli A, Martini A. Juvenile idiopathic arthritis. Lancet 2007; 369:767–78**

3 Symmons DP, Jones M, Osborne J et al. Pediatric rheumatology in the United Kingdom: data from the British Pediatric Rheumatology Group National Diagnostic Register. J Rheumatol 1996;23:1975–80

4 TA Griffin, MG Barnes, NT Ilowite et al. Gene expression signatures in polyarticular juvenile idiopathic arthritis demonstrate disease heterogeneity and offer a molecular classification of disease subsets. Arthritis Rheum 2009; 60:2113–23.

5 Prahalad S, Ryan MH, Shear ES et al. Twins concordant for juvenile rheumatoid arthritis. Arthritis Rheum 2000;43:2611–12.

6 Thompson SD, Moroldo MB, Guyer L et al. A genome-wide scan for juvenile rheumatoid arthritis in affected sibpair families provides evidence of linkage. Arthritis Care Res 2004;50:2920–30.

7 Thomson W, Donn R. Genetic epidemiology: juvenile idiopathic arthritis genetics – What's new? What's next? Arthritis Res 2004; 4:302.

8 **Hinks A, Cobb J, Marion MC et al.; Boston Children's JIA Registry; British Society of Paediatric and Adolescent Rheumatology (BSPAR) Study Group; Childhood Arthritis Prospective Study (CAPS); Childhood Arthritis Response to Medication Study (CHARMS); German Society for Pediatric Rheumatology (GKJR); JIA Gene Expression Study; NIAMS JIA Genetic Registry; TREAT Study; United Kingdom Juvenile Idiopathic Arthritis Genetics Consortium (UKJIAGC), Bohnsack JF, Haas JP, Glass DN et al. Dense genotyping of immune-related disease regions identifies 14 new susceptibility loci for juvenile idiopathic arthritis. Nat Genet. 2013 Jun;45:664–9.**

9 Prahalad S, Glass DN. A comprehensive review of the genetics of juvenile idiopathic arthritis. Pediatr Rheumatol Online J 2008;6:11.

10 Angeles-Han S, Prahalad S. The genetics of juvenile idiopathic arthritis: what is new in 2010. Curr Rheumatol Rep 2010;12:87–93.

11 **Hersh AO, Prahalad S. Immunogenetics of juvenile idiopathic arthritis: a comprehensive review. J Autoimmun 2015;64:113–24.**

12 Thomson W, Barrett JH, Donn R et al. Juvenile idiopathic arthritis classified by the ILAR criteria: HLA associations in UK patients. Rheumatology 2002;41:1183.

13 Vastert SJ, Kuis W, Grom AA. Systemic JIA: new developments in the understanding of the pathophysiology and therapy. Best Pract Res Clin Rheumatol 2009;23:655–64.

14 **Pascual V, Allantaz F, Arce E et al. Role of interleukin-1 (IL-1) in the pathogenesis of systemic onset juvenile idiopathic arthritis and clinical response to IL-1 blockade. J Exp Med 2005;201:1479–86.**

15 **De Benedetti F, Massa M, Pignatti P et al. Serum soluble interleukin 6 (IL-6) receptor and IL-6/soluble IL-6 receptor complex in systemic juvenile rheumatoid arthritis. J Clin Invest 1994;93:2114–19.**

16 De Jager W, Vastert SJ, Beekman JM et al. Defective phosphorylation of interleukin-18 receptor beta causes impaired natural killer cell function in systemic-onset juvenile idiopathic arthritis. Arthritis Rheum 2009;60:2782–93.

17 De Jager W, Hoppenreijs EP, Wulffraat NM et al. Blood and synovial fluid cytokine signatures in patients with juvenile idiopathic arthritis: a cross-sectional study. Ann Rheum Dis 2007;66:589–98.

18 **Quartier P, Allantaz F, Cimaz R et al. A multicentre, randomised, double-blind, placebo-controlled trial with the interleukin-1 receptor antagonist anakinra in patients with systemic-onset juvenile idiopathic arthritis (ANAJIS trial). Ann Rheum Dis 2011;70:747–54.**

19 **De Benedetti F, Brunner HI, Ruperto N et al.; PRINTO; PRCSG. Randomized trial of tocilizumab in systemic juvenile idiopathic arthritis. N Engl J Med 2012;367:2385–95.**

20 Ombrello MJ, Remmers EF, Tachmazidou I et al. HLA-DRB1*11 and variants of the MHC class II locus are strong risk factors for systemic juvenile idiopathic arthritis. Proc Natl Acad Sci U S A 2015; 112:15970–5.

21 Murray KJ, Luyrink L, Grom AA et al. Immunohistological characteristics of T cell infiltrates in different forms of childhood onset chronic arthritis. J Rheumatol 1996;23:2116.

22 Gregorio A, Gambini C, Gerloni V et al. Lymphoid neogenesis in juvenile idiopathic arthritis correlates with ANA positivity and plasma cells infiltration. Rheumatology 2007;46:308.

23 Nistala K, Moncrieffe H, Newton KR et al. Interleukin-17-producing T cells are enriched in the joints of children with arthritis, but have a reciprocal relationship to regulatory T cell numbers. Arthritis Rheum 2008;58:875–87.

24 Hunter PJ, Nistala K, Jina N et al. Biologic predictors of extension of oligoarticular juvenile idiopathic arthritis as determined from synovial fluid cellular composition and gene expression. Arthritis Rheum 2010;62:896–907

25 **De Benedetti F, Schneider R. Systemic juvenile idiopathic arthritis In: Petty RE, Laxer RM, Lindsley CB, Wedderburn LR (eds) Textbook of Pediatric Rheumatology, 7th edn. Philadelphia: Saunders Elsevier, 2016.**

26 Symmons DP, Jones M, Osborne J et al. Pediatric rheumatology in the United Kingdom: data from the British Pediatric Rheumatology Group National Diagnostic Register. J Rheumatol 1996;23:1975–80.

27 Behrens EM, Beukelman T, Gallo L et al. Evaluation of the presentation of systemic onset juvenile rheumatoid arthritis: data from the Pennsylvania systemic onset juvenile arthritis registry (PASOJAR). J Rheumatol 2008;35:343–8.

28 Schneider R, Laxer RM. Systemic onset juvenile rheumatoid arthritis. Baillieres Clin Rheumatol 1998;12:245–71.

29 Ravelli A. Macrophage activation syndrome. Curr Opin Rheumatol 2002;14:548–52.

30 **Ravelli A, Minoia F, Davì S et al.; Paediatric Rheumatology International Trials Organisation, the Childhood Arthritis and Rheumatology Research Alliance, the Pediatric Rheumatology Collaborative Study Group, and the Histiocyte Society. 2016 Classification Criteria for Macrophage Activation Syndrome Complicating Systemic Juvenile Idiopathic Arthritis: A European League Against Rheumatism/American College of Rheumatology/ Paediatric Rheumatology International Trials Organisation Collaborative Initiative. Ann Rheum Dis 2016;75:481–9.**

31 Schnitzer TJ, Ansell BM. Amyloidosis in juvenile chronic polyarthritis. Arthritis Rheum 1997;20:245.

32 Stoeber E. Prognosis in juvenile chronic arthritis. Follow-up of 433 chronic rheumatic children. Eur J Pediatr 1981;135:225.

33 Vastert SJ, van Wijk R, D'Urbano LE et al. Mutations in the perforin gene can be linked to macrophage activation syndrome in patients with systemic onset juvenile idiopathic arthritis. Rheumatology (Oxford) 2010;49:441–9.

34 Hazen MM, Woodward AL, Hofmann I et al. Mutations of the hemophagocytic lymphohistiocytosis-associated gene UNC13D in a patient with systemic juvenile idiopathic arthritis. Arthritis Rheum 2008;58:567–70.

35 Sen ES, Dick AD, Ramanan AV. Uveitis associated with juvenile idiopathic arthritis. Nat Rev Rheumatol 2015;11:338–48.

36 **Petty RE, Lindsley CB. Oligoarticular juvenile idiopathic arthritis. In: Petty RE, Laxer RM, Lindsley CB, Wedderburn LR (eds) Textbook of Pediatric Rheumatology, 7th edn. Philadelphia: Saunders Elsevier, 2016.**

37 **Rosenberg AM, Oen KG. Polyarticular juvenile idiopathic arthritis. In: Petty RE, Laxer RM, Lindsley CB, Wedderburn LR (eds) Textbook of Pediatric Rheumatology, 7th edn. Philadelphia: Saunders Elsevier, 2016.**

38 **Tse SML, Petty RE. Enthesitis related arthritis. In: Petty RE, Laxer RM, Lindsley CB, Wedderburn LR (eds) Textbook of Pediatric** Rheumatology, 7th edn. Philadelphia: Saunders Elsevier, 2016.

39 Ramanathan A, Srinivasalu H, Colbert RA. Update on juvenile spondyloarthritis. Rheum Dis Clin North Am 2013;39:767–88.

40 **Nigrovic PA, Sundel RP. Juvenile psoriatic arthritis. In: Petty RE, Laxer RM, Lindsley CB, Wedderburn LR (eds) Textbook of Pediatric Rheumatology, 7th edn. Philadelphia: Saunders Elsevier, 2016.**

41 Canna SW, de Jesus AA, Gouni S et al. An activating NLRC4 inflammasome mutation causes autoinflammation with recurrent macrophage activation syndrome. Nat Genet 2014;46:1140–6.

42 **Grom AA, Horne A, De Benedetti F. Macrophage activation syndrome in the era of biologic therapy. Nat Rev Rheumatol 2016;12:259–68.**

43 **Petty RE, Laxer RM, Wedderburn LR. Juvenile idiopathic arthritis. In: Petty RE, Laxer RM, Lindsley CB, Wedderburn LR (eds) Textbook of Pediatric Rheumatology, 7th edn. Philadelphia: Saunders Elsevier, 2016.**

44 Frosch M, Ahlmann M, Vogl T et al. The myeloid-related proteins 8 and 14 complex, a novel ligand of toll-like receptor 4, and interleukin-1beta form a positive feedback mechanism in systemic-onset juvenile idiopathic arthritis, Arthritis Rheum 2009;60:883–91.

45 **Horneff G, Foeldvari I, Minden K et al. Efficacy and safety of etanercept in patients with the enthesitis-related arthritis category of juvenile idiopathic arthritis: results from a phase III randomized, double-blind study. Arthritis Rheumatol 2015;67:2240–9.**

46 Lovell DJ, Reiff A, Jones OY et al. Pediatric Rheumatology Collaborative Study Group. Long-term safety and efficacy of etanercept in children with polyarticular-course juvenile rheumatoid arthritis. Arthritis Rheum 2006;54:1987–94.

47 **Lovell DJ, Giannini EH, Reiff A et al. Etanercept in children with polyarticular juvenile rheumatoid arthritis. Pediatric Rheumatology Collaborative Study Group. N Engl J Med 2000;342:763–9.**

48 Prince FH, Twilt M, Cate R et al. Long-term follow-up on effectiveness and safety of etanercept in juvenile idiopathic arthritis: the Dutch national register. Ann Rheum Dis 2009;68:635–41.

49 Lovell DJ, Reiff A, Ilowite NT et al. Pediatric Rheumatology Collaborative Study Group. Safety and efficacy of up to eight years of continuous etanercept therapy in patients with juvenile rheumatoid arthritis. Arthritis Rheum 2008;58:1496–504.

50 **Ungar W, Costa V, Burnett HF et al. The use of biologic response modifiers in polyarticular course juvenile idiopathic arthriits: a systematic review. Sem Arth Rheum 2013;42:597–618.**

51 Yokota S, Miyamae T, Imagawa T et al. Therapeutic efficacy of humanized recombinant anti-interleukin-6 receptor antibody in children with systemic-onset juvenile idiopathic arthritis. Arthritis Rheum 2005;52:818–25.

52 Yokota S, Miyamae T, Imagawa T et al. Clinical study of tocilizumab in children with systemic-onset juvenile idiopathic arthritis. Clin Rev Allergy Immunol 2005;28:231–8.

53 **Woo P, Wilkinson N, Prieur AM et al. Open label phase II trial of single, ascending doses of MRA in Caucasian children with severe systemic juvenile idiopathic arthritis: proof of principle of the efficacy of IL-6 receptor blockade in this type of arthritis and demonstration of prolonged clinical improvement. Arthritis Res Ther 2005;7:R1281–8.**

54 **Yokota S, Imagawa T, Mori M et al. Efficacy and safety of tocilizumab in patients with systemic-onset juvenile idiopathic arthritis: a randomised, double-blind, placebo-controlled, withdrawal phase III trial. Lancet 2008;371:998–1006.**

55 Yokota S, Kishimoto T. Tocilizumab: molecular intervention therapy in children with systemic juvenile idiopathic arthritis. Expert Rev Clin Immunol 2010;6:735–43.

56 **Ruperto N, Brunner HI, Quartier P et al. Two randomized trials of canakinumab in systemic juvenile idiopathic arthritis. N Engl J Med 2012;367:2396–406.**

57 **Ruperto N et al Abatacept in children with JIA – a randomised, double-blind, placebo-controlled withdrawal trial. Lancet 2008;372:383–91.**

58 Tappeiner C, Miserocchi E, Bodaghi B et al. Abatacept in the treatment of severe, longstanding, and refractory uveitis associated with juvenile idiopathic arthritis. J Rheumatol 2015;42:706–11.

59 **Lovell DJ, Ruperto N, Goodman S et al.; Pediatric Rheumatology Collaborative Study Group; Pediatric Rheumatology International Trials Organisation. Adalimumab with or without methotrexate in juvenile rheumatoid arthritis. N Engl J Med 2008;359:810–20.**

60 Castiblanco C, Meese H, Foster CS. Treatment of pediatric uveitis with adalimumab: the MERSI experience. J AAPOS 2016;20:145–7.

61 **Nigrovic PA, Mannion M, Prince FH et al. Anakinra as first-line disease-modifying therapy in systemic juvenile idiopathic arthritis: report of forty-six patients from an international multicenter series. Arthritis Rheum 2011;63:545–55**

62 **Wallace CA, Giannini EH, Spalding SJ et al.; Childhood Arthritis and Rheumatology Research Alliance. Trial of early aggressive**

therapy in polyarticular juvenile idiopathic arthritis. Arthritis Rheum 2012;64:2012–21.

63 Shenoi S, Wallace CA. Tumor necrosis factor inhibitors in the management of juvenile idiopathic arthritis: an evidence-based review. Paediatr Drugs 2010;12:367–77.

64 Ruperto N, Lovell DJ, Cuttica R et al. A randomized, placebo-controlled trial of infliximab plus methotrexate for the treatment of poly-articular-course juvenile rheumatoid arthritis. Arthritis Rheum 2007;56:3096–106.

65 Papadopoulou C, Eleftheriou D. How do I ensure safe use of biological agents in children and adolescents with rheumatic diseases? Paediatr Child Health 2015;24:264–8.

66 Hawkins MJ, Dick AD, Lee RJ et al. Managing juvenile idiopathic arthritis-associated uveitis. Surv Ophthalmol 2016;61:197–210.

67 Cohen SB, Emery P, Greenwald MW et al. Rituximab for rheumatoid arthritis refractory to anti-TNF: results of a randomized placebo-controlled double blind trial. Arthritis Rheum 2006;54:2793–806.

68 England N. Interim Clinical Commissioning Policy Statement: Biologic Therapies for the treatment of Juvenile Idiopathic Arthritis (JIA). 2015. Available from: https://www.engage.england.nhs.uk/consultation/specialised-services-policies/user_uploads/biolgcs-juvenl-idiop-arthrs-pol.pdf.

69 Brunner HI, Ruperto N, Zuber Z et al.; Paediatric Rheumatology International Trials Organisation PRINTO; Pediatric Rheumatology Collaborative Study Group (PRCSG). Efficacy and safety of tocilizumab in patients with polyarticular-course juvenile idiopathic arthritis: results from a phase 3, randomised, double-blind withdrawal trial. Ann Rheum Dis 2015;74:1110–7.

70 Webb K, Wedderburn LR. Advances in the treatment of polyarticular juvenile idiopathic arthritis. Curr Opin Rheumatol 2015;27:505–10.

71 McCullough CJ. Surgical management of the hip in juvenile chronic arthritis. Rheumatology 1994;33:178.

Systemic lupus erythematosus

Introduction. Systemic lupus erythematosus (SLE) is a severe, chronic, autoimmune disease, characterized by the presence of autoantibodies, which results in multiorgan inflammation and eventual damage [1]. When the disease presents in patients younger than 16 years old it is commonly referred to as juvenile SLE (JSLE) [2]. The dermatitis of SLE was described as early as the thirteenth century, the butterfly rash was recognized in 1845, and 7 years later the term *lupus erythemateux* was proposed [1].

Epidemiology and classification. JSLE is a rare disease, with an incidence of 10–20 in 100 000 Caucasian children [2]. The male:female ratio varies between 1:2 and 1:4.5 for the ages of 6 and 18 years, and the variation probably reflects racial differences in the population of the various reported epidemiological studies [1,3]. Similar to the adult disease, the incidence and prevalence rates are higher in Hispanic, Afro-Caribbean and South Asian populations. The diagnosis of SLE, whether affecting an adult or a child, is made based on a combination of clinical and laboratory features. The 1997 revised American College of Rheumatology (ACR) classification criteria [4] are commonly used by rheumatologists to diagnosis SLE, although these criteria were not specifically developed as diagnostic criteria (Box 149.4). Ferraz and colleagues examined the sensitivity and specificity of these criteria in a group of 103 paediatric patients with SLE and 101 children with other rheumatic diseases [5]. This group found that the most common criteria were positive ANA, arthritis, immunological disorder, haematological disorder, malar rash and photosensitivity. Sensitivity was 96% and specificity was 100% in this analysis [5]. In 2012, the Systemic Lupus International Collaborating Clinics (SLICC) classification criteria were introduced [6], and they have now surpassed the ACR classification criteria (Box 149.5). The performance of the new SLICC criteria in the paediatric population has been evaluated in a multicentre study and they have demonstrated a better sensitivity but a lower specificity compared with the ACR criteria [7].

Box 149.4 Revised criteria (1997) of the American College of Rheumatology for the 1982 classification of systemic lupus erythematosus (SLE) [4]

1. Malar rash
2. Discoid rash
3. Photosensitivity
4. Oral ulcers
5. Arthritis
6. Serositis:
   - Pleuritis or
   - Pericarditis
7. Renal disorder:
   - Proteinuria >0.5 g/24 h, or 3+ on urine dipstick
   - Cellular casts
8. Neurological disorders:
   - Seizures
   - Psychosis
9. Haematological disorders:
   - Haemolytic anaemia
   - Leucopenia $<4 \times 10^9$/L
   - Lymphopenia $<1.5 \times 10^9$/L on two or more occasions
   - Thrombocytopenia $<100 \times 10^9$/L
10. Immunological disorders:
    - Positive lupus erythematosus cell
    - Raised anti-DNA
    - Anti-Sm antibody
    - False-positive test for syphilis, present for 6 months
11. ANA in raised titre

The proposed classification is based on 11 criteria; disease is classified as SLE if any four or more of the 11 criteria are present simultaneously or not. ANA, antinuclear antibodies.

Pathogenesis. The pathogenesis of SLE is complex and not fully elucidated. SLE is likely to be the result of environmental factors such as exposure to sunlight, infections, drugs and chemicals in a genetically susceptible individual. Understanding the pathogenesis of SLE remains a considerable challenge. Both the innate and adaptive immune system have been described to be defective and, furthermore, immunological dysfunction precedes clinical presentation by many years [8]. In a small subgroup, SLE is associated with complement deficiencies and these patients are unable to handle immune complexes in an efficient manner [8]. Deficiency in the early components of the classic complement pathway is characteristically, but not always, associated with this disease. In particular, deficiencies in the C4A, C4B and C2 genes and some deficiency of the late components of complement (C6, C7) also manifest as lupus syndrome,

Box 149.5 Systemic Lupus International Collaborating Clinics (SLICC) classification criteria [6]

Clinical criteria

1. Acute or subacute cutaneous lupus
2. Chronic cutaneous lupus
3. Oral/nasal ulcers
4. Nonscarring alopecia
5. Inflammatory synovitis with physician-observed swelling of two or more joints *or* tender joints with morning stiffness
6. Serositis
7. Renal: urine protein/creatinine (or 24 h urine protein) representing at least 500 mg of protein/24 h or red blood cell casts
8. Neurological: seizures, psychosis, mononeuritis multiplex, myelitis, peripheral or cranial neuropathy, cerebritis (acute confusional state)
9. Haemolytic anaemia
10. Leucopenia (<4000/mm^3 at least once) *or* Lymphopenia (<1000/mm^3 at least once)
11. Thrombocytopenia (<100 000/mm^3) at least once

Immunological criteria

1. ANA above laboratory reference range
2. Anti-dsDNA above laboratory reference range (except ELISA: twice above laboratory reference range)
3. Anti-Sm
4. Antiphospholipid antibody (lupus anticoagulant, false-positive test for syphilis, anticardiolipin – at least twice normal or medium-high titre, anti-b2 glycoprotein 1)
5. Low complement (low C3, low C4, low CH50)
6. Direct Coombs test in absence of haemolytic anaemia

Criteria need not be present concurrently. A patient is classified as having SLE if the patient satisfies four of the criteria listed above, including at least one clinical criterion and one immunological criterion, *or* if the patient has biopsy-proven nephritis compatible with SLE and with ANA or anti-dsDNA antibodies.

ANA, antinuclear antibodies; anti-dsDNA, anti-double stranded DNA antibodies.

Source: Adapted from Petri et al. 2012 [6]. Reproduced with permission of John Wiley & Sons.

although the latter are usually associated more with susceptibility to *Neisseria* infections [8]. These complement-deficient patients often do not have high-titre ANA or double-stranded DNA antibodies. The majority of SLE patients, however, do have the characteristic antibodies as defined by the ACR criteria. Monoclonal anti-DNA antibodies have been found and cloned and shown to produce lupus nephritis in the severe combined immunodeficient (SCID) mouse [9]. In the last decade, our understanding of the genetic basis of SLE has rapidly improved through GWAS, which have identified over 40 susceptibility loci associated with SLE [10]. Most of these associated genes have roles in important pathways involved in the pathogenesis of SLE, such as immune complex processing, toll-like receptor signalling and type I interferon production [10]. SLE is strongly associated with HLA haplotypes such as class II HLA antigen DR3, the autoimmune haplotype DR3, C4QO and TNF-α2 polymorphisms [11]. In terms of contribution to environmental factors to the development of lupus, *in vitro* studies have revealed that exposure of keratinocytes to UV radiation (known to exacerbate skin or systemic disease in patients) leads to apoptosis, allowing membrane blebs containing self-antigens to appear on the cell surface and possibly lead to an autoimmune response [1]. Exposure to viruses, and in particular Epstein–Barr virus (EBV), has been suggested as a mechanism leading to lupus based on studies showing a higher exposure to EBV in SLE patients compared with controls, and uncontrolled reactivation of EBV as a mechanism for pathogenesis of the disease [12]. JSLE is recognized to have a more severe phenotype than adult-onset SLE, possibly caused by a greater contribution of genetic aetiological factors [13]. Next generation sequencing, a revolution in the field of molecular medicine, has led to the discovery of new monogenic causes of SLE, including: complement deficiencies, defects of apoptosis and genetic overproduction of interferon-α [13,14].

Clinical features. The clinical signs and symptoms of JSLE are summarized in Table 149.2. JSLE has more severe features at onset, and in addition there is significantly greater disease activity, accrued damage over time and mortality rates compared with adult disease [15]. Children with JSLE often present with constitutional symptoms such as fever, weight loss, diffuse hair loss, fatigue, generalized lymphadenopathy and hepatosplenomegaly, in addition to manifestations of specific organ involvement. Mucocutaneous, musculoskeletal and renal disease are the most common manifestations of paediatric lupus [1,16,17].

Table 149.2 Clinical features of juvenile systemic lupus erythematosus

Clinical signs/ symptoms	Within first year of diagnosis	At any time
Fever	35–90%	37–100%
Lymphadenopathy	11–45%	13–45%
Hepatosplenomegaly	16–42%	19–43%
Weight loss	20–30%	21–32%
Arthritis	60–88%	60–90%
Myositis	<5%	<5%
Any skin involvement	60–80%	60–90%
Malar rash	22–68%	30–80%
Discoid rash	<5%	<5%
Photosensitivity	12–45%	17–58%
Mucosal ulceration	25–32%	30–40%
Alopecia	10–30%	15–35%
Other rashes	40–52%	42–55%
Nephritis	20–80%	48–100%
Neuropsychiatric disease	5–30%	15–95%
Cardiovascular disease	5–30%	25–60%
Pulmonary disease	18–40%	18–81%
Gastrointestinal disease	14–30%	24–40%

Source: Adapted from Petty RE, Laxer RM, Lindsley CB, Wedderburn LR (eds) Textbook of Pediatric Rheumatology, 7th edn. Philadelphia: Saunders Elsevier, 2016.

Musculoskeletal disease

Arthritis and arthralgia are the most common symptoms in childhood and adolescent SLE, occurring in 60–90% of patients and commonly within the first year of disease [1,16]. This is usually a symmetrical polyarthritis and/or tenosynovitis affecting small peripheral joints, is episodic and generally less painful compared with the arthritis of JIA. Only 1–2% of patients have destructive radiographic changes [2]. There have been descriptions of conversion from systemic or polyarticular JIA to SLE [1]. Myalgia can be present in up to 30% of cases, but only fewer than 5% will have true myositis. The presence of myositis, in the context of skin involvement, makes it very difficult to distinguish it clinically from juvenile dermatomyositis.

Mucocutaneous involvement

The characteristic 'butterfly' rash of SLE is maculopapular in a malar distribution and it extends over the bridge of the nose with sparing of the nasolabial folds. It is often present on the chin with sparing of the area above the chin, features which help distinguish it from the sunburn rash (Fig. 149.5). The malar rash, present in 22–68% of children at diagnosis, is more common than in adults and it can be severe and photosensitive, but it usually heals without scarring [18]. The only other disease that can present with an identical rash, and is indistinguishable clinically or histologically, is juvenile dermatomyositis. A pink 'discoid-shaped' photosensitive rash can be present and affect parts of the body exposed to sunlight in around 30% of cases, but must be distinguished from the true discoid rash. Discoid lupus rash is very rare in SLE patients under 18 years of age, and it presents as a red, inflamed patch with a scaling and crusty appearance, often on the forehead or scalp, which heals with scarring, atrophy and residual discolouration [15]. Vasculitic rashes are seen in SLE and reported in 10–20% of patients [2,15]. Vasculitis of the skin affects the fingers and toes (Fig. 149.6), is painful, and can cause splinter haemorrhages and digital infarcts (Fig. 149.7). Oral or nasal ulceration can also occur (Fig. 149.8) [1,2,19]; oral changes involve often the hard palate, with erythema, petechial or true ulceration. Raynaud phenomenon, periungual

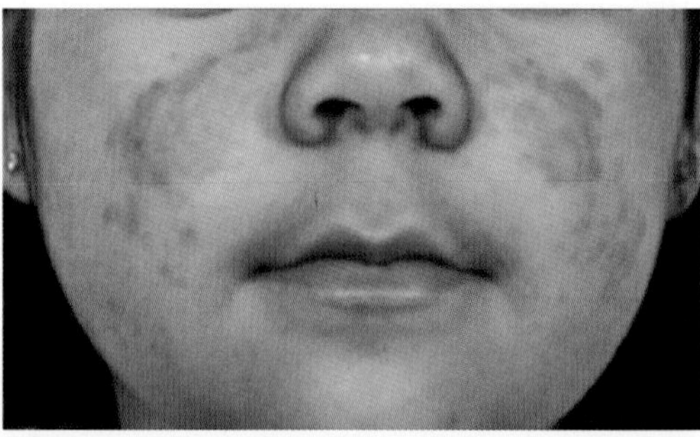

Fig. 149.5 Malar rash of systemic lupus erythematosus showing sparing of the nasolabial folds.

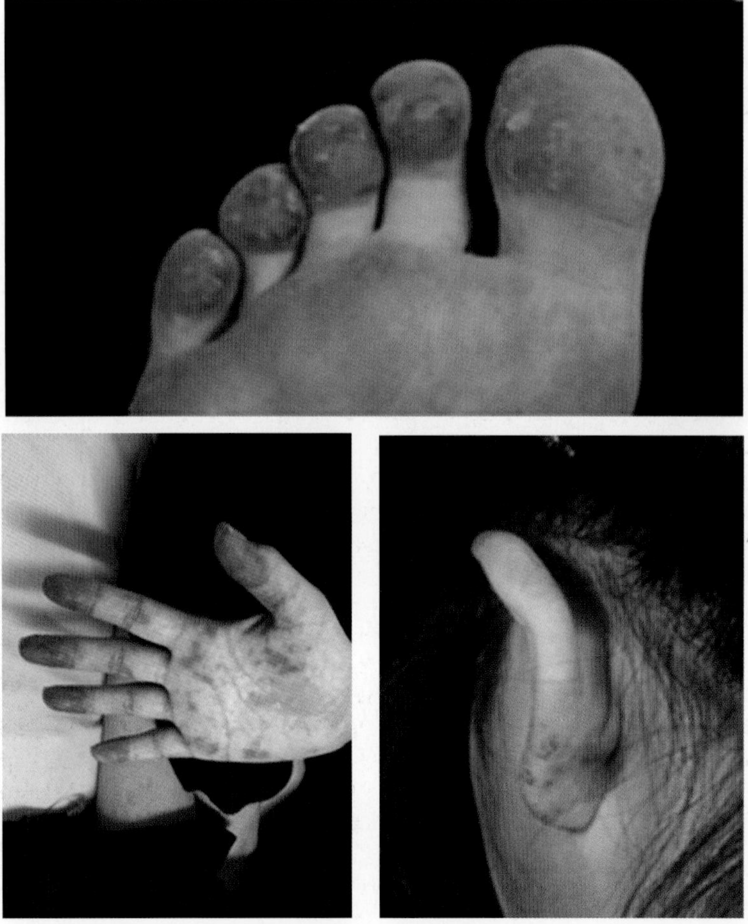

Fig. 149.6 Vasculitic rash of the fingers, palms, toes, earlobe and skin ulceration in a child with systemic lupus erythematosus.

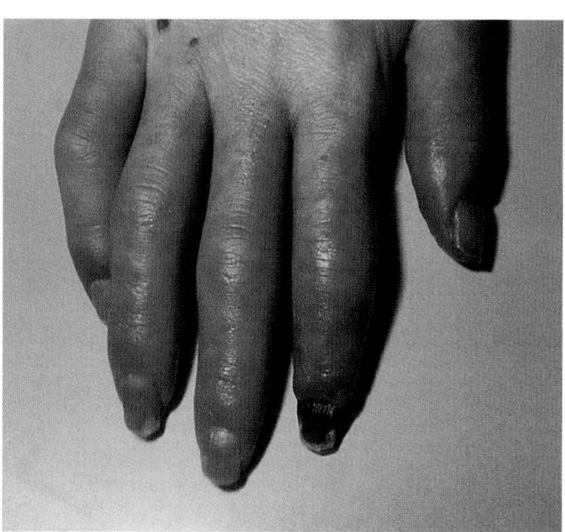

Fig. 149.7 Digital infarcts in systemic lupus erythematosus.

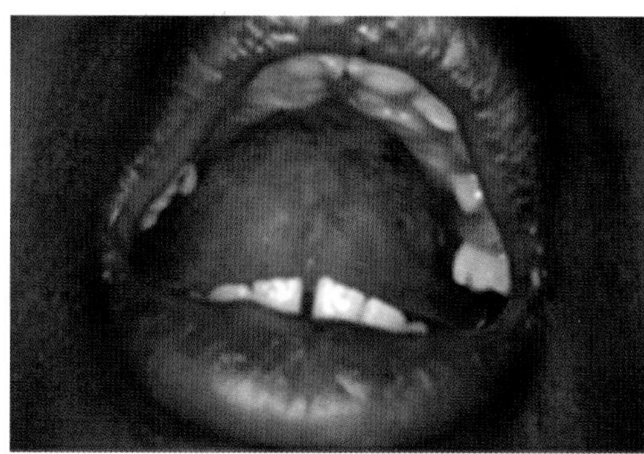

Fig. 149.8 Hard palate ulcers in a patient with systemic lupus erythematosus.

erythema and livedo reticularis can also be present, and other types of rashes have been reported, such as a follicular rash on the arms and trunk and generalized erythematous rash [20].

Neuropsychiatric systemic lupus erythematosus

Central nervous system (CNS) manifestations are a major cause of morbidity and mortality in JSLE [21]. Neuropsychiatric SLE (NP-SLE) encompasses both central and peripheral nervous system involvement and has been reported to occur in 10–95% of patients [16,21]. In 1999, a consensus conference developed the ACR Nomenclature and Case Definitions for Neuropsychiatric Lupus Syndromes and standardized the classification of adult patients with NP-SLE, which is useful for paediatric SLE (Table 149.3) [22]. The most common symptom of NP-SLE is headache, which is severe, unremitting, and occurs in 50–75% of patients [17,21]. Patients can present with affective or mood disorders, which are difficult to differentiate from the effects of steroids or reaction to the illness. Cognitive dysfunction may occur in up to 50% of children with SLE during the disease course, and in 12–30% within the first year of the disease [1]. Seizures occur in 10–15% of cases within the first year of diagnosis and in up to 50% at any time during the disease course. They are easily treatable with anticonvulsants [1]. Chorea is present in approximately 5% of patients and is almost universally associated with the presence of antiphospholipid antibodies [21]. In addition, NP-SLE can present with a spectrum of SLE-associated cerebral blood vessel abnormalities, ranging from inflammation of small arteries to cerebral vein thrombosis particularly in patients with antiphospholipid antibodies [23]. A true angiogram-positive large vessel vasculitis is uncommon but when present tends to present as a stroke [24]. Headaches and seizures are the most common symptoms and signs of CNS vasculitis. Cranial and peripheral neuropathies can occur. Paresis and transverse myelitis can also occur as a result of vasculitis. Magnetic resonance imaging (MRI) is the preferred study in patients with suspected CNS involvement. Lesions seen on MRI are frequently small, multifocal and bilateral with high signal intensity and the white matter is commonly affected [24]. Furthermore, multiple studies have demonstrated an association of anticardiolipin antibodies with CNS and peripheral nervous system disease [25,26]. The presence of antiphospholipid antibodies is associated with headache, cerebral vascular accidents, chorea and transverse myelitis [27].

Table 149.3 The 1999 American College of Rheumatology nomenclature and case definitions for neuropsychiatric systemic lupus erythematosus

Central nervous system	Peripheral nervous system
Aseptic meningitis	Guillain–Barré syndrome
Cerebrovascular disease	Autonomic disorder
Demyelinating syndrome	Mononeuropathy
Headache	Cranial neuropathy
Movement disorder	Myasthenia-like syndrome
Myelopathy	Plexopathy
Seizure disorder	Polyneuropathy
Acute confusional state	
Anxiety disorder	
Cognitive dysfunction	
Mood disorder/depression	
Psychosis	

Renal disease

Kidney disease is present in up to approximately 80% of children with lupus [16,17], and it is associated with significant morbidity and mortality, hence its presence has a major contribution to the choice of therapeutic agent. Clinically significant renal involvement ranges from asymptomatic haematuria or proteinuria to acute nephritic syndrome, nephrotic syndrome, gross haematuria and renal failure [28]. Most children with lupus nephritis present with proteinuria and/or persistent microscopic haematuria. Hypertension has been reported in 40% of patients and half of them have been shown to have reduced renal function [28]. Patients can have an identical clinical presentation and laboratory findings suggestive of renal involvement but the histological pattern can be significantly different, and therefore a renal biopsy is recommended for all patients with evidence of renal involvement. The World Health Organization (WHO) classification of lupus nephritis, introduced in 1974 and revised by the International Society of Nephrology/Renal Pathology Society in 2004, reflects our understanding of

Box 149.6 Abbreviated International Society of Nephrology/Renal Pathology Society (ISN/RPS) classification of lupus nephritis

- Class I: Minimal mesangial lupus nephritis
- Class II: Mesangial proliferative lupus nephritis
- Class III: Focal lupus nephritis[1]
- Class IV: Diffuse segmental (IV-S) or global (IV-G) lupus nephritis[2]
- Class V: Membranous lupus nephritis[3]
- Class VI: Advance sclerosing lupus nephritis

[1] Indicate the proportion of the glomeruli with active and with sclerotic lesions.
[2] Indicate the proportion of glomeruli with fibrinoid necrosis and cellular crescents.
[3] Class V may occur in combination with class III or IV in which case both will be diagnosed.

the pathogenesis of the various forms of renal injury in SLE nephritis [29,30] as summarized in Box 149.6. Renal biopsy is necessary to define the renal pathology and the degree of active and chronic damage.

The most common histopathological findings of lupus glomerulonephritis seen in JSLE are proliferative glomerulonephritis (Classes III and IV), followed by mesangial proliferative glomerulonephritis (Class II) and membranous nephropathy (Class V) [1].

Laboratory findings. SLE is characterized by the presence of autoantibodies; ANA are positive in virtually all lupus patients and anti-dsDNA antibodies are pathognomonic for SLE. Anti-Sm antibodies are also seen in SLE, often in association with anti-RNP; anti-Ro and anti-La are associated with risk of neonatal lupus for the newborn. Characteristically, the ESR is elevated and CRP is low; a raised CRP suggests the presence of serositis or infection. The complement levels (CH50, C4, C3) are low and indicative of disease activity. Haematological manifestations include isolated cytopenias or pancytopenia. Coombs haemolytic anaemia can be present, or a positive Coombs test in the absence of anaemia. The lipid profile in patients with SLE is often abnormal and dyslipidemia can contribute to the development of atherosclerosis in patients with JSLE. Other laboratory tests reflect the pattern of organ involvement and tissue biopsies or imaging can also provide significant information for diagnosis. NP-SLE is associated with the presence of antiphospholipid antibodies, in particular anti-β_2 glycoprotein I (anti-β_2 GPI), whilst lupus anticoagulant is present in patients with cerebral vein thrombosis or chorea.

Treatment. The severity spectrum of SLE is wide. Specific treatment should be individualized and take into consideration the extent and severity of the disease. Corticosteroids remain the backbone of treatment for SLE and are generally the first agents used, together with nonsteroidal anti-inflammatory medication [31]. The steroid dose varies depending on the severity of disease; in severe disease intravenous pulses of methylprednisolone at a dose of 15–30 mg/kg/day (maximum 1 g per dose) are used initially for 3 or more consecutive days, followed by oral steroids in severe disease. Mild disease with symptoms limited to arthralgia, rash or photosensitivity without evidence of significant internal organ involvement may be initially treated with low-dose oral prednisone and hydroxychloroquine [31]. Immunosuppressant medications are used either as a steroid-sparing agent in milder cases of lupus that are steroid dependent, or to improve outcomes in patients with organ involvement such as, for example, renal disease, NP-SLE, or lung disease. Addition of azathioprine is synergistic in the suppression of lupus manifestations, including lupus nephritis [31]. In fulminating lupus nephritis or NP-SLE, intravenous cyclophosphamide is preferred, given at approximately 500–750 mg/m^2/dose, up to a maximum total of 1 g; a total of six intravenous pulse cyclophosphamide doses with the first three given initially fortnightly or 3-weekly, followed by monthly pulses to put the disease into remission [32–34]. Patients then go on to maintenance azathioprine in order to allow further reduction of corticosteroid therapy in the case of remission [31]. Other immunosuppressant agents used for the treatment of adult and paediatric SLE are rituximab (chimeric monoclonal antibody against the protein CD20; B-cell depleting therapy), mycophenolate mofetil (MMF), methotrexate for SLE with arthritis or skin disease as a steroid-sparing agent, or ciclosporin reserved for SLE with membranous nephritis, MAS or severe skin disease refractory to other treatment. Rituximab has been shown to improve outcomes by a number of adult and paediatric studies; however, two randomized controlled trials (RCTs) of rituximab versus placebo ('Explorer' and 'Lunar') perhaps surprisingly failed to meet their endpoints [35,36]. In both RCTs there were no significant differences in outcomes for the experimental and placebo group; however, this could be because of the design of the trials which possibly did not allow for a statistically significant difference in outcomes between the two arms to be identified within the study period [35,36]. Furthermore, recent work has demonstrated that children with SLE respond well to the combination of rituximab and cyclophosphamide, with significant improvement in both systemic disease activity and renal parameters [37,38]. In addition, MMF has been used in lupus nephritis both for the induction phase and in the maintenance of remission. Seven adult clinical trials compared MMF with ciclosporin for the induction of remission in SLE nephritis, showing similar efficacy at 6 months from the initiation of treatment [39]. The paediatric data on the use of MMF have been mainly case reports or small trials of MMF use in SLE reported with promising results [40]. In addition to steroids and immunosuppressant medication, plasmapheresis is reserved for children presenting with very severe disease and devastating acute complications.

References

1 **Silverman ED, Eddy AA. Systemic lupus erythematosus. In: Petty RE, Laxer RM, Lindsley CB, Wedderburn LR (eds) Textbook of Pediatric Rheumatology, 7th edn. Philadelphia: Saunders Elsevier, 2016.**

2 Silverman ED, Eddy AA. Systemic lupus erythematosus in children. In: Maddison PT, Isenberg DA, Woo P et al. (eds) Oxford Textbook of Rheumatology, 2nd edn, Vol. 2. Oxford: Oxford University Press, 1998:1180–202.

3 **Lisnevskaia L, Murphy G, Isenberg D. Systemic lupus erythematosus. Lancet 2014;384(9957):1878–88.**
4 **Hochberg MC. Updating the American College of Rheumatology revised criteria for the classification of systemic lupus erythematosus. Arthritis Rheum 1997;40:1725.**
5 Ferraz MB, Goldenberg J, Hilario MO et al. Evaluation of the 1982 ARA lupus criteria data set in pediatric patients. Committees of Pediatric Rheumatology of the Brazilian Society of Pediatrics and the Brazilian Society of Rheumatology. Clin Exp Rheumatol 1994;12:83.
6 **Petri M, Orbai AM, Alarcón GS et al. Derivation and validation of the Systemic Lupus International Collaborating Clinics classification criteria for systemic lupus erythematosus. Arthritis Rheum 2012;64:2677–86.**
7 Sag E, Tartaglione A, Batu ED et al. Performance of the new SLICC classification criteria in childhood systemic lupus erythematosus: a multicentre study. Clin Exp Rheumatol 2014;32:440–4.
8 Mok CC, Lau CS. Pathogenesis of systemic lupus erythematosus. Br Med J 2003;56:481.
9 Mendlovic S, Brocke S, Shoenfeld Y et al. Induction of a systemic lupus erythematosus-like disease in mice by a common human anti-DNA idiotype. Proc Natl Acad Sci 1988;85:2260.
10 **Cui Y, Sheng Y, Zhang X. Genetic susceptibility to SLE: recent progress from GWAS. J Autoimmun 2013;41:25–33.**
11 Candore G, Lio D, Colonna Romano G, Caruso C. Pathogenesis of autoimmune diseases associated with 8.1 ancestral haplotype: effect of multiple gene interactions. Autoimmunity Rev 2002;1:29–35.
12 Draborg AH, Duus K, Houen G. epstein-barr virus and systemic lupus erythematosus. Clin Dev Immunol 2012;2012:370516.
13 **Belot A, Cimaz R. Monogenic forms of systemic lupus erythematosus: new insights into SLE pathogenesis. Pediatr Rheumatol Online J 2012;10:21.**
14 **Belot A, Kasher PR, Trotter EW et al. Protein kinase cδ deficiency causes mendelian systemic lupus erythematosus with B cell-defective apoptosis and hyperproliferation. Arthritis Rheum 2013;65:2161–71.**
15 Morgan TA, Watson L, McCann LJ, Beresford MW. Children and adolescents with SLE: not just little adults. Lupus 2013;22:1309–19.
16 **Watson L, Leone V, Pilkington C et al.; UK Juvenile-Onset Systemic Lupus Erythematosus Study Group. Disease activity, severity, and damage in the UK Juvenile-Onset Systemic Lupus Erythematosus Cohort. Arthritis Rheum 2012;64:2356–65.**
17 Levy DM, Kamphuis S. Systemic lupus erythematosus in children and adolescents. Pediatr Clin North Am 2012;59:345–64.
18 Mina R, Brunner HI. Pediatric lupus, are there differences in presentation, genetics, response to therapy, and damage accrual compared with adult lupus? Rheum Dis Clin N Am 2010;36:53–80.
19 Livingston B, Bonner A, Pope J. Differences in clinical manifestations between childhood-onset lupus and adult-onset lupus: a meta-analysis. Lupus 2011;20:1345–55.
20 **Weinstein C, Miller MH, Axtens R et al. Lupus and non-lupus cutaneous manifestations in systemic lupus erythematosus. Intern Med J 2008;17:501–6.**
21 Benseler SM, Silverman ED. Review: neuropsychiatric involvement in pediatric systemic lupus erythematosus. Lupus 2007;16:564.
22 **Karlson MD, Khoshbin S, Rogers MP. The American College of Rheumatology nomenclature and case definitions for neuropsychiatric lupus syndromes. Arthritis Rheum 1999;42:599–608.**
23 Stimmler MM, Coletti PM, Quismorio FP. Magnetic resonance imaging of the brain in neuropsychiatric systemic lupus erythematosus. Sem Arthritis Rheum 1993;22:335–49.
24 Böckle BC, Jara D, Aichhorn K et al. Cerebral large vessel vasculitis in systemic lupus erythematosus. Lupus 2014;23:1417–21.
25 Sanna G, Bertolaccini ML, Cuadrado MJ et al. Neuropsychiatric manifestations in systemic lupus erythematosus: prevalence and association with antiphospholipid antibodies. J Rheumatol 2003;30:985–92.
26 Sherer Y, Hassin S, Shoenfeld Y et al. Transverse myelitis in patients with antiphospholipid antibodies – the importance of early diagnosis and treatment. Clin Rheumatol 2002;21:207–10.
27 Harel L, Sandborg C, Lee T, von Scheven E. Neuropsychiatric manifestations in pediatric systemic lupus erythematosus and association with antiphospholipid antibodies. J Rheum 2006;33:1873–77.
28 Perfumo F, Martini A. Lupus nephritis in children. Lupus 2005;14:83.
29 Churg J, Bernstein J, Glassock RJ. Lupus nephritis. In: Churg J, Bernstein J, Glassock RJ (eds) Renal Diseases. Classification and Atlas of Glomerular Diseases. Igaku-Shoin: New York, 1995:127–49.
30 **Weening JJ, D'Agati VD, Schwartz MM et al. The classification of glomerulonephritis in systemic lupus erythematosus revisited. J Am Soc Nephrol 2004;15:241.**
31 MacDermott EJ, Adams A, Lehman T. Review: systemic lupus erythematosus in children: current and emerging therapies. Lupus 2007;16:677.
32 Thakur N, Rai N, Batra P. Pediatric lupus nephritis – review of literature. Curr Rheumatol Rev 2016;13:29–36.
33 Sinha R, Raut S. Pediatric lupus nephritis: management update. World J Nephrol 2014;3:16–23.
34 Baca V, Lavalle C, García R et al. Favorable response to intravenous methylprednisolone and cyclophosphamide in children with severe neuropsychiatric lupus. J Rheumatol 1999;26:432–9.
35 **Rovin BH, Furie R, Latinis K et al.; LUNAR Investigator Group. Efficacy and safety of rituximab in patients with active proliferative lupus nephritis: the Lupus Nephritis Assessment with Rituximab study. Arthritis Rheum 2012;64:1215–26.**
36 **Merrill JT, Neuwelt CM, Wallace DJ et al. Efficacy and safety of rituximab in moderately-to-severely active systemic lupus erythematosus: the randomized, double-blind, phase II/III systemic lupus erythematosus evaluation of rituximab trial. Arthritis Rheum 2010;62:222–33.**
37 Marks SD, Patey S, Brogan PA et al. B lymphocyte depletion therapy in children with refractory systemic lupus erythematosus. Arthritis Care Res 2005;52:3168–74.
38 Watson L, Beresford MW, Maynes C et al. The indications, efficacy and adverse events of rituximab in a large cohort of patients with juvenile-onset SLE. Lupus 2015;24:10–7.
39 Ward M. Recent clinical trials in lupus nephritis. Rheum Dis Clin North Am 2014; 40:519–35.
40 **Falcini F, Capannini S, Martini G et al. Mycophenolate mofetil for the treatment of juvenile onset SLE: a multicenter study. Lupus 2009;18:139–43.**

Juvenile dermatomyositis

Introduction. Juvenile dermatomyositis (JDM), the most common form of juvenile idiopathic inflammatory myopathies, is an immune-mediated vasculopathy which presents characteristically with skin rashes and proximal muscle weakness, but can involve other organs [1].

Epidemiology and classification. JDM is a rare disease, with an incidence of two to three cases per million children and some racial differences [2,3]. The peak age of presentation is between 6 and 9 years; however, around 35% of children present before their fifth birthday [4]. The diagnosis of JDM is still based on a combination of clinical and laboratory criteria as proposed by Bohan and Peter in 1975 [5]. Advances in imaging as a modality of detection for muscle inflammation and the inconsistent use of electromyography have been recognized as limitations for the Bohan and Peter diagnostic criteria. An international collaborative effort has been made to modify the diagnostic criteria for JDM for further validation, which is likely to also include MRI abnormalities suggestive of inflammatory myositis as a criterion [6] (Box 149.7).

Pathogenesis. JDM is an autoimmune vasculopathy which probably results from the interplay of environmental factors, immune dysfunction and the genetic makeup of the individual. The vasculopathy of JDM affects skeletal muscle, skin, the gastrointestinal tract and other tissues such as lungs, kidneys, eyes and heart [1]. Both HLA and non-HLA genetic relationships such as polymorphisms in cytokine genes have been reported to be disease-associated or protective [7]. A very recent genome-wide association study revealed HLA 8.1 ancestral haplotype alleles as major genetic risk factors for myositis phenotypes in both adults and children of European

Box 149.7 Modified Bohan and Peter criteria for the diagnosis of dermatomyositis in childhood [5,6]

- Characteristic rash
- Symmetrical proximal muscle weakness
- Elevated muscle-derived enzymes
- Characteristic muscle histopathology (inflammatory and atrophy)
- EMG changes of inflammatory myopathy
- MRI evidence of myositis

Definite juvenile dermatomyositis (JDM) is based on the presence of the rash plus three out of five other criteria, whereas probable JDM is defined based on the presence of rash plus two out of five other criteria. EMG, electromyographic; MRI, magnetic resonance imaging.

ancestry [8]. In Caucasians, the HLA allele HLA DRB1*0301 is the strongest HLA risk factor for JDM, and HLA-B*08, DRB1*0301, DQA1*0501 and HLA-DPB1*0101 are part of a haplotype that confers a risk of myositis in both adults and children [9]. Polymorphisms in proinflammatory cytokine genes such as TNFα, IL-1α and IL-1β, and the lymphocyte signalling gene *PTPN22* have been reported to increase the risk of JDM [9]. Gene expression profiling studies have shown upregulation of the interferon I pathway in JDM, providing significant insights into the pathogenesis of the disease [10]. There is scarce evidence on the presence of an infectious trigger. In two studies, most children with JDM had antecedent upper respiratory and gastrointestinal illnesses in the 3 months before the onset of symptoms [11,12]. Consequently, several infectious agents have been suggested to trigger the development of JDM, especially group A β-haemolytic streptococci, whilst coxsackievirus B, Toxoplasma, enterovirus and parvovirus have been linked to JDM inconsistently [1].

Clinical features and differential diagnosis. The hallmarks of the disease are proximal muscle weakness and cutaneous manifestations; however, organ involvement is not rare, including gastrointestinal involvement, interstitial lung disease or cardiac involvement. JDM has often an insidious onset, with fatigue, muscle pain and weakness, which interfere with the daily activities, and skin rashes. Rare adermatitic or amyopathic cases have also been described. In a number of patients, the disease onset can be acute with fever and it can mimic other conditions (Box 149.8). There is no correlation between the skin disease activity and muscle disease activity.

JDM is a rare disease, and international registries enrolling JDM patients have enabled a better characterization of the clinical features. The Juvenile Dermatomyositis National Registry and Repository (UK and Ireland) is the largest cohort with over 500 patients recruited to date, followed by the North American Childhood Arthritis and Rheumatology Research Alliance Registry (CARRA) which has enrolled over 500 patients [4,13–15]. It has become apparent that JDM is a heterogeneous condition and recent translational and clinical research studies have focused on dividing the disease into 'subphenotypes' based on clinical characteristics and the presence of novel autoantibodies which seem to correlate with certain clinical phenotypes [16].

Box 149.8 Differential diagnosis of childhood idiopathic inflammatory myopathies

Weakness alone

- Muscular dystrophies
- Limb-girdle dystrophies, dystrophinopathies, facioscapulohumeral dystrophy, other dystrophies
- Metabolic myopathies
- Muscle glycogenoses (glycogen storage diseases), lipid storage disorders, mitochondrial myopathies
- Endocrine myopathies
- Hypothyroidism, hyperthyroidism, Cushing syndrome or exogenous steroid myopathy, diabetes mellitus
- Drug-induced myopathy
- Consider for patients taking any of the following drugs or biologic treatments: statins, interferon α, glucocorticoids, hydroxychloroquine, diuretics, amphotericin b, caine anaesthetics, growth hormone, cimetidine and vincristine
- Neuromuscular transmission disorders
- Myasthenia gravis
- Motor neurone disorder
- Spinal muscular atrophy

Weakness with or without rash

- Viral enterovirus, influenza, coxsackievirus, echovirus, parvovirus, poliovirus, hepatitis B, human T-lymphotropic virus 1
- Bacterial and parasitic organisms: *Staphylococcus*, *Streptococcus*, toxoplasmosis, trichinosis, *Lyme borreliosis*
- Other rheumatic conditions
- Systemic lupus erythematosus, scleroderma, juvenile idiopathic arthritis, mixed connective tissue disease, idiopathic vasculitis
- Other inflammatory conditions
- Inflammatory bowel disease, coeliac disease

Rash without weakness

- Psoriasis, eczema, allergy

Source: Adapted from Feldman et al. 2008 [1].

Cutaneous involvement

The heliotrope rash can precede or follow the muscle weakness. It is characteristically violaceous and typically seen on the eyelid, over the bridge of the nose across the face (Fig. 149.9), over the joints of the fingers and the extensor knees. The rash is photosensitive and the skin changes, including violaceous papules known as Gottron's papules, with associated scaling, crusting or erosions, are often seen over the extensor aspect of the finger joints; Gottron's sign refers to macular lesions in the same distribution as Gottron's papules (Fig. 149.10). Telangiectasia are seen, characteristically, over the eyelids and nailfolds. The nailfolds have abnormally dilated capillaries with lower capillary density, areas of capillary dropout and cuticular overgrowth which can be seen most easily by capillaroscopy (Fig. 149.11) [17]. Cutaneous ulceration is considered a marker of severe disease, occurs during episodes of disease activity and warrants aggressive treatment. Twenty-five percent of patients in a

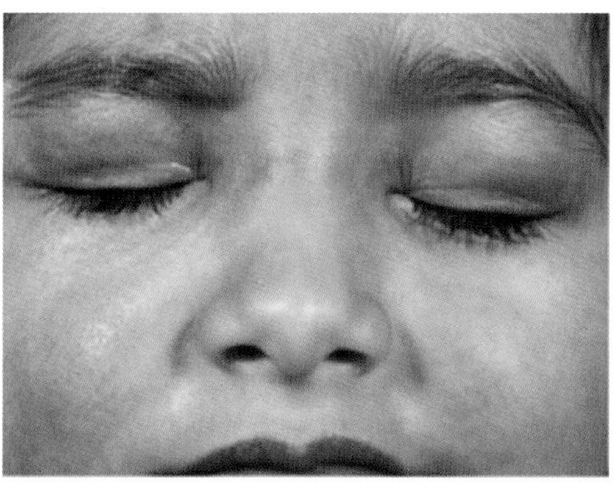

Fig. 149.9 Heliotrope rash and facial oedema in a child with juvenile dermatomyositis at initial presentation.

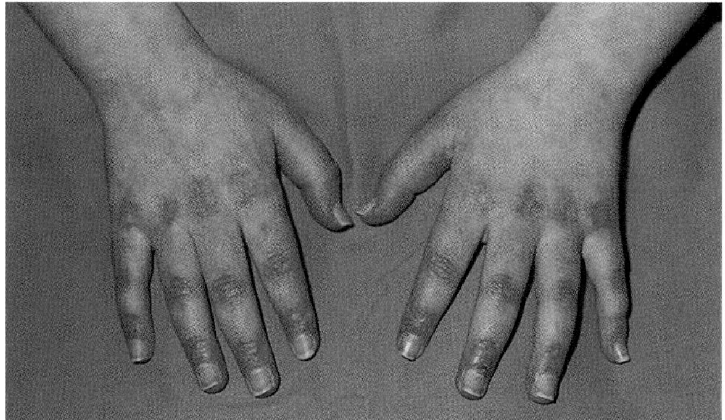

Fig. 149.10 Gottron's sign present on extensor surfaces of the small joints of the hands.

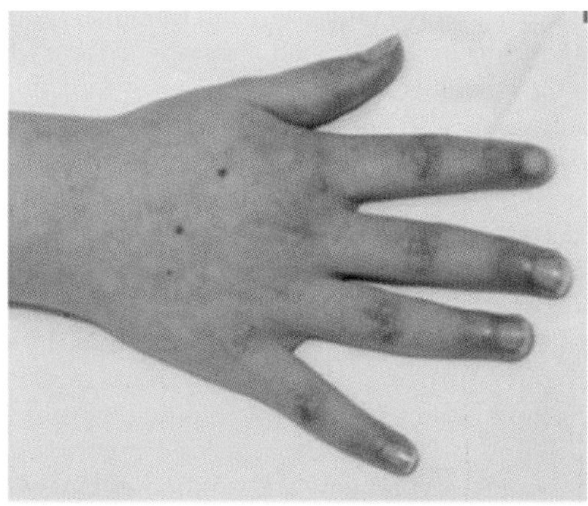

Fig. 149.11 Gottron's sign on extensor surfaces of the joints of the hand and dilated nailfold capillaries in a patient with juvenile dermatomyositis.

well-studied UK cohort were reported to have cutaneous ulceration around the time of initial presentation, whereas 30% develop ulceration within the first year of their disease course during flare ups [15], and skin ulceration was identified as a more common presentation in young children, under the age of 5 years [4]. Ulcerations typically occur at pressure points such as the elbows, the axillae, the lateral sides of the trunk and the corners of the eyes, where they can heal leaving atrophic scarring. Oedema can be seen at diagnosis or during exacerbation of the disease with generalized oedema felt to be a sign of a more severe disease course [18]. Other cutaneous manifestations of vasculopathy are livedo reticularis and erythema of the gingivae. Lipodystrophy is seen in 10–40% of patients, with generalized, partial or local variants, and can be associated with acanthosis nigricans [19,20]. Calcinosis is usually a sequelae of tissue damage and it may occur in muscles, skin, subcutaneous tissue and myofascia with a frequency of calcinosis in JDM of 30–70% [21]. It is often seen in cases with a delay in initiation of treatment or undertreated and is considered a marker for poor prognosis, requiring more aggressive treatment. The presence of calcinosis can result in significant cosmetic disfigurement, pain and limitation of movement, persistent ulceration with infection and muscle atrophy [21–23]. The presence of relatively recently described anti-NXP2 antibodies has been shown to increase the risk of calcinosis across all age groups in JDM and be associated with a phenotype with moderate to severe muscle disease [24].

Musculoskeletal disease

Muscle weakness initially occurs in the proximal muscle groups and the neck; abdominal flexors are the first to become weak and the last to recover. Problems with getting up from a chair or the floor, or climbing stairs, are other tell-tale signs of this disease. This weakness is associated with muscular tenderness and the child tends to hold the limb in flexion, thus promoting contractures. Diagnosis is made with the presence of abnormally high muscle enzymes, muscle histology from a biopsy and MRI findings. MRI is increasingly useful as a diagnostic tool to detect areas of inflammation which can be diffuse or patchy (Fig. 149.12), with involvement of myofascia or/and subcutaneous tissue [25,26], seen as high-signal intensity on fat-suppressed weighted and short tau inversion recovery (STIR) images, and it is a good test to follow progress, as well as being useful in identifying abnormal muscle for biopsy.

Arthritis often occurs in severe cases of JDM and osteoporosis occurs in untreated disease, although steroid therapy may also cause osteoporosis.

Gastrointestinal involvement

Decreased oesophageal motility with difficulty in swallowing, reflux with ulceration or aspiration pneumonia and a high-pitched nasal voice are all caused by myositis. In addition, vasculitis of the mesenteric vessels can cause small bowel angina, leading to infarction if untreated [27,28]. Abdominal pains in JDM patients should therefore be taken seriously, even if there is evidence of reflux and oesophageal ulceration. The areas most commonly affected are the duodenum and upper ileum [28]. Intestinal vasculopathy infrequently manifests as ulceration, haemorrhage, pneumatosis intestinalis or perforation [28,29]. Abdominal pain that is persistent, progressive or severe should be carefully assessed clinically and radiologically. Aggressive management with surgery and immunosuppression might have improved the outcome for this potentially life-threatening complication, because many old reports noted a high death rate.

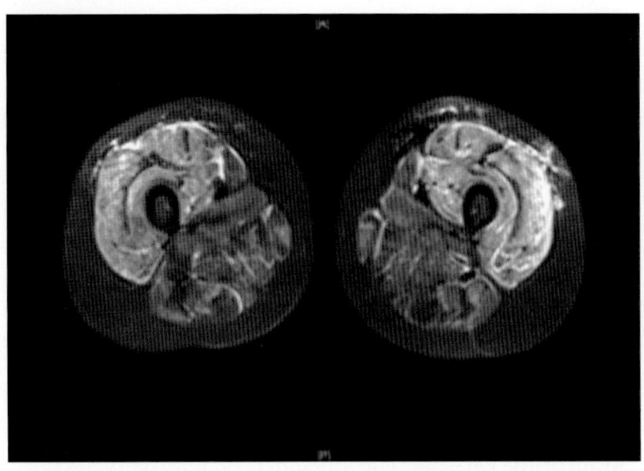

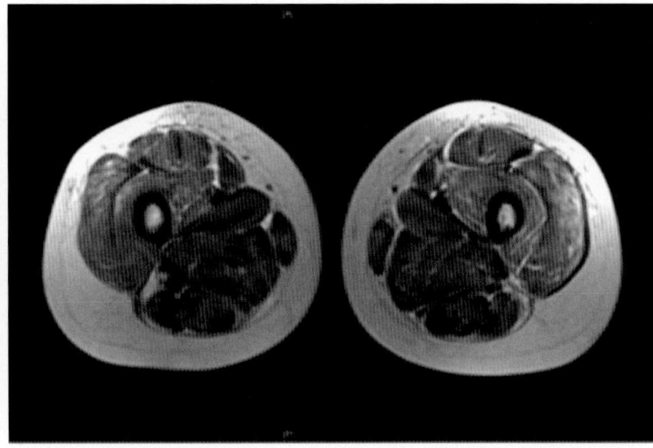

Fig. 149.12 Magnetic resonance imaging of the thigh of a girl with dermatomyositis showing widespread, severe inflammatory signal change throughout the musculature of the thighs, also inflammatory changes in the subcutaneous fat and fascial involvement.

Cardiorespiratory involvement

Interstitial lung disease is a well-recognized, but uncommon, manifestation of JDM that has been reported in case series with frequencies that range from 18.8 to 50% [29]; the presence of anti Jo-1 and newly discovered anti-MDA5 (Melanoma Differentiation-Associated protein 5) antibodies seems to correlate with a higher risk of interstitial lung disease in both adults and children, with the latter associated with a clinical subphenotype consisting of mild muscle disease and the presence of skin ulceration, lung disease and arthritis [30]. A reduction in ventilatory capacity in the absence of respiratory symptoms has been reported in 78% of JDM patients, mainly caused by muscle weakness [17]. Lung involvement is associated with a poor prognosis, can have a rapidly progressive course [1], and therefore these patients need to be targeted with aggressive treatment. Serious cardiac involvement is rare in JDM, but mainly includes pericarditis, myocardial inflammation, dilated cardiomyopathy, subclinical left ventricular diastolic dysfunction or conductive defects and first-degree heart block [1,31].

Genitourinary involvement

Renal ischaemia or vasculopathy can lead to renal failure and necrosis of the ureters has been reported [32,33].

Neurological involvement

Vasculitis can lead to vessel thrombosis in the retina and the eyelid [34]. CNS vascular involvement may lead to neuropsychiatric manifestations, as well as epileptic fits. However, severe CNS involvement is not common [35,36]. Areas of oedema are characteristic on MRI and are reversible with treatment.

Laboratory and histopathological findings. The laboratory investigations help to support the diagnosis of JDM and also rule out other differential diagnosis. The levels of muscle enzymes (creatine kinase, lactate dehydrogenase, aspartate transaminase, aldolase) are usually high at presentation but normalize rapidly after the initiation of treatment and in the absence of clinical improvement, and are therefore unreliable indicators of disease activity. ESR and CRP are usually elevated and correlate with disease activity, and von Villebrand factor can also be elevated. As described earlier in this chapter, MRI is now widely used to assist with the diagnosis of JDM; a recent study has shown that the severity of MRI changes or extent of muscle involvement do not correlate with the clinical outcome, but subcutaneous tissue involvement was specific for a severe disease course [37]. Diagnostic histopathological features include perifascicular atrophy, capillary pathology including complement deposition and capillary dropout, predominantly interstitial inflammation and electron microscopy tubuloreticular endothelial inclusions [1]. Other investigations can be directed towards investigation of gastrointestinal, respiratory, cardiac or CNS involvements. An international consensus working group has developed a scoring system for JDM muscle biopsies [38]. The score examines four domains: (i) endomysial, perivascular and perimysial inflammation; (ii) vascular changes; (iii) changes to muscle fibres including major histocompatibility complex (MHC) class I overexpression, atrophy of perifascicular and other muscle fibres, degeneration or regeneration, and the presence of neonatal myosin; and (iv) endomysial and perimysial fibrosis [11]. This scoring tool has been validated in a further study and shown to correlate well with clinical measures of disease activity [39].

In addition to the well-characterized myositis-specific autoantibodies, several new autoantibodies have recently been described in JDM, each associated with a distinct clinical phenotype (Table 149.4). The titres of these autoantibodies have been shown to fluctuate with the level of disease activity [43]. The detection and quantification of newly identified autoantibodies is done by immunoprecipitation and not yet routinely available in clinical laboratories.

Treatment. JDM is a rare disease, and therefore clinical trials are challenging in terms of patient recruitment and organization. There is limited evidence to assist the clinicians with treatment decisions; however, this is improving in recent years by well-organized collaborative networks which enable expert consensus conferences to

Table 149.4 Antibodies in patients with juvenile dermatomyositis [9,40–42]

Autoantibody	Autoantibody subtype	Antigen	Clinical associations
Myositis-specific antibodies			
Anti-ARS		Aminoacyl-tRNA synthetases	Moderate to severe weakness, may have arthritis, mechanics hands, Raynaud, fevers, interstitial lung disease
	Anti-Jo-1	Histidyl-tRNA synthetase	
	Anti-PL-12	Alanyl-tRNA synthetase	
	Anti-PL-7	Threonyl-tRNA synthetase	
	Anti-EJ	Glycyl-tRNA synthetase	
	Anti-OJ	Isoleucyl-tRNA synthetase	
	Anti-KS	Asparagynyl-tNRA synthetase	
	Anti-Ha	Tyrosyl-tRNA synthetase	
	Anti-Zo	Phenylalanyl-tRNA synthetase	
Other myositis-specific antibodies			
Anti-Mi-2		DNA helicase	Classical cutaneous JDM
Anti-SRP		Signal recognition particle	Necrotizing autoimmune myositis with severe weakness, very high creatine kinase and no rash
Recently identified myositis autoantibodies			
Anti-p155/140 or anti-p155		Transcriptional intermediary factor (TIF)-1 gamma protein	Severe cutaneous disease and lipodystrophy
Anti-p140 (MJ)		Thought to be the MJ autoantigen, nuclear matrix protein NXP2	Severe weakness, calcinosis, gastrointestinal bleeding, dysphagia and ulcers
Anti-MDA5		Melanoma Differentiation-associated protein 5	Clinically amyopathic dermatomyositis and rapidly progressive ILD in East Asian populations. Mild muscle disease, ulceration, arthritis, and ILD in Caucasian populations
Anti-HMGCR		3-hydroxy-3-methylglutaryl-coenzyme A reductase	Necrotizing autoimmune myositis *Rare in the paediatric population*
Anti-SAE		Small-ubiquitin-like modifier enzyme (SUMO)	May present as clinically amyopathic dermatomyositis then progress to muscle weakness *Rare in the paediatric population*
Myositis-associated antibodies			
Anti-U1-RNP		U1 ribonucleoprotein (snRNP)	Sclerodermatous overlap features
Anti-U3-RNP		U3 ribonucleoprotein (fibrillarin)	Sclerodermatous overlap features
Anti-PM-Scl		Nucleolar multiprotein complex	Sclerodermatous overlap features
Anti-Ro		52 or 60n>n>Kd ribonucleoproteins (hYRNA)	
Anti-La		Ribonucleoprotein	
Anti-Ku		p70/p80 heterodimer, DNA-associated proteins	
Anti-Topo		DNA topoisomerase 1	

ARS Aminoacyl-tRNA synthetases; ILD interstitial lung disease; JDM, juvenile dermatomyositis.

develop standardized therapy guidelines which will reduce the variation in JDM treatment between the centres. It is generally accepted that early and aggressive management of JDM results in improved prognosis. Standard treatment includes steroids and usually methotrexate, but ciclosporin or azathioprine have also been used. The North American Paediatric Rheumatology network defined the clinical features of patients with mild to moderate JDM and has recommended a corticosteroid regime for these patients starting at 2 mg/kg daily, weaning to 1 mg/kg by 14 weeks and stopping at 50 weeks [43]. With evidence of severe disease, intravenous methylprednisolone is preferable and is usually given as 3-day pulses of 30 mg/kg. If there is gastrointestinal involvement, intravenous steroids equivalent to oral doses should be given to ensure absorption in the early stages of the disease. Methotrexate is an important ancillary treatment for JDM. Early studies suggested that methotrexate improves muscular strength and reduces other signs of disease activity in nonresponsive (steroid-resistant) patients with acceptable side-effects and a steroid-sparing effect [44]. A recent international randomized controlled trial which compared prednisone versus prednisone plus methotrexate versus prednisone plus ciclosporin in patients with newly diagnosed JDM showed that combined treatment with prednisone and DMARD was more effective than prednisone alone, and the safety profile was higher for the combination of prednisone and methotrexate [45]. A first double-blind RCT with crossover design in idiopathic inflammatory myopathies which recruited both adults and children at sites in the USA and Canada was published in 2013, and studied the efficacy of rituximab [46]. The study did not detect a difference between patients treated 'early' or 'late' with rituximab, which can possibly reflect a slower effect of the drug than anticipated when the study was designed. However, in a subanalysis, the paediatric patients had better responses than adults but the numbers were too small to detect a statistically significant difference in this population [46]. A retrospective case control study of JDM showed effectiveness of intravenous immunoglobulin (IVIG) particularly in steroid-resistant patients [47]. A small retrospective case series of 12 patients with JDM treated with MMF showed encouraging results [48]. Cyclophosphamide is used as aggressive therapy for more severe disease such as ulcerative skin disease, lung involvement, very severe muscle disease or multiorgan involvement. It has been shown in a small case series to be well tolerated and effective [49]. Recently, anti-TNF therapies have been used with effect in pilot studies in resistant cases, and usually after other agents such as IVIG or cyclophosphamide have failed to control the disease [50]. Patients with calcinosis are particularly prone to *Staphylococcus* infection at these sites, which can be exacerbated by methotrexate. A number of treatments have been used to treat calcinosis with variable success, including aluminum hydroxide, diltiazem, probenecid, bisphosphonates, colchicines, local triamcinolone and infliximab [21,51].

In addition to the medical management, physiotherapy after the acute phase of the disease, in the form of passive stretches and graduated muscle strengthening, is important in assisting recovery and preventing contractures. Maillard and colleagues have shown that this regimen does not aggravate inflammation [52].

Outcome. Prior to treatment with corticosteroids, JDM had a high mortality rate (>30%) and left 50% of those who survived with serious permanent impairments [40]. After the introduction of corticosteroids, mortality rapidly dropped to less than 10%, and is currently reported to be less than 2–3% [53]. Because most children now survive this illness, there is greater interest in long-term outcomes such as physical function, quality of life, pain, educational and vocational achievement, patient satisfaction and ongoing disease activity [54]. Current efforts to identify key outcomes and validate measures for those outcomes will allow researchers in the future to provide this much needed information.

References

1 **Feldman BM, Rider LG, Reed AM, Pachman LM. Juvenile dermatomyositis and other idiopathic inflammatory myopathies of childhood. Lancet 2008;371:2201–12.**

2 Mendez EP, Lipton R, Ramsey-Goldman R et al., for the NIAMS Juvenile DM Registry Physician Referral Group et al. US incidence of juvenile dermatomyositis, 1995–1998: results from the National Institute of Arthritis and Musculoskeletal and Skin Diseases Registry. Arthritis Rheum 2003;49:300–5.

3 Symmons DP, Sills JA, Davis SM. The incidence of juvenile dermatomyositis: results from a nation-wide study. Br J Rheumatol 1995;34:732–6.

4 **Martin N, Krol P, Smith S et al. Juvenile Dermatomyositis Research Group (JDRG). Comparison of children with onset of juvenile dermatomyositis symptoms before or after their fifth birthday in a UK and Ireland juvenile dermatomyositis cohort study. Arthritis Care Res 2012;64:1665–72.**

5 **Bohan A, Peter JB. Polymyositis and dermatomyositis (first of two parts). N Engl J Med 1975;292:344–7.**

6 **Brown VE, Pilkington CA, Feldman BM, Davidson JE. An international consensus survey of the diagnostic criteria for juvenile dermatomyositis (JDM) Rheumatology (Oxford) 2006;45:990–3.**

7 **Rider LG, Lindsley CB, Miller FW. Juvenile dermatomyositis. In: Petty RE, Laxer RM, Lindsley CB, Wedderburn LR (eds) Textbook of Pediatric Rheumatology, 7th edn. Philadelphia: Saunders Elsevier, 2016.**

8 **Miller FW, Chen W, O'Hanlon TP et al.; Myositis Genetics Consortium. Genome-wide association study identifies HLA 8.1 ancestral haplotype alleles as major genetic risk factors for myositis phenotypes. Genes Immun 2015;16:470–80.**

9 Wedderburn LR, Rider LG. Juvenile dermatomyositis: new developments in pathogenesis, assessment and treatment. Best Pract Res Clin Rheumatol 2009;23:665–78.

10 Baechler EC, Bilgic H, Reed AM. Type I interferon pathway in adult and juvenile dermatomyositis. Arthritis Res Ther 2011;13:249.

11 Pachman LM, Hayford JR, Hochberg MC et al. New-onset juvenile dermatomyositis. Arthritis Rheum 1997;40:1526–33.

12 Pachman LM, Lipton R, Ramsey-Goldman R et al. History of infection before the onset of juvenile dermatomyositis: results from the National Institute of Arthritis and Musculoskeletal and Skin Diseases Research Registry. Arthritis Rheum 2005;53:166–72.

13 Martin N, Krol P, Smith S et al. Juvenile Dermatomyositis Research Group. A national registry for juvenile dermatomyositis and other paediatric idiopathic inflammatory myopathies: 10 years' experience; the Juvenile Dermatomyositis National (UK and Ireland) Cohort Biomarker Study and Repository for Idiopathic Inflammatory Myopathies. Rheumatology (Oxford) 2011;50:137–45.

14 **Robinson AB, Hoeltzel MF, Wahezi DM et al.; Juvenile Myositis CARRA Subgroup, for the CARRA Registry Investigators. Clinical characteristics of children with juvenile dermatomyositis: The Childhood Arthritis and Rheumatology Research Alliance Registry. Arthritis Care Res (Hoboken) 2014; 66:404–10.**

15 McCann LJ, Juggins AD, Maillard SM et al.; Juvenile Dermatomyositis Research Group. The Juvenile Dermatomyositis National Registry and Repository (UK and Ireland) – clinical characteristics of children recruited within the first 5 yr. Rheumatology (Oxford) 2006;45:1255–60.

16 Nistala K, Wedderburn LR. Update in juvenile myositis. Curr Opin Rheumatol 2013;25:742–6.

17 Lowry CA, Pilkington CA. Juvenile dermatomyositis: extramuscular manifestations and their management. Curr Opin Rheumatol 2009; 21:575.

18 Saygi S, Alehan F, Baskin E et al. Juvenile dermatomyositis presenting with anasarca. J Child Neurol 2008;23:1353.

19 Bingham A, Mamyrova G, Rother KI et al. Predictors of acquired lipodystrophy in juvenile-onset dermatomyositis and a gradient of severity. Medicine 2008;87:70.

20 **Dugan EM, Huber AM, Miller FW, Rider LG; International Myositis Assessment and Clinical Studies Group.Review of the classification and assessment of the cutaneous manifestations of the idiopathic inflammatory myopathies. Dermatol Online J 2009;15:2.**

21 **Saini I, Kalaivani M, Kabra SK. Calcinosis in juvenile dermatomyositis: frequency, risk factors and outcome. Rheumatol Int 2016;36:961–5.**

22 Hoeltzel MF, Oberle EJ, Buyun Robinson A et al. The presentation, assessment, pathogenesis, and treatment of calcinosis in juvenile dermatomyositis. Curr Rheumatol Rep 2014;16:467.

23 Mukamel M, Horev G, Mimouni M. New insight into calcinosis of juvenile dermatomyositis: a study of composition and treatment. J Pediatr 2001;138:763–6.

24 **Tansley SL, Betteridge ZE, Shaddick G et al. Juvenile Dermatomyositis Research Group. Calcinosis in juvenile dermatomyositis is influenced by both anti-NXP2 autoantibody status and age at disease onset. Rheumatology (Oxford) 2014;53:2204–8.**

25 **Malattia C, Damasio MB, Madeo A et al. Whole-body MRI in the assessment of disease activity in juvenile dermatomyositis. Ann Rheum Dis 2014;73:1083–90.**

26 **Davis WR, Halls JE, Offiah AC et al. Assessment of active inflammation in juvenile dermatomyositis: a novel magnetic resonance imaging-based scoring system. Rheumatology (Oxford) 2011;50:2237–44.**

27 Mamyrova G, Kleiner DE, James-Newton L et al. Late-onset gastrointestinal pain in juvenile dermatomyositis as a manifestation of ischemic ulceration from chronic endarteropathy. Arthritis Rheum 2007;57:881–84.

28 Wang IJ, Hsu WM, Shun CT et al. Juvenile dermatomyositis complicated with vasculitis and duodenal perforation. J Formos Med Assoc 2001;100:844–6.

29 Morinishi Y, Oh-Ishi T, Kabuki T, Joh K. Juvenile dermatomyositis: clinical characteristics and the relatively high risk of interstitial lung disease. Modern Rheumatol 2007;17:413–17.

30 Tansley SL, Betteridge ZE, Gunawardena H et al.; UK Juvenile Dermatomyositis Research Group. Anti-MDA5 autoantibodies in juvenile dermatomyositis identify a distinct clinical phenotype: a prospective cohort study. Arthritis Res Ther 2014;16:R138.

31 Karaca NE, Aksu G, Yeniay BS, Kutukculer N. Juvenile dermatomyositis with a rare and remarkable complication: sinus bradycardia. Rheumatol Int 2006;27:179–82.

32 Huang KH, Hsieh SC, Huang CY et al. Dermatomyositis associated with bilateral ureteral spontaneous rupture. J Formos Med Assoc 2007;106:251–4.

33 Borrelli M, Prado MJ, Cordeiro P et al. Ureteral necrosis in dermatomyositis. J Urol 1988;139:1275–7.

34 Cohen BH, Sedwick LA, Burde RM. Retinopathy of dermatomyositis. J Clin Neuroophthalmol 1985;5:177–9.

35 Ramanan AV, Sawhney S, Murray KJ. Central nervous system complications in two cases of juvenile onset dermatomyositis, Rheumatology (Oxford) 2001;40:1293–8.

36 Elst EF, Kamphuis SS, Prakken BJ et al. Case report: severe central nervous system involvement in juvenile dermatomyositis. J. Rheumatol 2003;30:2059–63.

37 Ladd PE, Emery KH, Salisbury SR et al. Juvenile dermatomyositis: correlation of MRI at presentation with clinical outcome. Am J Roentgenol 2011;197:W153–8.

38 **Wedderburn LR, Varsani H, Li CK et al. International consensus on a proposed score system for muscle biopsy evaluation in patients with juvenile dermatomyositis: a tool for potential use in clinical trials. Arthritis Rheum 2007;57:1192–201.**

39 **Varsani H, Charman SC, Li CK et al.; UK Juvenile Dermatomyositis Research Group. Validation of a score tool for measurement of histological severity in juvenile dermatomyositis and association with clinical severity of disease. Ann Rheum Dis 2015;74:204–10.**

40 **Shah M, Mamyrova G, Targoff IN et al., Childhood Myositis Heterogeneity Collaborative Study Group. The clinical phenotypes of the juvenile idiopathic inflammatory myopathies. Medicine (Baltimore) 2013;92:25–41.**

41 **Tansley SL, McHugh NJ. Serological subsets of juvenile idiopathic inflammatory myopathies - an update. Expert Rev Clin Immunol 2016;12:427–37.**

42 Stone KB, Oddis CV, Fertig N et al. Anti-Jo-1 antibody levels correlate with disease activity in idiopathic inflammatory myopathy. Arthritis Rheum 2007;56:3125–31.

43 **Huber AM, Robinson AB, Reed AM, et al. Consensus treatments for moderate juvenile dermatomyositis: beyond the first two months. Results of the second Childhood Arthritis and Rheumatology Research Alliance consensus conference. Arthritis Care Res (Hoboken) 2012;64:546–53.**

44 Miller LC, Sisson BA, Tucker LB et al. Methotrexate treatment of recalcitrant childhood dermatomyositis. Arthritis Care Res 1992; 35:1143–9.

45 **Ruperto N, Pistorio A, Oliveira S et al.; Paediatric Rheumatology International Trials Organisation (PRINTO). Prednisone versus prednisone plus ciclosporin versus prednisone plus methotrexate in new-onset juvenile dermatomyositis: a randomised trial. Lancet 2016;387(10019):671–8.**

46 **Oddis CV, Reed AM, Aggarwal R et al. Rituximab in the treatment of refractory adult and juvenile dermatomyositis and adult polymyositis: a randomized, placebo-phase trial. Arthritis Rheum 2013;65:314–24.**

47 **Lam CG, Manlhiot C, Pullenayegum EM et al. Efficacy of intravenous Ig therapy in juvenile dermatomyositis. Ann Rheum Dis 2011;70:2089–94.**

48 **Dagher R, Desjonqueres M, Duquesne A et al. Mycophenolate mofetil in juvenile dermatomyositis: a case series. Rheumatol Int 2012;32:711–16.**

49 **Riley P, Maillard SM, Wedderburn LR et al. Intravenous cyclophosphamide pulse therapy in juvenile dermatomyositis. A review of efficacy and safety. Rheumatology 2008;43:491–6.**

50 **Riley P, McCann LJ, Maillard SM et al. Effectiveness of infliximab in the treatment of refractory juvenile dermatomyositis with calcinosis. Rheumatology 2008;47:877–80.**

51 **Bilginer Y, Topaloglu R, Gonc N. Treatment of calcinosis with biphosphonates in juvenile dermatomyositis. Pediatr Rheumatol 2008;6:220.**

52 Maillard SM, Jones R, Owens CM et al. Quantitative assessments of the effects of a single exercise session on muscles in juvenile dermatomyositis. Arthritis Rheum 2005;53:558–64.

53 Laxer RM. Outcome in juvenile dermatomyositis. Br Med J 2005; 64(Suppl 3):105.

54 Huber A, Lang B, Leblanc CI et al. Medium- and long-term functional outcomes in a multicenter cohort of children with juvenile dermatomyositis. Arthritis Care Res 2000;43:541–9.

CHAPTER 150
Behçet Disease and Relapsing Polychondritis

Sibel Ersoy-Evans[1], *Ayşen Karaduman*[1] *& Seza Özen*[2]

[1]Department of Dermatology, Hacettepe University School of Medicine, Ankara, Turkey
[2]Department of Paediatric Rheumatology, Hacettepe University School of Medicine, Ankara, Turkey

Behçet disease, 1952	Relapsing polychondritis, 1958

Abstract

Behçet disease (BD) is a recurrent systemic disease that affects most organs. Clinically, there are some differences between paediatric and adult BD; in children gastrointestinal symptoms, neurological involvement and arthralgia are more common. As such, revised paediatric BD criteria have been proposed, which include neurological and vascular signs, and exclude the pathergy test; oral ulcers are not mandatory for diagnosis. Because of the lack of multicentre studies on childhood BD, there are no treatment guidelines for paediatric BD patients. Relapsing polychondritis (RP) is a multisystemic disease characterized by recurrent inflammation and cartilage destruction. The ears and nose are most commonly involved. In children with RP, respiratory tract involvement, costochondritis and atypical destructive arthritis are more severe and common than in adults. Diagnosis can be established based on clinical criteria. Treatment options include systemic steroids and immunosuppressive agents. Although the course of RP is variable, it can be a rapidly progressive and fulminating disease.

Key points

- **Behçet disease (BD) is an autoinflammatory disease.**
- **Gastrointestinal symptoms, neurological involvement and arthralgia are more common in children than in adults.**
- **Diagnostic criteria for paediatric BD differ from those for adults and include neurological and vascular signs, and exclude pathergy test results; oral ulcers are not mandatory for diagnosis.**

Behçet disease

Introduction. Behçet disease (BD) is a multisystemic disease that was first reported by a Turkish dermatologist, Hulusi Behçet, in 1937 [1]. He described BD as a triad: oral and genital ulcers, plus uveitis. The heterogeneity of the disease makes it difficult to diagnose. BD is a unique disease in many respects and is the only primary vasculitis that can affect vessels of any size with a type of inflammation that tends to cause thrombosis [2].

Epidemiology. BD is rare during childhood; therefore, data concerning its prevalence in children are scarce. A French study reported an estimated prevalence of BD as 1 in 600 000 children [3]. The highest prevalence of BD in adults was reported in the Turkish population (421 in 100 000) [4]. The prevalence of BD varies by country and ranges from 0.3 to 146.4 in 100 000. The disease does not exhibit a gender preference, but is generally more severe in males [5].

Aetiopathogenesis. The pathogenesis of BD is not fully understood; however, as are many rheumatological diseases, BD is a multifactorial disease associated with both genetic and environmental factors. A recent study by Mahr and colleagues [6] reported that the prevalence of BD among North Africans living in France was the same as in their countries of origin, suggesting that genetic factors may be more important than environmental factors. The role of genetics in BD is also supported by reports of familial cases, a high sibling recurrence and twin concordance rates, the well-known association between BD and HLA-B51, the frequency of BD among the population along the Silk Road (the ancient trade route linking the Far East to Europe), evidence of genetic anticipation, and recent genome-wide association studies (GWAS) [7–12].

Many studies have investigated the association between BD and polymorphisms in possible target molecules; however, most were small scale and lack statistical power or accompanying functional studies. Because BD is rare and has a heterogeneous presentation, reliable GWAS have been delayed. In 2010 two large GWAS [11,12] (1215 and 612 patients, respectively) replicated each other's findings that confirmed the association between BD and HLA-B51. In both studies the most significant non-HLA

Harper's Textbook of Pediatric Dermatology, Fourth Edition. Edited by Peter Hoeger, Veronica Kinsler and Albert Yan.

association was with the IL-10 and IL-23R loci, which is in agreement with recent reports on the pathogenesis of BD. The IL-10 variant associated with BD results in a low IL-10 level and is the same variant that is associated with juvenile rheumatoid arthritis [13]. Both studies [11,12] also showed that there is an association between BD and *IL23R/IL12RB2* genes. IL-23 is an immunoregulatory cytokine that shares a p40 subunit with IL-12 and stimulates the Th17 pathway [10,11].

An association study from Iran also confirmed the significance of IL-10 and *IL23R/IL12RB2* in 973 Iranian patients [14]. Subsequently, Kirino and colleagues [9] re-studied a cohort of 1209 Turkish patients with a GWAS of 779 465 single nucleotide polymorphisms with imputed genotypes, in order to discover new susceptibility loci for BD. They identified new associations between BD and CCR1-CCR3 (related to monocyte chemotaxis), STAT4 (a transcription factor in a signalling pathway related to such cytokines as IL-12, type I IFNs and IL-23), KLRK1-KLRKC1 (expressed on natural killer cells) and two single nucleotide polymorphisms in ERAP1. Furthermore, there was an epistatic interaction between ERAP1 and MHC Class I region; homozygosity for the putative ERAP1 introduced a threefold risk in HLA-B51-positive patients, whereas the risk was 1.48 for HLA-B51 negatives [9].

The association between BD and HLA-B51, in particular, HLA-B5101 and HLA-B5108, has been confirmed in many studies and in various populations; however, it is not the only genetic risk factor associated with BD (<20%) [13]. The precise nature of the association between HLA-B51 and BD remains unclear. HLA-B51 has low affinity to peptides [15]. The association between BD and infections has been linked to the behaviour of HLA-B51; however, recently published data suggest that the slow folding of HLA-B51 might play a critical role in the pathogenesis of BD. When HLA I class molecules bind to the peptide they must fold; unfolded protein response leads to endoplasmic stress and triggers inflammation through the IL-23/IL-17 pathway [16]. ERAP1 is an endoplasmic reticulum-expressed aminopeptidase that plays a role in processing and loading of peptides onto MHC class I molecules [17]. The endoplasmic reticulum-expressed aminopeptidase (ERAP) molecule can alter the folding characteristics of the HLA I molecule via its effect on peptide loading, resulting in a tendency to misfold. As recent genetic studies have demonstrated, the significance of the IL-23/IL-17 pathway in BD and the epistatic interaction between HLA-B51 and ERAP1, it is possible that ERAP1 plays a major role in the pathogenesis of BD via unfolded protein response and endoplasmic stress [9].

The aetiopathogenesis of BD is not only caused by genetic defects [18]; environmental triggers are thought to play a role in genetically susceptible individuals. Infectious agents, such as bacteria and viruses, have been investigated. *Streptococcus sanguinis* colonization in the oral flora in BD patients was observed to be elevated and induces BD-like symptoms in mice. Other bacteria implicated in the pathogenesis of BD include *Escherichia coli*, *Staphylococcus aureus*, *Mycoplasma*, *Helicobacter* and *Mycobacteria*. Because of the range of microorganisms associated with BD, it is hypothesized that T lymphocytes in BD patients are hyperreactive to all bacterial species [13]. Studies on the association between BD and viruses, especially herpes simplex virus (HSV), reported HSV DNA in blood cells, and in oral and genital ulcers in BD patients [19]; however, the lack of response to antiviral therapy indicates that HSV probably does not play a role in the pathogenesis of BD.

Heat shock proteins (HSP) protect cells against damage and premature death, and are synthesized in response to cellular stress. HSP60 is highly expressed in BD lesions [20]. Additionally, high levels of HSP70 and retinal S antigen antibodies were observed in BD patients [21,22]. As such, contemporary research is focusing on the role of HSPs in the pathogenesis of BD [13].

BD also have immune system dysfunction in which T lymphocytes (cytotoxic T cells (γδ subtype), Th1 cells, regulatory T cells, and Th17 cells) play a pivotal role. Neutrophil abnormalities, such as hyperactivation, and an increased chemotaxis, phagocytosis, superoxide generation and myeloperoxidase level, probably because of close communication between T cells and neutrophils, have also been reported in BD patients [13]. Additional abnormalities noted in BD patients include endothelial dysfunction and thrombosis [13].

The episodic nature of BD, involvement of the innate immune system and features similar to other monogenic autoinflammatory diseases indicate that there is a correlation between BD and autoinflammation. BD fits rather nicely under the umbrella of IL-17-related autoinflammation; however, as mentioned above, the adaptive immune system also apparently plays a role in the pathogenesis of BD [23].

Clinical features. BD is a recurrent systemic disease that affects virtually every organ in the body. Clinical presentation is variable and includes oral ulcers, genital ulcers, papulopustular lesions, erythema nodosum, necrotic folliculitis, ocular, vascular, neurological, cardiac and pulmonary lesions, arthritis and thrombophlebitis. There are some clinical differences between paediatric and adult BD. A study that compared 83 juvenile-onset BD patients with 536 adult-onset BD patients reported that the frequency of clinical findings was similar in both groups, except that neurological and gastrointestinal involvement was more common in the juvenile-onset BD group [24]. Another study reported that significantly more paediatric BD patients have gastrointestinal symptoms, neurological involvement and arthralgia, compared with adults [25]. Age of onset of childhood BD is variable and can occur even in neonates [26].

Mucocutaneous lesions

Recurrent oral ulcers (aphthae) are the most common finding, both in adult and paediatric BD patients [24]. Aphthae are localized on nonkeratinized mucosal membranes, primarily buccal mucosa, and the lateral and ventral surfaces of the tongue. Aphthae are painful lesions characterized by ulceration with an erythematous halo and are covered by a whitish pseudomembrane (Fig. 150.1).

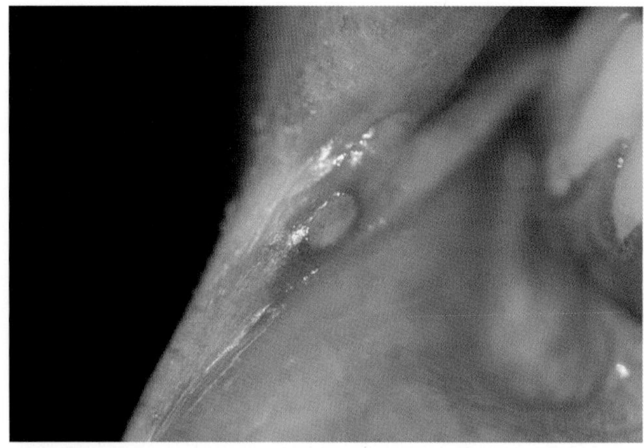

Fig. 150.1 Oral aphthae.

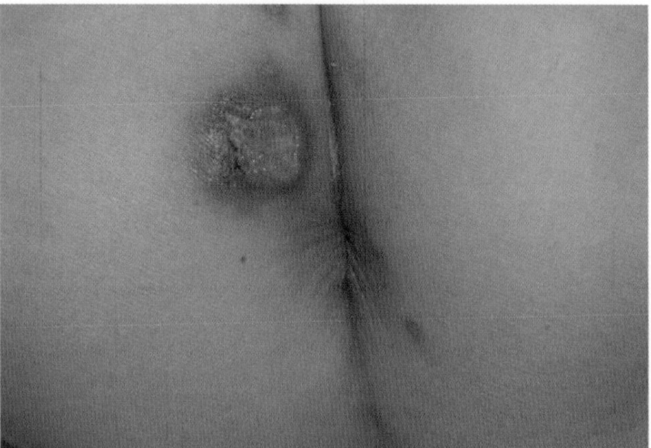

Fig. 150.2 Behçet disease with genital ulcer.

Genital ulcers initially present as papules that rapidly progresses to painful, deep ulcers with erythematous oedema at the periphery (Fig. 150.2). In males they are localized most commonly on the scrotum and inguinal area, versus the vulva and inguinal area in females. Healing occurs in 2–4 weeks and ulcers larger than 1 cm usually leave a scar. In females, ulcers of the labia minora and vestibule can heal without scar formation [27]. In children, the reported frequency of genital ulcers is 24–94% [24,28–32]. In a recent international study on paediatric BD, genital ulcers were more common in females [33].

Erythema nodosum (EN) is noted in approximately 50% of adult BD patients. EN lesions are localized symmetrically over the anterior lower extremities and characterized by painful, erythematous and warm subcutaneous nodules [27]. One study that included 219 children with BD reported that 18.7% of the patients had EN [33], whereas in another that included 83 children, EN frequency was reported as 51.8% [24].

Papulopustular lesions are reported to occur in 30–96% of adult BD patients and are more frequently observed in patients with arthritis [27]. These lesions present as papules or pustules localized in follicular or nonfollicular areas (Fig. 150.3). Although they are usually sterile, a recent study isolated coagulase-negative *Staphylococcus spp.* and *Prevotella spp.* from the lesions [34]. Other cutaneous findings of BD include necrotic folliculitis and Sweet syndrome-like lesions [28,31].

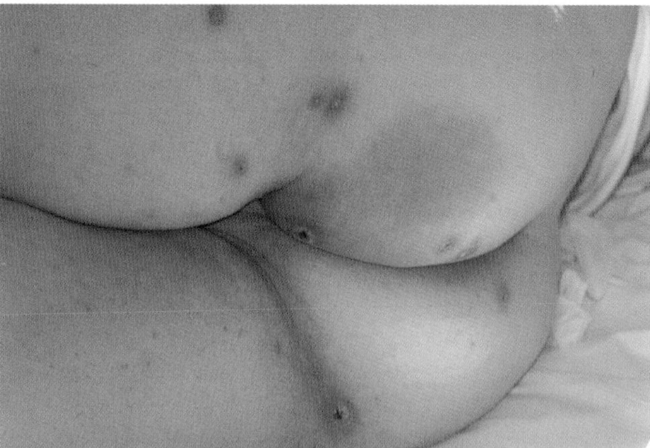

Fig. 150.3 Necrotic folliculitis.

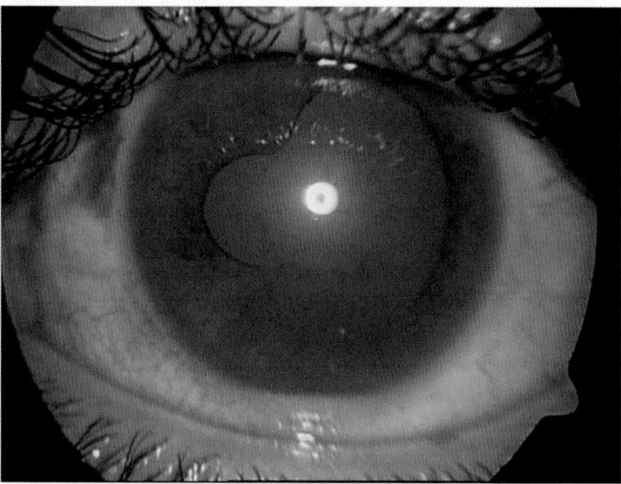

Fig. 150.4 Uveitis with posterior synechia and hypopyon. Source: Courtesy of Prof. Dr Sibel Kadayıfçılar.

Ocular involvement

The reported prevalence of ocular involvement in paediatric BD patients ranges from 30.9 to 61% [24,28,35]. Posterior and anterior uveitis are the most common ocular findings in children [28,33,35] (Fig. 150.4); however, one study reported that panuveitis was the most frequent ocular manifestation in children aged over 10 years and that a family history of BD was more common in BD patients younger than 10 years old [36]. The reported ocular prognosis in paediatric BD patients is inconsistent; one study reported that the course is severe, especially in males [28], whereas another study reported that the prognosis in children was better than in adults [37]. Other ocular findings of BD include conjunctivitis, hypopyon, posterior synechia, retinal vasculitis, retinitis, cataract, glaucoma and optic atrophy [25,33,35,36].

Vascular involvement

Vasculitis in BD patients is characteristically associated with arterial or venous thrombosis. The venous system is more frequently involved and usually occurs as thrombosis. Superficial or deep venous thrombosis is common in adults, but occur only in 5–15% of children. Additionally, arteritis and arterial aneurysms can occur [38–40]. Pulmonary artery thrombosis is rare, but is among the most severe features of BD and is associated with high morbidity and mortality rates [41,42]. Patients that develop superficial thrombophlebitis are more likely to develop major venous occlusions and must be carefully monitored. Vascular involvement was reported to be most common in non-European children [33].

Neurological involvement

Neurological involvement is the most devastating complication of BD. The reported frequency of neurological involvement in children varies from 7.2 to 15% [24,28]; however, when isolated headaches are included, the frequency can increase to 50% [43]. A large cohort study that included paediatric BD patients reported that neurological involvement was more common in European patients than in non-European patients [33]. There are two major forms of neurological involvement: vascular inflammatory central nervous system disease with parenchymal involvement (cranial nerve palsy, encephalomyelitis, seizures, hemiparesis and meningitis) and isolated cerebral venous sinus thrombosis (CVST) together with intracranial hypertension [44]. A comparative study that included children and adults with neuro-BD reported that in children the age of onset of neurological symptoms ranged between 11 and 15 years, males were more frequently affected than females and the most common type of neurological involvement was CVST, and that the prognosis was better in children than in adults. In adults, parenchymal involvement was the most common neurological finding [45]. As such, it was suggested that BD should be the first diagnosis to be excluded in adolescent males with CVST [44].

Gastrointestinal involvement

Gastrointestinal (GI) symptoms of BD are nonspecific and include abdominal pain, diarrhoea, vomiting and bleeding; therefore, they can easily be misdiagnosed as gastroenteritis, constipation or food allergy – all common childhood diseases. As such, for definitive diagnosis of intestinal BD, typical oval-shaped ulcers in the terminal ileum, or ulceration or inflammation of the small and large intestine must be observed, in addition to typical clinical findings after excluding tuberculosis, Crohn disease, nonspecific colitis and drug-associated colitis [46]. The frequency of GI involvement in paediatric BD patients ranges from 0 to 50% [47] and is reported to be more common in children than in adults [24,25]. Additionally, GI involvement is most common in European paediatric BD patients [33]. A study that included 20 children with BD reported that initial GI symptoms and intestinal ulcers were more commonly observed in the patients younger than 10 years old. Additionally, it was noted that patients with GI symptoms more frequently had skin involvement [47].

Joint involvement

Among adult BD patients, 50% have joint involvement [27]. Arthralgia or arthritis most commonly affect the knees, ankles, wrists and elbows. Arthritis in such patients does not cause deformity and resolves by itself. In children, the frequency of joint involvement ranges from 22.7 to 76% [24,28,32,33,35]; the knees and ankles are most commonly involved [28]. One study reported that articular symptoms were more common in European children than in non-European children [33].

Other features

Among adult BD patients, 7–46% have cardiac involvement [48]. Cardiac lesions in adults with BD were reviewed recently: 38.5% of such patients had pericarditis, 26.9% had endocarditis, 19.2% had intracardiac thrombosis, 17.3% had myocardial infarction and 1.9% had myocardial aneurysm, highlighting that BD must also be included in the differential of such lesions [49]. Moreover, fever can be observed in paediatric BD patients [33].

Diagnosis. Because of the lack of specific diagnostic laboratory tests, BD is diagnosed based on clinical features only. Diagnostic criteria (Table 150.1) proposed by the International Study Group in 1990 [50] have been widely accepted and used worldwide since their publication. In 2014 the same group published revised classification criteria [51]; however, diagnosis of BD in children remains challenging. As such, an international effort was initiated to collect all paediatric BD data, in order to delineate the features of childhood BD [52]. Initial findings show that 19% of paediatric BD patients have a positive family history of BD, indicating a high genetic burden in early onset BD. Additionally, only 1% of the children did not have oral ulcerations and not all of the paediatric patients fulfilled the adult criteria. Mounting evidence showing that some BD patients do not fulfil the diagnostic criteria, an increase in the importance of vascular and neurological features of BD and the genetic link in paediatric cases all suggest there was a need for revised diagnostic criteria for paediatric BD. Subsequently, in 2015, revised diagnostic criteria for paediatric BD were proposed which like adult criteria include neurological and vascular symptoms (Table 150.2). Moreover, they no longer include a positive pathergy test and although oral ulcers remain a diagnostic criterion, they are no longer mandatory for the diagnosis of paediatric BD; all symptom categories carry the same weight [33].

Table 150.1 International Study Group diagnostic criteria for Behçet disease [50]. Recurrent oral ulcers plus two of the four criteria are required for a diagnosis

Recurrent oral aphthous ulcers	>3 episodes/year
Recurrent genital ulcer or scar	
Eye lesions	Anterior/posterior uveitis, cells in vitreous humour via slit-lamp examination, retinal vasculitis
Skin lesions	Erythema nodosum, papulopustular lesions, pseudofolliculitis
Pathergy test positivity	

Source: Adapted from International Study Group for Behçet disease 1990 [50]. Reproduced with permission of Elsevier.

Table 150.2 Consensus classification of paediatric Behçet disease [33]. For diagnosis three of the six criteria must be fulfilled

Recurrent oral ulcers	≥3 episodes/year
Genital ulcers	Typically with scars
Skin lesions	Necrotic folliculitis, acneiform lesions, erythema nodosum
Ocular involvement	Anterior/posterior uveitis, retinal vasculitis
Neurological involvement	Except isolated headaches
Vascular involvement	Venous thrombosis, arterial thrombosis, arterial aneurysm

Source: Adapted from Koné-Paut et al. 2015 [33] by permission from BMJ Publishing Group Limited.

Pathergy test

A positive pathergy test is included in International Study Group criteria for diagnosing BD. The frequency of a positive pathergy test varies in adult populations according to geography and ranges from 0% (England) to 70% (Turkey) [53]. The frequency of a positive pathergy in children ranges from 18 to 44.7% [24,28,33]. Pathergy phenomenon occur when a needle prick triggers skin hyperreactivity with an inflammatory reaction, resulting in perivascular infiltration [54]. Unfortunately, there is no standard method for conducting the pathergy test; some investigators just prick the skin with a sterile needle (20 gauge), whereas others prefer to inject saline intradermally [55]. The test is performed on hairless forearm skin, because it was reported that the pathergy positivity rate was highest on the forearm [56]. A 20-gauge disposable needle is inserted at a 45° angle intradermally without disinfecting the skin. It was shown that the frequency and intensity of a positive pathergy test increase when using a reusable, sterilized blunt needle [57], as well as when two or more pricks are administered [58]. The test reaction is clinically assessed at 48 hours and a papule bigger than 2 mm in diameter is considered a positive test (Fig. 150.5).

Differential diagnosis. BD is a multisystemic disorder that is diagnosed according to clinical findings; therefore, other conditions, such as systemic lupus erythematosus (SLE), Crohn disease, ulcerative colitis, coeliac disease, sarcoidosis, hyper IgD syndrome (mevalonate kinase deficiency), cyclic neutropenia, SAPHO (synovitis, acne, pustulosis, hyperostosis, osteitis) syndrome, MAGIC (mouth and genital ulcers with inflamed cartilage) syndrome, antineutrophilic cytoplasmic antibody (ANCA)-positive vasculitis, multiple sclerosis, tuberculosis, AIDS and malignancies, should be excluded for a definitive diagnosis.

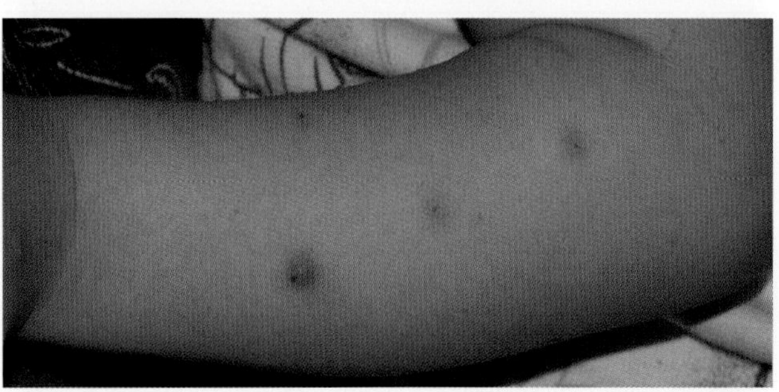

Fig. 150.5 Positive pathergy test.

Recurrent oral aphthae are the most common manifestation of BD; however, they can also be observed in SLE, spondyloarthropathies, rheumatoid arthritis, inflammatory bowel disease, hyperimmunoglobulin D syndrome, HSV and HIV infections, Stevens–Johnson syndrome, bullous skin disorders, lichen planus, cyclic neutropenia, and vitamin B12, iron and folic acid deficiency, as well as in response to drugs (methotrexate and chemotherapy drugs) [59], and as 'idiopathic' (minor or major type) aphthae.

Treatment. Unfortunately, because of the lack of multicentre studies on paediatric BD, there are no treatment guidelines for paediatric patients. Treatment recommendations for adult BD patients published by the European League Against Rheumatism (EULAR) [60] are used as a guideline for adults as well as for children with BD [61].

Oral and genital aphthae

Improving oral hygiene is the key to treating BD-related oral aphthae. Topical corticosteroids, sucralfate and chlorhexidine mouthwash should be tried first. Although findings concerning the efficacy of colchicine for treating oral and genital ulcers are inconsistent, when topical treatment fails, colchicine is the first-line treatment. Colchicine can also be used to treat genital ulcers when topical corticosteroids or sucralfate are not effective [59]. If colchicine fails, azathioprine is an alternative.

Skin lesions

One study showed that colchicine in women with BD reduced the frequency of genital ulcers, EN and arthritis, whereas in men it only reduced the frequency of arthritis [62]. A randomized, double-blind study reported that colchicine markedly improved oral and genital aphthae, pseudofolliculitis and EN [63]. Other effective agents for BD-related skin findings are azathioprine, anti-TNF therapy, IFN-α and thalidomide [59].

Ocular lesions

Azathioprine is the first-line treatment for BD-related uveitis and systemic corticosteroids are used for acute attacks. Cyclosporine is another alternative for ocular involvement and anti-TNF agents and IFN-α are used to treat refractory ocular disease [59].

Neurological involvement

Parenchymal disease associated with BD is treated with high-dose systemic steroids and azathioprine. Other alternatives for neurological involvement include methotrexate, mycophenolate mofetil, cyclophosphamide, tacrolimus and IFN-α. For severe cases, anti-TNF agents are a viable option. In cases of cerebrovascular thrombosis aggressive immunosuppression is required [59], whereas there is no evidence showing that anticoagulation is beneficial [61]. A case series that included paediatric BD patients with vascular involvement reported that azathioprine was effective [64].

GI involvement

GI disease associated with BD is usually treated empirically with steroids, mesalazine, azathioprine and anti-TNF agents. A case series that included paediatric BD patients with GI involvement reported that thalidomide markedly improved GI symptoms [65].

Prognosis. Paediatric BD patients have a better prognosis than adults with BD. Ocular, vascular and neurological involvement are associated with the highest morbidity and mortality rates in adult BD patients. It was reported that the mortality rate was 10-fold higher in Turkish males with BD aged 15–24 years than in age- and gender-matched controls [66]. Female BD patients with mucocutaneous involvement alone have a better prognosis [59].

References

1 Behçet H. Uber die rezidivierende ophthose durch ein reursachte Geschwure am Mund, am Auge und an den Genitalien. Dermatol Wochenschr 1937;105:1152.

2 Jennette JC, Falk RJ, Bacon PA et al. 2012 revised International Chapel Hill Consensus Conference Nomenclature of Vasculitides. Arthritis Rheum 2013;65:1–11.

3 Koné-Paut I, Bernard JL. Pediatric Behçet's disease in France. Arch Fr Pediatr 1993;50:561–5.

4 Azizlerli G, Köse AA, Sarıca R et al. Prevalance of Behçet's disease in Istanbul, Turkey. Int J Dermatol 2003;42:803–6.

5 Hatemi G, Yazıcı Y, Yazıcı H. Behçet's syndrome. Rheum Dis Clin N Am 2013;39:245–61.

6 Mahr A, Belarbi L, Wechsler B et al. Population-based prevalance study of Behcet disease: differences by ethnic origin and low variation by age at immigration. Arthritis Rheum 2008;58:3951–9.

7 Yazıcı H, Uğurlu S, Seyahi E. Behçet syndrome: is it one condition? Clin Rev Allergy Immunol 2012;43:275–80.

8 Hou S, Yang Z, Du L et al. Identification of a susceptibility locus in STAT4 for Behçet's disease in Han Chinese in a genome-wide association study. Arthritis Rheumatol 2012;64:4104–13.

9 Kirino Y, Bertsias G, Ishigatsubo Y et al. Genome-wide association analysis identifies new susceptibility loci for Behçet's disease and epistasis between HLA-B*51 and ERAP1. Nat Genet 2013;45:202–7.

10 Lee YJ, Horie Y, Wallace GR et al. Genome-wide association study identifies GIMAP as a novel susceptibility locus for Behcet's disease. Ann Rheum Dis 2013;72:1510–6.

11 Mizuki N, Meguro A, Ota M et al. Genome-wide association studies identify IL23R-IL12RB2 and IL10 as Behçet's disease susceptibility loci. Nat Genet 2010;42:703–6.

12 Remmers EF, Cosan F, Kirino Y et al. Genome-wide association study identifies variants in the MHC class I, IL10, and IL23R-IL12RB2 regions associated with Behçet's disease. Nat Genet 2010;42:698–702.

13 de Chambrun MP, Wechsler B, Geri G et al. New insights into the pathogenesis of Behçet's disease. Autoimmun Rev 2012;11:687–98.

14 Xavier JM, Shahram F, Davatchi F et al. Association study of IL10 and IL23R-IL12RB2 in Iranian patients with Behçet's disease. Arthritis Rheumatol 2012;64:2761–72.

15 Gül A, Ohno S. HLA-B*51 and Behçet Disease. Ocul Immunol Inflamm 2012;20:37–43.

16 DeLay ML, Turner MJ, Klenk EI et al. HLA-B27 misfolding and the unfolded protein response augment interleukin-23 production and are associated with Th17 activation in transgenic rats. Arthritis Rheumatol 2009;60:2633–43.

17 Zhang K, Kaufman RJ. From endoplasmic-reticulum stress to the inflammatory response. Nature 2008;454:455–62.

18 de Menthon M, Lavalley MP, Maldini C et al. HLA B51/B5 and the risk of Behçet's disease: a systematic review and meta-analysis of case-control genetic association studies. Arthritis Rheumatol 2009;61:1287–96.

19 Eglin RP, Lehner T, Subak-Sharpe JH. Detection of RNA complementary to herpes-simplex virus in mononuclear cells from patients with Behçet's syndrome and recurrent oral ulcers. Lancet 1982;2:1356–61.

20 Ergun T, İnce U, Ekşioğlu-Demiralp E et al. HSP 60 expression in mucocutaneous lesions of Behçet's disease. J Am Acad Dermatol 2001;45:904–9.

21 Direskeneli H, Saruhan-Direskeneli G. The role of heat shock proteins in Behçet's disease. Clin Exp Rheumatol 2003;21:S44–8.

22 Ermakova NA, Alekberova ZS, Prokaeova TB. Autoimmunity to S-antigen and retinal vasculitis in patients with Behçet's disease. Adv Exp Med Biol 2003;528:279–81.

23 Özen S, Eroğlu FK. Pediatric-onset Behçet's disease. Curr Opin Rheumatol 2013;25:636–42.

24 Karıncaoğlu Y, Borlu M, Çıkman Toker S et al. Demographic and clinical properties of juvenile-onset Behçet's diesase: a controlled multicenter study. J Am Acad Dermatol 2008;58:579–84.

25 Krause I, Uziel Y, Guedj M et al. Childhood Behçet's disease: clinical features and comparison with adult-onset. Rheumatology 1999;38:457–62.

26 Johnson EF, Hawkins DM, Gifford LK, Smidt AC. Recurrent oral and genital ulcers in an infant: neonatal presentation of pediatric Behçet disease. Pediatr Dermatol 2015;32:714–7.

27 Mat C, Göksügür N, Ergin B et al. The frequency of scarring after genital ulcers in Behçet's syndrome: a prospective study. Int J Dermatol 2006;45:554–6.

28 Koné-Paut I, Yurdakul S, Bahabri SA et al. Clinical features of Behçet's disease in children: an international collaborative study of 86 cases. J Pediatr 1998;132:721–5.

29 Yasui K, Komiyama A, Takabayashi Y et al. Behçet's disease in children. J Pediatr 1999;134;249–51.

30 Kari JA, Shah V, Dillon MJ. Behçet's disease in UK children: clinical features and treatment including thalidomide. Rheumatology 2001;40:933–8.

31 Koné-Paut I, Gorchakoff-Molinas A, Weschler B, Touitou I. Pediatric Behçet's disease in France. Ann Rheum Dis 2002;61:655–6.

32 Borlu M, Ukşal Ü, Ferahbaş A, Evereklioğlu C. Clinical features of Behçet's disease in children. Int J Dermatol 2006;45:713–6.

33 Koné-Paut I, Shahram F, Darce-Bello M et al. Consensus classification criteria for pediatric Behçet's disease from a prospective observational cohort: PEBD. Ann Rheum Dis 2015;0:1–7.

34 Hatemi G, Bahar H, Uysal S et al. The pustular skin lesions in Behçet's syndrome are not sterile. Ann Rheum Dis 2004;63:1450–2.

35 Atmaca L, Boyvat A, Yalçındağ FN et al. Behçet disease in children. Ocular Immunol Inflamm 2011;19:103–7.

36 Sungur GK, Hazırolan D, Yalvaç I et al. Clinical and demographics evaluation of Behçet disease among different pediatric age groups. Br J Ophthalmol 2009;93:83–7.

37 Kesen MR, Goldstein DA, Tessler HH. Uveitis associated pediatric Behçet disease in the American midwest. Am J Ophthalmol 2008;146:819–27.

38 Enoch BA, Castillo-Olivares JL, Khoo TCL et al. Major vascular complications in Behçet's syndrome. Postgrad Med J 1968;44:453–9.

39 Davies JD. Behçet's syndrome with haemoptysis and pulmonary lesions. J Pathol 1973;109:351–6.

40 Grenier P, Bletry O, Cornud F et al. Pulmonary involvement in Behçet's disease. Am J Roentgenol 1981;137:565–9.

41 Erkan F. Pulmonary involvement in Behçet disease. Curr Opin Pulm Med 1999;5:314–8.

42 Akdağ Kose A, Kayabalı M, Sarıca R et al. Pulmonary artery involvement in Behçet's disease. Adv Exp Med Biol 2003;528:419–22.

43 Bahabri SA, al-Mazyed A, al-Balaa S et al. Juvenile Behçet's disease in Arab children. Clin Exp Rheumatol 1996;14:331–5.

44 Siva A, Saip S. The spectrum of nervous system involvement in Behçet's syndrome and its differential diagnosis. J Neurol 2009;256:513–29.

45 Uludüz D, Kurtuncu M, Yapıcı Z et al. Clinical characteristics of pediatric-onset neuro-Behçet disease. Neurology 2011;77:1900–5.

46 Kobayashi K, Ueno F, Bito S et al. Development of consensus statements for the diagnosis and management of intestinal Behçet's disease using a modified Delphi approach. J Gastroenterol 2007;42: 737–45.

47 Hung CH, Lee JH, Chen ST et al. Young children with Behçet disease have more intestinal involvement. J Pediatr Gastroenterol Nutr 2013;57:225–9.

48 Demirelli S, Değirmenci H, İnci S, Arısoy A. Cardiac manifestations in Behçet's disease. Intr Rare Dis Res 2015;4:70–5.

49 Geri G, Wechsler B, Thi Huong du L et al. Spectrum of cardiac lesions in Behçet disease: a series of 52 patients and review of the literature. Medicine (Baltimore) 2012;91:25–34.

50 International Study Group for Behçet's disease. Criteria for diagnosis of Behçet's disease. Lancet 1990;335:1078–80.

51 International Team for the Revision of the International Criteria for Behçet's disease (ITR-BCD). The International Criteria for Behçet's

disease (ICBD): a collaborative study of 27 countrieas on the sensitivity and specificity of the new criteria. J Eur Acad Dermatol Venereol 2014;28:338–47.

52 **Kone-Paut I, Darce-Bello M, Shahram F et al. Registries in rheumatological and musculoskeletal conditions. Paediatric Behcet's disease: an international cohort study of 110 patients. One-year follow-up data. Rheumatology 2010;50:184–8.**

53 Yazıcı H, Chamberlain MA, Tüzün Y et al. A comprative study of the pathergy reaction among Turkish and British patients with Behçet's disease. Ann Rheum Dis 1984;43:74–5.

54 Gül A, Esin S, Dilsen N et al. Immunohistology of skin pathergy reaction in Behçet disease. Br J Dermatol 1995;132:901–7.

55 **Varol A, Seifert O, Anderson CD. The skin pathergy test:innately useful? Arch Dermatol Res 2010;302:155–68.**

56 **Özdemir M, Balevi S, Deniz F, Mevlitoğlu İ. Pathergy reaction in different body areas in Behçet's disease. Clin Exp Dermatol 2007;32:85–7.**

57 **Dilsen N, Konice M, Aral O et al. Comparative study of the skin pathergy test with blunt and sharp needles in Behçet's disease;confirmed specificity but decreased sensitivity with sharp needles. Ann Rheum Dis 1993;52:823–5.**

58 Özdemir M, Bodur S, Engin B, Baysal I. Evaluation of application of multiple needle pricks on the pathergy reaction. Int J Dermatol 2008;47:335–8.

59 Ambrose NL, Haskard DO. Differential diagnosis and management of Behçet syndrome. Nat Rev 2013;9:79–89.

60 Hatemi G,Silman A, Bang D et al. EULAR expert committee. EULAR recommendations for the management of Behçet's disease. Ann Rheum Dis 2008;67:1656–62.

61 **Özen S. Pediatric onset Behçet disease. Curr Opin Rheumatol 2010;22:585–9.**

62 Yurdakul S, Mat C, Tüzün Y et al. A double-blind trial of colchicine in Behçet's syndrome. Arthritis Rheumatol 2001;44:2686–92.

63 **Davatchi F, Sadeghi Abdollahi B, Tehrani Banihashemi A et al. Colchicine versus placebo in Behçet's disease;randomised, double-blind, controlled crossover trial. Mod Rheumatol 2009;19:542–9.**

64 **Özen S, Bilginer Y, Beşbaş N et al. Behçet disease: treatment of vascular involvement in children. Eur J Pediatr 2010;169:427–30.**

65 Yasui K, Uchida N, Akazawa Y et al. Thalidomide for treatment of intestinal involvement of juvenile-onset Behçet disease. Inflamm Bowel Dis 2008;14:396–400.

66 **Kural-Seyahi E, Fresko I, Seyahi N et al. The longterm mortality and morbidity of Behçet syndrome:a 2-decade outcome survey of 387 patients followed at a dedicated center. Medicine (Baltimore) 2003;82:60–76.**

Relapsing polychondritis

Key points

- **Relapsing polychondritis (RP) is characterized by recurrent inflammation and destruction of cartilage.**
- **RP most commonly affects the ears and nose.**
- **In children, respiratory tract involvement, costochondritis and atypical destructive arthritis are more severe and common than in adults.**
- **Diagnosis can be established based on clinical findings.**
- **RP can be a rapidly progressive and fulminating disease.**

Introduction. Relapsing polychondritis (RP) is a multisystemic disease characterized by recurrent inflammation and destruction of cartilage. The ears and nose are most commonly involved, but joints, the eyes, the cardiovascular system and the respiratory tract can also be affected [1]. With the exception of cartilage, proteoglycan-rich tissues, such as media of arteries, and the conjunctiva and sclera of the eyes are involved. In children, respiratory tract involvement, costochondritis and atypical destructive arthritis are more common and more severe than in adults [2].

History and epidemiology. RP was first described as 'polychondropathia' in 1923 by Jaksch-Wartenhorst [3] and was subsequently referred to as RP by Pearson and colleagues [1] in 1960 because of its episodic nature [4]. RP is a rare disease with an estimated incidence of 3.5 per 1 million adults [5]. White people and females are most frequently affected [1]. The literature includes only a few studies on paediatric RP and, as such, paediatric epidemiological data are limited. The age of onset in children varies from 1.7 months to 17 years [6].

Aetiopathogenesis. The aetipathogenesis of RP remains unknown. RP is associated with other autoimmune diseases (30%), it responds to systemic steroids and immunosuppressive treatments, its histopathology is characterized by infiltration of cartilage with CD4+ T lymphocytes and its association with antibodies against collagen type II, IX, XI, matrilin and COMP (cartilage oligomeric matrix proteins), all of which indicate an autoimmune hypothesis [7]. Although an association between RP and HLA-DR4 has been described, genetic factors do not appear to play a role in the pathogenesis of RP [8]. Cell-mediated immune response and activation of monocytes and macrophages were reported in a study that included 22 RP patients [9]. Factors that trigger RP include trauma, piercing, pregnancy, *Mycobacterium tuberculosis* and myxoma virus [7].

Clinical features. Auricular chondritis is the most common finding in adults (80–89%) [1,5] and is characterized by pain, tenderness, erythema (Fig. 150.6) and oedema of the pinna, typically sparing the earlobe. Recurrent attacks damage cartilage and result in flabby, droopy, or cauliflower ear. Auricular chondritis was reported in 27% of the 44 previously published paediatric RP case series [2].

Arthritis is the second most frequent clinical feature of RP, with involvement of the wrists, knees, hips, and metacarpophalangeal and proximal interphalangeal joints. In adults it manifests as migratory, non-erosive oligo/polyarthritis without deformity. Arthritis was reported to be the most common symptom (36%) in the largest study on childhood RP [2]. Additionally, RP-associated arthritis can be destructive and involve the epiphyseal plate [10].

Nasal chondritis is another common presentation in adults and children, which is acute and painful. Fullness in the nose, rhinorrhoea and epistaxis are the typical clinical manifestations. Because of destruction of nose cartilage, saddle nose deformity may occur [1]. Ocular involvement manifesting as episcleritis, scleritis, keratitis, conjunctivitis, uveitis or iritis occurs in 50–60% of both adult and paediatric RP patients [2].

Dermatological findings are observed in 17–36% of RP cases [11], including oral aphthae (most common), genital ulcer, purpura, vasculitis, erythema multiforme, erythema annulare centrifugum, erythema elevatum diutinum, panniculitis, urticarial lesions and Sweet syndrome [5,11]. Additionally, papular and annular fixed urticarial

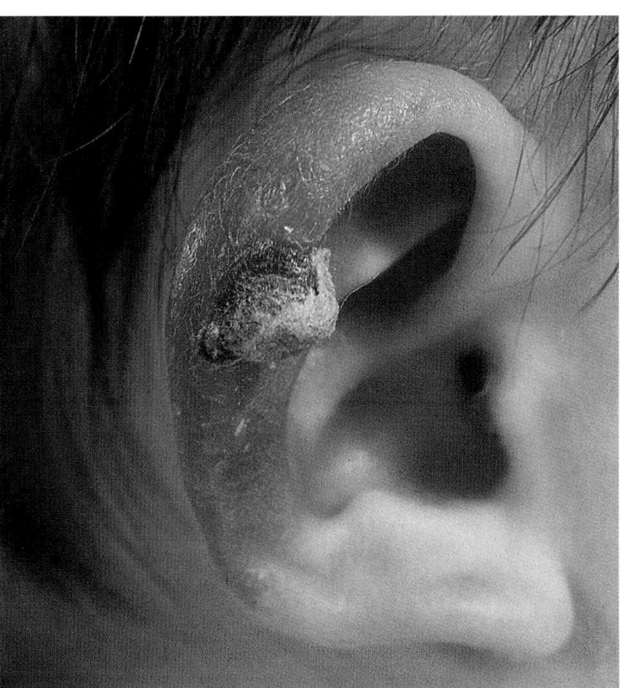

Fig. 150.6 Relapsing polychondritis with ear involvement. Source: Courtesy of Professor Paul A, Brogan, UCL Institute of Child Health, London, UK.

Table 150.3 Relapsing polychondritis diagnostic criteria

McAdam et al. [13]	For diagnosis ≥3 criteria must be fulfilled Bilateral auricular chondritis Nasal chondritis Respiratory chondritis Non-erosive seronegative arthritis Ocular inflammation Audiovestibular damage
Damiani and Levine [14]	Three of McAdam et al.'s criteria or One of McAdam et al.'s criteria + histopathological confirmation or Two of McAdam et al.'s criteria + positive response to dapsone or steroids
Michet et al. [15]	For diagnosis two major criteria or one major + two minor criteria must be fulfilled Major criteria: Auricular cartilage inflammation Nasal cartilage inflammation Laryngotracheal cartilage inflammation Minor criteria: Ocular inflammation Hearing loss Vestibular dysfunction Seronegative arthritis

eruption on the upper trunk with histopathological findings of lymphocytic vasculitis has been reported [12].

Cardiovascular involvement results in valvular insufficiency, arrhythmia, conduction defects, aortic aneurysm and pericarditis [1]; it occurs more commonly in males and is the second most common cause of mortality in RP patients [5]. Pulmonary disease occurs in 50% of adult RP patients, with involvement of the laryngo-bronchial structures. Pulmonary involvement can be very severe, with obstruction or stenosis of the larynx, trachea or bronchi. Presenting symptoms are cough, dyspnoea, stridor and wheezing. Subglottic inflammation caused by strictures, tracheal collapse and pulmonary infections can complicate the treatment of RP and lead to death. In fact, airway complications are the most common cause of death in patients with RP [1,5]. Respiratory tract involvement is more common and severe in paediatric RP patients than in adults [2] and tracheostomy is often necessary.

Neurological manifestations of RP primarily involve the cranial nerves and vasculitis has also been reported [1]. Renal involvement is rare and most commonly presents as IgA nephropathy or glomerulonephritis with a poor prognosis [1,5]. Audiovestibular involvement can lead, for example, to hearing loss (both conductive and sensory), tinnitus or vertigo [1].

Diagnosis. Unfortunately, there are no laboratory tests specifically designed for diagnosing RP. Histopathological examination is not specific for RP, but typically shows loss of basophilic staining of cartilaginous matrix, perichondrial inflammation and replacement of cartilage with fibrous tissue. Because biopsy is not specific and can cause cartilage damage, it is reserved for difficult to diagnose cases [1,2,5]. Nonetheless, RP can be diagnosed based on clinical criteria that were originally published by McAdam and colleagues [13] in 1976, expanded by Damiani and Levine [14] in 1979, and revised and modified by Michet and colleagues [15] in 1986 (Table 150.3).

The erythrocyte sedimentation rate can be elevated and correlated with disease activity. Anaemia, leucocytosis and eosinophilia can be observed. Urinary mucopolysaccharides can be high during flare-ups. Chest X-ray, pulmonary function tests, spiral CT, MRI and laryngotracheography can be used to evaluate airway involvement of RP [1,5]. Positron emission tomography/computed tomography is a good option for evaluating multisystem involvement, as well as disease activity [5].

Differential diagnosis. Auricular chondritis should be differentiated from bacterial cellulitis, erysipelas of the ear, trauma, insect bite, frostbite and congenital syphilis. Auricular chondritis is often bilateral and spares the earlobes. Saddle nose caused by nasal chondritis can also be seen in patients with leprosy, congenital syphilis, leishmaniasis, SLE, paracoccidioidomycosis, aspergillosis, rhinoscleroma, Wegener granulomatosis and lymphoma. RP-associated arthritis, which is non-erosive and transient, can mimic reactive arthritis. Airway involvement in RP patients mimics bronchial asthma or Wegener granulomatosis, whereas vascular involvement mimics polyarteritis nodosa, Takayasu arteritis, BD and antiphospholipid antibody syndrome [1,5].

Treatment. Because there are no randomized trials of RP treatments, all relevant data are derived from case reports and case series. Nonsteroidal anti-inflammatory drugs can be used for mild, localized disease. Systemic steroids (oral or pulse) remain the mainstay for treating acute flare-ups or organ-threatening disease. Steroid-sparing and immunosuppressive agents can also be used, including cyclophosphamide, azathioprine, methotrexate, cyclosporine and colchicine [1,2,5]. Additionally, anti-TNF agents, IL-1 receptor antagonist, tocilizumab, abatacept and infliximab have been successfully used to treat adult RP patients [16-19]. Remission has been reported in paediatric RP patients following administration of infliximab, adalimumab, anakinra and rituximab [16,20,21].

Prognosis. Although the course of RP is variable, it can be a rapidly progressive and fulminating disease. In adults mean survival is 5–7 years and the mortality rate is approximately 30%. In children, destructive chondritis, deafness, impaired vision and mortality have been reported. The cause of death in paediatric RP cases include tracheal collapse and acute valvular insufficiency [2,6].

References

1 **Rapini RP, Warner NB. Relapsing polychondritis. Clin Dermatol 2006;24:482–5.**

2 **Fonseca AR, de Oliveira SKF, Rodrigues MCF et al. Relapsing polychondritis in childhood: three case reports, comparison with adulthood disease and literature review. Rheumatol Int 2013;33: 1873–8.**

3 Jaksch-Wartenhorst R. Polychondropathia. Wien Arch Inn Med 1923;6:93–100.

4 Pearson CM, Kline HM, Newcomer VD. Relapsing polychondritis. New Engl J Med 1960;263:51–8.

5 **Cantarini L, Vitale A, Giuseppina Brizi M et al. Diagnosis and classification of relapsing polychondritis. J Autoimmun 2014;48–49:53–59.**

6 **Belot A, Duquesne A, Job-Deslandre C et al. Pediatric-onset relapsing polychondroitis: case series and systematic review. J Pediatr 2010;156:484–9.**

7 **Vitale A, Sota J, Rigante D et al. Relapsing polychondritis: an update on pathogenesis, clinical features, diagnostic tools, and therapeutic perspectives. Curr Rheumatol Rep 2016;18:3.**

8 **Zeuner B, Straub RH, Rauh G et al. Relapsing polychondritis: clinical and immunogenetic analysis of 62 patients. J Rheumatol 1997;24:96–101.**

9 Stabler T, Piette JC, Chevalier X et al. Serum cytokine profiles in relapsing polychondritis suggest monocyte/macrophage activation. Arthritis Rheum 2004;50:3663–7.

10 De Oliveira SKF, Fonseca AR, Domingues RC, Aymore IL. A unique articular manifestation in a child with relapsing polychondritis. J Rheumatol 2009;36:3.

11 **Frances C, El Rassi R, Laporte JL et al. Dermatologic manifestations of relapsing polychondritis. Medicine 2001;80:173–9.**

12 Tronquoy AF, de Quatrebarbes J, Picard D et al. Papular and annular fixed urticarial eruption: a characteristic skin manifestation in patients with relapsing chondritis. J Am Acad Dermatol 2011;65:1161–6.

13 McAdam LP, O'Hanlan MA, Bluestone R, Pearson CM. Relapsing polychondritis: prospective study of 23 patients and a review of literature. Medicine (Baltimore) 1976;55:193–215.

14 Damiani JM, Levine HL. Relapsing polychondroitis – report of ten cases. Laryngoscope 1979;89:929–46.

15 Michet Jr CJ, McKenna CH, Luthra HS, O'Fallon WM. Relapsing polychondritis: survival and predictive role of early disease manifestations. Ann Intern Med 1986;104:74–8.

16 Buonuomo PS, Bracaglia C, Campana A et al. Relapsing polychondritis: new therapeutic strategies with biological agents. Rheumatol Int 2010;30:691–3.

17 De Barros AP, Nakamura NA, Santana T de F et al. Infliximab in relapsing polychondritis. Rev Bras Reumatol 2010;50:211–6.

18 Peng SL, Rodriguez D. Abatacept in relapsing polychondritis. Ann Rheum Dis 2013;72:1427–9.

19 Wendling D, Godfrin-Valnet M, Prati C. Treatment of relapsing polychondritis with tocilizumab. J Rheumatol 2013;40:1232.

20 **Navarrete VM, Lebron CV, de Miera FJTS et al. Sustained remission of pediatric relapsing polychondritis. J Clin Rheumatol 2014;20:45–6.**

21 **Abdwani R, Kolethekkat AA, Al Abri R. Refractory relapsing polychondritis in a child treated with antiCD20 monoclonal antibody (rituximab): first case report. Int J Pediatr Otorhinol 2012;76:1061–4.**

CHAPTER 151
Erythromelalgia

Nedaa Skeik

Vascular Medicine Department, Minneapolis Heart Institute, Minneapolis, MN, USA

Abstract

Erythromelalgia is a very rare disease that can cause intermittent painful redness, heat and oedema affecting more commonly the lower extremities, mostly aggravated by heat and dependence, and can lead to significant disabilities. Whereas primary erythromelalgia is thought to be caused by familial or sporadic mutation in the *SCN9A* gene which encodes for the voltage-gated sodium channel, secondary erythromelalgia can be caused by different conditions including myeloproliferative, blood and autoimmune disorders. Differential diagnoses include peripheral neuropathy, complex regional pain syndrome, dermatitis, skin infections, autoimmune disease skin involvement, osteomyelitis, arterial or venous insufficiency and Fabry disease. Management for erythromelalgia can be very difficult and challenging and should have a multidisciplinary approach. There is no single effective treatment for erythromelalgia. Management includes patient education, controlling secondary and underlying factors, cooling techniques and selective medications such as aspirin in patients with myeloproliferative disorders.

Key points

- **Erythromelalgia is a very painful neurovascular disease that may be caused by a mutation of the *SCN9A* gene encoding for voltage-gated sodium channel leading to intermittent painful redness, heat and swelling of the affected extremity.**
- **Diagnosis is usually clinical and management can be very challenging.**

Definition. Erythromelalgia is a rare neurovascular condition characterized by intermittent redness, heat, pain and sometimes swelling more commonly affecting the lower extremities, but may also affect the upper extremities, face or other parts of the body [1]. Symptoms are mostly aggravated by heat and are commonly eased by cooling [1,2]. Erythromelalgia can be classified as either familial or sporadic, with the familial form inherited in an autosomal dominant manner [3,4]. Both of these may be further classified as either juvenile (manifests prior to the age of 20) or adult onset [3,4]. Reported secondary causes of erythromelalgia include myeloproliferative and blood disorders, drugs, infections, malignancies, connective tissue and autoimmune diseases [1].

History. Symptoms of hot and painful extremities were described by Graves in 1834 [5]. Erythromelalgia, or Mitchell disease, was then named by and after Weir Mitchell in 1878 from erythros (red), melos (extremity), and algos (pain) [6]. In 1932, Brown postulated five basic criteria for the diagnosis of the true primary variant of 'burning red congested extremities' [7,8]:

1. Attacks of bilateral or symmetrical burning pain in the hands and feet;
2. The attacks were initiated or aggravated by standing or exposure to heat;
3. Relief was obtained by elevation and exposure to cold;
4. During the attacks, the affected extremities were flushed and congested and exhibited increased local heat; and
5. The pathogenesis is unknown and there is no treatment available for primary erythermalgia.

Smith and Allen substituted the term erythromelalgia for erythermalgia to denote the importance of heat (therme) [9]. Other names used in the literature included acromelalgia from acro (extremity), erythralgia, erythermomelalgia, and erythroprosopalgia from prosopon (face) [10]. In 2004, *SCN9A* mutations were determined to be the main genetic predisposition for primary erythromelalgia [11].

Aetiology. Erythromelalgia can be classified as a primary or secondary disorder. Primary erythromelalgia is caused by a familial or sporadic mutation in the *SCN9A* gene which encodes for the voltage-gated sodium channel [1]. The familial form is inherited in an autosomal dominant manner. Both familial and sporadic forms may be further classified as either juvenile or adult onset. Juvenile onset occurs prior to the age of 20 years and frequently prior to the age 10 [1,3,12]. Reported secondary causes of erythromelalgia may include myeloproliferative disorders, blood dyscrasias, drugs, infections, malignancies, connective tissue and autoimmune disorders, cellular storage diseases, neuropathies and some ingested materials (Box 151.1) [1].

Harper's Textbook of Pediatric Dermatology, Fourth Edition. Edited by Peter Hoeger, Veronica Kinsler and Albert Yan.

Box 151.1 Reported causes of secondary erythromelalgia

Myeloproliferative diseases and blood disorders

Essential thrombocythemia
Polycythemia vera
Myelodysplastic syndrome
Pernicious anaemia
Thrombotic and immunological thrombocytopenic purpuras

Drugs

Cyclosporine
Verapamil
Nicardipine
Nifedipine
Norephedrine
Bromocriptine and pergolide

Infectious diseases

Human immunodeficiency virus
Hepatitis B vaccine
Influenza vaccine
Infectious mononucleosis
Pox virus

Connective tissue diseases

Systemic lupus erythematosus
Vasculitis

Neuropathic

Diabetic neuropathy
Peripheral neuropathies
Neurofibromatosis
Riley–Day syndrome
Multiple sclerosis

Neoplastic

Paraneoplastic syndrome
Astrocytoma
Malignant thymoma

Others

Mushroom ingestion
Mercury poisoning

Erythromelalgia is a very rare disease. A mean incidence of 1.3 per 100 000 was reported in Olmsted County, MN, USA in 2009, with slightly more prevalence in women [13]. Another study from New Zealand suggested an incidence rate as high as 15 per 100 000 [14].

Pathogenesis. The exact pathophysiology for erythromelalgia is not completely understood. However, it differs between the two main types [15]. There is enough literature to suggest that primary (inherited) erythromelalgia is an autosomal dominant disorder caused by gain-of-function mutations in the *SCN9A* gene encoding the $Na_v1.7$ sodium channel expressed mostly in the sympathetic and nociceptive small-diameter sensory neurons of the dorsal root ganglion that leads to altered function [1,16]. Around 20 mutations have been identified in patients with primary erythromelalgia [1]. Functionally, most of the studied primary erythromelalgia-related mutations were shown to produce a hyperpolarizing shift in activation and slow deactivation, and enhance the channel response to small depolarizing stimuli, changes that can confer hyperexcitability of cells harbouring these channels [1,17]. While the alteration of the function of sympathetic neurons leads to the microvascular symptoms, the alteration of the function of nociceptive neurons results in severe burning pain, which characterizes erythromelalgia [1,3]. Despite an increase in blood flow (as measured with laser Doppler), there is local hypoxia, reflected by low transcutaneous oxygen pressure ($TcPO_2$) values, which might be explained by arteriovenous shunting at a microvascular level [18]. The pathophysiology of the secondary type is poorly understood and thought to be caused by neuropathological and microvascular functional changes caused by the underlying condition [19].

Pathology. There have been no diagnostic pathology findings for erythromelalgia. Histopathological findings in skin biopsies from patients with primary congenital erythromelalgia are nonspecific, even showing the complete absence of any underlying disorder [20,21]. On the other hand, skin punch biopsy from a few patients with severe primary erythromelalgia revealed mild perivascular mononuclear infiltrate, vascular basement membrane thickening and significant perivascular oedema [22]. Other findings that have been reported included decreased density of acetylcholinesterase-positive and catecholamine-containing nerve terminals in the periarterial and sweat glandular plexuses [21,22].

Clinical features. Patients usually present with intermittent redness, pain, heat and swelling that can be exacerbated by warming, exercise and leg dependence, and relieved by cooling and elevation (Fig. 151.1) [2]. Erythromelalgia mainly involves the lower extremities, but occasionally affects the hands and very rarely the ears and face [23]. The pain is normally described as burning or piercing and sometimes can be very severe and disabling [1]. Symptoms are usually intermittent but can be constant, with changing intensity. Attacks can last for minutes or days [23]. Symptoms are more common in the summer and can be exacerbated by heat, ambulation, physical activity, sitting, leg dependence or wearing shoes or gloves [24]. A cool temperature may alleviate symptoms and in some cases abort an episode. Some patients seek relief by cooling the extremity in ice or cold water, exposing the limb to an air current, or elevating and uncovering the limb [25]. This may lead to ulceration, infection, limb ischaemia and even amputation [26,27].

A detailed history and physical examination are crucially important to make the diagnosis of erythromelalgia because there is no diagnostic laboratory test available at this time [1]. Vascular laboratory studies might reveal normal arterial Doppler signals, increased temperature and laser Doppler values in the presence of low $TcPO_2$ [28]. Autonomic reflex screen testing can be abnormal with small fibre disease [28]. Genetic testing can be helpful in making the diagnosis of the primary type [3,12]. There are no consensus guidelines on testing for *SCN9A*

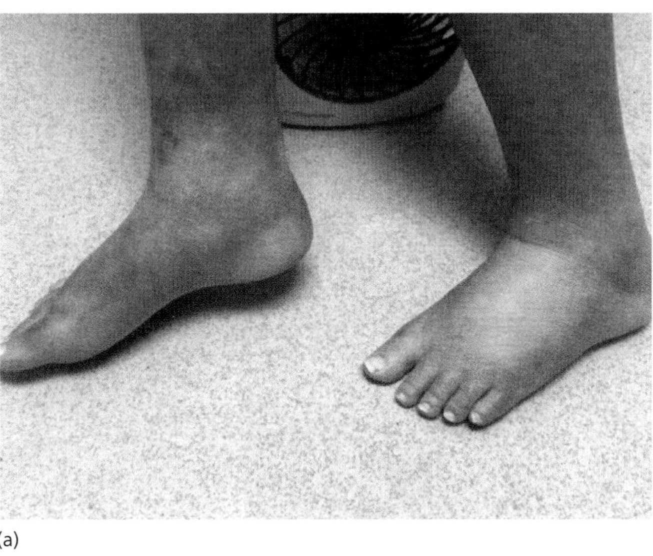
(a)

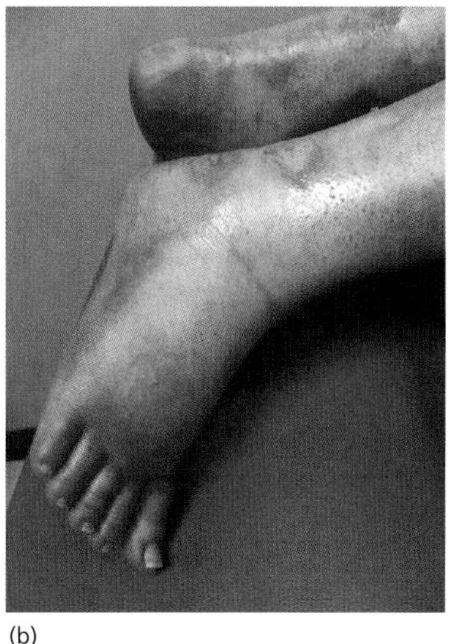
(b)

Fig. 151.1 Significant lower extremity erythema, swelling (a) and ulcerations (b) in a young girl with erythromelalgia.

mutations. Testing can be considered in young patients with positive family history when secondary aetiologies are less likely. Testing can also impact family planning because there is a 50% probability of inheriting the mutation and having a child with the same disease. Proving inherited rather than secondary erythromelalgia with genetic testing might also limit repeated extensive and expensive work-up in the search for secondary aetiologies [1].

Differential diagnosis. Peripheral neuropathy, complex regional pain syndrome, cellulitis, erysipelas, dermatitis, osteomyelitis, systemic lupus erythematosus, arterial or venous insufficiency, gout and Fabry disease may be included in the differential diagnosis [1,28].

Reflex sympathetic dystrophy is characterized by chronic disabling pain, swelling, vasomotor instability and a limited range of motion usually affecting the lower extremities. Patients usually present with cool, mottled and very painful extremities. Symptoms are not triggered by dependency and heat. Patients may benefit from sympathetic blockade [29,30].

Angiodyskinesia syndrome is predominantly a disease of young females which refers to a combination of early venous return, spastic arteries and pain affecting the lower extremities. Patients usually present with a blotchy erythema when standing that might be associated with paraesthesia or a burning pain. Management may include vasodilators and sympathectomy with equivocal results [29].

Fabry disease is an X-linked sphingolipid storage disorder characterized by α-galactosidase A deficiency resulting in angiokeratomas, corneal dystrophy, mitral valve disease and renal failure. It can present with acute painful crises following exercise, emotional stress and acute changes in temperature or humidity [29,31].

Treatment. Management can be very difficult and challenging. There is no single effective treatment for erythromelalgia. A multidisciplinary approach is recommended. Management includes patient education, controlling secondary and underlying factors, avoiding aggravating factors, cooling techniques and selective medication [1,32]. Aspirin can be effective in patients with secondary erythromelalgia caused by myeloproliferative disorders [28,32]. Based on case studies, intravenous sodium nitroprusside may be helpful in children and adolescents [33–36]. This works by relaxing both arteriolar and venous smooth muscle as well as inhibiting platelet aggregation. The reported used doses were initially 1 μg/kg/min increased up to 5 μg/kg/min [29]. Based on one report, four out of five patients had complete resolution of symptoms using this dosage [37]. There was no evidence of platelet count abnormalities or thiocyanate toxicity at the above dosage given continuously for several days. The maximum action of sodium nitroprusside was seen within 1–2 minutes [25,29]. Vasoactive drugs including β-blockers, magnesium, prostaglandin E1, iloprost (prostacyclin analog), and ergot alkaloids have been reported to relieve symptoms [28,32]. There are conflicting reports about the role of calcium channel blockers [28]. Neuroactive drugs including selective serotonin reuptake inhibitors (SSRIs), tricyclic antidepressants, gabapentin, pregabalin and benzodiazepines have also been reported to have some efficacy [28,32]. Careful use of nonsteroidal anti-inflammatory drugs (NSAIDs), other analgesics and narcotics may help in pain control [28]. Surgical procedures including sympathectomy and sympathetic nerve block can be tried in intractable cases [28,38]. There has been conflicting evidence for other therapies including acupuncture, biofeedback, hypnosis and magnets for adolescents and adults [19,39]. Work is ongoing to engineer an isoform-specific blocker that would target Na_v1.7 [11]. There has been some success in relieving neuropathic pain with gene therapy in rodent models. Using herpes simplex virus (HSV) as a vector, Na_v1.7 sequences have also been delivered to dorsal root ganglia (DRG) neurons in mice. This might open a new era for the management of erythromelalgia [40].

Prognosis. Unfortunately, the response to the currently available therapy has been poor. Many patients diagnosed in childhood have continued to have symptoms in adulthood. The disease might become chronic and disabling [19,29]. Conservative measures and aetiology-based therapy may result in remission especially in patients with secondary erythromelalgia. In contrast, there have been reported cases of amputation and self-harm, including suicide, because of pain intensity [22,41].

Antenatal diagnosis. DNA-based antenatal testing is available for families with a defined *SCN9A* mutation [29,42].

References

1 **Skeik N, Rooke TW, Davis MD et al. Severe case and literature review of primary erythromelalgia: a novel SCN9A gene mutation. Vasc Med 2012;17:44–9.**

2 Albuquerque LG, França ER, Kozmhinsky V et al. Primary erythromelalgia: case report. An Bras Dermatol 2011;86:131–4.

3 Novella SP, Hisama FM, Dib-Hajj SD et al. Case of inherited erythromelalgia. Nat Clin Pract Neurol 2007;3:229–34.

4 Klugbauer N, Lacinova L, Flockerzi V, et al. Structure and functional expression of a new member of the tetrodotoxin-sensitive voltage-activated sodium channel family from human neuroendocrine cells. EMBO J 1995;14:1084–90.

5 Graves RJ. Clinical Lectures on the Practice of Medicine. Dublin: Fannin, 1834.

6 Mitchell SW. On a rare vaso-motor neurosis of the extremities and on the maladies with which it may be confounded. Am J Med Sci 1878;76:17.

7 Brown GF. Erythromelalgia and other disturbances of the extremities accompanied by vasodilatation and burning. Am J Med Sci 1932; 183:468–85.

8 Michiels JJ. Aspirin resistant autosomal dominant familial erythermalgia: a congenital incurable neuropathic disorder caused by a gain of function mutation in exon 26 of the SCN9a gene on chromosome 2q24.3. J Hematol Thrombo Dis 2014;2: e113. doi:10.4172/2329-8790.1000e113.

9 Smith LA, Allen EV. Erythermalgia (erythromelalgia), of the extremities: a syndrome characterized by redness, heat and pain. Am Heart J 1938;16:175–88.

10 Lewis T. Clinical observation and experiments relating to burning pain in extremities and to so-called 'erythromelalgia' in particular. Clin Sci 1933;1:175–211.

11 Drenth JP, te Morsche RH, Guillet G et al. SCN9A mutations define primary erythermalgia as a neuropathic disorder of voltage gated sodium channels. J Invest Dermatol 2005;124:1333–8.

12 Dib-Hajj SD, Rush AM, Cummins TR et al. Gain-of-function mutation in Nav1.7 in familial erythromelalgia induces bursting of sensory neurons. Brain 2005;128:1847–54.

13 Reed KB, Davis MD. Incidence of erythromelalgia: a population-based study in Olmsted County, Minnesota. J Eur Acad Dermatol Venereol 2009;23:13–15.

14 Friberg D1, Chen T, Tarr G et al. Erythromelalgia? A clinical study of people who experience red, hot, painful feet in the community. Int J Vasc Med 2013;2013:864961.

15 Latessa V. Erythromelalgia: a rare microvascular disease. J Vasc Nurs 2010;28:67–71.

16 Sangameswaran LM, Fish BD, Koch DK, et al. A novel tetrodotoxin-sensitive, voltage-gated sodium channel expressed in rat and human dorsal root ganglia. J Biol Chem 1997;272:14805–9.

17 Dabby R, Sadeh M, Gilad R, et al. Chronic non-paroxysmal neuropathic pain – novel phenotype of mutation in the sodium channel SCN9A gene. J Neurol Sci 2011;301:90–2.

18 Klugbauer N, Lacinova L, Flockerzi V, Hofmann F. Structure and functional expression of a new member of the tetrodotoxin-sensitive voltage-activated sodium channel family from human neuroendocrine cells. EMBO J 1995;14:1084–90.

19 Cohen JS. Erythromelalgia: new theories and new therapies. J Am Acad Dermatol 2000;43:841–7.

20 Michiels JJ, van Joost T, Vuzevski VD. Idiopathic erythermalgia: a congenital disorder. J Am Acad Dermatol 1989;21:1128–30.

21 Drenth JP, Vuzevski V, Van Joost T et al. Cutaneous pathology in primary erythermalgia. Am J Dermatopathol 1996;18:30–4.

22 Uno H, Parker F. Autonomic innervation of skin in primary erythermalgia. Arch Dermatol 1983;119:65–71.

23 **Davis MDP, O'Fallon WM, Rogers RS et al. Natural history of erythromelalgia. Arch Dermatol 2000;136:330–6.**

24 Mørk C, Kalgaard OM, Kvernebo K. Erythromelalgia: a clinical study of 102 cases (abstract). Australas J Dermatol 1997;38(suppl 2):50.

25 Kvernebo K. Erythromelalgia: a condition caused by microvascular arteriovenous shunting. J Vasc Dis 1998(Suppl);51:1–39.

26 Michiels JJ, Abels J, Steketee J et al. Erythromelalgia caused by platelet-mediated arteriolar inflammation and thrombosis in thrombocythemia. Ann Intern Med 1985;102:466–71.

27 Mork C. Erythromelalgia: a mysterious condition. Arch Dermatol 2000;136:406–9.

28 **Davis MP, Rooke TW. Erythromelalgia. In: Creager MA, Dzau VJ, Loscalzo J (eds) Vascular Medicine: A Companion to Braunwald's Heart Disease. Philadelphia: Elsevier, 2006:711–21.**

29 **Daniels J. Erythromelalgia. In: Irvine A, Hoeger P, Yan A (eds) Harper's Textbook of Pediatric Dermatology, 3rd edn. Oxford: Blackwell Publishing, 2011: Chapter 166.**

30 Harden RN, Bruehl S, Stanton-Hicks M, Wilson PR. Proposed new diagnostic criteria for complex regional pain syndrome. Pain Med 2007;8:326.

31 Germain DP. Fabry disease. Orphanet J Rare Dis 2010;5:30.

32 **Davis MD, Rooke T. Erythromelalgia. Curr Treat Options Cardiovasc Med 2006;8:153–65.**

33 Stone JD, Rivey MP, Allington DR. Nitroprusside treatment of erythromelalgia in an adolescent female. Ann Pharmacother 1997; 31:590–2.

34 Kasapcopur O, Akkis S, Erdem A et al. Erythromelalgia associated with hypertension and leukocytoclastic vasculitis in a child. Clin Exp Rheum 1998;16:184–6.

35 Ozsoylu S, Caner H, Gokalp A. Successful treatment of erythromelalgia with sodium nitroprusside. J Pediatr 1979;94:619–21.

36 Catchpole BN. Erythromelalgia. Lancet 1964;1:909–11.

37 Drenth JPH, Michiels JJ. Clinical characteristics and pathophysiology of erythromelalgia and erythermalgia. Am J Med 1992;93:111–12.

38 Zhang L, Wang WH, Li LF, et al. Long-term remission of primary erythermalgia with R1151W polymorphism in SCN9A after chemical lumbar sympathectomy. Eur J Dermatol 2010;20:763–7.

39 Chakravarty K, Pharoah PDP, Scott DGI et al. Erythromelalgia: the role of hypnotherapy. Postgrad Med J 1992;68:44–6.

40 Waxman SG, Dib-Hajj S. Erythermalgia: molecular basis for an inherited pain syndrome. Trend Molec Med 2005;11:555–62.

41 Kalgaard OM, Seem E, Kvernebo K. Erythromelalgia: a clinical study of 87 cases. J Intern Med 1997;242:191–7.

42 McGraw T, Kosek P. Erythromelalgia pain managed with gabapentin. Anesthesiology 1997;86:988–90.

CHAPTER 152
Metabolic Disorders and the Skin

Fatma Al Jasmi[1], *Hassan Galadari*[1], *Peter T. Clayton*[2] *& Emma J. Footitt*[2]

[1] College of Medicine and Health Science, United Arab Emirates University, Al Ain, United Arab Emirates
[2] Institute of Child Health, University College London with Great Ormond Street Hospital for Children NHS Trust, London, UK

Introduction, 1965
Aminoacidopathies, 1967
Organic acidurias, 1971
Transport defects, 1973
Lysosomal storage diseases, 1973
Others metabolic deficiencies, 1979
Hyperlipoproteinaemia, 1980
Acrodermatitis enteropathica, 1981
Carotenaemia, 1982

Abstract

Metabolic disorders, both inherited and acquired, result from enzyme deficiency or overload, leading to accumulation or deficiency of a specific metabolite. These are generally multisystem disorders and frequently present with cutaneous features. Knowledge and recognition of these cutaneous features by the paediatric dermatologist can lead to early diagnosis and initiation of therapy, and there is evidence that early management may improve outcome in some diseases. This chapter discusses the cutaneous manifestations and management of metabolic diseases.

Key points

- Inborn errors of metabolism result from the deficiency of an enzyme or its cofactor.
- Most of inborn errors of metabolism are autosomal recessive disorders and may present at any age.
- The cutaneous manifestation of phenylketonuria is fair skin and hair resulting from impairment of melanin synthesis.
- The typical findings of tyrosinaemia type II are painful, well-demarcated hyperkeratosis lesions on the palms and soles.
- In alkaptonuria, the skin manifestations are the first diagnostic signs with axillae, groin and ears being most common sites of pigmentation in addition to the neck, nose and dorsum of the hands.
- Classical homocystinuria is a multisystem disease presenting with ectopis lentis, marfanoid habitus, premature osteoporosis, pectus carinatum, mental retardation, thromboembolic events, malar flush, fair skin and hair as well as thin brittle hair.
- Complications of propionic aciduria are alopecia, generalized candidiasis and acrodermatitis enteropathica-like syndrome as result of isoleucine deficiency.
- The clinical presentations of biotinidase deficiency are seizures, hypotonia, developmental delay, skin rash and alopecia.
- Photosensitivity, with a pellagra-like appearance, in childhood is usually the first sign of Hartnup disease.
- Gaucher disease type 2 may present with congenital ichthyosis. The dermatological manifestations precede severe neurological presentation and it ranges from mild skin peeling and scaling to a 'collodion baby' phenotype.
- Lysosomal storage diseases such as α-N-acetylgalactosaminidase deficiency, Fabry, fucosidosis and Farber may present with angiokeratomas.
- The mucopolysaccharidoses (MPS) patients have hirsutism and skin thickness.
- The skin marker of MPS II, which distinguished it from MPS I, is symmetrical, firm, nontender, discrete flesh coloured to ivory white papules and nodules in a reticular pattern typically in the scapulae area.
- The skin manifestations of transaldolase deficiency are dry skin, cutis laxa, ichthyosis, telangiectasias and haemangiomas.
- The hallmark of prolidase deficiency is severe, chronic, recalcitrant and painful skin ulcers on the lower extremities.
- The clinical features of familial hyperlipoproteinaemia are premature arteriosclerosis and xanthomatosis which may appear in childhood in homozygous familial hyperlipoproteinaemia patients.
- The classic triad of acrodermatitis enteropathica is acral dermatitis, alopecia and diarrhoea as a result of zinc deficiency.

Introduction

Inborn errors of metabolism (IEM) result from the absence or abnormality of an enzyme or its cofactor, leading to either accumulation or deficiency of a specific metabolite. Optimal outcome for patients with IEM depends upon early recognition of the signs and symptoms of metabolic disease and early management [1–3].

Most inborn errors of metabolism are autosomal recessive disorders. Patients may present at any age, *in utero*, in the neonatal period or later in infancy, or even in adolescence or adulthood. This chapter describes the key symptoms of IEM related to the skin and hair (Table 152.1 and Box 152.1). Porphyrias, hyperlipidaemias and the ichthyoses are described in detail elsewhere.

Harper's Textbook of Pediatric Dermatology, Fourth Edition. Edited by Peter Hoeger, Veronica Kinsler and Albert Yan.

Table 152.1 Skin symptoms of metabolic diseases and the associated metabolic disorders

Skin abnormalities	Type/location	Disease	First
Self mutilation	–	Lesch Nyhan syndrome	–
Retarded tooth eruption, loosening of teeth, mucosal pigmentation	–	Niemann–Pick disease	–
Bullae and erosions, reddening of teeth	–	CEP (congenital erythropoietic porphyria; Günther disease)	–
Varioliform scars, bullae, crusts, thickening of skin	–	EPP (erytropoietic protoporphyria)	–
Dental hypoplasia, rare syndrome epidermal naevus and warty growths (Oranje syndrome)	Rickets, vitamin D dependent	–	–
Yellow papules on the buttocks	Eruptive xanthomas	**Type I, IV and V hyperlipidaemia**	After childhood
Yellow–red papulonodular lesions on extensor aspect of the knees, elbows	Tuberous xanthomas	**Type II and III hyperlipidaemia**	Possible in childhood
Soft yellow plaques	Plane xanthomas (striatum palmare)	**Hyperlipidaemia in 50% of cases**	Possible in childhood
Decreased pigmentation, erythema/scaling, fair skin	Eczema, hypopigmentation	**Phenylketonuria**	Infancy
Dark urine, bluish pigmentation	Dark-grey/blue nappies	Alkaptonuria	Infancy
Hyperpigmentation	Hyperpigmentation in oral mucosa	**Adrenoleukodystrophy**	Childhood
Hyperpigmentation	Diffuse hyperpigmentation on face, neck and hands	**Gaucher disease**	Childhood
Yellow plaques; yellowish indurated skin; coarse facial features	Xanthomas in axillae, waxy induration of the trunk and legs	Niemann–Pick disease	Childhood
Palmoplantar hyperkeratosis and erosions	Keratoderma	**Tyrosinaemia II**	Childhood
Red cheeks	Malar flush, livido reticularis, ulceration	**Homocystinuria**	Childhood
Red pinpoint lesions around the navel and legs; pain in extremities and abdomen	Angiokeratomas	**Fabry disease**	Late childhood or adulthood
Red pinpoint lesions; coarse facial features	Angiokeratomas	Fucosidosis	Infancy
Red pinpoint lesions; coarse facial features	Angiokeratomas	β-mannosidosis	
Red pinpoint lesions, coarse facial features	Angiokeratomas	G_{M1} gangliosidosis	Childhood
Red pinpoint lesions, coarse facial features	Angiokeratomas	Galactosialidosis	Childhood
Red pinpoint lesions, coarse facial features	Angiokeratomas	Aspartylglucosaminuria	Childhood
Pink urine; skin erosions and poikiloderma (face, hands)	Pink nappies	Congenital erythropoietic porphyria	Infancy
Symmetrical circumorificial and acral vesicular erythematous lesions; alopecia	Acral located eczema	**Acrodermatitis enteropathica, (secondary) zinc deficiency**	Neonate
Neonatal erythroderma; erythema, sharply demarcated in the napkin and intertriginous areas	Erythroderma or seborrhoeic dermatitis-like	Holocarboxylase synthetase deficiency	Neonate
Alopecia, and same skin abnormalities as above	Acrodermatitis enteropathica-like	**Biotinidase deficiency**	Neonate
Erythematosquamous eruption in napkin, acral and periorificial areas; scalded skin	Seborrhoeic dermatitis or staphylococcal scalded skin–like eruption	**Propionic acidaemia**	Neonate
	–	**Methylmalonic acidaemia**	Neonate
Scaly skin at birth	Ichthyosis/collodion	Neuropathic Gaucher	Neonate
Scaly skin; small stature; hypogonadism; mental retardation; short stature	Ichthyosis, X-linked	Steroid sulphatase deficiency	Neonate to early childhood
Scaly skin; mental retardation; short stature	Ichthyosis	Multiple sulphatase deficiency	Neonate to early childhood
		Refsum disease	
Scaly skin at birth	Ichthyosis	Sjögren–Larsson syndrome; fatty alcohol oxidation defect	Neonate
Areas of scaling, circumscribed in lines or bands	Ichthyosis	Conradi–Hunermann syndrome or X-linked dominant chondrodysplasia punctata or CHILD syndrome	Neonate
Ichthyosis	Ichthyosis	**Serine synthesis defect**	
	Ichthyosis	Carbohydrate-deficient glycoprotein (CDG-1f)	
Ulcers; erythema; ecchymoses; purpura; telangiectasia	Ulcers of lower leg, erythematous purpuric	Prolidase deficiency	Neonate
Nodular swellings on ankle, wrist, elbow and friction sites	Granulomatous tumours	**Farber lipogranulomatosis (ceramidase deficiency)**	Early childhood

Table 152.1 *Continued*

Skin abnormalities	Type/location	Disease	First
Fat pads on buttocks, thickened skin; lipoatrophy (linear) on legs	Lipoatrophy, lipomatosis	Carbohydrate–deficient glycoprotein syndrome type I	Infancy
Ivory-coloured papules on the back; coarse face, thick nose, broad hands, short fingers	Skin infiltrations	**Mucopolysaccharidosis II**	–
Alopecia		**Acrodermatitis enteropathica**	Infancy
		Biotin-responsive multiple carboxylase deficiency	
		Calciferol metabolism defect	
		Congenital erythropoietic porphyria	
		Conradi-Hunermann syndrome	
		Essential fatty acid deficiencies	
		Menkes disease	
		Netherton syndrome	
		Methylmalonic and propionic aciduria	
Brittle hair; pili torti, trichorrhexis nodosa	Hair shaft abnormality	Menkes disease; copper deficiency	Infancy
Trichorrhexis nodosa		Netherton	Neonate
		Argininaemia	Early childhood
		Lysinuric protein intolerance	–
		Argininosuccinic aciduria	–
		CDG type I*	–

Treatable disorders are shown in boldface.
* Data from Silengo M, Valanzise M, Pagliardini S et al. Hair changes in congenital disorders of glycosylation (CDG type I). Eur J Pediatr 2003; 162: 114–15.

Box 152.1 Classification of inborn errors of metabolism

Aminoacidopathies

- Phenylketonuria
- Tyrosinaemia type II (Richner–Hanhart syndrome)
- Alkaptonuria
- Homocystinuria

Organic acidurias

- Propionic acidaemia
- Methylmalonic acidaemia
- Biotinidase deficiency

Transport defects

- Hartnup disease

Lysosomal storage diseases

- Gaucher
- α-NAGA deficiency/Schindler disease
- Fabry disease
- Fucosidosis
- Mucopolysaccharidoses
- GM1 type I gangliosidosis
- Farber lipogranulomatosis: ceramidase deficiency

Others:

- Transaldolase deficiency
- Prolidase deficiency

References

1 **Saudubray JM, Charpentier C. Clinical approach to inherited metabolic diseases. In: Scriver CR, Beaudet AL, Sly WS et al. (eds) The Metabolic and Molecular Bases of Inherited Disease. Clinical Phenotypes: Diagnosis/Algorithms, 8th edn. New York: McGraw-Hill, 2000:1327–407.**

2 Saudubray JM, Ogier de Baulny H, Charpentier C. Clinical approach to inherited metabolic diseases. In: Fernandes J, Saudubray JM, van den Berghe G (eds) Inborn Metabolic Diseases: Diagnosis and Treatment, 3rd revised edn. Berlin: Springer Verlag, 2000, pp. 3–41.

3 Saudubray JM, Ogier H, Bonnefont JP et al. Clinical approach to inherited metabolic disease in the neonatal period: a 20-year survey. J Inher Metab Dis 1989;12(Suppl 1):25–41.

Aminoacidopathies

Phenylketonuria

Definition. Phenylketonuria (PKU, OMIM #261600) is an autosomal recessively inherited aminoacidopathy, caused by deficiency of L-phenylalanine hydroxylase in the liver [1].

History. In the 1930s, Asbjørn Følling [2] identified raised levels of phenylalanine in the blood (hyperphenylalaninaemia) as the underlying cause of the neuropsychological deficits with a typical dermatitis on air-exposed skin, muscle hypotonia and green colouration of the urine after addition of ferrichloride. In the 1950s, Horst Bickel [3] introduced a low phenylalanine diet to treat PKU and in the 1960s, Robert Guthrie [4] introduced a newborn screening test for hyperphenylalaninaemia (the Guthrie test).

Pathogenesis. PKU is caused by mutations in the phenylalanine hydroxylase (*PAH*) gene. PAH converts phenylalanine into tyrosine and requires the cofactor tetrahydrobiopterin (BH4). Loss of PAH activity results in increased concentrations of phenylalanine in the blood and toxic concentrations in the brain, and leads to inhibition of tyrosinase which is responsible for decreased skin and hair pigmentation. A small group of patients (1–2%) with hyperphenylalaninaemia have defects of a cofactor that may result in a deficiency of neurotransmitters. Owing to the neurological sequelae, the name 'malignant PKU' is used for this group [5,6].

The prevalence of PKU varies between countries. In Turkey, its frequency is high (1 in 2600 live births) [7] but in Finland is very low (1 in 200 000 births) [5].

Clinical features. Neonates with PKU show no physical signs of the disease. When untreated, older children may present with microcephaly, seizures, a musty body odour, severe intellectual disability and behaviour problems, as well as structural brain changes visible on magnetic resonance imaging [5].

Fair skin and hair resulting from impairment of melanin synthesis is the most characteristic cutaneous manifestation of PKU. Patients often have photosensitivity, increased incidence of pyogenic infections, and increased incidence of keratosis pilaris, hair loss and eczema [8].

Untreated pregnant women with hyperphenylalaninaemia/PKU have a high risk of spontaneous miscarriage (maternal PKU syndrome); their offspring often show low birthweight, microcephaly, retarded development and cardiac malformations [5].

Prognosis. In classic PKU, early dietary treatment with a phenylalanine-restricted diet can prevent psychomotor delay and mental retardation.

Patients with defective biopterin biosynthesis should be carefully monitored for neurological symptoms. Some patients with these defects experience a rather benign course; however, some show severe neurological sequelae even if well treated. The long-term prognosis of these disorders is still unknown. Prevention of maternal PKU syndrome will be a main issue in the near future, because the generation of patients whose condition was detected early by newborn screening has now reached adulthood.

Differential diagnosis. In the neonatal period and in premature infants and patients with liver disease, plasma levels of phenylalanine can be abnormally high. This can lead to a false-positive PKU screening test caused by other metabolic defects, such as classic galactosaemia or tyrosinaemia (see later). The dermatological manifestations in PKU can mimic eczema and scleroderma-like lesions with pigment changes.

Screening and treatment. PKU screening is included in the national newborn screening programme in many countries. It can be detected in virtually 100% of cases by newborn screening utilizing the Guthrie card bloodspot obtained from a heel prick [9].

A low-phenylalanine, tyrosine-supplemented diet should be introduced as soon as the diagnosis of PKU is established. Vitamins, minerals and calcium should be added according to need and age. All patients should remain on this diet for life, or at least until they leave school; women of childbearing age should remain on the diet to prevent maternal PKU syndrome. Some centres institute a protein-restricted diet in adulthood. During treatment, patients' hair colour may darken as a result of tyrosine supplementation in the diet (Fig. 152.1) [5].

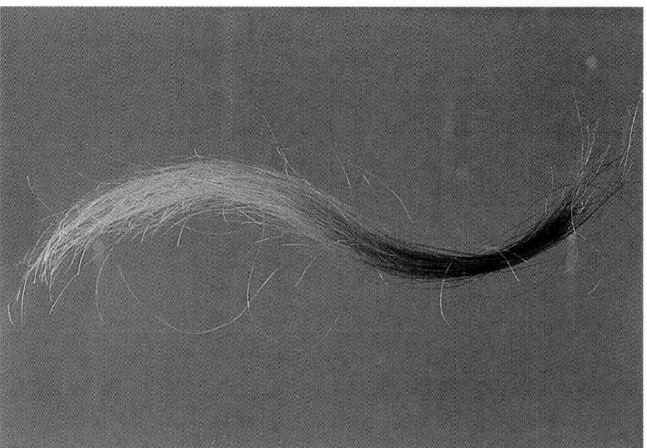

Fig. 152.1 Increase in hair pigmentation after the start of a phenylalanine-restricted, tyrosine-supplemented diet in a late-detected classic phenylketonuria patient. Source: Courtesy of Prof. F.J. van Sprang.

Tyrosinaemia type II

Definition. Tyrosinaemia type II (Richner–Hanhart syndrome, OMIM #276600) is the oculocutaneous form of tyrosine catabolism caused by a defect of hepatic cytosol aminotransferase [10]. Tyrosinaemia type II is an autosomal recessive disorder.

History. Richner in 1938 and Hanhart in 1947 recognized a distinctive oculocutaneous syndrome. In 1973, Goldsmith and colleagues [11] pointed out the similarity between the tyrosinaemia type II and the oculocutaneous syndrome.

Pathogenesis. It is caused by a deficiency of the hepatic, pyridoxal phosphate- dependent, cytosol enzyme, tyrosine aminotransferase. The enzyme catalyses the conversion of L-tyrosine into p-hydroxyphenylpyruvate [12]. As a consequence of tyrosine aminotransferase deficiency there is an accumulation of plasma tyrosine as well as of abnormal urinary tyrosine metabolites.

Intracellular crystallization is proposed as the mechanism for tissue damage. The levels of amino acids in the epidermis may exceed those in plasma, as tyrosine levels in plasma exceed saturation. The skin lesions are limited to volar surfaces and are associated with polymorphonuclear infiltrates.

Clinical features. Skin lesions occur in 80% of cases, and age of onset can range from the first week of life to the second decade [13]. The typical dermatological findings are painful, well-demarcated hyperkeratosis on the palms and soles, although the palms can be unaffected. On the palms the distribution usually involves the fingertips, and the thenar and hypothenar eminences (Fig. 152.2).

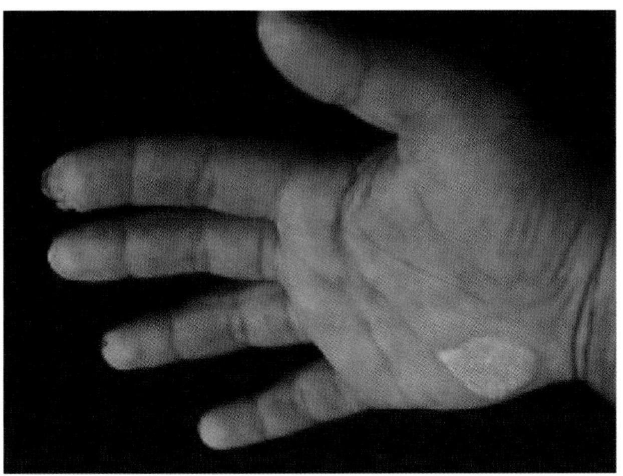

Fig. 152.2 Sharply demarcated yellowish white hyperkeratotic plaques located on the hypothenar eminence and on fingertips. Source: Charfeddine C et al. 2006 [14]. Reproduced with permission of Elsevier.

The lesions on the soles are found on the weight-bearing areas. The pain associated with the plantar lesions can be severe enough for the patient to refuse to walk. The lesions, which may begin as bullae and erosions that progress to crusted, hyperkeratotic plaques, are often associated with hyperhydrosis.

The eye lesions are often observed within the first year (but usually within the first decade) as bilateral erosions with photophobia or therapy-resistant keratitis. As a result, visual impairment can occur if correct diagnosis and treatment are delayed. Tyrosine crystals in the eye can also be observed on slit-lamp examination. Mental retardation and al abnormalities are highly variable features of tyrosinaemia type II [14].

Prognosis. Early institution of a diet low in phenylalanine and tyrosine will promptly reverse ocular and cutaneous abnormalities. With early detection, effective diet and careful biochemical surveillance, this disease can have a good prognosis. [15].

Differential diagnosis. Painful blisters in oculocutaneous tyrosinaemia should be considered as a differential diagnosis of various blistering diseases, such as different forms of epidermolysis bullosa.

Treatment. Oculocutaneous tyrosinaemia with eye crystals is treated with a phenylalanine- and tyrosine-restricted diet (the diet should also be low in phenylalanine because the conversion from the amino acid phenylalanine to tyrosine by l-phenylalanine hydroxylase is not hampered). Early dietary intervention is often successful in respect of oculocutaneous sequelae, growth and psychomotor development [15].

Alkaptonuria

Definition. Alkaptonuria (OMIM #03500) is an autosomal recessive hereditary disease with a deficiency of homogentisate 1,2-dioxygenase (EC 1.13.11.5). Owing to this effect, there is accumulation of homogentisic acid (HGA) in blood, tissue and it is excreted in the urine along with its oxidated form *alkapton* [16].

History. Studies on alkaptonuria have been of great importance in the development of ideas about inherited metabolic diseases. In 1908, Sir Archibald Garrod discussed alkaptonuria in one of the Croonian lectures [17]. The defect was narrowed down to HGA oxidase deficiency in a study published in 1958 [18]. The genetic basis was elucidated in 1996, when *HGD* mutations were demonstrated [19].

Pathogenesis. As a result of HGA oxidase enzyme deficiency, HGA accumulates and is excreted in the urine. HGA is an intermediary product in the tyrosine degradation pathway [16].

Clinical features. The three major features of alkaptonuria are the presence of HGA in the urine, ochronosis (bluish-black pigmentation in connective tissue), and arthritis of the spine and larger joints. Oxidation of the HGA excreted in the urine produces a melanin-like product and causes the urine to turn dark on standing. Ochronosis occurs only after age 30 years; arthritis often begins in the third decade. Other manifestations include palmoplantar hyperpigmentation, grey nail plate discolouration, darkened cerumen of the ears and perspiration, bluish pigmentation of the sclera, bluish pigmentation of ear cartilage in the concha and antihelix, calcification of the ear cartilage, aortic or mitral valve calcification or regurgitation and occasionally aortic dilatation, renal stones and prostate stones. The skin manifestations are the first diagnostic signs with axillae, groin and ears being the most common sites of pigmentation in addition to the neck, nose and dorsum of the hands [8]. A case of acrokeratoelastoidosis (hyperkeratotic linearly arranged blue papules along the lateral aspects of fingers of the hand and feet) has been reported in association with alkaptonuria [20].

Prognosis. The main impact is on quality of life; many people with alkaptonuria have disabling symptoms such as pain, poor sleep and breathing symptoms. These generally start in the fourth decade. The average age for joint replacement surgery is 50–55 years. They have a higher incidence of cardiovascular disease caused by arteriosclerosis.

Differential diagnosis. Ochronosis resulting from alkaptonuria may be confused with acquired, reversible pigmentary changes following prolonged use of carbolic acid dressings for chronic cutaneous ulcers [21]. Chemically induced ochronosis has also been described following long-term use of either the antimalarial agent Atabrine® [22], the skin-lightening agent hydroquinone or the antibiotic minocycline [23]. Chronic arthritis as a manifestation of long-standing alkaptonuria resembles gouty arthritis or rheumatoid arthritis.

Treatment. There is no evidence for long-term effects of ascorbate and/or protein restriction treatment, but improvement of symptoms has been reported with treatment with ascorbate 0.5–1 g/day and protein restricted to the minimum requirement for age [24]. Experimental treatment with nitisinone is another option for the management of alkaptonuria [25].

The symptomatic prevention of complications (joints, heart) seems to be the primary therapeutic goal.

Homocystinuria

Definition. Homocystinuria (OMIM #236200) caused by cystathionine β-synthase (CBS; EC 4.2.1.22) deficiency is the most common IEM metabolism [26].

History. The enzyme defect was identified in 1964 by Mudd and colleagues [27] after the first clinical description in 1962 by Gerritsen and colleagues [28].

Pathogenesis. CBS deficiency is a disorder of transsulphuration resulting in elevated plasma levels of homocyst(e)ine and methionine and a decreased level of cysteine [29]. CBS deficiency is inherited as an autosomal recessive trait. Enzyme activity may be higher in pyridoxine-responsive individuals than in those who are nonresponsive [30] but cannot reliably distinguish responders from nonresponders.

Clinical features. Affected patients have multisystem involvement, including eyes (ectopis lentis), skeleton (marfanoid habitus, premature osteoporosis, bone deformities, e.g. pectus carinatum, pectus excavatum), central nervous system (mental retardation, seizure and psychiatric symptoms), vascular system (thromboembolic events), fair skin and hair as well as malar flush. The hair is thin and brittle.

Reversible hypopigmentation in some treated homocystinuric patients has been reported; the mechanism is not clear, although some data suggest tyrosinase inhibition by homocyst(e)ine caused by interaction of homocyst(e)ine with copper at the active site of tyrosinase [31]. Malar flush in untreated patients manifests as roughening and red colouration of the skin of the cheeks, as seen in farmers (Fig. 152.3).

Prognosis. Clinical variability is present and mild cases may not be recognized until severe complications, such as thromboembolic accidents, develop. Even mild hyperhomocyst(e)inaemia has been related to higher risk of occlusive vascular disease, partly related to methylenetetrahydrofolate metabolism.

Differential diagnosis. The classic phenotype is often confused with Marfan syndrome, an autosomal dominantly inherited disease, and with eye lens dislocation, skeletal involvement and vascular complications (aneurysma of the aorta). Homocystinuria and Marfan syndrome are both systemic diseases with (different) collagen abnormalities. Mental retardation is not associated with Marfan syndrome, unlike homocystinuria.

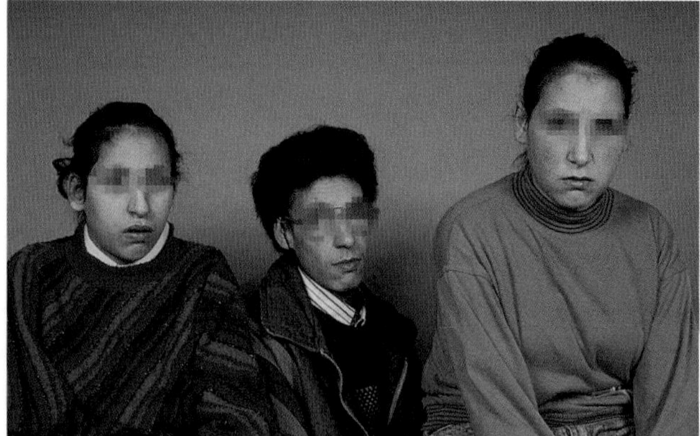

Fig. 152.3 Three Moroccan siblings with CBS (cystathionine β-synthase-deficient pyridoxine-responsive homocystinuria) before treatment. The boy's lenses have been extracted; the elder girl shows the facial malar flush.

Treatment. About half of the patients with homocystinuria caused by CBS deficiency respond to pharmacological doses of pyridoxine (three doses at 100–250 mg daily orally). Pyridoxal 5-phosphate is a cofactor for CBS and pyridoxine treatment (vitamin B_6) will increase the conversion of pyridoxine nonresponsive homocysteine to cysteine in patients with CBS deficiency. Betaine (dimethylglycine, as a methyl donor) is also used in the treatment of homocystinuria to stimulate the remethylation of homocysteine to methionine [29,32].

Other causes of hyperhomocysteinaemia can be caused by folic acid or vitamin B_{12} deficiency, or by inborn errors of cobalamin

References

1 Güttler F. Hyperphenylalaninaemia. Diagnosis and classification of the various types of phenylalanine hydroxylase deficiency in childhood. Acta Pediatr Scand 1980;280(Suppl):1–80.

2 Fölling A. Uber Ausscheidung von Phenylbrenztraubensaüre in den Harn als Stoffwechselanomalie in Verbindung mit Imbezillität. Höppe-Seylers Z Physiol Chem 1934;227:169.

3 Bickel H, Gerrad I, Hickmans EM. Influence of phenylalanine intake on phenylketonuria. Lancet 1953;ii:812.

4 Guthrie R, Susi A. A simple phenylalanine method for detecting phenylketonuria in large populations of newborn infants. Pediatrics 1963;32:338–43.

5 Scriver CR, Kaufman S. Hyperphenylalaninemia: phenylalanine hydroxylase deficiency. In: Scriver CR, Beaudet AL, Sly WS (eds) The Metabolic and Molecular Bases of Inherited Disease, 8th edn. New York: McGraw-Hill, 2001:1667–724.

6 Fitzpatrick TB, Miyamoto M. Competitive inhibition of mammalian tyrosinase by phenylalanine and its relationship to hair pigmentation in phenylketonuria. Nature 1957;179(4552):199–200.

7 Ozalp I, Coskun T, Ceyhan M et al. Incidence of phenylketonuria and hyperphenylalaninemia in a sample of the newborn population. J Inherit Metab Dis 1986;9(Suppl 2):237.

8 Urrets-Zavalía JA, Espósito E, Garay I et al. The eye and the skin in nonendocrine metabolic disorders. Clin Dermatol 2016;34:166–82.

9 Smith I, Cook B, Beasley M. Review of neonatal screening programme for phenylketonuria. BMJ 1991;303:333–5.

10 Paige DG, Clayton P, Bowron A et al. Richner–Hanhart syndrome (oculocutaneous tyrosinaemia type II). J Roy Soc Med 1992; 85:759–60.

11 Goldsmith LA, Kang ES, Bienfang DC et al. Tyrosinemia with plantar and palmer keratosis and keratitis. J Pediatr 1973;83:798–805.

12 Hargrove JL, Scoble HA, Mathews WR et al. The structure of tyrosine aminotransferase. J Biol Chem 1898;264:45e53.
13 Rabinowitz LG, Williams LR, Anderson CE et al. Painful keratoderma and photophobia: hallmarks of tyrosinemia type II. J Pediatr 1995; 126:266–9.
14 Charfeddine C, Monastiri K, Mokni M et al. Clinical and mutational investigations of tyrosinemia type II in Northern Tunisia: identification and structural characterization of two novel TAT mutations. Mol Genet Metab 2006;88:184–91.
15 Barr DGD, Kirk JM, Laing SC. Outcome of tyrosinaemia type II. Arch Dis Child 1991;66:1249–50.
16 Zatkova A. An update on molecular genetics of Alkaptonuria (AKU). J Inherit Metab Dis 2011;34:1127–36.
17 Garrod AE. The Croonian Lectures on inborn errors of metabolisms. Lecture II. Alkaptonuria. Lancet 1908;ii:73.
18 La Du BN, Zannoni VG, Laster L, Seegmiller JE. The nature of the defect in tyrosine metabolism in alkaptonuria. J Biol Chem 1958; 230:251–60.
19 Fernández-Cañón JM, Granadino B, Beltrán-Valero de Bernabé D,et al. The molecular basis of alkaptonuria. Nat Genet 1996;14:19–24.
20 Ramesh V, Avninder S. Endogenous ochronosis with a predominant acrokeratoelastoidosis-like presentation. Int J Dermatol 2008; 47:873–5.
21 La Du BN. Alkaptonuria. In: Scriver CR, Beaudet AL, Sly WS, Valle D, Vogelstein B (eds) The Metabolic and Molecular Bases of Inherited Disease, 8 edn. New York: McGraw-Hill, 2001:2109–23.
22 Ludwig GD, Toole JF, Wood JC. Ochronosis from quinacrine (atabrine). Ann Intern Med 1963;59:378–84.
23 Suwannarat P, Phornphutkul C, Bernardini I et al. Minocycline-induced hyperpigmentation masquerading as alkaptonuria in individuals with joint pain. Arthritis Rheum 2004;50:3698–701.
24 de Haas V, Carbasius Weber EC, de Klerk JB et al. The success of dietary protein restriction in alkaptonuria patients is age-dependent. J Inherit Metab Dis 1998;21:791–8.
25 Anikster Y, Nyhan WL, Gahl WA. NTBC and alkaptonuria. Am J Hum Genet 1998;63:920.
26 Mudd SH, Skovby F, Levy HL et al. The natural history of homocystinuria due to cystathionine β-synthase deficiency. Am J Hum Genet 1985;94:1–31.
27 Mudd SH, Finkelstein JD, Irreverre F, Laster L. Homocystinuria: an enzymatic defect. Science 1964;143:1443–5.
28 Gerritsen T, Vaughn JG, Waisman HA. The identification of homocystine in the urine. Biochem Biophys Res Commun 1962;9:493–6.
29 Mudd SH, Levy HL, Krans JP. Disorders of trans-sulfuration. In: Scriver CR, Beaudet AL, Sly WS et al. (eds) The Metabolic and Molecular Bases of Inherited Disease, 8th edn. New York: McGraw-Hill, 2001: 2007–56.
30 Chen X, Wang L, Fazlieva R, Kruger WD. Contrasting behaviors of mutant cystathionine beta-synthase enzymes associated with pyridoxine response. Hum Mutat 2006;27:474–82.
31 Rish O, Townsend D, Berry SA et al. Tyrosine inhibition due to interaction of homocysteine with copper: the mechanism for reversible hypopigmentation in homocystinuria due to cystathionine β-synthase deficiency. Am J Hum Genet 1995;57:127–32.
32 Wilcken DEN, Wilcken B, Dudman NPD et al. Homocystinuria – the effect of betaine in the treatment of patients not responsive to pyridoxine. N Engl J Med 1983;309:448–53.

Organic acidurias

Propionic acidaemia

Definition. Propionic acidaemia (OMIM #606054) is an autosomal recessively inherited inborn error of branched-chain amino acid metabolism.

History. In 1961, Childs described an infant with episodic metabolic ketoacidosis, protein intolerance and elevated plasma glycine concentrations. Many children with similar clinical and biochemical findings have since been described. Propionic acidaemia caused by a deficiency of propionyl co-enzyme A (CoA) carboxylase deficiency and different forms of methylmalonic acidaemia, all with markedly elevated plasma glycine concentrations, fit this description.

Pathogenesis. The essential amino acids, isoleucine, valine, methionine and threonine, are metabolized into propionyl CoA. Propionyl CoA is converted into methylmalonyl CoA by the enzyme propionyl CoA carboxylase. Deficiency of this enzyme causes propionic acidaemia [1].

Clinical features. The clinical characteristics of propionic acidaemia and methylmalonic acidaemia are similar. Patients are commonly seen in the first weeks of life with vomiting, metabolic acidosis, failure to thrive, hypotonia and mental retardation: neonatal death occurs.

In the course of propionic acidaemia (even under treatment), patients can develop large superficial desquamation of the skin, with epidermolysis that resembles staphylococcal scalded skin syndrome. This complication, potentially caused by nutrient or essential amino acid deficiency mainly caused by isoleucine deficiency, has recently been described as acrodermatitis enteropathica-like syndrome [2]. Generalized candidiasis often occurs. Alopecia often appears at the end of a period of decompensation and is reversible. In the case of severe protein deficiency, isoleucine supplementation 200–400 mg/kg/day is warranted. To decrease propionate production in the gut, metronidazole is advocated during periods of decompensation or once a week during a month. Pancytopenia, caused by bone marrow depression caused by the abnormal organic acids, is a common feature.

Prognosis. The acute neonatal form of propionic acidaemia has a poor prognosis. Symptomatic treatment with bicarbonate to correct the ketoacidosis and haemo- or peritoneal dialysis to remove the accumulated toxic metabolites can lead to survival in the neonatal period. However, at any age, each metabolic derangement is potentially life-threatening and severe psychomotor retardation is a common feature.

Patients affected with the late-onset form will often be on a lifelong dietary restriction of one or more essential amino acids, which in excess are the precursors of toxic metabolites. (Semi)synthetic formulas can provide the required daily intake of protein.

Differential diagnosis. The different syndromic forms of ketotic hyperglycinaemia, such as methylmalonic acidaemia and other organic acidaemias, should be ruled out by proper diagnosis by gas chromatography–mass spectrometry techniques.

Treatment. Propionyl CoA carboxylase requires biotin (10 mg daily) as a cofactor. Dietary treatment with special amino acid mixtures is available. Metronidazole, an antibiotic that inhibits colonic flora, has been found to be specifically effective in reducing urinary excretion of propionate metabolites. Supportive treatment with multivitamins and calcium is necessary. L-Carnitine supplementation, 100 mg/kg/day (secondary deficiency caused by urinary loss of esterified propionyl CoA), is indicated. Isoleucine 200–400 mg/day should be supplemented if deficient [3]. Growth hormone induces protein anabolism. For those patients with methylmalonic or propionic acidaemia, growth hormone treatment could be useful in the long term to allow a higher protein intake and better growth.

Some severe neonatal cases have been treated with liver transplantation; the outcome of this treatment seems to be promising regarding the physical condition and survival although the cognitive impairment is poor [4].

Methylmalonic acidaemia

Definition. Methylmalonic aciduria (OMIM #251000) is an autosomal recessive disease with deficiency of methylmalonyl CoA mutase activity. It is a genetically heterogeneous disorder caused by mutations at many different loci. Methylmalonic acidaemia is one of the most common organic acidurias.

History. In 1967, critically ill infants with metabolic ketoacidosis and developmental delay, with accumulated huge amounts of methylmalonate in blood and urine, were first described.

The early description, combined with new knowledge, has demonstrated that many different biochemical bases for inherited forms of methylmalonic acidaemia are present, among them defects of the mutase apoenzyme and defects of synthesis of adenosylcobalamin only.

Pathogenesis. It is caused by complete or partial deficiency of methylmalonyl-CoA mutase (mut0-enzymatic subtype or mut-enzymatic subtype, respectively), a defect in the transport or synthesis of its cofactor, adenosylcobalamin (cblA, cblB or cblD-MMA). Defects of cobalamin (vitamin B_{12}) transport or biosynthesis affecting the synthesis of both adenosylcobalamin and methylcobalamin are the main causes of this disease. Some children with distinct mutations designated as type C, D and F also show homocystinuria as a result of methyltetrahydrofolate involvement.

Clinical features. Presenting symptoms are similar to propionic acidaemia: vomiting, failure to thrive, lethargy, hypotonia and attacks of ketoacidosis and dehydration. Propionyl CoA metabolites, such as 1-methylcitrate, 3-hydroxypropionate and 3-hydroxyisovalerate, are usually found in urine with gas chromatographic analysis techniques. Vitamin B_{12} deficiency must be excluded.

As in propionic acidaemia, skin disorders can appear during decompensation periods [5,6]. Erythematosquamous eruptions around the orificia and acra, with lamellar desquamation, often with alopecia and candidiasis, can occur during metabolic decompensation.

Prognosis. Early diagnosis and dietary treatment influence the prognosis [7].

Treatment. A tentative treatment with pharmacological doses of vitamin B_{12}, a protein-restricted diet or a restriction of branched-chain amino acids (the precursors), in combination with supportive treatment with L-carnitine, is the therapy of choice. Fasting should be avoided to prevent ketoacidosis. In the near future, hepatic transplantation or hepatocyte transplantation could be an ultimate choice of treatment [8].

Biotinidase deficiency

Definition. Biotinidase deficiency (OMIM #253260) is an autosomal recessive rare disease and is diagnosed by demonstrating deficient enzyme activity in serum (less than 10% of normal serum activity) [9].

Clinical features. Presenting symptoms are seizures, hypotonia, ataxia, developmental delay, skin rash and alopecia. Other symptoms include optic atrophy, hearing loss, conjunctivitis and fungal infections, which are probably caused by abnormalities in immunoregulation.

Alopecia and/or skin eruption are the initial symptoms in about 20% of patients and are present during the clinical course in at least 60%. The alopecia is nonscarring. Perioral erosions, conjuctival erosions and crusts are frequent findings.

Prognosis. Early biotin therapy appears to prevent the development of neurological and cutaneous problems [10].

Differential diagnosis. Holocarboxylase deficiency and biotidinase deficiency can present with the same clinical features, such as vomiting, hypotonia, skin rash, alopecia, seizures, ataxia and metabolic ketoacidosis. Acrodermatitis entropathica is part of the differential diagnosis.

Treatment. Biotin, a member of the water-soluble B complex group, 10 mg daily orally, is the treatment of choice and can change the clinical picture dramatically.

References

1 **Fenton WA, Gravel RA, Rosenblatt DSLE. Disorders of propionate and methylmalonate metabolism. In: Scriver CR, Beaudet AL, Sly WS et al. (eds) The Metabolic and Molecular Bases of Inherited Disease, 8th edn. New York: McGraw-Hill, 2001:2165–94.**

2 De Raeve I, de Meirleir L, Ramet J et al. Acrodermatitis enteropathica-like cutaneous lesions in organic acidurias. J Pediatr 1994;124:416–20.

3 Touati G, Valayannopoulos V, Mention K et al. Methylmalonic and propionic acidurias: management without or with a few supplements of specific amino acid mixtures. J Inher Metab Dis 2006;29:288–99.

4 Leonard JV, Walter JH, McKiernan PJ. The management of organic acidaemias: the role of transplantation. J Inher Metab Dis 2001;24: 309–11.

5 Koopman RJJ, Happle R. Cutaneous manifestations of methylmalonic acidemia. Arch Dermatol Res 1990;282:272–3.

6 Bodemer C, de Prost Y, Bachollot B et al. Cutaneous manifestations of methylmalonic and propionic acidemia: a description of 38 cases. Br J Dermatol 1994;131:93–9

7 Burlina AB. Hepatocyte transplantation for inborn errors of metabolism. J Inher Metab Dis 2004;27:373–83.

8 Saudubray JM, Ogier H, Bonnefont JP et al. Clinical approach to inherited diseases in the neonatal period: a 20-year-survey. J Inher Met Dis 1989;12(Suppl 1):1 –17.
9 Wolf B, Heard GS, Weisbecker KA et al. Biotinidase deficiency: initial clinical features and rapid diagnosis. Ann Neurol 1985;18:614–17.
10 Jay AM, Conway RL, Feldman GL et al. Outcomes of individuals with profound and partial biotinidase deficiency ascertained by newborn screening in Michigan over 25 years. Genet Med 2015;17:205–9.

Transport defects

Hartnup disease

Definition. Hartnup disease (OMIM #234500) is an autosomal recessively inherited disorder leading to impaired transport of neutral amino acids, limited to kidneys and small intestine.

History. Hartnup disease was first described in two siblings of the Hartnup family in 1956. Soon after its initial description, it was suggested that Hartnup disease results from a tissue-specific failure to resorb neutral amino acids in the kidney and intestine.

Pathogenesis. Urinary amino acid analysis shows a typical neutral hyperaminoaciduria. The increased urinary loss of tryptophan and reduced absorption of tryptophan lead to a reduced synthesis of niacin owing to an impaired availability of tryptophan [1].

Clinical features. Most affected individuals remain asymptomatic. Photosensitivity is usually the first sign, with a pellagra-like appearance, and starts in childhood. The rash manifests as red and scaly, appearing predominantly on the sun-exposed areas of the body. Exposure to sunlight can cause blisters, appearing as sunburn blisters and burning pain appears after exposure to direct sunlight, followed by peeling, hyperkeratosis, fissuring and pigmentation. Neurological signs, such as intermittent cerebellar ataxia, pyramidal signs and psychotic behaviour, have been described. Some affected patients are mildly mentally retarded.

Prognosis. From prospective and retrospective studies of Hartnup disease patients identified by neonatal screening and with a long-term follow up, even without therapy, it has become clear that very few become symptomatic. The most recent hypothesis is that the cause of disease in the Hartnup disease is multifactorial [1]. It seems likely that Hartnup disease does not adversely affect pregnancy and is not damaging to the fetus.

Differential diagnosis. Photosensitivity in early childhood is seen in Bloom syndrome, Cockayne syndrome, xeroderma pigmentosum, lupus erythematosus and some forms of porphyria.

Treatment. Treatment with nicotinamide four to six times at 100–250 mg daily leads to clearing of the rash and may lead to disappearance of the ataxia.

Reference

1 Scriver ER, Mahon B, Levy HL et al. The Hartnup phenotype: mendelian transport disorder, multifactorial disease. Am J Hum Genet 1987;40:401.

Lysosomal storage diseases

Gaucher disease

Definition. Gaucher disease (GD, OMIM #230800, #230900, #231000), is the autosomal recessive inherited deficiency of the lysosomal enzyme glucocerebrosidase (EC 3.2.1.45). It encompasses a continuum of clinical findings from a perinatal lethal disorder to an asymptomatic type. There are three major clinical types (1, 2, and 3). Type 1 is distinguished from type 2 and type 3 by the lack of central nervous system involvement whereas type 2 is the acute neuronopathic and type 3 is the chronic neuronopathic type.

History. It was recognized by the French doctor Philippe Gaucher, who originally described it in 1882 [1]. The biochemical basis for the disease was elucidated in 1965 [2]. In 1988, ichthyosis and GD type 2 were described in two siblings of Lebanese origin from Australia [3]. The first effective treatment for GD type 1, the drug alglucerase (Ceredase), was approved by the US Food and Drug Administration (FDA) in April 1991. An improved drug, imiglucerase (Cerezyme), was approved by the FDA in May 1994 and has replaced Ceredase.

Pathogenesis. Deficiency of glucocerebrosidase leads to accumulation of glucocerebroside and other glycolipids within the lysosomes of macrophages [4].

Clinical features. GD type 1 presents with bone disease (osteopenia, focal lytic or sclerotic lesions, and osteonecrosis), hepatosplenomegaly, anaemia and thrombocytopenia, and lung disease. Disease with onset before age 2 years, limited psychomotor development and a rapidly progressive course with death by age 2–4 years is classified as GD type 2. Individuals with GD type 3 may have onset before age 2 years, but often have a more slowly progressive course, with survival into the third or fourth decade [4].

GD type 2 may present with congenital ichthyosis. The dermatological manifestations precede severe neurological presentation and it ranges from mild skin peeling and scaling that resolves quickly, to a 'collodion baby' phenotype. The term 'collodion baby' refer to the presentation of a newborn infant encased in cellophane-like skin wrapping. This tough shiny inelastic collodion-like membrane results in immobility of the limbs and causes ectropion of the eyelids. This membrane undergoes desquamation or peeling, which is usually complete by 2–3 weeks of life. The abnormal skin is erythematous and shiny and is present all over the body but predominantly over the palms and soles or in flexural folds. Skin biopsy shows dense hyperkeratosis, epidermal hyperplasia and inflammation. These changes were observed in patients with type 2

SECTION 32: SKIN AND SYSTEMIC DISEASE

Gaucher disease both with and without clinical evidence of ichthyosis. This pathology is thought to result from altered ratios of ceramides to glucosylceramides in the outermost layers of skin [5,6]. GD type 1 may rarely present with ichthyosis (personal observation)

Differential diagnosis. It depends upon the presenting symptoms and signs. Conditions including leukaemia, lymphoma, inflammatory diseases, such as rheumatoid arthritis, or other storage diseases, such as Niemann–Pick types A, B or C, and saposin C deficiency often are considered in the differential. The differentials for ichthyoses with neurological involvement are multiple sulfatase deficiency, Sjögren–Larsson syndrome and Refsum disease.

Prognosis. GD type 1 patients may live well into adulthood. The range and severity of symptoms can vary dramatically between patients depending on onset of disease and severity. GD type 2 patients usually die by age two whereas patients with GD type 3 often live into their early teen years and adulthood.

Treatment. The treatment for patients with GD type 1 is enzyme replacement therapy and/or substrate reduction therapy. The therapy for GD type 2 is primarily supportive. The enzyme replacement therapy does not cross the blood–brain barrier. Currently no therapy is available that will significantly alter the devastating neurological progression of disease.

α-*N*-acetylgalactosaminidase deficiency

Definition. Schindler disease (OMIM #609241) (α-*N*-acetylgalactosaminidase or α-NAGA deficiency) is a recently recognized lysosomal storage disease with a clinically heterogeneous picture [7].

History. In 1985, this neurodegenerative disease was first described by Schindler as being a lysosomal storage disease, in two affected brothers with primary neurological involvement.

Pathogenesis. In 1986, van Diggelen found the marked deficiency of α-NAGA in blood and cultured fibroblasts [7]. The deficient enzyme activity causes neuroaxonal pathology, presumably involving neuroaxonal transport, leading to dystrophy.

Clinical features. Two phenotypes have been identified. Type I disease is an infantile-onset neuroaxonal dystrophy with a rapid neurodegenerative course, with severe psychomotor retardation, blindness and myoclonic seizures. Type II disease was identified in an adult Japanese woman with mild mental retardation and angiokeratoma corporis diffusum [8]. Both forms of this disease have identical patterns of urinary glycopeptide accumulation caused by almost no detectable α-NAGA activity. Both types have an autosomal recessive inheritance.

Differential diagnosis. Similar structural lesions have been observed in Seitelberger disease, Hallervorden–Spatz disease and other forms of inherited neuroaxonal dystrophy. Type II disease should be differentiated from other diseases associated with angiokeratoma such as Fabry disease, sialidosis, GM_1 gangliosidosis and fucosidosis (see later).

Prognosis and treatment. Psychomotor retardation and seizures have been described. Appropriate supportive care as needed is the only treatment.

Fabry disease

Definition. Fabry disease (OMIM #301500) results from the defective activity of the lysosomal enzyme α-galactosidase A and is an inborn error of glycosphingolipid metabolism.

History. The first patients with angiokeratoma corporis diffusum were described by Anderson in England and Fabry in Germany in 1898 [9,10].

Pathogenesis. The enzymatic defect, transmitted by an X-linked recessive gene, leads to deposition of these glycosphingolipid substrates in body fluids and in many cell types in the heart, kidneys, eyes and other tissues [11].

Pathology. Angiokeratoma shows a histopathology pattern of numerous dilated, thin-walled, endothelium-lined, blood-engorged capillaries in the papillary dermis, with an overlying hyperkeratotic epidermis. Cytoplasmic vacuoles containing lipid may be present in the endothelial cells, fibroblasts and pericytes.

Clinical features. Clinical manifestations during childhood or adolescence are the onset of pain and paraesthesia in the extremities and angiokeratoma (telangiectases in the skin). Angiectases as an early manifestation may lead to diagnosis in childhood. With age, there is a progressive increase in the size and number of these cutaneous vascular lesions. The lesions may be flat and there is slight hyperkeratosis. The localization of the lesions is usually between the knees and the umbilicus. Hips, back, buttocks and scrotum are mostly involved. Hypohidrosis is reported in atypical variants; corneal and lenticular opacities are early findings.

The hallmark cutaneous manifestation of Fabry disease is angiokeratomas [12]. These develop in about 40% of male adolescents (14–16 years of age) with classic Fabry disease. With age, there is a progressive increase in the size and number of these cutaneous vascular lesions. Appearing as nonblanching red to blue–black lesions from 1 to 5 mm in diameter, they are not always covered by fine white scales as their name would suggest, being also macular or just palpable, tending to cluster around the umbilicus and swimming trunk regions. They can also present around the mouth or other parts of the body

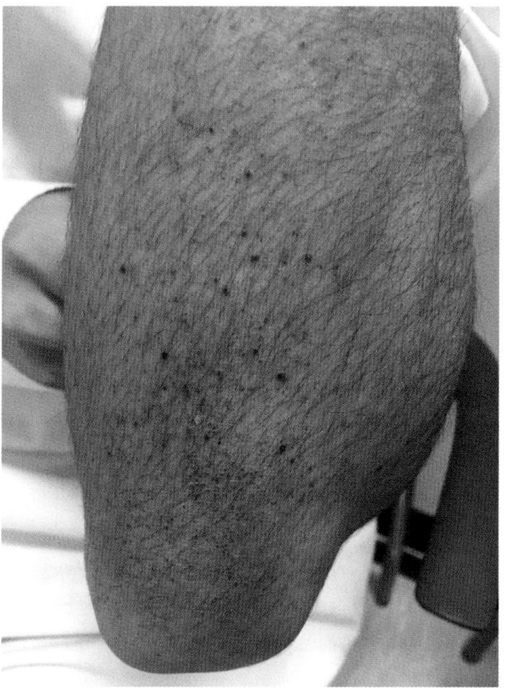
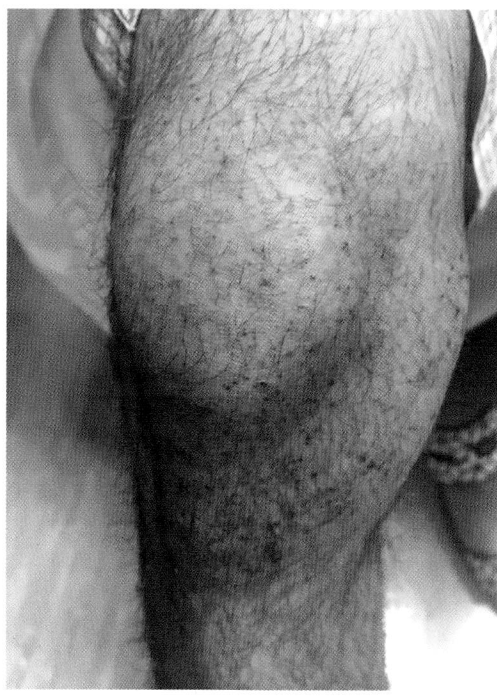

Fig. 152.4 Telangiectasia.

such as on the genitals, involving the penis, scrotum and groin in men. Later they can appear on the lips, umbilicus and periungual areas and palms [13]. A proportion of patients have no cutaneous vascular lesions, and others have macular angiomas (cherry angiomas) [14].

Telangiectasia is the second most common skin manifestation and occurs most commonly on photodamaged areas such as the face and the V of the neck. They appear later than angiokeratomas and may be seen at unusual sites such as the flanks, groins, elbow and knee flexures (Fig. 152.4) [15]. The presence of cutaneous vascular lesions (telangiectasias and/or angiokeratomas) has been associated with higher disease severity scores and a higher prevalence of major organ involvement [13]. Hypohidrosis (decreased sweating) is another common problem in Fabry disease, which has been attributed to both a main effect on the sweat glands and to autonomic neuropathy. More than 50% of men and 25% of women have hypohidrosis or/and heat intolerance in childhood [16].

Prognosis. Renal failure and cardiac or cerebrovascular disease are the main causes of death.

Differential diagnosis. Patients with Fabry disease should be distinguished from other patients with angiokeratoma corporis diffusum, such as Schindler disease, considering the X-linked inheritance.

Treatment. Angiokeratoma can be removed for cosmetic appearance by laser treatment, with little scarring [17]. Enzyme replacement therapy with intravenous recombinant enzyme supplementation is the treatment of choice to prevent cardiomyopathy and renal insufficiency.

Fucosidosis

Definition. Fucosidosis (OMIM #230000) is a lysosomal storage disease caused by a deficiency of α-fucosidase.

History. Fucosidosis was recognized in the late 1960s [18].

Pathogenesis. The deficiency of α-fucosidase results in accumulation of glycoproteins, glycolipids and oligosaccharides.

Pathology. Angiokeratomas of fucosidosis manifest as proliferative ectatic blood vessels that are lined by a flattened endothelium and are filled with erythrocytes. They are located in the papillary dermis underneath a thickened, papillomatous epidermis overlaid by a thickened horny layer. Electron microscopy examination may help to differentiate Fabry disease from fucosidosis. In Fabry disease there is electron-dense, lamellar (zebra-like) inclusions within endothelial and other cell types [19,20], whereas angiokeratoma of fucosidosis contain electron-lucent vacuoles in the skin as well as other tissues such as liver, peripheral nerves, rectal mucosa, eye and peripheral lymphocytes [18].

Clinical features. The severity of the disease is variable. The more severely affected patients present in infancy with growth retardation, psychomotor retardation, dysostosis multiplex and coarse facies.

Angiokeratoma is the main cutaneous feature present in 52% of patients [19]. It is mainly located over the lower abdomen, external genitalia and the perineum [22] (Fig. 152.5). Other cutaneous findings include widespread telangiectasias, acrocyanosis, purple transversal distal

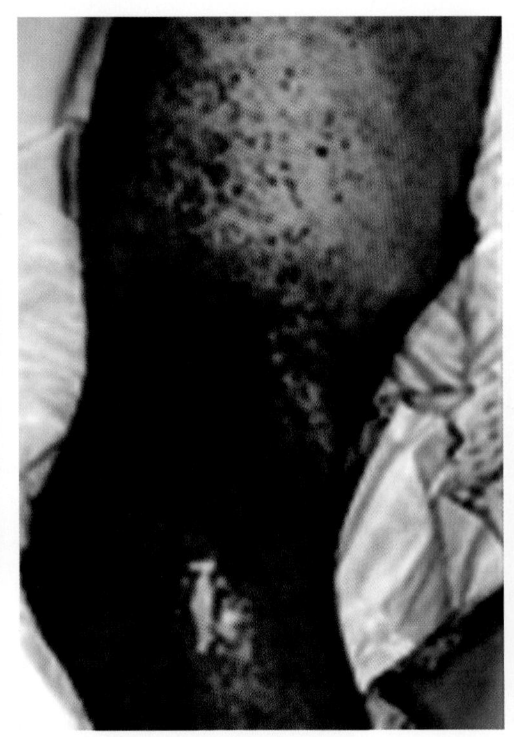

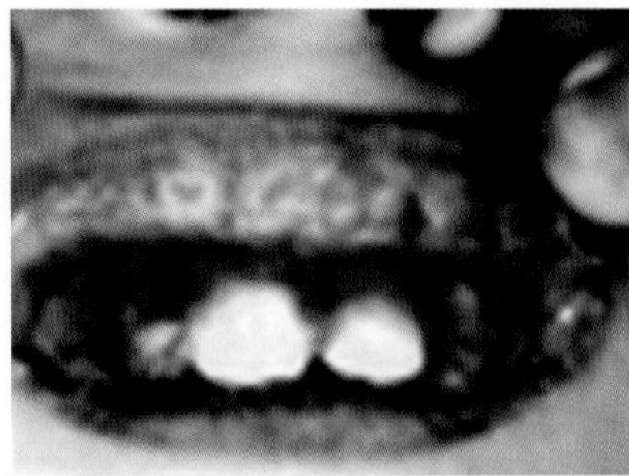

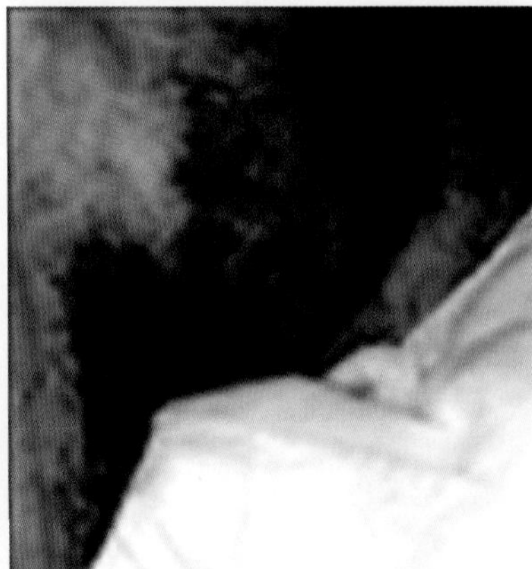

Fig. 152.5 Diffuse angiokeratoma lesions present on the trunk (left panel), the external genitalia (right lower panel), and the gums and lips (right upper panel). Source: From [24]. Reproduced with permission from John Wiley & Sons.

nail bands, increased palmoplantar vascularity, sweating abnormalities (hyper- or hypohidrosis) and dry, thin skin [23,24].

Prognosis. In one study, over 40% of the patients had died before the age of 10 years. A more normal sweat sodium chloride value is indicative of the milder phenotype. A review of 77 patients indicates a death rate of 41% after the age of 20 years [21].

Differential diagnosis. The angiokeratomas that occur in fucosidosis cannot be distinguished from those seen in adult-type α-NAGA deficiency.

Treatment. Stem cell transplantation is effective before the appearance of clinical neurological symptoms [25]. Prenatal diagnosis by mutation or biochemical analysis is reliable and has been demonstrated by analysis of chorionic villus biopsy samples or cultured amniotic fluid cells [26].

Mucopolysaccharidoses

Definition. The MPS are a group of lysosomal storage disorders caused by a deficiency of enzymes catalysing the stepwise degradation of mucopolysaccharides (glycosaminoglycans) (Table 152.2).

Depending on the enzymatic block, the catabolism of dermatan sulphate, heparan sulphate or keratan sulphate, singly or in combination, may be hampered; chondroitin sulphate may be involved.

Depending on the enzymatic deficiency, a different clinical picture exists.

History. The MPS are a group of disorders caused by a deficiency of lysosomal enzymes needed for the stepwise degradation of glucosaminoglycans (mucopolysaccharides) [27]. Hurler syndrome (MPS type I) and Hunter disease (MPS type II) were originally described as congenital dysostosis multiplex (and gargoylismus). Understanding of the classification of lysosomal storage diseases with mucopolysacchariduria in MPS came later.

Table 152.2 Classification of mucopolysaccharidoses

Type	Name	MPS product in urinary excretion
I H	Hurler	DS/HS
I S	Scheie	DS/HS
I H/S	Hurler–Scheie	DS/HS
II	Hunter	DS/HS
III A, B, C, D	Sanfilippo	HS
IV	Morquio	KS/CS
VI	Maroteaux–Lamy	DS
VII	Sly	DS/HS/CS

CS, chondroitin sulphate; DS, dermatan sulphate; HS, heparan sulphate; KS, keratan sulphate; MPS, mucopolysaccharidoses.

Pathogenesis. Accumulation of undegraded glycosaminoglycan molecules stored in lysosomes eventually results in tissue and organ dysfunction. Depending on the enzyme deficiency, a corresponding syndrome or syndrome subtype will develop.

Clinical features. The MPS share many clinical features with multisystem involvement, hepatosplenomegaly, dysostosis multiplex and coarse facies. Severe mental retardation is characteristic of Hurler syndrome, the severe form of Hunter syndrome and, later in infancy, of Sanfilippo syndrome (MPS type III). Morquio syndrome (MPS type IV) is predominantly related to the skeleton.

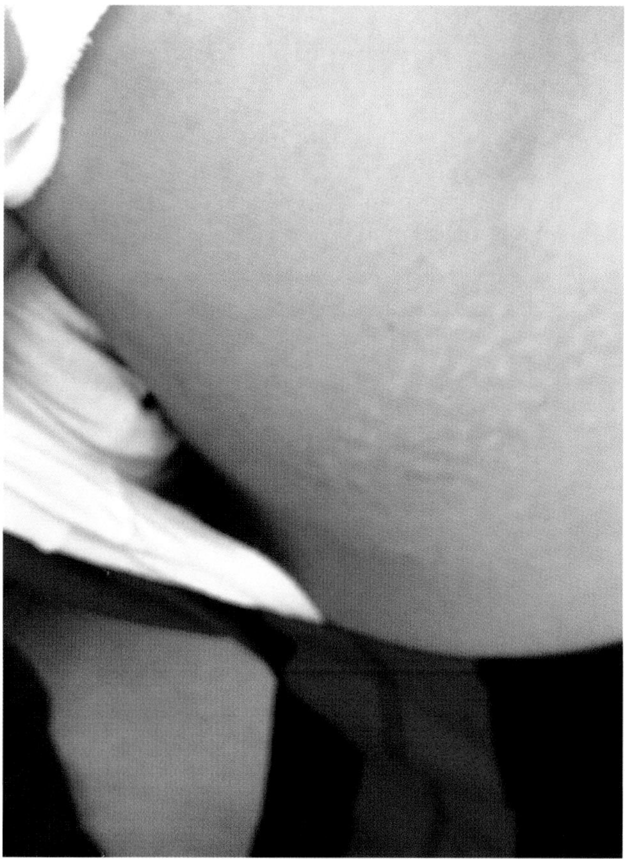

Fig. 152.6 Skin-coloured papules in a reticular pattern in Hunter's syndrome.

Short trunk, dwarfism, kyphosis and scoliosis are typical skeletal anomalies of Morquio syndrome.

MPS patients have hirsutism and increased skin thickness in the alae and the septum of the nares, for example. Patients with Hunter disease (MPS type II) have symmetrical, firm, nontender, discrete skin coloured to ivory white (hypopigmented) papules and nodules in a reticular pattern measuring 2–10 mm in diameter (Fig 152.6). They are located between the angles of the scapulae and posterior axillary lines, the pectoral regions on the chest, the neck and on the lateral aspect of the upper arm and thighs. This is a marker for the disease and distinguishes it from Hurler disease. They begin to appear in the second or third year of life, typically developing before the age of 10 and progress slowly, sometimes clearing spontaneously [28].

Extensive Mongolian spots have been noted in patients with MPS I, MPS II and GM1 gangliosidosis. It is thought to occur because normal migration of melanoblasts during embryonic development is arrested or interfered with by metabolic precursors that accumulate in these disorders [29].

Pathology. The lesion represents accumulations of extracellular mucopolysaccharides within the reticular dermis. It is believed that the papules result from the coalescence of cytoplasmic vacuoles that subsequently release their mucinous contents into the extracellular space to form the papules and nodules. These skin lesions are pathognomonic for Hunter disease but not all patients have them.

Prognosis. The disease takes a chronic and progressive course, with multisystem involvement. Mental retardation is a common feature, except in Morquio disease, Maroteaux–Lamy syndrome, Scheie and mild Hunter disease. Supportive management, with attention to respiratory and cardiovascular complications, can improve the quality of life of these patients.

Differential diagnosis. Analysis of urinary glycosaminoglycans can discriminate between the classes of glycosaminoglycans but not between subgroups. The easy spot test is inexpensive and useful for screening but can be either false positive or false negative. Definite diagnosis of MPS can be established only by enzyme assays. Mucoliposis and sialidosis should be considered if MPS investigations are negative.

Treatment. Bone marrow transplantation in MPS I and IV suggests that sufficient enzyme can be provided by haematopoietic cells.

Enzyme replacement therapy is available for MPS I (Hurler–Scheie disease), Hunter syndrome (MPS II) Maroteaux–Lamy syndrome (MPS VI) and recently for Morquio disease (MPS IV).

GM_1 gangliosidosis

Definition. GM_1 gangliosidosis (OMIM #230500, #230600) is a disorder involving the sphingolipids. There are two recognized types of this disorder in the paediatric age group. Type I is characterized by onset in early infancy, leading to death within 2 years. Type II occurs later in infancy, leading to death usually at 3–10 years of age.

History. GM_1 gangliosidosis was the second ganglioside storage disease described, the first one being Tay–Sachs disease. Originally, it was described as Landing disease: generalized neurovisceral lipidosis.

Pathogenesis. Accumulation of ganglioside GM_1 was documented by O'Brien and colleagues [30]. The primary defect is a severe deficiency of acid β-galactosidase. Intraneural storage is localized primarily to neurons of the basal ganglia.

Clinical features. The psychomotor development of an infant with GM_1 gangliosidosis is retarded in the first year of life. Many patients have facial abnormalities, including frontal bossing, large low-set ears, mild macroglossia and gum hypertrophy. Cherry-red spots, identical to those in Tay–Sachs disease, are present in about 50% of patients. Hepatomegaly is usually present after 6 months of life and splenomegaly occurs in the majority of patients. The skin is often thick, hirsute and rough.

Dermatological manifestations present at birth consisting of extensive and slate blue macules resembling Mongolian spots. It involves all area of skin except the face, scalp, palms and soles. A biopsy of a hyperpigmented macule showed melanocytic cells in the dermis consistent with a Monogolian spot but also a perivascular histiocytic infiltrate. Angiokeratoma was also reported in a patient [31,32].

Prognosis. Infantile GM_1 gangliosidosis presents with bone changes and neurological deterioration leading to early death. Progressive psychomotor deterioration with bony abnormalities is seen in juvenile GM_1 gangliosidosis.

Differential diagnosis. This includes lysosomal storage diseases with neurological symptoms.

Treatment. As far as is known, treatment can only be symptomatic.

Farber lipogranulomatosis: ceramidase deficiency

Definition. Farber disease (OMIM #228000) is an autosomal recessively inherited disorder of lipid metabolism associated with a deficiency of a lysosomal acid ceramidase and tissue accumulation of ceramide [33].

History. In 1952, the first case of 'Farber disease' was described by Sidney Farber in a 14-month-old infant. So far, the phenotype has been divided into six subtypes. It is likely that the diagnosis has frequently been missed because of the variability of the clinical picture.

Pathogenesis. Accumulation of ceramide has been reported in all well-documented cases. The granuloma formation and histiocytic response appear to be a consequence of ceramide accumulation.

Clinical features. Subcutaneous nodules near the joints and over pressure points, and progressively painful and deformed joints, are the main clinical manifestations. Hoarseness caused by laryngeal involvement can lead to aphonia, feeding and respiratory difficulties, failure to thrive and intermittent fever. Symptoms usually appear between the ages of 2 weeks and 4 months. Different subtypes have been described.

The diagnosis can be demonstrated by a deficiency of acid ceramidase in cultured skin fibroblasts or in white blood cells. Prenatal diagnosis by mutation analysis or measuring enzyme activity in cultured amniocytes has proved useful [33,34].

Prognosis. The disease often leads to death within the first few years; depending on the subtype, a longer lifespan can be observed.

Differential diagnosis. Juvenile rheumatoid arthritis and fibromatosis hyalinica multiplex can resemble the clinical picture of Farber disease [35]. Histopathological and enzymatic investigations are necessary to confirm the final diagnosis.

Treatment. The treatment is supportive. The development of enzyme replacement therapy is underway. Bone marrow transplantation may aid in early diagnosis before neurological involvement [36].

References

1 Gaucher PCE. De l'epithelioma primitif de la rate, hypertrophie idiopathique de la rate sans leucemie [academic thesis]. Paris, 1882.

2 Brady RO, Kanfer JN, Shapiro D. Metabolism of glucosylceramidase. II. Evidence of an enzymatic deficiency in Gaucher's disease. Biochem Biophys Res Commun 1965;18: 221–5.

3 Liu K, Commens C, Chong R, Jaworski R. Collodion babies with Gauchers disease. Arch Dis Child 1988;63:854–6.

4 Beutler E, Grabowski GA. Gaucher disease. In: Scriver CR, Beaudet AL, Sly WS, Valle D (eds) Metabolic and Molecular Bases of Inherited Disease. New York: McGraw-Hill, 2001:3635.

5 Stone DL, Carey WF, Christodoulou J et al. Type 2 Gaucher disease: the collodion baby phenotype revisited. Arch Dis Child Fetal Neonatal Ed 2000;82:F163–6.

6 Weiss K, Gonzalez A, Lopez G et al. the clinical management of type 2 Gaucher disease. Mol Genetics Metab 2015;114:110–22.

7 Van Diggelen OP, Schindler D, Kleijer WJ et al. Lysosomal α-N-acetylgalactosaminidase deficiency: a new inherited metabolic disease. Lancet 1987;ii:804.

8 Kanzaki T, Wang AM, Desnick RJ. Lysosomal α-N-acetylgalactosaminidase deficiency, the enzymatic defect in angiokeratoma corporis diffusum with glycopeptiduria. J Clin Invest 1991;88:707.

9 Anderson W. A case of angiokeratoma. Br J Dermatol 1898;10:113.

10 Fabry J. Ein Beitrag zur Kenntnis der Purpura haemorrhagica nodularis. Arch Dermatol Syph 1898;43:187.

11 Kint JA. Fabry's disease, α-galactosidase deficiency. Science 1970;167:1268.

12 Albano LM, Rivitti C, Bertola DR et al. Angiokeratoma: a cutaneous marker of Fabry's disease. Clin Exp Dermatol 2010;35:505–8.

13 Zampetti A, Orteu CH, Antuzzi D et al. Angiokeratoma: decision-making aid for the diagnosis of Fabry disease. Br J Dermatol. 2012;166:712–720.

14 Hogarth V, Dhoat S, Mehta AB et al. Late-onset Fabry disease associated with angiokeratoma of Fordyce and multiple cherry angiomas. Clin Exp Dermatol 2011;36:506–8.

15 Ries M, Ramaswami U, Parini R et al. The early clinical phenotype of Fabry disease: a study on 35 European children and adolescents. Eur J Pediatr 2003;162:767–72.

16 Lidove O, Ramaswami U, Jaussaud R et al. Hyperhidrosis: a new and often early symptom in Fabry disease. International experience and data from the Fabry Outcome Survey. Int J Clin Pract 2006;60:1053–9.

17 Newton JA, McGibbon HD. The treatment of multiple angiokeratoma with the argon laser. Clin Exp Dermatol 1987;12:23.

18 Durand P, Borrone C, Della Cella G. Fucosidosis. J Pediatr 1969;75:665–74.

19 Epinette W, Norins A, Drew A, Zeman W. Angiokeratoma Corporis Diffusum with a-L-fucosidase deficiency. Arch Dermatol 1973;107:754.

20 Kanzaki T. [Lysosomal storage diseases with angiokeratoma corporis diffusum]. Nippon Rinsho 1995;53:3062.

21 Willems PJ, Gatt R, Darby JK et al. Fucosidosis revisited: a review of 77 patients. Am J Med Genet 1991;38:111.

22 Porfiri B, Ricci R, Seminara D, Segni G. Ultrastructural studies of type II fucosidosis. Arch Dermatol Res 1981;270:57.

23 Fleming C, Rennie A, Fallowfield M, McHenry PM. Cutaneous manifestations of fucosidosis. Br J Dermatol 1997;136:594.

24 Kanitakis J, Allombert C, Doebelin B et al. Fucosidosis with angiokeratoma. Immunohistochemical and electronmicroscopic study of a new case and literature review. J Cutan Pathol 2005;32:506–11.

25 Miranda CO, Brites P, Mendes Sousa M, Teixeira CA. Advances and pitfalls of cell therapy in metabolic leukodystrophies. Cell Transplant 2013;22:189–204.

26 Butterworth J, Guy GJ. α-l-fucosidase of human skin fibroblasts and amniotic fluid cells in tissue culture. Clin Genet 1977;12:297.

27 Neufeld EF, Muenzer J. The mucopolysaccharidoses. In: Scriver CR, Beaudet AL, Sly WS et al. (eds) The Metabolic and Molecular Bases of Inherited Disease, 7th edn. New York: McGraw-Hill, 1995:2465–94.

28 Prystowsky SD, Maumenee IH, Freeman RG et al. A cutaneous marker in the Hunter syndrome a report of four cases. Arch Dermatol 1977;113:602–5.
29 Sapadin AN, Friedman IS. Extensive Mongolian spots associated with Hunter syndrome. J Am Acad Dermatol 1998;39:1013–5.
30 O'Brien JS, Stern MB, Landing BH et al. Generalized gangliosidosis. Am J Dis Child 1965;109:388.
31 Weissbluth M, Esterly NB, Caro WA. Report of an infant with GM1 gangliosidosis type I and extensive and unusual mongolian spots. Br J Dermatol 1981;104:195–200.
32 Beratis NG, Varvarigou-Frimas A, Beratis S, Sklower SL. Angiokeratoma corporis diffusum in GM1 gangliosidosis, Type 1. Clinical Genetics 1989;36:59–64.
33 Moser HW, Moser AB, Chen WW. Ceramidase deficiency: Farber lipogranulomatosis. In: Scriver CR, Beaudet AL, Sly WS et al. (eds) The Metabolic and Molecular Bases of Inherited Disease, 7th edn. New York: McGraw-Hill, 1995:1645–53.
34 Fensom AH, Benson PI, Neville BRG et al. Prenatal diagnosis of Farber's disease. Lancet 1979;ii:990.
35 Mancini GMS, Stojanov L, Willemsen R et al. Juvenile hyaline fibromatosis. Dermatology 1999;198:18–25.
36 Schuchman EH. Acid ceramidase and the treatment of ceramide diseases: the expanding role of enzyme replacement therapy. Biochim Biophys Acta 2016;1862:1459–71.

Others metabolic deficiencies

Transaldolase deficiency

Definition. Transaldolase deficiency (OMIM #606003) is an inborn error of the nonoxidative phase of the pentose phosphate pathway, which provides ribose-5-phosphate for nucleic acid synthesis and nicotinamide adenine dinucleotide phosphate (NADPH) for lipid biosynthesis [1].

History. This condition was first described in 2001, in a patient presenting with neonatal liver dysfunction and abnormal coagulation [1].

Pathogenesis. Transaldolase catalyses the reversible transfer of a three-carbon ketol unit from sedoheptulose 7-phosphate to glyceraldehyde 3-phosphate to form erythrose 4-phosphate and fructose 6-phosphate [2]. In transaldolase deficiency there is accumulation of sedoheptulose 7-phosphate and a failure to recycle ribose 5-phosphate, which leads to NADPH and glutathione (GSH) deficiency and an increased level of lipid hydroperoxides as well as the loss of the mitochondrial transmembrane potential [3].

Clinical features. Transaldolase deficient patients may present with a wide clinical phenotype including hydrops fetalis, hepatosplenomegaly, hepatic dysfunction, thrombocytopenia, anaemia, and renal, respiratory or cardiac abnormalities. The dysmorphic features include downward-slanting palpebral fissures, low-set ears and cutis laxa. All affected individuals have abnormal urinary polyol concentrations, which can be used as a biomarker for the diagnosis [1]. Most reported cases are from consanguineous families of Turkish or Arabic origin [4]. The severity of the symptoms and the outcome vary widely among patients. The skin manifestations are dry skin, cutis laxa, ichthyosis, telangiectasias and haemangiomas [5].

Prognosis. In general, it is variable and the lifespan of some patients is usually short because of liver failure

Differential diagnosis. It depends upon the presenting symptoms and signs

Treatment. Effective treatment for transaldolase deficiency remains elusive; patients might benefit from liver transplantation, although there is still a risk of disease recurrence. Hence, therapeutic approaches might be directed toward increasing the production of glutathione (GSH) using N-acetylcysteine and decreasing oxidative stress with antioxidants (e.g. vitamins C or E) [5].

Prolidase deficiency

Definition. Prolidase deficiency (OMIM #170100) is a rare, panethnic metabolic condition transmitted in an autosomal recessive manner and is caused by mutations in the *PEPD* gene [6].

History. Powell and colleagues studied two children with prolidase deficiency presented with chronic dermatitis, frequent infections, splenomegaly and massive imidodipeptiduria [7].

Pathogenesis. Prolidase catalyses hydrolysis of di- and oligopeptides with a C-terminal hydroxyproline or proline.

Clinical features. Prolidase deficiency is a multisystemic disorder, with varying clinical severity, ranging from asymptomatic individuals to severely affected patients. Mental retardation reported in two-thirds of patients and in some cases, subtle facial dysmorphic features.

The hallmark of prolidase deficiency is severe, chronic, recalcitrant and painful skin ulcers. The ulcers are located mainly on the lower extremities, particularly the feet. There are reported cases of: telangiectasias of the face, shoulders and hands; scaly, erythematous, maculopapular lesions; purpuric lesions in the absence of hematological abnormalities; and premature greying of the hair.

Prognosis. The severity is quite variable: in some individuals skin ulcerations lead to amputation of one or all toes, whereas others remain entirely asymptomatic.

Differential diagnosis. Sickle cell disease, Werner syndrome and acquired causes of lower-extremity ulcers including arterial insufficiency, venous insufficiency, pressure ulcers, vasculitis, systemic lupus erythematosus and infectious aetiologies, among others, should be considered.

Treatment. No curative treatment is available. The treatment of skin, lung and immunological manifestations is supportive.

References

1 Verhoeven NM, Huck JH, Roos B et al. Transaldolase deficiency: liver cirrho- sis associated with a new inborn error in the pentose phosphate pathway. Am J Hum Genet 2001;68:1086–92.
2 Heinrich PC, Morris HP, Weber G. Behavior of transaldolase (EC 2.2.1.2) and transketolase (EC 2.2.1.1) activities in normal, neoplastic, differentiating, and regenerating liver. Cancer Res 1976;36:3189–97.
3 Hanczko R, Fernandez DR, Doherty E et al. Prevention of hepatocarcinogenesis and increased susceptibility to acetaminophen-induced liver failure in transaldolase- deficient mice by N-acetylcysteine. J Clin Invest 2009;119:1546–57.
4 Tylki-Szymanska A, Stradomska TJ, Wamelink MM et al. Transaldolase deficiency in two new patients with a relative mild phenotype. Mol Genet Metab 2009;97:15–17.
5 **Al-Shamsi AM, Ben-Salem S, Hertecant J, Al-Jasmi F. Transaldolase deficiency caused by the homozygous p.R192C mutation of the TALDO1 gene in four Emirati patients with considerable phenotypic variability. Eur J Pediatr 2015;174:661–8.**
6 **Ferreira C, Wang H. Prolidase deficiency. June 25 2015. In: Pagon RA, Adam MP, Ardinger HH et al. (eds) GeneReviews® [Internet]. Seattle (WA): University of Washington, Seattle; 1993–2016. Available from http://www.ncbi.nlm.nih.gov/books/NBK299584/**
7 Powell GF, Rasco MA, Maniscalco RM. A prolidase deficiency in man with iminopeptiduria. Metabolism 1974;23:505–13.

Hyperlipoproteinaemia

Definition. Genetic hyperlipoproteinaemias are caused by defects of structural components of lipoproteins or receptors that affect the formation or removal of lipoproteins [1]. They consist of a group of disorders characterized by elevated serum cholesterol levels and/or elevated triglyceride levels.

History. Hyperlipoproteinaemias are usually grouped according to the classification of Fredricksen. They are all inherited disorders. Hyperlipoproteinaemias are classified into five groups, numbered I–V [2] (Table 152.3).

Aetiology. Lipoproteins are complexes that transport lipids within the blood: triglycerides, cholesterol (esterified and unesterified), phospholipids and fat-soluble vitamins. The major lipoprotein particles are chylomicrons, very low-density lipoproteins (VLDLs), low-density lipoproteins (LDLs) and high-density lipoproteins (HDLs).

The major consequences of lipoprotein disorders are premature arteriosclerosis and atherosclerosis in heterozygous or homozygous familial hypercholesterolaemia (FH). Life-threatening acute pancreatitis is the cause of death in untreated hypertriglyceridaemia and hyperchylomicronaemia caused by lipoprotein lipase deficiency (LPL) or apolipoprotein CII deficiency [3].

Pathology. Histopathological features consist of upper dermal infiltrates of non-xanthomized histiocytes, varying in appearance corresponding with clinical features, such as plane or more papular or nodular presentations. Based on the age of the lesion and differentiation, the infiltrate contains histiocytes, fully matured foam cells and Touton giant cells. In all forms of xanthomas, the lipid within the foam cells stains positively with fat stains such as oil red O, scarlet or Sudan red. These foam cells are characteristic of xanthomas. Depending upon the kind of xanthomas, the infiltrate is mixed with lymphocytes and neutrophils [4,5]. In tendinous xanthomas, older lesions are associated with fibrosis, but in plane xanthomas this is rare. Xanthomas, especially relevant in disseminated xanthomatosis, consist of non-Langerhans cell histiocytes, which are S100 protein negative [6,7].

Clinical features. The most important clinical features of FH are premature arteriosclerosis and xanthomatosis. Xanthomas tuberosa can occur in the Achilles tendon and the tendons around the elbows, knees and the back of the hand. The age at appearance depends on the heterozygous or homozygous state of the disease. Xanthelasma, which is lipid accumulation of the soft connective tissue on the eyelids, is also a recognizable clinical feature.

Xanthomas and xanthelasma appear between the third and fourth decades of life in heterozygous FH, whereas they can already be seen in early childhood in the homozygous FH patients (incidence 1 in 10^6 in the Caucasian population). LPL deficiency (Fredricksen type I) is characterized by attacks of acute abdominal pain caused by pancreatitis in untreated patients; the mortality rate is high.

Xanthomas consist of papules, nodules or tumours that contain lipid. There are several types: plane xanthomas, eruptive xanthomas, tendinous xanthomas (Fig. 152.7), tuberous xanthomas and xanthelasma (Fig. 152.8). A plane xanthoma is a flat or only slightly elevated plaque, commonly located in palmar and digital creases. An eruptive xanthoma is reddish-yellow and appears in crops. These xanthomas are mostly seen on the buttocks or extremities. A tendinous xanthoma is

Table 152.3 Hyperlipoproteinaemias according to Fredricksen types I–V

	I	II	III	IV	V
Inheritance	AR	AD	AR	AD	AR
Dermatology symptoms	Eruptive xanthomas	Tendinous, tuberous, plane xanthomas, xanthelasma	Plane, tendinous tuberous xanthomas	Eruptive, tuberous xanthomas	Eruptive, tuberous xanthomas
Age	Infants, teenagers	Children	Adults	Adults (obesity)	Adults (obesity)
Laboratory	VLDL, TG, CM raised; C, LDL raised		C, TG raised; LDL, HDL low or normal	VLDL, TG raised	VLDL, TG, CM raised

AD, autosomal dominant; AR, autosomal recessive; C, cholesterol; CM, chylomicron; HDL, high-density lipoprotein; LDL, low-density lipoprotein; TG, triglyceride; VLDL, very low-density lipoprotein.

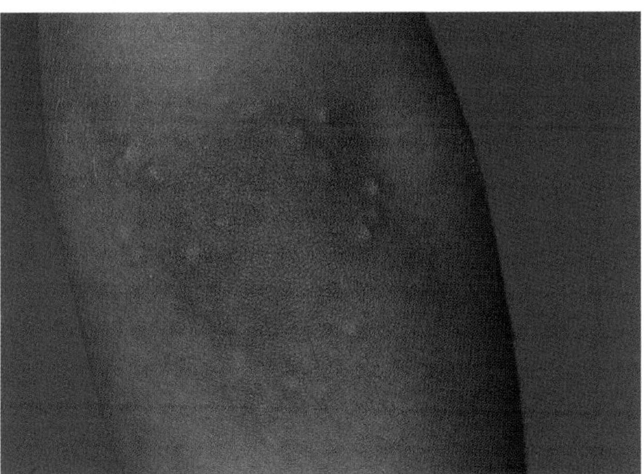

Fig. 152.7 Xanthomas in a boy with homozygous familial hypercholesterolaemia.

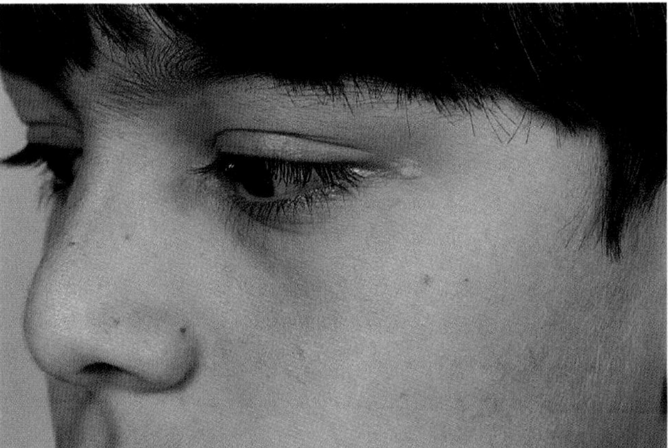

Fig. 152.8 Xanthelasma in a boy with homozygous familial hypercholesterolaemia, an extremely rare manifestation.

nodular and located on tendons especially of the elbows, hands, knees and feet. The tumour is skin coloured or yellow. A tuberous xanthoma is a nodule located on the extensor sites of the elbows, hands, buttocks or knees, and is skin coloured or yellow.

Prognosis. Untreated homozygous FH leads to early death in the second decade caused by coronary heart disease or cerebral vascular accident. Heterozygous FH leads to coronary heart disease and cerebral vascular accident between the third and fourth decades of life.

Differential diagnosis. Secondary causes of hyperlipidaemias, including hepatic disease, diabetes mellitus, nephrotic syndrome or hypothyroidism and drug-induced causes, must be excluded.

Treatment. In FH, a fat-restricted, linoleic acid-enriched diet should be advised by an experienced dietitian, combined with a fibre-rich diet. Physical exercise, an active nonsmoking lifestyle and prevention of obesity should be encouraged.

In homozygous FH, cholestyramine and hydroxymethylglutaryl CoA reductase (HMG CoA reductase) inhibitors, such as simvastatin or the very potent atorvastatin, are the drugs of choice, even at an early age. However, the majority of cases will require LDL apheresis. Liver transplantation is also being used in difficult cases [8]. Two new agents, oral lomitapide, a microsomal triglyceride transfer protein inhibitor, and injectable mipomersen, an antisense RNA therapy, both of which target hepatic production of atherogenic apoB-containing lipoproteins, were recently approved in the USA as adjunct therapy. Statin myopathy is now a well-known complication of statin users. Change of medication and control of creatine kinase is the treatment of choice [9].

In LPL deficiency, a fat-restricted, medium-chain triglyceride-enriched diet is the treatment of choice.

References

1 Brown MS, Goldstein JC. A receptor mediated pathway of cholesterol homeostasis. Science 1986;232:34–47.
2 Fredricksen DS, Lees RS. A system for phenotyping hyperlipoproteinaemia. Circulation 1965;31:321–7.
3 Santamarina-Fojo S. Genetic dyslipoproteinemias: role of lipoprotein lipase and apolipoprotein C-II. Curr Opin Lipidol 1992;3:186–95.
4 McKee P. Pathology of the Skin, 2nd edn. London: Mosby Wolfe, 1996:1–7, 10.
5 Crowe MJ, Gross DJ. Eruptive xanthoma. Cutis 1992;50:31–2.
6 Winkelmann RK. Cutaneous syndromes of non-X histiocytosis. A review of the macrophage–histiocyte diseases of the skin. Arch Dermatol 1981;117:667–72.
7 Soong VY, Rabkin MS, Thomas JM. Nodular lesions on the face and trunk: xanthoma disseminatum. Arch Dermatol 1991;1127:1717–22.
8 Wiegman A, Gidding SS, Watts GF et al. Familial hypercholesterolaemia in children and adolescents: gaining decades of life by optimizing detection and treatment. Eur Heart J 2015;36:2425–37.
9 Venero CV, Thompson PD. Managing statin myopathy. Endocrinol Metab Clin North Am 2009;38:121–36.

Acrodermatitis enteropathica

Definition. Acrodermatitis enteropathica is a biochemical disease of metal metabolism by zinc deficiency. There is an inability to absorb sufficient zinc from the diet.

History. Acrodermatitis enteropathica was recognized in 1936 by a Swedish dermatologist [1].

Aetiology and pathophysiology. Acrodermatitis enteropathica is an autosomal recessively inherited disease. Deficiency of zinc-dependent enzymes leads to the typical clinical features of hair, muscle and bone. The fact that a large number of enzymes require zinc as a cofactor is probably the basis of the heterogeneity of the symptoms.

Serum alkaline phosphatase is a zinc-containing enzyme and is decreased at all ages in patients with acrodermatitis enteropathica, but this is not an early indicator of the disease. The disturbance of zinc homeostasis results from a partial block in intestinal absorption [2].

Clinical features. Clinical symptoms of acrodermatitis enteropathica are those of zinc deficiency. They represent general symptoms such as failure to thrive, anorexia, tremor, diarrhoea and apathy, as well as local hair and skin symptoms. The classic triad is acral dermatitis, alopecia and diarrhoea. The patient presents with skin

SECTION 32: SKIN AND SYSTEMIC DISEASE

rash, alopecia, fine brittle hair and perioral and perianal vesiculobullous, pustular and hyperkeratotic dermatitis. Nail dystrophy may also occur [3]. Symptoms develop after the neonatal period (mostly after weaning). Laboratory findings show low plasma or serum zinc levels.

Prognosis. If the diagnosis is made correctly and in time, the prognosis in general is good.

Differential diagnosis. Biotinidase deficiency, malnutrition and several types of epidermolysis bullosa and severe seborrhoeic dermatitis must be considered. A skin biopsy is not always diagnostic. Essential fatty acid deficiency is one of the most common differential diagnoses. Some types of organic acidaemias caused by aberrant degration of branched-chain amino acids, such as propionic acidaemia and methylmalonic acidaemia [4,5] (see previously), cause acrodermatitis-like lesions. It should be noted that severe hypoalbuminaemia is associated with low serum zinc values.

Treatment. Zinc supplementation usually leads to a rapid improvement of the clinical features. At least double the normal daily requirement must be given initially. The therapy will need to be continued for life.

Acknowledgement

We acknowledge and thank Johannis B.C. de Klerk and Arnold P. Oranje for their contribution in the previous edition and for reuse of material and images.

References

1 Brandt T. Dermatitis in children with disturbances of general condition and absence of food. Acta Derm Venereol 1936;17:513–46.
2 Atherton DJ, Muller DPR, Aggett PJ et al. A defect in zinc uptake by jejunal biopsies in acrodermatitis enteropathica. Clin Sci 1970; 56:505–7.
3 Neldner KH, Hambridge KM, Walravens PA. Acrodermatitis enteropathica. Int J Dermatol 1978;17:380–7.
4 Koopman RJJ, Happle R. Cutaneous manifestations of methylmalonic acidemia. Arch Dermatol Res 1990;282:272–7.
5 Bodemer C, de Prost Y, Bachollet B et al. Cutaneous manifestations of methylmalonic acidemia and propionic acidemia: a description of 38 cases. Br J Dermatol 1994;131:93–8.

Carotenaemia

Definition. Carotenaemia is a condition in which the plasma concentration of carotenoids (principally β-carotene) is elevated, producing a yellowish discoloration of the skin (xanthodermia). Carotenoids are pigments that are synthesized by plants and are present in foods such as carrots and all green vegetables. They are generally C_{40} tetraterpenoids formed from eight isoprenoid units joined so that the configuration is reversed in the centre [1]. The most abundant carotenoid in the diet is β-carotene, the structure of which is shown in Fig. 152.9. Carotenoids are an important source of vitamin A. Normal plasma concentrations of β-carotene and vitamin A in children are given in Table 152.4 [2].

Table 152.4 Normal ranges for serum concentrations of β-carotene and vitamin A in children (0.025–0.975 fractiles

Analyte	Serum concentration	
	μmol/L	μg/L
β-Carotene	0.56–2.85	300–1530
Vitamin A	0.67–2.39	182–683

To convert μmol/L to μg/L, multiply by 537 for β-carotene and 286 for vitamin A (retinol).
Data from Malvy et al. 1993 [2].

History. Prior to the twentieth century, there were occasional observations on 'aurantiasis' and 'carotenosis cutis' as forms of xanthodermia that were different from jaundice. In 1926, Greene & Blackford [3] showed that it was possible to distinguish carotenaemia from jaundice by shaking serum with equal volumes of petroleum ether and absolute alcohol. Carotene colours the upper petroleum ether layer whereas bile pigments are found in the middle alcohol layer. The food rationing of the Second World War provided the background to a series of observations on dietary carotenaemia. In the UK, there was a successful campaign promoting the consumption of root vegetables (particularly carrots and swedes) and, in 1941, Almond & Logan [4] described four housewives who developed orange pigmentation of their palms and nasolabial folds following the ingestion of 2.7 kg of carrots weekly for 7 months. One of the four women was breastfeeding an infant and this infant also developed pigmentation, which disappeared following a change to bottle feeding. In 1958, Lord Cohen of Birkenhead [5] reported 50 cases of xanthodermia diagnosed in the war years in the UK and associated with a raw carrot intake of 1.8–3.6 kg daily. Xanthodermia appeared after 6–8 months, but if carrots were omitted from the diet the yellowish tinge faded in 2–6 weeks. Lord Cohen also described carotenaemia in hyperlipidaemic states (including diabetes mellitus, the nephrotic syndrome and myxoedema). He was the first to describe a case of carotenaemia with low plasma vitamin A concentration and postulate that this was because of an inborn error in the conversion of β-carotene to vitamin A [5].

Aetiology and pathogenesis. A normal intake of β-carotene is 900–1200 μg/day. Ingested carotene is largely converted to vitamin A (retinol) in the intestinal mucosa by carotenoid 15,15′-mono-oxygenase and retinaldehyde reductase (see Fig. 152.9). A small proportion is absorbed unchanged. The absorption of β-carotene is increased in subjects taking a high-fat diet. The highly lipid-soluble pigment is present in the lipoprotein fractions of plasma (LDL) and there is a close correlation between serum lipoprotein levels and serum β-carotene concentration [6]. Carotenaemia or hypercarotenaemia can therefore arise as a result of excessive ingestion of β-carotene, defective conversion to vitamin A (metabolic carotenaemia) or hyperlipidaemia. A recent case report

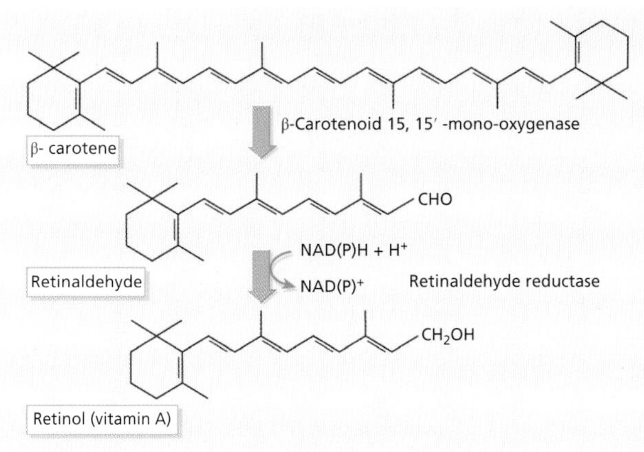

Fig. 152.9 Metabolism of β-carotene to vitamin A. Carotenoid 15, 15′-mono-oxygenase is located in the intestinal mucosa.

Table 152.5 Carotene content of foods

Moderate (50–250 μg/100 g)	High (300–600 μg/100 g)	Very high >600 μg/100 g)
Vegetables		
Aubergine	Asparagus	Cabbage (savoy)
Baked beans	Broccoli	Carrots
Broad beans	Brussels sprouts	Chilli (red)
Cauliflower	Courgette	Cress
Celery	Green beans	Curly kale
Fennel	French beans	Mange-tout
Marrow	Leeks	Peppers (red)
Peas (sugarsnap)	Peas (tinned/ frozen/fresh)	Parsley
Peppers (green/ yellow)	Petit pois	Pumpkin
Runner beans	Squash (acorn)	Spinach
Swede		Spring greens
Sweetcorn		Squash (butternut)
Sweet potato (white flesh)		Sweet potato (orange flesh)
		Tomato (fresh/tinned)[1]
		Tomato purée[1]
		Watercress
		Yam (yellow flesh)
Fruit		
Apricot (canned in syrup)	Peach (dried)	Apricot (dried)
Banana	Plum	Melon (canteloupe, flesh)
Blackberry		Watermelon[1]
Blackcurrant		
Orange		

[1] Major carotenoid is lycopene.

described acute onset of carotenaemia complicating immunoglobulin light chain amyloidosis [7]; the mechanism in this adult is not understood.

Excessive ingestion of carotene

Foods with a high content of β-carotene [8] are listed in Table 152.5. Ingestion of large amounts of any of these carotene-rich foods could give rise to carotenaemia. It is important to remember that β-carotene is also used as a food additive; its presence is usually declared on the package (as β-carotene or E160). Prince & Frisoli [9] have studied the accumulation of β-carotene in the plasma and skin in adult volunteers given a large daily dose of the pigment. The plasma concentration rises to a plateau over 9–10 days. Accumulation in the skin takes a further 2 weeks. On cessation of administration, plasma carotene concentrations decay, with a half-life of around 15 days [9].

Hyperlipidaemia

The concentration of β-carotene in the blood rises when the lipoprotein concentrations rise. The conditions which have been documented as giving rise to carotenaemia include diabetes mellitus (which usually gives rise to increased plasma VLDL), hypothyroidism (increased LDL) and the nephrotic syndrome (increased LDL and VLDL) [5]. Other causes of hyperlipoproteinaemia in childhood include obstructive jaundice, hepatic glycogenoses, renal dialysis, acute porphyria, cholesterol ester storage disease and the primary hyperlipidaemias [10]. It has also been reported in some patients with anorexia nervosa [11]. The mechanisms responsible for hyperlipidaemia in these conditions are beyond the scope of this chapter. In hypothyroidism the conversion of β-carotene to vitamin A is reduced so that this is an additional mechanism for the carotenaemia.

Metabolic carotenaemia

The combination of an elevated serum carotene concentration and low serum vitamin A suggests a defect in one of the enzymes responsible for conversion of carotene to vitamin A. To date, one such disorder has been described at a molecular genetic level and others require further clarification.

Carotenoid 15,15′-mono-oxygenase (*BCMO1, BCO1* or *CMO1*); gene locus 16q21-q23. Carotenoid 15,15′-mono-oxygenase (CMO) catalyses the first step in the conversion of dietary provitamin A carotenoids to vitamin A and a single patient with a confirmed mutation in this gene has been reported [12]. This subject, who did not ingest excess dietary carotene, had yellow discoloration of the skin but was otherwise healthy and had elevated serum β-carotene and low to normal serum vitamin A. A single T170M heterozygous missense mutation was identified resulting in a 90% loss of function of the *CMO1* enzyme. Although the function of this threonine residue is not understood, substitution of a small hydrophilic threonine with a large hydrophobic methionine residue severely attenuates enzyme activity. Because the mutation was only found in a single allele, other genes known to be involved in carotenoid metabolism and vitamin A synthesis were also analysed in this subject and were found to be normal (carotenoid 9′,10′-mono-oxygenase, cellular retinol binding protein I and II and retinol dehydrogenase types 11, 12 and 14). Thus, haploinsufficiency of *CMO1* may be enough to cause the clinical phenotype. Several other patients [13–16] with a similar clinical picture of orange-yellow skin pigmentation and biochemical hypercarotenaemia and hypovitaminosis A, which responds to supplementation, have been described but none has undergone mutational analysis of the *CMO1* gene.

A study in 2009 [17] showed that two nonsynonymous single nucleotide polymorphisms exist in the *CMO1* gene which alter β-carotene metabolism in healthy female volunteers. Those carrying either the 379V or the 267S +379V variants showed a reduced ability to convert β-carotene and had higher fasting β-carotene concentrations which may have implications for treatment of vitamin A deficiency states. A study in 2011 showed that single nucleotide polymorphisms upstream of the *CMO1* gene (rs6420424, rs11645428 and rs6564851) can also reduce conversion of β-carotene to vitamin A [18].

Retinol-binding protein 4 (*RBP4*) gene locus 10q24. Uncertainty remains as to whether RBP deficiency can cause isolated carotenaemia. Attard-Montalto and colleagues [19] described a 5-year-old girl with xanthodermia, elevated serum β-carotene and low serum vitamin A. The serum concentration of retinol-binding protein (RBP) was at the low end of the normal range and vitamin A supplements failed to correct the low serum vitamin A concentration. The authors proposed that the primary defect was in the RBP: deficiency of RBP was responsible for defective transport of vitamin A out of intestinal mucosal cells and hepatocytes. Accumulation of vitamin A within these cells resulted in defective conversion of β-carotene to vitamin A [19]. Direct proof of this hypothesis has not been obtained and genetic mutations in RBP4 have not been reported.

Two patients proven to have undetectable RBP caused by compound heterozygous mis-sense mutations in the *RBP4* gene were described by Seeliger and colleagues in 1999 [20]. They had low levels of serum vitamin A, night vision problems and 'fundus xerophthalicum' caused by progressive atrophy of the retinal pigment epithelium; they did not have xerophthalmia. The only dermatological manifestation described was acne and serum concentrations of β-carotene were not reported. This disorder is now known as the (autosomal recessive) retinal dystrophy, iris coloboma and comedogenic acne syndrome. Monoallelic mutations in *RBP4* can cause isolated microphthalmia with coloboma [21].

Pathology. When the concentration of β-carotene in the blood is high, it accumulates both in the epidermis and in the subcutaneous fat. Here it absorbs light with absorption maxima at 475, 490 and 510 nm, producing the orange-yellow discoloration [9]. There is no strong evidence that elevated concentrations of β-carotene have any adverse effects in the skin or in other tissues in which it accumulates. Shoenfeld and colleagues in 1982 [22] described a single patient, aged 21, who had mild neutropenia and gingival and buccal erosions while she was taking a high-carotene diet. The neutropenia resolved on a low-carotene diet and returned when ingestion of large amounts of carrot juice was resumed. Kaspar and colleagues in 1991 [23] reported two children with dietary carotenaemia and raised transaminases which fell when the dietary carotene intake was normalized. Gangakhedkar and colleagues described a child with dietary carotenaemia who developed hepatomegaly that resolved when the dietary intake of carotene was reduced [24]. However, it is by no means certain in these cases that liver damage was caused by high tissue concentrations of β-carotene or vitamin A and, in most cases of dietary carotenaemia, transaminases are normal (see later). Nishimura [25] in 1993 compared the serum carotene levels in 82 patients with 'biliary dyskinesia' with 27 control subjects. The patients with abnormal gallbladder contraction rates had a higher incidence of serum carotene levels (>5.6 μmol/L) than the control subjects. The carotenaemic patients were diagnosed as having metabolic or hyperlipidaemic carotenaemia. Nishimura [25] suggested that there was a close relationship between metabolic carotenaemia and biliary dyskinesia. These findings have not yet been confirmed by other investigators. Recently studies have been undertaken on animal models with knockouts of one of the two genes encoding enzymes involved in β-carotene metabolism (*BCMO1*, encoding β,β-carotene15,15′-monooxygenase 1; and *BCDO2*, encoding β,β-carotene-9,10-dioxygenase). These suggest that β-carotene conversion can influence retinoid-dependent processes in the mouse embryo and in adult tissues, and that pathological accumulation of these compounds can induce oxidative stress in mitochondria and cell signalling pathways related to disease [26]. However, evidence of serious adverse effects of carotenaemia in man is still lacking.

It is possible that high skin and tissue concentrations of β-carotene are in fact beneficial. Carotenoids are believed to protect cells against the harmful effects of free radicals. Someya and colleagues [27] have shown that, in the guinea pig, carotene supplementation prevents the skin lipid peroxidation caused by ultraviolet irradiation. Carotene supplementation is used in the treatment of erythropoietic protoporphyria and X-linked protoporphyria to improve tolerance to sunlight by inducing carotenoderma. It has been postulated that the free radical scavenging activity of carotenoids may help to prevent atherosclerosis and cancer. Individuals with blood β-carotene levels towards the upper limit of the normal range have a lower incidence of cancer and heart disease than those with lower β-carotene levels. Conversely, two studies have shown that supplementation with β-carotene does not prevent cancer and heart disease in well-nourished individuals and, indeed, in high-risk groups (smokers and people exposed to asbestos) the morbidity and mortality appear to be increased by supplementation. However, there were no excess cases of death and disease in those who attained the highest blood β-carotene levels during supplementation [28].

Dietary carotenaemia (and some cases of hyperlipidaemia) gives rise to mildly elevated plasma concentrations of vitamin A. The hypervitaminosis A is never sufficient to cause signs of intoxication; liver function tests are normal [29]. Metabolic carotenaemia may produce low plasma vitamin A concentrations. In such individuals it may be possible to show defective dark adaptation on careful visual testing [5]. In RBP deficiency, low levels of vitamin A in plasma cause night blindness but not xerophthalmia [20]. In theory, prolonged systemic vitamin A deficiency might lead to xerophthalmia, hyperkeratosis and increased susceptibility to infection. To date, these problems have never been documented, but that may be because metabolic carotenaemia has not been described in children from developing countries. It is important to remember that such children may already be predisposed to vitamin A deficiency by their poor dietary intake of vitamin A [30].

Clinical features. Carotenaemia produces a yellow-orange pigmentation of the skin that is usually most obvious on the palms, soles and nasolabial folds and is absent from the sclerae (Figs 152.10 and 152.11). The urine and stools have a normal colour.

Excessive ingestion

A careful dietary history should be taken. Carotenaemia has been documented in the first year of life in breastfed infants whose mothers ingest over 1.5 kg of carrots per week or more than 10 tangerines per day [31]. It has also been documented in infants whose parents were strict vegetarians and believed that carrot juice was better for their infant than milk. Such infants may also show evidence of failure to thrive. Carotenaemia may also occur in infants who are difficult to wean onto a balanced range of solids and show a marked preference for pureed carrots and green vegetables. It has been diagnosed in infants who ingested 2–4 tangerines per day for 4 weeks. Older children may select a vegetarian diet with a high content of β-carotene, and the clinician should consider the possibility that this is part of the anorexia nervosa syndrome [32]. Dietary carotenaemia has also been recorded in areas of West Africa where red palm oil (which has high carotene content) is used for cooking. Finally, it should be recalled that β-carotene has been used for treatment of photodermatoses such as porphyria and so a careful drug history must be taken. Laboratory investigations reveal an elevated plasma β-carotene concentration and a slightly elevated plasma vitamin A concentration.

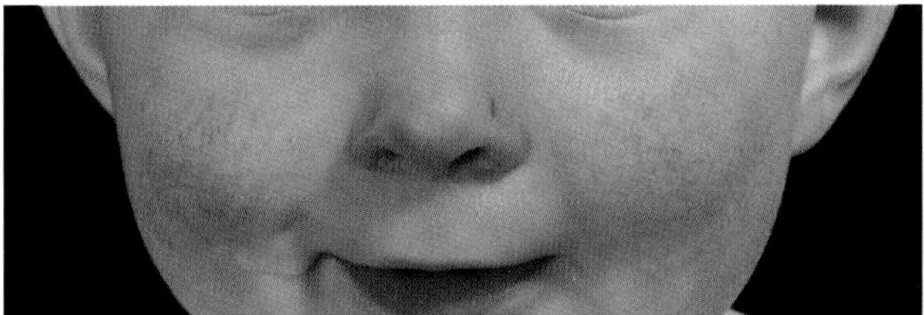

Fig. 152.10 Facies of an infant with metabolic carotenaemia. In this case the pigmentation was most obvious in the skin of the tip of the nose, the cheeks and the pinnae. Note the absence of pigmentation in the sclerae.

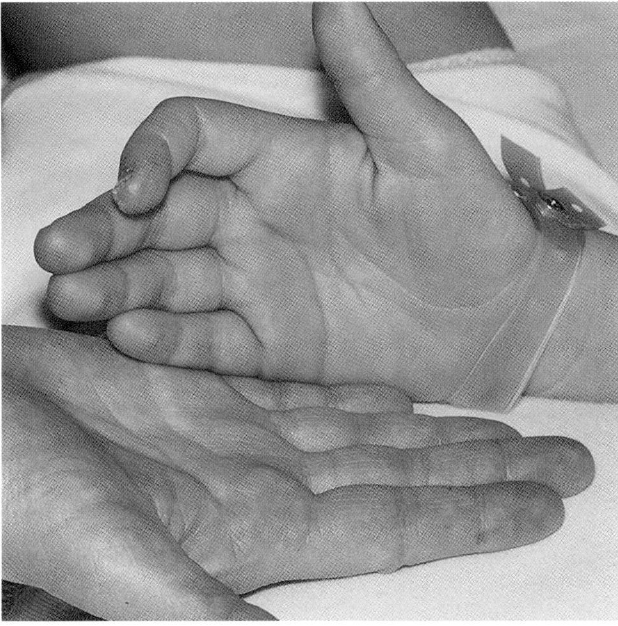

Fig. 152.11 Comparison of the skin colour of the palm of a child with carotenaemia (upper) and a normal palm (lower).

Hyperlipidaemias

A full medical history and examination (including urinalysis) should be undertaken. Weight loss could be the result of diabetes or anorexia nervosa. A history of polyuria and polydipsia points strongly to diabetes, which can be confirmed by testing the urine for sugar. A history of lethargy, developmental delay, constipation and poor linear growth should trigger a search for features of hypothyroidism such as the coarse facies, large tongue, umbilical hernia and bradycardia. A history of periorbital swelling should lead to a general search for oedema and ascites, and the urine should be checked for the heavy proteinuria that is characteristic of nephrotic syndrome. Symptoms of fasting hypoglycaemia (pallor, sweating, jitteriness, loss of consciousness, convulsions) and poor linear growth are suggestive of one of the hepatic glycogenoses and such a diagnosis will usually be obvious from massive hepatomegaly. The hyperlipidaemia of cholestasis and of homozygous familial hypercholesterolaemia may be associated with the presence of cutaneous xanthomas.

Investigations will be directed by the clinical findings but may include β-carotene, vitamin A, cholesterol, triglycerides, blood glucose, glycosylated haemoglobin, thyroid function, liver function, plasma albumin and renal function tests.

Inborn error(s) of carotene metabolism

The pigmentation is identical to that produced by excessive ingestion of carotene. The age at presentation ranges from 6 months to 24 years. The β-carotene intake is normal or low; some older patients have shown an aversion to β-carotene and have adopted a low-carotene diet [15]. Some parents of affected infants and toddlers have described loose stools regularly induced by ingestion of carotene-containing foods. There may be a family history of other affected individuals. The plasma concentration of β-carotene is elevated (5–22 μmol/L) and the plasma concentration of vitamin A may be normal or low. It is now possible to look for mutations in carotenoid 15,15′-mono-oxygenase [12] and RBP [20]. This should clarify whether genetic defects in these proteins are responsible for carotenaemia.

Table 152.6 Differential diagnosis of carotenaemia

Cause	Plasma carotene	Plasma vitamin A	Plasma cholesterol and/or triglycerides
Dietary carotenaemia	↑	↑	N
Metabolic carotenaemia	↑	N/↑	N
Hyperlipidaemia	↑	N/↑	↑

N, normal.

Prognosis. There are no proven adverse effects of dietary carotenaemia. The skin pigmentation can be eliminated by reducing the excessive carotene intake. In the occasional case in which there has been neutropenia or transaminaemia, these have also resolved. In children who have carotenaemia associated with hyperlipidaemia, discussion of the prognosis should focus on the cause of the hyperlipidaemia. Metabolic carotenaemia is a benign condition. Parents can be advised that any symptoms associated with ingestion of β-carotene will resolve when a low-carotene diet is instituted. Any potential effects of vitamin A deficiency can be avoided by a vitamin A supplement.

Differential diagnosis. Yellowish pigmentation of the skin (xanthodermia) is most commonly caused by jaundice. It is occasionally seen when substances such as picric acid, saffron and mepacrine are ingested and stain the skin. In all these conditions, in contrast to carotenaemia, the sclerae are also pigmented. The diagnosis of carotenaemia and its cause can often be elucidated from the history and examination (as indicated above) but differential diagnosis is aided by measurements of plasma concentrations of β-carotene, vitamin A and lipids (Table 152.6).

Treatment. Excessive ingestion of β-carotene should be managed by first reassuring the parents and the referring doctor that the child does not have jaundice or any other significant medical problem. General dietary advice should be given to ensure that the child will in future receive a balanced diet and the parents can also be told how they can eliminate the cutaneous pigmentation by cutting down the child's excessive intake of β-carotene.

Children with hyperlipidaemia should be treated on the basis of the underlying cause. Parents of children with metabolic carotenaemia should be reassured that it is a benign condition but that the pigmentation can be reduced or eliminated by the use of a low-carotene diet. This involves avoidance or restriction of certain vegetables and fruit and avoidance of foods which contain E160 carotenoid additives. The fruit and vegetables in Table 152.5 which have very high carotene content should be avoided altogether. Those with a high content should be restricted to a maximum of one portion per week, but two portions daily of those with a moderate content can be allowed. Children with metabolic carotenaemia should avoid carrot juice, apricot juice, mango juice, tomato juice and any squash or carbonated drinks with added β-carotene. Meat, fish, eggs and poultry can be used freely in the diet but ox liver should be avoided. Chilli, paprika, cayenne pepper and curry powder have high β-carotene content and should be omitted from the diet. Foods with a high content of cow's milk fat should also be avoided, as should butter and margarine (except for products with no added β-carotene). Flour, bread, pasta and breakfast cereals can be taken freely. Cakes and biscuits that are made with butter or margarine should be avoided, but those made with vegetable oil as the fat source can be used in the diet. Yellow-coloured sweets, desserts, preserves and so on should be checked for added β-carotene (e.g. lemon curd has a high content). If children with metabolic carotenaemia have a low plasma vitamin A concentration, this can usually be corrected by an oral vitamin A supplement (2500 units/day).

Acknowledgement

We are grateful to Marjorie Dixon, Chief Dietitian at Great Ormond Street Hospital, for valuable advice on the low-carotene diet.

References

1 Furr HC. Carotenoids. In: Macrae, R, Robinson, RK, Sadler, MJ (eds) Encyclopaedia of Food Science, Food Technology and Nutrition. London: Academic Press, 1993:707–18.
2 Malvy DJ, Burtschy B, Dostalova L et al. Serum retinol, β-carotene, β-tocopherol and cholesterol in healthy French children. Int J Epidemiol 1993;22:237–46.
3 Greene CH, Blackford L. Carotenemia. M Clin N Am 1926;10:733–44.
4 Almond S, Logan RFL. Carotinaemia. BMJ 1942;ii:239–41.
5 Cohen L. Observations on carotenaemia. Ann Intern Med 1958; 48:219–27.
6 Traber MG, Diamond SR, Lane JC et al. β-Carotene transport in human lipoproteins. Comparisons with β-tocopherol. Lipids 1994; 29:665–9.
7 Hůlková H, Svojanovský J, Sevela K et al. Systemic AL amyloidosis with unusual cutaneous presentation unmasked by carotenoderma. Amyloid 2014;21:57–6.
8 Holland B, Welch AA, Unwin ID et al. McCance and Widdowson's The Composition of Foods, 5th edn. London: HMSO, 1991.
9 Prince MR, Frisoli JK. Beta-carotene accumulation in serum and skin. Am J Clin Nutr 1993;57:175–81.
10 Lloyd JK. Plasma lipid disorders. In: Clayton, BE, Round, JM (eds) Chemical Pathology and the Sick Child. Oxford: Blackwell Scientific Publications, 1984.
11 Mordasini R, Klose G, Greten H. Secondary type II hyperlipoproteinemia in patients with anorexia nervosa. Metabolism 1978;27:71–9.
12 Lindqvist A, Sharvill J, Sharvill DE, Anderson S. Loss-of-function mutation in carotenoid 15,15′-monooxygenase identified in a patient with hypercarotenaemia and hypovitaminosis Am J Nutr 2007; 137:2346–50.
13 Sharvill DE. Familial hypercarotinaemia and hypovitaminosis A. Proc Roy Soc Med 1970;63:605–6.
14 McLaren DS, Zekian B. Failure of enzymic cleavage of β-carotene. The cause of vitamin A deficiency in a child. Am J Dis Child 1971; 121:278–80.
15 Monk BE. Metabolic carotenaemia. Br J Dermatol 1982;106:485–7.
16 Svensson A, Vahlquist A. Metabolic carotenemia and carotenoderma in a child. Acta Derm Venereol 1995;75:70–1.
17 Leung WC, Hessel S, Meplan C et al. Two common single nucleotide polymorphisms in the gene encoding beta-carotene 15,15′-monoxygenase alter beta-carotene metabolism in female volunteers. FASEB J 2009;23:1041–53.
18 Lietz G, Oxley A, Leung W, Hesketh J. Single nucleotide polymorphisms upstream from the β-carotene 15,15′-monoxygenase gene influence provitamin A conversion efficiency in female volunteers. J Nutr 2012;142:161S–5S.

19 Attard-Montalto S, Evans N, Sherwood RA. Carotenaemia with low vitamin A levels and low retinol-binding protein. J Inherit Metab Dis 1992;15:929–30.

20 Seeliger MW, Biesalski HK, Wissinger B et al. Phenotype in retinol deficiency due to a hereditary defect in retinol binding protein synthesis. Invest Ophthal Vis Sci 1999;40:3–11.

21 Chou CM, Nelson C, Tarle SA et al. Biochemical basis for dominant inheritance, variable penetrance, and maternal effects in RBP4 congenital eye disease. Cell 2015;161:634–46.

22 Shoenfeld Y, Shaklai M, Ben-Baruch N et al. Neutropenia induced by hypercarotenaemia. Lancet 1982;i:1245.

23 Kaspar P, Polsky A, Kudlova E et al. Carotenemia. Cesk-Pediatr 1991;46:275–7.

24 Gangakhedkar A, Somerville R, Jelleyman T. Carotenemia and hepatomegaly in an atopic child on an exclusion diet for a food allergy. Australas J Dermatol 2017;58:42–4.

25 Nishimura T. A correlation between carotenemia and biliary dyskinesia. J Dermatol 1993;20:287–92.

26 Lobo GP, Amengual J, Palczewski G et al. Mammalian carotenoid-oxygenases: key players for carotenoid function and homeostasis. Biochim Biophys Acta 2012;1821:78–87.

27 Someya K, Totsuka Y, Murakoshi M et al. The antioxidant effect of palm fruit carotene on skin lipid peroxidation in guinea pigs estimated by the chemiluminescence–HPLC method. J Nutr Sci Vitaminol Tokyo 1994;40:315–24.

28 Rowe PM. Beta-carotene takes a collective beating. Lancet 1996; 347:249.

29 Pollitt N. Beta-carotene and the photodermatoses. Br J Dermatol 1975;93:721–4.

30 Favaro RM, de-Souza NV, Batistal SM et al. Vitamin A status of young children in southern Brazil. Am J Clin Nutr 1986;43:852–8.

31 Honda T. Adverse effects of foods in genetic disorders. In: Jelliffe, EFP, Jelliffe, DB (eds) Adverse Effects of Foods. New York: Plenum Press, 1982:389–96.

32 Bilimoria S, Keczkes K, Williamson D et al. Hypercarotenaemia in weight watchers. Clin Exp Dermatol 1979;4:331–5.

CHAPTER 153
Cystic Fibrosis

Roderic J. Phillips
Royal Children's Hospital, Melbourne, Australia

Abstract

Cystic fibrosis is characterized by dysfunction of lungs, pancreas, skin and other organs. In some ethnic groups, it is the most common potentially lethal autosomal recessive disorder. In countries where neonatal screening for cystic fibrosis is routine, clinical problems can be anticipated and largely avoided. In other countries, one initial presentation of the disease may be in infancy with failure to thrive, oedema and well-demarcated, erythematous, scaly plaques covering most of the body. This presentation is related to kwashiorkor secondary to malabsorption and responds to pancreatic enzyme replacement. In older children, aquagenic wrinkling of palms can be seen in some children with cystic fibrosis and also in normal children. With current management protocols for cystic fibrosis, the life expectancy is now expected to be greater than 50 years.

Key points

- Clinical outcomes and life expectancy in children with cystic fibrosis are greatly improved if neonatal screening is available and if management is in a centre with specific expertise in this condition.
- Infants presenting with a difficult-to-diagnose rash with failure to thrive or oedema should have fecal testing for fat. If this is positive, a therapeutic trial of pancreatic enzymes should be given.
- Oral isotretinoin is safe and effective in adolescents with cystic fibrosis and acne.

Definition. Cystic fibrosis is an autosomal recessive disease characterized by abnormalities of chloride and sodium ion transport at epithelial surfaces in the lungs, pancreas, liver, gastrointestinal tract, skin and vas deferens. The principal clinical features are chronic suppurative lung disease, pancreatic exocrine deficiency and excessive salt loss from the skin.

Aetiology and pathogenesis. One of the striking medical achievements of the 1980s was a major international collaboration that led to the isolation and cloning of the 'cystic fibrosis gene' in 1989 [1]. This gene is located on the long arm of chromosome 7. One mutation, Phe508del, accounts for about 70% of cystic fibrosis gene mutations worldwide. Two thousand other mutations have been identified [2]. In populations of white Caucasians, cystic fibrosis is the most common serious inherited disease, with a gene frequency of 1 in 25 (i.e. 1 in 2500 births). It is significantly less common in other populations [2].

The cystic fibrosis gene codes for a protein, cystic fibrosis transmembrane conductance regulator (CFTR), that has several functions including regulation of chloride ion transport across epithelial cell membranes [3]. In sweat glands, chloride is normally reabsorbed as the sweat passes along the duct to the skin surface. In cystic fibrosis, this absorption is impaired, leading to increased salt loss in sweat.

In other organs, impaired transport of chloride into the ducts can lead to abnormally viscous secretions, duct obstruction and progressive organ dysfunction.

Clinical features. In countries where there is no neonatal screening programme, most children with cystic fibrosis present in the first 2 years of life with features of pancreatic insufficiency (e.g. greasy stools, poor weight gain and malnutrition). The 10–15% of children who retain adequate pancreatic function usually present during childhood with pulmonary or other symptoms. Clinical symptoms vary greatly from one child to another. Children with the same mutations exhibit considerable clinical variation, especially in lung problems, suggesting an influence of environmental and secondary genetic factors [3].

Gastrointestinal tract

Pancreatic exocrine insufficiency resulting in maldigestion and subsequent malabsorption of fat, protein and carbohydrate is a major manifestation of cystic fibrosis. Steatorrhoea and failure to thrive are usually apparent in the first few months of life. Malabsorption may be sufficiently severe in infancy to cause secondary anaemia and oedema [4]. Neonatal bowel obstruction (meconium ileus) secondary to thick meconium occurs in about 20% of cases. Partial or complete obstruction in older children can be caused by either intussusception or accumulation of faecal material in the lower bowel. Rectal prolapse can

Harper's Textbook of Pediatric Dermatology, Fourth Edition. Edited by Peter Hoeger, Veronica Kinsler and Albert Yan.

occur, and cystic fibrosis is the most common cause of this condition in childhood. Liver involvement with mucus plugs in bile ducts leading to focal biliary cirrhosis, widespread cirrhosis, portal vein obstruction and oesophageal varices occurs in about 10% of cases. Salivary glands can show inspissation of secretions in ducts but progressive fibrosis does not occur.

Respiratory

Deterioration in lung function in cystic fibrosis begins after birth and is progressive during infancy and childhood [5]. Symptoms begin with episodes of cough and wheeze due to occlusion of bronchioles by mucus. With time, the cough becomes increasingly persistent and purulent as bacterial infection becomes established. *Staphylococcus aureus* and *Haemophilus influenzae* are common early pathogens and *Pseudomonas aeruginosa* is increasingly common in later childhood. In later disease, bronchiectasis, gross hyperinflation and chronic hypoxaemia can lead to pulmonary hypertension, right heart failure and death. Nasal polyps in a child should always raise the suspicion of cystic fibrosis as they are common in this condition. Pansinusitis is commonly seen in older children.

Endocrine

Insulin-producing cells in the islets of Langerhans can be affected, leading to cystic fibrosis-related diabetes in 5–10% of adolescents with cystic fibrosis, and in a third or more of older adults [3]. Osteopenia in childhood and osteoporosis in adults are a complication of cystic fibrosis [3]. Virtually all males with cystic fibrosis have nonpatent vas deferens and are infertile.

Joints

With the considerably increased life expectancy as a result of treatment advances, more children with cystic fibrosis are developing joint complications. These occur in about 5% of children over 10 years old, usually as an episodic, nonerosive arthritis involving the large joints of the limbs [6]. Fleeting joint aches are also common.

Skin

An increased saltiness on the skin can be noted from shortly after birth. In hot weather, the increased salt loss can lead to collapse, with hyponatraemia, hypochloraemia and alkalosis. Some cystic fibrosis gene mutations can lead to abnormally high sweat salt concentrations without involvement of other organs [7]. Conversely, in rare cases, sweat salt levels are normal despite typical findings of cystic fibrosis in other organs [3]. Although high sweat salt levels in type 1 pseudohypoaldosteronism appear to be associated with damage and obstruction to the eccrine ducts [8], this has not been reported in cystic fibrosis, in which the skin is generally normal.

Cystic fibrosis presenting as rash

Case reports have described about 25 infants who presented with generalized erythematous rashes and who were subsequently found to have cystic fibrosis [9–24]. In this small subgroup of infants, the rash typically began as erythematous papules in the napkin area and was unresponsive to topical treatments. Over a period of weeks, this rash may become generalized and confluent, with well-demarcated, erythematous, scaly plaques covering most of the body (Figs 153.1 and 153.2). Papules and desquamation occur on palms and soles. Polycyclic psoriasiform plaques have been reported [22]. Associated findings at presentation typically include normal mucosal surfaces, sparse hair, oedema, lethargy, anaemia, severe hypoproteinaemia, raised liver enzymes and low levels of trace metals. This constellation of findings has been attributed to kwashiorkor secondary to unrecognized malabsorption [10]. The rash may be caused by free radical damage to mitochondrial and lipid membranes in the skin, in part due to multiple nutritional deficiencies, including zinc and essential fatty acids. Zinc replacement therapy without supplementation of enzymes or other minerals can lead to an improvement in the rash, suggesting that zinc deficiency is a factor in the induction of the rash [9,10,14]. This uncommon presentation of cystic fibrosis is not clearly related to a specific genotype. In 12 of the infants described, DNA analysis was used to confirm the diagnosis. Ten were homozygous for the phe508del mutation, one heterozygous for this mutation, and one had other mutations [9,10,21,23,24]. Thus the frequency of the phe508del mutation in infants with this presentation is consistent with its frequency in cystic fibrosis generally.

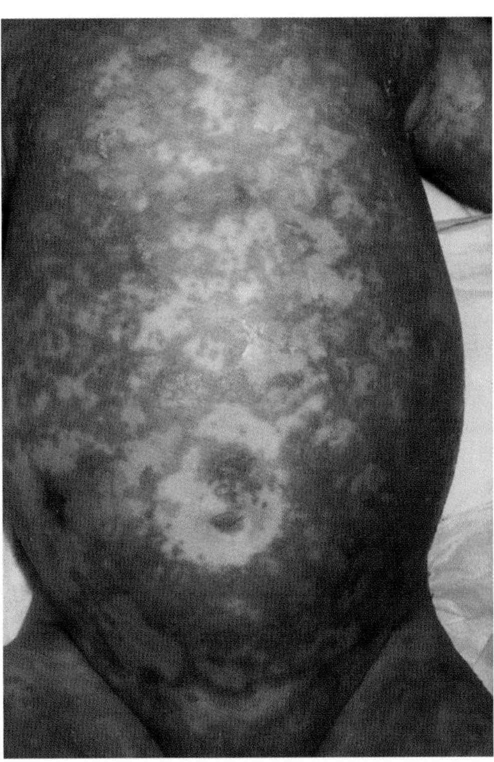

Fig. 153.1 Confluent, desquamating, erythematous rash on the abdomen of a 3-month-old boy subsequently diagnosed with cystic fibrosis. Source: Reproduced from Phillips et al. 1993 [10] with permission from the BMJ.

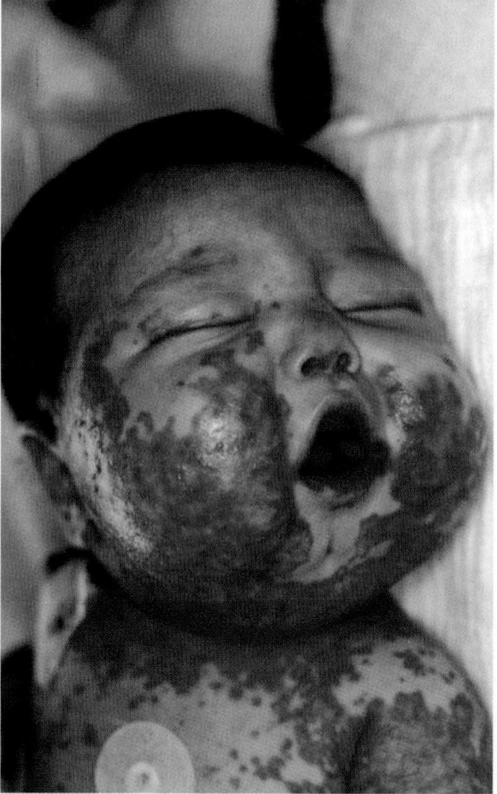

(a)

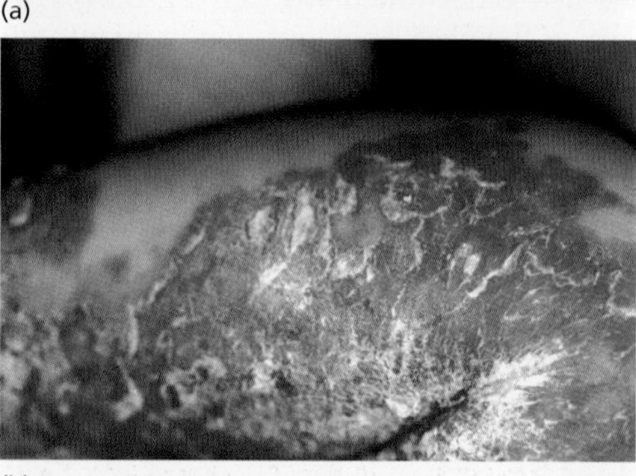

(b)

Fig. 153.2 A 4-month-old girl subsequently diagnosed with cystic fibrosis. (a) Desquamating erythematous patches on the face and chest with sparing of the mucous membranes. (b) Erythematous scaling eruption on the calf. Source: Courtesy of Dr J. Crone.

Cystic fibrosis and skin wrinkling in water

During the 1970s, many paediatricians reported that the skin of the hands and feet of children with cystic fibrosis would wrinkle much more rapidly than skin from control children when immersed in water, and suggested this as a useful diagnostic test for cystic fibrosis [25, 26]. In subsequent decades, this association was overlooked and many case reports appeared in the dermatological literature of children and adults who developed swelling and increased whitish wrinkling of the palms, often with a burning or itchy sensation, when exposed to water. Some were noted to have cystic fibrosis and/or hyperhidrosis [27]. This condition was given a variety of names, transient aquagenic palmar hyperwrinkling probably being the most accurate. A report described a 10-year-old boy with transient aquagenic palmar hyperwrinkling and a history of nasal polyps and diabetes who was found to have cystic fibrosis based on increased sweat chloride levels [25]. Transient aquagenic palmar hyperwrinkling has also been reported in children and adults who are heterozygous for a cystic fibrosis mutation.

Cystic fibrosis and skin wrinkling in alcohol gel

Rapid excessive skin wrinkling, possibly aquagenic in cause, has also been reported after exposure to various alcohol-based hand sanitizing gels [28].

Other skin manifestations

Infants newly diagnosed with cystic fibrosis typically develop a significant and sometimes erosive perianal dermatitis upon commencement of treatment with pancreatic enzymes. Enzymes being passed in stool are thought to contribute to this and it is self-limiting, just requiring barrier ointments. In older children on treatment for cystic fibrosis, the most common skin problems are erythematous or purpuric reactions secondary to the multiple antibiotics and other medications used in treatment regimes [29–31]. Palpable purpuric rashes indicative of vasculitis may be associated with vasculitis in other organs, including joints, kidney and brain [6]. Photosensitivity reactions from quinolone and tetracycline antibiotics are more common in children with cystic fibrosis and may be under-recognized. Up to 50% of adults with cystic fibrosis may develop photosensitivity with ciprofloxacin, and photosensitivity from this antibiotic induced by indoor fluorescent lighting has been reported in a 12-year-old girl [31].

About 40% of older children with treated cystic fibrosis who develop arthritis also have an associated rash. This is usually erythematous and maculopapular, but purpura, vasculitic nodules and erythema nodosum have also been observed [4,6,32]. Cutaneous reactivity to *Aspergillosis* species is common, particularly in children with more severe lung disease. The prevalence of cutaneous reactivity to other allergens used to test for atopy is the same as in the normal population [33–35]. The frequency and severity of acne in a group of 102 adolescents with cystic fibrosis at our institution were not higher than in the general population. In another study, a group of 100 children and adults with cystic fibrosis was shown to have a prevalence (not defined in the report) of acute urticaria of 9% and chronic urticaria of 7% [36].

Isolated associations between cystic fibrosis and Rothmund–Thomson syndrome [37], solar urticaria [38] and albinism [39] have been described and may be coincidental. Two children with cystic fibrosis and Kawasaki disease have been reported [40,41], but in both cases the diagnosis of Kawasaki disease is uncertain. Three teenage boys and a girl developed purpura on the lower limbs in conjunction with hypergammaglobulinaemia: all four died within 2 years of onset of purpura [42,43]. Mascaro and colleagues [44] described three siblings of consanguineous parents who had generalized follicular hamartoma and cystic fibrosis and suggested that there may be a genetic linkage between the two conditions.

Prognosis. Untreated, cystic fibrosis usually leads to death during infancy or childhood from malabsorption and/or pulmonary disease. With continued treatment, the quality and length of life are greatly improved. Most children live active childhoods and, in leading centres, life expectancy of patients born now is expected to be greater than 50 years [3]. Infants presenting with failure to thrive and a rash from malnutrition have been described as having a poor prognosis, leading to undertreatment [45]. This is not justified. These infants respond rapidly to adequate enzyme and other replacement therapy [46].

Diagnosis. The differential diagnosis depends on the clinical presentation and includes other causes of pulmonary disease, malabsorption or failure to thrive. In infants presenting with a widespread rash and failure to thrive, the differential diagnosis includes multiple causes of zinc, biotin, essential fatty acid, protein and amino acid deficiencies (e.g. inborn errors of metabolism, dietary deficiencies or increased losses from the gastrointestinal or urinary tracts) and immunodeficiency.

Many countries now routinely screen for cystic fibrosis by looking for elevated trypsinogen levels in neonatal heelprick blood. In these countries, diagnosis precedes the development of significant clinical problems and provides better short-term [47] and long-term [3] outcomes and is cost-effective [3,5,47]. In countries where neonatal screening is not routine, laboratory diagnosis after the onset of symptoms is either by DNA analysis or by pilocarpine iontophoresis (sweat test) carried out in an experienced centre. In conjunction with appropriate clinical findings, a sweat test is highly sensitive and specific. However, infants with cystic fibrosis who present with a desquamating rash and/or oedema commonly give false-negative sweat test results [4,12] and need to be retested after treatment of their malabsorption.

Transient aquagenic palmar hyperwrinkling detected in a child or adult without any other clinical features of cystic fibrosis has not been linked to the later development of cystic fibrosis-related symptoms. These individuals do not therefore require testing for cystic fibrosis. Testing them and their partner for cystic fibrosis carrier state can be considered if they are planning to have children.

Prevention. Families with a previous child with cystic fibrosis can be offered prenatal DNA or enzyme analysis for subsequent pregnancies. In populations with significant cystic fibrosis gene frequencies, families can elect to have gene testing before having children.

Treatment. Treatment requires effective management of maldigestion, pulmonary and other problems by a multidisciplinary team. Maldigestion is controlled by pancreatic enzyme replacement, a high-fat and high-protein diet and supplementation of fat-soluble vitamins. Pulmonary disease is treated with chest physiotherapy and antibiotics. Exacerbations of chest disease may require intravenous antibiotics for 10–14 days. The development of orally bioavailable small molecule drugs that target defective CFTR proteins is exciting. To date, each of these therapies is effective only for specific mutations [48]. Lung transplantation can be used for end-stage pulmonary disease in older children and adults. Gene replacement therapy remains a research project. With survival into adulthood now the rule, issues such as reproductive health, male infertility, delayed puberty, pregnancy and marriage all need to be addressed during childhood.

The severe erythematous desquamating rash occasionally seen in infants at diagnosis responds well to zinc [9,14] and is cured by correction of the underlying malabsorption [9–20]. However, specific treatment should not be delayed while waiting for a diagnosis. Pancreatic enzymes are safe. In countries where cystic fibrosis is prevalent but where there is no neonatal screening for this condition, all infants presenting with a difficult-to-diagnose rash with failure to thrive or oedema should have faecal testing for fat. If this is positive, a therapeutic trial of pancreatic enzymes should be given [46].

Generalized erythematous or urticarial drug reactions usually settle after ceasing or changing the causative medication, usually an antibiotic. Rechallenge to confirm the causal agent may be warranted. One child with a rash due to tobramycin was successfully desensitized using escalating doses, enabling the drug to be continued without further problems [49]. Antibiotics associated with photosensitivity reactions may need to be changed. However, if the reaction is mild, the use of sunscreen and minimizing light exposure may allow the antibiotic to be used again.

The presence of a palpable purpuric rash requires a search for the cause of vasculitis. This may be limited to the skin or may be disseminated and potentially fatal [6]. Possible causes include hypersensitivity reactions and connective tissue syndromes. Investigations may include skin histology, full blood count, erythrocyte sedimentation rate, antinuclear antibodies, antineutrophil cytoplasmic antibodies, assessment of renal function and brain magnetic resonance imaging [6]. Any medication suspected of causing a hypersensitivity reaction should be stopped. Systemic anti-inflammatory therapy may be required.

Acne in adolescents with cystic fibrosis may respond to conventional topical therapies. Most of these adolescents are already taking continuous antibiotics, and early introduction of oral isotretinoin is reasonable if significant acne develops. A case series of nine adolescents with cystic fibrosis and significant acne demonstrated that oral isotretinoin was effective with minimal side-effects [50]. Serum vitamin A levels are often low in cystic fibrosis, even with oral enzyme and vitamin supplementation [51] and may lead to ocular problems including impaired dark adaptation [52,53]. This is also a recognized side-effect of isotretinoin treatment. Home-based retinal function tests and vitamin A levels can be monitored during treatment with oral isotretinoin in cystic fibrosis [50]. A single case report raised the intriguing possibility that oral isotretinoin may improve pulmonary symptoms in cystic fibrosis [54].

References

1 Riordan JR, Rommens JM, Kerem B et al. Identification of the cystic fibrosis gene: cloning and characterization of complementary DNA. Science 1989;245:1066–73.

2 Cystic fibrosis mutations database at http://www.genet.sickkids.on.ca/.

3 O'Sullivan BP, Freedman SD. Cystic fibrosis. Lancet 2009;373: 1891–904.

4 Nielsen OH, Larsen BF. The incidence of anaemia, hypoalbuminaemia and oedema in infants as presenting symptoms of cystic fibrosis: a retrospective survey of the frequency of this symptom complex in 130 patients with cystic fibrosis. J Paediatr Gastroenterol Nutr 1982;1:355–9.

5 VanDevanter DR, Kahle JS, O'Sullivan AK et al. Cystic fibrosis in young children: a review of disease manifestation, progression, and response to early treatment. J Cyst Fibros 2016;15:147–57.

6 Turner MA, Baildam E, Patel L et al. Joint disorders in cystic fibrosis. J Roy Soc Med 1997;90(suppl 31):13–20.

7 Mickle JE, Macek M, Fulmer-Smentek SB et al. A mutation in the cystic fibrosis transmembrane conductance regulator gene associated with elevated sweat chloride concentrations in the absence of cystic fibrosis. Hum Mol Genet 1998;7:729–35.

8 Urbatsch A, Paller AS. Pustular miliaria rubra: a specific cutaneous finding of type 1 pseudohypoaldosteronism. Pediatr Dermatol 2002; 19:317–19.

9 Crone J, Huber W-D, Eichler I et al. Acrodermatitis enteropathica-like eruption as the presenting sign of cystic fibrosis – case report and review of the literature. Eur J Pediatr 2002;161:475–8.

10 Phillips RJ, Crock CM, Dillon MJ et al. Cystic fibrosis presenting as kwashiorkor with florid skin rash. Arch Dis Child 1993;69:446–8.

11 Dodge JA, Salter DG, Yassa JG. Essential fatty acid deficiency due to artificial diet in cystic fibrosis. BMJ 1975;2(5964):192–3.

12 Darmstadt GL, McGuire J, Ziboh VA. Malnutrition-associated rash of cystic fibrosis. Pediatr Dermatol 2000;17:337–47.

13 Hansen RC, Lemen R, Revsin B. Cystic fibrosis manifesting with acrodermatitis enteropathica-like eruption. Arch Dermatol 1983;119:51–5.

14 Mazzocchi C, Michel JL, Chalencon V et al. Zinc deficiency in mucoviscidosis. Arch Pediatrie 2000;7:1081–4.

15 Patrizi A, Bianchi F, Neri I, Specchia F. Acrodermatitis enteropathica like eruption: a sign of malabsorption in cystic fibrosis. Pediatr Dermatol 2003;20:187–8.

16 Muniz AE, Bartle S, Foster R. Edema, anemia, hypoproteinemia, and acrodermatitis enteropathica: an uncommon initial presentation of cystic fibrosis. Pediatr Emerg Care 2004;20:112–14.

17 Martin DP, Tangsinmankong N, Sleasman JW et al. Acrodermatitis enteropathica-like eruption and food allergy. Ann Allergy Asthma Immunol 2005;94:398–401.

18 Hussain W, Craven N, Swann I. An unwell child with a florid rash. Arch Dis Child 2005;90:1287.

19 O'Regan GM, Canny G, Irvine AD. 'Peeling paint' dermatitis as a presenting sign of cystic fibrosis. J Cystic Fibrosis 2006;5:257–9.

20 Lovett A, Kokta V, Maari C. Diffuse dermatitis: an unexpected initial presentation of cystic fibrosis. J Am Acad Dermatol 2008;58:S1–4.

21 Zedek D, Morrell DS, Graham M et al. Acrodermatitis enteropathica-like eruption and failure to thrive as presenting signs of cystic fibrosis. J Am Acad Dermatol 2008;58:S5–8.

22 Koch LH, Lewis DW, Williams JV. Necrolytic migratory erythema like presentation for cystic fibrosis. J Am Acad Dermatol 2008;58:S29–30.

23 Pekcan S, Kose M, Dogru D et al. A 4-month-old boy with acrodermatitis enteropathica-like symptoms. Eur J Pediatr 2009;168:119–21.

24 Wenk KS, Higgins KB, Greer KE. Cystic fibrosis presenting with dermatitis. Arch Dermatol 2010;146:171–4.

25 Seitz CS, Gaigl Z, Brocker EB, Trautmann A. Painful wrinkles in the bathtub: association with hyperhidrosis and cystic fibrosis. Dermatology 2008;21:222–6.

26 Berk DR, Ciliberto HM, Sweet SC et al. Aquagenic wrinkling of the palms in cystic fibrosis: comparison with controls and genotype-phenotype correlations. Arch Dermatol 2009;145:1296–9.

27 Phillips R. Aquagenic palmoplantar keratoderma: a new sign of cystic fibrosis? Br J Dermatol 2011;164:224–5.

28 Bhojani S, Sriskandan S, Bush A. Aquagenic wrinkling of palms on exposure to alcohol gel. Pediatr Pulmonol 2001;46:98–9.

29 Spigarelli MG, Hurwitz ME, Nasr SZ. Hypersensitivity to inhaled TOBI following reaction to gentamicin. Pediatr Pulmonol 2002;33:311–14.

30 Finnegan MJ, Hinchcliffe J, Russell-Jones D et al. Vasculitis complicating cystic fibrosis. Q J Med New Series 72 1989;267:609–21.

31 Jaffe A, Bush A. If you can't stand the rash, get out of the kitchen: an unusual adverse reaction to ciprofloxacin. Pediatr Pulmonol 1999; 28:449–50.

32 Vaze D. Episodic arthritis in cystic fibrosis. J Pediatr 1980;96:346.

33 Warner JO, Taylor BW, Norman AP et al. Association of cystic fibrosis with allergy. Arch Dis Child 1976;51:507–11.

34 Laufer P, Fink JN, Bruns WT et al. Allergic bronchopulmonary aspergillosis in cystic fibrosis. J Allergy Clin Immunol 1984;73:44–8.

35 Greally P, Cook AJ, Sampson AP et al. Atopic children with cystic fibrosis have increased urinary leukotriene E4 concentrations and more severe pulmonary disease. J Allergy Clin Immunol 1994;93:100–7.

36 Laufer P. Urticaria in cystic fibrosis. Cutis 1985;36:245–6.

37 Lewis MB. Rothmund–Thompson syndrome and fibrocystic disease. Aust J Dermatol 1972;13:105.

38 Laufer P, Laufer R. Solar urticaria in cystic fibrosis. Cutis 1983; 31:665–6.

39 Pruszewicz A, Sokolowski Z, Goncarzewicz A. Mucoviscidosis coexisting with generalised albinism. Otolaryngol Polska 1978;32:93–5.

40 Rivilla F, Lopez J. Meconium ileus equivalent and Kawasaki syndrome. Eur J Surg 1991;157:151–2.

41 Ciofu C, Laky D, Geormaneanu M. Kawasaki disease in an infant with cystic fibrosis. Rom J Morph Embryol 1992;38:63–6.

42 Nielsen HE, Lundh S, Jacobsen SV et al. Hypergammaglobulinemic purpura in cystic fibrosis. Acta Paediatr Scand 1978;67:443–7.

43 Soter NA, Mihm MC, Colten HR. Cutaneous necrotizing venulitis in patients with cystic fibrosis. J Pediatr 1979;95:197–201.

44 Mascaro JM, Ferrando J, Bombi JA et al. Congenital generalised follicular hamartoma associated with alopecia and cystic fibrosis in three siblings. Arch Dermatol 1995;131:454–8.

45 Zedek D, Morrell DS, Graham M et al. Acrodermatitis enteropathica-like eruption and failure to thrive as presenting signs of cystic fibrosis. J Am Acad Dermatol 2008;58:S5–8.

46 Phillips RJ. Malabsorption-related rash in cystic fibrosis does not portend a poor prognosis. J Am Acad Dermatol 2008;59:720.

47 Massie J. Re: Acrodermatitis enteropathica-like eruption and failure to thrive as presenting signs of cystic fibrosis. J Am Acad Dermatol 2008;59:720–1.

48 Quon BS, Rowe SM. New and emerging targeted therapies for cystic fibrosis. BMJ 2016;352:i859.

49 Spigarelli MG, Hurwitz ME, Nasr SZ. Hypersensitivity to inhaled TOBI following reaction to gentamicin. Pediatr Pulmonol 2002; 33:311–14.

50 Perera E, Massie J, Phillips RJ. Treatment of acne with oral isotretinoin in patients with cystic fibrosis. Arch Dis Child 2009;94:583–6.

51 Feranchak AP, Sontag MK, Wagener JS et al. Prospective, long-term study of fat-soluble vitamin status in children with cystic fibrosis identified by newborn screen. J Pediatr 1999;135:601–10.

52 Neugebauer MA, Vernon SA, Brimlow G et al. Nyctalopia and conjunctival xerosis indicating vitamin A deficiency in cystic fibrosis. Eye 1989;3:360–4.

53 Welsh BM, Smith AL, Elder JE et al. Night blindness precipitated by isotretinoin in the setting of hypovitaminosis A. Aust J Dermatol 1999;40:208–10.

54 Buckley JL, Chastain M, Rietschel R. Improvement of cystic fibrosis during treatment with isotretinoin. SKINmed 2006;5:252–5.

CHAPTER 154
Cutaneous Manifestations of Endocrine Disease

Devika Icecreamwala & Tor A. Shwayder
Department of Dermatology, Henry Ford Health System, Detroit, MI, USA

Alteration in thyroid hormone levels, 1993
Alterations in cortisol levels, 1996
Disorders of sex hormones, 1998
Dysfunction of parathyroid hormone, 2002
Pituitary dysfunction, 2004
Insulin-related disorders, 2005
Dermatological diseases with endocrine dysfunction, 2008

Abstract

Paediatric endocrine disease may result in changes of the skin, hair, nails and mucosa. Cutaneous signs of congenital and acquired hypothyroidism include xerosis, thickening and doughy appearance of the skin, and brittleness of the hair. Hyperthyroidism with goiter often have skin changes which include facial flushing, hyperhidrosis and warm, moist skin. Increased serum cortisol can cause facial plethora, broad and purple striae, acne, acanthosis nigricans and skin thinning. Hyperpigmentation is seen with adrenal insufficiency. Androgen excess can present with weight gain, pubic and facial hair growth, acne, body odour and muscular habitus. Gynaecomastia is associated with hyperoestrogenism. Wrinkling of skin especially around the eyes and mouth can be seen in hypopituitarism, whereas gigantism/acromegaly is associated with hyperpituitarism. Hypoparathyroidism can result in dry skin, alopecia and brittle nails. Primary hyperparathyroidism can cause dehydration with skin tenting, prolonged capillary refill time and dry mucous membranes.

Key points

- **Pediatric endocrine disease may result in changes of the skin, hair, nails and mucosa.**
- **Cutaneous signs of congenital and acquired hypothyroidism include xerosis, thickening and doughy appearance of the skin, and brittleness of the hair. Hyperthyroidism with goiter often have skin changes which include facial flushing, hyperhidrosis and warm, moist skin. Increased serum cortisol can cause facial plethora, broad and purple striae, acne, acanthosis nigricans and skin thinning. Hyperpigmentation is seen with adrenal insufficiency.**
- **Androgen excess can present with weight gain, pubic and facial hair growth, acne, body odour and muscular habitus.**
- **Gynaecomastia is associated with hyperoestrogenism.**
- **Wrinkling of skin especially around the eyes and mouth can be seen in hypopituitarism, whereas gigantism/acromegaly is associated with hyperpituitarism. Hypoparathyroidism can result in dry skin, alopecia and brittle nails.**
- **Primary hyperparathyroidism can cause dehydration with skin tenting, prolonged capillary refill time and dry mucous membranes.**

Alteration in thyroid hormone levels

Hypothyroidism

Pathogenesis. Congenital hypothyroidism most commonly results from agenesis, dysplasia or ectopy of the thyroid gland. It can also be caused by defects in thyroid receptors or enzymatic steps in thyroid hormone synthesis [1]. Unusual causes include endemic iodine deficiency [2], hypothalamopituitary dysfunction and infiltration of the thyroid gland such as with Langerhan's cell histiocytosis [3] and cystinosis [4]. Patients with multiple hepatic haemangiomas are predisposed to developing primary hypothyroidism caused by high levels of type 3-iodothyronine deiodinase activity [5].

Transient congenital hypothyroidism can occur from a variety of causes including transplacental transfer of antithyroid antibodies or thyroid hormone from mothers with thyroid dysfunction, certain medications such as antithyroid drugs, amiodorone or D-penicillamine ingested during pregnancy and cutaneous application of povidone iodine to open wounds in the neonatal period [6].

In older children, acquired hypothyroidism is most commonly caused by autoimmune destruction such as Hashimoto's thyroiditis [1]. Children with autoimmune diseases such as vitiligo and alopecia areata are at increased risk [7]

Clinical features. Various cutaneous manifestations are associated with congenital and acquired hypothyroidism. Thyroid hormone directly influences proteoglycan synthesis in the skin by stimulating fibroblasts. It is essential in hair formation, sebum production and in the conversion of beta-carotene to vitamin A [8].

The skin of hypothyroid infants is usually cool, dry and xerotic. Cutis marmorata, pallor and yellowing of the skin can be present. Eventually the skin will appear thickened and have a doughy, boggy feeling [8,9].

Harper's Textbook of Pediatric Dermatology, Fourth Edition. Edited by Peter Hoeger, Veronica Kinsler and Albert Yan.

The skin is cool and pale caused by the combined effects of anaemia, poor peripheral perfusion, and increased deposition of water and mucopolysaccharides in the dermis. Xerosis results from a combination of peripheral vasoconstriction, decreased epidermal sterol biosynthesis, diminished sebaceous gland secretion and hypohidrosis. Hypothermia in these infants can cause pronounced cutis marmorata. A yellowing of the skin is noticed because of carotene accumulation in the stratum corneum and prolonged neonatal jaundice. These patients have accumulation of glycosaminoglycan in the dermis that can result in thickened myxoedematous skin that is nonpitting. The thickening is usually most prominent around the eyes, lips and acral surfaces resulting in periorbital puffiness, thick lips and acral swelling. Accumulation of glycosaminoglycans in the tongue will result in macroglossia [8,9].

The infant's hair is often dry, lusterless and slow growing. Patchy alopecia and persistent lanugo hairs can be present. However, there have been reports of hypertrichosis in autoimmune thyroiditis. The nails tend to be brittle and slow growing. Other characteristic facies include a depressed nasal bridge, mild hypertelorism and delayed eruption of teeth [9].

Similar to congenital hypothyroidism, patients with acquired hypothyroidism can have cold, xerotic and pale skin. A yellowing of the palms, soles and nasolabial folds and development of 'pseudojaundice' with sparing of the conjunctivae can be noted. Periorbital oedema, broadened nose, swollen lips, macroglossia and a flat facial expression are characteristic. Ptosis may be appreciated caused by decreased sympathetic stimulation of the superior palpebral muscle. Scalp and body hair is commonly coarse and brittle and can result in diffuse or partial alopecia. Loss of the lateral third of the eyebrows is a distinct finding. A goitre may be visualized and/or palpated in the midpharyngeal area [10]. Delayed dentition, precocious puberty and galactorrhoea are associated [11].

Laboratory and histology findings. Serum thyrotropin (TSH), free thyroxine (T4), and total T4 should be ordered if suspecting hypothyroidism. Serum free and total T4 will be decreased in most cases of hypothyroidism. TSH level will be high in patients with primary hypothyroidism and low in patients with hypothyroidism secondary to hypothalamopituitary dysfunction. Measurement of triiodothyronine (T3) is not required [12].

Antithyroid antibodies may be found in neonates with transient hypothyroidism secondary to the transplacental transfer of maternal antibodies and in infants or children with autoimmune thyroiditis [13]. Ultrasound and radioisotope scanning may be useful in determining the cause of hypothyroidism and also in demonstrating absent or ectopic thyroid tissue [14].

Histological features of the skin in hypothyroidism include infiltration of the dermis with glycosaminoglycans. The infiltrate is prominent around appendageal structures. Mucin stains may be helpful to identify the infiltration [15].

Treatment and prevention. Treatment of congenital and acquired hypothyroidism is with levothyroxine (LaFranchi). The dose varies with age, weight and the cause of hypothyroidism. In congenital hypothyroidism, early diagnosis and thyroid hormone replacement is essential as delaying diagnosis and treatment can result in increased cognitive delay. Newborn screening programmes for congenital hypothyroidism have enabled early introduction of thyroxine replacement therapy. Optimal care includes diagnosis before the age of 10–13 days and normalization of serum thyroid hormone levels by 3 weeks of age [11,16,17]. Cutaneous signs often resolve once thyroid hormone levels normalize.

Hyperthyroidism

Pathogenesis. Hyperthyroidism is uncommon in paediatric patients. The most common cause is Graves disease. Rarely, hyperthyroidism can be caused by an overactive thyroid nodule, McCune–Albright syndrome, subacute thyroiditis, abnormal pituitary function, mutations in thyrotropin receptor, Hashimoto's thyroiditis in its earliest stage and increased iodine exposure [18]. Hyperthyroidism in neonates accounts for less than 1% of all cases of hyperthyroidism in paediatric patients. Neonatal hyperthyroidism is almost always secondary to transplacental passage of thyroid-stimulating immunoglobulin from mothers with Graves disease [19].

Clinical features. Ninety-nine percent of patients with Graves disease have a goitre present. Cutaneous findings include facial flushing, hyperhidrosis and warm, moist skin. Rare skin findings include thinning of the scalp hair, vitiligo, distal onycholysis of the fourth and fifth nail and hyperpigmentation [20–23]. Warm skin and flushing results from increased cutaneous blood flow and peripheral vasodilation. Skin moistness is attributed to a combination of peripheral cutaneous vasodilation and increased sebaceous gland secretion [8]. Hyperpigmentation is most often localized to the palmar creases, soles, gingiva and buccal mucosa. The hyperpigmentation is thought to be secondary to increased release of pituitary adrenocorticotropic hormones [24].

Graves dermopathy (pretibial myxoedema), severe ophthalmopathy and thyroid acropathy are extremely uncommon in children, developing in less than 2% of cases. Graves dermopathy develops from the deposition of hyaluronic acid in the dermis and presents as nonpitting plaques and nodules in the pretibial areas (Fig. 154.1). Although most of the cutaneous findings in hyperthyroidism are secondary to a hypermetabolic state, the development of Graves dermopathy does not correlate with thyroxine levels. Patients with Graves disease have a circulating factor that stimulates glycosaminoglycan production by fibroblasts in the pretibial and periorbital areas. Severe ophthalmopathy presents as exophthalmos and diminished eye movement caused by mucinous infiltration within the extraocular muscles and retroorbital tissue. Thyroid acropathy consists of clubbing and

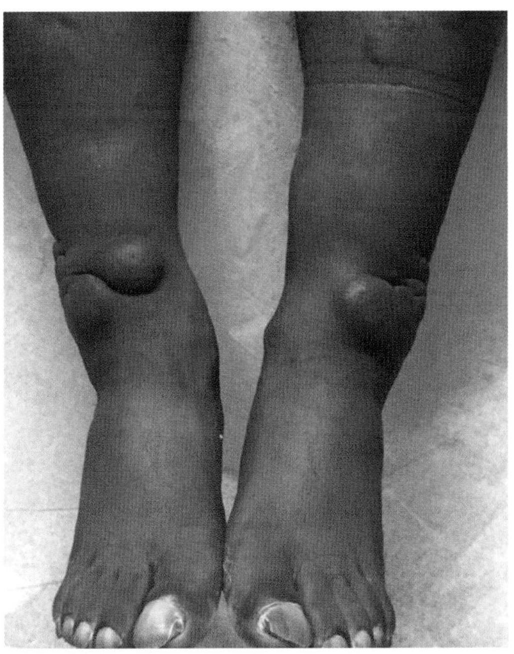

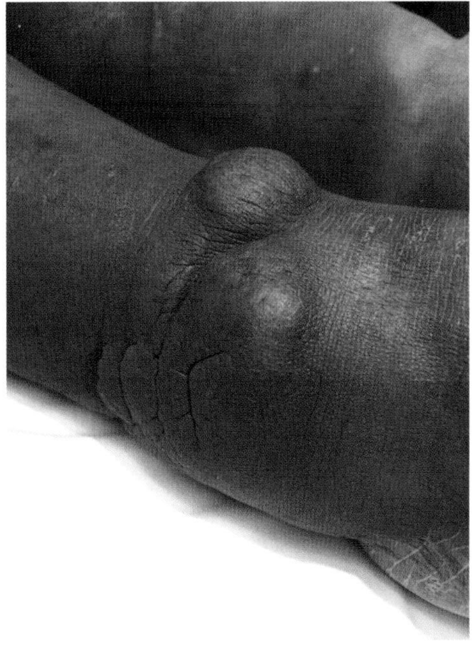

Fig. 154.1 Patient with long-standing hyperthyroidism who developed pretibial myxoedema in his early twenties.

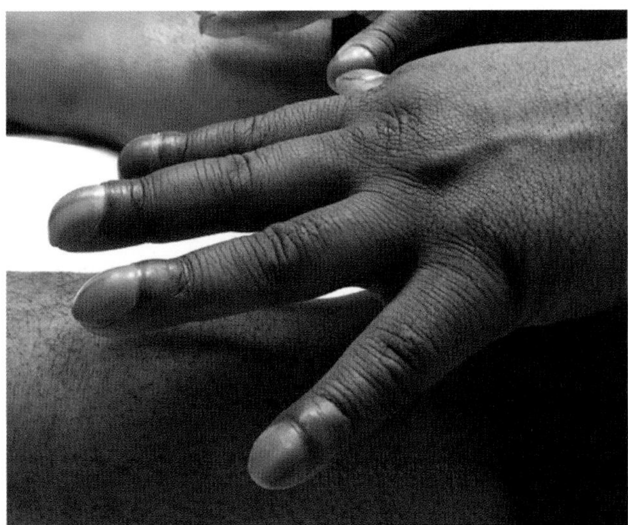

Fig. 154.2 Patient with long-standing hyperthyroidism who developed acropathy in his early twenties.

enlargement of the distal extremities caused by soft tissue hypertrophy and subperiosteal periostosis (Fig. 154.2). Neonatal hyperthyroidism can present with jaundice and a goiter [19].

Laboratory and histology findings. Laboratory testing needed to confirm the diagnosis includes free T4, T3, T3 resin uptake and TSH. Patients with Graves disease have increased T4, T3 and T3 resin uptake and decreased levels of TSH [18]. Patients with Graves disease will have circulating thyroid-stimulating antibodies.

Graves dermopathy is characterized by deposition of mucin in the mid- and reticular dermis. Mucin stains are helpful in histological confirmation [25]

Treatment and prevention. Treatment options include antithyroid medications, radioiodine ablation and thyroidectomy [26]. The treatment depends on the child's age and severity of disease. Monitoring for recurrent thyrotoxic symptoms or hypothyroidism is important.

The nonspecific symptoms and signs of hyperthyroidism will resolve when thyroxine levels return to normal. Graves dermopathy, severe ophthalmopathy and thyroid acropathy usually persist despite reduction in thyroxine levels. Treatment of Graves dermopathy is aimed at decreasing fibroblast production of hyaluronic acid [27]. Unfortunately, treatment is difficult. Topical steroids with occlusion and compression, intralesional steroids, systemic steroids, pentoxifylline, gamma globulin, plasmapheresis, surgical excision and immunotherapy have been used with varied success [28–30].

References

1 **Aversa T, Valenzise M, Corrias A et al. Underlying Hashimoto's thyroiditis negatively affects the evolution of subclinical hypothyroidism in children irrespectively of other concomitant risk factors. Thyroid 2015;25:183–7.**
2 Zimmerman MB, Boelaert K. Iodine deficiency and thyroid disorders. Lancet Diabetes Endocrinol 2015;3:286–95.
3 Yap WM, Chuah KL, Tan PH. Langerhans cell histiocytosis involving the thyroid and parathyroid gland. Mod Pathol 2001;14:111–5.
4 Gahl W, Thoenone J, Schneider J. Cystinosis. N Engl J Med 2002; 347:111–21.
5 Huang SA, Tu HM, Harney JW. Severe hypothyroidism caused by type 3-iodothyronine deiodinase in infantile hemangiomas. N Engl J Med 2000;343:185–9.
6 Parks, JS, Lin M, Grosse SD. The impact of transient hypothyroidism on the increasing rate of congenital hypothyroidism in the United States. Pediatrics 2010;125(Suppl 2):S54–63.
7 Pagovich OE, Silverberg JI, Freilich E. Thyroid abnormalities in pediatric patients with vitiligo in New York City. Cutis 2008;81:463–6.
8 **Daven N, Doshi MD, Marianna L. Cutaneous manifestations of thyroid disease. Clin Dermatol 2008;26:283–87.**

9 **Grant DB, Smith I, Fuggle PW et al. Congenital hypothyroidism detected by neonatal screening: relationship between biochemical severity and early clinical features. Arch Dis Child 1992;67:87–90.**

10 Leonhardt JM, Heymann WR. Thyroid disease and the skin. Dermatol Clin 2002;20:473–81.

11 Oerbeck B, Sundet K, Kase BF et al. Congenital hypothyroidism: influence of disease severity and L-thyroxine treatment on intellectual, motor, and school-associated outcomes in young adults. Pediatrics 2003;112:923–30.

12 LaFranchi SH, Austin J. How should we be treating children with congenital hypothyroidism? J Pediatr Endocrinol Metab 2007;20:559–78.

13 Zakarija M, McKenzie JM, Eidson MS. Transient neonatal hypothyroidism: characterization of maternal antibodies to the thyrotropin receptor. J Clin Endocrinol Metab 1990;70:1239–46.

14 Schoen EJ, Clapp W, To TT et al. The key role of newborn thyroid scintigraphy with isotopic iodide (123I) in defining and managing congenital hypothyroidism. Pediatrics 2004;114:683–8.

15 Gabrilove JL, Ludwig AW. The histogenesis of myxoedema. J Clin Endocrinol Metab 1957;17:925–32.

16 Bongers-Schokking JJ, Koot HM, Wiersma D et al. Influence of timing and dose of thyroid hormone replacement on development in infants with congenital hypothyroidism. J Pediatr 2000;136;293–7.

17 Donaldson M, Jones J. Optimizing outcome in congenital hypothyroidism; current opinions on best practice in initial assessment and subsequent management. J Clin Res Pediatr Endocrinol 2013; 5(Suppl 1):13–22.

18 **Bahn RS, Burch HB, Cooper DS et al. Hyperthyroidism and other causes of thyrotoxicosis: management guidelines of the American Thyroid Association and American Association of Clinical Endocrinologists. Endocr Pract 2011;17:456–520.**

19 **Zimmerman D. Fetal and neonatal hyperthyroidism. Thyroid 1999;9:727–33.**

20 Leonhardt JM, Heymann WR. Thyroid disease and the skin. Dermatol Clin 2002;20:473–81.

21 Vaidya VA, Bongiovanni AM, Parks JS et al. Twenty-two years experience in the medical management of juvenile thyrotoxicosis. Pediatrics 1974;54:565–70.

22 Barnes HV, Blizzard RM. Antithyroid drug therapy for toxic diffuse goiter (Graves' disease):thirty years experience in children and adolescents. J Pediatr 1977;91:313–20.

23 Gorton C, Sadeghi-Nejad A, Senior B. Remission in children with hyperthyroidism treated with propylthiouracil. Am J Dis Child 1987;141:1084–6.

24 Roberts CG, Ladenson PW. Hypothyroidism. Lancet 2004;363:1558.

25 Truhan AP, Roenigk HH Jr. The cutaneous mucinoses. J Am Acad Dermatol 1986;14:1–18.

26 US Preventative Service Task Force. Screening for thyroid disease: recommendation statement. Ann Intern Med 2004;140:125–7.

27 Ishizawa T, Sugiki H, Anzai S et al. Pretibial myxedema with Graves' disease: a case report and review of Japanese literature. J Dermatol 1998;25:264–8.

28 Chang CC, Chang SC, Kao SC et al. Pentoxyfilline inhibits the proliferation and glycosaminoglycan synthesis of cultured fibroblasts derived from patients with Graves ophthalmopathy and pretibial myxoedema. Acta Endocrinol 1993;129:322–7.

29 Antonelli A, Saracino A, Agastini S et al. Results of high-dose intravenous immunoglobulin treatment of patients with pretibial myxedema and Basedow's disease. Clin Ter 1992;141:63–8.

30 Pineda AM, Tianco EA, Tan JB et al. Oral pentoxifylline and topical clobetasol propionate ointment in the treatment of pretibial myxoedema, with concomitant improvement of Grave's ophthalmopathy. J Eur Acad Dermatol Venereol 2007;21:1441–3.

Alterations in cortisol levels

Cushing disease and Cushing syndrome

Pathogenesis. A Cushingoid appearance is caused from the effect of excessive glucocorticoids on body tissues. In Cushing disease, the adrenal gland overproduces glucocorticoids in response to an increased secretion of corticotrophin (ACTH) from a pituitary adenoma. Cushing syndrome results from an overproduction of glucocorticoids by the adrenal cortex caused by an adrenal tumour, hyperplasia or other autoimmune adrenal processes. Cushing syndrome can also be caused by an ectopic ACTH-secreting tumour [1]. Ectopic ACTH-producing tumours are rare in children and adolescents but have been reported in association with bronchial carcinoid, thymic carcinoid, pancreatic tumours, ganglioneuroblastoma, Wilm's tumour, Ewing's sarcoma and tumours of the kidney, liver, colon and ovary [2].

Features of Cushing syndrome can occur secondary to prolonged or increased use of oral, potent topical, intralesional, inhaled and/or intranasal corticosteroids [3,4].

Clinical features. The clinical features of Cushing syndrome, Cushing disease and steroid-induced Cushing syndrome are almost identical. Cutaneous findings include facial plethora, broad and purple striae, facial acne, skin fragility with poor wound healing and skin thinning with easy bruisability. Acanthosis nigricans can be seen caused by the associated glucose intolerance of the neck and axillae. Unlike in patients with Cushing disease, patients with Cushing syndrome will also develop androgen-mediated features such as fine downy facial lanugo hair, hirsutism and temporal scalp regression. Those with Cushing disease often develop hyperpigmentation [1,5].

Most of the cutaneous signs are caused by the direct effect of glucocorticoids on different body tissues. Superficial fungal infections such as tinea versicolor are more common in these patients secondary to cortisol-induced immune suppression and glucose intolerance. Striae form caused by interference in dermal collagen formation. The striae are often wide and purple, in contrast to the narrow and pink striae of rapid weight gain (Fig. 154.3). Hyperpigmentation in Cushing disease is caused by stimulation of melanocytes by increased ACTH production [1,5].

Weight gain, centripetal obesity, moon facies, buffalo hump and growth retardation are characteristic of Cushing disease, syndrome and steroid-induced syndrome [1,5].

Laboratory and histology findings. It is important to determine if the source of increase serum cortisol is endogenous or from exogenous corticosteroids. Cushing disease, syndrome and steroid-induced syndrome will have high levels of cortisol in the serum or urine. Methods to determine this include urinary free cortisol levels, the low dose dexamethasone suppression test, evening serum and salivary cortisol levels and the dexamethasone-corticotropin-releasing hormone test [1].

Measurement of ACTH levels can distinguish ACTH-dependent disease from adrenal-mediated disease. If serum ACTH levels are high, the high-dose dexamethasone suppression test, the corticotropin-releasing hormone (CRH) stimulation test, and inferior petrosal sinus sampling will distinguish pituitary and nonpituitary sources of ACTH. If plasma ACTH levels are normal or decreased and the high-dose dexamethasone suppression test does not reduce plasma cortisol levels, imaging is

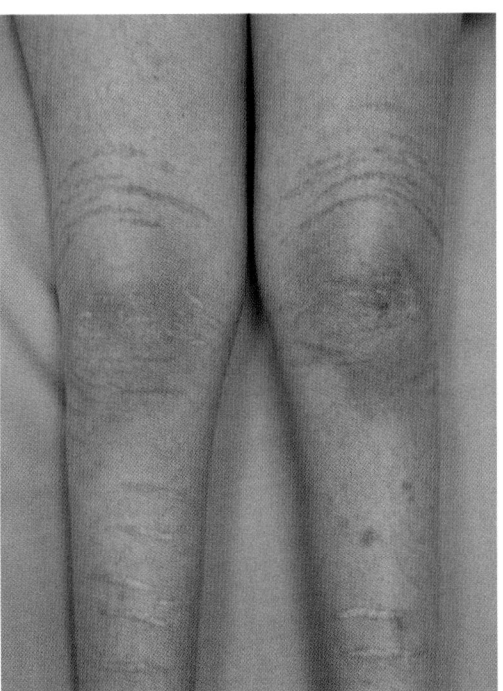

Fig. 154.3 A 12-year-old boy with Burkitt lymphoma who developed striae secondary to oral steroids.

required. An abdominal computed tomography (CT) scan is recommended if a primary adrenal pathology is suspected. If a pituitary source of excess ACTH is suspected, patients should undergo a contrast-enhanced magnetic resonance imaging (MRI) study of the pituitary. Chest and abdominal CT scans should be performed in patients with suspected ectopic ACTH production [1].

Treatment and prevention. Treatment depends on the underlying cause. Cushing disease caused by pituitary adenomas are often treated with transphenoidal surgery. Cushing syndrome is treated surgically if caused by adrenal hyperplasia, adrenal tumours, or ectopic ACTH tumours. Steroid-induced Cushing syndrome should be treated with a very slow taper of exogenous steroids. Although there are no consensus documents, several tapering regimens have been published so far. The goal is to rapidly reduce the therapeutic dose to a physiological level (equivalent to 8–10 mg/m^2/day of hydrocortisone equivalent) [6]. Most skin manifestations gradually resolve once cortisol levels are normalized. However, lightly pigmented striae may persist [5]. Treatment of striae is difficult. The use of topical tretinoin, topical silicone, chemical peels, dermabrasion, nonablative lasers, light therapy, radiofrequency devices and fractional resurfacing lasers have been reported to be helpful. Trofolastin cream, hyaluronic acid cream, cocoa butter products and olive oil have some evidence in preventing striae development [7].

Adrenal insufficiency

Pathogenesis. Hypocortisolism can be primary, which occurs when the adrenal glands are not functional (called Addison syndrome) or secondary, which occurs because of decreased secretion of ACTH from the pituitary gland. Acquired adrenal insufficiency can result from infection, haemorrhage, surgical removal of the adrenal glands, familial glucocorticoid deficiency or autoimmune causes such as polyglandular autoimmune syndrome. Long-term administration of glucocorticoids is the most common cause of paediatric Addison disease [8].

Clinical features. Hyperpigmentation of the skin and mucosal surfaces is associated with primary adrenal insufficiency caused by elevated ACTH levels (Fig. 154.4). The ACTH molecule contains the sequence of alpha-melanocyte-stimulating hormone, which stimulates melanocytes. The areolae, palmar creases, axillae, scars and areas of trauma are commonly affected with hyperpigmentation. Commonly affected mucosal surfaces include gingivae, tongue, hard palate, buccal mucosa, vagina and anus. Widespread hyperpigmentation can be accompanied by darkening of the hair, darkening of existing melanocytic naevi and development of longitudinal pigmented streaks in the nail plate. There may be hair loss in the axillae or pubic region because of lack of adrenal androgens. Vitiligo can accompany adrenal autoimmune disease [8–10].

Laboratory and histology findings. Hyponatraemia with or without hyperkalaemia is common in patients with primary adrenal insufficiency caused by deficient aldosterone secretion. Measurement of plasma ACTH and serum cortisol levels followed by an ACTH stimulation test will distinguish adrenal dysfunction from hypothalamopituitary dysfunction. Primary hypocortisolism will have elevated ACTH levels and decreased cortisol levels, whereas secondary hypocortisolism will have decreased ACTH and cortisol levels. Exogenous steroid-induced Addison's disease will have elevated ACTH levels. Measurement of antiadrenal antibodies can be helpful [8,10].

Abdominal CT may be normal but may show bilateral enlargement of adrenal glands in patients with Addison disease secondary to tuberculosis, fungal infections, adrenal haemorrhage or infiltrating diseases involving the adrenal glands. In idiopathic autoimmune Addison disease, the adrenal glands usually are atrophic [11].

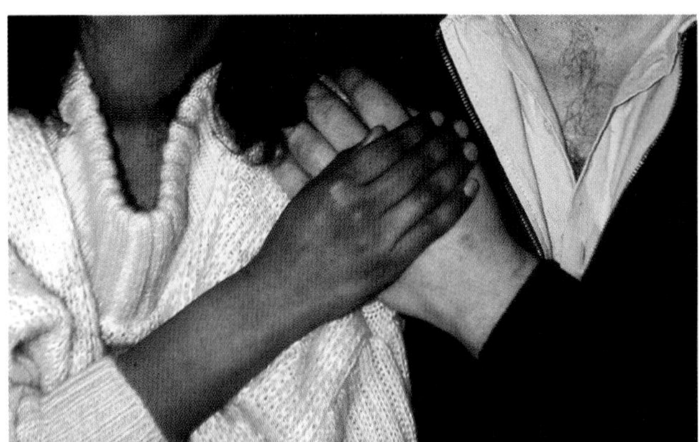

Fig. 154.4 Hyperpigmentation noted in a female with Addison disease, in contrast to her husband who has normal skin colour.

Treatment and prevention. Glucocorticoid replacement is necessary in all forms of hypocortisolism. Stress dosing of glucocorticoids should be administered in acute adrenal crisis. Mineralocorticoid replacement is necessary usually in only primary adrenal insufficiency. Most cutaneous findings will reverse once glucocorticoid and mineralocorticoid levels have normalized. Patients with circulating autoantibodies should be monitored for the development of other autoimmune diseases [8,10].

References

1 **Magiakou MA, Mastorakos G, Oldfield EH et al. Cushing syndrome in children and adolescents. Presentation, diagnosis and therapy. N Engl J Med 1994;331:629–36.**

2 More J, Young J, Reznik Y et al. Ectopic ACTH syndrome in children and adolescents. J Clin Endocrinol Metab 2011;96:1213–22.

3 Perry RJ, Findlay CA, Donaldson MD. Cushing's syndrome, growth impairment, and occult adrenal suppression associated with intranasal steroids. Arch Dis Chil 2002;87:14–8.

4 Siklar Z, Bostanci I, Atli O. An infantile Cushing syndrome due to misuse of topical steroid. Pediatr Dermal 2004;21:561–3.

5 **Stratakis CA, Mastorakos G, Mitsiades NS et al. Skin manifestations of Cushing disease in children and adolescents before and after the resolution of hypercortisolemia. Pediatr Dermatol 1998;15:253–8.**

6 **Alves C, Robazzi TC, Mendonca M et al. Withdrawal of glucosteroid therapy: clinical practice recommendations. J Pediatr 2008; 84:192–202.**

7 **Al-Himdani S, Ud-Din S, Gilmore S et al. Striae distensae: a comprehensive review and evidence-based evaluation of prophylaxis and treatment. Br J Dermatol 2014;170:527–47.**

8 **Perry R, Kecha O, Paquette J et al. Primary adrenal insufficiency in children: twenty years experience at the Sainte-Justine Hospital, Montreal. J Clin Endocrinol Metab 2005;90:3243–50.**

9 Lim YJ, Batch JA, Warne GL. Adrenal 21-hydroxylase deficiency in childhood: 25 years experience. J Paediatr Child Health 1995; 31:222–7.

10 **Grant DB, Barnes ND, Moncrieff MW et al. Clinical presentation, growth and pubertal development in Addison's disease. Arch Dis Child 1985;60:925–8.**

11 **Guo YK, Yang SG, Li Y et al. Addison's disease due to adrenal tuberculosis: contrast-enhanced CT features and clinical duration correlation. Eur J Radiol 2007;62:126–31.**

Disorders of sex hormones

Hypogonadism

Pathogenesis. Hypogonadism may occur if the hypothalamic–pituitary–gonadal axis is interrupted at any level. Hypergonadotropic hypogonadism occurs if the gonad does not produce the correct amount of sex hormone despite having adequate levels of luteinizing hormone (LH) and/or follicle-stimulating hormone (FSH). Turner syndrome is associated with hypergonadotropic hypogonadism. Hypogonadotropic hypogonadism occurs secondary to decreased levels of LH and/or FSH. Many genetic causes including Kallman and CHARGE syndrome may result in hypogonatropic hypogonadism [1]. Hypogonadotropic hypogonadism may also be seen in central nervous system tumours and postradiotherapy.

Clinical features. Hypogonadism manifests differently in male and females before and after the onset of puberty [1].

Hypogonadism in prepubertal females results in failure of breast development. They will still develop pubic and axillary hair, body odour, sebum production and acne caused by unaltered production and secretion of adrenal androgens. When hypogonadism occurs in postpubertal females, limited breast development occurs. Clues to Turner syndrome include short stature, webbing of the neck, short fourth metacarpals, widely spaced nipples and multiple pigmented naevi [1].

In males, hypogonadism *in utero* results in hypospadias, ambiguous genitalia or infants that appear phenotypically female (Figs 154.5 and 154.6). When hypogonadism occurs in prepubertal males, they will present with small genitalia, lack of scrotal rugae, eunuchoidism, decreased muscle mass, and delayed in epiphyseal closure resulting in long arms and legs. They will have decreased body hair, lack of acne and smooth, soft skin. If the androgen deficiency is not corrected by adolescence, the skin will retain its soft texture, the genitalia will enlarge, and body and facial hair will develop caused by the partial effect of adrenal androgens. If onset is postpubertal, clinical signs are subtle. The patient may notice not having to shave as frequently. Sebum production and acne vulgaris will improve, and the skin may become smooth [1].

Laboratory and histology findings. It is important to determine serum FSH, LH, prolactin, testosterone, oestrogen and thyroid levels. Decreased FSH, LH and sex hormone will lead you to hypogonadotropic hypogonadism. Hypergonadotropic hypogonadism will have normal FSH and LH levels but decreased sex hormone.

If suspecting a tumour, imaging may be necessary. If clinical signs point towards Klinefelter or Turner

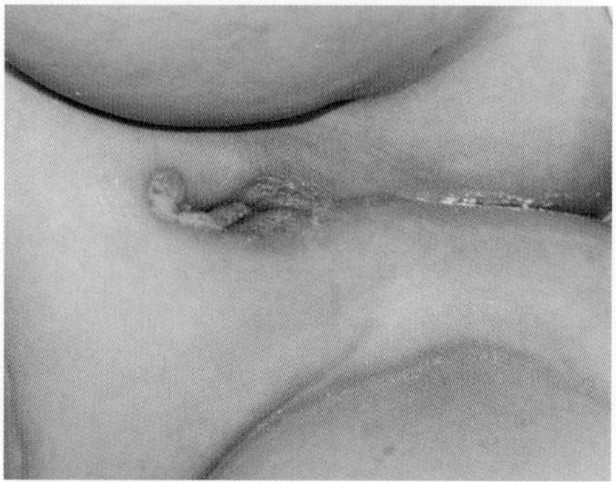

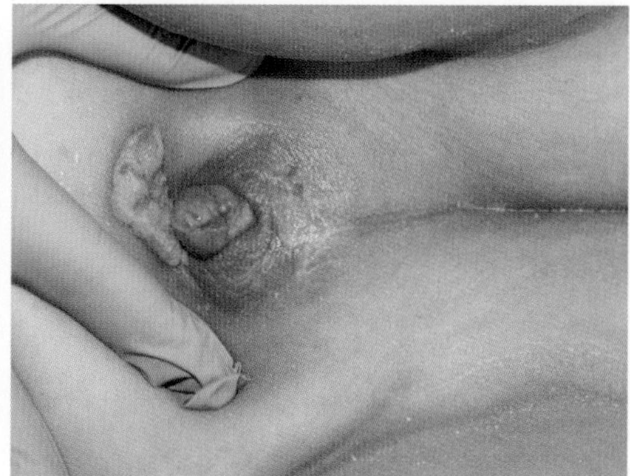

Fig. 154.5 An 8-year-old male presenting with ambiguous genitalia.

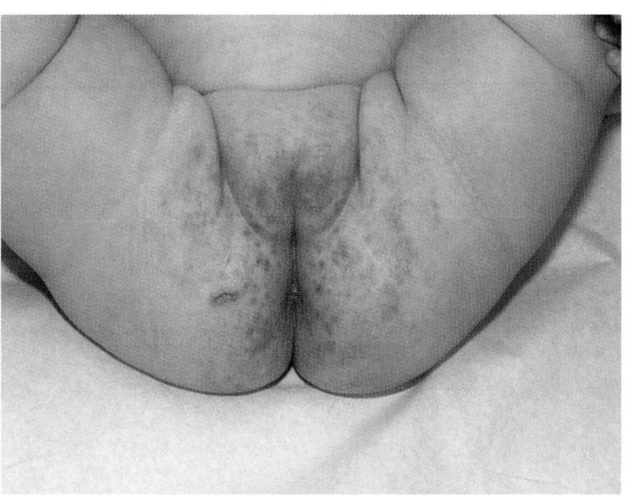

Fig. 154.6 Patient with XY genotype presenting with female phenotypic genitalia. Incidentally, the patient also presented with candidiasis.

syndrome or other genetic abnormalities, chromosomal studies will be helpful [2].

Treatment and prevention. Depending on the cause of the problem, treatment involves gonadotropin-releasing hormone, gonadotropins or sex hormone replacement therapy [2].

Turner syndrome

Turner syndrome is a common sporadic genetic disorder of girls, characterized by absence of either all or part of the second X chromosome. The defining clinical triad is short stature, impaired sexual development and infertility. Most female patients have gonadal dysgenesis and oestrogen deficiency. Turner syndrome may be first recognized by the affected individual's failure to undergo puberty; breast development is usually absent in an untreated patient. Short stature is the most common manifestation of Turner syndrome. Bone age is usually normal before adolescence but delayed after puberty as a result of decreased oestrogen. Lymphatic abnormalities including webbing of the neck, redundant neck folds, low hairline over the nape of the neck and acral congenital lymphoedema are common presentations of Turner syndrome. Lymphoedema can affect the nail anatomy, resulting in small hypoplastic fingernails. There is an increased incidence of benign melanocytic naevi noted in patients with Turner syndrome. Also, Turner syndrome patients have an increased tendency for hypertrophic scarring and keloid formation. Hair growth variation with unusual patches of short and long hair have been observed. Facial hirsutism can occur, although axillary and pubic hair is often scant. There is a decreased incidence of acne in Turner patients. Autoimmune disorders are common in Turner syndrome, with possible increased prevalence of hypothyroidism, early insulin resistance, inflammatory bowel disease, alopecia areata and vitiligo [3]. In childhood, growth hormone is often used to prevent short stature. Oestrogen therapy is started usually between the ages of 12 and 15 [4].

Klinefelter syndrome

Klinefelter syndrome is the most common chromosomal disorder associated with male hypogonadism and infertility. It is defined by a 47XXY karyotype, which represents either an excess X or Y chromosome. Infertility and gynaecomastia are the two most common symptoms that lead to a diagnosis of Klinefelter syndrome. Patients may lack secondary sexual characteristics because of decreased androgen production. This can result in sparse facial, pubic and axillary hair and a female fat distribution. During puberty, gynaecomastia develops secondary to elevated oestradiol levels. Leg ulcerations, likely caused by vascular disease, have been observed in Klinefelter syndrome. Treatment of Klinefelter is with androgen therapy to correct the androgen deficiency and to provide virilization [5].

Precocious puberty

Pathogenesis. Precocious puberty refers to the appearance of physical and hormonal signs of pubertal development at an earlier age than is considered normal caused by increased production of sex steroids. Girls with either breast development or pubic hair should be evaluated if this occurs before age 7 in white girls and before age 6 in African-American girls [6]. It can be classified as central precocious puberty and precocious pseudopuberty [7].

Central precocious puberty is gonadotropin dependent and caused by premature release of gonadotropins from the pituitary gland. Causes include central nervous system tumours, infections, head trauma, hydrocephalus, severe hypothyroidism and Addison disease. Precocious pseudopuberty is gonadotropin-independent and caused by the autonomous secretion of gender-appropriate sex hormones or administration of exogenous sex steroids. Examples of precocious pseudopuberty include congenital adrenal hyperplasia, gonad-secreting tumours, adrenal tumours and McCune–Albright syndrome [7,8].

Clinical features. In females, pubertal development is characterized, in order of appearance, by accelerated linear growth, breast enlargement, pubic and axillary hair development, and onset of menarche. In precocious puberty, these developments occur earlier than expected (Fig. 154.7). Females may have early development of severe acne vulgaris and body odour. Enlargement of the clitoris and change in colour of the vaginal mucosa from a deep-red colour to a moist pastel pink appearance results from increased androgen and oestrogen exposure [9,10].

In males, pubertal development is characterized, in order of appearance, by testicular enlargement, pubic hair development, penile enlargement, axillary and facial hair development, deepening of the voice and accelerated linear growth with an increase in muscle mass. Males will present usually with features of both adrenal and gonadal maturation. If there are signs of androgen excess in a boy without increased testicular size, consider causes of precocious pseudopuberty [9,10].

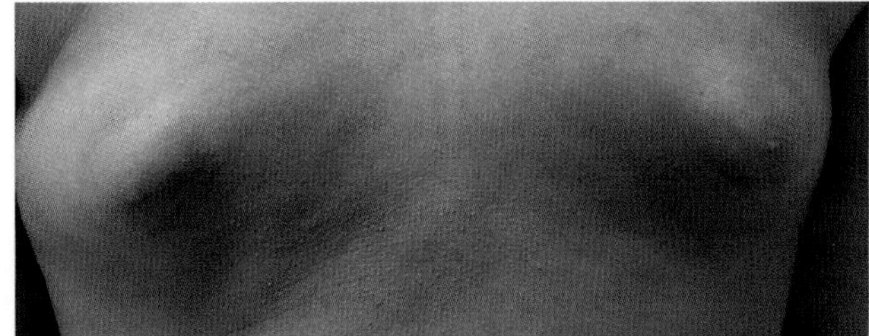

Fig. 154.7 An 8-year-old girl with early breast development, seen by an endocrinologist for precocious puberty.

Laboratory and histology findings. Serum LH, FSH, testosterone, oestrogen and thyroxine levels may help determine the cause of precocious puberty. Increased LH or FSH with increased sex hormones would suggest central precocious puberty. If LH and FSH levels are low but sex hormones are increased, precocious pseudopuberty is more likely. Measuring LH and FSH levels after stimulation with gonadotropin-releasing hormone is helpful for diagnosis. Head MRI is required if a tumour is suspected [11].

Treatment and prevention. If precocious puberty is caused by a tumour, surgical resection should be considered. Unfortunately, removal of the tumour rarely causes regression of the precocious puberty. Gonadotropin-releasing hormone analogs and progestins have been used in precocious pseudopuberty [10,11]. Congenital adrenal hyperplasia is treated with glucocorticoids. Testolactone, an inhibitor of the enzyme that converts androgens to oestrogens, has been used to treat McCune–Albright syndrome in females [12]. The acne often improves with reduction of sex hormone levels; standard acne vulgaris treatments can be also be tried to improve the precocious puberty-related acne [13].

Androgen excess

Pathogenesis. Androgen excess can be caused by oversecretion of androgens by adrenal or gonadal disease, hyperprolactinaemia, increased peripheral conversion of androstenedione to testosterone in obese patients and receptor defects resulting in increased secretion of ACTH [14]. Polycystic ovary syndrome and congenital adrenal hyperplasia present with hyperandrogenism [15].

Clinical features. Androgen excess can affect different tissues and organs, causing variable clinical features. Females usually will present with clitoromegaly, labial fusion and hirsutism (Fig. 154.8). They will have a delay in breast development and menarche. Males will present commonly with penile enlargement without enlargement of the testicles. Both sexes will have weight gain, pubic and facial hair growth, oily skin with severe acne, body odour, muscular habitus and deepening of the voice. They may develop early male-pattern baldness [14,16,17].

Androgens prolong the growth phase of hair and promote their conversion from vellus to terminal hairs. Androgens increase sebum production from the pilosebaceous unit causing acne and body odour [14,16,17].

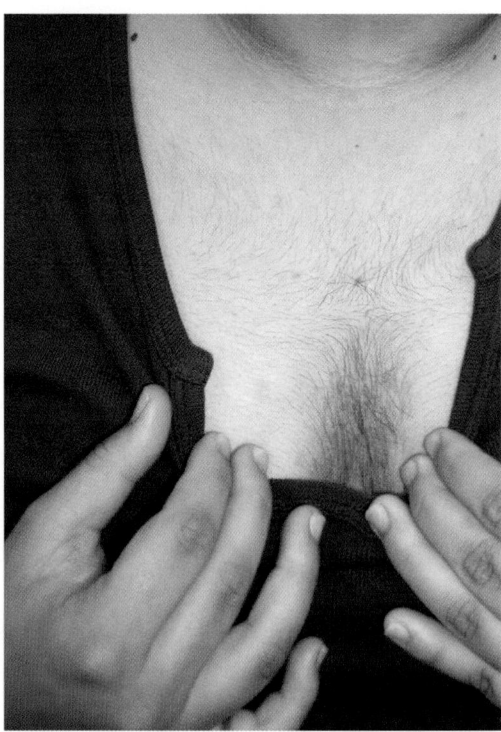

Fig. 154.8 A female with hyperandrogenism presenting with hirsutism.

Laboratory and histology findings. Laboratory testing includes measuring serum free testosterone, dehydroepiandrosterone (DHEAS) and androstenedione. Increased free plasma testosterone suggests a gonadal origin whereas increased DHEAS suggests an adrenal origin. An ultrasound, CT and/or MRI is required if a tumour is suspected [18].

Treatment and prevention. Treatment depends on the aetiology of hyperandrogenism. Tumours are often treated with surgical excision, chemotherapy and/or radiation. Ovarian-induced hyperandrogenism is treated with oestrogen-containing oral contraceptives [19]. Hirsutism can be treated with antiandrogen drugs, spironolactone, finasteride, gonadotropin-releasing antagonists and/or topical application of eflornithine [20]. Laser hair removal is also an option to treat the hirsutism.

Congenital adrenal hyperplasia

Congenital adrenal hyperplasia is caused by a deficiency in one of the enzymes involved in glucocorticoids and/or aldosterone synthesis. Decreased serum glucocorticoid or aldosterone results in increased secretion of ACTH. Accumulation of precursor molecules results in increased testosterone; therefore, congenital adrenal hyperplasia is a cause of hyperandrogenism. Most cases of congenital adrenal hyperplasia are caused by 21-hydroxylase deficiency, whereas the remaining cases are caused by 11B-hydroxylase deficiency or 3B-hydroxysteroid dehydrogenase deficiency [21].

Severe enzyme deficiencies in females with congenital adrenal hyperplasia will present with ambiguous genitalia and Addisonian crisis during infancy. Mild enzyme deficiency presents later with clinical signs later in life [15]. Affected male infants usually have normal genitalia, though the scrotum may be hyperpigmented.

An increase of 17-hydroxyprogesterone with an intravenous bolus of ACTH is diagnostic of congenital adrenal hyperplasia [21]. Congenital adrenal hyperplasia requires low-dose glucocorticoid therapy.

Polycystic ovary syndrome

The diagnostic criteria for polycystic ovary syndrome (PCOS) include one of the following three criteria: chronic anovulation, hyperandrogenism and polycystic ovaries. The full clinical spectrum of PCOS does not typically appear until puberty. Cutaneous symptoms include hirsutism, virilization, male-pattern hair loss, severe acne and acanthosis nigricans because of association with insulin insensitivity. These patients are often overweight and will have menstrual irregularities. Laboratory testing will show elevated free testosterone and an LH to FSH ratio of greater than 3. DHEAS may be normal or slightly above the normal range. First-line therapy is metformin (off-label) with or without oral contraceptive agents. Oral contraceptives increase sex hormone-binding globulin and thereby reduce the free testosterone level as well as suppress FSH and LH levels. Spironolactone, leuprolide and finasteride can be used for their antiandrogen properties. Selective oestrogen receptor modulators such as clomiphene can be used. Eflornithine is often used topically to treat the hirsutism [15].

Oestrogen excess

Pathogenesis. Elevated oestrogens in males can occur secondary to testicular feminization syndrome (also known as androgen insensitivity syndrome) or oestrogen-producing tumours by the adrenal gland or testes. Testicular feminization refers to failure of testosterone and dihydrotestosterone to bind adequately to the androgen receptor. The excess testosterone can be converted peripherally to oestrogen [22].

Elevated oestrogen levels in females can occur secondary to oral contraceptives, pregnancy or aetiologies causing precocious puberty such as McCune–Albright syndrome [23].

Clinical features. In testicular feminization syndrome, babies are born phenotypically female, but unilateral or bilateral masses in the inguinal canal may sometimes be appreciated. Adolescent patients will not develop pubic and axillary hair and will lack acne. Breast development, female fat distribution and the clitoris will appear phenotypically female as a result of conversion of testosterone to oestradiol. The inguinal masses will become more notable during adolescence, but they may be misdiagnosed as inguinal hernias [22].

Oestrogen-producing tumours in males result in gynaecomastia and pigmentation of the areolae. Several oestrogen tumours also produce androgens resulting in axillary and pubic hair growth, mild acne and penile enlargement [24].

Clinical signs of elevated oestrogen in paediatric females are discussed in the precocious puberty section.

Laboratory and histology findings. Laboratory tests to determine aetiology of hyperoestrogenism include serum testosterone, dihydrotestosterone, DHEA, androstenedione, LH, FSH and serum oestrogen. To diagnose testicular feminization syndrome, a karyotype is important. Pelvic ultrasound will reveal absent ovaries and fallopian tubes in testicular feminization syndrome [25]. A pregnancy test should also be obtained in females with clinical signs of hyperoestrogenism.

Treatment and prevention. Most patients with testicular feminization syndrome are raised as females. The testes should be removed to prevent malignancy and oestrogen replacement is usually started postoperatively. If patients have a more masculine appearance and have only partial androgen insensitivity syndrome, androgen replacement can be started [26–28]. Oestrogen-producing tumours can be removed surgically [24].

References

1 **Viswanathan V, Eugster EA. Etiology and treatment of hypogonadism in adolescents. Endocrinol Metab Clin North Am 2009;38:719–38.**

2 **Bhasin S, Cunningham GR, Hayes FJ et al. Testosterone therapy in men with androgen deficiency syndromes: an Endocrine Society clinical practice guideline. J Clin Endocrinol Metab 2010;95:2536–59.**

3 Lowenstein EJ, Kim KH, Glick SA. Turner's syndrome in dermatology. J Am Acad Dermatol 2004;50:767–76.

4 Ross JL, Quigley CA, Feuillan P et al. Growth hormone plus childhood low-dose estrogen in Turner's syndrome. N Engl J Med 2011;364:1230–42.

5 Visootsak J, Aylstock M, Graham JM et al. Klinefelter syndrome and its variants: an update and review for the primary pediatrician. Clin Pediatr 2011;40:639–51.

6 Kaplowitz PB, Oberfield SE. Reexamination of the age limit for defining when puberty is precocious in the United States: implications for evaluation and treatment. Drug and Therapeutic and Executive Committees of the Lawson Wilkins Pediatric Endocrine Society. Pediatrics 1999;104:936–41.

7 Wheeler MD, Styne DM. Diagnosis and management of precocious puberty. Pediatr Clin North Am 1990;37:1255–71.

8 Choi JH, Shin YL, Yoo HW. Predictive factors for organic central precocious puberty and utility of simplified gonadotropin-releasing hormone tests. Pediatr Int 2007;49:806–10.

9 **Kaplowitz P. Clinical characteristics of 104 children referred for evaluation of precocious puberty. J Clin Endocrinol Metab 2004; 89:3644–50.**

10 **Chemaitilly W, Merchant TE, Li Z et al. Central precocious puberty following the diagnosis and treatment of pediatric cancer and central nervous system tumors: presentation and long-term outcomes. Clin Endocrinol 2016;84:361–71.**

11 Armengoud JB, Charkaluk ML, Trivin C et al. Precocious pubarche: distinguishing late-onset congenital adrenal hyperplasia from premature adrenarche. J Clin Endocrinol Metab 2009;94:2835–40.

12 Feuillan PP, Foster CM, Pescovitz OH et al. Treatment of precocious puberty in the McCune–Albright syndrome with the aromatase inhibitor testolactone. N Engl J Med 1986;315:1115–19.

13 Eichenfield LF, Krakowki AC, Piggot C et al. Evidence-based recommendations for the diagnosis and treatment of pediatric acne. Pediatrics 2013;131:S163–86.

14 Azziz R, Sanchez LA, Knochenhauer ES et al. Androgen excess in women: experience with over 1000 consecutive patients. J Clin Endocrinol Metab 2004;89:453–62.

15 Cosma M, Swiglo BA, Flynn DN et al. Clinical review: Insulin sensitizers for the treatment of hirsutism: a systematic review and

metaanalyses of randomized controlled trials. J Clin Endocrinol Metab 2008;93:1135–42.
16 Hatch R, Rosenfield RL, Kim MH et al. Hirsutism: implications, etiology, and management. Am J Obstet Gynecol 1981;140:815–30.
17 Lowenstein EJ. Diagnosis and management of the dermatologic manifestations of the polycystic ovary syndrome. Dermatol Ther 2006;19:210–23.
18 Escobar-Morreale HF, Carmina E, Dewailly D et al. Epidemiology, diagnosis and management of hirsutism: a consensus statement by the Androgen Excess and Polycystic Ovary Syndrome Society. Hum Reprod Update 2012;18:146–70.
19 Rosenfield RL, Lucky AW. Acne, hirsutism and alopecia in adolescent girls. Endocrinol Metab Clin North Am 1993;22:507–32.
20 Shenenberger DW, Utecht LM. Removal of unwanted facial hair. Am Fam Physician 2002;66:1907–11.
21 Azziz R, Hincapie LA, Knochenhauer ES et al. Screening for 21-hydroxylase-deficient nonclassic adrenal hyperplasia among hyperandrogenic women: a prospective study. Fertil Steril 1999;72:915–25.
22 Solari A, Groisman B, Bidondo MP et al. Complete androgen insensitivity syndrome: diagnosis and clinical characteristics. Arch Argent Pediatr 2008;106:265–8.
23 Wong RC, Ellis CN. Physiologic skin changes in pregnancy. J Am Acad Dermatol 1984;10:929–40.
24 Nicol MR, Papacleovoulou G, Evans DB. Estrogen biosynthesis in human H296 adrenocortical carcinoma cells. Mol Cell Endocrinol 2009;300:115–20.
25 Dejager S, Bry-Gauillard H, Bruckert E et al. A comprehensive endocrine description of Kennedy's disease revealing androgen insensitivity linked to CAG repeat length. J Clin Endocrinol Metab 2002; 87:3893–901.
26 Hughes IA, Davies JD, Bunch TI et al. Androgen insensitivity syndrome. Lancet 2012;380:1419–28.
27 Winterborn MH, France NE, Raiti S. Incomplete testicular feminization. Arch Dis Child 1970;45:811–2.
28 Wierman ME, Basson R, Davis SR, et al. Androgen therapy in women: an Endocrine Society Clinical Practice guideline. J Clin Endocrinol Metab 2006;91:3697–710.

Dysfunction of parathyroid hormone

Hypoparathryoidism

Pathogenesis. Hypoparathyroidism occurs from defective synthesis or secretion of parathyroid hormone. Pseudohypoparathyroidism is described as end-organ resistance to parathyroid hormone. Hypoparathyroidism can occur caused by congenital absence of the parathyroid gland as in DiGeorge syndrome, antibodies against the parathyroid gland as in polyglandular autoimmune syndrome or iatrogenic removal during thyroid surgery [1]. McCune–Albright hereditary syndrome is characterized with pseudohypoparathyroidism.

Clinical features. Hyperreflexia and tetany caused by hypocalcaemia can occur. Cutaneous findings are rare but include dry skin and hair, patchy alopecia, thinning of the eyebrows and brittle nails [2].

Laboratory and histology findings. Serum calcium (total and ionized), phosphate, magnesium and intact parathyroid hormone should be measured. The calcium levels will be decreased in conjunction with increased serum phosphorus levels and reduced parathyroid hormone levels [1].

Treatment and prevention. Adequate replacement of calcium is necessary in symptomatic hypocalcaemia. Intravenous calcium may be required in the acute phase. Oral calcium and vitamin D can be used for long-term treatment. The use of parathyroid hormone (PTH) or PTH analogues are not currently recommended [1].

Polyglandular autoimmune syndrome

The three major components of polyglandular autoimmune syndrome I (polyglandular autoimmune polyendocrinopathy-candidiasis-ectodermal dystrophy) are autoimmune hypoparathyroidism, chronic mucocutaneous candidiasis and autoimmune adrenal insufficiency. The presence of all three components is not required to make a diagnosis, but at least two components have to present. Additional manifestations include type 1A diabetes, hypogonadism, pernicious anaemia, malabsorption, alopecia and vitiligo. It is a rare disease with autosomal recessive inheritance. Type II and III polyglandular autoimmune syndromes are rare in children and present mainly in adults [3].

Type 1 polyglandular autoimmune syndrome is also called polyendocrinopathy-candidiasis-ectodermal dystrophy. Candidiasis is usually the first clinical manifestation. It typically presents before the age of five with candida affecting primarily the skin, almost all nails, and oral and anal mucosa. Hypoparathyroidism occurs next, usually before the age of 10. Addison disease occurs last, usually before the age of 15. Hyperpigmentation occurs secondary to Addison disease. Other autoimmune cutaneous diseases can be associated including alopecia areata (29–40% of patients) and vitiligo (8–25% of patients). Other reported, but less well-characterized cutaneous associations include urticarial-like erythema with vasculitis, scleroderma, Sjögren syndrome and lichen planus. Type 1 polyglandular autoimmune syndrome does not have human leukocyte antigen (HLA) association, but it is strongly linked with a mutation in the autoimmune regulator AIRE. Type II polyglandular autoimmune syndrome is associated with HLA-DR3 and HLA-DR4 [3].

A serum endocrine autoantibody screen is helpful in diagnosis. The mucocutaneous candidiasis is treated with long-term oral antifungals such as fluconazole. Hypoparathyroidism is treated with oral calcium and vitamin D supplementation. Addison's disease is treated with low dose corticosteroids [3].

Pseudohypoparathyroidism

McCune–Albright hereditary osteodystrophy (polyostotic fibrous dysplasia) is characterized by PTH-resistant hypocalcaemia and hyperphosphataemia because of failure of peripheral tissues to respond to PTH. These patients will have short stature, rounded faces, brachydactyly (shortened fourth and fifth metacarpals), obesity, dental hypoplasia and soft tissue calcifications/ossifications. The calcification/ossification can be present at birth or may manifest during infancy or childhood as bluish macules, milia-like papules, nodules or plaques. There is predilection for periarticular skin and sites of pressure and trauma. Patients may also have café-au-lait macules located on the buttocks and lumbar regions. The café-au-lait macules usually do not cross the midline and tend to have a segmental distribution. The café-au-lait macules are often referred to as 'Coast of Maine'. The PTH and phosphorous levels will be elevated whereas calcium levels are low. Treatment is aimed at maintaining calcium levels with oral calcium and vitamin D supplementation [4]. The defect is in the *GNAS1* gene, which encodes the alpha subunit of the stimulatory G protein.

Hyperparathyroidism

Pathogenesis. Hyperparathyroidism is divided into primary, secondary and tertiary. Primary hyperparathyroidism can occur caused by genetic mutations, hyperplasia of the parathyroid, parathyroid adenoma, parathyroid carcinoma or neonatal severe hyperparathyroidism. Neonatal severe hyperparathyroidism is associated with inactivating mutations in the calcium-sensing receptor genes. Primary hyperparathyroidism can be caused by mucosal multiple endocrine neoplasia syndromes [5]. Secondary hyperparathyroidism occurs secondary to hypocalcaemia or hyperphosphataemia. Causes of secondary hyperparathyroidism include decreased intestinal absorption of calcium and vitamin D, chronic renal failure, insufficient vitamin D intake such as in rickets, cholestatic liver disease and iatrogenic causes. Tertiary hyperparathyroidism occurs when there is parathyroid hyperplasia so severe that removal of the underlying cause does not eliminate PTH secretion and hypertrophic chief cells become autonomous [5].

Clinical features. Hypercalcaemia in primary hyperparathyroidism can cause dehydration with skin tenting, prolonged capillary refill time and dry mucous membranes. Patients often have decreased muscle tone.

There are reports of metastatic calcinosis cutis and calciphylaxis developing in children with secondary hyperparathyroidism caused by end state renal disease. The metastatic calcinosis presented as erythematous, indurated firm nodules of different size (Fig. 154.9). Calciphylaxis presents initially with severe pain and livedo reticularis prior to cutaneous ulceration [6,7] (Fig. 154.10). Secondary hyperparathyroidism will often cause skeletal deformities, decreased muscle tone, bone pain and short stature [5].

Laboratory and histology findings. Serum calcium, phosphorous and PTH levels should be drawn. In primary disease, serum calcium and PTH will be elevated with low phosphorous. In secondary disease, calcium levels will be normal or low whereas PTH and phosphorous are increased [5].

Histology of calcinosis cutis will show amorphous and irregular basophilic deposits of calcium salts in the dermis. Von Kossa stain will be positive. In calciphylaxis, there will be mural calcification of the arteries and arterioles leading to vessel occlusion [6,7]. Some patients can have calcification of multiple internal vessels, so imaging for internal vascular disease may be necessary.

Treatment and prevention. Subtotal or total parathyroidectomy is first-line treatment for primary hyperparathyroidism. Medical management with or without

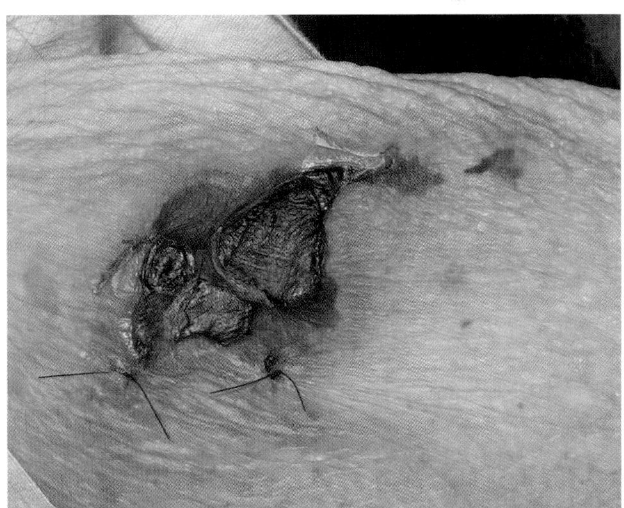

Fig. 154.10 Female diagnosed with calciphylaxis. Erythematous plaque with overlying eschar.

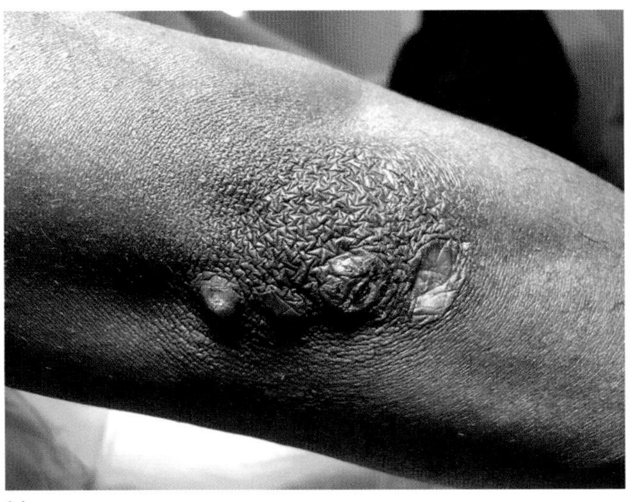

(a)

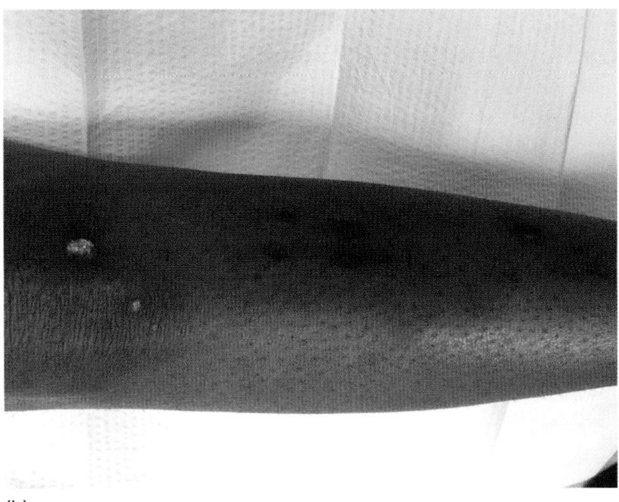

(b)

Fig. 154.9 Two patients presenting with calcinosis cutis. There are calcified nodules noted on the (a) elbow and (b) legs.

parathyroidectomy can be used for treatment of secondary hyperparathyroidism [5].

Calcinosis cutis and calciphylaxis may treated with surgical excision or with medical treatment that normalizes PTH levels and decreases the calcium–phosphorous ratio. Examples include sevelamer or other phosphate binders, vitamin D analogs, low-calcium dialysate in haemodialysis and dietary restrictions of phosphorus [6,7].

MEN syndrome

Multiple endocrine neoplasia syndrome (MEN syndrome) is divided into MEN 1, MEN 2a, and MEN 2b. In MEN 1 (Werner syndrome), there is hyperfunctioning of all four parathyroid glands, pancreatic islets and the anterior pituitary gland. MEN2a [8] is defined by medullary thyroid carcinoma, pheochromocytoma and hyperparathyroidism. MEN 2b (mucosal neuromata with endocrine tumours) has medullary thyroid cancer, pheochromocytoma, mucosal neuromas, marfanoid habitus and medullated corneal nerve fibres [9]. MEN 1 has a mutation in the *MEN1* gene, resulting in a defective menin nuclear protein. MEN 2 is caused by mutations in the RET proto-oncogene, which encodes a tyrosine kinase receptor.

Cutaneous findings associated with MEN 1 syndrome include lipomas, angiofibromas, and collagenomas. Multiple gingival papules, confetti-like hypopigmented macules, and café-au-lait macules can be seen less commonly. MEN2a is associated with macular and lichen amyloidosis, pruritus and notalgia paresthetica. The amyloid is secreted from the medullary thyroid cancer. MEN2b is characterized by multiple mucosal neuromas, especially on the eyelid, conjunctivae, lips and anterior tongue. The neuromas will give a pebbly and thickened appearance to the lips. The neuromas are present at birth and become pronounced during infancy and early childhood. There may be an increase in nerve fibres in normal skin. Lips and eyelids tend to be everted. Hyperpigmentation around the mouth and on the hands and feet can be seen. Circumoral lentigines, hypertrichosis and synophrys may be observed [9,10].

Genetic testing can confirm the diagnoses of MEN syndrome. Because early therapy improves the patient's prognosis in MEN syndrome, screening should be instituted in patients with risk factors [9].

MEN syndrome often needs to be treated both surgically and medically. The thyroid gland should be removed prophylactically in MEN2a and 2b. There are no definitive treatments for the cutaneous findings of MEN syndrome [9].

References

1 **Bollerslev J, Rejnmark L, Marcocci C et al. European Society of Endocrinology Clinical Guideline: treatment of chronic hypoparathyroidism in adults. Eur J Endocrinol 2015;173:G1–G20.**

2 Simpson JA. Dermatological changes in hypocalcaemia. Br J Dermatol 1954;66:1–15.

3 **LeBoeuf N, Garg A, Worobec S. The autoimmune polyendocrinopathy-candidiasis-ectodermal dystrophy syndrome. Pediatr Dermatol 2007;24:529–33.**

4 **Davies JH, Barton JS, Gregory JW et al. Infantile McCune-Albright syndrome. Pediatr Dermatol 2001;18:504–6.**

5 Burke JF, Chen H, Gosain A. Parathyroid conditions in childhood. Semin Pediatr Surg 2014;23:66–70.

6 Tan O, Atik B, Kizilkava A et al. Extensive skin calcifications in an infant with chronic renal failure: metastatic calcinosis cutis. Pediatr Dermatol 2006;23:235–8.

7 Feng J, Gohara M, Lazova R et al. Fatal childhood calciphylaxis in a 10-year-old and literature review. Pediatr Dermatol 2006;23:266–72.

8 Sipple, JH. The association of pheochromocytoma with carcinoma of the thyroid gland. Am J Med 1961;31:163–6.

9 **Brandi ML, Gagel RF, Angeli A, et al. Guidelines for diagnosis and therapy of MEN type 1 and type 2. J Clin Endocrinol Metab 2001; 86:5658–71.**

10 Darling, TN, Skarulis MC, Steinberg MC et al. Multiple facial angiofibromas and collagenomas in patients with multiple endocrine neoplasia type 1. Arch Dermatol 1997;133:853–7.

Pituitary dysfunction

Hypopituitarism

Pathogenesis. Hypopituitarism is partial or complete decrease of pituitary hormone secretion. Congenital causes include perinatal insults, interrupted pituitary stalk, absent or ectopic pituitary gland, defects in central nervous system development and Pallister–Hall syndrome [1]. Genetic causes include isolated growth hormone deficiency, multiple pituitary hormone deficiency, septo-optic dysplasia, isolated gonadotropin deficiency and Kallman syndrome [1,2].

Infiltrative disorders such as histiocytosis X, tuberculosis, sarcoidosis and lymphocytic hypophysitis can cause hypopituitarism. Tumours that can cause hypopituitarism include craniopharyngioma, germinoma, gliomas and pituitary adenomas. Cranial irradiation and haemochromatosis can also be the cause [1,2].

Clinical features. Clinical features are related to specific pituitary hormone deficiencies. Neonates will often present with microgenitalia, jaundice and pallor. Older children will have growth failure caused by growth hormone deficiency and delayed or absent puberty caused by gonadotropin deficiency. If hypopituitarism develops in the postpubertal period, puberty will fail to progress. Patients can have truncal obesity, normal head circumference, small facies and frontal bossing. Hypothyroidism and adrenal insufficiency can appear later in the course [3].

Skin findings are not specific and can include pallor, yellowish tinge, soft texture and wrinkling of skin especially around the eyes and mouth making the patient appear older. Absent terminal hair, decreased sebaceous gland activity, decreased hair and nail growth, onycholysis and longitudinal ridging of the nail plates can be present [3].

Laboratory and histology findings. All patients with hypopituitarism should have a brain MRI to rule out a tumour. Measurement of the plasma levels of the various pituitary hormones will be helpful in diagnosis [4].

Treatment and prevention. Most patients require lifelong hormone replacement. Surgical intervention may be necessary if aetiology is tumour-related [3].

Hyperpituitarism

Pathogenesis. Hyperpituitarism is rare in children. It typically occurs from a pituitary macroadenoma. The most common cause is a prolactinoma, followed by corticotropinoma and somatotropinoma. Hypersecretion of pituitary hormones caused by macroadenomas can interfere with other pituitary hormone functions [5].

Clinical features. Prolactinomas can cause hypogonadism and/or growth failure caused by suppression of gonadotropin and/or growth hormone secretion or local compression of the pituitary. Galactorrhoea and gynaecomastia can be noted in both males and females [5].

A Cushingoid appearance will develop with a corticotropinoma. Children will have generalized weight gain with growth failure. Pubertal arrest may occur [5].

Somatotropinomas secrete excess growth hormone. Gigantism occurs if the increase in growth hormone is before epiphyseal fusion. It is characterized by excessive linear growth without concomitant bone advancement age. Acromegaly and coarsening facial features occur if growth hormone excess occurs after closure of the epiphyseal plates. Acromegalic changes include enlargement of hands, feet, ears, nose, lips, tongue and mandible. The skin will also become thicker [5].

Laboratory and histology findings. Diagnosis should be made by measurement of pituitary hormones and imaging [5].

Treatment and prevention. Prolactinomas can be treated medically with dopamine agonists [5]. Surgery or ablation is recommended for corticotropinomas and somatotropinomas. Postoperative hormone replacement therapy is usually required [5].

References

1 Personnier C, Crosnier H, Meyer P et al. Prevalence of pituitary dysfunction after severe traumatic brain injury in children and adolescents: a large prospective study. J Clin Endocrinol Metab 2014;99:2052–60.

2 Sklar CA. Craniopharyngioma: endocrine abnormalities at presentation. Pediatr Neurosurg 1994;21(Suppl 1):18–20.

3 Toogood AA, Stewart PM. Hypopituitarism: clinical features, diagnosis, and management. Endocrinol Metab Clin North Am 2008; 37:235–61.

4 Argyropoulou MI, Kiortsis DN. MRI of the hypothalamic-pituitary axis in children. Pediatr Radiol 2005;35:1045–55.

5 Colao A, Loche S, Cappabianca P. Pituitary adenomas in children and adolescents. Clinical presentation, diagnosis, and therapeutic strategies. The Endocrinologist 2000;10:314–27.

Insulin-related disorders

Diabetes mellitus

Pathogenesis. Diabetes mellitus in paediatric patients is usually type 1 (insulin-dependent). However, the incidence of type 2 (noninsulin dependent) is increasing amongst the obese paediatric population [1]. Type 1 diabetes mellitus results from failure of the pancreatic islet cells to produce and secrete insulin. Causes of type 1 diabetes mellitus include genetic predisposition, viral illness, immunological factors or pancreatic destruction. Type 2 diabetes mellitus results from resistance to insulin action, inadequate insulin secretion and excessive or inappropriate glucagon secretion [1].

Clinical features. Clinical features of both type 1 and type 2 diabetes mellitus are similar with the exception of obesity-related signs in type 2. The cutaneous findings can be classified into four major groups: (i) skin diseases associated with diabetes, such as scleroderma-like changes of the hand, necrobiosis lipoidica (NLD) and diabetic dermopathy; (ii) cutaneous infections; (iii) cutaneous manifestations of diabetes complications; and (iv) skin reactions to diabetes treatment [2].

Skin dryness and ichythysiform skin changes are one of the earliest and most common manifestations of diabetes in paediatric patients. This is likely caused by the reduced hydration of the stratum corneum and decreased sebaceous gland activity [3]. Rubeosis faciei can occur caused by venular dilation of the cheeks and hyperglycaemia-induced sluggish microcirculation [4].

Limited joint mobility and waxy thickening of the skin occurs in about 28% of paediatric patients. The condition is characterized by flexion contractures of the proximal interphalangeal joint, which leads to an inability to press the palms together in a praying position. The severity of this disease can vary and larger joints can also be involved [5]. Those with pronounced joint immobility can have diffuse or discrete waxy thickening of the skin. The dorsum of the hands and fingers are typically affected. The skin thickness is caused by increased amounts of collagen that are heavily glycosylated [6].

NLD is also uncommon in paediatric patients. Lesions present as irregularly shaped plaques with a pink-red to reddish-violet periphery and central atrophy (Fig. 154.11). They tend to favour the anterior tibia but can present on other areas such as the trunk, limbs, face and scalp. The lesions are usually painless, symmetric, bilateral and can ulcerate [7,8]. The pathogenesis remains unknown. If the lesion is active, expanding or develops ulceration, treatment with topical or intralesional steroids can be helpful. Pentoxifylline, tretinoin, bovine collagen, hyperbaric oxygen and antiplatelet agents have been tried with varied improvement; overall, NLD is highly unresponsive to treatment [9].

Diabetic dermopathy has been reported only rarely in paediatric patients [10].

Obesity is strongly associated with type 2 diabetes mellitus. Patients with type 2 diabetes usually have acanthosis nigricans (AN), characterized by hyperpigmentation on posterior neck, axillae and flexural skin (Fig. 154.12). It is often confused with dirty skin. Stimulation of growth factor receptors are the cause of AN [11]. Multiple skin tags can be seen. Hypertriglyceridaemia in these overweight patients can result in development of eruptive xanthomas, particularly on the buttocks. Postpubertal females can develop hirsutism, difficult to control acne,

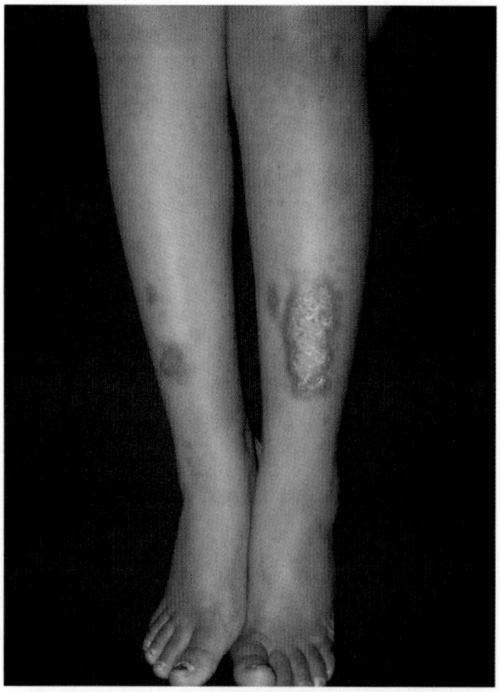

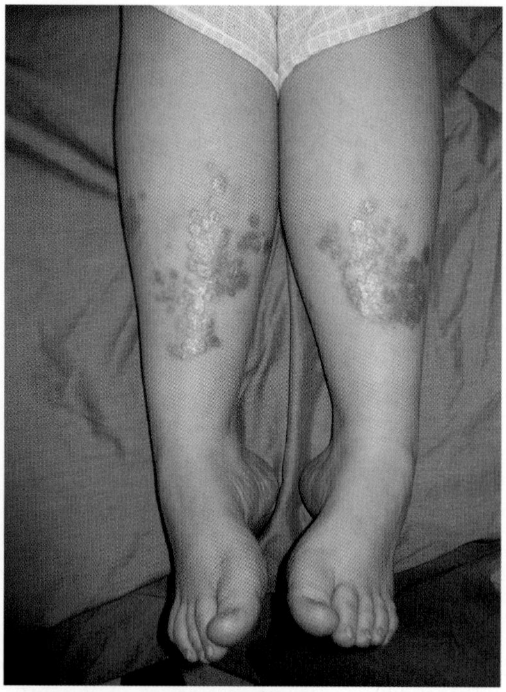

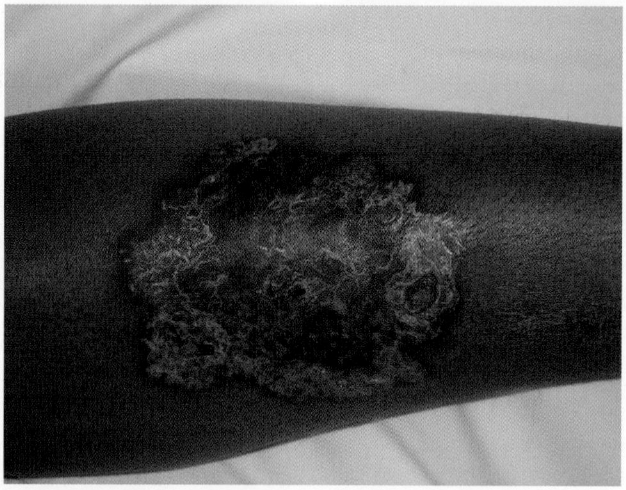

Fig. 154.11 Multiple patients with necrobiosis lipoidica diabeticorum. Well-circumscribed atrophic plaque with hyperpigmented border.

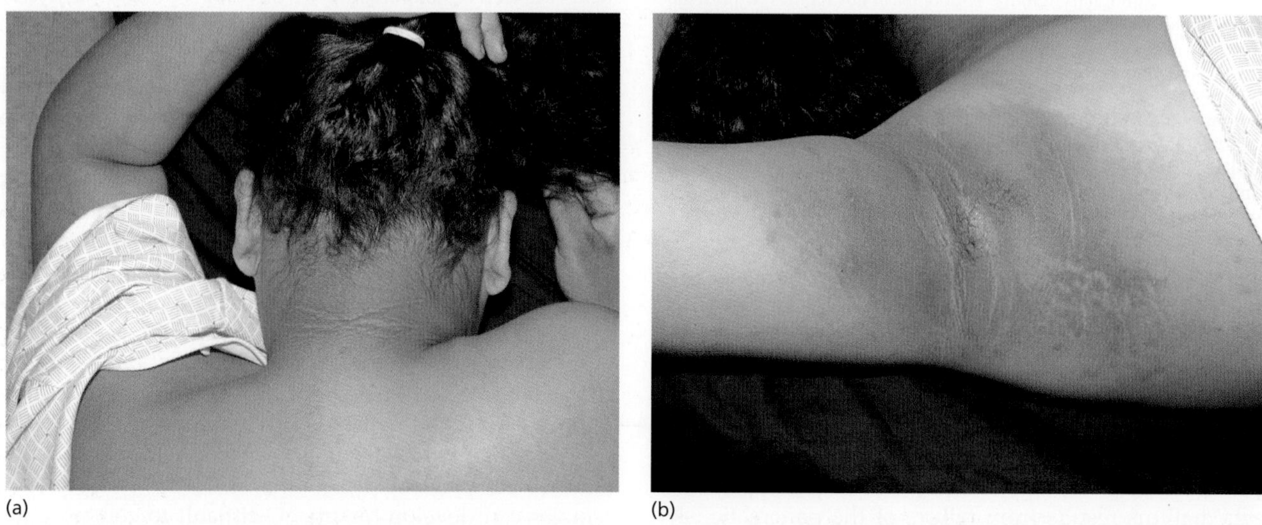

Fig. 154.12 Acanthosis nigricans of the (a) neck and (b) axillae in an 11-year-old girl with insulin resistance.

amenorrhoea and male-pattern hair loss because hyperinsulinaemia can be responsible for ovarian-derived hyperandrogenism [12].

Hyperglycaemia can impair immunity, therefore patients with poorly controlled diabetes are predisposed to developing infections [13]. Common cutaneous infections include impetigo, folliculitis, furunculosis, cellulitis and erysipelas. Erythrasma is common in obese patients. Severe malignant otitis external from *Pseudomonas aeruginosa* has been reported. *Candida albicans* commonly presents in these patients with vulvovaginitis, balanitis, angular cheilitis, intraoral candidiasis, intertrigo and/or paronychia. Children with poorly controlled diabetes are predisposed to mucormycosis presenting as a gangrenous ulcer in the upper respiratory tract [10,14].

The cutaneous manifestations of microangiopathy and neuropathy are rarely seen in children. Microangiopathy can present as cooling and mottling of the lower extremities while in a dependent position. Neuropathy in young patients may involve the autonomous nervous system resulting in anhidrosis with or without compensatory hyperhidrosis [10].

Local side effects of insulin therapy can manifest at the injection site as soft tissue hypertrophy, lipoatrophy or infection. Localized hypersensitivity reactions characterized by erthythema, pruritus and induration have been reported. Allergic reactions can be immediate or delayed. The diagnosis of insulin allergy can be confirmed by a positive skin prick test to insulin and the presence of serum immunoglobulin E antibodies to insulin [15].

The soft tissue hypertrophy from insulin injections presents with firm, nontender skin coloured nodules. Injection at different sites may or may not resolve the hypertrophy but counselling patients to inject at different sites from the start may prevent the hypertrophy. Children with diabetes favour areas of tissue hypertrophy as the injection site because of their hypoaesthetic nature. This should be discouraged because insulin absorption can be unpredictable from the sites of hypertrophy [5].

Lipoatrophy is now uncommon because of the use of highly purified insulin preparations [16]. A localized abscess, cellulitis or erysipelas can develop if a poor sterile technique is used for insulin injections. A generalized allergic reaction to insulin is extremely uncommon. The generalized systemic allergic reaction occurs shortly after starting or restarting treatment. Desensitization is necessary if insulin is required for treatment [17]. Useful adjuncts to managing allergic reaction include addition of desoximetasone to the insulin injection or a change in delivery system utilizing insulin pump therapy [18].

To our knowledge, bullosis diabeticorum has never been reported in the paediatric age group.

Laboratory and histology findings.
A random plasma glucose concentration of 200 mg/dL or more in association with polyuria, polydipsia or unexplained weight loss is diagnostic of diabetes. A serum glucose of 126 mg/dL or more or a 2-hour plasma glucose of 200 mg/dL or more during an oral glucose tolerance test is also diagnostic. Autoimmune markers such as glutamic acid decarboxylase and islet cell antibodies are usually positive in type 1 and negative in type 2. Fasting c-peptide is usually elevated in type 2.

Testing of type 2 diabetes mellitus is recommended for all paediatric patients that are overweight and have signs of insulin resistance [19].

Histological findings of waxy thickening of the skin reveals dermal thickening owing to increased amounts of collagen [6]. Histology of NLD will show granulomas arranged in a layered fashion and admixed areas of collagen degeneration in the dermis and subcutaneous tissue [9].

Infections may require cultures. The diagnosis of mucormycosis requires a biopsy revealing necrosis and nonbranching septate hyphae.

Treatment and prevention. Treatment for type 1 diabetes is with insulin therapy. Treatment for type 2 includes diet, exercise, weight loss, metformin and insulin if necessary. AN, eruptive xanthomas and hyperandrogenism associated with type 2 diabetes tend to improve weight loss.

Insulin resistance

Pathogenesis. Insulin resistance can be inherited or acquired. Hereditary causes include mutations in insulin receptors, antibodies blocking insulin receptors, defect in glucose transporters and abnormalities in signalling proteins [20]. Syndromes that are associated with inherited forms of insulin resistance include type A and B syndrome, Rabson–Mendenhall syndrome, lipodystrophic states, ataxia-telangiectasia, Werner syndrome and leprechaunism [21].

The most common cause of acquired insulin resistance is obesity [20]. Syndromes including polycystic ovary disease, Prader–Willi syndrome, myotonic dystrophy and streak gonads predispose patients to acquired insulin resistance. Other causes include gigantism/acromegaly, Cushing disease and hypothyroidism [21].

Clinical features. Central obesity is a good marker for insulin resistance [22]. Almost all causes of insulin resistance will present with AN in flexural and intertriginous areas because of high circulating levels of insulin or insulin-like growth factor on the skin. Females can present with hyperandrogenism. Patients can develop features related to hyperlipidaemia including eruptive xanthomas, xanthelasma and tuberous xanthomas.

Laboratory and histology findings. Insulin resistance can be detected by measuring plasma glucose, HbA1c and insulin levels. Other tests can be performed based on other clinical examination findings [23].

Treatment and prevention. Treatment depends on the underlying cause of insulin resistance. Metformin can enhance weight reduction, reduce hepatic glucose output and increase uptake of insulin by peripheral tissues. Other insulin-sensitizing drugs can also be used. Diet and exercise can decrease insulin levels if the cause of insulin resistance is acquired.

AN and signs of hyperandrogenism will improve with a decrease in serum insulin levels [24].

References

1 Dabelea D, Mayer-Davis EJ, Saydah S et al. Prevalence of type 1 and 2 diabetes among children and adolescents from 2001 to 2009. JAMA 2014;311:1778–86.

2 Ferringer T, Miller F 3rd. Cutaneous manifestation of diabetes mellitus. Dermatol Clin 2000:20;483–92.

3 Sakai S, Kikuchi K, Satoh J et al. Functional properties of the stratum corneum in patients with diabetes mellitus: similarities to senile xerosis. Br J Dermatol 2005;153:319–23.

4 Ngo BT, Hayes KD, DiMiao DJ et al. Manifestations of cutaneous diabetic microangiopathy. Am J Clin Dermatol 2005;225–37.

5 Kakourou T, Dacou-Voutetakis C, Kavadias G et al. Limited joint mobility and lipodstyrophy in children and adolescents with insulin-dependent diabetes mellitus. Pediatr Dermatol 1994;11:310–4.

6 Yosipovitch G, Hodak E, Vardi P et al. The prevalence of cutaneous manifestations in IDDM patients and their association with diabetic risk factors and microvascular complications. Diabetes Care 1998;21:506–9.

7 Lowitt MH, Dover JS. Necrobiosis lipoidica. J Am Acad Dermatol 1991;25:735–48.

8 Verotti A, Chiarelli F, Amerio P et al. Necrobiosis lipoidica diabeticorum in children and adolescents: a clue for underlying renal and retinal disease. Pediatr Dermatol 1995;12:220–3.

9 Szabo RM, Harris GD, Burke WA. Necrobiosis lipoidica in a 9-year-old girl with new-onset type II diabetes mellitus. Pediatr Dermatol 2001;18:316–9.

10 Eddin DV. Cutaneous manifestations of diabetes mellitus in children. Pediatr Dermatol 1985;2:161–79.

11 Fagot-Campagna A, Pettitt DJ, Engelgau MM et al. Type 2 diabetes among North American children and adolescents: an epidemiologic review and a public health perspective. J Pediatr 2000;136:664–72.

12 Grinstein G, Muzumdar R, Aponte L et al. Presentation and 5-year follow-up of type 2 diabetes mellitus in African American and Carribean-Hispanic adolescents. Horm Res 2003;60:121–6.

13 Clement S, Braithwaite SS, Magee MF et al. Management of diabetes and hyperglycemia in hospitals. Diabetes Care 2004;27:553–91.

14 Romano G, Moretti G, Benedetto A et al. Skin lesions in diabetes mellitus: prevalence and clinical correlation. Diabetes Res Clin Pract 1998;39:101–6.

15 Patterson R, Mellies CJ, Roberts M. Immunologic reactions against insulin to IgE anti-insulin, insulin allergy and combined IgE and IgG immunologic insulin resistance. J Immunol 1973;110:1135–45.

16 de Villiers FP. Lipohypertrophy: a complication of insulin injections. S Afr Med J 2005;95:858–9.

17 Lieberman P, Patterson R, Mertz R et al. Allergic reactions to insulin. JAMA 1971;215:1106–12.

18 Richardson T, Kerr D. Skin-related complications of insulin therapy: epidemiology and emerging management strategies. Am J Clin Dermatol 2003;4:661–7.

19 American Diabetes Association. Type 2 Diabetes in children and adolescents. Diabetes Care 2000;23;381–9.

20 Lutsey PL, Steffen LM, Stevens J. Dietary intake and the development of the metabolic syndrome: the Atherosclerosis Risk in Communities study. Circulation 2008;117:754–61.

21 Levy-Marchal C, Arslanian S, Cutfield W et al. Insulin resistance in children: consensus, perspective, and future directions. J Clin Endocrinol Metab 2010;95:5189–98.

22 Hirschler V, Ruiz A, Romero T et al. Comparison of different anthropometric indices for identifying insulin resistance in schoolchildren. Diabetes Technol Ther. 2009;11:615–21.

23 Katz A, Nambi SS, Mather K, et al. Quantitative insulin sensitivity check index: a simple, accurate method for assessing insulin sensitivity in humans. J Clin Endocrinol Metab 2000;85:2402–10.

24 Salpeter SR, Buckley NS, Kahn JA et al. Meta-analysis: metformin treatment in persons at risk for diabetes mellitus. Am J Med 2008;121:149–57.

Dermatological diseases with endocrine dysfunction

Insulin resistance and/or diabetes

Paediatric psoriasis patients have an increased risk for insulin resistance and metabolic syndrome compared with children without psoriasis. Early monitoring for metabolic syndrome and lifestyle modifications are recommended [1].

Congenital and acquired lipodystrophy syndromes are characterized by subcutaneous fat loss in either a generalized or partial pattern; these syndromes are commonly associated with insulin resistance [2].

There may be an association between subcutaneous granuloma annulare and insulin-dependent diabetes mellitus. There have been reports of the subcutaneous granuloma annulare resolving with treatment of the diabetes [3].

Type A insulin resistance syndrome presents in younger females with signs of virilization, increased growth, other signs of hyperandrogenism and acral enlargement. It is caused by defects in cell receptors for insulin. Type B is more common in adolescent females and is caused by circulating antibodies to the insulin receptors [4].

Rabson–Mendenhall syndrome is a rare autosomal recessive variant of type A insulin resistance. Patients present with classic features of insulin resistance, dental dysplasia and pineal hyperplasia.

Many syndromes that are associated with obesity may also have an insulin resistance and a diabetes association.

Hypothyroidism

Incontinentia pigmenti can present with congenital hypothyroidism [5]. Patients with Marfan syndrome can develop hypothyroidism.

Hypogonadism

IBIDS and PIBIDS are part of the trichothiodystrophy category. Both IBIDS (ichthyosis, brittle hair, impaired intelligence, decreased fertility and short stature) and PIBIDS (photosensitivity with IBIDS) have hair abnormalities. Infertility is caused by hypogonadism [6].

Hypopituitarism

Hypopituitarism caused by a partially empty sella turcica has been reported associated with PHACE syndrome (posterior fossa malformations, cervicofacial haemangiomas, arterial anomalies, cardiac defects, eye anomalies and midline/ventral defects) [7].

Oliver–McFarlane syndrome is characterized by trichomegaly, congenital hypopituitarism and retinal degeneration [8].

More than one associated endocrine dysfunction

Carney complex and its subsets LAMB syndrome and NAME syndrome are autosomal dominant syndromes that are characterized by endocrine overactivity and lentigines. Lentigines and hyperpigmentation are most frequently present on the lips, eyelids, conjunctivae and oral mucosa. The adrenal glands, gonads, thyroid and pancreas can be affected in these syndromes [9].

Cowden syndrome (also called multiple hamartoma syndrome) results in hamartomas in the skin such as trichilemmomas, papillomatous papules and acral keratosis. It can be associated with multinodular goitres, thyroid cancer, breast cancer and endometrial cancer [10].

Tuberous sclerosis is associated with angiofibromas, periungal fibromas, hypomelanotic macules, connective tissue naevi, gingival fibromas and confetti-like skin lesions. Tuberous sclerosis has been reported to occur with pituitary and parathyroid tumours, Cushing disease and pancreatic islet cell tumours, particularly insulinomas [11].

An increased incidence of central precocious puberty, diencephalic syndrome, growth hormone deficiency and growth hormone hypersecretion have been described in children with neurofibromatosis 1. These conditions may be a complication of optic gliomas but have also been reported in the absence of optic gliomas [12].

Langerhans cell histiocytosis can be associated with central diabetes insipidus caused by lack of posterior pituitary gland function. Growth hormone deficiency and hypogonadism have also been reported [13].

POEMS syndrome represents polyneuropathy, organomegaly, endocrinopathy, M protein and skin changes. The most common endocrinopathies are hypogonadism with gynaecomastia, insulin-dependent diabetes mellitus and primary hypothyroidism. Hyperpigmentation, hypertrichosis and skin thickening seem to be the most common skin features [14].

Rothmund–Thomson syndrome is characterized by poikilodermatous skin changes during infancy. Patients can have hypogonadism (25%), parathyroid adenomas, disturbed thyroid function and adrenal insufficiency [15].

IPEX syndrome (immune dysregulation, polyendocrinopathy, enteropathy, X-linked syndrome) can present with diabetes mellitus or thyroiditis. Cutaneous findings include atopic dermatitis-like lesions, psoriasiform dermatitis, ichthyosiform lesions, severe fissuring cheilitis, perioral oedema, urticaria and onychodystrophy [16].

H syndrome is an autosomal recessive autoinflammatory genodermatosis that presents with hyperpigmented hypertrichotic plaques with an underlying inflammatory infiltrate. These patients have hypogonadotropic hypogonadism, diabetes mellitus, short height and hallux valgus [17].

Woodhouse–Sakati syndrome is a rare autosomal recessive disorder characterized by alopecia, hypogonadism, diabetes mellitus, intellectual disability, sensorineural deafness, extrapyramidal signs and low insulin-like growth factor 1 levels [18].

Patients with vitiligo and/or alopecia areata have a higher incidence of developing other autoimmune diseases including hypothyroidism.

Endocrine tumours can present in several hereditary tumour syndromes such as neurofibromatosis 1, Peutz–Jeghers syndrome, Beckwith–Wiedemann syndrome, tuberous sclerosis, Li–Fraumeni syndrome, Gardner syndrome and Cowden syndrome (PTEN hamartoma syndrome) [19].

Down syndrome, Turner syndrome, Noonan syndrome, and Klinefelter syndrome can have both endocrine and dermatological manifestations.

Down syndrome

Down syndrome, which is characterized by trisomy 21, classically presents with short stature, epicanthal folds, flat nasal bridge, protruding tongue, growth retardation and short stature. There is a high incidence of gonadal malfunction and delayed puberty in Down syndrome. Girls often have a delay in menarche or adrenarche; boys may have ambiguous genitalia, cryptorchidism, micropenis and small testes. Hypothyroidism and growth hormone deficiency are often associated with Down syndrome [20].

References

1 Tom WL, Playford MP, Admani S et al. Characterization of lipoprotein composition and function in pediatric psoriasis reveals a more atherogenic profile. J Invest Dermatol 2016;136:67–73.
2 Akinci B, Koseoglu FD, Onay H et al. Acquired partial lipodystrophy is associated with increased risk for developing metabolic abnormalities. Metabolism 2015;64:1086–95.
3 Agrawal AK, Kammen BF, Guo H et al. An unusual presentation of subcutaneous granuloma annulare in association with juvenile-onset diabetes: case report and literature review. Pediatr Dermatol 2012; 29:202–5.
4 Kahn CR, White MF. The insulin receptor and the molecular mechanism of insulin action. J Clin Invest 1988;82:1151–6.
5 Poziomczyk CS, Bonamigo RR, Santa Maria FD et al. Clinical study of 20 patients with incontentia pigmenti. Int J Dermatol 2016;5:87–93.
6 Przedborski S, Ferster A, Goldman S et al. Trichothiodystrophy, mental retardation, short stature, ataxia, and gonadal dysfunction in three Moroccan siblilngs. Am J Med Genet 1990;35:566–73.
7 Goddard DS, Liang MG, Chamlin SL et al. Hypopituitarism in PHACES Association. Pediatr Dermatol 2006;23:476–80.
8 Hufnagel RB, Arno G, Hein ND et al. Neuropathy target esterase impairments cause Oliver-McFarlane and Laurence Moon syndromes. J Med Genet 2015;52:85–94.
9 McCarthy PM, Piehler JM, Schaff HV et al. The significance of multiple, recurrent, and 'complex' cardiac myxomas. J Thorac Cardiovasc Surg 1986;91:389–96.
10 Sardinoux M, Raingeard I, Bessis D et al. Cowden syndrome, or multiple hamartomatous tumor syndrome in clinical endocrinoloty. Ann Endocrinol 2010;71:264–73.
11 Dworakowska D, Grossman AB. Are neuroendocrine tumors a feature of tuberous sclerosis? A systematic review. Endocr Relat Cancer 2009;16:45–58.
12 Bizzarri C, Bottaro G. Endocrine implications of neurofibromatosis 1 in childhood. Horm Res Pediatr 2015;83:232–41.
13 Amato MC, Elias LL, Elias J et al. Endocrine disorders in pediatric-onset Langerhans cell histiocytosis. Horm Metab Res 2006;38:746–51.
14 Marina S, Broshilova V. POEMS in childhood. Pediatr Dermatol 2006; 23:145–8.
15 Vennos EM, Collins M, James WD. Rothmund-Thomson syndrome: review of the world literature. J Am Acad Dermatol 1992;27:750–62.
16 Halabi-Tawil M, Ruemmele FM, Fraitag S et al. Cutaneous manifestations of immune dysregulation, polyendocrinopathy, enteropathy, X-linked (IPEX) syndrome. Br J Dermatol 2009;160:645–51.
17 Gupta V, Patra S, Firdaus Ali M et al. Sclerodermoid hypertrichotic plaques with insulin-dependent diabetes mellitus. Pediatr Dermatol 2015;32:731–2.
18 Nanda A, Pasternack SM, Mahmoudi H et al. Alopecia and hypotrichosis as characteristic findings in Woodhouse-Sakati syndrome: report of a family with mutation in the C2orf37 gene. Pediatr Dermatol 2014;31:83–7.
19 Kalkan E, Waguespack SG. Endocrine tumors associated with neurofibromatosis type 1, peutz-jeghers syndrome and other familial neoplasia syndromes. Front Horm Res 2013;41:166–81.
20 Hawli Y, Nasrallah M, El-Haji Fuleihan G. Endocrine and musculoskeletal abnormalities in patients with Down syndrome. Nat Rev Endocrinol 2009;5:327–34.

CHAPTER 155
Autoinflammatory Diseases and Amyloidosis

Antonio Torrelo[1], Sergio Hernández-Ostiz[1] & Teri A. Kahn[2]

[1] Department of Dermatology, Hospital Infantil del Niño Jesús, Madrid, Spain
[2] Department of Dermatology, University of Maryland, MD, USA

Autoinflammatory diseases, 2010
Amyloidosis, 2023

Abstract

Autoinflammatory diseases (AIDs) are genetic diseases of the innate immune system causing a permanent state of inflammation with exacerbations caused by common triggers such as physical agents or infection. They are caused by heterogeneous gene mutations and present with many different clinical manifestations. However, most AIDs will have prominent cutaneous manifestations with an early onset of disease; these may consist of urticaria and oedemas, pustules, mucosal lesions, granulomatous skin lesions or vasculopathy. Any child with recurrent fevers, skin rash, elevation of acute phase reactants and systemic symptoms should be evaluated for an AID. Early recognition of AIDs is key because many of them can be effectively treated with targeted biologic therapy. Amyloidosis in children is usually the result of chronic inflammation and is related to long-standing or poorly controlled AIDs. Less commonly, genetic causes of amyloidosis or the well-known types usually occurring in adults can be seen in children.

Key points

- Autoinflammatory diseases (AIDs) are the result of mutations in many different genes regulating innate immunity.
- An early onset of recurrent fevers, skin rashes and systemic inflammation should raise an alert for an AID.
- AIDs should be rapidly recognized and treated with targeted biologic therapy.
- Amyloidosis is a severe complication of untreated AIDs.

Autoinflammatory diseases

Introduction

The immune system in humans provides protection against microbial infections, other external harmful molecules and cell waste or material from cell death. It is a complex structure involving a large number of defence molecules and cells. The most sophisticated branch of the immune system is called 'adaptive immunity' which has been the subject of intense research. Adaptive immunity provides protection for pluricellular individuals, and acts through recognition of antigens by T- or B-cell receptors, permitting adaption to new pathogens by complex genetic rearrangements and somatic mutations to create a repertoire of immune memory; it is thus directed against changing microbial molecules. Recently, another branch of immunity, common both to unicellular and pluricellular individuals, has gained considerable attention, and has been named 'innate immunity'. Innate immunity acts in an antigen-independent way and is activated by recognition of small pattern molecules associated with infectious pathogens (PAMPS, pathogen-associated molecular patterns) or damage (DAMPS, damage-associated molecular patterns). They are recognized both by extracellular receptors (Toll-like receptors) or intracellular receptors (NOD-like receptors or NLRP receptors), which activate multiple inflammatory signalling cascades and recruit cellular effectors of innate immunity, such as macrophages, neutrophils, mast cells and natural killer cells. Thus, innate immunity is not subject to adaptation or adjustment, does not change with age and is directed against invariable microbial or damage molecules that have been present for millions of years. Adaptive and innate immunity do not act separately but interact to provide a combined defence of maximal efficacy against external and internal agents [1].

Immune system pathology can be grouped under several broad headings. Firstly, related to states of insufficient protection, where the result will be immunodeficiency, either of the innate or the adaptive branches, or both. Secondly, an excessive 'response to self' by adaptive immunity will cause the production of autoantibodies that are mainly responsible for the well-known autoimmune diseases. Finally, an inappropriate hyperactive state of the innate immune system causes a continuous state of inflammation that is characteristic of a group of diseases collectively named 'autoinflammatory diseases'. This group of diseases is characterized by unexplained recurrent episodes of fever and severe

Harper's Textbook of Pediatric Dermatology, Fourth Edition. Edited by Peter Hoeger, Veronica Kinsler and Albert Yan.

localized inflammation without infections, neoplasms or high-titre autoantibodies [2]. It should be noted, however, that because both innate and adaptive immunity work in combination, a clear distinction between autoimmune and autoinflammatory diseases is an artifact, and there are many inflammatory disorders in which features of both types of diseases can be seen, with variable predominance of one or another.

Inflammation is a defensive reaction but causes local and systemic symptoms. The innate immune response needs fine regulation to permit a certain degree of self-damage to cells sufficient for elimination of the intruder pathogen with eventual cell survival or controlled cellular suicide, a phenomenon named pyroptosis. Furthermore, inhibitory mechanisms must be finely regulated to ensure the return to a noninflammatory state once the pathogen has been destroyed or cleared. Any disturbance in these fine mechanisms will lead to a disease of a constitutive proinflammatory state. In this state, usual triggers of autoinflammation (cold, stress, pathogens or toxic exposure) will lead to abnormally violent inflammatory attacks that may also take longer to subside. In humans, single gene mutations have been discovered as the cause of this group of autoinflammatory diseases (AIDs). They are of notable interest to the paediatric dermatologist, because most of these AIDs begin in infancy or early childhood, and have initial or prominent manifestations in the skin.

AIDs (Table 155.1) have been classified by different methods, according to the gene mutations responsible, the mechanisms involved or the organs involved. For this

Table 155.1 A summary of the main autoinflammatory diseases with their responsible mutations

Disease	Heredity	Genetic mutation	Mutated protein
Familial Mediterranean fever	AR	MEFV	Pyrin
Mevalonate kinase deficiency (hyper-IgD syndrome)	AR	*MVK*	Mevalonate kinase
Tumour necrosis factor receptor-associated periodic syndrome (TRAPS)	AD	TNFRSF1A	TNFR (TNF receptor) superfamily IA
Periodic fever with aphtous stomatitis, pharyngitis and adenitis syndrome (PFAPA)	Unknown	Unknown	Unknown
PLCG2-associated antibody deficiency and immune dysregulation (PLAID)/autoinflammation and PLCG2-associated antibody deficiency and immune dysregulation (APLAID)	AD	PLCG2	Phospholipase CG2 (PLCG2)
Familial cold autoinflammatory syndrome	AD	NLRP3/CIAS1	Cryopyrin
Muckle–Wells syndrome	AD	NLRP3/CIAS1	Cryopyrin
Neonatal onset multisystemic inflammatory disorder (NOMID)	AD	NLRP3/CIAS1	Cryopyrin
Deficiency of the interleukin-1 receptor antagonist (DIRA)	AR	IL-1RN	Interleukin-1 receptor antagonist
Deficiency of the interleukin-36 receptor antagonist (DITRA)	AR	IL-36RN	Interleukin-36 receptor antagonist
Pyogenic arthritis, pyoderma gangrenosum and acne syndrome (PAPA)	AD	PSTPIP1/CD2BP1	Proline/serine/threonine phosphatase-interacting protein 1
Majeed syndrome	AR	LPIN2	Lipin 2
Blau syndrome	AD	NOD2/CARD15	Nucleotide-binding oligomerization domain protein 2
H-syndrome	AR	SLC29A3	Human equilibrative nucleoside transporter 3 (hENT3)
Chronic atypical neutrophilic dermatosis with lipodystrophy and elevated temperature (CANDLE) syndrome	AR	PSMB8 PSMB4 PSMB9 PSMA3 POMP	i-proteasome β5i subunit Proteasome β7 subunit i-proteasome β1i subunit Preoteasome α3 subunit Proteasome maturation protein
Aicardi–Goutières syndrome	AR (rarely AD)	TREX1 (AGS1) RNASEH2 (AGS 2-4) SAMHD1 (AGS5) ADAR1 (AGS6) IFIH1 (AGS7)	3-prime repair exonuclease 1 RNASEH2 endonuclease complex SAM domain- and HD domain-containing protein 1 RNA-specific adenosine deaminase 1 interferon-induced helicase c domain-containing protein 1
Familial chilblain lupus	AD	TREX1 (AGS1) SAMHD1 (AGS5	3-prime repair exonuclease 1 SAM domain- and HD domain containing protein 1
STING-associated vasculopathy with onset in infancy (SAVI)	AD	TMEM173	Stimulator of interferon genes (STING)
Deficiency of adenosone deaminase 2 (DADA2)	AR	CECR1	Adenosine deaminase 2

AD, autosomal dominant; AR, autosomal recessive.

chapter, we will use a classification most useful to the paediatric dermatologist, based in the main type of skin manifestation, namely (i) urticarial and oedematous diseases; (ii) pustular diseases; (iii) mucosal diseases; (iv) histiocytic and granulomatous diseases; and (v) vasculopathic diseases.

References

1 Medzhitov R. Inflammation 2010: new adventures of an old flame. Cell 2010;140:771–6.

2 Dávila-Seijo P, Hernández-Martín A, Torrelo A. Autoinflammatory syndromes for the dermatologist. Clin Dermatol 2014;32:488–501.

Urticarial and oedematous diseases

In this group of AIDs, the main skin manifestations are recurrent skin swellings with erythema or oedematous wheals. It comprises a genetically heterogeneous group of diseases, although most of them are caused by mutations in the NLRP inflammasomes or in related regulatory proteins.

Cryopyrin-associated periodic syndromes

The cryopyrin-associated periodic syndromes (CAPS) or cryopyrinopathies, are caused by different mutations in the *NLRP3* gene (previously called *CIAS1*), which encodes a protein named cryopyrin. Cryopyrin activation leads to caspase 1 activation, which in turn converts pro-IL-1β and pro-IL-18 into IL-1β and IL-18, leading to biological proinflammatory effects. The CAPS are inherited in an autosomal dominant fashion, although cases caused by somatic mosaic mutations are well recognized [1]; in all cases, self-activating mutations lead to constitutive activation of the NLRP3 inflammasome.

Three main allelic diseases are included here.

Familial cold autoinflammatory syndrome

Familial cold autoinflammatory syndrome (FCAS) is the mildest of all CAPS [2,3]. Manifestations usually occur after 2–7 hours of generalized cold exposure. An urticarial rash is the main skin sign, which may itch, burn or sting. Contact with cold objects does not elicit the rash. Skin histopathology shows mild dermal oedema and a slight perivascular infiltrate rich in neutrophils; vasculitis is not seen [4,5]. The urticarial rash may be accompanied by fever, conjunctival infection, arthralgias, malaise, headache and myalgias. Episodes usually resolve in less than 24 hours after avoidance of cold. Transient leukocytosis is usually the only laboratory abnormality. In contrast with other CAPS, amyloidosis rarely occurs.

Muckle–Wells syndrome

Muckle–Wells syndrome (MWS) was formerly known as the triad of urticaria, deafness and amyloidosis syndrome. It shares many features with FCAS but shows a more severe phenotype. Onset usually occurs in early childhood and skin lesions are clinically and histopathologically similar to FCAS [4]. However, episodes last longer (up to 36 hours) and occur more frequently than in FCAS [6,7]. Cochlear and meningeal inflammation cause progressive sensorineural hearing loss in childhood that may evolve to complete deafness. The state of chronic inflammation is also supposed to be the cause of secondary amyloidosis, which occurs later in life in up to 25% of patients [6,7].

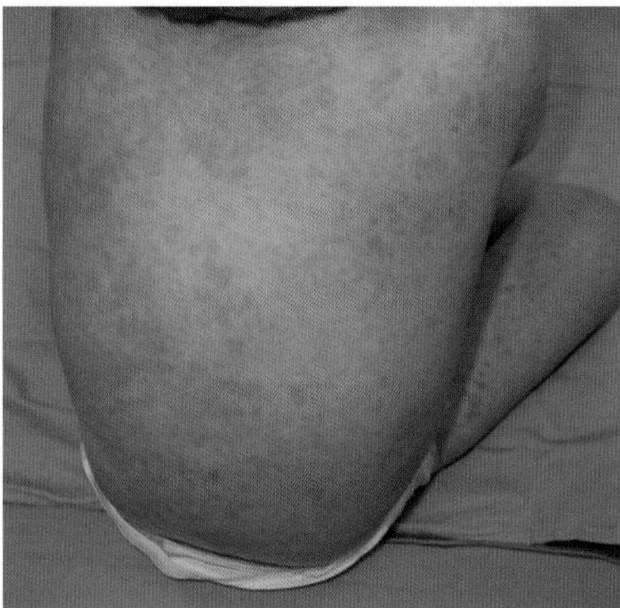

Fig. 155.1 Urticarial eruption in a child with neonatal onset multisystemic inflammatory disorder.

Neonatal onset multisystemic inflammatory disorder

Neonatal onset multisystemic inflammatory disorder (NOMID) is less commonly named CINCA (chronic infantile neurological cutaneous and articular syndrome). It is the most severe of the CAPS and can cause severe disability and mortality [8,9]. Onset is usually before 6 months of age and frequently during the neonatal period. The earliest sign consists of recurrent or continuous urticaria that can appear at birth in up to two-thirds of affected newborns (Fig. 155.1). Histopathology often shows superficial and deep perivascular infiltrates with lymphocytes, neuthrophils and some eosinophils [10], and in some instances neutrophilic eccrine hidradenitis can occur [11]. Certain facial features, such as flattened nasal bridge, frontal bossing and protruding eyes may provide an early clue to diagnosis [12]. The presence of urticaria with neutrophils on histopathology and abnormal facies in a newborn is highly suggestive of NOMID, and a genetic diagnosis must be obtained as soon as possible because early treatment can prevent serious manifestations. Short episodes of fever can occur but may appear later in life.

The most severe manifestations of NOMID appear progressively during life. Neurological manifestations include chronic aseptic meningitis, cerebral atrophy, sensorineural hearing loss, increased intracranial pressure and developmental delay. Anterior uveitis and papilloedema may lead to blindness [13]. Severe arthropathy can occur as early as 12 months of age in 50% of patients. Milder cases may only show pain and joint effusion, but severely affected children exhibit exuberant cartilaginous proliferations with secondary ossification resembling tumours [14]. Other features include enlarged lymph nodes, hepatosplenomegaly and secondary amyloidosis [4]. Laboratory analyses are usually relatively unhelpful, with only minor anomalies observed such as elevated erythrocyte sedimentation rate (ESR) and C-reactive protein (CRP), leukocytosis, thrombocytosis, eosinophilia and hyperglobulinaemia.

Therapy of CAPS

A considerable change in the prognosis of the most severe forms of CAPS has been achieved with the use of anti-IL-1 biologic agents. Anakinra, the IL-1 receptor antagonist, prevents attacks and decreases constitutive proinflammation, but requires daily subcutaneous injections. It also reduces the risk of secondary amyloidosis and there is evidence to suggest prevention of deafness. It should be administered as soon as a diagnosis is achieved, because its role in established manifestations of NOMID may be variable [15]. Canakinumab is a longer-lasting human anti-IL-1β monoclonal antibody that has shown sustained responses in CAPS, although at the expense of a possible increase in infections [15]. Rilonacept, a weekly subcutaneous IL-1 trap also appears to be an effective agent in CAPS [15].

Familial Mediterranean fever

Familial Mediterranean fever (FMF) is most commonly reported in Europe, North Africa and the Middle East [16]. It is a recessive disorder caused by homozygous or compound heterozygous mutations in the gene *MEFV* (MEditerranean FeVer), which encodes a protein named pyrin (or marenostrin). These mutations are usually missense and cause a loss of function of pyrin that acts as a main regulatory component of the NLRP3 inflammasome [17,18]. Up to 25% of patients, however, are heterozygous for *MEFV* mutations and present with milder clinical manifestations [19,20]. Certain environmental and genetic factors could modulate the manifestations of FMF [21].

FMF usually appears in childhood or adolescence [22]. The main skin manifestations are well-circumscribed, oedematous and erythematous plaques of up to 15 cm in diameter, mainly located on the lower extremities. These are termed erysipeloid-like lesions and appear in 15–20% of affected children [23,24]. Histopathology reveals a predominantly neutrophilic infiltrate with nuclear dust [25]. Other skin lesions in FMF include purpura and lobar panniculitis. Henoch–Schönlein purpura and polyarteritis nodosa seem to be more frequent in patients with FMF [26–29].

Systemic signs of FMF include episodic attacks of fever. They are accompanied by abdominal pain, pleurisy and mono- or oligoarticular arthritis or arthralgias [30]. Other less frequent signs are pericarditis or acute scrotal pain [31]. Attacks are self-limited, usually lasting less than 72 hours, and the patients remain asymptomatic between the attacks. These can be triggered by physical exercise, emotional stress, exposure to extreme temperatures and hormonal changes [30]. The most serious complication of FMF is amyloid A (AA) amyloidosis, which can lead to renal and hepatic dysfunction. Amyloidosis does not necessarily correlate with the frequency or intensity of the inflammatory attacks [21].

Laboratory investigations during acute attacks show elevation of ESR, CRP, beta-2 microglobulin, serum amyloid protein, fibrinogen and leukocytosis with increased neutrophil counts [30].

Continuous treatment with colchicine reduces the frequency, intensity and duration of the attacks. It has been associated with a decreased risk of amyloidosis. It should be started as soon as a diagnosis of FMF is made and maintained for life [30]. In colchicine-resistant patients, thalidomide, anti-TNFα agents such as etanercept and infliximab, and anakinra may be of use [32,33].

Mevalonate kinase deficiency

Mevalonate kinase deficiency (MKD) was formerly known as hyper-IgD syndrome (HIDS), but elevated IgD levels are not universally present in all patients and they do not seem to be responsible for any of the clinical manifestations. The gene responsible for MKD is the mevalonate kinase (*MVK*) gene [34], and the syndrome is caused by heterozygous mutations; the homozygous state, with complete absence of MK function, causes mevalonic aciduria [35]. MVK is an enzyme in the synthesis pathway of cholesterol/isoprenoids. It also acts as a negative regulator of caspase 1 in the NLRP3 inflammasome. *MVK* mutations in MKD produce a temperature-dependent MVK enzyme, whose activity is impaired at higher temperatures [36,37]. Thus, MKD attacks are triggered by events capable of inducing elevation in body temperature [38].

MKD usually appears during the first year of life. The skin manifestations in MKD are heterogeneous but appear in up to 80% of patients. The most frequent is a macular, erythematous eruption composed of solitary patches that may coalesce, usually located on the lower limbs and acral parts of the body. Other less common lesions include papules, erythematous nodules, urticarial lesions and petechiae. Histopathology usually shows endothelial swelling and perivascular inflammatory infiltrates. Description of skin diseases in patients with MKD have included Henoch–Schönlein purpura, erythema elevatum diutinum-like lesions, Sweet-like disease, cellulitis-like lesions and deep vasculitis [4,39,40].

In MKD, episodic attacks of fever last 4–7 days and occur every 4–8 weeks. They may be associated with prodromal symptoms such as headache, fatigue and nasal congestion. During the attacks, localized or generalized tender lymphadenopathy, abdominal pain, splenomegaly and polyarticular joint involvement may occur [39]. Joint involvement seldom causes joint destruction. Amyloidosis is an infrequent complication of MKD [40]. Patients remain asymptomatic between the attacks, although join and skin manifestations may last longer than the fevers [4,38]. Laboratory studies usually show elevated IgD and often IgA levels [39,41], but IgD levels can be normal.

Treatment of the attacks is based on nonsteroidal anti-inflammatory drugs (NSAIDs). Short courses of oral corticosteroids may be used in more severe instances.

Colchicine, cyclosporine, intravenous immunoglobulin G and thalidomide have been unsuccessful. Etanercept was used with variable results and a few cases have been treated successfully with anakinra [42].

Tumour necrosis factor receptor-associated periodic syndrome

Tumour necrosis factor receptor-associated periodic syndrome (TRAPS) or familial Hibernian fever is a dominantly inherited AID caused by a genetic mutation in the gene *TNFR* superfamily IA [43,44]. The tumour necrosis factor receptor (TNFR) acts as an antagonist to circulating TNF and plays a role in cellular functions related to pyrexia, cachexia, cytokine production, leukocyte activation, expression of adhesion molecules and resistance to cellular pathogens.

TRAPS symptoms may start from infancy to adulthood [45]. Patients with TRAPS suffer recurrent episodes of fever, myalgia with a characteristic distal migration, arthralgias, abdominal pain and conjunctivitis [4,46]. These attacks usually last less than one month. Most patients show skin lesions; the most frequent is called 'painful erythema' and consists of a centrifugally migrating erythema overlying the area with myalgia. Painful erythema typically migrates proximal to distal, accompanied by myalgia. Other less common lesions are urticarial lesions and erythematous macules and papules that may coalesce into an annular or serpiginous arrangement. Skin pathology shows perivascular and interstitial infiltrates of mononuclear cells. Small-vessel vasculitis and panniculitis may occur in TRAPS [47].

As with other AIDs, laboratory analyses only show elevated ESR and CRP during attacks. Antinuclear antibodies and rheumatoid factor are rarely present [46]. Systemic amyloidosis develops in up to 25% of patients [48].

TRAPS is responsive to oral corticosteroids, but not to colchicine. Anti-TNF drugs may induce variable responses. For example, etanercept can decrease but not eliminate the symptoms and infliximab can even precipitate paradoxical attacks. This suggests that the pathophysiology of TRAPS is complex and may be also related to intracellular aggregation of misfolded TNFR1 or other mechanisms leading to continuous signal activation [49]. In this way, the recombinant IL-1 receptor antagonist anakinra may show better results than anti-TNF agents.

Other urticarial and oedematous syndromes

AISLE (autoinflammatory syndrome with lymphoedema) is a syndrome featuring extensive urticarial eruption and fever, accompanied by progressive oedema of the scrotum and lower limbs. A decrease in the number and size of lymphatic vessels is seen on histopathology. AISLE is caused by mutations in the gene *MDFIC* (MyoD family inhibitor domain containing) [50].

Heterozygous gain-of-function mutations in the NLRC4 inflammasome cause a distinctive syndrome with erythematous skin nodules, urticaria, arthralgias and late-onset enterocholitis. Patients with this syndrome are partially responsive to anakinra [51].

PLAID (PLCG2-associated antibody deficiency and immune dysregulation) progresses with the combination of atypical cold urticaria with early onset and lifelong duration plus immunological defects, including antibody deficiency, recurrent infections and autoimmunity. Some patients suffer cutaneous granulomas. Patients with PLAID have heterozygous deletions in the *PLCG2* gene, located in a domain that normally prevents constitutive enzymatic function, thus resulting in a gain-of-function in phospholipase activity [52].

References

1 Tanaka T, Takahashi K, Yamane M et al. Induced pluripotent stem cells from CINCA syndrome patients as a model for dissecting somatic mosaicism and drug discovery. Blood 2012;120:1299–308.

2 Hoffman HM, Wanderer AA, Broide DH. Familial cold autoinflammatory syndrome: phenotype and genotype of an autosomal dominant periodic fever. J Allergy Clin Immunol 2001;108:615–20.

3 Doeglas HM, Bleumink E. Familial cold urticaria. Clinical findings. Arch Dermatol 1974;110:382–8.

4 Farasat S, Aksentijevich I, Toro JR. Autoinflammatory diseases: clinical and genetic advances. Arch Dermatol 2008;144:392–402.

5 Peroni A, Colato C, Zanoni G, Girolomoni G. Urticarial lesions: if not urticaria, what else? The differential diagnosis of urticaria: part II. Systemic diseases. J Am Acad Dermatol 2010;62:557–70; quiz 71–2.

6 Muckle TJ, Wells M. Urticaria, deafness, and amyloidosis: a new heredo-familial syndrome. Q J Med 1962;31:235–48.

7 Muckle TJ. The 'Muckle-Wells' syndrome. Br J Dermatol 1979; 100:87–92.

8 Aksentijevich I, Putnam CD, Remmers EF et al. The clinical continuum of cryopyrinopathies: novel CIAS1 mutations in North American patients and a new cryopyrin model. Arthritis Rheum 2007;56:1273–85.

9 Aksentijevich I, Nowak M, Mallah M et al. De novo CIAS1 mutations, cytokine activation, and evidence for genetic heterogeneity in patients with neonatal-onset multisystem inflammatory disease (NOMID): a new member of the expanding family of pyrin-associated autoinflammatory diseases. Arthritis Rheum 2002;46:3340–8.

10 Goldbach-Mansky R, Dailey NJ, Canna SW et al. Neonatal-onset multisystem inflammatory disease responsive to interleukin-1(beta) inhibition. N Engl J Med 2006;355:581–92.

11 Huttenlocher A, Frieden IJ, Emery H. Neonatal onset multisystem inflammatory disease. J Rheumatol 1995;22:1171–3.

12 Goldfinger S. The inherited autoinflammatory syndrome: a decade of discovery. Trans Am Clin Climatol Assoc 2009;120:413–8.

13 Ahmadi N, Brewer CC, Zalewski C et al. Cryopyrin-associated periodic syndromes: otolaryngologic and audiologic manifestations. Otolaryngol Head Neck Surg 2011;145:295–302.

14 Prieur AM. A recently recognised chronic inflammatory disease of early onset characterised by the triad of rash, central nervous system involvement and arthropathy. Clin Exp Rheumatol 2001; 19:103–6.

15 Nigrovic PA. Cryopyrin-associated periodic syndromes and related disorders. UpToDate 2017. ®2019.

16 Ben-Chetrit E, Touitou I. Familial mediterranean Fever in the world. Arthritis Rheum 2009;61:1447–53.

17 Ancient missense mutations in a new member of the RoRet gene family are likely to cause familial Mediterranean fever. The International FMF Consortium. Cell 1997;90:797–807.

18 French FMF Consortium. A candidate gene for familial Mediterranean fever. Nat Genet 1997;17:25–31.

19 Marek-Yagel D, Berkun Y, Padeh S et al. Clinical disease among patients heterozygous for familial Mediterranean fever. Arthritis Rheum 2009;60:1862–6.

20 Booty MG, Chae JJ, Masters SL et al. Familial Mediterranean fever with a single MEFV mutation: where is the second hit? Arthritis Rheum 2009;60:1851–61.

21 Pras M. Amyloidosis of familial mediterranean fever and the MEFV gene. Amyloid 2000;7:289–93.

22 Sohar E, Gafni J, Pras M, Heller H. Familial Mediterranean fever. A survey of 470 cases and review of the literature. Am J Med 1967;43:227–53.

23 Majeed HA, Quabazard Z, Hijazi Z et al. The cutaneous manifestations in children with familial Mediterranean fever (recurrent hereditary polyserositis). A six-year study. Q J Med 1990;75:607–16.
24 Rawashdeh MO, Majeed HA. Familial mediterranean fever in Arab children: the high prevalence and gene frequency. Eur J Pediatr 1996;155:540–4.
25 Barzilai A, Langevitz P, Goldberg I et al. Erysipelas-like erythema of familial Mediterranean fever: clinicopathologic correlation. J Am Acad Dermatol 2000;42:791–5.
26 Ozen S, Ben-Chetrit E, Bakkaloglu A et al. Polyarteritis nodosa in patients with Familial Mediterranean Fever (FMF): a concomitant disease or a feature of FMF? Semin Arthritis Rheum 2001;30:281–7.
27 Ozdogan H, Arisoy N, Kasapcapur O et al. Vasculitis in familial Mediterranean fever. J Rheumatol 1997;24:323–7.
28 Bosacki C, Richard O, Freycon F et al. [The association of polyarteritis nodosa and familial Mediterranean fever]. Presse Med 2003;32:24–6.
29 Tinaztepe K, Gucer S, Bakkaloglu A, Tinaztepe B. Familial Mediterranean fever and polyarteritis nodosa: experience of five paediatric cases. A causal relationship or coincidence? Eur J Pediatr 1997;156:505–6.
30 Ben-Chetrit A. Clinical manifestations and diagnosis of familial Mediterranean fever. UpToDate 2018. ©2019.
31 Kees S, Langevitz P, Zemer D et al. Attacks of pericarditis as a manifestation of familial Mediterranean fever (FMF). QJ Med 1997;90:643–7.
32 Ben-Chetrit A. Management of familial Mediterranean fever. UpToDate 2018. ©2019.
33 Seyahi E, Ozdogan H, Celik S et al. Treatment options in colchicine resistant familial Mediterranean fever patients: thalidomide and etanercept as adjunctive agents. Clin Exp Rheumatol 2006;24:S99–103.
34 Calligaris L, Marchetti F, Tommasini A, Ventura A. The efficacy of anakinra in an adolescent with colchicine-resistant familial Mediterranean fever. Eur J Pediatr 2008;167:695–6.
35 Drenth JP, Cuisset L, Grateau G et al. Mutations in the gene encoding mevalonate kinase cause hyper-IgD and periodic fever syndrome. International Hyper-IgD Study Group. Nat Genet 1999;22:178–81.
36 Houten SM, Frenkel J, Rijkers GT et al. Temperature dependence of mutant mevalonate kinase activity as a pathogenic factor in hyper-IgD and periodic fever syndrome. Hum Mol Genet 2002;11:3115–24.
37 Padeh YC, Rubinstein A. Hyperimmunoglobulin-D syndrome: Pathophysiology. UpToDate 2018. ©2019.
38 Drenth JP, Haagsma CJ, van der Meer JW. Hyperimmunoglobulinemia D and periodic fever syndrome. The clinical spectrum in a series of 50 patients. International Hyper-IgD Study Group. Medicine (Baltimore) 1994;73:133–44.
39 Drenth JP, Boom BW, Toonstra J, Van der Meer JW. Cutaneous manifestations and histologic findings in the hyperimmunoglobulinemia D syndrome. International Hyper IgD Study Group. Arch Dermatol 1994;130:59–65.
40 van der Hilst JC, Simon A, Drenth JP. Hereditary periodic fever and reactive amyloidosis. Clin Exp Med 2005;5:87–98.
41 Di Rocco M, Caruso U, Waterham HR et al. Mevalonate kinase deficiency in a child with periodic fever and without hyperimmunoglobulinaemia D. J Inherit Metab Dis 2001;24:411–2.
42 Padeh YC, Rubinstein A. Hyperimmunoglobulin-D syndrome: Management. UpToDate 2018. ©2019.
43 McDermott MF, Ogunkolade BW, McDermott EM et al. Linkage of familial Hibernian fever to chromosome 12p13. Am J Hum Genet 1998;62:1446–51.
44 Mulley J, Saar K, Hewitt G et al. Gene localization for an autosomal dominant familial periodic fever to 12p13. Am J Hum Genet 1998;62:884–9.
45 Kanazawa N, Furukawa F. Autoinflammatory syndromes with a dermatological perspective. J Dermatol 2007;34:601–18.
46 Hull KM, Drewe E, Aksentijevich I et al. The TNF receptor-associated periodic syndrome (TRAPS): emerging concepts of an autoinflammatory disorder. Medicine (Baltimore) 2002;81:349–68.
47 Toro JR, Aksentijevich I, Hull K et al. Tumor necrosis factor receptor-associated periodic syndrome: a novel syndrome with cutaneous manifestations. Arch Dermatol 2000;136:1487–94.
48 Kallinich T, Briese S, Roesler J et al. Two familial cases with tumor necrosis factor receptor-associated periodic syndrome caused by a non-cysteine mutation (T50M) in the TNFRSF1A gene associated with severe multiorganic amyloidosis. J Rheumatol 2004;31:2519–22.
49 Nigrovic PA. Tumor necrosis factor receptor-1 associated periodic syndrome (TRAPS). UpToDate 2018. ©2019.
50 Xirotagaros G, Hernández-Ostiz S, Aróstegui JI, Torrelo A. Newly described autoinflammatory diseases in pediatric dermatology. Pediatr Dermatol 2016;33:602–14.
51 Volker-Touw CM, de Koning HD, Giltay J et al. Erythematous nodes, urticarial rash and arthralgias in a large pedigree with NLRC4-related autoinflammatory disease, expansion of the phenotype. Br J Dermatol 2017;176:244–8.
52 Ombrello MJ, Remmers EF, Sun G et al. Cold urticaria, immunodeficiency, and autoimmunity related to PLCG2 deletions. New Eng J Med 2012;366:330–8.

Pustular diseases

Pustular eruptions can be the predominant manifestation of certain AIDs. They may appear as exanthematic pustular lesions overlying more or less diffuse erythema, and thus may resemble pustular psoriasis, both clinically and pathologically. In other diseases, acne-like, pyoderma-like, Sweet-like or pustular vasculopathy may be present.

Deficiency of the IL-1 receptor antagonist

This AID is caused by biallelic germ-line mutations in *IL1RN* [1,2], that disable the protein's antagonistic activity at the IL-1 receptor. Thus, absence of IL-1 signaling down-regulation leads to a continuous activation of IL-1 inflammatory pathways. Heterozygous carriers are usually asymptomatic or may have mild manifestations. Deficiency of the IL-1 receptor antagonist (DIRA) starts at birth or in early infancy, usually with skin lesions and fever. A generalized erythema with small overlying pustules that may eventually lead to diffuse desquamation simulates generalized pustular psoriasis. It often spares palms and soles, but nails often show pitting and onycomadesis. A vesicular stomatitis or mouth ulcers are also described. Some cases have shown pathergy [3,4]. Histopathology of skin lesions also resembles pustular psoriasis: parakeratosis with subcorneal microabscesses or spongiform neutrophilic pustules are seen, as well as a dermal neutrophilic infiltrate. Concomitant superficial folliculitis and/or neutrophilic eccrine hidradenitis may occur. Inmunofluorescence studies are negative [3,4].

With time, untreated patients develop extracutaneous manifestations. Chronic recurrent episodes of multifocal aseptic osteomyelitis and periostitis may occur very early. Other skeletal manifestations may ensue, which includes osteopenia, periarticular swelling, long-bone epiphyseal overgrowth, cervical vertebral fusion and widening of clavicle and anterior rib ends. Recurrent fever and failure to thrive also occur. Other less common manifestations of DIRA are respiratory distress, pulmonary infiltrates, thrombotic episodes and vasculitis. If untreated, DIRA may be fatal. Laboratory analyses barely show an increase in acute-phase reactants, mild anaemia and blood leukocytosis with neutrophilia [1–4].

The diagnosis of DIRA must be genetically confirmed, and immediate treatment with daily subcutaneous injections of anakinra, the recombinant analogue of IL-1RN, must be started. This treatment often leads to complete resolution of cutaneous and osteoarticular manifestations in most patients with DIRA and partial resolution in some of them [5]. Longer-acting anti-IL-1 such as canakinumab and rilonacept can be considered later in life, once clinical control is achieved, to avoid daily injections.

Deficiency of the IL-36 receptor antagonist

Deficiency of the IL-36 receptor antagonist (DITRA) is a disease similar to DIRA and is caused by mostly biallelic mutations in the IL-36 receptor antagonist (IL-36RN). Patients with these genetic abnormalities exhibit a phenotype of generalized or, less commonly, localized pustular psoriasis, usually without preceding plaque psoriatic lesions. It has also been recognized as the cause of many familial and sporadic cases of generalized pustular psoriasis [6,7]. In familial cases DITRA has an autosomal recessive inheritance. IL-36RN is a protein of the IL-1 cytokine family which is abundantly expressed in the skin. It acts as a competitive inhibitor of IL-36. In the absence of IL-36RN, proinflammatory IL-36-derived signalling cannot be downregulated, leading to continuous or recurring inflammation. IL-36 exerts varied actions and has an important role in the NF-κB pathway [6,7].

DITRA progresses with sudden and/or recurrent episodes of skin lesions that often are associated with fever, malaise and asthenia (Fig. 155.2). Involvement of other organs has been rarely reported. However, DITRA attacks may be life threatening and there is an increased risk of sepsis. Onset may occur during infancy or early childhood, but cases in the elderly have been reported. Triggers for the attacks include bacterial and viral infections, menstruation, pregnancy or drugs [6,7], and possibly psychological stress or trauma, amongst others. The skin lesions in DITRA are often indistinguishable from severe generalized pustular psoriasis; in fact, it is possible that a genetic study of all cases of recurrent generalized pustular psoriasis might show that IL-36RN mutations underlies a significant proportion of such cases. Other cases may be well explained by mutations in other genes, including *CARD14* [8]. A violent onset of a generalized pustular eruption occurs over deeply erythematous or violaceous skin. Psoriasis vulgaris lesions are generally lacking, but possible. Annular or arciform pustular lesions may appear in other cases. The morphology of skin lesions can be different in different attacks. Localized pustular eruptions and acral pustular lesions with nail destruction such as acrodermatitis continua of Hallopeau are recognized to be within the genetic spectrum of DITRA [9]. Histopathology of the skin shows the typical features of pustular psoriasis: spongiform pustules, psoriasiform acanthosis and parakeratosis in the stratum corneum [7].

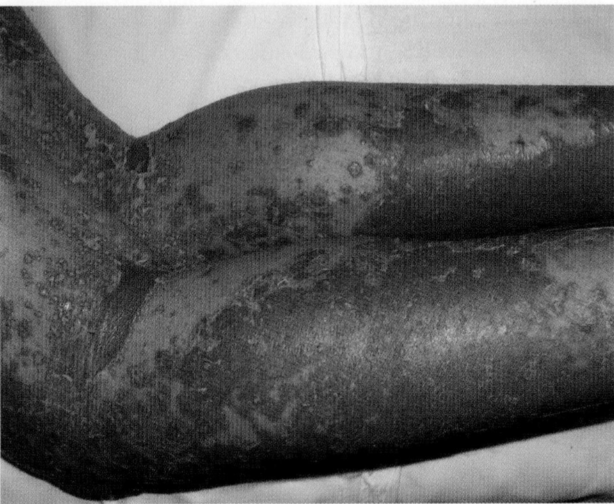

Fig. 155.2 Deficiency of the IL-36 receptor antagonist presenting as an acute attack of pustular psoriasis.

Treatment of DITRA is difficult and often unsatisfactory. Some cases may show transient improvement with acitretin, cyclosporin, corticosteroids or methotrexate. No specific biologic agent is currently available. Anakinra and adalimumab can induce good responses in some cases, but these may be transient.

Pyogenic arthritis, pyoderma gangrenosum and acne syndrome and related AIDS

Pyogenic arthritis, pyoderma gangrenosum and acne syndrome

Pyogenic arthritis, pyoderma gangrenosum and acne syndrome (PAPA) is an autosomal dominant disease caused by heterozygous mutations in the gene proline/serine/threonine phosphatase-interacting protein 1 (*PSTPIP1*). *PSTPIP1* is mainly expressed in haematopoietic cells and has modulatory actions on T-cell activation and cytoskeletal organization. Furthermore, *PSTPIP1* binds to pyrin, which in turn modulates the inflammasome NLRP3 and thus is a regulator of IL-1β release. PAPA-producing mutations in *PSTPIP1* increase its avidity for pyrin, which cannot bind the inflammasome and leads to IL-1β overproduction [10]. There are, however, other cases of PAPA without *PSTPIP1* mutations [11], and conversely *PSTPIP1* mutations have been described in an overlapping syndrome named PASH (pyoderma gangrenosum, acne and suppurative hidradenitis, see later) [12].

Clinically, PAPA progresses with skin pustular lesions and recurrent episodes of sterile arthritis, usually appearing during childhood. The skin lesions consist of severe cystic acne-like lesions, showing pathergy phenomenon. Also, recurrent sterile ulcers with undermined borders that mimic pyoderma gangrenosum occur; they leave a cribiform scarring. Some patients show milder manifestations resembling psoriasis and rosacea [10]. Arthritis is usually destructive. Other less common manifestations include recurrent otitis, pharyngeal papillomatosis, lymphadenopathy and splenomegaly. Laboratory analyses may show thrombocytopenia, hypergammaglobulinaemia, and haemolytic anaemia [10].

SAPHO syndrome (synovitis, acne, pustulosis, hyperostosis and osteitis) shares similar features with other neutrophilic AIDs. It occurs mainly in young adults and is self-limiting after an average of 4–5 years. A noninfectious, inflammatory osteitis is associated with cutaneous manifestations that include palmoplantar pustulosis, psoriasis, severe acne (conglobate or fulminans), pyoderma gangrenosum, Sweet syndrome and Sneddon–Wilkinson disease [13]. SAPHO syndrome has been reported associated with inflammatory bowel disease [14]. In spite of the existence of familial cases, a genetic cause has not been found for SAPHO syndrome. The genes *PSTPIP2*, *LPIN2*, *NOD2* and *IL1RNa* might be involved [13]. The proinflammatory cytokines IL-1β and TNF-α, seem likewise important in the pathogenesis of SAPHO [15]. It is possible that certain pathogens, such as Propionibacterium acnes could act as a trigger for an innate immune reaction [16] that could not be appropriately downregulated.

Anti-TNF drugs are the first-line therapy, but not all patients respond. Anakinra has shown variable results. Corticosteroids may be useful for arthritis, but not for skin lesions [10]. In SAPHO syndrome, doxycycline, anti-TNF-α agents and anakinra have been successfully used [17].

Majeed syndrome

This is an association of chronic recurrent multifocal osteomyelitis, congenital dyserythropoietic anaemia with microcytosis and an inflammatory dermatosis [18]. It starts early in life (earlier than 2 years of age), and progresses with clinical exacerbations that are associated with fever, pain and swelling, mainly around large joints. Patients also suffer growth delay and flexion contractures. Skin lesions in Majeed syndrome have been poorly described, mainly as 'Sweet syndrome', 'cutaneous pustulosis' and 'psoriasis'. Biallelic mutations in the gene *LPIN2* are responsible for Majeed syndrome, but the mechanisms by which such mutations cause the phenotype are unclear [19].

NSAIDs are the first-line therapy for Majeed syndrome. Oral corticosteroids are also helpful. Cases have been reported with a dramatic response to anakinra and canakinumab [20].

PASH, PAPASH and other related AIDs

Certain acronyms have been coined to describe a number of overlapping AIDs. These include PASH (pyoderma gangrenosum, acne and suppurative hidradenitis), PAPASH (pyogenic arthritis and PASH), and PsAPASH (featuring psoriasis) [21–23]. Although there is a clear clinical overlap of these syndromes with PAPA, a very few cases have been disclosed genetically. Whereas some patients with PAPASH bear *PSTPIP1* mutations that are also responsible for PAPA, mutations in other genes (*NCSTN*, *MEFV*, *NOD2*) have been described, but their significance is as yet uncertain [12].

Other rare pustular syndromes

APLAID, or autoinflammation and *PLCG2*-associated antibody deficiency and immune dysregulation is a disease allelic with PLAID (see previously), but caused by a heterozygous missense mutation in the *PLCG2* gene resulting in a gain of function [24]. Patients present with early-onset recurrent blistering skin lesions, resembling epidermolysis bullosa, but later develop erythematous plaques and vesiculopustular lesions. Skin biopsy shows a dense infiltrate mainly composed of neutrophils, as well as eosinophils, histiocytes and lymphocytes. Other associated features include interstitial pneumonitis, arthralgia, eye inflammation, enterocolitis and ulcerative colitis, corneal blisters and recurrent sinopulmonary infections. Laboratory studies show a decrease in circulating IgM and IgA antibodies, decreased numbers of class-switched memory B cells and decreased numbers of NK T cells.

A newly-described dominant syndrome featuring neutrophilic dermatosis with facial pustules and pyoderma gangrenosum-like lesions is known as PAAND (pyrin-associated autoinflammatory neutrophilic disease). Associated features include fever, elevated acute-phase reactants, arthralgia and myalgia/myositis [25]. It is caused by monoallelic mutations in the *MEFV* gene, involving a region that is the site of union of pyrin to a pyrin-inhibitory protein named 14-3-3. As a result, pyrin cannot be appropriately inhibited and leads to inflammasome-enhanced functioning.

References

1 Reddy S, Jia S, Geoffrey R et al. An autoinflammatory disease due to homozygous deletion of the IL1RN locus. N Engl J Med 2009;360:2438–44.

2 Aksentijevich I, Masters SL, Ferguson PJ et al. An autoinflammatory disease with deficiency of the interleukin-1-receptor antagonist. N Engl J Med 2009;360:2426–37.

3 Minkis K, Aksentijevich I, Goldbach-Mansky R et al. Interleukin 1 receptor antagonist deficiency presenting as infantile pustulosis mimicking infantile pustular psoriasis. Arch Dermatol 2012; 148:747–52.

4 Brau-Javier CN, Gonzales-Chavez J, Toro JR. Chronic cutaneous pustulosis due to a 175-kb deletion on chromosome 2q13: excellent response to anakinra. Arch Dermatol 2012;148:301–4.

5 Jesus AA, Osman M, Silva CA et al. A novel mutation of IL1RN in the deficiency of interleukin-1 receptor antagonist syndrome: description of two unrelated cases from Brazil. Arthritis Rheum 2011;63:4007–17.

6 Onoufriadis A, Simpson MA, Pink AE et al. Mutations in IL36RN/IL1F5 are associated with the severe episodic inflammatory skin disease known as generalized pustular psoriasis. Am J Hum Genet 2011;89:432–7.

7 Marrakchi S, Guigue P, Renshaw BR et al. Interleukin-36-receptor antagonist deficiency and generalized pustular psoriasis. N Engl J Med 2011;365:620–8.

8 Sugiura K. The genetic background of generalized pustular psoriasis: IL36RN mutations and CARD14 gain-of-function variants. J Dermatol Sci 2014;74:187–92.

9 Abbas O, Itani S, Ghosn S et al. Acrodermatitis continua of Hallopeau is a clinical phenotype of DITRA: evidence that it is a variant of pustular psoriasis. Dermatology 2013;226:28–31.

10 Demidowich AP, Freeman AF, Kuhns DB et al. Genotype, phenotype, and clinical course in five patients with PAPA syndrome (pyogenic sterile arthritis, pyoderma gangrenosum, and acne). Arthri Rheum 2012;64:2022–7.

11 Hong JB, Su YN, Chiu HC. Pyogenic arthritis, pyoderma gangrenosum, and acne syndrome (PAPA syndrome): report of a sporadic case without an identifiable mutation in the CD2BP1 gene. J Am Acad Dermatol 2009;61:533–5.

12 Calderón-Castrat X, Bancalari-Diaz D, Román-Curto C et al. PSTPIP1 Gene mutation in a pyoderma gangrenosum, acne and suppurative hidradenitis (PASH) syndrome. Br J Dermatol 2016;175:194–8.

13 Marzano AV, Borghi A, Meroni PL, Cugno M. Pyoderma gangrenosum and its syndromic forms: evidence for a link with autoinflammation. Br J Dermatol 2016;174:1–9.

14 Naves JE, Cabré E, Mañosa M et al. A systematic review of SAPHO syndrome and inflammatory bowel disease association. Dig Dis Sci 2013;58:2138–47.

15 Hurtado-Nedelec M, Chollet-Martin S, Nicaise-Roland P et al. Characterization of the immune response in the synovitis, acne, pustulosis, hyperostosis, osteitis (SAPHO) syndrome. Rheumatology (Oxford) 2008;47:1160–67.

16 Govoni M, Colina M, Massara A, Trotta F. SAPHO syndrome and infections. Autoimmun Rev 2009;8:256–59.
17 Firinu D, Murgia G, Lorrai MM et al. Biological treatments for SAPHO syndrome: an update. Inflamm Allergy Drug Targets 2014; 13:199–205.
18 Majeed HA, Al-Tarawna M, El-Shanti H et al. The syndrome of chronic recurrent multifocal osteomyelitis and congenital dyserythropoietic anaemia. Report of a new family and a review. Eur J Pediatr 2001;160:705–10.
19 Ferguson PJ, Chen S, Tayeh MK et al. Homozygous mutations in LPIN2 are responsible for the syndrome of chronic recurrent multifocal osteomyelitis and congenital dyserythropoietic anaemia (Majeed syndrome). J Med Genet 2005;42:551–7.
20 Herlin T, Fiirgaard B, Bjerre M et al. Efficacy of anti-IL-1 treatment in Majeed syndrome. Ann Rheum Dis 2012;72:410–3.
21 Duchatelet S, Miskinyte S, Join-Lambert O et al. First nicastrin mutation in PASH (pyoderma gangrenosum, acne and suppurative hidradenitis) syndrome. Br J Dermatol 2015;173:610–2.
22 Marzano AV, Trevisan V, Gattorno M et al. Pyogenic arthritis, pyoderma gangrenosum, acne, and hidradenitis suppurativa (PAPASH): a new autoinflammatory syndrome associated with a novel mutation of the PSTPIP1 gene. JAMA Dermatol 2013;149:762–4.
23 Saraceno R, Babino G, Chiricozzi A et al. PsAPASH: a new syn-drome associated with hidradenitis suppurativa with response to tumor necrosis factor inhibition. J Am Acad Dermatol 2015;72:e42–4.
24 Zhou Q, Lee G-S, Brady J et al. A hypermorphic missense mutation in PLCG2, encoding phospholipase C-gamma-2, causes a dominantly inherited autoinflammatory disease with immunodeficiency. Am J Hum Genet 2012;91:713–20.
25 Masters SL, Lagou V, Jéru I et al. Familial autoinflammation with neutrophilic dermatosis reveals a regulatory mechanism of pyrin activation. Sci Transl Med 2016;8:332ra45.

Mucosal diseases

In a number of AIDs, mucosal lesions are the hallmark of the disease. The most common manifestations are recurrent, painful oral or genital sores or aphthae. They are often associated with other skin manifestations.

Periodic fever with aphtous stomatitis, pharyngitis and adenitis syndrome

Periodic fever with aphtous stomatitis, pharyngitis and adenitis syndrome (PFAPA) is probably the most common of all periodic fever syndromes. However, no mutations have been identified so far in patients with PFAPA, but an activation of the innate immunity and an elevation of IL-1β secretion are likely to be involved [1,2]. It is a sporadic condition, with a few familal cases described [3].

In PFAPA, attacks commonly start between 2 and 5 years of age and resolve by the end of the first decade. Abrupt episodes of fever occur that last 3–6 days and recur every 3–4 weeks. Aphthous stomatitis, exudative or nonexudative pharyngitis, tender cervical lymphadenopathy, myalgias, headache and mild abdominal pain are most commonly associated with fever [4]. Aphthae are usually small, located on the lips or oral mucosa and heal without scarring. They are present in 40–70% of patients. A nonspecific 'skin rash' is at times reported during attacks [5]. Laboratory analyses during the attacks show moderate leukocytosis and elevation of ESR and CRP that return to normal when the attacks subside.

Because PFAPA is a self-healing condition and is usually a mild disease, therapy is not always indicated. NSAIDs are effective for fever. Systemic corticosteroids usually lead to rapid relief from fever and pharyngitis, but aphthae and lymphadenopathy are less responsive. Oral cimetidine has been beneficial in reducing recurrences in small case series. Colchicine might also induce longer episode-free intervals, but it is not routinely recommended. Tonsillectomy has been beneficial in most PFAPA patients, but not all, and recurrences are not eliminated. Also because of the benign course of the disease, tonsillectomy is not routinely recommended [5]

Behçet disease and other ulcerative disorders

Behçet disease, although not frequent in children, is one of the most common autoinflammatory diseases worldwide. It is discussed in Chapter 150.

Haploinsufficiency of protein A20 (HA20) is a rare disease caused by heterozygous, loss-of-function mutations in the *TNFAIP3* gene. Its product, protein A20, is a potent inhibitor of the NF-κB signalling pathway via its desubiquitinase activity [6]. Clinically, HA20 shares many features with paediatric-onset Behçet disease, including oral and genital ulcers and panniculitis [7].

Periodic fever, immunodeficiency and thrombocytopenia (PFIT) is caused by mutations in the actin regulatory gene *WDR1*, which controls actin cytoskeletal dynamics [8]. Skin manifestations are severe oral ulcers leading to disfiguring scarring and microstomy. Fevers, poor growth, infections and thrombocytopenia are associated features.

References

1 Thomas KT, Feder HM, Jr, Lawton AR, Edwards KM. Periodic fever syndrome in children. J Pediatr 1999;135:15–21.
2 Stojanov S, Hoffmann F, Kery A et al. Cytokine profile in PFAPA syndrome suggests continuous inflammation and reduced anti-inflammatory response. Eur Cytokine Netw 2006;17:90–7.
3 Valenzuela PM, Majerson D, Tapia JL, Talesnik E. Syndrome of periodic fever, aphthous stomatitis, pharyngitis, and adenitis (PFAPA) in siblings. Clin Rheumatol 2009;28:1235–7.
4 Padeh S, Brezniak N, Zemer D et al. Periodic fever, aphthous stomatitis, pharyngitis, and adenopathy syndrome: clinical characteristics and outcome. J Pediatr 1999;135:98–101.
5 Manthiram K. Periodic fever with aphthous stomatitis, pharyngitis and adenitis (PFAPA syndrome). UpToDate 2018. ©2019.
6 Zhou Q, Wang H, Schwartz DM et al. Loss-of-function mutations in TNFAIP3 leading to A20 haploinsufficiency cause an early-onset autoinflammatory disease. Nat Genet 2016;48:67–73.
7 Shigemura T, Kaneko N, Kobayashi N et al. Novel heterozygous C243Y A20/TNFAIP3 gene mutation is responsible for chronic inflammation in autosomal-dominant Behçet's disease. RMD Open 2016;2:e000223.
8 Brogan P. 8th International Congress of Familial Mediterranean Fever and Systemic Auto-Inflammatory Diseases, Dresden, 2015.

Histiocytic and granulomatous diseases

A predominant histiocytic response to innate immune stimulation is elicited in some AIDs. The pathomechanisms are varied as are the clinical phenotypes.

Blau syndrome

Blau syndrome shares many similarities with sarcoidosis, but shows an early onset, younger than 4 years of age. Blau syndrome is caused by mutations in the *NOD2* gene, but they have not been found in adult-onset sarcoidosis [1–3]. These are missense mutations that result in constitutive self-activation of NOD2 (nucleotide-binding oligomerization domain protein 2) [4]. NOD2 is a cytoplasmic receptor involved in innate immunity and functions as an inflammasome which, upon recognition of a PAMP or DAMP, activates the NFκB system, and leads to expression of proinflammatory genes [4]. Both heterozygous germline mutations and mosaic somatic mutations in *NOD2* are recognized as causing Blau syndrome [5].

The triad of early-onset polyarticular synovitis, granulomatous acute anterior uveitis and skin rash is characteristic [5]. Characteristic skin lesions are usually observed in early childhood and appear as asymptomatic, small, red or tan, papules (Fig. 155.3). They are usually generalized. Histopathology shows dermal and subcutaneous noncaseating granulomas with multiple epithelioid and multinucleated giant cells indistinguishable from sarcoidosis [5]. Other cutaneous manifestations described in Blau syndrome are recurrent lobar panniculitis, leukocytoclastic vasculitis and an ichthyosiform scaling mainly on the legs.

Joint disease usually begins before the age of 10, in the form of granulomatous synovial inflammation with giant multinucleated cells [6]. Clinically, slowly progressive joint deformities and cystic lesions appear mainly on the wrists, ankles, knees and elbows. Eye involvement mainly consists of recurrent episodes of anterior uveitis. Other manifestations described in Blau syndrome include fever, granulomatous lymphadenopathy, liver epithelioid granulomas, granulomatous infiltration of salivary glands, pneumonitis, granulomatous glomerulonephitis, interstitial nephritis and cranial neuropathy [6].

NSAIDs, corticosteroids, methotrexate and anti-TNF drugs are useful in Blau syndrome. Anakinra has been effective in anecdotal cases [7].

The H-syndrome

The name H-syndrome was coined because many of its main manifestations started with or contained the letter h: hyperpigmented and hypertrichotic plaques, hepatosplenomegaly, heart anomalies, hearing loss, hypogonadism, low height and hyperglycaemia [8].

Biallelic mutations in the gene *SLC29A3*, encoding the equilibrative nucleoside transporter hENT3 are responsible for the H-syndrome [9]. This protein mediates nucleoside transport from lysosomes to cytosol and is a key protein for the synthesis and recycling of nucleosides. hENT3 dysfunction causes accumulation of nucleosides within the lysosomes in macrophages, leading to macrophage dysfunction and accumulation and clinical manifestations. Furthermore, hENT3 is also localized in the mitochondria, and its dysfunction in the H-syndrome causes clinical manifestations not related to macrophage infiltration, such as hepatomegaly, heart disease and hyperglycaemia [9–11].

Pathognomonic skin manifestations of the H-syndrome are hyperpigmented, hypertrichotic and indurated plaques on the abdomen and lower limbs (Fig. 155.4). They appear insidiously during childhood and gradually progress. On skin biopsy, a dermal and hypodermal infiltrate of histiocytes is seen, showing focally emperipolesis.

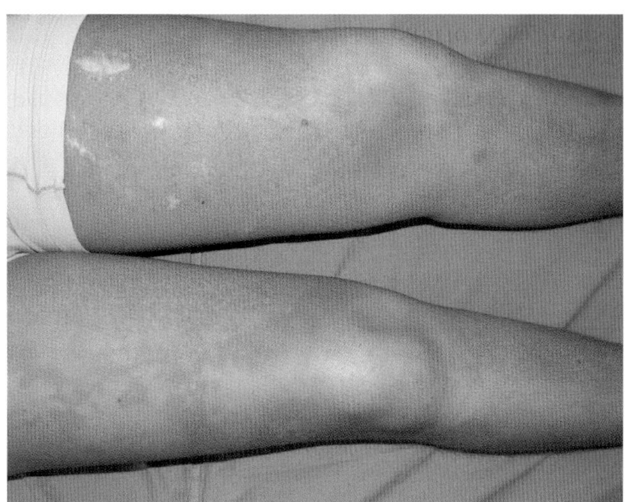

Fig. 155.4 Hyperpigmented, hypertrichotic, indurated plaques in the H-syndrome.

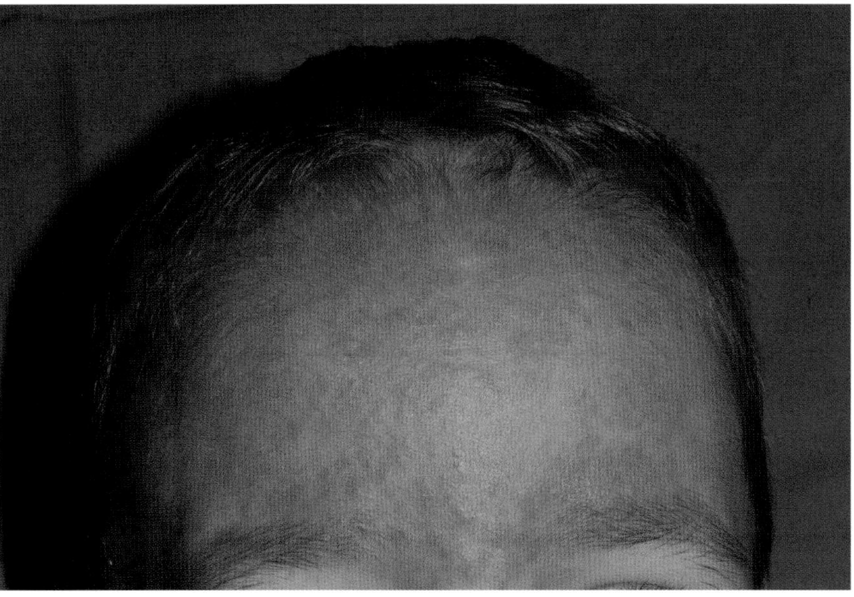

Fig. 155.3 Discrete erythematous papules in Blau syndrome.

Furthermore, the histiocytes stain for S-100 protein, and thus closely resemble Rosai–Dorfman histiocytosis [12].

Patients show a characteristic constellation of extracutaneous features [8]: sensorineural hearing loss, hepatosplenomegaly, short stature, heart abnormalities, angiopathy (varicose veins, dilated lateral scleral vessels and facial telangiectases), exophthalmos, gynaecomastia, mild mental impairment, scrotal masses, bilateral camptodactyly, hallux and contractures of the interphalangeal joints. Mild microcytic anaemia, elevated ESR, hyperglycaemia, growth hormone deficiency, relatively high gonadotropins and low normal testosterone are detected [8–11].

Treatment of the H-syndrome with oral corticosteroids and methotrexate has only induced partial remissions. The disease is progressive and disabling.

CANDLE syndrome

CANDLE is the acronym for chronic atypical neutrophilic dermatosis with lipodystrophy and elevated temperature (CANDLE) syndrome [13]. Although cells of the myeloid lineage are recruited in the attacks and they may be prominent in the skin and organ infiltrates, the molecular defect in CANDLE syndrome occurs mostly in macrophages. Also macrophages accumulate in the lesions, and this is also discussed here. CANDLE can be also discussed within the type I interferonopathies, because of the prominent IFN1 rubric it exhibits, but CANDLE is not an intrinsic defect in the IFN synthesis and pathway. In fact, CANDLE is the paradigm of proteasome/immunoproteasome dysfunction. Mutations in different protein subunits of the proteasome or immunoproteasome are responsible for CANDLE, and thus the disease can be monogenic or digenic. Most commonly mutations occur in the *PSMB8* gene encoding the subunit β5i of the immunoproteasome. Other less common mutations may occur in *PSMB4* (β7 subunit), *PSMB9* (β1i subunit) and *PSMA3* (α3 subunit) [14,15]. The proteasome and immunoproteasome are multicatalytic structures of all eukaryotic cells [16] and are formed by the ensembling of at least 28 protein subunits. They are responsible for the cleavage of protein substrates to generate short peptides that can be presented to the adaptive immune system, and also to remove waste proteins generated by cell metabolism. In the absence of normal function, waste proteins accumulate in the macrophages and cause cellular stress, leading to constitutive IFN1 excessive production. Common triggers such as cold, infections or stress cause further accumulation of metabolic waste in the cells, leading to massive IFN1 secretion and recruitment of myeloid cells in the tissues [14,15].

CANDLE syndrome starts in early infancy with recurrent fever and skin lesions. These are pathognomonic and consist of recurrent annular erythematous or violaceous plaques, affecting predominantly the trunk but also the face and the limbs, that progress to purpuric lesions and after several weeks remit with residual hyperpigmentation [13] (Fig. 155.5). Cold may act as a trigger and especially in young infants acral lesions may resemble pernio. Skin histopathology is equally pathognomonic and shows an interstitial and perivascular inflammatory infiltrate, mainly composed of mononuclear cells with atypical features and bizarre nuclei, without evidence of vasculitis. Mature polymorphonuclear cells can be seen and karyorrhexis [13]. Immunohistochemistry studies disclose myeloid cells positive for myeloperoxidase and CD163-positive macrophages. CD123-positive plasmacytoid dendritic cells, the most potent producers of type I interferons, are also prominently represented [17].

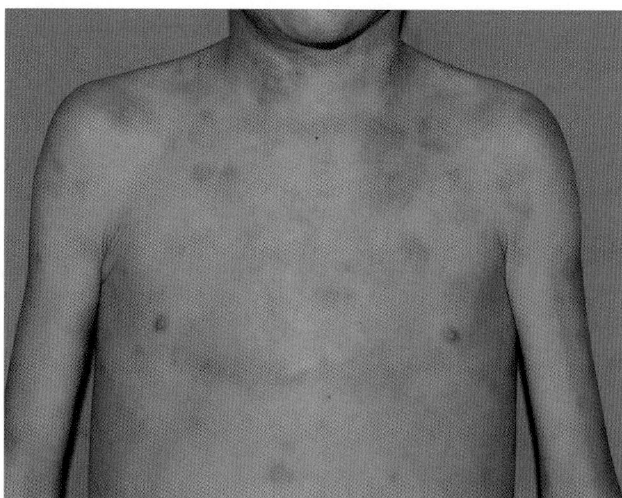

Fig. 155.5 Skin violaceous plaques in CANDLE (chronic atypical neutrophilic dermatosis with lipodystrophy and elevated temperature) syndrome.

The patients later develop peculiar features. Eyelids and lips are swollen with a typical violaceous hue [13]. Delayed physical development, progressive lipodystrophy, arthralgia without arthritis, hepatomegaly and splenomegaly occur. The loss of subcutaneous fat is a likely consequence of recurrent attacks of panniculitis. Other extracutaneous manifestations appear recurrently as multiorgan inflammatory attacks and include aseptic meningitis, conjunctivitis, nodular episcleritis, ear and nose chondritis, epididimitis, lymphadenopathy, otitis, nephritis and virtually any organ inflammation [13]. Acute inflammatory episodes can be fatal. The disease runs a chronic and progressive course, leading to delayed growth, muscle wastage, distal joint contractures, profound lipodystrophy of the whole body and face and considerable incapacity. Laboratory analyses barely show elevated ESR and CRP, chronic anaemia and mild elevation of liver enzymes.

So far, minimal improvement has been shown with oral corticosteroids and methotrexate in CANDLE syndrome. Clinical trials with the janus kinase (JAK) inhibitor baricitinib are showing promising results [18].

References

1 **Miceli-Richard C, Lesage S, Rybojad M et al. CARD15 mutations in Blau syndrome. Nat Genet 2001;29:19–20.**

2 Kanazawa N, Okafuji I, Kambe N et al. Early-onset sarcoidosis and CARD15 mutations with constitutive nuclear factor-(kappa)B activation: Common genetic etiology with Blau syndrome. Blood 2005;105:1195–7.

3 Rose CD, Doyle TM, McIlvain-Simpson G et al. Blau syndrome mutation of CARD15/NOD2 in sporadic early onset granulomatous arthritis. J Rheumatol 2005;32:373–5.
4 Kambe N, Nishikomori R, Kanazawa N. The cytosolic pattern-recognition receptor Nod2 and inflammatory granulomatous disorders. J Dermatol Sci 2005;39:71–80.
5 Rose CD, Arostegui JI, Martin TM et al. NOD2-associated pediatric granulomatous arthritis, an expanding phenotype: study of an international registry and a national cohort in Spain. Arthritis Rheum 2009;60:1797–803.
6 Manouvrier-Hanu S, Puech B, Piette F et al. Blau syndrome of granulomatous arthritis, iritis, and skin rash: A new family and review of the literature. Am J Med Genet 1998;76:217–21.
7 Arostegui JI, Arnal C, Merino R et al. NOD2 gene-associated pediatric granulomatous arthritis: clinical diversity, novel and recurrent mutations, and evidence of clinical improvement with interleukin-1 blockade in a Spanish cohort. Arthritis Rheum 2007;56:3805–13.
8 Molho-Pessach V, Agha Z, Aamar S et al. The H syndrome: a genodermatosis characterized by indurated, hyperpigmented, and hypertrichotic skin with systemic manifestations. J Am Acad Dermatol 2008;59:79–85.
9 Molho-Pessach V, Lerer I, Abeliovich D et al. The H syndrome is caused by mutations in the nucleoside transporter hENT3. Am J Hum Genet 2008;83:529–34.
10 Leung GP, Tse CM. The role of mitochondrial and plasma membrane nucleoside transporters in drug toxicity. Expert Opin Drug Metab Toxicol 2007;3:705–18.
11 Hsu CL, Lin W, Seshasayee D et al. Equilibrative nucleoside transporter 3 deficiency perturbs lysosome function and macrophage homeostasis. Science 2012;335:89–92.
12 Colmenero I, Molho-Pessach V, Torrelo A et al. Emperipolesis: an additional common histopathologic finding in H syndrome and Rosai-Dorfman disease. Am J Dermatopathol 2012;34:315–20.
13 Torrelo A, Patel S, Colmenero I et al. Chronic atypical neutrophilic dermatosis with lipodystrophy and elevated temperature (CANDLE) syndrome. J Am Acad Dermatol 2010;62:489–95.
14 Liu Y, Ramot Y, Torrelo A et al. Mutations in proteasome subunit β type 8 cause chronic atypical neutrophilic dermatosis with lipodystrophy and elevated temperature with evidence of genetic and phenotypic heterogeneity. Arthritis Rheum 2012;64:895–907.
15 Brehm A, Liu Y, Sheikh A et al. Additive loss-of-function proteasome subunit mutations in CANDLE/PRAAS patients promote type I IFN production. J Clin Invest 2015;125:4196–211.
16 Gomes AV. Genetics of proteasome diseases. Scientifica (Cairo) 2013;2013:637629.
17 Torrelo A, Colmenero I, Requena L et al. Histologic and immunohistochemical features of the skin lesions in CANDLE syndrome. Am J Dermatopathol 2015;37:517–22.
18 Xirotagaros G, Hernández-Ostiz S, Aróstegui JI, Torrelo A. Newly described autoinflammatory diseases in pediatric dermatology. Pediatr Dermatol 2016;33:602–14.

Vasculopathic diseases

This group of AIDs encompasses those syndromes in which main manifestations are a result of a direct vessel injury or resemble 'vascular collagen' disorders. In them, boundaries between adaptive immune system pathology (autoimmunity) and innate immune system (autoinflammation) are blurry, and the clinical picture is a mixture of both.

Type I interferonopathies

All type I IFNs signal through the membrane-associated receptor interferon-α receptor (IFNAR). Binding of type I IFNs to the IFNAR receptor triggers a signal by the JAK-STAT (signal transducer and activator of transcription) pathway, which results in the increased expression of hundreds of genes [1]. Type I IFNs are involved in immune response regulation. The type I interferonopathies are caused either by an inappropriate overstimulation of the type I IFN response pathway or by a defective downregulation of this pathway [1,2].

STING-associated vasculopathy with onset in infancy syndrome

STING-associated vasculopathy with onset in infancy (SAVI) syndrome is caused by heterozygous gain-of-function mutations in the *TMEM173* gene, leading to a constitutive activation of the stimulator of interferon genes (STING), a key molecule in the regulation of IFN secretion [3,4]. Recognition of cytosolic DNA leads to STING activation, which initiates the expression of interferon-inducible genes. In SAVI syndrome a chronic and sustained activation of the type I IFNs pathway occurs.

The cutaneous manifestations in SAVI syndrome consist of violaceous, scaling plaques and nodules on fingers, toes, nose, ears and cheeks that may progress to ulcers, necrosis, nail loss or dystrophy and nasal-septum perforation [2]. They can worsen if exposed to cold and other stimuli. Skin biopsies reveal vascular inflammation limited to capillaries, with deposition of IgM and C3 in scattered vessels. A mixed dermoepidermal interphase infiltrate can also appear [3].

Patients with SAVI syndrome may also present with severe interstitial lung disease, as well as widespread vasculopathy of the pulmonary vascular system. A systemic vasculopathic disorder can also occur. SAVI syndrome shows similarities with the so-called 'dermatopulmonary syndrome', an acquired disorder related to MD5 autoantibodies [5] which is currently considered as a subset of dermatomyositis. Elevated ESR and elevated levels of CRP are the main laboratory abnormalities in SAVI syndrome [3,4].

There is no effective treatment for SAVI syndrome. JAK inhibitors baricitinib or ruxolitinib may be potentially useful [3].

Aicardi–Goutiéres syndrome

Aicardi–Goutiéres syndrome (AGS) is a group of phenotypically similar disorders with a genetic heterogenous basis, encompassing up to seven different forms (AGS 1 to 7). AGS-causing mutations have been detected in genes encoding the 3-prime repair exonuclease 1 (*TREX1; AGS1*), the SAM domain- and HD domain-containing protein 1 (*SAMHD1; AGS5*), the three genes encoding the components of the RNASEH2 endonuclease complex (*AGS2-4*), the RNA-specific adenosine deaminase 1 (*ADAR1; AGS6*), and the interferon-induced helicase c domain-containing protein 1 (*IFIH1; AGS7*) [2]. Most of these are endonuclease enzymes that break down DNA and RNA molecules to avoid their recognition as foreign gene material, thus preventing the production of type I IFNs. Failed cellular processing of these nucleic acids will cause a permanent type I IFN immune activation and a defective downregulation of IFN response to viral infections [1,6].

AGS usually presents with an early-onset neurodegenerative disease, but there is considerable heterogeneity among both clinical and laboratory findings [6,7].

Skin lesions detected are the most prominent extraneurological features of the disease [8]. They consist of chilblain-like lesions and pernio, acrocyanosis and nail abnormalities with erythematous periungual skin lesions. An acral distribution on the extremities and the ear lobes is observed, and lesions worsen with cold exposure. Other cutaneous features include livedo reticularis and a blueberry-muffin rash in the newborn [2].

Calcification of the basal ganglia and white matter, cystic leukodystrophy, cortical-subcortical atrophy, atrophy of the corpus callosum, brainstem and cerebellum, chronic cerebrospinal fluid lymphocytosis and increased levels of IFN-α in plasma and cerebrospinal fluid are main clues to the diagnosis [8,9], but a definite diagnosis requires genetic confirmation.

Treatment of AGS is disappointing. Azathioprine, corticosteroids and intravenous immunoglobulin have been used. Anti-IFN-α monoclonal antibodies and reverse transcriptase inhibitors are being evaluated [10].

Familial chilblain lupus

Chilblain lupus is a rare form of cutaneous lupus erythematosus, usually sporadic. Familial chilblain lupus usually starts in early childhood and is inherited as an autosomal dominant trait. Disease-causing mutations in the *SAMHD1* and *TREX1* genes have been recently detected [11], and thus the disease is allelic with certain types of AGS. In some families, overlapping manifestations of both diseases occur.

Skin lesions appear mainly in acral sites such as fingers, toes, nose and ears. They consist of painful, cold-induced, bluish-red papules or nodules, and are similar to those seen in AGS. Arthralgia and arthritis can occur and antinuclear antibodies are occasionally detected.

Treatment has included topical corticosteroids, tacrolimus and pimecrolimus. For resistant lesions, oral antimalarials, corticosteroids, immunomodulators and calcium channel blockers may be tried [12].

C1q deficiency

In addition to C1q function for the activation of the complement cascade, C1q acts as an inhibitor of INF-α production by plasmacytoid dendritic cells and peripheral blood mononuclear cells [13].

Loss-of-function mutations in C1q are known to cause systemic lupus erythematosus (SLE)-like manifestations in most patients [14]. Skin lesions of C1q deficiency include a butterfly-like erythema on the face, discoid lupus-type lesions and Raynaud phenomenon [15,16]. Skin biopsies show findings similar to SLE, with hydropic degeneration of the basal layer and the presence of IgG, IgM, IgA and C3 deposits. C1q deficiency also causes segmental mesangiopathic glomerulonephritis and neurological symptoms similar to those detected in SLE. Furthermore, recurrent and severe infections caused by the deficiency in the classical pathway of complement are seen.

Laboratory analyses show CH50 activity and C1q plasma levels close to zero, but C2, C4 and C1 inactivator levels are usually normal or high. Antinuclear and anti-Sm antibodies are positive.

Treatment of C1q deficiency requires an immunodeficiency approach, but SLE manifestations may require immunosuppressants. A cure for the disease can be achieved with haematopoietic stem cell transplantation [17].

X-linked reticulate pigmentary disorder

X-linked reticulate pigmentary disorder (XLPDR) is caused by a hypomorphic mutation in the gene *POLA1*, encoding the catalytic subunit of DNA polymerase-α, a critical regulator of the type I IFN response [18]. POLA1 deficiency results in increased production of type I IFNs, and is thus included within the group of type I interferonopathies, even though a prominent vascular pathology is not seen.

The earliest manifestations appear in infancy. Patients suffer recurrent pneumonias, bronchiectasis, chronic diarrhoea and failure to thrive. An enterocolitis resembling inflammatory bowel disease appears later. On the skin, a characteristic diffuse and reticulated skin hyperpigmentation is evident from childhood [19]. Many patients also suffer from hypohidrosis and corneal inflammation. Characteristic facies are typical in affected males. Female carriers can present with linear hyperpigmentation following the lines of Blaschko [19].

Deficiency of adenosine deaminase 2

Adenosine deaminase 2 (ADA2) catalyses the conversion of deoxyadenosine into deoxyinosine. ADA2 is a secreted protein and also participates in the immune response through the differentiation of monocytes to macrophages. Furthermore, ADA2 also acts as a key endothelial growth factor for vascular development. Deficiency of ADA2 (DADA2) is caused by biallelic, loss-of-function mutations in the cat eye syndrome chromosome region candidate 1 gene (*CECR1*) [20]. Reduced or absent ADA2 activity causes systemic inflammation, vascular pathology and mild immunodeficiency [21].

The main skihnhn manifestations of DADA2 are livedo reticularis or livedo racemosa, Raynaud's phenomenon and necrosis. These are caused by small and medium-size vessel vasculopathy [20,21]. Systemic features include intermittent fevers, early-onset and recurrent strokes (ischaemic, haemorrhagic or lacunar), hepatosplenomegaly and systemic vasculopathy. MRI may reveal cerebral infarcts and ventricular haemorrhage. Aneurysms and stenoses of large abdominal arteries and renal cortex infarcts can be seen by angiography [20]. A striking overlap of the vascular component of DADA2 with polyarteritis nodosa is recognized [20].

Treatment with anti-TNF agents may be considered in DADA2. Replacement therapy with fresh-frozen plasma or recombinant ADA2 is a promising therapy [20].

References

1 **Crow YJ. Type I interferonopathies: a novel set of inborn errors of immunity. Ann N Y Acad Sci 2011;1238:91–8.**

2 Xirotagaros G, Hernández-Ostiz S, Aróstegui JI, Torrelo A. New autoinflammatory diseases in pediatric dermatology. Pediatr Dermatol 2016;33:602–14.

3 **Liu Y, Jesus AA, Marrero B et al. Activated STING in a vascular and pulmonary syndrome. N Engl J Med 2014;371:507–18.**

4 Abe J, Izawa K, Nishikomori R et al. Heterozygous TREX1 pAsp18Asn mutation can cause variable neurological symptoms in a family with Aicardi-Goutieres syndrome/familial chilblain lupus. Rheumatology 2013;52:406–8.
5 Chaisson NF, Paik J, Orbai AM. A novel dermato-pulmonary syndrome associated with MDA-5 antibodies: report of 2 cases and review of the literature. Medicine (Baltimore) 2012;91:220–8.
6 Dale RC, Gornall H, Singh-Grewal D et al. Familial Aicardi-Goutières syndrome due to SAMHD1 mutations is associated with chronic arthropathy and contractures. Am J Med Genet A 2010;152A:938–42.
7 Stephenson JB. Aicardi-Goutières syndrome (AGS). Eur J Paediatr Neurol 2008;12:355–8.
8 Juern A, Robbins A, Galbraith S, Drolet B. Aicardi-Goutières syndrome: cutaneous, laboratory, and radiologic findings: a case report. Pediatr Dermatol 2010;27:82–5.
9 Brisman S, Gonzalez M, Morel KD. Blueberry muffin rash as the presenting sign of Aicardi-Goutières syndrome. Pediatr Dermatol 2009;26:432–5.
10 Crow YJ, Vanderver A, Orcesi S et al. Therapies in Aicardi-Goutières syndrome. Clin Exp Immunol 2014;175:1–8.
11 Tüngler V, Silver RM, Walkenhorst H et al. Inherited or de novo mutation affecting aspartate 18 of TREX1 results in either familial chilblain lupus or Aicardi-Goutières syndrome. Br J Dermatol 2012;167:212–4.
12 Patel S, Hardo F. Chilblain lupus erythematosus BMJ Case Rep 2013 doi:10.1136/bcr-2013-201165.
13 Santer DM, Hall BE, George TC et al. C1q deficiency leads to the defective suppression of IFN-alpha in response to nucleoprotein containing immune complexes. J Immunol 2010;185:4738–49.
14 Botto M, Kirschfink M, Macor P et al. Complement in human diseases: lessons from complement deficiencies. Mol Immunol 2009;46:2774–83.
15 Roumenina LT, Sène D, Radanova M et al. Functional complement C1q abnormality leads to impaired immune complexes and apoptotic cell clearance. J Immunol 2011;187:4369–73.
16 Schejbel L, Skattum L, Hagelberg S et al. Molecular basis of hereditary C1q deficiency – revisited: identification of several novel disease-causing mutations. Genes Immun 2011;12:626–34.
17 Arkwright PD, Riley P, Hughes SM, Alachkar H, Wynn RF. Successful cure of C1q deficiency in human subjects treated with hematopoietic stem cell transplantation. J Allergy Clin Immunol 2014;133:265–7.
18 Starokadomskyy P, Gemelli T, Rios JJ et al. DNA polymerase-α regulates the activation of type I interferons through cytosolic RNA:DNA synthesis. Nat Immunol 2016;17:495–504.
19 Fernandez-Guarino M, Torrelo A, Fernandez-Lorente M et al. X-linked reticulate pigmentary disorder: report of a new family. Eur J Dermatol 2008;18:102–3.
20 Zhou Q, Yang D, Ombrello AK et al. Early-onset stroke and vasculopathy associated with mutations in ADA2. N Engl J Med 2014;370:911–20.
21 Navon Elkan P, Pierce SB, Segel R et al. Mutant adenosine deaminase 2 in a polyarteritis nodosa vasculopathy. N Engl J Med 2014; 370:921–31.

Amyloidosis

Definition. Amyloidosis, also known as the β-fibrilloses, comprises a diverse group of disease processes that result in the extracellular deposition of β-pleated protein-derived fibrils in various tissues [1–3]. The most common forms of amyloidosis consist of one of three major types of proteins within the fibrils: amyloid light chain protein, amyloid A (AA) protein or keratinocyte-derived amyloid (K amyloid) [1,2,4]. The quantity and site of amyloid deposition determine whether there is associated clinical disease or merely an incidental histological finding. Disease classification may be based on the location of the amyloid deposits (systemic versus localized), and whether the amyloid deposition is a primary or secondary disease process (Table 155.2). Cutaneous amyloidosis is extremely rare in children, and the most likely types of primary localized cutaneous amyloidosis (PLCA) to occur in this age group are lichen or macular amyloidosis. The systemic forms in children, which are even more uncommon, are usually the result of AIDs.

Table 155.2 Classification of amyloidoses

Type of amyloidosis	Origin of amyloid	Distribution of amyloid in tissue
Cutaneous amyloidosis		
PLCA	Keratinocyte	Papillary dermis
Lichenoid		
Macular		
Biphasic bullous		
Poikiloderma-like		
Nodular	Immunoglobulin AL protein	Papillary, reticular dermis, subcutaneous fat, eccrine glands and blood vessels
Secondary	Keratinocyte	Adjacent tissue Tumour associated
Systemic amyloidosis		
Primary	Immunoglobulin AL protein	Dermis, vessel walls, subcutaneous fat, eccrine glands and mesenchymal tissues
Secondary		
JRA, Hodgkin lymphoma, tuberculosis	SAA protein→AA protein	Subcutaneous fat, vessel walls, eccrine glands, parenchymal organs
Hereditary/familial		
Familial Mediterranean fever	SAA protein→AA protein	
Muckle–Wells syndrome	SAA protein→AA protein	
Neurotropic amyloidoses	Transthyretin (prealbumin)	

AA, amyloid A; AL, amyloid light chain; JRA, juvenile rheumatoid arthritis; PLCA, primary localized cutaneous amyloidosis; SAA, serum amyloid A.

Aetiology. Ultrastructurally, amyloid is composed of straight, nonbranching fibrils of 7.5–10.0 nm in diameter, arranged haphazardly in a 'felt-like' array [1–3,5]. The fibrils are arranged in an antiparallel (β-pleated) configuration, which is responsible for the affinity of amyloid to cotton dyes (e.g. Congo red) [1–3,5]. Several sources of amyloid fibrillar proteins have been identified. Plasma cells secrete amyloid light chain protein from intact immunoglobulin G (IgG) light chains (primarily λ) in three main disease states (immunocytic amyloidoses): primary systemic amyloidosis, amyloidosis associated with plasma cell dyscrasias (in particular, multiple myeloma) and localized nodular (tumefactive) amyloidosis of the skin or other organs [1,3,6]. Serum amyloid A (SAA) protein is a normal serum protein synthesized by the liver in association with serum high-density lipoprotein (HDL), and it behaves as an acute-phase reactant. During inflammatory states, macrophages phagocytose SAA and transform SAA into AA protein [1]. AA is present in both reactive (secondary) systemic amyloidosis and systemic heredofamilial amyloidosis [1]. Damaged and degenerating keratinocytes (e.g. caused by psoralens and ultraviolet A) [7] are the source of keratinoid amyloid, which is the principal amyloid protein in PLCA [4,8]. Transthyretin, a type of prealbumin that transports thyroxine and retinol-binding protein, is the source of amyloid in some of the heredofamilial neurotropic amyloidoses [9].

Cutaneous amyloidosis in children may be caused by genetic or environmental factors. Familial cutaneous lichen amyloidosis is autosomal dominant [10–14]. A form of lichen amyloidosis occurs in association with Sipple syndrome (multiple endocrine neoplasia [MEN] type 2A) [15–17], and a mutation of the *RET* proto-oncogene on chromosome 10 is believed to be responsible for this constellation of findings [18]. However, patients with familial cutaneous lichen amyloidosis do not have this gene mutation and therefore do not appear to be at risk of developing Sipple syndrome [19]. Macular amyloidosis is frequently an early form of lichen amyloidosis, but it may also occur because of friction from nylon brushes, backscratchers or sharp fingernails [20,21].

Pathology. Although amyloid is derived from many different sources, the different forms of amyloid are morphologically the same on histological sections [1–3,5,]. On haematoxylin and eosin staining amyloid appears as amorphous, eosinophilic extracellular aggregates, without accompanying inflammation [1–3,5]. Special stains are helpful when minimal amounts of amyloid are present. Amyloid stains metachromatically with toluidine blue, crystal violet or methyl violet [1–3,5,22]. Congo red and other cotton dyes produce an apple-green birefringence in polarized light and are the most specific stains for the detection of amyloid. With thioflavine T, fluorescent microscopy reveals a yellow–green fluorescence [1–3,5]. Under the electron microscope, amyloid deposits are seen as straight, nonbranching fibrils of 7.5–10.0 nm in diameter, arranged in a 'felt-like' array [1–3,5]. The fibril is composed of two twisted β-pleated sheet micelles, helically arranged in antiparallel conformation, as seen by X-ray crystallography [1–3,5].

Clinical features.

Cutaneous amyloidosis (Box 155.1)

Primary localized cutaneous amyloidosis

Lichen amyloidosis is the most common form of PLCA. Its peak incidence is between 40 and 60 years. However, it can occur in children, and where it does it usually occurs in adolescence [11–13]. It is most prevalent in Chinese people residing in Taiwan, Singapore and Indonesia [11–13]. Lichen amyloidosis presents with intensely pruritic flesh-coloured, grey or yellowish-brown papules ranging in size from 1 to 10 mm. They are most commonly located on the pretibial surfaces but may also occur on the extensor surfaces of the forearms, the trunk, shoulders and sacrum (Fig. 155.6).

Macular amyloidosis occurs more commonly in children than lichen amyloidosis [23] and is seen more frequently in people of Latin American, Asian or Middle Eastern origin [20–23]. Typically occurring during adolescence, the macular form presents as poorly delineated hyperpigmented patches or as a linear rippling of the skin by moderately pruritic, closely aggregated greyish-brown macules. This presentation most commonly involves the lower extremities but may also involve the mid-back or arms (Fig. 155.7). Rubbing the affected area with a nylon brush or backscratcher may lead to the macular form known as friction amyloidosis [20,21].

Diffuse biphasic amyloidosis is the existence of both macular and lichen amyloidosis in the same patient. Rubbing and scratching may transform the macular to the lichenoid form, and intralesional steroids may transform the lichenoid to the macular form [3–5,20,21].

Familial primary cutaneous amyloidosis (FPCA) is an autosomal dominant disorder with incomplete penetrance [10–14], caused by heterozygous missense mutations in the *OSMR* gene, encoding oncostatin M receptor beta (OSMRbeta), an interleukin-6 family cytokine receptor [24]. The onset is during puberty as either the macular or biphasic form of amyloidosis, and it progresses with age into the lichenoid form [10–14]. The most common

Box 155.1 Cutaneous amyloidosis in children

Primary localized cutaneous amyloidosis

Major types
- Lichenoid (sporadic/FPCA late stage)
- Macular (sporadic, 'friction' amyloidosis/FPCA early stage)
- Biphasic (sporadic/FPCA early stage)

Less common types
- FPCA associated with Sipple syndrome
- Poikiloderma-like
- Bullous
- Genodermatoses-associated macular variant

Secondary cutaneous amyloidosis
- Skin tumour associated

FPCA, familial primary cutaneous amyloidosis.

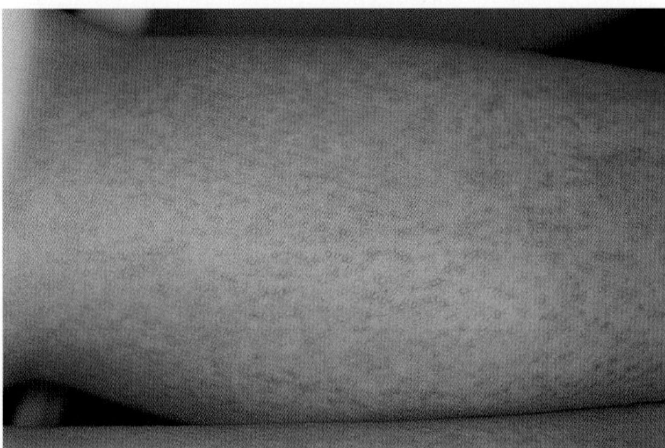

Fig. 155.6 Lichen amyloidosis. Flesh-coloured papules on the lower legs of a 17-year-old girl.

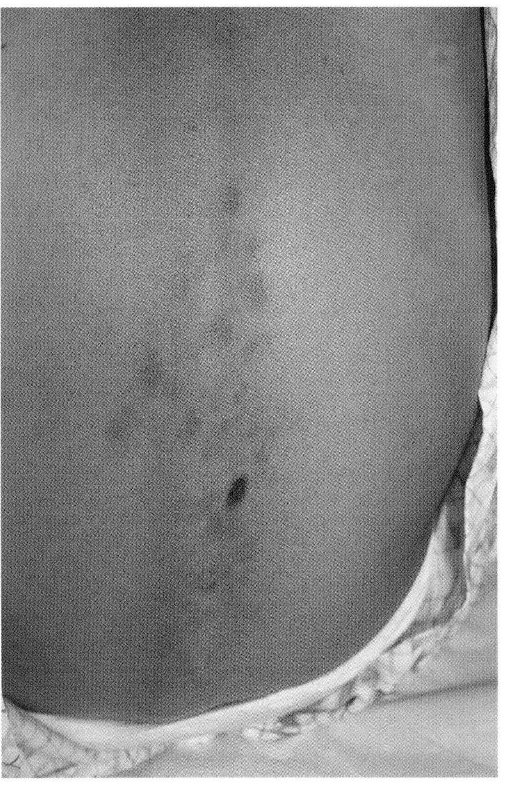

Fig. 155.7 Macular amyloidosis. Hyperpigmented patches with superficial erosion in a 12-year-old girl.

locations are the interscapular and pretibial areas, and the intensity of the pruritus is much greater than the clinical appearance [13].

In all of the sporadic and familial forms of lichenoid, macular or biphasic forms of amyloidosis, there is no risk of developing systemic amyloidosis [3,5]. However, there is one form of familial primary cutaneous amyloidosis in which the cutaneous lesions may signal the risk of developing Sipple syndrome or MEN 2A [15–17]. Sipple syndrome is an autosomal dominant disorder associated with the triad of parathyroid hyperplasia, phaeochromocytoma and medullary carcinoma of the thyroid. In some kindreds, cutaneous lichen or biphasic amyloidosis presents as an intensely pruritic plaque involving the interscapular area [15–17]. The cutaneous amyloidosis usually occurs in childhood or adolescence and frequently precedes the development of the neoplasms [15–17]. Therefore, young patients presenting with interscapular amyloidosis should be evaluated for the risk of developing MEN 2A, including the presence of the mutation for the *RET* proto-oncogene on chromosome 10 [18]. PLCA has also been reported in a family with medullary thyroid carcinoma, without other endocrinopathies [25].

Poikiloderma-like cutaneous amyloidosis is an extremely rare autosomal dominant disorder associated with poikiloderma, lichen amyloid papules, short stature and photosensitivity. The skin lesions appear early in life, and palmoplantar keratosis and blister formation may rarely occur. Amyloid deposition is present in both the poikilodermatous and the lichenoid lesions [21,26].

A single report of bullous amyloidosis describes bullous lesions around joints in adolescents, with onset of disease between 10 and 13 years of age. Biopsy confirmed the presence of amyloid within the bullae [27]. Nodular, anosacral and vitiliginous amyloidoses have not been reported to occur in children.

Genodermatosis-associated amyloidosis comprises several syndromes in which asymptomatic macular amyloid is found within cutaneous hyperpigmentation. Partington syndrome, or X-linked reticulate pigmentary disorder with systemic manifestations was formerly known as X-linked cutaneous amyloidosis [28] (see previously). Amyloid deposits were present in the pigmented skin of both sexes [28]. A 10-year follow-up study revealed that the amyloid deposits were not a consistent finding [29], and other reports have since confirmed that amyloid was not always found in identical clinical presentations, leading to the change in the name of the syndrome [30,31]. Other genodermatoses associated with asymptomatic macular amyloid include pachyonychia congenita (Tidman–Wells–MacDonald variant) [32], epidermolysis bullosa (Weber–Cockayne type) [33], dyskeratosis congenita [34] and the Nageli–Franceschetti–Jadassohn syndrome [35].

Secondary cutaneous amyloidosis

Skin tumour-associated amyloidosis is the asymptomatic deposition of amyloidosis withien and around tumours. In the paediatric population, these would include pilomatrixomas, porokeratosis of Mibelli and melanocytic naevi [3].

Systemic amyloidosis

Primary systemic or immunocytic amyloidosis is extremely rare in childhood [23,36]. Infiltration of amyloid in the tongue leads to macroglossia, and amyloid deposition within the blood vessel walls leads to 'pinch purpura' and purpura after the Valsalva manoeuvre. Waxy, smooth, shiny asymptomatic amber or yellow papules may occur in flexural areas, or on the central part of the face, lips and oral mucosa. A leonine facies may occur as well as sclerodermatous-type changes on the hands [3]. Rectal biopsy is often diagnostic for amyloidosis [3].

Reactive or secondary systemic amyloidosis is associated with chronic inflammatory diseases. These include juvenile rheumatoid arthritis, scleroderma, Hodgkin disease, tuberculosis and many of the AIDs discussed previously [37–41]. The amyloid deposits involve mainly the kidneys, spleen, liver, adrenal glands and heart, and skin findings are rare. Recessive dystrophic epidermolysis bullosa has been reported in association with systemic amyloidosis involving the heart, stomach, kidneys and thyroid gland [42].

Neurotropic amyloidoses are autosomal dominant disorders associated with amyloid neuropathy affecting Portuguese, Swedish and Finnish families [9,39,43]. Patients have the constellation of painless ulcers with eventual loss of digits, carpal tunnel syndrome, malabsorption, vitreous opacities and cardiac involvement. The neuropathy may occur in adolescence but the other skin changes, including hyperpigmented atrophic scars, hypotrichosis, blisters and sclerodermatous changes, do not appear until adulthood [9,23,37,43].

Prognosis. The localized cutaneous forms of amyloidosis persist unchanged or may slowly progress. In systemic amyloidosis, mortality is related to visceral involvement and is especially high with renal or cardiac amyloidosis.

Differential diagnosis. Lichen amyloidosis may be confused with lichen simplex chronicus, pretibial myxoedema, confluent and reticulated papillomatosis of Gougerot and Carteaud, lichen myxoedematosus, colloid milium, stasis dermatitis and lichen planus [21,23]. Macular amyloidosis may resemble stasis dermatitis, postinflammatory hyperpigmentation, pigmented purpuric dermatoses, pityriasis versicolour, erythema dyschromicum perstans and hyperpigmentation caused by endocrine disorders, drugs or heavy metals [44]. Poikiloderma-like cutaneous amyloidosis must be differentiated from Rothmund–Thomson syndrome, and Partington syndrome can clinically resemble incontinentia pigmenti. Histopathology and special stains are so specific and distinct that they can easily confirm the diagnosis of amyloidosis.

Treatment. Treatment is not totally satisfactory for localized cutaneous amyloidosis. Topical and intralesional corticosteroids offer some relief from the pruritus, often in conjunction with oral antihistamines [3,21–23]. Topical corticosteroids when used with ultraviolet B (UVB) or topical psoralens with ultraviolet A (PUVA) therapy may provide some benefit [45]. Cryosurgery, surgical excision and electrodesiccation have limited success. Dermabrasion or carbon dioxide laser may be helpful for some patients, although recurrences are common [40,46]. Topical dimethyl sulphoxide (DMSO) has a beneficial but transient effect on pruritus; however, its use is limited by its unpleasant garlic smell [47]. Acitretin may be effective for some patients with lichen amyloidosis [48,49] but is not recommended for female patients until after childbearing age. Oral cyclosporin has been reported to be beneficial for one patient who had lichen amyloidosis and severe atopic dermatitis [50].

Treatment for systemic amyloidosis is disease specific. Primary systemic amyloidosis is somewhat responsive to melphalan, prednisone and peritoneal dialysis [2,3]. Secondary systemic amyloidosis requires treatment of the underlying disease as well as cytotoxic or supportive care for the systemic amyloidosis. For familial Mediterranean fever, colchicine is a successful treatment for the renal amyloidosis [51].

References

1 Glenner GG. Amyloid deposits and amyloidosis. The beta-fibrilloses. Part 1. N Engl J Med 1980;302:1283–92.

2 Glenner GG. Amyloid deposits and amyloidosis. The beta-fibrilloses. Part 2. N Engl J Med 1980;302:1333–43.

3 Breathnach SM. Amyloid and amyloidosis. J Am Acad Dermatol 1988;18:1–16.

4 Kumakiri M, Hashimoto K. Histogenesis of primary localized cutaneous amyloidosis: sequential change of epidermal keratinocytes to amyloid via filamentous degeneration. J Invest Dermatol 1979;73:150–62.

5 Kyle RA. Amyloidosis. Part 1. Int J Dermatol 1980;19:537–9.

6 Glenner GG, Terry W, Harada M et al. Amyloid fibril proteins: proof of homology with immunoglobulin light chains by sequence analyses. Science 1971;172:1150–1.

7 Hashimoto K, Kumakiri M. Colloid-amyloid bodies in PUVA-treated human psoriatic patients. J Invest Dermatol 1979;72:70–80.

8 Hashimoto K. Progress in cutaneous amyloidosis. J Invest Dermatol 1984;82:1–3.

9 Benson MD. Inherited amyloidosis. J Med Genet 1991;28:73–8.

10 Sagher F, Shanon J. Amyloidosis cutis: familial occurrence in three generations. Arch Dermatol 1963;87:171–5.

11 Rajagopalan K, Tay CH. Familial lichen amyloidosis. Report of 19 cases in four generations of a Chinese family in Malaysia. Br J Dermatol 1972;87:123–9.

12 Ozaka M. Familial lichen amyloidosis. Int J Dermatol 1984;23:190–3.

13 Newton JA, Jagjivan A, Bhogal B et al. Familial primary cutaneous amyloidosis. Br J Dermatol 1985;112:201–8.

14 De Pietro WP. Primary familial cutaneous amyloidosis: a study of HLA antigens in a Puerto Rican family. Arch Dermatol 1981; 117:639–42.

15 Gagel RF, Levy ML, Donovan DT et al. Multiple endocrine neoplasia type 2A associated with cutaneous lichen amyloidosis. Ann Intern Med 1989;111:802–6.

16 Kousseff BG, Espinoza C, Zamore GA. Sipple syndrome with lichen amyloidosis as a paracrinopathy: pleiotropy, heterogeneity, or a contiguous gene? J Am Acad Dermatol 1991;25:651–7.

17 Robinson MF, Furst EJ, Nunziata V et al. Characterization of the clinical features of five families with hereditary primary cutaneous lichen amyloidosis and multiple endocrine neoplasia type 2. Henry Ford Hosp Med J 1992;40:249–52.

18 Mulligan LM, Kwok JBJ, Healey CS et al. Germ-line mutations of the RET proto-oncogene in multiple endocrine neoplasia type 2A. Nature 1993;363:458–60.

19 Hofstra RMW, Sijmons RH, Stelwagen T et al. RET mutation screening in familial cutaneous lichen amyloidosis and in skin amyloidosis associated with multiple endocrine neoplasia. J Invest Dermatol 1996;107:215–18.

20 Wong C-K, Lin C-S. Friction amyloidosis. Int J Dermatol 1988; 27:302–7.

21 Wang W-J. Clinical features of cutaneous amyloidoses. Clin Dermatol 1990;8:13–19.

22 Wong C-K. Cutaneous amyloidoses. Int J Dermatol 1987;26:273–7.

23 Mallory SB. Infiltrative diseases. In: Schachner LA, Hanson RC (eds) Pediatric Dermatology, Vol. 2. New York: Churchill Livingstone, 1988:859–61.

24 Arita K, South AP, Hans-Filho G et al. Oncostatin M receptor-beta mutations underlie familial primary localized cutaneous amyloidosis. Am J Hum Genet 2008;82:73–80.

25 Ferrer JP, Halperin I, Conget I et al. Primary localized cutaneous amyloidosis and familial medullary thyroid carcinoma. Clin Endocrinol 1991;34:435–9.

26 Ogino A, Tanaca S. Poikiloderma-like cutaneous amyloidosis. Dermatologica 1977;155:301–9.

27 DeSouza AR. Amiloidose cutanea bullosa familial. Observacao de 4 casos. Rev Hosp Clin Fac Med S Paulo 1963;18:413–17.

28 Partington MW, Marriott PJ, Prentice RS et al. Familial cutaneous amyloidosis with systemic manifestations in males. Am J Med Genet 1981;10:65–75.

29 Partington MW, Prentice RS. X-Linked cutaneous amyloidosis: further clinical and pathological observations. Am J Med Genet 1989;32:115–19.

30 Ades LC, Rogers M, Sillence DO. An X-linked reticulate pigmentary disorder with systemic manifestations: report of a second family. Pediatr Dermatol 1993;10:344–51.

31 Salmon JK, Frieden IJ. Congenital and genetic disorders of hyperpigmentation. Curr Prob Dermatol 1995;7:182–3.

32 Tidman MJ, Wells RS, Macdonald DM. Pachyonychia congenita with cutaneous amyloidosis and hyperpigmentation: a distinct variant. J Am Acad Dermatol 1987;16:935–40.

33 Kantor GR, Kasick JM, Bergfeld WF et al. Epidermolysis bullosa of the Weber–Cockayne type with macular amyloidosis. Cleve Clin Q 1985;52:425–8.

34 Llistosella E, Moreno A, deMoragas JM. Dyskeratosis congenita with macular cutaneous amyloid deposits. Arch Dermatol 1984;120:1381–2.

35 Frenk E, Mevorah B, Hohl D. The Nageli–Franceschetti–Jadassohn syndrome: a hereditary ectodermal defect leading to colloid–amyloid formation in the dermis. Dermatology 1993;187:169–73.

36 Pick AI, Versano I, Schreibman S et al. Agammaglobulinemia, plasma cell dyscrasia, and amyloidosis in a 12-year-old child. Am J Dis Child 1977;131:682–6.

37 Kyle RA. Amyloidosis. Part 3. Int J Dermatol 1981;20:75–80.

38 Ogiyama Y, Hayashi Y, Kou C et al. Cutaneous amyloidosis in patients with progressive systemic sclerosis. Cutis 1996;57:28–32.

39 Kutlay S, Civriz S, Ensari A et al. Development of amyloidosis in Behçet's syndrome with isolated mucocutaneous involvement. Rheumatol Int 2004;24:37–9.

40 Black MM, Albert S. Amyloidosis. In: Bolognia JL, Jorizzo JL, Rapini RP (eds) Dermatology, Vol. 1. London: C.V. Mosby, 2003:58–67.

41 Scarpioni R, Ricardi M, Albertazzi V. Secondary amyloidosis in autoinflammatory diseases and the role of inflammation in renal damage. World J Nephrol 2016;5:66–75.

42 Yi S, Naito K, Nogami R et al. Complicating systemic amyloidosis in dystrophic epidermolysis bullosa, recessive type. Pathology 1988;20:184–7.

43 Meretoja J. Familial systemic paramyloidosis with lattice dystrophy of the cornea, progressive cranial neuropathy, skin changes and various internal symptoms: a previously unrecognized heritable syndrome. Ann Clin Res 1969;1:314–24.

44 Wang C-K, Lee JY-Y. Macular amyloidosis with widespread diffuse pigmentation. Br J Dermatol 1996;135:135–8.

45 Jin AG, Por A, Wee LK et al. Comparative study of phototherapy (UVB) vs. photochemotherapy (PUVA) vs. topical steroids in the treatment of primary cutaneous lichen amyloidosis. Photodermatol Photoimmunol Photomed 2001;17:42–3.

46 Wong C-K, Li W-M. Dermabrasion for lichen amyloidosus. Arch Dermatol 1982;118:302–4.

47 Ozkaya-Bayazit E, Kavak A, Gungor H et al. Intermittent use of topical dimethyl sulfoxide in macular and papular amyloidosis. Int J Dermatol 1998;37:949–54.

48 Helander I, Hopsu-Havu VK. Treatment of lichen amyloidosus by etretinate. Clin Exp Dermatol 1986;11:574–7.

49 Hernandez-Nunez A, Dauden E, Moreno de Vega MJ et al. Widespread biphasic amyloidosis: response to acitretin. Clin Exp Dermatol 2001;26:256–9.

50 Behr FD, Levine N, Bangert J. Lichen amyloidosis associated with atopic dermatitis: clinical resolution with cyclosporine. Arch Dermatol 2001;137:553–5.

51 Zemer D, Pras M, Sohar E et al. Colchicine in the prevention and treatment of the amyloidosis of familial Mediterranean fever. N Engl J Med 1986;314:1001–5.

CHAPTER 156
Immunodeficiency Syndromes

Julie V. Schaffer[1], *Melanie Makhija*[2] *& Amy S. Paller*[2,3]

[1] Division of Pediatric and Adolescent Dermatology, Hackensack University Medical Center, Hackensack, NJ, USA
[2] Department of Pediatrics, Northwestern University, Feinberg School of Medicine, Chicago, IL, USA
[3] Department of Dermatology, Northwestern University, Feinberg School of Medicine, Chicago, IL, USA

Introduction, 2028
Ataxia telangiectasia, 2030
Cartilage–hair hypoplasia syndrome, 2033
Chédiak–Higashi syndrome, 2034
Chronic granulomatous disease, 2037
Chronic mucocutaneous candidiasis, 2041
Complement deficiency disorders, 2045
DiGeorge syndrome, 2051
Hyperimmunoglobulin E syndromes, 2052
Immunoglobulin deficiencies, 2056
IPEX syndrome, 2060
Leucocyte adhesion deficiency, 2060
Severe combined immunodeficiency, 2061
Wiskott–Aldrich syndrome, 2064

Abstract

Primary immunodeficiencies represent a heterogeneous group of disorders characterized by increased susceptibility to infection and often additional features such as autoimmunity, allergy and malignancy. Mucocutaneous manifestations are often a presenting sign, allowing one to suspect the diagnosis and initiate intervention. Improved understanding of the underlying genetic and molecular basis of many of these forms of immunodeficiency has led to reversal through stem cell transplantation or, in some cases, more targeted therapy.

Introduction

Primary immunodeficiencies represent a heterogeneous group of disorders characterized by increased susceptibility to infection, often together with additional features such as autoimmunity, allergy and malignancy (for reviews see references [1–4]). Since the 1990s, tremendous information has accrued to increase our understanding of the pathogenesis of primary immunodeficiencies. Immunodeficiencies are currently classified into nine major groups based on the main type of immune dysfunction [1]. These advances have substantially improved our ability to diagnose affected individuals and carriers, provide prognostic information and perform prenatal testing. Early diagnosis is key to optimal management and improved outcomes.

Immunodeficiency syndromes are often associated with prominent mucocutaneous abnormalities, which can facilitate early diagnosis [5,6]. In addition to mucocutaneous infections, which are most often caused by *Staphylococcus aureus*, *Candida* spp. and human papillomaviruses, noninfectious mucocutaneous features that are shared by several immunodeficiency syndromes include granulomas, eczematous dermatitis, lupus erythematosus-like lesions, small-vessel vasculitis and ulcers (Table 156.1) [7,8]. Other skin findings in patients with recurrent infections may suggest particular underlying diagnoses, such as the telangiectasias of ataxia telangiectasia and the silvery hair of Chédiak–Higashi and type 2 Griscelli syndromes.

In general, immunodeficiency should be suspected when patients have recurrent infections of increased duration and severity or caused by unusual organisms [9]. Incomplete clearance of infections or a poor response to antibiotic therapy may represent additional signs. Other frequent extracutaneous abnormalities in children with immunodeficiencies include failure to thrive, chronic diarrhoea, hepatosplenomegaly, lymphadenopathy or lack of expected nodes, and haematological abnormalities (especially immune thrombocytopenic purpura and autoimmune haemolytic anaemia). Malignancy is the second leading cause of death (after infection) in children and adults with congenital immunodeficiency disorders [10].

Diagnosis of specific forms of primary immunodeficiency has become easier with the availability of whole-exome sequencing, which has led to identification of mutations in new genes and has expedited mutation identification of known disorders. Newborn screening now is standard in many states in the USA. Definitive treatment for individuals with severe immunodeficiency through stem cell transplantation and gene therapy has become more successful with optimization [11,12].

Harper's Textbook of Pediatric Dermatology, Fourth Edition. Edited by Peter Hoeger, Veronica Kinsler and Albert Yan.

Table 156.1 Mucocutaneous findings in immunodeficiency syndromes

Disorder	*S. aureus* infections		CMC	Warts	Eczematous dermatitis	Granulomas (non-infectious)	LE	SVV	Ulcers (PG-like)	Other findings
	Superficial pyodermas	Abscesses								
Ataxia-telangiectasia	+	+			+	+ (often ulcerate)				Oculocutaneous telangiectasias, progeric changes, CALM, BCC
Cartilage–hair hypoplasia syndrome				+						Short-limbed dwarfism, varicella infections, BCC
Chédiak–Higashi syndrome	+	+							+	Pigmentary dilution, hyperpigmentation in sun-exposed sites, silvery hair, bleeding diathesis, gingivitis
Chronic granulomatous disease	++	++	+		+	++ (nodular, necrotic)	+		+	DLE in female carriers, Sweet syndrome, oral ulcers
CMC			++			(++) (candidal)				Dermatophyte infections, vitiligo, alopecia areata
Common variable immunodeficiency	+	+	+	+	+	++	+	+	+	Dermatophyte infections, vitiligo, alopecia areata
Complement deficiencies	+	+	+				++	+	+	Dermatomyositis, urticaria, lipodystrophy (C3), JIA
DiGeorge syndrome			+		+	+				
Hyper-IgE syndrome	++	++ (cold)	+	2	++					Infantile eosinophilic folliculitis[2]
Hyper-IgM syndrome	+	+		+		+	+		+	Oral ulcers
IgA deficiency	+	+	+		+		+	+	+	Vitiligo, lipodystrophia centrifugalis abdominalis
IgM deficiency	+	+		+	+		+			
IRAK4 deficiency	++	++ (cold)	+							
IPEX syndrome	+				+					Autoimmune enteropathy and endocrinopathies
Leucocyte adhesion deficiency		++ (necrotic)							++	Poor wound healing, delayed separation of the umbilical stump, gingivitis
SCID	+	+	+	+	+	+[1]				GVHD, erythroderma (Omenn syndrome)
TAP deficiency						++		+	+	
WHIM	+	+		++						
Wiskott–Aldrich syndrome	++	+			++	+		+		Bleeding diathesis
X-linked agammaglobulinaemia	+	++			+	+				Dermatomyositis-like eruption (due to echovirus); ecthyma gangrenosum

+, Occasional finding; ++ common finding.

BCC, basal cell carcinoma; CALM, café-au-lait macules; CMC, chronic mucocutaneous candidiasis; DLE, discoid lesions of lupus erythematosus; GVHD, graft-versus-host disease; IL, interleukin; IPEX, immune dysregulation, polyendocrinopathy, enteropathy, X-linked; IRAK4, IL-1 receptor associated kinase-4; JIA, juvenile idiopathic arthritis; SVV, small vessel vasculitis; LE, lupus erythematosus; PG, pyoderma gangrenosum; SCID, severe combined immunodeficiency; TAP, transporter associated with processing; WHIM, warts, hypogammaglobulinaemia, infections, and myelokathexis.

[1] Extensive cutaneous and extracutaneous granulomatous disease has been described in children with hypomorphic *RAG1* or *RAG2* mutations.

[2] Patients with the autosomal recessive form of hyper-IgE syndrome are also at increased risk of developing mucocutaneous squamous cell carcinomas and severe warts, molluscum contagiosum and herpes simplex or varicella-zoster viral infections.

Source: Adapted with permission from Bolognia JL, Schaffer JV, Cerroni L, eds. *Dermatology*, 4th edn. London: Elsevier, 2018.

References

1 Picard C, Gaspar HB, Al-Herz W et al. International Union of Immunological Societies: 2017 Primary Immunodeficiency Diseases Committee report on inborn errors of immunity. J Clin Immunol 2018;38:96–128.
2 Azizi G, Ghanavatinejad A, Abolhassani H et al. Autoimmunity in primary T-cell immunodeficiencies. Expert Rev Clin Immunol 2016;28:1–18.
3 Walkovich K, Connelly JA. Primary immunodeficiency in the neonate: early diagnosis and management. Semin Fetal Neonatal Med 2016;21:35–43.
4 Chan SK, Gelfand EW. Primary immunodeficiency masquerading as allergic disease. al. Immunol Allergy Clin North Am 2015; 35:767–78.
5 Sillevis Smitt JH, Kuijpers TW. Cutaneous manifestations of primary immunodeficiency. Curr Opin Pediatr 2013;25:492–7.
6 Relan M, Lehman HK. Common dermatologic manifestations of primary immune deficiencies. Curr Allergy Asthma Rep 2014;14:480.
7 Mitra A, Pollock B, Gooi J et al. Cutaneous granulomas associated with primary immunodeficiency disorders. Br J Dermatol 2005; 153:194–9.
8 Torrelo A, Vera A, Portugues M et al. Perforating neutrophilic and granulomatous dermatitis of the newborn: a clue to immunodeficiency. Pediatr Dermatol 2007;24:211–5.
9 Slatter MA, Gennery AR. An approach to the patient with recurrent infections in childhood. Clin Exp Immunol 2008;152:389–96.
10 Mueller BU, Pizzo PA. Cancer in children with primary or secondary immunodeficiencies. J Pediatr 1995;126:1–10.
11 Chinen J, Notarangelo LD, Shearer WT et al. Advances in basic and clinical immunology in 2014. J Allergy Clin Immunol 2015; 135:1132–41.
12 Fischer A, Hacein-Bey Abina S, Touzot F et al. Gene therapy for primary immunodeficiencies. Clin Genet 2015;88:507–15.

Ataxia telangiectasia

Key points

- Ataxia telangiectasia is an autosomal recessive disorder characterized by cerebella ataxia, telangectasias of the skin and conjunctivae.
- Patients are susceptible to recurrent infections, especially sinopulmonary infections.
- Chromosomal breakage syndrome with hypersensitivity to ionizing radiation and increased risk of malignancy, especially lymphoma, can occur.

Introduction and history. Ataxia telangiectasia (AT) was recognized as a distinct disease in the 1950s, based on reports of children with familial progressive cerebellar ataxia, oculocutaneous telangiectasias and frequent pulmonary infections. Soon after, it was found that these patients had a tendency to develop lymphoreticular malignancies and had a variable humoral immunodeficiency as well as thymic hypoplasia [1]. AT is an autosomal recessive disorder characterized by cerebellar ataxia beginning in infancy, progressive oculocutaneous telangiectasias, recurrent sinopulmonary infections and chromosomal instability with hypersensitivity to ionizing radiation.

Epidemiology and pathogenesis. The incidence of AT is estimated to be 1 in 50 000 to 1 in 100 000 births. Ataxia telangiectasia is caused by loss-of-function mutations in both copies of the *ataxia-telangiectasia mutated (ATM)* gene, which encodes a serine/threonine protein kinase that resembles phosphatidylinositol 3-kinases [2,3]. The MRE11-RAD50-NBS1 complex helps to recruit and activate the ATM protein in response to DNA damage, especially double-stranded breaks [4–6]. ATM subsequently phosphorylates (and thereby activates) multiple targets such as p53, BRCA1, FANCD2, Artemis, MRE11 and NBS1, which leads to cell cycle arrest at G_1/S and facilitates DNA repair or, in the event of severe DNA damage, apoptosis. DNA breaks occur not only upon exposure to ionizing radiation, but also during physiological processes such as V(D)J recombination in lymphocytes, telomere maintenance and meiosis, therefore explaining the sensitivity to ionizing radiation, immunodeficiency, premature ageing and defective spermatogenesis that are observed in patients with AT. The progressive neurological deterioration of AT is thought to result from defective DNA repair in this population of cells that are unable to replicate.

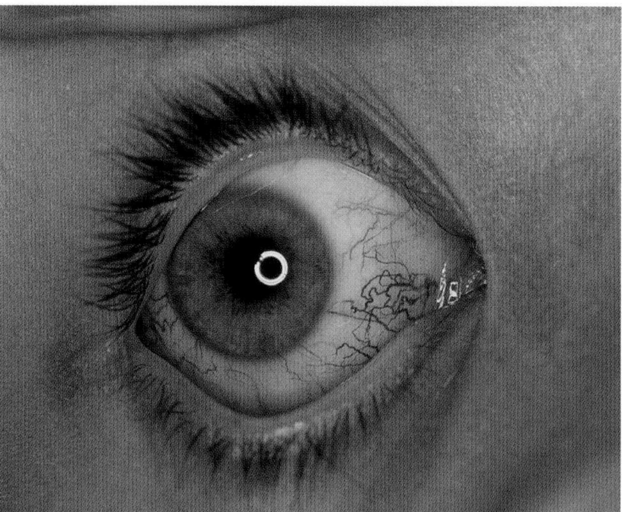

Fig. 156.1 Telangiectasias of the bulbar conjuctiva in ataxia telangiectasia are particularly prominent at the canthi.

Clinical features. The initial manifestation is usually ataxia, which typically becomes apparent when the child begins to walk. However, diagnosis of AT is often delayed until telangiectasias are noted, usually between 3 and 6 years of age. The telangiectasias first appear on the bulbar conjunctivae at the corners of the eyes and extend toward the iris as red symmetrical horizontal streaks (Fig. 156.1). During the next few years, patients begin to develop cutaneous telangiectasias, especially on the ears, eyelids, malar prominences, V of the neck and antecubital and popliteal fossae. Less commonly, telangiectasias are observed on the dorsal aspects of the hands and feet and the palate. Although the ocular telangiectasias are striking, the cutaneous telangiectasias may be subtle and resemble fine petechiae, especially in extrafacial sites.

Evidence of premature ageing of the skin and hair is noted in almost 90% of affected individuals [7].

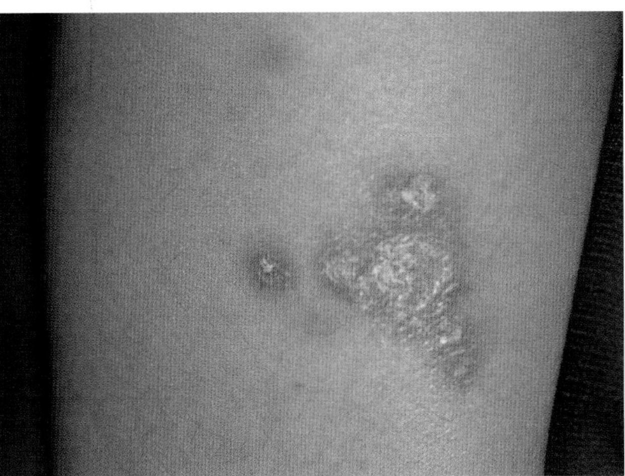

Fig. 156.2 Cutaneous granulomas in ataxia telangiectasia are persistent and may become ulcerated.

Subcutaneous fat is lost during childhood and facial skin tends to become atrophic and sclerotic. Grey hairs may be found in young children and diffuse greying of the hair often occurs by adolescence. Noninfectious cutaneous granulomas (Fig. 156.2) frequently develop and have a tendency to ulcerate [8]. Other skin findings associated with AT are large café-au-lait spots and other forms of 'pigmentary mosaicism' (presumably reflecting chromosomal instability), melanocytic naevi, facial papulosquamous rash, poikiloderma, hypertrichosis (especially on the forearms), seborrhoeic dermatitis with blepharitis and eczematous dermatitis [9,10].

The ataxia of AT is cerebellar in origin and characterized by swaying of the head and trunk. Myoclonic jerks, choreoathetosis, oculomotor abnormalities and dysarthric speech become prominent in older children. Ocular apraxia, the inability to follow an object with the eyes, is a typical neurological finding. Deterioration of vision and nystagmus also occur. Patients are usually confined to a wheelchair by the time they are 11 years old, despite relatively preserved muscular strength. A characteristic facies develops that is hypotonic and sad in appearance. Later, the face becomes mask-like when progeric changes ensue.

Chronic and recurrent sinopulmonary infections occur in up to 80% of patients with AT and represent the most common cause of death, which is usually from resultant bronchiectasis and respiratory failure [11,12]. Other manifestations of AT include retardation of somatic growth (70%), developmental delay and cognitive impairment (30%) and endocrine abnormalities, especially ovarian agenesis or gonadal failure in females and insulin-resistant diabetes mellitus [13]. Up to half of patients have evidence of glucose intolerance, hyperinsulinaemia and insulin resistance. Elevated serum transaminases are also observed in the majority of affected individuals.

Malignancy, most often a B-cell lymphoma or T-cell leukaemia, occurs in up to 40% of patients with AT who survive into their teenage years [14]. Gastric carcinomas have also been described in association with immunoglobulin A (IgA) deficiency in patients with AT, and basal cell carcinomas have been reported to develop after 20 years of age. Heterozygosity for the same *ATM* gene mutations that cause AT when biallelic occur in approximately 1% of the population and confer a two- to threefold increased risk of breast cancer in female carriers [15,16]. Monoallelic carriers of these mutations also have a two- to threefold increased risk of death from cancer, including malignancies of the stomach, colon and lung as well as the breast, with greater excess mortality in individuals younger than 50 years of age [15].

The median lifespan in patients with AT is 20–25 years [17,18]. More than half of patients die from progressive sinopulmonary disease and up to one-third succumb to malignancy or complications related to cancer treatment. Although the neurological manifestations of AT are typically progressive, some patients who survive into their thirties or forties experience stabilization of the disorder, with improvement in neurological and immunological status.

Differential diagnosis. The features of AT are similar to those of Nijmegen breakage syndrome (NBS), a rare autosomal recessive disorder caused by defects in the *NBS1* gene (see Pathogenesis). Nijmegen breakage syndrome features short stature, a 'bird-like' face, microcephaly, mental retardation and chromosomal instability. Patients with NBS have more severe immunodeficiency and a greater risk of malignancy than individuals with AT but no ataxia, telangiectasias or elevated α-fetoprotein levels. Ataxia telangiectasia-like disorder, which results from defects in the *MRE11* gene (see Pathogenesis), is characterized by radiosensitivity and neurological manifestations similar to AT but no telangiectasias, immunodeficiency, cancer predisposition or elevated α-fetoprotein levels. Lastly, the recently described RIDDLE syndrome presents with *r*adiosensitivity, *i*mmunodeficiency, facial *d*ysmorphism, *d*ifficulty *le*arning, abnormal motor control and short stature resulting from defects in RNF168 protein, which mediates ubiquitin-dependent signalling at sites of DNA double-stranded breaks.

Laboratory and histology findings. A variety of immunological abnormalities have been described in patients with AT [11,12]. Humoral defects include decreased or absent serum levels of immunoglobulin A (IgA) (70% of patients), IgG (especially IgG_2 and IgG_4; in 60% of patients) and IgE (in up to 80% of patients). Serum levels of IgM are occasionally increased [19], and 80% of patients have a low-molecular-weight (8S) serum IgM. Defective cell-mediated immunity occurs in approximately 70% of patients with AT and can include T- and B-cell lymphopenia, skin test anergy and deficient *in vitro* lymphoproliferative responses to antigens and mitogens. Patients tend to have a relative paucity of $CD4^+$ T cells, an excess of γ/δ T cells and an absent or hypoplastic thymus. Individuals with no ATM activity have more severe immunological deficits than those with low levels of ATM activity [12]. For children with significant T-cell lymphopenia, early detection has been reported through their identification after abnormal newborn screening for severe combined immunodeficiency (SCID), caused by low or absent T-cell receptor excision circles [20].

Spontaneous chromosomal abnormalities such as fragments, breaks, gaps and translocations occur 2–18 times more frequently than normal in AT patients. Rearrangements of chromosomes 7 and 14 are especially common, and some translocations (in particular those involving 14q32) result in a proliferative advantage and may predict the development of a lymphoid malignancy. DNA in fibroblasts from patients with AT is extremely sensitive to radiomimetic agents such as bleomycin as well as to ionizing radiation.

Almost all patients with AT have elevated serum levels of carcinoembryonic antigen and α-fetoprotein, and measurement of the latter can help to establish the diagnosis in children older than 2 years of age. Radiosensitivity testing with the colony survival assay, analysis of radioresistant DNA synthesis (indicating an abnormal S-phase checkpoint), karyotyping to identify 7;14 chromosomal translocations, immunoblotting for the ATM protein, assessment of ATM kinase activity and sequencing the *ATM* gene may be utilized to confirm the diagnosis of AT. DNA-based prenatal diagnosis can also be performed.

Treatment and prevention. The treatment of patients with AT is supportive. Infections must be treated with appropriate antibiotics and patients with severe immunodeficiency may benefit from prophylactic antibiotics and immunoglobulin replacement [21]. Avoidance of sun exposure and use of sunscreens may help to prevent actinically induced progeric changes. Physiotherapy should be instituted if there are signs of bronchiectasis and early physical therapy may help to prevent contractures related to neurological dysfunction. Patients should be screened for the development of malignancy. Although treatment of lymphoid malignancies in AT patients with standard-dose chemotherapy is more likely to achieve remission and increase survival than reduced-dose chemotherapy, radiomimetic chemotherapeutic agents such as bleomycin and radiation therapy should be avoided. If necessary, the radiation dosage should be restricted to fewer than 20 Gy, in fractions of fewer than 1 Gy. Patients with AT have decreased thresholds for postradiation erythema, tissue necrosis and radiation-induced cutaneous malignancy.

Bone marrow and fetothymic transplants have not resulted in clinical improvement in patients with AT. Aminoglycoside-induced read-through of premature termination codons has been found to restore production of functional ATM protein in cells from individuals with truncating mutations in the *ATM* gene, providing the basis for a possible therapeutic approach in AT patients with this type of mutation [22]. Oxidatative stress is thought to contribute to chromosomal instability, neurodegeneration and malignancy in AT, and treatment with antioxidants such as *N*-acetylcysteine has been shown to decrease the frequency of lymphomas and improve motor function in *ATM*-deficient mice. However, in a recent pilot study of antioxidant therapy (α-lipoic acid plus nicotinamide) for patients with AT, a trend toward increased lymphocyte counts was noted but no improvement in neurological or pulmonary function was observed [21].

References

1 Stiehm ER, Ochs HD, Winkelstein JD. Immunologic Disorders in Infants and Children, 5th edn. Philadelphia: Elsevier Saunders, 2004:512.

2 Savitsky K, Bar-Shira A, Gilad S et al. A single ataxia telangiectasia gene with a product similar to PI-3 kinase. Science 1995;268:1749–53.

3 Lavin MF. Ataxia–telangiectasia: from a rare disorder to a paradigm for cell signalling and cancer. Nat Rev Mol Cell Biol 2008; 9:759–69.

4 Ambrose M, Gatti RA. Pathogenesis of ataxia-telangiectasia: the next generation of ATM functions. Blood 2013;121:4036.

5 Lee JH, Paull TT. ATM activation by DNA double-stranded breaks through the Mre11-Rad50-Nbs1 complex. Science 2005;308:551–4.

6 Stracker TH, Roig I, Knobel PA et al. The ATM signaling network in development and disease. Fron Genet 2013;4:37.

7 Cohen LE, Tanner DJ, Schaefer HG et al. Common and uncommon cutaneous findings in patients with ataxia telangiectasia. J Am Acad Dermatol 1984;10:431–7.

8 Paller AS, Massey RB, Curtis MA et al. Cutaneous granulomatous lesions in patients with ataxia-telangiectasia. J Pediatr 1991; 119:917–22.

9 Khumalo NP, Joss DV, Huson SM, Burge S. Pigmentary anomalies in ataxia-telangiectasia: a clue to diagnosis and an example of twin spotting. Br J Dermatol 2001;144:369–71.

10 Greenberger S, Berkun Y, Ben-Zeev B et al. Dermatologic manifestations of ataxia-telangiectasia syndrome. J Am Acad Dermatol 2013;68:932–6.

11 Nowak-Wegrzyn A, Crawford TO, Winkelstein JA et al. Immunodeficiency and infections in ataxia-telangiectasia. J Pediatr 2004;144:505–11.

12 Staples ER, McDermott EM, Reiman A et al. Immunodeficiency in ataxia telangiectasia is correlated strongly with the presence of two null mutations in the ataxia telangiectasia mutated gene. Clin Exp Immunol 2008;153:214–20.

13 Nissenkorn A, Levy-Shraga Y, Banet-Levi Y. Endocrine abnormalities in ataxia telangiectasia: findings from a national cohort. Pediatr Res 2016;79:889–94.

14 Cabana MD, Crawford RO, Winkelstein JA et al. Consequences of the delayed diagnosis of ataxia-telangiectasia. Pediatrics 1998; 102:98–100.

15 Thompson D, Duedal S, Kirner J et al. Cancer risks and mortality in heterozygous ATM mutation carriers. J Natl Cancer Inst 2005; 97:813–22.

16 Renwick A, Thompson D, Seal S et al. ATM mutations that cause ataxia-telangiectasia are breast cancer susceptibility alleles. Nat Genet 2006;38:873–5.

17 Crawford TO, Skolasky RL, Fernandez R et al. Survival probability in ataxia telangiectasia. Arch Dis Child 2006;91:610–1.

18 Micol R, Ben Slama L, Suarez F et al. Morbidity and mortality from A-T are associated with ATM genotype. JACI 2011; 128:382–389.e381

19 Teresa de la Morena M. Clinical phenotypes of hyper-IgM syndromes. J Allergy Clin Immunol: In Pract 2016;4:1023–36.

20 Kwan A, Abraham RS, Currier R, Newborn screening for severe combined immune deficiency in 11 screening programs in the United States. JAMA 2014;312:729–38.

21 Lavin MF, Gueven N, Bottle S, Gatti RA. Current and potential therapeutic strategies for the treatment of ataxia-telangiectasia. Br Med Bull 2007;81–2:129–47.

22 Lai CH, Chun HH, Nahas SA et al. Correction of ATM gene function by aminoglycoside-induced read-through of premature termination codons. Proc Natl Acad Sci U S A 2004;10:16982.

Cartilage–hair hypoplasia syndrome

Key points

- **Cartilage–hair hypoplasia syndrome is an autosomal recessive disorder with a predominantly T-cell immunodeficiency.**
- **It is characterized by metaphyseal chondrodysplasia with normal head size and distinct hair abnormalities.**

Introduction and history. In 1964, McKusick described susceptibility to varicella infection in Amish children with dwarfism. He named the syndrome cartilage hair hypoplasia (CHH) [1]. CHH is an autosomal recessive disorder characterized by metaphyseal chondrodysplasia, a form of short-limbed dwarfism, with a variable predominantly T-cell immunodeficiency and light-coloured hair [1].

Epidemiology and pathogenesis. CHH syndrome is an autosomal recessive disorder with an incidence of 1 in 20 000 live births in Finland (the most affected European population) and 1.5 in 1000 births in the Amish population of the USA [2]. Cartilage–hair hypoplasia results from point mutations in the *RMRP* gene, mapped to chromosome 9p21-p12, which encodes the RNA component of ribonucleoprotein endoribonuclease MRP, which cleaves RNA primers responsible for DNA replication in mitochondria and processes pre-rRNA in the nucleolus [2–4].

Clinical features. Patients with CHH have fine, sparse, hypopigmented hair and metaphyseal dysostosis that results in short-limbed dwarfism. Affected individuals may also have soft doughy skin with degenerated elastic tissue [5]. Patients occasionally present with SCID (see later) and an Omenn syndrome-like phenotype of erythroderma, chronic diarrhoea, lymphadenopathy, hepatosplenomegaly and eosinophilia [6]. Anaemia (hypoplastic or autoimmune haemolytic), neutropenia (hypoplastic or autoimmune), autoimmune thyroid disease and Hirschsprung disease have also been described. Malignancy, most often non-Hodgkin lymphoma, occurs in 10% of patients. Affected individuals also have an increased risk of basal cell carcinoma [7].

Differential diagnosis. The differential diagnosis includes other autosomal recessive skeletal dysplasias with or without immunodeficiency, including anauxetic dysplasia, metaphyseal dysplasia without hyptrichosis, kyphomelic dysplasia, Shwachman–Diamond syndrome, ectodermal dysplasia with immunodeficiency and others.

Laboratory and histology findings. The majority of patients manifest some degree of defective cell-mediated immunity, which includes increased susceptibility to varicella [6,8]. Defective humoral immunity, most often deficiency of IgA or IgG, occurs in one-third of patients and may contribute to recurrent respiratory tract infections and resultant bronchiectasis [9]. In a Finnish study of 88 patients, laboratory findings included anaemia (primary or autoimmune) with or without macrocytosis in 86%, lymphopenia in 62% and neutropenia in 24% [10].

Treatment and prevention. Treatment of CHH depends on the manifestations present. All patients should receive all vaccinations including live viral vaccines if they have adequate T cell and antibody function. If T-cell levels and function are low, live viral vaccines should be avoided. If patients have antibody deficiency and hypogammaglobulinaemia, immunoglobulin replacement can be used. Varicella zoster immunoglobulin and antiviral drugs can be used for prevention and treatment. If patients have a SCID phenotype, stem cell transplantation may be curative but will not affect morphological features [11–13]. Newborn screening programmes for SCID help identify patients with RMRP mutations and severe immunodeficiency phenotype [14].

Individuals may have shortened lifespan caused by significant immunodeficiency in childhood or lymphoma/leukaemia in adulthood. Severe bronchiectasis may also shorten lifespan.

References

1 McKusick VA, Eldridge R, Hostetler JA et al. Dwarfism in the Amish. Ii. Cartilage-Hair Hypoplasia. Bull Johns Hopkins Hosp 1965;116:285–326.

2 Hermanns P, Bertuch AA, Bertin TK et al. Consequences of mutations in the non-coding RMRP RNA in cartilage-hair hypoplasia. Hum Mol Genet 2005;14:3723–40.

3 Rogler LE, Kosmyna B, Moskowitz D. Small RNAs derived from lncRNA RNase MRP have gen-silencing activity relevant to human cartilage-hair hypoplasia. Hum Mol Genet 2014;23:368–82.

4 Ridanpaa M, Van Eenennaam H, Pelin K et al. Mutations in the RNA component of RNase MRP cause a pleiotropic human disease, cartilage–hair hypoplasia. Cell 2001;104:195–203.

5 Brennan T, Pearson R. Abnormal elastic tissue in cartilage–hair hypoplasia. Arch Dermatol 1988;124:1411–14.

6 Kavadas FD, Giliani S, Gu Y et al. Variability of clinical and laboratory features among patients with ribonuclease mitochondrial RNA processing endoribonuclease gene mutations. J Allergy Clin Immunol 2008;122:1178–84.

7 Taskinen M, Ranki A, Pukkala E et al. Extended follow-up of the Finnish cartilage–hair hypoplasia cohort confirms high incidence of non-Hodgkin lymphoma and basal cell carcinoma. Am J Med Genet A 2008;146A:2370–5.

8 Notarangelo LD, Roifman CM, Giliani S. Cartilage–hair hypoplasia: molecular basis and heterogeneity of the immunological phenotype. Curr Opin Allergy Clin Immunol 2008;8:534.

9 Toivianen-Salo S, Kajosaari M, Piilonen A, Mäkitie O. Patients with cartilage hair hypoplasia have an increased risk for bronchiectasis. J Pediatr 2008;152:422–8.

10 Makitie O, Rajantie J, Kaitila I. Anemia and macrocytosis – unrecognized features in cartilage-hair hypoplasia. Acta Paediatr 1992;81:1026–9.

11 Guggenheim R, Somech R, Grunebaum E et al. Bone marrow transplantation for cartilage-hair-hypoplasia. Bone Marrow Transplant 2006;38:751–6.

12 Bordon V, Gennery AR, Slatter MA et al Clinical and immunologic outcome of patients with cartilage hair hypoplasia after hematopoietic stem cell transplantation. Blood 2010;116:27–35.

13 Ip W, Gaspar HB, Kleta R et al. Variable phenotype of severe immunodeficiencies associated with RMRP gene mutations. J Clin Immunol 2015;35:147–57.

14 Kwan A, Abraham RS, Currier R, Newborn screening for severe combined immune deficiency in 11 screening programs in the United States. JAMA 2014;312:729–38.

Chédiak–Higashi syndrome

Key points

- Chédiak–Higashi syndrome is an autosomal recessive disorder characterized by pigment abnormalities, silvery hair, severe recurrent infections and usually haemophagocytic lymphohistiocytosis.
- It is related to abnormality in vesicle trafficking.
- Examination of hair shafts to show pigment clumping and smears to show granules in white blood cells are quick screening tests.
- It must be distinguished from Griscelli syndrome, the other major disorder with silvery hair.
- Early stem cell transplantation is the treatment of choice.

Introduction and history. Chédiak–Higashi syndrome (CHS) is an autosomal recessive disorder of vesicle trafficking characterized by mild oculocutaneous albinism, silvery hair, severe recurrent infections and, in most patients, haemophagocytic lymphohistiocytosis [1–3].

Epidemiology and pathogenesis. This rare disorder is caused by mutations in the lysosomal trafficking regulator (*LYST*, also called *CHS1*) [4]. This results in dysregulated fission/fusion of intracellular lysosome-related organelles, which leads to the formation of large dysfunctional melanosomes, platelet-dense granules and leucocyte cytolytic granules. Because the giant leucocyte granules cannot properly discharge their proteolytic and peroxidative enzymes into phagocytic vacuoles, target cell killing is ineffective. Abnormal antigen presentation, regulation of T-cell activation and repair of plasma membranes may also contribute to the pathogenesis of CHS. *LYST* mutations that result in a truncated protein are associated with a severe phenotype and early death, whereas missense mutations produce milder disease with survival to adulthood [5].

Clinical features. Patients with CHS have a characteristic silvery metallic sheen to the hair and diffuse pigmentary dilution of the skin and eyes when compared with their family members. However, affected individuals with relatively dark constitutive pigmentation often develop bronze to slate-grey hyperpigmentation acrally and in other sun-exposed sites, and superimposed guttate hypopigmented macules may also be evident in these areas [3,6,7]. Photophobia, nystagmus and strabismus can occur because of decreased ocular pigment, but visual acuity is usually normal.

Recurrent infections typically begin to develop during infancy. Infectious episodes are associated with fever and primarily involve the skin, lungs and upper respiratory tract. The most common organisms are *S. aureus*, *Streptococcus pyogenes* and *Streptococcus pneumoniae*. Skin infections are usually superficial pyodermas, but deeper ulcerations resembling pyoderma gangrenosum have been reported. Inflammation and ulceration of the gingiva and other oral mucosal sites may also occur. Petechiae, easy bruising and epistaxis can result from the mild bleeding diathesis of CHS.

Up to 85% of patients with CHS undergo an 'accelerated phase' of haemophagocytic lymphohistiocytosis that is characterized by widespread visceral infiltration with lymphoid and histiocytic cells, which are sometimes atypical in appearance. Hepatosplenomegaly, lymphadenopathy, pancytopenia, jaundice, gingivitis and pseudomembranous sloughing of the buccal mucosa are associated features. Thrombocytopenia and decreased hepatic synthesis of coagulation factors lead to increased petechiae, bruising and gingival bleeding. Chédiak–Higashi syndrome is often fatal during childhood as a consequence of overwhelming infection or haemorrhage during the accelerated phase. Infection with Epstein–Barr virus has been implicated in the uncontrolled T-cell and macrophage activation of the accelerated phase [8].

Differential diagnosis. Chédiak–Higashi syndrome should be differentiated from Griscelli syndrome (GS) (Table 156.2), a group of autosomal recessive conditions that also present with silvery hair, mild diffuse pigmentary dilution and bronzing of sun-exposed skin [9]. Griscelli syndrome is a disorder of vesicle movement and transfer that is caused by defective attachment of lysosome-related organelles to the actin cytoskeleton via a protein complex that includes myosin Va, melanophilin and Rab27A within melanocytes [10–12].

Type 2 GS is caused by mutations in the *RAB27A* gene that is expressed in T cells as well as melanocytes; like CHS, it features recurrent infections and haemophagocytic lymphohistiocytosis. Patients with type 2 GS have hypogammaglobulinaemia in addition to impaired delayed-type hypersensitivity and NK cell activity, and they may develop secondary neurological dysfunction as a complication of the accelerated phase. Type 1 GS results from mutations in the myosin Va (*MYO5A)* gene that is expressed in neurons as well as melanocytes. It manifests with primary neurological abnormalities but not immunodeficiency. Elejalde syndrome (neuroectodermal melanolysosomal disease) presents with pigmentary features of GS plus severe neurological dysfunction and is thought to represent a variant of type 1 GS. Type 3 GS is caused by mutations in the melanophilin (*MLPH*) gene or deletion of the *MYO5A* F-exon, both of which are expressed primarily in melanocytes; as a consequence, the phenotype is limited to pigmentary findings [13,14].

Hermansky–Pudlak syndrome (HPS) is a group of autosomal recessive disorders with diffuse pigmentary dilution of the skin, hair and eyes together with platelet dysfunction. In particular, HPS2 (caused by mutations in *AP3B1*) has immune abnormalities in cytotoxic T and natural killer (NK) cells; haemophagocytic lymphohistiocytosis has also been reported [15–17]. Although the hair has a peculiar sheen, it is not the silver shade of CHS. Trichohepato-enteric syndrome (phenotypic diarrhoea of infancy) is an autosomal recessive disorder caused by mutations in the *TTC37* gene that can feature diffuse pigmentary dilution of the skin and hair, immunodeficiency

Table 156.2 Features of Chédiak–Higashi syndrome (CHS) and Griscelli syndromes (GS)

	CHS	GS1[1]	GS2	GS3
Gene defect	*LYST*	*MYO5A*	*RAB27A*	*MLPH*
Major sites of gene expression	Melanocytes, platelets, granulocytes, CNS	Melanocytes, CNS	Melanocytes, cytotoxic T cells	Melanocytes
Cellular defect	Vesicle trafficking (e.g. fission/fusion)		Vesicle movement and transfer	
Pigmentary dilution of the skin[2]	+	+	+	+
Silvery/metallic hair	+	+	+	+
Hair microscopy: clumps of melanin	Small, regularly spaced		Larger, irregularly distributed	
Melanocytes	Giant melanosomes		'Stuffed' with melanosomes	
Neutrophils	Giant granules		Normal-appearing granules	
Ocular findings	+	–	–	–
Bleeding diathesis	+	–	–	–
Recurrent infections	+	–	+	–
Accelerated phase	+	–	+	–
Primary neurological abnormalities	+	+	–[3]	–

CNS, central nervous system.
GS is caused by defective attachment of organelles to the actin cytoskeleton.
[1] Elejalde syndrome (neuroectodermal melanolysosomal disease), which presents with pigmentary features of GS plus severe neurological dysfunction, likely represents a variant of GS1. Elejalde syndrome is not associated with immunodeficiency.
[2] Often accompanied by hyperpigmentation +/– guttate hypopigmented macules in acral and sun-exposed sites.
[3] May develop neurological symptoms secondary to the haemophagocytic syndrome of the accelerated phase.
Patients with CHS who survive into the second decade of life develop progressive neurological deterioration, which typically presents with clumsiness, an abnormal gait and paraesthesias. Peripheral and cranial neuropathies, spinocerebellar degeneration, parkinsonism and dementia may complicate CHS in adults with otherwise mild disease or who underwent haematopoietic stem cell transplantation during childhood.
Source: Adapted with permission from Bolognia JL, Schaffer JV, Cerroni L, eds. *Dermatology*, 4th edn. London: Elsevier, 2018.

and platelet abnormalities; unlike CHS, it is also characterized by brittle hair with trichorrhexis nodosa, intractable diarrhoea during infancy, primary liver disease, facial dysmorphism and cardiac defects [18]. Additional inherited disorders characterized by lymphoproliferation in the context of immune dysregulation are summarized in Table 156.3. Silvery hair has also been described in a neonate with hypoproteinaemia from congenital hydrops fetalis; with clinical improvement, the hair spontaneously repigmented [19].

Laboratory and histology findings. The hallmark laboratory finding of CHS is giant granules within melanocytes (melanosomes), platelets (dense granules) and leucocytes (cytolytic granules). A peripheral blood smear showing giant granules in the perinuclear area of granulocytes can help to confirm the diagnosis. Microscopically, the silvery hair of CHS displays regularly spaced clumps of melanin. Immunological abnormalities in CHS patients include neutropenia, decreased leucocyte chemotaxis, impaired NK cell activity, diminished antibody-dependent cell-mediated cytotoxicity and reduced cytotoxic and regulatory T-cell function. Melanocytes from individuals with GS are 'stuffed' with numerous melanosomes, but neutrophils have normal-appearing granules. Microscopic examination of hair shafts from patients with GS shows clumps of melanin that tend to be larger and more irregularly distributed than those seen in patients with CHS.

Treatment and prevention. Haematopoietic stem cell transplantation (HSCT) can correct the immunodeficiency of CHS and prevent or (following immunochemotherapy with etoposide, corticosteroids and ciclosporin) treat the accelerated phase [20–23]. Reduced intensity conditioning has been used with success, especially in patients transplanted before the accelerated phase occurs. Absence of cytotoxic T-cell function has been touted to predict the later occurrence of haemophagocytic lymphohistiocytosis, and may be a biomarker for early transplantation [23]. Transplantation does not alter the pigmentary findings or halt neurological degeneration. Management of CHS is otherwise largely supportive, with use of prophylactic antibiotics to avoid recurrent infections.

References

1 Nagai K, Ochi F, Terui K et al. Clinical characteristics and outcomes of Chédiak-Higashi syndrome: a nationwide survey of Japan. Pediatr Blood Cancer 2013;60: 1582–6.
2 Introne WJ, Westbroek W, Golas GA et al. Chediak-Higashi syndrome. In: Pagon RA, Adam MP, Ardinger HH et al. (eds) GeneReviews® [Internet]. Seattle (WA): University of Washington, Seattle;1993–2016.
3 Anderson LL, Paller AS, Malpass D et al. Chediak–Higashi syndrome in a black child. Pediatr Dermatol 1992;9:31–6.
4 Barbosa MD, Nguyen QA, Tchernev VT et al. Identification of the homologous beige and Chediak–Higashi syndrome genes. Nature 1996;382:262–4.
5 Westbroek W, Adams D, Huizing M et al. Cellular defects in Chediak–Higashi syndrome correlate with the molecular genotype and clinical phenotype. J Invest Dermatol 2007;127:2674–7.
6 Al-Khenaizan S. Hyperpigmentation in Chediak–Higashi syndrome. J Am Acad Dermatol 2003;49:S244–6.
7 Raghuveer C, Murthy SC, Mithuna MN et al. Silvery hair with speckled dyspigmentation: Chediak-Higashi syndrome in three Indian siblings. Int J Trichology 2015;7:133–5.
8 Kinugawa N. Epstein–Barr virus infection in Chediak–Higashi syndrome mimicking acute lymphocytic leukemia. Am J Pediatr Hematol Oncol 1990;12:182–6.
9 Mancini AJ, Chan LS, Paller AS et al. Partial albinism with immunodeficiency. Griscelli syndrome: report of a case and review of the literature. J Am Acad Dermatol 1998;38:295–300.

Table 156.3 Inherited disorders characterized by immune dysregulation and lymphoproliferation

Disorder	Inheritance	Gene	Protein (function)	Clinical features
Chédiak–Higashi	AR	*LYST*	See text	See text
Griscelli type 2	AR	*RAB27A*		
Familial haemophagocytic lymphohistiocytosis	AR	*PRF1*	Perforin (major cytolytic granule protein of CTL and NK cells)	Haemophagocytic syndrome Absent NK cell cytotoxicity Fatal during early childhood without haematopoietic stem cell transplantation
	AR	*UNC13D*	Munc13–4 (primes cytolytic granules for secretion)	
	AR	*STX11*	Syntaxin 11 (involved in cytolytic granule trafficking and fusion)	
	AR	*STXBP2*	Munc 18–2 (involved in intracellular trafficking and release of cytoxic granules)	
X-linked lymphoproliferative syndrome (Duncan disease) and autosomal recessive EBV-associated lymphoproliferative syndrome	XR	*SH2D1A*	Signalling lymphocyte activation molecule-associated protein (adaptor protein that regulates B-, T- and NK-cell function; particularly important for immune responses to EBV)	Severe EBV-related infectious mononucleosis in childhood or adolescence (e.g. fever, pharyngitis, LAN, HSM), often associated with morbilliform eruptions, purpura, and/or jaundice Lack of NK T cells +/– Hypogammaglobulinaemia Fatal EBV-related B-cell lymphoma (not reported with XIAP defects) Lymphocytic vasculitis
	XR	*XIAP*	X-linked inhibitor of apoptosis	
	AR	*ITK*	IL-2-inducible T-cell kinase	
Autoimmune lymphoproliferative syndrome (Canale–Smith syndrome)	AD > AR	*TNFRSF6*	CD95 (Fas; cell-surface apoptosis receptor)	Massive LAN and/or splenomegaly Increased CD4$^-$/CD8$^-$ α/β T cells Autoimmune cytopenias, LE, small vessel vasculitis Recurrent bacterial and viral infections (*CASP* Increased risk of lymphoma
	AD	*TNFSF6*	CD95L (Fas ligand)	
	AD > AR	*CASP10*	Caspase 8 and 10 (proteases in intracellular apoptosis cascade)	
	AR	*CASP8*		
	AD	*NRAS*	NRAS (gain-of-function leads to decreased lymphocyte apoptosis)	
	AR	*PRKCD*	PRKCD (regulates B cell proliferation)	Lymphadenopathy and variable autoimmune manifestations
	AD	*CTLA4*	CTLA4 (costimulatory molecule on activated T cells)	Associated with autoimmune endocrine and rheumatic disorders
Immunodeficiency with lymphoid proliferation	AR	*IL2RA*	IL-2 receptor α chain (apoptosis of developing T cells in the thymus)	Bacterial, viral and fungal infections Extensive lymphocytic infiltration of the liver, lung, gut and bones Autoimmune endocrinopathies, enteropathy, cytopenias and eczematous dermatitis

AD, autosomal dominant; AR, autosomal recessive; CTL, cytotoxic T lymphocytes; EBV, Epstein–Barr virus; HSM, hepatosplenomegaly; LAN, lymphadenopathy; LE, lupus erythematosus; NK, natural killer; XR, X-linked recessive.
Source: Adapted with permission from Bolognia JL, Schaffer JV, Cerroni L, eds. *Dermatology*, 4th edn. London: Elsevier, 2018.

10 Menasche G, Pastural E, Feldmann J et al. Mutations in RAB27A cause Griscelli syndrome associated with haemophagocytic syndrome. Nat Genet 2000;25:173–6.
11 Pastural E, Barrat FJ, Dufourcq-Lagelouse R et al. Griscelli disease maps to chromosome 15q21 and is associated with mutations in the myosin-Va gene. Nat Genet 1997;16:289–92.
12 Ménasché G, Ho CH, Sanal O et al. Griscelli syndrome restricted to hypopigmentation results from a melanophilin defect (GS3) or a MYO5A F-exon deletion (GS1). J Clin Invest 2003;112:450–6.
13 Nouriel A, Zisquit J, Helfand AM et al. Griscelli Syndrome Type 3: two new cases and review of the literature. Pediatr Dermatol 2015;32:e245–8.
14 Westbroek W, Klar A, Cullinane AR et al. Cellular and clinical report of new Griscelli syndrome type III cases. Pigment Cell Melanoma Res 2012;25:47–56.
15 Enders A, Zieger B, Schwarz K et al. Lethal hemophagocytic lymphohistiocytosis in Hermansky–Pudlak syndrome type II. Blood 2006;108:81–7.
16 Gahl WA, Huizing M. Hermansky-Pudlak Syndrome. In: Pagon RA, Adam MP, Ardinger HH et al. (eds) GeneReviews® [Internet]. Seattle (WA): University of Washington, Seattle, 1993–2016.
17 Wei AH, Li W. Hermansky-Pudlak syndrome: pigmentary and non-pigmentary defects and their pathogenesis. Pigment Cell Melanoma Res 2013;26:176–92.
18 Hartley JL, Zachos NC, Dawood B et al. Mutations in TTC37 cause trichohepatoenteric syndrome (phenotypic diarrhea of infancy). Gastroenterology 2010;138:2388–98.
19 Galve J, Martín-Santiago A, Clavero C et al. Spontaneous repigmentation of silvery hair in an infant with congenital hydrops fetalis and hypoproteinemia. Cutis 2016;97:E1–5.
20 Umeda K, Adachi S, Horikoshi Y et al. Allogeneic hematopoietic stem cell transplantation for Chediak-Higashi syndrome. Pediatr Transplant 2016;20:271–5.
21 Hamidieh AA, Pourpak Z, Yari K et al. Hematopoietic stem cell transplantation with a reduced-intensity conditioning regimen in pediatric patients with Griscelli syndrome type 2. Pediatr Transplant 2013;17:487–91.
22 Trottestam H, Beutel K, Meeths M et al. Treatment of the X-linked lymphoproliferative, Griscelli and Chédiak–Higashi syndromes by HLH directed therapy. Pediatr Blood Cancer 2009;52:268–72.
23 Lozano ML, Rivera J, Sánchez-Guiu I et al. Towards the targeted management of Chediak-Higashi syndrome. Orphanet J Rare Dis 2014;9:132.

Chronic granulomatous disease

Key points

- **A group of X-linked and autosomal recessive disorders characterized by the inability to kill intracellular organisms through generation of oxidative metabolites.**
- **They are characterized by recurrent infections (especially of skin, lungs and perianal area), lymphadenopathy, hepatosplenomegaly, granuloma formation and other inflammatory manifestations (including cutaneous lupus erythematosus in some patients and female carriers of the X-linked form).**

Introduction. Chronic granulomatous disease (CGD) is a group of disorders characterized by severe, recurrent infections and inflammatory manifestations caused by an inability of leucocytes to kill phagocytosed organisms by generating oxidative metabolites. Reduced function of the nicotinamide adenine dinucleotide phosphate (NADPH) oxidase complex underlies all forms of CGD.

Epidemiology and pathogenesis. The incidence of this disease is estimated to be 1 in 200 000 live births. The disorder most often has an X-linked recessive pattern of inheritance, but several forms with autosomal recessive transmission also exist [1–3]. The molecular defects that underlie CGD involve five components of the phagocyte NADPH oxidase:

1 Membrane-bound gp91^{phox} encoded by the *CYBB* gene (~70% of patients, X-linked recessive);
2 Membrane-bound p22^{phox} encoded by the *CYBA* gene (≤5% of patients, autosomal recessive);
3 Cytoplasmic p47^{phox} encoded by the *NCF1* gene (~20% of patients, autosomal recessive);
4 Cytoplasmic p67^{phox} encoded by the *NCF2* gene (≤5% of patients, autosomal recessive); and
5 Cytoplasmic p40^{phox} encoded by the *NCF4* gene (rare, autosomal recessive).

The membrane-bound components represent subunits of flavocytochrome b_{558}, and upon activation of the NADPH oxidase they associate with the cytoplasmic components. Regardless of which component is affected, the presence of residual NADPH oxidase activity is associated with milder disease and longer survival [4,5].

The deficient microbial killing that characterizes CGD results from failure to rapidly generate toxic reactive oxygen species (ROS) via transfer of electrons from NADPH to molecular O_2 (the respiratory burst) following phagocytosis. The NADPH oxidase also has roles in activation of antimicrobial proteases within the phagosome and formation of microbicidal 'neutrophil extracellular traps' [6,7]. In addition to killing and degrading microorganisms, ROS produced through NADPH oxidase activity participate in induction of neutrophil apoptosis, which normally prevents tissue damage at sites of inflammation, and regulation of cytokine synthesis. Animal models of CGD have shown that the lack of ROS leads to excess inflammation via decreased regulatory T-cell activity, unrestrained γ/δ T-cell activity and augmented production of cytokines such as interleukin (IL)-1β, IL-8 and IL-17 [8,9]. NADPH oxidase also has a role in modulating MHC class II antigen presentation by B cells [10].

Clinical features. The areas of the body that are most often affected in CGD are those that are frequently challenged by bacteria, particularly the skin, lungs and perianal region. Organisms that commonly cause infections in patients with CGD include *S. aureus* (especially pyoderma, abscesses and adenitis), *Nocardia* spp., *Burkholderia cepacia*, *Klebsiella* spp., *Serratia marcescens* (especially osteomyelitis), *Candida* spp., *Aspergillus* spp. (especially pneumonia), and mycobacteria (including severe/disseminated bacillus Calmette-Guérin infection) [11]. The generation of ROS is necessary for phagocytic leucocytes to kill these organisms. The X-linked form of CGD tends to be more severe and to have a younger mean age at diagnosis (3 years) than autosomal recessive forms (8 years) [2].

The first manifestation of CGD is usually staphylococcal infections of the skin around the ears and nose in the neonatal period [12]. These localized pyodermas may progress during infancy to extensive purulent dermatitis with regional lymphadenopathy. Initial presentation of CGD as ecthyma gangrenosum in the neonatal period has also been described [13]. Cutaneous abscesses are common, especially in the perianal region, and are also most often caused by *S. aureus*. *S. marcescens* infection can also present with abscesses or chronic ulcers of the skin [14]. Cutaneous granulomas, which are nodular and often necrotic, occur less frequently than cutaneous infections. Purulent inflammatory reactions tend to develop at sites of minor skin trauma and heal slowly with scarring, and Sweet syndrome-like presentations have been reported [12]. Seborrhoeic dermatitis, folliculitis and ulcers of the oral mucosa (resembling aphthous stomatitis), perioral area and other cutaneous sites have also been described. Patients with CGD may develop cutaneous features of acute or chronic lupus erythematosus, especially discoid lesions [15]. In addition, female carriers of X-linked CGD occasionally present with discoid lupus erythematosus, photosensitive eruptions, Jessner lymphocytic infiltrate, Raynaud phenomenon, aphthous stomatitis and granulomatous cheilitis [16].

The extracutaneous organs typically involved in CGD are the lymph nodes, lungs, liver, spleen and gastrointestinal tract. Suppurative lymphadenitis most frequently affects the cervical lymph nodes, with abscess and fistula formation. Axillary, inguinal, mesenteric and mediastinal lymph nodes are often also involved. Pneumonia, which occurs in almost all children with CGD, responds inadequately to antibacterial therapy and can lead to abscess formation, cavitation and empyema. Hepatosplenomegaly is found in 80–90% of patients and more than one-third of affected individuals develop hepatic abscesses. Granulomas of the lungs, liver, spleen and gastrointestinal and genitourinary tracts are common and may manifest with bowel or urinary obstruction. Excessive inflammatory responses can result in additional noninfectious complications such as wound dehiscence, pneumonitis, haemophagocytic lymphohistiocytosis and clinical presentations mimicking inflammatory bowel disease (e.g. diarrhoea, anal fistulae; 40–80% of patients), sarcoidosis, rheumatoid arthritis and IgA nephropathy [1,15,17,18].

Differential diagnosis. Laboratory tests demonstrating a defective respiratory burst allow differentiation of CGD from other disorders characterized by increased susceptibility to bacterial and fungal infections. Additional inherited phagocyte disorders are summarized in Table 156.4.

Laboratory and histology findings. Laboratory abnormalities in patients with CGD include leucocytosis, anaemia, T-cell lymphopenia, hypergammaglobulinaemia and an elevated erythrocyte sedimentation rate. Skin testing for delayed-type hypersensitivity is normal, as are studies of chemotaxis and phagocytosis. The nitroblue tetrazolium (NBT) reduction assay can be useful in establishing the diagnosis of CGD. NBT is yellow in its soluble oxidized form; when reduced, the dye precipitates and becomes blue–black (formazan precipitate). Only 5–10% of leucocytes from patients with CGD are able to reduce NBT during phagocytosis, compared with 80–90% of leucocytes from unaffected individuals and approximately 50% of leucocytes from carriers of X-linked CGD. The dihydrorhodamine 123 assay and ferricytochrome *c* reduction assay are more accurate and quantitative in measuring the respiratory burst, and they can also be performed to verify the diagnosis [19].

Immunoblot analysis may demonstrate lack of the gp91^{phox} and p22^{phox} proteins; however, DNA analysis must be performed to ascertain which gene is affected, because mutations resulting in the absence of either protein lead to an absence of both proteins. In contrast, lack of the p47^{phox} or p67^{phox} protein by immunoblot analysis indicates the defective gene.

The NBT reduction and dihydrorhodamine 123 assays can be used to determine the carrier status of the sisters and other female relatives of patients with X-linked CGD, which is important to enable genetic counselling prior to pregnancy. Prenatal diagnosis of CGD using the aforementioned assays or DNA-based methods is also possible.

Treatment and prevention. The use of antibiotics has markedly reduced the morbidity and mortality of CGD [20,21]. Cutaneous and nodal infections are often readily apparent. However, localized internal infections, with or without associated fever, may be difficult to detect. Thorough periodic investigation of the lungs, liver and bones by radiography, ultrasonography, computed tomography (CT), magnetic resonance imaging (MRI), positron emission tomography (PET) and bone scans often uncovers occult foci of inflammation or infection. Cultures should be performed to determine the infectious agent, and invasive procedures may be required to obtain adequate tissue samples. While awaiting culture results or in instances when culture material cannot be obtained, patients with evidence of infection should be treated empirically with broad-spectrum parenteral antibiotics that cover *S. aureus* and Gram-negative bacteria. Intravenous therapy should be continued for at least 10–14 days and followed by a several-week course of oral antibiotics. Surgical interventions such as debridement, irrigation and prolonged drainage may be necessary for deeper infections.

Long-term prophylactic co-trimoxazole therapy decreases the incidence of bacterial infections in patients with CGD [22]. Likewise, prophylactic administration of itraconazole diminishes the frequency of *Aspergillus* infections [23]. Patients with CGD have shown clinical improvement after administration of γ-interferon [24], which likely augments oxidant-independent antimicrobial pathways. Granulocyte transfusions have been used in patients with rapidly progressive life-threatening infections [21]. Short courses of systemic corticosteroids can be beneficial in the management of obstructive granulomas of the bronchopulmonary, gastrointestinal or genitourinary tracts [20,21]. Additional immunomodulatory therapies with potential benefit for inflammatory manifestations of CGD include azathioprine, hydroxychloroquine, anakinra, thalidomide, pioglitazone (increases ROS production and efferocytosis), and possibly sirolimus [25,26]; antitumour necrosis factor (TNF) agents may improve colitis but increase the risk of infectious complications.

HSCT represents a potentially curative therapy for CGD, and its use in patients with this condition has increased in recent years [20,21,27–29]. Although younger patients without infection at the time of transplantation have better outcomes (survival >95%), utilization of reduced-intensity conditioning regimens has allowed successful treatment of higher-risk patients such as adults and individuals with recalcitrant infections or inflammation [30]. In children with CGD complicated by recurrent serious infections or corticosteroid-dependent inflammatory disease, transplant should be considered before irreversible organ damage ensues. Children with CGD who undergo transplantation have improved growth and fewer infections, surgical interventions and hospital admissions than those managed conservatively [31].

Gene therapy was first performed in five adults with the p47^{phox}-deficient form of CGD. A single infusion of transduced CD34^{+} peripheral blood stem cells led to peak levels of corrected granulocytes in 3–6 weeks, with persistence for as long as 6 months [32]. Subsequently, two young men with X-linked CGD were treated with nonmyeloablative conditioning prior to the infusion of CD34^{+} peripheral blood stem cells transduced *ex vivo* with a retroviral vector expressing gp91^{phox}. This led to sustained engraftment of functionally corrected phagocytes and initial resolution of infections. However, the transgene was silenced in both patients caused by viral promoter methylation, and within a few years they developed myelodysplasia caused by insertional activation of an ecotropic viral integration site [33]. To increase the

Table 156.4 Inherited defects in phagocytes and Toll-like receptor signalling

Disorder	Inheritance	Gene	Protein (defect or function)	Clinical features
Selected disorders featuring neutropenia or neutrophil defects				
Severe congenital neutropenia	AD	*ELANE*	Neutrophil elastase (abnormal elastase trafficking and accumulation)	Neutropenia MDS, AML
	AD	*GFI1*	Transcriptional repressor of elastase (abnormal elastase accumulation)	Neutropenia, lymphopenia Circulating myeloid progenitors
	AR	*HAX1*	Mitochondrial HS1-associated protein X1 (protects against apoptosis in myeloid cells)	Neutropenia Increased myeloid cell apoptosis Neurological abnormalities
	AD	*CSF3R*	Granulocyte colony-stimulating factor receptor	Neutropenia Severe myeloid hypoplasia
	AR	*G6PC3*	Glucose 6 phosphatase catalytic subunit 3 (glucose metabolism)	Neutropenia, thrombocytopenia Urogenital and cardiac malformations Ectatic veins on trunk/extremities
Cyclic neutropenia	AD	*ELANE*	Neutrophil elastase	Alternating 21 day cycles of neutropenia and monocytopenia Fever and oral ulcers at nadir
X-linked neutropenia	XL	*WASP*	WASP (gain-of-function; see text, Wiskott–Aldrich syndrome)	Neutropenia
p14 deficiency	AR	*LAMTOR2*	Endosomal adaptor protein 14 (p14; endosomal biogenesis)	Neutropenia Pneumococcal infections Diffuse pigmentary dilution of the skin and hair Short stature, coarse facies
Shwachman–Bodian–Diamond syndrome	AR	*SBDS*	SBDS protein (ribosomal RNA metabolism)	Neutropenia > pancytopenia MDS, AML Exocrine pancreatic insufficiency Chondrodysplasia
Poikiloderma with neutropenia, Clericuzio type	AR	*USB1*	U6 snRNA biogenesis phosphodiesterase 1	Neutropenia Dermatitis→poikiloderma, keratotic papules Recurrent skin & respiratory infections
Specific granule deficiency	AR	*CEBPE*	C/EBPε transcription factor (granulocyte differentiation)	Bilobed neutrophils Recurrent bacterial infections
Myeloperoxidase deficiency	AR	*MPO*	Myeloperoxidase (microbial killing by granulocytes)	*Candida* and *S. aureus* infections Often asymptomatic
Leucocyte adhesion deficiencies and related conditions				
Leucocyte adhesion deficiency I	AR	*ITGB2*	β2 integrin subunit of LFA-1, CR3 and p150 (see text)	Neutrophilia; ↓ tissue neutrophils Necrotic abscesses, ulcers
Leucocyte adhesion deficiency II	AR	*SLC35C1 (FUCT1)*	GDP-fucose transporter 1 (sialyl-Lewis X expression; see text)	Poor wound healing, delayed umbilical stump separation Gingivitis
Leucocyte adhesion deficiency III	AR	*FERMT3*	RAS guanyl releasing protein 2 (defective integrin activation; see text)	Bleeding diathesis (LAD-III) Osteopetrosis (LAD-III)
Rac2 deficiency	AD	*RAC2*	Rac2 GTPase (dysfunctional NADPH oxidase, integrin-dependent adhesion and neutrophil migration)	

(*Continued*)

Table 156.4 *Continued*

Disorder	Inheritance	Gene	Protein (defect or function)	Clinical features
Defects resulting in predisposition to specific infections				
Defects of the IL-12/IFN-γ axis	AR	*IL12B*	Subunit of IL-12 and IL-23 (stimulation of IFN-γ production)	Severe mycobacterial ± *Salmonella* infections
	AR	*IL12RB1*	IL-12 and IL-23 receptor β1 chain	Disseminated BCG infection
	AR, AD	*IFNGR1*	IFN-γ receptor (ligand binding)	Chronic mucocutaneous candidiasis (RORC, IL12RBA > IL12B)
	AR	*IFNFR2*	IFN-γ receptor (signalling)	Viral infections (STAT1, TYK2)
	AR, AD	*STAT*[1]	Signal transducer and activator of transcription (IFN-α/β/γ receptor signalling)	Hyper-IgE syndrome (variable in TYK2; see text)
	AR	*TYK2*	Tyrosine kinase 2 (IFN-α/β/γ, IL-12 and other cytokine signalling)	
	AD	*IRF8*	IFN regulatory factor 8 (IL-12 signalling)	
	AR	*ISG15*	IFN-α/β-inducible ubiquitin-like modifier	
	AR	*RORC*	RAR-related orphan receptor C (IFN- γ and IL-17 signalling)	
Defects in TLR signalling	AD	*TLR3*	TLR3 (signals IFN-α/β production)	Herpes simplex encephalitis (TLR3, TRAF3, TICAM1 and UNC-93B defects)
	AR	*UNC93B1*	UNC-93B (endoplasmic reticulum protein required for TLR3 signalling)	Recurrent pyogenic sinopulmonary and skin infections with *Streptococcus pneumoniae* and *S. aureus*, respectively (IRAK4 and MYD88 defects)
	AD	*TRAF3*	TNF receptor-associated protein 3 (TLR3 signalling)	
	AD, AR	*TICAM1 (TRIF)*	TLR-adaptor molecule 1 (TLR3/4 signalling)	
	AR	*IRAK4*	IRAK4 (IL-1 receptor and TLR signalling)	
	AR	*MYD88*	Myeloid differentiation primary response gene 88 (recruits IRAK4 to the IL-1 receptor and TLRs)	
MonoMAC syndrome/ GATA2 deficiency	AD	*GATA2*	GATA binding protein 2	Monocytopenia, B/NK lymphopenia, myelodysplasia, myeloid leukemia Mycobacterial and fungal (e.g. histoplasmosis) infections Recalcitrant warts Lymphedema Alveolar proteinosis

See Table 156.2 and the text for Chédiak–Higashi syndrome and chronic granulomatous disease.

AD, autosomal dominant; AML, acute myeloid leukemia; AR, autosomal recessive; BCG, bacillus Calmette–Guérin; IFN, interferon; IL, interleukin; IRAK4, IL-1 receptor associated kinase-4; LFA-1, lymphocyte function-associated antigen-1; MAP, mitogen-activated protein; MDS, myelodysplastic syndrome; STAT, signal transducer and activator of transcription; TLR, Toll-like receptor; WASP, Wiskott–Aldrich syndrome protein; XR, X-linked recessive.

[1] Defects in *STAT3* underlie AD hyper-IgE syndrome (see text), gain-of-function mutations in *STAT1* result in chronic mucocutaneous candidiasis (see text) and/or susceptibility to endemic dimorphic fungal infections, and defects in *STAT5B* (involved in IL-2 and growth hormone receptor signalling) lead to an AR syndrome of growth hormone insensitivity, decreased regulatory T cells, viral infections and eczematous dermatitis.

Source: Adapted with permission from Bolognia JL, Schaffer JV, Cerroni L, eds. *Dermatology*, 4th edn. London: Elsevier, 2018.

safety and efficacy of gene therapy for CGD, current investigations are utilizing approaches such as self-inactivating lentiviral vectors, targeted integration of transgenes into a genomic 'safe harbour' site, or the clustered regularly interspaced short palindromic repeat (CRISPR)-Cas9 site-specific nuclease system to encourage repair of the endogenous gene via homologous recombination [34,35].

References

1 Segal BH, Leto TL, Gallin JI et al. Genetic, biochemical, and clinical features of the chronic granulomatous disease. Medicine 2000;79:170–200.

2 Winkelstein JA, Marino MC, Johnston RB et al. Chronic granulomatous disease: report on a national registry of 368 patients. Medicine 2000;79:155–69.

3 Chiriaco M, Salfa I, Di Matteo G et al. Chronic granulomatous disease: clinical, molecular and therapeutic aspects. Pediatr Allergy Immunol 2016;27:242–53.

4 Kuhns DB, Alvord WG, Heller T et al. Residual NADPH oxidase and survival in chronic granulomatous disease. N Engl J Med 2010;363:2600–10.

5 Köker MY, Camcıoğlu Y, van Leeuwen K et al. Clinical, functional, and genetic characterization of chronic granulomatous disease in 89 Turkish patients. J Allergy Clin Immunol 2013;132:1156–63.

6 Rada BK, Geiszt M, Kaldi K et al. Dual role of phagocytic NADPH oxidase in bacterial killing. Blood 2004;104:2947–53.

7 Brinkmann V, Zychlinsky A. Beneficial suicide: why neutrophils die to make NETs. Nat Rev Microbiol 2007;5:577–82.

8 Romani L, Fallarino F, De Luca A et al. Defective tryptophan catabolism underlies inflammation in mouse chronic granulomatous disease. Nature 2008;451:211–6.

9 Lekstrom-Himes JA, Kuhns DB, Alvord WG, Gallin JI. Inhibition of human neutrophil IL-8 production by hydrogen peroxide and dysregulation in chronic granulomatous disease. J Immunol 2005; 174:411–7.

10 Crotzer VL, Matute JD, Arias AA et al. Cutting edge: NADPH oxidase modulates MHC class II antigen presentation by B cells. J Immunol 2012;189:3800–4.

11 Marciano BE, Spalding C, Fitzgerald A et al. Common severe infections in chronic granulomatous disease. Clin Infect Dis 2015;60:1176–83.

12 Sedel D, Huguet P, Lebbe C et al. Sweet syndrome as the presenting manifestation of chronic granulomatous disease in an infant. Pediatr Dermatol 1994;11:237–40.

13 Prindaville B, Nopper AJ, Lawrence H, Horii KA. Chronic granulomatous disease presenting with ecthyma gangrenosum in a neonate. J Am Acad Dermatol 2014;71:e44–5.

14 Friend JC, Hilligoss DM, Marquesen M et al. Skin ulcers and disseminated abscesses are characteristic of Serratia marcescens infection in older patients with chronic granulomatous disease. J Allergy Clin Immunol 2009;124:164–6.

15 De Ravin SS, Naumann N, Cowen EW et al. Chronic granulomatous disease as a risk factor for autoimmune disease. J Allergy Clin Immunol 2008;122:1097–103.

16 Cale CM, Morton L, Goldblatt D. Cutaneous and other lupus-like symptoms in carriers of X-linked chronic granulomatous disease: incidence and autoimmune serology. Clin Exp Immunol 2007;148:79–84.

17 Valentine G, Thomas TA, Nguyen T, Lai YC. Chronic granulomatous disease presenting as hemophagocytic lymphohistiocytosis: a case report. Pediatrics 2014;134:e1727–30.

18 Magnani A, Brosselin P, Beauté J et al. Inflammatory manifestations in a single-center cohort of patients with chronic granulomatous disease. J Allergy Clin Immunol 2014;134:655–62.

19 Jirapongsananuruk O, Malech HL, Kuhns DB et al. Diagnostic paradigm for evaluation of male patients with chronic granulomatous disease, based on the dihydrorhodamine 123 assay. J Allergy Clin Immunol 2003;111:374–9.

20 Kang EM, Malech HL. Advances in treatment for chronic granulomatous disease. Immunol Res 2009;43:77–84.

21 Seger RA. Modern management of chronic granulomatous disease. Br J Haematol 2008;140:255–66.

22 Margolis DM, Melnick DA, Alling DW et al. Trimethoprim-sulfamethoxazole prophylaxis in the management of chronic granulomatous disease. J Infect Dis 1990;162:723–6.

23 Gallin JI, Alling DW, Malech HL. Itraconazole to prevent fungal infections in chronic granulomatous disease. N Engl J Med 2003;348:2416–22.

24 International Chronic Granulomatous Disease Cooperative Study Group. A controlled trial of interferon gamma to prevent infection in chronic granulomatous disease. N Engl J Med 1991;324:509–16.

25 Noel N, Mahlaoui N, Blanche S et al. Efficacy and safety of thalidomide in patients with inflammatory manifestations of chronic granulomatous disease: a retrospective case series. J Allergy Clin Immunol 2013;132:997–1000.

26 Migliavacca M, Assanelli A, Ferrua F et al. Pioglitazone as a novel therapeutic approach in chronic granulomatous disease. J Allergy Clin Immunol 2016;137:1913–5.

27 Seger RA, Gungor T, Belohradsky BH et al. Treatment of chronic granulomatous disease with myeloablative conditioning and an unmodified hematopoietic allograft: a survey of the European experience, 1985–2000. Blood 2002;100:4344–50.

28 Del Guidice I, Iori AP, Mengarelli A et al. Allogeneic stem cell transplant from HLA-identical sibling for chronic granulomatous disease and review of the literature. Ann Hematol 2003;82:189–92.

29 Martinez CA, Shah S, Shearer WT et al. Excellent survival after sibling or unrelated donor stem cell transplantation for chronic granulomatous disease. J Allergy Clin Immunol 2012;129:176–83.

30 Güngör T, Teira P, Slatter M et al. Reduced-intensity conditioning and HLA-matched haemopoietic stem-cell transplantation in patients with chronic granulomatous disease: a prospective multicentre study. Lancet 2014;383:436–48.

31 Cole T, Pearce MS, Cant AJ et al. Clinical outcome in children with chronic granulomatous disease managed conservatively or with hematopoietic stem cell transplantation. J Allergy Clin Immunol 2013;132:1150–5.

32 Malech HL, Mapels PB, Whiting-Theoblad N et al. Prolonged production of NADPH oxidase-corrected granulocytes after gene therapy of chronic granulomatous disease. Proc Natl Acad Sci U S A 1997;94:12133–8.

33 Stein S, Ott MG, Schultze-Strasser S et al. Genomic instability and myelodysplasia with monosomy 7 consequent to EVI1 activation after gene therapy for chronic granulomatous disease. Nat Med 2010;16:198–204.

34 Kaufmann KB, Chiriaco M, Siler U et al. Gene therapy for chronic granulomatous disease: current status and future perspectives. Curr Gene Ther 2014:14:447–60.

35 De Ravin SS, Reik A, Liu PQ et al. Targeted gene addition in human CD34(+) hematopoietic cells for correction of X-linked chronic granulomatous disease. Nat Biotechnol 2016;34:424–9.

Chronic mucocutaneous candidiasis

Key points

- **A heterogeneous group of conditions characterized by recurrent and progressive candidal infections of the skin, nails and mucosae.**
- **They are caused by an impaired interleukin-17 response, which has a critical role in immune defence against *Candida*.**
- **Additional autoimmune and infectious manifestations may develop.**

Introduction. Chronic mucocutaneous candidiasis (CMC) represents a heterogeneous group of conditions characterized by recurrent, progressive infections of the skin, nails and mucous membranes with *Candida albicans* [1]. CMC reflects ineffective immune defence against *Candida*, and individuals with more profound immune defects tend to have an earlier onset and greater severity of cutaneous candidal infections.

Epidemiology and pathogenesis. Patients with CMC have a defective T-cell response to candidal organisms. In some individuals the deficiency is specific to *Candida*, and in others the immunological response to other organisms is also abnormal.

The autoimmune polyendocrinopathy–candidiasis–ectodermal dystrophy (APECED; also known as autoimmune polyendocrine syndrome, type I or APS1) syndrome has autosomal recessive inheritance and results from loss-of-function mutations in the autoimmune regulator gene (*AIRE*) [2,3]. The AIRE protein is a transcription factor that regulates ectopic expression of self-antigens in thymic medullary epithelial cells, thereby participating in the development of peripheral tolerance via negative selection of autoreactive T cells and generation of antigen-specific regulatory T cells [4–6]. In patients with APECED, failure to delete peripheral tissue-specific autoreactive T cells results in autoimmune disease [7].

The immune defects that underlie selective predisposition to *Candida* infections in both APECED and non-APECED CMC patients involve an impaired response by T helper 17 (Th17) cells, which have a critical role in immune defence against *Candida* [8,9]. Neutralizing autoantibodies targeting Th17-associated cytokines (e.g. IL-17A/F, IL-22) have been identified in APECED patients and individuals with thymoma-associated CMC [10,11]. Isolated CMC can be caused by heterozygous dominant-negative *IL17F* mutations that lead to IL-17F deficiency, biallelic *IL17RA* or *IL17RC* mutations that disrupt function of the IL-17 receptor, or biallelic loss-of-function *TRAF3IP2* (*ACT1*) mutations that prevent interaction between the IL-17 receptor and its TRAF3-interacting protein 2 adaptor molecule [12–14]. Heterozygous gain-of-function mutations in the signal transducer and activator of transcription 1 gene (*STAT1*) gene have emerged as the most common cause of CMC [9,15,16]. The resulting STAT1 activation leads to increased interferon-α/β and -γ signalling as well as repression of IL-17 production, and clinical manifestations can include predisposition to other infections, autoimmunity and aneurysms [17,18] (see Table 156.5).

In addition, biallelic mutations in the caspase recruitment domain family member-9 gene (*CARD9*) result in a predilection for both mucocutaneous and invasive infections with *Candida* spp. (especially of the central nervous system), dermatophytes and phaeohyphomycetes [19,20]. In another CMC variant, homozygous mutation in the gene encoding dectin-1 was identified in several siblings with recurrent vulvovaginal candidiasis and onychomycosis [21]. The dectin-1 pattern-recognition receptor (found on leucocytes and epithelial cells) binds to β-glucan in the *Candida* cell wall, which signals CARD9 to activate an immunological cascade that stimulates the development of IL-17-producing T cells. Decreased neutrophil function is also thought to contribute to invasive fungal infections in patients with CARD9 deficiency [20]. Additional aetiologies of CMC are listed in Table 156.5.

Clinical features. The severity and extent of involvement in CMC is variable, ranging from recurrent thrush (Fig. 156.3) to localized scaling plaques and a few dystrophic nails to severe widespread crusted granulomatous plaques (Fig. 156.4). Cutaneous plaques occur most commonly in intertriginous and periorificial sites and on the scalp, where involvement may result in scarring alopecia. Affected nails are thickened, brittle and discoloured (Fig. 156.5), and the paronychial areas are often erythematous, swollen and tender. The mouth is the most frequent site of mucosal alteration, typically manifesting as oral thrush with hyperkeratotic plaques. Genital, oesophageal and laryngeal mucosae may also be affected, and chronic infections in these locations can lead to stricture formation. Systemic candidiasis does not usually occur in patients with CMC.

Approximately 80% of patients with childhood-onset CMC experience recurrent or severe infections with organisms other than *Candida*, including bacterial septicaemia [22]. Patients with CMC are also especially susceptible to dermatophytosis. The clinical features of major types of CMC with onset in childhood and adolescence are presented in Table 156.5 [2,23,24]. Chronic mucocutaneous candidiasis in association with abnormal iron metabolism or (as noted previously) thymoma can also occur in adults.

Differential diagnosis. Candidal infections, especially thrush, are relatively common in infants. Recurrent thrush in young children may reflect changes in oral flora caused by frequent antibiotic treatment of conditions such as otitis media. Recurrent or recalcitrant candidal infections should prompt consideration of HIV infection as well as CMC.

IPEX (immune dysregulation, polyendocrinopathy, enteropathy, X-linked; see later) syndrome can present with autoimmune diseases and endocrinopathies together with recurrent infections, but the latter are usually bacterial rather than candidal [25]. Autoimmune endocrinopathies and a predisposition to bacterial, viral and fungal infections have also been reported as manifestations of IL-2 receptor α chain (CD25) deficiency (see Table 156.3) [26].

Laboratory and histology findings. Scrapings and cultures from cutaneous or mucosal lesions demonstrate candidal organisms. Histological examination of skin biopsy specimens from cutaneous plaques reveals hyperkeratosis, papillomatosis and infiltration of the dermis with lymphocytes, plasma cells, neutrophils and foreign body giant cells. The candidal organisms are typically confined to the stratum corneum.

Approximately 75% of patients with CMC have laboratory evidence of an immunological defect, including skin test anergy and deficient *in vitro* lymphoproliferation or cytokine release in response to *Candida* antigens as well as nonspecific findings such as abnormal leucocyte chemotaxis or phagocytosis, decreased IgA levels and complement dysfunction. The marked variability in these findings reflects the underlying heterogeneity of CMC. Candidal polysaccharides may act as serum factors that inhibit the immune response and delayed-type hypersensitivity to candidal antigens has been restored after

Table 156.5 Variants of chronic mucocutaneous candidiasis (CMC)

Mucocutaneous features	Other features
Autoimmune polyendocrinopathy–candidiasis–ectodermal dystrophy[1](APECED) syndrome (autoimmune polyendocrine syndrome, type 1)	
Onset of mucocutaneous candidal infections[2] at a mean age of 3 years Candidal granulomas Cutaneous autoimmune disorders • Alopecia areata (30%) • Vitiligo (20%) • Urticarial eruption[3] (up to 60%) • Lupus-like panniculitis	Autosomal recessive > dominant due to mutations in the *AIRE* gene Higher prevalence in Finns, Iranian Jews and Sardinians Autoimmune endocrinopathies (may not develop until adolescence or adulthood) • Hypoparathyroidism[2] (90%) • Addison disease[2] (80%) • Hypogonadism (30–50%) • Thyroid disease (20%) • Type 1 diabetes mellitus (20%) • Hypopituitarism (e.g. growth hormone deficiency; 15%) Other autoimmune disorders • Pernicious anaemia (20%) • Keratoconjunctivitis (20%) • Hepatitis (15–40%) • Hyposplenism (15%) • Pneumonitis (15–40%) • Sjögren-like syndrome (20–40%) Other manifestations • Dental enamel hypoplasia[1] (70%) • Chronic diarrhoea (20–80%) • Tubulointerstitial nephritis (10%) • Hypertension (15%) • Oral/oesophageal squamous cell carcinoma (10% of patients > age 25 years) Antitype I interferon antibodies (nearly 100%) Antiadrenal, thyroglobulin and parietal cell antibodies; rheumatoid factor Autosomal dominant CMC + autoimmune thyroid disease can occur due to a dominant-negative *AIRE* mutation and has also been linked to chromosome 2p in one family
Isolated CMC	Autosomal dominant due to mutations in the interleukin-17F gene (*IL17F*) Autosomal recessive due to mutations in the interleukin-17 receptor A or C gene (*IL17RA* or *IL17RC*) or TRAF3-interacting protein 2 gene (*TRAF3IP2*; *ACT1*)
CMC plus susceptibility to mycobacterial infections	Autosomal recessive due to mutations in the RAR-related orphan receptor C (*RORC*) gene that lead to decreased IL-17 and interferon-γ production
CMC due to increased STAT1 signalling Onset of mucocutaneous candidal infections at a mean age of 1 year – oropharynx (>95%), nails (60%), skin (50%) Dermatophyte infections of skin and/or nails (15%) Cutaneous autoimmune disorders (e.g. vitiligo, alopecia areata; 10%)	Autosomal dominant due to gain-of-function mutations in the *STAT1* gene[4] Autoimmunity (40%) • Thyroid disease (25%) • Type 1 diabetes mellitus (5%) • Cytopenias (5%) • Colitis or coeliac disease (5%) • Systemic lupus erythematosus (2%) • Hepatitis (2%) Other infections (variable) • Cutaneous with *Staphylococcus aureus* • Bacterial pneumonia (e.g. pneumococcal, *Pseudomonas*; 50%), otitis, sinusitis • Recurrent/severe viral (e.g. herpes simplex, varicella-zoster, EBV, CMV, orf; 40%) • Invasive fungal (e.g. *Candida*, *Aspergillus*, *Cryptococcus*, endemic dimorphic, mucormycosis, *Fusarium*; 10%) • Mycobacterial (tuberculosis, non-tuberculous; 5%) Aneurysms (e.g. cerebral, aortic; 5%) Squamous cell carcinoma (mucocutaneous; 5%) Dental enamel defects
CARD9 deficiency Chronic oral and vulvovaginal candidiasis Dermatophytosis	Autosomal recessive due to mutations in the *CARD9* gene Invasive fungal infections including candidiasis (especially of the brain), dermatophytosis and phaeohyphomycosis
Dectin-1 deficiency Chronic/recurrent vulvovaginal candidiasis Onychomycosis	Due to biallelic polymorphisms that result in a truncated dectin-1 protein
Chronic localized candidiasis ('candidal granuloma') Onset typically by age 5 years Thick plaques with adherent crusts favour the scalp and face Oral candidiasis common	

(*Continued*)

Table 156.5 *Continued*

Mucocutaneous features	Other features
Late-onset CMC	
Initial infections in later childhood or adolescence Milder course	Responses to *Candida* may normalize after effective therapy
Familial chronic nail candidiasis	
Onset in infancy of candidiasis limited to the nails of hands and feet	Autosomal dominant form of CMC mapped to 11p12-q12.1 in a five-generation Italian family Association with low serum levels of intracellular adhesion molecule-1
CMC associated with other syndromes	
Immunodeficiency disorders • Hyper-IgE syndromes due to STAT3 and DOCK8 deficiencies • Severe combined immunodeficiency • DiGeorge syndrome • Interleukin-12 receptor β1 and interleukin-12B (p40) deficiencies (see Table 156.4) • Autosomal dominant hypohidrotic ectodermal dysplasia with immunodeficiency (*NFKBIA* mutations) Metabolic disorders • Multiple carboxylase deficiency • Acrodermatitis enteropathica • Ectodermal dysplasia–ectrodactyly–clefting syndrome	

[1] 'Ectodermaly dystrophy' refers primarily to dental enamel hypoplasia.
[2] Two of these three manifestations are classically required for diagnosis.
[3] Mean onset at 1.5 years; histologically, shows focal vacuolar interface dermatitis plus superficial and deep dermal perivascular inflammation with mixed infiltrates including lymphocytes and neutrophils with karyorrhexis.
[4] Loss-of-function *STAT1* mutations lead to susceptibility to mycobacterial and viral infections (see Table 156.4), and gain-of-function *STAT1* mutations that impair responses to interferon-γ restimulation result in susceptibility to endemic dimorphic fungal infections.
Source: Adapted with permission from Bolognia JL, Schaffer JV, Cerroni L, eds. *Dermatology*, 4th edn. London: Elsevier, 2018.

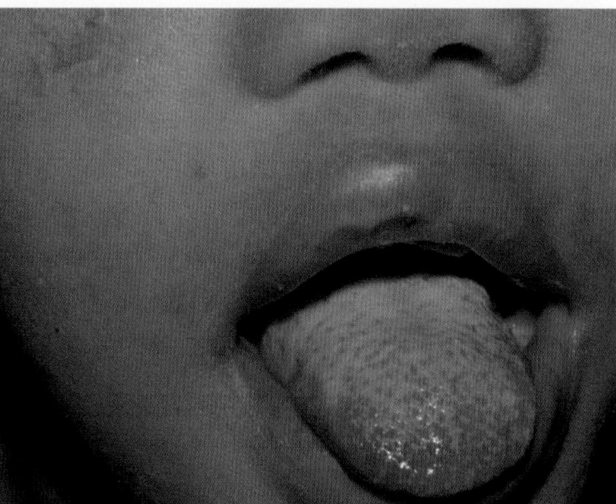

Fig. 156.3 Recurrent thrush and dermatophyte infections, together with failure-to-thrive, chronic diarrhoea, and autoimmune thrombocytopenia were the presenting manifestations in this 6-year-old with a heterozygous gain-of-function mutation in *STAT1*.

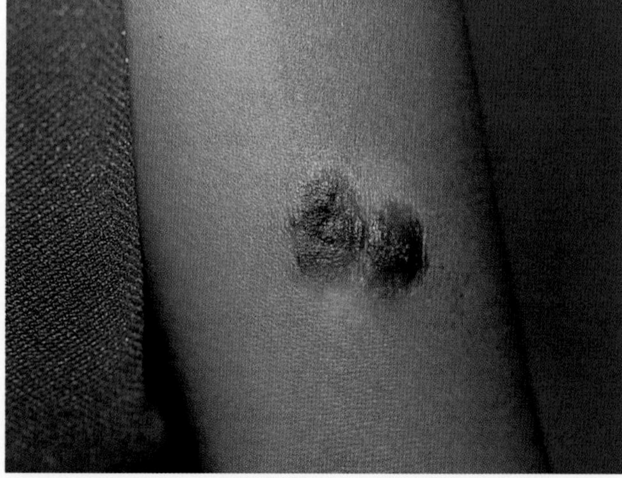

Fig. 156.4 Cutaneous candidal granulomas are a feature of severe forms of chronic mucocutaneous candidiasis.

antifungal therapy in some patients. Autoantibodies against type I interferons have been shown to represent a sensitive and specific marker for APECED [27].

Treatment and prevention. Patients with CMC do not respond adequately to topical antifungal medications and cutaneous granulomas are particularly difficult to treat. Most patients require long-term therapy with systemic antifungal agents such as fluconazole and itraconazole. Voriconazole (associated with phototoxicity), posaconazole, echinocandins and amphotericin B have been utilized for *Candida* isolates with decreased sensitivity to fluconazole [28,29]. Adjunctive therapy may include granulocyte-colony stimulating factor (may increase IL-17 production), nail avulsion, drainage of abscesses and debridement of thick crusted cutaneous plaques [30]. Treatment with a Janus kinases (JAK) inhibitor such as ruxolitinib may be of benefit for infectious and autoimmune disease in patients with gain-of-function *STAT1* mutations [31]. Patients should be evaluated at least annually for the development of endocrinopathies, especially if there is a family history of APECED syndrome.

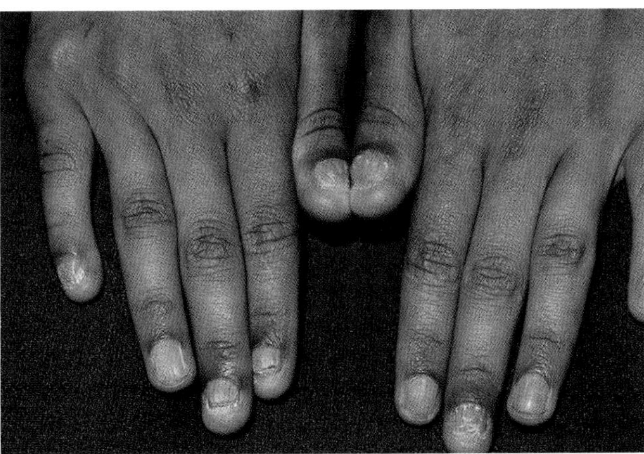

Fig. 156.5 Thickening, discolouration and dystrophy of all the fingernails resulting from candidal infection in a patient with APECED. Note the hyperpigmentation of the skin of the hands, particularly overlying the joints, related to his associated Addison disease.

References

1 Kirkpatrick CH. Chronic mucocutaneous candidiasis. Pediatr Infect Dis J 2001;20:197–206.

2 Ahonen P, Myllärniemi S, Sipilä I et al. Clinical variation of autoimmune polyendocrinopathy–candidiasis–ectodermal dystrophy (APECED) in a series of 68 patients. N Engl J Med 1990;322:1829–36.

3 Anonymous (Finnish–German APECED Consortium). An autoimmune disease, APECED, is caused by mutations in a novel gene featuring two PHD-type zinc-finger domains: autoimmune polyendocrinopathy–candidiasis–ectodermal dystrophy. Nat Genet 1997;17:399–403.

4 Liston A, Lesage S, Wilson J et al. Aire regulates negative selection of organ-specific T cells. Nat Immunol 2003;4:350–4.

5 Aschenbrenner K, D'Cruz LM, Vollmann EH et al. Selection of Foxp3(+) regulatory T cells specific for self antigen expressed and presented by Aire(+) medullary thymic epithelial cells. Nat Immunol 2007;8:351–8.

6 Anderson MS, Su MA. AIRE expands: new roles in immune tolerance and beyond. Nat Rev Immunol 2016;16:247–58.

7 Ferre EM, Rose SR, Rosenzweig SD et al. Redefined clinical features and diagnostic criteria in autoimmune polyendocrinopathy-candidiasis-ectodermal dystrophy. JCI Insight 2016;1:13.

8 Ng WF, von Delwig A, Carmichael AJ et al. Impaired T(H)17 responses in patients with chronic mucocutaneous candidiasis with and without autoimmune polyendocrinopathy-candidiasis-ectodermal dystrophy. J Allergy Clin Immunol 2010;126:1006–15.

9 Soltész B, Tóth B, Sarkadi AK et al. The evolving view of IL-17-mediated immunity in defense against mucocutaneous candidiasis in humans. Int Rev Immunol 2015;34:348–63.

10 Kisand K, Boe Wolff AS et al. Chronic mucocutaneous candidiasis in APECED or thymoma patients correlates with autoimmunity to Th17-associated cytokines. J Exp Med 2010;207:299–308.

11 Wolff AS, Sarkadi AK, Maródi L et al. Anti-cytokine autoantibodies preceding onset of autoimmune polyendocrine syndrome type I features in early childhood. J Clin Immunol 2013;33:1341–8.

12 Puel A, Cypowyj S, Bustamante J et al. Chronic mucocutaneous candidiasis in humans with inborn errors of interleukin-17 immunity. Science 2011;332:65–8.

13 Boisson B, Wang C, Pedergnana V et al. An ACT1 mutation selectively abolishes interleukin-17 responses in humans with chronic mucocutaneous candidiasis. Immunity 2013;39:676–86.

14 Ling Y, Cypowyj S, Aytekin C et al. Inherited IL-17RC deficiency in patients with chronic mucocutaneous candidiasis. J Exp Med 2015;212:619–31.

15 Liu L1, Okada S, Kong XF et al. Gain-of-function human STAT1 mutations impair IL-17 immunity and underlie chronic mucocutaneous candidiasis. J Exp Med 2011;208:1635–48.

16 van de Veerdonk FL, Plantinga TS, Hoischen A et al. STAT1 mutations in autosomal dominant chronic mucocutaneous candidiasis. N Engl J Med 2011;365:54–61.

17 Depner M, Fuchs S, Raabe J et al. The extended clinical phenotype of 26 patients with chronic mucocutaneous candidiasis due to gain-of-function mutations in STAT1. J Clin Immunol 2016;36:73–84.

18 Toubiana J, Okada S, Hiller J, et al. Heterozygous STAT1 gain-of-function mutations underlie an unexpectedly broad clinical phenotype. Blood 2016;127:3154–64.

19 Glocker EO, Hennigs A, Nabavi M et al. A homozygous CARD9 mutation in a family with susceptibility to fungal infections. N Engl J Med 2009;361:1727–35.

20 Alves de Medeiros AK, Lodewick E, Bogaert DJ et al. Chronic and invasive fungal infections in a family with CARD9 deficiency. J Clin Immunol 2016;36:204–9.

21 Ferwerda B, Ferwerda G, Plantinga TS et al. Human dectin-1 deficiency and mucocutaneous fungal infections. N Engl J Med 2009;361:1760–7.

22 Herrod HG. Chronic mucocutaneous candidiasis in childhood and complications of non-Candida infection: a report of the Pediatric Immunodeficiency Collaborative Study Group. J Pediatr 1990;116:377–82.

23 Perheentupa J. Autoimmune polyendocrinopathy–candidiasis–ectodermal dystrophy. J Clin Endocrinol Metab 2006;91:2843–50.

24 Collins SM, Dominguez M, Ilmarinen T et al. Dermatological manifestations of autoimmune polyendocrinopathy–candidiasis–ectodermal dystrophy syndrome. Br J Dermatol 2006;156:1088–93.

25 Halabi-Tawil M, Ruemmele FM, Fraitag S et al. Cutaneous manifestations of immune dysregulation, polyendocrinopathy, enteropathy, X-linked (IPEX) syndrome. Br J Dermatol 2009;160:645–51.

26 Caudy AA, Reddy ST, Chatila T et al. CD25 deficiency causes an immune dysregulation, polyendocrinopathy, enteropathy, X-linked-like syndrome, and defective IL-10 expression from CD4 lymphocytes. J Allergy Clin Immunol 2007;119:482–7.

27 Meloni A, Furcas M, Cetani F et al. Autoantibodies against type I interferons as an additional diagnostic criterion for autoimmune polyendocrine syndrome type 1. J Clin Endocrinol Metab 2008;93:4389–97.

28 Rautemaa R, Richardson M, Pfaller MA et al. Decreased susceptibility of Candida albicans to azole antifungals: a complication of long-term treatment in autoimmune polyendocrinopathy–candidiasis–ectodermal dystrophy (APECED) patients. J Antimicrob Chemother 2007;60:889–92.

29 van de Veerdonk FL, Netea MG. Treatment options for chronic mucocutaneous candidiasis. J Infect 2016;72 Suppl:S56–60.

30 Wildbaum G, Shahar E, Katz R et al. Continuous G-CSF therapy for isolated chronic mucocutaneous candidiasis: complete clinical remission with restoration of IL-17 secretion. J Allergy Clin Immunol 2013;132:761–4.

31 Higgins E, Al Shehri T, McAleer MA et al. Use of ruxolitinib to successfully treat chronic mucocutaneous candidiasis caused by gain-of-function signal transducer and activator of transcription 1 (STAT1) mutation. J Allergy Clin Immunol 2015;135:551–3.

Complement deficiency disorders

Key points

- **Deficiency or dysfunction of early complement components increases susceptibility to pyogenic infections caused by encapsulated bacteria and autoimmune disorders, especially systemic lupus erythematosus.**
- **Deficiency of late complement components leads to a markedly increased risk of meningococcal infections.**
- **Hereditary angioedema is an autosomal dominant disorder caused by deficiency or dysfunction of the complement C1 esterase inhibitor and, less often, by constitutive activation of factor XII; it features recurrent episodes of nonpruritic swelling of the face, extremities and gastrointestinal and respiratory tracts without associated urticaria.**

The complement system is an important effector of the innate immune response and has roles in defence against microbial pathogens, regulation of inflammation and coordination of a variety humoral and cellular immune functions. Three primary pathways can trigger

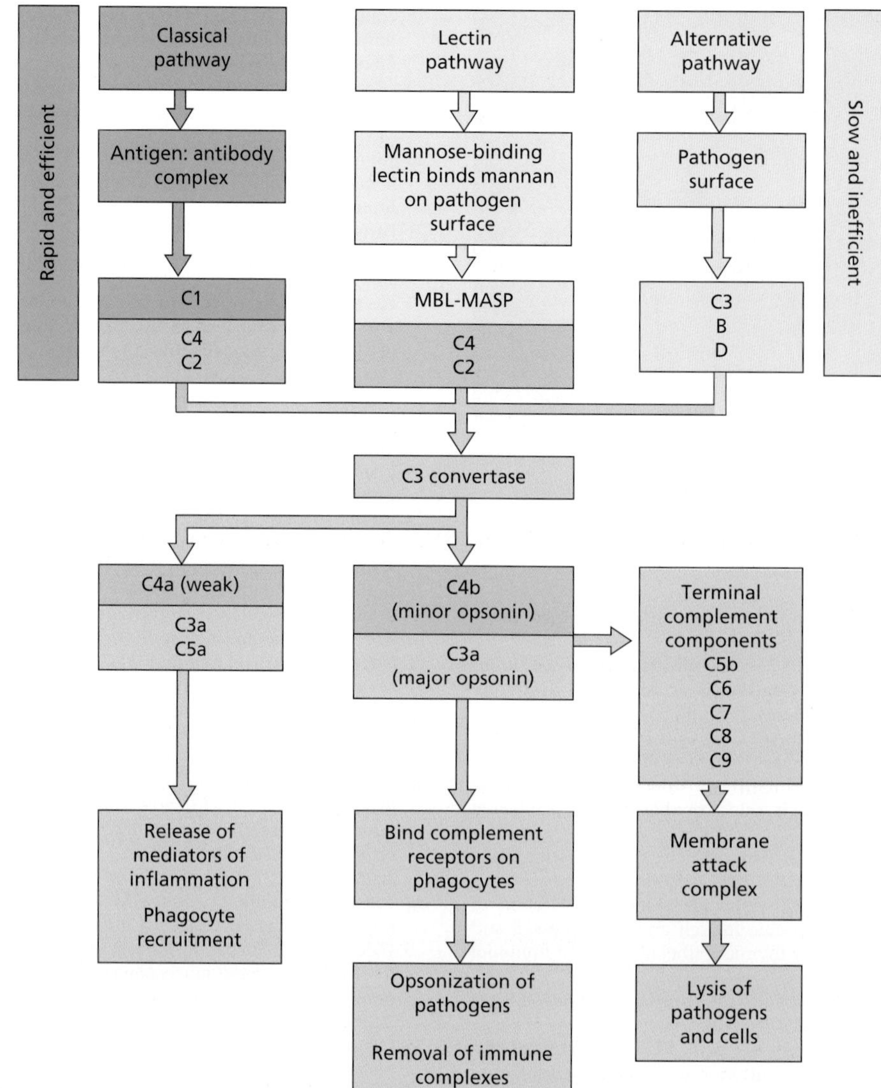

Fig. 156.6 The main components and effector actions of complement. The C3b bound to the C3 convertase binds C5, allowing the C3 convertase to generate C5b, which associates with the bacterial membrane and triggers the late events. MASP, MBL-associated serine protease; MBL, mannose-binding lectin. Source: Adapted from Janeway CA et al. 2005. Reproduced by permission of Garland Science/Taylor & Francis Group LLC.

an enzymatic cascade of complement activation: classic, alternative and lectin (Fig. 156.6). Isolated complement component deficiencies may result in autoimmune disorders as well as an increased susceptibility to infections with certain organisms [1–3].

C2 deficiency is the most common hereditary complement disorder, with the homozygous form of C2 deficiency occurring in 1 in 10 000 to 1 in 40 000 individuals. Homozygous deficiencies of C1q, C1r, C1s and C4 occur less frequently, but affected individuals are more likely to develop autoimmune disease than those with homozygous C2 deficiency [4]. Because heterozygosity for a complement deficiency is usually asymptomatic, most complement defects are inherited as autosomal recessive traits. Hereditary angioedema (HAE), a dominantly inherited disorder caused primarily by C1-esterase inhibitor (C1-INH) deficiency or dysfunction, represents an important exception and is discussed separately later.

In contrast to the relatively low prevalence and high clinical penetrance of homozygous deficiencies in components of the classic complement pathway [3], 5–10% of the population has polymorphisms in the *MBL2* gene that result in decreased function of mannose-binding lectin (MBL), which initiates the lectin pathway of complement activation [5]. Although affected individuals are often asymptomatic, MBL deficiency is thought to have substantial impact on immunity and autoimmunity on a population-wide level.

Hereditary angioedema

Introduction. HAE is a potentially lethal form of angioedema that is inherited as an autosomal dominant disorder with incomplete penetrance. The condition results from deficiency (type I; 85%) or dysfunction (type II; 15%) of complement C1-INH and is characterized by recurrent episodes of nonpruritic swelling of the face, extremities and gastrointestinal and respiratory tracts without associated urticaria [6–8]. The terms 'type III HAE' and 'oestrogen-dependent HAE' have previously been utilized for a rare, dominantly inherited form of angioedema in which the C1-INH is normal and almost all affected individuals are female [9]. This condition, now referred to as 'HAE with normal C1-INH', is caused by a heterozygous activating mutation in the gene that encodes coagulation factor XII in a subset of affected individuals [10].

Epidemiology and pathogenesis. HAE occurs in approximately 1 in 150 000 people, with a female:male ratio of 1.5:1 and a tendency for a more severe disease course in affected women [8]. Types I and II HAE are caused by heterozygous mutations in the serpin peptidase inhibitor G1 (*SERPING1*) gene, which encodes the C1-INH protein. In type I HAE, mutations result in a truncated or misfolded protein that is not efficiently secreted. The C1-INH level is typically only 5–30% of normal, suggesting that there is also decreased secretion or increased catabolism of the normal gene product. In type II HAE, missense mutations at or near the active site lead to a dysfunctional protein that is secreted normally.

The C1-INH has important roles in regulating vascular permeability and inflammation. Its diverse functions include inhibition of the following cascades: contact activation (factor XIIa and kallikrein); 'intrinsic' coagulation (factor XIa); fibrinolysis (plasmin); and the classic (C1r and C1s), alternative (C3bBb convertase) and lectin (MBL-associated serine proteases) complement pathways. Although the angioedema of HAE was previously thought to reflect uncontrolled activation of complement pathways, accumulated data suggest that the primary mediator is the contact activation product bradykinin, a potent inducer of vascular permeability that is generated in excess because of increased activity of factor XIIa and kallikrein [11,12].

Heterozygous gain-of-function mutations in the *F12* gene that produce a more readily activated form of factor XII underlie a subset of HAE with normal C1-INH [13–15]. As in types I and II HAE, this defect leads to increased production of bradykinin [13]. The transcription of the *F12* gene is augmented by oestrogens, which explains the marked female predominance in this form of HAE.

Clinical features. The first episode of angioedema often occurs during early childhood. Patients typically present with swelling of an extremity following trauma, which is commonly overlooked. The frequency and severity of attacks usually increases during adolescence. Although on average an untreated patient experiences an episode every 1–2 weeks, the frequency can range from every few days to once a decade [6,16]. No periodicity to the attacks is noted. Although attacks may be spontaneous, approximately 50% are precipitated by physical trauma, emotional stress or infection. Dental treatment of patients with HAE can trigger life-threatening laryngopharyngeal oedema, and the use of angiotensin-converting enzyme inhibitors can exacerbate the condition. Female patients commonly report an increased number of attacks in association with their menses or oral contraceptive use. However, during the last two trimesters of pregnancy the frequency of attacks usually wanes and the occurrence of angioedema at delivery is extremely rare.

Patients may experience fatigue, nausea or localized tingling of the skin prior to the onset of swelling, but the onset of angioedema can also be sudden without a prodrome. In up to 25% of attacks, a transient nonpruritic eruption of serpiginous erythematous patches resembling erythema marginatum precedes or accompanies the development of angioedema. However, typical urticaria is *not* a feature of HAE. Nonpruritic nonpitting oedema progressively increases for up to 24 hours, then stabilizes and gradually resolves over the next 2–3 days. Oedematous bullae are occasionally observed in association with severe dermal and subcutaneous swelling. Patients may experience a refractory period of days to weeks after an attack.

The most common sites of involvement are the extremities (50% of episodes, almost all patients), face (<5% of episodes, 75% of patients), genitals (<5% of episodes, approximately 50% of patients), gastrointestinal tract (50% of episodes, 90% of patients) and oropharyngeal mucosae (<2% of episodes, 50% of patients) [16]. Abdominal attacks often present with crampy or colicky pain that can mimic an acute abdomen. Upper gastrointestinal involvement frequently manifests with vomiting and signs of hypotension (e.g. lightheadedness) resulting from intravascular volume depletion, whereas lower gastrointestinal involvement tends to feature diarrhoea and abdominal distention [17]. Compromise of the airway from laryngeal oedema occurs most commonly in adults, and patients may be warned of impending obstruction by a voice change or dysphagia. Historically, approximately 25% of patients with HAE died from asphyxiation. Occasionally, oedema affecting the genitourinary tract, brain, pleura, muscles or joint space leads to urinary retention, headaches, pleuritic chest pain, myalgias or arthralgias in patients with HAE [16]. As in deficiencies of other complement system components (see below), HAE may also be associated with autoimmune manifestations such as systemic or discoid lupus erythematosus, Sjögren syndrome, scleroderma, partial lipodystrophy and glomerulonephritis.

Laboratory testing is required to confirm the diagnosis of HAE. Measurement of the serum C4 level, which is persistently low in virtually all untreated patients, is a sensitive screening test for types I and II HAE [9,18]. Subsequent determination of antigenic and functional C1-INH levels can confirm the diagnosis and differentiate between type I (low antigenic and functional levels) and type II (normal antigenic and low functional levels) [18]. However, the results of these tests are not reliable in very young children, especially those who are less than 1 year of age [19]. Of note, the total haemolytic complement (CH50) and levels of other complement components (e.g. C1q and C3) are typically normal in patients with HAE, although the two patients with homozygous C1-INH deficiency reported to date had low levels of C1q [20].

HAE with normal C1-INH has a later age of onset (usually in the second decade of life) and a higher frequency of facial angioedema than classic HAE [10,21]. In type III HAE, levels of C4 and C1-INH (both antigenic and functional) are normal.

Differential diagnosis. The diagnosis of HAE is easily made when a patient complains of angioedema with recurrent abdominal pain and reveals a positive family history. However, the possibility of HAE should be considered in all patients who present with recurrent angioedema without associated urticaria. Acquired angioedema usually occurs in adults with an underlying B-cell lymphoproliferative disorder and can be distinguished by extremely low levels of C1q as well as C4 and C1-INH (functional ± antigenic). The differential diagnosis of recurrent angioedema without urticaria may also include other rare inherited complement pathway defects (e.g. carboxypeptidase N or factor I deficiency), drug reactions (e.g. nonsteroidal anti-inflammatory drugs, angiotensin-converting enzyme inhibitors), episodic angioedema with eosinophilia (Gleich syndrome), capillary leak syndrome, vibratory angioedema and delayed pressure 'urticaria' as well as allergic and autoimmune (via histamine-releasing autoantibodies) aetiologies that usually result in urticaria in addition to angioedema.

Laboratory and histology findings. Laboratory testing is required to confirm the diagnosis of HAE. Measurement of the serum C4 level, which is persistently low in virtually all untreated patients, is a sensitive screening test for types I and II HAE [9,18]. Subsequent determination of antigenic and functional C1-INH levels can confirm the diagnosis and differentiate between type I (low antigenic and functional levels) and type II (normal antigenic and low functional levels) [18]. However, the results of these tests are not reliable in very young children, especially those who are younger than 1 year of age [19]. Of note, the total haemolytic complement (CH50) and levels of other complement components (e.g. C1q and C3) are typically normal in patients with HAE, although the two patients with homozygous C1-INH deficiency reported to date had low levels of C1q [20].

HAE with normal C1-INH has a later age of onset (usually in the second decade of life) and a higher frequency of facial angioedema than classic HAE [10,21]. In type III HAE, levels of C4 and C1-INH (both antigenic and functional) are normal.

Treatment and prevention. The morbidity and mortality of HAE can be reduced significantly by a therapeutic approach that includes short-term and (in patients with frequent severe attacks) long-term prophylaxis together with treatment of acute attacks [7,9,22,23]. Intravenous administration of C1-INH concentrate is indicated for short-term prophylaxis prior to dental work or invasive procedures. C1-INH is also highly effective for acute attacks, with improvement within 30–60 min of injection. Plasma-derived and recombinant forms of C1-INH concentrate are FDA-approved for intravenous use in acute attacks and (for the former) short- or long-term prophylaxis; self-administration at home is often utilized so treatment is not delayed [24]. Fresh-frozen plasma has been used in the past for acute attacks and short-term prophylaxis in patients with HAE, but it may contain contact activation proteins as well as C1-INH and can potentially exacerbate the condition. Other agents approved for the treatment of acute attacks of HAE include the kallikrein inhibitor ecallantide and the bradykinin B2 receptor antagonist icatibant [7,22,23]. Adrenaline administration is usually not helpful for acute attacks of HAE, although it may produce a mild transient decrease in swelling. Antihistamines and corticosteroids do not ameliorate or prevent attacks of HAE. Painful gastrointestinal oedema frequently necessitates aggressive fluid replacement and use of narcotic analgesics. Intubation or tracheotomy can be life-saving if medical therapy is not available or effective for airway involvement.

In addition to C1-INH administration every 3–4 days on an ongoing basis, there are two major groups of drugs that have been used for long-term treatment of HAE:

1 Antifibrinolytic agents such as ε-aminocaproic acid (EACA) and tranexamic acid; and
2 17α-alkylated ('attenuated') androgens such as danazol, stanozolol and oxandrolone [19,25,26].

Antifibrinolytic agents inhibit plasminogen activation and thereby reduce consumption of C1-INH. They have a relatively favourable risk/benefit profile, with potential side effects including gastrointestinal symptoms, muscle aches, postural hypotension and (rarely) thrombosis. By inducing mRNA synthesis in hepatocytes, androgens stimulate the synthesis of C1-INH and can reduce the frequency and severity of attacks in patients with HAE. Use of 17α-alkylated androgens during pregnancy is contraindicated, and adverse effects can include weight gain, hepatotoxicity, lipid abnormalities, menstrual irregularities, virilization and decreased linear growth in children.

Other complement deficiencies

Pathogenesis. Defects involving the early components of the classic complement pathway (C1, C4, C2) result in an increased risk of autoimmune disorders, especially systemic lupus erythematosus (SLE). The genes that encode these complement components, including four highly polymorphic genes for C4 (two each for C4A and C4B), are located within the HLA region on chromosome 6. C4-null alleles have been linked to SLE, and the C4A gene is deleted in the Caucasoid extended haplotype (HLA A1, B8, DR3) that is strongly associated with SLE.

Impaired clearance of apoptotic cells containing autoantigens may have a role in the pathogenesis of complement deficiency-related SLE [27,28]. When keratinocyes undergo UVB-induced apoptosis, the cells display autoantigens such as Ro in plasma membrane blebs. Binding of C1q to the blebs and the nucleolus leads to activation of the classic complement pathway and phagocytosis of the apoptotic cells [29]. In the absence of C1q, autoantibodies have the opportunity to bind to Ro, resulting in activation of B and T cells and loss of immune tolerance. Other complement functions that are relevant to SLE pathogenesis include elimination of self-reactive B cells during lymphocyte development, clearance of immune complexes and regulation of production of cytokines such as type I interferons.

The recurrent infections associated with complement deficiencies emphasize the central role of complement in defence against bacteria. Deficiencies of early classic components are associated with susceptibility to infections by encapsulated bacteria, especially *Strep. pneumoniae*. Opsonization of bacteria may be ineffective in these complement disorders because of slow inadequate formation of C3b. However, such classic pathway deficiencies do not typically manifest in overwhelming infections, because the lectin and alternative pathways can bypass early classic components to intersect with the cascade at the level of C3 (see Fig. 156.5). Patients with C5 deficiencies do not generate chemotactic factors normally and, as a result, neutrophil function may be inadequate. Individuals with C5–C9 (membrane attack complex; MAC), properdin and factor D deficiencies tend to develop recurrent neisserial infections in their teenage years. This reflects the importance of both the bactericidal MAC and the alternative complement pathway (which requires properdin and factor D) for defence against these organisms [30,31]. The mortality rate of meningococcal infections in the setting of MAC deficiency is actually lower than that in immunocompetent individuals, and it is postulated that a lack of serum lytic activity limits release of lipopolysaccharide and other bacterial products that can trigger a damaging cytokine response. In contrast, patients with a properdin or factor D deficiency are simply unable to clear *Neisseria* via opsonophagocytosis and have severe disease.

Clinical features. Individuals with homozygous deficiencies of the early components of the classic complement pathway (C1, C4, C2) have a risk of SLE that ranges from more than 90% for C1q to 10–20% for C2 [4]. C2 deficiency-associated SLE has a median age of onset of approximately 30 years (although children are commonly affected), favours female patients and typically features photosensitivity, skin lesions (especially subacute cutaneous lupus erythematosus), arthralgias/arthritis, fevers and anti-Ro antibodies [32]. Approximately half of patients develop oral ulcers and leucopenia. Although skin involvement is often extensive and resistant to therapy, the overall course of SLE in individuals with C2 deficiency is generally mild. Most patients have absent or low-titre ANA antibodies and minimal or no renal disease. In the setting of C1q/r/s or C4 deficiency, SLE usually develops during childhood, affects girls and boys equally, and is frequently associated with renal disease and palmoplantar keratoses as well as photosensitivity.

Some patients with deficiencies in classic complement components experience recurrent pneumonias caused by encapsulated organisms such as *Strep. pneumoniae*, with more severe infections in those with C3 deficiency. In a recent nationwide Danish study, 40% of children with unexplained recurrent invasive pneumococcal disease were found to have a C2 deficiency [33]. Individuals with deficiencies in properdin, factor D and MAC components have a propensity to develop recurrent neisserial infections beginning around puberty [34]. Exfoliative dermatitis in association with failure to thrive, chronic diarrhoea and recurrent infections during infancy (the 'Leiner phenotype') has been described in patients with C3 or C5 deficiency and in those with C5 dysfunction, but this constellation of clinical findings is not specific to these conditions. Additional autoimmune, inflammatory and infectious complications of complement deficiencies are summarized in Table 156.6.

The CH50 is markedly decreased or undetectable in complement deficiencies other than HAE. The alternative pathway lytic test (AP50) can be used to screen for deficiencies of components in this pathway, but it is less sensitive than the CH50. Immunoprecipitation assays (e.g. radial immunodiffusion or ELISA) can determine the levels of specific complement components and functional studies of individual components may be informative in the setting of normal antigenic levels [35,36].

Mannose-binding lectin deficiency may lead to an increased risk of acute respiratory infections in children aged 6–18 months who have lost their maternal antibodies but are not yet able to mount an effective antibody response to the carbohydrate antigens of encapsulated bacteria [5]. In some studies, MBL deficiency has been linked to an increased likelihood of developing SLE or dermatomyositis and a higher likelihood of infections in the setting of immunosuppressive therapy for SLE.

Treatment and prevention. Conservative therapy is often effective for patients with autoimmune manifestations of complement deficiency. The use of sun protection and topical corticosteroids may be sufficient to treat cutaneous lupus erythematosus. Antimalarial drugs, systemic corticosteroids and other immunosuppressive medications are required for patients with more severe skin disease or SLE, with consideration of the increased risk of infections that may be associated with complement deficiencies. The use of plasma transfusions to replace deficient complement components may paradoxically activate the cascade, accelerate immune complex deposition and promote inflammation. Early, aggressive antibiotic therapy is indicated for bacterial infections in patients with complement deficiencies. Pneumococcal vaccination is recommended for individuals with an early component complement deficiency and meningococcal vaccination for those with a C3, C5–C9, properdin, factor D, or factor H deficiency.

Table 156.6 Complement deficiencies

Complement component	Autoimmune/inflammatory disorders	Predisposition to infections
Classic pathway		
C1q	SLE (>90%), GN	Encapsulated bacteria
C1r, C1s	SLE (~50%), GN	Encapsulated bacteria
C1 esterase inhibitor	Hereditary angioedema >> SLE, GN, Sjögren syndrome, partial lipodystrophy, vasculitis	
C4	SLE (~75%) with palmoplantar keratoses and scarring, HSP, GN, urticaria, JIA (partial deficiency)	Encapsulated bacteria
C2[1]	SLE (10–20%), SCLE, DLE, dermatomyositis, HSP, other vasculitides, atrophoderma, cold urticaria, JIA (heterozygotes), IBD, atherosclerosis	Encapsulated bacteria, esp. *S. pneumoniae*
Lectin pathway		
MBL[2]	SLE, dermatomyositis, atherosclerosis, chronic pulmonary disease	Encapsulated bacteria, esp. *N. meningitides*
MASP-2	SLE, IBD	Encapsulated bacteria, esp. *S. pneumoniae*
C3 and alternative pathway		
C3	SLE, vasculitis, partial lipodystrophy, GN, 'Leiner phenotype'	Encapsulated bacteria (severe infections)
Factor H	SLE, HUS, GN, age-related macular degeneration	Encapsulated bacteria
Factor I (C3b inactivator)	SLE, HUS, aquagenic urticaria, angioedema	Encapsulated bacteria
Membrane cofactor protein	HUS	
Properdin[3]		*Neisseria* (fulminant meningococcal infections[4])
Factor D		*Neisseria*[4]
Membrane attack complex		
C5 dysfunction	'Leiner phenotype'	Gram-negative bacteria
C5 deficiency	SLE	*Neisseria*[4], *S. pneumoniae*
C6	SLE, JIA, GN	*Neisseria*[4], *Brucella, Toxoplasma*
C7	SLE, limited systemic sclerosis, ankylosing spondylitis	*Neisseria*[4]
C8α	SLE, fever with HSM, eosinophilia, hypergammaglobulinaemia	*Neisseria*[4]
C8β	SLE, JIA	*Neisseria*[4]
C9		*Neisseria*

Unless otherwise specified, affected individuals usually have biallelic defects. Encapsulated bacteria include *Streptococcus pneumoniae*, *Streptococcus pyogenes*, *Haemophilus influenzae* and *Neisseria meningitides*.
[1] Most common homozygous complement deficiency.
[2] Very low penetrance.
[3] X-linked recessive.
[4] >50% develop *N. meningitidis* infections, usually recurrent with onset around puberty.
DLE, discoid lupus erythematosus lesions; GN, glomerulonephritis; HSM, hepatosplenomegaly; HSP, Henoch–Schönlein purpura; HUS, haemolytic-uraemic syndrome; IBD, inflammatory bowel disease; INH, inhibitor; JIA, juvenile idiopathic arthritis; MBL, mannose-binding lectin; MASP, MBL-associated serum protease; SCLE, subacute cutaneous lupus erythematosus; SLE, systemic lupus erythematosus.
Source: Adapted with permission from Bolognia JL, Schaffer JV, Cerroni L, eds. *Dermatology*, 4th edn. London: Elsevier, 2018.

References

1 **Grumach AS, Kirschfink M. Are complement deficiencies really rare? Overview on prevalence, clinical importance and modern diagnostic approach. Mol Immunol 2014;61:110–7.**
2 Frank MM. Complement deficiencies. Pediatr Clin North Am 2000;47:1339–54.
3 **Truedsson L. Classical pathway deficiencies – a short analytical review. Mol Immunol 2015;68:14–9.**
4 **Macedo AC, Isaac L. Systemic lupus erythematosus and deficiencies of early components of the complement classical pathway. Front Immunol 2016;7:55.**
5 Casanova JL, Abel L. Human mannose-binding lectin in immunity: friend, foe, or both? J Exp Med 2004;199:1295–9.
6 Agostoni A, Cicardi M. Hereditary and acquired C1-inhibitor deficiency: biological and clinical characteristics in 235 patients. Medicine 1992;71:206–15.
7 **Zuraw BL. Hereditary angioedema. N Engl J Med 2008;359:1027–36.**
8 Nzeako UC, Frigas E, Tremaine WJ. Hereditary angioedema: a broad review for clinicians. Arch Intern Med 2001;161:2417–429.
9 Cicardi M, Aberer W, Banerji A et al. Classification, diagnosis, and approach to treatment for angioedema: consensus report from the Hereditary Angioedema International Working Group. Allergy 2014;69:602–16.
10 Bork K, Barnstedt SE, Koch P, Traupe H. Hereditary angioedema with normal C1-inhibitor activity in women. Lancet 2000;356:213–7.
11 Davis AE. Hereditary angioedema: a current state-of-the-art review, III: mechanisms of hereditary angioedema. Ann Allergy Asthma Immunol 2008;100:S7–12.
12 Joseph K, Tuscano TB, Kaplan AP. Studies of the mechanisms of bradykinin generation in hereditary angioedema plasma. Ann Allergy Asthma Immunol 2008;101:279–86.
13 Cinchon S, Martin L, Hennies HC et al. Increased activity of coagulation factor XII (Hageman factor) causes hereditary angioedema type III. Am J Hum Genet 2006;79:1098–104.
14 Björkqvist J, de Maat S, Lewandrowski U et al. Defective glycosylation of coagulation factor XII underlies hereditary angioedema type III. J Clin Invest 2015;125:3132–46.
15 de Maat S, Björkqvist J, Suffritti C et al. Plasmin is a natural trigger for bradykinin production in patients with hereditary angioedema with factor XII mutations. J Allergy Clin Immunol 2016;138:1414–23.
16 Bork K, Meng G, Staubach P, Hardt J. Hereditary angioedema: new findings concerning symptoms, affected organs, and course. Am J Med 2006;119:267–74.
17 Bork K, Staubach P, Eckardt AJ, Hardt J. Symptoms, course, and complications of abdominal attacks in hereditary angioedema due to C1-inhibitor deficiency. Am J Gastroenterol 2006;101:619–27.
18 Gompels MM, Lock RJ, Abinun M et al. C1-inhibitor deficiency: consensus document. Clin Exp Immunol 2005;139:379–94.
19 **Farkas H, Martinez-Saguer I, Bork K et al. International consensus on the diagnosis and management of pediatric patients with**

hereditary angioedema with C1 inhibitor deficiency. Allergy 2017; 72:300–13.
20 Blanch A, Roche O, Urrutia I et al. First case of homozygous C1-inhibitor deficiency. J Allergy Clin Immunol 2006;118:1330–5.
21 Deroux A, Boccon-Gibod I, Fain O et al. Hereditary angioedema with normal C1 inhibitor and factor XII mutation: a series of 57 patients from the French National Center of Reference for Angioedema. Clin Exp Immunol 2016;185:332–7.
22 Bork K. A decade of change: recent developments in pharmacotherapy of hereditary angioedema (HAE). Clin Rev Allergy Immunol 2016;51:183–92.
23 Craig T, Aygören-Pürsün E, Bork K et al. WAO Guideline for the Management of Hereditary Angioedema. World Allergy Organ J 2012;5:182–99.
24 Riedl MA, Bygum A, Lumry W et al. Safety and usage of C1-inhibitor in hereditary angioedema: Berinert Registry Data. J Allergy Clin Immunol Pract 2016;4:963–71.
25 Zuraw BL, Davis DK, Castaldo AJ, Christiansen SC.Tolerability and effectiveness of 17-α-alkylated androgen therapy for hereditary angioedema: a re-examination. J Allergy Clin Immunol Pract 2016;4:948–55.
26 Farkas H, Varga L, Széplaki G et al. Management of hereditary angioedema in pediatric patients. Pediatrics 2007;120:e713–22.
27 Cook HT, Botto M. The complement system and the pathogenesis of systemic lupus erythematosus. Nat Clin Pract Rheumatol 2006;2:330–7.
28 Sontheimer RD, Racila E, Racila DM. C1q: its functions within the innate and adaptive immune responses and its role in lupus autoimmunity. J Invest Dermatol 2005;125:14–23.
29 Cai Y, Teo BH, Yeo JG, Lu J. C1q protein binds to the apoptotic nucleolus and causes C1 protease degradation of nucleolar proteins. J Biol Chem 2015;290:22570–80.
30 Schneider MC, Exley RM, Ram S et al. Interactions between Neisseria meningitidis and the complement system. Trends Microbiol 2007;15:233–40.
31 Sprong T, Roos D, Weemaes C et al. Deficient alternative complement pathway activation due to factor D deficiency by 2 novel mutations in the complement factor D gene in a family with meningococcal infections. Blood 2006;107:4865–70.
32 Jönsson G, Sjöholm AG, Truedsson I et al. Rheumatological manifestations, organ damage and autoimmunity in hereditary C2 deficiency. Rheumatology 2007;46:1133–9.
33 Ingels H, Schejbel L, Lundstedt AC et al. Immunodeficiency among children with recurrent invasive pneumococcal disease. Pediatr Infect Dis J 2015;34:644–51.
34 Audemard-Verger A, Descloux E, Ponard D et al. Infections revealing complement deficiency in adults: a French nationwide study enrolling 41 patients. Medicine (Baltimore) 2016;95:e3548.
35 Frazer-Abel A, Sepiashvili L, Mbughuni MM, Willrich MA. Overview of laboratory testing and clinical presentations of complement deficiencies and dysregulation. Adv Clin Chem 2016;77:1–75.
36 Shih AR, Murali MR. Laboratory tests for disorders of complement and complement regulatory proteins. Am J Hematol 2015;90:1180–6.

DiGeorge syndrome

Key points

- **DiGeorge syndrome is a disorder that is part of the 22q11 deletion syndrome spectrum.**
- **Varying features include cardiac abnormalities, dysmorphic facies, thymic hypoplasia and hypocalcaemia caused by hypoparathyroidism.**
- **There is a variable degree of immunodeficiency.**

Introduction and history. Dr Angelo DiGeorge first described four patients with no thymus or parathyroid glands in 1965. One of these patients had absent T-cell immunity, normal immunoglobulins and poor antibody production [1]. DiGeorge Syndrome (DGS) is defined as a congenital T-cell immunodeficiency with a conotruncal cardiac abnormality, hypocalcaemia (and sometimes tetany), dysmorphic facies and thymic hypoplasia. The disorder may be underdiagnosed, because phenotypic findings may be mild in some patients. Patients with DGS can be divided into two subtypes – partial or complete DGS. Partial DGS encompasses most patients who have variable but not severe immune defects. Complete DGS patients have an SCID phenotype and no thymic tissue.

Epidemiology and pathogenesis. DGS is the most common chromosomal microdeletion syndrome with a reported incidence of 1 in 5950 births in the USA from a population-based study [2]. DGS belongs to a group of disorders (including velocardiofacial syndrome) caused by hemizygous deletion of chromosome 22q11.2 [3]. Such deletions lead to haploinsufficiency of the *TBX1* gene, which encodes a T-box transcription factor that is required for development of the fourth pharyngeal arch arteries [4]. In 2–5% of patients, heterozygous deletions in chromosome 10p13-14 (DGS II locus) have been found. These patients have more sensorineural hearing loss than DGS I but also have hypoparathyroidism, cardiac anomalies, renal anomalies and hypoparathyroidism [5,6].

Clinical features. DGS is characterized by abnormalities of the thymus and parathyroid glands (which are derived from the third and fourth pharyngeal pouches), conotruncal heart anomalies (especially tetrology of Fallot), cleft palate and facial dysmorphism (hypertelorism, a short philtrum and low-set malformed ears) [3]. Affected infants may present with hypocalcaemia and resultant tetany from parathyroid gland aplasia.

The thymic shadow is absent or reduced at birth in patients with DGS. T-cell abnormalities do not typically improve with age and range from mild ('partial DiGeorge') to severe [7]. Humoral immunity is usually normal. Patients often experience recurrent mucocutaneous candidal infections, often beginning soon after birth, and have increased susceptibility to viral, *Pneumocystis jiroveci* and other fungal infections. Graft-versus-host disease (GVHD) may develop in infants who receive nonirradiated blood products. Noninfectious cutaneous granulomas and eczematous eruptions characterized histologically by spongiotic dermatitis, satellite-cell necrosis and an infiltrate of eosinophils and oligoclonal autologous T cells have been described [8].

Other manifestations of DGS include autoimmunity caused by immune disregulation in 10% [9–11]. Malignancy, especially B-cell lymphomas, are more common in those with more profound T-cell defects. Other autoimmune diseases including juvenile idiopathic arthritis and cytopenias also appear to be more common in this population as do allergic diseases. Developmental and behavioural problems including language delay are common in DGS. Normal intelligence to moderate intellectual disability may occur. Adults with DGS may be predisposed to psychiatric problems including schizophrenia, schizoaffective disorder and major depression. Psychiatric or intellectual disability along with facial features or palatal abnormalities may be the presenting symptoms in adults who were not picked up as children [12].

Differential diagnosis. The differential diagnosis for DGS includes other congenital syndromes including 22q11 deletion syndrome, Zellweger syndrome, CHARGE (coloboma, heart, choanal atresia, retardation, genital and ear anomalies) and other forms of T-cell immunodeficiency including various forms of SCID.

Laboratory and histology findings. A neonate with suspected DGS should have an immediate cardiac evaluation, calcium and phosphorus levels and a parathyroid hormone assay. A CBC may indicate profound lymphopenia in complete DGS. Flow cytometric evaluation of B, T and NK cell subsets by fluorescence-activated cell sorting (FACS) and lymphoproliferative studies to evaluate T-cell function should be performed. In addition, immunoglobulin levels as well as antibody function testing is useful in older infants and children who have received their vaccinations. Genetic testing (fluorescence *in situ* hybridization [FISH] or microarray) for 22q11.2 deletion or a 10p deletion will establish a definitive diagnosis [13].

Treatment and prevention. Acute management of neonates with DGS includes management of cardiac issues, as well as management of hypocalcaemia and feeding and swallowing issues. Immunological management includes precautions against use of nonirradiated or cytomegalovirus-positive blood products. Thymic transplantation may be indicated if a patient has complete DGS. If not available or possible, HSCT may be performed. Patients with partial DGS should be followed for their immune deficiency. Live viral vaccines may be given if T-cell function is intact. Prognosis for patients with partial DGS is good. There is high mortality in complete DGS patients who do not undergo transplantation. Patients with low or absent T cells may be picked up by TREC (T-cell receptor excision circle) analysis used in newborn screening programmes for severe combined immunodeficiency [14–16].

References

1 Lischner HW, Dacou C, DiGeorge AM. Normal lymphocyte transfer (NLT) test: negative response in a patient with congenital absence of the thymus. Transplantation,1967;5:555–7.

2 Botto LD, May K, Fernhoff et al. A population-based study of the 22q11.2 deletion: phenotype, incidence, and contribution to major birth defects in the population. Pediatrics 2003;112:101–7.

3 Kobrynski LJ, Sullivan KE. Velocardiofacial syndrome, DiGeorge syndrome: the chromosome 22q11.2 deletion syndromes. Lancet 2007;370:1443–52.

4 Lindsay EA, Vitelli F, Su H et al. Tbx1 haploinsufficiency in the DiGeorge syndrome region causes aortic arch defects in mice. Nature 2001;410:97–101.

5 Lichtner P, Konig R, Hasegawa T et al. An HDR (hypoparathyroidism, deafness, renal dysplasia) syndrome locus maps distal to the DiGeorge syndrome region on 10p13/14. J Med Genet 2000:37:33–7.

6 Daw SC, Taylor C, Kraman M et al. A common region of 10p deleted in DiGeorge and velocardiofacial syndromes. Nat Genet 1996;13:458–60.

7 Markert ML, Hummell DS, Rosenblatt HM et al. Complete DiGeorge syndrome: persistence of profound immunodeficiency. J Pediatr 1998;132:15–21.

8 Selim MA, Markert ML, Burchette JL et al. The cutaneous manifestations of atypical complete DiGeorge syndrome: a histopathologic and immunohistochemical study. J Cutan Pathol 2008;35:380–5.

9 Piliero LM, Sanford AN, McDonald-McGinn DM et al., T-cell homeostasis in humans with thymic hypoplasia due to chromosome 22q11.2 deletion syndrome. Blood 2004;103:1020–5.

10 Chinen J, Rosenblatt HM, Smith EO et al. Long-term assessment of T-cell populations in DiGeorge syndrome. J Allergy Clin Immunol 2003;111:573–9.

11 Zemble R, Luning Prak E, McDonald K et al. Secondary immunologic consequences in chromosome 22q11.2 deletion syndrome (DiGeorge syndrome/velocardiofacial syndrome). Clin Immunol 2010;136:409–18.

12 Vogels A, Schevenels S, Cayenberghs R et al. Presenting symptoms in adults with the 22q11 deletion syndrome. Eur J Med Genet 2014;57:157.

13 Bassett AS, McDonald-McGinn DM, Devriendt K et al. Practical guidelines for managing patients with 22q11.2 deletion syndrome. J Pediatr 2011;159:332.

14 Kwan A, Abraham RS, Currier R et al. Newborn screening for severe combined immunodeficiency in 11 screening programs in the United States. JAMA 2014;312:729.

15 Lingman Framme J, Borte S, von Dobeln U et al. Retrospective analysis of TREC based newborn screening results and clinical phenotypes in infants with the 22q11 deletion syndrome. J Clin Immunol 2014;34:514.

16 Knutsen AP, Baker MW, Markert ML. Interpreting low T-cell receptor excision circles in newborns with DiGeorge anomaly: Importance of assessing naive T-cell markers. J Allergy Clin Immunol 2011;128:1375.

Hyperimmunoglobulin E syndromes

Key points

- **Most cases are autosomal dominant and result from mutations in STAT3, leading to inflammatory and infectious complications.**
- **They are characterized by recurrent cutaneous and sinopulmonary infections, early onset atopic dermatitis and extremely elevated IgE levels.**
- **Earliest manifestation is usually facial papules and pustules during infancy.**
- **The autosomal dominant form also features dental abnormalities, scoliosis and increased risk of fractures.**
- **Autosomal recessive forms typically have severe infections, particularly cutaneous viral infections and neurological complications.**

Introduction and history. Hyperimmunoglobulin E syndromes (HIES) are characterized by recurrent cutaneous and sinopulmonary infections, eczematous dermatitis beginning in infancy or early childhood, and extremely elevated IgE levels [1–3]. Job syndrome represents a subgroup of female patients with fair skin, red hair and hyperextensible joints in addition to the other features of HIES [3]. The classic form of HIES is an autosomal dominant disorder with variable expressivity. Clinically and molecularly distinct autosomal recessive forms of HIES (AR-HIES) have also been described [4–6].

Epidemiology and pathogenesis. The autosomal dominant form of HIES is caused by heterozygous mutations in the signal transducer and activator of the transcription 3 (*STAT3*) gene [7,8]. Receptor-associated JAKs and STAT proteins have key roles in the transduction of cytokine signals. Upon phosphorylation by JAKs, STAT proteins dimerize, translocate to the nucleus and activate transcription of target genes. The infectious and inflammatory complications that characterize HIES reflect disruption of the signal transduction pathways of certain cytokines. Impaired differentiation of IL-17-producing $CD4^+$ T cells (Th17 cells), which requires other STAT3-dependent cytokines (e.g. IL-6, IL-21 and IL-23), is thought to be especially important, contributing to HIES patients' susceptibility to bacterial and candidal infections [9]. A lack of stimulation of β-defensin production by IL-22 (which is produced by Th17 cells and signals via STAT3) may be a particular factor in recurrent infections at epithelial surfaces in HIES. STAT3 is also critical to other functions of IL-6 (which promotes acute phase responses and acts as a pyrogen) and to IL-10 (an anti-inflammatory cytokine), with decreased signalling by these cytokines providing a potential explanation for 'cold' abscesses and destructive inflammation (e.g. in the skin and lung), respectively. Increased proinflammatory activity is reflected in increased secretion of cytokines such as TNF-α and interferon-γ by leucocytes after stimulation with specific agonists [7,8]. The osteopenia of HIES is likely related to loss of STAT3-dependent downregulation of osteoclast differentiation. The precise mechanism underlying the extremely elevated IgE levels in HIES has not yet been determined, but it is thought to involve the interplay between cells of the immune system and the skin.

Biallelic mutations in the dedicator of cytokinesis 8 protein (*DOCK8*) gene have been identified in patients with AR-HIES [5,6]. The DOCK8 protein, a member of the DOCK180-related family of atypical guanine nucleotide exchange factors, is thought to regulate cytoskeletal rearrangements that have important roles in immune functions such T-cell expansion and antibody responses. Homozygous mutations in the tyrosine kinase 2 (*TYK2*) gene, which encodes a member of the JAK family, have been identified in a patient with an autosomal recessive condition resembling HIES [10]. This molecular defect also led to disruption of additional signalling pathways, including those for IL-12 and IFN-α/β (see Table 156.4). However, several other patients with TYK2 deficiency have had increased viral and mycobacterial infections but not HIES [11], suggesting that HIES is not an intrinsic feature of TYK2 deficiency. An HIES-like AR disorder with elevated IgE levels, atopy, autoimmunity and neurocognitive issues has been linked to biallelic mutations in phosphoglucomutase 3 (PGM3), a glycosylation enzyme [12–14].

Clinical features. During the first month of life, more than 80% of patients with HIES develop a noninfectious papulopustular eruption that favours the face, scalp, upper trunk, axillae and napkin area [15,16]. Chronic or recurrent cutaneous candidiasis may be the initial infectious manifestation of HIES and eventually affects approximately 85% of patients. Skin infections with *S. aureus* also begin during infancy and can present as crusted plaques, retroauricular fissures, pustules, furuncles, abscesses, cellulitis, lymphangitis and paronychia leading to nail dystrophy [17]. Cutaneous abscesses most commonly affect the neck (Fig. 156.7), scalp, periorbital area, axillae and groin. These lesions are often large but tend to be less erythematous, warm and tender than expected, leading to the designation 'cold abscesses'. Patients with abscesses and other infections are frequently afebrile or have only a slight temperature elevation. Recurrent skin infections with other organisms such as *Strep. pyogenes* may also develop.

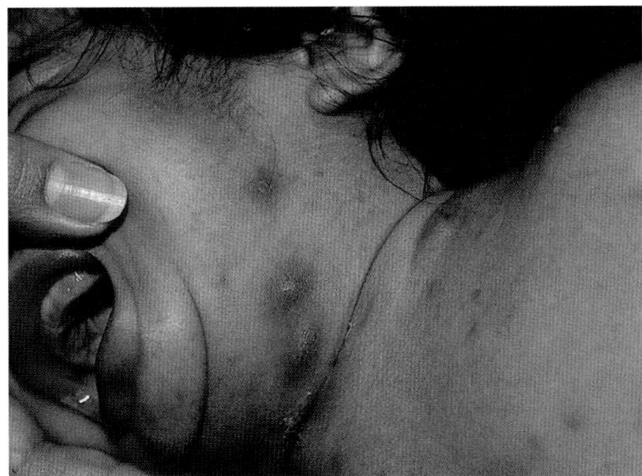

Fig. 156.7 Multiple staphylococcal abscesses on the neck of an infant with hyperimmunoglobulin E syndrome.

Most patients with HIES have recurrent bronchitis and pneumonias, which are usually caused by *S. aureus*, *Strep. pneumoniae* or *Haemophilus influenzae* and frequently result in empyema, bronchiectasis and pneumatocoele formation. *P. jiroveci* pneumonia can also occur in infants and children with HIES. Pneumatocoeles tend to persist and become the site of further infections with bacteria (often *P. aeruginosa*) or fungi (often *Aspergillus*), which are major causes of morbidity and mortality. Rarely, massive haemoptysis ensues. Other common sites of infection include the ears, oral mucosa, sinuses and eyes. Visceral infections other than pneumonia are unusual.

The eczematous dermatitis of HIES shares several clinical features with atopic dermatitis, including extreme pruritus and lichenification as well as staphylococcal superinfection. The dermatitis is virtually always present in infants and young children with HIES, but it may clear by adolescence or adulthood. Although other forms of atopy may occur, STAT3-deficient HIES is not strongly associated with hay fever or asthma [18], does not show a Th2 cell predominance and the IgE is not allergen-specific. In addition, skin barrier function has been found to be normal, in contrast to atopic dermatitis [19].

Patients with HIES develop an atypical facial appearance that may be partially caused by deforming facial abscesses, with progressive facial coarsening, a broad fleshy nose, deep-set eyes, a prominent forehead and irregularly proportioned cheeks and jaw; these facial changes usually become apparent by adolescence. Facial skin is often thick and doughy with large follicular ostia and pitted scarring. Osteopenia is a frequent finding and patients have an increased risk of bone fractures [20,21]; 60% of adolescents and adults with HIES have had at least three fractures of the long bones, ribs or pelvis, often resulting from unrecognized or minor trauma. Scoliosis occurs in 75% of patients aged 16 years of age or older, and joint hyperextensibility affects 70% of patients. Approximately half of affected individuals have a high-arched palate, and dental abnormalities associated with HIES include retention of primary teeth and lack of eruption of secondary teeth [22]. Chiari I malformations are present in approximately 20% of HIES patients. Coronary artery aneurysms and evidence of lacunar infarctions or focal white matter hyperintensities on brain MRI have been observed in patients with HIES, with the latter found in approximately 50% of patients 18 years of age or younger and approximately 80% of adult patients [23]. Hyperimmunoglobulin E syndrome is also associated with an increased risk of non-Hodgkin lymphomas of B-cell origin.

Autosomal recessive HIES is a separate condition that shares some findings with classic HIES, including markedly elevated serum IgE levels, peripheral eosinophilia, chronic eczematous dermatitis and recurrent staphylococcal infections of the skin (including cold abscesses) and respiratory tract [5,6]. However, instead of pneumatoceles, osteopenia and dental abnormalities, patients with AR-HIES are at risk of severe viral skin (e.g. molluscum contagiosum, warts, herpes simplex and varicella-zoster, overall in 44%) (Fig. 156.8) and opportunistic infections [10]. Mucocutaneous candidiasis occurs in only 28% of patients. The neonatal eruption has been described in only 24% of DOCK8-deficient HIES patients [17]. Food allergies (70%) [18], particularly to cow's milk and often leading to anaphylaxis, asthma (47%), autoimmunity, central nervous system vasculitis, mucocutaneous squamous cell carcinomas and lymphomas have also been described. Mortality in one series was 48%, due primarily to pneumonia and sepsis, with a median age of 10 years [24]; in another series, half of the patients died by 20 years of age, primarily from infection or cancer, and most had at least one life-threatening complication by 25 years, despite aggressive management with prophylactic antibiotics, intravenous immunoglobulin (IVIG) and IFNa [6].

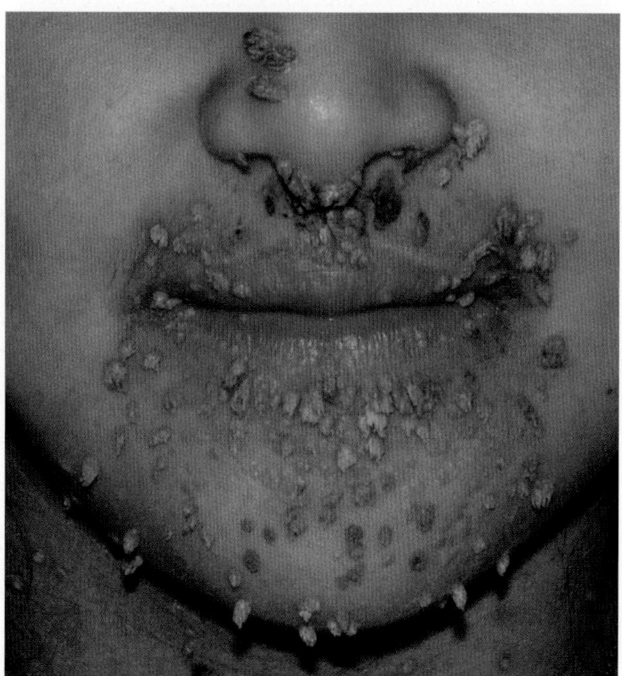

Fig. 156.8 Extensive warts on the face of a 10-year-old girl with DOCK8 deficiency.

Differential diagnosis. Hyperimmunoglobulin E syndrome must be differentiated from a number of other disorders that feature elevated IgE levels and dermatitis, including atopic dermatitis, Wiskott–Aldrich syndrome (WAS), Netherton syndrome, Omenn syndrome, DGS, IPEX syndrome, IL-1 receptor associated kinase-4 (IRAK-4) deficiency, prolidase deficiency and GVHD. Atopic dermatitis and WAS are most easily confused with HIES because of the frequent staphylococcal superinfections, eczematous dermatitis and often very high levels of IgE. The presence of coarse facial features, osteopenia, recurrent pneumonia and cold abscesses help to differentiate AD-HIES from these conditions, and platelet abnormalities also help to distinguish WAS. In a study of 70 paediatric patients over a 10-year period who had a serum IgE level of more than 2000 IU/ mL, 69% had atopic dermatitis and only 8% had HIES; no correlation was observed between the IgE level and diagnosis of HIES [25]. IRAK-4 deficiency leads to defective Toll-like receptor signalling and impaired antibody responses to vaccination. Affected individuals develop recurrent pyogenic sinopulmonary and skin infections, including cold abscesses, but not eczematous dermatitis. Early candida infections may raise the possibility of mucocutaneous candidiasis; interestingly, somatic mosaicism of STAT3 mutations can present with recurrent mucocutaneous candidiasis, even with normal Th17 cells [26]. Prolidase deficiency is an autosomal recessive disorder caused by defects in the gene encoding peptidase D. In addition to eczematous dermatitis and frequent pyogenic infections, prolidase deficiency features chronic leg ulcers, facial dysmorphism and developmental delay [27]. Although bacterial and candidal abscesses are features of chronic granulomatous disease and myeloperoxidase deficiency, these conditions are not characterized by elevated IgE levels.

Laboratory and histology findings. Diagnostic criteria for AD-HIES include IgE greater than 1000 IU/mL and a weighted score of five clinical features (typical newborn rash, recurrent pneumonia, pathological bone fractures, characteristic facies and a high palate) [28]; these characteristics plus a lack of Th17 cells or the detection of a heterozygous *STAT3* mutation allow for a probable or definitive diagnosis, respectively. Histological features of the pustular eruption in neonates and infants include eosinophilic spongiosis, eosinophilic folliculitis and a dermal perivascular infiltrate with abundant eosinophils. Patients with HIES have markedly elevated serum levels of polyclonal IgE, typically peaking at more than 2000 IU/mL and sometimes declining during adulthood.

Patients develop particularly high levels of antistaphylococcal and anticandidal IgE and often have immediate wheal-and-flare reactions upon skin prick testing with a variety of foods and inhaled allergens as well as bacterial and fungal antigens. Serum levels of IgG, IgA and IgM are usually normal. Many patients have eosinophilia of the peripheral blood and sputum, and abnormalities of neutrophil and monocyte chemotaxis are occasionally observed. Cell-mediated immunity is often abnormal, as manifested by anergy to skin testing and impaired *in vitro* lymphoproliferative responses to specific antigens. Th17 cell numbers are reduced.

AR-HIES is associated with a combined immunodeficiency that is characterized by lymphopenia (deficiency of CD4 T cells > CD8 T cells > B cells), low IgM levels and variable IgG levels as well as elevated IgE levels and peripheral eosinophilia. In contrast to STAT3-deficient HIES, there is a Th2 cell predominance [18]. Absence of DOCK8 expression can be demonstrated by flow cytometry [29].

Treatment and prevention. The mainstay of therapy for HIES is good skin care and the aggressive treatment of infections, particularly with antiseptics (e.g. dilute sodium hypochlorite baths), antibiotics (therapeutic and prophylactic), and incision and drainage of abscesses. Prophylactic antimicrobial administration (e.g. with fluconazole and cotrimoxazole) can be useful. Interferon-γ has been shown to increase neutrophil chemotaxis and potentially help control infections [30], and interferon-α has effectively treated the numerous warts [31] and severe herpetic infections [32,33] in DOCK8-deficient HIES. IVIG therapy may improve the dermatitis, reduce the incidence of bacterial pneumonia and lower IgE levels [34]. Alendronate has been administered for the osteopenia [21]. There have been anecdotal reports of improvement of the eczematous dermatitis of HIES with use of omalizumab, a monoclonal antibody directed against IgE [35]. Stem cell transplantation is generally reserved for DOCK8-deficient HIES [36–38] but has been successful in severe cases of STAT3-deficient HIES [39].

References

1 **Grimbacher B, Holland SM, Gallin JI et al. Hyper-IgE syndrome with recurrent infections: an autosomal dominant multisystem disorder. N Engl J Med 1999;340:692–702.**

2 **Farmand S, Sundin M et al Hyper-IgE syndromes: recent advances in pathogenesis, diagnostics and clinical care. Curr Opin Hematol 2015;22:12–22.**

3 **Chandesris MO, Melki I, Natividad A et al. Autosomal dominant STAT3 deficiency and hyper-IgE syndrome: molecular, cellular, and clinical features from a French national survey. Medicine 2012; 91:e1–e19.**

4 **Zhang Q, Davis JC, Lamborn IT et al. Combined immunodeficiency associated with DOCK8 mutations. N Engl J Med 2009;361:2046–55.**

5 **Engelhardt KR, Gertz ME, Keles S et al. The extended clinical phenotype of 64 patients with dedicator of cytokinesis 8 deficiency. J Allergy Clin Immunol 2015;136:402–12.**

6 **Aydin SE, Kilic SS, Aytekin C et al. DOCK8 deficiency: clinical and immunological phenotype and treatment options – a review of 136 patients. J Clin Immunol 2015;35:189–98.**

7 Holland SM, DeLeo FR, Elloumi HZ et al. STAT3 mutations in the hyper-IgE syndrome. N Engl J Med 2007;357:1608–19.

8 Minegishi Y, Saito M, Tsuchiya S et al. Dominant-negative mutations in the DNA-binding domain of STAT3 cause hyper-IgE syndrome. Nature 2007;448:1058–62.

9 Milner JD, Brenchley JM, Laurence A et al. Impaired T_H17 cell differentiation in subjects with autosomal dominant hyper-IgE syndrome. Nature 2008;452:773–6.

10 Minegishi Y, Saito M, Morio T et al. Human tyrosine kinase 2 deficiency reveals its requisite roles in multiple cytokine signals involved in innate and acquired immunity. Immunity 2006;25:745–55.

11 Kreins AY, Ciancanelli MJ, Okada S et al. Human TYK2 deficiency: mycobacterial and viral infections without hyper-IgE syndrome. J Exp Med 2015;212:1641–62.

12 Sassi A, Lazaroski S, Wu G et al. Hypomorphic homozygous mutations in phosphoglucomutase 3 (PGM3) impair immunity and increase serum IgE levels. J Allergy Clin Immunol 2014;133:1410–19.

13 Zhang Y, Yu X, Ichikawa M et al. Autosomal recessive phosphoglucomutase 3 (PGM3) mutations link glycosylation defects to atopy, immune deficiency, autoimmunity, and neurocognitive impairment. J Allergy Clin Immunol 2014;133:1400–9.

14 Yang L, Fliegauf M, Grimbacher B et al. Hyper-IgE syndromes: reviewing PGM3 deficiency. Curr Opin Pediatr 2014;26:697–703.

15 Chamlin SL, McCalmont TH, Cunningham BB et al. Cutaneous manifestations of hyper-IgE syndrome in infants and children. J Pediatr 2002;141:572–5.

16 Eberting CL, Davis J, Puck JM et al. Dermatitis and the newborn rash of hyper-IgE syndrome. Arch Dermatol 2004;140:1119–25.

17 Chu EY, Freeman AF, Jing H et al. Cutaneous manifestations of DOCK8 deficiency syndrome. Arch Dermatol 2012;148:79–84.

18 Boos AC, Hagl B, Schlesinger A et al. Atopic dermatitis, STAT3- and DOCK8-hyper-IgE syndromes differ in IgE-based sensitization pattern. Allergy 2014;69:943–53.

19 Mócsai G, Gáspár K, Dajnoki Z et al. Investigation of skin barrier functions and allergic sensitization in patients with hyper-IgE syndrome. J Clin Immunol 2015;35:681–8.

20 Sowerwine KJ, Shaw PA, Gu W et al. Bone density and fractures in autosomal dominant hyper IgE syndrome. J Clin Immunol 2014;34:260–4.

21 Scheuerman O, Hoffer V, Cohen AH et al. Reduced bone density in patients with autosomal dominant hyper-IgE syndrome. J Clin Immunol 2013;33:903–8.

22 Esposito L, Poletti L, Maspero C et al. Hyper-IgE syndrome: dental implications. Oral Surg Oral Med Oral Pathol Oral Radiol 2012;114:147–53.

23 Freeman AF, Collura-Burke CJ, Patronas NJ et al. Brain abnormalities in patients with hyperimmunoglobulin E syndrome. Pediatrics 2007;119:e1121–5.

24 Alsum Z, Hawwari A, Alsmadi O et al. Clinical, immunological and molecular characterization of DOCK8 and DOCK8-like deficient patients: single center experience of twenty-five patients. J Clin Immunol 2013;33:55–67.

25 Joshi AY, Iyer VN, Boyce TG et al. Elevated serum immunoglobulin E (IgE): when to suspect hyper-IgE syndrome: a 10-year pediatric tertiary care center experience. Allergy Asthma Proc 2009;30:23–7.

26 Hsu AP, Sowerwine KJ, Lawrence MG et al. Intermediate phenotypes in patients with autosomal dominant hyper-IgE syndrome caused by somatic mosaicism. J Allergy Clin Immunol 2013;131:1586–93.

27 Hershkovitz T, Hassoun G, Indelman M et al. A homozygous missense mutation in PEPD encoding peptidase D causes prolidase deficiency associated with hyper-IgE syndrome. Clin Exp Dermatol 2006;31:435–40.

28 Woellner C, Gertz EM, Schäffer AA et al. Mutations in STAT3 and diagnostic guidelines for hyper-IgE syndrome. J Allergy Clin Immunol 2010;125:424–32.

29 Pai SY, de Boer H, Massaad MJ et al. Flow cytometry diagnosis of dedicator of cytokinesis 8 (DOCK8) deficiency. J Allergy Clin Immunol 2014;134:221–3;e227.

30 Jeppson JD, Jaffe HS, Hill HR. Use of recombinant human interferon gamma to enhance neutrophil chemotactic responses in Job syndrome of hyperimmunoglobulinemia E and recurrent infections. J Pediatr 1991;118:383–7.

31 Al-Zahrani D, Raddadi A, Massaad M et al. Successful interferon-alpha 2b therapy for unremitting warts in a patient with DOCK8 deficiency. Clin Immunol 2014;153:104–8.

32 Keles S, Jabara HH, Reisli I et al. Plasmacytoid dendritic cell depletion in DOCK8 deficiency: rescue of severe herpetic infections with IFN-alpha 2b therapy. J Allergy Clin Immunol 2014;133:1753–5.e3.

33 Papan C, Hagl B, Heinz V et al. Beneficial IFN-alpha treatment of tumorous herpes simplex blepharoconjunctivitis in dedicator of cytokinesis 8 deficiency. J Allergy Clin Immunol 2014;133:1456–8.

34 Kimata H. High-dose intravenous gamma-globulin treatment for hyperimmunoglobulinemia E syndrome. J Allergy Clin Immunol 1995;95:771–4.
35 Bard S, Paravisini A, Avilés-Izquierdo JA et al. Eczematous dermatitis in the setting of hyper-IgE syndrome successfully treated with omalizumab. Arch Dermatol 2008;144:1662–3.
36 Cuellar-Rodriguez J, Freeman AF, Grossman J et al. Matched related and unrelated donor hematopoietic stem cell transplantation for DOCK8 deficiency. Biol Blood Marrow Transplant 2015;21:1037–45.
37 Gatz SA, Benninghoff U, Schutz C et al. Curative treatment of autosomal-recessive hyper-IgE syndrome by hematopoietic cell transplantation. Bone Marrow Transplant 2011;46:552–6.
38 Boztug H, Karitnig-Weiss C, Ausserer B et al. Clinical and immunological correction of DOCK8 deficiency by allogeneic hematopoietic stem cell transplantation following a reduced toxicity conditioning regimen. Pediatr Hematol Oncol 2012;29:585–94.
39 Patel NC, Gallagher JL, Torgerson TR et al. Successful haploidentical donor hematopoietic stem cell transplant and restoration of STAT3 function in an adolescent with autosomal dominant hyper-IgE syndrome. J Clin Immunol 2015;35:479–85.

Immunoglobulin deficiencies

Key points

- **Affected individuals suffer recurrent sinopulmonary bacterial infections.**
- **Antibody responses are poor or absent.**
- **It is a heterogenous group of B-cell or humoral immunodeficiencies including common variable immunodeficiency, IgA deficiency, hyper IgM syndrome, X-linked agammaglobulinemia and others.**

Several primary immunodeficiencies feature low levels of immunoglobulins. Affected individuals do not typically become symptomatic with recurrent bacterial infections until after 6 months of age, when levels of maternally transmitted antibodies wane. Major forms of immunoglobulin deficiency are discussed below and additional information on these and other entities is presented in Table 156.7 [1–3].

Immunoglobulin A deficiency

The most common immunoglobulin deficiency is selective IgA deficiency (sIgAD), with a range in prevalence around the world from approximately 1:143 in the Arabian Peninsula [4] to 1:18 500 in Japan [5]. In the USA, the frequency is estimated to be from 1:223 to 1:1000 in community studies and from 1:333 to 1:3000 among healthy blood donors [6]. Between 10 and 15% of affected individuals have clinical manifestations, usually bacterial sinopulmonary infections and *Giardia* gastroenteritis but also mucocutaneous candidiasis, autoimmune disorders and atopy. Selective IgA deficiency may progress to common variable immunodeficiency (CVID). Other immune deficiencies associated with IgA deficiency including ataxia-telangiectasia, DGS and SCID caused by RAG 1 and 2 deficiencies. sIgA deficiency is a diagnosis of exclusion in patients older than 4 years of age who have normal other immunoglobulin levels (IgG and IgM). Because half of patients have circulating anti-IgA antibodies, it is imperative that patients with sIgA deficiency do not receive IVIg or other blood products containing IgA-bearing lymphocytes. Fatal anaphylactic reactions have occurred from the administration of such blood products.

Hyperimmunoglobulin M syndromes

Hyperimmunoglobulin M syndromes (HIMS) represent a group of conditions characterized by defective immunoglobulin class switch recombination, which leads to increased production of IgM but decreased synthesis of other immunoglobulin isotypes [7–12]. Inheritance is most often the X-linked form of the disease caused by mutations in the CD40 ligand gene on chromosome Xq26.3, but autosomal recessive forms have also been described [13]. The estimated prevalence is 1: 1 000 000 [14]. Patients have recurrent skin, sinopulmonary and gastrointestinal infections with pyogenic bacteria and (in some forms of HIMS) opportunistic organisms. Other mucocutaneous manifestations include oral (Fig. 156.9) and anogenital ulcers, extensive warts and noninfectious granulomas [15]. Affected individuals are also predisposed to the development of autoimmune disorders, most often cytopenias [16], and have an increased risk of lymphoma. Hypohidrotic ectodermal dysplasia with immunodeficiency is a form of HIMS that is usually inherited in an X-linked recessive manner and caused by NF-κB essential modulator (*NEMO*) gene mutations that are less deleterious than the male-lethal *NEMO* defects that underlie incontinentia pigmenti. Other forms of primary immunodeficiency may also present with elevated IgM levels including AT, Nijmegen breakage syndrome, Cerunnos deficiency and congenital rubella syndrome [13].

Treatment is stem cell transplantation. Overall prognosis for patients with XHIGM is guarded with an average 20% survival by age 25 years and is not affected by stem cell transplantation [14].

Panhypogammaglobulinaemia

Panhypogammaglobulinaemia is found in approximately 1 in 25 000 people, and it is classified into two major subdivisions:

1 CVID: the most common, heterogenous B cell deficiency and;
2 Agammaglobulinaemia (90% representing the X-linked recessive Bruton variant) resulting from failure of B-cell differentiation [17,18].

CVID

CVID is the most prevalent form of humoral or B-cell immunodeficiencies in both children and adults. CVID can be inherited in an autosomal dominant or recessive manner, and it is characterized by variable defects in T-cell function as well as decreased levels of at least two classes of immunoglobulins (IgG, IgA > IgM) [19–21]. Only a small percentage (2–10%) of cases have a disease causing mutation in a single, nonredundant gene [22,23]. Whole exome sequencing is helpful in identifying immune pathways involved in patients with sporadic CVID [24]. Some patients with CVID have family members with selective IgA deficiency.

Table 156.7 Primary immunoglobulin deficiency disorders

Disorder	Gene	Protein (function)	Ig levels	B cells	Infectious organisms and extracutaneous manifestations	Cutaneous manifestations
Block in B-cell differentiation at the pro-B- to pre-B-cell transition						
X-linked (Bruton) agammaglobulinaemia	*BTK*	Bruton tyrosine kinase (pre-B-cell receptor [BCR] signalling)	All ↓	↓↓	Recurrent infections with *Streptococcus pneumoniae, Staphylococcus aureus, Moraxella catarrhalis, Haemophilus influenzae, Pseudomonas aeruginosa* and *Mycoplasma* spp. Hepatitis B and enteroviral infections Lymphomas (~5%)	Furuncles and cellulitis Ecthyma gangrenosum Eczematous dermatitis Papular dermatitis due to lymphohistiocytic infiltration Noninfectious granulomas Dermatomyositis-like disorder associated with chronic echoviral meningoencephalitis
AR agammaglobulinaemia	*IGHM*	μ heavy chain of IgM (component of pre-BCR)				
	CD79A, CD79B	Igα chain, Igβ chain (bind μ heavy chain)				
	IGLL1	λ5 (surrogate light chain of pre-BCR)				
	BLNK	B-cell linker protein (binds Bruton tyrosine kinase)				
AD agammaglobulinaemia	*LRRC8A*	Leucine-rich repeat-containing 8 family member A				
Defective class switch recombination (e.g. from IgM to IgG, IgA or IgE) and somatic hypermutation						
Common variable immunodeficiency (CVID)	*ICOS*	Inducible costimulator on activated T cells (T-cell help for B-cell differentiation)	IgG,A ↓; +/–IgM ↓	Nl or ↓	Sinopulmonary infections with encapsulated bacteria Gastroenteritis with *Giardi* and *Campylobacter* Autoimmune diseases, especially thrombocytopenic purpura and haemolytic anaemia Enteropathy Noninfectious granulomas/ lymphoproliferation in the lungs, liver, spleen, and GI tract Increased risk of lymphoma and gastric cancer	Pyodermas and mucocutaneous candidiasis Extensive warts (Fig. 156.10) and dermatophyte infections Eczematous dermatitis Noninfectious granulomas Autoimmune conditions such as vitiligo, alopecia areata and vasculitis Clonal $CD8^+$ lymphocytic infiltration of the skin
	TNFRSF13B (AD or AR)	Transmembrane activator and CAML interactor (TACI; B-cell isotype switching)				
	TNFRSF13C	B-cell activating factor receptor (BAFFR; B-cell isotype switching)				
	CD19[1]	CD19 antigen (B-cell survival and differentiation)				
	MSH5 (AD)	Mismatch repair protein (regulates class switch recombination)				
Selective IgA deficiency	*TNFRSF13B* (AD) *MSH5* (AD)	See above section	IgA ↓; anti-IgA antibodies in ~50%	Nl	Clinical manifestations in only 10–15% Similar to CVID Asthma and allergic rhinoconjunctivitis	Mucocutaneous candidiasis Eczematous dermatitis Autoimmune conditions such as SLE, vitiligo and lipodystrophia centrifugalis abdominalis
Selective IgM deficiency	?	?	IgM ↓	Nl	Recurrent bacterial infections Autoimmune diseases	Extensive warts Eczematous dermatitis SLE

(*Continued*)

Table 156.7 *Continued*

Disorder	Gene	Protein (function)	Ig levels	B cells	Infectious organisms and extracutaneous manifestations	Cutaneous manifestations
X-linked hyper-IgM syndrome AR hyper-IgM syndromes	*CD40LG* *CD40*	CD40 ligand (on T cells) CD40 (on B cells)	IgM ↑; isohaemagglutinins ↑; IgA,E,G ↓↓	Nl	Recurrent sinopulmonary and GI infections with pyogenic bacteria and opportunistic organisms (e.g. *Pneumocystis jiroveci*) Neutropenia Small lymph nodes Autoimmune diseases, especially cytopenias Increased risk of lymphoma and GI cancer	Pyodermas Extensive warts Oral (Fig. 156.9) and anogenital ulcers Noninfectious granulomas Autoimmune conditions such as SLE
	AICDA *UNG*	Activation-induced cytidine deaminase Uracil-DNA glycosylase			As above, but massive LAN (with germinal centres), HSM and *no* opportunistic infections	Pyodermas
Hypohidrotic ectodermal dysplasia with immunodeficiency	*IKBKG (NEMO)* (X-linked recessive)	NF-κB essential modulator (activates NF-κB, which is involved in CD40 signalling)	IgM ↑; +/–IgA ↑; +/–IgG ↓	Nl	Pyogenic bacterial and opportunistic infections Subset of *NEMO* patients Osteopetrosis Lymphoedema	Pyodermas Ectodermal dysplasia
	IKBA (*NFKBIA*; AD, gain of function)	Inhibitor of κBα (inhibits NF-κb)				
Abnormal DNA methylation leading to defective B-cell negative selection and terminal differentiation						
Immunodeficiency, centromeric instability and facial anomalies (ICF) syndrome	*DNMT3B*	DNA methyltransferase 3B	All ↓	Nl or ↓	Bacterial sinopulmonary and GI infections Abnormal facies, MR	Telangiectasias (uncommon) Naevoid hyperpigmentation
Aberrant chemokine signalling						
WHIM (warts, hypogammaglobulinaemia, infections, myelokathexis) syndrome	*CXCR4* (AD, gain-of-function)	CXC chemokine receptor 4 (binds CXCL12; key role in bone marrow homeostasis and lymphocyte trafficking)	IgG ↓; +/–IgA,M ↓	↓	Recurrent bacterial sinopulmonary infections Myelokathexis (mature neutrophils fail to exit the bone marrow)	Cellulitis and pyodermas Extensive verruca vulgaris and condyloma acuminate
Delayed maturation of helper T-cell function						
Transient hypo gammaglobulinaemia of infancy	?	?	IgG,A ↓ (resolves by age 2–3 years)	Nl	Failure to thrive in infancy Recurrent sinopulmonary and GI infections, usually beginning at ~6 months of age when maternal antibody levels wane	Recurrent pyodermas and abscesses

[1] CD81 is required for CD19 expression, and a homozygous mutation in the gene encoding *CD81* was reported in a patient with hypogammaglobulinemia and autoimmune vasculitis. Of note, a homozygous loss-of-function mutation in the *CD20* gene can result in recurrent sinopulmonary infections associated with low IgG levels, a normal total number of B cells, decreased memory B cells and poor T cell-independent antibody responses.

Autosomal recessive (AR) unless otherwise specified.

AD, autosomal dominant; CAML, calcium-modulating cyclophilin ligand; CNS, central nervous system; GI, gastrointestinal; HSM, hepatosplenomegaly; Ig, immunoglobulin; IKBKG, inhibitor of κ light polypeptide gene enhancer in B cells, kinase γ; LAN, lymphadenopathy; MR, mental retardation; Nl, normal; SLE, systemic lupus erythematosus.

Source: Adapted with permission from Bolognia JL, Schaffer JV, Cerroni L, eds. *Dermatology*, 4th edn. London: Elsevier, 2018.

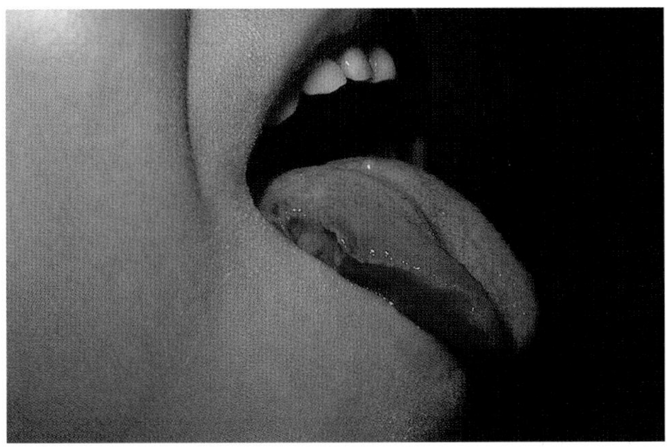

Fig. 156.9 Large ulceration on the side of the tongue in a young boy with X-linked hyperimmunoglobulin M syndrome. These oral ulcerations frequently occur during periods of neutropenia.

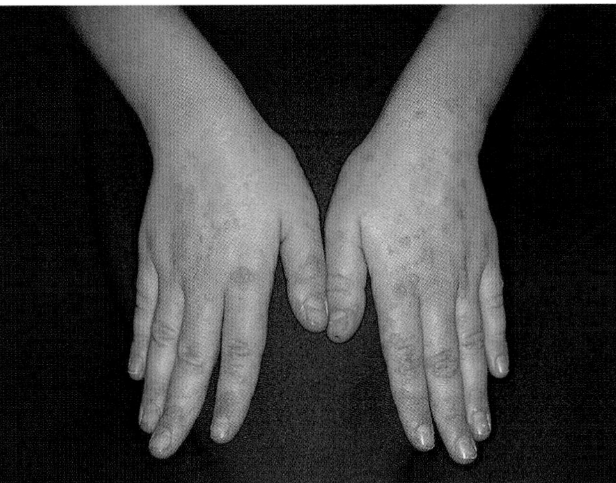

Fig. 156.10 Myriads of recalcitrant warts in a teenage girl with common variable immunodeficiency.

Clinical onset of CVID occurs in two peaks: one in school-aged children and the other in young adults [25]. It can present as early as 2 years of age, but distinguishing CVID from transient hypogammaglobulinaemia of infancy (see Table 156.7) may be difficult in young children. Patients with CVID are predisposed to the development of bacterial sinopulmonary infections, gastroenteritis (especially giardiasis) and skin infections including pyodermas, candidiasis, dermatophytosis and warts (Fig. 156.10). Additional manifestations include eczematous dermatitis, noninfectious granulomas of the skin and internal organs, autoimmune disorders (especially cytopenias) and inflammatory bowel disease [26].

Agammaglobulinaemia

Patients with agammaglobulinaemia typically develop recurrent bacterial infections during infancy, usually beginning at around 6 months of life. Ecthyma gangrenosum in the setting of *Pseudomonas* bacteraemia may be the presenting sign [27]. The skin is the most frequent site of infection, and other cutaneous manifestations include eczematous or granulomatous dermatitis and a dermatomyositis-like disorder associated with chronic echoviral meningoencephalitis. Common causes of infection include encapsulated bacteria (*Strep. pneumoniae, Haemophilus influenza, Pseudomonas*). Enteroviral infections such as echovirus and coxsackie viral infections are also common [28]. Lymphoma develops in approximately 5% of patients.

Flow cytometric analysis of lymphocytes revealing an absence of Bruton tyrosine kinase (BTK) can confirm the diagnosis of X-linked agammaglobulinaemia. Female carriers may be detected via analysis of B-cell X-inactivation patterns, which are skewed as a reflection of preferential survival of cells with inactivation of the mutated X chromosome. DNA-based prenatal diagnosis is possible when the genetic defect in affected family members is known. Differential diagnosis includes autosomal recessive agammaglobulinaemia especially in females and males who do not carry a BTK mutation.

Treatment of hypogammaglobulinaemia (agammaglobulinaemia and CVID) includes antibody replacement with IVIG or subcutaneous immunoglobulin and aggressive antibiotic therapy for infections [29,30]. TNF inhibitors have been successfully utilized to treat noninfectious granulomas in patients with CVID.

References

1 Conley ME. Genes required for B cell development. J Clin Invest 2003;112:1636–8.
2 Grimbacher B, Schäffer AA, Peter HH. The genetics of hypogammaglobulinemia. Curr Allergy Asthma Rep 2004;4:349–58.
3 Wood P, Stanworth S, Burton J et al. Recognition, clinical diagnosis and management of patients with primary antibody deficiencies: a systematic review. Clin Exp Immunol 2007;149:410–23.
4 Al-Attas RA, Rahi AH. Primary antibody deficiency in Arabs: first report from Eastern Saudi Arabia. J Clin Immunol 1998;18:368–71.
5 Kanoh T, Mizumoto T, Yasuda N et al. Selective IgA deficiency in Japanese blood donors: frequency and statistical analysis. Vox Sang 1986;50:81–6.
6 Cunningham-Rundles C. Physiology of IgA and IgA deficiency. J Clin Immunol 2001;21:303–9.
7 Korthäuser U, Graf D, Mages HW. Defective expression of T-cell CD40 ligand causes X-linked immunodeficiency with hyper-IgM. Nature 1993;361:539–40.
8 DiSanto JP, Bonnefoy JY, Gauchat JF et al. CD40 ligand mutations in X-linked immunodeficiency with hyper-IgM. Nature 1993;361:541–3.
9 Revy P, Muto T, Levy Y et al. Activation-induced cytidine deaminase (AIS) deficiency causes the autosomal recessive form of the hyper-IgM syndrome (HIGM2). Cell 2000;102:565–75.
10 Durandy A, Peron S, Fischer A. Hyper-IgM syndromes. Curr Opin Rheumatol 2006;18:369–76.
11 Lougaris V, Badolato R, Ferrari S, Plebani A. Hyper immunoglobulin M syndrome due to CD40 deficiency: clinical, molecular, and immunological features. Immunol Rev 2005;203:48–66.
12 Durandy A, Revy P, Imai K, Fischer A. Hyper-immunoglobulin M syndromes caused by intrinsic B-lymphocyte defects. Immunol Rev 2005;203:67–79.
13 Teresa de la Morena, M Clinical phenotypes of hyper-IgM syndromes JACI in Practice 2016;4:1023–36.
14 Winkelstein, JA, Marino MC, Ochs H et al. The X-linked hyper IGM syndrome: Clinical and immunologic features of 79 patients. Medicine (Baltimore) 2003;82: 373–84.
15 Chang MW, Romero R, Scholl PR et al. Mucocutaneous manifestations of the hyper-IgM Immunodeficiency syndrome. J Am Acad Dermatol 1998;38:191–6.
16 Jesus AA, Duarte AJ, Oliveira JB. Autoimmunity in hyper-IgM syndrome. J Clin Immunol 2008;28:S62–6.
17 Vetrie D, Vorechovsky I, Sideras P et al. The gene involved in X-linked agammaglobulinaemia is a member of the src family of protein-tyrosine kinases. Nature 1992;361:226–33.
18 Tsukada S, Saffran DC, Rawlings DJ et al. Deficient expression of a B cell cytoplasmic tyrosine kinase in human X-linked agammaglobulinemia. Cell 1993;72:279–90.

19 Castigli E, Wilson SA, Garibyan L et al. TACI is mutant in common variable immunodeficiency and IgA deficiency. Nat Genet 2005;37:829–34.
20 Park MA, Li JT, Hagan JB et al. Common variable immunodeficiency: a new look at an old disease. Lancet 2008;372:489–502.
21 Bonilla FA, Geha RS. Common variable immunodeficiency. Pediatr Res 2009;65:13–19R.
22 Bogaert D, Dullaers M, Labrecht BN et al. Genes associated with common variable immunodeficiency: one diagnosis to rule them all? J Med Genet 2016;53:575–90.
23 Chapel H. Common variable immunodeficiency. Diagnoses of exclusion, especially combined immune defects. J Allergy Clin Immunol: in Practice 2016;4:1158–9.
24 Maffucci P, Filion CA, Boisson B et al. Genetic diagnosis using whole exome sequencing in common variable immunodeficiency. Front Immunol 2016;7:220.
25 Glocker E, Ehl S, Grimbacher B. Common variable immunodeficiency in children. Curr Opin Pediatr 2007;19:685–92.
26 Cunningham-Rundles C, Bodian C. Common variable immunodeficiency: clinical and immunological features of 248 patients. Clin Immunol 1999;92:34–48.
27 Ng W, Tan CL, Yeow V et al. Ecthyma gangrenosum in a patient with hypogammaglobulinemia. J Infect 1998;36:331–5.
28 Bearden D, Collett M, Lan Quan P et al. Enteroviruses in X-linked agammaglobulimenia: update on epidemiology and therapy. J Allergy Clin Immunol: In Practice 2016;4:1059–65.
29 Ballow M. Immunoglobulin therapy: methods of delivery. J Allergy Clin Immunol 2008;122:1038–9.
30 Wasserman RL. The nuts and bolts of immunoglobulin treatment for antibody deficiency. J Allergy Clin Immunol: In Practice 2016; 4:1076–1081.e3.

IPEX syndrome

IPEX (immune dysregulation, polyendocrinopathy, enteropathy, X-linked) syndrome is an X-linked recessive disorder caused by *FOXP3* gene mutations that result in abnormal development of regulatory T cells. Affected individuals typically present during infancy with severe diarrhoea related to autoimmune enteropathy and develop a variety of autoimmune endocrinopathies, most often early-onset type 1 diabetes mellitus and thyroiditis, and cytopenias. Most IPEX patients develop widespread eczematous dermatitis and elevated IgE levels during early infancy, and this is often complicated by staphylococcal superinfections and sepsis. Cutaneous manifestations of IPEX can also include psoriasiform dermatitis, cheilitis, nail dystrophy and autoimmune skin conditions such as alopecia areata, chronic urticaria and bullous pemphigoid [1]. Autoimmune endocrinopathies, enteropathy and eczematous dermatitis have also been described in patients with IL-2 receptor α chain (CD25) deficiency (see Table 156.3) [2].

References

1 Halabi-Tawil M, Ruemmele FM, Fraitag S et al. Cutaneous manifestations of immune dysregulation, polyendocrinopathy, enteropathy, X-linked (IPEX) syndrome. Br J Dermatol 2009;160:645–51.
2 Caudy AA, Reddy ST, Chatila T et al. CD25 deficiency causes an immune dysregulation, polyendocrinopathy, enteropathy, X-linked-like syndrome, and defective IL-10 expression from CD4 lymphocytes. J Allergy Clin Immunol 2007;119:482–7.

Leucocyte adhesion deficiency

Leucocyte adhesion deficiency (LAD) is a group of autosomal recessive disorders that affect the ability of neutrophils, monocytes and T cells to adhere to vascular endothelial cells and migrate to sites of tissue injury and infection [1–3]. Three major subgroups have been described: LAD-I, LAD-II and LAD-III (also referred to as LAD-I variant).

Pathogenesis. The adherence of leucocytes involves a group of cell surface glycoproteins (integrins) that share a 95-kDa β_2 subunit (CD18). The CD18 β_2 integrin subunit can be linked to different α-chains to form three distinct cell surface glycoproteins: CD11a (lymphocyte function-associated antigen 1 [LFA-1]), CD11b (complement receptor type 3 [iC3b receptor or CR3], Mac-1) and CD11c (complement receptor type 4 [CR4], p150,95). The principal ligand for these glycoproteins is intracellular adhesion molecule 1 (ICAM-1), which has key functions in the initiation and evolution of inflammation in skin and other tissues. LAD-I is caused by mutations in the *ITGB2* gene that encodes CD18, and it presents with dysfunction of all three glycoproteins. This results in profound impairment of leucocyte firm adhesion to the vascular endothelium and extravasation into sites of inflammation as well as defective chemotaxis and phagocytosis by neutrophils and monocytes.

LAD II is caused by mutations in the *FUCT1* gene, which encodes a GDP-fucose transporter that is necessary for formation of sialyl-Lewis X [4]. Fucosylated sialyl-Lewis X on the surface of leucocytes normally interacts with E- and P-selectins on endothelial cells during processes of tethering and rolling, which target leucocytes to sites of inflammation. These contacts between leucocytes and the blood vessel wall are defective in patients with LAD-II.

In order to undergo firm adhesion and subsequently extravasate, circulating leucocytes need to activate cell-surface integrins *in situ* and thereby increase their affinity and avidity for endothelial ligands. Patients with LAD-III have impaired integrin activation in haematopoietic cells, which leads to defective leucocyte β_1 and platelet β_3 integrins as well as leucocyte β_2 integrins. Abnormalities in two genes on chromosome 11q13, both of which encode effectors of integrin activation in haematopoietic cells, have been identified in the same LAD-III patients from consanguineous Turkish kindreds:

1 A putative splice site mutation in RAS guanyl releasing protein 2 (*RASGRP2*); and
2 A nonsense mutation in kindlin-3 (*FERMT3*) [5,6].

However, other LAD-III patients were found to have nonsense mutations in *FERMT3* but no mutations in *RASGRP2*, demonstrating that *FERMT3* mutations are the cause of LAD-III [6].

Clinical features. Patients with LAD have frequent skin infections (most often of the face and perianal area), otitis media and pneumonias caused by pyogenic bacteria. Affected individuals often present with cellulitis and necrotic abscesses with relatively little purulence. Life-threatening bacterial, fungal or (less frequently) viral infections may develop. Approximately 80% of patients with severe LAD-I (<1% of normal CD18 levels) die within the first 5 years of life, whereas approximately half of those with moderate LAD-I (1–10% of normal CD18 levels) live to the age of 30 years [3].

The most frequent clinical manifestation of LAD is gingivitis with periodontitis, which may lead to loss of teeth. Patients also experience poor wound healing and atrophic scarring, and a history of delayed separation of the umbilical stump represents a clue to the diagnosis. Minor skin injuries can rapidly expand to form large chronic ulcers that resemble 'burnt out' pyoderma gangrenosum.

Patients with LAD-II have additional manifestations such as growth and mental retardation, microcephaly, hypotonia and facial dysmorphism [4,7]. LAD-III features a bleeding tendency, developmental delay, osteopetrosis and hepatosplenomegaly [8,9]. Dermal haematopoiesis may lead to a 'blueberry muffin' appearance in infants and children with LAD-III [8].

Differential diagnosis. A mutation in the gene encoding the Rac2 GTPase, which has a role in phagocyte NADPH oxidase activation as well as integrin-dependent adhesion and neutrophil migration, can lead to clinical features of LAD such as delayed separation of the umbilical stump, poor wound healing, neutrophilia and recurrent perirectal abscesses with minimal pus production (see Table 156.4).

Laboratory and histology findings. Leucocyte adhesion deficiency is characterized by striking peripheral blood neutrophilia (5- to 20-fold higher than normal) but a relative paucity of tissue neutrophils. Flow cytometric analysis reveals markedly decreased leucocyte CD18 expression in individuals with LAD-I. Patients with LAD-II have the Bombay red blood cell type because of a lack of the H blood group antigen, whereas those with LAD-III have abnormal platelet aggregation and (less often) anaemia.

Treatment. Soft tissue infections in LAD patients require prolonged antibiotic treatment and, in some cases, surgical debridement. Scrupulous dental hygiene is important in reducing the severity of periodontitis. Supplemental fucose administration may improve immune function in some patients with LAD-II [10]. HSCT currently represents the only definitive therapy for LAD, but its efficacy is limited by infectious complications and GVHD [1,11].

Two patients with severe LAD-I were treated without prior conditioning with an infusion of autologous haematopoietic stem cells that had been corrected *ex vivo* via a retroviral vector encoding CD18, but the $CD18^+$ cells persisted in the circulation for less than 2 months [3]. More recently, canine LAD-I was successfully treated with nonmyeloablative conditioning followed by infusion of autologous haematopoietic stem cells transduced *ex vivo* by a foamy virus vector expressing canine CD18 [12]. The dogs had complete reversal of the LAD phenotype, which was sustained for more than 2 years after the infusion. The foamy virus vector that was utilized is thought to have less potential for genotoxicity than the retroviral vectors previously used in gene therapy protocols.

References

1 Malech HL, Hickstein DD. Genetics, biology and clinical management of myeloid cell primary immune deficiencies: chronic granulomatous disease and leukocyte adhesion deficiency. Curr Opin Hematol 2007;14:29–36.
2 Bunting M, Harris ES, McIntyre TM et al. Leukocyte adhesion deficiency syndromes: adhesion and tethering defects involving β2 integrins and selectin ligands. Curr Opin Hematol 2002;9:30–5.
3 Bauer TR, Gu YC, Creevy KE et al. Leukocyte adhesion deficiency in children and Irish Setter dogs. Pediatr Res 2004;55:363–7.
4 Wild MK, Lühn K, Marquardt T et al. Leukocyte adhesion deficiency II: therapy and genetic defect. Cells Tissues Organs 2002;172:161–73.
5 Kuijpers TW, van de Vijver E, Weterman MA et al. LAD-1/variant syndrome is caused by mutations in FERMT3. Blood 2009;113:4740–6.
6 Svensson L, Howarth K, McDowall A et al. Leukocyte adhesion deficiency-III is caused by mutations in KINDLIN3 affecting integrin activation. Nat Med 2009;15:306–12.
7 Helmus Y, Denecke J, Yakubenia S et al. Leukocyte adhesion deficiency II patients with a dual defect of the GDP-fucose transporter. Blood 2006;107:3959–66.
8 Kuijpers TW, van Bruggen R, Kamerbeek N et al. Natural history and early diagnosis of LAD-1/variant syndrome. Blood 2007;109:3529–37.
9 Kilic SS, Etzioni A. The clinical spectrum of leukocyte adhesion deficiency (LAD) III due to defective CalDAG-GEF1. J Clin Immunol 2009;29:117–22.
10 Marquardt T, Luhn K, Srikrishna G et al. Correction of leukocyte adhesion deficiency type II with oral fucose. Blood 1999;94: 3976–85.
11 Qasim W, Cavazzana-Calvo M, Davies EG et al. Allogeneic haematopoietic stem-cell transplantation for leukocyte adhesion deficiency. Pediatrics 2009;123:836–40.
12 Bauer TR, Allen JM, Hai M et al. Successful treatment of canine leukocyte adhesion deficiency by foamy virus vectors. Nat Med 2008;14:93–7.

Severe combined immunodeficiency

Key points

- **SCID is a group of heterogenous, inherited immunodeficiencies which, if left untreated, lead to death early in life.**
- **Newborn screening programmes have greatly improved the prognosis for babies with SCID.**

Introduction and history. SCID is a heterogeneous group of disorders characterized by the markedly defective function of both cell-mediated and humoral immunity [1–3]. Patients with all types of SCID have profound T-cell immune defects and antibody impairment and present in the first few months of life with recurrent or persistent infections, chronic diarrhoea and failure to thrive.

Epidemiology and pathogenesis. A study of newborn screening programmes for SCID found an incidence of 1/58 000 (95% CI 1/46 000–1/80 000) for typical SCID, leaky SCID and OMENN syndrome [4]. In cultures where consanguinity is common, the incidence is thought to be higher, although epidemiological data is scarce [5]. Almost half of affected individuals have an X-linked recessive form of SCID, which is usually caused by defects in the gene encoding the common γ (γ_c) chain of the IL-12 receptor. Other forms of SCID have autosomal recessive inheritance and include adenosine deaminase (ADA) deficiency (20% of SCID) and JAK3 deficiency (approximately 5% of SCID). The molecular defects that can lead to a SCID phenotype are summarized in Table 156.8 [1,2,6].

Table 156.8 Severe combined immunodeficiency (SCID)

Disorder	Gene	Protein function ± specific clinical findings	Cells
Defects in cytokine receptors and their signalling			
X-linked SCID	*IL2RG*	Common γ chain (γ_c) of the receptors for IL-2, 4, 7, 9, 15 and 21	T⁻/B⁺/NK⁻
JAK3 deficiency	*JAK3*	Tyrosine kinase with a role in signal transduction via the receptors for IL-2, 4, 7, 9, 15 and 21	T⁻/B⁺/NK⁻
Interleukin-7 receptor deficiency	*IL7R*	α chain of the IL-7 receptor; critical for development and differentiation of T cells; occasionally Omenn-like phenotype	T⁻/B⁺/NK⁺
Increased apoptosis of lymphocytes ± other haematopoietic cells			
Accumulation of toxic metabolites due to purine pathway enzyme defects			
ADA deficiency	*ADA*	Enzyme in the purine salvage pathway; cupping/flaring of the costochondral junction on chest X-rays; occasionally Omenn-like phenotype	T⁻/B⁻/NK⁻
PNP deficiency	*PNP*	Enzyme in the purine salvage pathway that acts downstream of ADA	T⁻/B⁻/NK⁻
Defects disrupting mitochondrial energy production			
Reticular dysgenesis (aleucocytosis)	*AK2*	Adenylate kinase 2, a mitochondrial enzyme that regulates ADP levels in leucocytes; profound neutropenia and sensorineural deafness	T⁻/B⁻/NK⁻
Defects disrupting actin polymerization			
Coronin 1A deficiency	*CORO1A*	Actin regulator expressed in T-cell precursors	T⁻/B⁺/NK⁺
Defects in (pre-) TCRs +/–BCRs and their signalling			
Omenn syndrome	*RAG1* and *RAG2*	Mediate V(D)J recombination of genes that encode BCRs (immunoglobulins) and TCRs; exfoliative erythroderma, hepatosplenomegaly, lymphadenopathy, eosinophilia	T⁻/B⁻/NK⁺
Artemis deficiency	*DCLRE1C (Artemis)*	DNA cross-link repair protein that repairs DNA double-stranded breaks that occur during V(D)J recombination and upon exposure to ionizing radiation; sensitivity to ionizing radiation; occasionally Omenn-like phenotype	T⁻/B⁻/NK⁺
PRKDC deficiency	*PRKDC*	DNA-activated protein kinase catalytic subunit critical for V(D)J recombination; sensitivity to ionizing radiation	T⁻/B⁻/NK⁺
LIG4 syndrome	*LIG4*	Ligase component of DNA nonhomologous end-joining machinery required for repair of DNA double-stranded breaks; sensitivity to ionizing radiation; variable severity, occasionally Omenn-like phenotype; microcephaly, bird-like facies, photosensitivity and telangiectasias	T⁻/B⁻/NK⁺
NHEJ1 (Cernunnos) syndrome	*NHEJ1*	Nonhomologous end-joining factor required for the repair of DNA double-stranded breaks; sensitivity to ionizing radiation; variable severity; microcephaly and bird-like facies	T⁻/B⁻/NK⁺
TCR deficiencies	CD3γ, CD3δ, CD3ε and CD3ζ	TCR-associated proteins required for cell-surface expression of and signal transduction by the TCR; the T-cell defect is most severe with CD3δ defects	T⁻/B⁺/NK⁺
CD45 deficiency	*PTPRC*	Transmembrane tyrosine phosphatase with a role in TCR signalling	T⁻/B⁺/NK⁺
ZAP-70 deficiency	*ZAP-70*	Tyrosine kinase with a role in TCR signalling; lymphocytosis; variable severity and phenotype, occasionally Omenn-like	CD4⁺CD8⁻/B⁺/NK⁺
CD8 deficiency	*CD8A*	Co-receptor for TCRs recognizing MHC class I-associated peptides; role in TCR signalling; milder than true SCID	CD4⁺CD8⁻/B⁺/NK⁺
Calcium channel deficiency	*ORAI1*	Pore-forming subunit of calcium channel with a role in TCR signalling; hypohidrotic ectodermal dysplasia and myopathy	T⁺/B⁺/NK⁺
	STIM1	Calcium channel component with a role in TCR signalling; hepatosplenomegaly, lymphadenopathy, autoimmune cytopenias, dental dysplasia, myopathy	T⁺/B⁺/NK⁺
Antigen presentation defects (bare lymphocyte syndromes)			
MHC class II deficiency	*CIITA* *RFXANK* *RFX5* *RFXAP*	Transactivate the MHC class II promoter; MHC class II molecules are required for the positive selection of CD4⁺ T cells in the thymus as well as for antigen presentation to CD4⁺ T cells	T⁺/B⁺/NK⁺; fewer/dysfunctional CD4⁺ T cells
MHC class I deficiency	*TAP1*, *TAP2* and *TAPBP*	TAP and TAP binding protein (tapasin); translocate peptides from the cytosol to MHC class I molecules in the endoplasmic reticulum; milder than true SCID; cutaneous granulomas	CD4⁺CD8⁻/B⁺/NK⁺
Defective thymic development			
Winged helix nude (forkhead box N1) deficiency	*WHN (FOXN1)*	Transcription factor important to thymic development; congenital alopecia and nail dystrophy (human equivalent of 'nude' mice)	T⁻/B⁺/NK⁺

Cartilage–hair hypoplasia (see text) occasionally presents as SCID with an Omenn-like phenotype.
ADA, adenosine deaminase; BCR, B-cell receptor; IL, interleukin; MHC, major histocompatibility complex; NK, natural killer; PNP, purine nucleoside phosphorylase; TAP, transporter associated with antigen processing; TCR, T-cell receptor; V(D)J, variable/diversity/joining.
Source: Adapted with permission from Bolognia JL, Schaffer JV, Cerroni L, eds. *Dermatology*, 4th edn. London: Elsevier, 2018.

Clinical features. Patients with SCID typically begin to have recurrent infections, chronic diarrhoea and failure to thrive during the first few months of life. Early infections often include mucocutaneous candidiasis, persistent viral gastroenteritis and pneumonias resulting from bacteria, viruses or *P. jiroveci*. Skin infections are commonly caused by *S. aureus* and *Strep. pyogenes* as well as *Candida* spp. Despite their frequent infections, patients with SCID usually lack tonsillar buds and palpable lymphoid tissue.

Infants with SCID may present with morbilliform or seborrhoeic dermatitis-like eruptions [7,8], which often reflect maternofetal GVHD (see Chapter 157). Cutaneous GVHD in patients with SCID may also resemble lichen planus, acrodermatitis enteropathica, Langerhans cell histiocytosis, ichthyosiform erythroderma or scleroderma. Skin biopsy specimens show the histopathological characteristics of GVHD. Extensive eczematous dermatitis or severe exfoliative erythroderma, often associated with alopecia, may occur without GVHD in infants with Omenn syndrome. Additional features of Omenn syndrome include lymphadenopathy, hepatosplenomegaly and peripheral eosinophilia [9].

Maternal T-cell engraftment is detectable (requiring maternal cells to comprise ≥1% of peripheral blood leucocytes) in approximately 50% of infants with SCID [8]. In the majority of cases, the presence of these maternal T cells is asymptomatic; in 30–40% of patients, mild findings such as morbilliform eruptions, cutaneous erythema with scale, elevated hepatic transaminases and eosinophilia are evident. Fulminant or fatal maternofetal GVHD is rare, in contrast to the more severe GVHD that can occur secondary to postnatal inoculation of allogeneic lymphocytes via transfusion of nonirradiated blood products in SCID patients.

Differential diagnosis. Severe combined immunodeficiency must be distinguished from acquired forms of profound immunodeficiency. HIV infection can be differentiated by normal to increased immunoglobulin levels, a relative paucity of $CD4^+$ T cells and the presence of anti-HIV antibodies. Other combined immunodeficiencies are also on the differential including complete DGS, Zap-70 deficiency, WAS, X-linked hyper-IgM syndrome. Distinctive laboratory and clinical features help differentiate these forms of immunodeficiency. However, molecular testing is sometimes necessary.

Laboratory findings and histology. Most patients with SCID have a profound deficiency of T cells and a low absolute lymphocyte count. They also have poor T-cell function as measured by T-cell proliferation to mitogens and antigens. Patients are further classified by the results of fluorescent-activated cell sorter analysis into those with and without B and NK cells. Diagnosis of a particular form of SCID can be established by genetic testing, flow cytometric analysis of peripheral blood mononuclear cells with antibodies directed against a particular protein (e.g. γ_c or JAK3) that is missing from the cell surface, or measurement of red blood cell levels of a defective enzyme (e.g. ADA) or purine metabolites. In families with a previously affected sibling, prenatal diagnosis of SCID has been performed by fetal DNA analysis and ADA assays. TREC analysis (germline DNA that is excised and forms a stable DNA loop during gene rearrangement of T cells within the thymus or recent thymic emigrants) is the primary test used in newborn screening programmes. Newborn screening for SCID has been adopted by most of the USA and is now being implemented in countries around the world [4,10].

Treatment and prognosis. Patients with SCID usually die by 1 year of age without HSCT or other definitive therapy. Early diagnosis of SCID is imperative, if possible before the administration of live vaccines or nonirradiated blood products. With newborn screening and early identification and transplant of patients with SCID, prognosis is much improved [4,10]. Infants with SCID must be kept in protective isolation and monitored for signs of infection, which should prompt aggressive treatment. IVIG therapy and prophylaxis for *P. jirovecii* pneumonia should be given. Fluconozole prophylaxis or treatment, if oral candidiasis is present, should be used. Palivizumab, a monoclonal antibody against respiratory syncytial virus (RSV) should be given in RSV season [11]. Live viral vaccines should be avoided. All blood products must be irradiated, leukodepleted and cytomegalovirus negative.

HSCT during infancy is currently the treatment of choice for SCID [12–14]. This results in engraftment of donor T and NK cells, but usually not B cells. Because the patient's immune system is unable to reject the transplanted cells, myeloablative conditioning is not required. With an HLA-identical sibling donor, T-cell reconstitution usually occurs within 3–4 months, GVHD is uncommon, and the long-term survival rate is more than 90%. Transplantation of haploidentical parental stem cells, which can be depleted of post-thymic T cells to reduce the risk of GVHD, typically requires some chemotherapeutic conditioning to facilitate engraftment and results in survival rates of 80% or less. *In utero* injection of haploidentical $CD34^+$ cells has also been used to treat X-linked SCID [15]. SCID patients often require IVIG replacement therapy for persistent B-cell deficiency following HSCT, and T-cell function may decline over time. Virus-specific T lymphocytes from stem cell donors or third-party donors may be useful for the treatment and prevention of viral infectons after HSCT in patients with SCID [16].

Enzyme replacement via injection of polyethylene glycol-conjugated ADA has resulted in improved immune function in infants with ADA deficiency. Gene therapy utilizing *ex vivo* transduction of autologous $CD34^+$ cells with a retroviral vector has been successfully performed in more than 50 children with X-linked SCID or ADA deficiency [14,17–19]. Follow-up studies on 19 of these patients (4 months to 4 years after treatment) showed that the retrovirus preferentially integrated into transcriptional start sites and coding regions of active genes in both circulating T cells and preinfusion transduced $CD34^+$ cells. Approximately 25% of integrations in T cells were clustered at common sites, suggesting *in vivo* selection of transduced cells with a higher capacity for engraftment, survival and proliferation [20]. Although T- and NK-cell function was restored, at least five patients with X-linked SCID have developed T-cell leukaemias 2–6 years after treatment, which appears to be related to activation of proto-oncogenes such as *LM02* by the retroviral vector [21]. This has raised concerns regarding the safety of gene therapy, leading to protocol modifications and exploration of alternative approaches such as lentiviral vectors and *in situ* gene transfer.

References

1 Fischer A, Le Deist F, Hacein-Bey-Abina S et al. Severe combined immunodeficiency: a model disease for molecular immunology and therapy. Immunol Rev 2005;203:98–109.
2 Buckley RH. The multiple causes of human SCID. J Clin Invest 2004;10:1409–11.
3 Gaspar HB, Gilmour KC, Jones AM. Severe combined immunodeficiency: molecular pathogenesis and diagnosis. Arch Dis Child 2001;84:169–73.
4 Kwan A, Abraham RS, Currier R et al. Newborn screening for severe combined immunodeficiency in 11 screening programs in the United States. JAMA 2014;312:729–38.
5 Al-Herz, W, Al-Mousa H. Combined immunodeficiency: the Middle East experience. J Allergy Clin Immunol 2013;131:658–60.
6 Al-Herz W, Bousfiha A, Casanova JL et al. Primary immunodeficiency diseases: an update on the classification from the international union of immunological societies expert committee for primary immunodeficiency. Front Immunol 2014; 5:162.
7 Postigo Llorente C, Ivars Amorós J, Ortiz de Frutos FJ et al. Cutaneous lesion in severe combined immunodeficiency: two case reports and a review of the literature. Pediatr Dermatol 1991;8:314–21.
8 De Raeve L, Song M, Levy J et al. Cutaneous lesions as a clue to severe combined immunodeficiency. Pediatr Dermatol 1992;9:49–51.
9 Shearer WT, Dunn E, Notarangelo LD et al. Establishing diagnostic criteria for severe combined immunodeficiency disease (SCID), leaky SCID and Omenn Syndrome: the primary Immune Deficiency Treatment Consortium experience. J Allergy Clin Immunol 2014;133:1092.
10 Dion, ML, Sekaly RP, Cheynier R. Estimating thymic function through quantification of T-cell receptor excision circles. Methods Mol Biol 2007;380:197–213.
11 Papadopoulou-Alataki E, Hassan A, Davies EG. Prevention of infection in children and adolescents with primary immunodeficiency disorders. Asian Pac J Allergy Immunol 2012;30:239–58.
12 Buckley RH, Schiff SE, Schiff RI et al. Hematopoeietic stem cell transplantation for the treatment of severe combined immunodeficiency. N Engl J Med 1999;340:508–16.
13 Haddad E, Landais P, Friedrich W et al. Long-term immune reconstitution and outcome after HLA-non-identical T-cell depleted bone marrow reconstitution for severe combined immunodeficiency, a European retrospective study of 116 patients. Blood 1998;91:3646–53.
14 Thrasher AJ. Gene therapy for primary immunodeficiencies. Immunol Allergy Clin North Am 2008;28:457–71.
15 Flake AW, Roncarolo MG, Puck JM et al. Treatment of X-linked severe combined immunodeficiency by *in utero* transplantation of paternal bone marrow. N Engl J Med 1996;335:1806–10.
16 Naik S, Nicholas SK, Martinez CA et al. Adoptive immunotherapy for primary immunodeficiency disorders with virus-specific T lymphocytes. J Allergy Clin Immunol 2016;137:1498–505.
17 Cavazzana-Calvo M, Hacein-Bey S, de Saint Basile G et al. Gene therapy of human severe combined immunodeficiency (SCID)-X1 disease. Science 2000;288:669–72.
18 Aiuti A, Slavin S, Aker M et al. Correction of ADA-SCID by stem cell gene therapy combined with nonmyeloablative conditioning. Science 2002;296:2410–3.
19 Gaspar HB, Parsley KL, Howe S et al. Gene therapy of X-linked severe combined immunodeficiency by use of a pseudotyped gamma retroviral vector. Lancet 2004;364:2181–7.
20 Bushman FD. Retroviral integration and human gene therapy. J Clin Invest 2007;117:2083–6.
21 Hacein-Bey-Abina S, Garrigue A, Wang GP et al. Insertional oncogenesis in 4 patients after retrovirus-mediated gene therapy of SCID-X1. J Clin Invest 2008;117:3132–42.

Wiskott–Aldrich syndrome

Key points

- **Wiskott–Aldrich syndrome is an X-linked recessive disorder that classically manifests with recurrent bacterial and viral infections, bleeding from thrombocytopenia and platelet dysfunction, and recalcitrant atopic dermatitis.**
- **Early stem cell transplantation is the treatment of choice, although gene therapy approaches show promise.**

Introduction and history. WAS is a rare X-linked recessive disorder that classically manifests with recurrent pyogenic infections, bleeding resulting from thrombocytopenia and platelet dysfunction, and recalcitrant eczematous dermatitis [1,2]. This full triad develops in a minority of affected individuals, and platelet abnormalities are the most constant feature.

Epidemiology and pathogenesis. Most patients are boys, but girls are occasionally affected in settings of selective inactivation of the unaffected X chromosome or homozygosity for a mild mutation. The incidence of WAS is approximately 1 in 250 000 male births in European populations, and the condition is less common in Blacks and Asians.

WAS results from loss-of-function mutations in the *WASP* gene, which is constitutively expressed in cells of haematopoietic lineage. WAS protein (WASp) transduces signals from the cell surface to the actin cytoskeleton, and regulates its remodelling. This leads to activation of actin polymerization and facilitation of processes such as immune synapse formation, T-cell activation, phagocytosis and cellular polarization and migration [3]. WASp also has roles in homeostasis of peripheral B cells and activation of regulatory T cells, which promotes the development of the autoimmune manifestations of WAS [4–7].

Platelets from WAS patients are small and structurally abnormal, and they have a reduced half-life that is partly caused by increased destruction in the spleen. Some studies have shown that premature pro-platelets are released from the bone marrow because of defective podosome formation. Loss-of-function *WASP* mutations also underlie isolated X-linked recessive thrombocytopenia, whereas gain-of-function *WASP* mutations can cause X-linked recessive congenital neutropenia (see Table 156.4).

Clinical features. Thrombocytopenia and platelet dysfunction are present from birth, so early clinical signs of WAS often include epistaxis and petechiae (Fig. 156.11) or ecchymoses of the skin and oral mucosa. Haematemesis, melaena and haematuria are also frequent manifestations.

Eczematous dermatitis usually develops during the first few months of life and fulfils the diagnostic criteria for atopic dermatitis. The face, scalp and flexural areas are the most severely affected, although patients commonly

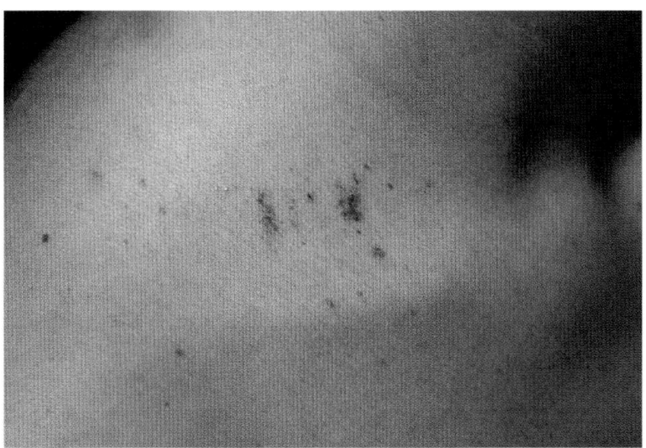

Fig. 156.11 Numerous petechiae in a boy with Wiskott–Aldrich syndrome, providing evidence of thrombocytopenia and platelet dysfunction.

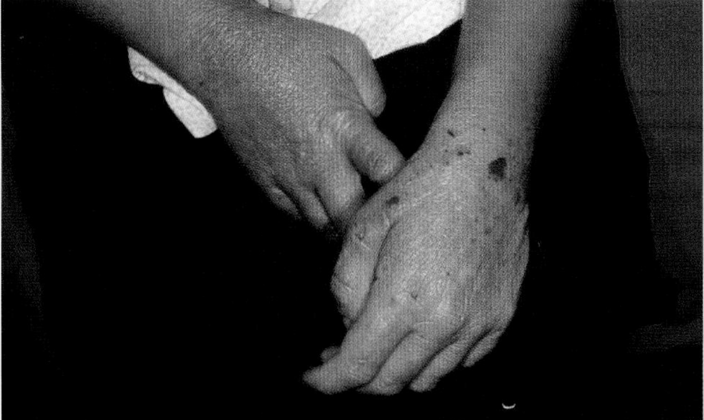

Fig. 156.12 Atopic dermatitis with marked lichenification and erosions covered with serosanguinous crust in a boy with Wiskott–Aldrich syndrome.

have widespread involvement with progressive lichenification (Fig. 156.12). Excoriated areas typically have serosanguinous crusting and petechiae or purpura. Secondary bacterial infections, eczema herpeticum and molluscum contagiosum represent additional complications.

Recurrent bacterial infections begin during infancy as levels of placentally transmitted maternal antibodies diminish, and encapsulated organisms such as *Strep. pneumoniae*, *H. influenzae* and *Neiserria meningitidis* predominate. Patients often develop furunculosis, otitis externa and media, pneumonia, sinusitis, conjunctivitis, meningitis and septicaemia. They also have increased susceptibility to infections with *P. jiroveci* and herpes simplex virus.

Most children with WAS develop one or more autoimmune diseases such as cutaneous small vessel vasculitis (frequently associated with painful oedema), arthritis, cytopenias, inflammatory bowel disease and central nervous system vasculitis [2,4]. Patients with WAS are also predisposed to the development of food allergies, asthma, hepatosplenomegaly and lymphadenopathy. Non-Hodgkin lymphoma occurs in approximately 20% of individuals with WAS, with a higher risk in adults and those with a history of autoimmune disorders. Diffuse large B-cell lymphomas with extranodal and brain involvement (similar to AIDS-related lymphomas) are particularly common.

The clinical course of WAS is progressive, usually resulting in death by adolescence. In patients who do not receive HSCT, the most common causes of death are infection (40%), bleeding (25%) and malignancy (25%) [7]. Patients with no detectable WASp in peripheral blood mononuclear cells upon flow cytometric or immunoblot analysis tend to have more severe disease and shorter survival.

Differential diagnosis. Several other immunodeficiencies are characterized by eczematous dermatitis as well as increased susceptibility to infections (see Table 156.1), but WAS can usually be distinguished by the bleeding tendency and laboratory evidence of microthrombocytopenia.

Laboratory and histology findings. WAS is characterized by persistent thrombocytopenia (typically 1000–80 000 platelets/mm^3) and a low mean platelet volume (3.5–5.0 fL). Lymphopenia and eosinophilia are occasional manifestations, and leucocyte chemotaxis is defective. Serum levels of IgM and IgG_2 are usually low, but levels of IgA, IgE and IgD tend to be elevated. Antibody responses to polysaccharide antigens are severely diminished, and older patients may develop skin test anergy and decreased *in vitro* responses to mitogens. Female carriers of WAS can be detected by their selective inactivation of the abnormal X chromosome in lymphocytes and platelets [8].

Treatment and prevention. HSCT is the treatment of choice for WAS. Full engraftment results in normal platelet number and function, normalization of immunological status and, if T cells engraft, clearance of the dermatitis [7,9–12]. Children younger than 5 years of age who receive a transplant from an HLA-identical donor (sibling or unrelated) have a survival rate of more than 85%; in contrast, older patients and those with mismatched donors have survival rates of approximately 50%. Clinical trials of gene therapy using lentivirally transduced, WAS-reconstituted, autologous $CD34^+$ cells have shown sustained clinical benefit in the majority of treated patients with reduction in resolution of dermatitis and susceptibility to infection, as well as improvement in autoimmunity [7,10,12]. Because of early trials in which leukaemia developed because of insertional oncogenesis, ongoing trials use self-inactivating lentiviral vectors. Most recently, induced pluripotent stem cells from a WAS patient were corrected using zinc finger nucleases, suggesting a nonviral approach to the correction of WAS cells [13].

Minimization of infectious and haemorrhagic complications is the major goal of supportive therapy for WAS. Prophylactic use of antibiotics and IVIG can decrease the incidence of serious infections and perhaps improve the eczematous dermatitis [4,8]. However, topical corticosteroids remain the mainstay for treatment of the latter.

Although splenectomy can reduce the bleeding diathesis of WAS, it increases the risk of infections with encapsulated organisms [14]. Platelet transfusions should be administered prior to surgical procedures and in instances of severe haemorrhage.

References

1 **Buchbinder D, Nugent DJ, Fillipovich AH et al. Wiskott-Aldrich syndrome: diagnosis, current management, and emerging treatments. App Clin Genet 2014; 7: 55–66.**

2 **Massaad MJ, Ramesh N, Geha RS et al Wiskott-Aldrich syndrome: a comprehensive review. Ann N Y Acad Sci 2013;1285:26–43.**

3 Cotta-de-Almeida V, Dupré L, Guipouy D et al. Signal integration during T lymphocyte activation and function: lessons from the Wiskott-Aldrich syndrome. Front Immunol 2015;6:47.

4 Dupuis-Girod S, Medioni J, Haddad E et al. Autoimmunity in Wiskott–Aldrich syndrome: risk factors, clinical features, and outcome in a single-center cohort of 55 patients. Pediatrics 2003;111:e622–7.

5 Dosanjh A. Autoimmunity and immunodeficiency. Pediatr Rev 2015;36:489–94.

6 Volpi S, Santori E, Abernethy K et al. N-WASP is required for B-cell-mediated autoimmunity in Wiskott-Aldrich syndrome. Blood 2016;127:216–20.

7 Pala F, Morbach H, Castiello MC et al. Lentiviral-mediated gene therapy restores B cell tolerance in Wiskott-Aldrich syndrome patients. J Clin Invest 2015;125:3941–51.

8 Winkelstein JA, Fearon E et al. Carrier detection of the X-linked primary immunodeficiency diseases using X-chromosome inactivation analysis. J Allergy Clin Immunol 1990;85:1090–7.

9 Worth AJ, Thrasher AJ. Current and emerging treatment options for Wiskott-Aldrich syndrome. Expert Rev Clin Immunol 2015; 11:1015–32.

10 Hacein-Bey Abina S, Gaspar HB, Blondeau J et al. Outcomes following gene therapy in patients with severe Wiskott-Aldrich syndrome. JAMA 2015;313:1550–63.

11 Braun CJ, Boztug K, Paruzynski A et al. Gene therapy for Wiskott-Aldrich syndrome – long-term efficacy and genotoxicity. Sci Transl Med 2014;6:227ra33.

12 Aiuti A, Biasco L, Scaramuzza S et al. Lentiviral hematopoietic stem cell gene therapy in patients with Wiskott-Aldrich syndrome. Science 2013;341:1233151.

13 Laskowski TJ, Van Caeneghem Y, Pourebrahim R et al. Gene correction of iPSCs from a Wiskott-Aldrich syndrome patient normalizes the lymphoid developmental and functional defects. Stem Cell Reports 2016;7:139–48.

14 Litzman J, Jones A, Hann I et al. Intravenous immunoglobulin, splenectomy, and antibiotic prophylaxis in Wiskott–Aldrich syndrome. Arch Dis Child 1996;75:436–9.

CHAPTER 157
Graft-Versus-Host Disease

John Harper[1] *& Paul Veys*[2]

[1] Paediatric Dermatology, Great Ormond Street Hospital for Children NHS Trust, London, UK
[2] Bone Marrow Transplantation Unit, Great Ormond Street Hospital for Children NHS Trust, London, UK

Abstract

In clinical practice, graft-versus-host disease (GVHD) is most frequently encountered in patients who receive a bone marrow transplant (BMT). Immune cells (white blood cells) in the donated tissue (the graft) recognize the recipient (the host) as foreign (non-self). The transplanted immune cells then attack the host's body cells. The essential criteria are: (i) a profound depression of cellular immunity of the recipient, otherwise the graft is rejected; (ii) the patient must have received an allograft of lymphoid immunocompetent cells in sufficient quantity and (iii) there is recognition by the graft of foreign antigens in the tissues of the host. GVHD is a common and often serious complication of haematopoietic cell transplantation. The cutaneous signs are usually the earliest manifestation of GVHD. Tissues that are primary targets are the skin, gastrointestinal tract and liver. Acute clinical features include: an erythematous rash, often involving the palms and soles, fever, diarrhoea and raised liver function tests, including hyperbilirubinaemia. Chronic skin manifestations of GVHD include lichen planus-like lesions, pigmentary skin changes and sclerosis. Chronic GVHD may also manifest as a variety of autoimmune or connective tissue diseases, sharing overlapping features with scleroderma, lupus erythematosus, dermatomyositis, polymyositis, Sjögren syndrome, vitiligo, primary biliary cirrhosis and chronic active hepatitis. There are published updated guidelines for the prevention and treatment of GVHD. In the past two decades, there have been significant advances in the management of acute GVHD, which has led to much improved outcomes for BMT. However, chronic GVHD still remains a challenge and current treatment relies on immunosuppression with a number of new treatments emerging, in particular extracorporeal photopheresis. Finally, GVHD may not be all bad news because it can be beneficial, when the donor cells attack leukaemia cells, known as the 'graft-versus-leukaemia effect'.

Key points

- In clinical practice, graft-versus-host disease (GVHD) is most frequently encountered in patients who receive a bone marrow transplant.
- The cutaneous signs are usually the earliest manifestation of GVHD.
- Tissues that are primary targets are the skin, gastrointestinal tract and liver.
- GVHD is divided into acute and chronic clinical manifestations.
- Acute clinical features include an erythematous rash, often involving the palms and soles.
- Chronic changes include lichen planus-like lesions, pigmentary skin changes and sclerosis and may also manifest as a variety of autoimmune or connective tissue diseases.
- GVHD may also have a beneficial 'graft-versus-leukaemia effect'.

Definition. Graft-versus-host disease (GVHD) is the term used to describe the clinical manifestations and histopathological features provoked by a graft-versus-host reaction (GVHR). A GVHR occurs when immunocompetent cells of the graft react with the tissues of an immunosuppressed histoincompatible recipient. Although this response has been known for many years and has been studied in several animal species, it has come to the fore as a clinical problem in humans as a major complication of haematopoietic cell transplantation (HCT), which is now widely used for the treatment of haematological malignancies, bone marrow failure, immunodeficiency, metabolic and gastrointestinal diseases.

Billingham [1] described the essential conditions for the occurrence of the reaction as follows.

1 There is a profound depression of cellular immunity of the recipient, otherwise the graft is rejected;
2 The patient must have received an allograft of lymphoid immunocompetent cells in sufficient quantity; and
3 There is recognition by the graft of foreign antigens in the tissues of the host.

Histoincompatibility differences may be major, carried on the histocompatibility antigens of the HLA system, the major histocompatibility complex (MHC) in humans, or there may be minor differences that are more difficult to

Harper's Textbook of Pediatric Dermatology, Fourth Edition. Edited by Peter Hoeger, Veronica Kinsler and Albert Yan.

define, as in the case of HLA-identical siblings in whom a GVHR may occur despite the graft and recipient having identical major HLA antigens.

Clinical situations in which GVHD may occur

GVHD may occur in a human fetus with a congenital cellular immunodeficiency caused by the transplacental passage of maternal lymphocytes (*maternal GVHD*) [2]. Lymphocytes are known to cross the placental barrier either before or during birth and may react against fetal antigens.

There may also be GVHD *in utero* following a blood transfusion for rhesus incompatibility (erythroblastosis fetalis) [3] (*transfusion GVHD*). In a neonate or infant with severe immune deficiency, transfusion GVHD may be provoked by administration of whole blood or blood products such as packed red cells, platelets and even fresh plasma [4,5]. Transfusion GVHD may also occur in patients with disseminated malignancies, who have a depressed immune system caused by the malignancy itself and to cytotoxic drugs [6,7]. This risk must be recognized in such susceptible individuals and all blood products should be irradiated to prevent a GVHR. The risk of transfusion GVHD may have been reduced in the UK as a result of leucocyte depletion for all red cell and platelet transfusions, which was introduced in 2001 to reduce the potential transmission of Creutzfeldt–Jakob disease.

GVHD occurs in patients who are given therapeutic grafts of haemopoietic cells, i.e. bone marrow, placental blood [8], liver and thymus. GVHD is a common and often serious complication of HCT, and it is in this clinical context that GVHD is most frequently encountered.

History.

Experimental animal models of GVHD

In 1916, Murphy [9] was the first to describe the GVHR. He observed that inoculation of the chorioallantoic membranes of young (7-day) chicken embryos with fragments of certain tissues (spleen and bone marrow) from adult chicken donors resulted in enlargement of the host spleen. The effect was misinterpreted as splenic stimulation and the implications of this were not fully realized until the 1950s.

When immunologically competent cells of an adult animal are injected into a newborn of a different strain, immunological immaturity of the recipient allows the graft to take, with the development of GVHD, which was originally described by Billingham and Brent [10] as *runt disease*.

A similar situation is brought about by injecting a first-generation hybrid, resulting from a cross between two pure strains, with lymphoid cells of either parent. The term *secondary disease* denotes GVHD in a lethally irradiated animal reconstituted by the administration of foreign haematological cells. This experimental model is called a *radiation chimera*.

The most studied animals are rodents: mice, rats and hamsters. In all of these experimental models of GVHD cutaneous lesions have been observed, the severity of which varies with the animal species.

Historical summary of human GVHD

The 1950s and 1960s saw the early attempts at human HCT, both autologous and allogeneic. Allogeneic HCT was initially plagued by the immunological problems of graft rejection and GVHD, and only 1 in 10 of the early allogeneic bone marrow transplants (BMTs) achieved a clinical improvement [11]. Much of the early pioneering work was performed by Thomas and colleagues [12] using dogs to develop effective total body irradiation schedules and introducing methotrexate to prevent GVHD. The characterization of the HLA system opened a new era in HCT, with transplants being carried out between matched sibling donor–recipient pairs.

Throughout the 1970s and 1980s, there was a rapid expansion in the number of allogeneic HCT procedures, facilitated by the introduction of ciclosporin prophylaxis against GVHD [13]. During the 1980s and 1990s, major advances occurred in the prophylaxis of GVHD, with the introduction of various negative depletion strategies to remove T-cells from the donor bone marrow. The major problem of GVHD in the haploidentical (parental) donor setting has been overcome by positive selection of $CD34^+$ progenitors from a large number of peripheral blood progenitor cells, indirectly achieving a very high level of T-cell depletion using a method of high-gradient magnetic-activated cell sorting (MACS) [14]. Finally, the anti-leukaemic properties of the GVHR have been recognized and a graft-versus-leukaemia (GVL) effect is deliberately employed in some patients with susceptible leukaemia.

Pathogenesis.

Acute disease

The essential hypothesis is that GVHD occurs as a result of an interaction of donor T lymphocytes with recipient histoincompatible antigens. The T lymphocytes become sensitized to recipient antigens, differentiate *in vivo* and then directly, or through secondary mechanisms, attack recipient cells, producing the clinical symptomatology of acute GVHD (aGVHD). In HCT, donor lymphocytes are infused into a host that has been profoundly damaged. The effects of the underlying disease, prior infection and the conditioning regime may result in substantial proinflammatory changes in endothelial and epithelial cells. Donor cells rapidly encounter not only a foreign environment, but also one that has been altered to promote the activation and proliferation of inflammatory cells by the increased expression of adhesion molecules [15], cytokines and cell surface recognition molecules [16]. Immune imbalance during recovery of immunity may also play a role in GVHD, as illustrated by an imbalance in T-cell subset recovery and the occurrence of skin GVHD following administration of ciclosporin to patients undergoing autologous transplantation [17].

The onset of aGVHD is determined by the time required for the infused lymphocytes to proliferate and differentiate. Mature donor T-cells recognize recipient peptide–HLA complexes (alloantigens) on the surface of antigen-presenting cells, in which both the HLA molecules and the bound peptides are foreign. The peptides represent minor histocompatibility antigens (mHAs), some of which have been identified [18–20]. In mouse models of GVHD, CD4$^+$ cells induce GVHD to MHC class II (HLA-DR, -DP, -DQ) differences, and CD8$^+$ cells induce GVHD to MHC class I (HLA-A, -B, -C) differences [21]. In HLA-matched HCTs, GVHD may be induced by either subset or simultaneously by both. Cytokines produced in response to alloantigens are predominantly secreted by the CD4$^+$ (T-helper type 1, or Th1) subset of T-cells [22]. Both interleukin 2 (IL-2) and interferon-γ (IFN-γ) play a central role in further T-cell activation, induction of cytotoxic T lymphocytes (CTLs) and natural killer (NK) cell responses, and the priming of additional donor and residual mononuclear phagocytes to produce IL-1 and tumour necrosis factor-α (TNF-α) [23]. The balance in Th1 and Th2 cytokines is critical for the development (or prevention) of aGVHD.

Keratinocytes have been shown to express HLA-DR antigen during early and established GVHD. Keratinocyte HLA-DR expression can be induced *in vitro* by IFN-γ [24], suggesting that during GVHD sensitized T lymphocytes release cytokines, which induce the expression of HLA-DR. The induced HLA-DR then becomes a target for CTLs directed against class II antigens.

The mechanism leading to tissue damage in GVHD is complex. As well as the cellular damage caused by CTLs and NK cells, inflammatory cytokines play an important role. TNF-α can cause direct tissue damage by inducing necrosis of target cells, or it may induce tissue destruction by apoptosis, or programmed cell death. The induction of apoptosis occurs after activation of the TNF-α–Fas antigen pathway [25].

The target organs of GVHD support the close relationship between infection and GVHD. The skin, gastrointestinal tract and liver all share exposure to endotoxin and other bacterial products that can trigger and amplify local inflammation. These tissues have a large proportion of antigen-presenting cells, such as macrophages and dendritic cells, that may enhance the GVHR. Similarly, viral infections, in particular cytomegalovirus (CMV), herpes viruses and Epstein–Barr virus, are frequent in patients undergoing HCT and may trigger or aggravate GVHD. Cells infected with a viral agent can induce neoantigens on their surface. The immune system may then recognize these cells as foreign and destroy them, even when both the infected cells and the immunologically competent donor cells have the same histocompatibility antigens.

Chronic disease

Chronic graft versus host disease (cGVHD) is a major cause of morbidity and mortality after allogeneic HCT [26]. Over the last 5 years, our understanding of cGVHD pathogenesis, based on mouse models and clinical studies, has significantly advanced. It is now thought that cGVHD is mediated by naive T cells, differentiating predominantly within highly inflammatory T-helper 17/T-cytotoxic 17 and T-follicular helper paradigms, with consequent thymic damage and impaired antigen presentation. This leads to aberrant T- and B-cell activation and differentiation, which cooperate to generate antibody-secreting cells that cause the deposition of antibodies to polymorphic recipient antigens (alloantibody) or nonpolymorphic antigens common to both recipient and donor (autoantibody) [27,28].

The mechanism of the sclerotic change in the skin most likely relates to the effect of cytokines on collagen synthesis. *In vitro* experiments have shown that collagen synthesis by fibroblasts is increased by the cytokines present in the supernatant of a phytohaemagglutinin (PHA)-stimulated lymphocyte culture [29,30,31]. Pathogenic B cell and macrophage reactions culminate in antibody formation and TGF-β secretion, respectively, leading to fibrosis [28].

Holmes and colleagues [32] reported a patient with disseminated carcinoma, who developed cutaneous and systemic features closely resembling those seen in cGVHD. The authors suggested the possibility that a GVH-like reaction was induced by alteration of 'self-antigens', consequent upon the malignancy. This case lends support to the suggestion that GVHRs are not simply limited to patients with bone marrow grafts or blood product transfusions but may develop in a situation in which there has been an alteration in self-antigens. Such a change in self-antigens could occur as a result of viral infections, malignant disease or certain drugs. This broader concept of GVHD may help to advance our understanding of the pathogenesis of the so-called 'idiopathic' disorders, i.e. lichen planus, toxic epidermal necrolysis (TEN) and scleroderma.

Pathology.

Histopathology

Histopathological features of a skin biopsy of GVHD are classified into four grades (Table 157.1). The earliest change is perivascular cuffing of lymphocytes, often seen around dilated blood vessels and swollen endothelial cells. These changes occur within the first 24 hours. The next stage is marked by a mild to moderate lymphocytic infiltrate in the upper dermis and dermoepidermal junction at sites of focal basal cell vacuolation. Established GVHD is characterized by more extensive basal cell vacuolation with disruption of the basement membrane,

Table 157.1 Histopathological grades of acute cutaneous graft-versus-host reaction

Grade	Definition
1	Focal or diffuse vacuolar alteration of basal epidermal cells
2	Vacuolar alteration of basal epidermal cells; spongiosis and dyskeratosis of epidermal cells
3	Formation of subepidermal cleft in association with spongiosis and dyskeratosis
4	Complete loss of epidermis

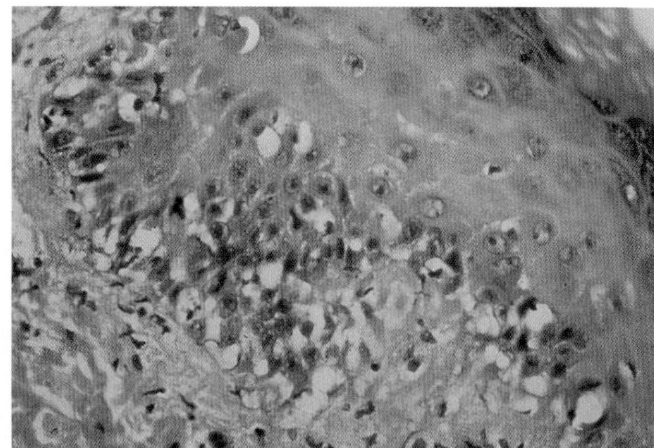

Fig. 157.1 Established graft-versus-host disease: histopathology of the skin, showing basal cell vacuolation, lymphocytic infiltrate and individual cell necrosis of keratinocytes (grade 2) (haematoxylin and eosin).

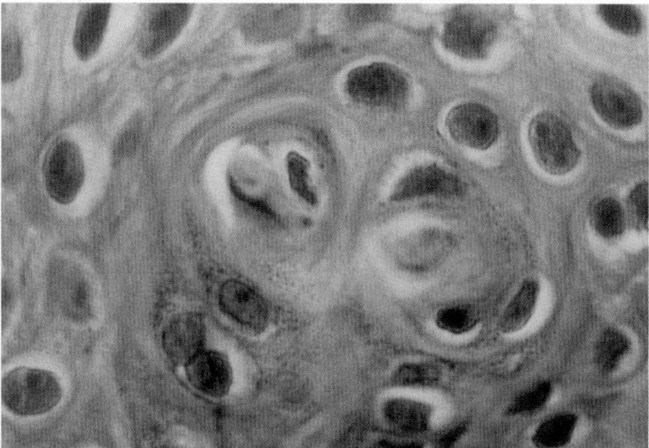

Fig. 157.2 Satellite cell necrosis in graft-versus-host disease (haematoxylin and eosin).

lymphocytes migrating into the epidermis and intercellular oedema of the epidermis (spongiosis) (Fig. 157.1). Degenerate keratinocytes (individual cell necrosis) are seen scattered throughout the epidermis, some with a pyknotic nucleus and eosinophilic, hyalinized cytoplasm. These necrotic keratinocytes are sometimes associated with one or more satellite lymphocytes, an association referred to as satellite cell necrosis [24] (Fig. 157.2). In fulminant GVHD there is separation of the epidermis at the dermoepidermal junction, with widespread desquamation of skin and necrosis of the overlying epidermis.

Histopathological features of cGVHD show the epidermis to be atrophic with hyperkeratosis, thickening of the basement membrane and condensed/homogeneous connective tissue in the upper dermis. Basal layer vacuolar degeneration, inflammation and eosinophilic body formation are rare or absent. The dermis shows thickened, hyalinized collagen bundles, together with destruction of the adnexal structures.

In the setting of BMT, a skin biopsy is the preferred method of establishing a diagnosis of GVHD and in monitoring its course. Although GVHD can be recognized early in its course as an erythematous maculopapular rash, there is no one clinical or pathological feature that is specifically diagnostic of GVHD [33]. Individual keratinocyte cell necrosis may be induced by total body irradiation [34] and various cytotoxic drugs [35,36]. Evidence that cytotoxic agents can produce mild epidermal damage, including necrosis of occasional keratinocytes in association with a sparse lymphocytic infiltrate and some vacuolar alteration of basal epidermal cells, comes from studies of psoriatic patients treated with methotrexate and hydroxyurea [37,38]. Similar changes have been described with bleomycin, adriamycin and cyclophosphamide [36]. The author's results showed 7 out of 17 pretransplant skin biopsies to be abnormal [39]. The specificity of the histological features of aGVHD was questioned by Sale and the Seattle team [36]. Some 49 skin biopsy specimens taken from marrow transplant patients, who received allogeneic, syngeneic or autologous marrow, were coded and studied 'blindly' by three pathologists. These authors concluded the following:

1 The early cutaneous histological changes do not permit a diagnosis of GVHD, except late in its evolution (after the 35th–40th day) when the effects of the cytotoxic agents have normally disappeared;
2 The presence of eosinophilic bodies, with or without satellite lymphocytes, is a necessary criterion, but is insufficient to confirm the diagnosis of GVHD because it can be caused by cytotoxic drugs. Their presence is, however, rare after the 19th day in patients who have received only cyclophosphamide and total body irradiation; and
3 Certain situations require the repetition of skin biopsies at intervals of a few days. If epidermal lesions persist, the probability that they are caused by cytotoxic agents decreases as the probability of GVHD increases. The histological diagnosis of GVHD therefore must take into account all other available relevant data. The author's findings stress the importance of taking a pretransplant skin biopsy as a baseline.

Immunopathology

In a study by the author (J.H.) and coworkers, 14 skin biopsies of GVHD [40] were examined by an indirect immunoperoxidase technique using a panel of monoclonal antibodies. Controls included pretransplant skin biopsies, skin from normal healthy volunteers and skin from patients with lichen planus and cutaneous T-cell lymphoma.

The results demonstrated the following immunopathological features of cutaneous GVHD:

1 The lymphoid infiltrate of aGVHD is composed of mainly T lymphocytes;
2 Helper ($CD4^+$) T lymphocytes, of donor origin, appear early and accumulate around blood vessels;
3 Suppressor/cytotoxic ($CD8^+$) T lymphocytes are found predominantly at the dermoepidermal junction and in the epidermis (Fig. 157.3);
4 There is a significant reduction in the number of detectable Langerhans cells in aGVHD;
5 Acute GVHD is associated with HLA-DR expression of keratinocytes (Fig. 157.4); and
6 There is a persistence of increased numbers of perivascular helper ($CD4^+$) T lymphocytes in cGVHD.

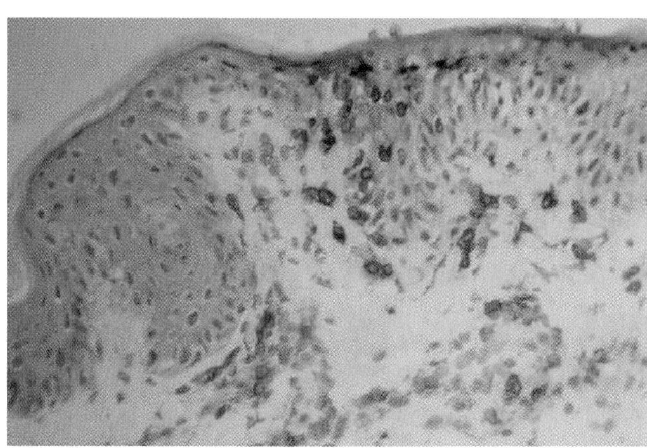

Fig. 157.3 CD8+ T lymphocytes at the dermoepidermal junction and in the epidermis demonstrated using an indirect immunoperoxidase technique.

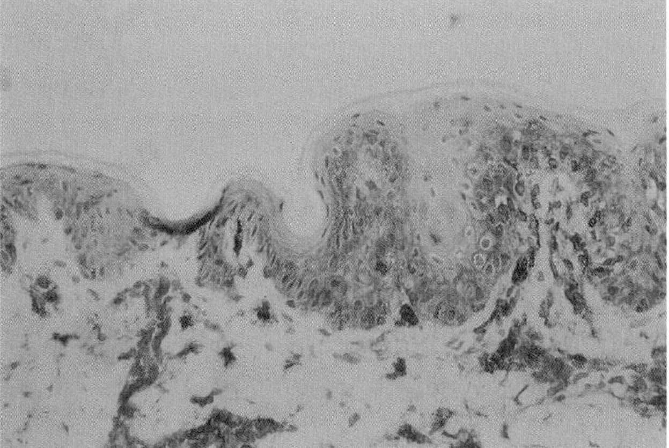

Fig. 157.4 HLA-DR expression of basal keratinocytes.

The presence of CD8+ cells in contact with destroyed keratinocytes strongly infers a cytopathic potential of these cells. Anti-Leu-7, which stains human NK cells as well as a subset of CD8+ cells, were few in number.

HLA-DR (Ia) staining of keratinocytes occurred in aGVHD, lichen planus and in two out of the six patients with cutaneous T-cell lymphoma. HLA-DR expression was not observed in normal or pretransplant skin biopsies. Studies in rats have shown that Ia staining can be induced in the skin during contact hypersensitivity reactions, but is absent following mechanical or chemical damage to the skin [41]. Scheynius and Tjernlund [42] have demonstrated the induction of HLA-DR on keratinocytes during the tuberculin reaction. These facts suggest that HLA-DR or Ia staining by keratinocytes is a consequence of cellular immunity. In a murine model of acute cutaneous GVHD, Breathnach and Katz [43] showed that the keratinocytes themselves synthesize Ia antigen in aGVHD.

The observation of a reduction in the number of Langerhans cells in aGVHD was first made by Lampert and colleagues [44] and Mason and colleagues. [45] in F1 hybrid rats and subsequently in human GVHD [46]. However, in these studies there were no controls. The author's studies (J.H.) confirmed that there is a significant decrease in the number of CD1+ dendritic (Langerhans) cells detectable in the skin biopsies of aGVHD, although there was a slight reduction in the number of Langerhans cells in pretransplant skin biopsies compared with the normal controls, presumably related to chemotherapy. These results suggest that the Langerhans cell could be a primary target in cutaneous GVHD [39,40]. When alemtuzumab (Campath-1H), a monoclonal antibody directed against CD52, is used *in vivo* to T-cell deplete the graft, it may also reduce GVHD by removing Langerhans cells from the recipient.

These immunopathological findings are reproduced in a more recent detailed study investigating the changing immune profile of the skin in seven patients undergoing sex-mismatched allogeneic HCT, using the technique of fluorescent *in situ* hybridization (FISH) and immunohistochemistry studies. Donor-derived cells were present and CD8+ cells increased in the epidermis at the time of aGVHD diagnosis. Donor cells were absent prior to the transplant, on day 14 post-transplant, at engraftment (unless aGVHD coincided with engraftment), and in aGVHD unaffected skin. Intraepidermal CD1a+ Langerhans cells were depleted in day 14 biopsies and were lowest in those receiving fully myeloablative transplant/total body irradiation; counts did not differ with the presence of aGVHD [47].

Clinical features. Tissues that are primary targets include the epithelium of the skin, gastrointestinal tract and liver. The cutaneous signs are usually the earliest manifestation of GVHD [39,48–50]. It was traditional to divide the clinical manifestations into acute and chronic phases, occurring before and after day 100 respectively; this distinction is difficult to define precisely as acute lesions can transform and progress imperceptibly into chronic lesions, and a syndrome resembling aGVHD may develop well after day 100 and has particularly been described following the recently introduced very-low-intensity BMT procedures. Diagnostic criteria have therefore defined cGVHD based on actual physical manifestations rather than by the timing of its occurrence [51].

Out of the 100 BMT patients studied by the author (J.H.) [39], 76 developed GVHD (Table 157.2). Fever and skin rash occurred in all 76 patients (100%); 46 patients (61%) had acute gastrointestinal symptoms, and 28 patients (37%) had hepatic involvement. Out of the 76 patients, 23 (30%) developed chronic skin changes of GVHD.

Table 157.2 Incidence of graft-versus-host disease in patients after bone marrow transplant

	No. of patients	GVHD
Aplastic anaemia	16	12
Leukaemias		
ALL	50	42
AML	5	3
Fanconi anaemia	3	3
Immunodeficiency diseases	11	4
Inborn errors of metabolism	15	12
Total	**100**	**76**

ALL, acute lymphocytic leukaemia; AML, acute myelocytic leukaemia.
Source: Harper 1985 [39].

Acute disease

The most common presentation is an erythematous maculopapular eruption on the trunk and limbs (Fig. 157.5), often starting on the face and affecting the palms and soles. Typically, aGVHD is seen at the time of haemopoietic reconstitution, 10–14 days post-transplant; in the author's series, this ranged from day 5 to day 60 post-graft. The more severe forms of aGVHD develop an erythroderma and subsequent epidermal separation, resulting in the appearance of bullae. The occurrence of TEN as a manifestation of fulminant aGVHD in humans was reported by Peck and colleagues [52] and was witnessed in 3 out of the author's 100 patients. This has a high mortality: of the 100 patients, one died as a result of overwhelming aGVHD and the other two died of septicaemia. In areas of blister formation, the separation is dermoepidermal, similar to that seen in drug-induced TEN. The severity of aGVHD is dependent on the degree of histoincompatibility and was inevitably worse when mismatched donors were used.

Other manifestations of aGVHD include fever and gastrointestinal and liver disturbance. Intestinal involvement is manifested by diarrhoea, nausea and vomiting. Abdominal pains and ileus are indicative of severe disease. Hepatic involvement causes an elevation in aspartate transaminase (AST) and alanine transaminase (ALT), hyperbilirubinaemia of the conjugated type and an elevation of alkaline phosphatase.

Individual organ system grading and calculation of an overall GVHD grade are shown in Tables 157.3 and 157.4, respectively. Patients with GVHD limited to grade I or II severity have a 6-month transplant-related mortality similar to patients with no GVHD. Patients with grade III GVHD, however, have a 50% risk of mortality at 6 months, whereas grade IV GVHD is usually fatal [53].

Although there remains a considerable degree of unpredictability in the occurrence of GVHD, there are many recognized risk factors. These include: HLA disparity between donor and recipient; minor MHC antigen differences, e.g. Y chromosome in male recipients of parous female marrow [54]; intensity of the pretransplant treatment [49,54]; increasing donor and recipient age; and viral infection after transplant [55]. Among recipients of umbilical cord blood (UCB) transplants there was no aGVHD of severity greater than grade I in recipients who were HLA matched or mismatched for one or two

Table 157.3 Clinician's grading of graft-versus-host disease: individual system

Skin (rash, % BSA)	GI tract (diarrhoea, mL/kg/day)	Liver (bilirubin, μmol/L)	Grade
<25	8–15	12–20	1
25–50	16–25	20–50	2
>50	>25	>50	3
Desquamation	Pain/ileus	Raised AST/ALT	4

ALT, alanine transaminase; AST, aspartate transaminase; BSA, body surface area: GI, gastrointestinal.

Table 157.4 Clinician's grading of graft-versus-host disease: overall grading

Skin	Gastrointestinal tract	Liver	Grade
1–2	–	–	I
1–3	1	1	II
2–3	2–3	2–3	III
2–4	2–4	2–4	IV

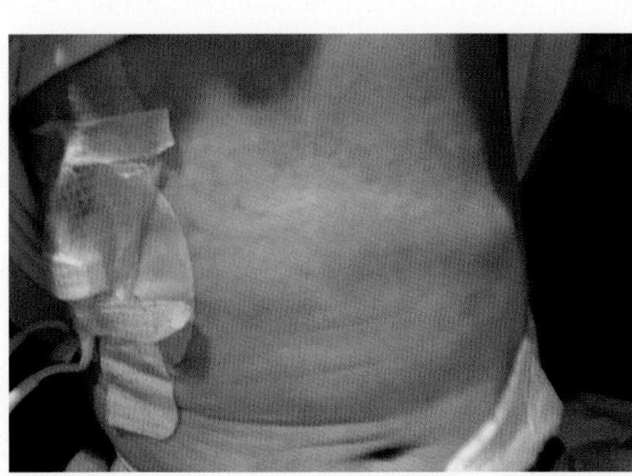

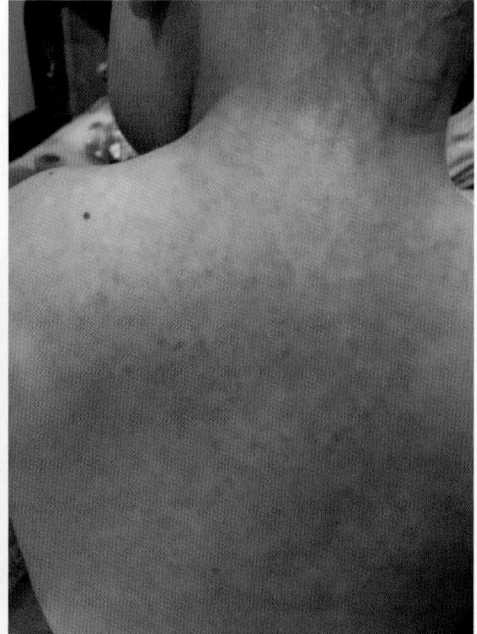

Fig. 157.5 Acute graft-versus-host disease: the early presentation of a morbilliform rash.

antigens [56]. Depending on all of these factors, the risk of GVHD can vary from 15 to 70% [57].

Chronic disease

Socié and Ritz published a review in 2014 highlighting advances that had been made in understanding the pathophysiology of cGVHD and in establishing precise criteria for diagnosis and classification of disease manifestations [58]. When patients survive aGVHD and other complications, especially infections, the cutaneous lesions either disappear completely or they gradually progress and evolve into the chronic manifestations of GVHD. The incidence of chronic cutaneous GVHD in the author's patients was 30%. All of the patients who developed chronic skin changes had experienced previous acute manifestations. In a series of transplant patients studied by the Seattle group [59], cGVHD proved to be a significant problem in 19 out of 92 patients (21%) surviving 150 days or more; in five individuals, cGVHD apparently occurred without a preceding acute reaction. Chronic skin manifestations of GVHD include lichen planus-like lesions, pigmentary changes and sclerosis.

In the author's series, a variety of lichenoid lesions occurred from day 29 to day 350 postgraft. Involvement of the buccal mucosa is a frequent finding. Saurat and Gluckman [60] stated that oral lesions always preceded the cutaneous lesions of cGVHD. However, this was not substantiated by this author's observations. The mucosal lesions are similar to those seen in idiopathic lichen planus, with a white reticulate pattern affecting the buccal mucosa, gingiva, tongue and palate. Lichen planus lesions of the genitalia have also been reported [59,60] and were seen in one patient in the author's series. The appearance of lichen planus papules on the skin shows similarities to that seen in idiopathic lichen planus [61–63], with polygonal, violaceous, shiny papules and Wickham's striae. More often, however, the lesions are less typical of lichen planus although remaining lichenoid in nature. Lesions are often seen in a reticulate configuration, especially on the limbs, suggesting some relationship with the underlying vascular network. The distribution, when widespread, does not tend to affect those areas of predilection seen in idiopathic lichen planus, such as the anterior aspects of the wrists.

Follicular lesions resembling lichen planopilaris are seen as an early manifestation of cGVHD. The lichenoid lesions exhibit the Koebner phenomenon, seen in two of the author's patients. It has been suggested that the lichenoid lesions occur more often in the zones previously affected by the aGVHD rash. The author observed no evidence to support this, although one patient in the series did develop tiny lichenoid papules on the palms, which is unusual in idiopathic lichen planus. Nail involvement occurred in two patients. Typically nails become brittle, crack and develop ridging [64]. Cicatricial alopecia has been reported by Touraine and colleagues [61] Saurat and colleagues [63] and Shulman and colleagues [59], but this was not noted in the author's study. Hair can become brittle and alopecia ensue even in children [65]. Premature greying of the hair is also common.

A frequent finding is hyperpigmentation, which can be diffuse, reticulate or follicular. Lesions may have a poikilodermatous appearance [59,61,66]. Less commonly, areas of hypopigmentation occur. Pigmentary changes precede the development of sclerosis.

Areas of induration and sclerosis of the skin develop as a late manifestation of GVHD. These sclerotic lesions tend to be localized [2,67,68], or progress to extensive sclerosis (generalized scleroderma). A nodular/keloid variant has been described [69]. Ulceration, particularly at pressure points [61,64,70], and flexion contractures with limitation of joint movement [71,72] may result. Four patients in the author's series developed morphoea-like areas of skin, and in one boy these were widespread. In these patients, the lesions have remained static or have gradually improved; none progressed to the more serious sequelae. This may be related to their long-term treatment with prednisolone and azathioprine. Saurat and colleagues [63] regard these late changes to be more like lichen sclerosus et atrophicus with, in particular, characteristic genital lesions. Shulman and colleagues [59] noted a phimosis in 2 of their 19 patients, an observation that could possibly reinforce Saurat's hypothesis. However, oesophageal involvement [73] and subcutaneous calcification [74] suggest that this disease process is more like scleroderma.

Other manifestations of chronic disease

Chronic GVHD may manifest as a variety of autoimmune or connective tissue diseases [29], sharing overlapping features with scleroderma, lupus erythematosus, dermatomyositis, polymyositis, primary biliary cirrhosis and chronic active hepatitis. The occurrence of Sjögren syndrome is well documented [59,74]. In the author's study xerophthalmia, conjunctivitis and xerostomia were observed in one patient, who also had lichenoid lesions of cGVHD. Gratwhol and colleagues [74] reported cutaneous lesions, which, clinically and histologically, resembled discoid lupus erythematosus in one patient, 19 months after transplantation. The author has seen vitiligo and polymyositis associated with cGVHD. Visceral manifestations of cGVHD are essentially malabsorption and chronic hepatitis. Chronic liver damage with progressive destruction of bile canaliculi may lead to primary biliary cirrhosis [75] or to a syndrome mimicking chronic active hepatitis. Most patients with cGVHD tend to have prolonged humoral and cellular immune defects, with an increased susceptibility to bacterial, viral and fungal infections. Laboratory tests in cGVHD may show abnormal liver function, eosinophilia, hypogammaglobulinaemia with polyclonal elevation of immunoglobulin G (IgG) or IgM, and a variety of circulating autoantibodies, especially antinuclear, antismooth muscle and antimitochondrial antibodies.

Differential diagnosis. The differential diagnosis of acute cutaneous GVHD includes the effects of radiotherapy, drug reactions, eczema, iron overload and infections. Usually, these can be distinguished clinically, but the major practical problems of diagnosis include: (i) drug-induced rashes, as a result of immunosuppressive or antibiotic therapy; and (ii) a viraemia caused by hepatitis B or CMV, which can exceptionally be responsible for an exanthematous eruption. As detailed in the section on histology, there are no features specifically diagnostic for GVHD; however, a skin biopsy may provide useful information to support the diagnosis. Candidate biomarkers have been identified that may be useful for the diagnosis and monitoring of cGVHD [76]. A more recent study [77] reviewed the accuracy of previously reported markers of cGVHD in a multicentre 'Chronic GVHD Consortium' and showed that a small subset of RNA biomarkers (IRS2, PLEKHF1 and IL1R2), when combined with specific clinical variables (recipient CMV serostatus and conditioning regimen intensity), can improve the accuracy for cGVHD diagnosis.

Treatment and prevention.

Prevention

There are some guidelines to the appropriate selection of prophylaxis against GVHD: identical twin transplants require no GVHD prophylaxis; ciclosporin and short-course methotrexate or mycophenolate mofetil (MMF) is adequate in standard risk-matched sibling donor transplants in children under 16 years of age [78], whereas *in vivo* T-cell depletion with alemtuzumab or anti-thymocyte globulin is usually required with unrelated donor transplants. For haplotype mismatched (parental) transplants, profound 4–5 log T-cell depletion is required, which is now readily achieved by CD34 selection techniques (e.g. CliniMACS), which usually ensure that no more than 1×10^5 $CD3^+$ cells/kg are returned with the graft. A more recent approach to haploidentical transplants has involved the administration of high-dose cyclophosphamide to the patient on day 3 and 4 after stem cell transplant (SCT) to achieve depletion of alloreactive cells *in vivo* [79]. In the absence of chronic GVHD, prophylactic immunosuppression can be discontinued at about 3–6 months after SCT without complications, indicating either that the originally infused T-cells, which recognize host alloantigens, have a limited lifespan, or that regulatory mechanisms develop to prevent the T-cells from causing immune damage. T-cells that develop in the host thymus after SCT do not cause GVHD because of induction of anergy and negative selection mediated by host thymic epithelial cells. A GVL effect may, to some extent, parallel GVHD, and complete abolition of GVHD may therefore not be desirable [80,81].

Acute disease

Several agents have been used to treat established aGVHD, with varying degrees of success. High-dose corticosteroids given as a bolus injection of intravenous methylprednisolone produce a dramatic effect on aGVHD and are used widely as first-line treatment [82]. Although skin GVHD responds rapidly, liver and gut GVHD can be resistant, and some patients become refractory to steroids. The treatment strategy for steroid-refractory GVHD [83] is less clear and outcomes remain unsatisfactory. Some responses have been achieved in refractory disease with anti-thymocyte globulin and various monoclonal antibodies including alemtuzumab, anti-IL2 receptor [84,85], anti-CD5 [86], anti-CD2 and anti-TNF (infliximab). With less aggressive disease, tacrolimus ointment can be substituted for ciclosporin [87], or indeed MMF added to either drug. More recently sirolimus (rapamycin) [88], mesenchymal stem/stromal cells [89] and the JAK1/2 inhibitor ruxolitinib [90] have been used with some benefit in steroid refractory GVHD.

Chronic disease

The treatment of cGVHD is intended to reduce the symptom burden, control manifestations and prevent damage and disability. The intensity of treatment required to control cGVHD decreases over time caused by the gradual development of immunological tolerance. There is therefore a risk of overtreatment, with associated toxicities, as well as undertreatment. The appropriate management of cGVHD therefore requires continuous recalibration using serial attempts to decrease the intensity of immunosuppressive treatment [91].

Local therapies may be sufficient to treat some cGVHD manifestations. In fact, if the cGVHD is mild according to NIH Consensus Criteria, the recommendation is to attempt local therapy in the first instance [51]. Preference for local therapies is also advised in patients with high-risk malignancies where a strong GVL effect is desired (see later). Topical treatments that are useful include ciclosporin in solution as a mouthwash [80,92], a potent corticosteroid as an inhaler (such as beclometasone) for oral erosive lichen planus and a potent or ultrapotent topical steroid ointment (clobetasol propionate) for phimosis or localized cGVHD elsewhere. Other approaches include the use of artificial tears for ocular involvement and the regular application of a sunscreen.

For patients with moderate or severe cGVHD, prednisolone is the treatment of choice, initiated at 1 mg/kg for 2 weeks with a taper to alternate-day prednisolone by 1–2 months. Azathioprine is often used as a steroid-sparing agent. Adding a calcineurin inhibitor, e.g. ciclosporin, may be beneficial as well [92]. Chronic GVHD occurring after stopping ciclosporin prophylaxis will often regress when the drug is reintroduced, but some patients develop cGVHD during adequate ciclosporin therapy [13]. Localized morphoea lesions may gradually improve [39]. However, the severe progressive wasting disease with immunodeficiency, liver damage and scleroderma is not always controllable; the sclerodermatous form may produce permanent deformity that persists after the GVHD process has burnt out, and requires aggressive ongoing physiotherapy and occupational health involvement.

When cGVHD fails to respond to first-line treatment there are a number of salvage therapies available where data mostly come from adult patients: rituximab [93]; sirolimus [94]; thalidomide [95,96]; and high-dose methylprednisolone [97]. Jacobsohn [92] reviewed salvage therapies for which data in children exist, including MMF [98], pentostatin [99] and hydroxychloroquine [100], all of which showed promise, with clinical responses of around 50% permitting reduction in steroid doses. However, the main drawback remains the potential for added infection, hence careful monitoring for infections; the use of adequate antiviral and antifungal agents is mandatory.

Ibrutinib is a new small molecule drug that binds to a protein, Bruton's tyrosine kinase (BTK), that is important for activation of B cells. It is used to treat chronic lymphocytic leukaemia, Waldenstrom macroglobulinaemia, and in August 2017 the US FDA approved ibrutinib to treat cGVHD in adults after failure of one or more other systemic treatments [101]. This is the first FDA-approved therapy for the treatment of cGVHD.

Extracorporeal photopheresis (ECP) has shown efficacy in children with steroid-refractory GVHD [102–105], both acute and chronic GVHD [106], and may be associated with less infection risk than other rescue therapies. ECP involves the infusion of autologous peripheral blood mononuclear cells collected by apheresis and incubated with the photoactive drug 8-methoxypsoralen, which induces apoptosis of treated lymphocytes. The immunological effect of ECP has been characterized by tolerogenic modulation, including induction of regulatory T (Treg) lymphocytes, which suppress GVHD activity without inducing further immunosuppression and facilitating reduction in concurrent immunosuppressive therapy [107].

Photochemotherapy (PUVA: psoralens and UVA) may be helpful for the treatment of lichenoid GVHD inadequately controlled by systemic therapy [108]. The efficacy of PUVA treatment for sclerodermatous GVHD is more controversial and there is a small but definite risk of developing skin malignancy [109].

The likelihood of treatment response depends upon whether single-organ or multiorgan systems are affected, and a platelet count with thrombocytopenia of fewer than 50×10^9/L carries a worse prognosis [110].

Graft-versus-leukaemia effect

There are several lines of evidence to suggest that alloreactive donor cells can exert an important antileukaemic action [111]. One mechanism of this GVL effect is mediated by cytotoxic T-cells recognizing major and/or minor histocompatibility antigen differences on recipient cells; hence it may also involve cells responsible for GVHD, although other GVL mechanisms may be more leukaemia-specific [112]. GVL reactions are more pronounced in the presence of GVHD and/or with increasing donor–recipient HLA disparity, for example in transplants from unrelated donors [113]. The GVL effect also appears to be disease specific, with the most powerful GVL effect being observed in chronic myeloid leukaemia, and the smallest effect in acute lymphoblastic leukaemia, presumably owing to coexpression or not of target antigens [114]. Gale and Fuchs [115] reviewed the subject and discuss whether GVL is immunologically specific to the leukaemia or results from donor immune cells reacting to disparate recipient HLA and non-HLA histocompatibility antigens on leukaemia cells or both.

Why is graft-versus-host disease important to the dermatologist

GVHD is a frequent complication of HCT and is responsible for significant mortality. The rash is usually the first sign of GVHD, and early recognition and treatment are imperative. The effect on the skin may be the chief morbid factor, such as TEN. Finally, GVHD is a biological model for other 'idiopathic' skin diseases such as lichen planus, TEN and morphoea/scleroderma. Knowledge of the mechanisms involved in GVHD will hopefully lead to a better understanding of the pathophysiology of these 'idiopathic' diseases.

References

1 **Billingham RE. The biology of graft versus host reactions. Harvey Lectures 1967;62:21–78.**

2 Grogan TM, Odom RB, Burgess JH. Graft versus host reaction. Arch Dermatol 1977;113:806–12.

3 Parkman R, Mosier D, Umansky I et al. Graft versus host disease after intrauterine and exchange transfusions for haemolytic disease of the newborn. N Engl J Med 1974;290:359–63.

4 Hathaway WE, Githens JH, Blackburn WR et al. Aplastic anaemia, histiocytosis and erythrodermia in immunologically deficient children: probable human runt disease. N Engl J Med 1965;273:953–8.

5 Park BH, Good RA, Gate J et al. Fatal graft versus host reaction following transfusion of allogenic blood and plasma in infants with combined immunodeficiency disease. Trans Proc 1974;6:385–8.

6 Von Fleidner V, Higby DJ, Kim U. Graft-versus-host reaction following blood product transfusion. Am J Med 1982;72:951–61.

7 Tolbert B, Kaufman CE, Burgdorf WHC et al. Graft-versus-host disease from leucocyte transfusions. J Am Acad Dermatol 1983;9:416–19.

8 Kurtzberg J, Laughlin M, Graham ML et al. Placental blood as a source of hematopoietic stem cells for transplantation into unrelated recipients. N Engl J Med 1996;335:157–66.

9 Murphy JB. The effect of adult chicken grafts on the chick embryo. J Exp Med 1916;24:1–6.

10 **Billingham RE, Brent L. A simple method for inducing tolerance of skin homografts in mice. Trans Bull 1957;4:67–71.**

11 Pegg DE. Allogeneic bone marrow transplantation in man. In: Pegg DE (ed.) Bone Marrow Transplantation. London: Lloyd-Luke Books, 1966;77–101.

12 **Thomas ED, Lochte HL, Lu WC et al. Intravenous infusion of bone marrow in patients receiving radiation and chemotherapy. N Engl J Med 1957;257:491.**

13 **Powles RL, Clink HM, Spence D et al. Cyclosporin A to prevent GvHD in man after allogeneic bone marrow transplantation. Lancet 1980;i:327–9.**

14 **Schumm M, Lang P, Taylor G et al. Isolation of highly purified autologous and allogeneic peripheral CD34[+] cells using the CliniMACS device. J Hematotherapy 1999;8:209–18.**

15 Behar E, Chao NJ, Hiraki DD et al. Polymorphism of adhesion molecule CD31 and its role in acute graft versus host disease. N Engl J Med 1996;334:286–91.

16 Vogelsang GB, Hess AD. Graft versus host disease: new directions for a persistent problem. J Am Soc Hematol 1994;84:2061–7.

17 Jones RJ1, Vogelsang GB, Hess AD et al. Induction of graft-versus-host disease after autologous bone marrow transplantation. Lancet 1989;1(8641):754–7.

18 Nichols W, Antin J, Lunetta K. Identification of non-HLA loci contributing to graft versus host disease. Blood 1995;86(Suppl. 1):630a.

19 Goulmy E, Schipper R, Pool J et al. Mismatches of minor histocompatibility antigens between HLA identical donors and recipients and the development of graft versus host disease after bone marrow transplantation. N Engl J Med 1996;334:281–5.

20 Den Haan JM, Sherman NE, Blokland E et al. Identification of a graft versus host disease-associated human minor histocompatibility antigen. Science 1995;268:1476–80.

21 Korngold R, Sprent J. T cell subsets in graft versus host disease. In: Burakoff SJ, Deeg HJ, Ferrara J et al. (eds) Graft Versus Host Disease: Immunology, Pathophysiology and Treatment. New York: Marcel Dekker, 1990:31–50.

22 Sad S, Marcotte R, Mosmann TR. Cytokine-induced differentiation of precursor mouse CD8+ T cells into cytotoxic CD8+ T cells secreting Th1 or Th2 cytokines. Immunity 1995;2:271–9.

23 Ferrara JLM. Paradigm shift for graft versus host disease. Bone Marrow Transplant 1994;14:183–4.

24 Morhenn VB, Nickoloff BJ, Merigan TC et al. The effect of gamma interferon on cultured human keratinocytes. J Invest Dermatol 1984;82:410 (abstract).

25 Laster SM, Wood JG, Gooding LR. Tumour necrosis factor can induce both apoptotic and necrotic forms of cell lysis. J Immunol 1988; 141:26–9.

26 Lee SJ Chronic graft-versus-host disease: classification systems for chronic graft-versus-host disease. Blood 2017;129:30–37.

27 MacDonald KP, Hill GR, Blazar BR. Chronic graft-versus-host disease: biological insights from preclinical and clinical studies. Blood 2017;129:13–21.

28 MacDonald KP, Blazar BR, Hill GR. Cytokine mediators of chronic graft-versus-host disease. J Clin Invest 2017;127:2452–63.

29 Harper JI. Graft versus host disease: aetiological and clinical aspects in connective tissue diseases. Semin Dermatol 1985;4:144–51.

30 Johnson RL, Ziff M. Lymphokine stimulation of collagen accumulation. J Clin Invest 1976;58:240–52.

31 Spielvogel RL, Goltz RW, Kersey JH. Mononuclear cell stimulation of fibroblast collagen synthesis. Clin Exp Dermatol 1977;3:25–35.

32 Holmes RC, Cooper CB, Jurecka W et al. Syndrome resembling graft-versus-host disease in a patient with disseminated carcinoma. J Roy Soc Med 1983;76:703–5.

33 Darmstadt GL, Donnenberg AD, Vogelsang GB et al. Clinical, laboratory, and histopathologic indicators of the development of progressive acute graft versus host disease. J Invest Dermatol 1992;99: 397–402.

34 Woodruff JM, Eltringham JR, Casey HW. Early secondary disease in the rhesus monkey. I. A comparative histologic study. Lab Invest 1969;20:499–511.

35 Woodruff JM, Hansen JA, Good RA et al. The pathology of the graft versus host reaction (GVHR) in adults receiving bone marrow transplants. Trans Proc 1976;8:675–84.

36 Sale GE, Lerner KG, Barker EA et al. The skin biopsy in the diagnosis of acute graft versus host disease in man. Am J Pathol 1977;89:621–35.

37 Smith C, Gelfant S. Effects of methotrexate and hydroxyurea on psoriatic epidermis. Preferential cytotoxic effects on psoriatic epidermis. Arch Dermatol 1974;110:70–2.

38 Kennedy BJ, Smith LR, Goltz RW. Skin changes secondary to hydroxyurea therapy. Arch Dermatol 1975;111:183–7.

39 Harper JI. A Clinicopathological Study of Cutaneous Graft Versus Host Disease. MD Thesis, University of London, 1985.

40 Harper JI, Zemelman V, Nagvekark NM et al. Graft versus host disease: T-lymphocyte subsets, Langerhans' cells and HLADR+ cells in the skin after human bone marrow transplantation. J Invest Dermatol 1984;82:562–3.

41 Suitters AJ, Lampert IA. Expression of la antigen on epidermal keratinocytes is a consequence of cellular immunity. Br J Exp Pathol 1982;63:207–13.

42 Scheynius A, Tjernlund U. Human keratinocytes express HLA-DR antigens in the tuberculin reaction. Scand J Immunol 1984;19:141–7.

43 Breathnach SM, Katz SI. Keratinocytes synthesize la antigen in acute cutaneous graft versus host disease. J Immunol 1983;131:2741–5.

44 Lampert IA, Suitters AJ, Chisholm PM. Expression of la antigen on epidermal keratinocytes in graft versus host disease. Nature 1981;293:149–50.

45 Mason DW, Dallman M, Barclay AN. Graft versus host disease induces expression of la antigen in rat epidermal cells and gut epithelium. Nature 1981;293:150–1.

46 Lampert IA, Janossy G, Suitters AJ et al. Immunological analysis of the skin in graft versus host disease. Clin Exp Immunol 1982; 50:123–31.

47 Stewart CL, Cornejo CM, Wanat KA et al. The immune reconstitution of the skin following sex mismatched allogeneic hematopoietic stem cell transplant: a prospective case series utilizing fluorescent in situ hybridization and immunohistochemistry. Br J Dermatol 2018;178:e55–6.

48 Dinulos JG, Levy M. Graft versus host disease in children. Semin Dermatol 1995;14:66–9.

49 Wu PA, Cowen EW. Cutaneous graft-versus-host disease – clinical considerations and management. Curr Probl Dermatol 2012; 43:101–15.

50 Strong Rodrigues K, Oliveira-Ribeiro C, de Abreu Fiuza Gomes S, Knobler R. Cutaneous graft-versus-host disease: diagnosis and treatment. Am J Clin Dermatol 2018;19:33–50.

51 Filipovich AH, Weisdorf D, Pavletic S et al. National Institutes of Health consensus development project on criteria for clinical trials in chronic graft-versus-host disease: I. Diagnosis and staging working group report. Biol Blood Marrow Transplant 2005;11:945–56.

52 Peck GL, Herzig GP, Elias PM. Toxic epidermal necrolysis in a patient with graft-vs-host reaction. Arch Dermatol 1972;105:561–9.

53 Martin P. Overview of marrow transplantation immunology. In: Forman SJ, Blume KG, Thomas ED (eds) Bone Marrow Transplantation. Oxford: Blackwell Scientific Publications, 1994;16–21.

54 Gale RP, Bortin MM, van Bekkum D et al. Risk factors for acute graft versus host disease. Br J Haematol 1987;67:397–406.

55 Lonqvist B, Ringden O, Wahren B et al. Cytomegalovirus infection associated with and preceding chronic graft versus host disease. Transplantation 1984;38:465–8.

56 Apperley JF. Umbilical cord blood progenitor cell transplantation. Bone Marrow Transplant 1994;14:187–96.

57 Weisdorf D, Hakke R, Blazar B et al. Risk factors for acute graft versus host disease in histocompatible donor bone marrow transplantation. Transplantation 1991;5:1197–203.

58 Socié G, Ritz J. Current issues in chronic graft-versus-host disease. Blood 2014;124:374–84

59 Shulman HM, Sale GE, Lerner KG et al. Chronic cutaneous graft versus host disease in man. Am J Pathol 1978;91:545–70.

60 Saurat JH, Gluckman E. Lichen planus-like eruption following bone marrow transplantation: a manifestation of the graft versus host disease. Clin Exp Dermatol 1977;2:335–44.

61 Touraine R, Revuz J, Dreyfus B et al. Graft versus host reaction and lichen planus. Br J Dermatol 1975;92:589.

62 Saurat JH, Didier-Jean L, Gluckman E et al. Graft versus host reaction and lichen planus-like eruption in man. Br J Dermatol 1975;92:591–2.

63 Saurat JH, Gluckman E, Bussel A et al. The lichen planus-like eruption after bone marrow transplantation. Br J Dermatol 1975;93:675–81.

64 Andrews M, Robertson I, Weedon D. Cutaneous manifestations of chronic graft-versus-host disease. Australas J Dermatol 1997;38:53–62.

65 Locatelli F, Giorgiani G, Pession A, Bozzola M. Late effects in children after bone marrow transplantation: a review. Haematologica 1993;78:319–28.

66 Spielvogel RL, Goltz RW, Keysey JH. Scleroderma-like changes in chronic graft versus host disease. Arch Dermatol 1977;113:1424–8.

67 Masters R, Hood A, Cosini A. Chronic cutaneous graft-vs-host reaction following bone marrow transplantation. Arch Dermatol 1975;111:1526.

68 Van Vloten WA, Scheffer E, Dooren LJ. Localised scleroderma-like lesions after bone marrow transplantation in man. Br J Dermatol 1977;96:337–41.

69 Prieto-Torres L, Boggio F, Gruber-Wackernagel A, Cerroni L. Nodular sclerodermatous chronic cutaneous graft-versus-host disease (GvHD): a new clinicopathological variant of cutaneous sclerodermatous GvHD resembling nodular/keloidal scleroderma. Am J Dermatopathol 2017;39:910–13.

70 Hood AF, Soter NA, Rappeport J et al. Graft versus host reaction. Cutaneous manifestations following bone marrow transplantation. Arch Dermatol 1977;113:1087–91.

71 Siimes MA, Johansson E, Rapola J. Scleroderma-like graft-versus-host disease as a late consequence of bone marrow grafting. Lancet 1977;ii:831–2.

72 Shulman HM, Sullivan KM, Weiden PL et al. Chronic graft-versus-host syndrome in man. A long-term clinicopathologic study of 20 Seattle patients. Am J Med 1980;69:204–17.

73 Roujeau JC, Revuz J, Touraine R. Graft versus host reactions. In: Rook A, Savin J (eds) Recent Advances in Dermatology, Vol. 5. Edinburgh: Churchill Livingstone, 1980:131–57.

74 Gratwhol AA, Moutsopoulos HM, Chused TM et al. Sjögren type syndrome after allogenic bone marrow transplantation. Ann Intern Med 1977;87:703–70.

75 Epstein O, Thomas HC, Sherlock S. Primary biliary cirrhosis is a dry gland syndrome with features of chronic graft versus host disease. Lancet 1980;i:1166–8.

76 Pidala J, Sarwal M, Roedder S, Lee SJ. Biologic markers of chronic GVHD. Bone Marrow Transplant 2014;49:324–31.

77 Pidala J, Sigdel TK, Wang A et al. A combined biomarker and clinical panel for chronic graft versus host disease diagnosis. J Pathol Clin Res 2016;29; 3: 3–16.

78 Poynton C. T cell depletion in bone marrow transplantation. In: Pegg DE (ed.) Bone Marrow Transplantation in Practice. Edinburgh: Churchill Livingstone, 1992;227–37.

79 Lznik L, Bolaños-Meade J, Zahurak M et al. High-dose cyclophosphamide as single-agent, short-course prophylaxis of graft-versus-host disease. Blood 2010;115:3224–30.

80 Sullivan KM, Weiden PL, Storb R et al. Influence of acute graft versus host disease after relapse and survival after bone marrow transplantation from HLA identical siblings as treatment of acute and chronic leukaemia. Blood 1989;73:1720–8.

81 Veys P, Sanders F, Calderwood S et al. The role of graft versus leukaemia in bone marrow transplantation for juvenile chronic myeloid leukaemia. Blood 1994;84(Suppl.):337A.

82 Kendra J, Barrett AJ, Lucas C et al. Response of graft versus host disease to high doses of methylprednisolone. Clin Lab Haematol 1981;3:19–26.

83 Deeg HJ. How I treat refractory acute GVHD. Blood 2007; 109:4119–26.

84 Hervé P, Wijdens J, Bergerat JP et al. Treatment of acute graft versus host disease with monoclonal antibody to the IL-2 receptor. Lancet 1988;ii:1072–3.

85 Przepiorka D, Kernan NA, Ippoliti C et al. Daclizumab, a humanized anti-interleukin-2 receptor alpha chain antibody, for treatment of acute graft-versus-host disease. Blood 2000;95:83–9.

86 Fay JW, Burkeholder S, Stone M. Treatment of allogeneic bone marrow with anti T cell antibody prior to transplantation. Bone Marrow Transplant 1987;2(Suppl. 2):127.

87 Kunitomi A, Iida H, Kamiya Y et al. Successful treatment using tacrolimus ointment for cutaneous graft-versus-host disease. Int J Hematol 2008;88:465–7.

88 Benito AI, Furlong T, Martin PJ et al. Sirolimus (rapamycin) for the treatment of steroid-refractory acute graft-versus-host disease. Transplantation 2001;72:1924–9.

89 Le Blanc K, Rasmusson I, Sundberg B et al. Treatment of severe acute graft-versus-host disease with third party haploidentical mesenchymal stem cells. Lancet 2004;363:1439–41.

90 Zeiser R, Burchert A, Lengerke C et al. Ruxolitinib in corticosteroid-refractory graft-versus-host disease after allogeneic stem cell transplantation: a multicenter survey. Leukemia 2015;29:2062–8.

91 Flowers MED, Martin PJ. How we treat chronic graft-versus-host disease. Blood 2015;125:606–15.

92 Jacobsohn DA. Optimal management of chronic graft-versus-host disease in children. Br J Haematol 2010;150:278–92.

93 Cutler C, Miklos D, Kim HT et al. Rituximab for steroid-refractory chronic graft-versus-host disease. Blood 2006;108:756–62.

94 Johnston LJ, Brown J, Shizuru JA et al. Rapamycin (sirolimus) for treatment of chronic graft-versus-host disease. Biol Blood Marrow Transplant 2005;11:47–55.

95 Vogelsang G, Farmer E, Hess A et al. Thalidomide for the treatment of chronic graft versus host disease. N Engl J Med 1992;326:1055–8.

96 Parker P, Chao N, Nademanee A et al. Thalidomide as salvage therapy for chronic graft versus host disease. Blood 1995;86:3604–9.

97 Akpek G, Lee SM, Anders V et al. A high-dose pulse steroid regimen for controlling active chronic graft-versus-host disease. Biol Blood Marrow Transplant 2001;7:495–502.

98 Busca A, Saroglia EM, Lanino E et al. Mycophenolate mofetil (MMF) as therapy for refractory chronic GVHD (cGVHD) in children receiving bone marrow transplantation. Bone Marrow Transplant 2000;25:1067–71.

99 Goldberg JD, Jacobsohn DA, Margolis J et al. Pentostatin for the treatment of chronic graft-versus-host disease in children. J Pediatr Hematol Oncol 2003;25:584–8.

100 Gilman AL, Chan KW, Mogul A et al. Hydroxychloroquine for the treatment of chronic graft-versus-host disease. Biol Blood Marrow Transplant 2000;6:327–34.

101 Miklos D, Cutler CS, Arora M et al. Ibrutinib for chronic graft-versus-host disease after failure of prior therapy. Blood 2017;130:2243–50.

102 Salvaneschi L, Perotti C, Zecca M et al. Extracorporeal photochemotherapy for treatment of acute and chronic GVHD in childhood. Transfusion 2001;41:1299–305.

103 Knobler R, Barr ML, Couriel DR et al. Extracorporeal photopheresis: past, present, and future. J Am Acad Dermatol 2009;61:652–65.

104 Alfred A, Taylor PC, Dignan F et al. The role of extracorporeal photopheresis in the management of cutaneous T-cell lymphoma, graft-versus-host disease and organ transplant rejection: a consensus statement update from the UK Photopheresis Society. Br J Haematol 2017;177:287–310.

105 Malik MI, Litzow M, Hogan W et al. Extracorporeal photopheresis for chronic graft-versus-host disease: a systematic review and meta-analysis. Blood Res 2014;49:100–6.

106 Abu-Dalle I, Reljic T, Nishihori T et al. Extracorporeal photopheresis in steroid-refractory acute or chronic graft-versus-host disease: results of a systematic review of prospective studies. Biol Blood Marrow Transplant 2014;20:1677–86.

107 Beattie B, Cole D, Nicholson L et al. Limited thymic recovery after extracorporeal photopheresis in a low-body-weight patient with acute graft-versus-host disease of the skin. J Allergy Clin Immunol 2016;137:1890–3.

108 Volc-Platzer A, Hönigsmann H, Hinterberger W et al. Photochemotherapy improves chronic cutaneous graft versus host disease. J Am Acad Dermatol 1990;23:220–8.

109 Altman R, Adler S. Development of multiple cutaneous squamous cell carcinomas during PUVA treatment for cutaneous chronic graft versus host disease. J Am Acad Dermatol 1994;31:505–7.

110 Sullivan KM, Witherspoon RP, Storb R et al. Prednisolone and azathioprine compared with prednisolone and placebo for treatment of chronic graft versus host disease: prognostic influence of prolonged thrombocytopenia after allogeneic bone marrow transplantation. Blood 1988;72:546–54.

111 Antin JH. Graft versus leukaemia: no longer an epiphenomenon. Blood 1993;82:2273–7.

112 Sullivan KM, Weiden PL, Storb R et al. Influence of acute and chronic graft versus host disease after relapse and survival after bone marrow transplantation from HLA matched siblings as treatment of acute and chronic leukaemia. Blood 1989;73:1720–8.

113 Gajewski JL, Champlin RE. Enhanced graft versus leukaemia effect in patients receiving matched unrelated donor bone marrow transplants. In: Champlin RE, Gale RP (eds) New Strategies in Bone Marrow Transplantation. New York: Wiley-Liss, 1991:281–4.

114 Horowitz MM, Gale RP, Sondel PM et al. Graft versus leukaemia reactions after bone marrow transplantation. Blood 1990;75:555–62.

115 Gale RP, Fuchs EJ. Is there really a specific graft-versus-leukaemia effect? Bone Marrow Transplant 2016;51:1413–15.

CHAPTER 158
The Oral Mucosa and Tongue

Jane Luker[1] & Crispian Scully[1,2]

[1] Bristol Dental Hospital, University Hospitals Bristol NHS Foundation Trust, Bristol, UK
[2] University College London, London, UK

Introduction, 2079
Mouth ulcers/sore mouth, 2079
White patches (leucoplakia), 2088
Red and pigmented lesions, 2091
Swellings/lumps in and around the mouth, 2094
Lesions of the tongue, 2099

Abstract

This chapter covers lesions of the oral mucosa, tongue and gingival mucosa which are either localized to the oral cavity or a manifestation of systemic diseases or infections. It describes some common conditions such as recurrent apthous stomatitis and how this may be differentiated from systemic conditions, and deficiencies that may exacerbate or cause oral ulceration. The chapter also describes some normal variants that may cause concern to parents of young children such as hairy tongue, erythema migrans and Fordyce spots, which may not be as familiar to medical practitioners.

Key points

- **The most common cause of recurrent oral ulceration in childhood is recurrent apthous stomatitis.**
- **Oral ulceration in children may be associated with acute infections and occasionally with a systemic disease or syndrome.**
- **Oral candidiasis in children may indicate an underlying haematological or immunological problem.**
- **Gingivitis in preschool children is unusual and systemic disease should be excluded.**
- **If in doubt about oral lesions, ask an oral physician (dentist) for an opinion.**

Introduction

Lesions of the oral mucosa may occur in isolation, as a specific disease entity or as a manifestation of a systemic disease process, or can be iatrogenic or induced by exogenous agents. Oral lesions may be the presenting or main feature of a systemic disease. This chapter describes oral conditions occurring in childhood, which may present to the dermatologist or may be noted on examination by the dermatologist. However, it is beyond the scope of this chapter to discuss all the conditions mentioned in great detail; these may be found in specialist textbooks on the oral mucosa. This chapter does not cover diseases affecting the teeth.

Mouth ulcers/sore mouth

Stomatitis is a term used for inflammatory diseases of the oral mucosa, be they either acute or chronic. The symptom of sore mouth is usually caused by some form of stomatitis, the most common of which is oral ulceration, defined as a local discontinuity of the oral epithelium, but occasionally there is soreness in the absence of any clinical signs of mucosal disease. This section deals with the various causes of oral ulceration, including those related to systemic disease.

Recurrent aphthous stomatitis

Definition. After dental caries, periodontal disease and traumatic ulceration, recurrent aphthous stomatitis (RAS) is the most common disease affecting the mouth, with up to 20% of the population being affected. The condition is characterized by painful shallow ulcers, which heal and recur at fairly regular intervals, and the onset is typically in childhood, with a natural history of regression by adult life. RAS affects only the mouth and, by definition, patients are otherwise clinically well. Ulcers that mimic RAS may be caused by a number of factors, and these ulcers are termed aphthous-like ulceration (ALU) seen for example in autoinflammatory conditions such as periodic syndromes.

Aetiology. The aetiology of RAS is not known [1]. There does appear to be a genetic predisposition, with one-third of patients having a positive family history, and an increased frequency of HLA-A2, HLA-A11, HLA-B12 and HLA-DR2. Reports of immunological phenomena are either unconfirmed or disputed. There is no evidence to suggest that RAS is a classic autoimmune disease. In some patients there appears to be a relationship with stress, and some females exhibit ulceration in the luteal phase of

Harper's Textbook of Pediatric Dermatology, Fourth Edition. Edited by Peter Hoeger, Veronica Kinsler and Albert Yan.

their menstrual cycle, suggesting a hormonal association. Some patients relate their RAS to the ingestion of particular foodstuffs, such as cheese or chocolate.

About 10–20% of patients investigated with ulcers have an underlying haematinic deficiency, usually a low serum ferritin, vitamin B_{12} or red cell folate [2]. Some 3% of patients with ALU have been found to have coeliac disease. Other gastrointestinal diseases that can cause malabsorption and present with ulcers include Crohn disease and pernicious anaemia. ALU has also been described in association with human immunodeficiency virus (HIV) infection, Behçet syndrome, autoinflammatory conditions and Sweet syndrome.

Pathology. Ulceration is thought to be preceded by lymphocytic infiltration of the basal cell layer and perivascular accumulation of monocytes in the connective tissue, although this is seldom seen. Once the epithelium has ulcerated, the surface of the ulcer is covered by a fibrinous exudate (slough) and there is a superficial infiltrate of neutrophils. Monocytes predominate more deeply.

Histopathology is not diagnostic and the diagnosis is primarily dependent upon the clinical history.

Clinical features. RAS can be divided into three clinical types, which are summarized in Table 158.1

Minor aphthous stomatitis

Syn.
Mikulicz ulcers

Minor aphthae are the most common, accounting for 80% of RAS. Ulceration usually begins in childhood or adolescence with a female sex predilection of 3:1. The lesions are usually of less than 10 mm, an average size being 3–4 mm in diameter, and they occur in crops of between one and five ulcers on nonkeratinized mobile mucosa, i.e. floor of mouth, buccal or labial mucosa. The ulcers are round or ovoid, are shallow and have a white slough with an erythematous inflammatory halo. They heal within 7–10 days and rarely cause scarring (8%). They recur at intervals of between 1 and 4 months. However, crops of ulceration may be so frequent that the patient may never be ulcer free. As the child gets older, minor RAS tends to occur less frequently and may cease to be a problem.

Table 158.1 Clinical features of recurrent aphthous stomatitis

	Minor	Major	Herpetiform
Incidence	80%	10%	10%
Age (years)	10–19	10–19	20–29
Sex (F:M)	1.3:1	0.8:1	2.6:1
Site membranes	Nonkeratinized mucosa	Anywhere	Anywhere
Number	1–5	1–5	1–100
Size	<10 mm	>10 mm	1–2 mm
Duration (days)	7–10	7–10	7–10
Scarring	8%	64%	32%
Recurrence	1–4 months	<1 month	>1 month
Duration of disease (years)	<5	>15	>5

Major aphthous stomatitis

Syn.
Sutton's ulcers, periadenitis mucosa necrotica recurrens

Major aphthae account for about 10% of all RAS. They are much larger than minor aphthae (being greater than 10 mm in diameter), typically 1.5–3.0 cm in diameter. They can occur anywhere in the mouth in crops of one to six ulcers and are much more painful than minor aphthae. They may have a firm raised margin but otherwise, apart from their size, have a similar clinical appearance to minor aphthae (Fig. 158.1). They take a month or more to heal. Healing often occurs with fibrosis, resulting in scarring (64%). Recurrence usually occurs after a shorter interval (within 4 weeks) than in the case of minor aphthae.

Herpetiform ulceration

Herpetiform ulceration affects a slightly older age group (20–29 years). The clinical features are shown in Table 158.1.

Differential diagnosis. The diagnosis of RAS is made on the clinical appearance of the lesions and the clinical history. It is important to eliminate any underlying predisposing factors such as haematinic deficiencies or coeliac disease, and to ask if genital ulceration is present in order to exclude Behçet syndrome. Biopsy is rarely indicated but may need to be carried out on major aphthae that have failed to heal, to eliminate neoplasia.

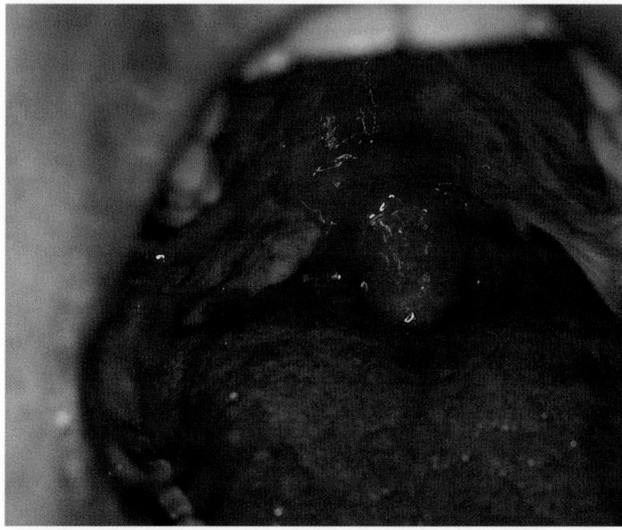

Fig. 158.1 Major aphthous ulceration of the palate.

Treatment. The management of RAS in children [3] is symptomatic and often unsuccessful, unless an underlying predisposing factor is identified and corrected. In the majority of patients, RAS resolves spontaneously with age. If symptomatic treatment is required, it is best to approach therapy systematically, working through a variety of topical agents, beginning with those that have few or no side-effects until one is found that provides symptomatic relief.

Chlorhexidine gluconate (0.2%) or benzydamine hydrochloride mouthwashes or sprays are a good starting point and often give good symptomatic relief. The spray forms of these agents are particularly useful in children.

Topical tetracycline mouthwash, made up from a 250 mg capsule of tetracycline in 5 mL of water, may be useful, particularly in herpetiform ulceration. However, it is unsuitable for young children because they may ingest some of the mouthwash which can cause tooth discolouration.

Topical steroids such as hydrocortisone hemisuccinate pellets (Corlan 2.5 mg four times daily) are often beneficial. Becotide inhaler (50 or 100 μg) may be used as a topical mouth spray four to six times per day. A mouthwash made up of soluble betametasone tablets (0.5 mg) in 15–20 mL of water and held in the mouth for 3 min four times a day may be of benefit to adolescents but is not suitable for young children.

Very occasionally, systemic steroids or other immunosuppressive agents such as azathioprine or colchicine have been necessary to control ulceration; their use in children must be carefully monitored and they should be used only as a last resort. There are multiple other 'therapies' available for RAS, including carbenoxolone, benzydamine, dapsone, cromoglycate, levamisole and anti-TNF agents such as pentoxyfylline or thalidomide and many others, but generally their efficacy has not been well proven or they have unacceptable adverse effects.

Autoinflammatory diseases

Autoinflammatory diseases are illnesses caused by primary dysfunction of the innate immune system and include a number of diseases, such as periodic syndromes, Crohn or Behcet disease, often presenting with oral ulceration and sometimes with recurrent attacks of fever, abdominal pain, arthritis or cutaneous signs, which may overlap and obscure an accurate diagnosis.

Behçet syndrome

Definition. Behçet syndrome is a multisystem disease in which the mouth is affected in most cases. Mouth lesions manifest as RAS. Other sites that may be affected include the genitals, eyes, skin and joints. There may be a number of other systemic or cutaneous manifestations. The clinical diagnosis of Behçet syndrome is dependent on the presence of at least three or more possible clinical manifestations, e.g. orogenital ulceration and uveitis (see Chapter 150).

Aetiology. The aetiology of Behçet syndrome is unknown. There is increasing evidence to suggest an immunological aetiology; however, immunological findings vary considerably and therefore cannot be used for the diagnosis or management of the disease. HLA-B5, HLA-BW51 and HLA-DR7 have been shown to be associated with Behçet syndrome.

Behçet syndrome can occur in any age group but most commonly affects adult males in their third decade, although it may occur in childhood. There is often a positive family history. There is also a higher prevalence of the disease in people from certain geographical areas, which include Japan, China, the Mediterranean and the Middle East [4].

Clinical features. The most common clinical feature is that of oral ulceration (90–100%), which may involve especially the posterior pharynx, and is indistinguishable clinically and histopathologically from RAS. Ulcers may occur at other sites, including the anus and genitals. Skin lesions such as erythema nodosum, pustules and pathergy are also common findings. The disease process is transient and subject to spontaneous remissions.

Differential diagnosis. Recurrent oral ulceration may be the first and only initial clinical feature of Behçet syndrome, but only a very few patients with recurrent oral ulcers develop Behçet syndrome; however, Behçet syndrome must always be excluded when considering a diagnosis of RAS because, unlike RAS, it is a systemic disorder and is not self-limiting.

Oral and genital ulceration may also result from folate deficiency and, together with ocular lesions, may occur in erythema multiforme and ulcerative colitis.

Treatment. Oral ulceration can be managed symptomatically as in RAS. Immunosuppressive treatment is required for those with other lesions. Results using ciclosporin and dapsone have been inconclusive, colchicine appears to be of value and thalidomide may be required in cases of recalcitrant orogenital ulceration but requires extreme caution because it is teratogenic.

MAGIC syndrome

This is a condition that overlaps with Behçet syndrome and causes large joint arthropathies. MAGIC is an acronym for mouth and genital ulcers with inflamed cartilage [5].

Local causes of mouth ulceration

Trauma, radiation, thermal or chemical agents may cause ulceration.

Traumatic ulceration

Trauma to the oral mucosa is common and may cause localized ulceration, which resolves as long as the causative agent is removed. It may be the result of sharp broken teeth, dental appliances or be self-inflicted, particularly with disorders such as congenital insensitivity to pain, Lesch–Nyhan syndrome, epilepsy, athetosis and learning impairment.

Clinical features. The clinical appearance of a traumatic ulcer is dependent upon the causative agent. Physical trauma gives rise to a localized ulcer that may resemble a minor or major aphthous ulcer. Tongue or cheek biting gives rise to a more irregularly shaped ulcer, often with a keratotic border. Thermal and chemical trauma caused by the ingestion of hot food or drinking caustic/acidic agents gives rise to more generalized ulceration, which tends to affect the tongue and palate. Ulcers may heal with scarring, especially if loss of connective tissue has occurred.

Oral ulceration may also be caused by nonaccidental injury. Oral ulceration caused by nonaccidental injury often occurs with other lesions extraorally or around the mouth and may involve the labial mucosa, particularly the labial fraenum, which may become torn and ulcerated by attempts to silence a child with a hand across the mouth.

Differential diagnosis. The possibility of other causes of oral ulceration should always be considered as described in this section.

Treatment. Usually no treatment is required other than reassurance. If soreness is a problem, benzydamine hydrochloride may be useful as either a mouthwash or a spray. If the ulcer has been caused by a sharp tooth or orthodontic appliance, appropriate modification should be carried out. If self-mutilation is a problem, the provision of polyvinyl occlusal splints may be useful. If an ulcer fails to heal within 2–3 weeks after the causative agent has been removed, a biopsy should be considered to exclude neoplasia.

If child abuse is suspected, appropriate action should be taken, which is usually dependent upon local guidelines.

Infections

A variety of infections may give rise to oral ulceration/stomatitis. These will be considered under three main groups: viral, fungal and bacterial.

Viral infections

The acute viral infections of childhood may give rise to oral ulceration and symptoms. The symptoms of acute viral infections affecting the mouth are all very similar, but the distribution of lesions may vary. Generally, if a viral infection is suspected, the diagnosis is made on clinical and epidemiological information. It is only where virus identification is of importance, such as in immunocompromised patients, that culture and polymerase chain reaction (PCR) studies to identify the virus are undertaken.

Herpetic gingivostomatitis (see Chapter 50)

Aetiology. Herpes simplex virus type 1 and increasingly type 2 cause primary herpetic gingivostomatitis. Primary herpes most commonly occurs in young children (2–4 years old) and is often subclinical; however, many children now reach maturity without acquiring immunity to the virus, giving rise to an increased incidence of primary herpes infections in young adults. Primary herpes infection is twice as common in lower socio-economic groups. Herpes simplex virus is found in the saliva in both primary and secondary infections, and may be spread in this way. The incubation period is 3–7 days.

Pathology. Well-defined fluid-filled vesicles form in the upper epithelium. The vesicles rupture, infecting the epithelium throughout its entire thickness. Ulceration is caused by shedding of the virus-damaged epithelial cells.

Clinical features. The lesions consist of well-defined vesicles of about 2 mm in diameter, which may coalesce to form larger irregular lesions that may be distributed over the entire oral mucosa and gingivae but are commonly seen on the dorsum of the tongue and the hard palate. The vesicles rapidly rupture to form circular, sharply defined shallow ulcers with a yellowish-grey floor and erythematous margin (Fig. 158.2). The ulcers are very painful. The gingival margins are usually enlarged and inflamed. There is often associated cervical lymphadenopathy, pyrexia and general malaise. Diagnosis is usually made on the clinical features.

Differential diagnosis. Acute ulcerative gingivitis, erythema multiforme and leukaemia may occasionally give a similar clinical appearance, as may hand, foot and mouth disease and herpangina (see later). Gingival enlargement may be seen in acute childhood leukaemia, particularly the myeloid type.

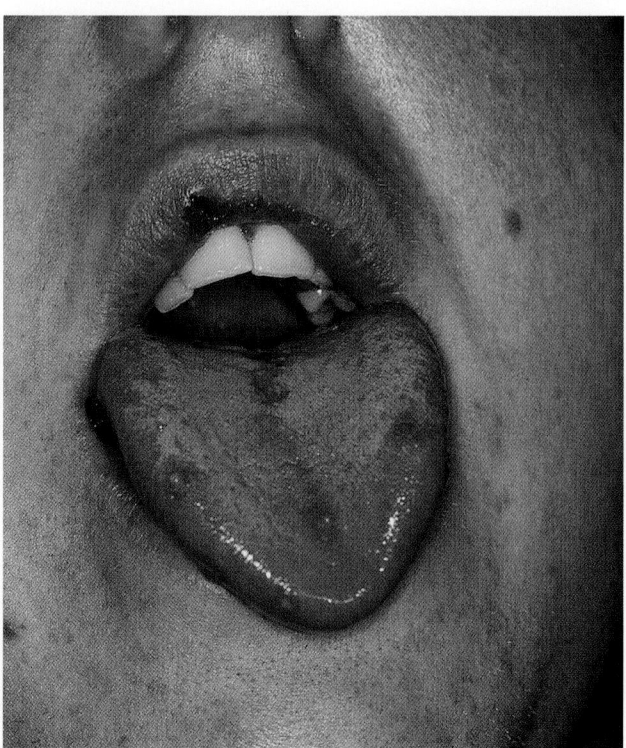

Fig. 158.2 Ulceration of the tongue and labial mucosa caused by primary herpes virus infection.

Treatment. In most cases, the infection resolves spontaneously with 7–10 days. For the majority of patients the management is supportive, with antipyretic analgesics (e.g. paracetamol/acetaminophen), bed rest and adequate fluid intake. Chlorhexidine gluconate 0.2% mouthwash or spray may help to prevent secondary infection of the ulcers.

Systemic aciclovir or similar antiviral agents hasten recovery but are only really useful if used in the first 3 days of onset, during the vesicular stage of infection [6]. Because most cases present in the ulcerative phase, this is of little benefit. Aciclovir does have a role to play if patients are immunocompromised, and in rare complications such as encephalitis and neuropathy.

Recurrent herpes simplex

Following primary infection, the herpes virus remains latent in the trigeminal ganglion. About one-third of patients experience recurrent herpes infections, the most common form of which is herpes labialis (cold sore) (Fig. 158.3). Typical triggering events include exposure to sunlight, infections such as the common cold, stress and trauma.

Intraoral recurrence often manifests as a dendritic ulcer on the tongue or palate. Chronic ulceration of this type or nodular lesions can occur in immunosuppressed individuals and may require treatment with systemic aciclovir.

Aciclovir-resistant herpes simplex infection

Severely immunocompromised children, such as those undergoing bone marrow transplantation, may develop aciclovir-resistant herpes simplex infections. The clinical appearance of this condition is almost pathognomonic of the infection (Figs 158.4 and 158.5). The lesions present as well-defined oral ulcers with a characteristic adherent greyish-white slough, which has a leathery texture [7].

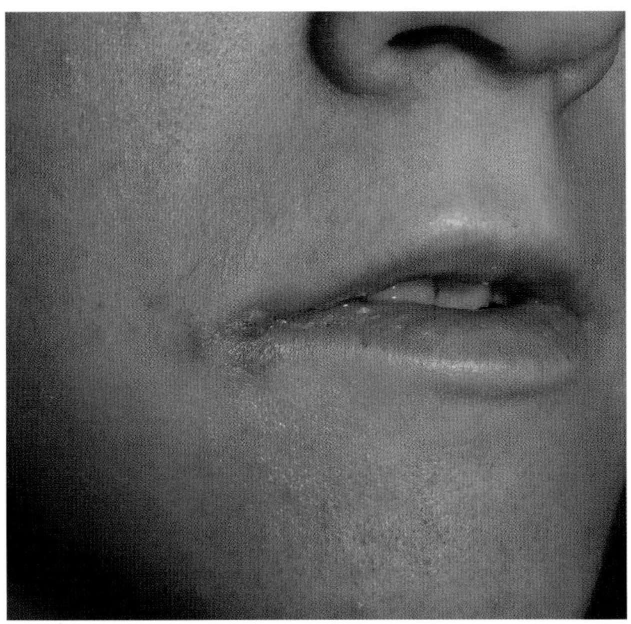

Fig. 158.3 Herpes labialis.

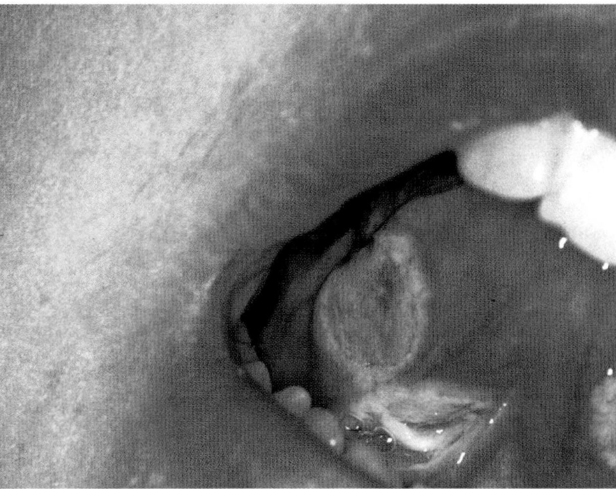

Fig. 158.4 Aciclovir-resistant herpes on the ventral surface of the tongue of a child following bone marrow transplantation. Note the well-defined lesion and the absence of an inflammatory reaction surrounding the lesion.

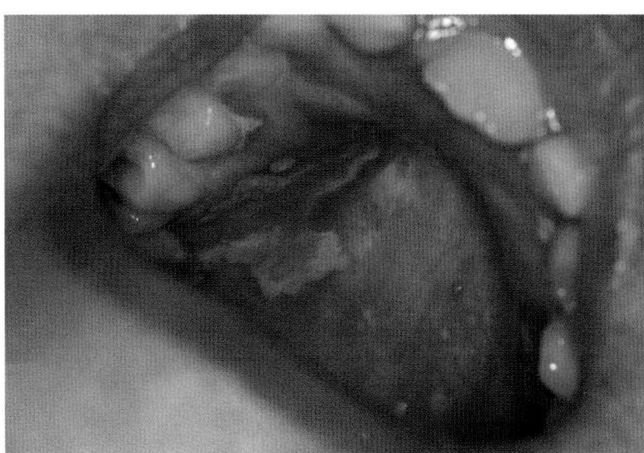

Fig. 158.5 Aciclovir-resistant herpes on the hard palate of a child following bone marrow transplantation.

The usual oral features of either primary or recurrent herpes are not usually present. The patients are nearly always on a prophylactic regimen of aciclovir and many have a history of previous herpes labialis [8]. The herpes virus may also be resistant to ganciclovir and foscarnet, which is nephrotoxic and has been used to treat the virus. Valaciclovir and cidofovir are alternative treatments. Aciclovir-resistant herpes simplex virus has also been reported in immune incompetence as a result of HIV infection and Wiskott–Aldrich syndrome [9].

Chickenpox

Chickenpox is caused by the varicella zoster virus. Lesions occur mainly over the trunk but may also occur intraorally. The oral lesions appear as vesicles, which break down to form discrete, well-defined ulcers. They are usually fewer in number than in primary herpes and there is no associated gingival enlargement.

Herpes zoster (shingles)

Herpes zoster may give rise to oral lesions if the maxillary or mandibular branch of the trigeminal nerve is involved. Ulcers appear in the distribution of the affected nerve; the lesions do not cross the midline and are preceded by a toothache-like pain. It is rare to see herpes zoster in childhood unless the child is immunocompromised or the mother was infected during pregnancy.

Chikungunya virus
Chikungunya virus (CHIKV) is a lavivirus transmitted mainly by mosquitoes, causing fever and joint pains, similar to Dengue fever. CHIKV can cause oral/nasal haemorrhagic lesions and more than 50% of CHIKV-infected people experience gingival bleeding.

Ebola virus
Ebola virus (EBOV) is highly lethal flavivirus infection, transmitted via bats and mammalian (monkey and ape) bush meat, causing haemorrhagic fever in humans and oral ulceration and bleeding.

Enteroviruses
At least 70 serotypes of enteroviruses (EV) that can infect humans have been identified, including mainly Coxsackie viruses (groups A and B), enteric cytopathic human orphan (ECHO) viruses and polioviruses. Recently, the EV genus has been reclassificated in five species: human enteroviruses A, B, C, and D and poliovirus. Enteroviruses are implicated in a range of diseases, some of which may affect the mouth, including herpangina and hand-foot and mouth disease (HFMD) which are common and in which complications including pneumonia, meningitis, or encephalitis are seen but rarely.

Herpangina. Herpangina is typically caused by Coxsackie viruses A1 to 6, 8, 10, and 22. Other cases are caused by Coxsackie group B (strains 1-4), ECHO viruses and other enteroviruses. Papulovesicular oropharyngeal lesions progress to ulcers and there is usually no rash.

Children with Coxsackie A2 infections mostly present with herpangina only and have fewer central nervous system complications and a better outcome than those with enterovirus 71 (EV71) infections.

The infection is usually confined to children and presents as an acute pharyngitis with lymphadenopathy and pyrexia. Oral lesions are localized to the soft palate; they resemble those of primary herpes. There is no gingival involvement. The infection resolves spontaneously in 10–14 days. Treatment is supportive, as described for primary herpes.

Hand, foot and mouth disease. Hand, foot and mouth disease (HRMD) often causes minor epidemics among school children. It is caused by a Coxsackie A virus, usually A10 or A16, or occasionally a Coxsackie B or other enterovirus.

HFMD is an exanthem on the hands and feet with associated fever and oral lesions. HFMD is typically a mild illness, caused mainly by Coxsackie virus A16 or EV71, occasionally by Coxsackie viruses A4–7, A9, A 10, B1–B3 or B5. Indeed, over 100 serotypes of enterovirus species may cause HFMD. EV71 is an important public health problem in Asia as it spreads easily to close contacts and may cause central nervous system involvement, serious illness and rarely death.

Clinically, the oral lesions resemble those of primary herpes, although they occur in much smaller numbers and cause few symptoms. As in herpangina, the gingivae are not involved. Cutaneous lesions affect the hands and feet and consist of small deep-seated vesicles, with surrounding erythema situated on the digits or base of the phalanges. Management is as for herpangina.

Infectious mononucleosis (Epstein–Barr viral infection)
Infectious mononucleosis is caused by the Epstein–Barr virus (EBV). In the Western world, it is more common in teenagers and young adults, but it may occur in children. Oral symptoms include sore throat, and palatal petechiae are often evident. Occasionally, there may be severe ulceration of the fauces; less severe nonspecific oral ulceration and pericoronitis may also occur.

Cytomegalovirus infection
Cytomegalovirus (CMV) may cause a glandular fever-type illness but rarely causes oral ulceration. CMV-induced ulcers have been described in immunosuppressed patients [10]. Persistent oral ulcers in immunosuppressed patients should be biopsied and sent for histopathology, microbiological culture and PCR DNA studies.

Human immunodeficiency virus
Oral ulceration may occur in children who are HIV positive. Clinically, they are often aphthous-like [11] and may be treated as such. However, the possibility of another infective cause should always be considered, e.g. CMV [12].

Zika virus
Zika virus (ZIKV) infection is a mosquito-borne flavivirus disease, associated mainly with Guillain-Barré syndrome. Fetal microcephaly and aphthous-type oral ulcers have been observed

Fungal infections

Oral fungal infections rarely cause ulceration of the oral mucosa in the Western world except in immunocompromised or debilitated patients. In the tropics, otherwise healthy individuals may occasionally present with oral ulcerated fungal lesions caused by endemic deep mycoses.

Deep mycoses
Deep mycotic infections are uncommon in the UK but are seen in Latin America and some parts of the southern USA. Oral lesions are most common in histoplasmosis and paracoccidioidomycosis but have been described in all mycoses. The oral lesions are not distinctive and diagnosis is usually made on biopsy.

The following deep mycoses may give rise to oral ulceration in the immunocompromised child, particularly those undergoing cytotoxic chemotherapy or bone marrow transplantation, or in patients with acquired immune deficiency syndrome (AIDS). They should always be

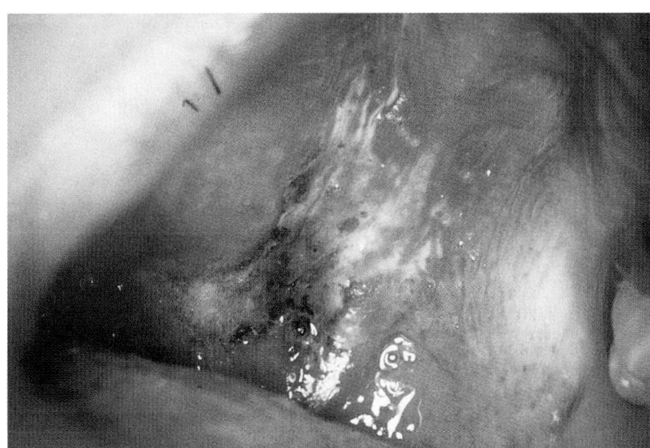

Fig. 158.6 Necrotic ulceration of the hard palate caused by antral aspergillosis in a child following bone marrow transplantation.

considered as part of the differential diagnosis in the immunocompromised and, if necessary, biopsied to exclude them as causative agents.

Aspergillosis may cause black necrotic ulceration of the palate (Fig. 158.6). The infection usually originates from infection in the maxillary sinuses and is caused by direct invasion of the palate. Diagnosis is made from biopsy and radiographic examination of the paranasal air sinuses. Treatment is usually with intravenous itraconazole or amphotericin.

Mucormycosis (zygomycosis, phycomycosis) is an infection with a fungus associated with mouldy bread, that may give rise to a similar clinical picture to aspergillosis. It is a condition that has been associated with uncontrolled diabetes mellitus.

Histoplasmosis oral lesions are uncommon and present as a nonspecific ulcer or lump. They are usually seen in chronic disseminated histoplasmosis.

Bacterial infections

Acute ulcerative gingivitis

Acute ulcerative gingivitis (AUG) is an uncommon disease in childhood and may be associated with immune deficiency such as AIDS and cytotoxic chemotherapy. In countries where nutrition is poor, it can manifest as cancrum oris (noma), causing massive soft tissue destruction. It is thought to be caused by a proliferation of two normal oral commensals, the Gram-negative anaerobes *Borrelia vincentii* and *Fusobacterium nucleatum*.

Classically, AUG begins on the tips of the interdental papillae, causing intense pain and halitosis. Spontaneous bleeding of the gingivae may occur. The ulceration spreads along the gingival margin but is well localized. In the immunocompromised child, the ulceration may be far more destructive and spread on to the palate and buccal sulci. Histologically, there is intense inflammation and destruction of the epithelium and connective tissue.

When occurring in a young child, primary herpetic gingivostomatitis may give a similar gingival appearance, but it is unusual for ulceration to be localized to the gingivae. Systemic upset is usually more severe in primary herpes.

AUG responds rapidly to metronidazole therapy three times daily for 3 days, the dose depending upon age. If the child is immunocompromised, a longer course and higher dose may be indicated. Local measures such as improving oral hygiene and the use of an antibacterial mouthwash (e.g. chlorhexidine gluconate 0.2%) should also be considered.

Other bacterial infections

Tuberculosis and syphilis are rare causes of chronic mouth ulcers.

Oral ulceration in association with neoplasia

Oral carcinoma is extremely rare in children. Very occasionally, oral ulceration may be the presenting feature of a malignant lesion, particularly lymphoma or histiocytosis. Any chronic oral ulcer in a child with no obvious causative factors should therefore be biopsied.

Oral ulceration associated with systemic disease

Oral ulceration may occasionally be the presenting feature of a systemic disease. The relationship of oral ulceration to systemic diseases will be discussed in this section with reference only to the systemic disease and oral features.

Haematological and immunological disorders

Haematinic deficiencies are discussed above. Immunodeficiencies, whether congenital or acquired, may also give rise to oral ulceration. These ulcers usually resemble recurrent aphthae but if a neutropenia is present, they lack the erythematous inflammatory halo, as in cyclic or hereditary benign neutropenias (Fig. 158.7).

Gastrointestinal disease

As discussed with RAS, haematinic deficiencies may give rise to oral ulceration, therefore any gastrointestinal disease causing malabsorption predisposes the child to oral ulceration.

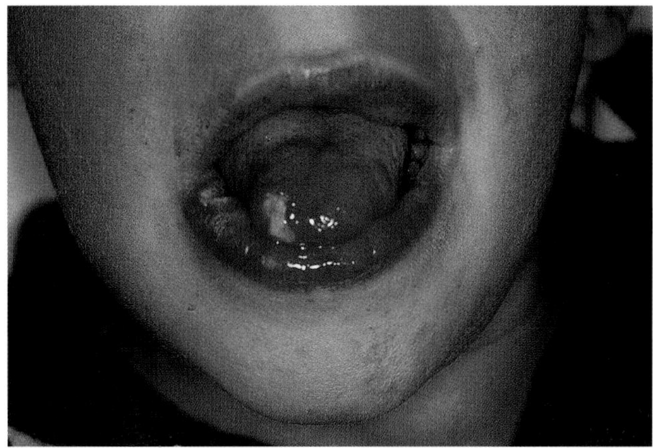

Fig. 158.7 Neutropenic ulcers in a child with familial chronic neutropenia. Note the lack of inflammation surrounding the ulcers.

Coeliac disease (gluten-sensitive enteropathy)

Older children and adolescents with undiagnosed coeliac disease may occasionally present with sore mouths. Oral manifestations include recurrent ulcers, glossitis, angular stomatitis and dental hypoplasia, related to underlying haematinic and vitamin deficiencies.

Inflammatory bowel diseases

This relates to the oral manifestations seen in Crohn disease and ulcerative colitis [13].

Crohn disease. Oral lesions related to Crohn disease are more prevalent in children and include facial or labial swelling (orofacial granulomatosis), oral ulcers, which may be large and ragged or linear in appearance, mucosal tagging or proliferation of the oral mucosa to give a 'cobblestone' appearance. Other lesions, such as ulcers and glossitis, may be caused by an associated nutritional deficiency caused by malabsorption or may be coincidental.

Oral lesions may occur prior to any gastrointestinal symptoms. Biopsy of the oral lesions will confirm the diagnosis, histology showing noncaseating granulomas in the corium with an overlying normal or ulcerated epithelium. Differential diagnosis includes orofacial granulomatosis, sarcoidosis and tuberculosis. Treatment of the oral lesions is dependent upon whether there is active gastrointestinal disease. If systemic corticosteroid or aminosalicylate therapy for active gastrointestinal disease is used, the oral lesions may also improve; if oral lesions remain symptomatic or occur in isolation, local measures to control the symptoms, such as those used in RAS, may be adequate.

Orofacial granulomatosis is a term given to labial or gingival swelling caused by a granulomatous reaction but without any detectable systemic cause, e.g. Crohn disease, sarcoidosis. Some patients with this diagnosis will go on to develop a systemic disease some time later. In other cases, the granulomatous reaction is thought to be caused by a food allergy, particularly to cinnamon-containing foodstuffs. Exclusion of cinnamon from the diet of these individuals may allow resolution of the lesions. A short course of high-dose or intralesional steroids may reduce the swelling [14].

Ulcerative colitis. Oral lesions associated with ulcerative colitis may occur in up to a third of children diagnosed with ulcerative colitis and include aphthous-type ulceration and glossitis, which may be associated with anaemia. Other oral lesions are rare and include: haemorrhagic ulceration of the mucosa; chronic oral ulceration; pyostomatitis gangrenosum and pyostomatitis vegetans, which clinically are analogous to cutaneous pyoderma gangrenosum and gives rise to hyperplastic folds of the oral mucosa between which microabscesses or fissures form with multiple yellowish pustules on the mucosa.

Behçet syndrome should be considered in the differential diagnosis of oral lesions. Treatment is the same as in Crohn disease, oral lesions being more apparent with exacerbations of bowel inflammation.

Dermatological disorders

Dermatological disorders rarely cause mouth ulcers in children; if they do occur, skin lesions can often aid diagnosis.

Lichen planus, lichenoid reactions and chronic graft-versus-host disease

Lichen planus is rare in childhood. It should be considered in the differential diagnosis of oral white lesions in children, particularly in children of Asian origin [15]. Drug-induced lichenoid lesions may occur; they are particularly associated with the use of anti-inflammatory agents, antihypertensives and antimalarial drugs. Graft-versus-host disease (GVHD) following organ or bone marrow transplantation may also give rise to lichenoid lesions.

Clinically, several forms of lichen planus may be observed. Reticular and papular lichen planus is usually asymptomatic and is usually symmetrically distributed on the buccal mucosa and lateral borders of the tongue. It may resemble oral thrush, particularly if it is plaque-like in appearance. These white forms of lichen planus often require no treatment if they are symptomless.

Atrophic or erosive lichen planus is symptomatic and may be seen in GVHD. It presents as erosive, often linear ulcers, which affect any site but commonly the tongue and buccal mucosa (Fig. 158.8). It is unlikely to be the only clinical manifestation of GVHD. Skin and liver GVHD are often concurrent, requiring the use of immunosuppressive therapy. The immunosuppressive therapy does not always resolve the oral GVHD, and topical steroid therapy using Becotide inhaler (50 or 100 μg) as a topical mouth spray four to six times per day, together with soluble betametasone 0.5 mg (Betnesol) used as a mouthwash (dissolved in 25 mL of water) and held in the mouth for 2–3 min four times per day, may aid healing and improve symptoms. Benzydamine hydrochloride mouthwash or spray may also be of symptomatic use. It is also important to keep the mouth as clean as possible to prevent secondary infection. Because tooth brushing may be painful, the use of chlorhexidine

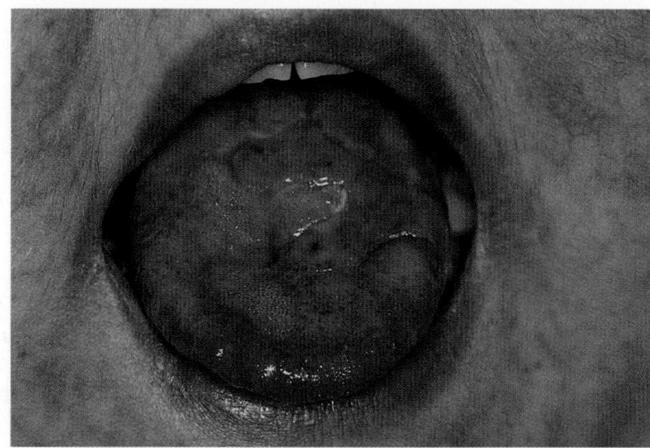

Fig. 158.8 Erosive lichen planus-like lesions of the tongue caused by graft-versus-host disease. Note also the depapillation of the tongue.

gluconate mouthwash 0.2% or spray twice daily may be helpful. As the GVHD responds to the immunosuppressive therapy, oral lesions usually resolve.

Vesiculobullous disorders

The dermatological conditions that cause vesiculobullous lesions in the mouth, such as pemphigus vulgaris and mucous membrane pemphigoid, are rare in childhood (see Chapter 74)

Epidermolysis bullosa

In most forms of epidermolysis bullosa, bullae will form on the oral mucosa. They usually appear in infancy and may be precipitated by suckling. The bullae break down to form ulcers, which heal slowly, usually with scarring. The tongue becomes depapillated. Because of the sensitivity of the mucosa to trauma, oral hygiene is usually poor and the incidence of caries and periodontal disease is therefore high. Epidermolysis bullosa is covered in more detail in Chapter 76.

Dermatitis herpetiformis and linear IgA disease

Dermatitis herpetiformis may occur in childhood and is often associated with gluten enteropathy. Oral lesions may occur and include erythematous papules and macules, petechiae, vesicles, bullae and erosions. Similar oral lesions may occur in linear immunoglobulin A (IgA) disease. Oral lesions rarely occur in isolation and will respond to therapy for cutaneous lesions, dapsone or sulfapyridine. Diagnosis is made on biopsy. Dermatitis herpetiformis is covered in more detail in Chapter 75.

Erythema multiforme

Oral features characteristically include swollen, bleeding, crusted lips and widespread oral ulceration. Oral ulcers are preceded by erythematous macules, which become vesicles. Intact vesicles are rarely seen as they rapidly break down to form ill-defined ulcers. The tongue is often furred and there may be regional lymphadenitis. Oral lesions may occur in isolation or with a skin rash, which characteristically consists of 'target' lesions and ocular involvement.

The combination of oral lesions, skin lesions and conjunctivitis is referred to as Stevens–Johnson syndrome.

Biopsy may be necessary in less characteristic cases and will exclude other vesiculobullous disorders and Behçet syndrome.

Aciclovir may be beneficial prophylactically in herpes-precipitated erythema multiforme.

Erythema multiforme is covered in more detail in Chapter 66.

Connective tissue disorders

Connective tissue disorders may give rise to oral ulceration, e.g. systemic and discoid lupus erythematosus. Juvenile idiopathic arthritis may be associated with anaemia, which may predispose to RAS. Felty syndrome is most likely to cause ulceration, presumably because of the associated neutropenia. Behçet syndrome may occur in childhood and is discussed above.

Iatrogenic oral ulceration

Oral ulceration may regularly be caused by certain drugs, e.g. cytotoxic agents. The ulceration is usually aphthous-like in appearance but may lack an inflammatory halo if associated with neutropenia. It is self-limiting and heals within 7–10 days. It is now less commonly seen in association with methotrexate as folic acid is now routinely given with methotrexate therapy. Aphthous-type ulceration can also occur in long-term use of some drugs, such as phenytoin or cotrimoxazole, which interfere with folate metabolism. Aplastic anaemia may also be drug induced and give rise to oral ulceration and purpura.

Radiation to the head and neck, and total body irradiation for bone marrow transplantation, gives rise to mucositis, which occurs 7–10 days after starting radiotherapy to the head and neck, and lasts for up to 4 weeks after completion of treatment. Those patients undergoing total body irradiation experience mucositis within 5–10 days and the mucositis heals within 2–3 weeks of treatment. Various agents have been used to decrease the amount of mucositis and improve healing; however, none has been particularly successful apart from oral cooling with ice. Treatment therefore remains symptomatic; benzydamine hydrochloride and chlorhexidine mouthwash may help alleviate symptoms.

References

1 Scully C, Gorsky M, Lozada-Nur F. The diagnosis and management of recurrent aphthous stomatitis: a consensus approach. J Am Dent Assoc 2003;134:200–7.
2 Field AE, Brookes V, Tyldesley W. Recurrent aphthous ulceration in children: a review. Int J Paediatr Dent 1992;2:1–10.
3 Montgomery-Cranny JA, Wallace A, Rogers HJ et al. Management of recurrent aphthous stomatitis in children. Dent Update 2015;42:564–6, 569–72.
4 Escudier M, Bagan J, Scully C. Behcets syndrome (Adamantiades syndrome). Oral Dis 2006;12:78–84.
5 Firestein GS, Gruber HE, Weisman MH et al. Mouth and genital ulcers with inflamed cartilage: MAGIC syndrome. Am J Med 1985;79:65–71.
6 Amir J, Harel L, Smetana Z et al. Treatment of herpes simplex gingivostomatitis with aciclovir in children: a randomized double blind placebo controlled study. BMJ 1997;314:1800–3.
7 Brooke AE, Eveson JW, Luker J et al. Oral presentation of a novel variant of herpes simplex in a group of bone marrow transplant patients: a report of five cases. Br J Dermatol 1999;141:381–3.
8 Venard V, Dauendorffer JN, Carrett AS et al. Infection due to aciclovir resistant herpes simplex virus in patients undergoing allogeneic haematopoetic stem cell transplantation. Pathol Biol 2001;49:553–8.
9 Saijo M, Suzutani T, Murono K et al. Recurrent aciclovir resistant herpes simplex in a child with Wiskott–Aldrich syndrome. Br J Dermatol 1998;139:311–14.
10 Epstein J, Scully C. Cytomegalovirus: a virus of increasing relevance to oral medicine. J Oral Pathol Med 1993;22:348–53.
11 Scully C, Laskaris G, Porter SR. Oral manifestations of HIV infection and their management. II. Less common lesions. Oral Surg Oral Med Oral Pathol 1991;71:167–71.
12 Scully C. The HIV global pandemic: the development, and emerging implications. Oral Dis 1997;3(suppl 1):1–6.
13 Katsanos KH, Torres J, Roda G et al. Review article: non-malignant oral manifestations in inflammatory bowel diseases. Aliment Pharmacol Ther 2015;42:40–60.
14 Grave B, McCullough M, Wiesenfeld D. Orofacial granulomatosis – a 20-year review. Oral Dis 2009;15:46–51.
15 Alam F, Hamburger J. Oral mucosal lichen planus in children. Int J Paediatr Dent 2001;11:209–14.

White patches (leucoplakia)

Definition of leucoplakia

The term 'leucoplakia' is often used clinically to describe a chronic white lesion of the oral mucosa. However, it should really be restricted to those white lesions for which there is no identifiable cause or underlying disease process.

Normal anatomy

Fordyce spots or granules

Fordyce spots are sebaceous glands that are present beneath the oral mucosa. Although they are present at birth, they do not usually become clinically apparent until puberty. They appear as asymptomatic, slightly raised yellowish nodules usually on the buccal mucosa, just inside the commissure or the labial and retromolar mucosa. They may be discrete or coalescent.

Diagnosis is made on the clinical appearance. Treatment involves reassurance that they are a normal feature of the oral mucosa.

Gingival cysts of infancy (Epstein pearls and Bohn nodules)

These cysts are commonly seen in the newborn. They either rupture spontaneously or involute and are rarely apparent after 3 months or age. They arise from remnants of the dental laminae on the alveolus (Epstein pearls) or epithelial inclusion at a site of fusion, e.g. midline of the palate (Bohn nodules). Clinically, they appear as 2–3 mm diameter white nodules on the crests of the alveolar ridge or the midline of the palate. Because they resolve spontaneously, no treatment is required.

Congenital/inherited causes of white patches

White sponge naevus (familial white folded gingivostomatitis)

This is a rare condition, inherited as an autosomal dominant trait, which results in the formation of widespread white plaques of the oral mucosa caused by abnormal tonofilament organization. Other mucosae may be affected. The epithelium appears hyperplastic and has a thick, irregular parakeratotic layer which, as a result of epithelial oedema, has a so-called 'basket-weave' appearance. White sponge naevus is caused by mutations in either the *KRT3* or *KRT14* gene.

The clinical appearance is very distinctive and is often first noticed in childhood. The oral mucosa is irregularly thickened, folded and appears white. Unlike other white lesions, there is no clear margin to the lesion and it merges imperceptibly with normal mucosa. The buccal mucosa is usually affected but the entire oral mucosa may be involved; the attached gingivae are usually spared. The clinical appearance is usually sufficient to diagnose the condition and a positive family history is helpful. Biopsy may be necessary to eliminate other causes of white patches in less classic cases. Because the condition is asymptomatic and benign, no treatment is required other than reassurance.

Darier–White disease (dyskeratosis follicularis)

Inherited as an autosomal dominant disorder of keratinization, this condition manifests in early adolescence (see Chapter 130). Oral lesions occur in about 50% of affected individuals and their appearance has no significance in relation to the intensity of skin involvement.

Clinically, the lesions consist of flattish initially erythematous papules, which coalesce to give a cobblestone appearance. The lesions become progressively paler until they are white. The lesions tend to occur on the tongue, palate and gingivae [1]. Palatal lesions can resemble nicotinic stomatitis.

Tylosis (palmoplantar keratoderma) and Clouston syndrome

Tylosis is inherited as an autosomal dominant trait and is discussed in Chapter 128. Orally, preleucoplakia lesions have been reported in most affected children [2]. These lesions are diffuse and greyish in colour; they go on to form nonspecific leucoplakia with increasing age and do not appear to be potentially malignant.

Clouston syndrome (hidrotic ectodermal dysplasia), which also causes palmoplantar hyperkeratosis, may give rise to oral leucoplakia [3].

Pachyonychia congenita

Pachyonychia congenita is discussed in Chapter 128. Oral lesions occur in 60% of affected individuals and present as focal or generalized greyish-white thickening of the oral mucosa. They do not have an increased malignant potential [4]. Vesicular and ulcerative oral lesions have also been described. Of affected individuals, 10% have angular cheilitis, and there is an increased risk of chronic candidiasis in this group. Natal or neonatal teeth may also be present in 16% of individuals [5].

Dyskeratosis congenita

This is a rare disorder with both a sex-linked and a recessive form. The main features include dysplastic lesions of the oral mucosa, dermal pigmentation, nail dystrophy and aplastic anaemia (see Chapter 140).

Oral lesions usually occur between the ages of 5 and 10 years and consist of white patches, usually affecting the palate or tongue, which may be preceded by vesicles or erosions [5,6]. Oral lesions may also manifest as small erythematous areas. Biopsy of the lesion shows dysplasia and there is a high risk of malignant change. Regular review and rebiopsy of lesions are essential.

Hereditary benign intraepithelial dyskeratosis

This is a very rare autosomal dominant condition in which oral lesions occur in childhood and become more obvious by adolescence. They consist of milky white, smooth translucent plaques that predominantly affect the buccal mucosa, lips and ventrum of the tongue. Biopsy may be necessary to differentiate from white sponge naevus and other white lesions. No treatment is required.

Acquired transient white lesions

Traumatic/frictional keratosis

Frictional keratosis is caused by chronic irritation of the oral epithelium, which causes hyperkeratosis. It is often caused by a sharp tooth or restoration, or by a habit such as cheek biting. Clinically, the relationship of the keratosis to a causative factor should be established. On removal of the causative agent or cessation of the habit, resolution of the keratosis should occur.

Chemical trauma to the oral mucosa may also lead to a transient white lesion. Children may occasionally ingest caustic or acidic agents, e.g. household cleaning agents, which cause epithelial cell death, clinically appearing as a soft white patch. Aspirin, which should not be administered to children, can cause burns as a result of an aspirin being placed next to a painful tooth. In this case, the white plaque is localized.

Materia alba

Debris collecting on the gingivae in uncleaned mouths may mimic thrush, and is termed materia alba.

Furred/hairy tongue

See Lesions of the tongue, later.

Koplik spots

Koplik spots are an oral manifestation of measles. They appear as small white lesions resembling grains of salt on the buccal mucosa. Their appearance may precede the cutaneous skin rash by 1–2 days. Measles is an uncommon childhood infectious illness in areas where there is a measles immunization programme.

Candidiasis (candidosis)

This is an acute or chronic infection of the oral mucosa caused by invasion of the epithelium by candidal hyphae, which usually induce a proliferative response and cause a plaque to form.

Candida species are isolated in about 50% of the population as a normal oral commensal organism, the most common species being *Candida albicans. Candida krusei, C. guilliermondii, C. tropicalis* and *C. parapsilosis* may also be implicated, especially in the immunocompromised patient. Should the balance of the oral environment be disturbed (e.g. systemic infection, use of an orthodontic or other dental appliance, suppression of cell-mediated immunity, iron deficiency, diabetes), candidal organisms may proliferate and give rise to infection. Candidiasis is the most common oral manifestation of HIV disease.

Chronic mucocutaneous candidiasis is characterized by persistent candidiasis, which usually begins in early childhood, involving the skin, mucous membranes and nails. About 50% of patients have an associated endocrinopathy, which is usually preceded by candidiasis. Of all patients, 20% have a family history.

The clinical features of oral candidiasis are dependent upon whether the infection is acute or chronic. The various clinical entities are discussed below.

Acute pseudo-membranous candidiasis (thrush)

Thrush is typically seen in the neonatal period when immune mechanisms have not fully developed. It may also be seen in children who are compromised in some way. The lesions are usually asymptomatic and manifest as thick creamy plaques which are easily wiped off the oral mucosa, leaving an erythematous area of mucosa. The lesions may occur in any area of the mouth but are commonly seen on the soft palate and fauces (Fig. 158.9).

On direct smear with a Gram or periodic acid–Schiff (PAS) stain, masses of candidal hyphae may be seen with a few yeast cells. The plaques are formed by proliferation of the epithelium in response to invasion by candidal hyphae. The plaque consists of epithelial cells that are separated by inflammatory infiltrate, making the plaque friable. The deeper epithelium is hyperplastic and there is an acute inflammatory reaction in the connective tissue. Sections stained with PAS show candidal hyphae growing downwards through the epithelium.

If no predisposing factor is evident, investigation should be undertaken to establish why candidiasis has occurred, e.g. anaemia, diabetes mellitus or immunodeficiency. If the child is known to be immunocompromised, it is important to culture the lesions for species other than *C. albicans*, such as *C. kruseii*, which is inherently resistant to some antifungal agents [7].

In the majority of cases, topical antifungal therapy is usually adequate to treat the infection. Nystatin suspension or pastilles can be used or amphotericin B lozenges or miconazole oral gel used four times per day for 10–14 days. If the lesions fail to respond to topical antifungals, systemic use of fluconazole or itraconazole should be considered.

Erythematous candidiasis

Candidal infection may cause erythematous lesions, such as in chronic denture stomatitis and candidiasis associated with xerostomia and the use of topical steroid inhalers. However, the term 'erythematous candidiasis' is now frequently used to describe the patchy erythematous lesions associated with HIV infection. Treatment is as for thrush.

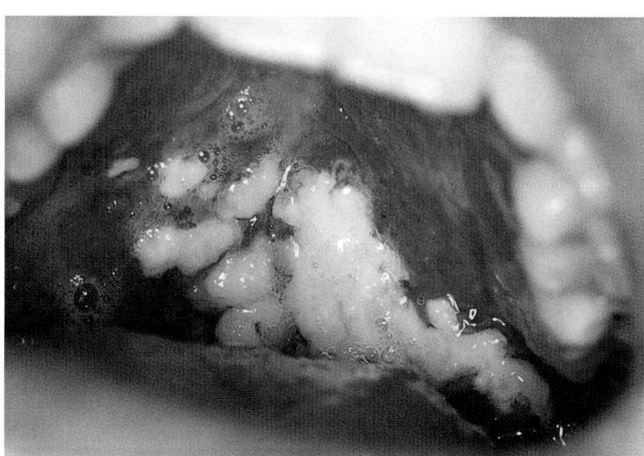

Fig. 158.9 Acute pseudo-membranous candidiasis in a child undergoing chemotherapy for acute leukaemia.

Chronic atrophic candidiasis (chronic denture stomatitis)

This condition is often seen under the fitting surface of upper dentures, hence the term 'denture-related stomatitis'. It may also occur under a removable orthodontic appliance. It is bright red in appearance and is clearly restricted to the area under the appliance. Candidal hyphae can be isolated from the mucosa and the porous acrylic surface of the appliance. The infection is caused by the continuous wearing of the appliance, which prevents debridement of the covered mucosa and forms a warm moist environment that favours the proliferation of candidal organisms.

Histologically, the epithelium exhibits acanthosis with an oedematous superficial layer. The underlying connective tissue contains a chronic inflammatory cell infiltrate.

Chronic atrophic candidiasis usually resolves if the appliance is removed from the mouth for a few hours each day, cleaned thoroughly and soaked in chlorhexidine or a mild hypochlorite solution, e.g. Milton. If this is not possible, miconazole gel can be applied to the mucosal surface of the appliance four times per day. When the appliance is no longer needed, the candidiasis will resolve spontaneously.

Angular stomatitis

Angular stomatitis describes an inflammatory lesion at the angle of the mouth. It is often bilateral and may be asymptomatic or painful. It can occur with any concurrent intraoral candidiasis but is not always caused by candidal infection. *Staphylococcus aureus* may also cause angular stomatitis, the organisms often originating from the nares. Angular stomatitis is typically seen where a dental appliance is being worn and, in the absence of this, an underlying immune or haematinic deficiency, or diabetes may be the cause (Fig. 158.10). Angular stomatitis may also be noninfective and may be caused by persistent dribbling causing maceration of the tissues.

Diagnosis of the causative organism will require a microbiological swab which should be cultured for *Staph. aureus* and *Candida* species.

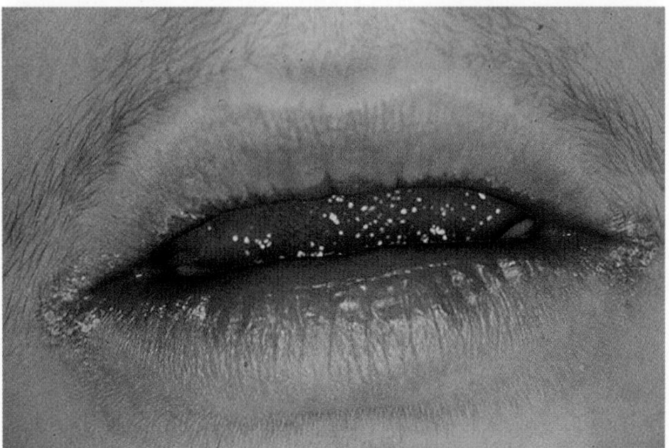

Fig. 158.10 Angular stomatitis which was related to diabetes.

Treatment is dependent on the causative factor [8]. Both candidal and *Staphylococcal* infections will respond to miconazole gel. If *Staphylococcus* is isolated, a more rapid resolution may occur with fusidic acid cream and the nose may also need to be treated. If no organisms are cultured and maceration is the cause, a barrier ointment may be of use.

Acquired persistent white lesions

Chronic hyperplastic candidiasis (candidal leucoplakia)

Chronic hyperplastic candidiasis in childhood is unusual and most often seen in mucocutaneous candidiasis, congenital immunodeficiencies and AIDS. Clinically, the oral lesions all have similar features: they are white, tough and firmly adherent to the underlying mucosa. They are often of irregular thickness and outline. Common sites include the buccal mucosa and dorsum of the tongue. There are four main clinical variants of chronic mucocutaneous candidiasis:

- candidal leucoplakia (idiopathic limited type)
- familial chronic mucocutaneous candidiasis
- diffuse-type chronic mucocutaneous candidiasis
- endocrine candidiasis syndrome.

All give rise to persistent candidiasis in which the mouth is the sole or main site of infection. The lesions do not respond to topical antifungal therapy.

Histologically, the features are similar to those seen in thrush. The plaques consist of thick layers of parakeratotic epithelium invaded by candidal hyphae. There is an inflammatory infiltrate within the plaque, which is concentrated at its base. The underlying epithelium is hyperplastic and there are chronic inflammatory changes in the dermis. Diagnosis of chronic hyperplastic candidiasis is confirmed by biopsy.

Treatment is difficult and topical antifungal agents are rarely of use. Systemic agents such as fluconazole and itraconazole are beneficial but may require continued prophylactic administration if mucocutaneous candidiasis syndrome is diagnosed. If recurrence occurs with the use of long-term azole antifungals, the recurrent lesions should be cultured to check for azole resistance.

Lichen planus, lichenoid lesions and chronic graft-versus-host disease

See Mouth ulcers, previously.

Psoriasis

Oral lesions are rare in psoriasis and may resemble erythema migrans (see later) or take the form of translucent plaques. Macules, diffuse erythema and pustules have also been reported.

Lupus erythematosus

This connective tissue disorder is rare in childhood but may give rise to oral lesions that resemble lichen planus, particularly the atrophic type. The lesions are not symmetrical in distribution and the white striae tend to radiate centrifugally.

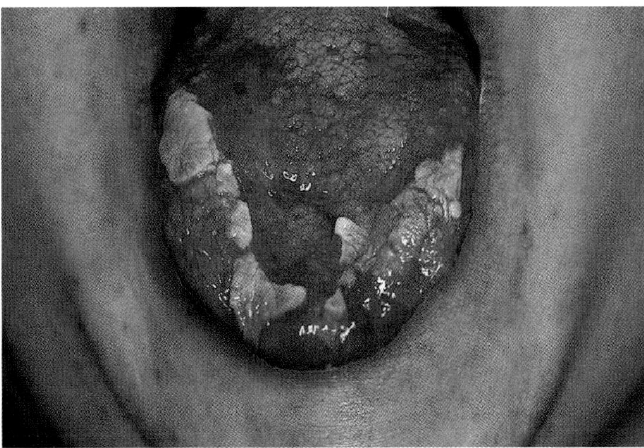

Fig. 158.11 Leucoplakia of the tongue. Clinically, this lesion resembles lichen planus but histologically showed only hyperkeratosis. The 17-year-old patient had undergone bone marrow transplantation 8 years previously, suggesting that the lesion may have been initially caused by graft-versus-host disease.

Hairy leucoplakia

Hairy leucoplakia may be seen in children with severe immune defects, particularly HIV infection. EBV has been shown to be present in the epithelium, and the lesions have been reported to regress with aciclovir therapy. Histological features include severe parakeratosis, hyperplasia, koilocyte-like cells and an absence of inflammatory infiltrate.

Clinically, the lesion appears more corrugated in appearance than hairy and is most often seen on the lateral borders of the tongue [9]. It is symptomless and no treatment is required. Biopsy may be necessary to confirm the diagnosis.

Chronic renal failure

Stomatitis is commonly seen in uraemic patients. Leucoplakias have also been reported [10]. Clinically, the lesions resemble congenital white sponge naevus, although the lesions have well-defined margins. The ventral surface of the tongue is often the main site affected.

Leucoplakia of unknown cause

Leucoplakia is uncommon in childhood. The clinical appearance is highly variable, as is the size of the lesion (Fig. 158.11). Histologically, the lesions range from simple hyperkeratosis to atrophic parakeratotic epithelium with severe dysplasia. Although the clinical appearance is no indication of the underlying histology, speckled lesions are more likely to show dysplastic changes.

Any leucoplakia of unknown cause should be biopsied and kept under regular 3-monthly review. If the lesion changes in character, it should be rebiopsied because of the risk of malignant change.

References

1 **Macleod RI, Munro CS. The incidence and distribution of oral lesions in patients with Darier's disease. Br Dent J 1991;177:133–6.**
2 **Tyldesley WR. Oral leukoplakia associated with tylosis and oesophageal carcinoma. J Oral Pathol 1974;3:62–70.**
3 **George DI, Escobar VH. Oral findings of Clouston's syndrome. Oral Surg Oral Med Oral Pathol 1984;57:258–62.**
4 Feinstein A, Friedman J, Schewach-Millet M. Pachyonychia congenita. J Am Acad Dermatol 1988;19:705–11.
5 Scully C, Langdon JD, Evans JH. A marathon of eponyms: Jadassohn Lewandowsky. Oral Dis 2010;16:310–11.
6 Cannell H. Dyskeratosis congenita. Br J Oral Surg 1971;9:8–20.
7 Johnson EM, Warnock DW, Luker J. Emergence of azole resistance in Candida species from HIV-infected patients receiving prolonged fluconazole therapy for oral candidosis. J Antimicrob Chemother 1995;35:103–14.
8 Scully C, El-Kabir M, Samaranayake LP. Candida and oral candidosis. Crit Rev Oral Biol Med 1994;5:124–58.
9 **Scully C, Laskaris G, Porter SR. Oral manifestations of HIV infection and their management. I. More common lesions. Oral Surg Oral Med Oral Pathol 1991;71:158–66.**
10 Kellet M. Oral white patches in uraemic patients. Br Dent J 1983:154:366–8.

Red and pigmented lesions

Localized lesions

Amalgam and graphite tattoos

Amalgam tattoos are the most common cause of localized oral pigmentation. They can occur at any age, and result from minor trauma to the oral mucosa during the placement of an amalgam restoration or during the extraction of a tooth containing an amalgam restoration, which allows amalgam particles to penetrate into the epithelium. The amalgam particles are deposited in the corium. A foreign body giant cell reaction or macrophage accumulation occurs in about 55% of cases.

Clinically, amalgam tattoos are most commonly seen on the gingivae, alveolar mucosa, floor of the mouth and buccal mucosa. They appear as symptomless blue-black macules, the margins of which may be well defined or diffuse. They may vary in size from 1 to 20 mm. Similar lesions may result from trauma from a pencil and are seen mainly in the palatal vault.

Radiography may aid the diagnosis because many lesions are radiopaque. If any doubt exists as to the diagnosis, biopsy should be performed.

Oral pigmented naevi

Melanocytic naevi are rare in the mouth when compared with the occurrence on the skin (see Chapter 105). They are twice as common in females and tend to occur in the 30–50-year-old age group, although they may be seen in childhood. They range in size from 1 to 30 mm, the majority being less than 6 mm. They may be grey, brown, black or blue in colour; about 20% are nonpigmented. The hard palate and buccal mucosa are the most common sites of occurrence.

Histologically, several types of naevi can be identified: junctional, compound, intramucosal, blue oral melanotic macule and melanoacanthoma. They are all benign. Malignant melanoma is rare in childhood. Diagnosis may be confirmed by biopsy.

Melanotic neuroectodermal tumour of infancy

This is a rare tumour occurring in the first year of life. It is thought to arise from neural crest tissue. Clinically, lesions occur in the anterior maxilla as painless, nontender enlarging dark masses. Growth may be rapid. Radiographical examination shows underlying radiolucency and displacement of developing teeth. The lesion is benign and conservative surgical excision is curative.

Peutz–Jeghers syndrome

This autosomal dominant syndrome comprises intestinal polyposis and melanotic pigmentation of the face and mouth (see Chapter 141). Oral pigmentation is usually confined to the lower lip and buccal mucosa.

Haemangiomas and vascular malformations

Haemangiomas in children are localized vascular tumours (described more fully in Chapter 119). Clinically, oral haemangiomas appear as superficial purple-bluish nodules or macules that blanch on pressure, the common sites of occurrence being the lips (Fig. 158.12), tongue, palate and buccal mucosa.

Intraoral capillary or capillary venous malformations are also associated with certain syndromes including Sturge–Weber syndrome (Fig. 158.13), Klippel–Trenaunay–Weber syndrome and Maffucci syndrome.

Excision or biopsy of the lesion may be necessary if the diagnosis is unclear or the lesion is enlarging, in order to eliminate neoplasia. Surgery or cryotherapy may be required if repeated haemorrhage is a problem. Very large venous malformations are difficult to treat surgically and sclerotherapy may be of benefit. Problematic haemangiomas respond well to oral propranolol (see Chapter 119).

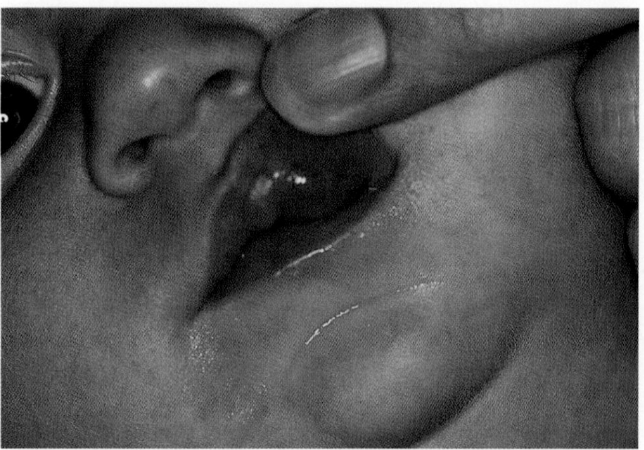

Fig. 158.12 Haemangioma of the upper lip in a 6-month-old baby.

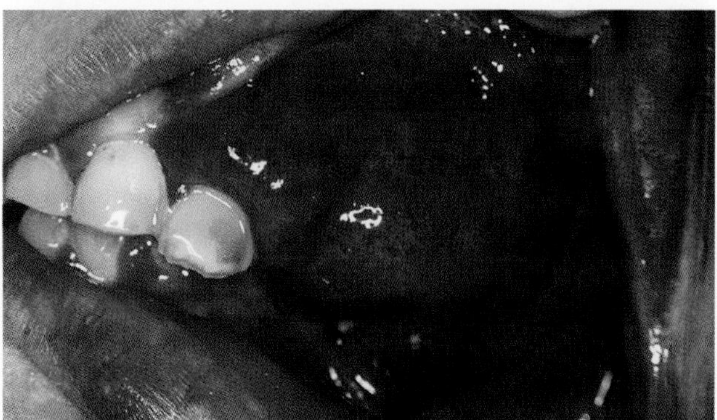

Fig. 158.13 Sturge–Weber syndrome; the child also suffered epilepsy and learning impairment.

Hereditary mucoepithelial dysplasia

This is a rare autosomal dominant trait that results in abnormal desmosome and gap junctions. Clinically, oral lesions appear in infancy as red macules or papules on the palate and gingivae. They are painless and may persist throughout life.

Erythema migrans

See Lesions of the tongue, later.

Kaposi sarcoma

Rarely, Kaposi sarcoma may occur intraorally in children who have contracted HIV/AIDS by nonsexual routes, particularly in Africa [1]. Lesions are most common on the palate or gingivae and present as purple-red macules or nodules. They rarely require specific treatment.

Chronic atrophic candidiasis

See Acquired transient white lesions (candidiasis), previously.

Gingivitis

Gingivitis is uncommon in preschool children (with the exception of acute viral infections), and an underlying systemic disease should always be considered in a differential diagnosis, particularly immunological deficiencies such as neutropenia (Fig. 158.14).

In older children, gingivitis is usually concurrent with poor oral hygiene; however, if associated with destruction of the periodontium (the supportive tissues of the teeth), underlying disease should be eliminated, particularly diabetes mellitus and immunodeficiency [2]. Other conditions such as Down syndrome, cathepsin C deficiency (Papillon–Lefevre syndrome), leucocyte adhesion deficiency (LAD) and hypophosphatasia underlie some cases.

Gingivitis presents clinically as redness of the gingivae surrounding the tooth; it is usually painless, but the child may report bleeding of the gingivae on tooth brushing. There is usually a heavy accumulation of plaque around the necks of the teeth.

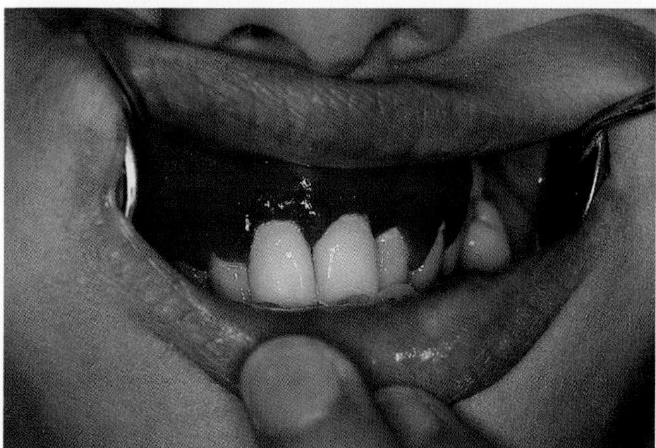

Fig. 158.14 Acute gingivitis and periodontitis in a child with familial chronic neutropenia.

Treatment involves removal of plaque, instigation of good oral hygiene and the use of chlorhexidine gluconate mouthwash 0.2% twice daily until gingivitis resolves.

Allergic gingivostomatitis

Occasionally, gingivitis may be caused by an allergic reaction. The gingivitis tends to be diffuse and oral hygiene is often very good. Common causative agents include cinnamon-containing toothpastes, some chewing gums and mints. The gingivitis resolves when the causal agent is removed and recurs when rechallenged.

Generalized lesions

Racial pigmentation is the most common cause of generalized pigmentation of the oral mucosa in both children and adults; however, other causes, such as those discussed later, should be eliminated from the differential diagnosis. Other rare causes of generalized oral pigmentation include haemochromatosis, neurofibromatosis and incontinentia pigmenti.

Racial pigmentation

Racial pigmentation mainly occurs in individuals of Black, Asian or Mediterranean descent and 5% of White people. It varies in colour from light brown to black and may occur anywhere in the mouth, particularly the gingivae and tongue.

Drug-induced hyperpigmentation

Drugs such as anticonvulsants, cytotoxic agents (especially busulphan), adrenocorticotrophic hormone (ACTH) therapy and oral contraceptives may cause brown oral pigmentation. Antimalarial drugs produce a range of mucosal pigmentation from yellow to blue-black, depending on the drug used. Minocycline may cause a blue-grey staining of the gingival margins [3].

Addison disease

Oral hyperpigmentation ranging from light brown to almost black may be seen in Addison disease or in ectopic ACTH production. The pigmentation is variable in its distribution but often affects the soft palate, buccal mucosa, lateral borders of the tongue, gingivae and lips. Addison disease may be associated with chronic mucocutaneous candidiasis (see above).

Albright syndrome

Pigmentation of the oral mucosa has been reported in Albright syndrome, which consists of polyostotic fibrous dysplasia (facial bones affected in 25% of cases), pigmentation of the skin and precocious puberty in females.

Hereditary haemorrhagic telangiectasia (Osler–Weber–Rendu disease)

This is an autosomal dominant trait characterized by multiple telangiectasia of the skin and mucous membranes. Lesions do not normally become apparent until the second or third decade. Any area of the mouth may be affected. The lesions appear as red spots or spider-like lesions, which empty on applying pressure; they are caused by the superficial dilation of small blood vessels [4]. If traumatized, they may cause bleeding, which may be difficult to control. Laser therapy to the lesions may be required.

Oral telangiectasia may also be seen in scleroderma, and after radiotherapy to the head and neck region.

Thrombocytopenic purpura

Thrombocytopenia, whatever its aetiology (idiopathic, drug induced, etc.), may cause oral purpura or petechiae at a platelet count of below 50×10^9/L. Lesions commonly occur on mucosa that is easily traumatized, such as the tongue, palate and buccal mucosa. They are reddish-purple in colour and vary in size (Fig. 158.15). They do not blanch on pressure. Oral purpura may be the first clinical manifestation of leukaemia, aplastic anaemia or HIV disease.

Pigmentation of the teeth

Pigmentation or discoloration of the teeth may be caused by intrinsic or extrinsic staining (Box 158.1, Fig. 158.16).

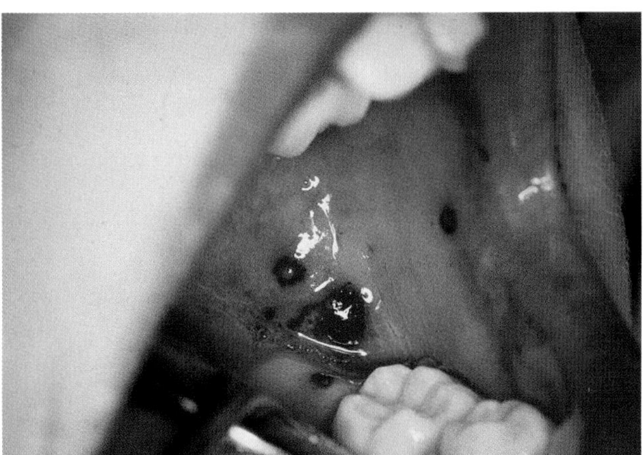

Fig. 158.15 Oral purpura in a child with thrombocytopenia caused by Wiskott–Aldrich syndrome.

Box 158.1 Causes of pigmentation of the teeth

Extrinsic

- Chromogenic bacteria
- Chlorhexidine gluconate
- Iron preparations

Intrinsic

- Amelogenesis imperfecta
- Dentinogenesis imperfecta
- Tetracycline staining
- Fluorosis
- Porphyria
- Erythroblastosis fetalis
- Chronological hypoplasia
- Trauma

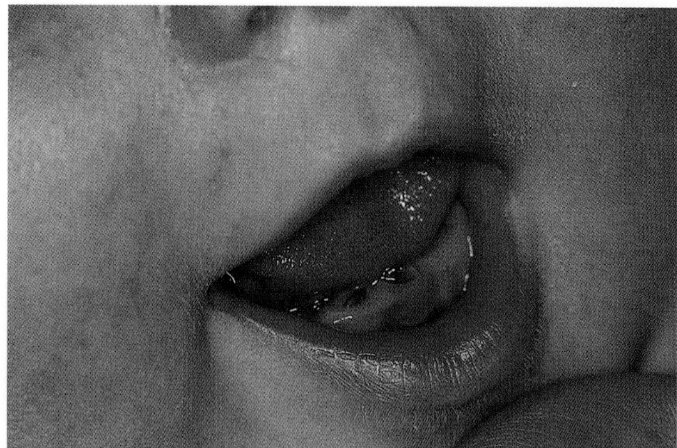

Fig. 158.16 Porphyria. A baby with the lower first deciduous incisors erupting. Note the red colour caused by porphyrin deposition in the dentine.

References

1 **Ficarra G, Berson AM, Silverman S et al. Kaposi's sarcoma of the oral cavity: a study of 134 patients with a review of the pathogenesis, epidemiology, clinical aspects and treatment. Oral Surg Oral Med Oral Pathol 1988;66:543–50.**
2 Hakki SS, Aprikyan AA, Yildirim S et al. Periodontal status in two siblings with severe congenital neutropenia: diagnosis and mutational analysis of the cases. J Periodontol 2005;75:837–44.
3 **Berger RS, Mandel EB, Hayes TJ et al. Minocycline staining of the oral cavity. J Am Acad Dermatol 1989;21:432–42.**
4 **Flint SR, Keith O, Scully C. Hereditary haemorrhagic telangiectasia: family study and review. Oral Surg Oral Med Oral Pathol 1988; 66:440–4.**

Swellings/lumps in and around the mouth

Lumps in the mouth may have a variety of causes ranging from normal anatomy to neoplasia. In this section, they are considered in three main groups: soft tissue swellings, bony swellings and gingival swelling.

Developmental soft tissue swellings

Congenital granular cell epulis of the newborn

The congenital epulis is a rare tumour occurring on the alveolar ridge and, as its name implies, is present at birth. It may form a soft, rounded, pedunculated swelling of a few millimetres in diameter or be so large as to protrude from the mouth. The aetiology is unclear but it is thought to be mesenchymal in origin and may be a hamartoma. Eighty percent of lesions occur in females, and they are more common on the maxillary alveolar ridge than the mandibular. Treatment is by excision and recurrence is very uncommon.

Lingual thyroid

See Lesions of the tongue, later.

Dermoid cyst

See Lesions of the tongue, later.

Lingual tonsil

See Lesions of the tongue, later.

Eruption cyst

Eruption cysts are soft tissue follicular cysts that form over the crowns of erupting teeth of children, particularly deciduous teeth or permanent molar teeth. They appear as rounded smooth bluish swellings on the alveolar ridge. They are usually asymptomatic and resolve spontaneously as the tooth erupts. If they cause symptoms or become infected, marsupialization may be necessary.

Lymphangioma

Lymphangiomas bear a close structural resemblance to cavernous haemangiomas but contain lymph instead of blood. They are often present at birth and usually manifest before 10 years of age. Intraoral lymphangiomas are uncommon but are most likely to occur on the tongue. Clinically, they appear as a sessile swelling with a pale translucent appearance and a finely nodular surface. They may appear to turn black if bleeding occurs into the lesion and then simulate a haemangioma. Treatment is required if the lesion is symptomatic and involves either sclerotherapy or surgical excision.

Haemangioma

See Red and pigmented lesions, previously.

Neurofibromatosis (see Chapter 142)

This syndrome comprises multiple neurofibromas, cutaneous pigmentation in the form of café-au-lait spots and skeletal abnormalities. Oral neurofibromas occur in about 10% of cases and may involve any oral soft tissues.

Tuberous sclerosis complex (epiloia) (see Chapter 143)

Oral lesions seen in tuberous sclerosis complex consist of fibrous outgrowths of the oral mucosa, affecting the anterior gingivae in particular [1].

Cowden syndrome (see Chapter 141)

Papillomatous outgrowths from the buccal mucosa and papular lesions of the palate, lips and gingivae have been described in this syndrome. Other oral lesions may include fissured tongue and hypoplasia of the maxillae, mandible and uvula.

Acquired soft tissue swellings

Abscesses

Intraoral abscesses are almost always dental in origin, usually originating from a carious tooth. They usually present as a painful fluctuant soft tissue swelling of the gingiva or buccal sulcus, occasionally in the palate (Fig. 158.17). An associated cellulitis may also occur, giving rise to facial swelling. The abscess is often preceded by toothache and the offending tooth is usually carious and tender to pressure.

The diagnosis is made on clinical findings and treatment involves draining the abscess via the tooth itself or the soft tissue. Antibiotics may be required if there is an associated regional lymphadenopathy or if treatment is delayed, because a general anaesthetic may be required to treat very young children.

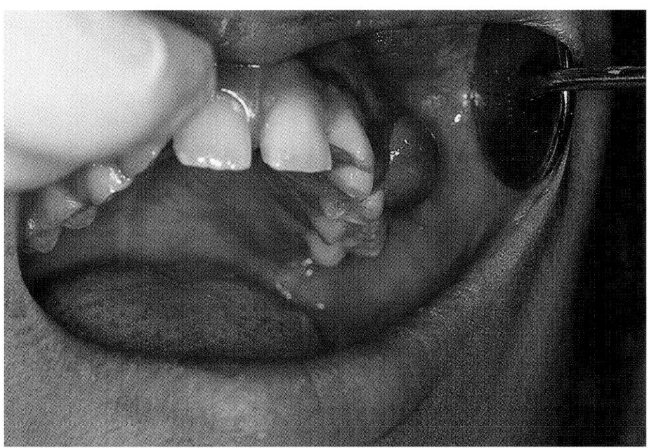

Fig. 158.17 Dental abscess causing soft tissue swelling in the upper left quadrant of a 12-year-old child.

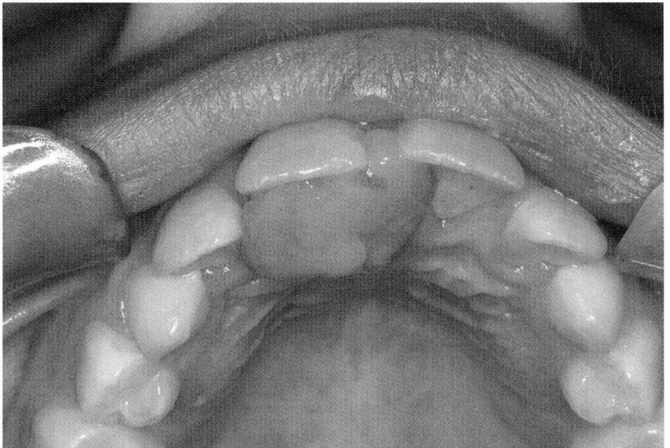

Fig. 158.18 Fibrous lump (epulis).

Fibroepithelial polyp/nodule

Fibroepithelial polyps or nodules are the most common type of tumour-like swelling found in the mouth (Fig. 158.18). They are usually considered to be caused by chronic low-grade trauma. Often a source of trauma cannot be found.

Histologically, these lesions consist of stratified squamous keratinized epithelium with underlying dense bundles of collagenous connective tissue in continuity with the corium. They are not encapsulated. There may be an inflammatory exudate and occasionally dystrophic calcification occurs.

Clinically, they appear as either sessile or pedunculated, soft, pink swellings. They may occur on the gingivae (where they are referred to as epulides), palate and buccal mucosa or tongue. They are usually painless. Treatment involves surgical excision with curettage of the underlying periostium to prevent recurrence.

Pyogenic granuloma

Pyogenic granulomas are soft tissue swellings that are highly vascular and have a tendency to haemorrhage. They are caused by a tissue reaction to nonspecific infection as a result of minor trauma to the oral mucosa.

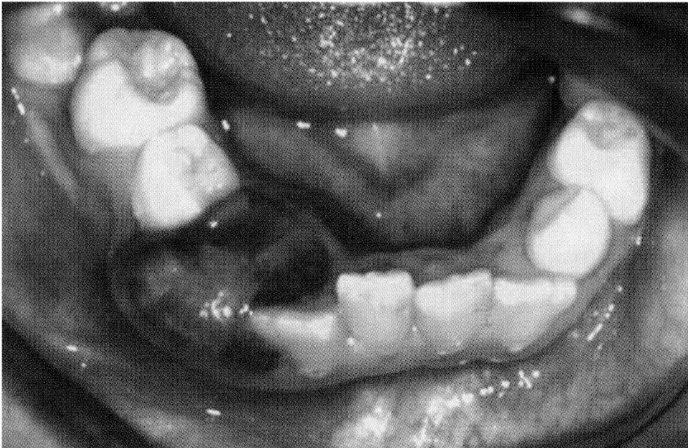

Fig. 158.19 Giant cell granuloma.

Histologically, they contain numerous thin-walled blood vessels in a loose, moderately cellular fibrous stroma.

Clinically, they usually present as a painless swelling on the gingival margin, but may occur at other sites, e.g. buccal mucosa, palate. The swelling may be sessile or pedunculated with a smooth, lobulated or warty surface. They are red in colour and soft to palpation. They are variable in size from a few millimetres to a few centimetres. Differential diagnosis includes a fibroepithelial polyp and giant cell epulis. Treatment is by surgical excision.

Giant cell epulis/granuloma

A giant cell granuloma is a non-neoplastic swelling of proliferating fibroblasts in a vascular stroma containing multinucleate giant cells. Its aetiology is unknown. It is more commonly seen in children than in adults and presents as a deep red-purple soft swelling, which often arises interdentally adjacent to permanent incisor or premolar teeth (Fig. 158.19). Hyperparathyroidism (brown tumours) should always be considered when a lesion containing giant cells is diagnosed. Treatment is by surgical excision and curettage of the underlying bone.

Squamous papillomas

Squamous cell papillomas are common benign oral lesions caused by human papillomavirus (HPV). They may occur at any age. Clinically, they present as a well-defined exophytic mass with a warty surface. If the surface epithelium is keratinized, they appear white. Although they may occur anywhere in the mouth, they are most commonly seen at the junction of the hard and soft palates. Oral papillomas should be excised and examined histologically to confirm the diagnosis, because they may resemble a fibroepithelial polyp. Treatment is by total excision to prevent recurrence.

Human papillomavirus may also cause common warts and oral papillomas, particularly on the lips, and is often seen in association with verruca vulgaris of the skin. HPV-13 and -32 are implicated in focal epithelial hyperplasia (Heck disease), which presents in certain racial groups, such as Inuits, as multiple sessile soft papules, usually on the lower labial and buccal mucosa.

Molluscum contagiosum (see Chapter 48)
Molluscum contagiosum may occasionally affect the mouth, particularly the lips, as a result of autoinoculation from cutaneous lesions. Facial and perioral molluscum contagiosum is frequently seen in patients with AIDS.

Orofacial granulomatosis and Crohn disease
See Gastrointestinal diseases, previously.

Melkersson–Rosenthal syndrome
See Lesions of the tongue, later.

Lymphoma
Lymphomas are the third most common malignant disease of childhood, although it is unusual for them to occur in the mouth and jaw (with the exception of Burkitt lymphoma). They may present as a soft tissue enlargement, nonhealing ulcer and occasionally loosening of the teeth. Radiographically, there may be evidence of bone resorption. Most lymphomas presenting in children younger than 10 years of age are of the non-Hodgkin type.

Any swelling of the oral tissues without obvious cause should be biopsied.

Burkitt lymphoma
African Burkitt lymphoma typically affects preteenage children and is strongly associated with EBV. The jaw, particularly the mandible, is a common site of presentation. Clinically, there is massive swelling, which may ulcerate into the mouth.

Langerhans cell histiocytosis (histiocytosis X, eosinophilic granuloma) (see Chapter 90)
This condition refers to a neoplastic-like proliferation of Langerhans cells. The spectrum of Langerhans cell histiocytosis ranges from isolated lesions, which spontaneously regress, to widespread fatal disease. Multifocal eosinophilic granuloma presents in young children and often gives rise to lytic lesions in the skull and mandible, which may involve oral soft tissue, resulting in swelling. Treatment is dependent upon the extent of dissemination of the disease and may involve surgery, chemotherapy and radiotherapy.

Sarcomas and related conditions
Oral facial sarcomas are rare tumours of childhood, the most common being rhabdomyosarcoma. Locally invasive tumours such as infantile fibromatosis may also give rise to intraoral swelling, which presents as a progressively enlarging mass. Biopsy of lesions of doubtful diagnosis should always be performed to eliminate neoplasia. Salivary gland tumours are also uncommon in childhood but should be considered in the differential diagnosis, particularly in swellings involving the upper lip, where mucocoeles are uncommon.

Bony swellings
The majority of intraoral bony swellings in children are caused by unerupted teeth, supernumerary teeth, cysts and odontomes.

Tori
Tori are slow-growing exostoses that are thought to be inherited as a dominant trait. The torus palatinus occurs in the midline of the hard palate and the torus mandibularis lingually in the premolar area of the mandible; 80% of cases are bilateral. Although they may be seen in childhood, the peak incidence is around 30 years of age.

Fibrous dysplasia
Fibrous dysplasias, which include familial fibrous dysplasia (cherubism) and monostotic or polyostotic fibrous dysplasia as in Albright syndrome, may all give rise to expansile lesions of the jaws. On skeletal maturation, the lesions tend to cease growth (see also Red and pigmented lesions, previously).

Odontogenic cysts
Odontogenic cysts refer to a group of jaw cysts that are derived from the epithelium of the dental laminae. Follicular cysts are the most common odontogenic cysts seen in childhood (see Eruption cyst, previously). Gorlin–Goltz syndrome, an autosomal dominant trait with variable expression, comprises multiple basal cell carcinomas, odontogenic keratocysts that may become apparent in childhood, bifid ribs and calcification of the falx cerebri (see Chapter 139).

Gardner syndrome
Gardner syndrome is an autosomal dominant trait consisting of colonic polyps, which often undergo malignant change, epidermoid or sebaceous cysts, dermoid tumours, multiple supernumerary and impacted teeth, and osteomas that may cause swellings of the jaw or cranium.

Bone cysts
Bone cysts, such as the aneurysmal bone cyst and solitary bone cyst, are seen almost exclusively in children and adolescents. They may occasionally present as a bony swelling of the mandible, but most are found as an incidental finding on routine radiography of the jaws.

Osteomyelitis
Osteomyelitis affecting the jaw is rare in the UK but is occasionally seen following radiotherapy to the head and neck as a result of endarteritis obliterans. Osteosarcoma may occur in the jaw of children who have undergone irradiation of the jaw for sarcomas.

Juvenile active ossifying fibroma
Juvenile active ossifying fibroma is occasionally seen in children younger than 15 years of age. Unlike the ossifying fibromas of adults, it is very cellular and locally aggressive.

Generalized gingival swelling

Gingivitis is the most common cause of generalized gingival enlargement. Gingival enlargement may be aggravated by local factors such as mouth breathing. Enlarged gingivae without evidence of poor oral hygiene

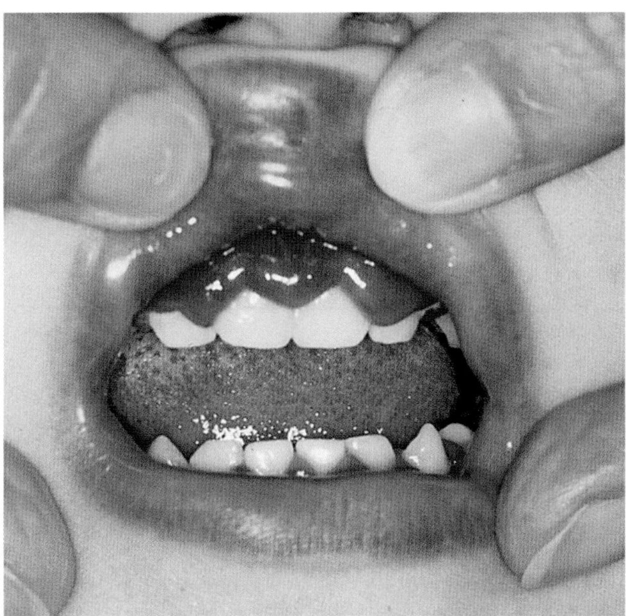

Fig. 158.20 Gingival enlargement caused by acute inflammation in a 3-year-old child with aplastic anaemia.

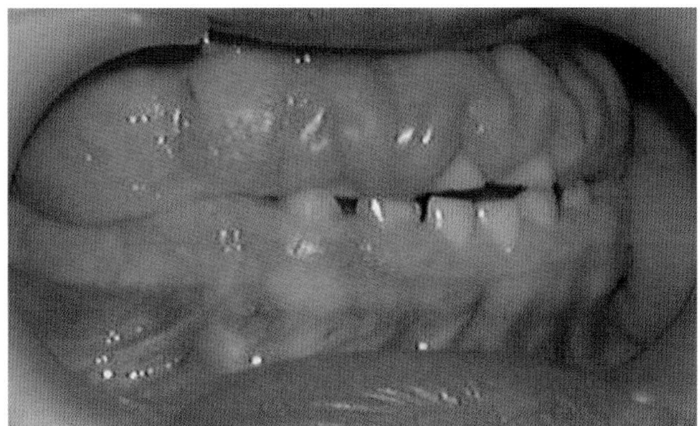

Fig. 158.21 Familial gingival hyperplasia (fibromatosis).

or in preschool children may be indicative of a systemic disorder, e.g. aplastic anaemia (Fig. 158.20) or sarcoidosis.

Hereditary gingival fibromatosis

Hereditary gingival fibromatosis is an autosomal dominant trait in which there is fibrous gingival enlargement, hypertrichosis and coarseness of facial features. It is occasionally associated with epilepsy, learning impairment and skeletal abnormalities [2]. Clinically, the gingivae begin to enlarge around the time of tooth eruption. The gingivae are usual firm, pink and stippled, although if oral hygiene is poor inflammation may be concurrent (Fig. 158.21). The teeth may eventually be buried by the gingivae. Treatment is by maintenance of good oral hygiene and, when aesthetically necessary, gingivectomy. Growth of the gingivae slows after puberty.

Drug-induced gingival hyperplasia

Drug-induced gingival hyperplasia is associated with several drugs, including phenytoin, ciclosporin and the calcium channel blockers such as nifedipine and diltiazem.

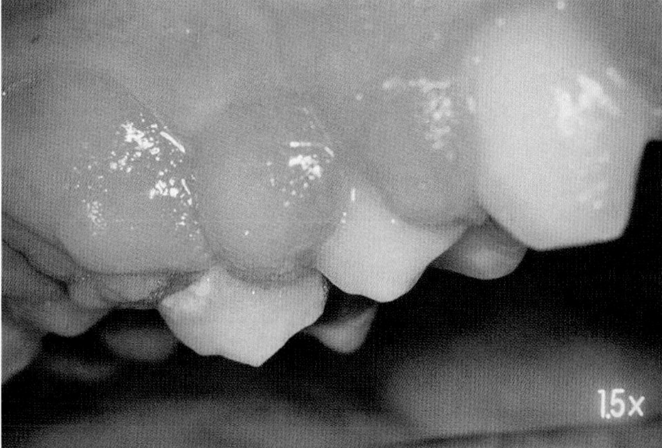

Fig. 158.22 Drug-induced (phenytoin) gingival hyperplasia. Note that the enlargement is particularly apparent at the interdental papillae.

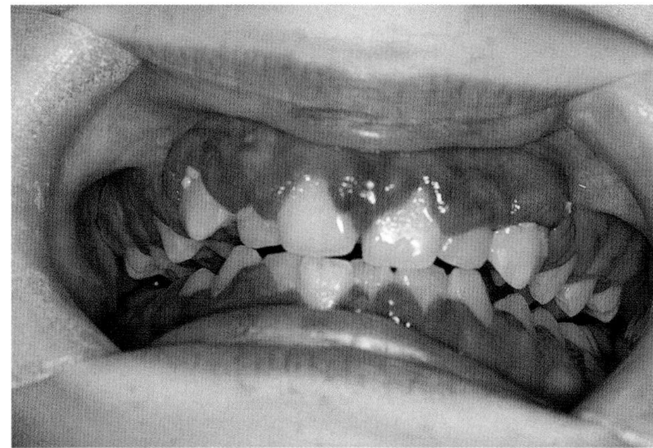

Fig. 158.23 Generalized gingival swelling in a child with acute myeloid leukaemia.

Clinically, the hyperplasia resembles that of hereditary gingival fibromatosis, although hyperplasia is particularly apparent at the interdental papillae and gingival stippling is exaggerated (Fig. 158.22). Poor oral hygiene aggravates the hyperplasia. The history and clinical features should help to distinguish it from the hereditary form.

Acute leukaemia

Generalized gingival swelling may occur with acute leukaemia [3]. It is more frequently reported in association with acute myeloid leukaemia but may also be apparent in other forms, e.g. acute lymphoblastic leukaemia. The swelling is produced by leukaemic cell infiltrate in response to bacteria in dental plaque. The gingivae appear swollen, soft and may have a bluish-purple colour (Fig. 158.23). The surrounding mucosa may be pale (anaemia) and there may be petechiae or purpura present (thrombocytopenia).

Salivary gland swelling

Historically, the most common cause of salivary gland swelling in children was mumps. However, with the introduction of the measles/mumps/rubella (MMR) vaccine in the Western world, mumps is now uncommon.

Box 158.2 Causes of salivary gland swelling in childhood

- Mumps
- Chronic recurrent sialadenitis
- Ascending parotitis
- Calculi
- HIV disease
- Cystic fibrosis
- Sjögren syndrome
- Sarcoidosis plus other granulomatosis
- Mikulicz disease
- Sialosis
- Drugs, e.g. chlorhexidine, sulphonamides, iodine
- Salivary gland neoplasia, e.g. juvenile haemangioma
- Lymphoma

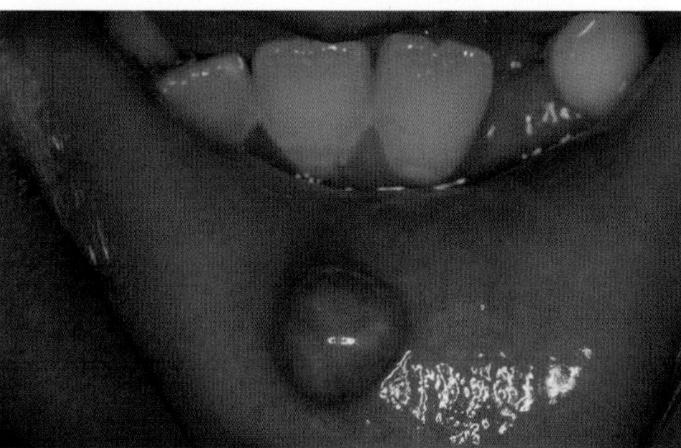

Fig. 158.24 Mucocoele in the most common site.

Mumps infections usually give rise to bilateral parotid swelling, causing eversion of the ear lobe. Occasionally, the swelling begins unilaterally. Parotitis may be caused by other viruses, including coxsackie A, ECHO virus, parainfluenza, EBV and CMV. Treatment is symptomatic. Other causes of salivary gland swelling are discussed in the following paragraphs and listed in Box 158.2 [4]. Salivary gland malignancy in childhood is rare [5].

Chronic recurrent sialadenitis

Chronic recurrent sialadenitis presents with recurrent painful swelling of one or more major salivary glands, usually the parotid. The attacks vary in frequency and the gland may remain enlarged between attacks. The aetiology is unclear but EBV may be involved. The condition usually resolves spontaneously at puberty.

Mucocoele/ranula

Mucocoeles are mucous extravasation cysts, often resulting from trauma to the minor salivary glands. They are common and usually occur on the lower lip (Fig. 158.24), but may occur on the palate, upper lip and buccal mucosa. They usually present as a tense, localized, fluid-filled swelling. The lesion may burst as a result of trauma from the teeth. Recurrence is common and may lead to fibrosis.

The diagnosis is usually made on the history and clinical appearance. Treatment is either by cryosurgery or surgical removal of the cyst together with the offending minor salivary gland.

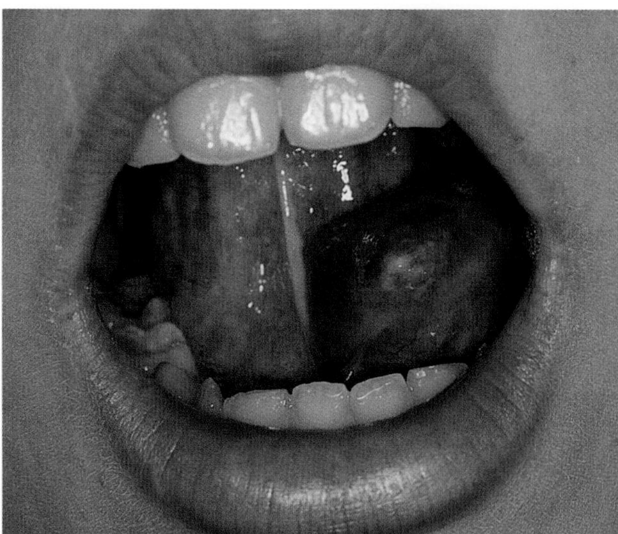

Fig. 158.25 A ranula – sublingual mucous retention cyst.

A ranula is a form of mucous retention cyst arising in the floor of the mouth, often involving the sublingual salivary gland. It may cause both intra- and extraoral swelling (Fig. 158.25). It is usually treated by marsupialization.

HIV infection

Cystic enlargement of the major salivary glands has been reported in HIV disease together with lymphocytic infiltration, giving a Sjögren syndrome appearance histologically, which may give rise to xerostomia. Swellings of this nature should be regularly observed because of the increased risk of lymphoma development.

Cystic fibrosis

Enlargement of the salivary glands, particularly the submandibular gland, may occasionally be seen in patients with cystic fibrosis.

Sarcoidosis

Sarcoidosis is a chronic granulomatous disease of unknown aetiology described more fully in Chapter 81. Sarcoidosis causes asymptomatic enlargement of the major salivary glands in 6% of cases and involvement of the facial nerve may lead to facial palsy. Gingival enlargement may also occur. Biopsy of affected gingivae or minor salivary glands shows typical granulomas.

References

1 Smith, D, Porter SR, Scully C. Gingival and other oral manifestations in tuberous sclerosis. Periodontal Clin Invest 1993;15:13–18.
2 Katz J, Guelmann M, Barak S. Hereditary gingival fibromatosis with distinct dental, skeletal and developmental abnormalities. Paediatr Dent 2002;24:253–6.
3 Francisconi CF, Caldas RJ, Oliveira M et al. Leukemic oral manifestations and their management. Asian Pac J Cancer Prev 2016;17:911–15.
4 Lamey PJ, Lewis MAO. Oral medicine in practice: salivary gland disease. Br Dent J 1990;168:237–43.
5 Baker SR, Malone B. Salivary gland malignancies in children. Cancer 1985;55:1730–6.

Lesions of the tongue

Congenital/developmental lesions

Macroglossia

The majority of cases of macroglossia, enlargement of the tongue, are congenital and most commonly associated with syndromes, e.g. congenital hypothyroidism, Down, Beckwith–Wiedemann (Fig. 158.26), Hurler and Rubenstein–Taybi syndrome. Congenital macroglossia is caused by muscle hypertrophy. Secondary macroglossia may occur and is caused by tumours, deposits or hamartomas, the most common of which in childhood is a lymphangioma. Congenital macroglossia is not usually treated, the only option being surgical.

Microglossia

Microglossia, small tongue, is a rare congenital anomaly that occasionally causes difficulty in talking and eating. Only a few cases of aglossia have ever been reported.

Ankyloglossia

Ankyloglossia or tongue tie affects up to 1.7% of children and is usually caused by a short lingual fraenum. Surgical intervention is rarely necessary because it is usually of little consequence and does not interfere with speech. However, the scavenging action of the tongue may be impaired.

Fissured/scrotal tongue

This is a tongue with multiple small fissures or grooves on the dorsal surface, which may have a scrotal appearance (Fig. 158.27). This is thought to be a developmental anomaly affecting about 1% of children, although it is rarely seen before the age of 4 years. In surveys of the adult population, the reported frequency is between 3 and 5%, suggesting that it may not be developmental. It has an increased frequency of occurrence in children who suffer from learning impairment, particularly Down syndrome.

Fissured tongue is one of the features of Melkersson syndrome; the other features include facial swelling and facial palsy.

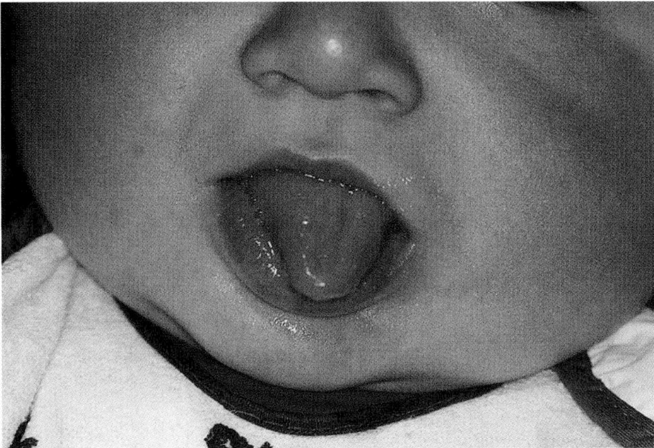

Fig. 158.26 Macroglossia in a baby with Beckwith–Wiedemann syndrome.

The histopathology of fissured tongue is essentially normal. Clinically, fissured tongue is usually asymptomatic except on occasions when food and debris collect in the fissures, giving rise to irritation. However, erythema migrans (geographic tongue) is very frequently found associated. If irritation occurs, food and debris should be removed by stretching and flattening the fissures and using a toothbrush, gauze or sponge to cleanse the surface.

Lingual thyroid

Ectopic thyroid tissue may occasionally be found at the base of the tongue at the site of the foramen caecum. Clinically, the lesion presents as a smooth-surfaced lump. Symptoms of dysphagia may occur, but the lesion is often asymptomatic. If surgery is indicated, it is important to establish that there is normal thyroid tissue in the neck.

Lingual tonsil

The lingual tonsil is a mass of lymphoid tissue, divided into two parts by a midline ligament, situated between the epiglottis and circumvallate papillae. If the lingual tonsil is enlarged, as in tonsillitis or in atopic individuals, symptoms such as a lump in the throat, dyspnoea and dysphonia may occur. The condition may be distinguished from other lesions of the tongue by its site, symmetry and midline ligament.

The foliate papillae on the lateral border also contain lymphoid tissue, which may undergo reactive hyperplasia during upper respiratory tract infections, causing the papillae to enlarge and rub against the teeth, causing inflammation (foliate papillitis).

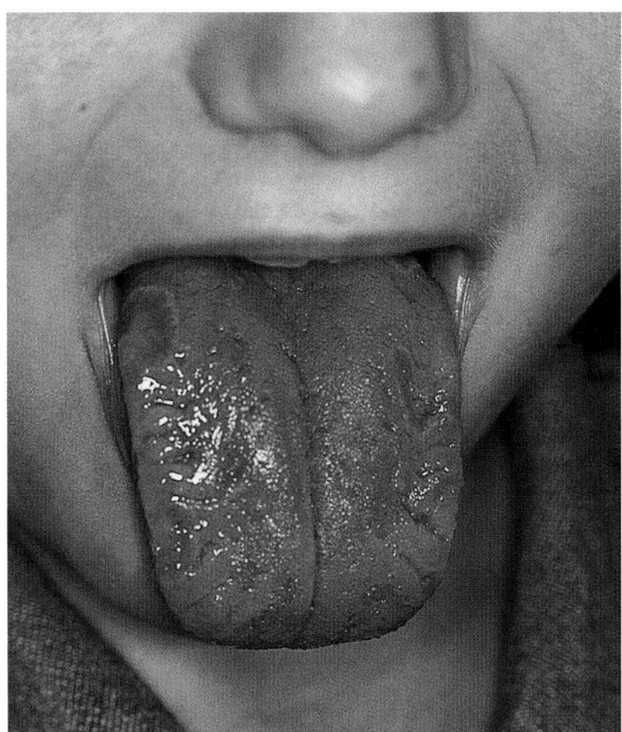

Fig. 158.27 A child with a mildly fissured tongue with concurrent erythema migrans, which is most evident on the right lateral border of the tongue, just anterior to the commissure.

Sublingual dermoid cyst

This is a developmental cyst derived from embryonic germinal epithelium. Sublingual dermoid cysts usually occur in the midline above the mylohyoid muscles. Although they do not occur in the tongue, they cause elevation of the tongue and may be associated with symptoms of dysphagia and dysphonia. Unlike other dermoid cysts, those arising in the floor of the mouth are seldom present at birth, becoming clinically obvious in the second decade.

The histological appearance of a dermoid cyst is very variable. It is usually lined by stratified squamous epithelium and surrounded by lymphoid tissue. The cyst wall may contain sweat and sebaceous glands and hair follicles. Its contents may include keratin, sebum and matted hair.

Clinically, the lesions are variable in size. They may be fluctuant to palpation or have a 'dough-like' feel, depending on the contents of the cyst.

Several lesions may resemble a sublingual dermoid cyst, including a ranula, obstruction of the submandibular duct, thyroglossal tract cyst, cystic hygroma, branchial cleft cyst and cellulitis of the floor of the mouth.

Oral-facial-digital syndrome

Oral-facial-digital type II or Mohr syndrome is characterized by facial deformities, median cleft of the upper lip, hand and feet deformities and tongue hamartomas. Tongue lipoma has also been reported in this condition [1].

Acquired lesions

Swollen tongue

The tongue may swell in allergic reactions (angioedema), inflammation, haematoma formation, deposits (e.g. amyloidosis) or neoplasms.

Glossitis

Glossitis describes an acute inflammatory reaction of the tongue. It may be localized to a particular area of the tongue or generalized. There may or may not be associated symptoms.

Median rhomboid glossitis

This is a central rhomboid-shaped area of depapillation anterior to the sulcus terminalis. It is rare in children.

Debate exists over the aetiology of median rhomboid glossitis, which affects 0.2% of the population. It was originally considered to be developmental in origin, resulting from the persistence of the tuberculum impar. However, because it is less commonly seen in children than in adults, this aetiology is unlikely. It is now thought to be infective in nature and caused by *Candida* (40% of lesions exhibit candidal colonization). The consistent positioning of this condition does, however, support a developmental aetiology, and it has been hypothesized that there may be a vascular anomaly in this area.

Histologically, the epithelium shows loss of papillae and parakeratosis of the epithelium, with acanthosis and downward growth of the rete ridges. Polymorphonuclear lymphocytes may be seen in the superficial epithelium and candidal hyphae may be present. The underlying connective tissue is vascular and infiltrated with chronic inflammatory cells.

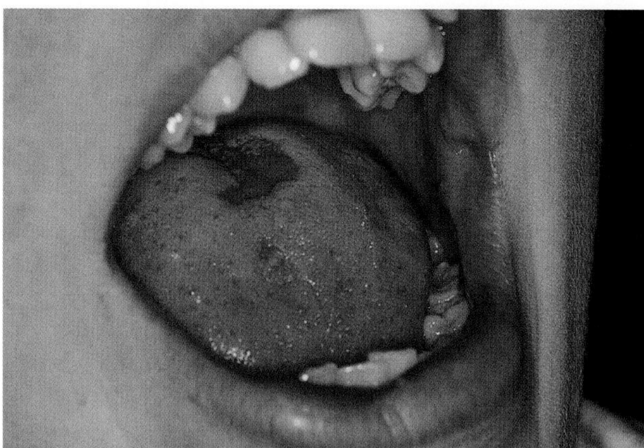

Fig. 158.28 Median rhomboid glossitis in a child using a steroid inhaler for asthma. In this case, the lesion is caused by candidal infection of the lingual mucosa.

The condition is usually asymptomatic but soreness may be reported, particularly after consumption of salty or spicy foods. The lesion presents as a rhomboid-shaped area of depapillation immediately anterior to the sulcus terminalis. It may vary in colour from pale pink to bright red. The surrounding lingual epithelium appears normal (Fig. 158.28).

A swab should be taken for candidal culture. If *Candida* is identified, a topical antifungal agent should be prescribed, e.g. miconazole gel, nystatin suspension or pastilles, or amphotericin B lozenges. If *Candida* is isolated, underlying systemic conditions predisposing to candidal infections should be eliminated.

Deficiency states

Nutritional deficiency in the Western world is rare in childhood and usually the result of malabsorption. Haematinic deficiencies (vitamin B_{12}, ferritin, folate) may give rise to a sore tongue and atrophic glossitis. The symptoms may precede the clinical features. Classically, vitamin B_{12} deficiency causes a raw beefy tongue. Clinically, other oral signs of deficiency may be apparent (see Oral ulceration and candidal infection, previously). If a nutritional deficiency is suspected, it is important to establish that the child is obtaining adequate dietary intake (is not vegetarian or anorexic) and to eliminate causes of malabsorption, e.g. Crohn disease, coeliac disease. If a deficiency is suspected, it may be prudent to measure full blood count, haemoglobin, serum ferritin, serum vitamin B_{12} and red cell folate, becasue a deficiency in a haematinic that has not yet given rise to anaemia may cause oral symptoms and produce glossitis.

Infections

Scarlet fever, *Streptococcus pyogenes* infection and Kawasaki disease (mucocutaneous lymph node syndrome [2]), of uncertain but possibly infectious aetiology, may cause furring of the tongue and prominence of the fungiform papillae, a so-called 'strawberry tongue' appearance.

In scarlet fever, the coating on the tongue is rapidly lost, and the tongue becomes smooth and deep red in colour (raspberry tongue). Infection with *Yersinnia pseudotuberculosis* has produced a similar clinical picture.

Erythema migrans (geographical tongue, benign migratory glossitis)

This is a benign condition which gives rise to well-defined areas of depapillation of the tongue, which heal and recur at a different site, hence the term migratory. Erythema migrans is a common condition affecting 1–2% of the population. The aetiology is unclear. There is often a positive family history and it is often associated with fissured tongue and possibly with psoriasis [3].

Histologically, erythema migrans bears a striking resemblance to oral psoriasis. The lesions exhibit thinning of the epithelium, elongation of the rete ridges and a polymorphonuclear infiltrate of the superficial epithelium. The lesions may occur at any age and are often symptomless. Soreness may be a presenting symptom, which is usually aggravated by eating salty or spicy foods. Typically, erythema migrans presents on the dorsum of the tongue as well-defined erythematous areas of depapillation, surrounded by a slightly raised white margin (see Fig. 158.27). The lesions are usually serpiginous in shape, giving rise to a map-like appearance; they may, however, be rounded or scalloped. The appearance of the lesions may change from day to day, hence the term 'migratory'. Rarely, erythema migrans has been described in other sites, such as the labial mucosa and the palate [4]. Usually, the diagnosis can be made from the history and clinical appearance of the lesions. If the lesions are causing symptoms then benzydamine hydrochloride mouth rinse or spray may be of use.

Localized enlargement of the tongue

The most common cause of localized enlargement of the tongue in children is acute inflammation caused by tongue biting. Persistent localized swellings are uncommon and are most likely to be caused by a lymphangioma (see Soft tissue swellings, previously) or a haemangioma (see Red and pigmented lesions, previously).

Hairy and furred tongue

Hairy tongue is not commonly seen in childhood; it results from excessive elongation of the filiform papillae of the posterior dorsum of the tongue, caused by chronic irritation, but may be idiopathic, particularly when seen in young children (Fig. 158.29). It is asymptomatic but if it is causing aesthetic problems, brushing the dorsum of the tongue with a toothbrush, sucking a peach stone or placing an effervescent vitamin C tablet on the tongue may be beneficial.

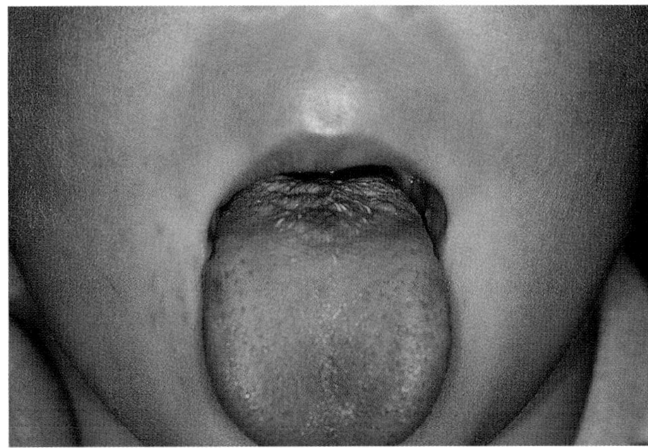

Fig. 158.29 Hairy tongue in a young preschool child.

Furring of the tongue resulting from an accumulation of squames rarely occurs in healthy children but is often seen in association with acute systemic illness, particularly scarlet fever. It results from a lack of mechanical debridement and changes in the oral flora. It may be precipitated by the use of broad-spectrum antimicrobial agents.

Brown or black discoloration may occur with either a furred or a coated tongue. The staining may be caused by chromogenic bacteria within the oral cavity or by extrinsic agents such as iron supplements or chlorhexidine gluconate, or coloured confectionery, tobacco or betel.

References

1 **Ghossainriant SN, Hadi U, Tawil A. Oral-facial-digital syndrome type II associated with congenital tongue lipoma. Oral Surg Oral Med Oral Pathol Oral Radiol Endod 2002;94:324–7.**
2 **Ogden GR, Kerr M. Kawasaki syndrome. Br Dent J 1988;165:327–8.**
3 Morris LF, Phillips CM, Binnie WH et al. Oral lesions in patients with psoriasis: a controlled study. Cutis 1992;49:339–44.
4 Luker J, Scully C. Erythema migrans affecting the palate. Br Dent J 1983;155:385.

SECTION 33: THE ORAL CAVITY

CHAPTER 159
Hair Disorders

Elise A. Olsen[1] *& Matilde Iorizzo*[2]

[1]Departments of Dermatology and Medicine, Duke University Medical Center, Durham, NC, USA
[2]Private Dermatology Practice, Bellinzona and Lugano, Switzerland

Introduction, 2103
Normal hair loss/growth in childhood, 2104
Hair loss, 2106
Hair shaft abnormalities presenting with hair breakage, 2112
Hair shaft abnormalities associated with unruly hair, 2120
Miscellaneous hair shaft abnormalities, 2123
Hair loss due to abnormal cycling, 2124
Miniaturization, 2128
Focal scarring and nonscarring causes of alopecia, 2129
Hypertrichosis, 2132

Abstract

This chapter is a comprehensive review of potential causes of alopecia or hair overgrowth that physicians may see in the paediatric population. It begins with an overview of the embryology and cycling of hair and then reviews the specifics of what is necessary to clinically diagnose a given hair disorder, i.e. the overall physical examination with particular reference to that of the scalp, microscopic evaluation of pulled or plucked hairs, the dermatoscopic examination and how and when to do a scalp biopsy. Hair loss is then addressed with various sections on abnormalities in the initiation of hair growth (examples include ectodermal dysplasias, follicular hyperkeratosis with scalp alopecia, syndromes with hypotrichosis); hair shaft abnormalities, including those presenting with hair breakage (examples include trichorrhexis nodosa, trichothiodystrophy, trichorrhexis invaginata, pili torti, monilethrix, etc.), hair shaft abnormalities associated with unruly hair (examples include uncombable hair syndrome, woolly hair, Marie–Unna type of hereditary hypotrichosis), and miscellaneous hair shaft abnormalities; hair loss due to abnormal cycling (examples include anagen and telogen effluvium, loose anagen syndrome); miniaturization of hair (androgenetic alopecia) and focal scarring and nonscarring causes of alopecia. The chapter then addresses causes of diffuse and local hypertrichosis. In each presentation of a type of hair loss or hypertrichosis, the clinical presentation, potential genetic association (if known) and available treatments are reviewed. Common conditions such as alopecia areata, trichotillomania and scalp infections/infestations are covered in other chapters.

Key points

- Hair loss presenting in childhood may be the clue to a genetic abnormality with variable phenotypic expression.
- An evaluation of the scalp by physical and dermatoscopic examination, microscopic analysis of pulled or plucked hairs and scalp biopsy may be necessary to completely characterize a given hair disorder.
- The hair, nails, teeth and potential for sweating should be evaluated in each child presenting with hair loss.
- Pili torti and trichorrhexis nodosa are not specific diagnoses but clinical clues to the presence of many different syndromes.
- Multiple gene abnormalities may lead to unruly hair: uncombable hair syndrome may be caused by at least three different genes, including PAD13, TGM3 and TCHH, and woolly hair by defects in keratin 74, LIPH, PTPN11 and HRAS.
- Patients with woolly hair should be evaluated for underlying cardiac abnormalities.
- Underlying metabolic problems such as argininosuccinic aciduria or citrullinaemia or certain inherited conditions leading to inability to absorb key dietary elements can lead to hair loss.
- For patients presenting with hypertrichosis, the location and length of excess hair, and the presence of any facial dysmorphism, dental abnormalities, gingival hypertrophy and mental or physical retardation should be noted as these will help separate out the potential genetic associations.
- Midback hypertrichosis may signal an underlying neurological abnormality and no excision or manipulation should be done without first evaluating the underlying cord and spinal column, probably best by imaging.

Introduction

Hair loss in childhood is usually accompanied by overwhelming parental concern that the condition will be permanent and/or leave psychological scars on the affected child. Conversely, physicians are more likely to focus on the potential relatedness of the hair loss to an underlying medical problem. The concerns of both are valid. There is great value in diagnosing a given case of childhood alopecia, as herein may be the necessary clue to an otherwise unfathomable multisystem illness or an explanation for an unexplained developmental delay. The hair loss presenting in childhood does include disorders for which no therapy yet exists, but there are many conditions in which specific treatment can either reverse

Harper's Textbook of Pediatric Dermatology, Fourth Edition. Edited by Peter Hoeger, Veronica Kinsler and Albert Yan.

the hair loss or make the hair more manageable and hence more cosmetically acceptable.

Hypertrichosis specifically refers to hair density or length beyond the accepted limits of normal for a particular age, race and sex and does not imply, as does the term hirsutism, a particular distribution of hair or a hormonal aetiology. Hypertrichosis may be generalized or localized, and may consist of lanugo, vellus or terminal hair. The presence of hypertrichosis in a child may signify an underlying physical abnormality, an associated metabolic disorder, a genetic multifocal syndrome or merely a cosmetic problem.

This chapter presents an effective approach to the diagnosis of the various types of alopecia and hypertrichosis presenting in childhood. Aetiologies of hair loss or hypertrichosis presented in detail in other chapters will be mentioned only briefly and the reader is referred to these other sources of information. Specifically, the common and potentially reversible alopecia areata is discussed in Chapter 160.

Normal hair loss/growth in childhood

To fully understand hair loss or excess hair growth in childhood, a basic working knowledge of normal hair growth is necessary, including the embryology and cycling of hair. Hair development begins *in utero* at 9–12 weeks, with the follicular units composed of a coordinated interdependent growth of epidermally derived cells that evolve into follicles and mesochymal cells that develop into papillae [1] (Fig. 159.1). By 18–20 weeks of gestation, fine lanugo hair (unpigmented, unmedullated fine hair, which may grow to several centimetres in length [2,3]) covers the scalp and proceeds to appear elsewhere in a cephalocaudal direction, eventually covering the entire fetus. This constitutes the first anagen (growth) wave, which is followed by telogen (resting phase) and, eventually, the actual shedding of the hair at the seventh or eighth month of gestation [2,4]. The lanugo hair is replaced by vellus hair on the body and vellus or terminal hair on the scalp.

The transition wave from anagen to telogen in the occipital scalp is delayed, however, and the expected telogen shedding in the occiput occurs at 2–3 months postpartum [2,4], accounting for the occipital alopecia normally seen in infants of this age (Fig. 159.2). Lanugo hair may also be seen on the limbs and shoulders of full-term, normally developed newborns, but this should be shed by 1–2 months of age.

For the remainder of the first year of life, scalp hair growth is synchronous, taking on the adult mosaic pattern only towards the end of the first year [2]. The number of follicles does not change after birth but, rather, the follicular density decreases as the skin expands to cover an increasing surface area [4,5]. There is a gradual transition from vellus (unmedullated, lightly pigmented hair with a final length less than 2 cm [5] to terminal (usually

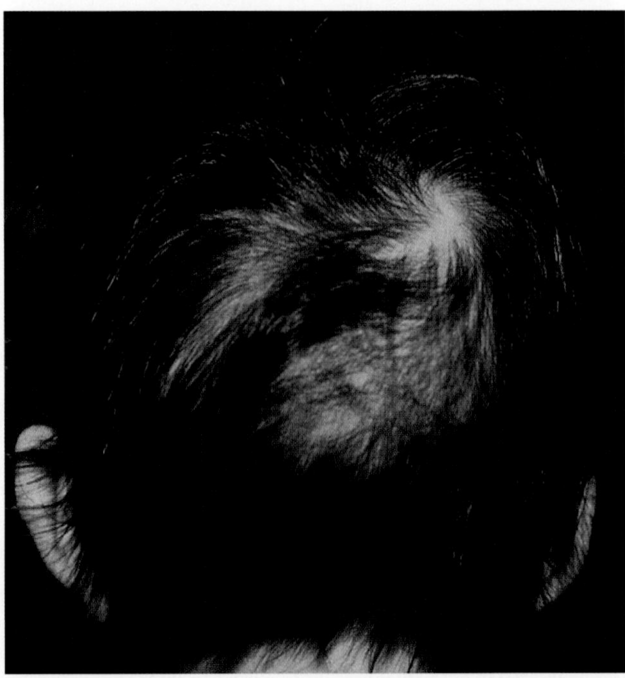

Fig. 159.2 Occipital alopecia in a 4-month-old infant.

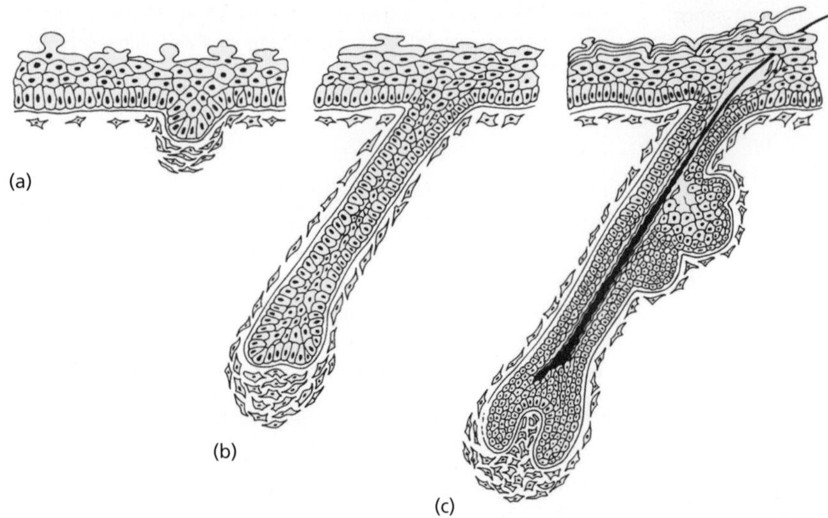

Fig. 159.1 Embryology of the hair follicle. (a) Follicular germ illustrating the condensing mesenchyme proximal to the epidermally derived follicle cells. (b) Follicle peg stage illustrating the organization of keratinocytes in the follicle and the mesenchyme of the follicle sheath and presumptive dermal papillae. (c) Bulbous hair peg stage illustrating the regions of the differentiated follicle. The upper bulge on the right represents the sebaceous gland and duct. The 'bulge' area where the arrector pili muscle will insert is below this.

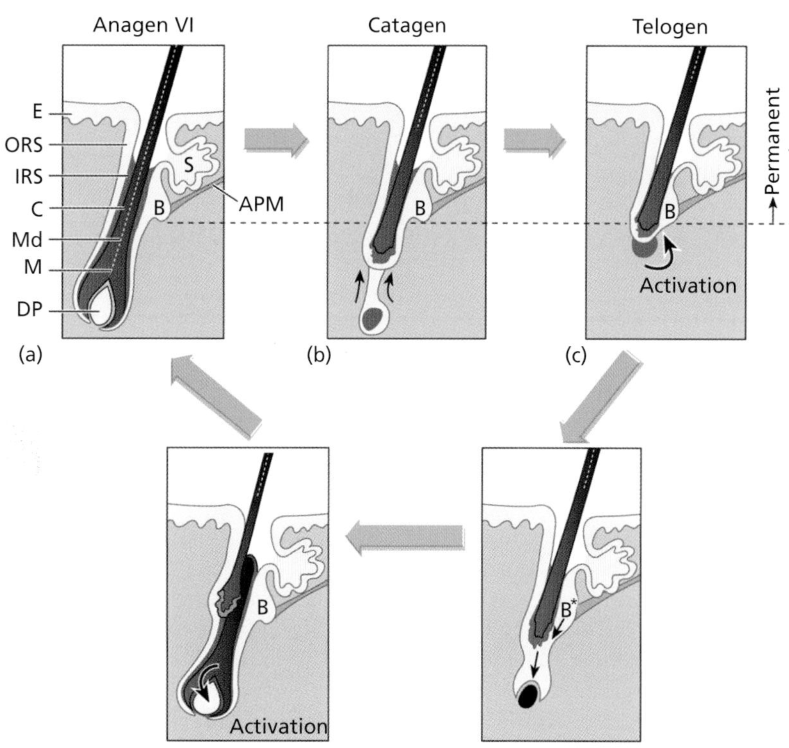

Fig. 159.3 (a–e) Normal cycling of hair. Follicular structures above the dashed line form the permanent part of the follicle. When the germinative epithelium undergoes downward proliferation and is once again in close approximation to the dermal papillae, the anagen growth cycle begins again. The preceding hair, if not lost by pressure or traction, will be shed as the new hair begins its growth phase. APM, arrector pili muscle; C, cortex; E, epidermis; IRS, inner root sheath; M, matrix; Md, medulla; ORS, outer root sheath; S, sebaceous gland.

pigmented, usually medullated, generally thicker shafts with longer anagen phase and thus longer ultimate length) hair over the scalp during the first year or two. Hair colour tends to darken with age [6].

All human scalp hairs regularly cycle through various stages of growth. In anagen, or the active growth phase, the follicular bulb embraces the dermal papillae in the dermis or subcutaneous tissue (Fig. 159.3). The division and maturation of the matrix (those cells in the centre of the hair bulb contiguous to the dermal papillae) produce columns of cells that stream superficially into the central portion of the bulb and then enter the straight linear portion of the follicle [7]. These proteins organize into keratin filaments and then into larger aggregates, which become progressively more compact as the shaft moves upwards and away from the bulb [8]. For much of the length of the follicle, the hair shaft is attached to layers of root sheaths, which serve both to anchor and to mould the newly formed hair. Anagen lasts for predetermined periods of time based on the area of the body the hair resides in; the normal time in anagen for scalp hair is longer and more variable than other body areas [9].

When a particular hair has completed its sojourn in anagen, it begins the process of transition to a resting (telogen) hair. The follicular bulb moves up in the dermis, with the dermal papillae no longer intimately associated but lagging behind (see Fig. 159.3). The transition phase between the end of anagen and the beginning of telogen is referred to as catagen and lasts 2–4 weeks. The time in telogen varies with body site, that in the normal scalp being 3–4 months. During telogen, there is a loosening of the attachment of the root sheaths to the hair shaft, meaning the hair can be dislodged by pressure or traction. Cells in the outer root sheath of the follicle at the base of the arrector pili insertion, the *bulge* region, are slow-cycling stem cells that are necessary for the recapitulation of anagen. Once telogen is completed, anagen begins again with downward growth of the follicle and regeneration of the matrix and lower follicle root sheaths [9,10]. The spontaneous loss of a telogen hair, termed exogen [11], generally signals the presence in the follicular canal of a new growing anagen hair.

References

1 Pinkus H. Embryology of hair. In: Montagna W, Ellis RA (eds) The Biology of Hair Growth. New York: Academic Press, 1958:1–32.
2 Barth JH. Normal hair growth in children. Pediatr Dermatol 1987;4:173–84.
3 Danforth CH. Studies on hair. Arch Dermatol Syph 1925;11:804–21.
4 Barman JM, Pecoraro V, Astore I et al. The first stage in the natural history of the human scalp hair cycle. J Invest Dermatol 1967;48:138–42.
5 Giacometti L. The anatomy of the human scalp. In: Montagna W (ed.) Advances in Biology of Skin, vol. 6. Oxford: Pergamon Press, 1965:97–120.
6 Price ML, Griffiths WAD. Normal body hair: a review. Clin Exp Dermatol 1985;10:87–97.
7 Cotsarelis G, Millar SE, Chan EF. Embryology and anatomy of the hair follicle. In: Olsen EA (ed.) Disorders of Hair Growth: Diagnosis and Treatment. New York: McGraw-Hill, 2003:1–21.
8 Bertolino A, O'Guin WM. Differentiation of the hair shaft. In: Olsen EA (ed.) Disorders of Hair Growth: Diagnosis and Treatment. New York: McGraw-Hill, 1994:22–5.
9 Lyle S, Cristofidou-Solomidou M, Liu Y et al. The C8/144B monoclonal antibody recognizes cytokeratin 15 and defines the location of human hair follicle stem cells. J Cell Sci 1998;111:3179–88.
10 Oshima H, Rochat A, Kedzia C et al. Morphogenesis and renewal of hair follicles from adult multipotent stem cells. Cell 2001;104: 233–45.
11 Milner Y, Sudnik J, Filippi M et al. Exogen, the shedding phase of the hair cycle: characterization of a mouse model. J Invest Dermatol 2002;119:639–44.

Hair loss

Evaluation of the child with hair loss

History. The evaluation of a child with scalp hair loss should always include a history, physical examination and microscopic examination of the hair bulb and/or shaft. Dermatoscopic evaluation offers additional information. The history should differentiate hair never coming in fully from hair that once covered the scalp but was later lost or shed. However, it is entirely within the range of normal for either the so-called second pelage (i.e. the second wave of anagen scalp hair) or the transition from vellus to terminal hair to be delayed up to 1 year of age, making it falsely appear that the affected child has congenital alopecia.

Diffuse scalp hair loss that has a hereditary basis usually manifests by the first or second year of life, but in some genetically based disorders, the associated hair loss becomes obvious only later (e.g. dyskeratosis congenita [1], Jorgensen syndrome [2], Beare pili torti [3], androgenetic alopecia). Obviously, family history is key in determining the exact mode of inheritance of a suspected genetic disorder, but family members may have only some of the features associated with a particular syndrome, and alopecia may not be one of them. Therefore, when a familial syndrome is suspected or when probing for a syndrome that has alopecia as one component of many potential abnormailities, one should inquire about multiorgan signs and symptoms. As the group of disorders collectively called ectodermal dysplasias commonly involve hair loss (and effects on the teeth, nails and sweating), this group of disorders should be sought in particular.

Examination.

Physical examination

A physical examination should be performed in all children with hair loss of uncertain aetiology. The possibility of a syndrome must be entertained and multisystem abnormalities sought for and catalogued; those of ectodermally derived organs (teeth, ears, eyes, central nervous system, mammary glands), bone, cleft lip and/or cleft palate are frequently associated with scalp hair loss. Particular attention should be paid to the child's facial features and whether a distinctive facies is present.

Hair and scalp examination

The scalp examination should first conclude whether the hair loss is diffuse (or global) or focal (Fig. 159.4). A diffuse loss could be secondary to an inherited abnormality in follicular or hair shaft development or a condition such as alopecia areata, anagen effluvium or telogen effluvium. Focal alopecia is less likely to be inherited and much more likely to be acquired.

The scalp in the areas of alopecia should be evaluated for the preservation of follicular openings (implying a nonscarring potentially reversible process; Fig. 159.5a) compared with smooth, poreless skin indicating attrition of follicular units and a potentially irreversible or scarring process (Fig. 159.5b). Dermatoscopic evaluation is helpful here as it shows loss of follicular openings with or without inflammation in cases of scarring or cicatricial alopecia. Scarring alopecia is rare in children in the absence of congenital focal scalp abnormalities, tumours or trauma.

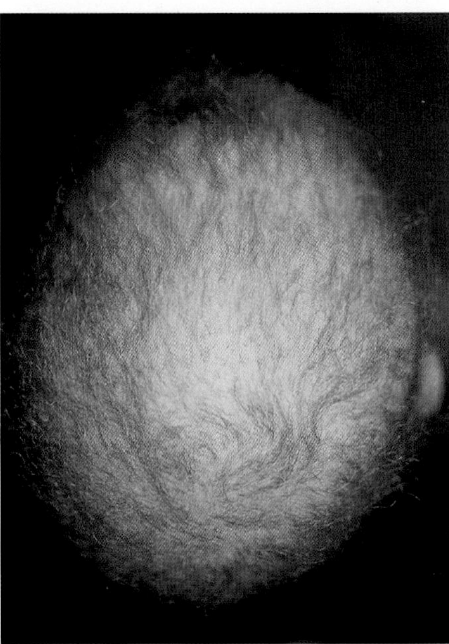

Fig. 159.4 Diffuse (global) hair loss in a child with Rosselli–Gulienetti syndrome (palate–popliteal pterygia syndrome) with subgroup type 1, 2, 3 and 4 ectodermal dysplasia.

Further differentiation can be made between hair growth abnormalities secondary to: (i) failure to initiate anagen; (ii) hair fragility leading to breakage; (iii) unruly hair; and (iv) premature curtailment or interruption of anagen (abnormality of hair cycle), leading to increased hair shedding. To determine if the hair growth rate is affected, a simple hair window can be performed. In this procedure, hair is clipped flush with the scalp in an arbitrarily determined target area (generally at the back of the scalp to prevent manipulation by the patient) and in a shape unlikely to occur naturally (such as a square or rectangle) and the hair length in this area observed a few weeks later. Even if there is an underlying hair shaft fragility problem that precludes the hair growing long, the hair should be able to attain a length of 0.5 cm in 2–3 weeks (1 cm/month is the normal hair growth rate).

To determine whether abnormal shedding is occurring, a simple hair pull is performed. Approximately 50–100 hairs are grasped at the base between the thumb and forefinger and gently pulled proximally to distally. This procedure should be repeated in at least five different areas of the scalp. The number and type of shed hairs are counted: there should normally be only telogen hairs. 'Loose anagen' hairs can be seen on hair pulls in very young children with otherwise normal hair if excessive tension is applied during the hair pull [4], whereas such hairs found on a hair pull in postpubescent children should trigger consideration of underlying hair pathology. A positive hair pull is considered more than three hairs/pull (assuming at least 50 hairs per pull) have been obtained from at least three

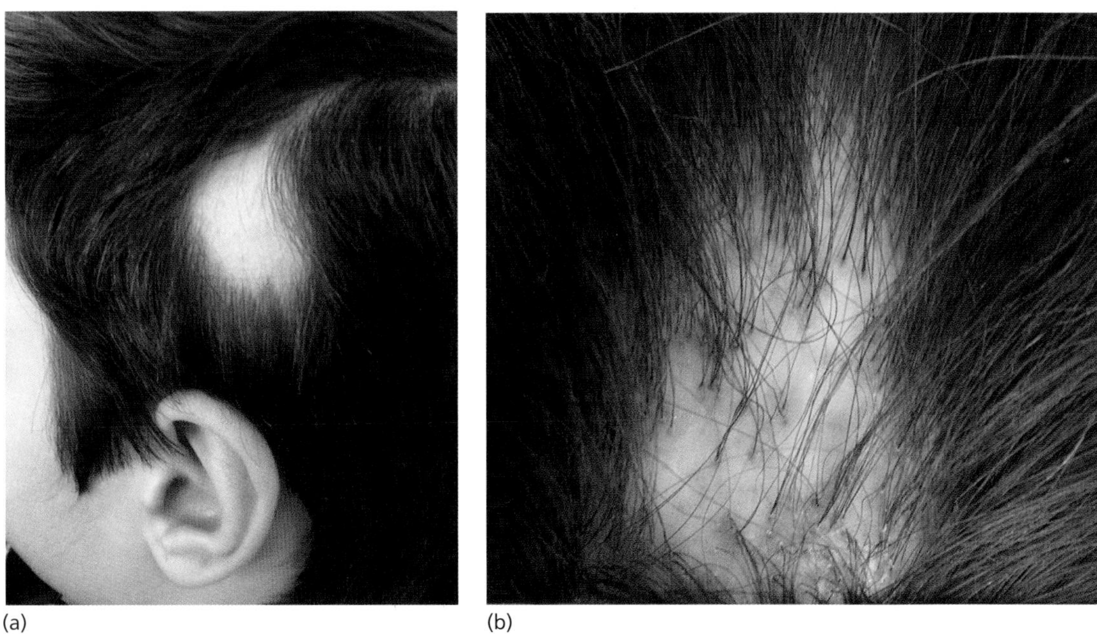

Fig. 159.5 (a) Focal, nonscarring hair loss of alopecia areata. (b) Scarring (permanent) hair loss in a child with lichen planopilaris.

of five hair pulls or >10 hairs total on five hair pulls from various sections of the scalp [5].

Microscopic examination of hairs

Light microscopic hair evaluation is a key first-line investigative tool for hair loss presenting in childhood [6,7]. If increased hair shedding is present, the proximal ends of hairs collected by a hair pull should be examined under the light microscope. One to two drops of cyanoacrylic glue are placed on a slide and the proximal hair shafts/bulbs are lined up in the glue and a coverslip placed over them: this decreases distortion and provides a permanent record of the hairs in question. The bulbs are then examined to determine if the hair loss is telogen or anagen. Telogen bulbs are unpigmented, rounded up and devoid of an attached root sheath (Fig. 159.6a). Normal anagen hairs are not readily obtained on a hair pull test but if one or two are, they generally have attached root sheaths (Fig. 159.6b). *Loose anagen hairs*, which can be seen in either normal young children as noted above, in patients with loose anagen syndrome or in patients with other causes of anagen hair dysfunction such as alopecia areata, are devoid of root sheaths and have a ruffled or floppy sock appearance of the attached cuticle (Figure 159.6c). Telogen versus anagen shedding should trigger very different types of work-up.

If there is no abnormal shedding, but instead the hair fractures with simple trauma (rubbing the hair between the fingers is one way of precipitating this in susceptible patients) or has an abnormal texture or dullness resulting in unruliness, a sample of affected hairs should be clipped and the distal portion examined under the microscope. Most hair shaft abnormalities can be diagnosed in this manner, although some will require further examination by scanning electron microscopy to confirm findings only hinted at under light microscopy (e.g. longitudinal grooving). Polariscopic examination is necessary in cases when the particular light microscopic findings of trichoschisis with or without trichorrhexis nodosa are seen, making the diagnosis of trichothiodystrophy a possibility. The aetiology of brittle hair can be further pursued by chemical analysis of the hair for sulphur content and/or quantification of individual amino acids.

Dermoscopic examination

In many situations, dermatoscopic examination can add key information that will facilitate a definitive diagnosis of hair loss in a child or will avoid the need for more invasive tests. It has been shown that the lens of the dermoscope (magnifications up to 160×) enables better appreciation of scalp/hair shaft patterns than the naked eye [8]. Moreover, if the dermoscope is connected to a camera, this permits capture and storage of the viewed images. In this way dermoscopy, a noninvasive and painless tool, is useful not only for diagnostic purposes but also to monitor progession of hair loss and efficacy of treatment, and to identify the preferred location of any potentially diagnostic biopsy.

There are three ways in which dermoscopy may be performed for the evaluation of hair disorders [9].

- *Nonpolarized dermoscopy*: this requires contact between the lens and the skin with a liquid interface placed between the two of them. This is the most widely used of the three methods and the first one utilized to describe diagnostic features of hair disorders [10]. However, because the liquid interface does not allow the evaluation of scalp scaling, this is not the preferred procedure in these cases.
- *Polarized dermoscopy* with cross-polarized filters allowing the reflected light from deeper layers to reach the observer's eye with contact between lens and skin.
- *Polarized dermoscopy* with cross-polarized filters without contact between lens and skin. This method is recommended for the evaluation of hair shaft abnormalities.

These methods are not equivalent but complementary.

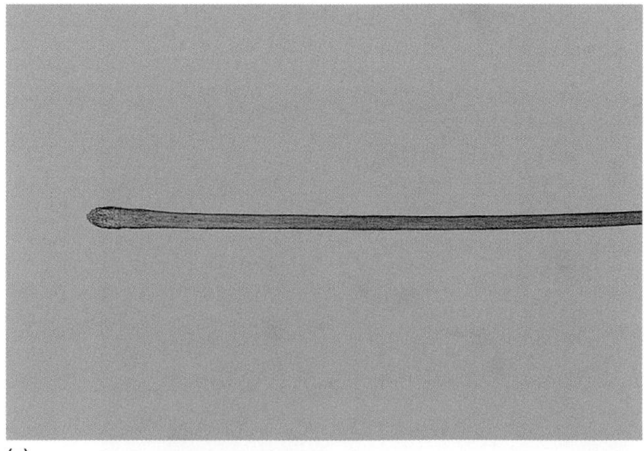

(a)

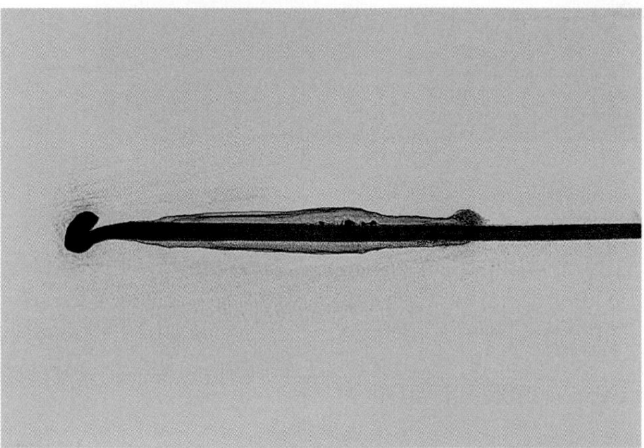

(b)

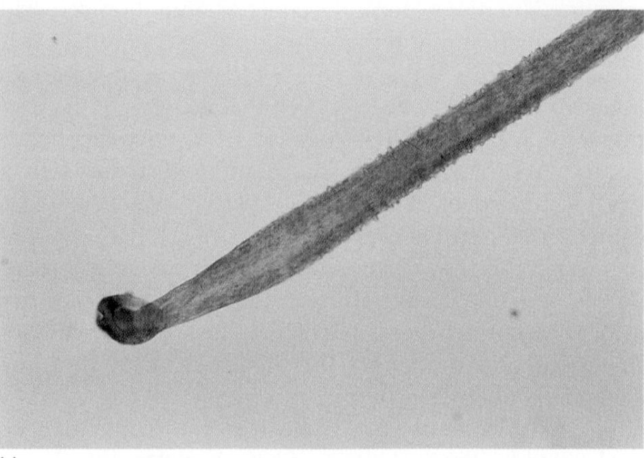

(c)

Fig. 159.6 (a) Telogen bulb (light micrograph, ×40). (b) Anagen bulb (light micrograph, ×40). (c) Loose anagen syndrome (light micrograph, ×100). Source: Reproduced from Olsen EA. Clinical tools for assessing hair loss. In: Olsen EA, ed. Disorders of Hair Growth: Diagnosis and Treatment, 2nd edn. New York: McGraw-Hill, 2003:59–69.

Scalp biopsy

A scalp biopsy performed in a representative area of the hair loss can determine the amount, type and location of inflammation present, whether there is follicular dropout, and if sectioned horizontally, the hair density, anagen/telogen ratio and terminal versus vellus hair. With a few exceptions, biopsies alone are rarely diagnostic of the hair loss condition, diagnosis being a clinicopathological correlation. Because of the pain involved in the procedure and potential uncooperative behaviour by the child, scalp biopsies are not commonly performed in children with hair loss.

Other procedures

Because the ectodermal dysplasias are such a large group of abnormalities and are defined by hair, teeth, nail and sweat abnormalities, dental radiographs may be necessary to exclude tooth involvement in the very young, and formal sweat testing may be necessary to document decreased sweating. Topical indicators such as iodinated starch or sodium alizarin sulphonate produce a dramatic colour change upon sweating and can probably establish anhidrosis but hypohidrosis may require thermal or chemical stimulatory tests to quantify sweat function plus/minus sweat gland number post induction [11–13].

Types of hair loss

Abnormality in initiation of hair growth

We are only now beginning to understand the genetic abnormalities associated with hair disorders. In several conditions, near or complete universal atrichia may be present at birth, or develop within the first 1–2 years of life. Caution should be exercised to ensure that the hair abnormality is isolated, as other associations may be unveiled only with time. For example, patients with mutations in the hairless gene may present with scalp alopecia alone [14] but develop characteristic keratin-filled epithelial cysts 3–18 years after the alopecia [15,16]. This syndrome (atrichia with papular lesions) is generally an autosomal recessive trait [17]. Total alopecia related to the hairless gene without other associated findings has been reported to be autosomal dominant, autosomal recessive or X-linked [14,18]. Patients with autosomal recessive hereditary vitamin D-dependent rickets (VDDRII) also present with total or near total hair loss within the first year of life but later develop rickets and cutaneous cysts [19]. The genetic abnormality is a mutation in the vitamin D receptor.

Universal alopecia may occur with (1) mental retardation as part of the alopecia-mental retardation syndrome (APMR), with *APMR1* mapped to chromosome 3q26.3-q27.3, *APMR2* mapped to chromosome 3q26.2-q26.31 and *APMR3* mapped to chromosome 18q11.2-q12.2, or (2) mental retardation and seizures as part of the Shokeir syndrome (alopecia, psychomotor epilepsy, pyorrhoea and mental subnormality) and the alopecia-mental retardation syndrome with convulsions and hypergonadotropic hypogonadism, both of uncertain aetiology [20]. Patients with the X-linked (Xq27.3–qter region) recessive condition Mendes da Costa–van der Valk genodermatosis present with universal alopecia at birth or within the first few months of life with reticular brown-red pigmentation on the face and extremities [20,21]. During the first few years of life, these patients develop recurrent nontraumatic intraepidermal blisters and may have associated acrocyanosis, microcephaly with mental retardation, dwarfism, short conic fingers and nail dystrophy [21,22].

Conditions in which follicular hyperkeratosis may be associated with total alopecia in infancy are presented in Table 159.1 [23].

Table 159.1 Follicular hyperkeratosis with scalp alopecia

	Inheritance	Hair	Teeth	Nails	Sweating	Skin	Other	References
Atrichia with papular lesions	AR	Born with normal, partial or absent scalp coverage but shed absent body hair	Normal	Normal	+/–	Keratin-filled epithelial cysts from age 2 years	Psychomotor retardation; ataxia; hypogonadism; all symptoms may be delayed a few years	[14–17]
Ichthyosis follicularis	AD or X-linked recessive	Sparse, short or absent scalp hair; sparse or absent lashes, brows and body hair	Normal	+/– Dystrophy in childhood (?secondary to infections)	Normal	Extensive follicular hyperkeratosis; chronic skin infections; hyperkeratotic plaques on extensor extremities, hands and groin	Marked photophobia +/– conjunctivitis, blepharitis, corneal abnormalities; +/– hearing loss	[24–26]
Keratosis follicularis spinulosa decalvans	X-linked recessive or AD	Progressive scarring; loss of scalp hair, lashes, brows and body hair during childhood and adolescence	Normal	Normal	Normal	Generalized follicular hyperkeratosis with marked plugging, especially head and dorsum of hands and fingers; these may become atrophic at puberty; palmoplantar hyperkeratosis; may develop telangiectatic pigmentation cheeks and brows late	Atopy; conjunctivitis; photophobia; corneal defects	[24,26–28]
Alopecia, keratosis pilaris, cataracts and psoriasis	AD	Childhood onset hair loss without preceding inflammation or lesions → scarring alopecia; sparse lashes, brows and body hair	Caries	Small and pitted	Normal	Childhood psoriasis; diffuse follicular hyperkeratosis sparing face and scalp	Keratoconjunctivitis; cataracts	[29]
Marie–Unna hypotrichosis	AD	Scalp hair sparse or absent at birth, coarse hair grows in early childhood, diffuse loss (especially over vertex) at puberty; hair shaft: cuticle abnormal, longitudinal ridging and irregular twisting; sparse or absent brows, lashes and body hair	No	Normal	Normal	Diffuse follicular hyperkeratosis with milia-like facial lesions	+/– Atopy	[30–33]
Perniola syndrome	AR	Near universal alopecia with sparse brittle lanugo hairs	Normal	Normal	Normal	Hyperkeratotic follicular papules	Seizures; +/– sensorineural deafness	[34]
Dwarfism, cerebral atrophy and keratosis pilaris	X-linked	Almost complete absence of hair	Delayed eruption	Normal	Normal	Generalized keratosis follicularis	Physical and psychomotor retardation, dwarfism	[35]
Keratitis–ichthyosiform erythroderma–deafness syndrome (KID syndrome)	AR and, AD reported	Diffuse, fine, sparse or absent scalp hair; +/– patchy, scarring alopecia; sparse lashes and brows; hair shaft: trichorrhexis nodosa	+/– Caries; brittle, malformed, delayed	Leuconychia, +/– thickend,hypoplastic	+/– decrease	Diffuse follicular hyperkeratosis; leathery erythroderma (not scaly) from birth including keratoderma; plaques on face in infancy; verrucous hyperkeratosis over knees	Neurosensory deafness; keratitis, increased susceptibility to mucocutaneous infections	[20,36–39]

(Continued)

Table 159.1 *Continued*

	Inheritance	Hair	Teeth	Nails	Sweating	Skin	Other	References
Onychotrichodysplasia with neutropenia (Cantu syndrome)	AR	Brittle, lustreless, sparse, short, curly scalp hair; scanty eyebrows, lashes and body hair; microscopic exam hair: trichorrhexis nodosa; sparse to absent pubic and axillary hair at puberty	Normal	Dystrophic; koilonychia and onychorrhexis	Normal	Follicular hyperkeratosis	Chronic neutropenia and recurrent infections; mild hypotonia	[3,40,41]
Pachyonychia congenita	AD	Generalized hypotrichosis, dry hair	Natal teeth; +/– caries; malformation	Yellowish-brown discoloration; thickened nails (distal 2/3) with pinched margins and upward tilt of distal tips (all cases); paronychial infections	Increased	Palmoplantar hyperkeratosis; follicular keratosis, especially knees and elbows; asteatosis; painful bullae or ulceration on palms and soles; verrucous lesions extremities; +/– epidermal cysts	Cataracts; hoarseness; +/– oral leucokeratosis; corneal dyskeratosis	[42–44]
Cystic eyelids, palmoplantar keratosis, hypodontia and hypotrichosis (Schöpf–Schulz–Passarge syndrome)	AR	Marked hypotrichosis, especially scalp; eyebrows and lashes coarse, sparse	Hypodontia; central incisors	Onychodystrophy; longitudinal ridging; splitting; onycholysis	Normal	Follicular hyperkeratosis; palmoplantar hyperkeratosis; late development eyelid aprocrine hidrocystomas		[23,45]
Monilethrix	AR, AD or spontaneous	Normal or absent hair at birth with development of brittle fractured hair in infancy; may include occiput only or extend to entire scalp, eyelashes, eyebrows and secondary sexual hair	Normal	Occasional fragility and splitting nails, longitudinal lines	Normal	Follicular hyperkeratosis on scalp and neck most commonly, also extensor limbs and periumbilical	± Physical retardation, syndactyly, juvenile cataracts	[46–48]

AD, autosomal dominant; AR, autosomal recessive.
Adapted from Olsen 2003 [23].

A few of the ectodermal dysplasias that present with universal or near total alopecia in infancy in which the genetic defect is known are listed below.

- Those associated with hair, nail and sweating abnormalities. Examples include odontoonychodysplasia with alopecia (mutation in WNT) [2,49,50], ichthyosis follicularis, alopecia and photophobia (IFAP syndrome: missense mutations in the membrane-bound transcription factor protease site 2 (*MBTPS2*) gene) [51] and ectodermal dysplasia/skin fragility syndrome (McGrath syndrome), caused by a mutation in the plakophilin-1 gene [20].
- Those associated with hair, teeth and sweating abnormalities under the hypohidrotic ectodermal dysplasia phenotype and related to genetic anomalies in the signalling cascade that leads to nuclear factor κB (NF-κB) activation. These include autosomal recessive or autosomal dominant mutations in the EDAR (ectodysplasin receptor) gene or EDAR-associated death domain gene EDARADD, respectively, or X-linked defects in the ectodysplasin A (EDA-1) gene, the receptor for EDA-2 and the NF-κB essential modulator (NEMO), the latter also associated with immune deficiency [52].
- Those associated with hair and nail abnormalities. An example is autosomal recessive palmoplantar keratoderma and congenital alopecia (also called cataracts-alopecia-sclerodactyly) [20,53].

Alopecia areata is the only potentially completely reversible universal alopecia that may present in infancy, but this is rare in the first year of life. This is discussed more fully in Chapter 160.

There is a very long list of conditions that present with hypotrichosis, but not complete alopecia, in infancy. The hypotrichosis may be secondary to follicular hypoplasia or to faulty hair shaft production and breakage. Hypotrichosis simplex of the scalp, related to a mutation in the gene that encodes corneodesmosin, begins in the mid first decade and is associated with almost complete hair loss by the third decade [20]. For example, individuals with autosomal recessive localized hypotrichosis (scalp hair, largely sparing secondary sexual hair) may have sparse hair at birth that regrows poorly or not at all: this may be related to a mutation in the *LIPH* (607365) gene on chromosome 3q27, *DGL4* on chromosome 18q12 or *P2RY5* on chromosome 13q14.12-q14.2 [20,54–56]. Other conditions may initiate hair loss a bit later.

Many of the ectodermal dysplasias are associated with hypotrichosis but, unfortunately, most of the hair shaft abnormalities have not been well characterized; the abnormal hair is generally described clinically only as 'brittle', 'sparse' or 'lustreless'. (The ectodermal dysplasias are discussed in detail in Chapter 134.)

Other nonectodermal dysplasia syndromes present in infancy with sparse, lustreless hair as one part of multiorgan abnormalities (example: cartilage-hair hypoplasia – mutation in the *RMRP* gene) [20,57]. Most of the multiple subtypes of orofaciodigital syndrome are autosomal recessive but type I is an X-linked dominant abnormality of the *CXORF5* gene. The hair in the latter is either dry and wiry or demonstrates diffuse or mosaic pattern of alopecia [20,58]. The diagnosis of the primary condition in these cases is rarely suggested by the hair abnormality, probably secondary to the dearth of available information on the hair.

There are, however, a number of conditions that *can* be diagnosed by microscopic evaluation of the hair shaft. Depending on the type of hair shaft abnormality, they generally present as fragile or unruly hair. These will be presented in the sections below according to their microscopic description.

References

1 Sirinavin C, Trowbridge AA. Dyskeratosis congenita: clinical features and genetic aspects: report of a family and review of the literature. J Med Genet 1975;12:339–54.

2 Freire-Maia N, Pinheiro M. Ectodermal Dysplasias: a Clinical and Genetic Study. New York: Alan R Liss, 1984.

3 Beare JM. Congenital pilar defect showing features of pili torti. Br J Dermatol 1952;64:366–72.

4 Olsen EA, Bettencourt MS, Coté N. The presence of loose anagen hairs obtained by hair pull in the normal population. J Invest Dermatol Symp Proc 1999;4:258–60.

5 Olsen EA, Roberts J, Sperling L et al. Objective outcome measures: collecting meaningful data on alopecia areata. J Am Acad Dermatol 2018;79:470–8.

6 Shao L, Newell B. Light microscopic hair abnormalities in children: retrospective review of 119 cases in a 10-year period. Pediatr Dev Pathol 2014:17: 36–43.

7 Olsen EA. Clinical tools for assessing hair loss. In: Olsen EA (ed.) Disorders of Hair Growth: Diagnosis and Treatment, 2nd edn. New York: McGraw-Hill, 2003:59–69.

8 Ross EK, Vincenzi C, Tosti A. Videodermoscopy in the evaluation of hair and scalp disorders. J Am Acad Dermatol 2006;55:799–806.

9 Nikam VV, Mehta HH. A nonrandomized study of trichoscopy patterns using nonpolarized (contact) and polarized (noncontact) dermatoscopy in hair and shaft disorders. Int J Trichol 2014;6(2):54–62.

10 Miteva M, Tosti A. Hair and scalp dermatoscopy. J Am Acad Dermatol 2012;67:1040–8.

11 Berg D, Weingold DH, Abson KG et al. Sweating in ectodermal dysplasia syndromes. Arch Dermatol 1990;6:1075–9.

12 Chia Ky, Tey HL. Approach to hypohidrosis. J Eur Acad Dermatol Venereol 2013:27:799–804.

13 Kim J, Farahmand M, Dunn C et al. Evaporimeter and bubble-imaging measures of sweat gland secretion rates. PLoS One 2016;11(10): e0165254.

14 Ahmad W, Zlotogorski A, Panteleyev AA et al. Genomic organization of the human hairless gene (HR) and identification of a mutation underlying congenital atrichia in an Arab Palestinian family. Genomics 1999;56:141–8.

15 Zlotogorski A, Panteleyev AA, Aita VM et al. Clinical and molecular diagnostic criteria of congenital atrichia with papular lesions. J Invest Dermatol 2001;117:1662–5.

16 Damsté TJ, Prakken JR. Atrichia with papular lesions, a variant of congenital ectodermal dysplasia. Dermatologica 1954;108:114–21.

17 Zlotogorski A, Martinez-Mir A, Green J et al. Evidence for pseudodominant inheritance of atrichia with papular lesions. J Invest Dermatol 2002;118:881–6.

18 Lundbäck H. Total congenital hereditary alopecia. Acta Dermatol Venereol 1945;25:189–206.

19 Miller J, Djabali K, Chen T et al. Atrichia caused by mutations in the vitamin D receptor gene is a phenocopy of generalized atrichia caused by mutations in the hairless gene. J Invest Dermatol 2001;117:612–17.

20 Online Mendelian Inheritance in Man, OMIM®. Johns Hopkins University, Baltimore, MD. https://omim.org/

21 Hassing JH, Doeglas HMG. Dystrophia bullosa hereditaria, typus maculatus (Mendes da Costa–van der Valk): a rare genodermatosis. Br J Dermatol 1980;102:474–6.

22 Carol WLL, Rooij R. Typus maculatus der bullosen hereditaren dystrophie. Acta Dermatol Venereol 1937;18:265–83.

23 Olsen EA. Hair loss in childhood. In: Olsen EA (ed.) Disorders of Hair Growth. Diagnosis and Treatment, 2nd edn. New York: McGraw-Hill, 2003:177–238.

24 Eramo LR, Esterly NB, Zieserl EJ et al. Ichthyosis follicularis with alopecia and photophobia. Arch Dermatol 1985;121:1167–74.

25 Rothe MJ, Weiss DS, Dubner BH et al. Ichthyosis follicularis in two girls: an autosomal dominant disorder. Pediatr Dermatol 1990;7:287–92.

26 **Rand R, Baden HP. Keratosis follicularis spinulosa decalvans: report of two cases and literature review. Arch Dermatol 1983;119:22–6.**

27 **Bellet JS, Kaplan AL, Selim MA, Olsen EA. Keratosis follicularis spinulosa decalvans in a family. J Am Acad Dermatol 2008;58(3):499–502.**

28 **Castori M, Covaciu C, Paradisi M, Zambruno G. Clinical and genetic heterogeneity in keratosis follicularis spinulosa decalvans. Eur J Med Genet 2009;52:53–8.**

29 Appell ML, Sherertz EF. A kindred with alopecia, keratosis pilaris, cataracts, and psoriasis. J Am Acad Dermatol 1987;16:89–95.

30 Stevanovic DV. Hereditary hypotrichosis congenita: Marie Unna type. Br J Dermatol 1970;83:331–7.

31 Wirth G, Bindewald I, Küster W et al. Hypotrichosis congenital hereditaria Marie Unna. Hautarzt 1985;36:577–80.

32 Mende B, Kreysel HW. Hypotrichosis congenita hereditaria Marie Unna mit Ehlers–Danlos-syndrom und atopie. Hautarzt 1987;38:532–5.

33 Solomon LM, Esterly NB, Medenica M. Hereditary trichodysplasia: Marie Unna's hypertrichosis. J Invest Dermatol 1971;57:389–400.

34 Perniola T, Krajewska G, Carnevali F et al. Congenital alopecia, psychomotor retardation, convulsions in two sibs of a consanguineous marriage. J Inheritable Metab Dis 1980;3:49–53.

35 Cantu JM, Hernandez A, Larracilla J et al. A new X-linked recessive disorder with dwarfism, cerebral atrophy, and generalized keratosis follicularis. J Pediatr 1974;84:564–7.

36 McGrae JD Jr. Keratitis, ichthyosis, and deafness (KID) syndrome. Int J Dermatol 1990;29:89–92.

37 Cram DL, Resneck JS, Jackson WB. A congenital ichthyosiform syndrome with deafness and keratitis. Arch Dermatol 1979;115:467–71.

38 Senter TP, Jones KL, Sakati N et al. Atypical ichthyosiform erythroderma and congenital neurosensory deafness: a distinct syndrome. J Pediatr 1978;92:68–72.

39 Rycroft RJG, Moynahan EJ, Wells RS. Atypical ichthyosiform erythroderma, deafness and keratitis. Br J Dermatol 1976;94:211–17.

40 Hernandez A, Olivares F, Cantu J-M. Autosomal recessive onychotrichodysplasia, chronic neutropenia and mild mental retardation. Clin Genet 1979;15:147–52.

41 Verhage J, Habbema L, Vrensen GF et al. A patient with onychotrichodysplasia, neutropenia and normal intelligence. Clin Genet 1987;31:374–80.

42 **Su WPD, Chun SI, Hammond DE et al. Pachyonychia congenita: a clinical study of 12 cases and review of the literature. Pediatr Dermatol 1990;7:33–8.**

43 Tidman MJ, Wells RS, MacDonald DM. Pachyonychia congenita with cutaneous amyloidosis and hyperpigmentation: a distinct variant. J Am Acad Dermatol 1987;16:935–40.

44 Feinstein A, Friedman J, Schewach-Millet M. Pachyonychia congenita. J Am Acad Dermatol 1988;19:705–11.

45 Burket JM, Burket BJ, Burket DA. Eyelid cysts, hypodontia, and hypotrichosis. J Am Acad Dermatol 1984;10:922–5.

46 **Zlotogorski A, Marek D, Horev L et al. An autosomal recessive form of monilethrix is caused by mutations in DSG4: clinical overlap with localized autosomal recessive hypotrichosis. J Invest Dermatol 2006;126:1292–6.**

47 Winter H, Rogers MA, Gebhardt M et al. A new mutation in the type II hair cortex keratin hHb1 involved in the inherited hair disorder monilethrix. Hum Genet 1997;101:165–9.

48 Karincaoglu Y, Coskun BK, Seyhan E et al. Monilethrix. Improvement with acitretin. Am J Clin Dermatol 2005;6:407–10.

49 Pinheiro M, Freire-Maia N, Gollop TR. Odonto-onychodysplasia with alopecia: a new pure ectodermal dysplasia with probable autosomal recessive inheritance. Am J Med Genet 1985;20:197–202.

50 **Adaimy L, Chouery, E, Mégarbané H et al. Mutation in WNT10A is associated with an autosomal recessive ectodermal dysplasia: the odonto-onycho-dermal dysplasia. Am J Hum Genet 2007;81:821–8.**

51 **Mégarbané H, André Mégarbané A. Ichthyosis follicularis, alopecia, and photophobia (IFAP) syndrome. Orphanet J Rare Dis 2011;6:29.**

52 **Smahi A, Courtois G, Rabia SH et al. The NF-kappaB signaling pathway in human diseases: from incontinentia pigment to ectodermal dysplasias and immune-deficiency syndromes. Hum Mol Genet 2002;11:2371–5.**

53 Wallis C, Ip FS, Beighton P. Cataracts, alopecia, and sclerodactyly: a previously apparently undescribed ectodermal dysplasia syndrome on the island of Rodrigues. Am J Med Genet 1989;32:500–3.

54 **Kazantseva A, Goltsov A, Zinchenko R et al. Hair growth deficiency is linked to a genetic defect in the phospholipase gene LIPH. Science 2006;314:982–5.**

55 **Rafiq MA, Ansar M, Mahmood S et al. A recurrent intragenic deletion mutation in DSG4 gene in three Pakistani families with autosomal recessive hypotrichosis. J Invest Dermatol 2004;123:247–8.**

56 **Kljuic A, Bazzi H, Sundberg JP et al. Desmoglein 4 in hair follicle differentiation and epidermal adhesion: evidence from inherited hypotrichosis and acquired pemphigus vulgaris. Cell 2003;113:249–60.**

57 Blackston RD, Brown AC. Cartilage–hair hypoplasia. In: Brown AC, Crounse RG (eds) Hair, Trace Elements and Human Illness. New York: Praeger, 1980:257–72.

58 Del Boente M, Primc N, Veliche H et al. A mosaic pattern of alopecia in the oral-facial-digital syndrome type I (Papillon-Léage and Psaume syndrome). Pediatr Dermatol 1999;5:367–70.

Hair shaft abnormalities presenting with hair breakage

Trichorrhexis nodosa

The most common defect of the hair shaft leading to hair breakage is trichorrhexis nodosa [1]. The primary abnormality is a focal loss of the cuticle, which leads to exposed and eventually frayed cortical fibres [2,3]. Initially, this appears microscopically as a nodal swelling and is followed by fracturing and splaying of the exposed fibres in a fan-like array (Fig. 159.7). Findings on dermoscopy mirror these changes and include multiple longitudinal splits in focal areas, white nodules along the hair shaft and frayed distal brush-like ends (Figure 159.8) [4]. Trichorrhexis nodosa can occur in normal hair that has been abused by excessive repetitive exposure to chemicals or physical trauma but more commonly occurs in inherently weak hairs after trivial trauma (e.g. brushing, combing).

Although trichorrhexis nodosa can present at birth as an isolated problem [5] or with teeth and/or nail abnormalities [6], its presence in an infant or young child should trigger a search for an underlying metabolic problem. One association is with argininosuccinic aciduria, an autosomal recessive disorder of the urea cycle caused by an abnormality in gene 7q11.21 [7] in which the absence of the enzyme argininosuccinate lyase (ASL), which normally splits argininosuccinic acid into arginine and fumaric acid, leads to acidosis, hyperammonaemia, low serum arginine, increased serum and urine citrulline and argininosuccinic acid (ASS) [8,9], the latter two findings being diagnostic of the condition [10]. Molecular genetic testing of ASL or ASL enzyme activity can be helpful when faced with equivocal biochemical results. In children with ASL deficiency, seizures and hepatomegaly may begin in infancy while symptoms of psychomotor retardation, ataxia and dull brittle hair (with microscopic trichorrhexis nodosa) may first manifest after the age of 2 years [11,12]. It has been proposed that the lack of ASL is linked with the reduced synthesis of nitric oxide and this could help to explain other symptoms of the disease (liver impairment, hypertension) present

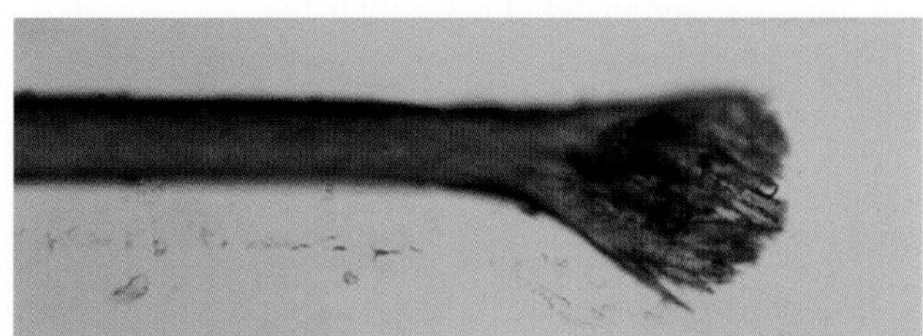

Fig. 159.7 Trichorrhexis nodosa (light micrograph, ×100).

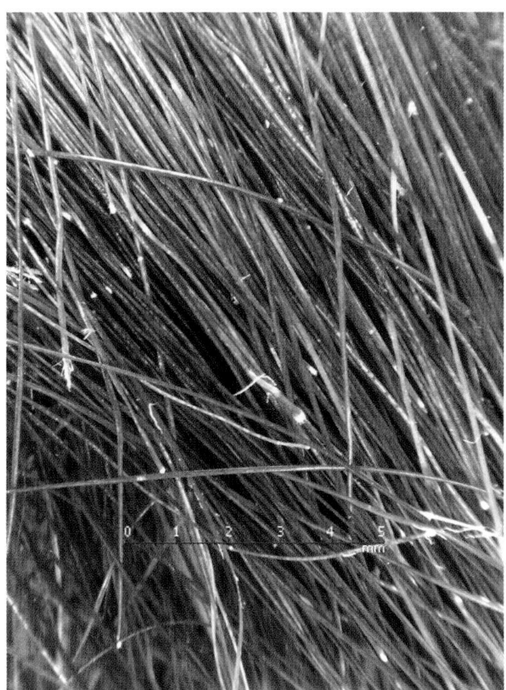

Fig. 159.8 Trichorrhexis nodosa seen at dermoscopy: white nodules along the hair shaft and frayed distal ends.

even with low or absent ammonaemia [13]. Dietary management with protein restriction and arginine supplementation, if initiated early, may ameliorate symptoms and has been shown in some cases to reverse the hair abnormality [10]. Other treatments include oral nitrogen scavenging treatment and/or orthotopic liver transplantation.

Another association of trichorrhexis nodosa is with citrullinaemia, in which affected children may also have increased serum citrulline and low arginine related to an abnormality of argininosuccinate synthase (ASS) [14]. Children with citrullinaemia may present with scaly skin eruption and hair fragility, with trichorrhexis nodosa and pili torti on microscopic examination of the hair [15–17].

Patients with Menkes syndrome, or trichopoliodystrophy, an X-linked disorder of copper transport, also have trichorrhexis nodosa and pili torti on microscopic examination of the hair [18,19]. The defective gene, *MKN* or *ATP7A*, encodes a copper-translocating membrane protein adenosine triphosphatase (ATPase) that disturbs intracellular copper homeostasis and the function of copper-requiring enzymes [20,21]. Systemic copper deficiency occurs from trapping of copper in some tissues, particularly the intestine, kidney, fibroblasts and red blood cells, leading to failure of copper delivery to other tissues [22–25]. In affected children, the hair is normal at birth but is replaced in early infancy by sparse, brittle, depigmented hair that feels like steel wool, hence the colloquial term of 'steely hair syndrome' [25–27] (Fig. 159.9). The skin is characteristically pale and lax, the face expressionless and the child drowsy and/or listless. There may be associated hypothermia, mental retardation and degeneration of cerebral, cerebellar, bone and connective tissue. A low serum ceruloplasmin is diagnostic of Menkes syndrome. Treatment with copper is usually ineffective

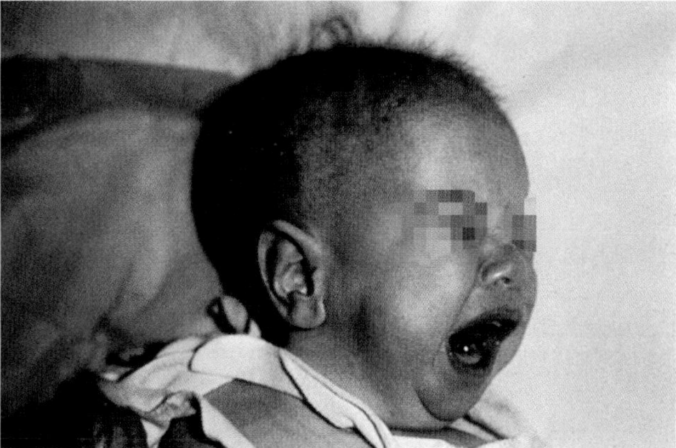

Fig. 159.9 Menkes syndrome. Source: Courtesy of Dr Janet L. Roberts.

and most affected children die by the age of 3 years [28]. Immediate postpartum treatment with copper-histidine has shown diminution in the severe neurodegeneration typical of the disease [20] but the genetic abnormalities causing Menkes disease cannot simply be corrected by copper replacement injections.

Other associations with trichorrhexis nodosa include trichohepatoenteric syndrome (mutations in both copies of *TTC37* or *SKIV2L*) [29], Kabuki syndrome [7] and biotinidase deficiency [30]. Trichorrhexis nodosa has also been reported in a patient treated with tumour necrosis factor-α for chronic plaque psoriasis [31].

Gentle hair care is the only treatment currently useful to improve the appearance of trichorrhexis nodosa.

Trichoschisis

Trichoschisis is a clear transverse fracture through the entire hair shaft (Fig. 159.10). Under the light microscope, the affected hairs often appear flat and may be folded over as well [32]. Trichorrhexis nodosa may also be present. Under scanning electron microscopy, the areas of fracture are associated with localized absence of the cuticle [32]. Trichoschisis, although not absolutely pathognomonic, is nonetheless seen with regularity only in the condition termed trichothiodystrophy.

Trichothiodystrophy is an autosomal recessive disorder characterized by sulphur-deficient brittle hair that may occur alone or in conjunction with other neuroectodermal abnormalities [33]. The hair abnormality identifies a group of genetic disorders in which acronyms or eponyms identify particular constellations of extratrichological findings (Table 159.2). Clinically, patients with trichothiodystrophy have, from early infancy, short brittle hair on the scalp, eyelashes or eyebrows (Fig. 159.11). The cystine content of the hair is about one-half of normal, primarily due to a major reduction and altered composition of the high sulphur matrix proteins [51–54]. Polariscopic examination of affected hairs characteristically shows alternating dark and light bands (tiger tail hair) (Fig. 159.12), presumably secondary to the alternating sulphur content [49]. Light microscopic and dermatoscopic changes are nonspecific although dermoscopy can be useful in identifying the specific hairs to be cut for examination, i.e. the hair with wavy contour and a 'grains

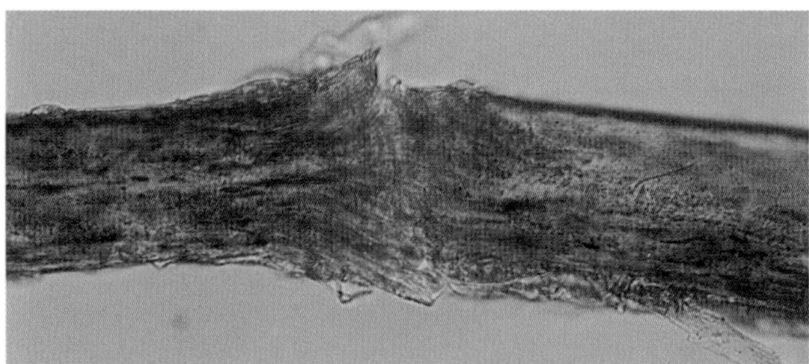

Fig. 159.10 Trichoschisis (light micrograph, ×400). Source: Reproduced from Whiting 2003 [57].

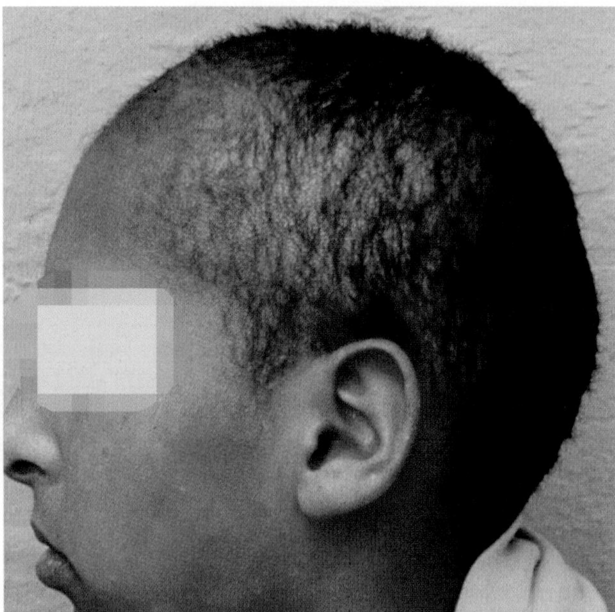

Fig. 159.11 Trichothiodystrophy. Reproduced from Whiting 2003 [1].

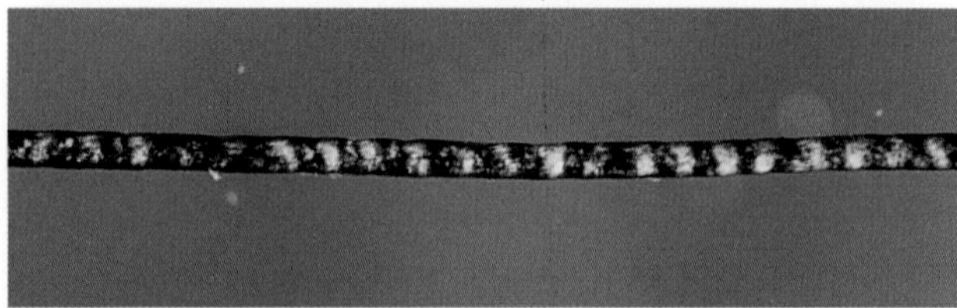

Fig. 159.12 Trichothiodystrophy (polariscopic micrograph, ×40). Note the alternating light and dark bands. Source: Courtesy of Dr David A. Whiting.

of sand' appearance [55]. Sulphur and/or amino acid analysis of the hair is diagnostic.

Other abnormalities should be sought in those patients with trichothiodystrophy (TTD) (see Table 159.2), particularly the presence of photosensitivity. Patients with TTD, particularly the 50% with photosensitivity, may have a defect in excision repair of ultraviolet damage but without an increased risk of skin cancer [56]. It has been determined that the various clinical presentations and DNA repair characteristics of both photosensitive TTD and xeroderma pigmentosum can be correlated with mutations found in the *ERCC2/XPD* locus on chromosome 19 that encodes the two-helicase subunits of transcription/repair factor TFIIH with trichothiodystrophy due primarily to mutations that affect the transcriptional role of *ERCC2* (TTD1) and xeroderma pigmentosum due to mutations that primarily alter the repair role of *ERCC2* [7,57]. Photosensitive trichothiodystrophy may also occasionally be associated with mutations in *ERCC3/XPB* on chromosome 2 (TTD2) and *TTD-A* (TFB5 gene; TTD3) on chromosome 6 [58]. The nonphotosensitive trichothiodystrophy mutations have been mapped to variations in the *C7ORF11* gene map locus 7p14 (TTD4), RNFII3A gene on chromosome X24 (TTD5) and GTF2E2 gene on chromosome 8p12 (TTD6) [7].

Trichorrhexis invaginata

Trichorrhexis invaginata (bamboo hair) clinically presents in infancy with short, brittle, often sparse hair [59] (Fig. 159.13). The primary defect appears to be abnormal keratinization of the hair shaft in the keratogenous zone allowing intussusception of the fully keratinized and hard distal shaft into the incompletely keratinized and soft proximal portion of the shaft [60,61].This leads to a proximal cup-like or socket-like expansion embracing a 'ball', the typical 'ball and socket' deformity (Fig. 159.14). Fracture of the shaft through this area is common, but there may also be disarticulation of the distal 'ball', leaving a golf-tee or tulip-shaped end to the abnormal hair [62] (Fig. 159.15). These changes may also be seen with dermoscopy as well as 'matchstick hairs' which are visible as short hair shafts with a bulging tip [63]. Pili torti and trichorrhexis nodosa may also be seen with trichorrhexis invaginata. Sulphur content is normal in trichorrhexis invaginata. Since the abnormal hairs may be present only in some sections of the scalp, many areas of the scalp may need to be evaluated to make a definitive diagnosis. The eyebrows and/or eyelashes should be evaluated if the scalp hair is unforthcoming for the suspected abnormality as they are frequently affected.

Trichorrhexis invaginata can rarely occur in traumatized, otherwise normal hair or with other congenital hair shaft abnormalities. Usually, however, the hair abnormality is associated with *Netherton syndrome,* an autosomal recessive inherited disorder that consists of the triad of ichthyosis, atopic diathesis and trichorrhexis invaginata [58,64,65]. The ichthyosis is most commonly ichthyosis linearis circumflexa, a polycyclic, ever-transforming scaly eruption with a double-edged scale on the leading edge [61,66] (Fig. 159.16). However, some cases of trichorrhexis invaginata have instead been associated with lamellar ichthyosis or, less commonly, ichthyosis vulgaris or X-linked ichthyosis [65,67]. The atopic diathesis usually includes persistent xerosis and may include erythroderma [64,68]. The diagnosis of Netherton syndrome should always be entertained in 'red scaly babies' who have sparse hair. Recurrent infections, short stature and mental retardation have been reported rarely in Netherton syndrome [69]. Netherton syndrome is caused by a mutation on chromosome 5q33.12 in the gene *SPINK5* which encodes lymphoepithelial Kazal-type inhibitor (LEKTI), a serine protease inhibitor of which various kallikreins are some of the targets [70]. It has been demonstrated that LEKTI deficiency leads to unapposed kallikrein 5 activity which in turn triggers stratum corneum detachment and

Table 159.2 Syndromes associated with trichothiodystrophy

Group	Brittle hair	Brittle nails	Intellectual impairment	Decreased fertility	Short stature	Ichthyosis	Photosensitivity	Neutropenia	Other findings	Acronym/eponym
(a) Isolated hair defect	+									Trichoschisis [34]
(b) Hair and nail dystrophy	+	+								Trichoschisis/onychodystrophy [32,35]
(c) Above and mental retardation and infertility	+	+	+	+					Astigmatism, pale optic discs, retinopathy	Sabina syndrome [36,37]
(d) Above and growth retardation	+	+	+	+	+				Quadriplegia, seizures, microcephaly	BIDS, Amish brittle hair syndrome [38,39]
(e) Above and ichthyosis	+	+	+	+	+	+			Abnormal teeth, tongue plaques, cataract, VSD	IBIDS [40,41], Tay syndrome [42,43], Pollitt syndrome [44]
(f) Above and photosensitivity	+	+	+	+	+	+	+		Abnormal repair of UV-induced DNA damage	PIBI(D)S [45–48]
(g) Most of above and chronic neutropenia	+	+	+		+	+		+	Recurrent infections, folliculitis, conjunctivitis	ONMR [38,49] Itin syndrome
(h) Marinesco–Sjögren syndrome	+	+	+		+				Ataxia, dysarthria, cataracts, abnormal teeth (primarily non-ectodermal)	Marinesco–Sjögren syndrome [15,16,50,51]

BIDS, brittle hair, impaired intelligence, decreased fertility and short shature; IBIDS, ichthyosis, brittle hair, impaired intelligence, decreased fertility and short stature; ONMR, onychotrichodysplasia, neutropenia, mental retardation; PIBI(D)S, photosensitivity, ichthyosis, brittle hair, impaired intelligence, (decreased fertility) and short stature; UV, ultraviolet; VSD, ventricular septal defect.
Adapted from Whiting 2003 [1].

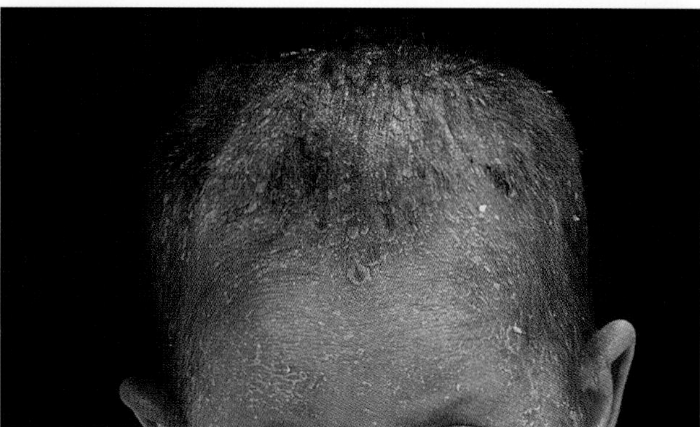

Fig. 159.13 Netherton syndrome. Source: Courtesy of Professor John Harper.

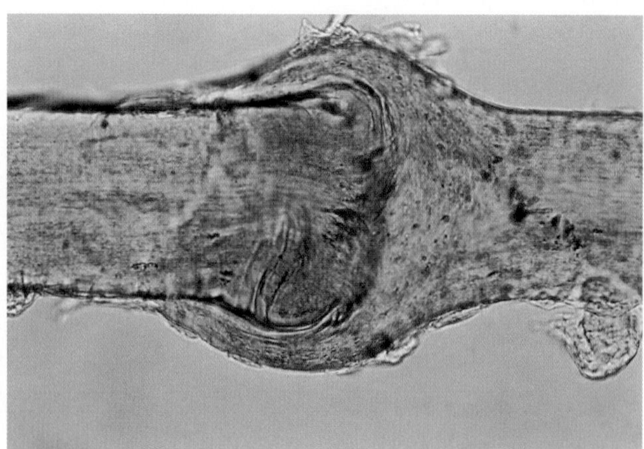

Fig. 159.14 Trichorrhexis invaginata (light micrograph, ×400). Source: Reproduced from Whiting 2003 [1].

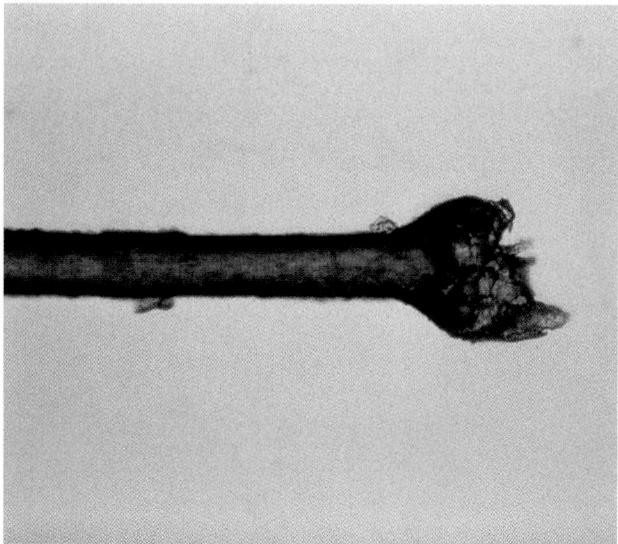

Fig. 159.15 Trichorrhexis invaginata, golf-tee fracture (light micrograph, ×200). Reproduced from Whiting 2003 [1].

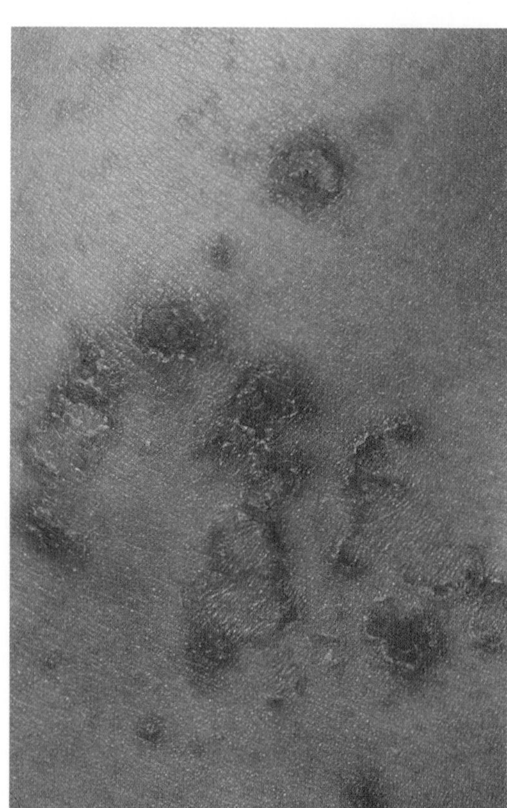

Fig. 159.16 Ichthyosis linearis circumflexa. Source: Courtesy of Dr Neil S. Prose.

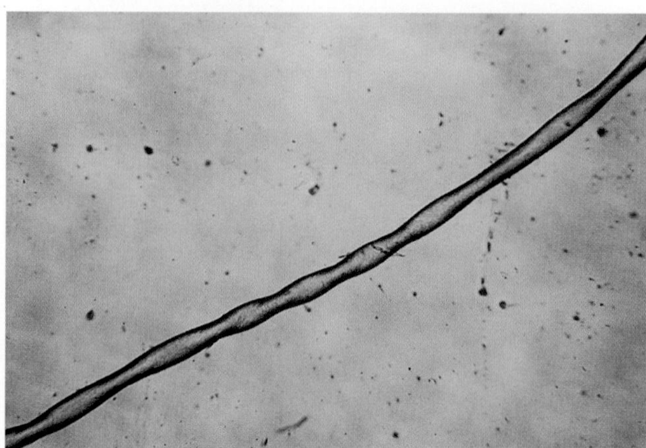

Fig. 159.17 Pili torti. Source: Reproduced from Whiting 2003 [1].

activates PAR-2 signalling, leading to the production of proallergic and proinflammatory mediators; this helps to explain the skin barrier defect and atopic diathesis [71].

There is no specific treatment for trichorrhexis invaginata. Retinoids (etretinate) and photochemotherapy (narrow-band UVB) have been reported to be of some value and the condition may spontaneously improve with age [72–74]. Newer treatments have suggested efficacy with omalizumab [75], infliximab [76], IVIG [71] and a topical ointment extemporaneously prepared with $NaHCO_3$, 40% zinc oxide in cod liver oil and lanolin postulated to act through kallikrein inhibition since skin proteases are inhibited by zinc and basic pH [77].

Pili torti

Patients with pili torti typically present with short, brittle scalp hair. It can also involve eyebrows and eyelashes [1,78]. Microscopically, the hair is flattened and twisted on its own axis, anywhere from 90° to 360° [79]. Twisted hairs on the scalp may normally be seen sporadically in Caucasians and are the norm in people of African descent and in the pubic/axillary hair of both races. For the

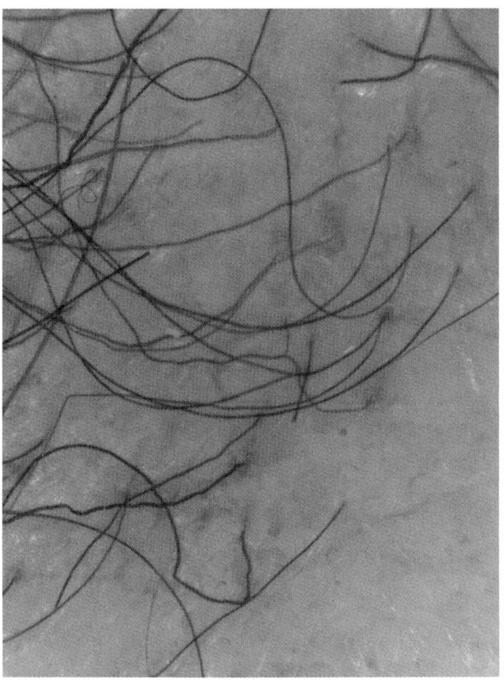

Fig. 159.18 Pili torti seen on dermoscopy.

diagnosis of pili torti, there must be multiple twists at irregular intervals on a given hair (Fig. 159.17) with each twist generally being 0.4-0.9 mm in width [79]. The same pattern of irregular twists is seen at dermoscopy (Fig. 159.18). The affected hairs generally fracture through the twists.

Pili torti may be an isolated finding or, like trichorrhexis nodosa, can occur in the presence of other hair shaft abnormalities as either an inherited or an acquired finding. It is also present in many different syndromes (Box 159.1). In the classic Ronchese type of pili torti, in which the isolated finding occurs in infancy primarily in blond hair, the inheritance is usually autosomal dominant, but autosomal recessive and sporadic inheritance have also been reported [82–85]. Pili torti has been reported to occur in association with monilethrix [86], pseudomonilethrix [87], woolly hair [88], longitudinal grooving [89], trichorrhexis nodosa [3] and trichorrhexis invaginata [90]. The hair abnormality usually presents in infancy [90]; however, as with many inherited hair abnormalities, the first and second pelages may be normal with the pili torti not developing until the second year. Sensorineural deafness has been described in a number of cases, and early auditory testing should be carried out in all children with pili torti [91,92].

Pili torti may persist indefinitely or improve at puberty. It may also present as a focal area of abnormal hair, usually secondary to trauma or to an underlying scarring condition of the scalp. It has been reported with the use of systemic retinoids in two patients with epidermolytic hyperkeratosis [93] and anorexia nervosa [94].

Monilethrix

Monilethrix may present at any time from infancy to the teens. The clinical picture of monilethrix can be very distinctive secondary to the appearance of extremely short brittle hairs emerging through keratotic follicular

Box 159.1 Infantile hair loss associated with pili torti

- Ectodermal dysplasia:
  - Rapp–Hodgkins syndrome
  - Solamon syndrome
  - Arthrogryposis and ectodermal dysplasia
  - Ectodermal dysplasia with syndactyly
  - Tricho-odonto-onychodysplasia with pili torti
  - Pili torti and enamel hypoplasia (Ronchese type)
  - Pili torti and onychodysplasia (Beare type)
  - Ankyloblepharon–ectodermal defects with cleft lip and palate syndrome
  - Trichodysplasia-xeroderma [7]
  - Palmoplantar keratoderma, mutilating, with periorificial keratotic plaques [80]
- Björnstad dysplasia
- Salti and Salem syndrome
- Crandall syndrome
- Menkes syndrome
- Tay syndrome and other cases of trichothiodystrophy
- Chondrodysplasia punctata
- Bazex syndrome
- Hypotrichosis with juvenile macular dystrophy [81]
- Citrullinaemia

Adapted from Olsen 2003 [95].

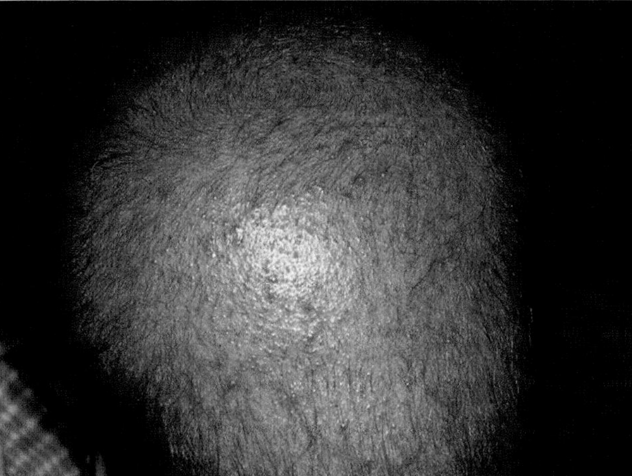

Fig. 159.19 Monilethrix. Source: Reproduced from Whiting 2003 [1].

papules (Fig. 159.19). The occiput and nape of the neck are especially affected and eyebrows and eyelashes may also be involved. Expression is variable with a spectrum of localized to global alopecia [96].

The diagnosis is entirely based on the microscopic findings. Because of this, it is important to take sufficient samples of short hairs from various parts of the scalp for evaluation; this should be done by cutting, not plucking the hairs, to reduce the potential for artifact being introduced in the assessment. Dermoscopy is valuable in choosing a suitable specimen for microscopic evaluation. Macroscopically, the hairs of monilethrix appear beaded, and with dermoscopy they look like a 'regularly bent ribbon' [55,97]. Microscopically, there are elliptical nodes occurring with regular periodicity every 0.7–1 mm [1]

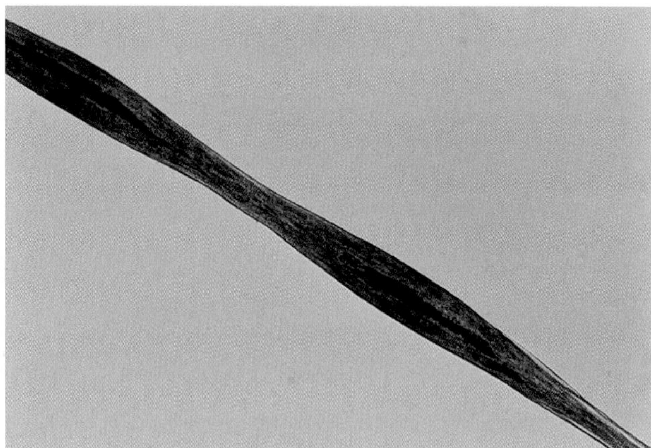

Fig. 159.20 Monilethrix (light micrograph, ×100). Source: Courtesy of Dr David A. Whiting.

(Fig. 159.20). In between the nodes, the hair shaft is constricted, and it is at these points that the hairs usually fracture. Pili torti is often mistaken for monilethrix by the uninitiated because of the microscopic illusion of variation in diameter of the shaft due to twisting. On scanning electron microscopy of monilethrix hairs, there are structural abnormalities of both the cortex and cuticle in the zone of keratinization [98].

Most pedigrees of monilethrix show autosomal dominant inheritance with high penetrance [85,99] and in these cases the disorder has been found to be closely linked to the type II keratin gene cluster on chromosome 12q13 (several mutations in the *KRT81*, *KRT83* and *KRT86* genes have been reported), implicating a mutation in the structure or regulation of a trichocyte keratin gene in the pathogenesis of this disorder [96]. Recessively inherited cases have been reported and are related to defects in the desmoglein 4 gene (*DSG4*), the same locus as autosomal recessive hypotrichosis [7,100,101].

The hair defect in monilethrix may occur alone or in association with keratosis pilaris, physical retardation, syndactyly, cataracts and nail/teeth abnormalities [102]. It has been reported in a child with Holt–Oram syndrome (limb and cardiovascular defects) [103]. Improvement in hair brittleness may occur during the summer and with age. Etretinate/acitretin and 2% topical minoxidil may be potentially useful therapies [104,105–108]. As in other hair shaft disorders characterized by fragility, protection against trauma such as excessive brushing, styling and braiding is key to limiting hair breakage.

Pseudomonilethrix

Pseudomonilethrix is microscopic irregular beading along the hair shaft as opposed to the regular beading seen in monilethrix [85]. Although it has been reported in patients with fragile hair [85,109], the appearance of pseudomonilethrix can be produced in normal hairs by compressing two hairs together between two glass slides [110,111]. It is likely that the nodes in pseudomonilethrix are artefactual [1].

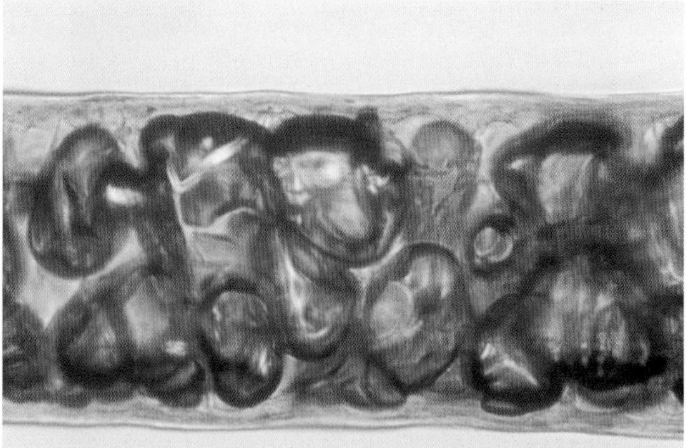

Fig. 159.21 Bubble hair; row of adjacent bubbles in shaft. Source: Reproduced from Whiting 2003 [1].

Bubble hair

Bubble hair is not a genetic abnormality in the hair but one of breakage caused by damage occuring during hair care. The resulting hairs have a characteristic microscopic appearance (Fig. 159.21). It has been possible to recapitulate the microscopic findings in normal hair by excessive heat [1,112]. Stopping the offending hair care practice usually resolves the problem.

References

1 **Whiting DA. Hair shaft defects. In: Olsen EA (ed.) Disorders of Hair Growth: Diagnosis and Treatment. New York: McGraw-Hill, 2003: 91–137.**

2 Dawber RPR, Comaish S. Scanning electron microscopy of normal and abnormal hair shafts. Arch Dermatol 1970;101:316–22.

3 Chernosky ME, Owens DW. Trichorrhexis nodosa: clinical and investigative studies. Arch Dermatol 1966;94:577–85.

4 **Miteva M, Tosti A. Dermatoscopy of hair shaft disorders. J Am Acad Dermatol 2013;68:473–81.**

5 Wolff HH, Vigl E, Braun-Falco O. Trichorrhexis congenita. Hautarzt 1975;26:576–80.

6 Rousset MJ. Genodermatose difficilement classable (trichorrhexis nodosa) predominant chez les males dans quatre generations. Bull Soc Fr Dermatol Syph 1952;59:298–300.

7 **Online Mendelian Inheritance in Man, OMIM®. Johns Hopkins University, Baltimore, MD. https://omim.org/**

8 Levin B, Mackay HMM, Oberholzer VG. Argininosuccinic aciduria, an inborn error of amino acid metabolism. Arch Dis Child 1961;36:622.

9 Batshaw ML, Thomas GH, Brusilow SW. New approaches to the diagnosis and treatment of inborn errors of urea synthesis. Pediatrics 1981;68:290–7.

10 **Nagamani SCS, Erez A, Lee B. Argininosuccinate lyase deficiency. Genet Med 2012:14(5):501–7.**

11 Shih VE. Early dietary management in an infant with argininosuccinase deficiency: preliminary report. J Pediatr 1972;80:645–8.

12 Rauschkolb EW, Chernosky ME, Knox JM et al. Trichorrhexis nodosa: an error of amino acid metabolism? J Invest Dermatol 1967;48:260–3.

13 Erez A, Nagamani SC, Shchelochkov OA et al. Requirement of argininosuccinate lyase for systemic nitric oxide production. Nat Med 2011;17 (12):1618–26.

14 Goldblum OM, Brusilow SW, Maldonado YA et al. Neonatal citrullinemia associated with cutaneous manifestations and arginine deficiency. J Am Acad Dermatol 1986;14:321–6.

15 Porter PS. The genetics of human hair growth. In: Bergsma D (ed.) Birth Defects, Original Article Series. Baltimore: Williams & Wilkins, 1972:69–85.

16 Danks DM, Tippett P, Zentner G. Severe neonatal citrullinemia. Arch Dis Child 1974;49:579–81.

17 Patel HP, Unis ME. Pili torti in association with citrullinemia. J Am Acad Dermatol 1985;12:203–6.

18 Menkes JH, Alter M, Steigleder GK et al. A sex-linked recessive disorder with retardation of growth, peculiar hair and focal cerebral and cerebellar degeneration. Pediatrics 1962;29:764–9.

19 Menkes JH. Kinky hair disease. Pediatrics 1972;50:181–3.

20 Tümer Z, Horn N, Tonnesen T et al. Early copper–histidine treatment for Menkes disease. Nature Genet 1996;12:11–13.

21 Davies K. Cloning the Menkes disease gene. Nature 1993;361:98.

22 Danks DM, Campbell PE, Walker-Smith J et al. Menkes' kinky hair syndrome. Lancet 1972;i:1100–3.

23 Horn N. Copper incorporation studies on cultured cells for prenatal diagnosis of Menkes' disease. Lancet 1976;i:1156–8.

24 Kodama H. Recent developments in Menkes disease. J Inherit Metab Dis 1993;16:791–9.

25 Danks DM, Campbell PE, Stevens BJ et al. Menkes' kinky hair syndrome. An inherited defect in copper absorption with widespread effects. Pediatrics 1972;50:188–201.

26 French JH, Sherard ES, Lubell H et al. Trichopoliodystrophy. Arch Neurol 1972;26:229–44.

27 Goka TJ, Stevenson RE, Hefferan PM et al. Menkes' disease: a biochemical abnormality in cultured human fibroblasts. Proc Natl Acad Sci USA 1976;73:604–6.

28 Wheeler EM, Roberts PF. Menkes's steely hair syndrome. Arch Dis Child 1976;51:269–74.

29 Hartley JL, Zachos NC, Dawood B et al. Mutations in TTC37 cause trichohepatoenteric syndrome (phenotypic diarrhea of infancy). Gastroenterology 2010; 138:2388–98.

30 Lünnemann L, Vogt A, Blume-Peytavi U, Garcia Bartels N. Hair-shaft abnormality in a 7-year-old girl. Trichorrhexis nodosa due to biotinidase deficiency. JAMA Dermatol 2013;149:357–63.

31 Mahendran P, George SAMC, Farrant PBJ. Trichorrhexis nododa: a distinctive presentation after tumour necrosis factor-α inhibitor therapy. Clin Exp Dermatol 2016;41:312–27.

32 Venning VA, Dawber RPR, Ferguson DJP et al. Weathering of hair in trichothiodystrophy [Abstract]. Br J Dermatol 1986;114:591–5.

33 Price VH, Odom RB, Ward WH et al. Trichothiodystrophy: sulfur deficient brittle hair as a marker for a neuroectodermal symptom complex. Arch Dermatol 1980;116:1375–84.

34 Brown AC, Belser RB, Crouses RG et al. A congenital hair defect: trichoschisis and alternating birefringence and low sulfur content. J Invest Dermatol 1970;54:496–509.

35 Van Neste D, Miller X, Bohnert E. Clinical symptoms associated with trichothiodystrophy. A review of the literature with special emphasis on light sensitivity and the association with xeroderma pigmentosum (complementation group D). In: Van Neste D, Lachapelle JM, Antoine JL (eds) Trends in Human Hair Growth and Alopecia Research. Dordrecht: Kluwer Academic, 1989:183–93.

36 Arbisser AI, Scott CI Jr, Howell RR et al. A syndrome manifested by brittle hair with morphologic and biochemical abnormalities, developmental delay and normal stature. Birth Defects 1976;12:219–28.

37 Howell RR, Collie WR, Cavados OI et al. The Sabinas brittle hair syndrome. In: Brown AC, Crounse RG (eds) Hair, Trace Elements and Human Illness. New York: Praeger: 1980:210–19.

38 Baden HP, Jackson CE, Weiss L et al. The physicochemical properties of hair in the BIDS syndrome. Am J Hum Genet 1976;28:514–21.

39 Jackson CE, Weiss L, Watson JHL. Brittle hair with short stature, intellectual impairment and decreased fertility: an autosomal recessive syndrome in an Amish kindred. Pediatrics 1974;54:201–7.

40 Jorizzo JL, Crounse RG, Wheeler CE Jr. Lamellar ichthyosis, dwarfism, mental retardation and hair shaft abnormalities; a link between the ichthyosis-associated and BIDS syndromes. J Am Acad Dermatol 1980;2:309–17.

41 Jorizzo JL, Atherton DJ, Crounse RG et al. Ichthyosis, brittle hair, impaired intelligence, decreased fertility and short stature (IBIDS syndrome). Br J Dermatol 1982;106:705–10.

42 Tay CH. Ichthyosiform erythroderma, hair shaft abnormalities, and mental and growth retardation: a new recessive disorder. Arch Dermatol 1971;104:4–13.

43 Happle R, Traupe H, Grobe H et al. The Tay syndrome (congenital ichthyosis with trichothiodystrophy). Eur J Pediatr 1984;141: 147–52.

44 Pollitt RJ, Jenner FA, Davies M. Sibs with mental and physical retardation and trichorrhexis nodosa with abnormal amino acid composition of the hair. Arch Dis Child 1968;43:211–16.

45 Crovato F, Borrone C, Rebora A. Trichothiodystrophy: BIDS, IBIDS and PIBIDS? Br J Dermatol 1983;108:247–51.

46 Crovato F, Rebora A. PIBI(D)S syndrome: a new entity with defect of the deoxyribonucleic acid excision repair system. J Am Acad Dermatol 1985;13:683–5.

47 Lucky PA, Kirsch N, Lucky AW et al. Low-sulfur hair syndrome associated with UVB photosensitivity and testicular failure. J Am Acad Dermatol 1984;11:340–6.

48 Rebora A, Guarrera M, Crovato F. Amino-acid analysis in hair from PIBI(D)S syndrome. J Am Acad Dermatol 1986;15:109–11.

49 Itin PH, Pittelkow MR. Trichothiodystrophy with chronic neutropenia and mild mental retardation. J Am Acad Dermatol 1991;24: 356–8.

50 Norwood WF. The Marinesco–Sjögren syndrome. J Pediatr 1964;65: 431–7.

51 Gillespie JM, Marshall RCA. Comparison of the proteins of normal and trichothiodystrophic human hair. J Invest Dermatol 1983;80:195–202.

52 Gummer CL, Dawber RPR, Price VH. Trichothiodystrophy: an electron-histochemical study of the hair shaft. Br J Dermatol 1984; 110:439–49.

53 Chen E, Cleaver JE, Weber CA et al. Trichothiodystrophy: clinical spectrum, central nervous system imaging, and biochemical characterization of two siblings. J Invest Dermatol 1994;103:154S–8S.

54 Gillespie JM, Marshall RC. Effect of mutations on the proteins of wool and hair. In: Rogers GE, Reis PJ, Ward KA et al. (eds) The Biology of Wool and Hair. London: Chapman & Hall, 1989:257–73.

55 Rakowska A, Slowinska M, Kowalska-Oledzka E, Rudnicka L. Trichoscopy in genetic hair shaft abnormalities. J Dermatol Case Rep 2008;2:14–20.

56 Takayama K, Salazar EP, Broughton BC et al. Defects in the DNA repair and transcription gene ERCC2 (XPD) in trichothiodystrophy. Am J Hum Genet 1996;58:263–70.

57 Faghri S, Tamura D, Kraemer KH, DiGiovanna JJ. Trichothiodystrophy: a systematic review of 112 published cases characterizes a wide spectrum of clinical manifestations. J Med Genet 2008;45:609–21.

58 Hashimoto S, Egly JM. Trichothiodystrophy view from the molecular basis of DNA repair/transcription factor TFIIH. Hum. Mole Genet 2009;18:R224–R230.

59 Netherton EW. A unique case of trichorrhexis nodosa: 'bamboo hairs'. Arch Dermatol 1958;78:483–7.

60 Ito M, Ito K, Hashimoto K. Pathogenesis in trichorrhexis invaginata (bamboo hair). J Invest Dermatol 1984;83:1–6.

61 Mevorah B, Frenk E. Ichthyosis linearis circumflexa Comel with trichorrhexis invaginata (Netherton's syndrome): a light microscopical study of the skin changes. Dermatologica 1974;149:193–200.

62 De Berker D, Paige D, Harper J et al. Golf tee hairs: a new sign in Netherton's syndrome. Br J Dermatol 1992;127(Suppl 40):30.

63 Goujon E, Beer F, Fraitag S et al. Matchstick eyebrow hairs: a dermoscopic clue to the diagnosis of Netherton syndrome. J Eur Acad Venereol 2010;24:740–1.

64 Wilkinson RD, Curtis GH, Hawk WA. Netherton's disease. Arch Dermatol 1964;89:106–13.

65 Greene SL, Muller SA. Netherton's syndrome. J Am Acad Dermatol 1985;13:329–37.

66 Comel M. Ichthyosis linearis circumflexa. Dermatologica 1949;98:133–6.

67 Hurwitz S, Kirsch N, McGuire J. Re-evaluation of ichthyosis and hair shaft abnormalities. Arch Dermatol 1971;103:266–71.

68 Krafchik BR. Netherton syndrome. Pediatr Dermatol 1992;9:158–60.

69 Greig D, Wishart J. Growth abnormality in Netherton's syndrome. Aust J Dermatol 1982;23:27–30.

70 Chavanas S, Garner C, Bodemer C et al. Localization of the Netherton syndrome gene to chromosome 5q32, by linkage analysis and homozygosity mapping. Am J Hum Genet 2000;66:914.

71 Furio L, Hovnanian A. Netherton syndrome: defective kallikrein inhibition in the skin leads to skin inflammation and allergy. Biol Chem 2014;385:945–58.

72 Hausser I, Anton-Lamprecht I, Hartschuh W et al. Netherton's syndrome. Ultrastructure of the active lesion under retinoid therapy. Arch Dermatol Res 1989;281:165–72.

73 Happle R, Traupe H. Etretinat bei Genodermatosen und Verschiedenen Entzundlichen Hautkrankheiten. In: Bauer RH, Gollnick H (eds) Retinoide in der Praxis. Berlin: Grosse, 1984:35–49.

74 Nagata T. Netherton's syndrome which responded to photochemotherapy. Dermatologica 1980;161:51–6.

75 Yalcin AD. A case of Netherton syndrome: successful treatment with omalizumab and pulse prednisolone and its effects on cytokines and immunoglobulin levels. Immunopharmacol Immunotoxicol 2016;38(2):162–6.

76 Fontao L, Laffitte E, Briot A et al. Infliximab infusions for Netherton syndrome: sustained clinical improvement correlates with a reduction of thymic stromal lymphopoietin levels in the skin. J Invest Dermatol 2011:131:1947–50.
77 Tiryakioglu No, Onal Z, Saygill SK et al. Treatment of ichthyosis and hyernatremia in a patient with Netherton syndrome with a SPINK5 c.153delT mutation using kallikrein inhibiting ointment. Int J Dermatol 2017;56:106–8.
78 Mirmirani P, Samimi SS, Mostow E. Pili torti: clinical findings, associated disorders, and new insights into mechanisms of hair twisting. Cutis 2009;84:143–7.
79 Whiting DA, Dy LC. Office diagnosis of hair shaft defects. Semin Cutan Med Surg 2006;25:24–34.
80 Mevorah B, Goldberg I, Sprecher E et al. Olmsted syndrome: mutilating palmoplantar keratoderma with periorificial keratotic plaques. J Am Acad Dermatol 2005;53:S266–S272.
81 Indelman M, Bergman R, Lurie R et al. A missense mutation in CDH3, encoding P-cadherin, causes hypotrichosis with juvenile macular dystrophy. J Invest Dermatol 2002;119:1210–13.
82 Hellier RR, Astbury WT, Bell FO. A case of pili torti. Br J Dermatol Syph 1940;52:173–82.
83 Ronchese F. Twisted hairs (pili torti). Arch Dermatol Syph 1932: 26:98–109.
84 Kurwa AR, Abdel-Aziz AM. Pili torti: congenital and acquired. Acta Dermatol Venereol 1973;53:385–92.
85 Lyon JB, Dawber RPR. A sporadic case of dystrophic pili torti. Br J Dermatol 1977;96:197–8.
86 Summerly R. Donaldson EM. Monilethrix: a family study. Br J Dermatol 1962;74:387–91.
87 Bentley-Phillips B, Bayles MAH. A previously undescribed hereditary hair anomaly (pseudo-monilethrix). Br J Dermatol 1973;89:159–67.
88 Hutchinson PE, Cairns RJ, Wells RS. Woolly hair: clinical and genetic aspects. Trans St John's Hosp Dermatol Soc 1974;60:160–77.
89 Peachey RDG, Wells RS. Hereditary hypotrichosis (Marie–Unna type). Trans St John's Hosp Dermatol Soc 1971;57:157–66.
90 Stevanovic DV. Multiple defects of the hair shaft in Netherton's disease; association with ichthyosis linearis circumflexa. Br J Dermatol 1969;81:851–7.
91 Björnstad R. Pili torti and sensory-neural loss of hearing. Proceedings of the 17th Meeting of the Fennoscandinavian Association of Dermatologists, Copenhagen, 1965:3.
92 Robinson GC, Johnston MM. Pili torti and sensory neural hearing loss. J Pediatr 1967;70:621–3.
93 Hays SB, Camisa C. Acquired pili torti in two patients treated with synthetic retinoids. Cutis 1985;35:466–8.
94 Lurie R, Danziger Y, Kaplan Y et al. Acquired pili torti – a structural hair shaft defect in anorexia nervosa. Cutis 1996;57(3):151–6.
95 Olsen EA. Hair loss in childhood. In: Olsen EA (ed.) Disorders of Hair Growth. Diagnosis and Treatment, 2nd edn. New York: McGraw-Hill, 2003:177–238.
96 Stevens HP, Kelsell DP, Bryant SP et al. Linkage of monilethrix to the trichocyte and epithelial keratin gene cluster on 12q11–q13. J Invest Dermatol 1996;106:795–7.
97 Rakowska A, Slowinska M, Czuwara J et al. Case reports: dermoscopy as a tool for rapid diagnosis of monilethrix. J Drugs Dermatol 2007;6:222–4.
98 Gummer CL, Dawber RPR, Swift JA. Monilethrix: an electron microscopic and electron histochemical study. Br J Dermatol 1981; 105:529–41.
99 Healy E, Holmes SC, Belgaid CE et al. A gene for monilethrix is closely linked to the type II keratin gene cluster at 12q13. Hum Mol Genet 1995;4:399–402.
100 Zlotogorski A, Marek D, Horev L et al. An autosomal recessive form of monilethrix is caused by mutations in DSG4: clinical overlap with localized autosomal recessive hypotrichosis. J Invest Dermatol 2006;126:1292–6.
101 Ullah A, Raza S, Ali RH et al. A novel deletion mutation in the DSG4 gene underlies autosomal recessive hypotrichosis with variable phenotype in two unrelated consanguineous families. Clin Exp Dermatol 2015;40:78–84.
102 Salamon T, Schnyder UW. Uber die Monilethrix. Arch Klin Exp Dermatol 1962;215:105.
103 Shah V, Tharini GK, Manoharan K. Monilethrix with Holt–Oram syndrome: case report of a rare association. Int J Trichol 2015; 7(1):33–5.
104 Karincaoglu Y, Coskun BK, Seyhan E et al. Monilethrix. Improvement with acitretin. Am J Clin Dermatol 2005;6:407–10.
105 Tamayo L. Monilethrix treated with the oral retinoid RO 10-9359 (Tegison). Clin Exp Dermatol 1983;8:393–6.
106 de Berker D, Dawber RPR. Monilethrix treated with oral retinoids. Clin Exp Dermatol 1990;16:226–8.
107 Saxena U, Ramesh V, Misra RS. Topical minoxidil in monilethrix [letter]. Dermatologica 1991;182:252–3.
108 Rossi A, Iorio A, Scali E, Fortuna MC, et al.Monilethrix treated with minoxidil. Int J Immunopathol Pharmacol 2011;24:239–42.
109 Bentley-Phillips B, Bayles MAH. Pseudo-monilethrix. Br J Dermatol 1975;92:113–15.
110 Zitelli JA. Pseudomonilethrix: an artifact. Arch Dermatol 1986;122:688–90.
111 Whiting DA. Structural abnormalities of hair shaft. J Am Acad Dermatol 1987;16:1–25.
112 Detwiler SP, Carson J, Woosley J et al. Bubble hair: case caused by an overheating hair dryer and reproducibility in normal hair with heat. J Am Acad Dermatol 1994;30:54.

Hair shaft abnormalities associated with unruly hair

Uncombable hair syndrome

Children with uncombable hair syndrome (UHS) present from infancy up to puberty with slow growing, silvery-blond 'spun-glass' hair that is disorderly and unmanageable [1–4] (Fig. 159.22). By itself, pili trianguli et canaliculi does not lead to hair fragility. Under light microscopy and dermoscopy, the hairs may appear normal or may have some midline darkening suggestive of the typical longitudinal grooves so clearly seen on scanning electron microscopy, the gold standard diagnostic method [5–7]. Longitudinal grooving in itself is a relatively common hair shaft abnormality, seen in normal hair and in many cases of ectodermal dysplasia along with other hair shaft abnormalities [8]. On scanning electron microscopy of hairs in the UHS syndrome, the longitudinal grooving is generally seen in conjunction with a cross-sectional triangular shape, the basis for the term pili trianguli et canaliculi [4] (Figs 159.23 and 159.24). UHS can be associated with ectodermal dysplasias, retinal dysplasia, juvenile cataract, digit abnormalities, tooth enamel anomalies, oligodontia and phalangoepiphyseal dysplasia.

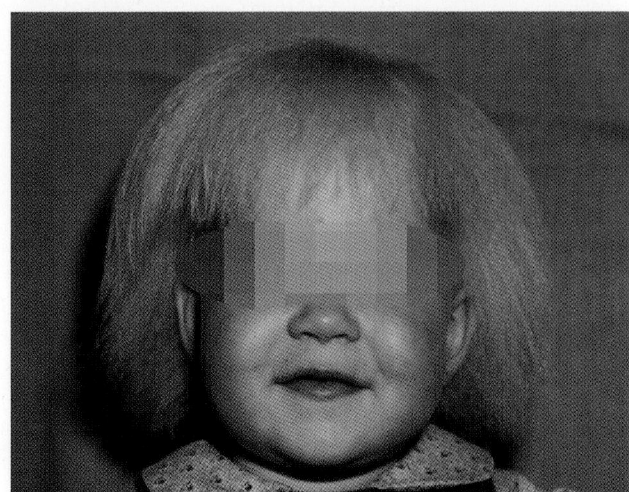

Fig. 159.22 Uncombable hair syndrome.

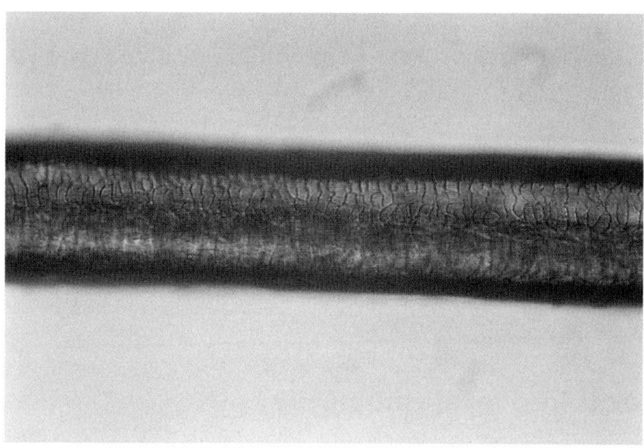

Fig. 159.23 Longitudinal grooving (light micrograph, ×400). Source: Courtesy of Dr David A. Whiting.

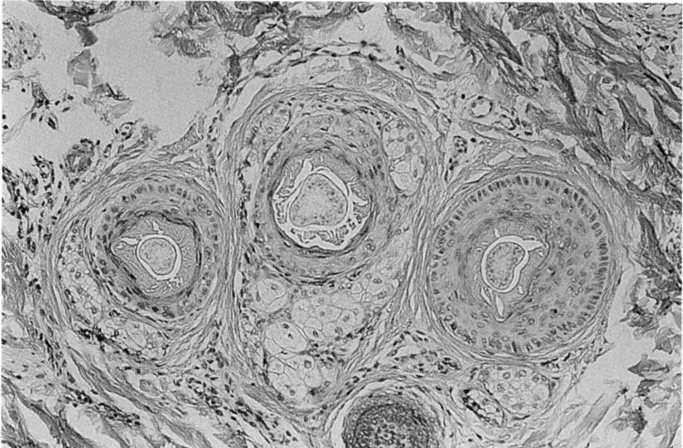

Fig. 159.24 Cross-section of hairs on a scalp biopsy of a child with uncombable hair syndrome. Note the triangular cross-section of an affected hair (horizontal section, haematoxylin and eosin stain). Source: Courtesy of Dr David A. Whiting.

Uncombable hair syndrome is autosomal recessive in the majority of cases although sporadic and autosomal dominant inheritance has been reported [5,9,10]. Recent investigation has shown causative mutations in at least three genes that encode for hair shaft proteins that display sequential interactions with each other: *PADI3* (UHS1) on chromosome 1p36, *TGM3* (UHS2) on chromosome 20p12 and *TCHH* (UHS3) on chromosome 1q21 [10]. The *PADI* gene encodes a member of the peptidyl arginine deiminase family of enzymes, which catalyse the posttranslational deimination of proteins by converting arginine residues into citrullines in the presence of calcium ions. The PADI3 enzyme modulates hair structural proteins, such as filaggrin in the hair follicle and trichohyalin in the inner root sheath, during hair follicle formation (www.ncbi.nlm.nih.gov/gene/51702). *TGM3* encodes transglutaminase 3 which is involved in the later stages of cell envelope formation in the epidermis and hair follicle (www.ncbi.nlm.nih.gov/gene/7053) and the protein encoded by *TCHH*, trichohyaline, forms cross-linked complexes with itself and keratin intermediate filaments to provide mechanical strength to the hair follicle inner root sheath. A recent report has shown an association of UHS and congenital anonychia with mutations in *RSPO4* and *PADI3* [11].

The condition of UHS may improve with age. Supplemental biotin was reported to be of use in one case [12] but generally does not affect the process. Conditioners are helpful.

Woolly hair

Woolly hair is the presence of hair that is similar to hair of people of African descent on the scalp of persons of other races. Microscopically, the hair is tightly coiled without generally going to the extremes of pili torti. However, pili torti and pili annulati (blond hair with both the clinical and microscopic findings of alternating bands of light and dark on the hair shaft) may be seen with this condition [13]. Although dermoscopic evaluation demonstrates broken hair shafts and a 'crawling snake' appearance [14], this method is not sufficient for the diagnosis and a detailed clinical evaluation is mandatory.

The hair in woolly hair is unruly only in the sense that it is difficult to manage, but probably not more so than the hair normally occurring in dark-skinned persons of African descent. The aberrant hair growth begins at birth or infancy with excessively tight curls, making the hair appear bushy or frizzy. Hair length may be decreased secondary to brittleness, which is common in the hair of people of African descent in general. Woolly hair may go from curly to wavy as the child ages. A diffuse partial woolly hair has been described in which scalp hair had two hair shaft populations, straight and wavy, intermingled [15]; this has been referred to as woolly hair naevus (WHN). An HRAS p G125 mutation has been found in the curly hair only in WHN associated with epidermal naevi [16] and a BRAF p.Lys601Asn mutation in phacomatosis pigmentokeratotica with WHN and epidermal naevi [17], suggesting that WHN represents a mosaic RASopathy with phenotype determined by location of mutation.

Woolly hair usually appears as a solitary problem. An autosomal dominant form (MIM 194300) has been reported with linkage to chromosome 12q13 (OMIM) and due to a defect in keratin 74 which encodes the inner root sheath (IRS) specific epithelial (soft) keratin 74 leading to disruption of keratin intermediate filaments [18,19]. An autosomal recessive form of woolly hair (MIM278150) with linkage to chromosome 17q21 and due to a defect in the *LIPH* gene (encoding a phospholipase that produces 2-acyl lysophosphatidic acid [LPA]) and *P2RY5/LPAR6* genes encoding a G-coupled receptor for LPA, both sets of genes expressed in the IRS [18], has also been noted. Woolly hair has also been reported in conjunction with enamel hypoplasia [20], ocular defects [21,22], deafness and ichthyosis vulgaris [23], keratosis pilaris atrophicans [24] and Noonan syndrome (short stature, facial dysmorphism and congenital heart defects related to a hetergenous mutation in *PTPN11*) [25,26].

Woolly hair, keratoderma and various cardiac abnormalities have been reported in Naxos syndrome (mutation in the plakoblobin gene, gene map locus 17q21, arrhythmogenic right ventricular cardiomyopathy) and in two syndromes associated with a mutation in the gene encoding desmoplakin, gene map locus 6p24: Carvajal syndrome (dilated cardiomyopathy) and the Naxos-like syndrome (arrhythmogenic right ventricular dysplasia) [8,26,27]. Curly hair, developmental delay, failure to thrive and cardiac abnormalities are seen in Costello syndrome and have been noted to be related to germline heterozygous HRAS mutation with phenotypic overlap with Noonan syndrome and cardiofaciocutaneous syndrome [26]. Skin fragility and woolly hair without cardiac abnormalities have been reported with another mutation of the desmoplakin gene [26].

With excessively curly hair in an infant who is not of African descent, one must also consider the following syndromes: trichodento-osseous syndrome (small widely spaced teeth, frontal bossing and dolichocephaly) [28] and CHAND (curly hair, ankyloblepheron and nail dysplasia) syndrome [29,30].

Marie–Unna type of hereditary hypotrichosis

Marie–Unna hereditary hypotrichosis (MUHH) is an autosomal dominant inherited condition which has a distinctive type of hair loss that varies with the child's age [31–34]. The hair is sparse or absent at birth with variable abnormal coarse scalp hair regrowth in childhood and potential scalp hair loss again at puberty (Fig. 159.25). There is associated general hypotrichosis of body hair. The coarse, wiry, twisted hair is very distinctive. Hair shaft examination shows irregular twisting and, on scanning electron microscopy, longitudinal ridging and peeling of the cuticle. Diffuse follicular hyperkeratosis with milia-like facial lesions may be present. Recent work confirms a mutation on chromosome 8p21 (MUHH1) of an inhibitory upstream ORF (U2HR) close to the gene encoding the human hairless homologue [8,35–37]. In addition, mutations have been identified. on chromosome 1p21-1q21.3 (MUHH2) [38].

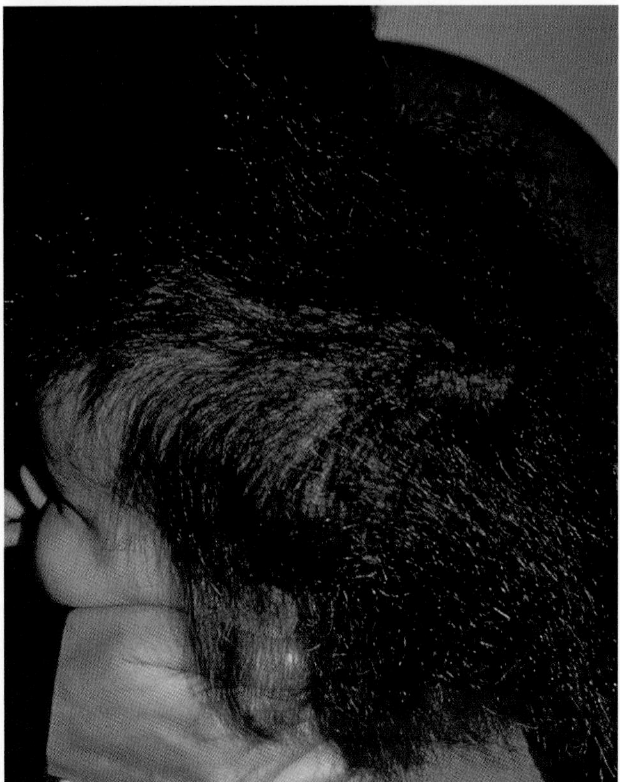

Fig. 159.25 Marie–Unna hypotrichosis.

Additional causes of wiry hair in childhood that can be lost after puberty include those conditions related to defects in the *TP63* gene at 3q27. These all are characterized by hypohidrosis and cleft lip/palate and have been designated by the other consistent abnormalities present: Rapp–Hodgkin (none), EEC3 (ectrodactyly) and AEC (ankyloblepharon) [8,39].

Acquired localized unruly hair

Four noninherited conditions may present as patches of scalp hair that differ from the normal texture/quality of hair for that individual. The most common is X-ray therapy related, with the hair that regrows after treatment (and epilation) being different in quality from that seen pretreatment. Localized woolly hair naevus, occurring only in people not of African descent, usually develops within the first 2 years of life (although this has been first reported in adolescence), with the affected hair being finer, lighter and more tightly curled than the rest of the scalp hair [40] (Fig. 159.26). Microscopically, the hairs may show trichorrhexis nodosa, longitudinal grooving, flattening and twisting [41–43]. Almost 50% of patients with woolly hair naevus have an underlying linear epidermal naevus or pigmented naevus, usually other than on the scalp [44,45].

Straight hair naevus, in which a localized portion of the normally curled or kinky hair is straight, has been noted only in persons of African descent. This may also have an association with an underlying epidermal naevus [46,47]. Acquired progressive kinking occurs after puberty, generally in males with androgenetic alopecia, and presents as gradual curling and darkening of the frontal, temporal, auricular and vertex hairs [48–51]. Microscopically, the hairs of acquired progressive kinking are short with kinks and twists, and may show longitudinal grooving.

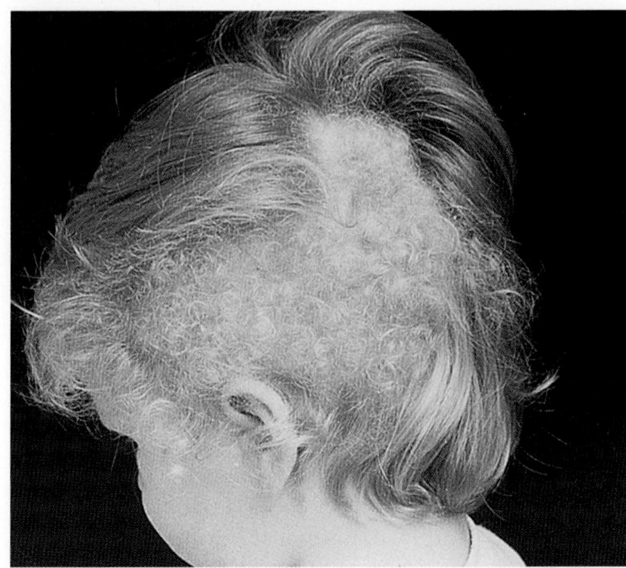

Fig. 159.26 Woolly hair naevus. Source: Courtesy of Dr Vera H. Price.

References

1 Dupre A, Rochiccidi P, Bonafe JL. 'Cheveux incoiffable': anomalie congenitale des cheveux. Bull Soc Fr Dermatol Syph 1973;80:111–12.
2 Stroud JD, Mehregan AH. 'Spun glass' hair. A clinicopathologic study of an unusual hair defect. In: Brown AC (ed.) The First Human Hair Symposium. New York: Medcom, 1974:103–7.
3 Dupre A, Bonafe JL, Litoux F et al. Le syndrome des cheveux incoiffables; pili tranguli et canaliculi. Ann Dermatol Vénéréol 1978;105:627–30.
4 Ferrando J, Fontarnau R, Gratacos MR et al. Pili canaliculi ('cheveux incoiffables' ou 'cheveux en fibre de verre'): dix nouveaux cas avec etude au microscope electronique a balayage. Ann Dermatol Vénéréol 1980;107:243–8.
5 Garty B, Metzker A, Mimouni M et al. Uncombable hair: a condition with autosomal dominant inheritance. Arch Dis Child 1982; 57:710–12.
6 Hebert AA, Charrow J, Esterly N et al. Uncombable hair (pili trianguli et canaliculi): evidence for dominant inheritance with complete penetrance based on scanning electron microscopy. Am J Med Genet 1987;28:185–93.
7 Matis WL, Baden H, Green R et al. Uncombable-hair syndrome. Pediatr Dermatol 1987;4:215–19.
8 Whiting DA. Hair shaft defects. In: Olsen EA (ed.) Disorders of Hair Growth: Diagnosis and Treatment. New York: McGraw-Hill, 2003:91–137.
9 Rest EB, Fretzin DF. Quantitative assessment of scanning electron microscope defects in uncombable-hair syndrome. Pediatr Dermatol 1990;7:93–6.
10 Basmanav FB, Cau L, Tafazzoli A. et al. Mutations in three genes encoding proteins involved in hair shaft formation cause uncombable hair syndrome. Am J Hum Genet 2016;99(6):1292–30.
11 Hsu CK, Romano MT, Nanda A et al. Congenital anonychia and uncombable hair syndrome: coinheritance of homozygous mutations in RSPO4 and PADI3. J Invest Dermatol 2017;137(5):1176–9.
12 Shelley WB, Shelley ED. Uncombable hair syndrome: observation on response to biotin and occurrence in siblings with ectodermal dysplasia. J Am Acad Dermatol 1985;13:97–102.
13 Lyon JB, Dawber RPR. A sporadic case of dystrophic pili torti. Br J Dermatol 1977;96:197–8.
14 Rakowska A, Slowinska M, Kowalska-Oledzka E, Rudnicka L. Trichoscopy in genetic hair shaft abnormalities. J Dermatol Case Rep 2008;2:14–20.
15 Lalević-Vasić BM, Nikolić MM, Polić DJ, Radosavljević B. Diffuse partial woolly hair. Dermatology 1993;187:243–7.
16 Levinsohn JL, Teng J, Craiglow BG et al. Somatic HRAS p.G12S mutation causes woolly hair and epidermal nevi. J Invest Dermatol 2014;134:1149–52.
17 Kuentz P, Mignot C, St-Onge J et al. Postzygotic BRAF p.Lys601Asn mutation in phacomatosis pigmentokeratotica with woolly hair nevus and focal cortical dysplasia. J Invest Dermatol 2016;136(5):1060–2.
18 Shimomura Y, Wajid M, Petukhova L et al. Autosomal -dominant woolly hair resulting from disruption of keratin 74(KRT74), a potential determinant of human hair texture. Am J Hum Genet 2010;86:632–8.
19 Wasif N, Naqvi SK, Basit S et al. Novel mutations in the keratin-74 (KRT74) gene underlie autosomal dominant woolly hair/hypotrichosis in Pakistani families. Hum Genet 2011;129:419–24.
20 Robinson GC, Miller JR. Hereditary enamel hypoplasia: its association with characteristic hair structure. Pediatrics 1966;37:498–502.
21 Jacobsen KU, Lowes M. Woolly hair nevus with ocular involvement. Report of a case. Dermatologica 1975;151:249–52.
22 Taylor AEM. Hereditary woolly hair with ocular involvement. Br J Dermatol 1990;123:523–5.
23 Verbov J. Woolly hair: study of a family. Dermatologica 1978;157:42–7.
24 McHenry PM, Nevin NC, Bingham EA. The association of keratosis pilaris atrophicans with hereditary woolly hair. Pediatr Dermatol 1990;7:202–4.
25 Neild VS, Pegum JS, Wells RS. The association of keratosis pilaris atrophicans and woolly hair, with and without Noonan's syndrome. Br J Dermatol 1984;110:357–62.
26 Online Mendelian Inheritance in Man, OMIM®. Johns Hopkins University, Baltimore, MD. https://omim.org/
27 Alcalai R, Metzger S, Rosenheck S et al. A recessive mutation in desmoplakin causes arrhythmogenic right ventricular dysplasia, skin disorder, and woolly hair. J Am Coll Cardiol 2003;42:319–27.
28 Lichtenstein J, Warson R, Jorgenson R et al. The tricho-dento-osseous (TDO) syndrome. Am J Hum Genet 1972;24:569–82.
29 Baughman FA. CHANDS: the curly hair–ankyloblepharon–nail dysplasia syndrome. Birth Defects 1971;7:100–2.
30 Gollasch B, Basmanav FB, Nanda A et al. Identification of a novel mutation in RIPK4 in a kindred with phenotypic features of Bartsocas-Papas and CHAND syndromes. Am J Med Genet A 2015;167A(11):2555–62.
31 Stevanovic DV. Hereditary hypotrichosis congenita: Marie Unna type. Br J Dermatol 1970;83:331–7.
32 Wirth G, Bindewald I, Küster W et al. Hypotrichosis congenital hereditaria Marie Unna. Hautarzt 1985;36:577–80.
33 Mende B, Kreysel HW. Hypotrichosis congenita hereditaria Marie Unna mit Ehlers–Danlos-syndrom und atopie. Hautarzt 1987;38:532–5.
34 Solomon LM, Esterly NB, Medenica M. Hereditary trichodysplasia: Marie Unna's hypertrichosis. J Invest Dermatol 1971;57:389–400.
35 Wen Y, Liu Y, Xu Y et al. Loss-of-function mutations of an inhibitory upstream ORF in the human hairless transcript cause Marie Unna hereditary hypotrichosis. Nat Gen 2009;41:228–33.
36 Cichon S, Kruse R, Hillmer AM et al. A distinct gene close to the hairless locus on chromosome 8p underlies hereditary Marie Unna type hypotrichosis in a German family. Br J Dermatol 2000;143:811–14.
37 Yun S-K, Cho Y-G, Song KH et al. Identification of a novel U2HR mutation in a Korean woman with Marie Unna hereditary hypotrichosis. Int J Dermatol 2014;53:1358–61.
38 Yang S, Gao M, Dui Y et al. Identification of a novel locus for Marie Unna hereditary hypotrichosis to a 17.5 cM interval at 1p21.1-1q21.3. J Invest Dermatol 2005;125:711–14.
39 Park S-W, Yong SL, Martinka et al. Rapp–Hodgkin syndrome: a review of the aspects of hair and hair color. J Am Acad Dermatol 2005;53:729–35.
40 Reda AM, Rogers RS, Peters MS. Woolly hair nevus. J Am Acad Dermatol 1990;22:337–80.
41 Crosti C, Menni S. Woolly hair nevus: osservazion sutre casi clinici. Minerva Dermatol 1979;114:45–9.
42 Harper MF, Klokke AH. Woolly hair nevus with triangular hairs [Abstract]. Br J Dermatol 1983;108:111–13.
43 Goldin HM, Branson DM, Fretzin DF. Woolly-hair nevus: a case report and study by scanning electron microscopy. Pediatr Dermatol 1984;2:41–4.
44 Wright S, Lemoine NR, Leigh IM. Woolly hair naevi with systematized linear epidermal naevus. Clin Exp Dermatol 1986;11:179–82.
45 Peteiro C, Oliva NP, Zulaica A et al. Woolly-hair nevus: report of a case associated with a verrucous epidermal nevus in the same area. Pediatr Dermatol 1989;6:188–90.
46 Day TI. Straight-hair nevus, ichthyosis hystrix, leukokeratosis of the tongue. Arch Dermatol 1967;96:606.
47 Gibbs RC, Berger RA. The straight hair nevus. Int J Dermatol 1970;9:47.
48 Coupe RL, Johnston MM. Acquired progressive kinking of the hair: structural changes and growth dynamics of affected hairs. Arch Dermatol 1969;100:191–5.
49 Mortimer PS, Gummer C, English J et al. Acquired progressive kinking of hair: report of six cases and review of literature. Arch Dermatol 1985;121:1031–3.
50 Balsa RE, Ingratta SM, Alvarez AG. Acquired kinking of the hair: a methodologic approach. J Am Acad Dermatol 1986;15:1133–6.
51 Esterly NB, Lavin MP, Garancis JC. Acquired progressive kinking of the hair. Arch Dermatol 1989;125:813–15.

Miscellaneous hair shaft abnormalities

Pili annulati

Pili annulati clinically has a ringed appearance only detectable in lightly pigmented hair and may appear any time during infancy [1]. It is an autosomal dominant or sporadic disorder usually occurring as an isolated anomaly although it has been seen with alopecia areata, woolly hair and blue naevus. Microscopic evalution of affected hairs reveals abnormal, air-filled cavities between the macrofibrillar units of the cortex, resulting in scattering of refected light. The hairs are generally not fragile but if they fracture, it is usually

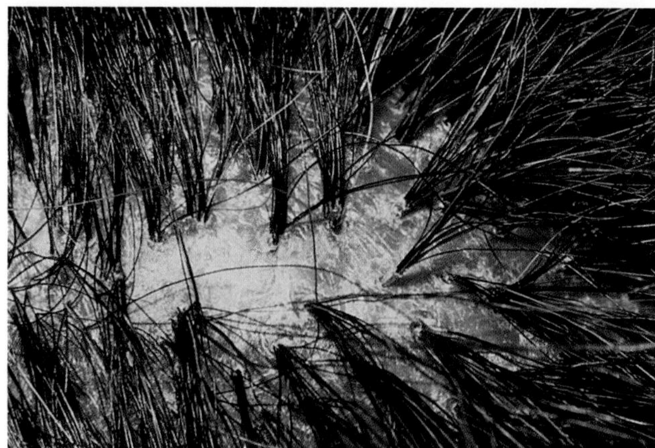

Fig. 159.27 Tufted folliculitis. Source: Tong and Baden 1989 [7]. Reproduced with permission from Elsevier.

through the abnormal bands. The gene locus has been mapped to chromosome 12q24.32-24.33 [2].

Pseudopili annulati

Pseudopili annulati is a variant of normal hair characterized by a banded appearance of the hair under reflective light [1]. It is usually only apparent in blond hair and there is no increased hair fragility. In pseudopili annulati, the banding is only seen with transverse illumination if the light strikes the hair at right angles to the long axis of the hair versus pili annulati in which the banding is seen regardless of which direction the light strikes the hair.

Localized tufts of hair

In pili multigemini, hairs from two to eight follicular bulbs, each with their own inner root sheath but surrounded by a common outer root sheath, emerge from one follicular canal [3]. In children, this condition may appear as an isolated scalp problem or may occur with classic pili torti [4] or in cleidocranial dysostosis [5]. Although compound follicles may appear similar to pili multigemini, in this condition two or three different hair shafts, each with their own inner root sheath and outer root sheath, eventually emerge from the same follicular opening. These two nonscarring entities must be differentiated from tufted folliculitis, in which scalp inflammation is prominent and leads to focal scarring with units of 10–15 hairs, each hair from its own follicle, emerging as tufts of hair from a single follicular canal [6,7] (Fig. 159.27).

References

1 **Whiting DA. Structural abnormalities of hair shaft. J Am Acad Dermatol 1987;16:1–25.**

2 **Giehl KA, Eckstein GN, Benet-Pages A et al. A gene locus responsible for the familial hair shaft abnormality pili annulati maps to chromosome 12q24.32–24.33. J Invest Dermatol 2004;123:1073–7.**

3 Pinkus H. Multiple hairs (Flemming–Giovannini): report of two cases of pili multigemini and discussion of some other anomalies of the pilary complex. J Invest Dermatol 1951;17:291–301.

4 Hellier RR, Astbury WT, Bell FO. A case of pili torti. Br J Dermatol Syph 1940;52:173–82.

5 Mehregan AH, Thompson WS. Pili multigemini: report of a case in association with cleidocranial dysostosis. Br J Dermatol 1979;100:315–22.

6 Dalziel KL, Telfer NR, Wilson CL et al. Tufted folliculitis: a specific bacterial disease? Am J Dermatopathol 1990;12:37–41.

7 Tong AKF, Baden HP. Tufted hair folliculitis. J Am Dermatol 1989; 21:1096–9.

Hair loss due to abnormal cycling

For the purposes of facilitating diagnosis, there are two main outcomes of premature disruption of anagen and, hence, there are two types of hair loss – anagen loss or telogen loss. Both should be suspected by the clinical presentation of abnormal shedding and confirmed by histological evaluation of the proximal hair shaft/bulb. The differential diagnosis and consequent evaluation and treatment vary greatly, however, between these two conditions.

Anagen loss

Anagen effluvium

Anagen loss is always abnormal and, with the exception of loose anagen syndrome and alopecia areata, scalp anagen hair loss generally implies a toxic exposure. The most common and easily recognizable cause of anagen loss (or effluvium) is X-ray therapy or chemotherapy. In both cases there may be a diminution of metabolic activity in the matrix, which results in weakening of the hair shaft and breakage a few millimetres from the scalp surface (Fig. 159.28). If exposure is persistent or particularly toxic, anagen may be interrupted entirely and the poorly anchored dystrophic hair shed. Hair loss is profound as up to 90% of scalp hair is normally in anagen at any given time, and the loss generally occurs within days to weeks of the insult. Telogen hairs may remain in place until their usual time of loss.

In general, the hair loss from chemotherapy is reversible when treatment stops; however, ultimately, this will depend on the specific agents utilized and the toxicities of the multiple agents used in a given regimen. The potential for regrowth after X-ray therapy will depend on the type, depth and dose fractionation of the X-rays. Regrowth after hair loss from either chemotherapy or X-ray therapy may produce hair that is different in colour, curl or texture from that seen pretreatment.

Other causes of anagen loss include loose anagen syndrome, alopecia areata and toxic exposure to boric acid or heavy metals. Loose anagen syndrome does not present

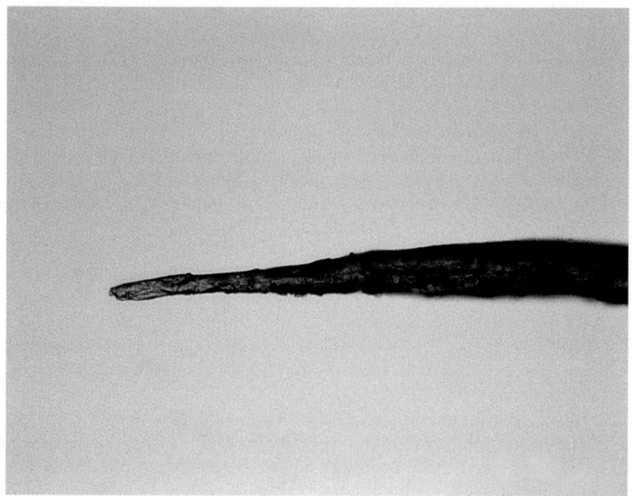

Fig. 159.28 Tapered proximal portion and point of breakage in hairs involved in an anagen effluvium (light micrograph, ×100). Source: Courtesy of Dr David A. Whiting.

as sudden diffuse shedding, but rarely alopecia areata does. Typically, alopecia areata may result in some focal hair loss or findings of exclamation point hairs that may help to distinguish this from other causes of anagen effluvium. Boric acid is the main ingredient in some common household pesticides and is also used as a preservative in some household products [1,2]. Boric acid poisoning is suggested by gastrointestinal, central nervous system and renal symptoms, skin findings of exfoliation, erythroderma and bullae, and a haemorrhagic diathesis [1,3,4]. Confirmation is by measuring blood boric acid levels [3].

Mercury intoxication is primarily through chronic industrial exposure, consumption of industrially polluted water or affected seafood, or inadvertent exposure to mercury used as a fungicide or antiseptic [5]. Hair loss may occur with or without the other common symptoms (particularly neurological) of mercury intoxication [6–8]. Acrodynia is a particular constellation of findings (pain in the abdomen, extremities and joints, pink scaly palms and soles, headache, photophobia, irritability, hyperhidrosis and hair loss) that can occur with chronic exposure to inorganic mercury [9]. Diagnosis of mercury intoxication is made by measuring urine, blood or hair levels of mercury [8,10].

Acute toxicity to arsenic may occur with suicidal or homicidal attempts or with accidental ingestion or exposure [5]. Inorganic arsenic compounds are found in insecticides, rodenticides, fungicides, herbicides and wood preservatives [10]. Acute arsenic toxification presents with gastrointestinal symptoms, hypotension, shortness of breath, central nervous system changes, haemolysis and acute tubular necrosis [11]. Approximately six weeks later, white transverse lines on all the nails (Mees' lines) may appear. The importance of hair in this diagnosis is not alopecia (which is rare) but, rather, that arsenic is concentrated in the hair and is detectable for months after exposure (as opposed to being detectable in urine for 7–10 days after exposure), facilitating a diagnosis even while symptoms improve or after the patient's demise [11,12].

The symptoms of acute thallium poisoning are insomnia, irritability, pain in the hands and feet and abdominal colic [13]. Two to three weeks after exposure, there is a precipitous loss of all scalp hair together with peripheral and autonomic nervous system symptoms. Mees' lines develop later. Blood and urine levels are diagnostic but must be measured as soon as possible as thallium levels tend to decrease rapidly.

Very severe protein malnutrition may also give rise to anagen effluvium, as can exposure to colchicine. Ingestion of some plants, such as *Lecythis ollaria* and *Leucaena glauca*, can also lead to anagen hair loss [5].

Loose anagen syndrome

The term loose anagen syndrome (LAS) was originally coined to describe a condition in children who had sparse hair that did not grow long, often with patches of dull, matted hair, in whom unusual anagen hairs were easily extracted. These anagen hairs had misshapen bulbs, absent root sheaths and ruffled cuticles [14–16]. The term loose anagen syndrome has also come to incorporate the

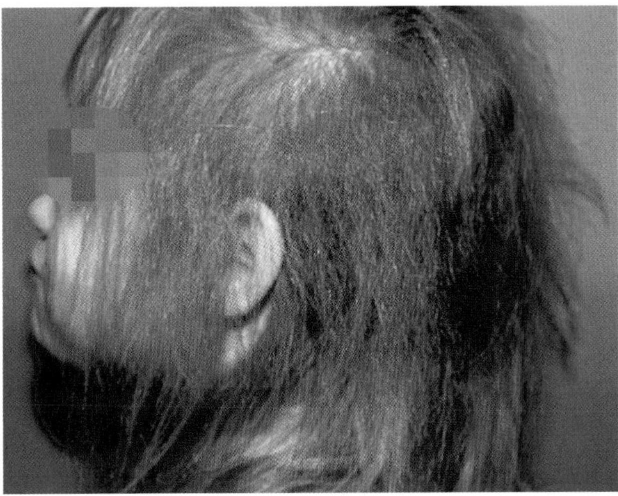

(a)

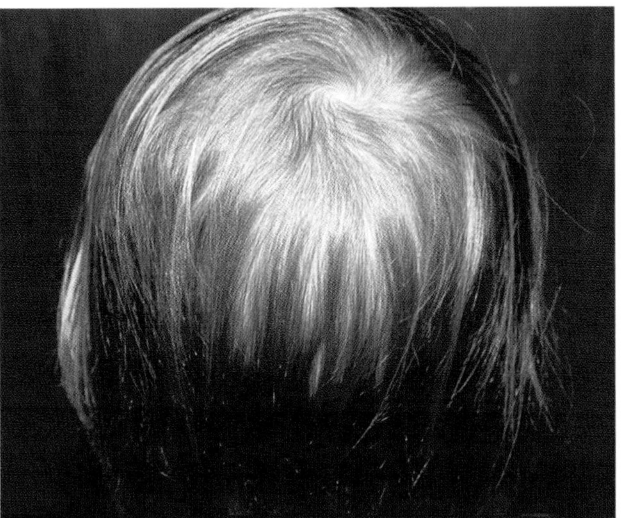

(b)

Fig. 159.29 Loose anagen syndrome in a child with (a) unruly hair and (b) easily extractable hair. Source: Olsen et al. 1999 [4]. Reproduced with permission from Elsevier.

easy extractability of these abnormal hairs in children with either patchy, unruly hair (LAS type B) (Fig. 159.29a) or otherwise clinically normal hair with increased shedding in subjects of any age (LAS types A and C) [17] (Fig. 159.29b). The underlying abnormality is a structural defect in the inner root sheath that normally anchors the anagen hair.

Loose anagen syndrome usually presents in children less than 6 years of age and is most common in girls (36:1 female to male ratio) [18], but this may be partly explained by the relatively short hairstyles of boys with less overall traction on hairs [19]. Most patients are Caucasian with blond or light brown hair although LAS has been reported in dark-skinned individuals [20]. Often the primary complaint is that the scalp hair is sparse and does not require cutting or will not grow long. Increased shedding is less common.

Loose anagen syndrome is considered an autosomal dominant condition with incomplete penetrance, although sporadic cases have been reported. Chapalain et al. reported on a K6HF keratin mutation that may be responsible for premature keratinization of the inner root sheath and leads to impaired adhesion between the cuticle of the inner root sheath and the companion layer [21]; whether this is the genetic abnormality in LAS remains to be confirmed. Whether loose anagen hairs are markers for a distinct disorder or a common endpoint seen in overlapping disorders is still unclear. LAS has been reported with a variety of syndromes including Noonan and Noonan-like syndrome with loose anagen hairs [18,22] but the definition of LAS utilized in each of the reports is unclear, or whether there may have been artifactual creation of loose anagen hairs by too much traction on a hair pull in very young children.

It is now clear that normal prepubescent children may have a few loose anagen hairs found on a gentle hair pull and that the criteria for diagnosis of LAS must include either a designated number of loose anagen hairs (3–10 per hair pull [17,23]) or a percentage of all hairs obtained on hair pull (50% has been suggested) [24]. Other hair shaft abnormalites may be seen in LAS other than loose anagen hairs, including trichorrhexis nodosa and tiger tail polarization [25]. Both LA hairs and dystrophic anagen hairs are commonly seen on hair pull in alopecia areata but the clinical presentations of LAS and alopecia areata are quite different except in the case of the diffuse subtype of the latter. Dermoscopy is useful in distinguishing LAS from alopecia areata and telogen effluvium: rectangular black granular structures are seen in 71% of cases of LAS, 8% of cases of alopecia areata and none in telogen effluvium; solitary yellow dots are seen in 50% of cases of LAS, 24% of cases of alopecia areata and 8% of cases of telogen effluvium [26]. Scalp biopsy can also be helpful in cases where diagnosis is unclear; the IRS in LAS is abnormal with tortuous and irregular swelling of the Henle layer, irregular keratinization of the cuticular cells and a swollen appearance of Huxley cells [27].

The differential diagnosis of loose anagen syndrome based on clinical presentation alone is dependent on the presenting phenotype [17]. In patients with type B LAS who present with patches of unruly hair, the primary differential diagnosis is woolly hair naevus. In those presenting with type A LAS, the primary differential diagnosis is short anagen syndrome [28]. Microscopic evaluation of hairs obtained by hair pull will differentiate the latter two conditions; the proximal ends of short anagen syndrome generally show an increased percentage of telogen hairs and the distal ends of hairs that have not been cut typically show tapered tips indicative of new growth, confirming that the shed hairs have had a shortened anagen phase.

Telogen loss or effluvium

The stress on the anagen hair follicle necessary to trigger telogen effluvium is milder than that with anagen effluvium and, instead of triggering damage to the matrix, it precipitates an abrupt transformation of anagen hairs to telogen hairs. In telogen effluvium, about 10–40%, rarely more, of the scalp anagen hairs suddenly move in concert through the physical transformation to telogen and are shed together after the usual obligatory time in telogen. Thus, a patient with telogen effluvium generally experiences a sudden increase in hair shedding diffusely over the scalp 3–4 months after an inciting event. In situations where the aetiological factor has been removed (e.g. recovery from a severe infection), the telogen loss would be followed by a recapitulation of anagen in the affected follicles and regrowth of hair over the ensuing 6–12 months. In cases where the aetiological factor remains (e.g. untreated thyroid disease), the continued effect on the anagen follicles would cause persistence of the increased percentage of hairs in telogen, and hence decreased scalp hair density, even while shed telogen hairs are being replaced in the normal cycle with anagen hairs. Once the inciting factor(s) is removed, a telogen effluvium will generally resolve over the next 6–12 months.

The diagnosis of telogen effluvium is confirmed by finding a positive hair pull from multiple areas of the scalp and the shed hairs all being telogen hairs. In total, 50–100 telogen hairs are normally shed per day, reflecting the 10–15% of scalp hairs in telogen at any one time [29]. In acute telogen effluvium, it is not uncommon for 200–300 hairs per day to be shed and 20–50% of the scalp hairs may be in telogen at a given time. Telogen effluvium is less common in children than in adults, and in children is more likely to be related to a sudden and transient illness than to the drugs and hormonal fluctuations that commonly trigger this in adults (Box 159.2). It must be emphasized that any drug can trigger a telogen effluvium, just as any drug can cause a cutaneous allergic reaction. However, some drugs cause this more commonly than others, and these are listed in Box 159.2.

Telogen effluvium is one of the few hair disorders in which blood tests may be helpful in determining a

Box 159.2 Causes of telogen effluvium in children and adolescents

- Medical illness
  - Severe infections, usually associated with high fever
  - Other systemic illnesses, acute or chronic
  - Hypo- or hyperthyroidism
- Postpartum
- Surgery
- Medications (including but not limited to):
  - Anticoagulants
  - β-Blockers
  - Lithium
  - Oral contraceptive pills: during use or after discontinuation
  - Retinoids and excess vitamin A
  - Valproic acid
- Nutritional
  - Precipitous diminution of calories or protein
  - Iron deficiency
  - Zinc deficiency
  - Essential fatty acid deficiency
  - Biotin deficiency
- Psychological stress

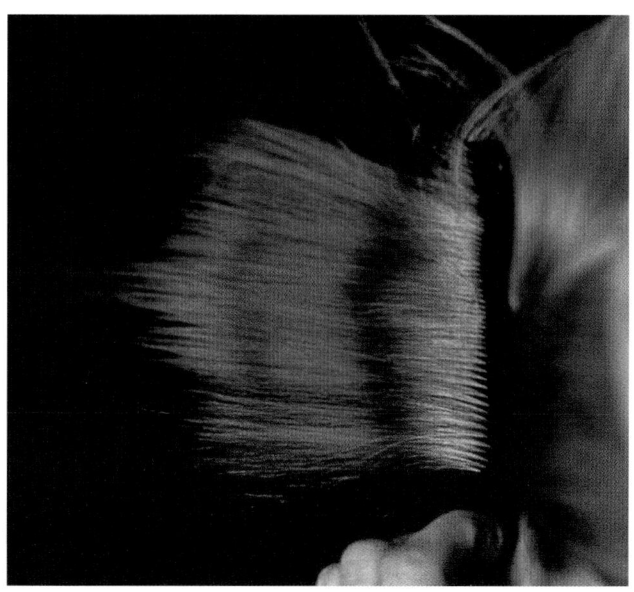

Fig. 159.30 Protein malnutrition: flag sign. Source: Courtesy of Dr Nancy B. Esterly.

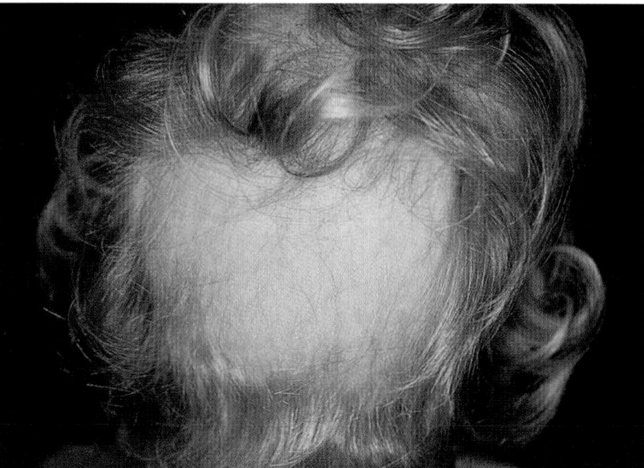

Fig. 159.31 Biotin deficiency. Source: Courtesy of Dr Nancy B. Esterly.

diagnosis; thyroid dysfunction, anaemia and iron deficiency should be screened for. Only those causes of telogen effluvium related to nutrition will be discussed further here.

Protein malnutrition (kwashiorkor) and caloric malnutrition (marasmus) usually occur concurrently and are common in children living in developing nations [30,31]. The hair in affected individuals is slow growing, sparse and dyspigmented (Fig. 159.30). The increased telogen percentage is accompanied by relative anagen bulb atrophy and a concomitant diminution in hair shaft diameter and stability [31–35].

Zinc deficiency in childhood can lead to sparse and slow hair growth. The low serum zinc levels are caused by an autosomal recessive inherited disorder of intestinal absorption of zinc (acrodermatitis enteropathica) or may be acquired in the situation of general intestinal malabsorption with inadequate zinc replacement [36]. The hair loss may be accompanied by acral and periorificial vesiculobullous or eczematoid plaques, glossitis, stomatitis, nail dystrophy and diarrhoea [37]. Oral zinc supplementation will reverse all findings.

Essential fatty acid deficiency in children usually occurs with prolonged parenteral alimentation with inadequate inclusion of supplemental essential fatty acids. The hair becomes sparse and less pigmented, and a generalized and periorificial dermatitis and thrombocytopenia may develop [38–41]. The skin returns to normal within weeks and the hair within months of either intravenous essential fatty acid replacement or treatment with topical linoleic acid [39].

Biotin deficiency may be secondary to either dietary deficiency, including that due to excessive dietary intake of avidin egg white glycoprotein that irreversibly binds biotin, or hereditary multiple carboxylase deficiency. The neonatal form, usually secondary to deficiency of holocarboxylase synthetase, is generally fatal, although rare cases with mild symptoms may present at several months of age [41,42]. The diagnosis is suggested by metabolic acidosis and organic aciduria; serum biotin levels may be normal [43–45]. In the late-onset, infantile form of multiple carboxylase deficiency, infants develop the first symptoms at 2–3 months of age [43,46–48].

The autosomal recessive genetic abnormality is most commonly a deficiency (<5% normal) of biotinidase leading to impaired biotin absorption and reutilization [46,48,49]. To date, over 100 mutations in the biotinidase gene on chromosome 3p25 have been noted [50]. Hair may be sparse and fine, and a distinctive, sharply marginated dermatitis of the face, groin and periorifical areas reminiscent of acrodermatitis entropathica may develop (Fig. 159.31), together with central nervous system dysfunction and recurrent infections. A partial deficiency (15–40% of normal) of biotinidase may exist and appears to be associated with lesser symptoms, i.e. mild hair loss and eczema [49]. The diagnosis is made by finding hyperammonuria, ketoacidosis and lactic acidosis and/or low serum biotin (however, the biotin level may be normal) [43,47]. The biotinidase deficiency can be overcome with biotin replacements, and most adverse effects are reversed if the biotin deficiency is treated early, although some neurological changes may be persistent [43,45].

References

1 Tan TG. Occupational toxic alopecia due to borax. Acta Dermatol Venereol 1970;50:55–8.
2 Schillinger BM, Berstein M, Goldberg LA et al. Boric acid poisoning. J Am Acad Dermatol 1982;7:667–73.
3 Stein KM, Odom RB, Justice GR et al. Toxic alopecia from ingestion of boric acid. Arch Dermatol 1973;108:95–7.
4 Rubenstein AD, Musher DM. Epidemic boric acid poisoning simulating staphylococcal toxic epidermal necrolysis of the newborn infant: Ritter's disease. J Pediatr 1970;77:884–7.
5 Sinclair R, Grossman KL, Kvedar JC. Anagen hair loss. In: Olsen EA (ed.) Disorders of Hair Growth: Diagnosis and Treatment, 2nd edn. New York: McGraw-Hill, 2003:275–302.
6 Pierard GE. Toxic effects of metals from the environment on hair growth and structure. J Cutan Pathol 1979;6:237–42.
7 Elhassani SB. The many faces of methylmercury poisoning. J Toxicol 1982;19:875–906.

8 National Research Council. An Assessment of Mercury in the Environment. A Report Prepared by the Panel on Mercury of the Coordinating Committee for Scientific and Technical Assessments of Environmental Pollutants, National Research Council. Washington: National Academy of Sciences, 1978.
9 Hirschman SZ, Feingold M, Boylen G. Mercury in house paint as a cause of acrodynia: effect of therapy with N-acetyl-d,l-penicillamine. N Engl J Med 1963;65:889–93.
10 Graef JW, Lovejoy FJ Jr. Heavy metal poisoning. In: Braunwald E, Isselbacher KJ, Petersdorf RG et al. (eds) Harrison's Principles of Internal Medicine, 11th edn. New York: McGraw-Hill, 1987:850–5.
11 Heyman A, Pfeiffer JB Jr, Willett RW et al. Peripheral neuropathy caused by arsenical intoxication. N Engl J Med 1956;254:401–9.
12 Peters HA, Croft WA, Woolson EA et al. Hematological, dermal and neuropsychological disease from burning and power sawing chromium–copper–arsenic (CCA)-treated wood. Acta Pharmacol Toxicol 1986;59:39–43.
13 Herrero F, Fernandez E, Gomez J et al. Thallium poisoning presenting with abdominal colic, paresthesia, and irritability. Clin Toxicol 1995; 33:261–4.
14 Nodl F, Zaun H, Zinn HK. Gesteigerte Epilierbarkeit von Anagenhaaren bei Kindernals Folge eines Reifungsdefekts der Follikel mit Gestorter Verhaftung von Haarschaft und Wurzelscheiden: Das Phanomen der Leicht Ausziehbaren Haare. Aktüel Dermatol 1986;12:55–7.
15 Hamm H, Traupe H. Loose anagen hair of childhood: the phenomenon of easily pluckable hair. J Am Acad Dermatol 1989;20:242–8.
16 Price VH, Gummer CL. Loose anagen syndrome. J Am Acad Dermatol 1989;20:249–56.
17 Olsen EA, Bettencourt MS, Coté N. The presence of loose anagen hairs obtained by hair pull in the normal population. J Invest Dermatol Symp Proc 1999;4:258–60.
18 Cantator-Francis JI, Orlow SJ. Practical guidelines in evaluation of loose anagen hair syndrome. Arch Dermatol 2009;145:1123–8.
19 Pham CM, Krejci-Manwaring J. Loose anagen hair syndrome: an underdiagnosed condition in males. Pediatr Dermatol 2010;27: 408–9.
20 Abdel-Raouf H, El-Din WH, Awad SS et al. Loose anagen syndrome in children of upper Egypt J Cosmet Dermatol 2009;8:103–7.
21 Chapalain V, Winter H, Langbein L et al. Is the loose anagen hair syndrome a keratin disorder? A clinical and molecular study. Arch Dermatol 2002;138:501–6.
22 Online Mendelian Inheritance in Man, OMIM®. Johns Hopkins University, Baltimore, MD. https://omim.org/
23 Balsa RE, Ingratta SM, Alvarez AG. Acquired kinking of the hair: a methodologic approach. J Am Acad Dermatol 1986;15:1133–6.
24 Coupe RL, Johnston MM. Acquired progressive kinking of the hair: structural changes and growth dynamics of affected hairs. Arch Dermatol 1969;100:191–5.
25 Tosti A, Peluso AM, Miscali C et al. Loose anagen hair. Arch Dermatol 1997;133:1089–93.
26 Rakowska A, Zadurska M, Czuwara J et al. Trichoscopy findings in loose anagen hair syndrome: rectangular granular structures and solitary yellow dots. J Dermatol Case Rep 2015;1:1–5.
27 Mirmirani P, Price VH. Abnormal inner root sheath of the hair follicle in the loose anagen syndrome: an ultrastructural study. J Am Acad Dermatol 2011;64l:129–34.
28 Antaya RJ, Sideridou E, Olsen EA. Short anagen syndrome. J Am Acad Dermatol 2005;53:130–4.
29 Olsen EA. Clinical tools for assessing hair loss. In: Olsen EA (ed.) Disorders of Hair Growth: Diagnosis and Treatment, 2nd edn. New York: McGraw-Hill, 2003:59–69.
30 Sims RT. Hair growth in kwashiorkor. Arch Dis Child 1967;42:397–400.
31 Bradfield RB, Jelliffe EFP. Early assessment of malnutrition. Nature 1970;225:283–4.
32 Bradfield RB, Baily MA, Cordano A. Hair-root changes in Andean Indian children during marasmic kwashiorkor. Lancet 1968;ii: 1169–70.
33 Bradfield RB, Cordano A, Graham GG. Hair-root adaptation to marasmus in Andean Indian children. Lancet 1969;ii:1395–7.
34 Bradfield RB, Bailey MA, Margen S. Morphological changes in human scalp hair roots during deprivation of protein. Science 1967;157:438–9.
35 Johnson AA, Latham MC, Roe DA. An evaluation of the use of changes in hair root morphology in the assessment of protein-calorie malnutrition. Am J Clin Nutr 1976;29:502–11.
36 Neldner KH, Hambidge KM, Walravens PA. Acrodermatitis enteropathica. Int J Dermatol 1978;17:380–7.
37 Tucker SB, Schroeter AL, Brown PW et al. Acquired zinc deficiency: cutaneous manifestions typical of acrodermatitis enteropathica. J Am Med Assoc 1976;235:2399–402.
38 Caldwell MD, Jonsson HT, Othersen HB Jr. Essential fatty acid deficiency in an infant receiving prolonged parenteral alimentation. J Pediatr 1972;81:894–8.
39 Skolnik P, Eaglstein WH, Ziboh VA. Human essential fatty acid deficiency: treatment by topical application of linoleic acid. Arch Dermatol 1977;113:939–41.
40 Hansen AE, Wiese HF, Boelsche AN et al. Role of linoleic acid in infant nutrition. Pediatrics 1963;31:171–92.
41 Burri BJ, Sweetman L, Nyhan WL. Mutant holocarboxylase synthetase. J Clin Invest 1981;68:1491–5.
42 Sherwood WB, Saunders M, Robinson BH et al. Lactic acidosis in biotin responsive multiple carboxylase deficiency caused by holocarboxylase synthetase deficiency of early and late onset. J Pediatr 1982;101:546–50.
43 Wolfe B, Heard GS, Jefferson LG et al. Neonatal screening for biotinidase deficiency: an update. J Inherited Metab Dis 1986;9(Suppl 2): 303–6.
44 Dupuis L, Leon Del-Rio A, Leclerc D et al. Clustering of mutations in the biotin-binding region of holocarboxylase synthetase in biotinresponsive multiple carboxylase deficiency. Hum Mol Genet 1996;5:1011–16.
45 Nyhan WL. Inborn errors of biotin metabolism. Arch Dermatol 1987;123:1696–8.
46 Burlina AB, Sherwood WG, Zacchello LF. Partial biotinidase deficiency associated with Coffin–Siris syndrome. Eur J Pediatr 1990; 149:628–9.
47 Williams ML, Packman S, Cowan MJ. Alopecia and periorificial dermatitis in biotin-responsive multiple carboxylase deficiency. J Am Acad Dermatol 1983;9:97–103.
48 Thoene J, Baker H, Yoshino M et al. Biotin-responsive carboxylase deficiency associated with subnormal plasma and urinary biotin. N Engl J Med 1981;304:817–20.
49 Burlina AB, Sherwood WG, Marchioro MV et al. Neonatal screening for biotinidase deficiency in north eastern Italy. Eur J Pediatr 1988;147:317–18.
50 Kasapkara CS, Akar M, Ozbek MN et al. Mutations in BTD gene causing biotinidase deficiency: a regional report. J Pediatr Endocrinol Metab 2015;28:421–4.

Miniaturization

Androgenetic alopecia

Androgenetic alopecia (AGA), or pattern hair loss, is characterized by a miniaturization of the dermal papillae and corresponding matrix, a decrease in anagen duration, an increase in the percentage in telogen and an associated lag phase after telogen that slows the onset of the next anagen cycle in the affected hair follicles [1]. Recent work has established that AGA is a complex polygenic disorder involving both the X-linked susceptibility androgen receptor (AR) gene and an androgen-independent autosomal locus on chromosome 20p11 [2,3]. Males who carry a risk allele of each locus have an odds ratio for developing AGA of >7, which implies a potential functional link between the two [3].

The initial presentation of AGA may occur immediately after puberty. Generally, hair loss presents in both boys and girls as central scalp hair thinning plus/minus frontal accentuation of hair loss. Dermoscopy represents a valid aid to avoid scalp biopsy in doubtful cases and to distinguish AGA from telogen effluvium. It has been stated that more than 20% hair diameter diversity is an early sign of AGA [4]. Rakowska et al. suggested trichoscopy criteria for AGA; the presence of two major criteria or one major plus two minor criteria diagnoses AGA with 98% specificity. Major criteria are (1) more than four yellow dots in four images in the frontal area; (2) lower average hair thickness in the frontal area compared with the occiput; (3) more than 10% of thin hairs (<0.03 mm) in the frontal area. Minor criteria are (1) increased frontal to occipital ratio of single-hair pilosebaceous units; (2) vellus hairs; (3) perifollicular discoloration [5]. In AGA the peripilar sign is frequently observed – a brown halo surrounding the follicular openings [6].

In girls, AGA should prompt a check for signs of hirsutism, severe acne and acanthosis nigricans and the performance of screening blood tests including thyroid function tests, complete blood count, free testosterone and dehydroepiandrosterone (DHEA) sulphate. If there is any confirmation of hyperandrogenism, a 17-OH progesterone test (best done on days 4–10 of the menstrual cycle and in the morning) and a 2 h glucose tolerance test with concomitant insulin levels should be performed to rule out diabetes and insulin resistance as part of the polycystic ovarian syndrome (PCOS): a baseline insulin level of >20 IU/mL or a glucose to insulin ratio of <4.5 are suggestive of insulin resistance [7]. A scalp biopsy can be helpful showing a terminal:vellus ratio of <3:1 in children compared to <4:1 in adults with AGA [8,9].

Treatment of AGA is a modification of that recommended for adults [10]. Treatment in adolescent boys should usually begin with topical minoxidil; this will both affect the miniaturization and increase the percentage of hairs in anagen. There is potential for systemic absorption with topical minoxidil and there may need to be adjustment of the maxiumum daily dose for size; the authors recommend starting with 2% topical minoxidil 1 mL once a day and titrating upwards to twice a day for those weighing less than 40 kg. The 5% topical minoxidil solution or foam is more effective than the 2% topical minoxidil solution and would be preferred for those adolescent males that are of adult size. Finasteride is FDA approved for for affected males at least 18 years of age and has been shown to markedly slow the rate of hair loss if used long term.

Treatment in girls should also begin with topical minoxidil as above. In those girls with hyperandrogenism, consideration should be given to treating the underlying condition, whether it be congenital adrenal hyperplasia, PCOS or another condition. Usually this involves putting the patient on an oral contraceptive pill that will both lower the androgen output from the ovary and prevent pregnancy while on a concomitant medication that may cause feminization of a male fetus (which all antiandrogens are at risk for doing). Spironolactone is the usual choice of antiandrogen in the United States and starting doses of 100 mg a day are reasonable, always making sure to check potassium levels after starting the drug to ensure no hyperkalaemia has resulted. Cyproterone acetate is available in Europe as an alternative oral antiandrogen, primarily of value in women with documented hyperandrogenism [11].

References

1 **Olsen EA. Pattern hair loss. In: Olsen EA (ed.) Disorders of Hair Growth: Diagnosis and Treatment. New York: McGraw-Hill, 2003:321–62.**

2 Hillmer AM, Brockschmidt FF, Hanneken S et al. Susceptibility variants for male-pattern baldness on chromosome 20p11. Nat Genet 2008;40:1279–81.

3 **Richards JB, Yuan X, Geller F et al. Male-pattern baldness susceptibility locus at 20p11. Nat Genet 2008;40:1282–4.**

4 de Lacharriere O, Deloche C, Misciali C et al. Hair diameter diversity: a clinical sign reflecting the follicle miniaturization. Arch Dermatol 2001;137:641–6.

5 Rakowska A, Slowinska M, Kowalska-Oledzka E et al. Dermoscopy in female androgenic alopecia: method standardization and diagnostic criteria. Int J Trichol 2009;1:123–30.

6 Deloche C, de Lacharriere O, Piraccini BM et al. Histological features of peripilar signs associated with androgenetic alopecia. Arch Dermatol Res 2004;295:422–8.

7 Legro RS, Myers ER, Barnhart HX et al. The pregnancy in polycystic ovary syndrome study: baseline characteristics of the randomized cohort including racial effects. Fertil Steril 2006;86(4):914–33.

8 **Tosti A, Iorizzo M, Piraccini BM. Androgenetic alopecia in children: report of 20 cases. Br J Dermatol 2005;152:556–9.**

9 **Whiting DA. Scalp biopsy as a diagnostic and prognostic tool in androgenetic alopecia. Dermatol Ther 1998;8:24–33.**

10 Olsen EA, Messenger AG, Shapiro J et al. Evaluation and treatment of male and female pattern hair loss. J Am Acad Dermatol 2004; 52:301–11.

11 Vexiau P, Chaspoux C, Boudou P, et al. Effects of minoxidil 2% vs cyproterone acetate treatment on female androgenetic alopecia: a controlled, 12-month randomized trial. Br J Dermatol 2002; 146(6):992–9.

Focal scarring and nonscarring causes of alopecia

Focal scarring alopecia

Focal alopecia can be of either a potentially transient nonscarring nature or a potentially permanent scarring nature. In an infant, there are five main causes of focal scarring hair loss: trauma (including prolonged pressure that results in ischaemia), an underlying naevus (or neoplasia), deep fungal infection, part of a syndrome, or aplasia cutis congenita. Those conditions associated with focal scarring alopecia are shown in Box 159.3 and aplasia cutis congenita is discussed in greater detail below.

Aplasia cutis congenita (ACC) is the focal absence of epidermis and/or other layers of the skin; the hair follicles are variably affected [1]. The incidence is estimated to be 3 in 10 000 births [2]. ACC presents on the scalp in 85% of cases, and 70% of patients have only a single lesion [1,3]. Usually, ACC lesions are small and round unless they are overlying one of the cranial suture lines, in which case they may be quite large and can extend to the dura or meninges. At birth, ACC may present with scalp ulcerations, crusting, scars or a parchment-like membrane secondary to *in utero* healing [1] (Fig. 159.32). Clinically, two different types of ACC may be distinguished: membranous ACC, due to an incomplete closure of ectodermal fusion lines and often with a 'hair collar', and nonmembranous ACC, which has been hypothesized to be due to a tension-induced disruption of the skin where tensile forces are greatest during brain development [2]. Familial ACC is generally of the nonmembranous type whereas membranous ACC is usually sporadic.

Box 159.3 Conditions associated with focal scarring hair loss in children

- Ankyloblepharon–ectodermal defects–cleft lip/palate syndrome
- Aplasia cutis congenita:
  - Single anomaly
  - Associated with other anomalies:
    associated with limb abnormalities
    46XY genotype/gonadal dysgenesis
    'lumpy' scalp syndrome
    trisomy 13
    4p syndrome
    ectodermal dysplasia of Carey
    ectodermal dysplasia of Tuffli
    Hallermann–Streiff syndrome
    ANOTHER syndrome
    focal dermal hypoplasia
    Johanson–Blizzard syndrome
- Birth trauma
- Congenital ectodermal dysplasia of the face
- Conradi–Hünermann chondrodysplasia punctata
- Epidermal or organoid naevus: CHILD syndrome (congenital hemidysplasia with ichthyosiform erythroderma and limb defects)
- Epidermolysis bullosa
- Incontinentia pigmenti
- Keratosis follicularis spinulosa decalvans
- Kerion
- KID syndrome (keratitis, ichthyosis, deafness)
- Neoplasia
- Prolonged pressure
- Primary cutaneous disease
- Tufted folliculitis

Source: Adapted from Olsen 2003 [21].

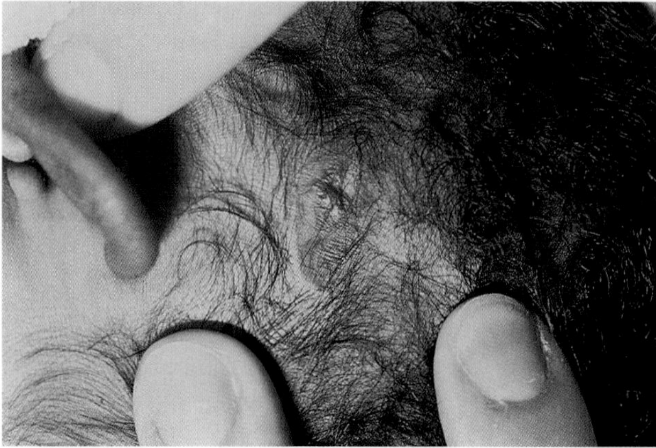

Fig. 159.32 Aplasia cutis congenita. Source: Courtesy of Dr Neil S. Prose.

The diagnosis of ACC is clinical, but the absence of yellow dots on dermatoscopic exam is useful to distinguish it from sebaceous naevus [4]. The dermatoscopic finding of elongated and radially arranged hair bulbs visible through the semitranslucent epidermis at the hair-bearing margin is specific to ACC [5].

Aplasia cutis congenita may present alone or with various other abnormalities including trisomy 13 syndrome, 4p syndrome, Adams–Oliver syndrome, oculocerebrocutaneous syndrome, SCALP syndrome, Setleis syndrome, epidermolysis bullosa, fetus papyraceus and various ectodermal dysplasias [2,6,7–18]. The Frieden classification system of ACC addresses many of these clinical associations (Box 159.4) [1]. It has also been suggested that there may be a relationship of ACC with *in utero* exposure to the antithyroid drug methimazole/carbimazole [19].

Box 159.4 Subtypes of ACC according to Frieden [1]

Group 1	Scalp ACC with other anomalies
Group 2	Scalp ACC with associated limb abnormalities (Adams–Oliver syndrome)
Group 3	ACC with associated epidermal or organoid naevi
Group 4	ACC overlying an embryological malformation such as a meningomyelocoele, gastroschisis or omphalocoele
Group 5	ACC with associated fetus papyraceus or placental infarct
Group 6	ACC associated with epidermolysis bullosa
Group 7	ACC localized to the extremities without blistering
Group 8	ACC caused by specific teratogens
Group 9	ACC with associated syndromes of malformations

Source: Adapted from Frieden 1986 [1]. Reproduced with permission of Elsevier.

Browning has suggested a treatment strategy based on associations and membranous versus nonmembranous subtypes of ACC [2]. Silberstein et al. have suggested treatment related to a classification system for ACC based on the size of the defect, the layers involved and the involvement of veins [20]. They suggest split-thickness skin grafts immediately for large defects or ones with large veins or sagittal sinus exposure.

Keratosis follicularis spinulosa decalvans

The most common primary cicatricial alopecias – lupus erythematosus, lichen planopilaris, folliculitis decalvans and pseudopelade of Brocq [22] – are rare in children. However, the group of disorders characterized by keratosis pilaris and scarring alopecia, termed *keratosis pilaris atrophicans* by Rand and Baden [23], typically have their onset in childhood. One of these, *keratosis follicularis spinulosa decalvans* (KFSD), begins with keratosis pilaris in infancy and is accompanied by photophobia, corneal changes, and progressive scarring alopecia of the scalp, eyebrows and/or eyelashes [23,24].

In the typical X-linked (locus Xp21.2-22.2) inheritance of KFSD [25], missense mutations have been identified in the responsible gene which encodes *MBTPS2*, a zinc metalloprotease whose function is required for cleavage of sterol regulatory element-binding proteins [26]. Mutations in *MBTPS2* have also been seen in IFAP syndrome and Olmsted syndrome [27]. An uncommon autosomal dominant form of KFSD has been reported [28,29]. Marked facial erythema, extensive folliculitis and onychodystrophy are typical of the autosomal dominant variant, while palmoplantar keratoderma and early onset seem more typical of the X-linked form. Recently, an increased level of the neuropeptide substance P has been identified in a patient with KFSP and severe scalp pruritus [30].

Multiple topical and systemic treatments have been tried without great success but among them, systemic isotretinoin seems the most promising [31].

Focal nonscarring hair loss

Most of the conditions that cause focal nonscarring hair loss are common and include alopecia areata, tinea capitis, traction alopecia and trichotillomania; these are discussed elsewhere in this textbook. Another less common cause of focal nonscarring hair loss is pityriasis amiantacea, which presents as localized scaling that is adherent to the involved hairs; this may be related to seborrhoeic dermatitis or psoriasis and usually responds to keratolytics and time [32]. However, parents need to be advised not to physically try to remove the pityriasis amiantacea scale as doing so can result in epilation of the involved hairs and permanent loss of the affected follicles. Pressure alopecia caused by prolonged and sustained pressure on a localized area of the scalp, usually in the operating room or the intensive care unit, is reversible unless ischaemia has occurred.

Triangular alopecia

Triangular alopecia is also a type of focal hair loss usually presenting in early childhood but potentially occurring at any age [33,34]. The temporal area is the most common location and the lesions may be unilateral or bilateral. The area of alopecia may be roughly triangular, oval or lancet shaped (Fig. 159.33) and may be hairless or vellus hair may be present. Histologically, there is a transition of hairs from terminal to vellus.

Clinically, differentiating triangular alopecia from alopecia areata or trichotillomania may be difficult, especially when the area is located close to the frontotemporal hair line. Dermoscopy is then very helpful in avoiding a biopsy; white hairs, diversity of hair diameter, empty follicles and white dots have been reported in triangular alopecia [35] as well as normal follicular openings containing long thin vellus hairs [36].

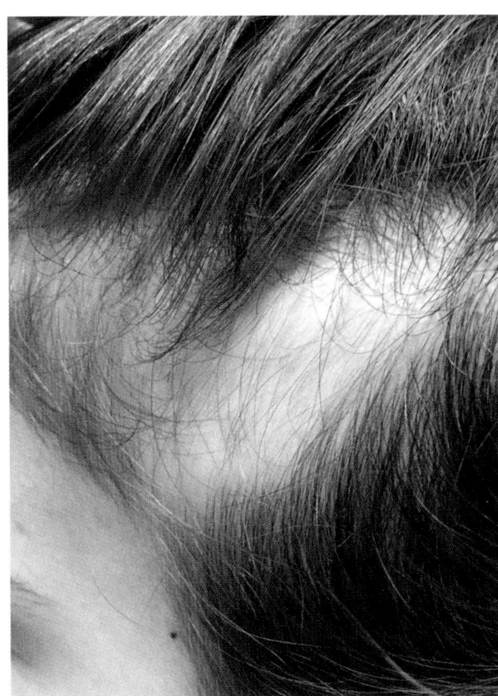

Fig. 159.33 Triangular alopecia.

The alopecia in triangular alopecia is usually persistent [37] but may improve with topical minoxidil [38].

Familial focal alopecia is the name proposed for patchy nonscarring areas of decreased hair density in the scalp in a mother and daughter [39]. On biopsy, there was telogen arrest, absence of inflammation and preservation of sebaceous epithelium.

References

1 **Frieden IJ. Aplasia cutis congenita: a clinical review and proposal for classification. J Am Acad Dermatol 1986;14:646–60.**

2 **Browning JC. Aplasia cutis congenita: approach to evaluation and management. Dermatol Ther 2013;26:439–44.**

3 Vexiau P, Chaspoux C, Boudou P et al. Effects of minoxidil 2% vs cyproterone acetate treatment on female androgenetic alopecia: a controlled, 12-month randomized trial. Br J Dermatol 2002;146(6): 992–9.

4 Neri I, Savoia F, Giacomini F et al. Usefulness of dermatoscopy for the early diagnosis of sebaceous naevus and differentiation from aplasia cutis congenita. Clin Exp Dermatol 2009;34:e50–2.

5 **Rakowska A, Maj M, Zadurska M et al. Trichoscopy of focal alopecia in children – new trichoscopic findings: hair bulbs arranged radially along hair-bearing margins in aplasia cutis congenital. Skin Appendage Disord 2016;2(1-2):1–6.**

6 **Freire-Maia N, Pinheiro M. Ectodermal Dysplasias: a Clinical and Genetic Study. New York: Alan R Liss, 1984.**

7 Peer LA, van Duyn J. Congenital defect of the scalp: report of a case with fatal termination. Plast Reconstr Surg 1948;3:722–6.

8 Ruiz-Maldonado R, Tamayo L. Aplasia cutis congenita, spastic paralysis, and mental retardation. Am J Dis Child 1974;128:699–701.

9 Sybert VP. Congenital scalp defects with distal limb anomalies (Adams–Oliver syndrome – McKusick 100300): further suggestion of autosomal recessive inheritance [Letter]. Am J Med Genet 1989;32:266–7.

10 Brosnan PG, Lewandowski RC, Toguri AG et al. A new familial syndrome of 45,XY gonadal dysgenesis with anomalies of ectodermal and mesodermal structures. J Pediatr 1980;97:586–90.

11 Finlay AY, Marks R. An hereditary syndrome of lumpy scalp, odd ears and rudimentary nipples. Br J Dermatol 1978;99:423–30.

12 Mardini MK, Ghandour M, Sakati NA et al. Johanson–Blizzard syndrome in a large inbred kindred with three involved members. Clin Genet 1978;14:247–50.

13 Zapata HH, Sletten LJ, Pierpont MEM. Congenital cardiac malformations in Adams–Oliver syndrome. Clin Genet 1995;47:80–4.

14 Baruchin AM, Nahieli O, Golan Y. Oculo-cerebro-cutaneous syndrome: first description in an adult. J Cranio-Maxillo-Facial Surg 1992;20:70–2.

15 Tuffli GA, Laxova R. Brief clinical report: new, autosomal dominant form of ectodermal dysplasia. Am J Med Genet 1983;14:381–4.

16 Pinheiro M, Penna FJ, Freire-Maia N. Two other cases of ANOTHER syndrome: family report and update. Clin Genet 1989;35:237–42.

17 Goltz RW, Henderson RR, Hitch JM et al. Focal dermal hypoplasia syndrome: a review of the literature and report of two cases. Arch Dermatol 1970;101:1–11.

18 Gershoni-Baruch R, Lerner A, Braun J et al. Johanson–Blizzard syndrome: clinical spectrum and further delineation of the syndrome. Am J Med Genet 1990;35:546–51.

19 Sachs C, Tebacher-Alt M, Mark M et al. Aplasia cutis congenital and antithyroid drugs during pregnancy; case series and literature review. Ann Dermatol Venereol 2016;143:423–35.

20 **Silberstein E, Pagkalos VA, Landau D et al. Aplasia cutis congenita: clinical management and a new classification system. Plast Reconstr Surg 2014:134(5):766e–774e.**

21 **Olsen EA. Hair loss in childhood. In: Olsen EA (ed.) Disorders of Hair Growth. Diagnosis and Treatment, 2nd edn. New York: McGraw-Hill, 2003:177–238.**

22 **Olsen E, Bergfeld W, Cotsarelis G et al. Summary of NAHRS sponsored workshop on cicatricial alopecia, Duke University Medical Center, February 10 and 11, 2001. J Am Acad Dermatol 2003;48:103–10.**

23 Rand R, Baden HP. Keratosis follicularis spinulosa decalvans. Report of two cases and literature review. Arch Dermatol 1983;119:22–6.
24 Herd RM, Benton EC. Keratosis follicularis spinulosa decalvans. Report of a new pedigree. Br J Dermatol 1996;134:138–42.
25 Oosterwijk JC, van der Wielen WJR, van de Osse E et al. Refinement of the localization of the X-linked keratosis follicularis spinulosa decalvans (KFSD) gene Xp22.13–p22.2. J Med Genet 1995;32:736–9.
26 Aten E, Brasz LC, Bornholdt D et al. Keratosis follicularis spinulosa decalvans is caused by mutations in MBTPS2. Hum Mutat 2010;31(10):1125–33.
27 Bornholdt D, Atkinson TP, Bouhadjar B et al. Genotype-phenotype correlations emerging from the identification of missense mutations in MBTPS2. Hum Mutat 2013;34:587094.
28 Castori M, Covaciu C, Paradisi M, Zambruno G. Clinical and genetic heterogeneity in keratosis follicularis spinulosa decalvans. Eur J Med Genet 2009;52:53–8.
29 Appell ML, Sherertz EF. A kindred with alopecia, keratosis pilaris, cataracts, and psoriasis. J Am Acad Dermatol 1987;16:89–95.
30 Doche I, Hordinsky M, Wilcox GL et al. Substance P in keratosis follicularis spinulosa decalvans. J Am Acad Case Rep 2015;1:327–8.
31 Gupta D, Kumari R, Bahunutula RK et al. Keratosis follicularis spinulosa decalvans showing excellent response to isotretinoin. Indian J Dermatol Venereol Leprol 2015;81:646–8.
32 Bettencourt MS, Olsen EA. Pityriasis amiantacea: a report of two cases in adults. Cutis 1999;64:187–90.
33 Kubba R, Rook A. Congenital triangular alopecia. Br J Dermatol 1976;95:657–9.
34 Trakimas C, Sperling LC, Skelton HG et al. Clinical and histologic findings in temporal triangular alopecia. J Am Acad Dermatol 1994;31:205–9.
35 Fernandez-Crehuet P, Vano-Galvan S, Martorell-Calatayud A et al. Clinical and trichoscopic characteristics of temporal triangular alopecia: a multicenter study. J Am Acad Dermatol 2016;75:634–7.
36 Iorizzo M. Videodermoscopy: a useful tool for diagnosing congenital triangular alopecia. Ped Dermatol 2008;25:652–4.
37 Minars N. Congenital temporal alopecia. Arch Dermatol 1974;109:395–6.
38 Bang C-Y, Byun J-W, Kang M-J et al. Successful treatment of temporal triancular alopecia with topical minoxidil. Ann Dermatol 2013; 25:387–8.
39 Headington JT, Astle N. Familial focal alopecia. A new disorder of hair growth clinically resembling pseudopelade. Arch Dermatol 1989;123:234–7.

Hypertrichosis

Generalized hypertrichosis

Hereditary generalized hypertrichosis

Congenital hypertrichosis lanuginosa implies a rare generalized and confluent overgrowth (or persistence) of lanugo hair in all hair-bearing areas [1–4]. The condition is thought to be of autosomal dominant inheritance with variable expressivity [4–6]. The excess hair is usually silvery-grey to blond in colour and is either apparent at birth or within the first few months of life (Fig. 159.34). Children are generally otherwise normal except for possible anomalous dental development [1]. The hypertrichosis may persist, decrease or increase with age [1].

The other types of generalized hereditary hypertrichosis seen in childhood do not generally have the even confluent hair growth seen in congenital hypertrichosis lanuginosa. There are three forms of what has been called *congenital generalized hypertrichosis* (abbreviated as HTC in Online Mendelian Inheritance of Man) [5]. Infants with the autosomal dominant HTC1 (Ambras syndrome) may have a generalized hypertrichosis at birth, but the hair is generally much longer and thicker on the face, ears and shoulders, and converges in the midline on the back [6]. Facial dysmorphism and dental abnormalities are common. HTC1 has been mapped to a de novo pericentric

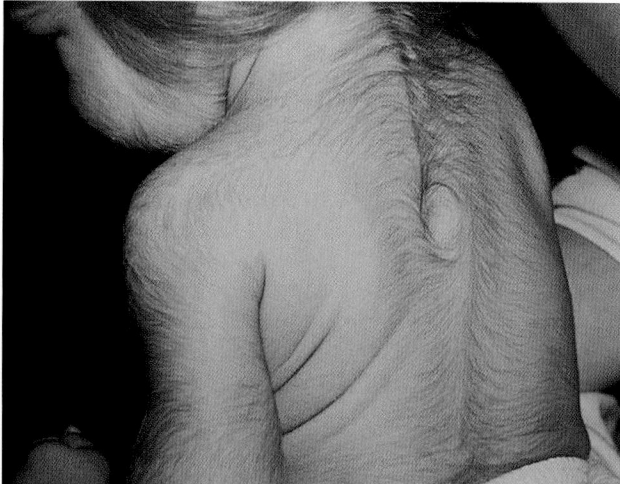

Fig. 159.34 Congenital hypertrichosis lanuginosa. Source: Reproduced from Olsen 2003 [7].

inversion of chromosome 8 with the suggestion that the phenotype is caused by a position effect versus a disruption of a gene [5]. Trichorhinophalangeal syndrome 1 (*TRPS1*), a second autosomal dominant form of HTC (HTC3 with or without gingival hyperplasia), presents with terminal hair primarily on the face with coarse facies. A microdeletion or microduplication on chromosome 17q24.2-q24.3 or a position effect of the *ABCA5* gene has been noted [5]. The X-linked congenital generalized hypertrichosis (HTC2) presents with excessive terminal hair on the face and upper body at birth, the hair shorter and curlier than that seen in Ambras syndrome and generally more excessive in males than females, who may show only patchy hypertrichosis. Deafness and dental abnormalities may occur. A 389 kb interchromosomal insertion in an extragenic palindrome site at Xq27.1 has also been reported [7].

Hereditary gingival fibromatosis characterized by marked gingival hypertrophy which usually appears in infancy [8–11] can be associated occasionally with excessive hair growth of the eyebrows, face, limbs and midback. The autosomal dominant *Zimmerman–Laband syndrome*, with hypoplastic phalanges, hepatosplenomegaly and facial dysmorphism [11], is best characterized as having an association with hypertrichosis and is related to missense mutations in the *KCNH1* gene on chromosome 1q32 and the *ATP6V1B2* gene on chromosome 8p21 [5].

The hypertrichosis in *Cornelia de Lange syndrome* (CDLS) is not as confluent as that seen in congenital hypertrichosis lanuginosa but consists of persistent excess lanugo hair over the forehead, nape of neck, back, shoulders and extremities [12–14]. The eyebrows are bushy and confluent and the lashes are very long. Children with CDLS have distinctive facies, mental and growth retardation, limb abnormalities and a low-pitched cry [15,16]. Typical laboratory findings are hyperglutamic acidaemia, hypoaminoaciduria and elevated serum and ketoglutarate. Eighty percent of cases of CDLS are determined to be of autosomal dominant inheritance and secondary to heterozygous mutations in the *NIPBL* gene on chromosome 5p13 (CDLS1) [5,14], and more recently a substantial proportion of apparently mutation-negative cases were found to be mosaic for mutations in the same gene [17]. Milder variants of CDLS have been identified: (1) autosomal dominant variants caused by a mutation in the *SMC3* gene (CDLS3) or the *RAD21* gene (CDLS4) and (2) X-linked variants caused by a mutation in the *SMC1A* gene (CDLS2) or the *HDAC8* gene (CDLS5), the vertebrate histone deacetylase of SMC3 [14]. All the mutations for CDLS encode components of the cohesin complex.

Children with the autosomal recessive *Hurler syndrome* also have distinctive 'gargoyle' facies, and their trunk and extremities may be covered with dense lanugo hair [18]; this is due to a homozygous or compound heterozygous mutation in the gene encoding α-L-iduronidase on chromosome 4p16 [5]. Two of the conditions within the 'histiocytosis-lymphadenopathy plus syndrome' or 'SLC29A3 spectrum disorder', caused by mutations in the *SLC29A3* gene which encodes the equilibrative nucleoside transposition hENT3, have an association with hypertrichosis: PHID (pigmented hypertrichosis with insulin-dependent diabetes mellitus) syndrome and 'H' syndrome (cutaneous *h*yperpigmentation, *h*ypertrichosis [in hyperpigmented indurated patches on the mid and lower body], *h*epatomegaly, *h*eart anomalies, *h*earing loss, *h*ypogonadism, low *h*eight, *h*allux valgus and fixed flexion contractures of the toe and proximal interphalangeal joints and occasional *h*yperglycaemia) [19].

Patients with different types of porphyria can develop generalized hypertrichosis. Children with the autosomal recessive erythropoietic protoporphyria usually develop widespread hypertrichosis by the age of 5–6 years [20]. The excess hair is usually mainly on the limbs and trunk, it may be downy or coarse, and is generally pigmented. Other cutaneous findings include photosensitivity and vesiculobullous lesions. Hypertrichosis is also common in porphyria cutanea tarda but presents on the temples, cheeks, eyebrows and hairline more than on the trunk and extremities [21]. Although the manifestations of this hereditary enzymatic disorder usually appear first in adulthood, an acquired form of porphyria cutanea tarda secondary to the inadvertent ingestion of hexachlorobenzene or chlorinated phenols may be seen at any age [21,22]. Variegate porphyria may cause similar cutaneous findings to those seen with porphyria cutanea tarda but is distinguished by intermittent gastrointestinal and neurological symptoms after exposure to certain provoking medications. Variegate porphyria has a different urine and stool porphyrin profile from porphyria cutanea tarda. Porphyrias are discussed in further detail in Chapter 78.

Acquired generalized hypertrichosis (drug related)

Generalized hypertrichosis, typically of vellus rather than lanugo hair, may be an acquired problem caused by several drugs. Minoxidil, a piperidinopyrimidine derivative used to treat hypertension, causes hypertrichosis in about 70% of users of the systemic drug [23,24]. The excess hair is especially prominent over the face, shoulders and extremities and develops weeks to months after starting treatment (Fig. 159.35). The hypertrichosis regresses within months of discontinuing the drug.

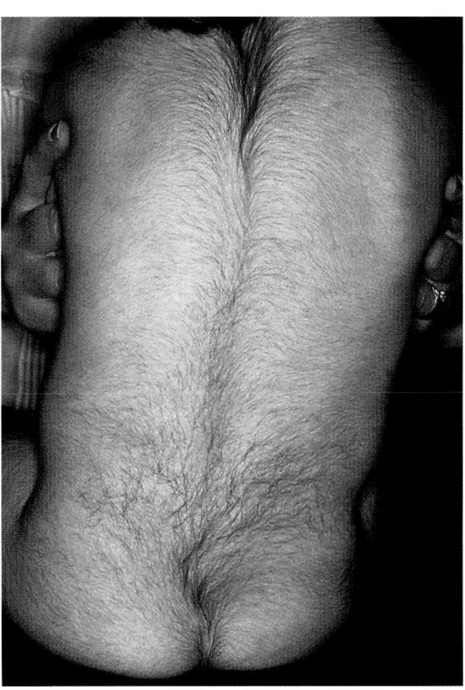

Fig. 159.35 Minoxidil-induced hypertrichosis. Source: Courtesy of Dr Nancy B. Esterly.

Hypertrichosis is seen in up to 60% of patients given ciclosporin to prevent organ rejection [25]. It is even more common in patients given ciclosporin to treat graft-versus-host disease or insulin-dependent diabetes mellitus [26,27]. The hair growth is diffuse and begins within 2–4 weeks of starting the drug. Children and adolescents are at the greatest risk of developing moderate to severe hypertrichosis [22]. Usually, the hypertrichosis resolves 1–2 months after discontinuing the drug [25,27].

Diazoxide is a benzothiadiazine used to treat idiopathic hypoglycaemia of childhood. Lanugo hair growth is commonly seen in children, usually beginning six weeks after the start of treatment, and is most prominent on the forehead, nape of the neck, eyebrows, eyelashes and dorsum of the trunk and limbs [28–31]. The excess hair growth usually regresses 2–5 months after discontinuation of the drug but may take longer. Infants born to women given diazoxide for hypertension during pregnancy have a high incidence of hair abnormalities, including hypertrichosis lanuginosa and focal alopecia [32].

Hypertrichosis occurs in 5–12% of patients on phenytoin, usually most prominently on the extremities rather than the face and trunk [33,34]. The hair growth usually regresses within one year after treatment stops but can persist [35,36].

Although uncommonly used in children, psoralens and ultraviolet A (PUVA) [37,38] and acetazolamide have both been reported to cause hypertrichosis [39]. Streptomycin used to treat tuberculosis has also been associated with hypertrichosis [40].

Other illnesses/conditions associated with hypertrichosis

Certain acquired medical conditions have been associated with diffuse hypertrichosis. *POEMS* is an acronym for *p*eripheral neuropathy, *o*rganomegaly, *en*docrine dysfunction, *m*onoclonal gammopathy and *s*kin changes, the last including hypertrichosis primarily on the extensor surfaces, malar region and forehead [41–43]. Patients with hypothyroidism, acrodynia (mercury poisoning), tuberculosis or head trauma may also exhibit a generalized increase in hair growth [3]. There have been several reports of hypertrichosis in children with a variety of gastrointestinal problems, including coeliac disease, infantile steatorrhoea and failure to thrive; the primary mechanism is unknown [3]. Children with juvenile dermatomyositis may have a concomitant hypertrichosis, which may diminish with treatment of the dermatomyositis [44,45].

Localized hypertrichosis

There are several causes of localized hypertrichosis in childhood, some of which are isolated anomalies while others are indicative of either underlying anatomical abnormalities or other anomalies.

Congenital localized hypertrichosis

Congenital hair on the elbows, usually lanugo at birth, may become terminal and denser in early childhood and then regress with age [46,47]. It is inherited as an autosomal dominant trait either as a singular defect or with multiple abnormalities (short stature, consistent facial features, intellectual deficiency and hypertrichosis on the back) in the Wiedemann–Steiner syndrome. The latter has been noted to be associated with a heterozygous mutation in the *MLL* (also called *KMT2A*) gene on chromosome 11q23 [5]. *Congenital hair on the external ears* in children can be seen as an isolated anomaly in some Pacific Islanders or in patients with XYY syndrome or the offspring of diabetic mothers [48–50]. *Congenital trichomegaly of the eyelashes* can occur as an isolated event or as part of one of several syndromes including Cornelia de Lange syndrome, Rubinstein–Taybi syndrome, congenital hypertrichosis lanuginosa and a syndrome described by Oliver and McFarlane which includes dwarfism, mental retardation and pigmentary degeneration of the retina [3,51].

A localized ring of dark hair surrounding congenital alopecic scalp lesions is termed the *hair collar sign*. These scalp lesions are often made up of heterotopic neural tissue that may communicate with the skull or brain and thus should trigger an imaging study before any biopsy is performed [52]. Naevoid hypertrichosis is an uncommon congenital disorder typically consisting of terminal hair growth in a solitary area but rarely in multiple patches of normal underlying skin [53]. However, localized hypertrichosis can be associated with underlying abnormalities and should be further evaluated by biopsy. Localized areas of either hypertrichosis or alopecia at birth can overlie primary cutaneous meningiomas [54]. These may occur on the scalp, midline or paravertebral area of the back or face. Histologically, these show polygonal to fusiform cells with syncytial appearance, eosinophilic cytoplasm and regular nuclei without psammoma bodies. Clinically, these are benign neoplasms.

Localized hypertrichosis and hyperpigmentation may be seen in both congenital smooth muscle hamartomas and congenital pigmented hairy naevi. These two conditions are easily distinguished both clinically and by biopsy [55]. *Congenital smooth muscle hamartomas* histologically show smooth muscle bundles varying in size, shape and orientation. Clinically, the lesions may be single or multiple (Fig. 159.36), are usually indurated and show transient raising upon rubbing (pseudo-Darier's sign) [55,56].

In contradistinction, *congenital hairy naevi* histologically demonstrate a naevocellular naevus on biopsy. They are usually solitary, are not indurated and have a negative pseudo-Darier's sign [3] (Fig. 159.37). Congenital hairy naevi tend to persist and have a potential for malignant degeneration.

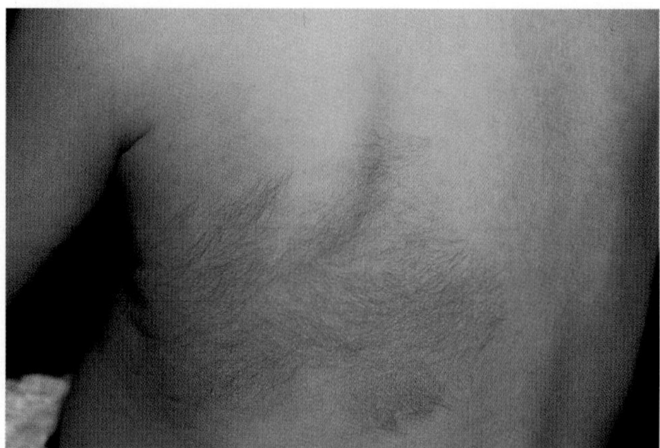

Fig. 159.36 Congenital smooth muscle hamartoma. Source: Courtesy of Dr Nancy B. Esterly.

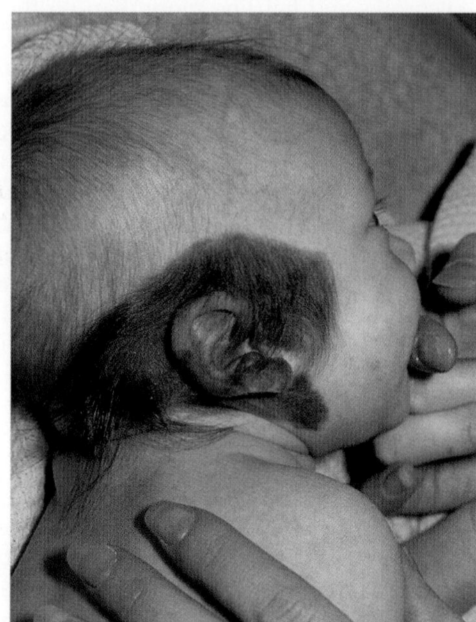

Fig. 159.37 Congenital hairy naevus. Source: Courtesy of Dr Nancy B. Esterly.

Patches of hypertrichosis have also been reported to occur in *Gorlin syndrome* [57]. The *Winchester syndrome* may also present with irregular patches of thickened skin, hyperpigmentation and hypertrichosis, but biopsy in this case shows fibroblastic proliferation with homogenized bundles of collagen [58]. Affected children will develop short stature secondary to osteoporosis, osteolysis and periarticular and intraarticular joint erosions. This is an autosomal recessive inheritance with a homozygous mutation in membrane type-1 metalloproteinase (MT1-MMP or MMP14) [59]. *Torg syndrome* is also related to mutations in a matrix metalloproteinase, in this case MMP2, and localized hypertrichosis has been reported as well [60].

The presence of *localized hypertrichosis over the spinal column*, most common in the lumbar or sacral area, is a cause for concern. Infants born with a so-called 'faun tail' (Fig. 159.38) may have an underlying spina bifida occulta, spina bifida, traction band or diastematomyelia [3,61]. A traction band can tether the cord or its appendages or the cauda equina to bone or skin through attachment to the meninges or through a tight filium terminale [62]. Diastematomyelia is the duplication or splitting of a portion of the spinal cord through which a bony spur or fibrous band passes and attaches to the vertebral body anteriorly or neural arch posteriorly [63]. In the last two conditions, neurological symptoms may not appear until the child is a toddler or older, when dissimilar growth of the cord and its bony housing causes the spinal cord to ascend in the vertebral column [62,63]. The localized hypertrichosis may not therefore be at the level of a neural defect if one occurs [64].

Midback hypertrichosis may accompany other cutaneous abnormalities that may signal either a primary or a secondary (from pressure) underlying neurological abnormality. Dermal sinuses, often associated with protrusion of hair from the sinus and pigmentation or port wine discoloration, can extend into the spinal canal or may expand into an epidermoid or dermal cyst. Midline lipomas are frequently attached to the cord, cauda equina, filum terminale or conus medullaris. Inadvertent manipulation of these lesions could lead to a portal of entry for infection into the central nervous system or neurological deficit. No excision or manipulation of an area of hypertrichosis over the spinal cord should be carried out without first evaluating the underlying cord or spinal column, preferably by noninvasive techniques.

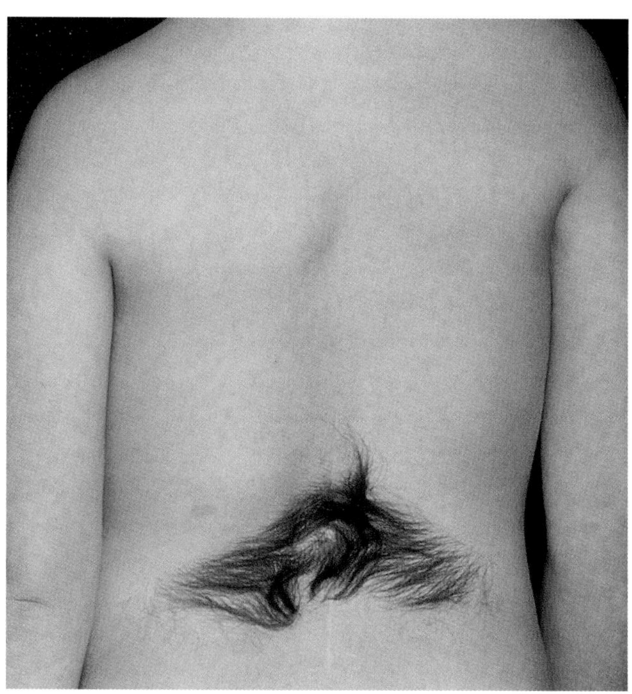

Fig. 159.38 Faun tail. Source: Courtesy of Dr Janet L. Roberts.

Acquired localized hypertrichosis

Any repeated irritation, inflammation or trauma may cause localized hypertrichosis by transformation of vellus to terminal hair [3]. The classic example is the localized hypertrichosis that develops under a casted appendage. The increased length of the hair that occurs in this situation is quickly lost when the cast is removed. Although localized hypertrichosis may be seen with morphoea [3], in general chronic dermatoses do *not* stimulate hair growth.

Scrotal hair in infants may occur with virilization (abnormal phallic size or testicular volume) or as a normal but uncommon variant without virilization. In the latter, scrotal hair appears at 2–7 months of age and then regresses by 18 months of age [65–67]. It is hypothesized to be related to the normal gonadotropin/androgen surge or 'mini puberty' that occurs in male infants at 1–6 months.

Interferon and ciclosporin have each been associated with localized hypertrichosis of the eyelashes, which in the case of ciclosporin is not surprising given that this drug is frequently associated with a diffuse hypertrichosis [68–70]. A localized increase in the length of hairs on the ear, eyebrows and/or eyelashes has also been reported in patients with acquired immune deficiency syndrome (AIDS), but the aetiology remains unclear [71–73]. Prostaglandin F analogues have been shown to induce eyelash growth when applied intraocularly or to the lid margin; topical bimatoprost is now FDA approved to treat inadequate eyelashes. When used for glaucoma, these prostaglandins can turn blue iris colour dark and induce periocular hyperpigmentation [74].

Becker's naevus usually first appears in adolescence but has been reported from infancy to middle age [75] (Fig. 159.39). These lesions may rarely have a familial incidence. The term 'naevus' is a misnomer as there are no naevus cells histologically, but rather variable hyperkeratosis and marked hyperpigmentation in the basal layers of the epidermis, with varying numbers of melanophages in the papillary dermis [75,76]. Hair follicles are normal or enlarged [75,77]. Some cases may also show an increase in smooth muscle bundles and in these cases, clinically one may see perifollicular papules [76,78]. The question of why these lesions appear in adolescence may be related to the presence of androgen

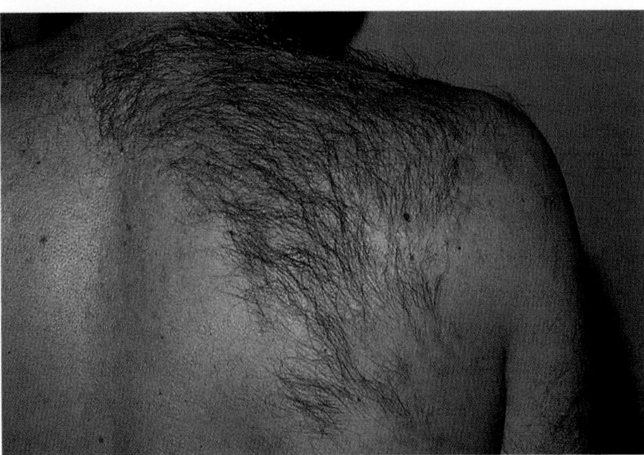

Fig. 159.39 Becker's naevus.

cytosol receptors in involved areas, similar to those in genital skin [79].

The hyperpigmentation of Becker's naevus usually appears first and may fade with time [78,80].The associated localized hypertrichosis may take years to develop [76,80]. Males are preferentially affected. Usually the lesions are single around the shoulders and at least palm sized, but occasionally an unusual size or location can cause confusion with a naevus. In most cases, there are no other associated problems or abnormalities, although hypoplasia of an ipsilateral limb or breast can occur, as can pectus carinatum, spina bifida and an accessory scrotum [3,75,81].

Treatment of hypertrichosis

In acquired hypertrichosis secondary to a drug or underlying disease, removal of the inciting cause will generally lead to loss of the increased hair growth and resumption of the normal type, length and cycle of hair. In the case of hereditary or developmental hypertrichosis, treatment must be directed at either psychological acceptance or cosmetic removal of the increased hair growth. Shaving and chemical depilatories serve to temporarily remove the offending hairs from sight without physically affecting the growth of the hairs. Plucking and wax epilation remove the hair only temporarily and can be quite painful. Each of these techniques runs the risk of pseudofolliculitis barbae in those with very curly or kinky hair and chemical depilatories can be very irritating.

Electrolysis refers to electrochemical destruction of the hair follicle, either through thermolysis (AC current with destruction of the hair by local heat production) or 'the blend', a combination of thermolysis and galvanic DC current (which produces destruction of the hair by local production of caustic lye and H_2 gas) [82,83]. The current used is generally low intensity and high frequency to minimize tissue destruction and pain. Electrolysis varies greatly in terms of technique, machines and probes used, and the potential for permanent hair removal varies widely. Potential but controllable side-effects are pain, scarring, infection and folliculitis.

Several different lasers (ruby, diode, alexandrite, Nd:YAG) have been introduced for hair removal [1,83]. The lasers vary in the active medium and hence the wavelength of the monochromatic light produced. All of these lasers remove hair by selectively targeting the contents of the follicular canal, either the melanin of the hair shaft in the case of the first three lasers listed above or a substance absorbed into the follicular canal in most cases of the Nd:YAG laser. In each case, the absorption of laser light by a specific chromophore transforms the energy into heat, which may translate into either temporary epilation or miniaturization or (and this requires long-term histological follow-up) destruction of the treated hairs. Usually, multiple treatments are needed to induce permanent hair reduction, the FDA definition of which is 'lasting reduction of treated hairs for a period greater than the complete cycle of hairs in a given treated area'. Although the lasers that target melanin do so indiscriminately, and thus epidermal melanin can be affected too, measures are available to minimize the effect on epidermal pigment and to target hair melanin more specifically. These include cooling of the epidermis immediately before laser treatment, prior use of topical hydroquinone and the use of lasers with longer target wavelengths. There is also a flashlamp-based system of hair removal that creates a broad rather than monochromatic wavelength spectrum of light pulses (which technically exempts it from laser status) that can be tailored by a set of filters to a narrower focus.

The potential side-effects of laser hair removal with any of the aforementioned devices, including the flashlamp device, are pain, local oedema and erythema and temporary hypopigmentation, blisters or purpura secondary to inadvertent effects on epidermal melanin.

References

1 Partridge JW. Congenital hypertrichosis lanuginosa: neonatal shaving. Arch Dis Child 1987;62:623–5.

2 Ravin JG, Hodge GP. Hypertrichosis portrayed in art. J Am Med Assoc 1969;207:533–5.

3 Olsen EA. Hypertrichosis. In: Olsen EA (ed.) Disorders of Hair Growth: Diagnosis and Treatment, 2nd edn. New York: McGraw-Hill, 2003:399–430.

4 Beighton P. Congenital hypertrichosis lanuginosa. Arch Dermatol 1970;101:669–72.

5 Online Mendelian Inheritance in Man, OMIM®. Johns Hopkins University, Baltimore, MD. https://omim.org/

6 Baumeister FAM, Egger J, Schildhauer MT et al. Ambras syndrome: delineation of a unique hypertrichosis universalis congenita and association with a balanced pericentric inversion (8) (p11.2;q22). Clin Genet 1993;44:121–8.

7 DeStefano GM, Fantauzzo KA, Petukhova L et al. Position effect on FGF13 associated with X-linked congenital generalized hypertrichosis. Proc Natl Acad Sci USA 2013;110:7790–5.

8 Laband PF, Habib G, Humphreys BS. Hereditary gingival fibromatosis: report of an affected family with associated splenomegaly and skeletal and soft-tissue abnormalities. Oral Pathol 1964;17:339–51.

9 Winter GB, Simpkiss MJ. Hypertrichosis with hereditary gingival hyperplasia. Arch Dis Child 1974;49:394–9.

10 Witkop CJ Jr. Heterogeneity in gingival fibromatosis. Birth Defects Orig Art Ser 1971;7:210–21.

11 LaCombe D, Bioulac-Sage P, Sibout M et al. Congenital marked hypertrichosis and Laband syndrome in a child: overlap between the gingival fibromatosis-hypertrichosis and Laband syndromes. Genet Counsel 1994;5:251–6.

12 De Lange C. Memoires originaux sur un type nouveau de dégénération (Typus Amstelodamensis). Arch Méd 1933;36:713–19.
13 Ptacek LJ, Opitz JM, Smith DW et al. The Cornelia de Lange syndrome. J Pediatr 1963;635:1000–20.
14 Boyle M I, Jespersgaard C, Brondum-Nielsen K et al. Cornelia de Lange syndrome. Clin Genet 2015;88:1–12.
15 Pashayan H, Whelan D, Guttman S et al. Variability of the de Lange syndrome: report of three cases and genetic analysis of 54 families. J Pediatr 1969;75:853–8.
16 Soderquist NA, Reed WB. Cornelia-de Lange syndrome. Cutis 1968;4:1333–5.
17 Ansari M, Poke G, Ferry Q et al. Genetic heterogeneity in Cornelia de Lange syndrome (CdLS) and CdLS-like phenotypes with observed and predicted levels of mosaicism. J Med Genet 2014; 51(10):659–68.
18 Hambrick GW Jr, Scheie HG. Studies of the skin in Hurler's syndrome. Arch Dermatol 1962;85:455–70.
19 Morgan NV, Morris MR, Cangul H et al. Mutations in SLC29A3 encoding an equilibrative nucleoside transporter ENT3, cause a familial histiocytosis syndrome (Faisalabad histiocytosis) and familial Rosai-Dorfman disease. PLoS Genet 2010;6:e1000833.
20 Magnus IA. The cutaneous porphyrias. Semin Hematol 1968;5: 380–408.
21 Grossman ME, Bickers DR, Poh-Fitzpatrick MB et al. Porphyria cutanea tarda: clinical features and laboratory findings in 40 patients. Am J Med 1979;67:277–85.
22 Bleiberg J, Wallen M, Brodkin R et al. Industrially acquired porphyria. Arch Dermatol 1964;89:793–7.
23 Earhart RN, Ball J, Nuss DD et al. Minoxidil-induced hypertrichosis: treatment with calcium thioglycolate depilatory. South Med J 1977;70:442–3.
24 Olsen EA, Weiner MS, Delong ER et al. Topical minoxidil in early male pattern baldness. J Am Acad Dermatol 1985;13:185–92.
25 Cohen DJ, Loertscher R, Rubin MF et al. Cyclosporine: a new immunosuppressive agent for organ transplantation. Ann Intern Med 1984;101:667–82.
26 Harper JI, Kendra JR, Desai S et al. Dermatological aspects of the use of cyclosporin A for prophylaxis of graft-versus-host disease. Br J Dermatol 1984;110:469–74.
27 Wysocki GP, Daley TD. Hypertrichosis in patients receiving cyclosporine therapy. Clin Exp Dermatol 1987;12:191–6.
28 Burton JL, Scutt WH, Caldwell IW. Hypertrichosis due to diazoxide. Br J Dermatol 1975;93:707–11.
29 Okun R, Russell RP, Wilson WR. Use of diazoxide with trichlormethiazide for hypertension. Arch Intern Med 1963;112:882–8.
30 Baker L, Kaye R, Root AW et al. Diazoxide treatment of idiopathic hypoglycemia of infancy. J Pediatr 1967;71:494–505.
31 Menter MA (for Wells RS). Hypertrichosis lanuginosa and a lichenoid eruption due to diazoxide therapy. Proc Roy Soc Med 1973;66:16–17.
32 Milner RDG, Chouksey SK. Effects of fetal exposure to diazoxide in man. Arch Dis Child 1972;47:537–43.
33 Herberg K-P. Effects of diphenylhydantoin in 41 epileptics institutionalized since childhood. South Med J 1977;70:19–24.
34 Livingston S, Pauli LL, Pruce I et al. Phenobarbital vs. phenytoin for grand mal epilepsy. Am Fam Phys 1980;22:123–7.
35 Livingston S, Petersen D, Boks LL. Hypertrichosis occurring in association with dilantin therapy. J Pediatr 1955;47:351–2.
36 Bartuska DG. Hypertrichosis in a brain damaged child. J Am Med Wom Assoc 1963;18:711–13.
37 Elliott JA Jr. Clinical experiences with methoxsalen in the treatment of vitiligo. J Invest Dermatol 1959;32:311–13.
38 Rampen FHJ. Hypertrichosis in PUVA-treated patients. Br J Dermatol 1983;109:657–60.
39 Weiss IS. Hirsutism after chronic administration of acetazolamide. Am J Ophthalmol 1974;78:327–8.
40 Fono R. Appearance of hypertrichosis during streptomycin treatment. Ann Paediatr 1950;174:389–92.
41 Bosco J, Pathmanathan R. POEMS syndrome presenting as systemic sclerosis. Am J Med 1988;84:524–8.
42 Feddersen RM, Burgdorf W, Foucark K et al. Plasma cell dyscrasia: a case of POEMS syndrome with a unique dermatologic presentation. J Am Acad Dermatol 1989;21:1061–8.
43 Viard J-P, Lesavre P, Boitard C et al. POEMS syndrome presenting as systemic sclerosis. Am J Med 1988;84:524–8.
44 Pope DN, Strimling RB, Mallory SB. Hypertrichosis in juvenile dermatomyositis. J Am Acad Dermatol 1994;31:383–7.
45 Fontenla MAF. Severe hypertrichosis as an uncommon feature of juvenile dermatomyositis. J Am Acad Dermatol 1995;33:691.
46 Andreev VC, Stransky L. Hairy elbows. Arch Dermatol 1979;115:761.
47 Beighton P. Familial hypertrichosis cubiti: hairy elbows syndrome. J Med Genet 1970;7:158–60.
48 Rafaat M. Hypertrichosis pinnae in babies of diabetic mothers [Letter]. Pediatrics 1981;65:745–6.
49 Singh M, Kumar A, Paul VK. Hairy pinna: a pathognomonic sign in infants of diabetic mothers. Indian Pediatr 1987;24:87–9.
50 Woods DL, Malan AF, Coetzee EJ. Intra-uterine growth in infants of diabetic mothers. S Afr Med J 1980;58:441–13.
51 Oliver GL, McFarlane DC. Congenital trichomegaly with associated pigmentary degeneration of the retina, dwarfism, and mental retardation. Arch Ophthalmol 1965;74:169–74.
52 Stevens C, Galen W. The hair collar sign. Am J Med Genet 2008; 146:484–7.
53 Rupert LS, Bechtel M, Pellegrini A. Nevoid hypertrichosis: multiple patches associated with premature graying of lesional hair. Pediatr Dermatol 1994;11:49–51.
54 Peñas PA, Jones-Caballero M, Amigo A et al. Cutaneous meningiomas underlying congenital localized hypertrichosis. J Am Acad Dermatol 1994;30:363–6.
55 Glover MT, Malone M, Atherton DJ. Michelin tire baby syndrome resulting from diffuse smooth muscle hamartoma. Pediatr Dermatol 1989;6:329–31.
56 Slifman NR, Harrist TJ, Rhodes AR. Congenital arrector pili hamartoma. Arch Dermatol 1985;121:1034–7.
57 Wilson LC1, Ajayi-Obe E, Bernhard B, Maas SM. Patched mutations and hairy skin patches: a new sign in Gorlin syndrome. Am J Med Genet A 2006;140(23):2625–30.
58 Cohen AH, Hollister DW, Reed WB. The skin in the Winchester syndrome. Arch Dermatol 1975;111:230–6.
59 Evans BR, Mosig RA, Lobl M et al. Mutation of membrane type-1 metalloproteinase, MT1-MMP, causes the muticentric osteolysis and arthritis disease Winchester syndrome. Am J Hum Genet 2012; 91:572–6.
60 Ekbote A, Danda S, Zankl A et al. Patient with mutation in the matrix metalloproteinase 2 (MMP2) gene – a case report and review of the literature. J Clin Res Pediatr Endocrinol 2014;6:40–6.
61 Harris HW, Miller OF. Midline cutaneous and spinal defects. Arch Dermatol 1976;112:1724–8.
62 Thursfield WRR, Ross AA. Faun tail (sacral hirsuties) and diastematomyelia. Br J Dermatol 1961;73:328–36.
63 James CCM, Lassman LP. Spinal dysraphism: an orthopaedic syndrome in children accompanying occult forms. Arch Dis Child 1960;35:315–27.
64 Perret G. Diagnosis and treatment of diastematomyelia. Surg Gynecol Obstet 1957;105:69–83.
65 Papadimitriou A, Beri D, Nicolaidou P. Isolated scrotal hair in infancy. J Ped 2006;148:690–1.
66 Slyper AH, Easterly NB. Non-progressive scrotal hair growth in two infants. Pediatr Dermatol 1993;10:34–5.
67 Francis JS, Ruvalcaba RH. Scrotal hair growth in infancy. Pediatr Dermatol 1993;10:389–90.
68 Berglund EF, Burton GV, Mills GM et al. Hypertrichosis of the eyelashes associated with interferon-⊠ therapy for chronic granulocytic leukemia. South Med J 1990;83:363.
69 Foon KA. Increased growth of eyelashes in a patient given leukocyte A interferon. N Engl J Med 1984;311:1259.
70 Weaver DT, Bartley GB. Cyclosporine-induced trichomegaly. Am J Ophthalmol 1990;109:239.
71 Casanova JM, Puig T, Rubio M. Hypertrichosis of the eyelashes in acquired immunodeficiency syndrome. Arch Dermatol 1987;123: 1599–601.
72 Tosti A, Gaddoni G, Peluso AM et al. Acquired hairy pinnae in a patient infected with the human immunodeficiency virus. J Am Acad Dermatol 1993;28:513.
73 Vélez A, Kindelán JM, García-Herola A et al. Acquired trichomegaly and hypertrichosis in metastatic adenocarcinoma. Clin Exp Dermatol 1995;20:237–9.
74 Johnstone MA. Hypertrichosis and increased pigmentation of eyelashes and adjacent hair in the region of the ipsilateral eyelids of patients treated with unitlateral topical latanoprost. Am J Ophthalmol 1997;124:544–7.
75 Glinick SE, Alper JC, Bogaars H et al. Becker's melanosis: associated abnormalities. J Am Acad Dermatol 1983;9:509–14.

76 Haneke E. The dermal component in melanosis naeviformis Becker. J Cutan Pathol 1979;5:53–8.
77 Poomeechaiwong S, Golitz LE. Hamartomas. Adv Dermatol 1990; 5:257–88.
78 Urbanek RD, Johnson WC. Smooth muscle hamartoma associated with Becker's nevus. Arch Dermatol 1978;114:104–6.
79 Person JR, Longcope C. Becker's nevus: an androgen-mediated hyperplasia with increased androgen receptors. J Am Acad Dermatol 1984;10:235–8.
80 Bhawan J, Chang WH. Becker's melanosis: an ultrastructural study. Dermatologica 1979;159:221–30.
81 Lambert JR, Willems P, Abs R et al. Becker's nevus associated with chromosomal mosaicism and congenital adrenal hyperplasia. J Am Acad Dermatol 1994;30:655–7.
82 Olsen EA. Methods of hair removal. J Am Acad Dermatol 1999; 40:143–55.
83 Dierickx C. Hair removal by lasers and intense pulsed light sources. Dermatol Clin 2002;20(1):135–46.

CHAPTER 160
Alopecia Areata

Kerstin Foitzik-Lau
Skin and Vein Clinic Winterhude, Hamburg, Germany

Abstract

Alopecia areata (AA) is an autoimmune disease with a genetic basis and environmental triggers. It presents as nonscarring hair loss ranging from few circular bald areas (patchy alopecia areata) to complete baldness of the head (alopecia totalis) or the entire body (alopecia universalis). Almost 2% of the population is affected once in a lifetime. The peak onset in childhood is before the age of 10. The genetic trait is complex and still not completely understood. Indeed, genome-wide association studies have given more insight into the pathogenesis of AA and opened new therapeutic options. It is now widely accepted that a collapse of the immune privilege of the hair follicle is responsible for AA activation which enables immune cells to attack the hair follicle. First studies using inhibitors of the JAK kinase pathway have shown promising results in the treatment of AA.

Key points

- Alopecia areata is an autoimmune disease with a genetic basis and environmental triggers.
- It is a nonscarring hair loss ranging from circular bald areas to complete baldness of the head and body.
- Almost 2% of the general population is affected, with peak onset in childhood before the age of 10.
- T-cell-driven collapse of the immune privilege is believed to be responsible for disease activation.
- Inhibition of JAK kinase has shown promising results in the treatment of AA.

Introduction. Alopecia areata (AA) is an autoimmune disease with a genetic basis and environmental triggers [1]. It is a nonscarring reversible hair growth disorder characterized by initially patchy hair loss, which can occur on any hair-bearing site of the body. It can be limited to a few circular bald areas (AAC) and can lead to complete baldness of the head (alopecia areata totalis, AAT) or the entire body (alopecia areata universalis, AAU). While patchy alopecia responds well to local treatments, the more severe forms are often resistant to treatment. Therefore, it is questioned whether these subtypes have distinct pathogenic mechanisms, or whether AAU and AAT are just exacerbated forms of AAC [2].

Epidemiology. Alopecia areata is a quite common hair growth disorder with a lifetime risk of almost 2% in the general population [3]. The lifetime risk in children of patients with AA is 6%, significantly higher than that seen among adults [4]. There is no male or female predilection and AA can affect persons of any age. Contrary to previous reports, the most common age of onset of AA is the third and fourth decade [5]. In children, opposite studies exist which report different peak incidences of AA between mean age of onset 1–5 years and 5–10 years [5,6]. However, early onset of the disease in known to present a more severe subtype with a higher extent of hair loss.

Genetics. Alopecia areata is an autoimmune disease with a genetic basis. The genetic trait is complex, multifactorial and still not completely understood, but genetic studies in the last decade have shed more light on the disease [2]. Family and twin studies support the hypothesis of a genetic background and heritable basis. Monozygotic twins have a concordance rate of 55% and show similar onset and hair loss pattern of AA [4]. In different studies, 10–40% of patients with AA report a positive family history of at least one relative [7]. The positive family history depends on the onset of AA. In patients with early onset, before the age of 30 years, the family history is higher (37%); in patients with later onset, after 30 years, the positive family history is only 7.1% [8]. Another study reported an estimated lifetime risk to develop AA in siblings of 7.1%, 7.8% in parents and 5.7% in offspring [9].

Several associations with human leucocyte antigen (HLA) have been reported in AA. Previous studies have shown that major histocompatibility complex (MHC) genes on chromosome 6p21 encoding HLAs are major determining loci for T-cell-mediated diseases, including AA [10]. Within the HLA-D genes, HLA-DQB1*03 seems to be the general susceptibility gene [11]. In sporadic AA, HLA-DQB1*03(*0301-*0305) alleles were present in 92% of patients AA with AAT/AAU and in 80% of all patients with AA. HLA-DRB1*1104 allele is also increased for all types of AA [12]. The nonclassic MHC class I chain-related gene A (MICA) is a stress-induced antigen and activates natural killer (NK) cells. NK cells are known to be increased in lesions of AA patients. MICA is associated with AA and other autoimmune diseases [13].

Harper's Textbook of Pediatric Dermatology, Fourth Edition. Edited by Peter Hoeger, Veronica Kinsler and Albert Yan.

Later performed family-based linkage studies and genome-wide association study (GWAS) analysis identified linkage or association on many other chromosomes [3], confirming that AA is a complex polygenetic disease.

Most of the individuals who carry the susceptibility MHC alleles do not develop AA, so MHC loci seem to be necessary but not sufficient for disease development. Wassermann et al. [14] postulated that other genes regulating the immune system could be responsible for the induction, maintenance and course of AA. Indeed, other non-HLA genes have been found to be associated with AA. Recent GWAS have identified several loci for genes with influence on immune responses. These genes also have been implicated in other autoimmune diseases like type 1 diabetes, psoriasis, rheumatoid arthritis and coeliac disease [2,15] supporting the common cause hypothesis of autoimmune diseases. Only ULBP3 and ULBP6, which are natural killer cell receptor D (NKG2D) ligands, are uniquely implicated in AA and not in other autoimmune diseases. This and the fact that CD8NKG2D+ T cells are the major effectors in AA suggest a key role for these genes in the pathogenesis of alopecia areata [3,16]. Also, IFN-γ chain cytokine and cytotoxic T-cell signatures were found in AA [2,3] which are mediated by JAK kinases.

Jabbari et al. hypothesized distinct gene expression in the AA subtypes and were able to develop an Alopecia Areata Disease Severity Index (ALADIN) that distinguishes AAC, AT, AU and normal control samples by distinct gene expressions metrics using microarray-based gene expression analysis [2]. They found high immune activity and higher concentration of CD8 T cells in AT and AU samples compared to AC samples and healthy controls. Using this index could be useful in the future to decide what kind of treatment is reasonable for the individual patient and what medication is recalcitrant.

Pathogenesis. The pathogenesis of alopecia areata is still incompletely understood and the evidence for AA being an autoimmune disease is still missing. The antigen targets have been hypothesized to be melanogenesis associated since melanogenesis is restricted to anagen hair bulbs and pigmented anagen hairs are more susceptible than grey hairs for AA [1].

Recent data suggest that triggering factors like viral infections, stress or vaccinations can induce in genetically predisposed patients a CD8+NKG2D+ T-cell-driven autoimmune disease. These T cells are thought to be a major agent responsible for disease initiation. IFN-γ released by T lymphocytes is responsible for the collapse of immune privilege of the hair follicle, inducing further production of interleukin (IL)-15 with subsequent attack of the hair follicle by cytotoxic cells which then results in acute hair loss [16,17].

Disease activation by loss of immune privilege

The loss of immune privilege in the hair follicle of AA patients as the key driver is now widely accepted [1]. While almost all nucleated cells of the body express MHC class I molecules in order to be recognized by NK cells, the hair follicles express only very low MHC I and no MHC class II molecules in the lower portion of anagen hair follicles. Potent immunosuppressants such as transforming growth factor β1 (TGF-β1), insulin-like growth factor 1 (IGF-1) and melanocyte-stimulating hormone α (α-MSH) build an immunoinhibitory milieu and prevent the presentation of autoantigens to NK cells (CD56+/NKG2D+) followed by destruction of the hair follicle [1]. The immune privilege is present during anagen but lost during catagen and telogen. So far, the immune privilege collapse is believed to occur only in immunogenetically predisposed individuals. IFN-γ has been shown in several studies to be the main contributor to immune privilege collapse by upregulating MHC I molecules [1,3,17]. Inhibitors of downstream signalling JAK/STAT kinases have been shown in initial studies to be effective in the treatment of AA patients [18].

However, recently AA lesions have been induced in healthy human scalp skin xenotransplants onto SCID mice while antigen-specific autoimmune attack of autoreactive T cells and a genetic predisposition were missing [19]. These results suggest that AA lesions could be a stereotypical response pattern that any anagen hair follicle will show whenever hair follicle immune privilege collapses and excessive IFN-γ signalling causes cytotoxic hair follicle damage [1,17] and this could happen without a genetic predisposition.

Regardless of these findings, the following events have to coincide to induce hair loss in AA [20].

- Occurrence of a perifollicular inflammation around the anagen hair bulb.
- Induction of hair follicle dystrophy, which leads to hair shaft shedding and production of dysfunctional hair shafts.
- Hair bulb immune privilege collapse by recognition of autoantigens within anagen hair follicles by CD8+ T cells and migration to and infiltration of hair follicles.

Clinical features. Alopecia areata shows a variety of clinical pattern. The most common is the sudden appearance of isolated,well-demarcated bald patches on the scalp that are asymptomatic, aside from occasional itching of the scalp and without any apparent clinical signs of inflammation. The anagen hair follicles undergo an abrupt conversion into telogen hair follicles [11,14]. Within the lesions are so-called exclamation mark hairs and black dots characteristic for AA. Exclamation mark hairs are short hairs with a dark expanded tip and black dots are hairs that are broken immediately after they have reached the skin surface. They are characteristic but not always present in AA. The patches can occur at any hair-bearing site of the body including eyelashes and eyebrows, but the scalp is the most frequently affected site (>90%) (Fig. 160.1) [11]. The patches can expand and affect the whole scalp (alopecia areata totalis, AAT) or involve also the body hair. Then, it is called alopecia areata universalis (AAU). The ophiasis type is a clinically differentiated type of AA, where hair loss extends along the posterior occipital and temporal scalp region and has a rather unfavourable prognosis. Some refer to the inverse form of

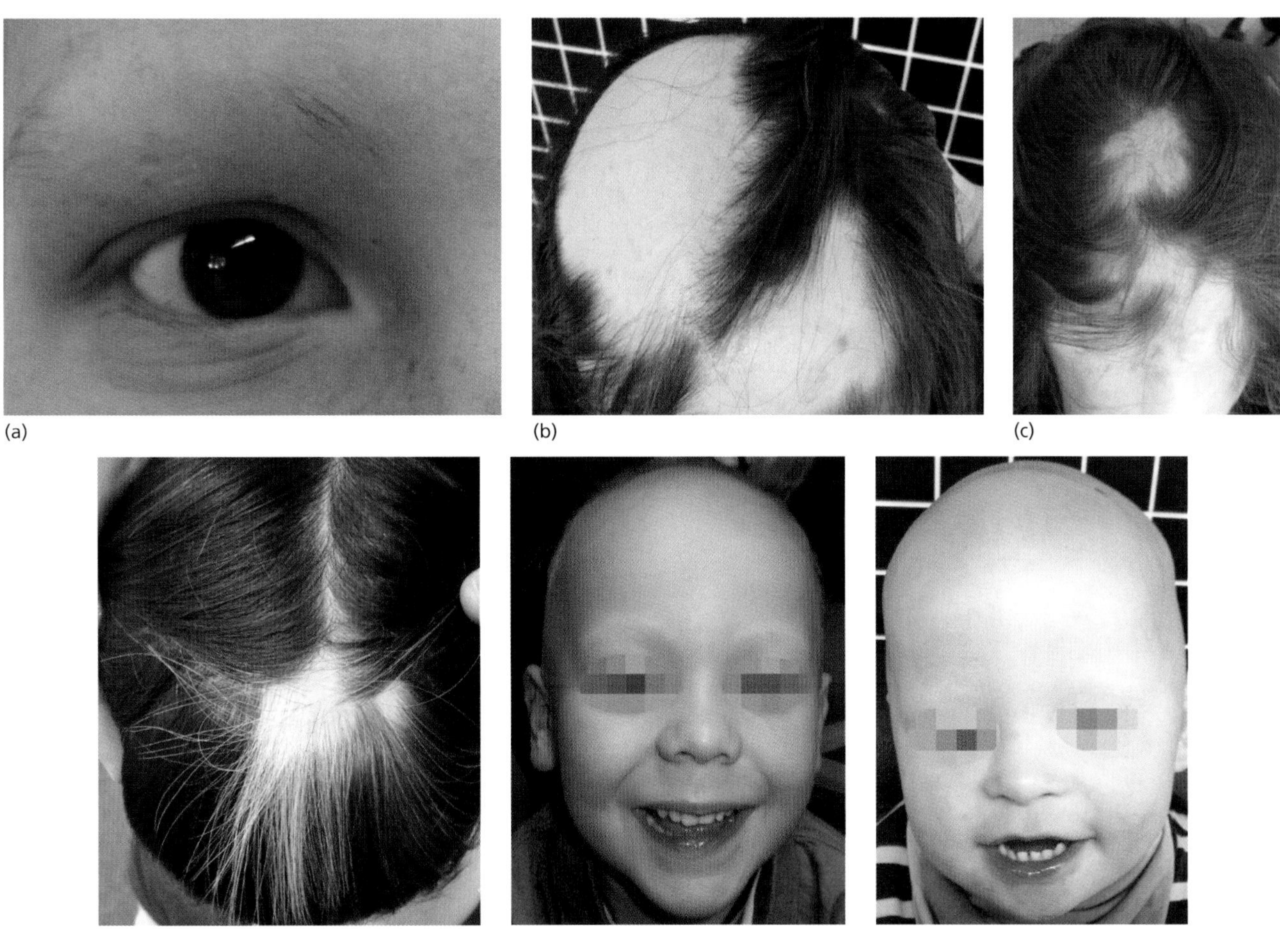

Fig. 160.1 (a) Alopecia areata (AA) of eyebrow and eyelashes. (b) Extensive AA circumscripta. (c) AA occipital. (d) AA with grey regrowing hairs. (e) AA totalis. (f) AA universalis in a patient with Down syndrome.

ophiasis as 'sisaihpo' (by reversing the letters of ophiasis). In rare cases, AA can look like telogen effluvium with diffuse thinning of the hair.

The regrowing hairs are often white at first and get darker with time. Obviously, melanocytes are affected by the inflammation and need time to recover. This is in line with the observation that pigmented hairs are more susceptible targets than white hairs. The reported overnight greying of hair in adults is the result of acute diffuse AA, which affects only pigmented hair while the white hairs are spared. This clinical and histological finding supports the hypothesis of melanocyte- and anagen-associated autoantigens as key players in the pathogenesis of AA [21]. However, because nonpigmented hair loss in AA is also reported, pigmented hair seems to be more susceptible but not exclusively affected.

Nail involvement is another feature of AA. Typical signs for AA are small pits, leuconychia punctata and vertical or longitudinal ridging. In severe forms, all 20 nails can be dystrophic. Nail involvement can precede or follow AA and often occurs in more widespread and recurring forms of AA.

The course of AA is unpredictable. Acute hair loss is often followed by spontaneous hair regrowth. As soon as one patch is gone, another can appear. The hair loss can persist for many years or for life. Alopecia areata is not scarring, hair follicles are usually preserved and hair can regrow even after many years. The prognosis depends on several factors (Box 160.1). Unfavourable prognostic factors include early onset of disease, positive family history, atopic dermatitis and extensive trachyonychia.

Box 160.1 Prognostic features for alopecia areata

- Positive family history
- First onset before puberty
- Atopic dermatitis
- Nail signs
- Long disease duration
- Ophiasis type
- Extent of hair loss
- Down syndrome
- HLA haplotype

Histological features. The typical characteristics of early AA are an increased number of catagen and telogen hair follicles. Around the lower hair follicle (peribulbar), an inflammatory lymphocytic infiltrate can be seen, which appears like a 'swarm of bees'. CD4+ T cells predominate in the infiltrate around the hair bulb, while CD8+ T cells reside within the hair follicles. The bulge region containing the hair follicle stem cells in the upper region of the hair follicle is spared. This is the reason why AA is not scarring, and hair follicles can potentially regrow even years later.

The infiltrate is mostly seen in terminal hair follicles reaching deep into the subcutaneous tissue. Affected anagen hair follicles rapidly enter telogen phase, the reason for sudden hair shedding. Afterwards, follicles reenter the next hair cycle but the lymphocytic infiltrate, which is still present, interrupts the anagen phase. Particularly in repeated episodes of AA, miniaturization of the hair follicle occurs [22]. In long-standing AA, the lymphocytic infiltrate can be variable and mostly miniaturized hair follicles are seen.

Differential diagnosis. In children, the most common differential diagnosis is tinea capitis, which often appears as isolated patchy hair loss of the scalp but here the skin typically shows scalding and signs of inflammation in contrast to AA. Also important to keep in mind is trichotillomania in children. Trichotillomania is the mechanical pulling of hair shafts, which can be a habituation or a sign of psychosomatic disorder. In trichotillomania, very short regrowing hair within the lesion can often be observed yielding a pattern in which hairs of multiple different lengths are seen and unusual or bizarre patterns that do not correlate with underlying anatomical or mosaic configurations. Traction alopecia is another differential diagnosis. Some types of hair styling using great pressure can be the reason for permanent patchy hair loss.

Associations

Alopecia areata is associated with autoimmune diseases such as Hashimoto thyroiditis, diabetes mellitus, rheumatoid arthritis, pernicious anaemia, lupus erythematosus, myasthenia gravis, lichen planus, coeliac disease and vitiligo. The prevalence of an autoimmune disease in patients with AA is 16%. Thyroid disease and vitiligo have the strongest relationship to AA. Atopic diseases such as asthma, atopic dermatitis and hay fever have been reported in 10–60% of patients [23,24]. A strong association with AA has also been observed in patients with Down syndrome (10%).

Treatment. The treatment of AA is still a therapeutic challenge and often frustrating, in small children even more than in adults. Immunosuppressive or immunomodulating agents have been used and are variably and at best temporarily effective in the treatment of AA, but there are still no definitive options to cure the disease or prevent relapses. Because of the high rate of spontaneous remission (34–50%) within one year, it is quite difficult to attribute successful regrowth to a particular treatment. In addition, there is an urgent need for double-blind placebo-controlled studies enrolling patients with extensive AA, AAT and AAU. In view of the high psychosocial impact of a stigmatizing disease in early childhood, psychological support is mandatory to help the child and family to cope with a disease which at present must be considered untreatable.

Table 160.1 Treatment options for alopecia areata in children

Age	Treatment
Children <10 years of age	Anthralin Topical corticosteroids Systemic steroids*
Children >10 years of age	Topical sensitizer Ultrapotent topical corticosteroids Intralesional cortiosteroids Anthralin Systemic steroids Ultraviolet light phototherapy (UVB) Low-dose methotrexate

*Only in rare cases with rapid recent onset of hair loss; only three courses.

Table 160.2 Treatments without efficacy

Treatment	Reference
Tacrolimus	[49]
Efalizumab	[58]
TNF-α blockers	[59]
Local latanoprost	[60]
5-Fluorouracil	[61]

In general, it is reasonable to choose the treatment depending on the extent and duration of alopecia and age of the child. While limited lesions of AA do not necessarily need therapy, they respond favourably to a variety of treatments; long-standing AAT and AAU as well as association with atopy, early onset and nail symptoms are less responsive and difficult to treat (Table 160.1). Corticosteroids exert a potent antiinflammatory effect and several ways of administration have been used: intralesional, topical and systemic. Therapeutic agents that have been shown to be ineffective in the treatment of AA are listed in Table 160.2.

Topical corticosteroids

Intralesional corticosteroids (e.g. triamcinolone acetonide) have been used for treatment of AA for the past five decades in adults and several studies have reported successful regrowth at the site of injection although placebo-controlled studies are lacking. In children, intralesional corticosteroid injection into the scalp has been described [25]. Eighty percent of children treated with intralesional corticosteroids in limited AA showed an improvement of >50%. However, skin atrophy is a possible side-effect, and intralesional injection is painful and therefore not generally suitable for children under the age of 12 years, particularly in view of the lack of a sustained response. Many studies reporting success with corticosteroids or other antiinflammatory agents either lacked a control group or did not report results of long-term follow-up.

Topically applied corticosteroids are very popular in the treatment of limited AA but there are only two placebo-controlled studies using 0.05% clobetasol ointment with or without occlusion in adults. In multifocal AA, 0.05% clobetasol foam was effective in 30%, while AAT and AAU did not respond. Using occlusion, 17% of patients with AAU and AAT responded to the treatment [26,27]. Another group compared the effect of clobetasol 0.05% with hydrocortisone 1.0% in 42 children with limited AA and showed a significant decrease in hair loss in the clobetasol group without any side-effects over a period of 24 weeks [28] Considering the difficulty of treating AAU and AAT at all, this is a good result. Another study reported that betamethasone valerate foam was an effective and well-tolerated treatment of mild-to-moderate AA [29]. In children, the risk of skin atrophy is higher than in adults and continuous uninterrupted treatment with a class IV corticosteroid for six months cannot be recommended. Therefore, further placebo-controlled studies with class II and III corticosteroids are needed.

Systemic corticosteroids

Treatment of AA with systemic corticosteroids has been known since 1952 [30]. Experience documented that daily administration of high-dose corticosteroids for several months resulted in multiple side-effects such as hypertension, diabetes, immunosuppression and osteoporosis. Therefore, different regimens involving pulse therapies were started in the 1970s in order to reduce potential side-effects. Corticosteroids were either administered intravenously or orally once a month for at least three courses. None of the studies were controlled and most of the patients who responded to therapy had patchy AA.

Only a very few studies exist investigating the effects of pulse therapy in children. Sharma and Muralidhar [31] studied 16 patients up to 18 years of age with widespread AA. Patients aged 12–18 years received 300 mg prednisolone in a monthly oral pulse; those aged 3–11 years received betamethasone sodium phosphate as soluble tablets or syrup equivalent to prednisolone 5 mg/kg bodyweight every month. The pulsed doses of corticosteroid were continued for a minimum of three doses or until cosmetically acceptable hair growth was obtained. Excellent hair growth was obtained in 9 (60%) of 15 patients evaluated at six months. Four patients out of 13 (>12 months follow-up) developed a localized relapse during mean follow-up of 16.4 and 33.7 months. Side-effects of pulsed corticosteroid were minimal and were recorded in two patients (one with transient giddiness and headache and one with epigastric burning). Kiesch et al. [32] treated seven children with severe, rapidly evolving AA with pulse steroid therapy. Alopecia areata had been present for 3–44 weeks and involved more than 30% of the scalp. One patient had AAT. Intravenous methylprednisolone (5 mg/kg twice a day) was administered for three days. No serious side-effects were noted. At 12-month follow-up, complete regrowth had occurred in five patients (71%). The patient with AAT had no regrowth.

Assouly et al. [33] enrolled 66 patients aged between 9 and 60 years with extensive AA. The administered treatment was methylprednisolone 500 mg/day for three days or 5 mg/kg twice per day for three days in children. These pulses were repeated after four and eight weeks. Ophiasic alopecia areata did not respond to treatment. One quarter of patients presenting with AAU had a good response (>80%) followed by a relapse in half the cases. Half of the patients presenting with AAT had a good response. Alopecia areata presented a good response in 63.8% (78% when it was a first episode and 90.5% if the treatment had been started less than three months before). The repetition of the pulses did not appear to increase the number of responders.

In conclusion, high-dose pulse therapy can be effective in extensive AA with rapid recent onset and did not show any serious side-effects in the patients reported in the studies reviewed. However, Smith et al. investigated whether methyprednisolone pulse therapy in 18 children with severe AA and with a short disease duration might show a benefit for the disease course. They confirmed the positive effect of hair regrowth in 75% after four months of treatment but observed a relapse in most patients after eight months [34]. Another group treated 65 children with AA more than 30% with oral dexamethasone (prednisolone 5 mg/kg equivalent) given once in four weeks. Patients received six, nine or 12 pulses. Clobetasol propionate 0.05% ointment under plastic wrap occlusion was applied six days a week. Six to twelve months after the therapy, 56.9% of patients had >75% hair regrowth [35].

Systemic corticosteroids are effective but have diverse side-effects and discontinuation of therapy often results in disease relapse. They could be important in the initial phase of treatment or at low dose in combination with other therapies.

Topical immunotherapy

Topical immunotherapy induces allergic contact eczema after application of contact allergens to the affected skin. The exact mechanism as to how contact sensitizers induce hair regrowth in AA remains unclear. The perifollicular lymphocytic infiltrate within the lesions is altered. While IFN-γ is reduced, IL-10 is increased after treatment with contact sensitizers. In addition, expression of MHC classes I and II is significantly downregulated in the hair follicle epithelium. These findings indicate that contact sensitizers might be able to restore the immune privilege of the hair follicle [14].

Topical sensitizers include squaric acid dibutyl ester (SADBE) and diphenylcyclopropenone (DPCP). Patients are first sensitized with a 2% solution on a small area of the scalp. Two weeks later, weekly half-headed treatments are started with increasing concentrations. The treatment is continued for several months until regrowth can be observed. Initial hair regrowth is usually seen after 8–12 weeks. Less serious side-effects include mild eczema and mild enlargement of retroauricular lymph nodes. More serious side-effects include vesicular or bullous reactions, dissemination of the allergic contact eczema, urticaria and erytheme multiforme-like reactions.

Contact sensitizers in the treatment of AA have been moderately effective in various studies. Cosmetically acceptable hair growth was observed in 30–70% of treated patients in different studies [36]. Relapse occurs in 50% of patients after cessation of therapy [36]. Studies involving children have been limited [37,38]. Schuttelaar et al. [37] observed cosmetically acceptable hair regrowth in 32% of 26 treated children. Cosmetically acceptable regrowth at the end of the study was seen in four of the 15 (27%) children with AAT and four of the 10 (40%) children with AA. In another study, 28 patients between 10 and 35 years of age with extensive AA were treated with DPCP for six months. Complete remission (90–100% terminal hair regrowth) was obtained in 22.2% (6/27) and partial remission (10–90% terminal hair regrowth) in 59.3% (16/27). Partial recurrence was observed in 50.9% (13/22) of these patients after 6–12 months of follow-up [39]. Tan et al. [25] treated 58 children between 6 and 15 years with SADBE. After six months, 74% achieved more than 50% hair regrowth. Side-effects in these young children included itchy dermatitis, blisters and lymphadenopathy.

Chiang et al. investigated how long DCP therapy should last. The median duration of DPCP treatment in their study was three years, with 47% patients experiencing their first regrowth in the first six months of DPCP therapy, 20% between six months and one year, and 8% at 1–2 years. More than 50% terminal hair regrowth was reached in 71% of alopecia totalis patients and 56% of alopecia universalis patients. Relapse was observed in 44% of patients. The authors suggest a duration of DPCP therapy for two years [40,41].

Kuin et al. reviewed 11 studies containing 500 patients, looking at quality of life and patient satisfaction. In half of the patients, DPCP appeared to be effective, with transient side-effects such as contact eczema, blistering, oedema of eyelids, headache and flu-like symptoms. If treatment was satisfactory, the effect was maintained for more than a year. Taken together, the authors found very low-quality evidence for the effectiveness of DCP treatment [42].

In general, the protocols are prepared for adults and children older than 10 years with 50% or more hair loss [42]. In addition, it should be noted that DPCP and SADBE represent off-label uses of these medications.

Anthralin

Anthralin is a topical irritant often used in the treatment of AA. So far, no placebo-controlled double-blind studies exist for the treatment of AA in children. In one study, 30 children with chronic, severe, treatment-refractory, extensive AA were treated with 1% anthralin ointment on one side of the scalp for 12 months. The mean time to first response in terms of new hair growth was three months and the mean time to maximal response was nine months. In the first 12-month period, 10 patients (33.4%) achieved complete response to treatment and 11 patients (36.6%) had a partial response. Of the 11 patients with partial response at the end of the first year, six achieved a complete response before the end of the study [43].

The effects of anthralin on hair growth have been studied in balding C3H/HeJ mice affected by an AA-like disease. Affected C3H/HeJ mice were treated daily for 10 weeks on half of the dorsal skin with 0.2% anthralin and the contralateral side was treated with the vehicle ointment. Hair regrowth was observed in 9/14 mice on the treated sides. Four mice displayed near complete replacement. Expression of TNF-α and TNF-β was inhibited by anthralin upon successful treatment [44]. Side-effects were pruritus, skin irritation, scaling and pigmentation.

For children under the age of 10 years, anthralin is a therapeutic option, but placebo-controlled studies are needed to further document safety and efficacy.

Minoxidil

Minoxidil is known for its potent hair growth-stimulating effect in androgenetic alopecia. Its effect in AA is very controversial. Several authors describe positive effects of topical 3% minoxidil solution in the treatment of AA. In a placebo-controlled study by Price et al. [45,46], 90 patients aged 7–63 years with extensive AA affecting 25–100% of the scalp were treated with minoxidil 3% for an entire year. Minoxidil-treated patients responded better than placebo-treated patients. The treatment was well tolerated and no blood pressure changes occurred [45,46]. However, in all placebo-controlled studies the effect of minoxodil was not significant compared with the placebo within the first three months of treatment [47,48]. Therefore, minoxidil cannot be routinely recommended for the treatment of AA in children.

Tacrolimus

Tacrolimus is a topical calcineurin inhibitor which has been shown to be ineffective in AA. In one study, none of the patients with AA affecting 10–75% of the scalp had terminal hair growth in response to tacrolimus ointment 0.1% applied twice daily for 24 weeks. Treatment failure may reflect insufficient depth of penetration of the ointment formulation and less than optimal patient selection [49].

Psoralen plus ultraviolet A

Several studies have been performed on the use of psoralen plus ultraviolet A (PUVA) in AA, with successful regrowth in 53–85% of treated patients in different studies. Besides the lack of controls in these studies and the recurrence of hair loss without continuous therapy, there is an increased risk of skin cancer that has been well documented in those receiving PUVA therapy. PUVA is therefore not a recommended treatment option in children.

Experience with UVB phototherapy has been more limited; some early data suggest some efficacy in a subset of patients who received UVB phototherapy in the form of narrow-band ultraviolet light laser therapy (308 or 311 nm) [50].

Methotrexate

Several studies in adults and children have been published showing a positive effect of systemic methotrexate on patients with recalcitrant alopecia areata [51]. Fourteen children (eight girls and six boys) aged between 8 and 18 years (mean 14.7) with AA present for a mean duration of 5.7 years were treated once weekly for 14.2 months. Thirteen children were assessable. In five out of 13 children, methotrexate treatment produced regrowth >50% of hair while the remaining eight children were treatment failures. No serious side-effects were reported. Thus, methotrexate can be considered as a treatment option in recalcitrant alopecia when other alternatives are missing [52]. However, the results of this study must be interpreted with caution since long-term follow-up results and outcome in an appropriate control group were not reported.

Hair prostheses

Some children do well with active nonintervention and can be fitted for social reasons with hairpieces. Organizations such as the Locks of Love in the USA can provide anatomically fitted hairpieces (prostheses) which can be provided at discounted rates based on financial need.

Outlook on future treatment options. Genetic association studies and several AA mouse models have revealed new insights into the pathogenesis of AA and downstream pathways of involved cells and cytokine receptors such as JAK/STAT kinases. This has created the possibility of new targeted therapeutic agents, some of which have already shown promising results in small studies.

JAK kinase inhibitors

An important therapeutic insight was the discovery that inhibition of JAK/STAT kinases could reverse AA in mice [16]. Three different JAK kinase inhibitors exist: ruxolitinib (JAK 1 and 2 inhibitor), the pan-JAK inhibitor tofacitinib and and the JAK 1 and 2 inhibitor bariticinib [3]. While oral treatment with ruxolitinib for three months results in 75% hair regrowth in treated patients [53], tofacitinib was also effective in two studies but to a lesser extent [54,55]. Discontinuation of therapy leads to relapse of hair loss in both studies. Therefore, larger placebo-controlled studies are needed to assess the efficacy and safety of these promising new drugs.

Antibodies and biologics

Phosphodiesterase inhibitor 4 (PDE4, apremilast) is known to decrease inflammatory cytokines such as IL-23 and IFN-γ. PDE4 successfully treated extensive AA in a small three-patient trial. [55]. Ongoing studies with abatacept, a CTLA4-Ig fusion protein which has been shown to prevent induction of AA in mouse models, IL-15 antibodies and IL-17, IL-23 antibodies (ustekinumab and secukinumab) are observed with interest. All of them influence downstream pathways of immune cells in the inflammatory infiltrate around the AA hair follicle bulb. Preliminary studies in mouse models and treatment of other diseases like psoriasis have shown positive effects in AA [3,56,57].

Cytokines that restore the immune privilege of the hair follicle such as α-MSH and IL-10 could also be interesting candidates for future treatment regimens by downregulation of MHC I molecules [1]. Also studies with platelet-rich plasma therapy in AA patients showed a benefit and need to be further elucidated.

Conclusion. Taken together, the therapeutic options for children with AA are still very limited and cure of the disease and relapse prevention are not currently available. Treatment options and side-effects have to be individually balanced depending on age, duration of the disease and extent of hair loss, but new molecular targeted therapeutic options are expected to be available in the near future. The psychological impact of the disease in young patients is often very high, and patients should be informed about support groups such as the National Alopecia Areata Foundation, the Child Alopecia Project and Locks of Love.

References

1 **Paus R, Bulfone-Paus S, Bertolini M. Hair Follicle Immune Privilege Revisited: The Key To Alopecia Areata Management. J Investig Dermatol Symp Proc 2018;19(1):S12–S17.**

2 **Jabbari A, Cerise JE, Chen JC et al. Molecular signatures define alopecia areata subtypes and transcriptional biomarkers. EBioMedicine 2016;7:240–7.**

3 **Pratt CH, King LE Jr, Messenger AG et al. Alopecia areata. Nat Rev Dis Primers 2017;3:17011.**

4 Dudda-Subramanya R, Alexis AF, Siu K, Sinha AA. Alopecia areata: genetic complexity underlies clinical heterogeneity. Eur J Dermatol 2007;17:367–74.

5 Villasante Fricke AC, Miteva M. Epidemiology and burden of alopecia areata: a systematic review. Clin Cosmet Invest Dermatol 2015; 8:397–403.

6 Kakourou T, Karachristou K, Chrousos G. A case series of alopecia areata in children: impact of personal and family history of stress and autoimmunity. J Eur Acad Dermatol Venereol 2007;21:356–9.

7 Barahmani N, Schabath MB, Duvic M, National Alopecia Areata Registry. History of atopy or autoimmunity increases risk of alopecia areata. J Am Acad Dermatol 2009;61:581–91.

8 Jackow C, Puffer N, Hordinsky M et al. Alopecia areata and cytomegalovirus infection in twins: genes versus environment? J Am Acad Dermatol 1998;38:418–25.

9 Blaumeiser B, van der Goot I, Fimmers R et al. Familial aggregation of alopecia areata. J Am Acad Dermatol 2006;54:627–32.

10 Martinez-Mir A, Zlotogorski A, Gordon D et al. Genomewide scan for linkage reveals evidence of several susceptibility loci for alopecia areata. Am J Hum Genet 2007;80:316–28.

11 Gilhar A, Paus R, Kalish RS. Lymphocytes, neuropeptides, and genes involved in alopecia areata. J Clin Invest 2007;117:2019–27.

12 Duvic M, Hordinsky MK, Fiedler VC et al. HLA-D locus associations in alopecia areata: DRw52a may confer disease resistance. Arch Dermatol 1991;27:64–8.

13 Barahmani N, de Andrade M, Slusser JP et al. Major histocompatibility complex class I chain-related gene A polymorphisms and extended haplotypes are associated with familial alopecia areata. J Invest Dermatol 2006;126:74–8.

14 Wasserman D, Guzman-Sanchez DA, Scott K, McMichael A. Alopecia areata. Int J Dermatol 2007;46:121–31.

15 Betz RC, Petukhova L, Ripke S. Genome-wide meta-analysis in alopecia areata resolves HLA associations and reveals two new susceptibility loci. Nat Commun 2015;6:5966.

16 Xing L, Dai Z, Jabbari A et al. Alopecia areata is driven by cytotoxic T lymphocytes and is reversed by JAK inhibition. Nat Med 2014;20: 1043–9.

17 McElwee K, Gilhar A, Tobin D et al. What causes alopecia areata? Exp Dermatol 2013;22:609–26.

18 Jabbari A, Dai Z, Xing L et al. Reversal of alopecia areata following treatment with the JAK1/2 inhibitor baricitinib. EBioMedicine 2015;2: 351–5.

19 Gilhar A, Schrum AG, Etzioni A et al. Alopecia areata: animal models illuminate autoimmune pathogenesis and novel immunotherapeutic strategies. Autoimmun Rev 2016;15:726–35.

20 **Gilhar A, Etzioni A, Paus R. Alopecia areata. N Engl J Med 2012; 366:1515–25.**

21 Paus R, Nickoloff BJ, Ito T. A 'hairy' privilege. Trends Immunol 2005;26:32–40.

22 Whiting DA. Histopathologic features of alopecia areata: a new look. Arch Dermatol 2003;139:1555–9.

23 Barahmani N, Schabath MB, Duvic M, National Alopecia Areata Registry. History of atopy or autoimmunity increases risk of alopecia areata. J Am Acad Dermatol 2009;61:581–91.

24 Goh C, Finkel M, Christos PJ, Sinha AA. Profile of 513 patients with alopecia areata: associations of disease subtypes with atopy, autoimmune disease and positive family history. J Eur Acad Dermatol Venereol 2006;20:1055–60.
25 Tan E, Tay YK, Goh CL, Chin Giam Y. The pattern and profile of alopecia areata in Singapore: a study of 219 Asians. Int J Dermatol 2002;41:748–53.
26 Tosti A, Iorizzo M, Botta GL, Milani M. Efficacy and safety of a new clobetasol propionate 0.05% foam in alopecia areata: a randomized, double-blind placebo-controlled trial. J Eur Acad Dermatol Venereol 2006;20:1243–7.
27 Tosti A, Piraccini BM, Pazzaglia M, Vincenzi C. Clobetasol propionate 0.05% under occlusion in the treatment of alopecia totalis/universalis. J Am Acad Dermatol 2003;49:96.
28 Lenane P, Macarthur C, Parkin PC et al. Clobetasol propionate, 0.05%, vs hydrocortisone, 1%, for alopecia areata in children: a randomized clinical trial. JAMA Dermatol 2014;150:47–50.
29 Mancuso G, Balducci A, Casadio C et al. Efficacy of betamethasone valerate foam formulation in comparison with betamethasone dipropionate lotion in the treatment of mild-to-moderate alopecia areata: a multicenter, prospective, randomized, controlled, investigatorblinded trial. Int J Dermatol 2003;42:572–5.
30 Dillaha CJ, Rothman S. Therapeutic experiments in alopecia areata with orally administered cortisone. J Am Med Assoc 1952;150:546–50.
31 Sharma VK, Muralidhar S. Treatment of widespread alopecia areata in young patients with monthly oral corticosteroid pulse. Pediatr Dermatol 1998;15:313–17.
32 Kiesch N, Stene JJ, Goens J et al. Pulse steroid therapy for children's severe alopecia areata? Dermatology 1997;194:395–7.
33 Assouly P, Reygagne P, Jouanique C et al. [Intravenous pulse methylprednisolone therapy for severe alopecia areata: an open study of 66 patients.] Ann Dermatol Venereol 2003;130:326–30.
34 Smith A, Trüeb RM, Theiler M et al. High relapse rates despite early intervention with intravenous methylprednisolone pulse therapy for severe childhood alopecia areata. Pediatr Dermatol 2015;32(4):481–7.
35 Lalosevic J, Gajic-Veljic M, Bonaci-Nikolic B, Nikolic M. Combined oral pulse and topical corticosteroid therapy for severe alopecia areata in children: a long-term follow-up study. Dermatol Ther 2015;28:309–17.
36 Happle R, Hausen BM, Wiesner-Menzel L. Diphencyprone in the treatment of alopecia areata. Acta Derm Venereol 1983;63:49–52.
37 Schuttelaar ML, Hamstra JJ, Plinck EP et al. Alopecia areata in children: treatment with diphencyprone. Br J Dermatol 1996;135: 581–5.
38 Weise K, Kretzschmar L, John SM, Hamm H. Topical immunotherapy in alopecia areata: anamnestic and clinical criteria of prognostic significance. Dermatology 1996;192:129–33.
39 Aghaei S. Topical immunotherapy of severe alopecia areata with diphenylcyclopropenone (DPCP): experience in an Iranian population. BMC Dermatol 2005;26:5–6.
40 Ross EK, Shapiro J. Management of hair loss. Dermatol Clin 2005;23: 227–43.
41 Chiang KS, Mesinkovska NA, Piliang MP, Bergfeld WF. Clinical efficacy of diphenylcyclopropenone in alopecia areata: retrospective data analysis of 50 patients. J Invest Dermatol Symp Proc 2015;17(2):50–5.
42 Kuin RA, Spuls PI, Limpens J, van Zuuren EJ. Diphenylcyclopropenone in patients with alopecia areata. A critically appraised topic. Br J Dermatol 2015;173(4):896–909.
43 Özdemir M, Balevi A. Bilateral half-head comparison of 1% anthralin ointment in children with alopecia areata. Pediatr Dermatol 2017; 34(2):128–32.
44 Tang L, Cao L, Sundberg JP, Lui H, Shapiro J. Restoration of hair growth in mice with an alopecia areata-like disease using topical anthralin. Exp Dermatol 2004;13:5–10.
45 Price VH. Topical minoxidil (3%) in extensive alopecia areata, including long-term efficacy. J Am Acad Dermatol 1987;16:737–44.
46 Price VH. Topical minoxidil in extensive alopecia areata, including 3-year follow-up. Dermatologica 1987;175(Suppl 2):36–41.
47 Fransway AF, Muller SA. 3 percent topical minoxidil compared with placebo for the treatment of chronic severe alopecia areata. Cutis 1988; 41:431–5.
48 Ranchoff RE, Bergfeld WF, Steck WD, Subichin SJ. Extensive alopecia areata: results of treatment with 3% topical minoxidil. Cleve Clin J Med 1989;56:149–54.
49 Price VH, Willey A, Chen BK. Topical tacrolimus in alopecia areata. J Am Acad Dermatol 2005;52:138–9.
50 Al-Mutairi N. 308-nm Excimer laser for the treatment of alopecia areata in children. Pediatr Dermatol 2009;26:547–50.
51 Lim SK, Lim CA, Kwon IS et al. Low-dose systemic methotrexate therapy for recalcitrant alopecia areata. Ann Dermatol 2017;29:263–7.
52 Royer M, Bodemer C, Vabres P et al. Efficacy and tolerability of methotrexate in severe childhood alopecia areata. Br J Dermatol 2011;165: 407–10.
53 Mackay-Wiggan J, Jabbari A, Nguyen N et al.Oral ruxolitinib induces hair regrowth in patients with moderate-to-severe alopecia areata. JCI Insight 2016;1:e89790.
54 Kennedy Crispin M, Ko JM, Craiglow BG et al. Safety and efficacy of the JAK inhibitor tofacitinib citrate in patients with alopecia areata. JCI Insight 2016;1:e89776.
55 Liu LY, Craiglow BG, Dai F, King BA. Tofacitinib for the treatment of severe alopecia areata and variants: a study of 90 patients. J Am Acad Dermatol 2017;76(1):22–8.
56 Guttman-Yassky E, Ungar B, Noda S et al. Extensive alopecia areata is reversed by IL-12/IL-23p40 cytokine antagonism. J Allergy Clin Immunol 2016;137(1):301–4.
57 Renert-Yuval Y, Guttman-Yassky E. The changing landscape of alopecia areata: the therapeutic paradigm.Adv Ther 2017;34(7):1594–609.
58 Price VH, Hordinsky MK, Olsen EA et al. Subcutaneous efalizumab is not effective in the treatment of alopecia areata. J Am Acad Dermatol 2008;58:395–402.
59 Abramovits W, Losornio M. Failure of two TNF-alpha blockers to influence the course of alopecia areata. Skinmed 2006;5:177–81.
60 Ochoa BE, Sah D, Wang G et al. Instilled bimatoprost ophthalmic solution in patients with eyelash alopecia areata. J Am Acad Dermatol 2009;61:530–2.
61 Kaplan AL, Olsen EA. Topical 5-fluorouracil is ineffective in the treatment of extensive alopecia areata. J Am Acad Dermatol 2004;50: 941–3.

CHAPTER 161

Nail Disorders

Antonella Tosti[1] *& Bianca Maria Piraccini*[2]

[1] Department of Dermatology and Cutaneous Surgery, Miller Medical School University of Miami, Miami, FL, USA
[2] Dermatology, Department of Experimental, Diagnostic and Specialty Medicine, University of Bologna, Bologna, Italy

Introduction, 2147
Nail anatomy and physiology, 2147
Common nail disorders, 2148
Uncommon nail disorders, 2153

Abstract

Although rare, nail diseases in children are a source of anxiety for patients and should be recognized and treated, if possible. They may be congenital and hereditary or may be acquired. In the first two cases, nail signs are present at birth or develop during neonatal life and may occasionally be a sign of a syndrome or a systemic disorder. Acquired nail dystrophies are typical of the age of 5–10 years and are commonly due to psoriasis or infective conditions. Nail tumours are rare.

Key points

- **Nail diseases in infants and children are uncommon.**
- **Congenital and hereditary nail disorders are present at birth or develop during neonatal life and may occasionally be a sign of a syndrome or a systemic disorder.**
- **Acquired nail dystrophies in children are usually due to inflammatory or infective diseases.**
- **Nail tumours are rare in children and malignant tumours exceptional.**
- **Treatment of nail disorders in children should consider age and severity of the condition.**

SECTION 34: HAIR, SCALP AND NAIL DISORDERS

Introduction

Nail diseases are a rather uncommon cause of dermatological consultation in children. They may be present at birth or be acquired. Nail signs of congenital and hereditary nail diseases usually develop early during childhood, and their presence may be a clue to the diagnosis of a syndrome or a systemic disorder. Although the acquired nail conditions observed in childhood are similar to those of adults, the prevalence of several diseases may vary in the different age groups [1]. For instance, there are some conditions, such as parakeratosis pustulosa and twenty-nail dystrophy (TND), which are exclusively or typically seen in children. Other disorders, such as onychomycosis, are encountered only exceptionally in the first 10 years of life. The common disorders and traumatic nail abnormalities account for 90–95% of all nail abnormalities in children.

This chapter reviews the nail disorders that are most commonly observed in childhood, and then reviews some nail diseases that, although uncommon, are of diagnostic significance.

Nail anatomy and physiology

The nail unit consists of four specialized epithelia: the nail matrix, the nail bed, the proximal nailfold and the hyponychium (Fig. 161.1). The nail matrix is a germinative epithelial structure that gives rise to a fully keratinized multilayered sheet of cornified cells: the nail plate. In longitudinal sections, the nail matrix consists of a proximal and a distal region. Because the vertical axes of the nail matrix cells are oriented diagonally and distally, proximal nail matrix keratinocytes produce the upper portion of the nail plate, whereas distal nail matrix keratinocytes produce the lower portion [2]. The peculiar kinetics of nail matrix keratinization explain why diseases of the proximal nail matrix result in nail plate surface abnormalities whereas diseases of the distal matrix result in abnormalities of the ventral nail plate or the nail free edge or both.

Nail plate corneocytes are tightly connected by desmosomes and complex digitations. The nail plate is a rectangular, translucent and transparent structure that appears pink because of the vessels of the underlying nail bed. The proximal part of the nail plate of the fingernails, especially those of the thumbs, shows a whitish, opaque, half-moon-shaped area, the lunula, that corresponds to the visible portion of the distal nail matrix. The shape of the lunula determines the shape of the free edge of the plate. The nail plate is firmly attached to the nail bed, which partially contributes to nail formation along its length. The longitudinal orientation of the capillary vessels in the nail bed explains the linear pattern of nail bed haemorrhages.

Proximally and laterally, the nail plate is surrounded by the nailfolds. The horny layer of the proximal nailfold forms

Harper's Textbook of Pediatric Dermatology, Fourth Edition. Edited by Peter Hoeger, Veronica Kinsler and Albert Yan.

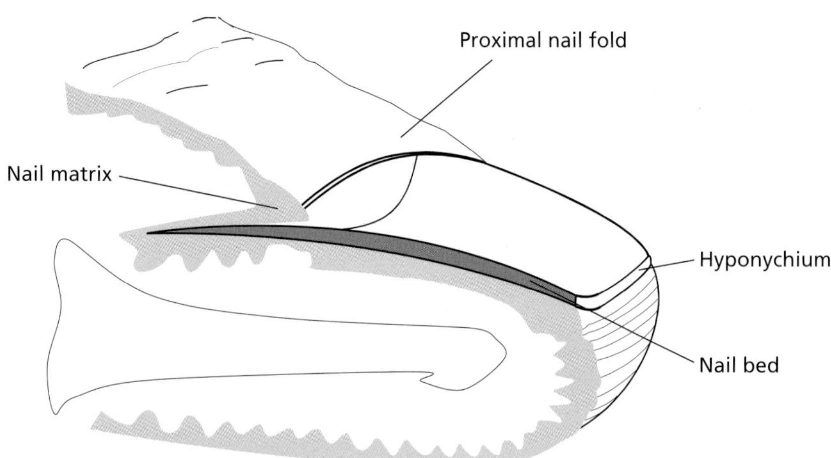

Fig. 161.1 Structure of the nail unit.

the cuticle, which adheres intimately to the underlying nail plate and prevents its separation from the proximal nailfold. Distally, the nail bed continues with the hyponychium, which marks the separation of the nail plate from the digit. The nail plate grows continuously and uniformly throughout life. Average nail growth is faster in fingernails (3mm per month) than in toenails (1–1.5mm per month).

The nails of newborns are thin and soft, and frequently present a certain degree of expected koilonychia that is especially evident in toenails. As the nail plate of the great toenail may be relatively short, a mild distal embedding is frequently observed as soon as the nail grows. This is transitory unless there is congenital malalignment. A transient light-brown or ochre pigmentation of the proximal nailfold is frequent in newborns and may persist for a few months [3,4].

Nail growth rate in children is similar to the values observed in young adults, the fastest values of nail growth (1.5mm per day) being reached between the ages of 10 and 14 years. The thickness and breadth of the nail plate increase rapidly in the first two decades of life [5]. The brief arrest of growth that characterizes the first days of life may involve the nail unit and result in a transitory arrest of the nail growth with development of Beau's lines, which become visible at the base of the nails after the age of about 4 weeks. These physiological lines, however, are an inconstant phenomenon that occurs in only about 20–25% of healthy newborns [6].

Common nail disorders

Transitory koilonychia

Key diagnostic criteria: thin, concave nails with everted edges

Key management features: no treatment necessary

Differentials: nail thinning due to trachyonychia

Transitory koilonychia is a physiological phenomenon of the toenails in children. The nail plate is flat, thin and soft with everted edges, resulting in a spoon-shaped appearance (Fig. 161.2). Lateral or distal embedding may occur and produce mild nail ingrowing. The condition spontaneously regresses when the nail plate thickens with age.

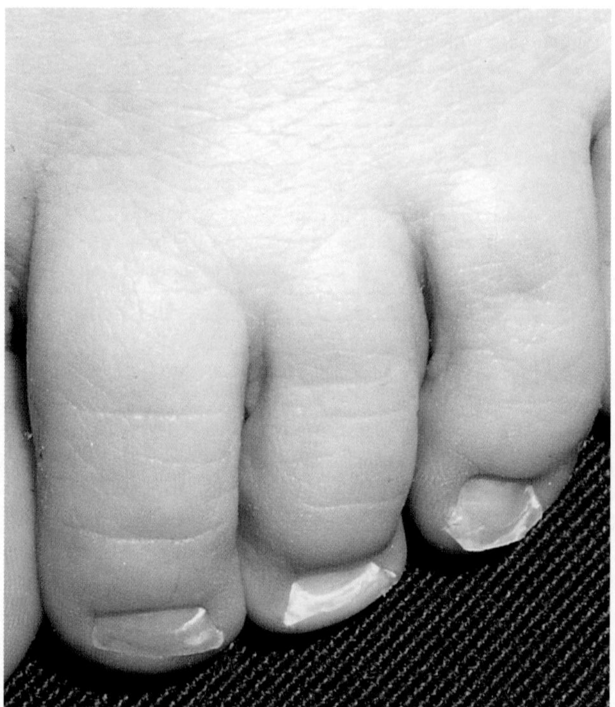

Fig. 161.2 Transitory koilonychia of the toenails in a young child. Thin and flat nail plates with everted edges, resulting in a spoon-shaped appearance.

Congenital malalignment of the big toenail

Key diagnostic criteria: the great toenail longitudinal axis is not parallel to that of the digit

Key management features: no treatment necessary except for surgery in very severe cases

Differentials: nail ingrowing

In congenital malalignment, the nail plate of the big toenail deviates laterally from the longitudinal axis of the distal phalanx [7,8]. The condition is always complicated by the development of lateral or distal nail embedding. The affected nail frequently shows dystrophic changes due to repetitive traumatic injuries: the nail plate may be thickened, yellow–brown in colour and present transverse ridging, Beau's lines and onychomadesis due to intermittent nail matrix damage (Fig. 161.3). Onycholysis

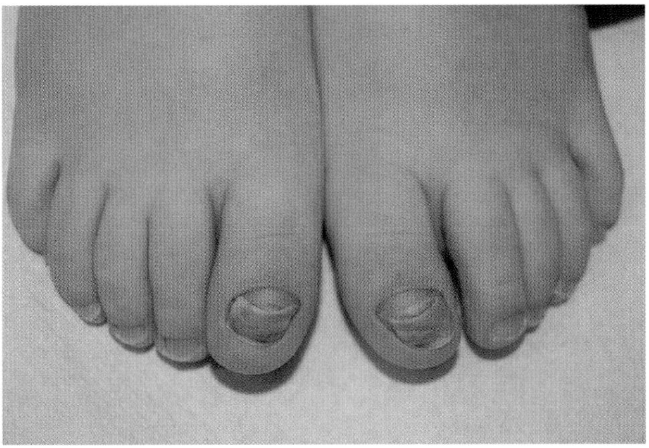

Fig. 161.3 Congenital malalignment of the toenails. The longitudinal axis of the toenails is deviated laterally and the nails are thickened, yellowish in colour with onychomadesis and onycholysis that follow trauma.

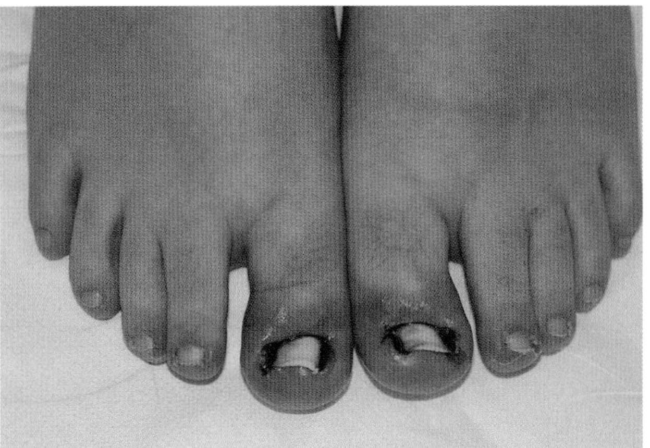

Fig. 161.4 Ingrown toenails. The lateral embedding of the nail plate induces marked inflammation of the lateral nailfolds with pyogenic granulomas. Note irregular distal edge of all toenails, indicating the child's habit of ripping them.

is frequent. This diagnosis should always be considered in children with dystrophic or ingrowing toenails.

Spontaneous improvement with complete resolution can occur. Surgical treatment produces the best results when performed before the age of 2 years [9].

Ingrown nails

Key diagnostic criteria: paronychia and pyogenic granuloma due to embedding of the nail edges into the lateral nailfold

Key management features: remove the spicula and treat the inflammation; lateral nail matrix phenolization

Differentials: nail pyogenic granulomas due to drugs or trauma

Ingrown nails are a common complaint and usually affect the great toe of teenagers and young adults. Predisposing factors include congenital malalignment of the great toenails and congenital hypertrophy of the lateral nailfolds. In the latter condition, the periungual soft tissues of the great toe are hypertrophic and partially cover the nail plate, favouring nail ingrowing [10]. The development of nail ingrowing is favoured by incorrect nail trimming, traumatic injuries and occlusive footwear. The clinical manifestations of ingrown toenails can be divided into three stages.

- *Stage 1.* Embedding of the nail spicula within the lateral nailfold produces painful erythema and swelling of the nailfold. Treatment is conservative with extraction of the embedded spicula and introduction of a package of nonabsorbent cotton under the lateral corner of the nail. This package should be replaced every few days. Patient-controlled taping, which allows constant pulling down of the lateral and distal folds, allowing disembedding of the nail plate, can be an alternative [11]
- *Stage 2.* This stage is characterized by the formation of granulation tissue, which covers the nail plate. The affected nail is very painful and the nailfold presents a pyogenic granuloma with seropurulent exudation; hyperhidrosis is common (Fig. 161.4). In this stage, the topical application of high-potency steroids under occlusion for a few days can reduce the overgrowth of granulation tissue. Conservative treatment as for stage 1 can then be utilized.
- *Stage 3.* The granulation tissue becomes covered by newly formed epidermis of the lateral nailfold. This stage requires selective destruction of the lateral horn of the nail matrix using surgery or chemical destruction with phenol.

Newborns can develop multiple ingrown fingernails with paronychia as a result of the grasp reflex [12]. The pathogenesis of the condition is the repeated compression of the soft tissues of the lateral nailfold by the lateral edges of the nails during grasping. The condition regresses spontaneously when the grasp reflex disappears, at about 3 months of age.

Herringbone (chevron) nails

This is a very common finding in fingernails of young children. The nail plate surface presents longitudinal ridges that cross its surface diagonally from the lunula to the distal margin with a V-shaped pattern [13].

Acute paronychia

Key diagnostic criteria: acute painful periungual inflammation, often with pus discharge

Key management features: pus drainage, topical antibiotics

Differentials: pustular psoriasis, herpes simplex infection

Acute paronychia is usually caused by *Staphylococcus aureus*, although other bacteria and herpes simplex virus may be responsible. A minor trauma commonly precedes the development of the infection. It is very common in children's fingernails, since the habit of biting the cuticle and finger sucking induces trauma and maceration of periungual skin. The affected digit shows acute inflammatory changes of the nailfolds, with erythema and swelling, more marked on one side, associated with pain, occasionally associated with abscess formation. Whenever possible, appropriate cultures should be taken to identify the responsible organism. Cytological examination with Tzanck smear is useful to exclude herpes and other causes of paronychia [14].

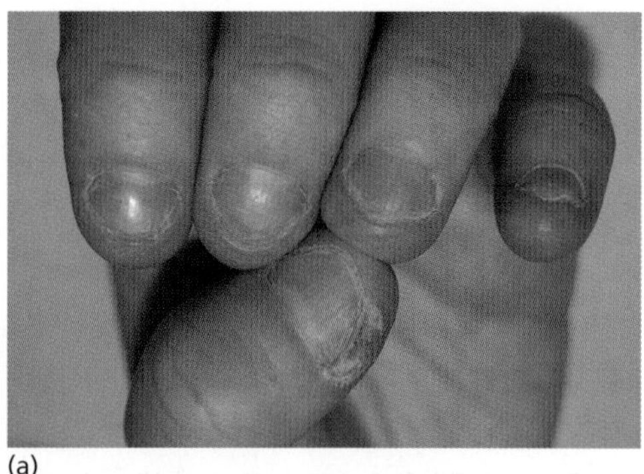
(a)

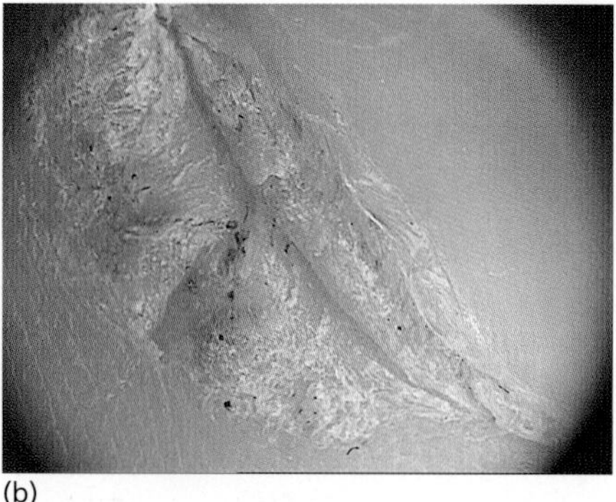
(b)

Fig. 161.5 Periungual wart of the first fingernail. Warty hyperkeratosis of the lateral nailfold (a). Dermoscopy shows irregular surface of a thickened epithelium with pointed haemorrhages (b). Note short nail plates due to nail biting, which favours transmission of warts from nail to nail.

Treatment includes prompt incision and drainage of the abscess [15], local medications with antiseptics and administration of systemic antibiotics or aciclovir, depending on the causative agent.

Warts

Key diagnostic criteria: warty papules of the nail folds or hyponychium
Key management features: topical keratolytics
Differentials: skin xerosis, subungual exostosis
Periungual and subungual warts are very common in children. Warts of this type often affect more than one digit and frequently recur. Nail biting facilitates the spread of periungual warts to several digits. Periungual warts may have the typical 'warty' exophytic appearance, or may present as a hyperkeratotic lesion of the nail folds (Fig. 161.5a). Dermoscopy can be very useful for diagnosis of very small warts, as it shows the irregular surface with pointed haemorrhages (Fig. 161.5b) [16]. Large subungual warts may cause lifting of the nail plate and result in pain.

In young children, surgical procedures should be avoided and treatment should be as conservative as possible, also because regression of warts is reported to occur in about 30% of cases [17]. Topical solutions containing salicylic and lactic acids are the treatment of choice. Topical immunotherapy with strong sensitizers (squaric acid dibutylester (SADBE) or diphenylcyclopropenone (DPCP)) is an effective and painless modality of treatment for multiple recalcitrant warts [18]. Intralesional bleomycin can be considered in recalcitrant cases. Similar to warts in other body sites, periungual warts may recur after cure.

Nail biting and onychotillomania

Key diagnostic criteria: paronychia with peeling scales and blood crusts, short irregular nails
Key management features: topical unpleasant-tasting preparations, *N*-acetylcysteine
Differentials: paronychia due to other causes
Nail biting is very common in childhood, especially after the age of 3–4 years, with a 25% prevalence at the age of 6 years. It occurs as a result of boredom or working on difficult problems rather than anxiety. Conversely, onychotillomania is rather uncommon in childhood and is usually associated with underlying psychological disorders. Nail biting produces short and irregular nails that show depressions and scratches and distal splitting (Fig 161.6; see also Fig. 161.5a). The habit of picking, breaking or chewing the skin over the proximal nailfold produces paronychia and nail matrix injury with nail plate surface abnormalities and melanonychia. Secondary bacterial infections of the periungual tissues are common, as are periungual warts. Other uncommon complications include change in the oral bacteria (Enterobacteriaceae), dental problems such as apical root resorption, alveolar destruction and malocclusions, temporomandibular disorders and gum injuries. Severe nail dystrophy due to biting also has negative social and psychological consequences for patients and their parents. Most children discontinue nail biting when they grow up. Frequent application of unpleasant-tasting topical preparations, usually containing capsicum, on the nail and periungual skin can discourage patients from biting and chewing their fingernails. *N*-acetylcysteine (NAC) 600 mg twice a day (60 mg/kg/day) can be a possible adjuvant therapy [19].

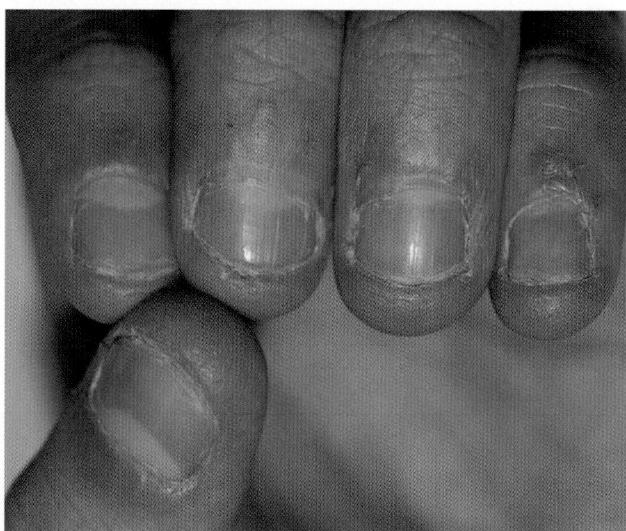

Fig. 161.6 Nail biting. Short nail plate with distal splitting and evident hyponychium. Note periungual scaling and haematic crusts due to picking the proximal nailfold skin.

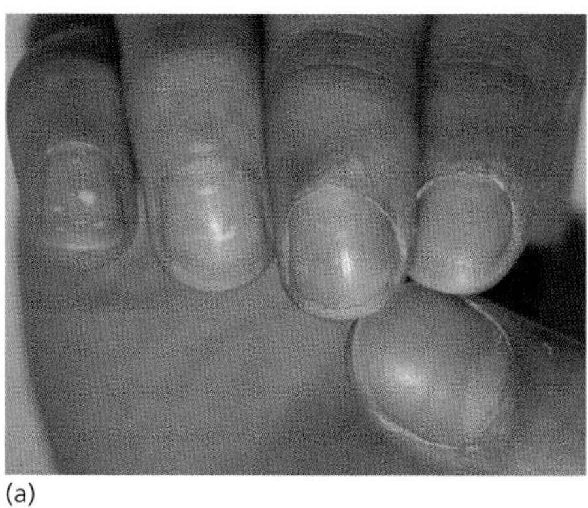
(a)

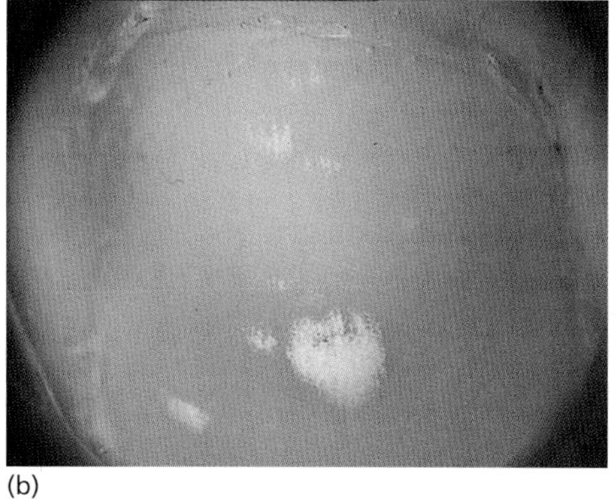
(b)

Fig. 161.7 Punctate leuconychia. Multiple small white spots (a) that at dermoscopy appear as clusters of white granules within the nail plate (b).

Punctate leuconychia

Key diagnostic criteria: small white spots on the fingernails
Key management features: treatment is not necessary
Differentials: drug-induced leuconychia

Punctate leuconychia is a traumatic fingernail abnormality that is almost exclusively seen in children. It is usually caused by repetitive minor traumatic injuries to the nail matrix. These occur because children's nails are thin. This process produces a disturbance in nail matrix keratinization and the development of parakeratotic cells in the ventral nail plate. These modify the transparency of the nail plate and appear as white spots. The affected nails show single or multiple small opaque white spots (Fig. 161.7a) that move distally with nail growth and usually disappear before reaching the distal edge. Dermoscopy of the white patch shows white granules corresponding to clusters of parakeratotic cells within the nail plate (Fig. 161.7b). Punctate leuconychia may involve a few or all the fingernails and there may be a variable number of white opaque spots. Although it is commonly believed to be caused by calcium deficiency, there is no known relationship between this condition and the calcium content of the nail.

Punctate leuconychia spontaneously regresses by avoiding trauma.

Atopic dermatitis

Key diagnostic criteria: hand and fingernail dermatitis including the periungual skin
Key management features: topical anti-inflammatory agents
Differentials: contact eczema

The nails in children with atopic dermatitis usually show eczema of the proximal nailfold (Fig. 161.8) that may be associated with nail plate surface abnormalities due to eczematous involvement of the nail matrix. These include irregular pitting and Beau's lines. Onycholysis may occasionally occur as a consequence of eczematous involvement of the fingertips.

Parakeratosis pustulosa

Key diagnostic criteria: one digit showing onycholysis and pulp scaling
Key management features: topical steroids
Differentials: psoriasis, eczema

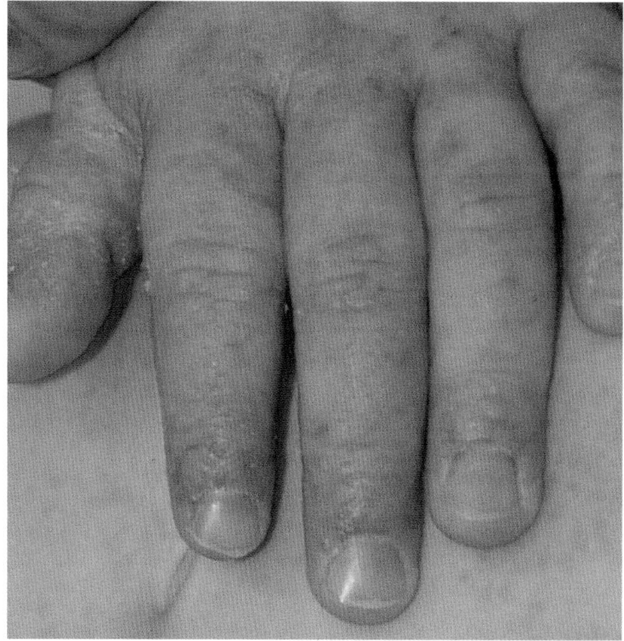

Fig. 161.8 Atopic dermatitis. Eczema of the skin of the dorsa of the hand and digits, with involvement of the proximal and lateral nailfolds.

Parakeratosis pustulosa is a chronic condition that exclusively affects children, usually between the ages of 5 and 7 years, and typically involves a single finger, most commonly the thumb or index finger [20]. In the early phases, the affected digit shows eczematous changes associated with mild distal subungual hyperkeratosis and onycholysis. Nail abnormalities are usually more marked on a corner of the nail (Fig. 161.9). Pitting of the nail plate may be present. Whether parakeratosis pustulosa is a limited form of nail psoriasis or a clinical manifestation of other conditions, such as contact and atopic dermatitis, is a matter of controversy. In the authors' experience, most children with parakeratosis pustulosa develop mild nail psoriasis when they become adults [21]. As parakeratosis pustulosa and nail psoriasis produce similar nail changes, the diagnosis of parakeratosis pustulosa is based on the localization of the disease to a single digit rather than on the morphology of the nail lesions. This diagnosis should always be considered in a child with psoriasiform nail

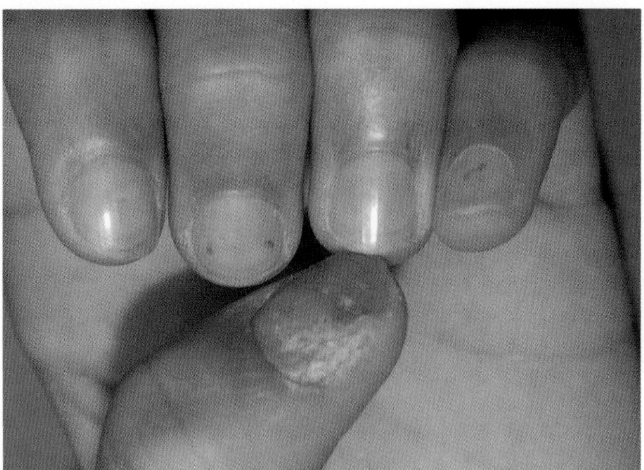

Fig. 161.9 Parakeratosis pustulosa. The first fingernail shows psoriasiform nail changes more marked on one side.

changes limited to a single finger. Patch tests can be useful to rule out contact dermatitis.

The nail lesions usually resolve spontaneously. Topical treatment with steroids and/or retinoic acid may induce partial remission of the nail changes.

Psoriasis

Key diagnostic criteria: irregular pitting, salmon patches of the nail bed, onycholysis with erythematous border
Key management features: topical vitamin D derivatives or tazarotene on the nail bed after cutting the detached nail plate
Differentials: onychomycosis, alopecia areata
In our experience, only 0.11% of children brought for a dermatological consultation and 15.5 (19.4%) of those affected by another clinical form of psoriasis have nail involvement [22].

The clinical manifestations of nail psoriasis in children are quite similar to those of adults, but in children they are usually mild and frequently go unnoticed by the child and parents [23]. Fingernails are much more commonly affected than toenails. Nail pitting is the most common sign of psoriasis in children. Pitting is the consequence of a focal psoriatic inflammatory involvement of the proximal nail matrix, which results in the persistence of clusters of parakeratotic cells within the upper layers of the nail plate. Pits usually look shiny because they reflect light. Psoriatic pits are usually large, deep and randomly scattered within the nail plate (Fig. 161.10). They are rarely found in toenails. Pits may be the sole manifestation of nail psoriasis or may be associated with distal onycholysis and salmon-pink patches of the nail bed.

The second common sign of nail psoriasis in children is onycholysis associated with subungual hyperkeratosis that may be seen in fingernails but is more evident in toenails. Onycholysis is the detachment of the nail plate from the nail bed. The onycholytic area looks whitish because of the presence of air under the detached nail plate. In psoriasis, the onycholytic area is typically separated from the normal nail plate by an erythematous border. The salmon-pink erythematous border (oil drop sign), usually surrounding the onycholytic area in psoriasis, may be

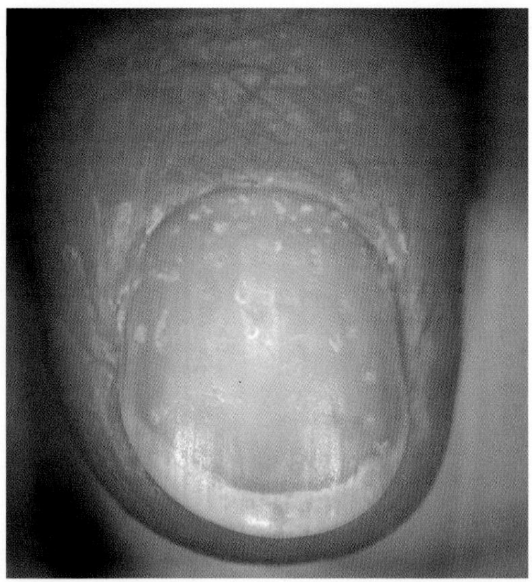

Fig. 161.10 Nail psoriasis. Psoriatic pits are irregular in size and distribution within the nail plate.

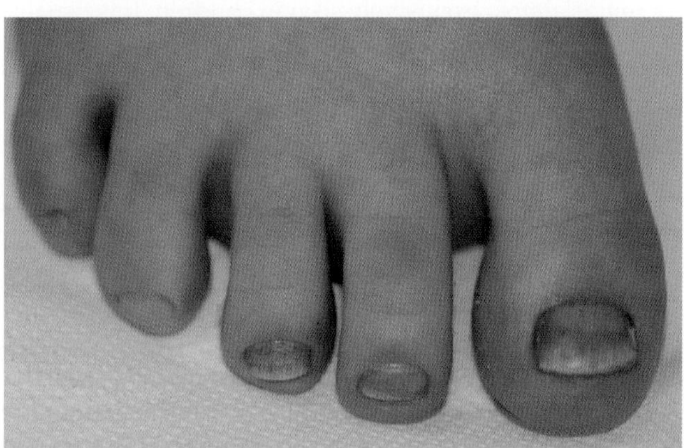

Fig. 161.11 Nail psoriasis. In the toenails, subungual hyperkeratosis with yellow discolouration and mild onycholysis are usually the sole symptoms.

absent or scarcely visible in children's toenails, making the diagnosis difficult in the absence of other skin features of psoriasis (Fig. 161.11).

Differential diagnosis with onychomycosis may require mycology or PAS examination of a nail clipping. Oily patches appear as yellowish or salmon-pink areas, easily visible through the transparent nail plate. They result from a focal psoriatic involvement of the nail bed. Splinter haemorrhages appear as longitudinal linear red-brown areas of haemorrhage. They are almost exclusively seen in fingernails and are usually located in the distal portion of the nail plate. Splinter haemorrhages are a consequence of psoriatic involvement of the nail bed capillary loops that run in a longitudinal direction along the nail bed dermal ridges.

The differential diagnosis of nail psoriasis in children mainly includes eczema and parakeratosis pustulosa. Although onychomycosis may produce nail changes very similar to nail bed psoriasis, this condition is rare in children.

Nail psoriasis has an unpredictable course, but in most cases the disease is chronic and complete remissions are uncommon. The beneficial effects of environmental factors such as sunlight are less certain than in skin psoriasis. Stressful events may precipitate relapses. There are no consistently effective treatments for nail psoriasis in children. Urea-containing creams or lacquers may help to reduce toenail thickening, while topical application of calcipotriol or tazarotene may be useful for nail bed psoriasis.

Twenty-nail dystrophy

Key diagnostic criteria: rough nail/s due to excessive longitudinal striations
Key management features: urea-containing emollients
Differentials: psoriasis, eczema

The term twenty-nail dystrophy (TND), or trachyonychia, describes a spectrum of nail plate surface abnormalities that produce nail plate roughness. Despite the name, the disease does not necessarily affect all the nails, and can even be limited to one nail. The affected nails show excessive longitudinal striations with loss of nail lustre (vertically striated sand-papered nails) (Fig. 161.12). Koilonychia and cuticle hyperkeratosis may be associated. This nail symptom is the clinical manifestation of several inflammatory nail diseases including alopecia areata, lichen planus and psoriasis. The nail histopathology permits definitive diagnosis by showing the typical features of lichen planus or psoriasis in trachyonychia due to these conditions, or spongiotic changes in trachyonychia due to alopecia areata [24,25].

Patients affected by TND may be divided into two major groups.

- Patients with a personal history or clinical evidence of alopecia areata. Up to 12% of children with alopecia areata present with this nail disorder, which may precede or follow the onset of hair loss by several years.
- Patients with isolated nail involvement (idiopathic trachyonychia). The frequency of idiopathic trachyonychia is unknown, but it is almost exclusively seen in children. It may possibly represent a variety of alopecia areata limited to the nails and is occasionally seen in association with other autoimmune diseases such as vitiligo. The disorder is symptomless and patients only complain of brittleness and cosmetic discomfort.

Twenty-nail dystrophy is a benign condition that usually regresses spontaneously over the years. Treatment is not necessary. Nail fragility may be improved by application of topical emollients.

Uncommon nail disorders

Lichen planus

Nail lichen planus (LP) is rare in children and is not usually associated with cutaneous or mucosal signs of the disease [26]. Lichen planus in children may have three different clinical presentations.

- Typical LP, similar to that seen in adults, is characterized by nail thinning with longitudinal ridging and splitting. Nail bed involvement produces onycholysis (Fig. 161.13). Dorsal pterygium, which appears as a V-shaped extension of the skin of the proximal nailfold, is rare.
- Trachyonychia (TND) resulting from nail LP is clinically similar to trachyonychia due to other inflammatory nail disorders. Even when due to LP, trachyonychia has a benign clinical course.
- Idiopathic atrophy of the nail is a rare, acute and rapidly progressing variety of nail LP that leads to painless diffuse nail destruction. It typically affects Indian patients. The nail plates are completely or almost completely absent due to the presence of dorsal pterygium and nail matrix atrophy [27].

The diagnosis of typical nail lichen planus should be considered when nail thinning is associated with longitudinal ridging and splitting. A nail biopsy is indicated for establishing the diagnosis before prescribing treatment, as differential diagnosis with nail psoriasis and other inflammatory conditions may be difficult. A longitudinal nail biopsy is always preferred, and needs patient compliance which in young children may be impossible without sedation. Systemic steroids (such as intramuscular triamcinolone acetonide 0.5 mg/kg per month for 3–6 months) can be effective in treating nail lichen planus and preventing destruction of the nail matrix [28].

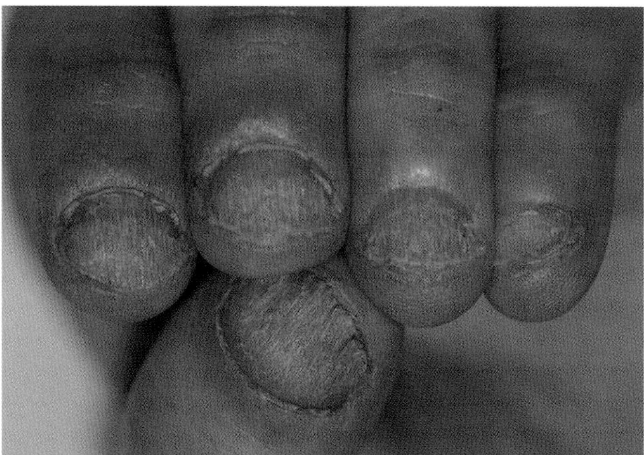

Fig. 161.12 Trachyonychia. The nails are thinned and opaque due to multiple longitudinal striations. Note associated koilonychia and cuticle hyperkeratosis.

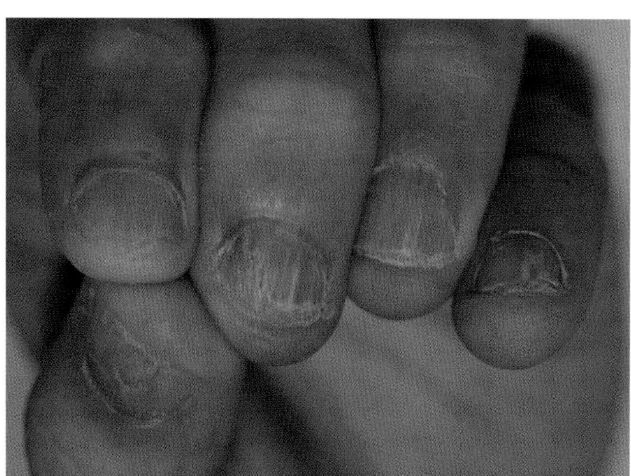

Fig. 161.13 Nail lichen planus. Nail thinning, longitudinal ridging and distal fissuring, due to nail matrix involvement, are associated with onycholysis due to nail bed involvement.

Treatment of TND due to LP is often not necessary, as this condition improves spontaneously and never produces scarring. Pterygium and idiopathic atrophy, however, are irreversible and treatment is not effective.

Lichen striatus

Nail lichen striatus is rare and almost exclusively seen in children. It is usually associated with typical skin lesions on the affected extremity but may occur in isolation [29]. It is almost always limited to a single nail. The nail abnormalities, consisting of nail thinning associated with longitudinal ridging and splitting, closely resemble those of nail matrix lichen planus but do not involve the whole nail plate, being most frequently restricted to its medial or lateral portion (Fig. 161.14). The presence of linearly arranged papules, sometimes with verrucous scales, along the affected extremity suggests the diagnosis. The nail pathology reveals changes similar to those of lichen planus in the nail matrix.

The nail lesions regress spontaneously in a few years although some cases with a long-lasting course have recently been reported [30]. Cutaneous changes may benefit from topical therapy with tacrolimus or combining a retinoid with a steroid [31].

Periungual fibromas

Periungual fibromas in children are usually a sign of tuberous sclerosis (Koenen tumour). They are more common in the toenails and usually arise from the proximal nailfold, appearing as pink filiform or nodular skin-coloured masses (Fig. 161.15). Compression of the underlying nail matrix produces a longitudinal groove in the nail plate. Subungual lesions can also occur. In tuberous sclerosis, Koenen tumours develop in up to 50% of cases, with onset occurring around puberty, and are a major diagnostic criterion, the diagnosis of tuberous sclerosis lying on the presence of two major features or one major feature plus two or more minor features.

Periungual fibromas are asymptomatic and usually require no treatment. Large lesions can be surgically excised.

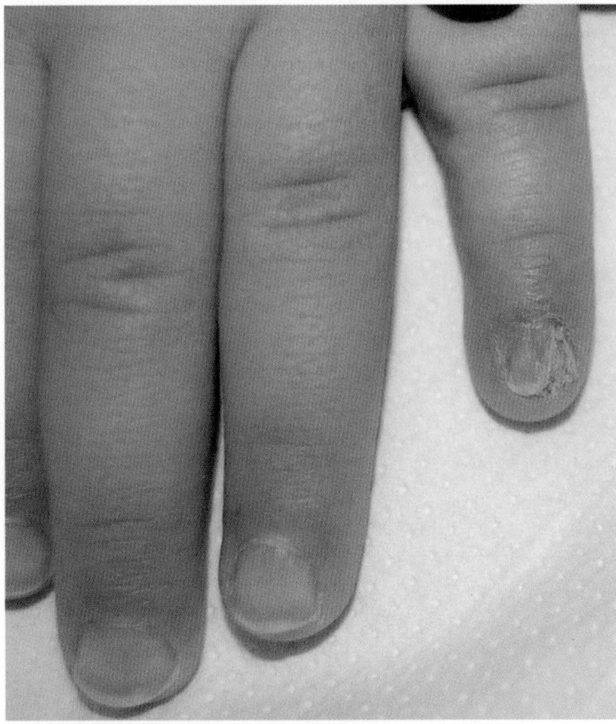

Fig. 161.14 Lichen striatus of the nail. The fifth fingernail shows nail thinning with longitudinal ridging and splitting limited to its lateral portion.

Subungual exostosis

Subungual exostoses are benign tumours of the bone of the distal phalanx. They are quite common in teenagers and are favoured by trauma. They almost exclusively involve the toenails, especially on the great toe, and are usually localized to the dorsomedial aspect of the distal phalanx. Subungual exostosis appears as a firm tender subungual nodule that elevates the nail plate and produces distal or lateral onycholysis (Fig. 161.16). The surface of the nodule is usually keratotic but may ulcerate in big lesions. Because of the gradual enlargement of the excess bone, the nail plate may be deformed or destroyed. Radiography, showing an exophytic lesion on the distal phalangeal bone, is diagnostic.

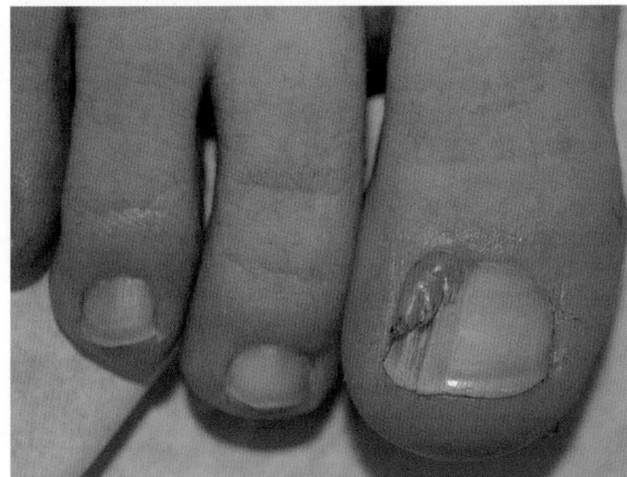

Fig. 161.15 Periungual fibroma. Elongated nodular lesion arising from the proximal nailfold, associated with nail plate longitudinal grooves due to compression of the nail matrix.

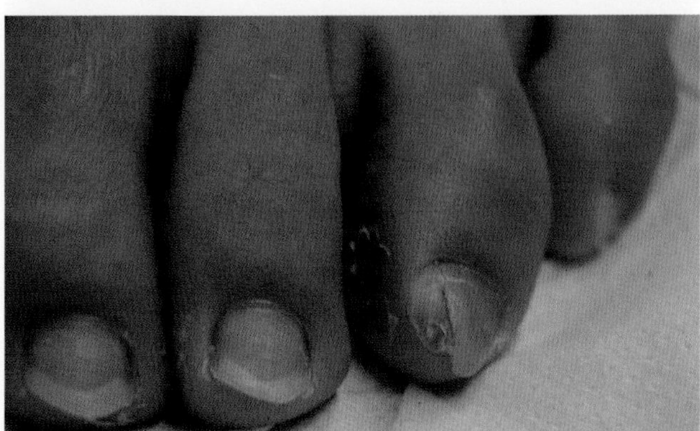

Fig. 161.16 Subungual exostosis of the fourth toenail. A subungual nodule with keratotic surface.

The lesion should be surgically excised, the best approach being complete marginal excision through a fish mouth. This technique has only 4% recurrence and good postoperative results [32].

Nail matrix naevi

Nail matrix naevi in Caucasians are uncommon but not exceptional, and are usually seen in childhood [33,34]. They may be congenital or develop at 2–4 years of age and usually produce a pigmented longitudinal band in the nail plate (longitudinal melanonychia) of a single digit (Fig. 161.17a). Nail matrix naevi occur more frequently in fingernails than in toenails, the thumb being affected in about half of cases. Nail plate pigmentation may be associated with a naevus of the periungual skin (benign Hutchinson's sign). The size and the degree of pigmentation of the band of longitudinal melanonychia vary considerably among patients. In most cases, the naevus produces a heavily pigmented band, but it can also cause a scarcely pigmented light or brown band that may even undergo spontaneous fading, especially in children, which indicates a decreased activity of the naevus cells [35]. Increased pigmentation of the band may also occur.

The diagnosis of a nail matrix nevus or lentigo should always be considered in a child with a band of longitudinal melanonychia of a single digit. Multiple bands of melanonychia involving fingernails and toenails are usually due to benign activation of melanocytes, which may be racial or due to drugs, most commonly hydroxyurea, which causes nail pigmentation in about 10% of thalassaemic children receiving the drug, cancer chemotherapeutic agents and zidovudine.

The clinical dermoscopy features utilized for evaluating melanic nail pigmentation of a single digit in adults [36] are not useful in children, where dermoscopy often shows irregular lines and black dots (Fig. 161.17b), which would be indicators of melanoma in adults [37]. A nail biopsy is necessary for definitive diagnosis, but is usually not advisable, as nail melanoma in children is exceptional, especially in Caucasians [38]. The authors advise excision of pigmented lesions only when they have particular clinical features (i.e. bands that enlarge and/or darken in a short time).

Anonychia/micronychia

Total or partial absence of the nail at birth is rare. It may be a consequence of fetal exposure to systemic medications in early pregnancy or a sign of a genetic syndrome. Hypoplasia of the nails and terminal phalanges can occur in children whose mothers have been exposed to anticonvulsant drugs, alcohol or warfarin. Congenital syndromes associated with anonychia include DOOR syndrome (deafness, onycho-osteodystrophy, mental retardation), Iso–Kikuchi syndrome and some ectodermal dysplasias.

Iso–Kikuchi syndrome

This congenital nail deformity affects one or both index fingers and occasionally other fingers [39,40]. The affected nails most commonly show micronychia or hemionychogryphosis. Anonychia may also be present. Diagnostic criteria include unilateral or bilateral hypoplasia of the index fingernails and/or other fingers, including toenails (up to total anonychia of hands and feet); radiographic abnormalities of the distal bony phalanx of the affected fingers; congenital occurrence, which can be both sporadic or hereditary. Lateral radiographic views show a Y-shaped bifurcation of the distal phalanx on lateral pictures.

Nail–patella syndrome

In this condition, which is due to a mutation of the *LMX1B* gene localized on chromosome 9q34.1 [41,42] and is inherited in an autosomal dominant pattern with variable expressivity, nail hypoplasia is associated with bone and kidney abnormalities. Nail abnormalities may be limited to the thumbs or affect all fingernails. When multiple nails are involved, the thumb is the most severely affected. The affected digits show absence or hypoplasia of the nail plate, usually more marked on the medial portion of the nail [43]. Triangular lunulae are also characteristic (Fig. 161.18). The bone abnormalities characteristic of nail–patella syndrome include absent or hypoplastic patella, radial head abnormalities and iliac crest exostosis. A pelvis X-ray identifying iliac crest exostosis permits diagnosis of nail–patella syndrome in children. In 40% of all cases of nail–patella

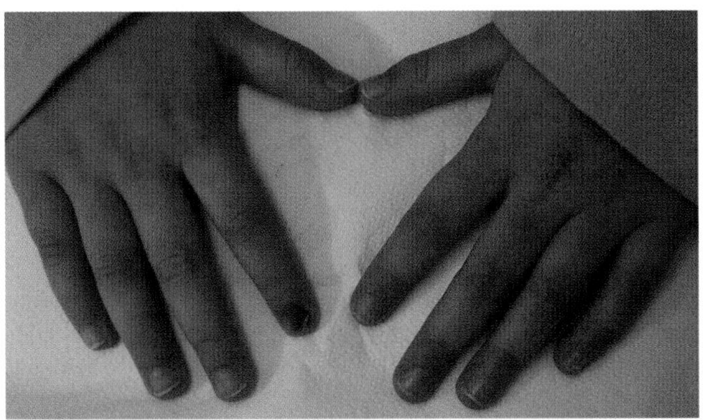

(a)

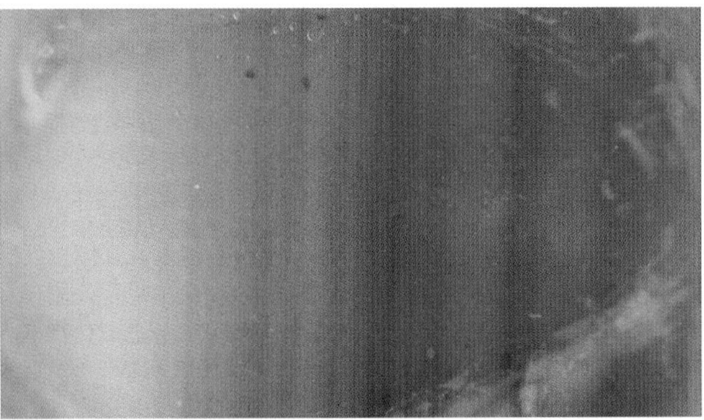

(b)

Fig. 161.17 Longitudinal melanonychia due to a nail matrix naevus of the second right fingernail. Black pigmentation that involves three quarters of the nail, associated with distal splitting (a). Dermoscopy (b) shows a brown background with blurred margins, multiple pigments that vary in thickness along their length, and granules of melanic pigment.

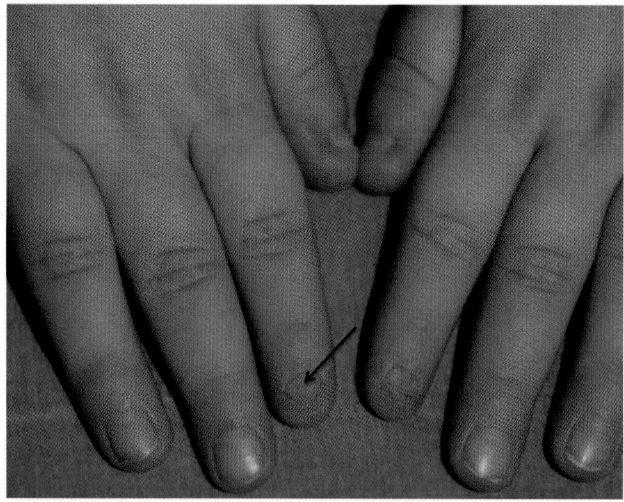

Fig. 161.18 Nail–patella syndrome: nail hypoplasia and triangular lunula. The thumb is more severely affected.

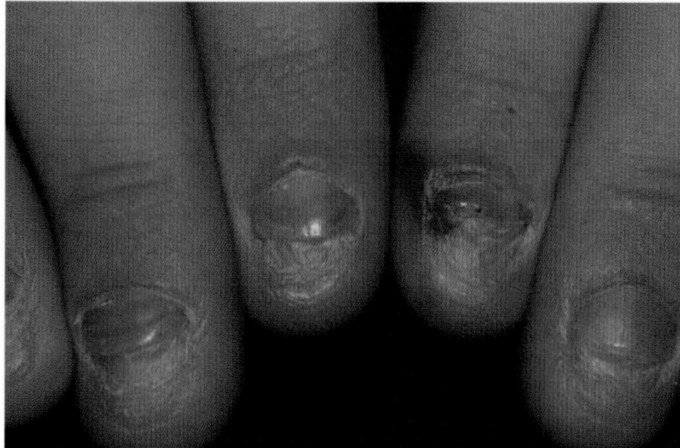

Fig. 161.19 Epidermolysis bullosa. Haemorrhagic blistering and short thick nails.

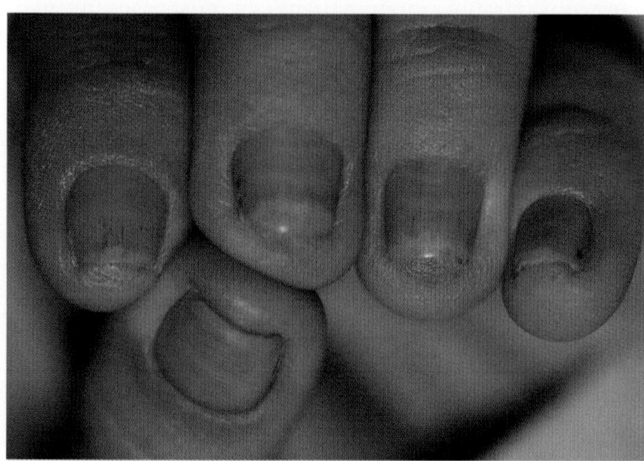

Fig. 161.20 Hidrotic ectodermal dysplasia (Clouston syndrome). The nails are short and thick, with transverse hypercurvature and mild onycholysis. Note multiple splinter haemorrhages.

syndrome, a nephropathy develops. In total, 5.5–8% of patients eventually require haemodialysis because of renal insufficiency.

Polydactyly

The frequency of polydactyly of the hands has been estimated to be 0.37%; it is more common than polydactyly of the feet. Duplication of the thumb is a manifestation of congenital polydactyly, one of the most common anomalies of the hand [44]. Patients with type 1 (bifid distal phalanx) and 2 (duplicated) thumb polydactyly may have two distinct nails separated by a longitudinal incision or a single nail with a central indentation of the distal margin. In that situation, bone duplication is limited to the distal phalanx [45]. Thumb polydactyly may be sporadic or transmitted as an autosomal dominant trait with variable expressivity. Radiography shows bone bifurcation.

Early surgical treatment is necessary to maximize functional restoration and correct disfigurement.

Epidermolysis bullosa

Epidermolysis bullosa includes a group of inherited blistering skin diseases, distinguished into three different types: epidermic, junction and dystrophic. The dominant epidermolysis bullosa starts at birth while recessive epidermolysis bullosa appears between the ages of 5 and 8 years. Nail abnormalities are common, but not specific for a particular type, as they result from blistering and scarring of nail matrix and nail bed, favoured by trauma. The most common signs include nail blisters, erosions, anonychia, nail atrophy, onychogryphosis, nail thickening and parrot beak nail deformity (Fig. 161.19) [46]. Extensive and repetitive blistering may produce permanent nail loss. Dystrophic or absent nails with periungual granulation tissue are suggestive for Herlitz EB. Dominant dystrophic epidermolysis bullosa may sometimes presents with isolated nail dystrophy, characterized by thickening and yellow discoloration of the nails [47]. Late-onset junctional epidermolysis bullosa is a subtype of autosomal recessive junctional EB, characterized by the onset of symptoms between the ages of 5 and 8 years. Nail lesions usually precede the other clinical manifestations of the disease. The nails appear thick and short, and develop recurrent periungual and subungual haemorrhagic blisters.

Ectodermal dysplasias

Patients with ectodermal dysplasia develop dystrophic nails, and the presence of nail abnormalities is a major criterion for the classification of these conditions (subclass 3). The nails show variable features, which depend on the exact form of ectodermal dysplasia. Nail hypoplasia is frequently associated with thickening of the nail plate (Fig. 161.20).

Pachyonychia congenita

Pachyonychia congenita is an autosomal dominant disorder due to mutations of four keratin genes (*KRT6A, 6B, 16, 17*), characterized by early development of nail thickening with an increased curvature due to nail bed hyperkeratosis, associated with painful plantar keratoderma. Nail and skin changes are present at birth in only 50% of the cases but by 5 years of age, they are seen in more than 75% of the children [48]. By the age of 10 years, pain is a

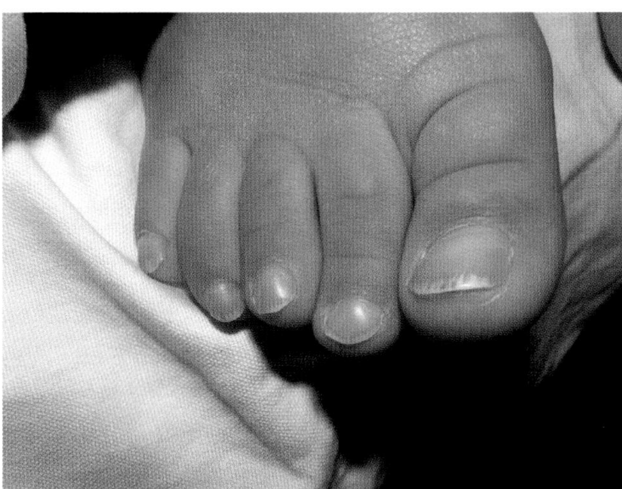

Fig. 161.21 Pachyonychia congenita. Mild nail thickening with subungual keratosis in a 6-month-old child.

commonly associated symptom and greatly impairs quality of life [49]. Toenail thickening is the most common finding, with severe subungual keratosis and difficulty in trimming nails (Fig. 161.21).

Yellow nail syndrome

The yellow nail syndrome (YNS) is a rare disorder characterized by the triad of yellow nails, respiratory problems and lymphoedema. The three features are not always present together and the diagnosis can be made when two are present and even nail changes alone can be enough for diagnosis. The pathogenesis is unknown. Nail signs diagnostic for YNS are arrested or slowed nail growth rate, nail plate thickening, lack of cuticles, yellow-green discoloration and increased transverse curvature of the nail plate. YNS in children is extremely rare and has been described as a congenital or acquired disease. Congenital YNS, transmitted as an autosomal dominant or recessive trait, is often associated with other anomalies, including nonimmune fetal hydrops, facial dysmorphism, mental retardation, seizures, inguinal hernia, deafness, cutis marmorata and eye changes [50]. Congenital YNS has also been reported in siblings, associated or not with mental retardation.

References

1 **Piraccini BM, Starace M. Nail disorders in infants and children. Curr Opin Pediatr 2014;26:440–5.**
2 Zaias N. The Nail in Health and Disease, 2nd edn. Norwalk, CT: Appleton and Lange, 1990.
3 Crespel E, Plantin P, Schoenlaub P et al. Hyperpigmentation of the distal phalanx in healthy Caucasian neonates. Eur J Dermatol 2001;11:120–21.
4 Iorizzo M, Oranje AP, Tosti A. Periungual hyperpigmentation in newborns. Pediatr Dermatol 2008;25:25–7.
5 Hamilton JB, Terada H, Mestler GE. Studies of growth throughout the lifespan in Japanese: growth and size of nails and their relationship to age, sex, heredity and other factors. J Gerontol 1995;10:401–15.
6 Sibinga MS. Observations on growth of fingernails in health and disease. Pediatrics 1959;24:225–33.
7 Wagner G, Sachse MM. Congenital malalignment of the big toe nail. J Dtsch Dermatol Ges 2012;10:326–30.
8 Fierro-Arias L, Morales-Martínez A, Zazueta-López RM et al. Congenital malalignment of the great toenail. Skinmed 2015;13:433–7.
9 Jellinek NJ. Flaps in nail surgery. Dermatol Ther 2012;25:535–44.
10 **Piraccini BM, Parente GL, Varotti E et al. Congenital hypertrophy of the lateral nail folds of the hallux: clinical features and follow-up of seven cases. Pediatr Dermatol 2000;17:348–51.**
11 Tsunoda M, Tsunoda K. Patient-controlled taping for the treatment of ingrown toenails. Ann Fam Med 2014;12:553–5.
12 Matsui T, Kidou M, Ono T. Infantile multiple ingrowing nails of the fingers induced by the grasp reflex: a new entity. Dermatology 2002;205:25–7.
13 Parry EJ. Chevron nail/herringbone nail. J Am Acad Dermatol 1999; 40:497–8.
14 **Durdu M, Ruocco V. Clinical and cytologic features of antibiotic-resistant acute paronychia. J Am Acad Dermatol 2014;70:120–6.**
15 Haneke E. Nail surgery. Clin Dermatol 2013;31:516–25.
16 **Piraccini BM, Bruni F, Starace M. Dermoscopy of nonskin cancer nail disorders. Dermatol Ther 2012;25:594–602.**
17 Tosti A, Piraccini BM. Warts of the nail unit: surgical and non surgical approaches. Dermatol Surg 2001;27:235–9.
18 Choi Y, Kim do H, Jin SY, et al. Topical immunotherapy with diphenylcyclopropenone is effective and preferred in the treatment of periungual warts. Ann Dermatol 2013;25:434–9.
19 Smith L, Tracy DK, Giaroli G. What future role might N-acetylcysteine have in the treatment of obsessive compulsive and grooming disorders? A systematic review. J Clin Psychopharmacol 2016;36: 57–62.
20 Hjorth N, Thomsen K. Parakeratosis pustulosa. Br J Dermatol 1967;79: 527–32.
21 **Tosti A, Peluso AM, Zucchelli V. Clinical features and long term follow-up of 2 cases of parakeratosis pustulosa. Pediatr Dermatol 1998;15:259–63.**
22 Piraccini BM, Triantafyllopoulou I, Prevezas C et al. Nail psoriasis in children: common or uncommon results from a 10-year double-center study. Skin App Dis 2015;1:43–8.
23 Al-Mutairi N, Manchanda Y, Nour-Eldin O. Nail changes in childhood psoriasis: a study from Kuwait. Pediatr Dermatol 2007;24:7–10.
24 **Gordon KA, Vega JM, Tosti A. Trachyonychia: a comprehensive review. Indian J Dermatol Venereol Leprol 2011;77:640–5.**
25 Tosti A, Piraccini BM. Trachyonychia or twenty-nail dystrophy. Curr Opin Dermatol 1996;3:83–6.
26 **Tosti A, Piraccini BM, Cambiaghi S et al. Nail lichen planus in children. Clinical features, response to treatment and long term follow up. Arch Dermatol 2001;137:1027–32.**
27 Tosti A, Piraccini BM, Fanti PA et al. Idiopathic atrophy of the nails: clinical and pathological study of 2 cases. Dermatology 1995;190:116–18.
28 Tosti A, Peluso AM, Fanti PA et al. Nail lichen planus: clinical study of 24 patients. J Am Acad Dermatol 1993;28:724–30.
29 **Tosti A, Peluso AM, Misciali C et al. Nail lichen striatus: clinical features and long-term follow-up of five cases. J Am Acad Dermatol 1997;36:908–13.**
30 Feely MA, Silverberg NB. Two cases of lichen striatus with prolonged active phase. Pediatr Dermatol 2014;31:e67–8.
31 Youssef SM, Teng JM. Effective topical combination therapy for treatment of lichen striatus in children: a case series and review. J Drugs Dermatol 2012;11:872–5.
32 **DaCambra MP, Gupta SK, Ferri-de-Barros F. Subungual exostosis of the toes: a systemic review. Clin Orthop Relat Res 2014;472:1251–9.**
33 **Tosti A, Baran R, Piraccini BM et al. Nail matrix nevi: a clinical and pathological study of 22 patients. J Am Acad Dermatol 1996;34: 765–71.**
34 Goettmann-Bonvallot S, Andre J, Belaich S. Longitudinal melanonychia in children: a clinical and histopathologic study of 4 cases. J Am Acad Dermatol 1999;41:17–22.
35 Tosti A, Baran R, Morelli R et al. Progressive fading of longitudinal melanonychia due to a nail matrix melanocytic nevus in a child. Arch Dermatol 1994;130:1076–7.
36 Ronger S, Touzet S, Ligeron C et al. Dermoscopic examination of nail pigmentation. Arch Dermatol 2002;138:1327–33.
37 **Tosti A, Piraccini BM, de Farias DC. Dealing with melanonychia. Semin Cutan Med Surg 2009;28:49–54.**
38 Iorizzo M, Tosti A, di Chiacchio N et al. Nail melanoma in children: differential diagnosis and management. Dermatol Surg 2008;34: 974–8.
39 Baran R. Syndrome d'Iso et Kikuchi. Ann Dermatol Vénéréol 1980; 107:431.
40 Valerio E, Favot F, Mattei I et al. Congenital isolated Iso–Kikuchi syndrome in a newborn. Clin Case Rep 2015;3:866–9.

41 McIntosh I, Dreyer SD, Clough MV et al. Mutation analysis of LMX1B gene in nail patella syndrome patients. Am J Hum Genet 1998;63: 1651–8.

42 Bongers EM, Gubler MC, Knoers NV. Nail–patella syndrome: overview on clinical and molecular findings. Pediatr Nephrol 2002;17: 703–12.

43 Neri I, Piccolo V, Balestri R et al. Median nail damage in nail–patella syndrome associated with triangular lunulae. Br J Dermatol 2015;173: 1559–61.

44 Little KJ, Cornwall R. Congenital anomalies of the hand – principles of management. Orthop Clin North Am 2016;47:153–68.

45 Tosti A, Paoluzzi P, Baran R. Doubled nail of the thumb: a rare form of polydactyly. Dermatology 1992;184:216–18.

46 Tosti A, de Farias DC, Murrell DF. Nail involvement in epidermolysis bullosa. Dermatol Clin 2010;28:153–7.

47 Dharma B, Moss C, McGrath JA et al. Dominant dystrophic epidermolysis bullosa presenting as familial nail dystrophy. Clin Exp Dermatol 2001;26:93–6.

48 Shah S, Boen M, Kenner-Bell B et al. Pachyonychia congenita in pediatric patients: natural history, features, and impact. JAMA Dermatol 2014;150:146–53.

49 Eliason MJ, Leachman SA, Feng BJ et al. A review of the clinical phenotype of 254 patients with genetically confirmed pachyonychia congenita. J Am Acad Dermatol 2012;67:680–6.

50 Dessart P, Deries X, Guérin-Moreau M et al. Yellow nail syndrome: two pediatric case reports. Ann Dermatol Venereol 2014;141:611–19.

CHAPTER 162

Genital Disease in Children

Gayle O. Fischer

The Northern Clinical School, The University of Sydney, Sydney, NSW, Australia

Introduction, 2159
Inflammatory dermatoses of the genital region, 2160
Lichen sclerosus in girls (syn. lichen sclerosus et atrophicus), 2164
Lichen sclerosus in boys (syn. balanitis xerotica obliterans), 2170
Birthmarks in the genital area, 2170
Vulvovaginitis, 2174
Nonsexually acquired genital infections in children, 2175
Sexually transmitted infections in children, 2179
Blisters and ulcers, 2179
Anatomical abnormalities, 2184
Foreign bodies, 2188
Neoplasia, 2188
Scrotal conditions, 2190
Genital signs of systemic disease, 2191
Psychological aspects of genital disease in children, 2193

Abstract

Genital skin disease in children comprises inflammatory dermatoses, infectious conditions, a range of congenital lesions including naevi and malformations, and neoplastic lesions. Although most of these conditions can be found on other parts of the skin, there are some that are most commonly found in the genital area and some that are specific to it. Genital inflammatory conditions such as atopic, irritant and seborrhoeic dermatitis and psoriasis may present differently in the macerated genital skin and may have different precipitants to the same condition on other parts of the skin, while lichen sclerosus is almost confined to genital skin in children. Infectious disease is uncommon and the range of infections differs to those found in adults, with group A *Streptococcus* dominating as the most common in both genders. Blistering and ulcerating conditions are rare but important to recognize, particularly where concern about child sexual abuse is a factor. It is important for dermatologists to have some knowledge of the possible anatomical abnormalities that may present in the genital area and of how systemic diseases and syndromes may present in this area. Finally, skin disease of the genital area presents a unique challenge in terms of its psychological importance to children, their parents and carers.

Key points

- The most common dermatoses of the genital area in children are eczema/dermatitis, psoriasis and lichen sclerosus.
- Genital candidiasis is rare in healthy prepubertal children; but common in babies with napkin dermatitis.
- Many innocent skin lesions and dermatoses are mistaken for signs of child sexual abuse.
- Lichen sclerosus in young girls may leave permanent scarring.
- Lichen sclerosus in girls cannot be expected to resolve at puberty.
- Lichen sclerosus in boys is a common cause of phimosis.
- The treatment of choice of lichen sclerosus is topical corticosteroid both to attain remission and to maintain it.
- The most common cause of infective genital disease in both sexes is group A *Streptococcus*.
- Fusion of the labia is not uncommon in young girls and usually self-resolving.
- Disease of the genital area carries a unique emotional significance.
- Child sexual abuse can present with no obvious physical signs.
- Crohn disease may present in the genital area and should be suspected in any case of persistent genital oedema.
- Hidradenitis suppurativa may begin before puberty.
- Atypical napkin dermatitis may present with nodules, vesicles and ulcers.
- Any bloodstained vaginal discharge in a prepubertal child should be investigated.
- Nonsexually acquired genital ulceration in girls is a type of aphthous ulceration which may present with acute and alarming vulval ulceration.

Introduction

Genital skin disease in children is less common than in adults and although many of the conditions that affect adults also affect children, there are some important differences between the two groups. In both adults and children of either sex, eczema/dermatitis and psoriasis are the most common causes of a chronic genital rash and, particularly in females, lichen sclerosus is also common [1]. However, acute, recurrent and chronic candidiasis are important components of female adult vulval disease that are not seen in the nonoestrogenized vulva and vagina of the child, and tinea of the groin, which is relatively common in men, is rare in children [2]. Birthmarks of the genital area, particularly haemangiomas, are an important issue in children but not in adults, in whom they are likely to have resolved long ago or have been diagnosed. Fusion of the labia is a self-limiting condition seen in small girls but it is seen in adults only in the setting of lichen sclerosus or severe lichen planus. Phimosis

Harper's Textbook of Pediatric Dermatology, Fourth Edition. Edited by Peter Hoeger, Veronica Kinsler and Albert Yan.

in boys is commonly due to lichen sclerosus of the prepuce and glans penis. Group A β-haemolytic streptococcal vulvovaginitis, balanitis and perianal cellulitis are diseases that affect mainly children but, apart from this, infective genital disease is rare in children. Sexual abuse is always an issue to be considered in any genital presentation in children but, in fact, is rarely a cause of genital skin disease. Malignancy of the skin of the genital skin is also very rare in children, as opposed to adults, in whom it is a real, if relatively uncommon, concern.

Within the paediatric age group, genital skin disease appears to be more common in girls than in boys. Very little work on the specific subject of paediatric genital disease has been published and even less on males than females. Most of what exists focuses on infective conditions, anatomical abnormalities and tumours. Anatomical abnormalities and tumours are in fact very rare in everyday practice, and even infection is unusual.

In articles on paediatric vulval disease, it is often asserted that the skin of the prepubertal vulva is fragile and sensitive because it is poorly oestrogenized. In fact, there is no evidence to back this up. It is physiological for a child's vulva to be low in oestrogen, and the fact that children have much less trouble with vulval rashes than do adults does not support the assumption that vulval skin of a child is prone to disease. The presence of oestrogen is in fact a liability that predisposes to the vaginitis, particularly candidiasis, seen in adults. Furthermore, oestrogen creams are often very irritating when applied to children.

Another common assertion is that genital and perianal disease in children is due to 'poor hygiene' and 'faecal contamination'. This is a facile statement that is also poorly supported, and which trivializes and stigmatizes this problem. In fact, mothers of small children are usually highly conscientious about genital hygiene and are more likely to be doing more washing than is necessary rather than too little.

When examining a child or adolescent with a genital problem, it is important to be sensitive to the probability that both the child and the parent will be not only embarrassed but also fearful. It is important to inform both of what you will do, to allow them control of the examination and in some cases, not to touch. This can be achieved by allowing the parent to aid in the examination by retracting the labia of a girl or the foreskin of a boy or in older children asking them to do this themselves. A small child is often best examined on the parent's lap. Telling a child you are just taking a look and that this is not going to hurt is an important reassurance to give before the start of the examination. Gaining a child's trust, particularly when the problem is one that will require ongoing surveillance, is very important.

References

1 Fischer GO. The commonest causes of symptomatic vulval disease: a dermatologist's perspective. Australas J Dermatol 1996;37:12–18.

2 Fischer GO, Rogers M. Vulvar disease in children: a clinical audit of 130 cases. Pediatr Dermatol 2000;17:1–6.

Inflammatory dermatoses of the genital region

Inflammation of the genital skin may be caused by any dermatosis occurring at this site in isolation or as part of a generalized eruption. In girls, there is often a mistaken diagnosis of a vaginal discharge when the skin is macerated and weeping due to the inflammatory changes, secondary infection and erosions of the affected epithelium, producing staining of underwear. The most common dermatological disorders affecting the genital skin in infancy and childhood are eczema/dermatitis, psoriasis and lichen sclerosus [1]. The eczema group includes irritant contact dermatitis, seborrhoeic eczema in infants and atopic eczema. Allergic contact eczema is rare relative to adults. It is important and helpful to examine other flexural sites, nails and scalp to see if there is evidence of these conditions elsewhere. Lichen sclerosus is the most common scarring skin disorder to affect this site exclusively as extragenital lesions are uncommon in children. Cutaneous lichen planus is very rare in childhood, with most of the cases reported occurring after the age of 10 years, and it is seen more commonly at this early age in Asian children and only a very few of these have genital involvement.

Dermatitis

Pathogenesis. Although it is a very common assumption that candidiasis is the usual cause of genital rashes, eczema/dermatitis is a much more common cause of genital pruritus and rashes in children. Although there are no published studies that confirm this in boys, at least 30% of children with pruritus vulvae have dermatitis, and 66% of these patients are atopic [1,2]. Despite this, the medical literature has largely neglected the subject of dermatitis specifically as it affects the genital area, and many cases are simply described as 'nonspecific' [3].

Older children wearing nappies at night may develop irritant contact dermatitis. Irritant contact dermatitis may also occur as a result of constant contact with faeces. This will most often happen in the context of the child with chronic diarrhoea or chronic constipation with soiling. Children who shower rather than bathe may miss washing the vulval area effectively, and children who wipe back to front may soil the vulval area with faeces. However, the most common causes of irritant contact dermatitis in children are overuse of soap or bubble bath, using shampoo in the bath and swimming in chlorinated swimming pools [1,2,4]. In some children, particularly those with urinary and faecal incontinence, persistent and atypical irritant contact dermatitis can occur. This goes by various names such as pseudoverrucous papules and nodules and granuloma gluteale infantum [5,6] (Fig. 162.1). It presents as nodules, papules and vesicles. The pathogenesis of atypical irritant contact dermatitis of the genital area (which also occurs in adults) is unclear and this histology is of nonspecific inflammation, without any true granulomas. In the past, granuloma gluteale infantum was attributed to the use

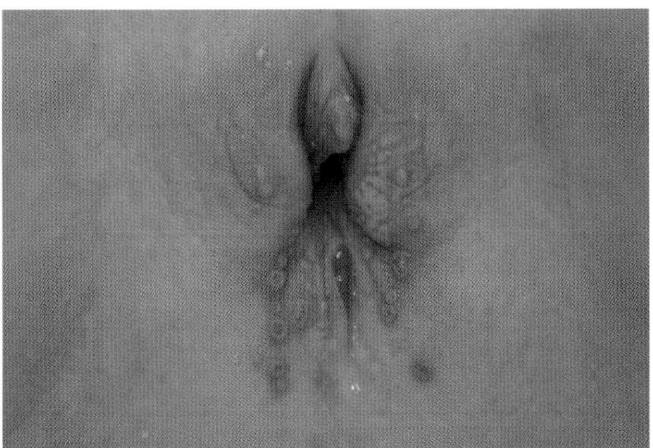

Fig. 162.1 Vesicular irritant contact dermatitis in an incontinent child.

of topical corticosteroids but a more recent view is that all of these conditions, including Jacquet erosive dermatitis (see below), are part of a disease spectrum [7]. Similar to other cases of irritant contact dermatitis, resolution occurs when the irritant is removed.

Irritation from overuse of medications and perfumed products is common in adults but less so in children, mainly because they are not exposed to nearly so many of these products. However, it is not uncommon for children to be treated with antifungal creams on the assumption that they have candidiasis, and these can be a cause of contact irritant dermatitis. True allergic contact dermatitis of the anogenital region is most often due to topical corticosteroids, preservatives and fragrances [8] and should be considered in any persistent, treatment-resistant case.

Clinical presentation. Because babies who suffer from atopic dermatitis rarely have signs of it in the well-hydrated skin under the nappy, the onset of vulval dermatitis is often delayed until the child is out of nappies.

Genital dermatitis presents with itching, stinging, soreness, dysuria and a fluctuating rash, which is often precipitated by contact with irritants and worsened by excessive washing and use of antifungal creams.The child's scratching behaviour is often a source of embarrassment for parents and of unwelcome attention at school. The symptoms can disturb sleep and it is common for children with vulval itching to wake in a distressed state at night with night terrors. Some girls complain of burning and stinging on urination and contact with bath water. The distribution of the rash is usually on the labia majora in girls and the base of the penis and the scrotum in boys.

Examination is often fairly unremarkable, and parents may have trouble convincing their doctor that there is anything wrong. Close inspection will reveal some erythema, scale and in girls slight rugosity of the labia majora, and increased erythema and desquamation of the minora (Fig. 162.2). In severe cases there is erythema, oedema, excoriation and fissuring. If the eruption is long standing there may be lichenification.The desquamation may stain the child's underwear and be misinterpreted as a vaginal discharge. If the rash is severe, it may extend to the inguinal areas and buttocks. Conversely, it can also be confined to the vestibule, particularly when there is an irritant such as bubble bath involved. Superinfection with *Staphylococcus aureus* may occur on the skin but there is no vaginitis, and vaginal swabs and urine culture are invariably negative.

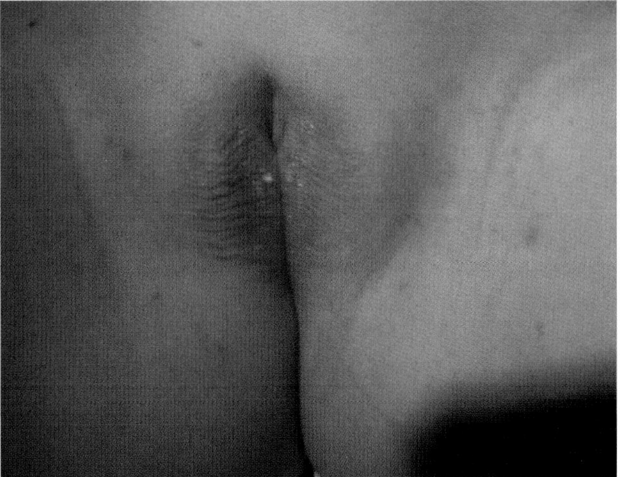

Fig. 162.2 Atopic dermatitis of the labia majora.

Differential diagnosis. The differential diagnosis of dermatitis of the genital area includes all of the conditions that can result in an erythematous, scaly eruption. This includes psoriasis, tinea, perianal streptococcal dermatitis and pinworm infestation. Treated lichen sclerosus may appear erythematous rather than white [9].

Where examination reveals little more than a scaly, erythematous, poorly defined rash, dermatitis is the most likely diagnosis, even if signs are subtle. When the rash is erythematous but well defined, and particularly when there is perianal involvement, it is important to look for signs of psoriasis and enquire about a family history [10].

Investigations. If weeping or pustules are present, a bacteriological swab from the affected area should be performed. If there appears to be a vaginal discharge, a swab from the introitus with a moistened cotton tip can be performed, but prepubertal children tolerate vaginal swabs poorly, and they are in general not indicated. If there is suspicion of a fungal infection, a fungal scraping should be performed. Urine culture is not required unless dysuria is present. Patch testing is rarely required.

Prognosis. The prognosis of genital dermatitis is excellent, particularly when simple irritancy from an identifiable source is present, which can be easily reversed. Even when there is an underlying tendency to atopic dermatitis, the condition can easily be controlled. Remissions and exacerbations are the rule, depending on irritant exposure, but most parents rapidly learn to deal with these situations. In children with a continence problem, the management is more challenging and prognosis is more guarded.

Management. Many cases of genital itching are due to dermatitis, either atopic or the result of irritation from clothing or applied substances. Often, a much greater emotional overlay is attached to any condition of the genital area than to conditions in other parts of the skin. As a result, the degree of distress experienced by the parents and sometimes the child may be out of proportion to the actual problem. There is still a tendency for genital disease to be poorly understood, and it is not uncommon for patients to visit many doctors without receiving what they consider a satisfactory explanation and effective treatment. As a result, parents are often angry and frustrated. This can make history taking difficult and leave the doctor wondering why the emotional reaction is so intense when there is so little to see.

The first step in treating genital dermatitis involves giving parents detailed environmental advice specific to the genital area. It is preferable to bathe rather than shower. No soap or bubble bath should be used; bath oil should be used in the bath and, if the child does shower, a soap substitute should be used and the parent needs to explain that the labia have to be parted and rinsed and, in boys over the age of 3 years, the foreskin retracted. This should be supervised. Shampoo should be rinsed out after the child gets out of the bath, or soap substitute used instead of shampoo.

If the child does any form of physical activity that involves wearing tight Lycra clothing, if possible this should be modified so that, at least during practice sessions, loose cotton clothes are worn. This, of course, is not possible for performances and competitions, but explain to the parents that some compromises have to be made. Even nylon tights worn as part of a school uniform may have to be discarded and parents may require a letter to take to the school.

If the child is going to swimming lessons, the chlorinated water can be a powerful irritant. Applying Vaseline® (petroleum jelly) or zinc cream before swimming is helpful, and the parents should be advised to always remove the costume straight after swimming and that the child should shower before going home.

If the child has an incontinence problem, either enuresis or constipation with overflow, this needs to be dealt with. Night nappies should be discarded if possible. Always actively ask about this; it is embarrassing, it is not always volunteered, and parents do not always make a connection between incontinence and the genital irritation.

Enquiry should be made concerning over-the-counter topical applications as these may not be volunteered, the parent seeing them only as unsuccessful treatment and not a potential problem. Ask about perfumed products, such as toilet paper and wet wipes, as well. The use of such products should be stopped.

In terms of ideal clothing, loose cotton underwear is desirable and underpants, particularly nylon ones, should be avoided at night.

Most cases of vulval dermatitis will respond to 1% hydrocortisone topically, as long as the environmental changes are also made. Ointment is preferable to creams, which may cause stinging. If the dermatitis is severe, a stronger, nonfluorinated topical steroid such as methylprednisolone aceponate 0.1% or desonide 0.05% can be used initially and continued until the dermatitis has settled. It should be possible to reduce to 1% hydrocortisone when the rash has settled. If this is not possible, consider an alternative diagnosis.

If suspected, the child should be treated for possible pinworm infestation.

Many parents are very apprehensive about using topical corticosteroids on their children, and even more so on the genital area where they are concerned that the preparations will 'thin the skin' or interfere with future sexual function and even fertility. In practice, the above treatment is very safe and it is wise to preempt any objections with strong reassurance.

If skin swabs show infection, which will usually be with *Staph. aureus*, a course of appropriate antibiotics should be given. A finding of β-haemolytic *Streptococcus* group A requires a 10-day course of penicillin or erythromycin.

Much stronger reassurance is often required when skin disease affects the genital area than when it is found on other skin areas, and it is important to enquire about fears of sexually transmitted disease and child abuse.

It is best to be matter of fact and help the parents to understand that the genital area is simply part of the skin and that their child has involvement in this area. Make them aware that children rapidly pick up their anxieties, and that an intelligent child may capitalize on this with attention-seeking or school-avoiding behaviour.

Psoriasis of the genital area

Incidence. The incidence and natural history of psoriasis in childhood are unknown. However, presentation of psoriasis in children and adults differs in type and pattern [11]. Also, few data exist on psoriasis of the genital area. It is an accepted fact that psoriasis may be confined to this part of the skin, with little evidence of the disease elsewhere.

If children with genital disease are taken as a group, psoriasis is a relatively common cause, representing about 10% of children presenting with vulval disease, and it should always be considered in the differential diagnosis of persistent genital rashes in both sexes [1,2,12]. A study in 2001 indicated that the genital area was involved in 8.9% of children with childhood psoriasis [11]. In children less than 2 years of age, the most common type of psoriasis is nappy rash with dissemination [11].

Clinical presentation. In babies, psoriasis may present for the first time as a persistent nappy rash. The features at this age include a well-demarcated edge and involvement of the inguinal folds, but the typical scale of psoriasis is lacking under the nappy. The rash may remain confined to the nappy area or may disseminate with typical psoriatic lesions on the trunk, limbs and scalp [1,2,4,13].

In older children, the morphology of the rash is much the same, with an itchy, red, well-demarcated, symmetrical plaque. Again, there is little scale; however, in girls this may be evident in the sulcus between the labia minora and majora. The vulva, penis, perineum, perianal area and often natal cleft may all be involved (Figs 162.3, 162.4 and 162.5). The rash may not be markedly symptomatic but parents may complain that the area is persistently erythematous [10,14].

If psoriasis is confined to the genital area, it is difficult to make a definite diagnosis unless other diagnostic clues are present. A history of cradle cap or difficult nappy rashes as a baby, nail pitting, postauricular or scalp rashes and a family history are all helpful [15].

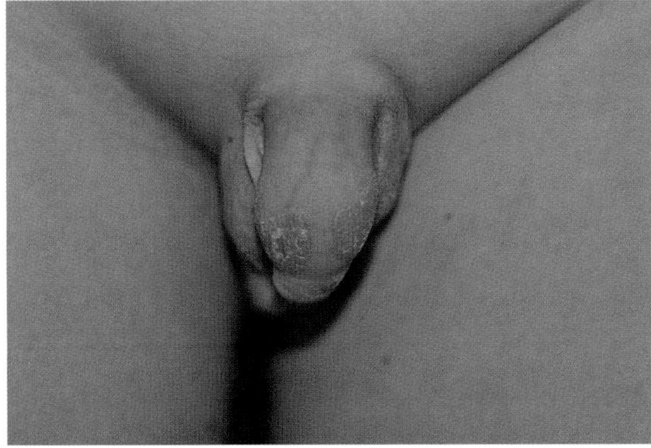

Fig. 162.3 Psoriasis of the penis.

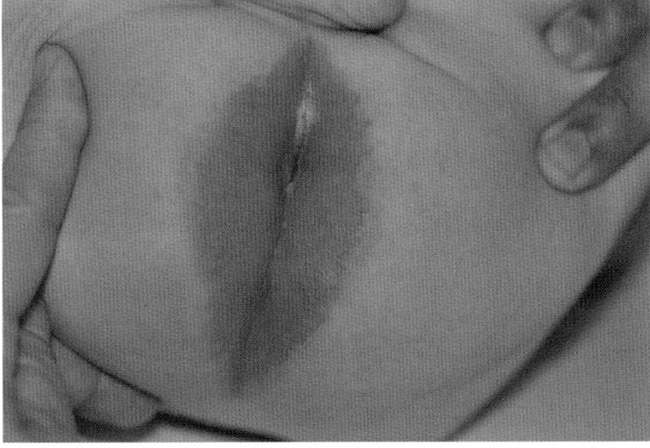

Fig. 162.4 Psoriasis of the perianal skin.

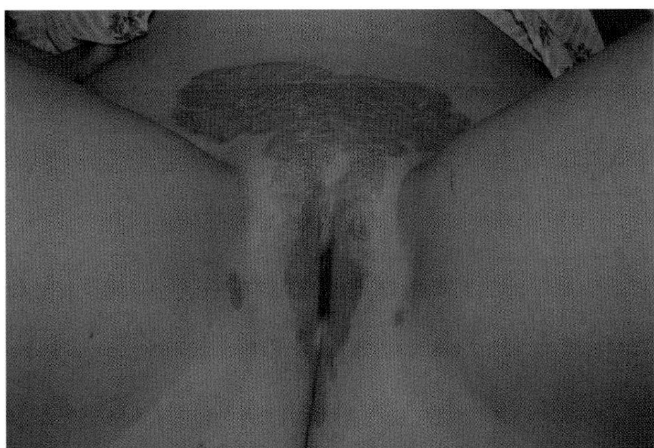

Fig. 162.5 Psoriasis of the vulva.

Investigations. If weeping or inflammation is present, a skin swab for bacteriology is indicated. Like psoriasis on other areas of the skin, infection of the genital area with group A *Streptococcus* will worsen the disease and create treatment resistance. Other investigations are not necessary.

Prognosis. Data are lacking on the outcome of childhood psoriasis. It is not known whether psoriatic nappy rash is a precursor to childhood or adult psoriasis, and the natural history of genital psoriasis in children is also not known [11].

Differential diagnosis. This includes dermatitis, erythematous lichen sclerosus and streptococcal perianal dermatitis.

Management. Psoriasis tends to be more difficult to treat than dermatitis. Even psoriatic nappy rash may not respond to 1% hydrocortisone. Although some cases do respond to the weaker corticosteroids that are usually recommended for the genital area, it is not uncommon for stronger corticosteroids to be required to achieve relief of itching [16]. Topical pimecrolimus and tacrolimus may be effective [17] but stinging is a significant side-effect in the genital area and initial control with topical corticosteroid is often required before other therapies can be initiated.

Low-concentration tar-containing preparations, such as 2% liquor carbonis detergens in an emollient base, are useful on the genital area, particularly for maintenance treatment. For thickened plaques, it is possible to use low-concentration dithranol with good effect. General skin care measures specific for the genital area (as outlined in Dermatitis, above) are also an adjunct to therapy.

References

1 **Fischer GO. Vulval disease in pre-pubertal girls. Australas J Dermatol 2001;42:225–34.**

2 **Fischer GO, Rogers M. Vulvar disease in children. A clinical audit of 130 cases. Pediatr Dermatol 2000;17:1–6.**

3 Paek SC, Merritt DF, Mallory SB. Pruritus vulvae in prepubertal children. J Am Acad Dermatol 2001;44:795–802.

4 Fischer G, Rogers M. Paediatric vulvovaginitis. In: Proceedings of the 3rd Symposium on Diseases of the Vulva and Vagina. Melbourne: Melbourne University, 1997:26–9.

5 Garrido-Ruiz MC, Rosales B, Rodriguez-Peralto J. Vulvar pseudoverrucous papules and nodules secondary to a urethral-vaginal fistula. Am J Dermatopahol 2011;33(4):410–12.

6 Dixit S, Scurry JP, Fischer G. A vesicular variant of pseudoverrucous papules and nodules in the genital area of an incontinent 4 year old. Australas J Dermatol 2013;54(4):e92–4.

7 Robson KJ, Maughan JA, Purcell SD et al. Erosive papulonodular dermatosis associated with topical benzocaine: a report of two cases and evidence that granuloma gluteale, pseudoverrucous papules, and Jacquet's erosive dermatitis are a disease spectrum. J Am Acad Dermatol 2006;55:S74–80.

8 **Warshaw EM, Furda LM, Maibach HI. Anogenital dermatitis in patients referred for patch testing: retrospective analysis of cross-sectional data from the North American Contact Dermatitis Group. Arch Dermatol 2008;144(6):749–55.**

9 Ridley CM. Genital lichen sclerosus (lichen sclerosus et atrophicus) in childhood and adolescence. J Roy Soc Med 1993;86:69–75.
10 Siegfried EC, Frasier LD. Anogenital skin disease in the pediatric population. Pediatr Ann 1997;26:321–31.
11 Morris A, Rogers M, Fischer G et al. Childhood psoriasis. A clinical review of 1262 cases. Pediatr Dermatol 2001;18:188–98.
12 Fischer G. Chronic vulvitis in pre-pubertal girls. Australas J Dermatol 2010;51:118–23.
13 Fischer GO. The commonest causes of symptomatic vulval disease: a dermatologist's perspective. Australas J Dermatol 1996;36:166–7.
14 Farber EM, Nall L. Genital psoriasis. Cutis 1992;50:263–6.
15 Ridley CM. Vulvar disease in the paediatric population. Semin Dermatol 1996;15:29–35.
16 Paek SC, Merritt DF, Mallory SB. Pruritus vulvae in prepubertal children. J Am Acad Dermatol 2001;44:795–802.
17 Amichai B. Psoriasis sof the glans penis in a child successfully treated with Elidel (pimecrolimus) cream. J Eur Acad Dermatol Venereol 2004;18(6):742–3.

Lichen sclerosus in girls (syn. lichen sclerosus et atrophicus)

Definition. Lichen sclerosus (LS) is a chronic, progressive inflammatory dermatosis characterized by shiny, white, atrophic patches with a predilection for the genital and perianal skin. It was originally described in 1887 by Hallopeau [1] as a variant of lichen planus. It is significantly more common in females than in males with a reported female to male ratio of 10:1 [2]. The peak ages of presentation are prepubertal children and menopausal women [3]. The prevalence has been estimated at 0.1% in prepubertal girls and 5–15% of all cases are estimated to occur in children [4,5]. In the paediatric setting, LS almost always affects the genital area, with only approximately 6% of patients having extragenital involvement [6]. A family history is found in 12–17% of cases [7,8].

Aetiology and pathogenesis. The aetiology is unknown, with autoimmune, genetic and possibly other factors postulated but not proven. Evidence is increasing that it is an autoimmune-related disorder, with many affected adult female patients having circulating autoantibodies to extracellular matrix protein and basement membrane zone components BP180/collagen XVII and BP230 as well as other organ-specific autoantibodies, in particular thyroid autoantobodies [9–11]. In a cohort of 70 patients, 15% were found to have concurrent autoimmune disease and 65% had a family history of autoimmune disease [3]. There is an association with other autoimmune disorders, the most frequently reported being vitiligo, alopecia areata and thyroid disease; however, it appears to be more common to find circulating antibodies than frank autoimmune dysfunction and the latter is uncommon in children.

Evidence for an association with particular HLA types in lichen sclerosus is conflicting, but an increased association with DQ7 has been found in adults and children [12]. More recently, researchers have described the coexistence of HLA B08 and HLA B18 in four siblings with LS, with a further unaffected sister not having these alleles [13]. Another group of researchers compared vulval LS tissue from 16 patients with tissue from 16 vulval control samples and found a significant increase of lipid peroxidation products, particularly within epidermal basal cells, colocalizing with ECM-1.17. The authors also demonstrated a significantly reduced expression of manganese superoxide dismutase, a mitochondrial enzyme that catalyses the reaction from superoxide anions to hydrogen peroxide. The enhanced oxidative stress caused by reduced enzyme expression could be a pathogenic factor in the autoimmune or neoplastic associations observed in some patients [14].

The reports of an association with *Borrelia burgdorferi* seem to depend on geographical location, but the association is still unclear and remains controversial [15]. Lichen sclerosus has been described as being common in Turner syndrome [16].

Pathology. The histopathological features were described first by Darier [17] and later by Hewitt [18]. The typical histological findings include a thinned, effaced epidermis, with or without an overlying hyperkeratosis. In the reticular dermis, immediately beneath the epidermis, there is a broad band of homogenized collagen. A lymphocytic infiltrate may be present just below the abnormal dermis (Fig. 162.6). In some areas, this infiltrate can be seen along the dermoepidermal junction, with areas of liquefactive degeneration similar to those changes seen in lichen planus.

Clinical features. The mean age of onset of LS in children is about 5 years of age. There is commonly a delay in diagnosis of up to 2 years.The main symptom in girls is itch and soreness, but dysuria and constipation are not uncommon when there is vulval or perianal fissuring. In about 5% it may be asymptomatic and found incidentally. The distribution is classically a figure of eight encircling the vulva, perineum and perianal skin but this is highly variable. It does not, however, involve the vagina (Fig. 162.7). Perianal involvement is not seen in boys.

In girls the initial cutaneous signs are erythema, excoriations and lichenification (Fig. 162.8) which progresses to a porcelain white, well-demarcated plaque with textural

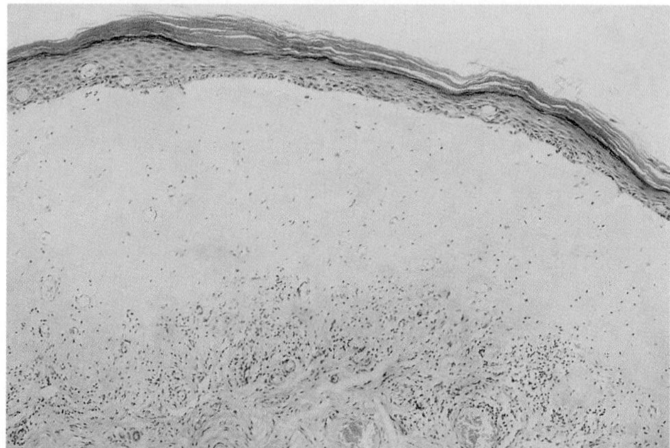

Fig. 162.6 Histology of lichen sclerosus. The epidermis is thinned and effaced. The superficial dermis is hyalinized and there is a lymphocytic infiltrate immediately beneath this zone.

change described in appearance as 'cigarette paper' wrinkling (Fig. 162.9). There may be blisters, purpura and extensive ecchymoses which can be mistaken for child abuse [19] (Fig. 162.10). This is not usually the case, but it must be appreciated that lichen sclerosus can koebnerize and, if a child was the subject of abuse, it could possibly exacerbate the symptoms and signs [20].

Although rare, milia may follow blister formation [21]. With time, untreated cases develop architectural distortion [22]. The labia minora may fail to develop or be lost due to scarring. The clitoral hood can become tethered to the glans of the clitoris and seal over completely. Fusion of the labia is described in association with lichen sclerosus in children [23]. Dysuria is common. If perianal involvement is severe, the associated fissuring results in painful defaecation, which can subsequently lead to constipation and faecal retention. Extragenital involvement is rare in children, occurring in less than 10%.

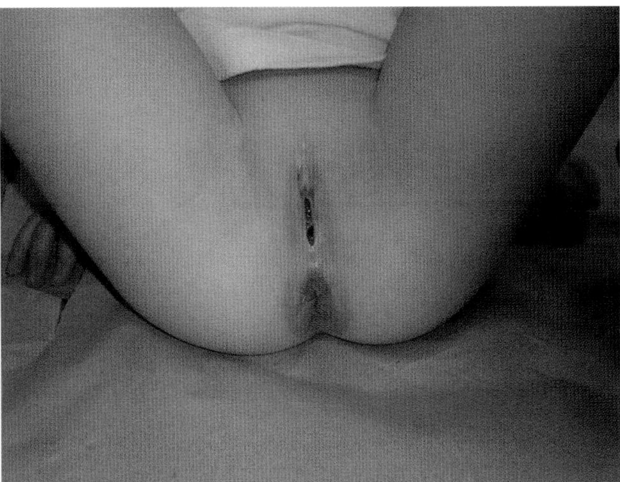

Fig. 162.7 Vulval lichen sclerosus showing classic figure of eight distribution.

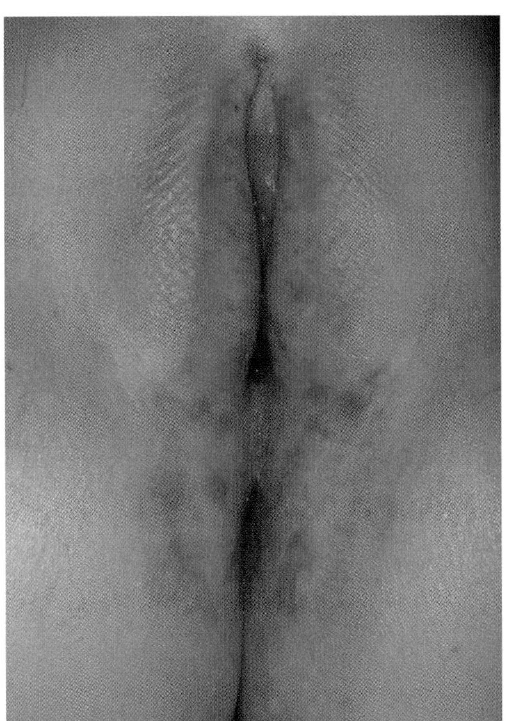

Fig. 162.8 Early, erythematous phase of lichen sclerosus involving the vulval and perianal skin in a figure of eight configuration.

Complications.

Scarring

Untreated, approximately 50% of children with LS of the vulva progress to scarring [22] with loss of the labia minora and clitoral substance. Fusion of the labia minora can result in loss of the introitus, causing difficulties with micturition. If there is significant introital narrowing, this may lead to problems with sexual intercourse in adult life [24]. This has been underappreciated in the literature on childhood vulval LS, but is of great importance. It can be halted by treatment and additionally early scarring can be reversed by treatment (see later in

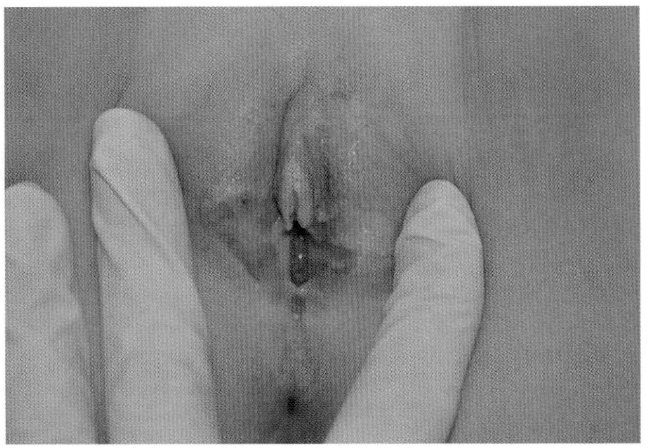

Fig. 162.9 Vulval lichen sclerosus with typical white 'cigarette paper' wrinkling and erosions.

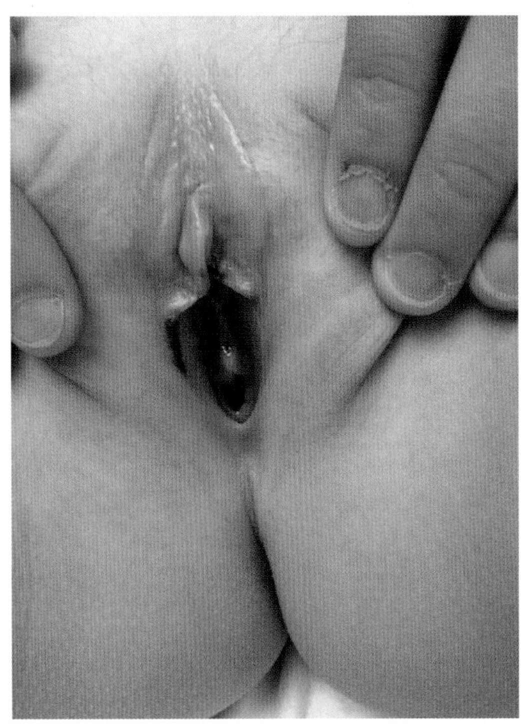

Fig. 162.10 Ecchymoses of introital skin.

this chapter). A pseudocyst of the clitoris may develop due to the accumulation of keratinous debris under the fused clitoral hood.

Malignancy

Squamous cell carcinoma (SCC) may occur on a background of genital lichen sclerosus with the incidence being 4–5% in adult women. The risk for children is unknown but is likely to be negligible. However, there are very rare case reports of SCC in young adults in their late teens and early twenties who may have had lichen sclerosus in childhood [3,25,26]. Melanoma has rarely been reported in association with vulval LS in children [27].

Prognosis. Children respond well to treatment but the previously held belief that the disease remits at puberty was challenged as early as 1987 [28]. There is no doubt that it may continue into adolescence [29]; indeed, studies have shown that although symptoms may improve, the condition persists in the majority, at least 75% [30]. If scarring and architectural changes have occurred prior to initiation of treatment, they are permanent [22]. In most cases, scarring does not interfere with future sexual function, pregnancy or normal vaginal delivery; however, it may have severe psychological effects associated with altered body image. Untreated, the disease can continue unremittingly for many years. Phimosis that does not respond to topical treatment will require a circumcision.

Differential diagnosis. In the early inflammatory stages, the disease can be mistaken for psoriasis or eczema but once the characteristic whitening occurs, these diseases can easily be excluded (Fig. 162.11). Psoriasis can coexist with LS, creating a confusing clinical picture with superimposed erythema. If blistering occurs, vulval bullous pemphigoid may be suspected. Vulval lichen planus is exceptionally rare in children but does come into the differential where scarring has distorted the vulval architecture on presentation. Vitiligo is white but does not result in a textural change in the skin or scarring (Fig. 162.12). Vitiligo and LS can occur together (Fig. 162.13). As already mentioned, if there are erosions and/or extensive ecchymoses, a mistaken diagnosis of child abuse may be made. A diagnosis of LS does not either rule out or prove sexual assault.

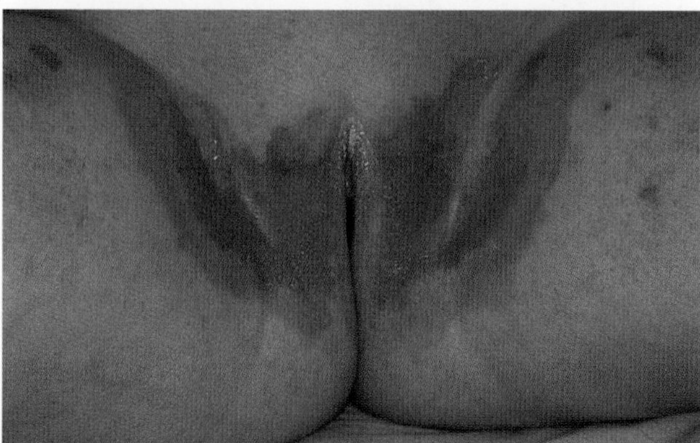

Fig. 162.11 Differential diagnosis: psoriasis extending into the genitocrural folds.

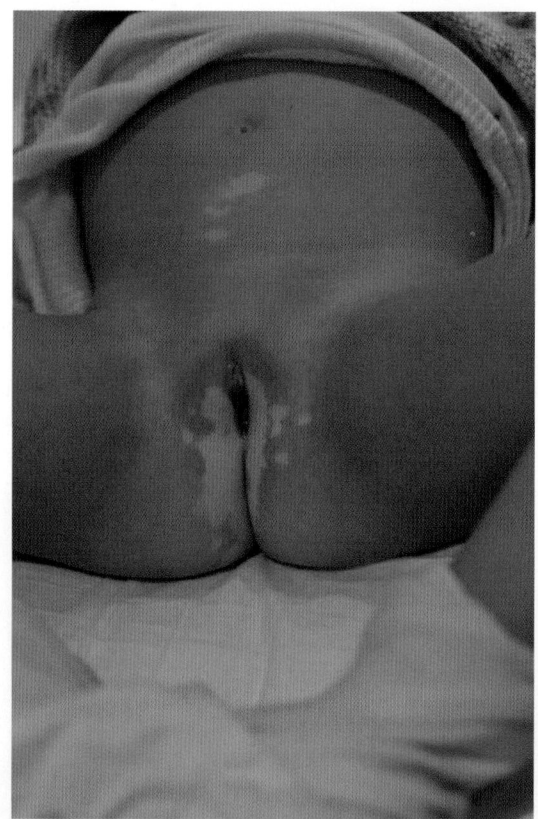

Fig. 162.12 Vitiligo.

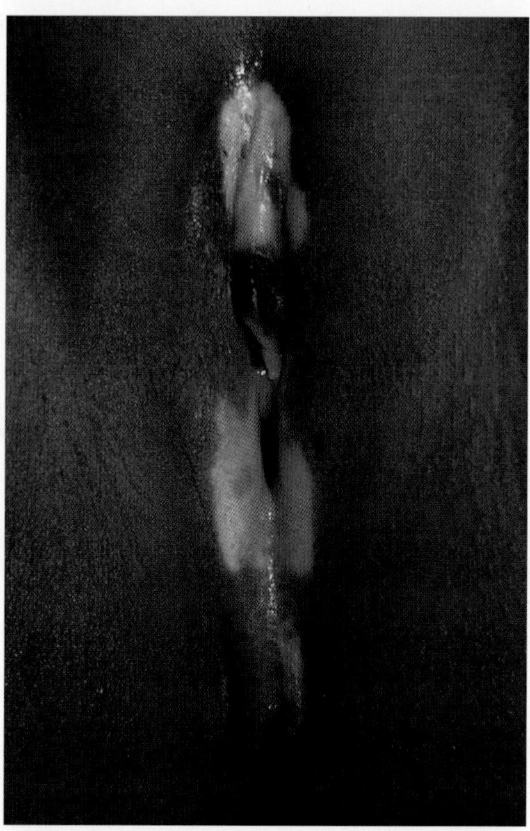

Fig. 162.13 Differential diagnosis: vitiligo results in loss of pigmentation only but on the right-hand side of the vulva, an area of textural change can be seen as the patient had lichen sclerosus as well as vitiligo.

Diagnosis. In children, LS is usually diagnosed clinically and a biopsy is only required if the diagnosis is in doubt. Although there are a number of differential diagnoses in adults, including malignancy, this is not the case in children.

Treatment.

Medical

Topical corticosteroids. The treatment of choice is a potent topical corticosteroid. The majority of studies have used clobetasol propionate 0.05% [31–34]; however, it is by no means the only effective medication and in most cases of unnecessary potency [22]. Because of the relative rarity of childhood LS, there are no randomized controlled trials comparing potency of steroid, frequency of application or length of treatment. What exists are case series which are not suitable for metaanalysis.

The first account of the use of superpotent topical corticosteroids to treat lichen sclerosus in adults was published in 1991 [35]. Prior to this, it had been considered inappropriate to use potent preparations on the vulva. Previous reported treatments with weak topical corticosteroids, topical testosterone and progesterone were ineffective, leaving the impression that LS was a very difficult condition to treat. Once it was discovered that vulval LS responded quickly and reliably to potent topical corticosteroid, many other authors confirmed this in subsequent studies and it is now considered gold standard treatment to obtain remission in children as well as adults. The majority of published studies have examined the use of clobetasol propionate, for no other reason than it was the subject of the first successful study in 1991. It is not necessary to use clobetasol to treat lichen sclerosus in children. Any potent topical corticosteroid will be effective.

Australian researchers were the first to describe the effective use of the potent topical corticosteroid betamethasone dipropionate 0.05% to successfully treat paediatric vulval LS in a cohort of 11 patients [36]. Susbequently, American researchers demonstrated the effectiveness of a 6–8-week course of twice-daily high-potency topical corticosteroids [37]. More recently, it has been confirmed by a large study of 327 patients, which included 74 girls, that ultrapotent topical corticosteroids are an effective treatment for vulval lichen sclerosus, relieving symptoms in most and completely reversing the skin changes in 23% of patients [38]. In this study, patients were treated for a minimum of three months with potent topical corticosteroids, including clobetasol propionate 0.05%, betamethasone 0.1% and clobetasone butyrate 0.05%. Of the 74 girls in the study, a reported response of symptoms to topical treatment was available in 36, with 26 (72%) of these girls graded as symptom free, nine girls (25%) graded as a partial response and one girl (3%) graded as a poor response. In another study, it was demonstrated that a 2–4-week course of clobetasol propionate is an effective and safe treatment for premenarchal vulval LS [39]. However, in this study population recurrences were common (82%), although most girls responded to retreatment. Only 18% had no recurrences, 46% had occasional relapses and 36% had frequent flares.

Although guidelines suggest an initial treatment of three months with an ultrapotent topical corticosteroid, it has been demonstrated that best outcomes occur when the aim of treatment is the disappearance of abnormal signs as well as the resolution of symptoms [22]. This may take longer than three months. While the disadvantage of prolonged treatment might be an increase in the adverse effects of local corticosteroids such as erythema and telangiectasia, these adverse effects always reverse with reduction of topical corticosteroid use.

Oral corticosteroids are not required nor are they effective, and failure to respond to the potent topical steroid ointment should raise the possibility of noncompliance, another diagnosis or sexual abuse. A soap substitute and emollient are useful adjuncts to treatment.

Topical calcineurin inhibitors. Calcineurin inhibitors, such as tacrolimus and pimecrolimus, have been described as potentially playing a role in the treatment of LS in children and adults. In 2006, a multicentre research group released the results of their phase II trial to assess the safety and efficacy of tacrolimus ointment 0.1% for the treatment of LS [40]; 84 patients (49 women, 32 men and three girls) aged between 5 and 85 years with longstanding, active disease were treated with topical tacrolimus ointment 0.1% twice daily. Clearance of active LS was reached by 43% of patients at 24 weeks of treatment and partial resolution was reached in a further 34% of patients. Maximal effects of therapy occurred between weeks 10 and 24 of treatment. There were no adverse events during the 18 months of follow-up.

In a double-blind, randomized prospective study evaluating topical clobetasol propionate 0.05% versus topical tacrolimus 0.1% in 55 patients with vulval lichen sclerosus, of whom five were under 18 years old, over a three-month period, both groups showed a decrease of symptoms and signs, but a significantly higher number of patients in the clobetasol group had an absence of signs and symptoms of lichen sclerosus [41]. With a condition that requires prolonged treatment, it is unknown whether calcineurin inhibitors are as safe as corticosteroids.

There is a theoretical risk of malignant transformation due to local immunosuppression, which is an important consideration given the well-described association of vulval LS and malignancy. SCC has been reported in an adult with LS in association with pimecrolimus and tacrolimus treatment [42,43]. There are insufficient data to recommend calcineurin inhibitors to treat LS, particularly given the safety of long-term low-potency corticosteroids in this condition.

Long-term maintenance treatment. Until recently, data on maintenance treatment of LS in children and also adults were lacking. The weakness of many published studies, particularly in children, has been inadequate length of follow-up. The data available on long-term treatment outcomes from previous studies in children suggest that although it is possible to suppress symptoms in about

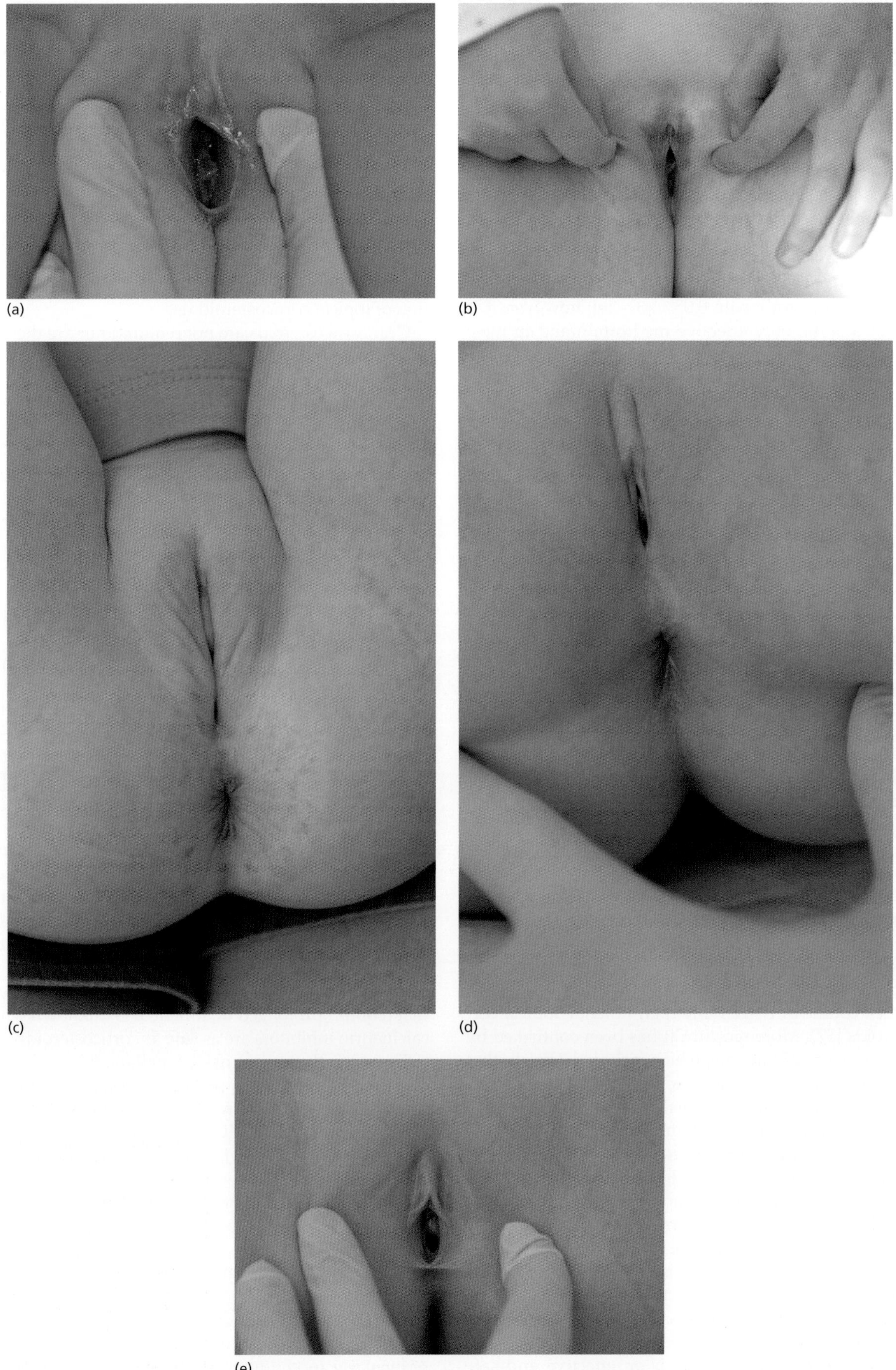

Fig. 162.14 Vulval lichen sclerosus with scarring (a) before treatment with potent topical corticosteroid and (b) during maintenance treatment with moderate topical corticosteroid. There is some erythema as a side-effect. (c–e) Vulval lichen sclerosus (c) before treatment and (d,e) during maintenance treatment with moderate topical corticosteroid.

75% of patients using treatment only when symptomatic, fewer than half of these treated patients achieve consistent disease control and about 40% develop scarring [22]. The psychological effects of abnormal vulval anatomy as a result of LS have never been studied but have the potential to be problematic.

Two recent studies, one in adults and one in children, have demonstrated the importance of maintenance treatment in LS and have shown that early intervention maintains normal skin and prevents scarring [22,44]. As remission at puberty is unlikely, parents need to understand the importance of long-term treatment from the outset. The issue of how to ensure ongoing compliance and surveillance in adolescents is difficult and many are lost to follow-up because of embarrassment.

The principle of maintaining remission is that topical corticosteroid potency should be titrated to individual patient requirements to achieve normal skin texture and colour. Once remission has been achieved with potent topical corticosteroid, the potency is reduced to a maintenance level over a period of 3–6 months. The patient is regularly reviewed to adjust dose. In the long term, it is often possible to maintain remission with weak to moderate-strength corticosteroids and in practice these have minimal side-effects, at the most mild erythema and telangiectasia (Fig. 162.14). Ideally, children should be seen once or twice a year to encourage compliance and adjust potency of medication [22]. Although there are no trials comparing topical corticosteroids, they are probably not necessary. What is important is the clinical response and any preparation that maintains normal skin is suitable.

Reassurance is also very important as parents now have access to medical information on the internet; some of the information is biased and may cause great concern. It is important to discuss these problems in consultations to avoid unnecessary concern. The majority of girls with well-managed lichen sclerosus should expect to have no problems with sexual intercourse in later life and to undergo a normal vaginal delivery at the end of any pregnancies.

Follow-up. When a prepubertal child presents with LS, it is important to realize that this patient will need long-term treatment and follow-up. Accordingly, realistic advice to these patients and their parents is that puberty may not be an endpoint to treatment. Adolescents find genital examination embarrassing and anxiety provoking and it is important that they have a trusting relationship, cemented prior to puberty, with their treating practitioner, which will allow ongoing follow-up throughout the teenage years even when apparent remission has been achieved.

Surgical

Only rarely is surgery indicated in the treatment of young girls with lichen sclerosus, as surgical excision may result in koebnerization and exacerbation of the disease postoperatively. In a very small number of cases, surgical division of persistently fused labia minora may be necessary if there is interference with micturition or menstruation; if a clitoral pseudocyst develops, surgical intervention is necessary to release the underlying collection of keratinous debris [45].

References

1 Hallopeau H. Lichen plan sclereux. Ann Dermatol Syph 1887;10: 447–9.

2 Meffert JJ, David BM, Grimwood RE. Lichen sclerosus. J Am Acad Dermatol 1995;32:393–416.

3 Wallace HJ. Lichen sclerosus et atrophicus. Trans St John's Dermatol Soc 1971;57:9–30.

4 Berth-Jones J, Graham-Brown RAC, Burns DA. Lichen sclerosus et atrophicus: a review of 15 cases in young girls. Clin Exp Dermatol 1991;16:14–17.

5 Fivozinsky KB, Laufer MR. Vulvar disorders in prepubertal girls. J Reprod Med 1998;48:763–73.

6 Powell J, Wojnarowska F. Childhood vulvar lichen sclerosus: an increasingly common problem. J Am Acad Dermatol 2001;44(5):803–6.

7 Sahn ES, Bluestein EL, Oliva S. Familial lichen sclerosus et atrophicus in childhood. Pediatr Dermatol 1994;11:160–3.

8 Sherman V, McPherson T, Baldo M et al. The high rate of familial lichen sclerosus suggests a genetic contribution: an observational cohort study. J Eur Acad Dermatol Venereol 2010;24(9):1031–4.

9 Chan I, Oyama N, Neill SM et al. Characterization of IgG autoantibodies to extracellular matrix protein 1 in lichen sclerosus. Clin Exp Dermatol 2004;29:499–504.

10 Goolamali SK, Barnes EW, Irvine WJ et al. Organ-specific antibodies in patients with lichen sclerosus. BMJ 1974;iv:78–9.

11 Howard A, Dean D, Cooper S et al. Circulating basement membrane zone antibodies are found in lichen sclerosus of the vulva. Australas. J Dermatol 2004;45:12–15.

12 Powell J, Wojnarowska F, Winsey S et al. Lichen sclerosus premenarche: autoimmunity and immunogenetics. Br J Dermatol 2000;142: 481–4.

13 Senturk N, Aydin F, Birinci A et al. Coexistence of HLA B08 and HLA B18 in four siblings with lichen sclerosus. Dermatology 2004;208: 64–6.

14 Sander CS, Ali I, Dean D et al. Oxidative stress is implicated in the pathogenesis of lichen sclerosus. Br J Dermatol 2004;151:627–35.

15 Edmonds E, Mavin S, Francis N et al. *Borrelia burgdorferi* is not associated with genital lichen sclerosus in men. Br J Dermatol 2009;160: 459–60.

16 Chakhtoura Z, Vigoureux S, Courtillot C et al. Vulvar lichen sclerosus is very frequent in women with Turner syndrome. J Clin Endocrinol Metabl 2014;99(4):1103–4.

17 Darier J. Lichen plan sclereux. Ann Dermatol Syph 1892;3:833–7.

18 Hewitt J. Histologic criteria for lichen sclerosus of the vulva. J Reprod Med 1986;31:781–7.

19 Handfield-Jones SE, Hinde FRJ, Kennedy CTC. Lichen sclerosus et atrophicus in children misdiagnosed as sexual abuse. BMJ 1987;294: 1404–5.

20 Warrington SA, San Lazaro C. Lichen sclerosus et atrophicus and sexual abuse. Arch Dis Child 1996;75:512–16.

21 Leppard B, Sneddon IB. Milia occurring in lichen sclerosus et atrophicus. Br J Dermatol 1975;92:711–14.

22 Ellis E, Fischer G. Prepubertal-onset vulvar lichen sclerosus: the importance of maintenance therapy in long-term outcomes. Pediatr Dermatol 2015;32(4):461–7.

23 Gibbon KL, Bewley AP, Salisbury JA. Labial fusion in children: a presenting feature of genital lichen sclerosus? Pediatr Dermatol 1991;16: 388–91.

24 Ridley CM. Genital lichen sclerosus (lichen sclerosus et atrophicus) in childhood and adolescence. J Roy Soc Med 1993;86:69–75.

25 Cario GM, House MJ, Paradinos FJ. Squamous cell carcinoma of the vulva in association with mixed vulvar dystrophy in an 18 yr old girl. Case report. Br J Obstet Gynaecol 1984;91:87–90.

26 Pelisse M. Lichen sclerosus. Ann Dermatol Venereol 1987;114:411–19.

27 La Spina M, Meli MC, de Pasquale R et al. Vulvar melanoma associated with lichen sclerosus in a child: case report and literature review. Pediatr Dermatol 2016;33(3):e190–4.

28 Ridley CM. Lichen sclerosus et atrophicus. Arch Dermatol 1987;123: 457–60.

29 Smith S, Fischer G. Childhood onset vulvar lichen sclerosus does not resolve at puberty: a prospective case series. Pediatr Dermatol 2009;26(6):725–9.

30 **Powell J, Wojnarowska F. Childhood vulvar lichen sclerosus: the course after puberty. J Reprod Med 2002;47:706–9.**
31 **Fischer G, Rogers M. Treatment of childhood vulvar lichen sclerosus with potent topical corticosteroid. Pediatr Dermatol 1997;14:235–8.**
32 Smith YR, Quint EH. Clobetasol propionate in the treatment of premenarchal vulvar lichen sclerosus. Obstet Gynecol 2001;98:588–91.
33 **Garzon MC, Paller AS. Ultrapotent topical corticosteroid treatment of childhood lichen sclerosus. Arch Dermatol 1999;135:525–8.**
34 Neill SM, Tatnall FM, Cox NH. Guidelines on the management of lichen sclerosus. Br J Dermatol 2002;147:640–9.
35 Dalziel KL, Millard PR, Wojnarowska F. The treatment of vulval lichen sclerosus with a very potent steroid (clobetasole propionate 0.05%) cream. Br J Dermatol 1991;124:461–4.
36 **Fischer G, Rogers M. Treatment of childhood vulvar lichen sclerosus with potent topical corticosteroid. Pediatr Dermatol 1997;14:235–8.**
37 **Garzon MC, Paller AS. Ultrapotent topical corticosteroid treatment of childhood genital lichen sclerosus. Arch Dermatol 1999;135:525–8.**
38 Cooper SM, Goa XH, Powell JJ, Wojnarowska F. Does treatment of vulvar lichen sclerosus influence its prognosis? Arch Dermatol 2004;140:702–6.
39 Smith YR, Quint EH. Clobetasol propionate in the treatment of premenarchal vulvar lichen sclerosus. Obstet Gynecol 2001;98:588–91.
40 Hengge UR, Krause W, Hofmann H et al. Multicentre, phase II trial on the safety and efficacy of topical tacrolimus ointment for the treatment of lichen sclerosus. Br J Dermatol 2006;155:1021–8.
41 Funaro D, Lovett A, Leroux N, Powell J. A double-blind, randomized prospective study evaluating topical clobetasol propionate 0.05% versus topical tacrolimus 0.1% in patients with vulvar lichen sclerosus. J Am Acad Dermatol 2014;71(1):84–91.
42 **Fischer G, Bradford J. Topical immunosuppressants, genital lichen sclerosus and the risk of squamous cell carcinoma: a case report. J Reprod Med 2007;52:329–31.**
43 **Ormerod AD. Topical tacrolimus and pimecrolimus and the risk of cancer: how much cause for concern? Br J Dermatol 2005;153:701–5.**
44 **Lee A, Bradford J, Fischer G. Long-term management of adult vulvar lichen sclerosus. A prospective cohort study of 507 women. JAMA Dermatol 2015;151(10):1061–7.**
45 Paniel BJ, Rouzier R. Surgical procedures in benign vulval disease. In: Neill S, Lewis F (eds) Ridley's The Vulva. Chichester: Wiley-Blackwell, 2009:235–6.

Lichen sclerosus in boys (syn. balanitis xerotica obliterans)

Lichen sclerosus in boys occurs most frequently on the prepuce and glans (Fig 162.15). The meatus and urethra may also be involved. It is said to be much less common than in girls; however, it may be underrecognized and is thought to be the main cause of acquired phimosis [1]. It is possible that it is more common than previously assumed, as not all circumcision specimens are examined histologically for lichen sclerosus [2].

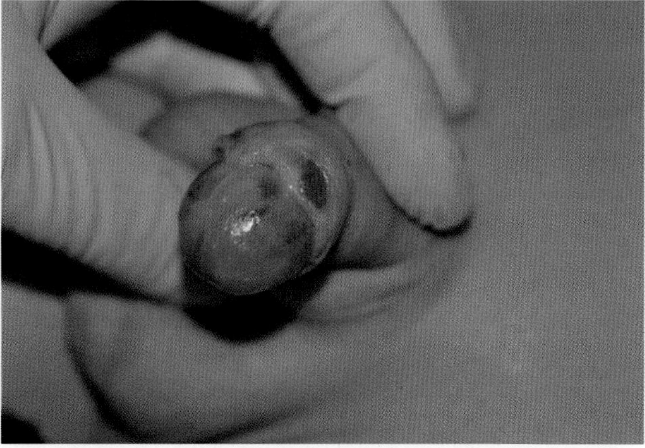

Fig. 162.15 Lichen sclerosus of the glans penis.

In boys, the disease is often asymptomatic; however, dysuria and acquired inability to retract the foreskin are the most common symptoms.

The clinical appearance is of a white sclerotic skin change of the distal prepuce. Scarring leads to progressive phimosis and attempts to retract reveal a white ring. If the foreskin is able to be retracted, it reveals the glans to be thickened and white, with retraction of the frenulum. In severe cases, stenosis of the urethral meatus occurs but extension into the urethra is rare.

Lichen sclerosus has been reported in brothers and in identical twins [2]; however, the literature contains very little evidence for familial occurrence. It is more common in boys with hypospadias [3]. Carcinoma of the penis is reported in 3–4% of adult males with LS but not in boys. In adult males, definitive management reduces this risk [4]. As in girls, it is unknown whether childhood-onset LS predisposes to early-onset genital carcinoma.

Lichen sclerosus is a disease of the uncircumcised male and it has been postulated that the moist environment under the foreskin contributes to pathogenesis [4,5]. This is supported by the fact that total (but not partial) circumcision has a high success rate [2].

Management. Lichen sclerosus in boys responds to potent topical corticosteroids; however, as in girls, this treatment often needs to be followed up with maintenance therapy. This is now first-line therapy with a success rate of 50–60% [4]. Circumcision is curative in the majority, but even after this recurrence is possible. Circumcision specimens should be submitted for histopathology and if there is evidence of lichen sclerosus, follow-up should be maintained. Cases of meatal stenosis without evident disease have been reported after circumcision [6].

References

1 **Becker K. Lichen sclerosus in boys. Dtsch Arztebl Int 2011;108(4): 53–8.**
2 Kiss A, Király L, Kutasy B, Merksz M. High incidence of balanitis xerotica obliterans in boys with phimosis: prospective 10-year study. Pediatr Dermatol 2005;22:305–8.
3 Mattioli G, Repetto P, Carlini C et al. LSA in children with phimosis and hypospadias. Pediatr Surg Int 2002;18:273–5.
4 **Edmonds V, Hunt S, Hawkins D et al. Clinical parameters in male genital lichen sclerosus: a case series of 329 patients. J Eur Acad Dermatol Venereol 2012;26(6):730–7.**
5 Gargollo PC, Kzakewich HP, Bauer SB et al. Balanitis xerotica obliterans in boys. J Urol 2005;174:1409–12.
6 Homer L. Buchanan KJ, Nasr B et al. Meatal stenosis in boys following circumcision for lichen sclerosus (balanitis xerotica obliterans). J Urol 2014;192(6):1784–8.

Birthmarks in the genital area

Special considerations in the genital area

Birthmarks may occur on the genital area as on any other part of the skin, but the importance of lesions in this location is that they may be mistaken for more sinister conditions. For example, pigmented naevi often raise queries of melanoma, where they might be ignored elsewhere, and epidermal naevi may be mistaken for warts or recalcitrant eczema. Any ulcerating lesion may cause queries about sexual abuse [1]. Haemangiomas and vascular malformations [2–11] are dealt with elsewhere in detail (see Chapters 118 and 119).

Melanocytic naevi

Pigmented naevi may occur on the genital and perianal area; they may be congenital lesions or appear at any stage of childhood (Fig. 162.16). The congenital lesions tend to be larger than late-onset ones. Pigmented naevi of the genital region rarely present a problem, but they do frequently raise fears of melanoma [4].

Despite this, melanoma in children is rare, and there have been very few reports of childhood genital melanoma [12]. There is no documented evidence that pigmented naevi of the genital area have a particular malignant potential [13]. Pigmented naevi with the histopathology of 'atypical naevi' occur on the genital skin, but a 2008 study confirms that they have a benign clinical course and cautions against overdiagnosis of melanoma [14].

Bannayan–Riley–Ruvalcaba syndrome (Ruvalcaba–Myhre–Smith syndrome) OMIM 153480

The PTEN hamartoma-tumour syndromes include at least two clinically different but overlapping cancer predisposition syndromes: Cowden syndrome and Bannayan–Riley–Ruvalcaba syndrome, both with autosomal dominant inheritance resulting from germline mutations in the *PTEN* tumour suppressor gene on chromosome 10q23.3 [15,16].

Bannayan–Riley–Ruvalcaba syndrome was first described in 1980 by Ruvalcaba et al. [17], as a classic triad of polyposis coli, pigmented macules of the penis and macrocephaly. The polyps, which may not appear until adult life, can occur throughout the gastrointestinal tract and have been reported on the tongue. They present with painless rectal bleeding and, sometimes, intussusception.

Other features described with the syndrome include developmental delay, hypotonia, myopathy, ocular abnormalities, café-au-lait macules, lipomas, haemangiomas and vascular malformations, facial verrucous or acanthosis nigricans-like lesions and multiple skin tags of the neck, axilla and groin [18]. Musculoskeletal changes and neuropathy have been reported [19].

The pigmented macules appear during childhood or adolescence and then persist and present as a speckled lentiginosis of the penis or vulva [20]. The syndrome can be differentiated from Peutz–Jeghers syndrome by the presence in the latter of pigmented macules of the lips and buccal mucosa.

Epidermal naevi

Epidermal naevi are uncommon and about 50% are not present at birth although most develop within the first year of life, seldom appearing after the age of 7. They may continue to extend for up to five years after they first appear [21]. They usually have a warty surface and are arranged in whorls or streaks, following the lines of Blaschko. Both verrucous and inflammatory epidermal naevi may involve the genital area. They may be localized or part of a larger lesion that extends to the leg and buttock.

Verrucous epidermal naevi have a warty, hyperkeratotic surface (Fig. 162.17). They are usually pigmented, but when they extend onto the macerated skin of the perineum or labia minora, they may have a white appearance. They may be papillomatous in some areas (Fig. 162.18).

Inflammatory epidermal naevi (ILVEN) are linear and have a scaly, erythematous surface. They are quite itchy and are therefore commonly mistaken for recalcitrant eczema. ILVEN have been rarely described involving the inguinogenital region [21,22]. In boys, ILVEN is described in the penoscrotal and inguingal skin region and in girls, on the vulva [23].

Because epidermal naevi have a tendency to extend with time, they may be confused with an inflammatory

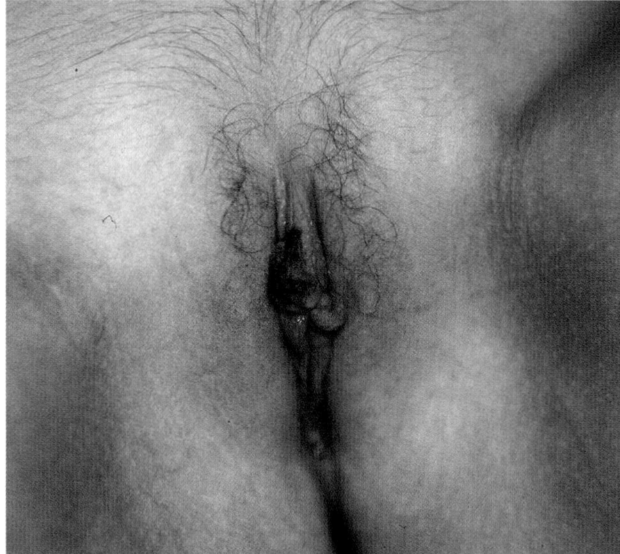

Fig. 162.16 Melanocytic naevus of the clitoris.

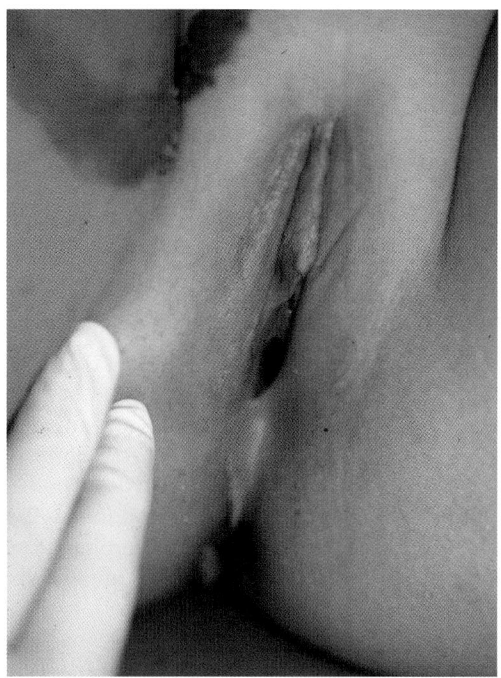

Fig. 162.17 Warty linear epidermal naevus.

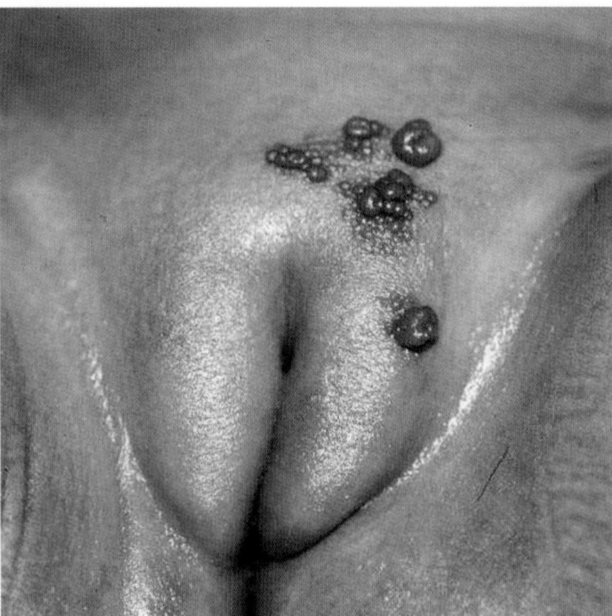

Fig. 162.18 Papillomatous epidermal naevus.

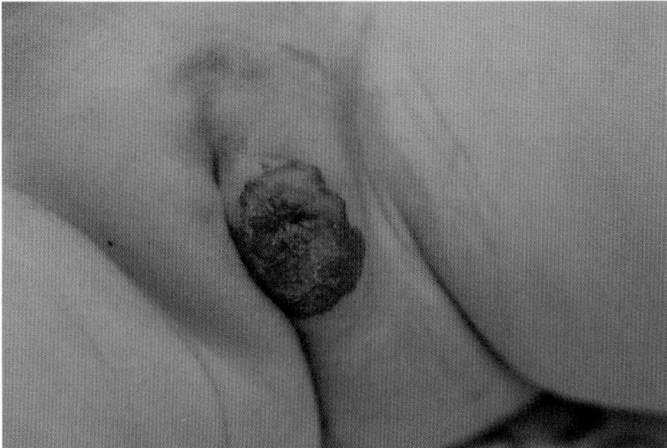

Fig. 162.19 Ulcerated haemangioma of infancy involving the vulva.

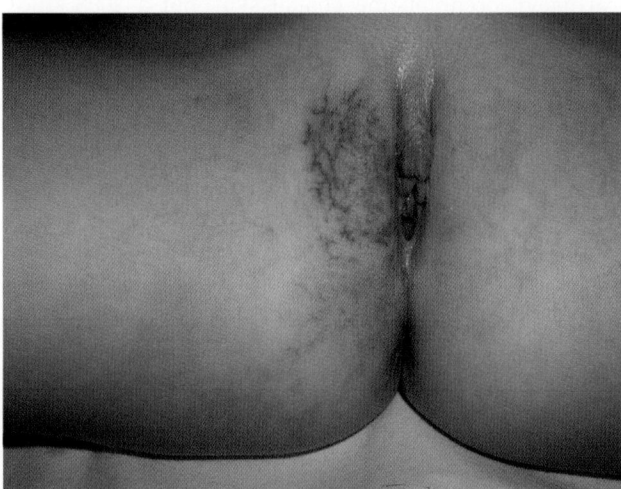

Fig. 162.20 Venous malformation of the vulva.

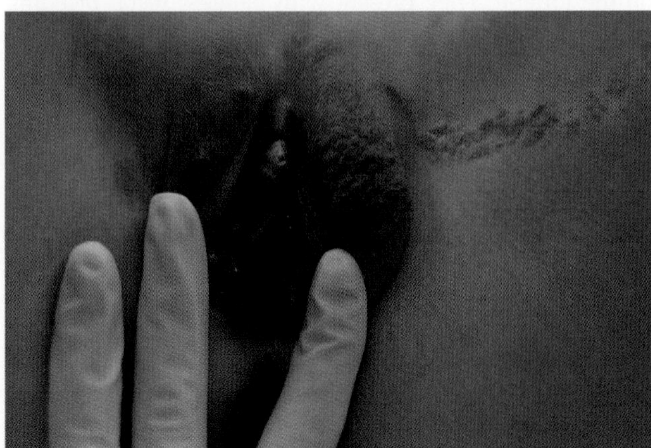

Fig. 162.21 Lymphatic malformation of the vulva with associated linear epidermal naevus.

dermatosis. If they become large, they can interfere with function, particularly in the perianal area. Epidermal naevi can be mistaken for warts, in turn giving rise to queries of child abuse. If they are itchy, they can be mistaken for treatment-resistant lichenified eczema or napkin dermatitis [4,22]. Naevus comedonicus has been reported on the vulva [24].

Management. Itchy genital epidermal naevi may be very resistant to topical therapy [22] and it is not uncommon for epidermal naevi of the genital region to cause enough trouble to require at least partial excision. For example, a warty perianal lesion is best removed, and sometimes recalcitrant itching is relieved only by surgically excising the lesion. However, if they are not causing problems, it is best just to reassure the patient and leave the lesions alone. There is no significant malignant potential.

Vascular naevi

Haemangioma of the genital area is common in both sexes and in a case series of genitourinary and perineal vascular anomalies, haemangioma was by far the most common lesion [25]. Ulceration is a common problem (Fig. 162.19). This can be so extensive that it obscures the original lesion and can be confused with child abuse. Details of haemangioma of infancy are discussed in Chapter 119.

Many genital vascular lesions have been described in children, including venous, lymphatic and mixed venolymphatic lesions (Figs 162.20, 162.21 and 162.22). Lymphangioma of the scrotum has been described [26,27]. These cases present with a scrotal mass and may be associated with other genital anomalies. Lymphangioma has also been described as a penile and a vulval lesion presenting with skin-coloured papules [28,29], and a single case of verrucous haemangioma of the glans penis has been described [30]. A haemangioma has been reported to cause clitoral hypertrophy [31].

In a large series of female patients with vascular anomalies, 2.6% were found to have lesions of the external genitalia. These presented with cutaneous macular stains, swelling, deformity, bleeding, fluid leakage and infection [32]. Vascular lesions may increase in size at puberty [33].

Patients with Klippel–Trenaunay syndrome, characterized by vascular malformation of capillary, venous and

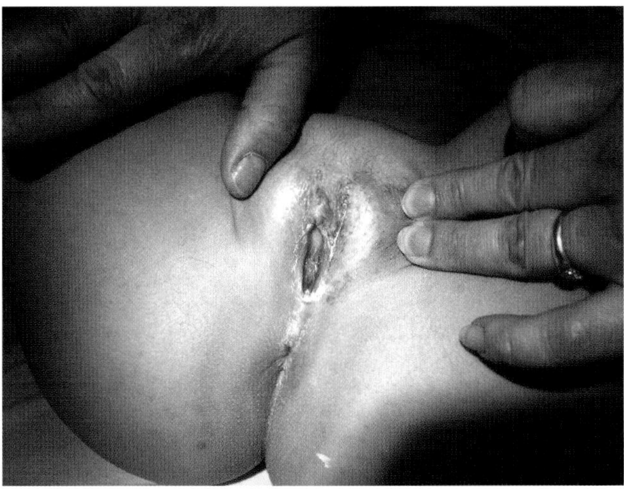

Fig. 162.22 Lymphangioma of the vulva.

lymphatic systems associated with soft tissue and bone hypertrophy, frequently have genitourinary involvement, including cutaneous and anatomical genital abnormalities, the overall incidence being reported to be 30%. Bleeding from genital lesions, as well as haematuria, may occur in these patients and approximately half of them eventually require surgical intervention for genitourinary complications [34,35].

Management. Genital vascular lesions other than localized haemangioma of infancy usually require magnetic resonance imaging, ultrasound, angiography and gynaecological exploration for full diagnostic clarification. Extension into the pelvis is common [25]. They can present a very difficult therapeutic challenge and are frequently devastating for the patient and family. Excision of these lesions may be very difficult; however, depending on the age of the patient surgical treatment may involve anything from local excision to vulvectomy [36]. Treatment with direct injection venography using sclerotherapy has been described as a successful treatment for vulval venous malformation [37]. Systemic sirolimus in the treatment of unresectable lymphatic malformations may be effective in the future for patients with inoperable genital lesions [38].

Papular acantholytic dyskeratosis of the vulva

Papular acantholytic dyskeratosis of the vulva is a rare condition that presents with a papular eruption of the vulva [39]. The lesions are scattered, skin-coloured to white, slightly keratotic papules associated with multiple grouped superficial erosions. The lesions are found on the labia majora.

Clinical features. The condition presents in childhood with white papules and erosions found bilaterally on the labia majora. There may be associated pruritus but it has also been described as asymptomatic [40]. Both the pruritus and clinical appearance may regress with time [41].

Most previous case reports have been in adults but the condition has been described in a child [41]. The condition does not appear to be familial.

Histology. Histopathology is distinctive, with hyperkeratosis, acantholysis, dyskeratotic cells resembling corps ronds and irregular proliferation of basaloid cells. Immunofluorescence is negative [41,42].

Differential diagnosis. This condition, although rare, is important as it may be confused with multiple flat genital warts or with papular lichen sclerosus. Histologically, it needs to be differentiated from Hailey–Hailey disease, Darier disease and warty dyskeratoma. Epidermal naevi, including those found on the vulva, may show acantholysis but are usually unilateral [43].

Management. This condition runs a chronic course. Treatment described so far has been disappointing. No specific treatment has been described in children and reassurance that this is a benign condition may be all that is required.

References

1 Hosteller BR, Jones CE, Miram D. Capillary hemangioma of the vulva mistaken for sexual abuse. Adolesc Pediatr Gynaecol 1994;7:44–6.
2 Bouchard S, Yazbeck S, Lallier M. Perineal hemangioma, anorectal malformation, and genital anomaly: a new association? J Plastic Surg 1999;34:1133–5.
3 Goldberg NS, Hebert AA, Esterly NB. Sacral hemangiomas and multiple congenital abnormalities. Arch Dermatol 1986;122:684–7.
4 Fischer GO. Vulval disease in pre-pubertal girls. Australas J Dermatol 2001;42:225–34.
5 Morelli JG, Tan OT, Yohn J et al. Treatment of ulcerated haemangiomas in infancy. Arch Pediatr Adolesc Med 1994;148:1104–5.
6 Alter GJ, Trengove-Jones G, Horton C. Haemangioma of the penis and scrotum. Urology 1993;42:205–8.
7 Young AE, Senapati A. Intra-abdominal and pelvic vascular malformations. In: Mulliken JB, Young AE (eds) Vascular Birthmarks. Philadelphia: W.B. Saunders, 1988:396.
8 Rodrigues D, Bourroul ML, Ferrer AP et al. Blue rubber bleb naevus syndrome. Rev Hosp Clin Fac Med Univ Sao Paulo 2000;55:29–34.
9 Khoudary KP, Nasrallah PF, Gordon DA. Glomus tumor of the penis. J Urol 1996;155:707.
10 Ramos LM, Payon EM, Barrilero AE. Venous malformation of the glans penis: efficacy of treatment with neodymium:yttrium aluminum-garnet laser. Urology 1999;53:779–83.
11 Norouzi BB, Shanberg AM. Laser treatment of large cavernous haemangiomas of the penis. J Urol 1998;160:60–2.
12 Egan CA, Bradley RR, Logsdon V et al. Vulvar melanoma in childhood. Arch Dermatol 1997;133:345–8.
13 Christensen WN, Friedman KJ, Woodruff JD et al. Histologic characteristics of vulvar nevocellular nevi. J Cutan Pathol 1987;14:87–91.
14 Gleason BC, Hirsch MS, Nucci MR et al. Atypical genital naevi. A clinicopathologic analysis of 56 cases. Am J Surg Pathol 2008;32(1):51–7.
15 Lachlan KL, Lucassen A, Bunyan D, Temple IK. Cowden syndrome and Bannayan Riley Ruvalcaba syndrome represent one condition with variable expression and age-related penetrance: results of a clinical study of PTEN mutation carriers. J Med Genet 2007;44(9):579–85.
16 Boccone L, Dessi V, Zappu A et al. Bannayan–Riley–Ruvalcab syndrome with reactive nodular lymphoid hyperplasia and autism and a PTEN mutation. Am J Med Genet 2006;140(18):1965–9.
17 Ruvalcaba RHA, Myhre S, Smith DW. Sotos syndrome with intestinal polyposis and pigmentary changes of the genitalia. Clin Genet 1980;8:413–16.
18 Bishop PR, Nowicki MJ, Parker PH. What syndrome is this? Pediatr Dermatol 2000;17:319–21.
19 Erkek E, Hizel S, Sanly C et al. Clinical and histopathological findings in Bannayan–Riley–Ruvalcaba syndrome. J Am Acad Dermatol 2005;53(4):639–43.

20 Blum RR, Rahimizadeh A, Kardon L et al. Genital lentigines in a 6-year-old boy with Cowden's disease. Clinical and genetic evidence of the genetic linkage between Bannayan–Riley–Ruvalcaba syndrome and Cowden's disease. J Cutan Med Surg 2001;5:228–30.
21 Rogers M, McCrossin I, Commens C. Epidermal naevi and the epidermal naevus syndrome: a review of 131 cases. J Am Acad Dermatol 1989;20:476–88.
22 Le K Wong L, Fischer G. Vulval and perianal inflammatory linear verrucous epidermal naevus. Australas J Dermatol 2009;50:115–17.
23 Bandyopadhyay D, Saha A. Genital/perigenital inflammatory and linear verrucous epidermal nevus: a case series. Indian J Dermatol 2015;60(6):592–5.
24 Gonzalez-Martinez R, Marin-Bertolin S, Martinez-Escribano J et al. Nevus comedonicus. Report of a case with genital involvement. Cutis 1996;58:418–19.
25 Willihnganz-Lawson K, Gordon J, Perkins J, Shnorhavorian M. Genitourinary and perineal vacular anomalies in children: a Seattle children's experience. J Pediatr Urol 2015;11(4):227.e–6.
26 Joshi AV, Gupta R, Parelkar S et al. An unusual congenital scrotal lymphatic malformation with absent corpora caver nosa: a case report. J Pediatr Surg 2008;43(9):1729–31.
27 Vikicevic J, Milobratovic D, Vukadinovic V et al. Lymphangioma scroti. Pediatr Dermatol 2007;24(6):654–6.
28 Shah A, Meacock L, More B, Chandran H. Lymphangioma of the penis: a rare anomaly. Pediatr Surg Int 2005;21(4):329–30.
29 Aggarwal K, Gupta S, Jain VK, Marwah N. Congenital lymphangioma circumscriptum of the vulva. Indian Pediatr 2009;46(5):428–9.
30 Akyol I, Jayanthi V, Luquette M. Verrucous hemangioma of the glans penis. Urology 2008;72(1):230.
31 Nayyar S, Liaqat N, Sultan N, Dar SH. Cavernous haemangioma mimicking as clitoral hypertrophy. African J Paediatr Surg 2014;11(1):65–6.
32 Vogel AM, Alesbury J, Burrows PE, Fishman SJ. Vascular anomalies of the female external genitalia. J Pediatr Surg 2006;41(5):993–9.
33 Kemoinarie A, de Raeve L, Roseeuw D et al. Capillary–venous maformation in the labia majora in a 12-year-old girl. Dermatology 1997; 194(4):405–7.
34 Husmann DA, Rathburn S, Driscoll DJ. Klippel–Trenaunay syndrome: incidence and treatment of genitourinary sequelae. J Urol 2007;177(4):1244–9.
35 Vicentini FC, Denes F, Gomes CM et al. Urogenital involvement in the Klippel–Trenaunay Weber syndrome. Treatment options and results. Int Braz J Urol 2006;32(6):697–703.
36 Kokcu A, Sari S, Kefeli B. Primary vulvar lymphangioma circumscriptum: a case report and review of the literature. J Lower Gen Tract Dis 2015;19(1):e1–5.
37 Herman AR, Morello F, Strickland JL. Vulvar venous malformations in an 11-year-old girl: a case report. J Pediatr Adolesc Gynecol 2004;17(3):179–81.
38 Laforgia N, Schettini F, de Mattia D et al. Lymphatic malformation in newborns as the first sign of diffuse lymphangiomatosis: successful treatment with sirolmus. Neonatology 2016;109:52–5.
39 Chorzelsky TP, Kudejko J, Jablonska S. Is papular acantholytic dyskeratosis of the vulva a new entity? Am J Dermatopathol 1984;6:557–9.
40 Bell HK, Farrar C, Curley RK. Papular acantholytic dyskeratosis of the vulva. Clin Exp Dermatol 2001;26:386–8.
41 Saenz AM, Cirocco A, Avendano M et al. Papular acantholytic dyskeratosis of the vulva. Pediatr Dermatol 2005;22(3):237–9.
42 Cooper P. Acantholytic dermatosis localized to the vulvocrural area. J Cutan Pathol 1989;16:81–4.
43 Cottoni F, Masala M, Cossu S. Acantholytic dyskeratotic epidermal naevus localized unilaterally in the cutaneous and genital areas. Br J Dermatol 1998;138:875–8.

Vulvovaginitis

Definition. Vulvovaginitis is defined as inflammation involving both the vulval and vaginal epithelia. However, in clinical practice, this term is often applied incorrectly to cases in which there is vulval inflammation alone, in other words vulvitis. Inflammation of the vagina (vaginitis) seldom occurs in isolation as the associated discharge that accompanies it usually results in contamination of the perineum with consequent irritation and inflammation of the vulva.

Vulvovaginitis associated with a vaginal discharge

Vaginal discharge can be physiological, such as that seen in the newborn whose vaginal epithelium is still under the influence of maternal oestrogens, or in the menarchal child. A physiological discharge is unlikely to be associated with inflammatory changes in either the vagina or vulva and when inflammation is present, there is likely to be pathology.

Pathological discharge can be associated with infection, chemical irritants such as bubble baths which cause weeping from the surface of the vestibule, congenital malformations, such as ectopic ureter when urine will be the cause of the discharge, rare tumours such lymphangioma producing lymph [1,2], endocrine abnormality or foreign body [3,4]. However, the majority of cases of vulvovaginitis in prepubertal girls are nonspecific, with an infectious cause found in about a third of cases [5]. The recognized pathogenic organisms include group A β-haemolytic *Streptococcus*, *Haemophilus influenzae*, *Escherichia coli* and on some occasions *Staphylococcus aureus* [5–9]. *Streptococcal* vaginitis has also been reported in association with constipation [10] and glomerulonephritis [11]. There have also been reports of an associated vulvovaginal inflammation with both echo and coxsackie virus infections [12]. The enteric pathogens associated with vulvovaginitis are *Shigella* [13], which can occur in the absence of diarrhoea, and *Yersinia* [14].

The microbiology of vulvovagintis changes as girls mature. Prior to puberty, group A β-haemolytic *Streptococcus* is the most common organism isolated, with *Candida* appearing at puberty just before menarche [15]. *Candida* infection is rarely the cause of problems prepubertally and is only seen in postpubertal children, due to the effects of oestrogen on the vaginal epithelium, increasing the glycogen content of the epithelial cells of both the vestibule and vagina and the presence of lactobacilli [16]. *Candida* may then be a normal vaginal commensal. The rare occurrence of *Candida* infection in the neonatal period may be explained by the fact that maternal oestrogens still exert an effect on the infant's mucosae from birth to 2 months. An overgrowth of *Candida* may, however, exacerbate a napkin dermatitis and/or vulval dermatitis in an older child, particularly if there is gastrointestinal carriage of the organism. Candidiasis in this situation is a secondary phenomenon and once the underlying dermatosis is treated, the *Candida* is no longer a problem.

Diagnosis. Any discharge must be fully investigated with samples for wet preparations and culture to examine for *Trichomonas*, *Gardnerella* and *Candida*, and further samples for Gram staining and bacterial culture. If herpes simplex is suspected, then viral culture and smear preparations for electron microscopy should be performed as well as serological testing. Any vaginal samples can be obtained without trauma using simple noninvasive techniques such as a swab from any discharge that has accumulated at the fourchette. If this is not possible, a vaginal specimen can be obtained using a neonatal suction catheter or a catheter within a catheter technique [17]. In this technique, the hub of a butterfly infusion set with only the first 11.25 cm of the tubing still attached to it, the needle end having been cut off, is threaded into the distal end of an FG no. 12 bladder catheter that has been shortened to 10 cm. The butterfly hub is then attached to a 1 mL syringe filled with sterile saline. The uncut proximal end of the catheter is inserted into the vagina and the saline is then gently flushed through and aspirated. This aspirate is then examined and cultured.

It is very important bearing in mind the confounding overlap between normal flora and potential pathogens that the finding of an organism does not necessarily mean that it is the cause of the discharge [2].

References

1 Allen-Davis JT, Russ P, Karrer FM et al. Cavernous lymphangioma presenting as a vaginal discharge in a six-year-old female: a case report. J Pediatr Adolesc Gynecol 1996;9:31–4.
2 Mulchahey K. Management quandary. Persistent discharge in a premenarchal child. J Pediatr Adolesc Gynecol 2000;13:187–8.
3 **Smith YR, Berman DR, Quint EH. Premenarchal vaginal discharge: findings of procedures to rule out foreign bodies. J Pediatr Adolesc Gynecol 2002;15:227–30.**
4 **Stricker T, Navratil F, Sennhauser FH. Vaginal foreign bodies. J Paediatr Child Health 2004;40:205–7.**
5 **Stricker T, Navratil F, Sennhauser FH. Vulvovaginitis in prepubertal girls. Arch Dis Child 2003;88:324–6.**
6 Gerstner GJ, Grunberger W, Boschitsch E, Rotter M. Vaginal organisms in prepubertal children with and without vulvovaginitis. A vaginoscopic study. Arch Gynecol 1982;231:247–52.
7 Jaquiery A, Stylianopoulos A, Hogg G, Grover S. Vulvovaginitis: clinical features, aetiology, and microbiology of the genital tract. Arch Dis Child 1999;81:64–7.
8 Donald FE, Slack DB, Colman G. *Streptococcus pyogenes* vulvovaginitis in children in Nottingham. Epidemiol Infect 1991;106:459–65.
9 Cox RA, Slack MP. Clinical and microbiological features of *Haemophilus influenzae* vulvovaginitis in young girls. J Clin Pathol 2002;55:961–4.
10 Van Neer PA, Korver CR. Constipation presenting as recurrent vulvovaginitis in prepubertal children. J Am Acad Dermatol 2000;43:718–19.
11 Nair S, Schoeneman MJ. Acute glomerulonephritis with group A streptococcal vulvovaginitis. Clin Pediatr 2000;39:721–2.
12 Heller RH, Joseph JM, Davis HJ. Vulvovaginitis in the premenarcheal child. J Pediatr 1969;74:370–7.
13 Murphy TV, Nelson JD. Shigella vaginitis: report of 38 patients and a review of the literature. Pediatrics 1979;63:511–16.
14 Watkins S, Quan L. Vulvovaginitis caused by *Yersinia enterocolitica*. Pediatr Infect Dis 1984;3:444–5.
15 **Yilmaz AE, Celik N, Soylu G et al. Comparison of clinical and microbiological features of vulvovaginitis in prepubertal and pubertal girls, J Formosan Med Assoc 2012; 111(7):392–6.**
16 **Fischer G. Vulval disease in pre-pubertal girls. Australas J Dermatol 2001;42:225–34.**
17 Pokorny SF, Stormer J. Atraumatic removal of secretion from the prepubertal vagina. Am J Obstet Gynecol 1987;156:581–2.

Nonsexually acquired genital infections in children

Streptococcal cellulitis, vulvovaginitis and balanitis

Pathogenesis. Group A β-haemolytic *Streptococcus* is the most common cause of acute vulvovaginitis and balanitis in prepubertal children [1]. Interestingly, adults are rarely prone to this and perianal dermatitis and balanitis caused by group A β-haemolytic *Streptococcus* has rarely been described in adults [2].

Perianal streptococcal dermatitis (also known as cellulitis) is a common cause of chronic and acute-on-chronic perianal rashes in children, more commonly in boys. Presentation is with persistent perianal erythema, swelling, scale and fissuring. It is not a true cellulitis. Symptoms include itch and pain. The rash is a noninfiltrated plaque that may extend several centimetres from the anal verge. Weeping from the surface may produce a persistent discharge, and pain on defaecation may result in chronic constipation which may in turn result in bleeding on defaecation [3].

In girls with vulvovaginitis, presentation is with sudden onset of an erythematous, swollen, painful vulva and vagina, with a thin mucoid discharge. In boys with balanitis, there is acute erythema of the glans (Fig. 162.23). There may have been a preceding throat infection with the same organism or preceding perianal dermatitis. Sometimes the infection can be low grade, similar to the perianal disease, presenting as a subacute vulvitis [4].

Recurrent disease has been reported as a result of chronic pharyngeal carriage [5]. This infection does not tend to self-resolve and symptoms tend to be persistent until a diagnosis is made and appropriate treatment initiated [6].

In general, patients with this condition are systemically well; however, fever and scarlatiniform rash, followed by acral desquamation in association with perianal disease, have been reported. In this case, a streptococcal pyrogenic exotoxin was assumed to be produced by the infective organism [7]. Guttate psoriasis may be precipitated by this infection in the genital region and genital psoriasis may be precipitated by genital streptococcal infection [8,9].

The infection is easily diagnosed by introital and perianal swabs. It is not necessary to insert the swab right into the vagina, which children usually find traumatic, particularly when the area is tender. A rapid antigen test may also be used [10].

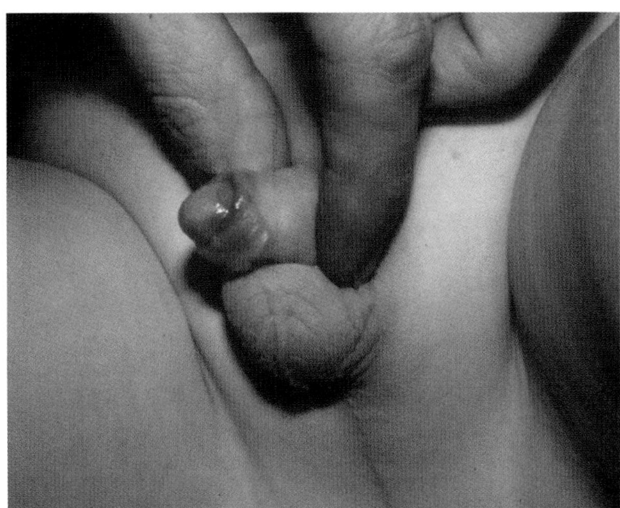

Fig. 162.23 Streptococcal balanitis.

Differential diagnosis. Although a differential diagnosis of acute candidiasis would be reasonable in an adult, this is not the case in children. Psoriasis and dermatitis are also in the differential diagnosis, particularly when the vulvitis is subacute. Recurrent streptococcal infections should raise the possibility of an intravaginal foreign body [1]. Also a blood-stained vaginal discharge may suggest a foreign body [11]. *Shigella* species may cause recurrent and chronic vulvovaginitis in association with diarrhoea. *Yersinia* vaginitis in conjunction with gastroenteritis has been reported [12].

Also in the differential diagnosis, but much rarer as a cause of acute vulvitis, is the fixed drug eruption. Erythema multiforme may also affect the vulva but is usually part of a generalized reaction in children.

Management. Any case of acute vulvitis or balanitis and any persistent perianal rash in a child should suggest this condition; swabs should be taken and the child commenced on either oral penicillin or amoxicillin, or a macrolide antibiotic if they are allergic to penicillin. The course must run for a full 10 days or recurrence may occur. Concurrent use of topical mupirocin will help to prevent recurrence. Apparent poor response to therapy, with ongoing symptoms despite resolution of infection, usually indicates an underlying condition such as dermatitis, psoriasis or vaginal foreign body [1,4]. A case report has drawn attention to recurrent disease as a result of chronic asymptomatic pharyngeal colonization which cleared with rifampicin and amoxicillin [5].

Recurrent toxin-mediated perineal erythema (scarlatina-like)

This condition, which was originally described in young men, presents with recurrent, asymptomatic erythema and desquamation of the perineum and groin area following acute pharyngitis (Fig. 162.24). The eruption may be associated with swelling, erythema and desquamation of the hands and feet, or a 'strawberry tongue'. Toxin-producing *Staph. aureus* or toxin-producing group A β-haemolytic *Streptococcus* is responsible for the eruption [13].

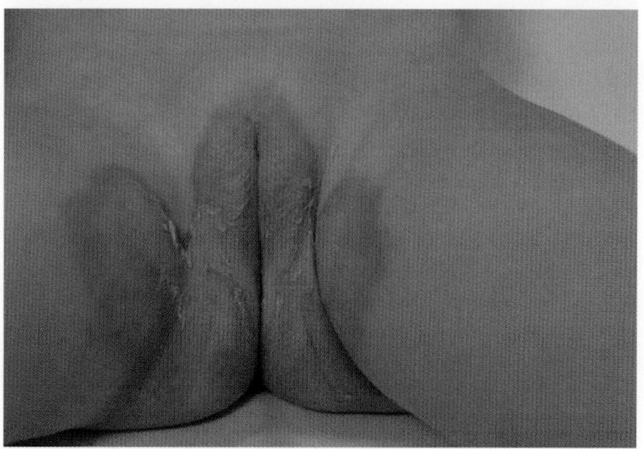

Fig. 162.24 Toxin-mediated perineal erythema with desquamation.

This phenomenon is assumed to be a superantigen-related disorder [14].

A series from 2001 reported 11 cases of this condition in children, seven boys and four girls presenting with acute onset of perineal erythema. In this series, four patients also had erythema of the hands and feet and seven had a strawberry tongue. Only three of these cases had recurrent disease. In all cases there was evidence of group A β-haemolytic *Streptococcus* infection, although this was not recovered from perineal culture and all were treated with oral antibiotics. All of the children were well and laboratory investigations normal [15].

In young children, this condition must be differentiated from Kawasaki syndrome.

Staphylococcal folliculitis and impetigo

Staphylococcal folliculitis is common on the buttocks of children, particularly those with eczema and those who are still in night nappies. It may sometimes spread to the vulva or groin or can be found there primarily (Fig. 162.25). Impetigo may also sometimes occur on the genital and perianal area.

The presentation is with pustules and crusted lesions, which are often more itchy and irritating rather than painful. The diagnosis is made with a bacterial swab.

Management. Although impetigo usually responds quickly to a course of appropriate antistaphylococcal antibiotics, folliculitis often represents a carrier state and can be very persistent. It is often better treated with topical agents, such as bath products containing chlorhexidine or triclosan and mupirocin 2% cream. Underwear and other garments in direct contact with genital skin, such as swimming costumes and pyjamas, sheets and towels, should be hot-washed, and every attempt made to discard night nappies. If there is underlying eczema, this should be treated.

Staphylococcal scalded skin syndrome

This is an exfoliative skin condition preceded by an often minor staphylococcal infection that produces an exfoliative toxin. The child presents with fever, irritability and usually a widespread erythematous eruption, with flexural accentuation. As the illness progresses, shallow blisters evolve to

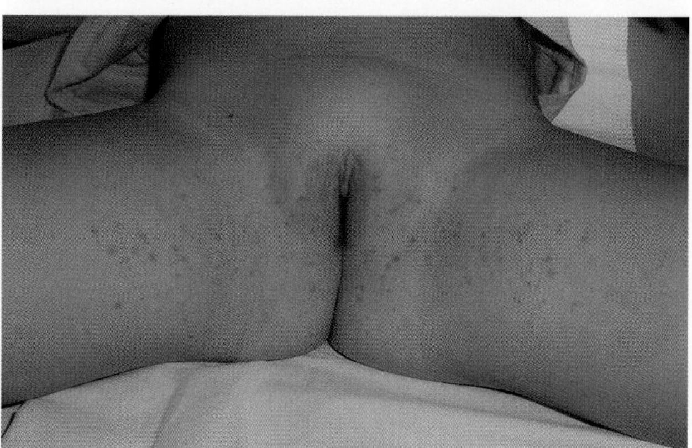

Fig. 162.25 Staphylococcal folliculitis.

raw, eroded areas, particularly in the perioral, axillary and genital areas. The eruption may begin in the genital area with a tender, erythematous eruption with superficial blistering (Fig 162.26) (see also Chapter 37).

Pinworm (*Enterobius vermicularis*)

Although many children with pinworm infestation are asymptomatic, symptoms are those of perianal and vulval itching, particularly at night, when the worms migrate onto the skin to lay eggs. An eczematous rash may occur, but the skin may be normal. Vaginal discharge and irritation may also occur. Pinworm is very well known as a cause of genital itching in children, and many children will already have been treated by their parents or their pharmacist before they see a doctor [16].

Diagnosis may be made by pressing the sticky side of clear tape to the perianal area first thing in the morning and then examining the tape under a microscope for the presence of ova (Fig 162.27). This test is not always reliable and if symptoms and signs are suggestive of infestation then this can be treated empirically.

Treatment requires oral mebendazole 100 mg or pyrantel pamoate 11 mg/kg up to 1 g. A further treatment in two weeks is recommended to kill worms that have hatched since the first treatment [17].

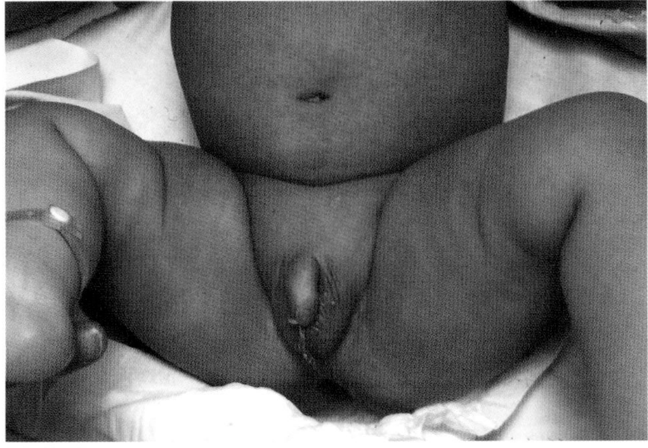

Fig. 162.26 Staphylococcal scalded skin syndrome presenting with an erythematous rash with superficial blistering.

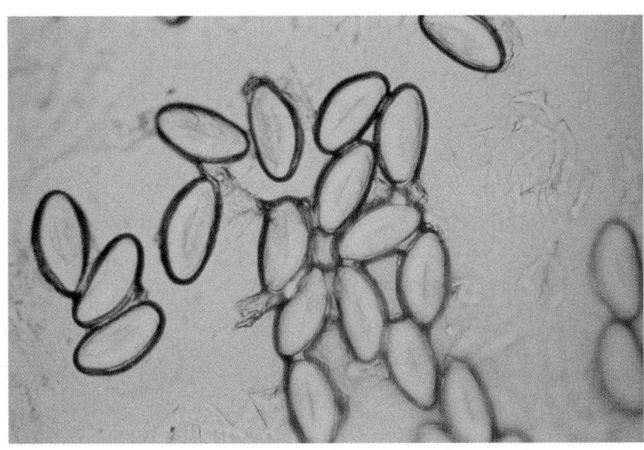

Fig. 162.27 Ova of *Enterobius vermicularis*.

Scabies

Scabetic nodules are common on the genital area, but are usually part of a generalized eruption. The irritable nodules occur on the vulva in girls and on the glans and scrotum in boys (Fig. 162.28).

Molluscum contagiosum

Molluscum contagiosum is a large double-stranded DNA poxvirus. DNA analysis has demonstrated four major viral types [18]. The virus codes for a number of proteins that enable it to evade the immune system by blocking immune recognition and clearance [19].

These viral lesions are very common in children. The virus is spread by close physical contact, fomites and autoinoculation. Transmission in water is well recognized, and this explains the predilection for the lower body where the child sits in the bath [20]. As a result, it is not uncommon for mollusca to be found on the genital area, often as part of a more generalized eruption [16] (Fig. 162.29).

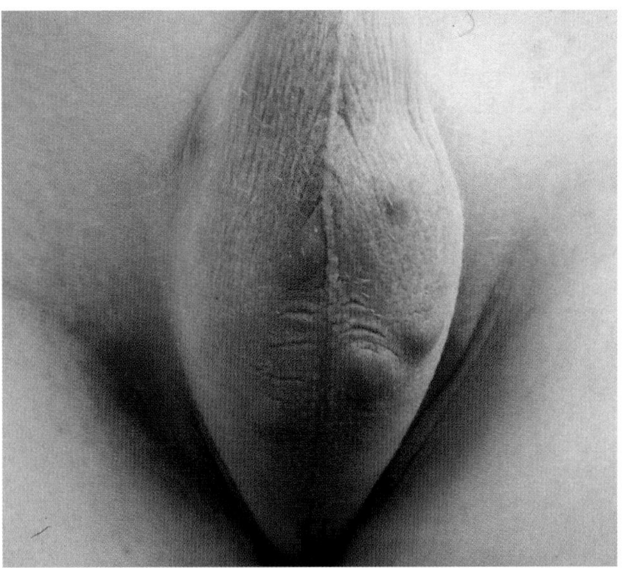

Fig. 162.28 Scabies nodules of the scrotum. Source: Courtesy of Dr M. Rogers.

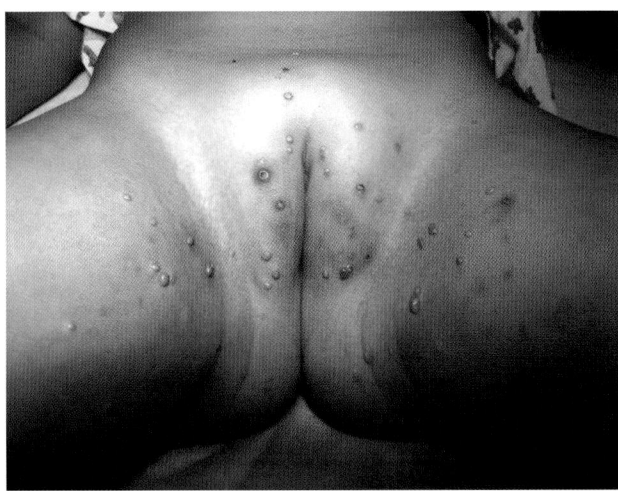

Fig. 162.29 Molluscum contagiosum of the vulva.

Sometimes vulval mollusca can be difficult to differentiate from condylomata acuminata, and close examination with a magnifier or a dermatoscope will be needed to see the typical central core. If there is doubt, the core may be examined as a smear stained with haematoxylin and eosin and a PCR technique has been described which can also genotype the virus [21]. It is important to be clear on this, as mollusca are generally not considered to be sexually transmitted in children, unlike condylomata acuminata. Sexual transmission of molluscum contagiosum is uncommon but possible [22,23]. Furthermore, studies have shown that the genotype found in children differs from that found in adults with sexually transmitted genital mollusca [24] and genital mollusca are rarely found in isolation without evidence of a more widespread infection of other parts of the skin. The appearance of these lesions can sometimes be very nonspecific, as a dermal papule without an obvious core, or as a large solitary skin tag.

Extensive, atypical lesions may be found in children with HIV disease and other forms of immunocompromise [25]. However, the majority even with extensive lesions are immunologically normal [26]. Giant genital mollusca are described in children [27].

In most cases, it is not necessary to treat genital mollusca. Methods that are used to extract the viral core from the centre, which may be tolerated on less sensitive parts of the skin, may prove to be very difficult. Avoidance of baths and swimming pools appears to reduce autoinoculation and topical corticosteroids reduce pruritus if present. Pimecrolimus and tacrolimus should be avoided as they have been reported to spread the lesions [28]. Spontaneous resolution invariably occurs. No study specifically examining the use of topical therapy for genital mollusca in children has been published to date.

Herpes zoster and simplex

Varicella frequently involves the genital area, and vesicles may occur on the mucosal surface, resulting in a blood-stained vaginal or penile discharge. The lesions may be localized to the area under the napkin, particularly when there is a napkin dermatitis or other dermatosis in this area, with little sign of blistering elsewhere (Fig. 162.30). Herpes zoster may also involve the genital area as a unilateral eruption.

Herpes simplex may complicate underlying dermatoses such as napkin dermatitis and atopic dermatitis or can occur alone on the genital area in children (Fig 162.31). It presents as small blisters which rapidly erode to leave superficial raw areas. Diagnosis is made by a positive PCR for the virus. The finding of genital herpes in a child is not necessarily sexually transmitted and may have been acquired from a parent or close contact with lesions on the face or fingers even when HSV2 is isolated. Nevertheless, it should raise the possibility particularly if HSV2 is isolated.

Fungal infections

Tinea is a common cause of groin rashes in men and sometimes causes vulval rashes in women, but is rarely found on the genital area in children. When it does occur,

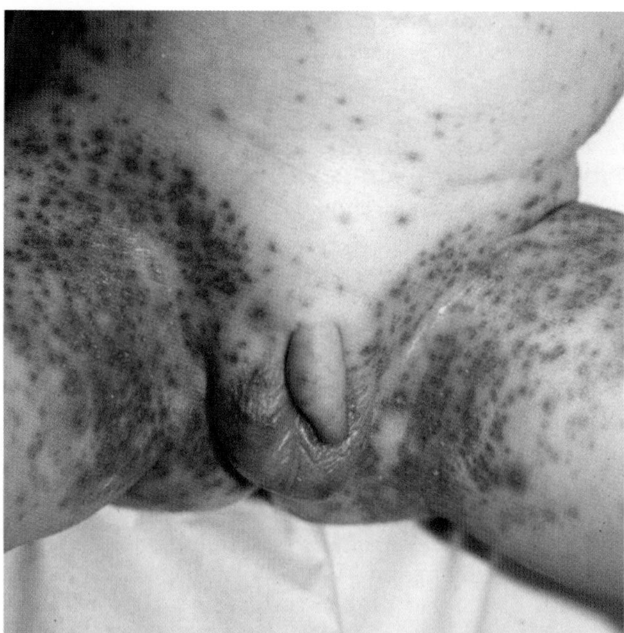

Fig. 162.30 Varicella localized to the area under the napkin. Source: Courtesy of Dr M. Rogers.

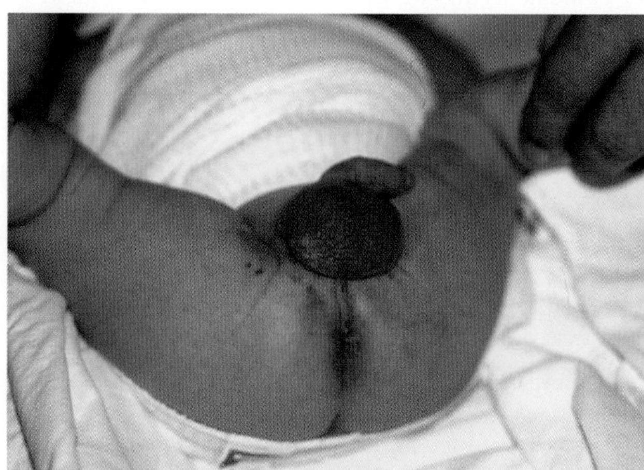

Fig. 162.31 Herpes simplex in a neonate.

it hardly ever has typical features, and this is often the result of treatment with topical corticosteroids. It is possible that it is more common than one would think, as so many cases of genital eruptions are assumed to be candidiasis and treated with imidazole creams. This would, in most childhood cases, fortuitously treat tinea.

In cases when no antifungal has been used and the rash is treated as dermatitis, tinea of the vulva, groin or under the napkin in a baby presents as a dermatitic rash that does not respond to treatment. The diagnosis requires a high index of suspicion but once thought of is easily confirmed by a skin scraping.

Candidiasis, on the other hand, does not occur in children out of nappies. In adult women with chronic vulval symptoms, about 15% have candidiasis, but this oestrogen-dependent condition is not seen after infancy in children with normal immune systems [29,30]. This is an important point, as it is common for children with skin diseases such as dermatitis and psoriasis to be diagnosed as having 'thrush' and treated with antifungal creams, which may cause irritation, particularly if dermatitis is present [31].

Mycobacterial infection

Tuberculosis of the penis and vulva, described as a genital tuberculid, has been reported in adults. However, a case report documents a case of lichen scrofulosorum of the vulva in an 11-year-old girl [32]. Vulval lepromatous leprosy has also been reported in a female infant [33].

References

1 **Fischer GO, Rogers M. Vulvar disease in children: a clinical audit of 130 cases. Pediatr Dermatol 2000;17:1–6.**
2 Neri I, Bardazzi F, Marzaduri I et al. Perianal streptococcal dermatitis in adults. Br J Dermatol 1996;135:796–8.
3 **Krol AL. Perianal streptococcal dermatitis. Pediatr Dermatol 1990;7: 97–100.**
4 **Dar V, Raker K, Adhmi Z et al. Streptococcal vulvovaginitis in girls. Pediatr Dermatol 1993;10:366–7.**
5 Hansen MT, Sanchez V, Eyster K, Hansen KA. Streptococcus pyognenes pharyngeal colonization resultig in recurent prepubertal vulvovaginitis. J Pediatr Adolesc Gynecol 2007;20(5):315–17.
6 **Mogielnicki NP, Schwartzman J, Elliott JA. Perineal group A streptococcal disease in a pediatric practice. Pediatrics 2000;106(2): 276–81.**
7 Velez A, Moreno JC. Febrile perianal streptococcal dermatitis. Pediatr Dermatol 1999;16:23–4.
8 **Herbst RA, Hoch O, Kapp A. Guttate psoriasis triggered by perianal streptococcal dermatitis in a 4 year old boy. J Am Acad Dermatol 2000;42:885–7.**
9 **Hernandez M, Simms-Dendan J, Zendell K. Guttate psoriasis following streptococcal vulvovagintis in a five-year-ole girl. J Pediatr Adolesc Gynecol 2015;28(5):e127–9.**
10 **Koskas M, Levy C, Romain O et al. Group A streptococcal perianal infection in children. Arch Pediatrie 2014;21 Suppl 2:S97–100.**
11 Gryngarten MG, Turco ML, Escobar ME et al. Shigella vulvovaginitis in prepubertal girls. Adolesc Pediatr Gynecol 1994;7:86–9.
12 Watkins S, Quan L. Vulvovaginitis caused by *Yersinia enterocolitica*. Pediatr Infect Dis 1984;3:444–5.
13 Manders SM. Toxin-mediated streptococcal and staphylococcal disease [review]. J Am Acad Dermatol 1998;39:383–98.
14 Manders SM, Heymann WR, Atillasoy E et al. Recurrent toxin-mediated perineal erythema. Arch Dermatol 1996;132:57–60.
15 **Patrizi A, Raone B, Savoia F et al. Recurrent toxin-mediated perineal erythema: eleven pediatric cases. Arch Dermatol 2008;144(2):239–43.**
16 Williams TS, Callen JP, Lafayette GO. Vulvar disorders in the prepubertal female. Pediatr Ann 1986;15:588–605.
17 St Georgiev V. Chemotherapy enterobiasis (oxyuriasis). Expert Opin Pharmacother 2001;2:267–75.
18 **Brown J, Janniger C, Schwartz RZ, Silverberg N. Childhood molluscum contagiosum. Int J Dermatol 2006;45:93.**
19 Agromayer M, Ortiz P, Lopez-Estebaranz JL et al. Molecular epidemiology of molluscum contagiosum virus and analysis of the host–serum antibody response in Spanish HIV-negative patients. J Med Virol 2002;66:151.
20 **Braue A, Ross G, Varigos G, Kelly H. Epidemiology and impact of molluscum contagiosum. Pediatr Dermatol 2005;22:287.**
21 Trama JP, Adelson M, Mordechai E. Idenfification and genotyping of molluscum contagiosum virus from genital swab samples by realtime PCR and pyrosequencing. J Clin Virol 2007;40:325.
22 Porter CD, Blake NW, Archard LC et al. Molluscum contagiosum virus types in genital and non-genital lesions. Br J Dermatol 1989;120: 37–41.
23 **Bargman H. Is genital molluscum contagiosum a cutaneous manifestation of sexual abuse in children? J Am Acad Dermatol 1986;14:847–9.**
24 Porter CD, Blake N, Archard L et al. Molluscum contagiosum virus types in genital and non-genital lesions. Br J Dermatol 1989;120:37.
25Gur I. The epidemiology of molluscum contagiosum in HIV seropositive patients: a unique entity or insignificant finding? Int J STD AIDS 2008;19:503.
26 **Dohil M, Lin P, Lee J et al. The epidemiology of molluscum contagiosum in children. J Am Acad Dermatol 2006;54:47.**
27 Kim SK, Do J, Kang HY et al. Giant molluscum contagiosum of immunocompetent children occurring on the genital area. Eur J Dermatol 2007;17:537.
28 Goksugar N, Ozbostanci B, Goksugar SB. Molluscum contagiosum infection associated with pimecrolimus use in pityriasis alba. Pediatr Dermatol 2007;23:574.
29 Vandeven AM, Emans SJ. Vulvovaginitis in the child and adolescent. Pediatr Rev 1993;14:141–7.
30 Farrington PF. Pediatric vulvovaginitis. Clin Obstet Gynecol 1997;40:135–40.
31 **Fischer G. Chronic vulvitis in pre-pubertal girls. Australas J Dermatol 2010;50:118–23.**
32 Pandhi D, Mehta S, Singal A. Genital tuberculid in a female child: a new entity (childhood vulval tuberculid). Pediatr Dermatol 2007;24(5):573–5.
33 Bodamyali P, Akay BN, Kundakci et al. Infantile lepromatous leprosy with vulval localization. Turkish J Pediatr 2011;53(2):213–15.

Sexually transmitted infections in children

Sexually transmitted infections are seen in sexually active teenagers or younger children who are being sexually abused (see Chapter 164). The most common bacterial pathogens in this situation are *Neisseria gonorrhoeae*, *Chlamydia trachomatis* and *Trichomonas*. The two viral infections seen are herpes simplex and human papillomavirus; when either is encountered in a child, there should be a high index of suspicion. However, it should also be appreciated that these viruses are not always sexually transmitted.

Blisters and ulcers

Blistering and ulcerative conditions of the genital area are unusual at any age, and are probably no rarer in children than in adults. Infection with *Staphylococcus aureus* and herpes simplex should be kept in the differential diagnosis.

Erosive and or blistering napkin eruption

Jacquet irritant erosive dermatitis describes a condition with ulcerated papules and pustules on the labia majora of the vulval skin of infants and is believed to be due to prolonged contact with soiled napkins (Fig. 162.32). This is seen less frequently with the use of disposable nappies and the improved absorbency of the materials used in their manufacture. Severe irritant contact dermatitis may also cause blistering (see Fig. 162.1).

Immunobullous disease – vulval bullous and cicatricial pemphigoid and linear IgA disease of childhood

Although bullous pemphigoid is very rare in children, when it does occur it may be localized to the vulva and penis [1,2]. The child presents with a history of painful and itchy blistering. The blistering lesions, which rapidly erode, occur around the labia minora and majora, glans penis and perianal area [3,4] (Fig. 162.33). Localized vulval bullous pemphigoid may be a distinct subtype of childhood bullous pemphigoid. It is a self-limited nonscarring disease with a good prognosis. It responds well to topical corticosteroids [2].

Bullous pemphigoid may be misdiagnosed as herpes simplex, lichen sclerosus or sexual abuse [5]. The biopsy appearance is typical of bullous pemphigoid at any site, with linear C3 and immunoglobulin G (IgG) [4].

Cicatricial pemphigoid or benign mucous membrane pemphigoid predominantly affects the mucosal surfaces, healing with scar formation. When it involves the vulva, scarring can lead to distortion of the vulval architecture with labial fusion and introital shrinkage that can mimic lichen sclerosus [6]. It has been described confined to the vulva in children [6]. Ophthalmological examination is essential to exclude ocular involvement.

In localized cases cicatricial pemphigoid is self-limiting and is easily controlled with potent topical steroid and topical tacrolimus [7]. However, severe cases may require systemic therapy with prednisone and immunosuppressive therapy [8].

Linear IgA disease (chronic bullous dermatosis of childhood) may also involve the genital area and in one study was present in 16 out of 20 girls with the condition, with a misdiagnosis of herpes simplex infection in one case and sexual abuse in another [9].

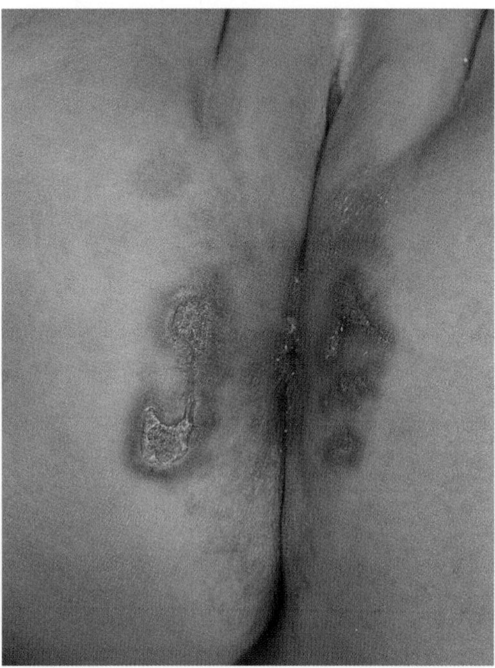

Fig. 162.32 Jacquet dermatitis, showing healing lesions that had been ulcerated nodules.

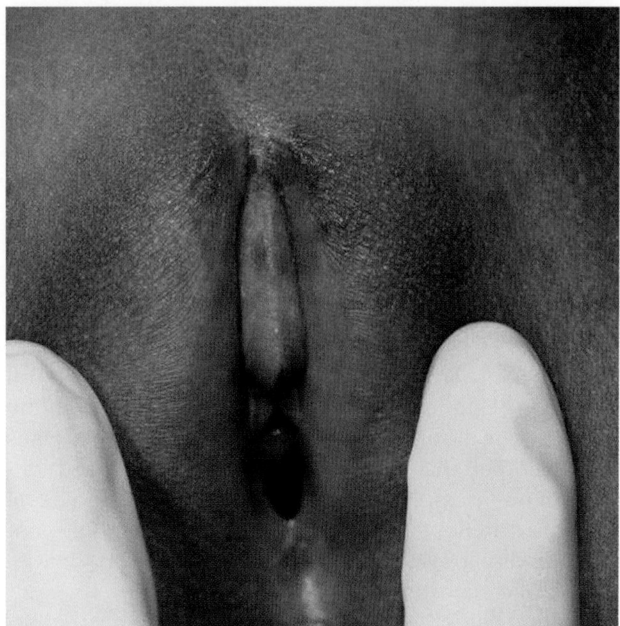

Fig. 162.33 Bullous pemphigoid of the vulva.

Nonsexually acquired acute genital ulcers (NSAGU)

Acute nonsexually acquired vulval ulcers were first described by Lipschutz in 1913; however, the literature on it was quite confusing until recent years when there has been increased interest in the subject.

Acute noninfectious ulceration can be either recurrent (most often thought to be due to aphthosis or associated with Behçet or Crohn disease) or a single event. This latter clinical situation has been termed 'Lipschutz ulcer', 'ulcus vulvae acutum', 'Miculicz ulcer' and 'Sutton's ulcer' [10].

The acute form of nonsexually acquired genital ulcers is usually seen in girls in the early adolescent age range, with one study finding the mean age to be 11.5 years [11]. The appearance is of a shallow, well-defined ulcer with a yellow, fibrinous base and a surrounding red halo. In some cases, the base may appear dark and necrotic (Fig. 162.34). These ulcers are of sudden onset and are usually preceded by fever [12]. They may be very large, up to 2 cm in diameter, severely painful and accompanied by oedema of the labia minora that makes examination very difficult without sedation. As a result, the ulceration may be missed. Pain may be so disabling that the patient is unable to urinate or walk and the lesions may take several weeks to months to heal, sometimes with scarring if the lesion has been deep and necrotic. The appearance is alarming and, not surprisingly, these girls are commonly assumed to have primary genital herpes, and are investigated for this and other sexually transmitted disease (Fig. 162.35).

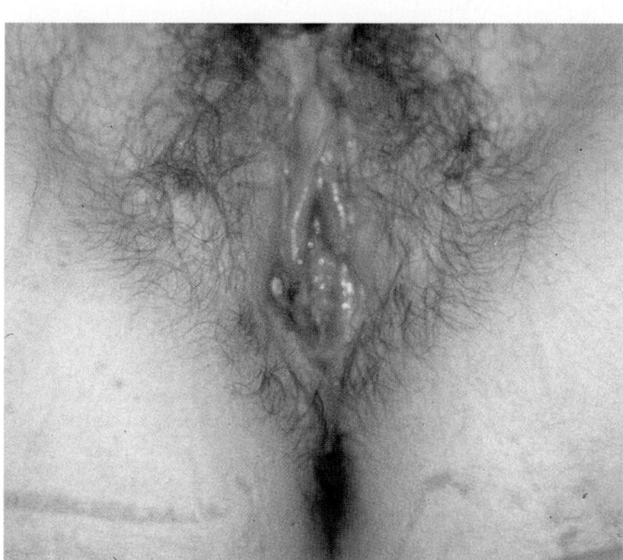

Fig. 162.34 Major aphthosis of the vulva.

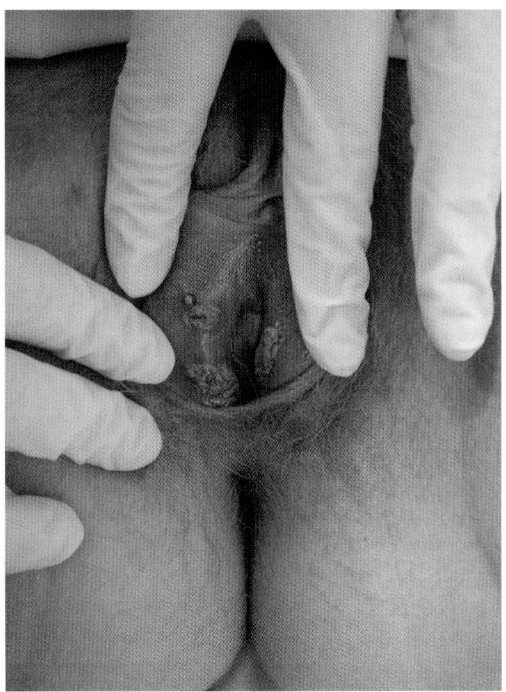

Fig. 162.35 Necrotic aphthous ulceration of the vulva.

Epstein–Barr virus (EBV) is often implicated in these lesions and a study of 13 cases reported it in four [12,13]. Epstein–Barr virus has been isolated from these ulcers by PCR. Serology is not always positive at the onset of the ulcer, which can precede other signs of infection. Other implicated infectious agents include mumps, cytomegalovirus, *Mycoplasma pneumoniae*, *Streptococcus*, enterovirus, parvovirus B19, paratyphoid fever and influenza A/B [14,15]. However, it is not uncommon for extensive work-up to fail to uncover a specific trigger. It would therefore appear that this is a reaction pattern seen with many precipitants.

The acute form of severe NSAGU which presents with ulceration following a febrile prodrome may be a different condition to aphthosis with less likelihood of recurrence [15]. Acute, nonsexually acquired genital ulceration is a clinical diagnosis. Biopsy is nonspecific and is not indicated. The importance of this condition is that is it underreported and underrecognized. This often leads to traumatic and unnecessary investigation for sexually transmitted infection and sexual abuse in these young girls. Acute genital ulceration in a girl this age should be a reason for urgent review by a dermatologist before any further action is taken. Investigation should be minimal, confined to bacterial swabs and viral PCR for herpes simplex.

Management usually involves hospitalization for analgesia and sometimes urinary catheterization. Oral prednisolone 0.5 mg/kg daily rapidly relieves pain and may hasten recovery [15,16] in severe cases; however, potent topical corticosteroids can be used if patients are not incapacitated.

Aphthous ulcers

Aphthous ulcers are usually small, painful lesions that may begin in childhood or adolescence, and subsequently recur at intervals that can be infrequent to frequent and disabling. Oral aphthous ulcers are very common, but uncommonly these lesions may also occur on the vulva or scrotum. It is important to recognize these lesions, as they are commonly mistaken for genital herpes simplex and other sexually transmitted infectious diseases [13,17].

Aetiology. Aphthous ulcers have been associated with iron, ferritin, folate and vitamin B_{12} deficiency, Behçet disease, Crohn disease, coeliac disease, cyclic neutropenia, PFAPA (periodic fever, aphthous ulcers, pharyngitis, adenitis) syndrome and HIV infection [18–22]. Severe, recurrent aphthae of the oral and genital mucosa, in the absence of systemic manifestations, is termed 'complex aphthosis'. It is possibly a *forme fruste* of Behçet disease [23] but this is speculative.

The pathogenesis of this disease is unknown. Various infectious agents, such as herpes simplex virus, cytomegalovirus, EBV, *Helicobacter pylori* and *Streptococcus* species, have been implicated but not reproducibly isolated [10,17].

Clinical presentation. The ulcers are usually small, round or oval, shallow lesions with a sharply defined edge and an erythematous margin. The base is yellow or grey. When they occur on the vulva, they are usually found on the mucosal surface of the labia minora. In males, they are found on the scrotum. They heal spontaneously in 1–2 weeks, without scarring. Genital aphthous ulcers are rare in children but in a series of 20 patients aged 10–19, five were premenarchal and in the same series half the patients had associated oral aphthae and a third had recurrent lesions [17].

Differential diagnosis. The diagnosis of aphthosis is a clinical one and an important one in a child presenting with a large painful genital ulcer, who is very likely to be traumatized by investigations for sexually transmitted disease, and to be subjected to unnecessary biopsy, which is nondiagnostic. Recurrent and major aphthosis should be differentiated from Behçet disease and Crohn disease. It is usually recommended that these patients be investigated for iron, folate and B_{12} deficiency but in the author's experience such investigations are often noncontributory. A history of bowel disease, systemic upset, joint pain and ocular symptoms should be obtained and further investigation for Behçet and Crohn disease undertaken if warranted. Other causes of recurrent genital ulceration in children include mucosal erythema multiforme, genital herpes and genital fixed drug eruption.

Management. Minor aphthosis can be managed with reassurance and topical potent corticosteroid or topical tetracycline. The situation of a child with a large, very painful genital lesion can be rapidly alleviated with oral prednisone at a dose of 0.5–1 mg/kg per day. Healing occurs within one week and the corticosteroid can then be rapidly tapered off.

Recurrent disease may be controlled with low-dose oral tetracycline in children not younger than 8 years of age

(British National Formulary recommends for use in children over the age of 12 years) or oral erythromycin in younger children. Other oral medications that have been considered useful include dapsone, colchicine and thalidomide [24].

Fixed drug eruption

Fixed drug eruption is an uncommon drug reaction which, when found on nongenital skin, presents as sharply demarcated round or oval plaques recurring at a fixed location. The eruption may vary from one to many involved areas. The offending drug has usually been administered within the last 12 hours and sometimes the eruption will occur within 30 minutes of ingestion. The plaques are usually asymmetrically distributed. During the recovery phase there is often hyperpigmentation.

Fixed drug eruption may occur on the genital area at any age. In this location, it presents in girls as a bilaterally symmetrical erosive eruption involving the vulva that may spread to the groins and buttocks. In boys, there is usually erythema and swelling and blistering of the penis and/or scrotum [25,26] (Fig. 162.36). The eruption is itchy and sore. It may be associated with dysuria and urinary retention. The onset is sudden, and it resolves spontaneously over a period of about two weeks. In the genital area, hyperpigmentation does not usually occur [27]. The symmetry of the eruption and the lack of postinflammatory pigmentation on the genital area may make the diagnosis difficult. When a drug is constantly administered, genital fixed drug eruption may present as a constant erosive eruption that is puzzlingly treatment resistant.

The differential diagnosis includes acute streptococcal vulvitis and balanitis, acute contact dermatitis and recurrent perineal erythema.

Drugs that have most often been implicated in children include paracetamol, co-trimoxazole, hydroxyzine and methylphenidate [25].

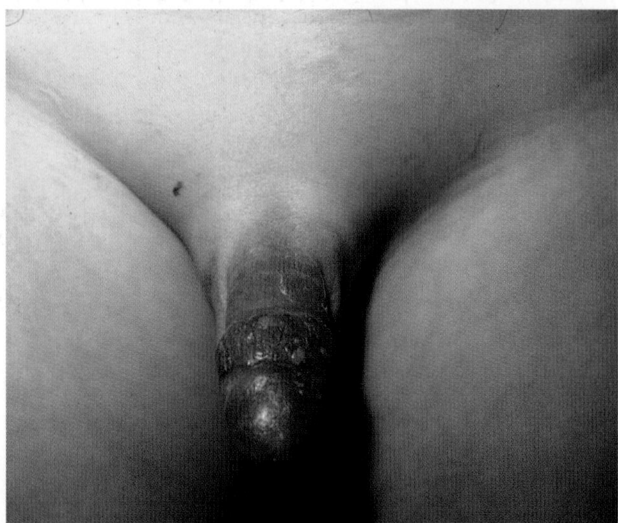

Fig. 162.36 Fixed drug eruption of the penis. Source: Courtesy of Dr M. Rogers.

Erythema multiforme and toxic epidermal necrolysis

Erythema multiforme major often involves mucosal surfaces in children and may do so in a recurrent fashion when precipitated by herpes simplex infection. Other precipitants include *Mycoplasma pneumoniae* infection and drug reactions. It is usually part of a generalized process but can involve mucosae only [28,29] (Fig. 162.37). The vulval involvement is an erosive vulvovaginitis. It has been postulated that the *M. pneumoniae*-induced form of erythema multiforme is a distinct entity with prominent mucositis and sparse skin disease. Urogenital lesions are reported in the majority of cases [30].

Toxic epidermal necrolysis is a much more severe, multisystem disease with severe skin blistering and erosions. It is, in most cases, a drug reaction. The genital changes are similar to those encountered in erythema multiforme.

If the mucosal surfaces are severely involved in either condition, vaginal adhesions may develop [31,32] and persistent mucosal erosions and ulceration have been reported to occur for over one year after the acute episode [33]. A case report of a child who required reconstructive vulvovaginal surgery as a result of toxic epidermal necrolysis at age 3 underlines the importance of attention to genital involvement during the acute phase, even in very young children [34].

Hidradenitis suppurativa

Hidradenitis suppurativa (HS) is a chronic suppurative scarring disease resulting from noninfective inflammation of apocrine sweat gland-bearing skin. It therefore favours the axilla and anogenital area but may occur on the buttocks, breast and scalp. Although it is usually seen in young adults and older people, it may occur in children, particularly those approaching and at puberty, and is estimated to occur in 2% of patients with HS. The condition is more common in girls than boys and the youngest reported patient is 5 years of age [35]. Children with HS are more likely to have a hormonal imbalance than adults with the disease and those with androgen excess from adrenal hyperplasia or metabolic syndrome, obesity

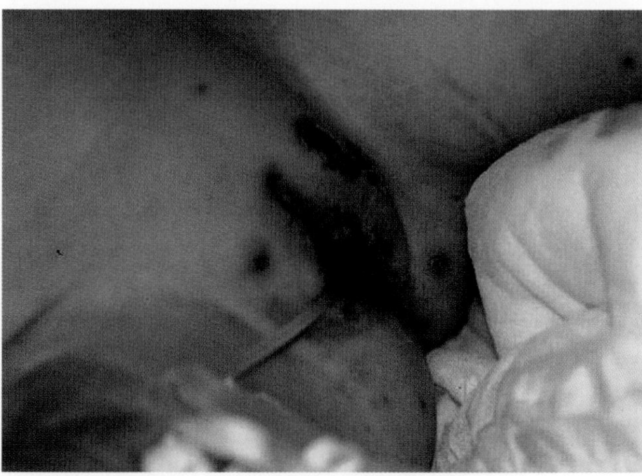

Fig. 162.37 Erythema multiforme major involving the vulva.

and premature adrenarche or puberty may suffer from it prematurely [36,37]. A positive family history of HS is also more common in early-onset disease [38].

Pathogenesis. Although the true aetiology of this disease remains unknown, it does appear that follicular occlusion in apocrine gland-bearing skin is the primary event. Rupture of the follicle creates a proinflammatory environment possibly accompanied by dysfunctional changes in the microbiome. Mutations in genes that impair Notch signalling in hair follicles have been implicated [39]. The disease in most cases appears to be androgen dependent, and it has been postulated that these patients have an end-organ hypersensitivity to androgens. Both obesity and smoking have been reported to be exacerbating factors [40]. The connection between smoking and this condition, seen in adults, can manifest in children who are passive smokers.

Clinical features. The earliest signs of the disease are tender dermal nodules that may progress to suppuration and scarring (Fig 162.38). With time, discharging sinus tracts, fistulae, comedones and fibrosing scars develop. Although bacterial swabs are usually negative, superinfection may result in recurrent cellulitis and oedema [41]. The disease may become debilitating, with constant painful nodules in the groin and axilla. Early-onset HS is associated with more widespread disease [39]. The Hurley severity staging which is used to grade disease severity in adults can also be applied to children.

Differential diagnosis. Particularly in children, in whom the disease may not be suspected, recurrent folliculitis or staphylococcal boils are usually diagnosed initially. However, repeated swabs do not reveal the expected staphylococcal infection and eventually the characteristic appearance declares itself.

Management. This condition may be very treatment resistant and has a severe impact on quality of life. Management should encompass firstly correction of any metabolic or endocrine disease and weight control. An endocrine evaluation should be undertaken. For children with mild Hurley stage I disease, topical clindamycin 1% and topical azaleic acid 15% are first line.

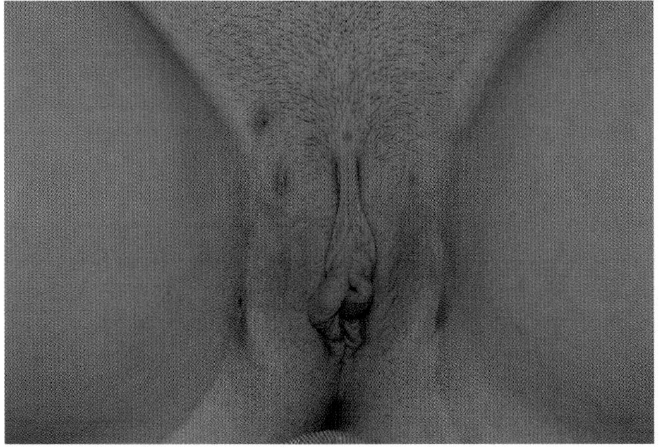

Fig. 162.38 Hidradenitis suppurativa in a child showing vulval nodules.

Oral antibiotics are used in children with moderate HS, Hurley stage II, with oral clindamycin 10–25 mg/kg/day in three divided doses being the most commonly prescribed [35]. The combination of rifampicin and clindamycin has been used successfully in adults and there are anecdotal reports in children [41]. In children over the age of 8 years old, doxycycline can be prescribed (British National Formulary recommends for use in children over the age of 12 years) and erythromycin can be used at all ages.There have been reports of the use of isotretinoin but results are disappointing. For severe disease, Hurley stage III, finasteride has been reported to be effective in three children, two of whom were prepubertal, with no side-effects [42].

Many biologic agents have been reported to be useful in treatment of HS and adalimumab (Humira®) is now approved for treatment of adults in some countries; however, trials are lacking in children [43]. Surgical and ablative laser treatment are second line and their use has been reported in children [35].

References

1 **Mirza A, Zamilpa I, Wilson JM. Localized penile bullous pemphigoid. J Pediatr Urol 2008;4(5):395–7.**
2 **Fisler RE, Saeb M, Liang MG et al. Childhood bullous pemphigoid: a clinicopathologic study and review of the literature. Am J Dermatopathol 2003;25(3):183–9.**
3 Farrell AM, Kirtschig G, Dalziel KL et al. Childhood vulval pemphigoid: a clinical and immunopathological study of five patients. Br J Dermatol 1999;140:308–12.
4 Saad RW, Domloge-Hultsch N, Yancey KB et al. Childhood localized vulvar pemphigoid is a true variant of bullous pemphigoid. Arch Dermatol 1992;128:807–10.
5 Levine V, Sanchez M, Nestor M. Localised vulvar pemphigoid in a child misdiagnosed as sexual abuse. Arch Dermatol 1992;128:804–6.
6 Hoque SR, Patel M, Farrell AM. Childhood cicatricial pemphigoid confined to the vulva. Clin Exp Dermatol 2005;31:63–4.
7 Lebeau S, Mainetti C, Masouye I et al. Localized childhood vulval pemphigoid treated with tacrolimus ointment. Dermatology 2004;208:273–5.
8 **Guenther LC, Shum D. Localised childhood vulvar pemphigoid. J Am Acad Dermatol 1990;22:762–4.**
9 **Marren P, Wojnarowska F, Venning V et al. Vulvar involvement in autoimmune blistering diseases. J Reprod Med 1993;38(2):101–7.**
10 Hernandez-Nunez A, Cordoba S, Romero-Mate A et al. Lipschutz ulcers – four cases. Pediatr Dermatol 2008;25(3):364–7.
11 Lehman JS, Bruce AJ, Wetter DA et al Reactive nonsexually related acute genital ulcers: review of cases evaluated at Mayo Clinic. J Am Acad Dermatol 2010;63(1):44–51.
12 **Farhi D, Wendling J, Molinari E et al. Non-sexually related acute genital ulcers in 13 pubertal girls: a clinical and microbiological study. Arch Dermatol 2009;145(1):38–45.**
13 **Ghate JV, Jorizzo MD. Behçet's disease and complex aphthosis. J Am Acad Dermatol 1999;40:1–18.**
14 Wetter DA, Bruce A, MacLaughlin KL et al. Ulcus vulvae acutum in a 13 year old girl after influenza A infection. Skinmed 2008;7(2):95–8.
15 **Rosman IS, Berk DR, Bayliss SJ et al. Acute genital ulcers in nonsexually active young girls: case series, review of the literature, and evaluation and management recommendations. Pediatr Dermatol 2012;29(2):147–53**
16 **Dixit S, Bradford J, Fischer G. Management of nonsexually acquired genital ulceration using oral and topical corticosteroids followed by doxycycline prophylaxis. J Am Acad Dermatol 2013;68(5):797–802.**
17 Huppert JS, Gerber M, Deitch HR et al. Vulvar ulcers in young females: a manifestation of aphthosis. J Pediatr Adolesc Gynecol 2006;19(3):195–204.
18 Rogers RS III. Recurrent aphthous stomatitis: clinical characteristics and associated systemic disorder. Semin Cutan Med Surg 1997;16: 278–83.

19 Unal M, Yildirim SV, Akbaba M. A recurrent aphthous stomatitis case due to paediatric Behçet's disease. J Laryngol Otol 2001;115:576–7.
20 Magalhaes MG, Bueno DF, Serra E et al. Oral manifestations of HIV positive children. J Clin Pediatr Dent 2001;25:103–6.
21 Bramanti E, Cicciu M, Matacena G et al Clinical evaluation of specific oral manifestation in Pediatric patients with ascertained versus potential coeliac disease: a cross-sectional study. Gastroenterol Res Pract 2014;2014:934159.
22 Lin CM, Wang CC, Lai CC et al. Genital ulcers as an unusual sign of periodic fever, aphthous stomatitis, pharyngotonsillitis, cervical adenopathy syndrome: a novel symptom? Pediatr Dermatol 2011;28(3):290–4.
23 Jorizzo JL, Taylor RS, Schmalstieg FC. Complex aphthosis: a forme fruste of Behçet's syndrome? J Am Acad Dermatol 1985;13:80–4.
24 Eisen D, Lynch DP. Selecting topical and systemic agents for recurrent aphthous stomatitis. Cutis 2001;68:201–6.
25 Nussinovitch M, Prais D, Ben-Amitai D et al. Fixed drug eruption in the genital area of 15 boys. Pediatr Dermatol 2002;19:216–19.
26 Morelli JG, Tay YK, Rogers M et al. Fixed drug eruptions in children. J Pediatr 1999;134:365–7.
27 Sehgal VH, Gangwani OP. Genital fixed drug eruptions. Genitourin Med 1986;62:56–8.
28 Salvado F, Furtado I. A case of erythema multiforme with only oro genital manifestations. Rev Port Estomatol Cirurg Maxilofac 1988;21: 19–24.
29 Latsch K, Girschick H, Abele-Horn M. Stevens–Johnson syndrome without skin lesions. J Med Microbiol 2007;56(12):1696–9.
30 Canavan TN, Mathes EF, Frieden I, Shinkai K. Mycoplasma pneumoniae-induced rash and mucositis as a syndrome distinct from Stevens-Johnson syndrome and erythema multiforme: a systematic review. J Am Acad Dermatol 2015;72(2):239–45.
31 Graham-Brown RA, Cochrane GW, Swinhoe JR et al. Vaginal stenosis due to bullous erythema multiforme (Stevens–Johnson syndrome). Br J Obstet Gynaecol 1981;88:115–16.
32 Bonafe JL, Thibaut I, Hoff J. Introital adhesions associated with the Stevens–Johnson syndrome. Clin Exp Dermatol 1990;15:356–7.
33 Sibaud V, Fricain J, Leaute-Labreze C et al. Persistent mucosal ulcerations: a rare complication of toxic epidermal necrolysis. Ann Dermatol Venereol 2005;132(8–9 Pt 1):682–5.
34 Pliskow S. Severe gynecologic sequelae of Stevens-Johnson syndrome and toxic epidermal necrolysis caused by ibuprofen: a case report. J Reprod Med 2013;58(7–8):354–6.
35 Liy-Wong C, Pope E, Lara-Corrales I. Hidradenitis suppurativa in the pediatric population. J Am Acad Dermatol 2015;73(5) Suppl:S36–41.
36 Palmer RA, Keefe M. Early onset hidradenitis suppurativa. Clin Exp Dermatol 2001;26:501–3.
37 Mengesha YM, Holcombe TC, Hansen RC. Prepubertal hidradenitis suppurativa: two case reports and review of the literature. Pediatr Dermatol 1999;16:292–6.
38 Deckers IE, vander Zee HH, Boer J, Prens EP. Correlation of early-onset hidradenitis suppurativa with stronger genetic susceptibility and more widespread involvement. J Am Dermatol 2015;72(3):485–8.
39 Pink AE, Simpson MA, Desai N et al. Gamma-secretase mutations in hidradenitis suppurativa: new insightsinto disease pathogenesis. J Invest Dermatol 2013;133:601–7.
40 Alikhan A, Lynch P, Eisen DB. Hidradenitis suppurativa: a comprehensive review. J Am Acad Dermatol 2009;60:539–61.
41 Scheinfeld N. Hidradenitis suppurativa in prepubescent and pubescent children. Clin Dermatol 2015;33:316–19.
42 Randhawa HK, Hamilton J, Pope E. Finasteride for the treatment of hidradenitis suppurativa in children and adolescents. JAMA Dermatol 2013;149(6):732–5.
43 Lee RA, Eisen DB. Treatment of hidradenitis suppurativa with biologic medications. J Am Acad Dermatol 2015;73(5)Suppl:S82–8.

Anatomical abnormalities

Vulval abnormalities

Abnormal-appearing genitalia present at birth in a girl has two most frequent causes: (1) masculinization due to congenital adrenocortical hyperplasia as a result of an inherited defect of steroid synthesis and (2) imperforate hymen. Although these problems would not normally present to a dermatologist, they come into the differential diagnosis of fusion of the labia as discussed below.

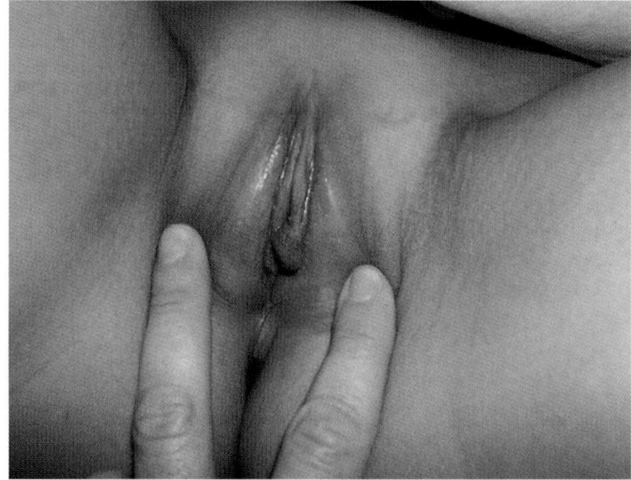

Fig. 162.39 Hypertrophy of the labia minora.

Agenesis of the labia minora and clitoris has been described as a congenital abnormality [1], as has agenesis of the scrotum and labia majora [2]. Hypertophy of the labia minora is a benign condition that may be unilateral or bilateral (Fig. 162.39). It is usually asymptomatic but very long labia may interfere with function [3]. Adolescent girls sometimes present with a great deal of anxiety about hypertrophic labia and asymmetrical labial growth may occur at puberty, also a cause for concern [4]. It is becoming more common for patients to seek a surgical solution as early as puberty [5]; however, it should be appreciated that the labia minora are highly innervated along their entire edge and that labioplasty runs the risk of sensory disturbance and may possibly affect sexual arousal [6]. Therefore any genital operation in the absence of real pathology is best deferred until adulthood.

Ambiguous genitalia should be a reason for referral to a paediatrician for assessment [7,8].

Penile abnormalities

Congenital hydrocoele caused by fluid trapped in the processus vaginalis, the tract through which the testes descend, is a common congenital abnormality. It results in mild scrotal swelling, which transilluminates. There is often an associated indirect inguinal hernia [9].

Chordee and penile hypospadias are also relatively common and produce abnormality of the appearance of the penis. Hypospadias is a ventral displacement of the urethral opening, which is usually associated with the presence of an incomplete foreskin with an absent ventral portion. Chordee results in a ventral curvature of the penis resulting from a deficiency of the ventral tissue distal to the abnormally placed meatus and fibrous tissue. It may occasionally occur without hypospadias. Both of these abnormalities may be associated with other abnormalities of the urinary tract [9,10].

CHARGE syndrome (OMIM 214800)

This syndrome, first described by Pagon [11], is a dominant disorder comprising coloboma, heart defects, atresia choanae, retarded growth and development, genital hypoplasia in boys, ear anomalies and deafness. Facial nerve palsy, tracheo-oesophageal fistula, hypocalcaemia and lymphopenia have also been described.

A gene mutation of *CHD7* on chromosome 8q12.1 is found in the majority of patients [12,13].

Although in girls hypoplastic uterus has been described, abnormalities of the external genitals have only been found in boys. Cryptorchism and micropenis are the most common anomalies [13].

Pearly penile papules

Pathogenesis. Pearly penile papules are small smooth excrescences projecting from the penile corona. They are not symptomatic and are a normal variant. They are more common after puberty but may be rarely seen in children. They are found in all races [14,15].

Histopathology. The pathology is reminiscent of an angiofibroma, with a core of connective tissue containing a vascular network and a mild lymphocytic infiltrate. The covering epidermis is normal and slightly acanthotic at the periphery [16].

Clinical presentation. The complaint is only of the appearance of the papules, which are usually assumed to be genital warts. There are one to three rings of lesions, partly or completely encircling the corona of the glans. Rarely, they may cover the entire glans [17]. The papules are usually small, 1–3 mm in diameter, and flesh-coloured to white. They are usually asymptomatic.

Management. None is indicated and parents should be reassured that this is not a disease at all. Some authors have suggested treatment of these lesions with CO_2 laser or cryotherapy. In the author's opinion this should be discouraged [15,18].

Fusion of the labia

Incidence. Fusion of the labia is sometimes seen in young children, with onset usually 3 years of age and under. It is not seen in adults, unless they have scarring skin diseases such as lichen sclerosus. It may be noticed from infancy to the age of 6 years, but the peak incidence is at 13–23 months of age. Once a child has had an adhesion, it may persist or recur until puberty [19].

Aetiology. The cause of labial adhesions is unknown but they are probably the result of inflammation and oedema associated with dermatological conditions such as dermatitis. Adhesions are commonly encountered with vulval lichen sclerosus and have been reported in association with calcinosis cutis [20]. Fusion of the labia is not a malformation and is acquired, but it may appear very early and has even been seen at birth.

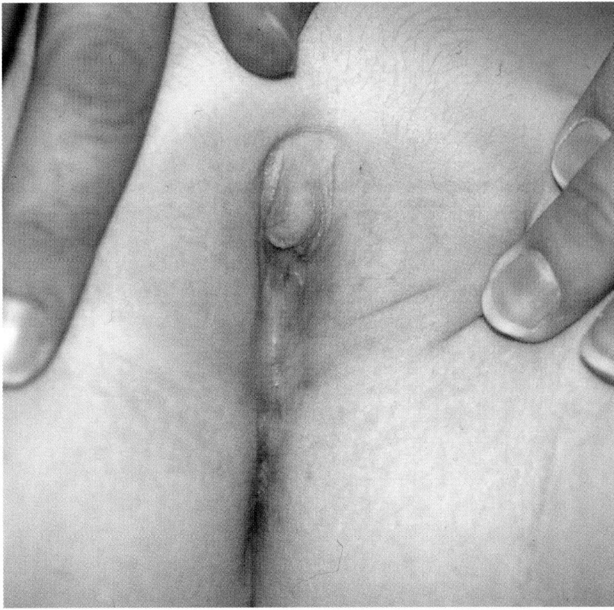

Fig. 162.40 Fusion of the labia minora.

Clinical presentation. The labia minora or majora are agglutinated in the midline to a variable degree from the tip of the clitoris to the posterior fourchette. This may result in an abnormal-looking vulva with no apparent vaginal opening or the vulva may look relatively normal but there appears to be a membrane across the vagina when the labia majora are parted [21] (Fig. 162.40).

Not all children with adhesions are symptomatic, but some experience soreness or itching. Urine can pool behind the fusion, causing irritating maceration. Urinary tract infections are, however, rarely a complicating factor.

Differential diagnosis. Fusion of the labia is important in the differential diagnosis of ambiguous genitalia and imperforate hymen and a gynaecological opinion should be sought if there is any doubt. The presence of a midline fusion line suggests the presence of this condition.

Management. This is the only condition for which oestrogen cream is acceptable treatment in a prepubertal child. The cream needs to be applied only once per day, and the fusion usually resolves over a 2–6-week period. Once the fusion has separated, ongoing treatment with soap avoidance, topical lubricants and 1% hydrocortisone is recommended. It is common for the fusion to reform and have to be retreated, particularly when the fusion is severe [22]. This can be a problem as oestrogen creams are irritating in children and they tend to sting, making cooperation difficult. Prolonged use of oestrogen creams in prepubertal girls may lead to breast budding and increased growth of hair [13,23]. Potent topical corticosteroid may also be effective and is less irritating than oestrogen and combining both may be slightly more effective than either alone [24]. Both will cause reversible erythema with prolonged use.

When the adhesion does not resolve with oestrogen treatment, manual separation may be required [25]. This should never be attempted without anaesthesia as it is very traumatic for the child. In some patients, surgical separation under local or general anaesthesia will be required, particularly where dense fibrous adhesions have formed. The condition tends to resolve spontaneously at puberty; however, surgery should only be undertaken if the condition is symptomatic. Dysuria, pain with activities, urinary retention and almost complete occlusion of the vestibule leading to a pinpoint opening with abnormal urinary stream are indications for such treatment [26].

The treatment of asymptomatic labial adhesions is controversial. Treatment is not always necessary if the child is asymptomatic and parents just need reassurance that eventual spontaneous recovery is the rule [27]. If the adhesion is small, nonintervention is probably justified. However, an almost complete adhesion could pose difficulties in the setting when a catheterization is required, and it has therefore been suggested that large adhesions should be treated even when there are no symptoms [28].

Clitoral cysts

Epidermal inclusion cysts are benign lesions found on any part of the skin. They are reported as an uncommon cause of clitoromegaly in children. They may follow trauma or arise spontaneously [29]. They have been described as relatively frequent following female genital mutilation [30]. The nature of the lesion can be confirmed on MRI imaging. The lesion can be removed surgically. In the differential diagnosis are clitoral vascular malformations, benign tumours and hair tourniquet syndrome.

Phimosis

At birth, the prepuce is adherent to the glans and cannot be easily retracted. Only 4% of boys have a retractable foreskin at birth, 15% at 6 months of age, 50% at 1 year and 80–90% at 3 years. It should be fully retractable by the age of 17 [31]. Dermatologists should be aware of this timeline, as inability to retract the foreskin, particularly when it has previously been retractable, may be a sign of inflammatory skin disease of the glans.

The degree of phimosis may vary from difficulty retracting the foreskin to a nonretractable pinpoint opening. Persistent phimosis after this age may lead to recurring balanitis.

Phimosis may be congenital or acquired. A study in 2002 found that among the group with congenital phimosis, 30% had lichen sclerosus, and in the group with acquired phimosis, this figure rose to 60%. The remainder of the boys showed inflammatory change on biopsy [32]. Thus, the aetiology of this condition, if lichen sclerosus is not present, may be similar to adhesion of the labia in girls. Phimosis has been associated with lichen planus of the glans [33]; however, lichen planus is very rare in children and this case was very unusual.

Management. Although circumcision has in the past been considered the treatment of choice for phimosis, more recent studies indicate that the use of moderately potent topical corticosteroids coupled with gentle retraction has a high success rate. This should now be considered as the first-line treatment for phimosis, prior to surgery [34–36].

Infantile pyramidal perineal protrusion

Although this has only quite recently been labelled as an entity in the medical literature [37], it is probably not rare. It is noticed in infancy as an asymptomatic soft protrusion of the median raphe, mostly in girls [38]. The lesion is usually anterior to the anus but may also be posterior (Fig. 162.41). The overlying skin is normal. Some cases have been seen in association with lichen sclerosus [39–41] and chronic constipation [42]. It has been reported in families [43].

Like many innocent genital lesions, this entity may be mistaken for genital warts or sexual abuse [42]. It also comes into the differential diagnosis of a sentinel tag.

No treatment is required. The natural history of the lesion in later childhood is unknown.

Median raphe cysts of the penis and scrotum

Cysts of the median raphe are embryological development anomalies of the male genitalia. They are usually present at birth but may not become noticeable until adult life [44]. They are considered to be congenital alterations in embryonal development.

Histology. The cysts are found in the dermis, and are lined by several layers of pseudo-stratified epithelium and contain amorphous material consisting of acid mucopolysaccharides [45].

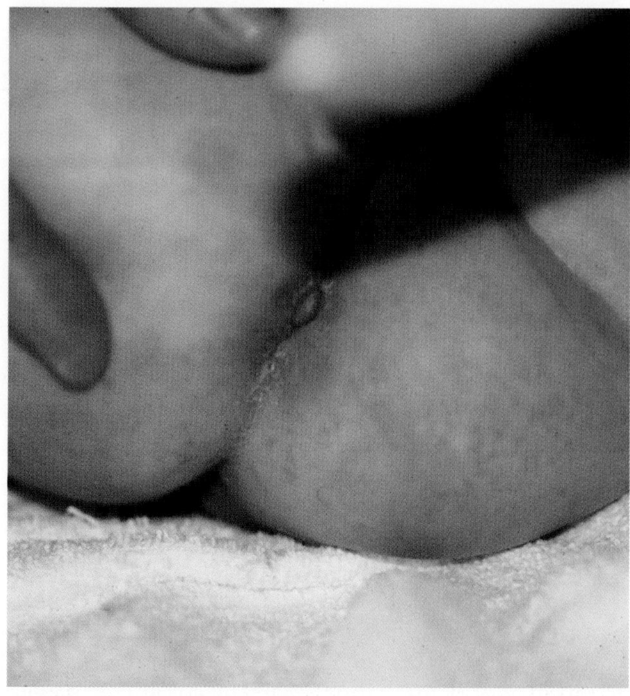

Fig. 162.41 Pyramidal perineal protrusion.

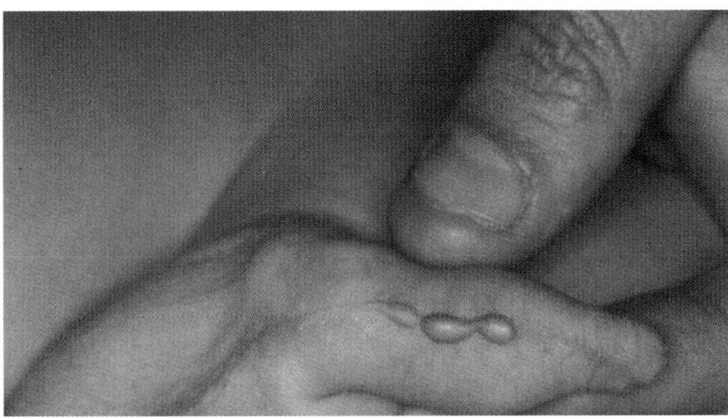

Fig. 162.42 Multiple median raphe cysts of the penis. Source: Courtesy of Dr M. Rogers.

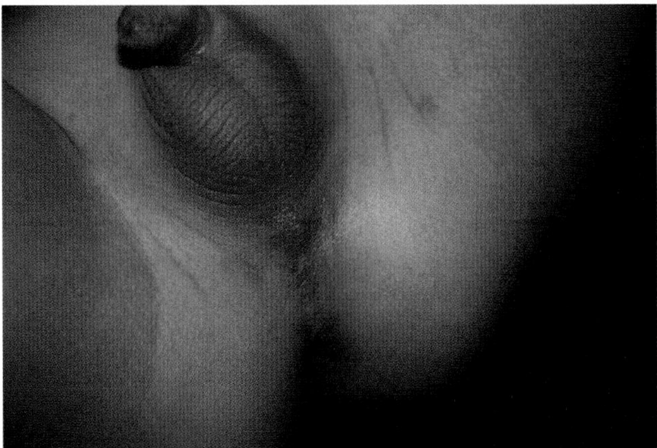

Fig. 162.43 Median raphe cyst of the perineum.

Clinical presentation. The cyst presents as a mobile swelling with translucent contents. It may be single or multiple (Fig. 162.42). The lesions may be found anywhere between the urinary meatus and the anus (Fig. 162.43). They are usually asymptomatic. Age at first presentation is usually after the first decade but the lesion has been reported in younger children [46,47].

Differential diagnosis. This includes epidermoid cyst, dermoid, urethral diverticulum and pilonidal cyst.

Management. Simple excision is recommended to avoid problems with friction in later life [48,49].

References

1 Martinon-Torres F, Martinon-Sanchez J, Martinon-Sanchez F. Clitoris and labia minora agenesis: an undescribed phenomenon. Clin Genet 2000;58(4):336–8.

2 Silay MS, Yesil G, Yildiz K et al. Congenital agenesis of the scrotum and labia majora in siblings. Urology 2013;81(2):421–3.

3 Schroeder B. Vulvar disorders in adolescents. Obstet Gynecol Clin 2000;27(1):5–48.

4 Pederiva F. A girl with labium majus swelling. Eur J Pediatr 2014; 173:401.

5 Rouzier R, Louis-Sylvestre C, Paniel BJ, Haddad B. Hypertrophy of labia minora: experience with 163 reductions. Am J Obstet Gynecol 2000;182(1 Pt 1):35–40.

6 Schober J, Cooney T, Pfaff D et al. Innervation of the labia minora in prepubertal girls. J Pedatr Adolesc Gynecol 2010;23(6):352–7.

7 Donahoe PK, Hendren WH. Evaluation of the newborn with ambiguous genitalia. Pediatr Clin North Am 1976;23:361–70.

8 Aaronson IA. The investigation and management of the infant with ambiguous genitalia: a surgeon's perspective. Curr Probl Pediatr 2001;31:168–94.

9 Lynch PJ, Edwards L. Pediatric problems. In: Genital Dermatology. New York: Churchill Livingstone, 1994:251–2.

10 Baskin LS. Hypospadias and urethral development. J Urol 2000;163:951.

11 Pagon RA, Graham J Jr, Zonana J, Yong SL. Coloboma, congenital heart disease and choanal atresia with multiple anomalies: CHARGE syndrome. J Pediatr 1981;99(2):223–7.

12 Aramaki M, Udaka T, Kosaki R et al. Phenotypic spectrum of CHARGE syndrome with CHD7 mutations. J Pediatr 2006;148(3):410–14.

13 Jongmans MC, Admiraal R, van der Donk KP et al. CHARGE syndrome: the phenotypic spectrum of mutations in the CHD7 gene. J Med Genet 2006;43(4):306–14.

14 Sonnex C, Dockerty WG. Pearly penile papules: a common cause of concern. Int J STD AIDS 1999;10:726–7.

15 Ackerman AB, Kronberg R. Pearly penile papules: acral angiofibromas. Arch Dermatol 1973;108:673–5.

16 Lane JE, Peterson CM, Ratz JL. Treatment of pearly penile papules with CO_2 laser. Dermatol Surg 2002;28:617–18.

17 Agarwal SK, Bhattacharya S, Singh N. Pearly penile papules: a review. Int J Dermatol 2004;43(3):199–201.

18 Porter WM, Bunker CB. Treatment of pearly penile papules with cryotherapy. Br J Dermatol 2000;142:847–8.

19 Carpraro VJ, Greenburg H. Adhesions of the labia minora. Obstet Gynecol 1972;39:65–9.

20 Bernardo BD, Huettner PC, Merritt DF et al. Idiopathic calcinosis cutis presenting as labial adhesions in children: report of two cases with literature review. J Pediatr Adolesc Gynecol 1999;12:157–60.

21 Bacon JL. Prepubertal labial adhesions. Evaluation of a referral population. Am J Obstet Gynecol 2002;187:327–32.

22 Granada C, Sokkary N, Sangi-Haghpeykar H, Ietrich JE. Labial adhesions and outcomes of office management. J Pediatr Adolesc Gynecol 2015;28(2):109–13.

23 Schober J, Dulabon L, Martin-Alguacil N et al. Significance of topical estrogens to labial fusion and vaginal introital integrity. J Pediatr Adolesc Gynecol 2006;19(5):337–9.

24 Eroglu E, Yip M, Oktar T et al. How should we treat prepubertal labial adhesions? Retrospective comparison of topial treatments: estrogen only, betamethasone only, and combination estrogen and betamethasone. J Pediatr Adolesc Gynecol 2011;24(6):389–91.

25 Soyer T. Topical estrogen therapy in labial adhesions in children: therapeutic or prophylactic? J Pediatr Adolesc Gynecol 2007;20:241–4.

26 Pokorny SF. Prepubertal vulvovaginopathies. Obstet Gynecol Clin North Am 1992;19:39–59.

27 Bacon JL, Romano ME, Quint EH. Clinical recommendation: labial adhesions. J Pediatr Adolesc Gynecol 2015;28(5):405–9.

28 Muram D. Treatment of prepubertal girls with labial adhesions. J Pediatr Adolesc Gynecol 1999;12:67–70.

29 Cetinkursun S, Narci A, Sahin O, Ozkaraca E. Epidermoid cyst causing clitoromegaly in a child. Int J Gynecol Obstet 2009;105(1):64.

30 Rouzi AA. Epidermal clitoral inclusion cysts: not a rare complication of female genital mutilation. Human Reprod 2010;25(7):1672–4.

31 Cold CJ, Taylor J. The prepuce. BJU Int 1999;83(suppl 1):34–44.

32 Mattioli G, Repetto P, Carlini C et al. Lichen sclerosus et atrophicus in children with phimosis and hypospadias. Pediatr Surg Int 2002;18:273–5.

33 Aste N, Pau M, Ferreli C et al. Lichen planus in a child requiring circumcision. Pediatr Dermatol 1997;14:129–30.

34 Orsola A, Caffaratti J, Garat JM. Conservative treatment of phimosis in children using a topical steroid. Urology 2000;5:307–10.

35 Ng WT, Fan N, Wong CK et al. Treatment of childhood phimosis with a moderately potent topical steroid. Aust NZ J Surg 2001;71:541–3.

36 Webster TM, Leonard MP. Topical steroid therapy for phimosis. Can J Urol 2002;9:1492–5.

37 Konta R, Hashimoto I, Takahashi M, Tamai K. Infantile perineal protrusion: a statistical, clinical and histopathologic study. Dermatology 2000;201(4):316–20.

38 Cruces MJ, de la Torre C, Losada A et al. Infantile perineal protrusion as a manifestation of lichen sclerosus et atrophicus. Arch Dermatol 1998;134(9):1118–20.

39 Hernandez-Machin B, Almeida P, Lukan D et al. Infantile pyramidal protrusion localized at the vulva as a manifestation of lichen sclerosus. J Am Acad Dermatol 2007;56(2 suppl):S49–50.

40 Kayashima KI, Kitoh M, Ono T. Infantile perianal pyramidal protrusion. Arch Dermatol 1996;132:1481–4.

41 Cruces MJ, de la Torre C, Losada A et al. Infantile pyramidal protrusion as a manifestation of lichen sclerosus et atrophicus. Arch Dermatol 1998;134:1118–20.
42 Khachemoune A, Guldbakke K, Ehrsam E. Infantile perineal protrusion. J Am Acad Dermatol 2006;54(6):1046–9.
43 Patrizi A, Raone B, Neri I et al. Infantile perianal protrusion: 13 new cases. Pediatr Dermatol 2002;19:15–18.
44 Krauel L, Tarrado X, Garcia-Aparicio L et al. Median raphe cysts of the perineum in children. Urology 2008;71(5):830–1.
45 Nagore E, Sanchez-Motilla J, Febrer MI et al. Median raphe cysts of the penis: a report of five cases. Pediatr Dermatol 1998;15:191–3.
46 Lever WF, Schaumberg-Lever G. Tumours and cysts of the epidermis. In: Lever WF, Schaumberg-Lever G (eds) Histopathology of the Skin, 7th edn. Philadelphia: J.B. Lippincott, 1990:540.
47 Otsuka T, Ueda Y, Terauchi M et al. Median raphe (parameatal) cysts of the penis. J Urol 1998;159:1918–20.
48 Asarch RG, Golitz LE, Sansker WF et al. Median raphe cysts of the penis. Arch Dermatol 1979;115:1084–6.
49 Little JS, Keating MA, Rink RC. Median raphe cysts of the genitalia. J Urol 1992;148:1872–3.

Foreign bodies

Although intravaginal foreign bodies are often mentioned as a cause of vulval disease in the medical literature, the fact is that they are not a common event. The foreign material is usually fragments of toilet paper or fluff. Small toys are less common [1].

The presence of vaginal bleeding in a prepubertal child is highly suggestive of a foreign body [2]. Another common presentation is a persistent purulent discharge heavy enough to cause maceration of the vulval skin. A crusted, erythematous or pigmented line along the tips of the labia majora may be the result of chronic maceration. Lichenification may occur. Swabs show recurrent bacterial infection, which responds to courses of antibiotics but rapidly recurs [3]. A study of 24 prepubertal girls presenting with vaginal discharge or bleeding found that a foreign body was responsible in seven cases; however, six girls had malignancies, three rhabdomyosarcomas and three endodermal sinus tumours, and a further two had benign mullerian papillomas [4].

A foreign body may be in place for weeks to years before symptoms develop [5].

Radiological and ultrasound techniques fail to detect most vaginal foreign bodies. It may be possible to lavage the vagina using saline solution as an office procedure; however, many children will require examination under anaesthesia with vaginoscopy and saline lavage. Often, there is very little to be seen on lavage, and it is likely that only small fragments can cause this clinical presentation [3,5,6]. All persistent, recurrent or blood-stained vaginal discharges resistant to treatment should be fully evaluated to rule out a foreign body or other vaginal or pelvic pathology.

Foreign bodies of the penile urethra are rare. Symptoms of dysuria, urethral discharge or bleeding may also occur. Endoscopic investigation may be required to locate and remove such objects and, rarely, surgery may be required [2].

Hair tourniquet

The hair tourniquet is a well-described condition where a hair or thread becomes tightly wrapped around an end perfusion appendage, causing hypoperfusion and reducing lymphatic draininge. This results in swelling, pain and sometimes necrosis leading to autoamputation of the strangulated structure. The genital area can be involved. This phenomenon has most often been described to involve the penis [7], clitoris [8] and labia [9]. When the clitoris is involved apparent clitoral hypertrophy can occur [10]. This is an emergency that requires prompt surgical intervention.

References

1 Pokorny SF. Prepubertal vulvovaginopathies. Obstet Gynecol Clin North Am 1992;19:39–58.
2 Di Meglio G. Genital foreign bodies. Pediatr Rev 1998;19:34.
3 Bacon JL. Pediatric vulvovaginitis. Adolesc Pediatr Gynecol 1989;2: 86–93.
4 Striegel AM, Myers J, Sorensen MD et al. Vaginal discharge and bleeding in girls younger than 6 years. J Urol 2006;176(6 Pt 1):2632–5.
5 Pokorny SF. Long term intravaginal presence of foreign bodies in children: a preliminary study. J Reprod Med 1994;39:931–5.
6 David VJ. What the paediatrician should know about paediatric and adolescent gynecology: the perspective of a gynaecologist. Pediatr Child Health 2003;8(8):491–5.
7 Dar NR, Siddiqui S, Qayyum R, Ghafoor T. Hair coil strangulation: an uncommon cause of penile edema. Pediatr Dermatol 2007;24(4):E33–5.
8 Alverson B. A genital hair tourniquet in a 9 year old girl. Pediatr Emerg Care 2007;23(3):169–70.
9 Bannier MA, Miedema CJ Hair tourniquet syndrome. Eur J Pediatr 2013;172(2):277.
10 Parlak M, Karakaya AE Hair-thread tourniquet syndrome of the hypertrophic clitoris in a 6-year-old girl. Pediatr Emerg Care 2015; 31(5):363–4.

Neoplasia

Neoplasia of the genitalia in children is a rare event. However, the differential diagnosis of an enlarging genital mass is wide and should be promptly investigated [1]. It includes a variety of tumours of mesenchymal origin, embryonic remnants and malignancies [1].

Malignancies

Langerhans cell histiocytosis may present as an erosive, purpuric and pustular recalcitrant nappy rash, usually with generalized lesions [2] (Fig 162.44). However, it has been reported as a genital ulceration alone and as such was confused with sexual abuse [3]. It has also been reported as a vulval eruption in an adolescent [4].

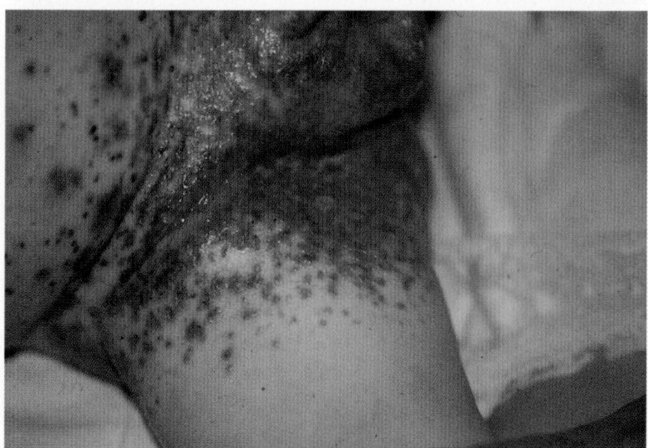

Fig. 162.44 Langerhans cell histiocytosis which was mistaken for recalcitrant napkin dermatitis.

Melanoma of the vulva has been rarely reported in children and adolescents, and in six cases this has been in association with childhood lichen sclerosus [5–7]. Rhabdomyoscarcoma is the most common tumour of the lower genitourinary tract in children and has been reported on the penis, perineum and vagina as a painless firm swelling or a protruding vaginal mass with vaginal bleeding [8,9]. A malignant schwannoma has been described on the penis [10].

Vulval intraepithelial neoplasia has been reported in children [8] and adolescents with abnormal cervical cytology [11]. Squamous cell carcinoma of the vulva in a setting of bowenoid papulosis has been reported in a 12-year-old girl with vertically acquired HIV disease [12] and in a 16-year-old liver transplant recipient [13]. In the latter case, uncommon human papillomavirus subtypes were extracted from the cancer, prompting a call for more careful vulval and cervical surveillance in immunosuppressed paediatric transplant recipients.

Primary malignant lymphoma is rare in the genital area, but a B-cell non-Hodgkin lymphoma has been reported involving the penis in a 4-year-old boy [14]. Vulval plasmablastic lymphoma has been reported in a HIV-positive child [15].

Benign tumours

Granular cell tumour is a rare benign soft tissue neoplasm originating from Schwann cells [16] that has been reported as a vulval, penile and scrotal lesion in children, presenting as slow-growing solitary nodules or plaques with a smooth or hyperkeratotic surface [16–20]. Syringomas of the vulva have been described in children [21] and multiple genital trichoepithelioma has been described in the setting of Bazex–Dupre–Christol syndrome [22]. A case of apocrine hidrocystoma has been described on the glans in a child [23]. Atyical fibroxanthoma, juvenile xanthogranuloma and solitary mastocytoma (Fig. 162.45) [24,25] may occur on the vulva [26].

Leiomyoma may occur on the glans penis, scrotum, vulva and prepuce, and myofibroma has been described on the penis in children [27,28].

Neuroendocrine tumours, such as small cell neuroendocrine carcinomas, are more common in the female than the male genital tract; however, they may uncommonly be found on the penis, scrotum and vulva, presenting as a mass [29]. Neurilemmoma may occur as multiple swellings of the penile shaft, and neurofibromas may be found on the penis and scrotum [30–32]. Benign schwannoma has been reported as a firm clitoral mass [33] and a labial mass [34]. Patients with neurofibromatosis may experience involvement of the genitals with plexiform neurofibroma [35]. The most frequent presenting sign of genital involvement of neurofibromatosis in females is clitoromegaly with pseudo-penis formation, and enlarged penis is the most common sign in males [36]. Rarely, in girls the labia may be involved [36].

A mesenchymal tumour which has been termed 'prepubertal vulval fibroma' has been described in prepubertal girls [37]. The presentation is with a nonspecific unilateral labial mass ranging in size from 2 to 8cm in diameter. This is a benign lesion showing the histopathology of spindle cells in a myxoid stroma, which can be locally recurrent after excision. Staining is positive for vimentin and CD34. The importance of this lesion is that it may be difficult to differentiate from soft tissue sarcoma histologically [38].

Epidermoid cysts are not uncommon on the genitals in adults and have been reported in children [39]. A ciliated cyst of the vulva has been reported in a child [40]. 'Smegma pearls' are benign collections of smegma in the subpreputial space of young uncircumcised boys. They are visible as a white domed lesion of the glans.The may collect if the foreskin is not regularly retracted to clean the glans and coronal sulcus. They may simulate a cyst but can be expressed manually [41].

Fibrous hamartoma of infancy is an uncommon subcutaneous proliferative lesion usually found on the trunk in the first two years of life. This lesion has also been reported on the vulva and scrotum [42].

Lipomas of the vulva have been described in girls as sharply circumscribed soft masses of the labia, pedunculated lesions or gross swelling of the vulva [43,44] and in boys as masses on the penis and perineum [45]. A case of congenital perineal lipoma has been reported as presenting as ambiguous genitalia [46]. Lipoma may be diagnosed by imaging and surgical excision is the treatment of choice. Lipoblastoma of the vulva has also been reported as an acquired, rapidly growing but benign lesion in a 13-month-old girl [47].

Prepubertal unilateral fibrous hyperplasia of the labium majus

This recently recognized condition presents with asymptomatic rapidly growing unilateral or occasionally bilateral enlargement of the labium majus [48,49].

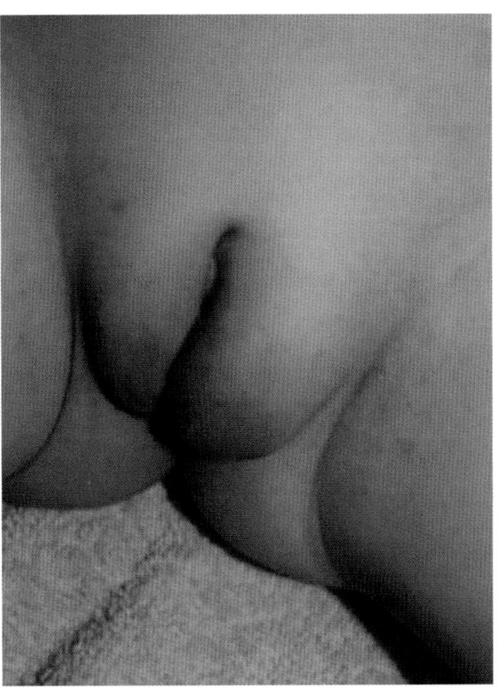

Fig. 162.45 Solitary mastocytoma of the vulva presenting as erythematous vulval swelling.

Clinical features. The mass is soft and has no palpable borders. The overlying skin is described as having a slightly hyperpigmented peau d'orange surface. It occurs around adrenarche and appears to be an asymmetrical physiological enlargement in response to hormonal surges of prepuberty and early puberty. It has been observed to regress if left untreated.

Histology. Histology shows hypocellular fibrous tissue. Oestrogen and progesterone receptors are identified on fibroblasts.

Differential diagnosis. This condition can mimic an infiltrative neoplasm because of its rapid growth [49].

References

1 **Lowry DL, Guido DS. The vulvar mass in the prepubertal child. J Pediatr Adolesc Gynecol 2000;13:75–8.**
2 **Otis CN, Fischer RA, Johnson N et al. Histiocytosis-X of the vulva: a case report and review of the literature. Obstet Gynecol 1990;75:555–8.**
3 Roche E, Pandya N, Munthali L, Atra A. Genital ulceration in a 4 year old: a case of safeguarding? From social services to pathology. BMJ Case Reports 2012;2012:ii.
4 Mottl H, Rob L, Stary J et al. Langerhans cell histiocytosis of vulva in adolescent. Int J Gynecol Cancer 2007;17(2):520–4.
5 Hassanein AM, Mrstik M, Hardt NS et al Malignant melanoma associated with lichen sclerosus in the vulva of a 10-year-old. Pediatr Dermatol 2004;21(4):473–6.
6 Egan CA, Bradley RR, Logsdon VK et al. Vulvar melanoma in childhood. Arch Dermatol 1997;133:345–8.
7 **La Spina M, Meli MC, de Pasquale R et al. Vulvar melanoma associated with lichen sclerosus in a child: case report and literature review. Pediatr Dermatol 2016;33(3):e190–4.**
8 Agrons GA, Wagner BJ, Lonergan JG et al. From the archives of the AFIP. Genitourinary myosarcoma in children: a radiologic-pathologic correlation. Radiographics 1997;17:919–37.
9 Youngstrom EA, Bartkowski DP. Vulvar embryonal rhabdomyosarcoma: a case report. J Pediatr Urol 2013;9(4):e144–6.
10 Mortell A, Amjad B, Breatnach F et al. Penile malignant peripheral nerve sheath tumour (schwannoma) in a three year old child without evidence of neurofibromatosis. Eur J Pediatr Surg 2007;17(6):428–30.
11 Lara-Torre E, Perlman S. Vulvar intraepithelial neoplasia in adolescents with abnormal Pap smear results: a series report. J Pediatr Adolesc Gynecol 2004;17(1):45–8.
12 Giaquinto C, del Mistro A, de Rossi A et al. Vulvar carcinoma in a 12 year old girl with vertically acquired human immunodeficiency virus infection. Pediatrics 2000;106(4):E57.
13 Kim NR, Lim S, Cho HY. Pediatr vulvar squamous cell carcinoma in a liver transplantation recipient: a case report. J Gynecol Oncol 2011; 22(3):207–11.
14 Wei CC, Peng C, Chiang IP, Wu KH. Primary B cell non-hodgkin lymphoma of the penis in a child. J Pediatr Hematol Oncol 2006; 28(7):479–80.
15 Chabay P, de Matteo E, Lorenzetti M et al. Vulvar plasmablastic lymphoma in a HIV-positive child: a novel extraoral localization. J Clin Pathol 2009;62(7):644–6.
16 Godoy G, Mufarrij PW, Tsou H et al. Granular cell tumour of scrotum: a rare tumor of the male external genitalia. Urology 2008;72(3):e7–9.
17 Yang JH, Mitchell K, Poppas DP. Granular cell tumor of the glans penis in a 9-year-old boy. Urology 2008;71(3):546.
18 Sidwell RU, Rouse P, Owen RA, Green JS. Granular cell tumour of the scrotum in a child with Noonan syndrome. Pediatr Dermatol 2008; 25(3):341–3.
19 Gentler L, Shimmed D. Granular cell tumour of the vulva. Pediatr Dermatol 1993;10:153–5.
20 Cohen Z, Kapuller V, Maor E et al. Granular cell tumour (myoblastoma) of the labia major: a rare benign tumour in childhood. J Pediatr Adolesc Gynecol 1999;12:155–6.
21 DiLernia V, Bisighini G. Localized vulvar syringomas. Pediatr Dermatol 1996;13:80–1.
22 Yung A, Newton-Bishop J. A case of Bazex–Dupre–Christol syndrome associated with multiple genital trichoepitheliomas. Br J Dermatol 2005;153(3):682–4.
23 Samplaski MK, Somani N, Palmer JS. Apocrine hidrocystoma on glans penis of a child. Urology 2009;73(4):800–1.
24 Shuangshoti S, Shuangshoti S, Pintong J et al. Solitary mastocytoma of the vulva: report of a case. Int J Gynecol Pathol 2003;22(4):401–3.
25 Serarslan G, Atik E, Zeteroglu S. Nodular mastocytosis of the vulva: an unusual localisation. Aust NZ J Obstet Gynecol 2005;45(4):335–6.
26 Berry T, Strand M, Smidt AD, Torrelo A. Localized mastocyoma of the vulva (review). Pediatr Dermatol 2014;31(1):111–13.
27 Redman JF, Liang X, Ferguson MA et al. Leiomyoma of the glans penis in a child. J Urol 2000;164:791.
28 Val-Bernal J, Fernando MD, Garijo M et al. Solitary cutaneous myofibroma of the glans penis. Am J Dermopathol 1996;19:317–21.
29 Eichhorn JH, Young RH. Neuroendocrine tumours of the genital tract. Am J Clin Pathol 2001;115(suppl):S94–112.
30 Pandit SK, Rattan KN, Gupta U et al. Multiple neurilemmomas of the penis. Pediatr Surg Int 2000;16:457.
31 Kousseff BG, Hoover DL. Penile neurofibromas. Am J Med Genet 1999;87:1–5.
32 Littlejohn JO, Belman AB, Selby D. Plexiform neurofibroma of the penis in a child. Urology 2000;56:669.
33 Yegane RA, Alaee MS, Khanicheh E. Congenital plexiform schwannoma of the clitoris. Saudi Med J 2008;29(4):600–2.
34 Santos LD, Currie B, Killingsworth MC. Case report: plexiform schwannoma of the vulva. Pathology 2001;33(4):526–31.
35 Mazdak H, Gharaati M. Plexiform neurofibroma of penis. Urol J 2007;4(1):52–3.
36 Pascual-Castroviejo I, Lopez-Pereira P, Savasta S. Neurofibromatosis type 1 with external genital involvement presentation in 4 patients. J Pediatr Surg 2008;43(11):1998–2003.
37 Iwasa Y, Fletcher C. Distinctive prepubertal vulval fibroma: a hitherto unrecognized mesenchymal tumour of prepubertal girls: analysis of 11 cases. Am J Surg Pathol 2004;28(12):1601–8.
38 Monajemzadeh M, Vasei M, Kalantari M et al. Vulvar fibrous hamartoma of infancy: a rare case report and review of the literature. J Lower Gen Tract Dis 2013;17(1):92–4.
39 Suwa M, Takeda M, Bilim V et al. Epidermoid cyst of the penis: case report and review of the literature. Int J Urol 2000;7:431–3.
40 Hamada M, Kiryu H, Ohta T, Furue M. Ciliated cyst of the vulva. Eur J Dermatol 2004;14(5):347–9.
41 Sonthalia S, Singal A. Smegma pearls in young uncircumcised boys. Pediatr Dermatol 2016;33(3):e186–9.
42 Stock JA, Niku SD, Packer MG et al. Fibrous hamartoma of infancy: a report of two cases in the genital region. Urology 1995;45:130–1.
43 Williams TS, Callen JP, Lafayette GO. Vulvar disorders in the prepubertal female. Pediatr Ann 1986;15:588–605.
44 **Oh JT, Choi SH, Ahn SG et al. Vulval lipomas in children: an analysis of 7 cases. J Pedatri Surg 2009;44(10):1920–3.**
45 Gao H, Wang C, Wang H et al. Lipomatosis of the penis and perineum in a 6-year-old boy. Eur J Pediatr 2005;164(2):115–16.
46 Chanda MN, Jamieson M, Poenaru D. Congenital perineal lipoma presenting as 'ambiguous genitalia': a case report. J Pediatr Adolesc Gynecol 2000;13(2):71–4.
47 Kirkham YA, Yarborough CM, Pippi Salle JL, Allen LM. A rare case of inguinolabial lipoblastoma in a 13 month old female. J Pediatr Urol 2013;9(1):e64–7.
48 Altcheck A, Deligdisch L, Norton K et al. Prepubertal unilateral fibrous hyperplasia of the labium majus: report of eight cases and review of the literature. Obstet Gynecol 2007;110(1):1039–8.
49 Vargas SO, Kozakewich H, Boyd TK et al. Childhood asymmetric labium majus enlargement: mimicking a neoplasm. Am J Surg Pathol 2005;29(8):1007–16.

Scrotal conditions

Idiopathic scrotal calcinosis

This condition may commence in childhood. Multiple firm, asymptomatic nodules, usually grey or white, appear on the scrotum. They may discharge chalky material from time to time [1,2].

There is no systemic metabolic disturbance, and calcium and phosphorus levels are normal.

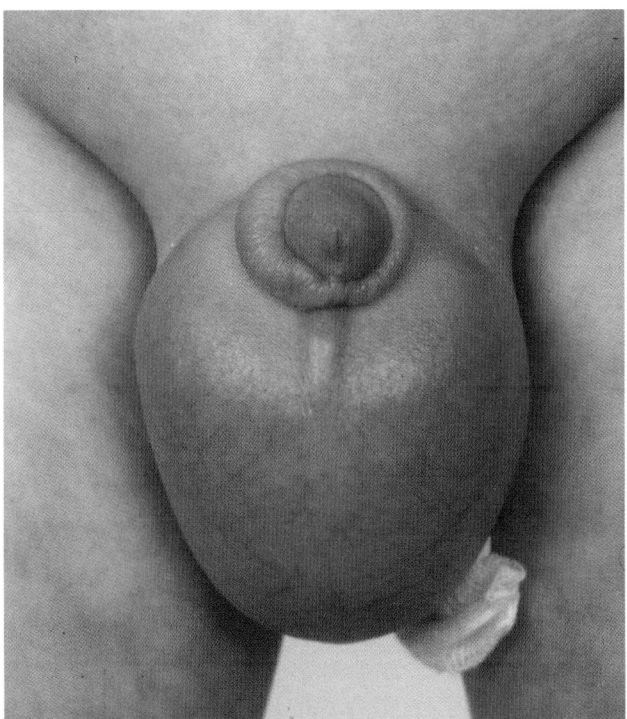

Fig. 162.46 Acute scrotal oedema in nephritic syndrome. Source: Courtesy of Dr M. Rogers.

Histopathology shows amorphous calcium deposits surrounded by a granulomatous reaction with foreign body giant cells.

Secondary dystrophic calcinosis may be the result of local trauma or infection.

The lesions may be excised surgically.

Acute scrotal oedema

Acute oedema and purpura of the scrotum may occur in Henoch–Schönlein purpura and acute haemorrhagic oedema of the newborn [3,4].

Painless bilateral scrotal oedema may be a presenting sign of nephrotic syndrome (Fig. 162.46).

Idiopathic scrotal oedema is an uncommon self-limited condition seen in prepubertal children. Painless or moderately painful swelling and erythema of the scrotum occur [5]. The condition may be unilateral or bilateral, and may be recurrent. This is the most common cause of acute disease of the scrotum in boys under the age of 10 years. It is probably an allergic phenomenon [6]. Ultrasound and Doppler studies show oedema of the scrotal skin but no increase in size of testicles and epididymis [7,8]. Patients with acute scrotal oedema must always be investigated for torsion of the testis.

References

1 **Gormally S, Dorman T, Powell FC. Calcinosis of the scrotum. Int J Dermatol 1992;31:75–9.**

2 Song DH, Lee KH, Kang WH. Idiopathic calcinosis of the scrotum. J Am Acad Dermatol 1998;19:1095–101.

3 Gomez Parada J, Puyol Pallas M, Vila Cots J et al. Acute scrotum and Schönlein–Henoch purpura: report of 2 new cases. Arch Esp Urol 2001;54:168–70.

4 Dubin BA, Bronson DM, Eng AN. Acute haemorrhagic edema of childhood: an unusual variant of leucocytoclastic vasculitis. J Am Acad Dermatol 1990;23:347–50.

5 **Van Langen AM, Gal S, Hulsmann AR et al. Acute idiopathic scrotal oedema: four cases and a short review. Eur J Pediatr 2001;160:455–6.**

6 Najmaldin A, Burge DM. Acute idiopathic scrotal oedema: incidence, manifestations and aetiology. Br J Surg 1987;74:634–5.

7 Planelles Gómez J, Beltrán Armada JR, Beamud Cortés M et al. Idiopathic scrotal edema: report of two cases. Arch Esp Urol 2007;60(7):799–802.

8 Coley B. Sonography of pediatric scrotal swelling. Semin Ultrasound CT MR 2007;28(4):297–306.

Genital signs of systemic disease

Crohn disease

Crohn disease, a chronic and relapsing inflammatory bowel disorder, is often associated with skin findings. Erythema nodosum and pyoderma gangrenosum may occur as nonspecific associations, but the same granulomatous process that affects the bowel may be found in the skin and can be confirmed histologically. The biopsy will demonstrate giant cells, macrophages, lymphocytes and plasma cells in sarcoidal granulomas. This is known as metastatic Crohn disease and is uncommon [1].

Crohn disease may affect the genital area in children and does so more commonly than in adults [2]. This can be contiguous with the bowel, with perianal lesions or on the genitalia [3,4]. It may also occur prior to and without gastrointestinal involvement [5]. The usual presentation is with discomfort and soreness, associated with firm oedema and hypertrophy of the labia in girls and the penis and scrotum in boys. Ulceration may occur. Perianal erosions and fissures, swelling, fistulae, skin tags and erythema are commonly found where there is genital involvement [6]. The sign of vulval oedema is particularly characteristic and can be the sole presenting sign [7]. It should always prompt a search for Crohn disease (Fig. 162.47). There may be a simultaneous cheilitis [8]. The vulval and perianal changes may precede gastrointestinal symptoms [2].

The condition must be differentiated from other processes that cause painless induration of the genital area, including filiariasis and lymphogranuloma venereum.

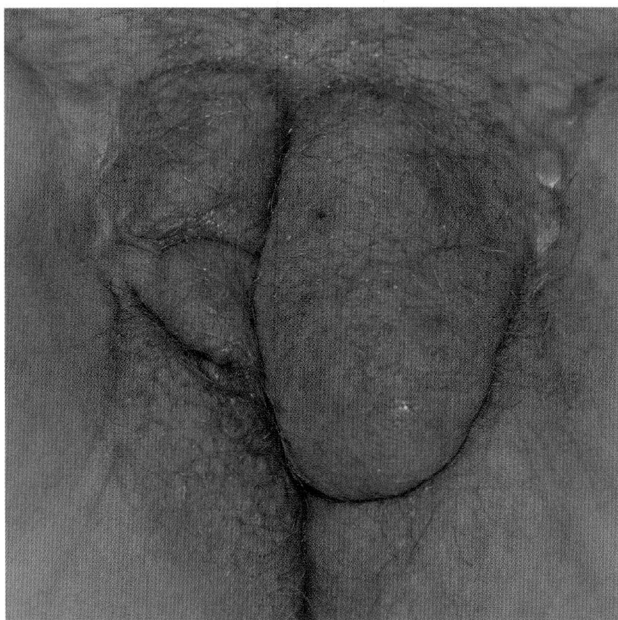

Fig. 162.47 Massive vulval oedema in Crohn disease.

Initial management of this condition should include referral to a gastroenterologist for investigation for bowel involvement. The skin lesions tend to be resistant to treatment with oral antibiotics, such as metronidazole and sulphasalazine, and prednisone is usually required to induce a remission. Topical tacrolimus has been reported as useful in children with genital Crohn disease [9]. In the long term, oral azathioprine may be required [2].

Orofacial granulomatosis and anogenital granulomatosis

In this group of children, painless induration of the lips associated with a similar induration of the penis, scrotum and perianal area occurs without bowel disease. Biopsy reveals sarcoidal granulomas with lymphangiectases [10]. Anogenital granulomatosis is the same condition histologically, presenting with diffuse penile, scrotal, vulval or anoperineal swelling [11].

This condition may be a forme fruste of Crohn disease [12] but some patients appear to be exhibiting a type IV hypersensitivity reaction to dietary allergens. This may be identified by patch testing [13].

Children with this condition should be investigated for Crohn disease. Treatment with topical and intralesional corticosteroids in association with dietary restriction is considered first-line management [14].

A report from 2002 documents three children with granulomatous periorificial dermatitis who also had involvement of the labia majora [15]. In these children, histopathology demonstrated noncaseating perifollicular granulomas. This condition presents with an erythematous papular eruption, rather than swelling and fissuring that is typical of Crohn disease, but may need to be differentiated from it because of the histological appearance. There is no systemic involvement.

Melkersson–Rosenthal syndrome is an uncommon granulomatous disease usually characterized by the triad of relapsing facial paralysis, orofacial swelling and fissured tongue. A case has been described in a 12-year-old boy who also had genital swelling with a biopsy showing noncaseating granuloma [16].

Behçet disease

Behçet disease is an autoinflammatory disease affecting vessels of all sizes but predominantly venules. It is characterized by recurrent oral ulcers, genital ulcers and ocular inflammatory disease. Joints, gastrointestinal tract, central nervous system and skin are other sites commonly involved in this multisystem disease. It is a heterogenous condition that varies depending on sex, country of origin and age of onset [17]. A variant, termed MAGIC syndrome (mouth and genital ulcers with inflamed cartilage), presents clinically as Behçet-like disease with inflammation of cartilage similar to relapsing polychondritis.

Behçet disease is reported in childhood and genital signs include epididymoorchitis [18] and genital ulceration [19,20]. Childhood-onset disease carries a strong genetic component.

The age of onset of juvenile Behçet disease is approximately 12 years and mucocutaneous and joint symptoms are the most common manifestations. One review showed that oral ulcers are present in all childhood cases and genital aphthous ulcers in over 90%, found on the vulva, scrotum and perianal region. Familial clustering was found in 45% of cases, significantly higher than in adult cases, but in other ways childhood Behçet disease presents similarly to adult cases and is treated in the same way [21]. TNF-α inhibitors are now the treatment of choice for severe disease and apremilast has shown promise. Azathioprine, colchicine, oral corticosteroids and other immunosuppressants have also been used to control inflammation [17].

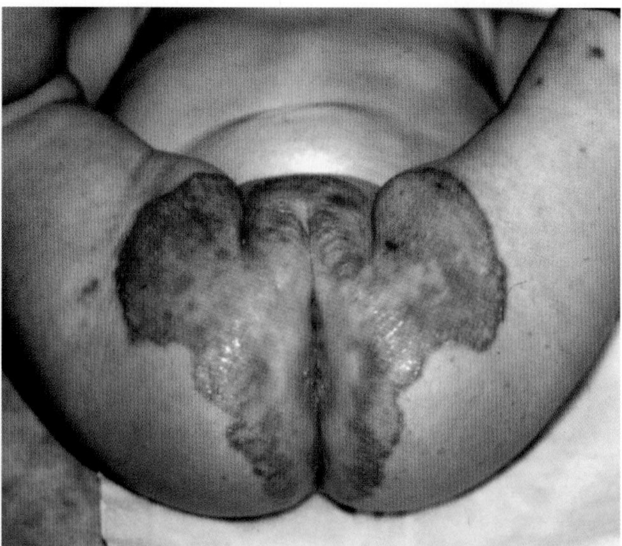

Fig. 162.48 The eroded, sharply demarcated eruption of acrodermatitis enteropathica.

Zinc deficiency

Zinc deficiency is seen either at birth or on weaning with acrodermatitis enteropathica, or at around 6–9 months in fully breastfed babies of mothers with low breast milk zinc. The appearance is with an eroded bilateral vulval rash with a very well-demarcated edge (Fig. 162.48). There is a similar perioral rash [22].

Henoch–Schönlein Purpura

Henoch–Schönlein purpura is an immune-mediated systemic vasculitis found most often in children. It presents with a vasculitic purpuric rash involving the lower limbs and buttocks most often, arthritis, abdominal pain and renal complications. In boys, oedema of the scrotum is common and the penile shaft and glans may also be involved, with purpuric lesions. Testicular torsion is a serious complication which may be difficult to differentiate [23].

References

1 Lehrnbecher T, Kontny H, Jeschke RJ. Metastatic Crohn's disease in a 9-year-old boy. Pediatr Gastroenterol Nutr 1999;28:321–3.

2 Ploysangam T, Heubi JE, Eisen D et al. Cutaneous Crohn's disease in children. J Am Acad Dermatol 1997;36:697–704.

3 Phillip SS, Baird DB, Joshi VV et al. Crohn's disease of the prepuce in a 12-year-old boy: a case report and review of the literature. Pediatr Pathol Lab Med 1997;17:497–502.

4 Tuffnell B, Buchan PC. Crohn's disease of the vulva in childhood. Br J Clin Pract 1991;45:159–60.

5 Bourrat E, Faure C, Vignon-Pennamen MD et al. Anitis, vulvar edema and macrocheilitis disclosing Crohn disease in a child: value of metronidazole. Ann Dermatol Venereol 1997;124(9):626–8.

6 Koluglu Z, Kansu A, Demirceken F et al. Crohn's disease of the vulva in a 10 year old girl. Turk J Pediatr 2008;50(2):197–9.

7 Corbett SL, Waslh CM, Spitzer RF et al Vulvar inflammation as the only clinical manifestation of Crohn disease in an 8-year-old girl. Pediatrics 2010;125(6):e1518–22.

8 Tatnall FM, Dodd HJ, Sarkany I. Crohn's disease with metastatic cutaneous involvement and granulomatous cheilitis. J Roy Soc Med 1987;80:49.

9 Al-Niami F, Lyon C. Vulval Crohn's disease in childhood. Dermatol Ther 2013;3(2):199–202.

10 Murphy M, Kogan B, Carlson JA. Granulomatous lymphangitis of the scrotum and penis: report of a case and review of the literature of genital swelling with sarcoidal granulomatous inflammation. J Cutan Pathol 2001;28:419–24.

11 Van de Scheur MR, van der Waal R, van der Waal I et al. Ano-genital granulomatosis: the counterpart of oro-facial granulo matosis. J Eur Acad Dermatol Venereol 2003;17(2):184–9.

12 Murphy MJ, Kogan B, Carlson JA. Granulomatous lymphangitis of the scrotum and penis. Report of a case and review of the literature of genital swelling with sarcoidal granulomatous inflammation. J Cutan Pathol 2001;28(8):419–24.

13 Armstrong BK, Biagioni P, Lamey PJ et al. Contact hypersensitivity in patients with orofacial granulomatosis. Am J Contact Dermatitis 1997;8:35–8.

14 Gibson J, Forsyth A, Milligan KA. Dietary and environmental allergens in patients with orofacial granulomatosis. J Dent Reserve 1996;75:334.

15 Urbatsch AJ, Frieden I, Williams ML et al. Extrafacial and generalised granulomatous periorificial dermatitis. Arch Dermatol 2002;138: 1354–8.

16 Chu Z, Liu Y, Zhang W, Geng S. Melkersson–Rosenthal syndrome with genitalia involved in a 12 year old boy. Ann Dermatol 2016;28(2):232–6.

17 Koné-Paut I. Behçet's disease in children: an overview. Pediatr Rheumatol 2016;14:10.

18 Pektas A, Devrim I, Besbas N et al. A child with Behcet's disease presenting with a spectrum of inflammatory manifestations including epididymoorchitis. Turk J Pediatr 2008;50(1):78–80.

19 Karincaoglu Y, Borlu M, Toker S et al. Demographic and clinical properties of juvenile-onset Behcet's disease: a controlled multicenter study. J Am Acad Dermatol 2008;58(4):579–84.

20 Yuksel Z, Schweizer J, Mourad-Baars PE et al. A toddler with recurrent oral and genital ulcers. Clin Rheumatol 2007;26:969–70.

21 Borlu M, Uksal U, Ferahbas A, Evereklioglu C. Clinical features of Behcet's disease in children. Int J Dermatol 2006;45(6):713–16.

22 Stapleton KM, O'Loughlin E, Relic JP. Transient zinc deficiency in a breast-fed premature infant. Australas J Dermatol 1995;36:157–9.

23 Dalpiaz A, Schwamb R, Miao Y et al. Urological manifestations of Henoch–Schonlein purpura: a review. Current Urol 2015;8(2):66–73.

Psychological aspects of genital disease in children

Among adults with genital complaints, a small but significant group presents with symptoms but with no apparent abnormality. Although some of this group have a psychiatric complaint which results in malingering behaviour or somatoform disorder there are many more who have a neuropathy or referred pain. Neuropathic vulval pain relieved by tricyclic antidepressant medication has also been reported in preadolescent girls, but is significantly less common than in adults [1]. Children who suffer from genuine neuropathic vulval pain describe it in a similar way to adults: intolerance of wearing tight clothes, stabbing, burning and aching. They may state that they relieve the pain by pressing on the painful spot.

When a child presents with symptoms but nothing to see, even after close examination when symptoms are maximal, it is more likely that there is no physical complaint, particularly when they do not give a consistent description that suggests neuropathy. A common scenario is the child who is presented because of a greenish discharge noticed as staining of the underwear. There are no symptoms other than the discharge and swabs and urine culture are normal. This situation appears to be a normal variant.

A somewhat less innocent situation occurs if a child constantly complains of vulval discomfort in the absence of findings and without any observable sign of being in pain. Children rapidly realize that complaining of genital pain, particularly at school or in public, attracts lots of adult attention and is a source of embarrassment for their parents. They may even find that they are rapidly sent home from school by teachers worried about sexual abuse allegations, and distraught parents are summoned to explain the behaviour. Children who do this have no idea how much real adult distress they are causing but know that it is an effective attention-seeking device. The best way to deal with it is usually to withdraw the attention, but occasionally psychiatric help is needed.

In some cases, a mother with a vulval problem may project her concerns onto the child, whether or not there is a real problem present. It may be helpful to enquire about this possibility when obtaining a family history. In some cases only reassurance is necessary, but a more deep-seated psychological problem may again require psychiatric help, not for the child but for the mother.

Children who masturbate, and whose parents are shocked by their behaviour, often learn to explain their actions to their parents by saying that they are in pain, and their parents may need to come to terms with the normality of their actions.

In most of these cases, nonintervention, reassurance and not giving in to attention-seeking behaviour is the best treatment. They represent a real trap for the unwary, however.

Most parents of a girl with a vulval condition of any sort will have considered the possibility of sexual abuse, even though they often do not tend to voice it, particularly at the first visit. It is reasonable for them to do so. Child sexual abuse and paedophilia have received enormous publicity in the lay press; however, details of the evidence for abuse are never provided, and this is therefore left to the readers' imagination. Professionals who deal with children are also made very aware of child abuse as an issue because of legal requirements to reveal criminal records as a condition of employment. It is therefore common for carers and teachers to have these concerns about children who scratch the vulval area constantly or complain of vulval pain. Their concern has to extend to the possibility that parents who suspect abuse in a child with a vulval condition may blame persons who care for the child in their absence.

Child sexual abuse is common, more so in girls than boys, with the peak age being 13–17. Although studies report varying rates, it is likely that about 20–30% of women and about 10% of men have experienced some form of unwanted sexual activity in childhood. Data suggest that over 95% of cases are never disclosed [2].

Even in expert hands, diagnosing sexual abuse is very difficult, and impossible to prove without a disclosure from the child or a relative. Even after investigation and interview in the child protection unit setting, many cases remain unresolved [3,4].

The fact is that most children who have been sexually abused do not have any physical signs, as trauma such as bruises resolve quickly, and abusive behaviour often does not necessarily involve attempts at penetration or infliction of trauma. Even when the latter is present, it may take on the form of 'dermatitis artefacta' with parents claiming that they have no idea how the lesions arose (Fig. 162.49) [2–4]. A finding of typical genital warts (Fig. 162.50) or genital herpes may suggest sexual abuse but does not confirm it as both can be acquired nonsexually. Physical examination cannot confirm or exclude non-acute sexual abuse as a cause of genital trauma in prepubertal girls [5]. The presence of a rash such as eczema, psoriasis or lichen sclerosus should not raise queries of abuse in the absence of other suspicious features.

When a child presents with a vulval rash, it is so common for parents to have unvoiced concern about sexual abuse that it is worth enquiring about this. Parents will usually be greatly relieved that their child simply has a skin problem. The medical literature contains many cases of skin conditions being mistaken for sexual abuse, and this includes lichen sclerosus, ulcerated haemangiomas and rarer skin conditions such as bullous pemphigoid, which may cause genital ulcers [6–9].

It is important to understand that lay people may attribute almost any vulval condition to sexual abuse. Although the presence of a skin condition does not rule it out, there would have to be other grounds to suspect it, based on household composition, parental concerns, presence of sexually acquired infections and behavioural abnormalities in the child.

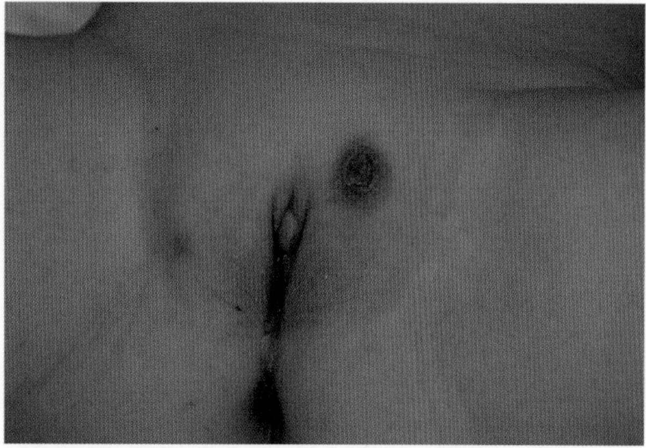

Fig. 162.49 Genital ulcers presumed to be cigarette burns.

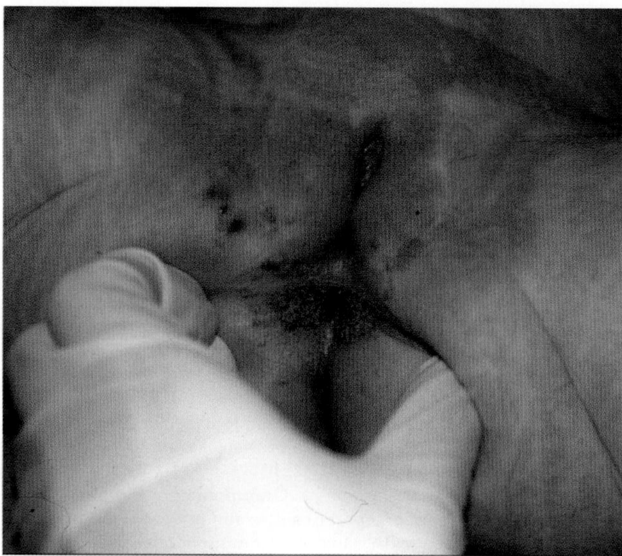

Fig. 162.50 Genital warts in a small child.

Acknowledgement

I would like to acknowledge and thank Dr Maureen Rogers, co-author of the original chapter, and Dr Sallie Neill, author of the original chapter on lichen sclerosus, for their previous contribution to the writing and illustration of this work.

References

1 **Reed BD, Cantoris L. Vulvodynia in preadolescent girls. J Lower Genital Tract Dis 2008;12(4):257–61.**

2 **Maratin EK, Silverstone PH. How much sexual abuse is "below the surface" and can we help adults identify it early? Front Psychiatry 2013;4:58.**

3 Tipton A. Child sexual abuse: physical examination techniques and interpretation of findings. Adolesc Pediatr Gynaecol 1989;2:10–25.

4 Weinberg R, Sybert VP, Feldman KW et al. Outcome of CPS referral for sexual abuse children with condylomata acuminata. J Pediatr Adolesc Gynecol 1994;7:19–24.

5 **Berkoff MC, Zolotor A, Makaroff KL et al. Has this prepubertal girl been sexually abused? JAMA 2008;300(23):2779–92.**

6 Jenny C, Kirby F, Fuquay D. Genital lichen sclerosus mistaken for child sexual abuse. Pediatrics 1989;4:597–9.

7 Wood PL, Bevan T. Child sexual abuse enquiries and unrecognised vulval lichen sclerosus et atrophica. BMJ 1999;319:899–900.

8 Hosteller BR, Jones CE, Miram D. Capillary hemangioma of the vulva mistaken for sexual abuse. Adolesc Pediatr Gynaecol 1994;7:44–6.

9 Levine V, Sanchez M, Nestor M. Localised vulvar pemphigoid in a child misdiagnosed as sexual abuse. Arch Dermatol 1992;128:804–6.

CHAPTER 163
Sexually Transmitted Diseases in Children and Adolescents

Arnold P. Oranje[1], *Robert A.C. Bilo*[2] *& Nico G. Hartwig*[3]

[1] Kinderhuid.nl, Rotterdam, Hair Clinic, Breda and Dermicis Skin Clinic, Alkmaar, The Netherlands
[2] Department of Forensic Medicine, Section on Forensic Pediatrics, Netherlands Forensic Institute, The Hague, The Netherlands
[3] Department of Pediatrics, Franciscus Gasthuis & Vlietland, Rotterdam, The Netherlands

Introduction, 2195
Syphilis, 2199
Gonorrhoea, 2204
***Chlamydia trachomatis* infections, 2209**
Condyloma acuminata, 2212
Hepatitis B in children, 2214
Genital herpes simplex virus infection, 2215
Human immunodeficiency virus, 2216
***Trichomonas vaginalis* infection, 2217**
Bacterial vaginitis, 2218

Abstract

Diseases that are defined in adults as sexually transmitted diseases can be transmitted in children in a nonsexual (e.g. intrauterine infections or vertical transmission) and sexual way (voluntary and unvoluntary sexual contacts). A better term for these diseases in children from a clinical and forensic medical point of view would be 'sexually transmittable diseases'. Dealing with a child with a STD requires particular care and expertise, concerning the diagnosis of the disease, the correct determination of the mode of transmission and the way in which the diagnosis and mode of transmission are discussed with the child and the parents.

Key points

- **Sexually transmitted diseases (STD) in children can be caused by intrauterine infection, vertical transmission, sexual abuse and voluntary sexual contact (in teenagers).**
- **The incubation periods in intrauterine and vertical transmission vary with the specific infections.**
- **In most STDs, there is no evidence to establish the age at which vertical transmission can be excluded with certainty.**
- **If a preadolescent child presents with an STD, sexual transmission should always be considered if congenital transmission and postnatal nonsexual transmission have been excluded.**
- **In pubertal children a consensual sexual contact should always be excluded before considering sexual abuse and/or before intervening because of a suspicion of sexual abuse.**
- **STDs are common among teenagers.**
- **Since 2015, the incidence of gonorrhoea and chlamydia is decreasing while the incidence of primary and secondary syphilis and consequently congenital syphilis is increasing.**

Introduction

In adults, sexually transmitted diseases (STDs) are almost exclusively transmitted through sexual contact. In childhood, however, STDs can occur as a result of nonsexual (e.g. intrauterine infections or vertical transmission) and sexual transmission (voluntary and unvoluntary sexual contacts) [1].

Sexually transmitted diseases have a special implication in pregnancy [2,3] and may cause premature birth due to chorioamnionitis or polyhydramnios. They may also pose a threat to the unborn and the newborn. A number of STDs (e.g. syphilis) are able to pass the placenta and may result in infection and damage to the fetus. The newborn may also become infected during passage through the birth canal. Important examples include *Chlamydia trachomatis* (CT), gonorrhoea, human immunodeficiency virus (HIV) and primary genital herpes simplex virus (HSV). The newborn may also acquire its infection via breastfeeding, as in HIV, or from bystanders, as in herpes labialis. Establishing a diagnosis of STD in a newborn forces investigation into the contacts and sexual partner(s) of the mother. It is evident that such an investigation may pose additional problems for the clinician.

Concerning postnatally acquired STDs, various modes of transmission must be considered. The child may acquire its infection through an everyday contact with an

Harper's Textbook of Pediatric Dermatology, Fourth Edition. Edited by Peter Hoeger, Veronica Kinsler and Albert Yan.

infected adult, for example through intimate but nonsexual physical contact or another nonsexual way of transmission [4]. Infections may also occur as a result of medical interventions. Thirdly, the child may acquire the infection through voluntary or nonvoluntary sexual contacts. Theoretically, STDs can also be transmitted during normal sexual exploratory behaviour between an infected and a noninfected child. An adolescent may also acquire STDs by voluntary sexual contact with another individual from their peer group. However, if STD is established in a young child, sexual abuse must always be considered. The occurrence of STDs in abused children has been reported to vary from 2% to 10% in the available literature [5–7]. Infection may sometimes be the presenting feature, although it is more often encountered during routine physical examination in suspected cases of child sexual abuse (CSA). Dealing with these problems requires particular care and expertise (see also Cutaneous signs of child maltreatment and sexual abuse, later in this chapter).

A number of factors influence the risk of acquiring a sexually transmitted disease during abuse. The risk is higher when abuse occurs outside the family than within the family. Furthermore, the occurrence of intercultural differences is an important factor in evaluating the way in which the child acquired the STD. Whittle et al. [8], for example, describe that at present horizontal transmission of hepatitis B from child to child is most common in certain developing countries, whereas vertical transmission from mother to child is more common in other countries, depending on the local epidemiology. HIV infections are described in Chapter 53.

In STDs in adults as well as in children and adolescents, one should always follow the 'CCC' rules [9,10]:

- correct diagnosis
- contact tracing if necessary; an abuser is not a partner, but should be treated
- counselling and education.

Policy on STDs in childhood

A full STD diagnostic work-up should be considered in all children with:

- suspected or proven CSA
- signs and symptoms of a STD
- unprotected consensual sexual contact
- anogenital injuries.

Sexually transmitted diseases in children have two important implications:

- it is essential that the correct diagnosis is made quickly and that adequate treatment is provided as soon as possible
- STDs provide a signal for imperative further investigation into the mode of transmission, in which sexual abuse must be considered. Therefore, a multidisciplinary approach is necessary in dealing with STDs in children (Box 163.1).

Tracing of (sexual) contacts should be undertaken for both public health and epidemiological reasons. The primary aim is the diagnosis and treatment of STDs and prevention of further spread [9,10].

Box 163.1 Policy on STDs in childhood

Phase 1

- Referral to a (paediatric) dermatologist and/or a paediatrician and eventually a (paediatric) gynaecologist
- If sexual abuse is suspected or cannot be excluded (Tables 163.1 and 163.2):
  - consultation with a child abuse doctor or consultant in forensic paediatrics
  - consultation with or report to child protection service (if immediate protection of the child is indicated)

Phase 2

- Examination, correct diagnosis and treatment of STD (Tables 163.3 and 163.4) by a (paediatric) dermatologist and/or a paediatrician and eventually a (paediatric) gynaecologist, concerning:
  - source of infection
  - mode of transmission
  - elimination of other STDs
  - examination of the parents and other members of the family
- Supplementary examination and diagnosis by a paediatrician in connection with other physical abnormalities and psychosocial problems, in cooperation with a (medical) social worker
- On indication:
  - hospitalization for observation, supplemented if appropriate by a paediatric psychological examination; and
  - gynaecological examination and investigation by a (paediatric) gynaecologist in older girls, to note any congenital abnormalities and abnormalities considered to be the result of sexual contacts/ sexual abuse

Phase 3

- If sexual abuse can not be excluded:
  - involvement of a child abuse doctor or consultant in forensic paediatrics for further investigation
  - report to child protection service

References

1 Workowski KA, Berman S, Centers for Disease Control and Prevention (CDC). Sexually transmitted diseases treatment guidelines, 2010. MMWR Recomm Rep 2010;59:1–110. Erratum (dosage error) in: MMWR Recomm Rep 2011;60:18.
2 Johnson HL, Ghanem KG, Zenilman JM, Erbelding EJ. Sexually transmitted infections and adverse pregnancy outcomes among women attending inner city public sexually transmitted diseases clinics. Sex Transm Dis 2011;38:167–71.
3 Seña AC, Hsu KK, Kellogg N et al. Sexual assault and sexually transmitted infections in adults, adolescents, and children. Clin Infect Dis 2015;61(Suppl 8):S856–64.
4 Zhang R, Jin H. Syphilis in an infant acquired by mouth to mouth transfer of prechewed food. Pediatr Dermatol 2016;33(6):e344–e345.
5 Hobbs CJ, Wynne JM. Child sexual abuse: an increasing rate of diagnosis. Lancet 1987;ii:837–41.
6 White ST, Leda FA, Ingram DL, Pearson A. Sexually transmitted diseases in sexually abused children. Pediatrics 1983;72:16–21.
7 Lowy G. Sexually transmitted diseases in children. Pediatr Dermatol 1992;9:329–34.
8 Whittle HC, Inskip H, Hall AJ et al. Vaccination against hepatitis B and protection against viral carriage in the Gambia. Lancet 1991; 337:747–50.
9 Radcliffe K. European STD Guidelines. Int J STD AIDS 2001;12 (Suppl 3):1–102.
10 Centers for Disease Control and Prevention. Sexually transmitted diseases: treatment guideline. CDC, 2015. www.cdc.gov/std/tg2015/default.htm
11 Royal College of Paediatrics and Child Health. The Physical Signs of Child Sexual Abuse – An Updated Evidence-Based Review and Guidance for Best Practice, 2nd edn. London: Royal College of Paediatrics and Child Health, 2015.

Table 163.1 Mode of transmission of sexually transmitted diseases (STD) [11]

	Prepubertal	Postpubertal	Vertical transmission*
Bacterial STD			
Chlamydia trachomatis (CT)	Sexual contact most likely. Confirmed CT: CSA likely	Sexual contact most likely. Consensual sexual activity should be considered	No evidence to establish the age at which vertical transmission can be excluded
Neisseria gonorrhoeae	Sexual contact most likely. Confirmed (nonophthalmic) gonorrhoea: CSA likely		
Treponema pallidum	Sexual contact most likely		Primary syphilis in a child older than 4 months or secondary syphilis in a child older than 2 years is most probably the result of an acquired infection
Bacterial vaginosis	Possibly sexual and nonsexual transmission		?
Viral STD			
Anogenital warts	CSA should always be considered	Sexual contact should always be considered. Consensual sexual activity should be considered	No evidence to establish the age at which vertical/perinatal transmission can be excluded
Herpes simplex virus	Autoinoculation and CSA should always be considered		
Hepatitis B and C virus	CSA should be considered if vertical/perinatal transmission, mother-to-child transmission or transmission by contaminated blood can be excluded		
Human immunodeficiency virus			
Other STD			
Trichomonas vaginalis (TV)	CSA should always be considered	Consensual sexual activity should be considered	No evidence to establish the age at which vertical transmission can be excluded. TV in a girl <2 months of age could be the result of a perinatal infection

*Positive diagnosis of STD in mother does not exclude CSA.
CSA, child sexual abuse.

Table 163.2 The relationship between sexually transmitted diseases (STDs) and child sexual abuse (CSA) and the implication of the diagnosis of a STD in a child [10,11]

	In sexually abused children?	If found, CSA confirmed in ...?	Implication
Bacterial STD			
Chlamydia trachomatis (CT)	Uncommon	Significant number of children with CT	Highly suspicious in children <13years: report to CPS*
Neisseria gonorrhoeae	Uncommon	Significant number of children with gonorrhoea	Highly suspicious: report to CPS*
Treponema pallidum	Uncommon	Significant number of children with syphilis	Highly suspicious: report to CPS*
Bacterial vaginosis	Very low prevalence in asymptomatic prepubertal girls. Slightly more often in sexually abused prepubertal girls with a discharge	Insufficient data to determine the significance in CSA	Medical follow-up
Viral STD			
Anogenital warts	Uncommon	Significant number of children with anogenital warts	Suspicious: consider report to CPS**
Herpes simplex virus (HSV)/genital herpes	Uncommon	Probably significant number of children with HSV	Suspicious: report to CPS***
Hepatitis B and C virus	Unknown	Insufficient data to determine the significance in CSA	Medical follow-up
Human immunodeficiency virus	Uncommon (depending on the prevalence in the local adult population)	Most children, if other modes are excluded	Highly suspicious: report to CPS*
Other STD			
Trichomonas vaginalis	Uncommon	Significant number of prepubertal girls	Highly suspicious in prepubertal children: report to CPS In postpubertal children: medical follow-up

*If not intrauterine or perinatally acquired. If so, medical follow-up.
**In most cases not sexually transmitted. If so, medical follow-up.
***Unless there is a clear history of autoinoculation. If so, medical follow-up.
CPS, child protection services.
Source: Adapted from CDC 2015 [10] and RCPCH 2015 [11].

Table 163.3 Quality standards for tests for the diagnosis of sexually transmitted diseases (STD) in children under the age of 16 years [11]

	Good	Medium	Poor
Bacterial STD			
Chlamydia trachomatis	NAAT confirmed Culture	Confirmed EIA/IF (positive only) NAAT unconfirmed	Negative EIA/ culture/IF
Neisseria gonorrhoeae	NAAT confirmed Culture	NAAT unconfirmed	Gram stain
Treponema pallidum	Full serology NAAT confirmed	Dark ground microscopy VDLR and/or EIA alone NAAT unconfirmed	
Bacterial vaginosis	Postpubertal: Amsell's criteria, Nugent score Prepubertal: any mention of clue cells, mixed anaerobes		*Gardnerella vaginalis*
Viral STD			
Anogenital warts	Macroscopic diagnosis		
Herpes simplex virus (HSV)	Culture NAAT confirmed	NAAT unconfirmed HSV 2 type-specific serology	Macroscopic HSV 1 type-specific serology
Hepatitis B and C virus	Serology NAAT confirmed		
Human immunodeficiency virus	Laboratory serology testing NAAT confirmed	Rapid serology testing	
Other STD			
Trichomonas vaginalis	Culture Wet prep microscopy NAAT confirmed	NAAT unconfirmed	Acridine orange

Source: Adapted from Royal College of Paediatrics and Child Health 2015 [11]. Reproduced with permission of the Royal College of Paediatrics and Child Health. The RCPCH is not responsible for any changes of practice since the date of original publication.
EIA, enzyme immunoassay; IF, immunofluorescence; NAAT, nucleic acid amplification test; VDRL, Venereal Disease Research Laboratory.

Table 163.4 Treatment of sexually transmitted diseases (STDs) in children aged less than 16 years [1,9–11]

	Treatment
Bacterial STD	
Chlamydia trachomatis (CT)	Children: • <8 years erythromycin 50 mg/kg/d 7–14 d • >8 years azithromycin 1 g single dose • doxycycline 100 mg bid 7 d (alternative)
Neonatal CT	• Erythromycin orally 50 mg/kg/d 10–14 d • Clarithromycin 15 mg/kg/daily 10–14 d • Azithromycin 20 mg/kg/daily (alternative)
Neisseria gonorrhoeae	Children: • weight <45 kg ceftriaxone 125 mg single dose • weight >45 kg ceftriaxone 250 mg single dose ciprofloxacin 20 mg/kg/d 5–7 d (alternative)
Gonococcal ophthalmia neonatorum	Ceftriaxone 25–50 mg/kg/IV or IM single dose
Treponema pallidum	See Box 163.4
Bacterial vaginosis	• 'Wait and see' (spontaneous recovery) • Metronidazole 30 mg/kg/day in 3 doses orally for 7 days • Amoxicillin 50 mg/kg/day in 4 doses for 7 days (alternative)
Viral STD	
Anogenital warts	• 'Wait and see' (75% spontaneous remission within 3 years) • 5% Imiquimod cream • Cryotherapy • For large (persisting) anogenital warts: CO_2 laser, pulsed-dye laser, surgical removal
Herpes simplex virus	None (uncomplicated cases)
Herpes genitalis	Valaciclovir 500 mg bid 5 d
Neonatal herpes	Aciclovir IV 20 mg/kg/8 h 14–21 d
Disseminated, central nervous system	Aciclovir IV 20 mg/kg/8 h 21 days
Skin, mucous membranes	Aciclovir IV 20 mg/kg/8 h 7–14 d
Hepatitis B and C virus	• Treatment by paediatrician with specialized expertise in infectious diseases
Human immunodeficiency virus	• Postexposure prophylaxis within 72 h after the insult and preferably sooner • Treatment by paediatrician with specialized expertise in infectious diseases
Other STD	
Trichomonas vaginalis	• Metronidazole 500 mg bid 5–7 d • Metronidazole 2 g single dose (alternative)

Syphilis

Definition. Syphilis is caused by infection with the bacterium *Treponema pallidum*. Syphilis is a multisystemic infection. The infection is classified as congenital or acquired.

History. Caspar Torella in 1498 suggested that syphilis in nursing infants was acquired from syphilitic wet nurses [1]. Paracelsus in the early part of the 16th century felt that syphilis could be acquired *in utero*, describing the condition as 'hereditary syphilis'. Even as late as 1901, Carpenter made reference to 'hereditary syphilis' [2]. The pathogenesis of congenital syphilis and a clear distinction between acquired and congenital syphilis were not understood until the identification of *T. pallidum* by Schaudinn and Hofman in 1905, and the development of a serological test for syphilis by von Wassermann in 1906. Published reports from 1906 until 1940 mostly described childhood syphilis in the first few years of life or after the initiation of sexual activity. Cases of syphilis in the first few years of life were either congenital or acquired. Most cases seen after the initiation of sexual activity were probably acquired and unlikely to be congenital.

However, if the presentation of syphilis is that of a neurological illness, the distinction between the sequelae of congenital syphilis and acquired syphilis is difficult to make based on serological tests. In the 1920s and 1930s, some but not all cases of syphilis described in children between the first year of life and the onset of sexual activity were reported to be associated with sexual abuse. A changing view of abuse requires a reinterpretation of these reports. It is likely that almost all cases of acquired syphilis in children were associated with abuse.

Although the incidence of gonorrhoea and chlamydia is decreasing, the incidence of primary and secondary syphilis is increasing [3,4]. Congenital syphilis follows this trend closely [3].

Pathology. Vasculitis and plasma cell infiltration are the hallmarks of infection with *T. pallidum*. However, atypical findings may be seen in early fetal death [5] or with secondary syphilis. Identification of *T. pallidum* in suspicious cases may clarify the issue [6].

Clinical features of congenital syphilis. Congenital syphilis is transplacentally acquired and presents either early (<2 years of age) or late (≥2 years of age). The presentation of congenital syphilis can be either a syphilitic stillbirth, an infant with signs and symptoms presenting at birth or an infant with delayed presentation who gradually develops signs and symptoms over the first few months of life. Late congenital syphilis presents with some characteristic finding such as interstitial keratitis. According to the older literature, it is possible to develop late congenital syphilis without any of the signs or symptoms of early congenital syphilis [7].

Congenital syphilis is an infection caused by maternal syphilis. If the mother lacks serological evidence of syphilis at delivery, then the signs and symptoms in her infant are not from congenital syphilis. While the presence of nontreponemal antibodies in an infant at birth suggests the diagnosis of passive transfer of maternal antibodies, the rate of false-positive and false-negative results in infant cord blood and serum would suggest that only a negative maternal test for syphilis at delivery should be used to eliminate congenital syphilis as a diagnostic possibility in the infant [8]. However, there are two flaws in this approach. If the maternal titre is extremely high, a false-negative result can be obtained (prozone effect). Thus, if an infant has signs and symptoms of congenital syphilis and the mother's serology is reported as negative, that test should be repeated after serial dilution. It is also possible that a mother incubating syphilis will have a negative serology but an infant infected with *T. pallidum*. However, that infant will not have symptoms at birth and by the time the infant presents with symptoms, the mother's serological test should be reactive [9].

In the penicillin era, almost all deaths from congenital syphilis are seen in either stillbirths or those infants who present at birth. While the diagnosis of delayed-onset congenital syphilis may not immediately be made, most often therapy is successful since the diagnosis is usually made before the infant becomes seriously ill. In the prepenicillin era, because therapy was not as effective as with penicillin, some infant deaths beyond the first few months of life were associated with early congenital syphilis. In the early 1900s, the death rate for congenital syphilis approached 80% [2].

The diagnosis of congenital syphilis in stillbirths can be made presumptively by performing a syphilis serology on all mothers who have had stillbirths. Serological titres that indicate recent syphilis (rapid plasmin reagin test >1:64) probably implicate syphilis as a cause of the fetal death [7]. However, syphilitic stillbirths can be associated with lower titres. Identification of *T. pallidum* in fetal tissue can be used to make a definitive diagnosis.

Syphilis is a multisystem disease. Congenital syphilis presents with similar features to secondary syphilis. Patients can have a rash, hepatosplenomegaly and central nervous system involvement. Although uncommon in secondary syphilis, bone findings are common in congenital syphilis and have been used to make a diagnosis before the other signs of congenital syphilis have developed [7].

The rash of congenital syphilis can resemble the papulosquamous eruption of secondary syphilis (Fig. 163.1) and features include condyloma lata. Involvement of the palms and soles (Fig. 163.2) may be prominent. In addition, unlike in secondary syphilis, the rash in congenital syphilis can be vesicular or bullous [3,10]. The presence of snuffles, a mucoid and sometimes bloody nasal discharge, was frequently reported in the prepenicillin era but has not been common in recent congenital syphilis outbreaks [11]. The skin lesions and nasal discharge will reveal the presence of *T. pallidum* and may be a source of infection; appropriate precautions should therefore be taken when examining or handling affected children. Hepatosplenomegaly and findings of abnormal levels of liver enzymes or evidence of cholestasis are seen in congenital syphilis [11]. Many now believe that the hepatic abnormalities are initially made

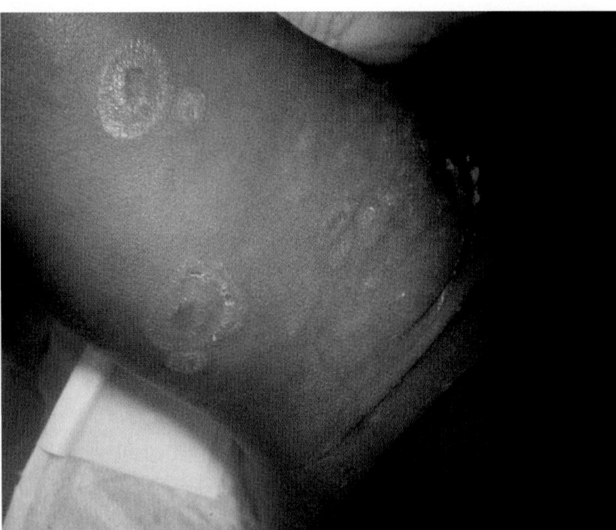

Fig. 163.1 Congenital syphilis: papulosquamous rash similar to secondary syphilis.

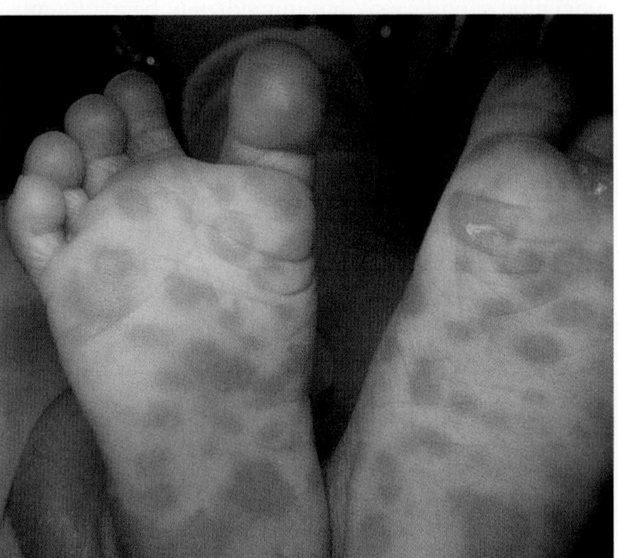

Fig. 163.2 Congenital syphilis: involvement of the soles.

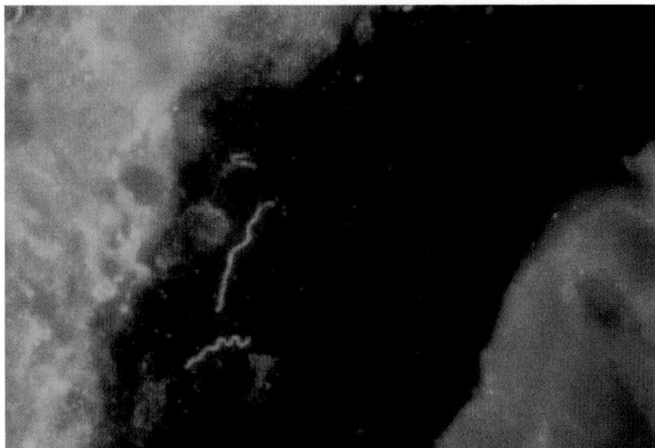

Fig. 163.3 Diagnosis by detection of *Treponema pallidum*.

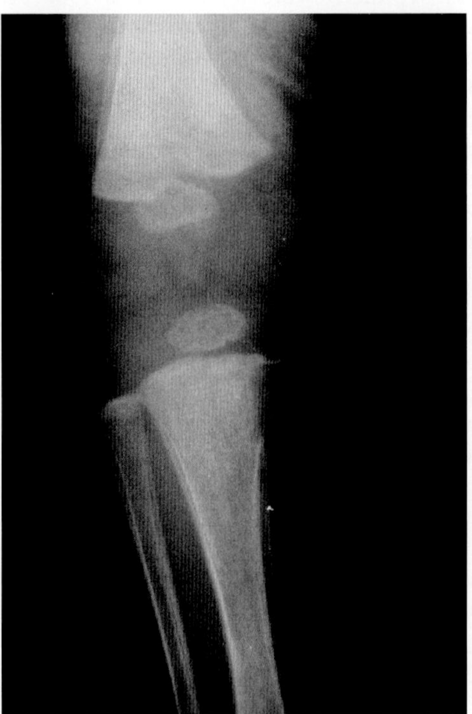

Fig. 163.4 Syphilitic periosteal involvement.

worse by therapy [12]. The liver findings are not specific enough to distinguish congenital syphilis from a number of other congenital infections.

A positive cerebrospinal fluid (CSF) VDRL test in a newborn establishes a diagnosis of congenital syphilis but the overlap between CSF cell counts and protein determinations in infants with and without syphilis is so broad as to make the cell count and protein determination of no value [13]. Detection of *T. pallidum* may also be diagnostic [14,15] (Fig. 163.3). The bone lesions of congenital syphilis are those of a metaphysitis with either lucency or increased density seen in the long bones. The development of further involvement with erosion is a later finding. Erosion of the tibia is known as the cat bite or Wimberger sign. Periosteal involvement is also seen with congenital syphilis [16] (Fig. 163.4). Inflammation of bone associated with congenital syphilis can cause pain and impairment of movement. This is known as the pseudoparalysis of Parrot. Occasionally, fractures are seen. Similar findings can be seen in child abuse. Diffuse bone involvement suggests congenital syphilis whilst an asymmetrical finding favours trauma [13]. A serological test for syphilis performed on the infant's serum will be reactive in cases of congenital syphilis associated with significant bone pathology.

Late-onset congenital syphilis is manifest by evidence of continuing infection or evidence of stigmata. Most stigmata of congenital syphilis should be avoidable by adequate treatment but since an infant with late-onset congenital syphilis may never exhibit the early signs of congenital syphilis, and since 60% of cases of late-onset congenital syphilis were initially detected by serology alone, stigmata could theoretically develop because of treatment failure or lack of therapy. The findings of late-onset congenital syphilis as summarized by the American public health service include the following.

- Interstitial keratitis, a condition which leads to bilateral blindness and tends to develop around the time of puberty.
- Hutchinson's teeth, a developmental abnormality of the upper and sometimes lower central incisors in which the teeth are notched and small, resulting in a gap between them.
- Mulberry molars in which the first molars show maldevelopment of the cusps and look like a mulberry.
- Eighth nerve deafness, which is infrequent and tends to develop around puberty.
- Neurosyphilis which has all the manifestations of neurosyphilis in acquired syphilis, including meningovascular, parenchymatous and gummatous neurosyphilis.
- Bone involvement which can be sclerotic (sabre shins, frontal bossing) or lytic (gummas resulting in destruction of the nasal bridge or the palate).
- Cutaneous involvement from healed syphilitic rhinitis (rhagades or cracks and fissures around the mouth).
- Cardiovascular lesions as seen in acquired lesions are reported but rare.
- Clutton's joints, the painless hydrarthrosis of the knees.

Hutchinson's triad consists of keratitis, dental abnormalities and deafness. Clutton's joints, interstitital keratitis and deafness are not infectious and do not respond to penicillin.

Clinical features of acquired syphilis. Postnatal transmission of *Treponema pallidum* can happen by direct contact with infected lesions. Usually, this will happen during a sexual contact but in theory, nonsexual transmission is possible when a primary chancre is identified at a nongenital site together with a plausible explanation such as a neck chancre from an innocent kiss. Another exception to sexual transmission is transmission during breastfeeding or transmission caused by contaminated blood.

Primary syphilis in a child older than 4 months or secondary syphilis in a child older than 2 years is most probably the result of an acquired infection. The symptoms in a child with an acquired infection resemble those in an adult. The following clinical descriptions of primary and secondary syphilis are based on data from adults, with specific examples from children cited when available.

Primary syphilis

The initial hallmark of acquired syphilis is the painless chancre. Chancres are seen at the site of contact. Since transmission is usually sexual, chancres are seen on the penis, vagina and anus. Lesions can also be seen on the lips and breasts. After an incubation period of between nine and 90 days (average three weeks), this usually single (but occasionally multiple) lesion develops at the site of initial infection. The chancre begins as an erythematous macule which becomes papular and then ulcerates. The resultant painless chancre has well-defined borders and a rubbery base. Associated with the chancre is regional nontender adenopathy. Without treatment, the chancre heals within 6–12 weeks [7]. In children, chancres are said to be smaller than in adults and less likely to be recognized. However, in adults, as in children, the presentation may be very atypical. Frequently, chancres are not recognized either because they are atypical or because they are hidden (e.g. cervical or anal).

Secondary syphilis

Six weeks after the development of a chancre (two weeks to six months), the rash of secondary syphilis develops as a consequence of generalized *T. pallidum* dissemination. The initial chancre may still be present when the secondary eruption occurs. The rash of secondary syphilis is macular, progressing to a papular eruption with a scaly component. The rash can be seen on both flexor and extensor surfaces. Associated with the rash are flat wart-like eruptions (condyloma lata) in intertriginous areas, especially the perineum. Alopecia is also associated with the secondary stage. Constitutional symptoms such as fever and malaise are common [10].

The descriptions of acquired syphilis in children include both papular and papulosquamous eruptions with a typical adult distribution including palms and soles as well as a description of moist verrucous plaques in the perianal area and mucous patches in the mouth [17–19]. Rash is a common initial complaint for paediatric patients with acquired syphilis. However, secondary syphilis can be asymptomatic [20].

Latent syphilis

By definition, syphilis becomes latent after the fading of the secondary rash. The stages are divided into early latent (<1 year) and late latent (>1 year), based on the lower level of transmissibility in late latent syphilis. Latent syphilis in children has not been well described.

Syphilis and child sexual abuse. If a child presents with syphilis, sexual transmission should always be considered if congenital transmission or postnatal nonsexual transmission can be excluded on plausible grounds. Acquired syphilis in children is infrequently reported [7,17,19,21–23]. Almost all cases of acquired syphilis in preadolescent children are associated with sexual transmission which by definition involves child sexual abuse. A few cases had a plausible nonabuse-related explanation for transmission. Since a modern interpretation of the older literature strongly suggests that most syphilis in children was associated with abuse, most evaluations of sexual abuse now involve an evaluation for syphilis.

Given the lag between infection and the presence of detectable nontreponemal antibodies, it is suggested that a syphilis serology be performed six weeks after an acute episode of sexual abuse to detect a serological response. However, since much sexual abuse is chronic, even a single serological test for syphilis would detect some cases of syphilis if the infection were commonly seen in abused children.

Rimsza and Niggemann [23] performed a medical evaluation on 311 sexually abused children who were seen in an emergency room over a three-year period. A Venereal Disease Research Laboratory (VDRL) test was obtained on any patient who was a victim of vaginal intercourse or sodomy. None of the 104 patients who had this test performed had a reactive test. No follow-up serological tests for syphilis were performed. It should be noted that antibiotics which could have had an effect on *T. pallidum* were given to 83 of the 311 patients.

De Jong [24] evaluated 532 victims of sexual abuse over a three-year period. Patients were evaluated for syphilis on the initial visit and at follow-up. Only one patient had syphilis.

White et al. [25] evaluated 409 cases of sexual abuse. In Wake County, North Carolina, 62 of 99 patients were evaluated for syphilis and in other counties, 46 of 310 were evaluated. Five patients had a diagnosis of syphilis in Wake County and one in the other counties. Tests were performed because of the presence of other sexually transmitted diseases in four of the children and because of a chancre in the other. Follow-up testing was not performed [25].

Diagnosis. Universal testing of women during pregnancy and at delivery will identify those with syphilis and infants at risk for congenital syphilis [26–28]. It is more difficult to eliminate the possible diagnosis of congenital syphilis in an infant born to a mother with a reactive test for syphilis, especially if previous test information is not available. Results of serological tests based on endemic treponematoses are not distinguishable from syphilis, and may lead to misinterpretation (see Chapter 44). Endemic treponematoses never lead to congenital infections. Those antibodies are always passively acquired. Without a careful history, neither reactive maternal serological findings nor the height of the maternal titre can determine infectivity [28,29]. By following the American Centers for Disease Control (CDC) criteria for STDs, one will overtreat some children but will almost never miss possible cases [7]. These criteria were developed to identify the still symptom-free infected infant (Box 163.2) [7].

A diagnosis of infection with *T. pallidum* is made by either detection of nonspecific antibodies (nontreponemal antibodies), with confirmation by the detection of specific antibodies (treponemal antibodies), or the detection of *T. pallidum*. Nontreponemal antibodies are detected using the rapid plasma reagin card or the VDRL test. The tests are reactive, a quantitative titre obtained and the results are confirmed with a specific treponemal test. The specific treponemal tests are considered as confirmatory.

Current tests include the fluorescent treponemal antibody absorbed (FTA-ABS) test or the microhaemagglutination assay for antibody to *T. pallidum* (MHA-TP). In Europe, immunoglobulin G (IgG) and IgM enzyme immunoassays (EIAs) are also used for the diagnosis of syphilis. Nonstandardized immunoblot assays are used by some investigators [14,15]. The IgM assays have the potential to detect cases of congenital syphilis as well as cases of acquired syphilis. The IgM test may not detect cases of congenital syphilis in which the patient has yet to develop symptoms [15]. In developing countries or in other sense hard-to-reach people, one may perform a point-of-care (POC) test for which you do not need laboratory equipment [30].

Treponema pallidum is detected by dark-field examination, immunofluorescent antigen detection, the polymerase chain reaction (PCR) or the rabbit infectivity test. These tests approach 100% specificity but have variable sensitivity. They are of most value in the diagnosis of the early stages of congenital and acquired syphilis. The rabbit infectivity test is a useful standard against which to measure these other tests but it is only available in a research setting. Infants suspected of highly probable disease should be thoroughly investigated (Box 163.3) [7].

Box 163.2 Congenital syphilis: diagnostic criteria according to Centers for Disease Control and Prevention Report on Sexually Transmitted Diseases 2015

Proven or highly probable congenital syphilis

Any neonate with:

- an abnormal physical examination that is consistent with congenital syphilis or
- a serum quantitative nontreponemal serological titre that is fourfold higher than the mother's titre (however, the absence of a fourfold or greater titre for a neonate does not exclude congenital syphilis) or
- a positive darkfield test or PCR of lesions or body fluid(s).

Possible congenital syphilis

Any neonate who has a normal physical examination and a serum quantitative nontreponemal serological titre equal to or less than fourfold the maternal titre and one of the following:

- mother was not treated, inadequately treated or has no documentation of having received treatment or
- mother was treated with erythromycin or a regimen other than those recommended in these guidelines (i.e. a nonpenicillin G regimen) (women treated with a regimen other than recommended in these guidelines should be considered untreated) or
- mother received recommended treatment <4 weeks before delivery

Congenital syphilis less likely

Any neonate who has a normal physical examination and a serum quantitative nontreponemal serological titre equal to or less than fourfold the maternal titre and both of the following are true:

- mother was treated during pregnancy, treatment was appropriate for the stage of infection, and treatment was administered >4 weeks before delivery and
- mother has no evidence of reinfection or relapse

Congenital syphilis unlikely

Any neonate who has a normal physical examination and a serum quantitative nontreponemal serological titre equal to or less than fourfold the maternal titre and both of the following are true:

- mother's treatment was adequate before pregnancy and
- mother's nontreponemal serological titre remained low and stable (i.e. serofast) before and during pregnancy and at delivery (VDRL <1:2; RPR <1:4)

Source: CDC, available from www.cdc.gov/std/tg2015/congenital.htm

Prognosis. Untreated congenital and acquired syphilis share some sequelae. Early and appropriate therapy results in a good outcome [28]. While there is not a large enough experience with late congenital syphilis to evaluate the effectiveness of penicillin therapy, case reports have not shown penicillin to be helpful [31]. Failures from appropriate therapy of congenital syphilis are not reported but there have been short-term failures of benzathine penicillin therapy. All patients have been

Box 163.3 Recommended evaluation of infants with proven or highly probable disease

- Direct darkfield examination or fluorescent antibody test or other specific test of skin lesions, lymph nodes or body fluids
- Serum quantitative nontreponemal and treponemal serological investigations. IgM serology is highly recommended
- Complete blood count and differential and platelet count
- Cerebrospinal fluid analysis for VDRL, cell count and protein
- Other tests as clinically indicated (long bone radiographs, chest radiograph, liver function tests, cranial ultrasound, ophthalmological examination)

retreated appropriately [32]. Careful follow-up of all infants at risk of congenital syphilis is essential to ensure that the treatment given was effective [7].

Differential diagnosis. Syphilis is the great imitator. When acquired syphilis in children presents with a primary chancre, the differential diagnosis should be considered for a suspected bacterial skin infection which does not respond to treatment. The differential diagnosis also includes HSV and chancroid. The rash of secondary syphilis can be confused with any of the papulosquamous disorders, with the greatest likelihood of confusion with pityriasis rosea. The systemic manifestations of acquired syphilis are nonspecific except for such findings as epitrochlear adenopathy.

Both congenital and acquired syphilis can present with a cerebrospinal pleocytosis. There are very few findings in the CSF that would specifically indicate syphilis other than tabes dorsalis.

The bullous skin findings of congenital syphilis can be confused with epidermolysis bullosa, dermatitis herpetiformis, staphylococcal infection or mastocytosis [33]. Hepatosplenomegaly can be seen in any of the congenital infections such as toxoplasmosis, rubella or cytomegalovirus. The anaemia of congenital syphilis can be seen in any other cause of hydrops fetalis, especially parvovirus infection. The bone lesions of congenital syphilis can be confused with either infection or child abuse.

Treatment (Box 163.4). Penicillin G, administered parenterally, is the preferred drug for treatment of all stages of syphilis [7,10]. First-choice treatment consists of benzathine penicillin G 50 000 units/kg IM, up to the adult dose of 2.4 million units in a single dose. Rarely, failures occur [31,32]. Patients who also have symptoms or signs suggesting neurological or ophthalmic disease should have an evaluation including CSF analysis and ocular slit-lamp examination. All patients should also be tested for HIV infection [8]. Administration of IM benzathine penicillin is painful; dilution of the penicillin with 1% lidocaine HCL may reduce pain symptoms [34].

Treatment of congenital syphilis involves:
- adequate treatment of the mother before pregnancy
- adequate treatment of the mother during pregnancy, preferably in the first half of pregnancy but definitely before the last month of pregnancy, or
- adequate treatment of the infant either at delivery or postnatally when symptoms develop.

Box 163.4 Recommended treatment regimens for children with acquired or congenital syphilis

Infants with congenital syphilis
Neonates with congenital syphilis: 200 000–250 000 units/kg/day penicillin G IV divided in 2 (first week), 3 (2–4 weeks) or 4 (>4 weeks) doses, for 14 days. Herxheimer reactions appear to be much less common in neonates compared to older infants and children.

Older children
Benzathin benzylpenicillin, 50 000 IE/kg/IM (maximal dose: 2.4 million IE/dose). No proven alternatives to penicillin are available. Erythromycin (in children) and doxycycline or tetracycline (only in adults) are claimed to be effective, but these drugs are not mentioned in the CDC STD guidelines. Ceftriaxone (children up to 12 years: 30–80 mg/kg/d, older children: 1–2 g/d IV, both in one dose for 10 days) is also an alternative, and there is no evidence in the literature that it is less efficient than penicillin [31]. In a recent metaanalysis it was concluded that ceftriaxone was a good alternative to penicillin in penicillin-allergic people [36].

Any strategy involving maternal therapy must involve therapy of all sexual partners or the treated mother will become reinfected. Adequate maternal therapy is defined as either one injection of benzathine penicillin (2.4 million units) for early syphilis (primary and secondary syphilis) or one injection per week for three weeks of benzathine penicillin to a total dose of 7.2 million units. As a result of this therapy, patients with early syphilis should show a fourfold decrease in nontreponemal titre or return to being negative. Patients with late syphilis should have stable or declining titres of less than or equal to 1:4 [10].

Most pregnant women with reactive syphilis serologies do not fit into any of these categories, frequently because an appropriate fall in titre is not documentable before delivery. Thus, many infants at risk for congenital syphilis are treated for congenital syphilis because adequate therapy in their mother cannot be established with certainty.

The therapy of congenital syphilis is 10–14 days of penicillin G (50 000/kg/dose every 12 h for the first week of life and every 8 h thereafter). Although therapy with intravenous penicillin G is one option, the authors' experience with procaine penicillin 50 000 units/kg given intramuscularly daily for 10 days has been good. There have been no reported treatment failures with either penicillin G or procaine penicillin while therapy with benzathine penicillin as a single injection has resulted in some treatment failures [31,32].

As in acquired syphilis, an appropriate fall in the nontreponemal serology is expected. Infants who are treated late in the course of their disease may never become seronegative. Fifteen percent of patients with early syphilis treated with the recommended therapy will not achieve a twofold dilution decline in nontreponemal titre [7,10]. Nonpenicillin therapies of congenital syphilis have not been evaluated and should not be used. Appropriate doses of ampicillin can be considered as equivalent to penicillin [7,10]. One should bear in mind that treatment failures can occur.

Screening for syphilis (repeated after 12 weeks) is recommended for victims of sexual abuse by high-risk individuals (previous STD infections, an infected sexual partner, HIV infection and more than four sex partners in the preceding year) [35].

References

1 Dennie CC. A History of Syphilis. Springfield, Illinois: C.C. Thomas, 1962.
2 Carpenter G. The Syphilis of Children in Every-Day Practice. New York: William Wood, 1901.
3 Smith L, Angarone MP. Sexually transmitted infections. Urol Clin North Am 2015;42:507–18.
4 Peterman TA, Bernstein KT, Weinstock H. Syphilis in the United States: on the rise? Expert Rev Anti Infect Ther 2015;13:161–8.
5 Harter CA, Benirschke K. Fetal syphilis in the first trimester. Obstet Gynecol 1976;124:705–11.
6 Jeerapaet P, Ackerman AB. Histologic patterns of secondary syphilis. Arch Dermatol 1973;107:373–7.
7 **Centers for Disease Control and Prevention. Sexually transmitted diseases: treatment guideline. CDC, 2015. www.cdc.gov/std/tg2015/default.htm**
8 Rawstron SA, Bromberg K. Comparison of maternal and newborn serologic tests for syphilis. Am J Dis Child 1991;145:1383–8.
9 Dorfman DR, Claser JH. Congenital syphilis presenting in infants after the newborn period. N Engl J Med 1990;323:1299–302.
10 Kent ME, Romanelli F. Reexamining syphilis: an update on epidemiology, clinical infection, and management. Ann Pharmacotherapeut 2008;42:226–36.
11 Rawstron SA, Jenkins S, Blanchard S et al. Maternal and congenital syphilis in Brooklyn, NY. Epidemiology, transmission, and diagnosis. Am J Dis Child 1983;147:727–31.
12 Shah MC, Barton LL. Congenital syphilitic hepatitis. Pediatr Infect Dis J 1989;8:891–2.
13 Fiser RH, Kaplan J, Holder JC. Congenital syphilis mimicking the battered child syndrome. how does one tell them apart? Clin Pediatr 1972;11:305–7.
14 Sanchez PJ, Wendel GD Jr, Grimprel E et al. Evaluation of molecular methodologies and rabbit infectivity testing for the diagnosis of congenital syphilis and neonatal central nervous system invasion by *Treponema pallidum*. J Infect Dis 1993;167:148–57.
15 Bromberg K, Rawstron S, Tannis G. Diagnosis of congenital syphilis by combining *Treponema pallidum*-specific IgM detection with immunofluorescent antigen detection for *T. pallidum*. J Infect Dis 1993;168:238–42.
16 Bilo RAC, Robben SGF, van Rijn RR. Forensic aspects of paediatric fractures. Differentiating accidental trauma from child abuse. Radiol Med 2011;116:671–2.
17 Zhang R, Jin H. Syphilis in an infant acquired by mouth to mouth transfer of prechewed food. Pediatr Dermatol 2016;33:e344–e345
18 Yu X, Zheng H. Syphilitic chancre of the lips transmitted by kissing: a case report and review of the literature. Medicine 2016;95:e3303.
19 Horowitz S, Chadwick DL. Syphilis as a sole indicator of sexual abuse: two cases with no intervention. Child Abuse Negl 1990;14:129–32.
20 Chapel TA. The signs and symptoms of secondary syphilis. Sex Transm Dis 1980;7(4):161–4.
21 Ackerman AB, Goldfaden G, Cosmides JC. Acquired syphilis in early childhood. Arch Dermatol 1972;106:92–3.
22 Schwarcz SK, Whittington WL. Sexual assault and sexually transmitted diseases: detection and management in adults and children. Rev Infect Dis 1990;12(Suppl 6):S682–90.
23 Rimsza ME, Niggemann EH. Medical evaluation of sexually abused children: a review of 311 cases. Pediatrics 1982;69:9–14.
24 De Jong AR. Sexually transmitted diseases in sexually abused children. Sex Transm Dis 1986;13:123–6.
25 White ST, Loda FA, Ingram DL et al. Sexually transmitted diseases in sexually abused children. Pediatrics 1983;72:16–21.
26 Boot JM, Oranje AP, de Groot R et al. Congenital syphilis. Int J STD AIDS 1992;3:161–7.
27 Boot JM, Menke HE, van Eijk RVW et al. Congenital syphilis in The Netherlands: cause and parental characteristics. Genito Urin Med 1988;64:298–302.
28 Boot JM, Oranje AP, Menke HE et al. Congenital syphilis in The Netherlands: diagnosis and clinical features. Genito Urin Med 1989;65:300–3.
29 Glaser JH. Centers for Disease Control prevention guidelines for congenital syphilis. J Pediatr 1996;129:488–90.
30 Peeling RW, Masey D. Point-of-care (POC) test for diagnosing infections in the developing world. Clin Microbiol Infect 2010;16:1062–9.
31 Causer LM, Kaldor JM, Conway DP. An evaluation of a novel dual treponemal/non-treponemal point-of-care test for syphilis as a tool to distinguish active from past treponemal infection. Clin Infect Dis 2015;61:184.
32 Beck-Sague C, Alexander ER. Failure of benzathine penicillin G treatment in early congenital syphilis. Pediatr Infect Dis 1987;6:1061–4.
33 Oranje AP, Soekanto W, Sukardi A et al. Diffuse cutaneous mastocytosis mimicking staphylococcal scalded-skin syndrome: report of three cases. Pediatr Dermatol 1991;8:147–51.
34 Amir J, Ginat S, Cohen YH, Marcus TE. Lidocaine as a diluent for administration of benzathine penicillin. Pediatr Infect Dis J 1998; 17(10):890–3.
35 Hardy JB, Hardy PH, Oppenheimer EH et al. Failure of penicillin in a newborn with congenital syphilis. JAMA 1970;212:1345–9.
36 Liang Z, Chen YP, Yang CS et al. Meta-analysis of ceftriaxone compared with penicillin for the treatment of syphilis. Int J Antimicrob Agents 2016;47:6–11.

Gonorrhoea

Definition. Gonorrhoea is caused by an infection with *Neisseria gonorrhoeae*. *Neisseria gonorrhoeae* (gonococci) are nonmotile, nonspore-forming Gram-negative diplococci (they grow in pairs). It is an infection with either an acute or a subacute course. The infection can be located in the genitalia, rectum or oropharynx.

History. Gonorrhoea is one of the oldest known human illnesses. While references to urethral discharge are made in the Old Testament, in the fourth and fifth centuries BCE Hippocrates wrote of gonorrhoea, although the term gonorrhoea ('flow of seed/semen') was not introduced until the second century by Galen. Neisser, who also discovered that the agent could be found in cases of ophthalmia neonatorum, finally identified the causal organism of gonorrhoea in 1879. Leistikow and Loeffler in 1882 were the first to culture the organism, and in 1881 Credé, who had been working on neonatal ophthalmia, started to use silver nitrate instillation into the eyes of newborns to prevent gonococcal ophthalmia, a common cause of blindness. The use of silver nitrate prophylaxis reduced the incidence of neonatal gonococcal ophthalmia from more than 10% to 0.5% [1].

Epidemic vulvovaginitis in girls was a common disease in the early 20th century before the advent of penicillin therapy, and was believed to be extremely contagious, requiring only superficial contact for transmission [2]. However, careful study of infected girls in controlled circumstances showed that gonococcal vulvovaginitis was not contagious (no transmission was seen from infected to noninfected girls on a ward, although there was no effective treatment at that time) [2]. The conclusion that transmission of the disease requires intimate contact between an infected adult or child and noninfected child remains today.

Aetiology and pathogenesis. Gonorrhoea is an infection which in adults can only be acquired by intimate contact, almost always sexual [3,4]. Humans are the only natural host and direct mucous membrane contact is necessary to spread disease [4–6].

Gonococcal infection in children is acquired either perinatally, from an infected mother to a newborn (vertical transmission), or by intimate contact (almost always sexual).

The role of fomites in the spread of disease is not clear, but is probably extremely uncommon. The only well-documented spread of gonococcal infection in a nonsexual manner was a hospital outbreak of neonatal gonococcal infection probably spread by contaminated rectal thermometers [7].

Pathology. Gonococcal infections start with the organism adhering to the mucosal cells which is mediated by pili and other surface proteins. Stratified squamous cells can resist invasion, but columnar epithelium is susceptible. This explains the distribution of infection: urethra, Skene and Bartholin glands, cervix and fallopian tubes in females; urethra, prostate, seminal vesicles and epididymis in males; and rectum, pharynx and conjunctivae in both sexes. Prepubertal girls are susceptible to vaginal infections with *N. gonorrhoeae* because of the alkaline pH and lack of oestrogenization, whereas postpubertal girls develop cervical but not vaginal infections. The organism is engulfed by endocytosis of the cell into vacuoles, where they may replicate and eventually exit from the basal surface of the epithelial cell to the subepithelial tissues [8]. There is a marked inflammatory response at the site of inoculation with a polymorphonuclear leucocyte response, purulent material being exuded from the surface and submucosal microabscess formation.

The pathology of the skin lesions in disseminated gonococcal infection (DGI) consists of haemorrhage, vasculitis and a moderately heavy inflammatory cell presence, mostly polymorphonuclear leucocytes but a variable presence of mononuclear cells [9]. Thrombosis of the small venules and arterioles of the dermis is common. Epidermal changes range from minimal oedema with few polymorphonuclear cells and red blood cells to intradermal vesicles or pustules. The organisms are only detected in the skin lesions by Gram stain or culture in about 10% of cases [10]. However, the presence of organisms can be detected in about 57% of skin lesions with the use of immunofluorescent stains [10].

Clinical features.

Infection in infants

In newborns, the disease is acquired perinatally from an infected mother during delivery through an infected birth canal with direct mucosal contact from infected cervical secretions of the mother to mucous membranes (conjunctiva, pharynx) of the baby.

Without prophylaxis, neonatal gonococcal conjunctivitis occurs in 42% of babies born to mothers with gonorrhoea, with 7% also having orogastric contamination with *N. gonorrhoeae* [11,12]. The prevalence of maternal disease varies depending on the prevalence of gonorrhoea in the community at any particular time. The rate of maternal gonorrhoea in most American populations is less than 5%, although rates in Africa are higher (5–10% or more). Prenatal care with screening and treatment is effective at preventing neonatal infections in high-risk populations. In addition, neonatal ocular prophylaxis can reduce the incidence of gonococcal ophthalmia in newborns with infected mothers by 83–93% [13]. However, universal screening of all pregnant women and neonatal ocular prophylaxis are not cost-effective when maternal gonococcal infections are infrequent (<1%), as is found in many industrialized countries. In the USA, both universal maternal screening and neonatal ocular prophylaxis are used to decrease the likelihood of neonatal infection, with neonatal ocular prophylaxis required by law in most states.

Conjunctivitis is the most common manifestation in newborns [14]. The conjunctivitis usually presents at 2–5 days of life (range 0–28 days), initially as a watery conjunctival exudate which rapidly becomes purulent and thick and may be blood-tinged. The conjunctiva and eyelid are oedematous and if the infection goes untreated, keratitis, iridocyclitis, corneal ulceration and perforation can ensue, with blindness as a consequence. Other manifestations seen at this age are other local infections such as scalp abscesses (associated with scalp electrodes) or systemic infections caused by gonococcaemia and subsequent seeding of organisms to other areas, for example sepsis, arthritis, meningitis and pneumonia.

Gonococcal infections may also be asymptomatic, with cultures positive from the oropharynx, genitalia/vagina and rectum. The most common manifestation of systemic infections in neonates is arthritis. This presents between one and four weeks after delivery. In the largest series [7], the neonates were often irritable and febrile, but neonates may also present with joint swelling alone, with no systemic findings [15]. Some had skin lesions (not described) and superficial abscesses before they developed arthritis. The arthritis was usually polyarticular, with wrists, knee and shoulder joints most commonly affected.

Older children

Gonococcal infections in older children are usually local infections (vaginitis, urethritis, conjunctivitis). Disseminated infections are uncommon but do occur in preadolescent children, with arthritis and DGI being the most common manifestations. However, many gonococcal infections are asymptomatic, with 15–44% of genital infections in children being asymptomatic [16,17].

The most common manifestation is vulvovaginitis. This usually presents as a profuse purulent vaginal discharge ranging from white, cream, yellow or green in colour which stains the underwear. However, the vaginal discharge may be minimal and confused with a benign discharge [18,19]. Associated pruritus, vulval erythema and dysuria may also be present [19,20]. Rarely, prepubertal girls may have lower abdominal pain and fever in association with gonococcal vaginitis, suggesting ascending pelvic infection [19–21]. Symptoms are usually present for less than a week (median three days), but some children have symptoms for more than two weeks or even months before they are brought for evaluation. Gonococcal infections are less frequent in boys and the usual presentation is a urethral discharge associated with urethritis [22]. The discharge may be copious or scant, and rarely may be associated with penile oedema [22] or the testicular swelling of epididymitis [20]. Dysuria may also be present.

Gonococcal conjunctivitis can also present outside the neonatal period, usually in association with autoinoculation from a genital infection in the same patient. Conjunctivitis is often severe with profuse purulent discharge, chemosis, eyelid oedema and ulcerative keratitis, and presentations may mimic orbital cellulitis [23]. On rare occasions, the conjunctivitis is the only gonococcal infection present, and the source of the infection is obviously from another person, often in the family [23,24]. The method of transmission in these cases is not clear, but nonsexual transmission is unlikely.

Pharyngeal and rectal infections are fairly common, but prevalence varies in different populations [20,25], probably reflecting sexual practices. Pharyngeal infections are seen in 15–54% of children with gonococcal infections [12,20,25–27]. Almost all pharyngeal and rectal infections are asymptomatic, and are detected by routinely screening these sites in children who are suspected to have been sexually abused or who have genital discharges [28]. Rarely, pharyngeal infections are symptomatic [24,29]. Rectal infections are common in girls, probably due to the proximity of the vagina and anus with the possibility of contamination of the anus with vaginal discharge. Rectal cultures may be positive in up to 50% of girls with positive vaginal gonococcal cultures [26]. Most rectal infections in girls are asymptomatic, but occasionally there are symptoms [30], usually a purulent rectal discharge with rectal pain, blood or mucus in the stools and perianal itching or burning. Symptomatic rectal infections are associated with penile–rectal penetration. Rectal infections are rarely seen in boys, and are associated with anal intercourse.

Infection in adolescents is very similar to that seen in adults. In girls, the presentation is with cervicitis, DGI, perihepatitis (Fitz–Hugh–Curtis syndrome), salpingitis and occasionally proctitis [31]. In boys, urethritis, epididymitis and occasionally proctitis are the usual presentations. The most serious potential complication of gonococcal infection in adolescent girls is salpingitis and pelvic inflammatory disease (PID), which is seen in about 15% of adolescent girls with gonococcal infections. DGI can be seen in the adolescent population, although it is more common in adults, with ages 15–35 years having the highest risk for DGI. DGI is more common in women than men, and more common during the first few days of menstruation and during pregnancy. DGI can result from a primary infection at any site including the cervix, urethra, anal canal, pharynx and conjunctiva. The presentation of DGI is usually with dermatitis, arthropathy or both. Skin involvement is seen in about 50–70% of patients with DGI [31,32]. The skin lesions are usually multiple, erythematous, maculopapular, vesicular, haemorrhagic, pustular or necrotic lesions. They often progress from papules to pustular, haemorrhagic or necrotic lesions, and the presence of lesions in different stages of evolution is typical of DGI [31,32]. The lesions are usually on the extremities and number from one to 40, and range in size from 1 to 20 mm [31,33].

Joint symptoms are seen at the initial presentation of DGI in more than 90% of patients [31,32]. The most commonly involved joints are the knees, ankles, wrists, elbows and the small joints of the hands and feet. Polyarthralgia is common and may be migratory. The symptoms range from mild to severe and include arthralgias with no inflammation to arthritis with synovial effusion and even joint destruction. Tenosynovitis is frequent [34]. It has been hypothesized that DGI consists of an early bacteraemic stage which if left untreated leads to a septic joint stage [31,32,34], although not all patients fit this picture. Some bacteriological findings are consistent with this hypothesis; for example, blood cultures are often positive in the early phase and joint fluid may be culture positive in the later stage. Positive blood and synovial fluid cultures are almost always mutually exclusive [34–36].

Gonorrhoea and child sexual abuse

Gonorrhoea is a relatively uncommon finding in sexually abused children and a very rare finding in nonabused children [37].

It is not possible to establish the age at which the possibility of vertical transmission can be excluded [37]. However, if vertical transmission can be excluded, the infection in prepubertal children is almost always sexually transmitted, usually by sexual abuse by an adult.

Gonorrhoea was found in 0–4% of sexually abused prepubertal children [38–41] and in 0% to almost 7% of sexually abused children between 0 and 18 years [17,42–44].

When children with gonorrhoea are evaluated for sexual abuse, a high number will have been abused. Sexual abuse was reported in around 35–80% of prepubertal children with gonorrhoea [16,38,41,45–48] and in 40–75% of children between 0 and 18 years with gonorrhoea [49,50]. The prevalence range seems to be a function of the prevalence of *N. gonorrhoeae* in the community. In addition, a heightened suspicion for sexual abuse in recent times has resulted in an apparent decreased prevalence due to more evaluations in asymptomatic children.

Careful interviewing enabled a history of sexual contact to be elicited in 44 of 45 1–9-year-old children with gonorrhoea [51]. Similarly, a history of sexual contact was obtained in 90–100% of children 5–12 years of age with gonorrhoea, and 35–75% of children 1–5 years of age [16,46]. Repeated interviews by empathic and skilled workers may be necessary to elicit a history of abuse [38]. Sometimes the history of abuse may not be revealed until years later [52].

In older postpubertal children, consensual sexual activity is the usual source of infection, although the sexual activity can still be associated with abuse [53].

If gonorrhoea is highly associated with sexual contact in verbal children, it follows that this is also the most likely mode of transmission in nonverbal children.

Possible child-to-child transmission, for example during sexual play between children, has been described [41,42], although in these cases abuse or exploitation of younger children by older ones who introduce the infection may play a role [54].

Diagnosis. Since the diagnosis of gonococcal infections in children has serious medicolegal implications, it is essential to use only standard culture systems for diagnostic purposes in children [35,36]. Nonculture gonococcal tests such as Gram-stained smears, EIA tests and DNA probes should not be used for diagnostic purposes in children. Although Gram-stained smears of specimens can be useful in clinical practice, and are recommended for screening, they are inadequate for definitive diagnostic purposes [35,36]. There is a need for an easy POC test for gonorrhoea [36]. However, a new gonorrhoea nucleic amplification acid testing system used as a POC test yielded many false-positive results [55].

Gonococci have complex growth requirements, but grow well on enriched chocolate agar. However, isolating gonococci from sites with many saprophytic bacteria is easier with selective media containing antimicrobial agents that inhibit the growth of saprophytic bacteria, but permit the growth of most gonococci. Therefore, specimens from the vagina, urethra, pharynx, rectum or conjunctiva should be streaked onto selective media for isolation of *N. gonorrhoeae*, such as Thayer–Martin media or modified Thayer–Martin media. Specimens from normally sterile sites such as synovial fluid, blood or CSF should only be inoculated onto nonselective media (enriched chocolate agar). Whenever possible, the culture plate should be inoculated immediately with the specimen at room temperature, and placed in a carbon dioxide-enriched environment (a candle extinction jar or carbon dioxide incubator) for incubation. Confirmation of isolates as *N. gonorrhoeae* should include at least two tests that include different principles, for example biochemical, enzyme substrate or serological. Misidentification of organisms as *N. gonorrhoeae* has occurred and confirmation of isolates is essential before action is taken regarding accusations of sexual abuse [56,57]. In addition, all isolates should be preserved to allow for repeated testing or additional testing in the future. This can be useful in individual cases or outbreak situations to indicate the likely source or perpetrator [4,6,20,35]. All gonococcal isolates should be tested for β-lactamase production and screened for additional resistance to penicillin and tetracycline.

Prognosis. The prognosis for most children with gonococcal disease is excellent, but complications can occur, especially when the child is not brought to medical attention promptly. In neonates with conjunctivitis, the prognosis for normal eyesight is excellent providing therapy is given in a timely fashion. Previously, neonatal gonococcal conjunctivitis was a significant cause of blindness, but this is no longer the case. The prognosis for preadolescent children with gonococcal infections from sexual abuse is again excellent. Young girls with gonococcal vaginitis rarely have any complications, although ascending pelvic infections have been described which responded well to parenteral antibiotics. Unfortunately, the psychological sequelae of sexual abuse and the turmoil in the family produced by suspicions and allegations are largely unknown, but are probably lifelong. The prognosis for gonococcal infections in adolescent girls is not as good. Many gonococcal infections are associated with salpingitis, and sequelae of this can include ectopic pregnancies and infertility. Sequelae of DGI are uncommon even with significant joint involvement.

Differential diagnosis. In the newborn period, gonococcal conjunctivitis may be confused with conjunctivitis caused by other bacteria or viruses or even chemical conjunctivitis secondary to prophylactic medication instilled in the eye at birth. The most common organism responsible for neonatal conjunctivitis is CT. Other bacteria responsible for neonatal conjunctivitis are *Staphylococcus aureus*, *Haemophilus* species, *Streptococcus pneumoniae*, *Streptococcus* group A, *Pseudomonas* and enteric Gram-negative organisms. Viral conjunctivitis can be caused by HSV type 1 and 2. It is more likely to be associated with keratitis.

The differential diagnosis of vulvovaginitis in prepubescent girls includes infection with group A *Streptococcus*, *N. meningitidis*, *H. influenzae*, pathogenic enteric organisms such as *Shigella* species and *Yersinia*, and nonspecific vaginitis caused by poor hygiene and growth of usually nonpathogenic bowel flora in the vagina. Foreign bodies in the vagina can also give a similar picture, as can threadworm (*Enterobius vermicularis*) infestation.

The differential diagnosis for urethritis and epididymitis in boys includes other STDs, such as CT and *Ureaplasma urealyticum*, as well as enteric Gram-negative infections.

Cervicitis, salpingitis and PID in adolescent girls can also be seen with infection with CT, and anaerobic infections.

Treatment. Penicillin was the treatment of choice until the spread of β-lactamase-producing gonorrhoea worldwide precluded this as an initial treatment option. However, third-generation cephalosporins are now first-line therapy in children and experience with these drugs has been very favourable. In adults, quinolones are also first-line therapy, but these are not approved for use in children less than 18 years of age due to effects on growth cartilage seen in animal experiments.

In infants with gonococcal ophthalmia neonatorum, the recommended regimen is ceftriaxone 25–50 mg/kg given intravenously or intramuscularly in a single dose not to exceed 125 mg [4,35,55,57–59]. Although one dose of ceftriaxone is sufficient for gonococcal conjunctivitis, some paediatricians prefer to continue the antibiotics until cultures are negative at 48–72 h. Frequent irrigation of the eye with topical saline is also recommended. Topical antibiotics are not necessary [35].

Disseminated gonococcal infection in infants is also treated with ceftriaxone 25–50 mg/kg/day given intravenously or intramuscularly in a single daily dose, but here treatment is continued for seven days, or 10–14 days if meningitis is documented. Alternative treatment is cefotaxime 25 mg/kg given intravenously every 12 h for seven days, with duration of 10–14 days if meningitis is documented [55,57–59].

Infants born to mothers with untreated gonococcal infections are at high risk for infection and it is therefore recommended that they receive prophylactic therapy with a single dose of ceftriaxone 25–50 mg/kg not exceeding 125 mg [55,57–59].

Prophylaxis for gonococcal ophthalmia neonatorum is recommended for all newborns in the USA, and is required by law in most American states. Recommended ocular prophylaxis includes erythromycin (0.5%) ophthalmic ointment or azithromycin (1%) ointment, each in a single application instilled into the eyes of every neonate as soon as possible after delivery, regardless of the type of delivery [35].

Gonococcal infections in older prepubertal children with uncomplicated vulvovaginitis, cervicitis, urethritis, pharyngitis or proctitis is with a single dose of ceftriaxone, 125 mg in those weighing less than 45 kg and 250 mg in those weighing more than 45 kg. An alternative regimen for patients allergic to ceftriaxone is spectinomycin 40 mg/kg (maximum 2 g) given intramuscularly in a single dose. The 2015 CDC guidelines advise combination therapy with ceftriaxone and azithromycin as first-line treatment, although this regimen may also lead to multiresistant gonococci [57].

In children who have DGI with bacteraemia, arthritis or meningitis, the recommended regimen for children weighing less than 45 kg is ceftriaxone 50 mg/kg/day (maximum 1 g) given intramuscularly or intravenously in a single dose daily for seven days. For children with meningitis, the maximum dose is 2 g and the duration is extended to 10–14 days [55,57–59].

Follow-up cultures from infected sites should be repeated to document adequate therapy. This is important since reinfection is not uncommon. Parenteral third-generation cephalosporins and spectinomycin are the only recommended therapies in children. Oral cephalosporins have been successfully used in adults, but have not been adequately evaluated to recommend their use in children. In addition to treatment for their gonococcal infection, children should be evaluted for coinfection with other STDs, particularly CT and syphilis [35].

References

1 Forbes GB, Forbes GM. Silver nitrate and the eyes of the newborn. Am J Dis Child 1971;121:1–4.
2 Rice JL, Cohn A, Steer A, Adler EL. Recent investigations on gonococcal vaginitis. JAMA 1941;117:1766–9.
3 Neinstein LS, Goldenring J, Carpenter S. Nonsexual transmission of sexually transmitted diseases: an infrequent occurrence. Pediatrics 1984;74:67–76.
4 **WHO Guidelines for the Treatment of Neisseria gonorrhoeae. Geneva: World Health Organization, 2016.**
5 Nazarian LF. The current prevalence of gonococcal infections in children. Pediatrics 1967;39:372–7.
6 **Creighton S. Gonorrhoea. BMJ Clin Evid 2011;2011:1604.**
7 Cooperman MB. Gonococcus arthritis in infancy. Am J Dis Child 1927;33:932–48.
8 Dallabetta G, Hook EW. Gonococcal infections. Infect Dis Clin North Am 1987;1:25–54.
9 Shapiro L, Teisch JA, Brownstein MH. Dermatopathology of chronic gonococcal sepsis. Arch Dermatol 1973;107:403–6.
10 Tronca E, Handsfield HH, Wiesner PJ et al. Demonstration of *N. gonorrhoeae* with fluorescent antibody in patients with disseminated gonococcal infection. J Infect Dis 1974;129:583–6.
11 Laga M, Nzanze H, Brunham R et al. Epidemiology of ophthalmia neonatorum in Kenya. Lancet 1986;ii:1145–9.
12 Woods CR. Gonococcal infections in neonates and young children. Semin Pediatr Infect Diseases 2005;16:258–70.
13 Laga M, Plummer FA, Piot P et al. Prophylaxis of gonococcal and chlamydial ophthalmia neonatorum. A comparison of silver nitrate and tetracycline. N Engl J Med 1988;318:653–7.
14 Desenclos J-C, Garrity D, Scaggs M et al. Gonococcal infection of the newborn in Florida, 1984–89. Sex Transm Dis J 1992;19:105–10.
15 Kleiman MB, Lamb GA. Gonococcal arthritis in a newborn infant. Pediatrics 1973;52:265–86.
16 Ingram DL, Everett VD, Lyna PR et al. Epidemiology of adult sexually transmitted disease agents in children being evaluated for sexual abuse. Pediatr Infect Dis J 1992;11:945–50.
17 De Jong AR. Sexually transmitted diseases in sexually abused children. Sex Transm Dis 1986;13:123–6.
18 Rimsza ME, Niggemann EH. Medical evaluation of sexually abused children: a review of 311 cases. Pediatrics 1982;69:8–14.
19 Michalowski B. Difficulties of diagnosis and treatment of gonorrhoea in young girls. Br J Vener Dis 1961;37:142–4.
20 Daval-Cotes M, Liberas S, Tristan A et al. Gonococcal vulvovaginitis in prepubertal girls: sexual abuse or acquired transmission? Acta Paediatr 2013;20:37–40.
21 Burry VF. Gonococcal vulvovaginitis and possible peritonitis in prepubertal girls. Am J Dis Child 1971;121:536–7.
22 Fleisher G, Hodge D, Cromie W. Penile edema in childhood gonorrhea. Ann Emerg Med 1908;9:314–15.
23 Lewis LS, Glauser TA, Joffe MD. Gonococcal conjunctivitis in prepubertal children. Am J Dis Child 1990;144:546–8.
24 Chan PA, Robinette A, Montgomery M et al. Extragenital infections caused by Chlamydia trachomatis and Neisseria gonorrhoeae: a review of the literature. Infect Dis Obstet Gynecol 2016;2016:5758387.
25 Oda K, Yano H, Okitsu N et al. Detection of Chlamydia trachomatis or Neisseria gonorrhoeae in otorhinolaryngology patients with pharyngeal symptoms. Sex Transm Infect 2014;90(2):99.
26 Nelson JD, Mohs E, Dajani A, Plotkin S. Gonorrhea in preschool and school-aged children. Report of the Prepubertal Gonorrhea Cooperative Study Group. JAMA 1976;236:1359–64.
27 Groothuis JR, Bischoff MC, Jauregui LE. Pharyngeal gonorrhea in young children. Pediatr Infect Dis J 1983;2:99–101.
28 Rawstron SA, Hammerschlag MR, Gullans C et al. Ceftriaxone treatment of penicillinase-producing *Neisseria gonorrhoeae* infections in children. Pediatr Infect Dis J 1989;8:445–8.
29 Abbott SL. Gonococcal tonsillitis–pharyngitis in a 5-year-old girl. Pediatrics 1973;52:287–9.
30 Speck WT, Lawsky AR. Symptomatic anorectal gonorrhea in an adolescent female. Am J Dis Child 1971;122:438–9.
31 Rice PA. Gonococcal arthritis (disseminated infection). Infect Dis Clin North Am 2005;19:853–61.
32 Ahmed H, Ilardi I, Antognoli A et al. An epidemic of Neisseria gonorrhoeae in a Somali orphanage. Int J STD AIDS 1992;3:52–3.
33 Barr J, Danielson D. Septic gonococcal dermatitis. BMJ 1971;1:482–5.
34 O'Brien JP, Goldenberg DL, Rice PA. Disseminated gonococcal infection: a prospective analysis of 49 patients and a review of pathophysiology and immune mechanisms. Medicine 1983;62:395–406
35 **Centers for Disease Control and Prevention. Recommendations for the laboratory-based detection of Chlamydia trachomatis and Neisseria gonorrhoeae – 2014. MMWR Recomm Rep 2014;63(RR-02):1–19.**
36 Herbst de Cortina S, Bristow CC, Joseph Davey D, Klausner JD. A systematic review of point of care testing for Chlamydia trachomatis, Neisseria gonorrhoeae, and Trichomonas vaginalis. Infect Dis Obstet Gynecol 2016;2016:4386127
37 **Royal College of Paediatrics and Child Health. The Physical Signs of Child Sexual Abuse – An Updated Evidence-Based Review and Guidance for Best Practice, 2nd edn. London: Royal College of Paediatrics and Child Health, 2015.**
38 Farrell MK, Billmire E, Shamroy JA, Hammond JG. Prepubertal gonorrhea: a multidisciplinary approach. Pediatrics 1981;67:151–3.
39 Dattel BJ, Landers DV, Coulter K et al. Isolation of Chlamydia trachomatis and Neisseria gonorrhoeae from the genital tract of sexually abused prepubertal females. J Pediatr Adolesc Gynecol 1989; 2(4):217–20.
40 Muram D, Speck PM, Dockter M. Child sexual abuse examination: is there a need for routine screening for N. gonorrhoeae? J Pediatr Adolesc Gynecol 1996;9(2):79–80.
41 Whaitiri S, Kelly P. Genital gonorrhoea in children: determining the source and mode of infection. Arch Dis Child 2011;96(3):247–51.
42 Potterat JJ, Markewich GS, King RD, Merecicky LR. Child-to-child transmission of gonorrhea: report of asymptomatic genital infection in a boy. Pediatrics 1986;78:711–12.
43 Gardner JJ. Comparison of the vaginal flora in sexually abused and nonabused girls. J Pediatr 1992;120(6):872–7.
44 Robinson AJ, Watkeys JE, Ridgway GL. Sexually transmitted organisms in sexually abused children. Arch Dis Child 1998;79(4):356–8.
45 Meek JM, Askari A, Belman AB. Prepubertal gonorrhea. J Urol 1979;122(4):532–4.
46 Ingram DL, White ST, Durfee MF, Pearson AW. Sexual contact in children with gonorrhea. Am J Dis Child 1982;136:994–6.

47 Shapiro RA, Schubert CJ, Myers PA. Vaginal discharge as an indicator of gonorrhea and Chlamydia infection in girls under 12 years old. Pediatr Emerg Care 1993;9(6):341–5.
48 Kelly P. Childhood gonorrhoea in Auckland. N Z Med J 2002; 115(1163):1–9.
49 Argent AC, Lachman PI, Hanslo D, Bass D. Sexually transmitted diseases in children and evidence of sexual abuse. Child Abuse Negl 1995;19(10):1303–10.
50 Siegel RM, Schubert CJ, Myers PA, Shapiro RA. The prevalence of sexually transmitted diseases in children and adolescents evaluated for sexual abuse in Cincinnati: rationale for limited STD testing in prepubertal girls. Pediatrics 1995;96(6):1090–4.
51 Branch G, Paxton R. A study of gonococcal infections among infants and children. Publ Health Rep 1965;80:347–52.
52 Ingram DL. The gonococcus and the toilet seat revisited. Pediatr Infect Dis J 1989;8:191.
53 Vermund SH, Alexander-Rodriguez T, Macleod S. History of sexual abuse in incarcerated adolescents with gonorrhea or syphilis. J Adolesc Health Care 1990;11:449–52.
54 Gunby P. Childhood gonorrhea – but no sexual abuse. JAMA 1980;244:1652.
55 Bennett A, Jeffery K, O'Neill E, Sherrard J. Outbreak or illusion: consequences of 'improved' diagnostics for gonorrhoea. Int J STD AIDS 2017;28:667–71.
56 Burstein GR, Berman SM, Blumer JL et al. Ciprofloxacin for the treatment of uncomplicated gonorrhoea infection in adolescents: does the benefit outweigh the risk? Clin Infect Dis 2002;35:S191–9.
57 Workowski KA, Bolan GA, Centers for Disease Control and Prevention. Sexually transmitted diseases treatment guidelines, 2015. MMWR Recomm Rep 2015;64 (RR-03):1–137. Erratum in: MMWR Recomm Rep 2015;64(33):924.
58 Kidd S, Workowski KA. Management of gonorrhea in adolescents and adults in the United States. Clin Infect Dis 2015;61(Suppl 8): S785–801.
59 Lancaster JW. Update treatment options for gonococcal infections. Pharmacotherapy 2015;35:856–68.

Chlamydia trachomatis infections

Definition and microbiology. *Chlamydia trachomatis* (CT) is a bacterial infection which causes urethritis in males and urethritis and cervicitis in females. Complications include ascending infections. The genus Chlamydiaceae is a group of obligate intracellular bacteria with a unique developmental cycle with morphologically distinct infectious and reproductive forms. All members of the genus have a Gram-negative envelope without peptidoglycan, share a genus-specific lipopolysaccharide antigen and utilize host adenosine triphosphate (ATP) for the synthesis of chlamydial protein [1]. The genus is separated from the chlamydophila to which *C. psittaci* and *C. pneumoniae* belong. There are 15 known serotypes of CT.

A chlamydial developmental cycle involves an infectious, metabolically inactive extracellular form (elementary body) and a noninfectious, metabolically active intracellular form (reticulate body). Elementary bodies, which are 200–400 nm in diameter, attach to the host cell by a process of electrostatic binding and are taken into the cell by endocytosis that is not dependent on the microtubule system. Within the host cell, the elementary body remains within a membrane-lined phagosome. Fusion of the phagosome with the host cell lysosome does not occur. The elementary bodies then differentiate into reticulate bodies that undergo binary fusion. After approximately 36 h, the reticulate bodies differentiate into elementary bodies. At about 48 h, release may occur by cytolysis or by a process of exocytosis or extrusion of the whole inclusion, leaving the host cell intact [1].

A CT infection in children is acquired either perinatally, from an infected mother to a newborn (vertical transmission), or by consensual or abusive sexual contact.

History. At the turn of the 20th century, there was no screening of expectant mothers for STDs, no instillation of prophylactic eyedrops and no antibiotic treatment for established infections. In this period, the term ophthalmia neonatorum was for all practical purposes synonymous with gonococcal conjunctivitis. As neonatal conjunctivitis came under control with silver nitrate prophylaxis, the importance of another form of ophthalmia neonatorum, termed 'inclusion blennorrhoea', was noted. The relationship between maternal genital infection and conjunctivitis of the newborn associated with inclusion bodies within epithelial cells was established by Lindner, Halberstader, von Prowazek and others [2]. It was not until the 1950s that CT was isolated from an infant with inclusion blennorrhoea [3]. In 1967, Schachter et al. further emphasized the relationship of sexual transmission of the infection in the parents of infants of inclusion conjunctivitis [4].

Respiratory infection in infants due to CT was probably first reported by Botsztejn in 1941 who described an entity he called pertussoid eosinophilic pneumonia [5]. However, it was not until 1975 that Schachter et al. [6] isolated CT from the respiratory tract of an infant with pneumonia. The syndrome of infantile chlamydial pneumonia was further characterized by Beem and Saxon in 1977 [7]. CT is probably the most prevalent curable sexually transmitted infection in the world today. The WHO estimated that in 2012, the number of CT infections among adults was around 131 million cases [8]. The prevalence of chlamydial infection is more weakly associated with socioeconomic status, urban/rural residence and race/ethnicity than gonorrhoea and syphilis. Prevalences of CT infection are consistently greater than 5% among sexually active, adolescent and young adult women attending outpatient clinics, regardless of the region of the country, location of the clinic (urban/rural) and the race or ethnicity of the population. Among sexually active adolescents, the prevalence commonly exceeds 10% and may exceed 20% [9,10]. Decreasing age at first intercourse and increasing age of marriage have contributed importantly to the higher prevalence of CT infection.

Clinical features.

Infections in infants

Pregnant women who have cervical infection with CT can transmit the infection to their infants who may subsequently develop neonatal conjunctivitis and pneumonia. Epidemiological evidence strongly suggests that the infant acquires chlamydial infection from the mother during vaginal delivery (transmission by contact with infected cervical secretions) [11,12]. Infection after caesarean section is rare and usually occurs after early rupture of an infected amniotic membrane. There is no evidence supporting postnatal acquisition from the mother or other family members. Approximately 50–75% of infants born to infected women will become infected at one or more anatomical sites, including the conjunctiva, nasopharynx, rectum and vagina.

Inclusion conjunctivitis

Chlamydia trachomatis is the most frequent identifiable infectious cause of neonatal conjunctivitis and the major clinical manifestation of neonatal chlamydial infection. Approximately 30–50% of infants born to *Chlamydia*-positive mothers will develop conjunctivitis. CT is identified in 30–40% of infants less than 1 month of age presenting with conjunctivitis [13–15]. The incubation period is 5–14 days after delivery, or earlier if there has been premature rupture of membranes. Infection is rare following caesarean section with intact membranes but can happen. At least 50% of infants with chlamydial conjunctivitis will also have nasopharyngeal infection. The presentation is extremely variable, ranging from mild conjunctival infection with scant mucoid discharge to severe conjunctivitis with copious purulent discharge, chemosis and pseudomembrane formation. The conjunctiva can be very friable and may bleed when stroked with a swab.

Chlamydial conjunctivitis needs to be differentiated from gonococcal ophthalmia in some infants, especially those born to mothers who did not receive any prenatal care, had gonorrhoea during pregnancy or abused drugs. There can be an overlap in both incubation periods and presentation. Besides, coinfection of CT and gonorrhoea is not uncommon in adult women, so also in infants.

Pneumonia

The nasopharynx is the most frequent site of perinatally acquired chlamydial infection. Approximately 70% of infected infants will have positive cultures at this site. The majority of these nasopharyngeal infections are asymptomatic and may persist for three years or more [11,15–17]. Chlamydial pneumonia develops in only about 30% of infants with nasopharyngeal infection. In those who develop pneumonia, the presentation and clinical findings are very characteristic. The children usually present between 4 and 12 weeks of age. A few cases have been reported presenting as early as 2 weeks of age, but no cases have been seen beyond 4 months. The infants frequently have a history of cough and congestion with an absence of fever. On physical examination, the infant is tachypnoeic and rales are heard on auscultation of the chest; wheezing is distinctly uncommon. There are no specific radiographic findings except hyperinflation [7,18]. Significant laboratory findings include peripheral eosinophilia (>300 cells/cm^3) and elevated serum immunoglobulins [18].

Infections at other sites

Infants born to *Chlamydia*-positive mothers may also become infected in the rectum and vagina [15,19]. Although infection at these sites appears to be totally asymptomatic, the infection may cause confusion if detected at a later date. Schachter et al. [19] reported finding subclinical rectal and vaginal infection in 14% of infants born to *Chlamydia*-positive women; some of these infants were still culture positive at 18 months of age. Harrison et al. [18] were able to follow 22 infants born to women with culture-proven chlamydial infections and found that positive cultures were detected in these children as late as 28.5 months after birth: this was the longest duration of perinatally acquired infection and it occurred in the nasopharynx or oropharynx. Nine infants had rectal or vaginal infections which persisted for slightly over 12 months. There are anecdotal reports of perinatally acquired rectal, vaginal and nasopharyngeal infections persisting for at least three years [16,20,21]. This needs to be kept in mind when evaluating children for suspected sexual abuse [16,21].

Infections in older children

Chlamydia trachomatis has not been associated with any specific clinical syndrome in older infants and children. Most attention to CT infection in these children has concentrated on the relationship to child sexual abuse. It has been suggested that isolation of CT from a rectal or genital site in children without prior sexual activity may be a marker of sexual abuse. Although evidence for other modes of spread, such as through fomites, is lacking for this organism, as previously mentioned, perinatal maternal–infant transmission resulting in vaginal and/or rectal infection has been documented with prolonged infection for periods of up to three years.

Chlamydia trachomatis ***infection and sexual abuse***

A sexual contact is the most likely mode of transmission in prepubertal and pubertal children with CT [22].

In pubertal children, consensual sexual contact should be considered as a mode of transmission [22]. The finding of CT in a prepubertal child should lead to a complete evaluation concerning sexual abuse. If children with CT are evaluated for sexual abuse, a large number will have been abused, as in gonorrhoea. Sexual transmission was reported in over 75% of the prepubertal children with CT [22].

However, *Chlamydia trachomatis* infection is, like gonorrhoea, an uncommon finding in sexually abused prepubertal children and a very rare finding in nonabused prepubertal children [22].

Vaginal infection with CT was uncommonly reported in prepubertal children before 1980. The possibility of sexual contact was frequently not even discussed. In 1981, Rettig and Nelson reported concurrent or subsequent chlamydial infection in nine of 33 (27%) episodes of gonorrhoea in a group of prepubertal children [23]. This compares with rates of concurrent infection in men and women of 11–62%, depending on the study. However, CT was not found in any of 31 children presenting with urethritis or vaginitis that was not gonococcal. No information was given by Rettig and Nelson about possible sexual activity. Studies have identified rectogenital chlamydial infection in 2–13% of sexually abused children, when these children were routinely cultured for the organism. The majority of those with chlamydial infection were asymptomatic.

In two early studies that had control groups, similar percentages of control patients were also infected [20,21]. The control group in one study consisted of children who were also referred for evaluation of possible sexual abuse but were found to have no history of sexual contact, and siblings of abused children. The mean age of this group was 4.5 years compared to 7.5 years for the group with a history of sexual contact, thus suggesting a bias related to the inability to elicit a history of sexual contact from young children. In the second study, the control group was selected from a well-child clinic. Three girls in this group were found to have positive chlamydial cultures; two who had positive vaginal cultures were sisters who had been sexually abused three years previously and had not received interim treatment with antibiotics. The implication of this observation was that these children were infected for at least three years and were totally asymptomatic. The remaining control child had CT isolated from her throat and rectum; no history of sexual contact could be elicited. A subsequent larger study by Ingram et al. [24,25] found a stronger association between vaginal chlamydial infection and a history of sexual abuse, but not with pharyngeal infection, which was found in a similar number of controls. Rectal infection was detected in only one of 124 abused children.

The possibility of prolonged perinatally acquired vaginal or rectal carriage in the sexually abused group was minimized in the study of Hammerschlag et al. [17] since the chlamydial cultures obtained at the initial examination were negative and the infection was only detected at follow-up examination 2–4 weeks later. However, the two abused girls who developed chlamydial infection were victims of a single assault by a stranger. In the setting of repeated abuse by a family member, over long periods of time, development of infection would be difficult to demonstrate. Even among adolescents and adults who are victims of sexual assault, acquisition of CT is uncommon – less than 2% over the rate found at baseline [20,26,27]. The 1993 STD treatment guidelines dropped the recommendation that cultures for CT be obtained routinely from the pharynx and urethra in children who are suspected as victims of sexual abuse [28,29]. The major reasons were the low yield from the urethra, the tendency for longer persistence of perinatally acquired pharyngeal infection and the potential confusion with *C. pneumoniae*.

Diagnosis. The 'gold standard' remains isolation by culture of CT from the conjunctiva, nasopharynx, vagina or rectum. *Chlamydia* culture was defined by the CDC in 1993 as isolation of the organism in tissue culture and confirmation by microscopic identification of the characteristic inclusions by fluorescent antibody staining [28]. Several nonculture methods have American Food and Drug Administration (FDA) approval for diagnosis of chlamydial conjunctivitis. They include EIA, specifically chlamydiazyme (Abbott Diagnostics, Illinois), Pathfinder (Sanofi-Pasteur, Minnesota) and SureCell (Kodak, New York), and direct fluorescent antibody tests (DFA) including Syva Micro Trak (Genetic Systems, Washington) and Pathfinder (Sanofi-Pasteur). These tests appear to perform very well with conjunctival specimens, with sensitivities over 90% and specificities over 95% compared to culture [30]. Unfortunately, the performance with nasopharyngeal specimens has not been as good, with sensitivities in infants with pneumonia at 79%, but only 30–60% in nasopharyngeal specimens from infants with conjunctivitis. The recently approved PCR assay Amplicor (Roche, New Jersey) has approval only for genital sites in adults.

Preliminary studies suggest that PCR is equivalent to culture for conjunctival specimens and possibly superior for respiratory specimens [31,32]. Nonculture tests should never be used for rectal or vaginal sites in children, or for any forensic purposes in adolescents and adults. Use of these tests for vaginal and rectal specimens has been associated with a large number of false-positive results [33–35]. Faecal material can give false-positive reactions with any EIA; none are approved for this site in adults. Common bowel organisms, including *Escherichia coli*, *Proteus* species, vaginal organisms such as group B *Streptococcus* and *Gardnerella vaginalis* and even some respiratory flora such as group A *Streptococcus*, can also give positive reactions with EIAs [35]. These types of test are best for screening infection in adolescents and adults in high-prevalence populations (prevalence of infection >7%) [28]. There are very few reports on the performance of the DNA probe, but it appears to be equivalent to most available EIAs, in terms of sensitivity and specificity compared to culture for genital specimens.

Another potential problem can occur with use of an EIA for respiratory specimens. As all the available EIAs use genus-specific antibodies, if used for respiratory specimens, these tests will also detect *C. pneumoniae*. Even though culture is considered the gold standard, culture of CT is not regulated and sensitivity may vary between laboratories [32].

Polymerase chain reaction techniques are currently more reliable [27]. PCR is the gold standard for diagnosis in adults. PCR or nucleic acid amplification tests (NAATs) are somewhat controversial. The CDC advises the isolation of CT from tissue culture as a standard determination in childhood cases of suspected sexual abuse [27]. Cultures may be positive after 2–7 days. Serological investigation in suspected childhood cases is not meaningful because of the limited reliability. Culturing samples from the pharynx for CT in children is also not meaningful considering the possibility of a persistent perinatal infection and confusion with *C. pneumoniae* [27,36].

In summary, nonculture tests for *Chlamydia* should not be used because of possible false-positive test results [36]. This is especially important because of the potential for a criminal investigation and legal proceedings for sexual abuse [29,37,38].

Treatment. Because of its long growth cycle, treatment of chlamydial infections requires multiple dose regimens. None of the currently recommended single-dose regimens for gonorrhoea is effective against CT.

Treatment of Chlamydia *conjunctivitis and pneumonia in infants*

Oral erythromycin suspension (ethylsuccinate or sterate) 50 mg/kg/day for 10–14 days is the therapy of choice. It provides better and faster resolution of the conjunctivitis

SECTION 35: ANOGENITAL DISEASE IN CHILDREN

as well as treating any concurrent nasopharyngeal infection, which will prevent the development of pneumonia. Treatment with clarithromycin (15 mg/kg/day in two doses for 14 days) also is effective [8,39]. Additional topical therapy is not needed [40]. The efficacy of this regimen has been reported to range from 80% to 90%, so as many as 20% of infants may require another course of therapy [40]. Erythromycin at the same dose for 2–3 weeks is the treatment of choice for pneumonia and does result in clinical improvement as well as elimination of the organism from the respiratory tract. Alternative therapy consists of azithromycin 20 mg/kg/daily in a single dose [8,30].

Treatment of older children

Chlamydial infections may be treated with oral erythromycin 50 mg/kg/day four times a day orally to a maximum of 2 g/day for 7–14 days. The macrolide antibiotic azithromycin is very effective as single-dose treatment for uncomplicated chlamydial urethral and cervical infection in men and nonpregnant women [8,28,29,37]. Single-dose azithromycin has also been shown to be effective in adolescents and older children [28,37]. In children aged 8 years and older, the treatment of choice is azithromycin 1 g orally in a single dose or doxycycline 100 mg orally twice a day for seven days.

References

1 Schachter J. The intracellular life of Chlamydia. Curr Top Microbiol Immunol 1988;138:109–39.
2 Thygeson P, Stone W. Epidemiology of inclusion conjunctivitis. Arch Ophthalmol 1942;27:91–122.
3 Jones BR, Collier LH, Smith CH et al. Isolation of virus from inclusion blennorrhoea. Lancet 1959;i:902–5.
4 Schachter J, Rose L, Dawson CR et al. Comparison of procedures for laboratory diagnosis of oculogenital infections with inclusion conjunctivitis agents. Am J Epidemiol 1967;85:443–8.
5 Botsztejn A. Die pertussoide, eosinophile pneumonie des Sauglings. Benigne subakute afebrile hilifugale pneumonie des untergewichtigen Sauglings im ersten trimeron mit starker eosinophilie und pertussisahnlichem husten. Ann Paediatr 1941;157:28–46.
6 Schachter J, Lum L, Gooding CA et al. Pneumonitis following inclusion blennorrhea. J Pediatr 1975;87:779–80.
7 Beem MO, Saxon EM. Respiratory tract colonization and a distinctive pneumonia syndrome in infants infected with Chlamydia trachomatis. N Engl J Med 1977;296:306–10.
8 WHO. Guidelines for the Treatment of Chlamydia trachomatis. Geneva: WHO, 2016.
9 Hammerschlag MR, Golden NH, Oh MK et al. Single dose azithromycin for the treatment of genital chlamydial infections in adolescents. J Pediatr 1993;122:961–5.
10 Geisler WM. Diagnosis and management of uncomplicated chlamydia trachomatis infections in adolescents and adults: summary of evidence reviewed for the 2015 Centers for Disease Control and Prevention Sexually Transmitted Diseases Treatment Guidelines. Clin Infect Dis 2015;61(Suppl 8):S774–84.
11 Alexander ER, Harrison HR. Role of Chlamydia trachomatis in perinatal infection. Rev Infect Dis 1983;5:713–19.
12 Darville T. Chlamydia trachomatis infections in neonates and young children.Semin Pediatr Infect Dis 2005;16:235–44.
13 Hammerschlag MR. Neonatal conjunctivitis. Pediatr Ann 1993; 22:346–51.
14 Zuppa AA, d'Andrea V, Catenazzi P et al. Ophthalmia neonatorum: what kind of prophylaxis? J Matern Fetal Neonat Med 2011; 24:769–73.
15 Choroszy-Krol I, Frej-Madrzak M, Hober M et al. Infections caused by Chlamydia pneumoniae. Adv Clin Exp Med 2014;23:123–6.
16 Bell TA, Stamm WE, Wang SP et al. Chronic Chlamydia trachomatis infections in infants. JAMA 1992;267:400–2.
17 Hammerschlag MR. Chlamydial infections. J Pediatr 1989;114:727–34.
18 Harrison HR, English MG, Lee CK et al. Chlamydia trachomatis infant pneumonitis: comparison with matched controls and other infant pneumonitis. N Engl J Med 1978;298:702–8.
19 Schachter J, Grossman M, Sweet RL et al. Prospective study of perinatal transmission of Chlamydia trachomatis. JAMA 1986; 255:3374–7.
20 Glaser JD, Schachter J, Benes S et al. Sexually transmitted diseases in postpubertal female rape victims. J Infect Dis 1991;167:726–30.
21 Hammerschlag MR, Doraiswamy B, Alexander ER et al. Are rectogenital chlamydial infections a marker of sexual abuse in children? Pediatr Infect Dis 1984;3:100–4.
22 Royal College of Paediatrics and Child Health. The Physical Signs of Child Sexual Abuse – An Updated Evidence-Based Review and Guidance for Best Practice, 2nd edn. London: Royal College of Paediatrics and Child Health, 2015.
23 Rettig PJ, Nelson JD. Genital tract infection with Chlamydia trachomatis in prepubertal children. J Pediatr 1981;99:206–10.
24 Ingram DL, Runyan DK, Collins AD et al. Vaginal Chlamydia trachomatis infection in children with sexual contact. Pediatr Infect Dis 1984;3:97–9.
25 Ingram DL, White ST, Occhiuti AR et al. Childhood vaginal infections: association of Chlamydia trachomatis with sexual contact. Pediatr Infect Dis 1986;5:226–9.
26 Jenny C, Hooton TM, Bowers A et al. Sexually transmitted diseases in victims of rape. N Engl J Med 1990;322:713–16.
27 Bechtel K. Sexual abuse and sexually transmitted infections in children and adolescents. Curr Opin Pediatr 2010;22(1):94–9.
28 Centers for Disease Control and Prevention. Recommendations for the prevention and management of Chlamydia trachomatis infections. MMWR 1993;42(RR-12):1–39.
29 Workowski KA, Bolan GA. Centers for Disease Control. 2015 Sexually transmitted diseases treatment guidelines. MMWR 2015; 64:1–140.
30 Hammerschlag MR. Treatment of Chlamydial infections. Exp Opin Pharmacother 2012;285:271–85.
31 Roblin PM, Sokolovskaya N, Gelling M. Comparison of Amplicor Chlamydia trachomatis test and culture for detection of Chlamydia trachomatis in ocular and nasopharynx of specimens from infants with conjunctivitis. Pediatr Res 1996;39:301A.
32 Pate MS, Hook EW III. Laboratory to laboratory variation in Chlamydia trachomatis culture practices. Sex Transm Dis 1995;22:322–6.
33 Hammerschlag MR, Rettig PJ, Shields ME. False positive results with the use of chlamydial antigen detection tests in the evaluation of suspected sexual abuse in children. Pediatr Infect Dis J 1988;7:11–14.
34 Hauger SB, Brown J, Agre F et al. Failure of direct fluorescent antibody staining to detect Chlamydia trachomatis from genital tract sites of prepubertal children at risk for sexual abuse. Pediatr Infect Dis J 1988;7:660–2.
35 Porder K, Sanchez N, Roblin PM et al. Lack of specificity of Chlamydiazyme for detection of vaginal chlamydia infection in prepubertal girls. Pediatr Infect Dis J 1989;8:358–60.
36 Lacey CJN. Sexually transmitted diseases in the prepubertal child. Clin Pediatr 1993;1:165–83.
37 Stary A. European guideline for the management of chlamydial infection. Int J STD AIDS 2001;12:30–3.
38 Seña AC, Hsu KK, Kellogg N et al. Sexual assault and sexually transmitted infections in adults, adolescents, and children. Clin Infect Dis 2015;61(Suppl 8):S856–64.
39 Zar HJ Neonatal chlamydial infections: prevention and treatment. Pediatr Drugs 2005;7:103–10.
40 Laming AC, Currie BJ, DiFrancesco M et al. A targeted, single-dose azithromycin strategy for trachoma. Med J Aust 2000;172(4):163–6.

Condyloma acuminata (see also Chapter 49)

Definition. Condyloma acuminata (CA) are anogenital warts (Fig. 163.5) caused by human papillomavirus (HPV) infection. Most commonly, these warts are caused by HPV types 6, 11, 16 and 18 and very rarely by HPV type 31. HPV type 2 is often found in children aged older than 3 years. In these children the infections are in most cases caused by manual transmission [1–3].

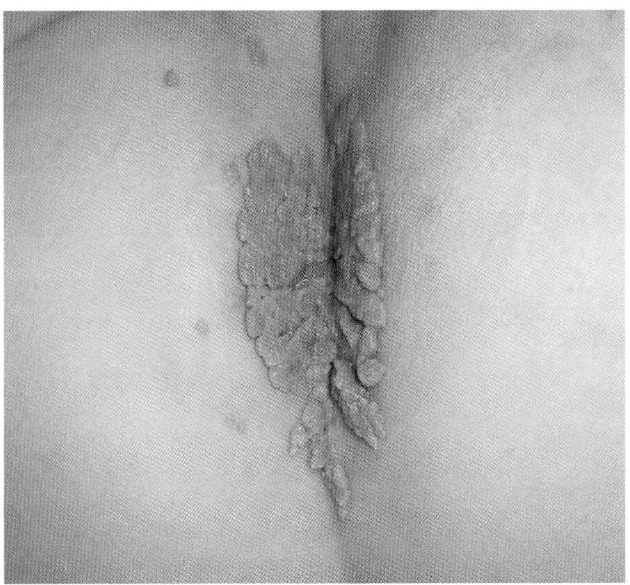

Fig. 163.5 Condyloma acuminata.

Aetiology. Human papillomavirus infections probably are the most common sexually transmittable disease in childhood, but in many cases the infection will not have been sexually transmitted. In the medical literature, vertical transmission, nonsexual transmission (autoinoculation and heteroinoculation) and sexual transmission are described as possible mechanisms of transmission in children [1].

The majority of the CA in children younger than 3 years is probably due to vertical transmission during vaginal delivery. However, within this age group, some CA will have been transmitted during child sexual abuse. The number of cases, however, is difficult to estimate. Nonsexual transmission via autoinoculation (manual transmission) from nongenital warts to the anogenital area has been described, for example in HPV type 2. Nonsexual transmission via child–child contact or sexual transmission via child–child exploratory sexual games is at least theoretically possible, as well as transmission via nonsexual intimate contacts between adults and children, such as hand–genital contact via an infected carer [1,4]. Inadequate hygiene, such as via contaminated objects such as a towel, is also theoretically possible.

Clinical features. The incubation period of HPV infections varies from 1.5 to eight months with a peak at three months. However, incubation periods of up to 20 months have been reported [2]. Such a long incubation period poses difficulty in establishing the exact aetiology [3]. The average incubation period from birth is about three months, with a maximum of about two years.

Usually, CA cause no complaints and are generally noticed by chance by the parents or by a doctor during physical examination [5]. CA are usually encountered in the mucocutaneous or intertriginous areas such as the anogenital region, the perineum, on the labia, around the vaginal entrance, around the anus and in the rectum. They are rarely found intravaginally in young girls. Moreover, CA may occur in and around the mouth, and in the throat cavity and between the toes. They are predominantly encountered in the perianal region (57% of CA in boys, 37% in girls). CA are seen on the labia in 23% of girls and on the penis and scrotum in 17% of boys [5]. They occur more frequently in girls than in boys (2.5:1). The majority are children younger than 3 years of age [6]. CA may also be encountered on the lips, tongue and palate because HPV can be transmitted via orogenital contact between the victim and the perpetrator [7].

The warts usually have the shape of a cauliflower or are stemmed, although flat forms may be encountered. They are red, pink or skin-coloured. Subclinical infections may occur in teenagers and adults. Probably, such infections also occur in children. Extremely large CA may occur in children with HIV infection [8].

Condyloma acuminata as a result of a perinatal infection occur in the larynx and the anogenital region. Juvenile papillomas of the respiratory tract (oral cavity, vocal chords, epiglottis, trachea and lungs) are a rare manifestation of such HPV infections. These are caused by HPV types 6 and 11 [9,10]. The majority of children with juvenile papillomas are diagnosed between the age of 1 and 3 years, although the disorder has been observed regularly in older children [1]. The infection presents as hoarseness or respiratory problems.

In any case, the virus may remain latent in apparently normal skin. Therefore, new lesions may develop several months after treatment [6].

Condyloma acuminata and child sexual abuse

Sexual transmission may happen during sexual abuse in prepubertal and pubertal children or during consensual sexual contact in pubertal children. A careful dermatological and paediatric examination is imperative in all children with CA.

Condylomata acuminata are found in less than 3.2% of sexually abused children (0–18 years of age) [11]. In 30–60% of children with CA, the infection was sexually transmissed [11]. The finding of CA in a prepubertal child should lead to a complete evaluation concerning sexual abuse. In pubertal children, the infection can be transmitted by consensual sexual contact.

All HPV types can infect the epithelium of the anogenital region, the mucous membranes in the mouth and the adjoining skin. Typing of HPV from the warts located in the anogenital region is therefore also indicated. This typing should be done with formalin-fixed or preferably cryobiopsies supplemented with PCR. If HPV types 6, 11, 16, 18 or (very rarely) 31 are found, then one may speak of a sexually transmissible form of the HPV types [1–3]. However, this is not proof of sexual contact or sexual abuse as mode of transmission.

In prepubertal children with anogenital warts, besides these HPV types, type 2 is commonly encountered. Usually, this type is also found in the warts on the hands and can be transmitted by hand–genital contact during child sexual abuse [1,3].

Treatment. The treatment of CA is difficult. It is questionable if it is really necessary. Commonly used therapeutic regimes like podophyllin toxin (toxic for infants) and liquid nitrogen are often painful, toxic (podophyllin) and of limited effectiveness. Because recurrence rates are also high, their use must be discouraged [1,12,13]. Imiquimod is an imidazoquinoline heterocyclic amine that is an immune response modifier. Topical 5% imiquimod cream has been used successfully to treat CA in adults [12]. In children, reports of successful treatment with 5% imiquimod cream have been published [13,14]. However, a 'wait and see' policy (nonintervention treatment) has the priority because CA show the same course of spontaneous regression as common warts (verrucae vulgares) [15]. The treatment of choice for extremely large CAs is surgery and cauterization or treatment with a CO_2 laser or pulsed dye laser [16]. Green tea extract (polyphenon E) has been successfully applied to genital wart, three times daily for at least 12–16 weeks, but this is still not the complete answer for treatment [17].

Prognosis. Condyloma acuminata disappear in more than half of cases spontaneously after three years so a 'wait and see' policy is possible [1,18]. Malignant transformation in young children has not been described. Human papillomavirus vaccinations will hopefully diminish the incidence of genital HPV infections [19].

References

1 Oranje AP, Waard-van der Spek FB de, Bilo RAC. Condylomata acuminata in children. Int J STD AIDS 1990;1:250–5.
2 Stewart D. Sexually transmitted diseases. In: Heger A, Emans SJ (eds) Evaluation of the Sexually Abused Child – A Medical Texbook and Photographic Atlas. Oxford: Oxford University Press, 1992:155–6.
3 Armstrong DKB. Anogenital warts in prepubertal children: pathogenesis, HPV typing and management. Int J STD AIDS 1997;8:78–81.
4 Herman-Giddens ME, Gutman LT, Berson NL. Association of coexisting vaginal infections and multiple abusers in female children with genital warts. Sex Transm Dis 1988;15:63–7.
5 Finkel MA, DeJong AR. Medical findings in child sexual abuse. In: Reece RM (ed.) Child Abuse – Medical Diagnosis and Management. Philadelphia: Lea and Febiger, 1994:229–30.
6 Lacey CJN. Sexually transmitted diseases in the prepubertal child. Clin Pediatr 1993;1:165–83.
7 Blackwell AL. Paediatric gonorrhoea: non venereal epidemic in a household. Genitourin Med 1986;62:228–9.
8 Shelton TB, Jerkins GR, Noe HN. Condylomata acuminata in the pediatric patient. J Urol 1986;135:548–9.
9 Lindeberg H, Elbrond O. Laryngeal papillomas: the epidemiology in a Danish subpopulation 1965–1984. Clin Otolaryngol 1990;15:125–31.
10 Terry RM, Lewis FA, Robertson S et al. Juvenile and adult laryngeal papillomata: classification by in-situ hybridization for human papilloma virus. Clin Otolaryngol 1989;14:135–9.
11 Royal College of Paediatrics and Child Health. The Physical Signs of Child Sexual Abuse – An Updated Evidence-Based Review and Guidance for Best Practice, 2nd edn. London: Royal College of Paediatrics and Child Health, 2015.
12 Vilata JJ, Badia X, ESCCRIM Group. Effectiveness, satisfaction and compliance with imiquimod in the treatment of external anogenital warts. Int J STD AIDS 2003;14:11–17.
13 Gruber PC,Wilkinson J. Successful treatment of perianal warts in a child with 5% imiquimod cream. J Dermatol Treat 2001;12(4):215–17.
14 Moresi JM, Herbert CR, Cohen BA. Treatment of anogenital warts in children with topical 0.05% podofilox gel and 5% imiquimod cream. Pediatr Dermatol 2001;18:448–50.
15 Allen AL, Siegfried EC. The natural history of condyloma in children. J Am Acad Dermatol 1998;39(6):951–5.
16 Tuncel A, Gorgu M, Ayhan M et al. Treatment of anogenital warts by pulsed dye laser. Dermatol Surg 2002;28(4):350–2.
17 Scheinfeld N. Update on the treatment of genital warts. Dermatol Online J 2013;19(6):18559.
18 Allen AL, Siegfried EC. The natural history of condyloma in children. J Am Acad Dermatol 1998;39(6):951–5.
19 Brotherton JM. HPV vaccination: where are we now? J Paediatr Child Health 2014;50:959–65.

Hepatitis B in children

Definition. Hepatitis B is an infection of the liver, which is caused by the hepatitis B virus (HBV). This virus belongs to the group of Hepadnaviridae. The presence of partially double-stranded DNA and the need for reverse transcriptase activity to replicate through RNA intermediates characterize this virus family. The intact and infectious HBV particle is spherical in shape and measures about 42 nm in diameter. The core particle contains RNA, the partially double-stranded DNA and the reverse transcriptase, wrapped in core proteins. An envelope surrounds the virus particle. The virus contains at least three antigenic components: hepatitis B surface antigen (HbsAg), hepatitis B core antigen (HBcAg) and hepatitis B early antigen (HbeAg). Antibodies generated against one or more of these components are helpful in determining chronic carrier state [1].

Aetiology and pathogenesis. Hepatitis B virus is one of the most clinically important viral infection in humans. About one third of the world's population has been infected by HBV, and more than 250 million people are chronically infected. HBV infections occur more often in Asia, southern Europe, Africa and South America.

Hepatitis B virus has specific tropism for human liver cells since they contain specific receptors through which they can enter the cell and start their replication. After entry, the virus produces no immediate clinical symptoms which only occur after the onset of some immune response in the host.

Hepatitis B virus transmission occurs through the exchange of body fluids such as blood, semen and vaginal secretions. Prior to blood donor screening, transfusion was a common route of transmission. Today, sexual transmission is the most common route. The incubation period varies from six weeks to six months.

Clinical features. Hepatitis B virus infection usually has an insidious onset including jaundice, malaise and urticaria. The jaundice may persist for weeks to months. Sometimes HBV infection is accompanied by arthralgia or arthritis. Three different courses of disease can be recognized. First, the immune response is of such a quality that the infection is cleared. This occurs in the majority of patients. Second, the infection may progress into a chronic infection, which occurs in about 10–20% of adult patients and in almost 90% of the neonates born to mothers with chronic active hepatitis B infection. Third, less than 1% will develop acute liver failure, often resulting in death or liver transplant.

Hepatitis B (and C) and child sexual abuse

In children, HBV infection occurs due to transplacental transmission, perinatal transmission, sexual and nonsexual transmission. Saliva and urine may contain small amounts of virus but this is usually too little for efficient transmission. Nonsexual transmission may occur by exposure of HBV to mucous membranes, abraded skin or unrecognized wounds. Occasionally, HBV can be transmitted through biting in daycare settings for the mentally handicapped. Most children acquire HBV infection via nonsexual contacts with infected individuals from their peer group or infected adults [2].

According to the 2015 RCPCH report, there is insufficient evidence to determine the significance of hepatitis B (and C) in relation to child sexual abuse [3]. However, sexual abuse should be considered in a child with hepatitis B (or C) if other modes of transmission have been excluded [3]. The criteria for testing children for HBV (or HCV) in suspected child sexual abuse are:

- a homosexual or heterosexual perpetrator with multiple sexual contacts with various partners, or
- a perpetrator who is an intravenous drug abuser or has a partner who is an intravenous drug abuser [2].

Diagnosis. An HBV infection is proven if HBV antigens (HbsAg, HbeAg, HBcAg) and/or antibodies to HBV antigens are demonstrated. Additionally, the virus can also be demonstrated and quantitated by means of PCR techniques on serum samples. In the majority of cases, anti-HBs antibodies are generated by the host soon after the onset of symptoms. Probably, they play a role in clearance of the virus. Patients with chronic HBV infection usually have no or low titres of circulating anti-HBs antibodies. In these circumstances, HbsAg and HbeAg are found for a prolonged period of time (many years).

In cases of suspected sexual abuse, it is not possible to demonstrate HBV antigens nor HBV antibodies immediately after the insult. After two months, HBV antigens can be demonstrated. A little later, antibodies may appear but then the child may already present clinical symptoms, if no measures were taken for passive immunization. If a child is tested HbsAg and HbeAg positive, the direct (nonsexual) contacts of the child should also be tested.

Prognosis. Chronic HBV infection may lead to chronic active hepatitis and eventually to cirrhosis and liver failure. Also, hepatocellular carcinoma is a well-known late complication. The incidence of chronic HBV infection is dependent on age at acquisition. Up to 90% of children acquiring HBV perinatally become chronic carriers, whereas 20% of older children do so. In adults 5–10% become chronic carriers after infection with HBV.

Treatment. Antiviral therapy for hepatitis B has made tremendous progress in recent years. Although most patients are still treated within experimental studies, cure has become within reach [4]. Passive and active immunization are by far the most effective prevention measures [5]. If risk factors for HBV transmission are present, passive immunization with HBV immunoglobulins followed by HBV vaccination is advised. Immunization and vaccination are standard in children born to HBV-positive mothers [6].

References

1 Lee WM. Hepatitis B virus infection. N Engl J Med 1997;337:1733–45.

2 Finkel MA, DeJong AR. Medical findings in child sexual abuse. In: Reece RM (ed.) Child Abuse – Medical Diagnosis and Management. Philadelphia: Lea and Febiger, 1994:229–30.

3 **Royal College of Paediatrics and Child Health. The Physical Signs of Child Sexual Abuse – An Updated Evidence-Based Review and Guidance for Best Practice, 2nd edn. London: Royal College of Paediatrics and Child Health, 2015.**

4 **Jonas MM, Lok AS, McMahon BJ et al. Antiviral therapy in management of chronic hepatitis B viral infection in children: a systematic review and meta-analysis. Hepatology 2016;63:307–18.**

5 Whittle HC, Inskip H, Hall AJ et al. Vaccination against hepatitis B and protection against viral carriage in the Gambia. Lancet 1991; 337:747–50.

6 Van Damme P, Vorsters A. Hepatitis B control in Europe by universal vaccination programmes: the situation in 2001. J Med Virol 2002; 67:262–4.

Genital herpes simplex virus infection

(see also Chapter 50)

Definition. Genital herpes simplex virus (HSV) infections are caused by HSV type 2 and less commonly type 1. Both types can cause genital and (peri)oral infections.

Aetiology. The transmission of HSV (both types) may occur by various methods such as intrauterine (transplacental or via an ascending infection), during delivery, after delivery via sexual contact or nonsexual contacts.

Transmission after birth occurs via close contact with an infected individual from an active lesion, mucosa or secretion. It is not necessary to have a clinically recognizable lesion to be infectious [1].

Autoinoculation via the fingers from the mouth to the genitalia is also possible. Autoinoculation is less probable if there has been recovery from the primary infection or in a recurrent infection [1]. In autoinoculation, the genital infection will occur simultaneously or soon after the oral infection. It should be noted that the simultaneous occurrence of an oral and a genital infection may also be the result of orogenital and genitogenital contact.

Herpes simplex virus can survive for some time, for example on a speculum, a glass slide or on plastic or rubber objects respectively for a maximum of 24h, 72h and 4h [2–4]. However, transmission in this manner is unlikely because for an infection, direct contact between live virus and the mucosa or damaged skin is essential [2]. HSV is rapidly inactivated at room temperature and through drying.

Clinical features.

Neonatal herpes

In a neonatal HSV infection, several days or weeks after delivery, the infant develops one or more of the following illnesses in which fever is not prominent:

- local skin infection (blisters), eyes (keratoconjunctivitis) and/or mouth
- disseminated infection with the appearance of neonatal sepsis
- meningoencephalitis with reduced consciousness, convulsions and/or general sickness
- pneumonia with (serious) respiratory problems (cough, tachypnoea) [5].

The last three disorders have a high mortality rate because the diagnosis of 'HSV infection' may be delayed and only considered after an unsuccessful clinical response to empirically chosen antibiotic treatment. The consequence is a delay in initiating adequate therapy [6]. In particular, residual abnormalities may be observed after meningoencephalitis or disseminated infection [7]. Moreover, it appeared that neurological damage still occurred in about 10% of cases after local infections without neurological abnormalities and with a normal CSF [7]. The residual complaints after an infection with HSV 2 are generally more severe than those after infection with HSV 1.

About 75% of children with neonatal herpes are born to mothers who are not known to have herpes genitalis [7]. Some neonatal infections are due to postnatal transmission of HSV.

Acquired HSV infection

The incubation period of acquired infection is 4–20 days. HSV causes painful vesicular or ulcerating lesions on the skin or mucosae, often with fever. Sometimes, there is pruritus.

An acquired infection in children is usually located around the mouth or on the fingers. Genital HSV infections are rare in children. An acute napkin rash and vulval ulceration have been reported.

Genital herpes simplex virus infection and child sexual abuse

Sexual contact, including child sexual abuse, should always be considered in acquired genital HSV infections in children, especially in prepubertal children (if other modes of transmission can be excluded on plausible grounds) [8]. According to the 2015 RCPCH report, sexual contact is the most prevalent mode of transmission in children. However, genital herpes has been reported in less than 1% of sexually abused children [8]. In case of a suspicion of child sexual abuse and a positive PCR, subtyping by culturing is not meaningful because both types are known to be transmitted sexually.

Diagnosis. In principle, the same diagnostics are used in children with an acquired HSV infection as are used in a neonatal infection (see Chapters 7 and 50).

Treatment. An uncomplicated genital HSV infection is usually not treated. A primary infection with severe symptoms is treated orally with 500 mg valaciclovir twice a day for five days. For very severe symptoms, including neonatal infection, intravenous treatment with aciclovir is mandatory (10 mg/kg/dose three times daily for 5–10 days). Neonatal herpes is always treated with aciclovir intravenously [9]. The recommended regimen for infants treated for known or suspected neonatal herpes is aciclovir 20 mg/kg bodyweight intravenously every 8 h for 21 days for disseminated and CNS disease or 14 days for disease limited to the skin and mucous membranes [9,10].

References

1 Finkel MA, DeJong AR. Medical findings in child sexual abuse. In: Reece RM (ed.) Child Abuse – Medical Diagnosis and Management. Philadelphia: Lea and Febiger, 1994:229–30.
2 Gardner M, Jones JG. Genital herpes acquired by sexual abuse of children. J Pediatr 1984;104:243–4.
3 Larson T, Bryson YJ. Fomites and herpes simplex virus (letter). J Infect Dis 1985;151:746–7.
4 Neinstein LS, Goldenring J, Carpenter S. Nonsexual transmission of sexually transmitted diseases: an infrequent occurrence. Pediatrics 1984;74:67–9.
5 Sullivan Bolyai JZ, Hull HF, Wilson C et al. Presentation of neonatal herpes simplex virus infections: implications for a change in therapeutic strategy. Pediatr Infect Dis J 1986;5:309–14.
6 Hubell C, Dominguez R, Kohl S. Neonatal herpes simplex pneumonitis. Rev Infect Dis 1988;10:431–8.
7 Whitley R, Arvin A, Prober C et al. Predictors of morbidity and mortality in neonates with herpes simplex virus infections. N Engl J Med 1991;324:450–4.
8 Royal College of Paediatrics and Child Health. The Physical Signs of Child Sexual Abuse – An Updated Evidence-Based Review and Guidance for Best Practice, 2nd edn. London: Royal College of Paediatrics and Child Health, 2015.
9 Centers for Disease Control. 2002 Sexually transmitted diseases treatment guidelines. MMWR 2002;51:1–78.
10 WHO. Guidelines for the Treatment of Chlamydia trachomatis. Geneva: WHO, 2016.

Human immunodeficiency virus (see also Chapter 53)

Definition. An infection with the human immunodeficiency virus can cause human immunodeficiency virus infection and paediatric acquired immune deficiency syndrome (HIV/(P)AIDS) in children.

Aetiology. Human immunodeficiency virus infection in children may be congenital, caused by intrauterine infection, vertical transmission, an acquired infection by mother-to-child transmission (breastfeeding) or after medical intervention such as administration of infected blood products, through intravenous drug abuse and through sexual contact. HIV is not transmitted via saliva or manually.

Human immunodeficiency virus infection in a child without proven vertical transmission or a history of uncontroled administration of blood products is highly suggestive for sexual transmission of the virus.

Clinical features. The incubation period between acquiring the infection and the first symptoms usually is many years, but may be shorter in children.

Initially, the HIV infection may present as an acute viral infection, but the symptoms may not be recognized. Eventually, the infection will develop into (P)AIDS, if not recognized and treated in time. (P)AIDS is defined as the presence of AIDS-defining conditions like wasting, emaciation, opportunistic infections, encephalopathy and malignicies [1].

Human immunodeficiency virus and child sexual abuse

Since 1989, several reports have been published in which attention has been drawn to the dangers of HIV infection through sexual abuse of children [2–4]. In most countries, the risk of acquiring HIV by sexual violence is still small, considering the epidemiological state [5].

The risk of acquiring HIV infection is slightly higher in girls than in women due to the thin vaginal epithelium before puberty and the cervical ectopy in adolescents. The risk of HIV transmission per exposure event for unprotected receptive vaginal intercourse is estimated to be 1 in 3000 to 1 in 10 000 cases, but is higher when trauma and mucous lacerations are present [6]. One should bear in mind that the same perpetrator may repeatedly have abused a specific child over a long period of time.

At present, there are no reasons for routinely testing for HIV in cases of suspected sexual abuse in countries with a low prevalence of HIV in the local adult population. Sexual contact (voluntary or nonvoluntary – sexual abuse) is the most likely mode of transmission in a child with HIV if mother–child transmission or a contact with contaminated blood can be excluded on plausible grounds [7]. In most of these cases sexual transmission can be proven [7].

The diagnosis of HIV may be essential on indication. The criteria for HIV testing in children [5] are as follows:
- a request from the victim, parents or guardians
- serious concern for the possibility of HIV infection
- the child has symptoms which may be due to HIV infection
- the suspicion or assurance of seropositivity of the perpetrator or risky sexual contacts of the perpetrator
- intravenous drug abuse by the perpetrator
- frequently occurring abuse with vaginal/anal contact
- additional 'unknown' perpetrators (e.g. in child prostitution)
- the suspicion or assurance that the perpetrator has been to high-risk areas such as Thailand and the Philippines and has had sexual contact there.

Treatment. One needs to realize that when a child is tested positive, no definite cure is available. Lifelong treatment is advised, which has many concurrent problems. Therefore, children should not be tested without extensive prior consultation with others and only when appropriate guidance is available. Testing may only be undertaken after either the parents or guardians have given permission.

Postexposure prophylaxis (PEP), instituted within 72 h after the insult and preferably sooner, is recommended to prevent transmission in cases where the perpetrator is known or suspected to have HIV infection [6]. PEP is usually given for 28 days and consists of 2–3 antiretroviral drugs, depending on local protocols. When PEP is given, a second HIV test should be performed after three months to determine whether HIV transmission had actually occurred.

The treatment of HIV infection in childhood must be left to a paediatrician with specialized expertise in infectious diseases. Cutaneous abnormalities should be referred to and treated by a paediatric dermatologist or a dermatologist experienced in paediatric skin diseases.

References

1 **Schneider E, Whitmore S, Glynn KM et al., Centers for Disease Control and Prevention (CDC). Revised surveillance case definitions for HIV infection among adults, adolescents, and children aged <18 months and for HIV infection and AIDS among children aged 18 months to <13 years – United States, 2008. MMWR Recomm Rep 2008;57(RR-10):1–12.**

2 Gellert GA, Mascola L. Rape and AIDS. Pediatrics 1989;83:644.

3 Gutman LT, St Claire KK, Weedy C et al. Human immunodeficiency virus transmission by child sexual abuse. Am J Dis Child 1991; 145:137–41.

4 Murtagh C, Hammill H. Sexual abuse of children: a new risk factor for HIV transmission. Adolesc Pediatr Gynecol 1993;6:33–5.

5 National Committee on the Prevention of AIDS. Children, HIV Infection and AIDS. Washington: NCAB, 1989.

6 Havens PL. Postexposure prophylaxis in children and adolescents for nonoccupational exposure to human immunodeficiency virus. Pediatrics 2003;111:1457–89.

7 **Royal College of Paediatrics and Child Health. The Physical Signs of Child Sexual Abuse – An Updated Evidence-Based Review and Guidance for Best Practice, 2nd edn. London: Royal College of Paediatrics and Child Health, 2015.**

Trichomonas vaginalis infection

Definition. Trichomoniasis is caused by an infection with *Trichomonas vaginalis* (TV). TV is a flagellated protozoon, which in adults is almost always sexually transmitted. TV is only found in the urogenital tract, unlike other species of *Trichomonas* which also occur in the oral cavity or in the intestines [1]. The period of incubation is not exactly known, but has been described to vary in adults from five to 28 days.

Aetiology. Pokorny [2] reported that the frequency of TV infections in adults had decreased to such an extent that one would be rarely confronted with such a problem in children. The Royal College of Physicians reported later that TV infection occurs very regularly in women after puberty [3]. There are several possible explanations for infections in children [3].

Contamination of the nose/throat cavity and also of the vagina may occur during delivery. It is not known how long TV may persist after vertical transmission, but an infection with TV in a girl under the age of 2 months may be the result of vertical transmission [4].

Acquired TV infections are rare before puberty because the environment in the prepubertal vagina (hypertrophic epithelium, nonglycogen-containing and alkaline environment) is a poor source of nutrition for TV. For that reason, growth and colonization are not possible. If acquired, the most prevalent mode of transmission is sexual contact (voluntary or nonvoluntary – sexual abuse). Nonsexual transmission in prepubertal children is probably very rare because the organism is highly location specific [2].

Nevertheless, in principle, nonsexual transmission because of inadequate hygiene should be excluded if sexual abuse is suspected; the organism of TV can survive for several hours on wet towels and clothing which have been used by infected women [2]. The organism also appeared to be able to survive in samples of urine and sperm even after they had been exposed to air for several hours [2].

Clinical features. Transient vulvovaginitis is the most probable complaint in prepubertal girls. In adolescent girls, there may be vulvovaginitis with purulent discharge, cervicitis, urethritis and cystitis. Pain in the lower abdomen may also be found. The genital area can be very red and swollen.

In boys, epididymitis can be found. In men, an infection with TV usually will lead to a transient infection, because TV requires oestrogenized mucosa to persist [4].

The infection may be asymptomatic, but screening of asymptomatic individuals is currently not recommended [1].

Trichomonas vaginalis *and child sexual abuse*

A sexual contact between a child and an adult should be suspected if a TV infection is encountered in a child between the age of 2 months and puberty. Moreover, it indicates that the contact has occurred recently because the organism of TV does not survive for long in the prepubertal vagina. TV has been reported in less than 3% of prepubertal and pubertal girls who were sexually abused [4]. If found, many children with TV are sexually abused [4].

Diagnosis. *Trichomonas vaginalis* is demonstrated by means of a direct preparation of the exudate to which physiological saline has been added (sampling with a moist cottonwool swab). The preparation must be evaluated immediately. The sensitivity of a direct preparation is moderate, but the specificity is very high; a TV culture has a sensitivity of 95% [5].

Treatment. In prepubertal girls, the infection almost always will resolve without treatment, because of the environment in the prepubertal vagina. If treatment is necessary, metronidazole 30 mg/kg/day in three doses given orally for seven days is the first choice. For children older than 12 years, the metronidazole dose is 500 mg orally twice daily for 5–7 days (first choice) or metronidazole 2 g orally (single dose) [6].

References

1 **Sherrard J, Donders G, White D, Jensen JS. European (IUSTI/WHO) guideline on the management of vaginal discharge, 2011. Int J STD AIDS 2011;22(8):4219.**

2 Pokorny SF. Child abuse and infections. Obstet Gynecol Clin North Am 1989;16:401–15.

3 Royal College of Physicians. Physical Signs of Sexual Abuse in Children. London: Royal College of Physicians of London, 1991.

4 **Royal College of Paediatrics and Child Health. The Physical Signs of Child Sexual Abuse – An Updated Evidence-Based Review and Guidance for Best Practice, 2nd edn. London: Royal College of Paediatrics and Child Health, 2015.**

5 Stewart D. Sexually transmitted diseases. In: Heger A, Emans SJ (eds) Evaluation of the Sexually Abused Child – A Medical Textbook and Photographic Atlas. Oxford: Oxford University Press, 1992:155–6.

6 Centers for Disease Control. 2002 Sexually transmitted diseases treatment guidelines. MMWR 2002;51:1–78.

Bacterial vaginitis

Definition and clinical features. Bacterial vaginitis (BV) is encountered regularly in adult women and is the most common cause of abnormal vaginal discharge in women of childbearing age [1]. BV is a polymicrobial disorder, in which various bacteria such as *G. vaginalis*, anaerobes (among others, *Bacteroides* and *Peptococcus* varieties), *Mobiluncus* species and *Mycoplasma hominis* are present in excess, whereas the number of lactobacilli is highly reduced.

The pathogenesis in both adults and children is only partially known. It is unclear whether BV can be transmitted during delivery. The length of time that BV can remain asymptomatic is also unclear. Complaints of vulvovaginitis, a thin, homogenous grey–white to yellow discharge or a typical odour may be the result of BV.

Bacterial vaginitis and child sexual abuse

Bacterial vaginitis has been reported in prepubertal girls, although the prevalence in these girls is extremely low [2]. The prevalence of BV in sexually abused prepubertal girls with a discharge is only slightly higher [2,3]. Because BV is encountered only slightly more often in sexually abused than in nonabused girls with a discharge, it cannot be regarded as strong evidence for abuse [2–6].

Diagnosis and treatment. Bacterial vaginitis is thought to be present if there is a homogenous discharge, a pH of higher than 4.5, a positive amine test and 'clue cells' in the physiological saline preparation. Measuring the vaginal pH is only meaningful in postpubertal girls. In younger girls, measuring the pH as a diagnostic criterion for BV is unreliable because the pH in these girls is always higher than 4.5. Demonstration of *G. vaginalis* in culture is unnecessary for the diagnosis. Spontaneous recovery is possible [1].

If treatment is considered, then the first choice is 30 mg/kg/day metronidazole in three doses given orally for seven days. Amoxicillin 50 mg/kg/day in four doses for seven days is an alternative choice.

Acknowledgement

We thank the authors of former editions: Kenneth Bromberg, Margaret Hammerschlag and Sarah A. Rawstron.

References

1 **Sherrard J, Donders G, White D, Jensen JS. European (IUSTI/WHO) guideline on the management of vaginal discharge, 2011. Int J STD AIDS 2011;22(8):421–9.**

2 **Royal College of Paediatrics and Child Health. The Physical Signs of Child Sexual Abuse – An Updated Evidence-Based Review and Guidance for Best Practice, 2nd edn. London: Royal College of Paediatrics and Child Health, 2015.**

3 Hammerschlag M, Cummings M, Doraiswamy B et al. Nonspecific vaginitis following sexual abuse in children. Pediatrics 1985; 75:1028–31.

4 Bartley DL, Morgan L, Rimsza M. *Gardnerella vaginalis* in prepubertal girls. Am J Dis Child 1987;141:1014–17.

5 Fernandez JP, Espana AR, Reus E. Isolation of *Gardnerella vaginalis* in the diagnosis of sexual abuse in children.[Article in Spanish] Child Abuse Negl 2000;24(6):861–6.

6 Centers for Disease Control. 2002 Sexually transmitted diseases treatment guidelines. MMWR 2002;51:1–78.

CHAPTER 164
Maltreatment, Physical and Sexual Abuse

Bernhard Herrmann
Child Protection Center, Pediatric and Adolescent Gynecology, Department of Pediatrics, Klinikum Kassel, Kassel, Germany

Definition, background and general considerations, 2219
Physical abuse, 2220
Child sexual abuse, 2229
Overall medical and multidisciplinary management, 2238

Abstract

Child abuse and neglect constitutes a prevalent and severe disorder of the child–caregiver relationship. Besides incurring physical harm, abused children and adolescents frequently suffer from severe psychological, emotional, cognitive and behavioural disorders that lead to significant mental and emotional distress and burdened lives. Physicians have a high responsibility to qualify in diagnosing and intervening in child abuse. Intervention requires a careful and thoughtful approach, always blending medical expertise with the concept of multiprofessional child protection. Medical findings in physical abuse have the highest potential for physicians to diagnose child abuse because the physician's knowledge about abuse-related findings and their differentiation from accidents and other medical conditions is pivotal. The fundamental approach is to evaluate if symptoms and findings are compatible with, and plausibly explained by, the history. In child sexual abuse the examination shows no physical evidence in the majority of cases and rarely serves for diagnostic or forensic purposes. The evaluation of the possibly sexually abused child is first and foremost the provision of medical care. The diagnosis mainly rests on history, gathered in a professional and nonsuggestive way. On the other hand, taking a history and performing a qualified and sensitive medical examination requires a high degree of specialized training.

Key points

- **Child abuse and neglect (CAN) leads to significant physical, mental and emotional harm and distress and long-lasting sequelae.**
- **CAN is far more prevalent than it is diagnosed, so a high index of suspicion needs to be maintained.**
- **Medical professionals play an important role in diagnosing CAN, evaluating suspicious injuries, excluding differential diagnosis and contributing to multiprofessional child protection.**
- **The critical appraisal of suspected cases of CAN requires attention and special education on the part of the physician and has evolved into a highly specialized medical field.**
- **In physical abuse it is crucial to critically evaluate the plausibility of injuries in the light of the history.**
- **In child sexual abuse the medical examination is first and foremost the provision of comprehensive medical care rather than checking for forensic evidence.**
- **The majority of victims have no findings so the medical examination has the purpose of detecting abnormality only in selected cases and rather serves to determine and reassure normality.**

Definition, background and general considerations

There is no universal definition of what constitutes child abuse. The understanding of what is acceptable interaction between adults and children concerning child development and parenting varies between social and cultural groups, different countries, across time and among professionals and agencies. *Abuse* and *maltreatment* are often used as interchangeable umbrella terms for the whole spectrum, frequently referred to as '*child abuse and neglect*' (CAN). CAN encompasses both acts of commission (abuse), meaning physical or emotional acts causing harm or potential harm, and acts of omission (neglect), defined as the failure to take care of basic physical, emotional or educational needs, or to protect a child from harm or potential harm. The World Health Organization (WHO) defines *child abuse* and *child maltreatment* as 'all forms of physical and/or emotional ill-treatment, sexual abuse, neglect or negligent treatment or commercial or other exploitation, resulting in actual or potential harm to the child's health, survival, development or dignity in the context of a relationship of responsibility, trust or power' [1]. Federal US laws define CAN in the Federal Child Abuse Prevention and Treatment Act (CAPTA) as (at minimum): 'Any recent act or failure to act on the part of a parent or caretaker which results in death, serious physical or emotional harm, sexual abuse or exploitation; or an act or failure to act, which presents an imminent risk of serious harm' (www.childwelfare.gov/topics/can/defining/federal/).

Harper's Textbook of Pediatric Dermatology, Fourth Edition. Edited by Peter Hoeger, Veronica Kinsler and Albert Yan.

CAN constitutes a far-reaching and severe disorder of the child–caregiver relationship, occurring mostly in families and less frequently in institutions. Besides the mostly treatable sequelae of physical harm and neglect, abused children and adolescents frequently suffer from severe psychological, emotional, cognitive and behavioural disorders. These disorders are related to significant mental and emotional suffering, insults and rejections, burdened lives and disruption of relationship-building abilities and participation in social life. CAN has severe effects on the ability to develop a secure attachment. Concerning mental health, it correlates with an unfavourable prognosis. Neurobiological research shows chronic derangements on electroencephalography and that chronic child maltreatment is a potent source of stress. The stress response, including dysregulation of the hypothalamic–pituitary–adrenal axis, affects brain development and actually leads to a reduction in brain volume [2]. In the WHO world report on violence and health, a significant amount of chronic physical and mental disorders in adults are shown to be results of child maltreatment in childhood, significantly contributing to the 'global burden of disease' [1]. Besides the toll of human misery, violence exacts substantial social and economic costs, although these are hard to quantify.

Epidemiology. Due to differing definitions, significant underreporting and underdiagnosis, the true extent of CAN is not known. According to reports to child protection services agencies in the USA, 3.24 million children received an investigation for child abuse or neglect, out of which 702 000 reports were substantiated. Three quarters (75.0%) of the victims were neglected, 17.0% were physically abused, and 8.3% were sexually abused. In 2014, a nationally estimated 1580 children died, which is equivalent to a rate of 2.13 per 100 000 children. More deaths were attributed to neglect than to physical abuse [3].

Role of medical professionals

Child abuse diagnosis and child protection in the medical context has emerged as a complex and challenging subspecialty. In the USA, the American Academy of Pediatrics (AAP) has established the board-certified 'Child Abuse Pediatrician'. The German Society for Child Protection in Medicine (Deutsche Gesellschaft für Kinderschutz in der Medizin, DGKiM) established a certificate and education for 'Child Protection Doctors' (Kinderschutzmediziner) and quality standards for child protection teams in 2017. Paediatricians and child protection teams in hospitals play a pivotal role in coordinating the expertise of a broad spectrum of health professionals. Their role and skills differ according to the respective forms of maltreatment and their field of expertise. Nevertheless, every physician caring for children needs basic knowledge to deal with cases of suspected CAN. Paediatric dermatologists may be involved in assessing a variety of skin findings that are allegedly, and not seldom, erroneously attributed to abuse. Due to far-reaching psychological, social and familial consequences, it is also of utmost importance to be aware of the potentially devastating consequences of an overlooked diagnosis of CAN for the child, as well as an erroneous diagnosis for the complete family. Physicians therefore have a high responsibility to make a knowledgeable and comprehensive contribution to multidisciplinary child protection [4]. In the USA, physicians have to be aware of mandatory reporting laws and regulations (www.childwelfare.gov/topics/systemwide/laws-policies/statutes/manda/).

References

1 World Health Organization (WHO). World report on violence and health, Chapter 3: Child abuse and neglect by parents and other caregivers. Geneva: World Health Organization, 2002. Available at: www.who.int/violence_injury_prevention/violence/global_campaign/en/chap3.pdf (accessed 17 February 2019).

2 Glaser D. Child abuse and neglect and the brain – a review. J Child Psychol Psychiatr 2000;41:97–116.

3 U.S. Department of Health and Human Services, Administration on Children, Youth and Families, Children's Bureau. Child maltreatment 2014. Available at: www.acf.hhs.gov/programs/cb/research-data-technology/statistics-research/child-maltreatment (accessed 17 February 2019).

4 **Herrmann B, Dettmeyer R, Banaschak S, Thyen U. Kindesmisshandlung. Medizinische Diagnostik, Intervention und rechtliche Grundlagen, 3rd revised edn. Heidelberg: Springer, 2016.**

Physical abuse

Diagnostic evaluation

Among all forms of child maltreatment, medical findings in physical abuse have the greatest diagnostic significance. Their assessment requires a careful and complete history, a thorough physical examination, meticulous verbatim and photographic documentation, the decision as to which additional diagnostic procedures are warranted, the knowledge of typical abuse-related findings and their differential diagnosis, formulating a thorough and defendable diagnosis, and cooperating with other, nonmedical professionals. The fundamental principle to diagnose or exclude child abuse is the critical appraisal of history concerning an alleged incident and to determine if the presenting symptoms and findings are compatible with, and plausibly explained by, the history [1,2].

History

Structured protocols may help to take a complete and thorough history, focusing on the exact circumstances, details and sequences in present illness or injury, possible witnesses, review of systems, past medical, developmental, social and family history, and prior contact with child protection services. Inappropriate, imprecise, vague or changing histories over time are unusual in cases where injury is accidental, as is a delayed presentation for medical help for significant injuries and should raise suspicion. In accidents, an appropriate history is given in the vast majority of cases. In child abuse it is completely missing in approximately 40%. It is not impossible for siblings to cause severe injuries but it is unusual. No evidence has so far been found to reconcile significant trauma such as fractures with an aetiology such as spontaneous turning or getting stuck between the bars of a cot [3].

SECTION 36: CUTANEOUS SIGNS OF CHILD MALTREATMENT

Medical examination

It is crucial always to perform a complete physical, neurological and anogenital examination of the completely undressed child, including growth parameters. All findings need to be described and documented in written form, as a drawing with measurements, and by photographs depicting location, type, size and extent, clustering, pattern and colour. All findings should be photographed using a professional measuring device, preferably a forensic ruler or photo scale such as the ABFO bite mark Scale No. 2 (www.crimetech.net/crime-scene-documentation-photo-scales-and-rulers/). Photo documentation should be performed following technical considerations and composition rules (i.e. a detailed photo and overview, indirect flash, vertical view, etc.).

Imaging and other diagnostic modalities

The role of imaging in cases of child abuse is to identify the type and extent of physical injury and to elucidate all imaging findings that point to alternative diagnoses. A complete radiographic skeletal survey is mandatory in all cases of suspected physical abuse in children younger than 2 years, following defined protocols according to current guidelines and suggestions as to what criteria justify a suspicion [4–6]. Cerebral computed tomography (cCT) without intravenous contrast should be performed as part of the initial evaluation for suspected acute abusive head trauma (AHT). In spite of some limitations in the acute-care setting, magnetic resonance imaging (MRI) remains the best modality for fully assessment of intracranial injury, including extra-axial collections, intraparenchymal haemorrhages, contusions, shear injuries, and brain swelling or oedema. Ultrasonography may be a helpful adjunct in cerebral and abdominal imaging, but is contraindicated as sole diagnostic procedure. A complete eye examination, including dilated pupils and indirect ophthalmoscopy by a qualified ophthalmologist is mandatory in all patients where there is suspicion of AHT. Laboratory tests play a limited role in excluding certain differential diagnoses such as disorders of coagulation or metabolic diseases and sometimes point to intra-abdominal trauma or intoxications in urine drug screening [7,8].

References

1 **Christian CW; Committee on Child Abuse and Neglect, American Academy of Pediatrics. The evaluation of suspected child physical abuse. Pediatrics 2015;135:e1337–54. Available at: pediatrics.aappublications.org/content/135/5/e1337 (accessed 22 February 2019).**

2 World Health Organization (WHO). World Report on Violence and Health, Chapter 3: Child abuse and neglect by parents and other caregivers. Geneva: World Health Organization, 2002. Available at: www.who.int/violence_injury_prevention/violence/global_campaign/en/chap3.pdf (accessed 22 February 2019).

3 Jackson AM, Jackson BM. Documenting the medical history in cases of possible physical child abuse. In: Jenny C (ed.) Child Abuse and Neglect: Diagnosis, Treatment and Evidence. St Louis: Elsevier Saunders, 2011:209–14.

4 American Academy of Pediatrics (AAP). Section on Radiology. Diagnostic imaging of child abuse. Policy Statement. Pediatrics 2009;123:1430–5. Available at: https://pediatrics.aappublications.org/content/123/5/1430.long (accessed 1 March 2019).

5 Borg K, Hodes D. Guidelines for skeletal survey in young children with fractures. Arch Dis Child Educ Pract Ed 2015;100:253–6. Available at: https://ep.bmj.com/content/100/5/253.long (accessed 1 March 2019).

6 Wood JN, Fakeye O, Mondestin V et al. Development of hospital-based guidelines for skeletal survey in young children with bruises. Pediatrics 2015;135:e312–20.

7 Anderst JD, Carpenter SL, Abshire TC; Section on Hematology/Oncology and Committee on Child Abuse and Neglect of the American Academy of Pediatrics. Evaluation for bleeding disorders in suspected child abuse. 2013;131:e1314–22. Available at: https://pediatrics.aappublications.org/content/131/4/e1314 (accessed 1 March 2019).

8 Kleinman P (ed.). Diagnostic Imaging of Child Abuse, 3rd edn. Cambridge, UK: Cambridge University Press, 2015.

Cutaneous signs of child abuse

Bruises

Bruises are the most prevalent injury and are diagnosed in approximately 60–90% of abused children. To assess the probability that bruises were inflicted, the criteria of location, distribution, type, configuration, size and extent, clustering, pattern and age of the patient are crucial. Multiple, large bruises in clusters and in unusual locations, bilateral bruises, patterned bruises, bruises with petechiae, and bruises in premobile infants have a strong predictive value. Recent research and systematic reviews have shown that there are no data for reliably determining the age of a bruise by its colour. Differently coloured bruises may be caused by a single event and still change colour at a different rate. The appearance and degradation of bruises depend on tissue properties and are differently visualized according to its depth. Perceptions differ between examiners. The only consistent colour indicator is that yellow has never been reported in bruises less than 18 hours old [1–3].

Accidental bruises – age and location

Accidental bruises are extremely rare in premobile infants ('Those who don't cruise, rarely bruise'), being reported in 0.6–1.5% of those aged <6 months, 1.7% <9 months and 2.2% of all premobile infants. The number of bruises and their size are usually small (<1 cm) and they are typically found on bony prominences of the frontal body. Twenty percent of crawlers and 50% of toddlers have accidental bruises, usually located on the lower extremities. Less than 2% are found on the chest, abdomen, pelvis, buttocks, chin, cheek, periorbital area, ears or neck. Typically located on the 'leading edges', accidental bruises are most prevalent on the knees and shins, back of the head, and the 'facial T' (forehead, nose, upper lip and chin; Fig. 164.1), caused by slips, trips and falls [2,4,5].

Bruises in child abuse

Inflicted bruises are found off the bony prominences, most frequently on the face (outside the 'facial T'), left cheek and left ear (Fig. 164.2), neck, upper arms, hands, thorax, back, frontal upper leg, buttocks (Fig. 164.3) and genitalia. Bruises of the trunk, ears or neck have a sensitivity of 97% and specificity of 84% according to systematic reviews. Multiple, large and clustered bruises (Fig. 164.4), and bruises with petechiae (Fig. 164.2), are significantly more prevalent (positive predictive value [PPV] 80%). In 25% of the cases there are additional fractures and/or injuries of the brain [1,3,6–8].

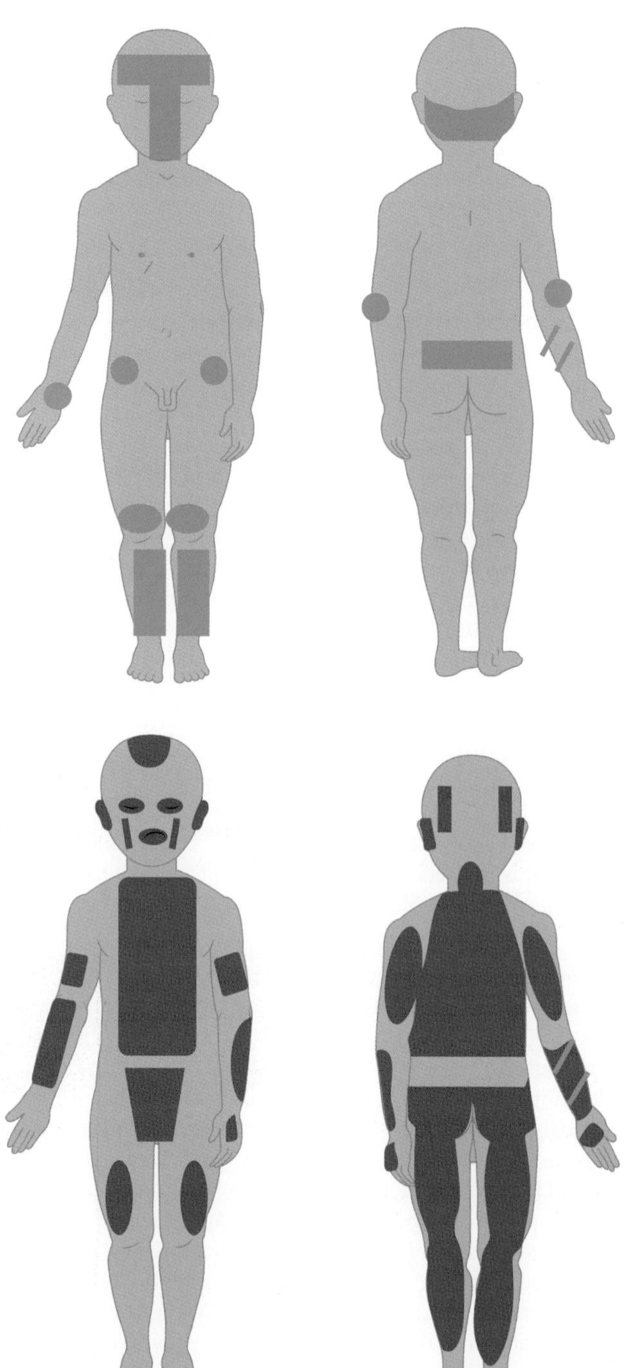

Fig. 164.1 Typical location of accidental versus inflicted bruises. Green, accidental; red, inflicted.

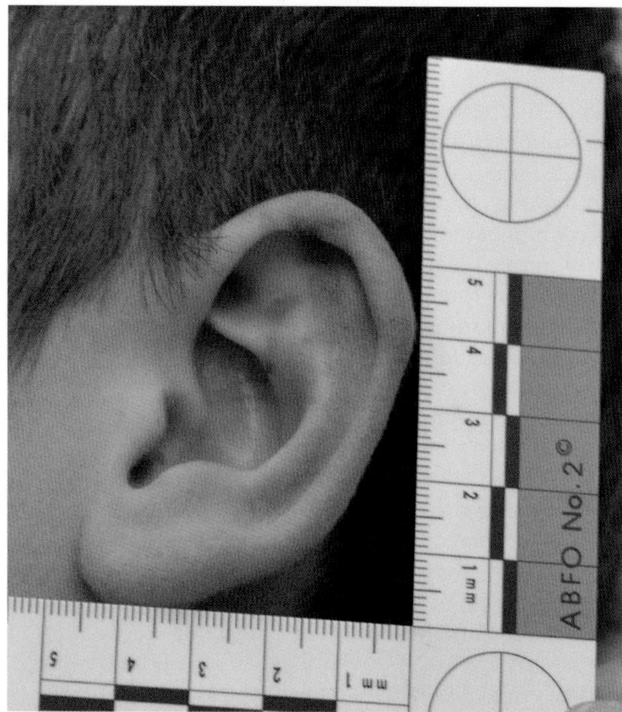

Fig. 164.2 Bruising to left ear caused by slap by right-handed perpetrator.

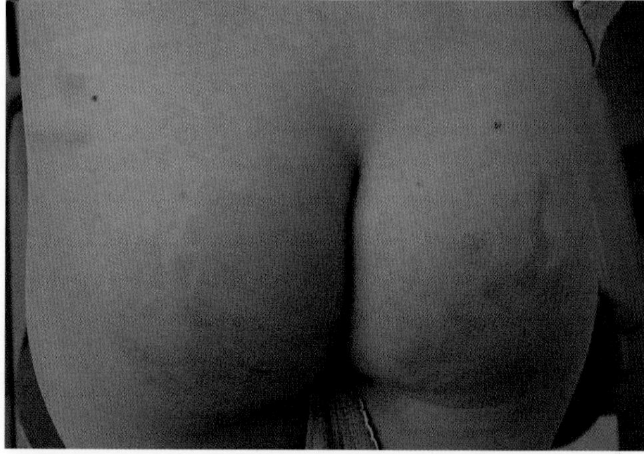

Fig. 164.3 Bruises on buttocks as typically inflicted injuries.

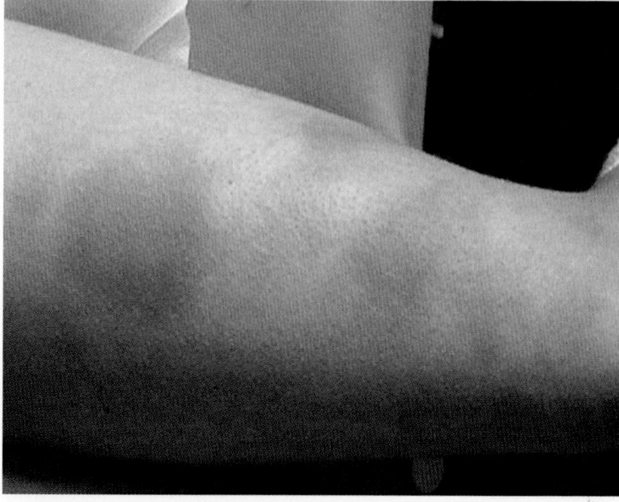

Fig. 164.4 Multiple, large and clustered bruises.

Bruising in children with physical disabilities

Children with disabilities show certain features which differ from the usual bruising characteristics described previously. Accidental bruises also frequently affect the knees but not the chin and shins. In contrast to nondisabled children, bruises are also found on usually suspicious locations such as hands, feet, arms, pelvis, abdomen and upper legs, partially caused by orthopaedic devices. In contrast, lower legs, ears, neck, chin, chest and genitalia are rarely involved in accidents. Depending on the type of disability, an individual determination of type and

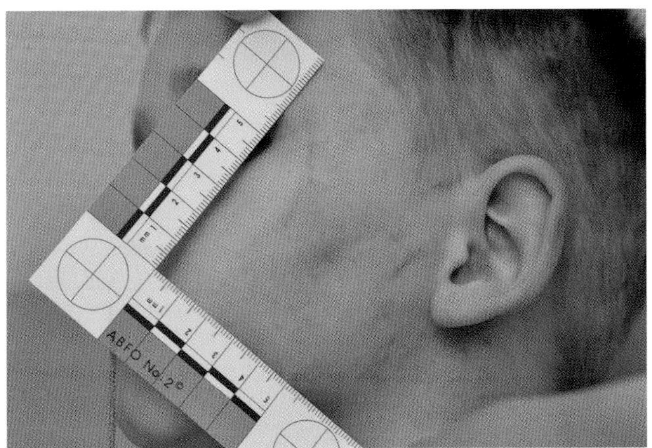

Fig. 164.5 Bruises on left cheek caused by right-handed perpetrator.

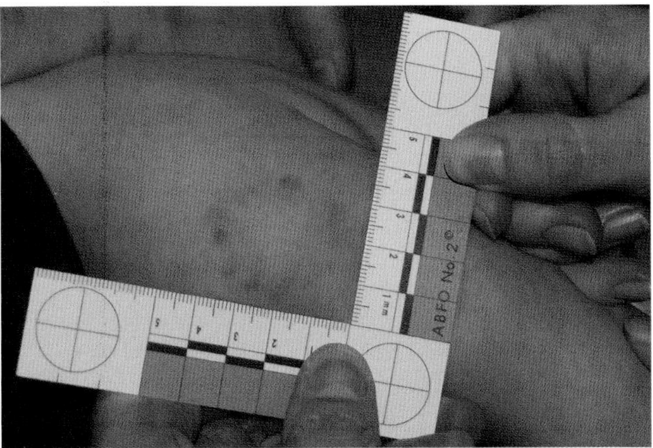

Fig. 164.6 Bite mark.

extent of mobility limitation has to be done in order to assess the plausibility of bruising [9].

Patterned bruises

Injuries inflicted with objects frequently leave a patterned mark that reflects the outline of the object or a hand – typically on the left cheek (except for lefthanders!) (Fig. 164.5). They are almost exclusively associated with abuse and reflect a variety of household or other objects. A stick leaves a typical double-contoured mark with a pale interior part and blood evacuating ruptured vessels forming the outer contour. Typical *bite marks* are a visual diagnosis, characterized by oval-shaped bruises consisting of two opposing half-moon configured arches with central sparing (Fig. 164.6). As a rule of thumb, in adult bites the intercanine distance is greater than 3 cm. Animal bite marks leave characteristic lacerations and puncture wounds, easily differentiated from the contusional bruise character of human bite marks. In fresh bite marks, gentle swabbing with sterile saline may permit recovery of genetic markers from saliva [10,11].

Abusive burns

Characteristics

Burns are regarded as a particularly severe form of child abuse. Due to their high degree of pain and disfiguring scarring, many abusive burns lead to significant physical and psycho-emotional sequelae. Mortality in abusive burns is up to 30%, in contrast to 2% in accidental burns. There are coexisting fractures in 15% of the cases, positive drug screening in urine in 14%, and coexisting injuries of the brain in 10%. Infant skin is almost half as thick as adult skin, reaching adult levels by 5 years of age. Systematic reviews have delineated typical features for a clear distinction between accidental and abusive burns [12,13].

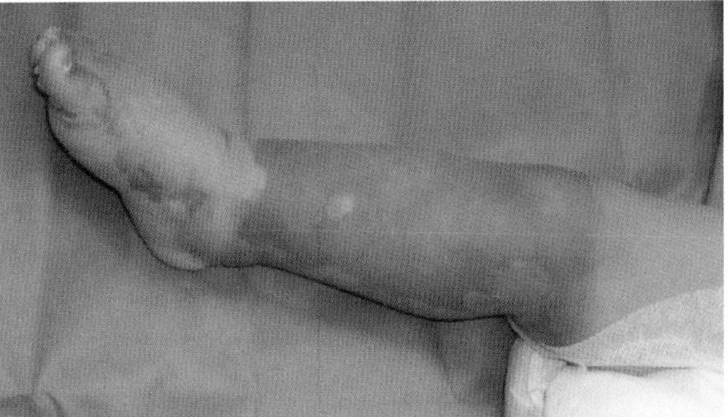

Fig. 164.7 Inflicted immersion burn.

Accidental scald burns

Typically, hot liquids from the kitchen (drinks, boiling cooking water rather than hot tap water) hitting a child from above cause irregular and often asymmetrical splash and drop patterned burns on anterior face, head, neck, anterior shoulder, upper arms and chest, becoming less intense downwards in the direction in which the liquid flows.

Abusive burns

These typically occur by forceful immersion into hot tap water. Typical are isolated immersion burns of the upper or lower extremities or the buttocks, characteristically producing a sharply demarcated, uniform and often symmetrical stocking or glove appearance on the hands, feet, arms, lower legs, trunk or genitalia with an absence of splash marks (Fig. 164.7). Sometimes buttocks, soles of the feet or the flexor creases may be spared. Highly suggestive of abuse are additional child abuse injuries, prior known abuse, domestic violence, a passive, introverted, fearful child, numerous prior accidental injuries, and a sibling blamed for the scald. Suspicious are previous burn injuries, neglect, differing historical accounts, lack of parental concern, triggers such as soiling or enuresis and child known to social services [12].

Abusive contact burns

These are produced by pressing a hot object on the skin, often on the back, shoulders, lower arms, backs of hands and buttocks, producing a typical patterned, often geometrical dry burn, delineating the object used. Inflicted cigarette burns are circular, of uniform size and depth, measuring approximately 8 mm with a range of 7.5–10 mm (Fig. 164.8). Other objects may include hair dryers, curling irons, domestic irons, etc. Accidental contact burns have less clear margins and tend to be more superficial and blurred [14].

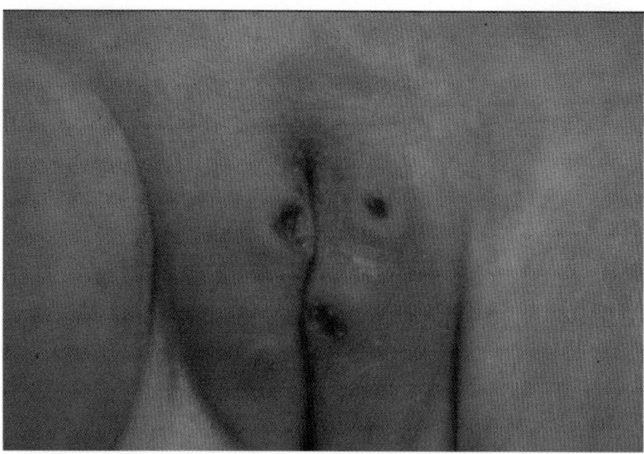

Fig. 164.8 Patterned burns caused by a cigarette.

References

1 Maguire SA, Mann MK, Sibert J, Kemp A. Can you age bruises accurately in children? A systematic review. Arch Dis Child 2005;90:187–9.

2 Bilo RAC, Oranje AP, Shwayder T, Hobbs CJ. Cutaneous Manifestations of Child Abuse and their Differential Diagnosis. Heidelberg: Springer Verlag, 2013.

3 Maguire S, Mann M. Systematic reviews of bruising in relation to child abuse—what have we learnt: an overview of review updates. Evid Based Child Health 2013;8:255–63.

4 Carpenter RE. The prevalence and distribution of bruising in babies. Arch Dis Childhood 1999;80:363–6.

5 Sugar NF, Taylor J, Feldman K. Bruises in infants and toddlers: Those who don't cruise rarely bruise. The Puget Sound Pediatric Research Network. Arch Pediatr Adolesc Med 1999;153:399–403.

6 Nayak K, Spencer N, Shenoy M et al. How useful is the presence of petechiae in distinguishing non-accidental from accidental injury? Child Abuse Negl 2006;30:549–55.

7 Pierce MC, Kaczor K, Aldridge S et al. Bruising characteristics discriminating physical child abuse from accidental trauma. Pediatrics 2010;125:67–74.

8 Harper NS, Feldman KW, Sugar NF et al. for the Examining Siblings to Recognize Abuse Investigators. Additional injuries in young infants with concern for abuse and apparently isolated bruises. J Pediatr 2014;165:383–8.

9 Goldberg AP, Tobin J, Daigneau J et al. Bruising frequency and patterns in children with physical disabilities. Pediatrics 2009;124:604–9.

10 Kemp AM, Maguire S A, Sibert J et al. Can we identify abusive bites on children? Arch Dis Child 2006;91:951.

11 Kemp AM, Jones S, Lawson Z, Maguire SA. Patterns of burns and scalds in children. Arch Dis Child 2015;99:316–21.

12 Maguire SA, Moynihan S, Mann M et al. A systematic review of the features that indicate intentional scalds in children. Burns 2008;34:1072–81.

13 Wibbenmeyer L, Liao J, Heard J et al. Factors related to child maltreatment in children presenting with burn injuries. J Burn Care Res 2014;35:374–81.

14 Kemp AM, Maguire SA, Lumb RC et al. Contact, cigarette and flame burns in physical abuse: a systematic review. Child Abuse Rev 2014;23:35–47.

Skin lesions confused with child abuse

A comprehensive and thoughtful differential diagnosis should be part of any child abuse evaluation. It has great potential to prevent unsubstantiated concerns of child maltreatment and can be looked upon as the essential task of the knowledgeable paediatrician or paediatric dermatologist.

Differential diagnosis of abusive bruises

A frequent area of concern (but not frequently occurring) are underlying disorders of coagulation, sometimes secondary to oncological disease (Fig. 164.9). They may be suspected clinically in some cases, but should be excluded on a routine basis with appropriate laboratory evaluations due to forensic reasons [1]. The most prevalent vasculitic disorder, *Henoch–Schönlein purpura* (HSP) (Fig. 164.9c), typically presents with a palpable rash on the bilateral lower extremities and buttocks but may show atypical presentations in less usual locations or appearance (scrotal haematoma, penile swelling or as haemorrhagic oedema of childhood, see Chapter 145) (Fig. 164.9d). Congenital conditions include haemangiomas and dermal melanosis (*Mongolian spots*; Fig. 164.9e). More commonly seen in children of certain ethnicities (Black, Latino, Asian, Near East, Native American), they can occur in any child and can be located anywhere on the body, including the scalp and not only in the typical lumbosacral and back location. *Disorders of pigmentation* potentially confused with bruises are naevus of Ota/Ito, incontinentia pigmenti, urticaria pigmentosa or mastocytosis. *Connective tissue diseases* such as Ehlers–Danlos syndrome may lead to easy bruising, haematomas, frequent lacerations, poor wound healing and multiple scars. Striae distensae have been confused with linear pattern bruising. Another group of differential diagnoses are *hypersensitivity syndromes* such as erythema multiforme, allergic contact dermatitis, panniculitis, erythema nodosum, perniosis (chilblains) and angioedema. Further concerns might arise from other conditions such as phytophotodermatitis (more commonly needing differentiation from burns), topical application of chemicals, ink or dye and discolouration of skin by clothing. Toe tourniquet syndrome (Fig. 164.10) is mostly seen due to accidental wrapping of a caregiver's hair around a toe (cases affecting the clitoris have also been described) causing strangulation. In single reports, however, it has also been linked to abuse.

The list of dermatological disorders possibly mimicking inflicted burns is quite long and listed in Box 164.1.

References

1 Anderst JD, Carpenter SL, Abshire TC; Section on Hematology/Oncology and Committee on Child Abuse and Neglect of the American Academy of Pediatrics. Evaluation for bleeding disorders in suspected child abuse. Pediatrics 2013;131:e1314–22. Available at: https://pediatrics.aappublications.org/content/131/4/e1314 (accessed 1 March 2019).

2 Makoroff KL, McGraw ML. Skin conditions confused with child abuse. In: Jenny C (ed.) Child Abuse and Neglect: Diagnosis, Treatment and Evidence. St.Louis: Elsevier Saunders, 2011:252–9.

3 Hymel K, Boos S. Conditions mistaken for child physical abuse. In: Reece RM, Christian CW (eds) Child Abuse: Medical Diagnosis and Management, 3rd edn. Elk Grove Village, IL: American Academy of Pediatrics, 2009:227–56.

Fractures in child abuse

In association with a missing plausible history of accidental trauma, multiple fractures, low age (especially under 18 months) and decreasing mobility are factors correlated with an increasing probability of child abuse. Multiple fractures in different stages of healing, metaphyseal fractures, rib fractures and fractures in infants, especially under 4 months of age, are highly suggestive of abuse.

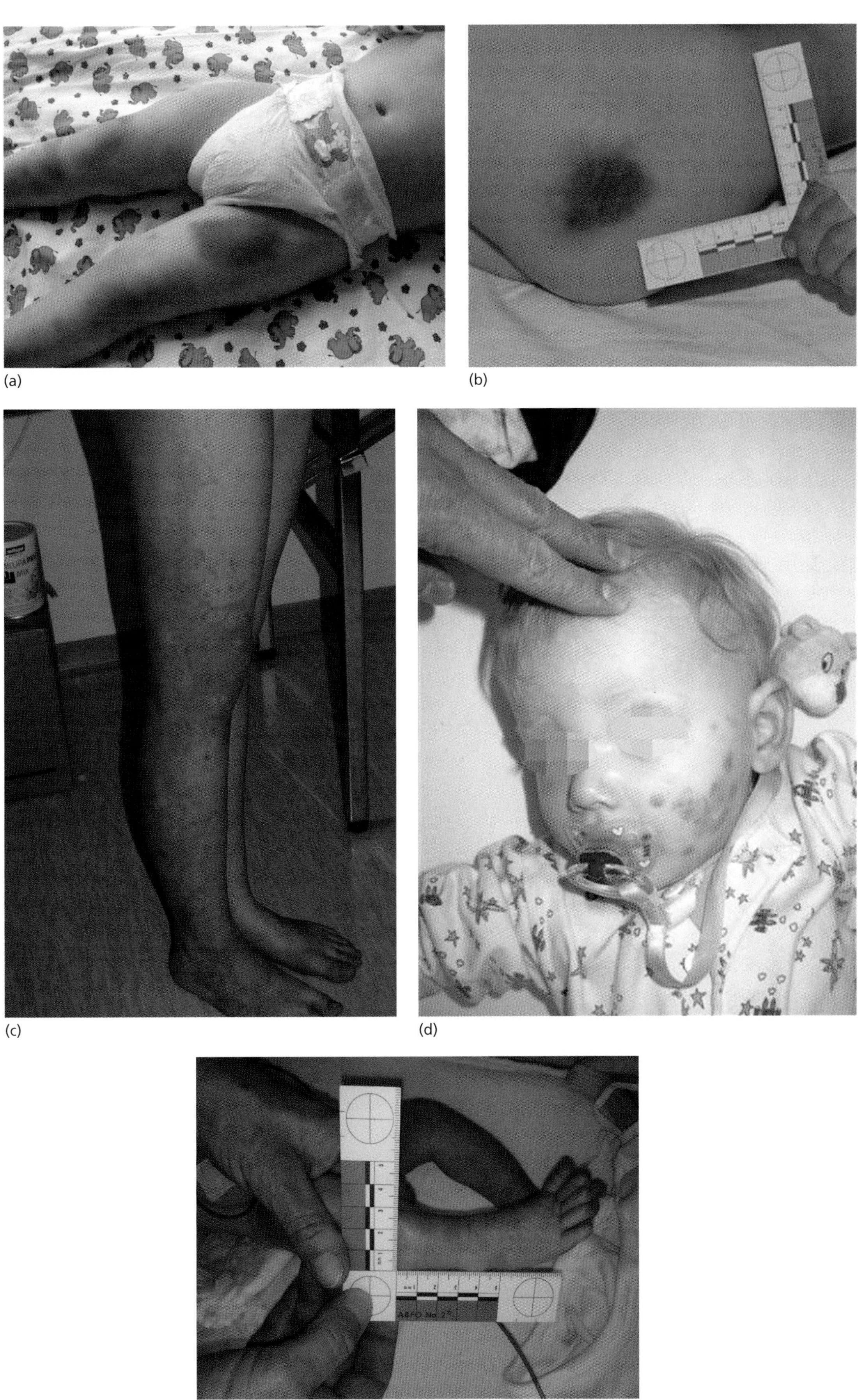

Fig. 164.9 Differential diagnosis of inflicted bruises: (a) idiopathic thrombocytopenic purpura; (b) acute lymphatic leukaemia; (c) Henoch–Schönlein purpura; (d) haemorrhagic oedema of childhood; (e) Mongolian spots.

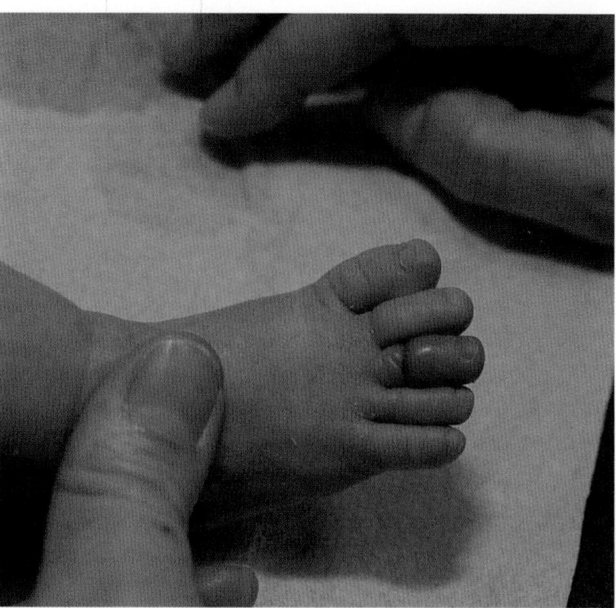

Fig. 164.10 Toe tourniquet syndrome.

Box 164.1 Dermatological conditions that may be mistaken for inflicted burns [2,3]

Dermatitis herpetiformis
Impetigo contagiosa
Ecthyma
Phytophotodermatitis
Drug eruption
Varicella
Guttate psoriasis
Pityriasis lichenoides
Contact dermatitis
Epidermolysis bullosa
Staphylococcal scalded skin syndrome
Stevens–Johnson syndrome
Pyoderma gangrenosum
Herpes zoster or simplex
Pemphigus
Insect bites

Forty percent of abusive fractures are clinically unexpected. There is a considerable coincidence with other manifestations of child abuse. Dating of fractures is imprecise, thus only rough time frames can be given to narrow their time of origin [1,2].

Epidemiology and evidence. Eight to twelve percent of fractures in children, 12–20% in infants and small children, and approximately 55–70% of all fractures in the first year of life are caused by child abuse, mostly in pre-mobile infants. Accidental fractures, however, are only reported in 2% of children under 18 months; 85% occur in children over 5 years of age. More than 50% of abused children with fractures have multiple fractures (three or more). Single accidental fractures occur in 80% and two fractures are found in 19% [3,4].

History. Fractures are severe injuries and require significant force. Falls from a napkin changing table (85–100 cm), sofas and beds have been reported to cause usually simple parietal fractures in 3–5% of cases, but very rarely lead to significant intracranial trauma (less than 1% in uncomplicated, small subdural haematomas –extremely rare incidents of fatal epidural haematomas). Fractures caused by spontaneous turning or by getting stuck in the bars of a cot have not been documented so far.

Metaphyseal fractures. (CML, classic metaphyseal lesion) as a result of accidental trauma have only been reported sporadically. They typically occur as a result of torsional and shearing strains on the metaphysis by pulling or twisting an extremity or by shaking. They are highly suggestive of abuse. Although depicted as a 'corner fracture' (or sometimes 'bucket handle fracture') radiologically, they do not represent an avulsion at the site of periosteal attachment as was previously thought, but rather a complete series of microfractures abutting the physis.

Periosteal reaction or subperiosteal new bone formation (SPNBF). without fracture of the bone reflects calcified subperiosteal haemorrhages caused by shaking, twisting or grabbing.

Spiral fractures. per se do not reflect a higher probability of abuse as was originally thought.

Skull fractures. are more commonly reported in accidents. Multiple, complex, diastatic fractures that cross sutures raise a higher index of suspicion, as they reflect higher forces.

Rib fractures. have the highest specificity and are due to abuse in 70% in the first and in 30% in the second year of life. Under 18 months, the positive predictive value (PPV) of rib fractures is 66%, the odds ratio (OR) 23.7. Rib fractures almost never occur as a result of cardiopulmonary resuscitation. Accidental rib fractures are rare and require significant forces such as severe motor vehicle accidents.

Humerus fractures. in a child under 18 months are significantly associated with abuse (P <0.001, PPV 43.8%, OR 2.3); the humerus is one of the most commonly affected bones.

Fractures of radius/ulna. are common injuries in childhood, but rarely occur in infants. Under 18 months they are suggestive of abuse (P <0.001).

Femur fractures: in a child under 18 months the PPV is 51.1%, OR 1.8. Sixty percent of these fractures in infants under 12 months are due to abuse.

Fractures of tibia and fibula. in child abuse are mostly diagnosed as distal metaphyseal fracture: OR (<18 months) 12.8, P <0.001. More than 50% of tibia fractures in infants are due to abuse [3–7].

Differential diagnosis. The most frequently considered differential diagnosis of child abuse fractures are true accidents. When children begin to ambulate, accidental (and occasionally unwitnessed) subtle spiral or oblique fractures of the tibia may occur from seemingly innocent trauma, called 'toddler's fracture'. A similar mechanism has been described for femur fractures. A broad spectrum of bone disorders has to be considered, with the often quoted osteogenesis imperfecta being rare. Taking into account all historical, radiographic and clinical information, the potential for a misdiagnosis is low. Subclinical hypovitaminosis D does not increase fracture rate [8].

References

1 Prosser I, Lawson Z, Evans A et al. A timetable for the radiologic features of fracture healing in young children. AJR 2012;198:1014–20.

2 Flaherty EG, Perez-Rossello JM, Levine MA, Hennrikus WL; American Academy of Pediatrics Committee on Child Abuse and Neglect; Section on Radiology, American Academy of Pediatrics; Section on Endocrinology, American Academy of Pediatrics; Section on Orthopaedics, American Academy of Pediatrics; Society for Pediatric Radiology. Evaluating children with fractures for child physical abuse. Pediatrics 2014;133:e47789. Available at: https://pediatrics.aappublications.org/content/133/2/e477 (accessed 1 March 2019).

3 Kemp AM, Dunstan F, Harrison S et al. Patterns of skeletal fractures in child abuse: systematic review. BMJ 2008;337: a1518.

4 Maguire S, Cowley L, Mann M, Kemp A. What does the recent literature add to the identification and investigation of fractures in child abuse: an overview of review updates 2005–2013. Evid Based Child Health 2013;8:2044–57.

5 Pierce MC, Bertocci GE, Janosky JE et al. Femur fractures resulting from stair falls among children: An injury plausibility model. Pediatrics 2005;115:1712–22.

6 Pandya NK, Baldwin KD, Wolfgruber H et al. Humerus fractures in the pediatric population: An algorithm to identify abuse. J Pediatr Orthopaed 2010;B19:535–41.

7 Kleinman P, Perez-Rossello JM, Newton AW et al. Prevalence of the classic metaphyseal lesion in infants at low versus high risk for abuse. AJR 2011;197:1005–8.

8 Schilling S, Wood JN, Levine MA et al. Vitamin D status in abused and nonabused children younger than 2 years old with fractures. Pediatrics 2011;127:835–41.

Injuries to the face, ear, nose and throat region

Of abused children, 65–75% have injuries of the face, neck, ear or inside of the mouth. External injuries and bruises of the cheeks (often patterned and containing petechiae) and of the ears due to slapping are most frequent. Both are more common on the left side (except for left-handed perpetrators!). Intraoral injuries such as mucosal lacerations, contusions of the inner part of the lips or gingiva and tears of labial or lingual frenulum are easily overlooked. According to systematic reviews, the latter are not per se diagnostic for abuse, but highly suspicious in infants. The only mechanism of injury recorded in the literature was a direct blow to the mouth. The most common recorded injury was laceration or bruising to the lip [1,2].

The teeth. may be affected by direct force or dental neglect. Direct blows can result in dental fractures leading to discolouration. Dental impressions into the maxilla may result from an accidental fall or abusive forceful intrusion of feeding devices. Dental extrusions by yanking out objects such as a pacifier are mostly abusive.

Dental neglect. as a variant of general physical neglect is characterized by caries in all studies, many of which were 'nursing bottle caries' or extensive early caries. Dental pain was an additional feature. Many children require extractions for dental caries, which included conditions that were painful or carried a risk of infection. Parental features are failure or delay in seeking dental treatment, failure to follow the dental advice given, and failure to provide basic oral care. It is not possible to define a precise threshold for dental neglect based on caries alone. However, a child who is experiencing pain, discomfort, social embarrassment or medical complications as a consequence of caries should be appropriately treated [3].

References

1 Maguire SA, Hunter B, Hunter LM et al. Diagnosing abuse: A systematic review of torn frenum and intra-oral injuries. Arch Dis Child 2007;92:1113–17. Erratum in Archives of Disease in Childhood. 2008;93(5):453.

2 Fisher-Owens SA, Lukefahr JA, Tate AR; American Academy of Pediatrics, Section on Oral Health, Committee on Child Abuse and Neglect; American Academy of Pediatric Dentistry, Council on Clinical Affairs, Council on Scientific Affairs; ad hoc Work Group on Child Abuse and Neglect. Oral and dental aspects of child abuse and neglect. Pediatrics 2017;140:e20171487. Available at: https://pediatrics.aappublications.org/content/140/2/e20171487 (accessed 1 March 2019).

3 Bhatia SK, Maguire SA, Chadwick BL et al. Characteristics of child dental neglect: A systematic review. J Dent 2014;42:229–39.

Abusive head trauma (AHT)

Abusive head injuries have the highest morbidity and mortality of all abuse injuries (66–75% of all child abuse fatalities; mortality 11–33%). They usually result from situations of intense frustration and anger of caregivers, mostly triggered by extensive crying of infants. Children younger than 1 year (mostly 2–5 months), male infants, children with regulation and bonding disorders, children in families with stressful and difficult circumstances, and children of young single mothers are at highest risk. The incidence ranges from 14 to 30 cases per 100 000 children during the first 2 years of life, and 36 per 100 000 in children under 6 months. Shaking is the most prevalent, but not the only, mechanism. Historical terms such as 'shaken baby syndrome' and others such as 'non-accidental head injury' (NAHI) have recently been replaced by 'abusive head trauma' (AHT). AHT with significant consecutive morbidity requires violent and forceful shaking of a child being held at the arms or chest. Perpetrator admissions confirm that shaking is commonly very violent and that symptoms occur immediately [1,2].

Diagnosis. AHT is a syndromic diagnosis, putting together historical, clinical, radiographic, ophthalmological and other pieces of information. The more components fit into the diagnosis, the less plausible are alternative diseases. Isolated findings such as retinal haemorrhages (RH) are not diagnostic. Characteristic features are traumatic encephalopathy with subdural haematomas (SDH) (77–90%), mostly extensive RH (74–92%) and frequently significant brain injury with an unfavourable outcome. Typical are missing or subtle external signs of trauma. A completely missing history in patients with traumatic brain injury has a 97% specificity and a 92% PPV for abuse [3,4].

AHT does not follow an all-or-nothing principle but is rather a continuum from mild, subclinical injury through severe impairment to death. In mild cases, symptoms may be nonspecific and lead to a misdiagnosis of irritability, gastrointestinal, viral or blood stream infection, apparent life-threatening event, etc. In one study, 31.2% of 173 children with AHT had been overlooked by physicians. Until the correct diagnosis was established, 27.8% were reinjured, with 40.7% experiencing medical complications. Four out of five deaths might have been prevented by earlier diagnosis [5]. Of anonymously questioned parents, 2.6–5.6% reported shaking their children at least once without seeking medical care. There are assumptions that a significant percentage of unclear neurological disabilities in children may thus be explained by AHT [6].

Evidence. SDH without a plausible accidental origin are strongly correlated with abuse (OR 9.18, $P < 0.00001$); in interhemispheric SDH the OR is 8.03 and in multiple SDH 6.01. In a child less than 3 years of age with intracranial injury and apnoea, the PPV is 93% (95% confidence interval [CI] 73–99%) and the odds ratio 17.1 (95%CI 5–58, $P < 0.001$). The combination with RH has a PPV of 71% (OR 3.5) and the combination with rib fractures (RF) has a PPV of 73% (OR 3). If RF or RH are combined with any of six factors (apnoea, RF, RH, long bone fractures, seizures, bruises in the head or neck region), the OR is >100, PPV >85%. Any combination of three or more findings was also calculated to have an OR of >100 and a PPV >85% [3,4]. Clinical decision rules use the four factors apnoea, haematomas of the head and neck region, bilateral or interhemispheric SDH, and any skull fracture that is not unilateral, parietal and isolated. Sensitivity was 96%, specificity 46%, PPV 55% and negative predictive value 93%, making it an especially helpful tool in screening out children where AHT is unlikely [7].

Symptoms and findings. Loss of appetite, poor feeding, inconsolability, irritability, lethargy, vomiting, muscular hypotonia, seizures, breathing difficulties, apnoea, unresponsiveness, coma and cardiorespiratory compromise are possible symptoms. External injuries are frequently missing, the exceptions are bruising of upper arms or chest and bruising of the scalp in shake impact. Findings are intracranial haemorrhages, mainly SDH (77–90%), occasionally skull fractures (in shake impact), RF (from chest compression), metaphyseal fractures (rotational trauma by shaking), RH (74–92%), vitreous haemorrhages, retinoschisis and haemorrhages of the optic nerve. RH are predominantly bilateral, but in 15% are unilateral and extensive (frequently too numerous to count), extending to the periphery and affecting pre-, intra-, and subretinal layers [8,9].

Pathophysiology and timing. Rotational and shearing forces cause tearing of bridging veins (leading to SDH) and retinal vessels (leading to RH). SDH and RH are clinical indicators, but insignificant for brain damage and outcome. An acute, significant and severe AHT is characterized by diffuse brain injury, which inevitably leads to acute neurological symptoms, apparently also recognizable to parents. Victims of moderate to severe AHT become rapidly, clearly and persistently ill [10]. Precise documentation of onset of symptoms has a higher degree of significance for timing than the rather imprecise MRI dating [10]. The mechanisms of brain damage are complex. Current understanding is that a combination of local and diffuse neuronal damage and traumatic apnoea caused by axonal injury in the cervicomedullary junction causes brain injury by complex neurometabolic cascades, vascular dysregulation and secondary inflammatory reactions, resulting in cerebral oedema and neuronal damage [11,12].

Diagnostic evaluation. In the acute setting, the cCT is the preferred imaging modality, especially in the critically ill child. Due to significantly higher sensitivity, MRI should follow promptly when the child is stable and after 2–3 months. Cerebral ultrasonography is not recommended for exclusion of the often rather subtle SDH. A complete eye examination and indirect ophthalmoscopy should be performed by an experienced ophthalmologist. A skeletal survey is mandatory in all children under 2 years.

Differential diagnosis.

Retinal haemorrhages. These are rare and commonly of lesser severity in accidents, disorders of coagulation, glutaric aciduria type 1, vascular disease, leukaemia, osteogenesis imperfecta, carbon monoxide intoxication, severe hypertension, severe meningitis and encephalitis, as well as cytomegalovirus retinitis. Birth-related RH affect 21–40% of all newborns; the vast majority disappear after 1–2 weeks.

Subdural hematomas. These are almost exclusively traumatic. Trivial falls (<1.2–1.5 m) result in uncomplicated, small SDH in <1% without neurological impairment. Clinically silent birth-related SDH occur in up to 25% and generally disappear after 4 weeks. Other differential diagnoses include disorders of coagulation (almost never SDH or RH as sole and leading symptom), late neonatal vitamin K deficiency haemorrhage, herpes virus encephalitis and glutaric aciduria type 1.

Outcome. Roughly one third of victims have severe neurological impairment, disruption of visual ability, hearing and speech, seizures, mental retardation and cerebral paralysis; 11–33% of victims die. Imaging shows brain atrophy, chronic SDH, subdural hygromas, microcephaly, multicystic encephalopathy and porencephaly. One third have moderate impairment, one third little or no impairment and only 15% are asymptomatic.

Even an uneventful early course may be followed by late consequences such as cognitive or behavioural disturbances, perceptual disorders, late seizures and hypopituitarism [13,14].

References

1 Adamsbaum C, Grabar S, Mejean N, Rey-Salmon C. Abusive head trauma: Judicial admissions highlight violent and repetitive shaking. Pediatrics 2010;126:546–55.

2 Christian CW, Block R; Committee on Child Abuse and Neglect; American Academy of Pediatrics. Abusive head trauma in infants and children. Pediatrics 2009;123:1409–11. Available at: https://pediatrics.aappublications.org/content/123/5/1409.long (accessed 1 March 2019).

3 Maguire S, Pickerd N, Farewell D et al. Which clinical features distinguish inflicted from non-inflicted brain injury? A systematic review. Arch Dis Child 2009;94:860–7.

4 Maguire SA, Kemp AM, Lumb RC, Farewell DM. Estimating the probability of abusive head trauma: a pooled analysis. Pediatrics 2011;128:e550–64.

5 Jenny C, Hymel KP, Ritzen A et al. Analysis of missed cases of abusive head trauma. JAMA 1999;281:621–6.

6 Greeley CS. Abusive head trauma: A review of the evidence base. Am J Radiol 2015;204:967–73.

7 Hymel KP, Armijo-Garcia V, Foster R et al. Validation of a clinical prediction rule for pediatric abusive head trauma. Pediatrics 2014;134:e1537–44.

8 Levin AV. Retinal hemorrhage in abusive head trauma. Pediatrics 2010;126:961–70.

9 Maguire SA, Watts PO, Shaw AD et al. Retinal haemorrhages and related findings in abusive and non-abusive head trauma: A systematic review. Eye 2013;27:28–36.

10 Adamsbaum C, Morel B, Ducot B et al. Dating the abusive head trauma episode and perpetrator statements: key points for imaging. Pediatr Radiol 2014;44(suppl 4): 578–88.

11 Kochanek PM, Berger RP, Gilles EE, Adelson PD. Biochemical, metabolic, and molecular responses in the brain after inflicted childhood neurotrauma. In: Reece RM, Nicholson CE (eds) Inflicted Childhood Neurotrauma. Elk Grove Village, IL: American Academy of Pediatrics, 2003:191–220.

12 Matschke J, Büttner A, Bergmann M et al. Encephalopathy and death in infants with abusive head trauma is due to hypoxic-ischemic injury following local brain trauma to vital brainstem centers. Int J Legal Med 2015;129:105–14.

13 Barlow KM, Thomson E, Johnson D, Minns RA. Late neurologic and cognitive sequelae of inflicted traumatic brain injury in infancy. Pediatrics 2005;116:e174–85.

14 Kaulfers A-M D, Backeljauw PF, Reifschneider K et al. Endocrine dysfunction following traumatic brain injury in children. J Pediatr 2010;157:894–9.

Abdominal trauma

After head injury, abdominal injuries are the second leading cause of death in child abuse. The mortality rate in abuse is 45–53%, whereas accidents have rates as low as 2–21%. Reasons for the high mortality are frequently delayed presentations with flawed history, generally missing external signs contrasting with significant visceral trauma and therefore delay in considering abdominal trauma in the medical setting. More than 90% of accident victims present within 3 hours whereas in 100% of abuse cases it is more than 3 hours. Anatomical reasons for severe injury include the relatively small abdomen of children with proportionately larger organs which lie close together and are less protected by the less developed abdominal wall musculature. Small children tend to have a higher degree of intraintestinal air due to more frequent crying, making them more susceptible to hollow organ perforation. Abuse victims are significantly younger (2.5 versus 7.7 years) and frequently show other signs of abuse [1,2].

Trauma is commonly caused by blunt force, punches or kicks, leading to contusions or lacerations of solid organs. In half of the cases perforations of hollow organs and intramural haematomas (mostly duodenum and proximal jejunum) occur, which are extremely rare in accidents. Liver lacerations (mostly left lobe) are the most common solid organ injuries. Pancreatic injuries are less common, often in conjunction with liver and duodenal injury; urinary tract and kidney injuries also occur. Marked elevations of liver enzymes (aspartate aminotransferase >450 U/L, alanine aminotransferase >250 U/L) are valid indicators of hepatic trauma [3], and urine should be screened for haematuria. Ultrasonography may depict intra-abdominal blood but is contraindicated as the sole imaging modality. Abdominal CT with double contrast is the method of choice; an alternative is MRI.

References

1 Barnes PM, Norton CM, Dunstan FD et al. Abdominal injury due to child abuse. Lancet 2005;366:234–5.

2 Maguire SA, Upadhyaya M, Evans A et al. A systematic review of abusive visceral injuries in childhood – their range and recognition. Child Abuse Negl 2013;37:430–45.

3 Lindberg DM, Shapiro RA, Blood EA et al.; ExSTRA investigators. Utility of hepatic transaminases in children with concern for abuse. Pediatrics 2013;131:268–75.

Child sexual abuse

Definition, background and general considerations

Child sexual abuse (CSA) is a serious health problem. Medical providers may get involved to interpret certain skin findings thought to be concerning for abuse, especially when these coincide with behavioural or mental health problems. Performing a comprehensive examination requires specialized training. In selected cases, the expertise of a paediatric dermatologist may be helpful to differentiate skin conditions not related to abuse and alleviate diagnostic insecurity and unjustified, stressful suspicions and procedures.

The vast majority (>90%) of sexually abused children and adolescents have no physical evidence, predominantly because widespread intrafamilial abuse (or by close, well-known individuals) tends to be physically less invasive. Findings are absent or may have healed completely when the examination is performed. Therefore the medical examination infrequently has a diagnostic or forensic purpose except for rare cases of acute assault. Nevertheless, the medical reassurance of physical normality and integrity has the potential to promote and support emotional recovery. The medical examination has the purpose of detecting abnormality as well as determining and reassuring normality and is first and foremost the provision of medical care.

The World Health Organization (WHO) defines CSA as 'the involvement of a child in sexual activity that he or she does not fully comprehend and is unable to give informed consent to, or for which the child is not developmentally prepared, or else that violate the laws or social taboos of society' [1].

Child sexual abuse (CSA) involves a wide spectrum of different sexual acts committed by adults on children or adolescents, from noninvasive acts ('hands off') to more or less invasive acts such as fondling ('hands on') to invasive, forceful penetration. More typical is a chronic sexualized relationship, mostly between close and well-known caregivers or other individuals and the victim. Strangers as offenders make up approximately 10% of all cases, more often accounting for single events, more accurately labelled as 'sexual assault' or 'rape'. Abuse may start in early childhood and continue into adolescence. Most cases of CSA are committed by men (approximately 90%), with higher numbers of female perpetrators when boys are victimized (up to 25%). At least 20–25% of perpetrators are juveniles, underscoring the importance of early intervention, including perpetrator treatment. Approximately 20% of adolescent internet users become victims of online sexual harassment. Current research and large systematic reviews indicate a global and worldwide prevalence of 12.7% (18–20% in girls and 7–8% in boys). Being within the percent range, CSA is far more prevalent than all malignancies in childhood (0.2%), juvenile diabetes (0.15%) and congenital heart disease (0.1%) combined [2–4]. In the 2014 report *Child Maltreatment* by the US Department of Health and Human Services, 8.3% of 702 000 substantiated victims of all child abuse and neglect were sexually abused [5].

For the victims, CSA is mostly frightening, emotionally and sexually confusing, and occasionally physically abusive and painful. Being sexually abused often creates profound feelings of guilt and shame and may lead to low self-esteem and familial and social isolation. CSA is associated with a marked increase in subsequent psychopathology, although long-term outcomes span from severe to asymptomatic (approximately 20%). Abuse varies significantly in severity and extent, the amount of physical force used, the relationship with the offender, and frequency and duration. Additional factors influencing outcome are the age of the child, pre-existing adverse psychosocial problems, coexisting physical abuse, or neglect in terms of additional vulnerability. The effects of professional intervention may be supportive or additionally traumatizing, if not performed in a gentle, noncoercive, professional and well-conceived manner. The outcome may also be modified and potentially at least partially compensated for by resilience factors, defined as an individual's ability to properly adapt to stress and adversity by intra- or extrafamilial support. A variety of reports have highlighted mental health problems (i.e. depression, suicide, multiple personality disorders, post-traumatic stress disorder, eating disorders, anxiety disorders, substance abuse), physical health problems (i.e. functional gastrointestinal disorders, chronic pelvic pain, dysmenorrhoea) and psychosexual dysfunction (i.e. excessive promiscuity, adolescent pregnancy, re-victimization, prostitution). Interpersonal close relationships may be difficult for CSA victims [6].

References

1 **World Health Organization. Guidelines for medico-legal care for victims of sexual violence. Geneva: WHO, updated 2003. Available from: www.who.int/violence_injury_prevention/publications/violence/med_leg_guidelines/en/ (accessed 21 February 2019).**

2 Pereda N, Guilerab G, Fornsa M, Gómez-Benito J. The international epidemiology of child sexual abuse: A continuation of Finkelhor (1994). Child Abuse Negl 2009;33:331–42.

3 Stoltenborgh M, van Ijzendoorn MH, Euser EM, Bakermans-Kranenburg MJ. A global perspective on child sexual abuse: Meta-analysis of prevalence around the world. Child Maltreat 2011;16:79–101.

4 Kaplan R, Adams JA, Starling SP, Giardino AP. Medical Response to Child Sexual Abuse. A Resource for Professionals Working with Children and Families. St Louis: STM Learning, 2011.

5 U.S. Department of Health & Human Services, Children's Bureau. Child Maltreatment 2014. Available at: www.acf.hhs.gov/cb/resource/child-maltreatment-2014 (accessed 21 February 2019).

6 Herrmann B, Navratil F. Sexual abuse in prepubertal children and adolescents. Endocr Dev 2012;22:112–37.

Medical aspects – potential and limitations

The paediatric and adolescent and forensic examination shows no physical evidence in the vast majority of victims (90–95%) – 'It's normal to be normal' [1]. Consequently the examination rarely serves for diagnostic or forensic purposes. The diagnosis mainly rests on history, gathered in a professional and nonsuggestive way. Rarely, in cases of acute assault, examination may provide evidence for diagnosis. In the majority of cases, however, abuse is of a physically lesser or noninvasive nature (which does not preclude significant emotional damage), not involving sufficient physical contact to produce physical sequelae. Additionally, victims mostly present at a long time interval after the last episode of abuse has occurred, when potential injuries have completely healed. Anogenital tissues furthermore have an enormous potential for rapid and complete healing, also contributing to the scarcity of findings. It is of utmost importance for medical providers to be aware of the conclusion that the absence of physical evidence is no evidence of the absence of abuse and to communicate this to all professionals caring for sexually abused children and adolescents [2].

Furthermore, most children do not have sufficient knowledge of their anatomy to describe appropriately what exactly has occurred. They may interpret any diffuse pain in the anogenital area as invasive or penetrative ('He stabbed a knife in my pipi!'). It is unknown at which age children are able to differentiate 'on' from 'in'. In addition, the medical understanding of 'penetration' is the penetration of an object beyond the hymenal membrane into the vagina; legally, however, it is viewed as even slight penetration between the labia majora. Finally, the outcome and traumatizing nature of child sexual abuse is not primarily affected by whether penetration has occurred or medical signs of trauma are evident. Another variable influencing the frequency of findings is the extent of professional qualification and training of the examiner and his or her capability and readiness to examine and interpret correctly. The risk of false positive findings seems to be greater in less well qualified examiners. Finally, organizational variables such as adequate and thoughtful preparation of the child, providing enough time, and the availability of technical aids (mainly a colposcope) may influence the outcome of an examination [3,4].

In selected cases a medical examination may aid in diagnosing CSA, treating associated injuries or infections or preventing the possibility of acquiring sexually transmitted infections (STI) or pregnancy (post exposure prophylaxis). Possibly an even greater opportunity to promote recovery after CSA is addressing concerns of physical abnormality in abused children and adolescents. The physician, as a known 'specialist for the body', has great potential to reassure children's normality and integrity after CSA and to integrate therapeutic messages into the procedure. The evaluation of the possibly sexually abused child is first and foremost the provision of medical care. Nonmedical professionals may misconceive the medical examination as inevitably intrusive and distressing for children, potentially causing 're-victimization'. On the other hand, they may misapprehend the potential of the examination to prove or exclude abuse by focusing on the integrity of the hymen. This underscores the need for thorough interprofessional communication and cooperation. The best outcome for a patient focuses on meeting the medical, mental health and protection needs of the child and the family. All children who are suspected victims of CSA should be offered an examination performed by a medical provider with specialized training in sexual abuse evaluation [5].

References

1 Adams JA, Harper K, Knudson S, Revilla J. Examination findings in legally confirmed child sexual abuse: it's normal to be normal. Pediatrics 1994;94:310–17.

2 Kaplan R, Adams JA, Starling SP, Giardino AP. Medical Response to Child Sexual Abuse. A Resource for Professionals Working with Children and Families. St. Louis: STM Learning, 2011.

3 Gallion HR, Milam LJ, Littrell LL. Genital findings in cases of child sexual abuse: genital vs vaginal penetration. J Pediatr Adolesc Gynecol 2016;29:604–11.

4 Herrmann B, Dettmeyer R, Banaschak S, Thyen U. Kindesmisshandlung. Medizinische Diagnostik, Intervention und rechtliche Grundlagen, 3rd revised edn. Heidelberg: Springer, 2016.

5 Finkel MA. Medical evaluation of an alleged childhood sexual abuse victim. In: Kaplan R, Adams JA, Starling SP, Giardino AP (eds) Medical Response to Child Sexual Abuse. A Resource for Professionals Working with Children and Families. St. Louis: STM Learning, 2011:41–57.

History and examination in child sexual abuse

When taking a history and performing a medical examination, it is crucial that the needs of the child have absolute priority over the desire to obtain forensic evidence. An essential prerequisite of examining possibly abused children in a nontraumatizing manner is to avoid any force or coercion.

The context of a patient's presentation may comprise perceived physical (mostly anogenital) abnormalities, mental and behavioural disorders, specific statements and rarely overt sexual assault. Anticipating and addressing children's fears concerning the medical examination are crucial for a successful examination. An essential prerequisite of examining possibly abused children is to avoid any force or coercion. A friendly and open attitude of the examiner and a gentle, objective and accepting atmosphere are important factors for making the examination a positive and beneficial experience. The experience of specialized child protection centres and a number of reports indicate that well-documented examinations help to avoid repeated examinations, and thereby may prevent further potential trauma. The emotional response to the medical examination is probably not only influenced by factors inherent to the examination situation itself, but also by many other variables, such as pre-existing factors (e.g. general anxiety, previous experiences with the medical system, the age and developmental status of the child) and on the other hand the characteristics and severity of the abuse. Several studies with small samples and the impression of experienced experts in the field indicate that most children seem to cope well with the examination [1].

History

History taking should avoid further trauma to the child and still gain a maximum of information. Depending on the extent of previous historical evaluations, it may not always be necessary to repeat questioning on all details of the abuse, which could be difficult or embarrassing for the child. In some cases, however, information on the specific details of what has happened may contribute to interpreting physical signs in the light of history. Recent research indicates that statements by a child may be promoted by the relationship of trust to the physician ('I can tell you, because you are a doctor…'). Paediatricians in particular have abundant experience in talking to children in difficult health situations. It is advisable to take a separate history from the child and the caregiver if possible. History taking includes emotional and mental status, behavioural symptoms, social situation, previously involved agencies, past medical history, review of systems, paediatric gynaecology issues and information about the abuse and current complaints (i.e. dysuria might point to recent fondling in the periurethral or vulvar area) [2,3].

Questions directed at the child should be simple, non-leading and not suggestive of the answer. Scrupulous and verbatim documentation is crucial for further court proceedings and the credibility of the child. In selected cases, children may disclose sexual abuse during the medical examination, for instance if they are asked if someone has ever touched them 'in this area' while the anogenital examination is performed. Taking history may also aid in assessing concerns, fears and the degree of self-blame related to the abuse, the latter being highly associated with emotional trauma symptoms. If sexual abuse already has been openly discussed, it can be addressed during the medical evaluation by integrating therapeutic messages in the procedure: 'It was good to tell', 'It is not children's fault when these things happen', 'I know more kids to whom this has happened, you are not the only one!' [4].

Medical examination

Recently published, revised and peer-reviewed guidelines on the evaluation of possibly abused children and adolescents have stressed the importance of urgency in prioritizing the medical evaluation as emergency, urgent or nonurgent, mainly depending on the amount of time since the last episode of abuse [5]. Most children present weeks, months or years after an abusive episode and it is important to differentiate the subjective emotional distress of caregivers or agencies caused by an acute disclosure from medical necessity. In most cases, the examination can and should be scheduled according to the needs of the child as well as those of the examining institution, potentially avoiding confronting a frightened child with an untrained (and maybe also frightened) examiner in the emergency department in the middle of the night. Reasons for emergency examinations are medical, psychological or safety concerns such as acute pain or bleeding, suicidal ideation, suspected human trafficking, or a recent assault within 24 hours in prepubertal children and 72 hours in adolescents with the necessity to collect forensic evidence, need for emergency contraception or post-exposure prophylaxis for STI or HIV. Follow-up evaluations should be considered if the examination was performed by an inexperienced examiner, when findings on the initial examination are unclear or questionable, for further testing for STI and for documentation of healing or resolution of acute findings [5,6]. The most recent revision of the so-called Adams Guidelines evolved into a new organization of classifying findings. Listed are three sections (physical findings, infections and findings diagnostic of sexual contact), each section again differentiated according to the probability and evidence for CSA [7].

Anticipating and addressing children's fears concerning the medical examination are crucial for a successful examination. Younger children rarely have problems with issues of shame. They are rather fearful of painful and unknown procedures. Any form of force or coercion is strictly contraindicated. The child should be given as much choice as possible in the procedure to ensure a sense of control. It is important to explain all steps of the examination in age-appropriate terminology. The child should be reassured that the purpose of the examination is to check if everything is 'alright', that it is healthy and 'okay'. Clinical experience indicates that at least for prepubertal children, the style and gentleness of the examination are far more important factors in the emotional impact than the gender of the examiner [8].

A complete head-to-toe examination is mandatory even for non-paediatricians to prevent focusing exclusively on the anogenital region. The anogenital examination in cases of suspected sexual abuse of the prepubertal child is principally an external visualization by varying techniques of separation, traction and positioning. It does not require anal or vaginal palpation or the use of specula, which in adolescents may be appropriate but usually not mandatory. The combination of the standard techniques (separation, labial traction and knee–chest position) significantly enhances the probability of perceiving findings and it is mandatory for a diagnosis of abuse according to recent guidelines. Including a colposcope for visualizing and documenting findings has become 'standard of care' and combines an excellent lighting source, optimal magnification and high-quality documentation (Fig. 164.11).

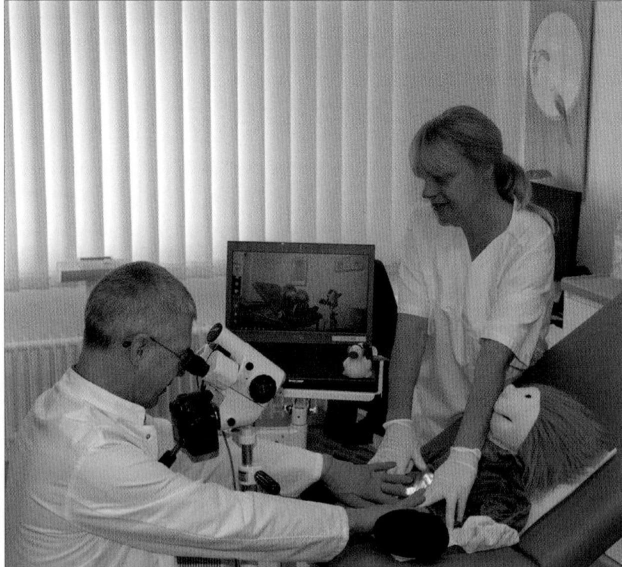

Fig. 164.11 Examination setting with colposcope and digital documentation.

This enables peer review (also required for a diagnosis of abuse), teaching and research, and prevents the necessity of repeat examinations.

References

1 **Jenny C, Crawford-Jakubiak JE; Committee on Child Abuse and Neglect; American Academy of Pediatrics. The evaluation of children in the primary care setting when sexual abuse is suspected. Pediatrics 2013;132:e558–67.**

2 DeLago C, Deblinger E, Schroeder C, Finkel MA. Girls who disclose sexual abuse: urogenital symptoms and signs after genital contact. Pediatrics 2008;122:e281–6.

3 Schaeffer P, Leventhal JM, Asnes AG. Children's disclosures of sexual abuse: Learning from direct inquiry. Child Abuse Negl 2011;35:343–52.

4 Melville JD, Kellogg ND, Perez N et al. Assessment for self-blame and trauma symptoms during the medical evaluation of suspected sexual abuse. Child Abuse Negl 2014;38:851.

5 Adams JA, Kellogg ND, Farst KJ et al. Updated guidelines for the medical assessment and care of children who may have been sexually abused. J Pediatr Adolesc Gynecol 2016;29:81–7. Available at: www.jpagonline.org/article/S1083-3188%2815%2900030-3/fulltext (accessed 21 February 2019).

6 Kaplan R, Adams JA, Starling SP, Giardino AP. Medical Response to Child Sexual Abuse. A Resource for Professionals Working with Children and Families. St Louis: STM Learning, 2011.

7 Adams JA, Farst KJ, Kellogg ND. Interpretation of medical findings in suspected child sexual abuse: an update for 2018. J Pediatr Adol Gynecol 2018;31:225–31. Available at: www.jpagonline.org/article/S1083-3188(17)30542-9/fulltext (accessed 1 March 2019).

8 Herrmann B, Navratil F. Sexual abuse in prepubertal children and adolescents. Endocr Dev 2012;22:112–37.

Anogenital findings in child sexual abuse

General considerations and normal findings

The evaluation of children for possible sexual abuse mandates a thorough understanding of the appearance of the anogenital anatomy both in abused and nonabused children. Anogenital findings should be described on the basis of a descriptive and standardized terminology. General terms such as 'normal genitalia' do not reflect the great variety of normal findings. 'Vulva' and 'pudenda' also lack specificity. 'Virgo intacta', 'virginal introitus', 'marital hymen', 'gaping vulva' or 'enlarged vaginal opening' are insufficient, imprecise and not descriptive terms and should be strictly avoided.

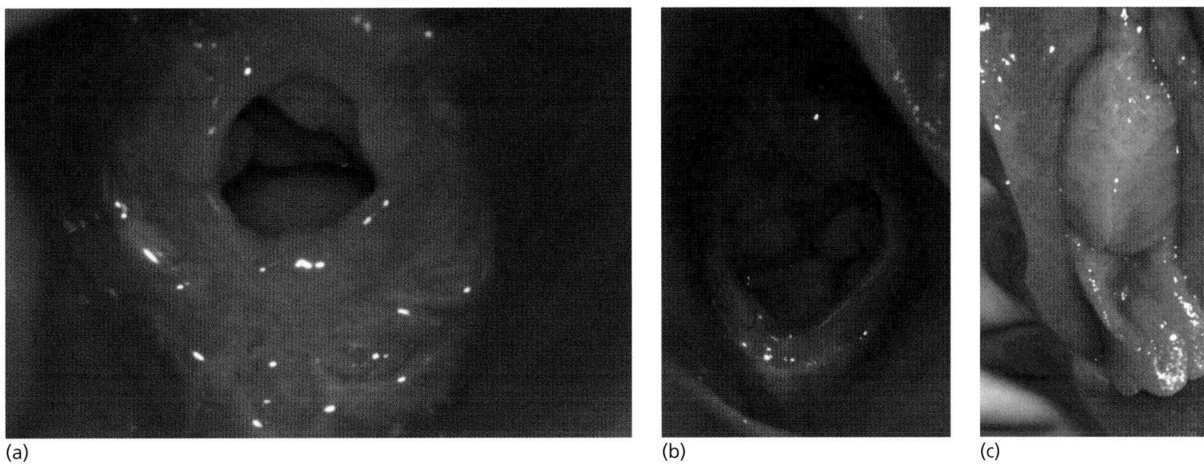

Fig. 164.12 (a) Normal annular hymen; (b) normal crescentic hymen; (c) normal oestrogenized, fimbriated hymen.

The appearance of the genitalia, especially the hymenal membrane, is quite variable and strongly influenced by age and hormonal factors but also by examination position, examination technique, amount of traction used and degree of relaxation of the child, thus potentially varying within the same examination. The whitish-pink hymen of newborn girls is mostly annular and rather thick and redundant due to maternal oestrogen influence. The appearance changes markedly due to withdrawal of oestrogen, thus creating the typical and most prevalent crescentic, semilunar configuration mostly found in children over 3 years of age. The hymen becomes a thin, more translucent and reddish membrane due to vascularization until pubertal raise of estrogen again creates a paler, redundant and fimbriated appearance. Typical hymenal configurations are:

- *Annular* (circumferential, concentric) – mostly seen in newborns and infants (Fig. 164.12a).
- *Crescentic* (semilunar, posterior rim type) – most frequent configuration in prepubertal girls (Fig. 164.12b).
- *Fimbriated* (denticular, oestrogenized) – mainly seen in newborns, small infants and at puberty (Fig. 164.12c).
- *Normal variants* include a sleeve-like (hymen altus), septate (Fig. 164.13) or microperforate hymen.

The hymen is a highly elastic tissue allowing the passage of a finger or even a penis without necessarily rupturing, depending on age and size. Unlike the common lay misconception it does not resemble a piece of paper irrevocably 'broken' by penetration or the idea of a complete membrane covering the vaginal introitus. The use of tampons may cause enlargement of the hymenal opening but, like masturbation, no injury. Physical activities such as gymnastics, running, jumping or splits do not lead to hymenal damage.

The abundance of normal congenital variants, findings commonly caused by other medical conditions and specific differential diagnosis with CSA need to be recognized (Adams Guidelines Class 1 findings [1–3]).

Findings associated with child sexual abuse

Specific findings that allow the diagnosis of CSA are only found in 3–8% of the victims. The main reason is that most abusive physical contacts are physically less invasive or involve fondling only and do not lead to significant and lasting trauma. Furthermore, anogenital tissues have an enormous potential for rapid and often complete healing. Disclosure is typically delayed and hence in many cases a significant amount of time has elapsed since the last episode, contributing to the paucity of findings. Findings vary considerably with the nature of the abuse, involved objects, the degree of force used, the age of the child and the frequency of the abuse. A short time span since the last event and a history of pain and/or bleeding increase the likelihood of detecting abnormal physical findings. In order to categorize anogenital findings, classification scales are intended to relate the findings to the probability of their abusive or alternative origin. They help to assess probabilities but must never be misinterpreted as rigid instructions on how to interpret anogenital findings. The current state of knowledge and its limitations have to be kept in mind and updated continuously, as in all other medical disciplines. In the last decade, the former Adams Classification has evolved into regularly reviewed and consensus-based 'Guidelines for the Medical Assessment and Care of Children Who

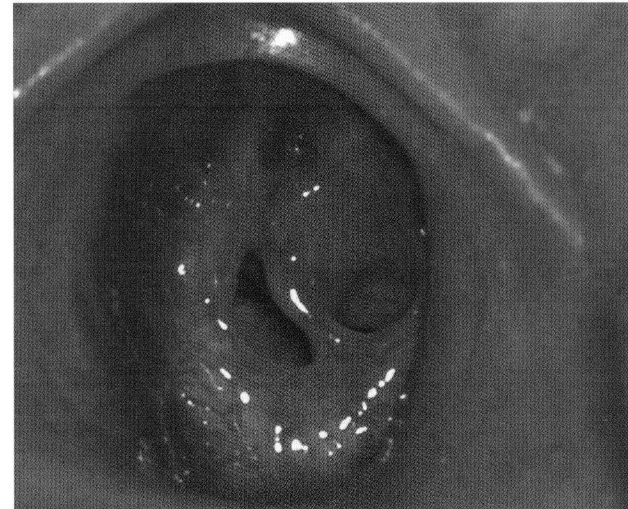

Fig. 164.13 Septate hymen.

May Have Been Sexually Abused'. Until 2016 findings were categorized as class I (normal or differential diagnosis), class II (no expert consensus; may support a child's disclosure of sexual abuse, if one is given, but should be interpreted with caution) and class III (findings caused by trauma and/or sexual contact; support a disclosure of sexual abuse and are highly suggestive of abuse even in the absence of a disclosure). In the 2018 guidelines the classification was reorganized, as mentioned above [3].

Normal findings after penetration

The gynaecological term 'virgo intacta' is frequently used to describe the clinical finding of a normal hymen. For nonmedical professionals and lay people this finding suggests that the possibility of previous sexual abuse and penetration is eliminated. A study by Kellogg et al. undermines this concept by finding that only two of 36 pregnant teenagers had a definite finding of previous penetrating injury; four girls showed indecisive findings ('Normal does not mean nothing happened' [4]). A Canadian study found penetration injuries in only 9% of a series of sexually assaulted adult virgins [5]. Another study only found 11% specific findings in paediatric and adolescent victims with a history of vaginal penetration, none of them in the prepubertal age group [6]. These and numerous other studies indicate that 'virgo intacta' is not only a misleading term but may also be dangerous for the credibility of victims in court and other circumstances and should be strictly avoided in this context.

Characteristics of anogenital findings in child sexual abuse

Abusive findings tend to be found in the lower/posterior segment, below the 9 to 3 o'clock line. The range of findings varies considerably, from superficial mucosal abrasions and scratches to clear transecting lacerations of anogenital tissues. Many of the resulting injuries tend to be superficial and heal rapidly, predominantly because the offender uses little physical force. Most of these findings resolve within 2–3 days after trauma. A retrospective longitudinal multicentre study has confirmed previous findings: nearly all nonhymenal and the majority of hymenal injuries heal rapidly and mostly completely. Of nonhymenal injuries, abrasions resolved within 2–3 days, petechiae within 24 hours and submucosal haemorrhages and haematoma within 7–14 days. Hymenal abrasions, petechiae, mild submucosal haemorrhages and haematomas healed completely in 2–3 days in most cases. Scars are infrequent in genital trauma and have never been documented after hymenal injuries. Seventy five percent of prepubertal incomplete tears of the hymen and 90% of those in puberty heal completely or leave a partial notch which changes its configuration due to healing from V-shaped to U-shaped. Both are also called concavities [7,8]. Superficial notches up to 50% of hymenal height are insignificant; deep notches more than 50% but less than 100% are class II findings, which are suspicious but not definite evidence. Complete posterior transections to the base of the hymen (Fig. 164.14) or extending into the vaginal wall have only been observed after penetrating trauma, which may be abusive or accidental. They leave a permanent defect or gap (Fig. 164.15). A narrow hymenal rim and the size of the hymenal opening (introitus) are not criteria for a diagnosis of child sexual abuse [1–3].

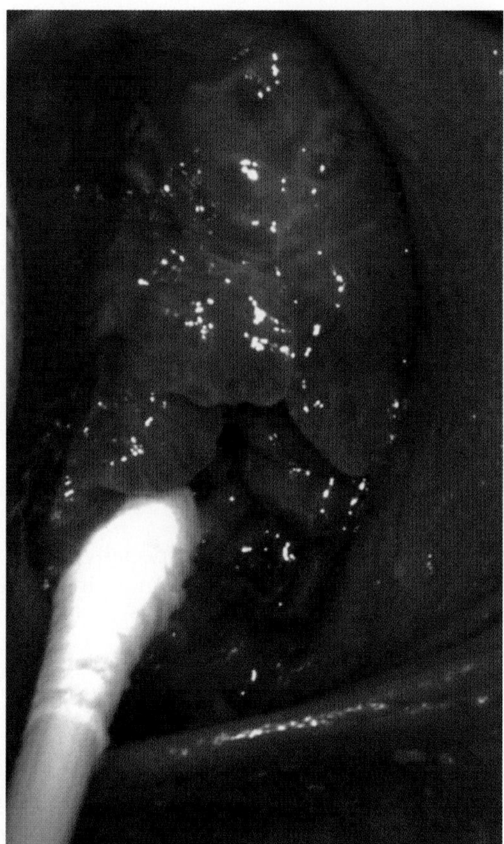

Fig. 164.14 Complete transection of hymen at 4 to 5 o'clock.

Acute and extensive anal findings such as deep lacerations and significant trauma to the anus are obvious results of anal penetration (Fig. 164.16). In these cases, anoscopy may aid in identifying internal injuries and collecting sperm. In the absence of acute findings, anoscopy is not indicated. The interpretation of chronic anal signs is far more controversial than genital signs of trauma. The ability of the external sphincter to dilate considerably when passing a large bolus of faecal matter without any injury to the anal tissues is a major contributing factor. Variables influencing the presence of physical signs include the size of the object introduced, the amount of force used, the age of the victim, the use of lubricants, frequency of episodes and time elapsed since the last episode. Particular controversy has evolved about the sign of 'reflex anal dilatation' (RAD). As an isolated sign, RAD should not be interpreted as diagnostic of CSA. Complete anal dilatation without visible stool is currently classified as a class II finding. Anal fissures are commonly caused by other medical conditions.

Findings caused by trauma and/or sexual contact comprise acute lacerations or bruising of anogenital tissues or

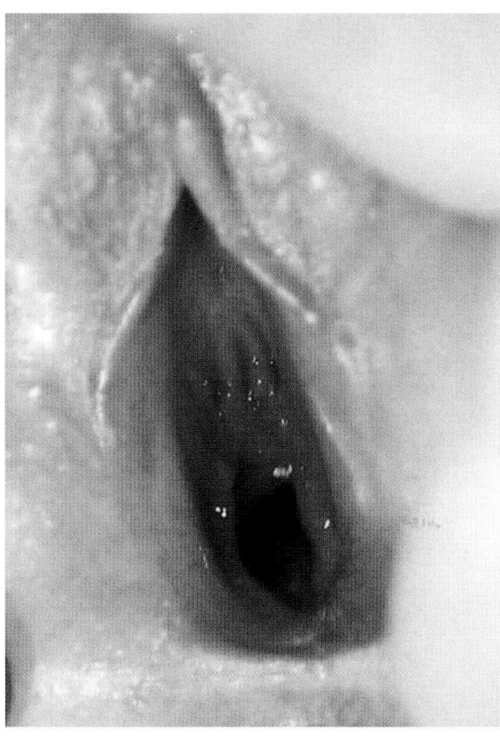

Fig. 164.15 Complete gap or defect of the hymen at 6 o'clock.

residual, healing injuries, including complete clefts of the hymen, certain infections, pregnancy and semen in forensic specimens taken directly from a child's body [1].

References

1 Jenny C, Crawford-Jakubiak JE; Committee on Child Abuse and Neglect; American Academy of Pediatrics. The evaluation of children in the primary care setting when sexual abuse is suspected. Pediatrics 2013;132:e558–67.

2 Kaplan R, Adams JA, Starling SP, Giardino AP. Medical Response to Child Sexual Abuse. A Resource for Professionals Working with Children and Families. St Louis: STM Learning, 2011.

3 **Adams JA, Farst KJ, Farst KJ, Kellogg ND. Interpretation of medical findings in suspected child sexual abuse: an update for 2018. J Pediatr Adolesc Gynecol 2018;31:225–31.**

4 Kellogg ND, Menard SW, Santos A. Genital anatomy in pregnant adolescents: "Normal" does not mean "Nothing happened." Pediatrics 2004;113:e67–9.

5 Biggs M, Stermac LE, Divinsky M. Genital injuries following sexual assault of women with and without prior sexual intercourse experience. CMAJ 1998;159:33–7.

6 Anderst J, Kellogg K, Jung I. Reports of repetitive penile-genital penetration often have no definitive evidence of penetration. Pediatrics 2009;124:e403–9.

7 McCann J, Miyamoto S, Boyle C, Rogers K. Healing of hymenal injuries in prepubertal and adolescent girls: a descriptive study. Pediatrics 2007;119:e1094–106.

8 McCann J, Miyamoto S, Boyle C, Rogers K. Healing of nonhymenal genital injuries in prepubertal and adolescent girls: A descriptive study. Pediatrics 2007;120, 1000–11.

Sexually transmitted infections

STI may be the only medical indicator of CSA in some cases. The diagnosis of an STI in a child beyond the neonatal period suggests CSA. The interpretation differs according to the respective disease. STI are diagnosed in 1–5% of abused children and 5–24% of abused

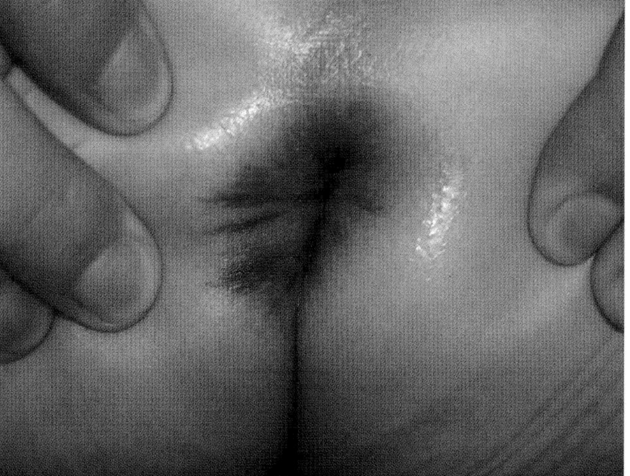

Fig. 164.16 Anal bruising secondary to trauma.

adolescents in US studies. Screening should only be performed in selected cases as the yield of positive results is very low in asymptomatic children. Selection criteria for screening include genital discharge at examination or in the recent history, a perpetrator with a known or suspected STI or with high-risk behaviour, anogenital findings indicating penetrative abuse, a history of genital-to-genital (or genital-to-anal) contact or penetration, concern of the patient or caregivers, or specific genital lesions. The screening formerly included vaginal and anal cultures for gonorrhoea (GO) and chlamydia (CT) and a vaginal smear for *Trichomonas vaginalis* (TV). Nuclear amplification techniques (NAAT) are becoming increasingly accepted as the diagnostic standard in children as well. For GO and CT, urine sampling seems to be effective. Screening in adolescents should be done with a lower threshold. Due to far-reaching legal and social implications, in case of positive results, confirmatory testing should be performed to exclude a possible false-positive result [1,2].

Except in documented congenital infections, confirmed results for GO or serological proof of acquired syphilis or HIV are definite evidence of CSA. Perinatally acquired infections with CT have been demonstrated to persist as long as 2 years in the genital area and up to 3 years in the pharynx. Infections appearing after the first 2 years of life are strong indicators of CSA, as are infections with TV, especially after the first year of life. Herpes type 1 or 2, confirmed by culture or polymerase chain reaction (PCR) testing, in the genital or anal area of a child with no other indicators of sexual abuse, is an indeterminate finding [3].

Genital warts, condylomata acuminata and human papillomavirus

Genital warts or condylomata acuminata (CA) (Fig. 164.17a and b) caused by human papillomavirus infection (HPV) are probably the most prevalent concern about CSA shared with the (paediatric) dermatologist. As HPV is primarily sexually transmitted in adults, concerns about sexual transmission by mucosal anogenital contact

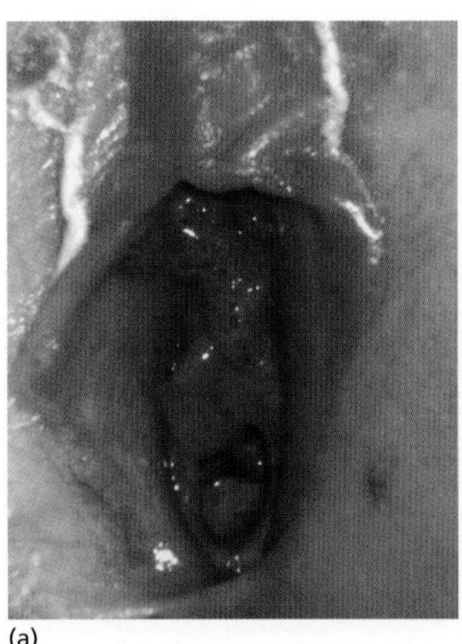
(a)

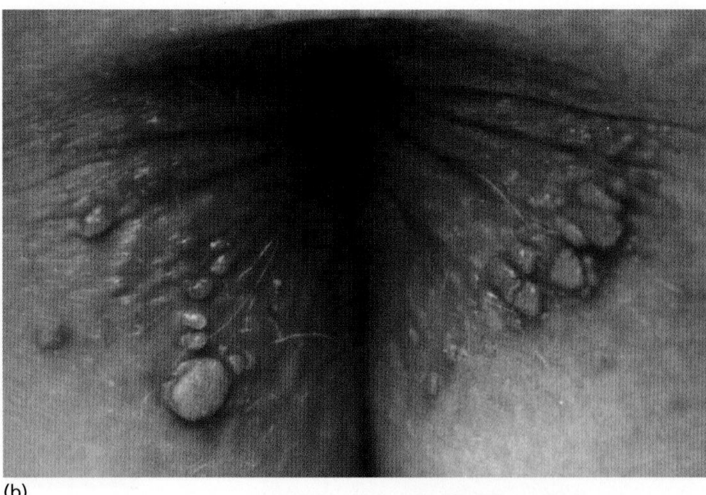
(b)

Fig. 164.17 (a) Genital warts or condylomata acuminata. (b) Anal warts or condylomata acuminata.

in children used to be high. Increasing evidence, however, points to alternative routes of transmission. Data about perinatal transmission and delayed infections up 3 years are conflicting, but indicate that vertical transmission is not frequent. As mothers may be asymptomatic and many infections are transient, there may often be no history of genital warts or abnormal Papanicolaou (PAP) smears. Transmission by household contacts and autoinoculation appear to be significant modes of transmission. A Norwegian study found HPV DNA in 3.4% of genital and 1.2% of anal swabs in nonabused 5- to 6-year-old girls. However, HPV is one of the most frequently diagnosed STI in sexually abused children [4,5].

Evaluation of a child presenting with anogenital warts should prompt consideration of CSA but never lead to a precocious assumption that abuse has occurred. Current guidelines state that genital or anal CA in the absence of other indicators of abuse are a class II finding, and that lesions appearing for the first time in a child older than 5 years may be more likely to be the result of sexual transmission [3]. It is recommended to perform a complete medical evaluation including a qualified anogenital examination for further signs of CSA, testing for additional STI, a child and caregiver interview about behavioural indicators, a maternal history of CA or abnormal PAP smears and a history of cutaneous warts affecting the child or household members.

HPV infections are associated with a wide range of cutaneous and mucosal infections in childhood. Different HPV types can cause common warts as well as genital warts. Diagnosis of anogenital CA is usually made clinically by visual inspection. Confirmation by biopsy is usually not indicated. There is no evidence about which of the different treatment options has greatest efficacy. Furthermore, genital warts have a high tendency to clear spontaneously and commonly recur regardless of treatment. Surgical removal, carbon dioxide laser surgery and cutaneous application of imiquimod (a topical immune enhancer) are frequently reported treatments; their use depends on age, extent and progression of lesions and the development of symptoms such as pruritus, pain or bleeding.

References

1 Girardet RG, Lahoti S, Howard LA et al. Epidemiology of sexually transmitted infections in suspected child victims of sexual assault. Pediatrics 2009;124:79–86.

2 Bechtel K. Sexual abuse and sexually transmitted infections in children and adolescents. Curr Opin Pediatr 2010;22:94–9.

3 Adams JA, Kellogg ND, Farst KJ et al. Updated guidelines for the medical assessment and care of children who may have been sexually abused. J Pediatr Adolesc Gynecol 2016;29:81–7. Available at: www.jpagonline.org/article/S1083-3188%2815%2900030-3/fulltext (accessed 21 February 2019).

4 Unger ER, Fajman NN, Maloney EM et al. Anogenital human papillomavirus in sexually abused and nonabused children: a multicenter study. Pediatrics 2011;128:e658.

5 Myhre AK, Dalen A, Berntzen K, Bratlid D. Anogenital human papillomavirus in non-abused preschool children. Acta Paediatr 2003;92:1445–52.

Differential diagnosis in child sexual abuse

Beside normal findings, normal variants and unspecific findings, there are a number of skin lesions and differential diagnoses to consider which may require paediatric dermatology expertise.

Accidental genital injuries. frequently cause concern that the history might be falsified and the injuries are caused by abuse. The pattern of injury and accompanying history, however, generally aid in the differentiation. Most accidents result from straddling, causing crushing injuries of the anogenital area, when children fall on hard objects such as a bicycle crossbar or the edge of a piece of furniture. The injuries mostly involve the labia majora and minora and the clitoral hood, and rarely involve the deeper and protected structures such as the hymen and the posterior fourchette. Accidental genital injuries tend to be mostly minor and superficial, located anteriorly, externally and unilaterally. In most cases of accidental injuries, except for rare cases of accidental penetrating injuries, the hymen usually is not injured (Fig. 164.18) [1].

Dermatological conditions. include erythema and excoriations in nonspecific skin irritation or infection, napkin dermatitis (Fig. 164.19), lack of hygiene, irritant substances (bubble bath, cosmetic care products), moniliasis,

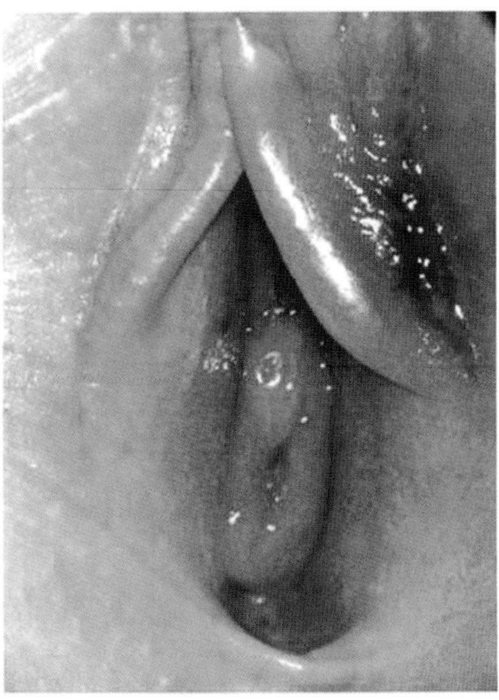

Fig. 164.18 Paralabial laceration as result of accidental genital injury.

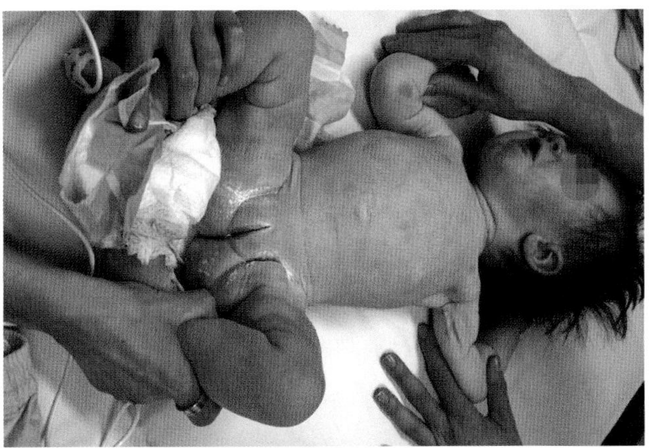

Fig. 164.19 Severely neglected child with napkin dermatitis.

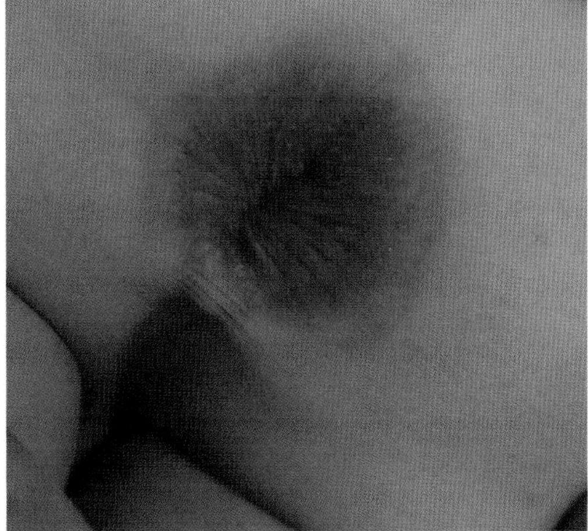

Fig. 164.20 Infection caused by group A β-haemolytic streptococci.

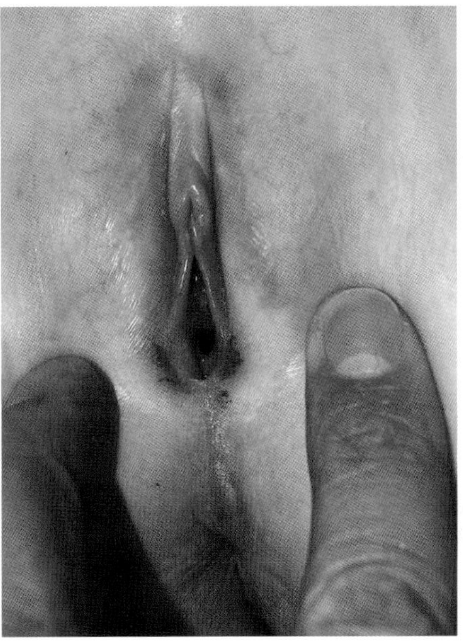

Fig. 164.21 Anogenital lichen sclerosus.

genital varicella and oxyuriasis. Recurrent vaginitis is often an area of concern, especially when expressed in the context of custody debates. The child returning with red genitals after a weekend visit with the separated father may equally have experienced a paternal lack of hygiene, or his aversion to properly cleaning the genital area because he fears allegations of sexual abuse. Although abuse is possible, and parental separation may result from nondisclosed abuse, the assumption is probably overstated. Vaginitis is the most prevalent paediatric gynaecological health problem and requires a systematic approach and broad differential diagnosis. Recurrent vaginitis of undetermined cause should warrant concern and further evaluation, possibly including vaginoscopy, but is never diagnostic per se [2].

An infection caused by Group A β-haemolytic streptococci (Fig. 164.20) may cause a fiery red, oedematous and tender vaginal or perianal inflammation, sometimes accompanied by various forms of discharge: thin, thick, serous, blood-tinged, creamy, white, yellow or green. Cultures have to be specifically requested as streptococci do not grow on routine media. Treatment is as for pharyngeal infections with a 7-day course of oral penicillin.

A frequently mistaken diagnosis of CSA occurs in children who present with anogenital lichen sclerosus (Fig. 164.21). After initial white papules that form white plaques, the skin becomes delicate and atrophic. It is extremely susceptible to minor trauma such as wiping with toilet paper, causing fissuring or alarming subepidermal haemorrhages and spontaneous bleeding. The typical presentation is with an 'hourglass or figure-of-eight configuration of decreased pigmentation around the labia majora and the anus.

Cutaneous bleeding. may also be caused by leukaemia, disseminated intravascular coagulation, purpura fulminans and other coagulation disorders.

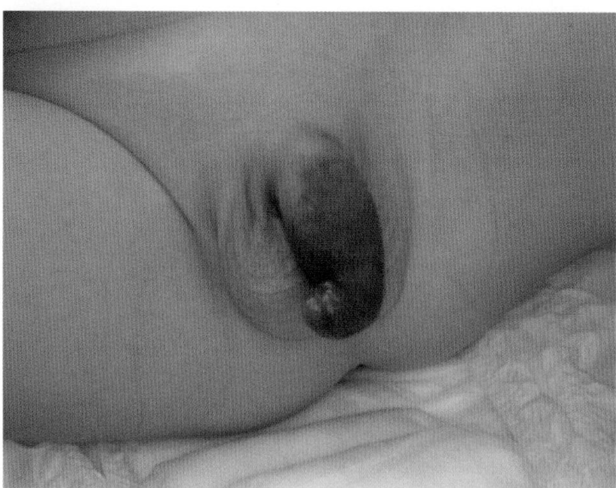

Fig. 164.22 Penile swelling and colour change as a result of atypical Henoch–Schönlein purpura.

Urethral bleeding. is more usually caused by urethral prolapse (more prevalent in African-American girls), polyps, haemangioma or papilloma than by CSA.

Vaginal bleeding. requires careful evaluation of the underlying causes. Most frequently it is caused by vaginitis (approximately 70%). Other less frequent causes include precocious puberty, sarcoma botryoides (embryonal rhabdomyosarcoma), internal or external application of hormones, or nonspecific, idiopathic bleeding [3].

Genital findings in boys. may be caused by sexual (sucking marks on the penis) or physical abuse (ligatures, pinch marks). Differential diagnoses include (as in girls) accidental injuries, infections and lichen sclerosus, causing bleeding into the prepuce. In Henoch–Schönlein purpura roughly 13% of boys develop scrotal haematoma which may be mistaken for abusive trauma or torsion. Single reports describe penile swelling and colour change with a purpuric rush (Fig. 164.22). Concomitant further skin signs may be missing or subtle [4].

Congenital conditions. mistaken for sexual abuse include haemangiomas of the hymen, vagina and labia. They may bleed or ulcerate. Failure of midline fusion is a congenital defect resembling scar tissue. Sometimes it is combined with an anteriorly located anus and also frequently creates confusion and misinterpretation as an abuse-related finding.

Anal findings. to be differentiated from abuse are fissures in chronic constipation, Crohn disease, rectal prolapse or Group A streptococcal cellulitis [2,3].

References

1 Sugar NF, Feldman KW. Perineal impalements in children: Distinguishing accidents from abuse. Pediatr Emerg Care 2007;23:605–16.

2 Kellogg ND, Frasier L. Conditions mistaken for child sexual abuse. In: Reece RM, Christian CW (eds) Child Abuse: Medical Diagnosis and Management, 3rd edn. Elk Grove Village, IL: American Academy of Pediatrics, 2009: 389–426.

3 Frasier L. Medical conditions that mimic sexual abuse. In: Kaplan R, Adams JA, Starling SP et al (eds) Medical Response to Child Sexual Abuse. A Resource for Professionals Working with Children and Families. St Louis: STM Learning, 2011:145–66.

4 Caliskan B, Guven A, Atabek C et al. Henoch-Schönlein purpura presenting with symptoms mimicking balanoposthitis. Pediatr Rep 2009;1:e5.

Overall assessment in child sexual abuse

Medical proof of abuse remains the exception, applicable only in acute anogenital trauma in the absence of a convincing history of accidental trauma, proof of gonorrhoea or syphilis (congenital infection excluded), pregnancy, proof of semen, sperm cells, acid phosphatase or sperm-specific glycoprotein p30 in or on the body of a child.

The overall assessment of the likelihood of CSA and the final conclusions have to be made conscientiously and need to include all physical findings, possible laboratory results and especially the history obtained from the child. The medical expert contributes a thoughtful and qualified piece of evidence to the multidisciplinary puzzle of evaluating children for possible CSA. Strictly medical interventions in CSA include treatment of injuries, infections or STI, and emergency contraception. Reassurance of physical intactness should be an integral part of the medical examination. Furthermore, the clinician participates in referral to therapy, emotional guidance of the family, and assisting the legal system in cases with confirmatory findings. It is crucial to develop extensive interdisciplinary and multidisciplinary cooperation and consultation in all cases.

Although we are constantly learning more about the role and significance of medical aspects in suspected CSA cases, the diagnosis of CSA primarily rests on the descriptive statements made by an abused child and obtained by a professionally qualified clinician.

Overall medical and multidisciplinary management

Any child with injuries or the suspicion for CSA needs to be carefully assessed and all physical, developmental and emotional abnormalities must be carefully documented and recorded in written form, with drawings and photographs, as well as the circumstances of the injuries and a detailed history. If appropriate, forensic specimens need to be obtained considering the chain of evidence. Any necessary treatment or prophylaxis has to be performed, as the abused child is first and foremost a patient to be taken care of.

Depending on the severity of injury, the obviousness of a CSA diagnosis and risk assessment concerning the child's safety, different strategies in order to react appropriately are possible. In private practice, sometimes rather subtle, subclinical injuries may warrant sharing concerns about possible problems with the caregivers and close monitoring in order to obtain more information. Consultation with respective specialists in child abuse paediatrics or forensic medicine may be helpful to clarify unclear findings and constellations. Children with more severe injuries or suspicions should be admitted to a hospital with a child protection team for a multidisciplinary approach and structured process of diagnosis and intervention. All cases with a justified suspicion or diagnosis of CAN must be taken care of in cooperation with child protection services and/or appropriate counselling agencies, with further possible necessity for therapy and rehabilitation. In some countries, such as the USA, physicians and other health professionals are mandated to report to child protection services by law. In most countries it is the responsibility of the medical and other child protection professionals to assess if a criminal court proceeding contributes to ensuring the child's safety and well-being or if other strategies such as family courts might be a more promising way to protect children. The most recent and comprehensive contribution to evidence-based child protection in medicine are the new German 2019 AWMF S3+ child abuse guidelines (*Leitlinie Kinderschutz*). Integrating relevant nonmedical professions it is a well-organized and profound description of diagnosis, diagnostic procedures, differential diagnosis, intervention and multidisciplinary cooperation (www.awmf.org/leitlinien/detail/ll/027-069.html; in German).

CHAPTER 165

Assessing and Scoring Life Quality

Andrew Y. Finlay

Division of Infection and Immunity, Cardiff University School of Medicine, Cardiff, UK

Introduction, 2241
What does 'quality of life' mean?, 2241
Why assessment of quality of life is important, 2242
Methods of quality of life assessment, 2242
Who should measure quality of life in children?, 2243
Validation of quality of life measures, 2244
Dermatology-specific quality of life measures, 2245
Disease-specific quality of life measures, 2245
Generic quality of life measures, 2250
Major life-changing decisions, 2251
Family impact, 2251
Utility measurement, 2252
Conclusion, 2252
Conflict of interest, 2252

Abstract

Measurement of the impact of skin disease on the quality of life of children is important to inform clinical decision taking, for research and audit purposes and to demonstrate the impact of skin disease compared to other conditions. Quality of life measures for children are designed to be disease specific, dermatology specialty specific or generic, usable across many specialties. There are measures for teenagers and for infants. Major life-changing decisions influenced by skin disease can be recorded. There are questionnaires to measure the secondary impact on the quality of life of other family members of having a child in the family with skin disease, a burden that is often unrecognized. These measures are also disease specific, dermatology specific or generic. Utility measures that allow calculation of economic impact of skin disease in children are being developed.

Key points

- Quality of life measurement is important in the clinic and for research, for audit and to demonstrate the importance of skin disease in children.
- There are disease-specific, specialty-specific and generic measures of the impact on the child, for use by children and their parents or carers.
- There is a similar range of measures to assess family impact of childhood skin disease.
- The most commonly used dermatology-specific quality of life measure for children is the Children's Dermatology Life Quality Index (CDLQI).

Introduction

Historically, the obvious impact of skin disease on the lives of affected children was an aspect of clinical practice that was largely ignored. There was a reasonable assumption that as the only way to improve this impact was to improve the skin condition, all the focus should be on the medical aspects of therapy. This thinking was coupled with an outlook that as there was no other way of improving quality of life (QoL), there was no point in dwelling on this aspect, far less trying to measure it.

But things have changed. There has been a major shift in orientation of medicine towards being 'patient centred'. There has also been a realization that the ability to measure information of relevance to physician and patient is essential to allow evidence-based progress in improving care of patients. For most children with skin disease, the impact of the disease on multiple aspects of their daily lives is critically important. This realization is the justification of the QoL measurement described in this chapter.

What does 'quality of life' mean?

It is crucial to assess the impact of skin disease on patients in order to address their real needs [1]. Although the concept of 'quality of life' seems simple and self-explanatory, it is not easy to define [2]. At its simplest, quality of life is judged by how an individual rates those aspects of their life that are of most importance to them. For simplicity and for practical reasons, an assumption is made that the things that matter to people are broadly the same. However, it should be remembered that in reality, every individual has their own set of values that underlies their attitudes towards what QoL means for them. Inevitably, any method of measuring such a concept, hugely influenced by age, cultural and personal attitudes, must be only an approximation to grasp what is arguably an unmeasurable idea. The related concept of health-related quality of life (HRQoL) concerns the specific impact of impaired health on QoL.

Harper's Textbook of Pediatric Dermatology, Fourth Edition. Edited by Peter Hoeger, Veronica Kinsler and Albert Yan.

If methods are used to measure QoL or HRQoL that result in scores, then information about the absolute meaning of the scores is required, along with the interpretation of change in scores.

Why assessment of quality of life is important

The assessment of the impact that skin disease has on children is important for clinical, research, audit and 'political' reasons related to allocation of resources. In the clinic, a realistic understanding of QoL impact is essential to inform appropriate management decision taking. Formal structured assessment may also identify areas in a child's life that need additional support. Including patient-reported outcome measures (PROMs), such as QoL measures, in the monitoring of children in the paediatric dermatology clinic gives a unique complementary and arguably most relevant indicator of the success or otherwise of therapy. The use of QoL measures in the clinic may enhance the doctor–patient relationship by clearly indicating to the patients and parents or carers that health professionals are interested in wider aspects of the child's well-being.

In the assessment of new therapies, such as new drugs for atopic eczema, and of novel ways of delivering care, such as the development of nurse-led clinics, the use of QoL measures gives an additional insight from the patient perspective into the effectiveness of such interventions. In the research context, QoL measures generally do not replace standard measures of signs or symptoms, but add to these measures, although there is no reason why QoL scores should not be used as a primary outcome measure. QoL measures have been used to assess the impact of educational interventions in children and adults [3].

When auditing a clinical service, it is important to use measures that are of relevance to service users, not simply process measures such as throughput of patients. QoL measures are ideal for this context, provided that they are short and easily completed.

In all healthcare fields, there is inevitably competition for limited resources. Often the area of skin disease has not fared well in such competition, partly because it has been difficult to provide evidence of the severe impact of skin disease on children and their families. Generic QoL measures can provide such evidence. Within dermatology, it could also be argued that more resources should be focused on support of and research into those conditions that have the greatest impact on QoL. As an example, molluscum contagiosum has not provoked widespread research interest, despite its high prevalence, but the evidence that over 10% of affected children experience a major impact on their QoL [4] may stimulate more focus on this subject.

The European Academy of Dermatology and Venereology Task Force of Quality of Life has identified ways in which measuring QoL in routine clinical practice in dermatology may be advantageous to both the doctor and the patient (Box 165.1) [5]. In a separate study, this Task Force reviewed the QoL measures available for children with skin disease [6]. A systematic review of generic and disease-related instruments in children and adolescents in 2008 [7] only identified two dermatology-specific instruments: the Children's Dermatology Life Quality Index (CDLQI) and the Infants' Dermatitis Quality of Life questionnaire (IDQoL).

Box 165.1 Key ways in which use of QoL measures in the clinic may be advantageous, as identified by the EADV Task Force [5]

Inform clinical decisions
Aid treatment decision taking
Guideline use
Shared decision making
Treatment goals
Treatment adjustment at follow-up
Discharge decisions

Clinician–patient communication
Clinician–patient relationship
Clinician–patient enhanced dialogue

Impact on clinician and on patient
Impact on clinician
Impact on patient

Informing the consultation
Prediction outcomes/prognosis
Adherence/compliance
Screening
Monitoring
Education
Referral to other services

Clinical service administration
Guideline development
Audit/clinical audit
Administration/policy

Clinician awareness comments
Background

Source: Finlay et al. [5]. Reproduced with permission of John Wiley & Sons Ltd.

There are several reviews summarizing QoL issues in paediatric dermatology and general paediatrics [8–10]. Three different dimensions of the impact of skin disease have been described [11] – the impact now (today), the impact in the long term and the impact on the lives of those closest to the patient – for children, parents and siblings (Fig. 165.1). There are methods for measuring all three of these dimensions.

Methods of quality of life assessment

Since the first dermatology disease-specific QoL measure was introduced in 1987 [12], a large variety of measures have been described, several specifically for use in children. The first generic dermatology QoL questionnaire for use by children with skin disease, the CDLQI [13], remains the most widely used measure [14]. A systematic review of randomized controlled trials of treatment for eczema has confirmed that the most common measures

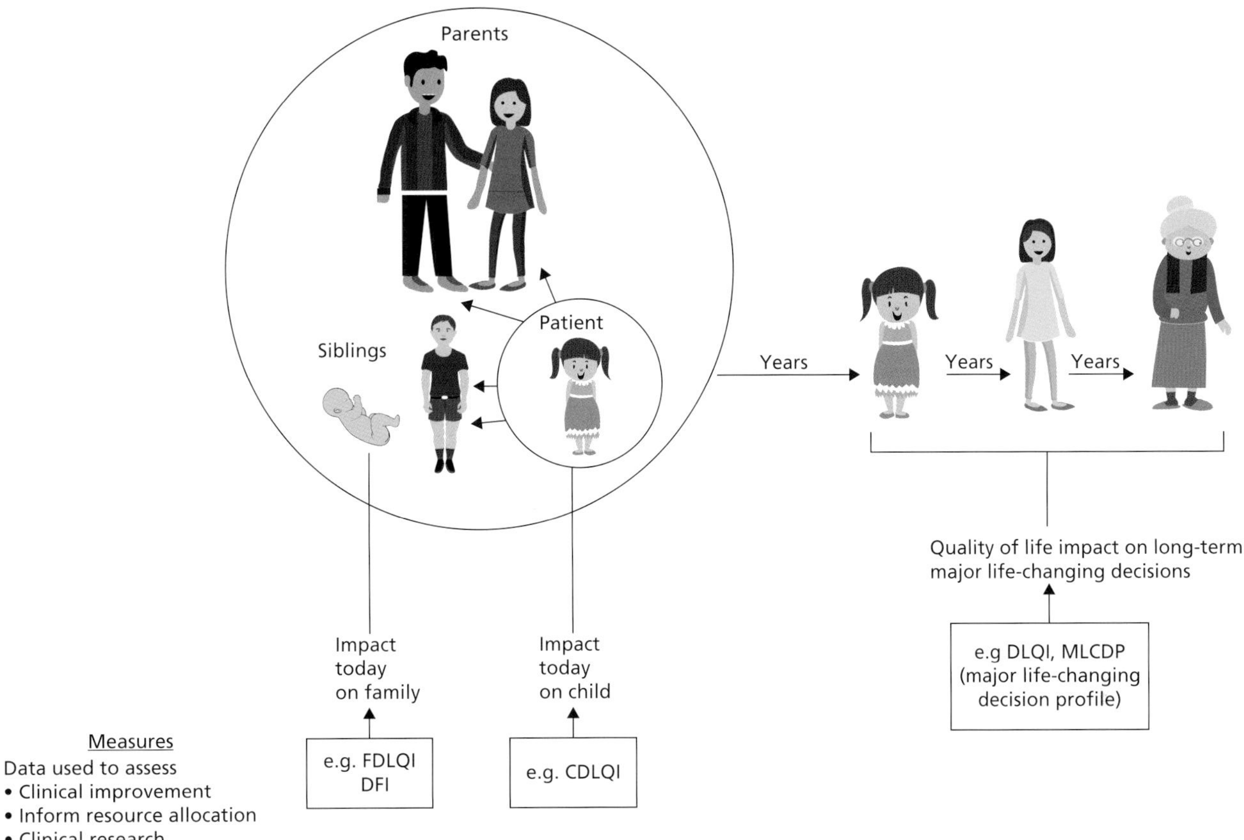

Fig. 165.1 The three dimensions of quality of life impact of skin disease in childhood: now, long term and family [11].

used in children and caregivers are the CDLQI, the IDQoL and the Dermatitis Family Impact (DFI) [15].

Quality of life assessment is usually carried out by means of questionnaires that are completed by the patient, by the patient with assistance from a parent or carer, or sometimes primarily by the parent or carer. The questionnaires are designed to be used specifically in a single disease, across a spectrum of conditions within a specialty (such as the CDLQI) or across all diseases.

As in many aspects of medical advance, there has been an initial focus on creating QoL measures for adults and the lessons learnt have only later been applied within a paediatric setting. A variety of utility measures, most notably based on the use of EQ-5D data and techniques such as standard gamble, have been developed for use in adults; utility measures for children are now being developed.

There are many challenges in trying to measure in children how QoL is affected by skin disease. The most obvious is that the lives of children are very different at different ages. Children develop at different rates and social and cultural factors have a profound influence on the details of how children live and of what is important to them. Any attempt therefore to use standard scales inevitably involves some compromise; there has to be a balance between developing multiple versions of scales to cater for every developmental stage or social setting, and the practical use of standard scales across widely differing circumstances. In view of this, perhaps surprisingly, there has been widespread acceptance of a simple generic dermatology measure (the CDLQI) across a wide age range and in vastly different cultural settings; this suggests that there may be core areas of experience of skin disease that are universal.

A separate problem relating to the measurement of QoL is that there is a poor standard of reporting of QoL data in the literature [16]. The names of QoL measures used may be omitted, the percentage change in scores may be given but not the absolute scores, making it difficult to judge whether a clinically relevant change has taken place or purely descriptive results may be reported, entirely omitting scores. Editors of dermatology journals should be encouraged to present data in a way that allows full interpretation by the reader, insisting for example that actual scores and identifiable names of measures used should be reported.

Who should measure quality of life in children?

Ideally, when measuring the impact of skin disease on the lives of children, the children themselves should be able to directly record their own views. The tools created to measure QoL impact should be designed to facilitate this. For paper and pen usage, the use of cartoons can make completion fun [17]. There is now a huge potential with electronic delivery of QoL measures to engage and encourage participants, especially children. Possible approaches are limited only by the imagination, and it is reasonable to hope for major advances in this area in coming years.

Infants obviously cannot complete questionnaires; for assessment at this very early age, questionnaires should be designed to be completed by the parent or carer. Very young children may not be able to complete a questionnaire but in conversation with their parents, questionnaires may be appropriately completed. Children of different abilities and ages will need varying amounts of adult input, with most older children completing questionnaires unaided, provided the design is appropriate.

Validation of quality of life measures

As illustrated in this chapter, there are many different QoL measures available for use in children with skin disease. The choice of which to use depends partly on the circumstances and practicality, but ideally only those measures which have been shown to fulfil certain aspects of validation should be considered. Key quality criteria are being set in the planning of a systematic review of QoL measures for use in eczema [18]. However, frequently measures are published and used without this assurance of quality having been reached. There may be an intention on the part of authors to carry out additional validation but this sometimes never happens or is not published.

Perhaps the most important initial concept in the creation of a QoL measure is the origin of the questions that are posed in the measure. The questions in some measures are created by 'experts', usually clinicians working with affected patients, or developed from the published literature. However, the only way to ensure that the content of a QoL questionnaire is appropriate and relevant is to primarily base the questions on information directly from patients themselves, preferably prospectively researched. Other sources of information can be used at a later stage to check that all areas are covered. When QoL measures are being developed, both factor analysis and Rasch analysis may be used to identify the most appropriate items to include. Factor analysis and Rasch analysis assist removal of redundant items that measure the same thing and test whether it is appropriate for scores to be combined in an overall score.

Important aspects of the validation of properties of health-related patient-reported outcomes are summarized within the COnsensus-based Standards for the selection of health status Measurement Instruments checklist (COSMIN), developed in an international Delphi study [19].

- *Internal consistency*: this concerns the interrelatedness between items.
- *Content validity*: the degree to which the content of a health-related PRO instrument is an adequate reflection of the construct to be measured.
- *Construct validity*: the degree to which the scores of a health-related PRO instrument are consistent with various hypotheses.
- *Hypotheses testing*: this is about whether the direction and magnitude of a correlation or difference is similar to what could be expected based on the construct(s) being measured.
- *Criterion validity*: the degree to which the scores of a health-related PRO instrument are an adequate reflection of a 'gold' standard.
- *Responsiveness*: the ability of a health-related PRO instrument to detect change over time in the construct to be measured.

Other aspects of validity include test–retest reliability, which is the stability of a scale when used repeatedly under the same conditions. Another is specificity, which is the ability of a questionnaire, where appropriate, to measure the impact of a specific disease or type of disease. As an example, there should be assurance that if a questionnaire is designed to measure the QoL impact of, say, psoriasis, then the questions should be worded to make it unlikely that the participant responds referring to the impact of another concomitant disease. There are many other issues that influence the practicality of use of QoL measures. These include face validity, which is how relevant and appropriate the questions appear to the user; ease of use, which is the burden placed on the user; availability of clear instructions for use; meaningful interpretability of the scores; and availability and cost.

The delivery of QoL questionnaires in electronic format raises further validity issues. Most QoL measures, originally designed for paper usage, when delivered electronically have not been validated in that format; there is simply an assumption that the measure will be completed similarly [20]. If a novel measure is developed de novo in an electronic format, then the validation will have taken place appropriately in that format and there is no problem. However, ideally there should be prospective confirmation that QoL measures delivered in different formats have similar measurement characteristics, as demonstrated for the cartoon CDLQI [17].

Quality of life measures not only need to be 'validated' when created, but they need to stay valid. Any written document when used by different people in different situations, especially when translated, runs the risk of being degraded by small but cumulative changes resulting from copying or translation inaccuracies or by new users adapting the questions. This is why maintenance of copyright is so important for a measure to gain and maintain widespread acceptance [21].

Medicine is an international science, and measurement techniques need to be used across different countries in a multitude of cultural settings and in many different languages. For multinational trials and for the interpretation of scores, scoring systems should ideally be valid and interchangeable between countries. For objective measurements, this is usually not a problem but in the measurement of QoL, cultural differences and translation issues have to be considered.

Concerning translation of QoL measures, it is not enough simply to carry out a single translation from the original language into a second language. Multiple errors can occur, not least because there is a temptation on behalf of the translator to 'improve' the wording and thereby alter the meaning of questions. Ideally, as a minimum requirement for a validated translation, the questionnaire should be independently translated by two separate translators, who then should confer and create an agreed translated version. This should then be back-translated independently by a third and a fourth translator; the two back-translations then need to be checked by the questionnaire originators. Nearly always, multiple errors are highlighted by this process, which needs to be repeated until the back-translations are as close as possible to the original.

More challenging is the creation of a 'culturally' validated translation. Some concepts in a questionnaire may not be relevant or appropriate in another culture, or other critical aspects in the other culture may be missed. A qualitative study is required involving patients in the 'other culture', seeking their views on the translated questionnaire and making changes where necessary.

Dermatology-specific quality of life measures

Children's Dermatology Life Quality Index

The CDLQI, introduced in 1995 [13], has 10 questions, each of which has four possible answers (Fig. 165.2). The questions are based on information given by children about how having a skin disease affected their lives; these are summarized in Box 165.2. The questionnaire takes about two minutes to complete. Children may complete it themselves or may be assisted by their parent or guardian. The cartoon version of the CDLQI [17] is preferred by younger children and is completed on average more quickly than the text-only version, in 1.5 minutes (Fig. 165.3). The CDLQI is available in over 44 languages, including six cultural adaptations; a cartoon version is available in 10 languages [22]. The CDLQI is validated for use in children aged from 4 to 16 years old. It has been used outside this age range; there is close correlation with adult DLQI scores between the ages of 16 and 18 years, although the mean score for the DLQI was slightly lower [23].

The CDLQI has been used in 28 countries in over 102 clinical studies [14]. It has been used in 14 skin conditions and in the assessment of 11 topical drugs, nine systemic drugs, 13 therapeutic interventions and two epidemiological and other studies. There is evidence of high internal consistency, test–retest reliability, responsiveness to change, and significant correlation with other subjective and objective measures [14].

The CDLQI score is calculated by summing each of the questions, giving a score range from 0 to 30, a higher score indicates a higher impact on QoL. Score descriptor bands have been described [24]; a score of greater than 13 means that a skin disease is having a very large effect on the child's life (Box 165.3). It is important to note that the CDLQI score descriptor bands are different from those validated for the adult DLQI [25] and that CDLQI scores should not be combined with DLQI scores [26]. The CDLQI score descriptor bands give clinical meaning to the scores and so make the CDLQI potentially useful clinically to support or inform clinical decision making concerning therapy.

It would be useful to know the minimal clinically important difference (MCID) of CDLQI scores; this information is not yet available, although it is likely that the MCID of the CDLQI will be of a similar order to that described for the adult DLQI [27], in the range of 3–5. In a survey of 67 studies using the CDLQI [28], most skin conditions had a mean 'small' impact on QoL (Fig. 165.4). However, the range of reported scores was wide and an important proportion of children with many common skin conditions experience a very large effect on QoL.

Teenagers

Many aspects of the lives of teenagers are clearly different from the lives of adults or of children [29]. The development of independent lives and of relationships and emerging sexuality are obvious aspects that may be affected by skin disease but may not be captured by QoL measures designed for children or adults. Skindex-Teen is a questionnaire designed for use in teenagers [30] and was based on clinical expertise, literature review and expert opinion, and was later piloted on adolescents themselves. Another separately developed questionnaire, Teenagers Quality of Life (T-QoL), was based on information directly from interviewing teenagers with skin disease [31].

Skindex-Teen

Skindex-Teen is a 21-item questionnaire that evaluates the impact of skin disease on the lives of adolescents between the ages of 12 and 17 years [30]. There is evidence of construct, content and face validity as well as test–retest reliability and responsiveness [30]. It has been used to assess the impact of tuberous sclerosis on affected individuals [32].

Teenagers Quality of Life

The T-QoL evaluates the impact of skin disease on the lives of adolescents between the ages of 12 and 19 years [31]. There are 18 items divided into three domains: self-image, physical well-being and the future, psychological impact and relationships (Box 165.4). There is evidence of convergent validity with Skindex-Teen, internal consistency, test–retest reliability and responsiveness to change.

Disease-specific quality of life measures

There are several dermatology disease-specific questionnaires for use in children, including for acne, infantile atopic eczema and infantile haemangiomas. The advantage of using a disease-specific questionnaire is that the questions are more likely to be specific to that particular disease and so patients perceive them as being relevant, appearing to be written with insight. However, the scores of disease-specific questionnaires can only be compared to scores from the same patient or other patients with the same disease and so the value of the data collected is limited.

CHILDREN'S DERMATOLOGY LIFE QUALITY INDEX

Hospital No
Name: Diagnosis: CDLQI SCORE: ☐
Age:
Address: Date:

The aim of this questionnaire is to measure how much your skin problem has affected you OVER THE LAST WEEK. Please tick ✓ on box for each question.

1. Over the last week, how **itchy**, **"scratchy"** **sore** or **painful** has your skin been?
   - Very much ☐
   - Quite a lot ☐
   - Only a little ☐
   - Not at all ☐

2. Over the last week, how **embarrassed** or **self conscious**, **upset** or **sad** have you been because of your skin?
   - Very much ☐
   - Quite a lot ☐
   - Only a little ☐
   - Not at all ☐

3. Over the last week, how much has your skin affected your **friendships**?
   - Very much ☐
   - Quite a lot ☐
   - Only a little ☐
   - Not at all ☐

4. Over the last week, how much have you changed or worn **different** or **special clothes/shoes** because of your skin?
   - Very much ☐
   - Quite a lot ☐
   - Only a little ☐
   - Not at all ☐

5. Over the last week, how much has your skin trouble affected **going out, playing,** or **doing hobbies**?
   - Very much ☐
   - Quite a lot ☐
   - Only a little ☐
   - Not at all ☐

6. Over the last week, how much have you avoided **swimming** or **other sports** because of your skin trouble?
   - Very much ☐
   - Quite a lot ☐
   - Only a little ☐
   - Not at all ☐

7. Last week, was it **school time**? ⇒ **If school time**: Over the last week, how much did your skin affect your **school work**?
   - Prevented school ☐
   - Very much ☐
   - Quite a lot ☐
   - Only a little ☐
   - Not at all ☐

   OR

   was it **holiday time**? ⇒ **If holiday time**: How much over the last week, has your skin problem interfered with your enjoyment of the **holiday**?
   - Very much ☐
   - Quite a lot ☐
   - Only a little ☐
   - Not at all ☐

8. Over the last week, how much trouble have you had because of your skin with other people **calling you names, teasing, bullying, asking questions** or **avoiding you**?
   - Very much ☐
   - Quite a lot ☐
   - Only a little ☐
   - Not at all ☐

9. Over the last week, how much has your **sleep** been affected by your skin problem?
   - Very much ☐
   - Quite a lot ☐
   - Only a little ☐
   - Not at all ☐

10. Over the last week, how much of a problem has the **treatment** for your skin been
    - Very much ☐
    - Quite a lot ☐
    - Only a little ☐
    - Not at all ☐

Please check that you have answered EVERY question. Thank you.

Fig. 165.2 The Children's Dermatology Life Quality Index © [13]. Reproduced with permission of the authors M.S. Lewis-Jones and A.Y. Finlay. More details and permission for use at www.cardiff.ac.uk/medicine/resources/quality-of-life-questionnaires/childrens-dermatology-life-quality-index [22].

Box 165.2 The 10 areas asked about in the CDLQI [13]. ©Lewis Jones SM, Finlay AY 1994

1. Symptoms
2. Embarrassment
3. Friendships
4. Clothes
5. Playing
6. Sports
7. School/holiday activities
8. Teasing
9. Sleep
10. Treatment

Adapted from Lewis-Jones and Finlay [13]. Reproduced with permission of John Wiley & Sons Ltd.

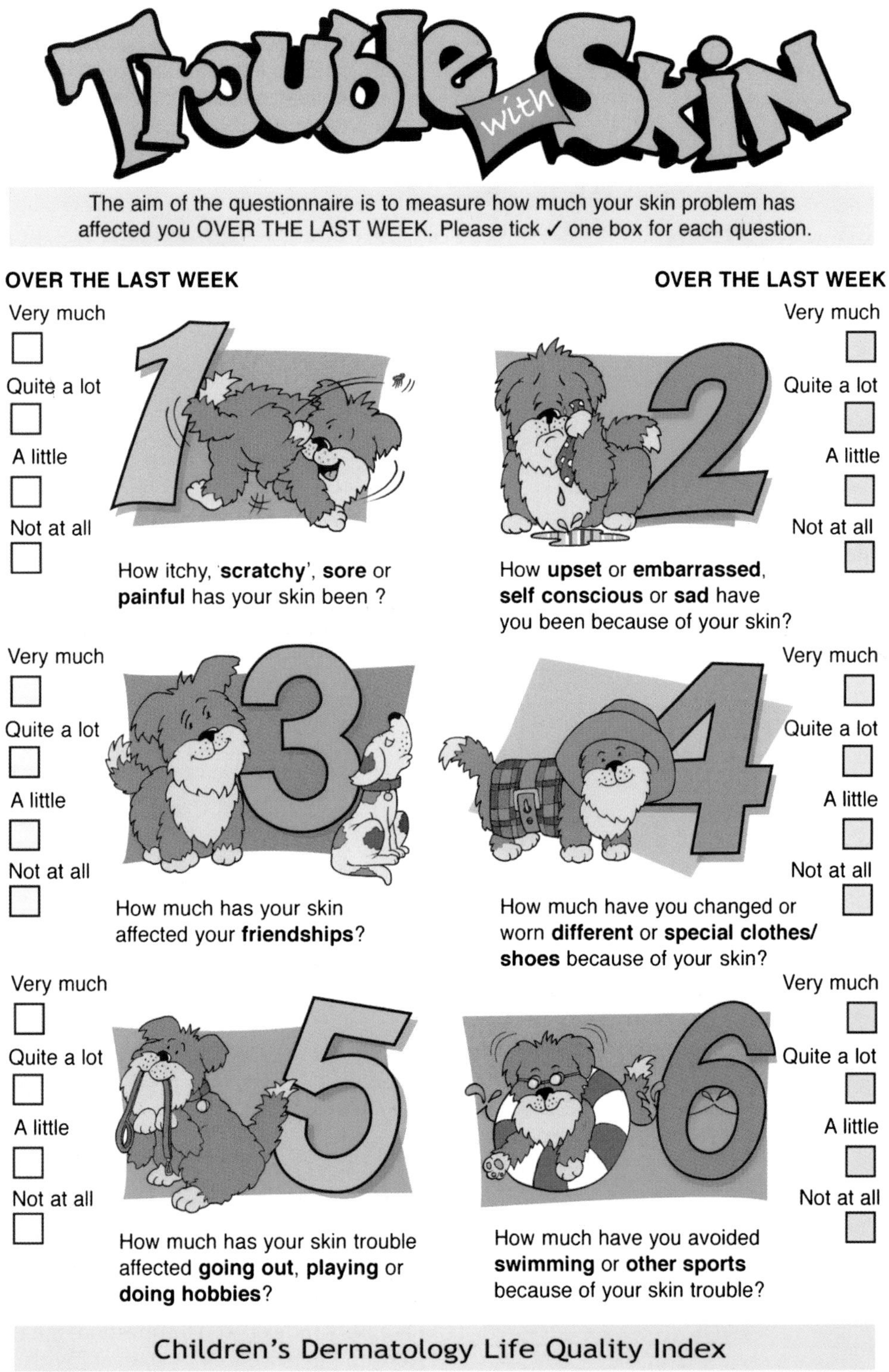

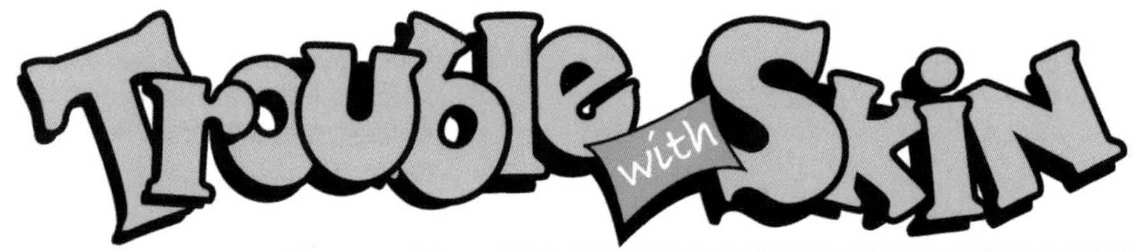

The aim of the questionnaire is to measure how much your skin problem has affected you OVER THE LAST WEEK. Please tick ✓ one box for each question.

OVER THE LAST WEEK

1. How itchy, '**scratchy**', **sore** or **painful** has your skin been ?
   Very much ☐ Quite a lot ☐ A little ☐ Not at all ☐

2. How **upset** or **embarrassed**, **self conscious** or **sad** have you been because of your skin?
   Very much ☐ Quite a lot ☐ A little ☐ Not at all ☐

3. How much has your skin affected your **friendships**?
   Very much ☐ Quite a lot ☐ A little ☐ Not at all ☐

4. How much have you changed or worn **different** or **special clothes/ shoes** because of your skin?
   Very much ☐ Quite a lot ☐ A little ☐ Not at all ☐

5. How much has your skin trouble affected **going out**, **playing** or **doing hobbies**?
   Very much ☐ Quite a lot ☐ A little ☐ Not at all ☐

6. How much have you avoided **swimming** or **other sports** because of your skin trouble?
   Very much ☐ Quite a lot ☐ A little ☐ Not at all ☐

Children's Dermatology Life Quality Index

Fig. 165.3 The cartoon version of the Children's Dermatology Life Quality Index © [17]. Reproduced with permission of the authors M.S. Lewis-Jones and A.Y. Finlay. More details and permission for use at www.cardiff.ac.uk/medicine/resources/quality-of-life-questionnaires/childrens-dermatology-life-quality-index [22].

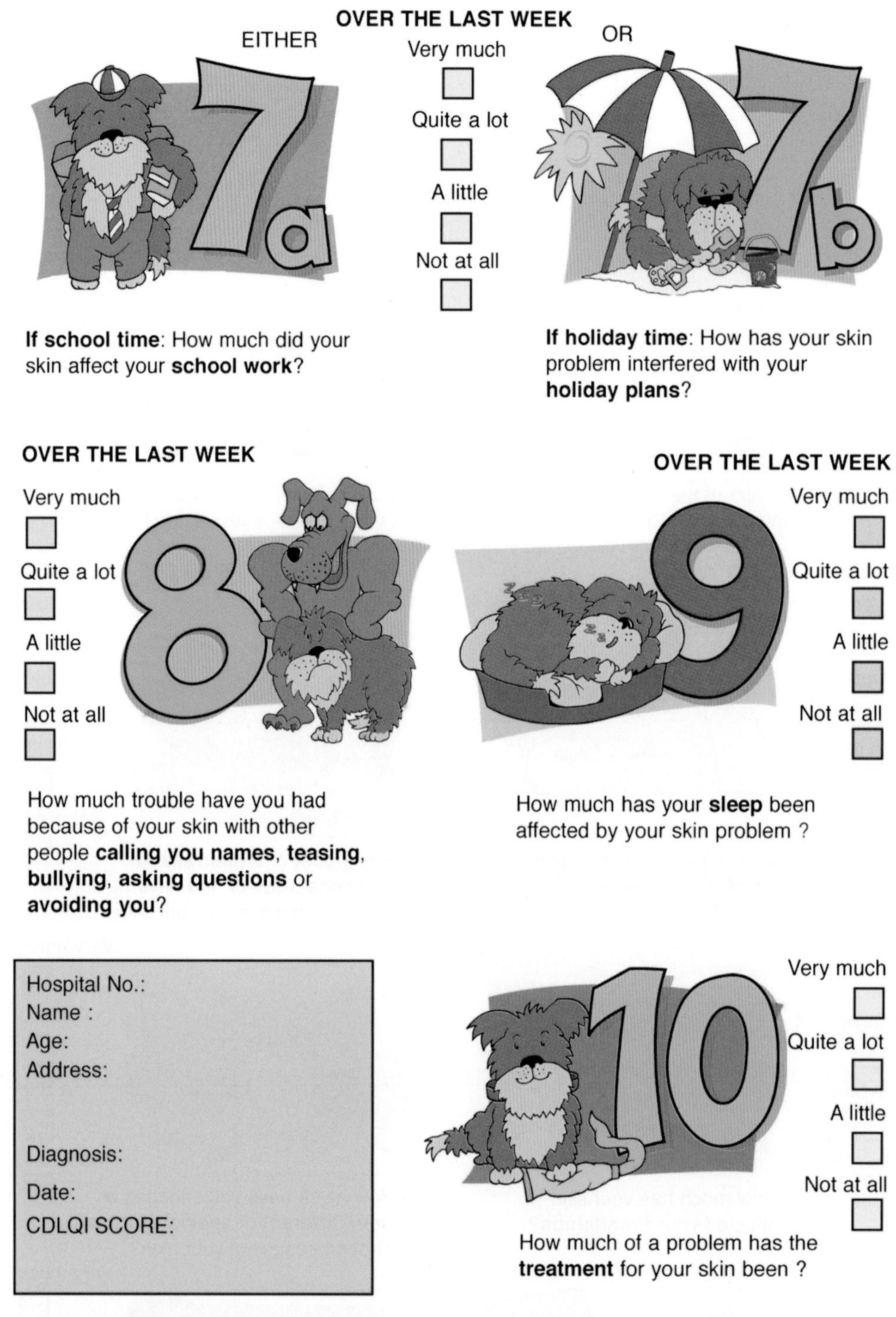
OVER THE LAST WEEK
EITHER
OR
Very much
Quite a lot
A little
Not at all
7a
7b
If school time: How much did your skin affect your school work?
If holiday time: How has your skin problem interfered with your holiday plans?
OVER THE LAST WEEK
Very much
Quite a lot
A little
Not at all
8
How much trouble have you had because of your skin with other people calling you names, teasing, bullying, asking questions or avoiding you?
OVER THE LAST WEEK
Very much
Quite a lot
A little
Not at all
9
How much has your sleep been affected by your skin problem ?
Hospital No.:
Name :
Age:
Address:
Diagnosis:
Date:
CDLQI SCORE:
10
Very much
Quite a lot
A little
Not at all
How much of a problem has the treatment for your skin been ?
Please check that you have answered EVERY question. Thank you.
© Children's Dermatology Life Quality Index. M S Lewis-Jones, A Y Finlay, June 1993.
Illustrations © Media Resources Centre, UWCM, Dec 1996.

Fig. 165.3 *(Continued)*

Box 165.3 The score descriptor bands of the CDLQI [24]

0–1 = no effect on child's life
2–6 = small effect
7–12 = moderate effect
13–18 = very large effect
19–30 = extremely large effect

Source: Waters et al. [24].

Cardiff Acne Disability Index (CADI)

The CADI is a simple five-item questionnaire [33], derived from the much longer and more complex Acne Disability Index [34]. The questions are therefore derived from the experiences of patients with acne. The questions address negative feelings, social life and relationships, use of public changing facilities, feelings about skin appearance and a question concerning perception

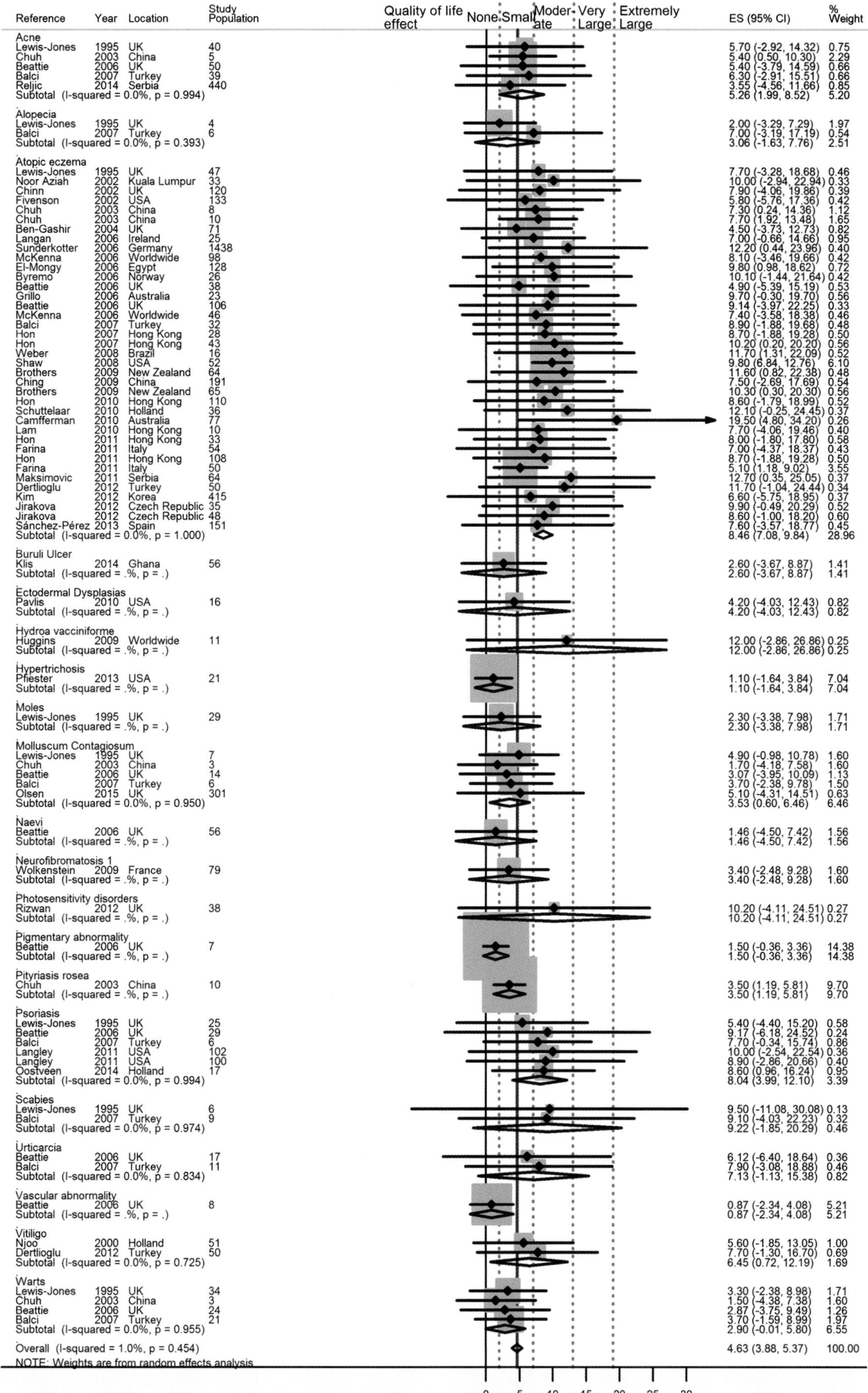

Reference Year Location Study Population
Quality of life effect
None
Small
Moderate
Very Large
Extremely Large
ES (95% CI)
% Weight
Acne
Lewis-Jones 1995 UK 40 5.70 (-2.92, 14.32) 0.75
Chuh 2003 China 5 5.40 (0.50, 10.30) 2.29
Beattie 2006 UK 50 5.40 (-3.79, 14.59) 0.66
Balci 2007 Turkey 39 6.30 (-2.91, 15.51) 0.66
Reljic 2014 Serbia 440 3.55 (-4.56, 11.66) 0.85
Subtotal (I-squared = 0.0%, p = 0.994) 5.26 (1.99, 8.52) 5.20
Alopecia
Lewis-Jones 1995 UK 4 2.00 (-3.29, 7.29) 1.97
Balci 2007 Turkey 6 7.00 (-3.19, 17.19) 0.54
Subtotal (I-squared = 0.0%, p = 0.393) 3.06 (-1.63, 7.76) 2.51
Atopic eczema
Lewis-Jones 1995 UK 47 7.70 (-3.28, 18.68) 0.46
Noor Aziah 2002 Kuala Lumpur 33 10.00 (-2.94, 22.94) 0.33
Chinn 2002 UK 120 7.90 (-4.06, 19.86) 0.39
Fivenson 2002 USA 133 5.80 (-5.76, 17.36) 0.42
Chuh 2003 China 8 7.30 (0.24, 14.36) 1.12
Chuh 2003 China 10 7.70 (1.92, 13.48) 1.65
Ben-Gashir 2004 UK 71 4.50 (-3.73, 12.73) 0.82
Langan 2006 Ireland 25 7.00 (-0.66, 14.66) 0.95
Sunderkotter 2006 Germany 1438 12.20 (0.44, 23.96) 0.40
McKenna 2006 Worldwide 98 8.10 (-3.46, 19.66) 0.42
El-Mongy 2006 Egypt 128 9.80 (0.98, 18.62) 0.72
Byremo 2006 Norway 26 10.10 (-1.44, 21.64) 0.42
Beattie 2006 UK 38 4.90 (-5.39, 15.19) 0.53
Grillo 2006 Australia 23 9.70 (-0.30, 19.70) 0.56
Beattie 2006 UK 106 9.14 (-3.97, 22.25) 0.33
McKenna 2006 Worldwide 46 7.40 (-3.58, 18.38) 0.46
Balci 2007 Turkey 32 8.90 (-1.88, 19.68) 0.48
Hon 2007 Hong Kong 28 8.70 (-1.88, 19.28) 0.50
Hon 2007 Hong Kong 43 10.20 (0.20, 20.20) 0.56
Weber 2008 Brazil 16 11.70 (1.31, 22.09) 0.52
Shaw 2008 USA 52 9.80 (6.84, 12.76) 6.10
Brothers 2009 New Zealand 64 11.60 (0.82, 22.38) 0.48
Ching 2009 China 191 7.50 (-2.69, 17.69) 0.54
Brothers 2009 New Zealand 65 10.30 (0.30, 20.30) 0.56
Hon 2010 Hong Kong 110 8.60 (-1.79, 18.99) 0.52
Schuttelaar 2010 Holland 36 12.10 (-0.25, 24.45) 0.37
Camfferman 2010 Australia 77 19.50 (4.80, 34.20) 0.26
Lam 2010 Hong Kong 10 7.70 (-4.06, 19.46) 0.40
Hon 2011 Hong Kong 33 8.00 (-1.80, 17.80) 0.58
Farina 2011 Italy 54 7.00 (-4.37, 18.37) 0.43
Hon 2011 Hong Kong 108 8.70 (-1.88, 19.28) 0.50
Farina 2011 Italy 50 5.10 (1.18, 9.02) 3.55
Maksimovic 2011 Serbia 64 12.70 (0.35, 25.05) 0.37
Dertlioglu 2012 Turkey 50 11.70 (-1.04, 24.44) 0.34
Kim 2012 Korea 415 6.60 (-5.75, 18.95) 0.37
Jirakova 2012 Czech Republic 35 9.90 (-0.49, 20.29) 0.52
Jirakova 2012 Czech Republic 48 8.60 (-1.00, 18.20) 0.60
Sánchez-Pérez 2013 Spain 151 7.60 (-3.57, 18.77) 0.45
Subtotal (I-squared = 0.0%, p = 1.000) 8.46 (7.08, 9.84) 28.96
Buruli Ulcer
Klis 2014 Ghana 56 2.60 (-3.67, 8.87) 1.41
Subtotal (I-squared = .%, p = .) 2.60 (-3.67, 8.87) 1.41
Ectodermal Dysplasias
Pavlis 2010 USA 16 4.20 (-4.03, 12.43) 0.82
Subtotal (I-squared = .%, p = .) 4.20 (-4.03, 12.43) 0.82
Hydroa vacciniforme
Huggins 2009 Worldwide 11 12.00 (-2.86, 26.86) 0.25
Subtotal (I-squared = .%, p = .) 12.00 (-2.86, 26.86) 0.25
Hypertrichosis
Pfiester 2013 USA 21 1.10 (-1.64, 3.84) 7.04
Subtotal (I-squared = .%, p = .) 1.10 (-1.64, 3.84) 7.04
Moles
Lewis-Jones 1995 UK 29 2.30 (-3.38, 7.98) 1.71
Subtotal (I-squared = .%, p = .) 2.30 (-3.38, 7.98) 1.71
Molluscum Contagiosum
Lewis-Jones 1995 UK 7 4.90 (-0.98, 10.78) 1.60
Chuh 2003 China 3 1.70 (-4.18, 7.58) 1.60
Beattie 2006 UK 14 3.07 (-3.95, 10.09) 1.13
Balci 2007 Turkey 6 3.70 (-2.38, 9.78) 1.50
Olsen 2015 UK 301 5.10 (-4.31, 14.51) 0.63
Subtotal (I-squared = 0.0%, p = 0.950) 3.53 (0.60, 6.46) 6.46
Naevi
Beattie 2006 UK 56 1.46 (-4.50, 7.42) 1.56
Subtotal (I-squared = .%, p = .) 1.46 (-4.50, 7.42) 1.56
Neurofibromatosis 1
Wolkenstein 2009 France 79 3.40 (-2.48, 9.28) 1.60
Subtotal (I-squared = .%, p = .) 3.40 (-2.48, 9.28) 1.60
Photosensitivity disorders
Rizwan 2012 UK 38 10.20 (-4.11, 24.51) 0.27
Subtotal (I-squared = .%, p = .) 10.20 (-4.11, 24.51) 0.27
Pigmentary abnormality
Beattie 2006 UK 7 1.50 (-0.36, 3.36) 14.38
Subtotal (I-squared = .%, p = .) 1.50 (-0.36, 3.36) 14.38
Pityriasis rosea
Chuh 2003 China 10 3.50 (1.19, 5.81) 9.70
Subtotal (I-squared = .%, p = .) 3.50 (1.19, 5.81) 9.70
Psoriasis
Lewis-Jones 1995 UK 25 5.40 (-4.40, 15.20) 0.58
Beattie 2006 UK 29 9.17 (-6.18, 24.52) 0.24
Balci 2007 Turkey 6 7.70 (-0.34, 15.74) 0.86
Langley 2011 USA 102 10.00 (-2.54, 22.54) 0.36
Langley 2011 USA 100 8.90 (-2.86, 20.66) 0.40
Oostveen 2014 Holland 17 8.60 (0.96, 16.24) 0.95
Subtotal (I-squared = 0.0%, p = 0.994) 8.04 (3.99, 12.10) 3.39
Scabies
Lewis-Jones 1995 UK 6 9.50 (-11.08, 30.08) 0.13
Balci 2007 Turkey 9 9.10 (-4.03, 22.23) 0.32
Subtotal (I-squared = 0.0%, p = 0.974) 9.22 (-1.85, 20.29) 0.46
Urticarcia
Beattie 2006 UK 17 6.12 (-6.40, 18.64) 0.36
Balci 2007 Turkey 11 7.90 (-3.08, 18.88) 0.46
Subtotal (I-squared = 0.0%, p = 0.834) 7.13 (-1.13, 15.38) 0.82
Vascular abnormality
Beattie 2006 UK 8 0.87 (-2.34, 4.08) 5.21
Subtotal (I-squared = .%, p = .) 0.87 (-2.34, 4.08) 5.21
Vitiligo
Njoo 2000 Holland 51 5.60 (-1.85, 13.05) 1.00
Dertlioglu 2012 Turkey 50 7.70 (-1.30, 16.70) 0.69
Subtotal (I-squared = 0.0%, p = 0.725) 6.45 (0.72, 12.19) 1.69
Warts
Lewis-Jones 1995 UK 34 3.30 (-2.38, 8.98) 1.71
Chuh 2003 China 3 1.50 (-4.38, 7.38) 1.60
Beattie 2006 UK 24 2.87 (-3.75, 9.49) 1.26
Balci 2007 Turkey 21 3.70 (-1.59, 8.99) 1.97
Subtotal (I-squared = 0.0%, p = 0.955) 2.90 (-0.01, 5.80) 6.55
Overall (I-squared = 1.0%, p = 0.454) 4.63 (3.88, 5.37) 100.00
NOTE: Weights are from random effects analysis
0 5 10 15 20 25 30

Fig. 165.4 Comparison of mean CDLQI scores by skin condition. Note: CDLQI scores reported in 67 studies. Each horizontal line represents the range of scores with the mean indicated. The solid vertical line represents the overall mean. The dotted vertical lines divide the score band descriptors (4): 0–1 = no effect on QoL, 2–6 small effect, 7–12 moderate effect, 13–18 very large effect, 19–30 extremely large effect. Source: Olsen et al. [28]. Reprinted with permission of John Wiley & Sons Ltd.

Box 165.4 The 18 aspects of the lives of teenagers asked about in the T-QoL questionnaire [31].

Self-image
Self-conscious
Upset
Look different
People stare
Embarrassed
Uncomfortable with people
Prevent going to places
Cover skin

Physical well-being and the future
Job/studies
Worry about future career
Pain/discomfort
Sleep

Psychological impact and relationships
Annoyed
Think about skin
Avoid meeting people
Unfriendly comments
Relationship with friends
Intimate relationships

Adapted from Basra et al. [31].

of severity. The CADI can be used in teenagers and in adults. It is available in 15 languages and has been used in over 15 countries [22].

Assessments of the Psychological and Social Effects of Acne (APSEA)

The APSEA questionnaire [35,36] has 15 questions, some of which relate to the overall impact of acne and some to the recent past.

Acne QoL Index

The Acne QoL index [37] is a 19-item questionnaire covering self-perception, role-emotional, role-social and acne symptoms. The total score is calculated by summing the scores from each of these sections; a higher score indicates better QoL.

Atopic dermatitis

There are several atopic dermatitis QoL measures designed for use in children, including CADIS [38,39], described in Chapter **000**. The use of QoL measures in the management of atopic dermatitis is described in guidelines [40]. The Parents' Index of Quality of Life in Atopic Dermatitis (PIQoL-AD) [41] is a 28-item questionnaire based on interviews with parents of affected children in three countries. The descriptor 'parents' in the title of this measure refers to it measuring the parent's assessment of the impact of the atopic dermatitis on the affected child, not the secondary impact on the parent.

Infants Dermatitis Quality of Life (IDQoL) questionnaire

The IDQoL was developed by interviewing parents of infants with atopic dermatitis and asking them how they thought their child's QoL was being affected by the skin disease [42]. This is therefore a 'surrogate' questionnaire in that the questions are derived from the parents' perception of the impact that the atopic dermatitis is having on their child's life, and it is also completed by parents, as of course the children are too young to participate.

Fifty-one publications using the IDQoL were reviewed [43]. The IDQoL has been translated into over 26 languages [22] and used in 18 countries, including two multinational studies. Thirty-one studies have demonstrated its psychometric properties, such as test–retest reliability, internal consistency, validity, responsiveness to change and interpretability. However, no studies have investigated dimensionality, carried out factor analysis or described the minimal clinically important difference of the tool. Eight studies used the IDQoL to assess the effectiveness of therapeutic interventions such as education programmes, consultations and wet-wrap therapy, while seven studies described the use of IDQoL in topical interventions [43].

Infantile haemangiomas

The Infantile Hemangioma Quality of Life instrument (IH-QoL) is a 29-item questionnaire to be completed by parents or carers of infants with haemangiomas [44]. There are four sections addressing child physical symptoms, child social interactions, parent emotional functioning and parent psychosocial functioning. The instrument therefore combines information about the child and about the parent rather than focusing on either the patient or the family members. Content validity and test–retest reliability have been established.

The TNO-AZL Quality of Life Questionnaire (TNO-AZL) is another haemangioma-specific tool, but with wider age ranges than the IH-QoL [45]. The TAPQoL is for children from 6 months to 6 years old and the TACQoL-CF is for children aged 6–15 years. Surprisingly, using these measures, children with haemangiomas had similar or better QoL scores than age-matched healthy children, perhaps because more attention was given to affected children.

Generic quality of life measures

There are a wide variety of generic tools that can be used to assess QoL in children with skin disease, or indeed any disease [7,8]. For example, the Pediatric Symptom Checklist [46], that consists of 35 questions answered by the parent, has been used for psychosocial screening in paediatric dermatology clinics.

Other generic measures available for use in children are reviewed and compared by Varni et al. [47] and include the Child Health Questionnaire (CHQ), the Child Health and Illness Profile (CHIP), the Functional Status measure

(FSII(R)) and the Pediatric Quality of Life Inventory (PedsQL™). Hullman et al. [48] give a helpful summary of the CHQ, PedsQL, DISABKIDS Chronic Generic Measure (DCGM), KINDL-R and Quality of My Life Questionnaire (QoML).

The conceptual content of generic measures designed for children has been critically reviewed [49], demonstrating high variability in emphasis of domains concerning body functions, activities and participation, and environment. Many instruments did not reflect World Health Organization definitions of QoL.

The advantage of using generic measures is that it is possible to compare scores with those of nondermatological patients. Such data may be useful when explaining the importance of skin disease, if scores for children with severe inflammatory skin disease, for example, are similar or greater than scores for children with systemic diseases. In addition, generic methods are generally more suitable on which to base utility calculations for economic analysis purposes (see Utility measures section below).

Major life-changing decisions

Nearly all methods of measuring the impact of disease on QoL focus on the current impact experienced by a patient; this is the immediate aspect to which attention is required in clinical practice and the most relevant approach if assessing change over the short term. However, skin disease can have a much longer lasting impact through its influence on major life-changing decisions (MLCDs), such as choice of school or university, choice of career or ability to develop expertise in sports [50,51]. A method of recording the number of MLCDs affected has been developed for use in adults, the MLCD Profile (MLCDP) [52]; the concept is of equal relevance to children but further exploration of this aspect is required. Influences on MLCDs are a key aspect of the concept of 'life course impairment' as applied to patients with chronic psoriasis [53,54].

Family impact

Skin disease not only affects the life of the child but may also have a profound effect on those closest to them, their parents, carers and siblings. In clinical practice, this is most obvious when parents seek help for their child's atopic dermatitis; they are often clearly exhausted and anxious and their own lives are disrupted by their child's condition [55]. However, this 'secondary' burden of childhood skin disease is not confined to atopic dermatitis; when family members of patients with other skin diseases are interviewed, many hidden aspects of this burden are revealed [56]. In clinical practice, the impact of disease on others is often largely ignored; the focus is on improving the patient with the assumption that this will reduce the secondary burden. However, it may be that by addressing some of the secondary issues, using a structured questionnaire, the doctor–patient relationship may be improved and compliance with therapy enhanced.

Methods of measurement of family impact

As for patient-completed QoL measures, there are disease-specific, dermatology-specific and generic measures designed to measure the impact on QoL of skin disease in family members, carers and (for adults) partners. In this context, the term 'carer' is generally taken to refer to family members who are carers, rather than to professional supporters.

Disease-specific family measures

Disease-specific measures include the Dermatitis Family Impact (DFI) questionnaire and the Quality of Life in Primary Caregivers of Children with Atopic Dermatitis (QPCAD) for use in atopic dermatitis, the Psoriasis Family Impact (PFI) questionnaire and the IH-QoL for infantile haemangioma.

Dermatitis Family Impact (DFI) questionnaire

The DFI was developed from interviews with 34 parents of children aged up to 3 years who had atopic dermatitis [55]. There are 10 questions, to be completed by an adult member of the affected child's family, about housework, food preparation, sleep, family leisure activity, shopping, expenditure, tiredness, emotional distress, relationships and the impact of helping with treatment on the main carer's life.

Up to 2012, the DFI had been used in 50 published studies [57]. There are 20 validated translations of the DFI [22] and it has been used in over 16 countries. There is evidence of test–retest reliability, internal consistency, sensitivity to change and convergent validity with other measures. Nine clinical studies using the DFI assessed the effectiveness of five different topical drugs and one probiotic supplement. Two studies assessed the effectiveness of care by dermatology nurses and dermatologists. In the previous absence of other similar measures, the DFI had been used inappropriately in other diseases; it is only validated for use in atopic dermatitis [57,58].

Other family measures in atopic dermatitis

In the CADIS scale [38,39], the QoL impact on both the child and the parent is measured. The QPCAD [59] is a 19-item questionnaire derived from interviews with 33 primary caregivers of children with atopic dermatitis. It has four categories: exhaustion, worry about atopic dermatitis, family cooperation and achievement. The Parents' Index of Quality of Life in Atopic Dermatitis (PIQoL-AD) [41] is a 28-item questionnaire based on interviews with parents of affected children in three countries. The descriptor 'parents' in the title of this measure refers to it measuring the parent's assessment of the impact of the atopic dermatitis on the affected child, not the secondary impact on the parent.

Psoriasis Family Impact (PFI) questionnaire

The PFI was developed by surveying 63 family members of adults with psoriasis [60]. The further validated PFI has 14 items [61]. Although therefore based on adults, the questions would on face value appear to be appropriate to use in adult family members of children; however, there is a need ideally for a new paediatric psoriasis family measure based on the experiences of families with a child with psoriasis.

Infantile haemangioma

Two of the four sections of the IH-QoL concern parental emotional functioning and parental psychosocial functioning [44].

Dermatology-specific measures

Initial exploration of the family impact of atopic dermatitis [55] led us to investigate whether there may be similar impacts caused by other skin diseases. We proposed the 'Greater Patient' concept, encompassing the patient and close family members, to highlight and focus attention on this massive and usually hidden burden of skin disease on family members and on partners of affected adults [56].

Family Dermatology Life Quality Index (FDLQI)

The FDLQI was created by interviewing 50 family members of patients with a wide variety of skin diseases [62]. The questionnaire is designed to be used by the adult family member or partner of any patient, including patients who are children. It has 10 items (Box 165.5) and has been further validated concerning internal consistency and convergent validity with other measures [63]. The FDLQI is available in over 17 languages [22] and has been used in several skin diseases, including in intervention studies as a secondary outcome measure.

Generic measures of family impact

In the development of QoL measures over the last four decades, the forerunners were generic measures such as the SF-36 or the Sickness Impact Profile. However, the progress of measures to capture family impact of disease has taken a reverse pattern with disease-specific measures being created before generic ones.

Box 165.5 The Family Dermatology Life Quality Index.Aspects covered in the 10 questions. © MKA Basra, AY Finlay, Cardiff University 2005

1. Emotional distress
2. Physical well-being
3. Personal relationships
4. Other people's reactions
5. Social life
6. Recreation/leisure activities
7. Time assisting therapy
8. Housework
9. Work/study
10. Expenditure

Adapted from Basra et al. 2007 [62]. Reproduced with permission of MKA Basra and AY Finlay.

Family Reported Outcome Measure (FROM-16)

This 16-item measure was created from information from interviews with 133 partners or family members of patients from across 26 medical specialties [64,65]. FROM-16 is designed to be completed by adult family members, but the affected person with skin disease may be of any age. As this measure was designed to be used across all medical specialties, it provides the potential to generate comparative data concerning the QoL impact on the family of having a family member with skin disease.

Utility measurement

In adult dermatology, the concept of utility measures is well established. For example, the calculation of QALYs, often based on EQ-5D data, is used in the assessment of new systemic therapies by regulatory agencies such as the National Institute for Health and Care Excellence [66]. However, in children, development of appropriate tools was slower [47], although the need for such utility measures and suggestions for possible approaches were recognized [67]. In the Aledan utility study [67], the three most important items identified by children were pets, favourite toy and playing with friends.

Stevens et al. [68] generated 16 health states from interviews with parents of children with atopic dermatitis. This health state classification and values can be used to calculate QALYs in the assessment of cost-effectiveness of interventions for children with atopic dermatitis. Two generic preference-based methods for assessing health-related QoL in adolescents, the Child Health Utility 9D (CHU9D) and the EuroQol five-dimensional questionnaire Youth version (EQ-5D-Y) [69], may be used as the basis for economic evaluation of interventions for adolescents [70]; these could potentially be used in dermatology.

Conclusion

The science of QoL assessment and scoring is still in its infancy or, more accurately, 'neonatal period'. However, it is now possible to measure the impact of skin disease on the lives of children and family members. There is already a wide range of methods available. The challenges for the development of this science are to ensure that methods used are appropriately developed (based on actual patient experience) and validated. If QoL measures are to be of clinical value, it is essential that the scores can be interpreted and are meaningful; raw scores by themselves are of little value in the clinical setting. The developing focus on QoL measurement in paediatric dermatology raises the prospect of improved and more appropriate therapy and frameworks of care delivery.

Conflict of interest

AYF is joint copyright owner of the DLQI, CDLQI, FDLQI, ADI, CADI, PDI, IDQoL, DFI, PFI, FROM-16 and MLCDP. These measures can be freely used for routine clinical purposes. Cardiff University and AYF gain royalties from the use of some of these measures.

References

1 Finlay AY. Dermatology patients: what do they really need? Clin Exp Dermatol 2000;25:444–50.

2 Naldi L. Health-related quality of life: from health economics to bedside. Dermatology 2007;215:273–6.

3 Pickett K, Loveman E, Kalita N et al. Educational interventions to improve quality of life in people with chronic inflammatory skin diseases: systematic reviews of clinical effectiveness and cost-effectiveness. Health Technol Assess 2015;19(86):1–176,v–vi.

4 Olsen JR, Gallacher J, Finlay AY et al. Time to resolution and effect on quality of life of molluscum contagiosum in children in the UK: a prospective community cohort study. Lancet Infect Dis 2015;15(2):190–5.

5 Finlay AY, Salek MS, Abeni D et al., for the EADV Task Force on Quality of Life. Why quality of life measurement is important in dermatology clinical practice. An expert-based Opinion Statement by the EADV Task Force on Quality of Life. J Eur Acad Dermatol Venereol 2016;31(3):424–31.

6 Chernyshov P, de Korte J, Tomas-Aragones L, Lewis-Jones S, for the EADV Quality of Life Task Force. EADV Task Force's recommendations on measurement of health-related quality of life in paediatric dermatology. J Eur Acad Dermatol Venereol 2015;29:2306–16.

7 Solans M, Pane S, Estrada M-D et al. Health-related quality of life measurement in children and adolescents: a systematic review of generic and disease-specific instruments. Value Health 2008;11:742–64.

8 Brown MM, Chamlin SL, Smidt AC. Quality of life in pediatric dermatology. Dermatol Clin 2013;31:211–21.

9 Matza LS, Swensen AR, Flood EM et al. Assessment of health-related quality of life in children: a review of conceptual, methodological, and regulatory issues. Value Health 2004;7:79–92.

10 Clarke S-A, Eiser C. The measurement of health-related quality of life (QOL) in paediatric clinical trials: a systematic review. Health Qual Life Outcomes 2004;2:66.

11 Finlay AY. The three dimensions of skin disease burden: 'now', 'long term' and 'family'. Br J Dermatol 2013;169:963–4.

12 Finlay AY, Kelly SE. Psoriasis – an index of disability. Clin Exp Dermatol 1987;12:8–11.

13 Lewis-Jones MS, Finlay AY. The Children's Dermatology Life Quality Index (CDLQI): initial validation and practical use. Br J Dermatol 1995;132:942–9.

14 Salek MS, Jung S, Brincat-Ruffini LA et al. Clinical experience and psychometric properties of the Children's Dermatology Life Quality Index (CDLQI), 1995–2012. Br J Dermatol 2013;169:734–59.

15 Heinl D, Chalmers J, Nankervis H, Apfelbacher CJ. Eczema trials: quality of life instruments used and their relation to patient-reported outcomes. A systematic review. Acta Dermatol Venereol 2016;96:596–601.

16 Finlay AY. Quality of life in dermatology: after 125 years, time for more rigorous reporting. Br J Dermatol 2014;170:4–6.

17 Holme SA, Man I, Sharpe SL et al. The Children's Dermatology Life Quality Index: validation of the cartoon version. Br J Dermatol 2003;148:285–90.

18 Heinl D, Prinsen CAC, Drucker AM et al. Measurement properties of quality of life measurement instruments for infants, children and adolescents with eczema: protocol for a systematic review. Syst Rev 2016;5:25.

19 Mokkink LB, Terwee CB, Knol DK et al. The COSMIN checklist for evaluating the methodological quality of studies on measurement properties: a clarification of its content. BMC Med Res Methodol 2010;10:22.

20 Campbell N, Ali F, Finlay AY, Salek SS. Equivalence of electronic and paper-based patient-reported outcome measures. Qual Life Res 2015;24:1949–61.

21 Finlay AY. © Copyright: why it matters. Br J Dermatol 2015;173:1115–16.

22 Cardiff University Department of Dermatology. Quality of life website. www.cardiff.ac.uk/medicine/resources/quality-of-life-questionnaires

23 van Geel MJ, Maatkamp M, Oostveen AM et al. Comparison of the Dermatology Life Quality Index and the Children's Dermatology Life Quality Index in assessment of quality of life in patients with psoriasis aged 16–17 years. Br J Dermatol 2016;174:152–7.

24 Waters A, Sandhu D, Beattie P et al. Severity stratification of Children's Dermatology Life Quality Index (CDLQI) scores. Br J Dermatol 2010;163(Suppl 1):121.

25 Hongbo Y, Thomas CL, Harrison MA et al. Translating the science of quality of life into practice: what do dermatology life quality index scores mean? J Invest Dermatol 2005;125:659–64.

26 Finlay AY, Basra MK. DLQI and CDLQI scores should not be combined. Br J Dermatol 2012;167:453–4.

27 Basra MK, Salek MS, Camilleri L et al. Determining the minimal clinically important difference and responsiveness of the Dermatology Life Quality Index (DLQI): further data. Dermatology 2015;230:27–33.

28 Olsen JR, Gallacher J, Finlay AY et al. Quality of life impact of childhood skin conditions measured using the Children's Dermatology Life Quality Index (CDLQI): a meta-analysis. Br J Dermatol 2016;174:853–61.

29 Golics CJ, Basra MK, Finlay AY, Salek MS. Adolescents with skin disease have specific quality of life issues. Dermatology 2009;218:357–66.

30 Smidt AC, Lai JS, Cella D et al. Development and validation of Skindex-Teen, a quality-of-life instrument for adolescents with skin disease. Arch Dermatol 2010;146:865–9.

31 Basra MKA, Salek MS, Fenech D, Finlay AY. Conceptualization, development and validation of T-QoL© (Teenagers' Quality of Life): a patient-focused measure to assess quality of life of adolescents with skin diseases. Br J Dermatol 2018;178:161–75.

32 Crall C, Valle M, Kapur K et al. Effect of angiofibromas on quality of life and access to care in tuberous sclerosis patients and their caregivers. Pediatr Dermatol 2016;33:518–25.

33 Motley RJ, Finlay AY. Practical use of a disability index in the routine management of acne. Clin Exp Dermatol 1992;17:1–3.

34 Motley RJ, Finlay AY. How much disability is caused by acne? Clin Exp Dermatol 1989;14:194–8.

35 Layton AM. Psychological assessment of skin disease. Interfaces Dermatol 1994;1:37–9.

36 Zauli S, Caracciolo S, Borghi A et al. Which factors influence quality of life in acne patients? J Eur Acad Dermatol Venereol 2014;28:46–50.

37 Gupta MA, Johnson AM, Gupta AK. The development of an acne quality of life scale: reliability, validity, and relation to subjective acne severity in mild to moderate acne vulgaris. Acta Derm Venereol 1998;78:451–6.

38 Chamlin SL, Frieden IJ, Williams ML, Chren MM. The effects of atopic dermatitis on young American children and their families. Pediatrics 2004;114:607–11.

39 Chamlin SL, Lai J-S, Cella D et al. Childhood Atopic Dermatitis Impact Scale. Reliability, discriminative and concurrent validity, and responsiveness. Arch Dermatol 2007;143:768–72.

40 Eichenfield LF, Tom WL, Chamlin SL et al. Guidelines of care for the management of atopic dermatitis: section 1. Diagnosis and assessment of atopic dermatitis. J Am Acad Dermatol 2014;70:338–51.

41 McKenna SP, Whalley D, Dewar AL et al. International development of the Parents' Index of Quality of Life in Atopic Dermatitis (PIQoL-AD). Qual Life Res 2005;14:231–41.

42 Lewis-Jones MS, Finlay AY, Dykes PJ. The Infant's Dermatitis Quality of Life Index. Br J Dermatol 2001;144:104–10.

43 Basra MK, Gada V, Ungaro S et al. Infants' Dermatitis Quality of Life Index: a decade of experience of validation and clinical application. Br J Dermatol 2013;169:760–8.

44 Chamlin SL, Mancini AJ, Lai JS et al. Development And Validation Of A Quality-Of-Life Instrument For Infantile Hemangiomas. J Invest Dermatol 2015;135:1533–9.

45 Hoornweg MJ, Grootenhuis MA, van der Horst CM. Health-related quality of life and impact of haemangiomas on children and their parents. J Plast Reconstr Aesthet Surg 2009;62:1265–71.

46 Rauch PK, Jellinek MS, Murphy JM et al. Screening for psychosocial dysfunction in pediatric dermatology practice. Clin Pediatr 1991;30:493–7.

47 Varni JW, Seid M, Kurtin PS. Pediatric health-related quality of life measurement technology: a guide for health care decision makers. J Clin Outcomes Manage 1999;6(4):33–40.

48 Hullmann SE, Ryan JL, Ramsey RR et al. Measures of general pediatric quality of life: Child Health Questionnaire (CHQ), DISABKIDS Chronic Generic Measure (DCGM), KINDL-R, Pediatric Quality of Life Inventory (PedsQL) 4.0 Generic Core Scales, and Quality of My Life Questionnaire (QoML). Arthritis Care Res 2011;63(Suppl 11):S420–30.

49 Fayed N, de Camargo OK, Kerr E et al. Generic patient-reported outcomes in child health research: a review of conceptual content using World Health Organization definitions. Dev Med Child Neurol 2012;54:1085–95.

50 Bhatti ZU, Salek MS, Finlay AY. Chronic diseases influence Major Life Changing Decisions, a new domain in quality of life research. J Roy Soc Med 2011;104:241–50.

51 Bhatti ZU, Finlay AY, Bolton CE et al. Chronic disease influences over 40 major life-changing decisions (MLCDs): a qualitative study in dermatology and general medicine. J Eur Acad Dermatol Venereol 2014;28:1344–55.
52 Bhatti ZU, Salek SM, Bolton CE et al. The development and validation of the Major Life Changing Decision Profile (MLCDP). Health Qual Life Outcomes 2013;11(1):78.
53 Kimball AB, Gieler U, Linder D et al. Psoriasis: is the impairment to a patient's life cumulative? J Eur Acad Dermatol Venereol 2010;24:989–1004.
54 Linder MD, Piaserico S, Augustin M et al. Psoriasis – the life course approach. Acta Derm Venereol 2016;96:102–8.
55 Lawson V, Lewis-Jones MS, Finlay AY et al. The family impact of childhood atopic dermatitis: the Dermatitis Family Impact questionnaire. Br J Dermatol 1998;138:107–13.
56 Basra MKA, Finlay AY. The family impact of skin diseases: the Greater Patient concept. Br J Dermatol 2007;156:929–37.
57 Dodington SR, Basra MK, Finlay AY, Salek MS. The Dermatitis Family Impact questionnaire: a review of its measurement properties and clinical application. Br J Dermatol 2013;169:31–46.
58 Finlay AY, Salek SS, Piguet V. Measuring family impact of skin diseases: FDLQI and FROM-16. Acta Derma Venereol 2015;95:1036.
59 Kondo-Endo K, Ohashi Y, Nakagawa H et al. Development and validation of a questionnaire measuring quality of life in primary caregivers of children with atopic dermatitis (QPCAD). Br J Dermatol 2009;161:617–25.
60 Eghlileb AM, Basra MKA, Finlay AY. The Psoriasis Family Index: preliminary results of validation of a quality of life instrument for family members of patients with psoriasis. Dermatology 2009;219:63–70.
61 Basra MK, Zammitt AM, Kamudoni P et al. PFI-14©: a Rasch analysis refinement of the Psoriasis Family Index. Dermatology 2015;231:15–23.
62 Basra MKA, Sue-Ho R, Finlay AY. The Family Dermatology Life Quality Index: measuring the secondary impact of skin disease. Br J Dermatol 2007;156:528–38. Erratum: Br J Dermatol 2007;156:791.
63 Basra MKA, Edmunds O, Salek MS, Finlay AY. Measurement of family impact of skin disease: further validation of the Family Dermatology Life Quality Index (FDLQI). J Eur Acad Dermatol Venereol 2008;22:813–21.
64 Golics CJ, Basra MKA, Salek MS, Finlay AY. The impact of patients' chronic disease on family quality of life: an experience from 26 specialties. Int J General Med 2013;6:787–98.
65 Golics CJ, Basra MK, Finlay AY, Salek S, for the the Family Quality of Life Research Group. The development and validation of the Family Reported Outcome Measure (FROM-16)© to assess the impact of disease on the partner or family member. Qual Life Res 2014;23:317–26.
66 Pereira FR, Basra MK, Finlay AY, Salek MS. The role of the EQ-5D in the economic evaluation of dermatological conditions and therapies. Dermatology 2012;225:45–53.
67 Aledan M, Gonzalez M, Finlay AY. Utility measure development for children with skin disease. J Eur Acad Dermatol Venereol 2000; 14(Suppl 1):281.
68 Stevens KJ, Brazier JE, McKenna SP et al. The development of a preference-based measure of health in children with atopic dermatitis. Br J Dermatol 2005;153:372–7.
69 Wille N, Badia X, Bonsel G et al. Development of the EQ-5D-Y: a child friendly version of the EQ-5D. Qual Life Res 2010;19:875–86.
70 Chen G, Flynn T, Stevens K et al. Assessing the health-related quality of life of Australian adolescents: an empirical comparison of the Child Health Utility 9D and EQ-5D-Y Instruments. Value Health 2015;18(4):432–8.

CHAPTER 166

Coping with the Burden of Disease

Sarah L. Chamlin

The Ann and Robert H. Lurie Children's Hospital of Chicago and Northwestern University, Feinberg School of Medicine, Chicago, IL, USA

Introduction, 2255
Paediatric skin disease burden, 2255
The family impact of paediatric skin disease, 2257
Biopsychosocial theory in skin disease, 2258
Coping strategies, 2258
Conclusion, 2259

Abstract

Paediatric skin disease may impart a psychological, physical and functional burden on afflicted children and their families. Much of the work on this burden of skin disease, both quantitative and qualitative, has been focused on atopic dermatitis, acne and infantile haemangiomas. Of note, burden varies based on the age of the affected child and the type of skin disease. Valuable resources for coping with disease burden include patient advocacy groups and psychology services.

Key points

- Skin disease is well documented to decrease quality of life of affected children and their families, and many quality-of-life scales exist to measure this burden.
- Symptomatic skin disease such as atopic dermatitis with related pruritus is reported to cause a greater impact on quality of life than other less symptomatic skin disease or skin lesions. Itch and sleep disruption are central to the quality of life impairment in atopic dermatitis.
- Adolescents with acne vulgaris report increased anxiety, embarrassment, social isolation and shame. Acne is also associated with increased rates of depression and suicidal ideation.
- Parents of children with infantile haemangiomas report social stigmatization along with feelings of panic and fear as their child's haemangioma proliferates. Accusations of child abuse are not uncommon for these parents.
- Many patient advocacy and support groups exist for patients with skin disease and are widely recognized to be of benefit. In some instances, such groups may be the primary source of support for a child and their family.
- Patients with skin disease may require support beyond the medical aspects of disease, and they often rely on their medical providers to refer for psychological services and support from advocacy groups.

Introduction

Quality of life, burden of disease and disease stigma are outcomes that are highly relevant to skin disease. Quality of life is a patient's ability to enjoy normal life activities. More precisely, health-related quality of life is an outcome that extends beyond traditional views of mortality and morbidity and includes the health dimensions of symptoms, functioning and social and psychological impact [1]. For paediatric patients, this outcome is not only relevant for the affected child but for their parents, caregivers and siblings as well. Burden of disease is how both quantity and quality of life are affected by a disease. Lastly, disease stigma describes the concept that someone is less valuable or disgraced because of their disease, and stigma measurement in skin disease is emerging as an important measureable outcome. Stigma is particularly relevant to appearance-changing skin disease. Clinicians caring for children with skin disease must help patients with coping strategies, both behavioural and psychological, to improve quality of life for the child and their family [2].

Paediatric skin disease burden

The effects of paediatric skin disease on children and their families can be measured using quality-of-life instruments. Quality-of-life instruments for children with skin disease address this outcome from a generic, skin-specific or disease-specific perspective [1]. In addition, for the paediatric population, many scales are age specific to allow more accurate measurement of disease impact. In recent years, many such scales have been developed and validated [2].

The Children's Dermatology Life Quality Index (CDLQI) is a skin-specific instrument that was developed to measure the effect of skin disease on children from 3 to 16 years of age and is widely used. With this scale, the greatest quality-of-life effects were reported in children with scabies, eczema, psoriasis and acne, compared to naevi [3]. This intuitively makes sense, with diseases with greater symptomatology having a higher impact on quality of life. Another skin-specific scale in Skindex-Teen. This scale has been validated in adolescents with skin disease from the ages of 12 to 17 years with the highest scores

SECTION 37: PSYCHOLOGICAL ASPECTS OF SKIN DISEASE

Harper's Textbook of Pediatric Dermatology, Fourth Edition. Edited by Peter Hoeger, Veronica Kinsler and Albert Yan.

(greatest impairment) reported for atopic eczema, morphea, acne and psoriasis [4].

Disease-specific quality-of-life scales have also been developed. For example, for atopic dermatitis, these include the Dermatitis Family Impact questionnaire (DFI), the Infants' Dermatitis Quality of Life Index (IDQOL), the Childhood Atopic Dermatitis Impact Scale (CADIS) and the Parents' Index of Quality of Life in Atopic Dermatitis (PIQoL-AD) [5–8]. Moreover, specifically, the impact of skin disease on the family can be quantified. The skin-specific Family Dermatology Life Quality Index (FDLQI) was developed for this purpose [9]. While disease-specific scales such as the DFI and CADIS measure the family impact of atopic dermatitis, the FDLQI scale can be used to measure this important outcome for any paediatric skin disease [5,7].

Measures of psychological disturbance are also used in paediatric and adult patients with skin disease. One such study which included teens and adults with acne, psoriasis and atopic dermatitis reported that individuals with skin disease exhibited higher levels of minor psychological disturbances and public self-consciousness, and were more neurotic than control patients [10]. This finding of increased self-consciousness has also been reported in several other investigations of individuals with skin disease.

The definition of self-esteem is the difference between how one actually sees oneself and how one would like to be [11], making this an important outcome for individuals with disease that affects their appearance. Self-esteem and other psychological sequelae have been investigated in adolescents and young adults with skin disease, acne vulgaris primarily, with reports describing low self-esteem, self-consciousness, frustration, anger, increased depressive symptoms, impaired self-image, feelings of uselessness, embarrassment, anxiety, fewer feelings of pride and lower self-worth [12,13]. Moreover, appearance-related teasing and bullying is a considerable problem for some children with acne, psoriasis and eczema and has been an underrecognized and seldom reported morbidity in this population [14]. In addition, suicidal ideation attributed to their skin disease has been reported by some patients [15].

The burden of atopic dermatitis

Atopic dermatitis (AD) is extremely common and presents early in childhood during a critical period for physical and psychosocial development [16]. AD presenting during this period may disrupt the establishment of normal sleep patterns, behaviour and relationships. The multidimensional effects of AD affect not only the afflicted child but the entire family. AD affects the child with symptoms (predominantly itch and sleep distrubance), activity limitations and behaviour changes, and affects the parents by causing sleep dysfunction, creating an emotional burden and imposing limitations on family and social functioning and activities [17]. Several disease-specific quality-of-life instruments have been developed to quantify this multidimensional impact on children and their families, as previously mentioned [5–8]. Of note, impairment in quality of life worsens with increasing disease severity [18].

Atopic dermatitis affects the emotions and behaviour of children in an age-dependent manner. The most commonly reported emotional symptoms for the young child with AD include irritability, fussiness and increased crying [17]. Parents most often attribute these emotions to the symptom of pruritus which may be central to quality-of-life impairment and the burden imposed by AD. For example, sleep disturbance from pruritus can affect daytime behaviour and productivity [19]. In addition, parents of young children with AD describe their children as being more clingy, fearful and frustrated, and wanting to be held more [17,20]. These psychological disturbances may increase with increasing severity of disease [20,21]. Of note, an association between attention deficit/hyperactivity disorder (ADHD) and eczema was suggested in a 2009 publication [22]. Although the authors recognize that this association may be secondary to other disease-related factors such as itching, sleep disturbance or other psychosocial impairment, this finding further defines the potential increased life burden of AD for the affected child and their family [23]. Further studies have since also reported this association between AD and ADHD [24–26].

Limited data exist describing the psychosocial effects of AD on adolescents. Adolescence is a critical time for the development of self-identity and self-esteem [27] and looking different due to skin disease adversely affects teens during this developmental stage. Adolescents affected by AD may have higher rates of mental health diagnoses such as depression, suicidal ideation, anxiety and conduct disorder [28,29].

Coincident with its impact on the child, childhood AD affects the emotional, financial and social well-being of their parents [30,31]. Mothers of young children with AD report a decrease in employment outside the home, poor social support, stress about parenting and difficulty with discipline [20]. In addition, parents of children with AD have many worries relating to disease triggers and medications use, including fear of using topical corticosteroids [32]. Increased AD disease severity is strongly associated with a higher impact on the family, and of note, family impact decreases as disease severity lessens [30,33]. In addition, the child's itching, sleeplessness and parent-perceived stress are strong predictors for a higher impairment in quality of life [34]. These findings highlight the importance of understanding and measuring the burden of disease on the entire family.

The burden of acne vulgaris

Acne is quite prevalent among adolescents and young adults, with over 90% of males and 80% of females being affected by the time they are 21 years old [35,36]. Adolescence is a critical period of life for the development of self-esteem, and when acne or other disfiguring disease occurs during this stage, there is often a negative effect on self-esteem, self-confidence and other psychological outcomes, as mentioned previously [37–40].

Adolescents and adults with acne vulgaris report increased anxiety, embarrassment, interpersonal difficulties, social isolation, shame and self-consciousness [37–39].

There is also an association with depression and suicidal ideation related to acne [15] and this has been shown in cases of both mild and moderate acne [41]. Additional psychosocial morbidity, including embarrassment with social inhibition and isolation, has also been reported [42]. Moreover, chronic stress and anxiety have been credited with exacerbating the disease process itself [43].

Quality of life has been measured in patients with acne using the disease-specific Cardiff Acne Disability Index (CADI), which was developed and tested for this purpose [44]. Skindex-Teen also suggested an impact equal to having psoriasis [4]. This scale and others, such as the Acne Disability Index and the Acne-QoL, have been used in clinical trials to evaluate response to treatment [44–47].

The burden of infantile haemangiomas and congenital malformations

Haemangiomas are among the most common congenital defects, with most lesions occurring in a visible location on the head and neck. One mother sadly described her experiences of having a child with a large facial haemangioma thus: 'Our first years were filled with doctor visits, staring strangers, rude comments and pitying looks. Comments like, "What did you do during your pregnancy to cause that?" were an everyday occurrence' [47].

Complex psychosocial issues exist for parents of children with congenital defects and for the child themselves, and having a child with a disfiguring haemangioma is probably comparable to having other congenital defects such as cleft lip/palate [48]. Drotar et al. have studied reaction patterns and coping mechanisms for parents of children with congenital malformations. In a study of 20 parents of children with various malformations, the authors noted a predictable course of parental reactions. Despite a wide variation in the type of underlying malformation, each parent evolved through five stages: shock, denial, sadness and anger, gradual adaptation and finally reorganization with variable time spent in each stage and varying success in the reorganization period. Some parents reported difficulties in becoming attached to these children and reported a fear of not being able to care for their child appropriately. Some continued to search endlessly for a cause and remained isolated from support while others accepted the malformation as a chance occurrence and were able to seek support from friends, family and support groups [49].

The feelings of parents immediately after the birth of children with malformations include grief, guilt, sadness and a sense of loss of their expected 'normal' child [49,50]. The heterogeneity of malformations and the uncertain and often unpredictable course may lead to feelings of anxiety and a loss of control. The reactions of strangers to children with congenital malformations are another significant source of stress and anxiety for parents. This parental anxiety, along with a perception that the child is more vulnerable due to their malformation, may trigger the development of indulgent and overprotective behaviours toward the affected child [51]. Studies investigating the impact of appearance on behaviour and self-esteem suggest that children with craniofacial anomalies are treated differently from children without these defects. The affected children have been shown to be more introverted and to express a more negative self-concept than unaffected children and these negative self-perceptions and lack of self-esteem continue to pose problems for those with congenital anomalies as they become adults [52,53]. These psychosocial difficulties have a negative impact on social functioning and quality of life.

Tanner et al. sought to understand the coping and adaptation mechanisms for children with haemangiomas and their parents [50]. The reactions of parents were similar to those observed by Drotar in parents of children with various malformations as outlined above, including feelings of loss and grief, despite the fact that haemangiomas generally follow a benign course with eventual involution. One particularly distressing aspect for parents noted in this and other similar studies was the reaction of strangers. In addition to negative reactions by strangers regarding the child's appearance, many parents have reported actual accusations of child abuse. Such social stigmatization, along with a sense of panic or fear associated with the presence of the haemangioma, has a significant psychological impact on these parents [54]. Parents may choose to minimize contact with strangers and maximize contact with familiar adults as a coping mechanism for both themselves and their children.

The adverse effects on the child and their parent's quality of life have been described and quantified using haemangioma-specific surveys [55–59]. One such validated survey, the Infantile Hemangioma Quality-of-Life Instrument (IH-QoL), reported a greater impact on quality of life for parents of young children with haemangiomas located on the head and neck, in the proliferative stage and those requiring treatment [58]. Additional work suggests that the psychological burden of having a haemangioma lessens for older children and their parents [57].

The family impact of paediatric skin disease

Parents, caregivers, siblings and extended family members are often affected by a child's skin disease. These effects can be emotional, physical and functional and may significantly impair healthy family functioning. Stress, anxiety, guilt and self-blame are often reported by parents and caregivers of children with skin disease. When a birthmark or skin disease is visible to strangers, these parents report a loss of anonymity due to the regular occurrence of stares and insensitive comments [47]. Some parents report the inability to effectively discipline a child afflicted with a disease [20]. In addition, the financial concerns may compound caregivers' stress. For example, the cost of office visits, medications and treatments, including over-the-counter remedies not covered by insurance, and the significant time associated with care can be especially burdensome on caregivers [60]. Time lost from work, decreased work productivity and the necessity to quit working have all been reported by parents of children with chronic skin conditions and have broader societal ramifications beyond the family unit.

Biopsychosocial theory in skin disease

Most parents expect and anticipate the birth of a healthy child and do not realistically understand the daily challenges and stress of raising a child. Moreover, when a life- or appearance-altering disorder is diagnosed, the expectation of this 'perfect' child is shattered and psychological adjustments must be made. As with any loss, the child, when old enough, and their parents usually go through a grieving process, best described by Elisabeth Kübler-Ross in her book *On Death and Dying* [61]. These stages of grief do not necessarily occur in a given sequence and include denial, anger, bargaining, depression and acceptance. They can be appropriately applied to the diagnosis of disease, as this is essentially the death of an ideal state of being, which affects not only the patient but also their loved ones. Passing through these stages may allow individuals to cope with the diagnosis and the subsequent life changes.

In 1977, George Engel, a psychiatrist, proposed the biopsychosocial model as a framework for addressing the multidimensional components of disease [62]. The model recognizes that disease involves more than just a pathophysiological process, or what is referred to as the biomedical model. The biopsychosocial model proposes that the biomedical outlook must be expanded to account for social, psychological and behavioural considerations. This robust view of the disease process provides a more comprehensive framework within which a physician can aid the healing process.

More recent models of coping and adjustment expand upon recognizing the significance of the biopsychosocial model by assessing the mechanisms which promote coping. Behaviours including early parental bonding have been associated with positive coping skills in stressful situations [63,64]. It has also been proposed that a child's self-esteem is linked to the parent–child relationship and how the parent reacts to the child's disease [65,66]. For children with skin disease, understanding and application of the biopsychosocial model are especially important. It ensures a wider vision of treatment, wherein the physician–caregiver–patient team recognizes the importance of a person-with-disease outlook, instead of mere treatment of the pathophysiological disease process. These models support the idea that intervention such as encouraging early parental bonding and positive parent–child relationships may improve or modify outcomes. Considering the potentially burdensome impact that paediatric dermatological diagnoses can have on the patient, family and society, a broader view of the disease course is required to achieve this.

In addition, it is also vital to recognize the natural resilience of children in coping with challenges and the factors that promote such resilience. Resilience is determined by the ability to access psychological, social and economic resources. Positive parental and family psychological well-being has been shown to lessen the likelihood of the affected child suffering from anxiety, depression and social withdrawal [65]. Promoting general well-being may decrease these burdensome negative effects.

Multidimensional care of paediatric skin disease begins during the clinical exam with assessment of disease severity in order to institute appropriate treatment. However, the role of the physician in improving quality of life is not purely based on medical treatment of disease. It is equally important to address the patient's and caregiver's psychosocial burden, assessing potential psychiatric comorbidity, especially anxiety and depression. Depending on the findings, a psychiatric referral may be advised. However, even if psychiatric referral is not deemed necessary, other supportive strategies may be appropriate.

Coping strategies

Many types of coping strategies exist and include problem-solving strategies – active efforts to alleviate a stressful occurrence – and emotion-focused coping strategies – efforts to regulate the emotional consequences of stressful events [67]. While most people use both types of strategies, one may predominate due to personal style and experience and the type of stressful event. Stressors that are less controllable, such as a chronic illness, often trigger the emotion-focused type of coping. In addition, coping can be active or avoidant with active strategies thought to be a better way to deal with stressful events [68].

While some suggest that increased emotional stress correlates with disease activity, others report a poor correlation between disease severity and quality of life [2]. Therefore, the approach to each patient and family should be individualized to account for different coping strategies. In addition to traditional medical therapy, psychosocial support, including education, patient advocacy groups and referral for formal psychiatric support and evaluation, can be offered to patients and families.

Extensive education regarding the disease process, treatment and outcomes is required for many families coping with chronic conditions. Without such education and support, patients may 'doctor shop' and experiment with nontraditional or unsafe therapy. Furthermore, when the most readily available sources of information are the internet, parents, friends and magazines, misconceptions are likely [69]. School-based peer education can be offered for children with disfiguring skin disease or congenital lesions as a change in physical appearance increases a child's risk of being bullied [70].

Patient advocacy groups

Although scant supportive evidence exists, patient advocacy and support groups are generally recognized by professionals and patients to be of benefit for children with chronic disease and their parents [71]. Many such groups exist, as seen in Table 166.1, and links to many such groups are available within disease-specific chapters in this book. Most patient advocacy groups offer education and support in multiple formats such as conferences, support groups, newsletters, pamphlets and trained staff. These groups may be the primary source of support for individuals with cutaneous disease, rare or complex, without access to tertiary care centres.

Table 166.1 Patient advocacy groups for children with skin disease and their families

Disease	Organization	Website
Albinism	National Organization for Albinism & Hypopigmentation (NOAH)	www.albinism.org
Alopecia areata	National Alopecia Areata Foundation (NAAF)	www.naaf.org
Basal cell carcinoma naevus syndrome/ Gorlin syndrome	BCCNS Life Support Network	www.bccns.org
Cicatricial alopecia	Cicatricial Alopecia Research Foundation (CARF)	www.carfinti.org
Cutaneous lymphoma	Cutaneous Lymphoma Foundation	www.clfoundation.org
Dystrophic epidermolysis bullosa	Dystrophic Epidermolysis Bullosa Research Association of America	www.debra.org
Ectodermal dysplasia	Ectodermal Dysplasia Society (ED) National Foundation for Ectodermal Dysplasias	www.ectodermaldysplasia.orgwww.nfed.org
Eczema/atopic dermatitis	National Eczema Association (NEA)	www.nationaleczema.org
Ehlers–Danlos syndrome	Ehlers–Danlos National Foundation	www.ednf.org
Epidermolysis bullosa	Epidermolysis Bullosa Medical Research Foundation EB Info World	www.ebkids.orgwww.ebinfoworld.com
Hidradenitis suppurativa	Hidradenitis Suppurativa Foundation, Inc.	www.hs-foundation.org
Ichthyosis	Foundation for Ichthyosis and Related Skin Types (FIRST)	www.firstskinfoundation.org
Incontinentia pigmenti	Incontinentia Pigmenti International Foundation	www.ipif.org
Klippel–Trenaunay syndrome	Klippel–Trenaunay Syndrome Support Group	www.k-t.org
Lupus erythematosus	Lupus Foundation of America	www.lupus.org
Mastocytosis	Pediatric Mastocytosis Organization	www.mastokids.org
Neurofibromatosis	National Neurofibromatosis Foundation	www.ctf.org
Naevi	Nevus Outreach Inc.	www.nevus.org
Pachyonychia congenita	Pachyonychia Congenita Project	www.pachyonychia.org
Parry–Romberg syndrome	Parry–Romberg Syndrome Resource	www.prsresource.com
Pediculosis/head lice	National Pediculosis Association	www.headlice.org
Pemphigus and pemphigoid	International Pemphigus Pemphigoid Foundation (IPPF)	www.pemphigus.org
PHACES syndrome	PHACES Syndrome Community	www.phacesyndromecommunity.org
Pityriasis rubra pilaris (PRP)	PRP Support Group	www.prp-support.org
Pseudoxanthoma elasticum (PXE)	National Association for Pseudoxanthoma Elasticum PXE International, Inc.	www.pxe.orgwww.napeusa.com
Psoriasis	National Psoriasis Foundation	www.psoriasis.org
Sturge–Weber syndrome	Sturge–Weber Foundation	www.sturge-weber.com
Tuberous sclerosis	Tuberous Sclerosis Alliance	www.tsalliance.org
Vascular anomalies	National Organzation of Vascular Anomalies (NOVA)	www.novanews.org
Vascular birthmarks	Vascular Birthmarks Foundation (VBF)	www.birthmark.org
Vitiligo	National Vitiligo Foundation, Inc. Vitiligo Support International	www.mynvfi.orgwww.vitiligosupport.org
Xeroderma pigmentosum	Xeroderma Pigmentosum Family Support Group	www.xpfamilysupport.org

Camps

In addition, in the USA, summer camps exist for children with skin disease [72,73]. Children with different skin diseases of varying severity can attend, as it is recognized that mild disease can still greatly affect a child's quality of life. Many children with chronic disease, skin or other, are not able to attend traditional summer camps because of their medical needs and such camps are of great potential benefit to children who otherwise would miss out on the summer camp experience. The benefits of camps for children with chronic disease have been studied and measured. Camps may enhance health-related quality of life for a period of time, including physical, psychosocial, cognitive and social effects, but further study is needed on this subject [74].

Conclusion

This chapter has described the burden of skin disease on affected individuals and their families with a focus on atopic dermatitis, acne and infantile haemangiomas. A multidimensional individualized approach to caring for patients and their families was suggested based on theory and practical experience with management of both medical and psychosocial needs to support the trend of patient-focused care. Strategies include support of parent bonding and strong parent–child relationships, family and school-based education, and advocacy groups and camps for affected children.

Acknowledgement

I gratefully acknowledge Dr Elisa S. Gallo for her contributions to the previous edition of this chapter.

References

1 VanBeek M, Beach S, Braslow JB et al. Highlights from the report of the working group on 'core measure of the burden of skin disease'. J Invest Dermatol 2007;127:2701–6.
2 Chren MM. Measurement of vital signs for skin diseases. J Invest Dermatol 2005;125:viii–ix.
3 **Lewis-Jones MS, Finlay AY. The Children's Dermatology Life Quality Index: initial validation and practical use. Br J Dermatol 1995;132:942–9.**

4 **Smidt AC, Lai JS, Cella D et al. Development and validation of Skindex-Teen, a quality-of-life instrument for adolescents with skin disease. Arch Dermatol 2010;146(8):865–9.**

5 Lawson V, Lewis-Jones MS, Finlay AY et al. The family impact of childhood atopic dermatitis: the Dermatitis Family Impact Questionnaire. Br J Dermatol 1998;138:107–13.

6 Lewis-Jones MS, Finlay AY, Dykes PJ. The Infant's Dermatitis Quality of Life Index. Br J Dermatol 2001;144:104–10.

7 Chamlin SL, Cella D, Frieden IJ et al. Development of the Childhood Atopic Dermatitis Impact Scale: initial validation of a quality-of-life measure for young children with atopic dermatitis and their families. J Invest Dermatol 2005;125:1106–11.

8 McKenna SP, Whalley D, Dewar AL et al. International development of the Parents' Index of Quality of Life in Atopic Dermatitis (PIQoL). Qual Life Res 2005;14(1):231–41.

9 Basra MKA, Sue-Ho R, Finlay AY. The family Dermatology Life Quality Index: measuring the secondary impact of skin disease. Br J Dermatol 2007;156:528–38.

10 Magin PJ, Pond CD, Smith WT et al. A cross-sectional study of psychological morbidity in patients with acne, psoriasis and atopic dermatitis in specialist dermatology and general practices. J Eur Acad Dermatol Venereol 2008;22:1435–44.

11 Higgins ET. Self-discrepancy: a theory relating to self and affect. Psychol Rev 1987;94:319–40.

12 **Dalgard F, Gieler U, Holm JO et al. Self-esteem and body satisfaction among late adolescents with acne: results from a population survey. J Am Acad Dermatol 2008;59:746–51.**

13 Magin P, Adams J, Heading G et al. Psychological sequelae of acne vulgaris: results of a qualitative study. Can Fam Physician 2006;52:978–9.

14 Magin P, Adams J, Heading G et al. Experiences of appearance-related teasing and bullying in skin disease and their psychological sequelae: results of a qualitative study. Scand J Caring Sci 2008;22:430–6.

15 **Gupta MA, Gupta AK. Depression and suicidal ideation in dermatology patients with acne, alopecia areata, atopic dermatitis and psoriasis. Br J Dermatol 1998;139:846–50.**

16 Laughter D, Istvan JA, Tofte SJ et al. The prevalence of atopic dermatitis in Oregon schoolchildren. J Am Acad Dermatol 2000;43:649–55.

17 **Chamlin SL, Frieden IJ, Williams ML et al. The effects of atopic dermatitis on young American children and their families. Pediatrics 2004;114:607–11.**

18 Hon KL, Pong NH, Poon TC et al. Quality of life and psychosocial issues are important outcome measures in eczema treatment. J Dermatol Treat 2015;26:83–9.

19 **Dahl RE, Bernhisel-Broadbent J, Scanlon-Holdford S et al. Sleep disturbances in children with atopic dermatitis. Arch Pediatr Adolesc Med 1995;149:856–60.**

20 **Daud LR, Garralda ME, David TJ. Psychosocial adjustment in preschool children with atopic eczema. Arch Dis Child 1993;69: 70–6.**

21 Absolon CM, Cottrell D, Eldridge SM et al. Psychological disturbance in atopic eczema: the extent of the problem in school-aged children. Br J Dermatol 1997;137:241–5.

22 **Schmitt J, Romanos M, Schmitt et al. Atopic eczema and attention-deficit/hyperactivity disorder in a population-based sample of children and adolescents. JAMA 2009;301:724–6.**

23 Moldofsky H. Evaluation of daytime sleepiness. Clin Chest Med 1992;3:417–25.

24 Romanos M, Gerlach M, Warnke A, Schmitt J. Association of attention-deficit/hyperactivity disorder and atopic eczema modified by sleep disturbance in a large population-based sample. J Epidemiol Community Health 2010;147(8):967–70.

25 Tsai JD, Chang SN, Mou CH et al. Association between atopic disease and attention-deficit/hyperactivity disorder in childhood: a population-based case-control study. Ann Epidemiol 2013;23(4):185–8.

26 Strom MA, Fishbein AB, Paller AS, Silverberg JL. Association between AD and attention deficit hyperactivity disorder in US children and adults. Br J Dermatol 2016;175:920–9.

27 Smith JA. The impact of skin disease on the quality of life adolescents. Adolesc Med State Art Rev 2001;12:343–53.

28 **Yaghmaie P, Koudelka CW, Simpson EL. Mental health comorbidity in patients with atopic dermatitis. J Allergy Clin Immunol 2013;131:428–33.**

29 **Halvorsen JA, Lien L, Dalgard F et al. Suicidal ideation, mental health problems, and social function n adolescents with eczema: a population-based study. J Invest Dermatol 2014;134:1847–54.**

30 Warschburger P, Buchholz HTh, Petermann F. Psychological adjustment in parents of young children with atopic dermatitis: which factors predict parental quality of life? Br J Dermatol 2004;150:304–11.

31 Balkrishnan R, Housman TS, Grummer S et al. The family impact of atopic dermatitis in children: the role of the parent caregiver. Pediatr Dermatol 2003;20:5–10.

32 Charman CR, Morris AD, Williams HC. Topical corticosteroid phobia in patients with atopic eczema. Br J Dermatol 2000;142:931–6.

33 Ben-Gashir MA, Seed PT, Hay RJ. Are quality of family life and disease severity related in childhood atopic dermatitis? J Eur Acad Dermatol Venereol 2002;16:455–62.

34 Pustisek N, Zivkovic MV, Situm M. Quality of life in families with children with atopic dermatitis. Pediatr Dermatol 2016;33(1):28–32.

35 **Smithard A, Glazebrook C, Williams HC. Acne prevalence, knowledge about acne and psychological morbidity in mid-adolescence: a community-based study. Br J Dermatol 2001;145:274–9.**

36 Rapp DA, Brenes GA, Feldman SR et al. Anger and acne: implications for quality of life, patient satisfaction and clinical care. Br J Dermatol 2004;151:183–9.

37 Jowett S, Ryan T. Skin disease and handicap: an analysis of the impact of skin conditions. Soc Sci Med 1985;20:425–9.

38 Wu SF, Kinder BN, Trunnell TN et al. Role of anxiety and anger in acne patients: a relationship with the severity of the disorder. J Am Acad Dermatol 1988;18:325–33.

39 Krowchuk DP, Stancin T, Keskinen R et al. The psychosocial effects of acne on adolescents. Pediatr Dermatol 1991;8:332–8.

40 **Nguyen CM, Koo J, Cordoro KM. Psychodermatologic effects of atopic dermatitis and acne: a review on self-esteem and identity. Pediatr Dermatol 2016;33(2):129–35.**

41 Thomas DR. Psychosocial effects of acne. J Cutan Med Surg 2005;8:3–6.

42 Rigopoulos D, Gregoriou S, Ifandi A et al. Coping with acne: beliefs and perceptions in a sample of secondary school Greek pupils. J Eur Acad Dermatol Venereol 2007;21:806–10.

43 Chiu A, Chon SY, Kimball AB. The response of skin disease to stress. Arch Dermatol 2003;139:897–900.

44 Salek MS, Khan GK, Finlay AY. Questionnaire techniques in assessing acne handicap: reliability and validity study. Qual Life Res 1996;5: 131–8.

45 Motley RJ, Finlay AY. How much disability is caused by acne? Clin Exper Dermatol 1989;14:194–8.

46 Martin AR, Lookingbill DP, Botek A et al. Health-related quality of life among patients with facial acne – assessment of a new acne-specific questionnaire. Clin Exper Dermatol 2001;26:380–5.

47 Gleason T. Summer's strawberry. J Am Acad Dermatol 2004;51: S53–4.

48 Pope AW, Ward J. Self-perceived facial appearance and psychosocial adjustment in preadolescents with craniofacial anomalies. Cleft Palate-Craniofac J 1997;34:396–401.

49 Drotar D, Baskiewicz A, Irvin N et al. The adaptation of parents to the birth of an infant with a congenital malformation: a hypothetical model. Pediatrics 1975;56(5):710–17.

50 **Tanner JL, Dechert, MP, Frieden IJ. Growing up with a facial hemangioma: parent and child coping and adaptation. Pediatrics 1998;101:446–52.**

51 Tomasgard M, Metz WP. The vulnerable child syndrome revisited. Dev Behav Pediatr 1995;16:47–53.

52 Horton KM, Renooy L, Forrest CR. Patients with facial difference: assessment of information and psychosocial support needs. Uni Toronto Med J 2000;78:8–11.

53 Dieterich-Miller CA, Cohen BA, Liggett J. Behavioral adjustment and self-concept of young children with hemangiomas. Pediatr Dermatol 1992;9:241–5.

54 Williams EF 3rd, Hochman M, Rodgers BJ et al. A psychological profile of children with hemangiomas and their families. Arch Facial Plast Surg 2003;5:229–34.

55 **Hoornweg MJ, Grootenhuis MA, van der Horst C. Health related quality of life and impact of haemangiomas on childrens and their parents. J Plast Reconstr Aesthet Surg 2009;62(10):1265–71.**

56 Zweegers J, van der Vleuten CJM. The psychosocial impact of an infantile haemangioma on the children and their parents. Arch Dis Child 2012;97:922–6.

57 Cohen-Barak E, Rozenman D, Adir AS. Infantile hemangiomas and quality of life. Arch Dis Child 2013;98:676–9.

58 **Chamlin SL, Mancini AJ, Lai JS et al. Development and validation of a quality-of-life instrument for infantile hemangiomas. J Invest Dermatol 2015;135:1533–9.**

59 Boccara O, Meni C, Leaute-Labreze C et al. Haemangioma family burden: creation of a specific questionnaire. Acta Derm Venereol 2015;95;78–82.

60 Mancini AJ, Kaulback K, Chamlin SL. The socioeconomic impact of atopic dermatitis in the United States: a systematic review. Pediatr Dermatol 2008;25:1–6.
61 Kübler-Ross E. On Death and Dying. New York: Simon and Schuster, 1969.
62 Engel GL. The need for a new medical model a challenge for biomedicine. Science 1977;196:129–36.
63 Wallander JL, Varni JW. Effects of pediatric chronic physical disorders on child and family adjustment. J Child Psychol Psychiatry 1998;39:29–46.
64 Thompson RJ Jr. Coping with the stress of chronic childhood illness. In: O'Quinn AN (ed.) Management of Chronic Disorders of Childhood. Boston: G.K. Hall, 1985:11–41.
65 Dennis H, Rostill H, Reed J et al. Factors promoting psychological adjustment to childhood atopic eczema. J Child Health Care 2006;10:126–39.
66 Harvey D, Greenway P. How parent attitudes and emotional reactions affect their handicapped child's self-concept. Psychol Med 1982;12:357–70.
67 Folkman S, Lazarus RS. An analysis of coping in a middle-aged community sample. J Health Soc Behav 1980;21:219–39.
68 Holahan CJ, Moos RH. Risk, resistance, and psychological distress: a longitudinal analysis with adults and children. J Abnormal Psychol 1987;96:3–13.
69 Tan JKL, Vasey K, Fung KY. Beliefs and perceptions of patients with acne. J Am Acad Dermatol 2001;44:439–45.
70 Pittet I, Berchtold A, Akre C et al. Are adolescents with chronic conditions particularly at risk of bullying? Arch Dis Child 2010;95:711–16.
71 Goh C, Lane AT, Bruckner AL. Support groups for children and their families in pediatric dermatology. Pediatr Dermatol 2007;24:302–5.
72 Sawin K, Lannon S, Austin J. Camp experience and attitude towards epilepsy. J Neurosci Nurs 2001;33:57–64.
73 Reddy KK, Reddy KK. Camp discovery: fifteen magical years. J Am Acad Dermatol 2007;56:677–8.
74 Epstein I, Stinson J, Stevens B. The effects of camp on health-related quality of life in children with chronic illness: a review of the literature. J Pediatr Oncol 2005;22:89–103.

CHAPTER 167

Physiological Habits, Self-Mutilation and Factitious Disorders

Arnold P. Oranje[1], *Jeroen Novak*[2] *& Robert A.C. Bilo*[3]

[1] Kinderhuid.nl, Rotterdam, Hair Clinic, Breda and Dermicis Skin Clinic, Alkmaar, The Netherlands
[2] GGZ Momentum, Breda, The Netherlands
[3] Department of Forensic Medicine, Section on Forensic Pediatrics, Netherlands Forensic Institute, The Hague, The Netherlands

Introduction, 2262
Physiological habits, 2263
Self-mutilation, 2267
Factitious disorders, 2273

Abstract

Skin findings which are not the result of a medical condition but rather of the behaviour of the child itself or of one of the parents or both parents/carers are a differential diagnostic challenge to doctors. In cases where there is a suspicion for this type of finding, dermatologists, paediatricians and (child) psychiatrists should all be involved. Physiological habits such as thumb sucking, hair pulling and nail biting are practised by most children of young age. In children and adolescents, this behaviour can become pathological and evolve into self-mutilative behaviour: obsessive thumb and finger sucking, onychotillomania, onychophagia, mutilation of the skin (dermatitis artefacta), trichotillomania, excessive obsessive hand washing and excoriated acne (acne excoriée de la jeune fille). Self-mutilative behaviour must be differentiated from factitious disorders. Self-mutilative behaviour is the deliberate alteration or destruction of one's own body tissue and fulfils an inner need without the intent of malingering. The behaviour in factitious disorders is meant to be deceptive and with the intent of malingering. The 'perpetrator' in factitious disorders can be the child itself (factitious disorder) or one of the parents/carers (factitious disorder by proxy).

Key points

- **Skin lesions caused by self-mutilation may occur in children who inflict the lesions consciously and knowingly, and in children who are satisfying a conscious or unconscious psychological need.**
- **In children and adolescents, thumb and finger sucking, onychotillomania, onychophagia, mutilation of the skin (dermatitis artefacta), trichotillomania, excessive obsessive hand washing and excoriated acne (acne excoriée de la jeune fille) are among the more common habits.**
- **Stereotypical self-mutilation is seen in children with mental retardation, autism and Gilles de la Tourette syndrome. In Gilles de la Tourette syndrome, familial occurrence is found in about 58% of the cases. It can also be observed as a symptom of neurobiological disorders, such as in Lesch–Nyhan syndrome, Prader–Willi syndrome, familial dysautonomia or de Lange syndrome.**

Introduction

Definition. The skin, mucous membranes (mouth and genitalia), hair and nails are the most visible parts of the human body. They are often also the most visible part of one's personality. Mostly, people are recognized by their fellow humans from certain characteristerics that are visible from the outside. It is no wonder that many people try to make that outside as beautiful as possible by using cosmetics, cosmetic surgery or tattoos and piercings. For that reason, it is not surprising that these body parts may also be direct targets for behavioural problems, in which one's aggression is directed towards oneself. This targeting may lead to visible lesions that can be observed by (paediatric) dermatologists.

Psychodermatology has emerged as an important subdiscipline of both dermatology and psychiatry. In many clinical situations, cooperation between the psychiatrist or the psychologist and the dermatologist is necessary for treatment.

Five main categories of dermatological disorders with psychological components are recognized [1,2].

1. Cutaneous disorders that result from underlying primary psychiatric disease.
2. Psychosomatic dermatoses that are mainly caused by pathological stress (such as lichen simplex chronicus).
3. Dermatological disorders in which the course is codetermined by emotional factors (e.g. atopic eczema).
4. Skin diseases caused or exacerbated by psychotropic medication.
5. Psychiatric effects of dermatological medications.

Self-mutilation and factitious disorders (fabricated or induced illnesses) belong to the first category. Skin lesions

Harper's Textbook of Pediatric Dermatology, Fourth Edition. Edited by Peter Hoeger, Veronica Kinsler and Albert Yan.

caused by self-mutilation may occur in children who inflict the lesions consciously and knowingly, and in children who are satisfying a conscious or unconscious psychological need.

Fabricated or induced illness, also known as factitious disorder or pathomimicry (simulation of a serious, known disease), was formerly termed Munchausen syndrome [2,3]. In children, a illness may be fabricated or induced by a parent or a parent figure: factitious disorder by proxy, fabricated or induced illness by a carer, paediatric condition falsification, medical child abuse (formerly known as Munchausen syndrome by proxy).

In children and adolescents, thumb and finger sucking, onychotillomania, onychophagia, mutilation of the skin (dermatitis artefacta), trichotillomania, excessive obsessive hand washing and excoriated acne (acne excoriée de la jeune fille) are most common [4].

In many children, hair pulling (trichotillomania), nail biting and thumb sucking are habitual activities that are practised spontaneously and inadvertently [5,6].

History. Prior to the 1950s, psychodermatology was confined to the study of the role of psychological factors in dermatological disorders. Diseases like urticaria and lichen simplex were the most frequent targets of studies [7]. After the 1950s and 1960s, the character of research changed from anecdotes and descriptions to analyses of large patient series evaluated through a standardized protocol [8].

The term trichotillomania was introduced by Hallopeau in 1889 (the Greek *thrix* means hair, *tillein* means to pull and *mania* means madness). Hallopeau considered trichotillomania to be a compulsive trait in otherwise healthy individuals [9].

Little is known about the history of dermatitis artefacta and self-mutilating behaviour. Tuke (1892) stated that self-mutilation was encountered 'not infrequently' [10]. It was concluded that such behaviour was observed mainly in psychotic or mentally retarded subjects. Although a relationship to eating disorders exists, it was described only incidentally [11].

In 1951, Asher used the term Munchausen syndrome to describe patients exhibiting questionable symptoms and a desire for extensive diagnostic evaluation [12]. Baron von Munchausen was an 18th-century mercenary who, after his return from the Russian–Turkish war, spent his remaining years concocting embellished tales of his adventures. Meadow introduced the term Munchausen syndrome by proxy to describe the behaviour of parents who fabricated or induced medical conditions in their children [13]. The term pathomimicry, as a synonym of Munchausen or Munchausen by proxy syndrome, was introduced by Millard in 1984 [14].

At the moment, factitious disorder (US) and fabricated or induced illness (UK) are used as synonyms for Munchausen syndrome. Paediatric condition falsification (US), medical child abuse (US) and fabricated or induced illness by a carer (UK) are the preferred terms instead of Munchausen syndrome by proxy.

References

1 Locala JA. Current concepts in psychodermatology. Curr Psychiatr Rep 2009;11(3):211–18.
2 Folks DG, Warnock JK. Psychocutaneous disorders. Curr Psychiatr Rep 2001;3:219–25.
3 Reece RM. Child Abuse: Medical Diagnosis and Management. Philadelphia: Lea & Febiger, 1994:266–78.
4 Koo JYM, Smith LL. Obsessive–compulsive disorders in the pediatric dermatology practice. Pediatr Dermatol 1991;8:107–13.
5 Oranje AP, Peereboom-Wynia JDR, de Raeymaecker DMJ. Trichotillomania in childhood. J Am Acad Dermatol 1986;15:614–19.
6 Duke DC, Keeley ML, Geffken GR, Storch EA. Trichotillomania: a current review. Clin Psychol Rev 2010;30:181–93.
7 Alexander F, French TM. Studies in Psychosomatic Medicine. New York: Ronald Press, 1948.
8 Musaph H. Itching and Scratching. Psychodynamics in Dermatology. Basel: Karger, 1964.
9 Hallopeau M. Alopecie par grattage (trichomanie ou trichotillomanie). Ann Dermatol Vénéréol 1889;10:440–1.
10 Tuke DH. A Dictionary of Psychological Medicine, vol. 2. Philadelphia: Blackiston, 1892.
11 Parry-Jones B, Parry-Jones WL. Self-mutilation in four historical cases of bulimia. Br J Psychiatr 1993;163:394–402.
12 Asher R. Munchausen syndrome. Lancet 1951;i:339–41.
13 Meadow R. Munchausen syndrome by proxy: the hinterland of child abuse. Lancet 1977;ii:343–5.
14 Millard LG. Dermatologic pathomimicry: a form of patient maladjustment. Lancet 1984;ii:969–71.

Physiological habits

Physiological habits can be defined as age-dependent behaviour that can be seen as a normal developmental stage at a certain age period. Thumb and finger sucking, for example, is very common in young children and soon becomes a habit, but only rarely continues to adulthood [1,2]. These habits are not rare, and are self-soothing and self-comforting behaviour. They can be seen at all times of day, for example whenever a child is getting tired, does not feel well or experiences stress. Some physiological habits can even be observed during sleep.

Physiological habits are never obsessive or compulsive. They disappear when they lose their function. Continuing after a certain age can be pathological. Physiological habits can result in skin lesions, caused by the habit itself or by complicating factors, such as the development of paronychia and warts in nail biting.

An overview of physiological habits and the moment they become pathological is given in Table 167.1 [1].

Thumb and finger sucking

Thumb and finger sucking develops as a habit in 13–45% of children [2]. The habit is physiological in infants from the early months to 4 years (peak age about 20 months).

Aetiology. The cause of thumb or finger(s) sucking is not fully understood [1]. It gives a feeling of warmth, pleasure and certainty. Trichotillomania in toddlers is often associated with thumb or finger sucking. In trichotillomania, thumb and finger sucking indicates the presence of inner conflicts.

Clinical features. Sucking of the thumb or fingers may cause maceration of the finger tips. In children, thumb sucking is the most common cause of paronychia. Digit sucking is also a cause of radial angular deformity, in

Table 167.1 Dermatitis artefacta, habit phenomenona and obsessive and compulsive disorders

Physiological habit/habit disorder	Age groups			
	Infancy	Childhood	Puberty	Adulthood
Body rocking, head banging, head rolling	++F	+P	–	–
Thumb sucking	++F	+F	+P	+P
Finger(s) sucking	++F	+F	+P	+P
Nail biting	+/–P	+F/P	++F/P	+P
Onychotillomania	–	+F/P	++F/P	+P
Trichotillomania	+P	++F/P	+P	+P
Lip licking/biting	–	+F/P	+F/P	+P
Cheek biting	–	–	+P	+P
Obsessive hand washing	–	+P	+P	+P
Dermatitis artefacta	–	+P	+P	+P
Excoriated acne	–	–	+P	+P
Teeth grinding (bruxism)	+	+	+P	+P

F, physiological; P, pathological; –, not occurring; +/–infrequent; +, common; ++, frequent.

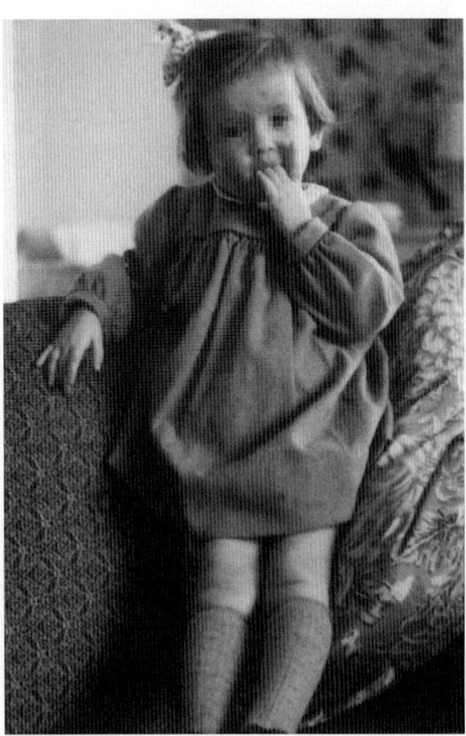

Fig. 167.1 Finger sucking in a girl aged 3 years.

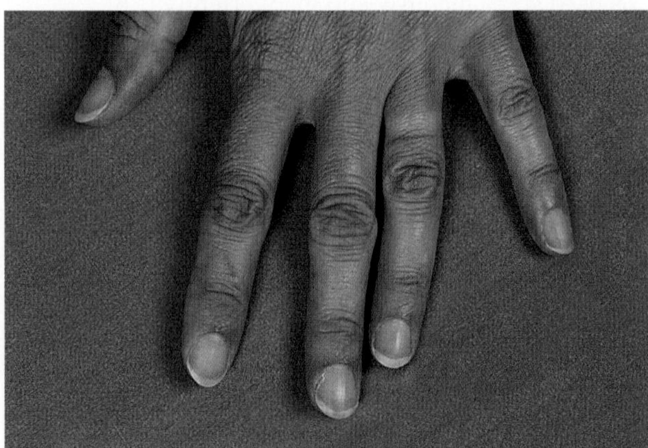

Fig. 167.2 Deformity of the fingers of the same girl (as an adult) as in Fig. 167.1 after prolonged sucking.

which a finger or the thumb is abnormally separated from the other fingers [1] (Figs 167.1 and 167.2).

If the habit persists, dental complications can develop [1]. Between the ages of 4 and 14 years, thumb and finger sucking may have a deleterious effect on dentofacial development [1,2]. A protective factor, especially against pacifier sucking, seems to be prolonged breast feeding [3].

Prognosis. The prognosis is usually excellent. Only rarely will the habit continue into adulthood.

Differential diagnosis. The diagnosis is very easy and simple because the habit is observed. There are no differential diagnostic problems.

Other physiological habits

In neonates, reflex smile, 'sobbing' inspirations and myoclonic twitches are physiological habits. From birth to 1 year of age, sucking of the thumb, finger(s), toe and lips is common. Other common habits are masturbation, rocking and rolling (head banging) and teeth grinding. Head banging is often dramatic and upsetting to other members of the family. Questions often asked by the parents are: (i) 'will it cause brain damage?' (the answer is always no) and (ii) 'is it associated with an emotional disorder?' (in most cases the answer is no) [1]. These habits are of pathological significance only when they persist beyond early childhood or occur in combination with other habits.

In children older than 1 year of age, nail biting, nose picking and habit tics may develop. Except for nail biting and nose picking, the symptoms warrant serious attention because they can be pathological. Males are more likely to have habit tics. Any stress factor needs to be identified and treated. Habit coughs are typical tics in adolescents. Chronic tic disorders can be the first signs of Gilles de la Tourette syndrome [4]. In this syndrome, motor and vocal tics of variable intensity develop between the ages of 2 and 15 years.

Prognosis. Many repetitive habits disappear with age and have no pathological importance. However, persistence of these repetitive behaviour problems may be a manifestation of psychological distress, side-effects of drugs or the first sign of physical disease.

Differential diagnosis. The diagnosis is most often simple because the habit is observed. The clinician must distinguish between physiological and pathological behaviour. It may be difficult to diagnose early Gilles de la Tourette syndrome [4].

Onychotillomania and onychophagia

Nail biting (onychophagia) and nail picking (onychotillomania) are very common, especially among children [5]. The incidence of nail biting has been reported to be 33% in children and 45% in teenagers [6–8]. Before the age of 10 years, the incidence of nail biting in the sexes is relatively equal. Thereafter, it is more common in boys [9]. Its incidence in adults is much lower.

Aetiology. Anxiety and stress play an important role in the aetiology of nail biting [6]. In most cases, nail biting cannot be categorized as a sign of psychological or psychiatric disease. Trichotillomania can be associated with nail biting, but rarely in children [10].

Clinical features. Damage to the cuticle, bleeding around the nails, distal onycholysis and short irregular nail plates are the clinical clues (Fig. 167.3). Nail dystrophy develops in more severe and persistent cases. Secondary periungual bacterial infection may occur as a complication.

Other sequelae of persistent nail biting are paronychia, periungual warts, melanonychia and osteomyelitis [5,11,12]. Nail biting may increase nail growth by 20% [6].

Rubbing the thumb nail and proximal nailfold with the index finger of the same hand results in characteristic median dystrophy. A longitudinal depression in the centre of the nail over its entire length is observed (Fig. 167.4).

Prognosis. The incidence is highest in children and teenagers. This habit normally disappears in early adult life.

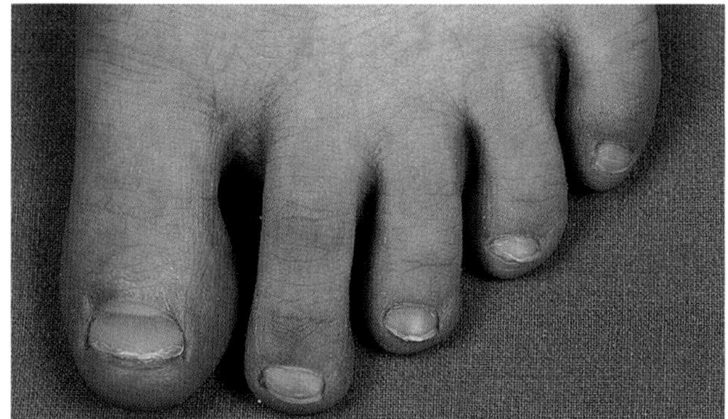

Fig. 167.3 Nail-biting of the toe nails.

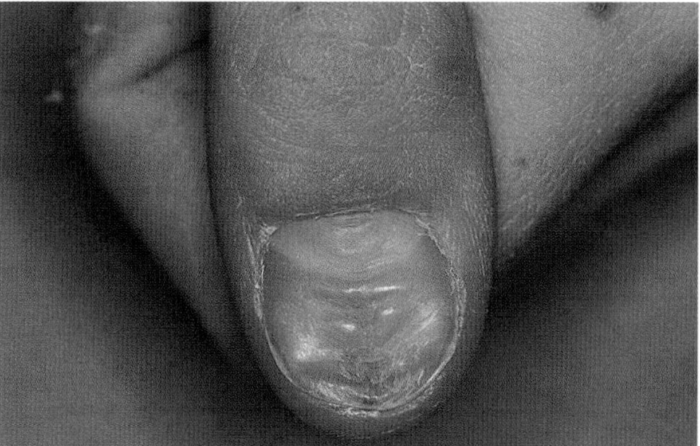

Fig. 167.4 Habit phenomenon resulting in median dystrophy.

Differential diagnosis. Nail changes because of biting should be distinguished from other physical or chemical trauma, as well as from congenital abnormalities and acquired disorders. Median nail dystrophia should be distinguished from congenital dystrophia mediana canaliformis [11]. In most cases it is not difficult; the history is most helpful.

Trichotillomania

Trichotillomania is seven times more common in children than in adults. It is 2.5 times more common in girls than in boys [13–15]. It is the most common form of artefactual disease after thumb or finger sucking [16]. The incidence is not really known, but at a child guidance clinic three cases of trichotillomania were diagnosed among 500 children [17].

Aetiology. Trichotillomania in young children is a habit phenomenon that is not usually a sign of serious emotional disturbance. It is comparable with thumb or finger(s) sucking and nail biting. Trichotillomania occurring later in life, especially of long duration, tends to be more serious from a psychological perspective. Hair is an important symbol of biological maturity. Therefore, trichotillomania may indicate an unconscious, symbolic effort to deny maturity [14].

Pathology. Microscopic examination of the hair roots (the trichogram), obtained using a standardized method, shows few telogen or catagen hairs, but there is an increase in dysplastic and/or dystrophic hair shapes [18].

Trichotillomania is characterized by the presence of empty hair follicles among completely normal hairs. Residual fragments of partially extracted hair provide evidence of trauma. Clumped melanin and keratinized material are seen within the disrupted hair follicles (trichomalacia) and this picture is considered pathognomonic [14,19]. Follicular plugging with keratin debris may also be present. Hair shafts within the lower follicular duct appear small and sometimes have a corkscrew appearance. Extravasated erythrocytes are sometimes visible in the epidermis and around the follicles. Usually, there is no infiltration of leucocytes, except when secondary

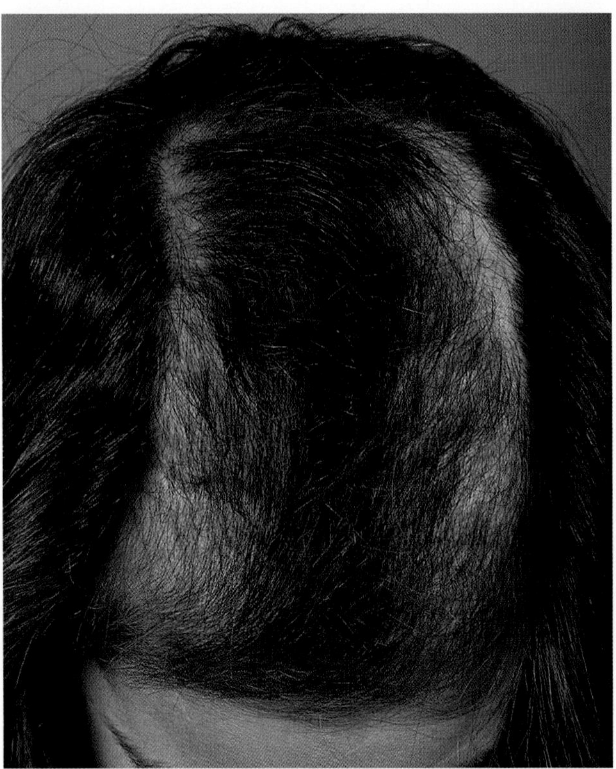

Fig. 167.5 Trichotillomania with 'Friar Tuck' sign.

infection develops. Completely normal anagen follicles are present in the affected areas.

Clinical features. One or more areas of the scalp are affected. The areas may be quite small or the process may involve almost the entire scalp [13]. In most cases, the areas of hair loss are not well demarcated. The eyebrows and eyelashes are sometimes affected. Most often, the areas of hair loss are contralateral to the handedness of the patient. Excoriation and crusts are sometimes visible on the scalp. The most typical pattern is an area of patchy alopecia surrounded by a rim of unaffected hair. This is called tonsure pattern alopecia or 'Friar Tuck' sign, for its resemblance to the hair style worn by monks [15,20] (Fig. 167.5).

Complications of trichotillomania are permanent damage to hair and hair ingestion (trichophagia) leading to a hairball (trichobezoar) in the stomach. Trichobezoar can lead to abdominal pain, nausea, vomiting, foul breath, anorexia, obstipation, flatulence, anaemia, gastric ulcer, bowel obstruction or perforation, intestinal bleeding, obstructive jaundice and pancreatitis [20]. Trichobezoars weighing up to 412 g have been described [21].

Although trichotillomania in children usually presents as an isolated symptom, it may be associated with serious psychopathology such as mental retardation, depression, borderline disorder, schizophrenia, autism, obsessive–compulsive disorder and drug abuse [20]. However, it is commonly an anxiety condition in toddlers and is easily cured [14].

Differential diagnosis. The differential diagnosis includes alopecia areata, psoriasis and tinea capitis. Clinical differential diagnosis between trichotillomania and alopecia areata may be difficult in some cases. History of hair pulling is often lacking, except in very young children, when the parents report the symptom [14]. The presence of an initial area of almost total hair loss favours alopecia areata. Exclamation hairs, a positive hair plucking test (loss of more than five hairs when pulled from the periphery of the bald area), pitting of the nails and depigmentation in regrowing hair in older children strongly support the diagnosis of alopecia areata. Laboratory examination will exclude tinea capitis.

Prognosis. In many cases this symptom disappears with appropriate emotional support and when the child gains insight into the underlying psychological problems. However, one should not assume that trichotillomania will disappear spontaneously, so careful follow-up is required to establish resolution [14]. In a selected population, one third of the patients required psychiatric treatment and guidance [14]. In serious and long-standing cases, psychological or psychiatric treatment is warranted.

Repeated manipulation of the hair in trichotillomania can lead to curly hair, trichorrhexis nodosa, other hair shaft fractures and, finally, to cicatricial alopecia.

Treatment. In cases where the symptoms do not disappear spontaneously, it is recommended that a psychiatrist and dermatologist join the treatment team. Behavioural therapy has a long-standing tradition of success in the treatment of trichotillomania. More recently, a variety of drug treatments have also been investigated. Psychopharmacological medications include antidepressants, serotonergic agents and antipsychotics. Selective serotonin reuptake inhibitors (SSRIs), which are known to be effective for depression, anxiety and obsessive–compulsive disorder, can also be effective in the treatment of trichotillomania [22]. In small children, oral medications will almost never be indicated or even necessary.

References

1 **Ellis CR. Childhood habit behaviors and stereotypic movement disorder. Emedicine.medscape 2015;1–9.**
2 Lubitz L. Nail biting, thumb sucking, and other irritating behaviours in childhood. Austr Fam Physician 1992;21:1090–4.
3 de Holanda AL, dos Santos SA, Fernandes de Sena M, Ferreira MA. Relationship between breast- and bottle-feeding and non-nutritive sucking habits. Oral Health Prev Dent 2009;7(4):331–7.
4 Regeur L, Pakkenberg B, Fog R et al. Clinical features and long-term treatment with pimozide in 65 patients with Gilles de la Tourette's syndrome. J Neurol Neurosurg Psychiatr 1986;49:791–5.
5 Oderick L, Brattstrom V. Nail biting: frequency and association with root resorption during orthodontic treatment. Br J Orthodont 1985; 12:78–81.
6 Leung AKC, Robson WLM. Nail biting. Clin Pediatr 1990;29:690–2.
7 Massler M, Malone AJ. Nail biting – a review. J Pediatr 1950; 36: 523–31.
8 Wechsler D. The incidence and significance of finger-nail biting in children. Psychoanal Rev 1931;18:201–8.
9 Malone AJ, Massler M. Index of nail biting in children. J Abnorm Soc Psychol 1952;47:193–202.
10 Dimino-Emme L, Carmisa CH. Trichotillomania associated with the 'Friar Tuck sign' and nail biting. Cutis 1991;47:107–10.
11 Tosti A, Peluso AM, Bardazzi F. Phalangeal osteomyelitis due to nail biting. Acta Derm Venereol 1994;74:206–7.

12 Baran R. Nail biting and picking as a possible cause of longitudinal melanonychia. Dermatologica 1990;181:126–8.
13 Stroud JD. Hair loss in children. Pediatr Clin North Am 1983;30: 641–57.
14 Oranje AP, Peereboom-Wynia JDR, de Raeymaecker DMJ. Trichotillomania in childhood. J Am Acad Dermatol 1986;15:614–19.
15 Muller SA. Trichotillomania. Dermatol Clin 1987;5:595–601.
16 Spraker MK. Cutaneous artifactual disease: an appeal for help. Pediatr Clin North Am 1983;30:659–68.
17 Anderson FW, Dean HC. Some aspects of child guidance clinic in policy and practice. Publ Health Rep 1956:71.
18 Peereboom-Wynia JDR. Hair root characteristics of the human scalp hair in health and disease. Thesis, Rotterdam, 1979.
19 Lachapelle JM, Pierard GE. Traumatic alopecia in trichotillomania. J Cutan Pathol 1977;4:51–67.
20 Hamdan-Allen G. Trichotillomania in childhood. Acta Psychiatr Scand 1991;83:241–3.
21 Ewert P, Keim L, Schulte-Markwort M. Der Trichobezoar. Monatsschr Kinderheilkd 1992;140:811–13.
22 Chamberlain SR, Menzies L, Sahakian BJ, Fineberg NA. Lifting the veil on trichotillomania. Am J Psychiatr 2007;164(4):568–74.

Self-mutilation

Self-mutilation is defined as the deliberate alteration or destruction of one's own body tissue without any conscious suicidal intent. The injury is done to oneself, without the aid of another person, and the injury is severe enough for tissue damage to result. Acts that are committed with conscious suicidal intent or are associated with sexual arousal are excluded [1,2].

Synonyms for self-mutilation are self-abusive behaviour, self-harm or self-injurious behaviour. A widely accepted term in dermatology is dermatitis artefacta as a synonym for self-mutilation. However, this is also used as a term for the skin lesions found in children which are inflicted by another person in factitious disorder by proxy.

Classification

Several subgroups exist. Hollender and Abram described three groups. The first group consists of patients with an autoaggressive habitual behaviour and recognized, plausible motives, or those who are neurotic pickers and who readily admit to damaging their skin. The second group consists of patients with hysterical and obsessive impulses. The third group encompasses mentally retarded or psychotic individuals who self-mutilate frequently and in the presence of others [3]. Patients with delusions of parasitosis may also self-mutilate.

The most accepted current classification of self-mutilation worldwide is the one developed by Favazza, namely superficial (compulsive and impulsive), stereotypic and major self-mutilation [4].

Comparing Hollender's subgroups with Favazza's classification shows that the first group consists of people/children with the impulsive type of superficial self-mutilation. Hollender's second group is comparable with the compulsive type of the superficial self-mutilation group, and the third group can be compared with the stereotypic self-mutilation group. The group of patients with delusions of parasitosis can belong to either the superficial or the major self-mutilation group.

Self-injurious behaviour (SIB) as seen in children with autism or developmental disabilities is not the same as self-mutilation because usually there is no deliberate intent to harm one's own body tissue.

Destruction of body tissue can be a result of repetitively stereotypical behaviour, stress due to over- or understimulation, impairment of communication skills, impairment of sensibility, somatic problems such as hearing problems or sight problems, and traumatization. The ontogenesis of SIB exhibited by young children with developmental disabilities is due to a complex interaction between neurobiological and environmental variables [5]. SIB in children with mental retardation starts at an early age: 68% starts before the age of 6 years. The prevalence of SIB in children with autism is 24–43%; the combination of both mental retardation and autism has a prevalence of more than 70% for SIB. Treatment involves behavioural therapy and/or psychomedication, depending on the likelihood of being able to change a patient's behaviour [6,7].

A new classification was proposed based on adult patients.

1 Dermatitis artefacta syndrome in the narrower sense of unconscious/dissociated self-injury.
2 Dermatitis para-artefacta syndrome: admitted self-injury.
3 Malingering: consciously simulated injuries and diseases to obtain material gain.
4 Special forms, such as the Gardner–Diamond syndrome, factitious disorder (Munchausen syndrome) and the paediatric condition of falsification syndrome by proxy [8].

The authors of this chapter are not sure that this classification is useful and suitable for children.

Superficial self-mutilation

Superficial self-mutilation is the most prevalent type of self-mutilation. It is estimated that the incidence is between 0.75% and 1.4% (750–1400 per 100 000 persons) per year [9,10]. The incidence in adolescents and young adults between the age of 15 and 35 years is estimated to be even higher at 1800 cases per 100 000 persons a year. The incidence among inpatient adolescents was estimated at about 40% [11].

Superficial self-mutilation has been described in a variety of populations with different ethnic and socioeconomic backgrounds. However, self-mutilation is three times more common in females than in males. The typical patient with self-mutilative behaviour is a Caucasian female, who started her behaviour in her teens and continues into her twenties or thirties, with a middle to upper class background.

In about 50% of cases there are also eating disorders [10]. A survey done by Ensink showed that about 35% of all women who were sexually abused and were to known to self-mutilate started before the age of 12, and in total almost 50% started before the age of 18 [12]. In medical literature, children (mostly child abuse victims) as young as 3 years are described with skin lesions as a result of superficial self-mutilation [13]. Van der Kolk et al. concluded that the earlier the abuse began, the more serious the self-mutilative behaviour will be [14].

Aetiology. Various hypotheses have been used to explain the aetiology of superficial self-mutilation. Psychoanalytical, developmental, personality and biochemical (serotonin) theories have been postulated [15]. The most serious forms of these disorders may be related to physical, emotional and sexual abuse [16].

The psychoanalytical theory stresses the importance of early emotional traumas such as illness, separation from parents and disturbances in the mother–child relationship [17]. Developmental difficulties (e.g. in school, coping problems, physical unattractiveness) also play a role. Van der Kolk et al. concluded that neglect is the most powerful predictor of self-destructive behaviour [14]. According to their opinion, childhood trauma contributes heavily to the initiation of self-destructive behaviour and the lack of secure attachments maintains it.

Developmental disturbances can lead to a poor self-image or lack of self-esteem. The child lacks positive feelings about their own body (even though they are not conscious of this problem). The child turns his aggression against himself [18].

In children, most cases are related to distortion of the parent–child relationship. Another important factor in children is violence between family members (physical, sexual or emotional) committed by an important person, like a parent, and double messages (e.g. loving caretaking and violent behaviour by the same person). The violence and the double messages lead to confusion and the loss or disruption of the relationship.

Motives. According to Malon and Berardi, there is a chain of feelings that leads to self-mutilation [19]. The start seems to be a threat of separation, rejection or disappointment. A feeling of overwhelming tension and isolation, resulting from fear of abandonment, self-hatred and apprehension about being unable to control one's own aggression, seems to take hold. The anxiety increases and culminates in a sense of unreality and emptiness that produces an emotional numbness or depersonalization [20]. The self-mutilation is a way to fight feelings of depersonalization and the immediate tension. It is also a way of dealing with feelings of anxiety, anger or sadness. It can be seen as an important coping mechanism [21]. The feeling of control is strengthened by a sense of calm that is the result of the stimulating effect of, for example, wrist cutting on the production of the body's endorphins [22,23].

Underlying psychiatric problems. There are many psychiatric problems in which self-mutilative behaviour can be observed. It has been described in, amongst others, personality disorders (borderline and antisocial personality disorders), posttraumatic stress disorder, eating disorders (anorexia, bulimia), mood disorders (depression, bipolar disorder), obsessive–compulsive disorders, dissociative disorders and impulse control disorders [15,24]. Many of these disorders have a link with adverse childhood experiences, such as (i) distortion within the parent–child relationship; (ii) violent disruptions in family life; and (iii) in children who have been the victims of physical, emotional and sexual abuse or emotional neglect.

Subforms of superficial self-mutilation. Two subforms of superficial self-mutilation can be recognized: compulsive and impulsive (episodic and repetitive) behaviour.

Compulsive self-mutilation

Compulsive self-mutilation is closely associated with obsessive–compulsive disorders [4]. Obsessive–compulsive disorders are characterized by obsessions and/or compulsions. An obsession is defined as an intrusive thought, urge or impulse that is experienced as repulsive, irrational and ego-dystonic. Compulsion is defined by repetitive, often ritualized or stylized behaviour [17,25]. The behaviour in obsessive–compulsive disorders is meant to relieve tension or to prevent negative events. The acts can be conscious or subconscious.

Obsessive–compulsive disorders may be difficult to distinguish from other causes of superficial self-mutilation [15]. Most observed behaviour in compulsive self-mutilation is trichotillomania, onychotillomania, onychophagia and acne excoriée, although these behaviours are only the result of obsessive and compulsive disorders in a small minority [18,24].

The obsessive–compulsive behaviour can be demonstrated in certain patients with trichotillomania, who pull out exact numbers of hairs, equally divided over each side of the head (front to back, left to right) to prevent negative events happening. Repeated hand washing is most often a form of obsessive–compulsive disorder, which may lead to irritative hand eczema. If this kind of hand-washing tendency suddenly develops, diabetes mellitus should be ruled out. Differential diagnosis of hand eczema also includes dermatophytic infection and allergic contact eczema. One percent of children and adolescents suffer from obsessive–compulsive disorders [26,27].

Although the behaviour is not life-threatening, the prognosis of compulsive self-mutilation and obsessive–compulsive disorder is poor, and the condition often worsens with age. The dermatologist should ask for the help of a paediatric psychiatrist in the diagnosis and treatment. Newer drug therapies, such as clomipramine and fluoxetine, have resulted in optimism regarding the treatment of obsessive–compulsive disorders [24].

Impulsive self-mutilation

Impulsive self-mutilation can be episodic or repetitive. The behaviour can start in early childhood and continue for many years.

Episodic self-mutilation is usually seen as a symptom of a psychological disorder. People who engage in episodic acts often do not see themselves as self-mutilators. The most common episodic acts are cutting, burning, needle sticking, bone breaking and interfering with wound healing.

Repetitive self-mutilation can be the result of episodic behaviour; if the episodic behaviour leads to relief of stress or the solving of other triggers, the patient may become convinced that it is the only way of solving their problems. It can lead to an 'addiction' to the self-mutilative behaviour where the patient cannot resist the impulse any longer. Instead of being a symptom of an underlying psychological disorder, the behaviour becomes a disorder in itself. The patient will see themselves as a self-mutilator. The acts are the same as in episodic behaviour.

Episodic and repetitive behaviour is impulsive in so far as it can be a response to any positive or negative trigger [15].

Differential diagnosis.

Tattooing and piercing

Some forms of self-mutilation are culturally and socially accepted. These can be defined as rituals and practices. Rituals reflect community traditions, very often with underlying symbolic meanings. Practices are used for cosmetic reasons or for (sub)cultural identification; they usually do not have an underlying symbolic meaning [4]. Tattoos and piercing can belong to both. These practices have varying levels of social acceptance and are seen by some as extremely mutilating. The behaviour, however, is not typical for self-mutilation. The majority of people who want to have a tattoo or piercing accept the pain of the process in order to attain a finished product. The person who shows self-mutilative behaviour seeks the pain for the purpose of feeling pain or seeing the blood as a way of escaping from unbearable feelings [28].

Suicidal behaviour

Suicide and self-mutilation seem to have the same purpose, namely stopping the pain. For people who commit suicide, the ultimate purpose is to end all feelings by killing oneself. For people who self-mutilate, it is not the ending of life that is the purpose but to feel better after the act of self-mutilating. Self-mutilating can be a coping mechanism and a means of surviving situations in which suicide seems to be inescapable and the only way out of pain [29].

Factitious disorder

Self-mutilation should be differentiated from factitious disorders. The motives for the behaviour in both situations are completely different. In self-mutilation, the act of mutilating is used to relieve pain. The act is committed in privacy and is usually kept private. In factitious disorders, the injuries are inflicted deliberately and are meant to produce symptoms that will attract attention from others, like doctors, and eventually lead to hospital admissions. The lesions are not kept private although the act itself will be denied by the patient.

Clinical features. Depending on the methods employed by the patient, the lesions in self-mutilation are characterized by excoriations, ulcerations, purpura or bullae [3,30] (Figs 167.6, 167.7, 167.8 and 167.9). Methods include mechanical (e.g. rubbing, sucking, biting, use of bottles, sucking cups, scratching, picking, cutting, slashing, gouging and puncturing), thermal (burning with objects) and chemical (e.g. the application of caustic or hot agents and injections of various substances, like milk) stimuli.

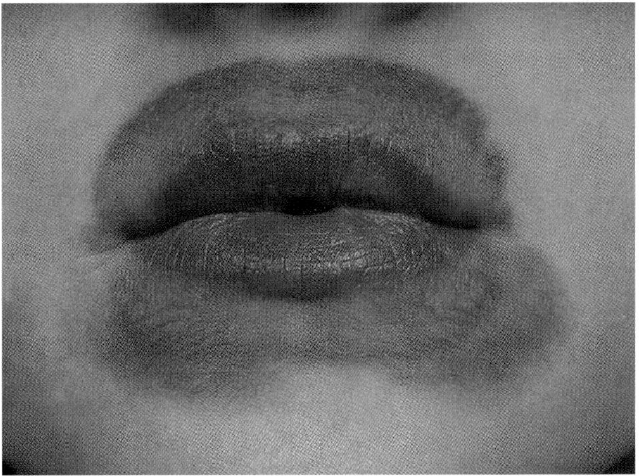

Fig. 167.6 Lip-lick dermatitis.

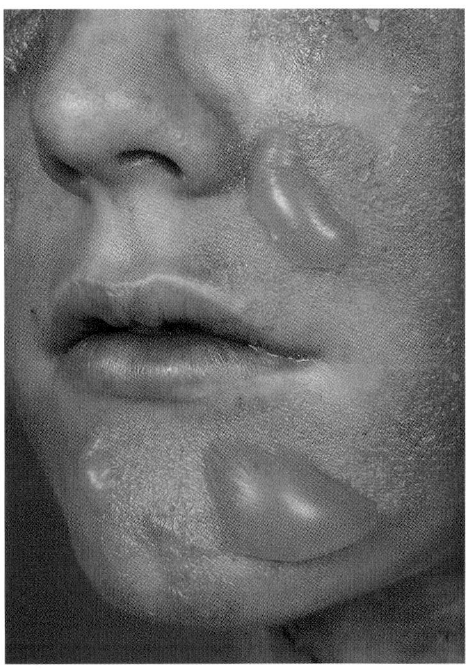

Fig. 167.7 Bullous dermatosis after application of caustic substances to the skin.

The lesions are single or multiple, and occur in an area accessible to the dominant hand. However, the lesions may be symmetrical and bilateral, especially after the patient has been confronted with the unilateral distribution of lesions. A significant sign is the presence of bizarre and angulated configurations. The lesions do not show any pre-stages.

The incidence is higher in females (adults and children) except for individuals involved in purposeful self-mutilation. The condition can be seen at any age, but is most common in adolescents and young adults [18]. The following are the main manifestations of self-mutilation.

- *Cutting*: the most common form of self-mutilation is probably cutting or carving of the whole body or, in particular, body parts like the wrists. Cutting can be done with sharp objects, such as razorblades and glass.

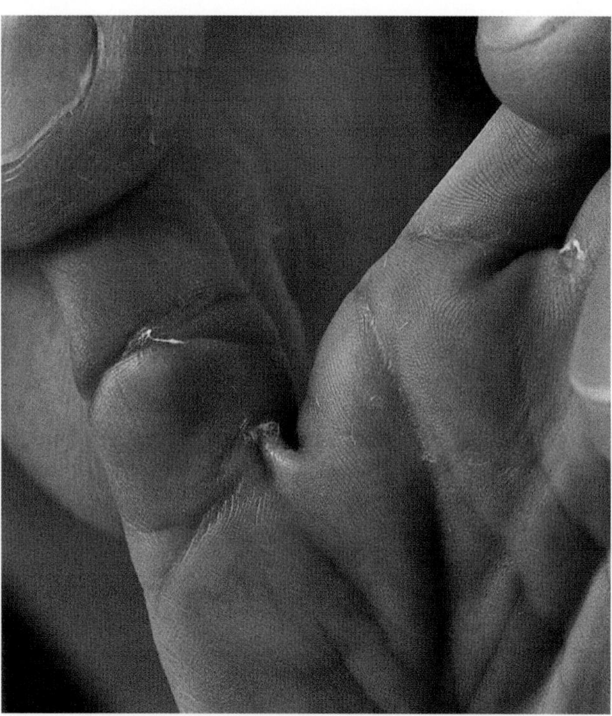

Fig. 167.8 Ligature around the thumb resulting in a demarcation.

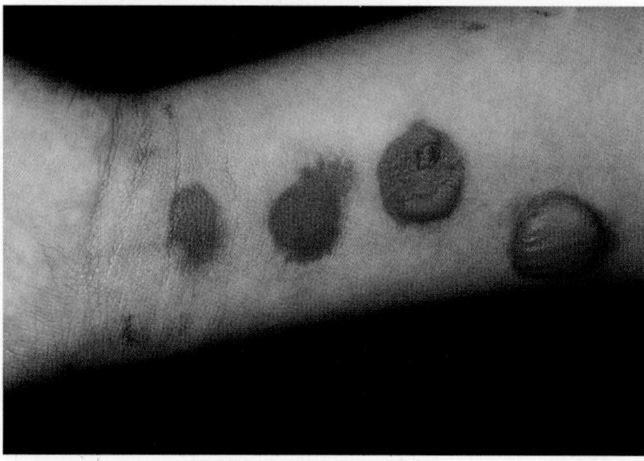

Fig. 167.9 Self-inflicted burns on the arms.

- *Excoriations*: excoriations are probably most common in self-mutilation. Lesions are sometimes deep enough to cause ulceration and scarring. Lesions are often localized (regional), sharply bordered, deep, linear and crusted.
- *Acne excoriée de la jeune fille (excoriated acne)*: acne patients often pick at their lesions. The majority of such patients are aware of and admit to their behaviour, and can be classified as neurotic excoriators. In extreme cases, the picking is more severe. Often, these patients are pubertal or adolescent girls who have only minimal acne. By manipulating their skin lesions, they transform them into excoriations or ulcers and cause scarring or postinflammatory hyperpigmentation.
- *Purpura*: purpura can be induced by sucking, cupping, rubbing or biting the skin, or with a bottle or a hard, rapidly moving object.
- *Burns*: self-induced burns are severe manifestations of a psychiatric disturbance. The skin is usually burned with a hot object, such as a cigarette. Most severe self-induced burns are observed in adolescents, although some occur in children [31]. Friction burns can also be observed. Burn-like lesions can be the result of the application of caustic or hot agents and injections of various substances [3]. Burns in children are usually inflicted by another individual and are manifestations of child abuse or Munchausen syndrome by proxy (see elsewhere in this chapter).
- *Other manifestations*: lip licking is a common and generally insignificant problem. Ligatures applied around a finger, extremity or penis may result in oedema, ulcerations or extreme demarcations and even amputations. Epistaxis and bleeding from other mucous surfaces, such as the gingiva, can be induced [32,33]. Also head banging or hitting the head or body against or with objects is seen. Self-inflicted injury of the eyes (irritation, wounding), nose, mouth or tongue can be observed. Genital mutilation, such as by scratching off the skin surrounding the vulva and anus or by inserting sharp objects into the vagina and/or anus, is rare.

Stereotypical self-mutilation

Stereotypical self-mutilation is the result of monotonous, repetitive, sometimes rhythmic acts like head banging. Some of the acts closely resemble behaviour described as physiological habits. Also, other acts like eye poking, self-beating and self-biting can be observed.

Stereotypical self-mutilation is seen in children with mental retardation, autism and Gilles de la Tourette syndrome. In Gilles de la Tourette syndrome, familial occurrence is found in about 58% of the cases [34]. It can also be observed as a symptom of neurobiological disorders, such as in Lesch–Nyhan syndrome, Prader–Willi syndrome, familial dysautonomia or de Lange syndrome [34–38]. In Lesch–Nyhan syndrome, lesions of the hands and lips can be seen in particular. Lesh–Nyhan syndrome is an X-linked recessive disorder caused by a deficiency of hypoxanthineguanine phosphoribosyltransferase activity [37]. The aetiology of Prader–Willi syndrome is unknown, but associations with abnormalities of chromosome 15 (of paternal origin) and paternal exposure to hydrocarbons have been reported [36,39].

According to Ellis et al., there is an inverse relationship between the prevalence of self-injurious behaviour and intellectual abilities: the more severe the level of mental retardation, the greater the prevalence of self-injurious behavior [37]. In a 1985 study of 10 000 mentally retarded persons by Griffin et al., 13.6% of the patients were found to engage in stereotypic self-mutilative behaviour [40]. Mostly, those affected are not aware of their behaviour, which does not seem to have any recognizable symbolic value. Sometimes, it can be interpreted as self-stimulating behaviour or as behaviour meant to suppress feelings of stress. This last idea is supported by the fact that one of the related factors seems to be institutionalization.

Major self-mutilation

Major self-mutilation is rare. It refers to self-injurious behaviour leading to substantial physical and lasting damage: self-castration, severe genital mutilation, eye enucleation or amputation of fingers, hand or complete limbs. Motives for the behaviour are themes related to (sub)culture or counterculture, religious guilt or sexual themes. Major self-mutilation is seen as part of psychiatric problems, like psychosis and acute alcohol and drug abuse, religious rites and sub- and countercultural habits, and transsexuality.

Major self-mutilation is very rare in minors, where it only occurs in combination with serious psychiatric problems or brain damage after a severe disease or trauma. In 1933, Goodhart and Savitsky described a 16-year-old girl who enucleated both her eyes without being able to explain her behaviour. She was known to have had chronic encephalitis eight years before the incident [41].

One of the problems in major self-mutilation is that there seems to be a 'by proxy' variant in which parents not only mutilate themselves but also their children, as in female genital mutilation, which is practised in some African countries as part of cultural rites [42].

General features of self-mutilation

Pathology. Self-mutilation shows no characteristic histopathological pattern. The abnormalities are compatible with irritant dermatitis. Severity depends on the techniques used by the patient.

Prognosis. Self-mutilation occurs in all age groups. It is more common in children, and has a significantly better prognosis. In some patients, the clinical symptoms and signs are present for years before the diagnosis is made. Careful follow-up is indicated in all cases. Sometimes, severe cases of self-mutilation in adults originate in childhood. However, in most children, the prognosis for complete recovery is excellent.

Diagnosis. The morphology of the lesions and the history will usually indicate the suspected diagnosis. Organic disturbances and systemic diseases should be ruled out. When self-mutilation is denied by the patient, it is possible to establish the diagnosis by careful observation.

Purpuric lesions can also be induced by stress, skin fragility, as side-effects of drugs and by ritualistic application of a device to the skin as a cultural healing practice (e.g. in Vietnam *cao gio* or coin rubbing). Purpura can be a symptom of thrombocytopenia, 'painful bruising' syndrome or vasculitis. It may also be the result of child abuse.

Treatment. There is no single treatment programme for self-mutilation, probably because self-mutilation is the result of many different causes and motives. Above all, it is the result of the complex interaction between the patient and their surroundings. Treatment approaches for self-mutilation can be divided into four categories:

- behavioural modification
- treatment devices and protective interventions
- pharmacological treatment
- psychotherapy.

Before choosing any treatment modality, it is first necessary to analyse the home and social environments, school and social influences and religious beliefs. Treatment should be directed at the causes of any precipitating stress [43,44]. Simple problems may be handled by the dermatologist [18]. A psychiatrist or psychologist should be consulted if the problem is more serious or if early therapeutic attempts are not successful.

Behavioural modification

The first step in behavioural modification is focused on building the child's self-confidence and self-esteem [43,44]. The next steps are:

- dispelling any threats of punishment
- improving insight and understanding
- maintaining authority
- tackling the symptoms
- recognizing positive self-actualizations.

The parents are important in these stages of treatment. Interaction between the parent(s) and the child should be monitored, and keeping a diary may be helpful. A schedule of tasks and a change in attitude may have a positive effect on behaviour [43].

Up to 6 years of age, the child undergoes the psychological development through which most children progress. During infancy and early childhood, oral habit phenomena are usually common, physiological and of relatively little importance [43]. In these cases, only limited therapeutic intervention is necessary. In trichotillomania, behavioural intervention may be successful [45]. In young children, trichotillomania is often accompanied by thumb sucking. The behavioural intervention may be aimed at the thumb sucking and include aversive taste treatment and response-dependent alarm [46,47]. Trichotillomania is, however, not always associated with thumb sucking. Behavioural therapy is still possible in these situations and can include hypnotherapy or intensive parent–child interaction (increased physical contact, frequent praise, avoiding criticism and discussing response prevention) [48]. Nail biting can be treated with bitter-tasting aversive substances and competing response therapies [49].

Use of devices and protective interventions

Use of devices is especially indicated in repetitive habit disorders. In trichotillomania, the child may be taught to pick hairs from a fuzzy toy [18]. Treatment of trichotillomania accompanied by thumb sucking may also include a response-disrupting thumb post [47]. Protective strategies (e.g. wearing a helmet in hand banging) are only supportive and do not add to learning more effective strategies for handling stress or inconvenience.

Pharmacological treatment

Drugs include clomipramine, desipramine, fluoxetine and pimozide. In a study in 25 serious nail-biting adults, clomipramine was superior to desipramine [50]. The same results were reported in the long-term treatment of serious trichotillomania [51]. Although anecdotal reports indicated that fluoxetine was effective, its efficacy could not be confirmed in a placebo-controlled, double-blind cross-over study in 21 adults with trichotillomania [52]. Several studies have suggested that oral N-acetylcysteine may be effective as an adjunct in the treatment of these behaviours given its purported effects on central glutamate metabolism although not all data are supportive [53–56]. Glutamatergic agents, which includes N-acetylcysteine, are of potential value for the treatment of obsessive-compulsive disorders in children and adolescents, according to a published systematic review of the literature [57].

Cognitive behavioural treatment can be combined with pharmacological modalities. This approach was reported to be successful, even in an autistic girl [58].

Psychotherapy

Psychotherapy is warranted in cases in which the above approaches are unsuccessful, or after thorough psychological analysis establishes the presence of serious psychopathology. Often, combined therapy with pharmacological agents and psychotherapy is used. Psychotherapy is more frequently indicated in cases of dermatitis artefacta and in obsessive–compulsive disorders.

References

1 Favazza AR, Rosenthal RJ. Diagnostic issues in self-mutilation. Hosp Comm Psychiatr 1993;44:134–40.
2 Winchel RM, Stanley M. Self-injurious behaviour: a review of the behavior and biology of self-mutilation. Am J Psychiatr 1991;148: 306–15.
3 Hollender MH, Abram HS. Dermatitis factitia. South Med J 1973; 66:1279.
4 Favazza AR. Bodies Under Siege – Self-Mutilation and Body Modification in Culture and Psychiatry, 2nd edn. Baltimore: Johns Hopkinis University Press, 1996.
5 Richman DM. Early intervention and prevention of self-injurious behaviour exhibited by young children with developmental disabilities. J Intellect Disabil Res 2008;52(1):3–17.
6 Parikh MS, Kolevzon A, Hollander E. Psychopharmacology of aggression in children and adolescents with autism: a critical review of efficacy and tolerability. J Child Adolesc Psychopharmacol 2008;18(2):157–78.
7 Matson JL, Lovullo SV. A review of behavioral treatments for self-injurious behaviors of persons with autism spectrum disorders. Behav Modif 2008;32(1):61–76.
8 Harth W, Taube KM, Gieler U. Facticious disorders in dermatology. J Dtsch Dermatol Ges 2010;8:361–72.
9 Timofeyev AV. Self mutilation. 2002. https://web.archive.org/web/20020607165049/http://wso.williams.edu/~atimofey/self_mutilation/Motivation/index.html
10 Favazza AR, Conterio K. Female habitual self-mutilators. Acta Psychiatr Scand 1989;78:283–9.
11 Suyemoto KL, MacDonald ML. Self-cutting in female adolescents. Psychotherapy 1995;32:162–71.
12 Ensink BJ. Confusing Realities: A Study on Child Sexual Abuse and Psychiatry. Amsterdam: VU University Press, 1992.
13 Hobbs CJ, Wynne JM. Physical Signs of Child Abuse – A Color Atlas, 2nd edn. Philadelphia: Saunders, 2001.
14 Van der Kolk BA, Perry JC, Herman JL. Childhood origins of self-destructive behavior. Am J Psychiatr 1991;148:1665–71.
15 Koblenzer C. Psychocutaneous Disease. Orlando: Grune-Stratton, 1987.
16 Gupta MA, Gupta AK. Dermatitis artefacta and sexual abuse. Int J Dermatol 1993;32:825–6.
17 Koo JYM, Smith LL. Obsessive–compulsive disorders in the pediatric dermatology practice. Pediatr Dermatol 1991;8:107–13.
18 Oranje AP, Peereboom-Wynia JDR, de Raeymaecker DMJ. Trichotillomania in childhood. J Am Acad Dermatol 1986;15:614–19.
19 Malon DW, Berardi D. Hypnosis with selfcutters. Am J Psychother 1987;50:531–41.
20 Cited in Martinson D. Self-injury: you are not the only one. 2002. https://web.archive.org/web/20120614084859/http://www.palace.net/~llama/psych/injury.html
21 Stanley B, Gameroff MJ, Michalsen V et al. Are suicide attempters who self-mutilate a unique population? Am J Psychiatr 2001;158:427–32.
22 Schetky DH. A review of literature on the long-term effects of childhood sexual abuse. In: Kluft RP (ed.) Incest-related Syndromes of Adult Psychopathology. Washington, DC: American Psychiatric Press, 1990:35–54.
23 Van der Kolk BA, Greenberg MS. The psychobiology of the trauma response: hyperarousal, constriction and addiction to traumatic reexposure. In: Van der Kolk BA (ed.) Psychological Trauma. Washington, DC: American Psychiatric Press, 1987:63–87.
24 Dulit RA, Fyer MR, Leon AC et al. Clinical correlates of self-mutilation in borderline personality disorder. Am J Psychiatr 1994;151:1305–11.
25 Stein DJ, Hollander E. Dermatology and conditions related to obsessive–compulsive disorder. J Am Acad Dermatol 1992;26:237–42.
26 Leonard HL, Rapoport JL. Pharmacotherapy of obsessive–compulsive disorders. Psychiatr Clin North Am 1989;12:963–70.
27 Rapoport JL. Annotation: childhood obsessive–compulsive disorder. J Child Psychol Psychiatr 1986;27:289–95.
28 Levenkron S. Cutting – Understanding and Overcoming Self-Mutilation. New York: Norton, 1998.
29 Favazza AR. The coming of age of self-mutilation. J Nerv Mental Dis 1998;186:259–68.
30 Spraker MK. Cutaneous artifactual disease: an appeal for help. Pediatr Clin North Am 1983;30:659–68.
31 Stoddard FJ. A psychiatric perspective on self-inflicted burns. J Burn Care Rehabil 1993;14:480–2.
32 Tunnessen WW, Chessar IJ. Factitious cutaneous bleeding. Am J Dis Child 1984;138:354–5.
33 Rodd HD. Self-inflicted gingival injury in a young girl. Br Dent J 1995;178:28–30.
34 Regeur L, Pakkenberg B, Fog R et al. Clinical features and long-term treatment with pimozide in 65 patients with Gilles de La Tourette's syndrome. J Neurol Neurosurg Psychiatr 1986;49:791–5.
35 Lesh M, Nyhan WL. A familiar disorder or uric acid metabolism and central nervous system function. Am J Med 1964;36:561–70.
36 Prader A, Labhart A, Willi H. Ein Syndrom von Adipositas, Kleinwuchs, Krytorchismus and Oligophrenie nach Myatonieartigem Zustand im Neugeborenalter. Schweiz Med Wochenschr 1956;86: 1260–1.
37 Ellis CR, Singh NN, Jackson EV. Problem behaviors in children with develomental disabilities. In: Parmelee DX (ed.) Child and Adolescent Psychiatry. St Louis: Mosby-Year Book, 1996:263–75.
38 Gadoth ME. Oro-dental self-mutilation in familial dysautonomia. J Oral Pathol Med 1994;23:273–6.
39 Butler MG, Palmer CG. Clinical and cytogenetic survey of 39 individuals with Prader–Labhart–Willi syndrome. Am J Med Genet 1986;23:793–809.
40 Griffin et al. cited in Timofeyev AV. Self mutilation. 2002. https://web.archive.org/web/20020607165049/http://wso.williams.edu/~atimofey/self_mutilation/Motivation/index.html
41 Goodhart S, Savitsky N. Self mutilation in chronic encephalitis. Am J Med Sci 1933;185:674–84.
42 Dorkenoo E. Cutting the Rose. Female Genital Mutilation – The Practice and Its Prevention. London: Minority Rights Publications, 1995.
43 Peterson JE, Schneider PE. Oral habits. A behavioral approach. Pediatr Oral Health 1991;38:1289–307.
44 Leung AKC, Robson WLM. Nail biting. Clin Pediatr 1990;29:690–2.
45 Blum NJ, Barone VJ, Friman PC. A simplified behavioral treatment for trichotillomania: report of two cases. Pediatrics 1993;75: 993–5.
46 Friman PC, Finney JW, Christophersen ER. Behavioral treatment of trichotillomania: an evaluative review. Behav Ther 1984;15:249–65.
47 Watson TS, Allen KD. Elimination of thumb-sucking as a treatment for severe trichotillomania. J Am Acad Child Adoles Psychiatr 1993;32:830–4.
48 Friman PC, Finney JW, Christophersen ER. Behavioral treatment of trichotillomania: an evaluative review. Behav Ther 1984;15:249–65.
49 Silber KP, Haynes CE. Treating nail biting: a comparative analysis of mild aversion and competing response therapies. Behav Res Ther 1992;30:15–22.

50 Leonard HL, Lenage MC, Swedo SE et al. A double-blind comparison of clomipramine and desipramine treatment of severe onychophagia (nail biting). Arch Gen Psychiatr 1991;48:821–7.
51 Swedo SE, Lenane MC, Leonard HL. Long-term treatment of trichotillomania (hair pulling). N Engl J Med 1993;329:141–2.
52 Christenson GA, Mackenzie TB, Mitchell JE et al. A placebo-controlled double-blind crossover study of fluoxetine in trichotillomania. Am J Psychiatr 1991;148:1566–71.
53 Deepmala, Slattery J, Kumar N et al. Clinical trials of N-acetylcysteine in psychiatry and neurology: a systematic review. Neurosci Biobehav Rev 2015;55:294–321.
54 Oliver G, Dean O, Camfield D et al. N-acetylcysteine in the treatment of obsessive compulsive and related disorders: a systematic review. Clin Psychopharmacol Neurosci 2015;13(1):12–24.
55 Grant JE, Odlaug BL, Kim SW. N-acetylcysteine, a glutamate modulator, in the treatment of trichotillomania: a double-blind, placebo-controlled study. Arch Gen Psychiatry 2009; 66(7):756–63.
56 Bloch MH, Panza KE, Grant JE et al. N-Acetylcysteine in the treatment of pediatric trichotillomania: a randomized, double-blind, placebo-controlled add-on trial. J Am Acad Child Adolesc Psychiatry 2013;52(3):231–40.
57 Mechler K, Häge A, Schweinfurth N et al. Glutamatergic agents in the treatment of compulsivity and impulsivity in child and adolescent psychiatry: a systematic review of the literature. Z Kinder Jugendpsychiatr Psychother 2018;46(3):246–263.
58 Holttum JR, Lubetsky MJ, Eastman LE. Comprehensive management of trichotillomania in a young autistic girl. J Am Acad Child Adolesc Psychiatr 1994;33:577–81.

Factitious disorders

Factitious disorder, formerly known as Munchausen syndrome

Munchausen syndrome was first described by Asher in 1951 [1]: 'Here is described a common syndrome which most doctors have seen, but about which little has been written. Like the famous Baron von Munchausen, the persons affected have always travelled widely; and their stories, like those attributed to him, are both dramatic and untruthful. Accordingly the syndrome is respectfully dedicated to the baron, and named after him'.

According to the American Psychiatric Association, factitious disorder is characterized by the following three criteria: (i) the patient intentionally feigns physical or mental signs or symptoms; (ii) the patient's apparent motive for this behaviour is to occupy the sick role; and (iii) there are no other motives such as found in malingering (financial gain, revenge or avoiding legal responsibility) [2]. The feigning can be done by consciously self-inflicting injuries and/or falsely reporting symptoms.

Until a few years ago, Munchausen syndrome was almost exclusively described in adults. Only a few cases were known from children and adolescents. Libow reviewed the literature and described 42 cases of illness falsification by children [3]. The most commonly reported falsified or induced conditions were fevers, ketoacidosis, purpura and infections. The fabrications ranged from false symptom reporting to active injections, bruising and ingestions. Libow stated: '... pediatricians (should) include illness falsification by the child-patient in the differential diagnosis of a persistent and unexplained medical condition, along with somatization, malingering, and Munchausen by proxy abuse'. This also applies to paediatric dermatologists. Libow concluded that better understanding and identification of children with illness falsification are likely to help prevent the development of chronic adult factitious disorders.

Some of the symptoms in fabricated or induced illness have been known for centuries. In 2001, Bjornson and Kirk reported a case of a 12-year-old girl with artificial haemoptysis [4]. Artificial haemoptysis was already known in the Middle Ages. Hysterics were known to place leeches in their mouth to simulate haemoptysis. They also abraded their skin to simulate dermatological disorders [5].

Factitious disorder by purposeful self-mutilation must be differentiated from self-mutilation that satisfies a psychological need (see earlier in this chapter).

Contagious self-mutilation behaviour in groups has been described in prisons, schools and psychiatric institutions. These epidemics are more common in females [6] and may occur in young people without clear psychopathology [7].

The relationship between factitious disorder and factitious disorder by proxy, as already mentioned by Libow, is illustrated by a case report of a mother with dermatitis artefacta on the forearm and lower legs who produced the same lesions on her child's face [8].

Factitious disorder by proxy, formerly known as Munchausen syndrome by proxy

Munchausen syndrome by proxy was first described by Meadow in 1977 [9]: 'Some patients consistently produce stories and fabricate evidence, so causing themselves needless hospital investigations and operations. Here are described parents who, by falsification, caused their children innumerable harmful hospital procedures – a sort of Munchausen syndrome by proxy'.

The term Munchausen syndrome by proxy has been replaced in the medical literature by terms like factitious disorder by proxy [2,10,11], factitious disorder imposed on another [12], paediatric condition falsification [11], medical child abuse [12] and fabricated or induced illness by carers [13]. According to Schreier [11], paediatric condition falsification describes the findings in the child and factitious disorder by proxy the behaviour of the parent/carer.

This form of child abuse can be described as a particular form of physical and psychological maltreatment whereby a disease is fabricated or induced in a child by a parent (mostly the mother) or someone who is responsible for the child's welfare. The behaviour of the perpetrator leads to repeated presentation of the child within the healthcare system, whereby repeated medical investigations and, eventually, interventions are performed. Signs and symptoms may be actively or passively induced. Passive induction includes the presentation of a fictitious medical history and/or the description of fictitious abnormalities. Active induction is possible by causing actual abnormalities or falsifying medical records [10].

According to the Royal College of Paediatrics and Child Health, fabricated or induced illness by carers (FII) involves a well child being presented by a carer as ill or disabled, or an ill or disabled child being presented with a more significant problem than he or she has in reality, and suffering harm as a consequence [14].

The American Psychiatric Association defines the following diagnostic criteria concerning factitious disorder imposed on another: (i) a pattern of falsification of physical or psychological signs or symptoms in another, associated with identified deception; (ii) a pattern of presenting another (victim) to others as ill or impaired; (iii) the behaviour is evident even in the absence of obvious external rewards; (iv) the behaviour is not better accounted for by another mental disorder such as delusional belief system or acute psychosis. According to the APA, all four criteria must be met to make this diagnosis and the perpetrator receives this diagnosis, not the victim.

If these factitious disorders/abnormalities involve the skin, then a wide range of findings may be present, varying from clearly recognizable self-mutilation lesions, through a suggestive history (for a dermatological disorder), to frequent, very persistent 'actual' dermatological disorders. As mentioned before, these disorders vary from easily recognizable artefacts to complicated cutaneous infections [10].

Abnormalities that have actually been observed by physicians or reported by the perpetrator and found on the skin and mucosa in paediatric condition falsification (and factitious disorder) include the following [10,12,14–18].

- Haemorrhagic tendency/coagulopathies/easy bruising.
- Cutaneous abscesses (sterile or infected).
- Cyanosis.
- Diaphoresis.
- Dermatitis artefacta/(cutaneous) rashes of unknown cause.
- Eczema.
- Erythema.
- Excoriations.
- Vaginal discharge and other abnormalities, such as vaginal or anal bleeding and/or abnormalities in the anogenital area.
- Abnormalities in the mouth.
- Oedema.
- Otitis externa.
- Vesicular eruptions (clustered, chronic).
- Cutaneous abnormalities in food allergy and other allergic reactions.
- Painting of the skin (may mimic cellulitis of purpura).

References

1 Asher R. Munchausen's syndrome. Lancet 1951;i:339–41.
2 American Psychiatric Association. DSM-IV-TR. Washington, DC: American Psychiatric Association, 2000.
3 Libow JA. Child and adolescent illness falsification. Pediatrics 2000;105:336–42.
4 Bjornson CL, Kirk VG. Munchausen's syndrome presenting as hemoptysis in a 12-year-old girl. Can Respir J 2001;8:439–42.
5 Tlacuilo-Parra JA, Guevara-Gutierrez E, Garcia-De La Torre I. Factitious disorders mimicking systemic lupus erythematosus. Clin Exp Rheumatol 2000;18(1):89–93.
6 Ross RR, McKay HB. Self-Mutilation. Lexiton, MA: DC Health, 1979.
7 Fennig S, Carlson GA, Fennig S. Contagious self-mutilation. J Am Acad Child Adolesc Psychiatr 1995;34:402–3.
8 Jones DPH. Dermatitis artefacta in a mother and baby as child abuse. Br J Psychiatr 1983;143:199–200.
9 Meadow R. Munchausen syndrome by proxy: the hinterland of child abuse. Lancet 1977;ii:343–5.
10 Bilo RAC. Forensic pediatric dermatology: my skin is only the top layer of the problem. In: Oranje AP, de Waard-van der Spek FB, Bilo RAC (eds) Dermatology from Young to Old. Zwolle: Isala Series No. 43, 2003:45–52.
11 Schreier HA. Munchausen by proxy defined. Pediatrics 2002;110(5): 985–8.
12 Roesler TA, Jenny C. Medical Child Abuse – Beyond Munchausen Syndrome by Proxy. Itasca: American Academy of Pediatrics, 2008.
13 American Psychiatric Association. DSM-V. Washington, DCL American Psychiatric Association, 2013.
14 Royal College of Paediatrics and Child Health. Fabricated or Induced Illness by Carers (FII): A Practical Guide for Paediatricians. London: RCPCH, 2009.
15 Rosenberg DA. Munchausen syndrome by proxy. In: Reece RM (ed.) Child Abuse: Medical Diagnosis and Management. Philadelphia: Lea & Febiger, 1994:266–78.
16 Stankler L. Factitious skin lesions in a mother and two sons. BMJ 1977;97:217.
17 Johnson CF. Dermatological manifestations. In: Levin AV, Sheridan MS (eds) Munchausen Syndrome by Proxy – Issues in Diagnosis and Treatment. New York: Lexington Books, 1995:189–200.
18 Schreier HA, Libow JA. Munchausen by proxy syndrome: a modern pediatric challenge. J Pediatr 1994;125:S110–15.

CHAPTER 168
Topical Therapy

Johannes Wohlrab

Department of Dermatology and Venereology and Institute of Applied Dermatopharmacy, Martin-Luther-University Halle-Wittenberg, Halle (Saale), Germany

Principles of therapy, 2275
Principles of topical pharmacokinetics, 2275
Pharmaceutical formulation and vehicle systems, 2277
Characteristics of paediatric dermatological therapy, 2278
Commonly used therapeutic agents, 2280

Abstract

Children's skin shows functional characteristics that are relevant to the topical application of active substances. Basic knowledge about the physicochemical properties of the stratum corneum, as well as about cutaneous pharmacokinetics, is essential for the professional use of topical preparations. Furthermore, basic concepts of pharmacological formulation and interactions are required in order to assess and avoid risks such as local intolerability, irritant effects, particularly from emulsifiers, and increased systemic bioavailability with toxicological relevance. Particular care has to be taken when using drugs that are not licensed for paediatric use (off-label use). Here, legal framework applies that calls for special diligence in choosing appropriate therapies.

Key points

- Cutaneous bioavailability of applied active substances depends not only on their physicochemical properties but on their interaction with the stratum corneum.
- The micromorphological conditions regarding both anatomical variations (thick and thin skin) and pathological alterations (epidermal proliferating or differentiating dysfunction) have a direct impact on the pharmacokinetic profile.
- After liberation (release) from a vehicle, active substances can diffuse into the stratum corneum (penetration) or pass through the stratum corneum (permeation).
- The optimum formulation and the application modalities of a topical preparation must always be customized for the specific dermatological situation.
- Prophylactic barrier protective therapy can be particularly effective, if adjusted to the special requirements of children's skin.
- Combining topical agents in one preparation should be avoided if possible.

Principles of therapy

It is less the morphological characteristics that distinguish children's skin from adult skin than the functional differences, which have great relevance for topical therapy [1–3]. In order to assess these functional distinctions, basic knowledge of the microanatomy of the skin is required, especially about the molecular structure of the stratum corneum (SC) as a boundary compartment between the topical preparation and the epidermis. The active substance with its characteristic physicochemical properties interacts with the vehicle system as well as with the skin. The therapeutic effect results from the synergy of cutaneous bioavailability and the concentration–time profile of the active substance in the target compartment plus the intrinsic effect of the vehicle system. Consequently, for optimal therapy, not only the appropriate active substance in the right concentration has to be chosen, but also a suitable vehicle, taking into account both its interaction with the active agent and its intrinsic effect.

Principles of topical pharmacokinetics

Cutaneous bioavailability of applied active substances depends not only on their physicochemical properties but primarily on their interaction with the SC [4]. From a pharmacological point of view, two contradictory features of the SC are essential for the activity of the agent: the barrier function and the reservoir function. The SC is not a homogeneous structure but has a compact layer following the stratum granulosum (the stratum compactum) that is then loosened by an enzyme-controlled desquamation process (stratum disjunctum) [5]. The maximum barrier function is assigned to the stratum compactum while the stratum disjunctum has the maximum reservoir function. The SC is thus the main acceptor for liberated phases from skin-applied preparations. This is important for the kinetics of the active agent since it reduces concentration peaks in deeper skin layers and slows down the penetration process. At the same time, large quantities of the active substance can be absorbed and become bioavailable

Harper's Textbook of Pediatric Dermatology, Fourth Edition. Edited by Peter Hoeger, Veronica Kinsler and Albert Yan.

even in a relatively short application time. It becomes clear that the micromorphological conditions regarding both anatomical variations (thick and thin skin) as well as pathological alterations (epidermal proliferating or differentiating dysfunction) have a direct impact on the pharmacokinetic profile [6].

Structure of the stratum corneum

The SC consists of three basic elements – separate microenvironments that together form the barrier [7]. The corneocytes, which result from differentiating keratinocytes, are highly metabolically active. They are surrounded by a complex membranous structure (the cornified envelope) that has a low permeability, especially for hydrophilic phases, and thus ensures the integrity of the corneocytes. In addition, the intercellular space is filled with a mixture of various lipids, proteins and water, whose physicochemical properties are relevant to barrier and reservoir function. The barrier function of the SC is a semi-permeable system set up by complex interaction between various molecular groups and cellular components [8]. According to present knowledge, not only the quantity and quality of the individual components but especially their molecular arrangement is essential for barrier function. Complex physicochemical and biological conditions influence the barrier under physiological conditions. For pathological skin conditions, the cutaneous alterations and the phase of the disease also have to be considered.

Lipophilic components of the SC

The lipid synthesis by keratinocytes is largely autonomous. Besides cholesterol and cholesterol derivates, free fatty acids with varying chain lengths and triglycerides are produced [9]. In addition, ceramides, which with their anisomeric molecular structure differ substantially from molecules of other lipid classes, are synthesized within the endoplasmic reticulum of keratinocytes. Due to electric charge differences within their long-chain molecules, ceramides are able to form spontaneously lyotrophic mesophases, such as liquid crystalline membrane structures. Unlike phospholipids, ceramides have two mobile alkyl chains that vary in length and, depending on the degree of hydration, in configuration. Various membrane models describe the complex network of membrane sections with their polymorphic phase behaviour. The dynamic organization of this complex system is increasingly understood by science and is gaining more and more importance for the development of advanced vehicle systems.

Hydrophilic phase of the SC

Another significant part of the barrier function is the quantity of the hydrophilic phase in microenvironments [10]. The water within the microcompartments of the SC exists in at least two forms: free water and bound water. The latter consists of fixed water, on one hand, and water that can be mobilized under certain circumstances on the other. The nomenclature is aiming here at the dynamic exchange of hydrophilic valences between the individual compartments. Fixed water is understood as the proportion of water that is bound by strong hygroscopic forces (conveyed by proteolytically generated amino acids). Its transport is subject to retardation. Under certain conditions, bound water can be mobilized by swellable membrane components and is then transferred into the free water phase. This is the functionally most significant water phase of the SC. The free water is held in the various microcompartments via hygroscopic molecules – the so-called 'natural moisturizing factor' (NMF) – and interacts with both the water phase of the epidermis and the environment (transepidermal water flow). Essential components of NMF are amino acids, pyrrolidine carboxylic acids, lactate, urea and inorganic ions [11].These are synthetized by keratinocytes and liberated depending on the degree of differentiation.

Pharmacokinetic processes

After liberation (release) from a vehicle, active substances can diffuse into the SC (penetration) or pass through the SC (permeation) (Fig. 168.1). Most substances permeate the SC along the numerous hydrophilic corneodesmosomal structures using the so-called intercellular pathway (Fig. 168.2). Lipophilic substances prefer to penetrate along the nonpolar, lipophilic route, via lateral diffusion along the lipophilic hydrocarbon chains of the SC lipids [12]. However, it is assumed that redistribution regarding the pathways can occur depending on the physicochemical properties of both the active substance and the vehicle, as well as the changing concentrations during penetration [5].

The main factors influencing penetration are described by Fick's laws of diffusion. Although there are also other factors that influence penetration (especially in colloidal vehicle systems), the crucial points in terms of pharmaceutical optimization are the difference in concentration between the preparation and the skin, the liberation of the active substance from the preparation, the properties of the skin regarding diffusion and the contact time between preparation and skin [13].

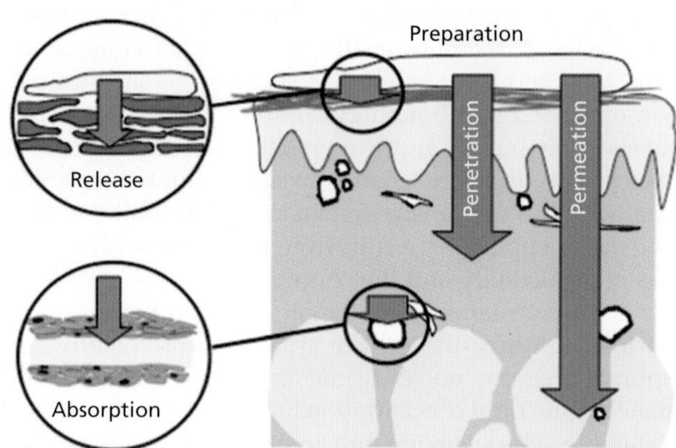

Fig. 168.1 Terms that describe the invasion of active substances into and through skin compartments during the diffusion process (liberation = release from a vehicle, penetration = diffuse into a layer, permeation = passing through a layer, absorption = uptake into blood or lymphatic vessels).

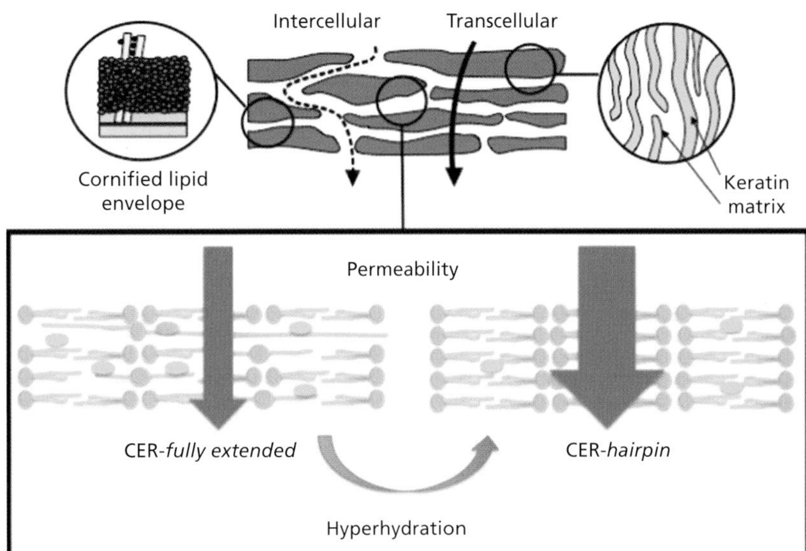

Fig. 168.2 Microenvironments of the stratum corneum, the main routes of penetration and the molecular order of ceramides (CER) depending on the grade of hydration (permeability).

General concept of topical preparations

In order to optimize bioavailability of active substances in the respective target compartments, specific vehicle systems can be designed which correspond with the molecular conditions and whose intrinsic effect is to effectively influence the overall physicochemical circumstances [14,15]. Choosing an optimized preparation for therapy requires a clear definition of the pathogenetic conditions of the respective dermatosis; that is, the pharmacological target compartment and the pharmaceutical formulation have to be determined. In addition, the physicochemical properties of the active substance have to be taken into account, in order to calculate the interactions between vehicle and skin. Here, cooperation between dermatological and pharmaceutical competences is needed. Besides finished medicinal products, so-called specialties and medical devices, there are pharmaceutical compounds that can be made individually for a patient. Furthermore, cosmetic preparations are recommended as basic therapy (also called supportive care therapy), to reduce the influence of external triggers and proactively suppress the disease activity with a barrier substitution.

Pharmaceutical formulation and vehicle systems

Detailed knowledge about the composition of vehicle systems and the possibilities for sensible and stable processing of active substances falls within the competence of pharmacists. Although in principle, physicians have the right to freely choose a therapy, they must not prescribe unreasonable, inefficient or obsolete individual pharmaceutical compounds. Therefore, there are precepts that regulate the use of vehicle systems for individually prepared formulations – the so-called standardized extemporaneous preparations. What makes things more difficult is the fact that the nomenclature for vehicle systems differs in pharmaceutical and dermatological parlance. This can be illustrated by the use of the term 'ointment', which by a pharmacist is considered to be a water-free mixture of lipids, whereas a dermatologist sees it rather as a lipophilic cream. The confusion is made worse by the fact that often the declaration of the ingredients of finished medicinal products do not correlate with the pharmaceutical nomenclature.

The formulation of a topical preparation determines the degree of cutaneous bioavailability of the active substance as well as its intrinsic effect. Basically, it can be said that the longer the topical therapy is applied, the stronger the intrinsic effect of the vehicle. Initially, a rapid bioavailability in the target compartment is desired, which means the vehicle should be able to liberate the active substance rapidly into the SC.

Vehicle systems

In daily clinical practice, a more pragmatic classification of vehicle types is used, which is geared towards therapeutic relevance rather than pharmaceutical details (Fig. 168.3).

Ointments are basically referred to as water-free preparations, namely, lipophilic ointments, water-free absorption bases and hydrophilic ointments. Creams, however, are understood as three-phase systems consisting of hydrophilic, oily and emulsifying phases. Depending on the type of continuous phase, hydrophilic creams (oil-in-water type), lipophilic creams (water-in-oil type) and amphiphilic creams (so-called bicontinuous creams with both oil-in-water and water-in-oil phases) are recognized. A special variant is the so-called quasi emulsion, also known as cold cream. These are stable at room temperature, highly viscous ointments with incorporated water droplets (without emulsifier). Applied on skin, the ointment melts and releases the water that evaporates with a cooling effect. Gels, on the other hand, consist of a matrix former – a three-dimensional structure which together with water or oil forms a semi-solid preparation of variable viscosity. Pastes have solid insoluble particles dispersed in an ointment or cream.

Apart from this, various other vehicle subtypes with significant pharmaceutical advantages exist, such as

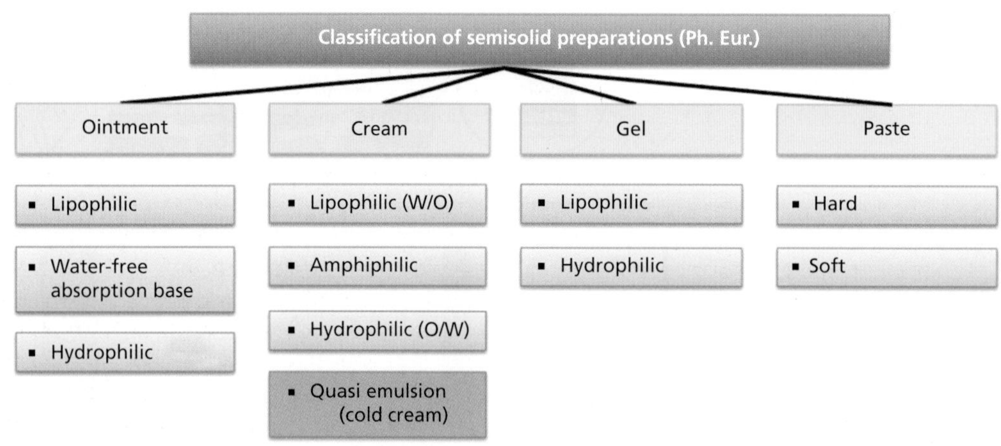

Fig. 168.3 Simplified depiction of classification of semi-solid formulations in accordance with the European Pharmacopoeia (Ph. Eur.). The information on solubility refers to properties of substances that can be incorporated. W/O, water in oil; O/W, oil in water.

colloidal systems. Liposomes are mostly aqueous phases encased in a lipid membrane and can show lamellar structures [16]. Microemulsions are so-called Newtonian fluids which consist of an aqueous and an oily phase plus an emulsifier/coemulsifier mixture and therefore have special thermodynamic properties [17]. Finally, nanoparticles have to be mentioned, which are mostly very small polymers that either encase droplets or absorb liquids in the form of sponge-like porous particles [18].

Intrinsic effect of vehicles

It is logical to allocate specific vehicle systems to certain clinical pictures [14,15]. It has been proven in practice that the use of hydrophilic vehicles for acute and lipophilic for chronic inflammatory conditions is sensible. However, professional therapy should give priority to the appropriate choice of the respective active substance. In some cases, it may be necessary to change the ingredients of the vehicle due to the particular physicochemical properties of the active substance. The optimum formulation and the application modalities of a topical preparation always have to be customized for the specific dermatological situation.

Characteristics of paediatric dermatological therapy

Apart from the first few months of life, healthy children's skin does not show clinically relevant distinctive features in morphology of the epidermis compared to adult skin [2]. With respect to topical application of active substances, however, functional limitations of the barrier can be postulated. In particular, there is a different sebaceous gland activity that can vary considerably depending on hormonal factors [19]. This has the potential for new specific strategies, especially for prophylactic basic therapy [20]. The focus of interest here is certain fatty acids with a strong antibacterial intrinsic effect [21].

Lower functional capacity

Even when reaching phenotypic equivalence with adult skin after the first year of life, the maturing of the infant epidermis is not yet completed [22]. The functional capacities of the system remain restricted, which is reflected in a higher permeability of the SC, a lower ability to compensate for environmental changes and a reduced reservoir function. Regarding the kinetics of applied substances, a higher maximum concentration can be expected, but with a shorter maintenance period of the effective concentration. Consequently, lower initial concentrations should be used, which in consequence have to be more frequently administered. External factors that influence the environment, such as emulsifiers, occlusion or change in hydration, should be used cautiously. By implication, this means also that prophylactic barrier protective therapy can be particularly effective, if adjusted to the special requirements of children's skin [23].

Risk of systemic toxicity

Penetration processes in pathological skin can differ dramatically compared to healthy skin, a fact that is especially relevant in all dermatoses with a pronounced barrier defect [24]. Also, bioavailability is more easily reached because of the characteristic body proportions of children. Children have up to 80% body water compared to adults with approximately 50–60%, which results in higher volumes of distribution and raises the proportion of extracellular fluid. This allows increased transcutaneous absorption and can therefore affect the safety profile of a substance [25]. Furthermore, the renal and hepatic capacity for elimination is significantly lower in infants than in adults. The degree of restriction is subject to large interindividual fluctuations until the age of 9 months. Consequently, it is not possible to make universal statements about pharmacokinetic and toxicological profiles – every case requires an individual risk–benefit assessment [26]. In principle, however, physicians should be cautious with topical therapy for infants, especially in preterm and newborn patients.

Increased permeability by heat application

Another possibility for modulating the barrier function is heating of the SC, which has received little attention in practice so far [27]. The exceedance of the phase transition temperature causes changes in phase behaviour of the lyotrophic mesophases and therefore increases the permeability especially for hydrophilic phases. When heating the SC above 42 °C, a relevant increase of permeability can be expected. On one hand, this may result in significant loss of moisture and therefore in functional decompensation. On the other hand, it alters the pharmacokinetic conditions, resulting in higher cutaneous and systemic bioavailability. This can be utilized purposefully but it also carries toxicological risks.

Irritant effect of emulsifiers

When combining hydrophilic and lipophilic phases, surface-active substances (tensides) are always needed in order to produce a stable compound. These so-called emulsifiers can be found in most multiphase systems. After application on skin, a dynamic process of physicochemical rearrangement is initiated, at the end of which the phases are reorganized [28]. In the course of this, the emulsifiers become bioactive and diffuse into the deeper skin layers. They compete with other tensidic structures within the SC or on the cell membranes. Depending on concentration, hydrophilicity-lipophilicity balance (HLB value) and environmental factors, irritant or even toxic effects may occur [29]. Clinicall,y they will appear as an inflammation or as triggering of an existing dermatosis. For use in children, the concentration of emulsifiers should therefore be limited to a necessary minimum. Besides that, qualities with good skin compatibility (e.g. sugar surfactants) should be preferred. When recommending cosmetics for use on pathological skin, only preparations that are especially designed for children should be chosen.

Substances with limited safety

In paediatric dermatology, substances are often used whose safety and harmlessness for children is likely but not certain. This applies especially for high concentrations and medium- and long-term use. Aiming at the safety of under-age patients, not all recommendations are toxicologically and allergologically verified. In particular, physicians must be warned against the use of salicylic acid, local anaesthetics, the antiseptics povidone-iodine (PVP), clioquinol, hexachlorophene and triclosan, and the antibiotics gentamicin and neomycin. Also, potentially irritant substances like urea, retinoids and dithranol should be used carefully in children. For almost all of these substances, appropriate alternatives exist, which should be preferred.

The latest knowledge about pharmacodynamic properties should always be kept in mind. Urea, for example, has been reevaluated lately, suggesting a better benefit–risk ratio than hitherto. Urea not only shows considerable hygroscopic effects but also has been identified as a potent factor for regulating the protein synthesis of keratinocytes [30]. The resulting effects open up new dimensions for the treatment of patients with atopic dermatitis. Besides, the crucial point is not the amount of urea administered, but the proportion that becomes bioavailable. Due to pharmacological characteristics, differences can appear between various preparations with identical urea content. A combination of urea and glycerol in concentrations up to 5%, as recommended by many physicians, seems to be an appropriate benchmark.

Moderate occlusion

Water-free vehicles like ointments or watertight patches and bandages severely affect the exchange of hydrophilic valences within the SC, between the SC and the environment and the SC and the epidermis [31]. Overhydration of the SC clinically manifests as maceration: the hydrophilic head groups of ceramides are pushed apart and molecules change their steric configuration. This process, also known as 'chain flip transition', transforms the diametric configuration of the lipophilic side chains (fully extended) into a parallel alignment (hair pin) [32]. This in turn results in a higher permeability, especially for hydrophilic substances.

In order to reduce the occlusive effect of lipophilic vehicles ('outer occlusion') whilst still providing a rich lipidic base, the principle of 'inner occlusion' has been developed [28]. Bipolar molecules whose properties are similar to those of ceramides (usually phospholipids) are processed into membranes using special high-pressure technology. The results are oblong, flat, oval liposomal structures that, after application, cause the phases to separate within the SC and thus form inner diffusion barriers. This principle has in practice been proven successful, especially in cases of deficient barrier function.

Cutaneous metabolism

In recent years, molecular biological studies have shown that keratinocytes are metabolically highly active cells [33]. They play an important role in the metabolic elimination of skin-applied substances. Depending on chemical structure, molecular weight and other factors including pathogenetic conditions, the activity pattern of catabolic enzymes changes. Of particular interest here is the cytochrome P450 system. For CYP2C19, a member of this system, activity patterns vary with age (but not with gender) [34]. It remains hypothetical whether this has an influence on the elimination rate of certain agents or not. Still, the possibility should be considered when using agents that are metabolized by CYP2C19 or that influence its activity.

Off-label use

In times of evidence-based medicine, the established criteria for quality-orientated medical practice naturally apply as well for paediatric therapy. Notoriously, most topical agents are not developed or licensed for paediatric use. Clinical trials in accordance with GCP guidelines are rare. The situation for the dermatologist is unsatisfactory from both a pharmacological and a legal point of view. The so-called 'off-label use' of pharmaceuticals remains a therapeutic option, which has to be considered within the context of ethical norms and national law. When all alternatives – including nontreatment – have been ruled out, the therapy should be chosen based on evidence and according to the latest guidelines. After an individual benefit–risk assessment considering child-specific pharmacology, the dosage should be adapted. Informed consent of the parents is compulsory. If possible, peers should be involved in the decision.

Fixed-dose combinations

Combining topical agents in one preparation should be avoided if possible. Fixed-dose combinations always bear the risk of unpredictable interactions and are therefore only acceptable in specific therapeutic settings. The problem here lies not only in the potential pharmacodynamic interactions and incompatibilities, but also in the necessary compromises regarding the formulation.

In some cases, however, the combined application of agents seems reasonable. Examples include the established topical treatment of acne vulgaris (benzoyl peroxide with clindamycin or adapalene), the therapy of severe inflammatory staphylococcal infections (glucocorticoid with antibiotic or antiseptic), the treatment for severe inflammatory dermatophytosis (glucocorticoid with fungicide) and some antipsoriatic therapies (glucocorticoid with vitamin D analogue or salicylic acid). Even when topical preparations containing different agents are administered sequentially to the same area, phases can get mixed on or within the skin, which may cause unwanted interactions. If separate preparations are used, an interval of at least 30 minutes between applications is therefore recommended. From a pharmacological point of view, the use of tri- or quadrivalent preparations (e.g. glucocorticoid with antibiotic/antiseptic and/or fungicide and/or local anaesthetic) is extremely questionable. Such therapeutic decisions make it impossible to calculate the risks, especially for medium- and long-term use.

Therapy planning

For an effective therapy, planning must be based on the current state of knowledge regarding efficacy and safety. Assessment should take into account the indication for treatment and the patient's individual situation (age, affected body area, acute or chronic state of disease, previous therapies, comorbidities, quality of life). The plan should include the choice of an agent/medicinal product, a dosing regime, safety aspects, potential off-label use, cost-effectiveness and measures to ensure patient compliance [35]. A transparent and comprehensible communication is essential for acceptance of the therapeutic plan by both physician and patient [36].

The priority is the choice of one or more active substances for topical application. Then an appropriate vehicle must be selected, which firstly allows the optimum cutaneous bioavailability of the actual agent and secondly, whose intrinsic effect substantially supports the therapy.

In the initial phase of the therapy, the choice of agent, dosage, frequency and period of application is geared towards an acute state of the disease. Often, this alone is sufficient for a permanent correction of a pathological skin condition. A subsequent maintenance phase involves the medium- and long-term application of an agent and/or a basic therapy. All above-mentioned criteria apply here as well.

Commonly used therapeutic agents

In summary, there are astringent, antiseptic, antipruritic, barrier protective, cooling, UV-protective and keratolytic therapies, which can be used as primary, adjunctive or follow-up medications. A topical active agent should be applied approximately 30 minutes prior to any other adjunctive therapy, so that any interactions may be avoided. Exceptions include keratolytic agents as a preliminary treatment for hyperkeratotic conditions in order to pave the way for other therapies, for example, antiinflammatory agents. Special indications may require special forms of application: agents can be delivered via wash or bath water, plaster, per occlusion, by touching or lacquering. Dosing and application aiding devices include combs, brushes, scoops and spatulas, vaporizers, foam spray and dosage dispensers. Active substances can be classified into (sometimes overlapping) categories. The following serve as examples: antiinflammatory agents (glucocorticoids, calcineurin inhibitors, antiinflammatory antibiotics, nonsteroidal antiinflammatory drugs, retinoids); antimicrobial agents (fungicides, antibiotics, antivirals, parasiticides, antiseptics); antiproliferative agents (vitamin D derivatives, dithranol); immune-modifying agents (so-called 'immune response modifier', cytotoxic agents).

References

1 Hoeger PH, Enzmann CC. Skin physiology of the neonate and young infant: a prospective study of functional skin parameters during early infancy. Pediatr Dermatol 2002;19(3):256–62.

2 Shwayder T, Akland T. Neonatal skin barrier: structure, function, and disorders. Dermatol Ther 2005;18(2):87–103.

3 Chiou YB, Blume-Peytavi U. Stratum corneum maturation. A review of neonatal skin function. Skin Pharmacol Physiol 2004;17(2):57–66.

4 Schaefer H, Jamoulle JC. Skin pharmacokinetics. Int J Dermatol 1988;27(6):351–9.

5 Trommer H, Neubert RH. Overcoming the stratum corneum: the modulation of skin penetration. A review. Skin Pharmacol Physiol 2006;19(2):106–21.

6 Wohlrab J. [Basics of topical therapy]. Hautarzt 2014;65(3):169–74.

7 Norlen L. Stratum corneum keratin structure, function and formation – a comprehensive review. Int J Cosmet Sci 2006;28(6):397–425.

8 Wartewig S, Neubert RH. Properties of ceramides and their impact on the stratum corneum structure: a review. Part 1: ceramides. Skin Pharmacol Physiol 2007;20(5):220–9.

9 Feingold KR. Thematic review series: skin lipids. The role of epidermal lipids in cutaneous permeability barrier homeostasis. J Lipid Res 2007;48(12):2531–46.

10 Verdier-Sevrain S, Bonte F. Skin hydration: a review on its molecular mechanisms. J Cosmet Dermatol 2007;6(2):75–82.

11 Robinson M, Visscher M, Laruffa A, Wickett R. Natural moisturizing factors (NMF) in the stratum corneum (SC). II. Regeneration of NMF over time after soaking. J Cosmet Sci 2010;61(1):23–9.

12 Engelbrecht TN, Schroeter A, Hauss T, Neubert RH. Lipophilic penetration enhancers and their impact to the bilayer structure of stratum corneum lipid model membranes: neutron diffraction studies based on the example oleic acid. Biochim Biophys Acta 2011;1808(12):2798–806.

13 Williams AC, Barry BW. Penetration enhancers. Advanced Drug Del Rev 2004;56(5):603–18.

14 Mollgaard B, Hoelgaard A. Vehicle effect on topical drug delivery. II. Concurrent skin transport of drugs and vehicle components. Acta Pharm Suec 1983;20(6):443–50.

15 Mollgaard B, Hoelgaard A. Vehicle effect on topical drug delivery. I. Influence of glycols and drug concentration on skin transport. Acta Pharm Suec 1983;20(6):433–42.

16 Vemuri S, Rhodes CT. Preparation and characterization of liposomes as therapeutic delivery systems: a review. Pharm Acta Helv 1995;70(2):95–111.
17 Ansari MJ, Kohli K, Dixit N. Microemulsions as potential drug delivery systems: a review. PDA J Pharm Sci Technol 2008;62(1):66–79.
18 Crosera M, Bovenzi M, Maina G et al. Nanoparticle dermal absorption and toxicity: a review of the literature. Int Arch Occup Environ Health 2009;82(9):1043–55.
19 Yamamoto A, Serizawa S, Ito M, Sato Y. Effect of aging on sebaceous gland activity and on the fatty acid composition of wax esters. J Invest Dermatol 1987;89(5):507–12.
20 Ness MJ, Davis DM, Careu WA. Neonatal skin care: a concise review. Int J Dermatol 2013;52(1):14–22.
21 Bibel DJ, Miller SJ, Brown BE et al. Antimicrobial activity of stratum corneum lipids from normal and essential fatty acid-deficient mice. J Invest Dermatol 1989;92(4):632–8.
22 Bharathi M, Sundaram V, Kumar P. Skin barrier therapy and neonatal mortality in preterm infants. Pediatrics 2009;123(2):e355; author reply e6.
23 Garcia Bartels N, Scheufele R, Prosch F et al. Effect of standardized skin care regimens on neonatal skin barrier function in different body areas. Pediatr Dermatol 2010;27(1):1–8.
24 Elias PM, Wakefield JS. Therapeutic implications of a barrier-based pathogenesis of atopic dermatitis. Clin Rev Allergy Immunol 2011; 41(3):282–95.
25 Derendorf H, Lesko LJ, Chaikin P et al. Pharmacokinetic/pharmacodynamic modeling in drug research and development. J Clin Pharmacol 2000;40(12 Pt 2):1399–418.
26 Derendorf H, Meibohm B. Modeling of pharmacokinetic/pharmacodynamic (PK/PD) relationships: concepts and perspectives. Pharmaceut Res 1999;16(2):176–85.
27 Oliveira G, Leverett JC, Emamzadeh M, Lane ME. The effects of heat on skin barrier function and in vivo dermal absorption. Int J Pharmaceut 2014;464(1-2):145–51.
28 Wohlrab J, Klapperstuck T, Reinhardt HW, Albrecht M. Interaction of epicutaneously applied lipids with stratum corneum depends on the presence of either emulsifiers or hydrogenated phosphatidylcholine. Skin Pharmacol Physiol 2010;23(6):298–305.
29 Wurbach G, Schiller F, Langguth K et al. [The modification of skin surface film by tensides. 1: Defatting as a function of concentration and constitution]. Dermatol Monatschr 1983;169(4):243–7.
30 Grether-Beck S, Felsner I, Brenden H et al. Urea uptake enhances barrier function and antimicrobial defense in humans by regulating epidermal gene expression. J Invest Dermatol 2012;132(6):1561–72.
31 Hafeez F, Maibach H. Occlusion Effect on in vivo percutaneous penetration of chemicals in man and monkey: partition coefficient effects. Skin Pharmacol Physiol 2013;26(2):85–91.
32 Kessner D, Ruettinger A, Kiselev MA et al. Properties of ceramides and their impact on the stratum corneum structure. Part 2: stratum corneum lipid model systems. Skin Pharmacol Physiol 2008;21(2): 58–74.
33 Gelardi A, Morini F, Dusatti F et al. Induction by xenobiotics of phase I and phase II enzyme activities in the human keratinocyte cell line NCTC 2544. Toxicol In Vitro 2001;15(6):701–11.
34 Bebia Z, Buch SC, Wilson JW et al. Bioequivalence revisited: influence of age and sex on CYP enzymes. Clin Pharmacol Therapeut 2004; 76(6):618–27.
35 Hanghoj S, Boisen KA. Self-reported barriers to medication adherence among chronically ill adolescents: a systematic review. J Adolesc Health 2014;54:121–38.
36 Hodari KT, Nanton JR, Carroll CL et al. Adherence in dermatology: a review of the last 20 years. J Dermatol Treat 2006;17(3):136–42.

CHAPTER 169
Systemic Therapy in Paediatric Dermatology

Blanca Rosa Del Pozzo-Magana[1] *& Irene Lara-Corrales*[2]

[1] London Health Sciences Center and Western University, London, ON, Canada
[2] Hospital for Sick Children, University of Toronto, Toronto, ON, Canada

Antibiotics, 2282
Antifungal therapy, 2285
Antivirals, 2286
Antiparasitic drugs, 2287
Corticosteroids, 2287
Antihistamines, 2288
Antimalarial agents, 2289
β-Blockers, 2289
Retinoids, 2290
Biologic agents, 2291
Chemotherapy and immunomodulators, 2293
Janus kinase (JAK) inhibitors, 2295
Miscellaneous, 2295

Abstract

While topical therapy is generally restricted to local effects based on site of application, systemic therapy may at times be advantageous due to its ability to distribute to various areas of the body, leading to a generally faster and more potent effect. Both oral medications (tablets, capsules, pills and syrups) and injectable solutions (intravenous, intramuscular or subcutaneous) are commonly used to treat or control skin disorders. When selecting a systemic medication, several variables must be considered, such as diagnosis, age, body surface area involved, cost, availability, contraindications and side-effects, among others. The list of medications used as systemic therapy in dermatology and more specifically in paediatric dermatology is extensive. This chapter reviews the most common groups of medications used in paediatric dermatology, their respective indications, and special considerations for their use in children.

Key points

- Beside their antibacterial effect, tetracyclines, sulfonamides and macrolides have anti-inflammatory properties and can be used in several noninfectious skin conditions including acne, rosacea, pityriasis lichenoides, periorificial dermatitis and pityriasis rosea.
- Currently, clindamycin and trimethoprim–sulfamethoxazole are first-line treatment options to treat methicillin-resistant *Staphylococcus aureus* (MRSA) skin infections.
- Patients with glucose-6-phosphate dehydrogenase (G6PD) deficiency have a higher risk of developing haemolysis when exposed to dapsone or other sulfone derivates.
- Systemic therapy for fungal infections in children should be limited to refractory infections or to conditions such tinea capitis, mucocutaneous candidiasis, onychomycoses, and systemic infections or immunocompromised patients.
- Systemic aciclovir indications include neonatal herpes, herpes gladiatorum, herpes labialis, herpetic gingivostomatitis, herpetic whitlow, Kaposi varicelliform eruption (eczema herpeticum) and prophylaxis of herpes simplex virus (HSV)-associated erythema multiforme.
- Safety and efficacy of ivermectin in children with scabies, pediculosis and larva migrans has been widely reported.
- Slow taper of corticosteroids for children receiving this treatment for more than 14 days is indicated, and live-viral vaccines should be avoided for up to 3 months after the treatment has been discontinued.
- H_1 antihistamines are the first-line treatment for chronic urticaria in children.
- β-Blockers are currently first-line treatment for the management of complicated infantile haemangiomas.
- Pregnancy is an absolute contraindication in female patients treated with systemic retinoids and patients should not become pregnant for at least 1–3 months after the drug has been discontinued.
- In children, etanercept, infliximab and rituximab are prescribed biologic agents used to treat cutaneous conditions. There are a number of new biologic agents in development. Dupilumab is the first biologic to be approved for the treatment of moderate-to-severe atopic dermatitis in adults. Clinical trials in children are currently underway.
- Weekly supplementation with folic acid in children treated with methotrexate reduces the risk of side-effects.
- Sirolimus has been shown to produce significant clinical improvement in children with complicated vascular anomalies such as kaposiform haemangioendothelioma with or without Kasabach–Merritt phenomenon.
- New emerging drugs such as Janus kinase (JAK) inhibitors seem to be a promising therapy for children with alopecia areata.

Antibiotics

Antibiotics are an important therapeutic resource in paediatric dermatology, used to treat both infectious and noninfectious skin conditions. These are part of a large group of chemical substances with a wide variety of molecular structures whose main purpose is either to inhibit the growth of or to destroy bacteria. In addition, some antibiotics also have well-recognized anti-inflammatory properties, thus expanding their use beyond strictly infectious dermatoses [1,2]

Skin and soft tissue infections are a common problem among children worldwide. The incidence of these

Harper's Textbook of Pediatric Dermatology, Fourth Edition. Edited by Peter Hoeger, Veronica Kinsler and Albert Yan.

conditions varies widely among hospital settings (in/outpatients) and geographical areas. Several reports show an incidence range between 12.1% and 43.5% [3–8]. Some of the bacterial skin infections commonly found in children include impetigo, folliculitis, furunculosis, carbuncles, wound infections, pyodermas, ecthymas, abscesses, cellulitis, erysipelas, scarlet fever, acute paronychia and staphylococcal scalded skin syndrome [9–12]. Overall, *Staphylococcus aureus* and *Streptococcus pyogenes* account for the majority of bacterial skin infections in children, and therefore empirical treatment should generally be directed towards these agents. However, the increase seen in the number of cases involving methicillin-resistant strains of *Staph.* (MRSA) may contribute to selection of specific agents targeting MRSA, depending on risk factors and local susceptibility patterns [13,14]. Antibiotics are also the mainstay of treatment for many of the sexually transmitted infections (STI) [15] (see Chapter 163).

In addition to antibacterial effects, several antibiotics possess anti-inflammatory and immune-modulatory characteristics. These properties were first described over 20 years ago in certain macrolide antibiotics used for the treatment of pulmonary disease (e.g. diffuse panbronchiolitis, chronic obstructive pulmonary disease [COPD], cystic fibrosis); currently, their use has spread to other areas of medicine including paediatric dermatology. Examples of skin conditions that benefit from the anti-inflammatory and immune-modulatory action of antibiotics include pityriasis rosea, seborrhoeic dermatitis, perioral dermatitis, acne, rosacea, neutrophilic dermatoses (pyoderma gangrenosum, subcorneal pustular dermatosis, Sweet syndrome), urticarial eruptions and various bullous disorders (pemphigus vulgaris, bullous pemphigoid, cicatricial pemphigoid, linear immunoglobulin A [IgA] dermatosis [chronic bullous disease of childhood], epidermolysis bullosa, dermatitis herpetiformis) [16].

β-Lactam antibiotics

β-Lactam antibiotics comprise a large group of medications widely used to treat a variety of infectious diseases. This group is composed of penicillins, cephalosporins and carbapenems. They share a common structure (β-lactam ring) and mechanism of action (inhibition of synthesis of the bacterial peptidoglycan cell wall) [17]. Although the numbers of β-lactam and methicillin-resistant bacterial strains have increased considerably, β-lactams continue to be useful in the treatment of specific infectious diseases (syphilis, Lyme disease, erysipeloid) and are often appropriate first-line agents when the suspected pathogen is methicillin-sensitive *Staph. aureus* or *Strep. pyogenes*, such as for impetigo, furunculosis, folliculitis, mild cellulitis and erysipelas, among others [9,13,17]. Use may be limited by the relative high frequency of adverse drug reactions; drug hypersensitivity to β-lactam antibiotics has been reported in 5–12% of children [18]. Other common side-effects include diarrhoea, nausea and vomiting [19].

Macrolides

Erythromycin and its semi-synthetic derivatives, clarithromycin, azithromycin and telithromycin, belong to the macrolide class of antibiotics. They contain a macrocyclic lactone ring attached to one or more deoxy sugars. These antibiotics are bacteriostatic agents that inhibit bacterial protein synthesis by binding reversibly to 50S ribosomal subunits. Aerobic Gram-positive cocci and bacilli, staphylococci and streptococci are susceptible to macrolides, although the emergence of resistant strains has limited their use. Even so, macrolides provide a reasonable alternative empirical treatment strategy for penicillin-allergic patients with erysipelas and cellulitis [20]. Additionally, azithromycin is useful in the treatment of certain STI caused by *Neisseria gonorrhoeae* and *Chlamydia trachomatis* [19]. Interestingly, macrolides also possess anti-inflammatory and immune-modulatory properties. They have been shown to inhibit the production of many pro-inflammatory cytokines, such as interleukin (IL)-1, IL-6, IL-8 and tumour necrosis factor-α. Several studies have demonstrated the utility of these antibiotics to treat inflammatory skin conditions such as acne, peri-orificial dermatitis, rosacea, pityriasis rosea and pityriasis lichenoides, among others [2,21–26]. Macrolides have the major disadvantage of being associated with gastrointestinal (GI) side-effects such as epigastric pain, nausea, vomiting and diarrhoea. Other undesirable effects include cholestatic hepatitis, cardiac arrhythmias and, less frequently, fever, eosinophilia and skin rash [20].

Tetracyclines

The use of tetracyclines in paediatric dermatology is restricted to older children (>8 years) and adolescents due to adverse effects reported in younger children, including discolouration of the teeth, delayed bone growth and pseudotumor cerebri [20]. The tetracycline antibiotics are formed by four fused, six-membered rings. Mechanism of action involves the inhibition of bacterial protein synthesis by binding to the 30S subunit of the bacterial ribosome, leading to bacteriostatic effects [27]. Common uses include the treatment of a wide range of infections, such as syphilis (*Treponema pallidum*), Lyme disease (*Borrelia borgdorferi*) and infections caused by strains of MRSA [28]. As with macrolides, tetracyclines have also demonstrated anti-inflammatory properties, with possible inhibition of COX-2-mediated prostaglandin E_2 and nitric oxide production [27]. Tetracyclines as anti-inflammatory agents have been used with varying degrees of success in the treatment of a variety of skin conditions, perhaps most commonly acne and rosacea, but their use in other inflammatory conditions such as bullous dermatoses, dystrophic epidermolysis bullosa, hidradenitis suppurativa and pityriasis lichenoides has been also reported [28]. Tetracycline, doxycycline and minocycline are the three tetracyclines that have been used and studied most extensively in dermatology. In addition to the side-effects reported in younger children, tetracyclines can produce GI upset including epigastric pain, nausea, vomiting and diarrhoea [20]. They also increase skin photosensitivity in patients exposed to sunlight. Onycholysis and pigmentation of the nails has also been reported [29].

Clindamycin

Clindamycin is a lincosamide, a derivate of the amino acid *trans* l-4-n propylhygrinic acid. It binds to the 50S subunit of bacterial ribosomes and suppresses protein synthesis. Antimicrobial activity is similar to erythromycin with susceptibility seen in strains of *Streptococcus pyogenes, Streptococcus viridans*, and meticillin-susceptible strains of *Staph. aureus*. It is therefore a reasonable alternative agent for the treatment of skin and soft tissue infections (SSTI), particularly in patients with β-lactam allergies or community-associated MRSA [20]. Recent studies have shown that clindamycin is superior to trimethoprim–sulfamethoxazole and β-lactams for the acute treatment and prevention of SSTI (in the case of recurrence); furthermore, bacterial resistance is lower for clindamycin than for other antibiotics [30]. Oral clindamycin combined with rifampicin has been shown to be effective in the treatment of hidradenitis suppurativa in adults and adolescents [31]. As with other antibiotics, clindamycin has been associated with GI side-effects, including its propensity to cause *Clostridium difficile*-associated diarrhoea. Skin rashes and hypersensitivity syndrome have also been reported in up to 10% of patients [32].

Trimethoprim–sulfamethoxazole

Trimethoprim–sulfamethoxazole (TMP-SMX) is a synergistic combination of two antibiotics that has shown efficacy against several infectious agents including *Corynebacterium diphtheriae, Strep. pneumoniae, Staph. aureus, Staph. epidermidis, Strep. pyogenes, Strep. viridans, Escherichia coli, Mycobacterium marinum/fortuitum* and *Nocardia asteroides*, among others [33]. Its mechanism of action is the result of the combination of both antibiotics. The sulfonamide inhibits the incorporation of *para*-aminobenzoic acid (PABA) into folic acid, and trimethoprim prevents the reduction of dihydrofolate to tetrahydrofolate, which is essential in bacterial nucleic acid synthesis [17]. Additionally, TMP-SMX may have anti-inflammatory and immune-modulatory properties. Some reports have shown that it reduces proliferation of lymphocytes [33]. Historically, the use of TMP-SMX decreased somewhat with the demonstration of severe adverse effects, including GI intolerance, cytopenias, severe systemic drug hypersensitivity syndromes, Stevens–Johnson syndrome (SJS) and toxic epidermal necrolysis (TEN) (Fig. 169.1); however, with the recent increased incidence of MRSA, TMP-SMX has re-emerged as an effective therapeutic option. Miller et al. studied the treatment of uncomplicated skin infections in 524 patients, notably with children comprising 30% of the study population, and found no significant difference between clindamycin and TMP-SMX regarding efficacy or side-effects [34]. It has been suggested that in areas with high rates of clindamycin resistance, TMP-SMX might be preferred as an empirical treatment option for skin infections [35]. There is little evidence regarding other dermatological indications for TMP-SMX in children. A recent review by Michalek et al. suggested that TMP-SMX may be prescribed as a first-line agent for nocardiosis, melioidiosis, *M. marinum* infections and cat scratch disease [33]. Other uses, when conventional therapy is ineffective, include acne vulgaris, granuloma inguinale, lymphogranuloma venereum and pyoderma gangrenosum.

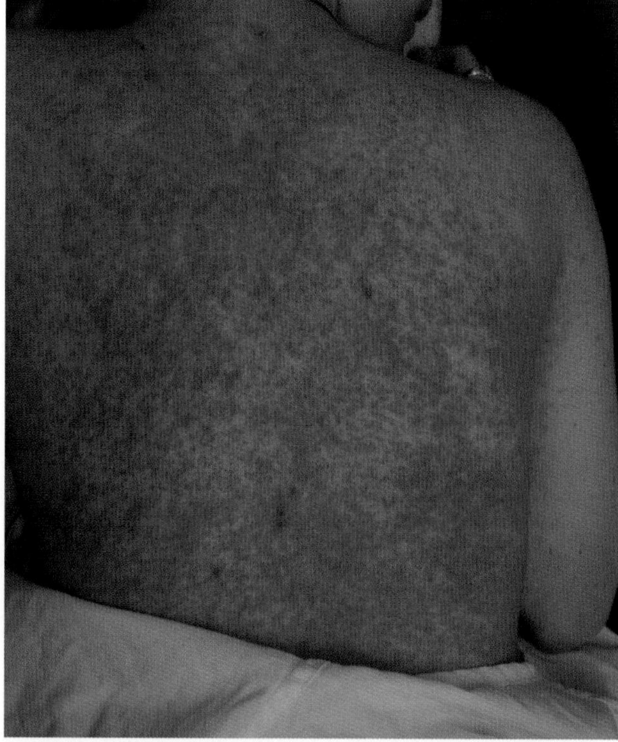

Fig. 169.1 Drug hypersensitivity syndrome secondary to trimethoprim–sulfamethoxazole.

Dapsone

Dapsone, also known as 4′-diaminodiphenylsulfone, belongs to the sulfonamide group of antibiotics. It is a structural analogue of PABA and a competitive inhibitor of dihydropteroate synthase in the folate pathway, with antibacterial, antiprotozoal, antifungal and anti-inflammatory properties. The latter are due to the inhibition of neutrophil myeloperoxidase and neutrophil lysosomal enzyme activity, neutralizing free radicals generated by neutrophils. It may also inhibit migration of neutrophils to inflammatory lesions [36]. Dapsone was initially used as antibiotic therapy for streptococcal infections, gonorrhoea, mycobacterial infections and leprosy. Later its use spread, due to its anti-inflammatory effects, to the treatment of dermatitis herpetiformis and other autoimmune dermatoses mediated by neutrophils [37,38]. Currently, dapsone is considered first-line treatment for dermatitis herpetiformis, subcorneal pustulosis, erythema elevatum diutinum, acropustulosis of infancy and linear IgA dermatosis [39]. Other conditions in children in which dapsone has demonstrated efficacy include Sweet syndrome, bullous systemic lupus erythematosus, pemphigus foliaceus and pustular psoriasis, among others [40–42]. A major disadvantage of this drug is its associations with haematological abnormalities such as haemolysis; patients with glucose-6-phosphate dehydrogenase (G6PD) deficiency have a higher risk of developing haemolysis when exposed to dapsone, and therefore this medication is contraindicated when known G6PD deficiency is present [43]. Methaemoglobinaemia is also a common adverse effect; less commonly, a genetic deficiency of the NADH-dependent methaemoglobin reductase can result in severe methaemoglobinaemia after administration of dapsone [36]. A dapsone hypersensitivity syndrome has also been described, characterized by fever, rash and systemic involvement (liver and blood abnormalities) [44]. Therefore, prophylactic administration of folic acid, iron and vitamin E in addition to close monitoring of laboratory (complete blood count, differential, liver function tests, renal function) and previous G6PD determinations are strongly recommended [37].

Antifungal therapy

Cutaneous fungal infections are a common presenting complaint to both paediatricians and dermatologists worldwide. Dermatophytes are the most common pathogens responsible for these infections, including *Trichophyton (tonsurans, violaceum, mentagrophytes, schoenleinii, soudanense, verrucosum)* and *Microsporum (canis, gallinae, audouinii, langeronii)* species. Dermatophyte infection may affect skin, hair and nails, but not mucosae. Candida (*C. albicans*), on the other hand, is a genus of yeast that is normally commensal in the human GI tract (including the mouth), becoming pathogenic when the host's normal immune system is altered [45]. Overall, fungal skin infections are generally not life-threatening and usually respond to topical therapy in immunocompetent hosts. Thus, the use of systemic antifungals for such infections in children should be limited to those fungal infections that are refractory to topical agents or where topical treatment is not sufficient to eradicate the infection. Typical conditions that require systemic treatment first-line include tinea capitis, mucocutaneous candidiasis, onychomycoses and systemic infections in severely ill or immunocompromised patients. Furthermore, deep mycoses such as sporotrichosis, histoplasmosis, cryptococcosis, coccidioidomycosis and aspergillosis, which are usually rare in developed countries but have become more common due to immunosuppression and globalization, also require systemic antifungal therapy [46]. There are numerous systemic agents available, although not all are recommended for paediatric use. Of these, the most common agents used in children and young adults include terbinafine, itraconazole, fluconazole and griseofulvin [47,48]. Choice of agent ultimately depends on local availability, cost and fungal susceptibility patterns.

Terbinafine

Terbinafine is an allylamine with fungicidal and fungistatic properties. Its mechanism of action is due to its ability to inhibit squalene epoxidase, which leads to reduced synthesis of ergosterol in fungal cell membranes and accumulation of squalene [45]. Terbinafine has been proven to be effective against dermatophytes and non-dermatophyte moulds with high cure rates, up to 80.4% in paediatric onychomycosis [49]. In tinea capitis, terbinafine proved to be superior to griseofulvin in infections caused by *Trichophyton* spp. [50] (Fig. 169.2). Although the efficacy and safety of terbinafine in children has been well documented, several reports (primarily in adults) have shown that it can cause liver damage with an estimated incidence of 1/120 000 [51]. For this reason, measurement of aspartate aminotransferase (AST) and alanine aminotransferase (ALT) is recommended by some physicians before starting systemic therapy [52]. Screening for associated co-morbid liver disease on history and physical examination may also be pertinent prior to initiating systemic terbinafine. Other adverse effects include allergic reactions, nasopharyngitis, headache, vomiting, SJS, exacerbation of systemic lupus erythematosus, depression and haematological abnormalities [45]. Terbinafine resistance of *Trichophyton* spp. is being increasingly reported, in particular in India.

Griseofulvin

Griseofulvin has been used for more than 50 years as a treatment of tinea capitis [53]. This drug is derived from *Penicillium griseofulvum*, a mould, and is active against dermatophytes such as *Trichophyton, Microsporum* and *Epidermophyton* species [54]. Griseofulvin is a mitotic

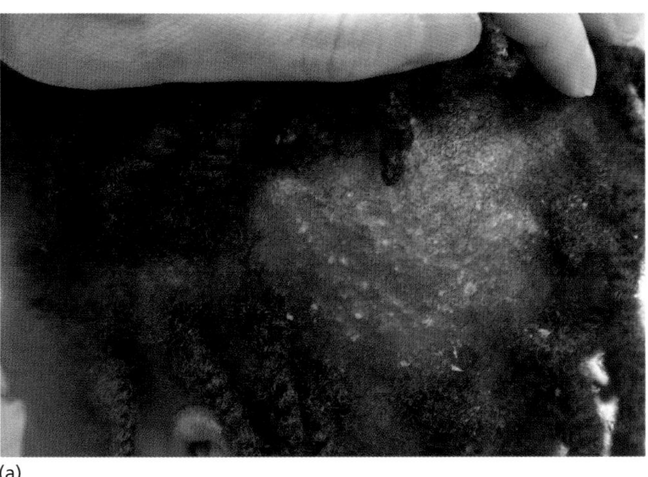
(a)

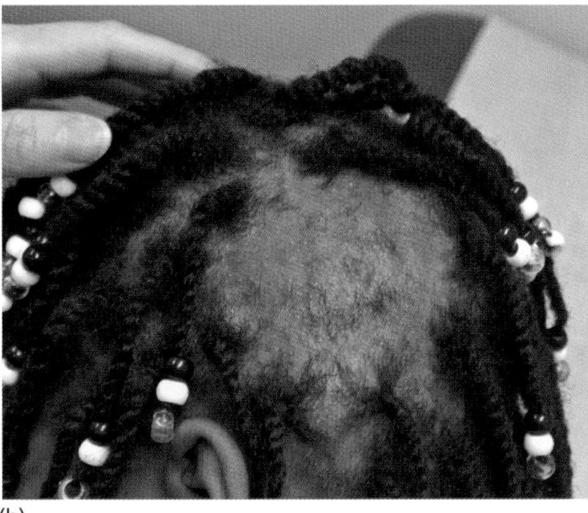
(b)

Fig. 169.2 Tinea capitis: (a) at diagnosis, and (b) 4 weeks after treatment with terbinafine.

inhibitor and interferes with nucleic acid, protein and cell wall synthesis of replicating dermatophyte cells. However, it cannot diffuse into the stratum corneum or hair follicle. Thus, several weeks of treatment, often more than six, are necessary to obtain clinical and mycological cure. Increasing resistance against griseofulvin has also led to the recommendation of higher doses of griseofulvin than previously used for the treatment of tinea capitis [45]. Recent studies have shown that griseofulvin continues to be an effective treatment for tinea capitis with cure rates of up to 96% [53], and it has been shown to be superior to terbinafine in tinea capitis caused by *Microsporum* spp. [50]. Griseofulvin is generally safe in children, with typically minor adverse effects: headaches, GI reactions and cutaneous eruptions are among those reported [55]. Griseofulvin increases the rate of metabolism of warfarin as a result of hepatic cytochromes P450 induction, thus the dose of warfarin must be adjusted in patients who are taking these medications simultaneously [56].

Itraconazole

Itraconazole is a fungistatic agent belonging to the azole group (triazoles) of antifungals. Its mechanism of action involves inhibition of lanosterol 14α-demethylase, which impairs the biosynthesis of ergosterol for the cytoplasmic membrane, thus inhibiting growth of the fungi [56]. Itraconazole has an extremely broad spectrum of activity against fungi including *Blastomyces dermatitidis, Histoplasma capsulatum, Paracoccidioides brasiliensis, Coccidioides immitis, Aspergillus* and dermatophytes [45,56]. It also has shown effectiveness in treating *Candida* infections [52]. A systematic review showed that itraconazole has similar cure rates to terbinafine (>80%) in paediatric patients treated for dermatophyte infections, particularly *Microsporum* spp. [49]. Itraconazole has also been shown to be effective as pulse therapy for the treatment of onychomycosis in children [57]. In adults, itraconazole has been associated with serious side-effects such as hepatotoxicity, drug interactions and cardiac failure; however, in children the frequency of adverse drug reactions is less than 2%, with documented side-effects including nausea, vomiting, skin rash, headache, dizziness, sleepiness and abnormal liver function (typically mild and transient) [49].

Amphotericin B

Amphotericin B (AmB) is one of some 200 polyene macrolide compounds with antifungal activity [56]. Its mechanism of action is based on the binding of the AmB molecule to ergosterol within the fungal cell membrane, producing an aggregate that creates a transmembrane channel, leading to leaking of the cytoplasm content and consequently cell death [58]. AmB has a wide clinical activity against *Candida* spp. and other fungal agents such as *Aspergillus* spp., *Sporothrix schenckii, Coccidioides* spp. and *P. brasiliensis*. It has also been shown to be effective against some protozoa such as *Leishmania* spp. [56]. In children, AmB has been used effectively in the treatment of neonatal candidiasis [59] and some forms of cutaneous and systemic leishmaniasis [60]. Despite its efficacy, the use of AmB has been limited due to its association with several adverse effects including fever, nausea, vomiting, nephrotoxicity, cardiac alterations, haemolysis and liver damage [61]. Several AmB lipid-based derivatives have been developed in an attempt to reduce adverse effects (AmB liposomal, AmB colloidal dispersion and AmB lipid complex), but their cost is extremely high compared to regular AmB [62].

Antivirals

Viral infections of the skin in children are very common. They can be localized (strictly mucocutaneous) or have multisystem involvement. Overall, viral infections of the skin are generally mild and self-limiting. However, when recurrent or associated with immunodeficiencies, viral infections may lead to serious complications and even life-threatening illness, particularly with the herpesviruses. Antiviral agents have been shown in these cases to reduce the duration of clinical illness, recurrences and consequently both morbidity and mortality [63–69]. Some of the agents frequently used in paediatric dermatology to treat herpesvirus infections include aciclovir and its derivatives, such as valaciclovir and famciclovir. Ribavirin (approved for the treatment of respiratory syncytial virus in children) has also been shown to be efficacious in the prevention and treatment of hand, foot and mouth disease in children (caused by various strains of the coxsackie virus) [70,71]. However, more evidence is necessary to establish its usefulness in this condition.

Aciclovir

Aciclovir selectively inhibits DNA replication in virus-infected cells. It binds to viral DNA polymerases in an irreversible complex, thus leaving the DNA polymerase inactive [72]. Aciclovir is currently used to treat several herpes simplex virus (HSV) and varicella zoster virus (VZV) infections including recurrent episodes of HSV in immunocompromised patients, severe initial episodes of genital HSV in immunocompetent patients, HSV encephalitis, VZV in immunocompromised or immunocompetent children and acute herpes zoster in immunocompetent children [73]. Specific paediatric HSV skin infections in which the use of aciclovir is indicated include neonatal herpes, herpes gladiatorum, herpes labialis, herpetic gingivostomatitis, herpetic whitlow, Kaposi varicelliform eruption (eczema herpeticum), prophylaxis of HSV-associated erythema multiforme, herpetic geometric glossitis, HSV infection in paediatric burn patients, and folliculitis attributable to HSV [63]. Although aciclovir is generally well tolerated, some infrequent minor adverse events have been reported such as nausea, diarrhoea, rash and headache. Rare severe reactions include leucopenia, renal insufficiency and neurotoxicity [74].

Valaciclovir

Valaciclovir is an L-valyl ester product of aciclovir. While its mechanism of action is comparable to aciclovir, valaciclovir has improved bioavailability [75], allowing for less frequent, and therefore more convenient, dosing [72,76]. The spectrum of activity of valaciclovir is identical to aciclovir, and it is similarly indicated for the treatment of initial or recurrent episodes of genital HSV, recurrent herpes labialis and VZV in immunocompromised patients [75]. A recent study comparing aciclovir and valaciclovir in the treatment of chickenpox in children demonstrated that while aciclovir was superior in reducing duration of fever, there was no significant difference between medications in the prevention of new lesions or rate of adverse effects [77]. The higher cost associated with valaciclovir compared with aciclovir may limit its use in certain populations.

Famciclovir

Famciclovir is a diacetyl 6-deoxy analogue of penciclovir which acts as an inhibitor of viral DNA synthesis [74]. It is effective against HSV-1, HSV-2 and VZV, and is therefore indicated for the treatment of herpes zoster, recurrent genital herpes and recurrent herpes labialis [75]. In children with active HSV and VZV disease, famciclovir has demonstrated resolution of symptoms in more than 90% of patients [78]. Adverse reactions are usually minor, and commonly include nausea, diarrhoea and headache [72]. Famciclovir has also been shown to be safe in infants [79].

Antiparasitic drugs

Parasitic diseases affect more than 2 billion people globally and cause substantial morbidity and mortality, particularly among the world's poorest populations [80]. Ectoparasites live on the outer surface of the host and generally attach themselves during feeding; organisms affecting the skin include a wide variety of arthropods and worms. In children, pediculosis capitis and scabies are the most common infections by ectoparasites worldwide and, although not life-threatening conditions, may cause high levels of discomfort due to itching and lead to secondary infections such as impetigo [81]. Other parasitic diseases with cutaneous involvement such as larva migrans, myiasis and tungiasis were classically restricted to tropical areas such as Africa, Latin America and the Caribbean; however, the increase in international trade, travel and immigration has led to their dissemination around the world [82]. Topical agents (pyrethrins, permethrin, malathion, sulphur and, previously, lindane) continue to be first-line treatment for many of these conditions, but the emergence of resistance and recurrence has led to alternative options such as oral albendazole and ivermectin [81,83].

Albendazole

Albendazole is a benzimidazole carbamate derivate. It has a wide spectrum of activity against intestinal nematodes (e.g. *Ascaris lumbricoides*), cestodes (e.g. neurocysticercosis) and systemic nematodes (e.g. cutaneous larva migrans) [84]. Its mechanism of action involves interaction with the eukaryotic cytoskeletal protein β-tubulin, inhibiting its polymerization intro microtubules [85]. Albendazole is considered first-line treatment for larva migrans in children and adults, especially in countries where ivermectin is not available [86]. Albendazole has been shown to be effective and safe in early infancy [87] and is well tolerated. Several authors have reported minimal side-effects, primarily stomach upset and bitter taste, when used to treat children with *Giardia lamblia* [88]; however, in patients exposed to high and prolonged doses (for example, in the treatment of hydatid disease) more significant effects, such as alopecia, skin rashes, headache, liver and haematological abnormalities, have been reported [84]. Tiabendazole, another antiparasitic usually indicated for strongyloidiasis, has also shown efficacy in the treatment of larva migrans and pediculosis capitis [89]. Tiabendazole has a similar mechanism of action to albendazole, but toxicity (particularly gastrointestinal) is more significant. In countries where albendazole and tiabendazole are not available, mebendazole, which is also a benzimidazole, has been used as a treatment option for patients with larva migrans; however, its poor oral bioavailability (less than 10% of the drug is absorbed systemically) makes it less effective than other agents, so the need to re-treat with either albendazole or ivermectin is not uncommon [86].

Ivermectin

Ivermectin is a synthetic derivative of a broad-spectrum antiparasitic class of macrocyclic lactones (avermectins). It has a similar structure to macrolides but has no antibacterial activity. Ivermectin acts on the chloride-dependent channels of both glutamate and γ-aminobutyric acid, interrupting neurotransmission of invertebrates [90]. Due to its wide antiparasitic activity, ivermectin is used to treat a wide range of endoparasitic and ectoparasitic infections in animals and humans worldwide. Dermatological interest in ivermectin has increased significantly since the demonstration of efficacy against scabies and head lice. Although ivermectin has been approved by several organizations for the treatment of worm infestations, it is not approved by the US Food and Drug Administration (FDA) for scabies and head lice despite known efficacy. In the USA and many other countries, its off-label use has increased [91]. Today, applications of ivermectin in dermatology include scabies, pediculosis, demodicosis, cutaneous larva migrans, cutaneous larva currens, myiasis, filariasis, onchocerciasis and loiasis [92]. Safety and efficacy specifically in children with scabies, pediculosis and larva migrans has been widely reported [86,90,93,94]. For mass drug administration in populations with endemic scabies, ivermectin has been shown to be more effective than permethrin for both primary scabies control and prevention of secondary impetigo [95]. Although no serious reactions have been documented, minor adverse effects reported include fever, headache, chills, arthralgia, rash, eosinophilia and anorexia. Caution in young children and pregnant women is recommended [96].

Corticosteroids

The use of systemic corticosteroids in children is usually limited to severe inflammatory and autoimmune disorders. Corticosteroids decrease the synthesis of pro-inflammatory molecules and inhibit prostaglandin and leukotriene production. They also have antiproliferative effects and impair monocyte and lymphocyte function. Their role as anti-inflammatories and immunosuppressants is wide and varied [97]. Potency of specific corticosteroids is determined both by extent of Na^+ retention (adrenal effects) and effect on glucose metabolism (anti-inflammatory effects), reflecting selective actions at distinct receptors. Corticosteroids are therefore divided into mineralocorticoids and glucocorticoids based on the primary site of action [98]. In dermatology, selecting a glucocorticoid with minimal mineralocorticoid activity, such as prednisone or prednisolone, is critical to maximizing the desired anti-inflammatory and immunosuppressive effect [99]. In paediatric dermatology, systemic therapy with corticosteroids has traditionally been used in the treatment of: moderate-to-severe adverse drug reactions including SJS and TEN; bullous conditions such as erythema multiforme, bullous dermatosis of childhood (linear IgA disease), bullous lichen planus, pemphigus and pemphigoid; acute allergic reactions such as anaphylactic shock, angioneurotic oedema, multiple bee or wasp stings, poisonous bites and severe contact dermatitis; cutaneous manifestations of connective tissue diseases, such as systemic lupus erythematosus, dermatomyositis and morphoea; vasculitis; neutrophilic dermatoses, including Sweet syndrome and pyoderma gangrenosum; and alopecia areata [97,100–104]. Although historically used first-line in the treatment of haemangiomas of infancy, oral steroids have largely been replaced by β-blockers, as these have been proven to be more effective and better tolerated [105]. In atopic dermatitis, use of systemic steroids is generally limited to the short term in isolated cases, and only while other systemic therapies or phototherapy are being initiated and/or optimized [106].

Although highly efficacious, long-term therapy with systemic corticosteroids is associated with a wide range of side-effects, and therefore assessment of risk–benefit ratios is critical prior to use. Of the extensive side-effects associated with systemic corticosteroids, some commonly reported adverse effects include gastritis, cataracts, psychological abnormalities (irritability, emotional lability, depression), hypothyroidism, amenorrhoea in women, fluid and electrolyte imbalances (oedema, hypertension and hypokalaemia), metabolic disturbances (increase of blood glucose, reduction of sensitivity to insulin, increase of gluconeogenesis), fat redistribution, hirsutism, acne, Cushing syndrome, osteoporosis and growth suppression (secondary to reduction of growth hormone) [107]. Several considerations may help minimize unwanted effects; these include selection of an agent with minimal mineralocorticoid effect, prolonged use of drugs with intermediate half-life and low affinity for the steroid receptor (such as prednisone), substitution of an agent with its biologically active form (for example prednisolone instead of prednisone), and use of methylprednisolone pulses (high potency with lower sodium retention) [108,109]. Administration in the morning, around 8:00 am, to reduce impairment of the hypothalamic–pituitary–adrenal axis, has been also recommended. For short-term courses, a dosing frequency of 2–3 times per day has proved to have better anti-inflammatory effect than once-daily dosing. For long-term courses, reducing frequency of administration to every other day can reduce the incidence of side-effects. Prior to discontinuing the steroid, a slow taper of the dose is indicated; however, when the therapy is shorter than 2–3 weeks, the reduction can be faster [97,110]. Children receiving systemic therapy with corticosteroids should avoid live-viral vaccines up to 3 months after the treatment has been discontinued [111].

Antihistamines

Antihistamines are drugs commonly used in dermatological practice to treat itch and other symptoms of allergic and/or inflammatory conditions. Antihistamines are antagonists of histamine receptors and act by competing with histamine for tissue receptors, thus preventing the normal pharmacological action of histamine [112]. Histamine is synthesized and released by different human cells (basophils, mast cells, platelets, histaminergic neurones, lymphocytes and enterochromaffin cells, among others) and exerts its effects by binding to its four receptors (H_1, H_2, H_3, H_4) which are localized in a wide variety of cell tissues such as nerve cells, airway and vascular smooth muscle, endothelial cells, eosinophils, bone marrow and peripheral haematopoietic cells, lungs, T and B cells, etc. [113]. Histamine regulates the expression of pruritic factors via the histamine H_1 receptor (H1R) and also plays a role in the induction of allergic inflammation by activating eosinophils, mast cells, basophils and Th2 cells via the histamine H_4 receptor (H4R). Traditionally, H_1 and H_2 antihistamines have been widely used in the treatment of several dermatological conditions with different degrees of effectiveness. Currently, a novel therapy targeting H4R (JNJ39758979, H4R antagonist) seems to have a promising effect against pruritus and allergic inflammation [114].

H_1 antihistamines

Initially classified by their chemical structure, the H_1 antihistamines were previously grouped as alkylamines (chlorphenamine), ethanolamines (diphenhydramine), ethylenediamines (prylamine), phenothiazines (promethazine), piperazines (hydroxyzine, cetirizine, levocetirizine) and piperidines (ketotifen, loratadine, desloratadine). Currently, H_1 antihistamines are usually divided into first- and second-generation [115].

First-generation H_1 antihistamines are lipophilic drugs that are rapidly absorbed and metabolized, necessitating dosing 3–4 times per day. They have poor receptor selectivity for H1R, occupying muscarinic, cholinergic, α-adrenergic, and serotonin receptors as well as ion channels [116]. They are also able to cross the blood–brain barrier, leading to characteristic central nervous system (CNS) effects such as sedation and somnolence [117]. Thus they have been commonly used as an adjuvant therapy in patients with itchy dermatitis to promote sleep and thereby reduce nocturnal scratching. Recent literature suggests that sedating antihistamines might have detrimental effects on quality of sleep, which can impair learning and work efficiency in both children and adults [118]. Currently, in children >2 years of age, first-generation H_1 antihistamines are used to treat pruritus secondary to atopic dermatitis, urticaria and other allergic reactions including insect bites. Some of the most commonly used agents include chlorphenamine, diphenhydramine, hydroxyzine and promethazine [116]. Doxepin, a tricyclic antidepressant, is also considered a first-generation H_1 antihistaminic drug. It is a potent H_1 antagonist and has important H_2 antagonist activity [119]. Doxepin has been shown to be effective in the treatment of some allergic conditions and seems to be more effective than other antihistamines such as diphenhydramine in adult patients with chronic urticaria and pruritus [120–122]. Doxepin also causes drowsiness, is associated with anticholinergic effects, and can cause cardiac dysrhythmias at higher doses, potentially limiting paediatric use. Furthermore, evidence supporting safety and efficacy for skin conditions in children is lacking.

Second-generation H_1 antihistamines have been well studied. They typically have a longer half-life than the first-generation H_1 antihistamines, facilitating once-daily dosing. In general, second-generation H_1 antihistamines act as a permeability glycoprotein (P-gp) substrate and have less sedating effects. However, dose-related (>10 mg) CNS effects including sedation have been reported with cetirizine in adults [115]. Second-generation H_1 antihistamines are noncompetitive inhibitors of histamine binding and because they have higher specificity for H1R, anticholinergic side-effects are infrequent [117]. Common second-generation H_1 antihistamines used in children include cetirizine, loratadine, fexofenadine, levocetirizine, desloratadine, olopatadine, acrivastine and azelastine. In children, cetirizine, loratadine and fexofenadine are considered first-line therapy for the management of urticaria secondary to food allergic reactions, allergic rhinitis and chronic spontaneous urticaria [116]. While there is controversy regarding the role of second-generation versus first-generation H_1 antihistamines as monotherapy for eczema/atopic dermatitis, some authors support the use of second-generation H_1 antihistamines for prevention of pruritus, without the impairment of sleep quality seen in first-generation agents [106,118,123]. Regarding systemic treatment for paediatric mastocytosis, several reviews suggest that treatment with either sedating and/or nonsedating H_1 antihistamines in combination with H_2 antihistamines is effective to control pruritus and wheal formation [124,125]. Reported adverse effects include hypersensitivity reactions, and interactions with other drugs (terfenadine, erythromycin and ketoconazole) have also been reported [113,126].

H_2 antihistamines

H_2 antihistamines (such as cimetidine and ranitidine) are generally indicated for the control of gastric acid secretion, and can be useful to protect vulnerable patients against gastric complications from prolonged systemic corticosteroid therapy. Various authors have shown that cimetidine may provide antipruritic activity and may enhance cell-mediated immunity [127]. Cimetidine has also been utilized in the treatment of common variable immunodeficiency [128,129], hyperimmunoglobulin E [130] and to reverse the cutaneous allergy associated with Crohn disease. Other dermatological conditions of childhood that may be responsive to cimetidine include mucocutaneous candidiasis [131], herpes zoster and a variety of HPV infections, ranging from plane warts to common warts and/or plantar warts [127,132]. Ranitidine, when used with an H_1-blocking antihistamine, is a useful adjunctive treatment for severe/symptomatic mastocytosis in infants [100].

Antimalarial agents

Chloroquine and hydroxychloroquine are two of the most common antimalarial agents used in the treatment of lupus erythematosus and other dermatological conditions such as dermatomyositis, polymorphous light eruption, porphyria cutanea tarda and sarcoidosis [36]. Antimalarial agents have traditionally been used in the treatment of malaria (*Plasmodium falciparum* infection); however, their broader use increased during the Second World War after improvement in symptoms of lupus in soldiers who received antimalarial prophylaxis was observed [133]. Their mechanism of action in autoimmune disorders is still not well understood, but it is known that they have immunomodulatory, anti-inflammatory, antiproliferative and photoprotective properties. Additionally these drugs have antithrombotic, lipid-lowering and glucose-lowering effects, as well as an influence on bone metabolism [134]. Currently, hydroxychloroquine and chloroquine continue to be first-line treatment of cutaneous lupus erythematosus and lupus erythematosus panniculitis in children and adults [133,135]. Common side-effects associated with chloroquine and hydroxychloroquine include GI upset (nausea, vomiting, diarrhoea), headache and skin pigmentation; these are seen in up to 30% of patients. Pigmentation typically appears on the face, hard palate, forearms and shins; hair and nails may also be affected. Less common, but severe side-effects include blurred vision, diplopia and retinopathy, and therefore ophthalmological assessment before and during treatment is recommended. In patients receiving high doses of antimalarial drugs, psychiatric effects (psychosis, irritability, depression, insomnia), haemolysis (G6PD deficiency), aplastic anaemia, leucopenia and myopathy have also been reported [134,136].

β-Blockers

β-Blockers (BB) are a group of drugs characterized by variable inhibition of β_1 (myocardium and kidneys) and β_2 (extracardiac vasculature, skeletal muscle and lungs) adrenergic receptors. In the heart, BB exert their action by partially activating the β receptors thus preventing the binding of norepinephrine and epinephrine, leading to decreased heart rate and contractility. BB also interfere with the increase of cyclic adenosine monophosphate (cAMP) and intracellular calcium in the vasculature, inducing smooth muscle relaxation. Although traditionally BB were only used in the treatment of cardiac conditions, current use has expanded due to newly described effects on vascular endothelial growth factor (VEGF) and basic fibroblast growth factor (bFGF), which play important roles in tumour-induced angiogenesis; their precise mechanism of action, however, is still not well understood [137]. The use of BB in paediatric dermatology was first described in 2008 by Léauté-Labrèze et al., who observed changes in the colour and consistency of a nasal infantile haemangioma (IH) in a child treated with propranolol to control the side-effects caused by oral corticosteroids [138]. Since then, propranolol has become the first-line treatment for IH, and other BB such as acebutolol, atenolol and nadolol have also been shown to be effective [139,140] (Fig. 169.3). IH are seen in 4% of infants and are the most common benign tumour in this age group. IH are characterized by massive proliferation of endothelial cells of blood vessels and, although they are self-involuting, several complications may arise including ulceration, scarring and disfigurement. Indications for systemic therapy are not standardized, but generally include life-threatening involvement of the airway, large haemangiomas of the face, ulceration and periorbital or nasal involvement, among others [141]. Efficacy of BB (mainly propanolol) in the treatment of children with IH has been demonstrated by multiple authors since it was first described, and although BB appear to be safe and well tolerated, long-term safety data are still pending [142,143]. In a retrospective study examining 635 children treated with propranolol, the overall incidence of side-effects was 2.1%; diarrhoea, hyperkalaemia and bradycardia were most commonly observed in this group [144]. Hypotension, hypoglycaemia and bronchospasm have also been reported in the literature [145]. A multicentre, randomized, double-blind study including 460 patients (1–5 months of age) confirmed that propranolol (3 mg/kg per day) was more effective (with few minor side-effects) than placebo in the treatment of IH [146]. Propranolol is highly lipophilic and can cross the blood–brain barrier, which has been postulated to account for reported CNS adverse effects, such as nightmares and sleep disturbances [147]. In a blinded cohort study comparing oral nadolol with propranolol in the treatment of IH, Pope et al. found nadolol to be superior to propanolol with minimal adverse events, and noted that nadolol is less fat soluble with theoretically decreased penetration of the CNS [140,148,149]. Atenolol, another long-acting BB, has also been found to be effective in the treatment of IH given once daily and is likewise thought to have fewer CNS effects given its lower lipophilicity [150]. Although they represent an effective and safe therapeutic option for IH, the indication for using a BB should be carefully considered, evaluating whether the benefits outweigh the risks.

Retinoids

Retinoids are synthetic and natural compounds with vitamin A-like biological activity. They bind to nuclear receptors and have an important role in division, cell proliferation and differentiation, bone growth, immune defence and tumour suppression [36]. Systemic retinoids used in paediatric dermatology include isotretinoin and acitretin. In children these have traditionally been used in the management of acne, psoriasis and a wide variety of disorders of keratinization [151].

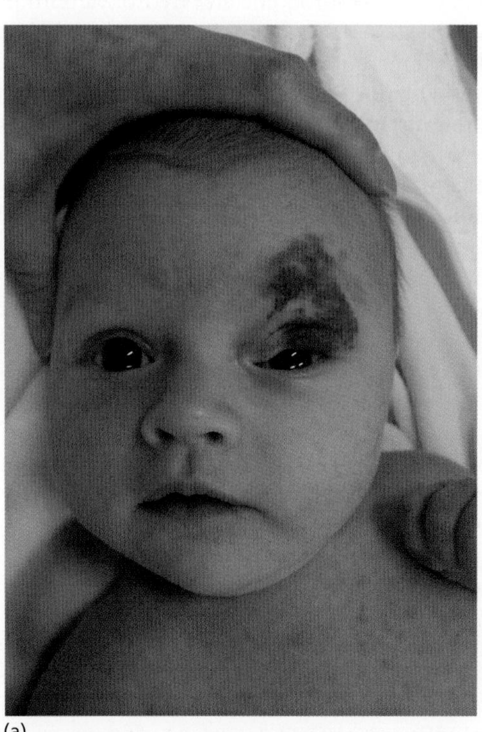
(a)

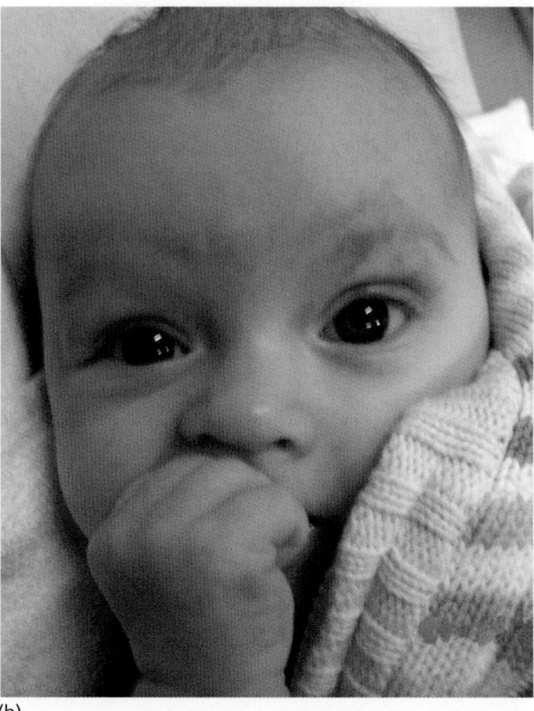
(b)

Fig. 169.3 Infantile haemangioma: (a) before the initiation of nadolol, and (b) 4 weeks after starting.

Isotretinoin

Isotretinoin (13-*cis*-retinoic acid) is a first-generation retinoid with a half-life of 10–20 hours. It is very effective in the treatment of severe, recalcitrant, nodulocystic acne and was approved by the FDA for this indication in 1982 [36]. Isotretinoin decreases the size of sebaceous glands and alters keratinization of the glandular acroinfundibulum. It also inhibits the release of arachidonic acid by macrophages portending an anti-inflammatory effect [152]. Eighty five percent of patients who receive a dose of 0.5–1.0 mg/kg per day are virtually clear of their acne by 16 weeks [153]. Relapses are more commonly observed in patients who complete a cumulative dose lower than 100–120 mg/kg [154]. For those who relapse, a second course of isotretinoin should be considered a minimum of 8 weeks after completion of the initial course, as ongoing improvement may be observed up to 2 months after cessation of therapy [151]. Other dermatological conditions for which isotretinoin may be effective include various ichthyoses and Darier disease [155]. Isotretinoin may be useful in the prevention of malignant skin tumours in individuals who are predisposed to skin cancers, including those previously exposed to arsenic insecticides, patients with naevoid basal cell carcinoma syndrome or those with xeroderma pigmentosum [156,157]. Isotretinoin is associated with a variety of skin and mucosal side-effects such as xerosis, cheilitis, conjunctival irritation, skin fragility and hair loss. Other potential side-effects include elevation of liver enzymes, hepatotoxicity, leucopenia, pseudotumor cerebri, papilloedema, nausea, vomiting, visual disturbances and arthralgia, which usually is a result of hyperostoses and tendinous calcifications. Other adverse events that have been linked to isotretinoin include flaring of severe acne during initiation of treatment (as seen with acne conglobata), inflammatory bowel disease, depression/anxiety/mood changes, cardiovascular sequelae (hypertriglyceridaemia), bone mineralization (premature epiphyseal closure and pathological fractures), scarring, and *Staph. aureus* colonization. However, to date there is insufficient evidence to prove causal association with these effects. Regardless, routine bloodwork (triglycerides, cholesterol and transaminases), and monitoring of growth, GI symptoms and mood changes is prudent [158]. The risk of teratogenicity is an extremely important factor to consider when prescribing systemic isotretinoin [155]. Pregnancy is an absolute contraindication and women should not become pregnant for at least 1 month after the drug has been discontinued. Literature describes several infants born with multiple major anomalies to women taking isotretinoin during pregnancy [159]. A specific syndrome that includes CNS, ear and great vessel abnormalities, along with hypoplasia of the thymus and parathyroid gland, has been described [160]. Additionally, elective surgical procedures should generally be avoided while on isotretinoin and up to 6–12 months after discontinuation of treatment; this recommendation arose out of several reports of abnormal scarring observed in patients treated with isotretinoin who also had cosmetic mechanical dermabrasion procedures. However, recent studies suggest that the previous reports could be idiosyncratic, and the recommendation to wait 6–12 months after treatment should be re-evaluated. The need for well-controlled studies to confirm this theory has been proposed [161,162].

Acitretin

Acitretin is a retinoid with an elimination half-life of about 55–60 hours; concurrent consumption of alcohol leads to reverse metabolization to the parent compound etretinate, which has a significantly prolonged half-life. It is therefore recommended that alcohol be avoided while taking this drug [152,163]. Acitretin is an effective treatment for severe psoriasis because of its effects on epidermal differentiation and keratinization. The medical board of the National Psoriasis Foundation considers acitretin a first-line agent for the treatment of pustular psoriasis [164]. A systematic review found that acitretin, ciclosporin and methotrexate are prescribed with equal frequencies for the treatment of paediatric pustular psoriasis, with no difference in their short-term effect [165]. Since acitretin has long-term storage and biological activity, its use for psoriasis in children should be undertaken with careful consideration, especially in adolescent girls, given the prolonged risk for teratogenicity. Isotretinoin could alternatively be considered, as it has a significantly more rapid clearance rate and its effectiveness in pustular psoriasis has also been reported [166]. Apart from psoriasis, a wide variety of disorders of keratinization are reported to be responsive to acitretin, including erythrokeratoderma variabilis [167], Papillon–Lefevre syndrome [168], epidermal naevus syndrome [169], keratitis–ichthyosis–deafness (KID) syndrome [170], pachyonychia congenita, epidermolytic hyperkeratosis [171], Darier disease, lamellar ichthyosis and non-bullous ichthyosiform erythroderma. Successful outcomes in cases of harlequin ichthyosis treated with acitretin have also been reported [172]. For some of these genetic conditions, chronic therapy may be necessary, as remission rates following discontinuation of treatment are not well characterized. Therefore the risk of remaining on long-term treatment must be weighed judiciously against the benefits of treatment. Overall, the use of acitretin is well tolerated, with a side-effect profile similar to that of isotretinoin; reported adverse effects include, but are not limited to, skin fragility, xerosis, transient hypertriglyceridaemia, mild liver enzyme elevation and teratogenicity [151]. Pardo et al. followed 12 patients with disorders of keratinization treated with systemic etretinate and acitretin for a period of 7–68 months. All patients developed cheilitis and dry skin, while less than 50% showed elevation in liver enzymes, all of which improved with time or dose reduction; no osseous or other severe adverse events were observed [171].

Biologic agents

Over the past decade, therapy for many autoimmune and inflammatory conditions has changed drastically with the introduction of biologic therapies. These agents are characterized by the targeting of specific mediators of inflammation, thereby stimulating or suppressing particular components of the immune response. In dermatology, biologics have been used and studied most extensively in psoriasis, but their use has currently expanded to over 40 different skin conditions, with ongoing new indications frequently described [173]. In children, etanercept, infliximab and rituximab are currently the most commonly prescribed agents used to treat conditions such as atopic dermatitis, juvenile pityriasis rubra pilaris, severe drug reactions (SJS/TEN), graft-versus-host disease (GVHD), hidradenitis suppurativa, pemphigus foliaceus, pemphigus vulgaris, bullous pemphigoid, primary cutaneous B-cell lymphoma, pyoderma gangrenosum, orofacial granulomatosis, and pyogenic arthritis, pyoderma gangrenosum and acne (PAPA) syndrome [174].

There are a number of new biologic agents in development. Dupilumab is the first biologic to be approved for the treatment of moderate-to-severe atopic dermatitis in adults. Clinical trials in children are currently underway (for more details refer to Chapter 19).

Although biologic agents seem to be useful in a wide spectrum of skin conditions, their use needs to be cautiously considered due to both potential side-effects and high cost, which can represent a heavy economic burden. It has been estimated that 1 year of treatment for psoriasis (including both induction and maintenance) may cost up to $55 000 US dollars for etanercept or ustekinumab [175].

Etanercept

Etanercept is a TNF-α inhibitor. Several studies have shown that it is relatively safe and efficacious in children and adolescents with moderate-to-severe psoriasis [176]. In a 48-week study conducted by Paller et al., children and adolescents received weekly treatment with 0.8 mg/kg. Reductions in disease severity were seen as early as 2 weeks after treatment initiation [177]. Etanercept has also been used successfully in the treatment of juvenile rheumatoid arthritis, psoriatic arthritis, juvenile pityriasis rubra pilaris and TEN [173,174]. Reported side-effects include upper respiratory tract infections (nasopharyngitis, streptococcal pharyngitis), bacterial sepsis, tuberculosis, pneumonia, local skin reactions, elevation of liver enzymes, headache, skin rash, nausea, vomiting, abdominal pain, blood dyscrasias such as leucopenia and thrombocytopenia, dizziness and hair loss [36,176,178]. Although the association of etanercept with increased risk of lymphoma in children remains controversial, close monitoring is recommended [179]. Longer-term safety data are needed in the paediatric population [180].

Infliximab

Infliximab is a chimeric IgG_1 monoclonal antibody to TNF-α and is approved by the FDA for children with Crohn disease and ulcerative colitis. Additional off-label indications include rheumatoid arthritis and ankylosing spondylitis. In paediatric dermatology several case reports and small case series have shown infliximab to be effective in the treatment of psoriatic arthritis, plaque psoriasis, hidradenitis suppurativa, Kawasaki disease, Behçet disease, pyoderma gangrenosum, atopic dermatitis and TEN [174,181–183]. Several clinical trials and large series of patients with juvenile idiopathic arthritis and inflammatory bowel disease have demonstrated that overall infliximab is well tolerated; however, Northcutt et al. reported a serious adverse event rate of at least 33.3%, with intra-abdominal abscess, appendicitis, pneumonia and pseudomembranous colitis among the reported complications [184]. Overall, the most frequent adverse events reported include upper respiratory tract and GI infections, opportunistic infections, GI upset, seizures, psoriasis, pharyngitis, infusion reactions, hepatitis B virus reactivation, hepatotoxicity, cytopenias and lupus-like syndrome [184,185]. In addition, the development of antinuclear or anti-ds DNA antibodies in 7.7–38% of patients on infliximab has been reported, and is associated with a loss of response to therapy [185]. Similar to etanercept, potential risk of malignancy has been reported and close monitoring is advised [186,187].

Rituximab

Rituximab is a chimeric monoclonal IgG antibody targeted against the CD20 epitope of mature, normal and malignant B lymphocytes. It depletes the B-cell population via apoptosis, cellular cytotoxicity and complement activation [188]. Rituximab has been traditionally used for the treatment of non-Hodgkin lymphoma, but its use has spread to several autoimmune conditions such as rheumatoid arthritis [189]. In paediatric skin conditions, rituximab has been shown to be effective in the treatment of bullous pemphigoid, GVHD, pemphigus vulgaris, pemphigus foliaceus, epidermolysis bullosa acquisita, juvenile dermatomyositis, primary cutaneous marginal B-cell lymphoma and nonhealing cutaneous ulcer with features of lymphomatoid granulomatosis [174,190,191]. Prevalence of side-effects in lymphoma patients treated with rituximab seems to be lower than in patients with autoimmune blistering disorders [187]. Some adverse events reported in children include local infusion reactions, severe infections, mortality secondary to sepsis, persistent hypogammaglobulinaemia and psoriasis [174,189,190,192]. Patients receiving rituximab require monitoring for tuberculosis and lymphoma. Contraindications include pregnancy, breastfeeding and active infections, among others, and patients should avoid live vaccines while on active treatment [188].

Intravenous immunoglobulin (IVIG)

Intravenous immunoglobulins (IVIG) consist of exogenous pooled human immunoglobulins, mainly IgG and a variable supply of IgA, IgE and IgM antibodies. Although its precise mechanism of action in autoimmune conditions is still unclear, it is postulated that IVIG has immunomodulatory activity [187]. Traditionally in children, IVIG has been used to treat Kawasaki disease. Over the last decade IVIG has gained popularity in the treatment of SJS and TEN. Initial data indicated that IVIG was superior to systemic corticosteroids in the management of severe drug reactions (SJS/TEN); however, additional studies showed conflicting results [193,194]. A systematic review of SJS/TEN treatment in children did not show a statistically significant difference in the outcome of patients receiving systemic steroids versus IVIG [195]. Despite this, IVIG remains one option in the treatment arsenal of SJS/TEN and although some controversy remains, it appears that IVIG in combination with systemic corticosteroids demonstrates overall efficacy and improved outcomes, such as decreased mortality [196,197]. Other dermatological conditions in which IVIG has been used include autoimmune bullous diseases (bullous pemphigoid, pemphigoid gestationis, cicatricial pemphigoid, epidermolysis bullosa acquisita, linear IgA dermatosis), connective tissue disease (dermatomyositis, systemic sclerosis), allergic disease (atopic dermatitis, chronic urticaria) and vasculitis (idiopathic thrombocytopenic purpura, pyoderma gangrenosum) [198]. IVIG has an overall risk of adverse reactions of approximately 10%, and although most are minor, such as infusion reactions (seen primarily in patients with hypogammaglobulinaemia), serious adverse reactions such as renal failure, aseptic meningitis, stroke, infection, haemolysis, deep venous thrombosis and anaphylaxis have been reported [199]. Symptoms of infusion reaction include headache, nausea, fever, vomiting, cough, malaise, muscle aches, arthralgia, abdominal pain, flushing, urticarial lesions and variations in heart rate/blood pressure [198].

Interferons

Interferons (IFN) are protein molecules that regulate cell growth based on their antigenic action, with antiviral, antiproliferative and immunomodulatory properties [200]. IFN can be further divided into IFN-α 2a and b. Some indications within the field of dermatology include HPV infections (warts), VZV and HSV infections, skin cancer (including melanoma) and other pigmentary disorders [201]. Additionally, paediatric patients with haemangiomas have been successfully treated with subcutaneous injections of IFN-α 2a and b [202,203]; however, it is now recognized that there is a long-term risk of neurological complications such as irreversible spastic diplegia when the medications are used in infants so their use for this indication has been abandoned.

Chemotherapy and immunomodulators

Methotrexate

Methotrexate (MTX) is an analogue of aminopterin, a folic acid antagonist, which has been used in the treatment of acute leukaemia in children and adults for more than six decades [204]. Its use in dermatology was first reported in 1958, when it was successfully used in the management of psoriasis [205]. Today, MTX is used in a wide variety of skin conditions including psoriasis, pityriasis rubra pilaris, cutaneous sarcoidosis, dermatomyositis, cutaneous lupus erythematosus, bullous pemphigoid, linear IgA dermatosis, pemphigus, Hailey–Hailey disease, cutaneous T-cell lymphoma, pityriasis lichenoides, lymphomatoid papulosis, atopic dermatitis, palmoplantar pustulosis, Behçet disease, morphoea, lichen planus, pyoderma gangrenosusm, alopecia areata universalis and vitiligo [206–210]. In addition to its antineoplastic effects, MTX has anti-inflammatory properties by inducing extracellular release of adenosine, leading to inhibition of neutrophil chemotaxis and adherence, superoxide anion formation and secretion of pro-inflammatory cytokines [205]. In paediatric dermatology, MTX is a recognized systemic agent for atopic dermatitis and psoriasis. Although the literature is not abundant, a systematic review recommended MTX as the treatment of choice in children with moderate-to-severe plaque psoriasis [211]. Kaur et al. reported 24 paediatric patients with severe forms of psoriasis (recalcitrant plaque psoriasis or erythroderma and generalized pustular psoriasis) who received systemic therapy with MTX, and all except two had an excellent response (>75% decrease in Psoriasis Area and Severity Index [PASI]) at the end of the treatment, showing 50% reduction in PASI during the first 5 weeks of treatment [212]. Beyond psoriasis, the American Academy of Dermatology currently recommends MTX as one treatment option for refractory atopic dermatitis [106]. A retrospective review of 31 patients with atopic dermatitis (<18 years) showed that MTX was effective in 75% of patients, with evidence of clinical improvement within 8–12 weeks and a mean duration of treatment in responders of 14 months (range 2–38 months) [213]. Unlike oncological indications, where high doses are utilized, low-dose MTX used in dermatological conditions is considered relatively safe [213,214]. The most commonly reported adverse effect is GI upset (nausea, vomiting, diarrhoea), but haematological abnormalities (including anaemia, leucopenia, thrombocytopenia and pancytopenia), hepatotoxicity, immunosuppression and severe drug reactions (such as TEN) have also been reported [206]. Supplementation with folic acid has been shown to reduce the risk of side-effects. Monitoring of complete blood counts and liver function tests while on treatment is advised [215].

Ciclosporin

Ciclosporin is a calcineurin inhibitor with potent immunosuppressive properties. It inhibits the phosphorylation of nuclear factor of activated T cells and its dependent cytokines, such as IL-2, which are required for full activation of the T-cell pathway [216]. In dermatology, ciclosporin is approved by the FDA for the treatment of psoriasis, but it has been used off-label in a variety of other skin conditions such as atopic dermatitis, alopecia areata, epidermolysis bullosa acquisita, pemphigus vulgaris, bullous pemphigoid, lichen planus, pyoderma gangrenosum, Sweet syndrome, chronic urticaria, cutaneous lupus erythematosus, dermatomyositis and SJS/TEN [217]. Literature supporting ciclosporine use in paediatric skin conditions is scarce, with the exception of its use in childhood psoriasis and atopic dermatitis. Di Lernia et al. described 38 paediatric patients with plaque psoriasis treated with ciclosporin, 39% of whom achieved complete clearance (>75% PASI) at week 16, with only minor side-effects reported [218]. Bulbul Baskan et al. similarly reported 17 of 22 paediatric patients with severe psoriasis treated with ciclosporin demonstrating excellent clinical response, with a median time to total clearance of 4 weeks [219]. Regarding atopic dermatitis, ciclosporin is considered by the American Academy of Dermatology as an effective off-label treatment option for patients with disease refractory to conventional topical treatment. Several studies have demonstrated that ciclosporin improves severity of atopic dermatitis within 2–6 weeks of treatment initiation [106]. Compared with other systemic treatments, ciclosporin appears to be as effective as MTX in reducing severity of atopic dermatitis in children [220]. Beyond psoriasis and atopic dermatitis, ciclosporin is emerging as an effective treatment option for SJS/TEN. Several studies have demonstrated efficacy in adults, and although literature in children is lacking; a few reports demonstrated that ciclosporin may be superior to IVIG in reducing associated complications and mortality [221]. Although ciclosporin at lower doses is considered safe and well tolerated, it has been associated with increases in serum creatinine, bilirubin, liver enzymes and blood urea, arterial hypertension, decreased magnesium, gingival hyperplasia, paraesthesia, headache, muscle aches and generalized hypertrichosis. Long-term therapy may be associated with development of lymphoproliferative disorders and other malignant tumours [217]. Additionally, as with other immunosuppressant drugs, the risk of bacterial, viral, fungal or other opportunistic agents may be increased [217]. Ciclosporin must be avoided in patients with abnormal renal function, uncontrolled hypertension, malignancy, hypersensitivity to ciclosporin and pregnancy. Live vaccines should be avoided during therapy [106]. To reduce the risk of nephrotoxicity and other side-effects in patients on long-term treatment, weekly maintenance therapy has been proposed as an effective alternative [222].

Sirolimus

Sirolimus is a derivate of *Streptomyces hygroscopicus* and was initially isolated as an antifungal agent against *Candida*. However, its antitumour and immunosuppressive properties were later demonstrated [223]. Sirolimus is a potent inhibitor of antigen-induced proliferation of T cells, B cells and antibody production. Its mechanism of action involves formation of immunosuppressive complexes with intracellular protein (FKBP12), which in turn blocks the activation of the cell cycle-specific kinase mammalian target of rapamycin (mTOR) resulting in the blockage of cell cycle progression at the juncture of G_1 and S phase. It further inhibits growth factor-mediated proliferation of non-immune cells, conferring significant antilymphangiogenic activity [223]. It has shown to be effective in patients with renal transplantation, some malignancies and patients with lymphatic metastases. Recent literature indicates that sirolimus might also play an important role in the treatment of complicated vascular anomalies such as kaposiform haemangioendothelioma with or without Kasabach–Merritt phenomenon [224]. Kai et al. reported six cases of children with kaposiform haemangioendothelioma who received sirolimus, all of whom showed significant clinical improvement with minimal side-effects, with an average response time of 5.3 ± 1 days and a length of treatment of 5.5 ± 5.5 months (ranging from 1 to 12 months), and without evidence of recurrence [225]. Sirolimus has also been used in the treatment of kaposiform lymphangiomatosis with promising results [226]. Other vascular lesions may also respond well to sirolimus; Kaylani et al. reported treatment of a child with PHACE syndrome (posterior fossa brain malformations, haemangiomas of the face, arterial anomalies, cardiac anomalies and eye abnormalities) in whom systemic corticosteroids, propranolol and vincristine had failed, but who responded to sirolimus [227]. There is also speculation that sirolimus may be useful in the management of the palmoplantar keratoderma of patients with pachyonychia congenita given the ability of sirolimus to inhibit expression of keratin 6a in keratinocytes [228]. Sirolimus is thought to be relatively well tolerated, as demonstrated in a large study including 61 patients (median age 8.1 years) with complicated vascular anomalies [224]. Adverse events include hypertriglyceridaemia, hyperglycaemia, hypercholesterolaemia, blood and bone marrow abnormalities (such as thrombocytopenia), GI symptoms (including nausea and diarrhoea) and pulmonary infections [224,229].

Azathioprine

Azathioprine is an immunomodulator historically used in the management of leukaemia and organ transplantation. It is a precursor to a purine analogue that impairs purine synthesis and selectively inhibits lymphocytes, particularly T lymphocytes [230]. Currently, azathioprine is utilized as a steroid-sparing agent for several autoimmune and inflammatory conditions including pemphigus vulgaris, bullous pemphigoid, dermatomyositis, atopic dermatitis, chronic actinic dermatitis, lupus erythematosus, psoriasis, pyoderma gangrenosum, vasculitis and Behçet disease [231,232]. In paediatric dermatology, azathioprine is additionally used off-label for the treatment of recalcitrant atopic dermatitis [106]. Although effective, azathioprine is associated with several side-effects including elevated liver enzymes, GI upset, potentially severe myelosuppression, and increased risk of infection; long-term therapy has also been associated with malignancy [215]. Complete blood counts and liver enzymes should therefore be monitored during treatment. Photoprotection is also recommended given increased photosensitivity to ultraviolet A (UVA) [28,215]. Azathioprine metabolism depends on the activity of the thiopurine methyl-transferase enzyme (TPMT). Patients with reduced TPMT activity have higher risk of severe immunosuppression and side-effects, whereas patients with increased activity may present with a lack of clinical improvement at typical doses. Baseline measurement of TPMT activity is therefore advised [230].

Others

Mycophenolate mofetil (MMF). This is an immunosuppressive agent traditionally used in renal transplantation. In dermatology it has proven to be effective particularly in skin diseases triggered by lymphocytes, including autoimmune bullous dermatoses, atopic dermatitis and psoriasis [233]. In children, MMF has specifically been used in patients with severe and recalcitrant atopic dermatitis [215]. In the

USA, registration for a risk evaluation and mitigation strategy (REMS) programme for girls and women of childbearing potential has been mandated due to risks of congenital malformations and pregnancy loss when taking this medication during pregnancy [234].

Vinblastine and etoposide. These derivatives of podophyllotoxin are very potent chemotherapeutic agents that can cause severe side-effects in children and should be used selectively. Both drugs have been reported to provide positive outcomes in children with multisystem Langerhans cell histiocytosis [235,236]. They appear to be equivalent in terms of response time and long-term remission of disease. Unfortunately, these agents can cause significant toxicity such as leucopenia, and long-term sequelae, including diabetes insipidus [235].

Vincristine. This is a vinca alkaloid that has antitumour properties (via inhibition of mitosis) and has proved to be an effective treatment for Kasabach–Merritt syndrome. Its use, however, has been associated with a number of side-effects including GI (abdominal pain, constipation, ileus, nausea, vomiting), neurological (autonomic neuropathy, loss of deep tendon reflex, peripheral paraesthesia, ataxia) and metabolic (hyponatraemia and syndrome of inappropriate antidiuretic hormone) complications [237]. Typically, vincristine requires administration through a central line, and is given as a once-weekly dose.

Janus kinase (JAK) inhibitors

JAK inhibitors are a new group of drugs that target the intracellular kinase JAK and have been demonstrated to be more effective than methotrexate and TNF inhibitors (adalimumab) in patients with rheumatoid arthritis [238]. At the time of writing, JAK inhibitors have not been approved for dermatological conditions, but several studies have shown their effectiveness in patients with alopecia areata, mostly in adults. In one study performed in children, Craiglow et al. treated 13 adolescents (12–17 years), with different variants of alopecia areata, with tofacitinib 5 mg twice daily. Clinical response was observed in 77% of patients, and 58% had more than 50% improvement [239]. Although no severe side-effects were reported, long-term safety has not been established; for now, JAK inhibitors seem to be a promising therapy for children with alopecia areata. The development of topical formulations of JAK inhibitors such as tofacitinib, ruxolitinib and baritinib, among others, is being evaluated in an effort to reduce systemic toxicity.

Miscellaneous

Colchicine

Colchicine is a tricyclic, lipid-soluble alkaloid with a half-life of 20–40 hours. It is known to have antimitotic properties which result from binding with free tubulin dimers, leading to disruption of microtubule polymerization and dissociation, thus inhibiting vesicle cell transport, cytokine secretion, phagocytosis, migration and cellular division [240]. Colchicine also has an anti-inflammatory effect by impairing neutrophil function by inhibiting intracellular signalling molecules and chemotaxis, thus obstructing T-lymphocyte activation and its adhesion to endothelial cells [241]. Additionally, colchicine has been shown to decrease the activation of caspase-1, thereby blocking the conversion of pro-interleukin (IL)-β to active IL-1β, and in turn decreasing cytokines such as TNF-α and IL-6 [240]. Furthermore, colchicine modulates pyrin expression, inhibits histamine release by mast cells, impairs cellular secretion of procollagen and increases collagenase activity [240,241]. Colchicine has proved to be useful in the management of familial Mediterranean fever, acute gouty arthritis and other inflammatory conditions including those affecting the skin. In children, colchicine is currently recommended as first-line treatment for Behçet disease [242]. Colchicine is additionally used as second-line treatment for a variety of conditions including linear IgA disease, recurrent aphthous stomatitis, PFAPA (periodic fever, aphthous stomatitis, pharyngitis and cervical adenitis) syndrome, Sweet syndrome, dermatitis herpetiformis, relapsing bullous Henoch–Schönlein purpura, scleroderma, amyloidosis, pyoderma gangrenosum and others [241,243,244]. Colchicine is overall well tolerated; commonly reported adverse events include GI side-effects (nausea, vomiting and diarrhoea), which are seen up to 10% of patients [240]. Symptoms of colchicine intoxication include GI upset, haemodynamic instability, prerenal failure, disseminated intravascular coagulation, pancytopenia and CNS effects (including mental depression, confusion, delirium, seizures, myoneuropathy and coma) [245].

Essential fatty acids

Essential fatty acids (EFA) are those acids that cannot be synthesized by humans and must therefore be consumed through diet. Major essential fatty acids found in humans are linoleic acid and its products, γ-linoleic acid and arachidonic acid.

Deficiency of EFA in the diet leads to a scaly dermatitis and impaired skin barrier function [246,247]. Oral intake may cause clinical improvement in the skin of patients with atopic dermatitis [248]. The eicosapentaenoic acids (EPA) are polyunsaturated fatty acids found in large quantities in fish oils. Long-term administration of fish oil, rich in omega-3 fatty acids, may modify the severity of psoriasis and enhance the efficacy of co-administered conventional psoriatic therapy. Oral and intravenous supplementations of omega-3 and omega-6 fatty acids have been found effective in adult psoriatic patients [249]. EPA have also been proposed as a supplementary treatment in patients who are receiving ciclosporin for psoriasis and other dermatoses because of their possible renal protective effects [250].

References

1 Crump T. Antibiotic Chart: Straight Healthcare; 2016. Available from: http://www.straighthealthcare.com/antibiotic-chart.html (accessed 28 February 2019).

2 **Alzolibani AA, Zedan K. Macrolides in chronic inflammatory skin disorders. Mediators Inflamm 2012;2012:159354.**

3 Kiprono SK, Muchunu JW, Masenga JE. Skin diseases in pediatric patients attending a tertiary dermatology hospital in Northern Tanzania: a cross-sectional study. BMC Dermatol 2015;15:16.
4 Patel JK, Vyas AP, Berman B, Vierra M. Incidence of childhood dermatosis in India. Skinmed 2010;8:136–42.
5 Landolt B, Staubli G, Lips U, Weibel L. Skin disorders encountered in a Swiss pediatric emergency department. Swiss Med Wkly 2013; 143:w13731.
6 Storan ER, McEvoy MT, Wetter DA et al. Pediatric hospital dermatology: experience with inpatient and consult services at the Mayo Clinic. Pediatr Dermatol 2013;30:433–7.
7 Casanova JM, Sanmartin V, Soria X et al. [Childhood dermatosis in a dermatology clinic of a general university hospital in Spain]. Actas Dermosifiliogr 2008;99:111–8.
8 Sacchidanand S, Sahana MS, Asha GS, Shilpa K. Pattern of pediatric dermatoses at a referral centre. Indian J Pediatr 2014;81:375–80.
9 Hedrick J. Acute bacterial skin infections in pediatric medicine: current issues in presentation and treatment. Paediatr Drugs 2003;5(suppl 1):35–46.
10 Hartman-Adams H, Banvard C, Juckett G. Impetigo: diagnosis and treatment. Am Fam Physician 2014;90:229–35.
11 Stevens DL, Bisno AL, Chambers HF et al. Practice guidelines for the diagnosis and management of skin and soft-tissue infections. Clin Infect Dis 2005;41:1373–406.
12 Cole C, Gazewood J. Diagnosis and treatment of impetigo. Am Fam Physician 2007;75:859–64. Pub
13 Moyano M, Peuchot A, Giachetti AC et al. [Skin and soft tissue infections in children: consensus on diagnosis and treatment]. Arch Argent Pediatr 2014;112:183–91.
14 Patel M. Community-associated meticillin-resistant Staphylococcus aureus infections: epidemiology, recognition and management. Drugs 2009;69:693–716.
15 Workowski KA, Bolan GA. Sexually Transmitted Diseases Treatment Guidelines, 2015. Centers for Disease Control and Prevention MMWR 2015/64(RR3);1–137.
16 Gordon RA, Mays R, Sambrano B et al. Antibiotics used in nonbacterial dermatologic conditions. Dermatol Ther 2012;25:38–54.
17 Petri WA. B-Lactam antibiotics. In: Brunton L, Chabner B, Knollman B (eds) Goodman and Gilman's The Pharmacological Basis of Therapeutics, 12th edn. McGraw-Hill, 2011:1477–503.
18 Matar R, Le Bourgeois M, Scheinmann P et al. Beta-lactam hypersensitivity in children with cystic fibrosis: a study in a specialized pediatric center for cystic fibrosis and drug allergy. Pediatr Allergy Immunol 2014;25:88–93.
19 Sanchez-Saldaña L, Saenz-Anduaga E, Pancorbo-Mendoza J et al. Systemic antibiotics in dermatology. Part 1: Betalactamics- Carbapenems - Aminoglucosides- Macrolides. Dermatol Peru 2004;14:7–20.
20 MacDougall C, Chambers HF. Protein synthesis inhibitors and miscellaneous antibacterial agents. In: Brunton L, Chabner B, Knollman B (eds) Goodman and Gilman's The Pharmacological Basis of Therapeutics, 12th edn. McGraw-Hill, 2011:1521–48.
21 Scheinfeld NS, Tutrone WD, Torres O, Weinberg JM. Macrolides in dermatology. Disease Mon 2004;50:350–68.
22 Lucas CR, Korman NJ, Gilliam AC. Granulomatous periorificial dermatitis: a variant of granulomatous rosacea in children? J Cutan Med Surg 2009;13:115–18.
23 Hapa A, Ersoy-Evans S, Karaduman A. Childhood pityriasis lichenoides and oral erythromycin. Pediatr Dermatol 2012;29:719–24.
24 De D, Kanwar AJ. Combination of low-dose isotretinoin and pulsed oral azithromycin in the management of moderate to severe acne: a preliminary open-label, prospective, non-comparative, single-centre study. Clin Drug Invest 2011;31:599–604.
25 Bardazzi F, Savoia F, Parente G et al. Azithromycin: a new therapeutical strategy for acne in adolescents. Dermatol Online J 2007;13:4.
26 Goel NS, Burkhart CN, Morrell DS. Pediatric periorificial dermatitis: clinical course and treatment outcomes in 222 patients. Pediatr Dermatol 2015;32:333–6.
27 Tsankov N, Broshtilova V, Kazandjieva J. Tetracyclines in dermatology. Clin Dermatol 2003;21:33–9.
28 Perret LJ, Tait CP. Non-antibiotic properties of tetracyclines and their clinical application in dermatology. Australas J Dermatol 2014;55:111–18.
29 Nag S, Weinstein M, Greenberg S. 14-year-old boy with painful nail changes. Pediatr Rev 2015;36:e8–10.
30 Williams DJ, Cooper WO, Kaltenbach LA et al. Comparative effectiveness of antibiotic treatment strategies for pediatric skin and soft-tissue infections. Pediatrics 2011;128:e479–87.
31 Danby FW. Current concepts in the management of hidradenitis suppurativa in children. Curr Opin Pediatr 2015;27:466–72.
32 Seitz CS, Brocker EB, Trautmann A. Allergy diagnostic testing in clindamycin-induced skin reactions. Int Arch Allergy Immunol 2009;149:246–50.
33 Michalek K, Lechowicz M, Pastuszczak M, Wojas-Pelc A. The use of trimethoprim and sulfamethoxazole (TMP-SMX) in dermatology. Folia Med Cracov 2015;55:35–41.
34 Miller LG, Daum RS, Creech CB et al. Clindamycin versus trimethoprim-sulfamethoxazole for uncomplicated skin infections. N Engl J Med 2015;372:1093–103.
35 Wessels MR. Choosing an antibiotic for skin infections. N Engl J Med2015;372:1164–5.
36 Burkhart CN, Morrell DS, Goldsmith L. Dermatological pharmacology. In: Brunton L, Chabner B, Knollman B (eds) Goodman and Gilman's The Pharmacological Basis of Therapeutics. McGraw-Hill, 2011:1803–32.
37 Miller MC, Moreno-Coutino G. Dapsone: Applications in dermatology. Dermatol Cosm Med Quir 2014;12:47–51.
38 Herrero-Gonzalez JE. [Clinical guidelines for the diagnosis and treatment of dermatitis herpetiformis]. Actas Dermosifiliogr 2010; 101:820–6.
39 Agrawal S, Agarwalla A. Dapsone hypersensitivity syndrome: a clinico-epidemiological review. J Dermatol 2005;32:883–9.
40 Liu KL, Shen JL, Yang CS, Chen YJ. Bullous systemic lupus erythematosus in a child responding to dapsone. Pediatr Dermatol 2014; 31:e104–6.
41 Garcia-Romero MT, Ho N. Pediatric Sweet syndrome. A retrospective study. Int J Dermatol 2015;54:518–22.
42 Garcia-Melendez ME, Eichelmann K, Salas-Alanis JC et al. Pemphigus foliaceus in an 11-year-old mexican girl with response to oral dapsone. Case Rep Pediatr 2013;2013:291256.
43 Poirot E, Vittinghoff E, Ishengoma D et al. Risks of hemolysis in glucose-6-phosphate dehydrogenase deficient infants exposed to chlorproguanil-dapsone, mefloquine and sulfadoxine-pyrimethamine as part of intermittent presumptive treatment of malaria in infants. PloS ONE 2015;10:e0142414.
44 Vinod KV, Arun K, Dutta TK. Dapsone hypersensitivity syndrome: A rare life threatening complication of dapsone therapy. J Pharmacol Pharmacother 2013;4:158–60.
45 Kelly BP. Superficial fungal infections. Pediatr Rev 2012;33:e22–37.
46 Fernandez-Flores A, Saeb-Lima M, Arenas-Guzman R. Morphological findings of deep cutaneous fungal infections. Am J Dermatopathol 2014;36:531–53; quiz 54–6.
47 Sethi A, Antaya R. Systemic antifungal therapy for cutaneous infections in children. Pediatr Infect Dis J 2006;25:643–4.
48 Kakourou T, Uksal U. Guidelines for the management of tinea capitis in children. Pediatr Dermatol 2010;27:226–8.
49 Gupta AK, Paquet M. Systemic antifungals to treat onychomycosis in children: a systematic review. Pediatr Dermatol 2013;30:294–302.
50 Gupta AK, Drummond-Main C. Meta-analysis of randomized, controlled trials comparing particular doses of griseofulvin and terbinafine for the treatment of tinea capitis. Pediatr Dermatol 2013;30:1–6.
51 Yan J, Wang X, Chen S. Systematic review of severe acute liver injury caused by terbinafine. Int J Clin Pharm 2014;36:679–83.
52 Feldstein S, Totri C, Friedlander SF. Antifungal therapy for onychomycosis in children. Clin Dermatol 2015;33:333–9.
53 Grover C, Arora P, Manchanda V. Comparative evaluation of griseofulvin, terbinafine and fluconazole in the treatment of tinea capitis. Int J Dermatol 2012;51:455–8.
54 Chan YC, Friedlander SF. New treatments for tinea capitis. Curr Opin Infect Dis 2004;17:97–103.
55 Develoux M. [Griseofulvin]. Ann Dermatol Venereol 2001;128: 1317–25.
56 Bennett JE. Antifungal agents. In: Brunton L, Chabner B, Knollman B (eds) Goodman and Gilman's The Pharmacological Basis of Therapeutics. McGraw-Hill, 2011:1571–92.
57 Huang PH, Paller AS. Itraconazole pulse therapy for dermatophyte onychomycosis in children. Arch Pediatr Adolesc Med 2000;154: 614–18.
58 Laniado-Laborin R, Cabrales-Vargas MN. Amphotericin B: side effects and toxicity. Rev Iberoam Micol 2009;26:223–7.
59 Carrasco Sanchez P, Castillo Montero ML, Bejarano Palma A et al. [Neonatal candidiasis and liposomal amphotericin B treatment: our experience]. An Esp Pediatr 1999;51:273–80.

60 Solomon M, Schwartz E, Pavlotsky F et al. Leishmania tropica in children: a retrospective study. J Am Acad Dermatol 2014;71:271–7.
61 Chavez-Fumagalli MA, Ribeiro TG, Castilho RO et al. New delivery systems for amphotericin B applied to the improvement of leishmaniasis treatment. Rev Soc Bras Med Trop 2015;48:235–42.
62 Bes DF, Sberna N, Rosanova MT. [Advantages and drawbacks of amphotericin formulations in children: literature review]. Arch Argent Pediatr 2012;110:46–51.
63 Trizna Z. Viral diseases of the skin: diagnosis and antiviral treatment. Paediatr Drugs 2002;4:9–19.
64 Nikkels AF, Pierard GE. Treatment of mucocutaneous presentations of herpes simplex virus infections. Am J Clin Dermatol 2002; 3:475–87.
65 Hoff NP, Gerber PA. Herpetic whitlow. CMAJ 2012;184:E924.
66 Usatine RP, Tinitigan R. Nongenital herpes simplex virus. Am Fam Physician 2010;82:1075–82.
67 Champet Lima AM, Llergo Valdez RJ, Garcia GR. Eccema herpético. Una urgencia dermatológica real. Comunicación de un caso. Dermatología Rev Mex 2010;54:141–4.
68 Rubio Jiménez ME, Losada Pajares A, Andrés Bartolomé A et al. Erupción variceliforme de Kaposi; descripción de dos casos. Rev Esp Pediatr 2014;70:8–11.
69 Amir J. Clinical aspects and antiviral therapy in primary herpetic gingivostomatitis. Paediatr Drugs 2001;3:593–7.
70 Zhang HP, Wang L, Qian JH et al. [Efficacy and safety of ribavirin aerosol in children with hand-foot-mouth disease]. 2014;16:272–6.
71 Pan S, Qian J, Gong X, Zhou Y. [Effects of ribavirin aerosol on viral exclusion of patients with hand-foot-mouth disease]. Zhonghua Yi Xue Za Zhi 2014;94:1563–6.
72 Lin P, Torres G, Tyring SK. Changing paradigms in dermatology: antivirals in dermatology. Clin Dermatol 2003;21:426–46.
73 Kimberlin DW. Acyclovir dosing in the neonatal period and beyond. J Pediatric Infect Dis Soc 2013;2:179–82.
74 Acosta EP, Flexner C. Antiviral agents (non-retroviral). In: Brunton L, Chabner B, Knollman B (eds) Goodman and Gilman's The Pharmacological Basis of Therapeutics. McGraw-Hill, 2011:1593–622.
75 Razonable RR. Antiviral drugs for viruses other than human immunodeficiency virus. Mayo Clin Proc 2011;86:1009–26.
76 Kimberlin DW, Jacobs RF, Weller S et al. Pharmacokinetics and safety of extemporaneously compounded valacyclovir oral suspension in pediatric patients from 1 month through 11 years of age. Clin Infect Dis 2010;50:221–8.
77 Canadian Agency for Drugs and Technologies in Health. Acyclovir versus valacyclovir for herpes virus in children and pregnant women: a review of the clinical evidence and guidelines [Internet]. CADTH Rapid Response Reports, 2014. Available at: https://www.ncbi.nlm.nih.gov/books/NBK253720/(accessed 1 March 2019).
78 Saez-Llorens X, Yogev R, Arguedas A et al. Pharmacokinetics and safety of famciclovir in children with herpes simplex or varicella-zoster virus infection. Antimicrob Agents Chemother 2009;53:1912–20.
79 Blumer J, Rodriguez A, Sanchez PJ et al. Single-dose pharmacokinetics of famciclovir in infants and population pharmacokinetic analysis in infants and children. Antimicrob Agents Chemother 2010;54:2032–41.
80 Kappagoda S, Singh U, Blackburn BG. Antiparasitic therapy. Mayo Clin Proc 2011;86:561–83.
81 Nordlund JJ. Cutaneous ectoparasites. Dermatol Ther 2009;22:503–17.
82 Davis RF, Johnston GA, Sladden MJ. Recognition and management of common ectoparasitic diseases in travelers. Am J Clin Dermato 2009;10:1–8.
83 Diaz JH. The epidemiology, diagnosis, management, and prevention of ectoparasitic diseases in travelers. J Travel Med 2006;13:100–11.
84 Aden Abdi Y, Gustafsson LL, Ericsson O, Hellgren U. Handbook of Drugs for Tropical Parasitic Infections, 2nd edn. London: Taylor and Francis, 2003:12–16.
85 Scholar EM, Pratt WB. Chemotherapy of helminthic diseases. In: The Antimicrobial Drugs, 2nd edn. New York: Oxford University Press, 2000: 458–80.
86 Kincaid L, Klowak M, Klowak S, Boggild AK. Management of imported cutaneous larva migrans: A case series and mini-review. Travel Med Infect Dis 2015;13:382–7.
87 Siddalingappa K, Murthy SC, Herakal K, Kusuma MR. Cutaneous larva migrans in early infancy. Indian J Dermatol 2015;60:522.
88 Risco M, Amaya I, Requena I et al. Utilidad terapéutica del albendazol en el tratamiento de niños infectados con Giardia lamblia. Saber 2013;25:73–82.
89 Namazi MR. Treatment of pediculosis capitis with thiabendazole: a pilot study. Int J Dermatol 2003;42:973–6.
90 Chosidow A, Gendrel D. [Safety of oral ivermectin in children]. Arch Pediatr 2016;23:204–9.
91 Currie BJ, McCarthy JS. Permethrin and ivermectin for scabies. N Engl J Med 2010;362:717–25.
92 Dourmishev AL, Dourmishev LA, Schwartz RA. Ivermectin: pharmacology and application in dermatology. Int J Dermatol 2005; 44:981–8.
93 Becourt C, Marguet C, Balguerie X, Joly P. Treatment of scabies with oral ivermectin in 15 infants: a retrospective study on tolerance and efficacy. Br J Dermatol 2013;169:931–3.
94 Ameen M, Arenas R, Villanueva-Reyes J et al. Oral ivermectin for treatment of pediculosis capitis. Pediatr Infect Dis J 2010;29:991–3.
95 Romani L, Whitfeld MJ, Koroivueta J et al. Mass drug administration for scabies control in a population with endemic disease. N Engl J Med 2015;373:2305–13.
96 Fawcett RS. Ivermectin use in scabies. Am Fam Physician 2003; 68:1089–92.
97 Torrelo A, Pérez-Gala S. Uso de corticoides orales en dermatología pediátrica. Dermatol Pediatr Lat 2005;3:71–82.
98 Schimmer BP, Funder JW. ACTH, adrenal steroids, and pharmacology of the adrenal cortex. In: Brunton L, Chabner B, Knollman B (eds) Goodman and Gilman's The Pharmacological Basis of Therapeutics. McGraw-Hill, 2011:1209–36.
99 Greaves MW, Gatti S. The use of glucocorticoids in dermatology. J Dermatolog Treat 1999;10:83–91.
100 West DP, Heath C, Haley AC et al. Principles of paediatric dermatological therapy. In: Irvine AD, Hoeger PH, Yan AC (eds) Harper's Textbook of Pediatric Dermatology, 3rd edn. Oxford: Wiley-Blackwell, 2011.
101 Friedland R, Tal R, Lapidoth M et al. Pulse corticosteroid therapy for alopecia areata in children: a retrospective study. Dermatology 2013;227:37–44.
102 Fritz KA, Weston WL. Systemic glucocorticosteroid therapy of skin disease in children. Pediatr Dermatol 1984;1:236–45.
103 Piram M, McCuaig CC, Saint-Cyr C et al. Short- and long-term outcome of linear morphoea in children. Br J Dermatol 2013;169: 1265–71.
104 Gupta G, Jain A, Narayanasetty N. Steroid pulse therapies in dermatology. Muller J Med Sci Res 2014;5:155–8.
105 Liu X, Qu X, Zheng J, Zhang L. Effectiveness and safety of oral propranolol versus other treatments for infantile hemangiomas: a meta-analysis. PloS One 2015;10:e0138100.
106 Sidbury R, Davis DM, Cohen DE et al. Guidelines of care for the management of atopic dermatitis: section 3. Management and treatment with phototherapy and systemic agents. J Am Acad Dermatol 2014;71:327–49.
107 Deshmukh CT. Minimizing side effects of systemic corticosteroids in children. Indian J Dermatol Venereol Leprol 2007;73:218–21.
108 Freitas THPd, Souza DAFd. Corticosteróides sistêmicos na prática dermatológica. Parte II: estratégias para minimizar os efeitos adversos. An Bras Dermatol 2007;82:177–82.
109 Sinha A, Bagga A. Pulse steroid therapy. Indian J Pediatr 2008;75: 1057–66.
110 Liu D, Ahmet A, Ward L et al. A practical guide to the monitoring and management of the complications of systemic corticosteroid therapy. Allergy Asthma Clin Immunol 2013;9:30.
111 Gupta P, Bhatia V. Corticosteroid physiology and principles of therapy. Indian J Pediatr 2008;75:1039–44.
112 Bruce RS. Antihistamine drugs. Postgrad Med J 1950;26:325–30.
113 Criado PR, Criado RF, Maruta CW et al. Histamine, histamine receptors and antihistamines: new concepts. An Bras Dermatol 2010;85:195–210.
114 Ohsawa Y, Hirasawa N. The role of histamine H1 and H4 receptors in atopic dermatitis: from basic research to clinical study. Allergol Int 2014;63:533–42.
115 Simons FE, Simons KJ. H1 antihistamines: current status and future directions. World Allergy Organ J 2008;1:145–55.
116 Fitzsimons R, van der Poel LA, Thornhill W et al. Antihistamine use in children. Arch Dis Child Educ Pract Ed 2015;100:122–31.
117 Schad CA, Skoner DP. Antihistamines in the pediatric population: achieving optimal outcomes when treating seasonal allergic rhinitis and chronic urticaria. Allergy Asthma Proc 2008;29:7–13.
118 Church MK, Maurer M. H1-Antihistamines and itch in atopic dermatitis. Exp Dermatol 2015;24:332–3.

119 Skidgel RA, Kaplan AP, Erdös EG. Histamine, bradikynin, and their antagonists. In: Brunton L, Chabner B, Knollman B (eds) Goodman and Gilman's The Pharmacological Basis of Therapeutics, 12th edn. McGraw-Hill, 2011:911–36.
120 Adhya Z, Karim Y. Doxepin may be a useful pharmacotherapeutic agent in chronic urticaria. Clin Exp Allergy 2015;45:1370.
121 Shohrati M, Davoudi SM, Keshavarz S et al. Cetirizine, doxepine, and hydroxyzine in the treatment of pruritus due to sulfur mustard: a randomized clinical trial. Cutan Ocul Toxicol 2007;26:249–55.
122 Smith PF, Corelli RL. Doxepin in the management of pruritus associated with allergic cutaneous reactions. Ann Pharmacother 1997;31:633–5.
123 van Zuuren EJ, Apfelbacher CJ, Fedorowicz Z et al. No high level evidence to support the use of oral H1 antihistamines as monotherapy for eczema: a summary of a Cochrane systematic review. Syst Rev 2014;3:25.
124 Castells M, Metcalfe DD, Escribano L. Diagnosis and treatment of cutaneous mastocytosis in children: practical recommendations. Am J Clin Dermatol 2011;12:259–70.
125 Azana JM, Torrelo A, Matito A. Update on mastocytosis (part 2): categories, prognosis, and treatment. Actas Dermosifiliogr 2016; 107:15–22.
126 Shakouri AA, Bahna SL. Hypersensitivity to antihistamines. Allergy Asthma Proc 2013;34:488–96.
127 Choi YS, Hann SK, Park YK. The effect of cimetidine on verruca plana juvenilis: clinical trials in six patients. J Dermatol 1993;20: 497–500. PubMed
128 Wershil DK, Mekery VA, Galli SJ. Cimetidine and common variable hypogammaglobulinemia. N Engl J Med 1985;313:264–6.
129 White WB, Ballow M. Modulation of suppressor-cell activity by cimetidine in patients with common variable hypogammaglobulinemia. N Engl J Med 1985;312:198–202.
130 Simon GL, Miller HG, Scott SJ. Cimetidine in the treatment of hyperimmunoglobulinemia E with impaired chemotaxis. J Infect Dis 1983;147:1121–2.
131 Jorizzo JL, Sams WM Jr, Jegasothy BV, Olansky AJ. Cimetidine as an immunomodulator: chronic mucocutaneous candidiasis as a model. Ann Intern Med 1980;92:192–5.
132 Gooptu C, Higgins CR, James MP. Treatment of viral warts with cimetidine: an open-label study. Clin Exp Dermatol 2000;25:183–5.
133 Sanchez-Montero D, Lopez-Castro J. Lupus eritematoso cutaneo subagudo de adecuada respuesta a hidroxicloroquina (plaquinol). Rev Med Cos Cen2013;605:129–39.
134 Rodriguez-Caruncho C, Bielsa Marsol I. Antimalarials in dermatology: mechanism of action, indications, and side effects. Actas Dermosifiliogr 2014;105:243–52.
135 Weingartner JS, Zedek DC, Burkhart CN, Morrell DS. Lupus erythematosus panniculitis in children: report of three cases and review of previously reported cases. Pediatr Dermatol 2012;29:169–76.
136 Skare T, Ribeiro CF, Souza FH et al. Antimalarial cutaneous side effects: a study in 209 users. Cutan Ocul Toxicol 2011;30:45–9.
137 Fernandez-Pineda I, Williams R, Ortega-Laureano L, Jones R. Cardiovascular drugs in the treatment of infantile hemangioma. World J Cardiol 2016;8:74–80.
138 Leaute-Labreze C, Dumas de la Roque E, Hubiche T et al. Propranolol for severe hemangiomas of infancy. N Engl J Med 2008;358:2649–51.
139 Baselga Torres E, Bernabeu Wittel J, van Esso Arbolave DL et al. [Spanish consensus on infantile haemangioma]. An Pediatr (Barc) 2016;85:256–65.
140 Pope E, Chakkittakandiyil A, Lara-Corrales I et al. Expanding the therapeutic repertoire of infantile haemangiomas: cohort-blinded study of oral nadolol compared with propranolol. Br J Dermatol 2013;168:222–4.
141 Kwon EK, Seefeldt M, Drolet BA. Infantile hemangiomas: an update. Am J Clin Dermatol 2013;14:111–23.
142 Chu DH, Castelo-Soccio L, Wan J et al. Retrospective analysis of beta-blocker instituted for treatment of hemangiomas (RABBIT study). Clin Pediatr 2014;53:1084–90.
143 Prey S, Voisard JJ, Delarue A et al. Safety of propranolol therapy for severe infantile hemangioma. Jama 2016;315:413–5.
144 Luo Y, Zeng Y, Zhou B, Tang J. A retrospective study of propranolol therapy in 635 infants with infantile hemangioma. Pediatr Dermatol 2015;32:151–2.
145 Raphael MF, Breur JM, Vlasveld FA et al. Treatment of infantile hemangiomas: therapeutic options in regard to side effects and adverse events – a review of the literature. Expert Opin Drug Saf 2016;15:199–214.
146 Leaute-Labreze C, Hoeger P, Mazereeuw-Hautier J et al. A randomized, controlled trial of oral propranolol in infantile hemangioma. N Engl J Med 2015;372:735–46.
147 de Graaf M, Breur JM, Raphael MF et al. Adverse effects of propranolol when used in the treatment of hemangiomas: a case series of 28 infants. J Am Acad Dermatol 2011;65:320–7.
148 Villalba-Moreno AM, Cotrina-Luque J, Del Vayo-Benito CA et al. Nadolol for the treatment of infantile hemangioma. Am J Health Syst Pharm 2015;72:44–6.
149 Bernabeu-Wittel J, Narvaez-Moreno B, de la Torre-Garcia JM et al. Oral nadolol for children with infantile hemangiomas and sleep disturbances with oral propranolol. Pediatr Dermatol 2015;32: 853–7.
150 Bayart CB, Tamburro JE, Vidimos AT et al. Atenolol versus propranolol for treatment of infantile hemangiomas during the proliferative phase: a retrospective noninferiority study. Pediatr Dermatol 2017;34:413–421.
151 Brecher AR, Orlow SJ. Oral retinoid therapy for dermatologic conditions in children and adolescents. J Am Acad Dermatol 2003;49:171–82; quiz 83–6.
152 DiGiovanna JJ. Isotretinoin effects on bone. J Am Acad Dermatol 2001;45:S176–82.
153 Layton A. The use of isotretinoin in acne. Dermatoendocrinol 2009;1:162–9.
154 Leyden JJ, Del Rosso JQ, Baum EW. The use of isotretinoin in the treatment of acne vulgaris: clinical considerations and future directions. J Clin Aesthet Dermatol 2014;7(2 suppl):S3–S21.
155 American Academy of Pediatrics Committee on Drugs. Retinoid therapy for severe dermatological disorders. Pediatrics 1992;90:119–20.
156 Kraemer KH, DiGiovanna JJ, Moshell AN et al. Prevention of skin cancer in xeroderma pigmentosum with the use of oral isotretinoin. N Engl J Med 1988;318:1633–7.
157 Peck GL, DiGiovanna JJ, Sarnoff DS et al. Treatment and prevention of basal cell carcinoma with oral isotretinoin. J Am Acad Dermatol 1988;19:176–85.
158 Zaenglein AL, Pathy AL, Schlosser BJ et al. Guidelines of care for the management of acne vulgaris. J Am Acad Dermatol 2016;74: 945–73 e33.
159 Autret-Leca E, Kreft-Jais C, Elefant E et al. Isotretinoin exposure during pregnancy: assessment of spontaneous reports in France. Drug Saf 2010;33:659–65.
160 Troncoso Sch M, Rojas HC, Bravo CE. [Isotretinoin embryopathy. Report of one case]. Rev Med Chil 2008;136:763–6.
161 Picosse FR, Yarak S, Cabral NC, Bagatin E. Early chemabrasion for acne scars after treatment with oral isotretinoin. Dermatol Surg 2012;38:1521–6.
162 Chandrashekar BS, Varsha DV, Vasanth V et al. Safety of performing invasive acne scar treatment and laser hair removal in patients on oral isotretinoin: a retrospective study of 110 patients. Int J Dermatol 2014;53:1281–5.
163 Berbis P. [Acitretine]. Ann Dermatol Venereol 2001;128:737–45.
164 Shah KN. Diagnosis and treatment of pediatric psoriasis: current and future. Am J Clin Dermatol 2013;14:195–213.
165 Posso-De Los Rios CJ, Pope E, Lara-Corrales I. A systematic review of systemic medications for pustular psoriasis in pediatrics. Pediatr Dermatol 2014;31:430–9.
166 Al-Shobaili H, Al-Khenaizan S. Childhood generalized pustular psoriasis: successful treatment with isotretinoin. Pediatr Dermatol 2007;24:563–4.
167 Graham-Brown RA, Chave TA. Acitretin for erythrokeratodermia variabilis in a 9-year-old girl. Pediatr Dermatol 2002;19:510–2.
168 Al-Khenaizan S. Papillon-Lefevre syndrome: the response to acitretin. Int J Dermatol 2002;41:938–41.
169 Pandhi D, Reddy BS. A rare association of epidermal nevus syndrome and ainhum-like digital constrictions. Pediatr Dermatol 2002;19:349–52.
170 Sahoo B, Handa S, Kaur I et al. KID syndrome: response to acitretin. J Dermatol 2002;29:499–502.
171 Pardo L, Torrelo A, Zambrano A. Seguimiento del tratamiento con retinoides en niños con trastornos importantes de la queratinización. Actas Dermosifiliogr 2002;93:190–4.
172 Singh S, Bhura M, Maheshwari A et al. Successful treatment of harlequin ichthyosis with acitretin. Int J Dermatol 2001;40:472–3.
173 Kerns MJ, Graves JE, Smith DI, Heffernan MP. Off-label uses of biologic agents in dermatology: a 2006 update. Semin Cutan Med Surg 2006;25:226–40.

174 Bellodi-Schmidt F, Shah KN. Beyond psoriasis: novel uses for biologic response modifiers in pediatric dermatology. Pediatr Dermatol 2016;33:18–27.

175 Fathi R, Armstrong AW. The role of biologic therapies in dermatology. Med Clin North Am 2015;99:1183–94.

176 Lofgren S, Krol A. New therapies in pediatric dermatology. Curr Opin Pediatr 2011;23:399–402.

177 Paller AS, Siegfried EC, Eichenfield LF et al. Long-term etanercept in pediatric patients with plaque psoriasis. J Am Acad Dermatol 2010;63:762–8.

178 Horneff G, Schmeling H, Biedermann T et al. The German etanercept registry for treatment of juvenile idiopathic arthritis. Ann Rheum Dis 2004;63:1638–44.

179 Hooper M, Wenkert D, Bitman B et al. Malignancies in children and young adults on etanercept: summary of cases from clinical trials and post marketing reports. Pediatr Rheumatol Online J 2013;11:35.

180 Paller AS, Siegfried EC, Langley RG et al. Etanercept treatment for children and adolescents with plaque psoriasis. N Engl J Med 2008;358:241–51.

181 Saji T, Takatsuki S, Kobayashi T. [Anti TNF-alpha (infliximab) treatment for intravenous immunoglobulin (IVIG) resistance patients with acute Kawasaki disease the effects of anticytokine therapy]. Nihon Rinsho 2014;72:1641–9.

182 Campos-Munoz L, Conde-Taboada A, Aleo E et al. Refractory pyoderma gangrenosum treated with infliximab in an infant. Clin Exp Dermatol 2014;39:336–9.

183 Ugras M, Ertem D, Celikel C, Pehlivanoglu E. Infliximab as an alternative treatment for Behcet disease when other therapies fail. J Pediatr Gastroenterol Nutr 2008;46:212–5.

184 Northcutt M, Al-Subu A, Bella B, Elitsur Y. Safety of infliximab in children with IBD: the experience of an academic center in WV. W V Med J 2014;110:26–9.

185 Bellodi Schmidt F, Shah KN. Biologic response modifiers and pediatric psoriasis. Pediatr Dermatol 2015;32:303–20.

186 Kui R, Gal B, Gaal M et al. Presence of antidrug antibodies correlates inversely with the plasma tumor necrosis factor (TNF)-alpha level and the efficacy of TNF-inhibitor therapy in psoriasis. J Dermatol 2016;43:1018–23.

187 Castelo-Soccio L, Van Voorhees AS. Long-term efficacy of biologics in dermatology. Dermatol Ther 2009;22:22–33.

188 Rosman Z, Shoenfeld Y, Zandman-Goddard G. Biologic therapy for autoimmune diseases: an update. BMC Med 2013;11:88.

189 Bennett DD, Ohanian M, Cable CT. Rituximab in severe skin diseases: target, disease, and dose. Clin Pharmacol 2010;2:135–41.

190 McKinley SK, Huang JT, Tan J et al. A case of recalcitrant epidermolysis bullosa acquisita responsive to rituximab therapy. Pediatr Dermatol 2014;31:241–4.

191 Cooper MA, Willingham DL, Brown DE et al. Rituximab for the treatment of juvenile dermatomyositis: a report of four pediatric patients. Arthritis Rheum 2007;56:3107–11.

192 Fiorillo L, Wang C, Hemmati I. Rituximab induced psoriasis in an infant. Pediatr Dermatol 2014;31:e149–51.

193 Bachot N, Revuz J, Roujeau JC. Intravenous immunoglobulin treatment for Stevens-Johnson syndrome and toxic epidermal necrolysis: a prospective noncomparative study showing no benefit on mortality or progression. Arch Dermatol 2003;139:33–6.

194 Lee HY, Lim YL, Thirumoorthy T, Pang SM. The role of intravenous immunoglobulin in toxic epidermal necrolysis: a retrospective analysis of 64 patients managed in a specialized centre. Br J Dermatol 2013;169:1304–9.

195 Del Pozzo-Magana BR, Lazo-Langner A, Carleton B et al. A systematic review of treatment of drug-induced Stevens-Johnson syndrome and toxic epidermal necrolysis in children. J Popul Ther Clin Pharmacol 2011;18:e121–33.

196 Lalosevic J, Nikolic M, Gajic-Veljic M et al. Stevens-Johnson syndrome and toxic epidermal necrolysis: a 20-year single-center experience. Int J Dermatol 2015;54:978–84.

197 Chen J, Wang B, Zeng Y, Xu H. High-dose intravenous immunoglobulins in the treatment of Stevens-Johnson syndrome and toxic epidermal necrolysis in Chinese patients: a retrospective study of 82 cases. Eur J Dermatol 2010;20:743–7.

198 Dourmishev LA, Guleva DV, Miteva LG. Intravenous immunoglobulins: mode of action and indications in autoimmune and inflammatory dermatoses. Int J Inflam 2016;2016:3523057.

199 Looney RJ, Huggins J. Use of intravenous immunoglobulin G (IVIG). Best Pract Res Clin Haematol 2006;19:3–25.

200 Levin D, Schneider WM, Hoffmann HH et al. Multifaceted activities of type I interferon are revealed by a receptor antagonist. Sci Signal 2014;7:ra50.

201 Moredo Romo E, Moreira Preciado M, Pérez López A. Uso de los interferones en Dermatología: experiencia con el alfa-interferon en la micosis fungoide. Rev Cubana Farm 2004;38:1.

202 Tryfonas GI, Tsikopoulos G, Liasidou E et al. Conservative treatment of hemangiomas in infancy and childhood with interferon-alpha 2a. Pediatr Surg Int 1998;13:590–3.

203 Garmendia G, Miranda N, Borroso S et al. Regression of infancy hemangiomas with recombinant IFN-alpha 2b. J Interferon Cytokine Res 2001;21:31–8.

204 Wojtuszkiewicz A, Peters GJ, van Woerden NL et al. Methotrexate resistance in relation to treatment outcome in childhood acute lymphoblastic leukemia. J Hematol Oncol 2015;8:61.

205 Puig L. Methotrexate: new therapeutic approaches. Actas Dermosifiliogr 2014;105:583–9.

206 Holliday AC, Moody MN, Berlingeri-Ramos A. Methotrexate: role of treatment in skin disease. Skin Therapy Lett 2013;18:4–9.

207 Alghamdi K, Khurrum H. Methotrexate for the treatment of generalized vitiligo. Saudi Pharm J 2013;21:423–4.

208 Hammerschmidt M, Mulinari Brenner F. Efficacy and safety of methotrexate in alopecia areata. An Bras Dermatol 2014;89:729–34.

209 Royer M, Bodemer C, Vabres P et al. Efficacy and tolerability of methotrexate in severe childhood alopecia areata. Br J Dermatol 2011;165:407–10.

210 Singh H, Kumaran MS, Bains A, Parsad D. A randomized comparative study of oral corticosteroid minipulse and low-dose oral methotrexate in the treatment of unstable vitiligo. Dermatology 2015;231:286–90.

211 de Jager ME, de Jong EM, van de Kerkhof PC, Seyger MM. Efficacy and safety of treatments for childhood psoriasis: a systematic literature review. J Am Acad Dermatol 2010;62:1013–30.

212 Kaur I, Dogra S, De D, Kanwar AJ. Systemic methotrexate treatment in childhood psoriasis: further experience in 24 children from India. Pediatr Dermatol 2008;25:184–8.

213 Deo M, Yung A, Hill S, Rademaker M. Methotrexate for treatment of atopic dermatitis in children and adolescents. Int J Dermatol 2014;53:1037–41.

214 van Geel MJ, Oostveen AM, Hoppenreijs EP, et al. Methotrexate in pediatric plaque-type psoriasis: Long-term daily clinical practice results from the Child-CAPTURE registry. J Dermatolog Treat 2015;26:406–12.

215 Slater NA, Morrell DS. Systemic therapy of childhood atopic dermatitis. Clin Dermatol 2015;33:289–99.

216 Krensky AM, Bennett WM, Vincenti F. Immunosuppressants, tolerogens and immunostimulants. In: Brunton L, Chabner B, Knollman B (eds) Goodman and Gilman's The Pharmacological Basis of Therapeutics. McGraw-Hill, 2011:1005–30.

217 Dehesa L, Abuchar A, Nuno-Gonzalez A et al. The use of cyclosporine in dermatology. J Drugs Dermatol 2012;11:979–87.

218 Di Lernia V, Stingeni L, Boccaletti V et al. Effectiveness and safety of cyclosporine in pediatric plaque psoriasis: A multicentric retrospective analysis. J Dermatolog Treat 2016;27:395–8.

219 Bulbul Baskan E, Yazici S, Tunali S, Saricaoglu H. Clinical experience with systemic cyclosporine A treatment in severe childhood psoriasis. J Dermatolog Treat 2016;27:328–31.

220 El-Khalawany MA, Hassan H, Shaaban D et al. Methotrexate versus cyclosporine in the treatment of severe atopic dermatitis in children: a multicenter experience from Egypt. Eur J Pediatr 2013;172:351–6.

221 Kirchhof MG, Miliszewski MA, Sikora S et al. Retrospective review of Stevens-Johnson syndrome/toxic epidermal necrolysis treatment comparing intravenous immunoglobulin with cyclosporine. J Am Acad Dermatol 2014;71:941–7.

222 Amor KT, Ryan C, Menter A. The use of cyclosporine in dermatology: part I. J Am Acad Dermatol 2010;63:925–46; quiz 47–8.

223 Sehgal SN. Sirolimus: its discovery, biological properties, and mechanism of action. Transplant Proc 2003;35(3 suppl):7S–14S.

224 Adams DM, Trenor CC 3rd, Hammill AM et al. Efficacy and safety of sirolimus in the treatment of complicated vascular anomalies. Pediatrics 2016;137:1–10.

225 Kai L, Wang Z, Yao W et al. Sirolimus, a promising treatment for refractory Kaposiform hemangioendothelioma. J Cancer Res Clin Oncol 2014;140:471–6.

226 Wang Z, Li K, Yao W et al. Successful treatment of kaposiform lymphangiomatosis with sirolimus. Pediatr Blood Cancer 2015; 62:1291–3.

227 Kaylani S, Theos AJ, Pressey JG. Treatment of infantile hemangiomas with sirolimus in a patient with PHACE syndrome. Pediatr Dermatol 2013;30:e194–7.

228 Hickerson RP, Leake D, Pho LN et al. Rapamycin selectively inhibits expression of an inducible keratin (K6a) in keratinocytes and improves symptoms in pachyonychia congenita patients. J Dermatol Sci 2009;56:82–88.

229 Curatolo P, Moavero R. mTOR inhibitors in tuberous sclerosis complex. Curr Neuropharmacol 2012;10:404–15.

230 Caufield M, Tom WL. Oral azathioprine for recalcitrant pediatric atopic dermatitis: clinical response and thiopurine monitoring. J Am Acad Dermatol 2013;68:29–35.

231 Meggitt SJ, Anstey AV, Mohd Mustapa MF et al. British Association of Dermatologists' guidelines for the safe and effective prescribing of azathioprine 2011. Br J Dermatol 2011;165:711–34.

232 Rumbo C. Azathioprine metabolite measurements: its use in current clinical practice. Pediatr Transplant 2004;8:606–8.

233 Eskin-Schwartz M, David M, Mimouni D. Mycophenolate mofetil for the management of autoimmune bullous diseases. Dermatol Clin 2011;29:555–9.

234 MYCOPHENOLATE REMS (Risk Evaluation and Mitigation Strategy). Available at: https://www.mycophenolaterems.com (accessed 1 March 2019).

235 Gadner H, Grois N, Arico M et al. A randomized trial of treatment for multisystem Langerhans' cell histiocytosis. J Pediatr 2001;138: 728–34.

236 Grifo AH. Langerhans cell histiocytosis in children. J Pediatr Oncol Nurs 2009;26:41–7.

237 Wang Z, Li K, Dong K et al. Successful treatment of Kasabach-Merritt phenomenon arising from Kaposiform hemangioendothelioma by sirolimus. J Pediatr Hematol Oncol 2015;37:72–3.

238 Yamaoka K. Janus kinase inhibitors for rheumatoid arthritis. Curr Opin Chem Biol 2016;32:29–33.

239 Craiglow BG, Liu LY, King BA. Tofacitinib for the treatment of alopecia areata and variants in adolescents. J Am Acad Dermatol 2017;76:29–32.

240 Slobodnick A, Shah B, Pillinger MH, Krasnokutsky S. Colchicine: old and new. Am J Med 2015;128:461–70.

241 Konda C, Rao AG. Colchicine in dermatology. Indian J Dermatol Venereol Leprol 2010;76:201–5.

242 Nanthapisal S, Klein NJ, Ambrose N et al. Paediatric Behcet's disease: a UK tertiary centre experience. Clin Rheumatol 2016;35: 2509–16.

243 Butbul Aviel Y, Tatour S, Gershoni Baruch R, Brik R. Colchicine as a therapeutic option in periodic fever, aphthous stomatitis, pharyngitis, cervical adenitis (PFAPA) syndrome. Semin Arthritis Rheum 2016;45: 471–4.

244 Ang P, Tay YK. Treatment of linear IgA bullous dermatosis of childhood with colchicine. Pediatr Dermatol 1999;16:50–2.

245 Bicer S, Soysal DD, Ctak A et al. Acute colchicine intoxication in a child: a case report. Pediatr Emerg Care 2007;23:314–17.

246 Skolnik P, Eaglstein WH, Ziboh VA. Human essential fatty acid deficiency: treatment by topical application of linoleic acid. Arch Dermatol 1977;113:939–41.

247 Tollesson A, Frithz A, Berg A, Karlman G. Essential fatty acids in infantile seborrheic dermatitis. J Am Acad Dermatol 1993;28: 957–61.

248 van Gool CJ, Thijs C, Henquet CJ et al. Gamma-linolenic acid supplementation for prophylaxis of atopic dermatitis—a randomized controlled trial in infants at high familial risk. Am J Clin Nutr 2003;77:943–51.

249 Silverberg NB. Pediatric psoriasis: an update. Ther Clin Risk Manag 2009;5:849–56.

250 Elzinga L, Kelley VE, Houghton DC, Bennett WM. Modification of experimental nephrotoxicity with fish oil as the vehicle for cyclosporine. Transplantation 1987;43:271–4.

CHAPTER 170

New Genetic Approaches to Treating Diseases of the Skin

Stephen Hart & Amy Walker

Experimental and Personalised Medicine, UCL GOS Institute of Child Health, London, UK

Introduction, 2301
Genetic therapies for skin diseases using viral vectors, 2302
Nanoparticles and nonviral approaches, 2303
Gene editing, 2305
Conclusion, 2307

Abstract

Gene therapy may be broadly defined as the transfer of nucleic acids for a therapeutic purpose. Gene transfer in the skin has many potential applications ranging from treatment or cure of known genetic skin diseases, to novel approaches to wound healing and vaccination. The field of genetic skin diseases is rapidly expanding, including not only the inherited genodermatoses but more recently the sporadic somatic mosaic conditions. Efficient delivery is key to the success of any gene therapy and the skin is an attractive target for topical application of therapeutic nucleic acids. However, the barrier properties of the stratum corneum limit the transfection efficiency of cells in the underlying epidermis and so a diverse range of approaches are under investigation to improve skin gene delivery. *In vivo*, topical approaches have largely focused on the use of nonviral methods including formulations of nucleic acids, for example with liposomes, polymeric nanoparticles or biomaterials, while intradermal injection and other physical methods of gene delivery, including ultrasound and electroporation, have largely focused on naked nucleic acids. The other major approach to skin gene therapy involves *ex vivo* gene modification of cells followed by expansion of cells for skin grafting. Retroviral and lentiviral vectors are the preferred modality for *ex vivo* modification of keratinocytes and epidermal stem cells for cell-mediated therapies. This approach has proven particularly beneficial for treating some forms of epidermolysis bullosa (EB) although this is highly labour intensive which might limit its deployment to larger numbers of patients.

Key points

- Gene delivery to the skin has potential applications in the treatment of monogenic diseases, cancers, chronic wounds and as a route of vaccination.
- The method of gene delivery remains the key technical barrier to successful gene therapy in the skin. Viral vectors and nanoparticle formulations are under investigation, each offering particular opportunities and advantages.
- *In vivo* approaches include topical application of nanoparticles, subdermal injection of viral vectors such as AAV and physical methods of delivery across the skin using ultrasound and electroporation to promote gene delivery.
- *Ex vivo* gene therapy involves correcting patient-derived keratinocytes in the laboratory with lentiviral or retroviral vectors, then expanding the cells into grafts which are applied to the patient. This approach has been successful for epidermolysis bulllosa.
- Gene editing offers prospects for new approaches to skin gene therapy provided safety and delivery isses can be addressed.

Introduction

The principles of gene therapy in the skin are the same as elsewhere in the body, and depend on the genetic basis of each disease. In the simplest terms, at the protein level, where a protein is missing it needs to be replaced, which can be achieved by correcting the DNA by gene editing, introducing a replacement gene (gene replacement therapy) or RNA (messenger RNA therapy), or replacing the protein itself. Where the protein is abnormal, it needs to be corrected, removed or silenced, which can be performed at the DNA or RNA level. This chapter will review the major molecular strategies and delivery vectors (Table 170.1) involved in gene therapy as applied to skin diseases, and major advances in the field to date.

Efficient delivery is key to the success of any gene therapy and the skin is an attractive target for topical application of therapeutic nucleic acids. However, the barrier properties of the stratum corneum limit the transfection efficiency of cells in the underlying epidermis and so a diverse range of approaches are under investigation to improve skin gene delivery. *In vivo*, topical approaches have largely focused on the use of nonviral methods including formulations of nucleic acids, for example with liposomes, polymeric nanoparticles or biomaterials, while intradermal injection and other physical methods of gene

Harper's Textbook of Pediatric Dermatology, Fourth Edition. Edited by Peter Hoeger, Veronica Kinsler and Albert Yan.

Table 170.1 Properties of vectors used for skin gene therapy

Feature	AAV	Retrovirus	Lentivirus	Nanoparticle
Genome	ssDNA	ssRNA	ssRNA	DNA or RNA
Infect nondividing cells	Yes	No	Yes	Yes
Genomic integration	Yes/No	Yes	Yes	No
Expression pattern	6–12 months	>12 months	>2 months	Days
Expression level	Moderate	Moderate	Moderate	Low
Cloning capacity	3.5–4 kb	7–8 kb	7–8 kb	Unlimited
Immune response	Low	Moderate	Low	Low
Viral titre/product yield	Low	Moderate	Moderate	High

AAV, adeno-associated virus; ss, single stranded.

delivery, including ultrasound and electroporation [1,2], have largely focused on naked nucleic acids.

The other major approach to skin gene therapy involves *ex vivo* gene modification of cells followed by expansion of cells for skin grafting [3,4]. Retroviral and lentiviral vectors are the preferred modality for *ex vivo* modification of keratinocytes and epidermal stem cells for cell-mediated therapies [5]. This approach has proven particularly beneficial for treating some forms of epidermolysis bullosa (EB) although it is highly labour-intensive which might limit its deployment to larger numbers of patients.

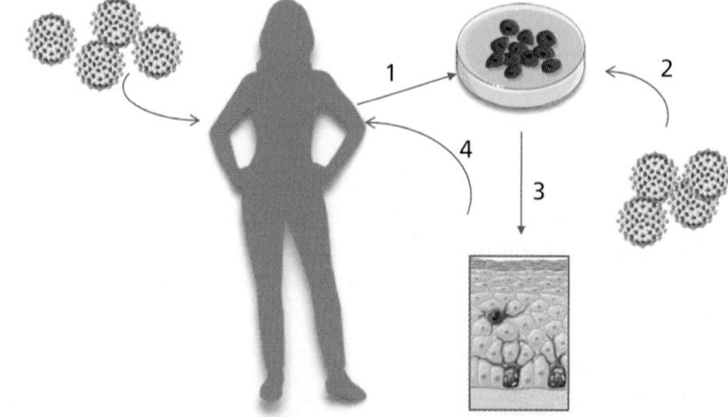

Fig. 170.1 *In vivo* and *ex vivo* gene therapy. In *ex vivo* gene therapy, a skin biopsy is first taken and epidermal stem cells are expanded in cell culture (1). Then the progenitor cells are transduced with an integrating virus, such as a retrovirus or lentivirus (2), and the population differentiated and expanded in cell culture to prepare a skin graft (3). The corrected, autologous skin graft is then applied to the patient's area of skin damage. *In vivo* gene therapy involves direct administration of the gene packaged in an AAV vector or a nanoparticle formulation where the cells are corrected *in situ* without the need for cell culture or skin grafting.

Genetic therapies for skin diseases using viral vectors

Retroviral and lentiviral vectors

Lentiviral vectors (LV) and retroviral vectors (RV; see Table 170.1) are mostly used for *ex vivo*, cell-mediated approaches to skin gene therapy [5] (Fig. 170.1). Transduction is the process of introducing genetic material into an organism using a viral vector. LV can transduce both dividing and nondividing cells, owing to the ability of the LV preintegration complex (PIC) to cross the nuclear envelope, while RV can only transduce mitotic cells. Both viruses have RNA genomes which are reverse transcribed into DNA and then integrated by the enzyme integrase into the genome of the transduced cells. RV and LV integration into the genome provides the benefits of long-term gene expression for the lifetime of the cell, but also presents risks of insertional oncogenesis, as occurred in an RV-based therapy for X-linked severe combined immunodeficiency disease (X-SCID) [6,7].

The latest generation of RVs and LVs, however, contain self-inactivating (SIN) long terminal repeats that reduce their ability to activate oncogenes in the genome, and have so far proven much safer [8,9]. Integration-deficient LVs, whose genetic material is reverse transcribed from RNA to DNA but does not integrate into the chromosome but rather is maintained in the nucleus episomally, have also been developed for *ex vivo* modification of keratinocytes by gene editing (discussed later in this chapter). For skin gene therapy, LVs and RVs have been used for *ex vivo* applications where keratinocytes or epidermal progenitor cells are obtained from punch biopsies, then transduced with the desired therapeutic gene and then expanded into grafts on plastic or fibrin sheets, and engrafted to the patient, such as reported for junctional epidermolysis bullosa (JEB) [3].

Ex vivo gene therapy for JEB was first demonstrated by transducing autologous keratinocytes from a patient with JEB with a murine Moloney leukaemia virus (MMLV) vector encoding *LAMB3*, the β_3 chain of the heterotrimeric protein known as laminin 332 or laminin 5 (LAM5). Transduced cells were expanded over several days and engrafted in a small area on the patient's legs [3]. Engraftment was complete after eight days with the restoration of an adherent epidermis that persisted for at least one year without blistering, infections or inflammation, and without an immune response to the graft. Synthesis of fully assembled, functional LAM5 (the missing protein in this instance) at normal levels was observed. This study was then followed up by a ground-breaking study in which the entire fully functional, epidermis derived from autologous epidermal stem cells, expanded *ex vivo*, was engrafted on a 7-year-old child with JEB [4]. The new epidermis was resistant to mechanical stress and remained healthy at a follow-up time of 21 months, demonstrating the enormous potential for *ex vivo* gene therapy of JEB, and proof of concept for the technique in other genetic skin diseases.

Adeno-associated virus

Adeno-associated virus (AAV) is a member of the parvovirus family and vectors derived from AAV are now one of the most widely used delivery systems for *in vivo* gene therapy in areas of medicine ranging from the liver for haemophilia [10] to the eye for retinitis pigmentosa [11]. They can transduce both dividing and nondividing cells with high efficiency with long-term gene expression. Unlike wild-type virus, AAV vectors have a very low chromosomal integration frequency but are maintained in the nucleus as episomes, DNA molecules independent of the chromosomes, and can achieve persistent expression, providing the therapeutic replacement protein for weeks to months [12]. An AAV therapy became the first EU-approved gene therapy product, Alipogene Tiparvovec or Glybera (uniQure N.V., The Netherlands), for the metabolic disease lipoprotein lipase deficiency, while recently the US FDA-approved Luxturna™, an AAV treatment for retinitis pigmentosa, a retinopathy caused by mutations in *RPE65*, was the first approved gene therapy product for a monogenic disease in the USA. AAV serotype 2 is the prototype AAV vector but many other serotypes have now been evaluated, which show tropisms for different tissues. For example, AAV serotype 6 (AAV6) achieved keratinocyte transduction frequency 5 logs higher than AAV2 [13]. The AAV capsid is also amenable to engineering so that artificial capsids can be engineered, further expanding tropism, including for human keratinocytes [14].

In vivo gene transfer by AAV in skin (see Fig. 170.1) was initially reported by intradermal injection of recombinant AAV particles into porcine skin, achieving transduction of epidermal keratinocytes, hair follicle epithelial cells and eccrine sweat glands with expression persisting for more than six weeks, although expression after readministration was less effective due to the immune response [15]. Other *in vivo* gene therapy studies were reported for diabetic wound models, by intradermal injection of AAV vectors, expressing vascular endothelial growth factor (VEGF)^{165} [16–18] or fibroblast growth factor-4 (FGF4) [19]. The immunogenicity of AAV may affect its clinical use in skin since preexisting immunity is widespread, with more than 90% of the population having preexisting immunity to the most common AAV serotypes, including AAV2 [20,21].

Adeno-associated virus also has potential for *ex vivo* skin gene therapy by gene editing of keratinocytes. A highly recombinogenic AAV serotype, AAV-DJ, was developed in a novel therapy for Herlitz-junctional epidermolysis bullosa (H-JEB) caused by autosomal recessive mutations in LAMA3 [22]. AAV-DJ-LAMA3 transduction of keratinocytes *ex vivo* achieved gene targeting at clinically relevant efficiencies with low rates of random, off-target integration. Correction of H-JEB patient cells restored their adhesion phenotype, thus eliminating the need for any further genetic selection and so enhancing the safety of this approach. This treatment fully reversed the blistering phenotype in skin grafts of corrected patient cells in nude mice [22].

Nanoparticles and nonviral approaches

Nanoparticles (see Table 170.1) are generally synthetic formulations of nucleic acids with different kinds of materials that enable the formation of particles, typically of the order of 100 nm in diameter, or 100 billionths of a metre! Typically, nonviral nanoparticles comprise self-assembling formulations of anionic nucleic acids with cationic reagents such as lipids, polymers and peptides [23–26]. Targeting properties may also be incorporated into nanoparticles using peptides, proteins, antibody fragments or carbohydrates designed to home to a particular cell surface receptor on a particular cell type [26]. By careful design of the formulation and methods of self-assembly, stable nanoparticles of approximately 100 nm or less may be prepared. Nanoparticle self-assembly is driven by electrostatic charge interactions, meaning that there are no specific size constraints on nucleic acid packaging as occur with viral vectors and so a diverse array of nucleic acid technologies may be delivered by nonviral methods, including plasmid and minicircle DNA [27–30], siRNA and mRNA [25,31–35], as well as CRISPR/Cas9 gene editing formulations [36,37]. Nanoparticles made of lipids and plasmid DNA (pDNA) have been described for topical delivery to the skin, as reviewed recently [2].

Compared to viral vectors, clinical and preclinical trials with liposomes, such as those for cystic fibrosis, have shown that nanoparticle formulations are safe, well tolerated and nonimmunogenic, although minor, transient inflammatory responses have been observed [38]. Although topical delivery to skin is attractive due to its noninvasive nature and potential to cover large surface areas, this approach is of low efficiency due to the stratum corneum which comprises a 'brick wall' structure of cornified, anuclear keratinocytes with a lipid-rich substance filling the spaces between them [1]. However, this barrier is not completely impermeable and improvements to nanoparticles such as those comprising gold cores coated with siRNA are increasing efficiency of nucleic acid delivery applied topically in moisturizer [39,40].

Topical application by spraying of liposomal pDNA encoding the reporter gene Green Fluorescent Protein (GFP) onto mouse or human skin once daily for three consecutive days showed that although messenger GFP mRNA and protein were detectable, fluorescent cells were not observed by fluorescence microscopy or flow cytometry [41]. In contrast, intradermal injection of liposomal pDNA was slightly better but still achieved only approximately 4% transfection efficiency. Combinations of nucleic acids with other biomaterials are under investigation to enhance skin transfection, such as the combination of an electrospun scaffold and a pDNA encoding keratinocyte growth factor (KGF) [42]. Animals receiving the KGF plasmid-loaded scaffold displayed better epithelial development, keratinocyte proliferation and granulation wound healing responses than pDNA without the scaffold [42]. In another example, chitosan wound dressings were combined with exosomes for microRNA (miRNA) delivery to a rat chronic wound model, demonstrating slow release of exosomes leading to healing of skin defects in a diabetic rat model [43].

Other promising approaches for plasmid delivery to skin reported the use of hollow nanoneedles to physically penetrate the skin and deposit antigen-encoding nucleic acids [44,45] and hollow microneedle devices have been reported for delivery of plasmid DNA by a hydrodynamic effect [46].

Minicircle DNA

Minicircle DNA differs from pDNA in that almost all bacterial DNA, including the antibiotic bacterial selection gene, is removed [30,47,48]. Minicircle DNA offers several benefits over plasmids, apart from smaller size, including reduced immunogenicity and increased transfection efficiency, and more persistent transgene gene expression *in vivo* as demonstrated in lung airway epithelial transfection experiments [27]. In skin, minicircles have been used to deliver VEGF with a nanoparticle formulated from an arginine-grafted, cationic polymeric dendrimer by subcutaneous injection into diabetes-related skin wounds in mice [49]. This resulted in high levels of transfected VEGF^{165} expression in actively proliferating cells in wound tissue, leading to wound healing within six days and the restoration of a well-ordered dermal structure. An alternative approach for minicircle delivery to diabetic wounds was demonstrated by subcutaneous injection of the naked minicircle encoding VEGF^{165}followed by ultrasound radiation, to promote localized minicircle uptake in the wound leading to accelerated wound repair [50]. Minicircle DNA encoding a peptide antigen, delivered by intradermal tattooing, elicited a more potent antigen-specific CD8+ T-cell response against *Listeria* in mice than a plasmid encoding the same antigen, suggesting its potential in vaccination [51].

A limitation of DNA-based therapeutics for gene therapy of skin diseases is transfecting the postmitotic or slowly dividing cells of the skin epithelium with pDNA, which is inefficient due to the need for the plasmid to enter the nucleus, and the highly selective nature of pDNA uptake through pores in the nuclear envelope [52,53]. However, RNA reagents such as siRNA, microRNA and messenger RNA are functional in the cytoplasm, and so offer the potential for greater activity than plasmids and better opportunities for skin therapeutics.

siRNA and spherical nucleic acids

RNA interference (RNAi) was discovered in the 1990s as a naturally occurring mechanism for regulating gene expression. This was quickly adapted to exploit the therapeutic potential of RNA with synthetic, double-stranded, short interfering RNA (siRNA) molecules. The mechanism of action has been well described elsewhere [54] but essentially, the siRNA guide strand is recruited into the RNA induced silencing complex (RISC), a cytoplasmic, multicomponent ribonucleoprotein complex in which the guide strand of the siRNA targets an intracellular mRNA by homologous base pairing, then cleaves the mRNA by the Argonaute protein component. The overall effect is that the specific mRNA corresponding to the mutant or undesired protein is degraded before it can be transcribed into protein.

SiRNA has been in clinical trials for cancers, genetic diseases and infections and it is anticipated that the first siRNA product, for the rare genetic disease transthyretin amyloidosis (TTR), will be licensed in 2018 [32]. In the skin, an allele-specific siRNA targeting the N171K mutant in the gene for keratin 6a (K6a) is in development for pachyonychia congenita (PC), a rare, autosomal dominant syndrome that involves a disabling plantar keratoderma [55]. In phase Ib clinical trials for treatment of PC, siRNA administered by intradermal injection specifically and potently silenced the K6a mutant mRNA without affecting the wild-type version, while calluses showed signs of regression in the siRNA- treated foot but not on the vehicle-treated foot [56]. This trial was the first to use an allele-specific siRNA in a clinical setting and the first to use siRNA in human skin.

In an alternative approach, siRNA was formulated as spherical nucleic acids (SNAs), which are chemically modified gold nanoparticles coated with dense layers of highly oriented siRNAs [40]. Epidermal growth factor receptor (EGFR) siRNA in SNA nanoconjugates (SNA-NCs), applied topically to hairless mice, almost completely silenced EGFR expression and reduced epidermal thickness by almost 40%, with similar results in human skin. The treatment had no adverse effects on the skin and was virtually undetectable in internal organs [40]. SNA-NCs applied topically in a moisturizer were also shown to deliver siRNAs that reversed impaired wound healing in diabetic mice by silencing of ganglioside GM3 synthase [39] and were also effective in the treatment of psoriasis by topical application of SNAs that silenced EGF and EGFR production, reducing cell proliferation [56].

MicroRNA (miRNA) is similar to siRNA but generally less sequence specific [54]. MiRNAs target semi-conserved 3′ untranslated regions of mRNAs so that many mRNAs sharing the same motif may be silenced. Moreover, the mechanism of silencing appears to be at the translational level (silencing the protein), rather than transcriptional levels (silencing the mRNA). MiRNAs play important roles in epidermal development, psoriasis, cutaneous squamous cell carcinoma and reepithelialization in the skin and thus have a wide range of opportunities as biomarkers and therapeutics, for example in skin wound repair [57–59]. Exosomes prepared from miR-126-3p-overexpressing synovium mesenchymal stem cells (SMSC-126-Exos) were shown to stimulate proliferation of human dermal fibroblasts and human dermal microvascular endothelial cells (HMEC-1) in a dose-dependent manner and also promoted migration and tube formation of HMEC-1 [43]. In a diabetic rat model, chitosan wound dressings incorporating SMSC-126-Exos enabled accelerated wound repair *in vivo*, demonstrating the wide potential of this approach [44].

In vitro transcribed mRNA

In vitro transcribed messenger RNA (mRNA) as a template for protein production is a relatively new approach to protein replacement therapy. The structure of mRNA from 5′ to 3′ comprises the 5′cap, 5′ untranslated region (UTR), coding region, 3′ UTR and polyadenosine (polyA) tail. Chemical modifications, particularly chemically modified bases such as pseudouridine, methylcytosine and others, have resulted in *in vitro* synthesis of mRNA with improved stability, translational efficiency and reduced immunogenicity [60]. Equally important have been the developments in the untranslated regions of the mRNA template, including the 5′-capping procedure using anti-reverse capping reagents (ARCA), capping analogues that reduce the rate of decapping [61], the structure of the 5′ and 3′ UTRs and polyA region, reviewed in Sahin et al. [62]. The coding region itself may be optimized for higher levels of expression by codon optimization in the template DNA; this ensures use of codons for which there is a higher concentration of transfer RNA (tRNA) with the relevant anticodon although, interestingly, this approach does not always lead to higher expression [63].

Translation of mRNA occurs in the cytoplasm so, unlike plasmid DNA, the nuclear envelope is not a barrier to transfection and so expression levels can be much higher. From a safety perspective, mRNA cannot integrate into the genome and so the risk of insertional mutagenesis is nullified, in contrast to plasmid DNA where there is a low but significant risk of insertional oncogenesis or germline transmission. Although chemical modifications to mRNA have reduced inflammatory toxicity [64] and improved stability [60], mRNA expression is short-lived compared to plasmid-based expression, necessitating administration at more frequent intervals. However, in skin, transient expression from mRNA can be used for vaccination applications [65] or wound repair [66].

Gene editing

Gene editing offers the potential for precise and specific gene repair for a variety of genetic diseases of the skin. The difficulties of delivery across the skin barrier *in vivo* mean that the *ex vivo* strategies are currently more likely to be effective in the short term. Gene editing may be performed with zinc finger nucleases (ZFN) and transcription activator-like effector nucleases (TALENs), both of which involve targeting by protein domains to specific DNA sequences. The targeting proteins are fused to dimeric *Fok*I nuclease which induces double strand breaks (DSB) [67].

Gene editing with clustered regularly interspaced palindromic repeats (CRISPR) and CRISPR-associated (Cas) nucleases (Fig. 170.2a) was first used in 2002 [68]. Targeted genome editing was realized by Charpentier Doudna [69] and shortly after that the use of CRISPR for engineering human cells was demonstrated [70]. CRISPR has advantages over ZFN and TALEN in that it is RNA guided, making it much simpler to use [67]. The CRISPR ribonucleoprotein complex is composed of a Cas9 nuclease, along with the noncoding RNA elements called the single guide RNA (sgRNA) which programme the specificity of the nucleic acid cleavage. Cas9 first binds to the protospacer adjacent motif (PAM) which in the *Streptococcus pyogenes* (SpCas9) type II CRISPR system is any 5′-NGG sequence, where 'N' is any nucleotide and 'GG' denotes two guanines and is located directly upstream [71]. After Cas9 recognition of a PAM sequence, the DNA unwinds upstream of the PAM, allowing guide RNA binding to the single-stranded DNA sequence. Upon guide RNA binding to the target sequence, Cas9 makes a DNA double-stranded break three bases upstream of the PAM sequence (see Fig. 170.2a).

All three gene editing methods introduce double-strand DNA breaks and in the absence of template DNA, the endogenous, nonhomologous end-joining (NHEJ) repair pathway mediates DNA repair, an imprecise pathway that can lead to insertion or deletion mutations (indels) in the DNA with the likelihood of premature termination codons inactivating the gene (Fig. 170.2b). In the presence of an exogenous template donor DNA, provided as a plasmid DNA, double-stranded or single-stranded oligonucleotide DNA [71] or by AAV [72], homology-directed repair (HDR) pathways may recruit the donor DNA at the cleavage site, with the potential to repair genetic mutations (see Fig. 170.2b). However, the HDR pathway is limited in its efficiency and is mainly active in mitotic cells [73]. Therefore, strategies that exploit non-HDR pathways are gaining more attention for *in vivo* gene editing, including PITCh (Precise Integration into Target Chromosomes), which exploits microhomology-mediated end joining [74], and HITI (Homology Independent Targeted Integration), which exploits the NHEJ pathway [75].

Gene editing for genetic diseases of the skin is at an early stage of development and to date has mainly involved methods of HDR to correct the genetic defect [76]. The potential of gene editing of keratinocytes was demonstrated with ZFN [77], with silencing of GFP while retaining the stem cell-like properties of the keratinocytes. In the next stage, targeted integration at the AAV integration site 1 (AAVS1) 'safe harbour' site of a GFP gene was achieved by ZFN-mediated homologous recombination [78]. Skin grafts in mice from unselected, ZFN-transduced keratinocytes were found to contain GFP-positive colonies with a high frequency of integration at the AAVS1 site in epithelial stem cells. It was proposed that gene-corrected autologous skin grafts could provide a safer approach than retroviral transduced keratinocyte-derived grafts for the treatment of genetic skin diseases [78].

Gene editing by TALENs has been explored for its potential to correct a defective type VII collagen gene (COL7A1) associated with recessive dystrophic epidermolysis bullosa (RDEB) by the NHEJ pathway [79] (79) and by HDR with a donor template DNA [80]. TALEN constructs were used to induce site-specific DSB with the goal of restoring the reading frame by indel formation in a proportion of cases A subset of indels did indeed restore the reading frame of COL7A1, resulting in expression of mutant or truncated collagen VII protein which was expressed in the skin dermoepidermal junction [79]. The HDR pathway was effective in inducible pluripotential stem cells (iPSC) derived from patients with RDEB which resulted in correction of the COL7A1 gene in primary fibroblasts [80].

In another study on RDEB, AAV was used to deliver TALENs and a donor DNA for gene editing repair of the

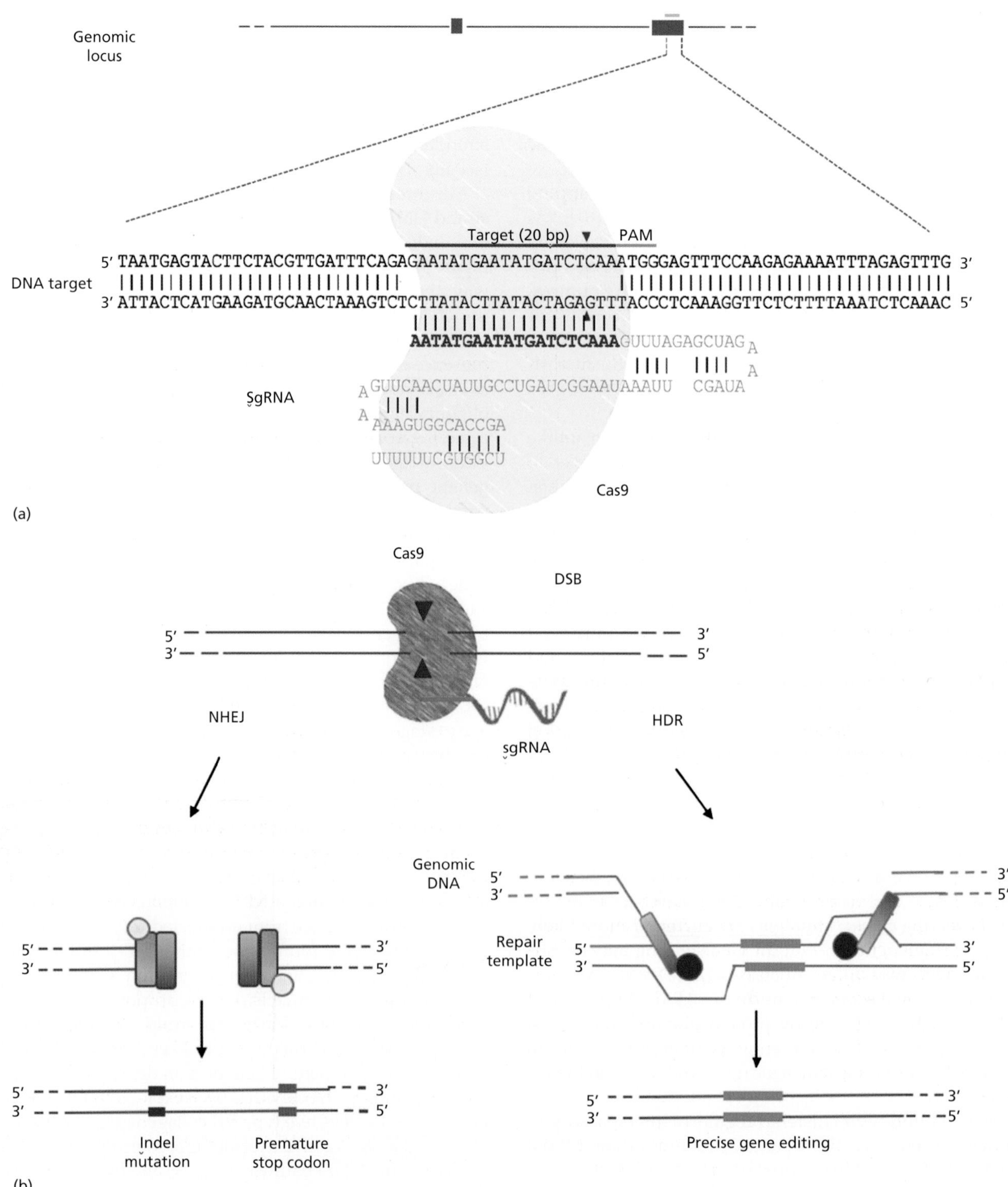

Fig. 170.2 Schematic of the RNA-guided Cas9 nuclease. The Cas9 (blue) is targeted to genomic DNA by an sgRNA consisting of a 20-nucleotide guide sequence (red) and a scaffold (blue). The guide sequence pairs with the DNA target directly upstream of a 5′-NGG protospacer adjacent motif (PAM). Cas9 mediates a double-strand break (DSB) 3 bp upstream of the PAM (red triangle) (a). DSBs induced by Cas9 (blue) are repaired via one of two pathways; in NHEJ, the ends are rejoined by endogenous DNA repair machinery, resulting in indel mutations at the junction site. Supplying a donor DNA template leverages the HDR pathway, allowing high fidelity and precise editing (b). Source: Adapted from Ran et al. [71]. Reproduced with permission of Springer.

disease-causing c.6527insC mutation in the COL7A1 gene [79]. Analysis of gene-edited clones showed physiologically relevant levels of COL7A1 mRNA and collagen VII protein. In addition, transduction of patient keratinocytes with TALENs without the donor template DNA resulted in indel generation (insertion/deletion mutations) by NHEJ close to the c.6527insC mutation, restoring the reading frame of COL7A1 in a proportion of cells, resulting in abundant expression of mutated or truncated collagen VII protein [79]. Keratinocyte clones corrected by

HDR or NHEJ were able to regenerate skin with collagen VII restored in the dermoepidermal junction. These novel approaches may offer opportunities for clinical studies in the future.

CRISPR/Cas9 gene editing has also been used to repair *COL7A1* by HDR by treatment of patient-derived keratinocytes, using either the wild-type Cas9 or D10A nickase [81]. Corrected single-cell clones were identified that produced levels of type VII collagen similar to control keratinocytes. Skin grafts from corrected keratinocytes in immunodeficient mice displayed typical localization of type VII collagen at the basement membrane in contrast to uncorrected keratinocytes, while skin layers showed normal differentiation and structures without blistering. Thus, gene editing either by TALENs or CRISPR has demonstrated the potential for *ex vivo* keratinocyte correction and subsequent fully functional skin grafting, offering a safer therapy with precise and specific gene correction.

Guide RNA and Cas9 may both be delivered by encoding plasmid DNA but, as noted above, the difficulties of transfecting the nondividing epithelium will limit efficiency *in vivo*. Synthetic gRNA delivered with Cas9 mRNA in a nanoparticle formulation may offer the best route to a gene editing strategy for skin since mRNA yields higher transient transfection efficiency than DNA. However, the template DNA will still be required for delivery into the nucleus. Short oligonucleotide templates will probably enter the nucleus more easily than plasmids and may provide higher HDR efficiencies [82] and specificities, while for larger DNA donors, minicircle DNA template is more efficient than plasmid DNA [75]. Viral vectors such as AAV may also be used to provide the template more efficiently [83], although this approach has the same problems of AAV immunogenicity.

Off-target effects are caused by DSBs occurring at alternative PAM sites, followed by NHEJ repair introducing indels. These can occur at sites downstream of potential PAMs bearing closer homology to the guide RNA. Whole genome sequencing suggested that the frequency of off-target effects was quite rare in mice [84] but simpler and cheaper genome screening methods have been described [85–88]. Genetically modified versions of Cas9 have been introduced that minimize off-target DSBs, including the 'double-nickase' approach where the Cas9 was engineered to cut one DNA strand rather than make DSBs. Thus, two guide RNAs on opposite strands are required to position the nucleases in close proximity to achieve a DSB, reducing the likelihood of off-target DSBs [89].

A recent approach that avoids DSBs altogether includes DNA base editing formulations [90,91]. In the first of these approaches, Cas9 fusion proteins were engineered to enable replacement of a mutant C with T, while Cas9 nickase fusions were made with cytidine deaminase, APOBEC1 and uracil glycosylase inhibitor (UGI) [92]. The deamination of cytosine (C) catalysed by cytidine deaminases results in generation of uracil (U), which behaves with base pairing properties of thymine (T). The UGI prevents U excision by cellular enzymes. The mutant Cas9 then nicks the unedited strand, which induces the cell's DNA repair mechanism, resulting in replacement of the G that originally paired with C into an A that pairs with the new T (U) [93]. In a further development, Cas9 fusion constructs were prepared with a tRNA adenosine deaminase that was selected by *in vitro* directed evolution, to convert adenine (A) in DNA to inosine, which acts like a G, pairing with C [91].

Thus, base editing constructs now enable the precise editing of the single bases, C to T, A to G, T to C and G to A, at much higher efficiencies than achievable by HDR and with much lower indel formation and off-target events. The use of this approach, however, is limited by the availability of a suitable PAM but may be overcome in future by the use of alternative nucleases to the original Cas9 that recognize unique PAM sequences with different sequences and lengths to that of *Sp* Cas9.

There are several different formats in which the CRISPR components can be delivered with plasmid DNA or virus encoding both Cas9 and guide RNA, or Cas9 nuclease may be delivered as the mRNA cotransfected with a synthetic guide RNA, or as a preassembled Cas9/gRNA ribonucleoprotein (RNP) complex [36,94]. There are also several ways, as described above, to package the DNA repair template, such as plasmid or minicircle DNA or by viral vector such as AAV.

Conclusion

The development of novel nucleic acid strategies including siRNA, mRNA and gene editing, as well as more traditional plasmid DNA and viral DNA therapies, is opening up the potential for new therapies for currently untreatable genetic skin diseases and chronic wounds, as well as vaccination. Overcoming barriers to *in vivo* delivery remains a major challenge although for some genetic conditions, approaches of *ex vivo* correction followed by cell expansion and skin grafting have offered spectacular insights into the future potential of skin gene therapy.

References

1 Chen X. Current and future technological advances in transdermal gene delivery. Adv Drug Deliv Rev 2018;127:85–105.

2 Zakrewsky M, Kumar S, Mitragotri S. Nucleic acid delivery into skin for the treatment of skin disease: proofs-of-concept, potential impact, and remaining challenges. J Control Release 2015;219:445–56.

3 Mavilio F, Pellegrini G, Ferrari S et al. Correction of junctional epidermolysis bullosa by transplantation of genetically modified epidermal stem cells. Nat Med 2006;12:1397–402.

4 Hirsch T, Rothoeft T, Teig N et al. Regeneration of the entire human epidermis using transgenic stem cells. Nature 2017;551:327–32.

5 Gorell E, Nguyen N, Lane A et al. Gene therapy for skin diseases. Perspect Med 2014;4:a015149.

6 Hacein-Bey-Abina S, von Kalle C, Schmidt M et al. A serious adverse event after successful gene therapy for X-linked severe combined immunodeficiency. N Engl J Med 2003;348:255–6.

7 Hacein-Bey-Abina S, von Kalle C, Schmidt M et al. LMO2-associated clonal T cell proliferation in two patients after gene therapy for SCID-X1. Science 2003;302:415–19.

8 Miyoshi H, Blomer U, Takahashi M et al. Development of a self-inactivating lentivirus vector. J Virol 1998;72:8150–7.

9 Montini E, Cesana D, Schmidt M et al. The genotoxic potential of retroviral vectors is strongly modulated by vector design and integration site selection in a mouse model of HSC gene therapy. J Clin Invest 2009;119:964–75.

10 High KH, Nathwani A, Spencer T et al. Current status of haemophilia gene therapy. Haemophilia 2014;20(Suppl 4):43 9.

11 Moore NA, Morral N, Ciulla TA et al. Gene therapy for inherited retinal and optic nerve degenerations. Expert Opin Biol Ther 2018;18:37–49.
12 Yang J, Zhou W, Zhang Y et al. Concatamerization of adeno-associated virus circular genomes occurs through intermolecular recombination. J Virol 1999;73:9468–77.
13 Petek LM, Fleckman P, Miller DG. Efficient KRT14 targeting and functional characterization of transplanted human keratinocytes for the treatment of epidermolysis bullosa simplex. Mol Ther 2010;18:1624–32.
14 Sallach J, di Pasquale G, Larcher F et al. Tropism-modified AAV vectors overcome barriers to successful cutaneous therapy. Mol Ther 2014;22:929–39.
15 Hengge UR, Mirmohammadsadegh A. Adeno-associated virus expresses transgenes in hair follicles and epidermis. Mol Ther 2000;2:188–94.
16 Deodato B, Arsic N, Zentilin L et al. Recombinant AAV vector encoding human VEGF165 enhances wound healing. Gene Ther 2002;9:777–85.
17 Galeano M, Deodato B, Altavilla D et al. Adeno-associated viral vector-mediated human vascular endothelial growth factor gene transfer stimulates angiogenesis and wound healing in the genetically diabetic mouse. Diabetologia 2003;46:546–55.
18 Keswani SG, Balaji S, Le L et al. Pseudotyped adeno-associated viral vector tropism and transduction efficiencies in murine wound healing. Wound Repair Regeneration 2012;20:592–600.
19 Jazwa A, Kucharzewska P, Leja J et al. Combined vascular endothelial growth factor-A and fibroblast growth factor 4 gene transfer improves wound healing in diabetic mice. Genetic Vaccines Ther 2010;8:6.
20 Masat E, Pavani G, Mingozzi F. Humoral immunity to AAV vectors in gene therapy: challenges and potential solutions. Discov Med 2013;15:379–89.
21 Halbert CL, Miller AD, McNamara S et al. Prevalence of neutralizing antibodies against adeno-associated virus (AAV) types 2, 5, and 6 in cystic fibrosis and normal populations: Implications for gene therapy using AAV vectors. Hum Gene Ther 2006;17:440–7.
22 Melo SP, Lisowski L, Bashkirova E et al. Somatic correction of junctional epidermolysis bullosa by a highly recombinogenic AAV variant. Mol Ther 2014;22:725–33.
23 Cullis PR, Hope MJ. Lipid nanoparticle systems for enabling gene therapies. Mol Ther 2017;25:1467–75.
24 Riley MK, Vermerris W. Recent advances in nanomaterials for gene delivery – a review. Nanomaterials 2017;7:94.
25 Tatiparti K, Sau S, Kashaw SK et al. siRNA delivery strategies: a comprehensive review of recent developments. Nanomaterials 2017;7:77.
26 Zylberberg C, Gaskill K, Pasley S et al. Engineering liposomal nanoparticles for targeted gene therapy. Gene Ther 2017;24:441–52.
27 Munye MM, Tagalakis AD, Barnes JL et al. Minicircle DNA provides enhanced and prolonged transgene expression following airway gene transfer. Sci Rep 2016;6:23125.
28 Vaysse L, Gregory LG, Harbottle RP et al. Nuclear-targeted minicircle to enhance gene transfer with non-viral vectors in vitro and in vivo. J Gene Med 2006;8:754–63.
29 Chen ZY, He CY, Ehrhardt A et al. Minicircle DNA vectors devoid of bacterial DNA result in persistent and high-level transgene expression in vivo. Mol Ther 2003;8:495–500.
30 Darquet AM, Rangara R, Kreiss P et al. Minicircle: an improved DNA molecule for in vitro and in vivo gene transfer. Gene Ther 1999;6:209–18.
31 Oberli MA, Reichmuth AM, Dorkin JR et al. Lipid nanoparticle assisted mRNA delivery for potent cancer immunotherapy. Nano Lett 2017;17:1326–35.
32 Kaczmarek JC, Kowalski PS, Anderson DG. Advances in the delivery of RNA therapeutics: from concept to clinical reality. Genome Med 2017;9:60.
33 Kauffman KJ, Webber MJ, Anderson DG. Materials for non-viral intracellular delivery of messenger RNA therapeutics. J Control Release 2016;240:227–34.
34 Fenton OS, Kauffman KJ, McClellan RL et al. Bioinspired alkenyl amino alcohol ionizable lipid materials for highly potent in vivo mRNA delivery. Adv Mater 2016;28:2939–43.
35 Dong Y, Dorkin JR, Wang W et al. Poly(glycoamidoamine) Brushes formulated nanomaterials for systemic siRNA and mRNA delivery in vivo. Nano Lett 2016;16:842–8.
36 Wang M, Zuris JA, Meng F et al. Efficient delivery of genome-editing proteins using bioreducible lipid nanoparticles. Proc Natl Acad Sci USA 2016;113:2868–73.
37 Zuris JA, Thompson DB, Shu Y et al. Cationic lipid-mediated delivery of proteins enables efficient protein-based genome editing in vitro and in vivo. Nat Biotechnol 2015;33:73–80.
38 Alton EW, Armstrong DK, Ashby D et al. Repeated nebulisation of non-viral CFTR gene therapy in patients with cystic fibrosis: a randomised, double-blind, placebo-controlled, phase 2b trial. Lancet Respir Med 2015;3:684–91.
39 Randeria PS, Seeger MA, Wang XQ et al. siRNA-based spherical nucleic acids reverse impaired wound healing in diabetic mice by ganglioside GM3 synthase knockdown. Proc Natl Acad Sci USA 2015;112:5573–8.
40 Zheng D, Giljohann DA, Chen DL et al. Topical delivery of siRNA-based spherical nucleic acid nanoparticle conjugates for gene regulation. Proc Natl Acad Sci USA 2012;109:11975–80.
41 Meykadeh N, Mirmohammadsadegh A, Wang Z et al. Topical application of plasmid DNA to mouse and human skin. J Mol Med 2005;83:897–903.
42 Kobsa S, Kristofik NJ, Sawyer AJ et al. An electrospun scaffold integrating nucleic acid delivery for treatment of full-thickness wounds. Biomaterials 2013;34:3891–901.
43 Tao SC, Guo SC, Li M et al. Chitosan wound dressings incorporating exosomes derived from microRNA-126-overexpressing synovium mesenchymal stem cells provide sustained release of exosomes and heal full-thickness skin defects in a diabetic rat model. Stem Cells Transl Med 2017;6:736–47.
44 Chen X, Kask AS, Crichton ML et al. Improved DNA vaccination by skin-targeted delivery using dry-coated densely-packed microprojection arrays. J Control Release 2010;148:327–33.
45 Kask AS, Chen X, Marshak JO et al. DNA vaccine delivery by densely-packed and short microprojection arrays to skin protects against vaginal HSV-2 challenge. Vaccine 2010;28:7483–91.
46 Dul M, Stefanidou M, Porta P et al. Hydrodynamic gene delivery in human skin using a hollow microneedle device. J Control Release 2017;265:120–31.
47 Bigger BW, Tolmachov O, Collombet JM et al. An araC-controlled bacterial cre expression system to produce DNA minicircle vectors for nuclear and mitochondrial gene therapy. J Biol Chem 2001;276:23018–27.
48 Chen ZY, He CY, Kay MA. Improved production and purification of minicircle DNA vector free of plasmid bacterial sequences and capable of persistent transgene expression in vivo. Hum Gene Ther 2005;16:126–31.
49 Kwon MJ, An S, Choi S et al. Effective healing of diabetic skin wounds by using nonviral gene therapy based on minicircle vascular endothelial growth factor DNA and a cationic dendrimer. J Gene Med 2012;14:272–8.
50 Yoon CS, Jung HS, Kwon MJ et al. Sonoporation of the minicircle-VEGF(165) for wound healing of diabetic mice. Pharm Res 2009;26:794–801.
51 Dietz WM, Skinner NE, Hamilton SE et al. Minicircle DNA is superior to plasmid DNA in eliciting antigen-specific CD8+ T-cell responses. Mol Ther 2013;21:1526–35.
52 Liu G, Li D, Pasumarthy MK et al. Nanoparticles of compacted DNA transfect postmitotic cells. J Biol Chem 2003;278:32578–86.
53 Meng Q, Robinson D, Jenkins RG et al. Efficient transfection of non-proliferating human airway epithelial cells with a synthetic vector formulated with EGTA. J Gene Med 2004;6:210–21.
54 Wilson RC, Doudna JA. Molecular mechanisms of RNA interference. Ann Rev Biophys 2013;42:217–39.
55 Leachman SA, Hickerson RP, Schwartz ME et al. First-in-human mutation-targeted siRNA phase Ib trial of an inherited skin disorder. Mol Ther 2010;18:442–6.
56 Nemati H, Ghahramani MH, Faridi-Majidi R et al. Using siRNA-based spherical nucleic acid nanoparticle conjugates for gene regulation in psoriasis. J Control Release 2017;268:259–68.
57 Luan A, Hu MS, Leavitt T et al. Noncoding RNAs in wound healing: a new and vast frontier. Adv Wound Care 2018;7:19–27.
58 Ross K. Towards topical microRNA-directed therapy for epidermal disorders. J Control Release 2018;269:136–47.
59 Li D, Landen NX. MicroRNAs in skin wound healing. Eur J Dermatol 2017;27:12–14.
60 Anderson BR, Muramatsu H, Jha BK et al. Nucleoside modifications in RNA limit activation of 2′-5′-oligoadenylate synthetase and increase resistance to cleavage by RNase L. Nucleic Acids Res 2011;39:9329–38.
61 Strenkowska M, Grzela R, Majewski M et al. Cap analogs modified with 1,2-dithiodiphosphate moiety protect mRNA from decapping and enhance its translational potential. Nucleic Acids Res 2016;44:9578–90.

62 Sahin U, Kariko K, Tureci O. mRNA-based therapeutics – developing a new class of drugs. Nat Rev Drug Discov 2014;13:759–80.
63 Mauro VP, Chappell SA. A critical analysis of codon optimization in human therapeutics. Trends Mol Med 2014;20:604–13.
64 Kariko K, Muramatsu H, Ludwig J et al. Generating the optimal mRNA for therapy: HPLC purification eliminates immune activation and improves translation of nucleoside-modified, protein-encoding mRNA. Nucleic Acids Res 2011;39:e142.
65 Probst J, Weide B, Scheel B et al. Spontaneous cellular uptake of exogenous messenger RNA in vivo is nucleic acid-specific, saturable and ion dependent. Gene Ther 2007;14:1175–80.
66 Schwarz KW, Murray MT, Sylora R et al. Augmentation of wound healing with translation initiation factor eIF4E mRNA. J Surg Res 2002;103:175–82.
67 Gaj T, Gersbach CA, Barbas CF 3rd. ZFN, TALEN, and CRISPR/Cas-based methods for genome engineering. Trends Biotechnol 2013;31: 397–405.
68 Jansen R, Embden JD, Gaastra W et al. Identification of genes that are associated with DNA repeats in prokaryotes. Mol Microbiol 2002;43: 1565–75.
69 Jinek M, Chylinski K, Fonfara I et al. A programmable dual-RNA-guided DNA endonuclease in adaptive bacterial immunity. Science 2012;337:816–21.
70 Mali P, Yang L, Esvelt KM et al. RNA-guided human genome engineering via Cas9. Science 2013;339:823–6.
71 Ran FA, Hsu PD, Wright J et al. Genome engineering using the CRISPR-Cas9 system. Nat Protocols 2013;8:2281–308.
72 Kaulich M, Dowdy SF. Combining CRISPR/Cas9 and rAAV Templates for efficient gene editing. Nucleic Acid Therapeut 2015;25:287–96.
73 Nishiyama J, Mikuni T, Yasuda R. Virus-mediated genome editing via homology-directed repair in mitotic and postmitotic cells in mammalian brain. Neuron 2017;96:755–68.
74 Sakuma T, Nakade S, Sakane Y et al. MMEJ-assisted gene knock-in using TALENs and CRISPR-Cas9 with the PITCh systems. Nat Protocols 2016;11:118–33.
75 Suzuki K, Tsunekawa Y, Hernandez-Benitez R et al. In vivo genome editing via CRISPR/Cas9 mediated homology-independent targeted integration. Nature 2016;540:144–9.
76 March OP, Reichelt J, Koller U. Gene editing for skin diseases: designer nucleases as tools for gene therapy of skin fragility disorders. Exp Physiol 2018;103:449–55.
77 Hoher T, Wallace L, Khan K et al. Highly efficient zinc-finger nuclease-mediated disruption of an eGFP transgene in keratinocyte stem cells without impairment of stem cell properties. Stem Cell Rev 2012; 8:426–34.
78 Coluccio A, Miselli F, Lombardo A et al. Targeted gene addition in human epithelial stem cells by zinc-finger nuclease-mediated homologous recombination. Mol Ther 2013;21:1695–704.
79 Chamorro C, Mencia A, Almarza D et al. Gene editing for the efficient correction of a recurrent COL7A1 mutation in recessive dystrophic epidermolysis bullosa keratinocytes. Mol Ther Nucleic Acids 2016;5:e307.
80 Osborn MJ, Starker CG, McElroy AN et al. TALEN-based gene correction for epidermolysis bullosa. Mol Ther 2013;21:1151–9.
81 Webber BR, Osborn MJ, McElroy AN et al. CRISPR/Cas9-based genetic correction for recessive dystrophic epidermolysis bullosa. NPJ Regen Med 2016;136:S66.
82 Richardson CD, Ray GJ, DeWitt MA et al. Enhancing homology-directed genome editing by catalytically active and inactive CRISPR-Cas9 using asymmetric donor DNA. Nat Biotechnol 2016; 34:339–44.
83 Mahiny AJ, Dewerth A, Mays LE et al. In vivo genome editing using nuclease-encoding mRNA corrects SP-B deficiency. Nat Biotechnol 2015;33:584–6.
84 Iyer V, Shen B, Zhang W et al. Off-target mutations are rare in Cas9-modified mice. Nat Methods 2015;12:479.
85 Tsai SQ, Nguyen NT, Malagon-Lopez J et al. CIRCLE-seq: a highly sensitive in vitro screen for genome-wide CRISPR-Cas9 nuclease off-targets. Nat Methods 2017;14:607–14.
86 Zhu LJ, Lawrence M, Gupta A et al. GUIDEseq: a bioconductor package to analyze GUIDE-Seq datasets for CRISPR-Cas nucleases. BMC Genomics 2017;18:379.
87 Kim D, Bae S, Park J et al. Digenome-seq: genome-wide profiling of CRISPR-Cas9 off-target effects in human cells. Nat Methods 2015;12:237–43.
88 Frock RL, Hu J, Meyers RM et al. Genome-wide detection of DNA double-stranded breaks induced by engineered nucleases. Nat Biotechnol 2015;33:179–86.
89 Ran FA, Hsu PD, Lin CY et al. Double nicking by RNA-guided CRISPR Cas9 for enhanced genome editing specificity. Cell 2013;154: 1380–9.
90 Komor AC, Badran AH, Liu DR. Editing the genome without double-stranded DNA breaks. ACS Chem Biol 2018;13:383–8.
91 Gaudelli NM, Komor AC, Rees HA et al. Programmable base editing of A*T to G*C in genomic DNA without DNA cleavage. Nature 2017;551:464–71.
92 Komor AC, Kim YB, Packer MS et al. Programmable editing of a target base in genomic DNA without double-stranded DNA cleavage. Nature 2016;533:420–4.
93 Kim YB, Komor AC, Levy JM et al. Increasing the genome-targeting scope and precision of base editing with engineered Cas9-cytidine deaminase fusions. Nat Biotechnol 2017;35:371–6.
94 Liu J, Gaj T, Yang Y et al. Efficient delivery of nuclease proteins for genome editing in human stem cells and primary cells. Nat Protocols 2015;10:1842–59.

CHAPTER 171

Surgical Therapy

Julianne A. Mann[1] *& Jane S. Bellet*[2]

[1] Dartmouth-Hitchcock Medical Center, Lebanon, NH, USA
[2] Duke University Medical Center, Durham, NC, USA

Introduction, 2310
Indications for paediatric dermatological surgery, 2312
Timing of elective (prophylactic) excisions, 2313
Bandaging, 2313
Procedures, 2314
Surgical complications, 2317
Conclusion, 2318

Abstract

Performing dermatological procedures in children requires patience, excellent communication skills, a knowledge of child development and a solid foundation in executing dermatological procedures. Many minor procedures can be performed with the aid of distraction and, if needed, local anaesthesia may be employed. General anaesthesia should be reserved for situations when the age of the child, the anatomical location or the extent of the surgery makes local anaesthesia inappropriate. Common indications for procedures include verruca vulgaris, congenital and acquired melanocytic naevi, naevus sebaceus, pilomatricomas, pyogenic granuloma, infantile haemangioma and epidermal naevi. A detailed knowledge of anatomy and proper surgical technique allow for a superior result and are crucial for minimizing the likelihood of postoperative complications.

Key points

- Performing paediatric dermatological procedures requires patience, excellent communication skills, an understanding of child development and surgical competence.
- Most paediatric dermatological procedures can be done under local anaesthesia with strategic use of distraction.
- The timing of elective (prophylactic) excision should take into account the potential cosmetic and psychosocial benefit of early surgical intervention as well as the theoretical risks of general anaesthesia exposure early in life.

Introduction

To perform dermatological procedures in children, the practitioner must not only learn a specialized technical skill set, but must also develop a compassionate, gentle, and encouraging approach with patients and their families. A simple punch biopsy is often a straightforward and simple procedure to perform on an adult but for a young child, just the idea of a biopsy may provoke substantial anxiety. Earning a child's trust through clear and honest communication, age-appropriate explanation and patience is of the utmost importance. A thorough understanding of child development enables the physician to most effectively employ a tailored combination of distraction, humour and anaesthesia to ensure that each patient has a positive experience.

Communication

When discussing a dermatological procedure with a paediatric patient and their family, it is important to keep in mind the age and developmental stage of the child. The procedure should be described in full to both the child and the parents ahead of time. Toddlers can be provided with a simple, reassuring message such as 'We're going to make your boo-boo go away. Your mom and dad will be right there with you, and you will be asleep the whole time. When you wake up you can have a Popsicle and go home'. Preschoolers and young school-aged children should be provided with slightly more detail, telling the truth but taking care to avoid using any words that might be frightening to the child (e.g. 'sharp', 'cut', 'shot'). This age group often responds well to integration of magical thinking into the explanation, such as making an analogy to Sleeping Beauty when talking about general anaesthesia (personal communication, Annette Wagner). Older school-aged children and adolescents may want a more detailed description of the planned procedure, although words should still be chosen with care to avoid frightening the patient. Patients of all ages should be given the opportunity to ask any questions and voice any concerns so that their fears can be allayed. Parents should be advised that siblings should not be brought to the procedure, as there will not be childcare available for them.

Harper's Textbook of Pediatric Dermatology, Fourth Edition. Edited by Peter Hoeger, Veronica Kinsler and Albert Yan.

Anaesthesia and distraction techniques

In almost all cases, minor procedures, such as a punch or shave biopsy, can be performed under local anaesthesia in the office. Larger lesions requiring excision can often be removed under local anaesthesia in school-aged children; however, lesions in sensitive areas (face, genital area) may be better suited to excision under general anaesthesia.

If a procedure is performed under local anesthesia, creating a calming and reassuring environment is of the utmost importance for all ages. The surgical tray should be covered with a towel before the procedure so that instruments and bandage materials are concealed. Allowing the child to watch a movie while waiting for the procedure to begin is an excellent way to help put the child and parents at ease. Even an adolescent will benefit from the distraction provided by an entertaining movie.

A DVD player mounted on a rolling cart with a library of DVDs or a streaming media device for all ages of patients to choose from is very useful (Fig. 171.1). During the procedure, the player can be placed close to the child on the side opposite the procedure being performed, and the parent should be positioned at their child's head on that side. The parent should be seated (not standing) as occasionally even experienced parents can feel light-headed when watching a procedure being done on their own child. The volume should be turned up so as to mask procedure-related noises such as metal instruments clinking or talk between the surgeon and assistant. Alternatively, a parent's smartphone or tablet can be used to play an entertaining video, soothing music or simple game. For short procedures such as cryotherapy of a small wart, bubbles or light-up magic wands held by the parent or an assistant can be helpful to distract young children.

For children between the ages of 2–12 years, a grape-sized dollop of eutectic lidocaine such as LMX® 4% cream applied under an occlusive dressing such as Tegaderm® 1–2 hours before the procedure anaesthetizes the skin so that injection with a 30 gauge needle cannot be felt by most children. LMX 4% cream and Tegaderm are sold together over the counter as a kit which can be readily purchased without a prescription online or at many pharmacies. Some physicians have parents apply the topical lidocaine-based anaesthetic cream at home 1–2 hours before a procedure, and others prefer to have their staff apply it in the office. Parents should be counselled about the correct amount of medication to apply to minimize the (low) risk of lidocaine toxicity. The physician should prepare the child for the injection by counting to 3 and then inserting the needle. Counting with the child again from 1 to 10 while the lidocaine is being injected is helpful and gives the child a sense of how long any stinging sensation will last. Lidocaine can be buffered, which reduces the amount of stinging felt as the anaesthetic is injected.

A treasure box of small prizes and stickers that the child can choose from after the procedure is complete can help motivate the child to cooperate, and ensures that the visit ends on a positive note.

Immobilization

Infants and toddlers may need to be immobilized during the procedure to keep the child and surgical team safe, and to allow the procedure to be done as quickly as possible. Parents should be counselled about the reasons for the immobilization prior to the beginning of the procedure. Immobilization should be performed by the physician and their assistants (not the parent) so that the parent may focus on soothing and distracting the child. Preschoolers and school-aged children can usually hold still if excellent distraction is provided, and furthermore are typically too large and strong to immobilize.

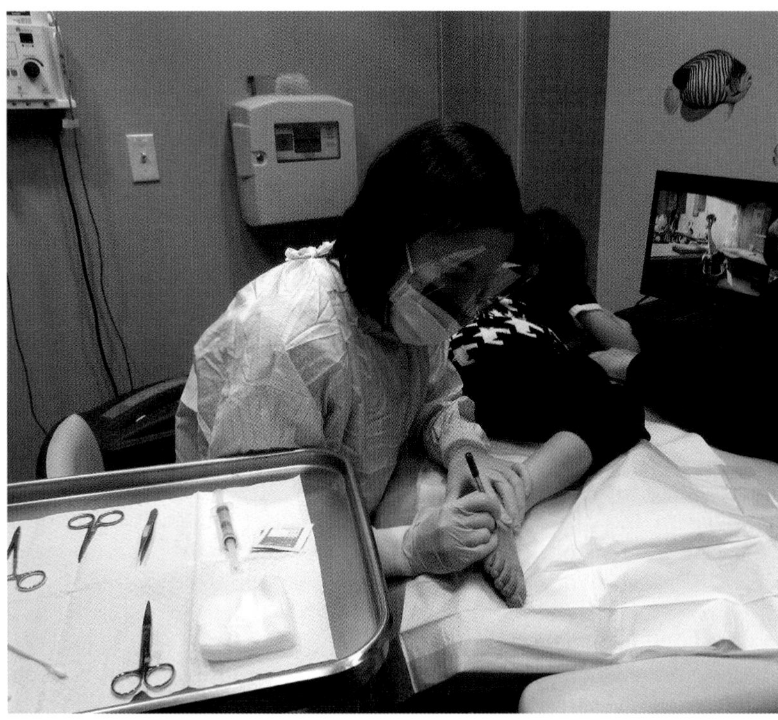

Fig. 171.1 DVD player and parent positioned close to the child's head, on the side opposite the procedure.

Indications for paediatric dermatological surgery

Verruca vulgaris

Verruca vulgaris (common warts) are commonly encountered by paediatric dermatologists, and can usually be effectively treated with cryotherapy or medical therapy. Shave removal with electrodesiccation can be considered for verrucae that are unresponsive to more conservative therapies or those that are in cosmetically distressing locations. Excision of verrucae is typically not advised given the fact that the vast majority of verruca vulgaris in children will spontaneously resolve within five years [1]. It is important to counsel parents that any surgical treatment of verrucae carries with it risks of scarring, while warts that resolve spontaneously or with medical therapy typically do so without scars.

Inflammatory or infectious skin conditions

A skin biopsy can be an invaluable tool if definitive diagnosis cannot be arrived at clinically. In most cases, a punch biopsy should be used as this allows sampling of the dermis and a portion of the subcutis. A punch biopsy of an induced blister is also critical in diagnosing epidermolysis bullosa.

Congenital melanocytic naevi

Indications for full-thickness excision of congenital naevi include the appearance of a rapidly growing papule or nodule within the naevus, a new area of ulceration, bleeding, pain or other significant change in appearance. These changes may signal the appearance of a melanoma within the naevus which, although rare in the paediatric population, can occur. The risk of developing melanoma within a congenital melanocytic neavus is proportional to its size, with large and giant congenital naevi having a higher risk [2]. Excisional biopsy removing the entire lesion is preferred but if this is not possible, the concerning area and at least a portion of the background naevus should be excised. This allows for more accurate pathological diagnosis than is possible with a smaller punch biopsy.

It is reasonable to excise small and medium-sized congenital naevi in cosmetically obvious areas if the child feels self-conscious or is being teased about the naevus. Some parents opt to have a congenital naevus removed early in childhood so the child does not have a lasting memory of the procedure, and so that the lesion is removed prior to the development of hypertrichosis and cobblestoning that can be socially distressing. Other parents prefer to delay potential excision until their child is old enough to make the decision about whether or not to proceed with removal as a young adult. Whenever possible, small and medium-sized congenital naevi should be removed in the office under local anaesthetic. Lesions occurring in areas of minimal tissue redundancy (scalp, face, lower legs, hands and feet) are most easily removed early in life when tissue elasticity is at its highest. Excision of large congenital naevi is typically performed by a plastic surgeon given that tissue expanders and multiple serial surgeries are usually necessary.

Acquired melanocytic naevi

Most melanocytic naevi in children are benign, but those with concerning features (including rapid growth, pain, bleeding, ulceration, change in shape or colour) should be biopsied. Biopsy technique depends upon the size of the naevus and the preference of the clinician and patient. Most small naevi can be effectively removed in full with a shave removal (also sometimes termed saucerization), so long as the clinician reaches the level of the deep dermis and includes a 1–2 mm margin of uninvolved skin at the periphery. A punch biopsy tool can be used to remove some melanocytic naevi (particularly those that have a more extensive dermal component), but to minimize the risk of recurrence the clinician should be sure to choose a trephine that is large enough to achieve a 1–2 mm margin of normal skin around the periphery of the naevus. Larger lesions or those that are very concerning for melanoma are generally better suited to traditional elliptical excision.

Removal of acquired naevi on the face solely for reasons of appearance should be approached with caution, particularly when the patient is school-aged or preadolescent. While some children do not like their facial naevi, this opinion often changes with age and maturity. It is difficult for most younger children to fully understand the inevitability of a permanent scar remaining after a naevus is removed. For these reasons, we recommend delaying cosmetic excision of benign facial naevi until late adolescence or early adulthood whenever possible.

It is worth noting that because many Spitz naevi have a substantial dermal component, we recommend excisional biopsy with intent to fully remove the lesion whenever possible. Some dermatologists feel that clinical observation is sufficient after a shave excision of a benign Spitz naevus is read as having positive margins, but it is generally recommended that any Spitz naevus with atypical histological features requires a complete excision with clear margins [3]. Initial excision minimizes the likelihood of a positive margin and thus the chances of a child having to undergo two separate procedures.

Naevus sebaceus

Some sebaceous naevi, particularly those on the face or the visible portions of the scalp, may cause psychosocial distress that prompts consideration of excision. This is particularly true at the onset of puberty, when many sebaceous naevi, develop a more raised, warty texture due to hormonal stimulation of sebaceous glands. Any new nodule appearing within a naevus sebaceus also merits excision, given the very low but potential risk of various types of carcinoma that can occur within these birthmarks. Basal cell carcinomas typically do not appear within sebaceous naevi until after puberty [4], so some families opt to have this birthmark removed prophylactically in infancy or childhood. Clinicians should be aware that statistically, a new nodule appearing within a naevus sebaceus is most likely to be a benign adnexal neoplasm, but as these are virtually impossible to distinguish from basal cell carcinomas clinically, biopsy is mandatory. Nearly one quarter of patients with untreated naevus sebaceus will develop adnexal tumours within them, typically in adulthood [4].

For elective excision of naevus sebaceus, the optimal timing of surgery remains somewhat controversial. Naevus sebaceus on the scalp that is wider than 1.5 cm in the newborn period typically requires staged excision if surgery is performed after 1 year of age (personal communication, Annette Wagner), whereas the greater scalp redundancy and elasticity may allow for a one-staged excision if performed at 6–12 months of age. Smaller sebaceous naevi may be excised under local anaesthesia later in childhood or adolescence, so long as the clinician's surgical suite is equipped to deal with the bleeding that often accompanies this procedure. Parents must be counselled about the inevitability of an alopecic scar after surgery, and the potential for significant scar spread on the scalp as the child grows.

Pilomatricoma (pilomatrixoma)

Pilomatricomas do not involute spontaneously, so the treatment of choice is surgical excision. These cysts typically continue to grow as long as they are present, and over time they may become inflamed and/or rupture. For these reasons, most paediatric dermatologists recommend excising pilomatricomas soon after they are diagnosed to minimize the length of the necessary scar, particularly if they are on the face. Cysts on the trunk and extremities can be monitored clinically if they are stable in size, so long as parents are informed about the risk of rupture and/or size increase.

Pyogenic granuloma (lobular capillary haemangioma)

Pyogenic granulomas typically grow rapidly and bleed frequently, making them bothersome and distressing to patients and their families. Most can be removed in the office with either a snip or shave removal, or punch excision followed by electrodesiccation. If punch or excisional biopsy is considered due to large size or location, it is important to treat any potential bacterial superinfection/colonization beforehand.

Infantile haemangioma

Propranolol therapy is highly effective for the treatment of proliferating infantile haemangiomas [5], with clinical response rates estimated to be as high as 98% [6]. As a result, only rarely now do these birthmarks need to be removed surgically in infancy. Untreated infantile haemangiomas (or those that were not treated until late infancy or toddlerhood) with a deep component may leave behind a fibrofatty residuum and/or scarring after involution that is cosmetically unacceptable.

When deciding upon the timing of excision of infantile haemangiomas, it is important to recognize that waiting until the haemangioma has fully involuted will allow for the smallest scar after excision. Although the traditional rule of thumb was that only 50% of haemangiomas were involuted by age 5 [7], newer analyses have suggested that most infantile haemangiomas do not improve substantially in appearance after 3.5 years of age [8]. Thus, if a haemangioma has left behind a large, exophytic, cosmetically obvious fibrofatty residuum, it is optimal from a psychosocial standpoint to excise it in the preschool years.

Epidermal naevus

Epidermal naevi in visible locations may pose cosmetic concerns, and surgical removal may be reasonable for small lesions. This can be performed as a simple elliptical excision in cases where the naevus is one contiguous plaque. For epidermal naevi that are composed of blaschkolinear arrangements of small papules, individual small papules can be anaesthetized and snipped. Electrodesiccation at the base of each snip removal reduces the likelihood of recurrence.

Timing of elective (prophylactic) excisions

For elective excisions, parents should be informed that wound healing and scar appearance are typically better the younger the age of the patient at the time of surgery. On the other hand, the potential risks of general anaesthesia must also be taken into account. Physicians should be aware that although general anaesthesia is considered to be very safe even in infants, particularly when performed by a paediatric anaesthesiologist [9–11], some studies suggest that anaesthesia exposure in the first 3–4 years of life, particularly if prolonged or repeated, may increase the risk of subsequent neurodevelopmental delay [12,13]. However, it is worth noting that studies which have looked at this issue are retrospective so cannot establish causation, and many are flawed by small sample sizes, insufficient power and poorly matched control groups [14]. Additionally, other authors point out that painful stimuli without anaesthesia and analgesia initiate a harmful stress response in young children which in and of itself can have deleterious effects on the developing brain [15]. Most excisional surgeries performed by a paediatric dermatologist are undertaken in one procedure, or at the most two, so the risk is extraordinarily low. A complete discussion of this issue is beyond the scope of this chapter, but it is prudent to review the current literature so as to be prepared for any questions that parents may pose.

Bandaging

Clear Tegaderm over a piece of gauze, or a combination of adhesive, Steri-Strips, and gauze, can be used for most surgical dressings on the face, trunk and extremities so that parents can visually monitor for the appearance of any bleeding, drainage and/or erythema (Fig. 171.2). For small excisions on the face, sometimes it may be appropriate to use just Steri-Strips or Vaseline®. Pressure dressings for scalp excisions are recommended (Fig. 171.3). Parents should be informed prior to the day of surgery that surgical dressings must be kept totally dry until they are removed 1–2 weeks later by the surgeon, so showers or baths must be avoided during this time. The exception is that on the scalp, the dressing is typically removed 48–72 hours after the surgery. Incisions on the scalp can then be washed once daily and petroleum jelly or antibiotic ointment applied.

Procedures

Cryosurgery

Cryosurgery is the use of liquid nitrogen to freeze and therefore destroy tissue. This method is useful in a number of dermatological conditions, including the treatment of verrucae (both common warts and flat warts). Some practitioners treat molluscum contagiosum as well as acrochordons with cryosurgery. Cryosurgery is best tolerated by older children, although children as young as 3 or 4 years are sometimes able to hold still. Treating lesions in which the diagnosis is in question with cryosurgery is not recommended because subsequent histological evaluation is not available.

Various application techniques can be employed: cotton-tipped applicator, forceps and spray. For young children, often the use of a cotton-tipped swab is the least threatening, and affords the highest likelihood that they will tolerate multiple applications. Although a swab is less frightening than a spray gun, some young children can still be frightened of the 'smoke' rising from a cup of liquid nitrogen. Allowing them to blow the smoke or holding their hand above the cup can be helpful prior to beginning the procedure. The applicator is first 'fluffed' by pulling the cotton. This allows the liquid nitrogen to penetrate the tip. The applicator is dipped into the cup and then applied to the lesion for 5–15 seconds, depending on its size. The applicator is then removed from the lesion [16]. Once the lesion has thawed, this is repeated. Usually several cycles of application at each visit (separated by 2–4-week intervals) are required for adequate treatment [17].

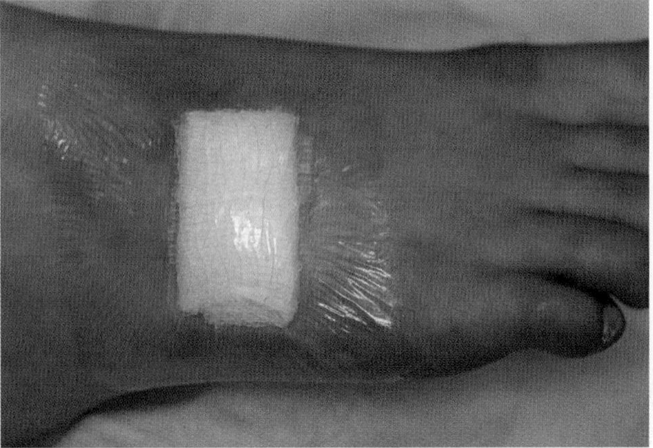

Fig. 171.2 Postoperative bandage consisting of Steri-Strips, gauze and Tegaderm.

The use of forceps is often useful for very small, pedunculated papules, especially on the face. Fine-tipped forceps such as Castro-Viejo or fine Adson forceps either with or without teeth are dipped in a cup of liquid nitrogen for 10 seconds, and then the base of the papule is grasped with the cold forceps. This is repeated multiple times, usually 3–15 (at 2–4-week intervals), depending on tissue response.

Spray cryotherapy is the most efficacious technique due to the amount of liquid nitrogen that can be applied, and can be used in older children and teenagers. Demonstrating the cold spray prior to treatment can allay any fears. Short pulses are applied until the lesion and the surrounding 1–2 mm of normal skin turns white. Thawing then takes place and the procedure is repeated. This is usually performed three times in succession. Parents and patients should be advised that the wart or other lesion may be a bit tender for 1–2 days and that a 'blood blister' or dark black haematoma may develop at the site of cryotherapy, especially for verrucae. This is normal and will

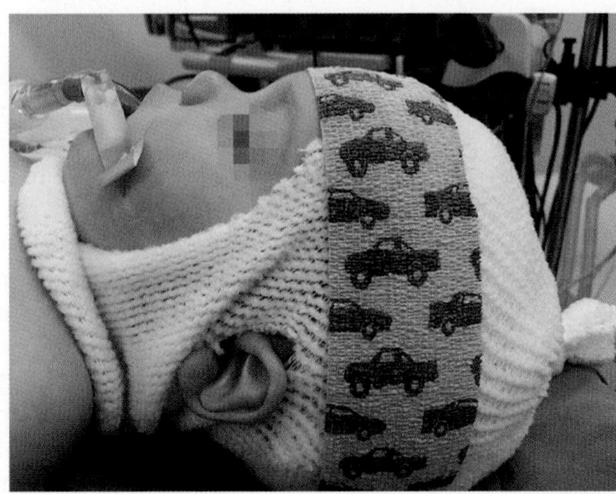

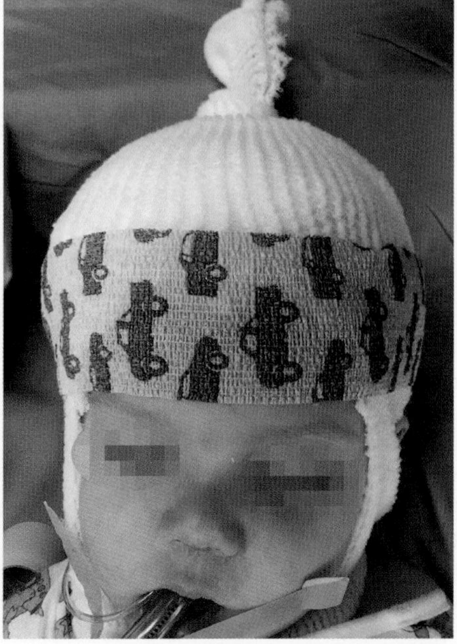

Fig. 171.3 Pressure dressing for the scalp consisting of petrolatum, a nonstick pad, rolled gauze, tubular net dressing and Coban® stretch wrap.

eventually resolve. Some verrucae will resolve with one treatment of cryosurgery, but most will require multiple visits. This can be frustrating to parents as well as physicians, which is why patience, as well as a combination approach, is often employed.

Biopsy (Box 171.1)

Skin biopsy can be very useful in determining a diagnosis, as the tissue can be examined microscopically, and may also be sent for culture (bacterial, viral, fungal or mycobacterial). In certain situations (when the lesion is <6 mm), the entire skin lesion can be removed for both diagnostic and therapeutic purposes. In other clinical scenarios (inflammatory or autoimmune skin conditions), the primary goal is to obtain tissue to enable a diagnosis. The depth of the lesion or process determines how deep the skin specimen needs to be. Usually, a punch biopsy is a good choice, since epidermis and dermis will be obtained, in addition to the top layer of fat in certain body locations. Attention to anatomy is critical, as even the smallest biopsy can cause significant problems if performed in inappropriate locations, such as over an open fontanelle on the scalp (risk of disruption of the meninges) or on the central nose (in the case of a potential nasal glioma). Congenital lesions on the midline are of particular concern for underlying dysraphism.

If a process involving the fat is suspected, a 'double punch' method may be employed, such that one specimen is first obtained and then through the same defect, a second, deeper specimen is also obtained [18]. This is often done with a larger-sized punch trephine first and then a smaller one through the defect, so that the hub does not become stuck on the epidermal rim of the initial defect. For example, a 6 mm trephine is used first, and then a 4 mmtrephine is utilized to obtain the second specimen. The specimens can be placed in separate formalin bottles. This method should only be used in areas of the body with ample subcutaneous fat, such as the abdomen, back or lateral aspects of the legs and arms. The dorsal hands and feet and the ankle do not have adequate subcutaneous tissue and the risk of nerve, vessel or tendon injury precludes this technique in those locations.

If the process appears to have multiple morphologies, it may be necessary to obtain specimens from each type of lesion seen. If a specimen is needed for tissue culture, it is of paramount importance that the tissue and instruments do not come in contact with formalin, as it will kill any organism, rendering the culture useless. Therefore, if specimens are needed for histology as well as culture, it is recommended that the culture specimen be obtained first, so that no inadvertent contamination occurs. The specimen should be placed in a sterile container on a piece of sterile gauze that has been soaked with nonbacteriostatic saline.

Once the specimen has been obtained, haemostasis is usually achieved with placement of sutures. In a neonate or young infant, often a 5-0 nonabsorbable suture such as nylon or polypropylene is used. Some providers use fast-absorbing chromic gut or poliglecaprone in a child so that suture removal is not required. For school-aged children and adolescents, 4-0 nonabsorbable suture is preferable to allow for adequate wound healing prior to removal. Some providers prefer to place Gelfoam; however, the time to place one or two sutures is usually negligible and may result in a smaller scar.

Shave biopsies can be useful for lesions that are not very deep, and only include the epidermis and superficial dermis. The resultant scar can be better than a full-thickness punch biopsy scar. There are certain pitfalls to shave biopsy, including a wider scar and subsequent longer scar if reexcision of the initial lesion is required. Exuberant granulation tissue is more likely to occur with a shave excision on the scalp, versus a punch biopsy.

Box 171.1 Skin punch biopsy

1. Choose the site. Take into consideration location, mobility of child, ability to hide resultant scar. Skin overlying the fontanelles should not be biopsied in a neonate or young infant without neurosurgical guidance, due to risk of disruption of the meninges. A punch biopsy on the dorsal hand or foot should not be performed in a child who will be difficult to restrain, due to the risk of damage to tendons in this area.
2. Immobilize the child.
3. Inject local anaesthetic.
4. Rotate the punch trephine firmly into the skin. Pay attention to depth, so that the specimen will be deep enough but not too deep. Only rarely is it necessary to use the full depth of the punch trephine in a child.
5. Pick up the base of the sample gently with forceps and cut the bottom attachment with sharp iris scissors.
6. Place the specimen in formalin for histology or in a urine cup with saline-soaked gauze for cultures or direct immunofluorescence. If splitting the specimen for both histology and culture, prepare the specimen for culture first to avoid exposing that specimen to formalin.
7. Place sutures for haemostasis. 5-0 Nonabsorbable suture is usually adequate; 4-0 can be used in older children.
8. Apply petroleum jelly or antibiotic ointment.
9. Place bandage.

Snip excision

Snip excision is useful for small, pedunculated papules such as pyogenic granulomas, acrochordons or epidermal naevi. Often, the resultant scar is much smaller than the lesion itself. After administration of local anaesthetic with epinephrine, waiting for at least 10 minutes to allow for adequate vasoconstriction is very useful. This enables haemostasis to be achieved much more swiftly than if the procedure is immediately performed after anaesthetic injection. Then, this author (JB) grasps the papule with fine forceps and snips the base of the papule using hypercurved scissors. Other scissors such as iris scissors can also be used. Haemostasis with electrocautery or aluminium chloride is usually all that is required before application of a bandage. This author (JAM) rolls a cotton swab soaked in aluminium chloride over acrochordons prior to snip excision, which often completely prevents any bleeding.

Elliptical excision

Elliptical excision is the most commonly used method to remove skin lesions. In this technique, local anaesthesia is administered (even if the patient is under general anaesthesia, as this allows for vasoconstriction and ensures that the patient does not feel any discomfort when they awaken). The lesion is measured and a margin of normal skin measured around it, depending on the diagnosis. For example, a 2 mm margin is frequently used for melanocytic naevi, and 4 mm for basal cell carcinoma or more concerning naevi. An ellipse following relaxed skin tension lines is then drawn on the skin using a marking pen and dotted lines. Traditionally, elliptical excisions are designed with a 3:1 length to width ratio; however, in children frequently the ratio only needs to be 2–2.5:1, secondary to greater skin elasticity. This results in a much smaller scar for the patient. In addition, the angle of the tips of the ellipse has traditionally been 30° but a much more acute angle often gives a better result [19,20]. Some physicians prefer to prepare the skin prior to marking the ellipse and others prefer to do it afterwards. A number of commercially available products are used, including some combination of chlorhexidine, betadine and isopropyl alcohol, which serve to decrease the bacterial load on the skin. There is some controversy as to whether elliptical excisions need to be done under sterile conditions or not [21,22].

Using a scalpel, often a 15 or 15c blade, the skin is incised to the subcutaneous fat, taking care to remember anatomy and take into account the thickness of the epidermis and dermis. In young infants, the top two layers of skin are very thin. On the scalp, the incision should be taken all the way down to the galea, so as to have a bloodless plane in which to work. The ellipse is then removed either using tenotomy scissors or with a scalpel, making sure to remain at the same depth and therefore in the same plane. The specimen should be placed in an appropriately labelled container of formalin and sent for histopathological evaluation.

The wound edges are everted with fine forceps or skin hooks grasping the dermis preferentially, so that wound healing is not impeded and permanent scars do not result from pinch marks on the epidermis. The edges are then undermined. We solely use tenotomy scissors for this purpose, first placing them into the subcutaneous fat perpendicular to the skin and opening the jaws of the scissors to stretch the tissue, and then reinserting them parallel and again spreading the tissue. There is less bleeding using this technique. Once the entire wound has been undermined, meticulous haemostasis with electrocautery should be obtained. This is usually done by having an assistant hold two skin hooks and lift the undermined edges to see if there are any active areas of bleeding, which are then cauterized. This author (JB) prefers using a needle tip for the cautery pencil as this allows for very accurate cauterization without destruction of adjacent tissue.

Once haemostasis is achieved, deep dissolvable sutures are placed to approximate the subcutaneous tissue. In most situations, only one deep layer of sutures is required, but sometimes two are required in wounds or areas of high tension, including the scalp, in which placing sutures through the galea can be helpful to approximate the defect. Different techniques are used to close the ellipse: by halves, from one end to the other, or setting the tips first and then moving from one end to the other. By setting the tips first, usually a dog ear will not need to be removed, even if one is present, as it can be 'sewn out' towards the centre of the wound using this method.

For approximation of the epidermis in wounds on the trunk and extremities, a subcuticular suture often results in a nice scar that does not have 'train tracks'. For the face, simple interrupted sutures are used to achieve precise epidermal approximation. Frequently, a nonabsorbable suture such as nylon or polypropylene is used, with size based on the body site. Some physicians use absorbable sutures such as poliglecaprone 25, so that the sutures do not need to be removed and a second suture packet does not need to be used. For the scalp, a running suture is often used. For the face and ears, interrupted sutures are typically preferred as they allow for more precise approximation of wound edges. For perfectly round lesions, such as residual fibrofatty tissue of a haemangioma, excising the lesion and placing a purse-string suture closure allows for a much smaller final scar than if the round lesion is excised using an elliptical shape. The initial scar can appear puckered but with time, this will usually settle and if necessary, a small revision can be done later to linearize the scar, if desired. In cases where the direction of relaxed skin tension lines is not clear, excising the lesion first and then assessing tissue mobility can be useful in determining which way to orient the closure.

Nail biopsy

A punch biopsy of the nail matrix or bed can be done to obtain tissue for histopathological evaluation. In the paediatric population, this technique is often used for longitudinal melanonychia (melanonychia striata). This can be done with or without nail avulsion. For most melanocytic nail lesions, a nail matrix biopsy is the technique of choice, which requires only partial nail avulsion. Sometimes it is preferable to submit the nail plate for histopathological evaluation, in which case a punch biopsy directly through nail plate to matrix or bed is performed. Otherwise, once a full or partial nail avulsion is done, adequate visualization of the area in question must be ascertained.

In order to visualize the matrix, reflecting incisions at the junction of the proximal and lateral nailfolds are often required bilaterally. These incisions run from the lateral proximal nailfold more proximolaterally on a diagonal (Fig. 171.4). The proximal nailfold is then gently loosened with a 15-blade scalpel or iris scissors and then skin hooks can be used to reflect the proximal nailfold and visualize the matrix. A 3 mm punch trephine is recommended for a punch biopsy of the matrix or bed. Closure of this small defect is usually not required, especially when the site is more distal. If reflecting incisions were placed, then the skin flaps should be returned to anatomical position and each side sutured using either 5-0 polypropylene or 5-0 fast-absorbing 910 polyglactin suture. Absorbable suture

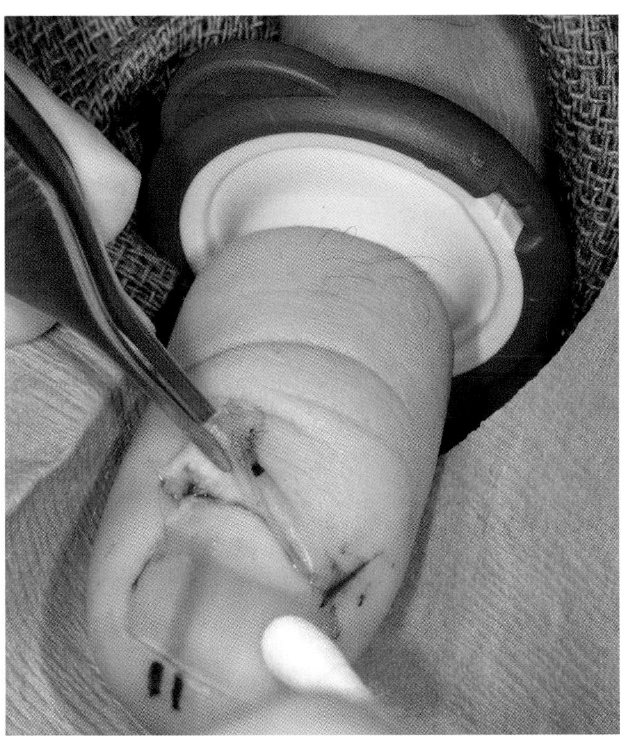

Fig. 171.4 T-ring tourniquet in place during nail matrix biopsy. Relaxing incisions placed at the junction of the proximal and lateral nailfolds in order to visualize the nail matrix.

is usually preferable as the patient does not need to return for suture removal. A larger size of trephine runs the risk of causing permanent dystrophy, especially if taken from the proximal matrix without careful approximation of the edges. If the lesion is larger than 3 mm, a different biopsy technique should be used.

Matrix shave

For lesions larger than 3 mm, the matrix shave is often a good option, as the nail matrix can be very superficially excised using the nail matrix shave technique as described by Haneke [23]. The matrix is exposed using the technique outlined above. The matrix is scored using a Teflon-coated 15-blade scalpel and then the specimen is cut at the base using the scalpel in a parallel fashion to the specimen, while gentle pressure is applied with a cotton-tipped applicator. The specimen is then oriented either directly on a nail diagram and/or inked and placed in a pathology cassette so that the orientation is preserved. A matrix shave does not require suture placement. The specimen is so superficial that there is not usually resultant dystrophy, particularly if the location is in the distal matrix.

Surgical complications

Intraoperative complications

Bleeding

Intraoperative bleeding can make visualization of the surgical site difficult, and can lengthen the duration of the surgery. The use of lidocaine with epinephrine can minimize oozing intraoperatively. A detailed knowledge of anatomy is crucial. In certain anatomical locations such as the lip, dorsal hands and feet, and shin, care should be taken to identify (and if possible avoid) large vessels, so as to avoid inadvertent transection of these arteries. It is critical to control any bleeding prior to closure to minimize the likelihood of haematoma formation. Small vessels can be cauterized while larger vessels (particularly those on the scalp) may need to be ligated; a figure-of-eight suture placed around the bleeding vessel is often effective.

Nerve damage

Parents should be counselled about the potential for damage to underlying structures during a surgical procedure. Although sensory nerves are inevitably transected during surgery, very few children will have notable sensory deficits postoperatively. Damage to motor nerves is of greater concern. To minimize this risk, the surgeon must have a detailed knowledge of the location of critical anatomical structures, particularly those in higher risk areas. Motor nerve injury is most likely to occur in certain well-defined 'danger zones,' including [24]:

- the zygomatic arch and temple (temporal branch of the facial nerve)
- the mid-mandible, near the facial artery (mandibular branch of the facial nerve)
- Erb's point in the posterior triangle of the neck (spinal accessory nerve).

Postoperative complications

The risk of postoperative wound infection can be minimized by applying a sterile surgical dressing that remains in place until sutures are removed. This avoids the possibility of the child touching the surgical incision during the first week or two of healing. The exception to this is that on the scalp, pressure dressings should be removed at 48–72 hours after surgery and the incision can be gently washed daily and Vaseline or antibiotic ointment applied.

Postoperative bleeding most often occurs on the scalp, and can be minimized by the application of a bulky pressure dressing that is left in place for 48 hours after the surgery.

Meticulous attention to haemostasis during surgical excisions can minimize the risk of haematoma formation postoperatively. Small haematomas can be left in place to absorb, while those larger than a golf ball are unlikely to self-resolve and should be surgically evacuated.

Wound dehiscence is of particular concern for toddlers and young children, for whom four weeks of postoperative activity restrictions is often difficult (Box 171.2). Performing elective surgeries during the winter months makes following these guidelines easier for most families.

Box 171.2 Postoperative activity restrictions following excision

- After the surgery is complete, the patient should be instructed to return home and rest quietly.
- No school for 1–2 days following the day of surgery.
- No sports or physical education for 2–4 weeks.
- No sleeping overnight at friends' houses for 2–4 weeks.
- No bathing until sutures or Steri-Strips are removed.

We recommend that all patients return to the dermatologist's office for suture removal so that the wound can be assessed for any potential signs of infection.

Unsatisfactory scarring

The possibility of track marks can be minimized by using running subcuticular stitches on the trunk and extremities. On the face, interrupted sutures should be removed 5–7 days postoperatively, as leaving them in longer than this increases the likelihood of residual marks.

Should hypertrophic or keloidal scarring occur, silicone gel sheeting, topical steroids or intralesional steroid injections can be helpful. Surgical scar revision may be considered if more conservative options fail.

Contact dermatitis

The most common cause of postoperative contact dermatitis is an irritant dermatitis reaction to the dressing adhesive. Less often, a true allergic contact dermatitis may occur to chlorhexidine, Mastisol®, tincture of benzoin or betadine. Allergic contact dermatitis must also be distinguished from postoperative infection.

Conclusion

With proper surgical training and knowledge, as well as good communication and patience, dermatological procedures can be safely performed in infants, children and adolescents. Thorough and compassionate communication before and during procedures is critical not only for creating a positive patient experience but also for optimizing surgical outcomes. An understanding of surgical indications, distraction and anaesthesia strategies and surgical techniques is essential. Excellent results can be achieved when all these components are in place.

Acknowledgement

Many thanks to Dr Annette Wagner, our mutual mentor, colleague and friend.

References

1 Williams HC, Pottier A, Strachan D. The descriptive epidemiology of warts in British schoolchildren. Br J Dermatol 1993;128(5):504–11.
2 Krengel S, Hauschild A, Schafer T. Melanoma risk in congenital melanocytic naevi: a systematic review. Br J Dermatol 2006;155(1):1–8.
3 Massi D, Tomasini C, Senetta R et al. Atypical Spitz tumors in patients younger than 18 years. J Am Acad Dermatol 2015;72(1):37–46.
4 Idriss MH, Elston DM. Secondary neoplasms associated with nevus sebaceus of Jadassohn: a study of 707 cases. J Am Acad Dermatol 2014;70(2):332–7.
5 Leaute-Labreze C, Hoeger P, Mazereeuw-Hautier J et al. A randomized, controlled trial of oral propranolol in infantile hemangioma. N Engl J Med 2015 372(8):735–46.
6 Marqueling AL, Oza V, Frieden IJ, Puttgen KB. Propranolol and infantile hemangiomas four years later: a systematic review. Pediatr Dermatol 2013;30(2):182–91.
7 Bowers RE, Graham EA, Tomlinson KM. The natural history of the strawberry nevus. Arch Dermatol 1960;82:667–80.
8 Couto RA, Maclellan RA, Zurakowski D, Greene AK. Infantile hemangioma: clinical assessment of the involuting phase and implications for management. Plast Reconstr Surg 2012;130(3):619–24.
9 Keenan RL, Shapiro JH, Dawson K. Frequency of anesthetic cardiac arrests in infants: effect of pediatric anesthesiologists. J Clin Anesth 1991;3(6):433–7.
10 Juern AM, Cassidy LD, Lyon VB. More evidence confirming the safety of general anesthesia in pediatric dermatologic surgery. Pediatr Dermatol 2010;27(4):355–60.
11 Cunningham BB, Gigler V, Wang K et al. General anesthesia for pediatric dermatologic procedures: risks and complications. Arch Dermatol 2005;141(5):573–6.
12 Lin EP, Soriano SG, Loepke AW. Anesthetic neurotoxicity. Anesthesiol Clin 2014;32(1):133–55.
13 Wang X, Xu Z, Miao CH. Current clinical evidence on the effect of general anesthesia on neurodevelopment in children: an updated systematic review with meta-regression. PLoS One 2014;9(1):e85760.
14 Crosby G, Davis PJ. General anesthesia in infancy is associated with learning disabilities – or not. Anesth Analg 2013;117(6):1270–2.
15 Ward CG, Loepke AW. Anesthetics and sedatives: toxic or protective for the developing brain? Pharmacol Res 2012;65(3):271–4.
16 Ahmed I, Agarwal S, Ilchyshyn A et al. Liquid nitrogen cryotherapy of common warts: cryo-spray vs. cotton wool bud. Br J Dermatol 2001;144(5):1006–9.
17 Bourke JF, Berth-Jones J, Hutchinson PE. Cryotherapy of common viral warts at intervals of 1, 2 and 3 weeks. Br J Dermatol 1995;132(3): 433–6.
18 Ha CT, Nousari HC. Surgical pearl: double-trephine punch biopsy technique for sampling subcutaneous tissue. J Am Acad Dermatol 2003;48(4):609–10.
19 Klapper M. The 30-degree angle revisited. J Am Acad Dermatol 2005;53(5):831–2.
20 Moody BR, McCarthy JE, Sengelmann RD. The apical angle: a mathematical analysis of the ellipse. Dermatol Surg 2001;27(1):61–3.
21 Nuzzi LC, Greene AK, Meara JG et al. Surgical site infection after skin excisions in children: is field sterility sufficient? Pediatr Dermatol 2016;33:136–41.
22 Heal C, Sriharan S, Buttner PG, Kimber D. Comparing non-sterile to sterile gloves for minor surgery: a prospective randomised controlled non-inferiority trial. Med J Aust 2015;202(1):27–31.
23 Haneke E, Baran R. Longitudinal melanonychia. Dermatol Surg 2001; 27(6):580–4.
24 Brown SM, Oliphant T, Langtry J. Motor nerves of the head and neck that are susceptible to damage during dermatological surgery. Clin Exp Dermatol 2014;39(6):677–2; quiz 681–2.

CHAPTER 172
Laser Therapy

Samira Batul Syed[1], Maria Gnarra[1] & Sean Lanigan[2]

[1] Great Ormond Street Hospital for Children NHS Trust, London, UK
[2] sk:n Limited, Birmingham, UK

Laser treatment of vascular lesions, 2319
Laser treatment of pigmented lesions, 2325
Ablative lasers, 2326
Hair removal by lasers, 2327

Abstract

The pulsed dye laser has revolutionized the treatment of vascular anomalies. More recently, the multiplex laser, a combination of pulsed dye and Nd:YAG, has been shown to be beneficial for recalcitrant port wine stains and other conditions. In addition to their use in treating port wine stains, lasers have also an important role in treating a number of childhood pigmentary disorders. These are primarily congenital naevi such as café-au-lait macules, naevus of Ito and some blue lesions.

Laser treatment is based on selective thermal destruction or damage to a targeted chromophore located in the skin, either that of blood, melanin or tissue water. Lasers have been shown to successfully treat vascular and pigmented lesions and also remove unwanted hair. They can also be used to remove verrucous lesions such as angiofibromas and epidermal naevi through vaporization.

Key points

- The pulsed dye laser is the treatment of choice for port wine stains.
- β-Blockers are the first-line treatment for complicated infantile haemangiomas; however, in certain circumstances, laser treatment is still indicated, especially for postregression telangiectasia.
- A variety of cutaneous pigmented lesions respond to laser treatment; most research is with high-energy short-pulsed (nanos) Q-switched lasers.
- Melanocytic naevi respond unpredictably to lasers, with risks of scarring and repigmentation.
- Long-term hair removal is possible with lasers even in pigmented skin.

Laser treatment of vascular lesions (S.B. Syed and M. Gnarra)

Introduction

At Great Ormond Street Hospital (GOSH), there is a designated Laser Unit for children which was established in 1994. Around 600 new patients are referred annually and to date 25 000 laser procedures have been performed. Children less than 5 years of age have procedures under general anaesthesia and older children are offered local anaesthesia, depending on the site and type of vascular lesion. All patients have pre- and postlaser review, either as an outpatient attendance or a telephone/email consultation whereby families have an opportunity to send photos to us for assessment and for comparison to pretreatment photos, prior to offering further treatment.

Laser treatment for all vascular birthmarks is best performed at an early age so that most, if not all, the treatment is completed before the child starts school. This may not always be possible but there is a clear advantage in terms of minimizing the potential psychological problems and also, the issue that younger children tend to be more compliant with the procedure [1,2].

Lasers treat vascular lesions via a process known as selective photothermolysis [3,4]. Laser light at different wavelengths will penetrate the skin with preferential absorption depending on the chromophore present, for example, oxyhaemoglobin of red blood cells within dilated superficial blood vessels or melanin within brown lesions. Different vascular pulsed-dye lasers (PDL) have varying parameters of wavelength, fluency and pulse width (Table 172.1). The laser spot size (diameter) is also relevant – newer lasers have a larger spot size (10–15 mm), enabling them to cover a larger area of skin [5,6]. In order to prevent any risk of damage to the surrounding skin caused by increased thermal exposure and heat dissipation, lasers also have an attached cooling device, some providing a targeted cryogenic spray to freeze the uppermost part of the skin a fraction of a second before the laser beam is delivered, others blowing cool air across the treatment site during and after the laser pulse. In some cases, an ice-cool gel is applied as a thin layer over the treatment zone prior to laser delivery.

Anaesthetic considerations

The decision to plan further treatment under general or topical anaesthetic depends on the site and size of the area to be treated as well as the patient's age and developmental ability to understand and cope with the procedure. In general, facial lesions on younger children will need a

Harper's Textbook of Pediatric Dermatology, Fourth Edition. Edited by Peter Hoeger, Veronica Kinsler and Albert Yan.

Table 172.1 Laser parameters for vascular lesions

	SPTL 1b	Scleroplus 1d	V beam	Perfecta V beam	Cynergy		
					PDL	Nd:YAG	Multiplex
WL (nm)	585	585–600	595	595	595	1064	595/1064
PW (msec)	0.45	1.5	0.45–40	0.45–40	0.5–40	0.5–300	0.5–40/0.5–300
Fluency (J/cm²)	3–10	3–15 (HP)	3–15 (30)	3–20 (40)	4–20	15–450	44–20/15–450
4Probes (mm²)	2,3,5,7	5,7,10,7 × 2	5,7,10,10 × 3	5,7,10,12,10 × 3	5,7,10,12	3,5,7,10,12,15	7,10
DCD	+/–	+	+	+		CRYO 6 Air cool system	

DCD, dynamic cooling device; HP, high power; Nd:YAG, neodymium:yttrium aluminium garnet; PDL, pulsed-dye laser; PW, pulse width; WL, wavelength.

general anaesthetic. Smaller lesions on the body in older children may be suitable for topical anaesthetic treatment: either EMLA® (Eutectic Mixture of Local Anaesthetics: 2.5% lignocaine and 2.5% prilocaine in an oil-in-water emulsion), which causes vasoconstriction, or Ametop® (3% amethocaine gel), which causes vasodilation and is therefore preferred for the treatment of vascular lesions, especially port wine stains [7,8].

Initial skin laser test

There are six different skin types. Each skin type responds differently to the laser and therefore it is important to do an initial skin laser test. An area of normal skin is selected either next to the birthmark or on the anterior aspect of the forearm. Topical anaesthesia is applied to this area of normal skin and to a small area on the vascular lesion 45 minutes beforehand. Two or three low laser fluence (energy) shots are fired at the area of normal skin and any skin reaction noted, in particular any purpura (Fig. 172.1). The fluence producing the earliest pupuric response is noted and multiplied by two to give an indication of the fluence needed for the test treatment of the vascular lesion. The small selected area on the vascular lesion is then treated (Fig. 172.2).

The timing of the skin laser test varies according to the protocol of the individual centre, either after the first birthday or, specifically at GOSH, after the second or third birthday. The child is then reviewed 2–3 months later. At this visit, the test sites are reviewed and there should be a full discussion with the parents on whether or not laser treatment is likely to be helpful, the risks, benefits and limitations of treatment, and to plan the timing of the first and subsequent treatment sessions.

Very small lesions (up to 10 dots in total needed) in older children do not require an initial laser test procedure and are directly treated, under local anaesthesia, although it is good practice to treat a small area of normal skin beforehand to ascertain the starting treatment fluence.

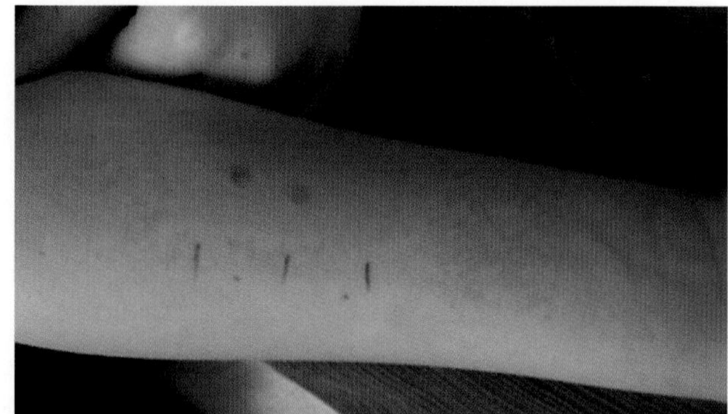

Fig. 172.1 Three laser shots to normal skin at low laser fluence of 3, 3.25 and 3.5 J/cm² and within a few seconds a purpuric response is noted at 3.25 and 3.5 J/cm².

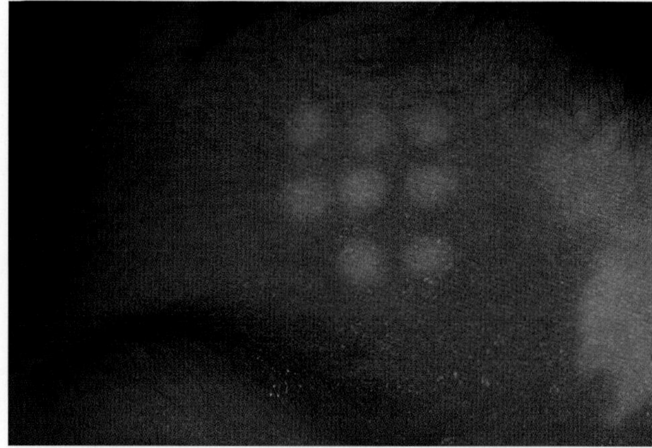

Fig. 172.2 Laser test treatment: a small test area is treated using local anaesthetic cream. This boy responded well to eight laser dots, at the lower end of the energy range. This picture was taken eight weeks after the test was performed.

Laser treatment

Once the laser test sites are assessed, if the decision is made to go ahead with treatment the family are given general advice, particularly regarding the before- and aftercare (see Chapter 177) and the commitment they will have to make if the child is to have repeated laser treatments. For children receiving treatment under general anaesthesia, a preoperative assessment is necessary prior to the operation. The treatments are at 4–6-monthly intervals and the child should be reviewed in the clinic before each treatment, so that the parents have an opportunity to discuss the results and any issues that might have arisen.

Treatment of periorbital lesions

Any lesion involving periorbital skin will require the insertion of an eye shield prior to the procedure, usually under general anaesthesia. In adolescents and adults, the eye shield can be inserted during a local anaesthesia procedure, using anaesthetic eye drops beforehand.

Further information
This can be found on the following website: www.gosh.nhs.uk/medical-information-0/procedures-and-treatments/laser-treatment-birthmarks

Adverse effects
Pulsed-dye lasers are a safe and effective treatment for vascular lesions of the skin. Adverse effects are minimal but include posttreatment swelling, postinflammatory hyper/hypopigmentation, immediate postlaser purpura (subsides within 5–10 days), occasional blistering and crusting and rarely scarring. Some lasers do not produce much bruising with a lower laser fluence and so care needs to be taken postoperatively.

Risks of general anaesthesia in infants and young children
Concern has been raised about the possible risks to neurocognitive development after general anaesthesia in young children, but studies of brief, single exposures for a relatively minor procedure are reassuring. Nevertheless, caution should be exercised with regard to treatment under general anaesthesia until further long-term evidence is available [9,10].

Capillary malformations (port wine stains)

A port wine stain is a capillary vascular malformation of developmental origin characterized pathologically by ectasia of superficial dermal capillaries and clinically by permanent macular erythema [11]. Port wine stains (PWS) affect three in 1000 newborns [12,13] and often present as part of congenital syndromes such as Sturge–Weber syndrome, Klippel–Trenaunay syndrome and limb overgrowth syndromes.

The PDL has revolutionized the treatment of PWS. Favourable factors for a good response to treatment include younger age, PWS of a pink/red colour (compared to dark purple) and certain anatomical sites [14]. PWS in the lateral facial region, forehead and neck respond better than those in the centrofacial region. In our experience, the least responsive PWS are those on the centre of the cheek. Published literature shows that PWS on the lower limbs respond least to treatment [15]. Due to their nature, PWS may recur after treatment.

The timing of laser treatment depends on the age at presentation to the specialist.

A recent survey demonstrated variation in consensus and practice across the UK with regard to the timing of PDL treatment of paediatric PWS [16]. Laser treatment is effective at any age but there are substantial benefits to early treatment, including better clearance, reduction in the risk of papules in adolescence and reduced thickening of the PWS. For this reason, the Birthmark Centre at GOSH is in favour of earlier referrals for assessment. This is also important if there is the possibility of any associated medical conditions such as Sturge–Weber syndrome and glaucoma, overgrowth or any other related problem essential to identify as early as possible. Another advantage of earlier referrals is the ability to recognize associated comorbidities, and to establish a multidisciplinary team approach to management.

Great Ormond Street Hospital receives more than 600 referrals for laser treatment annually. Of these, the vast majority are children with PWS. The results of laser treatment are assessed using a combination of standardized photography, a colour chart and dermospectrophotometry and recently we have used dermoscopy (subjective) and siascopy (objective). Seventy percent of children treated with the SPTL1b PDL (585 nm; 0.45 msec) showed an overall mean improvement of 70% lightening in colour compared to adjacent nonaffected skin, of which 43% showed more than 90% improvement, with some showing even near complete clearance (Fig. 172.3). Patients had between one and six treatments over a two-year period. Most then had a 2–4-year break, after which they were reassessed, looking for any recurrence of the PWS. In our experience, 10% of children showed some evidence of recurrence at the two-year follow-up [17].

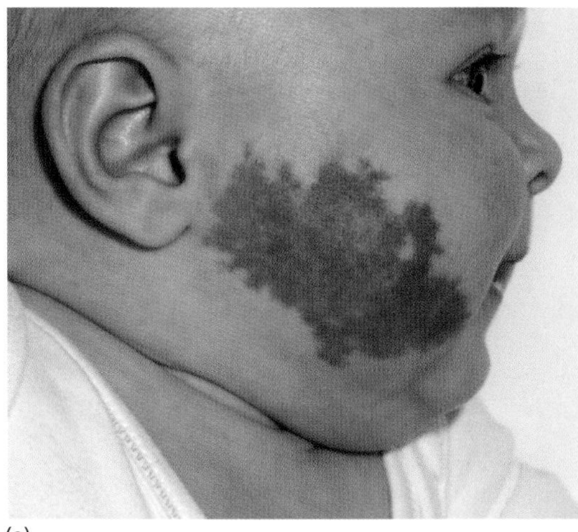
(a)

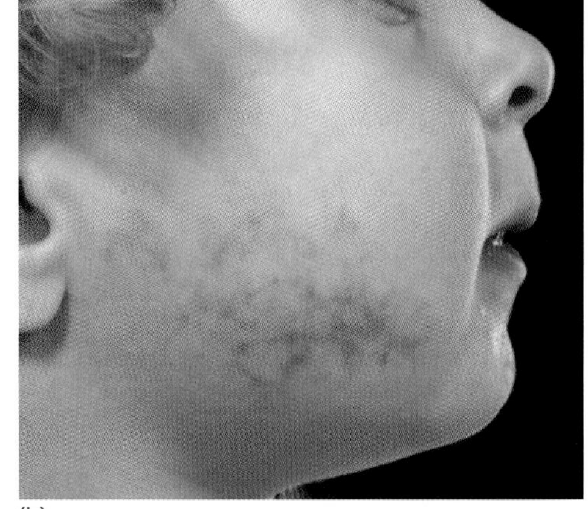
(b)

Fig. 172.3 PWS before (a) and after (b) laser treatment.

Our current practice is using the Perfecta V beam laser (595 nm; 1.5–40 msec). This has proven to be far superior to its predecessor, producing a 20–40% further improvement for recurrent and less responsive PWS. Our results indicate that a pulse width between 1.5 and 6 msec produces the optimum outcome [18]. The children are able to tolerate higher fluences with increased epidermal cooling.

Combination of PDL and medical therapy

Of recent interest is the successful use of combined PDL with topical rapamycin 0.5% ointment for the treatment of PWS, either as an isolated PWS or as part of the Sturge–Weber syndrome [19,20]. Another recent study reported no difference with PDL alone; however, the rapamycin used was only 0.1% [21].

Infantile haemangiomas

Infantile haemangiomas (IH) are common benign vascular tumours, affecting one in 10 children, and characterized by a spontaneous clinical involution within the first decade of life. The vast majority of IH do not require treatment. Most haemangiomas are not evident at birth but appear within the first few weeks of life and then increase in size over 3–6 months. First-line treatment for complicated IH is with nonselective β-blockers, such as propranolol (oral) [22] or timolol (topical), and very occasionally with additional steroids. β-Blocker therapy has been shown to be more effective than laser treatment as a first-line treatment [23]. However, in certain circumstances, laser treatment is still indicated, especially for postregression telangiectasia. The PDL results are usually excellent and treatment should be considered at any age but ideally from 5 to 10 years old.

Ulcerated haemangiomas

Ulceration is one of the most common complications of haemangiomas. In ulceration resistant to medical therapy, PDL treatment can be indicated. Risk factors for ulceration include rapid growth of the lesion causing localized areas of infarction, trauma, especially from scratching, and contact with irritant body fluids, especially with perioral and genital lesions.

Initial conservative treatment is daily nursing care which can usually be done by the parents and involves bathing the area with an antiseptic or astringent solution and a nonadhesive dressing covered with a dry dressing. At GOSH, we currently use Dermol 600® emollient to wash the area of ulceration, Mepitel®, Sorbisan® and gauze pads held in place with Mepitac® tape or a tubular bandage, depending on the site. In addition to the change of dressings, it is essential to ensure that the child has adequate analgesia. This conservative management would usually last for four weeks until further review.

Ulcerated haemangiomas also frequently become secondarily infected. In a retrospective study carried out at GOSH (2000–2006), the most common organisms cultured from ulcerated haemangiomas were *Pseudomonas* (30%) and *Staphylococcus aureus* (19%) (Fig. 172.4). Treatment of these organisms with the use of appropriate antibiotics helps heal the ulceration quicker.

Most ulcerations heal with conservative treatment and, if necessary, concomitant β-blocker therapy. However, a few may fail to heal and can be considered for laser therapy. In our experience, PDL is also an effective treatment in promoting the healing of these ulcers and reducing pain [24]. To maximize this effect, posttreatment nursing care is paramount.

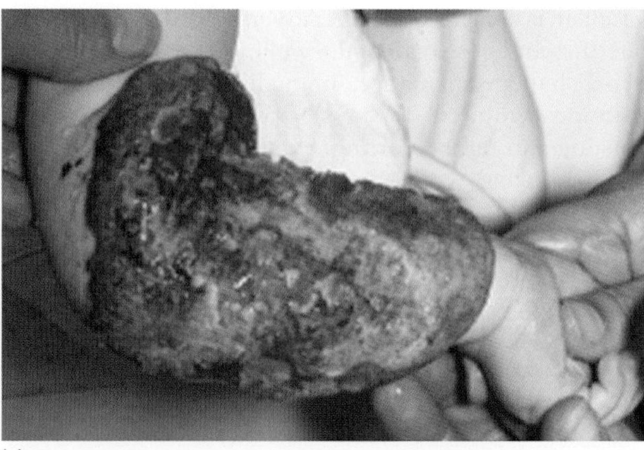

(a)

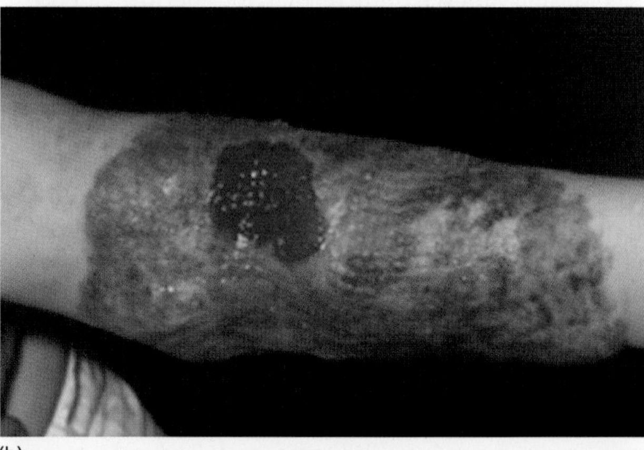

(b)

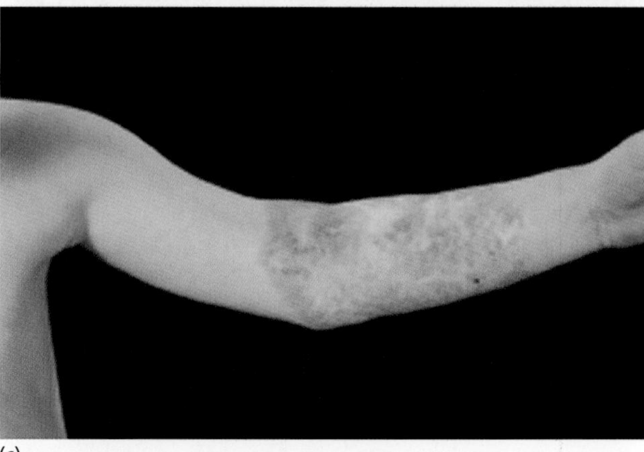

(c)

Fig. 172.4 (a) Large ulcerated haemangioma on the forearm that had failed to heal after several weeks of conservative treatment, including appropriate antibiotics and dressings (before treatment). (b) Same patient four weeks after laser treatment. (c) Same patient 18 months after laser treatment.

Telangiectasia

These are superficial, dilated blood vessels, the most common type being the spider naevus. They can occur on any site but are often seen in children on the cheeks and dorsum of the hands. Telangiectasia are also a feature of genetic disorders, including essential telangiectasia, Osler–Weber–Rendu syndrome, in which there are mucosal lesions and risk of gastrointestinal bleeding, and Rothmund–Thomson syndrome with poikiloderma. Another type is matt telangiectasia seen in genetic disorders such as capillary malformation-arteriovenous malformation (CM-AVM) (although laser treatment is contraindicated in CM-AVM due to the risk of activating the AVM). Most small superficial telangiectases respond well to treatment with the PDL and most disappear completely with one or two treatments.

Other skin disorders

Cutis marmorata telangiectatica congenita

Cutis marmorata telangiectatica congenita (CMTC) is a developmental vascular disorder present from birth and characterized by a purplish reticulate and mottled discolouration of the skin. It can involve circumscribed segments of the skin but is usually widespread. The lesions of CMTC may be associated with other medical problems, namely ulceration and localized lipoatrophy at the sites of vascular discolouration, as well as macrocephaly and hemihypertrophy. PDL therapy for this condition shows a variable response, often disappointing; 25 children have been treated at GOSH with an overall poor outcome. For that reason, PDL treatment for the reticulate vascular discolouration is not routinely offered, especially as the skin lesions tend to fade and become less conspicuous with age. The only exception is a capillary malformation of the upper lip, often a feature of this condition, which can respond well to laser treatment.

Angioma serpigiosum

This is a rare disorder affecting the small vessels of the upper dermis characterized clinically by red or purple punctuate lesions that cluster in a serpiginous pattern. It usually starts in childhood and is seen mainly in females. Typically, the lesions appear on the lower limbs and buttocks and are unilateral and asymptomatic [25]. They respond well to PDL therapy [26], although PDL does not have any effect on the progression of the condition and new lesions can continue to appear (Fig. 172.5).

Goltz syndrome

This condition is also known as focal dermal hypoplasia [27]. It is inherited as an X-linked dominant disorder. The skin features present as striate, atrophic and lipomatous lesions which are present from birth. Telangiectasia, hyper- and hypopigmentation can be associated with these lesions. Treatment with PDL removes the telangiectasia and can improve the cosmetic appearance, especially on the face.

Inflammatory epidermal naevus

Inflammatory linear verrucous epidermal naevus (ILVEN) can occur in childhood, often under the age of 1 year, and usually persists but can rarely resolve spontaneously. The lesions tend to be pruritic and are often cosmetically unacceptable. PDL treatment can improve these lesions by reducing and sometimes removing the erythematous component (Fig. 172.6) [28,29].

Angiofibromas in tuberous sclerosis

Twenty patients have been treated at GOSH with encouraging results. Lesions which are flat or only slightly raised do well, with diminution of their red colour. Those that are more papulonodular become less red and flatter with a reduced tendency to bleed. For these lesions, a combination

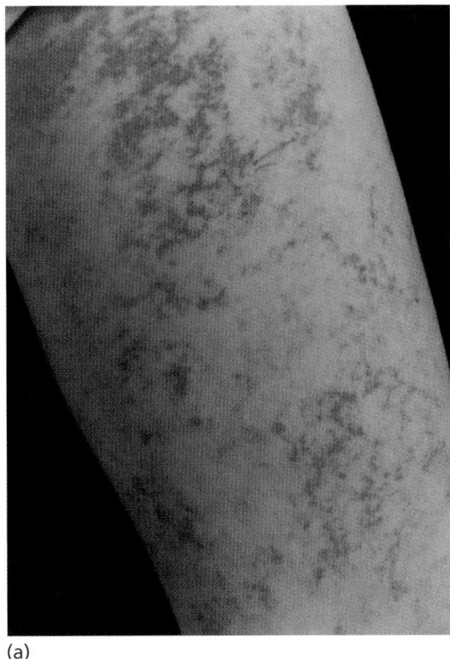
(a)

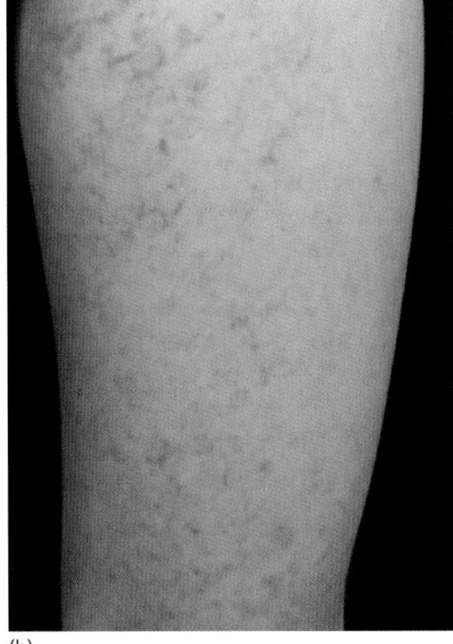
(b)

Fig. 172.5 Angioma serpiginosum before (a) and after (b) laser treatment.

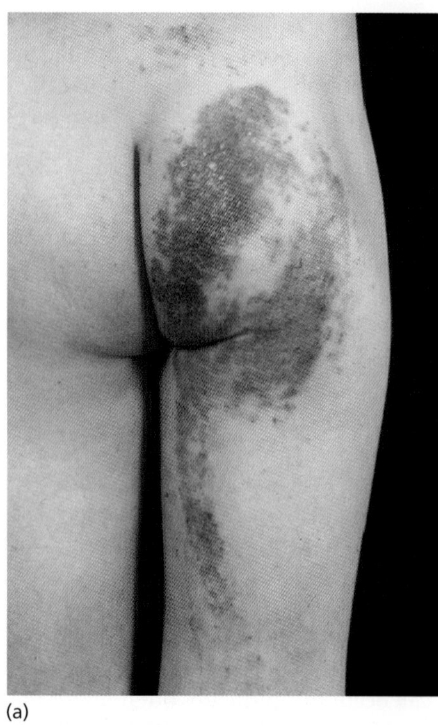
(a)

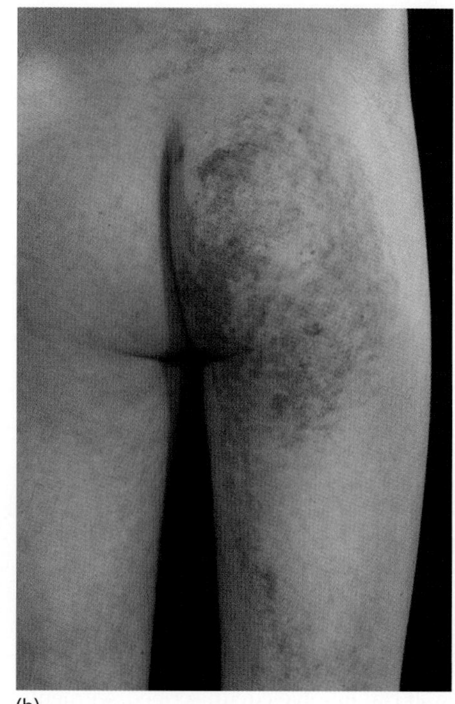
(b)

Fig. 172.6 ILVEN before (a) and after (b) laser treatment.

of CO^2 laser and the vascular PDL has been the preferred treatment. However, most children with this condition are now treated with sirolimus gel with an overall good outcome.

Hypertrophic, keloid and acne scars
These can be improved by PDL treatment with variable results, by reducing the erythema, flattening the scar and in many cases reducing the itch which is often the major problem, especially with vertical cardiothoracic scars over the sternum [30–32].

Verrucous haemangiomas (verrucous vascular malformations)/angiokeratomas
Laser treatment is undoubtedly helpful but will not remove the lesion. Prior to laser treatment, the overlying hyperkeratotic epidermis should be removed using a suitable keratolytic agent, such as salicylic ointment or urea cream. Our experience has shown that earlier treatment of this condition before the hyperkeratosis worsens shows a much improved outcome. After laser treatment, there is less tendency to develop hyperkeratosis, less bleeding and less discomfort.

Superficial cutaneous lymphangiomas
Laser treatment can be beneficial, especially for those lesions that contain blood by sealing the individual blebs and reducing lymph oozing and bleeding.

Chronic inflammatory skin conditions: psoriasis and eczema
There is evidence that psoriatic lesions can be improved following treatment with the vascular PDL [33]. An immunohistochemical study carried out to evaluate the role of the superficial capillary bed in the pathogenesis of psoriasis [34] demonstrated that selective photothermolysis following PDL therapy resulted in a reduction in endothelial cell proliferation and a reduction of the CD4+ and CD8+ T-cell infiltrate in the superficial papillary dermis. This study also found a corresponding reduction of the epidermal thickness, thus showing an association between epidermal hyperplasia and dermal angiogenesis. The effects of the vascular PDL on discoid areas of eczema had a similar positive result [35–37]. Thus, the PDL may offer another option for treatment of difficult refractory localized areas of both psoriasis and eczema. Further research is needed to define the optimum parameters as well as analysing long-term follow-up data.

Multiplex laser

The Cynergy multiplex laser system (Cynosure, Inc., Westford, MA, USA) delivers two different wavelengths, 595 (PDL) and 1064 nm (neodymium:yttrium aluminium garnet, Nd:YAG), at a specifically designed timed interval. It is useful for the treatment of refractory PWS, angiomas, venous malformations, difficult large thread veins, cutaneous small lymphatic lesions and other conditions. Advantages include better clearance, fewer treatments, 2–3 days of bruising and minimal pain and discomfort. The mechanism, confirmed by several studies, demonstrates that subtherapeutic (PDL) light doses alter the absorption characteristics of blood, making it a better target for the 1064 nm Nd:YAG component [38–41]. PDL conversion of blood to a combination of methaemoglobin and thrombus temporarily increases the absorbance at 1064 nm by approximately 3–5 times that of normal blood This synergistic approach provides an enhanced effect on the vascular lesions.

These higher-powered lasers carry an increased risk of scarring and should be used with caution. Other side-effects include hyper- or hypopigmentation, blistering, venous lake on the lip, infection with *Staphylococcus aureus* and hyperaemia.

Laser treatment of pigmented lesions (S. Lanigan)

Café-au-lait macules

Café-au-lait macules (CALM) are benign hyperpigmented areas, present at birth in 2% of all newborns. They can be markers of underlying disease such as neurofibromatosis, but isolated CALM are not an uncommon finding in many infants. The coffee-coloured brown discoloration can be reduced by treatment with any of the short-pulsed Q-switched lasers which selectively target melanosomes. Laser therapy for CALM is generally safe and treatment of affected children can be performed if required. Studies on the Q-switched Nd:YAG (532 nm or 1064 nm) (Fig. 172.7), the Q-switched alexandrite (755 nm) and the Q-switched ruby laser (694 nm) show that each of these lasers can be effective [42]. Approximately 50% of patients will obtain total clearing after repeated Q-switched laser treatments but recurrence and patchy pigmentation can occur in the other 50% [43]. It is generally agreed that results seen at 12 months after the last treatment are usually permanent [44,45].

Naevus of Ota

Naevus of Ota is a benign dermal melanocytic naevus seen most commonly in Asian and Japanese patients with a prevalence of 0.2–0.8% in the latter population. The naevus presents as blue/grey/black hyperpigmented macules and patches scattered unilaterally along the cutaneous distribution of the first and second divisions of the trigeminal nerve. Pigmentation of the conjunctiva or iris can be seen on the affected side. The disfigurement persists throughout life and can cause significant psychological distress.

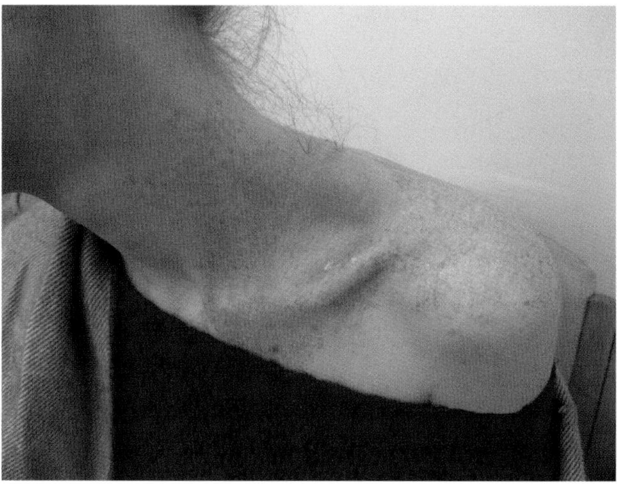

Fig. 172.7 Clearance of part of café-au-lait pigmentation with one treatment of QS Nd:YAG (532 nm).

Lasers have become the treatment of choice for the treatment of naevus of Ota [46], with multiple clinical studies over the past 15 years. Q-switched (QS) lasers have been most studied and can produce significant lightening or clearance of the cutaneous pigmentation. The QS ruby [47], alexandrite [48] and Nd:YAG lasers [49] can all be used. Of the three, the ruby laser is most strongly absorbed by melanin and has the shallowest penetration, the Nd:YAG laser has the weakest absorption by melanin and has the deepest penetration, with the alexandrite laser between the two. Unwanted epidermal pigment damage is more likely with the ruby laser [50] and it is recommended that this laser be restricted to skin phototypes I–III. For deeply situated lesions (which tend to look grey/black rather than blue), the deeply penetrating Nd:YAG laser is likely to be more appropriate. In 2003, Kono et al. reported on treatment with the QS ruby laser in different age groups with naevus of Ota [51]. The number of treatments needed for lesion clearance was significantly shorter in children compared to adults and the complication rate was significantly lower in children. Multiple treatments are necessary which in children may require general anaesthesia.

A useful comparative study has been performed, using three of the currently available QS lasers, including the Nd:YAG laser at 532 nm [52]. This green light laser has a relatively shallow depth of penetration. Interestingly, the authors did not detect any significant relationship between the laser used and level of improvement. After eight treatments, the mean improvement of those who completed treatment was 97% for QS Nd:YAG (1064 nm), 90% for QS Nd:YAG (532 nm) and 80% for QS alexandrite laser. The authors recommend test patches with a variety of available lasers to determine the most efficacious treatment for that individual.

Congenital melanocytic naevus

Congenital melanocytic naevi (CMN) are present from birth and affect approximately 1% of newborns. They may be cosmetically disfiguring and have the potential for malignant transformation. A variety of treatment modalities have been utilized with variable efficacy and the current treatment of choice, where possible, is surgical excision. However, some CMN occur in cosmetically sensitive areas, where a surgical scar is less acceptable, or in inoperable locations.

For these reasons, lasers have been investigated as potential alternative treatment modalities [53]. The lasers studied to date for the treatment of CMN can be grouped as pigment-specific lasers, including ruby (694 nm), alexandrite (755 nm) (Fig. 172.8) and Nd:YAG (1064 nm) (Fig. 172.9) targeting melanosomes, and ablative lasers such as the CO_2 (10 600 nm) and erbium:yttrium aluminium garnet (Er:YAG) (2940 nm). To date, ruby lasers have been studied most extensively in the treatment of CMN and have been shown to improve the cosmetic appearance of some CMN and can be considered for lesions where surgical excision is problematic. Unfortunately, there appears to be a high recurrence rate after treatment. Combined treatment with both the Q-switched and normal mode ruby laser may give better results but true comparative studies are lacking. An alternative approach is to remove the lesion nonselectively with an ablative laser. This can produce good results but has a higher risk of scarring [54,55].

Ablative lasers

Removal of the skin surface to improve blemishes and irregularities has been performed for many years. Before the advent of lasers, this was performed by deep chemical peels. The depth of the injury was often unpredictable and side-effects included toxicity and scarring.

Carbon dioxide and Er:YAG lasers have traditionally been used in ablative resurfacing procedures and are generally considered superior to chemical peels for deep regeneration. These infrared lasers heat up water rapidly in tissue which is converted to steam and superficial layers of skin are effectively vaporized to specific and varying depths. In this process, there is complete removal of the superficial skin surface, usually the whole epidermis and a superficial portion of the dermis.

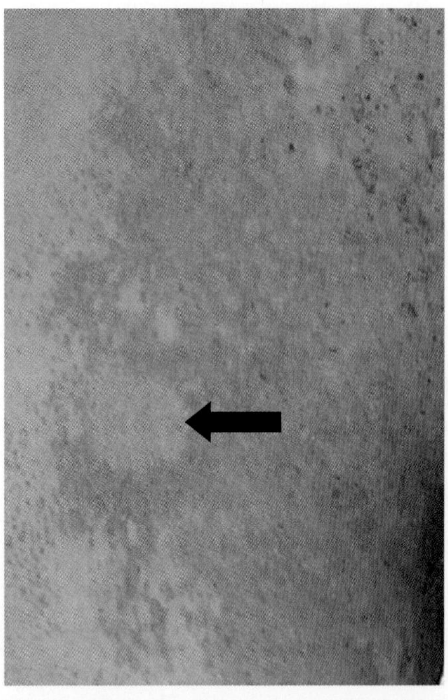

Fig. 172.8 Good response to treating a test area with the long pulsed alexandrite laser in congenital melanocytic naevus.

The CO_2 and Er:YAG lasers heat up tissue water so rapidly, in short pulses, that nearly all the energy of the laser beam is used up in forming steam and removing tissue. The Er:YAG laser is so efficient in doing this that the effects are almost entirely ablative, and this occurs very superficially in the skin. The CO_2 laser also has a small heating (thermal) effect, so that the surface of ablated skin has a small area of thermal injury.

There are advantages and advocates of both lasers. The Er:YAG produces a very superficial wound with no underlying thermal heating so ablation depth can be controlled. However, as ablation proceeds into the dermis, bleeding will occur which prevents any deeper ablation, and many consider this an advantage to prevent scarring. With the CO_2 laser, the small layer of thermally coagulated tissue will seal blood vessels and give the operator a clear field. It is thought that the small area of thermally damaged tissue will enhance new collagen formation. However, for the inexperienced practitioner, this extra layer of injury below the ablation field could increase side-effects. This haemostatic effect also allows the operator to use the CO_2 laser as a 'bloodless' scalpel when cutting tissue.

These lasers can be used for a variety of warty cutaneous lesions (Table 172.2). There are several case series on treatment of epidermal naevi in this way [56,57]. Epidermal naevi, which are frequently verrucous with secondary hyperpigmentation, have been notoriously difficult to treat due to their large size and often conspicuous location. Precise laser ablation can improve the verrucous nature of the lesion without complete clearance, leaving a good cosmetic result often at the expense of some hypopigmentation.

Facial angiofibromas are a manifestation of tuberous sclerosis. This autosomal dominant neurocutaneous syndrome exhibits a number of cutaneous signs as well as epilepsy and low intelligence. Treatment is often sought for the angiofibromas, which add to the stigmatization of the disorder. If the lesions have a significant vascular

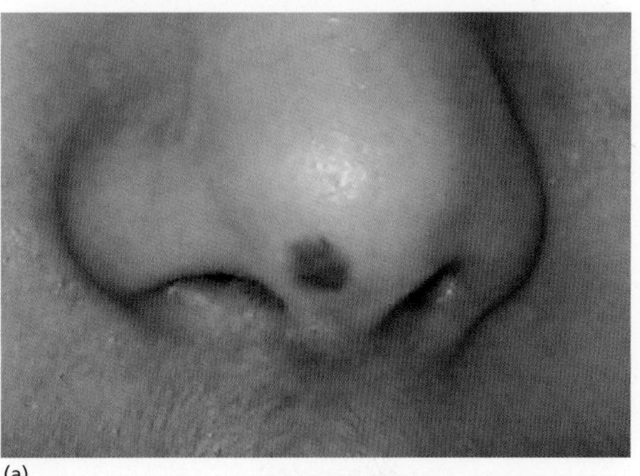

(a)

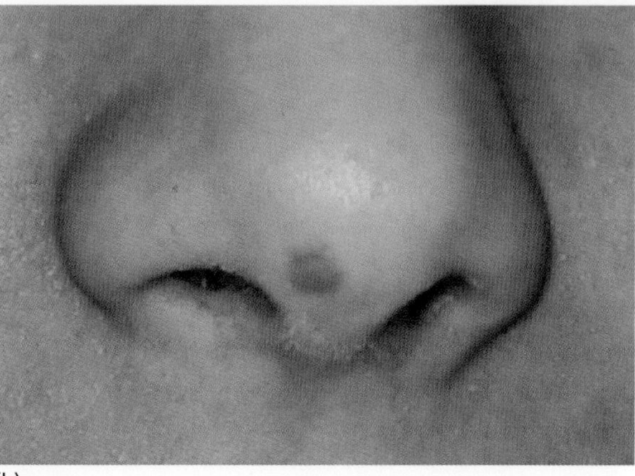

(b)

Fig. 172.9 (a,b) Partial response of small congenital melanocytic naevus to QS laser treatment.

component, the PDL can be used, but for verrucous lesions on the face, laser ablation with the CO_2 laser is the treatment of choice [58].

Large numbers of neurofibromas can be a major source of cosmetic disfigurement in a patient with peripheral neurofibromatosis. Lesions can be pedunculated, sessile or subcutaneous. Because of the large numbers, excisional surgery is impracticable and can be associated with undesirable scarring. It is possible to ablate these lesions with a CO_2 laser under general anaesthesia. The rapid removal of hundreds of lesions can be performed with minimal morbidity and an enhanced appearance with high patient satisfaction [59].

Resistant viral warts can be ablated with these lasers but the procedure is painful and can be associated with significant morbidity and cannot be routinely recommended [60]. In a retrospective review of 277 patients with recalcitrant warts treated with the PDL, there was a response rate of 86%. The authors recommending higher fluences than previously used, which can make the procedure very painful [61].

In recent years, new laser technology, fractional photothermolysis, has been introduced to specifically overcome the drawbacks of conventional resurfacing [62]. Instead of producing one large beam that causes uniform thermal damage to all tissue in its path (as with conventional resurfacing lasers), the output from fractional resurfacing devices consists of thousands of microscopic columns, which each produce thermal damage to a small volume of tissue. These can either be applied by ultrafast scanning of a stationary handpiece or scanned over the skin as the handpiece moves over the skin surface. There are two main ways of performing a fractional procedure: ablative and nonablative. Ablative fractionated lasers use CO_2 and Er:YAG laser technology to produce microscopic columns of tissue removal. Nonablative fractional lasers use wavelengths of light that heat up tissue water and hence tissue to produce coagulation but not sufficiently to cause ablation.

In the paediatric population, scar contractures can be very debilitating. Ablative fractional laser resurfacing is emerging as an adjunctive procedural option for scar contractures because of its potential efficacy and safety profile. Published studies are sparse but ablative fractional laser resurfacing may be a promising tool in the management of function-limiting scar contractures in children [63,64].

Table 172.2 Paediatric disorders reported as treatable by laser ablation

Epidermal lesions	Epidermal naevi
Dermal lesions	Neurofibromas Adenoma sebaceum Atrophic scars Hypertrophic scars Congenital melanocytic naevi
Vascular lesions	Port wine stains Pyogenic granulomas Angiofibromas Angiokeratomas Lymphangioma circumscriptum
Burn debridement	
Viral warts	

Hair removal by lasers

Lasers are well established as the most effective treatment for long-term hair reduction. Hair reduction by lasers has been achieved primarily by selective photothermolysis of pigment in hairs using lasers such as the long pulsed ruby (694 nm) and alexandrite (755 nm) lasers [65]. These wavelengths are well absorbed by melanin and have been shown to produce permanent hair reduction in dark hair in fair skin. Multiple treatments are required and in general a 60–70% reduction in hair growth can be achieved in this way. Alternatives to these lasers are the diode laser operating around 810 nm, the long pulsed Nd:YAG laser at 1064 nm and flashlamps, which are broadband light

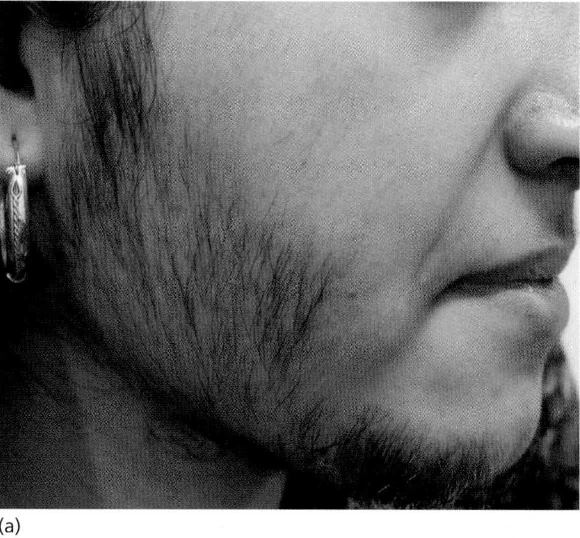
(a)

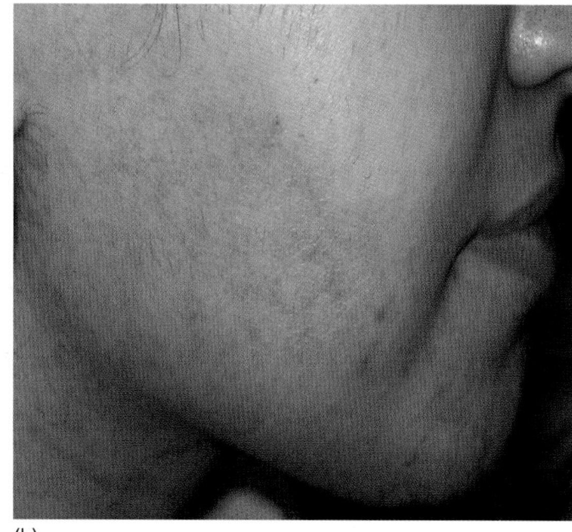
(b)

Fig. 172.10 (a,b) Excellent hair reduction in female skin type IV after long pulsed Nd:YAG laser treatment (before and after four treatments).

sources. The longer wavelengths of light are less avidly absorbed by melanin and penetrate more deeply.

While the long pulsed ruby (694 nm) and alexandrite (755 nm) lasers are very effective in achieving hair reduction in dark hair in fair skin, these wavelengths are associated with significant side-effects when used for hair reduction in darker skin types because of epidermal damage due to the absorption of laser light by epidermal melanin.

The Nd:YAG laser is an infrared laser at 1064 nm which when used with longer pulse durations (3–60 msec) has been to be shown efficacious in hair removal even in skin phototypes V–VI (Fig. 172.10). The side-effects when performing hair removal with this laser in darker skin types are significantly reduced compared to ruby and alexandrite laser therapy. Scarring is very rare with laser hair removal and very much less common than with electrolysis. Side-effects are most commonly due to thermal injury to skin and occur more commonly with shorter wavelength lasers and darker skin types or in tanned skin.

Laser hair removal can be safely performed in children. In a study by Rajpar et al. [66], constitutional hirsutism, polycystic ovarian syndrome, congenital melanocytic naevus, generalized hypertrichosis and naevoid hypertrichosis were all successfully treated in children under 16 years old.

Becker's naevus is a hamartomatous disorder which presents at puberty with spreading brown discolouration unilaterally overlying the chest, shoulder and upper back, associated with coarse dark terminal hair growth. While treatment of the pigmentation is frequently unsuccessful, laser hair removal can create a good cosmetic result for the affected individual [67].

References

1 **Lanigan S, Cottrill J. Psychological disabilities amongst patients with port wine stains. Br J Dermatol 1989;121(2):209–15.**
2 McClean K, Hanke W. The medical necessity for treatment of port wine stains. Dermatol Surg 1997;23:(8):663–7.
3 **Anderson RR, Parish JA. Selective photothermolysis: precise microsurgery by selective absorption of pulsed irradiation. Science 1983;220:524–7.**
4 **Tan OT, Sherwood K, Gilchrest BA. Treatment of children with port-wine stains using the flashlamp-pulsed tunable dye laser. N Engl J Med 1989;320(7):416–21.**
5 Tan OT, Motemedi M, Welch AJ, Kurban AK. Spotsize effects in guinea pig skin following pulsed irradiation. J Invest Dermatol 1988;90: 877–88.
6 Tan OT. Dye laser for benign cutaneous vascular lesions: clinical and technical development. In: Steiner R, Kaufmann R, Landthaler M, Braun-Falco O (eds) Lasers in Dermatology. Heidelberg: Springer-Verlag, 1991:60–72.
7 Tan OT, Stafford TJ. EMLA for laser treatment of port wine stain in children. Lasers Surg Med 1992;12:543–8.
8 Sherwood KA. The use of topical anaesthesia in removal of port wine stain in children. J Paediatr 1993;122:536–41.
9 **Smart T. Consensus Statement Supplement: On the Use of Anesthetic and Sedative Drugs in Infants and Toddlers. Available at: http://smarttots.org/consensus-statement-supplement/**
10 Rappaport B, Suresh S, Hertz S et al. Anesthetic neurotoxicity: clinical implications of animal models. N Engl J Med 2015;372:796–7.
11 Pratt AG. Birthmarks in infants. Arch Dermatol Syphilol 1953;67: 302–5.
12 **Jacobs AH, Walton RG. The incidence of birthmarks in the neonates. Pediatrics 1976;58:218–22.**
13 Mulliken JB, Young AE. Vascular Birthmarks: Hemangiomas and Malformations. Philadelphia: WB Saunders, 1988:179–95.
14 **Renfro L, Geronemus R. Anatomical differences of port wine stains in response to treatment with the pulsed dye laser. Arch Dermatol 1993;28:182–8.**
15 Lanigan SW. Port wine stains on the lower limb: response to pulsed dye laser therapy. Clin Exp Dermatol 1996;21:88–92.
16 **Beattie M, Widdowson D, Anderson W. Pulsed dye laser treatment of paediatric port wine stains – variations of practice in the UK (NHS). Lasers Med Sci 2016;31:597.**
17 Syed S, Linward J, Kennedy H et al. Ten years' experience of laser treatment for vascular birthmarks in children. 15th International Society for the Study of Vascular Anomalies (ISSVA), New Zealand, 2004; abstract T8:39.
18 Harper JI, Syed S, Linward L. Refractory port wine stains: improved response to higher fluence and longer pulsed width. 15th International Society for the Study of Vascular Anomalies (ISSVA), New Zealand, 2004; abstract T9:39.
19 Griffin TD Jr, Foshey J, Finney R, Saedi N. Port wine stain treated with a combination of pulsed dye laser and topical rapamycin ointment. Lasers Surg Med 2016;48(2):193–6.
20 Marques L, Nunez-Cordoba J, Aguado L et al. Topical rapamycin combined with pulsed dye laser in the treatment of capillary vascular malformations in Sturge Weber syndrome: phase II randomised double-blind intra-individual placebo-controlled clinical trial. J. Am Acad Dermatol 2015;72(1):151–8.
21 Greveling K, Prens E, van Doorn M. Treatment of port wine stains using pulsed dye laser, erbium YAG laser, and topical rapamycin (sirolimus) – a randomized controlled trial. Lasers Surg Med 2017; 49(1):104–9.
22 **Solman L, Murabit A, Gnarra M et al. Propranolol for infantile haemangiomas: a single centre experience of 250 cases and proposed therapeutic protocol. Arch Dis Child 2014;99(12):1132–6.**
23 Liu X, Qu X, Zheng J, Zhang L. Effectiveness and safety of oral propranolol versus other treatments for infantile haemangiomas: a meta-analysis. PLoS One 2015;10(9):e0138100.
24 Lacour M, Syed S, Linward J, Harper JI. Role of the pulsed dye laser in the management of ulcerated capillary haemangiomas. Arch Dis Child 1996;74:161–3.
25 Katta R, Wagner A. Angioma serpiginosum with extensive cutaneous involvement. J Am Acad Dermatol 2000;42:384–5.
26 Long C C, Lanigan S W. Treatment of angioma serpiginosum using pulsed dye laser. Br J Dermatol 1997;136(4):631–2.
27 Goltz RW, Peterson WC, Gorlin RJ et al. Focal dermal hypoplasia. Arch Dermatol 1962;86:708–17.
28 Sidwell R, Syed S, Harper JI. Pulsed dye laser treatment for inflammatory linear verrucous epidermal naevus. Br J Dermatol 2001;144: 1267–9.
29 Alster TS. Inflammatory linear verrucous epidermal naevus, successful treatment with the 585 nm flashlamp pulsed dye laser. J Am Acad Dermatol 1994;31:513–14.
30 Kono T, Erçöçen A, Nakazawa H et al. The flashlamp pumped pulsed dye laser (585 nm) treatment of hypertrophic scars in Asians. Ann Plast Surg 2003;51(4):366–71.
31 Alster TS, Taviji EL. Hypertrophic scars and keloids: etiology and management. Am J Clin Dermatol 2003;4(4):235–43.
32 Patel N, Clement M. Selective non ablasive treatment of acne scarring with 585 nm flashed pumped dye laser. Dermatol Surg 2002;28(10): 942–5.
33 Katugampola GA, Rees AM, Lanigan SW. Laser treatment of psoriasis. Br J Dermatol 1995;133:909–13.
34 Hern S, Allen MH, Sousa AR et al. Immunohistochemical evaluation wwof psoriatic plaques following selective photothermolysis of the superficial capillaries. Br J Dermatol 2001;145:45–53.
35 Zelickson BD, Mehregan DA, Wendelschfer-Crabb G et al. Clinical and histological evaluation of psoriatic plaques treated with flashlamp pulsed dye laser. J Am Acad Dermatol 1996;35:64–8.
36 Sidwell R, Syed S, Harper JI. Port wine stains and eczema. Br J Dermatol 2001;144:1269–70.
37 Syed S, Weibel L, Kennedy H, Harper JI. A pilot study showing pulsed dye laser treatment improves localized areas of chronic atopic dermatitis. Clin Exp Dermatol 2008;33(3):243–8.
38 Black JF, Barton JK. Time-domain optical and thermal analysis of blood undergoing laser photocoagulation. Proc SPIE 2001;4257: 341–54.
39 Mordon S, Brisot D, Fournier N. Using a 'non-uniform pulse sequence' can improve selective coagulation with a Nd:YAG laser (1.06 μm) thanks to Met-hemoglobin absorption: a clinical study on blue leg veins. Lasers Surg Med 2003;32:160–70.

40 Kuenstner JT, Norris KH. Spectrophotometry of human hemoglobin in the near infrared region from 1000 to 2500nm. J Near Infrared Spectrosc 1994;2:59–65.

41 Heger M, Beek JF, Moldovan NI et al. Towards optimization of selective photothermolysis: prothromic pharmaceutical agents as potential adjuvants in laser treatment of port wine stains – a theoretical study. Thromb Haemost 2005;93:242–56.

42 Grossman MC, Anderson RR, Farinelli W et al. Treatment of café au lait macules with lasers. A clinicopathologic correlation. Arch Dermatol 1995;131(12):1416–20.

43 Stratigos AJ, Dover JS, Arndt KA. Laser treatment of pigmented lesions – 2000: how far have we gone? Arch Dermatol 2000;136(7): 915–21.

44 Alster RS. Complete elimination of large café au lait birthmarks by the 510nm pulsed dye laser. Plast Reconstr Surg 1995;96:1660–4.

45 Levy JL, Mordon S, Pizzi-Anselme M. Treatment of individual café au lait macules with the Q-switched Nd: YAG: a clinicopathologic correlation. J Cutan Laser Ther 1999;1(4):217–23.

46 Shah VV, Bray FN, Aldahan AS et al. Lasers and nevus of Ota: a comprehensive review. Lasers Med Sci 2016;31(1):179–85.

47 Geronemus RG. Q-switched ruby laser therapy of nevus of Ota. Arch Dermatol 1992;128(12):1618–22.

48 Kang W, Lee E, Choi GS. Treatment of Ota's nevus by Q-switched alexandrite laser : therapeutic outcome in relation to clinical and histopathological findings. Eur J Dermatol 1999;9(8):639–43.

49 Polnikorn N, Tanrattanakorn S, Goldberg DJ. Treatment of Hori's nevus with the Q-switched Nd:YAG laser. Dermatol Surg 2000;26(5): 477–80.

50 Kono T, Nozaki M, Chan HH, Mikashima Y. A retrospective study looking at the long-term complications of Q-switched ruby laser in the treatment of nevus of Ota. Lasers Surg Med 2001;29(2):156–9.

51 Kono T, Chan HH, Erçöçen AR et al. Use of Q-switched ruby laser in the treatment of nevus of ota in different age groups. Lasers Surg Med 2003;32(5):391–5.

52 Felton SJ, Al-Niaimi F, Ferguson JE, Madan V. Our perspective of the treatment of naevus of Ota with 1,064-, 755- and 532-nm wavelength lasers. Lasers Med Sci 2014;29(5):1745–9.

53 Bray FN, Shah V, Nouri K. Laser treatment of congenital melanocytic nevi: a review of the literature. Lasers Med Sci 2016;31(1):197–204.

54 August PJ, Ferguson JE, Madan V. A study of the efficacy of carbon dioxide and pigment-specific lasers in the treatment of medium-sized congenital melanocytic naevi. Br J Dermatol 2011;164(5):1037–42.

55 A l-Hadithy N, Al-Nakib K, Quaba A. Outcomes of 52 patients with congenital melanocytic naevi treated with ultrapulse carbon dioxide and frequency doubled Q-switched Nd-Yag laser. J Plast Reconstr Aesthet Surg 2012;65(8):1019–28.

56 Ratz JL, Bailin PL, Wheeland RG. Carbon dioxide laser treatment of epidermal nevi. J Dermatol Surg Oncol 1986;12:567–70.

57 Hohenleutner U, Wlotzke U, Konz B, Landthaler M. Carbon dioxide laser therapy of a widespread epidermal nevus. Lasers Surg Med 1995;16:288–91.

58 Papadavid E, Markey A Bellaney G, Walker NP. Carbon dioxide and pulsed dye laser treatment of angiofibromas in 29 patients with tuberous sclerosis. Br J Dermatol 2002;147:337–42.

59 Becker DW Jr. Use of the carbon dioxide laser in treating multiple cutaneous neurofibromas. Ann Plast Surg 1991;26(6):582–6.

60 Logan RA, Zachary CB. Outcome of carbon dioxide laser therapy for persistent cutaneous viral warts. Br J Dermatol 1989;121(1):99–105.

61 Sparreboom EE, Luijks HG, Luiting-Welkenhuyzen HA et al. Pulsed-dye laser treatment for recalcitrant viral warts: a retrospective case series of 227 patients. Br J Dermatol 2014;171(5):1270–3.

62 Manstein D, Herron GS, Sink RK et al. Fractional photothermolysis: a new concept for cutaneous remodeling using microscopic patterns of thermal injury. Lasers Surg Med 2004;34(5):426–38.

63 Choi JE, Oh GN, Kim JY et al. Ablative fractional laser treatment for hypertrophic scars: comparison between Er:YAG and CO2 fractional lasers. J Dermatol Treat 2014;25(4):299–303.

64 Taudorf EH, Danielsen PL, Paulsen IF et al. Non-ablative fractional laser provides long-term improvement of mature burn scars – a randomized controlled trial with histological assessment. Lasers Surg Med 2015;47(2):141–7.

65 Dierickx C, Alora MB, Dover JS.A clinical overview of hair removal using lasers and light sources. Dermatol Clin 1999;17(2):357–66.

66 Rajpar SF, Hague JS, Abdullah A, Lanigan SW. Hair removal with the long-pulse alexandrite and long-pulse Nd:YAG lasers is safe and well tolerated in children. Clin Exp Dermatol 2009;34(6):684–7.

67 Choi JE, Kim JW, Seo SH et al. Treatment of Becker's nevi with a long-pulse alexandrite laser. Dermatol Surg 2009;35(7):1105–8.

CHAPTER 173

Sedation and Anaesthesia

Brenda M. Simpson[1], *Yuin-Chew Chan*[2] *& Lawrence F. Eichenfield*[3]

[1] El Paso Dermatology Center, El Paso, TX, USA
[2] Dermatology Associates, Gleneagles Medical Centre, Singapore
[3] Pediatric and Adolescent Dermatology, Rady Children's Hospital, San Diego University of California, San Diego School of Medicine, San Diego, CA, USA

Introduction, 2330
Local anaesthetics, 2331
Techniques to decrease the pain of injection, 2332
Perioperative analgesics, 2335
Sedation, 2335
Pharmacological agents, 2336
Other techniques, 2340

Abstract

Procedural pain control in children is essential as children of all ages, including infants, are able to experience pain, and painful physical experiences in children can have persisting physiological and psychological consequences. Anaesthetic options for paediatric patients undergoing dermatological and laser surgery are discussed. Techniques to decrease the pain of injection of local anaesthetics and to alleviate anxiety are essential. Topical anaesthetics are convenient, cost-effective and associated with few adverse effects. Sedation should be considered as a continuum within which a patient may drift from a state of consciousness to deep sedation and on to general anaesthesia. The potential influence of anaesthetic drugs on neurodevelopmental impairment is discussed.

Key points

- **Knowledge and utilization of anaesthetic options for paediatric patients can help reduce the anxiety and pain associated with dermatological procedures for both children and their caregivers.**
- **For children, no more than 1.5–2.0 mg/kg of lidocaine and 3.0–4.5 mg/kg of lidocaine with epinephrine should be administered in a single procedure.**
- **The safety and efficacy of codeine have recently been called into question, and use of alternative medications is encouraged.**
- **While long-term effects of anaesthesia in young children are under investigation, with inconclusive results, the risks and benefits of early treatment of dermatological conditions under general anaesthesia should be considered and individualized.**

Introduction

A sound knowledge of anaesthetic options for paediatric patients reduces the anxiety and pain associated with dermatological procedures for both children and their caregivers [1,2].

Pain perception

Children of all ages, including infants, perceive and remember pain. Multiple factors influence a child's response to pain during a surgical procedure. These include the type of painful stimulus, psychosocial factors, previous medical experiences and painful events in the past [3].

Previously, procedural pain control in young children was not given serious attention because of the misconception that their neuronal pain pathways were undeveloped. However, we now recognize that even neonates are able to experience pain. Moreover, intensely painful physical experiences in children can have long-term physiological and psychological ramifications. Therefore, the management of acute pain is essential [4–6].

The age of the child is a significant factor that determines the intensity of the experienced pain, as well as the anticipation of pain. Infants and young children often have a disproportionate fear of pain compared to older children and adults. This is due to anatomical (e.g. larger surface area for stimulation of sensory neurons) and neurophysiological (e.g. nonfunctional descending noradrenergic fibres at the spinal level) differences and because infants and young children may fail to fully comprehend the indication or necessity for the procedure. They are also more likely to have needle phobia and stranger anxiety. The child's anxiety may also be influenced by parental fear, so it is important to alleviate the apprehension of both the child and the parents, for instance by providing fun activities or having an aquarium in the waiting area.

References

1 Chen BK, Eichenfield LF. Pediatric anesthesia in dermatologic surgery: when hand-holding is not enough. Dermatol Surg 2001;27:1010–18.
2 Yeo LF, Eichenfield LF, Chan YC. Skin surgery in children: local anaesthesia and sedation techniques. Expert Opin Pharmacother 2007;8:317–27.

Harper's Textbook of Pediatric Dermatology, Fourth Edition. Edited by Peter Hoeger, Veronica Kinsler and Albert Yan.

3 Cunningham BB, Eichenfield LF. Decreasing the pain of procedures in children. Curr Prob Dermatol 1999;ii:1–36.
4 Anand KJS, Hickey PR. Pain and its effects in the human neonate and fetus. N Engl J Med 1987;317:1321.
5 Walco GA, Cassidy RC, Schechter NL. Pain, hurt and harm. The ethics of pain control in infants and children. N Engl J Med 1994;331:541–4.
6 Larsson BA. Pain management in neonates. Acta Paediatr 1999;88: 1301–10.

Local anaesthetics

History. The first topical anaesthetic was probably cocaine, the numbing qualities of which were noted in Peru some centuries ago. The first medical use was described in 1884 by Carl Koller, as a topical ophthalmic anaesthetic [1]. The first synthetic anaesthetic was procaine, an ester anaesthetic, which was developed in 1905. Lidocaine (also known as lignocaine), the first synthetic amide anaesthetic, was created in 1943 [2].

Mechanism of action. Sensory nerve conduction is mediated by the opening of voltage-gated sodium channels. When sufficient intracellular influx of sodium occurs, an action potential is propagated. Local anaesthetics inhibit the voltage-gated sodium channels in the neuronal cell membrane; this increases the threshold of excitatory potential and prevents the transmission of the noxious stimuli. The specific site of action of local anaesthetics is the intracellular portion of the sodium channel.

Local anaesthetics can be combined with vasoconstrictors, such as epinephrine, to provide improved haemostasis, reduce systemic toxicity and increase the duration of anaesthesia.

Classification of local anaesthetics. Local anaesthetics are weak bases that typically consist of three important components: an aromatic ring, an ester or amide linkage and a tertiary amine. The aromatic ring determines potency as lipid solubility allows it to permeate the neuronal membrane. The latter two parts are responsible for protein binding and hence duration of anaesthesia. Local anaesthetics are classified as either amide or ester based (Table 173.1). The ester-based anaesthetics include procaine, cocaine, chloroprocaine and benzocaine. They are metabolized by plasma cholinesterase and other nonspecific esterases. The amide-based anaesthetics include lidocaine, bupivacaine, prilocaine, mepivacaine, levobupivacaine and ropivacaine. These are primarily metabolized in the liver via microsomal enzymes. Variations exist in properties affecting lipophilic status, pK_a and protein binding that influence potency, speed of onset and duration of action, as well as potential toxicity [3].

Lidocaine. Lidocaine is usually administered as a 0.5–2% (5–20 mg/mL) solution. For children, no more than 1.5–2.0 mg/kg of lidocaine and 3.0–4.5 mg/kg of lidocaine with epinephrine should be administered in a single treatment [4]. Using 2.0 mg/kg (maximum dose lidocaine without epinephrine in children) is equivalent to a maximum volume of 0.2 mL of 1% lidocaine per kilogram of bodyweight [4].

The addition of epinephrine counteracts the natural vasodilatory effect of lidocaine and hence decreases the rate of lidocaine absorption, increases its duration of action and reduces the risk of systemic toxicity. As an added benefit, the localized vasoconstriction induced by epinephrine also decreases the amount of intraoperative bleeding during surgical excision. We recommend a maximum epinephrine dosage equivalence of 0.01 mg/mL (concentration of 1:100 000). The maximum recommended dose of lidocaine combined with epinephrine is 4.5 mg/kg, equivalent to a maximum volume of 0.45 mL per kilogram of bodyweight. For an average newborn weighing 4 kg, the maximum volume of lidocaine combined with epinephrine is only 1.8 mL. Traditionally, it was considered inadvisable to use epinephrine in procedures involving end-arterial structures, such as distal digits, penis or pinnae of the ear, due to vasoconstriction and necrosis risks, although recent guidelines have not supported this [4].

A disadvantage of lidocaine as a local anaesthetic is the pain associated with its injection. The addition of 8.4% sodium bicarbonate (1 mmol/mL) to 1% lidocaine (with or without epinephrine) in a ratio of 1:10 has been shown to decrease pain without significant alteration of onset, extent or duration of anaesthesia [5]. The increase in the

Table 173.1 Properties of selected local anaesthetics

Local anaesthetic	Onset of action (min)	Duration of action (h)		Maximum dose	
		With epinephrine	Without epinephrine	With epinephrine	Without epinephrine
Amides					
Lidocaine	2	1.0–6.5	0.5–2.0	4.5 mg/kg	2.0 mg/kg
Bupivacaine	5	4.0–8.0	2.0–4.0	3 m/kg	2.0 mg/kg
Others: prilocaine, mepivacaine, levobupivacaine, ropivacaine					
Esters					
Procaine	6–10	0.5–1.5	0.25–0.5	1 g in adults	
Tetracaine	Slow	4.0–8.0	2.0–4.0	Unknown	
Others: cocaine, benzocaine, chloroprocaine					

pH of the mixture, as well as faster nerve penetration as a result of an increase in the proportion of the uncharged and more lipophilic form of the amide molecule, may explain the reduction in pain. Lidocaine is more soluble and has a longer shelf-life at acid pH. After the addition of bicarbonate as a buffer, the mixture should be refrigerated and used within one week, as the concentration of lidocaine and epinephrine decreases at room temperature and with extended storage [6]. The average duration of anaesthesia with plain lidocaine is 40–60 min, and is decreased to 30 min with the addition of sodium bicarbonate [7]. For extended procedures, the addition of epinephrine to lidocaine is recommended.

Adverse effects. Local adverse effects related to the injection include pain, haematoma or ecchymosis, nerve damage and vasovagal syncope.

Ester anaesthetics are more likely than amide anaesthetics to cause allergic reactions. Allergic reactions to ester anaesthetics are related to their metabolism to paraaminobenzoic acid, a potential allergen. True allergic reactions to lidocaine and other amide anaesthetics are rare, making up less than 1% of adverse reactions [2]. Cross-reactivity of allergic reactions between the amide and ester anaesthetic classes is rare.

Injection into a highly vascularized area, accidental intravascular injection or overdosage can result in high, possibly toxic, systemic concentrations which may cause adverse central nervous system (CNS) and cardiovascular effects. Initially, stimulation of the nervous system occurs, causing perioral tingling and numbness, anxiety, apprehension, restlessness, nervousness, disorientation, confusion, dizziness, blurring of vision, twitching, shivering or seizures. At greater doses, neurodepression can occur, resulting in unconsciousness, respiratory depression or coma. Cardiovascular toxicity is generally noted after CNS symptoms have developed [8]. Effects include prolonged electrocardiographic intervals, bradycardia, hypotension, decreased myocardial contractility and cardiac arrest. Bupivacaine is especially associated with cardiac toxicity; an increase in PR interval and major widening of QRS usually precede arrhythmias (ventricular tachycardia, rarely torsades de pointes).

References

1 Calverley RK, Scheller MS. Anesthesia as a specialty: past, present and future. In: Barash PG, Cullen BF, Stoelting RK (eds) Clinical Anesthesia, 2nd edn. Philadelphia: JB Lippincott, 1992:3–33.

2 Grekin RC, Auletta MJ. Local anesthesia in dermatology surgery. J Am Acad Dermatol 1988;19:599–614.

3 Norris RL. Local anesthetics. Emerg Med Clin North Am 1992;10: 707–18.

4 **Kouba DJ, LoPiccolo MC, Alam M et al. Guidelines for the use of local anesthesia in office-based dermatologic surgery. J Am Acad Dermatol 2016;74:1201–19.**

5 **Glass JS, Hardy CL, Meeks NM et al. Acute pain management in dermatology. J Am Acad Dermatol 2015;73:533–40.**

6 Larson PO, Ragi G, Swandby M et al. Stability of buffered lidocaine and adrenaline used for local anesthesia. J Dermatol Surg Oncol 1991;17:411–14.

7 Holmes SG. Choosing a local anesthetic. Dermatol Clin 1994;12: 817–23.

Techniques to decrease the pain of injection

There are multiple techniques that may be employed to decrease the pain of lidocaine infiltration [1]. Prior treatment of the injection site with topical anaesthetics such as eutectic mixture of local anaesthetics (EMLA) cream or liposomal lidocaine (LMX cream), pH buffering of the anaesthetic solution, using small gauge needles (e.g. 30 gauge), warming of the anaesthetic to body temperature, cooling the injection site with ice or ethyl chloride spray, and a slow injection rate minimize the pain of the injection. Counterstimulation techniques, such as pinching, rubbing or vibrating the skin of the injection site prior to infiltration, may reduce the pain of injection by activating substance P fibres in the skin [2].

Topical anaesthetics

In order to gain access to the sensory nerve endings, cutaneous analgesics must diffuse through the stratum corneum, which is the major barrier preventing local anaesthetics from penetrating the deeper tissue layers [3]. None of the topical agents to date, even when used under occlusion, produces reliable anaesthesia of the palms and soles.

Topical anaesthetics are convenient, cost-effective and associated with few adverse effects. Novel anaesthetic formulations and transdermal delivery systems are promising and may result in even more effective and safer topical analgesia in the future [4].

Eutectic mixture of local anaesthetics (EMLA)

EMLA cream is a mixture of 2.5% lidocaine and 2.5% prilocaine. EMLA melts at a lower temperature than lidocaine or prilocaine alone, resulting in a stable cream at room temperature. It has been shown in numerous clinical trials to be safe and efficacious for needlestick, venepuncture, intravenous catheterization, lumbar puncture, debridement of ulcers, ablative treatment of molluscum contagiosum, laser treatment on skin and genital mucosa, and other superficial skin surgery [5]. EMLA cream alone does not appear to provide sufficient analgesia for deep biopsies or scalpel excision of skin. Standard usage requires application of the product on the skin surface with an occlusive wrap, such as Tegaderm™ or cellophane wrap, for 60–120 min. Patch preparations may allow easier application with equivalent efficacy [6]. The maximum recommended doses for EMLA on intact healthy skin in children are shown in Table 173.2. The depth and degree of analgesia are related to the duration of application. The maximum depth of analgesia is 5 mm. Mucous membranes, genital skin and diseased skin with an impaired skin barrier function absorb more rapidly, allowing for shorter application times (5–40 min). The recommended application times for EMLA cream in selected procedures are shown in Table 173.3.

EMLA commonly causes blanching or erythema at the site of application. It may occasionally cause transient, local irritation, swelling, purpura or pruritus. Periorbital application should be avoided as corneal ulceration and irritation

Table 173.2 Recommended eutectic mixture of local anaesthetics dosing on intact and healthy skin in children

Age/bodyweight	Maximum dose (g)	Maximum application area (cm²)	Maximum application time (h)
0–3 months old or <5 kg	1	10	1
2–12 months old and >5 kg	2	20	4
1–6 years old and >10 kg	10	100	4
7–12 years old and >20 kg	20	200	4

Table 173.3 Recommended application times for EMLA cream in selected procedures

Indication	Application time (min)
Molluscum contagiosum	30–60 (15 in children with atopic dermatitis)
Skin biopsy (pretreatment)	60
Condylomata acuminata	5–15
Port wine stain (pulsed-dye laser)	60
Leg ulcers (debridement)	30
Vaccination	60

Source: Adapted from Kearns et al. 2003 [36].

are possible adverse effects [7]. Methaemoglobinaemia due to the prilocaine component, a potentially life-threatening complication, has been reported, mainly in neonates and infants less than 3 months of age as their methaemoglobin reductase pathway is immature [8]. However, of 14 case reports since 1985, there were only five neonates, four toddlers with widespread molluscum, four patients who were applying EMLA to large surface areas followed by laser surgery, and a 7-month-old infant with prolonged use while receiving inhaled nitric oxide [9–11]. Use of medications associated with methaemoglobinaemia (including sulphonamides, dapsone, benzocaine and chloroquine) may increase the risk of EMLA-associated methaemoglobinaemia in infants. CNS toxicity has been reported after excessive application of EMLA over an extensive area [12].

Liposomal lidocaine

Liposomal lidocaine (LMX) is a topical anaesthetic encapsulated in a phospholipid-based carrier. Liposomal vehicles facilitate and improve diffusion of the local anaesthetic through the dermis. In a systematic review, topical liposomal anaesthetics were found to be effective prior to dermal instrumentation [13]. Liposome-encapsulated lidocaine is commercially available in both 4% and 5% preparations. In comparative clinical trials, LMX (applied for 30 min) and EMLA (applied for 60 min) were equally effective in reducing the pain associated with venepuncture and intravenous catheter insertion in children [14,15]. The faster onset of anaesthesia with LMX is an advantage in paediatric clinical practice. In studies carried out in adults, LMX has been shown to produce a longer duration of analgesia as the phospholipid carrier serves to maintain a longer localization of the anaesthetic [16–18].

While the absence of prilocaine prevents the risk of methaemoglobinaemia, there is still the risk for systemic toxicity with the use of LMX. An infant was reported who developed seizures, tachycardia, diffuse erythematous rash and locked jaw following application of 2.5 ampoules of 2 mL of 2% topical lidocaine, applied to the foreskin, translating to 100 mg, equivalent to a dose of 11 mg/kg in an area of rapid absorption. The patient recovered after midazolam and sodium thiopental, and required reintubation [19]. LMX should not be applied for more than 2 h in order to avoid excessive systemic levels of lidocaine. In children weighing less then 20 kg, LMX should not be applied to a surface area greater than 100 cm² [20].

Sensitization to lidocaine is increasing and has been associated with contact dermatitis. Retrospective review of patch testing results over a four-year period at the University of British Columbia revealed that the prevalence of allergic contact dermatitis to topical lidocaine is increasing, probably as a result of the addition of lidocaine and other amides in a variety of over-the-counter topical products [21]. A report of 16 cases of contact allergy to lidocaine stated definite relevance of positive intradermal delayed reactions in two cases, past, probable and unknown in one case each, and possible relevance in 11 cases [22]. In patients with patch tests positive to lidocaine, a rechallenge with intradermal lidocaine should be performed to help confirm clinical relevance [21].

Lidocaine ointment and spray

These lidocaine formulations work well as local anaesthetics when they are applied to mucosal surfaces such as those of the oropharynx, nose, vagina and cervix. However, they are not effective when applied to intact skin, as the lidocaine molecule is too big to penetrate the stratum corneum. Hence, EMLA cream is significantly more effective than 40% lidocaine ointment, even though the concentration of lidocaine in the latter formulation is many times greater [23].

Tetracaine formulations

Tetracaine is used in multiagent formulations for the repair of dermal lacerations. The first such agent, tetracaine/adrenaline/cocaine (TAC), was introduced in 1980. In recent years, other tetracaine-containing topical anaesthetics, such as lidocaine/epinephrine/tetracaine (LET), have replaced TAC due to the potential of cocaine to produce adverse effects [24]. Both tetracaine and liposomal tetracaine have been found to provide equivalent, if not greater, efficacy than EMLA for instrumentation of intact skin [25,26]. Pliaglis is a compounded mixture of 23% lidocaine and 7% tetracaine in ointment base that has become commonly used in laser therapy in adults, although it does not have paediatric indication [27]. Two cases of immediate vesicular eruption have been reported with resolution after one week and no reaction on rechallenge to LMX alone [27].

Lidocaine/tetracaine patch

A lidocaine/tetracaine patch is a topical agent that consists of a eutectic formulation of 70 mg lidocaine and 70 mg tetracaine and uses an oxygen-activated heating element to enhance delivery of the local anaesthetic. The temperature of the patch increases once removed from the package, which subsequently warms the underlying skin after application. In one study it provided appropriate analgesia after 20 min of application for venepuncture in children; only transient and minor side-effects, such as erythema and oedema, were noted [28].

Subcutaneous infusion anaesthesia

In the tumescent technique used for subcutaneous infusion anaesthesia, large volumes of highly diluted local anaesthetics, such as ropivacaine or prilocaine, are instilled into the subcutaneous layer by infusion pumps [29,30]. This provides profound perioperative anaesthesia owing to slow absorption from the relatively avascular subcutaneous fat. It also provides hydrodissection of the skin from underlying vessels and nerves, facilitating surgery. However, further studies need to be done to evaluate the feasibility of this technique in paediatric dermatological surgery [31].

Iontophoresis devices

Iontophoresis devices have been advocated for needleless delivery of local anaesthetics. A low-voltage direct current is applied to skin immersed in a local anaesthetic solution or placed under an anaesthetic-impregnated patch, facilitating transfer across the stratum corneum. Lidocaine iontophoresis has a rapid onset of anaesthesia (within 10 min) and appears to be as efficacious as EMLA cream and local lidocaine injection in providing pain relief for intravenous cannulation in children [32–35]. A study conducted in children 5–15 years of age found that the subjects tolerated iontophoresis well and systemic levels of lidocaine were low [36].

A prospective trial evaluating lignocaine iontophoresis in 60 children undergoing shave biopsy, curettage, injection and punch biopsy revealed that most of the subjects did not require any supplemental anaesthesia. No significant adverse events were reported [37].

Needle-free injection devices

Needle-free injection devices use high gas pressure to accelerate fine drug particles to supersonic speed and deliver them into the skin. Several clinical trials studying paediatric patients demonstrated the clinical efficacy of needle-free injections [38–40]. However, another study showed that a needle-free injection device is not completely painless or cost-effective [41].

Topical anaesthesia for mucosal surfaces

Topical Cetacaine® (benzocaine 14%, tetracaine 2%), benzocaine, viscous lidocaine, liposomal lidocaine and EMLA are effective topical agents for inducing mucosal anaesthesia. Anaesthetic effect is almost immediate upon application. These agents are useful for decreasing the pain of intralesional lidocaine injection, but are insufficient for scalpel surgery when used alone. In infants, the use of Cetacaine and benzocaine should be avoided because of the risk of methaemoglobinaemia [42]. While benzocaine is a known sensitizer, allergic contact dermatitis seldom occurs when it is used preoperatively, presumably because of lack of prior exposure and sensitization.

References

1 Eichenfield LF, Weilepp A. Pain control in pediatric procedures. Curr Opin Dermatol 1997;4:151–61.

2 Barnhill BJ, Holbert MD, Jackson NM, Erickson RS. Using pressure to decrease the pain of intramuscular injections. J Pain Symptom Manage 1996;12:52–8.

3 Friedman PM, Mafong EA, Friedman ES, Geronmus RG. Topical anesthetics update: EMLA and beyond. Dermatol Surg 2001;27: 1019–26.

4 Houck CS, Sethna NF. Transdermal analgesia with local anesthetics in children: review, update and future directions. Expert Rev Neurother 2005;5:625–34.

5 Garjraj NM, Pennant JH, Watcha MR. Eutectic mixture of local anesthetics (EMLA). Anesth Analg 1994;78:574–83.

6 Chang PC, O'Connor G, Rogers PJC et al. A multicentre randomized study of single-unit dose package of EMLA patch vs. EMLA cream 5% for venepuncture in children. Can J Anesth 1994;41:59–63.

7 McKinlay JR, Hofmeister E, Ross EV. EMLA cream-induced eye injury. Arch Dermatol 1999;135:855–6.

8 Jakobson B, Nilsson A. Methaemoglobinemia in children treated with prilocaine-lidocaine cream and trimethoprim-sulphamethoxazole. A case report. Acta Anaesth Scand 1985;29:453–5.

9 Touma S, Jackson JB. Lidocaine and prilocaine toxicity in a patient receiving treatment for mollusca contagiosa. J Am Acad Dermatol 2001;44:399–400.

10 Sinisterra S, Miravet E, Alfonso I et al. Methemoglobinemia in an infant receiving nitric oxide after the use of eutectic mixture of local anesthetic. J Pediatr 2002;141:285–6.

11 Shamriz O, Cohen-Glickman I, Reif S, Shteyer E. Methemoglobinemia induced by lidocaine-prilocaine cream. Isr Med Assoc J 2014;16: 250–4.

12 Rincon E, Baker RL, Iglesias AJ et al. CNS toxicity after topical application of EMLA cream on a toddler with molluscum contagiosum. Pediatr Emerg Care 2000;16:252–4.

13 Eidelman A, Weiss JM, Lau J, Carr DB. Topical anesthetics for dermal instrumentation: a systematic review of randomized, controlled trials. Ann Emerg Med 2005;46:343–51.

14 Eichenfield LF, Funk A, Fallon-Friedlander S et al. A clinical study to evaluate the efficacy of ELA-Max (4% liposomal lidocaine) as compared with eutectic mixture of local anesthetics cream for pain reduction of venepuncture in children. Pediatrics 2002;109:1093–9.

15 Kleiber C, Sorenson M, Whiteside K et al. Topical anesthetics for intravenous insertion in children: a randomized equivalency study. Pediatrics 2002;110:758–61.

16 Bucalo BD, Mirikitani EJ, Moy RL. Comparison of skin anesthetic effect of liposomal lidocaine, nonliposomal lidocaine, and EMLA using 30-minute application time. Dermatol Surg 1998;24:537–41.

17 el-Ridy MS, Khalil RM. Free versus liposome-encapsulated lignocaine hydrochloride topical applications. Pharmazie 1999;54:682–4.

18 Friedman PM, Fogelman JP, Nouri K et al. Comparative study of the efficacy of four topical anesthetics. Dermatol Surg 1999;25:950–4.

19 Özer AB, Erhan ÖL. Systemic toxicity to local anesthesia in an infant undergoing circumcision. Agri 2014;26(1):43–6.

20 Friedman PM, Mafong EA, Friedman ES, Geronmus RG. Topical anesthetics update: EMLA and beyond. Dermatol Surg 2001;27: 1019–26.

21 To D, Kossintseva I, de Gannes G. Lidocaine contact allergy is becoming more prevalent. Dermatol Surg 2014;40(12):1367–72.

22 Amado A, Sood A, Taylor JS. Contact allergy to lidocaine: a report of sixteen cases. Dermatitis 2007;18(4):215–20.

23 Hernandez E, Gonzalez S, Gonzalez E. Evaluation of topical anesthetics by laser-induced sensation: comparison of EMLA 5% cream and 40% lidocaine in an acid mantle ointment. Lasers Surg Med 1998; 23:167–71.

24 Bush S. Is cocaine needed in topical anaesthesia? Emerg Med J 2002; 19:418–22.

25 Carceles MD, Alonso JM, Garcia-Munoz M et al. Amethocaine-lidocaine cream, a new topical formulation for preventing venepuncture-induced pain in children. Reg Anesth Pain Med 2002;27:289–95.
26 Eidelman A, Weiss JM, Lau J, Carr DB. Topical anesthetics for dermal instrumentation: a systematic review of randomized, controlled trials. Ann Emerg Med 2005;46:343–51.
27 Vij A, Markus R. Immediate vesicular eruption caused by topical 23% lidocaine 7% tetracaine ointment in a patient scheduled for laser therapy: a new adverse drug reaction. J Cosmet Dermatol 2011;10(4):307–10.
28 Sethna NF, Verghese ST, Hannallah RS et al. A randomized controlled trial to evaluate S-Caine patch for reducing pain associated with vascular access in children. Anesthesiology 2005;102:403–8.
29 Moehrle M, Breuninger H. Dermatosurgery using subcutaneous infusion anesthesia with prilocaine and ropivacaine in children. Pediatr Dermatol 2001;18:469–72.
30 Breuninger H, Nogova L, Hobbach PS, Schimek F. Ropivacaine, an advantageous anesthetic for subcutaneous infusion anesthesia. Hautarzt 2000;51:759–62.
31 Dohil MA, Eichenfield LF. Subcutaneous infusion anesthesia for dermatologic surgery in children: are we ready? Pediatr Dermatol 2001; 18:532–3.
32 Zempsky WT, Anand KJ, Sullivan KM et al. Lidocaine iontophoresis for topical anesthesia before intravenous line placement in children. J Pediatr 1998;132:1061–3.
33 Galinkin JL, Rose JB, Harris K et al. Lidocaine iontophoresis versus eutectic mixture of local anesthetics (EMLA) for IV placement in children. Anesth Analg 2002;94:1484–8.
34 Kim MK, Kini NM, Troshynski TJ et al. A randomized clinical trial of dermal anesthesia by iontophoresis for peripheral intravenous catheter placement in children. Ann Emerg Med 1999;33:395–9.
35 Sherwin J, Awad IT, Sadler PJ et al. Analgesia during radial artery cannulation. Comparison of the effects of lidocaine applied by local injection iontophoresis. Anaesthesia 2003;58:474–6.
36 Kearns GL, Heacook J, Daly SJ et al. Percutaneous lidocaine administration via a new iontophoresis system in children: tolerability and absence of systemic bioavailability. Pediatrics 2003;112:578–82.
37 Zempsky WT, Parkinson TM. Lidocaine iontophoresis for topical anesthesia before dermatologic procedures in children: a randomized controlled trial. Pediatr Dermatol 2003;20:364–8.
38 Wolf AR, Stoddart PA, Murphy PJ et al. Rapid skin anaesthesia using high velocity lignocaine particles: a prospective placebo controlled trial. Arch Dis Child 2002;86:309–12.
39 Munshi AK, Hegde A, Bashir N. Clinical evaluation of the efficacy of anesthesia and patient preference using the needle-less jet syringe in pediatric dental practice. J Clin Pediatr Dent 2001;25:131–6.
40 Zempsky WT, Bean-Lijewski J, Kauffman RE et al. Needle-free powder lidocaine delivery system provides rapid effective analgesia for venipuncture or cannulation pain in children: randomized, double-blind Comparison of Venipuncture and Venous Cannulation Pain after Fast-Onset Needle-Free Powder Lidocaine or Placebo Treatment Trial. Pediatrics 2008;121(5):979–87.
41 Lysakowski C, Dumont L, Tramer MR, Tassonyi E. A needle-free jet injection system with lidocaine for peripheral intravenous cannula insertion: a randomized controlled trial with cost-effectiveness analysis. Anesth Analg 2003;96:215–19.
42 Nguyen ST, Cabrales RE, Bashour CA et al. Benzocaine-induced methemoglobinemia. Anesth Analg 2000;90:369–71.

Perioperative analgesics

Adjuvant agents can be used to provide perioperative analgesia for paediatric patients. The use of acetaminophen alone (15–20 mg/kg orally or 20 mg/kg per rectum) may be useful for perioperative pain.

Codeine has been utilized as a perioperative medication, although its safety and efficacy have been called into question. Codeine is converted into its active metabolite, morphine, by the cytochrome P450 isoenzyme 2D6 (CYP2D6). There is significant variability in the gene encoding for CYP2D6 which results in a wide range of phenotypes from poor metabolizers (slow rate of conversion to morphine) to ultra-rapid metabolizers [1]. A series of respiratory arrest in ultra-rapid metabolizing children treated with codeine after having just undergone adenotonsillectomy has been well documented by the Food and Drug Administration (FDA) which now strongly recommends against the use of codeine in children after a tonsillectomy and/or adenoidectomy and asks healthcare professionals to use an alternative pain reliever [2].

These are rare, yet catastrophic cases of rapid metabolizers with specific risk factors such as recent tonsillectomy and viral symptoms, but the benefit of codeine in general may not be worth the risk of these rare adverse events [3]. One randomized control trial found the percentage of poor metabolizers to be 46% in an urban population of children, and regardless of CYP2D6 phenotypes, all patients had subtherapeutic plasma levels of morphine within one hour after administration of codeine [4].

Alternatives to codeine, such as morphine, may be easier than codeine to titrate to an effective dose. Acetaminophen and nonsteroidal antiinflammatory agents lack the sedative properties of codeine but still can be effective analgesics that avoid respiratory risks. Hydrocodone may be utilized and, similar to codeine, may have a moderate sedative effect, which is particularly useful in young children. Nonsteroidal antiinflammatory agents such as ibuprofen and ketorolac may also be used, although their effects on platelet function and haemostasis should be considered.

Oral sucrose

The use of 24% oral sucrose solution administered to the anterior tip of the tongue via needleless syringe or a pacifier dip is an effective option for decreasing pain in infants undergoing brief minor painful procedures, such as intralesional corticosteroid treatment for infantile haemangioma [5].

References

1 Crews KR, Gaedigk A, Dunnenberger HM et al. Clinical pharmacogenetics implementation consortium guidelines for cytochrome P450 2D6 genotype and codeine therapy: 2014 Update. Clin Pharmacol Therapeut 2014;95:376–82.
2 FDA Drug Safety Communication. Safety review update of codeine use in children; new *Boxed Warning* and *Contraindication* on use after tonsillectomy and/or adenoidectomy. Released February 20, 2013. www.fda.gov/downloads/Drugs/DrugSafety/UCM339116.pdf
3 Racoosin JA, Roberson DW, Pacanowski MA, Nielsen DR. New evidence about an old drug – risk with codeine after adenotonsillectomy. N Engl J Med 2013;368(23):2155–7.
4 Williams DG, Patel A, Howard RF. Pharmacogenetics of codeine metabolism in an urban population of children and its implications for analgesic reliability. Br J Anaesth 2002;89(6):839–45.
5 Sorrell J, Carmichael C, Chamlin S. Oral sucrose for pain relief in young infants with hemangiomas treated with intralesional steroids. Pediatr Dermatol 2010;27:154–5.

Sedation

Sedation should be considered as a continuum within which a patient may drift from a state of consciousness to deep sedation and on to general anaesthesia. This continuum can be extremely variable and depends on individual response, age, health status and drug combinations used (Table 173.4).

Table 173.4 Continuum of depth of sedation

	Minimal sedation (anxiolysis)	Moderate sedation (conscious sedation)	Deep sedation/analgesia	General anaesthesia
Responsiveness	Normal response to verbal stimulation	Purposeful* response to verbal or tactile stimulation	Purposeful* response after repeated or painful stimulation	Unrousable, even with painful stimulus
Airway	Unaffected	No intervention required	Intervention may be required	Intervention often required
Spontaneous ventilation	Unaffected	Adequate	May be inadequate	Frequently inadequate
Cardiovascular function	Unaffected	Usually maintained	Usually maintained	May be impaired

*Reflex withdrawal from a painful stimulus is not considered a purposeful response.

Definitions relevant to sedation as proposed by the American Society of Anesthesiologists are listed below.

- *Minimal sedation ('anxiolysis')*: a drug-induced state during which patients respond normally to verbal commands. Although cognitive function and coordination may be impaired, ventilatory and cardiovascular functions are unaffected.
- *Moderate sedation ('conscious sedation')*: a drug-induced depression of consciousness during which patients respond purposefully to verbal commands, either alone or accompanied by light tactile stimulation. Reflex withdrawal from a painful stimulus is not considered a purposeful response. No interventions are required to maintain a patent airway, and spontaneous ventilation is adequate. Cardiovascular function is usually maintained.
- *Deep sedation/analgesia*: a drug-induced depression of consciousness during which patients cannot be easily aroused but respond purposefully following repeated or painful stimulation. The ability to independently maintain ventilatory function may be impaired. Patients may require assistance in maintaining a patent airway and spontaneous ventilation may be inadequate. Cardiovascular function is usually maintained. Reflex withdrawal from a painful stimulus is not considered a purposeful response.
- *Anaesthesia*: a drug-induced loss of consciousness during which patients are not arousable, even by painful stimulation. The ability to independently maintain ventilatory function is often impaired. Patients often require assistance in maintaining a patent airway, and positive pressure ventilation may be required because of depressed spontaneous ventilation or drug-induced depression of neuromuscular function. Cardiovascular function may be impaired.

To ensure the highest level of patient safety in the use of sedation for dermatological and diagnostic procedures in children in both office and hospital settings, providers should conform to the updated guidelines for the use of sedation established in collaboration by the American Academy of Pediatrics and the American Academy of Pediatric Dentistry [1]. These guidelines dictate the appropriate level of monitoring, equipment required, implementation of sedation protocols and staff training [1]. In general, deep sedation and general anaesthesia for dermatological procedures in children are most safely performed with the assistance of an anaesthetist. Moderate and deep sedation may be safely performed in an ambulatory setting if the facility and staff are appropriately equipped and trained.

Selecting an appropriate sedative technique requires preoperative assessment of the child's medical status, the degree of pain expected during the procedure, the duration of the procedure, the need or absence of need for the child to be motionless, the expertise of the practitioner performing the sedation, the facility resources for monitoring the patient and responding to adverse events, and knowledge of minimal levels of monitoring and personnel required for the level of sedation used [1]. Preoperative assessment must include the general health of the child, with the awareness that underlying systemic diseases and drug interactions may greatly increase the risk of adverse events. As protective airway reflexes may be compromised to varying degrees depending upon the type and dosage of sedative agents used, as well as the patient's baseline medical condition, adequate 'nil by mouth' status should be ensured for elective sedative procedures.

Monitoring requirements were updated in 2011 based on evidence that the use of capnography improves detection of respiratory depression and reduces the incidence of hypoventilation by capnography over pulse oximetry [2]. In addition to blood pressure and pulse oximetry, which continuously measure heart rate and arterial oxygen saturation using a spectrophotometric technique, capnography is now strongly recommended for moderate sedation and is required in addition to intravenous access for deep sedation [1].

References

1 Coté CJ, Wilson S, American Academy of Pediatrics, American Academy of Pediatric Dentistry. Guidelines for monitoring and management of pediatric patients before, during, and after sedation for diagnostic and therapeutic procedures: update 2016. Pediatrics 2016;138(1).

2 Waugh JB, Epps CA, Khodneva YA. Capnography enhances surveillance of respiratory events during procedural sedation: a meta-analysis. J Clin Anesth 2011;23:189–96.

Pharmacological agents

There is a broad array of medications that can be used as sedative, hypnotic, analgesic and anaesthetic agents. Analgesia refers to the relief of pain, amnesia to lack of memory, hypnosis to lack of consciousness and sedation to a decrease in consciousness. Anxiolytic agents decrease anxiety but have no analgesic effects. Local, topical or regional anaesthesia, together with sedatives that can induce amnesia, may produce the desired effect of a painless or minimally painful experience not remembered by the patient.

Benzodiazepines

Benzodiazepines are sedative agents with potent anxiolytic effects but no analgesic properties. They vary mainly based on duration and onset of action. Diazepam is becoming much less popular than midazolam due to its longer and more unpredictable duration of action [1].

Midazolam is a short-acting benzodiazepine that is useful for perioperative sedation in children. However, it is known to cause paradoxical reactions in children and is not recommended in premature infants or neonates [1]. After intravenous administration, the medication acts rapidly (1–5 min) and has a short duration of action (less than 2 h). Routes of administration include intravenous, oral, intramuscular and rectal. Intravenous dosing is 0.02–0.1 mg/kg, not exceeding 5 mg. Intranasal and oral routes require higher dosing owing to variable absorption: oral and nasal dosing is 0.2–0.5 mg/kg, up to 15 mg. Midazolam has potent anxiolytic effects and the anterograde amnesic effect is profound, making the agent useful for repetitive procedures (e.g. pulsed-dye laser treatment). Premedication with oral midazolam significantly reduces the pain of intravenous catheter insertion [2]. The addition of an analgesic agent, such as acetaminophen/codeine or fentanyl, may be reasonable, although the combination increases the risks of respiratory depression [3]. Pulse oximetry monitoring is recommended as higher doses of midazolam are associated with transient drops in transcutaneous oxygen saturation.

Remimazolam is a new benzodiazepine that has completed phase III clinical trials and has proven to be metabolized much faster than midazolam. It is metabolized by tissue esterases and thus has a rapid, predictable offset of action. Thus, it has potential for future use as a procedural sedative but is not yet available for use [4].

Flumazenil is the specific antagonist for benzodiazepines, and may reverse the depressant effects in a dose-dependent fashion. Incremental doses of 0.01 mg/kg can be administered intravenously over 15 seconds. There is risk of seizure, arrhythmia and resedation with this medication. Doses may be repeated every 60 seconds as needed to a maximum of four additional doses (0.05 mg/kg, maximum dose 1 mg).

Barbiturates

Barbiturates are potent sedative agents with amnesic effects. These medications are nonspecific CNS depressants and have more profound respiratory and cardiovascular depressant effects than benzodiazepines. Thiopental is the only barbiturate that is still used widely in other countries but is not available in the United States [1]. Barbiturates have no analgesic effect. Their use in paediatric procedures has decreased greatly as a result of the better safety profile of benzodiazepines.

Dexmedetomidine

One of the newest sedative drugs, dexmetomidine, an α2 agonist similar to clonidine, has favourable sedative and anxiolytic properties, fast onset and minimal cardiovascular or respiratory effects. It can be administered via many routes: mucosal (intranasal and buccal), oral and intravenous (bolus and infusion). It causes initial hypertension and bradycardia which then stabilize below baseline without treatment [5]. It is FDA approved in adults during mechanical ventilation, but is not currently approved for use in children. However, there are increasing reports of its off-label use in children and it may have potential for use in paediatric populations in the future.

Ketamine

Ketamine is an anaesthetic agent that may be given via the intramuscular or intravenous routes. It produces profound sedation, amnesia and analgesia, and induces a 'trance-like' state ('dissociative anaesthesia'). Onset is rapid: 1 min for the intravenous route (0.5 mg with an infusion of 0.01–0.2 mg/kg/min) and 5 min for the intramuscular route (0.5–1 mg/kg). Duration of sedation is quite variable, usually less than 90 min, but may be longer in some individuals [6]. It should be used together with an antisialagogue agent (e.g. atropine) at a dose of 0.01–0.02 mg/kg to attenuate the increase in salivary secretions. Postoperative nausea and prolonged unarousability are problems associated with its use. Ketamine may cause unpleasant dreams and emergence reactions. It is contraindicated in paediatric patients with active upper or lower airway disease, head injury, epilepsy or acute eye globe injury.

Opiates

Opiates are primarily used for analgesia, often as adjuncts to sedative agents. Morphine and fentanyl are potent analgesics. Morphine causes release of histamine, has a slower onset and longer duration of action. Fentanyl, a synthetic opiate agonist, has a rapid onset (within 5 min) and relatively short duration of action (30–60 min) when given intravenously (1–3 μg/kg), allowing titration of medication for pain relief with less risk of prolonged respiratory depression and hypotension. Fentanyl lozenges have been utilized for paediatric procedures, but studies to date report conflicting results with regard to its efficacy as a premedication [7–9]. Codeine is the least tolerated opiate and is no longer recommended because patients who are rapid metabolizers are at risk for severe adverse events, and contrarily 10% of patients lack the enzyme to metabolize it to its active form, which gives them no analgesic benefit [10].

Naloxone is the antidote for opiate overdosage. Incremental doses of 0.01 mg/kg can be administered intravenously and may be repeated every 2–3 min as needed. Patients who receive naloxone should be observed for at least 1 h to detect recurrence of sedation.

Chloral hydrate

Chloral hydrate is a sedative agent that has been used in children for several decades. Doses of 50–75 mg/kg (up to 100 mg/kg) are administered orally. Chloral hydrate has a slow onset (30–60 min) and induces sleep lasting 4–8 h, with amnesic effect. It requires prolonged monitoring both during and at the conclusion of a procedure. It lacks analgesic properties. Common adverse effects include nausea, vomiting and diarrhoea. Deaths have been reported from chloral hydrate use, most commonly from overdosage or its use in children with underlying cardiac or systemic disease. It has been reported to cause liver tumours, but there is no evidence that children receiving sedative dosages are at risk for this [11].

Propofol

Propofol is an intravenous anaesthetic that provides rapid onset of sedation; it is an aqueous formulation that appears milky in colour. The agent has an almost immediate onset of sedation, produces relatively limited haemodynamic instability and has a short duration of action, allowing a 'clean head wake-up' without the nausea or hangover effect commonly associated with traditional gas anaesthetics. Antiemetic properties have also been observed. The agent should not be given for prolonged periods of time at high doses as there is a risk of developing propofol-related infusion syndrome (PRIS) [1,12]. PRIS is often fatal and is characterized by refractory bradycardia leading to asystole in the presence of metabolic acidosis, rhabdomyolysis, hyperlipidaemia and/or liver enlargement.

There is some controversy regarding the nociceptive effect of propofol, but it does not have profound analgesic qualities and concurrent analgesics for painful procedures are appropriate. In a study of propofol anaesthesia in 48 children undergoing outpatient pulsed-dye laser treatment, 62% were calm and pain free upon awakening. The mean recovery time was 25 min, and none of the patients experienced emesis [13]. Propofol induction and halothane maintenance were shown to be associated with a lower incidence of adverse events during induction, postoperative nausea and vomiting, and postoperative delirium compared with sevoflurane anaesthesia [14]. Respiratory depression is dose dependent, and hypoxia and apnoea are not uncommon, thus limiting its use to well-equipped facilities with staff who are proficient in critical airway and ventilatory management.

Neurotoxicity caused by propofol is found in young nonhuman primates and rodents when administered early during brain development in the absence of noxious stimuli. The first report in 1999 was of newborn rats exposed within the first week of life to anaesthetic agents which induced widespread apoptotic neurodegeneration [15]. These early findings were extended to include other NMDA receptor antagonists such as nitrous oxide, and to γ-aminobutyric acid (GABA) receptor agonists, including isoflurane, propofol, benzodiazapines and barbiturates [16]. However, no neurotoxic effects have been found in humans and in fact, neuroprotective benefits are found when given during pathogenic situations.

Nitrous oxide

Nitrous oxide (N_2O) is a gas anaesthetic that has analgesic effects and rapidly induces a sedated, dissociative state with a euphoric feeling and profound amnesic effect. When used alone, 35–50% N_2O has analgesic properties with minimal respiratory and cardiovascular effects [17,18]. It is commonly administered with other agents to achieve general anaesthesia. There is an extensive history of its use in paediatric procedures. N_2O use requires extensive training and/or credentialling of personnel, a fail-safe system for oxygen/gas delivery to prevent anoxia, a scavenger device to eliminate gas traces and continuous oximetry monitoring.

Concerns have been raised about possible teratogenicity and spontaneous abortions from N_2O gas [19]. Nitrous oxide is a weak teratogen in rats that are exposed to it at high concentrations for long periods of time [20,21]. Large survey studies that evaluated outcomes in women who had anaesthesia, including nitrous oxide, for surgery during pregnancy suggested no increase in congenital anomalies, but rather an increase in the risk for abortions and low-birthweight neonates [22,23]. This increased risk was attributed to the requirement for surgery and not the anaesthesia. Despite the lack of clinical evidence, delaying the use of nitrous oxide in pregnant teenagers until the second trimester may reduce the risks for teratogenicity and spontaneous abortion.

General gas anaesthesia

The use of general gas anaesthesia is appropriate for painful but essential surgical procedures in children which cannot be safely or effectively performed with the use of local anaesthetics and sedative agents. The decision to utilize general anaesthesia has to be individualized and depends on the age and underlying health of the patient, the extent and location of the planned procedure and the need for a motionless patient, as well as on the medical and personnel resources available to induce and administer anaesthetic agents appropriately, including monitoring and ensuring safe postoperative recovery. Recommended preoperative fasting intervals for infant formula vary from 4 to 8 h. In healthy infants, formula may be consumed up to 4 h before surgery without any increase in gastric volume compared with infants who have not consumed formula 8 h before surgery [24]. A variety of anaesthetic gases are commonly used, including halothane, isoflurane, sevofluorane and N_2O. Children, especially infants, may be better served by paediatric anaesthetists who have considerable experience in working with this patient population [25].

The risks of general anaesthesia are dependent upon a variety of factors, including the age of the patient and underlying systemic conditions [26]. An increased risk of complications is associated with the use of general anaesthesia in the first year of life, with an even greater risk assigned to the first month of life [27–29]. New data regarding general anaesthesia and effects on the developing brain in animals have raised concerns regarding the potential for neurotoxic effects in young children. In animal studies, general anaesthesia medications at high doses during vulnerable times of rapid brain growth may impair brain development [30].

The findings in these animal studies cannot be directly translated to humans but have since inspired multiple studies to investigate the association between exposure to anaesthesia in early children and neurodevelopmental delay later in life [31–33]. While a systematic review summarizing epidemiological data suggested a potential influence of anaesthesia/surgery on later neurodevelopmental deficit affected by number of anaesthetic exposures before 4 years of age, the authors comment that the limitations of the study were many and that the possible association that was found 'should be taken cautiously in the context of the data upon which it is based' [34]. Other studies have not shown neurocognitive effects in children younger than 3 with a single general anesthesia event [31].

In December 2016, the United States Food and Drug Administration published guidance regarding the repeated or prolonged (>3h) use of medications for general anaesthesia and sedation. Mandated warning labels are now to be included when using these agents, and advice indicated delaying use of these agents for infants and children below 3 years of age or for pregnant mothers in their third trimester for procedures that are elective [35].

Impact of anaesthesia safety data in dermatology paediatric surgery

The short-term safety of general anaesthesia in healthy children undergoing paediatric dermatological surgery has enabled substantial growth of this field in the past 10 years, especially in the number of laser procedures done under general anaesthesia for the treatment of port wine stain (PWS), haemangiomas and disfiguring scars [36].

While long-term effects of anaesthesia in young children are under investigation, with inconclusive results, the risks and benefits of early treatment under general anaesthesia should be considered and individualized. Early dermatological procedures that lessen the degree of long-term functional impairment or deformity may be appropriate despite the need for multiple anaesthesic events. For example, in the treatment of facial PWS in children, one goal is to achieve the maximum amount of lightening early in life so as to lessen the psychological impact in adolescence [37]. Over time, PWS thickens, darkens and develops nodular blebs, all of which make the lesion less responsive to treatment. Early laser treatment of hypertrophic PWS was recently reviewed in a retrospective trial which found that initiation of treatment before the ages of 2 or 6 years allowed a significantly higher number to achieve at least 50% improvement [38]. Effective treatment may require multiple sessions to achieve the desired degree of lightening and it has been recommended that procedures might ideally be initiated prior to development of self-awareness [39].

Laser surgery of smaller lesions is often done using topical anaesthesics. However, inadequate management of procedural pain is known to negatively affect a child's response to pain and may have a long-term psychological impact [40], so multimodal methods of minimizing pain and anxiety may be reasonable, including perioperative pain medications or anxiolytics.

When weighing the risk of general anaesthesia in children versus delay in therapy, the psychosocial and functional effects of birthmarks, scars and other skin conditions must also be considered.

Laryngeal masks

Induction of anaesthesia with inhalational gases (halothane, isoflurane, desflurane, sevoflurane) is done with mask inhalation, followed by endotracheal visualization and intubation. Laryngeal masks are devices that allow placement of a hypopharyngeal airway, without the need for visualization or intubation of the trachea. After initial facemask induction of anaesthesia, the device – a deflated 'mask on a stick' – is placed in the mouth and pushed towards and below the epiglottis superior to the vocal cords. It is then inflated using a syringe (similar to a Foley catheter) and the breathing loop is connected to the exposed end. Both the effort of breathing by the patient and the procedural workload required of the anaesthetist associated with the insertion of the laryngeal mask compare favourably with endotracheal intubation [41,42]. The use of this device has gained widespread acceptance in paediatric surgical patients in whom there is no 'critical airway', and it has been used successfully for dermatological and laser surgery in children.

References

1 **Hansen TG. Sedative medications outside the operating room and the pharmacology of sedatives. Curr Opin Anesthesiol 2015;48:446–52.**
2 McErlean M, Bartfield JM, Karunakar TA et al. Midazolam syrup as a premedication to reduce the discomfort associated with pediatric intravenous catheter insertion. J Pediatr 2003;142:429–30.
3 Yaster M, Nichols DG, Desphande JK et al. Midazolam-fentanyl intravenous sedation in children: case report of respiratory arrest. Pediatrics 1990;86:463–7.
4 Gin T. Hypnotic and sedative drugs – anything new on the horizon? Curr Opin Anesthesiol 2013;26(4):409–13.
5 Kost S, Roy A. Procedural sedation and analgesia in the pediatric emergency department: a review of sedative pharmacology. Clin Pediatr Emerg Med 2010;11(4):233–43.
6 Green SM, Nakamura R, Johnson NE. Ketamine sedation for pediatric procedures. Part 1. A prospective series. Ann Emerg Med 1990;19: 1024–32.
7 Ashburn MA, Streisand JB, Tarver SD et al. Oral transmucosal fentanyl citrate for premedication in paediatric outpatients. Can J Anesth 1990;37:857–66.
8 Howell TK, Smith S, Rushman SC et al. A comparison of oral transmucosal fentanyl and oral midazolam for premedication in children. Anaesthesia 2002;57:798–805.
9 Klein EJ, Diekema DS, Paris CA et al. A randomized, clinical trial of oral midazolam plus placebo versus oral midazolam plus oral transmucosal fentanyl for sedation during laceration repair. Pediatrics 2002;109:894–7.
10 **Glass JM, Hardy CL, Meeks NM et al. Acute pain management in dermatology. J Am Acad Dermatol 2015;73:533–40.**
11 American Academy of Pediatrics Committee on Drugs and Committee on Environmental Health. Use of chloral hydrate for sedation in children. Pediatrics 1993;94:471–3.
12 Kam PC, Cardone D. Propofol infusion syndrome. Anaesthesia 2007; 62(7):690–701.
13 Vischoff D, Charest J. Propofol for pulsed dye laser treatments in pediatric outpatients. Can J Anesth 1994;41:728–32.
14 Moore JK, Moore EW, Elliott RA et al. Propofol and halothane versus sevoflurane in paediatric day-case surgery: induction and recovery characteristics. Br J Anaesth 2003;90:461–6.
15 Ikonomidou C, Bosch F, Miksa M et al. Blockade of NMDA receptors and apoptotic neurodegeneration in the developing brain. Science 1999;283(5398):70–4.

16 **Rappaport BA, Suresh S, Hertz S et al. Anesthetic neurotoxicity – clinical implications of animal models. N Engl J Med 2015;372(9):796–7.**
17 American Academy of Pediatrics. Guidelines for monitoring and management of pediatric patients during and after sedation for diagnostic and therapeutic procedures. Pediatrics 1992;89:1110–15.
18 Litman RS, Berkowitz RJ, Ward DS. Levels of consciousness and ventilatory parameters in young children during sedation with oral midazolam and nitrous oxide. Arch Pediatr Adolesc Med 1996; 150:671–5.
19 Rowland AS, Baird DD, Weinberg CR et al. Reduced fertility among women employed as dental assistants exposed to high levels of nitrous oxide. N Engl J Med 1992;327:993–7.
20 Keeling PA, Rocke DA, Nunn JF et al. Folinic acid protection against nitrous oxide teratogenicity in the rat. Br J Anaesth 1986;58:528–34.
21 Fujinaga M, Baden JM, Yhap EO et al. Reproductive and teratogenic effects of nitrous oxide, isoflurane, and their combination in Sprague Dawley rats. Anesthesiology 1987;67:960–4.
22 Mazze RI, Kallen B. Reproductive outcome after anesthesia and operation during pregnancy. A registry study of 5405 cases. Am J Obstet Gynecol 1989;161:1178–85.
23 Mazze RI, Kallen B. Appendectomy during pregnancy. A Swedish registry study of 778 cases. Obstet Gynecol 1991;77:835–40.
24 Cook-Sather SD, Harris KA, Chiavacci R et al. A liberalized fasting guideline for formula-fed infants does not increase average gastric fluid volume before elective surgery. Anesth Analg 2003;96:965–9.
25 Keenan RL, Shapiro JH, Dawson K. Frequency of anesthetic cardiac arrests in infants: effect of pediatric anesthesiologists. J Clin Anesth 1991;3:433–7.
26 Cohen MM, Cameron CB, Duncan PG. Pediatric anesthesia morbidity and mortality in the perioperative period. Anesth Analg 1990;70:160–7.
27 Tiret L, Nivoche Y, Hatton F et al. Complications related to anaesthesia in infants and children. A prospective survey of 40240 anaesthetics. Br J Anaesth 1988;61:263–9.
28 Holzman RS. Morbidity and mortality in pediatric anesthesia. Pediatr Clin North Am 1994;41:239–56.
29 Cohen MM, Cameron CB, Duncan PG. Pediatric anesthesia morbidity and mortality in the perioperative period. Anesth Analg 1990;70:160–7.
30 **Hays SR, Deshpande JK. Newly postulated neurodevelopmental risks of pediatric anesthesia. Curr Neurol Neurosci Rep 2011; 11(2):205–10.**
31 **Sun LS, Li G, Miller TL et al. Association between a single general anesthesia exposure before age 36 months and neurocognitive outcomes in later childhood. JAMA 2016;315(21):2312–20.**
32 Davison AJ, Disma N, de Graaff JC et al., for the GAS Consortium. Neurodevelopmental outcome at 2 years of age after general anaesthesia and awake-regional anaesthesia in infancy (GAS): an international multicentre, randomised controlled trial. Lancet 2016;387: 239–50.
33 Gleich SJ, Flick R, Hu D et al. Neurodevelopment of children exposed to anesthesia: design of the Mayo Anesthesia Safety in Kids (MASK) study. Contemp Clin 2015;25(1):65–72.
34 **Wang X, Xu Z, Miao CH. Current clinical evidence on the effect of general anesthesia on neurodevelopment in children: an updated systematic review with meta-regression. PLoS One 2014;9(1):e85760.**
35 US Food and Drug Administration. FDA Drug Safety Communication: FDA approves label changes for use of general anesthetic and sedation drugs in young children. www.fda.gov/Drugs/DrugSafety/ucm554634.htm
36 **Cunningham BB, Gigler V, Wang K et al. General anesthesia for pediatric dermatologic procedures: risks and complications. Arch Dermatol 2005;141:573–6.**
37 Van der Horst CM, de Borgie CA, Knopper JL, Bossuyt PM. Psychosocial adjustment of children and adults with port wine stains. Br J Plast Surg 1997;50(6):463–7.
38 Passeron T, Salhi A, Mazer JM et al. Prognosis and response to laser treatment of early-onset hypertrophic port-wine stains (PWS). J Am Acad Dermatol 2016;75:64–8.
39 Troilius A, Wrangsjö B, Ljunggren B. Potential psychological benefits from early treatment of port-wine stains in children. Br J Dermatol 1998;139(1):59–65.
40 Weisman SJ, Bernstein B, Schechter NL. Consequences of inadequate analgesia during painful procedures in children. Arch Pediatr Adolesc Med 1998;152(2):147–9.
41 Faberowski LW, Banner MJ. The imposed work of breathing is less with the laryngeal mask airway compared with endotracheal tubes. Anesth Analg 1999;89:644–6.
42 Weinger MB, Vredenburgh AG, Schumann CM et al. Quantitative description of the workload associated with airway management procedures. J Clin Anesth 2000;47:315–18.

Other techniques

Hypnosis

Hypnosis may be effective in decreasing the pain and anxiety of surgical procedures in older children. A variety of techniques, for example visual imagery, are used for distraction and to reduce awareness and perception of pain. Hypnosis has been useful for treatment of chronic pain as well as for acute management of painful injuries and procedures.

Other methods

These include the use of illustrated procedure books and dolls to display the planned procedure, concealment of the needle, draping of the surgical tray and constructing a curtain which obscures the procedure from the patient's field of view. For infants, cuddling, swaddling or using a pacifier may be soothing. In neonates, feeding a mixture of sucrose and water has been found to be as effective as EMLA cream for pain relief during venepuncture [1,2]. Distraction techniques involving visual imagery or deep breathing may be useful. In the older child, singing, storytelling and lively background music may be helpful [3,4]. For office procedures, allowing the child to choose a movie and watch it on a portable DVD player during the surgical procedure is an excellent distraction technique. Parents should be strongly discouraged from threatening to punish a child for not cooperating. The parent should be the key emotional support for the child during the procedure and should have both hands free and be fully focused on soothing the child. The doctor should have adequate assistance in restricting the child and should not ask the parents to fulfil this role. The use of positive reinforcement and reward is another key tool. Gifts of stickers, toys and sweets ensure that the child leaves feeling that they have done a great job, regardless of how difficult the procedure had been.

References

1 Gradin M, Eriksson M, Holmqvist G et al. Pain reduction at venipuncture in newborns: oral glucose compared with local anesthetic cream. Pediatrics 2002;110:1053–7.
2 Abad F, Diaz-Gomez NM, Domenech E et al. Oral sucrose compares favourably with lidocaine-prilocaine cream for pain relief during venepuncture in neonates. Acta Paediatr 2001;90:160–5.
3 Rothman KF. Pain management for dermatologic procedures in children. Adv Dermatol 1995;10:287–308.
4 Eichenfield LF, Weilepp A. Pain control in pediatric procedures. Curr Opin Dermatol 1997;4:157–61.

CHAPTER 174
Approach to the Paediatric Patient

Diana Purvis
Starship Children's Hospital, Auckland and Department of Paediatrics, University of Auckland, Auckland, New Zealand

Introduction, 2341
Approach to the neonate, 2342
Approach to the infant and child, 2344
Approach to the adolescent, 2347
Procedures in the paediatric patient, 2352
Adherence, 2352
End-of-life care in paediatrics, 2354

Abstract

Paediatric dermatology involves care of children from birth to the start of adult life. A knowledge of child development helps with approaching children and young people and their families in an appropriate and effective manner. This chapter covers aspects of development in neonates, infants, children and adolescents. An approach to paediatric procedures, adherence, end-of-life care and transition from paediatric to adult services will also be discussed.

Key points

- The provision of paediatric dermatology care is enhanced by good paediatric medical skills, the foundation of which is an understanding of child and adolescent growth and development.
- Involvement and collaboration with parents, family and caregivers are integral to all paediatric care.
- Neonates, particularly premature neonates, suffer physiological stress from even routine medical activities such as physical examination and minor procedures which can affect neurodevelopment. Minimizing stress and optimizing analgesia are important.
- History and examination of children should take into account their stage of development, and may require a less formal, more opportunistic approach.
- Adolescent patients have particular health needs related to their psychosocial and physical development. Clinical care needs to adapt to reflect their growing autonomy and legal rights.
- Transition describes the purposeful movement of adolescents with chronic health problems from child-centred to adult-oriented healthcare. Transition should be planned and can take a period of years.
- Poorly managed painful procedures in children can result in long-term adverse effects, including avoidance of healthcare. Nonpharmacological and pharmacological techniques should be used to minimize distress.
- Adherence refers to the extent to which a person's behaviour corresponds with recommendations from a healthcare provider and is affected by societal, financial, medical and patient factors. Optimizing adherence may have a greater impact on health than advances in medical treatments.
- The diagnosis of a terminal illness in a child due to dermatological disease is fortunately rare, but requires the dermatologist to communicate effectively and sensitively with the patient, family and other health professionals.

Introduction

'Children are not just small adults' (unknown)
'Adults are just obsolete children' (Dr Seuss)

Paediatric dermatology is different from adult dermatology. Firstly, the range, presentation and management of dermatological diseases in children are different. This is recognized in the evolution of paediatric dermatology as a distinct specialty and by the many chapters included in this textbook. But secondly and equally importantly, in paediatric dermatology the patients are different – physically, cognitively and socially. Therefore, medical skills in paediatrics can enhance the practice of paediatric dermatology.

Paediatrics is the branch of medicine dealing with the medical care of infants, children and adolescents. Descriptions of childhood illness are recorded in ancient history, yet paediatrics as a distinct discipline from adult medicine only began during the eighteenth and nineteenth centuries [1,2]. At that time, children often had a precarious existence, and death from perinatal events and infectious disease resulted in a high infant and child mortality rate. Most childhood illnesses lacked effective treatment and so initial interventions were focused on public health measures, hygiene and nutrition. The twentieth century saw great advances in medical science and technology with corresponding improvements in child morbidity and mortality, and as we enter the twenty-first century the way in which medicine is practised continues to change and adapt.

Improvements in public health and hygiene, as well as the benefit of widespread immunization programmes, mean that the role of infections in paediatric disease has been greatly reduced. However, there has been an increase in chronic diseases. This includes behavioural disorders

Harper's Textbook of Pediatric Dermatology, Fourth Edition. Edited by Peter Hoeger, Veronica Kinsler and Albert Yan.

(such as autism and attention deficit/hyperactivity disorder), allergic diseases (such as food allergy and asthma) as well as chronic disease in survivors of previously fatal childhood conditions (such as congenital heart disease, immune deficiencies, childhood cancers and endocrine/metabolic disease).

Society's expectations of child health have also changed over the last century. It is no longer sufficient to merely survive until adulthood. Optimal cognitive and physical development has become the desired outcome, to allow the child to compete successfully in the adult workforce and social life. Cosmetic outcome has also increased in importance and there has been an extension of elective cosmetic practice from antiageing procedures in mature adults to procedures performed in teenagers and young adults designed to 'optimize' physical appearance.

The foundation of good paediatric care is the understanding of child development as this allows the clinician to approach the child in an age-appropriate way, recognize factors which may impact on health and disease at each stage and identify when there is variance from normal development.

Involvement of the parents and family is integral to the practice of paediatrics and clinicians need to offer care in a collaborative way which takes into account the wishes and health beliefs of the child and family. Children, for the most part, are not able to make decisions for themselves regarding treatment and need guidance and assistance from adults with accessing medical care, the administration of medication and application of topical agents. At times, treatment and procedures may need to be performed which cause distress to a child but which are in their best interests overall. Issues regarding guardianship, legal responsibility, assent and informed consent must also be considered by any doctor caring for children.

This chapter aims to give a broad overview of the assessment of neonatal, paediatric and adolescent patients, including their growth and development and the effect this has on delivery of healthcare. The paediatric dermatologist needs to be equipped to deal with all children, from the extremely premature neonate in the neonatal intensive care unit (NICU), through to the adolescent beginning to act as an independent adult. The approach here is a suggested one and individual clinicians need to use their own judgement and experience in how best to work with their paediatric patients and families.

Approach to the neonate

Introduction

Dermatologists may be asked to see neonates with a variety of problems, from minor self-resolving eruptions such as erythema toxicum, to birthmarks with permanent cosmetic implications, to life-threatening genetic disorders. To new parents, all of these problems may initially raise an equal degree of concern about the well-being of their baby, and it is important that the dermatologist listens to their concerns, and competently and confidently speaks with them about the care their child needs.

Table 174.1 Age terminology in paediatrics [3]

Age description	Definition
Extremely preterm	Born <28 weeks gestation
Very preterm	Born 28 to <32 weeks gestation
Preterm	Born 32 to <37 weeks gestation
Term	Born >37 weeks gestation
Neonate	A newborn infant <28 days old
Infant	Age 1 month to 12 months*
Toddler	Age 1 year to 3 years
Preschooler	Age 3 years to 5 years
School age	Age 5 years to 12 years
Adolescent	Age 10 years to 19 years
Young person	Age 10 years to 24 years

*Some groups define infant as 1–24 months.

The neonatal period is defined as the first 28 days of life (Table 174.1). However, life can start before completing a nine-month pregnancy. With advances in neonatal care, particularly with the use of incubators and the development of specialized neonatal units with highly trained neonatologists and nurses, infants are now surviving from birth as early as 23 weeks gestation.

Immediately after birth is a time of immense physiological change necessary for adaptation to life outside the womb. Major changes to the cardiovascular circulation and respiratory system take place to allow effective oxygenation, the digestive system has to adapt to exogenous nutrition, the immune system acts to defend the infant from infections and the neurological system and special senses have to cope with an onslaught of stimulation. The skin also has to adapt to the external environment (see Chapter 4).

Newborn infants are at high risk of morbidity and mortality, not only from a failure to adapt to the outside world, but it is also a time when development anomalies and genetic and metabolic diseases can present. Neonates are also at risk of developing life-threatening infection, both vertically transmitted while *in utero* and from their environment.

Neonatal development

Neonates are grouped as term, preterm, very preterm or extremely preterm depending on their gestational age at birth (see Table 174.1). Gestational age refers to the number of weeks since the last menstrual period and is usually expressed as weeks plus days out of a total of 40 weeks, for example 33+2/40. Chronological age refers to the time (days, weeks, months or years) since birth. Prematurely born children also have a corrected gestational age, which is their chronological age reduced by the number of weeks born before 40 weeks gestation and is used up until the age of 3 years. Corrected gestational age adjusts for the effect of preterm birth on the timing of developmental milestones. For example, an infant who was born at 34 weeks gestation who is now 12 weeks old has a chronological age of 12 weeks but a corrected gestational age of six weeks [3].

Prematurely born infants still need to progress through periods of neurological development that would normally have occurred *in utero*. Developmental care refers to a range of measures taken in NICUs that aim to promote infant neurodevelopment by increasing comfort levels and sleep and reducing stress [4]. It is recognized that infants experiencing discomfort and painful procedures suffer physiological stress and this has the potential to adversely affect infant neurodevelopment [5]. This needs to be considered whenever a neonate is examined or undergoes a procedure.

Behavioural and motor development [6]

Extremely preterm infants (less than 28 weeks gestation) have a very limited range of behaviours [6]. They have very weak muscle tone and are unable to control their posture. Movements are limited to twitches and jerks and these may become more frequent during painful procedures. These infants easily become physiologically stressed by handling and procedures and can become medically unstable. Over the next eight weeks, infants progressively develop muscle tone and strength so that by 36 weeks they are able to demonstrate the typical flexed posture and spontaneous movements of the term infant. Even at full term, babies continue to have poor head control and need support when being lifted or turned.

By 28–32 weeks, infants are able to exhibit behaviours including periods of deep sleep and crying in response to painful stimuli. However, handling for physical examination and care such as washing and changing can still be tiring and should be timed to allow for periods of sleep. The transition between sleep and wake becomes progressively more distinct and by term, infants are able to settle into a regular sleep–wake pattern and offer cues to signal hunger and tiredness. Infants can gradually tolerate care and procedures more easily, but staff and parents continue to need to watch for signs of fatigue and physiological stress.

Vision, hearing, taste and smell [6]

The eyelids may still be fused until 25 weeks gestational age and the cornea cloudy until 27 weeks. Despite this, infants will respond to visual stimulation with signs of physiological stress. Infants may not be able to reliably close the eyelids tightly in response to visual stimulation until 33 weeks and so require protection against bright light. By 36 weeks, infants can begin to focus on near objects and may start to show a preference for the human face.

The inner ear is fully developed by 24 weeks gestation. Infants respond to loud noises by exhibiting physiological stress, but even at early gestations can demonstrate a preference for the soft human voice, particularly their mother's voice.

At 24 weeks, taste and olfactory receptors seem to be functional and infants can demonstrate responses to noxious smells. The development of a coordinated suck and swallow does not typically begin until after 33 weeks and infants will need support with either parenteral or enteral nutrition that may continue until 36 weeks or more.

The neonatal consultation

Setting

Premature or unwell neonates will usually be cared for in a NICU. NICUs provide different levels of supportive care depending on the requirements of the infant. Very and extremely premature neonates, or neonates of any age with severe illness, are typically nursed in an incubator. These provide warmth and humidity to help maintain stable temperature and prevent dehydration due to loss of water through immature skin. Infants may have intraumbilical or central vascular access for parenteral feeds, medication and monitoring and can be provided with respiratory support by continuous positive airways pressure (CPAP) or ventilation via endotracheal tube. Phototherapy for neonatal jaundice can be provided. When the infant is old enough to maintain a stable temperature and well enough to not require close observation and monitoring, they can be dressed and moved to a conventional cot.

Neonatal intensive care units aim to provide developmentally appropriate care to optimize neurodevelopment and actively involve families in infants' care [4,6,7] (Box 174.1). Lighting is kept dimmed to the lowest level to allow clinical activity without causing too much stimulation to the infant. Where increased lighting is required for procedures or phototherapy then infants' eyes are covered to shield them from the light. Noise levels in NICUs are kept low. Monitors and alarms can startle infants and increase stress so are kept at a low volume. Voices should be quiet and calm, and longer discussions within medical teams and with families are ideally held away from the cotside.

Family-centred care is encouraged, and parents should be encouraged to take part in routine cares such as changing, feeding and bathing. Parents can also begin to learn how to apply topical therapies to ready them for when the baby is able to go home. Kangaroo care refers to the practice of placing the infant vertically skin to skin on the chest of the parent with a supportive wrap around them. This enhances the bonding of the parent and child and improves the infant's physiological stability as well as promoting breast feeding. In settings without access to incubators, kangaroo care has been shown to improve

Box 174.1 Neonatal unit etiquette

- Wash your hands on entry to the NICU
- Introduce yourself and your team to staff and family members
- Keep voices low
- Always check with staff and parents before approaching the baby
- Keep lights dim, or protect the baby's eyes from bright light
- Do not put items on the incubator as the noise is amplified for the baby
- Ask the neonatal nurse to assist with handling, turning and procedures
- Keep the baby warm during examination
- Ensure adequate analgesia is given for painful procedures
- Be prepared to stop if the baby is becoming distressed
- Communicate diagnosis and plan with the neonatal team and the family

survival of small neonates [8]. The opportunity for family members to hold and nurture their baby can be immensely important emotionally and, if done carefully, is usually possible even for infants with severe forms of epidermolysis bullosa or ichthyosis.

Routine care such as turning, weighing and changing nappies can all increase physiological stress. Staff in the NICU aim to minimize handling of infants and time routine care to allow for periods of natural sleep.

History

Relevant history is largely taken from the parents with supplementary information from other family members, midwives, neonatal staff and others involved with the infant's care. It may be necessary to find a private place to talk away from the cotside if the baby is in a neonatal unit.

Attention should be paid to periconceptual and gestational events such as illnesses that may suggest antenatal infection. Family history of disease may also be relevant and consanguinity should be asked about.

The neonatal period is often one of intense emotional and social upheaval for families, especially if the baby is unwell or has a major congenital malformation. Fatigue and physical illness may also affect the parent's ability to participate and communicate, particularly if the mother has had a complicated delivery. It is important to be sensitive to this, and sometimes it is prudent to allow the family to rest.

Examination

Examination of a neonate should be conducted with the permission of the parents if possible. If the infant is in a NICU, always check with nursing staff before examining, as they will know if it is a suitable time and be able to help minimize the stress of examination for the baby.

Ideally, the baby should not be woken from sleep for examination. Ensure voices are low and only necessary lighting is used. Minimal handling of premature or sick infants is ideal, and the nurse can help with turning and undressing to reduce stress. Neonates have poor thermoregulation so where possible the incubator should be kept closed or the baby covered. If the infant is sleeping or becomes stressed during the examination, it may be necessary to return at a later time.

Procedures

It is clear that neonates can experience pain in the same way older people do. Pain is evident in changes of facial expression, cries and physiological changes such as increase in heart and respiration rate and apnoea. There is also evidence that exposure to painful events in the newborn period can be associated with long-term adverse effects on neurodevelopment and somatosensory and stress responses which can persist into childhood [5,9,10]. Therefore, pain relief should be used for all neonates undergoing painful procedures.

Procedures such as dressing changes, laser treatment and skin biopsies can cause significant stress to a newborn infant, particularly if these are performed repeatedly. So careful thought needs to be given to the necessity and timing of these. Ideally, procedures should be limited to those providing immediate health benefit or clinically relevant information for the newborn's current care. Very small premature neonates also have a very small blood volume so requesting multiple blood tests can result in significant anaemia necessitating transfusion. Nonurgent tests and procedures (for example, procedures performed to improve cosmetic outcome) should be deferred until a more appropriate time.

For minor procedures such as injection of local anaesthetic or blood taking, use of nonpharmacological measures or oral sucrose solutions may be helpful in reducing pain scores. Nonpharmacological measures include breast feeding the infant, nonnutritive sucking (pacifier use), swaddling or providing skin-to-skin contact. Sensorial stimulation (stroking the face or back, talking to the infant while administering oral sucrose/glucose) also reduces pain scores [9]. Oral sucrose has a calming effect due to the release of endogenous endorphins but it remains unclear whether it acts more as a soothing rather than anaesthetic agent [11]. Topical local anaesthetic creams have not been shown to reduce pain with heelprick tests although they have with lumbar puncture. There are concerns about the use of topical anaesthetics in infants less than 3 months of age, particularly premature neonates who have reduced skin barrier function and a risk of increased percutaneous absorption. Concerns include the development of methaemoglobinaemia, local skin irritation and toxicity [9,12].

For more painful procedures or for procedures in a medically unstable neonate, liaison with the neonatologist or paediatrician is appropriate. It is essential to recognize that there are differences in drug handling in this age group. Oral analgesics such as paracetamol and codeine, intravenous opiates and local and regional anaesthesia can all potentially be used in neonates but require an experienced prescriber [9,12].

There are concerns as to whether general anaesthesia in infancy may affect neurodevelopment, although this is still being investigated. General anaesthesia should be used thoughtfully and only when it is considered to be the most appropriate way to allow a neonate to undergo a procedure safely. It seems the greatest risk may be with children exposed before the age of 3 years, or exposed to multiple general anaesthetics [13–15].

Approach to the infant and child

There are only two things a child will share willingly: communicable diseases and his mother's age.' (Dr Benjamin Spock)

Parents who have watched their own child grow will know that the developmental changes that take place during the first 10 years of life are phenomenal. The pace of change is particularly rapid during infancy, and then proceeds steadily through childhood and into adolescence.

A dermatologist does not usually require a detailed knowledge of child development, but a broad understanding of the physical, social and cognitive changes during childhood is important for anyone who works with children. Not only does it allow the dermatologist to adapt their consultation style in an age-appropriate way, but it also allows them to identify children whose development is not progressing as it should and refer them appropriately.

Infant and child development

Child development is considered broadly under the four domains of gross motor, fine motor, language and social development. Evaluation of development involves assessment of the child's abilities by both history and examination. Children with abnormal development may progress more slowly or in a different pattern due to physical, cognitive or behavioural problems. Development may be affected in one or two or all of the four domains, depending on the cause [16–19].

Detailed assessment of development requires specialized skills, equipment and more time than is typically available to the dermatologist. However, a brief developmental screen will often detect children with possible developmental problems (Table 174.2).

The paediatric consultation

Setting

Children with dermatology problems may be seen in a wide variety of settings depending on the severity and acuity of the problem, their age and the presence of comorbid diseases. Making the environment child friendly can aid in the consultation process by keeping the child and family comfortable and relaxed [20].

Office/clinic setting

The majority of paediatric dermatology patients will be seen in a clinic or office setting, often alongside adult patients. Children are usually accompanied by one or two adult relatives and often by a number of siblings.

Clinic rooms should be clean and bright with sufficient space to accommodate the child and family and their accompanying paraphernalia. Young children typically crawl on the floor so it is important this is kept clean and rugs or carpets may be more suitable. Children placed on examination tables may need to be relocated if parental attention strays in order to avoid accidental falls. Children often actively explore their environment. A good selection of toys may be helpful in keeping them occupied, but it is essential to ensure the whole room is childproof. This entails keeping dangerous items such as medications, chemicals and sharps out of reach – either up high or locked away. An active toddler will often turn on taps and empty boxes of tissues or gloves that are in reach.

A variety of toys and decorations such as pictures and mobiles can have a useful role in assessing development by observing the child's play or asking them to name colours or objects. These can also act as a distraction during the physical examination and minor procedures.

Hospital ward

Hospital-based dermatologists will often see children who are inpatients on a hospital ward. Hospitalization is very stressful for the child and their family and there is a level of anxiety related to being in an unfamiliar environment to add to the discomfort of the illness and fears about its outcome. Many children and families will also be sleep deprived and there may be stress related to other matters such as care of siblings, employment and financial concerns.

It is important to approach children gently and in a nonthreatening manner. If possible, speak with the nurse or medical team caring for the child who can assist with introductions. The child's nurse can often be a source of useful information regarding their clinical condition and relevant social information. Families may reveal concerns and anxieties to nursing staff that they do not feel comfortable expressing to doctors.

Table 174.2 Guide to child development screening [16–18]

Age	Social development	Language development	Fine motor development	Gross motor development
3 months	Smiles Regards own hand	Squeals and laughs Turns to sound	Looks at and follows face past midline Brings hands together in midline	Lifts head Holds head steady
6 months	Works to reach a toy Feeds self	Turns to voice Imitates speech sounds	Looks at small objects Reaches Transfers hand to hand	Rolls over Sits with support
9 months	Waves bye-bye Fear of strangers	Combines syllables	Thumb-finger grasp Picks up small objects	Sits unsupported Stands holding on Crawls
12 months	Indicates wants Fear of strangers	Mama/Dada specific One or two single words Follows simple instructions	Bangs objects together	Stands alone Nearly walking
2 years	Takes off clothes Brushes teeth with help Tantrums	Speech half understandable Names body parts	Builds a tower of 4–6 cubes	Kicks and throws ball Runs and jumps
5 years	Dresses and brushes teeth without assistance Plays board games	Speech all understandable	Draws a person (6 body parts) Copies letters	Hops Balances on each foot for 4 seconds Rides a tricycle

A child's hospital room should be considered a safe place for them to be. Therefore, if painful procedures such as blood tests are required, it is better for these to be performed elsewhere. Many children's wards have a dedicated procedure room for this purpose.

History

The patient's history remains the cornerstone of medicine and there are many benefits to be obtained from taking a good history. Not only is the history most important in formulating a differential diagnosis, but it also gives the dermatologist a better understanding of the child's circumstances. The child and family's psychological, emotional, social, financial and cultural background may potentially influence disease and affect management strategies. History taking is also an important time for establishing a therapeutic relationship with the child and family. By listening to the child's and parents' concerns, the dermatologist can help to build a trusting relationship which will allow the child to permit physical examination more easily, and the family to agree upon a management plan [20].

Guidance and a structure for the dermatologist taking a paediatric history are offered in Table 174.3, while recognizing that a comprehensive history may not be possible or appropriate in every consultation. History taking needs to be tailored to the nature of the presenting complaint, the age of the patient and the time available.

A consultation should always begin with introducing the medical team to the patient and family and identifying who is accompanying the child and their relationship to them.

The child should be allowed to feel involved in the consultation. Talk with them about something familiar such as a toy or an interesting item they are wearing. For older children, asking them about school or recent holidays may be appropriate. Use the child's name when speaking with them and try to use language that they will understand. Young children are often quite shy initially but may become more comfortable during the consultation. Therefore, it is usually helpful to start with history taking before moving to physical examination.

A parent or caregiver will usually give the history of an illness for infants and preschoolers. Parents have an important role in describing their interpretation of subjective symptoms such as pain and itch in their child, which the child is unable to express. Parents are generally good observers of their children and are frequently able to give detailed descriptions of the effects of an illness or skin condition on their child. However, parents' ability to give an accurate history may be compromised by anxiety, misinterpretation or because the child's day-to-day care is shared with others (for example, extended family, nannies or childcare facilities).

By early school age, a child will often be able to describe some of their symptoms and treatments, but this will usually need to be supplemented by information from a parent. Address some simple medical questions to the child and allow them to participate in the discussion where it is appropriate. As they get older, the child will be able to give more of the history and a motivated adolescent will typically be capable of offering a medical history of similar quality to an adult patient. However, even in the teenage years, a parent or caregiver may still be needed to give support, for example with offering a history of medical events in early life or a family history of illness.

During the consultation, allow younger children to play with toys so that parents are able to talk with fewer interruptions. While they are playing, it is also an opportunity for observation of their behaviour and development.

Table 174.3 Guide to the paediatric history [20]

History	Remarks
History of the presenting complaint	Time of onset of problem Appearance – location, colour, size, etc. Symptoms – itch, pain, fever, etc. Evolution with time – precipitating and relieving factors Previous and current treatments – response Impact of problem on child and family
Past medical history	Other known medical problems and previous surgery Other professionals involved in the child's care
Pre- and periconception	Maternal health Maternal medication and illegal drug use
Antenatal	Maternal health during pregnancy – infections, medication and drug use Results of antenatal testing and ultrasound scans
Delivery and postnatal period	Gestational age Mode of delivery Apgar score Birth weight Birth complications Requirement for intensive or special care
Growth and nutrition	Growth during infancy and childhood (often recorded as part of well-child monitoring) Mode of infant feeding – breast, bottle Current nutrition – food avoidances, food allergies
Development	See Table 174.2
Medication history	Prescribed medications – adherence and quantities used Over-the-counter medications Complementary and alternative medications Drug allergies
Immunization history	Timing of routine and additional vaccinations
Family medical history	Known medical disorders in immediate family members Presence of inheritable disease History of consanguinity
Social history	Family members Carers Housing School – academic progress, socialization, bullying Involvement in activities and sports Psychosocial problems
Finally	'Is there anything else you'd like to tell me?'

Examination

Examination of infants and children generally requires a less formal, more opportunistic approach than in adults. Much can be learned from standing back and observing the child during the history taking and examination, including information about the child's developmental progress, the quality of their relationship with their parents, and the presence of itch or pain and visible disease [20].

It is normal for children to feel anxious about strangers from around 9 months. This fear of strangers and anxiety about separation from parents is particularly strong around the age of 12–18 months and then gradually subsides [18]. However, in unfamiliar settings like a doctor's office or hospital, these feelings of anxiety can often be exhibited until school age and beyond. This has particular implications for the way children should be approached during examination.

Infants and young children usually feel more comfortable when close to their parents. For infants and preschoolers, this may entail conducting much of the examination while the child is sitting on the parent's lap. If the child is on a bed or examination couch, invite the parent to stand next to them.

Ask the parent, or child if they are old enough, to remove clothing to allow examination. Nappies and underwear are usually best kept in place apart from the period of time that observation of that area is required, as much for hygiene as modesty.

Infants and preschoolers are naturally shy and may find examination frightening. Distracting the child with the parent's assistance can be very helpful. There are many ways to do this: start by asking to hold their hand, count their fingers, ask them if they can point to various body parts, use toys or books for the child to look at and hold while the examination takes place around them. Portions of the examination that require the child to be quiet and still, for example auscultation of the heart, are often best performed at the start of the examination. Otherwise, begin by looking at the area of concern first while the child is most likely to be cooperative. If the child is comfortable and relaxed, the examination can be performed quickly and effectively. If the child becomes upset and uncooperative then examination can be very challenging and it may be necessary to just focus on the most important aspects rather than conducting a complete physical examination. Any uncomfortable aspects should be left until last.

Growth and nutrition

An important part of paediatric examination is assessment of the child's growth and nutrition. Normal growth is usually an indicator of overall good health, whereas faltering growth can be a marker of disease. In many countries, children's growth is monitored as part of well-child checks, and parents may have a record of their child's previous growth [21].

Children should have their weight and height or length measured as part of a physical examination and serially plotted on a growth chart [22,23]. Normal growth is usually evident by relative symmetry between weight and height centiles and by serial measurements that follow a centile curve. One-off measurements may be misleading; for example, a weight measurement on the third centile may represent concerning weight loss for a child previously measured on the 25th centile, pleasing improvement in a child previously less than the third centile or appropriate growth in a child whose previous weight and height measurements are also on the third centile.

After infancy, height velocity gradually slows until the pubertal growth spurt begins. Thus pubertal assessment becomes an important aspect of growth assessment in older childhood [21].

Growth charts can be accessed at: www.rcpch.ac.uk/growthcharts

Approach to the adolescent

Adolescence spans the time between childhood and adulthood. It is characterized by a period of rapid physical growth, sexual development and psychosocial changes. It is a stage of development that takes place between the ages of 10 years and the early 20s and eventually leads to functional independence in adult life [24].

Adolescents have particular health needs in the ways in which care is delivered that distinguish them from child and adult populations. There are few diseases unique to adolescence, but young people can be affected by both late presentation of paediatric diseases and early presentation of adult illness. In addition, improved medical care means that increasing numbers of children are surviving into adolescence with chronic illnesses as a result of genetic disorders, malformations (such as congenital heart disease) and childhood malignancy. Skin conditions, particularly those which result in a visible difference, can have a particularly high impact during adolescence due to increased self-consciousness, high desire to conform with peers and issues with body image [25].

Although adolescence is usually a period of relative good physical health, morbidity and mortality from social and psychological causes increase. A recent World Health Organization survey of the global burden of disease in young people found that injury is the leading cause of mortality in teenagers, reflecting an increase in risky behaviours related to driving, fighting, alcohol and drug use, as well as mood issues and self-harm. However, it should be noted that skin and soft tissue complaints were one of the leading causes of morbidity in adolescence [26].

The development of mental health issues (mood disorders, psychiatric disorders, suicide), sexual health issues (unplanned pregnancy and sexually transmitted infections) and risk factors for adult morbidity (smoking, diabetes, obesity, physical inactivity) often start in adolescence and continue into adult life, making this an important time for health promotion. The dermatologist may be well placed to engage with young people in a health context, and has the potential to identify nondermatological health issues that may require intervention.

In adolescence, the psychological and social changes mean the dynamic of clinical care needs to evolve to reflect the growing autonomy, understanding, wishes and legal rights of the young person as they move into adulthood.

Specialized clinical skills in adolescent health may allow the clinician to engage with the young person and their family in a way that promotes accurate history taking, sympathetic clinical examination and the formation of a management plan while respecting the privacy and confidentiality of the young person and their relationship with their family.

Adolescent development

Adolescent development reflects the physical changes caused by the hormonal surges of puberty and the psychological effects of maturation and myelination of the brain (Table 174.4) [27–30].

The physical changes of puberty may begin as early as 8 years of age and continue as late as the early 20s and result in physical growth and the development of secondary sexual characteristics.

After infancy, growth in childhood usually progresses at a relatively steady rate until puberty. The timing of onset of the pubertal growth spurt naturally varies between individuals and is affected by factors such as genetics, nutrition, chronic illness and psychosocial factors. It usually begins between 8 and 13 years of age in females and 9 and 15 years in males. In females, the onset of puberty is signalled by the beginning of breast and pubic hair development (adrenarche), followed by a surge in growth and then the onset of menses (menarche). In males, an increase in testicular volume is the first sign of puberty. The pubertal growth spurt in males generally starts later than females and continues for longer, with the development of facial hair and deepening of the voice occurring towards the end of puberty and musculoskeletal growth continuing into the early 20s.

Brain maturation, particularly of the prefrontal cortex, limbic system and white matter, continues throughout puberty and is not completed until the mid-20s. This process has a significant influence on behaviour, for instance, through effects on risk and reward assessment and impulsivity. Thinking progresses from concrete to abstract and from egocentric to decentred. Social development is influenced by the physical and cognitive changes of puberty, and also by the cultural expectations of the family and broader society [31].

It is important to recognize that there may be dissonance between physical and psychological changes. A young teenager with early onset of puberty who has reached physical maturity may still have the cognitive processes of a child and conversely a young person with delayed onset of puberty may have the physical appearance of a child while being cognitively and socially mature.

Adolescent consultation

Adolescents should be able to access healthcare that meets their needs, in a format they understand and can participate in, from an appropriately trained provider. Training specific to adolescent health is increasingly included within paediatric training programmes [32].

History

Information gathered as a part of history taking should change as a child reaches adolescence and needs to reflect the activities and problems seen in this age group. As well as taking a general medical history (see Table 174.3), obtaining information related to psychosocial issues can be helpful in understanding the young person and the effect of illness on their lives. A structured approach to psychosocial history taking during adolescence is provided by the HEADSS assessment (Table 174.5) [27,30,33].

Table 174.4 The changes of adolescence [27,28]

	Early adolescence (8–14 years)	Mid adolescence (12–17 years)	Late adolescence (>17 years)
Biological	Females: breast bud and pubic hair growth Growth spurt begins Males: testicular enlargement and beginning of genital growth	Females: completion of growth and breast development Female body shape Menarche Males: voice breaking Spermarche Growth spurt begins	Males: completion of pubertal growth Ongoing effects of androgens on hair and muscle development
Psychological/ cognitive	Concrete thinking Difficulty understanding effects of immediate behaviours on long-term outcome Sexual identity and orientation development	Abstract and rational thinking ability increasing Development of morality and ideology (religious and political opinions) Views self as invulnerable/'bullet-proof' Takes risks without fear of consequences	Complex abstract thinking Improved impulse control Further development of personal identity, morality and ideology
Social	Adjusting to puberty and physical changes Beginning of separation of self from parents Start of strong identification with peers Beginning of risk-taking behaviours	Establishing separation of self from parents Strong peer influence, fear of exclusion Health risk behaviours often begin (drinking, smoking, drugs, sex) Behaviours driven by short-term rewards Privacy and confidentiality important	Education and career progression Start of economic independence Development of intimate and mutually caring relationships Mature interdependent relationship with family Concept of future, delayed gratification

Source: Adapted from Viner 2008 [27] with permission of Elsevier, and Bennet and Robards 2013 [28].

Table 174.5 The HEADSS assessment: an approach to the psychosocial history in adolescence [27,30,33]

Domain			Example questions
H	Home	Family members Household members Quality of relationships Quality of housing	Where do you live? Who do you live with? Do you feel safe at home? Who could you turn to if you had a problem?
E	Education and employment	School Academic achievement Vocational goals Truancy/attendance Bullying	What do you like/dislike about school? How are your grades and attendance? How do you get along with other students?
A	Activities	Sport Cultural activities Music Hobbies	What do you do for fun? With whom? Where? Do you go to parties? What exercise do you do?
D	Drugs	Exposure to and use of legal and illicit drugs	Some young people experiment with smoking, drinking or drugs, do you know anyone doing that? Have you tried any? How often? Have they caused you any problems?
S	Sex	Sexual activity Contraception Sexually transmitted infections Sexual orientation Nonconsensual sex	How do you feel about relationships/dating? Some people your age start to get physically involved, have you? Has anyone ever touched you in a way that makes you uncomfortable or forced you to have sex?
S	Suicide	Mood symptoms – anxiety, depression Self-harm thoughts and behaviours	How do you feel at the moment? Do you ever feel really sad or worried? How often? What do you do when you feel bad? Some people think about hurting or killing themselves when they feel bad, have you? Have you ever tried to hurt yourself or kill yourself?

Taking a full psychosocial history requires obtaining the trust of the young person, reassuring them regarding confidentiality, taking time and most importantly listening to them [32]. It may be best done over the course of a number of consultations when there is also the opportunity to develop a good doctor–patient relationship. Generally, it is best to start taking a psychosocial history by asking about more neutral topics that are less likely to be upsetting or difficult to discuss. Often, but not always, school and activities are good starting points and then the consultation may be allowed to flow into other areas. These are also good starting points for identifying resiliency factors – those positive influences that help a young person cope with adversity. Resiliencies include having good relationships within the family and with peers, engagement in school and cultural activities, religious belief [34].

Although home is often a safe and comfortable environment, this may not be the case for all young people. Homes may harbour problems such as domestic violence, sexual and psychological abuse, drug and alcohol use which make life difficult for the young person. It may be particularly important to be able to speak to the young person confidentially about some of these issues without the presence of a parent or family member. Young people may also not wish to reveal some of their activities to a parent for fear of punishment.

Young people with skin conditions such as acne, eczema and psoriasis are at a higher risk of mood disorders such as depression, anxiety and suicidal behaviours and talking with young people about these can identify opportunities to help with management of some of these issues [25,35–38]. Knowledge of local services for the care of mental health problems and how to refer to them is valuable. Young people are unlikely to reveal information about mood issues if they are not asked about them. It is important to ask about suicide and self-harm directly as suicide risk is not always associated with the presence of a mood disorder [37,38].

Sexual intercourse often begins during adolescence. The mean age of sexual debut has some variation between countries and genders but often takes place between 16 and 18 years of age, with perhaps a third having had sex by age 16 years and as many as 10–18% engaging in sexual intercourse before the age of 15 years [30,39–41]. Studies among adolescents with chronic illnesses suggest that sexual debut may occur earlier than in their healthy peers at a mean of 15 years [42]. Sexual risk behaviours such as unprotected sex are also more common in adolescents with chronic illness, with consequently higher risk of sexually transmitted infection and pregnancy. About a quarter of girls do not use condoms at their first sexual encounter, and fewer than 70% of teens regularly use condoms [30]. This can have important implications when prescribing medications, particularly to young women. Therefore, it is important to offer young people the opportunity to discuss sex and contraception in a nonjudgemental and confidential way, so that they may get appropriate advice.

Adolescents with a chronic illness are also as likely or more likely than their healthy peers to smoke, drink or use illegal drugs, and these activities may have the potential to cause more harm in the context of their illness or medications [42]. Again, talking with the young person regarding these activities nonjudgementally can aid with identifying risky behaviours and discussing how to continue to support their social life and peer relationships while minimizing the potential impact on their health.

Examination

Physical examination of an adolescent is in many ways the same as examination of an adult patient. However, adolescence is a time of heightened sensitivity to their appearance and a strong desire for privacy.

Take the time to explain to the young person what the physical examination involves. Ensure they are able to have adequate privacy to remain comfortable by limiting the number of people in the room and using gowns and screens. A chaperone may be necessary for the comfort and protection of both clinician and patient.

Confidentiality and consent in adolescence

Confidentiality is a central tenet of the doctor–patient relationship [43,44]. It is also a major factor affecting young people's engagement with healthcare services, particularly for matters involving sexual and mental health or substance abuse [45]. Where a service is perceived to be confidential, young people are more likely to disclose sensitive health information and to return for follow-up [46]. Perceived lack of confidentiality has been found to affect young people's decision to seek medical care [47,48].

Confidential healthcare should be offered to adolescents who are considered competent to make decisions regarding their own health. The landmark case in Britain of *Gillick v West Norfolk and Wisbech Area Health Authority* has shaped the concept of competence. The judgement in this case stated that an adolescent under 18 years of age is capable of giving informed consent when they have 'a sufficient understanding and intelligence to enable him or her to understand fully what is proposed' [49].

Young people of 14 years of age have demonstrated levels of competence around medical decision making equivalent to adults [50]. Nevertheless, competence is not purely based upon chronological age and is also strongly linked to cognitive ability and social experience.

Cultural expectations of young people's behaviour and independence can also be relevant, and at times can result in conflict between parents and young people as to the young person's ability to make their own healthcare decisions. The complexity of the medical problem is also pertinent. Health professionals should make themselves aware of legal guidance regarding competency and consent local to their country or state.

Health professionals need to balance the rights of the young person for privacy and confidentiality and their desire for independence, against allowing the family sufficient information and involvement to provide the support the young person needs [44,45]. When possible, young people should be offered the opportunity to be seen separately from their parents, at least for part of the consultation [32,34]. Parents may need reassurance that the aim of these independent visits is to improve healthcare engagement and support the growing capabilities of the teenager. Ongoing involvement of parents in supporting the young person's health, and respectful communication between the young person and their parent is to be encouraged alongside supporting the development of independence. Having a secure loving relationship with family is important to a young person's well-being and their parents' ongoing practical and emotional support is vital.

Communication may be helped by assuring the young person of confidentiality at the start of the consultation [44,47]. This may allow them to speak about matters they may not wish to share with others [46]. However, there are some circumstances where confidentiality should not be maintained [51].

- When the young person is at risk of harm. This includes serious risk of physical, sexual or emotional abuse from others, or self-harm.
- The young person is at risk of harming others.
- Where there is a legal requirement for disclosure. Examples of this include notifiable diseases, and information required for court proceedings.
- When it is necessary for the young person's well-being, such as communication between members of the treating team or in an emergency.

Whenever possible, the young person's agreement to share information should be obtained by explaining who the information is to be given to, what information is to be shared and the purpose of that.

Chronic illness or disfigurement during adolescence

Adolescence may be one of the most difficult times in life to adjust to having a chronic illness or disfigurement [31]. The normal goals of adolescence of achieving a sense of identity, developing personal relationships, a career and independence can all be adversely affected by the impact of illness.

Chronic illness of any type may have unfavourable effects on adolescent development. Physical growth and puberty in a young person with a chronic physical illness may be delayed well into the late teens or early 20s. Growth failure may be due to chronic inflammation, malnutrition or the effects of medications such as glucocorticoids. Impaired physical growth may have effects on the development of self-image and sexuality, and delay social independence.

In addition, a young person with a chronic illness, particularly a skin problem, may need to grapple with the effects of looking visibly different at a time when the need for conformity and acceptance by peers is high.

Time away from school to attend appointments or due to illness can adversely affect educational performance and result in long-term effects on vocational choice and financial well-being. It can also impact on the formation and maintenance of friendships in the school environment. Physical problems or self-consciousness may limit the ability to take part in social and sporting activities, further adding to social isolation. Conversely, many normal adolescent social behaviours, such as experimenting with alcohol, drugs and sexuality, may have an increased adverse impact because of illness [42,52].

Adolescence is usually a time of increasing independence but young people with a chronic illness may be forced to maintain dependence on parents to assist with their medical needs such as administering medication and attending appointments. They may also struggle with accepting advice from clinicians at a time of life normally associated with rebellion against authority figures [53].

Actively supporting young people with chronic illness to maintain normal growth and development is important to their overall well-being. This includes monitoring growth and pubertal development and intervening when needed. The dermatologist can help by aiming to optimize disease control and nutrition while minimizing exposure to medications affecting growth. Inducing onset of puberty through use of exogenous hormones or managing growth impairment due to growth hormone deficiency may require the involvement of a paediatric endocrinologist.

Listening to the young person regarding the impact of their condition on their ability to participate in activities and on social functioning is necessary to be able to address those issues which are important to them [32]. Linking the young person's goals to correct use of medical treatment can help their motivation with adherence. Physical appearance can also be a major concern for some young people and addressing that can be an important part of care. Prioritizing involvement in education and achievement of vocational and self-care goals is valuable in promoting eventual independence in adult life, even if the young person does not prioritize this at the time [52].

Transition from paediatric to adult services

The Society for Adolescent Medicine defines transition as 'The purposeful planned movement of adolescents and young adults with chronic physical and medical conditions from child-centred to adult-oriented health care systems' [54].

Transition from a paediatric to an adult-oriented model of care can be a challenge for young people with chronic health needs but is essential to provision of good-quality care [55]. Some of these young people may have been engaged with paediatric health services for most or all of their lives and transition requires moving from familiar trusted services to unfamiliar new services [56,57]. Transfer to adult services usually occurs between the ages of 16 and 20 years, a time of life when many other major changes may be taking place: leaving school, leaving home, developing social and financial independence. Studies of young people in a variety of services (oncology, haematology, cardiology, gastroenterology, endocrinology and more) have shown the time of transition from paediatric to adult care to be one where the young person is vulnerable to poorer health outcomes and being 'lost' to follow-up [55,58–60].

Services for adult patients differ from paediatric services in many ways. The young person is expected to be independent and manage their own healthcare. However, everyday matters such as transport to and from clinic, having blood tests and paying for prescriptions can be a challenge for some young people. Adult services may also be less proactive in identifying problems and young people are expected to speak out about issues that are troubling them. Young people and their families need to be given time to adjust to these differences, learn to negotiate new systems and environments and form relationships with new healthcare providers [56,57].

There is a paucity of medical literature on transition in dermatology. A transition process for young people with epidermolysis bullosa in the UK has been described [61]. The process of transition begins in childhood or early teens with the discussion of available adult services and the formation of an agreement with the patient and family regarding the process of transition. Young people are encouraged to take a progressively more active role in consultations to allow the development of self-reliance. There are opportunities to visit adult centres for epidermolysis bullosa and to meet staff on a number of occasions before formal transfer of care takes place, typically between 16 and 18 years of age. Review of progress after transition also occurs.

For many young people with complex chronic dermatology problems, a formal transition process may not be available. This may be due to the rarity of their disorder and the absence of appropriate specialized or multidisciplinary adult services. In these instances, the young person and their family are likely to require additional support in transferring to a range of adult specialty providers. However, many dermatologists provide care to both paediatric and adult patients and so transition to another service is not needed, although a change to an adult model of care needs to take place [62]. As paediatric dermatology grows as a subspecialty, more consideration needs to be given to the changing services we offer for our patients.

Recommendations for transition services include the following [55–57,62,63].

- Provide care for the young person in the environment best suited to both their chronological age and psychosocial development.
- Create written transition plans in collaboration with the young person and their family before the age of 14 years, with the aim of undertaking the transition process over several years.
- Have a designated professional responsible for coordinating the process of transition.
- Address aspects of health relevant to all adolescents – growth and development, sexuality, mental health, substance use, education and vocational skills.
- Enhance autonomy and self-efficacy. This includes providing self-management skills training to the young person such as understanding their disease and medications, forming a partnership with healthcare providers, managing practicalities (e.g. filling prescriptions, making appointments), and general healthcare around diet, exercise and stress management [64].
- Provide support individualized to the young person's needs.
- Support development of services for adult survivors of childhood disease.

Procedures in the paediatric patient

Performing uncomfortable procedures in children can result in significant distress and anxiety for the child, their family and also medical staff. In the past, it was thought that very young children did not experience pain, or at least did not remember it, and that experience of pain was in some way character building [65]. However, there is increasing evidence that experience of poorly managed painful procedures in childhood can have long-term adverse effects.

- Adverse neurodevelopment, particularly following painful experiences in early neonatal life [5].
- Pain sensitization/hyperalgesia, meaning subsequent experiences are even more painful and difficult to manage [10].
- Development of procedural anxiety or needle phobia. Many adults experience procedural anxiety or needle phobia which affects their ability to interact or engage with medical care and can often date it back to a traumatic experience in childhood [65].
- Posttraumatic stress disorder following very distressing experiences.

An approach to performing procedures in children is presented in Table 174.6.

There are a variety of nonpharmacological techniques that can be helpful in procedural management [65]. Distraction uses music, toys, videos or games to draw the child's attention away from the uncomfortable or frightening procedure, and can help not only with pain but also with the distress and anxiety that accompany a procedure. Distraction can be used alongside most pharmacological methods. Deep breathing, muscle relaxation, guided imagery and forms of hypnosis can also be used. Many paediatric departments have play or child life specialists who are trained in use of these techniques.

The pharmacological methods such as topical and infiltrated local anaesthetics and sedation are addressed in Chapter 173.

General anaesthesia should be considered for procedures causing significant pain or requiring a longer period of cooperation, particularly in children less than 12 years of age. The choice of pain management technique will depend upon the nature of the procedure as well as the temperament, understanding and previous experiences of the child.

Table 174.6 Procedural management of paediatric patients [65]

Action	Remarks
Child-centred approach	Listen to the needs of the child and family Don't rush Allow the child and family to be active participants Use parents for positive assistance, not negative restraint
Optimize the procedure	Only perform procedures that are clinically necessary Use the least invasive techniques Use experienced personnel when possible, or ensure close supervision of trainees Ensure all necessary equipment is available before starting Perform procedures in a child-friendly environment away from the child's bed
Minimize anticipatory anxiety	Allow the child time to be prepared for the procedure Don't wait too long as anxiety can escalate Aim to manage pain and anxiety well for the first procedure to make subsequent procedures easier
Encourage helpful support behaviour	Nonprocedural talk (e.g. parties, friends, pets) Distracting activities (e,g. bubbles, games, music, TV, playing tablet/smartphone game) Breathing techniques Use experienced play therapists or paediatric nurses to assist when possible
Discourage unhelpful support behaviour	Avoid comments which draw attention to the procedure (e.g. 'sorry you have to go through this', 'you'll be all right', explanations of what is happening) Avoid lying (e.g. 'this won't hurt a bit') Avoid bargaining (e.g. 'if you do this you'll get a Playstation') Avoid giving the child control over the procedure (e.g. 'tell us when you're ready')
Optimize pain interventions	Use a combination of nonpharmacological and pharmacological techniques Choose technique based upon procedural and child factors Distraction can be used alone or alongside other techniques Do not use sedation without appropriate experience, monitoring and resuscitation equipment Sedation does not provide analgesia Reassess adequacy of pain management interventions throughout the procedure and adjust as necessary

Source: Data from Paediatrics & Child Health Division 2005 [65].

Adherence

Adherence has been defined as 'the extent to which a person's behaviour – taking medication, following a diet and/or executing lifestyle changes – corresponds with agreed recommendations from a healthcare provider' [53]. Nonadherence generally refers to being adherent less than 80% of the time.

Adherence to treatment advice is important for optimizing treatment effectiveness, safety and health outcomes. Reduced adherence in children with chronic illness has been shown to be associated with increased healthcare use and health costs [66]. Thus, addressing factors that reduce adherence should be an important goal of healthcare providors. It has been suggested that improving adherence may have a greater impact on the health of the general population than advances in specific medical treatments [67].

Adherence rates

Global studies of chronic diseases such as hypertension, asthma and diabetes show adherence rates as low as 50% [53]. It is thought that adherence to treatment with topical therapies is likely to be even lower [68].

In clinical trials of psoriasis therapies, adherence rates to topical therapies are around 50–60% [69–71]. Interestingly, patient self-report of adherence over the same period may be significantly higher than objectively measured adherence, as high as 90–100% [71]. Even during short-term interventions, adherence can be surprisingly poor [72].

Outside clinical trial settings, adherence is generally lower. A study of topical corticosteroid adherence in eczema patients found average adherence with twice-daily application over an eight-week period to be just 32% [73]. Adherence was generally better in the days just before or after clinical assessment.

Although adherence during adolescence is generally considered to be poor, a review of studies of adherence to acne therapies showed rates of around 76% for both oral and topical therapies, although a number of the studies included had used subjective measures of adherence which may overreport use [68]. Disappointingly, a study in the United States found that as many as 27% of acne patients did not even fill their prescription [74].

Factors affecting adherence

It is worth considering the factors that affect adherence. It is often too easy to focus on or even blame the patient and family, but there are many reasons for nonadherence. These include not only factors related to the patient, their disease and its treatment, but also broader societal factors related to accessibility of healthcare and training of healthcare providers (Table 174.7).

Factors associated with poor adherence to topical therapies include frustration that treatment is not meeting expectations and fear of side-effects, such as corticosteroid phobia [70,75]. Patient and parent education may be helpful in addressing these issues in advance.

Inconvenience can be a significant factor for more complex and time-consuming treatments. Especially for conditions such as generalized childhood eczema that require frequent and widespread application of multiple topical agents, the time spent performing treatments can be considerable. Many patients and families also become confused regarding the purpose of their various medicaments and providing a written treatment plan can be a useful memory aid. Unsurprisingly, simplifying treatment programmes appears to be helpful in improving adherence [76]. Topical therapies also have a number of aspects related to consistency, feel and smell which may affect patients' use of them. Taking into account a patient's personal preferences and creating an individualized treatment programme may help with their engagement and adherence.

Adherence seems to be improved with better clinician–patient relationships, patient education and counselling about the disease and expected effects of treatment. Therapeutic patient education and nurse-led clinics could potentially improve outcomes and medication use for a number of dermatological conditions [68,77–79]. More frequent follow-up with health professionals also has a beneficial effect [71,80].

Goal setting and use of rewards such as tokens or sticker charts can be used to improve adherence in school-age children. Adolescents may be a more difficult group to motivate. Long-term consequences may not be a concern due to their stage of cognitive development, and focus on the short-term benefits of adherence in terms of well-being and appearance may be more effective. Forgetfulness is a commonly reported reason for nonadherence [68]. There are an increasing number of smartphone applications designed to aid adherence. Unfortunately, the use of electronic or text reminders in improving adherence for acne therapy seems disappointing to date [80,81].

A recent Cochrane review has shown that to date, the methods used in studies to improve adherence are

Table 174.7 Factors affecting adherence to treatment [53]

Factors	Potential intervention
Social and economic related	
Low socioeconomic status Poor education, illiteracy Poverty Work/education commitments Living conditions, transportation High cost of medical care High cost of medications	Public policy improving access to health and education
Healthcare system and provider related	
Poorly developed systems for care of chronic diseases Lack of reimbursement or recognition for adherence interventions Lack of provider knowledge/skills in adherence interventions Short consultation times Lack of continuity Poor communication between professionals Lack of support in community	Closing gaps in care for chronic diseases Prioritizing funding of adherence activities, e.g. education programmes, community support Development of clinician education and clinical tools for addressing adherence Use of nurse-led education programmes Adequate consultation times Frequent follow-up Continuity of care to allow development of effective therapeutic relationship Community-based support programmes
Disease related	
Severity of symptoms Level of disability Patient's risk perception	Patient education about disease Use of handouts and websites Patient support organizations
Treatment related	
Complexity of treatment Immediacy of benefit Duration of treatment Previous treatment experiences Adverse effects	Simplified treatment programmes Written and verbal advice about use of treatments Education about expected outcome Education and support around adverse effects Use of better tolerated therapies Involvement of patient in treatment choices
Patient related	
Knowledge of illness Personal and cultural health beliefs Confidence, self-efficacy Motivation to treat Social and family support for treatment Forgetfulness	Education regarding disease Adapting treatment programme to fit with personal and cultural beliefs Support of patient in self-management Peer support – use of patient organizations Encouragement of ongoing family support for adolescents Use of reminder strategies and reward systems (e.g. sticker charts)

Source: Data from Sabaté 2003 [53].

generally complex, expensive and difficult to compare [82]. Unfortunately, the methods used also do not seem to be very effective in improving health outcomes. Further research into adherence, with particular attention to health improvements, is needed if more benefit is to be gained from existing therapies.

End-of-life care in paediatrics

Unfortunately, there are a number of dermatological conditions that may result in the death of children in early life, quite often in the neonatal period; these include junctional epidermolysis bullosa, harlequin ichthyosis, severe vascular anomalies and some tumours and infections. The dermatologist may have an integral role as part of a multidisciplinary team in caring for these patients and families in their final days.

The dermatologist will often play an important role in establishing a diagnosis for infants with life-limiting cutaneous disease. A diagnosis may give an understanding of prognosis and assist with recognizing when life-prolonging interventions may be futile. Working closely with the neonatal/paediatric team as well as colleagues in genetics and other specialties both locally and internationally may be necessary. Guidance can also be offered regarding skin care and medications needed to keep the child comfortable.

At some stage, a decision may need to be made to no longer undertake life-prolonging interventions and take a palliative approach, and this is best done by a multidisciplinary team in conjunction with the family. It is not uncommon for clinicians find it difficult to reach this decision and support from colleagues can be helpful [83,84].

Good communication at this time is very important as the family will remember the caring and compassion of health professionals involved with their child, as well as any insensitivity. The main priorities should be the comfort and dignity of the child, and allowing the family to spend precious time together [85]. It is important that families are reassured that the medical team will continue to be actively involved in their child's care now that the goal is comfort rather than cure [83].

When breaking bad news, ensure that this is done in a quiet private place, free from interruptions. Parents may feel supported by the presence of family, known health professionals, a social worker or counsellor when bad news is given. Use simple unambiguous language and avoid euphemisms (for example, say 'died' rather than 'passed away'). Do not hurry and ensure the family have time to process information and ask questions. It is normal for families to return to matters discussed previously as it can take time for them to assimilate information given at this time.

Reactions of parents and family members to being told their child is terminally ill will vary. Grief often begins at the time that the family are told there is no curative treatment and continues through the illness to the end of the child's life as well as for many years after their death. The family may experience shock, anger, denial, numbness, guilt and great sadness. Staff should be empathetic and understanding. It is also important to remember that health professionals may experience many of these emotions too, particularly with a child they have known for some time.

Older children and adolescents will have their own fears and questions about dying which need to be addressed in a sensitive way. Anxieties may be based around the fear of separation from loved ones, and what will happen to their family once they have died. Children may feel they are in some way to blame for their illness and the distress that it is causing. Specialized psychological support may be helpful in assisting with processing of these thoughts and feelings [83].

Respect should be given to the wishes of the child, parents and family about the care they would like in the days/weeks leading up to the child's death and in the time after. Many will want an opportunity for family and friends to visit and say goodbye. Involvement of religious figures can help with providing baptism, blessings and prayers as well as caring for the family's emotional and spiritual needs.

Some families may wish to move the child to a less medicalized setting or take them home to be looked after once intensive care has been withdrawn. Practical support with pain relief and nursing may be needed to allow this. Many centres have expert multidisciplinary teams that specialize in paediatric palliative care who can be instrumental in supporting effective care and symptom control.

After a child dies, it can be helpful for families to receive acknowledgement of that from the professionals involved in the child's care. Health professionals can often find it difficult to speak with families after their child has died. They may feel that speaking of the child will reopen wounds, and they may find their own emotions difficult to manage. However, most families appreciate contact from a health professional with whom they have had a relationship and this can be as simple as a card, a telephone call or attendance at a funeral or memorial service [86].

A follow-up appointment should be offered to the family 1–2 months after death. This should involve senior medical and nursing staff involved with the child and other relevant professionals such as social workers. This can be an opportunity to discuss the diagnosis again and address any questions that the family may have. Issues related to heritability and genetic investigations can be discussed and the family referred to genetic counselling if they so wish. Involvement of specialized genetic services and counsellors may be helpful in discussing options such as testing of family members, recurrence risk and prenatal testing.

It is important that the child's outcome is communicated to the family's general practitioner and other professionals involved in the child's care. The general practitioner will have an important role in the follow-up of the family, particularly monitoring the mood and well-being of the parents and siblings, and ensuring that referral for prenatal or antenatal testing occurs for future pregnancies.

References

1 Gillis J, Loughlan P. Not just small adults: the metaphors of paediatrics. Arch Dis Child 2007;92(11):946–7.
2 https://en.wikipedia.org/wiki/Pediatrics
3 Committee on Fetus and Newborn. Age terminology during the perinatal period. Pediatrics 2004;114:1362–4.
4 Symington AJ, Pinelli J. Developmental care for promoting development and preventing morbidity in preterm infants. Cochrane Database Syst Rev 2006;2:CD001814.
5 Anand KJS, Scalzo FM. Can adverse neonatal experiences alter brain development and subsequent behavior? Biol Neonate 2000;77:69–82.
6 Auckland District Health Board Newborn Services. Developmental care. Available at: www.adhb.govt.nz/newborn/Guidelines/Developmental/DevelopmentalCare.htm
7 Als H, Duffy FH, McAnulty GB et al. Early experience alters brain function and structure. Pediatrics 2004;113(4):846–57.
8 Conde-Agudelo A, Díaz-Rossello JL. Kangaroo mother care to reduce morbidity and mortality in low birthweight infants. Cochrane Database Syst Rev 2014;4:CD002771.
9 AAP Committee on Fetus and Newborn and Section on Anesthesiology and Pain Medicine. Prevention and management of procedural pain in the neonate: an update. Pediatrics 2016;137(2):e20154271.
10 Taddio A, Katz J, Ilersich AL, Koren G. Effects of neonatal circumcision on pain response during subsequent routine vaccination. Lancet 1997;340:599–603.
11 Stevens B, Yamada J, Lee GY, Ohlsson A. Sucrose for analgesia in newborn infants undergoing painful procedures. Cochrane Database Syst Rev 2013;1:CD001069.
12 Haidon JL, Cunliffe M. Analgesia for neonates. Contin Educ Anaesth Crit Care Pain 2010;10(4):123–7.
13 Wang X, Xu Z, Miao C-H. Current clinical evidence on the effect of general anesthesia on neurodevelopment in children: an updated systematic review with meta-regression. PLoS One 2014;9(1):e85760.
14 Zhang H, Du L, Du Z et al. Association between childhood exposure to single general anesthesia and neurodevelopment: a systematic review and meta-analysis of cohort study. J Anesth 2015;29(5):749–57.
15 Davidson AJ, Disma N, de Graaff JC et al. Neurodevelopmental outcome at 2 years of age after general anaesthesia and awake-regional anaesthesia in infancy (GAS): an international multicentre, randomised controlled trial. Lancet 2016;387(10015):239–50.
16 Feigelman S. The first year. In: Kleigman RM, Behrman RE, Jenson HB, Stanton BF (eds) Nelson Textbook of Pediatrics, 18th edn. Philadelphia: Saunders Elsevier, 2007.
17 Feigelman S. The second year. In: Kleigman RM, Behrman RE, Jenson HB, Stanton BF (eds) Nelson Textbook of Pediatrics, 18th edn. Philadelphia: Saunders Elsevier, 2007.
18 Feigelman S. The preschool years. In: Kleigman RM, Behrman RE, Jenson HB, Stanton BF (eds) Nelson Textbook of Pediatrics, 18th edn. Philadelphia: Saunders Elsevier, 2007.
19 Feigelman S. Middle childhood. In: Kleigman RM, Behrman RE, Jenson HB, Stanton BF (eds) Nelson Textbook of Pediatrics, 18th edn. Philadelphia: Saunders Elsevier, 2007.
20 Becher J, Laing I. History, examination, basic investigation and procedures. In: McIntosh N, Helms P, Smyth R, Logan S (eds) Forfar and Arneil's Textbook of Paediatrics, 7th edn. Oxford: Elsevier, 2008.
21 Keane V. Assessment of growth. In: Kleigman RM, Behrman RE, Jenson HB, Stanton BF (eds) Nelson Textbook of Pediatrics, 18th edn. Philadelphia: Saunders Elsevier, 2007.
22 WHO Child Growth Standards. Available at: www.who.int/childgrowth/en/
23 Royal College of Paediatrics and Child Health. UK-WHO growth charts 0–18 years. Available at: www.rcpch.ac.uk/growthcharts
24 Joint Working Party on Adolescent Health of the Royal Medical and Nursing Colleges of the UK. Bridging the Gaps: Healthcare for Adolescents. London: Royal College of Paediatrics and Child Health, 2003.
25 Rodway C, Tham S, Ibrahim S et al. Suicide in children and young people in England: a consecutive case series. Lancet Psychiatry 2016;3:751–9.
26 Mokdad AH, Forouzanfar MH, Daoud F et al. Global burden of diseases, injuries, and risk factors for young people's health during 1990–2013: a systematic analysis for the Global Burden of Disease Study 2013. Lancet 2016;387:2383–401.
27 Viner R. Adolescent medicine. In: McIntosh N, Helms P, Smyth R, Logan S (eds) Forfar and Arneil's Textbook of Paediatrics, 7th edn. Oxford: Elsevier, 2008.
28 Bennett DL, Robards F. What is adolescence and who are adolescents? In: Kang M, Skinner SR, Sanci LA, Sawyer SM (eds) Youth Health and Adolescent Medicine. Melbourne: IP Communications, 2013.
29 Rosen DS. Physiological growth and development during adolescence. Paediatr Rev 2004;25(6):194–9.
30 Marcell AV. Adolescence. In: Kleigman RM, Behrman RE, Jenson HB, Stanton BF (eds) Nelson Textbook of Pediatrics, 18th edn. Philadelphia: Saunders Elsevier, 2007.
31 Ullrich G. The teenage brain. In: McDonagh JE, White PH (eds) Adolescent Rheumatology. Oxford: Informa Healthcare, 2008.
32 McDonagh JE. Creating a listening culture: communication with young people. In: McDonagh JE, White PH (eds) Adolescent Rheumatology. Oxford: Informa Healthcare, 2008.
33 Goldenring JM, Rosen DS. Getting into adolescents' heads: an essential update. Contemp Pediatr 2004;21(1):64.
34 Mackenzie RG. Communication with adolescents. In: Steinbeck K, Kohn M (eds) A Clinical Handbook in Adolescent Medicine: A Guide for Health Professionals Who Work with Adolescents and Young Adults. Singapore: World Scientific Publishing, 2013.
35 Halvorsen JA, Lien L, Dalgard F et al. Suicidal ideation, mental health problems, and social function in adolescents with eczema: a population-based study. J Invest Dermatol 2014;134(7):1847–54.
36 Remrod C, Sjostrom K, Svensson A. Psychological differences between early- and late-onset psoriasis: a study of personality traits, anxiety and depression in psoriasis. Br J Dermatol 2013;169(2):344–50.
37 Halvorsen JA, Stern RS, Dalgard F et al. Suicidal ideation, mental health problems, and social impairment are increased in adolescents with acne: a population-based study. J Invest Dermatol 2011;131:363–70.
38 Purvis DJ, Robinson E, Merry S, Watson P. Acne, anxiety, depression and suicide in teenagers: a cross-sectional survey of New Zealand secondary school students. J Paediatr Child Health 2006;42(12):793–6.
39 Wellings K, Collumbien M, Slaymaker E et al. Sexual behaviour in context: a global perspective. Lancet 2006;368 (9548):1706–28.
40 Ramiro L, Windlin B, Reis M et al. Gendered trends in early and very early sex and condom use in 20 European countries from 2002 to 2010. Eur J Public Health 2015;25(2):65–8.
41 Crochard A, Luyts D, di Nicola S, Gonçalves MAG. Self-reported sexual debut and behavior in young adults aged 18–24 years in seven European countries: implications for HPV vaccination programs. Gynecol Oncol 2009;115:S7–S14.
42 Suris J, Parera N. Sex, drugs and chronic illness: health behaviours among chronically ill youth. Eur J Public Health 2005;15(5):484–8.
43 Yeo M. Consent and confidentiality. In: Steinbeck K, Kohn M (eds) A Clinical Handbook in Adolescent Medicine: A Guide for Health Professionals Who Work with Adolescents and Young Adults. Singapore: World Scientific Publishing, 2013.
44 Larcher V. Consent, competence and confidentiality. BMJ 2005;330(7487):353–6.
45 Sanci LA, Sawyer SM, Kang MS-L et al. Confidential health care for adolescents: reconciling clinical evidence with family values. Med J Aust 2005;183:410–14.
46 Ford CA, Millstein SG, Halpern-Felsher BL, Irwin C. Influence of physician confidentiality assurances on adolescents' willingness to disclose information and seek future health care. A randomized controlled trial. JAMA 1997;278:1029–34.
47 Lehrer JA, Pantell R, Tebb K, Shafer M. Forgone health care among U.S. adolescents: associations between risk characteristics and confidentiality concern. J Adolesc Health 2007;40:218–26.
48 Cheng TL, Savageau JA, Sattler AL, DeWitt TG. Confidentiality in health care: a survey of knowledge, perceptions and attitudes among high school students. JAMA 1993;269:1404–7.
49 Gillick v West Norfolk and Wisbech Area Health Authority (1986) AC 112 at 189
50 Kuther TL. Medical decision-making and minors: issues of consent and assent. Adolescence 2003;38(150):343–58.
51 RACP Joint Adolescent Health Committee. Confidential Health Care for Adolescents and Young People (12–24 years). September 2010. Available at: www.racp.edu.au/docs/default-source/advocacy-library/confidential-health-care-for-adolescents-and-young-people.pdf
52 White PD. Transition to adulthood. Curr Opin Rheumatol 1999;11:408–11.
53 Sabaté E. Adherence to long-term therapies – evidence for action. WHO, 2003. Available at: https://apps.who.int/iris/bitstream/handle/10665/42682/9241545992.pdf;jsessionid=DAC193ED8E8A02562A3E08D12248E043?sequence=1

54 Society for Adolescent Medicine. Transition from pediatric to adult-oriented health care systems for adolescents with chronic conditions. A position paper. J Adolesc Health 1993;14:570–6.

55 Viner RM. Transition of care from paediatric to adult services: one part of improved health services for adolescents. Arch Dis Child 2008;93:160–3.

56 Hergenroeder AC, Wiemann CM, Cohen MB. Current issues in transitioning from paediatric to adult-based care for youth with chronic health needs. J Pediatr 2015;167(6):1196–201.

57 White PH. Growing up: transition from adolescence to adulthood. In: McDonagh JE, White PH (eds) Adolescent Rheumatology. Oxford: Informa Healthcare, 2008.

58 Kapellen TM, Kiess W. Transition of adolescents and young adults with endocrine diseases to adult health care. [Review] Best Pract Res Clin Endocrinol Metab 2015;29(3):505–13.

59 Moceri P, Goossens E, Hascoet S et al. From adolescents to adults with congenital heart disease: the role of transition. [Review] Eur J Paediatr 2015;174(7):847–54.

60 Kerkar N, Annunziato R. Transitional care in solid organ transplantation. [Review] Semin Pediatr Surg 2015;24(2):83–7.

61 Foster L, Holmes Y. Transition from paediatric to adult service in epidermolysis bullosa. Br J Nursing 2007;16(4):244–6.

62 American Academy of Pediatrics, American Academy of Family Physicians, and American College of Physicians, Transitions Clinical Report Authoring Group. Supporting the health care transition from adolescence to adulthood in the medical home. Pediatrics 2011;128(1):182–200.

63 Rosen DS, Blum RW, Britto M et al. Transition to adult health care for adolescents and young adults with chronic conditions. Position paper for the Society for Adolescent Medicine. J Adolesc Health 2003;33:309–11.

64 Henry HKM, Schor EL. Supporting self-management of chronic health problems. Pediatrics 2015;135(5):789–92.

65 Paediatrics & Child Health Division, Royal Australasian College of Physicians. Guideline Statement: Management of Procedure-related Pain in Children and Adolescents. Sydney: Royal Australasian College of Physicians, 2005.

66 McGrady ME, Hommel KA. Medication adherence and health care utilization in pediatric chronic illness: a systematic review. Pediatrics 2013;132:730–40.

67 Haynes RB. Interventions for helping patients to follow prescriptions for medications. Cochrane Database Syst Rev 2002;2:CD00011.

68 Snyder S, Crandell I, Davis SA, Feldman SR. Medical adherence to acne therapy: a systematic review. Am J Clin Dermatol 2014;15:87–94.

69 van de Kerkhof PC, de Hoop D, de Korte J et al. Patient compliance and disease management in the treatment of psoriasis in the Netherlands. Dermatology 2000;200:292–8.

70 Brown KK, Rehmus WE, Kimball AB. Determining the relative importance of patient motivations for nonadherence to topical corticosteroid therapy in psoriasis. J Am Acad Dermatol 2006; 55(4):607–13.

71 Carroll CL, Feldman SR, Camacho FT et al. Adherence to topical therapy decreases during the course of an 8-week psoriasis clinical trial: commonly used methods of measuring adherence to topical therapy overestimate actual use. J Am Acad Dermatol 2004;51:212–16.

72 Hix E, Gustafson CJ, O'Neill JL et al. Adherence to a five day treatment course of topical fluocinonide 0.1% cream in atopic dermatitis. Dermatol Online J 2013;19(10):20029.

73 Krejci-Manwaring J, Tusa MG, Carroll C et al. Stealth monitoring of adherence to topical medication: adherence is very poor in children with atopic dermatitis. J Am Acad Dermatol 2007;56(2):211–16.

74 Anderson KL, Dothard EH, Huang KE, Feldman SR. Frequency of primary nonadherence to acne treatment. JAMA Dermatol 2015;151(6): 623–6.

75 Charman CR, Morris AD, Williams HC. Topical corticosteroid phobia in patients with atopic eczema. Br J Dermatol 2000;142:931–6.

76 Ryan R, Santesso N, Lowe D et al. Interventions to improve safe and effective medicines use by consumers: an overview of systematic reviews. Cochrane Database Syst Rev 2014;4:CD007768.

77 Thiboutot D, Dreno B, Layton A. Acne counseling to improve adherence. Cutis 2008;81(1):81–6.

78 Eichenfield LF, Totri C. Optimizing outcomes for paediatric atopic dermatitis. Br J Dermatol 2014;170(Suppl. s1):31–7.

79 Moore E, Williams A, Manias E, Varigos G. Nurse-led clinics reduce severity of childhood atopic eczema: a review of the literature. Br J Dermatol 2006;155(6):1242–8.

80 Park C, Kim G, Patel I et al. Improving adherence to acne treatment: the emerging role of application software. J Clin Cosmet Invest Dermatol 2014;7:65–72.

81 Boker A, Armstrong A, Feetham HJ et al. A multicenter, randomized, controlled, evaluator-blinded pilot study to evaluate the effect of automated text reminders on patients compliance with topical medications and its efficacy on disease control in adolescents and adults with mild to moderate acne. J Am Acad Dermatol 2012;66(4)S1:AB83.

82 Nieuwlaat R, Wilczynski N, Navarro T et al. Interventions for enhancing medication adherence. Cochrane Database Syst Rev 2014;11:CD00011.

83 Liben S. The care of children with life-limiting illness. In: Kleigman RM, Behrman RE, Jenson HB, Stanton BF (eds) Nelson Textbook of Pediatrics, 18th edn. Philadelphia: Saunders Elsevier, 2007.

84 Wender E and the AAP Committee on Psychosocial Aspects of Child and Family Health. Supporting the family after the death of a child. Pediatrics 2012;130(6):1164–9.

85 McHaffie H E. Crucial Decisions at the Beginning of Life. Abingdon: Radcliffe Medical Press, 2001.

86 Macdonald ME, Liben S, Carnevale FA et al. Parental perspectives on hospital staff members' acts of kindness and commemoration after a child's death. Pediatrics 2005;116(4):884–90.

CHAPTER 175

Dermoscopy of Melanocytic Lesions in the Paediatric Population

Maria L. Marino[1], *Jennifer L. DeFazio*[1], *Ralph P. Braun*[2] *& Ashfaq A. Marghoob*[1]

[1] Department of Dermatology, Memorial Sloan-Kettering Cancer Center, New York, USA
[2] Dermatology Clinic, University Hospital Zürich, Zürich, Switzerland

Introduction, 2357
Congenital melanocytic naevi, 2360
Acquired melanocytic naevi, 2365
Halo naevi, 2368
Differentiating benign naevi from melanoma, 2368
Spitz naevi, 2369
Conclusion, 2376

Abstract

This chapter addresses dermoscopic features of melanocytic lesions, both benign and malignant, in the paediatric population. While the majority of melanocytic lesions in children are benign, on rare occasions melanoma can develop and it is critical that clinicians are able to identify these malignancies while the cancer is in its early evolutionary stages. To avoid missing a melanoma, many clinicians resort to the biopsy of many naevi, with over 600 naevi being biopsied in children for every melanoma found. In an effort to improve the ability to differentiate naevi from melanoma, clinicians can use technologies such as dermoscopy. It has been shown that dermoscopy improves the clinician's diagnostic accuracy, helps detect melanomas at an earlier stage, and correctly identifies banal naevi, preventing the biopsy of many of these lesions. To adequately use and interpret the dermoscopic findings to know when to biopsy and when it is safe to monitor a lesion does require training. In this chapter, we highlight the salient features seen with dermoscopy that are important in differentiating certain naevi from melanoma. The two-step dermoscopy algorithm and dermoscopic features of congenital melanocytic naevi, acquired naevi, halo naevi, Spitz naevi and melanoma are reviewed. When evaluating melanocytic lesions in children, it is also important to remember that as opposed to the adult population, the process of naevogenesis in children is more dynamic, with new naevi forming, evolving/growing and involuting. In this chapter, we will also describe the dermoscopic features of normal evolving melanocytic naevi. While melanomas in children can have morphological features associated with superficial spreading melanoma, many have features associated with nodular and amelanotic melanomas. The clinical and dermoscopic features of paediatric melanoma are reviewed. In summary, this chapter provides a framework for the dermoscopic evaluation of melanocytic lesions in children.

Key points

- **The vast majority of melanocytic lesions in the paediatric population are benign.**
- **Identifying certain melanoma subtypes can be challenging and differentiating them from some naevi, including Spitz naevi, can be extremely difficult. Dermoscopy, however, can improve the clinician's diagnostic accuracy.**
- **Dermoscopy offers additional information when assessing melanocytic lesions but requires training.**
- **Dermoscopic features to help differentiate naevi from melanoma are outlined.**
- **Growing naevi in children are commonly encountered and the dermoscopic features are discussed.**
- **The overlapping dermoscopic features of Spitz naevi and melanoma are highlighted.**

Introduction

Melanocytic neoplasms comprise one of the most common tumours encountered in the skin of children. Some of these neoplasms are evident at birth while many others develop, become visible and/or change during life's most biologically dynamic growth periods, namely infancy into childhood and childhood into adolescence. Although the vast majority of pigmented skin lesions in children are benign and of no consequence, some may herald a phenotype with an increased predisposition towards melanoma, others may be potential precursors to melanoma, while a few will unfortunately be malignant. The challenge for clinicians is to distinguish between these melanocytic lesions so as to appropriately direct prevention education and targeted screening to populations that will derive the most benefit from such efforts, while at the same time correctly differentiating benign naevi from melanoma. This challenge is compounded by the fact that many melanocytic naevi in childhood and adolescence are new and evolving lesions that have not yet undergone senescence.

Harper's Textbook of Pediatric Dermatology, Fourth Edition. Edited by Peter Hoeger, Veronica Kinsler and Albert Yan.

Although the presence of a new melanocytic lesion or a change within a preexisting melanocytic lesion may be a sensitive and specific sign for melanoma in older adults, this is not true in children. Thus, clinicians evaluating melanocytic lesions in children need to be aware of not only the primary static morphology patterns of benign naevi, but also the normal dynamic morphology of changing naevi. This knowledge may help them identify outlier lesions that do not conform to benign naevus patterns or growth characteristics, thereby indirectly helping them to isolate potential malignant lesions.

A patient's history of symptoms, analytical analysis of the lesion, differential recognition and comparative recognition may all play a role in improving diagnostic accuracy [1]. Although the patient's history is very important, this is often not easily obtainable in a reliable fashion from young children. Hence, thorough cutaneous examination with attention to primary morphology becomes critically important, as it is often the only information available for rendering a diagnosis. Unfortunately, relying purely upon the primary clinical morphology has proven to be a challenge since many melanomas arising in children are reported to lack the conventional ABCD features associated with melanoma (asymmetry, border irregularity, colour variegation, and diameter greater than 6 mm or dark-coloured lesion) [2]. In fact, it has been proposed that melanomas in children more often manifest a different set of ABCD features, namely amelanotic, bump/bleeding, colour homogeneity and de novo (revised ABCD or rABCD) [2].

Recent work by our group has assimilated a collection of clinical and dermoscopic images of paediatric melanomas from around the world. Analysis of these images reveals that paediatric melanomas can manifest either the conventional ABCD features associated with adult melanomas or the revised rABCD features associated with paediatric melanomas. Thus, the two mnemonics complement each other and should both be used in the evaluation of lesions in children. Unfortunately, many benign naevi in children can also manifest one or more of the ABCD or rABCD features. The use of dermoscopy can aid in differentiating naevi from melanoma by allowing the physician to assess both the surface macroscopic and subsurface microscopic primary morphology of skin lesions. By analysing a lesion's dermoscopic colours, structures and patterns, clinicians can enhance their diagnostic accuracy. This in turn will lead to the timely biopsy of potentially fatal cutaneous malignancies, while at the same time decreasing the unnecessary removal of many clinically atypical but benign naevi.

Dermoscopy is a noninvasive, *in vivo* technique that allows the clinician to visualize colours and structures located at the epidermis, dermoepidermal (DE) junction and upper dermis that are otherwise not routinely visible to the unaided eye. This technique affords dermatologists an additional tool in their armamentarium to more accurately evaluate and diagnose skin lesions. Multiple studies have documented the ability of dermoscopy to improve the clinician's sensitivity, specificity and diagnostic accuracy [3–7].

Two types of dermoscopes are available, one utilizing standard light-emitting diode (LED) illumination (nonpolarized dermoscopy) and the other utilizing cross-polarized LED light (polarized dermoscopy). The nonpolarized dermatoscope utilizes standard LED illumination, requiring a liquid interface and direct contact between the glass plate of the dermatoscope and the lesion. The most commonly used liquids applied to the skin are isopropyl alcohol, ultrasound gel and mineral oil. In contrast, the polarized dermatoscope does not require a liquid interface nor does it require direct skin contact as the cross-polarized light minimizes light reflectance from the cutaneous surface, allowing visualization of light reflected from deeper tissue [8,9]. In the paediatric examination, noncontact dermoscopy is often better tolerated and less traumatizing given that the instrument does not touch the patient.

The presence or absence of specific dermoscopic structures and their distribution can assist in correctly classifying most skin lesions (Table 175.1). Many of the colours and structures seen on dermoscopy have been correlated with histopathological findings, supporting the role of dermoscopy as a bridge between gross clinical inspection and histopathological analysis [10–12] (see Table 175.1). Since visualizing lesions with a dermoscope poses neither physical discomfort nor emotional stress, it serves as the ideal looking glass to examine paediatric skin lesions. Its use, in turn, can help the clinician identify subtle clinical clues, confirm naked-eye clinical diagnoses and assist in monitoring lesions [13,14]. Needless to say, diagnostic precision is not only crucial for the proper management of the patient, but it also helps in allaying the anxieties of parents, especially when the decision to perform a surgical procedure is contemplated.

Dermoscopy helps in the evaluation of neoplasms (benign and malignant), inflammatory conditions such as psoriasis, infections such as molluscum and warts, infestations such as scabies and lice, just to mention a few. This chapter will focus on the key dermoscopic features of melanocytic lesions commonly encountered in the paediatric population, including small congenital melanocytic naevi, acquired naevi, halo naevi and Spitz naevi. In addition, the dermoscopic features of melanoma will be discussed. Furthermore, this chapter will focus on lesions located on the torso and extremities. It will not discuss the dermoscopic features of lesions located on so-called special sites of the palms, soles, nails, face and mucosal surfaces.

Before applying dermoscopy to differentiate naevi from melanoma, it is important to first decide whether the lesion under investigation is in fact a melanocytic tumour. The two-step dermoscopy algorithm was created to help differentiate melanocytic from nonmelanocytic neoplasms (Fig. 175.1). The first step of the algorithm requires that the observer decide whether the lesion is of melanocytic origin or not. If the lesion is considered to be a melanocytic lesion then one proceeds to the second step. In the second step, the observer decides whether the melanocytic lesion is benign and can be monitored or is suspect enough to warrant a biopsy. With few exceptions, lesions displaying any of the following dermoscopic structures are considered to be of melanocytic origin: pigment network, negative network, streaks, aggregated

Table 175.1 Dermoscopic structures and their histopathological correlations

Dermoscopic structures	Definition	Histopathological correlation
Pigment network (reticulation)	Grid-like network consisting of pigmented 'lines' and hypopigmented 'holes'	The lines of the network are due to melanin in keratinocytes and/or melanocytes along the epidermal rete ridges. The holes of the network correspond to the suprapapillary plate
Pseudo-network	In facial lesions, diffuse pigmentation interrupted by nonpigmented follicular openings, appearing similar to a network	Pigment in the epidermis or dermis interrupted by follicular and adnexal openings of the face
Negative network	The 'negative' of the pigment network, consisting of hypopigmented lines making up the grid and dark areas filling up the 'holes'. Sometimes the negative network resembles multiple, clustered, elongated, irregular globules, each of which is surrounded by hypopigmentation	It is believed to represent thin elongated rete ridges and large tubular melanocytic nests within a widened papillary dermis. However, it may also represent bridging of rete ridges
Structureless (homogeneous) areas	Areas devoid of dermoscopic structures but without signs of regression. These areas can be hypopigmented, but they cannot be depigmented. If the area is uniformly dark, it is referred to as a 'blotch' (see below). If the area is depigmented then it is referred to as a scar-like area or regression structure (see below)	Structureless hypopigmented areas are due to decreased melanin concentration or simply the fact that the areas are devoid of discernible structures. Structureless hyperpigmented areas are known as blotches and they correspond to the presence of melanin in all layers of the skin
Blotches	Dark brown to black, usually homogeneous areas of pigment that obscure the ability to see any underlying structures	Aggregates of melanin in the stratum corneum, epidermis and upper dermis
Dots	Small, round structures that are less than 0.1 mm in diameter. They may be black, brown, grey or bluish in colour	Aggregates of melanocytes or melanin granules. Black dots represent pigment in the upper epidermis or stratum corneum. Brown dots represent pigment at the dermoepidermal (DE) junction. Grey-blue dots represent pigment in the papillary dermis
Globules	Round to oval structures that may be brown, black, white or bluish in colour. They differ from dots by having a diameter greater than 0.1 mm	Nests of melanocytes in the dermis or along the DE junction. Brown globules represent naevomelanocytic nests in the upper dermis. Bluish globules represent naevomelanocytic nests in the deeper dermis. The bluish hue is due to the Tyndall effect. Black globules are due to heavily melanized naevomelanocytic nests in the upper dermis. White globules are seen in balloon cell naevi
Peppering or granularity	Tiny, blue-grey granules	Melanin deposited as intracellular (mostly within melanophages) or extracellular particles in the upper dermis
Streaks (pseudopods, radial streaming)	Radially arranged projections of dark pigment (brown to black) at the periphery of the lesion. These projections emanate from the main tumour body and extend away from the main tumour body towards uninvolved skin	Confluent junctional nests of melanocytes at the periphery of the lesion. They usually reflect radial growth of the lesion
Regression structures. Also known as blue-white veil over flat areas or blue-white structure over flat areas or scar-like depigmentation	White, scar-like depigmentation, which is lighter than the surrounding skin and appears shiny white under polarized dermoscopy. It is frequently associated with a blue-white veil with adjacent blue-grey areas or peppering	Scar-like changes including fibrotic papillary dermis, lymphocytic infiltrates and/or variable numbers of melanophages
Blue-white veil over raised areas. Also known as blue-white structures over raised areas	Irregular, confluent blue pigmentation with an overlying white 'ground glass' haze	Aggregation of heavily pigmented cells in the dermis in combination with compact orthokeratosis of the stratum corneum
Vascular pattern	The morphology of blood vessels in melanocytic lesions includes comma vessels, dotted vessels, linear vessels, serpentine vessels, corkscrew or torturous vessels and polymorphous vessels. In addition, the milky red area (also known as the pink veil or red globules) is also considered to be a vascular structure	The blood vessels may represent tumour neoangiogenesis or may simply represent normal dilated blood vessels in the papillary dermis. The milky red area reflects an increased vascular volume
Milia-like cysts	Round whitish or yellowish structures that shine brightly (like 'stars in the sky') under nonpolarized dermoscopy	Intraepidermal keratin cysts

(Continued)

Table 175.1 *Continued*

Dermoscopic structures	Definition	Histopathological correlation
Comedo-like openings	'Blackhead'-like plugs on the surface of the lesion	Concave clefts in the surface of the epidermis, often filled with keratin
Fingerprint-like structures	Thin, light brown parallel running lines	Probably represent thin, elongated pigmented epidermal rete ridges
Ridges and fissures. Also known as gyri and sulci	An undulating and thickened epidermal surface creates gyri (ridges) and sulci (fissures). This often gives the lesion a cerebriform appearance	Wedge-shaped clefts of the surface of the epidermis often filled with keratin (fissures)
Moth-eaten border	Concave invaginations of the lesion border	Not available
Leaf-like areas	Brown to grey-blue discrete bulbous structures that form a pattern resembling a leaf	Irregular-shaped tumour islands of pigmented basal cell carcinoma at or near the DE junction
Spoke-wheel-like structures or concentric globules	Well-circumscribed brown to grey-blue-brown radial projections meeting at a darker central hub	Tumour nests of basal cell carcinoma at or near the DE junction
Large blue-grey ovoid nests	Large, well-circumscribed bluish areas that are larger than globules	Large round to oval tumour nests of basal cell carcinoma in the dermis
Multiple blue-grey globules	Nonaggregated round well-circumscribed structures which, in the absence of a pigment network, suggest basal cell carcinoma	Small tumour nests of basal cell carcinoma in the dermis
Lacunae	Red, maroon or black lagoons	Dilated vascular spaces
Parallel patterns	On volar surfaces, parallel rows of pigmentation following the furrows (naevi) or ridges (melanoma) of the dermatoglyphics	Pigmented melanocytes in the furrows (crista limitants) or ridges (crista intermedia) of acral skin
Shiny white structures (lines, blotches, strands and rosettes)	Bright white linear orthogonal lines that are seen only with polarized dermoscopy	Collagen in the dermis

globules, peripheral rim of globules, homogeneous blue colour (blue naevus), parallel pattern (palms and soles) or pseudo-network (face) (Fig. 175.1, level 1). In addition, lesions without any of the aforementioned structures and without the structures commonly seen in nonmelanocytic tumours (Fig. 175.1, levels 2–6) are by default also considered to be of melanocytic origin (Fig. 175.1, levels 7–8). While many dermoscopic feature-poor lesions can be correctly diagnosed based on evaluation of the vascular structures (Fig. 175.1, levels 6–7), some lesions are completely nonspecific in their dermoscopic morphology (these lesions are also called featureless or structureless) and all such lesions (Fig. 175.1, level 8) are also considered to be of melanocytic origin, helping to mitigate the chances of missing the diagnosis of featureless melanomas.

Congenital melanocytic naevi

The presence of congenital melanocytic naevi (CMN) is determined *in utero* [15]. Depending on a multitude of factors including timing of proliferation, senescence, melanin synthesis and melanin transfer, these naevi may be visible at birth or become apparent months to years thereafter. The aforementioned factors probably also exert an influence on the clinical morphology manifested by the CMN. Although the majority of senescent CMN will not change significantly over time, some may develop focal changes, the most feared of which is the development of melanoma.

The classification of CMN divides lesions into categories primarily based on size: small (<1.5 cm), medium (M1 1.5–10 cm, M2 > 10–20 cm), large (L1 > 20–30 cm, L2 > 30–40 cm) and giant (G1 > 40–60 cm, G2 > 60 cm). Other features that factor into the classification of CMN include number of satellite naevi, anatomical location, colour variegation, surface rugosity, nodularity and extent of hypertrichosis [16]. These features may all factor into melanoma risk stratification. However, while melanoma may develop in association with any CMN irrespective of size and morphology, the risk appears greatest for individuals with bulkier large to giant CMN [17,18]. The location and age of onset of melanoma appear to differ between small and large CMN. Melanomas developing in smaller CMN tend to appear after puberty and are more likely to be located at the DE junction and towards the peripheral edge of the CMN [19,20]. In contrast, melanomas occurring in large CMN develop earlier in life and are frequently located below the DE junction [19].

Besides melanoma, other malignancies such as rhabdomyosarcomas and benign tumours such as proliferative nodules can develop in association with CMN and the risk for developing these tumours also appears to correlate with CMN size. In addition, patients with multiple CMN are at risk for neurocutaneous melanocytosis [21].

From the aforementioned clinical observations, it is clear that there are biological differences between the subtypes of CMN. In fact, the hypothesis that small and large CMN may be biologically distinct subsets of naevi is now being confirmed at the molecular level. Studies investigating the mutation profile of small and large CMN are revealing that large to giant CMN often harbour NRAS mutations while small CMN usually harbour BRAF mutations [22]. Since the molecular profile correlates with phenotype, it is not unreasonable to speculate that the molecular profile of CMN may someday be used to refine risk stratification.

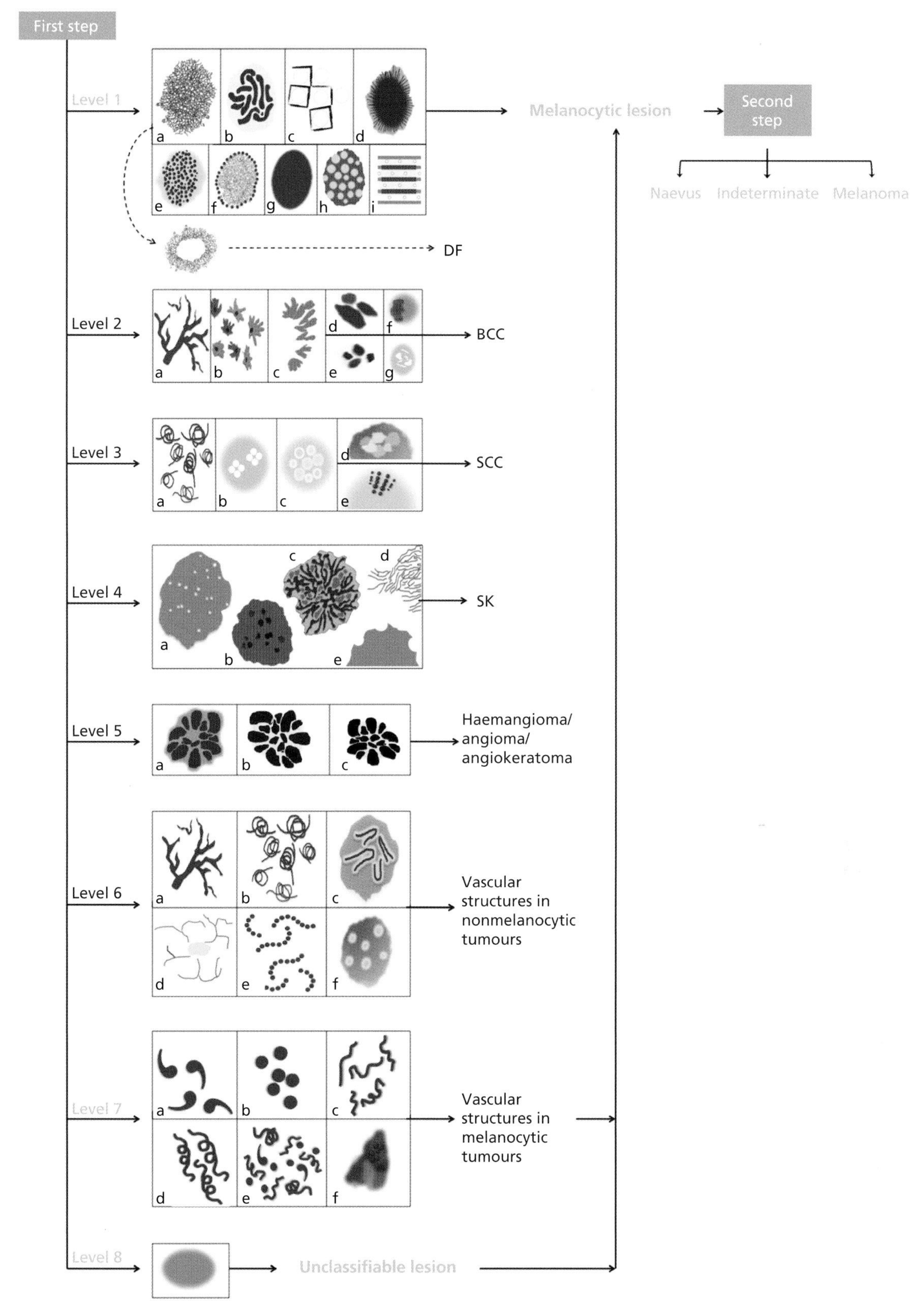

Fig. 175.1 Schematic of the two-step dermoscopy algorithm.

Current management options for CMN include close clinical follow-up with or without baseline photographs, partial or complete prophylactic surgical excision, dermabrasion and laser therapy [19,23]. The eventual management and treatment path chosen must be individualized, taking into account the CMN phenotype, its location, cultural issues, physician and patient belief systems, anxiety and quality of life factors. With that said, many physicians and patients are electing to follow CMN, especially those that have a homogeneous clinical appearance and are small to medium in size, by periodic follow-up examinations.

Dermoscopy has improved our ability to clinically monitor CMN [24]. Knowledge of the dermoscopic structures and patterns common to CMN can aid physicians in following these lesions and recognizing aberrancy that may be suggestive of melanoma. In other words, if the dermoscopic pattern does not conform to one of the commonly encountered CMN patterns or if focal atypical dermoscopic structural changes are observed, then a biopsy or excision may be warranted. It is important to acknowledge that although most small and medium CMN are fairly homogeneous both clinically and dermoscopically, large CMN are often heterogeneous, displaying multiple 'islands' of colour and irregular topography. However, each 'island' within the large CMN tends to be fairly homogeneous in its appearance.

Dermoscopic evaluation of a CMN begins by analysing the dermoscopic features present in the lesion, including network, globules and diffuse pigmentation (Table 175.2) [25]. A *network* describes a honeycomb-like network of brown pigment in which pigmented lines correspond to hypermelanotic rete ridges and the open holes correspond to the suprapapillary plate or dermal papillae (Fig. 175.2) [26–28]. A network is the hallmark of melanocytic lesions and may also be seen in thin superficial spreading melanomas and benign acquired melanocytic naevi [29,30].

A network, as seen in CMN, is characterized by its:

- *quality*, which can be fine and/or thick
- *distribution*, in which the network can be present homogeneously throughout the lesion, or present focally (patchy), or may be present only at the periphery
- *specific type*, linear network fragments or branched streaks that resemble hyphal elements (i.e. resemblance to the tubular branching of fungal hyphae) (Fig. 175.3) [25].

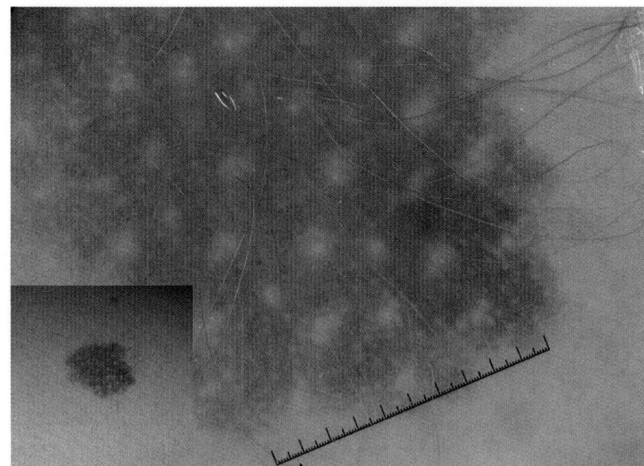

Fig. 175.2 This CMN has a network pattern. It also has hypertrichosis and perifollicular hypopigmentation, both features commonly seen in CMN. A few centrally located scattered globules can also be seen.

Globules consist of sharply circumscribed, round to oval aggregates that represent nests of melanin-containing naevus cells within the dermis (Fig. 175.4) [28,31]. Their colour can vary, based on their depth within the dermis, from light brown to dark brown to black to blue due to the Tyndall effect. Globules in CMN are characterized by their:

- *quality*, which can be small and/or large
- *distribution*, in which the globules can be present diffusely throughout the lesion in a sparse or dense distribution, or can cluster centrally with surrounding network

Table 175.2 Dermoscopic structures observed in CMN

Pattern	Definition	Characteristics
Pigment network	Honeycomb-like network of brown-black pigment	*Quality* • Fine • Thick *Distribution* Homogeneously throughout • Patchy throughout • Peripheral *Specific type* • Linear fragments (hyphal-like)
Globules	Sharply circumscribed, round to oval aggregates of brown-black pigment	*Quality* • Small • Large *Distribution* • Diffusely throughout (sparse or dense concentration) • Central *Specific type* • Cobblestone • Target
Diffuse background pigmentation	Diffuse distribution of brown background pigment	*Remnant structures* • Network fragments • Few globules

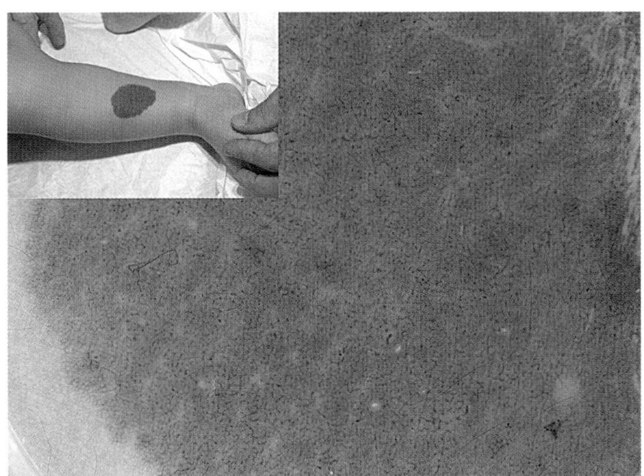

Fig. 175.3 This CMN has network fragments resembling hyphal elements. The lesion also has a few milia cysts, which are commonly seen in CMN.

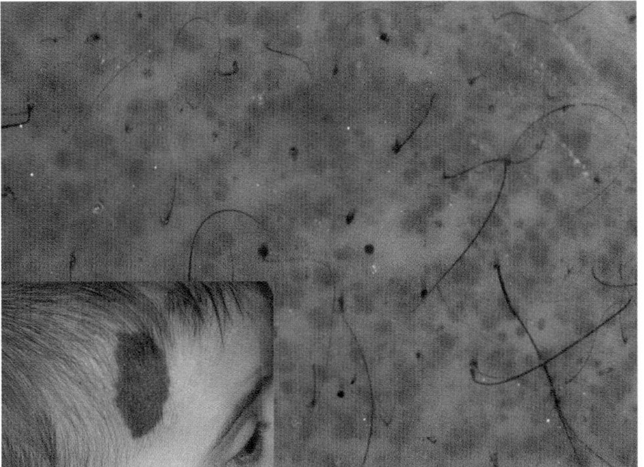

Fig. 175.4 CMN with brown and a few bluish globules throughout the entire lesion. This lesion also has hypertrichosis.

- *specific type*, in which the globules are somewhat polygonal in shape, creating a cobblestone-like arrangement (Fig. 175.5), or in which the globules appear to be surrounded by a halo, producing a target-like appearance (Fig. 175.6). The target-like appearance is created when the globule is centred in the 'hole' of the network, and this corresponds to nests of melanocytes in the dermal papillae (see Fig. 175.6).

The *diffuse background pigmentation* is due to the diffuse distribution of brown pigment across the entire lesion, corresponding to the presence of epidermal or dermal melanin pigment (Fig. 175.7) [28].These CMN are often relatively featureless, in that one cannot see any discernible dermoscopic structures, but on close inspection some may reveal a few scattered network fragments and/or small globules.

Other dermoscopic structures frequently observed in CMN include milia-like cysts, hypertrichosis, perifollicular pigment changes and polymorphous vascular structures (Table 175.3). *Milia-like cysts* are white to yellow, rounded, often hazy structures that correlate histologically with intraepidermal keratin cysts and horn pseudocysts (see Fig. 175.3) [32]. They derive their name from their resemblance to the small seeds or millets of various grain grasses. Although milia-like cysts are one of the dermoscopic hallmarks of seborrhoeic keratosis, they may also be seen in papillomatous dermal naevi, CMN and, rarely, in melanomas. Some mammillated CMN can even display keratin-filled invaginations resembling

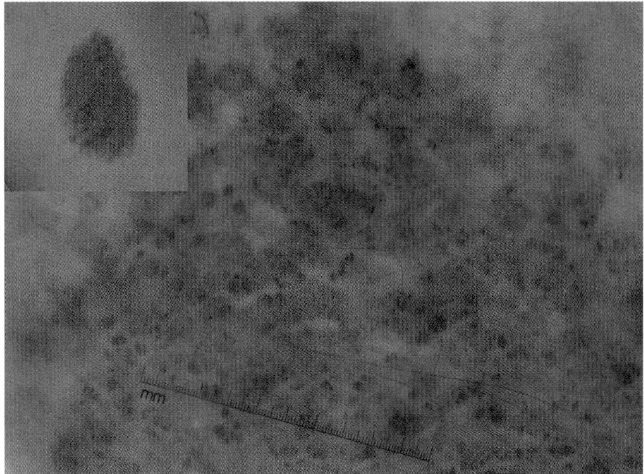

Fig. 175.5 CMN with a cobblestone globular pattern.

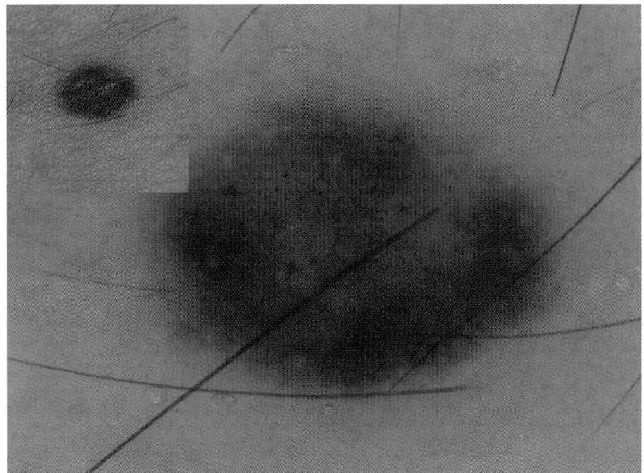

Fig. 175.6 This CMN has focal target globules.

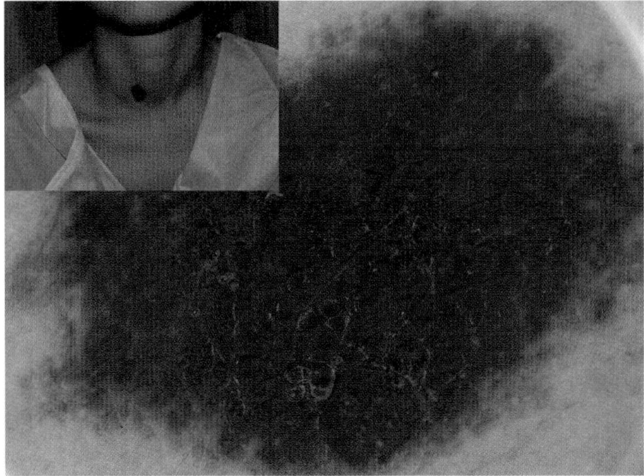

Fig. 175.7 Homogeneous CMN with a diffuse brown background colour pattern.

Table 175.3 Other dermoscopic features seen in CMN

Feature	Definition
Milia-like cysts	White to yellow, rounded, often hazy structures resembling the small seeds or millets of various grain grasses
Hypertrichosis	Increased number of thicker hairs
Perifollicular pigment changes	Hypopigmentation or hyperpigmentation occurring around the hair follicles
Vascular structures	Blood vessels of differing shapes, including comma vessels, dotted vessels and serpentine vessels, can be seen in CMN. In addition, target network with vessels, consisting of a network in which the hole of the network contains a blood vessel, can also be seen in CMN

Table 175.4 CMN dermoscopic patterns

Global pattern	Definition
Reticular	Primarily network pattern
Globular	Primarily globular in pattern
Reticulo-globular	Peripheral network in conjunction with central globules (symmetrical)
Diffuse brown pigmentation	Primarily diffuse structureless pattern with or without network fragments and/or a few focal small globules
Multicomponent	Symmetrically or asymmetrically distributed globules, network, blotches, dots, veil, regression structures and/or structureless areas (three or more of these need to be present)

comedo-like openings or crypts, which are more commonly seen in seborrheic keratosis. *Hypertrichosis* (see Figs 175.2 and 175.4) is characteristic of CMN and is often accompanied by *perifollicular hyperpigmentation* or *hypopigmentation* (see Fig. 175.2). *Vascular structures* are seen in around 70% of CMN with dermoscopy [32]. These include comma vessels, dotted vessels, serpentine vessels and target network with vessels (see Table 175.3). The target network with vessels consists of a blood vessel centred in the 'hole' of the network, and corresponds to vessels in the dermal papillae.

After identifying the local dermoscopic features commonly seen in CMN, it becomes apparent that these naevi often form specific dermoscopic patterns (Table 175.4). These patterns are composed of structures that are generally distributed in an organized and symmetrical manner. The five primary global patterns are reticular, globular, reticulo-globular (symmetrical), diffuse brown pigmentation and multicomponent (Fig. 175.8). Some CMNs are either primarily *reticular* (see Fig. 175.2) or primarily *globular* (see Figs 175.4 and 175.5). Others exhibit peripheral reticulation in conjunction with central globules, and are designated *reticulo-globular* (Fig. 175.9). As noted earlier, CMN that primarily have *diffuse brown pigmentation* are often structureless but some may contain focal network fragments and/or a few scattered globules. CMN with a *multicomponent* pattern are difficult to differentiate from melanoma since they often have blotches, structureless areas, globules and reticulation distributed asymmetrically (Fig. 175.10).

It has been observed that anatomical location dictates, to a great extent, the dermoscopic pattern observed in congenital naevi [32]. CMN on the extremities usually have a reticular pattern and CMN on the torso, head and neck

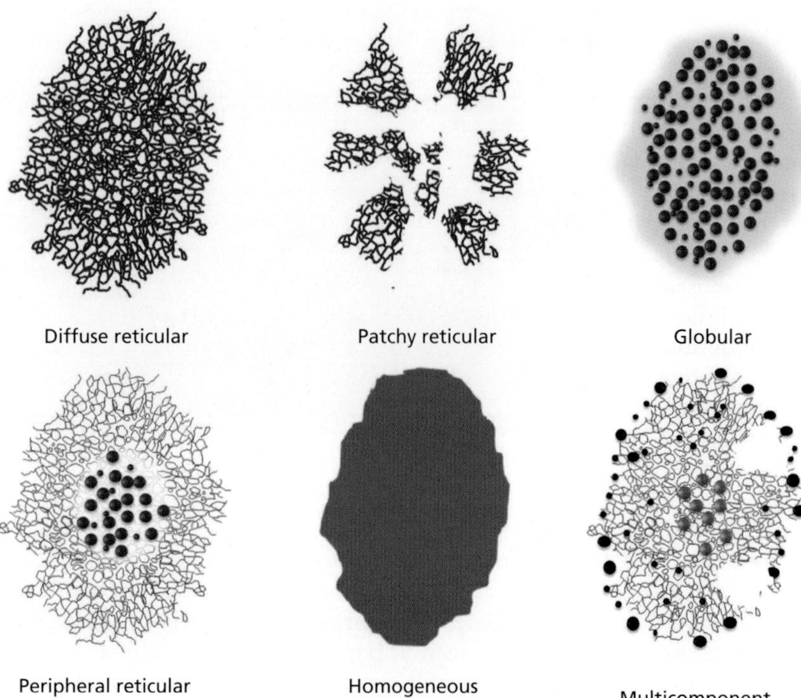

Fig. 175.8 A schematic of the most frequently encountered patterns in CMN.

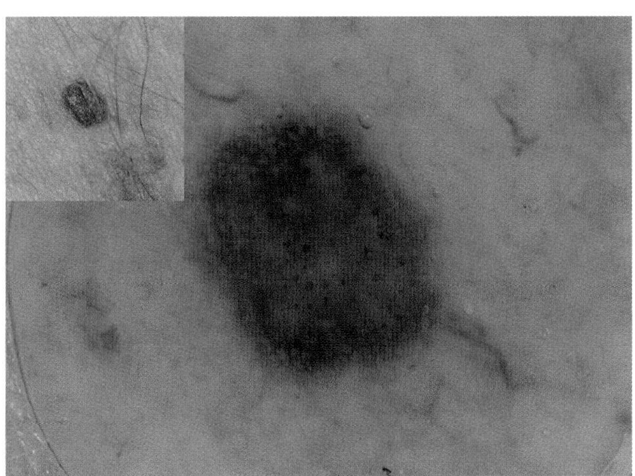

Fig. 175.9 This small CMN has a peripheral network with central globular pattern.

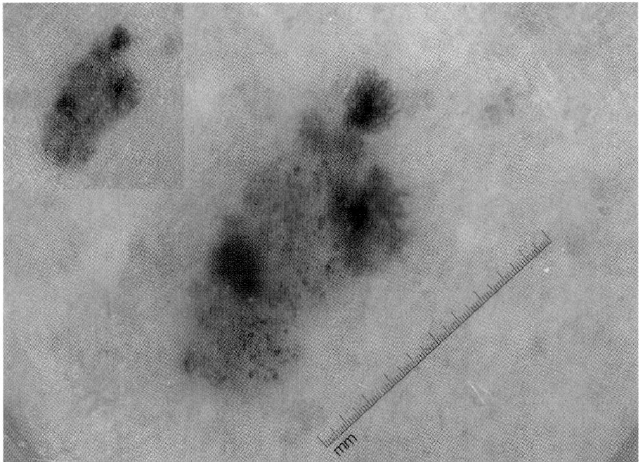

Fig. 175.10 This CMN has an asymmetrical multicomponent pattern with irregular blotches, globules and reticulation. Such lesions are difficult to differentiate from melanoma. This lesion also has milia cysts.

usually have a globular pattern [32,33]. The theory to account for the variation in dermoscopic pattern related to anatomical location hinges on presumed migratory pathways that melanoblasts may take during embryogenesis [34]. Melanoblasts destined for the skin of the extremities are presumed to preferentially migrate along the dorsolateral route, which happens to be more 'superficial', thus accounting for the predominant reticular pattern seen in CMN located on the extremity. In contrast, melanoblasts destined for the skin of the torso, head and neck are presumed to preferentially migrate along the ventral route, which happens to correspond to the pathway of nerve trunks. The ventral pathway is 'deeper' and this helps explain why CMN in these locations often have a component.

Although Unna's theory of naevogenesis has long been used to explain the origin of junctional, compound and intradermal naevi, dermoscopic observations have brought into question Unna's 'Abtropfung' theory of naevogenesis [35]. The current opinion is that there are at least two pathways for naevogenesis. One, known as the congenital or endogenous pathway, is believed to be related to mutations in genes such as *c-kit*, *c-met* and *NRAS*. These mutations occur *in utero*, leading to melanoblast migration arrest in the dermis or epidermis. Based on location of migration arrest, rate of proliferation and timing of senescence, these melanocytic naevi can manifest a globular, reticular or reticulo-globular appearance (see Fig. 175.8). Those naevi in which no dermoscopic structures can be visualized are classified as having diffuse brown pigment (homogeneous) (see Fig. 175.8). Unlike acquired naevi, which frequently regress with age, once CMN undergo senescence they rarely regress and thus they are usually visible on the skin for the life of the individual [36]. The second conduit to naevogenesis is called the acquired or exogenous pathway and is discussed in the next section.

Acquired melanocytic naevi

Current belief posits that acquired naevi result from ultraviolet radiation-induced mutations, such as BRAF, in melanocytes residing along the DE junction, resulting in their proliferation. Depending on the patient's phenotype, these acquired naevi usually manifest a reticular (diffuse or patchy) (Fig. 175.11; see also Fig. 175.8), peripheral reticular with central hyperpigmentation (Figs 175.12 and 175.13), peripheral reticular with central hypopigmentation (Fig. 175.14; see also Fig. 175.12) or homogeneous pattern (see Fig. 175.8) [37]. Research is starting to reveal that there are biologically distinct subsets of naevi that differ from each other on both the morphological and molecular level. For example, globular pattern naevi were associated with single nucleotide polymorphism (SNPs) in IRF4 and TERT, while reticular pattern naevi were associated with SNPs in PARP1, MTAP and CDKN1B [38].

Histological evaluation of acquired naevi has shown that it is common for small junctional naevomelanocytic nests to develop at the tips of the rete ridges. These nests can be seen with dermoscopy as brown dots or small globules overlying the network lines (see Fig. 175.11), which is a dermoscopic feature suggestive of a benign

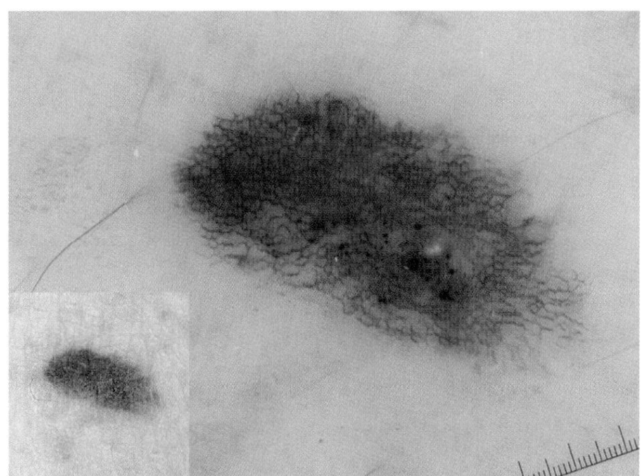

Fig. 175.11 This acquired naevus has a reticular pattern. It also has brown dots and small globules that are overlying the network lines. These dots represent small junctional naevomelanocytic nests at the tips of rete ridges.

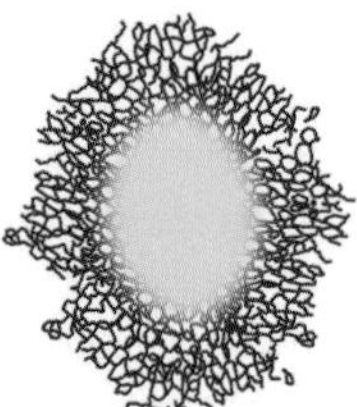
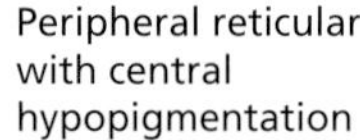
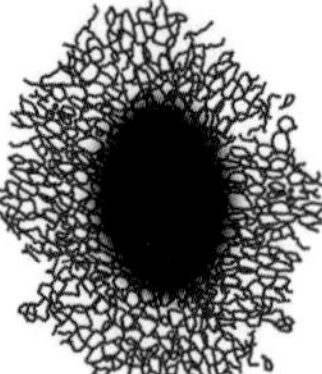
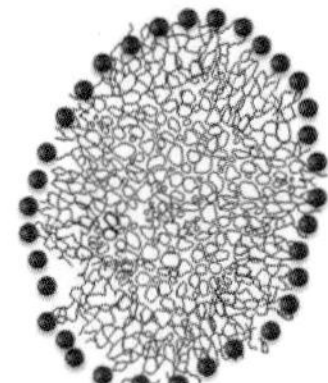
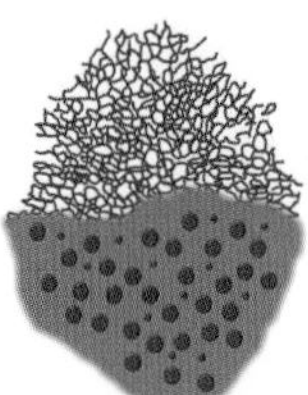

Fig. 175.12 The benign patterns of acquired naevi are those depicted in this schematic and the one in Fig. 175.8.

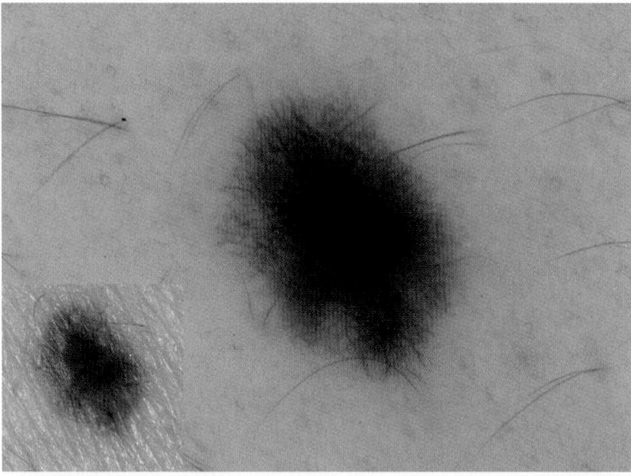

Fig. 175.13 This naevus has a peripheral reticular and central hyperpigmentation pattern.

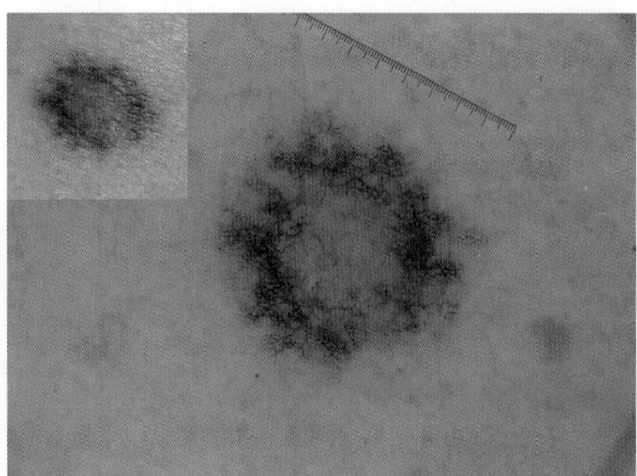

Fig. 175.14 This naevus has a peripheral reticular with central hypopigmentation pattern.

naevus. Junctional nests observed around the perimeter of a naevus, corresponding dermoscopically to the peripheral globular pattern, represent the radial growth phase of one subset of acquired naevi know as dysplastic naevi/Clark's naevi/large acquired naevi (see Fig. 175.12) [39]. These lesions tend to grow in a symmetrical manner for approximately 4–5 years, during which time the peripheral globules become progressively more sparse and eventually disappear, and once senescence occurs, the naevus usually manifests a reticular or homogeneous pattern (Fig. 175.15) [39].

Recognizing the benign pattern seen with dermoscopy affects management. For example, the knowledge that a symmetrical peripheral globular pattern in childhood represents a benign growing naevus may help prevent the lesion from undergoing a biopsy. While change is a sensitive sign for identifying potential melanomas, the specificity is quite low since naevi in childhood frequently undergo change [39,40]. In fact, one study showed that approximately 75% of children developed new naevi and approximately 28% had naevi that became smaller and disappeared over three years of follow-up [41]. In addition, it was interesting to note that approximately 80% of baseline naevi were observed to manifest changes (i.e. larger or smaller). However, despite observing these changes, the overall dermoscopic naevus pattern for most of these naevi did not change [42]. From a management perspective, it is reassuring to know that changing lesions such as those manifesting a symmetrical peripheral globular pattern are indeed benign and do not require biopsy (see Fig. 175.15).

Other benign naevus patterns include the two-component pattern (see Fig. 175.12) and the organized symmetrical multicomponent pattern (see Fig. 175.8). The two-component naevi can present in one of three ways: reticular-globular, reticular-homogeneous or globular-homogeneous. In these naevi, one half of the lesion manifests one pattern while the other half of the lesion manifests a different pattern (Fig. 175.16). The benign multicomponent pattern consists of organized and symmetrically distributed globules, reticulation, blotches, dots, veil, regression structures and/or structureless areas (three or more of these need to be present) (Fig. 175.17). It is important to underscore here that although the organized multicomponent pattern is considered a benign pattern, it should always be evaluated in the context of the patient's other lesions and patient history. While a stable organized multicomponent pattern naevus present in a sea of similar-appearing naevi is reassuring, an isolated and changing multicomponent pattern lesion should raise concern.

It is well known that the presence of a large number of naevi, presence of naevi with an atypical clinical morphology, and fair phenotype are risk factors for melanoma. As an aside, it is interesting to note that naevus count appears to correlate with polymorphisms, including MTAP rs10757257, PLA2G6 rs132985 and IRF4 rs12203592 [38,43]. In childhood, the presence of acquired naevi on the scalp may herald the atypical mole syndrome phenotype [44–47], another risk factor for melanoma.

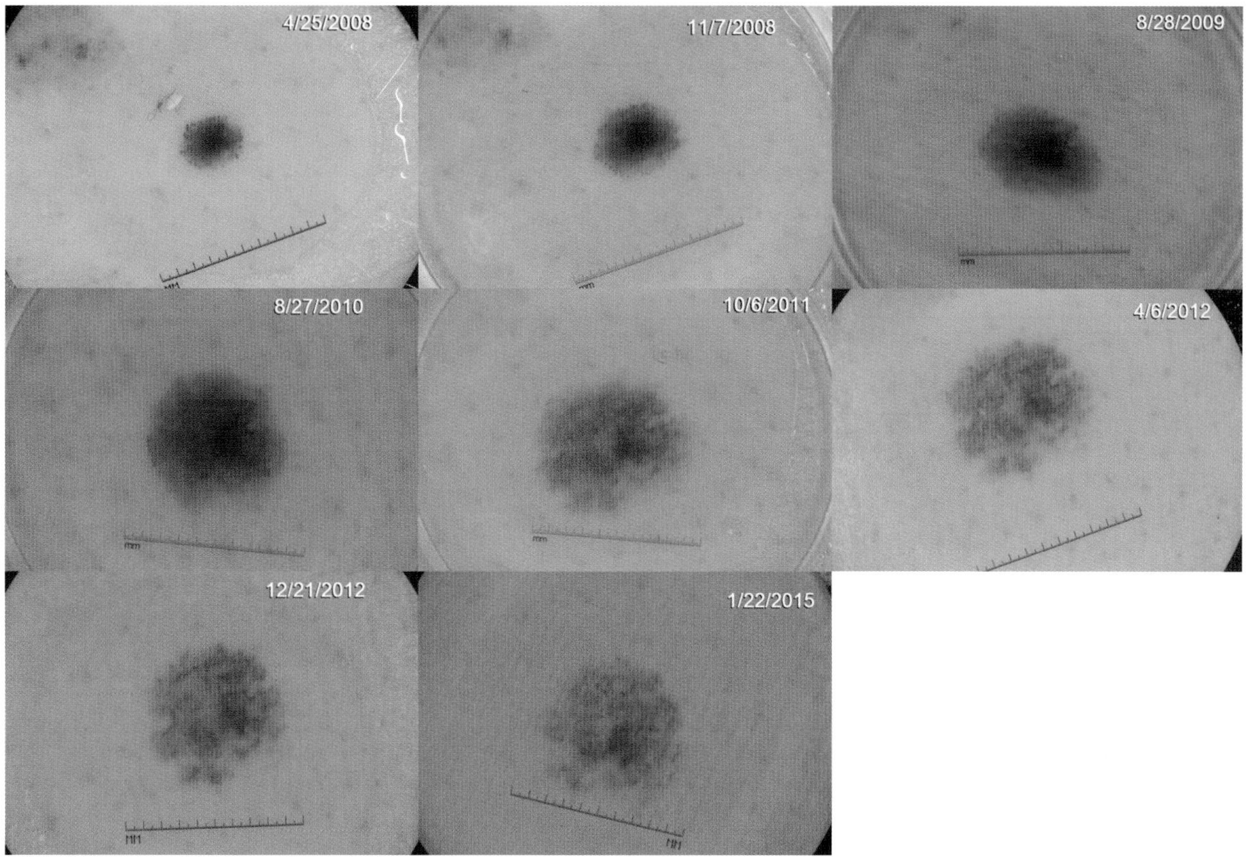

Fig. 175.15 This lesion originally had a peripheral globular pattern. The lesion was sequentially followed. Note that the lesion has enlarged symmetrically and the peripheral globules have become more sparse over time.

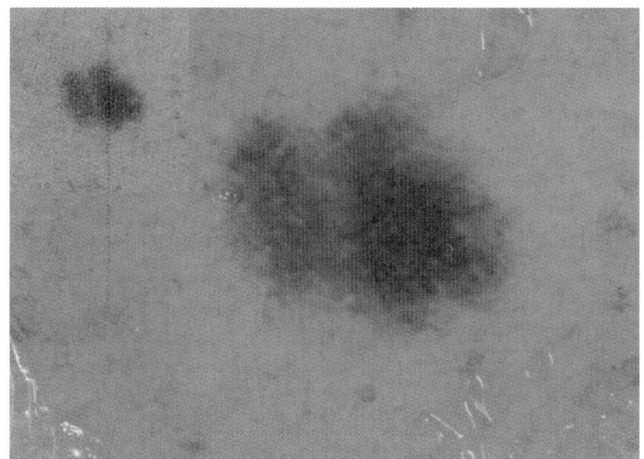

Fig. 175.16 This benign naevus has a two-component pattern.

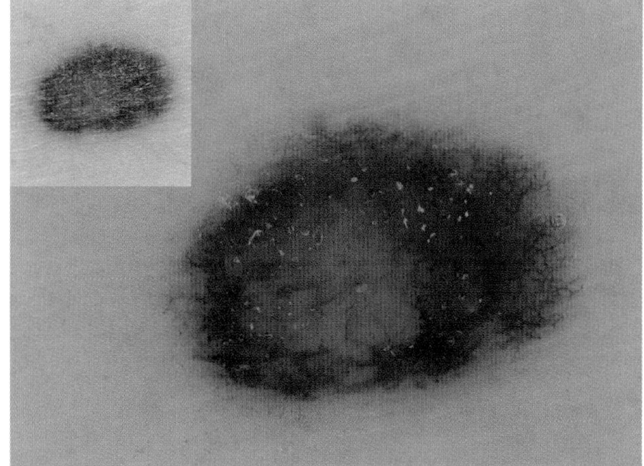

Fig. 175.17 This benign naevus has a multicomponent pattern. It has a symmetrically distributed network (reticulation), homogeneous areas and brown dots.

Further refinements of melanoma risk stratification may be possible with the use of dermoscopy. It has been shown that most individuals harbour a limited number of dermoscopic naevus patterns, a concept known as 'moles breed true' or 'signature naevus pattern' [48]. In other words, if a given mole in an individual manifests a reticular pattern with central hypopigmentation then it is highly probable that most of their other naevi will reveal a similar pattern. Preliminary observations indicate that individuals possessing an overall complex mole pattern (e.g. patients without a signature naevus pattern) with naevi of varying dermoscopic patterns may be at higher risk for developing melanoma [48]. Furthermore, it has been observed that most individual naevi manifest a simple dermoscopic pattern (i.e. diffuse reticular, patchy reticular, peripheral reticular with central hypopigmentation, peripheral reticular with central hyperpigmentation, globular or homogeneous). However, some individual naevi possess a complex dermoscopic pattern (i.e. one that contains both network and globules) and a pilot study concluded that a 'complex' dermoscopic naevus pattern was more prevalent in patients with melanoma compared to controls [49].

Knowledge of all the aforementioned risk factors can assist in identifying individuals who may benefit most from focused education efforts regarding prevention and early detection of melanoma. In addition, these individuals may benefit from periodic skin cancer surveillance examinations.

Halo naevi

Isolated or multiple halo naevi are frequently encountered in children. A halo naevus consists of a melanocytic naevus with a surrounding peripheral zone of hypopigmentation, resembling a halo. This type of naevus was first described by Sutton in 1916 [50]. Halo naevi occur most commonly in individuals under the age of 20, with a mean age of onset of 15 years [51]. In a study of the dermoscopic features of naevi surrounded by a halo, globular and homogeneous patterns were most common [52]. Decreasing size of these naevi was observed over time, with a mean reduction in naevus area of 2.2% per month (Fig. 175.18). Interestingly, the structural pattern of these regressing naevi remained relatively unchanged as they became smaller. Although the halo of a halo naevus may persist for some time, the naevus component eventually involutes until it can no longer be seen clinically or dermoscopically [52]. The duration from onset of halo reaction to complete involution of the naevus to repigmentation of the halo takes approximately eight years. Typical halo nevi do not need to be biopsied. However, a halo surrounding a pigmented lesion manifesting a pattern other than a globular or homogeneous pattern should be considered suspicious.

Differentiating benign naevi from melanoma

While melanoma in children is very uncommon, its incidence increased in the period 1973–2001. However, in the last decade, its incidence is reported to be decreasing [53,54]. According to the National Cancer Institute SEER database, there was a decrease in the incidence (11.58% per year) in the years 2004–2010 [54]. There were 1185 cases of melanoma in persons ≤20 years of age, with only 124 cases in children under the age of 10 between the years 2000–2010 [54]. Superficial spreading melanoma was the most common histological subtype in children older than 10 years of age but in younger patients, the proportions of nodular and superficial spreading melanoma were similar [54]. Paediatric melanoma is slightly more common in girls [54–56] and individuals over the age of 10 [54,55]. In adolescents (15–19 year olds), melanoma is most commonly found on the trunk [54], while melanomas located on the head and neck region are more common in younger patients [54–56]. While many melanomas manifest the classic ABCD features (asymmetry, border irregularity, colour

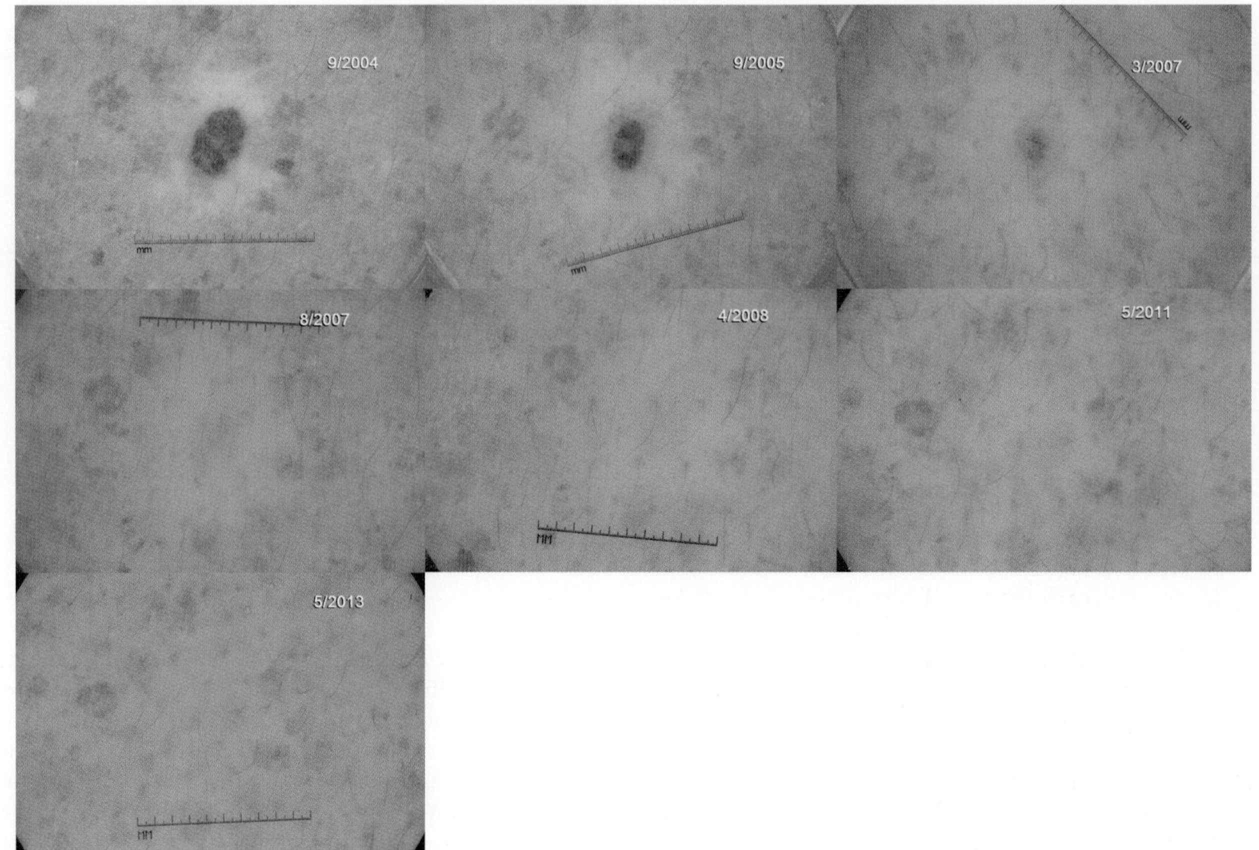

Fig. 175.18 This globular halo naevus was followed sequentially. Notice that the naevus pattern remains unchanged over follow-up. The naevus becomes smaller until it completely disappears.

Table 175.5 Benign dermoscopic patterns (see Figs 175.8 and 175.12)

Global pattern	Definition
Reticular diffuse	Diffuse homogeneous network with minimal variation in the thickness and colour of lines. The holes of the network are of relatively uniform size. The network tends to fade at the periphery. This pattern can be seen in congenital naevi, especially those located on the lower extremity, and in acquired naevi
Reticular patchy	Homogeneous network with uniform thickness and colour of lines. However, the network is not contiguous due to the presence of intervening homogeneous structureless areas. This pattern can be seen in congenital naevi, especially those located on the lower extremity, and in acquired naevi
Peripheral reticular with central hypopigmentation	A relatively uniform network at the periphery of the lesion with a central homogeneous and hypopigmented structureless area. This type of acquired naevus is more common in fair skin phenotypes
Peripheral reticular with central hyperpigmentation	A relatively uniform network at the periphery of the lesion with a central homogeneous and hyperpigmented blotch. This type of acquired naevus is more common in darker skin phenotypes
Globular	Globules of similar shape, size and colour distributed symmetrically throughout the lesion. This pattern is seen most commonly in congenital naevi
Peripheral reticular with central globules	A relatively uniform network at the periphery of the lesion with central globules. This pattern is seen most often in naevi with a congenital histopathology pattern
Peripheral globules with central network or homogeneous area	The central component of this type of naevus is either reticular or homogeneous. Relatively uniform globules surround the entire perimeter of the lesion. This represents a radially growing (enlarging) naevus that has not yet undergone senescence
Homogeneous tan, brown or blue pigmentation	Primarily diffuse structureless pattern with or without focal reticular network fragments and/or few scattered globules. When tan in colour, they usually represent acquired naevi in fair skin phenotypes. When brown in colour, they usually represent congenital naevi. When blue in colour, they represent blue naevi
Two-component	These lesions can reveal one of three different patterns (reticular-globular, reticular-homogeneous or globular-homogeneous). One half of the lesion manifests one pattern while the other half manifests a different pattern
Multicomponent	Symmetrically distributed globules, reticulation, blotches, dots, veil, regression structures and/or structureless areas (three or more of these need to be present)
Starburst	Streaks (radial streaming or pseudopods) present around the perimeter of the lesion giving the appearance of an exploding star

variegation, and diameter >6 mm), many paediatric melanomas lack the classic ABCD characteristics [2,57]. Over 40% are amelanotic and more than 50% are symmetrical lesions with well-defined borders [58]. The majority of melanomas arise de novo with an increased proportion of nodular melanomas occurring in the paediatric population [58,59]. Given the rarity of melanoma in childhood coupled with an often atypical presentation in children, misdiagnosis and delay in treatment are not uncommon [60,61].

Melanocytic lesions manifesting one of the benign dermoscopic patterns listed in Table 175.5 and in which the dermoscopic structures are distributed in an organized and symmetrical manner (see Figs 175.8 and 175.12) can safely be monitored. Lesions displaying a pattern that deviates from the benign patterns listed in Table 175.5 should be viewed with caution, especially if any of the melanoma-specific structures listed in Table 175.6 are also seen (Fig. 175.19). On rare occasions, melanomas will display a symmetrical and organized pattern; however, this apparently banal-appearing pattern will not adhere to one of the benign patterns listed in Table 175.5 (Figs 175.20 and 175.21).

It is important to remember that melanomas developing in children are often nodular, spitzoid and/or amelanotic. These melanomas are often difficult to diagnose but the presence of irregular blood vessels, shiny white structures seen with polarized light and/or a negative network seen with dermoscopy can assist in their identification (Figs 175.22 and 175.23) [62].

Lastly, the greatest melanoma masquerader encountered in the paediatric population is the Spitz naevus (including Reed naevus). It should be noted that any dermoscopic structure encountered in melanoma (see Table 175.6) can also be seen in Spitz naevi, with the exception of peripheral tan structureless areas and regression structures.

Spitz naevi

Spitz naevi are biologically benign melanocytic naevi, which can be confused with melanoma both clinically and histopathologically. A deeply pigmented variant of this naevus is referred to as a Reed naevus or pigmented spindle cell naevus of Reed. Spitz naevi are made up of epithelioid and/or spindled melanocytes and they often have little to no pigmentation. Classically, the lesions appear pink-red in colour. In contrast, the Reed naevus contains spindled melanocytes with heavy pigmentation, with a brown-black clinical appearance. While most Spitz naevi appear as solitary lesions, they can also appear as grouped (clustered) or disseminated lesions [63,64].

Diagnostic accuracy of Spitz naevi has been shown to increase from 56% to 93% with the utilization of dermoscopy [65]. There are several dermoscopic patterns that can be appreciated in Spitz–Reed naevi (Fig. 175.24). The patterns include thick (atypical) reticular, atypical globular, starburst, homogeneous (pink or black lamella), negative network and atypical/multicomponent [26,65–69]. The archetypal Spitz naevus pattern is the starburst pattern, a pattern that resembles an exploding star. In fact, over 50%

Table 175.6 Histopathological correlates of dermoscopic structures found in superficial spreading melanoma

Dermoscopic structure	Description	Histopathological correlate
Atypical pigment network	Reticulated grid of brown lines with broadened, thickened or darkened areas that may end abruptly at the periphery	Atypical lentiginous or nested melanocytic proliferation along the dermoepidermal junction
Streaks	Linear, radially oriented pigmented projections at the periphery of a lesion	Confluent junctional nests of pigmented melanoma cells at the periphery (radial growth phase)
Negative network	The 'negative' of the pigment network, consisting of hypopigmented lines making up the grid and dark areas filling up the 'holes'	It is believed to represent thin elongated rete ridges and large tubular melanocytic nests within a widened papillary dermis. However, it may also represent bridging of rete ridges
Shiny white lines	Fine, white, shiny streaks within a lesion, visible only under polarized light dermoscopy	Remodelled matrix or new dermal collagen
Atypical dots and globules	Dark, punctate or round to oval structures of varying shape, size, colour and distribution within a lesion	Junctional or dermal nests of melanocytes; dots can also represent pagetoid nests
Irregular blotches	Dark areas of diffuse pigmentation with irregular shapes, sharp margins or eccentric locations	Melanin pigmentation throughout the epidermis or dermis or both
Blue-white structures over raised areas	White areas, blue areas or both, overlying raised or thick portions of a lesion	Compact orthokeratosis overlying melanophages, melanocytes or free melanin in the papillary dermis
Regression structures	White areas, grey granularity/peppering or both, overlying flat portions of a lesion	Fibrosis within the papillary dermis and melanosis (melanophages and free melanin 'dust' within the dermis)
Atypical vascular structures	Milky red areas, dotted, serpentine, linear or twisted red structures with differing sizes	Tumour-induced neoangiogenesis
Peripheral brown structureless areas	Peripherally arranged light brown or tan areas of variable shape lacking perceptible structures	Flattening of the rete ridges with pagetoid spread of atypical melanocytes

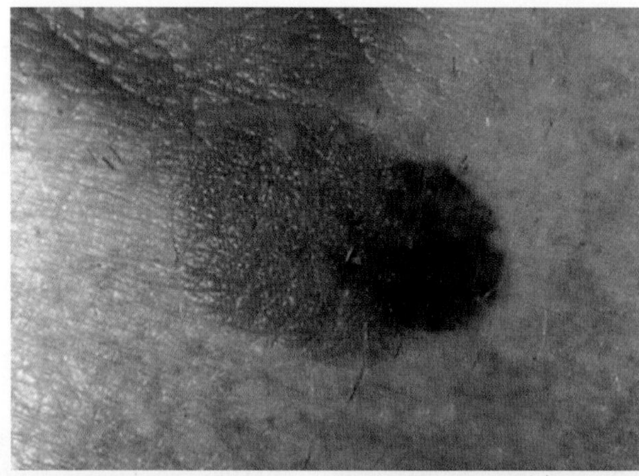

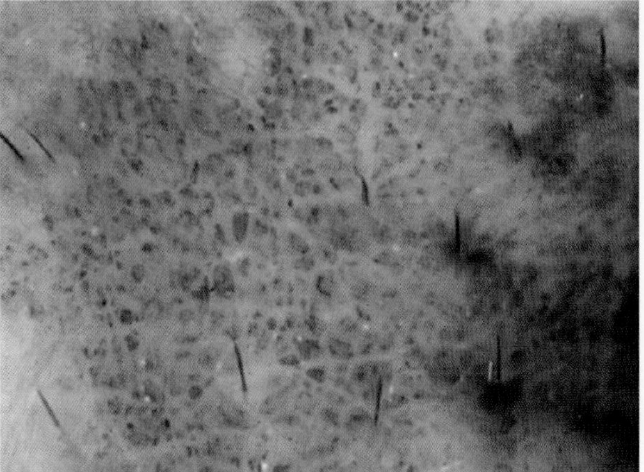

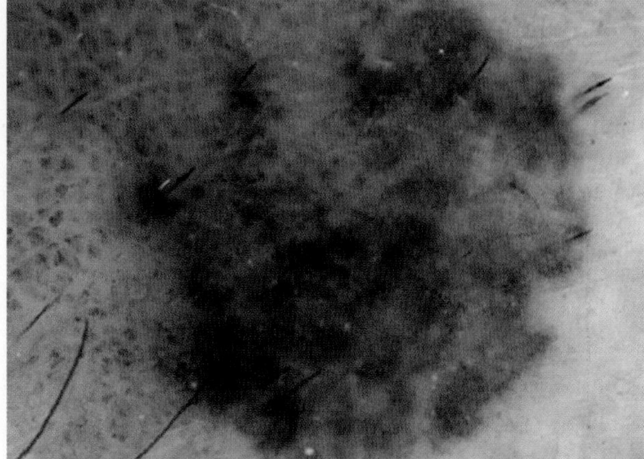

Fig. 175.19 This lesion has a pattern that deviates from the known benign naevus patterns. It has a cobblestone globular pattern. However, at the peripheral edge there is an area with irregular dots and network. This represents a melanoma developing in association with a CMN.

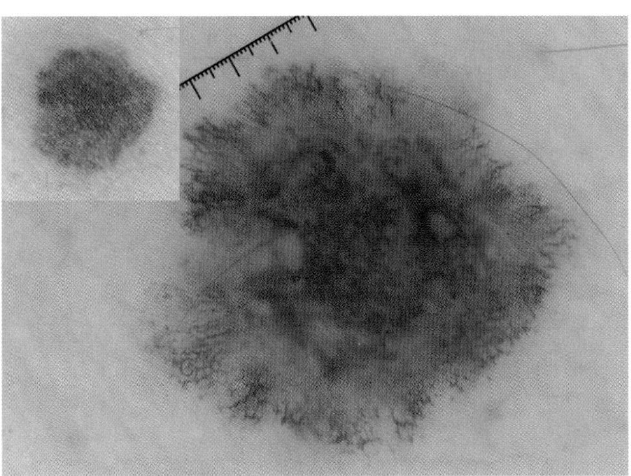

Fig. 175.20 This melanoma has a symmetrical and organized pattern but it is not one of the known benign patterns. In addition, it has a negative network in the centre and a focal blue-white veil.

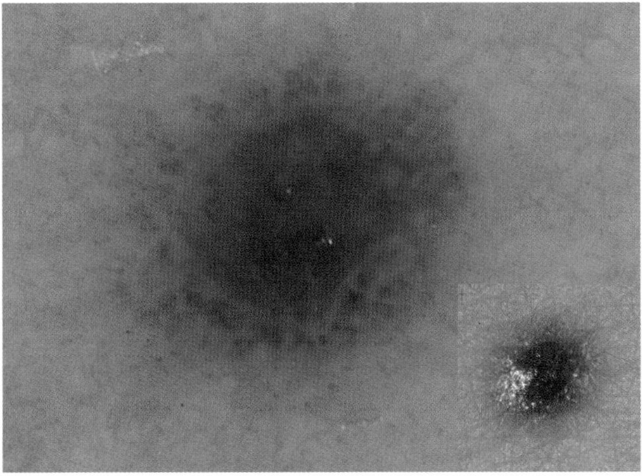

Fig. 175.21 This symmetrical and organized-appearing melanoma does not adhere to the known benign naevus patterns. It also has a central raised blue-white veil and irregular globules at the periphery.

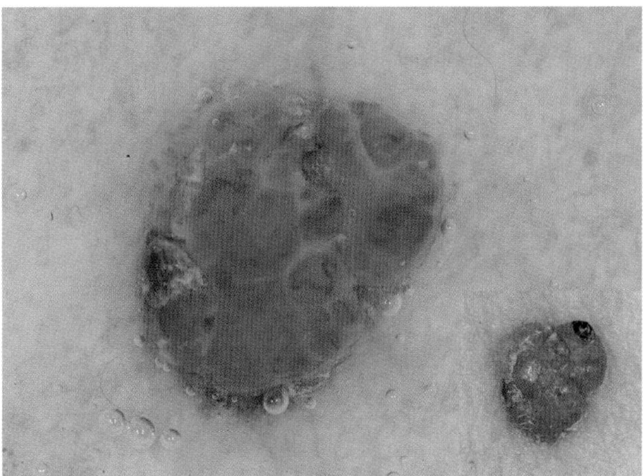

Fig. 175.22 This lesion does not reveal any network, aggregated globules or streaks. It lacks features diagnostic of one of the nonmelanocytic lesions. However, it does have irregular, serpentine vessels, helping to correctly diagnose it as a malignant melanoma.

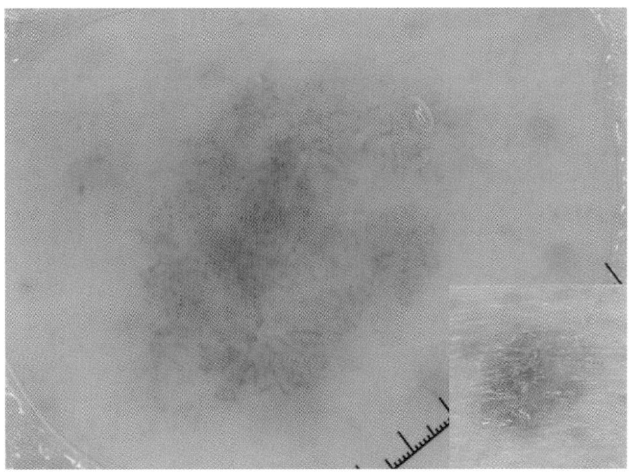

Fig. 175.23 This seemingly featureless lesion has dotted and serpentine vessels. The presence of these vessels helped to correctly identify this lesion as a melanoma.

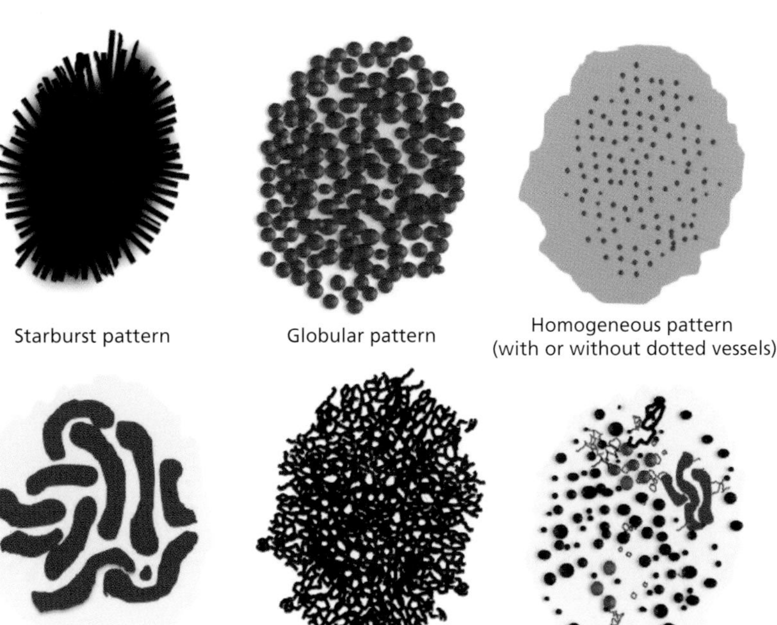

Fig. 175.24 The schematic illustrates the most common patterns seen in Spitz naevi.

of the biopsied Reed naevi had the starburst pattern [70]. In the starburst pattern, the lesion has a homogeneously distributed pattern of streaks, pseudopods and/or tiered globules around the entire perimeter of the lesion (Figs 175.25, 175.26 and 175.27). Tiered globules around the naevus create a starburst pattern composed of multiple rows of peripheral globules [25,70]. This pattern has similarity to the peripheral globular pattern seen in growing naevi with the difference that in Spitz, there are multiple rows of globules and in nonSpitz growing naevi there is a single row (Fig. 175.28) [70].

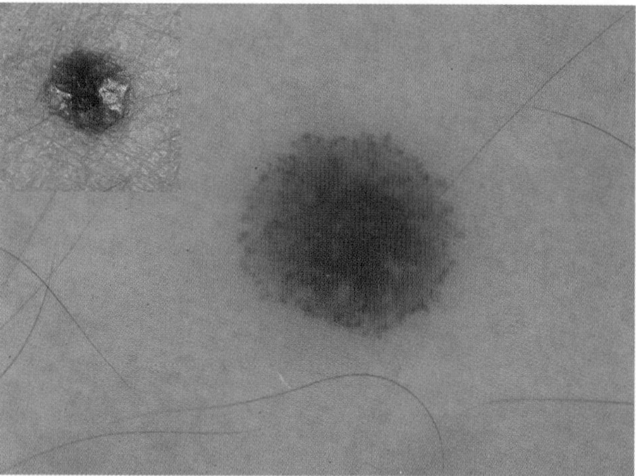

Fig. 175.25 Classic starburst pattern of a Spitz naevus with globules and streaks.

The central part of these naevi usually displays a homogeneous pattern ranging in colour from blue-grey to blue-white to brown or brown-black. Histopathology reveals discrete junctional fascicles and nests of pigmented spindle cells with melanin and melanophages in the papillary dermis [26,27,66,71,72]. Over 50% of Spitz–Reed naevi present with the starburst pattern. When present, this pattern has been reported to allow for a diagnostic sensitivity of 96% [10].

Spitz naevi can present with a thickened and dark network pattern (Fig. 175.29). The reticular pattern consists of a predominantly black, sometimes dark brown network. The network can appear thickened. Centrally, there may be bluish-grey hue. On histopathology, there are nests of epithelioid and spindle cells of varying degrees of pigmentation located along the epidermal rete ridges [26,27,66,71,72].

The negative network pattern, with or without shiny white line structures, is another pattern encountered in Spitz naevi (Figs 175.30, 175.31 and 175.32). The negative network results from relatively hypopigmented and narrow rete ridges, and large melanocytic nests residing in a widened dermal papillae. The negative network consists of light areas making up the 'grid' of the network, with the dark areas presenting as the 'holes'. While Spitz naevi

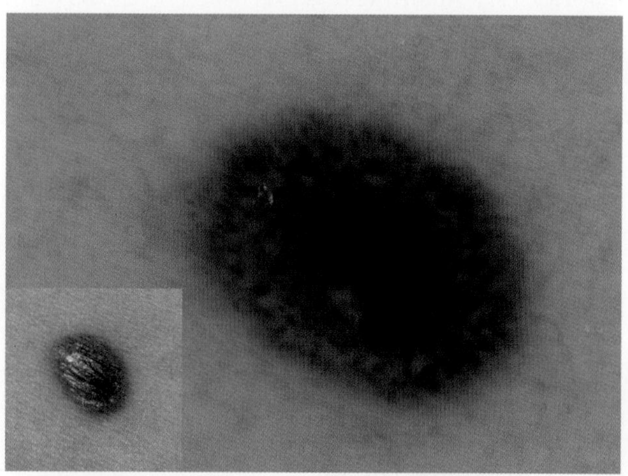

Fig. 175.26 Classic starburst pattern of a Spitz naevus with streaks.

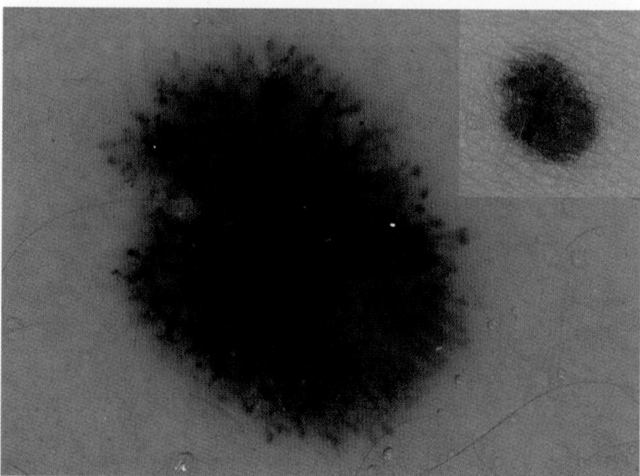

Fig. 175.27 This lesion has a starburst pattern with streaks. The differential diagnosis is Spitz naevi versus malignant melanoma. This lesion was a Spitz naevus.

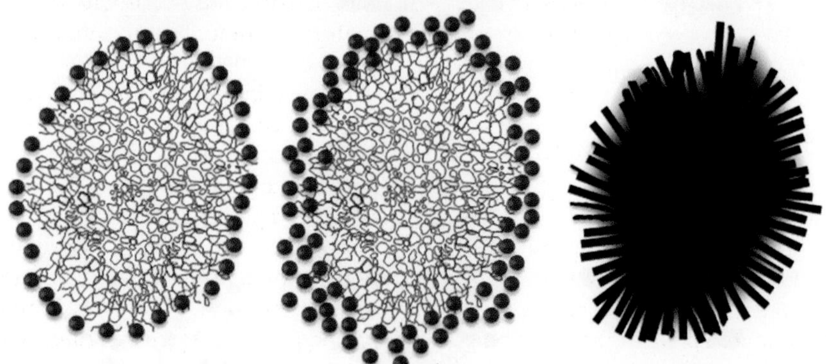

Fig. 175.28 The schematic on the left corresponds to a growing nonspitz naevus and the schematic on the right corresponds to a growing Reed naevus. The central schematic depicts the tiered globular pattern. Naevi with this pattern tend to have a spitzoid morphology on histopathology.

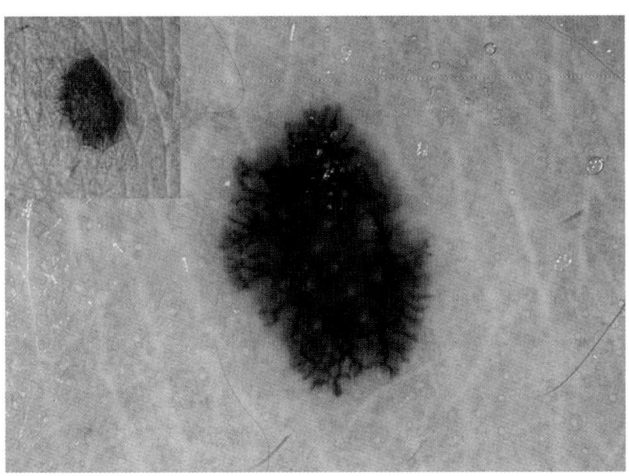

Fig. 175.29 Black network over grey background is present in this Spitz naevus. Source: Courtesy of Dr Ralph Braun.

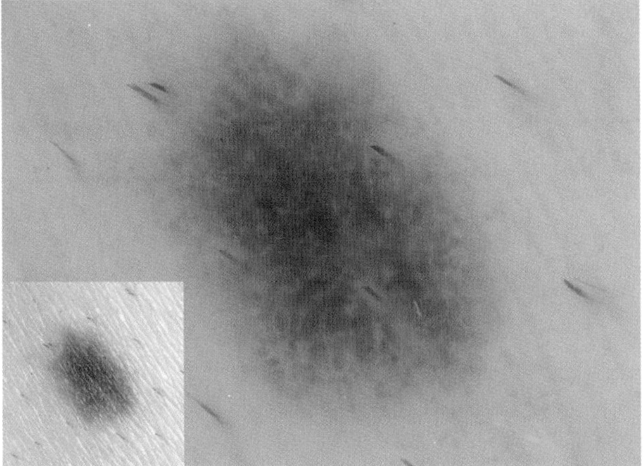

Fig. 175.30 This Spitz naevus has a negative network pattern.

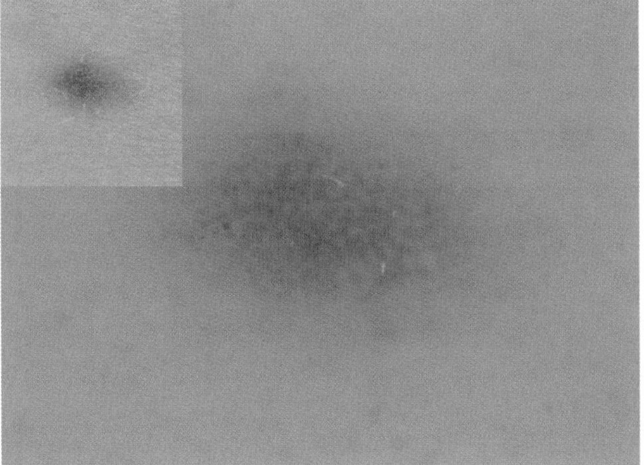

Fig. 175.31 This Spitz naevus has a negative network pattern.

tend to have a symmetrically distributed negative network and melanomas an asymmetrically or eccentrically distributed negative network, the overlap is significant enough that the quality of the negative network and its distribution cannot be used to reliably differentiate Spitz naevi from melanoma [70]. The shiny white lines (also known as crystalline structures) consist of bright white orthogonally oriented lines and correlate with altered papillary dermal collagen. Since collagen is birefringent, the shiny white lines can easily be seen with polarized light dermoscopy and are not visible when viewed with standard nonpolarized light dermoscopy (Fig. 175.33). Focal shiny white lines can be seen in any Spitz naevus, irrespective of its global pattern (see Fig. 175.33).

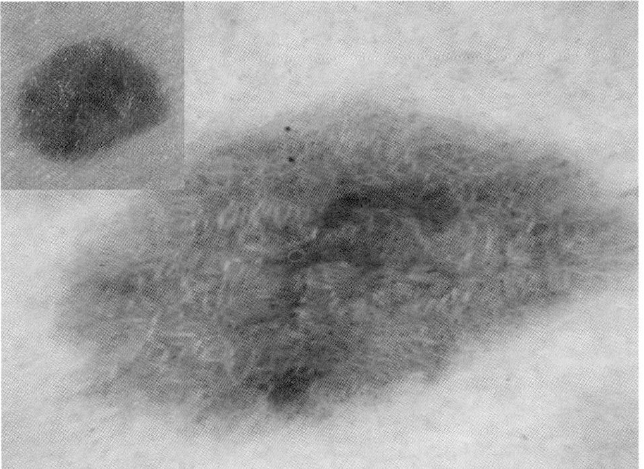

Fig. 175.32 This Spitz naevus has shiny white lines, consisting of linear, white, orthogonal streaks. They can be seen only with polarized light. Source: Courtesy of Dr Harold Rabinovitz.

The globular Spitz naevus pattern consists of globules that can vary in size and colour (see Fig. 175.33). The colours of the globules range from brown-black to blue-grey. Approximately 22% of Spitz naevi manifest a globular pattern [73]. These globules tend to be distributed throughout the lesion with prominence of central grey-blue-white pigmentation.

The homogeneous pattern usually consists of a pink (Fig. 175.34) or black (black lamella) lesion (Fig. 175.35). Although in most homogeneous Spitz tumours one cannot discern any dermoscopic structures, in some pink Spitz naevi one can see dotted or irregular vessels (Fig. 175.36). Pink Spitz naevi that possess dotted or irregular vessels cannot clinically be differentiated from melanoma with confidence [26,27,66,71,72]. In addition, there exists another group of Spitz naevi that manifest an atypical dermoscopic pattern. These lesions are often dermoscopically asymmetrical and/or appear to have a disorganized architecture (Fig. 175.37). Many of these lesions will have an asymmetrical multicomponent pattern and will manifest features commonly associated with melanoma (Fig. 175.38).

Due to the overlapping of clinical, dermoscopic and histopathological features, it is currently clinically impossible to differentiate an atypical Spitz naevus from melanoma [74]. It is interesting to note that 53% of Spitz lesions with an atypical dermoscopic pattern were found to be atypical on histopathology as well [73]. Guidelines created for management of spitzoid lesions by Ferrara et al. suggest that spitzoid lesions in prepubertal children that are dome-shaped or plaque-type lesions manifesting an organized/symmetrical dermoscopic pattern can be

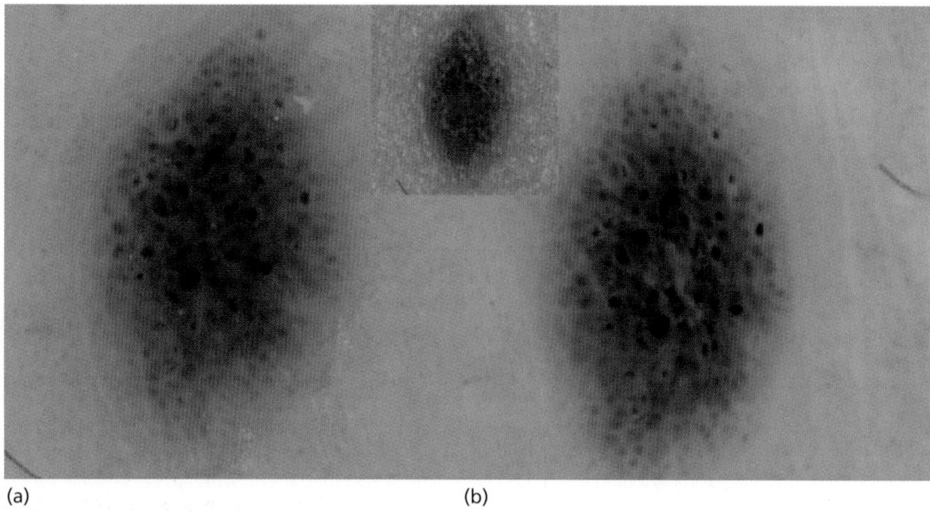

Fig. 175.33 This Spitz naevus has a globular pattern. Image (a) is taken with nonpolarized light dermoscopy. Image (b) is taken with polarized light. Note that shiny white lines can only be seen with polarized light.

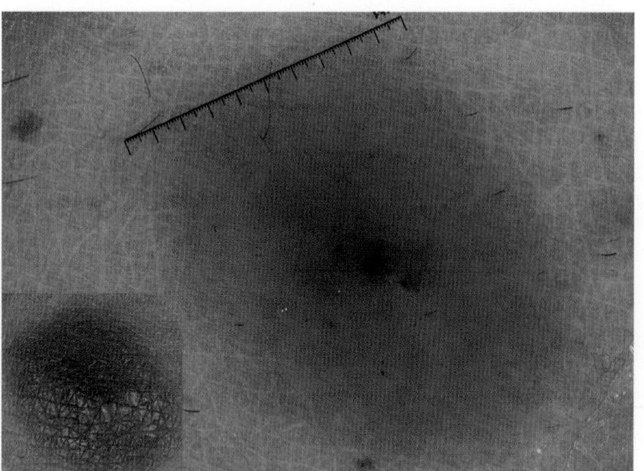

Fig. 175.34 Homogeneous, pink Spitz naevus pattern.

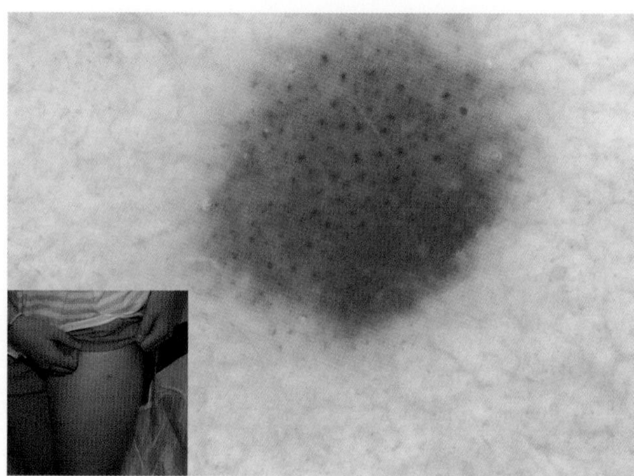

Fig. 175.36 This homogeneous, pink Spitz naevus reveals dotted vessels. A similar pattern can also be seen in amelanotic melanoma.

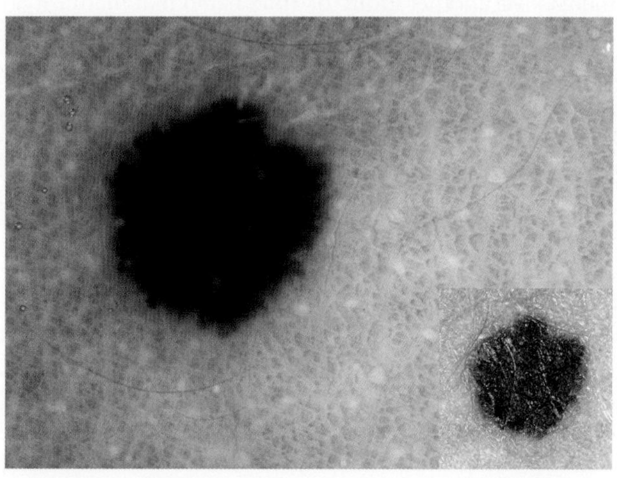

Fig. 175.35 Homogeneous, black lamella Spitz naevus pattern.

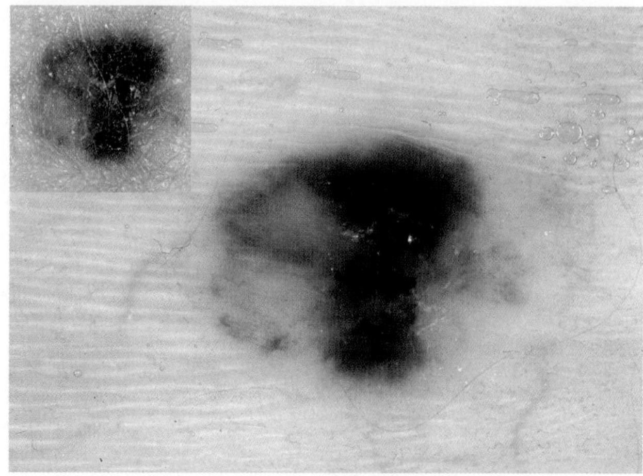

Fig. 175.37 This Spitz naevus reveals an asymmetrical, disorganized, multicomponent pattern. It is impossible to differentiate such Spitz naevi from malignant melanoma via dermoscopy.

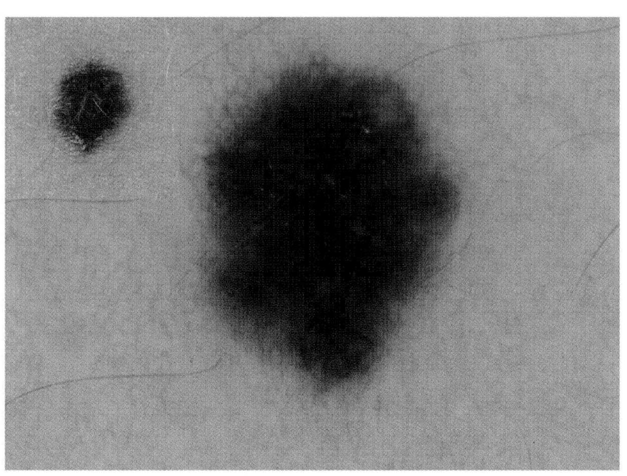

Fig. 175.38 This Spitz naevus has a focal atypical network and irregular globules located focally at the periphery. It is virtually impossible to rule out melanoma in this lesion via dermoscopy.

monitored via sequential digital dermoscopy imaging [75,76]. These lesions can be followed as long as they remain stable or grow in a symmetrical manner without developing any melanoma-specific structures. However, complete excision is recommended for lesions that are nodular, larger than 10 mm, ulcerated or have an atypical growth pattern [76].

Since atypical Spitz naevi may share many histological features of melanoma, the challenge in distinguishing them is not limited to the clinical examination alone. Investigation in the molecular realm (CGH, sequencing, gene expression profiling) may aid in the distinction between melanoma and Spitz naevi. Comparative genomic hybridization (CGH) is a technique that helps detect chromosomal copy number changes or aberrations in cells [77–79]. In addition, direct DNA sequencing has helped isolate specific mutations. For example, it has been found that up to 25.8% of Spitz naevi harbour HRAS genetic alterations due to mutations or copy number gains [77,80–82]. Chromosomal changes in primary cutaneous melanoma have been reported to include frequent deletions of chromosome 9p and 10q with gains of chromosomes 7, 8q and 6p [83]. Spitz naevi lack chromosomal abnormalities, with the exception of a subset of Spitz naevi that possess an increased copy number of chromosome 11p [77].

Recently, kinase fusion proteins involving serine-threonine kinase BRAF or the receptor tyrosine kinases ALK, NTRK1, RET and ROS1 have been associated with benign and malignant spitz tumours [84,85]. Moreover, Wititsuwannakul et al. described the expression of Neuropilin-2 (NRP2) in 100% (n = 19) of spitzoid malignant melanoma cases but in only 26% (n = 5) of Spitz naevi

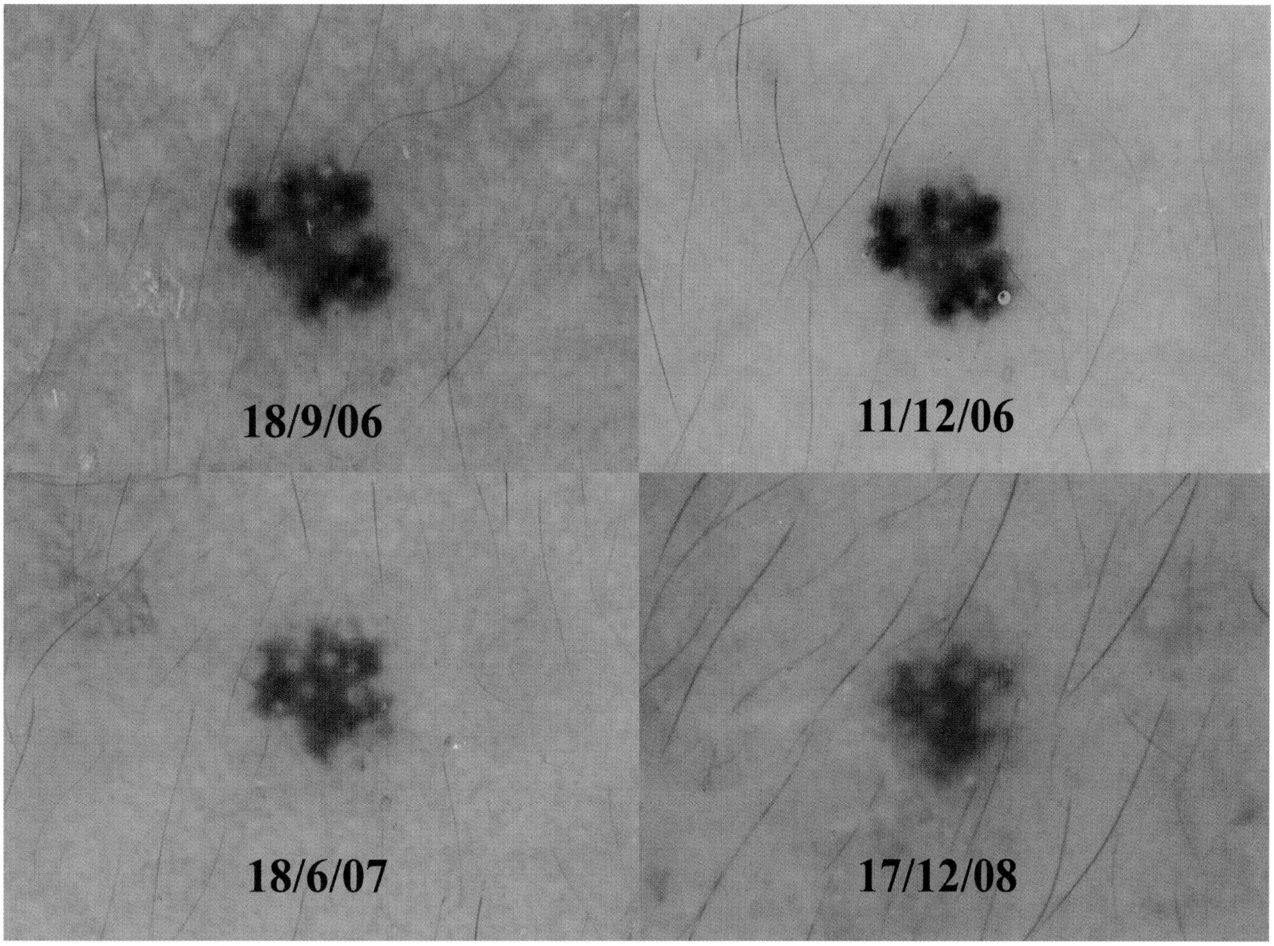

Fig. 175.39 This presumed Spitz naevus on the face of a 14-year-old girl involuted over a follow-up of 27 months.

cases [86]. Future molecular studies may help provide the basis for a technique to improve diagnostic accuracy in spitzoid tumours [77].

It has been suggested that some Spitz naevi can change their pattern over time. The changing patterns are believed to represent various stages of naevogenesis. In the early stage of a Spitz–Reed naevus a globular pattern can be appreciated. As the lesion continues to mature, the classic starburst pattern can be observed. This is considered to be an intermediate stage in the radial growth phase of a Spitz–Reed naevus [67]. As the naevus proceeds in maturation, a homogeneous pattern emerges, presenting as diffuse brown pigmentation with a central bluish hue [69,87,88]. It has been suggested that the final stage in evolution of some Spitz naevi may be complete involution of the lesion (Fig. 175.39) [69,87].

Conclusion

While the majority of pigmented lesions in children are benign, the challenge lies in correctly identifying high-risk pigmented lesions and malignant melanoma. Dermoscopy is a noninvasive, *in vivo* technique that gives the clinician an additional tool to help evaluate and diagnose pigmented lesions more accurately. This chapter offers the clinician a framework for assessing dermoscopic structures within pigmented lesions. When used together, both the clinical and dermoscopic morphology can greatly assist the clinician in evaluating pigmented lesions in children.

References

1 Marghoob AA, Scope A. The complexity of diagnosing melanoma. J Invest Dermatol 2009;129(1):11–13.

2 Cordoro KM, Gupta D, Frieden IJ et al. Pediatric melanoma: results of a large cohort study and proposal for modified ABCD detection criteria for children. J Am Acad Dermatol 2013;68(6):913–25.

3 Binder M, Puespoeck-Schwarz M, Steiner A et al. Epiluminescence microscopy of small pigmented skin lesions: short-term formal training improves the diagnostic performance of dermatologists. J Am Acad Dermatol 1997;36(2 Pt 1):197–202.

4 Pagnanelli G, Soyer HP, Argenziano G et al. Diagnosis of pigmented skin lesions by dermoscopy: web-based training improves diagnostic performance of non-experts. Br J Dermatol 2003;148(4):698–702.

5 Kittler H, Pehamberger H, Wolff K, Binder M. Diagnostic accuracy of dermoscopy. Lancet Oncol 2002;3(3):159–65.

6 Bafounta ML, Beauchet A, Aegerter P, Saiag P. Is dermoscopy (epiluminescence microscopy) useful for the diagnosis of melanoma? Results of a meta-analysis using techniques adapted to the evaluation of diagnostic tests. Arch Dermatol 2001;137(10):1343–50.

7 Vestergaard ME, Macaskill P, Holt PE, Menzies SW. Dermoscopy compared with naked eye examination for the diagnosis of primary melanoma: a meta-analysis of studies performed in a clinical setting. Br J Dermatol 2008;159(3):669–76.

8 Pan Y, Gareau DS, Scope A et al. Polarized and nonpolarized dermoscopy: the explanation for the observed differences. Arch Dermatol 2008;144(6):828–9.

9 Benvenuto-Andrade C, Dusza SW, Agero AL et al. Differences between polarized light dermoscopy and immersion contact dermoscopy for the evaluation of skin lesions. Arch Dermatol 2007;143(3): 329–38.

10 Yadav S, Vossaert KA, Kopf AW et al. Histopathologic correlates of structures seen on dermoscopy (epiluminescence microscopy). Am J Dermatopathol 1993;15(4):297–305.

11 Rezze GG, Scramim AP, Neves RI, Landman G. Structural correlations between dermoscopic features of cutaneous melanomas and histopathology using transverse sections. Am J Dermatopathol 2006;28(1):13–20.

12 Massi D, de Giorgi V, Soyer HP. Histopathologic correlates of dermoscopic criteria. Dermatol Clin 2001;19(2):259–68, vii.

13 Menzies SW, Gutenev A, Avramidis M et al. Short-term digital surface microscopic monitoring of atypical or changing melanocytic lesions. Arch Dermatol 2001;137(12):1583–9.

14 Benvenuto-Andrade C, Marghood AA. Ten reasons why dermoscopy is beneficial for the evaluation of skin lesions. Exp Rev Dermatol 2006;1(3):369–74.

15 Cramer SF, Salgado CM, Reyes-Mugica M. The high multiplicity of prenatal (congenital type) naevi in adolescents and adults. Evidence for the intradermal origin of prenatal naevi. Pediatr Dev Pathol 2016;19(5):409–16.

16 Krengel S, Scope A, Dusza SW et al. New recommendations for the categorization of cutaneous features of congenital melanocytic naevi. J Am Acad Dermatol 2013;68(3):441–51.

17 Krengel S, Hauschild A, Schafer T. Melanoma risk in congenital melanocytic naevi: a systematic review. Br J Dermatol 2006;155(1):1–8.

18 Kinsler VA, Chong WK, Aylett SE, Atherton DJ. Complications of congenital melanocytic naevi in children: analysis of 16 years' experience and clinical practice. Br J Dermatol 2008;159(4):907–14.

19 Krengel S, Marghoob AA. Current management approaches for congenital melanocytic naevi. Dermatol Clin 2012;30(3):377–87.

20 Alikhan A, Ibrahimi OA, Eisen DB. Congenital melanocytic naevi: where are we now? Part I. Clinical presentation, epidemiology, pathogenesis, histology, malignant transformation, and neurocutaneous melanosis. J Am Acad Dermatol 2012;67(4):495.e1–17; quiz 512–14.

21 Slutsky JB, Barr JM, Femia AN, Marghoob AA. Large congenital melanocytic naevi: associated risks and management considerations. Semin Cutan Med Surg 2010;29(2):79–84.

22 Charbel C, Fontaine RH, Malouf GG et al. NRAS mutation is the sole recurrent somatic mutation in large congenital melanocytic naevi. J Invest Dermatol 2014;134(4):1067–74.

23 Schaffer JV. Update on melanocytic naevi in children. Clin Dermatol 2015;33(3):368–86.

24 Braun RP, Calza AM, Krischer J, Saurat JH. The use of digital dermoscopy for the follow-up of congenital naevi: a pilot study. Pediatr Dermatol 2001;18(4):277–81.

25 Haliasos EC, Kerner M, Jaimes N et al. Dermoscopy for the pediatric dermatologist part III: dermoscopy of melanocytic lesions. Pediatr Dermatol 2013;30(3):281–93.

26 Marghoob AA, Braun RP, Malvehy J. Atlas of Dermoscopy, 2nd edn. New York: Informa Healthcare, 2012.

27 Soyer HP, Kenet RO, Wolf IH et al. Clinicopathological correlation of pigmented skin lesions using dermoscopy. Eur J Dermatol 2000; 10(1):22–8.

28 Soyer HP, Smolle J, Hodl S et al. Surface microscopy. A new approach to the diagnosis of cutaneous pigmented tumors. Am J Dermatopathol 1989;11(1):1–10.

29 Kenet RO, Kang S, Kenet BJ et al. Clinical diagnosis of pigmented lesions using digital epiluminescence microscopy. Grading protocol and atlas. Arch Dermatol 1993;129(2):157–74.

30 Seidenari S, Ferrari C, Borsari S et al. The dermoscopic variability of pigment network in melanoma in situ. Melanoma Res 2012; 22(2):151–7.

31 Soyer HP, Argenziano G, Chimenti S, Ruocco V. Dermoscopy of pigmented skin lesions. Eur J Dermatol 2001;11(3):270–6; quiz 2777.

32 Changchien L, Dusza SW, Agero AL et al. Age- and site-specific variation in the dermoscopic patterns of congenital melanocytic naevi: an aid to accurate classification and assessment of melanocytic naevi. Arch Dermatol 2007;143(8):1007–14.

33 Seidenari S, Pellacani G, Martella A et al. Instrument-, age- and site-dependent variations of dermoscopic patterns of congenital melanocytic naevi: a multicentre study. Br J Dermatol 2006;155(1):56–61.

34 Nordlund JJ. The lives of pigment cells. Dermatol Clin 1986; 4(3):407–18.

35 Zalaudek I, Hofmann-Wellenhof R, Kittler H et al. A dual concept of nevogenesis: theoretical considerations based on dermoscopic features of melanocytic naevi. J Deutsch Dermatol Ges 2007;5(11):985–92.

36 Strauss RM, Newton Bishop JA. Spontaneous involution of congenital melanocytic naevi of the scalp. J Am Acad Dermatol 2008;58(3):508–11.

37 Zalaudek I, Argenziano G, Mordente I et al. Nevus type in dermoscopy is related to skin type in white persons. Arch Dermatol 2007; 143(3):351–6.

38 Orlow I, Satagopan JM, Berwick M et al. Genetic factors associated with naevus count and dermoscopic patterns: preliminary results from the Study of Naevi in Children (SONIC). Br J Dermatol 2015;172(4):1081–9.

39 **Bajaj S, Dusza SW, Marchetti MA et al. Growth-curve modeling of naevi with a peripheral globular pattern. JAMA Dermatol 2015;151(12):1338–45.**

40 Banky JP, Kelly JW, English DR et al. Incidence of new and changed naevi and melanomas detected using baseline images and dermoscopy in patients at high risk for melanoma. Arch Dermatol 2005;141(8):998–1006.

41 **Scope A, Dusza SW, Marghoob AA et al. Clinical and dermoscopic stability and volatility of melanocytic naevi in a population-based cohort of children in Framingham school system. J Invest Dermatol 2011;131(8):1615–21.**

42 LaVigne EA, Oliveria SA, Dusza SW et al. Clinical and dermoscopic changes in common melanocytic naevi in school children: the Framingham school nevus study. Dermatology 2005;211(3):234–9.

43 Kvaskoff M, Whiteman DC, Zhao ZZ et al. Polymorphisms in nevus-associated genes MTAP, PLA2G6, and IRF4 and the risk of invasive cutaneous melanoma. Twin Res Human Genet 2011;14(5):422–32.

44 Tucker MA, Greene MH, Clark WH Jr et al. Dysplastic naevi on the scalp of prepubertal children from melanoma-prone families. J Pediatr 1983;103(1):65–9.

45 Fernandez M, Raimer SS, Sanchez RL. Dysplastic naevi of the scalp and forehead in children. Pediatr Dermatol 2001;18(1):5–8.

46 Gupta M, Berk DR, Gray C et al. Morphologic features and natural history of scalp naevi in children. Arch Dermatol 2010;146(5):506–11.

47 Aguilera P, Puig S, Guilabert A et al. Prevalence study of naevi in children from Barcelona. Dermoscopy, constitutional and environmental factors. Dermatology 2009;218(3):203–14.

48 Scope A, Burroni M, Agero AL et al. Predominant dermoscopic patterns observed among naevi. J Cutan Med Surg 2006;10(4):170–4.

49 Lipoff JB, Scope A, Dusza SW et al. Complex dermoscopic pattern: a potential risk marker for melanoma. Br J Dermatol 2008;158(4):821–4.

50 Sutton R. An unusual variety of vitiligo (leucoderma acquisitum centrifugum). J Cutan Dis 1916;34:797–800.

51 Barnhill RL, Rabinovitz H. Benign melanocytic neoplasms: halo nevus. In: Bolognia J, Schaffer JV, Duncan KO, Ko CJ (eds) Dermatology Essentials, 2nd edn. London: Mosby Elsevier, 2008: 1725–6.

52 Kolm I, di Stefani A, Hofmann-Wellenhof R et al. Dermoscopy patterns of halo naevi. Arch Dermatol 2006;142(12):1627–32.

53 Siegel DA, King J, Tai E et al. Cancer incidence rates and trends among children and adolescents in the United States, 2001–2009. Pediatrics. 2014;134(4):e945–55.

54 Campbell LB, Kreicher KL, Gittleman HR et al. Melanoma incidence in children and adolescents: decreasing trends in the United States. J Pediatr 2015;166(6):1505–13.

55 Lange JR, Palis BE, Chang DC et al. Melanoma in children and teenagers: an analysis of patients from the National Cancer Data Base. J Clin Oncol 2007;25(11):1363–8.

56 Hamre MR, Chuba P, Bakhshi S et al. Cutaneous melanoma in childhood and adolescence. Pediatr Hematol Oncol 2002;19(5):309–17.

57 Yagerman SE, Chen L, Jaimes N et al. 'Do UC the melanoma?' Recognising the importance of different lesions displaying unevenness or having a history of change for early melanoma detection. Australas J Dermatol 2014;55(2):119–24.

58 Ferrari A, Bono A, Baldi M et al. Does melanoma behave differently in younger children than in adults? A retrospective study of 33 cases of childhood melanoma from a single institution. Pediatrics 2005;115(3):649–54.

59 Jafarian F, Powell J, Kokta V et al. Malignant melanoma in childhood and adolescence: report of 13 cases. J Am Acad Dermatol 2005; 53(5):816–22.

60 Linabery AM, Ross JA. Childhood and adolescent cancer survival in the US by race and ethnicity for the diagnostic period 1975–1999. Cancer 2008;113(9):2575–96.

61 Saenz NC, Saenz-Badillos J, Busam K et al. Childhood melanoma survival. Cancer 1999;85(3):750–4.

62 **Menzies SW, Kreusch J, Byth K et al. Dermoscopic evaluation of amelanotic and hypomelanotic melanoma. Arch Dermatol 2008; 144(9):1120–7.**

63 Zayour M, Bolognia JL, Lazova R. Multiple Spitz naevi: a clinicopathologic study of 9 patients. J Am Acad Dermatol 2012;67(3):451–8, 8.e1–2.

64 **Moscarella E, Lallas A, Kyrgidis A et al. Clinical and dermoscopic features of atypical Spitz tumors: a multicenter, retrospective, case-control study. J Am Acad Dermatol 2015;73(5):777–84.**

65 Steiner A, Pehamberger H, Binder M, Wolff K. Pigmented Spitz naevi: improvement of the diagnostic accuracy by epiluminescence microscopy. J Am Acad Dermatol 1992;27(5 Pt 1):697–701.

66 **Argenziano G, Scalvenzi M, Staibano S et al. Dermatoscopic pitfalls in differentiating pigmented Spitz naevi from cutaneous melanomas. Br J Dermatol 1999;141(5):788–93.**

67 Pizzichetta MA, Argenziano G, Grandi G et al. Morphologic changes of a pigmented Spitz nevus assessed by dermoscopy. J Am Acad Dermatol 2002;47(1):137–9.

68 Pellacani G, Cesinaro AM, Seidenari S. Morphological features of Spitz naevus as observed by digital videomicroscopy. Acta Dermato-Venereol 2000;80(2):117–21.

69 Ferrara G, Moscarella E, Giorgio C, Argenziano G. Spitz nevus and its variants. In: Argenziano G, Hofmann-Wellenhof R, Johr R (eds) Color Atlas of Melanocytic Lesions of the Skin. Berlin: Springer, 2007:151–63.

70 Kerner M, Jaimes N, Scope A, Marghoob AA. Spitz naevi: a bridge between dermoscopic morphology and histopathology. Dermatol Clin 2013;31(2):327–35.

71 Walsh N, Crotty K, Palmer A, McCarthy S. Spitz nevus versus spitzoid malignant melanoma: an evaluation of the current distinguishing histopathologic criteria. Human Pathol 1998;29(10):1105–12.

72 Suster S. Hyalinizing spindle and epithelioid cell nevus. A study of five cases of a distinctive histologic variant of Spitz's nevus. Am J Dermatopathol 1994;16(6):593–8.

73 **Ferrara G, Argenziano G, Soyer HP et al. The spectrum of Spitz naevi: a clinicopathologic study of 83 cases. Arch Dermatol 2005; 141(11):1381–7.**

74 Moscarella E, Al Jalbout S, Piana S et al. The stars within the melanocytic garden: unusual variants of Spitz naevi. Br J Dermatol 2015; 172(4):1045–51.

75 Ferrara G, Zalaudek I, Savarese I et al. Pediatric atypical spitzoid neoplasms: a review with emphasis on 'red' ('spitz') tumors and 'blue' ('blitz') tumors. Dermatology 2010;220(4):306–10.

76 Ferrara G, Cavicchini S, Corradin MT. Hypopigmented atypical Spitzoid neoplasms (atypical Spitz naevi, atypical Spitz tumors, Spitzoid melanoma): a clinicopathological update. Dermatol Pract Concept 2015;5(1):45–52.

77 Bastian BC, Wesselmann U, Pinkel D, Leboit PE. Molecular cytogenetic analysis of Spitz naevi shows clear differences to melanoma. J Invest Dermatol 1999;113(6):1065–9.

78 Harvell JD, Kohler S, Zhu S et al. High-resolution array-based comparative genomic hybridization for distinguishing paraffin-embedded Spitz nevi and melanomas. Diagn Mol Pathol: Am J Surg Pathol B 2004;13(1):22–5.

79 Bastian BC. Molecular cytogenetics as a diagnostic tool for typing melanocytic tumors. Recent Results Cancer Res 2002;160:92–9.

80 Roh MR, Eliades P, Gupta S, Tsao H. Genetics of melanocytic naevi. Pigment Cell Melanoma Res 2015;28(6):661–72.

81 van Engen-van Grunsven AC, van Dijk MC, Ruiter DJ et al. HRAS-mutated Spitz tumors: a subtype of Spitz tumors with distinct features. Am J Surg Pathol 2010;34(10):1436–41.

82 Bastian BC, LeBoit PE, Pinkel D. Mutations and copy number increase of HRAS in Spitz naevi with distinctive histopathological features. Am J Pathol 2000;157(3):967–72.

83 Bastian BC, LeBoit PE, Hamm H et al. Chromosomal gains and losses in primary cutaneous melanomas detected by comparative genomic hybridization. Cancer Res 1998;58(10):2170–5.

84 Wiesner T, He J, Yelensky R et al. Kinase fusions are frequent in Spitz tumours and spitzoid melanomas. Nature Commun 2014;5:3116.

85 Busam KJ, Kutzner H, Cerroni L, Wiesner T. Clinical and pathologic findings of Spitz naevi and atypical Spitz tumors with ALK fusions. Am J Surg Pathol 2014;38(7):925–33.

86 Wititsuwannakul J, Mason AR, Klump VR, Lazova R. Neuropilin-2 as a useful marker in the differentiation between Spitzoid malignant melanoma and Spitz nevus. J Am Acad Dermatol 2013; 68(1):129–37.

87 **Argenziano G, Zalaudek I, Ferrara G et al. Involution: the natural evolution of pigmented Spitz and Reed naevi? Arch Dermatol 2007;143(4):549–51.**

88 Piccolo D, Ferrari A, Peris K. Sequential dermoscopic evolution of pigmented Spitz nevus in childhood. J Am Acad Dermatol 2003; 49(3):556–8.

CHAPTER 176

The Role of Histopathology and Molecular Techniques in Paediatric Dermatology

Lori Prok[1] & Adnan Mir[2]

[1] University of Colorado Denver and Children's Hospital Colorado, Denver, CO, USA
[2] University of Texas Southwestern Medical Center and Children's Medical Center Dallas, Dallas, TX, USA

Introduction, 2378
Rashes, 2379
Lumps and bumps, 2383
Vascular lesions, 2384
Melanocytic lesions, 2386
Molecular diagnostic techniques, 2389
The 'normal' biopsy, 2390

Abstract

Histopathological evaluation of skin biopsies is a powerful tool that aids in the diagnosis and management of paediatric skin conditions. While definitive diagnoses can often be rendered based on histology alone, clinicopathological correlation is often necessary to differentiate entities with overlapping features, and requires communication between the clinician and the pathologist. Where routine histopathology is insufficient, ancillary studies such as immunohistochemistry, genetic testing and cytogenetics can be helpful.

Key points

- **Skin biopsies are an ancillary test that can aid in the diagnosis and management of dermatological conditions, but often require clinicopathological correlation.**
- **Understanding the different inflammatory reaction patterns can help provide specific diagnoses for paediatric inflammatory skin conditions.**
- **Differentiating benign and malignant neoplastic conditions based on histopathology alone is not always possible, and often requires ancillary laboratory testing.**

Introduction

Histopathological examination of a skin biopsy specimen is an essential tool in the investigation of many paediatric dermatological conditions. Although biopsy findings may not be specifically diagnostic when viewed in isolation, when discussed at a clinicopathological multidisciplinary meeting where microscopic findings are placed in the context of the history and clinical photographs, a definitive diagnosis often can be reached. Similar histological findings may require different interpretation according to the clinical circumstances, particularly in the paediatric population.

A skin biopsy may be performed for many reasons: to confirm a clinical suspicion; to distinguish between two or more possibilities that look similar clinically; as a screening test to direct further investigation; as a diagnostic test; to assess response to treatment; to follow the natural history of a disease and, if possible, determine the prognosis. With these goals in mind, several guiding principles can aid the clinician in determining when and how to biopsy the skin in order to provide the pathologist, and ultimately the patient and family, with the most useful and diagnostic information.

- A good clinical history and indication for the biopsy, together with some suggested diagnoses, are very helpful to the pathologist. If there are any special investigations that need to be performed, it is beneficial to discuss these in advance in case the specimen needs special handling. An algorithmic approach to the microscopic examination of the specimen and meticulous attention to detail will often reward the pathologist with the ability to categorize the disease process and frequently to name it precisely.
- Site selection for biopsy can be critical in the correct interpretation of skin disease. In the case of inflammatory processes, biopsy of lesional skin with minimal secondary change (i.e. ulceration, crust, hemorrhage) is best. For blistering disorders, biopsy of the edge of the blister, to include both blistered and normal skin, is preferred. For suspected vasculitis, the 'freshest' lesional petechial or purpuric lesion should be biopsied; older, crusted lesions or those with secondary

SECTION 39: DIAGNOSTIC PROCEDURES IN DERMATOLOGY

Harper's Textbook of Pediatric Dermatology, Fourth Edition. Edited by Peter Hoeger, Veronica Kinsler and Albert Yan.

changes are less likely to be diagnostic. When choosing a biopsy site for direct immunofluorescence investigation of a suspected autoimmune blistering disease, perilesional normal skin (approximately 1 cm away from an active lesion) is most high-yield; lesional skin may be quite inflammatory, and immunoreactants can be locally degraded and difficult to identify.

- Shave, punch and excisional biopsies all have roles in the diagnosis of skin disease. In general, shave biopsies are preferred for superficial inflammatory processes and papular lesions, as they allow adequate evaluation of the epidermis, dermoepidermal junction and superficial dermis, with minimal invasion and wound care for the patient. Broad and deep shave biopsies are also preferred for most pigmented lesions; punch biopsies of small pigmented lesions may be adequate, but many punch specimens are too narrow, allowing for evaluation of only a portion of the centre of the melanocytic lesion, rather than the entire breadth [1]. If there is strong clinical suspicion for melanoma or high-grade atypia in a melanocytic lesion, complete excisional biopsy is preferred, to ensure the entire lesion is examined. Punch or excisional biopsies are best for suspected disorders of dermal collagen, panniculitis, vasculitis and dermal/subcutaneous nodules.
- Some cutaneous eruptions do not have specific findings. In these cases, biopsy will not be definitive or diagnostic. For example, distinguishing between drug eruptions, viral exanthems and urticaria is often not possible without clinicopathological correlation. Similarly, distinguishing between various types of eczematous dermatitis (i.e. irritant contact dermatitis, allergic contact dermatitis and atopic dermatitis) is difficult in most cases.
- Certain in-office procedures can provide very useful and diagnostic information, and alleviate the need for more invasive skin biopsy. Skin scraping with potassium hydroxide preparation is fast and diagnostic of cutaneous fungal infection. Allowing the KOH-treated specimen to 'rest' for 5–10 minutes prior to microscopic evaluation allows easier identification of the fungal organisms. Addition of one drop of chlorazol black, a dye that highlights fungal hyphae, can also make interpretation much easier [2]. Similarly, skin scraping with mineral oil preparation can often isolate scabies mites and ova without need for invasive biopsy. For suspected onychomycosis, a clipping of the involved nail can be sent in a sterile container to the laboratory and stained with H&E and PAS; this technique is considered the gold standard for diagnosis of onychomycosis (Fig. 176.1). The 'turnaround time' for results is much more rapid than fungal nail culture, and can identify fungal hyphae in the nail plate with greater than 90% sensitivity [3].

The remainder of this chapter discusses some of the more common clinical scenarios encountered by the paediatric dermatologist and dermatopathologist, with illustrative examples.

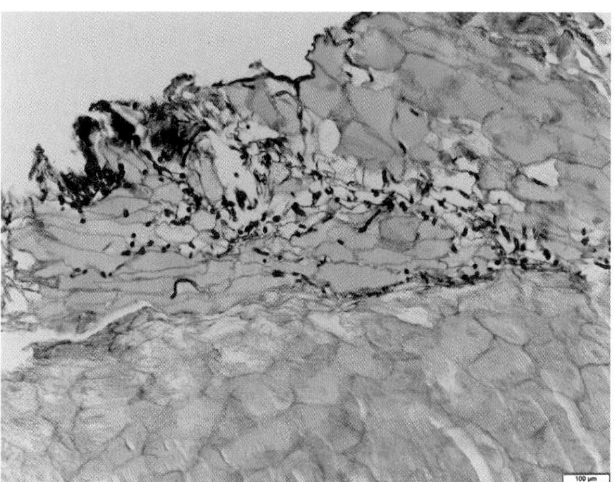

Fig. 176.1 Nail plate stained with PAS, demonstrating fungal hyphae.

References

1 **Armour K, Mann S, Lee S. Dysplastic naevi: to shave or not to shave? A retrospective study of the use of the shave biopsy technique in the initial management of dysplastic naevi. Australas J Dermatol 2005;46(2):70–5.**

2 Shi VY, Lio PA. In-office diagnosis of cutaneous mycosis: a comparison of potassium hydroxide, Swartz-Lamkins, and chlorazol black E fungal stains. Cutis 2013;92(6):E8–10.

3 Jeelani S, Ahmed Q, Lanker A et al. Histopathological examination of nail clippings using PAS staining (HPE-PAS): gold standard in diagnosis of onychomycosis. Mycoses 2015;58(1):27–32.

Rashes

While histological features of 'rashes' or inflammatory conditions of the skin may be nonspecific in some cases, there are several commonly encountered reaction patterns that can provide a specific diagnosis of inflammatory skin disease in the paediatric age group, and help distinguish between similar clinical entities.

Lichenoid dermatoses

Lichen planus involves a cell-mediated immune reaction that damages basilar epithelial cells. The classic reaction shows hyperkeratosis, wedge-shaped hypergranulosis, irregular acanthosis with pointing of rete ridges, basal vacuolar change, dyskeratotic keratinocytes and an underlying band-like lymphocytic infiltrate which often obscures the dermal-epidermal junction (Fig. 176.2). These findings may also be seen in fixed drug eruption and lichenoid drug eruptions. In the latter, eosinophils and pigmentary incontinence are usually more prominent.

In erythema multiforme, lesional skin also demonstrates basal vacuolar change, dyskeratotic keratinocytes and lymphocytic inflammation at the dermoepidermal junction. T-cell lymphocytes predominate and satellite cell necrosis (lymphocytic inflammation of individual necrotic keratinocytes) may be present. Perivascular lymphocytic inflammation is present in the papillary dermis. Spongiosis, vesiculation and necrosis may be a feature in acute lesions (Fig. 176.3). A 'zonal' quality to the epidermal and dermal changes may be appreciated, reflecting the targetoid appearance of the clinical lesions.

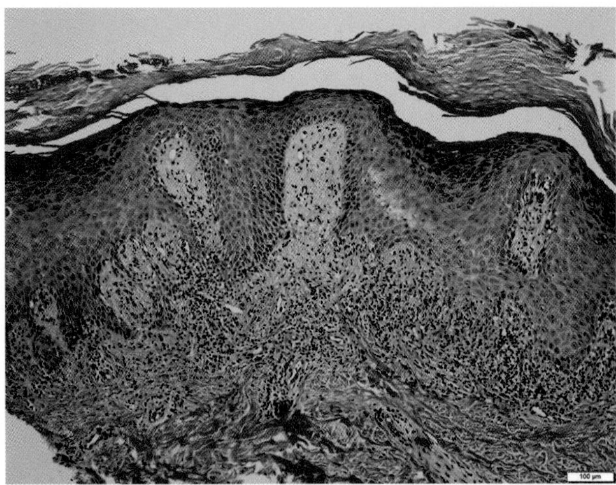

Fig. 176.2 Classic histological features of lichen planus, with epidermal hyperplasia and hyperkeratosis, wedge-shaped hypergranulosis, vacuolar change, dyskeratosis and band-like lymphocytic inflammation.

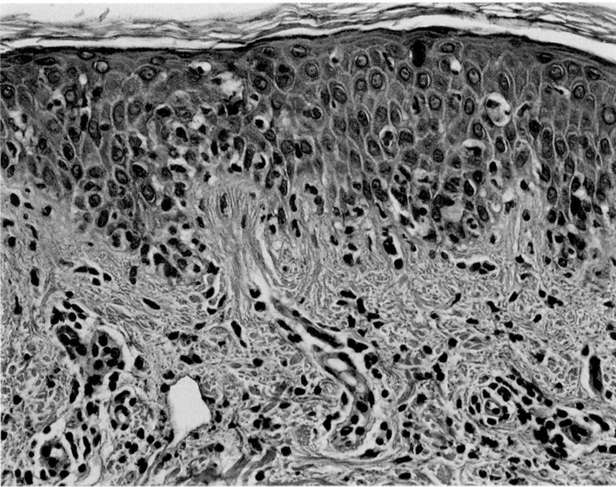

Fig. 176.3 Both spongiosis and interface changes characterize acute erythema multiforme.

While biopsy of Stevens–Johnson syndrome and toxic epidermal necrolysis may show vacuolar changes, the infiltrate is sparse and necrosis is more prominent. Cell-poor necrosis, vacuolar change, keratinocyte apoptosis and subepidermal blister formation characterize Stevens–Johnson syndrome (SJS) and toxic epidermal necrolysis (TEN).

Pityriasis lichenoides is essentially a lymphocytic vasculitis in which the associated T-cell inflammatory cell infiltrate shows exocytosis into the epidermis with obscuring of the dermoepidermal junction, with some 'lichenoid' features histologically. Haemorrhage in the dermal papillae is a common feature (Fig. 176.4). In the chronic form, the infiltrate is less dense and more superficial and the epidermal changes are much less pronounced. The overlap with early mycosis fungoides may be impossible to resolve solely on morphological features and may necessitate molecular genetic studies of T-cell clonality [1].

Spongiotic disorders

The histological features present in atopic dermatitis, contact dermatitis, nummular eczema, eczematous drug eruptions and other similar spongiotic dermatoses are not specific. However, several features may help distinguish acute allergic contact dermatitis (Fig. 176.5), including:

- intense epidermal spongiosis
- spongiotic microvesicle formation, which may show a 'flask-like' shape in the upper epidermis and associated Langerhans cells
- overlying orthokeratosis, indicating acute onset
- lymphocyte exocytosis
- papillary dermal oedema
- numerous eosinophils.

In more chronic cases, and in cases of irritant contact dermatitis and atopic dermatitis, the features listed above are often blunted, with less intense spongiosis and presence of parakeratosis, hypergranulosis and psoriasiform hyperplasia (indicating chronicity).

Guttate psoriasis, a common presentation of psoriasis in children, may also present with epidermal spongiosis,

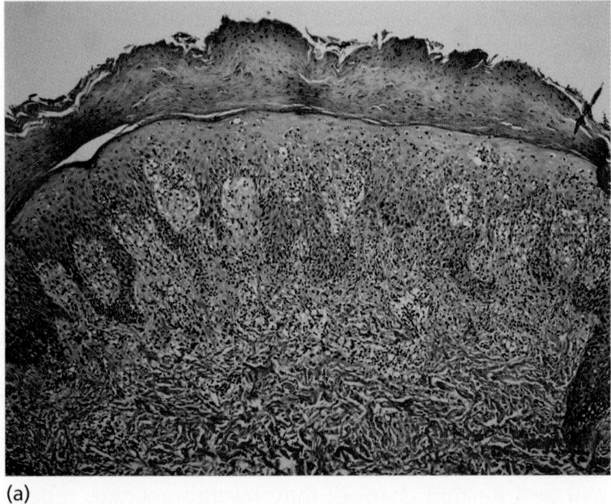

(a)

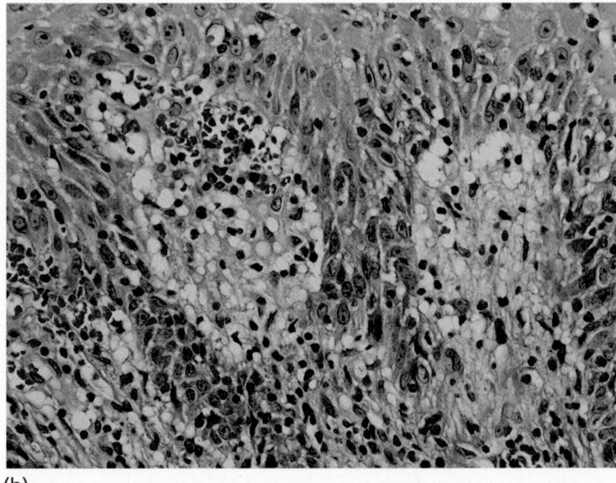

(b)

Fig. 176.4 Low-power (a) and high-power (b) views of pityriasis lichenoides, with vacuolar change, dense lymphocytic inflammation with exocytosis and focal haemorrhage.

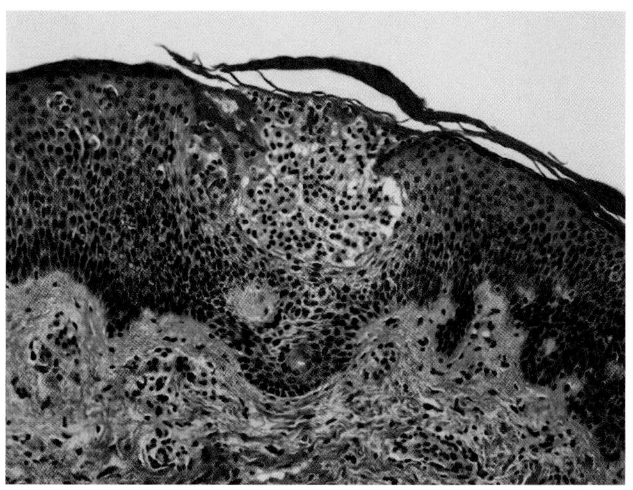

Fig. 176.5 Spongiosis in acute allergic contact dermatitis, with 'flask-shaped' spongiotic microvesicle associated with lymphocytes and Langerhans cells.

and is accompanied by subtle acanthosis, mounding parakeratosis with or without neutrophils, papillary dermal telangiectasia, scant haemorrhage and perivascular lymphocytic inflammation. Eosinophils are absent in the dermal infiltrate.

Bullous dermatoses

Bullous impetigo is characterized by a subcorneal or intragranular blister, reflecting impairment of the target antigen, desmoglein 1, from bacteria-derived toxin. Acantholysis is often present. Neutrophils and bacteria are present within the blister cavity, and the surrounding epidermis is spongiotic (Figs 176.6 and 176.7).

Pemphigus foliaceous (PF) results from an autoimmune dysfunction of the same target, desmoglein 1, and can present with identical histological features as those seen in bullous impetigo. In PF, acantholysis is usually more prominent and neutrophilic inflammation is minimal. Bacteria are not expected, unless the lesion is superinfected. However, in difficult cases, immunofluorescent studies are indicated to distinguish the two diseases.

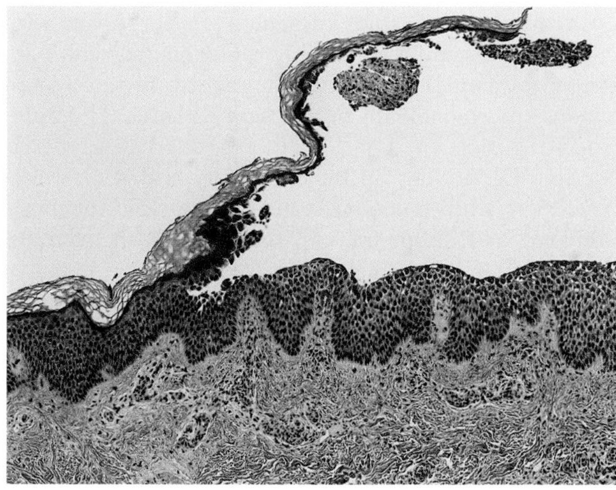

Fig. 176.6 Bullous impetigo, demonstrating subcorneal blister with acanthoysis.

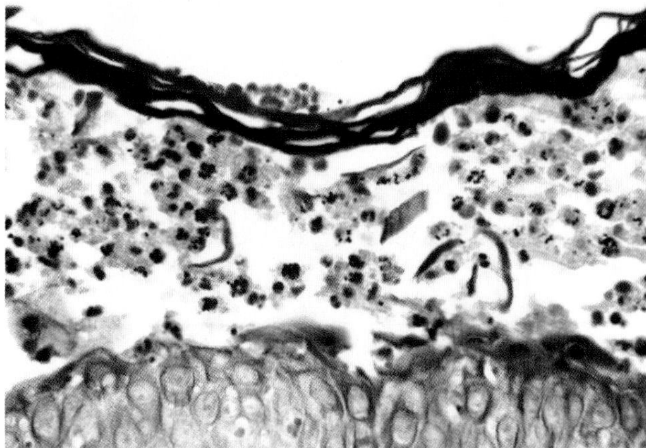

Fig. 176.7 Bacteria highlighted by Gram stain in bullous impetigo.

Like most cases of bullous impetigo, staphylococcal scalded skin syndrome (SSSS) results from infection with *Staphylococcus aureus* and the action of exfoliative toxins on the skin. While in bullous impetigo exotoxins are released and act locally from direct cutaneous bacterial infection, in cases of SSSS the nidus of infection is remote from the skin. Haematogenous spread of exotoxin results in indirect epidermal cleavage; the skin itself is not infected. Biopsy of affected skin will demonstrate a pauci-inflammatory subcorneal or intragranular blister. Bacteria are not present. SSSS and SJS/TEN can be distinguished histologically by the location of the blister plane (subcorneal in SSSS, subepidermal in SJS/TEN). Vacuolar changes are not a feature of SSSS.

Chronic bullous dermatosis of childhood (CBDC) is an acquired autoimmune subepidermal blistering disease of childhood. The target antigen in most cases of linear IgA disease (LAD) and CBDC is a 97 kDa secretory protein of BP180, although other antigens have been implicated, including a 120 kDa protein fragment of BP180 [2]. Cleavage in this area of the hemidesmosomal complex leads to subepidermal blistering. Light microscopy shows subepidermal blistering with neutrophilic inflammation. Neutrophils may cluster in the dermal papillae, mimicking dermatitis herpetiformis. Neutrophils that 'line up' at the dermoepidermal junction are more specific for CBDC. Direct immunofluorescence of perilesional demonstrates strong linear IgA at the basement membrane (Fig. 176.8). Some patients have detectable low titre circulating anti-IgA antibodies on indirect immunofluorescent studies [3].

Dermatitis herpetiformis lesions are characterized by aggregates of neutrophils and microabscesses in the papillary dermis (Fig. 176.9). Within the dermal papillae, neutrophilic clusters will typically be separated from the dermoepidermal junction by a small clear cleft. True vesiculation may be present. Eosinophils are often identified within the infiltrate and nuclear dust is classically present. Vasculitis is not a feature. Direct immunofluorescence shows granular IgA deposits along the basement membrane zone and in the dermal papillae. Indirect immunofluorescence is negative for circulating IgA autoantibodies directed toward skin, but some patients

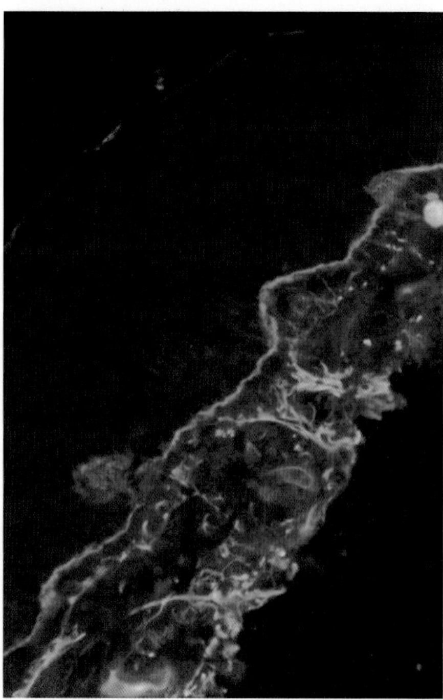

Fig. 176.8 Direct immunofluorescence of chronic bullous disease of childhood, demonstrating a linear band of IgA at the dermal-epidermal junction.

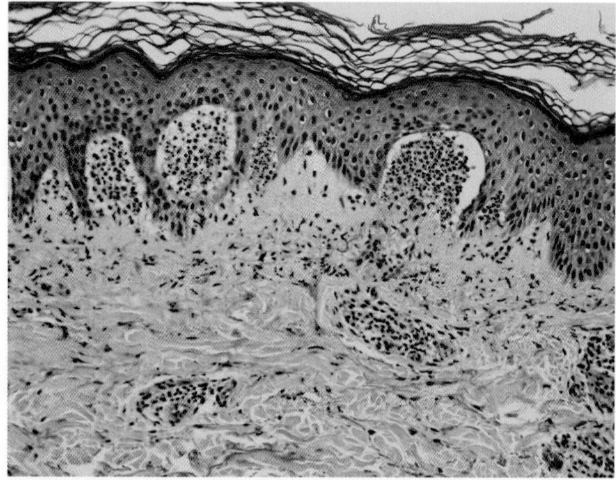

Fig. 176.9 Classic findings in dermatitis herpetiformis, with neutrophilic aggregates in the dermal papillae, separated from the basement membrane zone by a thin cleft.

show IgA endomysial antibodies and/or IgA-containing complexes in the serum.

Vasculitis

In practical paediatric dermatopathology, there is a common question: is this a vasculitis? The postcapillary venules in the dermal papillae are an important functional site for disease processes in the skin. In the case of the vasculitides, serious morbidity and even mortality may result. In most vasculitides, the age of the lesion biopsied may influence the type and intensity of the inflammatory response. In *urticarial vasculitis*, the only clue may be mild interstitial oedema of the papillary dermis, dilation of small blood vessels with swelling of endothelial cells and a mild perivascular lymphocytic infiltrate with occasional eosinophils.

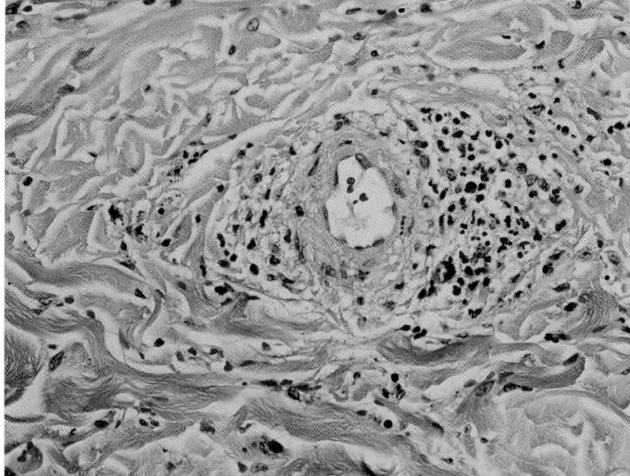

Fig. 176.10 Neutrophilic infiltration of blood vessel epithelium in leucocytoclastic vasculitis.

Leucocytoclastic vasculitis is associated with neutrophil infiltration of vessel walls, swollen and sometimes degenerate endothelial cells, and vascular fibrin deposition (Fig. 176.10). The neutrophils undergo degeneration with the formation of nuclear dust. In the later stages, perivascular lymphocytes and macrophages are a feature.

Immunohistochemistry in inflammatory skin conditions

The use of immunohistochemistry to evaluate skin specimens has increased significantly in recent years, and can aid the dermatopathologist in distinguishing between similar disorders and confirming specific diagnoses. For example, CD117 (c-kit) is a marker of mast cells, and easy to interpret in comparison to older special staining techniques (such as Giemsa). CD203 (Langerin) is a marker of Langerhans cells, and is more specific for Langerhans cell disease than S-100 or CD1a. This can be quite useful in distinguishing Langerhans cell histiocytosis from very inflammatory disorders that recruit numerous antigen-presenting CD1a cells, such as scabies infestation [4]. Herpes and varicella infection cannot be reliably differentiated with light microscopy alone, but specific immunohistochemical preparations are available for herpes simplex virus (HSV) and varicella zoster virus (VZV) if a specific diagnosis is required. Depending on the laboratory and clinical scenario, these studies may also allow more rapid diagnosis compared to PCR or culture. Immunohistochemistry is often critical when characterizing T-cell infiltrates in mycosis fungoides and lymphomatoid papulosis.

References

1 Vonderheid EC, Kadin ME, Telang GH. Commentary about papular mycosis fungoides, lymphomatoid papulosis, and lymphomatoidpityriasis lichenoides: more similarities than differences. J Cutan Pathol 2016;43:303–12.

2 Schumann H, Baetge J, Tasanen K et al. The shed ectodomain of collagen XVII/BP180 is targeted by autoantibodies in different blistering skin diseases. Am J Pathol 2000;156(2):685–95.

3 Monia K, Aida K, Amel K et al. Linear IgA bullous dermatosis in Tunisian children: 31 cases. Indian J Dermatol 2011;56(2):153–9.
4 Bhattacharjee P, Glusac EJ. Langerhans cell hyperplasia in scabies: a mimic of Langerhans cell histiocytosis. J Cutan Pathol 2007;34(9): 716–20.

Lumps and bumps

The dermal nodule carries a wide differential diagnosis both clinically and histologically. The most commonly encountered in the paediatric age group is the *pilomatricoma*, which has a characteristic histological appearance with nests of basaloid cells and eosinophilic ghost cells. Calcification occurs in more than two thirds, and is usually in the ghost cells. A foreign body giant cell reaction is common (Fig. 176.11).

Spindle cell lesions carry a wide histological differential diagnosis and may need immunostaining for confirmation. *Neural tumours* can usually be diagnosed without difficulty, and express S-100 protein (Fig. 176.12). The *dermatofibroma* (also called fibrous histiocytoma) can show a wide variety of appearances depending on which components predominate: fibroblast-like cells, histiocytes, some of which may be xanthomatous or multinucleate, or blood vessels. *Juvenile xanthogranulomas* show different appearances depending on the age of the lesion, with early lesions being predominantly mononuclear followed by the classic Touton cell-rich stage and finally a stage with a spindle cell pattern and a variable component of mononuclear and multinucleated cells (Fig. 176.13). Immunostaining shows positivity for CD68, factor XIIIa and CD163, the latter of which may help distinguish these lesions from fibrous histiocytomas [1].

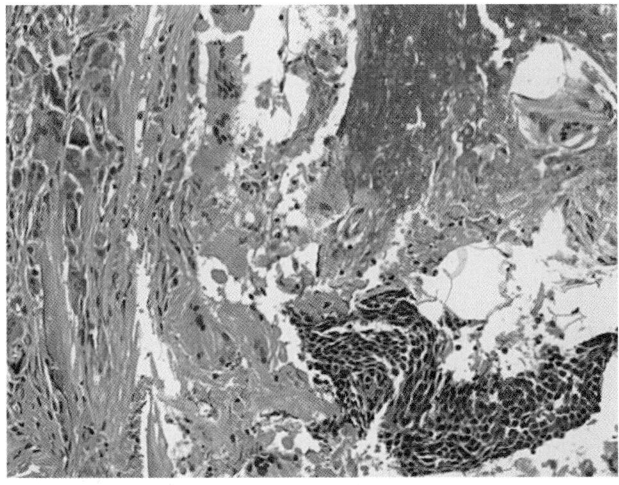

Fig. 176.11 High-power field from a pilomatricoma showing an island of basophilic cells, lightly calcified ghost cells and foreign body giant cells.

The *myofibroma* consists of characteristic short fascicles of plump spindle-shaped cells separated by thin bundles of collagen. Vascular spaces resembling those of a haemangiopericytoma are often found in the centre, giving most lesions a biphasic pattern. This vascular component may lead to the clinical diagnosis of a haemangioma or other vascular tumour [2]. Necrosis, hyalinization, calcification, mucin deposition and focal haemorrhage may also be present in the centre. Immunostaining is positive for vimentin and smooth muscle actin. *Dermatofibrosarcoma protuberans* and its more common variant in children, the *giant cell fibroblastoma*, extend into the subcutis and are composed of bundles of small spindle cells with plump nuclei in a characteristic storiform or cartwheel pattern. Scattered mitoses are present but atypical mitoses are rare. Giant cell fibroblastomas often demonstrate floret-like giant cells with intermixed pseudovascular spaces, hyalinzed areas and tight 'onion-skin' perivascular lymphocytes. Immunostaining for CD34 shows 50–100% of cells to be positive. Staining for factor XIIIa is negative [3].

Granuloma annulare demonstrates one or more areas of necrobiosis surrounded by histiocytes and lymphocytes in the superficial and mid-dermis (Fig. 176.14). Variable numbers of multinucleate giant cells are present. In some cases, the histological changes are subtle and there are no formed areas of necrobiosis ('interstitial granuloma annulare').

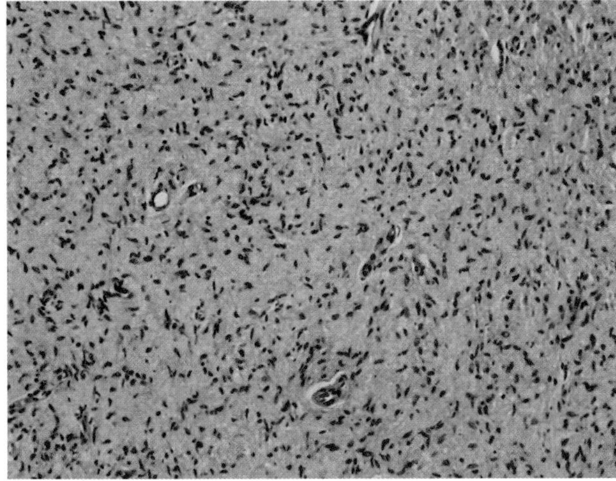

Fig. 176.12 Neurofibroma demonstrating delicate spindle cells arranged haphazardly in a loose collagenous stroma.

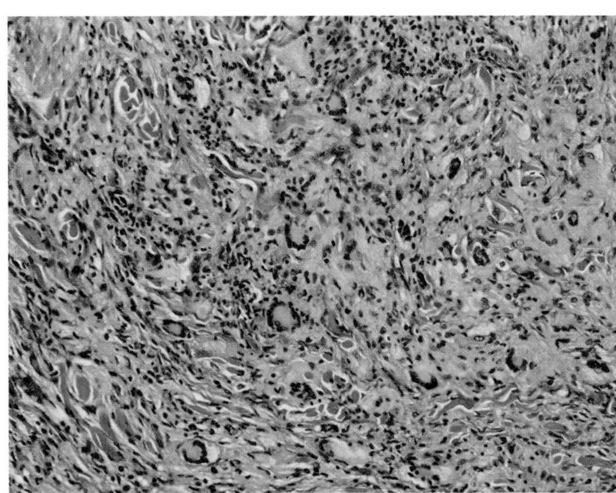

Fig. 176.13 Classic Touton-type giant cells in juvenile xanthogranuloma.

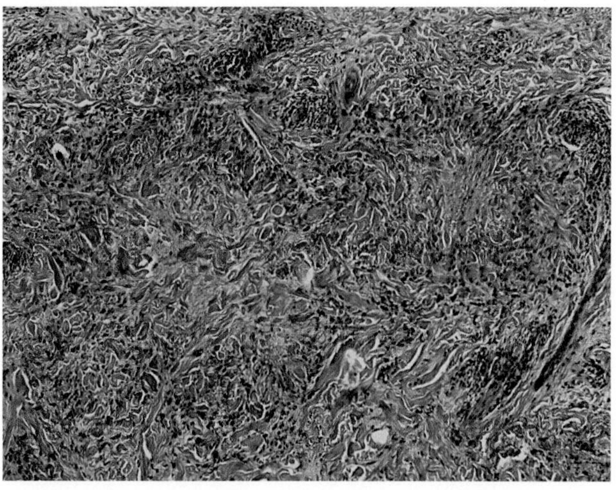

Fig. 176.14 Granuloma annulare, demonstrating central collagen necrobiosis and mucin deposition, with surrounding palisaded histiocytes and lymphocytes.

References

1 Sandell RF, Carter JM, Folpe AL. Solitary (juvenile) xanthogranuloma: a comprehensive immunohistochemical study emphasizing recently developed markers of histiocytic lineage. Hum Pathol 2015;46(9): 1390–7.

2 Friedman BJ, Shah K, Taylor J, Rubin A. Congenital myofibroma masquerading as an ulcerated infantile hemangioma in a neonate. Pediatr Dermatol 2008;30(6):e248–9.

3 Jafarian F, McCuaig C, Kokta V et al. Dermatofibromasarcoma protuberans in childhood and adolescence: report of eight patients. Pediatr Dermatol 2008;25(3):317–25.

Vascular lesions

An important part of paediatric dermatopathology is the diagnosis of cutaneous vascular lesions, which are often sampled by dermatologists, surgeons and interventional radiologists in the absence of an obvious clinical diagnosis. The International Society for Vascular Anomalies classification has previously identified two main categories of superficial vascular anomalies in infancy and childhood: vascular malformations and vascular tumors (Table 176.1). Many of these entities have overlapping histopathological features and must be interpreted within their clinical contexts. However, advances in the understanding of the pathophysiology of many vascular lesions have identified specific immunohistochemical markers that can reliably differentiate among different cell types and disease entities (Table 176.2).

Table 176.1 Classification scheme and major histopathological findings of vascular lesions [1]

Classification	Findings		
Vascular malformations	Low-flow	Capillary malformation	Dilated dermal capillaries and postcapillary venules
		Venous malformation	Dilated, thin-walled vascular channels lined by flattened endothelial cells
		Glomuvenous malformation	Ectatic vascular spaces lined by cuboidal cells, positive for smooth muscle actin
		Lymphatic malformation	Dilated, thin-walled vascular channels often containing eosinophilic lymph fluid, positive for D2-40
		Mixed malformation	Any combination of the features above
	High-flow	Arteriovenous malformation	Admixed thick- and thin-walled vessels representing arteries and veins
Vascular tumours	Benign	Infantile haemangioma	Proliferating phase: cellular proliferation of plump endothelial cells with small, interspersed lumens Regressive phase: replacement of endothelial cells with fat and fibrosis Endothelial cells are positive for GLUT-1, Lewis Y antigen and merosin
		Congenital haemangioma	Lobular capillary proliferation, negative for GLUT-1
		Tufted angioma	Multinodular dermal proliferation of capillaries, with semilunar, D2-40-positive lymphatic channels around each nodule
		Lobular capillary haemangioma (pyogenic granuloma)	Lobular, cellular capillary proliferation with epidermal collarette
		Glomus tumour	Proliferation of monomorphous glomus cells with uniform, round nuclei, with associated interspersed dilated blood vessels. Glomus cells are positive for smooth muscle actin
	Locally aggressive/ borderline	Kaposiform haemangioendothelioma	Infiltrative tumour with lobular angiomatous areas – positive for CD31 and other endothelial markers – and fascicles of D2-40-positive spindle cells
		Papillary intralymphatic angioendothelioma (Dabska tumour)	Dilated, thin-walled vascular channels lined by hobnailed endothelial cells, with intravascular papillary projections and prominent lymphoid aggregates
		Kaposi sarcoma	Multiple morphologies ranging from inconspicuous increase in dermal vessels with minimal atypia in patch stage to highly cellular spindle cell proliferations with slit-like vascular spaces and extravasated red blood cells. All stages are positive for HHV-8
	Malignant	Angiosarcoma	Infiltrative tumour with a network of interanastamosing vessels which dissect through collagen. More advanced lesions may show poorly differentiated features with high degrees of nuclear atypia, and may resemble carcinomas or other malignancies

Source: Adapted from Wassef et al. 2015 [1].
GLUT, glucose transporter; HHV, human herpesvirus.

Table 176.2 Important immunohistochemical markers in vascular lesions [3–5]

Marker	Clinical application
CD31	Endothelial marker, stains blood and lymphatic vessels
D2-40	Lymphatic endothelial cell marker
GLUT-1	Positive in infantile haemangiomas, negative in congenital haemangiomas and other vascular tumours
Prox1	Lymphatic endothelial maker, also positive in Kaposi sarcoma, kaposiform haemangioendothelioma, tufted angioma and some angiosarcomas
WT-1	Positive in vascular tumours, negative in malformations (except arteriovenous malformations)

Vascular malformations are divided into two groups, fast-flow and slow-flow, based on clinical and radiological findings, and are classified histologically according to the predominant type of vessel involved: lymphatic, venous, capillary, or mixed – involving any combination. Most fast-flow cutaneous malformations are arteriovenous malformations. Microscopic examination shows distorted arteries and veins, stromal fibrosis and a variable admixture of capillaries. Prior embolization results in occlusion of vessels by the embolic agent, thrombus formation and secondary recanalization, haemosiderin deposition and fibrosis. Venous malformations show a histologically poorly circumscribed lesion containing ectatic, thin-walled channels lined by flattened endothelial cells forming a complex network which dissects through normal tissues (Fig. 176.15). There is frequent microcalcification and there may be admixed capillaries, and thrombi which are sometimes recanalized. Glomuvenous malformations (formerly known as glomangiomas), of which 65% are autosomal dominantly inherited, account for 5% of venous malformations. Microscopy shows irregular ectatic vascular channels surrounded by bland cuboidal glomus cells which stain positively for smooth muscle actin, and may be very sparse in some cases. Blue rubber bleb naevus syndrome is characterized by cutaneous and gastrointestinal venous malformations. Histopathological examination shows irregular, widely dilated, thin-walled venous channels in the deep dermis and subcutis with positive immunostaining for smooth muscle actin within vessel walls. Lymphatic malformations consist of dilated, thin-walled vascular channels which show positive immunostaining for D2-40 in endothelial cells (Fig. 176.16). Sensitivity of the immunostain is variable and is more consistent in smaller lymphatic channels. Capillary malformations (including port wine stains, naevus simplex, cutis marmorata telangiectasia congenita and others) show subtle-to-marked dilation of capillaries and postcapillary venules in the superficial dermis. Complex combined vascular malformations associated with limb overgrowth show anomalous veins with deformed, insufficient or absent valves and fibromuscular anomalies of venous walls. There may also be dilated lymphatics with associated lymphoedema.

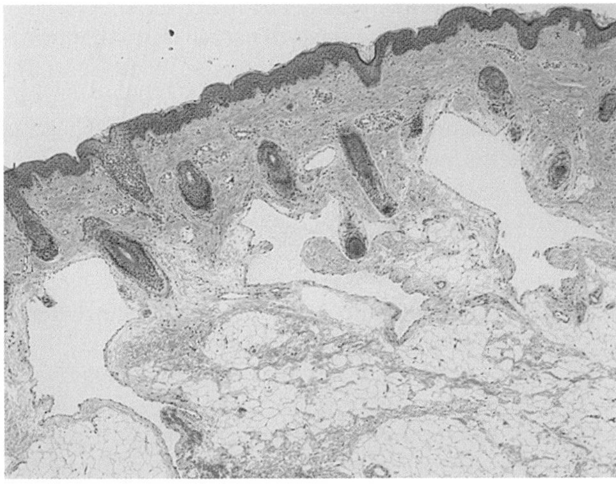

Fig. 176.15 Venous malformation in which the dermis shows ectatic thin-walled vessels. Immunostaining for D2-40 was negative.

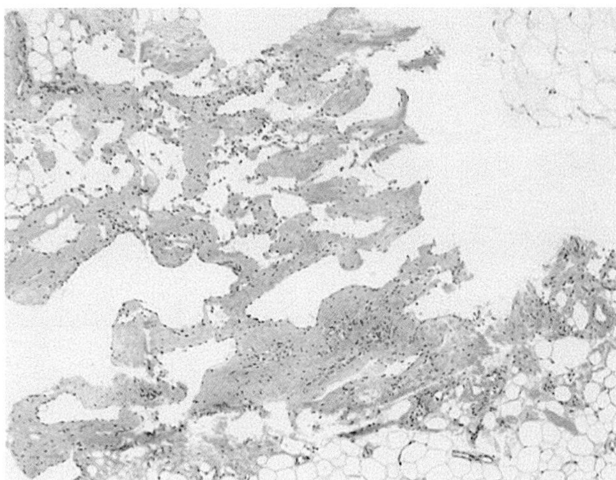

Fig. 176.16 Needle biopsy specimen from a lymphatic malformation showing anastomosing thin-walled vascular channels within the dermal collagen. Immunostaining for D2-40 was positive.

Vascular tumours are divided by their biological potential – benign, locally aggressive or borderline, and malignant. The most common vascular tumour of childhood is the infantile haemangioma, in which the appearance depends on the stage. Microscopic evaluation of early lesions in the proliferative stage shows sheets of plump endothelial cells in solid cords. In the involutional stage, endothelial cells flatten and vascular channels become more ectatic. The lesion consists of abnormal thin-walled vessels separated by islands of fat and fibrous tissue. The fully involuted lesion shows scattered capillary-like vessels with larger feeding vessels and draining veins in a stroma of fatty and fibrous tissue and collagen fibres.

Immunohistochemistry shows positive staining of endothelial cells for the glucose transporter protein, GLUT1, which is diagnostic in this context. GLUT1 staining differentiates infantile haemangioma from other vascular tumours such as congenital haemangioma, tufted haemangioma and pyogenic granuloma, as well as vascular malformations (Fig. 176.17).

Congenital haemangiomas are of two varieties – rapidly involuting (RICH) and noninvoluting (NICH). Both types show lobules of capillaries in a fibrous tissue stroma with

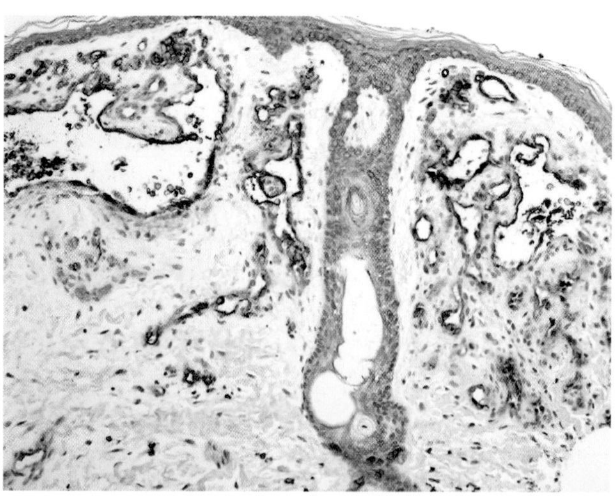

Fig. 176.17 Photomicrograph of an infantile haemangioma displaying endothelial GLUT1 expression by immunohistochemistry.

abnormal-appearing arteries and veins towards the centre. Immunostaining for GLUT1 and D2-40 is negative. Tufted angioma, which is associated with Kasabach–Merritt phenomenon, consists microscopically of small circumscribed angiomatous tufts and lobules in the mid-dermis, which are formed of central whorled nodules of tightly packed endothelial cells with dilated vessels peripherally (Fig. 176.18). Immunostaining for D2-40 shows partial positivity in the surrounding dilated vessels and is negative in the cannonball-like proliferative capillaries [2]. The lobular capillary haemangioma, or pyogenic granuloma, shows a well-developed epidermal collarette at the margin while the dermis contains lobules of infantile haemangioma-like angiomatous tissue separated by fibrous septae. Immunostaining for GLUT1 is negative.

The glomus tumour is a well-circumscribed solid tumour within the dermis. Distinct lobules are composed of monomorphous cells with plump or round-oval nuclei and scant cytoplasm. Immunostaining shows the cells to be positive for smooth muscle actin and negative for endothelial markers. Kaposiform huemangioendothelioma is frequently associated with Kasabach–Merritt phenomenon. Biopsy shows lobular angiomatous areas and spindle cells in fascicles. Immunostaining for D2-40 shows strong reactivity in the spindle cell areas and is negative in the surrounding dilated vessels.

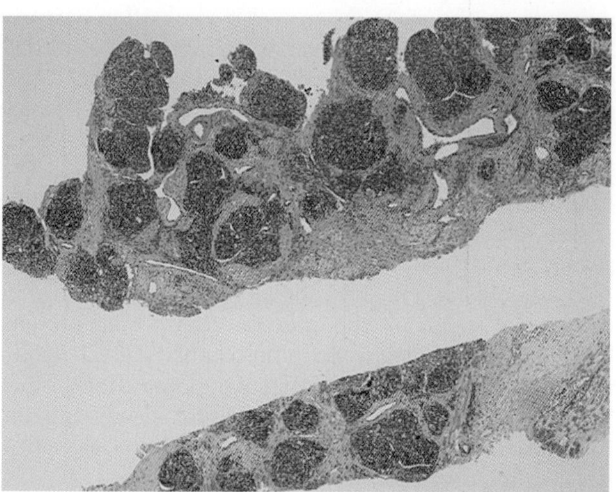

Fig. 176.18 Photomicrograph of a needle biopsy specimen from a tufted angioma, showing well-circumscribed angiomatous nodules formed of tightly packed endothelial cells with dilated vessels peripherally.

References

1 **Wassef M, Blei F, Adams D et al. Vascular anomalies classification: recommendations from the International Society for the Study of Vascular Anomalies. Pediatrics 2015;136:e203–14.**

2 Arai E, Kuramochi A, Tsuchida T et al. Usefulness of D2-40 immunohistochemistry for differentiation between Kaposiform hemangioendothelioma and tufted angioma. J Cutan Pathol 2006;33:492–7.

3 McCalmont TH. Vessels making loud sounds. J Cutan Pathol 2014;41:414–16.

4 Markku M, Wang ZF. Prox1 transcription factor as a marker for vascular tumors-evaluation of 314 vascular endothelial and 1086 nonvascular tumors. Am J Surg Pathol 2012;36:351–9.

5 Trindade F, Tellechea O, Torrelo A et al. Wilms tumor 1 expression in vascular neoplasms and vascular malformations. Am J Dermatopathol 2011;33:569–72.

Melanocytic lesions

The occurrence of malignancy in pigmented lesions of childhood is quite low. Nevertheless, they are often removed for reasons including the presence of concerning clinical features, exposure to recurrent trauma based on location and morphology, obviating the risk of malignancy and cosmetic considerations. When evaluating the histopathology of a paediatric pigmented lesion, it is important to bear in mind that features that are cause for alarm in an elderly individual may not hold the same significance in a young child. Additionally, the clinical course of melanoma in children differs greatly from that in adults, and the utility of prognostic factors such as depth of invasion, presence of regional nodal metastasis and mitotic index is not clear.

Congenital naevi may be junctional, compound or intradermal, depending on the age at which they are removed. The presence of melanocytes in the lower two thirds of the dermis, extension of cells between collagen bundles or in single file, and extension of cells around nerves, vessels and adnexae are characteristic of congenital naevi. Some large melanocytic naevi show peripheral nerve sheath differentiation with nerve fascicle-like structures closely resembling authentic nerve fascicles [1]. Structures resembling Meissner's corpuscles and Verocay body-like structures may be present. Large naevi showing these patterns may be associated with neurocutaneous melanosis, and magnetic resonance imaging (MRI) of the brain and spinal cord should be considered. Proliferative nodules may develop within congenital naevi and are often excised to exclude melanoma, which develops in less than 1% of small and medium congenital naevi and less than 5% of large and giant congenital naevi [2].

Histopathological features that favour a diagnosis of melanoma are very high mitotic index, the presence of atypical mitotic figures, surface ulceration, focal necrosis and the presence of certain cytogenetic abnormalities [3,4].

Spitzoid neoplasms are a distinct group of melanocytic lesions with a spectrum of biological potential. The Spitz naevus is a benign, pink, skin-coloured or brown papule that occurs most commonly on the face or lower extremities, but may occur on any part of the body. Characteristic histological features include a mixture of spindled and epithelioid melanocytes and presence of Kamino bodies (dull eosinophilic globules representing reduplicated basement membrane zone) (Fig. 176.19). The pigmented spindle cell naevus (of Reed) is a variant of a Spitz naevus with distinct symmetrical architecture, predominantly spindled cells and heavy pigmentation (Fig. 176.20). Atypical Spitz tumours have intermediate or indeterminate malignant potential, often spreading to regional lymph nodes without distant metastasis, and can present a diagnostic challenge in differentiating from malignant spitzoid melanomas (Fig. 176.21). Features suggestive of malignancy in a spitzoid neoplasm are age over 10 years, diameter greater than 1 cm, the presence of ulceration and of deep atypical mitoses [5] (Fig. 176.22).

While conventional histopathology remains the cornerstone of diagnosis of melanocytic lesions, there is an expanding role for ancillary studies such as immunohistochemistry. Differences in the expression of markers such as p16, neuropilin-2, BAP1 and many others have shown variable promise in differentiating between challenging benign and malignant lesions [6–8]. Recent advances in cytogenetics have given dermatopathologists additional tools to aid in the distinction between atypical spitzoid tumours and spitzoid melanomas, and will be discussed in more detail below.

Acquired melanocytic naevi undergo progressive maturation with age. Initially, the acquired melanocytic naevus is a macular lesion in which nests of proliferating melanocytes are confined to the dermoepidermal junction (junctional naevus). The lesion becomes progressively more elevated as nests of melanocytes proliferate in the underlying dermis (compound naevus). With further

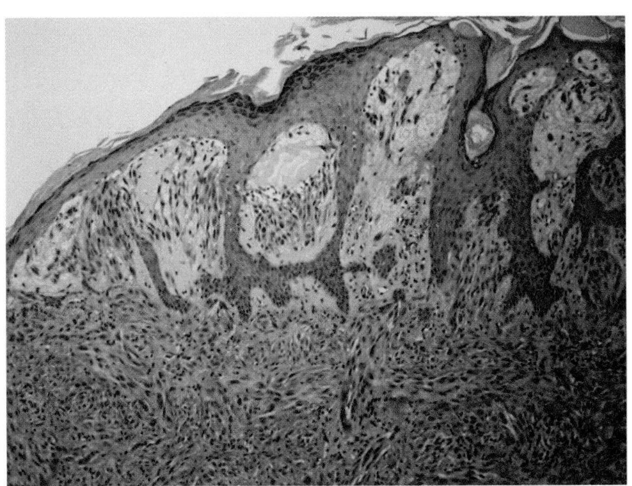

Fig. 176.19 Compound Spitz naevus, demonstrating epidermal hyperplasia, plump spindled and epithelioid melanocytes, junctional cleavage of cells away from the epidermal basement membrane zone and numerous Kamino bodies.

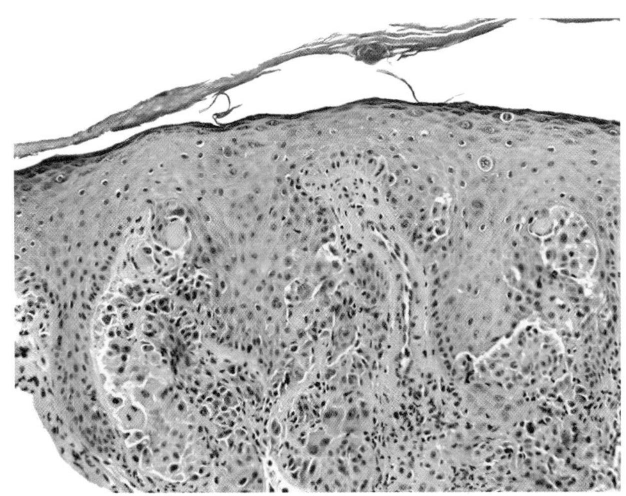

Fig. 176.21 This Spitz naevus demonstrates atypical features, including nuclear pleomorphism and pagetoid extension of cells. Several mitoses were present in the superficial portion.

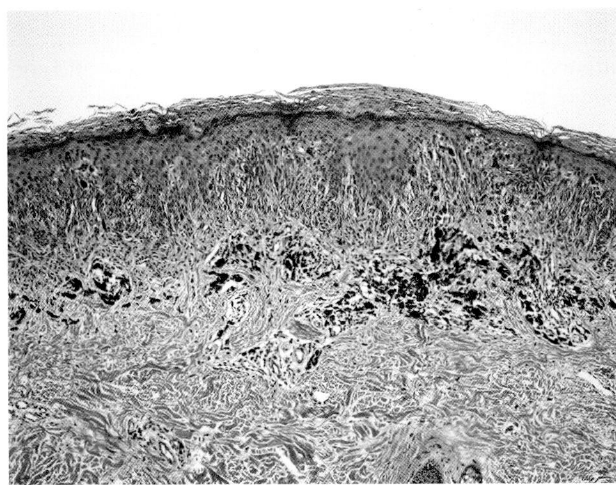

Fig. 176.20 Heavily pigmented spindled melanocytes arranged in large, vertically oriented nests, characterize the pigmented spindle cell naevus of Reed.

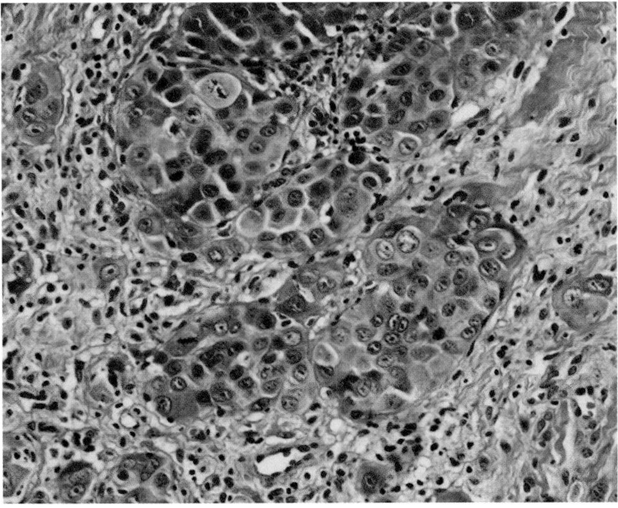

Fig. 176.22 High-power section of 'spitzoid' melanoma with deep atypical mitoses. This lesion presented as 1.1 cm papule in a 14 year old.

maturation, junctional activity ceases and the lesion is composed only of dermal naevus cells (intradermal naevus) (Figs 176.23 and 176.24). In compound naevi, the cells in the upper dermis are usually cuboidal with melanin pigment in the cytoplasm. Deeper cells are often smaller and contain less melanin. Atypical compound naevi may arise in adolescents and show lateral extension of junctional activity beyond the dermal component, elongation of rete ridges with bridging of naevus cells between them, pagetoid spread and cytological atypia. Large, bizarrely shaped nests may be scattered in a disorderly fashion along the junctional zone. Mitoses are rare. Many cases show a mild lymphocytic infiltrate. Deep penetrating naevus is a variant of compound naevus found in young adults in which loosely arranged nests and fascicles of spindle and epithelioid naevus cells interspersed with melanophages may extend deep into the dermis [9].

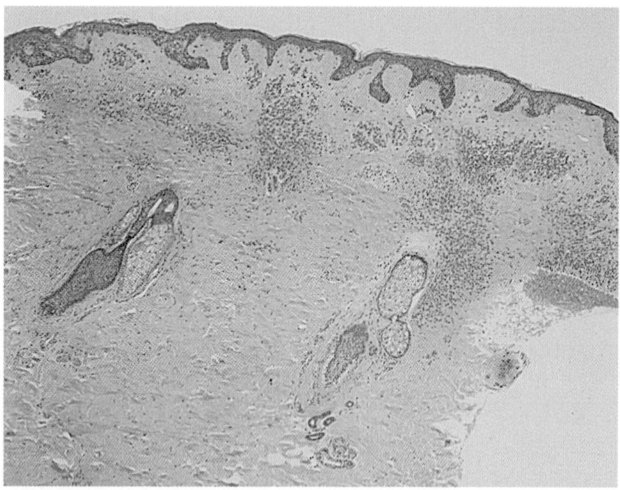

Fig. 176.23 Photomicrograph of a congenital melanocytic naevus of intradermal type showing collections of melanocytes in the dermis and surrounding a pilosebaceous unit.

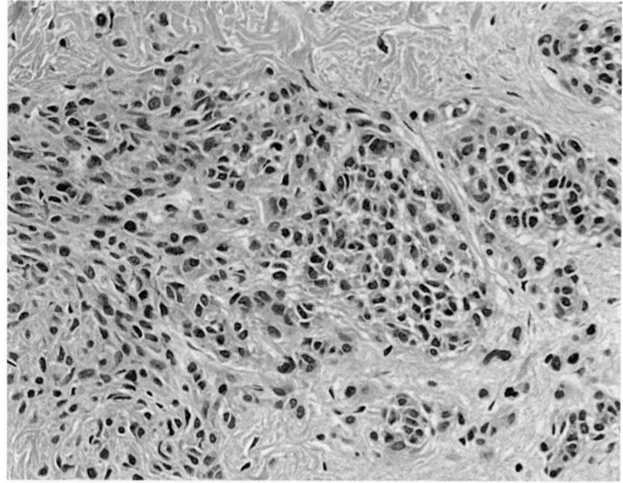

Fig. 176.24 High-power view of melanocytes in the dermis showing regular cells with monomorphic dense nuclei and ample pale eosinophilic cytoplasm.

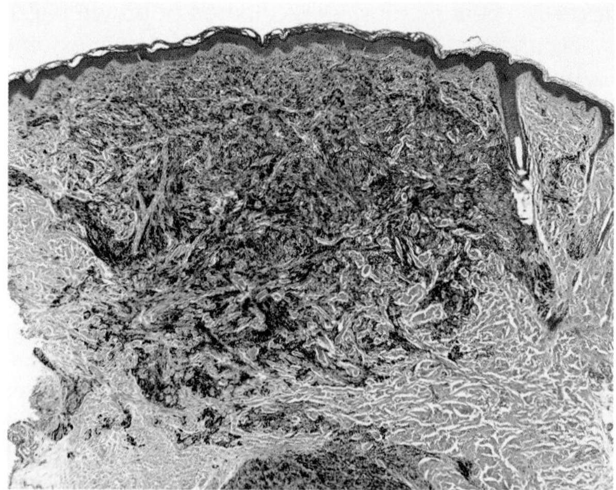

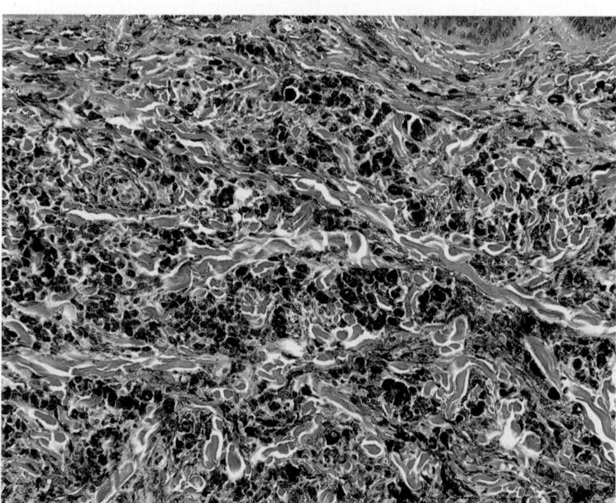

Fig. 176.25 Low-power (a) and high-power (b) images of a blue naevus showing a well-demarcated, heavily pigmented neoplasm composed of an admixture of finely pigmented melanocytes and heavily pigmented melanophages.

The blue naevus is a dermal lesion composed of finely branching melanocytes containing cytoplasmic melanin granules situated between the collagen bundles of the upper and mid-dermis, with admixed heavily pigmented macrophages (Fig. 176.25). The cellular variant is a much larger nodular lesion often found on the buttocks and consisting of nests and fascicles of pale-staining melanocytes together with islands and bundles of spindle and epithelioid cells with abundant cytoplasm and little pigment.

References

1 Mirago N. The relationship between melanocytic and peripheral nerve sheath cells. Part 1: melanocytic nevus (excluding so-called 'blue nevus') with peripheral nerve sheath differentiation. Am J Dermatopathol 2000;22:217–29.

2 Schaffer JV. Update on melanocytic nevi in children. Clin Dermatol 2015;33:368–86.

3 Herron MD, Vanderhooft SL, Smock K et al. Proliferative nodules in congenital melanocytic nevi: a clinicopathologic and immunohistochemical analysis. Am J Surg Pathol 2004;28:1017–25.

4 Oriol Y, Arva NC, Obregon R. A comparative study of proliferative nodules and lethal melanomas in congenital nevi from children. Am J Surg Pathol 2015;39:405–15.

5 Barnhill RL, Cerroni L, Cook M et al. State of the art, nomenclature, and points of consensus and controversy concerning benign melanocytic

lesions: outcome of an international workshop. Adv Anat Pathol 2010;17:73–90.
6 George E, Polissar NL, Wick M. Immunohistochemical evaluation of p16INK4A, E-cadherin, and cyclin D1 expression in melanoma and Spitz tumors. Am J Clin Pathol 2010;133:370–9.
7 Wititsuwannakul J, Mason AR, Klump VR, Lazova R. Neuropilin-2 as a useful marker in the differentiation between Spitzoid malignant melanoma and Spitz nevus. J Am Acad Dermatol 2012;68:129–37.
8 Piris A, Mihm MC, Hoang MP. BAP1 and BRAFV600E expression in benign and malignant melanocytic proliferations. Hum Pathol 2015;46:239–45.
9 Magro CM, Crowson AN, Mihm MC Jr et al. The dermal-based melanocytic tumor: a categorical approach. J Am Acad Dermatol 2010;62:469–79.

Molecular diagnostic techniques

The use of molecular techniques is a relatively recent development in diagnostic medicine. While the results of such studies must be viewed in the context of the clinical and histopathological setting, certain assays provide a cost-effective and rapid benefit. An example is the highly sensitive polymerase chain reaction (PCR) for detection of specific microbes such as HSV [1]. Cytogenetic and gene expression profiling studies have been useful in providing diagnostic and prognostic information when standard histopathology and immunohistochemistry fall short. Cytogenetics refers to the microscopic visualization of chromosome number and structure, while gene expression profiling examines the phenotype of a cell based on which genes are transcribed (Table 176.3).

Molecular diagnostic techniques have been particularly useful in the diagnosis and management of melanocytic lesions. The discovery of the high frequency of mutation of the mitogen-activated protein kinase (MAPK) pathway member BRAF has led to significant advancement in understanding the pathophysiology of melanoma and breakthroughs in its treatment.

These techniques have also become critical in the diagnosis and management of spitzoid neoplasms. As discussed above, spitzoid neoplasms follow a distinct clinical course which makes sentinel lymph node biopsy less useful than in conventional melanoma. Atypical spitzoid tumours may present with local nodal metastasis but do not progress, whereas spitzoid melanoma has the potential for extranodal spread. Fluorescence *in situ* hybridization (FISH) studies, which use probes to detect specific genomic DNA sequences, have identified several cytogenetic abnormalities that portend an aggressive clinical course, most notably homozygous loss of 9p21 [2,3]. Comparative genomic hybridization has the ability to detect gains or losses of chromosomal segments across the entire genome, and has been used to differentiate between benign and malignant spitzoid neoplasms – benign tumours have few copy number aberrations and melanomas may have multiple [4]. A more recently discovered prognostic factor in conventional and spitzoid melanoma is the detection of mutations in the TERT promoter, which are thought to confer increased telomerase activity, potentiating an aggressive clinical course with distant tumour spread [5,6]. Gene expression profiling has shown some promise in diagnostic and prognostic testing of melanocytic lesions. Commercially available tests such as myPath® Melanoma and DecisionDx-Melanoma are becoming more commonly used for adult lesions, but further validation is necessary before they become widely applicable in paediatric tumours.

Cytogenetic analysis is routinely used in many paediatric soft tissue tumours which may present in the skin. Giant cell fibroblastoma, a mesenchymal neoplasm seen primarily in children, bears a t(17;22) translocation. It is thought to be on a spectrum with dermatofibrosarcoma protuberans, which shares the same translocation. This is

Table 176.3 Common molecular diagnostic techniques

Technique	Method and uses	Common clinical applications
Immunohistochemistry	Visualization of protein expression in standard histopathological specimens	Differentiating between histologically similar conditions by identification of cell types Characterization and subclassification of known entities for diagnostic, prognostic and treatment considerations
Polymerase chain reaction	Bulk amplification of a specific DNA fragment to detect its presence or absence	Detection of microbes
Gene sequencing	Determination of nucleotide sequence of a DNA fragment	Diagnosis of genetic conditions Identification of mutations within a tumour
Gene expression profiling	Detection of actively transcribed genes in a tissue to assess cellular identity and function	Diagnostic and prognostic information on target tumours
Whole-exome sequencing	Determination of nucleotide sequence of all protein-encoding portions of an individual's genome	Identification of causative genes in rare genetic conditions or those in which an expected mutation is absent
Fluorescence *in situ* hybridization (FISH)	Detection of specific chromosomal aberrations – very high resolution but requires a specific target	Diagnostic confirmation of conditions with known cytogenetic abnormalities (e.g. t(17:22) in DFSP) Detection of prognostic cytogenetic abnormalities (e.g. detection of 9p21 copy loss in spitzoid tumours)
Comparative genomic hybridization	Detection of chromosomal aberrations – lower resolution than FISH but detects changes across the entire genome	Cytogenetic characterization of tumours

DFSP, dermatofibrosarcoma protuberans.

important from both a diagnostic and management standpoint, as the translocation leads to a fusion protein of COL1A1 and PDGFB, which can be targeted by the drug imatinib in cases not amenable to complete resection. Ewing sarcoma, alveolar soft part sarcoma, congenital infantile fibrosarcoma and extrarenal malignant rhabdoid tumour are malignancies that are uncommonly encountered in the skin, and are strongly associated with specific translocations (Table 176.4).

Molecular diagnostics are a critical component in the diagnosis of cutaneous T-cell lymphomas (CTCL). Although the diagnosis of mycosis fungoides (MF) can often be reliably made based on histopathological changes alone, the highly variable nature of CTCL can pose diagnostic challenges. Immunohistochemical analysis to evaluate the subtypes and cell surface markers of lymphocytes in an infiltrate can be useful, but must be interpreted with a critical eye as features may overlap with those of a number of benign entities. Similarly, evaluation for T-cell clonality by T-cell gene rearrangement is a powerful adjunct test, but a positive result does not necessarily equate with malignancy, as many benign dermatoses such as lichen planus, lymphomatoid papulosis and pityriasis lichenoides may display clonality. Conversely, in the early stages of CTCL, the host immune response to atypical cells may lead to false-negative T-cell gene rearrangement testing. The use of other molecular studies such as cytogenetics and gene expression profiling is still investigational and has not come into widespread diagnostic use.

Perhaps the most frequently used molecular diagnostic technique is gene sequencing in the diagnosis of heritable conditions. The complete sequencing of the human genome, along with advances in molecular genetic techniques, has led to the identification of causative genes in thousands of diseases. This has been particularly important in paediatric dermatology, where disorders of cornification, bullous diseases and developmental anomalies have broad phenotypic variation. Whole exome sequencing, which focuses on the parts of DNA that encode proteins, has become essential in identifying causative genes of many rare conditions, and has been used on a case-by-case basis to identify novel mutations in patients in whom expected mutations were not identified by conventional methods.

Table 176.4 Important molecular abnormalities in paediatric melanocytic and soft tissue tumours

Tumour	Aberrations (method)
Spitzoid melanoma (to differentiate from atypical spitzoid tumors)	Homozygous loss of 9p21 (FISH) TERT promoter mutation (gene sequencing) Multiple copy number aberrations (CGH)
Giant cell fibroblastoma	t(17;22)
Dermatofibrosarcoma protuberans	t(17;22)
Ewing sarcoma	t(11;22)
Alveolar soft part sarcoma	t(X;17)
Congenital infantile fibrosarcoma	t(12;15)
Extrarenal malignant rhabdoid tumour	22q11.2 inactivation (by deletion or other mutations)

CGH, comparative genomic hybridization; FISH, fluorescence *in situ* hybridization.

References

1 Aurelius E, Johansson B, Sköldenberg B et al. Rapid diagnosis of herpes simplex encephalitis by nested polymerase chain reaction assay of cerebrospinal fluid. Lancet 1991;337:189–92.

2 Gerami P, Cooper C, Bajaj S et al. Outcomes of atypical Spitz tumors with chromosomal copy number aberrations and conventional melanomas in children. Am J Surg Pathol 2013;37:1387–94.

3 Gerami P, Scolyer RA, Xu X et al. Risk assessment for atypical Spitzoid melanocytic neoplasms using FISH to identify chromosomal copy number aberrations. Am J Surg Pathol 2013;37:676–84.

4 Ali L, Helm T, Cheney R et al. Correlating array comparative genomic hybridization findings with histology and outcome in Spitzoid melanocytic neoplasms. Int J Clin Exp Pathol 2010;3:593–9.

5 Horn S, Figl A, Rachakonda PS et al. TERT promoter mutations in familial and sporadic melanoma. Science 2013;399:959–61.

6 Lee S, Barnhill RL, Dummer R et al. TERT promoter mutations are predictive of aggressive clinical behavior in patients with Spitzoid melanocytic neoplasms. Sci Rep 2015;10:11200.

The 'normal' biopsy

Histopathological changes in skin biopsies may be remarkably subtle even when the clinical features are striking. Examination of the specimen at multiple levels often reveals changes not apparent in the initial sections. Staining for fungi may demonstrate fungal hyphae or spores in the superficial corneal layers. The linear epidermal naevus and the connective tissue nevus may be very subtle, the former consisting of a localized area of hyperkeratosis with papillomatosis (Fig. 176.26), and the latter showing a localized area of thickened dermal collagen which may be more easily appreciated on an elastic stain. Biopsies from children with superficial morphoea and

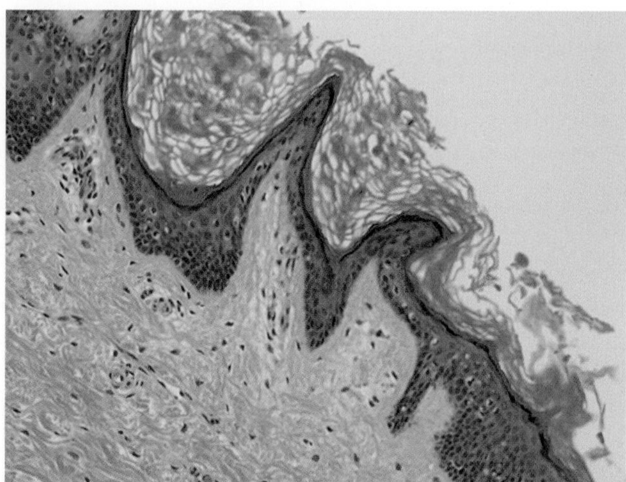

Fig. 176.26 High-power view of a skin biopsy from a patient with a linear epidermal nevus showing hyperkeratosis and papillomatosis.

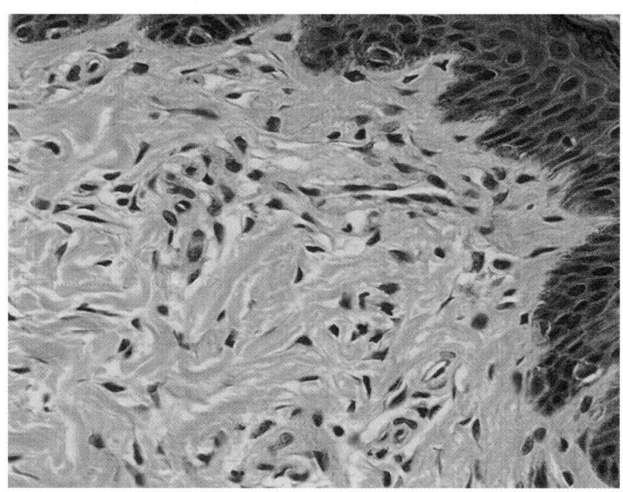

Fig. 176.27 High-power view of a skin biopsy from a patient with a clinically life-threatening severe vasculitis in which the histological changes are subtle. Note the endothelial swelling and mild lymphocytic infiltration of vessel walls. This biopsy was taken early in the clinical course. A biopsy taken a few weeks later showed a full-blown leucocytoclastic vasculitis.

localized scleroderma may also show subtle changes of dermal collagen, the former more likely to be associated with an inflammatory infiltrate in the early stages. Biopsies in the early stages of a vasculitis or in the involutional stages of a haemangioma may show little more than dilation of dermal capillaries (Fig. 176.27). Lastly, the possibility that the lesion has been missed should be borne in mind, and a further biopsy requested if clinically indicated.

In conclusion, skin biopsy is a diagnostic tool that must be interpreted by the clinician within the given clinical context. Communication of clinical findings and considerations to the dermatopathologist is essential. A collaborative approach between the clinician and the pathologist is the most likely means to obtain an accurate and specific diagnosis.

CHAPTER 177

Nursing Care of the Skin in Children

Bisola Laguda[1], Hilary Kennedy[2], Jackie Denyer[2], Heulwen Wyatt[3], Jean Robinson[4] & Karen Pett[5]

[1] Chelsea and Westminster Hospital, London, UK
[2] Great Ormond Street Hospital, London, UK
[3] St Woolos Hospital, Newport, UK
[4] Royal London Hospital, London, UK
[5] West Hertfordshire Hospitals NHS Trust, St Albans, UK

Introduction, 2393
Collodion baby and harlequin ichthyosis, 2393
The newborn with epidermolysis bullosa, 2395
Eczema: wet wrap dressings, paste bandages and therapeutic clothing, 2396
Bleach baths for eczema, 2399
Psoriasis, 2400
Infections and infestations, 2402
Vascular birthmarks, 2402
Systemic treatment, 2406
Intensive care, 2409
Safeguarding issues in paediatric dermatology, 2410
Conclusion, 2413

Abstract

This chapter details the nursing care of selected paediatric skin conditions. It varies from providing advice and guidance to parents in the clinic, through monitoring of children on systemic medication, to the treatment of children with more serious skin conditions in hospital. It would be impossible to cover all aspects of nursing care. This chapter is intended to be of practical value to nurses, paediatricians and dermatologists.

Key points

- **Nursing care is an integral part of management of paediatric skin diseases.**
- **Erythroderma can be a manifestation of many diseases but whatever the underlying cause, the acute symptoms of the impaired skin barrier function must be recognized.**
- **Nursing care of harlequin/collodion babies should take place in a humidified incubator to reduce transepidermal water loss.**
- **Safeguarding issues are the responsibility of all healthcare professionals.**
- **Children with severe adverse life-threatening cutaneous reactions, such as Stevens–Johnson syndrome and toxic epidermal necrolysis, should be admitted to specialized paediatric intensive care units or burns units.**
- **Systemic drug monitoring should be according to published guidelines.**

Introduction

The nursing management of many skin conditions is an essential part of the management of children with various dermatological conditions. This varies from providing advice and guidance to parents in the clinic, through monitoring of children on systemic medication, to the treatment of children with more serious skin conditions in hospital. It would be impossible to cover all aspects of nursing care, but in this chapter we have included guidelines for the nursing care of selected conditions used by various paediatric dermatology departments which we hope will be of practical value to nurses, paediatricians and dermatologists.

The skin care regimens that are listed should be viewed as personal practice and we appreciate that there are many different approaches to treatment. It may well be that our suggestions could be improved and we are willing to update our ideas. Nevertheless, the purpose of this section is to provide a basic plan of management that can be used by other nurses/doctors.

Collodion baby and harlequin ichthyosis

Collodion baby

Management of the baby born with a collodion membrane is detailed in Chapters 10 and 129. The nursing aspects are listed in Table 177.1. The severely compromised skin barrier presents the greatest challenge during the neonatal period and previously high mortality rates were mainly due to temperature instability, hypernatraemic dehydration and sepsis [1,2] but advances in neonatal care have greatly improved the prognosis. The baby should be nursed in a high-humidity incubator in a neonatal intensive care unit. A multidisciplinary team of paediatrician, dermatologist and ophthalmologist should be involved in the baby's care [1,2].

Harper's Textbook of Pediatric Dermatology, Fourth Edition. Edited by Peter Hoeger, Veronica Kinsler and Albert Yan.

Table 177.1 Nursing care of the collodion baby and harlequin ichthyosis (HI)

Action	Rationale
General measures	
Record vital signs and temperature	
Monitor respiratory rate and effort and oxygen saturation	Respiratory difficulties may result from restriction of chest movement in babies with HI [2,4] and blockage of nasal passages by collodion membrane [1]
Barrier nurse in humidified incubator with a minimum of 50% humidity with adjustments as needed and lower temperature 32–34 °C [5], aiming to keep baby's temperature at 36.5–37 °C	Transepidermal water loss (TEWL) is up to 7 times greater than normal skin due to severe loss of skin barrier function [6]. TEWL essentially ceases at 80% relative humidity or above so controlling incubator humidity in the range of 50–70% is reasonable to decrease TEWL and associated energy expenditure [4]. Incubator use helps prevent hypernatraemic dehydration and hypothermia as a result of increased TEWL. Monitor electrolytes initially daily [1]. High humidity settings can promote the growth of candidiasis and *Pseudomonas* [2] Hypohidrosis due to a functional inhibition of the baby's sweat glands [7] and overheating can occur so incubator temperatures should be kept lower than usual (32–34 °C) and adjusted in correlation with the baby's temperature [2,4]. The use of greasy skin treatments may also affect the baby's temperature regulation
Record length and weight on admission and weigh daily	To help in assessment of fluid balance and growth; also for calculating drug doses
Minimize invasive procedures where possible [1,2] and observe for signs of infection in intravenous cannulas and skin, particularly when collodion membrane shedding or harlequin 'coat of armour' splits	High risk of sepsis; early detection and treatment important
Pain should be measured using an appropriate assessment tool. Administer analgesia when indicated – this may include opiates [2,4]	Fissured truncal skin in babies with HI can reduce respiratory effort due to pain and increases the risk of pulmonary complications. Deep fissures in HI are painful especially when bathing the baby [2,4]
Skin management	
Clinical assessment of the skin and record in the nursing notes	To assess the extent of the condition, provide baseline and monitor progress
Observe digits closely	Constricting bands can cause ischaemia [2]
Liberal applications of 50:50 white soft paraffin/liquid paraffin [2,4]	To reduce fluid loss, soften skin, promote desquamation, increase mobility and comfort and prevent fissures; it also allows for increased chest movement and deeper respirations [2,4]
Use a new sterile tongue blade or clean utensil to retrieve emollient from container with each use [2]	Reduced risk of contamination
When the baby's condition allows, daily baths with an oily emollient [2,4,5]	To cleanse, increase hydration of the skin and promote the softening and shedding of the collodion membrane and plaques in HI
Use a soap substitute, such as aqueous cream or emulsifying ointment	Normal soap is astringent
Allow the collodion membrane or plaques in HI to shed spontaneously – do not cut or attempt to remove	Cutting membranes or plaques increases the risk of infection
Avoid the use of medicated ointments, e.g. those containing urea or salicylic acid	Due to the disrupted epidermal barrier, there is a risk of percutaneous absorption and systemic intoxication [1,2,4,7]
Pressure areas: nurse on infant pressure-relieving mattress, turn regularly and monitor pressure areas	To relieve pressure to the skin and alleviate pain from fissured areas
Eyes: ophthalmological evaluation of ectropion (everted eyelids). Four-hourly eye care with saline; apply eye ointment/emollient eye drops as prescribed [1,4]	To prevent dryness and infection in the presence of ectropion
For severe ectropion, especially in babies with HI in whom the eyes are usually closed, use eye drops and apply ointment to the eyelids	To prevent damage to the mucosal lining of the eyelids
Ears: ENT/otorhinolaryngology evaluation	External ear canals can be obstructed with debris, affecting hearing [1,4]
Mouth: two-hourly mouth care if limited oral intake and marked eclabium (eversion of the lips)	To prevent dry, cracked and sore lips and mouth
Oral retinoid treatment	
Babies with HI may be treated with acitretin (vitamin A derivative) [1–4] which requires careful handling	Accelerates shedding of hyperkeratotic plates and continued use reduces scaling, improving ectropion and eclabium. An oil-based liquid formulation is available but this has a short half-life and is unstable in daylight. Teratogenic and so gloves should be worn by female nurses and the child's mother when handling [7]
Nutrition	
Dietitian for assessment and guidance [1,2]	Increased metabolic demands due to severe TEWL and chronic inflammation. May require as much as 25% more calories [4]. This is likely to be an ongoing problem in children with HI
Vitamin D supplementation [3]	Defective vitamin D synthesis in HI
Initiate oral feeding as soon as possible. Encourage breastfeeding if possible [8]	To ensure optimum intake, leading to adequate hydration and weight gain and promote maternal/baby bonding [3]

Table 177.1 *Continued*

Action	Rationale
Consider the use of a Haberman feeder with a specially designed teat which is activated by tongue and gum pressure rather than sucking, imitating the mechanics of breastfeeding	Allows for decreased sucking due to eclabium and possible jaw immobility in HI [3]
If a nasogastric tube is required, secure with a tubular bandage, such as Tubifast around the tube and the baby's head	Adhesive tape may damage the skin and is difficult to secure due to greasy emollients
Family support	
Encourage parental contact; handling baby on infant mattress may make this easier. Encourage parents and carers to participate in the baby's care as soon as possible [1,4,7] and educate them on how to care for the baby's skin	To promote bonding; baby may be difficult to handle owing to greasy emollients
Give practical and emotional support to the family. Provide the families with written information about the condition and details of relevant family support groups (in the UK, it is the Ichthyosis Support Group: www.isg.org.uk)	The appearance of babies with HI is striking and shocking for staff, but most importantly for parents [4], and they will need support and information. Parents generally find compromised skin status difficult to understand [1]. Accurate information needs to be given by professionals who have experience in looking after these babies [1,4]. In collodion babies, it is particularly challenging to communicate regarding the actual diagnosis as this can't be assessed initially [1].
Discharge planning	
Set up a mechanism for rapid access to medical treatment	Children can rapidly become unwell due to dehydration and sepsis
Teach parents and carers the emollient therapy to be continued at home and any additional care that the baby may require	To maintain progress
Follow-up required with paediatrician, dermatologist, ophthalmologist and otolaryngologist and allied therapists as needed [5]	To monitor ongoing progress and discuss further management and prognosis. Children will go on to live with a chronic skin disease that needs daily input. Many children with HI will have problems with their hair and nails, eyes and ears and gastrointestinal tract, poor growth and some degree of locomotor problems. Developmental delay has also been reported in some children [3]
Genetic counselling should be organized	These conditions are inherited as autosomal recessive. Prenatal diagnostic testing is now available in specialist centres [3]
Ensure health visitor support in place for routine immunizations and developmental checks. Set up local community nurse support and input from social care as needed. Forward planning for the child's educational needs is essential and health providers should liaise with education providers as the child grows	To ensure adequate support and practical assistance for the family after discharge from hospital. Many families will need professional help to organize the extra support their child needs at nursery and school. Ongoing laborious treatments are needed with social and financial implications for these children and their families [5,7–9]
Refer to psychological services as needed	
In the UK, Changing Faces is a charity support group which is particularly helpful for children who are having psychological problems coping with their appearance (www.changingfaces.org.uk)	

Harlequin ichthyosis

Harlequin ichthyosis (HI) is the most rare and most severe form of congenital ichthyosis with a previous high mortality mainly due to sepsis and respiratory failure [3]. Improvements in neonatal care and the early introduction of the oral retinoid acitretin (Neotigason®), a vitamin A derivative, have improved survival and HI should now be regarded as a severe chronic disease that is not invariably fatal [3]. It is described in detail in Chapter 129. Nursing management shares some commonalities with that of collodion babies. These babies should be nursed in a neonatal intensive care unit with input from a multidisciplinary team of paediatrician, dermatologist, ophthalmologist and otolaryngologist [2–4] (see Table 177.1).

References

1 Prado R, Ellis LZ, Gamble R et al. Collodion baby: an update with a focus on practical management. J Am Acad Dermatol 2012;67(6):1362–74.
2 Dyer JA, Spraker M, Williams M. Care of the newborn with ichthyosis. Dermatol Therapy 2013;26:1–15.
3 Rajpopat S, Moss C, Mellerio J et al. Harlequin ichthyosis: a review of clinical and molecular findings in 45 cases. Arch Dermatol 2011;147:681–6.
4 Harvey HB, Shaw MG, Morrell S. Perinatal management of harlequin ichthyosis: a case report and literature review. J Perinatol 2010;30:66–72.
5 Oji V, Traupe H. Ichthyosis: clinical manifestations and practical treatment options. Am J Clin Dermatol 2009;10(6):351–64.
6 Buyse L, Graves C, Marks R et al. Collodion baby dehydration: the danger of high transepidermal water loss. Br J Dermatol 1993;129(1):86–8.
7 Vahlquist A, Gånemo A, Virtanen M. Congenital ichthyosis: an overview of current and emerging therapies. Acta Derm Venereol 2008;88(1):4–14.
8 Gånemo A, Lindholm C, Lindberg M et al. Quality of life in adults with congenital ichthyosis. J Adv Nurs 2003;44(4):412–19.
9 Dreyfus I, Pauwels C, Bourrat E et al Burden of inherited ichthyosis: a French national survey. Acta Derm Venereol 2015;95(3):326–8.

The newborn with epidermolysis bullosa

These babies have fragile skin and are prone to blistering and wounds. In many of those severely affected, extensive wounds resulting from intrauterine movements and birth trauma are present at delivery. Recognition of this

Table 177.2 Immediate nursing care of the newborn with epidermolysis bullosa

Action	Rationale
Remove cord clamp and replace with ligature	To avoid trauma to the surrounding skin
Nurse in cot/bassinette unless incubator required for reasons such as prematurity	To avoid additional blistering from heat and humidity within incubator
Skin treatment	
Avoid wearing gloves or if local policy dictates, lubricate finger tips with greasy emollient	To avoid friction and trauma
Lance all blisters with a sterile needle	To prevent blisters from enlarging
Leave the roof on the blister	To protect the underlying skin
Dust area with cornflour	To dry the blisters and limit their spread
Wound management[a]	
Ensure adequate analgesia given prior to dressing changes	
Apply a nonadherent primary dressing such as polymeric membrane, soft silicone or lipido-colloid	To avoid trauma to the wound and surrounding skin and to encourage healing
Cover primary dressing (with the exemption of polymeric membrane which does not require a secondary dressing) with soft silicone foam and antimicrobial agent	To provide padding to avoid trauma, to absorb exudate and avoid critical colonization
Dress fingers and toes individually	To avoid digital fusion
Secure with tubular bandage	To avoid using adhesive tape that will tear the skin
Fixation of cannula	
If IV cannula required, secure with soft silicone rather than adhesive-based tape	To ensure skin integrity on removal
Removal of adhesive products	
Use silicone medical adhesive remover to dissolve adhesive	To avoid skin stripping
Napkin area	
Cleanse skin with 50% liquid paraffin/50% white soft paraffin rather than water	To avoid friction and reduce pain
Cover open or blistered areas with hydrogel-impregnated gauze dressing	To assist healing and avoid contamination
Line disposable nappy with soft liner	To prevent edges of nappy from rubbing the skin
Feeding	
Use Haberman special needs feeder if not breastfed	To avoid further mucosal blistering from traditional teats
Apply teething gel to teat	To reduce pain from oral lesions and allow infant to suck
Protect lips with petroleum jelly	To avoid the teat sticking to the lips and tearing the skin
Avoid nasogastric tube if possible	To avoid damage to mucosa
If essential, use tube suitable for long-term feeding and secure with soft silicone tape	To minimize mucosal and skin damage
Handling	
Lift on soft pad; use a roll-and-lift technique	Shearing forces from traditional handling can result in skin loss
Avoid bathing until intrauterine and birth damage have healed	When naked, the infant will kick legs together and remove skin from healing areas
Clothing	
Dress in front-fastening baby suit; turn clothing inside out	To protect skin; to prevent seams from rubbing

[a] When recommended products are not available, use a nonadherent dressing but apply 50% liquid paraffin/50% white soft paraffin over the dressing to reduce adhesion and minimize skin damage.
IV, intravenous.

condition is of primary importance so that these babies can be handled with care and the appropriate measures taken to look after their skin. Management is by assessment and guidance from a specialized multidisciplinary team. An outreach service is available in the UK by clinical nurse specialists to avoid the transportation of vulnerable neonates.

Epidermolysis bullosa comprises a group of genetic disorders with a number of different subtypes that vary in severity. The most severe forms are dystrophic epidermolysis bullosa and junctional epidermolysis bullosa (see Chapter 76). Nursing care for the newborn suspected of having epidermolysis bullosa is summarized in Table 177.2.

Eczema: wet wrap dressings, paste bandages and therapeutic clothing

Wet wrap dressings, bandages and therapeutic clothing can be helpful in breaking the 'itch–scratch' cycle for children with atopic eczema. They are especially useful at night by protecting the skin from the damage of subconscious night-time scratching. They are not stand-alone treatments, but are used as part of the stepped-up care plan of treatments recommended by the UK National Institute for Health and Care Excellence (NICE) for atopic eczema.

Dry and wet wrap dressings

Dry dressings are cotton/viscose-based tubular bandages that are cut to size to fit the limbs or trunk, or therapeutic garments that are available in child and adult sizes. They provide a protective layer over the skin and help with temperature control, prevent damage from scratching and improve the absorption of topical medication and emollient. They also help cut down the soiling of clothes and bedlinen from blood and exudate from scratching. They can be worn under clothes such as school uniform in the day or under nightwear at night.

Wet wrap dressings (Fig. 177.1) are the same bandages or garments but worn in a double layer. The inner layer is usually soaked in a dilute steroid (the wet layer) and the outer layer remains dry. Some centres dampen the inner layer with water. They should not be used over eczema that is infected as the wraps create a warm, humid environment that encourages bacteria and spreads infection [1–3].

The gradual drying of the wet layer has a cooling therapeutic effect on the skin which helps to reduce itching and discomfort. The occlusion of the skin allows time for the skin to heal and breaks the constant itching and scratching.

Two methods have been described; one is used exclusively in hospital for the treatment of an acute exacerbation of eczema (Table 177.3) and the other has been adapted mainly for use at home (Table 177.4). If wet wrap dressings are used at home, they should be limited to 1–2 weeks to help during flares of eczema and once the eczema is under control, the dressings should be discontinued.

Paste bandages

These are bandages impregnated with a paste containing substances such as zinc oxide (Zipzoc®) or ichthamol (Ichthopaste®), which are anti-inflammatory and soothing on the skin providing some relief from irritation. They are particularly helpful for treating areas of stubborn lichenified eczema.

Paste bandages are messy and a second dry layer of bandage is required. There are several methods of securing the paste bandage, such as Coban® or similar elasticated bandage (not advisable if there is a known latex allergy) or a tubular bandage such as Comfifast® or Tubifast®, which is generally better tolerated by children (Fig. 177.2). The method of application is detailed in Table 177.5.

Paste bandages can be used for either a whole or part of a limb, in areas such as the wrist or ankle. They should be left in place for at least 48 hours and, depending on the

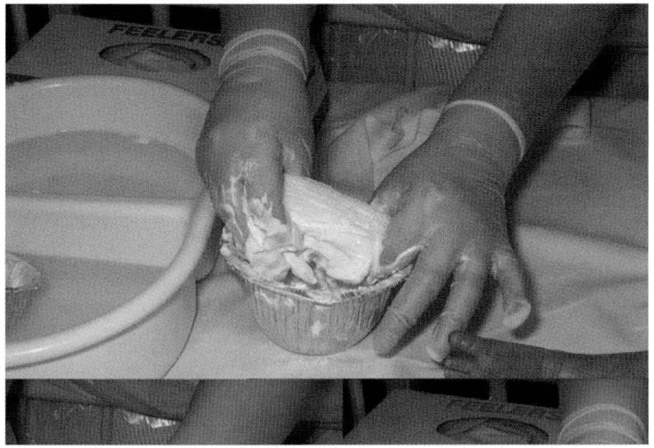
(a)

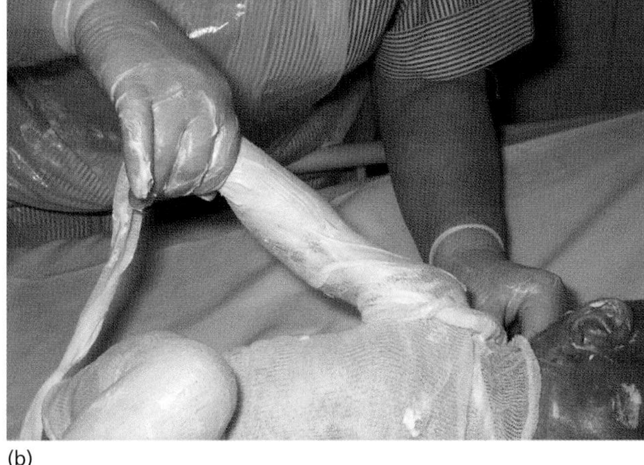
(b)

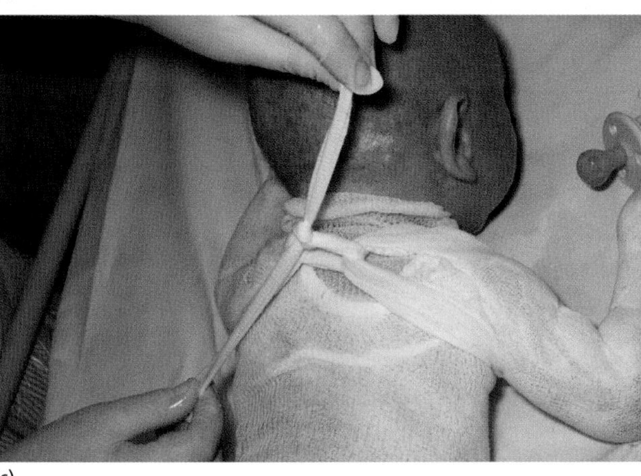
(c)

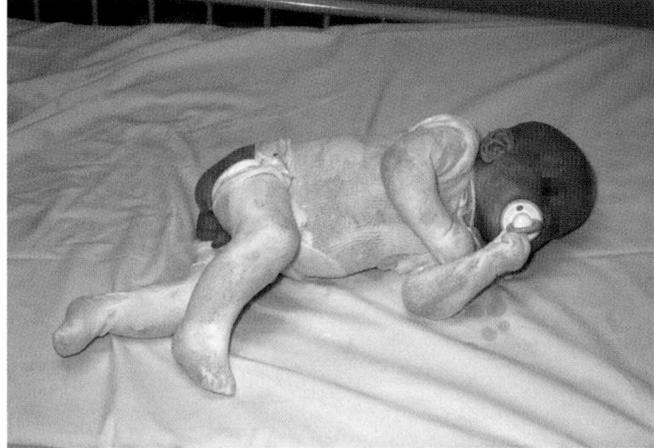
(d)

Fig. 177.1 (a–d) Wet dressings for inpatient treatment using Tubegauz.

Table 177.3 Wet dressings for inpatient treatment using Tubegauz® (Fig. 177.1)

Action	Rationale
Initial assessment on admission	
Nose, throat and skin swabs for MC&S	To detect secondary infection
MRSA screen if previous hospitalization and/or recurrent antibiotic therapy	To ensure early detection, increased susceptibility
Baseline temperature, pulse, respiratory rate and blood pressure; increase frequency as indicated	To obtain baseline values
Length and weight	To monitor growth and calculate drug doses
Assess skin and record findings	To assess severity of eczema and monitor progress with treatment
Treatment procedure	
Cut appropriately sized pieces of the cotton tubular bandage (Tubegauz) for the arms, legs and trunk	The technique involves two layers of bandaging
Soak the individual pieces of Tubegauz (suit 1) in the steroid cream[a] (not water)	To produce the first 'wet' layer
Put on the first layer of 'wet' Tubegauz; tie the arm and leg pieces to the trunk	This enables all affected areas on the limbs and trunk to be covered by a dressing impregnated with a weak steroid cream
Then apply the second 'dry' suit over the top of the wet layer, securing the arm and leg pieces to the trunk section	This completes the dressing
Keep hands covered; if the child is a thumb-sucker a small hole can be cut in the bandage	To minimize damage from scratching
Treatment regimen	
Dressings are changed twice daily by the nursing staff, usually for 3 days	There is usually a rapid improvement, and in most cases >90% clearance of eczema in this period of time
Apply separate topical preparation to face and neck as prescribed	Areas not covered by the wet dressings
Treatment immediately after the application of wet dressings	
The child is kept in hospital for a further 1–2 days and the residual or recurrent areas of eczema are treated with an appropriate topical steroid ointment[b] (without the use of dressings) once or twice daily, as needed	Treatment is then continued after discharge from hospital at home; it allows for the skin condition to stabilize
The use of a moisturizing agent at other times during the day to all areas of dry skin (2–3 times daily)	To maintain the integrity of the skin barrier
General measures	
Twice-daily cool baths with an oily bath emollient	To cleanse and hydrate the skin
Use a soap substitute, such as aqueous cream or emulsifying ointment, to wash	Normal soap too drying and can irritate the skin
If there is any suspicion of secondary bacterial infection, oral antibiotics should be prescribed[c]	Skin infection may be responsible for the exacerbation of eczema
A sedative antihistamine is also helpful in this situation and should be given as prescribed	To help settle the child
Loose cotton pyjamas should be worn over wet dressings	To prevent child becoming cold
Discharge planning	
Educate caregivers on treatment and management at home; support with written instructions	Essential so that the control of eczema is maintained
Liaise with GP and community paediatric nursing team as appropriate	To ensure child and caregiver are supported locally
Outpatient follow-up appointment within 2–3 weeks	To closely monitor progress and review long-term treatment plan

MC&S, microscopy, culture and antibiotic sensitivity; MRSA, meticillin-resistant *Staphylococcus aureus*.

[a] Currently we use, for babies under 1 year, 0.5% hydrocortisone cream; for children over 1 year, betamethasone valerate 0.01% cream (Betnovate® diluted 1:10). Both hydrocortisone and Betnovate can be diluted with either aqueous or cetomacrogol cream.

[b] Currently we use, for babies under 1 year, 1% hydrocortisone ointment; for children over 1 year, betamethasone valerate 0.025% ointment (Betnovate-RD®).

[c] If there is overt impetiginization then wet dressings should be delayed until 48–72 h after commencing antibiotics and when appropriate treatment has been confirmed from the skin swab results. If eczema herpeticum is suspected then this is an absolute contraindication to the use of wet dressings.

method and covering used, can be left *in situ* for 5–7 days and renewed repeatedly until the eczema has cleared.

The disadvantage of paste bandages is that they are messy and time consuming to apply. Children are often embarrassed by the appearance of them and cannot participate in sports or swimming at school whilst they are in place; cooperation by the child is essential. Parents can get round these issues by applying them only at weekends or in school holidays.

Therapeutic clothing

There is a wide range of companies that supply cotton and silk clothing and garments for wet wrap dressings. Various items such as vests, leggings, socks and gloves are available both on prescription and to buy online and over the counter. The garments are easier to apply than bandages and should be used over topical treatments as normal. As cotton and silk are both natural fibres, they are well tolerated by children with eczema. They can be used

Table 177.4 Wet dressings more suitable for use at home using Tubifast

Action	Rationale
Treatment procedure	
Apply the weak topical steroid ointment, beclomethasone dipropionate 0.0025% (Propaderm® in a dilution of 1 in 10) to the affected areas	To reduce inflammation
Apply 50:50 white soft paraffin/liquid paraffin liberally to the unaffected areas	As a moisturizing agent and to maintain the integrity of the skin barrier
Apply a suit of Tubifast bandages (one wet layer and one dry layer). Tubifast has a tighter fit than Tubegauz. The wet layer uses water and needs to be kept damp using a sponge or spray	To reduce itching and prevent damage from scratching, as well as maintaining an appropriate skin temperature
Then apply the second 'dry' suit over the top of the wet layer, securing the arm and leg pieces to the trunk section	This completes the dressing
Treatment regimen	
For use in hospital, dressings are changed twice daily for 3–5 days	This will produce a significant improvement, sufficient for the child to be discharged
Continue nightly wet wraps at home for up to two weeks and then review. Some dermatologists use them for longer and gradually reduce the frequency	Stopping wet wraps abruptly can induce a flare of eczema

The initial assessment on admission, general measures and discharge planning are similar to those described with the other method (see Table 177.3).
A set of Tubifast garments (Mölnlycke Health Care) includes long-sleeved vests, tights/leggings, mittens and socks, in different sizes, which makes it easier for the family, and they can be washed and reused.

in the day under clothes or at night under nightwear. Unlike paste bandages or wet wrapping, they can be used long term for comfort and to help relieve irritation and reduce scratching.

The disadvantages of therapeutic clothing are that they are expensive and there is little therapeutic evidence to support their clinical effectiveness.They require a special washing detergent and need replacing regularly.

Bleach baths for eczema

Children with eczema are often colonized with *Staphylococcus aureus*. This may produce overt signs such as weeping, crusting and folliculitis but may also be responsible for aggravating the eczema due to the production of superantigens and proteases. The use of sodium hypochlorite baths with nasal mupirocin has been shown to decrease the severity of eczema in patients with signs of bacterial infection [4,5].

The ideal formula for bleach baths in the UK is Milton sterilizing fluid (MSF) which contains 2% sodium hypochlorite. Other household bleaches contain additives such as surfactants and perfumes that may exacerbate eczema. Patients are instructed to bath twice a week in the chlorinated water for 5–10 minutes and the rinse thoroughly with clean water. Patients continue their normal emollient and steroid regime. They are also asked to use nasal mupirocin in both nostrils, three times a day for five consecutive days a month.

Instructions for bleach baths

1 Add lukewarm water to fill the tub completely (about 120 litres of water).
2 Add 250 mL of MSF using a kitchen measuring jug. This contains 2% sodium hypochlorite and can be obtained from any supermarket. The amount of Milton fluid added may need to be adjusted depending on size of the tub and amount of water used.
3 Stir the mixture with the jug to make sure that the bleach is completely diluted in the bath water.
4 The patient should soak in the chlorinated water for 5–10 minutes.
5 Thoroughly rinse the skin with lukewarm fresh water at the end of the bleach bath to prevent dryness and irritation.
6 As soon as the bath is over, pat the child dry. Do not rub dry as this may irritate the skin.
7 Immediately apply any prescribed medication/emollients.
8 Repeat bleach baths twice weekly or as prescribed.

Cautions

- Do not use undiluted bleach directly on the skin. Even diluted bleach can potentially cause dryness and irritation.
- Do not use bleach baths if there are many breaks or open areas on the skin (may provoke stinging and burning).
- Do not use bleach baths if there is a known contact allergy to chlorine.

References

1 **Goodyear HM, Spowart K, Harper JI. 'Wet-wrap' dressings for the treatment of atopic eczema in children. Br J Dermatol 1991;125(6):604.**
2 Goodyear HM, Harper JI. 'Wet wrap' dressings for eczema: an effective treatment but not to be misused. Br J Dermatol 2002;146(1):159.
3 **Oranje AP, Devillers AC, Kunz B et al. Treatment of patients with atopic dermatitis using wet-wrap dressings with diluted steroids and/or emollients. An expert panel's opinion and review of the literature. J Eur Acad Dermatol Venereol 2006;20(10):1277–86.**
4 **Huang JT, Rademaker A, Paller AS. Dilute bleach baths for Staphylococcus aureus colonization in atopic dermatitis to decrease disease severity. Arch Dermatol 2011;147(2):246–7.**
5 Kaplan SL, Forbes A, Hammerman WA. Randomized trial of 'bleach baths' plus routine hygienic measures vs. routine hygienic measures alone for prevention of recurrent infections. Clin Infect Dis 2014; 58(5):679–82.

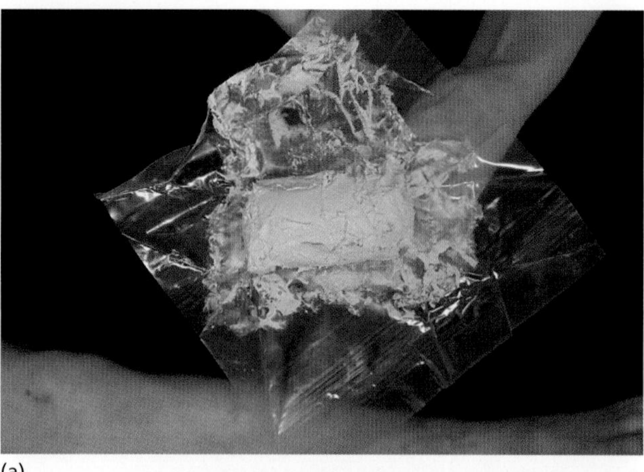

(a)

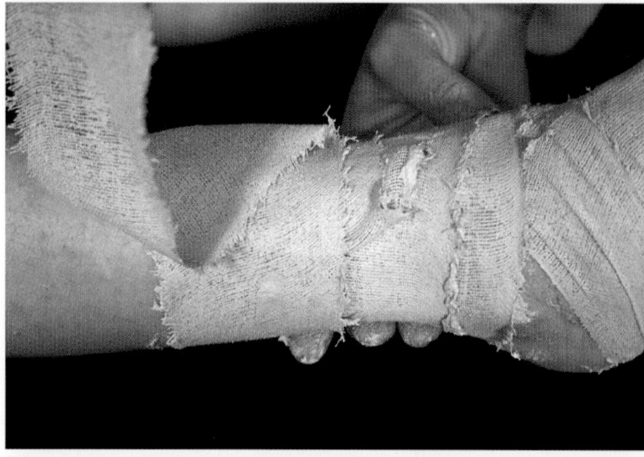

(b)

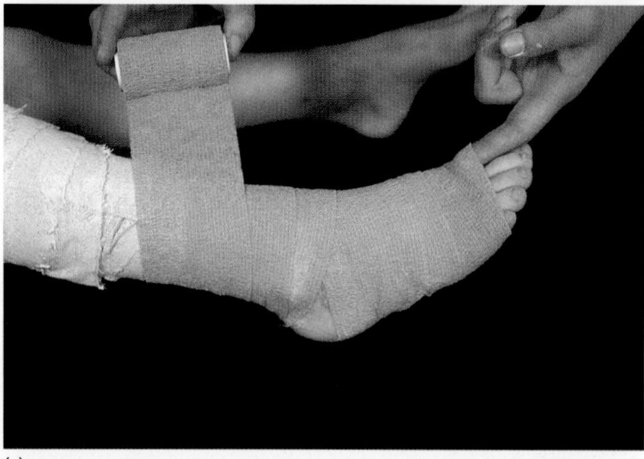

(c)

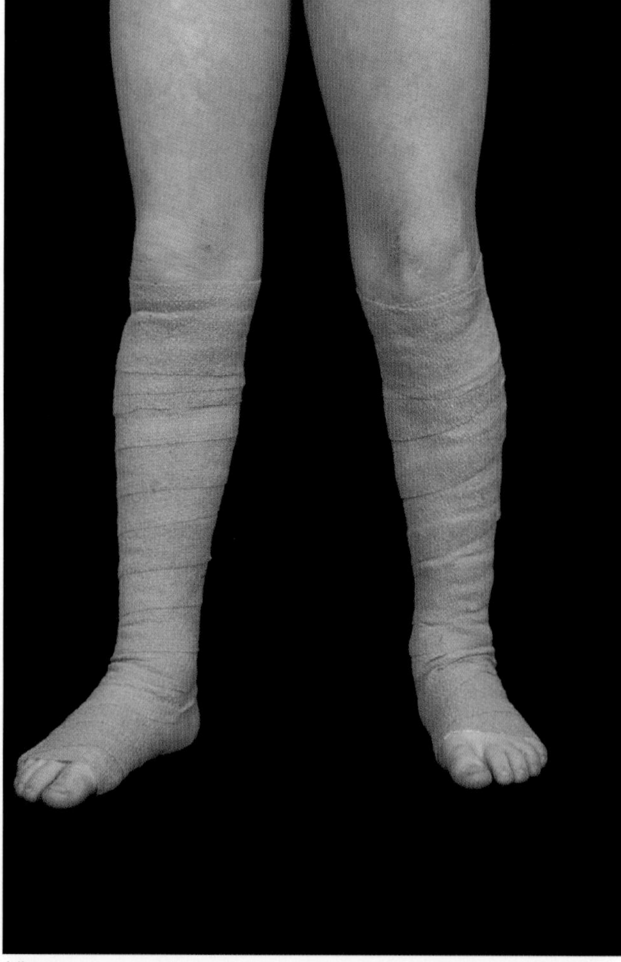

(d)

Fig. 177.2 (a–d) The application of Ichthopaste and Coban bandages.

Psoriasis

Dithranol preparations

Dithranol is a time-honoured treatment for plaque psoriasis (see Chapter 31). Traditionally, it has been used as an inpatient treatment incorporated at varying strengths (usually 0.05–2%) in Lassar's paste (zinc and salicylic acid paste BP). It is left on for a defined period of time, dependent on the thickness of the psoriasis, the individual skin sensitivity and age of the child, usually from 30 min to 2 h. It must be explained to the family that dithranol produces a temporary brownish-purple staining of the skin and may 'burn' the normal surrounding skin if this is not protected.

'Short-contact' therapy can be undertaken as a day-attender at the hospital. For children, therapy should be supervised in a hospital unit by nurses experienced in applying dithranol preparations. In certain situations, when parents are taught the treatment regimen, it can be carried out at home with caution. Other formulations available include Dithrocream® 0.1–2%. The nursing procedure is detailed in Table 177.6.

Table 177.5 The application of Ichthopaste and Coban bandages (Fig. 177.2)

Action	Rationale
Preparation	
Explain the procedure to patient and caregiver, including why it is indicated; use photographs and a doll if appropriate	To alleviate anxiety, determine the level of cooperation and ensure that informed consent to treatment is given
Ensure the topical treatments are prescribed on the patient's prescription chart	To adhere to the medication policy
Assemble and prepare the following: Ichthopaste roll, Coban bandage, emollient/topical treatment to be applied to the skin, round-ended scissors	
Select appropriate distraction toys for the child as they will be required to sit still during the treatment	To avoid boredom and anxiety during treatment
Apply the emollient/topical therapy to the affected area	To reduce inflammation and maximize comfort
Legs and feet	
Wind the Ichthopaste bandage around the foot, overlapping one-half of the width of the bandage; bandage the ankle separately in the same fashion; work up the leg, occasionally reversing the direction of winding in order to make a pleat	This allows for shrinkage and maximum mobility; pleating and overlapping prevent a tourniquet effect from occurring
Arms and hands	
Using approximately 15 cm lengths, cover the palms and backs of hands; fingers can be bandaged separately as required; work up the arms, winding the Ichthopaste bandage around the arm, occasionally reversing the direction in order to make a pleat	As with the legs and feet
Coban bandage	
Apply the Coban bandage on top of the Ichthopaste bandage, winding around the limb, leaving a small section of Ichthopaste showing at both ends	To secure the underlying Ichthopaste bandage and protect clothing
Release most of the tension from the bandage during use	
General measures	
Usually left *in situ* for 12–48 h, but can be left for longer	To prevent constriction
For home use: ensure that the carer is competent in the application following demonstration	To ensure correct application
Support with written instructions; advise that treatment may stain clothing/ bedding	To support verbal instructions

Table 177.6 The application of dithranol preparations

Action	Rationale
Preparation	
Explain the procedure to the family, including why it is indicated; use photographs if appropriate	To alleviate anxiety, determine the level of cooperation and ensure informed consent to treatment
Ensure that the treatments are prescribed on the patient's prescription chart and check each preparation	To adhere to the medication policy and ensure correct strength is used
Assemble and prepare the following: disposable gloves (for the nurse), dithranol preparation, white soft paraffin, talcum powder, arachis oil[a], bath emollient, moisturizer, orange sticks and spatula, gauze squares, old pyjamas/gown or Tubegauz suit	
Select appropriate distraction toys for the child as they will be required to sit still during the treatment	Can be a lengthy treatment; need to prevent boredom and anxiety
Administration	
Apply white soft paraffin to all areas of healthy skin surrounding the psoriasis plaques	To prevent the dithranol burning healthy skin
Use either an orange stick or spatula (depending on size of plaque) to apply the dithranol preparation to the areas of psoriasis	To ensure the dithranol is applied carefully and accurately
Check the time of application	To ensure the dithranol is left on for the correct amount of time
Dust treated skin with talcum powder	To help keep the dithranol preparation *in situ* and prevent smearing
Dress the child in old pyjamas/gown or Tubegauz suit	Dithranol will stain all clothing and other contacts
Removal	
After the allocated time, remove the dithranol using gauze squares and arachis oil[a]	
Follow with a bath using an oily bath emollient	
Use a soap substitute to cleanse the skin, such as emulsifying ointment	

[a] Olive oil can be used in cases of peanut allergy.

Table 177.7 The application of scalp preparations for psoriasis

Action	Rationale
Preparation	
Assess the patient's scalp psoriasis and record extent and severity	To monitor effectiveness of therapy
Explain the procedure to the family, including why it is indicated; use photographs if appropriate	To alleviate anxiety, determine the level of cooperation and ensure informed consent to treatment is given
Ensure the treatments are prescribed on the patient's prescription chart and check against the preparations	To adhere to the medications policy and ensure that the correct treatments are administered
Assemble and prepare the following equipment: disposable gloves, plastic comb, scalp ointment, shampoo	
Select appropriate distraction tools for the child, as they will be required to sit still during the treatment	To prevent boredom and anxiety
Administration	
The scalp ointment should be applied in a methodical manner by parting the hair in sections; part the hair with a comb and apply a smear of the ointment along the parting; use the comb to gently encourage any scale to lift from the scalp; reapply the ointment to the thickened encrusted areas; part the hair, 1 cm from the treated area, and repeat until the whole scalp is treated	This technique ensures adequate coverage of the whole scalp
Leave *in situ* for the required time; a shower cap/scarf may be used	The longer it is left on, the more effective it is, ideally overnight
If left overnight, pillow cases should be covered	The treatment may stain pillow cases
After the allocated time, wash the hair with the prescribed shampoo	To gently remove the loosened scale/crust
Comb the hair against its natural fall	To gently lift any remaining scale, being careful not to pull out any scalp hairs
Review the scalp with each treatment	To monitor effectiveness

Scalp treatment

A traditional treatment for scalp psoriasis is the use of Sebco® (coal tar solution 12%, salicylic acid 2%, precipitated sulphur 4%, in a coconut oil emollient base). This is massaged into the scalp, left on for a defined period of time and then washed off with a prescribed shampoo, usually one containing coal tar (Table 177.7).

As the scalp improves, the duration of treatment and frequency can be reduced. At home, it may be more practical to apply the scalp ointment at teatime, when the child returns home from school, leave it on for 2–4 h and wash off prior to going to bed.

Infections and infestations

Care of the dermatology inpatient with MRSA

The prevalence of meticillin-resistant *Staphylococcus aureus* (MRSA) in the hospital setting, as well as the community, is an ongoing concern. This is part of a much wider problem of antibiotic resistance. The carriage of MRSA is particularly relevant to children with chronic skin disease. In the community, skin colonization is not as much of an issue as it is in a hospital environment, where it can be transmitted to other patients, some of whom would be at risk because of immunosuppression. Often these strains are resistant to most common antibiotics, which can include fucidic acid (Fucidin®) and mupirocin (Bactroban®). Antibiotic treatment of MRSA infection may be required in the outpatient setting; clindamycin, trimethoprim/sulfamethoxazole and linezolid could be effective based on culture results. In the inpatient setting, intravenous antibiotics such as teicoplanin and vancomycin are used. Other drugs now available include daptomycin and tigecycline. There are strict infection control measures to prevent cross-infection within the hospital setting (Table 177.8).

Staphylococcal scalded skin syndrome

Certain strains of *S. aureus* produce toxins, which can cause widespread skin peeling (Chapter 37). The source of infection is often the nasopharynx, umbilicus, skin wound, blood or as a result of breastfeeding. The symptoms develop within a few hours to a few days. The upper part of the epidermis peels off like wet tissue paper. Affected children can be very unwell and require high-dependency nursing care (Table 177.9). Treatment includes intravenous fluids, antibiotics and adequate analgesia.

Scabies

Scabies is a highly contagious mite infestation transmitted by close physical contact. All members of the family and close contacts should be treated simultaneously. Written instructions given to the family increase the likelihood of the correct procedure being followed (Table 177.10). There are a number of different topically applied treatments that can be used, which include permethrin 5% cream (Lyclear®) and malathion 0.5% in an aqueous base (Derbac-M®). For more details see Chapter 59.

Vascular birthmarks

Skin care after laser therapy for port wine stains

Laser treatment for port wine stains is described in detail in Chapter 172. Meticulous attention to skin care after laser treatment is essential and minimizes the risk of scarring and postoperative pigmentary changes (Table 177.11).

Table 177.8 Care of the dermatology inpatient with meticillin-resistant *Staphylococcus aureus* (MRSA) infection

Action	Rationale
Environment	
Nurse in an isolation cubicle with an infection precautions sign clearly visible	To prevent transmission of MRSA to others and to alert those entering the cubicle
Keep the door closed at all times	MRSA can be airborne
Remove excess equipment from the cubicle before the patient is isolated	To prevent unnecessary items being contaminated
When bathing is required, if possible limit use of bathroom to MRSA patient only or clean thoroughly following each use	To prevent cross-infection
Ensure the bath is rinsed thoroughly after cleaning	To prevent skin irritation to next patient
The isolation room should be cleaned regularly during use and surfaces should be kept clean and dry	Reduces the risk of contamination
Staff/visitors	
Ensure MRSA status is recorded confidentially in all the patient's relevant medical and nursing documentation	Essential information
Limit the number of staff/visitors entering the cubicle at the same time	Reduces the risk of cross-infection
Prior to entry into isolation cubicle: wear plastic apron; wash hands; wear disposable gloves; collect all equipment required	To protect clothing and to prevent cross-infection
Prior to exiting isolation cubicle: remove plastic apron and gloves; wash hands	
Involve play specialist for activities	Child will be bored in cubicle; no access to playroom
Skin care	
In cases of colonization only, normal skin care regime should continue	
When attending to wound/skin care, hands should be washed before and after, and gloves should be worn	
Equipment	
Where possible, allocate equipment for sole patient use	Reduces the risk of cross-infection
Equipment should be kept clean and dry	Less likely to become contaminated
Do not take into the cubicle unnecessary equipment, including pens, notes and personal stethoscopes	To avoid unnecessary contamination
Clean/disinfect all equipment before removing from the room	To prevent cross-infection
General measures	
Give practical and reassuring support to the family	Acknowledging the stigma of MRSA status, and parental concerns
After discharge from hospital	
Thorough cleaning of the cubicle according to a strict hospital protocol	

Nursing aspects of haemangiomas

Haemangiomas are common birthmarks and the majority do not require any intervention. However, if medical treatment is needed, propranolol is now first-line treatment in preference to oral steroids [1–6]. Topical treatment with timolol is also increasingly used for smaller haemangiomas. The main medical complication of haemangiomas is bleeding from trauma. In certain situations, they can become necrotic on the surface and ulcerate, which may be slow to heal and give rise to local problems, depending on the site. Haemangiomas are discussed in detail in Chapter 119 but we have included protocols for both propranolol and timolol in this chapter

Propranolol for the treatment of infantile haemangiomas

Haemangiomas of infancy (HI) are vascular tumours that undergo a proliferative phase followed by stabilization and eventual spontaneous involution. Early recognition and treatment of problematic lesions help to minimize complications. Propranolol, a nonselective β-blocker, has been used to treat haemangiomas that are causing, or are likely to cause, clinically significant impairment of function or, if untreated, could lead to significant permanent disfigurement. Propranolol produces clinical improvement through vasoconstriction, apoptosis and reduced expression of proangiogenic factors.

Before starting propranolol

- Take a careful history with full clinical examination, including cardiovascular and respiratory assessment.
- Examination should include heart rate, blood pressure and peripheral capillary oxygen saturation measurement.
- Document any history of hypoglycaemia, episodes of bronchospasm, arrhythmias, family history of arrhythmias or maternal connective tissue disease.
- Clinical photography.
- Echocardiogram (ECHO) and electrocardiogram (ECG) if there is any cause for concern, in particular patients with one or more large haemangiomas (more than 10 cm in diameter); more than five cutaneous haemangiomas or known liver haemangioma; a history, symptoms or

Table 177.9 Nursing care of staphylococcal scalded skin syndrome

Action	Rationale
On admission	
Nose, throat and skin swabs for culture and antibiotic sensitivities, including a specific request for an MRSA screen	For early detection of infection
Baseline temperature, pulse, respiratory rate and blood pressure; increase frequency as indicated	To obtain the normal range and detect deterioration of condition
Height and weight	To assess fluid loss, monitor weight loss and calculate drug doses
Assess skin and record	To assess extent of condition and monitor progress
Skin care	
Daily bathing/washes; dependent on mobility and fragility of the skin	To clean the skin
Use an oily emollient in the water	To prevent dryness
Use a gentle cream soap substitute	Normal soap too astringent
Dress denuded areas with Vaseline Gauze® soaked liberally in a 50:50 mixture of white soft paraffin/liquid paraffin. These are changed every 12–24 h	For comfort, to promote healing and to protect denuded areas from infection and further trauma
Secure with a loose Tubegauz suit	To keep dressings *in situ*
Apply the 50:50 paraffin mix to all exposed areas, in particular the face and napkin area	To protect these areas and prevent further trauma
As the dressings dry out, reapply the 50:50 paraffin mix to the Vaseline Gauze	To maximize effectiveness of dressings
Eyes: at least 4-hourly eye care in the acute period; apply eye ointment/drops as prescribed	To prevent damage, infection and long-term complications
Mouth: 2-hourly mouth care if limited oral intake and in the presence of mucosal and lip involvement	To prevent and/or improve mucosal and lip involvement
Pressure areas: nurse on a pressure-relieving mattress, monitor pressure areas and position patient appropriately	To relieve pressure on the skin and alleviate pain
Fluid and electrolyte balance	
Administer IV replacement fluid as prescribed	To correct fluid, electrolyte and protein loss and prevent dehydration, renal failure and shock
Secure cannula with nonadhesive tape/dressing and bandage well	Adhesive tapes/Band-Aid plasters will damage fragile skin
Careful fluid balance monitoring essential	To ensure correct fluid balance and to observe for urinary retention
Consider urinary catheter for painful micturition and/or urine retention	To normalize urine output and reduce pain on micturition
Nutrition	
Encourage/initiate enteral feeding	To prevent weight loss, protein loss and promote wound healing
If a nasogastric tube is required, secure with a tubular bandage or nonadhesive tape	Adhesive tape will damage fragile skin
Involve dietitian for assessment and guidance	To ensure optimum dietary intake
Pain relief	
Ensure adequate analgesia is administered; consider IV analgesics with extensive skin involvement	To ensure child is pain free; extensive skin loss causes high levels of pain that may be difficult to control with oral analgesics alone
General measures	
Minimal handling	To prevent pain and damage to the skin
Provide constant environmental temperature where possible (30–32 °C is optimum)	Temperature regulation is compromised due to extensive skin loss
Monitor core temperature closely	Skin temperature is unreliable; at risk of hypothermia because of excess heat loss
Nurse under strict infectious and protective precautions in a cubicle	To protect against further sepsis
Give practical and emotional support to the child and family	Child and family may experience high levels of distress
Discharge planning	
Teach the parents/carer the skin care regimen to be continued at home	To sustain recovery

IV, intravenous ; MRSA, meticillin-resistant *Staphylococcus aureus*.

signs of cardiovascular disease and plaque/segmental haemangiomas/PHACES syndrome. If the heart rate is below normal for age, that is less than 80/min in an infant under 1 year old, then an ECG is mandatory.

Dosage regime

- Week 1: 1 mg/kg/day in three divided doses. First dose given under medical supervision, monitoring heart rate and blood pressure every 30 min over a 2-hperiod. Babies who are premature, those with comorbidities and all patients weighing less than 3.5 kg must be admitted and monitored for longer, if necessary. Special care also needs to be taken in babies with PHACES syndrome.
- Week 2: 1.5 mg/kg/day in three divided doses.
- Week 3: 2 mg/kg/day in three divided doses, which is usually the optimum dose.
- Thereafter the dose is increased at monthly intervals in line with weight gain. Heart rate and blood pressure to be checked 24 h after each increase in dose.

Table 177.10 Treatment of scabies

Action	Rationale
Pretreatment	
Contact tracing should include all close/prolonged skin-to-skin contacts over the previous six weeks, even if asymptomatic	Clinical manifestations may not appear for at least one month after initial infestation
Ensure that treatments are coordinated to treat all contacts on the same day or avoid interaction until treatment is administered	In order to avoid reinfection
Application	
Always read the advice leaflet before applying the treatment	In order to apply the treatment correctly; preparations may vary
Ensure that the skin is kept cool and dry	Increased absorption can occur when the skin is damp
Do not bathe before applying the cream	Hot baths can increase absorption of the cream into the bloodstream
The cream or lotion should be applied to the entire body surface area	Missing areas will prevent complete eradication
Apply particularly thoroughly to behind the ears, axillae, external genitalia, inner thighs, backs of knees and under the nails	
Always treat the face and scalp in infants, young children and the immunocompromised	The head and face are commonly affected within these groups
Avoid application around the eyes and mucous membranes	Will be an irritant
The treatment should be left *in situ* for 8–12 h or overnight	In order to allow time for the cream/lotion to penetrate the burrows and skin
Mittens should be used on the hands of thumb-sucking infants and toddlers	To avoid ingestion and removal of the treatment
Gloves should be worn when applied by an unaffected person	To avoid further cases of infection
If hands are washed during treatment, more cream should be applied	Otherwise hands will be left untreated
After the allocated time the application should be washed off with cool, plain water	
After treatment	
A normal bath should follow treatment	Mites can continue to live for 72 h following separation from skin
All clothes and any items worn next to the skin should be turned inside out and washed using a hot wash cycle; any items that cannot be laundered should be stored away for at least three days	
Additional points	
Patients should be advised that itching may continue for at least two weeks and that scabietic nodules can take several months to resolve	As mites die, they release allergen that can cause pruritus; avoid unnecessary retreatments, which can cause a contact irritant dermatitis
Antihistamines, emollients and/or topical steroid preparations can be considered	To alleviate symptoms
Observe for secondary bacterial infection	Can occur due to broken skin and scratching
Patients must be given full written and verbal instructions on treatment guidelines	In order to achieve optimal treatment and compliance
Always provide reassurance and practical and emotional support	To alleviate anxiety and minimize distress
If infestations occur within the hospital setting, involve the infection control team	To avoid further transmission

Table 177.11 Skin care after laser therapy

Action	Rationale
Immediately after laser treatment	
Any discomfort can be relieved with the use of ice packs	Laser treatment produces local heat in the skin at the point of treatment; ice cools the area and makes the skin feel more comfortable
Give the child analgesia, if needed. This is usually administered during the operation whilst under general anaesthesia	To ensure that there is no pain postoperatively
After discharge from hospital	
A moisturizing cream should be applied to the treated area at least four times daily; after laser treatment, the skin tends to be dry and may feel itchy	To prevent trauma from rubbing or scratching to the laser-treated area, which could result in scarring
Avoid soap, shampoo or bubble baths for three weeks after laser treatment	These will dry the area and may cause further scratching
No swimming in chlorinated water for three weeks	Chlorine dries the skin and may cause itching

- Propranolol treatment is usually continued until the age of around 1 year but occasionally it may need to continue for longer.
- When the decision is made to stop propranolol, our practice has been to reduce the dose by half over a two-week period, but dose reduction is not absolutely necessary.

Potential adverse effects

These must be explained to the parents/guardian before commencing propranolol therapy.

- Bradycardia
- Hypotension
- Hypoglycaemia
- Bronchospasm

- Peripheral vasoconstriction/cold/mottled extremities
- Sleep disturbance
- Gastrointestinal disturbance

Propranolol may need to be temporarily discontinued during an episode of viral-induced wheeze or chest infection, during intercurrent illness with restricted oral intake or if the infant will be undergoing procedures requiring fasting.

Care should be taken with products containing lidocaine, including Bonjela, Dentinox® and Calgel® teething gels as concurrent use of propranolol increases the risk of lidocaine toxicity. Propranolol should not be given with salbutamol or any other β2 agonists. If bronchodilation is needed, ipratropium bromide (Atrovent®) should be used.

Topical timolol for the treatment of early superficial infantile haemangiomas

A few reports have proposed the beneficial effect of topical β-blockers for the treatment of small, minimally raised infantile haemangiomas [6–10]. Topical β-blockers have been shown to be safe in treating high ocular pressure in the paediatric population. Topical β-blockers may be absorbed [4], so the amount applied must be controlled, particularly in young infants.

Treatment is with Timoptol® LA 0.5% timolol (as maleate) w/v gel-forming eye drops solution. The off-label use of this medication must be explained to the parents and information leaflet provided. The parents are instructed to apply the gel, one drop twice daily, to the surface of the haemangioma using their finger tip.

Systemic side-effects would not be expected, but care needs to be taken if used on premature babies. The same potential side-effects as for oral propranolol need to be explained to the parents beforehand.

Topical timolol is an effective treatment for small superficial infantile haemangiomas, with no significant adverse effects so far noted. However, larger randomized controlled studies are needed.

Ulcerated haemangiomas

Ulcerated haemangiomas occur most commonly in the napkin area and around the mouth. They easily become secondarily infected and can be difficult to heal. The child may be distressed, feed poorly and fail to thrive. First-line treatment is conservative daily nursing care together with β-blocker therapy if appropriate. If this fails after a period of 1–2 weeks then laser treatment should be considered.

Nursing aspects of nonulcerated and ulcerated haemangiomas are detailed in Tables 177.12 and 177.13 respectively.

References

1 **Léauté-Labrèze C, Dumas de la Roque E, Hubiche T et al. Propranolol for severe hemangiomas of infancy. N Engl J Med 2008;358(24):264951.**
2 Drolet BA, Frommelt PC, Chamlin SL et al. Initiation and use of propranolol for infantile hemangioma: report of a consensus conference. Pediatrics 2013;131(1):12840.
3 **Léauté-Labrèze C, Hoeger P, Mazereeuw-Hautier J et al. A randomized, controlled trial of oral propranolol in infantile hemangioma. N Engl J Med 2015;372(8):735–46.**
4 **Hoeger PH, Harper JI, Baselga E et al. Treatment of infantile haemangiomas: recommendations of a European expert group. Eur J Pediatr 2015;174(7):855–65.**
5 Léaute-Labrèze C, Boccara O, Degrugillier-Chopinet C et al. Safety of oral propranolol for the treatment of infantile hemangioma: a systematic review. Pediatrics 2016;138(4):ii.
6 **Léauté-Labrèze C, Harper JI, Hoeger PH. Infantile haemangioma. Lancet 2017;390(10089):85–94.**
7 **Püttgen K, Lucky A, Adams D et al. Topical timolol maleate treatment of infantile hemangiomas. Pediatrics 2016;138(3):ii.**
8 **Khan M, Boyce A, Prieto-Merino D et al. The role of topical timolol in the treatment of infantile hemangiomas: a systematic review and meta-analysis. Acta Derm Venereol 2017;97(10):1167–71.**
9 Danarti R, Ariwibowo L, Radiono S, Budiyanto A. Topical timolol maleate 0.5% for infantile hemangioma: its effectiveness compared to ultrapotent topical corticosteroids – a single-center experience of 278 cases. Dermatology 2016;232(5):566–71.
10 Weibel L, Barysch MJ, Scheer HS et al. Topical timolol for infantile hemangiomas: evidence for efficacy and degree of systemic absorption. Pediatr Dermatol 2016;33(2):184–90.

Systemic treatment

Systemic drug therapy monitoring

There has been an increase in the use of systemic drug therapy for widespread and incapacitating dermatological disease. Dermatology nurses have an important role in the monitoring of patients undergoing systemic therapy, and nurse-led monitoring clinics are a valuable and cost-effective resource. Successful monitoring is dependent on commitment, monitoring for adverse

Table 177.12 Nursing aspects of nonulcerated haemangiomas

Action	Rationale
Cut fingernails – nails need to be cut twice weekly and the edges buffed	To prevent trauma from scratching
Apply a thin layer of moisturizing ointment (such as Vaseline) over the surface of the haemangioma at least once daily	The overlying skin is often dry
Use Vaseline on the dummy (pacifier) and teat, for haemangiomas around the mouth or on the lips. Apply Vaseline around the nipple if the baby is breastfed	To lubricate and prevent any trauma to the haemangioma
Application of a tubular bandage (Tubifast) for large haemangiomas on the chest or arms, in the form of a vest or sleeve	To protect and prevent trauma from scratching or when picking up the child
If the haemangioma bleeds, apply firm pressure for 5 min without release	To stop bleeding
If bleeding persists after 5 min of pressure, reapply pressure and seek medical advice	May require surgical intervention

SECTION 40: NURSING CARE OF CUTANEOUS DISORDERS

Table 177.13 Nursing aspects of ulcerated haemangiomas

Action	Rationale
Preparation	
Assemble and prepare the following: sterile dressing pack; extra gauze swabs; nonadherent silicone dressing of appropriate size, such as Mepitel®; alginate dressing or similar, such as Sorbsan®; an oil-based cleansing solution such as Dermol 600® or similar; cotton bandage and adhesive silicone tape such as Mepitac®	
Method	
Take a wound swab for microbiology	To identify any infection
Analgesia: 30–45 min prior to dressing	Pain relief enables the dressing to be performed with least possible stress to the child
Remove any dressing already *in situ*; if it is adherent, irrigate with the cleansing solution	To clean the ulcer
Allow the haemangioma to dry naturally or use a hair dryer on a cool setting at arm's length; do not wipe or pat dry	A dry wound is less likely to become infected
Apply the Mepitel dressing to the ulcerated area; if an antibiotic or antiseptic ointment has been prescribed then this should be applied to the dressing (not directly on the ulcer) before it is put in place	Mepitel is a nonadherent perforated dressing that allows exudate to soak through
Over the Mepitel, place the Sorbsan dressing, then the gauze swabs, held in place with a bandage and Mepitac silicone tape	To provide padding and a secure dressing
Dressings should be changed once or twice daily	The frequency depends on various factors, which include infection, site and extent/depth of ulceration
Support	
Make arrangements for the dressings to be applied at home by either the parents or paediatric community nurses	It is best if the parents can apply the dressings at home, but they may need some supervision initially
Review the child weekly at first	Close monitoring needed
Give the parents/carer written information on haemangiomas, a contact telephone number and the website of any relevant family support group, such as the Birthmark Support Group in the UK	Information and support are an essential part of management

Table 177.14 Examples of drugs that require monitoring

Drug	Indication	Essential monitoring requirements
Prednisolone	Severe atopic dermatitis, bullous dermatoses, connective tissue disorders, vasculitis	BP, weight, growth, urine dipstick for glucose, baseline electrolytes, varicella antibodies
Ciclosporin	Severe atopic dermatitis, psoriasis	BP, weight, height, full blood count, urea and electrolytes, liver function tests, varicella antibodies, GFR within six months
Azathioprine	Severe atopic dermatitis/ steroid-sparing drug	Weight, thiopurine methyltransferase prior to starting, full blood count, urea and electrolytes, liver function tests including ALT, varicella antibodies
Acitretin	Severe forms of ichthyosis/other disorders of keratinization, psoriasis	Weight, height, full blood count, urea and electrolytes, liver function tests, fasting cholesterol and triglyceride, targeted X-ray investigation as required, DEXA scan yearly
Methotrexate	Psoriasis, morphoea	Weight, height, surface area, full blood count, urea and electrolytes, liver function tests including ALT, varicella antibodies
Propranolol	Haemangioma	Monitor according to recommended guidelines
Roaccutane® (isotretinoin)	Acne	Weight, height, full blood count, urea and electrolytes, liver function tests, fasting cholesterol and triglyceride Pretreatment pregnancy test if female of child-bearing age, monthly HCG and five weeks after stopping treatment
Thalidomide	Behçet disease, vasculitis	Baseline and six-monthly nerve conduction studies, effective contraception, registry
Biologics (administer according to manufacturer's guidelines)	Psoriasis	PASI/DLQ1, assessment for latent TB including chest X-ray, full blood count, urea and electrolytes, liver function tests, hepatitis B, C, HIV (in those at risk), varicella antibodies, cardiac and neurological assessments
Sulfapyridine/dapsone	Bullous dermatoses	Weight, full blood count, urea and electrolytes, liver function tests
Hydroxychloroquine	Systemic lupus erythematosus	Renal and liver function at baseline, enquire about visual impairment

ALT, alanine transaminase; BP, blood pressure; DEXA, dual-energy X-ray absorptiometry; DLQI, Dermatology Life Quality Index; GFR, glomerular filtration rate; HCG, human chorionic gonadotropin; PASI, Psoriasis Area and Severity Index.

effects, patient education and support. Examples of drugs requiring monitoring are listed in Table 177.14.

Systemic therapy should be monitored according to published guidelines or as recommended by the pharmaceutical company. What needs to be done will vary according to the specific medication and condition, but some basic principles of management are listed in Table 177.15.

Table 177.15 Basic principles of systemic drug therapy monitoring

Action	Rationale
Prior to treatment	
Carry out baseline blood tests, urinalysis and vital sign monitoring as required. Measure weight, height and calculate surface area if needed	To ensure that the child is suitable for treatment and to provide baseline data prior to treatment
Check chickenpox (varicella) status if applicable	Relevant to immunosuppressive treatments
Ensure that the patient and/or carer is fully informed about the treatment, including indication for use, side-effects, complications and monitoring required	To ensure informed consent is given to treatment
Give written information about the treatment, allow time for this to be read and allocate time for questions	To ensure patient/carer is fully informed and given sufficient time
Ensure written/verbal consent is obtained as required	To record consent for treatment
Provide a booklet for the parent/carer in order to have a written hand-held record; this should include contact telephone numbers, details of medication, i.e. name of drug, dose, frequency, mode of administration, date of commencement; monitoring required; baseline vital signs and blood tests; steroid card if applicable	To ensure appropriate monitoring is carried out and recorded
Ensure carer is competent in handling and administering medication correctly; discuss appropriate management in those who are/may become pregnant where relevant	To ensure medication is handled and administered safely
On commencement of treatment	
Ensure that GP, referring physician and any other relevant healthcare professionals are informed of treatment in writing	To initiate good communication
Ensure that processes in place for relevant monitoring to be carried out	For safe monitoring
Record blood results, urinalysis and blood pressure as applicable in patient's hand-held record	Baseline data are required to observe for any changes
Ensure that an appropriate healthcare professional is allocated to check blood results as a routine during treatment	For safe monitoring
Troubleshooting	
In event of the following: medication is vomited shortly after administration; the child has vomiting and/or diarrhoea and may not be absorbing medication; a dose is forgotten	Carers need instruction on what action to take if this occurs
If any adverse effects are noted the parent/carer should seek urgent advice from relevant healthcare professional	Reducing or stopping treatment may be necessary, but stopping abruptly may be detrimental for some medications
Follow-up	
Ensure that the family/patient has a follow-up appointment	The patient must be followed up on a regular basis
Give adequate supplies of the medication and instructions on how to obtain a repeat prescription	To continue supply
Advise parent/carer to ensure they do not run out of the medication	This may be detrimental
Advise parent/carer to bring hand-held record to all appointments	For monitoring and communication
Give practical and emotional support to the child and family	The child and family may experience high levels of anxiety
Discharge planning	
Teach the parents/carer the skin care regimen to be continued at home	To sustain recovery
Assess need for psychological support	The severity of the illness and hospitalization will have a long-term psychological impact on the child and the family

Administration of methylprednisolone

Intravenous bolus infusions of methylprednisolone are used to treat a number of severe inflammatory conditions, including connective tissue disorders, such as systemic lupus erythematosus, dermatomyositis and mixed connective tissue disease (Chapter 149); graft-versus-host disease (Chapter 157); vasculitis (Chapter 148) and morphoea (Chapter 99). It is usually used to treat the acute phase of the illness and the child is then established on maintenance treatment, the nature of which depends on the diagnosis, but often this would include oral prednisolone, at least initially.

Traditionally, methylprednisolone is given as daily infusions for three consecutive days and then repeated one week later (Table 177.16). This regimen can be varied according to clinical circumstances.

The dose used is usually 30 mg/kg or 0.5 g if the bodyweight exceeds 15 kg, given over 2 hours in 30 mL of normal saline (0.9%).

Monitoring of isotretinoin for acne

Acne is a condition that is usually associated with adolescents although it may be seen in both young children and adults. For individuals with severe acne not responding

Table 177.16 The administration of intravenous methylprednisolone

Action	Rationale
Preparation	
Ensure child and family are fully informed of reason for treatment, administration and possible side-effects	To ensure that informed consent is given to treatment and that child and family are fully prepared
Obtain baseline temperature, pulse, respiratory rate and blood pressure; discuss with medical staff if vital signs are outside the normal range	To ensure child is fit for treatment and to obtain baseline parameters in order to monitor side-effects
Record blood pressure cuff size on vital signs chart	To prevent variations in future recordings
Obtain baseline urinalysis; discuss with medical staff if any abnormalities, in particular evidence of glycosuria	Treatment can cause glycosuria
Negotiate when to commence infusion with child and family	To fit in with the child's routine
Administration	
Check dose and route of administration according to IV guidelines	In order to give treatment safely
Administer the infusion over at least 2 h	To minimize side-effects
Ensure that the child stays in bed and is occupied with quiet activities throughout the infusion	To minimize side-effects and prevent boredom/anxiety
Monitor temperature, pulse, respiratory rate and blood pressure every 15 min for the first hour and then every 30 min	To ensure early detection of changes to vital signs
Observe for side-effects such as hypotension, hypertension, tachycardia, blurred vision, flushing, sweating, headaches, metallic taste in mouth and mood changes; discuss any occurrence with medical staff	For early detection and to alleviate symptoms; to discuss action
After completion, monitor temperature, pulse, respiratory rate and blood pressure at 2 h, 4 h and then 4-hourly until next infusion	Methylprednisolone may continue to affect vital signs despite completion of infusion
Discuss any significant changes in vital signs with medical staff immediately	To discuss action
After infusion	
Check urinalysis daily and prior to discharge	To detect glycosuria
Ensure cannula is flushed with heparin 10 units/mL	To keep cannula patent
On discharge	
Ensure vital signs and urinalysis are within normal limits	To make sure that child is fit for discharge
Ensure oral prednisolone is started/restarted if prescribed	To avoid omission/confusion
Give contact numbers and procedure for parents to follow should the child become unwell at home	In case of emergency
Ensure child has follow-up clinic appointment date/admission date for next pulse	To ensure adequate follow-up/continuation of treatment

IV, intravenous.

to other conventional treatments, isotretinoin may be appropriate. Due to the potential side-effects, careful monitoring is required and this is a role where the nurse can take increasing responsibility (Table 177.17).

Intensive care

Stevens–Johnson syndrome and toxic epidermal necrolysis

Stevens–Johnson syndrome (SJS) and toxic epidermal necrolysis (TEN) are rare severe adverse reactions involving predominantly the skin and mucous membranes (see Chapter 66) [1,2]. In children, a common cause of SJS is *Mycoplasma pneumoniae* but most cases are drug induced, in particular by sulphonamides, cephalosporins, penicillins and nonsteroidal anti-inflammatory drugs. The most important aspects of care are immediate withdrawal of any suspected offending drug(s) and optimal supportive therapy. These children should be admitted to a paediatric intensive care unit and managed by a multidisciplinary team comprising ideally a paediatric intensivist, dermatologist and ophthalmologist. Details of their nursing care are summarized in Table 177.18.

Erythroderma

Erythroderma is defined as generalized skin erythema affecting at least 90% of the body. This is not specific for one diagnosis. Erythroderma without fever can be seen in a variety of dermatological conditions including psoriasis, eczema and ichthyosis [4,5]. In neonates, it can be the primary manifestation of some immune deficiencies and some metabolic conditions [5]. Erythroderma and fever may be a manifestation of a variety of illnesses, including infections, toxin-mediated diseases and drug-related reactions. Whatever the underlying cause, acute symptoms of impaired skin barrier function (hypothermia, dehydration and sepsis) must be recognized and treated adequately [6,7] (Table 177.19). This may include intravenous rehydration and antibiotic therapy. The underlying condition will also require diagnosis and management.

References

1 Ferrandiz-Pulido C, Garcia-Patos V. A review of causes of Stevens–Johnson syndrome and toxic epidermal necrolysis in children. Arch Dis Child 2013;98:998–1003.
2 Quirke KP, Beck A, Gamelli R, Mosier M. A 15-year review of pediatric toxic epidermal necrolysis. J Burn Care Res 2014;36:130–6.

Table 177.17 Monitoring of isotretinoin

Potential side-effects	Nursing implication and rationale
Teratogenicity	All sexually active females must use two forms of contraception, for example the oral contraceptive pill and barrier. A monthly pregnancy test must be performed on the unit by two members of staff. The nurse must ensure that a fresh urine specimen is obtained and that the pregnancy test is not performed by the patient themselves. The manufacture code and expiry date must be documented in the patient notes. The nurse should discuss contraception at each appointment. The patient should avoid donating blood whilst on treatment, to avoid the risk of transfusion to a pregnant female
Dry lips and mucosal membranes	Lip balm should be used frequently and regularly though the day. A moisturizing cream may be required for dry skin. A bland ointment, such as Vaseline, may be applied in and around the nostrils if nose bleeds occur
Muscle aching	Advice to reduce sports and intense exercise. Commencement of treatment may be delayed until change of sporting season. Mild analgesia usually adequate
Photosensitivity	Avoid sunbeds and sunbathing and consider delaying treatment if a holiday is imminent
Hepatotoxicity	Blood monitoring before or during the course of treatment depending on patient history and local guidelines. The nurse to counsel regarding importance of abstaining from alcohol for the duration of treatment
Mood swings and depression	Ascertain if any previous history of depression, self-harming, suicidal intent or psychiatric illness. Observe for signs of previous self-harm and general demeanour. Ensure that the parent/guardian is aware of observing mood swings. Provide contact details so that urgent advice and help may be sought. A strong warning against taking any nonprescribed or hallucinogenic drugs such as cannabis, Ecstasy, etc.
Skin fragility	Explain that skin healing is delayed for up to a year after stopping medication. Nonessential surgery should be avoided. Explain that new piercings, tattoos and waxing preferably should be avoided for a year
Hair changes	There may be temporary thinning of the hair whilst on medication and the nurse should advise against perms and tight braiding

3 **Creamer D, Walsh SA, Dziewulski LS et al. U.K. guidelines for the management of Stevens–Johnson syndrome/toxic epidermal necrolysis in adults. Br J Dermatol 2016;174:1194–227.**

4 Ott H, Hütten M, Baron J et al Neonatal and infantile erythrodermas. J Deutsch Dermatol Ges 2008;6:1070–86.

5 **Hoeger PH, Harper JI. Neonatal erythroderma: differential diagnosis and management of the 'red baby'. Arch Dis Child 1998; 79:186–91.**

6 Byer RL, Bachur RG. Clinical deterioration among patients with fever and erythroderma. Pediatrics 2006;118(116):2450–60.

7 Ott H, Grothaus J. Red, scaly baby: a pediatric dermatological emergency. Clinical and differential diagnoses of neonatal erythroderma. Hautarzt 2017;68(10):796–802.

Safeguarding issues in paediatric dermatology

Safeguarding of children is a responsibility for all professionals, especially those within the field of paediatrics. Government guidelines recognize that safeguarding and promoting the welfare of children is a shared responsibility and medical and nursing staff need to work to ensure that the child's safety is the paramount concern [1].

It is estimated that one child in 14 experiences physical abuse at some point during their childhood [2]. While there are almost 50 000 children subject to child protection plans in England alone, it is estimated that unidentified or unrecorded abuse probably accounts for eight times as many children being harmed [3]. Children under the age of 2 are more likely to present with fractures or having been shaken and the older child is more likely to present with skin manifestations of physical abuse. These may be found fortuitously while examining the skin during a dermatological consultation and the practitioner should be aware of when abuse can mimic more innocent presentations.

Bruises

Innocently acquired bruises are common in the young child and normally present on the anterior surfaces over bony prominences. Bruising to the forehead is regularly seen in young children pulling themselves to stand. However, bruising in nonindependently mobile infants is rarely seen and of considerable concern. It is recognized that bruising in noncruising infants is rare and likely to be an indicator of physical abuse. Maguire (2010) identified that abusive bruising is often found on the head and neck, while bruising on the trunk and upper limbs may indicate that the child has tried to defend themselves from blows [4].

Mongolian blue spots are often confused with bruising and it is important that such innocent lesions are documented within the child's care records. When concerns are identified regarding the diagnosis of such bruise-like appearances, clinical photographs should be taken. The child may then be reexamined a week later. Bruises are likely to have disappeared or changed significantly in that time while Mongolian blue spots will still be present (Table 177.20). If bruises are observed, local guidelines for safeguarding children should be observed and a referral made to Social Services.

Cigarette burns

Cigarette burns are inflicted injuries that result in annular scars. They often produce crater-like scars as the centre of the cigarette is the hottest area and results in a deeper burn.

As cigarette burns heal, they may develop secondary crusting that may be confused with impetigo (Table 177.21). Impetigo will result in golden crusted lesions but these will vary in size and appearance.

Table 177.18 Nursing care of toxic epidermal necrolysis/Stevens–Johnson syndrome

Action	Rationale
Observe respiratory effort, rate, skin and mucosal colour and vital signs, including oxygen saturation	Oxygen and mechanical ventilation required by many children
Monitor temperature	Skin temperature control unreliable due to extensive skin loss; at risk of hypothermia due to excessive heat loss
Nurse in cubicle controlled for humidity with ambient temperature raised to between 25 and 28 °C	At room temperature energy expenditure increases; a raised ambient temperature leads to reduced energy consumption and associated metabolic stress
Barrier nurse	Prone to infection due to loss of epidermis
Circulation	
Fluid resuscitation if clinically indicated and daily review of requirements linked to overall condition Daily weight Careful monitoring of fluid balance	Extensive epidermal detachment results in large insensible transcutaneous fluid losses usually compounded by reduced oral intake due to disease involvement of the mouth
Administer IV replacement fluid as prescribed	To correct these fluid, electrolyte and protein losses and prevent dehydration, shock and end-organ hypoperfusion
Monitor urinary and bowel output carefully	To aid in monitoring fluid balance
Consider urinary catheter for dysuria and/or urinary retention with urogenital involvement	To reduce pain on micturition, maintain patency of urethra, restore and enable accurate measurement of output
Skin care	
Assess skin and record	To assess extent of condition and monitor progress
Regularly cleanse all the skin, at least daily, with warmed sterile water, saline or an antimicrobial agent	To clean the skin
Apply a greasy emollient, e.g. 50:50 white soft paraffin and liquid paraffin, over the whole skin, including the denuded areas	To protect these areas and reduce fluid loss
Apply a topical antimicrobial agent to potentially infected areas on microbiological advice	This acts as biological dressing
Decompose blisters by piercing and expressing tissue fluid. Leave detached lesional epidermis *in situ*	
Apply nonadherent dressings to denuded dermis; suitable dressings include Mepitel (Mölnlycke Health Care) or Telfa® (Covidien)	For comfort, to promote healing and to protect denuded areas from infection and further trauma
Secondary foam or burn dressing should be used to collect exudate (suitable dressings include Exu-Dry® (Smith and Nephew)	
Secure with Tubegauz suit if necessary.	To keep dressings *in situ*
Clinical deterioration with extension of epidermal detachment, subepidermal pus, local sepsis, delayed healing may require supplementation of conservative approach with surgical approach	Conservative management insufficient
Site intravenous lines through nonlesional skin where possible	Avoid further trauma
Secure cannula with nonadhesive tape/dressing and bandage well	Adhesive tapes/Band-Aid plasters will cause further trauma
Nurse on a pressure-relieving mattress, monitor pressure areas	
Administer passive exercises	Prevent development of contractures
Minimize shearing forces when moving child	Fragile skin liable to peel away to leave areas of denuded skin
Early intervention from ophthalmology and daily ophthalmology review. The ophthalmologist needs to carry out daily eye hygiene to remove inflammatory debris and remove any conjunctival adhesions	Ocular sequelae are one of most prevalent long-term complications, which include corneal and conjunctival scarring and dry eyes
Two-hourly ocular surface lubrication, e.g. nonpreserved carmellose eye drops and conjunctival hygiene in the acute period	To reduce the risk of ulceration and infection
Administration of topical antibiotic therapy as either prophylaxis or treatment of corneal infection	May reduce ocular surface damage but may mask the signs of corneal infection
Topical corticosteroid drops, e.g. nonpreserved dexamethasone 0.1% if prescribed	
Avoid use of cotton buds or glass rods	Potentially cause damage
Administration of topical local anaesthetic prior to cleaning	Painful procedure
Mouth: daily examination after initial assessment, especially if limited oral intake and in the presence of mucosal and lip involvement: two-hourly application of white soft paraffin ointment to the lips and clean the mouth with warm saline mouthwashes with oral sponges. Anti-inflammatory and antibacterial rinses may be indicated	Oral involvement is a frequent problem; tongue and palate frequently affected, painful mucosal erythema with subsequent blistering and ulceration and can have long-term issues with scarring and restricted mouth opening and difficulty speaking and swallowing [3]
Infection	
Monitor temperature	For prompt detection of infection
Change peripheral venous cannulas every 48 h	Reduce risk of sepsis

(Continued)

SECTION 40: NURSING CARE OF CUTANEOUS DISORDERS

Table 177.18 *Continued*

Action	Rationale
Nutrition regimen	
Nutritional support with increased energy requirement Involve dietitian early	Conditions characterized by increased metabolic response with increased energy expenditure. In extensive epidermal detachment, there is a loss of large amounts of albumin and protein from blister fluid
Nasogastric feeding through silicone tube	Condition of mouth often precludes normal oral intake and plastic tubes may lead to further trauma [3]
Secure nasogastric tube with tubular bandage or nonadhesive tape	To prevent pain and damage to skin
Analgesia	
Daily assessment of pain using appropriate paediatric tool	To ensure that the child is pain free and comfortable at rest; extensive skin loss causes high levels of pain that may be difficult to control with oral analgesics alone
Supplementary opiates are often needed. May require additional doses prior to dressing changes, handling or repositioning	
Parents/carers	
Give practical and emotional support to the child and family Encourage family to help with care where possible	The child and family may experience high levels of distress
Discharge planning	
Teach parents/carer the skin care regimen to be continued at home	Ongoing skin and eye care will be required
Ensure ophthalmology, dermatology and paediatric follow-up is organized	To monitor for ophthalmic and other complications long term, as many children suffer long-term sequelae
Assess the need for ongoing psychological support	The severity of the illness and hospitalization will have a long-term psychological impact on the child and the family
Give family written information about drug(s) to avoid Encourage older children to wear Medic-Alert bracelet Document drug allergy in patient's written and electronic notes and inform all doctors involved in the child's care Report episode to national pharmacovigilance authority *Diagnostic testing*: not recommended routinely but could be considered if the culprit is unknown or where medication avoidance is detrimental to the child	Ensure child is not exposed to responsible drug again if identified

Table 177.19 Nursing care of erythroderma

Action	Rationale
Babies should be nursed in an incubator Older children should be nursed in a cubicle controlled for humidity with ambient temperature raised to between 25 and 28 °C Monitor vital signs	Skin temperature control unreliable due to vasodilation and impaired skin barrier function; at risk of hypothermia due to excessive heat loss
Monitor fluid balance with careful recording of input and output Administer prescribed intravenous fluids and oral intake as tolerated, to meet requirements Monitor electrolytes	Risk of hypernatraemic dehydration due to impaired skin barrier and increased transepidermal water loss
Apply ointment-based emollients liberally and repeatedly to all areas	Hydrate and soften the skin, making it more supple, reducing pain and also reducing fluid and heat loss

Table 177.20 Mongolian blue spots compared to bruises

Mongolian blue spots	Bruises
Slate grey macules	Blue/purple changing to green and yellow
Typically on lumbosacral area but may extend to wrist and ankle.	Can be anywhere – normal bruising in toddlers on anterior surfaces and bony prominences
No tenderness or discomfort	Area may be painful or tender
Consistent in appearance from day to day – resolve over many months	Change considerably on a daily basis and usually resolve within a few weeks

Table 177.21 Cigarette burns compared to impetigo

Cigarette burns	Impetigo
Annular crater-like lesions approximately 7 mm in diameter Clear history must be taken Clinical photographs Application of greasy emollient will help reduce development of scab	Golden crusted lesions that develop spontaneously over a few days Swabs should be taken to confirm diagnosis Crusted lesions should be softened with an emollient and washed off before administration/application of topical antibiotic

If impetigo is suspected, swabs should be taken to confirm the presence of *Staphylococcus aureus* but it must be recognized that healing cigarette burns may also be colonized with *Staphylococcus aureus*.

Human bites

Human bites result in paired crescent-shaped bruises. Clinical photographs must be taken and a clear history obtained. The size of the bite imprint may indicate the age of the perpetrator. Young children often bite each other as a sign of frustration and anger but bites from primary teeth are easily recognized from the size of the intercanine distance.

Perineal warts

Most perineal warts in young children are acquired innocently, especially if one of the parents has warts on their hands. However, there is a risk that genital warts in children may be an indication of child sexual abuse. If there is any suspicion, the family should be referred to Social Services so that further investigations may be undertaken.

The role of the nurse in safeguarding examinations

When a referral is made to Social Services, they would then instigate a review by a designated medical practitioner. Such consultations can take place in outpatients or on the ward, if the child presents with severe injuries. The child will need accurate measurements of height, weight and head circumference, especially if neglect is suspected.

The nurse is an essential part of the team (Table 177.22) and should always be aware that the priority is the child. One element of the nurse's role is to be a chaperone while any examination is being undertaken. The nurse should also be an impartial and nonjudgemental witness of the consultation. Observations of the parental interactions with both the child and any other family member may be invaluable.

It is essential that an explanation is given to the child of all procedures, in terms appropriate to the age and development of the child, who is likely to be wary of adults. If sexual abuse is suspected, intimate examination is required, often with swabs and colposcopy, and the nurse should help calm the child's fears while ensuring that the examination is as rapid, dignified and pain free as possible. Blood samples may be required to ensure that there is no underlying medical or haematological condition that could confuse the diagnosis.

Table 177.22 The role of the nurse in safeguarding examinations

Action	Rationale
Provide correct documentation Observe the consultation Obtain blood samples and swabs as required Contact colleagues from medical illustration Provide explanations of procedures to parents/carers and child	Correct procedures must be carried out during a safeguarding investigation to prevent accusation of abuse or being challenged on technicalities Provide impartial opinion regarding the family dynamics and relationship between child and parent/carers Pathological samples help confirm or dismiss concerns and exclude any underlying medical condition Photographic evidence is crucial, especially for physical manifestations of abuse when the appearance of an injury may be transient Many referrals to Social Services automatically result in examination by a medical officer. Colposcopy, swabs, physical examination, bone scans and blood tests are undertaken routinely as indicated but may cause considerable anxiety

References

1 HM Government. Working Together to Safeguard Children. A Guide to Inter-Agency Working to Safeguard and Promote the Welfare of Children. Nottingham: Department for Education, 2010.
2 NSPCC. Preventing Child Abuse and Neglect. Available at: www.nspcc.org.uk/preventing-abuse/child-abuse-and-neglect/
3 NSPCC. Statistics on Child Abuse. Available at: https://learning.nspcc.org.uk/statistics-child-abuse/
4 Maguire S. Which injuries may indicate child abuse? Arch Dis Child Educ Pract 2010;95:170–7.

Conclusion

Nurses play a vital role in the management of children with skin disease. This is particularly relevant to those with more severe disease requiring either admission to hospital or regular outpatient attendance. The scope of involvement in patient care of the clinical nurse specialist continues to develop; in the UK, the clinical nurse specialist role now includes nurse-led clinics and nurse prescribing and is recognized as an expert nursing resource. The British Dermatological Nursing Group (BDNG) is an affiliated group of the British Association of Dermatologists and is at the forefront of dermatological nursing development, encompassing research and evidence-based practice.

Index

Note: Page numbers in *italics* refer to figures, those in **bold** refer to tables and boxes.

AA *see* alopecia areata
AAV *see* adeno-associated virus
abacavir hypersensitivity, HIV infection 653
abdominal trauma, child abuse and neglect (CAN) 2229
ablative lasers, laser therapy 2326–2327
abscesses
  oral mucosa 2094, *2095*
  tuberculous metastatic abscess 489–490, *491*
absorption, percutaneous *see* percutaneous absorption
abuse *see* child abuse and neglect; child sexual abuse
abusive head trauma (AHT) 2227–2229
  diagnosis 2227–2228
  diagnostic evaluation 2228
  differential diagnosis 2228
  evidence 2228
  outcome 2228–2229
  pathophysiology and timing 2228
  symptoms and findings 2228
ACA *see* acrodermatitis chronica atrophicans
acanthamoeba infection, HIV infection 653
acantholytic EB due to desmoplakin deficiency 917
acantholytic EB due to plakoglobin deficiency 917
acanthosis nigricans (AN) 844–846
  aetiology 845–846
  clinical features 845
  diabetes mellitus 2005, *2006*
  diagnosis 845
  differential diagnosis 845
  epidemiology 845
  histopathology 845
  management 846
  metabolic syndrome (MetS) 844–846
  pathogenesis 845–846
  prevalence 845
ACC *see* aplasia cutis congenita
accessory tragi 103
  aetiology 103
  clinical features 103
  pathology 103
  treatment 103
ACD *see* allergic contact dermatitis; amyloidosis cutis dyschromica
α-N-acetylgalactosaminidase deficiency 1974
  clinical features 1974
  definition 1974
  differential diagnosis 1974
  history 1974
  pathogenesis 1974
  prognosis 1974
  treatment 1974
aciclovir
  antiviral agents 2286
  erythema multiforme (EM) 783
  herpes simplex virus (HSV) infections 605–607
aciclovir-resistant herpes simplex infection, oral mucosa 2083
acitretin, systemic therapies 2291
Ackerman syndrome **1631**
acne 803–819
  acne infantum (infantile acne) **135**, 814–815
  acrocephalosyndactyly 816–817
  apert syndrome 816–817
  autoinflammatory disorders with acne 816
  cutaneous microbiome 52
  drug-induced acneiform eruptions 817, **818**
  gram-negative folliculitis 817
  infantile acne (acne infantum) **135**, 814–815
  inflammatory acne, differential diagnosis **819**
  neonatal acne, differential diagnosis **819**
  paediatric differential diagnosis 819
  PAPA (pyogenic arthritis, pyoderma gangrenosum and acne) 816
  PASH (pyoderma gangrenosum, acne and suppurative hidradenitis) 816
  SAPHO (synovitis, acne, pustulosis, hyperostosis and osteitis), 816
acne conglobata 807, *808*
acne excoriée de la jeune fille (excoriated acne) 819
  superficial self-mutilation 2270
acne fulminans 816
acneiform eruption induced by epidermal growth factor receptor inhibitors 818
acne in endocrine abnormalities associated with insulin resistance 815
  androgens abuse 815
  hyperandrogenism, insulin resistance and acanthosis nigricans (HAIR-AN) syndrome 815
  polycystic ovary syndrome (PCOS) 815
acne infantum (infantile acne) **135**, 814–815
acne inversa *see* hidradenitis suppurativa (HS)
acne mechanica 817
acne neonatorum 814
Acne QoL Index 2250
acne scars, laser therapy 2324
acne variants 814–819
acne vermoulante *see* atrophoderma vermiculata
acne vulgaris 803–812
  acne conglobata 807, *808*
  Acne QoL Index 2250
  aetiology 804–805
  antiandrogens 811
  Assessments of the Psychological and Social Effects of Acne (APSEA) 2250
  azelaic acid 809
  benzoyl peroxide 808–809
  burden of disease 2256–2257
  Cardiff Acne Disability Index (CADI) 2248–2250
  clinical features 806–807

acne vulgaris (*cont'd*)
combined oral contraceptives (COC) 811
comedogenesis 805
comedonal acne 806–807, **819**
corticosteroids 811
dapsone (diaminodiphenylsulfone) 809
definition 803
dietary interventions 811
doxycycline 809
epidemiology 803–804
follicular hyperkeratinization 805
genetics 804
hormonal agents 811
hormonal influences 804–805
inflammation 804–805
inflammatory lesions 806
isotretinoin 2408–2409, **2410**
isotretinoin, systemic 809–810
macrolides 809
matrix metalloproteinases (MMPs) 805
minocycline 809
noninflammatory (comedonal) lesions 805–806
oral antibiotics: overview 809
oral isotretinoin 809–810
oral treatments 809–811
papulopustular acne 807
pathogenesis 804–805
pathology 805–806
physical approaches 811–812
postinflammatory lesions 806
prognosis 807
Propionibacterium acnes 805
suicide/suicide ideation, isoretinoin-induced 810
tetracyclines 809
topical antibiotics 809
topical retinoids 808
topical therapy 808–809
treatment 807–812
acquired cutis laxa 1135–1136
acquired generalized hypertrichosis (drug related) 2133
acquired generalized lipoatrophy (AGL) 1224–1225
acquired hypopigmentation *1493*, 1496–1498
acquired lesions, tongue 2100
acquired lipodystrophies 1224–1225
acquired localized hypertrichosis 2135
acquired localized unruly hair 2122
acquired melanocytic naevi (AMN) 1252–1255, 2365–2368
see also congenital melanocytic naevi (CMN)
associations 1253–1254
blue naevi 1254
clinical features 1253
dermoscopic patterns 2365–2368
epidemiology 1252–1253
histopathology 1254
management 1254
naevus spilus 1255
natural history 1253
pathogenesis 1252–1253
surgical therapy 2312
acquired neonatal infections, neonates 86–91
acquired protein C or S deficiency caused by drugs or specific diseases, purpura fulminans 1896
acral peeling skin syndrome 916
acral vasospasm, systemic sclerosis (SSc) **1184**, 1188
acrocyanosis, transient skin disorders in neonates and young infants 76
acrodermatitis chronica atrophicans (ACA), lyme borreliosis (LB)/lyme disease 467–468
acrodermatitis enteropathica 1981–1982
aetiology 1981
clinical features 1981–1982
definition 1981
differential diagnosis 1982
napkin dermatitis 277
pathophysiology 1981
prognosis 1982
treatment 1982
acro-dermato-ungual-lacrimal- tooth syndrome (ADULT syndrome) **1632**
ectodermal dysplasias (EDs) 1682
acrokeratoelastoidosis *see* marginal papular keratoderma
acrometageria 1731–1732
clinical features 1732
differential diagnosis 1732
epidemiology 1732
histology findings 1732
history 1731–1732
laboratory findings 1732
pathogenesis 1732
treatment 1732
acropustulosis of infancy **135**
acrorenal field defect, ectodermal dysplasia, lipoatrophic diabetes (AREDYLD) syndrome **1631**
actinic lichen planus (ALP) 395
actinic prurigo (AP) 947–949
clinical features 947–948
differential diagnosis 948
epidemiology 947
histology findings 948
history 947
key features **947**
laboratory findings 948
pathogenesis 947
prevention 948
treatment 948
actinomycetoma 563–564
clinical features 563–564
differential diagnosis 563–564
epidemiology 563
histology findings 564
laboratory findings 564
pathogenesis 563
prevention 564
treatment 564
actinomycosis 574–575
clinical features 574
differential diagnosis 574
epidemiology 574
histology findings 574
laboratory findings 574–575
pathogenesis 574
prevention 575
treatment 575
acute, eruptive lichen planus 396
acute erythematous atrophic candidosis 547
acute generalized exanthematous pustulosis (AGEP), hypersensitivity reactions to drugs 792–793
acute haemorrhagic oedema of infancy (AHEI) 1870–1872
cf. Henoch-Schonlein purpura (HSP) **1871**
clinical features 1870–1871
differential diagnosis 1871
epidemiology 1870
histology 1871
history 1870
laboratory findings 1871
pathogenesis 1870
prognosis 1872
treatment 1872
acute infectious purpura fulminans 1892–1895, 1900–1901
acute inflammation at the site of prior bacillus Calmette–Guerin (BCG) vaccination, Kawasaki disease (KD) 1911
acute intermittent porphyria **959**, **960**, 965, **967**
acute leukaemia, oral mucosa 2097
acute lymphoblastic leukaemia (ALL) 1063–1066
clinical features 1064–1066
dermatological manifestations 1063
differential diagnosis 1064–1066
differential diagnosis of inflicted bruises *2225*
epidemiology 1063–1064
histology findings 1066
laboratory findings 1066
pathogenesis 1063–1064
prevention 1066
treatment 1066
acute myeloid leukaemia (AML) 1063–1066
clinical features 1064–1066
dermatological manifestations 1063
differential diagnosis 1064–1066
epidemiology 1063–1064
histology findings 1066
laboratory findings 1066
pathogenesis 1063–1064
prevention 1066
treatment 1066
acute nonallergic urticaria 757
acute nonpurulent cervical adenopathy, Kawasaki disease (KD) 1910–1911
acute paronychia, nail disorders 2149–2150
acute porphyric attack 960
acute pseudomembranous candidosis (thrush) 546–547
oral mucosa 2089
acute rheumatic fever (ARF), erythema marginatum **768**
acute scrotal oedema 2191

acute spontaneous urticaria 754, 757, **758**, 759–760
acute ulcerative gingivitis (AUG), oral mucosa 2085
AD *see* atopic dermatitis
ADA2 *see* adenosine deaminase 2
adalimumab, psoriasis 372–373
Adams–Oliver syndrome 1418
ADCL *see* anergic diffuse cutaneous leishmaniasis; autosomal dominant cutis laxa
Addison disease, oral mucosa 2093
Addison syndrome *see* adrenal insufficiency
adeno-associated virus (AAV), genetic therapies 2303
adenosine deaminase 2 (ADA2), deficiency 2022
Aden ulcer *see* tropical skin ulcer
adherence 2352–2354
  adherence rates 2352–2353
  approach to the paediatric patient 2352–2354
  factors affecting adherence 2353–2354
adhesiotherapy (occlusotherapy), human papillomaviruses (HPV) 594
adhesive tape damage, iatrogenic disorders of the newborn 163
adjuvant therapy, hidradenitis suppurativa (HS) (acne inversa) 827–828
adnexal disorders 1325–1337
  inflammatory diseases 1325–1328
  tumours 1329–1337
adnexal polyp, transient skin disorders in neonates and young infants 81
adolescents
  adolescent development 2348
  approach to the patient 2347–2351
  changes of adolescence **2348**
  chronic illness or disfigurement during adolescence 2350–2351
  confidentiality and consent 2350
  consultation 2348
  HEADSS assessment 2348–2349
  striae 1172
adolescent seborrhoeic dermatitis (SD) 279–284
  clinical features 280–281
  differential diagnosis 281–282
  epidemiology 279–280
  histological findings 282
  history 279
  Malassezia spp. (*Pityrosporum* spp.) 280–281, 284
  pathogenesis 280
  prevention 282–284
  treatment 282–284
adrenal insufficiency 1997–1998
  clinical features 1997
  cutaneous manifestations 1997–1998
  histology findings 1997
  laboratory findings 1997
  pathogenesis 1997
  prevention 1998
  treatment 1998
ADULT syndrome *see* acro-dermato-ungual-lacrimal- tooth syndrome
adult T-cell leukaemia/lymphoma 1049
adverse drug reactions (ADR)
  see also hypersensitivity reactions to drugs
  definition 785
  epidemiology 785
  neonatal erythroderma 129–130
  vesiculobullous lesions 866
adverse effects
  laser therapy 2321
  local anaesthetics 2332
  propranolol 2405–2406
  sunscreens 978
AEC syndrome (Hay–Wells syndrome)
  clinical features 1678–1681
  craniofacial features 1681
  definition 1678
  differential diagnosis 1681
  ectodermal dysplasias (EDs) 1678–1681
  ectodermal structures 1680–1681
  hair features 1678–1679
  history 1678
  nails features 1679–1680
  pathology 1678
  prognosis 1681
  skin features 1680
  sweat glands features 1680
  teeth features 1679
  treatment 1681
AEI *see* annular epidermolytic ichthyosis
AGA *see* androgenetic alopecia
AGEP *see* acute generalized exanthematous pustulosis
AGL *see* acquired generalized lipoatrophy
AGS *see* Aicardi–Goutiéres syndrome
AHEI *see* acute haemorrhagic oedema of infancy
AHO *see* Albright hereditary osteodystrophy
AHT *see* abusive head trauma
AIBDs *see* autoimmune blistering diseases
Aicardi–Goutiéres syndrome (AGS) 2021–2022
AIDs *see* autoinflammatory diseases
airborne allergens and pollution, atopic dermatitis (AD) 260
airway haemangiomas, infantile haemangiomas (IH) 1430
AISLE *see* autoinflammatory syndrome with lymphoedema
albendazole, antiparasitic drugs 2287
albinism 1486–1490
  associated genes **1487**
  Chédiak–Higashi syndrome 1489–1490
  Cross syndrome 1490
  Griscelli–Pruniéras syndromes 1490
  Hermansky–Pudlak syndrome 1489
  oculocutaneous albinism (OCA) 1486–1489, **1803**
Albright hereditary osteodystrophy (AHO) 1347–1348
  clinical features 1348
  differential diagnosis 1348
  epidemiology 1348
  laboratory studies 1348
  pathogenesis 1348
  treatment 1348
Albright syndrome, oral mucosa 2093
alefacept, atopic dermatitis (AD) 260
ALHE *see* angiolymphoid hyperplasia with eosinophilia
alkaptonuria 1969–1970
  clinical features 1969
  definition 1969
  differential diagnosis 1969
  history 1969
  pathogenesis 1969
  prognosis 1969
  treatment 1970
ALL *see* acute lymphoblastic leukaemia
allelic disease: Haim–Munk syndrome (HMS) *see* palmoplantar keratoderma with periodontitis
allergens, allergic contact dermatitis (ACD) 306–310
allergen testing and immunotherapy, insects/insect bites 737
allergic complications, meningococcal disease 444
allergic contact dermatitis (ACD) 300–312
  allergens 306–310
  clinical features 303
  emerging concepts 311–312
  epidemiology 300–302
  patch testing in children 304–306
  pathogenesis 302–303
  primary interventions 310–311
  review of 2010–2015 paediatric patch test studies 300, **301**
allergic contact napkin dermatitis 267–268, 270
allergic gingivostomatitis, oral mucosa 2093
allergy
  atopic dermatitis (AD) 256, 260–261
  contact allergy 256
allopurinol, leishmaniasis 699
allylamines, dermatophytoses 541
alopecia
  androgenetic alopecia (AGA) 2128–2129
  focal scarring alopecia 2129–2130
  focal scarring and nonscarring causes of alopecia 2129–2131
  follicular hyperkeratosis with scalp alopecia **2109–2110**
  odontoonychodysplasia with alopecia 2111
  triangular alopecia 2131
  universal alopecia 2108
alopecia, keratosis pilaris, cataracts and psoriasis **2109**
alopecia–anosmia– deafness–hypogonadism syndrome **1632**
alopecia areata (AA) 2106, 2107, 2111, 2139–2145
  anthralin (cignolin, dithranol) 2144
  antibodies and biologics 2145
  associations 2142
  clinical features 2140–2141
  differential diagnosis 2142

alopecia areata (AA) (*cont'd*)
disease activation by loss of immune privilege 2140
epidemiology 2139
genetics 2139–2140
hair loss 2111
hair prostheses 2145
histology findings 2141–2142
janus kinase (JAK) inhibitors 2145
methotrexate (MTX) 2144–2145
minoxidil 2144
outlook on future treatment options 2145
pathogenesis 2140
phosphodiesterase inhibitor 4 (PDE4, apremilast) 2145
psoralen plus ultraviolet A 2144
systemic corticosteroids 2143
tacrolimus 2144
topical corticosteroids (TCS) 2142–2143
topical immunotherapy 2143–2144
treatment 2142–2145
alopecia–onychodysplasia–hypohidrosis **1632**
alopecia–onychodysplasia–hypohidrosis–deafness **1632**
alopecia universalis congenita *see* atrichia with papular lesions
alopecia universalis congenita (ALUNC; generalized atrichia) **1633**
alopecia universalis–onychodystrophy–total vitiligo **1633**
ALP *see* actinic lichen planus
alternative therapies, pediculosis 729
alveolar soft part sarcoma (ASPS) 1391
aetiology 1391
clinical features 1391
definition 1391
differential diagnosis 1391
epidemiology 1391
pathogenesis 1391
pathology 1391
treatment 1391
amalgam and graphite tattoos, oral mucosa 2091
AmB *see* amphotericin B
amelo onycho hypohidrotic dysplasia **1633**
amenamevir, herpes simplex virus (HSV) infections 607
American histoplasmosis 565–567
aminoacidopathies 1967–1970
δ-aminolaevulinic acid dehydratase deficiency porphyria **959**, **960**, 966
AML *see* acute myeloid leukaemia
AMN *see* acquired melanocytic naevi
amniocentesis, iatrogenic disorders of the newborn 156
amnion rupture sequence *see* amniotic constriction band
amniotic constriction band (amnion rupture sequence) 118–119
aetiology 118
clinical features 119
definition 118
differential diagnosis 119
treatment 119
amphotericin B (AmB), antifungal therapy 2286
amphotericin B deoxycholate, leishmaniasis 699
amplification-refractory mutation system (ARMS), molecular genetics 45
amyloidosis 2023–2026
aetiology 2023–2024
classification **2023**
clinical features 2024–2026
cutaneous amyloidosis 2024–2025
definition 2023
differential diagnosis 2026
familial primary cutaneous localized amyloidosis 1470
hyperpigmentation 1466, 1470
pathology 2024
primary localized cutaneous amyloidosis 2024–2025
prognosis 2026
secondary cutaneous amyloidosis **2024**, 2025
systemic amyloidosis 2025–2026
treatment 2026
amyloidosis cutis dyschromica (ACD) 1507–1509
differential diagnosis 1508–1509
epidemiology 1507
histopathology 1509
history 1507
pathogenesis 1507–1508
treatment 1510
AN *see* acanthosis nigricans
anaemia
see also Fanconi anaemia
dystrophic epidermolysis bullosa (DEB) 922, 931
parvovirus B19 665
anaesthesia 2330–2340
see also sedation
barbiturates 2337
benzodiazepines 2337
chloral hydrate 2337–2338
dexmedetomidine 2337
dystrophic epidermolysis bullosa (DEB) 930–931
general gas anaesthesia 2338–2339
hypnosis 2340
impact of anaesthesia safety data in dermatology paediatric surgery 2339
iontophoresis devices 2334
ketamine 2337
laryngeal masks 2339
laser therapy 2319–2320
local anaesthetics 2331–2332
needle-free injection devices 2334
nitrous oxide (N2O) 2338
opiates 2337
pain perception 2330
perioperative analgesics 2335
pharmacological agents 2336–2339
propofol 2338
risks of general anaesthesia in infants and young children 2321
sedation 2335–2336
subcutaneous infusion anaesthesia 2334
surgical therapy 2311
techniques to decrease the pain of injection 2332–2334
topical anaesthetics 2332–2334
anagen effluvium, hair loss 2124–2125
anagen loss, hair loss 2124–2126
anatomical abnormalities, genital disease 2184–2187
androgenetic alopecia (AGA) 2128–2129
androgen excess 2000–2001
clinical features 2000
congenital adrenal hyperplasia 2000–2001
cutaneous manifestations 2000–2001
histology findings 2000
laboratory findings 2000
pathogenesis 2000
polycystic ovary syndrome (PCOS) 2001
prevention 2000–2001
treatment 2000–2001
anemones/corals (Anthozoa) 741
anergic diffuse cutaneous leishmaniasis (ADCL) 695, 697–698
anetoderma 1151–1155
aetiology 1152–1153
anetoderma of prematurity 1153
autoimmune disorders 1153
classification **1152**
clinical features 1153–1154
definition 1151
differential diagnosis 1154, 1715
histopathology 1154
history 1151
infections 1152–1153
localized dermatoses 1153
postinflammatory elastolysis and cutis laxa 1155
primary anetoderma 1152
secondary anetoderma 1152
treatment 1155
'angel kiss,' transient skin disorders in neonates and young infants 75
angioedema
hypersensitivity reactions to drugs 787
urticaria 751, 752, *753*, 754–755, **758**, 787
vibratory urticaria (angioedema) 759
angiofibromas in tuberous sclerosis, laser therapy 2323–2324
angiokeratomas 1417
Fabry disease 1974–1975, *1976*
angiolipoma
characteristics **1196**
histological features **1196**
angiolymphoid hyperplasia with eosinophilia (ALHE) 1350–1353
cf. Kimura disease 1351–1352
clinical features 1351
definition 1350
dermoscopic features 1352
differential diagnosis 1351–1352
epidemiology 1350
histology findings 1352–1353

history 1350
laboratory tests 1352
pathogenesis 1350–1351
prognosis 1353
radiological examination 1352
treatment 1353
angioma serpiginosum with oesophageal papillomatosis, differential diagnosis 1715
angioma serpigiosum, laser therapy 2323
angiosarcoma 1388, 1448
aetiology 1388
clinical features 1388
definition 1388
differential diagnosis 1388
epidemiology 1388
pathogenesis 1388
pathology 1388
treatment 1388
angora hair naevus 1266
angular stomatitis, oral mucosa 2090
animal mites, pseudoscabies 720
ankyloblepharon–ectodermal defects–cleft lip and palate (AEC) syndrome **1633**
ankyloglossia 2099
annular epidermolytic ichthyosis (AEI) 1570
annular erythema of infancy **765**, 769–770
clinical features 769
epidemiology 769
history 769
laboratory findings 769–770
pathogenesis 769
pathology 769–770
treatment 770
annular erythemas 764–770
annular erythema of infancy **765**, 769–770
erythema annulare centrifugum 764–766
erythema gyratum repens **765**, 767
erythema marginatum **765**, 767–768
erythema migrans **765**, 769
annular psoriasis 356
anogenital findings, child sexual abuse (CSA) 2232–2235
anogenital granulomatosis, genital signs of systemic disease 2192
anogenital warts: condylomas, human papillomaviruses (HPV) 593
anonychia/micronychia, nail disorders 2155
anonychia–onychodystrophy with brachydactyly type b and ectrodactyly **1633**
anonychia with flexural pigmentation **1633**
Anoplura 734
see also pediculosis
anorexia nervosa/bulimia 839
antenatal procedures, iatrogenic disorders of the newborn 156–157
anthralin (cignolin, dithranol)
alopecia areata (AA) 2144
psoriasis 369–370, *373*
antiandrogens, acne vulgaris 811
antibiotic resistance, pseudomonal skin disease 448
antibiotics
see also topical antibiotics
hidradenitis suppurativa (HS) (acne inversa) 828
lyme borreliosis (LB)/lyme disease 470, **471**
systemic therapies 2282–2285
antibodies and biologics, alopecia areata (AA) 2145
antibodies in patients with juvenile dermatomyositis **1949**
antibody (humoral) deficiencies, immunocompromised children 686
antifungal therapy 2285–2286
see also fungal infections
amphotericin B (AmB) 2286
griseofulvin 2285–2286
itraconazole 2286
systemic therapies 2285–2286
terbinafine 2285
antihistamines 2288–2289
dermatitis herpetiformis (DH) 904
H_1 antihistamines 2288–2289
H_2 antihistamines 2289
systemic therapies 2288–2289
antimalarial agents
chloroquine 2289
hydroxychloroquine 2289
systemic therapies 2289
antimicrobial agents, orofacial granulomatosis (OFG) 1020
antineutrophil cytoplasmic antibody (ANCA)-associated vasculitides (AAV) 1882–1883
eosinophilic granulomatosis with polyangiitis (EGPA) 1883
granulomatosis with polyangiitis (GPA) 1882, 1924–1930
histology findings 1928–1929
laboratory findings 1928–1929
microscopic polyangiitis (MPA) 1882–1883
pathogenesis 1925
prognosis 1930
antiparasitic drugs
albendazole 2287
ivermectin 2287
systemic therapies 2287
α1-antitrypsin deficiency 1218–1219
clinical features 1218–1219
epidemiology 1218
histopathology 1219
pathogenesis 1218
treatment 1219
antitubercular therapy (ATT), cutaneous tuberculosis 495
antiviral agents
aciclovir 2286
famciclovir 2287
molluscum contagiosum (MC) 585
systemic therapies 2286–2287
valaciclovir 2286–2287
antiviral chemotherapy, herpes simplex virus (HSV) infections 605–607
ants (formicidae) 736–737
AP *see* actinic prurigo
APECED syndrome *see* autoimmune polyendocrinopathy–candidiasis–ectodermal dystrophy syndrome
aphthous ulcers
aetiology 2181
clinical presentation 2181
differential diagnosis 2181
genital disease 2181–2182
management 2181–2182
apids (honey bees, bumble bees) 736
APLAID *see* autoinflammation and PLCG2-associated antibody deficiency and immune dysregulation
aplasia cutis congenita (ACC) **139**, 150, 2129–2130
aetiology 116
clinical features 116–118
definition 116
differential diagnosis 118
pathology 116
treatment 118
apocrine differentiation tumours 1331–1333
apocrine hidrocystoma 1331
aetiology 1331
diagnosis 1331
differential diagnosis 1331
epidemiology 1331
pathology 1331
presentation 1331
prognosis 1331
treatment 1331
apocrine miliaria *see* Fox–Fordyce disease
apocrine naevi 1281, 1333
aetiology 1333
diagnosis 1333
differential diagnosis 1333
epidemiology 1333
pathology 1333
presentation 1333
treatment 1333
APP *see* Atrophoderma of Pasini and Pierini
appendage formation, developing human skin 23–24
appendages, neonates 61
approach to the adolescent 2347–2351
adolescent development 2348
changes of adolescence **2348**
chronic illness or disfigurement during adolescence 2350–2351
confidentiality and consent 2350
consultation 2348
examination 2350
HEADSS assessment 2348–2349
history 2348–2350
transition from paediatric to adult services 2351
approach to the infant and child 2344–2347
consultation setting 2345–2346
examination 2346–2347
growth and nutrition 2347
history 2346
infant and child development 2345

approach to the neonate 2342–2344
age terminology in paediatrics **2342**
consultation setting 2343–2344
examination 2344
history 2344
neonatal development 2342–2343
neonatal unit etiquette 2343–2344
procedures 2344
approach to the paediatric patient 2341–2354
adherence 2352–2354
adolescents 2347–2351
end-of-life care in paediatrics 2354
infants and children 2344–2347
neonates 2342–2344
procedures in the paediatric patient 2352
APSEA *see* Assessments of the Psychological and Social Effects of Acne
aquagenic reactive papulotranslucent keratoderma *see* transient aquagenic keratoderma
aquagenic syringeal acrokeratoderma *see* transient aquagenic keratoderma
aquagenic urticaria 759
aquagenic wrinkling of the palms *see* transient aquagenic keratoderma
aquatic dermatoses 746–749
cercarial dermatitis 746–748
seabather's eruption/Cnidaria dermatitis 748–749
toxic seaweed dermatitis 749
Arachnids 738–739
arboviruses 676–679
chikungunya virus (CHIKV) 678–679
dengue 676–677
Zika 677–678
ARCI *see* autosomal recessive congenital ichthyoses
ARCL type I, cutis laxa **1134**, 1135
ARCL type II, cutis laxa **1134**, 1135
ARCL type III (De Barsy syndrome), cutis laxa **1134**, 1135
ARC syndrome *see* arthrogryposis renal dysfunction cholestasis syndrome
ARF *see* acute rheumatic fever
ARKID *see* autosomal recessive keratoderma, ichthyosis and deafness
ARMS *see* amplification-refractory mutation system
array techniques, molecular genetics 42–43
arterial catheterization, iatrogenic disorders of the newborn 160–161
arterial tortuosity syndrome (ATS), cutis laxa *1134*, 1135
arteriovenous malformations (AVM) 1399–1405
Bannayan–Riley–Ruvalcaba syndrome (BRRS) 1403
Bonnet–Dechaume–Blanc syndrome 1401
capillary malformation-arteriovenous malformation (CM-AVM) 1402–1403
clinical features 1400–1403
Cobb syndrome 1401
Cowden syndrome 1403
differential diagnosis 1403
epidemiology 1399
hereditary haemorrhagic telangiectasia (HHT) 1401–1402
histology findings 1403–1404
laboratory findings 1403–1404
localized or extensive AVM 1400–1403
Parkes Weber syndrome 1401
pathogenesis 1399–1400
prevention 1404
PTEN hamartoma tumour syndrome (PHTS) 1403
superselective arterial embolization 1404
surgical resection 1404–1405
treatment 1404–1405
Wyburn–Mason syndrome 1401
artesunate, herpes simplex virus (HSV) infections 607
arthrogryposis and ectodermal dysplasia **1634**
arthrogryposis renal dysfunction cholestasis (ARC) syndrome 1589
arthropods 733–740
vesiculobullous lesions 864
aspergillosis 572–574
clinical features 573
differential diagnosis 573
epidemiology 573
histology findings 573
laboratory findings 573
oral mucosa 2085
pathogenesis 573
prevention 573–574
treatment 573–574
Aspergillus spp., neonates **87**
ASPS *see* alveolar soft part sarcoma
Assessments of the Psychological and Social Effects of Acne (APSEA) 2250
associated disorders, dermatitis herpetiformis (DH) 901
asymmetrical periflexural exanthem of childhood 675
clinical features 675
differential diagnosis 675
epidemiology 675
laboratory findings 675
prevention 675
treatment 675
AT *see* ataxia telangiectasia; Louis–Bar syndrome
ataxia telangiectasia (AT) **1804**, 2030–2032
see also telangiectases
clinical features 2030–2031
differential diagnosis 2031
epidemiology 2030
histology findings 2031–2032
history 2030
laboratory findings 2031–2032
pathogenesis 2030
prevention 2032
treatment 2032
athlete's foot (*Tinea pedis*) 535–536, 540, 542–543
atopic dermatitis (AD)
see also eczema
aetiology 184–191
age studies 172
airborne allergens and pollution 260
alefacept 260
allergic sensitization and the 'atopic march' 178–179
allergy 256, 260–261
associated physical signs 197
atmospheric pollutants 179–180
azathioprine **257**, 258
bacterial infections 200–201, 245–246
bathing 254
binary vs continuous definitions 206–207
biologics 259–260
breastfeeding 177
burden of disease 2256
cheilitis 196
ciclosporin **257**, 258–259
classification *204*
clinical features 193–202
clinical trials 213, 215–218
complications 200–201, 245–251
contact allergy 256
continuous vs binary definitions 206–207
cost 171–172
cutaneous microbiome 51–52
cutaneous 'minor' signs 198–199
definition 168–170, 184–185, 206–211
Dennie–Morgan lines 197–198
descriptive epidemiology 171–173
diagnostic criteria **168**, **193**, 203–211
diagnostic criteria, applying 206
diagnostic criteria, systematic review 208–209
differential diagnosis 201–202
diffuse 'dry type' AD 199–200
discoid atopic dermatitis 199, *200*, 235–236
distribution 194–196
dupilumab 259
dyshidrotic eczema 231–234
eczema herpeticum (EH) 247–248
eczema subtypes/phenotypes 200
education and general advice 253–254
emollients 70, 254
environmental risk factors 179–180
epidemiology 167–183
etanercept 260
ethnic group studies 172–173
exfoliative dermatitis 201
family size studies 173
fetal predictors 176
food allergy 260
general advice and education 253–254
genetic basis 185
genetic dissection 185–186
genetics 175–176, 184–191
geographical variation 173
gut microflora role 176–177
hygiene hypothesis 177
incidence 171
infant feeding 177
infantile seborrhoeic dermatitis (SD) 237–239

infection 178
infection management 256
infliximab 260
initial therapy 254–256
irritants and washing 178
janus kinase (JAK) inhibitors 256
key requirements of a disease definition for AD 207–208
lebrikizumab 260
lichen simplex chronicus (LSC) 240–241
Malassezia-associated diseases 554
management 253–261
management of infection 256
mental health disorders 250–251
mepolizumab 260
metabolic syndrome (MetS) 858
methotrexate (MTX) 257–258
migrant studies 172–173
molluscum infections *248*
morbidity 171
morphology 197
mycophenolate mofetil (MMF) **257**, 259
nail disorders 2151
napkin dermatitis 274
natural history 172
nemolizumab 260
neonatal erythroderma 123–124
neonatal skin care 70
new cases, defining 206
nomenclature 203–204
nummular dermatitis 199, *200*, 235–236
nursing and infant feeding 177
ocular complications 197–198, 251
omalizumab 259
Patient-Oriented Eczema Measure (POEM) 219, *220–221*
periocular and ocular signs 197–198
pets 178
phosphodiesterase 4 (PDE4) inhibitors 256
phototherapy 256–257
pityriasis alba (PA) 228–230
pollutants, atmospheric 179–180
pollution and airborne allergens 260
pompholyx 231–234
prevalence 171
prevalence, effects of low disease prevalence 205
prevention 182, 261
probiotics and nutritional intervention 261
progressive nosology 206–207
prurigo nodularis (PN) 242–243
prurigo pigmentosa (PP) 244
pruritus 261
psychological impact 261
psychosocial complications 249–250
quality of life (QoL) assessment 219–225
racially pigmented skin types 199
related disorders 228–244
risk factors 175–180
rituximab 259
secular trends 173
sensitive vs specific criteria in different study types 204–205
severity 171, 205
severity scoring 212–219
sex studies 172
silk therapeutic clothing 255
skin barrier enhancement 261
skin microbiome role 176–177
sleep disturbance 248–249
social class studies 173
systemic corticosteroids 257
systemic therapies 257–259
terminology 185
tocilizumab 260
topical calcineurin inhibitors (TCI) 255–256
topical corticosteroids (TCS) 254–255
tralokinumab 260
unresponsive disease 256–257
ustekinumab 260
validation studies 207, 210–211
verrucae vulgaris *248*
viral infections 201, 247–248
visible flexural dermatitis 168, *169*
washing and irritants 178
wet wraps 255
atopic napkin rash **268**
atretic (rudimentary, sequestrated) meningocoele 112
atrichia with papular lesions **1634**, **2109**
atrichia with papular lesions; alopecia universalis congenita 1690
clinical features 1690
definition 1690
differential diagnosis 1690
history 1690
pathology 1690
prognosis 1690
treatment 1690
atrophic lichen planus 396
Atrophoderma of Pasini and Pierini (APP) 1157–1158
aetiology 1157
clinical features 1158
definition 1157
diagnosis 1158
history 1157
pathology 1158
treatment 1158
atrophoderma reticulata symmetrica faciei *see* atrophoderma vermiculata
atrophoderma reticulatum *see* atrophoderma vermiculata
atrophodermas 1157–1161
associated diseases 1159–1160
Atrophoderma of Pasini and Pierini (APP) 1157–1158
atrophoderma vermiculata (AV) 1159
Bazex–Dupré–Christol syndrome 1160
chondrodysplasia punctata (X-linked form) 1160
Conradi–Hünermann–Happle syndrome 1160
diffuse congenital ichthyosis 1160
focal dermal hypoplasia (FDH) (Goltz syndrome) 1160
focal facial dermal dysplasias (FFDD) 1160–1161
follicular atrophoderma 1159–1160
generalized and diffuse nonscarring hypotrichosis 1160
Goltz syndrome (focal dermal hypoplasia (FDH)) 1160
Happle–Tinschert syndrome 1160
linear atrophoderma 1160
linear atrophoderma of Moulin (LAM) 1158–1159
marked hypohidrosis and woolly hair 1160
patchy follicular atrophoderma 1160
atrophoderma vermiculata (AV) 1159
keratosis pilaris 1601
atropho-scleroderma superficialis *see* Atrophoderma of Pasini and Pierini
ATS *see* arterial tortuosity syndrome
ATT *see* antitubercular therapy
AUG *see* acute ulcerative gingivitis
autoimmune blistering diseases (AIBDs) 868–888
other subepidermal blistering diseases 885–888
pemphigoid diseases 874–885
pemphigus diseases 869–874
prevalence **870**
target antigens **869**
autoimmune causes
erosive or ulcerative skin lesions **139**
vesiculobullous lesions 866, *867*
vesiculopustular and bullous skin lesions **136–137**, 146–147
autoimmune diseases, hyperpigmentation 1467
autoimmune disorders, panniculitis 1216
autoimmune lymphoproliferative syndrome (Canale–Smith syndrome) **2036**
autoimmune polyendocrinopathy–candidiasis–ectodermal dystrophy (APECED) syndrome **1634**
autoimmune polyendocrinopathy–candidiasis–ectodermal dystrophy1 (APECED) syndrome (autoimmune polyendocrine syndrome, type 1), chronic mucocutaneous candidiasis (CMC) **2043**
autoimmunity, morphoea 1176
autoinflammation and PLCG2-associated antibody deficiency and immune dysregulation (APLAID) 2017
autoinflammatory diseases (AIDs) 2010–2022
adenosine deaminase 2 (ADA2), deficiency 2022
Aicardi–Goutiéres syndrome (AGS) 2021–2022
AISLE (autoinflammatory syndrome with lymphoedema) 2014
autoinflammation and PLCG2-associated antibody deficiency and immune dysregulation (APLAID) 2017
Behçet disease (BD) 2018
Blau syndrome/early-onset sarcoidosis (EOS) 2018–2019
C1q deficiency 2022

autoinflammatory diseases (AIDs) (*cont'd*)
  chronic atypical neutrophilic dermatosis with lipodystrophy and elevated temperature (CANDLE) syndrome 2019–2020
  cryopyrin-associated periodic syndromes (CAPS) 2012–2013
  deficiency of the IL-1 receptor antagonist (DIRA) 2015–2016
  deficiency of the IL-36 receptor antagonist (DITRA) 2016
  familial chilblain lupus 2022
  haploinsufficiency of protein A20 (HA20) 2018
  histiocytic and granulomatous diseases 2018–2020
  H-syndrome 2019–2020
  Majeed syndrome 2017
  mevalonate kinase deficiency (MKD) 2013–2014
  mucosal diseases 2018
  mutations **2011**
  PASH, PAPASH and other related AIDs 2017
  periodic fever, immunodeficiency and thrombocytopenia (PFIT) 2018
  periodic fever with aphtous stomatitis, pharyngitis and adenitis syndrome (PFAPA) 2018
  PLCG2-associated antibody deficiency and immune dysregulation (PLAID) 2014
  pustular diseases 2014–2017
  pyogenic arthritis, pyoderma gangrenosum and acne syndrome (PAPA) 2016–2017
  STING-associated vasculopathy with onset in infancy (SAVI) syndrome 2021
  tumour necrosis factor receptor-associated periodic syndrome (TRAPS) 2014
  type I interferonopathies 2021–2022
  urticarial and oedematous diseases 2012–2014
  vasculopathic diseases 2021–2022
  X-linked reticulate pigmentary disorder (XLPDR) 2022
autoinflammatory syndrome with lymphoedema (AISLE) 2014
autoinoculation, human papillomaviruses (HPV) 590
autosomal dominant anhidrotic ED with T cell immunodeficiency 1675
autosomal dominant cutis laxa (ADCL) 1133–1135
autosomal dominant lipodystrophies 1223–1224
autosomal recessive congenital ichthyoses (ARCI) 1557–1566
  see also specific ichthyoses
  epidemiology 1557
  pathogenesis 1557
autosomal recessive EBV-associated lymphoproliferative syndrome **2036**
autosomal recessive epidermolysis bullosa simplex due to keratin 14 mutations 914–915
autosomal recessive keratoderma, ichthyosis and deafness (ARKID) 1537
  clinical features 1537, *1538*
  differential diagnosis 1537
  epidemiology 1537
  histology findings 1537
  history 1537
  laboratory findings 1537
  pathogenesis 1537
autosomal recessive lipodystrophies 1223
AV *see* atrophoderma vermiculata
AVM *see* arteriovenous malformations
azathioprine
  atopic dermatitis (AD) **257**, 258
  systemic therapies 2294
azelaic acid, acne vulgaris 809
azoles, dermatophytoses 540

bacillary angiomatosis 475–478
  clinical features 476–477
  differential diagnosis 477
  epidemiology 476
  histology findings 477–478
  history 475–476
  laboratory findings 477–478
  pathogenesis 476
  treatment 478
bacteria, cutaneous *see* cutaneous microbiome
bacterial infections
  acute ulcerative gingivitis (AUG) 2085
  atopic dermatitis (AD) 200–201, 245–246
  congenital infections 85–86, **87**, **88**, 89–90
  HIV infection 650
  immunocompromised children 686–687, 689–690
  neonates 85–86, **87**, **88**, 89–90
  oral mucosa 2085
  vesiculobullous lesions 864
bacterial toxin-mediated syndromes 430–433
  recurrent toxin-mediated perineal erythema (RPE) 433
  staphylococcal scalded skin syndrome (SSSS) 430–431
  staphylococcal toxic shock syndrome 431–432
  streptococcal scarlet fever 432
  streptococcal toxic shock syndrome (STSS) 432
  toxic shock syndrome (TSS) 431–432
bacterial vaginitis (BV) 2218
  child sexual abuse (CSA) 2218
  clinical features 2218
  definition 2218
  diagnosis 2218
  treatment 2218
Baisch syndrome **1634**
balanitis, streptococcal cellulitis, vulvovaginitis and balanitis 2175–2176
balanitis xerotica obliterans *see* lichen sclerosus in boys
balneotherapy, congenital ichthyoses (CI) 1594
bamboo hair *see* trichorrhexis invaginata
bandaging, surgical therapy 2313–2314
Bannayan–Riley–Ruvalcaba syndrome (BRRS) 1403, **1806**
  see also Cowden syndrome; *PTEN* (Phosphatase and TENsin homologue) hamartoma tumour syndrome (PHTS)
  birthmarks in the genital area 2171
  characteristics **1199**
  clinical features **1199**, 1201
  differential diagnosis 1201
BAP1 tumour predisposition syndrome *see* familial atypical mole–malignant melanoma syndrome
barbiturates, anaesthesia 2337
Bartonella infections 475–482
  bacillary angiomatosis 475–478
  bartonellosis 480–482
  cat scratch disease 478–480
bartonellosis 480–482
  clinical features 480–481
  differential diagnosis 481
  epidemiology 480
  histology findings 481–482
  history 480
  laboratory findings 481–482
  pathogenesis 480
  prevention 482
  treatment 482
Bart–Pumphrey syndrome 1695
basal cell carcinoma (BCC) 1370–1373
  carcinogens 1371
  clinical features 1372
  differential diagnosis 1372
  epidemiology 1370–1371
  histology findings 1372
  immunosuppression 1372
  pathogenesis 1371–1372
  predisposing genodermatoses 1371–1372
  prevention 1373
  risk factors **1371**
  treatment 1372–1373
basal cell epithelioma *see* basal cell carcinoma
basaloid follicular hamartoma 1280
Basan syndrome **1631**
bathing, atopic dermatitis (AD) 254
bathing suit icthyosis (BSI) 1560–1561
  clinical features 1561
  definition 1560
  histology findings 1561
  laboratory findings 1561
  pathogenesis 1560–1561
  treatment 1561
  ultrastructure 1561
Bazex–Dupré–Christol syndrome (BDCS) 1160, 1802–1803
  clinical features 1802–1803
  differential diagnosis 1803
  pathogenesis 1802
BB *see* β-blockers; mid-borderline leprosy
BCC *see* basal cell carcinoma
BCG vaccine, cutaneous tuberculosis 494

BCH *see* benign cephalic histiocytosis
BD *see* Behçet disease
BDCS *see* Bazex–Dupré–Christol syndrome
BDD *see* blistering distal dactylitis
Becker naevus (BN) 1265–1266, 1304
  associated syndrome 1266, 1304
  clinical features 1265
  histopathology 1265
  history 1265
  hypertrichosis 2135–2136
  pathogenesis 1265
  treatment 1265–1266
Becker naevus syndrome 1266, 1304
Beckwith–Wiedemann syndrome (BWS) **1805**, 1807–1808
  clinical features 1807–1808
  pathogenesis 1807
  treatment 1808
bedbug infestation *see* cimicosis
behavioural modification, self-mutilation 2271
Behçet disease (BD) 1952–1957, 2018
  aetiopathogenesis 1952–1953
  clinical features 1953–1955
  diagnosis 1955–1956
  differential diagnosis 1956
  epidemiology 1952
  gastrointestinal involvement 1955, 1957
  genital signs 2192
  joint involvement 1955
  mucocutaneous lesions 1953–1954
  neurological involvement 1955, 1956
  ocular involvement 1954
  ocular lesions 1956
  oral and genital aphthae 1956
  pathergy test 1956
  prognosis 1957
  skin lesions 1956
  transplacental 98–99
  treatment 1956–1957
  vascular involvement 1954–1955
Behçet syndrome 2081
  aetiology 2081
  clinical features 2081
  definition 2081
  differential diagnosis 2081
  oral mucosa 2081
  treatment 2081
Bell's palsy, herpes simplex virus (HSV) infections 604
benign (or transient) neonatal pustular melanosis **135**
benign anteromedial plantar nodules, transient skin disorders in neonates and young infants 81
benign cephalic histiocytosis (BCH) 1086–1087
  clinical features 1086
  differential diagnosis 1086
  epidemiology 1086
  histology findings 1086–1087
  history 1086
  pathogenesis 1086
  treatment 1087
benign conditions, vesiculobullous lesions 864
benign dermoscopic patterns, melanocytic lesions 2369
benign fibrous histiocytoma *see* dermatofibroma
benign migratory glossitis 2101
benign or neonatal cephalic pustulosis *see* neonatal cephalic pustulosis
benign summer light eruption *see* polymorphous light eruption
benign symmetric lipomatosis
  see also multiple symmetric lipomatosis
  characteristics **1199**
  clinical features **1199**
benign tumours, neoplasia, genital disease 2189
benzalkonium chloride, allergic contact dermatitis (ACD) 310
benzodiazepines, anaesthesia 2337
benzoyl peroxide, acne vulgaris 808–809
Berardinelli–Seip congenital lipodystrophy (BSCL) 1223
BHDS *see* Birt–Hogg–Dubé syndrome
bilateral conjunctival injection, Kawasaki disease (KD) 1909
biologic agents
  atopic dermatitis (AD) 259–260
  etanercept 2292
  infliximab 2292
  interferons (IFN) 2293
  intravenous immunoglobulin (IVIG) 2292–2293
  juvenile idiopathic arthritis (JIA) 1937–1938
  pityriasis rubra pilaris (PRP) 384
  psoriasis 372–374
  rituximab 2292
  systemic therapies 2291–2293
biologics and antibodies, alopecia areata (AA) 2145
biopsy
  see also histopathology
  nail biopsy 2316–2317
  'normal' biopsy 2390
  principles 2378–2379
  reasons 2378
  scalp biopsy, hair loss 2108
  skin biopsy, genetic investigation of mosaic disorders 1234
  skin biopsy, rickettsial disease 511
  skin biopsy, vasculitis *2391*
  skin punch biopsy, surgical therapy 2315
  skin punch biopsy, vesiculobullous lesions 862
  small bowel biopsy, dermatitis herpetiformis (DH) 903
  surgical therapy 2315, 2316–2317
biopsychosocial theory in skin disease, burden of disease 2258
biotin deficiency, hair loss 2127
biotinidase deficiency 1972
  clinical features 1972
  definition 1972
  differential diagnosis 1972
  prognosis 1972
  treatment 1972
bird mites, pseudoscabies 720–721
birthmarks in the genital area 2170–2173
  Bannayan–Riley–Ruvalcaba syndrome (Ruvalcaba–Myhre–Smith syndrome) 2171
  epidermal naevi 2171–2172
  melanocytic naevi 2171
  papular acantholytic dyskeratosis of the vulva 2173
  vascular naevi 2172–2173
Birt–Hogg–Dubé syndrome (BHDS) **1805**, 1808–1809
  clinical features 1808–1809
  differential diagnosis 1809
  pathogenesis 1808
  pathology 1808
  treatment 1809
bitemporal aplasia cutis congenita 1160–1161
bitemporal forceps marks syndrome 1160–1161
bitemporal scars with abnormal eyelashes 1160–1161
BL *see* borderline lepromatous leprosy
black piedra 556
  clinical features 556
  diagnosis 556
  treatment 556
blastomycosis 567–568
  clinical features 567–568
  differential diagnosis 567–568
  epidemiology 567
  histology findings 568
  laboratory findings 568
  pathogenesis 567
  prevention 568
  treatment 568
blastomycosis-like pyoderma 428–429
Blau syndrome/early-onset sarcoidosis (EOS) 1000–1004, 2018–2019
  vs classic sarcoidosis **996**
  clinical features 1002–1003
  cutaneous manifestations 1002
  differential diagnosis 1003
  epidemiology 1001
  expanded manifestations 1003
  extracutaneous manifestations 1002–1003
  history 1001
  NOD2 in nuclear factor-κβ (NF-κβ) signalling 1001–1002
  pathogenesis 1001
  pathology 1002
  prognosis 1003
  treatment 1003–1004
bleach baths, eczema 2399
bleeding, surgical therapy 2317
blepharocheilodontic syndrome **1634**
blistering diseases in infancy and childhood, vesiculobullous lesions 865–867
blistering distal dactylitis (BDD) 429
blisters and ulcers 2179–2183
  aphthous ulcers 2181–2182
  erosive and or blistering napkin eruption 2179, *2180*
  erythema multiforme and toxic epidermal necrolysis 2182
  fixed drug eruption (FDE) 2182

blisters and ulcers (*cont'd*)
genital area 2179–2183
hidradenitis suppurativa (HS) (acne inversa) 2182–2183
immunobullous disease – vulval bullous and cicatricial pemphigoid and linear IgA disease of childhood 2179–2180
nonsexually acquired acute genital ulcers (NSAGU) 2180–2181
β-blockers (BB)
infantile haemangiomas (IH) 1435–1436, 2290
systemic therapies 2289–2290
Bloom syndrome (BS) 1791–1793, **1805**
clinical features 1792–1793
differential diagnosis 1793
epidemiology 1791–1792
histology findings 1793
history 1791
laboratory findings 1793
pathogenesis 1791–1792
prevention 1793
treatment 1793
'blueberry muffin rash' (dermal extramedullary erythropoiesis)
neonates 85, **86**
rubella 663
blue naevi
acquired melanocytic naevi (AMN) 1254
histopathology 2388
blue rubber bleb naevus syndrome of Bean 1407
BN *see* Becker naevus
body lice *see* pediculosis
Bohn nodules, transient skin disorders in neonates and young infants 77–78
Bohn nodules and Epstein pearls (gingival cysts of infancy), oral mucosa 2088
bone cysts, oral mucosa 2096
Bonnet–Dechaume–Blanc syndrome 1401
bony swellings, oral mucosa 2096
book dysplasia **1635**
borderline lepromatous leprosy (BL) **497**
borderline tuberculoid leprosy (BT) **497**, **498**, **499**
Borrelia burgdorferi, neonates **87**
borrelial lymphocytoma (lymphadenosis benigna cutis), lyme borreliosis (LB)/lyme disease 467
BOS *see* Buschke–Ollendorff syndrome
botryomycosis 428
bovine vaccinia **625**, 638
clinical features 638
epidemiology 638
history 638
pathogenesis 638
bowenoid papulosis, human papillomaviruses (HPV) 592
BP *see* bullous pemphigoid
brachymetapody–anodontia–hypotrichosis–albinoidism **1635**
branchial cysts, sinuses and fistulae 104–105
aetiology 104
clinical features 105
pathology 104–105
treatment 105
Brauer syndrome 1160–1161
Brazilian or South American blastomycosis (paracoccidioidomycosis) *see* paracoccidioidomycosis
breast and nipple abnormalities 106–107
breast milk, cutaneous microbiome 48–49
brincidofovir, herpes simplex virus (HSV) infections 607
brivudine, herpes simplex virus (HSV) infections 605–607
Brooke-Spiegler syndrome (BSS), multiple familial trichoepitheliomas and familial cylindromatosis **1804**, 1810–1811
clinical features 1810
histology findings 1810–1811
pathogenesis 1810
treatment 1811
BRRS *see* Bannayan–Riley–Ruvalcaba syndrome
bruises
child abuse and neglect (CAN) 2221–2223, *2225*
differential diagnosis of inflicted bruises 2224, *2225*
Mongolian spots, differential diagnosis *2225*, **2412**
safeguarding issues in paediatric dermatology 2410
BS *see* Bloom syndrome
BSCL *see* Berardinelli–Seip congenital lipodystrophy
BSI *see* bathing suit icthyosis
BSS *see* Brooke-Spiegler syndrome
BT *see* borderline tuberculoid leprosy
bubble hair, hair disorders 2118
buffalopox **625**, 642–643
clinical features 642
differential diagnosis 642
epidemiology 642
histology findings 643
history 642
laboratory findings 643
pathogenesis 642
prevention 643
treatment 643
bullae in the newborn due to maternal autoimmune blistering disorders 146–147
clinical features 146
differential diagnosis 146–147
epidemiology 146
histology findings 147
laboratory findings 147
pathogenesis 146
prevention 147
treatment 147
bullous and diffuse cutaneous mastocytosis *see* diffuse cutaneous mastocytosis
bullous and vesiculopustular skin lesions *see* vesiculopustular and bullous skin lesions
bullous congenital ichthyosiform erythroderma *see* epidermolytic ichthyosis
bullous congenital ichthyosiform erythroderma of Brocq *see* epidermolytic ichthyosis
bullous dermatoses
see also linear immunoglobulin IgA bullous dermatosis
histopathology 2381–2382
superficial self-mutilation *2269*
bullous dermolysis of the newborn 920
bullous drug eruptions, hypersensitivity reactions to drugs 794–795
bullous impetigo, infectious napkin dermatitis **268**, 273
bullous lichen planus 396–397
bullous mastocytosis **137**
bullous neonatal lupus erythematosus (NLE) **137**
bullous pemphigoid (BP) 879–882
clinical features 880–881
differential diagnosis 881
epidemiology 879–880
histology findings 881
laboratory findings 881
neonates **136**
pathogenesis 880
prevention 881
treatment 881
bullous systemic lupus erythematosus (SLE) 888
see also systemic lupus erythematosus (SLE)
clinical features 888
differential diagnosis 888
epidemiology 888
laboratory findings 888
pathogenesis 888
treatment 888
bumps and lumps, histopathology 2383, *2384*
burden of disease 2255–2259
acne vulgaris 2256–2257
atopic dermatitis (AD) 2256
biopsychosocial theory in skin disease 2258
camps for children 2259
Children's Dermatology Life Quality Index (CDLQI) 2255–2256
congenital malformations 2257
coping strategies 2258–2259
coping with the 2255–2259
family impact 2257
haemangiomas 2257
paediatric skin disease 2255–2256
patient advocacy groups 2258–**2259**
quality of life (QoL) assessment 2255–2256
Bureau–Barriere–Thomas (palmoplantar keratoderma with clubbing of the fingers and toes and skeletal deformity) 1548
Burkitt lymphoma, oral mucosa 2096
burns
abusive burns 2223, *2224*, **2226**, 2410–2413
chemical burns 992–993

cigarette burns 2410–2413, **2413**
superficial self-mutilation 2270
thermal burns 991–992
burn wound infections, pseudomonal skin disease 449–450
Buruli ulcer 500–501
Buschke–Ollendorff syndrome (BOS) 1139–1141, 1278–1279
aetiology 1140
clinical features 1140–1141, 1278–1279
definition 1139
differential diagnosis 1141, 1279
epidemiology 1278
history 1139–1140, 1278
pathogenesis 1140, 1278
pathology 1141
treatment 1141, 1279
Butcher's warts, human papillomaviruses (HPV) 591–592
BV *see* bacterial vaginitis
BWS *see* Beckwith–Wiedemann syndrome

C1q deficiency, autoinflammatory diseases (AIDs) 2022
CA *see* condyloma acuminata
CAD *see* chronic actinic dermatitis
CADI *see* Cardiff Acne Disability Index
CADIS *see* Childhood Atopic Dermatitis Impact Scale
Caesarean section delivery
cutaneous microbiome 48
iatrogenic disorders of the newborn 158
café-au-lait macules (CALM), laser therapy 2325
CAHMR syndrome *see* cataract, hypertrichosis, mental retardation syndrome
calcification and ossification in the skin 1338–1349
aberrant calcification and ossification of the skin 1339–1340
calcitonin 1339
calcium regulation 1338–1339
causes **1339–1340**
classification **1339–1340**
connective tissue diseases 1343–1344
CREST syndrome 1343
cutaneous ossification 1346–1349
dermatomyositis 1343
dystrophic calcification 1343–1344
Ehlers–Danlos syndromes (EDS) 1344
iatrogenic calcinosis cutis 1345
idiopathic calcification 1340–1342
idiopathic calcinosis of the scrotum/vulva 1340–1341
infections 1344
inherited disorders 1344
lobular panniculitis 1343–1344
metastatic calcification 1345
milia-like idiopathic calcinosis cutis 1341
miliary osteoma cutis of the face 1349
panniculitis 1343–1344
parathyroid hormone 1338–1339
phosphate regulation 1338–1339
phosphatonins 1339
platelike osteoma cutis (OC) 1348–1349
pseudoxanthoma elasticum (PXE) 1344
scleroderma 1343
subepidermal calcified nodule 1340
trauma 1344
tumoral calcinosis 1341–1342
tumours 1344
vitamin D 1339
Werner syndrome (WS) 1344
calcifying aponeurotic fibroma 1366–1367
clinical features 1366–1367
differential diagnosis 1366–1367
epidemiology 1366
pathogenesis 1366
pathology 1367
treatment 1367
calcifying fibroma *see* calcifying aponeurotic fibroma
calcifying fibrous pseudotumour 1361
clinical features 1361
differential diagnosis 1361
epidemiology 1361
history 1361
pathogenesis 1361
pathology 1361
treatment 1361
calcineurin inhibitors
see also topical calcineurin inhibitors
psoriasis 369, *373*
calcinosis cutis, iatrogenic 1345
calciphylaxis 1219–1220
calcitonin, calcification and ossification in the skin 1339
calcium regulation, calcification and ossification in the skin 1338–1339
C-ALCL *see* cutaneous anaplastic large cell lymphoma; primary cutaneous anaplastic large cell lymphoma
CALM *see* café-au-lait macules
CALMs
neurofibromatosis type 1 (NF1) 1825, 1830
neurofibromatosis type 2 (NF2) 1833
Camarena syndrome **1635**
camelpox **625**
Camisa variant of Vohwinkel syndrome *see* loricrin keratoderma
camps for children, burden of disease 2259
CAN *see* child abuse and neglect
Canale–Smith syndrome (autoimmune lymphoproliferative syndrome) **2036**
Candida albicans
napkin dermatitis 267
neonates **87**
Candida antigen immunotherapy, molluscum contagiosum (MC) 585
candida granuloma 548
candidal (monilial) napkin dermatitis **268**
infectious napkin dermatitis 271–272
Candida leucoplakia (chronic hyperplastic candidosis) 547
oral mucosa 2090
candidiasis *see* candidosis
candidosis (candidiasis) **138**, 545–550, 569–570
see also chronic mucocutaneous candidiasis
acute erythematous atrophic candidosis 547
acute pseudo-membranous candidiasis (thrush) 2089
acute pseudomembranous candidosis (thrush) 546–547
aetiology 545–546
angular stomatitis 2090
candida granuloma 548
Candida leucoplakia (chronic hyperplastic candidosis) 547
chronic atrophic candidiasis (chronic denture stomatitis) 2090
chronic denture stomatitis (chronic atrophic candidiasis) 2090
chronic erythematous candidosis 547
chronic hyperplastic candidosis (*Candida leucoplakia*) 547
clinical features 546–548, 569
congenital cutaneous candidosis 547
cutaneous candidosis 549
diagnosis 548–549
differential diagnosis 549, 569
epidemiology 569
erythematous candidiasis 2089
histology findings 569–570
history 545
laboratory findings 569–570
molecular diagnostics 549
nails 548
napkin dermatitis 547
onychia 547, 549
oral candidosis 546–547, 549
oral lesions 548
oral mucosa 2089–2090
paronychia 547, 549
pathogenesis 545–546, 569
pathology 546
prevention 570
prognosis 548
skin lesions 548
thrush (acute pseudomembranous candidosis) 546–547, 2089
treatment 549, 570
white patches (leucoplakia), oral mucosa 2089–2090
CANDLE syndrome *see* chronic atypical neutrophilic dermatosis with lipodystrophy and elevated temperature syndrome
cantharidin, molluscum contagiosum (MC) 584
Cantu syndrome *see* onychotrichodysplasia with neutropenia
CAPB *see* cocamidopropyl betaine
capillary malformation 1412–1414
clinical features 1412–1413
differential diagnosis 1413
epidemiology 1412
histology findings 1413–1414
laboratory findings 1413–1414
occult spinal dysraphism and midline capillary malformations 1413

capillary malformation (*cont'd*)
pathogenesis 1412
'port-wine stain' (localized or extensive capillary malformation) 1412–1413, 2321–2322
prevention 1414
prognosis 1414
treatment 1414
capillary malformation-arteriovenous malformation (CM-AVM) 1402–1403
CAPS *see* cryopyrin-associated periodic syndromes
carba mix/carbamates, allergic contact dermatitis (ACD) 308–309
carcinomas of the skin 1370–1376
basal cell carcinoma (BCC) 1370–1373
Merkel cell carcinoma 1375–1376
pilomatrix carcinoma 1374–1375
sebaceous carcinoma 1375
squamous cell carcinoma (SCC) 1373–1374
CARD9 deficiency, chronic mucocutaneous candidiasis (CMC) **2043**
cardiac complications, dystrophic epidermolysis bullosa (DEB) 922
cardiac disease, systemic sclerosis (SSc) **1191**, 1192
cardiac failure, infantile haemangiomas (IH) 1430
cardiac findings, tuberous sclerosis complex (TSC) 1848–1849
Cardiff Acne Disability Index (CADI) 2248–2250
cardiofaciocutaneous syndrome (CFCS) **1601**, **1635**, **1806**, 1860–1861
see also Noonan syndrome
aetiology 1860
clinical features 1860–1861
definition 1860
diagnosis 1861
history 1860
summary of RASopathies **1858**
treatment 1861
cardiopulmonary manifestations, systemic sclerosis (SSc) **1191**
cardiorespiratory involvement, juvenile dermatomyositis (JDM) 1948
cardiovascular and other complications, Kawasaki disease (KD) 1912–1913
care of the skin *see* neonatal skin care; nursing care of the skin
Carey syndrome **1636**
carotenaemia 1982–1986
aetiology 1982–1984
carotene content of foods **1983**
carotenoid 15,15′-mono-oxygenase (*BCMO1, BCO1 or CMO1*); gene locus 16q21-q23 1983–1984
clinical features 1985
definition 1982
differential diagnosis 1986
excessive ingestion 1985
excessive ingestion of carotene 1983
history 1982
hyperlipidaemias 1983, 1985
inborn error(s) of carotene metabolism 1985
metabolic carotenaemia 1983
pathogenesis 1982–1984
pathology 1984–1985
prognosis 1986
retinol-binding protein 4 (*RBP4*) gene locus 10q24 1984
treatment 1986
cartilage–hair hypoplasia syndrome (CHH) **1636**, **1804**, 2033
clinical features 2033
differential diagnosis 2033
epidemiology 2033
histology findings 2033
history 2033
laboratory findings 2033
pathogenesis 2033
prevention 2033
treatment 2033
Carvajal syndrome (PPK with left ventricular cardiomyopathy and woolly hair) **1636**, 1701
cataract, hypertrichosis, mental retardation (CAHMR) syndrome **1636**
cataract–alopecia–sclerodactyly syndrome **1636**
caterpillars and moths (Lepidoptera) 738
cat scratch disease 478–480
clinical features 479
differential diagnosis 479
epidemiology 478–479
histology findings 479–480
history 478
laboratory findings 479–480
pathogenesis 478–479
treatment 480
CAV1-associated lipodystrophy 1737
clinical features 1737
differential diagnosis 1737
epidemiology 1737
histology findings 1737
history 1737
laboratory findings 1737
pathogenesis 1737
treatment 1737
CCC *see* congenital cutaneous candidiasis
CD4+/CD56+ haematodermic neoplasm (blastic plasmacytoid dendritic cell neoplasm) 1056
clinical features 1056
definition 1056
epidemiology 1056
genetic features 1056
histopathology 1056
immunophenotype 1056
precursor haematological neoplasm 1056
predictive factors 1056
prognosis 1056
treatment 1056
CDLQI *see* Children's Dermatology Life Quality Index
CDLS *see* Cornelia de Lange syndrome
CDP *see* chondrodysplasia punctata
CDPX2 *see* type 2 chondrodysplasia punctata
CDS *see* Chanarin–Dorfman syndrome
CEDNIK *see* cerebral dysgenesis, neuropathy, ichthyosis and palmoplantar keratoderma syndrome
cellular DNA repair systems
direct reversion 1744
excision repair 1744
multistep cancer theory 1744
translesional synthesis 1744
xeroderma pigmentosum and related diseases 1743–1744, 1765–1766
cellular senescence, xeroderma pigmentosum and related diseases 1766–1767
cellulitis 428
centipedes (Chilopoda) 739
cephalocoeles 111
cercarial dermatitis 746–748
clinical features 747
differential diagnosis 747
epidemiology 746–747
histology findings 747
history 746
laboratory findings 747
lifecycle 747
pathogenesis 746–747
prevention 747–748
treatment 747–748
cerebral dysgenesis, neuropathy, ichthyosis and palmoplantar keratoderma syndrome (CEDNIK) 1536–1537, 1589
clinical features 1536
differential diagnosis 1536
epidemiology 1536
histology findings 1537
history 1536
laboratory findings 1537
pathogenesis 1536
treatment 1537
cerebro-oculo-facio-skeletal syndrome (COFS syndrome) 1763
UV-sensitive syndrome, COFS/TTD and CS/TTD 1763
cervicofacial lymphadenopathy 500
CEVD *see* congenital erosive and vesicular dermatosis with reticulated supple scarring
CFCS *see* cardiofaciocutaneous syndrome
CGD *see* chronic granulomatous disease
CGL *see* congenital generalized lipoatrophy
CH *see* congenital haemangiomas
Chanarin–Dorfman syndrome *see* neutral lipid storage disease with ichthyosis
Chanarin–Dorfman syndrome (CDS) 126
CHAND syndrome *see* curly hair–ankyloblepharon–nail dysplasia syndrome
changes of adolescence, approach to the adolescent **2348**
CHARGE syndrome, anatomical abnormalities 2184–2185

Chédiak–Higashi syndrome (CHS) 1489–1490, 2034–2035, **2036**
clinical features 1490, 2034
differential diagnosis 2034–2035
epidemiology 1489, 2034
histology findings 2035
history 2034
laboratory findings 1490, 2035
pathogenesis 1489, 2034
prevention 1490, 2035
treatment 1490, 2035
cheilitis, atopic dermatitis (AD) 196
chemical irritant contact dermatitis 984–985
chemoprophylaxis, lyme borreliosis (LB)/lyme disease 472
chemotherapy, specific antiviral, herpes simplex virus (HSV) infections 605–607
chemotherapy and immunomodulators 2293–2295
azathioprine 2294
ciclosporin 2293–2294
methotrexate (MTX) 2293
mycophenolate mofetil (MMF) 2294–2295
sirolimus 2294
systemic therapies 2293–2295
vinblastine 2295
vincristine 2295
chevron (herringbone) nails, nail disorders 2149
CHH *see* cartilage–hair hypoplasia syndrome
chickenpox
oral mucosa 2083
varicella zoster virus (VZV) infections 615–617
chikungunya virus (CHIKV) 678–679
clinical features 678–679
laboratory findings 679
oral mucosa 2084
chilblains 989–990
child abuse and neglect (CAN) 2219–2229
see also child sexual abuse
abdominal trauma 2229
abusive burns 2223, *2224*, **2226**
abusive head trauma (AHT) 2227–2229
bruises 2221–2223, *2225*
burns, abusive 2223, *2224*, **2226**
cutaneous signs of child abuse 2221–2223
definition 2219–2220
dental neglect 2227
diagnostic evaluation 2220
differential diagnosis of inflicted bruises 2224, *2225*
epidemiology 2220
fractures 2224–2227
history 2220
imaging and other diagnostic modalities 2221
injuries to the face, ear, nose and throat region 2227
medical examination 2221
napkin dermatitis 278, *2237*
role of medical professionals 2220
skin lesions confused with child abuse 2224
teeth 2227
toe tourniquet syndrome 2224, *2225*
Childhood Atopic Dermatitis Impact Scale (CADIS) 223
Childhood Impact of Atopic Dermatitis (CIAD) 223
childhood rosacea 821–824
clinical presentation 821–822
comorbidity 823–824
differential diagnosis 822–823
epidemiology 821
ocular rosacea 822
pathogenesis 821
treatment 823
Children's Dermatology Life Quality Index (CDLQI)
atopic dermatitis (AD) 222–223
burden of disease 2255–2256
quality of life (QoL) assessment 2242–2243, 2245, *2246–2248*, *2249*
child sexual abuse (CSA) 2229–2239
see also child abuse and neglect
anogenital findings 2232–2235
background 2229–2230
bacterial vaginitis (BV) 2218
characteristics of anogenital findings in child sexual abuse 2234–2235
Chlamydia trachomatis infections 2210–2211
condyloma acuminata (CA) 2213
definition 2229–2230
differential diagnosis 2236–2238
findings associated with child sexual abuse 2233–2234
general considerations 2229–2230
general considerations and normal findings 2232–2233
genital herpes simplex virus infection 2216
gonorrhoea 2206
hepatitis B 2214–2215
history 2231
HIV infection 2216–2217
medical aspects – potential and limitations 2230–2231
medical examination 2231–2232
normal findings after penetration 2234
overall assessment 2238
overall medical and multidisciplinary management 2238–2239
psychological aspects of genital disease in children 2193–2194
sexually transmitted diseases (STDs) **2197**
sexually transmitted infections (STIs) 2235–2236
syphilis 2201–2202
Trichomonas vaginalis infection 2218
CHILD syndrome *see* congenital hemidysplasia with ichthyosiform naevus and limb defects syndrome
Chilopoda (centipedes) 739
chimaerism, mosaicism 1231–1232
CHIME syndrome *see* coloboma, heart defect, ichthyosiform dermatosis, mental retardation, ear anomalies syndrome
CHIP-seq *see* chromatin immunoprecipitation sequencing
Chlamydia trachomatis infections 2209–2212
child sexual abuse (CSA) 2210–2211
clinical features 2209–2211
definition 2209
diagnosis 2211
history 2209
inclusion conjunctivitis 2210, 2211–2212
infections at other sites 2210
infections in infants 2209–2210
infections in older children 2210–2211
microbiology 2209
pneumonia 2210, 2211–2212
sexually transmitted diseases (STDs) 2209–2212
treatment 2211–2212
chloral hydrate, anaesthesia 2337–2338
chloroquine, antimalarial agents 2289
cholinergic urticaria 755–756, 758
chondrodysplasia punctata (CDP)
neonates 96
type 2 (CDPX2) 126
X-linked form 1160
choriocarcinoma 1396–1397
aetiology 1397
clinical features 1397
definition 1396
differential diagnosis 1397
epidemiology 1396
history 1396
laboratory studies 1397
pathogenesis 1397
pathology 1397
prognosis 1397
treatment 1397
chorionic villus sampling (CVS), iatrogenic disorders of the newborn 156
CHP *see* cytophagic histiocytic panniculitis
chromatin immunoprecipitation sequencing (CHIP-seq), molecular genetics 42
chromoblastomycosis 561–562
clinical features 562
differential diagnosis 562
epidemiology 561–562
histology findings 562
laboratory findings 562
pathogenesis 561–562
prevention 562
treatment 562
chromosomal mosaicism and chimaerism, fine and whorled Blaschkolinear hypoand hyperpigmentation (incorporating hypomelanosis of Ito, and linear and whorled naevoid hypermelanosis) 1299
chronic actinic dermatitis (CAD) 953–954
clinical features 954
differential diagnosis 954
epidemiology 953
history 953
laboratory investigation 954
microscopy 954
pathogenesis 953
prevention 954
treatment 954

chronic atrophic candidiasis (chronic denture stomatitis), oral mucosa 2090
chronic atypical neutrophilic dermatosis with lipodystrophy and elevated temperature (CANDLE) syndrome 2019–2020
chronic circumscribed nodular lichenification *see* prurigo nodularis
chronic denture stomatitis (chronic atrophic candidiasis), oral mucosa 2090
chronic erythematous candidosis 547
chronic graft-versus-host disease, oral mucosa 2086–2087
chronic granulomatous disease (CGD) 2037–2041
  clinical features 2037–2038
  differential diagnosis 2038, **2039–2040**
  epidemiology 2037
  histology findings 2038
  immunocompromised children 687
  laboratory findings 2038
  pathogenesis 2037
  prevention 2038–2041
  treatment 2038–2041
chronic hyperplastic candidosis (*Candida leucoplakia*) 547
  oral mucosa 2090
chronic illness or disfigurement during adolescence, approach to the adolescent 2350–2351
chronic inducible urticaria subtypes 755–762
chronic infantile neurological cutaneous and articular syndrome (CINCA) *see* neonatal onset multisystemic inflammatory disorder
chronic inflammatory skin conditions: psoriasis and eczema, laser therapy 2324
chronic localized candidiasis ('candidal granuloma'), chronic mucocutaneous candidiasis (CMC) **2043**
'chronic lyme disease,' lyme borreliosis (LB)/lyme disease 471
chronic meningococcaemia 444
chronic mucocutaneous candidiasis (CMC) 547–548, 549–550, 2041–2045
  autoimmune polyendocrinopathy–candidiasis–ectodermal dystrophy1 (APECED) syndrome (autoimmune polyendocrine syndrome, type 1) **2043**
  CARD9 deficiency **2043**
  chronic localized candidiasis ('candidal granuloma') **2043**
  clinical features 2042
  CMC associated with other syndromes **2044**
  CMC due to increased STAT1 signalling **2043**
  CMC plus susceptibility to mycobacterial infections **2043**
  dectin-1 deficiency **2043**
  differential diagnosis 2042
  epidemiology 2042
  familial chronic nail candidiasis **2044**
  histology findings 2042–2044
  isolated CMC **2043**
  laboratory findings 2042–2044
  late-onset CMC **2044**
  pathogenesis 2042
  variants **2043–2044**
chronic plaque psoriasis **364**
chronic recurrent sialadenitis, oral mucosa 2098
chronic renal failure, white patches (leucoplakia), oral mucosa 2091
chronic spontaneous urticaria 754–755, 757, **758**, 760–761
chronic urticaria **760**
CHS *see* Chédiak–Higashi syndrome
CI *see* congenital ichthyoses
CIAD *see* Childhood Impact of Atopic Dermatitis
ciclosporin
  atopic dermatitis (AD) **257**, 258–259
  psoriasis 371
  systemic therapies 2293–2294
cidofovir, herpes simplex virus (HSV) infections 607
CIDs *see* combined immunodeficiencies
CIE *see* congenital ichthyosiform erythroderma
cigarette burns
  vs impetigo **2413**
  safeguarding issues in paediatric dermatology 2410–2413
cignolin (dithranol, anthralin), psoriasis 369–370, *373*
CIL-F *see* congenital infiltrating lipomatosis of the face
cimicosis (bedbug infestation) 731–732, 734–735
  aetiology 731
  clinical features 732
  diagnosis 732
  epidemiology 731
  pathogenesis 731
  treatment 732
CINCA (chronic infantile neurological cutaneous and articular syndrome) *see* neonatal onset multisystemic inflammatory disorder
CIPA *see* congenital insensitivity to pain with anhidrosis
circumscribed hyperpigmentation 1463–1465
  drug-induced circumscribed hyperpigmentation 1464–1465
  infective causes 1463
  postinflammatory hyperpigmentation 1463–1464
CL *see* cutaneous leishmaniasis
CLAPO syndrome
  PIK3CA-related overgrowth spectrum (PROS) 1291
  syndromic vascular anomalies 1415
Clarke–Howell–Evans–McConnell syndrome *see* tylosis with oesophageal cancer (TOC)
classic sarcoidosis 995–999
  vs Blau syndrome/early-onset sarcoidosis (EOS) **996**
  clinical features 997–998
  cutaneous manifestations 997–998
  differential diagnosis 999
  epidemiology 995–996
  extracutaneous manifestations 998
  history 995
  laboratory findings 998
  pathogenesis 996–997
  pathology 997
  prognosis 998–999
  treatment 999
cleft lip/palate–ectodermal dysplasia syndrome (CLEPD) **1636**
CLEPD syndrome *see* cleft lip/palate–ectodermal dysplasia syndrome
clindamycin, systemic therapies 2284
clitoral cysts 2186
CLM *see* cutaneous larva migrans
Clouston syndrome *see* hidrotic ectodermal dysplasia
CLOVE syndrome *see* congenital lipomatous overgrowth, vascular malformations and epidermal naevus
CM-AVM *see* capillary malformation-arteriovenous malformation
CMC *see* chronic mucocutaneous candidiasis
CMC associated with other syndromes, chronic mucocutaneous candidiasis (CMC) **2044**
CMC due to increased STAT1 signalling, chronic mucocutaneous candidiasis (CMC) **2043**
CMC plus susceptibility to mycobacterial infections, chronic mucocutaneous candidiasis (CMC) **2043**
CMN *see* congenital melanocytic naevi
CMTC *see* van Lohuizen syndrome
CMV *see* cytomegalovirus
Cnidaria 740–742
Cnidaria dermatitis/seabather's eruption 748–749
  clinical features 748
  differential diagnosis 748
  epidemiology 748
  histology findings 748
  laboratory findings 748
  pathogenesis 748
  prevention 748–749
  treatment 748–749
CNVs *see* copy number variations
cobalt, allergic contact dermatitis (ACD) 307
Cobb syndrome 1401
COC *see* combined oral contraceptives
cocamidopropyl betaine (CAPB), allergic contact dermatitis (ACD) 309
coccidioidomycosis 564–565
  clinical features 564–565
  differential diagnosis 564–565
  epidemiology 564
  histology findings 565
  laboratory findings 565
  pathogenesis 564
  prevention 565
  treatment 565
Cockayne syndrome (CS) 1729, 1756–1760

clinical features 1756–1758
clinical tests 1759
differential diagnosis 1758–1759
epidemiology 1756
histopathology 1758
history 1756
laboratory tests 1759
pathogenesis 1756
prevention 1759–1760
treatment 1759–1760
UV-sensitive syndrome, COFS/TTD and CS/TTD 1763
XP/CS complex 1760
coeliac disease (gluten-sensitive enteropathy), oral mucosa 2086
Coffin–Siris syndrome **1637**
COFS syndrome *see* cerebro-oculo-facio-skeletal syndrome
colchicine, systemic therapies 2295
cold-induced skin lesions 989–991
cold panniculitis 1211
clinical features 1211
differential diagnosis 1211
epidemiology 1211
histology findings 1211
pathogenesis 1211
prevention 1211
treatment 1211
cold urticaria 756, 758
Cole disease 1547
clinical features 1547
epidemiology 1547
history 1547
pathogenesis 1547
collagen vascular diseases 1883–1884
collodion baby, nursing care of the skin 2393, **2394–2395**
collodion baby and self-improving congenital ichthyosis 1560, 1596
clinical features 1560
definition 1560
differential diagnosis 1560
pathogenesis 1560
treatment 1560
coloboma, heart defect, ichthyosiform dermatosis, mental retardation, ear anomalies (CHIME) syndrome 1590
clinical features 1590
definition 1590
pathogenesis 1590
treatment 1590
combination therapies, human papillomaviruses (HPV) 596
combined (macrocystic and microcystic) LM, lymphatic malformations (LMs) 1453, **1453**, 1457–1458
combined immunodeficiencies (CIDs), immunocompromised children 685
combined oral contraceptives (COC), acne vulgaris 811
comedogenesis, acne vulgaris 805
comedonal acne 806–807
differential diagnosis **819**
Comel–Netherton syndrome *see* Netherton syndrome (NS)
common skin papules and cysts in childhood, differential diagnosis **1317**
common warts, human papillomaviruses (HPV) 590–591, 596
communication, surgical therapy 2310
comorbidity, metabolic syndrome (MetS) 853–857
complement deficiency disorders 2045–2050
clinical features 2049, **2050**
hereditary angioedema (HAE) 2046–2048
pathogenesis 2048–2049
prevention 2049–2050
treatment 2049–2050
compulsive self-mutilation 2268
conductive deafness, with ptosis and skeletal anomalies **1637**
condyloma acuminata (CA) 2212–2214
aetiology 2213
child sexual abuse (CSA) 2213
clinical features 2213
definition 2212
prognosis 2214
treatment 2213–2214
confidentiality and consent, approach to the adolescent 2350
congenital abnormalities, dermatoglyphics 119
congenital abnormalities of dermatoglyphics 119
congenital adrenal hyperplasia, cutaneous manifestations 2000–2001
congenital and infantile fibrosarcomas 1368–1369
clinical features 1368
differential diagnosis 1368
epidemiology 1368
pathogenesis 1368
pathology 1369
treatment 1369
congenital cartilaginous rests of the neck (wattles) 103–104
congenital cutaneous candidiasis (CCC), neonatal erythroderma 129
congenital cutaneous candidosis 547
congenital/developmental lesions, tongue 2099–2100
congenital disorders, vesiculobullous lesions 864–865
congenital ectodermal dysplasia of the face 1160–1161
congenital eosinophilia 317
congenital erosive and vesicular dermatosis with reticulated supple scarring (CEVD)
clinical features 150
differential diagnosis 150
histology findings 150–151
laboratory findings 150–151
neonates **139**, 150–151
prevention 151
treatment 151
congenital erythropoietic porphyria **137**, **959**, **960**, 963–964, **967**
congenital fascial dystrophy 1168
congenital generalized lipoatrophy (CGL) 1223
congenital granular cell epulis of the newborn, oral mucosa 2094
congenital haemangiomas (CH) 1440–1442
noninvoluting congenital haemangioma (NICH) 1440–1442
rapidly involuting congenital haemangioma (RICH) 1440–1442
congenital hair on the elbows 2134
congenital hairy naevi 2134
congenital hemidysplasia with ichthyosiform naevus and limb defects (CHILD syndrome) 1271–1272, 1577
clinical features 1272
differential diagnosis 1272
histopathology 1272
history 1271
pathogenesis 1272
treatment 1272
congenital hypertrichosis lanuginosa 2132–2133
congenital hypopigmentation 1492–1496
congenital hypotrichosis with juvenile macular dystrophy (HJMD) **1637**
congenital ichthyoses (CI) 1592–1597
balneotherapy 1594
collodion baby and self-improving congenital ichthyosis 1596
ear, nose and throat (ENT) aspects 1595
emollients 1592–1593
future directions 1597
general aspects of therapy 1592
harlequin ichthyosis (HI) 1596
keratolytic agents 1593–1594
lifestyle recommendations 1596
management 1592–1597
nutritional issues and growth 1595–1596
ophthalmological aspects 1595
patient organizations and other resources 1596–1597
psychosocial aspects 1596
scalp therapy 1595
systemic therapies 1594–1595
topical therapies 1592–1594
congenital ichthyosiform erythroderma (CIE) 1561–1566
clinical features 1563–1566
definition 1561
epidemiology 1561–1563
genetic analyses 1566
histology 1566
laboratory findings 1566
pathogenesis 1561–1563
ultrastructure 1566
congenital idiopathic gingival fibromatosis *see* gingival fibromatosis
congenital inclusion dermoid cysts 113–114
see also dermoid cysts
aetiology 113
clinical features 113–114
differential diagnosis 114
pathology 113
treatment 114

congenital infections
bacterial infections 85–86, **87**, **88**, 89–90
fungal infections 86, **87**, **88**, 90
neonates 84–86, **87**
protozoal infections 86, **87**
viral infections 85, **86**, 88
congenital infiltrating lipomatosis of the face (CIL-F) 1198–1200
characteristics **1199**
clinical features **1199**, 1200
differential diagnosis 1200
epidemiology 1200
histology findings 1200
laboratory findings 1200
pathogenesis 1200
prevention 1200
treatment 1200
congenital insensitivity to pain with anhidrosis (CIPA) **1637**
congenital lipomatous overgrowth, vascular malformations and epidermal naevus (CLOVE syndrome) 1269
lymphatic malformations (LMs) **1453**, 1455, 1460
PIK3CA-related overgrowth spectrum (PROS) 1290
syndromic vascular anomalies 1415
congenital lip pits 106
congenital localized hypertrichosis 2134–2135
congenital malalignment of the big toenail 2148–2149
congenital malformations, burden of disease 2257
congenital melanocytic naevi (CMN) 1237–1255, 1304, 2360–2365
see also acquired melanocytic naevi (AMN)
associations 1243–1245
benign proliferations 1237–1240
classification 1240–1243, 2360
classification for practical clinical management 1242–1243
classification for research, publication and accurate sharing of data 1240–1242
clinical features 1237–1240
CMN number and satellites 1240
CMN surface characteristics and benign proliferations 1237–1240
CMN syndrome – extracutaneous features 1242, 1304
colour and lightening 1237
cosmetic aspects of CMN 1252
cutaneous features 1240–1242
dermoscopic features 2362–2365
dermoscopic patterns 2362–2365
dermoscopic structures 2362–2365
endocrinological disorders 1245
epidemiology 1243
extracutaneous features – CMN syndrome 1242, 1304
facial features 1244–1245
genetic counselling 1252
genetic testing 1247–1248
genotype 1242
histopathology 1246
intraparenchymal melanosis 1244
laser therapy 2325–2326
management 1248–1252
melanoma arising in the CNS 1250–1252
melanoma arising in the skin 1250, **1252**
melanoma in CMN 1245
metabolic disorders 1245
multiple CMN management 1249, *1250*
naevus spilus-type CMN 1240, *1241*
neurological abnormalities 1243–1244
new lump or cutaneous change within a CMN 1249–1250, *1251*
new neurological presentation in a patient with CMN 1250, *1251*
other abnormalities of the CNS 1244
other tumours in CMN 1245–1246
pathogenesis 1246–1247
phenotypic subtypes 1240
potential germline predisposition 1247–1248
primary melanoma of the CNS 1245
rhabdomyosarcoma (RMS) 1245–1246
single CMN management 1248–1249
skin care of CMN 1248
surface characteristics 1237–1240
surgical therapy 2312
tardive CMN 1240
congenital midline cervical cleft 105
congenital muscular fibromatosis *see* fibromatosis colli
congenital psoriasis **366**
congenital purpura fulminans caused by defects in the protein C or S pathway 1896
congenital reticular ichthyosiform erythroderma (CRIE) **1568**, 1572
clinical features 1572
differential diagnosis 1572
epidemiology 1572
genetic findings 1572
histology findings 1572
laboratory findings 1572
pathogenesis 1572
prevention 1572
treatment 1572
congenital self-healing reticulo-histiocytosis **139**
congenital smooth muscle hamartoma (CSMH) 110
aetiology 110
clinical features 110
definition 110
differential diagnosis 110
hypertrichosis 2134
pathology 110
treatment 110
congenital syphilis **136**
infectious napkin dermatitis 273–274
connective tissue diseases
calcification and ossification in the skin 1343–1344
oral mucosa 2087
panniculitis 1215–1216
connective tissue naevi (CTN) 1276–1278
clinical features 1277
differential diagnosis 1277
epidemiology 1276
histology findings 1277–1278
intervention 1278
laboratory findings 1277–1278
pathogenesis 1276
treatment 1278
Conradi–Hünermann–Happle syndrome 126, 1160
clinical features 1576
differential diagnosis 1576
pathogenesis 1576
treatment 1576–1577
consent and confidentiality, approach to the adolescent 2350
consent for genetic testing and incidental findings 38
constipation, dystrophic epidermolysis bullosa (DEB) 921–922, 930
constitutional mismatch repair deficiency syndrome *see* Muir–Torre syndrome
consultation settings
approach to the infant and child 2345–2346
approach to the neonate 2343–2344
contact allergy, atopic dermatitis (AD) 256
contact dermatitis, surgical therapy 2318
contact napkin dermatitis **268**, 269–270
contact sensitizers, human papillomaviruses (HPV) 595
contact urticaria 756, **758**, 759
Cook syndrome **1638**
coping strategies, burden of disease 2258–2259
copper deficiency 838
copy number variations (CNVs), molecular genetics 42
corals/anemones (Anthozoa) 741
corals/jellyfish (Hydrozoa) 741
Cornelia de Lange syndrome (CDLS), hypertrichosis 2132–2133
corneodermato-osseous syndrome **1638**
corticosteroids
see also systemic corticosteroids; topical corticosteroids
acne vulgaris 811
allergic contact dermatitis (ACD) 309
dermatitis herpetiformis (DH) 904
infantile haemangiomas (IH) 1436
systemic therapies 2287–2288
cortisol levels alterations, cutaneous manifestations 1996–1998
cosmetic camouflage, vitiligo 1484
Costello syndrome 1740, **1806**, 1861–1862
aetiology 1740, 1861
clinical features 1740, 1861
definition 1740, 1861
diagnosis 1861
differential diagnosis 1740
history 1740, 1861
management 1861–1862
pathogenesis 1740

pathology 1740
prognosis 1740
summary of RASopathies **1858**
surveillance 1862
treatment 1740
Cowden syndrome 1403, **1806**
see also Bannayan–Riley–Ruvalcaba syndrome (BRRS); *PTEN* (Phosphatase and TENsin homologue) hamartoma tumour syndrome (PHTS)
characteristics **1199**
clinical features **1199**, 1201
differential diagnosis 1201
endocrine dysfunction 2009
oral mucosa 2094
cowpox **625**, 638–640
clinical features 638–639
differential diagnosis 639
epidemiology 638
histology findings 639–640
history 638
laboratory findings 639–640
pathogenesis 638
prevention 640
treatment 640
coxsackie-type enterovirus **136**
coxsackievirus A4, neonates **86**
cranial dysraphism
aetiology 111
clinical features 111
cutaneous signs 111
definition 111
differential diagnosis 111
treatment 111
cranial neural tube defect 111
aetiology 111
clinical features 111
definition 111
differential diagnosis 111
treatment 111
cranio-ectodermal syndrome **1638**
CREST syndrome
calcification and ossification in the skin 1343
systemic sclerosis (SSc) 1183, 1184
CRIE *see* congenital reticular ichthyosiform erythroderma
Crohn disease
cutaneous microbiome 52–53
genital signs 2191–2192
oral mucosa 2086
perioral dermatitis with extrafacial genital manifestations and metastatic Crohn disease, napkin dermatitis 276
Cross syndrome 1490
Crowe's sign (skinfold freckling), neurofibromatosis type 1 (NF1) 1825
crusted (Norwegian) scabies, scabies 714–715
cryopyrin-associated periodic syndromes (CAPS) 2012–2013
urticaria 753, **754**, **758**
cryosurgery 2314–2315
cryotherapy, human papillomaviruses (HPV) 594
cryotherapy and curettage, molluscum contagiosum (MC) 584
cryptococcosis 570–571
clinical features 570–571
differential diagnosis 570–571
epidemiology 570
histology findings 571
laboratory findings 571
pathogenesis 570
prevention 571
treatment 571
cryptorchidism, recessive X-linked ichthyosis (RXLI) 1556
CS *see* Cockayne syndrome
CSA *see* child sexual abuse
CSMH *see* congenital smooth muscle hamartoma
CTCL *see* cutaneous T-cell lymphomas
CTN *see* connective tissue naevi
curettage and surgical treatment, human papillomaviruses (HPV) 594
curly hair–ankyloblepharon–nail dysplasia syndrome (CHAND syndrome) **1639**
Cushing disease and Cushing syndrome 1996–1997
clinical features 1996
cutaneous manifestations 1996–1997
histology findings 1996–1997
laboratory findings 1996–1997
pathogenesis 1996
prevention 1997
striae 1173
treatment 1997
cutaneous anaplastic large cell lymphoma (C-ALCL) 1050–1051
clinical features 1050
definition 1050
epidemiology 1050
genetic features 1051
histopathology 1050
immunophenotype 1050–1051
predictive factors 1051
prognosis 1051
treatment 1051
cutaneous and mucocutaneous non-Langerhans cell histiocytoses: the nonxanthogranuloma family (C Group) 1087–1088
cutaneous and mucocutaneous non-Langerhans cell histiocytoses: the xanthogranuloma family (C Group) 1080–1087
benign cephalic histiocytosis (BCH) 1086–1087
generalized eruptive histiocytosis (GEH) 1087
giant cell reticulohistiocytoma (GCRH) 1084
juvenile xanthogranuloma (JXG) 1080–1082
monomorphic types 1082–1087
multicentric reticulohistiocytosis (MRH) 1084–1085
papular xanthoma (PX) 1082–1083
polymorphic type 1080–1082
progressive nodular histiocytosis (PNH) 1085–1086
spindle cell xanthogranuloma 1085
xanthoma disseminatum (XD) 1083–1084
cutaneous B-cell lymphomas 1054–1056
intravascular large B-cell lymphoma 1056
primary cutaneous diffuse large B-cell lymphoma (PCDLBCL) 1055–1056
primary cutaneous follicle centre lymphoma (PCFCL) 1055
primary cutaneous marginal zone B-cell lymphoma (PCMZL) 1054–1055
cutaneous bronchogenic cysts 105
cutaneous candidosis 549
cutaneous defences, endogenous photoprotection 975
cutaneous diseases and the microbiome 51–53
cutaneous Ewing sarcoma 1388–1389
aetiology 1389
clinical features 1389
definition 1388–1389
diagnosis 1389
differential diagnosis 1389
epidemiology 1388–1389
pathogenesis 1389
pathology 1389
treatment 1389
cutaneous larva migrans (CLM) 705–707
aetiology 705
clinical features 705–706
definition 705
diagnosis 706
differential diagnosis 706
epidemiology 705
history 705
pathogenesis 705
prevention 707
prognosis 707
treatment 707
cutaneous leishmaniasis (CL) 693, 695
cutaneous lymphoma, primary *see* primary cutaneous lymphoma
cutaneous mastocytosis 1097–1098, **1104**
cutaneous microbiome 46–55
acne 52
adults 49
analysis methods 50–51
atopic dermatitis (AD) 51–52
breast milk 48–49
Caesarean section delivery 48
collection methods 50–51
commonly encountered cutaneous bacteria **47**
Crohn disease 52–53
cutaneous diseases and the microbiome 51–53
evolution 47–49
exposures affecting the microbiome 47–49
first exposures contribute to the microbiome 47–49
fungal microbiota 54–55
infants 47–49
mode of delivery 48
neonates 47–49
parasites 54–55

cutaneous microbiome (*cont'd*)
  preadolescents and adolescents 49
  psoriasis 52–53
  skin inflammation 49
  terminology **47**
  virome 54–55
cutaneous ossification
  Albright hereditary osteodystrophy (AHO) 1347–1348
  calcification and ossification in the skin 1346–1349
  progressive osseous heteroplasia (POH) 1347
cutaneous polyarteritis nodosa 1879–1882
cutaneous porphyrias 961–965
cutaneous reactions to plants 983–989
cutaneous Rosai–Dorfman disease (C Group) *see* Rosai–Dorfman disease
cutaneous skeletal hypophosphatemia syndrome, naevus sebaceous 1262–1263
cutaneous T-cell and NK cell lymphomas 1045–1054
  mycosis fungoides (MF) 1045–1054
cutaneous T-cell lymphomas (CTCL) 1045–1054
  molecular diagnostics 2390
cutaneous tuberculosis 486–496
  antitubercular therapy (ATT) 495
  BCG vaccine 494
  classification 486–494
  culture 494
  diagnosis 494–495
  drug resistance 495–496
  epidemiology 486
  erythema induratum of Bazin (EIB) 493
  erythema nodosum 494
  histopathology 494
  lichen scrofulosorum (LS) 490–492
  lupus vulgaris (LV) 486–487, *490*
  multidrug resistance (MDR) 495–496
  orificial tuberculosis 490
  papulonecrotic tuberculid (PNT) 492–493
  polymerase chain reaction (PCR) 494–495
  screening 494
  scrofuloderma (SFD) 488, *490*
  sporotrichoid cutaneous tuberculosis 490
  treatment 495–496
  tuberculids 490
  tuberculosis verrucosa cutis 489, *490*
  tuberculous gumma 489–490, *491*
  tuberculous metastatic abscess 489–490, *491*
  warty tuberculosis 489, *490*
cutaneous vasculitis 1865–1884
  acute haemorrhagic oedema of infancy (AHEI) 1870–1872
  antineutrophil cytoplasmic antibody (ANCA)-associated vasculitides (AAV) 1882–1883
  classification **1866**
  collagen vascular diseases 1883–1884
  cutaneous polyarteritis nodosa (PAN) 1879–1882
  erythema elevatum diutinum (EED) 1874–1876
  Henoch-Schonlein purpura (HSP) 1866–1870
  histological classification **1866**
  itching purpura 1878–1879
  Kawasaki disease (KD) 1883
  leukocytoclastic vasculitis 1865–1876
  lichen aureus/lichen purpuricus 1878
  Majocchi disease 1878
  medium vessel vasculitis 1883
  mixed connective tissue disease (MCTD) 1884
  pigmented purpuras 1876–1879
  polyarteritis nodosa (PAN) 1879–1882
  Schamberg disease 1877–1878
  Sjögren–Larsson syndrome (SLS) 1884
  systemic diseases with secondary cutaneous vasculitis 1882–1884
  systemic lupus erythematosus (SLE) 1883–1884
  systemic PAN 1883
  urticarial vasculitis 1872–1874
cutaneovisceral angiomatosis *see* multifocal lymphangioendotheliomatosis (also known as cutaneovisceral angiomatosis) with thrombocytopenia (MLT/CAT)
cutis laxa 1132–1137, 1738
  acquired cutis laxa 1135–1136
  additional inherited conditions with cutis laxa-like phenotypes 1135
  ARCL type I **1134**, 1135
  ARCL type II **1134**, 1135
  ARCL type III (De Barsy syndrome) **1134**, 1135
  arterial tortuosity syndrome (ATS) *1134*, 1135
  autosomal dominant cutis laxa (ADCL) 1133–1135
  clinical features 1132–1136
  differential diagnosis 1136–1137
  histopathology 1136
  inherited forms 1133, **1134**
  laboratory findings 1136
  macrocephaly, alopecia, cutis laxa and scoliosis syndrome (MACS syndrome) **1134**, 1135
  pathogenesis 1132
  postinflammatory elastolysis 1136
  postinflammatory elastolysis and cutis laxa 1155
  treatment 1137
  X-linked cutis laxa (XLCL) **1134**, 1135
cutis marmorata, transient skin disorders in neonates and young infants 75
cutis marmorata telangiectatica congenita (CMTC), laser therapy 2323
cutis tricolor 1505–1506
  clinical features 1506
  differential diagnosis 1506
  epidemiology 1505
  histopathology 1506
  history 1505
  pathogenesis 1506
cutis verticis gyrata (CVG)
  aetiology 101–102
  clinical features 102–103
  definition 101
  developmental anomalies 101–103
  pathology 102
  treatment 103
cutting, superficial self-mutilation 2269
CVG *see* cutis verticis gyrata
CVS *see* chorionic villus sampling
cyclic neutropenia **2039**
cystic eyelids, palmoplantar keratosis, hypodontia and hypotrichosis (Schöpf–Schulz–Passarge syndrome) **1663**, **2110**
cystic fibrosis 1988–1991
  aetiology 1988
  clinical features 1988–1990
  cystic fibrosis and skin wrinkling in alcohol gel 1990
  cystic fibrosis and skin wrinkling in water 1990
  cystic fibrosis presenting as a rash 1989
  definition 1988
  diagnosis 1991
  endocrine manifesations 1989
  gastrointestinal tract 1988–1989
  joints manifesations 1989
  oral mucosa 2098
  pathogenesis 1988
  prevention 1991
  prognosis 1991
  respiratory manifesations 1989
  skin manifesations 1989, 1990–1991
  treatment 1991
cystic warts, human papillomaviruses (HPV) 591
cytokeratins
  ectodermal dysplasias (EDs) 1697
  overview of basic biology 1697
cytomegalovirus (CMV)
  HIV infection 651–652
  neonates 85, **86**
  oral mucosa 2084
cytomegalovirus (CMV or HHV-5) 672–673
  clinical features 672–673
  differential diagnosis 673
  epidemiology 672
  laboratory findings 673
  pathogenesis 672
  prevention 673
  treatment 673
cytophagic histiocytic panniculitis (CHP) 1216–1217
  clinical features 1217
  epidemiology 1216–1217
  histopathology 1217
  pathogenesis 1216–1217
  treatment 1217

dapsone, systemic therapies 2284–2285
dapsone (diaminodiphenylsulfone)
  acne vulgaris 809
  dermatitis herpetiformis (DH) 903–904
Darier disease (DD) 1603–1606
  associated conditions 1605

clinical features 1603–1604
complications 1604–1605
definition 1603
differential diagnosis 1605–1606
epidemiology 1603
histology findings 1605–1606
history 1603
pathogenesis 1603
prognosis 1605
treatment 1606
Darier's sign, mastocytosis 1103
Darier–White disease (dyskeratosis follicularis), oral mucosa 2088
Darling disease 565–567
DBS *see* DeBarsy syndrome
DC *see* dyskeratosis congenita
DCM *see* diffuse cutaneous mastocytosis
dcSSc *see* diffuse cutaneous SSc
DD *see* Darier disease
deafness, onychodystrophy, osteodystrophy, mental retardation and seizures syndrome (DOOR syndrome) **1639**
deafness and onychodystrophy **1639**
DEB *see* dystrophic epidermolysis bullosa
DeBarsy syndrome (DBS) 1730–1731
clinical features 1731
differential diagnosis 1731
epidemiology 1731
histology findings 1731
history 1730–1731
laboratory findings 1731
pathogenesis 1731
treatment 1731
dectin-1 deficiency, chronic mucocutaneous candidiasis (CMC) **2043**
deep fungal infections 560–575
opportunistic mycoses 569–575
subcutaneous mycoses 561–564
systemic mycoses 564–569
deep morphoea 1178
deep mycoses, oral mucosa 2085–2086
deep plantar warts/myrmecia, human papillomaviruses (HPV) 591
deep vein thrombosis (DVT), Proteus syndrome (PS) 1286–1287
deficiency of interleukin-1 receptor antagonist (DIRA) **137**
deficiency of the IL-1 receptor antagonist (DIRA) 2015–2016
deficiency of the IL-36 receptor antagonist (DITRA) 2016
deficiency states, tongue 2100
degranulation, mastocytosis 1102
delayed pressure urticaria 759
dendritic and histiocyte cell lineage, Langerhans cell histiocytosis (LCH) 1071–1072, 1078–1080
dengue 676–677
clinical features 677
differential diagnosis 677
epidemiology 676
laboratory findings 677
pathogenesis 676
prevention 677
treatment 677
Dennie–Morgan lines, atopic dermatitis (AD) 197–198
dental abnormalities, Proteus syndrome (PS) 1286
dental lamina cysts, transient skin disorders in neonates and young infants 78
dental neglect, child abuse and neglect (CAN) 2227
dentition, ectodermal dysplasias (EDs) **1705**
dermatitis, genital area 2160–2162
clinical presentation 2161
differential diagnosis 2161
investigations 2161
management 2162
pathogenesis 2160–2161
prognosis 2161
dermatitis artefacta, physiological habits **2264**
Dermatitis Family Impact (DFI) questionnaire, quality of life (QoL) assessment 2243, 2251
dermatitis herpetiformis (DH) 898–904
age of onset 900
antihistamines 904
associated disorders 901
clinical features 900–901
corticosteroids 904
dapsone (diaminodiphenylsulfone) 903–904
definition 898
diagnostic tests **902**
differential diagnosis 901
distribution of the rash 900
epidemiology 899
follow-up 904
gastrointestinal manifestations 901
gluten-free diet (GFD) 903
histology findings 901–903
history 898–899
laboratory findings 901–903
morphology of the rash 900–901
oral mucosa 2087
pathogenesis 899–900
prevention 904
prognosis 904
screening for autoimmune diseases 903
serological findings 902–903
sex distribution 900
small bowel biopsy 903
sulfapyridine 904
sulfasalazine 904
testing of HLA haplotypes 903
treatment 903–904
vesiculobullous lesions 866, *867*
dermatofibroma
clinical features 1318–1319
course and prognosis 1319
definition 1318
differential diagnosis **1317**
pathogenesis 1318
treatment 1319
dermatofibrosarcoma protuberans (DFSP) 1392–1394
aetiology 1392–1393
clinical features 1393
differential diagnosis 1393
pathogenesis 1392–1393
pathology 1393
treatment 1393–1394
dermatoglyphics, congenital abnormalities 119
dermatographic (dermographic) urticaria 755, 758
dermatological diseases with endocrine dysfunction 2008–2009
see also endocrine disease cutaneous manifestations
Cowden syndrome 2009
Down syndrome 2009
hereditary tumour syndromes 2009
H-syndrome 2009
hypogonadism 2008
hypopituitarism 2008
hypothyroidism 2008
immune dysregulation, polyendocrinopathy, enteropathy, X-linked syndrome (IPEX syndrome) 2009
insulin resistance 2008
LAMB syndrome 2008
Langerhans cell histiocytosis (LCH) 2009
NAME syndrome 2008
Oliver–McFarlane syndrome 2008
POEMS syndrome 2009
Rabson–Mendenhall syndrome 2008
Rothmund–Thomson syndrome 2009
tuberous sclerosis complex (TSC) 2009
Woodhouse–Sakati syndrome 2009
dermatomyositis 1215–1216
calcification and ossification in the skin 1343
histology findings 1215–1216
laboratory findings 1215–1216
panniculitis 1215–1216
treatment 1216
dermatopathia pigmentosa reticularis **1639**
see also Naegeli–Franceschetti–Jadassohn syndrome
hyperpigmentation 1471, *1472*, 1517–1518
keratin disorders 1471, *1472*, 1517–1518
dermatophytoses 527–543
aetiology 528
allylamines 541
athlete's foot (*Tinea pedis*) 535–536, 540, 542–543
azoles 540
clinical features 532–537
collection of specimens 537
culture 538–539
definition 527
diagnosis 537–540
differential diagnosis 540
ecology **528**
endothrix infections 532–534
epidemiology 528, 529–530
fluconazole 540–542
griseofulvin 540, **543**
history 527–528
itraconazole 540–542, **543**

dermatophytoses (*cont'd*)
large-spored ectothrix infections 532
microscopy 537, *538*
molecular diagnostics 539–540
morpholines 541
onychomycosis 536–537
pathogenesis 528, 530–531
pathology 531–532
scalp ringworm 532
small-spored ectothrix infections 532
terbinafine **543**
Tinea capitis 532, *533*, 540, 541–542
Tinea corporis 534, 540, 542
Tinea cruris 535, 540, 542
Tinea faciei 534
Tinea imbricata 535
Tinea incognito 534–535
Tinea manuum 536, 540
Tinea pedis (athlete's foot) 535–536, 540, 542–543
Tinea unguium 536–537, 540, 543
transmission and source of infection 530
treatment 540–543
dermis
embryonic–fetal transition 14–15
neonates 61
dermographic (dermatographic) urticaria 755, 758
dermoid cysts 1320
see also congenital inclusion dermoid cysts
clinical features 1320
course and prognosis 1320
definition 1320
pathogenesis 1320
treatment 1320
dermo-odonto-dysplasia **1639**
dermoscopic structures and their histopathological correlations **2359–2360**
dermoscopy algorithm, melanocytic lesions 2358–2360, *2361*
dermotrichic syndrome **1640**
desmoplastic trichoepithelioma (DTE) 1329–1330
aetiology 1329
diagnosis 1330
differential diagnosis 1330
epidemiology 1329
pathology 1330
presentation 1329–1330
treatment 1330
desmosomes, ectodermal dysplasias (EDs) 1699, *1700*
developing human skin, unique features *see* unique features of developing human skin
developmental anomalies 101–119
accessory tragi 103
amniotic constriction band (amnion rupture sequence) 118–119
aplasia cutis congenita (ACC) 116–118
atretic (rudimentary, sequestrated) meningocoele 112
branchial cysts, sinuses and fistulae 104–105
breast and nipple abnormalities 106–107
cephalocoeles 111
congenital abnormalities of dermatoglyphics 119
congenital cartilaginous rests of the neck (wattles) 103–104
congenital inclusion dermoid cysts 113–114
congenital lip pits 106
congenital midline cervical cleft 105
congenital smooth muscle hamartoma (CSMH) 110
cranial dysraphism 111
cutaneous bronchogenic cysts 105
cutis verticis gyrata (CVG) 101–103
encephalocoele 111
infantile perineal (perianal) protrusion (IPP) 108–109
median raphe cysts and canals of the penis 108
meningoencephalocoele 111
nasal glioma (nasal cerebral heterotopia) 112–113
nipple and breast abnormalities 106–107
polythelia (supernumerary nipples) 106–107
preauricular cysts and sinuses 104
precalcaneal congenital fibrolipomatous hamartoma (PCFH) 109–110
rhabdomyomatous mesenchymal hamartoma (RMH) 110–111
rudimentary (atretic, sequestrated) meningocoele 112
sequestrated, (rudimentary, atretic) meningocoele 112
skin dimples 106
spinal dysraphism 114–116
supernumerary nipples (polythelia) 106–107
thyroglossal duct cysts 105
transverse nasal line 106
umbilicus developmental abnormalities 107–108
developmental soft tissue swellings, oral mucosa 2094
dexmedetomidine, anaesthesia 2337
DFI questionnaire *see* Dermatitis Family Impact questionnaire
DFSP *see* dermatofibrosarcoma protuberans; giant cell fibroblastoma and dermatofibrosarcoma protuberans
DGS *see* DiGeorge syndrome
DH *see* dermatitis herpetiformis
diabetes mellitus 2005–2007
acanthosis nigricans (AN) 2005, *2006*
clinical features 2005–2007
cutaneous manifestations 2005–2007
histology findings 2007
laboratory findings 2007
metabolic syndrome (MetS) 850–852
necrobiosis lipoidica diabeticorum (NLD) 2005, *2006*
pathogenesis 2005
prevention 2007
psoriasis 360
treatment 2007
4′-diaminodiphenylsulfone, systemic therapies 2284–2285
diaper/napkin care, neonatal skin care 65
dietary interventions
acne vulgaris 811
orofacial granulomatosis (OFG) 1019
differential diagnosis, skin nodules and cysts 1313–1323
common skin papules and cysts in childhood **1317**
cutaneous lumps by colour **1315**
cutaneous lumps by surface appearance **1315**
cutaneous lumps by texture **1315**
dermatofibroma **1317**
epidermal cyst **1317**
histological diagnoses of 775 superficial lumps excised in children **1314**
juvenile xanthogranuloma (JXG) **1317**
mastocytoma **1317**
nonvascular nodules and cysts 1316–1322
pilomatricoma (pilomatrixoma) 1316, **1317**
pyogenic granuloma **1317**
skin lumps that are itchy **1316**
skin lumps that may be tender/painful **1316**
spitz naevus **1317**
diffuse congenital ichthyosis 1160
diffuse cutaneous mastocytosis (DCM) **139**, 1101–1102
clinical features 149–150
differential diagnosis 150
epidemiology 149
histology findings 150
laboratory findings 150
neonatal blistering 149–150
neonatal erythroderma 127
pathogenesis 149
prevention 150
treatment 150
diffuse cutaneous SSc (dcSSc) **1185**, *1189*
diffuse 'dry type' atopic dermatitis (AD) 199–200
diffuse epidermolytic palmoplantar keratoderma 1525–1526
clinical features 1526
differential diagnosis 1526
epidemiology 1525–1526
histology findings 1526
history 1525
laboratory findings 1526
pathogenesis 1525–1526
treatment 1526
diffuse hereditary palmoplantar keratodermas with associated features 1529–1537
diffuse hyperpigmentation 1467, 1469–1470
diffuse nonepidermolytic palmoplantar keratoderma 1527–1529
DiGeorge syndrome (DGS) 2051–2052
clinical features 2051–2052

differential diagnosis 2052
epidemiology 2051
histology findings 2052
history 2051
laboratory findings 2052
pathogenesis 2051
prevention 2052
treatment 2052
digital fusion and contracture, dystrophic epidermolysis bullosa (DEB) 927, *928*
Diplopoda (millipedes) 739–740
Diptera (flies) 735–736
DIRA *see* deficiency of interleukin-1 receptor antagonist; deficiency of the IL-1 receptor antagonist
DISABKIDS Atopic Dermatitis Module (DISABKIDS-ADM), quality of life (QoL) assessment, atopic dermatitis (AD) 223
disabling pansclerotic morphoea 1178
discoid atopic dermatitis 199, *200*, 235–236
disease-specific quality of life measures, quality of life (QoL) assessment 2245–2250
disperse dyes, allergic contact dermatitis (ACD) 310
disseminated HSV infection, herpes simplex virus (HSV) infections 603
disseminated superficial actinic porokeratosis 1624
distal and lateral subungual onychomycosis 536
distraction and anaesthesia techniques, surgical therapy 2311
dithranol (anthralin, cignolin), psoriasis 369–370, *373*, 2400, **2401**
DITRA *see* deficiency of the IL-36 receptor antagonist
Divry–van Bogaert syndrome 1418
DNA mutations, molecular genetics 38
DNA repair systems, cellular *see* cellular DNA repair systems
docosanol, herpes simplex virus (HSV) infections 607
DOOR syndrome *see* deafness, onychodystrophy, osteodystrophy, mental retardation and seizures syndrome
doughnut/ring warts, human papillomaviruses (HPV) 591
Dowling–Degos disease (DDD)
hyperpigmentation 1471
keratin disorders 1518
Down syndrome, endocrine dysfunction 2009
doxycycline, acne vulgaris 809
DP *see* dyschromatosis ptychotropica
DRESS *see* drug rash with eosinophilia and systemic symptoms
drug-induced circumscribed hyperpigmentation 1464–1465
drug-induced diffuse hyperpigmentation 1467
drug-induced gingival hyperplasia, oral mucosa 2097
drug-induced hyperpigmentation, oral mucosa 2093
drug rash with eosinophilia and systemic symptoms (DRESS), hypersensitivity reactions to drugs 790–791
drug reactions, HIV infection 653
drug resistance
see also meticillin-resistant *Staphylococcus aureus*
cutaneous tuberculosis 495–496
drugs and nutrients complications, iatrogenic disorders of the newborn 161
drugs that require monitoring 2406–2409, **2407**
dry skin, neonatal skin care 68–70
DSH *see* dyschromatosis symmetrica hereditaria
DTE *see* desmoplastic trichoepithelioma
Dubowitz syndrome **1640**
duck itch 746–748
duck worms 746–748
duct tape, molluscum contagiosum (MC) 585
DUH *see* dyschromatosis universalis hereditaria
Duncan disease (X-linked lymphoproliferative syndrome) **2036**
dupilumab, atopic dermatitis (AD) 259
DVT *see* deep vein thrombosis
dwarfism, cerebral atrophy and keratosis pilaris **2109**
dysbiosis, hidradenitis suppurativa (HS) (acne inversa) 826
dyschromatosis 1499–1510
amyloidosis cutis dyschromica (ACD) 1507–1509, 1510
cutis tricolor 1505–1506
dyschromatosis ptychotropica (DP) 1509
dyschromatosis symmetrica hereditaria (DSH) 1500–1502, 1510
dyschromatosis universalis hereditaria (DUH) 1502–1504, 1510
familial progressive hyperpigmentation and hypopigmentation (FPHH) 1504–1505
other entities associated with dyschromia 1509, *1510*
treatment 1510
Westerhof syndrome 1506–1507
dyschromatosis ptychotropica (DP) 1509
dyschromatosis symmetrica hereditaria (DSH) 1500–1502
clinical features 1501
differential diagnosis **1500**, 1501–1502
epidemiology 1500
histopathology 1502
history 1500
pathogenesis 1500–1501
treatment 1510
dyschromatosis universalis hereditaria (DUH) 1502–1504
clinical features 1502–1504
differential diagnosis 1504
epidemiology 1502
histopathology 1504
history 1502
pathogenesis 1502
treatment 1510
dyschromic and atrophic variation of scleroderma *see* Atrophoderma of Pasini and Pierini
dyshidrotic eczema 231–234
dyskeratosis congenita (autosomal recessive) **1641**
dyskeratosis congenita (DC) 1729, 1793–1795, **1804**
clinical features 1794–1795
differential diagnosis 1795
epidemiology 1794
hereditary benign intraepithelial dyskeratosis 2088
histology findings 1795
history 1793–1794
hyperpigmentation 1471, *1472*
laboratory findings 1795
oral mucosa 2088
pathogenesis 1794
prevention 1795
squamous cell carcinoma (SCC) *1472*
treatment 1795
dyskeratosis congenita, autosomal dominant (Scoggins type) **1641**
dyskeratosis congenita, X-linked **1641**
dyskeratosis follicularis (Darier–White disease), oral mucosa 2088
dyskeratotic and acantholytic epidermal naevus 1270
clinical features 1270
differential diagnosis 1270
histopathology 1270
history 1270
pathogenesis 1270
treatment 1270
dyslipidaemia
metabolic syndrome (MetS) 849–850
psoriasis 359–360
dysphagia, dystrophic epidermolysis bullosa (DEB) 928–930
dysregulated immune response, hidradenitis suppurativa (HS) (acne inversa) 826
dystrophic calcification, calcification and ossification in the skin 1343–1344
dystrophic epidermolysis bullosa (DEB) 907, *908*, 917–932
aetiology 917–918
anaemia 922, 931
anaesthesia 930–931
bullous dermolysis of the newborn 920
cardiac complications 922
classification **910**
clinical features 918–922
complications 922, 927–932
constipation 921–922, 930
definition 917
differential diagnosis 922–923
digital fusion and contracture 927, *928*
dysphagia 928–930
epidermolysis bullosa pruriginosa 920
eyes 922, 931–932
gastrointestinal tract features 921–922
gastro-oesophageal reflux 930

dystrophic epidermolysis bullosa (DEB) (*cont'd*)
  gene, cell and protein therapy 926–927
  genitourinary tract 922
  growth problems 922
  hands features 920–921
  inversa dystrophic epidermolysis bullosa 920
  nail problems 928
  nails features 921
  nutrition 928–930
  nutritional problems 922
  ocular complications 922
  osteoporosis 928
  pain 931
  pathogenesis 917–918
  pathology 918
  physiotherapy and maintenance of mobility 928
  pretibial epidermolysis bullosa 920
  prevention of complications 927–932
  prognosis 922
  renal complications 922
  skin bio-equivalents 926
  skin care 923–925
  skin features 918–920
  systemic therapies 926–927
  teeth 931
  teeth features 922
  topical antimicrobials 925–926
  topical therapies 926–927
  treatment 923–932
  treatment of complications 927–932

ear, nose and throat (ENT) aspects, congenital ichthyoses (CI) 1595
early-onset sarcoidosis *see* Blau syndrome/early-onset sarcoidosis
eating disorders 839–840
  anorexia nervosa/bulimia 839
  obesity 839–840
EB *see* epidermolysis bullosa
EBA *see* epidermolysis bullosa acquisita
Ebola virus (EBOV), oral mucosa 2084
EBS *see* epidermolysis bullosa simplex
EBV *see* Epstein–Barr virus (EBV or HHV-4)
ECCL *see* encephalocraniocutaneous lipomatosis
eccrine angiomatous hamartomas 1281
eccrine differentiation tumours 1333–1336
eccrine naevi 1281, 1335–1336
  aetiology 1335
  diagnosis 1336
  differential diagnosis 1336
  epidemiology 1335
  pathology 1336
  presentation 1336
  prognosis 1336
  treatment 1336
eccrine naevus/mucinous eccrine naevus 1266
eccrine poroma (EP) 1334–1335
  aetiology 1334–1335
  diagnosis 1335
  differential diagnosis 1335
  epidemiology 1334
  pathology 1335
  presentation 1335
  prognosis 1335
  treatment 1335
eccrine sweat gland formation, developing human skin 25–28
ECD *see* Erdheim–Chester disease
Echinoidea (sea-urchins) 742
echovirus, neonates **86**
ecthyma 427
ecthyma gangrenosum **139**
  pseudomonal skin disease *447*, 449
ectodermal defect with skeletal abnormalities **1642**
ectodermal dysplasia 4; pure hair and nail type **1643**
ectodermal dysplasia 10A, hypohidrotic/hair/nail type, autosomal dominant; includes Jorgenson syndrome **1650**
ectodermal dysplasia 10B, hypohidrotic/hair/tooth type, autosomal recessive **1650**
ectodermal dysplasia and neurosensory deafness **1642**
ectodermal dysplasias (EDs) 1629–1705
  Ackerman syndrome **1631**
  acro-dermato-ungual-lacrimal- tooth syndrome (ADULT syndrome) **1632**, 1682
  acrorenal field defect, ectodermal dysplasia, lipoatrophic diabetes (AREDYLD) syndrome **1631**
  ADULT syndrome 1682
  AEC syndrome (Hay–Wells syndrome) 1678–1681
  alopecia–anosmia– deafness–hypogonadism syndrome **1632**
  alopecia–onychodysplasia–hypohidrosis **1632**
  alopecia–onychodysplasia–hypohidrosis–deafness **1632**
  alopecia universalis congenita (ALUNC; generalized atrichia) **1633**
  alopecia universalis–onychodystrophy–total vitiligo **1633**
  amelo onycho hypohidrotic dysplasia **1633**
  ankyloblepharon–ectodermal defects–cleft lip and palate (AEC) syndrome **1633**
  anonychia–onychodystrophy with brachydactyly type b and ectrodactyly **1633**
  anonychia with flexural pigmentation **1633**
  arthrogryposis and ectodermal dysplasia **1634**
  atrichia with papular lesions **1634**
  atrichia with papular lesions; alopecia universalis congenita 1690
  autoimmune polyendocrinopathy–candidiasis–ectodermal dystrophy (APECED) syndrome **1634**
  autosomal dominant anhidrotic ED with T cell immunodeficiency 1675
  Baisch syndrome **1634**
  Bart–Pumphrey syndrome 1695
  Basan syndrome **1631**
  blepharocheilodontic syndrome **1634**
  book dysplasia **1635**
  brachymetapody–anodontia–hypotrichosis–albinoidism **1635**
  Camarena syndrome **1635**
  cardiofaciocutaneous syndrome **1635**
  Carey syndrome **1636**
  cartilage–hair hypoplasia syndrome **1636**
  Carvajal syndrome **1636**
  Carvajal syndrome (PPK with left ventricular cardiomyopathy and woolly hair) 1701
  cataract, hypertrichosis, mental retardation (CAHMR) syndrome **1636**
  cataract–alopecia–sclerodactyly syndrome **1636**
  classification 1630–1669
  cleft lip/palate–ectodermal dysplasia syndrome (CLEPD) **1636**
  clinical characteristics 1630–1669
  Coffin–Siris syndrome **1637**
  conductive deafness, with ptosis and skeletal anomalies **1637**
  congenital hypotrichosis with juvenile macular dystrophy (HJMD) **1637**
  congenital insensitivity to pain with anhidrosis (CIPA) **1637**
  Cook syndrome **1638**
  corneodermato-osseous syndrome **1638**
  cranio-ectodermal syndrome **1638**
  curly hair–ankyloblepharon–nail dysplasia syndrome (CHAND syndrome) **1639**
  cytokeratins 1697
  deafness, onychodystrophy, osteodystrophy, mental retardation and seizures syndrome (DOOR syndrome) **1639**
  deafness and onychodystrophy **1639**
  definition 1630
  dentition **1705**
  dermatopathia pigmentosa reticularis **1639**
  dermo-odonto-dysplasia **1639**
  dermotrichic syndrome **1640**
  desmosomes 1699, *1700*
  Dubowitz syndrome **1640**
  dyskeratosis congenita (autosomal recessive) **1641**
  dyskeratosis congenita, autosomal dominant (Scoggins type) **1641**
  dyskeratosis congenita, X-linked **1641**
  ectodermal defect with skeletal abnormalities **1642**
  ectodermal dysplasia 4; pure hair and nail type **1643**
  ectodermal dysplasia 10A, hypohidrotic/hair/nail type, autosomal dominant; includes Jorgenson syndrome **1650**
  ectodermal dysplasia 10B, hypohidrotic/hair/tooth type, autosomal recessive **1650**

ectodermal dysplasia and neurosensory deafness **1642**
ectodermal dysplasias caused by mutations in tumour necrosis factor like/NF-κB signalling pathways 1669–1675
ectodermal dysplasia with adrenal cyst **1643**
ectodermal dysplasia with distinctive facies and preaxial polydactyly of feet **1643**
ectodermal dysplasia with ectrodactyly and macular dystrophy (EEM syndrome) **1643**
ectodermal dysplasia with mental retardation and syndactyly **1643**
ectodermal dysplasia with natal teeth **1642**
ectodermal dysplasia with palatal paralysis **1642**
ectodermal dysplasia with severe mental retardation **1642**
ectodermal dysplasia with short stature **1642**
ectodermal dysplasia with syndactyly **1643**
ectrodactyly and ectodermal dysplasia without cleft lip/palate (eec without cleft lip/ palate) **1644**
ectrodactyly–ectodermal dysplasia-cleft lip/palate (EEC1) syndrome **1644**
ectrodactyly–ectodermal dysplasia-cleft lip/palate syndrome (EEC3) **1643**
EEC syndrome 1681–1682
EGFR-related ectodermal dysplasia-like disease 1684
Ellis–van Creveld syndrome **1644–1645**
essential aspects 1630
Fischer syndrome (Fischer–Volavsek syndrome) **1645**
focal dermal hypoplasia (FDH) (Goltz syndrome) 1689–1690
focal dermal hypoplasia syndrome **1645**
focal facial dermal dysplasia, type I (FFDD type I) **1646**
focal facial dermal dysplasia, type II (FFDD type II) **1646**
focal facial dermal dysplasia, type III **1646**
focal facial dermal dysplasia, type IV **1646**
focal nonepidermolytic PPK 1698
fried tooth and nail syndrome **1646**
gap junction proteins 1691–1695
gingival fibromatosis and hypertrichosis **1646**
gingival fibromatosis–sparse hair–malposition of teeth **1646**
Gorlin–Chaudhry–Moss syndrome **1647**
growth retardation–alopecia–pseudoanodontia–optic atrophy (GAPO) **1647**
Haim–Munk syndrome (HMS) **1647**
hair loss 2111
Hallerman–Streiff syndrome **1648**
Hayden syndrome **1648**
Hay–Wells syndrome (AEC syndrome) 1678–1681
hereditary mucoepithelial dysplasia **1648**
hidrotic ectodermal dysplasia (Clouston syndrome, ED2) **1649**, 1692–1693
hidrotic ectodermal dysplasia, Christianson– Fourie type **1649**
hypertrichosis and dental defects **1649**
hypohidrotic ectodermal dysplasia (HED) with deafness **1650**
hypohidrotic ectodermal dysplasia (HED) with hypothyroidism and agenesis of the corpus callosum **1651**
hypohidrotic ectodermal dysplasia (HED) with hypothyroidism and ciliary dyskinesia (HEDH syndrome) **1650–1651**
hypohidrotic ectodermal dysplasia (HED) with immune deficiency **1650**
hypohidrotic ectodermal dysplasia (HED) with immune deficiency, osteopetrosis and lymphoedema **1650**
hypohidrotic ectodermal dysplasia (HED) with immunodeficiency 1675
hypohidrotic ectodermal dysplasia (HED) with immunodeficiency with osteopetrosis and lymphoedema 1675
hypohidrotic ectodermal dysplasia (HED) -X-linked (ED1) **1649**
hypotrichosis and recurrent skin vesicles **1651**, 1701–1702
hypotrichosis–osteolysis–periodontitis–palmoplantar keratoderma syndrome (HOPP syndrome) **1651**
hypotrichosis simplex **1651**
hypotrichosis simplex of the scalp 1702
hypotrichosis with juvenile macular degeneration 1702
ichthyosis follicularis, atrichia and photophobia syndrome (IFAP syndrome) **1652**
immune dysfunction with T-cell inactivation due to calcium entry defect 1 and 2 (immunodeficiency 9 and 10) **1652**
incontinentia pigmenti (IP) **1652**
Johanson–Blizzard syndrome **1652–1653**
keratin disorders 1520
keratitis ichthyosis deafness syndrome (KID syndrome) **1653**, 1693–1694
keratosis palmoplantaris striata I (PPKS1) **1653**, 1701
keratosis palmoplantaris striata II (PPKS2) **1653**
keratosis palmoplantaris striata III (PPKS3) **1653**, 1699
keratosis palmoplantaris striata type II (PPKS2) 1701
Kirghizian dermato-osteolysis **1653**
Kohlschutter–Tonz syndrome **1633**
Lelis syndrome **1654**
limb–mammary syndrome **1654**
LMS syndrome 1682
localized autosomal recessive hypotrichosis, type 1 (LAH1) **1654**, 1701
localized autosomal recessive hypotrichosis, type 2 (LAH2) **1655**
localized autosomal recessive hypotrichosis, type 3 (LAH3) **1655**
management 1704–1705
Margarita Island ED (allelic to cleft lip/palate–ectodermal dysplasia syndrome [CLEPD1]) **1655**
Marshall syndrome (allelic to Stickler syndrome [108300], but no ectodermal dysplasia in Stickler syndrome) **1655**
McGrath syndrome **1655**
melanoleucoderma, infantilism, mental retardation, hypodontia, hypotrichosis **1656**
mesomelic dwarfism–skeletal abnormalities–ectodermal dysplasia **1656**
molecular basis 1630–1669
molecular pathways 1669–1671
monilethrix **1656**, 1697–1698
mutations in structural and adhesive molecules, disorders caused by 1697–1702
Naegeli–Franceschetti–Jadassohn syndrome (NFJS) **1657**, 1698–1699
nail disorders 2156
Naxos disease **1657**, 1700–1701
neonatal erythroderma 127
nonsyndromic SHFM 1682
oculodentodigital dysplasia 1695
oculo-dentodigital dysplasia (ODDD) syndrome, autosomal dominant **1657**
oculo-dentodigital dysplasia (ODDD) syndrome, autosomal recessive **1657–1658**
oculotrichodysplasia **1658**
odontomicronychial dysplasia **1658**
odonto-onycho-dermal dysplasia syndrome (OODD syndrome) **1658**, 1686–1688
oligodontia-colorectal cancer syndrome **1658**
onychotrichodysplasia and neutropenia **1658**
orofaciodigital (OFD) syndrome type 1 **1659**
pachyonychia congenita (PC) 1698
pachyonychia congenita, autosomal recessive type **1659**
pachyonychia congenita type 2 **1659**
palmoplantar hyperkeratosis with congenital alopecia **1659**
palmoplantar keratoderma with deafness **1660**
Papillon–Lefevre syndrome **1660**

ectodermal dysplasias (EDs) (*cont'd*)
pili torti and developmental delay **1660**
pili torti and onychodysplasia **1660**
pilodental dysplasia with refractive errors **1660**
poikiloderma with neutropenia **1660**
polyposis, skin pigmentation, alopecia and fingernail changes **1661**
'pure' hair-nail type 1520, 1698
Rapp–Hodgkin syndrome **1661**
Rosselli–Gulienetti syndrome **1661**
Rothmund–Thomson syndrome (RTS) **1661**
Sabina brittle hair and mental deficiency syndrome **1662**
scalp–ear–nipple syndrome **1662**
Schinzel–Giedion midface retraction syndrome **1662–1663**
Schöpf–Schulz–Passarge syndrome (cystic eyelids, palmoplantar keratosis, hypodontia and hypotrichosis) **1663**
Sener syndrome **1663**
sensorineural hearing loss, enamel hypoplasia and nail defects **1663**
short-limb skeletal dysplasia with severe combined immunodeficiency **1631**
skeletal anomalies–ectodermal dysplasia–growth and mental retardation **1663**
skin fragility syndrome (McGrath syndrome) 916–917, 1699–1700
skin fragility–woolly hair syndrome **1664**, 1701
split hand-foot malformation (SHFM1) **1664**
split hand-foot malformation 4 **1664**
SSP syndrome (SSPS) 1688–1689
steatocystoma multiplex 1698
taurodontia, absent teeth and sparse hair **1664**
TDO syndrome 1683
tetramelic deficiencies, ectodermal dysplasia, deformed ears and other abnormalities **1664**
thumb deformity and alopecia **1665**
TP63-related phenotypes: overview of molecular pathway 1677–1678
transcription factors and homeobox genes: major regulators of gene expression 1677–1684
transcription factors other than *p63* 1682–1683
trichodental dysplasia **1665**
trichodento-osseous syndrome **1665**
tricho-odonto-onychial dysplasia **1665**
tricho-odonto-onychial dysplasia with bone deficiency **1666**
tricho-odonto-onycho dermal syndrome **1665**
tricho-onycho-dental (TOD) dysplasia **1666**
trichorhinophalangeal syndrome type II **1666**
trichorhinophalangeal syndrome types I and III **1666**
trichothiodystropy 4, nonphotosensitive **1667**
TRPS type I, II, III syndromes 1683–1684
ulnar mammary syndrome **1667**
uncombable hair, retinal pigmentary dystrophy, dental anomalies and brachydactyly **1667**
uncombable hair syndrome (UHS 1) 1699
Vohwinkel syndrome (VS) 1694–1695
Weyer acrofacial dysostosis **1667**
Witkop syndrome **1667**
Wnt-β-catenin pathway 1686–1690
woolly hair, hypotrichosis, everted lower lip and outstanding ears **1668**
xeroderma–talipes–enamel defect (XTE syndrome) **1668**
X-linked, autosomal dominant and recessive HED 1671–1675
X-linked tooth agenesis **1668**
Zanier–Roubicek syndrome **1668**
ectodermal dysplasia/skin fragility syndrome (McGrath syndrome) 916–917, 1699–1700
hair loss 2111
ectodermal dysplasia with adrenal cyst **1643**
ectodermal dysplasia with distinctive facies and preaxial polydactyly of feet **1643**
ectodermal dysplasia with ectrodactyly and macular dystrophy (EEM syndrome) **1643**
ectodermal dysplasia with mental retardation and syndactyly **1643**
ectodermal dysplasia with natal teeth **1642**
ectodermal dysplasia with palatal paralysis **1642**
ectodermal dysplasia with severe mental retardation **1642**
ectodermal dysplasia with short stature **1642**
ectodermal dysplasia with syndactyly **1643**
ectodysplasin A (EDA-1) gene, hair loss 2111
ectrodactyly, ectodermal dysplasia and cleft lip/ palate (EEC) syndrome 1681–1682
clinical features 1681–1682
craniofacial features 1681
definition 1681
differential diagnosis 1682
ectodermal structures 1681
hair features 1681
history 1681
nails features 1681
pathology 1681
prognosis 1682
skin features 1681
sweat glands features 1681
teeth features 1681
treatment 1682
ectrodactyly and ectodermal dysplasia without cleft lip/palate (EEC without cleft lip/ palate) **1644**
ectrodactyly–ectodermal dysplasia-cleft lip/palate (EEC1) syndrome **1644**
ectrodactyly–ectodermal dysplasia-cleft lip/palate syndrome (EEC3) **1643**
eczema
see also atopic dermatitis (AD)
aetiology 187–190
association studies 185–190
bleach baths 2399
filaggrin (filament aggregating protein; FLG) 187–189
future directions 190–191
GARP (glycoprotein A repetitions predominant)/LRRC32 (leucine-rich repeat-containing protein 32) 190
genes implicated in aetiology 187–190
genetic basis 185
genetic dissection 185–186
laser therapy 2324
nursing care of the skin 2396–2399
paste bandages 2397–2398, *2400*, **2401**
subtypes/phenotypes 200
terminology 185
T-helper 2 (Th2) cytokine cluster 189–190
therapeutic clothing 2398–2399
wet wrap dressings 2397, **2398**, **2399**
eczema herpeticum (EH)
atopic dermatitis (AD) 247–248
differential diagnosis 629, **630**
herpes simplex virus (HSV) infections 604
eczema-psoriasis overlap 356
eczematoid- like purpura of Doucas and Kapetanakis *see* itching purpura
eczematous dermatitis, HTLV-1 infection **656**
eczematous/papulosquamous napkin dermatitis **269**
eczematous psoriasis 356
EDAR-associated death domain gene, hair loss 2111
EDM *see* extensive or atypical dermal melanocytosis
EDP *see* erythema dyschromicum perstans
EDs *see* ectodermal dysplasias
EDS *see* Ehlers–Danlos syndromes
EDV *see* epidermodysplasia verruciformis
EEC syndrome *see* ectrodactyly, ectodermal dysplasia and cleft lip/ palate syndrome
EED *see* erythema elevatum diutinum
EEM syndrome *see* ectodermal dysplasia with ectrodactyly and macular dystrophy syndrome
EF *see* eosinophilic fasciitis
EFA *see* essential fatty acids
EGFR-related ectodermal dysplasia-like disease 1684
EGPA *see* eosinophilic granulomatosis with polyangiitis
EGW *see* external genital warts
EH *see* eczema herpeticum
Ehlers–Danlos, progeroid type 1741–1742
aetiology 1741
clinical features 1741–1742

definition 1741
differential diagnosis 1742
history 1741
pathogenesis 1741
pathology 1741
prognosis 1742
treatment 1742
Ehlers–Danlos syndromes (EDS) 1111–1122
arthrochalasia type (previously types VIIA and B) 1112, 1119–1120
Beighton scoring system **1117**
brittle cornea syndrome 1113, 1121
calcification and ossification in the skin 1344
cardiac-valvular type 1113, 1121
cardiovascular aspects 1116
classical-like type 1113, 1121
classical type (previously types I and II) 1112, 1118
classification **1113–1114**
clinical features 1113–1121
cutaneous aspects 1113–1115
dental and oral aspects 1117
dermatosparaxis type (previously type VIIC) 1112, 1120
diagnostic investigations 1121
differential diagnosis 1117–1118
epidemiology 1111–1113
gastrointestinal aspects 1117
genetic features **1113–1114**
genitourinary aspects 1116
history 1111
hypermobility type (previously type III) 1112, 1118
kyphoscoliotic type (previously type VIA) 1112, 1119
musculocontractural type (previously type VIB) 1112, 1119
musculoskeletal aspects 1115–1116
myopathic type 1113, 1121
neurological aspects 1116–1117
obstetric complications 1117
ocular aspects 1117
pathogenesis 1111–1113
periodontal type (previously type VIII) 1112, 1120
spondylodysplastic type 1112–1113, 1120–1121
subtypes 1118–1121
treatment 1121–1122
vascular type (previously type IV) 1112, 1115, *1116*, 1118–1119
EI *see* epidermolytic ichthyosis; erythema infectiosum
EIB *see* erythema induratum of Bazin
EKV *see* erythrokeratoderma variabilis
EKVP *see* erythrokeratoderma variabilis progressiva
electromagnetic spectrum *970*, *971*
electrosurgery, molluscum contagiosum (MC) 584
ELISA *see* enzyme-linked immunosorbent assay
elliptical excision, surgical therapy 2316
Ellis–van Creveld syndrome **1644–1645**
EM *see* erythema migrans; erythema multiforme
embolization, infantile haemangiomas (IH) 1437
embryogenesis of the skin 1–33
embryonic–fetal transition 10–15
embryonic skin 3–9
fetal skin 16–19
time-scale of skin development 2, *3*
unique features of developing human skin 20–33
embryonic–fetal transition 10–15
dermis 14–15
embryogenesis of the skin 10–15
hypodermis 15
intermediate cells 11–12
keratinocytes 11–12, *13*
Langerhans cells 13
melanocytes *11*, 12–13
Merkel cells 13
periderm 11–12
subcutaneous tissue *11*, 14–15
embryonic skin 3–9
embryogenesis of the skin 3–9
epidermis 3–9
Langerhans cells 4–5, *6*
Merkel cells 6, *9*
EMLA *see* eutectic mixture of local anaesthetics
emollients
atopic dermatitis (AD) 70, 254
congenital ichthyoses (CI) 1592–1593
neonatal skin care 68–70
potentially irritant or hazardous components **69**
emulsifiers, neonatal skin care 69
EN *see* epidermal naevi; erythema nodosum
encephalocoele 111
encephalocraniocutaneous lipomatosis (ECCL) 1200–1201, 1280–1281
characteristics **1199**
clinical features **1199**, 1200
differential diagnosis 1200–1201
epidemiology 1200
histology findings 1201
laboratory findings 1201
pathogenesis 1200
prevention 1201
treatment 1201
en coup de sabre morphoea 1177, *1178*
endemic pemphigus 873
endemic syphilis 515–521
aetiology 515, 516
characteristics **519**
differential diagnosis 519, **520**
distribution 516
history 515–516
laboratory tests 519–520
pathology 517
prognosis 521
treatment 520–521
endemic treponematoses 515–521
endocrine and metabolic disorders, hyperpigmentation 1467
endocrine disease cutaneous manifestations 1993–2009
see also dermatological diseases with endocrine dysfunction
adrenal insufficiency 1997–1998
androgen excess 2000–2001
cortisol levels alterations 1996–1998
Cushing disease and Cushing syndrome 1996–1997
dermatological diseases with endocrine dysfunction 2008–2009
diabetes mellitus 2005–2007
hyperparathyroidism 2003–2004
hyperpituitarism 2005
hyperthyroidism 1994–1995
hypogonadism 1998–1999
hypoparathyroidism 2002–2004
hypopituitarism 2004
hypothyroidism 1993–1994
insulin-related disorders 2005–2008
insulin resistance 2007–2008
Klinefelter syndrome 1999
oestrogen excess 2001
parathyroid hormone dysfunction 2002–2004
pituitary dysfunction 2004–2005
precocious puberty 1999–2000
sex hormones disorders 1998–2001
thyroid hormone levels alterations 1993–1995
Turner syndrome 1999
endocrinological disorders, congenital melanocytic naevi (CMN) 1245
end-of-life care in paediatrics, approach to the paediatric patient 2354
endogenous photoprotection 975
cutaneous defences 975
skin phototypes 975
endonyx onychomycosis 536
endothrix infections 532–534
ENS *see* epidermal naevus syndromes
ENT aspects *see* ear, nose and throat (ENT) aspects
enteroviral infections 668–670
enteroviruses (EV), oral mucosa 2084
enthesitis-related arthritis, juvenile idiopathic arthritis (JIA) 1936
environmental factors affecting epidermal integrity, neonatal skin care 64
environmental or plant mites, pseudoscabies 721
environmental risk factors
atopic dermatitis (AD) 179–180
psoriasis 351
enzyme-linked immunosorbent assay (ELISA)
lyme borreliosis (LB)/lyme disease 470
rickettsial disease 511
eosinophilia in older children 318
eosinophilic cellulitis (Wells syndrome) 328–330
eosinophilic fasciitis (EF) 331–332, 1178
clinical features 332
differential diagnosis 332
epidemiology 331–332
histology findings 332
history 331
laboratory findings 332
pathogenesis 331–332
treatment 332
eosinophilic granulomatosis with polyangiitis (EGPA), antineutrophil cytoplasmic antibody (ANCA)-associated vasculitides (AAV) 1883

eosinophilic panniculitis 333–334
clinical features 333
differential diagnosis 333
epidemiology 333
histology findings 333
pathogenesis 333
prevention 334
treatment 334
eosinophilic pustular folliculitis in infancy and childhood 318–322
clinical features 320
differential diagnosis 320–321
epidemiology 318–320
histopathology 321–322
history 318
laboratory findings 321
pathogenesis 318–320
treatment 322
EP *see* eccrine poroma
EPDS *see* erosive pustular dermatosis of the scalp
epidermal cyst 1319
clinical features 1319
course and prognosis 1319
definition 1319
differential diagnosis **1317**
pathogenesis 1319
treatment 1319
epidermal homeostasis disorders, neonatal erythroderma 126–127
epidermal naevi (EN) 1260–1272
angora hair naevus 1266
Becker naevus (BN) 1265–1266
birthmarks in the genital area 2171–2172
congenital hemidysplasia with ichthyosiform naevus and limb defects (CHILD syndrome) 1271–1272
cutaneous mosaicism 1260
dyskeratotic and acantholytic epidermal naevus 1270
eccrine naevus/mucinous eccrine naevus 1266
epidermal naevus syndrome (ENS) 1260–1261
epidermolytic hyperkeratotic epidermal naevus 1270
ILVEN 1270–1271
keratinocytic epidermal naevus (KEN) 1267–1269
linear Cowden naevus 1269
naevus comedonicus (NC) 1263–1264
naevus marginatus 1272
naevus sebaceous 1261–1263
naevus trichilemnocysticus 1266–1267
nonorganoid epidermal naevi 1267–1272
organoid epidermal naevi 1261–1267
papular epidermal naevus with skyline basal cell layer (PENS) 1269–1270
porokeratotic eccrine ostial and dermal duct naevus (PEODDN) 1264–1265
Proteus syndrome (PS) 1269
segmentally arranged basaloid follicular hamartomas 1267
surgical therapy 2313
woolly hair naevus 1266
epidermal naevus syndromes (ENS) 1260–1261
epidermal necrolysis *see* toxic epidermal necrolysis (TEN)
epidermis
embryonic skin 3–9
environmental factors affecting epidermal integrity 64
neonates 57–60, 64
epidermodysplasia verruciformis (EDV) **1803**, 1811–1812
clinical features 1811–1812
differential diagnosis 1812
histology findings 1812
human papillomaviruses (HPV) 592
pathogenesis 1811
treatment 1812
epidermoid carcinoma *see* squamous cell carcinoma
epidermolysis bullosa (EB) **137**, **140**, 907–935
see also junctional epidermolysis bullosa (JEB); Kindler syndrome
classification 907–909, **910**
diagnosis 907–909
nail disorders 2156
neonates 2395–2396
nursing care of the skin 2395–2396
oral mucosa 2087
epidermolysis bullosa, recessive dystrophic **1803**
epidermolysis bullosa acquisita (EBA) 882–885
clinical features 883, *885*, *886*
differential diagnosis 883
epidemiology 883
histology findings 883–884
laboratory findings 883–884, *887*
neonates 98
pathogenesis 883
prevention 885
treatment 885
epidermolysis bullosa pruriginosa 920
epidermolysis bullosa simplex (EBS) 907, *908*
acantholytic EB due to desmoplakin deficiency 917
acantholytic EB due to plakoglobin deficiency 917
acral peeling skin syndrome 916
aetiology 909–910
autosomal recessive epidermolysis bullosa simplex due to keratin 14 mutations 914–915
classification **910**
clinical features 910–912
definition 909
differential diagnosis 913
EBS due to BP230 mutations 915
EBS due to exophilin 5 mutations 915
EBS generalized intermediate (Köbner) 911
EBS generalized severe (Dowling–Meara) 911–912, *913*
EBS Ogna type 915–916
EBS with mottled pigmentation 914
EBS with muscular dystrophy 915
EBS with pyloric atresia 915
epidermolysis bullosa superficialis 916
keratin disorders 1517
localized (Weber–Cockayne) epidermolysis bullosa simplex 910–911
pathogenesis 909–910
pathology 910
prognosis 912–913
skin fragility–ectodermal dysplasia syndrome 916–917
skin fragility–woolly hair syndrome due to desmoplakin deficiency 917
skin fragility–woolly hair syndrome due to plakoglobin deficiency 917
suprabasal epidermolysis bullosa simplex 916–917
treatment 913–914
variations 909
epidermolytic hyperkeratosis *see* epidermolytic ichthyosis
epidermolytic hyperkeratotic epidermal naevus 1270
clinical features 1270
differential diagnosis 1270
histopathology 1270
pathogenesis 1270
treatment 1270
epidermolytic ichthyosis (EI) 125–126, **138**, **140**, 1518–1520, 1567–1570
clinical features 1567–1570
epidemiology 1567
pathogenesis 1567
epidermolytic naevi (mosaic epidermolytic ichthyosis) 1570–1571
differential diagnosis 1570–1571
genetic findings 1571
histology findings 1571
laboratory findings 1571
prevention 1571
treatment 1571
epiloia *see* tuberous sclerosis complex
episodic urticaria **758**
epithelial cyst *see* epidermal cyst
epithelioid sarcoma (ES) 1387
aetiology 1387
clinical features 1387
definition 1387
differential diagnosis 1387
epidemiology 1387
pathogenesis 1387
pathology 1387
treatment 1387
epithelioma calcificans Malherbe *see* pilomatricoma
EPP *see* erythropoietic protoporphyria
Epstein–Barr viral infection, oral mucosa 2084
Epstein–Barr virus (EBV or HHV-4), infectious mononucleosis (IM) 671–672, 2084
Epstein pearls, transient skin disorders in neonates and young infants 77
Epstein pearls and Bohn nodules (gingival cysts of infancy), oral mucosa 2088

Erdheim–Chester disease (ECD) 1091
clinical features 1091
differential diagnosis 1091
epidemiology 1091
histology findings 1091
history 1091
pathogenesis 1091
prognosis 1091
treatment 1091
erosive and or blistering napkin eruption 2179, *2180*
erosive or ulcerative skin lesions
autoimmune causes **139**
causes **138–139**
differential diagnosis **138–139**
genodermatoses **140**
infective causes **138–139**
mechanical and/or iatrogenic causes **138**
neonates 150–151
erosive pustular dermatosis of the scalp (EPDS)
clinical features 146
differential diagnosis 146
epidemiology 146
histology findings 146
laboratory findings 146
neonates 145–146
pathogenesis 146
prevention 146
treatment 146
eruption cyst
oral mucosa 2094
transient skin disorders in neonates and young infants 78–79
eruptive, acute lichen planus 396
eruptive hypomelanosis 681–683
aetiology 682
atypical presentations 682
clinical features 682
definition 681
differential diagnosis 682–683
epidemiology 681–682
history 681
pathology 682
treatment 683
eruptive pseudoangiomatosis 676
clinical features 676, 677
differential diagnosis 676, 677
laboratory findings 676, 677
prevention 676, 677
treatment 676, 677
eruptive vellus hair cysts 1320–1321
clinical features 1321
course and prognosis 1321
definition 1320
pathogenesis 1320
pathology 1321
treatment 1321
erysipelas 428
erysipeloid 460–462
clinical features 460–461
diagnosis 461
differential diagnosis 461
epidemiology 460
laboratory findings 461
pathogenesis 460
prevention 462
treatment 462
erythema, generalized, HTLV-1 infection **656**
erythema annulare centrifugum 764–766
clinical features 765–766
differential diagnosis 765–766
epidemiology 764–765
histology findings 766
history 764
laboratory findings 766
pathogenesis 764–765
treatment 766
erythema dyschromicum perstans (EDP), hyperpigmentation 1465
erythema elevatum diutinum (EED) 1874–1876
clinical manifestations 1875
definition 1874–1875
differential diagnosis 1875
epidemiology 1875
histology 1875
history 1874–1875
laboratory findings 1875
pathogenesis 1875, *1876*
prognosis 1876
treatment 1876
erythema gyratum repens **765**, 767
clinical features 767
differential diagnosis 767
epidemiology 767
histology findings 767
history 767
laboratory findings 767
pathogenesis 767
treatment 767
erythema induratum of Bazin (EIB) 493
erythema infectiosum (EI) 665–666
clinical features 665
differential diagnosis 666
epidemiology 665
laboratory findings 666
pathogenesis 665
prevention 666
treatment 666
erythema marginatum **765**, 767–768
acute rheumatic fever (ARF) **768**
clinical features 767–768
epidemiology 767, **768**
histology findings 768
history 767
Jones Criteria 767, **768**
laboratory findings 768
pathogenesis 767, **768**
treatment 768
erythema migrans (EM) **765**, 769
lyme borreliosis (LB)/lyme disease 466–467
tongue 2101
erythema multiforme (EM) 777–780, 782–784
aciclovir 783
classification 777–778
drugs associated 778–779
epidemiology 778
eye care 782–783
intravenous immunoglobulin (IVIG) 783
management 782–784
medication controversy 783
oral mucosa 2087
pathogenesis 778–779
systemic corticosteroids 783
erythema multiforme and toxic epidermal necrolysis, genital disease 2182
erythema neonatorum, transient skin disorders in neonates and young infants 76
erythema nodosum (EN) 494, 1213–1214
causes **1213**
clinical features 1213, **1214**
differential diagnosis 1213
epidemiology 1213
histology findings 1213–1214
laboratory findings 1213–1214
pathogenesis 1213, **1214**
treatment 1214
erythematosquamous skin diseases
atopic dermatitis 123–124
infantile seborrhoeic dermatitis (SD) 123
neonatal erythroderma 123–125
pityriasis rubra pilaris (PRP) 124–125
psoriasis 124
erythematous candidiasis, oral mucosa 2089
erythema toxicum neonatorum (ETN) **135**
clinical features 142
differential diagnosis 142
epidemiology 141–142
histology findings 142
laboratory findings 142
neonates 76, 141–142
pathogenesis 141–142
prevention 142
transient skin disorders in neonates and young infants 76
treatment 142
erythrasma 458–460
clinical features 459
differential diagnosis 459
epidemiology 459
histology findings 459–460
history 458
pathogenesis 459
prevention 460
treatment 460
erythroderma, neonatal *see* neonatal erythroderma
erythrodermic psoriasis 358, *359*, **366**
erythrokeratodermas 1575, 1608–1611
clinical features 1609–1610
differential diagnosis 1610
epidemiology 1608–1609
erythrokeratoderma variabilis (EKV) 1608
erythrokeratoderma variabilis progressiva (EKVP) 1608–1611
histology findings 1610–1611
history 1608
laboratory findings 1610–1611
pathogenesis 1608–1609
progressive symmetric erythrokeratoderma (PSEK) 1608
treatment 1611

erythrokeratoderma variabilis (EKV) 1608
see also erythrokeratodermas
erythrokeratoderma variabilis progressiva (EKVP) 1608–1611
see also erythrokeratodermas
erythromelalgia 1961–1964
aetiology 1961–1962
antenatal diagnosis 1964
clinical features 1962–1963
definition 1961
differential diagnosis 1963
history 1961
pathogenesis 1962
pathology 1962
prognosis 1964
treatment 1963
erythropoietic protoporphyria (EPP) **959**, **960**, 962–963, **967**
ES *see* epithelioid sarcoma
ESFT *see* Ewing sarcoma family of tumours
essential fatty acids (EFA)
deficiency 2295
deficiency, hair loss 2127
systemic therapies 2295
etanercept
atopic dermatitis (AD) 260
biologic agents 2292
psoriasis 372, *373*
ETN *see* erythema toxicum neonatorum
eumycetoma 562–563
clinical features 563
differential diagnosis 563
epidemiology 563
histology findings 563
laboratory findings 563
pathogenesis 563
prevention 563
treatment 563
eutectic mixture of local anaesthetics (EMLA) 2332–2333
EV *see* enteroviruses; epidermodysplasia verruciformis
Ewing sarcoma family of tumours (ESFT), cutaneous Ewing sarcoma 1388–1389
exanthema subitum *see* roseola infantum
excoriations, superficial self-mutilation 2270
exfoliative dermatitis, atopic dermatitis (AD) 201
exfoliative ichthyosis 1574
see also peeling skin syndrome (PSS)
clinical features 1574
differential diagnosis 1574
histology findings 1574
laboratory findings 1574
pathogenesis 1574
treatment 1574
exogenous photoprotection 975–980
inorganic sunscreens 975–976
organic sunscreens 976
personal behaviour changes 979, *980*
physical photoprotection 978–979, *980*
recommendations *980*
sunscreen controversies 976–977
sunscreen efficacy 977
sunscreen ingredients **976**
sunscreen recommended usage 977–978
sunscreens 975
sunscreens adverse effects 978
systemic photoprotective agents 978
topical photoprotective agents 978
exomphalos-macroglossia-gigantism syndrome *see* Beckwith–Wiedemann syndrome
extensive or atypical dermal melanocytosis (EDM) 1303–1304
associated abnormalities 1303–1304
clinical features 1303
differential diagnosis 1303
epidemiology 1303
histology 1303
management 1303–1304
pathogenesis 1304
external genital warts (EGW), human papillomaviruses (HPV) 596
extranodal NK/T-cell lymphoma, nasal type 1053–1054
extravasation injuries, iatrogenic disorders of the newborn 161–162
ex vivo gene therapy 2302, 2303
eyes
see also ocular complications; ophthalmological aspects
dystrophic epidermolysis bullosa (DEB) 922, 931–932
erythema multiforme (EM) 782–783
Stevens–Johnson syndrome (SJS) 782–783
toxic epidermal necrolysis (TEN) 782–783

FA *see* Fanconi anaemia
Fabry disease 1974–1975
angiokeratomas 1974–1975, *1976*
clinical features 1974–1975
definition 1974
differential diagnosis 1975
history 1974
pathogenesis 1974
pathology 1974
prognosis 1975
telangiectasia 1974–1975
treatment 1975
facial angiofibromas, tuberous sclerosis complex (TSC) 1853–1854
facial infiltrating lipomatosis *see* congenital infiltrating lipomatosis of the face
facial psoriasis 355
factitial panniculitis 1220
factitious disorder 2273
differential diagnosis 2269
factitious disorder by proxy 2273–2274
famciclovir
antiviral agents 2287
herpes simplex virus (HSV) infections 606
familial and sporadic Rosai–Dorfman disease (R Group) 1087–1088
familial atypical mole–malignant melanoma (FAMMM) syndrome **1804**
familial cerebral 'cavernous' malformation 1408
familial chilblain lupus 2022
familial chronic nail candidiasis, chronic mucocutaneous candidiasis (CMC) **2044**
familial chronic neutropenia, oral mucosa *2085*, *2092*
familial cold autoinflammatory syndrome (FCAS) 2012
familial haemophagocytic lymphohistiocytosis **2036**
familial Hibernian fever *see* tumour necrosis factor receptor-associated periodic syndrome
familial mastocytosis + gastrointestinal stromal tumours (GIST) **1805**
Familial Mediterranean fever (FMF) 2013
familial multiple lipomatosis
characteristics **1199**
clinical features **1199**
familial multiple lipomatosis (FML) 1204
clinical features 1204
differential diagnosis 1204
epidemiology 1204
histology findings 1204
laboratory findings 1204
pathogenesis 1204
prevention 1204
treatment 1204
familial partial lipodystrophies (FPLD) 1223–1224
familial progressive hyperpigmentation 1469–1470
familial progressive hyperpigmentation and hypopigmentation (FPHH) 1504–1505
clinical features 1505
differential diagnosis 1505
epidemiology 1504
histopathology 1505
history 1504
pathogenesis 1504–1505
familial white folded gingivostomatitis (white sponge naevus), oral mucosa 2088
Family Dermatology Life Quality Index (FDLQI) 2252
family impact
burden of disease 2257
quality of life (QoL) assessment 2251–2252
Family Reported Outcome Measure (FROM-16), QoL (quality of life) assessment 2252
FAMMM syndrome *see* familial atypical mole–malignant melanoma syndrome
Fanconi anaemia (FA) 1796–1798, **1805**
clinical features 1796–1797
differential diagnosis 1797
epidemiology 1796
histology findings 1797
history 1796
hyperpigmentation 1471
laboratory findings 1797

pathogenesis 1796
prevention 1797–1798
treatment 1797–1798
Farber lipogranulomatosis: ceramidase deficiency 1978
clinical features 1978
definition 1978
differential diagnosis 1978
history 1978
pathogenesis 1978
prognosis 1978
treatment 1978
fatty acid deficiency 835
FCAS *see* familial cold autoinflammatory syndrome
FDE *see* fixed drug eruption
FDH *see* focal dermal hypoplasia (FDH) (Goltz syndrome)
FDLQI *see* Family Dermatology Life Quality Index
femur fractures 2226
Ferguson–Smith syndrome *see* multiple self-healing squamous epitheliomas
fetal monitoring, iatrogenic disorders of the newborn 157
fetal skin 16–19
conclusion of the first trimester 16
embryogenesis of the skin 16–19
second-trimester fetal skin 16–18, *19*
third-trimester fetal skin 18–19
fetal wound healing, iatrogenic disorders of the newborn 155
FFD *see* Fox–Fordyce disease
FFDD *see* focal facial dermal dysplasias
fibroepithelial polyp/nodule, oral mucosa 2095
fibromatoses 1356–1369
calcifying aponeurotic fibroma 1366–1367
calcifying fibrous pseudotumour 1361
congenital and infantile fibrosarcomas 1368–1369
fibromatosis colli 1359
fibrous hamartoma of infancy 1359–1361
giant cell fibroblastoma and dermatofibrosarcoma protuberans (DFSP) 1367–1368
gingival fibromatosis 1364–1365
infantile (desmoid-type) fibromatosis 1362–1363
infantile digital fibromatosis 1365–1366
lesions with a generally indolent course **1356**, 1357–1362
lesions with potential for a locally aggressive course **1356**, 1362–1369
myofibroma/myofibromatosis 1357–1358
nodular fasciitis 1362
palmar–plantar fibromatosis 1363–1364
fibromatosis colli 1359
clinical features 1359
differential diagnosis 1359
epidemiology 1359
history 1359
pathogenesis 1359
pathology 1359
treatment 1359
fibrosarcoma 1386
clinical features 1386
definition 1386
differential diagnosis 1386
epidemiology 1386
pathology 1386
prognosis 1386
treatment 1386
fibrous dysplasia, oral mucosa 2096
fibrous hamartoma of infancy 1359–1361
clinical features 1360
differential diagnosis 1360
epidemiology 1360
history 1359–1360
pathogenesis 1360
pathology 1360–1361
treatment 1361
filaggrin (filament aggregating protein; FLG), eczema 187–189
filariasis 708–710
aetiology 708
clinical features 708, **709**
definition 708
diagnosis 708
distribution **709**
epidemiology 708
history 708
new therapies 710
pathogenesis 708
prevention 710
sites of infection **709**
treatment 708–710
Wuchereria bancrofti lifecycle *709*
filiform/digitate warts, human papillomaviruses (HPV) 591
fine and whorled Blaschkolinear hypoand hyperpigmentation (incorporating hypomelanosis of Ito, and linear and whorled naevoid hypermelanosis) 1297–1300
chromosomal mosaicism and chimaerism 1299
clinical features 1297
differential diagnosis 1299–1300
epidemiology 1297
histology findings 1298
management 1297–1298
mosaic *KITLG* mutations 1299–1300
mosaic *MTOR* mutations 1299
mosaic *TP63* mutations 1299
Pallister–Killian syndrome (PKS) 1299
pathogenesis 1298–1299
single gene mosaicism 1299–1300
terminology 1297
Fischer syndrome (Fischer–Volavsek syndrome) **1645**
FISH *see* fluorescence in situ hybridization
Fishman syndrome *see* encephalocraniocutaneous lipomatosis
fissured/scrotal tongue 2099
fixed drug eruption (FDE)
genital disease 2182
hypersensitivity reactions to drugs 794–795
fleas 734
flexural psoriasis 362
FLG *see* filaggrin (filament aggregating protein)
flies (Diptera) 735–736
fluconazole
dermatophytoses 540–542
leishmaniasis 699
fluorescence in situ hybridization (FISH), molecular genetics 44
FMF *see* Familial Mediterranean fever
FML *see* familial multiple lipomatosis
focal acral hyperkeratosis *see* marginal papular keratoderma
focal dermal hypoplasia (FDH) (Goltz syndrome) 1160, **1645**, 1706–1715
atrophic, striate and lipomatous lesions 1714
central nervous system 1713
clinical features 148, 1706–1713
congenital aplasia 1714
definition 1689–1690
differential diagnosis 148–149, 1714–1715
epidemiology 148, 1706–1707
eye features 1713
face features 1712
genetics 1706–1707
growth and lifespan 1713
gynecological features 1713
hair features 1712
histology findings 149
histopathology 1713–1714
inflammatory lesions 1714
laboratory findings 149
laser therapy 2323
nails features 1713
neonatal blistering **140**, 148–149
papillomas 1709–1710, 1714
pathogenesis 148, 1706–1707
PORCN gene diagram **1708**
prevention 149
skeletal system 1710–1712
skin features 1706–1709
teeth features 1712
treatment 149, 1715
focal epithelial hyperplasia (Heck disease), human papillomaviruses (HPV) 592
focal facial dermal dysplasias (FFDD) 1160–1161
clinical features 1160–1161
definition 1160
history 1160
type I (FFDD type I) **1646**
type II (FFDD type II) **1646**
type III **1646**
type IV **1646**
focal NEPPK *see* pachyonychia congenita (PC)
focal nonepidermolytic PPK, ectodermal dysplasias (EDs) 1698
focal nonscarring hair loss 2131
focal scarring alopecia 2129–2130
focal scarring and nonscarring causes of alopecia 2129–2131
follicular atrophoderma 1159–1160

follicular hyperkeratinization, acne vulgaris 805
follicular hyperkeratosis with scalp alopecia **2109–2110**
follicular lichen planus 393–394
folliculear differentiation tumours 1329–1331
folliculitis 427
 gram-negative folliculitis 451
 pseudomonal skin disease 449
folliculotropic mycosis fungoides 1048–1049
food allergy, atopic dermatitis (AD) 260
forceps deliveries, iatrogenic disorders of the newborn 158
Fordyce spots or granules, oral mucosa 2088
foreign bodies, genital disease 2188
formaldehyde, allergic contact dermatitis (ACD) 309
formicidae (ants) 736–737
foscarnet, herpes simplex virus (HSV) infections 606–607
Fox–Fordyce disease (FFD) 1328
 aetiology 1328
 diagnosis 1328
 differential diagnosis 1328
 epidemiology 1328
 pathology 1328
 presentation 1328
 treatment 1328
FPHH *see* familial progressive hyperpigmentation and hypopigmentation
FPLD *see* familial partial lipodystrophies
fractures 2224–2227
 child abuse and neglect (CAN) 2224–2227
 differential diagnosis 2227
 epidemiology and evidence 2226
 femur fractures 2226
 history 2226
 humerus fractures 2226
 metaphyseal fractures 2226
 periosteal reaction or subperiosteal new bone formation (SPNBF) 2226
 radius/ulna fractures 2226
 rib fractures 2226
 skull fractures 2226
 spiral fractures 2226
 tibia and fibula fractures 2226
fragrances, allergic contact dermatitis (ACD) 307–308
frictional/traumatic keratosis, oral mucosa 2089
fried tooth and nail syndrome **1646**
FROM-16 *see* Family Reported Outcome Measure
frostbite 990–991
frostnip 991
fucosidosis 1975–1976
 clinical features 1975–1976
 definition 1975
 differential diagnosis 1976
 pathogenesis 1975
 pathology 1975
 prognosis 1976
 treatment 1976
fumaric acid esters, psoriasis 371–372, *373*
fungal infections
 see also antifungal therapy; deep fungal infections; superficial fungal infections
 aspergillosis 2085
 congenital infections 86, **87**, **88**, 90
 deep mycoses 2085–2086
 genital area 2178–2179
 histoplasmosis 2085
 HIV infection 650–651
 immunocompromised children 686, 687, 690
 mucormycosis (zygomycosis, phycomycosis) 2085
 neonates 86, **87**, **88**, 90
 oral mucosa 2084–2085
 vesiculobullous lesions 864
fungal microbiota, cutaneous microbiome 54–55
furuncular myiasis (warble) 703
furunculosis 427–428
fusion of the labia 2185–2186
 aetiology 2185
 clinical presentation 2185
 differential diagnosis 2185
 incidence 2185
 management 2185–2186
Futcher lines *see* pigmentary demarcation lines

GA *see* granuloma annulare
Galli-Galli disease, hyperpigmentation 1471
gap junction proteins, ectodermal dysplasias (EDs) 1691–1695
GAPO *see* growth retardation–alopecia–pseudoanodontia–optic atrophy
Gardner syndrome **1805**, 1812–1813
 characteristics **1199**
 clinical features **1199**, 1812–1813
 differential diagnosis 1813
 histology findings 1813
 oral mucosa 2096
 pathogenesis 1812
 treatment 1813
Garin–Bujadoux–Bannwarth (GBB) syndrome, lyme borreliosis (LB)/lyme disease 468
GARP (glycoprotein A repetitions predominant)/LRRC32 (leucine-rich repeat-containing protein 32), eczema 190
GAS disease *see* Group A *Streptococcus*
gastrointestinal disease, oral mucosa 2085–2086
gastrointestinal involvement
 Behçet disease (BD) 1955, 1957
 juvenile dermatomyositis (JDM) 1947
gastrointestinal manifestations, dermatitis herpetiformis (DH) 901
gastrointestinal tract, systemic sclerosis (SSc) 1190
gastrointestinal tract features, dystrophic epidermolysis bullosa (DEB) 921–922
gastro-oesophageal reflux, dystrophic epidermolysis bullosa (DEB) 930
Gaucher disease (GD) 1973–1974
 clinical features 1973–1974
 definition 1973
 differential diagnosis 1974
 history 1973
 pathogenesis 1973
 prognosis 1974
 treatment 1974
Gaucher disease type II 1589
GBB syndrome *see* Garin–Bujadoux–Bannwarth syndrome
GCRH *see* giant cell reticulohistiocytoma
GCS *see* Gianotti–Crosti syndrome
GD *see* Gaucher disease
GEH *see* generalized eruptive histiocytosis
gene, cell and protein therapy, dystrophic epidermolysis bullosa (DEB) 926–927
gene editing, genetic therapies 2305–2307
general gas anaesthesia 2338–2339
generalized and diffuse nonscarring hypotrichosis 1160
generalized eruptive histiocytosis (GEH) 1087
 clinical features 1087
 differential diagnosis 1087
 epidemiology 1087
 histology findings 1087
 history 1087
 pathogenesis 1087
 treatment 1087
generalized gingival swelling, oral mucosa 2096–2097
generalized granuloma annulare (GA) **1008**, 1010
generalized hypertrichosis 2132–2133
generalized hypertrophy of the gums *see* gingival fibromatosis
generalized lesions, oral mucosa 2093
generalized lymphatic anomaly (GLA), lymphatic malformations (LMs) **1453**, 1455, 1460
generalized morphoea 1178
genetic aspects, porphyrias **959**
genetic basis, eczema 185
genetic counselling
 congenital melanocytic naevi (CMN) 1252
 genetic testing 39
genetic disorders predisposing to malignancy 1802–1821
genetic dissection, eczema 185–186
genetic features
 Ehlers–Danlos syndromes (EDS) **1113–1114**
 mycosis fungoides (MF) 1048
genetic investigation of mosaic disorders 1233–1234
 blood samples 1234
 choosing the right test 1234
 formalin-fixed paraffin-embedded tissue 1234

sampling and testing the right tissue 1233–1234
skin biopsy 1234
genetic mechanisms, mosaicism/mosaic disorders 1231
genetics
atopic dermatitis (AD) 175–176, 184–191
hidradenitis suppurativa (HS) (acne inversa) 827
morphoea 1176
neurofibromatosis type 1 (NF1) 1824
PIK3CA-related overgrowth spectrum (PROS) 1292
Proteus syndrome (PS) 1287
pseudoxanthoma elasticum (PXE) 1126
genetics and inheritance in brief 36–38
genetic susceptibility, vitiligo 1476–1477
genetic testing 38–40
see also molecular genetics
blood DNA 39
cheek swab or saliva DNA 39
congenital melanocytic naevi (CMN) 1247–1248
consent and incidental findings 38
genetic counselling 39
interpreting results 39
neurofibromatosis type 2 (NF2) 1833–1834
personalized medicine 39–40
samples to take 39
skin DNA 39
terminology 39
vesiculobullous lesions 862
genetic therapies 2301–2307
adeno-associated virus (AAV) 2303
ex vivo gene therapy 2302, 2303
gene editing 2305–2307
lentiviral vectors (LV) 2302–2303, **2302**
messenger RNA (mRNA) 2304–2305
minicircle DNA 2304
nanoparticles and nonviral approaches **2302**, 2303–2305
nonviral approaches and nanoparticles **2302**, 2303–2305
retroviral vectors (RV) 2302–2303, **2302**
short interfering RNA (siRNA) 2304
spherical nucleic acids (SNA) 2304
vectors used for skin gene therapy **2302**
viral vectors 2302–2303, **2302**
in vitro transcribed messenger RNA (mRNA) 2304–2305
in vivo gene therapy 2301, *2302*, 2303
genital disease 2159–2194
acute scrotal oedema 2191
anatomical abnormalities 2184–2187
aphthous ulcers 2181–2182
benign tumours 2189
birthmarks in the genital area 2170–2173
blisters and ulcers 2179–2183
CHARGE syndrome 2184–2185
clitoral cysts 2186
dermatitis, genital area 2160–2162
Enterobius vermicularis (pinworm) 2177
erosive and or blistering napkin eruption 2179, *2180*
erythema multiforme and toxic epidermal necrolysis 2182
fixed drug eruption (FDE) 2182
foreign bodies 2188
fungal infections 2178–2179
fusion of the labia 2185–2186
genital signs of systemic disease 2191–2192
hair tourniquet 2188
Herpes zoster and simplex 2178
hidradenitis suppurativa (HS) (acne inversa) 2182–2183
idiopathic scrotal calcinosis 2190–2191
immunobullous disease – vulval bullous and cicatricial pemphigoid and linear IgA disease of childhood 2179–2180
infantile pyramidal perineal protrusion 2186
inflammatory dermatoses of the genital region 2160–2163
lichen sclerosus in boys (syn. balanitis xerotica obliterans) 2170
lichen sclerosus in girls (syn. lichen sclerosus et atrophicus) 2164–2169
malignancies 2188–2189
median raphe cysts of the penis and scrotum 2186–2187
molluscum contagiosum (MC) 2177–2178
mycobacterial infection 2179
neoplasia 2188–2190
nonsexually acquired acute genital ulcers (NSAGU) 2180–2181
nonsexually acquired genital infections in children 2175–2179
pearly penile papules 2185
penile abnormalities 2184
phimosis 2186
pinworm (*Enterobius vermicularis*) 2177
prepubertal unilateral fibrous hyperplasia of the labium majus 2189–2190
psoriasis, genital area 2162–2163
psychological aspects of genital disease in children 2193–2194
recurrent toxin-mediated perineal erythema (scarlatina-like) 2176
scabies 2177
scrotal conditions 2190–2191
sexually transmitted infections in children 2179
staphylococcal folliculitis and impetigo 2176
staphylococcal scalded skin syndrome (SSSS) 2176–2177
streptococcal cellulitis, vulvovaginitis and balanitis 2175–2176
vulval abnormalities 2184
vulvovaginitis 2174–2175
genital herpes simplex virus infection (herpes genitalis) 2215–2216
acquired HSV infection 2216
aetiology 2215
child sexual abuse (CSA) 2216
clinical features 2215–2216
definition 2215
diagnosis 2216
herpes simplex virus (HSV) infections 602
treatment 2216
genital HPV infection, human papillomaviruses (HPV) 593
genital/penoscrotal porokeratosis 1625
genital signs of systemic disease 2191–2192
Behçet disease (BD) 2192
Crohn disease 2191–2192
Group A *Streptococcus* (GAS) *2237*
Henoch-Schonlein purpura (HSP) 2192, *2238*
lichen sclerosus (LS) *2237*
orofacial granulomatosis and anogenital granulomatosis 2192
zinc deficiency 2192
genitourinary involvement, juvenile dermatomyositis (JDM) 1948
genitourinary tract, dystrophic epidermolysis bullosa (DEB) 922
genodermatoses
ectodermal dysplasia 127
epidermal homeostasis disorders 126–127
erosive or ulcerative skin lesions **140**
neonatal blistering **137–138**, 147–149
neonatal erythroderma 125–127
nonsyndromic ichthyoses 125–126
syndromic ichthyoses 126
genome-wide association studies (GWAS), molecular genetics 44–45
geographical tongue 2101
German measles *see* rubella
geroderma osteodysplastica (GO) 1739–1740
aetiology 1739
clinical features 1739
definition 1739
differential diagnosis 1739–1740
history 1739
pathogenesis 1739
pathology 1739
prognosis 1739
treatment 1739
gestational pemphigoid, neonates 98
Gianotti–Crosti syndrome (GCS) 771–775
definition 771
diagnostic criteria **774**
differential diagnosis 774, **775**
history 771
HIV infection 652
pathogenesis 771–772
pathology 772–774
prognosis 774
treatment 774–775
vaccines associated with GCS **772**

giant cell epulis/granuloma, oral mucosa 2095
giant cell fibroblastoma and dermatofibrosarcoma protuberans (DFSP) 1367–1368
  clinical features 1367
  differential diagnosis 1367
  epidemiology 1367
  pathogenesis 1367
  pathology 1367–1368
  treatment 1368
giant cell reticulohistiocytoma (GCRH) 1084
  clinical features 1084
  differential diagnosis 1084
  epidemiology 1084
  histology findings 1084
  history 1084
  pathogenesis 1084
  treatment 1084
Gilchrist disease *see* blastomycosis
gingival cysts of infancy (Epstein pearls and Bohn nodules), oral mucosa 2088
gingival elephantiasis *see* gingival fibromatosis
gingival fibromatosis 1364–1365
  clinical features 1364
  differential diagnosis 1364
  epidemiology 1364
  history 1364
  pathogenesis 1364
  pathology 1364–1365
  treatment 1365
gingival fibromatosis and hypertrichosis **1646**
gingival fibromatosis–sparse hair–malposition of teeth **1646**
gingivitis, oral mucosa 2092–2093
GIST *see* familial mastocytosis + gastrointestinal stromal tumours
glomus tumour (glomuvenous malformation) 1323, 1407–1408
  clinical features 1323
  course and prognosis 1323
  definition 1323
  glomangioma *1323*
  pathogenesis 1323
  treatment 1323
glomuvenous malformation (GVM) *see* glomus tumour
glossitis, tongue 2100
glucose metabolism, metabolic syndrome (MetS) 850–852
gluten-free diet (GFD), dermatitis herpetiformis (DH) 903
gluten-sensitive enteropathy (coeliac disease), oral mucosa 2086
GM_1 gangliosidosis 1977–1978
  clinical features 1977–1978
  definition 1977
  differential diagnosis 1978
  history 1977
  pathogenesis 1977
  prognosis 1978
  treatment 1978
GO *see* geroderma osteodysplastica
gold, allergic contact dermatitis (ACD) 307
Goltz syndrome *see* focal dermal hypoplasia (FDH)
gonorrhoea 2204–2208
  aetiology 2204–2205
  child sexual abuse (CSA) 2206
  clinical features 2205–2206
  definition 2204
  diagnosis 2206–2207
  differential diagnosis 2207
  history 2204
  infection in infants 2205
  infection in older children 2205–2206
  pathogenesis 2204–2205
  pathology 2205
  prognosis 2207
  treatment 2207–2208
Gorham–Stout disease (GSD), lymphatic malformations (LMs) 1411, **1453**, 1455, 1460
Gorlin–Chaudhry–Moss syndrome **1647**
Gorlin syndrome 1769–1783, **1804**
  aetiology 1770–1772
  clinical features 1773–1779
  confirmation of diagnosis by mutation analysis 1780
  definition 1769
  diagnosis 1779
  diagnostic criteria 1779–1780
  differential diagnosis 1780–1781
  ectopic calcification 1776–1777, *1778*
  family history 1779
  histology of BCCs 1772
  histology of jaw cysts 1772
  history 1769–1770
  hypertrichosis 2135
  jaw cysts 1783
  local treatment 1781–1782
  naevi 1776
  naevi and BCCs 1776
  naevoid BCCs 1776
  natural history 1773–1779
  palmar and plantar pits 1772
  patched gene and the hedgehog signalling pathway 1770
  pathogenesis 1770–1772
  pathology 1772–1773
  photodynamic therapy (PDT) 1783
  physical examination 1779
  prognosis 1780
  prophylaxis 1781
  radiation response 1772
  radiography and imaging investigations 1779
  skeletal radiographs 1776, *1777–1778*
  small molecule inactivators of SMO 1783
  spectrum of mutations 1770–1772
  surveillance 1781
  systemic retinoids 1782–1783
  treatment 1781–1783
  treatment by radiation 1782
  ultraviolet radiation 1772–1773
graft-versus- host-disease (GVHD) 2067–2075
  acute disease 2068–2069, 2072–2073, 2074
  chronic disease 2069, 2073, 2074–2075
  chronic graft-versus-host disease 2086–2087
  clinical features 2071–2073
  clinical situations in which GVHD may occur 2068
  definition 2067–2068
  differential diagnosis 2073–2074
  experimental animal models of GVHD 2068
  graft-versus-leukaemia effect 2075
  histopathology 2069–2070
  historical summary of human GVHD 2068
  history 2068
  immunopathology 2070–2071
  importance of GVHD to the dermatologist 2075
  incidence **2071**
  neonatal erythroderma 130–131
  oral mucosa 2086–2087
  pathogenesis 2068–2069
  pathology 2069–2071
  prevention 2074–2075
  treatment 2074–2075
gram-negative folliculitis 451
gram-negative infections, cutaneous manifestations 434–451
gram-negative septicaemia, neonates **87**
gram-negative soft tissue infections 450–451
granular cell tumour 1321–1322
  clinical features 1321–1322
  course and prognosis 1322
  definition 1321
  pathogenesis 1321
  treatment 1322
granuloma annulare (GA) 851–852, 1006–1013
  aetiology 851, 1007
  associations 1007–1008
  clinical features 1008–1012
  clinical symptoms 851
  diagnosis 851
  differential diagnosis 851, 1012
  epidemiology 1007
  generalized GA **1008**, 1010
  histology findings 1011–1012
  history 1006
  immunophenotype 1012
  linear GA **1008**, 1011
  localized GA **1008**, 1009
  management 1012–1013
  metabolic syndrome (MetS) 851–852
  papular umbilicated GA **1008**, 1010–1011
  pathogenesis 1007–1008
  perforating GA **1008**, 1010
  prevention 1012–1013
  prognosis 851–852
  segmental GA **1008**, 1011
  subcutaneous GA **1008**, 1009–1010
  therapeutic options **1013**
  treatment 852, 1012–1013
granuloma gluteale infantum, napkin dermatitis 271

granulomatosis with polyangiitis (GPA) 1924–1930
antineutrophil cytoplasmic antibody (ANCA)-associated vasculitides (AAV) 1882, 1924–1930
clinical features 1925–1928
comparison of features **1928**
differential diagnosis **1928**
epidemiology 1925
histology findings 1929
history 1924–1925
pathogenesis 1925
radiological findings 1929
treatment 1929–1930
granulomatous slack skin (GSS) 1049
green nail syndrome, pseudomonal skin disease 448
Griscelli–Pruniéras syndromes 1490
clinical features 1490
clinical variants 1490
epidemiology 1490
laboratory findings 1490
pathogenesis 1490
prevention 1490
treatment 1490
Griscelli syndrome (GS) **2035**, **2036**
griseofulvin
antifungal therapy 2285–2286
dermatophytoses 540, **543**
Group A *Streptococcus* (GAS) 423–424, 425, 427, 429
genital signs of systemic disease *2237*
Group B streptococci, neonates **87**
growth and nutrition, approach to the infant and child 2347
growth problems, dystrophic epidermolysis bullosa (DEB) 922
growth retardation–alopecia–pseudoanodontia–optic atrophy (GAPO) **1647**
GS *see* Griscelli syndrome
GSS *see* granulomatous slack skin
guttate psoriasis 357, 362, **364**
GVHD *see* graft-versus- host-disease
GVM *see* glomus tumour (glomuvenous malformation)
GWAS *see* genome-wide association studies

H_1 antihistamines 2288–2289
H_2 antihistamines 2289
HA20 *see* haploinsufficiency of protein A20
Haberland syndrome *see* encephalocraniocutaneous lipomatosis
habit phenomena, physiological habits **2264**
HAE *see* hereditary angioedema
haemangiomas
see also infantile haemangiomas (IH)
burden of disease 2257
nursing care of the skin 2403–2406
ulcerated haemangiomas 2406, **2407**
haemangiomas and vascular malformations, oral mucosa 2092
haemangiopericytoma (HPC) 1394–1395
aetiology 1394
clinical features 1394
definition 1394
differential diagnosis 1394
pathogenesis 1394
pathology 1394
treatment 1394–1395
haematological and immunological disorders, oral mucosa 2085
haem biosynthesis, porphyrias 957–958
haemophagocytic lymphohistiocytosis (HLH) (H Group) 1089–1090
clinical features 1089
diagnosis 1090
epidemiology 1089
histology findings 1089–1090
history 1089
laboratory findings 1089
pathogenesis 1089
prognosis 1090
treatment 1090
haemorrhagic oedema of childhood, differential diagnosis of inflicted bruises *2225*
Haim–Munk syndrome (HMS) **1647**
see also palmoplantar keratoderma with periodontitis
hair disorders 2103–2136
see also hair loss
acquired localized unruly hair 2122
alopecia, focal scarring and nonscarring causes 2129–2131
androgenetic alopecia (AGA) 2128–2129
aplasia cutis congenita (ACC) 2129–2130
bubble hair 2118
focal nonscarring hair loss 2131
focal scarring alopecia 2129–2130
focal scarring and nonscarring causes of alopecia 2129–2131
hair shaft abnormalities presenting with hair breakage 2112–2118
hypertrichosis 2132–2136
ichthyosis linearis circumflexa (ILC) 2114, *2116*
keratosis follicularis spinulosa decalvans 2130–2131
localized tufts of hair 2124
Marie–Unna hereditary hypotrichosis (MUHH) 2122
miniaturization 2128–2129
miscellaneous hair shaft abnormalities 2123–2124
monilethrix 2117–2118
Netherton syndrome (NS) *2116*
normal hair loss/growth in childhood 2104–2105
occipital alopecia 2103–2104
pili annulati 2123–2124
pili torti 2116–2117
pseudomonilethrix 2118
pseudopili annulati 2124
triangular alopecia 2131
trichopoliodystrophy (Menkes syndrome) 2113
trichorrhexis invaginata (bamboo hair) 2114–2116
trichorrhexis nodosa 2112–2113
trichoschisis 2113
trichothiodystrophy (TTD) 2113–2114
uncombable hair syndrome (UHS) 2120–2121
woolly hair 2121–2122
hair follicle naevus 1330–1331
aetiology 1330
diagnosis 1330
differential diagnosis 1331
epidemiology 1330
pathology 1331
presentation 1330
prognosis 1331
treatment 1331
hair loss 2106–2111
see also hair disorders
abnormality in initiation of hair growth 2108–2111
alopecia, keratosis pilaris, cataracts and psoriasis **2109**
alopecia areata 2106, 2107, 2111
anagen effluvium 2124–2125
anagen loss 2124–2126
atrichia with papular lesions **2109**
biotin deficiency 2127
Cantu syndrome (onychotrichodysplasia with neutropenia) **2110**
cystic eyelids, palmoplantar keratosis, hypodontia and hypotrichosis (Schöpf–Schulz–Passarge syndrome) **2110**
dermoscopic examination 2107–2108
dwarfism, cerebral atrophy and keratosis pilaris **2109**
ectodermal dysplasias 2111
ectodermal dysplasia/skin fragility syndrome (McGrath syndrome) 2111
ectodysplasin A (EDA-1) gene 2111
EDAR-associated death domain gene 2111
essential fatty acid deficiency 2127
evaluation of the child with hair loss 2106–2108
examination 2106–2108
follicular hyperkeratosis with scalp alopecia **2109–2110**
hair and scalp examination 2106–2107
hair loss due to abnormal cycling 2124–2127
history 2106
ichthyosis follicularis **2109**
ichthyosis follicularis, with atrichia and photophobia (IFAP) syndrome 2111
keratitis ichthyosis deafness syndrome (KID syndrome) **2109**
keratosis follicularis spinulosa decalvans **2109**
loose anagen syndrome (LAS) 2125–2126
Marie–Unna hypotrichosis **2109**
microscopic examination of hairs 2107, *2108*
monilethrix **2110**
NF-κB essential modulator (NEMO) 2111

hair loss (*cont'd*)
odontoonychodysplasia with alopecia 2111
onychotrichodysplasia with neutropenia (Cantu syndrome) **2110**
pachyonychia congenita (PC) **2110**
perniola syndrome **2109**
physical examination 2106
protein malnutrition (kwashiorkor) 2127
scalp biopsy 2108
Schöpf–Schulz–Passarge syndrome (cystic eyelids, palmoplantar keratosis, hypodontia and hypotrichosis) **2110**
telogen loss or effluvium 2126–2127
types 2108–2111
universal alopecia 2108
zinc deficiency 2127
hair prostheses, alopecia areata (AA) 2145
hair removal, laser therapy 828, 2327–2328
hair tourniquet, genital disease 2188
hairy and furred tongue 2101
hairy leucoplakia
HIV infection 652
oral mucosa 652, 2091
Hallerman–Streiff syndrome **1648**
halo naevi 1255, 2368
hamartomas 1279–1281
apocrine naevi 1281
basaloid follicular hamartoma 1280
eccrine angiomatous hamartomas 1281
eccrine naevi 1281
encephalocraniocutaneous lipomatosis (ECCL) **1199**, 1200–1201, 1280–1281
mixed hamartomas 1280
mucinous eccrine naevi 1281
smooth muscle hamartoma 1279
hand, foot and mouth disease (HFMD) 668–670
clinical features 669
differential diagnosis 669
epidemiology 668–669
laboratory findings 669–670
oral mucosa 2084
pathogenesis 668–669
prevention 670
treatment 670
hands features, dystrophic epidermolysis bullosa (DEB) 920–921
haploinsufficiency of protein A20 (HA20) 2018
Happle–Tinschert syndrome 1160
harlequin colour change, transient skin disorders in neonates and young infants 75–76
harlequin ichthyosis (HI) 1558–1559, 1596
clinical features 1559
epidemiology 1558–1559
histology 1559
nursing care of the skin **2394–2395**, 2395
pathogenesis 1558–1559
treatment 1559
ultrastructure 1559
Hartnup disease 1973
clinical features 1973
definition 1973
differential diagnosis 1973
history 1973
pathogenesis 1973
prognosis 1973
treatment 1973
Hayden syndrome **1648**
Hay–Wells syndrome *see* AEC syndrome
HCP *see* hereditary coproporphyria
head lice *see* pediculosis
HEADSS assessment, adolescents 2348–2349
heat urticaria 758
Heck disease (focal epithelial hyperplasia), human papillomaviruses (HPV) 592
HED *see* hypohidrotic ectodermal dysplasia
HEDH syndrome *see* hypohidrotic ectodermal dysplasia with hypothyroidism and ciliary dyskinesia
heelprick marks, iatrogenic disorders of the newborn 164
helminthic Infections 702–710
cutaneous larva migrans (CLM) 705–707
filariasis 708–710
myiasis 702–704
hemihyperplasia multiple lipomatosis syndrome
characteristics **1199**
clinical features **1199**
hemihyperplasia–multiple lipomatosis syndrome (HHML) 1202–1203
clinical features 1202–1203
differential diagnosis 1203
epidemiology 1202
pathogenesis 1202
prevention 1203
treatment 1203
Henoch-Schonlein purpura (HSP) 1866–1870
arthritis and arthralgia 1869
cf. acute haemorrhagic oedema of infancy (AHEI) **1871**
classification **1867**
clinical features 1867–1869
cutaneous findings 1867–1868
definition 1866–1867
differential diagnosis 1869
differential diagnosis of inflicted bruises *2225*
epidemiology 1867
gastrointestinal manifestations 1868–1869
genital signs 2192
genital signs of systemic disease *2238*
histology 1869
history 1866–1867
laboratory findings 1869
prognosis 1869–1870
renal involvement 1869
treatment 1869–1870
HEP *see* hepatoerythropoietic porphyria
hepatitis B 2214–2215
aetiology 2214
child sexual abuse (CSA) 2214–2215
clinical features 2214–2215
definition 2214
diagnosis 2215
pathogenesis 2214
prognosis 2215
sexually transmitted diseases (STDs) 2214–2215
treatment 2215
hepatoerythropoietic porphyria (HEP) **959**, **960**, 964, **967**
hereditary angioedema (HAE) 2046–2048
clinical features 2047–2048
differential diagnosis 2048
epidemiology 2047
histology findings 2048
laboratory findings 2048
pathogenesis 2047
prevention 2048
treatment 2048
hereditary benign intraepithelial dyskeratosis, oral mucosa 2088
hereditary congenital hypopigmented and hyperpigmented macules *see* Westerhof syndrome
hereditary coproporphyria (HCP) **959**, **960**, 964–965
hereditary disorders associated with mucocutaneous malignancies **1803**
hereditary generalized hypertrichosis 2132–2133
hereditary gingival fibromatosis
hypertrichosis 2132
oral mucosa 2097
hereditary gingival hyperplasia *see* gingival fibromatosis
hereditary haemorrhagic telangiectasia (HHT) 1401–1402
Curaçao criteria **1402**
oral mucosa 2093
subtypes **1401**
hereditary leiomyomatosis and renal cell cancer (HLRCC) syndrome 1813–1814
clinical features 1814
differential diagnosis 1814
pathogenesis 1813–1814
pathology 1814
treatment 1814
hereditary mucoepithelial dysplasia **1648**
oral mucosa 2092
hereditary multiple lipomas
see also familial multiple lipomatosis
characteristics **1199**
clinical features **1199**
hereditary skin disorders associated with extracutaneous malignancies **1805**
hereditary skin disorders associated with mucocutaneous and extracutaneous malignancies **1804**
hereditary symmetrical systemic aplastic naevi 1160–1161
hereditary tumour syndromes, endocrine dysfunction 2009

heredopathia atactica polyneuritiformis *see* Refsum disease (RD)
Hermansky–Pudlak syndrome 1489
clinical features 1489
epidemiology 1489
laboratory findings 1489
pathogenesis 1489
prevention 1489
treatment 1489
herpangina 670
clinical features 670
differential diagnosis 670
epidemiology 670
laboratory findings 670
oral mucosa 2084
pathogenesis 670
prevention 670
treatment 670
herpes genitalis (genital herpes simplex virus infection), herpes simplex virus (HSV) infections 602
herpes keratitis, herpes simplex virus (HSV) infections 603
herpes labialis, herpes simplex virus (HSV) infections 600–601
herpes simplex encephalitis, herpes simplex virus (HSV) infections 603
herpes simplex virus (HSV) infections **135**, **138**, 598–608
aciclovir 605–607
amenamevir 607
antiviral chemotherapy 605–607
artesunate 607
Bell's palsy 604
brincidofovir 607
brivudine 605–607
chemotherapy, specific antiviral 605–607
cidofovir 607
clinical features 600–604
differential diagnosis 604
disseminated HSV infection 603
docosanol 607
eczema herpeticum 604
epidemiology 598–599
famciclovir 606
foscarnet 606–607
genital herpes simplex virus infection 2215–2216
genital herpes simplex virus infection (herpes genitalis) 602
herpes genitalis (genital herpes simplex virus infection) 602
herpes keratitis 603
herpes labialis 600–601
herpes simplex encephalitis 603
herpetic whitlow and hand lesions 601–602
histology findings 604–605
history 598
HIV infection 651
human herpesviruses (HHV) infections 671–674
immunocompromised children 603–604, 689
immunology 599–600
Kaposi varicelliform eruption 604
laboratory findings 604–605
napkin dermatitis *278*
pathogenesis 598–599
prevention 608
primary herpes gingivostomatitis 600–601
pritelivir 607
recurrent attacks 607–608
recurrent herpes gingivostomatitis 601
supportive therapy 605
surgery 607
topical preparations 607
treatment 605–608
trifluridine 607
herpes simplex virus (HSV) types I and II, neonates **86**
Herpes zoster, varicella zoster virus (VZV) infections 617–618
Herpes zoster (shingles), oral mucosa 2083–2084
Herpes zoster and simplex, genital area 2178
herpetic gingivostomatitis 2082–2083
aetiology 2082
clinical features 2082
differential diagnosis 2082
pathology 2082
treatment 2083
herpetic whitlow and hand lesions, herpes simplex virus (HSV) infections 601–602
herringbone (chevron) nails, nail disorders 2149
heteroinoculation and iatrogenic transmission, human papillomaviruses (HPV) 590
HFMD *see* hand, foot and mouth disease
HFS *see* hyaline fibromatosis syndrome
HHML *see* hemihyperplasia multiple lipomatosis syndrome
HHT *see* hereditary haemorrhagic telangiectasia
HHV *see* human herpesviruses infections
HHV-5 *see* cytomegalovirus
HHV-8 *see* human herpesvirus-8
HI *see* harlequin ichthyosis
hibernoma
characteristics **1196**
clinical features 1197
epidemiology 1197
histological features **1196**
histology findings 1197
laboratory findings 1197
pathogenesis 1197
treatment 1197
hidradenitis suppurativa (HS) (acne inversa) 818–819, 825–829, 1326–1327, 2182–2183
adjuvant therapy 827–828
aetiology 1326–1327
antibiotics 828
clinical features 827, 1327, 2183
combined approach 828–829
differential diagnosis 827, 1327, 2183
dysbiosis 826
dysregulated immune response 826
epidemiology 826, 1326
genetics 827
histology 1327
histology findings 827
hormones 828
Hurley score 827
immunosuppressants 828
laboratory findings 827
lasers and intense pulsed light for hair removal 828
management 1327, 2183
metabolic syndrome (MetS) 853–854
pathogenesis 826–827, 2183
prognosis 1327
surgery 828
systemic retinoids 828
systemic therapies 828
topical therapies 828
treatment 827–829
hidrotic ectodermal dysplasia (Clouston syndrome, ED2) **1649**, 1692–1693
clinical features 1692–1693
definition 1692
differential diagnosis 1693
history 1692
oral mucosa 2088
pathology 1692
prognosis 1693
treatment 1693
hidrotic ectodermal dysplasia, Christianson–Fourie type **1649**
HIES *see* hyperimmunoglobulin E syndrome; hyperimmunoglobulin E syndromes
high-resolution melt PCR (HRM), molecular genetics 45
histiocyte and dendritic cell lineage, Langerhans cell histiocytosis (LCH) 1071–1072, 1078–1080
histiocytic and granulomatous diseases 2018–2020
histiocytoma *see* dermatofibroma
histiocytoses 1078–1091
see also Langerhans cell histiocytosis
classification **1079**
histological diagnoses of 775 superficial lumps excised in children **1314**
histopathological correlates of dermoscopic structures found in superficial spreading melanoma 2369, **2370**
histopathology 2378–2388
see also biopsy
biopsy reasons and principles 2378–2379
blue naevi 2388
bullous dermatoses 2381–2382
lichenoid dermatoses 2379–2380
lumps and bumps 2383, *2384*
melanocytic lesions 2386–2388
rashes 2379–2382
Spitz melanomas 2386–2387
Spitz naevi 2386–2387
spongiotic disorders 2380–2381
vascular lesions 2384–2386
vasculitis 2382
histoplasmosis 565–567
clinical features 566
differential diagnosis 566
epidemiology 565

histoplasmosis (*cont'd*)
histology findings 566–567
laboratory findings 566–567
oral mucosa 2085
pathogenesis 565–566
prevention 567
treatment 567
HIV infection 649–654, 2216–2217
abacavir hypersensitivity 653
acanthamoeba infection 653
acute HIV infection 650
aetiology 2216
bacterial infections 650
child sexual abuse (CSA) 2216–2217
clinical features 650–654, 2216–2217
cutaneous manifestations 650–651
cytomegalovirus (CMV) 651–652
definition 649, 2216
differential diagnosis 654
drug reactions 653
epidemiology 649–650
fungal infections 650–651
Gianotti–Crosti syndrome 652
hairy leucoplakia 652
herpes simplex virus (HSV) infections 651
history 649
human papillomaviruses (HPV) 652
infectious napkin dermatitis 274
infestations 652–653
inflammatory disorders 653
Kaposi sarcoma 653–654
lipodystrophies 1225
measles (rubeola) 651
molluscum contagiosum (MC) 652
neonates **86**
neoplasms 653–654
oral hairy leucoplakia 652
oral mucosa 2084, 2098
parasitic infections 653
prognosis 654
sexually transmitted diseases (STDs) 2216–2217
treatment 654, 2217
varicella zoster virus (VZV) infections 651
viral infections 651–652
HJMD *see* congenital hypotrichosis with juvenile macular dystrophy
HLH *see* haemophagocytic lymphohistiocytosis
HLRCC syndrome *see* hereditary leiomyomatosis and renal cell cancer syndrome
HMS (Haim–Munk syndrome) *see* palmoplantar keratoderma with periodontitis
Hodgkin disease 1067–1068
clinical features 1067–1068
epidemiology 1067
histology findings 1068
laboratory findings 1068
pathogenesis 1067
prevention 1068
treatment 1068
Hoffmann–Zurhelle (naevus lipomatosus cutaneous superficialis), differential diagnosis 1715
hoi con 746–748
holocarboxylase synthetase deficiency (HSD), neonatal erythroderma 132
homocystinuria 1970
clinical features 1970
definition 1970
differential diagnosis 1970
history 1970
pathogenesis 1970
prognosis 1970
treatment 1970
homozygous hereditary coproporphyria 964–965
honey bees, bumble bees (apids) 736
honeycomb atrophy *see* atrophoderma vermiculata
HOPP syndrome *see* hypotrichosis–osteolysis–periodontitis–palmoplantar keratoderma syndrome
hormonal agents, acne vulgaris 811
hormonal influences, acne vulgaris 804–805
hormones, hidradenitis suppurativa (HS) (acne inversa) 828
Howell–Evans syndrome *see* tylosis with oesophageal cancer (TOC)
HPC *see* haemangiopericytoma
HPV *see* human papillomaviruses
HPV genotyping, human papillomaviruses (HPV) 594
HPV infections of the aerodigestive tract, human papillomaviruses (HPV) 592–593
HPV infections of the skin, human papillomaviruses (HPV) 590–592
HRM (high-resolution melt PCR), molecular genetics 45
HS *see* hidradenitis suppurativa
HSD *see* holocarboxylase synthetase deficiency
HSP *see* Henoch-Schonlein purpura
HSV *see* herpes simplex virus infections
H-syndrome
autoinflammatory diseases (AIDs) 2019–2020
endocrine dysfunction 2009
HTLV-1 infection 654–657
see also infective dermatitis (ID)
clinical features 655
definition 654
diagnosis 655
diagnostic criteria **657**
differential diagnosis 657
eczematous dermatitis **656**
epidemiology 654
erythema, generalized **656**
histopathology 655–657
history 654
pathogenic mechanism *655*
pathophysiology 655
prognosis 657
treatment 657
human herpesvirus-8 (HHV-8) 673–674
clinical features 674
epidemiology 674
laboratory findings 674
pathogenesis 674
prevention 674
treatment 674
human herpesviruses (HHV) infections 671–674
cytomegalovirus (CMV or HHV-5) 672–673
human herpesvirus-8 (HHV-8) 673–674
infectious mononucleosis (IM) 671–672
human immunodeficiency virus (HIV) infection *see* HIV infection
human papillomaviruses (HPV) 588–596
adhesiotherapy (occlusotherapy) 594
anogenital warts: condylomas 593
autoinoculation 590
bowenoid papulosis 592
Butcher's warts 591–592
classification 588–589
clinical features 590–593
combination therapies 596
common warts 590–591, 596
contact sensitizers 595
cryotherapy 594
curettage and surgical treatment 594
cystic warts 591
deep plantar warts/myrmecia 591
differential diagnosis 594
doughnut/ring warts 591
epidemiology 589
epidermodysplasia verruciformis (EDV) 592
external genital warts (EGW) 596
factors to consider in the treatment of warts in children 596
filiform/digitate warts 591
focal epithelial hyperplasia (Heck disease) 592
genital HPV infection 593
Heck disease (focal epithelial hyperplasia) 592
heteroinoculation and iatrogenic transmission 590
histology 593–594
HIV infection 652
HPV genotyping 594
HPV infections of the aerodigestive tract 592–593
HPV infections of the skin 590–592
imiquimod 595
immune stimulation and modulation 595
immunocompromised children 688–689
ingenol mebutate 595
interferons (IFN) 595
intralesional agents 595
keratoacanthomas 592
keratolytic agents 594
laser treatment 594
management of common warts 596
mode of transmission 589–590
mosaic warts 591
occlusotherapy (adhesiotherapy) 594
pathogenesis 589
penile warts 593
periungual and subungual warts 591, *592*
phototherapies 596

polyphenon E (sinecatechins) 595
prevention 594–596
punctate warts 591
recurrent respiratory papillomatosis (RRP) 592–593
sexual transmission 590
sinecatechins (polyphenon E) 595
subclinical and latent forms 589–590
systemic immune stimulation 595
treatment 594–596
vaccinations 595–596
verrucae planae/plane warts/flat warts 591
vertical transmission 590
virucidal therapy 595
vulvovaginal warts 593
WHIM syndrome 589
humerus fractures 2226
humoral (antibody) deficiencies, immunocompromised children 686
Huriez syndrome *see* palmoplantar keratoderma with scleroatrophy
Hurler syndrome, hypertrichosis 2133
Hurley score, hidradenitis suppurativa (HS) (acne inversa) 827
Hutchinson–Gilford progeria syndrome (HGPS) 1725–1727
clinical features 1726–1727
differential diagnosis 1727
epidemiology 1725–1726
history 1725
pathogenesis 1725–1726
pathology 1726
prognosis 1727
HV *see* hydroa vacciniforme
HVL *see* hydroa vacciniforme-like cutaneous T-cell lymphoma
hyaline fibromatosis syndrome (HFS) 1164–1166
aetiology 1164
clinical features 1164–1166
definition 1164
differential diagnosis 1166
pathology 1164
prognosis 1166
treatment 1166
hyalinoses 1164–1166
hyalinosis cutis et mucosae 1166–1167
hydroa vacciniforme (HV) 952–953
clinical features 952–953
differential diagnosis 953
epidemiology 952
histology findings 953
history 952
key features **952**
laboratory findings 953
pathogenesis 952
prevention 953
treatment 953
hydroa vacciniforme-like cutaneous T-cell lymphoma (HVL) 1054
clinical features 1054
definition 1054
epidemiology 1054
histopathology 1054
immunophenotype 1054
prognosis 1054
treatment 1054
hydroxychloroquine, antimalarial agents 2289
hymenopterids 736–737
hymenopterid venoms 737
hypereosinophilic disorders 316–334
congenital eosinophilia 317
eosinophilia in older children 318
eosinophilic cellulitis (Wells syndrome) 328–330
eosinophilic fasciitis 331–332
eosinophilic panniculitis 333–334
eosinophilic pustular folliculitis in infancy and childhood 318–322
hypereosinophilic syndrome 324–327
infantile eosinophilia 317
neonatal eosinophilia 317
hypereosinophilic syndrome 324–327
clinical features 324–325
differential diagnosis 325–327
epidemiology 324
treatment 327
hyperimmunoglobulin E syndrome (HIES) **137**
hyperimmunoglobulin E syndromes (HIES) 2052–2055
clinical features 2053–2054
differential diagnosis 2054
DOCK8-deficient HIES patients 2054
epidemiology 2052–2053
histology findings 2054–2055
history 2052
laboratory findings 2054–2055
pathogenesis 2052–2053
prevention 2055
treatment 2055
hyperlipidaemias, carotenaemia 1983, 1985
hyperlipoproteinaemia 1980–1981
aetiology 1980
clinical features 1980–1981
definition 1980
differential diagnosis 1981
history 1980
pathology 1980
prognosis 1981
treatment 1981
types **1980**
hypernatraemic dehydration, Netherton syndrome (NS) 1618
hyperparathyroidism 2003–2004
clinical features 2003
cutaneous manifestations 2003–2004
histology findings 2003
laboratory findings 2003
multiple endocrine neoplasia syndrome (MEN syndrome) 2004
pathogenesis 2003
prevention 2003–2004
treatment 2003–2004
hyperpigmentation 1463–1471, *1472*
see also pigmentation
acquired hyperpigmentation 1463–1469
amyloidosis 1466, 1470
autoimmune diseases 1467
circumscribed hyperpigmentation 1463–1465
dermatopathia pigmentosa reticularis 1471, *1472*, 1517–1518
diffuse hyperpigmentation 1467, 1469–1470
Dowling–Degos disease (DDD) 1471
drug-induced circumscribed hyperpigmentation 1464–1465
drug-induced diffuse hyperpigmentation 1467
dyskeratosis congenita (DC) 1471, *1472*
endocrine and metabolic disorders 1467
erythema dyschromicum perstans (EDP) 1465
familial primary cutaneous localized amyloidosis 1470
familial progressive hyperpigmentation 1469–1470
Fanconi anaemia 1471
Galli-Galli disease 1471
incontinentia pigmenti (IP) 1470
inherited disorders of pigmentation 1469–1471
linear and whorled naevoid hypermelanosis (LWNH) 1470–1471
linear hyperpigmentation 1468, 1470–1471
mastocytosis 1465
melasma 1465–1466
minocycline **1465**
miscellaneous disorders 1468
Naegeli–Franceschetti–Jadassohn syndrome (NFJS) 1471, *1472*, 1517–1518
nail dystrophy *1472*
nutritional abnormalities 1467
periorbital hyperpigmentation 1465
pigmentary demarcation lines 1468
postinflammatory hyperpigmentation 1463–1464
primary cutaneous localized amyloidosis 1466
reticulate acropigmentation of Kitamura 1471
reticulated hyperpigmentation 1468–1469
reticulate hyperpigmentation 1471, *1472*
X-linked reticulate pigmentary disorder 1471
hyperpituitarism 2005
clinical features 2005
cutaneous manifestations 2005
histology findings 2005
laboratory findings 2005
pathogenesis 2005
prevention 2005
treatment 2005
hypersensitivity reactions to drugs 785–801
see also adverse drug reactions (ADR)
acute generalized exanthematous pustulosis (AGEP) 792–793
angioedema 787
bullous drug eruptions 794–795
classification **785**
clinical manifestations 786
diagnostic approach 800
drug rash with eosinophilia and systemic symptoms (DRESS) 790–791

hypersensitivity reactions to drugs (*cont'd*)
- fixed drug eruption (FDE) 794–795
- Gell and Coombs classification **785**
- maculopapular drug eruptions or exanthems (MPDEs) 789–791
- management 800
- pustular eruptions 792–793
- serum sickness-like reaction (SSLR) 788
- staphylococcal scalded skin syndrome (SSSS) 797
- Stevens–Johnson syndrome (SJS) 795–798
- toxic epidermal necrolysis (TEN) 795–798
- urticaria 787
- urticarial infections 787–788

hypertension, psoriasis 360
hyperthyroidism 1994–1995
- clinical features 1994–1995
- cutaneous manifestations 1994–1995
- histology findings 1995
- laboratory findings 1995
- pathogenesis 1994
- prevention 1995
- treatment 1995

hypertrichosis 2132–2136
- acquired generalized hypertrichosis (drug related) 2133
- acquired localized hypertrichosis 2135
- Becker naevus (BN) 2135–2136
- congenital hair on the elbows 2134
- congenital hairy naevi 2134
- congenital hypertrichosis lanuginosa 2132–2133
- congenital localized hypertrichosis 2134–2135
- congenital smooth muscle hamartomas 2134
- Cornelia de Lange syndrome (CDLS) 2132–2133
- generalized hypertrichosis 2132–2133
- Gorlin syndrome 2135
- hereditary generalized hypertrichosis 2132–2133
- hereditary gingival fibromatosis 2132
- Hurler syndrome 2133
- localized hypertrichosis 2134–2136
- localized hypertrichosis over the spinal column 2135
- minoxidil-induced hypertrichosis 2133
- other illnesses/conditions associated with hypertrichosis 2134
- porphyria 2133
- treatment 2136
- Winchester syndrome 2135

hypertrichosis and dental defects **1649**
hypertrophic lichen planus 395, *396*
hypertrophic scars, laser therapy 2324
hypnosis 2340
hypodermis, embryonic–fetal transition 15
hypogonadism 1998–1999
- clinical features 1998
- cutaneous manifestations 1998–1999
- histology findings 1998–1999
- Klinefelter syndrome 1999
- laboratory findings 1998–1999
- pathogenesis 1998
- prevention 1999
- treatment 1999
- Turner syndrome 1999

hypohidrotic ectodermal dysplasia (HED)
- with deafness **1650**
- HED-X-linked (ED1) **1649**
- with hypothyroidism and agenesis of the corpus callosum **1651**
- with hypothyroidism and ciliary dyskinesia (HEDH syndrome) **1650–1651**
- with immune deficiency **1650**
- with immune deficiency, osteopetrosis and lymphoedema **1650**
- with immunodeficiency 1675
- with immunodeficiency with osteopetrosis and lymphoedema 1675

hypoparathyroidism 2002–2004
- clinical features 2002
- cutaneous manifestations 2002–2004
- histology findings 2002
- laboratory findings 2002
- McCune–Albright syndrome (MAS) 2002–2003
- pathogenesis 2002
- polyglandular autoimmune syndrome 2002
- prevention 2002–2003
- pseudohypoparathyroidism 2002–2003
- treatment 2002–2003

hypopigmentation 1492–1498
- acquired hypopigmentation *1493*, 1496–1498
- congenital hypopigmentation 1492–1496
- lichen sclerosus (LS) 1497
- localized congenital hypopigmentation 1495–1496
- mycosis fungoides (MF) 1497–1498
- other conditions associated with acquired hypopigmentation 1498
- overview **1493**
- piebaldism 1493–1494
- pityriasis alba (PA) 1496–1497
- Waardenburg syndrome (WS) 1495

hypopituitarism 2004
- clinical features 2004
- cutaneous manifestations 2004
- histology findings 2004
- laboratory findings 2004
- pathogenesis 2004
- prevention 2004
- treatment 2004

hypothermia, Netherton syndrome (NS) 1618
hypothyroidism 1993–1994
- clinical features 1993–1994
- cutaneous manifestations 1993–1994
- histology findings 1994
- laboratory findings 1994
- pathogenesis 1993
- prevention 1994
- treatment 1994

hypotrichosis and recurrent skin vesicles **1651**, 1701–1702
hypotrichosis–osteolysis–periodontitis–palmoplantar keratoderma syndrome (HOPP syndrome) 1544, **1651**
- clinical features 1544
- differential diagnosis 1544
- epidemiology 1544
- history 1544
- pathogenesis 1544
- treatment 1544

hypotrichosis simplex **1651**
hypotrichosis simplex of the scalp 1702
hypotrichosis with juvenile macular degeneration 1702

IA *see* infantile acropustulosis
iatrogenic calcinosis cutis, calcification and ossification in the skin 1345
iatrogenic disorders of the newborn 154–164
- adhesive tape damage 163
- amniocentesis 156
- antenatal procedures 156–157
- arterial catheterization 160–161
- Caesarean section delivery 158
- chorionic villus sampling (CVS) 156
- drugs and nutrients complications 161
- extravasation injuries 161–162
- fetal monitoring 157
- fetal wound healing 155
- forceps deliveries 158
- heelprick marks 164
- injuries acquired during normal or operative deliveries 157–158
- injuries during labour 157–158
- injury during pregnancy 156–157
- intensive care monitoring 163
- needle marks 163
- phototherapy complications 164
- respiratory function damage 160
- scar formation in postnatal skin 154–156
- skin disorders after birth 159–164
- surgical scars 164
- total parenteral nutrition (TPN) 161–162
- transcutaneous monitoring 163
- transillumination burns 163
- vaccinations 164
- vacuum extractors 158

iatrogenic oral ulceration 2087
iatrogenic panniculitis 1220
iatrogenic scalp birth injuries **138**
ICD *see* irritant contact dermatitis
ichthyoses 1549–1597
- annular epidermolytic ichthyosis (AEI) 1570
- arthrogryposis renal dysfunction cholestasis (ARC) syndrome 1589
- autosomal recessive congenital ichthyoses (ARCI) 1557–1566
- bathing suit icthyosis (BSI) 1560–1561
- CEDNIK 1589
- Chanarin–Dorfman syndrome (neutral lipid storage disease with ichthyosis) 1580–1581

classification 1549–1550, **1551**
collodion baby and self-improving congenital ichthyosis 1560
coloboma, heart defect, ichthyosiform dermatosis, mental retardation, ear anomalies (CHIME) syndrome 1590
complex and ultra-rare neuroichthyotic syndromes 1589
congenital hemidysplasia–ichthyosiform naevus-limb defect syndrome (CHILD) syndrome 1577
congenital ichthyoses (CI) 1592–1597
congenital ichthyosiform erythroderma (CIE) 1561–1566
congenital reticular ichthyosiform erythroderma (CRIE) **1568**
Conradi–Hünermann–Happle syndrome 1576–1577
epidermolytic ichthyosis (EI) 125–126, **138**, **140**, 1518–1520, 1567–1570
epidermolytic naevi (mosaic epidermolytic ichthyosis) 1570–1571
erythrokeratoderma 1575
exfoliative ichthyosis 1574–1575
Gaucher disease type II 1589
harlequin ichthyosis (HI) 1558–1559
history 1549
ichthyoses with hair abnormalities, gastrointestinal or respiratory symptoms 1581–1584
ichthyosis, spastic quadriplegia and mental retardation (ISQMR) syndrome 1589
ichthyosis Curth–Macklin (ICM) **1568**
ichthyosis follicularis, with atrichia and photophobia (IFAP) syndrome 1578
ichthyosis hypotrichosis syndrome 1581
ichthyosis prematurity syndrome (IPS) 1583–1584
ichthyosis vulgaris (IV) 1551–1554
keratinopathic ichthyoses (KPI) 1567
keratitis ichthyosis deafness syndrome (KID syndrome) 1586–1587
keratosis linearis with ichthyosis congenita and sclerosing keratoderma (KLICK) syndrome 1531, 1575
lamellar ichthyosis (LI) 1561–1566
loricrin keratoderma 1575
management of congenital ichthyoses 1592–1597
mental retardation-enteropathy-deafness-neuropathy-ichthyosis-keratodermia (MEDNIK) syndrome 1589
multiple sulphatase deficiency (MSD) 1591–1592
neonatal ichthyosis-sclerosing cholangitis (NISCH) syndrome 1581–1583
Netherton syndrome (NS) 1579
Neu-Laxova syndrome (NLS) 1590
neuroichthyotic syndromes 1585–1589
neutral lipid storage disease with ichthyosis (Chanarin–Dorfman syndrome) 1580–1581
nonsyndromic ichthyoses 1551–1576
nosology 1549–1550
pathophysiological aspects 1550–1551
peeling skin syndrome (PSS) 1575
recessive X-linked ichthyosis (RXLI) 1554–1556
Refsum disease (RD) 1591
severe dermatitis, multiple allergies, metabolic wasting syndrome (SAM) syndrome 1579–1580
Sjögren–Larsson syndrome (SLS) 1585–1586
Stormorken syndrome 1589
superficial epidermolytic ichthyosis (SEI) **1568**, 1571–1572
syndromic ichthyoses 1576–1592
trichothiodystrophy (TTD) 1587–1589
ultra-rare neuroichthyotic syndromes with later disease presentations 1591–1592
X-chromosomal ichthyosis syndromes 1576–1581
ichthyosiform mycosis fungoides (IMF) 1049
ichthyosis, spastic quadriplegia and mental retardation (ISQMR) syndrome 1589
ichthyosis bullosa of Siemens *see* epidermolytic ichthyosis; superficial epidermolytic ichthyosis
ichthyosis Curth–Macklin (ICM) **1568**, 1572–1573
clinical features 1573
differential diagnosis 1573
epidemiology 1572
genetic findings 1573
histology findings 1573
laboratory findings 1573
pathogenesis 1572
prevention 1573
treatment 1573
ichthyosis follicularis **2109**
ichthyosis follicularis, with atrichia and photophobia (IFAP) syndrome 1578, **1652**
clinical features 1578
differential diagnosis 1578
hair loss 2111
pathogenesis 1578
treatment 1578
ichthyosis hypotrichosis syndrome 1581
definition 1581
pathogenesis 1581
ichthyosis linearis circumflexa (ILC), hair disorders 2114, *2116*
ichthyosis prematurity syndrome (IPS) 1583–1584, **1583**
clinical features 1583
differential diagnosis 1583, *1584*
laboratory findings 1584
pathogenesis 1583
prevention 1584
treatment 1584
ultrastructure 1584
ichthyosis vulgaris (IV) 1551–1554
clinical features 1552–1553
differential diagnosis 1553
epidemiology 1551–1552
histology findings 1553–1554
laboratory findings 1553–1554
pathogenesis 1551–1552
prevention 1554
treatment 1554
ichthyosis with hypotrichosis **1583**
ICM *see* ichthyosis Curth–Macklin
ID *see* infective dermatitis
idiopathic calcinosis of the scrotum/vulva 1340–1341, 2190–2191
clinical features 1340–1341
differential diagnosis 1341
epidemiology 1340
histopathology 1341
pathogenesis 1340
treatment 1341
idiopathic photodermatoses and skin testing 943–956
actinic prurigo (AP) 947–949
chronic actinic dermatitis (CAD) 953–954
hydroa vacciniforme (HV) 952–953
idiopathic solar urticaria 949–951
polymorphous light eruption (syn. polymorphic light eruption, benign summer light eruption, lucite estivale bénigne) 944–946
skin testing 954–956
solar urticaria, idiopathic 949–951
idiopathic scrotal calcinosis *see* idiopathic calcinosis of the scrotum/vulva
idiopathic solar urticaria 949–951
clinical features 950
differential diagnosis 950
epidemiology 949–950
histology findings 950
key features **950**
laboratory findings 950
pathogenesis 949–950
prevention 950–951
treatment 950–951
idiopathic thrombocytopenic purpura, differential diagnosis of inflicted bruises *2225*
IDQoL *see* Infants' Dermatitis Quality of Life questionnaire
IEM *see* inborn errors of metabolism
IFAP syndrome *see* ichthyosis follicularis, with atrichia and photophobia syndrome
IFN *see* interferons
IH *see* infantile haemangiomas
IH-QoL *see* Infantile Hemangioma Quality of Life instrument
IL *see* indeterminate leprosy
IL-12/IFN-γ axis, defects **2040**
ILC *see* ichthyosis linearis circumflexa
ILVEN *see* inflammatory linear verrucous epidermal naevus
IM *see* infectious mononucleosis
imaging, diagnostic, pseudoxanthoma elasticum (PXE) 1130
imaging findings, lipodystrophies 1225–1226
imaging studies, infantile haemangiomas (IH) 1431
IMF *see* ichthyosiform mycosis fungoides

imiquimod, human papillomaviruses (HPV) 595
immobilization, surgical therapy 2311
immune dysfunction, systemic sclerosis (SSc) 1185
immune dysfunction with T-cell inactivation due to calcium entry defect 1 and 2 (immunodeficiency 9 and 10) **1652**
immune dysregulation, polyendocrinopathy, enteropathy, X-linked syndrome (IPEX syndrome) 2060
  endocrine dysfunction 2009
immune modulators., molluscum contagiosum (MC) 585
immune stimulation and modulation, human papillomaviruses (HPV) 595
immune system, vitiligo 1477–1478
immunobullous disease – vulval bullous and cicatricial pemphigoid and linear IgA disease of childhood 2179–2180
immunocompromised children 684–690
  antibody (humoral) deficiencies 686
  bacterial infections 686–687, 689–690
  chronic granulomatous disease (CGD) 687
  combined immunodeficiencies (CIDs) 685
  cutaneous infections 684–690
  fungal infections 686, 687, 690
  herpes simplex virus (HSV) infections 603–604, 689
  human papillomaviruses (HPV) 688–689
  humoral (antibody) deficiencies 686
  mycobacterial infections 685–686
  phagocytic defects 687
  primary immunodeficiencies 685–687
  pyogenic infections 686
  secondary immunodeficiencies 687–690
  varicella zoster viruses (VZV) 689
  viral infections 686, 688–689
immunodeficiencies, primary, neonatal erythroderma 131
immunodeficiency syndromes 2028–2066
  ataxia telangiectasia (AT) 2030–2032
  autoimmune lymphoproliferative syndrome (Canale–Smith syndrome) **2036**
  autosomal recessive EBV-associated lymphoproliferative syndrome **2036**
  Canale–Smith syndrome (autoimmune lymphoproliferative syndrome) **2036**
  cartilage–hair hypoplasia syndrome (CHH) 2033
  Chediak–Higashi syndrome (CHS) 2034–2035
  chronic granulomatous disease (CGD) 2037–2041
  chronic mucocutaneous candidiasis (CMC) 2041–2045
  complement deficiency disorders 2045–2050
  DiGeorge syndrome (DGS) 2051–2052
  Duncan disease (X-linked lymphoproliferative syndrome) **2036**
  familial haemophagocytic lymphohistiocytosis **2036**
  Griscelli syndrome (GS) **2036**
  hereditary angioedema (HAE) 2046–2048
  hyperimmunoglobulin E syndromes (HIES) 2052–2055
  immune dysregulation, polyendocrinopathy, enteropathy, X-linked syndrome (IPEX syndrome) 2060
  immunoglobulin deficiencies 2056–2059
  leucocyte adhesion deficiency (LAD) 2060–2061
  mucocutaneous findings **2029**
  severe combined immunodeficiency (SCID) 2061–2064
  Wiskott–Aldrich syndrome (WAS) 2064–2066
  X-linked lymphoproliferative syndrome (Duncan disease) **2036**
immunodeficiency with lymphoid proliferation **2036**
immunofluorescence assay (IFA), rickettsial disease 511
immunoglobulin, intravenous *see* intravenous immunoglobulin
immunoglobulin deficiencies 2056–2059
  aberrant chemokine signalling **2058**
  abnormal DNA methylation leading to defective B-cell negative selection and terminal differentiation **2058**
  agammaglobulinaemia 2059
  block in B-cell differentiation at the pro-B- to pre-B-cell transition **2057**
  CVID 2056–2059
  defective class switch recombination (e.g. from IgM to IgG, IgA or IgE) and somatic hypermutation **2057**
  delayed maturation of helper T-cell function **2058**
  hyperimmunoglobulin M syndromes (HIMS) 2056
  immunoglobulin A deficiency 2056
  panhypogammaglobulinaemia 2056–2059
immunohistochemical markers, vascular lesions **2385**
immunohistochemical staining, rickettsial disease 511
immunohistochemistry, inflammatory skin conditions 2382
immunological alterations, ultraviolet radiation (UVR) 974
immunological disorders, neonatal erythroderma 130–132
immunomodulators
  see also chemotherapy and immunomodulators
  topical immunomodulators, irritant contact dermatitis (ICD) 296
  vitiligo 1483
immunophenotype, granuloma annulare (GA) 1012
immunosuppressants, hidradenitis suppurativa (HS) (acne inversa) 828
immunosuppressants and TNF-α inhibitors, systemic, orofacial granulomatosis (OFG) 1020
immunosuppression, systemic sclerosis (SSc) 1193
immunotherapy and allergen testing, insects/insect bites 737
impetigo 426–427
  vs cigarette burns **2413**
impulsive self-mutilation 2268–2269
inborn errors of metabolism (IEM) 1965–1967
  see also metabolic disorders
  carotenaemia 1985
  classification **1967**
  neonatal erythroderma 132
inclusion body fibromatosis *see* infantile digital fibromatosis
inclusion conjunctivitis, *Chlamydia trachomatis* infections 2210, 2211–2212
incontinentia pigmenti (IP) **138**, **1652**, 1718–1723
  breast and nipple abnormalities 1721
  clinical features 148, 1719–1721
  diagnostic criteria 1722
  differential diagnosis 148, 1714, 1722
  epidemiology 147–148, 1718–1719
  eye features 1721
  genetic testing 1722
  hair features 1721
  histology 1722
  histology findings 148
  hyperpigmentation 1470
  laboratory findings 148, 1722
  medical surveillance and treatment 1722–1723
  nails features 1720–1721
  neonatal blistering **140**, 147–148
  neurological signs 1721
  pathogenesis 147–148, 1718–1719
  prevention 148
  skin features 1719–1720
  teeth features 1721
  treatment 148
indeterminate cell histiocytosis 1090–1091
  clinical features 1090–1091
  differential diagnosis 1091
  epidemiology 1090
  histology findings 1091
  history 1090
  pathogenesis 1090
  treatment 1091
indeterminate leprosy (IL) **497**, **499**
indications for paediatric dermatological surgery 2312–2313
indirect immunoperoxidase assay, rickettsial disease 511
indolent systemic mastocytosis (ISM) **1104**
infantile (desmoid-type) fibromatosis 1362–1363
  clinical features 1363

differential diagnosis 1363
epidemiology 1363
history 1362
pathogenesis 1363
pathology 1363
treatment 1363
infantile acne (acne infantum) **135**, 814–815
infantile acropustulosis (IA) 144–145
clinical features 144
differential diagnosis 144
epidemiology 144
histology findings 144
laboratory findings 144
pathogenesis 144
prevention 144–145
treatment 144–145
infantile dermal fibromatosis *see* infantile digital fibromatosis
infantile digital fibromatosis 1365–1366
clinical features 1365
differential diagnosis 1365
epidemiology 1365
history 1365
pathogenesis 1365
pathology 1365
treatment 1365–1366
infantile eosinophilia 317
infantile haemangiomas (IH) 1425–1437
active non-intervention 1435
airway haemangiomas 1430
associations 1431–1435
β-blockers (BB) 1435–1436, 2290
cardiac failure 1430
classification **1426**
clinical features 1426–1428
complications 1429–1431, **1435**
corticosteroids 1436
differential diagnosis 1431
disfigurement 1431
embolization 1437
epidemiology 1425–1426
histopathology 1426
imaging studies 1431
laser therapy 1436–1437, 2322
lower body haemangiomas and structural malformations (PELVIS/SACRAL/LUMBAR syndrome) 1433–1434
multifocal infantile haemangiomas 1434–1435
ophthalmological complications 1430
pathogenesis 1425–1426
PELVIS/SACRAL/LUMBAR syndrome (lower body haemangiomas and structural malformations) 1433–1434
PHACES syndrome 1432–1433
prognosis 1428–1429
propranolol 1435–1436, 2403–2406
quality of life (QoL) assessment 2252
surgery 1437
surgical therapy 2313
systemic corticosteroids 1436
systemic therapies 1436
topical therapies 1436
topical timolol 2406
treatment 1435
ulceration 1429–1430
Infantile Hemangioma Quality of Life instrument (IH-QoL) 2250
infantile perineal (perianal) protrusion (IPP) 108–109
aetiology 108
clinical features 109
definition 108
differential diagnosis 109
pathology 108–109
treatment 109
infantile pyramidal perineal protrusion 2186
infantile seborrhoeic dermatitis (SD)
atopic dermatitis (AD) 237–239
clinical features 238
definition 237
differential diagnosis 238–239
epidemiology 237–238
erythematosquamous skin diseases 123
napkin dermatitis **269**, 274, 275
neonatal erythroderma 123
pathology 238
prognosis 239
treatment 239
infantile systemic hyalinosis (ISH) 1164–1166
infants
see also neonates; transient skin disorders in neonates and young infants
cutaneous microbiome 47–49
infants and children, approach to the paediatric patient 2344–2347
Infants' Dermatitis Quality of Life questionnaire (IDQoL)
atopic dermatitis (AD) 223
quality of life (QoL) assessment 2242–2243, 2250
infections
calcification and ossification in the skin 1344
tongue 2100–2101
infections and infestations, nursing care of the skin 2402
infectious causes of blistering, vesiculobullous lesions 863–864
infectious mononucleosis (IM) 671–672
see also Epstein–Barr virus (EBV or HHV-4)
clinical features 671–672
differential diagnosis 672
epidemiology 671
laboratory findings 672
oral mucosa 2084
pathogenesis 671
prevention 672
treatment 672
infectious napkin dermatitis 271–274
bullous impetigo 273
candidal (monilial) napkin dermatitis 271–272
congenital syphilis 273–274
HIV infection 274
perianal streptococcal disease 272–273
scabies 273
streptococcal intertrigo 272–273
infective dermatitis (ID) 654–657, *655*
see also HTLV-1 infection
definition 654
diagnostic criteria **657**
infective panniculitis 1220
infestations and infections
HIV infection 652–653
nursing care of the skin 2402
inflammation of the skin, cutaneous microbiome 49
inflammatory acne, differential diagnosis **819**
inflammatory bowel diseases, oral mucosa 2086
inflammatory dermatoses of the genital region 2160–2163
inflammatory diseases, adnexal disorders 1325–1328
inflammatory disorders
HIV infection 653
vesiculobullous lesions 865–866
inflammatory linear verrucous epidermal naevus (ILVEN) 1270–1271
clinical features 1271
differential diagnosis 1271
histopathology 1271
history 1270
laser therapy 2323
pathogenesis 1271
treatment 1271
inflammatory or infectious skin conditions, surgical therapy 2312
inflammatory skin conditions, immunohistochemistry 2382
infliximab
atopic dermatitis (AD) 260
biologic agents 2292
infundibular cyst *see* epidermal cyst
ingenol mebutate, human papillomaviruses (HPV) 595
ingrown nails 2149
inheritance and genetics in brief 36–38
inheritance potential, mosaicism/mosaic disorders 1229–1231
inherited causes, vesiculobullous lesions 866
inherited connective tissue disorders, striae xref, 1173
inherited disorders, calcification and ossification in the skin 1344
insect repellents 735–736
insects/insect bites 734
irritant contact dermatitis (ICD) 291
insulin metabolism and the skin, metabolic syndrome (MetS) 843–844
insulin-related disorders, cutaneous manifestations 2005–2008
insulin resistance 2007–2008
clinical features 2007
cutaneous manifestations 2007–2008
endocrine dysfunction 2008
histology findings 2007
laboratory findings 2007
pathogenesis 2007
prevention 2007–2008
treatment 2007–2008

'insulin signalling' genes, lipodystrophies 1224
intensive care
neonatal erythroderma 2409
nursing care of the skin 2409
Stevens–Johnson syndrome (SJS) 2409
toxic epidermal necrolysis (TEN) 2409
intensive care monitoring, iatrogenic disorders of the newborn 163
interferons (IFN)
biologic agents 2293
human papillomaviruses (HPV) 595
intermediate cells, embryonic–fetal transition 11–12
internet resources, tuberous sclerosis complex (TSC) **1854**
intertrigo napkin rash **268**, 270–271
intralesional agents, human papillomaviruses (HPV) 595
intralesional corticosteroids, orofacial granulomatosis (OFG) 1019–1020
intraoperative complications, surgical therapy 2317
intraparenchymal melanosis, congenital melanocytic naevi (CMN) 1244
intravascular large B-cell lymphoma 1056
intravenous immunoglobulin (IVIG)
biologic agents 2292–2293
erythema multiforme (EM) 783
Stevens–Johnson syndrome (SJS) 783
toxic epidermal necrolysis (TEN) 783
inversa dystrophic epidermolysis bullosa 920
inverse lichen planus 397
inverse psoriasis 357, 362, **365**
in vitro transcribed messenger RNA (mRNA), genetic therapies 2304–2305
in vivo gene therapy 2301, *2302*, 2303
IP *see* incontinentia pigmenti
IPEX syndrome *see* immune dysregulation, polyendocrinopathy, enteropathy, X-linked syndrome
IPP *see* infantile perineal (perianal) protrusion
IPS *see* ichthyosis prematurity syndrome
irritant contact dermatitis (ICD) 287–298
acute care 295
antiseptics 292
body fluids 291
clinical features 288–294
clinical types 288–289
definition 287–288
diagnosis 294–295
differential diagnosis 294–295
epidemiology 288
food 293
hobbies and recreations 292–293
household products 291
insects/insect bites 291
investigations 295
irritants 290–294
management 295–296
medical devices 292
medications 291–292
minimizing contact with irritants 295
monitoring for complications 296
pathogenesis 288
patient characteristics 289–290
phototherapy 296
physical irritants 293–294
plants 291
prevention of recurrences 296
skin care products 292, **293**
skin care to enhance recovery 296
topical corticosteroids (TCS) 296
topical immunomodulators 296
treatment 296
irritant reactions to plants 984–986
chemical irritant contact dermatitis 984–985
mechanical irritant contact dermatitis 984
ISH *see* infantile systemic hyalinosis
ISM *see* indolent systemic mastocytosis
Iso–Kikuchi syndrome, nail disorders 2155
isolated CMC, chronic mucocutaneous candidiasis (CMC) **2043**
isotretinoin
acne vulgaris 809–810, 2408–2409, **2410**
monitoring 2408–2409, **2410**
isotretinoin, systemic 2291
acne vulgaris 809–810
suicide/suicide ideation, isoretinoin-induced 810
ISQMR syndrome *see* ichthyosis, spastic quadriplegia and mental retardation syndrome
itching purpura 1878–1879
clinical overview 1878
prognosis 1879
treatment 1879
Ito lines *see* pigmentary demarcation lines
itraconazole
antifungal therapy 2286
dermatophytoses 540–542, **543**
leishmaniasis 699
IV *see* ichthyosis vulgaris
ivermectin
antiparasitic drugs 2287
scabies 717, 718
IVIG *see* intravenous immunoglobulin
ixodid tick bites, lyme borreliosis (LB)/lyme disease 466

Jackson–Lawler syndrome *see* pachyonychia congenita (PC)
Jadassohn–Lewandowsky syndrome *see* pachyonychia congenita (PC)
janus kinase (JAK) inhibitors
alopecia areata (AA) 2145
atopic dermatitis (AD) 256
systemic therapies 2295
jaundice, physiological jaundice, transient skin disorders in neonates and young infants 74–75
JDM *see* juvenile dermatomyositis
JEB *see* junctional epidermolysis bullosa
jellyfish (Cubozoa) 741
jellyfish (Scyphozoa) 741–742
jellyfish/corals (Hydrozoa) 741
Jessner lymphocytic infiltrate (JLI) 1040–1042
aetiology 1040
clinical features 1041–1042
definition 1040
differential diagnosis 1042
histopathology 1041
history 1040
pathogenesis 1040
prognosis 1042
treatment 1042
JHF *see* juvenile hyaline fibromatosis
JIA *see* juvenile idiopathic arthritis
JLI *see* Jessner lymphocytic infiltrate
Johanson–Blizzard syndrome **1652–1653**
joint involvement, Behçet disease (BD) 1955
Jones Criteria, erythema marginatum 767, **768**
JPD *see* juvenile plantar dermatosis
JSSc *see* juvenile-onset SSc; systemic sclerosis
junctional epidermolysis bullosa (JEB) 907, *908*, 932–935
aetiology 932
classification **910**
clinical features 932–934
definition 932
differential diagnosis 934
junctional epidermolysis bullosa generalized intermediate 934
junctional epidermolysis bullosa generalized severe 932–933, *934*
junctional epidermolysis bullosa with pyloric atresia 934
junctional epidermolysis bullosa with respiratory and renal disease 935
laryngo-onycho-cutaneous (Shabbir) syndrome 934
pathogenesis 932
pathology 932
prognosis 934
treatment 934–935
jungle rot *see* tropical skin ulcer
juvenile active ossifying fibroma, oral mucosa 2096
juvenile aponeurotic fibroma *see* calcifying aponeurotic fibroma
juvenile dermatomyositis (JDM) 1945–1950
antibodies in patients with juvenile dermatomyositis **1949**
cardiorespiratory involvement 1948
classification 1945
clinical features 1946–1948
cutaneous involvement 1946–1947
diagnosis **1946**
differential diagnosis **1946**
epidemiology 1945
gastrointestinal involvement 1947
genitourinary involvement 1948
histopathological findings 1948
laboratory findings 1948
musculoskeletal disease 1947, **1948**
neurological involvement 1948
outcome 1950
pathogenesis 1945–1946
treatment 1948–1950
juvenile hyaline fibromatosis (JHF) 1164–1166

juvenile idiopathic arthritis (JIA) 1933–1938
  biologic therapies 1937–1938
  classification 1933–1935
  clinical features 1935–1937
  differential diagnosis **1934**, 1937
  enthesitis-related arthritis 1936
  epidemiology 1933–1935
  laboratory findings 1937
  oligoarthritis 1936
  pathogenesis 1933–1935
  polyarthritis, rheumatoid factor negative 1936
  polyarthritis, rheumatoid factor positive 1936
  prevention 1937–1938
  psoriatic arthritis 1937
  treatment 1937–1938
juvenile-onset SSc (JSSc) *see* systemic sclerosis
juvenile plantar dermatosis (JPD) 335–337
  clinical features 336
  differential diagnosis 336
  epidemiology 335–336
  histology findings 336
  history 335
  laboratory findings 336
  pathogenesis 335–336
  prevention 336–337
  treatment 336–337
juvenile xanthogranuloma (JXG) 1080–1082
  clinical features 1081–1082
  differential diagnosis 1082, **1317**
  epidemiology 1080–1081
  histology findings 1082
  history 1080–1081
  pathogenesis 1081
  treatment 1082
juvenile xanthoma *see* juvenile xanthogranuloma

kala-azar, leishmaniasis 693
kaposiform haemangioendothelioma (KHE) 1444–1445
  see also tufted angioma
kaposiform lymphangiomatosis (KLA) 1449
Kaposi sarcoma
  HIV infection 653–654
  oral mucosa 2092
Kaposi varicelliform eruption, herpes simplex virus (HSV) infections 604
karyotype testing, molecular genetics 40
Kasabach–Merritt phenomenon (KMP) 1446–1448
  diagnosis 1447
  prognosis 1447
  therapeutic options 1447–1448
Kawasaki disease (KD) 1883, 1906–1915
  acute inflammation at the site of prior bacillus Calmette–Guerin (BCG) vaccination 1911
  acute nonpurulent cervical adenopathy 1910–1911
  aetiology 1907
  bilateral conjunctival injection 1909
  cardiovascular and other complications 1912–1913
  changes in lips and oral cavity 1909, *1910*
  changes in peripheral extremities 1908
  clinical features 1907–1911
  diagnosis 1907–1911
  differential diagnosis 1911–1912
  early detection of incomplete Kawasaki disease 1912
  epidemiology 1906–1907
  history 1906
  incomplete cases 1912
  laboratory findings 1912
  management 1914
  napkin dermatitis 276
  other cutaneous findings 1911
  pathogenesis 1907
  polymorphous skin eruption 1908–1909
  prognosis 1914–1915
  tongue 2100–2101
  treatment 1914
  unique feature 1911
keloid scars, laser therapy 2324
KEN *see* keratinocytic epidermal naevus
keratin disorders 1515–1521
  congenital reticular ichthyosiform erythroderma (CRIE) **1568**, 1572
  dermatopathia pigmentosa reticularis 1471, *1472*, 1517–1518
  Dowling–Degos disease (DDD) 1518
  ectodermal dysplasia, 'pure' hair-nail types 1520, 1698
  epidermolysis bullosa simplex (EBS) 1517
  epidermolytic ichthyosis (EI) 125–126, **138**, **140**, 1518–1520, 1567–1570
  ichthyosis Curth–Macklin (ICM) **1568**, 1572–1573
  keratin biology 1515–1517
  monilethrix 1520, *1521*
  Naegeli–Franceschetti–Jadassohn syndrome (NFJS) 1471, *1472*, 1517–1518
  palmoplantar keratodermas 1520
  pseudo-folliculitis barbae 1521
  superficial epidermolytic ichthyosis (SEI) **1568**, 1571–1572
  white sponge 'naevus' of Cannon 1520
keratinization, developing human skin 23
keratinocytes, embryonic–fetal transition 11–12, *13*
keratinocytic epidermal naevus (KEN) 1267–1269
  associated syndromes 1268–1269
  clinical features 1267, *1268*
  CLOVE syndrome (congenital lipomatous overgrowth, vascular malformations and epidermal naevus) 1269
  histopathology 1268
  history 1267
  pathogenesis 1267, *1268*
  treatment 1268
keratinopathic ichthyoses (KPI) 1567
  definition 1567
  epidemiology 1567
  pathogenesis 1567
keratitis ichthyosis deafness syndrome (KID syndrome) 1586–1587, **1653**, **1803**
  clinical features 1586–1587, 1694
  definition 1693
  differential diagnosis 1587, 1694
  epidemiology 1586
  genetic findings 1587
  hair loss **2109**
  histology findings 1587
  laboratory findings 1587
  pathogenesis 1586
  pathology 1694
  porokeratotic eccrine naevus (PEN) 1587
  prevention 1587
  prognosis 1694
  treatment 1587, 1694
keratoacanthomas, human papillomaviruses (HPV) 592
keratoderma palmoplantaris transgrediens *see* Mal de Meleda
keratodermas *see* palmoplantar keratodermas (PPKs)
keratolytic agents
  congenital ichthyoses (CI) 1593–1594
  human papillomaviruses (HPV) 594
keratolytics, molluscum contagiosum (MC) 584
keratosis extremitatum hereditaria transgrediens et progrediens *see* Mal de Meleda
keratosis follicularis spinulosa decalvans (KFSD) 1601–1602, **2109**, 2130–2131
keratosis linearis with ichthyosis congenita and sclerosing keratoderma (KLICK) syndrome 1531, 1575
  clinical features 1531
  differential diagnosis 1531
  epidemiology 1531
  history 1531
  laboratory investigation 1531
  pathogenesis 1531
  pathology 1531
  treatment 1531
keratosis palmoplantaris areata et striata *see* striate palmoplantar keratoderma
keratosis palmoplantaris papillomatosa et verrucosa Jakac–Wolf 1548
keratosis palmoplantaris striata I (PPKS1) **1653**, 1701
keratosis palmoplantaris striata II (PPKS2) **1653**, 1701
keratosis palmoplantaris striata III (PPKS3) **1653**, 1699
keratosis palmoplantaris varians Siemens–Wachters *see* striate palmoplantar keratoderma
keratosis pilaris 1599–1602
  aetiology 1600
  atrophoderma vermiculata 1601
  cardiofaciocutaneous syndrome **1601**
  clinical features 1600–1602

keratosis pilaris (*cont'd*)
definition 1599
differential diagnosis 1602
history 1599–1600
keratosis follicularis spinulosa decalvans (KFSD) 1601–1602
keratosis pilaris atrophicans 1601–1602
pathogenesis 1600
pathology 1600
phrynoderma 1602
prognosis 1602
treatment 1602
keratosis pilaris atrophicans 1601–1602
keratosis punctate palmoplantaris type Buschke–Fischer–Brauer *see* punctate palmoplantar keratoderma
ketamine, anaesthesia 2337
ketoconazole, leishmaniasis 699
KFSD *see* keratosis follicularis spinulosa decalvans
KHE *see* kaposiform haemangioendothelioma
KID syndrome *see* keratitis ichthyosis deafness syndrome
Kimura disease, cf. angiolymphoid hyperplasia with eosinophilia (ALHE) 1351–1352
Kindler syndrome 907, *908*, 935–937
see also epidermolysis bullosa (EB)
classification **910**
clinical features 936
definition 935
diagnostic criteria **137**
differential diagnosis 936–937
history 935
molecular basis 935
pathology 935–936
prognosis 936
treatment 937
Kirghizian dermato-osteolysis **1653**
KIT mutations, mastocytosis 1098–1099
KLA *see* kaposiform lymphangiomatosis
KLICK syndrome *see* keratosis linearis with ichthyosis congenita and sclerosing keratoderma syndrome
Klinefelter syndrome, cutaneous manifestations 1999
Klippel–Trenaunay syndrome (KTS)
lymphatic malformations (LMs) **1453**, *1456*, 1460–1461
PIK3CA-related overgrowth spectrum (PROS) 1291
syndromic vascular anomalies 1415
KMP *see* Kasabach–Merritt phenomenon
koganbyo 746–748
Kohlschutter–Tonz syndrome **1633**
KPI *see* keratinopathic ichthyoses
KTS *see* Klippel–Trenaunay syndrome
kwashiorkor (protein malnutrition) 831–834
hair loss 2127
marasmus–kwashiorkor 831–834

LABD *see* linear immunoglobulin IgA bullous dermatosis
β-lactam antibiotics, systemic therapies 2283
LAD *see* leucocyte adhesion deficiency; linear IgA dermatosis
LAM *see* linear atrophoderma of Moulin
LAMB syndrome, endocrine dysfunction 2008
lamellar ichthyosis (LI) 1561–1566
clinical features 1563–1566
definition 1561
epidemiology 1561–1563
genetic analyses 1566
histology 1566
laboratory findings 1566
pathogenesis 1561–1563
ultrastructure 1566
Langerhans cell histiocytosis (LCH) **137**, **139**, 1071–1076
see also non-Langerhans cell histiocytoses
classification 1072
clinical features 1072–1074
dendritic and histiocyte cell lineage 1071–1072, 1078–1080
diagnostic investigations 1074, *1075*
endocrine dysfunction 2009
epidemiology 1072
evaluation 1074–1075
histiocyte and dendritic cell lineage 1071–1072, 1078–1080
history 1072
napkin dermatitis 276–277
oral mucosa 2096
pathogenesis 1072
prognosis 1074
treatment 1075–1076
Langerhans cells
embryonic–fetal transition 13
embryonic skin 4–5, *6*
lanolin
allergic contact dermatitis (ACD) 308
neonatal skin care 69
lanugo, transient skin disorders in neonates and young infants 73
large-spored ectothrix infections 532
laryngeal masks, anaesthesia 2339
LAS *see* loose anagen syndrome
lasers and intense pulsed light for hair removal 2327–2328
hidradenitis suppurativa (HS) (acne inversa) 828
laser therapy 2319–2328
ablative lasers 2326–2327
acne scars 2324
adverse effects 2321
anaesthetic considerations 2319–2320
angiofibromas in tuberous sclerosis 2323–2324
angioma serpigiosum 2323
café-au-lait macules (CALM) 2325
capillary malformations (port wine stains) 2321–2322
chronic inflammatory skin conditions: psoriasis and eczema 2324
congenital melanocytic naevi (CMN) 2325–2326
cutis marmorata telangiectatica congenita (CMTC) 2323
eczema 2324
focal dermal hypoplasia (FDH (Goltz syndrome)) 2323
hair removal 828, 2327–2328
hypertrophic scars 2324
infantile haemangiomas (IH) 1436–1437, 2322
inflammatory linear verrucous epidermal naevus (ILVEN) 2323
initial skin laser test 2320
keloid scars 2324
laser parameters for vascular lesions **2320**
laser treatment 2320–2321
multiplex laser 2324–2325
naevus of Ota 2325
nursing care of the skin 2402, **2405**
periorbital lesions 2320–2321
pigmented lesions 2325–2326
porokeratosis 1627
'port-wine stain' (localized or extensive capillary malformation) 2321–2322
psoriasis 2324
risks of general anaesthesia in infants and young children 2321
superficial cutaneous lymphangiomas 2324
telangiectasia 2323
ulcerated haemangiomas 2322
vascular lesions 2319–2325
verrucous haemangiomas (verrucous vascular malformations)/ angiokeratomas 2324
laser treatment
human papillomaviruses (HPV) 594
molluscum contagiosum (MC) 584
late-onset CMC, chronic mucocutaneous candidiasis (CMC) **2044**
Launois–Bensaude syndrome
see also multiple symmetric lipomatosis
characteristics **1199**
clinical features **1199**
LB *see* lyme borreliosis (LB)/lyme disease
LCH *see* Langerhans cell histiocytosis
lcSSc (limited cutaneous SSc) **1185**
learning disabilities, neurofibromatosis type 1 (NF1) 1828
lebrikizumab, atopic dermatitis (AD) 260
leiomyomatosis, cutaneous and uterine (Reed syndrome) *see* hereditary leiomyomatosis and renal cell cancer syndrome
leiomyomatosis cutis et uteri *see* hereditary leiomyomatosis and renal cell cancer syndrome
leiomyosarcoma 1391–1392
aetiology 1392
clinical features 1392
definition 1391–1392
differential diagnosis 1392
epidemiology 1391–1392
pathogenesis 1392
pathology 1392
treatment 1392

leishmaniasis 693–699
  aetiopathogenesis 694–695
  allopurinol 699
  amphotericin B deoxycholate 699
  anergic diffuse cutaneous leishmaniasis (ADCL) 695, 697–698
  clinical syndromes 695–697
  cutaneous leishmaniasis (CL) 693, 695
  diagnosis 697–698
  differential diagnosis 697
  epidemiology 693–694
  fluconazole 699
  histopathology 697–698
  incidence 693
  itraconazole 699
  kala-azar 693
  ketoconazole 699
  miltefosine 699
  mucocutaneous leishmaniasis (MCL) 693–699
  paromomycin 699
  pentamidine 699
  pentavalent antimonials 699
  post-kala-azar dermal leishmaniasis (PKDL) 697
  prevention 699
  treatment 698–699
  visceral leishmaniasis (VL) 693, 695
Lelis syndrome **1654**
Lenaerts syndrome 1736
  clinical features 1736
  differential diagnosis 1736
  epidemiology 1736
  histology findings 1736
  history 1736
  laboratory findings 1736
  pathogenesis 1736
  treatment 1736
lentiviral vectors (LV), genetic therapies 2302–2303, **2302**
Lenz–Majewski syndrome (LMS) 1734–1735
  clinical features 1734
  differential diagnosis 1735
  epidemiology 1734
  histology findings 1735
  history 1734
  laboratory findings 1735
  pathogenesis 1734
  treatment 1735
LEOPARD syndrome *see* Noonan syndrome with multiple lentigines
Lepidoptera (caterpillars and moths) 738
lepromatous leprosy (LL) **497**
leprosy in children 496–497
  BCG vaccine 497
  borderline lepromatous leprosy (BL) **497**, **498**, **499**
  borderline tuberculoid leprosy (BT) **497**
  clinical spectrum 496, **497**
  diagnosis 496
  epidemiology 496
  indeterminate leprosy (IL) **497**, **499**
  lepromatous leprosy (LL) **497**
  mid-borderline leprosy (BB) **497**, **499**
  treatment 497, **500**
  tuberculoid leprosy (TT) **497**
Letterer–Siwe disease *see* Langerhans cell histiocytosis
leucocyte adhesion deficiency (LAD) 2060–2061
  clinical features 2060–2061
  differential diagnosis 2061
  histology findings 2061
  laboratory findings 2061
  LAD I **2039**
  LAD II **2039**
  LAD III **2039**
  pathogenesis 2060
  treatment 2061
leucoplakia
  see also white patches (leucoplakia), oral mucosa
  definition 2088
leukaemia 1063–1066
  clinical features 1064–1066
  dermatological manifestations 1063
  differential diagnosis 1064–1066
  epidemiology 1063–1064
  histology findings 1066
  laboratory findings 1066
  pathogenesis 1063–1064
  prevention 1066
  treatment 1066
leukocytoclastic vasculitis 1865–1876
LI *see* lamellar ichthyosis
lice 734
  see also pediculosis
lichen aureus/lichen purpuricus 1878
  clinical overview 1878, *1879*
  histology 1878
  prognosis 1878
  treatment 1878
lichen nitidus (LN) 403–406
  associated diseases **405**
  clinical features 404–405
  differential diagnosis **405**
  epidemiology 403
  history 403
  laboratory findings 405–406
  pathogenesis 403–404
  pathology findings 405–406
  prognosis 406
lichenoid dermatoses, histopathology 2379–2380
lichenoid drug eruptions 397
lichenoid or lichen planus-like graft-versus-host disease 397
lichenoid reactions 397
  oral mucosa 2086–2087
lichenoid sarcoidosis *see* Blau syndrome/early-onset sarcoidosis
lichen planopilaris (LPP) 393–394
lichen planus (LP) 390–400
  actinic lichen planus (ALP) 395
  acute, eruptive lichen planus 396
  aetiology 390–391
  associated diseases **392**
  atrophic lichen planus 396
  bullous lichen planus 396–397
  clinical presentation 392–397
  clinical variants 393–397
  diagnosis 397–400
  differential diagnosis 397, **398–399**
  drugs implicated **398**
  epidemiology 391–392
  eruptive, acute lichen planus 396
  follicular lichen planus 393–394
  history 390
  hypertrophic lichen planus 395, *396*
  inverse lichen planus 397
  lichenoid drug eruptions 397
  lichenoid or lichen planus-like graft-versus-host disease 397
  lichenoid reactions 397
  lichen planopilaris (LPP) 393–394
  linear lichen planus 396
  nail disorders 2153–2154
  nail lichen planus (NLP) 393, *394*, 2153–2154
  ocular lichen planus 395
  oral lichen planus 394–395
  oral mucosa 2086–2087
  pathogenesis 390–391
  treatment 400
  Wickham's striae 390, 392
lichen planus (LP) pemphigoides 396–397, 887–888
  clinical features 887
  differential diagnosis 887
  epidemiology 887
  laboratory findings 888
  pathogenesis 887
  treatment 888
lichen planus-like or lichenoid graft-versus-host disease 397
lichen planus–lupus erythematosus (lupus planus) overlap 397
lichen planus pigmentosus 397
lichen sclerosus (LS) 1497
  genital signs of systemic disease *2237*
lichen sclerosus in boys (syn. balanitis xerotica obliterans) 2170
lichen sclerosus in girls (syn. lichen sclerosus et atrophicus) 2164–2169
  aetiology 2164
  clinical features 2164–2165
  complications 2165–2166
  definition 2164
  diagnosis 2167
  differential diagnosis 2166
  follow-up 2169
  long-term maintenance treatment 2167–2169
  malignancy 2166
  pathogenesis 2164
  pathology 2164
  prognosis 2166
  scarring 2165–2166
  surgery 2169
  topical calcineurin inhibitors (TCI) 2167
  topical corticosteroids (TCS) 2167
  treatment 2167–2169
lichen scrofulosorum (LS) 490–492
lichen simplex chronicus (LSC) 240–241
  clinical features 241
  definition 240
  differential diagnosis 241
  epidemiology 240
  pathogenesis 240
  pathology 240
  prognosis 241
  treatment 241

lichen striatus (LS) 408–414
clinical features 409–412
differential diagnosis 412–413
epidemiology 408–409
histology findings 413–414
history 408
nail disorders 2154
pathogenesis 409
prognosis 412
treatment 414
lidocaine, local anaesthetic 2331–2332
lidocaine ointment and spray, topical anaesthetics 2333
lidocaine/tetracaine patch, topical anaesthetics 2334
life expectancy
PIK3CA-related overgrowth spectrum (PROS) 1292
Proteus syndrome (PS) 1287
lifestyle recommendations, congenital ichthyoses (CI) 1596
limb–mammary syndrome **1654**
limited cutaneous SSc (lcSSc) **1185**
lindane, scabies 717
linear and whorled naevoid hypermelanosis (LWNH) 1470–1471
linear atrophoderma 1160
linear atrophoderma of Moulin (LAM) 1158–1159
aetiology 1158–1159
clinical features 1159
definition 1158
diagnosis 1159
history 1158
pathology 1159
treatment 1159
linear Cowden naevus 1269
linear granuloma annulare (GA) **1008**, 1011
linear hyperpigmentation 1468, 1470–1471
linear IgA dermatosis (LAD) 874–879
clinical features 878
differential diagnosis 878
epidemiology 875–877
oral mucosa 2087
pathogenesis 877
prevention 878–879
treatment 878–879
linear immunoglobulin IgA bullous dermatosis (LABD) **137**
see also bullous dermatoses
clinical features 147
differential diagnosis 147
epidemiology 147
histology findings 147
laboratory findings 147
neonates 147
pathogenesis 147
treatment 147
linear lichen planus 396
linear morphoea 1177, *1178*
linear porokeratosis 1624
linear psoriasis 356
lingual thyroid, tongue 2099
lingual tonsil, tongue 2099
lip-lick dermatitis, superficial self-mutilation *2269*
lipoblastoma
characteristics **1196**
clinical features 1197
epidemiology 1196–1197
histological features **1196**
histology findings 1197
laboratory findings 1197
pathogenesis 1196–1197
treatment 1197
lipodystrophies 1221–1226
acquired generalized lipoatrophy (AGL) 1224–1225
acquired lipodystrophies 1224–1225
autoimmune markers 1226
autosomal dominant lipodystrophies 1223–1224
autosomal recessive lipodystrophies 1223
classification **1222**
clinical features 1222–1223
congenital generalized lipoatrophy (CGL) 1223
differential diagnosis 1222–1223
epidemiology 1223–1225
familial partial lipodystrophies (FPLD) 1223–1224
genetic lipodystrophy syndromes **1222**
haematological markers 1226
HIV infection 1225
imaging findings 1225–1226
'insulin signalling' genes 1224
laboratory findings 1225–1226
lipodystrophy in complex syndromes 1224
LMNA mutations 1223–1224
localized lipodystrophies 1225, *1226*
pathogenesis 1223–1225
PPARG mutations 1224
prevention 1226
treatment 1226
whole body irradiation 1225
lipodystrophy in complex syndromes 1224
lipoid proteinosis 1166–1167
aetiology 1167
clinical features 1167
definition 1166–1167
differential diagnosis 1167
pathology 1167
prognosis 1167
treatment 1167
lipoma 1195–1204
characteristics 1196
clinical features 1195–1196
epidemiology 1195
histological findings 1196
laboratory findings 1196
pathogenesis 1195
prevention 1196
treatment 1196
lipomatosis 1198–1204
Bannayan–Riley–Ruvalcaba syndrome **1199**, 1201
benign symmetric lipomatosis **1199**
characteristics **1196**, **1199**
clinical features **1199**
congenital infiltrating lipomatosis of the face (CIL-F) 1198–1200, **1199**
Cowden syndrome **1199**
encephalocraniocutaneous lipomatosis (ECCL) **1199**, 1200–1201
familial multiple lipomatosis **1199**
Gardner syndrome **1199**
hemihyperplasia multiple lipomatosis syndrome **1199**
hereditary multiple lipomas **1199**
histological features **1196**
Launois–Bensaude syndrome **1199**
Medelung's disease **1199**
multiple symmetric lipomatosis **1199**
nasopalpebral lipoma coloboma syndrome **1199**
Proteus syndrome (PS) **1199**
PTEN (Phosphatase and TENsin homologue) hamartoma tumour syndrome **1199**
liposarcaoma 1197–1198
clinical features 1198
epidemiology 1198
histology findings 1198
laboratory findings 1198
pathogenesis 1198
treatment 1198
liposarcoma 1385–1386
aetiology 1385
clinical features 1385
definition 1385
differential diagnosis 1385
epidemiology 1385
myxoid liposarcoma **1196**, 1197–1198, 1385
pathogenesis 1385
pathology 1385
treatment 1385–1386
liposomal lidocaine (LMX), topical anaesthetic 2333
Listeria monocytogenes, neonates **87**, **136**, **139**
LL *see* lepromatous leprosy
LM-associated overgrowth syndromes, lymphatic malformations (LMs) 1455, 1460–1461
LMNA mutations, lipodystrophies 1223–1224
LMS *see* Lenz–Majewski syndrome
LMs *see* lymphatic malformations
LMS syndrome, ectodermal dysplasias (EDs) 1682
LMX *see* liposomal lidocaine
LN *see* lichen nitidus
lobster claw deformity *see* ectrodactyly, ectodermal dysplasia and cleft lip/palate (EEC) syndrome
lobular capillary haemangioma *see* pyogenic granuloma
lobular panniculitis, calcification and ossification in the skin 1343–1344
local anaesthetics 2331–2332
adverse effects 2332
classification 2331
history 2331
lidocaine 2331–2332
mechanism of action 2331

localized (Weber–Cockayne) epidermolysis bullosa simplex 910–911
localized angiokeratomas, lymphatic malformations (LMs) 1411
localized autosomal recessive hypotrichosis, type 1 (LAH1) **1654**, 1701
localized autosomal recessive hypotrichosis, type 2 (LAH2) **1655**
localized autosomal recessive hypotrichosis, type 3 (LAH3) **1655**
localized congenital hypopigmentation 1495–1496
localized granuloma annulare (GA) **1008**, 1009
localized hypertrichosis 2134–2136
localized hypertrichosis over the spinal column 2135
localized scleroderma (LSc) *see* morphoea
localized telangiectatic vascular malformation 1417
localized tufts of hair 2124
loose anagen syndrome (LAS), hair loss 2125–2126
loricrin keratoderma 1529–1530, 1575
  clinical features 1530
  differential diagnosis 1530
  epidemiology 1530
  histology findings 1530
  history 1529–1530
  laboratory findings 1530
  pathogenesis 1530
  treatment 1530
Louis–Bar syndrome (AT) 1418
lower body haemangiomas and structural malformations (PELVIS/SACRAL/LUMBAR syndrome), infantile haemangiomas (IH) 1433–1434
LP *see* lupus panniculitis
LPP *see* lichen planopilaris
LS *see* lichen sclerosus; lichen scrofulosorum; lichen striatus
LSC *see* lichen simplex chronicus
LSc (localized scleroderma) *see* morphoea
lucite estivale bénigne *see* polymorphous light eruption
LUMBAR/PELVIS/SACRAL syndrome (lower body haemangiomas and structural malformations), infantile haemangiomas (IH) 1433–1434
lumps and bumps, histopathology 2383, *2384*
lupus erythematosus, oral mucosa 2090
lupus erythematosus profundus *see* lupus panniculitis
lupus panniculitis (LP) 1215
  clinical features 1215
  histology findings 1215
  laboratory findings 1215
  treatment 1215
lupus vulgaris (LV) 486–487, *490*
LV *see* lentiviral vectors; lupus vulgaris
LWNH *see* linear and whorled naevoid hypermelanosis
lyme borreliosis (LB)/lyme disease 463–472
  acrodermatitis chronica atrophicans (ACA) 467–468
  antibiotics 470, **471**
  arthritis 469
  associated infections 472
  borrelial lymphocytoma (lymphadenosis benigna cutis) 467
  causative organisms 465–466
  cause 463
  chemoprophylaxis 472
  'chronic lyme disease' 471
  clinical features 466–469
  definition 463
  diagnosis 469–470
  diagnostic tests that are not recommended 470
  direct detection methods 469
  enzyme-linked immunosorbent assay (ELISA) 470
  epidemiology 464–465
  erythema migrans (EM) 466–467
  Garin–Bujadoux–Bannwarth (GBB) syndrome 468
  history 463
  indirect diagnostic methods 469–470
  ixodid tick bites 466
  lymphadenosis benigna cutis (borrelial lymphocytoma) 467
  meningoencephalitis 468
  musculoskeletal manifestations 468–469
  nervous system manifestations 468
  neuroborreliosis 468
  pathogenetic factors 465–466
  pregnancy 469
  prevention 471–472
  prognosis 470–471
  skin manifestations 466–468
  southern tick-associated rash illness (STARI) 472
  tick removal 472
  treatment 470, **471**
lymphadenosis benigna cutis (borrelial lymphocytoma), lyme borreliosis (LB)/lyme disease 467
lymphangioendotheliomatosis. *see* multifocal lymphangioendotheliomatosis (also known as cutaneovisceral angiomatosis) with thrombocytopenia (MLT/CAT)
lymphangioma, oral mucosa 2094
lymphatic malformations (LMs) 1409–1412, 1452–1461
  aetiopathogenesis 1452
  clinical features 1410–1411, 1452–1455
  CLOVE syndrome (congenital lipomatous overgrowth, vascular malformations and epidermal naevus) **1453**, 1455, 1460
  combined (macrocystic and microcystic) LM 1453, **1453**, 1457–1458
  differential diagnosis 1411
  epidemiology 1410
  generalized lymphatic anomalies 1411
  generalized lymphatic anomaly (GLA) **1453**, 1455, 1460
  Gorham–Stout disease (GSD) 1411, **1453**, 1455, 1460
  histology findings 1411–1412
  histopathology 1455–1457
  imaging 1455–1457
  Klippel–Trenaunay syndrome (KTS) **1453**, *1456*, 1460–1461
  laboratory findings 1411
  LM-associated overgrowth syndromes 1455, 1460–1461
  localized angiokeratomas 1411
  lymphoedema 1411, 1453–1455, **1453**, 1459–1460
  macrocystic LM 1452–1453, **1453**, 1457–1458
  management 1457–1461
  microcystic LM 1453, **1453**, *1454*, 1458–1459
  pathogenesis 1410
  phenotypes **1453**
  prevention 1412
  primary (idiopathic) lymphoedema 1453–1455, **1453**, 1459–1460
  treatment 1412
lymphoedema 1411, 1453–1455, **1453**, 1459–1460
  primary (idiopathic) lymphoedema 1453–1455, **1453**, 1459–1460
lymphoma
  see also Burkitt lymphoma; cutaneous anaplastic large cell lymphoma; Hodgkin disease; hydroa vacciniforme-like cutaneous T-cell lymphoma (HVL); primary cutaneous follicle centre lymphoma; subcutaneous panniculitis-like T-cell lymphoma
  oral mucosa 2096
lymphomatoid papulosis (LyP) 1051–1053
  clinical features 1051
  definition 1051
  epidemiology 1051
  histopathology 1051–1052
  immunophenotype 1052
  predictive factors 1052–1053
  prognosis 1052–1053
  treatment 1053
Lyngbya dermatitis 749
LyP *see* lymphomatoid papulosis
lysosomal storage diseases 1973–1978

macrocephaly, alopecia, cutis laxa and scoliosis syndrome (MACS syndrome) **1134**, 1135, 1739
macrocystic LM, lymphatic malformations (LMs) **1453**, 1457–1458
macroglossia 2099
macrolides
  acne vulgaris 809
  systemic therapies 2283
MACS *see* macrocephaly, alopecia, cutis laxa and scoliosis syndrome

maculopapular cutaneous mastocytosis (MPCM) 1100–1101
maculopapular drug eruptions or exanthems (MPDEs), hypersensitivity reactions to drugs 789–791
MAD *see* mandibuloacral dysplasia
Madelung's disease *see* multiple symmetric lipomatosis
Maffucci syndrome 1407, **1805**
MAGIC syndrome, oral mucosa 2081
Majeed syndrome 2017
Majocchi disease 1878
  clinical overview 1878
  prognosis 1878
  treatment 1878
Malabar ulcer *see* tropical skin ulcer
Malassezia (*Pityrosporum*) folliculitis 553–554
Malassezia (*Pityrosporum*) yeasts in seborrhoeic dermatitis 554
Malassezia-associated diseases 550–555
  atopic dermatitis (AD) 554
  neonatal cephalic pustulosis 554
  pityriasis versicolor 550–553
Malassezia fungaemia and invasive infection 554–555
Malassezia spp. (*Pityrosporum* spp.)
  adolescent seborrhoeic dermatitis (SD) 280–281, 284
  neonates **87**
Mal de Meleda 1528–1529
  clinical features 1529
  differential diagnosis 1529
  epidemiology 1529
  histology findings 1529
  history 1528
  laboratory findings 1529
  pathogenesis 1529
  treatment 1529
Mal de Mljet *see* Mal de Meleda
malignancy
  lichen sclerosus in girls (syn. lichen sclerosus et atrophicus) 2166
  neoplasia, genital disease 2188–2189
malignant histiocytosis (M Group) 1089
malignant tumours of neural crest and germ cell origin 1395–1397
mandibular hypoplasia, deafness, progeroid features and lipodystrophy (MDPL) syndrome 1736
  clinical features 1736
  differential diagnosis 1736
  epidemiology 1736
  histology findings 1736
  history 1736
  laboratory findings 1736
  pathogenesis 1736
  treatment 1736
mandibuloacral dysplasia (MAD) 1733
  clinical features 1733
  differential diagnosis 1733
  epidemiology 1733
  histology findings 1733
  history 1733
  laboratory findings 1733
  pathogenesis 1733
  treatment 1733
maple syrup urine disease (MSUD), neonatal erythroderma 132
marasmus 831–834
marasmus–kwashiorkor 831–833
Marfanoid progeria–lipodystrophy syndrome 1737
  clinical features 1737
  differential diagnosis 1737
  epidemiology 1737
  histology findings 1737
  history 1737
  laboratory findings 1737
  pathogenesis 1737
  treatment 1737
Marfan syndrome (MFS) 1143–1145
  associated diseases **1143**
  cardiovascular manifestations 1144
  clinical features 1144–1145
  cutaneous manifestations 1144–1145
  definition 1143
  diagnosis 1145
  history 1143
  management 1145
  musculoskeletal features 1144
  ocular manifestations 1144
  pathogenesis 1143–1144
Margarita Island ED (allelic to cleft lip/palate–ectodermal dysplasia syndrome [CLEPD1]) **1655**
marginal papular keratoderma 1546, *1547*
Marie–Unna hereditary hypotrichosis (MUHH) 2122
Marie–Unna hypotrichosis **2109**
marine envenomations 740–743
marked hypohidrosis and woolly hair 1160
Marshall syndrome (allelic to Stickler syndrome, but no ectodermal dysplasia in Stickler syndrome) **1655**
MAS *see* McCune–Albright syndrome
mast cell leukaemia **1104**
mast cell lineage cells, mastocytosis **1106**
mast cell sarcoma (MCS) 1102–1103, **1104**
mast cell tumour *see* mast cell sarcoma; mastocytoma; mastocytosis
mastocytoma **1317**, 2189
  mastocytosis 1100
mastocytosis 1097–1107
  classification 1097, **1098**, **1104**
  clinical features 1100–1103
  cutaneous manifestations 1100–1102
  cutaneous mastocytosis 1097–1098, **1104**
  Darier's sign 1103
  degranulation 1102
  diagnosis **1105**
  diagnostic criteria **1098**
  differential diagnosis 1103
  diffuse cutaneous mastocytosis (DCM) 1101–1102
  epidemiology 1098
  histology findings 1103–1106
  hyperpigmentation 1465
  indolent systemic mastocytosis (ISM) **1104**
  KIT mutations 1098–1099
  laboratory findings 1103
  maculopapular cutaneous mastocytosis (MPCM) 1100–1101
  mast cell degranulators **1100**
  mast cell leukaemia **1104**
  mast cell lineage cells **1106**
  mast cell mediators 1099–1100
  mast cell products **1100**
  mast cell sarcoma (MCS) 1102–1103, **1104**
  mastocytoma 1100
  pathogenesis 1098–1100
  prognosis 1107
  smouldering systemic mastocytosis (SSM) **1104**
  systemic mastocytosis 1097–1098, 1102, **1104**
  telangiectasia macularis eruptiva perstans (TMEP) 1102
  therapeutic options for patients with advanced mastocytosis 1107
  therapeutic options for patients with cutaneous mastocytosis and ISM 1106–1107
  treatment 1106–1107
  urticaria pigmentosa 1100–1101
materia alba, oral mucosa 2089
matrix metalloproteinases (MMPs), acne vulgaris 805
matrix shave, surgical therapy 2317
MC *see* molluscum contagiosum
McCune–Albright syndrome (MAS) 1300–1301
  clinical features 1300
  cutaneous manifestations 2002–2003
  epidemiology 1300
  histology findings 1300–1301
  management 1300
  pathogenesis 1301
McGrath syndrome (ectodermal dysplasia/skin fragility syndrome) 916–917, **1655**, 1699–1700
MCI/MI *see* methylchloroisothiazolinone/methylisothiazolinone
MCL *see* mucocutaneous leishmaniasis
MCS *see* mast cell sarcoma
MCTD *see* mixed connective tissue disease
MDPL syndrome *see* mandibular hypoplasia, deafness, progeroid features and lipodystrophy syndrome
MDR *see* multidrug resistance
measles (rubeola) 660–662
  clinical features 661–662
  differential diagnosis 662
  epidemiology 661
  HIV infection 651
  laboratory findings 662
  pathogenesis 661
  prevention 662
  treatment 662
mechanical damage avoidance
  neonatal skin care 66–67
  premature infants 66–67

mechanical irritant contact dermatitis 984
Medelung's disease
  characteristics **1199**
  clinical features **1199**
median raphe cysts and canals of the penis 108
median raphe cysts of the penis and scrotum 2186–2187
  clinical presentation 2187
  differential diagnosis 2187
  histology 2186–2187
  management 2187
median rhomboid glossitis, tongue 2100
medication controversy
  erythema multiforme (EM) 783
  Stevens–Johnson syndrome (SJS) 783
  toxic epidermal necrolysis (TEN) 783
MeDIP-seq *see* methylated DNA immunoprecipitation
medium vessel vasculitis 1883
MEDNIK syndrome *see* mental retardation-enteropathy- deafness-neuropathy-ichthyosis-keratodermia syndrome
MEDOC (Mendelian Disorders of Cornification) *see* ichthyoses; keratodermas
Megalencephaly CAPillary malformation syndrome (MCAP), *PIK3CA*-related overgrowth spectrum (PROS) 1291
Megarbane–Loiselet neonatal progeroid syndrome 1734
  differential diagnosis 1734
  epidemiology 1734
  histology findings 1734
  history 1734
  laboratory findings 1734
  pathogenesis 1734
melanocyte loss, vitiligo 1477
melanocytes, embryonic–fetal transition *11*, 12–13
melanocytic lesions 2357–2376
  acquired melanocytic naevi (AMN) 1252–1255, 2365–2368
  benign dermoscopic patterns 2369
  congenital melanocytic naevi (CMN) 2360–2365
  dermoscopic structures and their histopathological correlations **2359–2360**
  dermoscopy 2357–2376
  dermoscopy algorithm 2358–2360, *2361*
  differentiating benign naevi from melanoma 2368–2369
  halo naevi 1255, 2368
  histopathological correlates of dermoscopic structures found in superficial spreading melanoma 2369, **2370**
  histopathology 2386–2388
  Spitz naevi 1254–1255, **1317**, 2369–2376, 2386–2387
melanocytic naevi, birthmarks in the genital area 2171
melanoleucoderma, infantilism, mental retardation, hypodontia, hypotrichosis **1656**
melanoma 1377–1380
  clinical features 1378–1379
  differential diagnosis 1378–1379
  epidemiology 1377–1378
  histology findings 1379–1380
  history 1377
  laboratory findings 1379–1380
  pathogenesis 1377–1378
  prevention 1380
  risk of development 1378
  Spitz melanomas 1377, 1378–1380
  transplacental 98–99
  treatment 1380
  xeroderma pigmentosum 1378
melanoma arising in the CNS, congenital melanocytic naevi (CMN) 1250–1252
melanoma arising in the skin, congenital melanocytic naevi (CMN) 1250, **1252**
melanoma in CMN, congenital melanocytic naevi (CMN) 1245
melanosis universalis hereditaria *see* familial progressive hyperpigmentation
melanotic neuroectodermal tumour of infancy, oral mucosa 2091–2092
melasma 1465–1466
  clinical features 1466
  differential diagnosis 1466
  hyperpigmentation 1465–1466
  pathology 1466
  prognosis 1466
  treatment 1466
Meleda disease *see* Mal de Meleda
MEN 1A *see* multiple endocrine neoplasia 1A
MEN 2A *see* multiple endocrine neoplasia 2A
MEN 3A *see* multiple endocrine neoplasia 3A
Mendelian Disorders of Cornification (MEDOC) *see* ichthyoses; palmoplantar keratodermas (PPKs)
meningococcal disease 434–446
  aetiology 435
  allergic complications 444
  antibiotic choice 439
  chemoprophylaxis 444
  chronic meningococcaemia 444
  clinical features 437–439, *441*, *442*, *443*, *444*
  differential diagnosis 439, *446*
  epidemiology 435
  laboratory diagnosis 439
  management of acute meningococcal septicaemia 439–444, *445*
  management of the skin lesions 440–441
  outcome of skin disease 442–444
  pathophysiology 435–437, *438*, *439*, *440*
  prevention 444–446
  recognition and initial therapy 439
  supportive care 439
  surgical intervention 441–442, *446*
  vaccines 446
meningoencephalitis, lyme borreliosis (LB)/lyme disease 468
meningoencephalocoele 111
Menkes syndrome *see* trichopoliodystrophy
MEN syndrome *see* multiple endocrine neoplasia syndrome
mental health disorders, atopic dermatitis (AD) 250–251
mental retardation-enteropathy-deafness-neuropathy-ichthyosis-keratodermia (MEDNIK) syndrome 1589
mepolizumab, atopic dermatitis (AD) 260
Merkel cell carcinoma 1375–1376
Merkel cells
  embryonic–fetal transition 13
  embryonic skin 6, *9*
mesomelic dwarfism–skeletal abnormalities–ectodermal dysplasia **1656**
messenger RNA (mRNA), genetic therapies 2304–2305
metabolic and cardiovascular obesity, psoriasis 359
metabolic carotenaemia 1983
metabolic disorders 1965–1986
  α-N-acetylgalactosaminidase deficiency 1974
  acrodermatitis enteropathica 1981–1982
  alkaptonuria 1969–1970
  aminoacidopathies 1967–1970
  biotinidase deficiency 1972
  carotenaemia 1982–1986
  classification **1967**
  congenital melanocytic naevi (CMN) 1245
  Fabry disease 1974–1975
  Farber lipogranulomatosis: ceramidase deficiency 1978
  fucosidosis 1975–1976
  Gaucher disease (GD) 1973–1974
  GM_1 gangliosidosis 1977–1978
  Hartnup disease 1973
  homocystinuria 1970
  hyperlipoproteinaemia 1980–1981
  lysosomal storage diseases 1973–1978
  methylmalonic acidaemia 1972
  mucopolysaccharidoses (MPS) 1976–1977
  organic acidurias 1971–1972
  phenylketonuria (PKU) 1967–1968
  prolidase deficiency 1979
  propionic acidaemia 1971–1972
  skin symptoms **1966–1967**
  transaldolase deficiency 1979
  transport defects 1973
  tyrosinaemia type II 1968–1969
metabolic napkin conditions 277
metabolic syndrome (MetS) 841–858
  acanthosis nigricans (AN) 844–846
  atopic dermatitis (AD) 858
  comorbidity 853–857
  diabetes mellitus 850–852

metabolic syndrome (MetS) (*cont'd*)
diagnosis **842**
dyslipidaemia 849–850
glucose metabolism 850–852
granuloma annulare (GA) 851–852
hidradenitis suppurativa (HS) (acne inversa) 853–854
insulin metabolism and the skin 843–844
necrobiosis lipoidica (NL) 852
plantar hyperkeratoses 847–848
polycystic ovary syndrome (PCOS) 854–856
psoriasis 856–857
skin associations *842*
skin tags (soft fibroma, fibroma pendulans) 849
'stretch marks' 847–848
striae distensae (SD) 847–848
xanthelasma 849–850
xanthomas 849–850
metaphyseal fractures 2226
metastatic calcification, calcification and ossification in the skin 1345
methotrexate (MTX)
alopecia areata (AA) 2144–2145
atopic dermatitis (AD) 257–258
pityriasis rubra pilaris (PRP) 384
psoriasis 370–371, *373*
systemic therapies 2293
methylated DNA immunoprecipitation (MeDIP-seq), molecular genetics 42
methylchloroisothiazolinone/ methylisothiazolinone (MCI/MI), allergic contact dermatitis (ACD) 310
methylmalonic acidaemia 1972
clinical features 1972
definition 1972
history 1972
pathogenesis 1972
prognosis 1972
treatment 1972
methylmalonic acidaemias (MMA) **139**
neonatal erythroderma 132
methylprednisolone, administration 2408, **2409**
meticillin-resistant *Staphylococcus aureus* (MRSA)
nursing care of the skin 2402, **2403**
pathophysiology 424–425
MetS *see* metabolic syndrome
mevalonate kinase deficiency (MKD) 2013–2014
MF *see* mycosis fungoides
MFS *see* Marfan syndrome
microbiological studies, vesiculobullous lesions 862
microbiome, cutaneous *see* cutaneous microbiome
microcystic LM, lymphatic malformations (LMs) **1453**, *1454*, 1458–1459
microglossia 2099
microphthalmia with linear skin defects, differential diagnosis 1715
microscopic polyangiitis (MPA) 1931–1932
antineutrophil cytoplasmic antibody (ANCA)-associated vasculitides (AAV) 1882–1883
clinical features 1931–1932
differential diagnosis 1931–1932
epidemiology 1931
histology findings 1932
laboratory findings 1932
pathogenesis 1925, 1931
prognosis 1932
treatment 1929–1930, 1932
mid-borderline leprosy (BB) **497**, **499**
mid-childhood acne 815
migratory myiasis 703–704
milia
epidemiology 134
laboratory findings 141
neonates 134–141
pathogenesis 134
prevention 141
transient skin disorders in neonates and young infants 74
treatment 141
milia-like idiopathic calcinosis cutis 1341
clinical features 1341
epidemiology 1341
pathogenesis 1341
miliaria
clinical features 141
differential diagnosis 141
epidemiology 141
histology findings 141
laboratory findings 141
napkin dermatitis 275
neonates 141
pathogenesis 141
prevention 141
treatment 141
miliaria crystallina **135**
miliaria rubra **135**
miliary osteoma cutis of the face 1349
milker's nodule (pseudocowpox) **625**, 646–647
millipedes (Diplopoda) 739–740
miltefosine, leishmaniasis 699
mineral deficiencies 837–839
copper 838
selenium 838
trichopoliodystrophy (Menkes syndrome) 838
zinc 838–839
mineral oils, neonatal skin care 69
miniature puberty, transient skin disorders in neonates and young infants 74
miniaturization, hair disorders 2128–2129
minicircle DNA, genetic therapies 2304
minocycline
acne vulgaris 809
hyperpigmentation **1465**
minoxidil, alopecia areata (AA) 2144
minoxidil-induced hypertrichosis 2133
mites and ticks 738
mitochondrial repair, xeroderma pigmentosum and related diseases 1767–1768
mixed connective tissue disease (MCTD) 1884
mixed epidermolysis bullosa *see* Kindler syndrome
mixed hamartomas 1280
mixed morphoea 1178
mixed napkin dermatitis 275
MKD *see* mevalonate kinase deficiency
MLPA *see* multiplex ligation-dependent probe amplification
MLT/CAT *see* multifocal lymphangioendotheliomatosis (also known as cutaneovisceral angiomatosis) with thrombocytopenia
MMF xmycophenolate mofetil
MMP *see* mucous membrane pemphigoid
MMPs *see* matrix metalloproteinases
molecular basis
ectodermal dysplasias (EDs) 1630–1669
Kindler syndrome 935
molecular diagnostics
candidosis (candidiasis) 549
cutaneous T-cell lymphomas (CTCL) 2390
dermatophytoses 539–540
pityriasis versicolor 553
techniques 2389–2391
molecular genetics 36–45
see also genetic testing
amplification-refractory mutation system (ARMS) 45
array techniques 42–43
chromatin immunoprecipitation sequencing (CHIP-seq) 42
consent for genetic testing and incidental findings 38
copy number variations (CNVs) 42
DNA mutations 38
fluorescence in situ hybridization (FISH) 44
genetics and inheritance in brief 36–38
genome-wide association studies (GWAS) 44–45
high-resolution melt PCR (HRM) 45
karyotype testing 40
methods for genotyping specific base pair changes 45
methylated DNA immunoprecipitation (MeDIP-seq) 42
multiplex ligation-dependent probe amplification (MLPA) 43
mutation identification by DNA sequencing 40
next-generation sequencing (NGS) of DNA 40–42
polymerase chain reaction (PCR) 43–45
psoriasis 351–352
quantitative real-time PCR (qRT-PCR) 43–44
restriction fragment length polymorphisms (RFLPs) 45
Sanger sequencing 40
techniques 40–45

terminology **37**
molecular genetic testing, neurofibromatosis type 1 (NF1) 1829–1830
molluscipoxvirus **625**
molluscs 742
molluscum contagiosum, neonates **86**
molluscum contagiosum (MC) 579–585
aetiology 579
antiviral agents 585
Candida antigen immunotherapy 585
cantharidin 584
clinical features 581–583
cryotherapy and curettage 584
diagnosis 583–584
duct tape 585
electrosurgery 584
epidemiology 579–580
genital area 2177–2178
HIV infection 652
immune modulators. 585
immune response 581
keratolytics 584
laser treatment 584
oral mucosa 2096
pathology 580–581, *582*
relation to disease state 580
topical cytotoxic therapy 585
topical potassium hydroxide 584
treatment 584–585
molluscum infections, atopic dermatitis (AD) *248*
Mongolian spots
differential diagnosis of inflicted bruises *2225*, **2412**
nursing care of the skin **2412**
transient skin disorders in neonates and young infants 79
monilethrix **1656**
ectodermal dysplasias (EDs) 1697–1698
hair disorders 2117–2118
hair loss **2110**
keratin disorders 1520, *1521*
monkeypox **625**, 640–642
clinical features 641
differential diagnosis 642
epidemiology 640–641
histology findings 642
history 640
laboratory findings 642
pathogenesis 640–641
prevention 642
treatment 642
monogenic autoinflammatory diseases and primary immune deficiency 1211–1213
clinical features 1212
epidemiology 1212
histology 1212
panniculitis 1211–1213
pathogenesis 1212
treatment 1212
monoMAC syndrome/ GATA2 deficiency **2040**
Moorea producens 749
morphoea 1175–1180
aetiopathogenesis 1175–1176
associated diseases 1178–1179
autoimmunity 1176
classification 1176–1177
clinical features 1176–1178
deep morphoea 1178
differential diagnosis 1176–1178
disabling pansclerotic morphoea 1178
disease monitoring 1179
en coup de sabre morphoea 1177, *1178*
eosinophilic fasciitis 1178
epidemiology 1175–1176
generalized morphoea 1178
genetics 1176
histology findings 1179
history 1175
inflammatory response 1176
laboratory findings 1179
linear morphoea 1177, *1178*
mixed morphoea 1178
Parry Romberg 1178
plaque morphoea 1177
prevention 1180
prognosis 1179
progressive facial hemiatrophy 1178
treatment 1180
triggers 1175
morphoea plana atrophica *see* Atrophoderma of Pasini and Pierini
morpholines, dermatophytoses 541
mosaic disorders of pigmentation 1296–1307
Becker naevi 1304
Becker naevus syndrome 1304
CMN syndrome 1304
congenital melanocytic naevi (CMN) 1304
extensive or atypical dermal melanocytosis (EDM) 1303–1304
fine and whorled Blaschkolinear hypoand hyperpigmentation (incorporating hypomelanosis of Ito, and linear and whorled naevoid hypermelanosis) 1297–1300
McCune–Albright syndrome (MAS) 1300–1301
mosaic Legius syndrome 1307
mosaic neurofibromatosis type 1 (NF1) 1306–1307
naevus depigmentosus (ND) 1306
naevus of Ito 1303–1304
naevus of Ota 1303–1304
phakomatosis pigmentokeratotica (PPK) 1304
phakomatosis pigmentovascularis (PPV) 1301–1303
phylloid hypo- and hypermelanosis 1300
speckled lentiginous naevus (SLN) 1304–1306
mosaic epidermolytic ichthyosis *see* epidermolytic naevi
mosaicism/mosaic disorders 1229–1234
cell type affected by the mutation 1233
chimaerism 1231–1232
classification 1229–1231
conditions mimicking mosaicism 1231–1232
definition 1229
gene expression, spatial and temporal patterns 1233
genetic investigation of mosaic disorders 1233–1234
genetic mechanisms 1231
germline genotype of the affected individual 1233
inheritance potential 1229–1231
Mendelian disorders, in the context of 1231, *1232*
patterns 1233, *1234*
phenotype of mosaic disorders 1232–1233
revertant mosaicism 1231
specificity of the mutated genotype 1233
sporadic mosaic disorders 1231
timing of the mutation 1232–1233
mosaic *KITLG* mutations, fine and whorled Blaschkolinear hypoand hyperpigmentation (incorporating hypomelanosis of Ito, and linear and whorled naevoid hypermelanosis) 1299–1300
mosaic Legius syndrome, mosaic neurofibromatosis type 1 (NF1) 1307
mosaic *MTOR* mutations, fine and whorled Blaschkolinear hypoand hyperpigmentation (incorporating hypomelanosis of Ito, and linear and whorled naevoid hypermelanosis) 1299
mosaic neurofibromatosis type 1 (NF1) 1306–1307
associated features 1306–1307
classification 1306
cutaneous features 1306
differential diagnosis 1307
epidemiology 1306
genetic investigation and risk to offspring 1307
management 1306–1307
mosaic Legius syndrome 1307
pathogenesis 1306
mosaic *TP63* mutations, fine and whorled Blaschkolinear hypoand hyperpigmentation (incorporating hypomelanosis of Ito, and linear and whorled naevoid hypermelanosis) 1299
mosaic warts, human papillomaviruses (HPV) 591
mosquitoes 735–736
moths and caterpillars (Lepidoptera) 738
mouth *see* oral…; tongue
MPA *see* microscopic polyangiitis
MPCM *see* maculopapular cutaneous mastocytosis
MPDEs *see* maculopapular drug eruptions or exanthems
MPS *see* mucopolysaccharidoses
MRH *see* multicentric reticulohistiocytosis

mRNA *see* messenger RNA
MRSA *see* meticillin-resistant Staphylococcus aureus
MSD *see* multiple sulphatase deficiency
MSL *see* multiple symmetric lipomatosis
MSS *see* Mulvihill–Smith syndrome
MSUD *see* maple syrup urine disease
MTS *see* Muir–Torre syndrome
MTX *see* methotrexate
mucinous eccrine naevi 1281
Muckle–Wells syndrome (MWS) 2012
mucocoele/ranula, oral mucosa 2098
mucocutaneous involvement, systemic lupus erythematosus (SLE) 1942–1943
mucocutaneous leishmaniasis (MCL) 693, 695
mucocutaneous lymph node syndrome, tongue 2100–2101
mucopolysaccharidoses (MPS) 1976–1977
  classification **1976**
  clinical features 1976–1977
  definition 1976
  differential diagnosis 1977
  history 1976
  pathogenesis 1976
  pathology 1977
  prognosis 1977
  treatment 1977
mucormycosis (zygomycosis, phycomycosis), oral mucosa 2085
mucosal diseases 2018
mucosal surfaces, topical anaesthetics 2334
mucous membrane pemphigoid (MMP) 885–887
  clinical features 886–887
  differential diagnosis 887
  epidemiology 885
  laboratory findings 887
  pathogenesis 885–886
  treatment 887
MUHH *see* Marie–Unna hereditary hypotrichosis
Muir–Torre syndrome (MTS) **1805**, 1815–1816
  clinical features 1815–1816
  differential diagnosis 1816
  histology findings 1816
  pathogenesis 1815
  treatment 1816
multicentric reticulohistiocytosis (MRH) 1084–1085
  clinical features 1085
  differential diagnosis 1085
  epidemiology 1084–1085
  histology findings 1085
  history 1084–1085
  pathogenesis 1085
  treatment 1085
multidrug resistance (MDR)
  see also meticillin-resistant *Staphylococcus aureus*
  cutaneous tuberculosis 495–496
multifocal infantile haemangiomas 1434–1435
multifocal lymphangioendotheliomatosis (also known as cutaneovisceral angiomatosis) with thrombocytopenia (MLT/CAT) 1448
multiple circumscribed lipomas *see* familial multiple lipomatosis
multiple cutaneous and uterine leiomyomatosis syndrome *see* hereditary leiomyomatosis and renal cell cancer syndrome
multiple endocrine neoplasia (MEN) 1A **1805**
multiple endocrine neoplasia (MEN) 2A **1805**
multiple endocrine neoplasia syndrome (MEN syndrome), cutaneous manifestations 2004
multiple familial lipomatosis *see* familial multiple lipomatosis
multiple self-healing squamous epitheliomas (Ferguson–Smith syndrome) **1803**
multiple sulphatase deficiency (MSD) 1591–1592
  clinical features 1591–1592
  definition 1591
  extracutaneous findings 1592
  pathogenesis 1591
  prevention 1592
  treatment 1592
multiple symmetric lipomatosis (MSL) 1203–1204
  characteristics **1199**
  clinical features **1199**, 1203–1204
  differential diagnosis 1204
  epidemiology 1203
  histology findings 1204
  laboratory findings 1204
  pathogenesis 1203
  prevention 1204
  treatment 1204
multiplex laser, laser therapy 2324–2325
multiplex ligation-dependent probe amplification (MLPA), molecular genetics 43
Mulvihill–Smith syndrome (MSS) 1735
  clinical features 1735
  differential diagnosis 1735
  epidemiology 1735
  histology findings 1735
  history 1735
  laboratory findings 1735
  pathogenesis 1735
  treatment 1735
Munchausen syndrome *see* factitious disorder
Munchausen syndrome by proxy *see* factitious disorder by proxy
musculoskeletal disease
  juvenile dermatomyositis (JDM) 1947, **1948**
  systemic lupus erythematosus (SLE) 1942
musculoskeletal manifestations, lyme borreliosis (LB)/lyme disease 468–469
musculoskeletal system, systemic sclerosis (SSc) 1192
mutations
  autosomal recessive epidermolysis bullosa simplex due to keratin 14 mutations 914–915
  DNA mutations 38
  ectodermal dysplasias (EDs) 1697–1702
  ectodermal dysplasias caused by mutations in tumour necrosis factor like/NF-κB signalling pathways 1669–1675
  KIT mutations 1098–1099
  LMNA mutations 1223–1224
  mosaicism/mosaic disorders 1232–1233
  mosaic *KITLG* mutations 1299–1300
  mosaic *MTOR* mutations 1299
  mosaic *TP63* mutations 1299
  mutation identification by DNA sequencing 40
  PPARG mutations 1224
  structural and adhesive molecules 1697–1702
mutilating palmoplantar keratoderma with periorificial keratotic plaques (Olmsted syndrome) 1533–1534
  clinical features 1534
  differential diagnosis 1534
  epidemiology 1533–1534
  histology findings 1534
  history 1533
  laboratory findings 1534
  pathogenesis 1533–1534
  treatment 1534
MWS *see* Muckle–Wells syndrome
mycetoma 562–564
  actinomycetoma 563–564
  eumycetoma 562–563
mycobacteria, classification 485–486
mycobacterial skin infections 485–501
  cutaneous tuberculosis 486–496
  genital area 2179
  immunocompromised children 685–686
  leprosy in children 496–497
  nontuberculous mycobacterial infections (NTM) 497–501
Mycobacterium marinum infection 501
Mycobacterium tuberculosis, neonates **87**
mycophenolate mofetil (MMF)
  atopic dermatitis (AD) **257**, 259
  systemic therapies 2294–2295
Mycoplasma hominis, M. pneumoniae, neonates **87**
mycosis fungoides (MF) 1045–1054, 1497–1498
  adult T-cell leukaemia/lymphoma 1049
  clinical features 1045–1047
  clinical presentation 1497–1498
  cutaneous anaplastic large cell lymphoma (C-ALCL) 1050–1051
  cutaneous T-cell and NK cell lymphomas 1045–1054
  definition 1045
  differential diagnosis 1047, **1048**
  epidemiology 1045, 1497

extranodal NK/T-cell lymphoma, nasal type 1053–1054
folliculotropic mycosis fungoides 1048–1049
genetic features 1048
granulomatous slack skin (GSS) 1049
histopathology 1047
hydroa vacciniforme-like cutaneous T-cell lymphoma (HVL) 1054
ichthyosiform mycosis fungoides (IMF) 1049
immunophenotype 1047–1048
lymphomatoid papulosis (LyP) 1051–1053
pagetoid reticulosis (PR) 1049
predictive factors 1048
primary cutaneous anaplastic large cell lymphoma (C-ALCL) 1050–1051
primary cutaneous CD30+ lymphoproliferative disorders 1050
prognosis 1048
Sézary syndrome (SS) 1049
subcutaneous panniculitis-like T-cell lymphoma (SPTL) 1053
treatment 1048
myeloperoxidase deficiency **2039**
myiasis 702–704
aetiology 703
clinical features 703–704
definition 702
diagnosis 704
differential diagnosis 704
epidemiology 702–703
furuncular myiasis (warble) 703
history 702–703
migratory myiasis 703–704
pathogenesis 703
prevention 704
prognosis 704
traumatic cutaneous myiasis 704
treatment 704
wound myiasis 704
Mykids 536–537
myofibroma/myofibromatosis 1357–1358
clinical features 1357–1358
differential diagnosis 1357–1358
epidemiology 1357
history 1357
pathogenesis 1357
pathology 1358
treatment 1358
myxoid liposarcoma 1197–1198, 1385
characteristics **1196**
histological features **1196**

Naegeli–Franceschetti–Jadassohn syndrome (NFJS) **1657**
ectodermal dysplasias (EDs) 1698–1699
hyperpigmentation 1471, *1472*, 1517–1518
keratin disorders 1471, *1472*, 1517–1518
naevoid basal cell carcinoma *see* Gorlin syndrome
naevo-xanthoendothelioma *see* juvenile xanthogranuloma
naevus comedonicus (NC) 1263–1264
associated syndrome 1264
clinical features 1263
histopathology 1263–1264
history 1263
pathogenesis 1263
treatment 1264
naevus depigmentosus (ND) 1306
naevus lipomatosus cutaneous superficialis (Hoffmann–Zurhelle), differential diagnosis 1715
naevus lipomatosus superficialis (NLS) 1280
naevus marginatus 1272
naevus of Ito, extensive or atypical dermal melanocytosis (EDM) 1303–1304
naevus of Ota
extensive or atypical dermal melanocytosis (EDM) 1303–1304
laser therapy 2325
naevus sebaceous 1261–1263
associated syndromes 1262–1263
clinical features 1261–1262
cutaneous skeletal hypophosphatemia syndrome 1262–1263
differential diagnosis 1261–1262
epidemiology 1261
histopathology 1262
history 1261
pathogenesis 1261
phacomatosis pigmentokeratotica 1262–1263
Schimmelpenning syndrome 1262–1263
surgical therapy 2312–2313
treatment 1262
naevus simplex, transient skin disorders in neonates and young infants 75
naevus spilus, acquired melanocytic naevi (AMN) 1255
naevus spilus-type CMN, congenital melanocytic naevi (CMN) 1240, *1241*
naevus trichilemnocysticus 1266–1267
NAFLD *see* nonalcoholic fatty liver disease
Naga sore *see* tropical skin ulcer
nail biopsy, surgical therapy 2316–2317
nail biting (onychophagia) 2150, 2265
nail disorders 2147–2157
see also onychomycosis
acute paronychia 2149–2150
anonychia/micronychia 2155
atopic dermatitis (AD) 2151
common nail disorders 2148–2153
congenital malalignment of the big toenail 2148–2149
ectodermal dysplasias (EDs) 2156
epidermolysis bullosa (EB) 2156
herringbone (chevron) nails 2149
ingrown nails 2149
Iso–Kikuchi syndrome 2155
lichen planus (LP) 2153–2154
lichen striatus (LS) 2154
nail anatomy and physiology 2147–2148
nail biting and onychotillomania 2150
nail lichen planus (NLP) 393, *394*, 2153–2154
nail matrix naevi 2155
nail–patella syndrome 2155–2156
nail psoriasis 346, 357–358, 362, **365**, 2152–2153
onychotillomania and nail biting 2150
pachyonychia congenita (PC) 2156–2157
parakeratosis pustulosa 2151–2152
periungual fibromas 2154
polydactyly 2156
psoriasis 2152–2153
punctate leuconychia 2151
subungual exostosis 2154–2155
transitory koilonychia 2148
twenty-nail dystrophy (TND) 2153
warts 2150
yellow nail syndrome (YNS) 2157
nail dystrophy, hyperpigmentation *1472*
nail formation, developing human skin 24–25
nail lichen planus (NLP) 393, *394*, 2153–2154
nail matrix naevi, nail disorders 2155
nail–patella syndrome 2155–2156
nail picking (onychotillomania) 2150, 2265
nail problems, dystrophic epidermolysis bullosa (DEB) 928
nail psoriasis 346, 357–358, 362, **365**, 2152–2153
nails features, dystrophic epidermolysis bullosa (DEB) 921
NAME syndrome, endocrine dysfunction 2008
nanoparticles and nonviral approaches, genetic therapies **2302**, 2303–2305
napkin/anogenital psoriasis 357, **365**
napkin dermatitis 265–278, 547
acrodermatitis enteropathica 277
aetiology 265, 266–268, *266*
allergic contact napkin dermatitis 267–268, 270
allergy 267–268
atopic dermatitis (AD) 274
atopic napkin rash **268**
bullous impetigo 273
bullous impetigo napkin rash **268**
Candida albicans 267
candidal (monilial) napkin dermatitis 271–272
candidal napkin rash **268**
chemical irritants 267
child abuse and neglect (CAN) 278, *2237*
clinical diagnosis 268–269
clinical presentation 265
congenital syphilis 273–274
contact napkin dermatitis **268**, 269–270
definition 265
differential diagnosis 268–269, **269**
eczematous/papulosquamous **269**
faeces 266–267
friction 267
granuloma gluteale infantum 271
herpes simplex virus (HSV) infections *278*

napkin dermatitis (*cont'd*)
history 265–266
HIV infection 274
hydration 267
infantile seborrhoeic dermatitis (SD) **269**, 274, 275
infectious napkin dermatitis 271–274
inflammatory conditions 274–276
intertrigo napkin rash **268**, 270–271
Kawasaki disease (KD) 276
Langerhans cell histiocytosis (LCH) 276–277
metabolic napkin conditions 277
microorganisms 267
miliaria 275
mixed napkin dermatitis 275
napkins/diapers role 266
neoplastic napkin conditions 276–277
nodular **269**
'perianal pseudoverrucous papules and nodules' entity 275–276
perianal streptococcal disease 272–273
perioral dermatitis with extrafacial genital manifestations and metastatic Crohn disease 276
primary and secondary inflammatory conditions 274–276
primary irritant napkin rash **268**, 269–270
psoriasis 275
scabies 273
streptococcal intertrigo 272–273
temperature 267
types **268**
urine 267
verrucous **269**
vesiculobullous disorders 278
vesiculobullous/erosive **269**
napkin/diaper care, neonatal skin care 65
nasal cerebral heterotopia *see* nasal glioma
nasal glioma (nasal cerebral heterotopia) 112–113
aetiology 112
clinical features 112–113
definition 112
differential diagnosis 113
pathology 112
treatment 113
nasopalpebral lipoma coloboma syndrome
characteristics **1199**
clinical features **1199**
natal and neonatal teeth, transient skin disorders in neonates and young infants 78
Naxos disease **1657**, 1700–1701
NC *see* naevus comedonicus
NCIE (nonbullous congenital ichthyosiform erythroderma) 125
NCP *see* benign or neonatal cephalic pustulosis
ND *see* naevus depigmentosus
necrobiosis lipoidica (NL)
aetiology 852
clinical symptoms 852
definition 852
diagnosis 852
epidemiology 852
metabolic syndrome (MetS) 852
pathogenesis 852
treatment 852
necrobiosis lipoidica diabeticorum (NLD), diabetes mellitus 2005, *2006*
necrobiotic xanthogranuloma with paraproteinaemia (NXG) 1088
clinical features 1088
epidemiology 1088
histology findings 1088
history 1088
treatment 1088
necrotizing fasciitis (NF) 429
necrotizing skin and soft tissue infections 450–451
needle marks, iatrogenic disorders of the newborn 163
Neisseria gonorrhoeae, neonates **87**
NEMO (NF-κB essential modulator), hair loss 2111
nemolizumab, atopic dermatitis (AD) 260
neomycin, allergic contact dermatitis (ACD) 307
neonatal acne, differential diagnosis **819**
neonatal blistering
diffuse cutaneous mastocytosis (DCM) 149–150
focal dermal hypoplasia (FDH) (Goltz syndrome) **140**, 148–149
genodermatoses **137–138**, 147–149
incontinentia pigmenti (IP) **140**, 147–148
restrictive dermopathy (RD) 149
vesiculobullous lesions 864–865
neonatal bullous autoimmune disorders, transplacental 97–98
neonatal bullous neutrophilic dermatosis *see* Sweet syndrome
neonatal cephalic pustulosis, *Malassezia*-associated diseases 554
neonatal cephalic pustulosis (NCP) **135**, 145
clinical features 145
differential diagnosis 145
epidemiology 145
histology findings 145
laboratory findings 145
pathogenesis 145
prevention 145
treatment 145
neonatal development
approach to the neonate 2342–2343
behavioural and motor development 2343
vision, hearing, taste and smell 2343
neonatal eosinophilia 317
neonatal eosinophilic pustulosis (NEP)
clinical features 143
differential diagnosis 143
epidemiology 143
histology findings 143
laboratory findings 143
neonates 142–144
pathogenesis 143
prevention 143–144
treatment 143–144
neonatal eosinophilic pustulosis/pustular folliculitis **135**
neonatal erythroderma 121–133
adverse drug reactions (ADR) 129–130
atopic dermatitis (AD) 123–124
congenital cutaneous candidiasis (CCC) 129
cutaneous disorders 123–128
diagnostic algorithm *122*
diagnostic work-up 133
differential diagnosis 121–133
diffuse cutaneous mastocytosis (DCM) 127
ectodermal dysplasia 127
epidermal homeostasis disorders 126–127
erythematosquamous skin diseases 123–125
genodermatoses 125–127
graft-versus- host-disease (GVHD) 130–131
holocarboxylase synthetase deficiency (HSD) 132
immunodeficiencies, primary 131
immunological disorders 130–132
inborn errors of metabolism 132
infantile seborrhoeic dermatitis (SD) 123
infections and toxicities 128–129
intensive care 2409
maple syrup urine disease (MSUD) 132
methylmalonic acidaemias (MMA) 132
nonsyndromic ichthyoses 125–126
nursing care of the skin **2412**
Omenn syndrome (OS) 130
pityriasis rubra pilaris (PRP) 124–125
red man syndrome 130
scabies 127–128
staphylococcal scalded skin syndrome (SSSS) 128–129
Stevens–Johnson syndrome (SJS) 129–130
syndromic ichthyoses 126
toxic epidermal necrolysis (TEN) 129–130
neonatal ichthyosis-sclerosing cholangitis (NISCH) syndrome 1581–1583, **1583**
clinical features 1581–1583, *1584*
laboratory findings 1583
pathogenesis 1581
neonatal lupus erythematosus (NLE) 93–97
transplacental 93–97
neonatal onset multisystemic inflammatory disorder (NOMID) 2012–2013
neonatal pemphigus 874
neonatal pemphigus vulgaris 98
neonatal skin care 63–71
see also nursing care of the skin
aims 63
atopic dermatitis (AD) 70

dry skin 68–70
emollients 68–70
emulsifiers 69
environmental factors affecting epidermal integrity 64
lanolin 69
mechanical damage avoidance 66–67
mineral oils 69
napkin/diaper care 65
olive oil 69
percutaneous absorption 71
polyethylene glycols (PEG) 69
premature infants 66–67
skin care immediately after birth and in the first 2–3 days 64
sodium lauryl sulfate (SLS) 69
term neonates and infants 67–70
transepidermal water loss (TEWL) 66
umbilical cord care 65
urea 69
vegetable oils 69
washing and bathing 64–65

neonatal unit etiquette, approach to the neonate 2343–2344

neonates
see also infants; neonatal skin care; premature infants; transient skin disorders in neonates and young infants
acquired neonatal infections 86–91
appendages 61
approach to the paediatric patient 2342–2344
bacterial infections 85–86, **87**, **88**, 89–90
benign or neonatal cephalic pustulosis 145
'blueberry muffin rash' (dermal extramedullary erythropoiesis) 85, **86**
bullous pemphigoid (BP) **136**
common acquired infections **88**
congenital erosive and vesicular dermatosis with reticulated supple scarring (CEVD) **139**, 150–151
congenital infections 84–86, **87**
cutaneous microbiome 47–49
cytomegalovirus (CMV) 85, **86**
dermis 61
epidermis 57–60, 64
epidermolysis bullosa (EB) 2395–2396
epidermolysis bullosa acquisita (EBA) 98
erosive or ulcerative skin lesions **138–140**, 150–151
erosive pustular dermatosis of the scalp (EPDS) 145–146
erythema toxicum neonatorum (ETN) 76, 141–142
fungal infections 86, **87**, **88**, 90
gestational pemphigoid 98
infantile acropustulosis (IA) 144–145
linear immunoglobulin IgA bullous dermatosis (LABD) 147
Listeria monocytogenes **87**, **136**, **139**
milia 134–141
miliaria 141
neonatal cephalic pustulosis (NCP) 145
neonatal eosinophilic pustulosis (NEP) 142–144
neonatal pemphigus vulgaris 98
nursing care of the skin 2395–2396
parasitic infections 90–91
pemphigoid gestationis (PG) 98, **136**
pemphigus foliaceus (PF) 98, **136**, **139**
percutaneous respiration 61
physiology of neonatal skin 56–61
protozoal infections 86, **87**
pustular eruptions **89**
scabies 90–91
sebaceous gland activity 61
skin anatomy comparison **57**
skin roughness 60
skin surface pH 59–60
stratum corneum hydration 60
Streptococcus pyogenes **135**
thermoregulation 61
transepidermal water loss (TEWL) 58–60
transient neonatal pustular melanosis (TNPM) 142
transient skin disorders 72–81
transplacentally acquired dermatoses 93–99
varicella zoster virus (VZV) infections 85, **86**, **139**
vernix caseosa 56, 72–73
vesiculopustular and bullous skin lesions 134–151
viral infections 85, **86**, 88
wound healing 61

neoplasia, genital disease 2188–2190
benign tumours 2189
malignancies 2188–2189
prepubertal unilateral fibrous hyperplasia of the labium majus 2189–2190

neoplasms, HIV infection 653–654

Neoscytalidium infections 557–558
clinical features 558
diagnosis by morphology 558
treatment 558

NEP *see* neonatal eosinophilic pustulosis

nerve damage, surgical therapy 2317

Nestor–Guillermo syndrome 1737–1738
clinical features 1738
differential diagnosis 1738
epidemiology 1737
histology findings 1738
history 1737
laboratory findings 1738
pathogenesis 1737
treatment 1738

Netherton syndrome (NS) 1579, 1613–1620
aetiology 1613–1614
atopic manifestations and allergy 1617
clinical features 1615–1618
diagnosis 1618–1619
differential diagnosis 1579
growth and development 1618
hair abnormalities 1616–1617
hair disorders *2116*
history 1613
hypernatraemic dehydration 1618
hypothermia 1618
immunological abnormalities and infections 1617–1618
pathogenesis 1613–1614
pathology 1615
presentation in infancy 1615
prognosis 1619–1620
skin manifestations 1615–1616
treatment 1619

Neu-Laxova syndrome (NLS) 1590
clinical features 1590
definition 1590
differential diagnosis 1590
pathogenesis 1590
prevention 1590
treatment 1590

neuroblastoma 1395–1396
aetiology 1395
clinical features 1395
definition 1395
differential diagnosis 1396
epidemiology 1395
laboratory studies and images 1396
pathogenesis 1395
pathology 1396
treatment 1396

neuroborreliosis, lyme borreliosis (LB)/lyme disease 468

neurofibromas, neurofibromatosis type 1 (NF1) 1826, 1830

neurofibromatoses 1823–1834
neurofibromatosis type 1 (NF1) 1823–1831
neurofibromatosis type 2 (NF2) 1832–1834
oral mucosa 2094
segmental or mosaic neurofibromatosis type 1 1831–1832

neurofibromatosis type 1 (NF1) **1804**, 1823–1831
age of onset **1825**
CALMs 1825, 1830
clinical features 1824–1828, **1829**
cutaneous features **1824**
dermatological features 1825, 1827
diagnostic criteria 1824–1825
differential diagnosis 1828–1829
epidemiology 1823–1824
frequency of common clinical features **1825**
gene/chromosome **1824**
genetics 1824, **1829**
histology findings 1830
incidence **1824**
inheritance **1824**
laboratory findings 1829–1830
learning disabilities 1828
management 1830–1831
molecular genetic testing 1829–1830
neurofibromas 1826, 1830
NF1 gene and neurofibromin 1824
nondermatological features 1827–1828
ophthalmological manifestations 1827–1828
orthopaedic manifestations 1827

neurofibromatosis type 1 (NF1) (*cont'd*)
  pathogenesis 1823–1824
  PNFs 1830
  protein **1824**
  segmental or mosaic neurofibromatosis type 1 1831–1832
  skinfold freckling (Crowe's sign) 1825
neurofibromatosis type 2 (NF2) 1832–1834
  CALMs 1833
  clinical features 1832–1834
  dermatological features 1833
  differential diagnosis 1833
  epidemiology 1832
  genetic testing 1833–1834
  NIH diagnostic criteria 1832–1834
  non-dermatological features 1833
  pathogenesis 1832
  pathology 1834
  peripheral nerve tumours 1833
  prevention 1834
  treatment 1834
neuroichthyotic syndromes 1585–1589
neurological disease, Proteus syndrome (PS) 1285–1286
neurological findings, tuberous sclerosis complex (TSC) 1844–1846
neurological involvement
  Behçet disease (BD) 1955, 1956
  juvenile dermatomyositis (JDM) 1948
neuropsychiatric systemic lupus erythematosus 1943
neutral lipid storage disease with ichthyosis (Chanarin–Dorfman syndrome) 1580–1581
  clinical features 1580
  definition 1580
  epidemiology 1580
  extracutaneous findings 1580
  laboratory findings 1580, *1581*
  pathogenesis 1580
next-generation sequencing (NGS) of DNA, molecular genetics 40–42
NF *see* necrotizing fasciitis
NF1 *see* neurofibromatosis type 1
NF1 gene and neurofibromin, neurofibromatosis type 1 (NF1) 1824
NFJS *see* Naegeli–Franceschetti–Jadassohn syndrome
NF-κB essential modulator (NEMO), hair loss 2111
NGS of DNA *see* next-generation sequencing of DNA
NICH *see* noninvoluting congenital haemangioma
nickel, allergic contact dermatitis (ACD) 306–307
nipple and breast abnormalities 106–107
NISCH syndrome *see* neonatal ichthyosis-sclerosing cholangitis syndrome
nitrous oxide (N_2O), anaesthesia 2338
NL *see* necrobiosis lipoidica; neonatal lupus erythematosus
NLD *see* necrobiosis lipoidica diabeticorum
NLE *see* neonatal lupus erythematosus
NLP *see* nail lichen planus
NLS *see* naevus lipomatosus superficialis; Neu-Laxova syndrome
nocardiosis 574
  clinical features 574
  differential diagnosis 574
  epidemiology 574
  histology findings 574
  laboratory findings 574
  pathogenesis 574
  prevention 574
  treatment 574
NOD2 in nuclear factor-κβ (NF-κβ) signalling, Blau syndrome/early-onset sarcoidosis (EOS) 1001–1002
nodular fasciitis 1362
  clinical features 1362
  epidemiology 1362
  history 1362
  pathogenesis 1362
  pathology 1362
  treatment 1362
nodular napkin dermatitis **269**
NOMID *see* neonatal onset multisystemic inflammatory disorder
nonalcoholic fatty liver disease (NAFLD), psoriasis 360
nonbullous congenital ichthyosiform erythroderma (NCIE) 125
noncutaneous porphyrias 965–966
nonepidermolytic palmoplantar tylosis *see* nonepidermolytic PPK type Bothnia
nonepidermolytic PPK type Bothnia 1527
  clinical features 1527
  differential diagnosis 1527
  epidemiology 1527
  histology findings 1527
  history 1527
  laboratory findings 1527
  pathogenesis 1527
  treatment 1527
nonepidermolytic PPK type Nagashima (PPKN) 1528
  clinical features 1528
  differential diagnosis 1528
  epidemiology 1528
  histology findings 1528
  history 1528
  laboratory findings 1528
  pathogenesis 1528
  treatment 1528
noninflammatory (comedonal) lesions, acne vulgaris 805–806
noninvoluting congenital haemangioma (NICH) 1440–1442
non-Langerhans cell histiocytoses 1078–1091
  see also Langerhans cell histiocytosis
nonorganoid epidermal naevi 1267–1272
nonrenal hamartoma, tuberous sclerosis complex (TSC) 1849
nonsexually acquired acute genital ulcers (NSAGU) 2180–2181
nonsexually acquired genital infections in children 2175–2179
nonspecific viral eruptions 675
nonsyndromic ichthyoses, neonatal erythroderma 125–126
nonsyndromic SHFM, ectodermal dysplasias (EDs) 1682
nontuberculous mycobacterial infections (NTM) 497–501
  Buruli ulcer 500–501
  cervicofacial lymphadenopathy 500
  clinical spectrum 500–501
  epidemiology 497–500
  Mycobacterium marinum infection 501
  skin and soft tissue infections 500–501
nonvascular nodules and cysts, differential diagnosis 1316–1322
nonviral approaches and nanoparticles, genetic therapies **2302**, 2303–2305
Noonan syndrome (NS) **1806**, 1857–1859
  see also cardiofaciocutaneous syndrome
  aetiology 1857–1858
  clinical features 1859
  clinical variants 1859
  cutaneous features 1859
  definition 1857–1858
  diagnosis 1859
  history 1857–1858
  Noonan syndrome-like disorder with or without juvenile myelomonocytic leukaemia 1859
  other features 1859
  summary of RASopathies **1858**
  treatment 1859
Noonan syndrome-like disorder with or without juvenile myelomonocytic leukaemia 1859
Noonan syndrome with multiple lentigines (LEOPARD syndrome) **1806**, 1859–1860
  aetiology 1859
  clinical features 1860
  definition 1859
  diagnosis 1860
  history 1859
  summary of RASopathies **1858**
  treatment 1860
Norbotten-type palmoplantar keratoderma *see* diffuse epidermolytic palmoplantar keratoderma
North American blastomycosis *see* blastomycosis
Norwegian (crusted) scabies 714–715
novel therapeutic strategies/DNA repair creams, xeroderma pigmentosum and related diseases 1768
NS *see* Netherton syndrome; Noonan syndrome
NSAGU *see* nonsexually acquired acute genital ulcers
NSML *see* Noonan syndrome with multiple lentigines (LEOPARD syndrome)
nucleotide excision repair
  nucleotide excision repair pathway 1745–1747

UV-induced DNA damage 1745
xeroderma pigmentosum and related diseases 1744–1747
nucleotide excision repair defective syndromes, xeroderma pigmentosum and related diseases 1748–1763, 1768
nummular dermatitis 199, *200*, 235–236
clinical features 235, *236*
definition 235
differential diagnosis 236
epidemiology 235
pathogenesis 235
pathology 235
prognosis 236
treatment 236
nurses' role, safeguarding examinations 2413
nursing care of the skin 2393–2413
see also neonatal skin care
bleach baths 2399
collodion baby 2393, **2394–2395**
eczema 2396–2399
epidermolysis bullosa (EB) 2395–2396
haemangiomas 2403–2406
harlequin ichthyosis (HI) **2394–2395**, 2395
infections and infestations 2402
intensive care 2409
laser therapy 2402, **2405**
meticillin-resistant *Staphylococcus aureus* (MRSA) 2402, **2403**
Mongolian spots **2412**
neonatal erythroderma **2412**
neonates 2395–2396
paste bandages 2397–2398, *2400*, **2401**
'port-wine stain' (localized or extensive capillary malformation) 2402, **2405**
psoriasis 2400–2402
scabies 2402, **2405**
staphylococcal scalded skin syndrome (SSSS) 2402, **2404**
Stevens–Johnson syndrome (SJS) 2409, **2411–2412**
systemic therapies 2406–2409
therapeutic clothing 2398–2399
toxic epidermal necrolysis (TEN) 2409, **2411–2412**
ulcerated haemangiomas 2406, **2407**
vascular birthmarks 2402–2406
wet wrap dressings 2397, **2398**, **2399**
nutrition, dystrophic epidermolysis bullosa (DEB) 928–930
nutritional abnormalities, hyperpigmentation 1467
nutritional deficiency, tongue 2100
nutritional disorders 831–840
eating disorders 839–840
fatty acid deficiency 835
mineral deficiencies 837–839
protein-energy malnutrition (severe acute malnutrition) 831–834
vitamin deficiencies 835–837
nutritional issues and growth, congenital ichthyoses (CI) 1595–1596
nutritional problems, dystrophic epidermolysis bullosa (DEB) 922
NXG *see* necrobiotic xanthogranuloma with paraproteinaemia

obesity 839–840
obsessive and compulsive disorders, physiological habits **2264**
OC *see* miliary osteoma cutis of the face; platelike osteoma cutis
OCA *see* oculocutaneous albinism
occipital alopecia 2103–2104
occlusotherapy (adhesiotherapy), human papillomaviruses (HPV) 594
occult spinal dysraphism (OSD) 114–116
OSD and midline capillary malformations 1413
ocular complications
see also eyes; ophthalmological aspects
atopic dermatitis (AD) 197–198, 251
dystrophic epidermolysis bullosa (DEB) 922
ocular involvement, Behçet disease (BD) 1954
ocular lesions, Behçet disease (BD) 1956
ocular lichen planus 395
oculocutaneous albinism (OCA) 1486–1489
clinical features 1487–1488
differential diagnosis 1488
epidemiology 1486–1487
laboratory findings 1488–1489
pathogenesis 1486–1487
prevention 1489
treatment 1489
oculo-dentodigital dysplasia (ODDD) syndrome 1695
autosomal dominant **1657**
autosomal recessive **1657–1658**
clinical features 1695
definition 1695
differential diagnosis 1695
history 1695
pathology 1695
prognosis 1695
treatment 1695
oculodento-osseous dysplasia *see* oculo-dentodigital dysplasia syndrome
oculotrichodysplasia **1658**
odontogenic cysts, oral mucosa 2096
odontomicronychial dysplasia **1658**
odonto-onycho-dermal dysplasia syndrome (OODD syndrome) 1532–1533, **1658**, 1686–1688
clinical features 1532–1533, 1687–1688
definition 1686–1687
differential diagnosis 1533, 1688
history 1532, 1687
laboratory investigation 1533
pathogenesis 1532
pathology 1533, 1687
prognosis 1688
treatment 1533, 1688
odontoonychodysplasia with alopecia, hair loss 2111
oestrogen excess 2001
clinical features 2001
cutaneous manifestations 2001
histology findings 2001
laboratory findings 2001
pathogenesis 2001
prevention 2001
treatment 2001
OFG *see* orofacial granulomatosis
Ofuji disease *see* eosinophilic pustular folliculitis in infancy and childhood
Ohio Valley fever 565–567
OI *see* osteogenesis imperfecta
oligoarthritis, juvenile idiopathic arthritis (JIA) 1936
oligodontia-colorectal cancer syndrome **1658**
olive oil, neonatal skin care 69
Oliver–McFarlane syndrome, endocrine dysfunction 2008
Olmsted syndrome *see* mutilating palmoplantar keratoderma with periorificial keratotic plaques
omalizumab, atopic dermatitis (AD) 259
Omenn syndrome (OS), neonatal erythroderma 130
omphalitis, pseudomonal skin disease 449
onychia 547, 549
onychomycosis 536–537
see also nail disorders
distal and lateral subungual onychomycosis 536
endonyx onychomycosis 536
Mykids 536–537
proximal subungual onychomycosis 536
superficial white onychomycosis 536
total dystrophic onychomycosis 536
onychophagia (nail biting) 2150, 2265
onychotillomania (nail picking) 2150, 2265
onychotrichodysplasia with neutropenia (Cantu syndrome) **1658**, **2110**
OODD *see* odonto-onycho-dermal dysplasia syndrome
ophthalmological aspects
see also eyes; ocular complications
congenital ichthyoses (CI) 1595
ophthalmological complications, infantile haemangiomas (IH) 1430
ophthalmological findings, tuberous sclerosis complex (TSC) 1846–1847
ophthalmological manifestations, neurofibromatosis type 1 (NF1) 1827–1828
opiates, anaesthesia 2337
optical properties of skin 971–972
oral and genital aphthae, Behçet disease (BD) 1956
oral candidosis 546–547, 549
oral-facial-digital syndrome, tongue 2100
oral hairy leucoplakia 2091
HIV infection 652
oral isotretinoin, acne vulgaris 809–810

oral lesions
Bohn nodules 77–78
dental lamina cysts 78
Epstein pearls 77
eruption cyst 78–79
natal and neonatal teeth 78
sucking pads of the lips 79
transient skin disorders in neonates and young infants 77–79
oral lichen planus 394–395
oral mucosa 2079–2098
see also tongue; white patches (leucoplakia), oral mucosa
abscesses 2094, *2095*
aciclovir-resistant herpes simplex infection 2083
acquired soft tissue swellings 2094–2096
acute leukaemia 2097
acute pseudo-membranous candidiasis (thrush) 2089
acute ulcerative gingivitis (AUG) 2085
Addison disease 2093
Albright syndrome 2093
allergic gingivostomatitis 2093
amalgam and graphite tattoos 2091
angular stomatitis 2090
aspergillosis 2085
autoinflammatory diseases 2081
bacterial infections 2085
Behçet syndrome 2081
Bohn nodules and Epstein pearls (gingival cysts of infancy) 2088
bone cysts 2096
bony swellings 2096
Burkitt lymphoma 2096
candidal leucoplakia (chronic hyperplastic candidiasis) 2090
candidosis (candidiasis) 2089–2090
chickenpox 2083
chikungunya virus (CHIKV) 2084
chronic atrophic candidiasis (chronic denture stomatitis) 2090
chronic denture stomatitis (chronic atrophic candidiasis) 2090
chronic graft-versus-host disease 2086–2087
chronic hyperplastic candidiasis (candidal leucoplakia) 2090
chronic recurrent sialadenitis 2098
coeliac disease (gluten-sensitive enteropathy) 2086
congenital granular cell epulis of the newborn 2094
connective tissue diseases 2087
Cowden syndrome 2094
Crohn disease 2086
cystic fibrosis 2098
cytomegalovirus (CMV) 2084
Darier–White disease (dyskeratosis follicularis) 2088
deep mycoses 2085–2086
dermatitis herpetiformis (DH) 2087
developmental soft tissue swellings 2094
drug-induced gingival hyperplasia 2097
drug-induced hyperpigmentation 2093
dyskeratosis congenita (DC) 2088
dyskeratosis follicularis (Darier–White disease) 2088
Ebola virus (EBOV) 2084
enteroviruses (EV) 2084
epidermolysis bullosa (EB) 2087
epiloia 2094
Epstein–Barr viral infection 2084
Epstein pearls and Bohn nodules (gingival cysts of infancy) 2088
eruption cyst 2094
erythema multiforme (EM) 2087
erythematous candidiasis 2089
familial chronic neutropenia *2085, 2092*
familial white folded gingivostomatitis (white sponge naevus) 2088
fibroepithelial polyp/nodule 2095
fibrous dysplasia 2096
Fordyce spots or granules 2088
frictional/traumatic keratosis 2089
fungal infections 2084–2085
Gardner syndrome 2096
gastrointestinal disease 2085–2086
generalized gingival swelling 2096–2097
generalized lesions 2093
giant cell epulis/granuloma 2095
gingival cysts of infancy (Epstein pearls and Bohn nodules) 2088
gingivitis 2092–2093
graft-versus- host-disease (GVHD) 2086–2087
haemangiomas and vascular malformations 2092
haematological and immunological disorders 2085
hairy leucoplakia 652, 2091
hand, foot and oral mucosa disease (HFMD) 2084
hereditary benign intraepithelial dyskeratosis 2088
hereditary gingival fibromatosis 2097
hereditary haemorrhagic telangiectasia (HHT) 2093
hereditary mucoepithelial dysplasia 2092
herpangina 2084
Herpes zoster (shingles) 2083–2084
herpetic gingivostomatitis 2082–2083
hidrotic ectodermal dysplasia (Clouston syndrome, ED2) 2088
histoplasmosis 2085
HIV infection 2084, 2098
iatrogenic oral ulceration 2087
infections 2082–2085
infectious mononucleosis (IM) 2084
inflammatory bowel diseases 2086
juvenile active ossifying fibroma 2096
Kaposi sarcoma 2092
Langerhans cell histiocytosis (LCH) 2096
lichenoid reactions 2086–2087
lichen planus (LP) 2086–2087
linear IgA dermatosis (LAD) 2087
local causes of oral mucosa ulceration 2081–2082
lupus erythematosus 2090
lymphangioma 2094
lymphoma 2096
MAGIC syndrome 2081
materia alba 2089
melanotic neuroectodermal tumour of infancy 2091–2092
molluscum contagiosum (MC) 2096
mucocoele/ranula 2098
mucormycosis (zygomycosis, phycomycosis) 2085
neurofibromatoses 2094
odontogenic cysts 2096
oral mucosa ulcers/sore oral mucosa 2079–2087
oral pigmented naevi 2091
oral ulceration associated with systemic disease 2085
oral ulceration in association with neoplasia 2085
osteomyelitis 2096
pachyonychia congenita (PC) 2088
palmoplantar keratoderma (tylosis) 2088
Peutz–Jeghers syndrome 2092
pigmentation of the teeth 2093
porphyrias *2094*
psoriasis 2090
pyogenic granuloma (PG) (lobular capillary haemangioma) 2095
racial pigmentation 2093
recurrent aphthous stomatitis (RAS) 2079–2081
red and pigmented lesions 2091–2094
salivary gland swelling 2097–2098
sarcoidosis 2098
sarcomas and related conditions 2096
squamous papillomas 2095
Sturge–Weber syndrome (SWS) 2092
swellings/lumps in and around the oral mucosa 2094–2098
thrombocytopenic purpura 2093
thrush (acute pseudo-membranous candidiasis) 2089
tori 2096
traumatic/frictional keratosis 2089
traumatic ulceration 2081–2082
tuberous sclerosis complex (TSC) 2094
tylosis (palmoplantar keratoderma) 2088
ulcerative colitis 2086
vesiculobullous disorders 2087
viral infections 2082–2084
white patches (leucoplakia) 2088–2091
white sponge naevus (familial white folded gingivostomatitis) 2088
Wiskott–Aldrich syndrome (WAS) 2093
Zika virus (ZIKV) infection 2084
oral pigmented naevi, oral mucosa 2091
oral sucrose, perioperative analgesics 2335
oral therapies, porokeratosis 1626–1627
oral treatments, pediculosis 728–729
orf **625**, 643–646

clinical features 643–645
clinical stages **643**
differential diagnosis 645
epidemiology 643
histology findings 645
history 643
laboratory findings 645
pathogenesis 643
prevention 646
treatment 646
organic acidurias 1971–1972
organoid epidermal naevi 1261–1267
orificial tuberculosis 490
orofacial granulomatosis (OFG) 1017–1020
antimicrobial agents 1020
clinical features 1018–1019
diagnostic studies 1018–1019
dietary interventions 1019
differential diagnosis 1018–1019
epidemiology 1017–1018
genital signs of systemic disease 2192
histology findings 1019
history 1017
immunosuppressants and TNF-α inhibitors, systemic 1020
intralesional corticosteroids 1019–1020
laboratory findings 1019
pathogenesis 1017–1018
surgery 1020
systemic corticosteroids 1019–1020
systemic immunosuppressants and TNF-α inhibitors 1020
topical therapies 1019
treatment 1019–1020
orofacial granulomatosis and anogenital granulomatosis, genital signs of systemic disease 2192
orofaciodigital (OFD) syndrome type 1 **1659**
Oroya fever 480–482
orthopaedic manifestations, neurofibromatosis type 1 (NF1) 1827
orthopoxvirus **625**
orthopoxvirus infection 626–643
OS *see* Omenn syndrome
OSD *see* occult spinal dysraphism
Osler–Weber–Rendu disease *see* hereditary haemorrhagic telangiectasia
ossification in the skin *see* calcification and ossification in the skin
osteogenesis imperfecta (OI) 1147–1149
classification **1148**
clinical features 1148–1149
common variable OI – OI type 4 1148–1149
definition 1147
differential diagnosis 1149
history 1147
OI with calcification in interosseous membranes – OI type 5 1149
pathogenesis 1147–1148
perinatally lethal OI syndromes – OI type 2 1148
progressively deforming OI – OI type 3 1148
treatment 1149
osteomyelitis, oral mucosa 2096
osteoporosis, dystrophic epidermolysis bullosa (DEB) 928
otitis externa, pseudomonal skin disease 448–449
overlap SSc, systemic sclerosis (SSc) **1185**

p14 deficiency **2039**
PA *see* pityriasis alba
pachyonychia congenita (PC) 1541–1543, 1698, **2110**
clinical features 1541–1543
differential diagnosis 1543
epidemiology 1541
histology findings 1543
history 1541
laboratory findings 1543
nail disorders 2156–2157
oral mucosa 2088
pathogenesis 1541
treatment 1543
pachyonychia congenita, autosomal recessive type **1659**
pachyonychia congenita type 2 **1659**
pagetoid reticulosis (PR) 1049
pain, dystrophic epidermolysis bullosa (DEB) 931
pain perception *see* anaesthesia
Pallister–Killian syndrome (PKS), fine and whorled Blaschkolinear hypoand hyperpigmentation (incorporating hypomelanosis of Ito, and linear and whorled naevoid hypermelanosis) 1299
palmar–plantar fibromatosis 1363–1364
clinical features 1364
differential diagnosis 1364
epidemiology 1363
history 1363
pathogenesis 1363
pathology 1364
treatment 1364
palmoplantar hidradenitis 1325–1326
aetiology 1325–1326
clinical presentation 1326
differential diagnosis 1326
epidemiology 1325
histology 1326
management 1326
palmoplantar hyperkeratosis and true hermaphroditism *see* palmoplantar hyperkeratosis with squamous cell carcinoma of skin and sex reversal
palmoplantar hyperkeratosis with congenital alopecia **1659**
palmoplantar hyperkeratosis with squamous cell carcinoma of skin and sex reversal 1532, **1803**
clinical features 1532
differential diagnosis 1532
epidemiology 1532
history 1532
laboratory investigation 1532
pathogenesis 1532
pathology 1532
treatment 1532
palmoplantar keratoderma (tylosis), oral mucosa 2088
palmoplantar keratoderma, and cutaneous SCC **1803**
palmoplantar keratoderma, leukonychia and exuberant scalp hair 1537
clinical features 1537
history 1537
palmoplantar keratoderma cum degeneratione granulosa Vorner *see* diffuse epidermolytic palmoplantar keratoderma
palmoplantar keratoderma-deafness syndromes 1544–1545
clinical features 1545
differential diagnosis 1545
epidemiology 1544–1545
history 1544
pathogenesis 1544–1545
treatment 1545
palmoplantar keratoderma punctate type 1 (PPKP1) *see* punctate palmoplantar keratoderma
palmoplantar keratoderma punctate type 3 (PPKP3) *see* marginal papular keratoderma
palmoplantar keratodermas (PPKs) 1524–1548
autosomal recessive keratoderma, ichthyosis and deafness (ARKID) 1537
Bureau–Barriere–Thomas (palmoplantar keratoderma with clubbing of the fingers and toes and skeletal deformity) 1548
cerebral dysgenesis, neuropathy, ichthyosis and palmoplantar keratoderma syndrome (CEDNIK) 1536–1537
classification 1524–1525
clinical examination 1525
Cole disease 1547
diffuse epidermolytic palmoplantar keratoderma 1525–1526
diffuse hereditary palmoplantar keratodermas with associated features 1529–1537
diffuse nonepidermolytic palmoplantar keratoderma 1527–1529
focal hereditary palmoplantar keratodermas with associated features 1539–1545
focal hereditary palmoplantar keratodermas without associated features 1537–1539
generic management 1525
genetic diagnosis 1525
history 1525
hypotrichosis–osteolysis–periodontitis– palmoplantar keratoderma syndrome (HOPP) 1544
keratin disorders 1520

palmoplantar keratodermas (PPKs) (*cont'd*)
keratosis linearis with ichthyosis congenita and sclerosing keratoderma (KLICK) syndrome 1531
keratosis palmoplantaris papillomatosa et verrucosa Jakac–Wolf 1548
loricrin keratoderma 1529–1530
Mal de Meleda 1528–1529
marginal papular keratoderma 1546, *1547*
mutilating palmoplantar keratoderma with periorificial keratotic plaques (Olmsted syndrome) 1533–1534
nonepidermolytic PPK type Bothnia 1527
nonepidermolytic PPK type Nagashima 1528
odonto-onycho-dermal dysplasia spectrum (OODD) 1532–1533
pachyonychia congenita (PC) 1541–1543
palmoplantar hyperkeratosis with squamous cell carcinoma of skin and sex reversal 1532
palmoplantar keratoderma, leukonychia and exuberant scalp hair 1537
palmoplantar keratoderma-deafness syndromes 1544–1545
palmoplantar keratodermas of uncertain identity 1548
palmoplantar keratoderma with clubbing of the fingers and toes and skeletal deformity (Bureau–Barriere–Thomas) 1548
palmoplantar keratoderma with periodontitis 1534–1536
palmoplantar keratoderma with scleroatrophy (Huriez syndrome) 1531
papular hereditary palmoplantar keratodermas with associated features 1547–1548
papular hereditary palmoplantar keratodermas without associated features 1545–1547
PLACK syndrome 1548
PPK associated with hearing loss 1694–1695
punctate palmoplantar keratoderma 1545–1546
striate palmoplantar keratoderma 1537–1539
transient aquagenic keratoderma 1547
tylosis with oesophageal cancer (TOC) 1539–1545
tyrosinaemia type II 1540–1541
Vohwinkel syndrome (VS) 1694–1695
palmoplantar keratoderma type Thost *see* diffuse epidermolytic palmoplantar keratoderma
palmoplantar keratoderma type Unna *see* diffuse epidermolytic palmoplantar keratoderma
palmoplantar keratoderma with clubbing of the fingers and toes and skeletal deformity (Bureau–Barriere–Thomas) 1548
palmoplantar keratoderma with deafness **1660**
palmoplantar keratoderma with oesophageal cancer *see* tylosis with oesophageal cancer (TOC)
palmoplantar keratoderma with periodontitis 1534–1536, **1804**
clinical features 1535–1536
differential diagnosis 1536
epidemiology 1535
histology findings 1536
history 1534
laboratory findings 1536
pathogenesis 1535
treatment 1536
palmoplantar keratoderma with scleroatrophy (Huriez syndrome) 1531
clinical features 1531
epidemiology 1531
history 1531
laboratory investigation 1531
pathogenesis 1531
pathology 1531
treatment 1531
palmoplantar psoriasis 356, 363
PAN *see* polyarteritis nodosa
pancreatic panniculitis 1219
clinical features 1219
epidemiology 1219
histopathology 1219
pathogenesis 1219
treatment 1219
panniculitis 1207–1220
aetiology **1208**
autoimmune disorders 1216
calcification and ossification in the skin 1343–1344
calciphylaxis 1219–1220
classification **1208**
clinical features 1208–1209
cold panniculitis 1211
connective tissue diseases 1215–1216
cytophagic histiocytic panniculitis (CHP) 1216–1217
dermatomyositis 1215–1216
diagnosis 1208–1209
epidemiology 1207–1208
erythema nodosum (EN) 1213–1214
factitial panniculitis 1220
history 1207
iatrogenic panniculitis 1220
infective panniculitis 1220
lobular panniculitis 1343–1344
lupus panniculitis (LP) 1215
monogenic autoinflammatory diseases and primary immune deficiency 1211–1213
pancreatic panniculitis 1219
pathogenesis 1207–1208
poststeroid panniculitis 1210–1211
primary immune deficiency 1212–1213
sclerema neonatorum 1210
subcutaneous fat necrosis of the newborn (SCFN) 1209–1210
subcutaneous panniculitis-like T-cell lymphoma (SPTCL) 1217–1218
traumatic panniculitis 1220
vasculitis 1215–1216
α1-antitrypsin deficiency 1218–1219
PAPA *see* pyogenic arthritis, pyoderma gangrenosum and acne syndrome
papillary intralymphatic angioendothelioma (PILA) 1397–1398
clinical features 1397
definition 1397
differential diagnosis 1398
pathology 1397–1398
treatment 1398
papillomavirus, neonates **86**
Papillon–Lefevre syndrome **1660**
Papillon–Lefèvre syndrome (PLS) *see* palmoplantar keratoderma with periodontitis
papular acantholytic dyskeratosis of the vulva 2173
clinical features 2173
differential diagnosis 2173
histology findings 2173
management 2173
papular epidermal naevus with skyline basal cell layer (PENS) 1269–1270
associated syndromes 1270
clinical features 1269–1270
differential diagnosis 1269–1270
histopathology 1270
pathogenesis 1269
treatment 1270
papular hereditary palmoplantar keratodermas with associated features 1547–1548
papular-purpuric gloves-and socks syndrome (PPGSS) 667–668
clinical features 667–668
differential diagnosis 668
epidemiology 667
laboratory findings 668
pathogenesis 667
prevention 668
treatment 668
papular umbilicated granuloma annulare (GA) **1008**, 1010–1011
papular xanthoma (PX) 1082–1083
clinical features 1082
differential diagnosis 1083
epidemiology 1082
histology findings 1083
pathogenesis 1082
treatment 1083
papulonecrotic tuberculid (PNT) 492–493
papulopustular acne 807
paracoccidioidomycosis (South American or Brazilian blastomycosis) 568–569
clinical features 568
differential diagnosis 568
epidemiology 568
histology findings 568–569
laboratory findings 568–569

pathogenesis 568
prevention 569
treatment 569
parakeratosis pustulosa, nail disorders 2151–2152
paraneoplastic pemphigus 874
para-phenylenediamine (PPD), allergic contact dermatitis (ACD) 309
parapoxvirus **625**, 626
parapoxvirus infection 643–647
parasites, cutaneous microbiome 54–55
parasitic infections
see also antiparasitic drugs
HIV infection 653
neonates 90–91
vesiculobullous lesions 864
parathyroid hormone, calcification and ossification in the skin 1338–1339
parathyroid hormone dysfunction, cutaneous manifestations 2002–2004
paravaccinia *see* milker's nodule
Parkes Weber syndrome 1401
paromomycin, leishmaniasis 699
paronychia 547, 549
Parry Romberg, morphoea 1178
parvovirus B19 665–666
anaemia 665
differential diagnosis 666
laboratory findings 666
neonates **86**
prevention 666
treatment 666
PASH, PAPASH and other related AIDs 2017
PASI *see* Psoriasis Area and Severity Index
paste bandages, eczema 2397–2398, *2400*, **2401**
patch testing in children, allergic contact dermatitis (ACD) 304–306
patchy follicular atrophoderma 1160
pathophysiology
meningococcal disease 435–437, *438*, *439*, *440*
meticillin-resistant *Staphylococcus aureus* (MRSA) 424–425
staphylococci 424
streptococci 423–424
patient advocacy groups, burden of disease 2258–**2259**
patient organizations and other resources, congenital ichthyoses (CI) 1596–1597
Patient-Oriented Eczema Measure (POEM), atopic dermatitis (AD) 219, *220–221*
PC *see* pachyonychia congenita
PC1 and PC2 *see* pachyonychia congenita (PC)
PCDLBCL *see* primary cutaneous diffuse large B-cell lymphoma
PCFCL *see* primary cutaneous follicle centre lymphoma
PCFH *see* precalcaneal congenital fibrolipomatous hamartoma
PCL *see* primary cutaneous lymphoma
PCMZL *see* primary cutaneous marginal zone B-cell lymphoma
PCOS *see* polycystic ovary syndrome
PCR *see* polymerase chain reaction
PCT *see* porphyria cutanea tarda
PDE4 *see* phosphodiesterase 4 inhibitors
PDE4, apremilast *see* phosphodiesterase inhibitor 4
PE *see* pulmonary embolism
pearly penile papules 2185
clinical presentation 2185
histopathology 2185
management 2185
pathogenesis 2185
pedal papules of infancy, transient skin disorders in neonates and young infants 81
pediculosis 723–730
aetiology 724–726
alternative therapies 729
body lice 729
clinical features 726–727
control 730
diagnosis 727
differential diagnosis 727
distinguishing features **724**
epidemiology 724
history 723–724
lifecycle, head louse 725–726
oral treatments 728–729
pathogenesis 724–726
pediculosis capitis 726
pediculosis corporis 726
pediculosis pubis 726–727
prevention 730
pubic lice 729–730
resistance to pediculicides 730
topical therapies 728, **729**
treatment 727–730
peeling skin syndrome (PSS) 1575
see also exfoliative ichthyosis
clinical features 1575
definition 1575
differential diagnosis 1575
histology investigations 1575
laboratory findings 1575
pathogenesis 1575
treatment 1575
PELVIS/SACRAL/LUMBAR syndrome (lower body haemangiomas and structural malformations), infantile haemangiomas (IH) 1433–1434
pemphigoid diseases 874–885
bullous pemphigoid (BP) 879–882
epidermolysis bullosa acquisita (EBA) 882–885
linear IgA dermatosis (LAD) 874–879
pemphigoid gestationis (PG), neonates 98, **136**
pemphigus diseases 869–874
endemic pemphigus 873
neonatal pemphigus 874
paraneoplastic pemphigus 874
pemphigus foliaceus (PF) 872–873
pemphigus herpetiformis 874
pemphigus vulgaris (PV) 870–872
rare pemphigus variants 873–874
pemphigus foliaceus (PF) 872–873
clinical features 873
differential diagnosis 873
epidemiology 873
histology findings 873
laboratory findings 873
neonates 98, **136**, **139**
pathogenesis 873
prevention 873
treatment 873
pemphigus herpetiformis 874
pemphigus vulgaris (PV) **136**, **139**, 870–872
clinical features 871
differential diagnosis 871–872
epidemiology 870–871
histology findings 872
laboratory findings 872
pathogenesis 871
prevention 872
treatment 872
PEN *see* porokeratotic eccrine naevus
penile abnormalities
anatomical abnormalities 2184
median raphe cysts of the penis and scrotum 2186–2187
pearly penile papules 2185
phimosis 2186
penile warts, human papillomaviruses (HPV) 593
PENS *see* papular epidermal naevus with skyline basal cell layer
pentamidine, leishmaniasis 699
pentavalent antimonials, leishmaniasis 699
Penttinen progeroid disorder 1734
PEODDN *see* porokeratotic eccrine ostial and dermal duct naevus
percutaneous absorption
neonatal skin care 71
potential hazards **71**
percutaneous intralesional sclerotherapy, venous anomalies 1409
percutaneous respiration, neonates 61
perforating granuloma annulare (GA) **1008**, 1010
'perianal pseudoverrucous papules and nodules' entity, napkin dermatitis 275–276
perianal streptococcal dermatitis 429
perianal streptococcal disease, infectious napkin dermatitis 272–273
periderm, embryonic–fetal transition 11–12
perineal groove, transient skin disorders in neonates and young infants 81
periodic fever, immunodeficiency and thrombocytopenia (PFIT) 2018
periodic fever with aphtous stomatitis, pharyngitis and adenitis syndrome (PFAPA) 2018
perioperative analgesics 2335
oral sucrose 2335
perioral dermatitis 338–341
clinical features 339
differential diagnosis 339–340
epidemiology 338–339
histology findings 340
history 338
laboratory findings 340
pathogenesis 338–339
prevention 340–341
treatment 340–341

perioral dermatitis with extrafacial genital manifestations and metastatic Crohn disease, napkin dermatitis 276
periorbital hyperpigmentation 1465
periorbital lesions, laser therapy 2320–2321
periorificial lentiginosis *see* Peutz–Jeghers syndrome
periosteal reaction or subperiosteal new bone formation (SPNBF) 2226
peripheral nerve tumours, neurofibromatosis type 2 (NF2) 1833
periungual and subungual warts, human papillomaviruses (HPV) 591, *592*
periungual fibromas, nail disorders 2154
periungual hyperpigmentation, transient skin disorders in neonates and young infants 79–80
permethrin, scabies 716–717
perniola syndrome **2109**
perniosis 989–990
personal behaviour changes, photoprotection 979, *980*
personalized medicine, genetic testing 39–40
Petty syndrome 1738
  clinical features 1738
  differential diagnosis 1738
  epidemiology 1738
  histology findings 1738
  history 1738
  laboratory findings 1738
  pathogenesis 1738
Peutz–Jeghers syndrome **1805**, 1816–1817
  clinical features 1817
  differential diagnosis 1201
  oral mucosa 2092
  pathogenesis 1817
  treatment 1817
PF *see* pemphigus foliaceus
PFAPA *see* periodic fever with aphtous stomatitis, pharyngitis and adenitis syndrome
PFI *see* Psoriasis Family Impact questionnaire
PFIT *see* periodic fever, immunodeficiency and thrombocytopenia
PG *see* pemphigoid gestationis; pyoderma gangrenosum; pyogenic granuloma
PGA *see* Physician Global Assessment
PHACES syndrome, infantile haemangiomas (IH) 1432–1433
phacomatosis pigmentokeratotica, naevus sebaceous 1262–1263
phacomatosis pigmentovascularis A and B, syndromic vascular anomalies 1414–1415, **1415**
phagocytic defects, immunocompromised children 687
phakomatosis pigmentokeratotica (PPK) 1304
phakomatosis pigmentovascularis (PPV) 1293, 1301–1303
  associated abnormalities 1301–1303
  classification **1301**
  clinical features 1301, *1302*
  epidemiology 1301
  management 1301–1303
  pathogenesis 1303
  phenotypic subclassifications **1301**
pharmaceutical formulation, topical therapies 2277–2278
pharmacokinetic processes, topical pharmacokinetics 2276, *2277*
pharmacological agents, anaesthesia 2336–2339
phenotypes, lymphatic malformations (LMs) **1453**
phenylketonuria (PKU) 1967–1968
  clinical features 1968
  definition 1967
  differential diagnosis 1968
  history 1967
  pathogenesis 1967–1968
  prognosis 1968
  screening 1968
  treatment 1968
phimosis 2186
phosphate regulation, calcification and ossification in the skin 1338–1339
phosphatonins, calcification and ossification in the skin 1339
phosphodiesterase inhibitor 4 (PDE4, apremilast)
  alopecia areata (AA) 2145
  atopic dermatitis (AD) 256
photoageing, ultraviolet radiation (UVR) 974
photocarcinogenesis, ultraviolet radiation (UVR) 974–975
photopatch test, skin testing 955–956
photophytodermatitis 986–988
photoprotection 969–980
  see also sunscreens
  cutaneous effects of UV radiation 971–975
  endogenous photoprotection 975
  exogenous photoprotection 975–980
  solar radiation properties 970
  UV radiation sources 970–971
  vitiligo 1484
phototherapy
  atopic dermatitis (AD) 256–257
  human papillomaviruses (HPV) 596
  irritant contact dermatitis (ICD) 296
  pityriasis rubra pilaris (PRP) 384
  psoriasis 370
  vitiligo 1483
phototherapy complications, iatrogenic disorders of the newborn 164
phototoxic reactions to plants 986–988
phrynoderma, keratosis pilaris 1602
PHTS *see PTEN* (Phosphatase and TENsin homologue) hamartoma tumour syndrome
phylloid hypo- and hypermelanosis 1300
physical approaches, acne vulgaris 811–812
physical photoprotection 978–979
  photoprotection *980*
physical trauma, vesiculobullous lesions 866
Physician Global Assessment (PGA), psoriasis 363
physiological desquamation, transient skin disorders in neonates and young infants 73
physiological habits 2263–2266
  dermatitis artefacta **2264**
  habit phenomena **2264**
  nail biting (onychophagia) 2265
  nail picking (onychotillomania) 2265
  obsessive and compulsive disorders **2264**
  psychodermatology 2263–2266
  thumb and finger sucking 2263–2266
  trichotillomania 2265–2266
physiological jaundice, transient skin disorders in neonates and young infants 74–75
physiological skin findings, transient skin disorders in neonates and young infants 72–75
physiology of neonatal skin 56–61
  appendages 61
  dermis 61
  epidermis 57–60
  percutaneous respiration 61
  sebaceous gland activity 61
  skin anatomy comparison **57**
  skin roughness 60
  skin surface pH 59–60
  stratum corneum hydration 60
  thermoregulation 61
  transepidermal water loss (TEWL) 58–60
  vernix caseosa 56
  wound healing 61
physiotherapy and maintenance of mobility, dystrophic epidermolysis bullosa (DEB) 928
Picker's nodules *see* prurigo nodularis
piebaldism 1493–1494
  clinical features 1494
  differential diagnosis 1494
  epidemiology 1494
  histology findings 1494
  history 1494
  laboratory findings 1494
  pathogenesis 1494
  prevention 1494
  treatment 1494
piedra 556
pigmentary demarcation lines, hyperpigmentation 1468
pigmentary lines of newborns, transient skin disorders in neonates and young infants 79
pigmentary skin lesions
  Mongolian spots 79
  periungual hyperpigmentation 79–80
  pigmentary lines of newborns 79
  transient skin disorders in neonates and young infants 79–80
pigmentation
  see also hyperpigmentation
  ultraviolet radiation (UVR) 973–974
pigmentation of the teeth 2093

pigmented lesions, laser
therapy 2325–2326
pigmented purpuras 1876–1879
PIK3CA-related overgrowth spectrum
(PROS) 1289–1293
CLAPO syndrome 1291
clinical features 1289–1291
CLOVE syndrome (congenital
lipomatous overgrowth, vascular
malformations and epidermal
naevus) 1290
complications 1291
diagnostic criteria **1290**
epidemiology 1289
genetics 1292
histopathology 1292
Klippel–Trenaunay syndrome
(KTS) 1291
laboratory findings 1292
life expectancy 1292
management 1292
Megalencephaly CAPillary
malformation syndrome
(MCAP) 1291
pathogenesis 1289
specific syndromic clinical diagnoses
within PROS 1290–1291
syndromic vascular
anomalies 1416–1417
targeted medical therapy 1292–1293
thromboembolic disease 1291
tumour risk 1291
PILA *see* papillary intralymphatic
angioendothelioma
pilar cyst *see* trichilemmal cyst
pili annulati 2123–2124
pili torti
developmental delay **1660**
hair disorders 2116–2117
onychodysplasia **1660**
pilodental dysplasia with refractive
errors **1660**
pilomatricoma (pilomatrixoma)
clinical features 1316
course and prognosis 1316
definition 1316
differential diagnosis 1316, **1317**
pathogenesis 1316
surgical therapy 2313
treatment 1316
pilomatrix carcinoma 1374–1375
clinical features 1375
differential diagnosis 1375
epidemiology 1374
histology findings 1375
pathogenesis 1374
risk factors **1374**
treatment 1375
pilosebaceous apparatus formation,
developing human skin 28–32
pinta 515–521
aetiology 515, 516
characteristics **519**
clinical features 519
differential diagnosis 519, **520**
distribution 516
endemic syphilis 519
history 515–516
laboratory tests 519–520
pathology 517
prognosis 521
treatment 520–521
pitted keratolysis (PK) 456–458
clinical features 457
diagnosis 457–458
differential diagnosis 458
epidemiology 457
histology findings 457
history 456–457
microbiology 457
pathogenesis 457
prevention 458
treatment 458
pituitary dysfunction, cutaneous
manifestations 2004–2005
pityriasis alba (PA) 228–230, 1496–1497
clinical features 229
clinical presentation 1496–1497
definition 228
differential diagnosis 229–230
epidemiology 228, 1496
management 1497
pathogenesis 229, 1497
pathology 229
prognosis 229
treatment 230
pityriasis lichenoides (PL) 1035–1038
clinical features 1036–1037
differential diagnosis 1037
epidemiology 1035–1036
histology findings 1037–1038
history 1035
laboratory findings 1037–1038
pathogenesis 1035–1036
prevention 1038
treatment 1038
pityriasis rosea 416–420
aetiology 417
atypical presentations 418–419
classification 419
clinical features 418
definition 416
diagnostic criteria 419
differential diagnosis 419
drug-induced pityriasis rosea-like
rashes 419
epidemiology 416–417
history 416
pathology 417–418
treatment 419–420
pityriasis rubra pilaris (PRP) 377–385
associated diseases 381
biologics 384
classification **379**
clinical features 378–381
differential diagnosis 382–383
epidemiology 377–378
histopathology 381–382
history 377
laboratory findings 381–382
management 383–385
methotrexate (MTX) 384
neonatal erythroderma 124–125
other treatments 384–385
pathogenesis 378
phototherapy 384
vs psoriasis **382**
retinoids 384
systemic therapies 384
topical therapies 383–384
type I PRP: classic adult 378–379
type II PRP: atypical adult 379
type III PRP: classic juvenile 379–380
type IV PRP: circumscribed
juvenile 380–381
type V: atypical juvenile 381
type VI: HIV-associated 381
pityriasis versicolor 550–553
aetiology 551–552
clinical features 552–553
definition 550
diagnosis 553
history 550–551
molecular diagnostics 553
pathogenesis 551–552
pathology 552
treatment 553
Pityrosporum (*Malassezia*)
folliculitis 553–554
Pityrosporum (*Malassezia*) yeasts in
seborrhoeic dermatitis 554
PK *see* pitted keratolysis
PKS *see* Pallister–Killian syndrome
PKU *see* phenylketonuria
PL *see* pityriasis lichenoides
PLACK syndrome 1548
clinical features 1548
epidemiology 1548
history 1548
pathogenesis 1548
PLAID *see* PLCG2-associated antibody
deficiency and immune
dysregulation
plantar hyperkeratoses, metabolic
syndrome (MetS) 847–848
plantar psoriasis 356, 363
plant or environmental mites,
pseudoscabies 721
plants 983–989
cutaneous reactions 983–989
irritant reactions 984–986
phototoxic reactions 986–988
plaque morphoea 1177
plaque psoriasis 354–355, **364**
platelet-mediated purpura fulminans
occurring during heparin
therapy 1897
platelike osteoma cutis (OC)
1348–1349
PLCG2-associated antibody deficiency
and immune dysregulation
(PLAID) 2014
PLE *see* polymorphous light eruption
PLS (Papillon–Lefèvre syndrome) *see*
palmoplantar keratoderma with
periodontitis
PN *see* poikiloderma with neutropenia;
prurigo nodularis
pneumonia
Chlamydia trachomatis infections 2210,
2211–2212
Mycoplasma hominis, *M. pneumoniae* **87**
PNFs, neurofibromatosis type 1
(NF1) 1830

PNH *see* progressive nodular histiocytosis
PNT *see* papulonecrotic tuberculid
POEMS syndrome, endocrine dysfunction 2009
POH *see* progressive osseous heteroplasia
poikiloderma with neutropenia (PN) **1660**, 1798–1800
  clinical features 1798–1800
  differential diagnosis 1800
  epidemiology 1798
  histology findings 1800
  history 1798
  laboratory findings 1800
  pathogenesis 1798
  pathogenic allelic variants 1798
  prevention 1800
  treatment 1800
poikiloderma with neutropenia, Clericuzio type **2039**
policy on STDs in childhood 2196
pollution and airborne allergens, atopic dermatitis (AD) 260
polyarteritis nodosa (PAN) 1879–1882, 1918–1923
  classification 1918–1919
  clinical features 1919–1920, **1921**
  clinical manifestations 1879–1881
  comparison of systemic vasculitides **1881**
  cutaneous nodules 1879–1880
  cutaneous ulcerations and ischaemic injury 1880–1881
  differential diagnosis 1881, **1921**
  epidemiology 1879, 1918–1919
  extracutaneous manifestations 1881
  histology 1881–1882
  histology findings 1920–1921, *1922*
  history 1879, 1918
  laboratory findings 1881, 1920–1921, *1922*
  livedo reticularis 1880
  pathogenesis 1879, 1919
  prognosis 1882, 1922–1923
  treatment 1882, 1922–1923
polyarthritis, rheumatoid factor negative, juvenile idiopathic arthritis (JIA) 1936
polyarthritis, rheumatoid factor positive, juvenile idiopathic arthritis (JIA) 1936
polycystic ovary syndrome (PCOS) 854–856
  acne in endocrine abnormalities associated with insulin resistance 815
  cutaneous manifestations 2001
  cutaneous signs of hyperandrogenism 855–856
  diagnosis 854–855
  metabolic syndrome (MetS) 854–856
  pathogenesis 854–855
polydactyly, nail disorders 2156
polyethylene glycols (PEG), neonatal skin care 69
polyglandular autoimmune syndrome, cutaneous manifestations 2002
polymerase chain reaction (PCR)
  high-resolution melt PCR (HRM) 45
  molecular genetics 43–45
  quantitative real-time PCR (qRT-PCR) 43–44
  rickettsial disease 511
polymorphic light eruption *see* polymorphous light eruption
polymorphous light eruption (PLE) 944–946
  clinical features 944–945
  differential diagnosis 945–946
  epidemiology 944
  history 944
  laboratory investigation 946
  microscopy 946
  pathogenesis 944
  prevention 946
  treatment 946
polymorphous skin eruption, Kawasaki disease (KD) 1908–1909
polyostotic fibrous dysplasia *see* McCune–Albright syndrome (MAS)
polyphenon E (sinecatechins), human papillomaviruses (HPV) 595
polyposis, skin pigmentation, alopecia and fingernail changes **1661**
polythelia (supernumerary nipples) 106–107
pompholyx 231–234
  clinical features 232–233
  definition 231
  differential diagnosis 233–234
  epidemiology 231
  pathogenesis 231–232
  pathology 232
  prognosis 233
  treatment 234
porokeratosis 1623–1627, **1803**
  aetiology 1623
  clinical variants 1624–1625
  definition 1623
  diagnosis 1625
  disseminated superficial actinic porokeratosis 1624
  genital/penoscrotal porokeratosis 1625
  laser and light therapies 1627
  linear porokeratosis 1624
  management 1625–1627
  oral therapies 1626–1627
  porokeratosis of Mibelli 1624
  porokeratosis palmaris and plantaris disseminata 1624–1625
  porokeratosis ptychotropica 1625
  punctate porokeratosis 1625
  surgical management 1626
  topical therapies 1626
porokeratotic eccrine naevus (PEN)
  see also porokeratotic eccrine ostial and dermal duct naevus
  keratitis ichthyosis deafness syndrome (KID syndrome) 1587
porokeratotic eccrine ostial and dermal duct naevus (PEODDN) 1264–1265, 1336
  aetiology 1336
  associated syndrome 1265
  clinical features 1264–1265
  diagnosis 1336
  differential diagnosis 1336
  epidemiology 1336
  histopathology 1265
  history 1264
  pathogenesis 1264
  pathology 1336
  presentation 1336
  prognosis 1336
  treatment 1265, 1336
porphyria cutanea tarda (PCT) **959**, **960**, 961–962, **967**
porphyrias 957–968
  acute intermittent porphyria **959**, **960**, 965, **967**
  acute porphyric attack, pathogenesis 960
  biochemical characteristics **960**
  classification **958**, **959**
  clinical symptoms *961*
  congenital erythropoietic porphyria **959**, **960**, 963–964, **967**
  cutaneous porphyrias 961–965
  cutaneous symptoms, pathogenesis 958–959
  diagnosis 960–961
  diagnosis algorithms *961*
  differential diagnosis of the noncutaneous porphyrias 966
  epidemiology 958
  erythropoietic protoporphyria (EPP) **959**, **960**, 962–963, **967**
  genetic aspects **959**
  haem biosynthesis 957–958
  hepatoerythropoietic porphyria (HEP) **959**, **960**, 964, **967**
  hereditary coproporphyria (HCP) **959**, **960**, 964–965
  history 957–958
  homozygous hereditary coproporphyria 964–965
  hypertrichosis 2133
  laboratory findings 960–961
  noncutaneous porphyrias 965–966
  oral mucosa *2094*
  pathogenesis 958–960
  porphyria cutanea tarda (PCT) **959**, **960**, 961–962, **967**
  prevention 966–967
  therapy of acute attacks in the noncutaneous porphyrias 967
  therapy of the cutaneous porphyrias 966–967
  treatment 966–967
  variegate porphyria (VP) **959**, **960**, 964, **967**
  X-linked dominant protoporphyria (XLDPP) **959**, **960**, 963, **967**
  δ-aminolaevulinic acid dehydratase deficiency porphyria **959**, **960**, 966, **967**
'port-wine stain' (localized or extensive capillary malformation) 1412–1413
  laser therapy 2321–2322
postinfectious purpura fulminans *1892*, 1895, *1896*, 1901

postinflammatory elastolysis, cutis laxa 1136
postinflammatory hyperpigmentation 1463–1464
  treatment 1464
post-kala-azar dermal leishmaniasis (PKDL) 697
postoperative complications, surgical therapy 2317–2318
poststeroid panniculitis 1210–1211
  clinical features 1211
  epidemiology 1210–1211
  histology findings 1211
  pathogenesis 1210–1211
  treatment 1211
potassium dichromate, allergic contact dermatitis (ACD) 308
poxvirus infections 624–648
  classification 624
  diagnosis 624–626
  orthopoxvirus infection 626–643
  parapoxvirus infection 643–647
  yatapoxvirus infection 647–648
PP *see* prurigo pigmentosa
PPARG mutations, lipodystrophies 1224
PPD *see* para-phenylenediamine
PPGSS *see* papular-purpuric gloves-and socks syndrome
PPK *see* phakomatosis pigmentokeratotica
PPKN *see* nonepidermolytic PPK type Nagashima
PPKP1 (palmoplantar keratderma punctate type 1) *see* punctate palmoplantar keratoderma
PPKP3 (palmoplantar keratderma punctate type 1) *see* marginal papular keratoderma
PPKs *see* palmoplantar keratodermas
PPV *see* phakomatosis pigmentovascularis
PR *see* pagetoid reticulosis
preadolescents and adolescents, cutaneous microbiome 49
preauricular cysts and sinuses 104
  aetiology 104
  clinical features 104
  pathology 104
  treatment 104
precalcaneal congenital fibrolipomatous hamartoma (PCFH) 109–110
  aetiology 109
  clinical features 109–110
  definition 109
  differential diagnosis 110
  pathology 109
  treatment 110
precalcaneal congenital fibrolipomatous hamartomas, transient skin disorders in neonates and young infants 81
precocious puberty 1999–2000
  clinical features 1999, *2000*
  cutaneous manifestations 1999–2000
  histology findings 2000
  laboratory findings 2000
  pathogenesis 1999
  prevention 2000
  treatment 2000
precursor haematological neoplasm 1056
  CD4+/CD56+ haematodermic neoplasm (blastic plasmacytoid dendritic cell neoplasm) 1056
premature ageing syndromes 1725–1742
  acrometageria 1731–1732
  CAV1-associated lipodystrophy 1737
  Cockayne syndrome (CS) 1729, 1756–1760
  conditions in which individuals appear aged 1735–1738
  conditions with skin atrophy/lipoatrophy 1729–1735
  conditions with skin laxity 1738–1742
  Costello syndrome 1740
  cutis laxa 1738
  DeBarsy syndrome (DBS) 1730–1731
  dyskeratosis congenita (DC) 1471, *1472*, **1641**, 1729, 1793–1795
  Ehlers–Danlos, progeroid type 1741–1742
  geroderma osteodysplastica (GO) 1739–1740
  Hutchinson–Gilford progeria syndrome (HGPS) 1725–1727
  Lenaerts syndrome 1736
  Lenz–Majewski syndrome (LMS) 1734–1735
  macrocephaly, alopecia, cutis laxa and scoliosis syndrome (MACS syndrome) **1134**, 1135, 1739
  mandibuloacral dysplasia (MAD) 1733
  Marfanoid progeria–lipodystrophy syndrome 1737
  MDPL syndrome 1736
  Megarbane–Loiselet neonatal progeroid syndrome 1734
  Mulvihill–Smith syndrome (MSS) 1735
  Nestor–Guillermo syndrome 1737–1738
  Penttinen progeroid disorder 1734
  Petty syndrome 1738
  Rothmund–Thomson syndrome (RTS) **1661**, 1714–1715, 1729
  Werner syndrome (WS) 1344, 1727–1728
  Wiedemann–Rautenstrauch syndrome (WRS) 1729–1730
premature infants
  see also neonates
  mechanical damage avoidance 66–67
  skin care 66–67
  transepidermal water loss (TEWL) 66
prepubertal unilateral fibrous hyperplasia of the labium majus 2189–2190
  clinical features 2190
  differential diagnosis 2190
  histology 2190
preschool sarcoidosis *see* Blau syndrome/early-onset sarcoidosis
prescleroderma/limited SSc, systemic sclerosis (SSc) **1185**
pretibial epidermolysis bullosa 920
primary (idiopathic) lymphoedema, lymphatic malformations (LMs) 1453–1455, **1453**, 1459–1460
primary cutaneous anaplastic large cell lymphoma *see* cutaneous anaplastic large cell lymphoma
primary cutaneous aspergillosis **139**
primary cutaneous CD30+ lymphoproliferative disorders 1050
primary cutaneous diffuse large B-cell lymphoma (PCDLBCL) 1055–1056
primary cutaneous follicle centre lymphoma (PCFCL) 1055
  clinical features 1055
  definition 1055
  epidemiology 1055
  genetic features 1055
  histopathology 1055
  immunophenotype 1055
  predictive factors 1055
  prognosis 1055
  treatment 1055
primary cutaneous localized amyloidosis, hyperpigmentation 1466
primary cutaneous lymphoma (PCL) 1044–1057
  classification of cutaneous lymphomas 1044, **1044**
  cutaneous B-cell lymphomas 1054–1056
  cutaneous T-cell and NK cell lymphomas 1045–1054
  cutaneous T-cell lymphomas (CTCL) 1045–1054
  diagnosis 1056–1057
  epidemiology in the paediatric age group 1044–1045
  precursor haematological neoplasm 1056
primary cutaneous marginal zone B-cell lymphoma (PCMZL) 1054–1055
  clinical features 1054
  definition 1054
  epidemiology 1054
  histopathology 1054–1055
  immunophenotype 1055
  predictive factors 1055
  prognosis 1055
  treatment 1055
primary herpes gingivostomatitis, herpes simplex virus (HSV) infections 600–601
primary immune deficiency, panniculitis 1212–1213
primary immunodeficiencies, immunocompromised children 685–687
primary irritant napkin rash **268**, 269–270
primary localized cutaneous amyloidosis 2024–2025
primary melanoma of the CNS, congenital melanocytic naevi (CMN) 1245
pritelivir, herpes simplex virus (HSV) infections 607
probiotics and nutritional intervention, atopic dermatitis (AD) 261

procedures
  approach to the neonate 2344
  approach to the paediatric patient 2352
  surgical therapy 2314–2318
progressive facial hemiatrophy 1178
progressive nodular histiocytosis (PNH) 1085–1086
  clinical features 1085–1086
  differential diagnosis 1086
  epidemiology 1085
  histology findings 1086
  history 1085
  treatment 1086
progressive osseous heteroplasia (POH) 1347
  clinical features 1347
  differential diagnosis 1347
  epidemiology 1347
  histopathology 1347
  laboratory studies 1347
  pathogenesis 1347
  treatment 1347
progressive symmetrical erythrokeratoderma (PSEK) *see* erythrokeratodermas; loricrin keratoderma
prolidase deficiency 1979
  clinical features 1979
  definition 1979
  differential diagnosis 1979
  history 1979
  pathogenesis 1979
  prognosis 1979
  treatment 1979
Propionibacterium acnes, acne vulgaris 805
propionic acidaemia 1971–1972
  clinical features 1971
  definition 1971
  differential diagnosis 1971
  history 1971
  pathogenesis 1971
  prognosis 1971
  treatment 1971–1972
propofol, anaesthesia 2338
propranolol
  adverse effects 2405–2406
  infantile haemangiomas (IH) 1435–1436, 2403–2406
propylene glycol, allergic contact dermatitis (ACD) 310
PROS *see* PIK3CA-related overgrowth spectrum
protein-energy malnutrition (severe acute malnutrition) 831–834
  aetiology 832
  classification 831–832
  cutaneous manifestations 832–833
  management 833–834
  prognosis 834
protein malnutrition (kwashiorkor) 831–834
  hair loss 2127
Proteus syndrome (PS) 1269, 1284–1288, **1806**
  characteristics **1199**
  clinical features **1199**, 1202, 1284–1286
  complications 1286–1287
  cutaneous features 1284–1285
  deep vein thrombosis (DVT) 1286–1287
  dental abnormalities 1286
  diagnostic criteria 1284, **1285**
  differential diagnosis 1202
  epidemiology 1284
  genetics 1287
  histopathology 1287
  laboratory findings 1287
  life expectancy 1287
  management 1287–1288
  neurological disease 1285–1286
  other abnormalities 1286
  pathogenesis 1284
  prevention 1202
  pulmonary disease 1285
  pulmonary embolism (PE) 1286–1287
  skeletal overgrowth 1285, *1286*
  spectrum of AKT1-mosaicism 1286
  targeted medical therapy 1288
  thromboembolic disease 1286–1287
  treatment 1202
  tumour risk 1287
protozoal infections
  congenital infections 86, **87**
  neonates 86, **87**
proximal subungual onychomycosis 536
PRP *see* pityriasis rubra pilaris
prurigo nodularis (PN) 242–243
  clinical features 242–243
  definition 242
  differential diagnosis 243
  epidemiology 242
  pathogenesis 242
  pathology 242
  prognosis 243
  treatment 243
prurigo pigmentosa (PP) 244
  clinical features 244
  differential diagnosis 244
  pathogenesis 244
  pathology 244
  treatment 244
pruritus
  atopic dermatitis (AD) 261
  management 261
PS *see* Proteus syndrome
PSEK (progressive symmetrical erythrokeratoderma) *see* loricrin keratoderma
pseudocowpox *see* milker's nodule
pseudo-folliculitis barbae, keratin disorders 1521
pseudohypoparathyroidism, cutaneous manifestations 2002–2003
pseudomonal skin disease 446–450
  aetiology 447
  antibiotic resistance 448
  burn wound infections 449–450
  carriage 447
  clinical features 448–449
  cutaneous manifestations of systemic infection 449
  ecthyma gangrenosum *447*, 449
  epidemiology 447
  folliculitis 449
  green nail syndrome 448
  omphalitis 449
  otitis externa 448–449
  pathophysiology 447–448
  primary skin infections 448–449
  toe web infections 448
  treatment 449–450
pseudomonilethrix, hair disorders 2118
pseudopili annulati 2124
pseudoscabies 720–721
  animal mites 720
  bird mites 720–721
  environmental or plant mites 721
  plant or environmental mites 721
pseudotumour of infancy *see* fibromatosis colli
pseudoxanthoma elasticum (PXE) 1125–1131
  calcification and ossification in the skin 1344
  cardiovascular manifestations 1128
  clinical features 1127–1129
  diagnosis 1130
  diagnostic imaging 1130
  differential diagnosis 1129
  disorders resembling PXE **1129**
  epidemiology 1126–1131
  genetics 1126
  histopathology 1129–1130
  laboratory findings 1130
  metabolic hypothesis 1126–1127
  ocular manifestations 1128
  paediatric clinical features 1129
  pathogenesis 1126–1127
  phenocopies **1129**
  skin manifestations 1128
  treatment 1130–1131
psoralen plus ultraviolet, alopecia areata (AA) A 2144
psoriasiform eczema 356
psoriasis
  adalimumab 372–373
  aetiology 350–353
  annular psoriasis 356
  anthralin (cignolin, dithranol) 369–370, *373*
  biologics 372–374
  calcineurin inhibitors 369, *373*
  chronic plaque psoriasis **364**
  ciclosporin 371
  cignolin (dithranol, anthralin) 369–370, *373*
  classification 362–363
  clinical features 354–359
  clinical presentations 345–346
  comorbidity 346–348, 359–360
  congenital psoriasis **366**
  cutaneous microbiome 52–53
  diabetes 360
  diagnosis 363, **366**
  differential diagnosis **382**
  dithranol (anthralin, cignolin) 369–370, *373*, 2400, **2401**
  dyslipidaemia 359–360
  eczema-psoriasis overlap 356
  eczematous psoriasis 356
  environmental risk factors 351
  epidemiology 343–348

erythrodermic psoriasis 358, *359*, **366**
etanercept 372, *373*
facial psoriasis 355
flexural psoriasis 362
fumaric acid esters 371–372, *373*
gender distribution 345
genetic epidemiology 350–351
guttate psoriasis 357, 362, **364**
hypertension 360
immunopathogenesis model 352–353
incidence 345
inverse psoriasis 357, 362, **365**
investigations **366**
laser therapy 2324
linear psoriasis 356
management 368–374
metabolic and cardiovascular obesity 359
metabolic syndrome (MetS) 856–857
methotrexate (MTX) 370–371, *373*
molecular genetics 351–352
nail psoriasis 346, 357–358, 362, **365**, 2152–2153
napkin/anogenital psoriasis 357, **365**
napkin dermatitis 275
neonatal erythroderma 124
nonalcoholic fatty liver disease (NAFLD) 360
nursing care of the skin 2400–2402
oral mucosa 2090
palmoplantar psoriasis 356, 363
pathogenesis 350–353
pathogenetic mechanisms 351–352
pathogenetic model 352–353
phototherapy 370
Physician Global Assessment (PGA) 363
vs pityriasis rubra pilaris (PRP) **382**
plantar psoriasis 356, 363
plaque psoriasis 354–355, **364**
pretreatment 369
prevalence 344–345
psoriasiform eczema 356
Psoriasis Area and Severity Index (PASI) 363
Psoriasis Family Impact (PFI) questionnaire 2251–2252
psoriatic arthritis 359, 363
psychosocial effects 360
pustular psoriasis 353, 358, 362–363, **366**
retinoids 371
scalp preparations **2402**
scalp psoriasis 355, 362, **364**, **2402**
scores 363, **364–366**
screening 359, 360
systemic therapies 370–374
topical corticosteroids (TCS) 369, *373*
topical therapies 368–370
treatments 368–374
ustekinumab 373–374
vitamin D analogues and combination with corticosteroids 369, *373*
von Zumbusch pustular psoriasis 353, 358
psoriasis, genital area 2162–2163
clinical presentation 2162–2163
differential diagnosis 2163
incidence 2162
investigations 2163
management 2163
prognosis 2163
Psoriasis Area and Severity Index (PASI) 363
Psoriasis Family Impact (PFI) questionnaire 2251–2252
psoriatic arthritis 359, 363
juvenile idiopathic arthritis (JIA) 1937
PSS *see* peeling skin syndrome
psychodermatology 2262–2274
categories of dermatological disorders with psychological components 2262–2263
definition 2262–2263
history 2263
physiological habits 2263–2266
self-mutilation 2267–2272
psychological aspects of genital disease in children 2193–2194
psychological effects, vitiligo 1478
psychological impact, atopic dermatitis (AD) 261
psychosocial aspects, congenital ichthyoses (CI) 1596
psychosocial complications, atopic dermatitis (AD) 249–250
psychosocial effects, psoriasis 360
psychotherapy, self-mutilation 2272
PTEN (Phosphatase and TENsin homologue) hamartoma tumour syndrome (PHTS) 1403, 1818–1821
see also Bannayan–Riley–Ruvalcaba syndrome (BRRS); Cowden syndrome
characteristics **1199**
clinical features **1199**, 1818–1820
diagnostic criteria **1820**
differential diagnosis 1820
epidemiology 1201
pathogenesis 1201, 1818
pathology 1820
treatment 1820–1821
puberty, miniature puberty, transient skin disorders in neonates and young infants 74
pubic lice *see* pediculosis
pulmonary disease, Proteus syndrome (PS) 1285
pulmonary embolism (PE), Proteus syndrome (PS) 1286–1287
pulmonary findings, tuberous sclerosis complex (TSC) 1849
pulmonary involvement, systemic sclerosis (SSc) 1190–1192
pulmonary LAM, tuberous sclerosis complex (TSC) 1852–1853
punctate leuconychia, nail disorders 2151
punctate palmoplantar keratoderma 1545–1546
clinical features 1546
differential diagnosis 1546
epidemiology 1545–1546
histology findings 1546
history 1545
laboratory findings 1546
pathogenesis 1545–1546
treatment 1546
punctate porokeratosis 1625
punctate warts, human papillomaviruses (HPV) 591
purpura annularis telangiectoides *see* Majocchi disease
purpura fulminans 1891–1903
acquired protein C or S deficiency caused by drugs or specific diseases 1896
acute infectious purpura fulminans 1892–1895, 1900–1901
classification 1892–1897
clinical features 1897–1899
congenital purpura fulminans caused by defects in the protein C or S pathway 1896
definition 1891, *1892*
differential diagnosis 1903
histology *1897*
history 1891
pathology 1897
platelet-mediated purpura fulminans occurring during heparin therapy 1897
postinfectious purpura fulminans *1892*, 1895, *1896*, 1901
prognosis 1899–1900
purpura fulminans associated with the antiphospholipid antibody syndrome 1896–1897
purpura fulminans associated with the antiphospholipid syndrome or systemic vasculitides 1902
purpura fulminans following bites or envenomation 1897
specific treatment for individual subgroups 1900–1903
superficial self-mutilation 2270
surgical, orthopaedic and other aspects of treatment 1902–1903
treatment 1900–1903
pustular dermatosis of myelodysplasia in Down syndrome **137**
pustular diseases 2014–2017
pustular eruptions
hypersensitivity reactions to drugs 792–793
neonates **89**
pustular psoriasis 353, 358, 362–363, **366**
PV *see* pemphigus vulgaris
PX *see* papular xanthoma
PXE *see* pseudoxanthoma elasticum
pyoderma gangrenosum (PG) 1027–1031
associated diseases 1028–1030
clinical features 1028–1030
differential diagnosis 1028–1030
epidemiology 1027–1028
history 1027
pathogenesis 1027–1028
systemic therapies 1031
topical therapies 1031

pyodermas 426–430
blastomycosis-like pyoderma 428–429
blistering distal dactylitis (BDD) 429
botryomycosis 428
cellulitis 428
ecthyma 427
erysipelas 428
folliculitis 427
furunculosis 427–428
impetigo 426–427
necrotizing fasciitis (NF) 429
perianal streptococcal dermatitis 429
streptococcal intertrigo 429–430
pyogenic arthritis, pyoderma gangrenosum and acne syndrome (PAPA) 2016–2017
pyogenic granuloma (PG) (lobular capillary haemangioma) 1322–1323, 1443–1444
clinical diagnosis 1443–1444
clinical features 1322
course and prognosis 1322
definition 1322
differential diagnosis **1317**
histology 1444
oral mucosa 2095
pathogenesis 1322, 1443
surgical therapy 2313
treatment 1322, 1444
pyogenic infections, immunocompromised children 686

QoL *see* quality of life assessment
qRT-PCR *see* quantitative real-time PCR
quality of life (QoL) assessment 2241–2252
Acne QoL Index 2250
Assessments of the Psychological and Social Effects of Acne (APSEA) 2250
assessors 2243–2244
burden of disease 2255–2256
Cardiff Acne Disability Index (CADI) 2248–2250
Children's Dermatology Life Quality Index (CDLQI) 2242–2243, 2245, *2246–2248, 2249*
Dermatitis Family Impact (DFI) questionnaire 2243, 2251
dermatology-specific quality of life measures 2245, 2252
disease-specific family measures 2251
disease-specific quality of life measures 2245–2250
Family Dermatology Life Quality Index (FDLQI) 2252
family impact 2251–2252
Family Reported Outcome Measure (FROM-16) 2252
generic measures of family impact 2252
generic quality of life measures 2250–2251
importance of assessment 2242
infantile haemangiomas (IH) 2252
Infantile Hemangioma Quality of Life instrument (IH-QoL) 2250
Infants' Dermatitis Quality of Life questionnaire (IDQoL) 2242–2243, 2250
major life-changing decisions 2251
meaning of 'quality of life' 2241–2242
methods 2242–2243
methods of measurement of family impact 2251
Skindex-Teen 2245
teenagers 2245
Teenagers Quality of Life (T-QoL) 2245, **2250**
utility measurement 2252
validation of quality of life measures 2244–2245
quality of life (QoL) assessment, atopic dermatitis (AD) 219–225, 2250
Childhood Atopic Dermatitis Impact Scale (CADIS) 223
Childhood Impact of Atopic Dermatitis (CIAD) 223
Children's Dermatology Life Quality Index (CDLQI) 222–223
clinical trials 213
dermatology-specific instruments 222–223
DISABKIDS Atopic Dermatitis Module (DISABKIDS-ADM) 223
disease-specific instruments 223
evaluation of instruments 222
family impact measurementt 224, 2251
generic QoL instruments 221–222
Infants' Dermatitis Quality of Life Index (IDQoL) 223
instrument quality 223
instrument types 221
measuring instruments 213–215
outcome reporting, standardization 224
proxy-reported instruments 222
Psoriasis Family Impact (PFI) questionnaire 2251–2252
specific instruments 222
systematic review 223–224
quantitative real-time PCR (qRT-PCR), molecular genetics 43–44

RAC2 deficiency **2039**
racial pigmentation, oral mucosa 2093
radius/ulna fractures 2226
rapidly involuting congenital haemangioma (RICH) 1440–1442
Rapp–Hodgkin syndrome **1661**
rare noninfectious disorders, vesiculobullous lesions 865
rare pemphigus variants 873–874
RAS *see* recurrent aphthous stomatitis
RAS gene associated mosaicism 1293
rashes, histopathology 2379–2382
RASopathies 1857–1862
see also recurrent aphthous stomatitis; *individual conditions*
Ras/MAPK signal transduction pathway *1858*
summary of RASopathies **1858**
RD *see* Refsum disease; restrictive dermopathy
RDD *see* Rosai–Dorfman disease
recessive X-linked ichthyosis (RXLI) 1554–1556
clinical features 1555–1556
contiguity syndromes 1556
cryptorchidism 1556
definition 1554
differential diagnosis 1556
epidemiology 1554–1555
extracutaneous findings 1556
genetic findings 1556
histology findings 1556
laboratory findings 1556
pathogenesis 1554–1555
treatment 1556
recurrent aphthous stomatitis (RAS) 2079–2081
see also RASopathies
aetiology 2079–2080
clinical features 2080
definition 2079
differential diagnosis 2080
herpetiform ulceration 2080
major aphthous stomatitis 2080
minor aphthous stomatitis 2080
pathology 2080
treatment 2081
recurrent attacks, herpes simplex virus (HSV) infections 607–608
recurrent digital fibromatosis *see* infantile digital fibromatosis
recurrent herpes gingivostomatitis, herpes simplex virus (HSV) infections 601
recurrent herpes simplex, oral mucosa 2083
recurrent respiratory papillomatosis (RRP), human papillomaviruses (HPV) 592–593
recurrent toxin-mediated perineal erythema (RPE) 433
recurrent toxin-mediated perineal erythema (scarlatina-like) 2176
red man syndrome, neonatal erythroderma 130
Reed naevus *see* Spitz naevi
Reed syndrome *see* hereditary leiomyomatosis and renal cell cancer syndrome; leiomyomatosis, cutaneous and uterine
Refsum disease (RD) 1591
clinical features 1591
definition 1591
differential diagnosis 1591
extracutaneous findings 1591
histology findings 1591
laboratory findings 1591
pathogenesis 1591
prevention 1591
treatment 1591
regionalization in developing skin 22–23
relapsing polychondritis (RP) 1958–1959
aetiopathogenesis 1958
clinical features 1958–1959
diagnosis 1959
differential diagnosis 1959
epidemiology 1958
history 1958

prognosis 1960
treatment 1959–1960
renal angiomyolipomas, tuberous sclerosis complex (TSC) 1851–1852
renal complications, dystrophic epidermolysis bullosa (DEB) 922
renal disease
systemic lupus erythematosus (SLE) 1943–1944
systemic sclerosis (SSc) 1192
renal findings, tuberous sclerosis complex (TSC) 1847–1848
repigmentation, vitiligo 1480
research opportunities, tuberous sclerosis complex (TSC) **1854**
respiratory function damage, iatrogenic disorders of the newborn 160
restriction fragment length polymorphisms (RFLPs), molecular genetics 45
restrictive dermopathy (RD) **140**, 1168–1170
clinical features 1169–1170
definition 1168
differential diagnosis 1170
history 1168
neonatal blistering 149
pathogenesis 1168–1169
pathology 1169
prenatal diagnosis 1170
prognosis 1170
treatment 1170
reticulate acropigmentation of Kitamura, hyperpigmentation 1471
reticulated hyperpigmentation 1468–1469
reticulate hyperpigmentation 1471, *1472*
retinoids
acitretin 2291
isotretinoin 2291
pityriasis rubra pilaris (PRP) 384
psoriasis 371
systemic therapies 2290–2291
retroviral vectors (RV), genetic therapies 2302–2303, **2302**
RFLPs (restriction fragment length polymorphisms), molecular genetics 45
rhabdomyomatous mesenchymal hamartoma (RMH) 110–111
aetiology 110
clinical features 110
definition 110
differential diagnosis 110–111
pathology 110
treatment 111
rhabdomyosarcoma (RMS) 1382–1384
aetiology 1383
clinical features 1383–1384
congenital melanocytic naevi (CMN) 1245–1246
definition 1382–1383
diagnosis 1384
differential diagnosis 1384
epidemiology 1382–1383
pathogenesis 1383
pathology 1384
prognosis 1384
treatment 1384
Rhus tree (*Toxicodendron*), allergic contact dermatitis (ACD) 310
rib fractures 2226
RICH *see* rapidly involuting congenital haemangioma
Richner–Hanhart syndrome *see* tyrosinaemia type II
rickettsial disease 503–514
agent 504
childhood disease 509–510
clinical features 506–510
complications **510**
cutaneous features 506–509
diagnosis 510–511
differential diagnosis 511, **512**
environment **504**, 505
enzyme-linked immunosorbent assay (ELISA) 511
epidemiology 503–505
future directions 513–514
histopathology 511
host 504–505
host immune response 506
immunofluorescence assay (IFA) 511
immunohistochemical staining 511
indirect immunoperoxidase assay 511
laboratory tests 511
pathogenesis 505–506, *507*
polymerase chain reaction (PCR) 511
prevention 513
prognosis 511–512
rickettsial species **504**
risk factors 511–512
skin biopsy 511
systemic features 509, **510**
transmission **504**, 505
treatment 512–513
Weil–Felix test 511
rituximab
atopic dermatitis (AD) 259
biologic agents 2292
RMH *see* rhabdomyomatous mesenchymal hamartoma
RMS *see* rhabdomyosarcoma
rosacea, childhood *see* childhood rosacea
Rosai–Dorfman disease (RDD) 1087–1088
clinical features 1087–1088
epidemiology 1087
histology findings 1088
history 1087
pathogenesis 1087
treatment 1088
roseola infantum 666–667
clinical features 667
differential diagnosis 667
epidemiology 666–667
laboratory findings 667
pathogenesis 666–667
prevention 667
treatment 667
Rosselli–Gulienetti syndrome **1661**
Rothmund–Thomson syndrome (RTS) **1661**, 1729, 1786–1790, **1804**
clinical features 1787–1789
differential diagnosis 1714–1715, 1788–1790
endocrine dysfunction 2009
epidemiology 1787
histology findings 1789–1790
laboratory findings 1789–1790
pathogenesis 1787
prevention 1789–1790
treatment 1789–1790
RP *see* relapsing polychondritis
RPE *see* recurrent toxin-mediated perineal erythema
RRP *see* recurrent respiratory papillomatosis
RTS *see* Rothmund–Thomson syndrome
rubella 663–664
'blueberry muffin rash' (dermal extramedullary erythropoiesis) 663
clinical features 663–664
complications 663–664
differential diagnosis 664
epidemiology 663
laboratory findings 664
pathogenesis 663
prevention 664
treatment 664
rubella virus, neonates **86**
rubeola *see* measles
rudimentary (atretic, sequestrated) meningocoele 112
aetiology 112
clinical features 112
definition 112
differential diagnosis 112
pathology 112
treatment 112
Ruvalcaba–Myhre–Smith syndrome *see* Bannayan–Riley–Ruvalcaba syndrome
RV *see* retroviral vectors
RXLI *see* recessive X-linked ichthyosis

Sabina brittle hair and mental deficiency syndrome **1662**
SACRAL/LUMBAR/PELVIS syndrome (lower body haemangiomas and structural malformations), infantile haemangiomas (IH) 1433–1434
safeguarding issues in paediatric dermatology 2410–2413
bruises 2410
cigarette burns 2410–2413
human bites 2413
nurses' role 2413
perineal warts 2413
salivary gland swelling, oral mucosa 2097–2098
salmon patch, transient skin disorders in neonates and young infants 75
SAM syndrome *see* severe dermatitis, multiple allergies, metabolic wasting syndrome
Sanger sequencing, molecular genetics 40
San Joaquin Valley fever 564–565
sarcoidosis 995–1004
Blau syndrome/early-onset sarcoidosis (EOS) 1000–1004
classic sarcoidosis 995–999
oral mucosa 2098
sarcomas and related conditions, oral mucosa 2096

Sarcoptes scabiei, neonates **87**
sawah itch 746–748
SC *see* stratum corneum
scabies **136**, 711–721
  aetiology 712
  clinical features 712–715
  crusted (Norwegian) scabies 714–715
  definition 711
  differential diagnosis 715
  genital area 2177
  history 711–712
  infectious napkin dermatitis 273
  ivermectin 717, 718
  laboratory testing 715–716
  lindane 717
  microscopic view of scabies mite *712*
  neonatal erythroderma 127–128
  neonates 90–91
  nursing care of the skin 2402, **2405**
  pathogenesis 712
  pathology 716
  permethrin 716–717
  prognosis 718–719
  pseudoscabies 720–721
  sulphur 717
  systemic therapies 718–719
  topical ivermectin 717
  topical therapies 716–718
  treatment 716
  treatment procedure 717–718
scalp biopsy, hair loss 2108
scalp–ear–nipple syndrome **1662**
scalp preparations, psoriasis **2402**
scalp psoriasis 355, 362, **364**, **2402**
scalp ringworm 532
scalp therapy, congenital ichthyoses (CI) 1595
scar formation in postnatal skin, iatrogenic disorders of the newborn 154–156
scarlet fever, tongue 2100–2101
scarlet fever, streptococcal 432
scarring
  lichen sclerosus in girls (syn. lichen sclerosus et atrophicus) 2165–2166
  surgical therapy 2318
SCC *see* squamous cell carcinoma
SCFN *see* subcutaneous fat necrosis
SCH *see* spindle cell haemangioma
Schamberg disease 1877–1878
  aetiology 1877
  clinical manifestations 1877
  epidemiology 1877
  histology 1878
  history 1877
  laboratory findings 1877–1878
  prognosis 1878
  treatment 1878
Schimmelpenning syndrome, naevus sebaceous 1262–1263
Schindler disease *see* α-N-acetylgalactosaminidase deficiency
Schinzel–Giedion midface retraction syndrome **1662–1663**
Schöpf–Schulz–Passarge syndrome (cystic eyelids, palmoplantar keratosis, hypodontia and hypotrichosis) **1663**, **2110**
Schulman syndrome 331–332
SCID *see* severe combined immunodeficiency
sclerema neonatorum 1210
  aetiology 1210
  clinical features 1210
  epidemiology 1210
  histology 1210
  treatment 1210
scleroderma
  see also systemic sclerosis
  calcification and ossification in the skin 1343
sclerodermie atrophique d'emblee *see* Atrophoderma of Pasini and Pierini
sclerodermie atypique liliacee non induree (Gougerot) *see* Atrophoderma of Pasini and Pierini
sclerosing haemangioma *see* dermatofibroma
sclerotylosis *see* palmoplantar keratoderma with periodontitis
scorpions 739
screening
  autoimmune diseases 903
  cutaneous tuberculosis 494
  dermatitis herpetiformis (DH) 903
  phenylketonuria (PKU) 1968
  psoriasis 359, 360
scrofuloderma (SFD) 488, *490*
scrotal conditions 2190–2191
  acute scrotal oedema 2191
  idiopathic scrotal calcinosis 1340–1341, 2190–2191
  median raphe cysts of the penis and scrotum 2186–2187
SD *see* seborrhoeic dermatitis; striae distensae
seabather's eruption *see* Cnidaria dermatitis/seabather's eruption
sealpox **625**
sea snakes 743
sea-urchins (Echinoidea) 742
sebaceous carcinoma 1375
  clinical features 1375
  differential diagnosis 1375
  epidemiology 1375
  histology 1375
  pathogenesis 1375
  treatment 1375
sebaceous differentiation tumours 1337
sebaceous gland activity, neonates 61
sebaceous gland hyperplasia, transient skin disorders in neonates and young infants 73–74
sebaceous hyperplasia 1337
  aetiology 1337
  diagnosis 1337
  differential diagnosis 1337
  epidemiology 1337
  pathology 1337
  presentation 1337
  prognosis 1337
  treatment 1337
sebaceous naevus syndrome, differential diagnosis 1200
seborrhoeic dermatitis (SD) *see* adolescent seborrhoeic dermatitis; infantile seborrhoeic dermatitis
secondary cutaneous amyloidosis **2024**, 2025
secondary immunodeficiencies, immunocompromised children 687–690
sedation 2335–2336
  see also anaesthesia
  continuum of depth of sedation 2335–2336
  definitions 2336
SEGA *see* subependymal giant cell astrocytoma
segmental granuloma annulare (GA) **1008**, 1011
segmentally arranged basaloid follicular hamartomas 1267
segmental or mosaic neurofibromatosis type 1 1831–1832
  clinical features 1831–1832
  differential diagnosis 1832
  epidemiology 1831
  pathogenesis 1831
  prevention 1832
  treatment 1832
segmental vitiligo *1477*, 1478, 1481
SEI *see* superficial epidermolytic ichthyosis
selenium deficiency 838
self-mutilation 2267–2272
  see also superficial self-mutilation
  behavioural modification 2271
  classification 2267
  diagnosis 2271
  general features 2271
  major self-mutilation 2271
  pathology 2271
  pharmacological treatment 2271–2272
  prognosis 2271
  psychotherapy 2272
  stereotypical self-mutilation 2270
  superficial self-mutilation 2267–2270
  treatment 2271–2272
  use of devices and protective interventions 2271
Sener syndrome **1663**
senescence, cellular *see* cellular senescence
sensorineural hearing loss, enamel hypoplasia and nail defects **1663**
sequestrated, (rudimentary, atretic) meningocoele 112
serological analysis, vesiculobullous lesions 862
serological findings, dermatitis herpetiformis (DH) 902–903
serum sickness-like reaction (SSLR), hypersensitivity reactions to drugs 788
Setleis syndrome 1160–1161
severe acute malnutrition (protein-energy malnutrition) 831–834
  aetiology 832
  classification 831–832
  cutaneous manifestations 832–833
  management 833–834
  prognosis 834

severe combined immunodeficiency (SCID) 2061–2064
  clinical features 2063
  differential diagnosis 2063
  epidemiology 2061–**2062**
  histology findings 2063
  history 2061
  laboratory findings 2063
  pathogenesis 2061–**2062**
  prognosis 2063–2064
  SCID mouse model, varicella zoster virus (VZV) infections 613–614
  treatment 2063–2064
severe congenital neutropenia **2039**
severe dermatitis, multiple allergies, metabolic wasting syndrome (SAM) syndrome 1579–1580
  clinical features 1579
  differential diagnosis 1579–1580
  epidemiology 1579
  genetic findings 1580
  histology findings 1580
  laboratory findings 1580
  pathogenesis 1579
  prevention 1580
  treatment 1580
severity scoring, atopic dermatitis (AD) 212–219
  clinical trials 213, 215–218
  evidence-based recommendations 215–218, 219
  global measurement instruments 218
  measuring instruments 213–215
  Patient-Oriented Eczema Measure (POEM) 219, *220–221*
sex hormones disorders, cutaneous manifestations 1998–2001
sexual abuse *see* child sexual abuse
sexually transmitted diseases (STDs) 2195–2218
  bacterial vaginitis (BV) 2218
  child sexual abuse (CSA) **2197**
  Chlamydia trachomatis infections 2209–2212
  condyloma acuminata (CA) 2212–2214
  diagnosis **2198**
  genital herpes simplex virus infection 2215–2216
  gonorrhoea 2204–2208
  hepatitis B 2214–2215
  HIV infection 2216–2217
  mode of transmission **2197**
  policy on STDs in childhood 2196
  quality standards for tests for the diagnosis **2197**
  syphilis 2199–2204
  treatment **2198**
  Trichomonas vaginalis infection 2217–2218
sexually transmitted infections (STIs) 2179
  child sexual abuse (CSA) 2235–2236
sexual transmission, human papillomaviruses (HPV) 590
Sézary syndrome (SS) 1049
SFD *see* scrofuloderma
SFT *see* solitary fibrous tumour
short interfering RNA (siRNA), genetic therapies 2304
short-limb skeletal dysplasia with severe combined immunodeficiency **1631**
Shwachman–Bodian–Diamond syndrome **2039**
silk therapeutic clothing, atopic dermatitis (AD) 255
sinecatechins (polyphenon E), human papillomaviruses (HPV) 595
single gene mosaicism, fine and whorled Blaschkolinear hypoand hyperpigmentation (incorporating hypomelanosis of Ito, and linear and whorled naevoid hypermelanosis) 1299–1300
siRNA *see* short interfering RNA
sirolimus, systemic therapies 2294
sixth disease *see* roseola infantum
Sjögren–Larsson syndrome (SLS) 126, 1585–1586, 1884
  clinical features 1585
  definition 1585
  differential diagnosis 1585
  epidemiology 1585
  extracutaneous symptoms 1585
  laboratory findings 1585
  pathogenesis 1585
  prevention 1586
  treatment 1586
SJS *see* Stevens–Johnson syndrome
skeletal anomalies–ectodermal dysplasia–growth and mental retardation **1663**
skeletal findings, tuberous sclerosis complex (TSC) 1850
skeletal overgrowth, Proteus syndrome (PS) 1285, *1286*
skin anatomy comparison, neonates **57**
skin barrier enhancement, atopic dermatitis (AD) 261
skin bio-equivalents, dystrophic epidermolysis bullosa (DEB) 926
skin biopsy
  see also skin punch biopsy
  genetic investigation of mosaic disorders 1234
  rickettsial disease 511
skin care *see* neonatal skin care; nursing care of the skin
Skindex-Teen, quality of life (QoL) assessment 2245
skin dimples 106
skinfold freckling (Crowe's sign), neurofibromatosis type 1 (NF1) 1825
skin fragility–ectodermal dysplasia syndrome 916–917, 1699–1700
skin fragility–woolly hair syndrome **1664**, 1701
  due to desmoplakin deficiency 917
  due to plakoglobin deficiency 917
skin lumps that are itchy, differential diagnosis **1316**
skin lumps that may be tender/painful, differential diagnosis **1316**
skin nodules and cysts, differential diagnosis 1313–1323
skin phototypes, endogenous photoprotection 975
skin punch biopsy
  see also skin biopsy
  surgical therapy 2315
  vesiculobullous lesions 862
skin roughness, neonates 60
skin sclerosis, systemic sclerosis (SSc) **1184**
skin surface pH, neonates 59–60
skin tags (soft fibroma, fibroma pendulans), metabolic syndrome (MetS) 849
skin testing 954–956
  determination of threshold doses 955
  idiopathic photodermatoses and skin testing 954–956
  photopatch test 955–956
  provocative skin testing 955
skin thickening, ultraviolet radiation (UVR) 974
skull fractures 2226
SLE *see* systemic lupus erythematosus
sleep disturbance, atopic dermatitis (AD) 248–249
SLN *see* speckled lentiginous naevus
SLS *see* Sjögren–Larsson syndrome
small bowel biopsy, dermatitis herpetiformis (DH) 903
smallpox (variola) **625**, 626–630
  classification **627**
  clinical features 627–629
  differential diagnosis 629, **630**
  epidemiology 626–627
  histology findings 629–630
  history 626
  implications of the use of smallpox as a bioterrorist weapon 637
  laboratory findings 629–630
  pathogenesis 626–627
  pathology 630
  treatment 630
small-spored ectothrix infections 532
smooth muscle hamartoma 1279
  clinical features 1279
  differential diagnosis 1279
  epidemiology 1279
  histology findings 1279
  laboratory findings 1279
  pathogenesis 1279
  prevention 1279
  treatment 1279
smouldering systemic mastocytosis (SSM) **1104**
SNA *see* spherical nucleic acids
snake bites 740
snip excision, surgical therapy 2315
sodium lauryl sulfate (SLS), neonatal skin care 69
SOLAMEN syndrome *see* Proteus syndrome
solar radiation, properties 970
solar urticaria 756, 758–759
solar urticaria, idiopathic *see* idiopathic solar urticaria
solitary fibrous tumour (SFT) 1394–1395
South American or Brazilian blastomycosis (paracoccidioidomycosis) *see* paracoccidioidomycosis

southern tick-associated rash illness (STARI), lyme borreliosis (LB)/lyme disease 472
SP *see* syringocystadenoma papilliferum
specific granule deficiency **2039**
speckled lentiginous naevus (SLN) 1304–1306
spectrum of AKT1-mosaicism, Proteus syndrome (PS) 1286
spherical nucleic acids (SNA), genetic therapies 2304
spiders 738–739
spinal dysraphism
 aetiology 114
 clinical features 114–116
 cutaneous signs 114–116
 definition 114
 differential diagnosis 116
 treatment 116
spindle cell haemangioma (SCH) 1443
spindle cell lipoma
 characteristics **1196**
 histological features **1196**
spindle cell xanthogranuloma 1085
 clinical features 1085
 differential diagnosis 1085
 histology findings 1085
 treatment 1085
spiral fractures 2226
Spitz melanomas 1377, 1378–1380
 differential diagnosis **1317**, 1378–1379
 histopathology 2386–2387
Spitz naevi 1254–1255, 1377, 1378–1380, 2369–2376
 differential diagnosis **1317**, 1378–1379
 histopathology 2386–2387
split hand-foot malformation (SHFM1) **1664**
split hand-foot malformation (SHFM4) **1664**
SPNBF *see* periosteal reaction or subperiosteal new bone formation
sponges 742
spongiotic disorders, histopathology 2380–2381
sporotrichoid cutaneous tuberculosis 490
sporotrichosis 561
 clinical features 561
 differential diagnosis 561
 epidemiology 561
 histology findings 561
 laboratory findings 561
 pathogenesis 561
 prevention 561
 treatment 561
SPTCL/SPTL *see* subcutaneous panniculitis-like T-cell lymphoma
squamous cell carcinoma (SCC) 1373–1374
 clinical features 1374
 differential diagnosis 1374
 dyskeratosis congenita (DC) *1472*
 epidemiology 1373
 histology findings 1374
 pathogenesis 1373–1374
 prevention 1374
 risk factors **1371, 1374**
 treatment 1374
squamous papillomas, oral mucosa 2095
SS *see* Sézary syndrome; Sweet syndrome; synovial sarcoma
SSc *see* systemic sclerosis
SSLR *see* serum sickness-like reaction
SSM *see* smouldering systemic mastocytosis
SSP syndrome (SSPS) 1688–1689
 clinical features 1688–1689
 definition 1688
 differential diagnosis 1689
 history 1688
 pathology 1688
 prognosis 1689
 treatment 1689
SSS *see* stiff skin syndrome
SSSS *see* staphylococcal scalded skin syndrome
staphylococcal folliculitis and impetigo 2176
staphylococcal scalded skin syndrome (SSSS) **138**, 430–431, 2176–2177
 hypersensitivity reactions to drugs 797
 neonatal erythroderma 128–129
 nursing care of the skin 2402, **2404**
staphylococcal toxic shock syndrome 431–432
staphylococci **135**
 epidemiology 425–426
 meticillin-resistant *Staphylococcus aureus* (MRSA) 424–425
 pathophysiology 424
Staphylococcus aureus, neonates **87**
STARI *see* southern tick-associated rash illness
STDs *see* sexually transmitted diseases
steatocystoma multiplex, ectodermal dysplasias (EDs) 1698
stereotypical self-mutilation 2270
sternocleidomastoid tumour *see* fibromatosis colli
steroid-induced striae 1172–1173
Stevens–Johnson syndrome (SJS) 777–784
 classification 777–778
 drugs associated 778–779
 epidemiology 778
 eye care 782–783
 hypersensitivity reactions to drugs 795–798
 intensive care 2409
 intravenous immunoglobulin (IVIG) 783
 management 782–784
 medication controversy 783
 neonatal erythroderma 129–130
 nursing care of the skin 2409, **2411–2412**
 pathogenesis 778–779
 Stevens–Johnson syndrome/toxic epidermal necrolysis overlap and toxic epidermal necrolysis 781–782
 systemic corticosteroids 783
stiff skin syndrome (SSS) 1168
 aetiology 1168
 clinical features 1168
 definition 1168
 differential diagnosis 1168
 history 1168
 pathology 1168
 prognosis 1168
 treatment 1168
STING-associated vasculopathy with onset in infancy (SAVI) syndrome 2021
stingrays 743
STIs *see* sexually transmitted infections
'stork bite,' transient skin disorders in neonates and young infants 75
Stormorken syndrome 1589
stratum corneum (SC)
 hydration, neonates 60
 hydrophilic phase 2276
 lipophilic components 2276
 structure 2276
 topical therapies 2276
streptococcal cellulitis, vulvovaginitis and balanitis 2175–2176
 differential diagnosis 2176
 genital area 2175–2176
 management 2176
 pathogenesis 2175
streptococcal intertrigo 429–430
 infectious napkin dermatitis 272–273
streptococcal scarlet fever 432
streptococcal toxic shock syndrome (STSS) 432
streptococci
 epidemiology 425
 Group A *Streptococcus* (GAS) 423–424, 425, 427, 429
 Group B streptococci **87**
 pathophysiology 423–424
Streptococcus pyogenes, neonates **87, 135**
Streptococcus pyogenes infection, tongue 2100–2101
'stretch marks' *see* striae
striae 1172–1174
 see also striae distensae
 adolescents striae 1172
 aetiology 1172–1173
 clinical features 1173
 Cushing syndrome 1173
 definition 1172
 differential diagnosis 1173
 history 1172
 inherited connective tissue disorders 1173
 metabolic syndrome (MetS) 847–848
 pathogenesis 1173
 pathology 1173
 prognosis 1174
 steroid-induced striae 1172–1173
 striae atrophicans 1172
 striae gravidarum 1172
 treatment 1173–1174
 weight gain 1173
 Wickham's striae 390, 392
striae distensae (SD) 847–848
 see also striae
 aetiology 847
 diagnosis 847
 differential diagnosis 848
 epidemiology 847
 evaluation and severity 848
 histopathology 847–848

metabolic syndrome (MetS) 847–848
pathogenesis 847
treatment 848
striate palmoplantar keratoderma 1537–1539
clinical features 1538, *1539*
differential diagnosis 1538–1539
epidemiology 1538
histology findings 1539
history 1537–1538
laboratory findings 1539
pathogenesis 1538
STSS *see* streptococcal toxic shock syndrome
Sturge–Weber syndrome (SWS) 1293
oral mucosa 2092
syndromic vascular anomalies 1416
subclinical and latent forms, human papillomaviruses (HPV) 589–590
subcutaneous fat necrosis of the newborn (SCFN) 80–81, 1209–1210
clinical features 1209
differential diagnosis 1209
epidemiology *1208*, 1209
histology 1209
pathogenesis *1208*, 1209
prevention 1210
treatment 1210
subcutaneous granuloma annulare (GA) **1008**, 1009–1010
subcutaneous panniculitis-like T-cell lymphoma (SPTCL) 1053, 1217–1218
clinical features 1053, 1218
definition 1053
epidemiology 1053, 1217–1218
genetic features 1053
histopathology 1053, 1218
immunophenotype 1053
pathogenesis 1217–1218
predictive factors 1053
prognosis 1053
treatment 1053, 1218
subcutaneous tissue, embryonic–fetal transition *11*, 14–15
subdermal fibromatous tumour of infancy *see* infantile digital fibromatosis
subependymal giant cell astrocytoma (SEGA), tuberous sclerosis complex (TSC) 1845–1846, 1851
subepidermal calcified nodule 1340
clinical features 1340
differential diagnosis 1340
epidemiology 1340
histopathology 1340
pathogenesis 1340
treatment 1340
sublingual dermoid cyst, tongue 2100
subungual exostosis, nail disorders 2154–2155
sucking blisters, erosions and calluses **138**
transient skin disorders in neonates and young infants 80–81
sucking pads of the lips, transient skin disorders in neonates and young infants 79
suicidal behaviour, differential diagnosis 2269
suicide/suicide ideation, isoretinoin-induced, acne vulgaris 810
sulfapyridine, dermatitis herpetiformis (DH) 904
sulfasalazine, dermatitis herpetiformis (DH) 904
sulphur, scabies 717
sunburn, ultraviolet radiation (UVR) 972–973
sunscreens 975
see also photoprotection
adverse effects 978
controversies 976–977
efficacy 977
ingredients **976**
inorganic sunscreens 975–976
organic sunscreens 976
recommended usage 977–978
superficial cutaneous lymphangiomas, laser therapy 2324
superficial epidermolytic ichthyosis (SEI) **138**, **140**, **1568**, 1571–1572
clinical features 1571, *1572*
differential diagnosis 1571
epidemiology 1571
laboratory findings 1571
pathogenesis 1571
prevention 1572
treatment 1572
superficial fibromatosis *see* palmar–plantar fibromatosis
superficial fungal infections 527–559
candidosis (candidiasis) 545–550
dermatophytoses 527–543
Malassezia-associated diseases 550–555
Neoscytalidium infections 557–558
piedra 556
Tinea nigra 556–557
superficial self-mutilation
see also self-mutilation
acne excoriée de la jeune fille (excoriated acne) 2270
aetiology 2268
bullous dermatosis *2269*
burns 2270
clinical features 2269–2270
compulsive self-mutilation 2268
cutting 2269
differential diagnosis 2269
excoriations 2270
impulsive self-mutilation 2268–2269
lip-lick dermatitis *2269*
motives 2268
purpura fulminans 2270
sub-forms 2268–2269
underlying psychiatric problems 2268
superficial white onychomycosis 536
supernumerary nipples (polythelia) 106–107
supportive therapy, herpes simplex virus (HSV) infections 605
suprabasal epidermolysis bullosa simplex 916–917
surgery
herpes simplex virus (HSV) infections 607
hidradenitis suppurativa (HS) (acne inversa) 828
infantile haemangiomas (IH) 1437
orofacial granulomatosis (OFG) 1020
surgical complications
bleeding 2317
contact dermatitis 2318
intraoperative complications 2317
nerve damage 2317
postoperative complications 2317–2318
scarring, unsatisfactory 2318
surgical therapy 2317
surgical management, porokeratosis 1626
surgical resection
arteriovenous malformations (AVM) 1404–1405
venous anomalies 1409
surgical scars, iatrogenic disorders of the newborn 164
surgical therapy 2310–2318
acquired melanocytic naevi (AMN) 2312
anaesthesia and distraction techniques 2311
bandaging 2313–2314
biopsy 2315, 2316–2317
bleeding 2317
communication 2310
congenital melanocytic naevi (CMN) 2312
contact dermatitis 2318
cryosurgery 2314–2315
distraction and anaesthesia techniques 2311
elliptical excision 2316
epidermal naevi (EN) 2313
immobilization 2311
indications for paediatric dermatological surgery 2312–2313
infantile haemangiomas (IH) 2313
inflammatory or infectious skin conditions 2312
intraoperative complications 2317
matrix shave 2317
naevus sebaceous 2312–2313
nail biopsy 2316–2317
nerve damage 2317
pilomatricoma (pilomatrixoma) 2313
postoperative complications 2317–2318
procedures 2314–2318
pyogenic granuloma (PG) (lobular capillary haemangioma) 2313
scarring, unsatisfactory 2318
skin punch biopsy 2315
snip excision 2315
surgical complications 2317
timing of elective (prophylactic) excisions 2313
verrucae vulgaris (common warts) 2312

Sweet syndrome (SS) **137**, 1023–1026
  associated diseases 1024–1025, 1026
  clinical features 1024–1025
  diagnostic criteria 1025, **1026**
  differential diagnosis 1024–1025
  epidemiology 1023–1024
  extracutaneous disease 1024
  histology findings 1025
  history 1023
  laboratory findings 1025
  occurrence **1025**
  pathogenesis 1023–1024
  prognosis 1026
  treatment 1026
swimmer's itch 746–748
swollen tongue 2100
SWS *see* Sturge–Weber syndrome
syndromic angiokeratomas (angiokeratoma corporis diffusum and lysosomal storage disorders) 1417
syndromic ichthyoses, neonatal erythroderma 126
syndromic vascular anomalies 1414–1417
  CLAPO syndrome 1415
  clinical features 1414–1415
  CLOVE syndrome (congenital lipomatous overgrowth, vascular malformations and epidermal naevus) 1415
  differential diagnosis 1415
  epidemiology 1414
  histology findings 1416
  KTS 1415
  laboratory findings 1415–1416
  pathogenesis 1414
  phacomatosis pigmentovascularis A and B **1415**
  PIK3CA-related overgrowth spectrum (PROS) 1416–1417
  PPV 1414–1415
  prognosis 1416
  Sturge–Weber syndrome (SWS) 1416
  treatment 1416–1417
syndromic venous malformation Maffucci syndrome 1407
synovial sarcoma (SS) 1390
  aetiology 1390
  clinical features 1390
  definition 1390
  differential diagnosis 1390
  epidemiology 1390
  pathogenesis 1390
  pathology 1390
  treatment 1390
syphilis 2199–2204
  see also congenital syphilis; endemic syphilis
  child sexual abuse (CSA) 2201–2202
  clinical features of acquired syphilis 2201
  clinical features of congenital syphilis 2199–2201
  definition 2199
  diagnosis 2202
  differential diagnosis 2203
  history 2199
  latent syphilis 2201
  pathology 2199
  primary syphilis 2201
  prognosis 2202–2203
  secondary syphilis 2201
  treatment 2203–2204
syringocystadenoma papilliferum (SP) 1332
  aetiology 1332
  diagnosis 1332
  differential diagnosis 1332
  epidemiology 1332
  pathology 1332
  presentation 1332
  prognosis 1332
  treatment 1332
syringoma 1333–1334
  aetiology 1333–1334
  diagnosis 1334
  differential diagnosis 1334
  epidemiology 1333
  pathology 1334
  presentation 1334
  prognosis 1334
  treatment 1334
systemic corticosteroids 2287–2288
  alopecia areata (AA) 2143
  atopic dermatitis (AD) 257
  erythema multiforme (EM) 783
  infantile haemangiomas (IH) 1436
  orofacial granulomatosis (OFG) 1019–1020
  Stevens–Johnson syndrome (SJS) 783
  toxic epidermal necrolysis (TEN) 783
systemic diseases with secondary cutaneous vasculitis 1882–1884
systemic immune stimulation, human papillomaviruses (HPV) 595
systemic immunosuppressants and TNF-α inhibitors, orofacial granulomatosis (OFG) 1020
systemic lupus erythematosus (SLE) 1883–1884, 1940–1944
  see also bullous systemic lupus erythematosus
  classification 1940, **1941**
  clinical features 1941–1944
  epidemiology 1940
  laboratory findings 1944
  mucocutaneous involvement 1942–1943
  musculoskeletal disease 1942
  neuropsychiatric systemic lupus erythematosus 1943
  pathogenesis 1940–1941
  renal disease 1943–1944
  treatment 1944
systemic mastocytosis 1097–1098, 1102, **1104**
  diagnosis **1105**
systemic PAN 1883
systemic photoprotective agents 978
systemic retinoids, hidradenitis suppurativa (HS) (acne inversa) 828
systemic sclerosis (SSc) 1183–1193
  acral vasospasm **1184**, 1188
  aetiology 1184–1188
  autoantibodies **1186**
  cardiac disease **1191**, 1192
  cardiopulmonary manifestations **1191**
  cellular interplay in pathogenesis 1185–1187
  cellular pathogenesis *1187*, 1188
  characteristic findings in the early and late stages **1186**
  classification **1189**
  clinical features **1185**, 1188–1192
  CREST syndrome 1183, 1184
  differential diagnosis **1184**
  diffuse cutaneous SSc (dcSSc) **1185**, *1189*
  drug treatment 1192–1193
  gastrointestinal tract 1190
  immune dysfunction 1185
  immunosuppression 1193
  limited cutaneous SSc (lcSSc) **1185**
  musculoskeletal system 1192
  overlap SSc **1185**
  pathogenesis 1184–1188
  prescleroderma/limited SSc **1185**
  pulmonary involvement 1190–1192
  renal disease 1192
  skin sclerosis **1184**
  systemic features 1189–1190
  systemic sclerosis sine scleroderma **1185**
  treatment 1192–1193
  vascular aspects 1193
  vascular lesions 1188
systemic sclerosis sine scleroderma **1185**
systemic steroids, vitiligo 1483
systemic therapies 2282–2295
  antibiotics 2282–2285
  antifungal therapy 2285–2286
  antihistamines 2288–2289
  antimalarial agents 2289
  antiparasitic drugs 2287
  antiviral agents 2286–2287
  atopic dermatitis (AD) 257–259
  biologic agents 2291–2293
  β-blockers (BB) 2289–2290
  chemotherapy and immunomodulators 2293–2295
  clindamycin 2284
  colchicine 2295
  congenital ichthyoses (CI) 1594–1595
  corticosteroids 2287–2288
  dapsone 2284–2285
  4′-diaminodiphenylsulfone 2284–2285
  dystrophic epidermolysis bullosa (DEB) 926–927
  essential fatty acids (EFA) 2295
  hidradenitis suppurativa (HS) (acne inversa) 828
  infantile haemangiomas (IH) 1436
  janus kinase (JAK) inhibitors 2295
  β-lactam antibiotics 2283
  macrolides 2283
  nursing care of the skin 2406–2409
  pityriasis rubra pilaris (PRP) 384
  psoriasis 370–374

pyoderma gangrenosum (PG) 1031
retinoids 2290–2291
tetracyclines 2283
trimethoprim–sulfamethoxazole (TMP-SMX) 2284

tacrolimus, alopecia areata (AA) 2144
tanapox **625**, 647–648
clinical features 648
differential diagnosis 648
epidemiology 647
history 647
investigations 648
treatment 648
tardive CMN, congenital melanocytic naevi (CMN) 1240
taterapox **625**
tattooing and piercing, differential diagnosis 2269
taurodontia, absent teeth and sparse hair **1664**
TCI *see* topical calcineurin inhibitors
TCS *see* topical corticosteroids
TDO syndrome *see* trichodento-osseous syndrome
Teenagers Quality of Life (T-QoL), quality of life (QoL) assessment 2245, **2250**
teeth
child abuse and neglect (CAN) 2227
dystrophic epidermolysis bullosa (DEB) 931
teeth features, dystrophic epidermolysis bullosa (DEB) 922
telangiectases 1417–1418
see also ataxia telangiectasia
Adams–Oliver syndrome 1418
angiokeratomas 1417
clinical features 1417–1418
CMTC (van Lohuizen syndrome) 1417–1418
differential diagnosis 1418
Divry–van Bogaert syndrome 1418
epidemiology 1417
Fabry disease 1974–1975
histology findings 1418
laboratory findings 1418
laser therapy 2323
localized telangiectatic vascular malformation 1417
AT (Louis–Bar syndrome) 1418
Louis–Bar syndrome (AT) 1418
pathogenesis 1417
syndromic angiokeratomas (angiokeratoma corporis diffusum and lysosomal storage disorders) 1417
treatment 1418
van Lohuizen syndrome (CMTC) 1417–1418
telangiectasia macularis eruptiva perstans (TMEP) 1102
telogen loss or effluvium, hair loss 2126–2127
TEN *see* toxic epidermal necrolysis
terbinafine
antifungal therapy 2285
dermatophytoses **543**
terminology
age terminology in paediatrics **2342**
atopic dermatitis (AD) 185
cutaneous microbiome **47**
eczema 185
genetic testing 39
molecular genetics **37**
term neonates and infants, neonatal skin care 67–70
tetracaine formulations, topical anaesthetics 2333
tetracyclines
acne vulgaris 809
systemic therapies 2283
tetramelic deficiencies, ectodermal dysplasia, deformed ears and other abnormalities **1664**
TEWL *see* transepidermal water loss
T-helper 2 (Th2) cytokine cluster, eczema 189–190
therapeutic clothing, eczema 2398–2399
thermal injuries 989–992
chemical burns 992–993
chilblains 989–990
cold-induced skin lesions 989–991
frostbite 990–991
frostnip 991
perniosis 989–990
thermal burns 991–992
thermoregulation, neonates 61
thiomersal (thimerosal), allergic contact dermatitis (ACD) 309–310
thrombocytopenic purpura, oral mucosa 2093
thromboembolic disease
PIK3CA-related overgrowth spectrum (PROS) 1291
Proteus syndrome (PS) 1286–1287
thrush (acute pseudo-membranous candidiasis), oral mucosa 2089
thrush (acute pseudomembranous candidosis) 546–547
thumb and finger sucking 2263–2266
aetiology 2263–2265
clinical features 2263–2264
differential diagnosis 2264
prognosis 2264
thumb deformity and alopecia **1665**
thyroglossal duct cysts 105
thyroid hormone levels alteration, cutaneous manifestations 1993–1995
tibia and fibula fractures 2226
ticks and mites 738
time-scale of skin development *2*, *3*
timing of elective (prophylactic) excisions 2313
timolol, topical, infantile haemangiomas (IH) 2406
Tinea capitis 532, *533*, 540, 541–542
Tinea corporis 534, 540, 542
Tinea cruris 535, 540, 542
Tinea faciei 534
Tinea imbricata 535
Tinea incognito 534–535
Tinea manuum 536, 540
Tinea nigra 556–557
clinical features 557
differential diagnosis 557
treatment 557
Tinea pedis (athlete's foot) 535–536, 540, 542–543
Tinea unguium 536–537, **540**, 543
TLR signalling defects **2040**
TMEP *see* telangiectasia macularis eruptiva perstans
TMP-SMX *see* trimethoprim–sulfamethoxazole
TND *see* twenty-nail dystrophy
TNPM *see* transient neonatal pustular melanosis
TOC *see* tylosis with oesophageal cancer
tocilizumab, atopic dermatitis (AD) 260
toe web infections, pseudomonal skin disease 448
tongue 2099–2101
see also oral…
acquired lesions 2100
ankyloglossia 2099
benign migratory glossitis 2101
congenital/developmental lesions 2099–2100
deficiency states 2100
erythema migrans (geographical tongue, benign migratory glossitis) 2101
fissured/scrotal tongue 2099
geographical tongue 2101
glossitis 2100
hairy and furred tongue 2101
infections 2100–2101
Kawasaki disease (KD) 2100–2101
lingual thyroid 2099
lingual tonsil 2099
localized enlargement of the tongue 2101
macroglossia 2099
median rhomboid glossitis 2100
microglossia 2099
mucocutaneous lymph node syndrome 2100–2101
nutritional deficiency 2100
oral-facial-digital syndrome 2100
scarlet fever 2100–2101
Streptococcus pyogenes infection 2100–2101
sublingual dermoid cyst 2100
swollen tongue 2100
topical anaesthetics
eutectic mixture of local anaesthetics (EMLA) 2332–2333
lidocaine ointment and spray 2333
lidocaine/tetracaine patch 2334
liposomal lidocaine (LMX) 2333
mucosal surfaces 2334
tetracaine formulations 2333
topical antibiotics
acne vulgaris 809
allergic contact dermatitis (ACD) 307
topical antimicrobials, dystrophic epidermolysis bullosa (DEB) 925–926

topical calcineurin inhibitors (TCI)
  atopic dermatitis (AD) 255–256
  lichen sclerosus in girls (syn. lichen sclerosus et atrophicus) 2167
topical corticosteroids (TCS)
  allergic contact dermatitis (ACD) 309
  alopecia areata (AA) 2142–2143
  atopic dermatitis (AD) 254–255
  irritant contact dermatitis (ICD) 296
  lichen sclerosus in girls (syn. lichen sclerosus et atrophicus) 2167
  psoriasis 369, *373*
  vitiligo 1483
topical cytotoxic therapy, molluscum contagiosum (MC) 585
topical immunomodulators, irritant contact dermatitis (ICD) 296
topical immunotherapy, alopecia areata (AA) 2143–2144
topical ivermectin, scabies 717
topical pharmacokinetics
  hydrophilic phase of the SC 2276
  lipophilic components of the SC 2276
  pharmacokinetic processes 2276, *2277*
  structure of the stratum corneum (SC) 2276
topical photoprotective agents 978
topical potassium hydroxide, molluscum contagiosum (MC) 584
topical preparations, herpes simplex virus (HSV) infections 607
topical retinoids, acne vulgaris 808
topical therapies 2275–2280
  acne vulgaris 808–809
  characteristics of paediatric dermatological therapy 2278–2280
  commonly used therapeutic agents 2280
  congenital ichthyoses (CI) 1592–1594
  cutaneous metabolism 2279
  dystrophic epidermolysis bullosa (DEB) 926–927
  fixed-dose combinations 2280
  general concept of topical preparations *2277*
  hidradenitis suppurativa (HS) (acne inversa) 828
  increased permeability by heat application 2278–2279
  infantile haemangiomas (IH) 1436
  irritant effect of emulsifiers 2279
  lower functional capacity 2278
  moderate occlusion 2279
  off-label use 2279–2280
  orofacial granulomatosis (OFG) 1019
  pediculosis 728, **729**
  pharmaceutical formulation 2277–2278
  porokeratosis 1626
  principles of therapy 2275
  principles of topical pharmacokinetics 2275–2277
  pyoderma gangrenosum (PG) 1031
  risk of systemic toxicity 2278
  substances with limited safety 2279
  therapy planning 2280
  vehicle systems 2277–2278
topical timolol, infantile haemangiomas (IH) 2406
tori, oral mucosa 2096
total dystrophic onychomycosis 536
total parenteral nutrition (TPN), iatrogenic disorders of the newborn 161–162
toxic epidermal necrolysis (TEN) 777–784
  classification 777–778
  drugs associated 778–779
  epidemiology 778
  eye care 782–783
  hypersensitivity reactions to drugs 795–798
  intensive care 2409
  intravenous immunoglobulin (IVIG) 783
  management 782–784
  medication controversy 783
  neonatal erythroderma 129–130
  nursing care of the skin 2409, **2411–2412**
  pathogenesis 778–779
  systemic corticosteroids 783
toxic seaweed dermatitis 749
  clinical features 749
  differential diagnosis 749
  epidemiology 749
  histology findings 749
  laboratory findings 749
  pathogenesis 749
  prevention 749
  treatment 749
toxic shock syndrome (TSS) 431–432
Toxoplasma gondii, neonates **87**
TP63-related phenotypes: overview of molecular pathway, ectodermal dysplasias (EDs) 1677–1678
TPN (total parenteral nutrition), iatrogenic disorders of the newborn 161–162
T-QoL *see* Teenagers Quality of Life
tralokinumab, atopic dermatitis (AD) 260
transaldolase deficiency 1979
  clinical features 1979
  definition 1979
  differential diagnosis 1979
  history 1979
  pathogenesis 1979
  prognosis 1979
  treatment 1979
transcription factors and homeobox genes: major regulators of gene expression, ectodermal dysplasias (EDs) 1677–1684
transcription factors other than *p63*, ectodermal dysplasias (EDs) 1682–1683
transcutaneous monitoring, iatrogenic disorders of the newborn 163
transepidermal water loss (TEWL)
  neonatal skin care 66
  neonates 58–60
  premature infants 66
transient aquagenic keratoderma 1547
  clinical features 1547
  epidemiology 1547
  history 1547
  pathogenesis 1547
  treatment 1547
transient neonatal pustular melanosis (TNPM)
  clinical features 142
  differential diagnosis 142
  epidemiology 142
  histology findings 142
  laboratory findings 142
  neonates 142
  pathogenesis 142
  prevention 142
  transient skin disorders in neonates and young infants 76–77
  treatment 142
transient skin disorders in neonates and young infants 72–81
  acrocyanosis 76
  adnexal polyp 81
  'angel kiss' 75
  benign anteromedial plantar nodules 81
  Bohn nodules 77–78
  cutis marmorata 75
  dental lamina cysts 78
  Epstein pearls 77
  eruption cyst 78–79
  erythema neonatorum 76
  erythema toxicum neonatorum (ETN) 76
  harlequin colour change 75–76
  lanugo 73
  milia 74
  miniature puberty 74
  Mongolian spots 79
  naevus simplex 75
  natal and neonatal teeth 78
  oral lesions 77–79
  pedal papules of infancy 81
  perineal groove 81
  periungual hyperpigmentation 79–80
  physiological desquamation 73
  physiological jaundice 74–75
  physiological skin findings 72–75
  pigmentary lines of newborns 79
  pigmentary skin lesions 79–80
  precalcaneal congenital fibrolipomatous hamartomas 81
  salmon patch 75
  sebaceous gland hyperplasia 73–74
  'stork bite,' 75
  subcutaneous fat necrosis 80–81
  sucking blisters, erosions and calluses 80–81
  sucking pads of the lips 79
  transient neonatal pustular melanosis 76–77
  transient vascular physiological changes 75–76
  transient vesicopustular eruptions 76–77
  Unna naevus 75

vernix caseosa 72–73
transient vascular physiological changes, transient skin disorders in neonates and young infants 75–76
transient vesicopustular eruptions, transient skin disorders in neonates and young infants 76–77
transillumination burns, iatrogenic disorders of the newborn 163
transition from paediatric to adult services, approach to the adolescent 2351
transitory koilonychia, nail disorders 2148
transplacentally acquired dermatoses 93–99
Behçet disease (BD) 98–99
melanoma 98–99
neonatal bullous autoimmune disorders 97–98
neonatal lupus erythematosus (NLE) 93–97
transplantation methods, vitiligo 1483
transport defects, metabolic disorders 1973
transverse nasal line 106
TRAPS *see* tumour necrosis factor receptor-associated periodic syndrome
trauma, calcification and ossification in the skin 1344
traumatic cutaneous myiasis 704
traumatic/frictional keratosis, oral mucosa 2089
traumatic panniculitis 1220
traumatic ulceration, oral mucosa 2081–2082
clinical features 2082
differential diagnosis 2082
treatment 2082
Treponema pallidum, neonates **87**
triangular alopecia 2131
trichilemmal cyst 1319
clinical features 1319
course and prognosis 1319
definition 1319
pathogenesis 1319
treatment 1319
trichodental dysplasia **1665**
trichodento-osseous (TDO) syndrome **1665**
clinical features 1683
definition 1683
differential diagnosis 1683
ectodermal dysplasias (EDs) 1683
history 1683
pathology 1683
prognosis 1683
treatment 1683
trichofolliculoma 1329
aetiology 1329
diagnosis 1329
differential diagnosis 1329
epidemiology 1329
pathology 1329
presentation 1329
prognosis 1329
Trichomonas vaginalis infection 2217–2218
aetiology 2217
child sexual abuse (CSA) 2218
clinical features 2217–2218
definition 2217
diagnosis 2218
treatment 2218
tricho-odonto-onychial dysplasia **1665**
tricho-odonto-onychial dysplasia with bone deficiency **1666**
tricho-odonto-onycho dermal syndrome **1665**
tricho-onycho-dental (TOD) dysplasia **1666**
Trichophyton rubrum, neonates **87**
trichopoliodystrophy (Menkes syndrome)
copper deficiency 838
hair disorders 2113
mineral deficiencies 838
trichorhinophalangeal syndrome (TRPS) types I, II, III **1666**, 1683–1684
clinical features 1684
definition 1683
trichorrhexis invaginata (bamboo hair) 2114–2116
trichorrhexis nodosa 2112–2113
trichoschisis, hair disorders 2113
trichothiodystrophy (TTD) 1587–1589, 1760–1763
clinical features 1588, 1760–1762
differential diagnosis 1588, 1762
epidemiology 1587–1588
genetic classification 1762–1763
genetic findings 1588–1589
hair disorders 2113–2114
hair phenotype 1761–1762
histology findings 1588–1589
history 1760
laboratory findings 1588–1589
laboratory tests 1762
nonphotosensitive **1667**
pathogenesis 1587–1588
prevention 1589
syndromes associated with **2115**
treatment 1589, 1762
UV-sensitive syndrome, COFS/TTD and CS/TTD 1763
XP/TTD complex 1763
trichotillomania 2265–2266
aetiology 2265
clinical features 2266
differential diagnosis 2266
pathology 2265–2266
prognosis 2266
treatment 2266
trifluridine, herpes simplex virus (HSV) infections 607
trimethoprim–sulfamethoxazole (TMP-SMX), systemic therapies 2284
tropical phagedena *see* tropical skin ulcer
tropical skin ulcer (TU) 523–526
acute leg ulcers **526**
chronic leg ulcers **526**
clinical features 524–525
complications 525
definition 523
diagnosis 525
differential diagnosis 525, **526**
epidemiology 524
history 523–524
pathogenesis 524
predisposing factors **524**
treatment 525–526
TRPS syndrome *see* trichorhinophalangeal syndrome
TSC *see* tuberous sclerosis complex
TSS *see* toxic shock syndrome
TT *see* tuberculoid leprosy
TTD *see* trichothiodystrophy
TU *see* tropical skin ulcer
tuberculids 490
tuberculoid leprosy (TT) **497**
tuberculosis verrucosa cutis 489, *490*
tuberculous gumma 489–490, *491*
tuberculous metastatic abscess 489–490, *491*
tuberous sclerosis **1805**
tuberous sclerosis complex (TSC) 1837–1854
cardiac findings 1848–1849
clinical features 1841–1850
dermatological findings 1841–1844
diagnostic approach 1840–1841
diagnostic criteria **1838**
differential diagnosis 1841
endocrine dysfunction 2009
epidemiology 1838, **1838**
epilepsy 1850–1851
facial angiofibromas 1853–1854
historical perspective 1837–1838
internet resources **1854**
management and surveillance recommendations **1850**
moving foward 1854
neurological findings 1844–1846
nonrenal hamartoma 1849
ophthalmological findings 1846–1847
oral mucosa 2094
pathogenesis 1838–1839
pathophysiology 1839–1840
pulmonary findings 1849
pulmonary LAM 1852–1853
renal angiomyolipomas 1851–1852
renal findings 1847–1848
research opportunities **1854**
skeletal findings 1850
subependymal giant cell astrocytoma (SEGA) 1845–1846, 1851
surveillance and management recommendations **1850**
treatment 1850–1854
tufted angioma 1443, 1444–1445, *1446*
see also kaposiform haemangioendothelioma
tumoral calcinosis 1341–1342
clinical features 1341–1342
epidemiology 1341
histopathology 1342
laboratory studies 1342
pathogenesis 1341
treatment 1342
tumour necrosis factor receptor-associated periodic syndrome (TRAPS) 2014

tumour risk
PIK3CA-related overgrowth spectrum (PROS) 1291
Proteus syndrome (PS) 1287
tumours
see also vascular tumours
adnexal disorders 1329–1337
apocrine differentiation 1331–1333
apocrine hidrocystoma 1331
apocrine naevi 1281, 1333
calcification and ossification in the skin 1344
desmoplastic trichoepithelioma (DTE) 1329–1330
eccrine differentiation 1333–1336
eccrine naevi 1281, 1335–1336
eccrine poroma (EP) 1334–1335
folliculear differentiation 1329–1331
hair follicle naevus 1330–1331
porokeratotic eccrine ostial and dermal duct naevus (PEODDN) 1336
sebaceous differentiation 1337
sebaceous hyperplasia 1337
syringocystadenoma papilliferum (SP) 1332
syringoma 1333–1334
trichofolliculoma 1329
Turner syndrome, cutaneous manifestations 1999
twenty-nail dystrophy (TND), nail disorders 2153
tylosis *see* tylosis with oesophageal cancer (TOC)
tylosis (palmoplantar keratoderma), oral mucosa 2088
tylosis with oesophageal cancer (TOC) 1539–1545, **1805**
clinical features 1539–1540
differential diagnosis 1540
epidemiology 1539
histology findings 1540
history 1539
laboratory findings 1540
pathogenesis 1539
treatment 1540
type 2 chondrodysplasia punctata (CDPX2) 126
type I interferonopathies 2021–2022
tyrosinaemia type II 1540–1541, 1968–1969
clinical features 1540–1541, 1968–1969
definition 1968
differential diagnosis 1969
epidemiology 1540
histology findings 1541
history 1540, 1968
laboratory findings 1541
pathogenesis 1540, 1968
prognosis 1969
treatment 1541, 1969
tyrosine transaminase deficiency *see* tyrosinaemia type II

UHS *see* uncombable hair syndrome
ulcerated haemangiomas
laser therapy 2322
nursing care of the skin 2406, **2407**
ulceration, infantile haemangiomas (IH) 1429–1430
ulcerative colitis, oral mucosa 2086
ulcers and blisters *see* blisters and ulcers
ulcus tropicum *see* tropical skin ulcer
ulerythema acneiforme *see* atrophoderma vermiculata
ulnar mammary syndrome **1667**
ultra-rare neuroichthyotic syndromes with later disease presentations 1591–1592
ultraviolet light addiction 975
ultraviolet radiation (UVR)
artificial sources 970–971
cutaneous effects 971–975
early effects on skin 972–974
endogenous photoprotection 975
exogenous photoprotection 975–980
immunological alterations 974
late effects 974–975
optical properties of skin 971–972
photoageing 974
photocarcinogenesis 974–975
pigmentation 973–974
skin thickening 974
solar radiation 970
sources 970–971
sunburn 972–973
ultraviolet light addiction 975
UV index recommendations **971**
UV-sensitive syndrome, COFS/TTD and CS/TTD 1763
vitamin D synthesis 972
umbilical cord care, neonatal skin care 65
umbilicus developmental abnormalities 107–108
uncombable hair syndrome (UHS) 2120–2121
ectodermal dysplasias (EDs) 1699
retinal pigmentary dystrophy, dental anomalies and brachydactyly **1667**
unique features of developing human skin 20–33
appendage formation 23–24
eccrine sweat gland formation 25–28
keratinization 23
nail formation 24–25
periderm 20–22
pilosebaceous apparatus formation 28–32
regionalization in developing skin 22–23
Unna naevus, transient skin disorders in neonates and young infants 75
unresponsive disease, atopic dermatitis (AD) 256–257
Urbach–Wiethe syndrome 1166–1167
urea, neonatal skin care 69
urticaria 751–762, 988, *989*
acute nonallergic urticaria 757
acute spontaneous urticaria 754, 757, **758**, 759–760
aetiology 756–759
angioedema 751, 752, *753*, 754–755, **758**, 787
angioedema (vibratory urticaria) 759
aquagenic urticaria 759
cholinergic urticaria 755–756, 758
chronic inducible urticaria **758**
chronic inducible urticaria subtypes 755–756, 757–758, 761–762
chronic spontaneous urticaria 754–755, 757, **758**, 760–761
chronic urticaria **760**
classification 752
clinical presentation 754–756
cold urticaria 756, 758
contact urticaria 756, **758**, 759
cryopyrin-associated periodic syndromes (CAPS) 753, **754**, **758**
definition 752
delayed pressure urticaria 759
dermographic (dermatographic) urticaria 755, 758
diagnostic procedures **758**
differential diagnosis 752–753, **754**
epidemiology 751–752
episodic urticaria **758**
heat urticaria 758
histology findings 756–759
history 751
hypersensitivity reactions to drugs 787
laboratory findings 756–759
pathogenesis 751–752
prevention 759–762
prognosis 759–762
solar urticaria 756, 758–759
treatment 759–762
urticaria mimickers 752–753, **753**
vibratory urticaria (angioedema) 759
urticarial and oedematous diseases 2012–2014
urticarial infections, hypersensitivity reactions to drugs 787–788
urticarial vasculitis **758**, 1872–1874
clinical manifestations 1873
definition 1872
diagnostic criteria for hypocomplementemic urticarial vasculitis syndrome **1873**
differential diagnosis 1873
epidemiology 1872
histology 1874
history 1872
imaging findings 1874
laboratory findings 1874
pathogenesis 1872–1873
prognosis 1874
treatment 1874
urticaria pigmentosa, mastocytosis 1100–1101
ustekinumab
atopic dermatitis (AD) 260
psoriasis 373–374
utility measurement, quality of life (QoL) assessment 2252

vaccinations
see also vaccinia
clinical features 631–633
history 631
human papillomaviruses (HPV) 595–596
iatrogenic disorders of the newborn 164

vaccines
  meningococcal disease 446
  vaccines associated with Gianotti–Crosti syndrome (GCS) **772**
vaccinia 631–637
  see also vaccinations
  adverse reactions to vaccinia vaccination 633–637
  bovine vaccinia **625**, 638
  complications of vaccination with vaccinia 633–637
  history 631
  implications of the use of smallpox as a bioterrorist weapon 637
  modern vaccination 631
  protective immune responses to variola and vaccinia 633
  treatment of severe complications of vaccinia vaccination 636–637
  vaccinia immune globulin treatment for complications of smallpox vaccination 636–637
vacuum extractors, iatrogenic disorders of the newborn 158
valaciclovir, antiviral agents 2286–2287
'vanishing bone disease' *see* Gorham–Stout disease
van Lohuizen syndrome (CMTC) 1417–1418
varicella zoster virus (VZV) infections **136**, 612–620
  chickenpox 615–617
  clinical features 615–618
  differential diagnosis 615–618
  epidemiology 612–613
  Herpes zoster 617–618
  histology findings 614, 618–619
  history 612
  HIV infection 651
  immunocompromised children 689
  laboratory findings 618–619
  neonates 85, **86**, **139**
  pathogenesis 613–615
  prevention 619–620
  SCID mouse model 613–614
  transmission 614
  treatment 619–620
  vaccine 620
variegate porphyria (VP) **959**, **960**, 964, **967**
variola *see* smallpox
vascular aspects, systemic sclerosis (SSc) 1193
vascular birthmarks, nursing care of the skin 2402–2406
vascular involvement, Behçet disease (BD) 1954–1955
vascular lesions
  classification **2384**
  histopathology 2384–2386
  immunohistochemical markers **2385**
  laser therapy 2319–2325
vascular malformations 1399–1418
  arteriovenous malformations (AVM) 1399–1405
  capillary malformation 1412–1414
  classification **1400**
  fast-flow vascular malformations 1399–1405
  lymphatic malformations (LMs) 1409–1412
  slow-flow vascular malformations 1405–1418
  syndromic vascular anomalies 1414–1417
  telangiectases 1417–1418
  venous anomalies 1405–1409
vascular naevi, birthmarks in the genital area 2172–2173
vascular neoplasms 1322–1323
vascular tumours 1440–1449
  angiosarcoma 1388, 1448
  benign vascular tumours 1440–1444
  classification **1441**
  congenital haemangiomas (CH) 1440–1442
  kaposiform haemangioendothelioma (KHE) 1444–1445
  kaposiform lymphangiomatosis (KLA) 1449
  Kasabach–Merritt phenomenon (KMP) 1446–1448
  locally aggressive or borderline vascular tumours 1444–1448
  malignant vascular tumours 1448
  multifocal lymphangioendotheliomatosis (also known as cutaneovisceral angiomatosis) with thrombocytopenia (MLT/CAT) 1448
  provisionally unclassified vascular anomalies 1448–1449
  pyogenic granulomas (PG) 1443–1444
  spindle cell haemangioma (SCH) 1443
  tufted angioma 1443
vasculitis
  histopathology 2382
  panniculitis 1215–1216
  skin biopsy *2391*
vasculopathic diseases 2021–2022
vegetable oils, neonatal skin care 69
vehicle systems
  intrinsic effect of vehicles 2278
  topical therapies 2277–2278
venom immunotherapy (VIT), insects/insect bites 737
venom toxic reactions, insects/insect bites 737
venous anomalies
  blue rubber bleb naevus syndrome of Bean 1407
  clinical features 1406–1408
  differential diagnosis 1408
  epidemiology 1405
  familial cerebral 'cavernous' malformation 1408
  glomuvenous malformation (GVM) 1407–1408
  histology findings 1409
  laboratory findings 1408–1409
  localized or extensive venous malformations 1406–1407
  Maffucci syndrome 1407
  pathogenesis 1405–1406
  percutaneous intralesional sclerotherapy 1409
  prevention 1409
  surgical resection 1409
  syndromic venous malformation Maffucci syndrome 1407
  treatment 1409
  venous malformation, multiple cutaneous and mucosal (VMCM) 1407
venous malformation, multiple cutaneous and mucosal (VMCM) 1407
ventouses (vacuum extractors) 158
vernix caseosa
  neonates 56, 72–73
  transient skin disorders in neonates and young infants 72–73
verrucae planae/plane warts/flat warts, human papillomaviruses (HPV) 591
verrucae vulgaris (common warts)
  atopic dermatitis (AD) *248*
  surgical therapy 2312
verrucous haemangiomas (verrucous vascular malformations)/angiokeratomas, laser therapy 2324
verrucous napkin dermatitis **269**
verruga peruana 480–482
vertebrates 742–743
vertical transmission, human papillomaviruses (HPV) 590
vesiculobullous disorders
  napkin dermatitis 278
  oral mucosa 2087
vesiculobullous/erosive napkin dermatitis **269**
vesiculobullous lesions 859–867
  adverse drug reactions (ADR) 866
  arthropods 864
  autoimmune causes 866, *867*
  bacterial infections 864
  benign conditions 864
  blistering diseases in infancy and childhood 865–867
  clinical findings 860–861
  congenital disorders 864–865
  definition of lesions 859–860
  dermatitis herpetiformis 866, *867*
  diagnostic approach 860–861
  differential diagnosis 859–867
  fungal infections 864
  genetic testing 862
  infectious causes of blistering 863–864
  inflammatory disorders 865–866
  inherited causes 866
  laboratory tests 861–862
  microbiological studies 862
  neonatal blistering 864–865
  parasitic infections 864
  physical trauma 866
  rare noninfectious disorders 865
  red flags 862, *862*
  serological analysis 862
  skin and mucosal surfaces 867
  skin punch biopsy 862
  urgent considerations 862, *862*
  viral infections 863
vesiculopustular and bullous skin lesions
  autoimmune causes **136–137**, 146–147
  differential diagnosis **135–138**
  infective causes **135–136**
  neonates 134–151

vespids (wasps, yellow-jacket and hornets) 736
vibratory urticaria (angioedema) 759
vinblastine, systemic therapies 2295
vincristine, systemic therapies 2295
viral exanthems 660–680
  arboviruses 676–679
  classic viral exanthems 660–667
  eruptions considered viral but without exact aetiology 675–676
  other well-recognized viral eruptions 667–675
viral infections
  atopic dermatitis (AD) 201, 247–248
  'blueberry muffin rash' (dermal extramedullary erythropoiesis) 85, **86**
  congenital infections 85, **86**, 88
  cytomegalovirus (CMV) 85, **86**
  eczema herpeticum (EH) 247–248
  herpes simplex virus (HSV) infections 598–698
  HIV infection 651–652
  human papillomaviruses (HPV) 588–596
  immunocompromised children 686, 688–689
  molluscum contagiosum (MC) 579–585
  molluscum infections *248*
  neonates 85, **86**, 88
  oral mucosa 2082–2084
  varicella zoster virus (VZV) infections 85, **86**, 612–620
  verrucae vulgaris *248*
  vesiculobullous lesions 863
viral vectors, genetic therapies 2302–2303, **2302**
virome, cutaneous microbiome 54–55
virucidal therapy, human papillomaviruses (HPV) 595
visceral leishmaniasis (VL) 693, 695
visible flexural dermatitis, atopic dermatitis (AD) 168, *169*
VIT *see* venom immunotherapy
vitamin D
  calcification and ossification in the skin 1339
  synthesis, ultraviolet radiation (UVR) 972
vitamin D analogues and combination with corticosteroids, psoriasis 369, *373*
vitamin deficiencies 835–837
  B group vitamins 835–837
  vitamin A 835
  vitamin B1 (biotin) 837
  vitamin B2 (riboflavin) 835–836
  vitamin B3 (vitamin PP, nicotinamide, niacin) 836
  vitamin B6 (pyridoxine) 836–837
  vitamin B12 (cyanocobalamin) 837
  vitamin C (ascorbic acid) 837
vitiligo 1476–1484
  aetiology 1476–1478
  age of onset 1478
  associated diseases 1481
  associated skin conditions 1481
  choice of treatment 1484
  classification 1478–1481
  clinical features 1478
  cosmetic camouflage 1484
  differential diagnosis 1481–1482
  distribution 1478–1481
  extent of involvement 1479–1480
  familial background 1481
  gender 1478
  genetic susceptibility 1476–1477
  immune system 1477–1478
  immunomodulatory drugs 1483
  melanocyte loss 1477
  morphology 1478
  pathogenesis 1476–1478
  pathology 1478
  photoprotection 1484
  phototherapy 1483
  prevalence 1478
  prognosis 1482
  progression 1480
  psychological effects 1478
  race 1478
  repigmentation 1480
  segmental vitiligo *1477*, 1478, 1481
  systemic steroids 1483
  topical corticosteroids (TCS) 1483
  transplantation methods 1483
  treatment 1482–1484
VL *see* visceral leishmaniasis
VMCM *see* venous malformation, multiple cutaneous and mucosal
Vohwinkel syndrome (VS) 1694–1695
Voigt lines *see* pigmentary demarcation lines
von Hippel–Lindau disease **1806**
von Recklinghausen disease *see* neurofibromatosis type 1
von Zumbusch pustular psoriasis 353, 358
VP *see* variegate porphyria
VS *see* Vohwinkel syndrome
vulval abnormalities
  anatomical abnormalities 2184
  clitoral cysts 2186
  fusion of the labia 2185–2186
vulvovaginal warts, human papillomaviruses (HPV) 593
vulvovaginitis 2174–2175
  definition 2174
  diagnosis 2174–2175
  streptococcal cellulitis, vulvovaginitis and balanitis 2175–2176
  vulvovaginitis associated with a vaginal discharge 2174–2175
VZV *see* varicella zoster virus infections

Waardenburg syndrome (WS) 1495
  clinical features 1495
  differential diagnosis 1495
  epidemiology 1495
  histology findings 1495
  history 1495
  laboratory findings 1495
  pathogenesis 1495
  prevention 1495
  subtypes **1495**
  treatment 1495
warble (furuncular myiasis) 703
warts, nail disorders 2150
warty tuberculosis 489, *490*
WAS *see* Wiskott–Aldrich syndrome
washing and bathing, neonatal skin care 64–65
wasps, yellow-jacket and hornets (vespids) 736
wattles *see* congenital cartilaginous rests of the neck
Wegener's granulomatosis *see* granulomatosis with polyangiitis (GPA)
weight gain, striae 1173
Weil–Felix test, rickettsial disease 511
Wells syndrome (eosinophilic cellulitis) 328–330
Werner syndrome (WS) 1727–1728, **1806**
  calcification and ossification in the skin 1344
  clinical features 1728
  differential diagnosis 1728
  epidemiology 1728
  history 1727–1728
  pathogenesis 1728
  pathology 1728
  prognosis 1728
  treatment 1728
Westerhof syndrome 1506–1507
  clinical features 1507
  differential diagnosis 1507
  epidemiology 1507
  histopathology 1507
  pathogenesis 1507
wet wrap dressings
  atopic dermatitis (AD) 255
  eczema 2397, **2398**, **2399**
Weyer acrofacial dysostosis **1667**
WHIM syndrome, human papillomaviruses (HPV) 589
white patches (leucoplakia), oral mucosa 2088–2091
  acquired transient white lesions 2089–2090
  Bohn nodules and Epstein pearls (gingival cysts of infancy) 2088
  candidal leucoplakia (chronic hyperplastic candidiasis) 2090
  candidosis (candidiasis) 2089–2090
  chronic hyperplastic candidiasis (candidal leucoplakia) 2090
  chronic renal failure 2091
  Clouston syndrome 2088
  congenital/inherited causes 2088
  Darier–White disease (dyskeratosis follicularis) 2088
  definition 2088
  dyskeratosis congenita (DC) 2088
  dyskeratosis follicularis (Darier–White disease) 2088
  Epstein pearls and Bohn nodules (gingival cysts of infancy) 2088
  familial white folded gingivostomatitis (white sponge naevus) 2088
  Fordyce spots or granules 2088
  gingival cysts of infancy (Epstein pearls and Bohn nodules) 2088

hairy leucoplakia 2091
hereditary benign intraepithelial dyskeratosis 2088
hidrotic ectodermal dysplasia (Clouston syndrome, ED2) 2088
Koplik spots 2089
leucoplakia of unknown cause 2091
lupus erythematosus 2090
materia alba 2089
pachyonychia congenita (PC) 2088
palmoplantar keratoderma (tylosis) 2088
psoriasis 2090
traumatic/frictional keratosis 2089
tylosis (palmoplantar keratoderma) 2088
white sponge naevus (familial white folded gingivostomatitis) 2088
white piedra 556
clinical features 556
differential diagnosis 556
white sponge naevus (familial white folded gingivostomatitis), oral mucosa 2088
white sponge 'naevus' of Cannon, keratin disorders 1520
Wiedemann–Rautenstrauch syndrome (WRS) 1729–1730
clinical features 1730
differential diagnosis 1730
epidemiology 1729–1730
histology findings 1730
history 1729
laboratory findings 1730
pathogenesis 1729–1730
treatment 1730
Winchester syndrome, hypertrichosis 2135
Wiskott–Aldrich syndrome (WAS) **1806**, 2064–2066
clinical features 2064–2065
differential diagnosis 2065
epidemiology 2064
histology findings 2065
history 2064
laboratory findings 2065
oral mucosa 2093
pathogenesis 2064
prevention 2065–2066
treatment 2065–2066
Witkop syndrome **1667**
Wnt-β-catenin pathway
ectodermal dysplasias (EDs) 1686–1690
overview *1687*
Woodhouse–Sakati syndrome, endocrine dysfunction 2009
woolly hair 2121–2122
woolly hair, hypotrichosis, everted lower lip and outstanding ears **1668**
woolly hair naevus 1266
World Allergy Organization (WAO), atopic dermatitis (AD), nomenclature 203–204
wound healing
fetal wound healing, iatrogenic disorders of the newborn 155
neonates 61
wound myiasis 704
WRS *see* Wiedemann–Rautenstrauch syndrome
WS *see* Waardenburg syndrome; Werner syndrome
Wuchereria bancrofti
filariasis *709*
lifecycle *709*
Wyburn–Mason syndrome 1401

xanthelasma 849–850
clinical presentation 849–850
diagnosis 849–850
differential diagnosis 850
epidemiology 849
histopathology 850
laboratory findings 850
metabolic syndrome (MetS) 849–850
prevention 850
treatment 850
xanthogranuloma family 1078–1091
cutaneous and mucocutaneous non-Langerhans cell histiocytoses: the nonxanthogranuloma family (C Group) 1087–1088
cutaneous and mucocutaneous non-Langerhans cell histiocytoses: the xanthogranuloma family (C Group) 1080–1087
haemophagocytic lymphohistiocytosis (HLH) (H Group) 1089–1090
malignant histiocytosis (M Group) 1089
xanthoma disseminatum (XD) 1083–1084
clinical features 1083
differential diagnosis 1084
epidemiology 1083
histology 1084
history 1083
pathogenesis 1083
treatment 1084
xanthoma multiplex *see* juvenile xanthogranuloma
xanthomas 849–850
clinical presentation 849–850
diagnosis 849–850
differential diagnosis 850
epidemiology 849
histopathology 850
laboratory findings 850
metabolic syndrome (MetS) 849–850
prevention 850
treatment 850
X-chromosomal ichthyosis syndromes 1576–1581
XD *see* xanthoma disseminatum
xeroderma pigmentosum (XP) 1748–1756, *1757*, **1804**
clinical features 1748–1752
complementation groups 1753–1756
differential diagnosis 1752
epidemiology 1748
histopathology 1752
history 1748
internal neoplasias 1751–1752
laboratory tests 1752
melanoma 1378
neurological symptoms 1751
ocular manifestations 1750–1751
pathogenesis 1748
prevention 1753–1756
treatment 1753–1756
variant form of XP 1756
XP/CS complex 1760
XP/TTD complex 1763
xeroderma pigmentosum and related diseases 1743–1768
cellular DNA repair systems 1743–1744, 1765–1766
cellular senescence 1766–1767
disease susceptibility in heterozygous carriers of defective DNA repair genes 1765–1766
mitochondrial repair 1767–1768
novel therapeutic strategies/DNA repair creams 1768
nucleotide excision repair 1744–1747
nucleotide excision repair defective syndromes 1748–1763, 1768
xeroderma–talipes–enamel defect (XTE syndrome) **1668**
XLDPP *see* X-linked dominant protoporphyria
X-linked, autosomal dominant and recessive HED 1671–1675
clinical features 1672–1674
definition 1671
differential diagnosis 1674
history 1671
pathology 1672
prognosis 1674
treatment 1674–1675
X-linked cutis laxa (XLCL) **1134**, 1135
X-linked dominant chondrodysplasia type II/CDPX2 *see* Conradi–Hünermann–Happle syndrome
X-linked dominant protoporphyria (XLDPP) **959**, **960**, 963, **967**
X-linked lymphoproliferative syndrome (Duncan disease) **2036**
X-linked neutropenia **2039**
X-linked reticulate pigmentary disorder, hyperpigmentation 1471
X-linked reticulate pigmentary disorder (XLPDR) 2022
X-linked tooth agenesis **1668**
XLPDR *see* X-linked reticulate pigmentary disorder
XP *see* xeroderma pigmentosum

yatapox **625**
yatapoxvirus infection 647–648
yaws 515–521
aetiology 515, 516
characteristics **519**
clinical features 517–518
differential diagnosis 519, **520**
distribution 516
history 515–516
laboratory tests 519–520
pathology 516, *517*
prognosis 521
treatment 520–521
yellow nail syndrome (YNS), nail disorders 2157

Zanier–Roubicek syndrome **1668**
Zika virus (ZIKV) infection 677–678
  clinical features 678
  differential diagnosis 678
  laboratory findings 678
  oral mucosa 2084
  prevention 678
  treatment 678
zinc deficiency 838–839
  genital signs 2192
  hair loss 2127
Zunich's neuroectodermal syndrome *see* coloboma, heart defect, ichthyosiform dermatosis, mental retardation, ear anomalies (CHIME) syndrome
zygomycosis 571–572
  clinical features 572
  differential diagnosis 572
  epidemiology 571–572
  histology findingsn 572
  laboratory findings 572
  pathogenesis 571–572
  prevention 572
  treatment 572